Classroom

- Detailed lecture notes organized by learning outcome
- Suggestions for classroom activities
- Guide to relevant additional resources
- Comprehensive PowerPoint™ presentations integrating lecture, images, animations, and videos
- Classroom Response questions
- Image Gallery
- Video and Animation Gallery
- Online course management systems complete with instructor tools and student activities available in a variety of formats

PEARSON
mynursinglab™

- Saves instructors time by providing quality feedback, ongoing formative assessments and customized remediation for students.
- Provides easy, one-stop access to a wealth of teaching resources, such as test item files, PowerPoint™ slides, and video suggestions.
- A built-in electronic gradebook tracks students' progress on assessment and remediation activities.

Clinical

- Suggestions for Clinical Activities and other clinical resources organized by learning outcome

Real Nursing Simulations Facilitator's Guide: Institutional Edition

- 25 simulation scenarios that span the nursing curriculum
- Consistent format includes learning objectives, case flow, instructions for set up, student debriefing questions and more!
- Companion online course cartridge with student exercises, activities, videos, skill checklists, and reflective questions also available for adoption

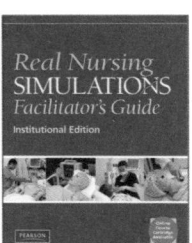

NCLEX-RN®

- Test Item Files with NCLEX®-style questions and complete rationales for correct and incorrect answers mapped to learning outcomes. *available in TestGen, Par Test, and MS Word*

Instructor Resources

BRIEF CONTENTS

Your steps to success.

STEP 1: Register

All you need to get started is a valid email address and the access code below. To register, simply:

1. Go to **www.mynursingkit.com**.
2. Select "**Student**."
3. Find and click on the appropriate book cover. Cover must match the textbook edition being used for your class.
4. On the new page click "**I have an access code**."
5. Read the **License Agreement** and **Privacy Policy**. If you accept, click "**I Accept**."
6. Leave "**No**" selected under "Do you have a Pearson account?"
7. Using a coin scratch off the silver coating below to reveal your access code. Do not use a knife or other sharp object, which can damage the code.
8. Enter your access code in lowercase or uppercase.
9. Follow the on-screen instructions to complete registration.

During registration, you will establish a personal login name and password to use for logging into the Website. You will also be sent a registration confirmation email that contains your login name and password. Be sure to save this email. You must respond to the confirmation e-mail to activate the account correctly.

Your Access Code is:

*Note: If there is no silver foil covering the access code, it may already have been redeemed, and therefore may no longer be valid. In that case, you can purchase access online using a major credit card. To do so, go to www.mynursingkit.com. Click "Students" under "First Time Users," find the cover of your textbook, then click "**Buy Access**," and follow the on-screen instructions.*

STEP 2: Log in

1. Go to **www.mynursingkit.com** and click "**Students**."
2. Find and click on the appropriate book cover. Cover must match the textbook edition being used for your class.
3. Enter the login name and password that you created during registration. If unsure of this information, refer to your registration confirmation email.
4. Click "**Login**."

Got technical questions?

Customer Technical Support: To obtain support, please visit us online anytime at http://247pearsoned.custhelp.com where you can search our knowledgebase for common solutions, view product alerts, and review all options for additional assistance.

SYSTEM REQUIREMENTS

For the latest updates on System Requirements, go to www.mynursingkit.com. Click "**Support**" and choose "**System Requirements**." Click on "**Need help**" at bottom of page for site requirements and other frequently asked questions.

Important: Please read the Subscription and End-User License agreement, accessible from the book Website's login page, before using the *mynursingkit* Website. By using the Website, you indicate that you have read, understood, and accepted the terms of this agreement.

0-13-159714-0

MEDICAL-SURGICAL NURSING

Preparation for Practice

Volume 1

Kathleen S. Osborn, RN, MS, EdD
California State University
Sacramento, California

Cheryl E. Wraa, RN, MSN
University of California, Davis Medical Center
California State University
Sacramento, California

Annita B. Watson, RN, MS, DNSc
California State University
Sacramento, California

Pearson
Boston   Columbus   Indianapolis   New York   San Francisco   Upper Saddle River
Amsterdam   Cape Town   Dubai   London   Madrid   Milan   Munich   Paris   Montreal   Toronto
Delhi   Mexico City   Sao Paulo   Sydney   Hong Kong   Seoul   Singapore   Taipei   Tokyo

Library of Congress Cataloging-in-Publication Data

Osborn, Kathleen S.

   Medical-surgical nursing: preparation for practice/Kathleen S. Osborn, Cheryl E. Wraa, Annita B. Watson.

     p. ; cm.

   Includes bibliographical references and index.

   ISBN-13: 978-0-13-178102-3

   ISBN-10: 0-13-178102-2

   1. Nursing. 2. Surgical nursing. I. Wraa, Cheryl E. II. Watson, Annita B., III. Title.

   [DNLM: 1. Perioperative Nursing—methods. 2. Nurse's Role. 3. Nursing Care—methods. WY 161 O81m 2010]

   RT41.O68 2010

   610.73—dc22

                                                   2009002926

Publisher: Julie Levin Alexander

Publisher's Assistant: Regina Bruno

Editor-in-Chief: Maura Connor

Executive Acquisitions Editor: Pamela Fuller

Development Editor: iD8 Publishing Services, Marion Waldman

Editorial Assistant: Jennifer Aranda

Managing Production Editor: Patrick Walsh

Production Liaison: Cathy O'Connell

Production Editor: Emily Bush, S4Carlisle Publishing Services

Manufacturing Manager: Ilene Sanford

Creative Director: John Christiana, Design Development Services

Interior and Cover Design: Mary Siener, Design Development Services

Cover and Interior Illustration: A.k.A., Anthony Robinson

Director of Marketing: Karen Allman

Senior Marketing Manager: Francisco Del Castillo

Marketing Specialist: Michael Sirinides

Marketing Assistant: Crystal Gonzalez

Digital Media Product Manager: Travis Moses-Westphal

Media Project Manager: Deb O'Connell, All Things Media

Media Project Manager: Rachel Collett

Manager, Rights and Permissions: Zina Arabia

Manager, Visual Research: Beth Brenzel

Image Permission Coordinator: Fran Toepfer

Composition: S4Carlisle Publishing Services

Printer/Binder: Courier/Kendallville

Cover Printer: Lehigh-Phoenix Color/Hagerstown

Cover Photos: A.k.A., Anthony Robinson, Shayle Keating

Notice: Care has been taken to confirm the accuracy of information presented in this book. The authors, editors, and the publisher, however, cannot accept any responsibility for errors or omissions or for consequences from application of the information in this book and make no warranty, express or implied, with respect to its contents.

    The authors and publisher have exerted every effort to ensure that drug selections and dosages set forth in this text are in accord with current recommendations and practice at time of publication. However, in view of ongoing research, changes in government regulations, and the constant flow of information relating to drug therapy and drug reactions, the reader is urged to check the package inserts of all drugs for any change in indications of dosage and for added warnings and precautions. This is particularly important when the recommended agent is a new and/or infrequently employed drug.

www.pearsonhighered.com

10 9 8 7 6 5 4 3

ISBN-10:   0-13-159714-0

ISBN-13:   978-0-13-159714-3

KATHLEEN S. OSBORN

Dr. Kathleen Osborn was first introduced to the profession of nursing at St. Francis School of Nursing in San Francisco, where she received her diploma. She went on to obtain a bachelor's degree in nursing from Sacramento State University, a master of science degree from the University of California, San Francisco, and a doctorate in educational leadership from the University of Southern California. Her clinical practice is in critical care, including cardiac, burn, neurological, and respiratory specialties. She has more than 29 years of experience teaching bachelor and master's degree students, as well as teaching nurses in hospital in-service and continuing education programs. Dr. Osborn's expertise includes program and course development, didactic lecturing, and clinical supervision of undergraduate and graduate students. She also has been actively involved in nursing research and publication throughout her clinical and teaching career. Since 1999, Dr. Osborn has participated as a nurse educator on humanitarian surgical missions to Laos, Africa, Vietnam, Honduras, Bangladesh, and Ecuador. She received the "Heroes in Healthcare" Community Service Award for her humanitarian work from the Coalition for Excellence in Healthcare, a division of the Health Communication Research Institute of Northern California. She also received the Community Service Award from Sacramento State University for her humanitarian work and her service to student development. In 1995, a perpetual faculty award was begun in her honor by the graduating class: The Guiding Light Award for Outstanding Performance by a Nursing Faculty.

This book is dedicated to the important people in my life. I want to thank my husband John for his devotion, patience, and understanding during this project. I also want to thank our children, Christopher and his wife Toni, Patrick, Staci, and Mike for their ongoing understanding of my time away from them. Finally, I want to thank all of the nursing students whom I have had the pleasure of teaching and the patients around the world that I have cared for. You have made my career fulfilling and happy.

—Kathleen Osborn

CHERYL E. WRAA

Cheryl Wraa received her nursing diploma from the Kaiser Foundation School of Nursing in Oakland, California. She went on to obtain a bachelor's degree, and master of science degree in nursing from California State University, Sacramento. Her clinical career has focused on critical care nursing, leadership, and education. Ms. Wraa's clinical practice includes the medical intensive care unit, emergency department, and flight nursing. She is currently the trauma program manager at a level 1 trauma center and clinical faculty for advanced medical–surgical nursing students in a baccalaureate program. Ms. Wraa is also an educator for Interplast and has participated on surgical missions to Vietnam, Bangladesh, and Ghana. She has been active in education and publication throughout her career and is currently a senior clinical editor for the *Journal of Emergency Nursing*. She is past president of the Air and Surface Transport Nurses Association, and president-elect of the Trauma Managers Association of California. Ms. Wraa received the Barbara A. Hess Award for her contributions to education in the air medical and ground transport field.

I dedicate this book to my parents for sharing their incredible faith, zest for life, and unconditional love— I miss you. To my mentors for sharing their wisdom— I would not be where I am without you. To my students for keeping the thirst for knowledge alive and, most importantly, to my family and friends for their unending support and love—I would not have survived this without you.

—Cheryl Wraa

ANNITA B. WATSON

Dr. Annita Watson began her nursing career in Jamestown, New York, at WCA Hospital School of Nursing. She completed her bachelor's degree at Teachers College, Columbia University, and her master's and doctorate in nursing at the University of California, San Francisco. Her graduate focus was medical–surgical nursing and leadership and administration in the service and educational settings. Dr. Watson began her teaching career in 1970 at California State University, Sacramento, where she currently teaches at both the undergraduate and graduate levels. Her areas of practice include medical–surgical nursing, intensive care, long-term care, and community health. Throughout her career, she has served as a national consultant to health care agencies and educational programs on topics related to development of management systems, quality improvement of patient care, curriculum development and evaluation, and implementation of accreditation processes. She has published in like areas, and made numerous professional preparations. Research interests focus on measurement of patient and student outcomes. Currently Dr. Watson assumes a leadership role on several local and regional community boards, focusing on health services for vulnerable populations, for example, children, the elderly, and people who have been abused. Nationally, she serves as an accreditation site evaluator for the Commission on Collegiate Nursing Education. In 2008, she was awarded the Life Time Achievement Award for community service by California State University, Sacramento, recognizing her contributions to the health of the community and her ability to foster community-based learning experiences for students.

To my family, friends, colleagues, and students who supported me in completing this project. Thank you for your existence, endurance, and encouragement. I could not have completed this project without you. Your inspiration and guidance remain in my thoughts and prayers.

—Annita Watson

We extend a heartfelt thanks to our contributors, who gave their time, effort, and expertise so tirelessly to the development and writing of chapters and resources that helped foster our goal of preparing student nurses for evidence-based practice.

Text Contributors

Jaynce Agruss, PhD, APN/CNP
Coordinator, Family Nurse Practitioner Program
Rush University Medical Center
Chicago, Illinois
Chapter 62

Mary Alexander, MA, RN, CRNI, CAE
Chief Executive Officer
Education Manager
Infusion Nurses Society
Norwood, Massachusetts
Chapter 22

Nancy Ames, RN, MSN, CCRN
Critical Care Clinical Specialist
National Institutes of Health, Clinical Center
Nursing and Patient Care Services
Bethesda, Maryland
Chapter 36

Sue Apple, RN, DNSc
Assistant Professor
School of Nursing and Health Studies
Georgetown University
Washington, D.C.
Chapter 39

Jane Ashley, PhD, RN
Associate Professor
Connell School of Nursing
Boston College
Boston, Massachusetts
Chapters 25 and 27

Laurie Baker, RN, MS, APRN, BC, ANP
Coordinator, Barrow Neurosurgical Spine Assessment Clinic
Barrow Neurosurgical Associates
Phoenix, Arizona
Chapter 34

Patricia Baker, RN
Skills Lab Coordinator
School of Nursing and Health Studies
Georgetown University
Washington, D.C.
Chapters 24 and 32

Doris Ballard-Ferguson, RN, PhD
Professor
School of Nursing
Florida A&M University
Tallahassee, Florida
Chapter 7

Karen Bawel Brinkley, RN, PhD
Associate Professor
Chair, Advanced Medical-Surgical Nursing
School of Nursing
San Jose State University
San Jose, California
Chapter 55

Patricia Benner, RN, PhD, FAAN
Thelma Shobe Endowed Chair in Ethics and Spirituality in Nursing
University of California San Francisco
San Francisco, California
Chapter 2
The Foreword

Deborah Benvenuto, BS, CRNI
Education Manager
Infusion Nurses Society
Norwood, Massachusetts
Chapter 22

Debra Brady, DNP, RN, CNS
Assistant Professor of Nursing
California State University Sacramento
Sacramento, California
Chapters 59 and 60

Krista Margaret Brecht, RN, MSc(A)N
Nurse Specialist
Pain Programs
McGill University Health Centre
Montreal General Hospital
Montreal, QC
Chapter 26

Claudia Campbell, RN, BSN, CCRN
Manager of Pain Services LDS Hospital
Intermountain Healthcare
Salt Lake City, Utah
Chapter 15

Ann Cashion, RN, PhD
Chair and Associate Professor, Acute and Chronic Care Department
Robert Wood Johnson Executive Nurse Fellow
Director, Center for Health Evaluation and Lifestyle Promotion
University of Tennessee Health Science Center
Memphis, Tennessee
Chapter 11

Patricia Caudle, DNSc, CNM, FNP
Faculty
Frontier School of Midwifery and Family Nursing
Heber Springs, Arizona
Chapters 48 and 50

Donna York Clark, RN, MS, CFRN, CMTE
Senior Account Manager
Golden Hour Data Systems
Carmel, Indiana
Chapter 1

Jan Clark, BSN, RN, CWOCN
Wound, Ostomy, Continence Consultant
Wilford Hall Medical Center
Lackland Air Force Base
San Antonio, Texas
Chapter 67

Karen Cooper, RN, MSN, CCRN, CNS, WOCN
Assistant Manager ICU
Kaiser Permanente
Sacramento, California
Chapters 33 and 57

Ellen DeLuca, RN, PhD
Professor of Nursing
Lynchburg College
Lynchburg, Virginia
Chapter 35

Jeromy D. Dyer, PA-C, MPAS
Orthopedic Surgery Specialist
Sutter General Hospital
Sutter Medical Group
Sacramento, California
Chapter 55

Lucie Elfervig, DNS, MSN, BSN, APRN-CS, CRNO, FAAN
Ophthalmic Consultant, Clinician, Researcher, Educator,
and Electrophysiologist
Eye Specialty Group
Memphis, Tennessee
Chapter 71

Peggy Ellis, PhD, RN, ANP, FNP, BC
Associate Professor
Associate Dean, School of Nursing,
Director, DNP Program
Doisy College of Health Sciences
St. Louis University
St. Louis, Missouri
Chapters 20, 65, and 66

Harold Engle, RN, BSN, BS
Program Director
Memorial Hermann Northeast Wound Care Center (R)
Humble, Texas
Chapter 67

Gina Flaharty, RN, BSN, FNP
President & Owner
Passport Health of Northern California
Sacramento, California
Chapter 40

Darlene M. Gilcreast, PhD, RN, MSN, BSN, CLNC
Partner, Diabetes Educator
Gilcreast & Associates, LLC
San Antonio, Texas
Chapter 18

J. Carolyn Graff, PhD, RN, FAAIDD
Associate Professor, College of Nursing
Director, College of Graduate Health Sciences
Chief of Nursing, Boling Center for Developmental Disabilities
University of Tennessee Health Science Center
Memphis, Tennessee
Chapter 11

Michele Grigaitis, MS, FNP-BC, CNRN
Nurse Practitioner, Adult Neurosurgical Services
Barrow Neurological Institute
Phoenix, AZ
Chapter 28

Ginny Wacker Guido, JD, MSN, RN
Associate Dean and Director of Graduate Studies
College of Nursing
University of North Dakota
Grand Forks, North Dakota
Chapter 4

Kori Harder, RN, MS
Clinical Nurse Specialist, Cardiology
Nurse Manager, Cardiovascular
University of California Davis Heart Center
Sacramento, CA
Chapter 40

Ann Harley, EdD, RN
Former Dean/Chair
Nursing Behavioral Health
Carson-Newman College
Jefferson City, Tennessee
Chapter 21

Corinne Harmon, RN, MS, EdD, AOCN
Assistant Professor
Clemson University
Clemson, South Carolina
Chapter 51

Helene Harris, RN, MSN
Instructor
Temple College
Temple, Texas
Chapters 54 and 55

Abby M. Heydman, PhD, RN
Interim President
Samuel Merritt College
Oakland, California
Chapter 52

Reneé Semonin Holleran, RN, PhD, CEN, CCRN, CFRN, CTRN, FAEN
Staff Nurse
Emergency Department
Intermountain Medical Center
Salt Lake City, Utah
Chapters 61 and 73

Rich Keegan, RN, MSN
Lecturer
Division of Nursing
Sacramento State University
Sacramento, California
Chapter 9

Katherine Kelly, RN, MSN, FNP-C, CEN
Lecturer
Sacramento School of Nursing
California State University
Sacramento, California
Chapter 17

Gale Kittle, RN, MPH
Research Nurse Coordinator
Barrow Neurological Institute
Arizona Alzheimer's Center
Phoenix, Arizona
Chapter 30

Dawn Lambie, RN, MSN, CHPN
Clinical Nurse Educator
Clinical Education
Kaiser Permanente
Roseville, California
Chapter 64

Kristine L'ecuyer, MSN, RN
Continuing Nursing Education Director Associate Professor
School of Nursing
Saint Louis University
St. Louis, Missouri
Chapter 37

Joseph Lindsay Jr, MD, FACC
Professor of Medicine
The George Washington University School of Medicine
Director, Emeritus, Division of Cardiology
Washington Hospital Center
Washington, D.C.
Chapter 39

Dawna Martich, RN, BSN, MSN
Director, Education
MCN Healthcare, Inc.
Denver, Colorado
Chapter 70

Bonnie McCracken, RN, NP
UC Davis Medical Center
Sacramento, CA
Chapter 44

Brenda McCulloch, RN, MSN, CNS
Sutter Heart and Vascular Institute
Sutter Medical Center
Sacramento, California
Chapter 43

Arlene McGory, DNSc, RN
Research Nurse
Massachusetts Eye and Ear Infirmary
Boston, Massachusetts
Chapter 69

Joyce Mikal-Flynn, RN, FNP, EdD
California State University, Sacramento
Sacramento, California
Chapter 7

Barbara Moyer, BSN, MS, EdD
DeSales University
Center Valley, Pennsylvania
Chapter 70

Teri A. Murray, PhD, RN
Doisy College of Health Sciences
St. Louis University
St. Louis, Missouri
Chapters 20, 65, and 66

Krisna Ogerio, RN, BScN, CPN(C)
McGill University Health Centre
Royal Victoria Hospital
Montreal, QC
Chapter 26

John Osborn, MD, FACS
Senior Surgeon, The Plastic Surgery Center
Clinical Professor, Department of Surgery
University of California Davis School of Medicine
Sacramento, California
Chapter 49

M. Miki Patterson, PhD, RN, PNP, ONP-C
Past President-National Association of Orthopedic Nurses
UMass Memorial Orthopedics
North Worcester, Massachusetts
Chapter 56

Laurie Quinn, BSN, MSN, PhD
Clinical Associate Professor
College of Nursing
University of Illinois
Chicago, Illinois
Chapter 53

Kismet Rasmusson, FNP-BC, FAHA
Heart Failure Prevention and Treatment Program, NP-Program Development
Intermountain Healthcare
College of Nursing
University of Utah
Salt Lake City, Utah
Chapter 42

Kathleen Richerson
Chief Nursing Officer
North Bay Healthcare
VacaValley Hospital
Vacaville, California
Chapter 3

Katherine Ricossa, MS, RN
Director of Education
Kaiser Permanente San Jose Medical Center
San Jose, California
Chapter 58

Leslie Rittenmeyer, RN, CNS, PsyD
Associate Professor of Nursing
Purdue University Calumet School of Nursing
Hammond, Indiana
Chapter 13

Carol Robinson, RN, MPA, CNAA, FAAN
Director of Nursing/Chief Patient Care Services Officer
University of California Davis Health System
Sacramento, California
Chapter 5

Denita Ryan, MN, RN, ANP-C, CNRN
Nurse Practitioner, Adult Neurosurgical Service
Barrow Neurological Institute
St. Joseph's Hospital and Medical Center
Phoenix, Arizona
Chapters 29 and 30

Ann Sievers, RN, MA, CORLN
Clinical Nurse Specialist
University California Davis Medical Center
University of California Davis
Sacramento, California
Chapter 34

Karen Silady, RN, MN, CNS, CEN
Staff Nurse
East Jefferson General Hospital
Metairie, Louisiana
Chapter 72

Donna Stanbridge, BScN, MA, CPN(C)
Clinical Nurse Specialist
Minimally Invasive Surgery and Surgical Innovation
McGill University Health Centre
Montreal General Hospital
Montreal, QC
Chapter 26

James Stotts, RN, MS
Director
PCS, Practice and Education
Stanford University Medical Center
Stanford, California
Chapter 40

Douglas Sutton, APRN, EdD
Assistant Professor,
Christine E. Lynn College of Nursing
Florida Atlantic University
Boca Raton, Florida
Chapters 45 and 46

Debera Thomas, DNS, RN, CS, ARNP
Assistant Dean and Associate Professor,
Christine E. Lynn College of Nursing
Florida Atlantic University
Boca Raton, Florida
Chapters 45 and 46

Gail Thurkauf, RN, MS
Director of the Department of Nursing Quality
Georgetown University Hospital
Washington, D.C.
Chapter 19

Eileen Trigoboff, RN, APRN/PMH-BC, DNS, DABFN
Clinical Nurse Specialist
Buffalo Psychiatric Center
Buffalo, New York
Chapter 16

Sheila Tucker, MA, RD
Nutritionist, Dining Services
Part Time Faculty, School of Nursing and Lynch School of Education
Boston College
Boston, Massachusetts
Chapter 14

Danielle Vigeant, MScN, CPN(C)
Nurse Manager
Peri-operative Services
McGill University Health Centre
Royal Victoria Hospital
Montreal, QC
Chapter 26

Laurie Walsh, NP
Kaiser Permanente
Sacramento, CA
Chapter 10

Suzanne Watt, RN, MSc(A), CON(C)
McGill University Health Centre
Royal Victoria Hospital
Montreal, QC
Chapter 26
Kathy Yeates, BSN, RN, CCRN
Mercy General Hospital
Sacramento, California
Chapter 60

Supplement Contributors

Sandra N, Berryman, RN, MSN, APN-BC
Assistant Professor
University of Arkansas, College of Nursing
Little Rock, Arkansas
Instructor's Resource Manual
Tracy Blanc, RN, BSN
Nursing Instructor
Ivy Tech Community College
Terre Haute, Indiana
Instructor's Resource Manual
Monica G. Cashiotta-Munn, RN, MFT
Instructor
National University
La Jolla, CA
Instructor's Resource Manual
Kim Cooper, RN, MSN
Nursing Department Chair
Ivy Tech Community College
Terre Haute, Indiana
Instructor's Resource Manual
Test Item File
Karlynne Galczyk, RN, MSN, MPH
Lecturer
Widener University School of Nursing
Chester, Pennsylvania
Instructor's Resource Manual
Test Item File
Rhonda Hutton Gann, RN, MSN
Nursing Informatics Lab Manager
State Fair Community College
Sedalia, Missouri
Test Item File
Margaret Gingrich, RN, MSN
Professor
Harrisburg Area Community College
Harrisburg, Pennsylvania
Instructor's Resource Manual
Test Item File
R. Sue Lasiter PhD (c), RN
Assistant Professor
University of Central Missouri
Warrensburg, Missouri
Instructor's Resource Manual
Wanda K. Lawrence, PhD, RNC, MSN
Assistant Professor of Nursing
Winston-Salem State University
Winston-Salem, North Carolina
Instructor's Resource Manual
Denice Kirchoff, MSN, APRN, BC
Assistant Professor of Nursing
Fairmont State University
Fairmont, West Virginia
Test Item File
Andrea R. Mann, MSN, RN
Instructor and Third Level Chair
Frankford Hospital School of Nursing
Philadelphia, Pennsylvania
Test Item File

Dawna Martich, RN, BSN, MSN
Director, Education
MCN Healthcare, Inc.
Denver, Colorado
Test Item File
Joyce Mikal-Flynn
Assistant Professor
Division of Nursing
Sacramento State University
Sacramento, California
Instructor's Resource Manual
Donna Russo, RN, MSN, CCRN, CNE
Nursing Instructor
Frankford Hospital School of Nursing
Philadelphia, Pennsylvania
Test Item File
Barbara Kim Stevens, MSN, RN
Professor of Nursing
University of Rio Grande
Rio Grande, Ohio
Instructor's Resource Manual
Betsy Swinny MSN, RN, CCRN
Critical Care Educator
St. Lukes Baptist Hospital
San Antonio, Texas
Test Item File
Jane Walker BBA, RN MSN
Walters State Community College
Morristown, Tennessee
Test Item File

REVIEWERS. Our heartfelt thanks go out to our colleagues from schools of nursing across the country who have given their time generously to help create this exciting new medical-surgical nursing textbook. These individuals helped us plan and shape our book and resources by reviewing chapters, art, design, and more. *Medical-Surgical Nursing: Preparation for Practice* has reaped the benefit of your collective knowledge and experience as nurses and teachers, and we have improved the materials due to your efforts, suggestions, objections, endorsements, and inspiration. Among those who gave their time generously to help us are the following:

UNIT REVIEWERS. We are so grateful to our Unit Reviewers, who contributed their valuable time, knowledge, and insight to ensure that the Units are written to the highest standard of accuracy and consistency.

Christi DeLemos, RN, MSN, ACNP-c
UC Davis Medical Center, Department of Neurological Surgery, Sacramento, California
Unit 6
Heidi A. Hotz, RN
Cedars-Sinai Medical Center, Los Angeles, California
Unit 16
Dawn Lambie, RN, MSN, CHPN
Kaiser Permanente, Roseville, California
Immunological, Inflammatory and Hematological Disorders
Units 5, 13, and 14
Mary McDermott, MS, RN
Hospital for Special Surgery, New York, New York
Unit 12
Charlotte Miller, RN
Cool, California
Units 1, 2, and 8
Kim Moody, PhD, RN
University of Southern Maine School of Nursing, Portland, ME
Unit 8
Donna York, RN, MS, CFRN, CMTE
Indiana University School of Nursing, Indianapolis, Indiana
Units 3 and 4
Kelly Karr, BA, MA
Sacramento, California

Academic Reviewers

Faisal H. Aboul-Enein, RN, MSN, MPH, NP, BC
Texas Woman's University College of Nursing, Houston, Texas
Joy Ache-Reed, RN, MSN
Indiana Wesleyan University, Marion, Indiana
Betty N. Adams, PhD
Prairie View A & M University, Houston, Texas
Sheila A. Alexander, RN, PhD
University of Pittsburgh, Pittsburgh, Pennsylvania
Cheryl Alt, RN, MSN
Great Falls College of Technology, Great Falls, Montana
Ella R. Anaya, RN, MSN, CNS
Kent State University, Kent, Ohio
Beverly Anderson, MSN, RN
Salt Lake Community College, Salt Lake City, Utah
Cheryl Anema, RN, MSN
Trinity Christian College, Palos Heights, Illinois
Gail Armstrong, RN, ND
University of Colorado–Denver, Denver, Colorado
Karen Sue Bailey, RN, MSN, APRN-BC-FNP
Marshall University, Huntington, West Virginia
L. Antoinette Bargagliotti, DNSc, RN, ANEF
University of Memphis, Memphis, Tennessee
Shirley Sperinde Baxter, RN, BSN, MSN
University of California Davis Medical Center, Sacramento, California
Randal D. Beaton, PhD, EMT
University of Washington, Seattle, Washington
Julie A. Beck, RN, DEd, CNE
York College of Pennsylvania, York, Pennsylvania
Deborah Becker, PhD, RN, ACNP-BC
University of Pennsylvania, Philadelphia, Pennsylvania
William T. Bester, MSN, RN
The University of Texas at Austin, Austin, Texas
Cynthia Ann Blum, PhD, RN, CNE
Florida Atlantic University, Boca Raton, Florida
Donna W. Bohmfalk, MSN, RN
The University of Texas Medical Branch, Galveston, Texas
Joanne Bonesteel, MS, RN
Excelsior College, Albany, New York
Portia A. Botchway, MSN, RN
Clemson University, Clemson, South Carolina
Sharon McFadden Bradley, MSN, RN, CNL
University of Florida College of Nursing, Gainesville, Florida
Janet Witucki Brown, RN, PhD
University of Tennessee, Knoxville, Knoxville, Tennessee
Cindy L. Brubaker, EdD, RN
Bradley University, Peoria, Illinois
Tammy Bryant, RN, BSN
Southwest Georgia Technical College, Thomasville, Georgia
Kathleen Burke, PhD, RN
Ramapo College, Mahwah, New Jersey
Dorothy Burns, RN, PhD, MS
Hampton University, Hampton, Virginia
Dorothy Stano Carlson, DEd, RN
Edinboro University of Pennsylvania, Edinboro, Pennsylvania
Tracy Carlson, MSN, RN
Kent State University, Kent, Ohio
Monica G. Cashiotta-Munn, RN, MFT, MSN
National University, La Jolla, California
Olivia Catolico, PhD, RN, BC
Dominican University of California, San Rafael, California
Donna York Clark, RN, MS, CFRN, CMTE
Golden Hour Data Systems, San Diego, California
Patricia Clark, RN, PhD
Abraham Baldwin College, Tifton, Georgia
Pamela S. Combs, MSN, RN
University of Louisville, Louisville, Kentucky
Cathy Cormier, PhD, RN
Southeastern Louisiana University, Hammond, Louisiana
Nancy Dentlinger, RN, AS, BS, MS, EdD
Redlands Community College, El Reno, Oklahoma
Susan DeSanto-Madeya, DNSc, RN
University of Massachusetts, Boston, Massachusetts

Patricia Brown Dominguez, RN, MSN
Houston Baptist University, Houston, Texas
Nancy Duffy, RN, CEN, MSN
Medical University of South Carolina, Charleston, North Carolina
Jaibun Earp, FNP, PhD, MA, BSN
Florida Agricultural and Mechanical University, Quincy, Florida
Sandra Eggenberger, PhD
Minnesota State University Mankato, Mankato, Minnesota
Jeanette Embry, RN, MS, PhD
West Texas A&M University, College Station, Texas
Deborah Erickson, PhD, RN
Bradley University, Peoria, Illinois
Geralyn M. Frandsen, EdD, RN
Maryville University, St. Louis, Missouri
Kathy Frum, RN, MSN
West Virginia University at Parkersburg, Parkersburg, West Virginia
Kay E. Gaehle, RN, PhD
Southern Illinois University, Edwardsville, Illinois
Karlynne Galczyk, RN, MSN, MPH
Widener University, Chester, Pennsylvania
Donna Gauthier, PhD, RN, CNE
University of Louisiana, Lafayette, Louisiana
Rebecca Gesler, MSN, RN
Spalding University, Louisville, Kentucky
Margaret M. Gingrich, RN, MSN
Harrisburg Area Community College, Harrisburg, Pennsylvania
Donna Glankler, MSN, RN
College of Mount St. Joseph, Cincinnati, Ohio
Sharron Guillett, PhD, RN
Marymount University, Arlington, Virginia
Susan Sweat Gunby, RN, PhD
Mercer University, Atlanta, Georgia
Polly C. Haigler, PhD, RN
University of South Carolina, Columbia, South Carolina
Lori Rae Hamilton, RN, MSN
Otero Junior College, La Junta, Colorado
Jenny Hamner, DSN
Auburn University, Auburn, Alabama
Chris Hawkins, PhD, RN
Texas Woman's University, Denton, Texas
Connie S. Heflin, MSN, RN, CNE
West Kentucky Community and Technical College, Paducah, Kentucky
Carol Heim, MA, RN
Mount Mercy College, Cedar Rapids, Iowa
Jan Herren, MSN, RNC
Southern Arkansas University, Magnolia, Arkansas
Susan Holmes, RN, MSN, CRNP
Auburn University, Auburn, Alabama
Gail M. Holtzman, MSN, CCRN, CNE
University of Alaska, Anchorage, Alaska
Linda Howe, PhD, CNS, CNE
Clemson University, Clemson, South Carolina
Trinity Ingram, MSN, APRN, CPNP, PCNS
South University and Savannah Technical College, Savannah, Georgia
Pamela B. James, RN, BSN, MSN
Fayetteville Technical Community College, Fayetteville, North Carolina
Cindy K. Jenness, BSN, MAE, MSN
Allen College, Waterloo, Iowa
Michelle Johnson, MSN, RN
Northern Michigan University, Marquette, Michigan
Pam Johnson, MSN, RN, APRN, BC
Viterbo University, LaCrosse, Wisconsin
Karin Jones, RN, PhD
Grambling State University, Grambling, Louisiana
Peggy Kalowes, RN, MSN, CNRN, CNS
California State University, Los Angeles, California
Tamara Kear, MSN, RN, CNN
Gwynedd-Mercy College, Gwynedd Valley, Pennsylvania
Frances Keen, DNSc, RN
Villanova University, Villanova, Pennsylvania
Deborah Kern, MSN, RNCS, FNP
Montana State University, Bozeman, Montana
Joan E. King, PhD, ACNP-BC, ANP-BC
Vanderbilt University, Nashville, Tennessee

Kenn M. Kirksey, RN, PhD, APRN, BC
California State University, Fresno, California
Ina Koerner, RN, MS, PhD
University of Louisiana, Lafayette, Louisiana
Cheryl Lacasse, PhDc, RN, OCN
University of Arizona, Tucson, Arizona
Dawn Lambie, RN, MSN, CHPN
Kaiser Permanente, Roseville, California
R. Shelly Lancaster, MSN, RN
University of Wisconsin, Oshkosh, Wisconsin
Karen M. Lavallee, RNC, CS, ARNP
New Hampshire Technical Institute, Concord, New Hampshire
Wanda K. Lawrence, PhD, RN, MSN
Winston-Salem State University, Winston-Salem, North Carolina
Theresa Gunter Lawson, MS, APRN, FNP-BC
Lander University, Greenwood, South Carolina
Patricia Price Lea, PhD, RNC, MSN, MSEd, BSN
North Carolina Agricultural & Technical State University, Greensboro, North
Carolina
Barbara Lee, MSN, RN, BC, MEd, CWOCN
Bellarmine University, Louisville, Kentucky
Elizabeth Lee, MSN, APRN, BC
Harding University, Searcy, Arkansas
Manon Lemonde, RN, PhD, BScN, MScN
University of Ontario Institute of Technology, Ontario, Canada
Linda Lichty, RN
Cosumnes Community Fire Service District, Elks Grove, California
Cynthia A. Logan, PhD, RN
Southeastern Louisiana University, Hammond, Louisiana
Gayla Love, RN, MS, BSN, CCM
Griffin Technical College, Griffin, Georgia
Naomi Lungstrom, MN, FNP
Washington State University, Pullman, Washington
Susan Luparell, PhD, CNS-BC, CNE
Montana State University, Bozeman, Montana
Amy Ma, DNP, APRN, FNP-BC
Long Island University, Brooklyn, New York
Bernadette Madara, BC, EdD, APRN
Southern Connecticut State University, New Haven, Connecticut
Cecilia Jane Maier, MS, RN
Mount Carmel College of Nursing, Columbus, Ohio
Andrea R. Mann, MSN, RN
Frankford Hospital School of Nursing, Philadelphia, Pennsylvania
Bradley J. Manuel, RN, MSN, CNOR(E)
Texas Woman's University, Houston, Texas
Karen S. March, PhD, RN, CCRN, ACNS-BC
York College of Pennsylvania, York, Pennsylvania
Suzanne Marnocha, RN, MSN, PhD, CCRN
University of Wisconsin, Oshkosh, Wisconsin
Janet G. Marshall, PhD, RN
Florida A&M University School of Nursing, Tallahassee, Florida
Brenda Mason, MSN, BSN, RN-FNP
Alderson-Broaddus College, Philippi, West Virginia
Dotti Mathers, MSN, RN
Pennsylvania College of Technology, Williamsport, Pennsylvania
Amy McClune, PhD, RN, BC
Edinboro University of Pennsylvania, Edinboro, Pennsylvania
Emily McClung, RN, MSN
Kent State University College of Nursing, Kent, Ohio
Mary McDermott, MS, RN, APN, NE-C
Hospital for Special Surgery, New York, New York
Barbara McGraw, MSN, RN, CNE
Central Community College, Grand Island, Nebraska
Phyllis McKiernan, MSN, APN-C, RN
Hackensack University Medical Center, Hackensack, New Jersey
Melody McKinney, DNS, RN
Indiana State University, Terre Haute, Indiana
Tara McMillan-Queen, RN, MN, APRN, BC
Mercy School of Nursing, Charlotte, North Carolina
Debbie Metzler, MSN, APNP, GNP-BC
Bellin College of Nursing, Green Bay, Wisconsin
Rita Miller, MSN, RN
Idaho State University–Pocatello, Boise, Idaho

Connie Miller, MSN, FNP-C
University of Northern Colorado, Greeley, Colorado
Donna Molyneaux, PhD
Gwynedd-Mercy College, Gwynedd Valley, Pennsylvania
Kimberly Moody, PhD, RN-CS, ANP
University of Southern Maine, Portland, Maine
Judy K. Moren, BM, RN
California State University, Sacramento, California
Martha C. Morris, PhD, RN
The University of Southern Mississippi, Hattiesburg, Mississippi
Deborah R. Murphy, RN, MSN
West Virginia University at Parkersburg, Parkersburg, West Virginia
Janice A. Neil, RN, PhD
East Carolina University, Greenville, North Carolina
Nancy Noble, RN, MSN, ACNS-BC
Marian University, Fond du Lac, Wisconsin
Catherine M. Nosek, RN, PhD
Winona State University, Winona, Minnesota
Elizabeth Palmer, PhD, RN, CNE
Indiana University of Pennsylvania, Indiana, Pennsylvania
Laurie J. Palmer, RN, MS, AOCN
Monroe Community College, Rochester, New York
Denise Panosky, MSN, RN, CCHP
University of Connecticut, Storrs, Connecticut
Barbara Patterson, RN, PhD
Widener University, Chester, Pennsylvania
Jo Ann Pelaez-Fisher, MSHA, BSN, RN
The College of Southern Nevada, Las Vegas, Nevada
Linda Honan Pellico, MSN, PhD, RN
Yale University, New Haven, Connecticut
Sheila Perrault, MSN
Salem State College, Salem, Massachusetts
Kathleen Perrin, PhD, RN, CCRN
Saint Anselm College, Manchester, New Hampshire
Rebecca Phillip, PhD, RN
The University of Oklahoma Health Sciences Center, Oklahoma City, Oklahoma
Jennifer Ponto, RN, BSN
South Plains College, Levelland, Texas
Christopher B. Powe, PhD(c), ACNP
University of Mississippi Medical Center, Jackson, Mississippi
Rorey D. Pritchard, RN, MSN, CNOR
Chippewa Valley Technical College, Eau Claire, Wisconsin
Anne Purvis, RN, MSN
Gordon College, Barnesville, Georgia
Colleen M. Quinn, RN, MSN
Broward College, Pembroke Pines, Florida
Valeria Ramdin, MS, APRN-BC
Northeastern University, Boston, Massachusetts
Carol Delia Ratta, RN, MS, CCRN
Stony Brook University, Stony Brook, New York
Kathleen M. Rayman, PhD, RN
East Tennessee State University, Johnson City, Tennessee
Anita K. Reed, MSN, RN
Saint Joseph's College, Lafayette, Indiana
Joy Reed, MS, BSS, ADN
Indiana Wesleyan University, Marion, Indiana
Mattie L. Rhodes, RN, PhD, CNS
State University of New York at Buffalo, Buffalo, New York
Gwendolyn E. Richardson, APRN, MN
Midlands Technical College, Columbia, South Carolina
Margaret Richbourg, MSN, BSN, ASN, AA
Florida State University, Tallahassee, Florida
Michelle Robnett, BA, BSN, MA, MBA, PhD
University of Iowa, Iowa City, Iowa
Cheryl Ross, MS, RN
Oklahoma City University, Oklahoma City, Oklahoma
Donna Russo, RN, MSN, CCRN, CNE
Frankford Hospital School of Nursing, Philadelphia, Pennsylvania
Arlene Saliba, MS, RNCS
Andrews University, Berrien Springs, Michigan
Buckie Sasser, RN, MSN
South Georgia College, Douglas, Georgia
Jacalyn M. Schaefer, MSN, RN, CNOR
The Ohio State University, Columbus, Ohio

Diane K. Daddario, MSNc, RN, BC, CMSRN
Pennsylvania College of Technology, Williamsport, Pennsylvania
Yvonne D'Arcy, MS, CRNP, CNS
Suburban Hospital, Bethesda, Maryland
Sherri Davidson, RN, MSN, CS, ACNP
Central Texas Neurological Association, Waco, Texas
Christi DeLemos, RN, MSN, ACNP-c
UC Davis Medical Center, Department of Neurological Surgery,
Sacramento, California
Lisa Duquette, BSN, CCRN, CEN, CFRN, EMT-P
Hartford Hospital, Hartford, Connecticut
Tracey C. Gaslin, RN, MSN, CRNI, CPNP
University of Louisville, Louisville, Kentucky
Barbara Gercke, MSN, FNP
San Diego State Student Health Services, San Diego, California
Denice E. Gibson, MSN
Banner Good Samaritan Medical Center, Phoenix, Arizona
Jean G. Gisler, RN, MSN, FNP-c, CDE
University of Texas Health Science Center at San Antonio, San Antonio, Texas
Theresa M. Glessner, RN, MSN, NP, BC, CCRN
Rochester General Hospital, Rochester, New York
Karen Diane Groller, MSN, RN, BC, CMSRN
Lehigh Valley Hospital, Allentown, Pennsylvania
Melody H. Hale, MSN, APRN-BC
New River Family Health, Scarbro, West Virginia
Lori Harris, RN, BSN, CNOR, CLNC
Mercy Health Center, Oklahoma City, Oklahoma
Amy Herrington, RN, MSN, CEN, NR-EMT-B
Bluegrass Community and Technical College, Lexington, Kentucky
Ellen S. Kane, MSN, RN, CDE
Banner Good Samaritan Medical Center, Phoenix, Arizona
Mary Knudtson, DNSc, NP
University of California Irvine, Irvine, California
Dawn Lambie, RN, MSN, CHPN
Kaiser Permanente, Roseville, California
Marilyn Leshko, RN
Lehigh Valley Hospital, Allentown, Pennsylvania
Patricia Lewis, MSN, FNP, CVN
Bassett Healthcare, Cooperstown, New York
Lori Kennedy Madden, MS, RN, ACNP, CCRN, CNRN
University of California, Davis, Sacramento, California
Kathleen-McCaffrey, RN, MSN
New York University Medical Center, New York, New York

Mary McDermott, MS, RN, NE-BC, APRN
Hospital for Special Surgery, New York, New York
Phyllis McKiernan, MSN, APN-C, RN
Hackensack University Medical Center, Hackensack, New Jersey
Ann McSwain, RN, MSN, CCRN, APRN, BC
St. Mary's Health Center, Jefferson City, Missouri
Peggy Tidikis Menck, PhD, RN
Independent Consultant
Barry M. Mitchneck, RN, MSN, CEN
Lehigh Valley Hospital, Allentown, Pennsylvania
Judy K. Moren, BM, RN
Nursing Education and Collections Training Manager, BloodSource,
Sacramento, California
Maxine L. Morris, BSN
New York Medical Center, New York, New York
Agnes Oblas, ANP-C
Ray Road Medical Center, Phoenix, Arizona
Jaime L. Peters, ADN
Lehigh Valley Hospital, Bethlehem, Pennsylvania
Sherri Reese, RN, BSN, CIC
University of California Davis Medical Center, Sacramento, California
Lory Anne F. Robles, BSN, MSN, RN
Stanford University Hospital, Palo Alto, California
Bonnie Smith Rosario, RN
Assumption Rural Health Clinic, Napoleonville, Louisiana
Sande Rowlee, MS, RN, CNS, ACNP-BC
Sacramento Bariatric Medical Associates, Carmichael, California
Jeremy Sabatino, BSN
Trinitas Hospital, Elizabeth, New Jersey
Debby Skroch, BSN, RN
John C. Lincoln North Mountain Hospital, Phoenix, Arizona
Leonard Sterling, RN, BSN
University of California Davis Medical Center, Sacramento, California
Ann D. Stoltz, PhD, RN
California State University, Sacramento, California
Belinda J. Swearingen, RN, MSN, FNP-C
Corrigan Medical Center, Corrigan, Texas
William E. Trumbore, III, RN, CEN, PHRN, AAS, BSPA
Lehigh Valley Hospital, Allentown, Pennsylvania
Deborah Tuggle, RN, MN, CCNS
Jewish Hospital-St. Mary's Healthcare, Louisville, Kentucky
Patricia Walters, RN, ACNP, CCRN, ACLS, BCLS
Hackensack University Medical Center, Hackensack, New Jersey

Authors Kathleen Osborn, Cheryl Wraa, and Annita Watson and their contributors have written an integrative and comprehensive textbook for preparing basic nursing students for evidence-based practice in medical–surgical nursing. This text places caring practices as conceptualized by the nurse theorist Sr. Simone Roach (1984) at the center of excellent nursing practice. Caring includes six essential components: compassion, competence, confidence, conscience, commitment, and comportment. The authors also place clinical judgment and critical thinking within the context of best evidence-based practice, recognizing that nursing and medicine are subject to ever-changing modes of scientific discovery and validation and that a particular patient may not easily fit into statistical norms. Therefore, the nurse must exercise good clinical reasoning, evaluation of evidence, and critical thinking.

This text invites the student to begin a lifelong journey of learning and clinical knowledge development while providing a clear road map beginning with the general and moving to more complex medical–surgical nursing care. The ability to recognize the nature of an ambiguous, under-determined clinical situation is at the heart of good clinical reasoning and care. The Critical Alert boxes throughout the text help the student focus on essential nursing interventions for attending to a particular patient with specific clinical conditions. Mastering this text will facilitate students' learning so they begin to think like a nurse in a broad range of clinical situations.

The authors are to be commended for fostering a comprehensive and holistic view of nursing practice, as caregiver, patient advocate, educator, researcher, and leader. Clinical vignettes and nurse interviews are included so that the student can develop a clinical imagination for the care of patients with specific clinical conditions and sociocultural characteristics. I highly recommend this book for all nursing students! Studying this text is a great way to gain visions and examples of excellent nursing practice, research, patient advocacy, leadership, and education.

PATRICIA BENNER, RN, PhD, FAAN
Thelma Shobe Endowed Chair in Ethics and Spirituality
University of California, San Francisco,
Department of Social and Behavioral Sciences

As the 21st century evolves, nursing and its place in health care are also evolving. This era is characterized by rapid change, including a growing multicultural population, longer life spans, arrival of new illnesses, and poor health conditions. Explosive advances in technology, ever-changing work settings, and a complex health care environment that is costly and competitive contribute to nursing's evolving environment. The burgeoning level of information affects decision making, and newer, faster modes of communication add to the environment's complexity. The definitions of roles and responsibilities for health care providers are changing; new boundaries are defined in which accountabilities are different, quality indicators are vital, and evidence-based practice is the standard. Ethical considerations must be balanced as nurses are called on to think quickly in establishing short- and long-term goals with the patient and family, in collaboration with the health care team and the community.

Never before in the history of nursing has the profession faced greater challenges to produce enough qualified nurses to practice in such a rapidly changing environment. And at a time when the need for professional nurses is overwhelming, we face a deficit in qualified nurses. Thus, it is time for professional scrutiny, self-determination, and innovation; nursing education is challenged to be innovative in preparing nurses for practice now and in the future. The challenge is to prepare nurses who can provide cognitively skilled care, in a caring manner, with a diverse patient population, and in innovative health care settings.

The authors' vision for this textbook is to meet that challenge. This textbook prepares the learner to be a knowledgeable, caring health care professional. It is a foundation on which to build the nursing practice of today and tomorrow, incorporating the cognitive, affective, and psychomotor skills necessary to practice. This book is not a destination to be achieved, but the beginning of lifelong learning.

Goals

The goal of this book is to expose the learner to concepts basic to the practice of professional nursing, including caring, critical thinking, research, nursing process, and health promotion. Caring is the foundation of nursing practice because of its impact on patients and their families. The authors have adopted Roach's (1984) theory of caring, which includes six components: compassion, competence, confidence, conscience, commitment, and comportment. Within the chapter features the authors have applied these six components when describing the nursing care needed for each of the physical disorders. This helps learners develop their understanding of how to be a caring nurse and makes them aware of these qualities in fellow health care professionals' practice and when advocating for the patient.

The nursing process is used to develop critical thinking and clinical reasoning skills, providing the framework for applying evidenced-based practice. Research is discussed throughout the text, providing opportunities for the reader to examine current research topics and their application to nursing practice.

Health promotion, one of the primary roles of the nurse, is woven throughout the book, so learners will understand the importance of educating the patient/family about healthy habits and lifestyles that prevent illnesses and injuries.

Readers will become active participants in learning about nursing as they progress through the book contents. Learners should be able to demonstrate understanding of the concepts of medical–surgical nursing in a variety of settings by collaborating with the authors in defining requisite content for patient care, arriving at patient diagnoses, and developing plans of care.

The concepts of experiential learning shape the book contents. The intention is that learners will engage in reflective thought and analysis of their practice as they apply the principles and concepts incorporated in the book to clinical practice, using the book as a resource for validating perceptions, expanding their knowledge base, and evaluating their approaches to patient care. The book is organized to introduce learners to the basic concepts of health care in general, and to nursing specifically, before moving on to the concepts underlying health promotion and disease management and the common physiological disorders that are encountered in medical–surgical nursing practice.

The units and chapters are grouped to lead the learner from general concepts to the more complex concepts and challenges of disease management. The information is sequenced to enhance critical thinking skills, thereby promoting the development of clinical judgment.

Knowledge acquisition is enhanced by application, analysis, and evaluation. Thus, this text provides numerous opportunities for learners to participate in activities designed to develop critical thinking and problem-solving skills in collaboration with the nursing experts who have contributed to the book. These learning activities include preparing clinical preparation plans, establishing priorities for care, developing patient care plans, and evaluating knowledge in the affective, cognitive, and psychomotor domains of practice. As learners complete these experiential and interactive activities, they will achieve a holistic, scientific, and caring approach to professional nursing practice for now and the future.

Organization

The book consists of 16 units sequenced from simple, basic concepts to complex, medical–surgical disorders. Units 1 and 2 introduce the reader to general concepts related to health care delivery, followed by basic concepts related to nursing practice. The next two units cover physiological concepts and the theoretical basis of skills that are germane to all areas of nursing practice. Units 5 through 16 focus on physiological disorders common to medical–surgical nursing. Each disorder unit opens with an assessment chapter that provides a template to assess the presenting patient within the specific body system.

THE TEXT FEATURES were designed to highlight the concepts that form the framework for this textbook and that are basic to professional nursing: **caring, research, critical thinking, the nursing process,** and **health promotion.** The capstone feature in each disorders chapter, **Clinical Preparation,** offers learners the opportunity to bring all of the concepts into one summary exercise and thus prepares learners for safe and knowledgeable clinical practice in their future work as professional nurses.

Caring

Profiles in Nursing. Each unit opens with a portrait of a nurse who describes "a day in the life" of working in a given specialty area. This profile includes a snapshot of a typical day and highlights the nurse's application of the six components of caring into his or her specialty. The information helps nursing students learn about the possibilities open to them when they are deciding where to spend concentrated clinical rotations or contemplating a job change.

Research

RESEARCH OPPORTUNITIES AND CLINICAL IMPACT RELATED TO CORONARY ARTERY DISEASE

Research Area	Clinical Impact
Stem cell injection after acute myocardial infarction.	Stimulate new growth of myocardial cells and increase myocardial viability.
Gene therapy for chronic CAD patients who have no other alternatives.	Stimulate angiogenesis, thereby decreasing symptoms and increasing quality of life.
Facilitated percutaneous intervention for acute myocardial infarction.	Conjoined mechanical and pharmacologic interventions for AMI will decrease mortality and increase myocardial salvage.
Establish heart-healthy food supplements.	Decrease hyperlipidemia, thereby providing risk factor modification for some predisposed risk factors.
Identify predictors of vulnerable plaque and their impact.	Provide ability to manage plaque and prevent plaque rupture, thus future coronary events.
Establish standard of providing fibrinolytic therapy in the field.	Increase survival for acute myocardial infarction patient.
Effect of community awareness programs on patients with ACS emphasizing early symptom recognition and treatment.	Decrease adverse cardiovascular events and increase survival from out-of-hospital events.
Effect of immediately triaging women with ACS-like symptoms to chest pain unit.	Increase survival in the female population and bring awareness because their symptoms are often missed.
Behavior modification techniques and their effect on CAD and its events.	Lower all modifiable risk factors, thereby decreasing cardiovascular events in a high-risk population.
Effect on established grammar and high school education program teaching about CAD; i.e., signs and symptoms, treatments, outcomes.	Establish an aware and healthier population early on, thereby decreasing total cardiovascular events.

Research Opportunities and Clinical Impact. Current research topics and their clinical impact introduces the learner to prospective research needs that are designed to potentially improve patient care. The purpose is to help the learner focus on future research needs and potential projects to improve patient care.

EVIDENCE-BASED PRACTICE

Heart Failure

Clinical Problem

Heart failure (HF) remains the most common discharge diagnosis in elderly patients, accounting for almost a quarter of all cardiovascular hospitalizations (Stewart et al., 2002). Heart failure patients commonly experience readmissions due to noncompliance, lack of understanding of self-management principles, inadequate treatment, and/or progressive disease. Although a number of pharmacologic treatments have been shown to improve outcomes in patients with HF (Jessup & Brozena, 2003), the prognosis of these patients remains poor (MacIntyre et al., 2000), resulting in frequent readmission to the hospital. Thus, there is a need for other approaches to management.

Research Findings

McAlister, Stewart, Ferrua, & McMurray (2004) conducted a study to determine whether multidisciplinary strategies improve outcomes for HF patients. The researchers searched electronic databases, bibliographies, and contacted experts to find multidisciplinary management programs in HF. Twenty-nine trials (5,039 patients) were identified. The researchers independently reviewed the results of the search strategy and selected all studies reporting the impact of outpatient-based multidisciplinary management strategies on mortality or hospitalization rates in patients with HF. Each type of intervention was then independently assigned to one of four groups: (1) multidisciplinary HF clinic; (2) multidisciplinary team providing specialized follow-up but not in a hospital or practice-based clinic; (3) telephone follow-up or telemonitoring and enhanced communication with primary care physician (including advice to deteriorating patients to see their regular physician); or (4) educational programs designed to enhance patient self-care activities.

The study results reveal that these programs are associated with a 27% reduction in HF hospitalization rates and a 43% reduction in total number of HF hospitalizations. Those strategies that incorporate specialized follow-up by a multidisciplinary team or in a multidisciplinary HF clinic also reduce all-cause mortality by approximately one-quarter and all-cause hospitalizations by one-fifth.

Implications for Nursing Practice

In order to assist the patient in getting ready for discharge from the hospital, it is essential that the nurse have an understanding of the symptoms, diagnosis, and management (medical, device, and self-management). The nurse must stress the importance of compliance with every aspect of care. If the patient has been cared for using a multidisciplinary approach, the nurse typically coordinates each member of the team. The nurse must reinforce teaching and determine the patient/family's understanding of the disease and its management.

When doing discharge planning, the nurse must ask the patient about her resources and support system. A plan needs to be developed that is realistic and manageable for the patient and family. Assistance for patients who may have difficulties taking or obtaining their medications must be provided. Ensure patients have access to urgent care, outside emergency department settings. It could be beneficial if a system for postdischarge telephone follow-up were instituted for these patients.

Critical Thinking Questions

1. Your patient was discharged from the hospital 3 days ago after a heart failure hospitalization. You are the nurse calling him to see how he is feeling since discharge. He states that his daughter was supposed to pick up his medications, but had a family emergency and forgot. He still does not have his medications, and he was discharged 5 days ago. What do you do?

2. You are the nurse in a clinic, and a patient with heart failure says she is taking her medications appropriately and following a low-salt, fluid-restricted diet. Your patient's weight continues to rise, and symptoms are worsening. What do you do to help this patient?

3. Your patient is readmitted for heart failure 2 weeks after his last heart failure hospitalization. What can you do to understand what went wrong at home, and how you can prevent a third admission?

References

Jessup, M., & Brozena, S. (2003). Medical progress heart failure. *The New England Journal of Medicine, 348,* 2007–2018.

Macintyre, K., Capewell, S., Stewart, S., et al. (2000). Evidence of improving prognosis in heart failure trends in case fatality in 66,547 patients hospitalized between 1986 and 1995. *Circulation, 102,* 1126–1131.

McAlister, F. A., Stewart, S., Ferrua, S., & McMurray, J. J. (2004). Multidisciplinary strategies for the management of heart failure patients at high risk for admission: A systematic review of randomized trials. *Journal of the American College of Cardiology, 44*(4), 810–819.

Stewart, S., Jenkins, A., Buchan, S., McGuire, A., Capewell, S., & McMurray, J. J. V. (2002). The current cost of heart failure to the National Health Service in the UK. *European Journal of Heart Failure, 4,* 361–371.

Evidence-Based Practice. This feature presents examples of evidence and how the studies impact nursing interventions, patient teaching, skills, and professional guidelines. Learners have an opportunity to test their understanding by responding to the critical thinking questions provided for each Evidence-Based Practice feature.

ETHICAL ISSUES for Pain Management at End of Life

Management of pain at the end of life is the right of the patient and the duty of the caregiver. Many families state that their loved ones suffered from untreated pain at the end of their life (Jackson & Abrahm, 2005). Failure to treat the pain adequately can arise from the caregiver's fear of violating ethical and moral tenets in the administration of pain medication to the dying patient.

At the end of life, the use of opioids, benzodiazepines, and other medications in doses high enough to control the patient's symptoms may unintentionally hasten death. This is referred to as double effect, where an action may have two possible effects, one good and one bad. The action is not considered immoral if it is undertaken with the intention of achieving the good effect without intending the bad effect, even though it may be foreseen. At the end of life not administering a drug to relieve symptoms because it may hasten death would be viewed as causing the patient harm and increased suffering.

Ethical Issues. This feature highlights the diverse ethical dilemmas that nurses face in clinical practice daily.

GERONTOLOGICAL CONSIDERATIONS Weight Management

Adults over age 65 years can benefit from weight management with improved day-to-day functioning and reduced cardiovascular risk. Before weight loss is recommended or attempted, however, a thorough nutrition assessment should be considered because of the high prevalence of malnutrition among older adults. Improper dieting attempts could unwittingly contribute to increased risk of malnutrition. Patients should be evaluated for their individual risks and benefits associated with potential weight loss. Specific attention should be given to preservation of muscle mass with physical activity. Appropriate referrals should be made for monitoring nutrition and exercise in the elderly.

Gerontological Considerations. The special needs of the fastest growing population are considered in order to help prevent complications and improve the prognoses for elderly patients.

CULTURAL CONSIDERATIONS for Therapeutic Communications

Munoz and Luckmann (2005) provide a rationale for the growing need for transcultural communication. They cite the increasing ethnic, racial, and cultural diversity of the United States; the increase in the number of patients who represent different culturally influenced patterns of health behavior; the different cultural meanings of health care; the different ways in which patients and families respond to health care; the multicultural nature of health care settings; and the nursing profession's commitment to culturally competent humanistic care. They further contend that talking to strangers about deeply personal issues is often difficult and may be particularly so for patients who are from different cultural backgrounds. They identify several behaviors on the part of nurses that are necessary to encourage patents to talk about themselves. Nurses must convey empathy, show respect, build trust, establish rapport, listen actively, provide appropriate feedback, and demonstrate genuine interest (p. 148). They also identify barriers to effective transcultural communication as follows: nurses' lack of knowledge, bias, ethnocentrism, prejudice, and stereotyping. Further, language differences, differences in the understanding of terminology, and differences in perceptions and expectations also create barriers (p. 162).

Cultural Considerations. These topics teach the learner to be sensitive to the needs of patients with different ethnic/cultural backgrounds, religious practices, and beliefs about health care and end of life, thereby enabling the learner to develop a multicultural approach to care.

GENETIC CONSIDERATIONS Implications for Weight Management

Speculation about the genetic implications in weight management has existed for some time. The specific roles of genetics as related to risk of obesity and eating disorders are being investigated. Risk factors for the development of eating disorders have been linked to genetic phenotypes for other disorders, such as the traits for obsessive-compulsive disorder and disturbances of dopamine systems (Kaye et al., 2004; Shinohara et al., 2004).

The role of genetics and the possibility of genetic manipulation have been heavily researched in the hope of identifying obesity risk factors and treatment options. Substances involved in appetite regulation, such as neuropeptide Y and ghrelin, proteins involved in thermogenesis, and leptin, and their relation to obesity are among the areas of research (Campion, Milagro, & Martinez, 2004; Marti, Moreno-Aliaga, Hebebrand, & Martinez, 2004). Although the topic of genetic influence on the development of both eating disorders and obesity is intriguing, it is difficult to draw firm conclusions without further research into these areas (Bulik, Sullivan, Wade, & Kendler, 2000; Kaye et al., 2004).

Genetic Considerations. This box contributes vital information about risk factors, therapies, research, legal implications, and counseling/ screening, as appropriate.

COMPLEMENTARY & ALTERNATIVE THERAPIES — Music Therapy

BEHAVIORAL MEDICINE, psychologists, and nurses have focused on prevention and psychosocial influences of cardiovascular diseases for the past 30 years. Music therapy is a viable collaborative, complementary method in the psychosocial arena for alleviating risks and motivating rehabilitation from cardiac events. For the most part, music is listened to via headphones during hospitalization. Cardiac units should stock headphones, CD or other varieties of players, and a wide selection of musical CDs, ranging from country-western to rock and roll to classical scores. Patients can be encouraged to use their music of choice on an outpatient basis prior to discharge.

Research Support:
Research supports the use of music to modulate heart health measurements such as heart rate and blood pressure, to enhance exercise programs, and to relieve stress symptoms. One study (Metzger, 2004) involved administering a music therapy survey to determine current use and preference for music in a cardiac rehabilitation program. Patients attending sessions in a large city hospital completed a survey on which they rated their level of use of music for exercise, relaxation, and enjoyment. Information was also gathered about musical preferences, musical experiences, and pertinent demographics. Patients, mostly white males over the age of 60, showed positive responses to the aesthetically pleasurable aspects of music. The results suggest that education about and development of music therapy in a cardiac rehabilitation program are warranted.

A German study with coronary patients (Vollert et al., 2003) concluded that music is able to lower stress and fear, contributing to relaxation in spite of physical exercise. Fifteen patients in a coronary sports unit listened to relaxation music while doing their heart-frequency-adapted exercises. Before the exercises and after listening to music, blood pressures were measured and blood was collected for determination of beta-endorphin. Simultaneous to blood collection, the participants had to perform two psychometric tests: the Perceived Stress Questionnaire (PSQ) of Levenstein, to measure the graduation of subjective perceived stress, and the State-Trait Anxiety

Inquiry (STAI) of Spielberger, as an indicator of coping. The whole protocol was performed one week prior to the mean trial, but without listening to music and without blood collections and blood pressure measurements. In the test trial without music, there were no significant changes in PSQ data. In the mean trial, under the influence of music, values in the section "worries" decreased as a sign of lower worries. STAI values were significantly lower as a sign of reduced fear after listening to music. Beta-endorphin concentration and systolic blood pressure decreased significantly after listening to music. These researchers conclude that in worries and fear, patients benefit by the intervention of music (Vollert et al., 2003).

The use of music therapy has been shown to reduce pain, anxiety, and physiological parameters in patients having surgical procedures. One study (Sendelbach et al., 2006) used an experimental design to compare the effects of music therapy versus a quiet, uninterrupted rest period on pain intensity, anxiety, physiological parameters, and opioid consumption after cardiac surgery. A sample of 86 patients was randomized to 1 of 2 groups receiving either 20 minutes of music (intervention) or 20 minutes of rest in bed (control). A significant reduction in anxiety and pain was demonstrated in the group that received music compared with the control group, but no difference was observed in systolic blood pressure, diastolic blood pressure, or heart rate. No reduction in opioid usage occurred in the 2 groups.

References
Metzger, L. K. (2004). Assessment of use of music by patients participating in cardiac rehabilitation. *Journal of Music Therapy, 41*(1), 55–69.

Sendelbach, S. E., Halm, M. A., Doran, K. A., Miller, E. H., & Gaillard, P. (2006). Effects of music therapy on physiological and psychological outcomes for patients undergoing cardiac surgery. *Journal of Cardiovascular Nursing, 21*(3), 194–200.

Vollert, J. O., Stork, T., Rose, M., & Mockel, M. (2003). Music as adjuvant therapy for coronary heart disease. Therapeutic music lowers anxiety, stress and beta-endorphin concentrations in patients from a coronary sport group. *Dtsch Med Wochenschr, 128*(51–52), 2712–2716.

Complementary and Alternative Therapies. The content of this feature introduces the learner to a variety of therapies used by patients that augment mainstream medicine. An understanding of the interactions of these therapies with more traditional therapies is essential for patient safety.

Nursing Process

PHARMACOLOGY Summary of Medications to Treat Inflammatory Heart Disease

Medication Category	Action	Application/Indication	Nursing Responsibility
Inflammatory Heart Disease **Antibiotics** Erythromycin Penicillin Specific type depends on the organism	Inhibits protein synthesis of microorganisms by binding reversibly to a ribosome, thus interfering with transmission of genetic information.	*Rheumatic fever:* treats Lancefield group A beta-hemolytic streptococcus. *Pericarditis and myocarditis:* indicated if it is a bacterial infection. *Endocarditis:* indicated if infecting organism is bacterial and prophylactic for invasive procedures and dental work.	Assessment of history of drug allergies prior to administration. Assessment of clinical manifestations of allergic reaction. Assessment of relief of clinical manifestations to determine drug effectiveness. Patient education regarding need to complete the entire regimen and report any clinical manifestations of drug allergy.
Nonsteroidal Anti-Inflammatory Agents (NSAIDs) Indomethacin (Indocin) Ibuprofen Aspirin	Inhibits cyclooxygenase, an enzyme responsible for the formation of prostaglandins. When cyclooxygenase is inhibited, inflammation and pain are reduced.	*Rheumatic fever:* joint pain and fever. *Pericarditis:* chest pain and swelling. *Myocarditis:* pain. *Endocarditis:* fever.	Assess pain before and after administration to determine effectiveness. Medications should not be taken on an empty stomach. Monitor renal and liver function tests for abnormalities related to drug side effects. Assessment of bleeding and gastric ulcer development.
Steroids Solu-Cortef Cortisone Solu-Medrol	Stabilizes leukocyte lysosomal membrane; inhibits phagocytosis and release of allergic substances; reduces capillary dilation and permeability. Modifies immune response to various stimuli.	*Myocarditis:* to prevent cardiac damage when the cause is autoimmune.	Careful assessment of relief of clinical manifestations. Assessment of side effects: Infection due to depressed immune response. Blood glucose monitoring. Gastric bleeding. Emotional lability. Lack of wound healing. Patient education regarding need to eventually reduce dosage.
Cardiac Medications **ACE inhibitors:** Lisinopril Enalapril Ramipril Captopril	ACE inhibitor: Lowers peripheral resistance and reduces blood volume by enhancing the excretion of sodium by inhibition of angiotensin-converting enzyme.	*Myocarditis:* heart failure. *Rheumatic fever, pericarditis, and myocarditis:* to control atrial and ventricular dysrhythmias caused by inflammation and stretching of myocardium.	Monitor blood pressure carefully after first dose for hypotension. Educate patient that it takes 2 weeks for therapeutic effect. May experience dizziness.
Antiarrhythmic Agents Adenosine Amiodarone Atropine sulfate Sotalol	Alters the electrophysiological properties of the heart by either blocking flow through the channels or altering autonomic activity.	To control dysrhythmias.	There is a narrow margin between therapeutic effect and toxicity; therefore, careful and ongoing cardiac monitoring is essential. Patient teaching includes avoiding the use of alcohol, drugs, and tobacco.
Diuretics Furosemide Torsemide	Blocks reabsorption of sodium and chloride in the loop of Henle. Reduces edema associated with heart failure.	*Myocarditis:* heart failure.	Potassium levels also need monitoring because low levels are a side effect of certain diuretics, especially furosemide. May need potassium replacement. Measure urine output prior to administration to gauge the response to the medication.

Pharmacology Summary Tables. These four-column tables offer a comprehensive overview of the pharmacology for the chapter disorders, organized by drug categories, and include medications, actions, applications and indications, and the nursing responsibilities.

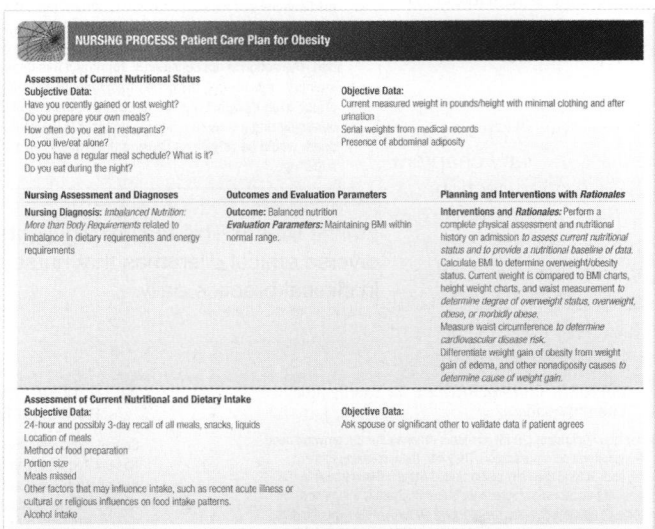

NURSING PROCESS: Patient Care Plan for Obesity

Assessment of Current Nutritional Status

Subjective Data:
Have you recently gained or lost weight?
Do you prepare your own meals?
How often do you eat in restaurants?
Do you live/eat alone?
Do you have a regular meal schedule? What is it?
Do you eat during the night?

Objective Data:
Current measured weight in pounds/height with minimal clothing and after urination
Serial weights from medical records
Presence of abdominal adiposity

Nursing Assessment and Diagnoses	Outcomes and Evaluation Parameters	Planning and Interventions with Rationales
Nursing Diagnosis: *Imbalanced Nutrition: More than Body Requirements* related to imbalance in dietary requirements and energy requirements	Outcome: Balanced nutrition *Evaluation Parameters:* Maintaining BMI within normal range.	Interventions and *Rationales:* Perform a complete physical assessment and nutritional history on admission *to assess current nutritional status and to provide a nutritional baseline of data.* Calculate BMI to determine overweight/obesity status. Current weight is compared to BMI charts, height weight charts, and waist measurement *to determine degree of overweight status, overweight, obese, or morbidly obese.* Measure waist circumference *to determine cardiovascular disease risk.* Differentiate weight gain of obesity from weight gain of edema, and other nonadiposity causes *to determine cause of weight gain.*

Assessment of Current Nutritional and Dietary Intake

Subjective Data:
24-hour and possibly 3-day recall of all meals, snacks, liquids
Location of meals
Method of food preparation
Portion size
Meals missed
Other factors that may influence intake, such as recent acute illness or cultural or religious influences on food intake patterns.
Alcohol intake

Objective Data:
Ask spouse or significant other to validate data if patient agrees

Nursing Process: Patient Care Plan. The nursing process care plan provides the learner with an easy-to-follow, easy-to-apply, succinct way of organizing nursing care, guided by nursing diagnosis, assessment, intervention, and outcome evaluation. It is designed to assist the learner in developing a plan of care specific to the patient with desired patient outcomes and specific nursing interventions for a given diagnosis.

Critical Alerts. This feature alerts the learner to the immediate need for a nursing intervention that will prevent complications and promote learning. The learner will differentiate the critical nature of various clinical situations and determine the need to prioritize interventions.

DIAGNOSTIC TESTS for Cardiac Valve Disease

Test and Normal Values	Expected Abnormality	Rationale for Abnormality
Echocardiogram and transesophageal echocardiography (TEE) Echocardiogram (ultrasound): *Normal chamber size and normal cardiac structures*	Abnormal structure and function of heart valves, able to identify thickened valve leaflets, vegetative growths, myocardial function, and chamber size. TEE is particularly useful not only for diagnosing but also for tracking the progression of the disease.	Vegetative growths and infection cause a thinning of valve leaflets leading to abnormal function.
Chest x-ray: *Clear lungs and normal heart size*	Pulmonary congestion, cardiac hypertrophy, chamber and great vessel enlargement, and calcification of the valves.	Abnormal valve function causes a change in blood flow leading to changes in chamber size and valve structure.
Cardiac catheterization: *Normal coronary artery blood flow, chamber size, and valve function*	The size of the valve opening and pressure gradients across valve surfaces is abnormal. Pressure in the heart chambers and pulmonary system is increased. Cardiac output typically is decreased.	Abnormal valve structure causes changes in openings leading to increased pressures in the cardiac chambers and decreased cardiac output.
Electrocardiogram (ECG): *Normal conduction time intervals*	Conduction delays, atrial and ventricular dysrhythmias, because of cardiac ischemia. Is useful in detecting increased ischemia and the presence of life-threatening dysrhythmias.	Changes occur due to diminished blood flow to the myocardium due to decreased cardiac output caused by abnormal valvular function.
Cardiac MRI (CMR): *Normal heart valve function*	Valve size and competence.	Abnormal valve structure causes changes in openings, leading to increased pressures in the cardiac chambers and decreased cardiac output.

Diagnostic Tests. These tables inform the learner about the relevant diagnostic tests for the disorder under discussion. Normal result ranges are included, as well as expected abnormalities with rationales.

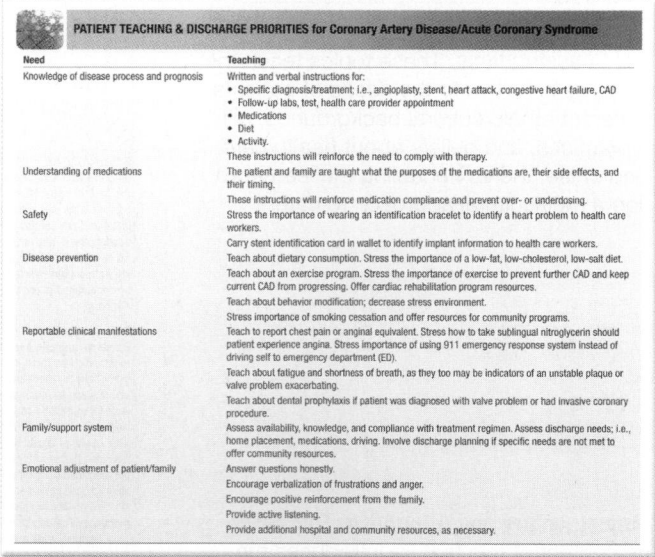

PATIENT TEACHING & DISCHARGE PRIORITIES for Coronary Artery Disease/Acute Coronary Syndrome

Need	Teaching
Knowledge of disease process and prognosis	Written and verbal instructions for: • Specific diagnosis/treatment; i.e., angioplasty, stent, heart attack, congestive heart failure, CAD • Follow-up labs, test, health care provider appointment • Medications • Diet • Activity. These instructions will reinforce the need to comply with therapy.
Understanding of medications	The patient and family are taught what the purposes of the medications are, their side effects, and their timing. These instructions will reinforce medication compliance and prevent over- or underdosing.
Safety	Stress the importance of wearing an identification bracelet to identify a heart problem to health care workers. Carry stent identification card in wallet to identify implant information to health care workers.
Disease prevention	Teach about dietary consumption. Stress the importance of a low-fat, low-cholesterol, low-salt diet. Teach about an exercise program. Stress the importance of exercise to prevent further CAD and keep current CAD from progressing. Offer cardiac rehabilitation program resources. Teach about behavior modification; decrease stress environment. Stress importance of smoking cessation and offer resources for community programs.
Reportable clinical manifestations	Teach to report chest pain or anginal equivalent. Stress how to take sublingual nitroglycerin should patient experience angina. Stress importance of using 911 emergency response system instead of driving self to emergency department (ED). Teach about fatigue and shortness of breath, as they too may be indicators of an unstable plaque or valve problem exacerbating. Teach about dental prophylaxis if patient was diagnosed with valve problem or had invasive coronary procedure.
Family/support system	Assess availability, knowledge, and compliance with treatment regimen. Assess discharge needs; i.e., home placement, medications, driving. Involve discharge planning if specific needs are not met to offer community resources.
Emotional adjustment of patient/family	Answer questions honestly. Encourage verbalization of frustrations and anger. Encourage positive reinforcement from the family. Provide active listening. Provide additional hospital and community resources, as necessary.

Patient Teaching & Discharge Priorities. This table helps identify priorities for discharge planning while integrating patient teaching with home and community care.

Health Promotion

Risk Factors. These boxes highlight particular items in the patient history and interview that should alert the nurse to possible problems.

Health Promotion. Found as appropriate in many chapters, Health Promotion sections call the learner's attention to one of the primary roles of the nurse, that of educating the patient and family about healthy habits and lifestyles, thereby preventing or ameliorating unhealthy conditions.

National Guidelines. These guidelines are integrated throughout the chapters where appropriate to provide pertinent, specific objectives to increase the awareness of the learner of the need for uniformity of care on national and international levels (i.e., *Healthy People 2010,* HIPAA, and AHA).

Preparation for Practice

Clinical Preparation. This exercise is presented at the end of each disorder chapter to present the learner with a reality-oriented approach to patient assessment and diagnosis. The learner will complete the assignment on the Web in MyNursingKit.

Clinical Preparation Assignments. The assignment helps the learner develop a problem-solving approach to nursing care. By completing the assignments presented at the end of the chapters, the learner will gain experience in critical thinking skills and develop a systematic method for determining a patient's health problem, devising a plan of care, developing evaluation criteria, and determining expected outcomes. The Clinical Preparation assignments also help the learner articulate the patient's needs and learn how to write effective evaluation statements. This, in turn, significantly improves documentation skills and the ability to communicate with other health care team members to provide the safest, most effective, and holistic care for the patient.

ACKNOWLEDGMENTS

In addition to the individuals mentioned in our dedications, we would also like to thank people who were instrumental in the development of the book. The following people assisted us in bringing this project to fruition:

- *Marion Waldman, the development editor, for being the glue that kept the project moving in a positive direction. For listening and being patient with our never ending list of questions. We could not have done it without her.*
- *Kelly Karr for her editing expertise and for the long hours she dedicated to making sure each chapter was error free.*
- *Susan Poirier for her exacting work in developing, formatting, and editing the pharmacology tables.*
- *Charlotte Miller for precise review of units to ensure consistency of content, developing the Kardex format, and placing URLs in the chapters.*
- *Linda Cooke for developing the clinical preparation framework, hand printing the Kardexs, and patiently guiding the authors to ensure consistency.*
- *Judy Tanner for her endless support, diligence, and patience in the detailed editing of chapters in the first page proofs.*
- *Mary Ann Shahdi, Jennifer FitzGerald, Andrea Perry, Sonia Garcia, Kathleen Budesa, and Jolie Tietz, nursing students, who generously shared their thoughts and feelings about caring behavior observed in nurses, presented in Chapter 1.*
- *Mike Osborn, Maddison Thivierge, and Adam Jonathan Davis for very short notice assistance with finalizing content for the book; it was greatly appreciated.*

CONTENTS

UNIT 2

General Concepts Related to Nursing Practice   146

UNIT 5

Nursing Management of the Surgical Patient 584

UNIT 6

Nursing Management of Patients with Neurological Disorders 692

UNIT 9

Nursing Management of Patients with Gastrointestinal, Renal, and Urinary Disorders   1364

UNIT 10

Nursing Management of Patients with Reproductive Disorders   1502

CHAPTER 48
Nursing Assessment of Patients with Reproductive Disorders   1504

CHAPTER 49
Caring for the Patient with Female Reproductive Disorders   1518

CHAPTER 50
Caring for the Patient with Male Reproductive Disorders   1566

UNIT 11

Nursing Management of Patients with Endocrine Disorders   1594

CHAPTER 51
Nursing Assessment of Patients with Endocrine Disorders   1596

CHAPTER 52
Caring for the Patient with Glandular and Hormonal Disorders   1613

UNIT 13

Nursing Management of Patients with Immunologic, Inflammatory, and Hematologic Disorders 1862

MEDICAL-SURGICAL NURSING
Preparation for Practice

UNIT 1

Concepts Related to Health Care Delivery and Nursing Practice

KATHY My name is Kathy and my nursing role is that of senior management leader for nursing services with the title of Vice President, Chief Nursing Officer, for two nonprofit, independent community acute care hospitals that offer a full range of services. I oversee all inpatient nursing units, including emergency/trauma, perioperative, women's/children's, cardiopulmonary, medical–surgical units, and physician hospitalist programs. Specifically I am responsible for staffing/scheduling functions, strategic direction, environment of practice, quality/patient safety, standards of care, and collaborative relationships with other disciplines providing care to patients. I also oversee the financial planning for operating and capital budgets that support the provision of care and the resources needed to meet the demands of our services. This role allows me to interface at many levels including governing board meetings, unit-based staff meetings, medical staff committees, and various state and community forums. One of my essential responsibilities is to ensure high-quality, safe patient care while balancing the financial needs of the organization.

I begin my day catching up on e-mail and voice mail communications because I know it is important for people to get timely responses. I keep my door open when I am in my office for "drop-in" conversations and "face time" with my team. Visibility is a key component of my job because staff, physicians, and the nursing management team need to know that I am listening to their concerns. A technique I use to increase my visibility is that when I need information I go to the person or department to communicate with them directly. This way I can check in with people as I travel the hallways and I can observe the environment. My **commitment** to being available to staff and my leadership team is important to ensure I understand their needs in order to represent them well.

The majority of my work is done in groups and team meetings to discuss, debate, and make decisions on policy and direction for the hospitals. My **comportment** is important in order to adequately represent nurses as credible leaders. I must be knowledgeable about issues such as quality and patient safety standards so I can contribute to discussions for improvement. My individual meetings are with the people who report directly so I can guide and mentor them in their roles.

The hardest part of my day is adjusting to changing priorities and schedules. At any moment a disaster can occur. For example, one day a pipe burst, causing water to be shut down in the main part of the hospital, which caused the closure of the surgery unit and required emergency plans to make sure the needs of staff, patients, and visitors were met. You must be very calm and considerate at these times as people deal with no running water, electricity, or functioning toilets. The **competence** to remain calm and direct the activities of a hospital during crises like this only comes from years of experience. Every situation gives me new insight into how things work and different solutions for unexpected events.

Another aspect of my job is dealing with complaints, which can be related to the quality of care and/or its aftermath, when patients receive their bills. It is very important to show **compassion** and to let the patients or their families know that I value their opinion and am committed to working with them to solve the problem. While care may have been delivered appropriately, if the caregiver failed to have the right attitude it will impact the recipients of that care. One vivid incident I remember was a woman whose husband had died. He had a terminal diagnosis, but they thought they had months to deal with his eventual death. Instead he became septic and died quickly. During the hospitalization she kept trying to get people to understand that she was confused and scared, yet everyone was so busy taking care of him, no one was listening to her. She was devastated by the experience and fearful that her husband's last moments were painful and chaotic. Incidents like these weigh heavy on my **conscience** and I work hard to help the staff know that their behavior and attitude can greatly affect the people they serve.

Working on committees with physicians and other allied health providers has helped me to understand the political dynamics of the hospital and how those dynamics interface with the community. I have to understand the internal workings of these committees, their level of authority to make decisions that affect patient care and nursing practice, and how the members perceive their responsibilities. This is very complex and requires study and preparation to be able to help the process along. First I must be sure that my **clinical reasoning** is sound so that I can debate on an appropriate level. My **critical thinking skills** are used to prepare appropriate responses and to offer solutions.

Although my days are busy, I enjoy the challenges of my job. Working in the global realm of the hospital allows me to use all of the components of the nursing process.

> "Every situation gives me new insight into how things work and different solutions for unexpected events."

Preparation for Practice

Kathleen Osborn, Cheryl Wraa, Annita Watson

With contributions by:
Donna York-Clark (Roles of the Nurse)

Outcome-Based Learning Objectives

After studying this chapter, the learner will be able to:

1. Distinguish the characteristics of nursing as defined in the roles of caregiver, advocate, educator, researcher, and leader.
2. Apply the six components of caring as defined by Roach to nursing practice.
3. Describe the roles of the professional nurse within the health care delivery system.
4. Compare and contrast the nursing role in the care delivery models for nursing practice.
5. Explain the importance of cultural competence as defined by Campinha-Bacote.

Research Collaboration Health Promotion Nursing Process Caring Critical Thinking

THE UNIQUENESS of nursing as a professional career lies in its diversity of practice and the opportunity for lifelong learning. The relatively fluid nature of the profession allows nurses to move from one setting to the next, thereby expanding knowledge, skills, and interest in their profession. The goal of nursing is to mobilize human and environmental resources to support healing, maintain well-being, prevent illness, and promote health. In every setting or specialty, the core of practice is the nursing process: assessment, diagnosis, planning, implementation, and rationales, and evaluation (Carpenito-Moyet, 2007). The American Nurses Association (ANA) states that "the essence of nursing is that nurses combine the art of caring with the science of health care. Nursing places its focus not only on a particular health problem, but on the whole patient and his or her response to treatment. Care of the patient and a firm base of scientific knowledge are indispensable elements" (ANA, 2008, p. 1).

There are approximately 2.8 million licensed nurses in the United States who deliver patient care in all locations where care is provided, including hospitals, ambulatory care centers, nursing homes, private homes, schools, and employee workplaces (Institute of Medicine [IOM], 2004). Patients within the health care system often turn to nurses for assistance, because nurses are the health care providers the patients are most likely to encounter and the ones with whom the patients spend the greatest amount of time. As America moves forward to improve the health care delivery system, nurses will contribute in many ways. The ANA publication ***Nursing's Agenda for the Future*** (2002) states:

> Nursing is the pivotal health care profession, highly valued for its specialized knowledge, skill and caring in improving the health status of the public and ensuring safe, effective, quality care.
>
> The profession mirrors the diverse population it serves and provides leadership to create positive changes in health policy and delivery systems.

As health care in America changes, nurses must have a strong voice in cultivating a stable workforce and be key participants in developing a viable health care system.

Medical–Surgical Nursing

The Academy of Medical–Surgical Nurses (AMSN) is a professional organization committed to promoting nursing practice in the areas of health promotion and prevention of illness in adults. Within its position statement, *Identification of the Registered Nurse in the Workplace* (AMSN, 2004), the organization offers a description of medical–surgical nursing:

> The nurse provides leadership for the provision of [medical surgical] care based on current research, nursing judgment, and careful analysis of each individual patient's unique situation. The nursing process is the decision-producing model for the selection of nursing interventions. The nurse as a direct or indirect practitioner selects, executes, performs, delegates, directs and supervises, and evaluates nursing actions. It is in the performance of these activities that the nurse is distinguished from other health care professionals.

Nurses play a pivotal role in health care, and research is beginning to document that how well patients are cared for by nurses affects their health (IOM, 2004). Advances in health care and technology have allowed more patients to receive care in venues other than the hospital. However, the acuity of patients within the hospital setting has risen. Patients who would have been cared for in an intensive care unit a few years ago are now being cared for on medical–surgical floors or in the home (American Association of Critical Care Nurses [AACN], 2004).

Nurses develop a partnership with the patient and assist patients in learning how to cope with circumstances in order to develop an environment that promotes health, prevents illness, and facilitates recovery (Figure 1–1 ■). One of the stated goals of the ANA (2004a) is to "implement new ways in which nursing services can be delivered to respond to current and future demands for cost-effective, quality health care."

FIGURE 1–1 ■ The nurse–patient partnership is critical to help the patient cope with illness.
Source: Chip Henderson/Photolibrary.com

Components of the Nursing Role

Certain commonalities are a part of every nursing role. The commonalities included in the nursing role are as follows: caregiver, advocate, educator, researcher, and leader. Each of these components is discussed next.

Caregiver

The nurse provides care based on current research, nursing judgment, and careful analysis of each individual patient's unique situation. The nursing process is the decision-producing model for the selection of nursing interventions (AMSN, 2004). Caring is the most central and unifying concept in nursing. In 1988, Jean Watson identified human care as an intersubjective human process and a moral ideal for nursing. She stated that the necessary conditions for caring to occur are knowledge and awareness about the need for care, an intention to act, action's based on knowledge, and a positive change that results from caring (Watson, 1988).

Advocate

As patients enter the health care system, they are often overwhelmed and unprepared to make informed decisions regarding their care. Also, patients may be so ill that they are unable to communicate their wishes. Part of the nurse–patient relationship is the nurse's assessment of the patient's and family's understanding regarding the diagnosis and plan of care, identification of educational needs, and communicating with other members of the health care team to advocate for the patient's rights to autonomy, free choice, and the ability to make informed decisions.

Nurses play a key role by serving as change agents within the health care system. Advocacy is more than just understanding an issue; it requires involvement and collaboration to provide a strong unified voice for nursing through legislative and regulatory representation. The American Nurses Association has federal and state advocacy web pages that track the status of current issues that are affecting health care. The ANA has also developed the Nurses Strategic Action Team (N-STAT). N-STAT is a grassroots network for nurses that alerts members to the progress of key bills as they move through Congress and who to contact regarding support or opposition (ANA, 2007a). The nurse as advocate supports excellence of care through patient, family, and community education, communication with other health care team members, and participation in health policy formulation.

Educator

The nurse not only provides education for patients and families, but also participates in the education of the community. Health education determines how well patients, families, and communities are able to develop behaviors that are beneficial to optimal self-care. The ANA's *Standards of Clinical Nursing Practice* (1998) and all state nurse practice acts include teaching as a function of nursing practice.

The emphasis in nursing education is on health promotion and maintenance. Nurses promote health by teaching, by modeling lifestyles that promote wellness, and by providing information regarding the characteristics and consequences of diseases, including risk factors and ways to decrease health risks. The U.S. Department of Health and Human Services (DHHS) has published national health objectives for the year 2010 (DHHS,

MyNursingKit | Healthy People

2000). The focus areas represent an opportunity for healthy lifestyle choices and encourage clinicians to incorporate prevention into their practice. An overview of the focus areas of *Healthy People 2010* occurs later in this chapter.

Researcher

The American Nurses Association (1997) believes that nurses from all levels of educational preparation are capable of participating in research activities, from the design of the study to interpretation of results. Nurses not only investigate issues of relevance to the practice of nursing, but also participate in interdisciplinary collaborations to research common health care issues. Collaborative and interdisciplinary research fosters communication and mutual respect and enhances collaborative practice. The National Institute of Nursing Research (NINR, 2001) believes that with more interdisciplinary collaborations, nursing can provide a more comprehensive approach to research in health promotion, illness, and disabling conditions. Chapter 8 ⊙ explores the role of research in nursing practice.

Leader

There are many definitions of the word *leadership*. One example states that leadership refers to the use of personal traits and personal power to constructively and ethically influence patients, families, and others toward an end point vision or goal (Yoder-Wise, 2008). All nurses are leaders as they model time management, priority setting, patient and family teaching, evaluation of the quality of care, precepting of students, mentoring of colleagues, and development of community outreach programs. A leader has the ability to tie together the support, collaboration, and enthusiasm of people to meet specific goals and objectives, whether it is a patient and his family or an entire organization.

Throughout this book, the learner is presented with a body of knowledge and skills that, with experience, will assist the nurse to create relationships and environments that are healing, humane, and caring. Professional nurses practice with compassion and respect for the inherent dignity, worth, and uniqueness of every individual, despite social or economic status, personal attributes, or the nature of health problems.

■ Framework for Nursing Practice

The framework for nursing practice is that it is an evidence-based profession that is guided by the ANA Code of Ethics for nurses (ANA, 2001a). The practice of nursing requires knowledge, critical thinking skills, and clinical judgment, and uses the nursing process to apply these concepts to patient care situations. All aspects of nursing practice are shaped and guided by a caring approach to patient care. Additionally, nurses have a responsibility to promote health and wellness for individuals and communities. Nursing as a profession was one of the first to understand the need for primary health care and prevention. As gaps in health care have occurred over the years, nurses have been able to fill them and provide high-quality service. This is true in all areas of nursing: acute care, specialty nursing, advanced practice, community nursing, and education. The nursing profession also has actively cared for disadvantaged socioeconomic groups. Because the breadth of nursing practice

is so great, the profession is in a good position to impact health care policy and decisions. In this time of tremendous health care transition, nurses must rise to the challenge of providing accessibility to quality patient care. The tenets of the framework for nursing practice are discussed next.

Nursing Process

The **nursing process** is a thinking and doing approach to patient care that provides the nurse with a systematic means of identifying, preventing, and treating actual and potential health problems (Carpenito-Moyet, 2007). According to the American Nurses Association (2007b), the nursing process is defined as a variation of scientific reasoning and is used to diagnose and to treat human responses to potential and actual health problems. The nursing process provides a patient-centered approach to care that is an essential part of the patient care plan. It is the framework that provides nurses with a concise method of organizing patient care. The nursing process promotes communication and collaboration with the health care team because it is an established approach that is understood and used by nurses to identify and treat patients' problems.

The nursing process includes the following steps: assessment, diagnosis, outcome identification, planning, implementation, and evaluation. These steps are ordered to facilitate the process of identifying patient problems and desired outcomes in an efficient, consistent manner. Each step depends on the activity of the previous step. In practice, the steps of the nursing process overlap with each other. For example, while performing interventions, the nurse continues to assess the patient. The new data that result from the assessment are used to determine desired outcomes, to identify and plan interventions, and to evaluate them. The evaluation phase overlaps all phases of the nursing process because the nurse is constantly evaluating nursing care (Wilkinson, 2009). Chapter 7 ⊙ contains an in-depth discussion of the nursing process.

Critical Thinking

Nursing is a highly complex and challenging profession that exists within a rapidly changing health care environment. The essence of nursing lies not in the special environments or amid the special equipment, but in the nurse's decision-making process and willingness to act on these decisions. In other words, the nurse must have the ability to think critically, possess sound clinical judgment, and effectively apply these concepts in multiple health care arenas and complex patient care situations. Critical thinking is not a separate body of knowledge to be learned, but, like reading and writing, critical thinking is a process that occurs in all areas of life and learning. Critical thinking is typically described as a purposeful, two-dimensional, goal-directed, self-regulatory process that is context bound (Lipe & Beasley, 2006). An international group of nursing experts consisting of 72 participants from nine countries developed a definition of critical thinking as it applies to nursing:

Critical thinking in nursing is an essential component of professional accountability and quality nursing care. Critical thinkers in nursing exhibit these habits of the mind: confidence, contextual perspective, creativity, flexibility, inquisitiveness, intellectual integrity, intuition, open-mindedness, perseverance, and reflection. Critical thinkers in nursing practice the cognitive skills of analyzing, applying standards, discriminating, information seeking, logical reasoning, predicting and transforming knowledge. (Gendrop & Eisenhauer, 1996)

Two dimensions are necessary for the development of critical thinking: the cognitive, which entails reflective, reasoned thinking, and the affective, which consists of being open-minded to divergent perspectives and having an inquisitive spirit (Lipe & Beasley, 2006). In addition to the cognitive and affective abilities, effective critical thinking skills evolve with time, knowledge, professional practice, and structured feedback (Benner, Tanner, & Chesla, 1996). Critical thinking skills develop in tandem with intellectual and ethical development (L'Eplattenier, 2001). Chart 1–1 identifies key critical thinking skills.

Critical thinking is necessary to begin the problem solving necessary for complex patient care situations. Critical thinking, however, is not *just* problem solving; it is also an application of logic that evolves from an understanding of the need to question conventions and habits and to base decisions on sound reasoning (D'Amico & Barbarito, 2007; Lipe & Beasley, 2006). Critical thinking is cultivated by questioning the norms and avoiding an acceptance of the biases. According to D'Amico and Barbarito, five essential elements are involved in the critical thinking process:

- Collection of information
- Analysis of the situation
- Generation of alternatives
- Selection of alternatives
- Evaluation.

Critical thinking skills are needed in order to observe, gather, organize, and analyze data accurately because interpretation of patient's symptoms can be complex and diverse. When applied to patient care situations critical thinking promotes health and assists the patient to achieve the desired outcomes of care (Fesler-Birch, 2005).

The process of developing critical thinking skills begins during the nurse's education process. The American Association of Colleges of Nursing (2007) requires that critical thinking be reflected within academic nursing programs as a core competency for program accreditation. However, the evolution and refinement of critical thinking continue as the nurse gains experience through practice (Brunt, 2005). To think critically, the nurse needs to apply experience and knowledge to patient care situations. Benner (2001) asserts that as nurses gain experience and knowledge in practice they progress through five distinct stages of skill acquisition, from novice to expert nurse. A complete description of these stages is discussed as outlined in Chapter 2 🔗 .

The goal of nursing education is to holistically prepare the learner for the profession by not only providing the necessary critical thinking skills, but also by providing socialization to the role of nursing. Central to role socialization is the development of **clinical judgment**, which is defined as a complex skill involving several cognitive phases and integrative processes. Critical thinking skills overlap with the conceptual boundaries of clinical judgment (Fesler-Birch, 2005).

Christine Tanner (1983), an identified expert in the study of clinical judgment, defines clinical judgment skills as follows:

- Making decisions regarding what to observe in the patient situation
- Making inferential decisions by deriving meaning from data observed
- Making decisions regarding actions to be taken that will be of optimal benefit to the patient.

After reviewing more than 200 studies on clinical judgment, Tanner (2006) identified five conclusions about a nurse's ability to develop and refine clinical judgment skills:

- Clinical judgment is more influenced by what nurses bring to the situation than the objective data about the situation at hand.
- Sound clinical judgment rests to some degree on knowing the patient's typical pattern of responses, as well as an engagement with the patient and her concerns.
- Clinical judgments are influenced by the context in which the situation occurs and the culture of the nursing care unit.
- Nurses use a variety of reasoning patterns alone or in combination.
- Reflection on practice is often triggered by a breakdown in clinical judgment, and therefore is critical in the development of clinical knowledge and improvement in clinical reasoning skills.

Tanner (2006) states that nurses' backgrounds, the context of situations, and nurses' relationships with their patients are central to what nurses notice and how they interpret findings, respond to those findings, and reflect on their responses. Assumptions basic to an integrated critical thinking model for clinical judgment development are that it is a multidimensional concept and that every act of clinical judgment in nursing has diagnostic, therapeutic, and ethical dimensions. Therefore, sound clinical judgment, which is a requirement for expertise in nursing, is derived from an ability to think critically.

Development of Critical Thinking Skills

As stated earlier, the acquisition of both critical thinking and subsequent clinical judgment skills begins with the education

---

CHART 1–1	**Critical Thinking Skills**

- Be inquisitive by asking pertinent questions.
- Assess what information is necessary to determine a solution to the problem.
- Gather the facts and validate the information.
- Consider available options.
- Be flexible and open-minded about all options.
- Draw on past experiences and knowledge.
- Formulate creative decisions and test their effectiveness.
- Be open-minded to dissonance and ambiguity.

process. During all phases of nursing education, learners are initially taught theory in the classroom followed by psychomotor skill demonstrations, which are practiced in simulated situations. To further refine decision-making and problem-solving skills, the student must then transfer and apply the theoretical knowledge to the clinical setting in a variety of patient care situations (Walsh & Seldomridge, 2006). It is imperative for the nurse to reflect on attitudes such as curiosity, fair-mindedness, humility, courage, and perseverance, which facilitate critical thinking in each patient care situation. Additionally, it is beneficial to reflect on previous patient care situations in which decisions were made and then assess the outcome of those decisions. This reflective thinking process identifies areas of strengths and weaknesses in a given situation, and gives direction to the nurse for future development and refinement of critical thinking and clinical judgment skills. Being open-minded to dissonance and ambiguity is essential if the nurse is going to expand critical thinking skills. If possible, any final decision should be suspended until all sides of an issue have been evaluated; note, however, that emergency situations do not allow for delay. This is why experienced nurses typically function more effectively in emergent situations—they have the thinking and judgment skills to effectively function with minimal delay.

Creating an environment where critical thinking is encouraged and nurtured is the responsibility of the nursing leadership. Differences in opinions and examination of various solutions must be tolerated and encouraged. Independent, individual, and divergent thinking skills are necessary to avoid "group thinking" and the pressure to defer to group decisions. If nurses are aware of their critical thinking skills, while they are doing the *thinking*, they can detect errors in judgment. Experiencing both negative and positive outcomes promotes the development of these skills. One example of clinical setting analysis occurs in some trauma centers where emergency resuscitation situations are videotaped and subsequently analyzed by the staff to determine the effectiveness of the resuscitation efforts. This is an excellent way of reflecting on the thinking and decision making that was done in a high-stress, complex patient care situation. The purpose of this reflective effort is to promote more effective patient care outcomes. But, it also presents an opportunity to enhance and refine high-level critical thinking and clinical judgment skills through experience.

Six Components of Caring

When a family member is being treated, families often do not remember the medications and the machines as much as they remember the caring spirit of the nurses. Nursing is a caring discipline with a foundation of nursing science guided by the application of moral and ethical principles of care and responsibility. **Caring**, which is directly derived from the ethical principle of beneficence, is the core of nursing and constitutes the essence of nursing regardless of the level at which nursing is practiced and conceptualized. Caring represents the unique aspect of nursing and is reflected in conscience, confidence, compassion, commitment, competence, and comportment (Roach, 1984). Without these components, nursing is a scientific and technical skill-based body of knowledge. Adding the components of caring to this body of knowledge enables nursing to be identified as a holistic profession. Without caring the nurse will

not see the psychological and spiritual sufferings of the patient (DeWolf-Bosek & Savage, 2007). The definition of each component of caring is outlined here:

- *Conscience* is possessing a moral sense of what is right and wrong. The nurse's conscience guides the nurse's practice and serves as a strong deterrent to providing minimal or inappropriate care. Conscience is not easily displayed, but every action is led by the conscience. The conscience helps nurses decide right from wrong and guides the *care* nurses give to patients.

- *Confidence* is defined as having a full belief in the trustworthiness or reliability of a person. Confidence in oneself is the belief in your own knowledge and skills and the ability to use them when necessary. Confidence in a fellow nurse means that you are totally secure in the accuracy and efficiency of your colleague. Being confident in both yourself and your colleagues minimizes conflict and provides an optimal working environment that ultimately benefits the patient.

- *Compassion* is having a sympathetic feeling for another with an aspiration to help that individual. This is not just a feeling one possesses; it is accompanied by an action to do good. Effective holistic nursing requires a feeling of compassion for people who are sick and injured.

- *Commitment* means being obligated to see something through to completion. Nurses must value their profession and be committed to delivering the highest level of nursing care. Professional commitment is manifested in different ways. To achieve positive outcomes, nurses must be committed to their patients as well as their institution. The institution also has a duty to be supportive of its nurses, to assist them in increasing their knowledge and skills, and to provide current monitoring equipment that promotes a safe patient care environment.

- *Competence* refers to being capable and qualified to perform a job. Caring as it relates to nursing is not simply a matter of good intentions or warm regard; there also must be a foundation of knowledge. The nurse has a responsibility to the patient to be knowledgeable about the disease process and about the skills necessary to ensure safe patient care.

- *Comportment* means that one is aware of one's conduct and behavior around others. Professional comportment is an essential aspect of nursing because it is representative of the level of professionalism being exhibited. Additionally, it instills confidence in the patient and provides an atmosphere that alleviates anxiety. Nurses must conduct themselves professionally with their patients as well as their fellow health care workers. Being respectful of each other is germane to creating a positive work environment that promotes team building (Roach, 1984).

The nurse manifests caring as she assists health care consumers in preventing or adapting to actual and potential health problems. Without caring, nursing becomes mechanical and lacking in warmth. It takes much skill and devotion on the nurse's part to ensure that every patient is afforded the components just listed to make certain that patient care is as nurturing and positive as possible. The manner in which nurses choose to implement the six components of caring in clinical practice greatly influences how well the patient is able to adapt to the environment. Caring "sets up the conditions of trust that enables the [patient] to accept the help offered and to *feel* cared for" (Benner & Wrubel, 1989, p. 4).

Development of Caring Skills

During the educational process it is essential that learners perceive caring as critical to their socialization to the professional nursing field. Therefore, it is incumbent on educators to incorporate the concept of caring with its component parts in all aspects of the curriculum. It is not enough to incorporate the content of caring into didactic materials; the concept also must be communicated as a guide for practice and modeled by the faculty. Caring must become a measurable outcome of learner performance comparable to the measurement of scientific knowledge and psychomotor skills. To illustrate this point, excerpts from learners' clinical assignments in which they were asked to observe an example of nurses demonstrating caring behaviors are listed here:

- **Conscience**
  An example of staff working by their conscience during my shift was when a young patient came in and we had to treat him. He was brought in after driving drunk, hitting a car, and fleeing the scene. After hitting the first car, he hit a second car and attempted to flee that scene as well and was finally caught. We knew the damage he had done and we knew that when he was released, he was being released to the police and placed under arrest. However, this did not stop us from providing him with the best treatment we could. We did a full assessment, cleaned him up and controlled his pain just as we did with all of the other patients that we cared for.
  Source: Courtesy of Jennifer Fitzgerald, Sacramento, CA

- **Confidence**
  In the emergency department all of the nurses displayed confidence in their skills and procedures. The nurse established a level of trust right from the beginning. A patient displayed confidence in the nurse when he asked for something and the nurse answered that she could not do that. The patient was not happy with the answer but he had confidence in the nurse to know that she knew what needed to be done for his treatment, and he accepted the answer without question.
  Source: Courtesy of Sonia Garcia

- **Compassion**
  Possibly one of the most important components of caring is compassion. As a medical professional it may become easy to simply detach oneself from the plight of patients in pain or in need; however remaining compassionate is crucial to good patient care. It is the best way to build trust with your patient and to facilitate a caring environment, which is especially important in the emergency department where patients are often afraid and in severe pain. I saw many people exhibit compassion throughout the shift; for example, when a patient complained of severe leg pain that did not respond to the two doses of morphine his nurse had already given him, the RN went to the physician and requested a stronger pain medicine which finally put the patient at ease.
  Source: Courtesy of Maryam Shahdi, Sacramento, CA

- **Commitment**
  The nurse that I worked with in the Post Anesthesia Care Unit (PACU) had actually been called in that day after another nurse had called in sick. I guess he had been called in because nobody from the night shift wanted to stay and they were anticipating a very busy day in surgery. Since the level of acuity is so high in the PACU, it is necessary to have plenty of nurses on every shift. He told me he did not mind coming in on his day off though, because he really enjoyed his job and liked to come to work. One could say with absolutely no hesitation that this employee was very committed to his job and to his patients.
  Source: Courtesy of Jolie Tietz, Sacramento, CA

- **Competence**
  The nurse I was assigned to in the emergency department had four patients within a half hour that needed IVs placed. In previous experiences, I have seen nurses try three or four times, wiggling the needle around in the poor patient's arm before finding a vein. However, this nurse efficiently and almost painlessly started the IVs one after the other. I know the patients appreciated her accuracy, and she probably did not even think about how simply she had started the things.
  Source: Courtesy of Andrea Perry

- **Comportment**
  The Post Anesthesia Care Unit (PACU) nurse I worked with showed comportment to our patients, especially when they were first waking up. When the patient with a nasopharyngeal tube became more awake, he began to move and flail his arms around. He then began to try to take out the nasopharyngeal tube. The nurse and I carefully took his arms and held them so he would not pull out any lines or hurt himself. My nurse very calmly explained to the patient that the surgery was over, that it went well, and that he was in the PACU. He also explained who we were, what time it was, and why there was a tube in his nose. The nurse's demeanor helped the patient to calm down. The nurse also explained to the patient that the "spacey feeling" he was having was due to the anesthesia because of the fact that our bodies are not used to it. He reassured the patient that the feeling would soon wear off. My nurse handled the situation beautifully, and his caring behavior positively impacted the patient.
  Source: Courtesy of Kathleen Budesa, Sacramento, CA

Health and Wellness Promotion

In the last two decades, the concept of health and wellness promotion has come to the forefront of health care issues. The focus has shifted from disease treatment to a holistic approach of disease prevention and promotion of wellness. People are more aware than ever before how the relationship between healthy lifestyles and habits impacts disease prevention. For example, most individuals regularly monitor their cholesterol and triglycerides and understand that lifestyle changes are necessary when the levels become elevated. Regular exercise programs and a well-balanced healthy diet have become a way of life for many individuals.

In 1979 the surgeon general's office published its first health promotion and disease guidelines in *Healthy People*. This first report was followed in 1990 by a second edition, titled *Healthy People 2000*, which emphasized health promotion, health protection, and preventive service strategies (DHHS, 1991). The report was once again updated in the year 2000. This current report, *Healthy People 2010*, outlines a 10-year strategy for promoting health, preventing illness, disability, and premature death

(DHHS, 2000). The report also identified two major goals that are reflective of the changing demographics in the United States:

- Increase quality and years of healthy life.
- Eliminate health disparities.

Healthy People 2010 outlines 27 focus areas for improving health and meeting these two major objectives (Chart 1–2).

Healthy People 2010 also outlined the leading health concerns for the beginning of the 21st century, as listed in Chart 1–3. These indicators illuminate individual behaviors, physical and social environmental factors, and important health system issues that greatly affect the health of individuals and communities. Indicators are identified to help in the development of action plans for dealing with each indicator (DHHS, 2000, p. 24). For each leading health indicator, specific objectives have been identified that can be used to track progress and provide a snapshot of the health of the nation. The goal is to improve the health of both the individual and the community.

CHART 1–2   *Healthy People 2010:* **Focus Areas for Improving Health**

- Access to quality health care services
- Arthritis, osteoporosis, and chronic back conditions
- Cancer
- Chronic kidney disease
- Diabetes
- Disability and secondary conditions
- Educational and community-based programs
- Environmental health
- Family planning
- Food safety
- Health communication
- Heart disease and stroke
- HIV
- Immunization and infectious diseases
- Injury and violence prevention
- Maternal, infant, and child health
- Medical product safety
- Mental health and mental disorders
- Nutrition and overweight
- Occupational safety and health
- Oral health
- Physical activity and fitness
- Public health infrastructure
- Respiratory diseases
- Sexually transmitted infections
- Tobacco use
- Vision and screening

Source: U.S. Department of Health and Human Services. (1991). *Healthy people 2000: National health promotion and disease prevention objectives* (DHHS Publication No. 91-5021). Washington, DC: U.S. Government Printing Office; U.S. Department of Health and Human Services. (2000). *Healthy people 2010.* Retrieved May 1, 2004, from http://www.health.gov/healthpeople.

A vital part of the nurse's role today is to promote health and wellness through teaching and modeling of healthy behaviors based on the health indicators. For consistency and comprehensiveness, it is helpful to develop a template for health education. The components of this template include an understandable description of the cause of the disease or disorder, what habits will slow or stop progression, medication actions, side effects, and prognosis. As part of the plan, the nurse should provide written material and other resources such as websites and support organizations. It is important to provide the patient and family with an opportunity to ask questions and air feelings about the diagnosis. The nurse also needs to tailor the education to be culturally sensitive. This is especially true when it comes to dietary teaching, because food selection is heavily dependent on cultural customs. In summary, teaching as a function of the nursing role is included in the ANA's *Standards of Clinical Nursing Practice* (1998) and in all state nurse practice acts (ANA, 2004b).

Standards of Nursing Practice

Nurses are accountable to the public for their practice. Therefore, the ANA has developed standards for nursing practice and articulated the scope of practice (DeWolf-Bosek & Savage, 2007). **Standards of nursing practice** are authoritative statements by which the nursing profession describes the common level of performance or care by which the quality of practice can be determined, and responsibilities for which its practitioners are accountable (ANA, 2004b, p. 1). There are two parts to the standards of practice: standards of care and standards of professional performance. Charts 1–4 (p. 12) and 1–5 (p. 13), respectively, outline the ANA standards of care and standards of professional performance. In addition to the general standards the ANA also publishes standards for many specialty areas. The **standards of care** are guidelines for nursing practice and are general to any setting or specialty, and follow the nursing process with the broad categories of assessment, diagnosis, outcomes identification, planning, implementation, and evaluation (ANA, 2004b). **Standards of professional performance** address the professional nursing role with regard to education, ethics, research, collegiality, and resource utilization (ANA, 2004b). Standards of practice and performance focus on the nurse as the provider of patient care. They are process oriented and relate to what is expected of the provider. Each state has its own nurse practice act that defines the scope of nursing practice in that state. They have evolved as criteria against which care is measured for quality purposes.

It is essential that institutions where nurses practice provide an environment that is conducive to safe nursing practice and facilitates nurses' abilities to adhere to the standards of practice. Nurses are required to maintain currency in the knowledge and skills needed to practice in a given setting. This is accomplished in part by reading current professional journals, attending education classes related to their area of practice, and collaborating with fellow colleagues to share knowledge. Many states mandate continuing education classes in order to retain licensure. Professional organizations offer programs and conferences that nurses can attend to maintain currency.

CHART 1–3	*Healthy People 2010* Leading Health Indicators

Leading Health Indicator	Rationale
Physical activity	Regular physical activity throughout life is important for maintaining a healthy body, enhancing psychological well-being, and preventing premature death.
Overweight and obesity	Overweight and obesity are major contributors to many preventable causes of death. On average, higher body weights are associated with higher death rates. The number of overweight children, adolescents, and adults has risen over the past four decades.
Tobacco use	Cigarette smoking is the single most preventable cause of disease and death in the United States. Smoking results in more deaths each year in the United States than AIDS, alcohol, cocaine, heroin, homicide, suicide, motor vehicle crashes, and fires—combined.
Substance abuse	Alcohol and illicit drug use are associated with many of this country's most serious problems, including violence, injury, and HIV infection. The annual economic costs to the United States from alcohol abuse were estimated to be $167 billion in 1995, and the costs from drug abuse were estimated to be $110 billion.
Responsible sexual behavior	Unintended pregnancies and sexually transmitted infections (STIs), including infection with the human immunodeficiency virus that causes AIDS, can result from unprotected sexual behaviors. Abstinence is the only method of complete protection. Condoms, if used correctly and consistently, can help prevent both unintended pregnancy and STIs.
Mental health	Approximately 20 percent of the U.S. population is affected by mental illness during a given year; no one is immune. Of all mental illnesses, depression is the most common disorder. More than 19 million adults in the United States suffer from depression. Major depression is the leading cause of disability and is the cause of more than two-thirds of suicides each year.
Injury and violence	More than 400 Americans die each day from injuries due primarily to motor vehicle crashes, firearms, poisonings, suffocation, falls, fires, and drowning.
Environmental quality	An estimated 25 percent of preventable illnesses worldwide can be attributed to poor environmental quality. In the United States, air pollution alone is estimated to be associated with 50,000 premature deaths and an estimated $40 billion to $50 billion in health-related costs annually. Two indicators of air quality are ozone (outdoor) and environmental tobacco smoke (indoor).
Immunization	Vaccines are among the greatest public health achievements of the 20th century. Immunizations can prevent disability and death from infectious diseases for individuals and can help control the spread of infections within communities.
Access to health care	Strong predictors of access to quality health care include having health insurance, a higher income level, and a regular primary care provider or other source of ongoing health care. Use of clinical preventive services, such as early prenatal care, can serve as indicators of access to quality health care services.

Source: U.S. Department of Health and Human Services. (2000). *Healthy people 2010.* Retrieved May 1, 2004, from http://www.health.gov/healthpeople.

MyNursingKit | Video: Healthy People 2010

Code of Ethics for Nurses

A **code of ethics** is a formal statement by a group that expresses the group's ideals and values. A code of ethics for an organization is a set of ethical principles that have been agreed on by the organization's members that reflect their moral judgments, define expectations, and serve as a standard for their professional actions (DeWolf-Bosek & Savage, 2007). Codes of ethics, although not legally enforceable, typically have more stringent requirements than legal standards. Codes of ethics must not be stagnant; they must be revised as a given profession changes and evolves.

The purposes of nursing's code of ethics include the following:

- Inform the public about the minimum standards of the profession and help them understand professional nursing conduct.
- Provide a sign of the profession's commitment to public service.
- Outline the major ethical considerations of the profession.
- Provide ethical standards for professional behavior.
- Guide the profession in self-regulation.

- Remind nurses about the special responsibility they assume when caring for the sick.

Fundamental to the practice of nursing is a respect for human dignity and the uniqueness of each patient, without regard for social and economic status, the cause of the illness, or personal attributes. Therefore, it is the responsibility of every educator to ensure that an integral part of socializing the learner to the profession of nursing is to incorporate the code of ethics into the learner's value set (DeWolf-Bosek & Savage, 2007). The principles contained within the code serve to guide the learner in formulating the ethical values necessary for practicing nursing.

Values are freely chosen beliefs or attitudes about the worth of an individual or object. Values influence decisions and actions including ethical decision making. A value set is an internal group of beliefs that have been formulated and prioritized based on past experiences, education, and influences from others. This system of values gives direction to life and determines behavior, especially when decisions and choices are required. When learners enter a professional nursing program they do so with an

CHART 1–4	**American Nurses Association Standards of Care**

STANDARD I. ASSESSMENT

The Nurse Collects Patient Health Data

Measurement Criteria

1. Data collection involves the patient, family, and other health care providers as appropriate.
2. The priority of data collection is determined by the patient's immediate condition or needs.
3. Pertinent data are collected using appropriate assessment techniques and instruments.
4. Relevant data are documented in a retrievable form.
5. The data collection process is systematic and ongoing.

STANDARD II. DIAGNOSIS

The Nurse Analyzes the Assessment Data in Determining Diagnoses

Measurement Criteria

1. Diagnoses are derived from the assessment data.
2. Diagnoses are validated with the patient, family, and other health care providers, when possible and appropriate.
3. Diagnoses are documented in a manner that facilitates the determination of expected outcomes and plan of care.

STANDARD III. OUTCOME IDENTIFICATION

The Nurse Identifies Expected Outcomes Individualized to the Patient

Measurement Criteria

1. Outcomes are derived from the diagnoses.
2. Outcomes are mutually formulated with the patient, family, and other health care providers, when possible and appropriate.
3. Outcomes are culturally appropriate and realistic in relation to the patient's present and potential capabilities.
4. Outcomes are attainable in relation to resources available to the patient.
5. Outcomes include a time estimate for attainment.
6. Outcomes provide direction for continuity of care.
7. Outcomes are documented as measurable goals.

STANDARD IV. PLANNING

The Nurse Develops a Plan of Care that Prescribes Interventions to Attain Expected Outcomes

Measurement Criteria

1. The plan is individualized to the patient (e.g., age appropriate, culturally sensitive) and the patient's condition or needs.
2. The plan is developed with the patient, family, and other health care providers, as appropriate.
3. The plan reflects current nursing practice.
4. The plan provides for continuity of care.
5. Priorities for care are established.
6. The plan is documented.

STANDARD V. IMPLEMENTATION

The Nurse Implements the Interventions Identified in the Plan of Care

Measurement Criteria

1. Interventions are consistent with the established plan of care.
2. Interventions are implemented in a safe, timely, and appropriate manner.
3. Interventions are documented.

STANDARD VI. EVALUATION

The Nurse Evaluates the Patient's Progress toward Attainment of Outcomes

Measurement Criteria

1. Evaluation is systematic, ongoing, and criterion based.
2. The patient, family, and other health care providers are involved in the evaluation process, as appropriate.
3. Ongoing assessment data are used to revise diagnoses, outcomes, and the plan of care, as needed.
4. Revisions in diagnoses, outcomes, and the plan of care are documented.
5. The effectiveness of interventions is evaluated in relation to outcomes.
6. The patient's responses to intervention are documented.

Source: American Nurses Association. (2004b). *Nursing: Scope & Standards of Practice.* Silver Spring, MD: Nursebooks pp. 21–31. Reprinted with permission from American Nurses Association, Nursing: Scope and Standards of Practice, © 2004 nursesbooks.org, Silver Spring, MD.

inherent set of values. It is the responsibility of the education system to assist learners in socializing to the nursing profession and adopting its code of ethics and values. This also is true of the nurse practicing in a health care organization where comparable values are essential. The organization has its own set of values, as does the nurse, and those values must be compatible in order for the nurse to provide appropriate and comprehensive patient care.

Codes of ethics have been established by international, national, and state nursing associations. Nursing's first code of ethics is believed to be the Florence Nightingale pledge that was written by Lystra Gretter in 1893 (Chart 1–6, p. 14). It is apparent even in that early code that nurses understood the impor-

tance of patient privacy that is still stressed today in health care, although it is also apparent in that first code that there was a dependence on physicians. Today, nursing has become more autonomous, which is why codes of ethics are revised to keep pace with current practice. It is essential that codes of ethics be updated as situations change with time (Tschudin, 2006). An updated code of ethics was not adopted until 1950 (DeWolf-Bosek & Savage, 2007). The code of ethics was again revised in 1956, 1960, 1968, 1976, and 2001.

The ANA represents the interests of the nation's registered nurses through its 54 constituent state and territorial associations. The ANA advances the nursing profession by fostering high standards of nursing practice, promoting the economic

| CHART 1–5 | American Nurses Association Standards of Professional Performance |

STANDARD I. QUALITY OF CARE

The Nurse Systematically Evaluates the Quality and Effectiveness of Nursing Practice

Measurement Criteria

1. The nurse participates in quality of care activities as appropriate to the nurse's education and position. Such activities may include:
   - Identification of aspects of care important for quality monitoring.
   - Analysis of quality data to identify opportunities for improving care.
   - Development of policies, procedures, and proactive guidelines to improve quality of care.
   - Identification of indicators used to monitor quality and effectiveness of nursing care.
   - Collection of data to monitor quality and effectiveness of nursing care.
   - Formulation of recommendations to improve nursing practice or patient outcomes.
   - Implementation of activities to enhance the quality of nursing practice.
   - Participation on interdisciplinary teams that evaluate clinical practice or health services.
2. The nurse uses the results of quality of care activities to initiate changes in nursing practice.
3. The nurse uses the results of quality of care activities to initiate changes throughout the health care delivery system, as appropriate.

STANDARD II. PERFORMANCE APPRAISAL

The Nurse Evaluates One's Own Nursing Practice in Relation to Professional Practice Standards and Relevant Statutes and Regulation

Measurement Criteria

1. The nurse engages in performance appraisal on a regular basis, identifying areas of strength as well as areas for professional development.
2. The nurse seeks constructive feedback regarding one's own practice.
3. The nurse takes action to achieve goals identified during performance appraisal.
4. The nurse participates in peer review as appropriate.
5. The nurse's practice reflects knowledge of current professional practice standards, laws, regulations.

STANDARD III. EDUCATION

The Nurse Acquires and Maintains Current Knowledge and Competency in Nursing Practice

Measurement Criteria

1. The nurse participates in ongoing educational activities related to clinical knowledge and professional issues.
2. The nurse seeks experience to maintain current clinical skills and competence.

3. The nurse acquires knowledge and skills appropriate to the specialty area and practice setting.

STANDARD IV. COLLEGIALITY

The Nurse Interacts with, and Contributes to, the Professional Development of Peers and Other Health Care Providers as Colleagues

Measurement Criteria

1. The nurse shares knowledge and skills with colleagues.
2. The nurse provides peers with constructive feedback regarding their practice.
3. The nurse acquires knowledge and skills appropriate to the security area and practice setting.
4. The nurse contributes to an environment that is conductive to clinical education of nursing learners, other health care learners, and other employees, as appropriate.
5. The nurse contributes to a supportive and healthy work environment.

STANDARD V. ETHICS

The Nurse's Decisions and Actions on Behalf of Patients Are Determined in an Ethical Manner

Measurement Criteria

1. The nurse's practice is guided by the *Code for Nurses.*
2. The nurse maintains patient confidentiality within legal and regulatory parameters.
3. The nurse acts as a patient advocate and assists patients in developing skills to advocate for themselves.
4. The nurse delivers care in a nonjudgmental and nondiscriminatory manner that is sensitive to patient diversity.
5. The nurse delivers care in a manner that preserves patient autonomy, dignity, and rights.
6. The nurse seeks available resources to formulate ethical decisions.

STANDARD VI. COLLABORATION

The Nurse Collaborates with the Patient, Family, and Other Health Care Providers in Providing Patient Care

Measurement Criteria

1. The nurse communicates with the patient, family, and other health care providers regarding patient care and nursing's role in the provision of care.
2. The nurse collaborates with the patient, family, and other health care providers in the formulation of overall goals, the plan of care, and decisions related to care and the delivery of services.
3. The nurse consults with other health care providers for patient care, as needed.
4. The nurse makes referrals, including provisions for continuity of care, as needed.

(continued)

CHART 1–5 | **American Nurses Association Standards of Professional Performance—*Continued***

STANDARD VII. RESEARCH

The Nurse Uses Research Findings in Practice

Measurement Criteria

1. The nurse utilizes available research to develop the plan of care and interventions.

2. The nurse participates in research activities as appropriate to the nurse's education and position. Such activities may include:
   - Identifying clinical problems suitable for nursing research.
   - Participating in data collection.
   - Participating in a unit, organization, or community research committee or program.
   - Sharing of research activities with others.
   - Conducting research.
   - Critiquing research for application to practice.
   - Using research findings in the development of policies, procedures, and practice guidelines for patient care.

STANDARD VIII. RESOURCE UTILIZATION

The Nurse Considers Factors Related to Safety, Effectiveness, and Cost in Planning and Delivering Patient Care

Measurement Criteria

1. The nurse evaluates factors related to safety, effectiveness, availability, and cost when choosing between two or more practice options that would result in the same expected patient outcome.

2. The nurse assists the patient and family in identifying and securing appropriate and available services to address health-related needs.

3. The nurse assigns or delegates tasks as defined by the state nurse practice act and according to the knowledge and skills of the designated caregiver.

4. If the nurse assigns or delegates tasks, the delegation is based on the needs and conditions of the patient, the potential for harm, the stability of the patient's condition, the complexity of the task, and the predictability of the outcome.

5. The nurse assists the patient and family in becoming informed consumers about the cost, risks, and benefits of treatment and care.

Source: American Nurses Association. (2004b). *Nursing: Scope & Standards of Practice.* Silver Spring, MD: Nursebooks pp. 33–44. Reprinted with permission from American Nurses Association, Nursing: Scope and Standards of Practice, © 2004 nursesbooks.org, Silver Spring, MD.

CHART 1–6 | **Florence Nightingale Pledge**

I solemnly pledge myself before God and in the presence of this assembly, to pass my life in purity and to practice my profession faithfully. I will abstain from whatever is deleterious and mischievous, and will not take or knowingly administer any harmful drug. I will do all in my power to maintain and elevate the standard of my profession, and will hold in confidence all personal matters committed to my keeping and all family affairs coming to my knowledge in the practice of my calling. With loyalty will I endeavor to aid the physician, in his work, and devote myself to the welfare of those committed to my care.

Source: Retrieved October 29, 2007, from http://www.countryjoe.com/nightingale/pledge.htm.

and general welfare of nurses in the workplace, projecting a positive and realistic view of nursing, and by lobbying the Congress and regulatory agencies on health care issues affecting nurses and the general public. The most recent revision of the ANA code of ethics was adopted in July 2001 and is shown in Chart 1–7.

Guiding Ethical Principles

Ethical principles guide nurses in making determinations about what is and is not ethical in nursing and medicine (DeWolf-Bosek & Savage, 2007; Guido, 2006; Mathes, 2005a). There are four cornerstone principles of bioethics from which many other ethical principles can be derived. These principles do not always exist in harmony and there is not a generally accepted ranking system (DeWolf-Bosek & Savage, 2007). These principles are used by nurses as tools for moral reflection and to aid them in decision making when controversy exists. The four cornerstone principles are (1) nonmaleficence, (2) beneficence, (3) autonomy, and (4) justice. These and other ethical principles are discussed in detail in Chapter 4 .

Roles of the Nurse

As stated, the professional nurse embodies many roles. Throughout history, nursing has continuously adapted to the ever-changing needs of patients and the health care delivery system. There are roles that interface with patients throughout the entire health care continuum and these roles continue to grow. The spectrum of nursing roles includes practice in acute and nonacute care, advanced practice, and practice in a number of new and evolving arenas. All nursing practice roles rely on the nursing process as a framework for patient care delivery.

Acute Care Nurses

Acute care nurses practice in the hospital setting. These nurses care for patients with actual and potential health problems related to any body system and any age group. The types of patients an acute care nurse works with will vary depending on the individual hospital's mission, goals, and specialty areas provided.

Staff Nurse

The staff nurse has the primary responsibility to care for a specific patient or group of patients for an assigned period of time. Patient care assignments vary among organizations depending on the nursing care delivery model being used. The nursing care delivery models are discussed in Chapter 5 . These models define the workload distribution and job description for each member of the nursing health care team. Organization and coordination are inherent in the role of the nurse regardless of the type of patient care delivery model due to the variety of diagnoses and complexity of patient care. Therefore, the staff nurse uses critical nursing judgments in determining patient interventions according to assigned responsibilities. Regardless of which care delivery model is used, certain components are common to all of them, including nursing management and administration, which are described next.

American Nurses Association Code of Ethics for Nurses

CHART 1-7

1. The nurse in all professional relationships practices with compassion and respect for the inherent dignity, worth, and uniqueness of every individual, unrestricted by considerations of social or economic status, personal attributes, or the nature of health problems, and restoration of health; the prevention of illness; and the alleviation of suffering in the care of clients.

2. The nurse's primary commitment is to the patient, whether an individual, family, group, or community.

3. The nurse promotes, advocates for, and strives to protect the health, safety, and rights of the patient.

4. The nurse is responsible and accountable for individual nursing practice and determines the appropriate delegation of tasks consistent with the nurse's obligation to provide optimum patient care.

5. The nurse owes the same duties to self as to others, including the responsibly to preserve integrity and safety, to maintain competence, and to continue personal and professional growth.

6. The nurse participates in establishing, maintaining, and improving health care environments and conditions of employment conducive to the provision of quality health care and consistent with the values of the profession through individual and collective action.

7. The nurse participates in the advancement of the profession through contributions to practice, education, administration, and knowledge development.

8. The nurse collaborates with other health professionals and the public in promoting community, national, and international efforts to meet health needs.

9. The profession of nursing, as represented by associations and their members, is responsible for articulating nursing values, for maintaining the integrity of the profession and its practice, and for shaping social policy.

Source: Reprinted with permission from American Nurses Association, Code of Ethics for Nurses with Interpretive Statements, © 2001 nursesbooks.org, Silver Spring, MD.

Nurse Manager

The role of nurse managers is to coordinate and ensure the delivery of quality nursing care in their area of responsibility. Their role encompasses personnel management, staff development, and ensuring the availability of supplies, other resources, and processes that allow the nurses they manage to provide care. In most settings a nurse manager has 24-hour accountability for a specific patient care arena.

Nurse Administrator

Nurse administrators have a greater scope of responsibility than nurse managers. The ultimate role of a nurse administrator is to support the achievement of the standards that the organization has set for nursing practice and the guidelines of care that outline how care is to be delivered in a setting.

Nurse Researcher

Research is the never-ending quest for information and validation that lead to evidenced-based nursing practice. Nurse researcher roles are multifaceted and involve many aspects of pharmaceutical, medical, and nursing research. Nurses serve as investigators, monitors, auditors, data managers, clinical coordinators, or research professionals. Research nurses monitor patient responses and other critical parameters.

Factors to consider as a research nurse are regulatory developments and trends, clinical research management, protocol design and implementation, and ethical issues in human research. Educational preparation varies depending on the role and setting in which one practices. Some nurses involved in research may be educationally prepared as ADN, diploma, or BSN nurses. Some nurses accomplish PhD preparation and serve as primary scientific investigators. Chapter 8 ♂ provides a complete description of the role of nurses in research.

Nurse Educator

Nurse educators are a critical component to the success of nurses and their patients. The role of educator varies from organization to organization and department to department. Many in-hospital educator roles include responsibilities such as teaching of patients and staff, research, and direct patient care. Core competencies for the role of educator are strong clinical skills and effective teaching skills.

The nurse educator may be responsible for developing educational content for presentation, written delivery, or multimedia applications. Nurse educators also participate in the evaluation of learners (staff or patients) and serve as consultants to staff and patients. The ultimate goal of a nurse educator is to ensure quality patient care by providing education to patients and nurses and assessing the competency of those who practice.

Nonacute Care Nursing

Nonacute nurses practice outside of a hospital setting. For example, nurses perform a variety of roles in the community setting. Each role requires special training and expertise, which can be acquired through formal education and on-the-job training. With the goal of providing nursing care and preventive health care, nurses in these settings have to be flexible and creative when providing their nursing care. Examples of common nonacute nursing roles are discussed in the following subsections.

Community-Based Home Health Nurse

Community-based home health nurses are employed by government agencies, private enterprises, hospitals, and a myriad of other clinics or health care–focused organizations. These nurses provide care to patients in the community by making home visits to patients, operating mobile clinics, and staffing various types of health screening events. Home health nurses concentrate on providing care and educating patients and their significant others regarding health care issues.

These nurses may be specialists who focus on specific populations or generalists who work with families to improve the overall health of communities. Each agency operates with the concepts of disease prevention, nutrition, and child care and elder care as constructs on which to build healthy communities. Home health nurses integrate into the community and work in concert with community leaders, teachers, parents, and physicians to promote community health education.

Parish Nurse

Parish nursing is a form of community nursing that concentrates on the population of a church and the members of the congregation. The health care provided by a parish nurse is very similar to that provided by a home health/community health nurse. The parish nurse serves as a consultant and facilitator for the health care needs of the parish's congregation. Many parish nurse programs provide preventive health screening such as blood pressure and cholesterol clinics.

Long-Term Care Nurse

Long-term care is not a subset of acute care; it is a distinct entity with special needs, functions, and care providers. A variety of medical and social services are provided to help people who have disabilities or chronic care needs. Services may be short or long term and may be provided in a person's home, in the community, or in residential facilities (e.g., nursing homes or assisted living facilities). Care is provided in the form of medical and support services to persons who have lost some or all of the capacity to function due to an illness or disability. Most long-term care clients are older and require care due to diagnoses such as stroke or Alzheimer's disease. However, long-term care is not limited to those who are elderly. Younger patients may require long-term care for a chronic disease such as multiple sclerosis or conditions resulting from trauma such as spinal cord injury or traumatic brain injury. A source for more information on long-term care is the American Society for Long-Term Care Nurses.

Assisted Living Nurse

Assisted living is defined as a setting in which patients are provided long-term assisted care in a residential setting. Assisted living settings provide care to patients who have needs that are beyond the scope of home care, but do not require the level of services provided in nursing homes. Assisted living programs take on many forms; however, the most encompassing description is any group residential program not licensed as a nursing home that provides care to residents through trained staff available to respond to unscheduled calls for assistance.

Assisted living services support the resident in all activities of daily living (ADLs). Examples of activities where staff assist residents include bathing, grooming, taking medications, transferring assistance, and toileting. The assisted living setting provides a "homey" environment for people requiring or potentially requiring assistance with ADLs, but for which 24-hour nursing care is not a necessity.

Nurses' roles in assisted living facilities are multifaceted. Nurses provide direct care in some, oversee medication administration, and participate with the staff in evaluating and planning to meet the needs of residents. Unlike their acute care counterparts, nurses who care for residents in assisted living facilities are often called on to participate in decisions that impact the quality of care and quality of life of the resident (Day, 2005).

Occupational Health and Industrial Nurse

Occupational health and *industrial nursing* are terms that have been used interchangeably. This practice integrates concepts of public health nursing theory, holistic evaluation, primary prevention, surveillance, and compliance. The American Association of Occupational Health Nurses describes occupational nursing as a practice that focuses on promotion and restoration of health, prevention of illness and injury, and protection from work-related and environmental hazards.

The occupational health nurse has two primary objectives: (1) participating in the management of workers' health to mitigate health issues that may adversely affect work productivity and (2) ensuring that the employer's practices are compliant with the requirements of the Occupational Safety and Health Act.

The occupational health nurse practices in many settings, including factories, corporations, or hospitals. This type of nurse may provide direct nursing care to employees, manage workers' compensation records, conduct environmental surveillance for health hazards, and provide health education or counsel employees.

School Nurse

School nursing practice strives to advance the well-being, academic performance, and lifelong achievement of students. School nurses interact with students to foster positive responses to normal growth and development and promote health and safety practices. School nurses get involved with actual and potential health problems. In some situations a school nurse may be called on to provide case management services. These nurses actively collaborate with the student, administration, teachers, parents, and legal entities to build student and family capacity for adaptation to health care needs and self-management of issues, to promote self advocacy, and to foster learning of health-related concepts. A source of information regarding school nursing is the National Association of School Nurses.

Clinic Nurse

Clinic nurses provide patient care and support within the setting of an office building, a clinic, or a surgery center. They are routinely responsible for preparing patients for examination, administering injections, and performing clerical duties. Clinic nurses are the physician's most important professional adjunct. In this role, nurses facilitate the delivery of care to patients and manage the daily operation of the office. A source of information regarding clinic nursing is the American Association of Office Nurses.

Hospice Nurse

Hospice nurses provide care for the physical and emotional needs of dying patients and their significant others. Interventions may include pain management, palliative care, symptom management, and emotional support. A source of information regarding hospice nursing is the Hospice and Palliative Nurses Association. Chapter 17 provides a detailed description of the role of hospice nurses.

Gerontologic Nurse

Gerontologic nurses provide for the physical and psychosocial needs of older adults both in the acute care and community setting. These specialized nurses work with their patient's insurance carrier, such as health maintenance organizations, to maximize functional ability while working with the patient to maintain and restore the patient's physical and mental health. The arena of gerontologic nursing is growing because older adults have begun to represent an increasingly greater component of the population.

Age-related health issues and typically a limited ability to navigate the health care system could result in inadequate health maintenance, especially for the frail elderly. Gerontologic nurses are specially trained to deal with the special needs of this population. This training can be either in the form of an advanced degree or on-the-job training. Care specific to the elder patient is discussed in Chapter 10 ◎. One source of information regarding gerontologic nursing is the National Gerontological Nurses Association.

Advanced Practice Nursing Roles

Advanced practice nursing roles have grown in response to a societal need to improve the distribution of health care services and to decrease the costs of health care. The development of advanced practice roles such as nurse practitioners, clinical nurse specialists, certified nurse midwives, certified registered nurse anesthetists, and academic nurse educators occurred as a direct response to patient needs, specifically the need for access and cost-effective care.

Research has demonstrated that the use of advanced practice nurses has improved patient outcomes and reduced health care costs. Key factors that led to this success were the interpersonal skills of the nurse, knowledge and expertise in the area of practice, and a level of trust when working with physicians, nursing staff, vendors, pharmacists, insurance companies, and other health care providers. Successful enactment of the role required being a facilitator for patients and families with the health care team (Canam, 2005; MacDonald, Herbert, & Thilbeault, 2006).

These nurses provide direct care to patients through independent practice, practice within a health care agency, or in collaboration with a health care provider. As in all professions, advancements in technology and the incredible access to information have resulted in the various advanced practice roles becoming more and more specific. The most rapidly growing sectors of advanced practice nursing are the roles of nurse practitioner and clinical nurse specialist.

Nurse Practitioner

Nurse practitioners (NP) focus on individualized care. Nurse practitioners interact with patients of all ages as they examine the impact of illness on the lives of patients and their support networks. NPs practice in both acute and nonacute care settings, are eligible for Medicare reimbursement, and, in some states, have prescriptive authority.

NPs formulate their actions and interventions with a focus on prevention, wellness, and patient education. The impact of these priorities often results in fewer prescriptions and potentially less expensive medical care. NPs collaborate with their patients by fostering the acquisition of knowledge and encouraging participation in decision making related to their health care needs. The role of the NP is not limited to the delivery of health care; many are active participants in research, whereas others are active in patient advocacy work, such as development of support groups for a specific diagnosis.

Nurse practitioner programs classically specialize in an area such as family practice, internal medicine, or women's health. The advanced practice degree can be granted by a number of academic institutions. The variety of educational paths for NPs is a result of the historical development of the role. In 1965, the profession of nurse practitioner was introduced with a requirement of a master's degree. After successful completion of the education program, the NP candidates must achieve licensure in the state in which they plan to practice. The state boards of nursing regulate nurse practitioners, and each state has its own licensing and certification criteria. In general, the criteria include completion of an accredited advanced practice program and clinical experience. Depending on the requirements of the various state boards, nurse practitioners may have to fulfill additional requirements such as certification by the American Nurses Credentialing Center (ANCC) or a specialty nursing organization. Terms of licensure also vary from state to state.

Clinical Nurse Specialist

The National Association of Clinical Nurse Specialists (NACNS) defines a clinical nurse specialist (CNS) as a licensed registered nurse who has graduate preparation (master's degree or doctorate) in nursing as a CNS. CNS practice usually takes place in a hospital setting and involves interactions with patients all across the health care continuum. CNSs practice within a prescribed area of care, and define their role as having five components: clinical practice, education, management, consultation, and research. These advanced practice nurses deliver direct patient care, educate staff and patients, consult with other health care professionals, do research, and provide leadership and supervision in the workplace. Depending on the state in which they practice, the institutional policies, and the clinical specialty they choose, clinical nurse specialists may have extended scope of practice authority.

CNSs are expert nurses in a specialized area of clinical practice. According to the NACNS, the specialty may be identified in different ways. The CNS practice may be focused on a specific type of problem (e.g., pain, wounds, and stress), a defined patient population (e.g., pediatrics, geriatrics, women's health), or a setting (e.g., critical care, emergency department). Other practice focuses include medical subspecialty (e.g., diabetes, oncology) and types of care (e.g., psychiatric, rehabilitation). Although most CNSs do practice in the hospital setting, some practice in other health care settings.

In addition to providing direct patient care, the CNS influences care outcomes by providing expert consultation for nursing staff and by implementing improvements in health care delivery systems. The practice of a CNS integrates expert nursing practice, which focuses on assisting patients in the prevention or resolution of illness, with a medical diagnosis and treatment of disease, injury, and disability. It is believed that CNSs improve outcomes such as better pain management, reduced medical complications in hospitalized patients, and reduced frequency of emergency visits.

As advanced practice roles continue to grow, more need for clarification of roles and responsibilities has been required. Many states have amended their nurse practice acts to authorize nurses to perform functions that were previously restricted to the practice of physicians. Examples of these expanded functions include diagnosis, treatment, performance of selected invasive procedures, and prescription of medications and treatments. Each state regulates practices differently. In all states, the board of nursing controls these functions.

The differences in the role of nurse practitioner and clinical nurse specialist are often unclear, especially in hospital settings. This lack of distinction is very confusing to the health care consumer, other health care providers, and nurses. There is a need for clear universal definitions of the roles and responsibilities of advanced practice nurses. Nurses who pursue these roles often discuss the benefits in terms of interdependent function with other health care professionals and the establishment of peer relationships with physicians. As health care systems continue to develop, the roles of these advanced practice nurses will continue to adapt and change.

Nurse-Midwife

A nurse-midwife is defined as a nurse who has undergone special training and has received certification on child birthing (labor and delivery). Nurse-midwives can perform most of the same tasks as physicians, although they typically have emergency physician backup when they deliver a baby.

Nurse-midwives have been contributing to the birth process of millions of women and families during the past 300 years. The American College of Nurse-Midwives (ACNM) reported in 2005 that there were 6,200 nurse-midwives in clinical practice and 43 accredited ACNM nurse-midwifery programs in the United States. Of these programs, 4 are postbaccalaureate certificate programs and 39 are graduate degree programs. This advanced practice role is lawful in all 50 states and in the District of Columbia. According to an ACNM fact sheet (2005) more than 50% of certified nurse-midwives list physician practices or hospitals as their principal employer.

Certified Registered Nurse Anesthetist

The American Association of Nurse Anesthetists (2007) states "Nurse anesthesia is an advanced clinical nursing specialty. As anesthesia specialists, certified registered nurse anesthetists (CRNA) administer approximately 65% of the 26 million anesthetics given to patients in the United States each year." CRNAs provide care to patients in collaboration with other health care professionals including anesthesiologists, surgeons, and dentists.

The consistent functions of a CRNA include providing care of a patient's anesthesia needs before, during, and after surgery or the delivery of a baby. The CRNA's responsibilities are to assess, participate in operative teaching, prepare the operative area for anesthetic management, administer anesthesia, and maintain anesthesia during the operative procedure.

A CRNA is a registered nurse who is prepared through a formal nurse anesthesia didactic and clinical program. This education process prepares the CRNA candidate to sit for a national certification examination. This exam is administered by the Council on Certification of Nurse Anesthetists (CCNA). The mission of CCNA is to protect the public by ensuring that individuals who are credentialed have met predetermined qualifications or standards for providing nurse anesthesia services. All nurse anesthesia programs are graduate or postgraduate degree programs.

It is clear that initial care, ambulatory health care, and anticipatory guidance are all becoming increasingly important in nursing practice. Advanced practice roles enable nurses to function interdependently with other health care professionals and to establish a more collegial relationship with physicians. As changes in health care delivery continue, the role of advanced practice nurses, especially in primary care settings, is expected to increase in terms of scope, responsibility, and recognition.

Academic Nurse Educator

College and continuing education nursing instruction must be provided by nurses prepared at the master's or doctoral level. All **academic nurse educators** practice as faculty in colleges, universities, hospital-based schools of nursing or technical schools, or as staff development educators in health care facilities. The continuum of students these educators instruct ranges from entry into nursing practice, professional nurses in pursuit of advanced degrees, and practicing nurses interested in expanding their knowledge and skills related to care of individuals, families, and communities (*Nurses for a Healthier Tomorrow*, 2007).

■ Nursing Care Delivery Models

The assignment of nursing care staff to patients is a basic activity of health care systems. **Assignment** is defined as the transfer of a task and the accountability for the outcome (Huber, 2006). Assignments are the method by which the division of labor is accomplished within the structure of a health care system. A determination of the parts of an assignment that will be transferred from an RN to an assistant is *delegation*. Organizations use the concept of delegation in nursing when determining the nursing care model, or system of nursing care delivery, that will be established for the work unit.

Nurses deliver and coordinate patient care within the framework of the organizational structure and model of the nursing care delivery system. The model of care selected has a direct correlation to the allocation of control over decisions about patient care. This, in turn, has implications for job satisfaction, the character of professional practice, and the amount of authority that is actually transferred to the staff (Huber, 2006).

A nursing care model is the method of organizing and delivering nursing care to meet patients' needs. The basic elements of nursing care delivery models are work allocation, clinical decision making, communication, and management. These are fully described in Chapter 5 for the four traditional models of nursing care delivery: case method, functional nursing, team nursing, and primary nursing. The practice model also may be thought of as a link between the problems presented by the patient population, the purposes of professional occupations, and the purposes of health care organizations.

For any practice model, there needs to be consistency between the degree of integration of the nursing care given to a patient, the degree of continuity in assignment of care to a patient, and the type of coordination used to plan or organize the patient's care based on general patient characteristics, available nursing resources, and the organizational support available to nursing (Huber, 2006). There is no one correct way of structuring patient care delivery. All models have advantages and disadvantages. Any specific model may be better suited to one set of environmental circumstances than another. It is, therefore, important to have an understanding of the models of patient care delivery.

Models of Organizing Patient Care

The four primary means of organizing nursing care for patient care delivery are (1) case method, (2) functional nursing, (3) team and modular nursing, and (4) primary nursing. (Marquis & Huston, 2007). Each of these basic types has undergone many modifications, often resulting in new terminology. For example, *primary nursing* now is frequently referred to as a *professional practice model*, and *team nursing* often is termed *partners in care* or *patient service partners* or other similar names.

When closely examined many of the newer models of patient care delivery systems are recycled, modified, or retitled versions of older models. In fact, it is difficult to find a "pure" delivery model; the models have become blended with most having parts of others in their design. Choosing the most appropriate organizational mode to deliver patient care for each unit or organization depends on the skill and expertise of the staff, the availability of RNs, the economic resources of the organization, the acuity of the patients, and the complexity of the tasks to be completed. These factors may change over time within an organization contingent on external environmental factors (e.g., the nursing shortage, technological advances, population factors), in which case, the nursing care delivery model also may change.

We discuss the four primary means of organizing patient care mentioned above, along with some other methods and new methods, in the following subsections.

Case Method

Case method is the oldest model of organizing care. In this method nurses assume total responsibility for meeting all of the needs of assigned patients during their time on duty. Initially, case method, sometimes referred to as case management, was provided in the patient's home, and the nurse was responsible for cooking, house cleaning, and other activities specific to the patient and family, in addition to traditional nursing care (Nelson, 2000). This type of care also was called *private duty nursing*. When people could no longer afford home care, during the depression of the 1930s, they began using hospitals for care that had been performed by private duty nurses in the home. As hospitals grew during the 1930s and 1940s, case method continued as the primary means of organizing patient care.

As mentioned above, case method nursing is sometimes referred to as a total patient care assignment because patients were assigned as cases—much like contemporary private duty nursing is carried out. Nurses are responsible for the care of a patient but only for the hours in which that specific nurse is present. The distinguishing feature of case method is the shift-only accountability for care. The term has come to mean the assignment of each patient to a nurse who plans and delivers care during a typical 8- to 12-hour per shift workweek. Within this context case method has been termed a "form of primary nursing" (Marquis & Huston, 2007). This method of assignment still is widely used in hospitals and home health agencies. Its uses and advantages and disadvantages are discussed in Chapter 5 .

Functional Nursing

Functional nursing has been defined as work assignment by functions or tasks, such as passing medications, doing dressing changes, giving baths, or doing vital signs. Philosophically, functional nursing is not oriented to individualized and holistic patient care, but is more oriented to task accomplishment, as patterned after the industrial concepts of scientific management. Under functional nursing the nurse identifies the tasks to be done for a shift. The work is divided up and assigned to personnel who focus on completing the assigned tasks. Functional nursing has the advantage of being efficient for taking care of the tasks related to handling a large number of patients. It is also

considered to be an economical means of providing care with efficiency (Marquis & Huston, 2007). The historical development of functional nursing and the advantages and disadvantages of this care delivery model are discussed in Chapter 5 .

Team Nursing/Modular Nursing

Team nursing is a care model that involves a group of people led by a knowledgeable nurse. It was developed in the 1950s in an effort to decrease the problems associated with the functional organization of patient care, the intent being to reduce the fragmentation that accompanied functional nursing. In team nursing, ancillary personnel collaborate in providing care to a group of patients under the direction of a professional nurse. As the team leader, the nurse is responsible for knowing the conditions and needs of all patients assigned to the team and for planning individual care.

This care delivery model usually is associated with democratic leadership, and allows team members to contribute their own special expertise. Group members are given as much autonomy as possible when performing assigned tasks, although the team shares responsibility and accountability collectively. Team leaders should use their knowledge about each member's abilities when making patient assignments. Recognizing each member's worth and giving team members autonomy results in high job satisfaction. The advantages and disadvantages of team nursing are discussed in Chapter 5 . Recent attempts to refine and improve team nursing have resulted in the concept of "modular" nursing, as discussed next (Marquis & Huston, 2007).

Modular Nursing

Modular nursing is a type of team nursing that involves a small team of two to three persons. It is predicated by a facility's layout and actual structural and spatial changes that enable nurses to stay near the bedside. Nurses are stationed near their patients, and a wider range of responsibility is delegated to them. The open designs and convenient access architectures of modular nursing provide for geographic decentralization of care delivery and enhanced communication (Huber, 2006).

Primary Nursing

Primary nursing was developed in the early 1970s to overcome the discontent associated with the emphasis of the functional and team nursing methods on tasks and discrete functions. Primary nursing uses some of the concepts of case method to bring the registered nurse back to the bedside to provide clinical care (Marquis & Huston, 2007). This goes along with a societal trend toward accountability and nursing's rising level of professionalism. As originally designed, primary nursing requires a nursing staff comprised totally of RNs. The RN primary nurse assumes 24-hour responsibility for planning the care of one or more patients from admission or the start of treatment to discharge or the treatment's end.

Although designed for use in hospitals, the structure lends itself well to home health nursing, hospice nursing, and other health care delivery systems. An integral responsibility of the primary nurse is to establish clear communication among the patient and family, the physician, associate nurses, and other team members. Although the primary nurse establishes the plan of care, input is sought from others in coordinating the patient's care. Clear and consistent communication among the group and consistent, direct patient care by relatively few nursing staff allows for holistic, high-quality patient care. The primary nursing care delivery model is discussed in Chapter 5 ☺, including its advantages and disadvantages.

New Types of Care Delivery Models

Evolving or new types of nursing care delivery models can be found in the literature. In general, these new types are mixed models, revisited primary care, or professional practice models that emphasize outcomes management, collaboration, use of a variety of caregivers with variable competencies and preparation, and integrated practice. "The terms *case management* and *managed care* are joined with concepts of accountability, cost containment, effectiveness, seamless continuum of care, integration, multidisciplinary collaboration, new roles, alteration in skill mix, and new assignment systems" (Huber, 2003, p. 525). All seek to reconfigure nursing's work within resource constraints, care needs, and current ideas about professional nursing practice.

Among the new types of models are partnership models such as interdisciplinary teams and patient-focused care. These models are designed to meet the needs of organizations that are reengineered to be more cost effective and competitive. Due to the nature of complex knowledge, work models are needed that enhance the professional practice of all disciplines, clarify accountability for outcomes, and focus decision making at the point of service. As organizations integrate, partnership concepts become important as a way to create relationships and horizontal links that will make the system effective. Teams are no longer a mechanism for assigning work. Nor are they even composed of just nursing personnel. Rather, they form the core strategy for managing interdependency to address the complexity of health care service delivery.

Patient-Centered Care

The **patient-centered care** model, also referred to as *patient-focused care*, is part of a redesign effort to realign the structure and processes involved in delivering care to center around the patient to improve efficiency and resource use. This approach adopts the perspective of the person receiving care and strives to establish mutual goals to meet unique needs. The advantage of patient-centered care redesigns is that they center systems and services closer to the patient. This strong customer focus tends to increase patient satisfaction, which can conserve resources (Marquis & Huston, 2007).

Case Management

Case management is the latest work design proposed to meet patient needs. It is a collaborative process that assesses, plans, implements, coordinates, monitors, and evaluates options and services to meet an individual's health needs through communication and available resources to promote quality, cost-effective outcomes (Cesta & Tahan, 2003; Huber, 2006; Marquis & Huston, 2007). The focus in case management is on individual patients, not populations of patients. Case managers handle each case individually, identifying the most cost-effective providers, treatments, and care settings for insured individuals (Finkelman, 2001).

Some health care organizations use the term *case management* to define a patient-centered model of care. The American Nurses Association first defined nursing case management as a

system of health assessment, planking, service procurement, service delivery, service coordination, and monitoring through which the multiple service needs of clients are met (ANA, 1988). Case management within the hospital setting is seen as a way to incorporate the strengths of earlier care models yet provide a professional practice model. Case management in acute care hospital nursing has been defined as a system of patient care delivery that focuses on the achievement of patient outcomes within effective and appropriate time frames and resources (Marquis & Huston, 2007). It focuses on an entire episode of illness, crossing all sections in which the patient receives care. A case manager directs care; however, the case manager may or may not be a nurse.

Community-Based Care

A community is a "locally-based entity composed of formal organizations reflecting societal institutions, informal groups, and aggregates. These components are interdependent, and function to meet a wide variety of collective needs" (Schuster & Goeppinger, 1996, p. 290). The community is considered to be the client when the nursing focus is on the collective or common good rather than the health of an individual. Thus, **community-based care**, also called *community-based nursing practice*, is directed toward health changes for the whole community's benefit. The unit of service may be individuals, families, groups, aggregates, institutions, or communities, but the purpose is to affect the entire community. The term *community* denotes a local entity, whereas the term *population* refers to an aggregate with any common characteristic, not necessarily tied to a place.

Within this context community-based nursing describes a setting for practice and a philosophy of care applicable to all nurses in all settings. It reflects how nursing care is provided, is typically not confined to one practice setting, is directed toward individuals and families within any community setting, and is designed to assist patients as they move among health care settings. Community-based nursing occurs in places where people spend their time, for example, in the home, in shelters, in long-term care residences, at work, in senior citizen centers, in ambulatory settings, and in hospitals (Berman, Snyder, Kozier, & Erb, 2008).

Legislative, regulatory, and social changes in the health care system as a result of health care reform initiatives of the 1990s have increased the need to move services out of the hospital and into community-based alternative health care settings. The numbers and kinds of agencies that provide care in the home and community have expanded because of the increasing needs of patients. As more health care delivery shifts into the community, more nurses are working in public health and community-based settings.

Community-based nurses are challenged as patients with complex nursing care needs are discharged from acute care settings early in the recovery process. Such patients include those who are elderly and have multiple-system problems. Medical technologies that were once thought to be useful in the hospital setting only have been adapted to the home and community settings. As a result, the community-based care setting is becoming one of the largest practice areas for nursing.

Within these settings nurses often deliver care without direct supervision or the support of other health care personnel. They must be self-directed, flexible, adaptable, and tolerant of various lifestyles and living conditions. Expertise in independent decision making, critical thinking, assessment, health education, and competence in basic nursing care are essential to function effectively in community-based settings.

Community Health Nursing

The phrase *community-based nursing* often is interchanged with *community health nursing*, but a distinction should be made. The phrase **community health nursing** has generally been equated with *public health nursing*, a specialty focused on special populations although care may be given to individuals. The term *community health* means meeting the collective needs of a group by identifying problems and managing interactions both within the community and among communities that make up the larger society. Community-based nursing is broader and may incorporate community health/public health nursing.

Population-Based Care

Population-based care is focused on aggregates and communities. Williams (1996) defined a population as "a collection of individuals who have in common one or more personal or environmental characteristics" (p. 25). Also called an aggregate, the members of a community are defined in terms of geography, special interest, disease state, or other common characteristics. The research-related term is target population. In community health, population-focused practice is directed toward care for defined populations or subpopulations as opposed to care for individual patients. Population-based case management is defined as the integration and coordination of health services for a specified population. This concept is implemented by providing a continuum of care from many health care organizations, and it is sometimes referred to as disease management.

Disease Management

More typically, the term *disease management* refers to a comprehensive, integrated approach to care and reimbursement based on a disease's natural course. The goal is to address the disease condition with maximum effectiveness and efficiency. Huber (2006) describes this as addressing a high-cost, chronic illness or condition, such as diabetes, with maximum efficiency across treatment settings regardless of typical reimbursement patterns. Thus, a continuum of chronic illness care is established that includes early detection and early intervention. This prevents or reduces exacerbation of the disease, acute episodes, and the use of expensive resources such as hospital inpatient care. Prevention and proactive case management are two major aspects of disease management programs. Additionally, disease management programs include comprehensive tracking of patient outcomes. Thus, the goals for disease management are focused on integrating components and improving long-term outcomes (Marquis & Huston, 2007).

Community-Based Care Versus Acute Care

Although there are noted differences between community-based care and acute care, there also are similarities. Practice in the acute care setting, where the patient is defined by disease or condition, typically takes place in specialized units where family access and patient autonomy are regulated by agency policies. Health is viewed as the opposite of illness, and the focus of care

is to eliminate illness. Nursing activities are geared toward short-term interventions. In the community setting, the patient is seen within the context of family and social network, and is treated in one's own environment, typically where the patient is more at ease. Illness is seen as a part of life, and the purpose of care is to limit patient disability and to improve functional capacity and quality of life. Nursing practice in the community has greater autonomy with therapeutic interventions, usually defined by clinician and patient who hold the patient's values central to the care performed.

Although traditional values and ways in which we think about each area of practice differ, nursing does not require widely different skills and knowledge. In both settings, nurses apply principles of interpersonal communication and caring skills to the patient, family, and other caregivers. Similarly, in each setting, nurses use leadership skills to plan, organize, coordinate, delegate, and evaluate care of patients. In both, nurses provide effective physical care. General principles of community-based care include advocating self-care; focusing on prevention; family, culture, and community; and continuity of care. Within the framework of these principles, when patient self-care, prevention, collaboration, continuity, and care within the context of family, culture, and community are emphasized, the nurse is participating in community-based nursing. It truly becomes a philosophy of care about *how* nurses practice—not *where* they work—and it can be incorporated into any type of work setting.

The Future and Workplace Design

The preceding discussion allows one to conclude that there is no one single way to organize patient care delivery systems. The method of workplace design depends on the internal and external environmental factors currently in play. They are not static, but in a constant state of flux.

It is well known that forces and pressures outside of nursing influence nursing care delivery models; however, it is not known which form is the best care model for each setting (Marquis & Huston, 2007). Although we have knowledge about the advantages of different model types, there is a lack of research evidence about which setting is most appropriate for which care model, where each is most cost effective, or which one is going to produce a higher quality of care delivery. Restructuring today means looking at new care models as they relate to a cost–quality balance. In the restructuring process, the desired outcomes are that patient care be delivered more efficiently, people be more satisfied, and costs be minimized. What is clear is that with all models, nurses must collaborate with each other and other members of the health care team in order to provide health care to the current and future generations.

Collaborative Care

Collaboration among health care professionals becomes increasingly important as the roles and boundaries change and merge. Some practitioners have begun to specialize in progressively more narrow areas of expertise, whereas others have taken on the role of generalist. Over time the legal scope of practice of each health care profession may change. To deliver optimum comprehensive care to the patient, nurses must work as a member of a team, collaborating in a collegial manner with other health care providers. This requires discussing patients' diagnoses and cooperating in the management and delivery of care (ANA, 1992).

Nurses as collaborators in patient care delivery also may be involved in determining and resolving bioethical issues, speaking out on legislation, participating in health-related research, and working with professional organizations. In fulfilling a collaborative role, nurses need to assume accountability and increased authority in practice areas. Key elements necessary for collaboration include effective communication skills, mutual respect, trust, and a decision-making process.

Some institutions use the collaborative practice model. Nurses, physicians, and ancillary health personnel function within a decentralized organizational structure and collaborate when making clinical decisions. A joint practice committee, with representation from all care providers, may function at the unit level to monitor, support, and foster collaboration (Berman et al., 2008; Marquis & Huston, 2007). The collaborative model of care, or some variation of it, should be a primary goal for nursing. This model promotes shared participation, responsibility, and accountability in a health care environment that is striving to meet the complex health care needs of the public with an increasing array of health care workers.

■ Influences in Health Care Delivery

The health care delivery system of the 21st century is undergoing a major transformation. A new system is emerging in response to the social, economic, technological, scientific, and political forces challenging the century. Among the most significant of these changes are the changing population demographics, changes in health care needs, and changing expectations of the consumers of health care.

The characteristics of the 21st-century health care system include short-term stays, fast patient turnover, advanced technology, flexibility, early engagement, mobility, and the involvement of family members as primary caregivers. These changes along with the environmental changes previously discussed will influence how nursing care is delivered, as well as who will deliver the care and when this will occur (Huber, 2006; Sullivan & Decker, 2005; Yoder-Wise, 2008).

Population Demographics

Population changes in general are having a direct impact on health care delivery. The 2000 U.S. census data indicated that the United States population is 281.4 million people. This figure indicates that people are living longer, possibly due to improved health services and improved nutrition. In 2004, the U.S. Census Bureau completed an estimate of general demographic characteristics. At that time the total U.S. population was estimated to be 299,398,484, with a small majority being female.

Most sources agree that not only is the population increasing and living longer, but it is also changing in composition. The decline in birth rate and the increase in life span attributed to improved health care have resulted in fewer school-age children and more senior citizens, most of whom are women. People re-

side in areas dictated by age and ethnicity. Much of the population resides in highly congested urban areas, with a steady migration of minority groups to the inner cities and migration of middle-class people to suburban areas. The culturally diverse population is growing, as is the homeless population.

These population shifts, joined by major concerns about emerging infectious diseases, trauma, and bioterrorism, are changing the focus of health care and, therefore, the roles of health care providers. The focus is shifting more to prevention, health promotion, and management of chronic conditions than in the prior century. This shift in focus coincides with a nationwide emphasis on cost control and resource management directed toward providing cost-effective and efficient health services for all (Dower, 2002).

Aging Population

Advances in technology, discoveries of cures for diseases, new treatment modalities, and the push for wellness have all had an impact on life span, significantly increasing the proportion of the population who grow to old age. According to some projections, by the year 2010, the baby boomers will turn 65 plus. In the next decade the proportion of society over 65 years of age will nearly double, and the health of older Americans will become a critical health care issue during this century (Administration on Aging [AoA], 2004). However, as the population of older adults dramatically increases, a few signs indicate that adequate resources will not be available to meet the challenge of providing health care and good quality of life for these older adults and their families. The aging population currently accounts for 12.4% of the entire U.S. population. The projection by the year 2030 is that the older U.S. population will double to about 71 million and account for 20% of the population (AoA, 2004). The "oldest-old" Americans, those 85 years and older, are the fastest growing group in the United States. This population is projected to increase from 4.6 million in 2002 to 9.6 million in 2030 (National Center for Health Statistics, 2007).

Although demographic projections for the coming decades include growth in the population of older adults, particularly those over age 85, a decrease in younger age groups is projected, a reflection of lower fertility rates and delayed childbearing among baby boomers. The dependency ratio often is cited as a determining factor in care for older adults, and is projected to reach unprecedented heights, having grown from 9.1 older adults per 100 workers in 1930 to 35.7 in 2030 (Centers for Disease Control and Prevention [CDC], 2004; U.S. Census Bureau, 2000). The concern is that this will create a functional scarcity among younger generations, with higher demand on fewer people for informal caregiving and proportionately lower contributions to Social Security benefits (AoA, 2004).

Other trends may also influence the availability of family caregivers. For example, fewer women are at home to provide care because of the growing number of female heads of households and two-income families. In the future there will be more childless elders, based on a higher percentage of currently childless women in the 40- to 45-year-old age group. It is important to consider that the oldest-old individuals are most likely to have disabilities, use multiple medications, or need consistent caregiving. Also important to note is that many older adults will be from ethnically diverse cultures. Hispanic elders, now 5.6% of the elderly population, will increase to 16.4% of the elderly population in the next 50 years (CDC, 2004). These trends are important to those planning health care services for the future because they suggest an increasing demand on formal services, a pattern already in evidence during the past decade. The health care needs of the aging, availability of health care resources, and the nurse's role in caring for the aging are discussed in detail in Chapter 10 🔗.

Informed Consumers

In addition to age, other demographic factors are developing that will affect health care in the 21st century. The majority of the consumers of health care will be well educated and, hence, better able to obtain and use the information needed for maintaining health (Baker, Wagner, Singer, & Bundorf, 2003). They will be able to use the Internet to assist them in learning about their illness or health issues, and they will be better able to make informed decisions regarding their health care. Consumers also will be more diverse, requiring a multicultural sensitivity.

The roles of women and the family will change. There will be an increase in single-parent families and an increase in multiple-family combinations. Parents will be older with fewer children. More women will work outside the home and choose to remain in the workplace after having children. Society will place a higher value on children. Such demographic variables have a significant impact on health care, economics, public policy, and quality of life, including the delivery of health care (Dower, 2002; Getzen, 2006; Mechanic, Rogut, & Colby, 2005; Shortell & Kaluzny, 2005).

Cultural Diversity

Diversity is a word that means something different to each and every person. **Cultural diversity** refers to the variations among groups of people with respect to the habits, values, preferences, beliefs, taboos, and rules determined to be appropriate for individuals and social interaction (Huber, 2006). It represents the variety and differences in the customs and practices of defined social groups. The changing demographics and economics of our growing multicultural world and the long-standing disparities in the health status of people from culturally diverse backgrounds have challenged health care providers and organizations to consider cultural diversity as a priority.

As with aging, cultural diversity is increasing at a rapid speed (U.S. Census Bureau, 2002). Some projections indicate that by 2030 racial and ethnic minority groups will comprise 40% of the U.S. population. With increased immigration, this figure could rise to 50% by the year 2030. As the cultural composition of the population changes, it becomes increasingly important to address cultural considerations in the delivery of health care. Patients from diverse sociocultural groups bring different health care beliefs, values, and practices to the health care setting, as well as different risk factors for some disease conditions. They also respond to treatment uniquely. These factors significantly affect the way one responds to health care problems or illness, to those who provide the care, and to the care itself. It is understood that an appreciation of the diverse characteristics and needs of individuals from varied ethnic and cultural backgrounds is important in health care and nursing. Unless these

factors are understood and respected by health care providers, the care delivered may be ineffective and health care outcomes may be negatively affected.

In addressing cultural diversity, health care providers must realize that it goes beyond knowing the values, beliefs, customs, and practices of racial groups, such as African Americans, Asians, Hispanics/Latinos, Native Americans, and Pacific Islanders. Religious affiliation, language, physical size, gender, sexual orientation, age, disability, political orientation, socioeconomic status, occupational status, and geographic location also represent a few of the faces of diversity (Campinha-Bacote, 2003).

To understand cultural diversity, it is necessary to understand **culture**. Culture refers to a complex of learned patterns of behavior, beliefs, and values that can be attributed to a particular group of people. These learned behaviors, beliefs, and values guide thinking, decisions, and actions. Included among the many characteristics that distinguish cultural groups are the manner of dress, language spoken, values, rules or norms of behavior, gender-specific practices, economics, politics, laws and social control, artifact, technology, dietary practices, and health beliefs and practices. Health promotion, illness prevention, causes of sickness, treatment, coping, caring, dying, and death are all a part of the health-related component of every culture. Individuals have a unique belief and value system, which has, in part, been shaped by their cultural environment. This value system influences and guides the individual's response to illness and to health care. It is incumbent on the health care delivery system to consider these individual needs by providing practitioners who are culturally competent and providing organizational structures that are sensitive to cultural diversity.

Cultural Competence

Health care service policies, protocols, and regulations call for **cultural competence**, which is the act of providing care effectively to persons from a multiplicity of cultures. Cultural competence is an ongoing evolution of knowing, respecting, and incorporating the values of others. It means being open to the cultural beliefs and behaviors of others. It is a crucial link to practicing empathy, understanding, communicating, valuing, and caring in health care.

To achieve cultural competence one must possess a set of congruent behaviors, attitudes, and policies that come together in a system, agency, or among professionals and enables that system, agency, or those professionals to work effectively in cross-cultural situations. The word *competence* implies having the capacity to function effectively (Campinha-Bacote, 2003). Because cultural differences are learned, cultural sensitivity and competence also can be learned. The four identified components needed to become more culturally competent are cultural awareness, cultural knowledge, cultural skill, and cultural encounters.

Campinha-Bacote (2003) believes that all people belong to the same human race, with all of the same basic needs. However, she stresses that it is important to remember that these needs may be expressed differently, and that quality health care services may mean something different to each person. It is critically important for the health care delivery system to recognize the increasing diversity of those who seek care and make provisions for those who practice in the system to become culturally competent. It is equally important for health care professionals to apply the concepts of cultural competence to the patients they care for. Because every person comes from a unique and different background, the individual needs and values must be taken into account to make hospital stays as comfortable as possible. For example, the nurse should consider which room numbers mean bad luck to Asian Americans, what foods are comfort foods to Hispanics, or how to bring comfort and caring to a Muslim individual. Cultural competence will enable the health care system to improve the quality of care as measured by patient outcomes and to meet state and national licensure and accreditation standards.

Changing Disease Patterns

The health problems of Americans have changed significantly during the past 50 years. Many infectious diseases have been controlled or eradicated; others, such as tuberculosis, acquired immunodeficiency syndrome (AIDS), and sexually transmitted infections are on the rise. An increasing number of infection agents are becoming resistant to antibiotics. Conditions that once were treated easily have become complex and difficult to treat—some have even become life threatening.

The increasing life span of the general population is contributing significantly to the increase in chronic disease and disability (CDC, 2004). Also, the successful treatment options for conditions such as cancer and human immunodeficiency virus (HIV) allow people with these conditions to live decades longer than in earlier years. People with chronic illnesses are the largest group of health care consumers in the United States (CDC, 2004). Due to the heavy incidence of chronic conditions, many people are learning how to protect and maximize their health within the constraints of chronic illness and disability. As chronic conditions increase, health care broadens from a focus on cure and eradication of disease to include the prevention or rapid treatment of exacerbations of chronic conditions. The shifting changes in disease patterns support the need for increased emphasis on community-based care, rather than acute care.

In discussing changing disease patterns, it is necessary also to address globalization and health for all. Those entering the United States through travel and immigration are bringing many new diseases with them. Current society exists in a world where global infectious disease cannot be controlled by border patrols. One of the new diseases, West Nile virus, was first detected in the United States in 1999. By 2002, West Nile virus had spread to most of the continental United States. The first human case of this virus was reported in early July 2003, with three deaths due to the virus reported by August. In 2005 alone, there were 3,000 human cases and 119 deaths linked to infection, up from 2,539 cases and 100 deaths in 2004 (Medline Plus, 2006). Severe acute respiratory syndrome (SARS) is another example of a new viral disease that was first identified in China, Hong Kong, and Vietnam in 2003. This disease has spread to the United States, and at the time of this writing, there were more than 200 suspected cases in the United States (National Institute of Allergy and Infectious Diseases, 2005). According to the World Health Organization, 8,098 people worldwide became

sick with SARS during the 2003 outbreak. Of these, 774 died. In the United States only 8 people had laboratory evidence of SARS-CoV infection; no deaths were reported (CDC, 2006).

Now, society is faced with the avian flu and methicillin-resistant *Staphylococcus aureus* (MRSA). Avian influenza virus refers to influenza A viruses found chiefly in birds, but infections with these viruses can occur in humans. Although the risk for human infection is low, confirmed cases of human infection from several subtypes of avian influenza infection have been reported since 1997. Most cases of avian influenza infection in humans have resulted from contact with infected poultry (e.g., domesticated chicken, ducks, and turkeys) or surfaces contaminated with secretion/excretions from infected birds.

Of the few avian influenza viruses that have crossed the species barrier to infect humans, H5N1 has caused the largest number of detected cases of severe disease and death in humans. However, it is possible that those cases in the most severely ill people are more likely to be diagnosed and reported, while milder cases go unreported (CDC, 2007). Of the human cases associated with the ongoing H5N1 outbreaks in poultry and wild birds in Asia and parts of Europe, the Near East, and Africa, more than half of those people reported infected with the virus have died. Most cases have occurred in previously healthy children and young adults and have resulted from direct or close contact with H5N1-infected poultry or H5N1-contaminated surfaces.

Although there has been some human-to-human spread of H5N1, it has been limited, inefficient, and unsustained. Nonetheless, because all influenza viruses have the ability to change, scientists are concerned that one day the H5N1 virus could be able to infect humans and spread easily from one person to another. Because these viruses do not commonly infect humans, there is little or no immune protection against them in the human population. If the H5N1 virus were to gain the capacity to spread easily from person to person, an influenza pandemic (worldwide outbreak of disease) could begin. No one can predict when a pandemic might occur. However, experts from around the world are watching the H5N1 situation in Asia and Europe very closely and are preparing for the possibility that the virus may begin to spread more easily and widely from person to person.

MRSA joins avian flu, West Nile virus, SARS, and HIV as a potentially deadly infectious disease that seems to be becoming more prevalent (Mayo Clinic, 2007). Worldwide, an estimated 2 billion people carry some form of *S. aureus*; of these, up to 53 million (2.7% of carriers) are thought to carry MRSA. In the United States, 95 million carry *S. aureus* in their noses; of these, 2.5 million (2.6% of carriers) carry MRSA.

Increasing numbers of outbreaks of community-acquired MRSA colonization and infection through skin contact in locker rooms and gymnasiums, even among healthy populations, have been reported. MRSA causes as many as 20% of *S. aureus* infections in populations that use intravenous drugs. These out-of-hospital strains, or community-acquired (CA)-MRSA, are more easily treated, even though they are more virulent, than hospital-aquired (HA)-MRSA. CA-MRSA apparently did not evolve *de novo* in the community but represents a hybrid between MRSA that spread from the hospital environment and strains that were once easily treatable in the community. Most of the hybrid strains also acquired a factor that increases their virulence, resulting in the development of deep tissue infections from minor scrapes and cuts, as well as many cases of fatal pneumonia.

The spread of HIV/AIDS and other catastrophic illnesses threatens both personal and political viability. Lack of access to safe reproductive health puts hundreds of millions of people at risk and also contributes to the burgeoning global population growth and migration. Poor child health and nutrition rob future generations of human potential and years of life. Health for all continues to be a call for equity and social justice, a global issue that must be dealt with at the local level in communities around the world.

Complementary and Alternative Therapy

Health care in the 21st century requires that nurses not only care for the critically ill, elderly, and infirm, but also that they recognize and incorporate new and evolving methods to enhance the health of those who choose alternative or complementary therapies. This evidence-based, integrative style of care originates from holistic nursing, a precursor and philosophical framework for many of the now popular alternative and complementary therapies. Holistic nursing is simply defined as caring for the whole person—body, mind, and spirit—in an ever-changing environment.

Complementary or Alternative: What Is the Difference?

The words *complementary* and *alternative* are sometimes used interchangeably, but they are not the same. **Complementary therapy** refers to a therapy used in addition to a conventional therapy. For example, a nurse might use touch therapies, music, or guided imagery for pain control in addition to the prescribed drug therapy.

Alternative therapy, sometimes called *unconventional therapy*, refers to a therapy used instead of conventional or mainstream therapy. An example is the use of acupuncture instead of analgesics.

Integration of Complementary and Alternative Systems into Traditional American Health Care

Until recently, in North America, the primary system of medicine was simply called *medicine*, although some refer to it as **allopathic medicine**. In the past two decades a number of schools of thought and philosophies have become intertwined with traditional medicine. The most frequently seen new systems include Ayurvedic, Chinese, chiropractic, naturopathic, Native American, and osteopathic medicine. Each of these systems can stand alone, or be used in combination with other systems (Chart 1–8, p. 26).

Safety and Effectiveness of Alternative Therapies

Safety generally is interpreted to mean "freedom from danger" in which the benefits of alternative therapy outweigh the risks. If the patient is interested in using an alternative or complementary therapy, the nurse should first counsel the person about the benefits and risks and advise her to ask the practitioner of the therapy about the safety and effectiveness of the treatment.

Complementary and alternative medicine (CAM) therapies can be dangerous if used improperly. As for any medical endeavor, practitioners must be trained and, with some therapies, licensed or certified. The most prevalent deficit of CAM therapies is seen when patients use them instead of conventional therapy and do not seek traditional diagnosis and treatment. People who choose CAM therapies first and continue to use them for symptom treatment may delay diagnosis of treatable cancers as well as a huge array of curable conditions. Thus, most CAM therapies are best used alongside conventional medicine. The positive effects of these therapies used to augment allopathic medicine are presented in the Complementary and Alternative Therapies feature boxes that appear in most of the forthcoming disorder chapters in this text.

When assessing patients the nurse should ask if they use any nontraditional therapies and, if so, what their response is to them. The nurse should try to eliminate any preconceived notions she may have about a certain therapy. Patients typically will feel more comfortable discussing nontraditional therapies if they feel the nurse understands the treatment and why they have decided to use it. If patients are unfamiliar with alternative or complementary therapies (Chart 1–9, p. 27), they may ask the nurse questions about specific treatments or therapies. Following are some sample questions that patients may ask:

- What will this therapy do for me?
- What are the advantages of this therapy?
- What are the disadvantages?
- Are there side effects?
- What risks are associated with this therapy?
- How much will it cost?
- How long will it take? How many treatments will be necessary?
- How will it interact with my other therapies?

The use of alternative and complementary therapies is proliferating. Nurses who have additional training in specific CAM therapies can use many of them to provide better care for patients. When patients use complementary therapies, nurses should consider the usage an attempt to increase potential health benefits and not as signs of distress or dissatisfaction with their current care. Throughout this text in the chapters that cover disorders, Complementary and Alternative Therapies features highlight single or occasionally multiple therapies that will work with one of the conditions referred to in the chapter. These boxed features may be used as an example of how nurses can incorporate CAM into their care.

Advances in Technology and Genetics

Advances in technology and genetics have occurred with greater frequency in the last several decades than ever before. They are causing changes in all health care settings and in the roles and responsibilities of all health care providers.

Technological Changes

Biomedical technology, information technology, telecommunications, and the Internet have changed the delivery of health care into a national and even international system. The previous state of the art is being replaced by new high-tech developments at an ever-increasing rate. The advances have enabled practitioners to make faster diagnoses, treat illnesses more quickly,

CHART 1–8	Systems of Health Care Services

System	Description
Allopathic/Western medicine	The most common name for allopathic medicine is *Western medicine*. Other terms for Western medicine are *conventional medicine* and *mainstream medicine*. Many people have not heard the term *allopathic* because most health care professionals do not refer to themselves or their practice with this name. Practitioners of other systems of medicine more often use the term when referring to what can be called Western medicine or mainstream medicine. Allopathy is a method of treating disease with remedies that produce effects different from those caused by the disease itself. This system of medicine uses scientific data to determine the validity of a diagnosis and the effectiveness of treatment. It is evidence-based medicine. Practitioners use a variety of therapies including drugs, surgery, and radiation therapy. Western medicine practitioners have made most of the significant advances and developments in modern medicine.
Ayurvedic medicine	Ayurveda is the ancient Hindu system of medicine from India. Its main goals are to maintain the health of healthy people and cure the illnesses of sick people. Ayurveda maintains that illness is the result of falling out of balance with nature. Diagnosis is based on three metabolic body types call *doshas*. The Ayurvedic doctor determines the doshas type as vata, pitta, and kapha. Treatment usually involves prescribing a diet, herbal remedies, breathwork, physical exercise, yoga, meditation, massage, and a rejuvenation or detoxification program.
Traditional Chinese medicine	Traditional Chinese medicine is thousands of years old and involves such techniques and practices as acupuncture, acupressure, herbs, massage, and qi gong. The diagnosis and treatment of disturbances of qi (pronounced "chee")—or vital energy—are distinctive characteristics of Chinese medicine. Acupuncturists, one type of traditional Chinese medicine practitioner, access patients' health by checking pulses, looking at the color of the tongue, checking facial color, assessing voice and smell, and asking a variety of questions. To treat patients, acupuncturists insert a needle(s) along the meridians (pathways) where qi flows. Many acupuncturists also prescribe herbs.
Chiropractic	The main treatment modality of chiropractors is manual adjustment and manipulation of the vertebral column and the extremities. They use direct hand contact and mechanical and electrical treatment methods in the course of treatment. Chiropractors primarily treat back pain, neck pain, and headaches. They do not perform surgery, nor do they prescribe drugs.
Homeopathic medicine	Homeopathy is based on the principle that "like cures like," in which tiny doses of a substance that create the symptoms of disease in a healthy person will relieve those symptoms in a sick person.
Naturopathic medicine	Naturopathy primarily uses natural therapies such as nutrition, botanical medicine, hydrotherapy, counseling, physical medicine, and homeopathy to treat disease, promote healing, and prevent illness. Naturopathic physicians have a doctor of naturopathy (ND) degree and must be licensed.
Native American healing	Native American medicine practices vary from tribe to tribe. In general, Native American medicine is a community-based system with rituals and practices: the sweat lodge, use of herbal remedies, the medicine wheel, sacred hoop, the "sing," and shamanistic healing. For example, an ill person may be placed in a small, enclosed sweat lodge. While singing or chanting is done outside the lodge, it is believed that toxic substances will come out in the sweat of the person inside the lodge. After the ceremony, the ill person may be placed on a cot outside and be prayed over.
Osteopathic medicine	This practice of medicine emphasizes the interrelationship of the body's nerves, muscles, bones, and organs. The osteopathic philosophy involves treating the whole person, recognizes the body's ability to heal itself, and stresses the importance of diet, exercise, and fitness with a focus on prevention.

make decisions faster, and communicate more quickly and effectively with all members of the health care team.

Biomedical Technology

Biomedical technology is used for physiological monitoring, diagnostic testing, drug administration, and therapeutic treatments. Developments in biomedical technology include the use of implantable devices such as automated defibrillators, artificial organ transplants, gene therapy, and the use of robotics for people who have disabilities. Biomedical technologies also have revolutionized surgery, making it convenient and cost effective for many surgical procedures to be performed on an outpatient basis. Robotic inventions have invaded health care settings. They currently are being used in surgery, and in some institutions they provide patient care.

The health care industry also has benefited from the advanced technologies developed for space travel. These technologies have been adapted to produce health care aids such as Viewstar (an aid for people with visual impairments), the insulin infusion pump, the voice-controlled wheelchair, magnetic resonance imaging, laser surgery, filtering devices for intravenous fluid control devices, and monitoring systems for intensive care.

Information Technology

Information technology refers to those systems used to manage and process information. This involves the computer, other equipment, and processes used to store, organize, retrieve, and communicate data with accuracy and speed. Most health care delivery systems use computers and computer programs to pro-

CHART 1–9	Categories and Types of Alternative and Complementary Therapies
Category of Therapy	**Types of Individual Therapies**
Herbal medicine and nutritional supplements	Herbal medicine Nutrition and special diet therapies Nutritional supplements
Mind–body therapies	Psychology Art therapy Music/sound therapies Guided imagery Hypnosis and hypnotherapy Meditation and relaxation
Posture and mobility	Movement therapies T'ai chi and qi gong Yoga
Touch therapies and body work	Massage and related massage therapies Acupressure
Energetic therapies	Biofeedback Healing touch Magnet therapy Polarity therapy Reiki Spiritual healing Therapeutic touch
Miscellaneous therapies	Aquatherapy/hydrotherapy Aromatherapy Chanting Chelation therapy Colon therapy Kinesiology Light therapy Pet therapy

vide accounting, clinical, and administrative functions. Clinical nursing information systems and medical information systems manage clinical information required for the practice of nursing and medicine, respectively.

The use of information technology is growing at an exponential rate, in part because the federal government and third-party payers are supporting new technologies to reduce costs. Much of the growth in information technology has been spearheaded by an executive order that created the Office of the National Coordinator for Health Information Technology (DHHS, 2004). A 10-year plan was developed to transform the delivery of health care by building a new health information infrastructure, including electronic health records and a new network to link health records nationwide. Health information technology is believed to improve quality of care and reduce medical errors, even as it lowers administrative costs (DHHS, 2004).

The use of health information technology is really just getting started, with much growth anticipated in the next 10 years, resulting in many changes in the way health care is implemented, documented, and monitored. However, the phenomenon of information overload also can develop. According to some the adoption of information technology (IT) has been slow and the results have been mixed. If not implemented correctly, IT systems without well-conceived process improvements can hinder the efficiency, accuracy, and effectiveness of the health care system, leading to critical delays or mistakes (Klein, 2006). Another potential problem to be considered is "information overload." It is possible to move from a century in which there was a deficit of patient information to a century in which there is a surplus of patient information. The question is raised, "Can health care workers assimilate the volume of information becoming available to them?"

Longitudinal computerized patient records, telecommunications, and devices that store health history data are technologies that will grow in the future. Computerized charting and scheduling of procedures already are the norm. Hospital reimbursement systems have resulted in the redesign of patient care plans to clinical pathways that detail the interventions needed day by day to achieve the outcomes of discharge by the final approved day. Data from the clinical pathway form the basis of the episode of care in the computerized patient record. The federal government has mandated use of a computerized patient record. Credit card–like devices called smart cards store a limited number of pages of data on a computer chip. The implementation of computer-based health information systems will lead to computer networks that will store health records across local, state, national, and international boundaries. The smart card serves as a bridge between the clinician terminal and the central repository, making patient information available to the caregiver quickly and cheaply at the point of service because the patients bring it with them. This will help coordinate care, improve quality of care decisions, and reduce risk, waste, and duplication of effort (Sullivan & Decker, 2005). The challenge for nurses is to use data to create information and then change information into knowledge, which will improve the health outlook for all. This emerging body of knowledge is known as informatics.

Informatics Informatics is a combination of computer science, information science, and health care science that is designed to assist in the management and delivery of health care. Nursing informatics facilitates the integration of data, information, and knowledge and is used to assist the nurse in decision making in all roles and settings. This support is accomplished through the use of information structures, information processes, and information technology (ANA, 2001b). According to the ANA, the beginning nurse "is expected to have fundamental information management and computer literacy skills" (p. 25). Nurses must be proficient in the use of computer hardware and software. They may participate in computer utilization at varying levels of competency, although it is recognized that the level of skill needed may vary among nurses.

In many health care settings nurses will be expected to use integrated delivery systems as facilities become paperless (Huber, 2006; Marquis & Huston, 2007). The move toward increased use of information technology systems is supported strongly by The Joint Commission.

Telecommunications

Telecommunications and systems technology facilitate clinical oversight of health care via telephone or cable lines, remote monitoring, information links, and the Internet. Telehealth is the use of modern telecommunications and information technologies for the provision of health care to individuals at a distance and the transmission of information to provide that care.

This is accomplished through the use of two-way interactive videoconferencing and high-speed telephone lines, fiber-optic cable, and satellite transmissions. Patients sitting in front of the teleconference camera can be diagnosed, treated, monitored, and educated by nurses and physicians. Electrocardiograms and x-ray films can be viewed and transmitted. Sophisticated electronic stethoscopes and dermascopes allow nurses and physicians to hear heart, lung, and bowel sounds and to look closely at wounds, eyes, ears, and skin. Ready access to expert advice and patient information is available no matter where the patient or information is located, which is of particular benefit to patients in rural areas and prisons.

Advances in telemedicine already can be evidenced by home monitoring systems, where the sound of a patient's heart or a patient's blood pressure readings are transmitted over telephone lines to off-site physicians; by transmission of x-ray images over a modem to specialized physicians in other states; and by videoconferencing in which physicians consult with patients or other physicians. Telecommunications also are being used to teach physicians and nurses how to treat patients and how to provide patient care.

Internet

Another vehicle for health information is the Internet. The Internet can provide health education and health information. Health care providers and patients alike can use it to retrieve and share information. The Internet also provides a system of communication between health care provider and patients and can be a very effective means of delivering health services to people (Baker et al., 2003).

Future Projections

Technological advances in the future health care environment will stress wellness, health promotion, illness management, and the linking of local and global communities. Care in this era will focus on empowering patients and their families through information and education. Clinicians will move beyond the traditional walls of health care facilities to become skilled with wellness maintenance activities and prevention methods as well as direct care delivery. Technology will become the bond that links people and information. Nurses need to prepare for this future in which developments and refinements such as portable computers, handheld terminals, voice input, videodisc technology, expert systems, artificial intelligence, and more advanced decision support and modeling systems will continue to augment their practice. There will be greater connectedness and outreach linkages. Matching payment strategies with the technology evolution will continue to challenge the heath care system.

Nurses will be using information technology for effective outcome measurement and for capturing information at the point of care that is then distributed instantly to other users. Systems can then be mined in real time for data on quality and cost targets. Point-of-care technology can transform nurses' work processes. For example, wireless or radio frequency technology, tablet personal computers, locking/docking stations, and barcode readers constitute technological advances for nursing (Huber, 2006; Marquis & Huston, 2007).

Not only do nurses need to know how to use this technology and to access data in order to do their jobs, they need to function

as information brokers and advocates for patients. As more people use the computer and the Internet to access health-related information, it becomes incumbent on the nurse to assist them in sorting out relevant, valid, and reliable information. This becomes a part of the nurse educator role. The nurse also must assume the ethical responsibility of safeguarding the integrity and confidentiality of patient information, which is now mandated by the 1996 Health Insurance Portability and Accountability Act (HIPAA) (Sullivan & Decker, 2005). HIPAA is discussed in Chapters 3, 4, & 6 ☻ as it relates to the specific content area.

Genetics

Within the last decade the body of knowledge called genetics has exploded, largely due to the result of identifying the human genome through the Human Genome Project (HGP). The HGP was funded by Congress in 1988, and is the result of a collaborative, coordinated research effort in human genetics planned by the Department of Energy and the National Institutes of Health (Drell & Adamson, 2003). The HGP has been instrumental in fostering a multidisciplinary approach to research with an expectation of openness and sharing of discoveries via information technology. The achievement of uncovering the full genome sequence is regarded as a historic scientific event. The HGP has provided knowledge and insights into many diseases and development of improved methods for diagnosis and prevention.

As the pace of genetic knowledge continues to progress at a rapid rate, the private and public sectors have become increasingly interested. The private sector is interested in building markets on the information available from the HGP and offering commercialization of genetic diagnostics and services. Molecular medicine and information-based targeted health care are attracting entrepreneurial companies to consider the role of proactive prediction and prevention of disease risk based on an individuated genetic profile. Optimum goals of the HGP for the 2009 and beyond include a catalog of variations in the human DNA sequence, faster/cheaper technology, a focus on gene function, and continued attention to the implications of such knowledge for society.

The new discoveries in genetics are being publicized in all forms of mass media. Health care consumers are becoming more aware of gene-based tests and therapies and the technologies that make them possible. As genetic-based testing becomes more commonplace, individuals and their families will approach health care providers with questions about testing, resources for having testing done, interpretation of results, and requests for specialized services in genetic centers. Because nurses are widely accessible to the public, they are regarded as a group of health care providers who can begin to provide basic information and referrals for appropriate assistance. The ANA (1999) has adopted the position that the nurse, as "a provider in all health settings must have a strong knowledge base in genetics to be able to accurately assess, provide information, and make referrals for patients and families with genetic concerns" (p. 1). Chapter 11 ☻ contains a complete discussion of genetics.

Economics

During the past 20 years, health care costs in the United States have skyrocketed and are expected to continue to rise. It is projected that by 2010 they will consume 13% of the gross domestic product, the highest percentage among the five other industrialized nations (Congressional Budget Office, 2003). Health care spending continues to outstrip inflation and be a source of concern for insured and uninsured alike. New medical technology, expanding insurance coverage, increased spending for prescription drugs, and the aging of the population account for the greatest increases in spending in recent years. As overall health care costs have spiraled upward, so have employers' health care costs, thereby causing many employers to decrease the coverage provided for employees or increase the amount that employees must contribute toward their health care.

With rising costs and an unstable economy, the number of uninsured Americans continues to grow (Dower, 2002; Sullivan & Decker, 2005). Studies have shown that those who are uninsured often go without necessary medical care and are more likely to be sicker and in an emergency room when they do seek care. Hospitals must cope with higher indigent medical care expenses, additional regulatory fees, and escalating equipment and supply costs. These factors have led to higher patient care charges, which means higher costs for third-party payers. This, in turn, means higher health care insurance premiums, which then leads to a greater number of uninsured.

Demand for health services has expanded along with medical costs (U.S. Census Bureau, 2002). This is occurring at a time when there is a shortage of many health care personnel to provide needed services, and when patient expectations of medical care also are at higher levels. Patients want access to the latest and greatest technology, the most modern prescription drugs available, and all forms of alternative medicine. They expect services to be provided in a timely manner. If a health care facility cannot offer such services, patients may choose to go elsewhere. It has been found that health care corporations that achieve positive patient satisfaction results do so because they have created a customer service culture and infrastructure that enables them to respond to the ever-changing demands of customers (Marquis & Huston, 2007). Patient satisfaction is significant because health care organizations are operating in an extremely competitive environment, and patient satisfaction has become key to gaining and maintaining market share. Though employers, legislators, insurers, and health care providers continue to collaborate in efforts to resolve the issues affecting the costs of health care, a solution has not yet been found. A comprehensive discussion of health care economics is found in Chapter 3.

Demand for Quality Care

With rising health care costs, consumers and third-party payers alike are questioning the quality of service provided by health care providers and organizations. The general public has become increasingly aware of health care options and health promotion. An increased knowledge base has been generated by television, magazines, periodicals, newspapers and other communications media, and by political debate. Consumers have become more active in pursuing health care in an organization that measures and reports quality of care behaviors and outcomes. Regulatory agencies and third-party payers also are basing approval and acceptance behaviors on the ability of health care organizations to produce quality of care indicators and outcomes. The demand for quality from a consumer and regulatory perspective is fully discussed in Chapter 3.

Summary

Nursing offers a career path in which opportunity abounds for all interested. As the population ages and the need for nurses continues to sky rocket, the practice of nursing will grow and evolve. The work of nurses will continue to change. Many hypothesize that nurses will become much more active in the fields of prevention and health screening as they reach further out into the fabric of the community in which patients live. Others suggest that nursing will continue to grow in the technology of interventional patient care, translating the high-tech information and educating those involved to care for those who have received these interventions in the home environment.

This also is a time of incredible tension as the need for change in the U.S. health care delivery system continues to expand. What will nursing be in 10 years? Advancements in the science of clinical practice, including imaging, pharmaceutical agents, and technology, keep adding to the demands of nursing. These advancements also result in changes in patients' expectations and knowledge. Nurses continue to serve the role of integrator of patients into health care systems. Their practice will be based on scientific and caring concepts, and they will develop from novice to expert through experiential learning as discussed in Chapter 2.

The future is unclear, but the diversity and adaptability of nursing is a constant. There is one certainty: Nurses will continue to be a critical component of health care delivery and the opportunities are limitless for those who join the ranks of the nursing profession.

REVIEW QUESTIONS

1. One of the characteristics of nursing is defined in the role of nursing education. In providing information regarding the characteristics and consequences of disease, promoting and modeling healthy lifestyle, the professional nurse is emphasizing which of the following?
   1. Health promotion and maintenance
   2. Advocacy
   3. Complementary therapies
   4. Physiological adaptation

2. Roach identified six components of caring that are reflected in conscience, confidence, commitment, competence, and comportment. Without caring, the nurse will not see what type needs of the client?
   1. Physical and comfort
   2. Psychological and spiritual
   3. Physiological
   4. Ethics and moral

3. When deciding on a delivery model for nursing practice, nursing administration determined that a method of assignment with nurses having accountability for a specific 'case load' of patients for a defined shift was appropriate for the department.

   This describes which delivery model?

   1. Functional nursing
   2. Modular nursing
   3. Primary care nursing
   4. Total patient care nursing

4. The staff nurse has the primary responsibility to care for a specific patient or group of patients for an assigned period. Organization and coordination are inherent in the role due to which of the following?

   1. The need to support the achievement of practice standards
   2. Patient advocacy
   3. Variety of client diagnoses and complexities of patient care
   4. The requirement for 24-hour accountability

5. Cultural competence will enable the health care system to improve the quality of care as measured in patient outcomes. Campinha-Bacote defines four components of this model. They are cultural awareness, cultural knowledge, cultural skills, and

   1. Cultural encounters
   2. Cultural studies
   3. Cultural diversity
   4. Culture

Answers for review questions appear in Appendix D

KEY TERMS

academic nurse educator *p.18*
acute care nurse *p.14*
advanced practice nursing *p.17*
allopathic medicine *p.25*
alternative therapy *p.25*
assignment *p.18*
assisted living *p.16*
caring *p.8*
clinical judgment *p.7*

code of ethics *p.11*
community-based care *p.20*
community health nursing *p.21*
complementary therapy *p.25*
cultural competence *p.23*
cultural diversity *p.23*
culture *p.23*
information technology *p.26*

nursing process *p.6*
Nursing's Agenda for the Future p.4
patient-centered care *p.20*
population-based care *p.21*
standards of care *p.10*
standards of nursing practice *p.10*
standards of professional performance *p.10*
values *p.11*

PEARSON
EXPLORE **mynursingkit**™

MyNursingKit is your one stop for online chapter review materials and resources. Prepare for success with additional NCLEX®-style practice questions, interactive assignments and activities, web links, animations and videos, and more!

Register your access code from the front of your book at
www.mynursingkit.com

REFERENCES

Academy of Medical–Surgical Nurses. (2004). *Identification of the registered nurse in the workplace.* Retrieved May 23, 2004, from http://www.medsurgnurse.org/position/workprnt.htm

Administration on Aging. (2004). *Statistics: Aging into the 21st century.* Retrieved October 10, 2007, from http://www.aoa.gov/prof/Statistics/future_growth/aging21/summary.asp

American Association of Colleges of Nursing. (2007). *The essentials of baccalaureate education for professional nursing practice (draft).* Retrieved October 9, 2007, from http://www.aacn.nche.edu/Education/pdf/BEdraft8-1-07.pdf

American Association of Critical Care Nurses. (2004). *About critical care nursing.* Retrieved May 31, 2004, from http://www.aacn.org

American Association of Nurse Anesthetists. (2007). *About AANA.* Retrieved April 8, 2008, from http://www.aana.com

American College of Nurse-Midwives. (2005). *About ACNM.* Retrieved from http://www.midwife.org/about.cfm

American Nurses Association. (1988). *Nursing case management* (Publication No. NS-32). Kansas City, MO: Author.

American Nurses Association. (1992). *House of delegates report: 1992 convention, Las Vegas, Nevada* (pp. 104–120). Kansas City, MO: Author.

American Nurses Association. (1997). *Education for participation in nursing research.* Retrieved May 31, 2003, from http://www.ana.org

American Nurses Association. (1998). *Standards of clinical nursing practice* (2nd ed.). Silver Spring, MD: Author.

American Nurses Association. (1999). *House of delegates action report: Nursing and genetics.* Retrieved April 22, 2004, from http://www.ana.org

American Nurses Association. (2001a). *Code of ethics for nurses with interpretive statements.* Washington, DC: American Nurses Publishing.

American Nurses Association. (2001b). *Scope and standards of nursing informatics practice.* Washington, DC: American Nurses Publishing.

American Nurses Association. (2002). *Nursing's agenda for the future.* Retrieved May 23, 2004, from http://www.ana.org

American Nurses Association. (2003). *Nursing's social policy statement 2003.* Washington, DC: American Nurses Publishing.

American Nurses Association. (2004a). American nurses association (ANA) & you: Nursing on the move. In *ANA Stakeholders Report.* Silver Spring, MD: Author.

American Nurses Association. (2004b). *Nursing scope & standards of practice.* Silver Spring, MD: Author.

American Nurses Association. (2007a). *Let's make nurses' voice heard! Sign up for N-STAT today.* Retrieved April 8, 2008, from http://rnaction.org/politicalpower/join.html

American Nurses Association. (2007b). *The nursing process: A common thread amongst all nurses.* Retrieved September 16, 2007, from http://nursingworld.org/EspeciallyForYou/StudentNurses/Thenursingprocess.aspx

American Nurses Association. (2008). *What is nursing.* Retrieved April 18, 2008 from http://nursingworld.org/EspeciallyForYou/StudentNurses/WhatisNursing.aspx

Baker, L., Wagner, T. H., Singer, S., & Bundorf, K. (2003). Use of the Internet and e-mail for health care information. *Journal of the American Medical Association, 289*(19), 2400–2406.

Benner, P. (2001). *From novice to expert: Excellence and power in clinical nursing practice. A commemorative edition.* Upper Saddle River, NJ: Pearson Prentice Hall.

Benner, P., Tanner, C., & Chesla, C. (1996). *Expertise in nursing practice; Caring, clinical judgment, and ethics.* New York: Springer.

Benner, P., & Wrubel, J. (1989). *The primacy of caring: Stress and coping in health and illness.* Menlo Park, CA: Addison-Wesley.

Berman, A., Snyder, S. J., Kozier, B., & Erb, G. (2008). *Kozier & Erb's fundamentals of nursing: Concepts, process, and practice* (8th ed.). Upper Saddle River, NJ: Pearson Prentice Hall.

Brunt, B. A. (2005). Models, measurement, and strategies in developing critical-thinking skills. *Journal of Continuing Education in Nursing, 36*(6), 255–262, 283–284.

Campinha-Bacote, J. (2003). Many faces: Addressing diversity in health care. *Online Journal of Issues in Nursing, 8*(1). Retrieved April 8, 2008, from http://nursingworld.org/MainMenuCategories/ANAMarketplace/ANAPeriodicals/OJIN/TableofContents/Volume82003/Num1Jan31_2003/AddressingDiversityinHealthCare.aspx

Canam, C. (2005). Illuminating the clinical nurse specialist role of advanced practice nursing: A qualitative study. *Canadian Journal of Nursing Leadership, 18*(4), 70–89.

Carpenito-Moyet, L. J. (2007). *Nursing diagnosis: Application to clinical practice* (12th ed.). Philadelphia: Lippincott Williams & Wilkins.

Centers for Disease Control and Prevention. (2004). *Health care in America: Trends in utilization* (DHHS Publication No. 2004-1031). Washington, DC: U.S. Government Printing Office.

Centers for Disease Control and Prevention. (2006). *Severe acute respiratory syndrome (SARS).* Retrieved July 28, 2006, from http://www.cdc.gov/NCIDOD/SARS/factsheet.htm

Centers for Disease Control and Prevention. (2007). *Key facts about avian influenza (bird flu) and avian influenza A (HRN1).* Retrieved October 24, 2007, from http://www.cec.gov/flu/avian/gen-info/facts.htm

Cesta, T. G., & Tahan, H. A. (2003). *The case manager's survival guide: Winning strategies for clinical practice* (2nd ed.). St. Louis: Mosby.

Congressional Budget Office. (2003, March 20). Testimony to the Senate Special Committee on Aging.

D'Amico, D., & Barbarito C. (2007). *Health and physical assessment in nursing.* Upper Saddle River, NJ: Pearson Prentice Hall.

DeWolf-Bosek, M. S., & Savage, T. A. (2007). *The ethical component of nursing education.* Philadelphia: Lippincott Williams & Wilkins.

Dower, C. (2002). *Status of changes in patient care delivery: How can we meet demand for health care workers?* San Francisco: Center for the Health Professions, University of California, San Francisco.

Drell, D., & Adamson, A. (2003). *Fast forward to 2020: What to expect in molecular medicine.* Retrieved January 20, 2008, from http://www.ornl.gov/sci/ techresourcxews/Human+Genome/ medicine/tnty.shtml

Fesler-Birch, D. M. (2005). Critical thinking and patient outcomes: A review. *Nursing Outlook, 53,* 59–65.

Finkelman, A. W. (2001). *Managed care: A nursing perspective.* Upper Saddle River, NJ: Pearson Prentice Hall.

Gendrop, S., & Eisenhauer, L. (1996). A transactional perspective on critical thinking. *Scholarly Inquiry into Nursing Practice: International Journal, 10,* 329–342.

Getzen, T. E. (2006). *Health economics and financing* (3rd ed.). Indianapolis: John Wiley & Sons.

Guido, G. W. (2006). *Legal and ethical issues in nursing* (4th ed.). Upper Saddle River, NJ: Pearson Prentice Hall.

Huber, D. (2003). *Leadership and nursing care management* (2nd ed.). Philadelphia: W. B. Saunders.

Huber, D. (2006). *Leadership and nursing care management* (3rd ed.). Philadelphia: W. B. Saunders.

Institute of Medicine. (2004). *Keeping patients safe: Transforming the work environment of nurses.* Washington, DC: National Academies Press.

Klein, M. (2006, May 15). Will technology improve healthcare delivery? *Wisconsin Technology Network.* Retrieved July 23, 2006, from http://wistechnololgy.com/printarticle.php?id+2961

L'Eplattenier, N. (2001). Tracing the development of critical thinking in baccalaureate nursing learners. *Journal of the New York Nurses Association, 32*(2), 27–32.

Lipe, S., & Beasley, S. (2006) *Critical thinking in nursing: A cognitive skills workbook.* Philadelphia: Lippincott Williams & Wilkins.

MacDonald, J. A., Herbert, R., & Thilbeault, C. (2006). Advanced practice nursing: Unification through a common identity. *Journal of Professional Nursing, 22*(3), 172–179.

Marquis, B. L., & Huston, C. J. (2007). *Leadership roles and management functions in nursing theory & application* (5th ed.). Philadelphia: Lippincott Williams & Wilkins.

Mathes, M. (2005a). Ethical decision making and nursing. *Dermatology Nursing, 17*(6), 444–458.

Mayo Clinic Staff. (2007). *MRSA Infection.* Retrieved January 20, 2008, from http://www.mayoclinic.com/health/mrsa/DS00735

Mechanic, H., Rogut, L., & Colby, D. C. (2005). *Policy challenges in modern health care.* Piscataway, NJ: Rutgers University Press.

Medline Plus. (2006). West Nile laying low, so far. *Scout News.* Retrieved July 28, 2006, from http://www.nlkn.nih.gov/medlineplus/news/fullstory_36096.html

National Center for Health Statistics. (2007). *Professional vital statistics for April 2007 Released.* Retrieved January 20, 2008, from http://www.ced.gov/nchs

National Institute of Allergy and Infectious Diseases. (2005). *NIAID research on severe acute respiratory syndrome (SARS).* Retrieved January 20, 2008, from http://www.niaid.nih.gov/factsheets/sars.htm

National Institute of Nursing Research. (2001). *Mission statement.* Retrieved May 31, 2004, from http:// www.nih.gov/ninr/research/diversity/mission.html

Nelson, J. W. (2000). Models of nursing care: A century of vacillation. *Journal of Nursing Administration, 30*(4), 156, 184.

Nurses for a Healthier Tomorrow. (2007) Retrieved June 29, 2007, from http://www.nursesource.org/nurse-educator.html

Roach, M. (1984). *Caring the human mode of being: Implications for nursing.* Toronto, Canada: University of Toronto Press.

Shortell, S., & Kaluzny, A. D. (2005). *Health care management: Organization design and behavior* (5th ed.). Clifton Park, NY: Delmar Cengage Learning.

Sullivan, E. J., & Decker, P. J. (2005). *Effective leadership & management in nursing* (6th ed.). Upper Saddle River, NJ: Pearson Prentice Hall.

Tanner, C. (1983). Research on clinical judgment. In W. Holzemer (Ed.), *Review of research in nursing education.* Thorofare, NJ: Charles B. Slack.

Tanner, C. (2006). *Thinking like a nurse: A research-based model of clinical judgment in nursing. Journal of Nursing Education, 45*(6).

Tschudin, V. (2006). How nursing ethics as a subject changes: An analysis of the first 11 years of publications of the journal of nursing ethics. *Nursing Ethics, 13*(1), 65–75.

U.S. Census Bureau. (2000). *Profile of older Americans: 2000. Population projections of the United States by age, sex, race, and Hispanic origin 1995–2050* (Current Population Reports, P25-1130). Washington, DC: Author.

U.S. Census Bureau. (2002). *National population projections summary tables.* Retrieved May 19, 2004, from: http://www.census.gov/population/www/projections/natproj.html

U.S. Department of Health and Human Services. (1991). *Healthy people 2000: National health promotion and disease prevention objectives* (DHHS Publication No. 91-5021). Washington, DC: U.S. Government Printing Office.

U.S. Department of Health and Human Services. (2000). *Healthy people 2010.* Retrieved May 1, 2004, from http://www.health.gov/healthpeople

U.S. Department of Health and Human Services. (2004, July 21). *Thompson launches decade of health information technology.* Press release retrieved July 28, 2006, from http://www.hhs.gov/news/press//2004pres/20049721a.html

Walsh, C. M., & Seldomridge, L. A. (2006). Critical thinking: Back to square two. *Journal of Nursing Education, 45*(6), 212–219.

Watson, J. (1988). *Nursing: Human science and human care. A theory of nursing.* New York: National League for Nursing.

Wilkinson, J. (2009). *Nursing process and critical thinking* (3rd ed.) Upper Saddle River NJ: Pearson Prentice Hall.

Williams, C. A. (1996). Community-based population-focused practice: The foundation of specialization in public health nursing. In M. Stanhope & J. Lancaster (Eds.), *Community health nursing: Promoting health of aggregates, families, and individuals* (4th ed., pp. 21–33). St. Louis: Mosby.

Yoder-Wise, P. S. (2008). *Leading and managing in nursing* (4th ed.). St. Louis: Mosby.

2

Experiential Learning: Skill Acquisition and Gaining Clinical Knowledge

Patricia Benner

Outcome-Based Learning Objectives

After studying this chapter, the learner will be able to:

1. Recognize and describe their own clinical learning in the form of an experience-near first person narrative account.

2. Give at least three examples of practical and theoretical knowledge related to adult medical-surgical nursing.

3. Give two examples of clinical interventions that can be standardized and two examples of clinical interventions that cannot be standardized.

4. Give an example of phronesis or clinical judgment that illustrates adjusting to transitions in the patient's clinical condition, or the clinician's understanding of the patient's clinical condition.

5. Give two clinical examples of how the nurse's relationship with the patient may alter the nurse's clinical judgment.

6. Explain how and why the nurse's moral agency might change with experience, according to the Dreyfus Model of Skill Acquisition.

7. Characterize three distinct differences between competent and expert clinical nursing practice.

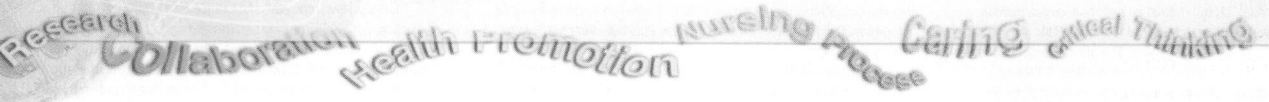

Nursing like medicine, involves a rich, socially embedded clinical know-how that encompasses perceptual skills, transitional understandings across time, and understanding of the particular in relation to the general. Clinical knowledge is a form of engaged reasoning that follows modus operandi thinking, in relation to patients' and clinical populations' particular manifestations of disease, dysfunction, response to treatment and recovery trajectories. Clinical knowledge is necessarily configurational, historical (by historical, I mean the immediate and long-term histories of particular patients and clinical populations), contextual, perceptual, and based upon knowledge gained in transitions. . . . [Through articulation], clinical understanding becomes increasingly articulate and translatable at least by clinical examples, narratives and puzzles encountered in practice. (Benner, 1994, p. 139)

BECOMING A NURSE requires more than mastery of technical and scientific knowledge. It also requires ongoing experiential learning, reflection on practice, and continuous improvement in practice as science and technology and experiential knowledge change. A metaphor of "mastery" is somewhat misleading in any professional endeavor because it projects the imagined possibility that the field is stable and can be completely "mastered" or learned at any one point in time. Fields like nursing and medicine, however, are constantly changing, self-correcting, and the study of these fields never completely covers what actually might be encountered in clinical practice. Another way of saying this is that clinical practice is open ended and un-

derdetermined. Underdetermined here, means that more than one thing may be going on, and more than one or two outcomes may occur, and that the situation is practical and necessarily ambiguous and historical. For example, the nurse's action may well alter the course and outcome of the situation in ways that are not necessarily predetermined, or uninfluenced by the patient's response, and the timing of the intervention. Clinical practice knowledge includes learning experientially and directly by engaging in practice situations. Relational knowledge (skills of engaging with patients and patient situations), skilled know-how in actual practice situations, and patient interventions based on patients' responses to their illnesses and therapies are all examples of experiential clinical learning.

Types of Knowledge and Learning Experiences

Clinical knowledge (a type of phronesis), which includes recognizing signs and symptoms of physiological and emotional distress and changes in a patient's vital signs and knowing how to titrate an intravenous (IV) rate, **clinical judgment**, and many more aspects of engaging in nursing are all forms of **practical knowledge**. For example, having a sense of **salience**, that is, having some things stand out as more or less important in a practical situation, is a form of practical knowledge that is learned after having many concrete clinical experiences in which a range of relevant clinical issues stand out as high priority, such as reestablishing IV access in a critically ill patient whose IV has become occluded or attending to opening an airway and providing respiration for a patient who is not breathing. The preceding two examples work well because they are obvious, but with experience other clinical aspects will stand out as salient—not just as one more fact among many equally relevant facts. With time, any highly salient clinical demands begins to seem obvious to the expert clinician.

Skills of engagement with both patients and their families and with clinical problems are learned experientially and are also forms of practical knowledge. For example, learning how to be attuned to a patient's emotional responses and concerns and knowing when and how to communicate about concerns and feelings associated with illness and recovery require experiential learning of **skills of involvement**. The skill of perceiving, that is, noticing relevant changes or nuances in clinical situations, also is experientially learned and forms part of a nurse's practical clinical knowledge.

Practical knowledge is shaped by a nurse's knowledge of the discipline and practice, the science and technology relevant to the situation at hand. But scientific, formal knowledge is not sufficient for good clinical practice, whether the discipline is law, medicine, nursing, teaching, or social work. Practitioners still have to learn when and how to use scientific knowledge in practical situations.

Clinical reasoning, a form of practical knowledge, also is distinct from scientific reasoning even though it draws on science. Clinical judgment requires clinical reasoning across time about a particular patient. Clinical judgment is very different from the scientific reasoning used in doing clinical or bench research. Scientific experiments use formal criteria to develop "yes" and "no" judgments under controlled circumstances at specific points in time. Scientific reasoning is closer to static snapshot reasoning than clinical reasoning, which is reasoning across time about the particular situation through changes in the clinician's understanding or changes in the patient's condition (Taylor, 1993). Practical knowledge may be compared to, though not completely separated from, theoretical knowledge. For example, knowledge of growth and development are essential to developing practical knowledge about working with young children, just as normal physiology and pathophysiology are essential for understanding clinical signs and symptoms. Discovery and experiential learning favor the prepared knowledgeable practitioner who is engaged in learning both practical and theoretical knowledge.

Because nurses are involved in assisting patients and families as they cope with the demands of an illness in the context of their social world (lifeworld), nurses need to learn much practical knowledge about human concerns and functioning in diverse social worlds. Learning how patients and families cope and how to assist them with specific transitions in recovery and rehabilitation or even as they face death requires both practical and theoretical learning in nursing. The nurse can learn much from each patient's concerns and strategies in dealing with an illness and recovery, as well as what illness and recovery trajectories look like in different patients. This kind of experiential learning of nurses in caring for many patients needs to be captured and made accessible for reflection and study. The practice of nursing gives many unique windows on a large range of human experience that remain sources of experiential learning to the curious and reflective nurse.

Given the range of practical knowledge and experiential learning required in nursing, one begin's to understand why reducing rationality to the kind offered by scientific experiments is too narrow. **Rationality** includes reasoning across time with changes in the patient's condition and concerns. Practical rationality, as illustrated in clinical judgment, includes noticing subtle changes and informed emotional responses, such as those that happen when a patient's condition changes, but the changes are not limited to explicit vital signs and may not show up immediately in the vital sign trends. For example, in early impending shock due to blood loss, the patient usually compensates at first, so the actual changes in vital signs are delayed and are best detected by assessing the patient's distress and following vital sign trends, rather than an isolated finding.

A contrast also can be made between what can be standardized and replicated, described by the early Greeks as **techne** (the know-how and skill of producing things), and what requires productive thinking, adjustment, and judgment in particular cases. Aristotle called the latter *practice* or *praxis* that requires *phronesis,* something qualitatively distinct from techne. Clinical judgment is a prime example of phronesis. This distinction is similar to the distinction between scientific and clinical reasoning. Scientific experiments must be capable of replication under precise conditions, whereas clinical reasoning is applied to a practice that occurs in real time, is uncontrolled, often about a single case, and is almost always underdetermined. The professions of nursing, medicine, and law all require a socially embedded form of knowledge that has notions of the good internal to the practice. For example, holding the patient's best interests and choices as central to clinical decisions is internal to the practice of nursing and medicine. Aristotle's example of the use of phronesis was that of a statesman who had to develop character, skilled know-how, practical reasoning, and comportment, all of which include appropriate emotional responses and relationships.

This contrast form of rationality and skill-based character, called **phronesis**, is a good example of clinical judgment and stands in contrast to rational-technical thinking. A rational-technical mode (techne), sometimes called rational technicality, separates means and ends and focuses on achieving prespecified outcomes. Rational-technical thought is a powerful strategy for those areas of science and technology that can be standardized and routinized. Nursing and medicine use techne, such as blood pressure measurements and dosage ranges for medication, but when clinical judgment, relationship, perception (or noticing), timing, and skilled know-how are involved, then more than techne or rational calculation is required. Guignon (1983) points out that separating means and outcomes often devalues or does violence to the means, especially where means and ends are closely interwoven. For example, it is not sensible to separate means and ends in human situations such as birth, comfort, health promotion, or end-of-life care. In each of these caring practices, means and ends are not separable. The picture is further complicated by the fact that most often there are multiple means and ends at stake in any clinical encounter.

As an example, consider caregiving relationships. Such relationships may open up possibilities or close them down. But even with the best intentions and comportment, the person cared for may not be able to respond to care. "Outcomes" in caregiving relationships are necessarily interdependent and mutual. Some types of influence are morally unacceptable. Manipulation, coercion, or misuse of professional influence in persuading a patient to accept a treatment is unethical. When things go well and the patient or family is able to respond to caring practices, the practitioner cannot attribute the good outcome solely to the efficacy of some technique she may have used. The focus on "prespecified outcomes" and identifying and evaluating nursing outcomes in case management are based on the premise that only technique is involved in health care, that one knows the outcomes to expect, and that all things can be "fixed." The problem is further complicated by institutional constraints to good caregiving. Meeting and responding to the patient or family may clash with the bureaucratic goals of care for the many in the most cost-efficient manner. For all of these reasons, developing moral agency and the skills of involvement that are required for the development and use of good clinical judgment present ongoing demands for experiential learning and character development in nursing. Viewing nursing as a basic human encounter and as a practice that requires phronesis has major implications for nursing education and the moral development of practitioners.

Technical care and restorative care are not mutually exclusive for the nurse or physician. One way to create more equal partners between technical medicine and human lifeworlds is to understand medicine, nursing, and other health care practices as *practices* that encompass more than the science and technologies that they use to effect cures.

■ The Nature of Practice: A Socially Embedded Form of Knowledge

As noted earlier, a socially organized practice such as nursing has notions of *good* internal to the practice (Dreyfus, 1992). For example, attentiveness, not neglect, and recognition practices, not depersonalization, are notions of good internal to the practice of nursing. A nurse educated to be an excellent nurse can recognize, in most instances, good and poor nursing care, even though it would be impossible to formally list all of the precise behaviors and comportments of excellent nursing care.

In philosophy, the inability to make explicit or formal all elements of a social practice is called the **limits of formalization** (Dreyfus, 1992). Likewise, the practical knowledge embedded in the traditions of science cannot be made completely formal and explicit (Benner, Tanner, & Chesla, 1996; Lave & Wenger, 1991). Every complex social practice has a foreground of focused attention and a background of comportment, practical skills, and understanding of the social practice. Science and technology have

extensive traditions of formalizing the reasoning and knowledge associated with scientific experiments. Consequently, it can appear to the naïve scientific practitioner that thinking within a particular scientific discipline is restricted to what can be formalized. However, as Thomas Kuhn (1970) demonstrated through historical examples, every science has nonrational (not *irrational)* aspects of thinking such as the use of metaphors, understandings about what constitutes an interesting scientific problem, and skillful know-how in conducting experiments. The practice of a particular discipline such as nursing or a science such as crystal growing or genomics contains the **ethos** or notions of what counts as good nursing or good scientific practice. In practice disciplines such as nursing and medicine, the ethos of the practice shapes and is shaped by relevant science. Knowledge development occurs in science and in experiential learning directly from practice. Practice is a way of knowing in its own right, in this nontechnological understanding of what constitutes a practice (Benner & Wrubel, 1982; Dunne, 1997).

To make good clinical judgments, the nurse must be skillful in moral and clinical perception (Benner & Wrubel, 1982; Dunne, 1997; Vetleson, 1994). Although conceptual knowledge is essential, it is not sufficient to ensure that the nurse will form relationships with patients that lead to salient disclosures, or that the nurse will notice and correctly identify an instance of pulmonary edema, despair, or pain when the nurse sees it, even though the nurse may know conceptually what the formal characteristics of these patient conditions are in principle. Perceptual recognition skills, skills of involvement, and moral agency are required for good clinical judgment and acting on behalf of the patient based on one's judgment.

In the practice of medicine and nursing, science and technology are used to increase certainty about the measurement of signs and symptoms. The practice of objective measurement of signs and symptoms reduces errors and improves clinical judgment. No one would recommend going back to guessing body temperatures by palpation alone. However, even the most formal measurements cannot replace the perceptual skill of the clinician in recognizing when a measurement is relevant or the meaning of a particular measurement. Also, following the course of a patient's development of signs and symptoms (the trajectory or evolution of signs and symptoms) improves the clinician's understanding of the meaning of the signs and symptoms. This may seem patently obvious to any practicing clinician, yet current strategies for applying algorithms or making particular clinical judgments based on aggregate outcomes data alone ignore the clinical know-how, relational skills, and need for clinical judgment as reasoning across time (Halpern, 2001).

Good nursing practice requires ongoing development of clinical knowledge through experiential learning. Experiential learning is not automatic. It requires openness, attentiveness, reflection on practice, and active engaged learning on the part of the practitioner. Here a distinction is being made between detached, disengaged reflection and engaged thinking-in-action (Guignon, 1983). Standing outside of a situation and reflecting back on it is a powerful critical-thinking strategy for improving practice, especially in situations of breakdown and error (Schon, 1987). However, being emotionally attuned to the patient and family and the demands of the situation in the immediate moment is also required for well-timed expert performance (Figure 2–1 ■).

FIGURE 2–1 ■ A nurse must always be emotionally attuned to the demands of a specific situation.
Source: © Timothy Tadder/CORBIS All Rights Reserved

Doctoring and nursing particular patients require relational and communication skills and art. The relationship between the patient and nurse, for example, determines what will be disclosed by the patient, what can be thought about and talked about together, and what level of acceptance and endorsement of the therapies will be acceptable to patients and clinicians alike. Patients often rehearse their most fearful concerns with nurses who they expect to be more approachable than a physician and also effective in helping them communicate with physicians. Technique alone cannot address the interpersonal and relational responsibilities, discernment, and situated possibilities required when caring for persons made vulnerable by illness and injury. Phronesis (clinical judgment and the ability to act on good clinical judgment) is required. Means and ends are inextricably related when caring for people who are ill. Clinician and patient bend and respond to the other so that new horizons appear or are reconstituted, leading to the emergence of new possibilities. On the patient's side, healing and recovery of one's embodied relationship with the world is lived rather than mastered and requires relationship, openness, and trust.

The clinician must always intelligently appraise the relevance of the best evidence for a particular patient in addition to critically evaluating the "best evidence" itself. Qualitative distinctions must be made about the patient's concerns, actual responses to therapies, and the disease or injury processes. Clinical judgment, when not requiring instantaneous action (e.g., titrating a vasopressor IV medication to keep the patient's blood pressure within safe parameters), must be communicated and adjudicated by other clinicians. If a nurse recognizes early signs of deterioration in a patient's clinical condition, she must be able to document and communicate the evidence for the changes. This requires social skills and experiential wisdom in communicating with other clinicians so that the evidence can be verified.

Dreyfus Model of Skill Acquisition

The **Dreyfus model of skill acquisition** is based on determining the level of practice evident in particular situations (Benner, 1984, 2001; Dreyfus, 1979; Dreyfus & Dreyfus, with Athanasiou, 1986). It elucidates strengths as well as problems. Situated practice ca-

pacities are described rather than traits or talents of the practitioners. At each stage of experiential learning (novice, advanced beginner, competent, proficient, expert), clinicians can perform at their best. For example, one can be the best advanced beginner possible, typically during the first year of practice. However, no practitioner can be beyond experience regardless of the level of skill acquisition in most clinical situations and despite the necessary attempts to make practice as clear and explicit as possible. If the nurse has never encountered a particular clinical situation, experiential learning is required. For example, referring to critical pathways is not the same as recognizing when and how these pathways are relevant or must be adapted to particular patients. Experiential learning that leads to individualization and clinical discernment is required to render the use of critical pathways sensible and safe. Such individualization requires clinical discernment based on experience with past whole concrete clinical situations. This ability to make clinical comparisons between whole concrete clinical cases without decomposing the whole situation into its analytical components is a hallmark of expert clinical nursing practice (Benner & Wrubel, 1982; Ruddick, 1989).

A renewing, coherent, recognizable identity requires that practitioners develop notions of good that are constantly being worked out and extended through experiential learning in local and larger practice communities. Practice is a way of knowing, as well as a way of being in the world (Dunne, 1997; Ruddick, 1989; Taylor, 1993, 1994). A self-renewing practice directs the development, implementation, and evaluation of science and technology. Clinical judgment requires **moral agency** (defined as the ability to effect and influence situations), relationship, perceptual acuity, skilled know-how, and narrative reasoning across time about particular patient transitions (Benner & Wrubel, 1982; Guignon, 1983). As Joseph Dunne notes:

> A practice is not just a surface on which one can display instant virtuosity. It grounds one in a tradition that has been formed through an elaborate development and that exists at any juncture only in the dispositions (slowly and perhaps painfully acquired) of its recognized practitioners. (Dunne, 1997, p. 378)

The Dreyfus model of skill acquisition has illuminated ongoing research on skill acquisition and articulation of knowledge embedded in expert practice in nursing (Dreyfus, 1982; Dreyfus & Dreyfus, 1977, 1979, 1980). The Dreyfus model is developmental, based on situated performance and experiential learning. Three studies of skill acquisition in nursing that were guided by the Dreyfus model of skill acquisition have been conducted. Hubert and Stuart Dreyfus served as consultants in each of these three studies (Benner, 1982, 1984; Benner, Hooper-Kyriakidis, & Stannard, 1999; Benner, Tanner, & Chesla, 1992).

The first study, conducted from 1978 to 1981 (Benner, 1982, 1984), was based on 21 paired interviews with newly graduated nurses and their preceptors. In addition, interviews or participant observations were conducted with 51 additional experienced nurse clinicians, 11 newly graduated nurses, and 5 senior nursing students to further delineate and describe characteristics of nurse performance at different levels of education and experience. The small-group and individual interviews were conducted in six hospitals: two private community hospitals, two community teaching hospitals, one university medical center, and one inner-city general hospital.

A second study of skill acquisition and clinical knowledge of critical care nurses was conducted between 1988 and 1994 (Benner et al., 1992; Benner, Tanner, Chesla with Dreyfus and Dreyfus and Rubin 1996). The study population was made up of 130 nurses practicing in intensive care units and general floor units from eight hospitals, seven of which are located in two far Western and one in the Eastern region of the country. Small-group narrative interviews, individual interviews, and participant observation were used as data collection strategies. The two aims of the study relevant to this discussion were to (1) describe the nature of skill acquisition in critical care nursing practice and (2) delineate the practical knowledge embedded in expert practice.

The third study was an extension of this study, conducted from 1996 to 1997 to include other critical care areas (including emergency departments, flight nursing, home health, the operating room, and postanesthesia care units; $N = 75$ nurses) and enlarge the sample of advanced practice nurses.[1] This chapter synthesizes the findings of these three studies using data from each of the studies.

Nursing, like other practice disciplines, is not merely an "applied" field in the sense that the practice is complex, varied, and underdetermined. Good practice requires that the nurse develop skillful ethical comportment as a practitioner and that the nurse use good clinical judgment informed by scientific evidence and technological development. The sciences of medicine and nursing are broad and multidisciplinary and require translation into the particular practice situation. Basic sciences such as biochemical; physical, biological, and physiological processes; research and development of specific therapies and technologies; and finally clinical trials and more make up a broad range of relevant science used in the practice of medicine and nursing.

Monitoring the quality of care and preventing imminent breakdown in practice quality require social communication skills and effective moral agency, both of which are the patient's frontline defense against errors and the hazards of hospitalization. For example, in the operating room (OR), it is the requirement of anyone in the OR to immediately and verbally identify a break in sterile technique, just as it is the nurse's job to provide early warnings of changes in a patient's clinical condition. Moral agency requires more than the intent to do good or to *be* a good practitioner; it requires the experiential skill to recognize when an ethical breach in practice has occurred and the social and communication skills to effectively intervene on behalf of the patient.

■ Skill Acquisition and Experiential Learning

The clinician's capacity for moral agency literally changes with the growth of clinical judgment, perceptiveness, communication skills, and skillful comportment. The skill of involvement

both with the patient and engagement with the clinical situation are also learned developmentally over time and change with level of skill acquisition. The stages of skill acquisition as uncovered in research on clinical nursing practice are described in this chapter with a focus on the development of the relational skills of involvement and the skills of moral agency in the clinician.

Experience, as defined here, is an active process (Gadamer, 1960/1975). **Experiential learning** requires a turning around of preconceptions, or an adding of nuances to one's understanding. Experiential learning also requires the stance of an engaged learner, rather than the stance of one expert in techne who skillfully applies well-established knowledge in prespecified clear circumstances. To improve practice over time, experiential learning requires openness and responsiveness by the learner. The learner who develops an attuned, response-based practice learns to recognize whole situations in terms of past concrete experiences as pointed out by the Dreyfus model.

The researchers found that recognizing the situation as an "instance of particular concerns" is central to the logic of excellent practice. For example, consider a situation of heart "pump" failure or fluid depletion (Benner, 2001; Benner, Hooper-Kyriakidis & Stannard, 1999). Deciding which intervention to implement depends on clarifying and confirming the nature of the clinical situation at hand. The skillful practitioner learns to keep background understandings fluid or semipermeable so that he can recognize when these tacit expectations are not met. For example, a nurse with expertise in detecting heart arrhythmias on a unit where all patients' cardiac functioning is monitored will only notice aberrations in sound patterns, rather than attending to the familiar sounds in the foreground of attention. Recognizing the unexpected, that is, recognizing when tacit global expectations of patients' recovery are not met, is a hallmark of expert practice.

Major Shifts in the Style of Practice with the Development of Expertise

As noted earlier, the nurse's capacity for effective moral agency changes with developing practice skills and insights from experience. Also the skills of problem and person engagement grow more attuned. The development of moral agency and skills of involvement should be considered at each stage of skill acquisition, from novice to expert. The nurse increasingly is able to recognize when she does not have a good grasp of the clinical situation, and this lack of a sense of understanding guides the nurse's questioning and problem solving. Over time, an increased grasp of the nature of particular clinical situations, including opportunities and constraints, guides the nurse's actions and interactions. Consequently, responses to patients become more contextualized and attuned.

Recognition of clinical situations moves from abstract textbook accounts of general features to comparisons with past whole concrete cases. These real comparisons can include qualitative distinctions and more subtle variations. Having a grasp of the situation, with all of its various possibilities and constraints, enables the nurse to move from rule-governed thinking to an intuitive grasp of the situation (Dreyfus & Dreyfus with Athanasiou, 1986). This intuitive grasp is experienced based and not based on "extrasensory" powers or wild hunches. It is situated in

[1]The first study was sponsored by a grant from the U.S. Department of Health and Human Services, Public Health Service, Division of Nursing, Bureau of Health Professions (Grant No. 7 D10 NU 29104-03). The second and third studies were funded by the Helene Fuld Health Trust.

the clinician's grasp of the situation based upon experience with prior similar situations. Improved skills of involvement create disclosive spaces where all patients and families express their concerns, and allow the nurse to notice and respond to the most plausible actions to be discovered and taken in particular situations. Relational skills are schooled by learning to be "at home" in a highly differentiated clinical world where some actions are plausible and effective, and others are experienced as "ill timed" or implausible. A sense of salience develops over time so that some things stand out as more plausible and appropriate than others.

The practitioner develops a richer sense of the possibilities of practice based on shared notions of good practice within the profession (Rubin, 1996). Because the Dreyfus model of skill acquisition is a situated and descriptive phenomenological account of the development of skill over time, it does not point to isolated competencies nor enabling traits or talent. Consequently, a practitioner may be at different levels of skill in different areas of practice based on the particular practitioner's background experience and knowledge. For example, a practitioner skilled in caring for adults at an expert level will not be at that level of skill when caring for young children or premature infants. The patient populations that nurses care for determine the nurses' opportunities for experiential learning. Chart 2–1 lists the stages of skill acquisition in the Dreyfus model. The stages are also discussed in the following subsections.

Novice: First Year of Education

The novice stage of skill acquisition occurs in areas where the student has no experiential background on which to base an understanding of clinical situations. For example, the art and skill required for a range of medical and nursing interventions on particular patients will be new. The educator must offer good descriptions of features and attributes of the situation that the novice can recognize. For example, to determine fluid balance students are given clear parameters and guidelines:

> To determine fluid balance, check the patient's morning weights and daily intake and output for the past three days. Weight gain and an intake that is consistently greater than 500 mls could indicate water retention, in which case fluid restriction should be started until the cause of the imbalance can be found. (Benner, 1984, p. 21)

An experienced clinician can immediately think of the many situations where this evaluation would be inappropriate or too stringent. But the novice is given clear directions about safe ways to proceed until the significance of fluid balance for different clinical conditions can be learned.

| CHART 2–1 | **Major Characteristics of Dreyfus Model of Skill Acquisition Found in Nursing** |

NOVICE: BEGINNING NURSING STUDENT

- Little or no experiential background understanding
- Recognizes attributes and features
- Requires rules and broad guidelines to organize task world
- Matches actual cases with textbook descriptions

ADVANCED BEGINNER, NEWLY GRADUATED NURSE

- Developing a perspective on clinical patient situations
- Legitimizing and evaluating the discomfort of patients
- Establishing boundaries of the role and expectations of the nurse
- Finding credible sources of information and teaching

COMPETENT STAGE—ONE TO TWO YEARS OF PRACTICE

- A time of planning and analysis
- Limit the unexpected through planning and prediction
- Anxious times now more tailored to situation
- Clinical forethought and clinical grasp developing
- Cushion of inexperience, cannot know what you don't know
- Work world can seem like a bunch of Multiple and competing tasks
- Matching examples with textbook accounts with new kinds of patients
- Limits of formal knowledge; Now knows that not everything is in procedure book or text books
- Choosing a perspective for clinical work is now required for organization
- Pattern recognition based upon experience developing
- Encountering the patient anew; now recognizes patient's plight and suffering anew

PROFICIENCY: A TRANSITION TO EXPERTISE

- A QUALITATIVE LEAP in way work is organized
- Sees the "big" picture of the patient's world and clinical situation
- Takes situated action, as orderly as the situation requires
- Gains a differentiated world of practice
- Recognizes changing relevance where changes in treatment goals or patient's clinical condition changes the meanings and interpretation of signs and symptoms
- Situation speaks to practitioner. Practice is becoming more situated, patient-response based
- Gains differentiated skill of involvement based on differing concerns and needs of patient

EXPERTISE...PRACTICE NOW EXCELLENT

- Uses both techne and phronesis appropriately
- Practice takes up theories and ends of practice in multiple ways that fit the situation
- Attunement; Skilled know-how is related to particular patients
- Skill of involvement varied and suited to individual patients need
- The particularities of clinical situations now more discernible
- New clinical knowledge is developed from practice
- Makes qualitative distinctions about patients' conditions, signs, and symptoms
- Moral dilemmas are articulated and made more visible to the work group

---

Source: Adapted from Benner, P., Tanner, C. A., Chesla, C. A. *Expertise in nursing practice: Caring, clinical judgment, and ethics.* New York: Springer Publishers. 1996.

Note that the rules and guidelines must not require prior experience for their recognition. They must provide a safe beginning point for specific, situated learning in a clinical situation. Fluid balance is salient, but what must be learned is the particular salience for particular patients. The rule-governed behavior of the novice is extremely limited and inflexible. The student is coached in comparing and matching textbook examples with actual clinical cases. Skills that are performed easily on a mannequin in a skills lab require adaptation along with communication and reassurance skills when performed on patients whose attitudes range from calm to highly anxious. Students have a limited ability to forecast immediate futures because they have not yet lived through many of them; usually they must instead rely on textbook forecasts.

The best clinical educators are good ethnographers who can give students access to the culture and expectations of the clinical units where they are gaining clinical experience. Clinical educators should offer broad guidelines and timelines to guide their students' understanding of the task world and the expectations of a particular unit (Figure 2–2 ■). Good informants are identified as resources for the new students on the unit. In addition, the clinical supervisor is "on call" to deal with questions or emergencies encountered by the student.

Advanced Beginner: New Graduate

The newly graduated nurse has usually functioned very close to the level of a beginning staff nurse in his final year of nursing education. Typically, newly graduated nurses will not have functioned in any administrative or managerial functions, though they will have studied principles and practices related to these roles. The striking change for the newly graduated nurse is that

FIGURE 2–2 ■ A clinical educator presents a broad overview of the experiences students can expect in a particular unit.
Source: John M. Osborn, M.D, FACS

she now has full legal and professional responsibility for patients. This new level of responsibility and entitlement brings with it changes in the way nurses experience themselves and the practice environment. They no longer feel that they can always look to other nurses to tell them what to do or to bear their responsibility. This level of individual and team professional responsibility heightens new nurses' sense of engagement with patients and their clinical problems. Nurses look to patients and family members to fill in expectations of them in their newly forming role. This heightened and qualitatively different kind of engagement encourages experiential learning and spurs the development of a sense of moral agency in the professional role (Benner et al., 1996, p. 93).

The quality of learning is quite different for new as opposed to more experienced nurses. Beginners have a level of trust in the environment and in the legitimacy of coworkers' knowledge, which allows them to absorb information as fact. This trust sets up qualities of freedom and exhilaration in learning that are probably only available to those who do not yet comprehend the contingent nature of both the situation and what is known about it. This freedom in learning is furthered because advanced beginners do not yet feel responsible for managing clinical situations with which they are unfamiliar.

In what follows, an advanced beginner evidences this "lightness of being" about learning as he describes a postoperative patient who had undergone complex gastrointestinal (GI) surgery. His entire statement was delivered in an excited, enthusiastic tone:

> I had learned so much. There are two clinical nurse specialists involved right now. There are people on the unit who are CNII's and CNIII's who are just really knowledgeable on major GI surgery on infants. I talked to all these people and pediatric surgery were really helpful, and our attendings and fellows were . . . I mean, I just learned so much in the last three days, I couldn't even tell you. (Benner et al., 1996, p. 52)

Advanced beginners have a heightened awareness of any feedback on performance and pay close attention to the practice of colleagues. They actively search for credible sources of good and useful information. In the preceding situation, clinical nurse specialists assisted with the care of the infant but also engaged in intensive teaching of the new nurse.

The advanced beginner can experience each situation as a myriad of competing tasks, all of which may feel of equal priority to the new nurse. Anxiety and excessive fatigue are frequently experienced by new nurses. Worry and anxiety tend to be more global because the advanced beginner does not yet have a sense of salience in a range of situations, and the anxiety of learning to perform new tasks is ever present:

> And I just talked to myself and I had a great night because this was the first time I did it. . . . I was (saying to myself) "Okay. Just take it one step at a time. You're only human, do one thing then go onto the next thing. It will all get done, it will get done easier if you're calm and because you think better that way." . . . And the shift went great. (Benner et al., 1996, p. 50).

Much of the experiential learning required of an advanced beginner has to do with developing a perspective on particular situations and developing a sense of salience in particular clinical assignments and situations. In coaching an advanced beginner, strategies for keeping anxiety at bay and staying calm enhance performance capacity because the anxiety is so general. The sense of foreboding and anxiousness over particular clinical situations is not yet very attuned to the demands, possibilities, and constraints of the situation simply due to a lack of experience.

Anxiety is also ameliorated by this very lack of attunement and sense of salience. Advanced beginners have a secondary ignorance, or "cushion of inexperience," in that they have few past high-warning situations. Consequently, the advanced beginner in a new clinical setting may feel less concerned over lack of knowledge of specific clinical situations than an expert nurse transferring to a novel practice setting where the expert nurse is keenly aware of missing practice knowledge and lack of knowledge of resources.

Advanced beginners rely on textbook accounts of patient signs and symptoms related to diseases, injuries, and therapies, but they may have difficulty recognizing subtle variations. In addition, they cannot gauge the level of severity based on past experiences simply because they have not had enough experiences. For example, advanced beginners collect their assessment data carefully and then consult about the meanings of the numbers and signs and symptoms in a particular case. They will need to ask "Is this the usual amount of bleeding or is this a frank hemorrhage in a postoperative or obstetrical patient? Drainage from wounds and tubes must be evaluated in relation to the "usual" quantities and qualities. But the "usual" quantities may vary with specific procedures, patient conditions, and characteristics. The range and variations cannot be captured fully in textbooks. (Remember the discussion earlier in this chapter of the "limits of formalism.")

The perceptual skills associated with recognizing fuzzy or "family resemblances," qualitative distinctions, and real-life presentations complete with their range of manifestations cannot be captured in textbooks or single case presentations. The difficulty in recognizing fuzzy resemblances and the need for situated coaching from clinical mentors is vividly illustrated in the following nursing student's account of a clinical emergency:

> This man is a very pleasant fellow, very bright, very alert and awake, and was unfortunately requiring tracheal suctioning approximately every hour to two hours for moderate amounts of tracheal secretions which were relatively tenacious in character, relatively white tannish in color. He unfortunately did not tolerate the suctioning extremely well. It was relatively uncomfortable for him, caused a moderate amount of cough and gag reflex, which in turn caused a transient increase in blood pressure. Following suctioning on one occasion, as I was replacing his tracheal mist mask, he began coughing up very copious amounts of bright red blood per mouth. I mildly panicked, called for help from the nurse next door, placed him in a moderate Trendelenburg position, opened his I.V. to a rapid rate, and continued to experience mild panic. Perhaps more like moderate panic. (Benner, 1984, p. 19)

This advanced beginner nurse performed well considering the enormity of the situation. The student wonders tacitly whether his suctioning technique was too traumatic and, therefore, caused the bleeding. But notice that the advanced beginner cannot know this because he has had little experience with patients with similar compromised situations and with the skill of suctioning itself. The story is told with extraneous details, and the language is couched in textbook terms. The student's account responds to the immediate situation with little or no forecasting of the future. He gives a full account of his own anxiety in the situation that results in part from his lack of experiential knowledge about what can be done in the situation. Like the novice, the advanced beginner is dependent on others to provide them with experience-based comparisons, interpretations, and qualitative distinctions. In a later section, this episode is contrasted with the account from the expert's perspective.

Competent Stage: 1 to 2 Years of Practice

Developing skill and clinical judgment in particular cases is dependent on experiential learning. Consequently, how fast someone can gain competence depends on how varied and complex his patient population is. Obviously, nurses working in a high-volume heart surgery center where the patient population is the same will gain more experience sooner about typical patterns in a specific patient population than a nurse working on a general medical–surgical floor. But even in the high-volume center, it is usually some time before the newer nurse is assigned complete responsibility for complicated postoperative patients.

Competence with particular patient populations will develop unevenly depending on experience with that population and with the quality of clinical teaching available in the institution. The competent stage of skill acquisition is typically a time of heightened planning for what are now more predictable immediate futures. The competent nurse tries to limit the unexpected through planning and analysis and by forecasting the needs and contingencies of the immediate future. Anxiety is no longer just general anxiety; it is now more attuned to the particular situation as illustrated in the following example in which a nurse describes her discovery (experiential learning) that a post–heart transplant surgery patient could not maintain good oxygenation when placed on the nonoperative side, a physiological principle that the new graduate would probably recognize in a formal, written test, but which is more ambiguous to her in the actual situation:

> I was being a good nurse and turning him every two hours and he had really bad breath sounds on his left side. So I gave him P.T., elevated his left side so he could drain, had him cough. But it took me a couple of times to realize that when I turned him on his left side, with his bad lung down and his good lung up, his oxygen saturations showed great readings and his heart rate was wonderful, and then I would turn him on his back, or turn him up on his right side and within a few minutes, he would go into bursts of SVT [*supraventricular tachycardia*] and his [*oxygen*] saturations would drop. I had called the doctors and they didn't seem too concerned about it. They said: "Relax, he has a healthy heart." I said, if he has a healthy heart, why is he doing this? It spontaneously resolved after I turned him off his side. And I said okay, now I know what's going on. I'll keep him off that side. It was just a hypoxic reaction because he wasn't oxygenating well enough with his bad lung . . . It could be a bad situation if we left this so now we

know that we just have to work on that lung and get it back aerating again, and he did fine. He's out walking around. (Benner et al., 1996, p. 155)

In reflecting on the above experiential learning, the competent level nurse comments:

Nurse: It kind of humbles you. At one point, I'm feeling like I have things straight now, and I can handle the situations, and when something like this happens, I think, well, I still have a lot of learning to do. I can handle the situations that are status quo; it's the unexpected that I have to learn to deal with now. But then I think back to situations when I was brand new. Things that are status quo now weren't back then. Things I can troubleshoot and solve now were much different back then. I usually needed help. (Benner et al., 1996, p. 172)

This nurse's anxiety is now more tailored to the particular situation. Coaching at this point should encourage a competent-level nurse to follow through on her sense that things seem out of the ordinary or even her vague feelings of foreboding or anxiety. The nurse now has an experiential base from which these emotional responses serve to activate a "fuzzy" recognition of similar or dissimilar past clinical situations.

Nurses at this stage feel exhilarated when they perform well, and remorse when they recognize that their performance could have been more effective or more prescient. These emotional responses are the formative stages of aesthetic appreciation of good practice. Feelings of satisfaction and uneasiness with performance act as a moral compass that guides experiential ethical and clinical learning. There is a built-in tension between the strategies of organizing, planning, and prediction and the development of a more response-based practice as pointed out in our study of critical care nurses:

Not needing help, ordering the task world, and planning based on goals and predictions structure what the nurse notices, and what are considered issues. It is not accidental that this vision of performance and agency is institutionally rewarded and encouraged as "standard."

Structuring the day by goals and plans, however, interferes with perceiving the demands of the situation and with timing interventions in response to the patient's responses and readiness. The competent nurse seldom sees changing relevance in a clinical situation. Their skill of seeing is hampered by the need to organize data collection and to achieve goals. Inevitably the clinical situation intrudes by not matching the goals and plans and the nurse must adapt. Conceptual descriptions do not automatically lead to recognition of actual signs, and varied responses require time to assimilate and interpret. Slavishly following one's plans and holding on to preset expectations can limit perceptual grasp of when the situation has changed significantly. This was illustrated in the nurse's discovery of the cause of the heart transplant patient's supraventricular tachycardia.

The nurse's lack of prior experience with this particular situation calls for new experiential learning in order for her to realize that turning the patient so that his good or less compromised lung was compressed from lying on his right side, and his left lung (compromised lung) when placed up, was not able to compensate for the loss of aeration from the right long (Benner et al., 1996, pp. 155–172). In the future, no doubt, this common problem with post operative heart patients will be more recognizable to this nurse.

Experiential learning based on past patient care enables the nurse to develop a greater sense of salience. As illustrated in the preceding nurse's statement, there is an increasing sense of when the nurse has or does not have a good clinical grasp of the situation. Nurses can use their sense of confusion or questioning to propel their understanding of the clinical situation. Because they have now lived through more clinical futures, they can now better predict immediate likely events and the resulting patient needs and better plan for them.

Toward the upper limits of competent performance, nurses may begin to apprehend the limits of formal and practical knowledge. Nurses can now recognize that not everyone is a proficient or expert clinician, just at the point that they realize that they must develop a perspective on the situation in order to perform well in the situation. They typically buy more comprehensive reference works and medical and nursing textbooks at this point because loss of confidence in the advice of specific others may be overgeneralized and, consequently, the nurse may feel hyper-responsible. This inability to trust colleagues can be aggravated if incompetence, accompanied by a lack of social integration and informal coaching, is encountered on a particular clinical unit.

Proficiency: The Transition to Expertise

It is the felt crisis in the limits of formalism, the limits of planning and prediction, and an enhanced ability to read a situation that may propel the nurse into the proficient stage of performance. Whereas skill development up until this point has been incremental, now, in order to progress, learners must make a qualitative leap in the way they engage and perform in any given situation. They must literally learn to situate themselves differently in relation to their work. At this stage, experience-near first-person narratives (Geertz, 1987) often take the form of describing changes in their perspectives on a situation. The narrative structure is often something like "I went into the situation thinking that I knew what was going on or that this particular thing was going on," only to have it disconfirmed by the patient's responses to their assessment. This is evidence for developing the ability to let reading the situation guide their patient assessment:

Nurse: You're with the patient, you take care of them and you see them hour to hour exactly. [The physicians] don't see every little drop in the blood pressure or every little change in the rhythm. They just kind of get an overview, [whereas] you are in there constantly. . . . They [The physicians] can go read the chart; you're in there. You're turning this patient, you're doing this, and you're seeing every little aspect.

This excerpt illustrates a new level of skill of seeing and interpreting patient responses. The interviewer asks the nurse quoted above:

Interviewer: Can you give a specific example of when you saw something very differently?

Nurse: [The physicians] come in and look at the flow sheet and we don't, you can't write every, every change you know.

Everyone always says, you may take hourly signs that you put on the chart, but if we had a little computer in our head that really wrote down every little blood pressure or heart rate we looked at for the day, it might be just fine. So they might come in and say, "He looks stable, why don't we take him off the dopamine." And we say, well, wait a minute, I didn't write everything down. I turned him and his blood pressure dropped.

You don't know that. "Let's give him some Lasix." "No, he's not ready for that." . . . I notice that [the physicians are] good about talking to you before making decisions.

The nurse is now synthesizing the meaning of the patient's responses through time. She imagines that a computer could capture all of her readings, but she fails to recognize that her understanding of the patient is now situated and based on a practical understanding of the patient's responses and qualitative changes made over time rather than a collection of data points. The clinician struggles with articulating this practical grasp:

Nurse: I had drawn a [blood] gas on a person and the gas was pretty poor and I took another gas to the house officer and he looked at it and said: "I don't believe this gas, the patient hasn't changed. And at that point—it takes a while to get to this point, but I felt comfortable in saying to him: "What do you mean, this patient hasn't changed?" This patient's blood pressure has gone up to 200, and I presented him with a picture of this patient that he had obviously overlooked. It takes a while to get to the point where you can feel comfortable saying this to the doctor and feeling comfortable, feeling that you can go with your instincts.

Interviewer: What happened in that situation?

Nurse: I was right. . . .

Interviewer: How did you learn that the objective signs that you were seeing were correlated with blood gas?

Nurse: Just experience and seeing different patients and different breathing patterns and knowing by looking at the patient that this breathing pattern is effective and this one isn't, knowing whether there is air exchange there or not. These breaths aren't effective and he's wearing himself out and that could be the cause of his deterioration in his gas, and just experience and seeing different cases and how people adjust to physical things that are going on.

Though difficult to articulate, this practical grasp is not mystical. It reflects the skill of seeing the practical manifestations of changed physiological states and patient responses and engaging in practical reasoning about these changes. The nurse actively interprets the direction of the change and keeps track of what can be ruled in or ruled out. Practical grasp is perceptually grounded and response based and requires being open to correction and to having one's thinking disconfirmed as the situation unfolds. The clinician is always in the situation with some practical understanding, and it is that practical understanding that is revised or confirmed.

In situations where patterns and trends are clear and have definitive interventions associated with the clinical trend, the practitioner can make quick decisive responses. When the practitioner's grasp of the patient's clinical situation is jarred by changes or un-

expected patient responses, the practitioner searches for a new grasp and, if all goes well, experiential clinical learning occurs. Engaged reasoning through transitions requires being open to correction and disconfirmation. The ethos of openness, rather than prediction and control, and fidelity to what one sees and hears, rather than excessive suggestibility and confusion, are embodied and linked to emotional responses to the situation. Thus, one's skilled emotional responsiveness guides perceptual acuity *and* responsiveness to changes in the situation (Benner et al., 1996, pp. 116–117).

The nurse operates in a much more differentiated world of practice at the proficient level. The nurse feels increasingly at home in the situation and can now recognize changing relevance. The following excerpt demonstrates this new comfort level by describing open heart surgery patients' trajectories:

Nurse: I feel pretty comfortable, and you learn when they're warming to start giving the volume and when to stop because now maybe they need a little bit of Levophed to keep their blood pressure up, when to shut off the Levophed because they're waking up and you know their catecholamines have kicked in and that kind of thing. It's almost routine, whereas before it took a lot of trial and asking questions.

This change is based on procedural knowledge and protocols, but the transition being described is the flexible recognition of patient changes in particular situations. These decisions cannot be based on quantitative physiological measures alone, but must be based on understanding the relationship between the numbers and the way the patient looks and responds. This form of response-based action is crucial for performing well in a rapidly changing emergency (Benner et al., 1996, p. 232).

Because the proficient-level nurse is learning to adjust her responses to the situation more, the skill of both problem and person engagement becomes more differentiated and attuned. Observing nurses across situations reveals that they vary their relationships with patients and families based on their understanding of what the situation requires. Timing becomes much more refined, and recognizing opportunities in the situation for patient learning or for supporting a patient is now more attuned to the needs and concerns of the patient.

Nurse: Transplant patients become so dependent on you for everything—Can I brush my teeth now? Do you think I should do this? And you have to really encourage them to take control back. It's a hard concept for a lot of them because they need to be dependent—because it's safe for them to be dependent. . . . I've learned how to give them control back slowly and how to encourage them to take that control back over their own [lives].

Qualitative distinctions are laden with tone, emotional and attitudinal qualities as well as action and contextual qualities. In the context of extreme fatigue or the beginning of rejection or infection, the transplant patient may have to relinquish most independence, but with astute coaching the patient can often retain control over information and participation in decision making may be retained even in extreme periods of dependency (Benner et al., 1996, pp. 125–126). Once begun, the proficient nurse usually continues to refine his reading of particular situations.

Expertise: Phronesis

Once a nurse has progressed to proficiency, the style of being a more situated, response-based performer propels experiential learning and the ability to switch from taking for granted tacit expectations to focusing on aspects of the situation that are changing and creating an altered sense of the situation. The expert nurse is response based in using techne and phronesis. The expert is able to take up theories and ends or goals and notions of *good* in the practice in multiple ways, often creating new possibilities (Taylor, 1991). These situated practical innovations seem intuitively obvious to the practitioner and might not be captured easily in a narrative description of the situation. This is why observation and informal interviewing in actual situations are required to discover and describe all levels of practice, but particularly proficient and expert levels of practice. As noted in our research, ways of seeing the situation increasingly just call for appropriate actions.

Intuitive links develop between seeing and responding to the most relevant issues. This is revealed by observing the nurse in the situation, and is partially captured in the following account of an emergency situation in which a patient who was hemorrhaging stopped breathing. The links between the patient's condition and action are sufficiently strong that the nurse attends primarily to actions rather than assessment of signs and symptoms. This is reasonable since, in extreme circumstances, the possible responses are fewer, but experience is required to make this shift in performance:

> *Nurse:* So we didn't even call the code. We just called the doc[tor] stat [emergency] and got him up there. [They had sufficient people available to resuscitate the patient, so no formal page for additional help was needed.] I looked at his heart rate and I said: "O.K. he is bradying down. Someone want to give me some atropine?" I just started calling out the drugs that I needed to get for this guy, so we started to push these drugs in. In the meantime, I said, "Can we have some more blood?" I was just barking out this stuff [the things that were needed and had to be done]. I can't even tell you the sequence. I was saying, "We need this." I needed to anticipate what was going to happen and I could do this because I had been through this a week before with this guy and knew what we had done [and what had worked]. The anesthesiologist came in and did a good intubation. He asks: "What kind of [IV] lines do we have?" I said, we have a triple lumen and we have blood. All [IV] ports are taken. We need another kind of line. He's got no veins left." He goes, "O.K., fine, give me a cut-down tray...."

The recognition and assessment language are minimal, in part, because the number of actions per problem are limited, but also because recognition and assessment language become so linked with actions and outcomes that they become self-evident or "obvious" for the expert practitioner. In this situation, the response was fluid and knowing because this nurse had taken care of this patient during a previous successful resuscitation where she had learned, firsthand, what worked and what did not. This is not just a rote repetition of the previous resuscitation; rather her responses are based on the understanding gained in the previous situation (Benner et al., 1996, pp. 142–143).

Based on enriched experiential learning spawned by an increasing ability to read the current situation in terms of past whole concrete cases, nurses develop a sense of whether or not they have a good (better or poorer) grasp of the situation. They describe the frustrating situation of "chasing a problem" and never being quite "in synch" with the situation when they do not have a good perceptual grasp of the situation at hand (Benner et al., 1996, pp. 146–147; 1999, pp. 23–87). Skilled "know-how" now allows for more fluid and rapid performance of procedures. Narratives often focus on new clinical learning or troubling moral dilemmas or conflicts in the situation. Qualitative distinctions associated with nuanced responses allow nurses to know and do more than they can tell or think to describe (Polanyi, 1958/1962).

Attunement allows for flexible fusion of thought, feeling, and action. Seeing the unexpected based on having a rich set of expectations as well as a rich sense of the particular situation requires engagement with the patient, openness to noticing when things do not go as implicitly expected, and evidence that disconfirms one's assumptions (Benner et al., 1999, pp. 85–86). Exhibiting the relational skill of attunement to the patient's concerns and clinical situation creates the possibility that patients and family members will disclose or reveal their concerns and fears to the nurse and allows for the nurse to notice changes in the patient/family across time (transitions). The qualities of attentiveness and relationship literally create different disclosive spaces and moods for the patient and family so that different clinical issues are noticed based on qualitatively different disclosive possibilities.

Now, let's return to the example in the advanced beginner discussion in which a patient developed a carotid hemorrhage. Now compare the expert's narrative of the event with the advanced beginner's version:

> I had worked late and was just about ready to go home, when a nurse preceptor said to me, "Jolene, come here." Her voice had urgency in it, but not Code Blue. I walked in and I looked at the patient and his heart rate was about 120, and he was on the respirator and breathing. And I asked her: "What's wrong?" There was a new graduate taking care of him. And he just pointed down to the patient who was lying in a pool of blood. There was a big stream of blood drooling out of his mouth. This man's diagnosis was mandibular cancer, which had been resected, and about a week previous to that he had had a carotid bleed from external carotid, which had been ligated secondary to radiation erosion. That wound had become septic and he had developed respiratory failure and he was in the ICU for that. So I looked at the dressing and it was dry, the blood was coming out of his mouth. The man had a tracheostomy because of the type of surgery that had been done. He also had an NG tube in for feedings, and I got to thinking that it might be the innominate or the carotid artery that had eroded. So we took him off the ventilator to see if anything was going to pump out of his trach. There was a little blood, but it looked mostly like it had come down from the pharynx into the lungs. So we began ventilating him, trying to figure what was inside his mouth that was pumping out this tremendous amount of blood.... (Benner, 1984, p. 17).

This nurse went on to describe her quick actions to draw blood for a cross-match and typing and preparing the man for an immediate transfer to the OR after marshalling all of the resources for the surgical team. She gives us an immediate, direct grasp of the nature of the situation. Action, thought, and feeling are fused. She evaluates the resistance in the lungs by hand ventilating the patient. Fortunately, because of her rapid responses, the patient survived the hemorrhage.

Expert practice by its very nature is comprised of local specific knowledge, know-how, and technical and scientific knowledge, which are transferable to other practice contexts. Because practice is a way of knowing through experiential learning and embodied know-how, it is highly valuable to study and articulate the knowledge embedded in complex practices such as nursing and medicine. Articulation of the knowledge embedded in proficient and expert practice, plus articulation of the range of practical knowledge learned by beginning practitioners in local settings creates the possibility of self-improving practice based on making experiential learning public and, therefore, open to development so that experiential learning and practical wisdom become cumulative and shared.

◼ Summary

Nursing is a practice discipline that is comprised of both practical and theoretical knowledge. Nursing, like medicine, is an underdetermined complex practice that requires clinical judgment and discernment in particular situations. Clinical reasoning calls for reasoning across time about changes in the patient and changes in the clinician's understanding of the situation. Nursing and medicine cannot be reduced to techne (or technique), but must include phronesis, wise skillful judgment, and practice by excellent practitioners.

Every professional nurse is engaged in ongoing experiential learning, clinical inquiry, and clinical knowledge development. Clinicians need to keep track of their experiential learning over time, reflect on it, and make it public and accessible for examination and further studies. Clinical practice is a way of knowing in its own right, but this experiential clinical knowledge development needs to be made accessible to others, and extended by further studies and confirmation in diverse clinical situations.

Each of the studies on skill acquisition conducted by Benner and colleagues was based on extensive experience-near first-person narrative accounts of clinical situations that stood out in the participants' minds. In addition a subsample of participants was observed and informally interviewed in their practice. The nurse researchers deliberately sampled nurses with a range of experience and reported skillfulness, and interviewed nurses with like backgrounds in small-group narrative interviews. They created an open dialogue with the tenets of the Dreyfus model of skill acquisition and the philosophical basis for this model. The researchers found that the model was predictive and descriptive of distinct stages of skill acquisition in nursing practice, and added nuances to the model in terms of the development of moral agency and the influence of emotional engagement with the person and the problem, as well as emotional climate on skill acquisition. They found that nurses who had some difficulty with understanding the ends of practice, and difficulty with their skills of interpersonal and problem engagement did not go on to become expert nurses.

The model was also useful in helping articulate knowledge and skill embedded in the practice of nursing. The rational-technical vision of performance is that of a practitioner or technical expert developing mastery of a body of knowledge and applying that knowledge in prespecified ways to arrive at prespecified outcomes. The rational-technical model does not account for development of relational, perceptual, or skillful comportment over time. It also does not account for the role of experiential learning in learning to practice in a dynamic, underdetermined, and complex practice such as nursing and medicine. A strict technical application of knowledge does not take into account the skills required for discerning the nature of the situation and its possibilities and constraints. Even the expert in the Dreyfus model of skill acquisition must stay attuned to the situation and remain open to the unexpected. Practitioners must remain open to experiential learning and reading changes in transitions in fast-paced, open-ended environments. In the Dreyfus model, the practitioner is assumed to dwell with increasing skill and finesse in a meaningful, intelligible but changing world.

REVIEW QUESTIONS

1. After assisting with care for a patient with a sudden gastrointestinal bleed, the nurse states "I learned so much from watching all of the other nurses and doctors help this patient." Which of the following levels of experience is this nurse most likely to be?
   1. Novice
   2. Advanced Beginner
   3. Competent
   4. Proficient

2. The nurse provides oxygen at 2 liters via nasal cannula to a patient whose pulse oximetry measurement is 95% on room air. One reason for this administration of oxygen would be:
   1. The patient requested oxygen.
   2. The patient expressed anger for being admitted to the hospital.
   3. The patient's glucose level is elevated.
   4. The patient's hemoglobin and hematocrit levels are low.

3. While being transferred from the bed to a chair, a patient who is day 2 total knee replacement experiences a gush of bright red blood from the incision site. The nurse, following the care map for a total knee replacement, should:
   1. Place the patient in the chair.
   2. Return the patient to the bed.
   3. Measure the patient's blood pressure once situated in the chair.
   4. Reinforce the dressing once the patient is situated in the chair.

4. A newly admitted patient repeatedly responds inappropriately to health related questions. Which of the following should the nurse do first to assist this patient?
   1. Contact the physician and suggest a neurological evaluation for a stroke.
   2. Repeat the questions to evaluate the patient's hearing.
   3. Determine if the patient is becoming combative and apply wrist restraints per organizational policy.
   4. Measure the patient's blood pressure and heart rate.

5. A patient, admitted with a sudden onset of lower extremity edema and multiple spontaneous leg wounds, demonstrated breathlessness when asking for the bedpan. Which of the following should the nurse do first?

1. Culture the leg wound exudate.

2. Elevate the patient's legs.

3. Further explore the patient's breathlessness.

4. Ambulate the patient to the bathroom.

Answers to review questions appear in Appendix D

KEY TERMS

clinical judgment *p.32*
clinical knowledge *p.32*
Dreyfus model of skill acquisition *p.35*
ethos *p.34*
experience *p.36*

experiential learning *p.36*
limits of formalization *p.34*
moral agency *p.35*
phronesis *p.33*
practical knowledge *p.32*

rationality *p.33*
salience *p.32*
skills of involvement *p.33*
techne *p.33*

PEARSON

EXPLORE mynursingkit™

MyNursingKit is your one stop for online chapter review materials and resources. Prepare for success with additional NCLEX®-style practice questions, interactive assignments and activities, web links, animations and videos, and more!

Register your access code from the front of your book at
www.mynursingkit.com

REFERENCES

Benner, P. (1982). From novice to expert. *American Journal of Nursing, 82,* 402–407.

Benner, P. (1984). *From novice to expert: Excellence and power in clinical nursing practice.* (Commemorative ed.) Menlo Park, CA: Addison-Wesley.

Benner, P. (1994). The role of articulation in understanding practice and experience as sources of knowledge in clinical nursing. In J. Tully (Ed.), *Philosophy in an age of pluralism: The philosophy of Charles Taylor in question* (pp. 136–155). New York: Cambridge University.

Benner, P. (2001). *From novice to expert: Excellence and power in clinical nursing practice.* (Commemorative ed.) Menlo Park, CA: Addison-Wesley.

Benner, P., Chelsa, C., Dreyfus, H. L., Dreyfus, S. E., and Rubin, J. (1996). *Expertise in Nursing Practice: Caring, Clinical Judgment & Ethics.* New York, NY: Springer Publishing Company.

Benner, P., Hooper-Kyriakidis, P., & Stannard, D. (1999). *Clinical wisdom and interventions in critical care: A thinking-in-action approach.* Philadelphia: W. B. Saunders.

Benner, P., Tanner, C., & Chesla, C. (1992). From beginner to expert: Gaining a differentiated clinical world in critical care nursing. *Advances in Nursing Science, 14*(3), 13–28.

Benner, P., Tanner, C. A., & Chesla, C. A. (1996). *Expertise in nursing practice: Caring, clinical judgment, and ethics.* New York: Springer.

Benner, P., & Wrubel, J. (1982). Clinical knowledge development: The value of perceptual awareness. *Nurse Educator, 7,* 11–17.

Dreyfus, H. L. (1979). *What computers can't do: The limits of artificial intelligence.* (Rev. ed.). New York: Harper & Row.

Dreyfus, H. L. (1992). *What computers still can't do: A critique of artificial reason.* Cambridge, MA: The MIT Press.

Dreyfus, H. L., & Dreyfus, S. E. (1977, March). *Uses and abuses of multi-attribute and multi-aspect model of decision making.* Unpublished manuscript, Department of Industrial Engineering and Operations Research, University of California at Berkeley.

Dreyfus, H. L., & Dreyfus, S. E.., with Athanasiou, T. (1986). *Mind over machine, the power of human intuition and expertise in the era of the computer.* New York: The Free Press.

Dreyfus, S. E. (1982). Formal models vs. human situational understanding: Inherent limitations on the modeling of business expertise. *Office: Technology and People, 1,* 1133–1155.

Dreyfus, S. E., & Dreyfus, H. L. (1979, February). *The scope, limits, and training implications of three models of aircraft pilot emergency response behavior.* Unpublished report supported by the Air Force Office of Scientific Research, USAF (Grant AFOSR-78-3594), University of California at Berkeley.

Dreyfus, S. E., & Dreyfus, H. L. (1980, February). *A five-stage model of the mental activities involved in directed skill acquisition.* Unpublished report supported by the Air Force Office of Scientific Research, USAF (Contract F49620-79-C-0063), University of California at Berkeley.

Dunne, J. (1997). *Back to the rough ground, practical judgment and the lure of technique.* Notre Dame, IN: University of Notre Dame Press.

Gadamer, H. (1960/1975). *Truth and method* (G. Barden & J. Cumming, Trans.). New York: Seabury.

Geertz, C. (1987). Deep play: Notes on the Balinese cockfight. In P. Rabinow & W. Sullivan (Eds.), *Interpretive social science: A second look.* Berkeley, CA: University of California.

Guignon, C. B. (1983). *Heidegger and the problem of knowledge.* Indianapolis, IN: Hackett.

Halpern, J. (2001). *From detached concern to empathy. Humanizing medical care.* Oxford: Oxford University Press.

Kuhn, T. S. (1970). *The structure of scientific revolutions* (2nd ed.). Chicago: University of Chicago Press.

Lave, J., & Wenger, E. (1991). *Situated learning: Legitimate peripheral perspectives (Learning in doing: Social, cognitive and computational perspectives.)* Cambridge, UK: Cambridge University Press.

Polanyi, M. (1958/1962). *Personal knowledge: Towards a post-critical philosophy.* Chicago: University of Chicago Press.

Rubin, J. (1996). Impediments to the development of clinical knowledge and ethical judgment in critical care nursing. In P. Benner, C. Tanner, & C. Chesla (Eds.), *Expertise in nursing practice, caring, clinical judgment and ethics* (pp. 170–192). New York: Springer.

Ruddick, S. (1989). *Maternal thinking: Toward a politics of peace.* New York: Ballantine.

Schon, D. (1987). *The reflective practitioner: How professionals think in action.* New York: Basic Books.

Taylor, C., (1991). *Ethics of authenticity.* Cambridge, MA: Harvard University Press.

Taylor, C. (1993). Explanation and practical reason. In M. Nussbaum & A. Sen (Eds.), *The quality of life.* Oxford: Clarendon Press.

Taylor, C. (1994). Philosophical reflections on caring practices. In S. S. Phillips & P. Benner (Eds.), *The crisis of care: Affirming and restoring caring practices in the helping professions* (pp. 174–187). Washington, DC: Georgetown University Press.

Vetleson, A. J. (1994). *Perception, empathy, and judgment: An inquiry into the preconditions of moral performance.* University Park, PA: Pennsylvania State University Press.

Health Care Trends and Regulatory Aspects of Health Care Delivery

Kathleen Richerson
With contributions by: Annita Watson

Outcome-Based Learning Objectives

After studying this chapter, the learner will be able to:

1. Discuss how major trends in health care quality and patient safety are related to nursing practice.
2. Compare the differences between the types of managed care plans: health maintenance organizations, preferred provider organizations, Medicare, and Medicaid.
3. Describe the key components of the budget process for hospitals and health care systems.
4. Explain the nurse's role in assisting patients with insurance and financial issues.
5. Differentiate between the three types of standards used to measure quality in health care settings.
6. Compare and contrast the impact of licensure, regulation, and accreditation on health care delivery systems.
7. Differentiate between the types of advance directives for health care and describe the nurse's responsibility in advocating and documenting the patient's wishes related to an advance directive.
8. Explain the patient's rights with regard to his or her medical record according to the legal principles of documentation in the patient's medical record.
9. Identify the three main components of the Health Insurance Portability and Accountability Act.
10. Identify the components of case management in the hospital and the associated acute care nursing responsibilities.

HEALTH CARE at the federal and state level is highly regulated to ensure that care is delivered safely, access to care is available, and patient rights are secure. Consumer demand for assurances about the quality of the care they receive and the right to choose their care providers has greatly influenced legislation regarding health care funding and programs. It is important for nurses to understand from a global perspective the forces at work in the health care environment that affect nursing practice, patient care, delivery of service, and advancements in science and technology. As discussed in Chapter 5 nurses play a vital role in managing these challenges by providing leadership in the management of patient care and design of patient care delivery models.

This chapter provides an overview of legal, financial, and social forces that influence the way health care is provided in organizations and how it is delivered to patients. The issues discussed directly and indirectly affect the practice of nursing, the way in which nurses contribute to the health of patients, the organizations for which they work, and the communities in which they live.

▌ Health Care Delivery Systems

A **health care delivery system** is a set of services designed to deliver professional health care and to promote health and wellness to constituents in a given society (Barber et al., (1998). Basically, it is all the activities of a society that are designed to protect or restore health, whether directed at the individual, society, or the environment. These activities include services from personnel engaged in medical occupations, physical plants, capital, and other goods and services.

Health care delivery systems in the United States have evolved significantly during the past two decades. Historically, people in the United States received health care through personal physicians and locally owned and operated community hospitals. However, highly competitive, expanding health care delivery systems are replacing that model. This transformation of the health care industry is being molded by increasing delivery costs, changing reimbursement requirements, standardization of diagnoses and treatment methods, contracted care, rising liability issues, and emerging technologies. Other influencing factors include increased severity of illness in inpatient facilities, major cost reductions and restructuring, emerging new illnesses, changing population demographics, and an exploding global community.

Within the context of these changes, delivery systems have moved from a horizontal organizational model to a vertically integrated model and more recently are evolving into a model of virtual networks. In **horizontal organizational models**, hospitals were aligned to form multiple-hospital systems, with a focus on traditional acute care services. With the transition to **vertically integrated models**, services have been aligned to provide a continuum of care. This model includes the integration of physician, hospital, and ancillary services. Integrated systems can offer a broad range of services pre- and post-hospitalization from primary care to long-term care (Wolper, 2004).

Health care delivery models have most recently evolved into networks of integrated systems and services that are virtually connected by relationships through contracts rather than ownership. Within the virtually integrated model, technology plays a critical part in linking the network. The concept of e-health, which provides a computer-based framework for communication and a central repository for data and information, has been introduced. This central framework allows virtual patient access. For instance, patient-specific health information is available at any time to providers within the network and to the patients themselves (Harris et al., 2003). As this model develops, patients and their families will begin to rely on nurses to assist them with accessing care within these complex systems. Linking to resources such as financial counseling, social services, and case management may be required to provide specific support for patients. Such links are especially important when preparing the patient for discharge and transition to other care and services outside the hospital.

Future Delivery Implications

High consumer demand and increasing health care costs are dominant forces influencing the future structure of health care delivery. Joining these prevailing forces is a heightened scrutiny around the quality and safety of care delivered to patients as well as how patients access that care. Evidence of this influence is the growth of agencies that provide ratings and benchmarking for health care systems locally, regionally, and nationally, most of which are publicly available and Internet-based for easy access. Consumers can use ratings information to evaluate the services and quality outcomes of organizations before making choices about health plans or providers. This major trend is driving health care organizations to shift to consumer-directed service cultures (Scalise, 2005).

In the future, health care providers will be challenged to incorporate new advances in technology and treatment. This challenge will come primarily from consumers and payers seeking new services and cost-effective care. Traditional inpatient hospital services are evolving into more sophisticated outpatient-focused services that will allow more consumer control in terms of the selection of treatments and services (Abramson & Tyler, 2006). One such example of the transition from inpatient to outpatient is general surgery laparoscopic procedures.

Hospital Organizations

Currently, according to the American Hospital Association (2006) there are four categories of hospital organizations: general acute care, specialty, rehabilitative, and psychiatric. General acute care hospitals provide diagnostic and therapeutic services for a range of health conditions. General acute care hospitals range from small rural facilities to large multicampus academic med-

ical centers. The types of services vary depending on community needs, competition with other organizations in the immediate market area, and the specific mission of the organization.

Specialty organizations focus on specific medical conditions or procedures. Some specialty organizations provide outpatient services only or short-stay 24-hour service. Some examples of organizations in this category are cardiovascular, orthopedic, plastic/cosmetic surgery, and women's services (McKinley, 2005). Rehabilitative and chronic disease facilities provide care for people who have disabilities. Their patients receive restorative or adjustive care on either a short-term or long-term basis. Examples of these types of agencies include Alzheimer and memory loss care centers and skilled nursing or long-term care centers. Finally, psychiatric care facilities provide inpatient and outpatient care for psychiatric-related illnesses (American Hospital Association [AHA], 2007). These are freestanding facilities that may or may not be associated with an acute care facility. Chart 3–1 outlines the various types of hospital organizations. Each type of health care organization is subject to increasing health care costs and survival as a health care delivery system.

■ Health Care Costs

Health care costs have steadily increased during the past two decades, spiraling to a higher figure than that spent on national defense (California HealthCare Foundation, 2004). Costs are expected to continue their unparalleled growth in the future. As a result of these increasing costs, many employers have decreased the coverage provided to employees or increased the amount that employees contribute toward their health care costs, thereby contributing to the numbers of uninsured Americans. On the other hand, even as health care costs have escalated, so have patients' demands for health care services, due largely in part to the growing numbers of elderly and the request for the latest technological and pharmaceutical advances in medical care (U.S. Census Bureau, 2002). Health care organizations are striving to meet patients' expectations in order to survive in a very competitive marketplace.

Historical Development of Health Care Economics

The current economics of health care have developed as a result of the historical impact of social, cultural, political, and economic issues in the United States. Prior to the 1940s, the U.S. government's role in health care delivery was limited to the local level. Almshouses and poorhouses were built for those with insurance, people who had chronic disabilities, and people who were mentally ill. Other individuals requiring health care paid their local doctor out of pocket and they usually were cared for in their homes. Private-duty nurses often were hired to provide nursing care at home because there was little insurance to pay for hospital care. Care was provided under a fee-for-service arrangement; the patient or the insurer paid for the type and amount of care provided based on a cost reimbursement system.

Since the 1940s, several major legislative acts have led to an increased role for the federal government. Market forces also have helped to replace fee-for-service plans with prospective contracted insurance plans, referred to as managed care, for most working Americans. Enacted in 1946, post–World War II,

| CHART 3–1 | **Hospital Organizations** |

Type of Hospital Organization	**Description**
General acute care	Functions to provide patient care, diagnostic and therapeutic services for a variety of medical conditions. Includes • Diagnostic imaging • Clinical laboratory • Operating rooms.
Specialty	Functions to provide diagnostic and treatment services for specified medical conditions. Includes • Appropriate diagnostic and treatment services for the specialty • Clinical laboratory capable of providing tissue diagnosis when offering pregnancy termination services.
Rehabilitative	Functions to provide diagnostic and treatment services to individuals with handicaps or disabilities who require restorative and adjustive care. Includes • Arrangements for diagnostic imaging services • Arrangements for clinical laboratory services • Arrangements for operating room services if required • Physical therapy service • Occupational therapy service • Psychological and social work services on a regular basis • Arrangements for educational and vocational services on a regular basis • Transfer agreements with a general acute care hospital for transfer of patients requiring a higher level of care.
Psychiatric	Functions to provide diagnostic and treatment services for patients who have psychiatric-related illnesses. Includes • Arrangements for clinical laboratory services • Arrangements for diagnostic imaging services • Psychiatric, psychological, and social services • Arrangements for electroencephalograph services on a regular basis • Transfer agreements with a general acute care hospital for transfer of patients requiring a higher level of care.

Source: American Hospital Association. (2007). Guide to the health care field—2007 edition.

the Hill-Burton program was established to fund the construction of hospitals. The program required facilities that were receiving federal funds to make their services available to all persons residing in the facility's service area without discrimination. Although the program meant that health care services would be available to all who lived in that community, it did not dictate how hospitals would charge for their services or how people would pay for them (Grohar-Murray & DiCroce, 2003).

In the 1960s Medicare and Medicaid legislation was passed as an amendment to the Social Security Act. The **Medicare** portion of the act provides insurance for people over age 65 and payment for their hospitalization, physicians' fees, and diagnostic tests. Medicare also provides coverage for persons with disabilities and those with permanent kidney failure. As an entitlement for older adults, Medicare essentially provides universal coverage for hospitalization and outpatient care. Together these services account for more than half of all Medicare expenditures (Centers for Medicare & Medicaid Services [CMS], 2007). The other portion, **Medicaid**, funds health care to the dependent population and is administered by each state. The state determines eligibility and level of coverage, establishes the rate of payment for services, and retains the right and power to determine the type, amount, duration, and scope of services.

The role of insurance companies as third-party payers evolved as a part of these new reimbursement procedures. Employers began providing health care benefits to workers as part of a total employment package, and organized labor aggressively negotiated for better packages. The relationship between hospitals, physicians, and patients changed, as everyone became aware that the insurance companies, rather than the patients, were paying most health care bills.

Because the medical world was aware that the insurance companies and government would pay for all reasonable costs of health care, expenses skyrocketed in the early 1980s. Abuses and fraud have been widely publicized, especially those involving Medicare and Medicaid. Also, rapid technological advances contributed to the increased cost of care, as more knowledgeable patients came to expect the latest and best of diagnostic and interventional care. Malpractice fears also influenced the diagnostic test-ordering practices of primary care providers and the cost of health care. Although the overall quality of life of the elderly population has improved, the goal of providing cost-effective health care through these programs has not been achieved.

In the 1980s public attention became focused on the spiraling costs of health care. The philosophy that all citizens had the right to comprehensive quality health care prompted governmental concerns about the spiraling costs and the wide variation in charges among providers. The government was no longer able to pay for care that was delivered without defined limits or costs (Sullivan & Decker, 2005). In the face of huge budget deficits, the federal government moved to gain control of spiraling Medicare costs by enacting legislation to change Medicare payments from retrospective fee-for-service schedules to prospective fee schedules based on diagnostic categories. A payment system was adopted, based on diagnostic-related groups, that organizes diagnoses- and procedure-related conditions into categories or groups. Payment is based on national averages for cost and length of stay for these groups. *Length of stay* refers to the number of days a patient is hospitalized.

Managed Care and the Current Status of Reimbursement Practices

Within the complex American health care system, changes in reimbursement practices have led to changes in the way health care is delivered or "managed." *Managed care* is a generic term for a system that attempts to control and influence the way health care is financed and delivered. Managed care has affected the health care industry significantly since the early 1980s by changing the standards, the cost structure of medical care, and many aspects of access to care. The development of managed care has been aimed at balancing the three elements of access, cost, and quality. Under the fee-for-service system, health care costs increased dramatically due to high utilization of services. Other factors that have continued to contribute to high costs include new technology, cost shifting, the aging population, legal pressures, and administrative costs (Wolper, 2004).

Discussions and debate over time have tried to determine the effect of managed care plans on the quality of health care in light of managed care's cost-cutting strategies and tight controls on utilization of services. The National Committee for Quality Assurance (NCQA) found that plans do vary in their approach to prevention and treatment, but that performance of the plans in contrast to fee-for-service plans was equivalent or better under managed care. In addition, patients may be more likely to comply with the health risk screenings and preventive treatments that are the focus of managed care. They also reported that patients are satisfied with the actual care, but complain about the administrative services (NCQA, 2006). The managed care system and health plans will continue to evolve along with the dynamics of social and environmental change. Consumers are demanding more choice in selection of health care providers and seem to be willing to pay higher premiums for this flexibility.

It is important to understand the basic plan designs that provide coverage for health care within the United States. Plans differ in the aspects of care that are covered and funding for that care. Chart 3–2 defines the types of insurance plans that are common throughout the country.

Forms of Managed Care

A number of abbreviations are used to describe the various types of managed care. These include HMO, IPA, PPO, and EPO. An HMO refers to a health maintenance organization, IPA refers to an independent/individual practice association, PPO refers to a preferred provider organization, and EPO refers to an exclusive provider organization. An EPO has a contract with a single entity or group of physicians rather than a network of independent providers as seen in a PPO. Chart 3–3 outlines the most common forms of managed care.

The HMOs and PPOs pay a fixed rate per day per patient for providing care, regardless of equipment, supplies, or number of procedures or services required. Per case or per stay reimburses providers a fixed sum regardless of the length of stay. Capitation arrangements pay the hospital a fixed amount each month per member enrolled.

Many managed care organizations, regardless of whether the member uses the hospital, physician, or other services, have in-

---

CHART 3–2	**Definitions of Health Insurance Plans**

Type of Health Plan	Definition
Traditional insurance	*Indemnity:* The insured individual is indemnified against financial losses for health care costs. The insured is not restricted in terms of which providers they can access and they are reimbursed directly for any costs.
	Service plans: The plan contracts with providers to accept payment based on a fee schedule. The insured may have some restrictions on providers, and the provider is paid directly by the plan.
Government programs	*Medicare:* National health insurance program for individuals age 65 or older, under age 65 with disabilities, and those with end-stage renal disease.
	Medicaid: Medical assistance for individuals and families with low incomes. Each state will set regulations about eligibility and services.
	Military, civil service, federal employees, and veterans programs also fall under this category.
Self-funded plans	Under the Employee Retirement Income Security Act companies can cover their employees for medical costs instead of providing commercial insurance plans.
Health maintenance organization (HMO)	The organization provides comprehensive health care to individuals who prepay through premiums for the coverage. A primary care physician generally directs care within a network of providers.
Preferred provider organization (PPO)	The organization has a network of providers under contract. The insured can use the network providers or—for a higher deductible—access providers outside the network.

Sources: Data from HCAB, 2003; Grohar-Murray, M. E., & DiCroce, H. R. (2003). *Leadership and management in nursing.* Upper Saddle River, NJ: Pearson Prentice Hall; Wolper, L. F. (2004). *Health care administration: Planning, implementing, and managing organized delivery systems* (4th ed.). Sudbury, MA: Jones and Bartlett.

CHART 3–3	**Common Forms of Managed Care**
Health maintenance organization (HMO)	A group health care agency that provides basic and supplemental health maintenance and treatment services to voluntary enrollees. A fee is set without regard to the amount or kind of service provided.
Independent practice association (IPA)	A group of physicians who are in practice for themselves join together to form an associate offering a full spectrum of services to managed care organizations. IPAs will take capitated payment from HMOs and distribute a fee-for-service arrangement within the association. IPAs provide an opportunity for physicians who want to remain in individual practices to form an association that can interact and negotiate with HMOs.
Preferred provider organization (PPO)	Consists of a group of physicians, and perhaps a health care agency, that provide an insurance company or an employer with health services at a discounted rate. Employers and insurance companies set up standards and criteria for practices. When joining the organization the physician agrees to abide by those standards and abide by the reimbursement structure. An advantage of a PPO is that it provides the patient with a choice of health care providers and services.
Exclusive provider organization (EPO)	The physician organization becomes the exclusive provider of care. Participants are not allowed to receive coverage from any other providers. By developing an exclusive provider situation, an exclusive employer provider can negotiate better rates because the system can guarantee a certain volume of business.

ducements for maintaining wellness through health screenings and patient education. This emphasis is believed to decrease the number of inpatient hospital days per admission and can have a positive effect on a hospital margin.

Another way in which managed care plans control costs is to require prior approval for many types of care. Referrals by an individual's primary care provider also are often required. Although "true emergencies" are covered, many visits to the emergency department fall into nonemergent categories and coverage for these visits can be denied. The issue of prior approval also can arise before a patient can receive prescription drug benefits for certain drugs. Formularies of lists of drugs that are covered actually help to decrease skyrocketing drug costs by providing therapeutic, cost-effective choices for the practitioner. However, these limits also may delay care in an attempt to get approval for non-formulary drugs and patients may be required to pay any costs not covered by the insurance plan. These additional costs are based on the contract prices and selections health care providers have negotiated with the pharmaceutical distributors. Additionally, practitioners in groups often are given financial incentives for keeping their members healthy and out of the hospital.

Managed care today is in the mode of creating a delivery system that manages both costs and care along with methods of documenting cost-effective care. As such, quality improvement activities are now mandated, and health care organizations must meet the standards of the NCQA with the Health Plan Employer Data and Information Set.

Health Maintenance Organization

Health maintenance organizations (HMOs) were the earliest form of managed care, and are now the most common. HMOs deliver comprehensive health services for fixed, prepaid fees or capitation. Comprehensive health care usually includes procedures that focus on preventive care and early detection, such as annual physicals, mammography, proctoscopy, immunizations, and well-baby visits. HMOs manage services and costs through utilization review/management, restriction of access to a specific network of providers, and incentives for physicians.

Various HMO models and structures are available based on the relationship of the HMO and the providers. A group model is one in which a medical group or organization contracts to provide care exclusively to the HMO's members. In return, the HMO pays the medical group on a capitated basis, which is a set amount per member per month. An example of this model is Kaiser Permanente. In a network model, the HMO has a nonexclusive contract with two or more physician groups and allows the physicians to treat HMO as well as non-HMO patients (HCAB, 2003b).

Independent Practice Association

An **independent practice association (IPA)** contracts on the behalf of individual physicians or groups of physicians to provide health care to the members of an HMO. In this model the physicians remain independent contractors with separate practices. Another model is a staff model in which the HMO employs physicians to provide care to its members (HCAB, 2003b).

Preferred Provider Organization

A **preferred provider organization (PPO)** differs from an HMO in several ways. PPOs provide a coordinated care plan that provides medical care by contracting with a network of providers. These providers agree to accept a set reimbursement rate for care covered by the plan. PPOs also provide reimbursement for covered care to noncontracted providers, but the level of reimbursement may differ from their contracted providers, and the member may have to pay a higher deductible.

PPOs also differ from HMOs in that they do not rely on strict utilization management and other controls common with HMOs (Grohar-Murray & DiCroce, 2003). Instead, they usually attempt to contain costs by negotiating with individual providers and health care organizations to provide certain kinds of health care at an agreed-on price. This price is usually lower than the price that a patient would pay for the same medical services outside of the PPO.

Government Programs

The Medicare and Medicaid programs were established by the Social Security Act in 1965. Medicare is the national health insurance program that covers people 65 years or older, some people under 65 years with disabilities, and people with end-stage renal disease. In the mid-1980s Congress adopted a prospective payment system based on the use of diagnosis-related groups

(DRGs) as a reimbursement method for hospitalized Medicare patients. A DRG refers to a like classification of diagnoses. The hospital is paid a certain capped amount per DRG category. A fixed payment has been predetermined for more than 470 possible diagnostic categories, covering the majority of medical diagnoses of all patients admitted to the hospital.

The switch to the DRG payment schedule effectively predetermined the amount that a hospital is reimbursed for the treatment of a Medicare patient diagnosed with a particular condition. DRGs shifted the payment unit from total charges or "days in the hospital" to the patient's diagnosis. The purpose of the DRG was, and still is, to ease the burden of Medicare financing and to control delivery of care. The advent of DRGs has served as an incentive for hospitals to place greater emphasis on reducing costs, utilization of services, and length of patient stay.

Under the DRG prospective payment system, hospitals and extended care facilities have had to develop length-of-stay (LOS) estimates for a variety of diagnoses. These estimates help determine, on average, the LOS beyond which the facility will not be reimbursed for the patient's care. A subspecialty of nursing, called *discharge planners,* has evolved to help plan patient discharges in a timely manner. Discharge planning nurses also help provide some assurance that the patient's needs will be met after discharge. At discharge, arrangements are made for family teaching, home care, or extended care.

With an emphasis on patient days, discharge planners have focused on care management and clinical pathways. Consequently, patient acuity levels in hospitals are now higher, and those discharged are sicker than ever before (Dower, 2002; Shortell & Kaluzny, 2005). Patients are sometimes discharged to their homes before it is appropriate, and equipment and services are not always adequate to meet all of their needs. This situation has led to the emergence of subacute, transitional rehabilitation units in long-term care facilities. These facilities have had to train their staff to care for much sicker patients than they usually care for, patients who often require intravenous therapy and complex nursing interventions previously provided only in the acute care setting. Also, it is not unusual for those patients who have returned home to be treated with intravenous therapy, respiratory care, wound care, and various rehabilitation therapies. Much of the home care is dependent on the availability of family members, who may have to take unpaid time from work to care for their loved ones. The care that family and friends provide is not without cost, even though it is not reimbursed. Critics of the DRG system believe that while prospective payment may ease the burden of Medicare financing, it does not necessarily reduce the overall cost of health care, especially when these costs are calculated from the point of view of society as a whole. It is worth noting that high hospital readmission rates are seen in cases of patients sent home too early or those sent home without appropriate care and support. To guarantee Medicare reimbursement for the readmission, these patients are sometimes readmitted with a different diagnosis than the initial admission (Dower, 2002).

Medicaid is a state-administered program that provides medical assistance for certain individuals and families (dependents) with low incomes and resources. The federal agency that is responsible for oversight of the programs is the Centers for Medicare and Medicaid Services. CMS also establishes guidelines for state Medicaid programs; however, program requirements are set by the individual state and administration of the state program may differ by county. These coverage plans may be administered by a managed care contract through an HMO or PPO to provide care for patients (CMS, 2006).

Future Economic Projections

Managed care as a model for health care delivery is not going to go away (Marquis & Huston, 2007; Rosenbaum, 1998). It permeates the current health care delivery system and is likely to grow in magnitude regarding the number of subscribers to its plans as well as its impact on the entire health care system. Although managed care continues to dominate markets, it is evolving in ways that have diminished its potential to control costs and promote quality. As health care premiums continue to rise and labor markets slacken, consumers are likely to face growing financial burden for the cost of care. These developments could have the positive effect of making consumers more cost conscious in their use of health care services. Conversely, they may result in increased disparities in the health system, with further stratification based on the ability to pay and greater burden on those who have chronic illnesses for the cost of their care (Dower, 2002; Marquis & Huston, 2007; Shortell & Kaluzny, 2005).

Currently, Americans spend more on their health care than any other Western industrialized nation. The United States is the only one of this group of nations that does not offer basic benefits globally to all citizens (Woolf, Johnson, & Geiger, 2006). The many barriers created by the current health care system affect access to care for individuals and specific population groups such as the elderly and rural residents. According to the American Hospital Association, consumers worry about insurance cost increases, that their income will not keep pace with these rising costs, and that insurance plans may decrease health care quality and access to cut their operating expenses. There is further concern that as these issues go unchecked, consumers may be influenced to go without insurance or the care they need. Inappropriate use of hospital emergency departments and the inability of patients to pay increased costs for health care is forcing hospitals to offset these losses by raising prices for services, drugs, and supplies. The consequences of these trends may include higher rates of chronic illnesses, more frequent and severe disease complications, and overall adverse effects on access to health care for children (Woolf et al., 2006).

It is expected that out-of-pocket costs, or those expenses not covered by health plans, will grow rapidly for consumers. This is primarily due to higher premiums for health plan coverage, which are based on higher medical care costs. These higher premiums have forced employers to share the added burden with their employees. To combat these competing cost structures, which seem to be increasing without end, reform initiatives are being proposed on many fronts. Certainly the government is looking at reducing expenses within the Medicare and Medicaid programs. Additionally, coverage programs are being developed to give consumers more choice about what their health plan will include and to align incentives among all parties to focus on access, appropriate care, and reduced costs (Samuel, Raleigh, Hower, & Schwartz, 2003).

Nurses should assess their patient's health care coverage or insurance plan for potential referrals for financial assistance or counseling. Patients may be concerned about their current coverage or may lack coverage altogether. This concern can cause significant stress that may affect the patient's ability to rest and recover. Referrals may be made to the hospital's financial department or social services to assist in resolving any payment or coverage issues.

The cost and financing of health care will continue to drive the development of health care delivery models based on the premise that more should be provided for less. This focus will influence how health care professionals, including nurses, are used in the future. This pressure will continue until the consumers (individual, employer, and insurance provider) are comfortable that the health care product (service) they are receiving is balanced by its availability and cost. Along with changes in health care finances and managed care, other important trends are affecting the future of health care delivery systems and the financial configuration of health care organizations.

■ Financial Aspects of Health Care Organizations

Health care organizations, especially hospitals, are structured financially in one of two ways. **For-profit or proprietary organizations** focus their mission and structure on earning a profit from their operations. The profits are then distributed to the owners of the organization or the investors who have purchased shares of the organization (Finkler & Kovner, 2000). The excess earnings of a **not-for-profit organization** must be used for public rather than private gain. The mission of the not-for-profit organization is to earn a profit, but those profits are generally used to improve the physical facility and services offered by the agency (Wolper, 2004).

Regardless of whether a hospital uses a for-profit or not-for-profit structure, it cannot turn patients away who require emergency care services and it cannot refuse to care for patients. The **Emergency Medical Treatment and Labor Act (EMTALA)** was enacted in 1986 to ensure public access to emergency services regardless of patients' ability to pay. When patients are not able to pay for care, they fall under the hospital's charity care policy. Charity care is accounted for in annual budgets based on the organization's history and the demographic projections for the population they serve. Charity care is considered a loss from the organization's operations. Programs are available to assist hospitals that are adversely affected by their patient population's inability to pay; however, this assistance does not cover all costs incurred by the organization. Charity care can contribute to higher costs for insured or self-pay patients if the hospital has to structure its financial plan to make up for large losses. Chapter 73 ⊙ includes an in-depth discussion of emergency department regulations.

Budgeting Process for Health Care Institutions

Budgets have three main components:

- Revenue is the money an organization receives or is entitled to receive to cover the costs of providing services or goods.

- Expenses are costs of operating the organization and include salaries, benefits, supplies, utilities, purchased services, and administrative costs.
- Capital refers to equipment purchased by the organization or construction projects.

Chart 3–4 (p. 52) outlines the basic structure of a hospital-based budget.

A budget is basically a plan for a future period that is defined in measurable terms and expected outcomes. The process begins with the forecasting of revenue and expense projections for the next budget period. This period is referred to as a fiscal year and is generally a calendar year, but may begin at any time during the year, and lasts for 12 consecutive months. For instance, some organizations budget January through December, whereas others may define their fiscal year as July through June.

Forecasting involves a review of the organization's assets, which includes their property, equipment cash on hand, and the amount of money calculated as outstanding from billing. Organizations will next look at the trends in reimbursement for services and population demographics for growth or change. Reimbursement is the payment received for health or medical care from a health plan (insurance) or payer source. The amount of payment is often discounted from the actual charges for the service. Historical data also are reviewed for volume trends and patterns of service that may be seasonal in nature such as higher patient admissions during winter months.

All of this information is calculated to provide a projection for potential revenue, which must be compared to the estimated expenses. The comparison takes into account the bottom line or the outcome of revenue divided by expense. Usually this is a positive outcome, but at times organizations will project a loss or a break-even scenario based on their analysis of all of these factors. The administration and the governing body of the organization generally approve budgets before they are implemented. The budget is monitored continuously throughout the year and appropriate adjustments are made as necessary.

Capital budgets determine the organization's ability to purchase equipment and to upgrade or expand facilities. The capital budget is based on a calculation from the operating budget, or an estimate of what the organization can afford. Projections range from the next fiscal year to multiple years out into the future. Capital equipment needs generally fall into the categories of needing replacement, upgrading of existing equipment or systems, or purchasing of a new business or service opportunity. Facility needs usually are based on the age of the building, technology, and expansion for population growth or new services (Wolper, 2004).

Funding for the capital budget comes from the estimated revenue from operations or a percentage of expected income or loans. Some capital equipment can be leased to avoid an outright purchase if purchasing funds are not available. Some leases allow the organization to rent equipment with an option to buy at the end of a set period for a discounted price or to allow payments for large pieces of equipment to be billed over several years.

Nursing professionals play an important part in the budget process through their observations of the environment, equipment, and changing needs of patients. Their input to the management structure provides important information for making

CHART 3–4	**Hospital Budget Components**	
Major Category	**Component**	**Definition**
Revenue	Volume	Volume for hospitals overall is based on units of service. The overall hospital generally looks at patient days, and departments look at relative statistics for the type of work they do. *Examples:* Inpatient unit = patient days Surgery = surgery minutes Respiratory therapy = procedures or treatments Laboratory = tests or procedures Emergency department = patient visits
	Charges	Charges are based on the cost of supplies or services. They take into consideration the price paid to the vendor and a markup for processing, staff time, and organizational overhead.
	Deductions from revenue	These deductions are any decrease in revenue from charity care or payer contracts.
	Nonoperating revenue	Includes adjustments that may come from investment income or legal actions in favor of the organization.
Operating expenses (controllable expenses)	Salaries/wages	These expenses include regular salaries for staff, premium pay such as overtime, benefits, and temporary labor. Benefits can include medical care coverage, vacation/sick time, training/orientation, and travel reimbursement.
	Supplies	Examples include disposable and reusable supplies, minor medical equipment, and office supplies.
	Purchased services	Examples include maintenance agreements for large equipment, equipment rentals, repair costs, and vendor contracts for services.
Non-Discretionary expenses	Overhead	This category covers system costs for depreciation of the buildings and equipment, administrative positions and expenses, and interest on loans. Administrative costs are for nonrevenue-generating departments such as finance, human resources, and housekeeping.

Sources: Data from Finkler, S. A., & Kovner, C. T. (2000). *Financial management for nurse managers and executives.* Philadelphia: W. B. Saunders; Wolper, L. F. (2004). *Health care administration: Planning, implementing, and managing organized delivery systems* (4th ed.). Sudbury, MA: Jones and Bartlett.

decisions about the allocation of resources, the control of expenses, and planning for future growth. It is also important for nurses to take an active role in containing costs through judicial use of supplies, awareness of equipment safety and maintenance, and appropriate adjustments to staffing and workload.

■ Health Care Trends

Several major trends are affecting and changing health care in the United States:

- Evidence-based practice guidelines and research are creating a shift in approach to care that is more systematic and clear.
- Quality and patient safety standards have been a main focus of consumer watchdog groups and regulatory bodies and are influencing the purchase of health care insurance and the selection of medical care providers.
- Threats of potential major events such as bioterrorism attacks or widespread epidemics are requiring health care organizations to set priorities and plan their responses.
- Advancements in technology and science are enhancing medical care now and in the future.

These and other trends are discussed in the following subsections.

Evidence-Based Practice

Evidence-based practice can be described broadly as an approach that integrates current research evidence with clinical expertise and patients' needs. Evidence-based practice has come about as a response to the demand for grounded clinical decision making that critically examines the benefits and costs of treatments and interventions.

Factors that form a framework for decision making with this approach include understanding patients' needs, their concerns, and their values, building on the clinical expertise or experience of the professional nurse, and seeking relevant clinical data and best practices (Malloch & Porter-O'Grady, 2006). Best practices are defined as proven processes that produce consistent, high-quality results. In nursing there are many sources of knowledge that guide critical thinking about care, including the applicability of nursing interventions and intuition about approaches and interactions with patients. Data and research are also becoming more available through the use of Internet resources in the practice arena. Internet resources provide instant access for caregivers. Information systems used in health care organizations often provide immediate access to concise resources and guidelines for practice. It is important for nurses to keep current with relevant literature in their area of practice and be competent in accessing available resources.

Hospital Report Cards

Consumer-oriented hospital report cards are available to the public through periodicals and on the Internet. They provide a wealth of information on quality outcome measurements and the experience of organizations in providing care (Richard, Rawal, & Martin, 2005). The development of these tools was intended to help improve the quality of care by providing feedback and benchmarking practice standards. Benchmarking offers qualitative or quantitative measurement of specific data related to reported outcome information. Benchmark information often is displayed as a range and includes the best practice reported by participants. This can be of interest to patients or patient groups with specific health problems or chronic diseases who are making a selection of physicians or health care institutions (Werner & Asch, 2005).

Patient Safety Standards

There is heightened awareness in the United States regarding the safety of patients in the health care environment. Major efforts are under way to focus on measuring, reporting, and improving patient safety. Organizations conducting such research include the Institute of Medicine, the Leapfrog Group, and the Joint Commission.

The **Institute of Medicine (IOM)** provides science-based advice on medicine and health in an effort to improve health. It provides unbiased, evidence-based, and authoritative information to policy makers, professionals, and the public at large (IOM, 1999). In 1999 IOM produced the study, *To Err Is Human: Building a Safer Health System*, which indicated that preventable errors in hospitals are the eighth leading cause of death in the United States. Following the recommendations of the IOM report, hospitals were required to assess their practices and institute changes to ensure the reduction of preventable errors. Reports from the investigation of medical errors found that errors were not necessarily the result of carelessness, but were instead the result of systems and processes that did not provide the appropriate checks to prevent the errors (Leapfrog Group, 2006).

The **Leapfrog Group** was established by a coalition of public and private organizations that provide health care benefits. The group focuses on collecting data about medical errors and setting standards that will reduce errors. In addition, information is provided to consumers that assist them in making more informed choices about hospitals and health care systems. The Leapfrog Group has developed platforms for improving patient safety including (1) computer physician order entry (CPOE), (2) evidence-based hospital referral, (3) intensive care unit (ICU) physician staffing or the use of intensivists, and (4) National Quality Forum–endorsed safe practices.

CPOE is aimed at eliminating errors from the process of transcribing physician orders that are handwritten or given verbally. CPOE requires that the prescribing physician or allied health care provider personally enter orders into the computer system. It is well known that illegible handwriting has been one of the root causes of medication and therapy error. According to the Leapfrog Group, if this practice were implemented in all urban hospitals in the United States as many as 907,600 serious medication errors could be prevented each year. In addition, CPOE has been shown to reduce patient length of stay and du-

plicate orders for procedures and tests (Leapfrog Group, 2006). Computer system software programs are also available that help to prevent prescribing errors by providing alerts to incompatibilities with medications.

Evidence-based hospital referral is aimed at guiding patients to hospitals and clinical teams that are more likely to produce better outcomes for specific treatments and procedures. Information provided on Leapfrog Group web pages offers data on hospital volume, geographic specifics, risk-adjusted outcomes, and benchmarking among providers. Currently the Leapfrog Group collects data on eight high-risk conditions or procedures and three maternal high-risk delivery outcomes.

The group also advocates for dedicated physician staffing in ICUs. This type of program provides physicians who specialize in critical care and managing complex patients. Studies have shown that when this system is in place there is a 30% reduction in overall hospital mortality and a 40% reduction in mortality in the intensive care environment (Leapfrog Group, 2006). These intensivist programs in the ICU can also be used to provide remote monitoring of acutely ill patients (Nathans et al., 2006). Remote coverage is provided via computer monitoring of clinical data from specific diagnostic equipment and the ongoing review of test results and recorded documentation. Some systems provide video surveillance of the patient from the bedside linked to intensivists at a central location. Benefits of using an intensivist model include reduced mortality rates, reduced inappropriate admissions, shorter ICU stays, faster weaning from mechanical ventilators, early detection of hemodynamic complications, fewer consultations with other specialists, and an overall reduction in hospital costs (Fuchs, Berenholtz, & Dorman, 2005).

The National Quality Forum is a public–private partnership created to develop and implement a national strategy for health care quality measurement and reporting. The organization has established an agenda to implement proven patient safety practices (National Quality Forum, 2006). National patient safety goals and practices have been endorsed by other organizations such as the Joint Commission and the Leapfrog Group who have formed a partnership to collaborate on patient-safety standards. In addition, the CMS (2006) is also joining with the Leapfrog Group to provide information for their consumers about the initiatives and hospital-specific ratings that are now available.

The Joint Commission (**Joint Commission**), the accrediting body for hospitals and health care organizations, is an independent, private, not-for-profit organization. The Joint Commission focuses on setting standards for patient care and safety, competency of staff, and responsibilities of the administration and governing board. It evaluates and certifies or accredits health care organizations and programs in the United States. The Joint Commission's patient safety standards took effect in July 2001 and are generally updated or expanded on an annual basis. Hospitals must take all of these standards and initiatives into consideration as they plan quality activities and develop policies and procedures (Joint Commission, 2006).

Emergency Preparedness

Hospitals must develop disaster or emergency preparedness plans to ensure that the organization can respond rapidly and function under extreme conditions. These plans are required by licensing and accreditation agencies. Accreditation agencies evaluate and certify organizations on specific standards or regulations. The plans must address fire, utility failures, terrorism, and natural disasters. A committee generally oversees the development and periodic revision of the plan, as well as the conduction of drills to test the training and readiness of the staff to respond (Wolper, 2004).

Nurses have a vital role in the response to these emergency situations. Patients in the hospital may need to be evacuated to a safe area or triaged based on their current status. Triage involves skilled evaluation of the patient's condition, stability, and ongoing need for treatment. In a community-wide disaster, beds in the acute care hospital will need to be made available for patients with immediate life-threatening needs. To ensure maximum bed capacity, patients may be discharged to lower levels of care or be sent home to recover. Assessment of the patient's home environment and evaluation of the competency of surrogate caregivers are essential functions of the nurse in these instances.

With the advent of the September 11, 2001, terrorist attacks in New York City and Washington, D.C., and the events surrounding the mailing of anthrax to citizens, the standards for hospital emergency planning changed dramatically:

- Hospitals have been engaged in training and readiness planning for all types of bioterrorism, which include threats of biological, chemical, or radiological exposures (Zinkovich, Malvey, Hamby, & Fottler, 2005).
- Community-wide and institutional drills are required to test and train staff members on the current plans to ensure readiness on an ongoing basis.
- Hospitals must be able to identify infections such as anthrax, smallpox, plague, and other communicable diseases as part of heightened surveillance.
- Hospitals must be aware of the worldwide concern for potential pandemics from diseases such as influenza and avian flu.
- Natural disasters, such as floods, earthquakes, fires, and storms, will trigger similar responses.

Procedures have also been put in place to handle mass casualties and to lock down facilities to prevent contamination from the environment should a chemical or radiological event occur. In the future hospitals will be required to have advanced systems and processes in place to provide for staff, patient, and community safety (Hsu et al., 2006). Disasters and bioterrorism are discussed in detail in Chapter 72 🔗.

Scientific and Technical Advancements
Telemedicine
Telemedicine refers to systems or programs that use video or computer-based equipment to link providers or to monitor patients electronically. Telemedicine was actually first given a trial in the 1930s when television technology began. Now it is used throughout the world to provide videoconferencing in a variety of health care settings. This technology is used to improve access to higher levels of care for advice and direction, especially in rural areas, prison health care, psychiatry, and home health.

Telecommunication capabilities for diagnostic imaging examinations, such as digital x-rays and computerized tomography (CAT) scans, are common in institutions. These capabilities are particularly useful for emergency departments to link physicians remotely to diagnose patient conditions or obtain specialty consultations (Heinzelmann, Lugn, & Kvedar, 2005).

Other applications for telemedicine include its use in accessing consultations in distant clinic settings, which saves the patient time and expense for travel to specialists. Through videoconferencing, physicians and technicians can engage in assessment, view procedures, and review data concurrently while communicating directly with the patient. The use of telecommunications is discussed at length in Chapter 1 🔗.

Minimally Invasive Surgery
Minimally invasive surgery depicts a surgical technique that uses laparoscopic or video equipment to perform procedures without directly opening the body's cavities. Small incisions are made to introduce probes, video devices, and instruments. The technique has been described as telemanipulation, because the surgeon is physically separated from the surgical site and operates equipment using tactile cues and intuitive dexterity (Darzi & Mackay, 2002). It has been estimated that in the near future 70% of all surgical procedures will involve minimally invasive techniques. Surgeries now being performed in this manner include removal of esophageal tumors, treatment of morbid obesity, excision of malignant liver tumors, removal of gallbladders and colon tumors, and a variety of gynecologic procedures (Fuchs, 2002). Benefits of minimally invasive surgery include reduced pain, quicker return to oral intake, and less scarring. This results in shorter hospitalizations and an increased use of outpatient centers for these procedures (Robinson & Stiegmann, 2004).

Robotics
Robotics used in surgery is described as computer-controlled manipulators that have artificial sensory abilities. These manipulators can be programmed to perform surgical tasks using tools or instruments (Satava, 2004). Surgical robots are used passively to consistently hold a position or to actively move instruments in the surgical area. Benefits of the use of robotics include minimized surgical trauma, improved precision, decreased invasiveness, and fewer complications. It is also estimated that patients recover faster following the use of robotics techniques than other traditional or open procedures. Surgical procedures can be performed long distance, and the same type of robotics have been used to perform nonsurgical procedures in space (Chandra & Frank, 2003).

Robotics also is being used to perform internal examinations through the use of pills or capsules that contain video cameras and light sources. One such device, a video pill, can perform endoscopic examinations for the small and large bowel (Baines, 2003). Lastly, according to Marketing Health Services (2003), a robot has been developed to assist with some aspects of patient care. The robot can provide mobile communication and videoconferencing and will be able to transport patients and eventually to take temperatures and draw blood.

Gene Therapy
Genes are located in the nuclei of all cells and control hereditary traits and cell functions. Genes are attached end to end in long, double-stranded helical molecules of DNA. The study of genes

has been aimed at identifying them individually, their functions, how they work, and what happens when they do not work. Scientists have been able to identify the human genetic code and the sequencing of 100% of the human genome (Human Genome Project, 2008). This research is helping to determine gene function and even how to stop a gene from functioning if it produces disease or adverse conditions. Ongoing studies are focused on understanding the other elements of the biological processes of genes (Medem Medical Library, 2006).

Ethical and legal issues surround the field of gene therapy and the ongoing research in this area. Patients undergoing gene research face social dilemmas, especially if there is the potential to predict a debilitating disease. Personal conflicts may arise when disease is detected, but not yet manifested. Although gene therapy will continue to be a major part of future health research, it is extremely expensive and thus questions arise about access to therapy and payment for associated services. See Chapter 11 💿 for a complete discussion on genetics.

Inpatient to Outpatient Shift

As mentioned earlier, one overall trend in health care service is a shift from inpatient care to outpatient care settings for many procedures and treatment modalities. Even though the predicted growth of inpatient bed needs is 10% to 15% during the next decade (HCAB, 2003c) the need for more outpatient beds is even more crucial. Factors affecting this growth include population growth, aging of the population, new technologies to manage chronic diseases, and less invasive procedures, which will reduce length of stay. Specialty centers are becoming more prevalent and are offering alternatives to the acute care hospital. Outpatient settings have advantages over the hospital in that they provide increased efficiency and reduced costs per procedure. Outpatient specialty centers have been developed for spine surgery, incontinence treatment, diagnostic testing, endoscopic procedures, surgical specialties like orthopedics, and cardiac services (HCAB, 2003c).

Health Care Worker Shortages

Shortages of physicians, nurses, and other health care–related specialists are affecting the delivery of care and services in the United States and elsewhere in the world. In hospitals shortages of nurses, radiology technicians, pharmacists, medical record personnel, housekeepers, and food service personnel are becoming severe. A report released by the American Hospital Association (2006) indicated that the many open nursing positions in hospitals in the United States equate to an 8.5% vacancy rate. Nursing education programs turned away 147,000 qualified applicants in 2005 due to shortages of faculty (American Association of Colleges of Nursing [AACN], 2006).

Factors affecting the recruitment and retention of health care workers include aging of the workforce, workload concerns, pay and benefits, and the work environment (Buerhaus et al., 2005). In 2006 *Nursing Management* magazine's Aging Workforce Survey indicated that 55% of the respondents were planning on retiring before 2020. The Health Resources and Services Administration (HRSA) further indicated in an April 2006 survey it conducted that the shortfall of registered nurses will be 17% in 2010 and will grow to 36% in 2020. Hospitals are implementing strategies to retain and recruit health care staff; however, the benefits and overall effect of these strategies will not be felt for years. In addition, nursing education programs and health care service organizations are collaborating on new models for boosting the enrollment in and graduation from nursing schools (AACN, 2006; HRSA, 2006).

Hospitalist Programs

Inpatient hospital care has become a specialty for physicians, called **hospitalists**, who concentrate their practice in the acute care environment. The use of hospitalists is designed to provide 24-hour coverage for patients. Hospitalists may be contracted to provide care to inpatients by primary care physicians who do not provide inpatient care or by patients who do not have a physician at the time of hospitalization. Internists and family practice physicians are turning the care of their patients who need hospitalization over to these specialists (Freed, 2004).

The benefits of using a hospitalist program include decreases in length of stay, improved outcomes, and enhanced efficiency (Cowan et al., 2006). Continuity of care is improved, and there is increased development and adherence to clinical pathways and guidelines because the hospitalist is readily available to assess the patient's progress and make adjustments to the medical plan of care. These benefits also help to reduce inpatient costs and provide a higher level of inpatient care. Hospitalists become assimilated as part of the hospital staff, working well with the nursing staff and other providers to develop relationships and trust (Amin & Owen, 2006).

Information Technology

The growth of information management technology in health care has been an ongoing trend. New systems span the continuum of care and provide resources that are immediately available to practitioners and patients. Electronic medical records and clinical information systems that integrate departmental functions and facilitate reporting and tracking of data and observations are being increasingly used. Clinical information systems also link providers to individual patient data and appropriate clinical reference material (Harrison & Palacio, 2006). Some of these systems allow patients to schedule appointments for therapy and follow-up and also communicate with health care professionals regarding their questions or concerns.

Connections through the Internet or a telephone also are used to monitor and interact with patients who have chronic disease disorders such as heart failure and diabetes. Disease management programs are successful in reducing emergency department visits and acute admissions to the hospital. In the future most data collection and documentation will be electronic and integrated for use in caring for patients. Integrated electronic documentation is expected to improve quality, reduce costs, and enhance work flow. It also creates better clinical collaboration and fosters evidence-based decision making and the use of best practices (Halamka, 2006). Chapter 6 💿 discusses the use of electronic medical records and documentation in detail.

Demand for Quality Care

Four driving forces underlie health care system policies and decisions: cost, equity, access, and quality. Thus, quality is an important factor in public policy regarding health care delivery. Quality, the definition and interpretation of such, has become critically important as the general public has become increasingly aware of health care options and as health care moves forward in the 21st century (Marquis & Huston, 2007).

Quality Defined

Quality refers to the characteristics of and the pursuit of excellence. Excellence may be established by determining whether the outcomes compare favorably to the standards that were set. **Quality of care** is the degree to which health services for individuals and populations increase the likelihood of desired health outcomes and are consistent with current professional knowledge. Donabedian (1980) has defined health care–related quality as the balance of health benefits and harms to a patient. Quality also may be defined in terms of effectiveness and efficiency, benefits and harm, or appropriateness of care, as is the case in a service setting. It has been described as consisting of two interdependent parts: quality in fact and quality in perception. **Quality in fact** is defined as conforming to standards and meeting one's own expectations. **Quality in perception** is meeting the customer's expectations. Within the framework of continuous quality improvement, quality is defined as meeting or exceeding customer requirements. The Joint Commission has considered quality to increase the probability of desired outcomes and reduce the probability of undesired outcomes (Huber, 2006; Joint Commission, 2007).

Quality processes in which health care delivery systems engage have been categorized as quality assurance programs, quality improvement programs, total quality management, and continuous quality improvement. Each of these terms and the current state of utilization are described next in order to understand the impact of quality demands on health care delivery systems:

- Quality assurance generally refers to an organization's effort or ability to provide services according to accepted professional standards and in a manner acceptable to the patient. Quality assurance builds on quality assessment, the measurement of quality, taking evaluative action to ensure a designated level of quality (Huber, 2006). Thus, quality assurance activities are intended to guarantee or ensure quality of care. Most health care organizations do not use this interpretation of quality anymore because they do not endorse the concept that quality can be assured. The term *quality assurance* has been replaced with *quality assessment, improvement,* or *management.*

- Quality improvement programs function as organizational umbrellas that extend into many areas for the purpose of accountability to the consumer and payer. The program is a continuous, ongoing measurement and evaluation process that includes structure, process, and outcomes. The quality improvement process uses preestablished criteria and standards and then follows the evaluation of care with an appropriate change for the purpose of improvement. Thus, quality improvement is a process of attaining a new level of performance that is superior to the previous level (Marquis & Huston, 2007). Many health care organizations have endorsed the concept of quality improvement and have adopted standards of care designed to improve quality of care.

- Total quality management (TQM), sometimes called the total quality process, is a way to ensure customer satisfaction by involving all employees in the improvement of the quality of every product or service. All systems and processes are evaluated and improved. The goal of TQM is to reduce the waste and cost of poor quality. TQM has been defined as a structured system for involving an entire organization in a continuous quality improvement process targeted to meet and exceed customer expectations (Marquis & Huston, 2007; Sullivan & Decker, 2005). Many health care systems subscribe to this process of defining and measuring quality.

- Continuous quality improvement (CQI) is a process of continuously improving a system by gathering data on performance and using multidisciplinary teams to analyze the system, collect measurements, and propose changes. The four main principles are (1) a customer focus, (2) the identification of key processes to improve quality, (3) the use of quality tools and statistics, and (4) the involvement of all people and departments in problem solving (Huber, 2006; Sullivan & Decker, 2005). CQI is endorsed by many health care agencies.

With the paradigm shift from the assurance of quality to quality assessment, there has been a value shift from a focus on the provider's values to a focus on the customer's (patient's) values. At the level of the individual nurse and patient, the quality improvement process is an appraisal of how the nurse is performing in taking care of patients. At the unit level, concurrent and retrospective audits, clinical pathway variances, and other data analyses may be used to examine the process and outcomes of care (Huber, 2006).

Regulatory Agency Impact

Standard setting occurs outside the professional arena in three areas: (1) federal and state government regulation (via Medicare and Medicaid reimbursement regulations), (2) state licensure, and (3) private accreditation. All are concerned with quality, usually at a minimum level. Federal reimbursement regulations for Medicare are administered through the Centers for Medicare and Medicaid Services. Individual states promulgate Medicaid rules and regulations. They also regulate segments of the health care system, such as skilled nursing facilities or capital expenditures. Since the Joint Commission's founding in 1951, it has become the principal, but not exclusive, standard setter for health care facilities (Joint Commission, 2007).

Other major accreditation initiatives are those of the National Committee for Quality Assurance. The NCQA is the not-for-profit accrediting body for managed care organizations. The NCQA has developed a core set of 60 health plan performance measures. These measures that cover the areas of quality access, patient satisfaction, membership, utilization, and finance, as found in the 1993 version of the Health Plan Employer Data and Information Set (HEDIS). HEDIS represents a major effort to standardize and systematize the quality measurement process, thereby allowing for national comparison of performance and benchmarking. Technical quality of care, access to services, and enrollee satisfaction are measured. HEDIS measures are evaluated every 3 years, and new standards are added as appropriate. NCQA has a national database for comparison and benchmarking, referred to as the Quality Compass (NCQA, 2006).

The CMS has mandated the use of the standardized Outcome and Assessment Information Set (OASIS) for home health care for both Medicare and non-Medicare patients. OASIS is a series of questions for collecting data on the quality of home care. Clinical, financial, and administrative data are included. For all of the accreditation and regulation systems, the goals are to improve the quality of care and collect data for comparisons.

Quality Measurement

The measurement of quality is founded on several principles: Quality can be measured; quality measures results against a standard or some degree of excellence; and excellence is determined either by validating standards of care or by measuring professional actions in caring for patients. Standards essentially define quality, against which outcomes and performance are measured. Because standards establish the baseline against which an evaluation is conducted, they need to be reliable and valid. Standards take three different approaches or forms: structure, process, and outcomes (Huber, 2006):

- **Structure standards**, or measures, focus on the internal characteristics of the organization and its personnel. They answer the questions "Is a structure in place that will allow quality to exist?" and "Is the structure of the organization set up to allow quality of care?"
- **Process standards** focus on whether the activities within an organization are being conducted appropriately. Process measures focus on the behaviors of the provider of care. Process standards look at activities, interventions, and the sequence of caregiving events.
- **Outcome standards** refer to whether the services provided by the organization make any difference. They answer questions about the services that nurses provide and whether they make a difference to the patients or to the health status of the population. Outcome standards address physical health status, mental health status, social and physical functioning, health attitudes/knowledge/ behavior, utilization of services, and the patient's perception of quality care. Outcome refers to a change in the current or future health status attributed to antecedent health care and patient attributes of health care. Outcomes present the possibility of measuring the effectiveness, quality, and time allocated for care.

In measuring quality, both structure and process parameters are important, but they are not sufficient in determining whether the care made a difference or whether the patient learned, recovered, or improved his health status. It is important for the care to make a difference and that the care is not above a certain cost. In addition, measuring nursing care outcomes as related to cost would assist in establishing the value of nursing care. Chart 3–5 provides a definition of the three types of standards and examples corresponding to each.

Quality Improvement and Research Studies

Research and quality assessment/management both rely on evaluation and are applications of the problem-solving process. However, they are distinct and separate processes. Highly controlled experimental research is on one end of the spectrum, and day-to-day quality assessment evaluation is on the other. Research studies manipulate variables, may introduce new nursing

CHART 3–5	Quality Standards and Measurement Examples	
Type of Standard	**Measurement Example**
Structure standards focus on the internal characteristics of the organization and its personnel. These standards regulate the environment to ensure quality and answer the question "Is a structure in place that will allow quality to exist?"	Nursing department provides in-service opportunities for staff development. Agency will staff at least one RN for every six patient visits.
Process standards focus on whether the activities within an organization are being appropriately conducted. These standards target behaviors, activities, interventions, and the sequence of caregiving events.	A nursing assessment will be completed on each patient within 2 hours of admission. Vital signs will be taken every hour.
Outcome standards refer to whether the services provided make any difference. These standards address physical health status, mental health status, social and physical function, health attitudes/knowledge/behavior, utilization of services, and the patient's perception of care.	Ambulates without assistance. Breath sounds are clear, free of rales and rhonchi.

procedures, and may not have an immediate application to practice. In contrast, quality improvement studies do not withhold an intervention to see if it made a difference. In a quality improvement study an intervention that is not commonly accepted would not be introduced.

Quality improvement studies are necessary for the institution's patient care management. They are not designed to manipulate variables, withhold interventions, or introduce new techniques. They are designed for measuring what exists with the idea of determining how it measures against standards, so that patient care can be managed and improved. The purpose of nursing research is generalizable knowledge; the purpose of quality improvement is determining effectiveness, efficiency, and appropriateness of care. Research utilization and other research activities can contribute to quality improvement, whereas the contribution of quality assessment to the research process is through problem identification. A key challenge for the future is to integrate research, clinical practice, and evaluation methods. Chapter 8 ☞ includes a complete description of research and quality assessment.

Licensure, Regulations, and Accreditation of Health Care Organizations

Licensure refers to the process for approving a health care organization to provide medical care and services. Licensing is generally accomplished at the state level through a department of health services. The purpose of the licensure process is generally to ensure access to care and the quality of the care provided. Regulations on licensure differ from state to state as does the process for credentialing an organization. Requirements generally cover business practices, building codes, facility maintenance, aspects of safety, evaluation and planning activities, and delivery of care including the credentials and competency of employees. States also determine licensure for professionals and describe the scope of practice for various levels of caregivers.

The state agency responsible for licensing will survey the organization periodically for compliance with regulations. Regulations are rules or laws that govern delivery of care or maintenance of the facility or work environment. A compliance survey focuses on all aspects of the facility's operations in addition to the quality improvement program. State agencies are enforcement bodies that can levy fines and other restrictions on health care organizations that do not meet the intent of the regulations or show a history of deficiencies or noncompliance with requirements or the organization's own policies.

Federal and state governmental agencies regulate the delivery of health care in specific areas such as safety, facility structural requirements, and disease prevention and control. These agencies have some jurisdiction over hospitals and other health care delivery organizations to ensure compliance with standards and to assist with problems that may occur in those environments.

Occupational Safety and Health Administration

The **Occupational Safety and Health Administration (OSHA)** is an agency that oversees environmental safety. It was established under the U.S. Department of Labor by the Occupational Safety and Health Act of 1970. This agency works through federal and state partnerships to inspect and enforce safety standards in the workplace. OSHA oversees numerous health and safety requirements within health care facilities. Examples of this oversight include bloodborne pathogen control programs, control of biological hazards, ergonomic health/safety issues, and chemical and radiological safety. It also is concerned with medical equipment, mechanical maintenance, food and laundry services, and housekeeping standards.

OSHA produces guidelines and reports that help hospitals and other care facilities meet state and national regulatory standards. OSHA personnel provide consultation services on health and safety issues, and they survey or inspect facilities if complaints are received regarding regulations under their jurisdiction. If facilities do not meet OSHA regulations, the organization can be fined or have its licensure affected (OSHA, 2006).

Fire and Life Safety Standards

Health care facilities must also meet fire and life safety standards and regulations. These regulations vary by state and community. Inspections are generally made on a routine basis by the fire marshal, or other appropriate officials, to check for building code compliance and the training of staff to respond to emergency situations. Inspections also occur whenever new regulations or standards are enacted, during construction and remodeling, or after any significant structural damage. Facilities must maintain compliance with regulations or be subject to evacuation of employees and patients and possibly closure of affected areas.

Infection and Disease Control

The **Centers for Disease Control and Prevention (CDC)** is an agency under the U.S. Department of Health and Human Services. This agency focuses on protecting the health and safety of people within and outside of health care environments. The CDC accomplishes this charge through the development and application of disease prevention and control, promotion of environmental health, and education. The CDC provides guidelines and alerts, which are communicated to health care organizations usually through the infection control department of a health agency. These communications are aimed at assisting organizations with policy development, screening of patients, and reporting requirements if specific diseases are detected. The CDC responds to significant outbreaks and threats to assist health care organizations in taking appropriate actions (CDC, 2006). Chapter 20 ♋ provides a full discussion of infection control policies and procedures.

Professional Practice Oversight

Certain agencies oversee the practice of professionally licensed care providers. For example, there are professional licensing boards for physicians, nurses, pharmacists, and radiology and laboratory technicians. These boards will set the specific requirements for initial licensure, ongoing or continuing education hours and courses, the scope of practice for the particular discipline, and the disciplinary action processes should a professional act outside of the scope of practice or behavioral requirements.

The requirements may differ from state to state as to the curriculum and number of clinical hours required from educational programs and the acceptable scores for passing licensing examinations. Compliance with licensing standards is reviewed with the professional's periodic recertification or renewal of license and during surveys of the organization by regulatory and accreditation agencies. Professional practice oversight is discussed in more detail in Chapter 4 ♋.

Accreditation

Accreditation is the process of evaluating actual care delivered to patients, performance of the hospital as an organization, and the outcomes of treatment for patients. The leading accreditation body for health care providers in the United States is the Joint Commission. The Joint Commission accredits about 80% of the nation's health care organizations, which includes hospitals, home health agencies, health care networks, ambulatory care facilities, long-term care facilities, behavioral health agencies, and clinical laboratories (Joint Commission, 2006).

The concept of accreditation for health care agencies dates back to 1910 when Ernest Codman, MD, proposed a process to evaluate the outcomes of ineffective treatments. He called this concept the "end result system of hospital standardization." Several years later the American College of Surgeons (ACS) adopted this methodology to develop minimum standards for hospitals, which included on-site surveys. In 1952 the ACS forwarded this responsibility to a new organization called the Joint Commission on Accreditation of Hospitals. This organization evolved during the next 30 years and transitioned to the current expanded form of the Joint Commission (Joint Commission, 2006).

An approved accrediting body must certify hospitals and other health care organizations that want to participate in the federal Medicare and state Medicaid programs. This requirement from the CMS is termed *conditions of participation.* Through the accreditation process, organizations must develop and maintain a quality assessment and performance improvement program. Organizations also must provide ongoing monitoring of key clinical indicators and be able to demonstrate assessment of the data and appropriate actions taken to improve results (*Federal Register*, 2003).

The Joint Commission generally conducts accreditation surveys every 3 years. Prior to 2004 these surveys were prescheduled and consisted of reviewing written material provided by the health care organization on policies, procedures, and data regarding compliance with standards, and a site inspection of the organization to look at current practice and retrospectively review past practice. Beginning in 2004 a new process was implemented using a "tracer" methodology, which is designed to monitor a specific patient through his or her hospitalization and evaluate policies along with the patient's interactions and experience with all services. In 2005 the survey process initiated unannounced survey visits (Joint Commission, 2006). Standards are organized into functions of the organization, which delineate specific criteria that must be met. Chart 3–6 outlines the functional areas for which the Joint Commission has developed standards.

Hospitals also are held to the Joint Commission patient safety standards and national indicators called *core measures.* Hospital-specific data regarding compliance with these criteria are incorporated into the survey process. Hospitals are required to collect data and report performance outcomes from sets of identified core measures. Examples of current core measures categories set by the Joint Commission include acute myocardial infarction, heart failure, community-acquired pneumonia, and pregnancy and related conditions. These core measures are part of the Joint Commission's initiative focusing on the integration of outcomes and performance measurement into the accreditation process (Joint Commission, 2006).

The Joint Commission also publishes sentinel event alerts that advise hospitals of process or system failures that have resulted in significant errors. **Sentinel events** are unexpected occurrences that have the potential to cause, or actually result in, death or serious physical or psychological injury. Serious injury specifically includes loss of limb or function. The hospital must review the sentinel event alerts, then address their own policies and procedures to be sure they have measures in place to reduce risk. Examples of recent alerts from the Joint Commission include prevention of fires in surgical areas, misadministration of concentrated potassium chloride, and prevention of ventilator-related infections and deaths. The alerts contain a root-cause analysis that defines actual causes of errors or events that threaten patient and staff safety. Risk reduction strategies are provided to assist hospitals with policy and procedure development to prevent error (Joint Commission, 2006).

■ Legal Aspects of Health Care

Having an understanding of the legal aspects of health care is important for the staff nurse's role of advocacy for patients and their families. Laws and regulations that guide practice and guard the rights of patients can be complex and change frequently. Nurse practice acts that define the scope of nursing responsibility and expectations for the delivery of care support the nurse's role in meeting legal requirements for communication with patients/families, reporting and recording of observations related to patients' conditions and their safety, and the limitations of practice for each discipline caring for the patient.

Nurses are held accountable for their performance within the scope of their practice. It is imperative that nurses be familiar with the policies and procedures of their organization and maintain competency as defined by those standards. Should a nurse fail to perform appropriately, the nurse could be held subject to malpractice or negligence claims. Health care organizations provide malpractice insurance to cover staff performing under the professional standards of those of the organization. It is generally recommended that professionals also carry personal malpractice insurance to cover any risks outside of their employment area. Chapter 4 ☜ includes a discussion of the legal principles that guide nursing practice.

Nurses also have a role in the management of problems or risk in the health care environment. **Risk management** encompasses the identification of real or potential risks to employees, patients, and the public. Real or potential risks usually are formally identified through the use of incident or unusual occurrence reports. These reports are submitted by any individual who identifies a problem or risk. The forms used assist with gathering important data about the issue and help with follow-up investigation and resolution of the issue. Hospitals have formalized risk management programs that create comprehensive

CHART 3–6	The Joint Commission's Hospital Standards	
Section	**Standards**
1. Patient-focused functions	• Ethics, rights, and responsibilities
	• Provision of care, treatment, and services
	• Medication management
	• Surveillance, prevention, and control of infection
2. Organization functions	• Improving organization performance
	• Leadership
	• Management of the environment of care
	• Management of human resources
	• Management of information
3. Structures with functions	• Medical staff
	• Nursing

Source: © Joint Commission Resources (2006). Hospital Accreditation Standards. Oakbrook Terrace, IL: Joint Commission on Accreditation of Healthcare Organizations. Available at http://www.jointcommission. Accessed October 21, 2006. Reprinted with permission.

plans for preventing risk and taking appropriate actions when adverse events take place. Risks to an organization can also be financial in nature related to business failures, property damage, and the resulting liability for negative patient outcomes (Grohar-Murray & DiCroce, 2003).

Advance Directives

Advance directives are instructions individuals can give, in advance of a health problem, to guide caregivers in the event the individuals are no longer able to speak for themselves. Advance directives were enhanced with the federal Patient Self-Determination Act of 1989, which was implemented in December 1991. This act requires that individuals under Medicare and Medicaid be provided with information about their rights to determine health care decisions. It was the intention of this legislation to increase the use of advance directives, thus improving appropriateness of care and ensuring the patient's right to make decisions (American Medical Association, 2006; Salmond & David, 2005).

With advancements in medical knowledge and technology, end-of-life decisions have become more and more complex. For patients who are considering making decisions regarding medical care, there are three possible goals: cure, stabilization of functioning, and preparing for a comfortable and dignified death. These goals may change over a person's lifetime depending on the status of the individual's health and age. Advance directives can be used at any time to establish a plan to meet goals regarding medical care. For example a young, healthy person may establish an advance directive to guide decisions should she suffer an irreversible condition following a catastrophic event. Another person who has been diagnosed with a potentially terminal disease may document choices about pain management, terminal care, or life-sustaining measures. Advance directives can be changed as the individuals needs and goals change. Chart 3–7 discusses the differences between the various types of advance directives.

Patient and Caregiver Issues and Concerns

The nurse should be aware of certain issues and concerns for patients establishing advance directives and the ability to have them carried out. First, not all health care professionals are comfortable or knowledgeable about advance directives and sometimes fail to discuss this aspect of care with the patient. The nurse should query patients regarding any discussions or decisions they may have made. If a patient has not dealt with this issue, it should be brought to the attention of the attending health care professionals. A lack of formal education, barriers to communication, or personal opinions may also interfere with the process. Not all patients wish to be fully informed about their diagnosis or condition. It may be helpful to determine the patient's preferences for receiving information (Keating, Nayeem, Gilmartin, & O'Keeffe, 2005). The patient or family can be given a referral to appropriate resources such as social services to aid them in understanding these issues.

Second, cultural or situational factors may influence an individual's decision about executing an advance directive. This seems to be more prevalent in the younger, healthy population than in the elderly or those dealing with disabilities or chronic illness (Rosnick & Reynolds, 2003). Although considerable information has been presented to the public about advance directives, a significant number of individuals have not followed

CHART 3–7   Types of Health Care Advance Directives

Type of Directive	Key Points
Health care advance directive	Documented instructions about your health care if you cannot speak for yourself. *Written:* Witnessed document, which requires the individual's signature and those of the witnesses. *Oral:* Instructions given to the individual's physician during the course of treatment, illness, or stay in a hospital. This directive is documented in the patient's medical record.
Living will	Formal written documents that communicate the wishes of the individual about life-sustaining medical treatments should she become terminally ill. They are dependent on the caregiver's willingness to follow the wishes stated and they may have no legal effect.
Health care power of attorney, durable health care power of attorney	Legal document that establishes a surrogate decision maker to make medical treatment decisions for the individual should he become incapacitated.
Do-not-resuscitate order	Organizations will usually have policies that describe resuscitation orders and options. These can be implemented by the patient surrogate or family telling the physician, by an advance directive, or by a durable power of attorney for health care.

Sources: Data from American Association of Colleges of Nursing. (2006). *Nursing shortage resource.* Retrieved December 15, 2006, from http://www.aacn.nche.edu; Healthguide. (2006). *Advance directives.* Retrieved October 21, 2006, from http://www.healthguide.org; Stein, J. (2003). The ethics of advance directives: A rehabilitation perspective. *American Journal of Physical Medicine and Rehabilitation, 82*(2), 152–157.

through to complete the process. For those dealing with disabilities or chronic illness, knowledge about treatments and alternatives is necessary before the individual can articulate appropriate choices, including the desire to have an advance directive. For example, an individual may need to choose among palliative care, aggressive chemotherapy, or refusing treatment altogether. In the latter case, an advance directive should be executed.

Third, the advance directive may not be present at the time it is needed due to an emergency situation, or the patient may not have given a copy of it to the health care provider. Patients should be encouraged to have documents readily available in their home to guide prehospital caregivers, such as emergency medical technicians (EMTs), should they respond to an emergency situation for the patient. The documentation contained within the patient's medical record and the placement of the advance directive in the record affect the ability of the physician and other caregivers to use the information at critical times (Williams & Haywood, 2003).

In some situations family members may disagree with the treatment plan and the patient's stated wishes. This can present an ethical dilemma for the nurse in advocating for the patient and assisting the family through appropriate decision making. At this point the nurse should seek consultation with the health care provider and an administrative representative of the organization regarding a plan of action.

If the patient is not able to advocate for himself, the case may need to be referred to social services or the appropriate committee within the organization for discussion and counsel. Bioethics or biomedical ethics involves obtaining relevant factual information, assessing its reliability, identifying moral problems, and recommending alternative solutions to problems that have been identified. In medicine this specifically relates to problems identified with making decisions about a patient's care and treatment. The bioethics process in most hospital organizations includes a committee or an ad hoc group that can quickly assemble to review a case and provide advice and counsel on a course of action. A case conference with the caregivers, family, and patient, if appropriate, can be called to discuss openly all of the facts. Nurses can be integral to this process because they may have firsthand knowledge of the patient's wishes or can offer information regarding the patient's present condition. Health care providers are obligated to follow an advance directive or the patient's wishes regarding care and treatment. If there is any doubt or conflict it should be referred to the appropriate authority for resolution (Williams & Haywood, 2003).

- *It is the nurse's responsibility to know the policies and procedures for identifying and referring a bioethical issue.*
- *The nurse must manage disputes regarding the patient's care and treatment plan and assist to diffuse situations that may be detrimental to the patient's immediate environment.*
- *The nurse should notify the health care provider and the organizational leadership when disputes arise.*
- *The nurse must be prepared to participate in conferences to discuss a case and advocate for the patient per her assessment and knowledge of the patient's wishes.*

Documentation and Legal Requirements

Health care directives are legal in all states, but the requirements for their content and authorization may differ. An advance directive has two parts: appointment of an agent or surrogate decision maker and specific instructions about care and treatment preferences. The patient has the option to complete either or both parts. Most states have legal forms and witnessing requirements. An advance directive can be canceled or changed at any time. If an advance directive is changed, all copies of the previous directive should be destroyed and replaced with the new ones to avoid confusion. In the acute care setting, the nurse has a key role in ensuring that documentation has been done regarding the presence of a directive, actions taken if no directive is available, and any ongoing issues regarding the status of the patient's wishes.

Nursing responsibilities include:

- *Query the patient regarding the existence of an advance directive.*
- *Document the existence in the medical record:*
    a. *If there is a prestanding directive from a previous admission, the nurse should query the patient regarding any changes and confirm the date of the directive.*
    b. *If the patient is submitting the document to a health care provider for the first time, it should be placed in the medical record per policy.*
    c. *If the patient has a directive, but did not bring it with him, it should be documented as such and efforts should be made to have the document brought in as soon as possible.*
- *If the patient wishes to make an oral directive, the health care provider should be notified.*
- *After discussion with the patient, the health care provider must document in the medical record the results of the discussion with the patient.*
- *If the patient does not have a directive, information should be given to the patient and, if appropriate, a referral made to a resource such as social services. The actions taken should be clearly documented in the medical record.*

Legal Aspects of Documentation

Documentation of patient care and interactions is important for many aspects of health care. For example, it provides a vehicle for communication between health care providers, promotes continuity of care, meets insurance requirements, ensures compliance with regulations, and helps create a health history for the patient. Clear documentation also assists with accurate coding of the patient's care and treatment process for appropriate billing and maximum reimbursement for the organization. Chapter 6 🌐 provides detailed information on nursing documentation.

Nursing documentation is critical from a legal perspective to describe the care the patient received and the actions taken by the caregivers. It is estimated that nurses spend 13% to 28% of their time on documentation (Clancy, Delany, Morrison, & Gunn, 2006). Studies have shown, however, that nursing documentation sometimes fails to provide a clear record due to the following reasons:

- Lack of understanding of the importance of documentation for medical and legal reasons
- Time constraints on care delivery and the time needed for documentation
- Discrepancies between observations and their interpretation from the patient's, nurse's, or other caregiver's perspectives.

Other documentation issues include the redundancy of information on multiple forms and the location of records in multiple places, inconsistent and irregular systems, and a lack of standardization in how information is written (Taylor, 2003).

Trends in Documentation

To address concerns with documentation, several initiatives have been advanced over time, including charting by exception, interdisciplinary assessment forms, and computerized documentation systems. These models or systems are aimed at saving nursing time and reducing redundancy in the patient's medical record.

One major trend in health care documentation is the implementation of clinical information systems. These systems allow documentation by multiple providers to be retrieved from a central database or repository. Information is consistent and readily available 24 hours a day, 7 days per week. Systems can also allow care to be summarized and trends in data to be detected over time. An additional benefit is the ability to conduct quality and outcome studies concurrently and retrospectively directly from the data repository (Doyle, 2006).

The Medical Record

The patient's medical record is a legal document that is the property of the institution providing care and services to the patient. Patients do, however, have a right to view and copy their records and enter their own information into them as they see fit. Care providers are legally required to compile and maintain an accurate record of a patient's care and treatment. This is important to guide ongoing care needs and to support decisions and actions taken should litigation occur.

Health care licensing agencies and accreditation bodies have established standards and requirements for adequacy and completeness of records as well as where they are stored and how long they must be kept. During health care organizational surveys to evaluate performance, the legibility, currency, and completeness of medical records are scrutinized (Wolper, 2004). The content and sequencing, or order, of medical records fall under general guidelines that are organization specific. Documentation or entries in the medical record should accurately reflect the care provided and any events that occur during the course of hospitalization or treatment.

- *The patient should be clearly identified on each record form or upon accessing the record electronically. This will prevent errors in charting that could lead to care decisions that may harm the patient.*
- *Observations should be objective and factual. Opinions regarding care or decisions are not appropriate for the legal record.*
- *Entries should be accurate and legible using only approved terms and abbreviations. It is essential that other caregivers be able to translate the information and for the caregiver to be able to accurately recall the information he has entered.*
- *Observations should be entered as close to the time they occurred as possible. This prevents loss of information and makes critical information available to others who may assume care of the patient.*
- *All entries should be authenticated with the name and title of the caregiver.*

Health Insurance Portability and Accountability Act

The **Health Insurance Portability and Accountability Act (HIPAA)** became law in 1996. The intent of this act was to improve health insurance portability and continuity of coverage for individuals. The three central goals of this law are (1) to create standards and a framework for health information, (2) to prevent inappropriate access to health information, and (3) to give patients control over their health information and how it is used.

In December 2001 the Administrative Simplification Compliance Act became law. Its goal is to add administrative efficiencies into the transmission of health information by standardizing electronic transactions. These laws affect almost every aspect of health care and have required organizations to make significant changes in the way they conduct business and provide patient care (Banks, 2006; Department of Health and Human Services [DHHS], 2006).

Impact of HIPAA Standards

Organizations must take the implementation of and compliance with HIPAA standards seriously. Penalties for noncompliance—whether intentional or unintentional—are assessed. Unintentional violations may result in fines of up to $25,000 for each incident. Intentional violations can result in imprisonment of up to 10 years and fines of $250,000 (HIPAAcomply, 2007).

The implementation of HIPAA impacts the delivery of nursing care in many ways. Nurses must be educated regarding the details of the regulations and the policies governing their specific health care organization. All health care providers are held individually responsible for preventing indiscriminate or unauthorized review or disclosure of personal information, medical or otherwise, from any source the patient has expressly prohibited. The guiding principle for caregivers is the "minimum necessary" rule, which means that the information disclosed will be only that which is minimally required for the specified purpose. Patients will be asked to make known their preferences about disclosure at the time of admission or when beginning a relationship with a health care provider (DHHS, 2006).

Case Management

Case management is an approach to coordinating care for patients in the hospital or in an outpatient setting. The Case Management Society of America (CMSA) defines case management as a collaborative process that assesses, plans, implements, coordinates, monitors, and evaluates the options and services required to meet an individual's health needs, using communication and available resources to promote quality, cost-effective outcomes. This occurs across a continuum of care and addresses ongoing individual needs (CMSA, 2006). Acute care hospitals generally have case management services that provide oversight and management of discharge planning, social services, and utilization review. Chart 3–8 provides an overview of key functions of the components of hospital-based case management.

CHART 3–8	Components of Hospital-Based Case Management
Component	**Key Functions**
Discharge planning	• Assess discharge needs.
	• Coordinate referrals.
	• Assign expected length of stay.
	• Evaluate progress toward discharge.
	• Provide consultation to the patient and family on placement alternatives if appropriate.
	• Arrange for health assistance or durable medical equipment and supplies as necessary.
Social services	• Assess referral needs.
	• Assist with application for aid if needed.
	• Provide links to financial counseling/consultation.
	• Evaluate discharge environment and caregiver support.
Utilization review	• Track length-of-stay data.
	• Review resources and services used.
	• Evaluate appropriate placement and level of care.

Sources: Centers for Medicare and Medicaid Services. (2006). *Programs, guidelines and regulations.* Retrieved December 15, 2006, from http://www.cms.gov; Cohen, E. L., & Cresta, T. (2004). *Nursing case management: From essentials to advanced practice applications* (4th ed.). St. Louis: Mosby; HCAB (2003b) *HMOs' impact on health care quality.*

Focus of Case Management in the Hospital

Hospital case managers focus on potential admissions for their appropriateness in the acute care setting and on length of stay (LOS). LOS is an important measure because it is an indicator of quality and risk, and many payers limit reimbursement by benchmarked standards for hospital stays. Many institutions have implemented case management in the emergency department to assist with determining appropriate placement of patients either to admit them to the hospital or transfer them to other hospitals or levels of care. A benefit of this approach is that potentially high-risk patients can be identified early and tracked for utilization of services and special referral needs (Bristow & Herrick, 2002). Case managers also work closely with physicians and other care providers to determine ongoing needs for the patient and potential modifications to their lifestyle and home environment after discharge. This includes identifying the need for caregivers to assist the patient at home and the ability of the patient's support system to provide needed care.

Staff Nurse Case Management Responsibilities

Case managers interface with the nursing staff to help assess discharge needs and to establish a plan for discharge. Discharge planning begins when the patient is admitted and continues to be evaluated throughout the patient's stay. The interface between the staff nurse providing direct care and the case manager is crucial in assessing the need for referral to specialty services and in determining financial concerns for ongoing care and progress toward the discharge goals.

Another form of case management is performed by or on the part of the payer source for patients' medical care. It is focused on continuity of care and **repatriation**, or the return of patients to appropriate levels of care or contracted institutions. Patients with long-term needs for care such as mental health services, chronic disease management, or rehabilitation are also assigned case managers who are agents of the payer source or a contracted service for the payer (Cohen & Cresta, 2004).

Case Management by Health Plans

Case review from these nonhospital-based managers may be accomplished by telephone from a central office or by on-site reviewers. The reviewers ensure that the patient's case is progressing as expected. If the patient is not progressing, the manager may authorize continued or additional care. If the reviewer determines that the patient no longer needs hospitalization at a specific level of care, he will issue a denial of payment for services (Wolper, 2004). The institution and the payer will work through these issues via a process of case review and appeals to determine a financial outcome.

■ Summary

It is evident from both historical and current perspectives that social and economic forces influence the types and availability of health care delivery systems. Consumers are not only vulnerable to these influences, but also are in a position to dictate and determine how the future of health care should be delivered. The new consumer-driven health care model that is emerging focuses on the quality of services as well as their costs. In developing new models of health care delivery, nurses will play a key role in determining how the future evolution of health care will meet the needs of a changing society.

REVIEW QUESTIONS

1. A nurse is planning the care for a patient using the best practice approach. Which of the following best describes this approach?
   1. It integrates current research evidence with clinical expertise and patient's needs.
   2. It is a proven process that produces consistent high quality results.
   3. It offers qualitative or quantitative measurement of specific data related to reported outcome information.
   4. It focuses on collecting data about medical errors and setting standards that will reduce errors.

2. A nurse is analyzing the revenue category of the annual budget. Which of the following is a component of this category?
   1. Salaries/wages
   2. Supplies
   3. Overhead
   4. Volume

3. When preparing to change a patient's dressing, the nurse has several choices for supplies. Which of the following would be the most cost effective choice for the nurse to make?
   1. Use some supplies that have already been charged to another patient.
   2. Select supplies that can be used over a period of time for less cost.
   3. Select the supplies the patient needs making sure there are supplies left over for the next dressing change.
   4. Create a dressing changing area within the patient's room that is fully stocked with multiple supply items so everyone can use the supplies at any time.

4. Individuals from an accrediting body arrive at a health care organization, requesting to conduct a "tracer" visit. The accrediting body is most likely:
   1. OSHA.
   2. The Joint Commission.
   3. The CDC.
   4. The state board of nursing.

5. A patient tells the nurse that he has a paper that says that his wife is supposed to make decisions about his health care if he becomes unable to do so himself. This patient is describing:
   1. Living will.
   2. Oral advance directive.
   3. Health care power of attorney.
   4. Written advance directive.

Answers for review questions appear in Appendix D

KEY TERMS

accreditation *p.58*
case management *p.62*
Centers for Disease Control and Prevention (CDC) *p.58*
Emergency Medical Treatment and Labor Act (EMTALA) *p.51*
evidence-based practice *p.52*
for-profit (proprietary) organization *p.51*
health care delivery system *p.45*
Health Insurance Portability and Accountability Act (HIPAA) *p.62*
health maintenance organization (HMO) *p.49*

horizontal organizational model *p.46*
hospitalist *p.55*
independent practice association (IPA) *p.49*
Institute of Medicine (IOM) *p.53*
Joint Commission *p.53*
Leapfrog Group *p.53*
licensure *p.57*
Medicaid *p.47*
Medicare *p.47*
not-for-profit organization *p.51*
Occupational Safety and Health Administration (OSHA) *p.58*
outcome standards *p.57*

preferred provider organization (PPO) *p.49*
process standards *p.57*
quality *p.56*
quality in fact *p.56*
quality in perception *p.56*
quality of care *p.56*
repatriation *p.63*
risk management *p.59*
robotics *p.54*
sentinel event *p.59*
structure standards *p.57*
telemedicine *p.54*
vertically integrated models *p.46*

REFERENCES

Abramson, S. M., & Tyler, D. (2006). Margin alert: Time to revisit your outpatient strategy. *Healthcare Financial Management, 60*(4), 106–108, 110, 112–113.

American Association of Colleges of Nursing. (2006). *Nursing shortage resource.* Retrieved December 15, 2006, from http://www.aacn.nche.edu

American Hospital Association. (2006). *Healthcare consumer research.* Retrieved December 10, 2006, from http://www.aha.org

American Hospital Association. (2007). *Guide to the health care field—2007 edition* (page A3). Chicago: Author.

American Medical Association. (2006). *Resources/standards, policy statement on provision of life-sustaining medical treatment.* Retrieved December 15, 2006, from http://www.ama-assn.org

Amin, A. N., & Owen, M. M. (2006). Productive interdisciplinary team relationships: The hospitalist and the case manager. *Lippincott's Case Management, 11*(3), 160–164.

Baines, E. (2003, April 14). Pill-sized robot is reinventing endoscopy. *General Practitioner.*

Banks, D. L. (2006). The Health Insurance Portability and Accountability Act: Does it live up to the promise? *Journal of Medical Systems, 30*(1), 45–50.

Barber, J., Koch, K. E., Parente, K., Mark, J., Davis K. M. (1998). Evolution of an Integrated Health System: A Life Cycle Framework. *Journal of Healthcare Management, 43*(4), 361–375.

Bristow, D. P., & Herrick, C. A. (2002). Emergency department case management: The dyad team of nurse case manager and social worker improve discharge planning and patient and staff satisfaction while decreasing inappropriate admissions and costs: A literature review. *Lippincott's Case Management, 7*(6), 243–251.

Buerhaus, P. I., Donelan, K., Ulrich, B. T., Norman, L., Williams, M., & Dittus, R. (2005). Hospital RNs' and CNOs' perceptions of the impact of the nursing shortage on the quality of care. *Nursing Economics, 23*(5), 214–221.

California HealthCare Foundation. (2004). *Preventing unnecessary hospitalizations in Medi-Cal: Comparing fee-for-service with managed care.* Retrieved February 13, 2007 from University of California San Francisco's Primary Care Research website: http://www.chcf.org/topics/medi-cal

Case Management Society of America. (2006). *What is case management?* Retrieved February 13, 2007, from http://www.cmsa.org

Centers for Disease Control and Prevention. (2006). *Guidelines and alerts.* Retrieved December 15, 2006, from http://www.cdc.gov

Centers for Medicare and Medicaid Services. (2006). *Programs, guidelines and regulations.* Retrieved December 15, 2006, from http://www.cms.gov

Centers for Medicare and Medicaid Services. (2007). *Brief summaries of Medicare*Medicaid, Title XVIII and Title XIX of the Social Security Act as of November 1, 2007.* Retrieved January 23, 2008, from http://search.cms.hhs.gov/search?q+Ependitures+2002+reference&site=cms_collection&...

Chandra, A., & Frank, Z. D. (2003). Use of robotics in health procedures—Are we ready for it? *Hospital Topics, 81*(1).

Clancy, T. R., Delany, C. W., Morrison, B., & Gunn, J. K. (2006). The benefits of standardized nursing languages in complex adaptive systems such as hospitals. *Journal of Nursing Administration, 36*(9), 426–434.

Cohen, E. L., & Cresta, T. (2004). *Nursing case management: From essentials to advanced practice applications* (4th ed.). St. Louis: Mosby.

Cowan, M. J., Shapiro, M., Hays, R. D., Afifi, A., Vazirani, S., Ward, C. R., et al. (2006). The effect of a multidisciplinary hospitalist/physician and advance practice nurse collaboration on hospital costs. *Journal of Nursing Administration, 36*(2), 79–85.

Darzi, A., & Mackay, S. (2002). Recent advances in minimal access surgery. *British Medical Journal, 324*(7328).

Donabedian, A. (1980). *Explanations in quality assessment and monitoring: The definition of quality and approaches to its assessment* (Vol. 1). Ann Arbor, MI: Health Administration Press.

Dower, C. (2002). *Status of changes in patient care delivery: How can we meet demand for health care workers?* San Francisco: The Center for the Health Professions, University of California, San Francisco.

Doyle, M. (2006). Promoting standardized nursing language using an electronic medical record system. *AORN Journal, 83*(6), 1336–1342.

Federal Register. (2003). Medicare and Medicaid programs; hospital conditions of participation: Quality assessment and performance improvement final rule. *68*(16), 3435–3455.

Finkler, S. A., & Kovner, C. T. (2000). *Financial management for nurse managers and executives.* Philadelphia: W. B. Saunders.

Freed, D. H. (2004). Hospitalists: Evolution, evidence, and eventualities. *Health Care Management, 23*(3), 238–256.

Fuchs, K. H. (2002). Minimally invasive surgery. *Endoscopy, 3*(42), 154–159.

Fuchs, R. J., Berenholtz, S. M., & Dorman, T. (2005). Do intensivists in ICU improve outcomes? *Best Practice and Research. Clinical Anaesthesiology, 19*(1), 125–135.

Grohar-Murray, M. E., & DiCroce, H. R. (2003). *Leadership and management in nursing.* Upper Saddle River, NJ: Pearson Prentice Hall.

Halamka, J. (2006). The perfect storm for electronic health records. *Journal of Healthcare Information Management, 20*(3), 25–27.

Harris, C. M., Burns, J., Gregorich, T., Kall, G., Piar, P. M., Miller, H. D., et al. (2003). Managing technology in a complex healthcare delivery system. *Journal of Healthcare Information Management, 17*(2), 37–41.

Harrison, J. P., & Palacio, C. (2006). The role of clinical information systems in health care quality improvement. *Health Care Management, 25*(3), 206–212.

Health Care Advisory Board. (2003b, March 25). *HMOs' impact on health care quality* (pp. 1–4).

Health Care Advisory Board. (2003c, July 9). *Rising costs place financial burden on patients and employers.*

Health Resources and Services Administration. (2006). *What is behind HRSA's projected supply, demand, and shortage of registered nurses?* Retrieved December 15, 2006, from http://hrsa.gov

Heinzelmann, P. J., Lugn, N. D., & Kvedar, J. C. (2005). Telemedicine in the future. *Journal of Telemedicine and Telecare, 11*(8), 384–390.

HIPAAcomply. (2007). *HIPAA FAQs.* Retrieved February 13, 2007, from http://www.hipaacomply.com

Hsu, E. B., Thomas, T. L., Bass, E. B., Whyne, D., Kelen, G. D., & Green, G. B. (2006, March 20). Healthcare worker competencies for disaster training. *Biomedical Central Medical Education,* pp. 6–19.

Huber, D. (2006). *Leadership and nursing care management* (3rd ed.). Philadelphia: W. B. Saunders.

Human Genome Project. (2008). Frequently Asked Questions. Retrieved April 26, 2008, from http://www.ornl.gov

Institute of Medicine. (1999). *To err is human: Building a safer health system.* Retrieved October 21, 2006, from http://www.iom.edu

Joint Commission on Accreditation of Healthcare Organizations. (2006). *Hospital accreditation standards.* Retrieved October 21, 2006, from http://www.jointcommission

Joint Commission on Accreditation of Healthcare Organizations. (2007). *Setting the standard.* Oakbrook Terrace, IL: Author.

Keating, D. T., Nayeem, K., Gilmartin, J. J., & O'Keeffe, S. T. (2005). Advance directives for truth disclosure. *Chest, 128*(2), 1037–1039.

Leapfrog Group. (2006). *Patient safety initiatives.* Retrieved October 21, 2006, from http://www.leapfroggroup.org

Malloch, K., & Porter-O'Grady, T. (2006). *Introduction to evidence-based practice in nursing and healthcare.* Sudbury, MA: Jones and Bartlett.

Marketing Health Services. (2003). *Robots to the Rescue*, Summer 2003: 23(2).

Marquis, B. L., & Huston, C. J. (2007). *Leadership roles and management functions in nursing theory & application* (5th ed.). Philadelphia: Lippincott Williams & Wilkins.

Medem Medical Library. (2006). *Gene therapy.* Retrieved December 15, 2006, from http://medem.com

McKinley, A. (2005, December 31). Health care providers and facilities: Health facilities—2005 (End of year issue brief). *Issue Brief Health Policy Tracking Service*, pp. 1–10.

Nathans, A. B., Rivara, F. P., Mackenzie, E. J., Maier, R. V., Wang, J., Egleston, B., et al. (2006). The impact of an intensivist-model ICU on trauma-related mortality. *Annals of Surgery, 244*(4), 545–554.

National Committee for Quality Assurance. (2006). *Measurement improves healthcare quality for 70 million American's, but gaps remain.* Retrieved November 2, 2006, from http://ncqa.org

National Quality Forum. (2006). *Health care quality measurement and reporting.* Retrieved October 21, 2006, from http://www.qualityforum.org

Occupational Safety and Health Administration. (2006). *Safety and health regulations and guidelines.* Retrieved December 15, 2006, from http://www.osha.gov

Richard, S. A., Rawal, S., & Martin, D. K. (2005). An ethical framework for cardiac report cards: A qualitative study. *BioMedical Central Medical Ethics, 28*(6), E3.

Robinson, T. N., & Stiegmann, G. V. (2004). Minimally invasive surgery. *Endoscopy, 36*(1), 48–50.

Rosenbaum, S. (1998). Negotiating the new health system: Purchasing publicly accountable managed care. *American Journal of Preventive Medicine, 14*(3S), 67–71.

Rosnick, C. B., & Reynolds, S. L. (2003). Thinking ahead: Factors associated with executing advance directives. *Journal of Aging and Health, 15*(2), 409–429.

Salmond, S. W., & David, E. (2005). Attitudes toward advance directives and advance directives completion rates. *Orthopaedic Nursing, 24*(2), 117–127.

Samuel, T. W., Raleigh, S. G., Hower, J. M., & Schwartz, R. W. (2003). The next stage in the health care economy: Aligning the interests of patients, providers, and third-party payers through consumer driven health care plans. *American Journal of Surgery, 186*(2),117–124.

Satava, R. M. (2004). Future trends in the design and application of surgical robots. *Seminars in Laparoscopic Surgery, 11*(2),129–135.

Scalise, D. (2005). Building a consumer-directed service culture. *Hospitals and Health Networks, 79*(12), 53–59.

Shortell, S., & Kaluzny, A. D. (2005). *Health care management: Organization design and behavior* (5th ed.). Clifton Park, NY: Delmar Cengage Learning.

Sullivan, E. J., & Decker, P. J. (2005). *Effective leadership & management in nursing* (6th ed.). Upper Saddle River, NJ: Pearson Prentice Hall.

Taylor, H. (2003). An exploration of the factors that affect nurses' record keeping. *British Journal of Nursing, 12*(12), 751–754, 756–758.

U.S. Census Bureau. (2002). *National population projections summary tables.* Retrieved May 19, 2004, from http://www.census.gov/population/www/projections/natproj.html

U.S. Department of Health and Human Services. (2006). *Medical privacy—National standards to protect the privacy of personal health information.* Retrieved December 15, 2006, from http://www.hhs.gov

Werner, R. M., & Asch, D. A. (2005). The unintended consequences of publicly reporting quality information. *Journal of the American Medical Association, 293*(10), 1239–1244.

Williams, M. A., & Haywood, C., Jr. (2003). Critical care research on patients with advance directives or do-not-resuscitate status: Ethical challenges of clinician-investigators. *Critical Care Medicine, 31*(3), 167–171.

Wolper, L. F. (2004). *Health care administration: Planning, implementing, and managing organized delivery systems* (4th ed.). Sudbury, MA: Jones and Bartlett.

Woolf, S. H., Johnson, R. E., & Geiger, H. J. (2006, October 31). The rising prevalence of severe poverty in America, a growing threat to public health. *American Journal of Preventive Medicine*, No. 4, pp. 332–341.

Zinkovich, L., Malvey, D., Hamby, E., & Fottler, M. (2005). Bioterror events: Preemptive strategies for healthcare executives. *Hospital Topics, 83*(3), 9–15.

4

Ethical and Legal Guidelines for Nursing Practice

Ginny Wacker Guido and Annita Watson

Outcome-Based Learning Objectives

After studying this chapter, the learner will be able to:

1. Explain how ethical theories and principles influence nursing practice in a clinical setting.
2. Identify and apply the steps of the MORAL model in ethical decision making.
3. Compare and contrast the three distinct structures that ethics committees demonstrate in health care institutions.
4. Explain how the state nurse practice act governs and guides nursing practice.
5. Distinguish among the types of laws that typically affect nursing practice: common, civil, tort, contract, and criminal.
6. Identify the six elements of malpractice law as described in the chapter.
7. Discuss the importance of standards of care and how they are differentiated between internal and external standards.
8. Distinguish between regional and national norms.
9. Identify the three most common intentional torts and three most common quasi-intentional torts seen in health care settings and explain the defenses against them.
10. Explain the doctrine of informed consent as it relates to the use of implied consent in nursing settings.
11. Explain actions that the nurse may take to avoid or prevent possible liabilities.

Research   Collaboration   Health Promotion   Nursing Process   Caring   Critical Thinking

THIS CHAPTER highlights the continuing influence that ethical and legal concepts have on the professional practice of nursing. Professional accountability and responsibility continue to gather additional prominence, especially as nurses become more autonomous and practice settings expand from acute care facilities to community, ambulatory, and long-term settings and as consumers of health care become more knowledgeable about their rights and options for care.

It is not sufficient, though, to know and understand ethical and legal concepts. Nurses must blend these important aspects with competent, skilled nursing diagnoses and interventions. To perform this high-quality nursing care, nurses must also understand the concepts of critical thinking and clinical judgment, for without these latter concepts one is not able to fully appreciate the application of legal and ethical concepts in professional practice settings. Thus, this chapter first explores ethics and legal concepts and issues that impact professional nursing practice and concludes with a section on critical thinking and clinical judgment. Knowing about and using these concepts and issues moves nursing from merely a "hands-on" skills performance role to that of a truly professional practice.

Ethics and Nursing

Ethics is the science relating to moral actions and individual value systems. It is the systematic study of what a person's conduct and actions ought to be with regard to self, other human beings, and the environment. Many nurses envision ethics as dealing with principles of morality and what is right or wrong (Yoder-Wise, 2007). Applied ethics requires application of normative ethical theory to everyday problems. Normative ethical theory for each profession provides the foundation and filter from which ethical decisions are made (Marquis & Huston, 2006). Thus, from a nursing perspective, a broader conceptual definition of ethics is that ethics is concerned with motives and attitudes and the relationship of these attitudes to the overall care of the individual. It is the justification of what is right or wrong, and the study of what one's life and relationships ought to be, not what they are (Marquis & Huston, 2006).

Morality concerns the social nature of the community, codes of behavior, and community expectations (Hall, 2000; Perle, 2004). Morality provides the means for ascertaining if certain actions are right or wrong and whether the consequences of actions are good or bad. Thus, morals are ways of behaving to accomplish ethical practices. Ethics is the broader, more reflective endeavor and begins when a person goes beyond the acceptance and internalization of traditional rules, or normative behaviors, of the social group. The ultimate goal of ethics is to provide a reasoned and best solution to situations that arise in everyday clinical practice.

As a beginning step in the application of ethics to everyday clinical practice, nurses should first determine the essential or underlying issue. Does the issue concern a situation that the patient or the patient's family views as wrong, such as the discontinuance of nonextraordinary life-support measures? For many, the removal of a feeding tube that is delivering to the patient essential fluids and nutritional support would be considered a violation of a moral duty. Or does the issue involve a treatment or therapy that could or could not be instituted, such as whether to initiate full life-support measures in a geriatric patient who is terminally ill?

The implementation of ethics is internal to one's self, looks to the good of an individual rather than society as a whole, and concerns the "why" of one's actions. Ethics asks questions about motives and actions. Why did the person act as she did and what was the final outcome of acting as she did? Was the outcome satisfactory to the individual?

Ethical Theories

Many different ethical theories have evolved to justify existing moral principles. These theories are considered normative because they describe the norms or standards of behavior and value that are ultimately applied to daily life. Normative ethics concerns human actions and the outcomes of those actions. Most normative approaches to ethics fall under the three broad theoretical categories discussed next.

Deontological Theories

Deontological (from the Greek *deon*, or "duty") **theories** derive norms and rules from the duties human beings owe to one another by virtue of commitments made and roles assumed. Generally, deontologists hold that a sense of duty consists of rational respect for the fulfilling of one's obligations to other human beings, rather than looking at the rewards of one's actions. The greatest strength of this theory is its emphasis on the dignity of human beings. Deontological theory looks not to the end or consequences of an action, but to the intention of the action. It is one's good intentions, the intentions to do a moral duty that ultimately determine the praiseworthiness of the action.

Duty-based, rights-based, and intuitionist ethical reasoning derive their framework from deontological theory. Deontological ethics have sometimes been subdivided into situation or "love" ethics, wherein the decision making takes into account the unique characteristics of each individual, the caring relationship between the person and the caregiver, and the most humanistic course of action given the circumstances (Butts & Rich, 2005). Examples of this theory in action in the health care setting abound when making these types of decisions:

- Decisions about forgoing life-sustaining treatment that may conflict with religious beliefs
- Decisions not to pursue aggressive treatment while waiting to see what outcome God wants or trusting that conservative treatment will work if God so intends

- Decisions to bow to a higher order, given by divine command, such as in the case of Jehovah's Witnesses, who do not ingest blood and, therefore, refuse blood transfusions even if they will lose their lives or the lives of their children (DeWolf-Bosek & Savage, 2007).

Teleological Theories

Teleological (from the Greek *telos*, for "end") **theories** derive norms or rules for conduct from the consequences of actions. Right consists of actions that have good consequences, and wrong consists of actions that have bad consequences. Teleologists disagree, though, about how to determine the goodness or badness of the consequences of actions. Teleological theories support decisions that favor the common good. An alternate way of viewing this theory is that the usefulness of an action is determined by the amount of happiness it brings. An example of a decision using this approach is that of allowing individual family members to make the difficult choices for their loved ones rather than mandating that all patients in persistent vegetative states must be given parenteral nutrition.

This theory frequently is referred to as utilitarianism; what makes an action right or wrong is its utility, and useful actions bring the greatest amount of happiness and satisfaction into existence (Butts & Rich, 2005). Teleological theories are used to support utilitarianism. Utilitarian ethics can be subdivided into rule and act utilitarianism. Rule utilitarianism seeks the greatest happiness for all; it appeals to public agreement as a basis for objective judgment about the nature of happiness. Act utilitarianism tries to determine in a particular situation which course of action will bring about the greatest happiness, or the least harm and suffering, to a single person. As such, act utilitarianism makes happiness subjective, basing decisions on what is the best for the greatest number of people (Guido, 2006; Marquis & Huston, 2006).

Principlism

A third ethical theory has slowly been evolving over the past 25 years and, although not yet given the full status of a theory, it does assist nurses and health care providers who are struggling with difficult ethical issues. Called **principlism**, this emerging theory incorporates existing ethical principles and attempts to resolve conflicts by applying one or more of those ethical principles (Beauchamp & Childress, 2001). Ethical principles actually control ethical decision making much more than do ethical theories, since principles encompass the basic premises from which rules are developed. Principles are moral norms that nurses demand and strive to implement daily in clinical settings. In the case of principlism, four principles form the basis for decision making: respect for autonomy, nonmaleficence, beneficence, and justice. Each of the principles can be used individually, although it is much more common to encounter two or more ethical principles used in concert or to see two or more principles coming into conflict in a specific patient situation.

Ethical theories are important because they form the essential base of knowledge from which to proceed. Without ethical theories, decisions revolve around personal emotions. Because most health care providers do not ascribe to either deontology or teleology exclusively, principlism is growing in popularity among health care professionals in today's society.

Ethical Principles

There are eight ethical principles that nurses encounter when making decisions in clinical settings. Chart 4–1 outlines these principles and gives a short definition for each principle.

Autonomy

The principle of **autonomy** addresses personal freedom and the right to choose what will happen to one's own person. The legal doctrine of informed consent is a direct reflection of this principle. Autonomy involves health care deliverers' respect for patients' rights even if the health care deliverer does not agree with the decisions made. For example, autonomy issues often arise when parents of young children refuse immunizations. Most health care deliverers would advocate for their need in preventing possible complications should the child later be exposed to what could have been a preventable disease.

Beneficence

The principle of **beneficence** states that the actions a person takes should promote good. In caring for patients, good can be defined in many ways, including allowing a person to die without advanced life support and in the company of loved ones. Good may prompt the nurse to encourage the patient to undergo extensive, painful treatment procedures especially if these procedures will increase both the quality and quantity of life. Good also may extend to the patient's family by prompting family members to leave a patient's bedside so that they can get some needed rest.

Nonmaleficence

The corollary of beneficence, the principle of **nonmaleficence**, states that a person should do no harm. Many nurses find it difficult to follow this principle when performing treatments and procedures that bring discomfort and pain to patients. Health care providers often use the concept of a detrimental-benefit analysis when the issue of nonmaleficence is raised. Using this analysis, the focus of the projected treatment or procedure is on the consequences of the benefits to the patient and not on the harm that occurs at the time of the intervention. For example, the nurse may use this analysis when medicating a postoperative patient. Even though the injection causes some level of discomfort and suffering, the overall benefit is less postoperative pain. A second example is the need to change and reapply dressings for patients who have sustained severe burns. Though extremely painful, not performing this needed intervention would cause more serious complications for the patient. Thus, the principle of nonmaleficence may be chosen because even pain and suffering can bring about a desirable outcome for the patient.

Veracity

Veracity concerns truth telling and incorporates the concept that individuals should always tell the truth. This principle also compels that the truth be told completely. Nurses and other health care providers exemplify this principle when they give all of the facts of a situation truthfully and then assist patients and their loved ones to make appropriate decisions. For example, patients must be told of all options in terms that they can understand and then be allowed to make their own decisions.

The principle of veracity compels health care members to fully inform patients about all aspects of care, both the desirable effects as well as the more negative effects. Without the entire truth, patients cannot make informed choices. This also is true of nursing management. For instance, a manager who believes deception is morally acceptable if it is done with the objective of beneficence may tell all rejected job applicants that they were highly considered, whether they had been or not. Another management example is that of the nurse manager who, in the event of a low patient census (i.e., a slow period on a unit), relays all of the options to staff and lets them make their own decisions about floating to other units, taking vacation time, or taking a day without pay, contingent on agency policy.

Justice

Justice concerns the issue that persons should be treated equally and fairly. This principle usually arises in times of short supplies or when there is competition for resources or benefits. This principle most often is considered when patient census is high and two patients are equally qualified to be cared for in a specific unit, such as an intensive care or cardiac care unit, or when there is an organ available for transplantation and two patients are equally appropriate candidates for the organ transplant.

Justice also demands that the same quality of care be given to all patients, regardless of their ethnicity, socio-economic status, or lifestyle. Thus, the health care team must be vigilant concerning decisions that are made about why one candidate would be the more appropriate recipient of an available transplant organ and how the care of the second potential recipient will be delivered. Acceptable reasons for selecting one candidate over a second potential recipient could be compliance with recommended therapies and the supportive role of family members.

Paternalism

The principle of **paternalism** sometimes referred to as parentialism, allows one to make decisions for another and often has been viewed as a negative or undesirable principle. Used appropriately, however, paternalism assists persons to make decisions when they do not have sufficient data or expertise to make a decision. Staff members frequently use some degree of paternalism when they assist patients and their family members to decide if surgical procedures should be undertaken or if medical management is a better option. Paternalism becomes undesirable when the entire decision is taken from the patient or family member.

CHART 4–1	**Ethical Principles**
Principle	**Definition**
Autonomy	Personal freedom, right of self-determination
Beneficence	Duty to perform good actions
Nonmaleficence	Duty to prevent harm from occurring
Veracity	Truth-telling
Justice	Fairness, treating all equally
Paternalism	Allows another to make decisions for individual patients
Fidelity	Duty to keep one's promises and commitments
Respect for others	Duty to treat all respectfully and without prejudice

Fidelity

Fidelity means keeping one's promises or commitments. Staff members know not to make promises to patients that they may not be able to keep, such as assuring the patient that no code will be performed before consulting with the patient's physician for such an order or that the patient will be able to return home at a specific time frame. Fidelity also prevents health care deliverers from promising that the patient will be given sufficient pain medication after a surgical procedure so that the patient is totally pain free. Rather, nurses reinforce that such freedom from pain is a goal that the health care team will work to achieve.

Hamric (2002) suggests that it is helpful to view the "nurse in the middle" phenomenon from a fidelity perspective. Although nurses have multiple fidelity duties to the patient, physician organization, profession, and self that at times may conflict with one another, the American Nurses Association (ANA) Code of Ethics is clear than one duty "dominates" over all others, namely, the nurse's commitment to the patient.

Respect for Others

Many think the principle of **respect for others** is the highest principle and incorporates all other principles. Respect for others acknowledges the right of individuals to make decisions and to live by these decisions. Respect for others also transcends cultural differences, gender issues, and racial concerns. Nurses positively reinforce this principle daily when giving competent nursing care to all patients for whom they care. Nurses also reinforce these principles when they incorporate Watson's (2003) theory of caring into their interactions with patients and peers. For example, caring for a very demanding, verbally abusive patient is difficult, and nurses might elect not to be as attentive to her needs as a patient who is pleasant and cooperative. The principle of respect for others, however, demands that appropriate and competent care be given to both patients.

Ethical Decision Making

In clinical practice, ethical principles differ among the individuals involved in patient care settings. Frequently, the ethical principles and values of family members differ from patients' values or from health care providers' values. For example, an elderly, but independent patient may value his independence and ability to remain in an independent living situation (autonomy), whereas his family and the staff caring for him may feel that he needs closer supervision and desire that the patient be relocated to an assisted living center (beneficence). Resolving such issues is the goal of understanding ethical dilemmas and ethical decision making.

Ethical Dilemma

When such disagreements occur, an ethical dilemma emerges. **Ethical dilemmas** by definition involve two or more unfavorable alternatives to a given situation. For example, in the preceding scenario, the elderly gentleman may be at risk for injury when living by himself at his home, but his ability to be independent will be hampered by living at an assisted living center. One means of addressing such situations is to use ethical decision-making models. **Ethical decision making** involves asking the following questions:

1. Who should make the choices?
2. What are the possible options or courses of action?
3. What are the available and reasonable alternatives?
4. What are the consequences, both positive and negative, of all possible options?
5. Which rules, obligations, and values should direct the choices?
6. What are the desired goals and outcomes in the given situation?

When making decisions, health care providers must use an orderly, systematic, and objective method to find the best solution. Various ethical decision-making models are available to assist with ethical decision making. These models are based on a process of steps and vary from 5 to 20 steps, depending on the specific model. The decision maker moves from step to step in an attempt to decide the best course of action given the specifics of the situation. Perhaps one of the easiest ethical decision-making models to use in clinical settings is the **MORAL model** (Thiroux, 1977). The MORAL model was developed by Thiroux (1977) and then subsequently, applied to nursing situations. Since that time, the MORAL model has been further refined and utilized by Crisham (1990). The MORAL model of decision making is shown in Chart 4–2.

Ethical decision making is always a process and the steps of the process remain fluid and flexible. As health care providers

---

CHART 4–2	**MORAL Model of Ethical Decision Making**

The letters of the acronym remind users of the steps of the model

Acronym Request	Example	
M	Massage the dilemma.	Issues are identified and defined, taking into consideration the value systems and principles of all major players in the dilemma.
O	Outline the options.	Options are fully examined, including those that are less realistic.
R	Resolve the dilemma.	Issues and options are reviewed and basic ethical principles are applied to each of the identified options. A decision is made concerning the plan of action that will be taken.
A	Act by applying the chosen option.	Requires implementation by all members of the health care team and family members.
L	Look back and evaluate.	Process of reviewing and reexamining whether desired outcomes were attained and whether new options need to be implemented.

move through any model's various steps, they may find that they need to return to a previous step and redefine the issue or that a major player's values were not taken into consideration when making the final decision. Sufficient time must be allowed for making decisions so that all players in the dilemma reach a conclusion that they can support.

Accountability and responsibility for making ethical decisions varies depending on the dilemma encountered. For the ethical decisions that must be addressed on a daily basis, such as helping family members understand the full extent of their loved one's prognosis or assisting a patient with understanding why a nurse cannot give more pain medication when the patient continues to have pain, the nurses working directly with the patients are generally responsible for these ethical dilemmas. For issues that involve the entire health care team, such as assisting family members to determine if a feeding tube should be placed for nutritional support in an elderly patient who is terminal, the hospital ethics committee is generally responsible for making such decisions.

 It is not uncommon in the practice of nursing to encounter situations in which a patient and family members must make decisions about lifesaving measures: Should they or should they not be used? The resulting conflict may compromise how nurses choose to provide care to the patient/family and how that care is rendered, keeping in mind that the nurse has an ethical duty to provide the minimum standard of care. It is essential that nurses know what resources are available to them in the agency where they work to help them solve this dilemma and meet the normal standard of care for the given situation.

Ethics Committees

With the increasing complexity of ethical issues in health care, ethics committees have been created to assist in making ethical decisions in clinical settings. Ethical committees can:

1. Provide structure and guidelines for potential problems.
2. Serve as an open forum for discussion and debate.
3. Function as a patient advocate by placing the patient at the core of the committee's deliberations.

Committee Structures

Ethics committees generally follow one of three distinct structures, though in some institutions these structures are blended. The autonomy model facilitates decision making for the competent patient. The patient benefit model uses **substituted judgment** (what the person would have done if she were capable of making a decision) and facilitates decision making for the incompetent patient. The social justice model considers broad social issues that may arise within the institution; in this model, many ethics committees hold ethical grand rounds.

Ethical grand rounds usually are conducted on a monthly basis and allow staff members to begin to be more involved in ethical decision making by presenting cases that involve a variety of ethical issues. The purpose of ethical grand rounds is to assist health care providers with future ethical decision making by making them more knowledgeable about ethical principles and the MORAL model. For example, presenting the case of the elderly gentleman who desires to remain in his own home rather than move to an assisted living center helps nurses to fully ex-

amine both sides of the issue. The nurses are then able to more quickly and competently address this same type of issue in the future. Such case presentations also allow nurses to become more fully versed on both sides of controversies and better understand their own ethical values and principles.

Legal Concepts in Nursing

Legal concepts are equally important as ethics concepts in forming a framework for practice in health care settings. A general definition of **law** is that it concerns rules and regulations by which a society is governed. These rules and regulations are made by individuals and are capable of being changed or modified. Legal issues differ from ethical issues in that laws are external to the individual because they entail the rules and regulations of society as a whole, and laws are concerned with one's conduct and actions as opposed to the motives and values of the individual. The question asked is "What did the person do or fail to do?" rather than "Why did the person act as he did?" Finally, the enforcement of laws is much stronger that enforcement of ethics; laws are enforced through courts of law, statutes, and state boards of nursing.

Sources of Law

The most basic source of law is constitutional law, which is a system of fundamental laws or principles for the governance of a nation, society, or other aggregate of individuals. Statutory laws are those rules and regulations enacted by the legislative branch of the government. Nurses are usually familiar with this source of law because the nurse practice act is an example of statutory law. Administrative laws are enacted through the decisions and rules of administrative agencies, which are specific governing bodies charged with implementing selected legislation. When statutory laws are enacted, administrative agencies are given the authority to implement the specific intentions of the statutes, creating rules and regulations that enforce the statutory law. Boards of nursing are examples of administrative law agencies. Finally, judicial laws are created by courts of law, interpreting legal issues that are in dispute.

All laws, regardless of origin, are subject to change. Constitutional laws may be amended; statutory laws may be amended, repealed, or expanded; administrative agencies may be dissolved, expanded, or redefined; and judicial laws may be modified or completely altered by subsequent court decisions.

Nurse Practice Acts

An example of statutory and administrative law is the state nurse practice act. The state **nurse practice act** is the single most important piece of legislation for nursing because the practice act affects all aspects of nursing practice. The act defines nurses' **scope of practice**, those actions and duties that are allowable by a profession, and establishes standards for nurses in a given state or territory. Requirements for licensure and entry into practice, empowerment of a board of nursing to oversee practice, and means for disciplinary action are part of the nurse practice act. The act is the law within the state or territory, and state boards of nursing cannot grant exceptions, waive the act's provisions, or expand practice outside the act's specific provisions.

Nurse practice acts typically define three categories of nurses: licensed practical or vocational nurses, licensed registered nurses, and advanced practice nurses. The nurse practice act, in concert with common law, sets educational and examination requirements, provides for licensing by individuals who have met these requirements, defines the functions of each category of nurse, and may include a section on mandatory continuing education hours for renewal of licenses. Additionally, nurse practice acts state any exceptions that may occur, such as that nursing students may function in clinical settings as an exception to required licensure. The state nurse practice act also may include help for those affected by addiction, for example, diversion programs for registered nurses with drug and alcohol and mental illness problems. Many acts also provide assistance for nurses undergoing rehabilitation for a chemical dependency.

Individual differences in nurse practice acts among states are seen. For instance, some states have separate acts for licensed practical or vocational nurses and some states do not define advanced practice roles. Five states have separate boards for the licensing of practical or vocational nurses and registered nurses: California, Georgia, Louisiana, Texas, and West Virginia.

Each state practice act establishes a board of nursing. This board ensures enforcement of the act, regulation of those who come under its provisions and prevention of those not addressed by the act from practicing nursing, and protection of the public. Qualifications for board members, terms of office, and specific duties of board members are defined in the state practice act.

Although the nurse practice act is a statutory law, judicial law may become involved in its application. The application of judicial law actually helps define the meaning of the act for practicing nurses. In selected court decisions, the interpretation of the nurse practice act has assisted nurses in understanding the full application of the law. For example, landmark court cases in 1983 upheld the right of nurses to practice as advanced nurse practitioners (*Sermchief v. Gonzales*) and in 1985 allowed a board of nursing to set educational standards for advanced nurse practitioners (*Bellegie v. Board of Nurse Examiners*).

Nurses should be aware that when courts or legislatures expand the nurse's role, the legal accountability of nurses also increases. Thus, nurses have an obligation to continually remain current on issues that affect their practice. Means of remaining current include reading professional nursing journals, accessing the state board of nursing website for changes in the state nurse practice act, and being active in professional nursing organizations. Many states require mandatory continuing education in order to renew the registered nurse license.

Divisions or Types of Law

There are different types or divisions of law that affect nursing practice. Each type or division of law uses different processes to determine guilt or innocence.

Common and Civil Law

Common law, which initiated in England, is a system of law that is derived from judges' decisions (which arise from the judicial branch of the government), rather than statutes or constitutions (which are derived from the legislative branch of government)

(Garner, 2004). Common law is derived from principles rather than rules and regulations. Common law is based on justice, reason, and common sense. It represents law made by judges through decisions in specific cases. These case-by-case decisions are used again and again in similar cases, thereby becoming customary or "common" to all people living under the authority of the court of law. Common law in modern America continues to be the product of generations of judicial decisions. Principles that govern the use of human subjects in research and the composition and function of an institutional review board are examples of common law (DeWolf-Bosek & Savage, 2007).

Civil law, or continental law, is the predominant system of law in the world. In contrast to common law, civil law was promulgated after the French Revolution in France and is based on rules and regulations that became normative principles. These normative principles are codified in codes and statutes. In countries with civil law, legislation is seen as the primary source of law. By default, courts thus base their judgments on the provision of codes and statutes from which solutions in particular cases are to be derived. The terms *common law* and *civil law* often are used interchangeably to describe law that affects individuals rather than state entities. However, the main difference is that common law draws abstract rules from specific cases, whereas civil law starts with abstract rules, which judges must then apply to the various cases before them (Guido, 2006). Common and civil law are divided into a variety of legal specializations, including tort law and contract law (Guido, 2006).

Tort Law

Nurses are more likely to become involved in civil litigation rather than criminal litigation. Such litigation usually comes under the category of tort law. A tort is a wrongful act committed against another person or the person's property. These wrongful acts result in an injury or harm, thereby, constituting the basis for a claim by the injured party. Although some torts are crimes punishable by imprisonment, the primary aim of **tort law** is to provide relief for the damages incurred and to deter others from committing the same harms. The injured person may sue for an injunction to prevent the continuation of the tortuous conduct or for monetary damages (Stanford Encyclopedia of Philosophy, 2003). Examples of such tort actions include negligence, malpractice, assault and battery, false imprisonment, defamation, invasion of privacy, and breach of confidentiality. Each of these types of actions is covered in subsequent sections.

Lawsuits involving tort law usually are broken down into intentional, nonintentional, or quasi-intentional wrongs. **Intentional torts** are those that occur when the person acting knew or should have known a wrong would result from his conduct. A **nonintentional tort** is a wrong that would result from a person's negligent conduct. A tort becomes **quasi-intentional** when intent is lacking, but there is a volitional or willful action and direct causation.

Contract Law

Contracts are promises that the law will enforce. Contract law is that which governs the formation of these promises or agreements between two or more parties, in relation to a particular subject. Contracts can cover a broad range of matters, including the sale of goods or real property, the terms of employment or of an independent contractor relationship, the settlement of a dispute, and ownership of intellectual property developed as part of a work for hire (Larson, 2003). The law provides remedies if a promise is breached or recognizes the performance of a promise as a duty. Contracts arise when a duty does or may come into existence because of a promise made by one of the parties. To be legally binding as a contract, a promise must be exchanged for adequate consideration. Adequate consideration is a benefit or determinant that a party receives which reasonably and fairly induces them to make the promise (i.e., contract).

Contracts are mainly governed by state statutory and common (judge-made) law and private law. Private law principally includes the terms of the agreement between the parties who are exchanging promises. This private law may override many of the rules otherwise established by state law. Statutory law may require some contracts to be put in writing and executed with particular formality. In certain situations, the parties may enter into a binding agreement without signing a formal written document. Typically, in order to be enforceable, a contract must involve the following elements: mutual consent, offer and acceptance, mutual consideration, performance or delivery, good faith, and no violation of public policy. Given these stipulations it is important to remember that an agreement, or contract, between parties can be a verbal agreement. This is referred to as an oral contract.

 Though an oral contract is legal, it can be very difficult to prove that an oral contract exists. Absent proof of the terms of the contract, a party may be unable to enforce the contract or may be forced to settle for less than the original bargain. Thus, even when there is no opportunity to draft a formal contract, it is always good practice to put something in writing, signed by both parties, to capture the key terms of an agreement.

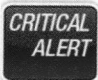 *Because contracts are promises that the law will enforce, the law provides remedies if a promise is breached or the court recognizes the performance of a promise as a duty. Consider these very good reasons to avoid breaching a contract:*

- *Your business or professional reputation could be damaged.*
- *You could sever your business or professional relationship with the other party.*
- *You could be sued. If sued, you could be forced to spend valuable time away from your business or practice in order to respond to factors of litigation: discovery requests, depositions, court appearances.*
- *You could incur legal fees.*
- *You could be ordered by the court to perform your obligations under the contract. If you do not obey the court's order, you could be held in contempt of court, fined, and/or imprisoned.*
- *You could be forced to pay money damages to the nonbreaching party, in an amount that puts that party in as good a position as it would have been in were it not for the breach.*
- *You could be forced to pay punitive damages, which are not limited by the amount of the other party's losses and can be very significant.*
- *You could end up spending much more time, money, and mental and physical energy resolving the breach than you would have spent performing your obligations under the contract.*

Criminal Law

Criminal law, sometimes called public law, refers to laws that affect the state in its political capacity and that affect society as a whole. Criminal law involves prosecution by the government of a person for an act that has been classified as a crime. This is in contrast to a civil case, which involves individuals and organizations seeking to resolve legal disputes. In a criminal case, the state, through a prosecutor, initiates the suit; whereas in a civil case, the victim brings the suit. A crime is any act or omission to act that violates public law either in forbidding or commanding it. Most crimes are established by local, state, and federal governments; thus, criminal laws vary from state to state. Criminal law may be divided into misdemeanors, or lesser crimes, and felonies, or more serious crimes that involve fines of more than $1,000 and are punishable by prison terms of greater than 1 year or death.

Sources of Civil and Criminal Litigation for Nurses

Nurses and other health care professionals may become involved with either the civil or criminal justice systems. The most frequent means by which a nurse incurs criminal action is by failure to renew one's nursing license in a timely manner. Once a nursing license has expired, the nurse is then practicing nursing without a license, which is a direct violation of state nurse practice acts. Other actions against nurses that are examples of criminal law frequently involve substance abuse, particularly if the nurse is illegally acquiring medications from clinical settings (e.g., when patients' prescribed narcotics are diverted to support a nurse's substance abuse and the patients are given placebos instead). Less frequently, nurses have been charged with either intentionally or unintentionally causing the death of a patient.

Negligence and Malpractice

Negligence and malpractice are the common terms for nonintentional torts. **Negligence** is the commission of an act that a reasonable and prudent person would not perform or the omission of something that a reasonable and prudent person would do in a given situation. In these situations reasonableness is described as acceptable and according to common sense or normal practice. It connotes sensibility and rational thought. Negligence thus denotes conduct that is lacking in care and is usually seen as carelessness on the part of the care provider.

Malpractice, sometimes referred to as professional negligence, evolves from negligence law and the premise that all individuals are responsible for the consequences of their actions or inactions (Negligence, 2007). It refers to any misconduct or lack of skill in carrying out professional responsibilities in a reasonable and prudent manner. Issues of malpractice have become increasingly important to the nurse as the authority, accountability, and autonomy of nurses have increased. As roles have expanded, nurses have begun performing duties traditionally reserved for medical practice. As a result of an increased scope of practice, many nurses now carry individual malpractice insurance, which is considered by some to be a double-edged sword. Nurses need malpractice insurance because of their expanded role, but they also incur a greater likelihood of being sued if they have malpractice insurance, because insured parties tend to seek damages from as many individuals with financial resources as possible (Marquis & Huston, 2006). The National Practitioner Data Bank reveals that the number of malpractice payments made by nurses has increased during the past several years and the trend shows no sign of stopping (Croke, 2003).

In all liability suits, there is a plaintiff and a defendant. In malpractice cases, the plaintiff is the injured party and the defendant is the professional who is alleged to have caused the injury. Essentially, six elements must be presented in a successful malpractice suit; all of these factors must be proven before the court will find liability against the nurse and/or institution (Guido, 2006). These six elements are duty owed the patient, breach of the duty owed the patient, foreseeability of harm, causation, injury, and damages. Chart 4–3 outlines these elements in greater detail and each of these elements is further expanded in the subsections that follow.

Elements of Malpractice

To understand how the law applies each element of malpractice to specific court cases, we use the following scenario: A nurse employed by a state medical center has been assigned to care for Mr. Gee, a patient admitted for a right hip replacement. Mr. Gee is 89 years old, weighs 255 pounds, is in relatively good health, and is competent mentally. He is to have surgery tomorrow and requires assistance in ambulating to and from the bathroom. While caring for Mr. Gee, the nurse fails to obtain the assistance of a second person when walking Mr. Gee to the bathroom, and he falls. Mr. Gee sustains a broken left hip and a mild concussion. He will be hospitalized for several additional days because he must now undergo bilateral hip replacement and physical therapy. Additionally, he will spend 2 days in the neurological step-down unit because of the concussion.

Duty Owed the Patient

The first element of malpractice is duty owed the patient and involves both the existence of the duty and the nature of the duty. That a nurse owes a duty of care to a patient is usually not hard to establish. Often this is established merely by showing the valid employment of the nurse within the institution. The more difficult part is the nature of the duty, which involves standards of care that represent the minimum requirements that define acceptable practice (internal standards). In the preceding scenario,

the applicable standard of care is taken from the institution's policy and procedure manual and concerns the standard of care owed the elderly patient regarding safety issues. In this instance, the specific standard of care relates to the need for two attendants to safely assist Mr. Gee to the bathroom. Standards of care are established by reviewing the institution's policy and procedure manual, the individual's job description, and the practitioner's education and skills, as well as the pertinent standards as established by professional organizations, journal articles, standing orders and protocols, and national and community expectations (or standards) for this type of care.

Several sources can be used to determine the applicable standard of care. The American Nurses Association, as well as a cadre of specialty organizations, publishes standards for nursing practice. The overall framework of these external standards is the nursing process. In 1988, the ANA first published its standards for nurse administrators, a series of nine standards incorporating the responsibilities of nurse administrators across all practice settings. Since that time, additional standards have been published that describe nursing care for a variety of patient populations and in selected nursing settings (ANA, 2001). A list of current ANA nursing practice standards is shown in Chart 4–4 (p. 74). Accreditation standards, especially those published yearly by the the Joint Commission (2007), also assist in establishing the acceptable standards of care for health care facilities.

Breach of the Duty Owed the Patient

The second element of malpractice is breach of the duty of care owed the patient, or failure to meet the standard of care. Once the standard of care has been established, the breach of or failure to provide the standard of care is often easy to show. But establishing the standard of care may be difficult because the various parties to the suit may not be able to agree on the applicable standard of care, depending on whether the injured party or the hospital's attorney is trying to establish the standard of care for the given circumstances. The injured party will attempt to show that the acceptable standard of care is a higher standard

CHART 4–3 Elements of Malpractice and Examples of Nursing Actions That May Result in Malpractice

Element	Explanation	Examples of Nursing Actions
Duty owed the person	Care should be given under the circumstances (what the prudent nurse would have done).	Failing to monitor a patient for postoperative bleeding
Breach of duty owed the patient	Not giving the care that should be given under the circumstances.	Failing to observe and report changes in a patient's condition
Foreseeability of harm	The nurse must have reasonable access to information about whether the possibility of harm exists.	Failing to act as a patient advocate, for example, the drug handbook specifies that the wrong route of dosage may cause injury. The nurse acts on behalf of the patient to clarify the correct route of administration.
Causation (a direct relationship exists between failure to meet the standard of care and injury and can be proven)	Patient is harmed because proper care is not given.	Failing to question an inappropriate order
Injury	Actual harm results to patient.	Failing to provide patient education and discharge planning
Damages	Based on pain and suffering, expenses, emotional damages, or malicious damages.	Giving the patient incorrect medications

ANA Nursing Standards

- Corrections Nursing: Scope and Standards of Practice
- Faith Community Nursing: Scope and Standards of Practice
- Genetics/Genomics Nursing: Scope and Standards of Practice
- HIV/AIDS Nursing: Scope and Standards of Practice
- Holistic Nursing: Scope and Standards of Practice
- Home Health Nursing: Scope and Standards of Practice
- Hospice and Palliative Nursing: Scope and Standards of Practice
- Intellectual and Developmental Disabilities Nursing: Scope and Standards of Practice
- Legal Nurse Consulting: Scope and Standards of Practice
- Neonatal Nursing: Scope and Standards of Practice
- Nursing Informatics: Scope and Standards of Practice
- Nursing: Scope and Standards of Practice
- Pain Management Nursing: Scope and Standards of Practice
- Plastic Surgery Nursing: Scope and Standards of Practice
- Psychiatric–Mental Health: Scope and Standards of Practice
- Public Health Nursing: Scope and Standards of Practice
- Radiology Nursing: Scope and Standards of Practice
- School Nursing: Scope and Standards of Practice
- Scope and Standards for Nurse Administrators, Second Edition
- Scope and Standards of Addictions Nursing Practice
- Scope and Standards of Diabetes Nursing Practice (2nd Edition)
- Scope and Standards of Gerontological Nursing Practice, 2nd Edition
- Scope and Standards of Neuroscience Nursing Practice
- Scope and Standards of Practice for Nursing Professional Development
- Scope and Standards of Vascular Nursing Practice

Source: Nursing World/Nurses online Bookstore: ANA Nursing Standards. Retrieved May 18, 2007 from http://nursingworld.org/books/pdescr.cfm?cnum=15. American Nurses Association. ANA Nursing standards, April 14, 2008 from www.nursingworld.org

of care than that shown by the defendant hospital and staff. Each of these two sides to the dispute help determine the standard of care through the testimony of expert witnesses. Expert witnesses give testimony in court to determine the applicable and acceptable standard of care on a case-by-case basis and to assist the judge and jury in understanding nursing standards of care. In the scenario involving Mr. Gee, the injured party's expert witness would quote the institution's policy manual, and the nurse's expert witness would note any viable exceptions to the stated policy.

An example case that remains the standard for the distinction in standards of care is *Sabol v. Richmond Heights General Hospital* (1996). In *Sabol*, a patient was admitted to a general acute care hospital for treatment after attempting suicide by drug overdose. While in the acute care facility, the patient became increasingly paranoid and delusional. A nurse sat with the patient and tried to calm him. Restraints were not applied because the staff feared this would compound the situation by raising his level of paranoia and agitation. The patient got out of bed, knocked down the nurse who was in his room, fought his way past two nurses in the hallway, ran off the unit, and jumped from a third-story window, fracturing his arm and sustaining other relatively minor injuries.

Expert witnesses for the patient introduced standards of care pertinent to psychiatric patients, specifically those patients hospitalized in psychiatric facilities or in acute care hospitals with separate psychiatric units. The court ruled that the nurses in this general acute care situation were not negligent in this patient's care. The court stated that the nurses' actions were consistent with basic professional standards of practice for medical–surgical nurses in an acute care hospital. They did not have, nor were they expected to have, specialized psychiatric nursing training and would not be judged as if they did.

Foreseeability of Harm

The third element of malpractice, **foreseeability of harm**, involves the concept that certain events may reasonably be expected to cause specific results. The nurse must have prior knowledge or information that failure to meet a standard of care may result in harm. The challenge is to show what was foreseeable given the facts of the case at the time of the occurrence, not when the case finally comes to court. In the given scenario, it was foreseeable that the patient could fall and harm himself if fewer than two people attempted to assist with ambulation.

Causation

The fourth element of malpractice is causation, which means that the nurse's action or lack of action directly caused the patient's harm and not merely that the patient had some type of harm. There must be a direct relationship between the failure to meet the standard of care and the patient's injury. Stated differently, causation means that it is not sufficient that a patient was harmed (Guido, 2006; Nursing malpractice, 2003)—the patient must be able to show that the nurse's action or lack of action was the direct reason for the injury that resulted. In the given scenario, Mr. Gee suffered a broken hip and a concussion as a result of his fall.

Injury

The resultant injury, the fifth element of malpractice, must be physical, not merely psychological or transient. In other words, the patient must incur some physical harm before malpractice will be found against the health care provider. In the given scenario, Mr. Gee came to harm as a direct result of ambulating to the bathroom, and he incurred the physical injuries of both a broken hip and a concussion.

Damages

Finally, the injured party must be able to prove damages, the sixth element of malpractice. The term *damages* refers to financial harm incurred by the injured party. The ability to prove damages is vital in a malpractice suit because malpractice is nonintentional and unintended. Thus, the patient must show financial harm before the courts will allow a finding of liability against the defendant nurse and/or hospital. Mr. Gee, in the given scenario, would be able to show damages that include additional hospital costs related to the second hip replacement surgery, physical therapy needs, and admission to the step-down unit. Further medical needs may arise based on these injuries, such as a need for long-term physical therapy and temporary admission to a skilled nursing facility.

Liability for Negligence by Students

Nursing students have the ultimate responsibility for their own actions and may be liable for their own negligence. Student liability holds true even if the student is not an adult under state law. The often used adage that a student practices under the instructor's license is not a true or valid statement because only the individual awarded the license practices on the license. The individual student always retains accountability, and nurse practice acts allow students to perform professional actions without being awarded a license to practice nursing, thus according them the opportunity to learn how to practice nursing.

The standard of care to which the nursing student is held is the same as that for the reasonably prudent practicing professional nurse. As such, the student and the instructor must know hospital policies and procedures and remain current in medical and nursing knowledge. The licensure exception further requires that unprepared nursing students or those who need additional supervision inform the faculty instructor of their special needs or lack of preparedness for clinical practice. Thus, nursing students remain accountable for their knowledge and skills, and faculty or staff may become accountable for individual student incompetence or lack of preparedness (Guido, 2006).

Regional and National Norms for Standards of Care

Sometimes the issue of whether standards of care follow a **regional (locality) rule** or national norm becomes an issue in courts of law. **National standards of care** are based on reasonableness and are the average degree of skill, care, and diligence exercised by members of the same profession. Such national standards mean that nurses in all settings, urban and rural, must meet the same standards when caring for patients in clinical settings.

National standards of care have slowly replaced the previously used regional or locality standard of care, which allowed the standard of care to be viewed from the perspective of care within a given geographical area or "similar community." There are two important reasons for national standards of care. With the advent of educational programs and videos, a better ability to transport individuals to national conferences or to consult in small, more rural areas, and the use of telemedicine and virtual diagnostics, all areas with health care delivery systems have access to the same information and educational opportunities. A second reason is that all patients have the right to quality health care, whether hospitalized in a small community setting or in a major medical center.

Intentional Torts

Nurses also may be found liable for intentional torts, which are generally defined as actions that violate another person's rights. In such actions, the nurse's actions must intend to interfere with the patient or property, the nurse must intend to bring about the consequences of the act, and the act must be a substantial factor in bringing about the consequences or outcomes. Note that, unlike negligence and malpractice, no actual harm is necessary for this tort; it is the violation of another person's rights that creates the cause of action. The more commonly seen intentional torts in

health care settings are assault, battery, and false imprisonment (Guido, 2006; Nursing malpractice, 2003), as discussed next.

Assault, Battery, and False Imprisonment

Assault places the patient in apprehension of being touched in an offensive, insulting, or physically injurious manner, such as when one threatens the patient with an injection or the placement of a nasogastric tube. **Battery** is the actual contact with another person or the person's property. Examples of batteries include forcing patients to ambulate against their wishes and restraining a patient so that a procedure can be implemented. For assault or battery to occur, there must be an absence of legal consent on the part of the patient.

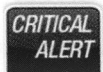 *With assault, no actual touching of the person is required; it is the fear or apprehension of being touched that constitutes the intentional tort. Thus, a nurse cannot assault a sleeping or unconscious patient, because no matter how angry or violent the nurse might be or how irrational the nurse's actions might be, the patient has no knowledge of the potential contact and is, therefore, not apprehensive of the potential contact.*

With battery, however, a single touch, regardless of how fleeting or faint, is sufficient for a tort to have occurred. The patient does not need to experience any harm, injury, or pain in order for battery to occur. Also, in contrast to assault, the patient need not be aware of the battery for tort to have occurred. Taking the pulse of a sleeping person could be considered battery. The nurse also may commit battery by the unwarranted touching of the patient's clothes or an article held by the patient, such as a purse or suitcase. For purposes of battery, anything that is connected with the patient's person is viewed as part of the person.

False imprisonment is the unjustified detention of a person without the legal right to confine the person, such as when one prevents a patient from leaving against medical advice or when nurses restrain a person in a confined space. Use of medications that alter a patient's ability to leave the health care setting can also create this tort. As with assault and battery, consent is a vital element in this tort; patients who are compromised mentally and are restrained to prevent their harm are not falsely imprisoned because consent is implied (Guido, 2006).

 The patient must be aware of the detention or restraint (the act) for a successful false imprisonment lawsuit. False imprisonment also may occur if the act is directed at the patient's family or possessions, such as keys, clothing, or a purse. Sedated patients who are incapable of realizing their confinement do not have a suit for false imprisonment. Likewise, future threats are not enough to sustain the tort of false imprisonment. It is, however, prudent to realize that state law must be followed to the letter when a person's liberty is at stake; if it is not the citizen can sue for false imprisonment.

Quasi-Intentional Torts

Tort law also recognizes quasi-intentional torts. The difference between quasi-intentional and intentional torts is that there is no intent to injure or cause distress to another person; there is, however, an intentional (volitional) action that causes injury or distress. Two quasi-intentional torts are recognized in health care settings: defamation of character and invasion of privacy, which includes the subset of breach of confidentiality.

Defamation of Character

Defamation of character, also known as libel and slander, is harming another's reputation by diminishing the esteem, respect, goodwill, or level of confidence that others have for that person. Individuals have the right to their good name. Defamation often occurs in medical record documentation, and nurses are cautioned about what and how to record patient data and descriptions in the medical record. For example, charting that a patient is a prostitute or acts "crazy" may raise potential liability issues for the nurse and agency. If there is no reason to include a statement, such as the comment about a person's lifestyle or occupation, then it should not be included in the official record. If, however, a record is needed to validate a patient's mental state or actions, the nurse should chart actual patient behaviors or statements rather than making a subjective appraisal of the patient. The nurse should state exactly what the patient said and not the nurse's interpretation of the statement. A rule that assists nurses in this area is to write in the medical record as though the patient and her family will be reading the record. The documentation should always be truthful (Nursing malpractice, 2003).

Invasion of Privacy

Invasion of privacy is a violation of a person's right to protection against unreasonable and unwarranted interference with his personal life. To show that invasion of privacy has occurred, the person must show that the nurse intruded on the patient's privacy, the intrusion would be objectionable to a prudent and reasonable person, the intrusion concerns private or unpublished facts or pictures of a private nature, and that public disclosure of private facts was made. Examples of invasion of privacy include the taking of photographs without the patient's permission, disclosure of medical facts to persons not entitled to those facts, and publishing information that misrepresents the patient's condition.

Breach of Confidentiality

Breach of confidentiality, a part of invasion of privacy, concerns facts that are presented in the medical record. The majority of the cases concerning breach of confidentiality concern privileged conversations that are included in the patient's medical record and the faxing or electronic conveyance of medical records. Health care professionals are cautioned to have procedures in place that allow for the disclosure of confidential data; the patient's written authorization to reveal selected information prevents a cause of action concerning invasion of privacy and breach of confidentiality.

Health Insurance Portability and Accountability Act (HIPAA)

A newer application of invasion of privacy is the recently enacted Health Insurance Portability and Accountability Act of 1996 (HIPAA; Public Law 104-191), which is further elaborated on in Chapters 3, 6, and 8 😊. The HIPAA regulations greatly expand the patient's right to confidentiality in all health care settings. Prior to the enforcement of this act, federal law did not protect patient confidentiality in the medical record and individual states offered only limited protection of these records.

The HIPAA legislation includes comprehensive standards regarding the transmission of medical data, administrative records, and financial records. Significant fines and penalties are included to enable enforcement of the act against those who violate its provisions, so organizations must take the implementation of and compliance with HIPAA standards seriously. Unintentional violations may result in fines of up to $25,000 for each incident. Intentional violations can result in imprisonment of up to 10 years and fines of $250,000 (HIPAAdvisory, 2006). Only "covered entities" come under the HIPAA regulations and such covered entities include health care plans that employ greater than 50 participants and who transmit health care information in an electronic format (45 *Code of Federal Regulations*, Sections 160.102 and 160.103, 1996).

One of the most important reasons for this act was the concept that patients retained a right to their medical information. Before HIPAA was enacted, information could be shared with other entities; now, patients have the right to either allow the disclosure or deny the disclosure. To ensure that medical information is protected, the act defines protected health information (PHI), which includes 18 possible identifiers that relate to the past, present, or future physical or mental health of the person. PHI includes the following: names of the individual or initials; addresses, including street, e-mail, and Internet addresses; dates, including birth dates and dates of services received; telephone and fax numbers; Social Security or other personal identification numbers; medical record numbers; health plan identification numbers; license or certificate numbers; medical device identifiers; biometric identifiers such as fingerprints or photographic images; or any other unique identifying characteristic or code (45 *Code of Federal Regulations*, Section 160.103, 1996).

The HIPAA standards limit how information will be used or shared, mandate safeguards for the protection of health information, and shift control of health information from providers to the patient. Covered health care facilities must provide patients with a document entitled Notice of Privacy Practices, which explains how the PHI will be used or shared with other entities. The document also alerts patients to the process for complaints if they determine that their information rights were violated. Chart 4–5 provides a concise overview of the components of the HIPAA.

Consent

Generally, the health care provider's right to treat a patient, barring true emergency conditions or unanticipated occurrences, is based on a contractual relationship that arises through the mutual consent of parties to the relationship. This relationship is formed when the health care provider performing the therapy or treatment provides the patient with needed information and the patient voluntarily consents to the therapy or treatment. This fulfills the provisions of contracts: (1) agreements made between two or more persons or entities for the performance of an action; (2) mutual understanding of the terms and meanings of the contract; (3) compensation in the terms of something of value; and (4) fulfillment of a lawful purpose (Guido, 2006). This concept is discussed under the previous section on contract law and in Chapter 6 😊.

Consent is the voluntary authorization by a patient or the patient's legal representative to do something to the patient. It is based on the mutual consent of all parties involved, and the key to true and valid consent is patient comprehension. Consent may be given orally or in writing. Unless state law mandates written consent, the law views oral and written consent as

CHART 4–5	Overview of HIPAA

Provision	Requirements
Electronic data interchange	• Implement standardized transactions, which includes forms and content. • Implement use of standard code sets for documenting care, drugs, and services. • Implement use of individual and unique identifiers for the patient, the provider, and the insurance plan.
Security	• Develop administrative policies and procedures. • Provide physical safeguards for health information. • Provide technical security and mechanisms for health information.
Privacy	• Limit disclosure of information to appropriate sources. • Define information use and authorization for access to health information. • Establish business associate agreements.

Sources: HIPAA privacy rule and public health. Guidance from CDC and the U.S. Department of Health and Human Services. (2003). *Morbidity and Mortality Weekly Report, 5*(2; Suppl), 1–17; Indian Health Service. (2008). HIPAA. Retrieved April 18, 2008, from http://www.ihs.gov/Adminmngrresources/HIPAA/index.cfm.

CHART 4–6	Information Necessary for Informed Consent

1. A brief, but complete explanation of the treatment or procedure to be performed.
2. The name and qualifications of the person who will perform the procedure and, if others will assist, the names and qualifications of those assistants.
3. An explanation of any serious harm that may occur during the procedure, including death if that is a realistic outcome. Pain and discomforting side effects both during the procedure and following the procedure also should be discussed.
4. An explanation of alternative therapies to the procedure or treatment, including the risk of doing nothing at all.
5. An explanation that the patient can refuse the therapy or procedure without having alternative care or support discontinued.
6. The fact that the patient can still refuse, even after the procedure or therapy has begun. For example, all of the suggested radiation treatments need not be completed.

Informed Consent

Consent, technically, is an easy yes or no: "Yes, I will allow the surgery" or "No, I want to try medications first, then maybe I will allow the surgery." The law concerning consent in health care situations is based on informed consent. The doctrine of **informed consent** has developed from negligence law as the courts began to realize that although consent may have been given, not enough information was imparted to form the foundation of an informed decision. Informed consent mandates to the physician or independent health care provider the separate legal duty to disclose needed material facts in terms that the patient can reasonably understand so that the patient can make an informed choice. There should also be a description of the available alternatives to the proposed treatment and the risks and dangers involved in each alternative. Failure to disclose the needed facts in understandable terms does not negate the consent, but it does place potential liability on the practitioner for malpractice. To be informed, the patient must receive, in terms he can understand and comprehend, specific information (American Medical Association, 2007), as shown in Chart 4–6.

Nurses may become involved in the process of obtaining informed consent in one of several ways. When one realizes that consent must be obtained for all procedures and treatments, not just medical procedures, one realizes the vast impact of this doctrine. This does not mean that nurses have to obtain written consent each time they give an injection or turn a patient. Most nursing interventions rely on oral expressed consent or implied consent that may be readily inferred through the patient's actions.

What the doctrine of informed consent means is that nurses must continually communicate with patients. What it also means is that the patient's refusal to allow a certain procedure must be respected. If the patient is unable to communicate, permission may be derived from the patient's admission to the hospital or obtained from the patient's legal representative.

A second way to enhance understanding is to allow time between the actual giving of information and when the patient

equally valid. As a precaution, health care providers should recognize that oral consent is much more difficult to prove should consent or lack of consent become a legal issue. As a convenience and to prevent such court issues, most health care institutions require written consent, primarily for invasive procedures, surgical interventions, and selected medication regimes.

Consent becomes an important issue from a legal perspective in that the patient may sue for a battery (unconsented touching) if she does not consent to the procedure or treatment and the health care provider goes ahead with the procedure or treatment. This means that the patient may bring a lawsuit and be awarded damages even if the patient was helped by the procedure or treatment. The more current trend, though, is to argue consent under a negligence or malpractice cause of action because generally the patient has given consent for the procedure, an adverse outcome has occurred, and the issue of consent is argued secondary to the adverse outcome (harm) that occurred.

The right to consent and the right to refuse consent are based on a long-recognized, common law right of persons to be free from harmful or offensive touching of their bodies. Consent is not contingent on a request for information or clarification by the patient, but must be actively given by health care providers.

Consent may be obtained in a variety of ways. Perhaps the easiest means of obtaining informed consent is when the consent is expressed. Expressed consent is consent given by direct words, either written or oral. For example, after the nurse informs the patient that she is going to start an intravenous infusion, the patient says, "Okay, but could you put the needle in my left hand, as I am right-handed?" As a rule, expressed consent is the type most often sought and received by health care providers, particularly nurses.

must make a decision. Such time intervals allow patients to consider what has been suggested, to put into words their questions and concerns, and then make the final decision and sign the informed consent forms.

Implied Consent

Implied consent is consent that may be inferred by the patient's conduct or that may legally be presumed in emergency situations. Many patients hold out their arm and roll up their sleeve when the nurse approaches with a stethoscope and blood pressure cuff. This is an example of implied consent because a reasonable person would infer by the patient's action that she is consenting to the procedure. Or the patient extends his left shoulder for an injection after the nurse explains why the medication is being given. Nurses most often obtain implied consent for minor procedures and routine care.

Implied consent may be presumed to exist in true emergency situations and is known as the **emergency doctrine**. For such consent, the patient must not be able to make his wishes known, and a delay in providing care would result in the loss of life or limb. An important element in allowing emergency consent is that the health care provider must not have any reason to know or believe that consent would *not* be given were the patient able to deny consent. For example, a health care provider cannot wait until a patient loses consciousness to order treatment that the patient had previously refused, such as a blood transfusion for a patient who is known to be a Jehovah's Witness. Implied consent is frequently relied on during surgery or in critical care units when an untoward event occurs and an immediate decision must be made to prevent further injury to the patient.

Revocation of Consent

The nurse also has an important role if the patient subsequently wishes to revoke his or her prior consent or if it becomes obvious that the patient's already signed, informed consent form does not meet the institution's standards for informed consent. Most nurses have been faced with the problem of what to do when it becomes all too clear that the patient does not understand the procedure to be performed or believes that there are no major risks or adverse consequences inherent to the procedure. It is important to remember that the nurse and the hospital may incur liability if there is reason to know that the standards of informed consent have not been met. In such a case, it is the nurse's responsibility to contact his immediate supervisor and the responsible physician. Both entities need to be informed of the patient's change of mind or lack of comprehension.

Signing of a Consent Form

Equally as important as the patient being given all material facts needed on which to base an informed choice is that the correct person(s) consent to the procedure or therapy. Informed consent becomes a moot point if the wrong signature is obtained. The basic rule is that if the patient is a competent adult according to state law, only that adult can give or refuse consent. Most states recognize 18 as the age at which one becomes an adult, although some actions might serve to classify the person as an adult prior to the legal age, for example, marriage or termination of parental rights. The adult giving or refusing consent must be competent to either sign or refuse to sign the necessary consent forms. Competency at law means that (1) the court has not declared the person to be incompetent and (2) the person is generally able to understand the consequences of her actions. There is a strong legal presumption of continuing competency.

Some persons are never adjudicated or judged to be incompetent by a court of law, but they become incompetent to give informed consent based on their current medical condition. Many states allow the patient's family members to make decisions for the incompetent patient. For example, an automobile accident may render the patient incapable of making decisions and giving consent, and the physician will frequently ask the family about medical matters for the unconscious patient. The order of selection for most states usually is (1) spouse, (2) adult children or grandchildren, (3) parents, (4) grandparents, (5) adult brothers and sisters, and (6) adult nieces and nephews.

Most states recognize the child under 18 as a minor. Parental or guardian consent is necessary for medical therapies unless (1) the emergency doctrine applies, (2) the individual is an emancipated (liberated) minor or mature minor, (3) there is a court order to proceed with the therapy, or (4) the law recognizes the minor as having the ability to consent to the therapy. Some states also follow the *in loco parentis* doctrine, which refers to the ability of a person or the state to stand in the place of the parents. Look to the individual state statutory laws to see who may consent in the absence of a parent and what constitutes emancipated status because there is no general consensus on these issues. Such laws can be accessed through the individual state governmental website. If there is a family consent doctrine, it will generally be a grandparent, adult brother or sister, or adult aunt or uncle.

Emancipated minors are persons under the legal age of an adult who are no longer under their parent's control and regulation and who are managing their own financial affairs. Some states require the parent to completely surrender the right of care and custody of the child to prevent runaways from coming under this classification. Such emancipated minors may validly consent for their own medical therapies. Examples of emancipated minors are married persons, underage parents, or those in the armed service of their country. In some states pregnant adolescents are considered emancipated for the purposes of giving or refusing medical treatment for themselves and their fetuses. However, after the infant is born, the adolescent mother may only make decisions for the infant or for herself unless she is married. Some states allow college students living away from their parents to fall in the category of emancipated minor. Individual nurses should consult agency policies and state regulations for information regarding emancipated minors.

Mature minors also may consent to some medical care. The concept of a mature minor is a relatively new one that is gaining legal recognition (DeWolf-Bosek & Savage, 2007; Driggs, 2002; Guido, 2006). The mature minor is a minor between the ages of 14 and 17 who is able to understand the nature and consequences of the proposed therapy, is making his own decisions on a daily basis, and is independent. The health care provider is encouraged to seek parental consent along with the consent of the mature minor in most circumstances. Such a practice aids in limiting potential liability and encourages family involvement. It is necessary to consult agency policy for further information regarding this concept and the state statutes that govern the interpretation of mature minors.

The law also recognizes the right of the minor to consent to some selected therapies without informing parents of the treatment. The reason for these exceptions is to encourage the minor to seek needed treatment. Informing the parents of the treatment might prevent the minor from receiving the necessary therapy. Instances for which the minor may give valid consent include (1) diagnosis and treatment of infectious, contagious, or communicable diseases; (2) diagnosis and treatment of drug dependency, drug addiction, or any condition directly related to drug usage; (3) obtaining birth control devices; and (4) treatment during a pregnancy as long as the care concerns the pregnancy.

 *There is no foolproof method for determining maturity among minors. It is a subjective and arbitrary process depending to a great degree on the perceptions of the evaluator. Also, state courts are inconsistent in the use of a standard of proof that is required for application of the mature minor doctrine.*

Preventing Possible Liability

Nurses and other health care providers often ask what they can do to prevent potential lawsuits. Understanding and applying the legal concepts involved are two means of preventing possible liability. For example, ensuring that standards of care are fully implemented each time a nurse administers nursing care will help prevent potential lawsuits. Two other areas where nurses can have the most impact in reducing their potential legal liability involve the nurse–patient relationship and patient rights.

Nurse–Patient Relationship

One of the most fundamental aspects of malpractice law involves relationships. For a duty to be owed the patient, one must first establish that a nurse–patient relationship exists. This may be accomplished by showing that a reliance relationship exists: One person (the patient) is depending on another person (the nurse) for competent, quality nursing care.

The core of any reliance relationship is trust and communication. Establishing rapport with a patient, informing patients honestly and openly of all aspects of their care, and allowing patients to make decisions for themselves have always been credited to nurses as one means of preventing potential liability. Nursing is a caring profession; part of caring is maintaining communications and ensuring that trust is established and continues throughout the interactions between the nurse and the patient.

Patient Rights

Health care providers are becoming increasingly more aware and respective of patient rights. In 1959, the National League for Nursing wrote one of the earliest statements regarding patients' rights (National League for Nursing, 1959). In the early 1970s, the American Hospital Association (AHA) published *A Patient's Bill of Rights*, enumerating 12 rights that were to be afforded all hospitalized patients. These rights primarily concerned the patient's right to considerate and respectful care; informed consent concepts, including making treatment decisions based on informed choice; considerations of privacy; the right to know who will provide care; and the right to information about advance directives. The docu-

ment was revised in 1992, and more recently in 2003, and now presents patients' rights, expectations, and responsibilities. The latest document (2003) emphasizes a collaborative approach to patient care in which the patients' responsibilities are explicit. In return, patients may expect a certain level of care delivery. This statement is entitled The Patient Care Partnership: Understanding Expectations, Rights, and Responsibilities, and an abridged version is shown in Chart 4–7 (p. 80). The full text may be obtained from the American Hospital Association. See Chart 4–7 (p. 80) for the current provisions of *A Patient's Bill of Rights* (AHA, 2003).

Today, nurses are much more cognizant of the rights of patients, including those not enumerated on the various published documents. For example, the patient has the right to be cared for in a facility that ensures the safety rights of the patients. Observing and enforcing these patient rights prevents possible lawsuits. In this regard, nurses serve as patients' advocates by defending their legal and ethical rights.

Nursing has identified three models of advocacy that are employed in clinical practice settings. The rights protection model is perhaps the best known model of advocacy. Nurses assist patients in asserting their autonomy rights; for example, a nurse might help an individual patient successfully convince health care providers that he does not desire surgical intervention for coronary artery disease, but will comply with medical management. The third principle in the ANA's Code of Ethics (2001) reinforces this mandate: "The nurse promotes, advocates for, and strives to protect the health, safety, and rights of the patient."

A second approach to advocacy is the values-based decision model. Using this approach, the nurse assists the patient by discussing her needs and desires and helps the patient make choices that are most consistent with the patient's values, lifestyle, and desires. This model is predicated on sharing information and assisting the individual to become empowered to speak on her own behalf. Using this approach, the patient is assisted to exert her right to autonomy and self-determination.

The third model is the respect for persons model, which is sometimes known as the patient-advocate model. This approach centers on the inherent human dignity that is deserving of respect. In this model, the nurse acts to protect the rights, dignity, and choices of the patient. If the patient cannot assist in making decisions about his care and treatments, the nurse advocates for the best interests of the patient. The ultimate goal of this model is to promote the autonomy and individual uniqueness of the patient.

Defenses Against Torts

In the event that a legal claim or lawsuit is filed, nurses and other health care providers can use certain legal defenses to negate liability. Defenses are arguments in support of or arguments used for justification. Defenses may be based on statutory law, common law, or the doctrine of precedent, in which decisions are left to stand based on prior decisions made by a court (Guido, 2006). Defenses also can be classified by the type of cause of action, or tort, filed against the health care personnel: intentional, quasi-intentional, or nonintentional.

Defenses Against Intentional Torts

Defenses against intentional torts are most commonly consent, self-defense, defense of others, and necessity. Consent, as

CHART 4–7	The Patient Care Partnership: Understanding Expectations, Rights and Responsibilities

Our goal is for you and your family to have the same care and attention we would want for our families and ourselves. The sections explain some of the basics about how you can expect to be treated during your hospital stay. They also cover what we will need from you to care for you better. If you have questions at any time, please ask them. Unasked or unanswered questions can add to the stress of being in the hospital.

WHAT TO EXPECT DURING YOUR HOSPITAL STAY

- **High quality hospital care.** Our first priority is to provide you the care you need, when you need it, with skill, compassion, and respect. Tell your caregivers if you have concerns about your care or if you have pain. You have the right to know the identity of doctors, nurses and others involved in your care.

- **A clean and safe environment.** We use special policies and procedures to avoid mistakes in your care and keep you free from abuse or neglect. If anything unexpected and significant happens during your hospital stay, you will be told what happened, and any resulting changes in your care will be discussed with you.

- **Involvement in your care.** Please tell your caregivers if you need more information about treatment choices. When decision-making takes place, it should include:
  - *Discussing your medical condition and information about medically appropriate treatment choices.* To make informed decisions with your doctor, you need to understand:
    - The benefits and risks of each treatment, and whether the treatment is experimental or part of a research study.
    - What you can reasonably expect from your treatment and any long-term effects it might have on your quality of life.
    - What you and your family will need to do after you leave the hospital.
    - The financial consequences of using uncovered services or out-of-network providers.
  - *Discussing your treatment plan.* When you enter the hospital, you sign a general consent to treatment. In some cases, such as surgery or experimental treatment, you may be asked to confirm in writing that you understand what is planned and agree to it.

- *Getting information from you.* Your caregivers need complete and correct information about your health and coverage so that they can make good decisions about your care. That includes:
  - Past illnesses, surgeries or hospital stays; past allergic reactions; any medicines or dietary supplements (such as vitamins and herbs) that you are taking; and any network or admission requirements under your health plan.
- *Understanding your health care goals and values.* Make sure your doctor, your family and your care team know your wishes.
- *Understanding who should make decisions when you cannot.* If you have signed a health care power of attorney stating who should speak for you if you become unable to make health care decisions for yourself, or a "living will" or "advance directive" that states your wishes about end-of-life care; give copies to your doctor, your family and your care team.

- **Protection of your privacy.** State and federal laws and hospital operating policies protect the privacy of your medical information. You will receive a Notice of Privacy Practices that describes the ways that we use, disclose and safeguard patient information and that explains how you can obtain a copy of information from our records about your care.

- **Preparing you and your family for when you leave the hospital.** The success of your treatment often depends on your efforts to follow medication, diet and therapy plans. You can expect us to help you identify sources of follow-up care and to let you know if our hospital has a financial interest in any referrals. You can also expect to receive information and, where possible, training about the self-care you will need when you go home.

- **Help with your bill and filing insurance claims.** Our staff will file claims for you with health care insurers or other programs, such as Medicare and Medicaid. If you have questions about your bill, contact our business office. If you need help understanding your insurance coverage or health plan, start with your insurance company or health benefits manager. If you do not have health coverage, we will try to help you and your family find financial help or make other arrangements.

Source: American Hospital Association. (2003). *A patient's bill of rights.* Chicago, IL: Author. This is an abridged text. Full text is available at www.aha.org. © 2003 American Hospital Association. All rights reserved.

previously discussed, may be oral, implied by law, or expressed. Self-defense and defense of others may be justifiable to protect oneself and others from harm, for example, in the case of a combative patient. Defense of others can be extended to include the patient as well. The overriding caveat is that one can only use reasonable force—that which is necessary to defend oneself or others from injury. Necessity allows the nurse to interfere with the patient's property rights to avoid threatened injury, for example, an attack with a knife. The two overriding caveats in this situation are that a defense of necessity (1) does not allow the nurse the right to search the patient's property and (2) stipulates that the patient's property must be the threatening factor.

Defenses Against Quasi-Intentional Torts

The primary defenses against quasi-intentional torts are consent, truth, privilege, qualified privilege, and disclosure statutes. Consent

may be a defense against the quasi-intentional torts of defamation and invasion of privacy as well as to the intentional torts. Truth is a valid defense against defamatory statements; however, nurses should be aware that in using this defense the entire statement must be true, not merely parts of the statement (Guido, 2006).

Privilege is a disclosure that might otherwise be considered defamatory under different circumstances, however, such disclosure may be allowable to protect or further private or public interests recognized by law. An example of such would be the legal mandate to report persons with certain diagnoses or diseases or those suspected of abusing others. Qualified privilege prevails when the person making the allegedly defamatory statements has a legal duty to do so, as in the case of a manager reporting the professional performance of an employee. Qualified privilege legally negates any inference of malice because of the overriding public policy interest. When the quality of medical care is at issue, the reputation rights of health care professionals may concede to the greater social need. Liability will not be imposed, even if the communications are false, as long as there is no malice and the communications are made in good faith to those persons who need to know such facts. Three caveats of qualified privilege need to be observed: The communication must be made through appropriate channels to persons needing the information, liability may be granted for untruthful communications released with malice, and the communications should be worded in objective and observable behavioral terms rather than judgmental descriptions.

Both federal and state laws require the reporting of certain types of health-related information to protect the public at large. These laws are referred to as disclosure statutes. These statutes require that health care providers submit certain information to the proper agency. The most common example of reporting statutes is vital statistics. All states require births and deaths to be reported, and a majority of states require an accounting of neonatal deaths and abortions. Public health agencies may require a variety of disease states to be reported, for example, communicable and venereal disease must be reported to protect the public. In addition, some states require that patients suffering any type of seizure disorder be reported to the state driver's licensing agency. Also, cancer and other related diseases are to be reported in some states. If providers disclose only the limited information they are required to disclose by law, there is no liability for the disclosure under either a defamation or invasion of privacy lawsuit. Thus, the statutes serve as a defense against both defamation and invasion of privacy (Guido, 2006).

Defenses Against Nonintentional Torts

Defenses against nonintentional torts or negligent actions include release, contributory or comparative negligence, assumption of the risk, unavoidable accident, defense of the fact, and immunity statutes. A release may be signed during the process of settling a claim to prevent any and all future claims arising from the same incident. Once signed, the release bars future suits. In medical malpractice claims, a release is frequently a part of the "out-of-court" settlement. Effectively, the plaintiff states that the agreed-on settlement is the only compensation for the negligent action. Contributory and comparative negligence serve as defenses and in essence hold injured parties accountable for their part in the injury. Such fault by the plaintiff may occur for failure to follow prescribed treatments or if incorrect treatment is given based on the patient's false information to the physician. Similarly, the assumption of risk defense states that plaintiffs are partially responsible for consequences if they understood the risk involved when they proceeded with the action (Guido, 2006).

The defense of unavoidable accident comes into play when nothing other than an accident could have caused the person's injury. An unavoidable accident is an inevitable occurrence that cannot be foreseen or prevented by vigilance, care, and attention and not occasioned by or contributed to in any manner by an act or omission of the party claiming the accident was unavoidable (Dawson, 2007; Guido, 2006). The defense of the fact is used when there is no indication, direct or otherwise, that the health care provider's actions were the cause of the patient's injury or untoward outcome (e.g., the patient who receives an injection in his right arm and then begins to experience numbness and tingling in his left leg). There is no connection between the two events; thus, the defense is defense of fact.

Immunity

Immunity statutes have been enacted in some states that serve to dismiss certain causes of action. A good example of a state immunity statute is the Good Samaritan statute. Because of these laws, negligent actions against health care providers at scenes of accidents are rare. Good Samaritan laws are enacted to allow health care personnel and citizens who are trained in first aid to deliver needed medical care in an emergency without unnecessary fear of incurring criminal and civil liability (Garner, 2004). Most states require that the care be given in good faith and that it be gratuitous. Guidelines that govern the interpretation of Good Samaritan laws are shown in Chart 4–8 (p. 82).

■ Critical Thinking, Decision Making, and Clinical Judgment

Nurses in today's professional world must do more than merely understand legal and ethical concepts. Nurses must blend these important aspects with competent, skilled nursing diagnoses and interventions. To perform such high-quality nursing care, nurses must understand the concepts of critical thinking and clinical judgment, for without these latter concepts one is not able to fully appreciate the application of legal and ethical concepts in professional practice settings. For this reason, the concepts of critical thinking, decision making, and clinical judgment are discussed in depth in Chapters 1, 2, and 7 ⚙. National guidelines that may be used in assisting nurses with making legal and ethical decisions are shown in the National Guidelines box. Research possibilities for ethics and legal concepts are suggested in the Research Opportunities and Clinical Impact box (p. 82).

| CHART 4–8 | **Good Samaritan Laws** |

1. Make your decision quickly as to whether you will stay and help. There is no common law duty to stop and render aid; however, once you begin to provide care, you incur the legal duty to maintain a standard of reasonable emergency care.

2. Ask the injured person or family members for permission to help. Do not force your services once refused.

3. Care for the injured party where you can do so safely, in the vehicle or at the exact site where the victim is found. Only move the injured party if you must do so without causing further harm and as needed to prevent further harm.

4. Apply the rules of first aid. Assess for and prevent major bleeding, assess for the need to initiate cardiopulmonary resuscitation, cover the injured party with a blanket or coat, and so forth.

5. Assess and reassess the person continuously for additional injuries, and communicate findings of your assessment to the injured person and family.

6. Have someone call or go for additional help while you stay with the injured person.

7. Stay with the injured person until equally or more qualified help arrives. Prevent unskilled persons from treating or moving the injured party.

8. Provide the police or emergency medical personnel with as complete a description as possible of the care that you have rendered so that continuity of care exists. Give family members or police any personal items such as dentures, eyeglasses, and the like.

9. Do not accept any compensation of any kind offered by the injured party or family members as this may change your status into a fee-for-service situation and cause you to lose your Good Samaritan protection.

10. Should you choose not to stop and render aid, stop at the nearest phone and report the accident to proper authorities so that the injured party may be aided.

Source: Guido, G. W. *Legal and ethical issues in nursing* (4th ed.) © 2006. Electronically reproduced by permission of Pearson Education Inc., Upper Saddle River, New Jersey.

NATIONAL GUIDELINES for Interpretation of Ethical and Legal Issues

- American Hospital Association *A Patient's Bill of Rights* (1992)
- American Medical Association statement of informed consent (2007)
- American Nurses Association Code of Ethics (2001)
- American Nurses Association Nursing Practice Standards (1998)
- Health Insurance Portability and Accountability Act (HIPAA) (1996)
- Joint Commission *Accreditation Manual for Hospitals* (2007)

RESEARCH OPPORTUNITIES AND CLINICAL IMPACT RELATED TO PROFESSIONAL CONCEPTS

Research Opportunity	Clinical Impact
Ethical Concepts	
Means by which nurses make ethical decisions	Improve the knowledge base of nurses concerning ethical principles so that they can make more effective ethical decisions in clinical practice settings.
Identification of ethical dilemmas by nurses in clinical practice settings	
Knowledge base of nurses regarding ethical principles	Explore why nurses are not on ethics committees and the vital need to include nurses in this aspect of patient care.
Involvement of nurses in institutional ethics committees	
Legal Concepts	
Knowledge base of practicing nurses regarding legal issues	Understand the extent of lawsuits filed against nurses, the causes of actions in the filed lawsuits, and the legal knowledge of practicing and student nurses to hopefully prevent further lawsuits.
Numbers of malpractice lawsuits in which nurses are named as defendants	
Numbers of legal courses in schools of nursing	
Critical Thinking, Decision Making, and Clinical Judgment	
Descriptive and qualitative studies on how nurses make decisions and their critical thinking abilities	Improve nurses' decision-making and critical thinking skills with the goal of improving patient outcomes.
Use of clinical pathways and clinical judgment in multiple clinical practice settings	Determine the effectiveness of critical pathways currently being used and the need for modifications, as applicable.
Patient outcomes studies to determine the effectiveness of clinical pathways	

REVIEW QUESTIONS

1. During the course of one day, a nurse will support one patient's decision to not receive a particular medication, suggest family members of another patient go home to get rest, promise one patient that the injection will only pinch for a second, and will spend equal amounts of time with each patient on her assignment. Which ethical theory is this nurse demonstrating?
   1. Deontology
   2. Principlism
   3. Rule utilitarianism
   4. Act utilitarianism

2. The hospital ethics committee is currently studying all of the options available to them to address an ethical dilemma. In which step of the MORAL model is this committee functioning?
   1. Identify issues
   2. Resolve
   3. Options
   4. Evaluate

3. The Ethics Committee schedules Ethics Grand Rounds to be held the Friday of every month. This committee is demonstrating which type of ethics committee structure?
   1. Autonomy model
   2. Social justice model
   3. Fidelity model
   4. Patient benefit model

4. A nurse that just recently passed the state board examination has questions about what she can and cannot do regarding patient care. This nurse should:
   1. Read the state nurse practice act.
   2. Study the organization's standards of patient care.
   3. Contact the school in which she earned her nursing education.
   4. Assume she can provide all aspects of care since she did pass the state board examination.

5. A patient cannot find his dentures and claims the nurse threw them away when they were left on a meal tray. In which of the following types of laws would this situation be addressed?
   1. Common
   2. Civil
   3. Contract
   4. Tort

Answers for review questions appear in Appendix D

KEY TERMS

assault *p.75*
autonomy *p.68*
battery *p.75*
beneficence *p.68*
breach of confidentiality *p.76*
civil law *p.71*
common law *p.71*
criminal law *p.72*
defamation of character *p.75*
deontological theories *p.67*
emancipated minors *p.78*
emergency doctrine *p.78*
ethical decision making *p.69*
ethical dilemma *p.69*
ethics *p.66*

false imprisonment *p.75*
fidelity *p.69*
foreseeability of harm *p.74*
implied consent *p.78*
informed consent *p.77*
intentional torts *p.71*
invasion of privacy *p.76*
justice *p.68*
law *p.70*
malpractice *p.72*
mature minors *p.78*
MORAL model *p.69*
morality *p.66*
national standards of care *p.75*

negligence *p.72*
nonintentional torts *p.71*
nonmaleficence *p.68*
nurse practice acts *p.70*
paternalism *p.68*
principlism *p.67*
quasi-intentional torts *p.71*
regional (locality) rule *p.75*
respect for others *p.69*
scope of practice *p.70*
substituted judgment *p.70*
teleological theories *p.67*
tort law *p.71*
veracity *p.68*

REFERENCES

American Hospital Association. (1992). *A patient's bill of rights*. Chicago, IL: Author.

American Medical Association. (2007). Informed consent. *AMA Legal Issues*. Retrieved June 3, 2007, from http://www.ama-assn.org/ama/pub/category/print/4608.html

American Nurses Association. (2001). *Code of ethics with interpretive statements*. Silver Spring, MD: Author.

Beauchamp, T. L., & Childress, J. G. (2001). *Principles of biomedical ethics* (5th ed.). New York: Oxford University Press.

Butts, J. B., & Rich, K. L. (2005). *Nursing ethics across the curriculum and into practice*. Sudbury, MA: Jones and Bartlett.

Crisham, N. (1990). Living wills: Controversy and certainty. *Journal of Professional Nursing, 6*(6), 321.

Croke, F. M. (2003). Nurses, negligence, and malpractice. *American Journal of Nursing, 103*(9), 54–64.

Dawson, J. (2007). *Negligence oversimplified*. Retrieved June 3, 2007, from University of Vermont website: http://asci.uvm.edu/equine/law/articles/neg12.htm

DeWolf-Bosek, M. S., & Savage, T. A. (2007). *The ethical component of nursing education*. Philadelphia: Lippincott Williams & Wilkins.

Driggs, A. E. (2002). *The mature minor doctrine: Do adolescents have the right to die?* Columbus, OH: Case Western Reserve University School of Law.

Garner, B. A. (2004). *Black's law dictionary* (8th ed.). Berkeley, CA: West Group Publishing.

Guido, G. W. (2006). *Legal and ethical issues in nursing* (4th ed.). Upper Saddle River, NJ: Pearson Prentice Hall.

Hall, R. T. (2000). *An introduction to health care organizational ethics*. New York: Oxford University Press.

Hamric, A. B. (2002). Bridging the gap between ethics and clinical practice. *Nursing Outlook, 50*(5), 176–178.

HIPAAdvisory. (2006). *Status of HIPAA regulations compliance calendar*. Retrieved November 8, 2007, from http://www.hipaadvisory.com/Regs/com;loiancecal.htm

Joint Commission. (2007). *Accreditation manual for hospitals*. Oak Terrace, IL: Author.

Larson, A. (2003). *Contract law—An introduction, expert law*. Retrieved May 9, 2007, from http://www.expertlaw.com/library/business/contract_law.html

Marquis, B. L., & Huston, C. J. (2006). *Leadership roles an management functions in nursing* (5th ed.). Philadelphia: Lippincott Raven Publishers.

National League for Nursing. (1959). *Patients' rights*. New York: Author.

Negligence. (2007). *The Columbia Electronic Encyclopedia* (6th ed.). New York: Columbia University Press.

Nursing malpractice: Understanding the risks [Special issue]. (2003, June). *Travel Nursing 2003*, pp. 7–12.

Perle, S. (2004). Morality and ethics: An introduction.11(4). Retrieved April 29, 2008 from The American Academy of Anti-Aging Medicine, In. website: http://www.chiroweb.com/archives/22/06/16.html

Sabol v. Richmond Heights General Hospital, 676 N.E.2nd 958 (Ohio App. 1996).

Stanford Encyclopedia of Philosophy (2003). Theories of Tort Law. Retrieved August 14, 2008 from http://plato.stanford-edu/entries/tort-theories/

Thiroux, J. (1977). *Ethics: Theory and practice*. Philadelphia: Macmillan.

Watson, J. (2003, July–September). Love and caring: Ethics face and hand—An invitation to return to the heart and soul of nursing and our deep humanity. *Nursing Administration Quarterly, 27*(3), 197–202.

Yoder-Wise, P. S. (2007). *Leading and managing in nursing* (4th ed.). St. Louis: Mosby.

45 Code of Federal Regulations, Sections 160.102 and 160.103. (1996). General Adminstrative Requirements. Retrieved August 14, 2008 from http://www. hhs.gov/OCR/regtext.html.

Nursing Care Delivery Systems

Carol Robinson

Outcome-Based Learning Objectives

After studying this chapter, the learner will be able to:

1. Identify the four types of nursing care delivery systems most commonly used in health care settings.

2. Analyze the influences of each nursing care delivery system on professional nurse satisfaction, patient satisfaction, and quality of care delivered.

3. Explain the delegation responsibilities of the registered nurse for each nursing care delivery system.

4. Distinguish among the economic variables influencing the selection of a nursing care delivery system.

5. Differentiate the roles of advanced practice nurses and case managers within the context of the four nursing care delivery systems identified in this chapter.

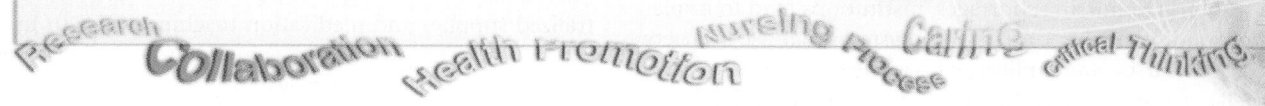

NURSING AND hospital administrators have struggled for more than 100 years with the question of how to deliver appropriate nursing care to patients in an efficient and effective manner. **Nursing care delivery systems** were developed to describe a structure for the organization of nursing work, to identify the types of health care workers providing the nursing care, and to define the boundaries for the delegation of authority.

Nursing Care Delivery Systems: Past to Present

Registered nurses work in several different settings and have many different job titles, responsibilities, and credentials. (As new roles for nurses develop in the health care setting, many nursing professionals describe these innovations in care modalities as nursing care delivery systems.) This chapter will discuss the innovations and advancements in health care delivery as evolutionary adaptations of the four basic nursing delivery systems using Marie Manthey's (1990) definition of a nursing care delivery system. Manthey describes nursing care delivery systems as ". . . a set of concepts defining four basic organizational elements. The definitions of these elements are based on principles that are in turn based on fundamental values. These fundamental values will ultimately determine the quality of the

product. These four fundamental values or elements are clinical decision making, work allocation, communication, and management" (Manthey, 1990, p. 203). Marie Manthey's definitions of nursing care delivery systems published in 1990 are still widely accepted (Tiedeman & Lookinland, 2004).

Historical Influence

Nursing care delivery systems are complex and subject to the economic, social, political, and technological influences of the time period. World wars, the Industrial Revolution, the Great Depression, the development of diagnosis-related groups (DRGs), and managed care have sparked changes in health care delivery and challenged the way the profession of nursing is practiced (Marquis & Huston, 2006). (See Chapter 1 ⦿ .)

The pressure to reduce unnecessary costs resulted in the development of several different types of managed care organizations such as the health maintenance organization (HMO). Managed care is a form of health care delivery that uses financial incentives to direct patients to the most cost-effective and efficient treatment center. HMOs focus resources on prevention of illness and the avoidance of the use of costly hospital resources. Managed care has resulted in shorter lengths of stay for hospitalized patients. Conversely, it has caused more patients to require home health services and utilize outpatient clinics, and

MyNursingKit | Video: Leadership: Care Delivery—Leadership and Management Introduction it has created a dire need for the coordination of care (Roussel, 2006). The complexity of how health care is financed has a great impact on who delivers the care and how the care delivery is organized (Finkler & Kovner, 2000). Chapter 3 🖉 discussed health care finance issues.

Current Influence

The nursing shortage has historically influenced the types of nursing care delivery systems used in many health care settings, and the shortage continues to drive the search for the ideal nursing care delivery system. It is predicted that there may be a shortage of as many as 800,000 nurses by the year 2020, and an unprecedented shortage of registered nurses by 2030 if dramatic interventions are not taken (Buerhaus, Donelan, Ulrich, Norman, & Dittus, 2006). The decision to implement a particular nursing care delivery system will increasingly depend on the complexity and variability within the health care setting. The availability of the labor pool, the acuity of patients, and the financial health of the institution are important variables to consider when selecting a nursing care delivery system. The term **acuity** refers to the measurement of patient severity of illness and the amount of nursing care required by the patient (Finkler & Kovner, 2000). It is an important variable that must be considered when determining the skill level needed to provide appropriate care, and it takes into account patients' needs, technology required to care for patients, and the amount of interdisciplinary support needed by the nurse (Hinshaw & McClure, 2002; Ritter-Teitel, 2004).

In response to nursing shortages, institutions tend to implement or modify nursing care delivery systems that use a variety of licensed nurses and unlicensed assistive personnel (UAP) (Formella & Rovin, 2004). Because RN salaries have increased due to the decreased supply of nurses and the increased demand for nurses, many health care institutions have changed the skill mix by hiring UAP in an effort to reduce labor costs. Organized labor unions have responded to managements' cost savings efforts by introducing legislation in several states to enact mandatory staffing ratios as a patient safety initiative and to force hospitals to increase the number of licensed nurses. In January 2004 California was the first state to mandate licensed nurse staffing ratios (Clarke & Aiken, 2003; Haugh, 2005). A literature review in 2004 of more that 490 articles and a detailed analysis of 43 articles revealed that there is ". . . no support for specific, minimum nurse–patient ratios for acute care hospitals, especially in the absence of adjustments for skill and patient mix. . . ." This study found probable relationships between richer RN staffing and nurse satisfaction, lower failure to rescue rates, lower inpatient mortality, and shorter lengths of stay" (Lang, Hodge, Olson, Romano, & Kravitz, 2004, p. 326). The legislation by the state of California has opened debate and fueled a call for more research to clearly identify the relationship of quality patient outcomes to skill mix. In the meantime, many states have legislation pending in an attempt to attract and retain RNs in the face of increasing acuity and the nursing shortage. The Joint Commission on Accreditation of Healthcare Organizations, the national accrediting body for hospitals and health systems, has set standards for nurse staffing and assignment of patient care. These must be adhered to in order to maintain accreditation

NATIONAL GUIDELINES for The Joint Commission

The Joint Commission is an accrediting body for hospitals and health systems. Information on staffing requirements can be found in the September 2006 document titled *Comprehensive Accreditation Manual for Hospitals, The Official Handbook, Update 2,* but can only be accessed through an organization that has purchased the reference. Limited free information can be found on the Joint Commission's official website: http://www.jointcommission.org.

and to meet quality of care standards. These guidelines are described in the National Guidelines box.

The physical design of the patient care areas and the experience and competency of the personnel might also influence the choice or modification of a nursing care delivery system (Daditch, 2003). Nursing units designed in circles, squares, or rectangles with central or decentralized medication and supply services may require different configurations of staff to safely provide observation and care. The creation of smaller sections where patient care is delivered may increase the ability of staff to obtain assistance when needed (Kalisch & Begeny, 2005). The American Institute of Architects (AIA) published design standards in 2006 that emphasize safety for patients and staff. These guidelines recommend a unit layout that can reduce the time nurses spend walking and thereby reduce the fatigue factor that leads to errors (AIA, 2006). The National Guidelines box provides more information about the AIA guidelines. Units designed to have decentralized supplies and medication machines close to the patient care activities are referred to as modular units (Ulrich & Quan, 2004). Increased support from ancillary departments is critical for modular units to succeed. "The intent behind any nursing unit design must be to reduce time spent performing non-nursing tasks" (Institute of Medicine [IOM], 2004, p. 101).

Evidenced-Based Management Practices

Traditional delivery systems form a framework that can be modified to meet the uniqueness of the particular agency setting; however, measuring the effectiveness of such a system is complex and difficult. The efficiency and effectiveness of any system usually is evaluated by measuring four factors: quality patient care, patient satisfaction, nursing job satisfaction, and cost effectiveness for the health care organization. The Joint Commission (2006) has adopted a standard definition of quality patient care as "the degree to which health services for individuals and populations increase the likelihood of desired health outcomes and

NATIONAL GUIDELINES for the American Institute of Architects

Guidelines for Design and Construction of Health Care Facilities is a publication of the American Institute of Architects. The guidelines were developed in 2006 with the assistance of the U.S. Department of Health and Human Services. Federal agencies, the Joint Commission, and 42 states use this information to plan and guide new construction or remodels of patient care areas.

are consistent with current professional knowledge" (p. GL-20). Desired outcomes that might be measured include fewer medication errors and fewer pressure ulcers. Undesired outcomes might be the failure of the RN to rescue the patient before the patient's condition causes irreparable harm or death (Huber, 2006; IOM, 2004).

The California Nursing Outcomes Coalition is a self-funded organization that was created by the Association of California Nurse Leaders and the American Nurses Association. The purpose of this organization is to develop a database of patient outcomes and hospital statistics. Data on nurse staffing, patient days, patient falls, pressure ulcer prevalence, and patient satisfaction scores are captured, and the data are used to provide evidence for practice changes (Brown, 2002). There is potential for future research as more hospitals elect to contribute to this database.

The outcome variable of patient satisfaction measures the degree of coordination of care, the degree to which emotional and spiritual needs are met, and the degree of safety in the care provided. The outcome variable of nurse job satisfaction measures the degree to which nursing care delivery systems acknowledge, nurture, and protect the practice of the professional nurse. Common indicators of nurse job satisfaction are the degree of job autonomy, the accountability of the professional nurse, and the presence of meaningful work (Aiken, Clarke, Sloane, Sochalski, & Silber, 2002; Deutschendorf, 2003; Kramer & Schmalenberg, 2002).

The cost-effective measurement of nursing care delivery systems is difficult to achieve. Identifying the best care for the lowest cost may be deemed a cost-effective choice (Finkler & Kovner, 2000). Deutschendorf (2003) studied care delivery, but concluded that all models need to be uniquely developed while balancing fiscal responsibility. A review of the research in the Institute of Medicine's 2004 report *Keeping Patients Safe* did not identify a particular nursing care delivery system that stood out from all others. The complexity of the nursing work environment today involves leadership resources, availability of technology, culture, and measures of workload. Nursing researchers are still testing nursing care delivery systems, but have not achieved success in identifying specific cost-effective systems.

Houser (2003) tested a model of demands on nursing in an attempt to measure the multivariate nature of the nursing work environment. This research was a first step toward evaluating the complex issues of maintaining a competent, satisfied workforce and providing acceptable patient care at a reasonable cost. Further evidence relating nursing workload to patient outcomes is needed to make the management decisions necessary to achieve the desired results. Nursing researchers such as Aiken, Buerhaus, Kramer, and Needleman have contributed to a body of knowledge about work hours, work environment, satisfaction, patient outcomes, and educational preparation that begins to answer some of management's questions about professional practice, but falls short of identifying effective delivery systems. Citing the lack of evidence to support a specific delivery system, the IOM and others support the selection of care delivery system models that can be tailored to the unit's unique design, availability of resources, and quality of professional staff (Deutschendorf, 2003; Formella & Rovin, 2004; IOM, 2004). Subsequent to the IOM report, Needleman and Buerhaus (2006) found that in-

creases in the proportion of nurses while keeping the number of hours of care the same can reduce unnecessary deaths and shorten lengths of stay.

Integration of RN Roles in Care Delivery Systems

There are four well-defined and widely used traditional nursing care delivery systems encountered in acute, outpatient, and long-term health care settings. Each of these systems—the case method, functional nursing, team nursing, and primary nursing—takes advantage of a variety of caregivers with licenses or certifications and different education levels. Different roles for **registered nurses (RNs)** have been developed over the years to complement and support nurses and physicians delivering care at the bedside (Bryant-Lukosius, DiCenso, Browne, & Pinelli, 2004). These roles include the advanced practice nurse, certified registered nurse anesthetist, clinical nurse specialist, certified nurse midwife, nurse practitioner, and the new role of clinical nurse leader. These roles are discussed within the context of each of the delivery systems.

An **advanced practice nurse (APRN)** is a registered nurse with advanced education, knowledge, and skills. APRNs might also have additional certifications, and their practice can vary depending on the scope of practice defined by the state board of registered nursing in which they work. APRNs are increasingly being used in the clinical setting and may be used in all nursing care delivery systems without changing the basic structure or philosophy of the delivery system. Advanced practice nurses include nurses with the titles **certified registered nurse anesthetist (CRNA), clinical nurse specialist (CNS), certified nurse midwife (CNM),** and **nurse practitioner (NP).** Economic, social, political, and technologic factors influence the acceptability and demand for these roles in much the same way as nursing care delivery models are influenced (Bryant-Lukosius et al., 2004). Chapter 1 🔗 includes an in-depth discussion of advanced practice roles.

A new role for an RN at the bedside is currently being evaluated. The role of **clinical nurse leader (CNL)** is intended to manage patient services across multidisciplinary boundaries at the bedside and to be a resource to the bedside nurse. The American Association of Colleges of Nursing (AACN) determined that a new role was needed to differentiate the education of nurses and entry levels into nursing without differentiating existing practice levels. CNLs are envisioned as coordinators of care and leaders with the authority to function as part of the clinical health care team. CNLs, by virtue of their advanced education and ability to manage complex systems of care, would be responsible for evaluating outcomes and leading change at the point of care (AACN, 2005; Drenkard & Cohen, 2004). Several institutions are piloting this role; however, research is not complete as to the effectiveness of such a role (Begun, Hamilton, Tornabeni, & White, 2006). Another, more widely accepted approach to coordinating and managing complex systems has been the delegation of these responsibilities to administrative nurses without direct clinical care duties.

The introduction of managed care in the early 1990s resulted in a new position being created within the health care setting titled **case manager.** Managed care requires close coordination of care across all health care settings and therefore affects the role of the RN in the delivery of care. Some institutions, however, do not always use RNs (Huber, 2006). The chief function of the case manager is to collaboratively plan, coordinate, and evaluate services in a cost-effective manner. Nurse case managers interact with health care team members to reduce fragmentation and improve outcomes. In many settings, case managers do not provide direct patient care (American Nurses Credentialing Center, 2006; White & Hall, 2006). In others, case management is considered to be a care delivery model.

Care Delivery Models

The delivery of health care to the patient is a multidisciplinary process that must take into account the availability of resources, the educational preparation of the nurse, the competencies of staff, the needs of the patient, and the cost implications for the institution or health system (McCauley & Irwin, 2006). Models of care delivery are continually being modified to adjust for the many variables in the health care setting. The traditional models are presented next to provide a baseline understanding of the structured work of nursing in a health care setting.

Case Method

The **case method** of delivering nursing care is simply defined, and sometimes referred to as **total patient care.** The RN is responsible for the patient and has total care responsibility for the patient during the shift worked.

Work Allocation

All patients have an RN assigned to them, and this type of delivery system requires exclusive use of an all RN staff (Figure 5–1 ■). There is no assignment requirement that the RN have the same patient day after day nor is there a consistent coordinator to ensure continuity of care during the course of the hospitalization (Tomey, 2004). The case method is frequently practiced in the intensive care setting or in the home health setting (Huber, 2006).

Clinical Decision Making

The RN assumes responsibility for the total care of the patient and may have several assigned patients. In addition to being responsible for the nursing process, the RN is responsible for all indirect and direct patient care functions. Care planning and goal setting occur between family, patient, and nurse during the specific shift. The charge nurse may have a patient load or may assist where needed. The role of the charge nurse is to manage the shift activities, provide consultation to staff, and make patient assignments according to the resources available.

Communication

The RN communicates changes, needs, and requests for assistance to the charge nurse. The RN is generally expected to communicate with physicians and other disciplines regarding patient care needs. Communication and coordination of care between shifts is dependent on the efforts of the individual shift nurse.

Management

The advantages of the case method are considered to be holistic and comprehensive care delivered by a registered nurse. The cost of RNs, the lack of continuity between shifts, and the dependence on an adequate supply of nurses are considered to be disadvantages of this system (Daditch, 2003).

The disadvantages to the case method of nursing care delivery can be mitigated through the use of advanced practice nurses and case managers. Advanced practice nurses typically work side by side in settings where the case method is implemented. The clinical nurse leader would serve to coordinate care between the other disciplines in this delivery care system. The use of the CNS or NP in the intensive care unit may provide specialty expertise and education for the nursing staff or extend the physician's capabilities and provide additional consultative support for the bedside nurse (Whitcomb et al., 2002). The use of advance practice nurses as part of the health care team provides continuity of care and can reduce the length of stay and mortality rate (Cowan et al., 2006). Case managers may place patients with a specific diagnosis on a clinical pathway. In situations where case managers are used, the planning, coordinating, and evaluating of the care responsibilities of the bedside nurse are assumed by the case manager. The bedside nurse then is responsible for the assessment and intervention components of patient care (Marquis & Huston, 2006). A collaborative effort between the bedside nurse, the case manager, and the physician ensures continuity of care for the patient as the patient progresses to different levels of care. This collaborative partnership is outcome

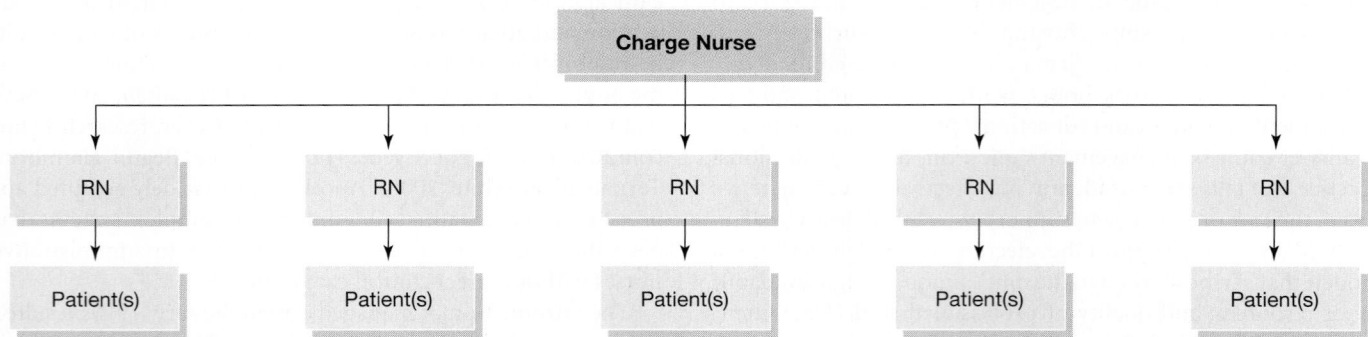

FIGURE 5–1 ■ Sample staffing assignments for the case method of nursing care delivery.

driven and offers the added benefit of providing care to a defined group of patients with limited resources (Cortes, Noyes, & Brennan, 2000). (Case management is discussed in more detail in Chapter 3 🔗.)

Functional Nursing

The functional nursing care delivery system was first developed in response to the increasing demand for hospital nursing in the late 1800s and it resurfaced due to the sporadic nursing shortages resulting from World War II (Daditch, 2003). A **functional nursing** care delivery system is defined as a task-oriented system in which individual caregivers are not given patient assignments, but are expected to perform specific assigned tasks within their capability for all patients in a given area. This method of providing care to the patient involves both licensed nursing staff and unlicensed assistive personnel. "**Unlicensed assistive personnel** are health care personnel who are not licensed and may be technicians or certified nurses' aides or nursing assistants" (Daditch, 2003 p. 255). Several variations may be used in health care settings today, but all functional models depend on a hierarchical structure that requires strict definition of roles and responsibilities and control of tasks (Tomey, 2004).

Work Allocation

Figure 5–2 ■ shows a standard flowchart for the functional nursing care delivery system. The charge nurse may be responsible for both administrative and clinical functions such as taking orders, contacting physicians for patient needs, assisting personnel with difficult or emergent patient care needs, adjusting staffing schedules, and evaluating or orienting staff. The task of medication administration is usually assigned to an RN in the role of **medication nurse.** The use of a medication nurse is not a common practice in acute care facilities today, but it is a useful function in long-term care facilities. This role may be assigned in

acute care settings, however, during disasters or other emergent situations when the patient-to-staff ratio is higher than usual.

In situations where there is a shortage of RNs, a **licensed vocational/practical nurse (LVN/LPN)** may be assigned to administer oral and parenteral medications while the charge RN administers the IV medications (Daditch, 2003). LVN/LPNs receive 1 to 2 years of practical training to deliver basic nursing care and are licensed according to state practice acts.

A treatment nurse is assigned the responsibility of providing treatments. This nurse is frequently an LVN/LPN and the assignment of tasks is dependent on the scope of practice of the LVN/LPN and the complexity of patients' needs. The scope of practice may change according to state law and regulations. It also is dependent on agency policy, wherein the agency may be more restrictive than the law allows.

UAP are assigned to take vital signs, assist the patients with basic hygiene tasks, and provide comfort measures. This variation in the functional delivery system may work well in skilled nursing facilities or facilities with lower acuity patients (Tomey, 2004).

Clinical Decision Making

In a typical functional model, an RN is assigned to be in charge and coordinate the care of all patients. The clinical decision making for all patients rests with the charge nurse since that individual is responsible for collecting all pertinent information about the patients. The RN is responsible for delegating tasks to personnel consistent with the applicable state nurse practice act. **Delegation** is defined as being accountable for outcomes of work that is shared with others (Daditch, 2003). "To delegate is to transfer authority to a competent individual for completing selected nursing tasks/activities/functions" (National Council of State Boards of Nursing [NCSBN], 2005).

 Delegation by an RN requires clinical judgment and knowledge of the applicable state's nurse practice act, which authorizes the scope of responsibility and grants the authority to delegate. All RNs must know how to prioritize patients' needs and assign tasks based on the competency of the personnel, but they also must know how to supervise the personnel and intervene when necessary.

The RN must consider qualifications, job descriptions, and competency when delegating tasks to various caregivers. Qualifications are generally determined by state licensure or certification, and the RN may reference hospital policies and procedures, job descriptions, published state practice acts, or unit guidelines if unfamiliar with specific qualifications (Koloroutis, 2004). For instance, an LVN/LPN may be permitted by license to draw blood in some states. In other states the LVN/LPN must have an additional certification to draw blood.

State practice acts address these qualifications in published regulations, and hospital job descriptions delineate the roles and responsibilities of individuals within a specific agency. Many workers may be unlicensed and have only basic training in health care. The nurse needs to be familiar with each job description and confident about the competency of the worker before assigning tasks. The authority and accountability for the outcome of the worker's performance still rests with the RN (Potter & Grant, 2004). (The functions of state nursing practice acts are discussed in more detail in Chapter 4 🔗.)

MEDICAL OR SURGICAL 30 BED UNIT

FIGURE 5–2 ■ Sample staffing assignments for the functional method of nursing care delivery.

Competency to perform a task or procedure may be measured by tests, clinical observation, or certification by a training facility. Nursing assistants may be certified by the state or may have a certificate from a training facility. Certifications specifically identify the types of procedures or tasks that the individual has been trained to perform. RNs and LVN/LPNs also may be certified to perform specific procedures. The RN must be knowledgeable about the competence of the individual before delegating tasks, and the hospital must keep records documenting the competence of the individuals performing those tasks.

Delegating a task to an individual who is not competent has serious implications for the RN, the RN's license, and the institution should the patient suffer an adverse outcome. The RN should assess the patients' needs and consider situations where the outcome is uncertain or the potential for harm is high. Tasks should not be delegated under those circumstances. Nursing assessment and judgment may not be delegated. In addition to considering qualifications, job descriptions, competence, and patient needs, the RN must evaluate the effectiveness of the delegation and whether the desired outcome was achieved (Corbo, 2006; NCSBN, 2005).

Communication

The members of the staff are responsible for communicating changes to the charge nurse. It is the charge nurse's ultimate responsibility to communicate patient needs and coordinate the care with other disciplines. On busy or large patient care units, there is a possibility that patient needs will be overlooked (Huber, 2006). The increased number of personnel performing specific tasks for the individual patient intentionally fragments care. The functional nursing model is an industrial efficiency model that demands a high level of coordination and communication. The overall assessment of the patient from beginning to end may be incomplete and cause critical changes to go unnoticed (Daditch, 2003).

Management

Functional care delivery systems are implemented by management when the desired outcomes for nursing are efficiency in completing a large number of tasks. The ability to train unskilled personnel to complete limited specific tasks and to avoid high labor costs by using lower paid workers are incentives for health care facilities interested in the industrial model of efficiency (Huber, 2006). Institutions that embrace the industrial model of efficiency do not tend to modify the nursing care delivery system to provide better coordinated care by using advanced practice nurses or case managers. Nurse practitioners or nurse midwives might be used as physician extenders in these facilities.

The disadvantages of functional nursing are fragmented patient care, low job satisfaction, and low patient satisfaction. Nurses report a lack of satisfaction with their work because tasks are boring or because there is difficulty identifying the effect of their work on their patients. Functional nursing resembles assembly-line tasking and the fragmentation of tasks results in a perceived lack of accountability and increased frustration (Tiedeman & Lookinland, 2004; Tomey, 2004). Reduced patient satisfaction is linked to fragmented care and the resultant lack of confidence in the caregivers (Huber, 2006).

Charge nurses working with a functional nursing care delivery system must be knowledgeable about the RN and LVN/LPN practice laws in the state in which they are practicing. The delegation of tasks must be consistent with the state training and licensure or certification regulations. The UAP performing patient care tasks may face misdemeanor charges or penalties for practicing nursing without a license in states where mandatory licensure protects the title of registered nurse and the actions are protected by the state nursing practice act (Guido, 2006; NCSBN, 2005). The nursing practice act and its functions as related to regulations are discussed at length in Chapter 4 🔗.

Team Nursing

Team nursing was developed in the early 1950s in response to complaints that functional nursing created a fragmented care delivery system and resulted in nursing and patient dissatisfaction with care (Marquis & Huston, 2006). In the team nursing care delivery system, patients are assigned to a nursing team, which usually is led by an RN. The team may include RNs, LVN/LPNs, respiratory therapists, dieticians, and UAP. Small teams may be assigned to care for patients. These teams include an LVN/LPN and UAP. These types of teams may be called care partners, modular teams, patient-focused teams, or any name that incorporates the concept of a work redesign with the skill mix intended to be used.

Work Allocation

A typical unit with 30 patients may have a charge nurse, two team leaders, and usually two to four team members per team (Figure 5–3 ■), but no more than five members per team (Marquis & Huston, 2006). Assignments are based on the acuity of the patients and the skill level and experience of the caregivers (Huber, 2006). The team leader assigns all patients to team members and may delegate additional tasks according to the team members' competence (Daditch, 2003). The team assign-

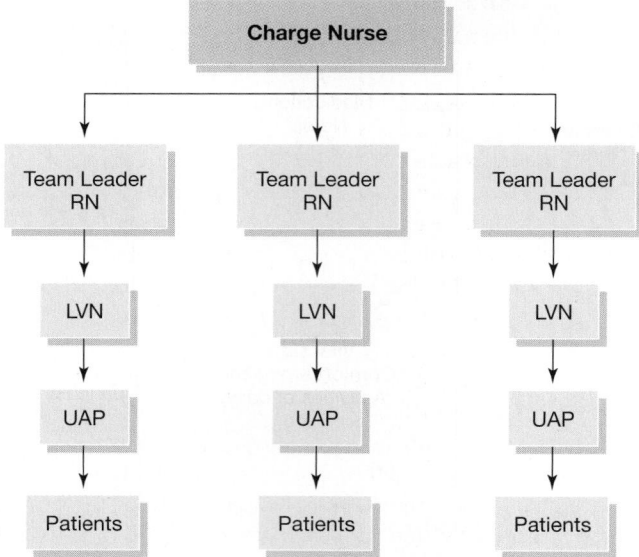

MEDICAL OR SURGICAL UNIT

FIGURE 5–3 ■ Sample staffing assignments for the team method of nursing care delivery.

ments may sometimes mirror a functional approach to care when the team leader is the only RN or licensed person on the team (Marquis & Huston, 2006). The team leader would assume responsibility for administering all medications and IV solutions to patients on the team and delegate remaining responsibilities to the team members.

Clinical Decision Making

The charge nurse is responsible for assigning groups of patients and caregivers to the team leaders and for facilitating communications between multidisciplinary caregivers. Decision making is delegated to several team leaders versus a single charge nurse, and team members work collaboratively toward common goals. Team leaders are responsible for making the individual patient assignments to their team members. Team leaders plan the care, delegate tasks, and monitor the work of the team to ensure quality. As time permits, the team leader may coordinate care conferences for patients with complex health care needs. Daily conferences are the ideal, but frequently time constraints prevent completion of conferences.

Communication

Team nursing is difficult to implement without extensive team communication (Daditch, 2003). Nursing shortages and high turnover among unlicensed assistive personnel can make communication between ever-changing team members a challenge. Research has documented RN dissatisfaction with communication and teamwork when UAP are used. Research also suggests that how personnel are assigned may mitigate these concerns (Potter & Grant, 2004). Experienced RNs with good communication, organization, and leadership skills are necessary (Marquis & Huston, 2006). Numerous formal and informal structures for communication among team members are available. Written care plans, written assignment responsibilities, and team conferences encourage coordinated care (Yoder-Wise, 2007).

Management

Team nursing has advantages because it uses individual team members' strengths to the greatest advantage for a large number of patients (Huber, 2006). Responsibility for the delegation of tasks remains the same as in the functional nursing care delivery system. Unlicensed assistive personnel may not practice nursing without a license, and nursing responsibilities are delineated in the state nursing practice act. All team members need specific role definition and communication skills to ensure that care is not fragmented, because fragmentation of care may decrease job satisfaction and contribute to decreased quality of care. It also has been reported that high-level teams working toward common goals and focused missions can experience increased job satisfaction (Kalisch & Begeny, 2005).

Complex, time-intensive training is essential to ensure that team members can function within a team structure and effectively communicate. Clinical nurse specialists and nurse practitioners can provide consultative support in a team nursing care delivery system. The clinical nurse leader role could be useful in this type of delivery system because the CNL would provide coordination within multidisciplinary teams and provide consistent information to the patient as well as the team. The use of APRNs can complement nursing care of patients with complex

needs and provide advanced educational support (Deutschendorf, 2003).

Primary Nursing

Primary nursing was developed as a nursing care delivery system in the late 1960s or early 1970s in response to the unhappiness of the professional nurse with the lack of autonomy and the declining quality of patient care (Daditch, 2003). **Primary nursing** is defined as a system in which each patient is assigned to a nurse who has 24-hour responsibility for the nursing care delivered to the patient (Tomey, 2004).

Work Allocation

Figure 5–4 ■ (p. 92) shows a typical flowchart for the primary nursing care method. The primary nurse is responsible for planning for the patient's care and delegating the care during the hours that the nurse is not present and also is accountable for the coordination and continuity of care from admission to discharge. The nurse who assists the primary nurse during off-duty hours is called an **associate nurse** or **associate caregiver.** The associate nurse follows the plan of care, communicates pertinent information or changes in the patient status to the primary nurse, and provides direct patient care when the primary nurse is not present. An associate caregiver may be an LVN/LPN or UAP (Manthey, 2002). A nurse may be a primary nurse for a small caseload of patients and also may be an associate nurse for other patients.

Clinical Decision Making

The three major responsibilities of the primary nurse can be simplified into (1) clear communication among all care disciplines, (2) development of a plan of care using the nursing process, and (3) discharge planning from the time of admission to discharge (Marquis & Huston, 2006). The primary nurse is held accountable for collecting and communicating important patient information during the patient's hospitalization. The primary nurse provides direct patient care because this nurse is in the best position to plan the care (Manthey, 2002; Roussel, 2006). Involving the patient in the collection of information, eliciting patient expectations for the outcomes of care, and encouraging participation in the development of goals is a significant part of the process (Daditch, 2003).

The nurse develops the plan of care using whatever documentation method the health care facility may have developed to direct all care providers. Instruments such as Kardex care plans, care pathways, care maps, nursing admission forms, guidelines, and multidisciplinary education forms can be used. Planning for the discharge of the patient is facilitated by the process of fulfilling the first two responsibilities: identifying the expected outcomes on admission and keeping the health care team on target with the plan of care (Manthey, 2002; Roussel, 2006). The primary nurse may use institutional resources such as discharge planning nurses, case managers, or social services to assist the patient in discharge from the health care facility.

Communication

Consistent and accurate communication of information between shifts and appropriate delegation of care planning activities between associate nurses and primary nurses eliminate the charge nurse from the communication chain between physician

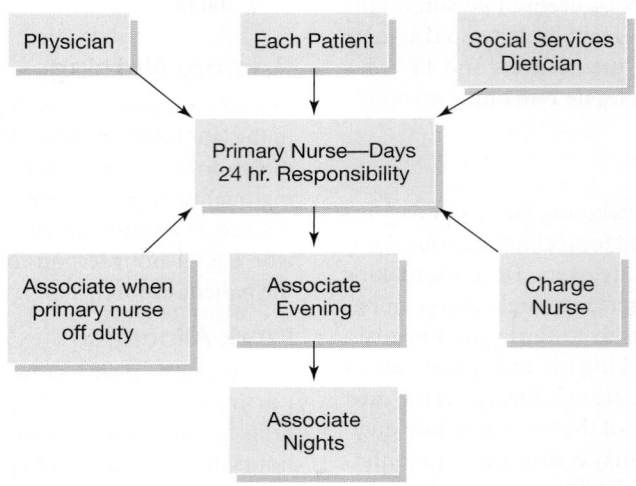

MEDICAL OR SURGICAL 28 BED UNIT

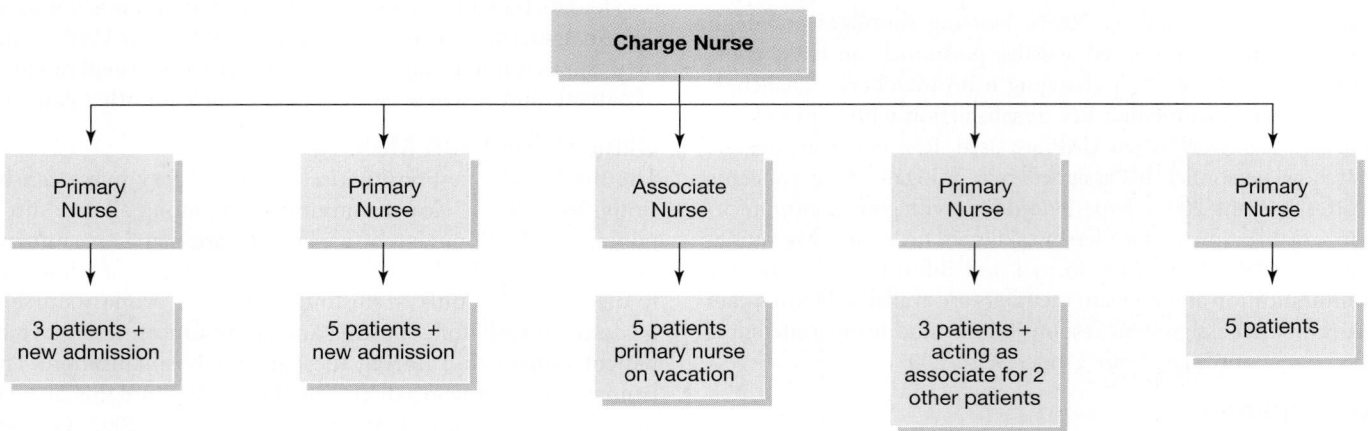

ASSIGNMENT PATTERN
DAY SHIFT–23 PATIENTS ON 30 BED UNIT

FIGURE 5–4   ■   Sample staffing assignments for the primary nursing method of nursing care delivery.

and caregiver (Roussel, 2006; Swansburg & Swansburg, 2002). Direct communication improves the rapport and trust between the primary nurse, the patient, and the physician, creating a therapeutic relationship. The charge nurse is then able to support the activities of the unit and provide consultation for the primary nurse.

Management

The use of an associate caregiver is not inconsistent with the intent of the primary nursing care delivery system, which is to provide patient-focused care in an environment where the professional nurse is held accountable for practice. The associate caregiver may be task focused, but the care continues to be coordinated and monitored on a 24-hour basis by the primary nurse.

The advantages of the primary nursing care delivery system are the increased nurse perception of autonomy, the continuity of care, and the patient focus. Research also suggests that the outcomes of care are better and nurse satisfaction is higher (Tomey, 2004). Although the research does not support a spe-

cific patient care delivery model, many studies suggest that richer RN staffing levels result in lower lengths of stay, fewer patient deaths, and lower failure-to-rescue rates (Aiken, Clarke, & Sloane, 2000; Needleman et al., 2002; Sovie et al., 2000). Patient satisfaction has been correlated with nurse satisfaction and quality of care in several basic studies (Hegyvary & Haussman, 1976; Weisman & Nathanson, 1985). Recent studies suggest a link between nurse burnout and decreased patient satisfaction (Vahey, Aiken, Sloane, Clarke, & Vargas, 2004). Other research suggests that there are higher levels of nurse satisfaction, greater continuity of care, positive patient outcomes, and improved nurse retention with the use of primary nursing care delivery systems (Huber, 2006; Kramer & Schmalenberg, 2002).

The primary nursing care delivery system uses many hospital resources, but places the control and authorization of such resources in the hands of the primary nurse. The primary nurse is responsible for developing the plan of care and prioritizing the daily activities to achieve the mutually agreed-on goals in the plan. For instance, because the primary nurse understands the sleeping and eating preferences of a particular patient who has cancer, routines and treatments can be adjusted to meet the patient's basic needs. If the patient and family need complex information from the physicians or other members of the health care team about the prognosis and treatment options of chemotherapy and radiation, the primary nurse may coordinate a care conference and identify the desired outcomes to realize a productive meeting. The primary nurse may advocate for scheduling placement of central lines for chemotherapy with patient and family schedules. Chemotherapy treatments may be managed to coincide with family support. All of these activities are the responsibility of the primary nurse providing care at the bedside.

Nurse practitioners can function within this system as physician extenders and consultants to the primary nurse. Clinical nurse specialists are valuable in providing clinical expertise and education to the primary nurse. The use of case managers may be redundant because of the primary nurse's accountability for the entire patient experience. This also may be true of the clinical nurse leader role, depending on the interpretation of primary nursing used, since the primary nurse is responsible for all of the functions that a clinical nurse leader normally would assume in one of the other types of nursing care delivery models. This may not be true in all agencies, depending again on the interpretation and usage of primary nursing.

A primary nursing care delivery system may not be the preferred system during downturns in the economy and cyclical nursing shortages. There is a perception that labor costs are high because primary nursing requires a large number of RNs, although cost studies have disputed this perception (Daditch, 2003). Additional research is needed to determine whether a primary nursing care delivery system shields an institution from the impact of a nursing shortage by attracting and retaining nurses and improving patient outcomes.

Relationship-Based Care

Primary care is enjoying renewed popularity as a nursing care delivery system because of an evolution described as *relationship-based care*. Relationship-based care incorporates the structure of primary nursing with the principles and values of a professional nursing practice environment. "The purpose of relationship-based care is to establish a therapeutic relationship between nurses, patients, and their families during their episode of care, to accomplish essential nursing interventions, and to maximize collaborative interdisciplinary practice" (Person, 2004, p. 159).

The professional nursing practice environment is best defined by research conducted in the early 1990s by Linda Aiken, Margaret McClure, Margaret Sovie, Marlene Kramer, Donna Havens, Heather Laschinger, and others. A professional nursing practice environment facilitates professional autonomy and control over individual practice, while encouraging collaborative relationships. These researchers and many others identified specific professional nursing practice attributes in hospitals that were successful in retaining and attracting nurses. These hospitals were labeled **magnet hospitals.** Research on magnet hospitals indicates that there is improved quality of care, improved patient satisfaction, and improved nursing satisfaction within hospitals meeting the magnet standards (Aiken, 2002; Kramer & Schmalenberg, 2004). The national standards for magnet hospitals are shown in the National Guidelines box.

The primary nursing care delivery system that has evolved using the principles of relationship-based care reinforces the professional practice environment. This system builds on healing relationships that can be tailored to individual units with varying staffing patterns or standardized health care settings to meet the unique needs of patients and families. This structure may be attractive to health care settings trying to attract and retain nurses while improving the quality of care, improving patient satisfaction, and improving patient safety. There is increasing pressure from third-party payers to reduce medical errors, hospital-acquired infections, patient falls, and pressure ulcers, and the search has begun to discover the links between the environment and the safe delivery of health care.

■ Providing Safe Patient Care

The IOM published its report *Keeping Patients Safe: Transforming the Work Environment of Nurses* in 2004. It speaks to the importance of providing safe patient care in a complex health system. Safe patient care depends on evidence-based nursing

---

NATIONAL GUIDELINES for Magnet Hospitals

Hospitals are recognized and formally designated by the American Nurses Credentialing Center as magnet hospitals when they have demonstrated, to the satisfaction of specially trained external appraisers, that the 14 forces of magnetism or standards are evident throughout the facility. Designation is valid for 4 years and hospitals must provide annual documentation of continued compliance with the forces.

The 14 forces of magnetism are listed below:

1. Quality of nursing leadership
2. Organizational structure
3. Management style
4. Personnel policies and programs
5. Professional models of care
6. Quality of care
7. Quality improvement
8. Consultation and resources
9. Autonomy
10. Community and the hospital
11. Nurses as teachers
12. Image of nursing
13. Interdisciplinary relationships
14. Professional development

Detailed information on the magnet recognition program can be found at the following website: http://www.nursecredentialing.org/magnet/forces.html.

care delivery systems. Nurses are critical elements of the overall health system and how care is organized, how work is designed, how much staffing is allocated, and how the multidisciplinary teams work together will determine whether quality care can be delivered with minimal errors to the patient (IOM, 2004).

Four nursing care delivery systems have historically provided a basic structure for organizing and delivering nursing care, but the research appears to support a model that uses a richer mix of RNs. The primary nursing model discussed in this chapter uses a richer mix of RNs, with its emphasis on relationship-based care, and creates new possibilities for collaborative success. Leaders in health care are searching for the components and processes to make patient care safe, and the ability of the RN to coordinate, communicate, and manage the multidisciplinary team of health care workers will be very important.

REVIEW QUESTIONS

1. A nurse is responsible for providing total care to a patient during the entire scheduled shift. The nurse is functioning within which of the following care delivery systems?
   1. Case method
   2. Functional
   3. Team
   4. Primary

2. Which of the following statements best describes the quality of care patients receive on a unit that utilizes functional nursing?
   1. Holistic and comprehensive
   2. Maximum use of individual caregivers' strengths for a large number of patients
   3. Better care outcomes and greater nurse satisfaction
   4. Intentional fragmentation of care

3. In a functional nursing care delivery system, a registered nurse is in charge and is responsible for delegating activities and tasks to unlicensed assistive personnel. This same approach to delegating tasks to unlicensed assistive personnel is seen in which of the following care delivery systems?
   1. Case Method
   2. Team
   3. Primary
   4. Primary Care

4. An organizational committee is considering changing the current care delivery system to one that is more cost-effective. Which of the following characteristics should be considered when selecting a cost-effective method to provide patient care?
   1. Highest quality for the lowest cost
   2. Amount of job autonomy
   3. Nurse accountability
   4. Patient acuity

5. Which of the following care areas would be the least likely to utilize advance practice nurses or case managers to assist with patient care needs?
   1. Case method
   2. Functional
   3. Team
   4. Primary

Answers for review questions appear in Appendix D

KEY TERMS

acuity *p.86*
advanced practice nurse (APRN) *p.87*
associate caregiver *p.91*
associate nurse *p.91*
case manager *p.87*
case method *p.88*
certified nurse midwife (CNM) *p.87*
certified registered nurse anesthetist (CRNA) *p.87*

clinical nurse leader (CNL) *p.87*
clinical nurse specialist (CNS) *p.87*
delegation *p.89*
functional nursing *p.89*
licensed vocational/practical nurse (LVN/LPN) *p.89*
magnet hospital *p.93*
medication nurse *p.89*

nurse practitioner (NP) *p.87*
nursing care delivery systems *p.85*
primary nursing *p.91*
registered nurse (RN) *p.87*
team nursing *p.90*
total patient care *p.88*
unlicensed assistive personnel *p.89*

REFERENCES

Aiken, L. H. (2002). Superior outcomes for magnet hospitals: The evidence base. In M. McClure & A. S. Hinshaw (Eds.), *Magnet hospitals revisited* (pp. 61–81). Washington, DC: American Nurses Association.

Aiken, L. H., Clarke, S. P., & Sloane, D. M. (2000). Hospital restructuring: Does it adversely affect care and outcomes? *Journal of Nursing Administration, 30,* 457–465.

Aiken, L. H., Clarke, S. P., Sloane, D. M., Sochalski, J., & Silber, J. H. (2002). Hospital nurse staffing and patient mortality, nurse burnout, and job dissatisfaction. *Journal of the American Medical Association, 288*(16), 1987–1993.

American Association of Colleges of Nursing. (2005). *Fact sheet: The clinical nurse leader.* Retrieved January 15, 2007, from http://www.aacn.nche.edu/Media/FactSheets/CNLFactSheet

American Institute of Architects. (2006). *Private rooms are new standard in guidelines for design and construction of health care facilities.* Retrieved January 15, 2007, from http://www.aia.org/release_071906_healthcare

American Nurses Credentialing Center. (2006). Retrieved January 15, 2007, from http://www.nursingworld.org/ancc/cert/eligibility/CaseMgmt

Begun, J. W., Hamilton, J. A., Tornabeni, J., & White, K. R. (2006). Opportunities for improving patient care through lateral integration: The clinical nurse leader. *Journal of Healthcare Management, 51*(1) 19–25.

Brown, D. (2002). *Linking quality measurement and evidence-based practice research for hospitals and long-term care.* CalNOC Director's Report. Retrieved February 28, 2007, from http://nurseweb.ucsf.edu/conf/cripc/calnocDirRep.html

Bryant-Lukosius, D., DiCenso, A., Browne, G., & Pinelli, J. (2004) Advanced practice nursing roles: Development, implementation and evaluation. *Journal of Advanced Nursing, 48*(5), 519–529.

Buerhaus, P. I., Donelan, K., Ulrich, B. T., Norman, L., & Dittus, R. (2006). State of the register nurse workforce in the United States. *Nursing Economics, 24*(1), 6–12.

Clarke, S. P., & Aiken, L. H. (2003). Failure to rescue: Needless deaths are prime examples of the need for more nurses at the bedside. *American Journal of Nursing, 103*(1), 42–47.

Corbo, S. A. (2006). Delegation defined: Examining the principles of this tool as both an art and a science. *Advance for Nurses, 8*(16), 21.

Cortes, T., Noyes, B., & Brennan, E. (2000). Is now the time to design new care delivery models? *Journal of Nursing Administration, 30*(9), 403–404.

Cowan, M. J., Shapiro, M., Hays, R. D., Afifi, A., Vasirani, S., Ward, C. R., et al. (2006). The effect of a multidisciplinary hospitalist/physician and advanced practice nurse collaboration on hospital costs. *Journal of Nursing Administration, 36*(2), 79–85.

Daditch, K. (2003). Care delivery strategies. In P. S. Yoder-Wise (Ed.), *Leading and managing in nursing* (3rd ed.). St. Louis: Mosby.

Deutschendorf, A. L. (2003). From past paradigms to future frontiers: Unique care delivery models to facilitate nursing work and quality outcomes. *Journal of Nursing Administration, 33*(1), 52–59.

Drenkard, K., & Cohen, E. (2004). Clinical nurse leader: Moving toward the future. *Journal of Nursing Administration, 34*(6) 257–269.

Finkler, S. A., & Kovner, C. T. (2000). *Financial management for nurse managers and executives* (2nd ed.). Philadelphia: W. B. Saunders.

Formella, N., & Rovin, S. (2004). Creating a desirable future for nursing, part 2: The issues. *Journal of Nursing Administration, 34*(6), 264–267.

Guido, G. W. (2006). *Legal and ethical issues in nursing* (4th ed.). Upper Saddle River, NJ: Pearson Prentice Hall.

Haugh, R. (2005 , February). California: Can this sinking ship be saved? *Hospitals and Health Networks,* pp. 54–60.

Hegyvary, S. T., & Haussman, R. K. (1976). Correlates of the quality of nursing care. *Journal of Nursing Administration, 6*(9), 22–27.

Hinshaw, A. S. (2002). Building magnetism into organizations. In M. McClure & A. S. Hinshaw (Eds.), *Magnet hospitals revisited* (pp. 83–102). Washington, DC: American Nurses Association.

Houser, J. (2003). A model for evaluating the context of nursing care delivery. *Journal of Nursing Administration, 33*(1), 39–47.

Huber, D. (2006). *Leadership and nursing care management* (3rd ed.). Philadelphia: W. B. Saunders.

Institute of Medicine. (2004). *Keeping patients safe: Transforming the work environment of nurses.* Washington, DC: National Academies Press.

Joint Commission. (2006, September). *Comprehensive accreditation manual for hospitals: The official handbook. Update 2.* Retrieved on February 27, 2007, from http://www.Jointcommission.org

Kalisch, B. J., & Begeny, S. M. (2005). Improving nursing unit teamwork. *Journal of Nursing Administration, 35*(12), 550–556.

Koloroutis, M. (2004). Professional nursing practice. In M. Koloroutis (Ed.), *Relationship-based care* (pp. 117–158). Minneapolis, MN: Creative Health Care Management.

Kramer, M., & Schmalenberg, C. (2002). Staff nurses identify essentials of magnetism. In M. McClure & A. S. Hinshaw (Eds.), *Magnet hospitals revisited* (pp. 25–55). Washington, DC: American Nurses Association.

Kramer, M., & Schmalenberg, C. (2004). Development and evaluation of essentials of magnetism tool. *Journal of Nursing Administration, 34*(7/8), 365–378.

Lang, T. A., Hodge, M., Olson, V., Romano, P. S., & Kravitz, R. L. (2004). Nurse–patient ratios: A systematic review on the effects of nurse staffing on patient, nurse employee, and hospital outcomes. *Journal of Nursing Administration, 34*(7/8), 326–337.

Manthey, M. (1990). Definitions and basic elements of a patient care delivery system with an emphasis on primary nursing. In G. G. Mayer, M. J. Madden, & E. Lawrenz (Eds.), *Patient care delivery models* (pp. 201–211). Rockville, MD: Aspen Publishers.

Manthey, M. (2002). *The practice of primary nursing* (2nd ed.). Boston: Blackwell Scientific Publications.

Marquis, B. L., & Huston, C. J. (2006). *Leadership roles and management functions in nursing* (5th ed.). Philadelphia: Lippincott Williams & Wilkins.

McCauley, K., & Irwin, R. S. (2006). Changing the work environment in ICUs to achieve patient-focused care. *Chest, 130*(5), 1571–1578.

National Council of State Boards of Nursing. (2005). *Working with others: A position paper.* Retrieved January 15, 2007, from http://www.NCSBN.org/pdfs/workingwithothers.pdf

Needleman, J., & Buerhaus, P. (2006). Nurse staffing in hospitals: Is there a business case for quality? *Health Affairs, 25*(1), 204–211.

Needleman, J., Buerhaus, P. I., Mattke, S., Stewart, M., Zelevinsky, K. (2002). Nurse staffing levels and the quality of care in hospitals. *New England Journal of Medicine, 346,* 1715–2722.

Person, C. (2004). Patient care delivery. In M. Koloroutis (Ed.), *Relationship-based care* (pp. 159–182). Minneapolis, MN: Creative Health Care Management.

Potter, P., & Grant, E. (2004). Understanding RN and unlicensed assistive personnel working relationships in designing care delivery strategies. *Journal of Nursing Administration, 34*(1), 19–25.

Ritter-Teitel, L. (2004). Registered nurse hours worked per patient day. The key to assessing staffing effectiveness and ensuring patient safety. *Journal of Nursing Administration, 34*(4), 167–169.

Roussel, L. (2006). Conceptualization of nursing administration: Theory and concepts. In L. Roussel (Ed.) with R. C. Swansburg & R. J. Swansburg, *Management and leadership for nurse administrators.* Sudbury, MA: Jones and Bartlett.

Sovie, M. D., Gift, A., Jawad, A. F., Stratton, L., Wallace, PL., Aiken, L. (2000). *Hospital restructuring's impact on outcomes. Final report* (NIH Grant 5 R01 NR04285-03). Bethesda, MD: National Institute of Nursing Research.

Swansburg, R. C., & Swansburg R. J. (2002). *Introduction to management and leadership for nurse managers* (3rd ed.). Sudbury, MA: Jones and Bartlett.

Tiedeman, M. E., & Lookinland, S. (2004). Traditional models of care delivery. What have we learned? *Journal of Nursing Administration, 34*(6), 291–297.

Tomey, A. M. (2004). *Guide to nursing management and leadership* (6th ed.). St. Louis: Mosby.

Ulrich, R., & Quan, X. (2004). *The role of the physical environment in the hospital of the 21st century: A once-in-a-lifetime opportunity. The Center for Health Design for Designing the 21st Century Hospital Project.* Princeton, NJ: Robert Wood Johnson Foundation.

Vahey, D. C., Aiken, L. H., Sloane, D. M., Clark S. P., & Vargas, D. (2004). Nurse burnout and patient satisfaction. *Medical Care, 42*(2), 11-57–11-66.

Weisman, C. S., & Nathanson, C. A. (1985). Professional satisfaction and client outcomes. *Medical Care, 23*(10) 1179–1192.

Whitcomb, R., Wilson, S., Chang-Dawkins, S., Durand, J., Pitcher, D., Lauzon, C., et al. (2002). Advanced practice nursing: Acute care model in progress. *Journal of Nursing Administration, 32*(3), 123–125.

White, P., & Hall, M. E. (2006). Mapping the literature of case management of nursing. *Journal of the Medical Library Association, 94,* E99–E106.

Yoder-Wise, P. S. (2007). Delegation: An art of professional practice. In P. S. Yoder-Wise (Ed.), *Leading and managing in nursing* (4th ed.). St. Louis: Mosby.

6

Nursing Documentation

Cheryl Wraa

Outcome-Based Learning Objectives

After studying this chapter, the learner will be able to:

1. Explain regulatory and professional standards for patient care documentation.
2. List general principles that guide documentation.
3. Differentiate advantages and disadvantages of different documentation systems.
4. Apply the nursings process to the Preparation for Practice exercises.

NURSES COLLECT data from multiple sources that they analyze and integrate to formulate nursing care plans, implement care decisions, evaluate patient response, and communicate the information to other members of the health care team. The most familiar way in which the information is conveyed is through the patient's **medical record,** which is the legal document for all information regarding a patient's hospital course and evidence for the extent of care provided and the outcome of that care. The medical record also describes anticipated treatment and educational needs (Austin, 2006; Lee, 2005). The patient's medical record is not only used to verify the care given, but to convey the quality of care, ensure continuity of care, assist with reimbursement, demonstrate compliance with regulations and policies, provide evidence in a court of law, and provide data for research and education (Austin, 2006; Childers, 2005).

Documentation Standards

Accrediting organizations, federal and state agencies, and professional organizations and institutions all set standards that guide nursing documentation in the particular places in which nurses practice.

Accreditation Standards

Nursing documentation must comply with the standards established through accrediting and licensing organizations, such as the Joint Commission, formerly known as the Joint Commission on Accreditation of Healthcare Organizations or JCAHO. The commission surveys facilities to measure compliance with its standards for safe health care. This accreditation could be jeopardized by inadequate or poor documentation. Loss of accreditation can affect reimbursement eligibility for Medicare, Medicaid, and managed care plans. The Joint Commission's standards do not require traditional nursing care plans, but do require documentation of an individualized plan of care for each patient. Here are some selected standards that should be reflected within the nursing documentation:

- Staff members integrate the information from various assessments of the patient to identify and assign priorities to their care needs.
- A registered nurse assesses the patient's need for nursing care in all settings where nursing care is provided.
- The assessment process for an infant, a child, or an adolescent patient is individualized.
- The assessment process addresses the special needs of patients who are receiving treatment for alcoholism or other drug dependencies.
- The assessment process addresses the special needs of patients who are receiving treatment for emotional or behavioral disorders.

- The assessment process addresses the special needs of patients who are possible victims of abuse.
- Each patient is reassessed at points designated in hospital policy.
- Care is planned and provided in an interdisciplinary, collaborative manner by qualified individuals.
- Care, treatment, and rehabilitation are planned to ensure that they are appropriate to the patient's needs and severity of disease, condition, impairment, or disability.
- The patient's progress is periodically evaluated against care goals and the plan of care and, when indicated, the plan or goals are revised.
- Continuing care at the time of discharge is based on the patient's assessed needs.
- Functional rehabilitation status is assessed to determine the current level of functioning, self-care, self-responsibility, independence, and quality of life.
- Restraint or seclusion use is limited to situations with adequate, appropriate, clinical justification.
- Patients are educated about pain and pain management.

Accrediting organizations will periodically review medical records to ensure that the standard of care is consistent throughout. The Joint Commission currently uses a *tracer methodology* during accreditation visits. The site surveyor will choose a patient who is currently hospitalized and use the patient's clinical record as a "road map." The surveyor reviews the care documented to determine if the organization has complied with standards and systems for providing care. The Joint Commission also requires that health care facilities regularly monitor, evaluate, and explore ways to improve the quality of care given to patients.

Each year the Joint Commission publishes patient safety goals that need to be addressed by health care facilities to improve patient care (Joint Commission, 2008). They are listed on the Joint Commission website for the current year. One example of a patient safety goal is the 2008 goal to "improve the effectiveness of communications among caregivers," which includes a standardized list of abbreviations, acronyms, symbols, and dose designations that are *not* to be used throughout the organization. The Joint Commission (2008) has stated that the following abbreviations are banned from use:

Abbreviation	Alternative
• U	unit(s)
• IU	international unit(s)
• QD	daily
• QOD	every other day
• Always use leading zero	Use 0.X mg (example: 0.5 mg)
• Never use a trailing zero	Use X mg (example: 5 mg)
• MS	Morphine sulfate or morphine
• MSO₄	Morphine sulfate or morphine
• MgSO₄	Magnesium sulfate

State, Federal, and Professional Standards

Documentation must also follow guidelines set by state and federal agencies such as the Health Care Financing Administration (HCFA), insurance companies, professional organizations such as the American Nurses Association, and the policies of the institution where the nurse is employed. In general, they require documentation to include initial and ongoing assessments, any change in the patient's condition, therapies given and the patient's response, patient teaching, and relevant statements made by the patient (Duclos-Miller, 2004).

State boards of nursing control the practice of nursing by development of state **nurse practice acts** that establish guidelines to ensure safe practice. The standards set by the practice acts are based on the nursing process, which is a systematic method of planning and providing care to the patient, and requires compliance as evidenced in documentation. State nurse practice acts are revised frequently and, as such, documentation requirements may also change. What the nurse documents in the medical record shows compliance with the standards set by the health care facility, state law, and professional organizations (Austin, 2006).

 It is important to be familiar with the nurse practice act of the state in which you work. Most state boards of nursing have a website for reference.

Health Insurance Portability and Accountability Act

The Health Insurance Portability and Accountability Act (HIPAA) of 1996 requires the Department of Health and Human Services (DHHS) to adopt standards for electronic health care transactions. DHHS published a Privacy Rule in December 2000 that became effective on April 14, 2001. The Privacy Rule set national standards for the protection of health information. It was modified in March 2002 and again in August 2002. Further information is found in Chapter 3 ☺ .

The rule affects documentation in that only the patient or those health care team members involved with the patient's care have a legal right to review the medical record. Release of patient information without the consent of the patient is a violation of the patient's privacy and a violation of HIPAA. If a health care facility is found to be in violation of HIPAA, the facility must pay a fine and is in jeopardy of losing Medicare and Medicaid funding. The person responsible for the violation may face immediate dismissal.

■ Documentation Principles

To be effective, documentation needs to be systematic, timely, and accurate and give a clear account of the nursing care that was provided. The standards and guidelines for documentation differ among health care facilities and specific patient populations, but certain fundamental principles guide all forms of documentation:

- Write legibly.
- Date and time each entry.
- Use only approved abbreviations.

- Document in chronological order.
- Document information promptly.
- Document all observations objectively.
- Use institutional policy to correct written errors.
- Ensure that documentation is complete, concise, and accurate.
- Sign all documents per your institutional policy and include your professional credentials.

Complete, Concise, and Accurate

It is important to document your observations as clearly as possible. Document only facts: what you see, hear, and do. Describe what you see and do not be vague. For example, "Drainage from the surgical wound soaked three 4×4s in 10 minutes. Surgeon notified" is more accurate than "Drainage from surgical wound increased."

Chart relevant information that relates to the patient's care and the nursing process. The documentation should clearly differentiate the nurse's actions from those of the other health care team members. It should reflect nursing actions and the patient outcomes indicating the progress of the patient. Incomplete documentation negates the purpose of documentation. If incomplete, the document cannot stand as sound evidence in a court of law, quality of care cannot be evaluated, continuity of care may be broken, coordination of care may be compromised, and reimbursements may be rejected. The patient record is a legal document, so the nurse should never:

- Document procedures or medication administration in advance.
- Chart for another person without signing his name.
- Add information at a later date unless the nurse indicates that he did so.
- Add inaccurate information.
- Refer to staff conflicts or staffing problems.
- Document that you filed an "incident report."
- Destroy records.

 CRITICAL ALERT *In a court of law, the general rule is if it was not documented, it was not done.*

Objectivity

Document accurately what happened and your findings. Describe the factual occurrences that you can see, hear, smell, or touch. Be objective and avoid vague statements that are subjective. Instead of documenting that a patient "appears short of breath" or "breathing appears labored," document statements such as these:

- Patient is complaining of shortness of breath.
- Patient is able to speak only in 1- or 2-word sentences.
- Inspiratory and expiratory wheezes heard.

The example "patient appears short of breath" is subjective and could be manipulated later should your treatment or judgment be challenged. Instead of using the word "appears" as a shortcut, fac-

tually describe what you see that makes you come to the conclusion that the patient "appears" short of breath. For example, "Patient noted to have increased respiratory rate with use of accessory muscles and nasal flaring."

Any information you obtain from the patient or family should be documented in that context to preserve your credibility. For example, if the nurse writes "Patient fell from standing position," but did not observe this actually happening, it is not accurate. It should be documented as follows "Per patient (or witness), patient walking on uneven surface, fell from standing position." Complete, factual, accurate documentation is difficult to misinterpret and will give a clear account of the patient's care.

Timeliness

Documentation should flow so that the person reading it can picture exactly what is occurring. Timeliness includes these aspects: (1) Document as soon as possible after an observation is made or care is provided. Documentation that is done concurrently with the care provided is more likely to be accurate and complete. (2) Document date and time of each entry. Documenting the sequence of events and changes in patient condition is essential. Timed occurrences followed by nursing actions and patient response can help prevent misinterpretation. Failure to act or improper action can lead to a malpractice suit. The expectation is that you practice at the same level as any other competent registered nurse in the same situation. Deviation from the standard of care or poor documentation of care can lead to allegations of negligence. Frequent, accurate updates verify the nursing care that was given. If you have forgotten to document something, or need to add important information, add the entry on the first available line and record the current date and time, label it *late entry,* and record the date and time when the entry should have been made.

Military time is used by many facilities to alleviate confusion over a.m. and p.m. entries. Military time is expressed in 24 one-hour-long periods per day, rather than two sets of 12 one-hour periods. Chart 6–1 compares military time to regular time.

CHART 6–1   Military Time

Military Time	a.m.	Military Time	p.m.
0100 hours	1 a.m.	1300 hours	1 p.m.
0200 hours	2 a.m.	1400 hours	2 p.m.
0300 hours	3 a.m.	1500 hours	3 p.m.
0400 hours	4 a.m.	1600 hours	4 p.m.
0500 hours	5 a.m.	1700 hours	5 p.m.
0600 hours	6 a.m.	1800 hours	6 p.m.
0700 hours	7 a.m.	1900 hours	7 p.m.
0800 hours	8 a.m.	2000 hours	8 p.m.
0900 hours	9 a.m.	2100 hours	9 p.m.
1000 hours	10 a.m.	2200 hours	10 p.m.
1100 hours	11 a.m.	2300 hours	11 p.m.
1200 hours	12 noon	2400 hours	12 midnight

Legibility

One of the main purposes of the patient medical record is to communicate with other members of the health care team. Documentation that is sloppy or difficult to read wastes time and puts the patient in jeopardy because critical information may be missing or misinterpreted. Incorrect grammar and misspelled words can create the same negative impression as sloppy handwriting. Even if you gave excellent care to the patient, the attorney or jury in a court of law may interpret it as below the acceptable standard of care if the documentation is sloppy or incomplete (Austin, 2006; Childers, 2005).

The medical record is a legal, permanent document and should be completed in colored ink that is easily photocopied. If a nurse's cursive writing is difficult to read, then the nurse should print instead.

Abbreviations

Accrediting bodies and state regulation stipulate that health care facilities must develop an approved list of abbreviations to be used for documentation. Use of unapproved abbreviations can lead to serious errors. For instance, what does the abbreviation "BS" mean? Are you documenting information regarding the patient's breath sounds or their bowel sounds? Does "pt" stand for patient, physical therapy, or prothrombin time?

 Be sure that you know and use your institution's approved abbreviations. If you are not sure the abbreviation is correct, spell the word out.

Corrections

Documentation errors may occur. When a nurse has made a documentation error, she should correct it immediately by drawing a single line through the entry, identifying it as an error, and adding the date, time, and her signature. The nurse should never try to obliterate the error with ink or correction fluid because this appears as if she is trying to hide something.

If you are documenting on a computerized record, follow the protocol developed by your facility for correction of entries. As with handwritten entries, once notes are entered into the computerized record, they become a part of that permanent record and should not be deleted or changed without explanation, date, time, and signature. If using an electronic medical record, the date, time, and signature will be placed automatically.

 Changing a patient care record in any way is illegal and constitutes tampering.

Effective documentation is clear, concise, objective recording of the care given, including any significant events, presented in a legible, organized manner that is representative of the nursing process.

Legal Situations

Certain procedures or legal situations in which the nurse is involved require special documentation. You should be aware of these and know how to document them.

Consent Forms

Prior to most procedures or treatments, the procedure must be explained to the patient and the patient must agree to have the procedure or treatment. Included in this explanation are the risks and benefits. Most facilities have a standard form that is used to obtain consent. The legal responsibility for obtaining informed consent is with the physician, but the nurse may be asked to witness the consent. The requirement for obtaining informed consent can be waived in two situations: (1) if the patient who is mentally competent states that he does not want to hear the details of the treatment or procedure (2) if the patient is in extremis and an immediate medical or surgical treatment is needed to save her life.

If the patient asks questions after the physician has explained the procedure, answer only those questions that fall within your scope of practice. Document the information that you gave the patient. When you witness a consent, it is important to evaluate the patient to make sure the person is competent, awake, alert, and aware of what he is being told.

 Patients who have received sedation or pain medication should never be allowed to sign an informed consent. The patient may not be able to understand the risks and benefits associated with the procedure, and the consent will be invalid, putting the institution and the nurse at legal risk.

Advance Directives

The Patient Self-Determination Act requires that health care facilities provide information about the patient's right to refuse treatment. It is the nurse's responsibility to document that the patient received the information. The facility is also required to ask if the patient has advance directives, which are legal documents that state the patient's wishes regarding life-sustaining medical care. If the patient has advance directives, the nurse should ascertain if the patient brought them to the hospital. Whenever a patient has an advance directive, a copy should be placed in the patient's medical record. Common types of advance directives include durable powers of attorney for health care, living wills, and do-not-resuscitate orders.

Using Restraints

Most facilities have special forms for physical restraint orders. Such orders must contain the date and time of the order, reason for restraint use, duration of restraint use, type of restraint, and the physician's signature. The order must be reviewed and renewed every 24 hours. It is the nurse's responsibility to observe the patient frequently for any problem that might be related to the restraint, such as skin breakdown or decreased distal circulation. Additionally, the nurse should perform range-of-motion exercises on all extremities, and document observations and care.

Leaving Against Medical Advice

A patient who is mentally competent has the right to refuse treatment and leave the hospital at any time. If a patient chooses to leave, it should be clearly documented that the patient has been advised that she is leaving against medical advice (AMA), understands the risks of leaving, and understands that she can come back.

An AMA form should be signed by the patient and includes this information:

- Names of those notified of the patient's decision
- The risks of leaving as told to the patient
- Name of person accompanying the patient and any discharge instructions given
- The patient's destination, if known.

This protects the facility, physician, and nurse if problems arise after the patient leaves. If the patient refuses to sign or leaves without telling anyone, an incident report should be completed.

Incident Reports

Whenever an adverse event occurs, an incident report should be completed. An incident report is not part of the patient's medical record; it is a mechanism for informing administration about an incident. The incident report can alert the administration to a potential claim and, therefore, the need to gather more detail. It also assists the administration in identifying possible areas for performance improvement. Only those who witnessed the incident should complete and sign the form, and each witness should file a separate form. When completing the form, include, in quotes, any statements made by the patient or family members regarding the incident.

Documentation of the incident in the patient's medical record should be factual and include follow-up treatment and the patient's response. Do not document in the patient record that an incident report was completed, because this negates the confidential nature of the report. Most facilities have specific forms for legal situations. If you are not familiar with the form, be sure to ask for assistance in order to protect yourself and the facility.

Nursing Process

The nursing process is a systematic method of planning and providing care to patients and is the foundation for nursing documentation. It is also the basic organizing system for the National Council Licensure Examination for registered nurses (NCLEX-RN®). The nursing process contains six phases or steps: assessment; nursing diagnosis, which describes an actual or potential health problem that a nurse can legally manage; outcome identification; planning; implementation; and evaluation (Hendler, Kovach, & Sciarra, 2005; White, 2003). (Note that one of the steps discussed here, outcome identification, is often considered part of the diagnosis phase; see further discussion in Chapter 7 🔗 .) The steps build on each other, but are not linear. Steps overlap and the process changes as new information is gathered and the patient's responses are evaluated. The nursing process requires critical thinking skills to evaluate findings, identify assumptions, examine alternatives, and understand various points of view. Critical thinking is an integral part of each step of the nursing process.

The steps in the nursing process are briefly discussed next. Chapter 7 🔗 covers the nursing process in more detail.

Assessment

Assessment initiates the nursing process. It begins when the patient arrives at the facility and continues throughout the hospi-

talization. During the assessment, important information is collected from various sources to assist the nurse in formulating nursing diagnoses.

Documentation of assessment findings is very important because it serves as a communication tool for the other health care team members.

Nursing Diagnosis

A nursing diagnosis differs from a medical diagnosis in that doctors are licensed to diagnose and treat illnesses, and nurses are licensed to diagnose and treat the patient's response to illness and need for education. Nursing diagnosis should be documented in order of priority with the highest priorities being those related to immediate physical care needs.

Outcome Identification

The goal is to assist the patient to reach the highest functional level possible. Expected outcomes should be realistic, measurable, and documented with target dates. When documenting outcome statements, the following should be included:

- The desired behavior that is to be observed
- Criteria for measuring the behavior
- The conditions under which the behavior should occur
- When the behavior should occur.

Planning

The plan of action or nursing care plan is developed to help deliver quality patient care. The plan includes nursing diagnoses, expected outcomes, and nursing interventions. The documented plan of care becomes a permanent part of the medical record, and often guides daily documentation of the patient's progress.

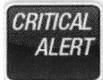 *Patients' problems can change during their hospitalization. Review the plan of care often and make changes as needed.*

In some specialized areas, such as intensive care units, the nursing care plan has been replaced by plans that are developed by multidisciplinary teams. These plans, called **critical pathways,** are comprehensive plans of care for specific patient situations or disease processes. Critical pathways include nursing interventions, medical interventions, and expected timelines for patient outcomes. The critical pathway is placed on a flow sheet for documentation purposes. A sample critical pathway is provided on the accompanying Student CD-ROM.

Implementation

Implementation refers to the actual nursing interventions delivered. The interventions must be directed toward the "related to" clause of the identified nursing diagnoses. To write interventions clearly, state when and how the intervention is to be performed. Be sure the intervention fits the patient's age, condition, developmental level, and values. Also, keep the patient's safety in mind, consider other health care activities, and use available resources. Documentation should be outcome oriented, so it is important to document when an intervention has been performed and the patient's response.

Evaluation

Documentation standards include an evaluation of the patient's progress toward the expected outcomes within the plan of care. An evaluation statement is one that includes the details of the care provided, with objective evidence of the patient's response. The evaluation should indicate whether the expected outcome criterion from the plan of care was achieved.

The nursing process allows for an organized method of planning and delivering nursing care. Using the nursing process for the basis of your documentation demonstrates that the standard of care has been met.

◼ Documentation Systems

Health care facilities select documentation systems to meet the needs of their specific patient care areas and to comply with legal and regulatory requirements. An acute care facility may have multiple systems in different areas of the hospital. Chart 6–2 provides brief comparisons of the different documentation systems.

Narrative System

Narrative documentation is used across most health care settings. It consists of narrative progress notes that describe a chronologi-

cal account of the patient's status, interventions performed, and response to interventions. Advantages to narrative documentation are that it is flexible, descriptive and gives the reader a picture of what has occurred over an extended period of time. Key elements of this system are knowing when to document, what to document, and how to organize the data. A disadvantage to narrative documentation is the tendency to chart everything that happens. This can make the documentation long and repetitive.

Flow sheets are often used in conjunction with narrative documentation. They are used to document routine observations such as assessments. This allows the reader to observe significant changes or trends. Samples that you can use to practice your documentation skills are located in the Student CD-ROM Toolbox. Please go to the accompanying CD-ROM to access this useful information.

Problem-Oriented Medical Record

The problem-oriented medical record (POMR) is most effective in acute and long-term settings. This system consists of five components that are discussed further: baseline data, a problem list, a plan of care for each problem, multidisciplinary progress notes, and a discharge summary. This system was developed by physicians and later adapted by nurses.

CHART 6–2 Documentation Systems Comparison			
System	**Parts of Record**	**Description**	**Nurse's Notes Format**
Narrative	Nurse's notes / Flow sheets to supplement care plan	Each discipline writes narrative progress notes in segregated areas of the medical record.	Narration with time of entry
Problem-oriented medical record (POMR)	Nurse's notes / Database / Nursing care plan / Problem list / Discharge summary	Consists of gathering baseline data and creating a problem list and plan of care for each identified problem.	SOAP, SOAPIE, or SOAPIER
Problem, intervention, evaluation (PIE)	Nurse's notes / Assessment flow sheets / Problem list	Uses a problem, intervention, evaluation format to describe patient problems, intervention, and evaluation of responses to interventions.	Problem / Intervention / Evaluation
Focus	Nurse's notes / Flow sheets / Checklists	Uses a data–action–response format to identify focus areas of concern, plan care, and evaluate response to care.	Data / Action / Response
Charting by exception (CBE)	Nurse's notes / Flow sheets with patient teaching records and discharge notes / Care plan / Graphic record	Only requires documentation of abnormal or significant findings and events.	SOAPIE or SOAPIER
Flow sheet, assessment, concise, timely (FACT)	Nurse's notes / Flow sheets / Assessment sheet	Uses a baseline assessment and data, action, response format to evaluate problems identified in the nursing diagnosis care plan.	Data / Action / Response
Electronic medical record (EMR)	Nurse's notes / Flow sheets / Nursing care plan / Database / Teaching plan	Uses a database, outcome-based plan of care.	Evaluative statements / Expected outcomes / Learning outcomes

Source: From Duclos-Miller, P. A. (2004). Managing documentation risk: A guide for nurse managers. Marblehead, MA: HCPro, Inc.

Database

Nurses most commonly complete the database or admission assessment. This initial assessment is very important, because it is the basis for the patient's plan of care. The database includes the reason for hospitalization, past medical history, allergies, current medications, physical assessment, psychosocial findings, self-care abilities, educational needs, and discharge planning needs. From this information, the problem list is formed.

Problem List

The problem list contains the patient's current medical problems in chronological order of when each was identified, not in order of acuteness or priority. The list provides the nurse with an overview of the patient's health status. Each problem is then given a number. Documentation on the initial plan, progress notes, and discharge summary will correspond to these numbers. When a problem has been resolved, the problem remains on the list, but is then highlighted to show that it has been resolved.

Initial Plan

From the problem list, an initial plan is developed that includes expected outcomes, plans for further data collection, patient care, and teaching plans. The nurse should include the patient in goal setting as the plan is developed.

Progress Notes

Progress notes are written using the SOAP, SOAPIE, or SOAPIER format. This format documents the following information for each problem:

- **S–subjective data:** Information that the patient or significant others tell the nurse. It can be stated as a complaint or an impression if not from the patient.
- **O–objective data:** Measurable information the nurse gathers during the assessment, such as vital signs, laboratory test results, and signs and symptoms noted.
- **A–assessment data:** This is stated as the patient problem or nursing diagnosis that the nurse derived from the subjective and objective data that was gathered. This is a dynamic process and will change as more information is gathered.
- **P–plan:** The plan describes the interventions planned to resolve each problem. The plan should include short-term and long-term goals.
- **I–interventions:** This documents the measures that are taken to achieve an expected outcome. Teaching and documentation of the patient's understanding of the plan would be placed here.
- **E–evaluation:** Evaluation of the patient's response to the interventions.
- **R–revision:** Documentation of any change of plan for a particular problem.

Discharge Summary

The discharge summary notes whether each problem on the list is resolved. This is the place in the SOAPIE note for the nurse to discuss unresolved problems and document the plan for addressing the problem after discharge. It is also the place to note any communication with an outside facility, agency, or the patient's family.

CHART 6–3 Sample of SOAPIE Documentation

1/12/09 0800

S: The patient states "I am having chest pain."

O: Patient in telemetry bed, skin pale and moist, monitor shows sinus rhythm with elevated T waves and occasional unifocal PVCs. Blood pressure 170/98, heart rate 66, respiratory rate 24, patient rates pain at a 6.

A: Patient appears in moderate distress

P: Follow physician orders for chest pain, page primary physician.

1/12/09 0810

I: Placed patient on oxygen at 2L per nasal cannula, 4 mg of morphine given IV, 12-lead ECG completed, Dr. Johnson at bedside.

E: Patient states pain has decreased to a 3. Skin now dry with good color. Monitor shows sinus rhythm without ectopy, T waves remain elevated.

A sample of documentation using the SOAPIE method is shown in Chart 6–3.

One disadvantage of the problem-oriented system is that it lists the problems in chronological order, rather than by priority.

Problem, Intervention, Evaluation System

The problem, intervention, evaluation (PIE) system works well in areas where the patient's condition can change rapidly. This system lists the patient's problem first, followed by the interventions taken to alleviate the problem, and last, the evaluation of the patient's response to the intervention. This system organizes the information according to the patient's problems and integrates the plan of care into the progress notes. A daily assessment flow sheet is used to document routine care and monitoring measures, with detailed information documented in the progress note. Chart 6–4 shows an example of PIE documentation.

Problem

After an initial assessment is done, nursing diagnoses are identified and form the "problem" piece of the documentation system. Most facilities will develop a list of accepted nursing diagnoses that usually correspond to those approved by the North American Nursing Diagnosis Association (NANDA). Each problem is then numbered for future reference.

CHART 6–4 Sample of PIE Nursing Progress Notes

1/12/09 2200

P#1: Pain related to fractured femur

IP#1: Pain identified as 8 out of 10. Pain medication given per physician orders. Reassess pain level at 2230. Continue to assess pain every 4 hours using pain scale.

1/12/09 2230

EP#1: Pain identified as 4 out of 10.

Intervention

Nursing actions that are taken to alleviate a problem are documented for each nursing diagnosis. Each "I" should be labeled with the corresponding problem number.

Evaluation

Following the interventions, the patient's responses should be documented. As with the interventions, the "E" should be labeled with the corresponding problem number.

One disadvantage of the PIE system is that each problem needs to be evaluated once each shift. The PIE system also does not document the planning step in the nursing process, which addresses expected outcomes.

Focus System

The Focus system includes a detailed patient assessment leading to the development of patient-centered problems or foci of concern. Each problem is written as a nursing diagnosis or may refer directly to a specific sign or symptom, patient behavior, or significant event such as an invasive procedure. The Focus system is flexible, centers on the nursing process, and allows the reader to easily locate information about a specific problem. A daily assessment flow sheet is used to document routine care and monitoring measures.

The Focus documentation is completed in the progress notes in a data–action–response format, as shown in Chart 6–5. The problem focus is identified and then followed by:

- **D–data:** The data include both subjective and objective information regarding the problem.
- **A–action:** The action includes current and future nursing actions based on the assessment of the patient.
- **R–response:** The response describes the patient's response to the action.

Charting by Exception System

Charting by exception (CBE) is used to eliminate lengthy or repetitive documentation. It departs from traditional types of systems by documenting only significant or abnormal findings. To use the CBE system, the nurse must be using critical pathway or interdisciplinary plans of care that address every possible patient problem. The format contains baseline data and a problem-oriented plan of care. Preprinted guidelines are prepared for each body system and the initial and ongoing assessments are documented only as exceptions to these guidelines. Flow sheets provide a normal assessment to chart against. For each body system the nurse would document within normal limits or document what is not normal. The different types of flow sheets needed for the CBE system are:

- Physician's order flow sheet
- Nursing order flow sheet
- Graphic form
- Patient teaching record
- Patient discharge note
- Supplemental nurse's progress notes.

The CBE system saves time and decreases the amount of documentation needed. The flow sheets are nursing focused and improve documentation because the format highlights care interventions and requires a documented evaluation of the patient's response. A disadvantage of the CBE system is the time it takes to develop the guidelines and standards of care. These must be in place and taught to all nursing staff for this system to be effective.

FACT System

The FACT system uses assessment and action flow sheets with nursing progress notes. The flow sheets may be patient specific or follow the CBE format of normal assessment parameters for each body system. The nursing progress notes use the data–action–response format discussed earlier. The FACT acronym stands for the four key elements of the system:

- **F**–Flow sheets that are individualized to specific services
- **A**–Assessment features that are standardized with baseline parameters
- **C**–Concise, integrated nursing progress notes and flow sheets that document the patient's condition and response to treatments
- **T**–Timely entries that can be documented when care is given.

As with CBE, the FACT system eliminates repetition and promotes consistent language. It encourages immediate recording of data because the system is readily accessible. Disadvantages include the time commitment needed to develop the standards and the training needed to implement the system.

Electronic Medical Record

One of the most significant recent changes in documentation has been the introduction of computerized charting systems. The ability to have universal access to patient records is necessary to the delivery of safe and effective health care. For example, a patient's medication history is readily accessible throughout the health care system and each change can be updated whether the change is made by telephone or via an office visit. The electronic medical record (EMR) is legible, decreases recording time and costs, decreases errors, improves communication between health care providers, and provides better access to medical data for patient care, education, performance improvement activities, and

| CHART 6–5 | Sample of Focus Charting |

Date	Time	Focus	Nursing Progress Notes
1/12/09	1000	Pain	D: Patient complains of pain to abd. incision. Rates pain as 6 out of 10. Abdominal incision clean dry and intact. No redness or drainage noted. Abdomen soft with moderate tenderness near the incision. A: Patient given pain medication per physician order.
1/12/09	1030		R: Patient states pain is now 3 out of 10.

research (Duclos-Miller, 2004). Another advantage to the EMR is the use of standard terminology, which promotes better communication among providers.

As just stated, the EMR allows a patient's medication history to be accessible throughout the health care system. Complications from drug reactions account for approximately 4.7% of admissions to hospitals in the United States with the estimated associated costs being $3.8 million per hospital per year (Varkey et al., 2007). Because of these adverse reactions, the Institute for Healthcare Improvement's 100,000 Lives Campaign and the Joint Commission identified the prevention of adverse drug reactions as a priority for national action and have required institutions to perform **medication reconciliation,** which is the process of identifying an accurate list of all medications the patient is taking and using this list to provide correct medications for the patient anywhere in the health care system. The initial list is developed by either the primary care provider or on admission to the hospital. When a patient is admitted to the hospital, any new medication prescribed is added to the EMR or any medication stopped during the hospitalization is marked as deleted. The EMR medication list is then reconciled by the health care team daily. It is of great importance to reconcile the medication list prior to the patient's discharge. The nurse will review and be sure that the patient understands all changes.

Depending on the type of computer and software that is used by a facility, patient information may be accessed by voice recognition, a keyboard, light pen, touch screen, or mouse. Most facilities place computers or terminals at workstations or patient bedsides to allow quick access by the health care team to patient information.

Privacy rights and confidentiality need to be addressed through institutional policies specific to the EMR. Security can be monitored by assigning electronic log-in names to each user and creating audit trails.

Nursing Care Documentation

Most EMRs provide a menu of words and phrases from which to choose to document in a standard format. You can further elaborate on a problem or clarify flow sheet documentation in the comment section of the form.

Nursing information systems (NIS) software programs have been developed that allow you to select and record nursing actions in the EMR. These systems contain most of the components of the nursing process and therefore adhere to the Joint Commission standards for documentation. Most NIS have features that allow customization of forms to allow specific institutional requirements. Some newer systems are interactive and, as data are entered, will prompt you with questions and suggestions regarding your data. These systems will also suggest nursing diagnoses for the care plan based on the assessment data that were entered.

The advantages of an EMR are the ability to retrieve information quickly and easily. It helps to link different sources of patient information such as clinic notes, laboratory results, consults, and diagnostic results. The EMR uses standard terminology and the documentation is legible, which improves communication among health care providers. Disadvantages are that not all health care providers are comfortable with computer

technology and extensive training may be necessary; lack of security measures can threaten patient confidentiality; if the system is "down," then information is unavailable unless hard copies are used and readily accessible; and initial implementation of the system is expensive.

Regardless of the system that is used where you practice, knowing the components of that system and understanding the basic principles of documentation are essential. The patient's medical record demonstrates that the care given was based on accepted professional and regulatory standards. When you complete your documentation, ask yourself the following questions:

- Is it factual?
- Does it document all the care given?
- If it is read 2 years from now, will it demonstrate that the care given met the standard of care?
- Does it show the sequence of events accurately, including the patient's response to treatment?
- Does it contain subjective statements or personal opinions?
- Does it clearly identify when information was obtained from the patient, family, or other caregivers?
- Is it legible?
- Are errors corrected in the approved manner?

Your documentation will show the quality of the care given, the outcome of that care, and collaboration among the members of the health care team and also describe future interventions and education needed. Documentation that is accurate and complete protects both the patient and the caregiver.

■ Preparation for Practice

As stated earlier, the development of a nursing plan of care using the nursing process requires critical thinking skills to evaluate findings, identify assumptions, examine alternatives, and understand various points of view. Critical thinking is an integral part of each step of the nursing process. To assist you in the development of your critical thinking skills, each chapter that covers a disorder has a real-life vignette at the end, followed by several questions to stimulate critical thinking. Using the same vignette, you will proceed to the accompanying MyNursingkit to view:

1. **The patient care Kardex.** The Kardex contains information regarding the patient's name, age, religion, medical diagnoses, past medical history, surgeries and major procedures since admission, current medications, treatments, diet, intravenous therapy, diagnostic tests, and procedures. The Kardex will also include the permitted level of activity, functional limitations, and assistance that may be needed.

2. **Three days of laboratory results.** This will allow you to look for abnormal values and trends.

From this information you will be asked to complete several forms that would assist you in preparing to care for the patient:

- **Summary of hospitalization.** This includes pertinent information regarding the patient such as age, admitting diagnosis, past medical history, surgeries or major procedures since admission, history of current illness or injury, vital signs and physical findings from the previous 24 hours, and the basic nursing care needed for the patient.

- **Pathophysiology.** This includes detailed pathophysiology for the current illness. Included are common signs and symptoms, and possible complications. This will help you to anticipate the patient's needs, possible complications, and knowledge deficits.
- **Laboratory results explanations.** All abnormal lab values or significant trends should be listed. Next to the result you will write a brief explanation of what the cause of the abnormality might be for this patient and the significance of the finding. This will help you to become familiar with trends for specific disease processes and hone your interpretive skills.
- **Medication administration record.** This form includes the usual dose, route, frequency, class, and action of the drug, the rationale for administration, side effects with nursing implications, and assessment data that indicate effectiveness. This will help you to become familiar with different classes of drugs, the nursing interventions and assessments necessary for safe administration, and the evaluations necessary to determine effectiveness.
- **Concept map.** The concept map assists the learner in the development of the nursing plan of care using the nursing process. The primary and secondary diagnoses are listed. For the primary diagnosis, list the critical assessments that are a priority for the patient. Follow the primary and secondary nursing diagnoses with high-risk potential problems. For each nursing diagnosis, list all assessment findings that sup-

port the diagnosis such as vital signs, lab results, and physical assessment findings. Then list medical and nursing interventions aimed at improving the problem. Following the nursing process, list the knowledge deficits and educational needs for the patient and family. In the last section, describe what the patient must be able to do before discharge or transfer, including appropriate community referrals.

The assignment assists the learner in the development of a problem-solving approach to nursing care. By doing this, the learner will gain experience in critical thinking skills and develop a systematic method for determining a patient's health problem, devising a plan of care, developing evaluation criteria, and knowing expected outcomes. The Preparation for Practice assignments will also help the learner to articulate the patient's needs and learn how to write effective evaluation statements. This, in turn, will significantly improve documentation skills and the ability to communicate with other health care team members to provide the safest most effective and holistic care for the patient.

■ Summary

Accurate, concise documentation takes practice. Remember, the patient's medical record is not only used to verify the care given, but to convey the quality of care. The record ensures continuity of care, assists with reimbursement, demonstrates compliance with regulations and policies, provides evidence in a court of law, and provides data for research and education. The patient's medical record is a powerful communication tool. Developing the ability to articulate the patient's condition and potential problems assists in creating a collaborative plan of care.

REVIEW QUESTIONS

1. The nurse is reviewing the latest National Patient Safety Goals. The regulatory body that publishes these goals is:
   1. Medicare.
   2. Medicaid.
   3. The Joint Commission.
   4. The State Board of Nursing.

2. The nurse makes a mistake while documenting in a patient's medical record. What should this nurse do?
   1. Rip out the page in the record and start over.
   2. Draw a single line through the entry, write the word error, date, time, and sign the entry.
   3. Use liquid paper to white out the entry.
   4. Use heavy black ink to darken the entry.

3. The nurse is documenting, using the narrative method. One disadvantage of using this method is:
   1. The time needed to develop standards.
   2. Problems are listed in chronological order.
   3. Problems need to be evaluated once per shift.
   4. There is a tendency to document everything.

4. Which of the following tools helps the nurse prepare a plan of care using the nursing process?
   1. Kardex
   2. Concept Map
   3. Medication Administration Record
   4. Past Medical History

Answers for review questions appear in Appendix D

KEY TERMS

critical pathways *p.100*
medical record *p.96*

medication reconciliation *p.104*
nurse practice act *p.91*

EXPLORE PEARSON **mynursingkit**™

MyNursingKit is your one stop for online chapter review materials and resources. Prepare for success with additional NCLEX®-style practice questions, interactive assignments and activities, web links, animations and videos, and more!

Register your access code from the front of your book at
www.mynursingkit.com

REFERENCES

Austin, S. (2006). Ladies and gentlemen of the jury, I present the nursing documentation. *Nursing 2006, 36*(1), 56–62.

Childers, K. P. (2005). Paying a price for poor documentation. *Nursing 2005, 35*(11).

Duclos-Miller, P. A. (2004). *Managing documentation risk: A guide for nurse managers.* Marblehead, MA: HCPro, Inc.

Hendler, C., Kovach, P., & Sciarra, J. (Eds.). (2005). *Charting made incredibly easy* (3rd ed.). Philadelphia: Springhouse.

Joint Commission. (2008). *Facts about the 2008 national patient safety goals.* Retrieved April 22, 2008, from http://www.jointcommission.org/PatientSafety/NationalPatientSafetyGoals/08_npsg_facts.htm

Lee, T. (2005). Nursing diagnoses: Factors affecting their use in charting standardized care plans. *Journal of Clinical Nursing, 14,* 640–647.

Varkey, P., Cunningham, J., O'Meara, J., Bonacci, R., Desai, N., & Sheeler, R. (2007). Multidisciplinary approach to inpatient medication reconciliation in an academic setting. *American Journal of Health-System Pharmacists, 64*(8), 850–854.

White, L. (2003). *Documentation & the nursing process.* New York: Thomson.

Nursing Process

Doris Ballard Ferguson, Annita Watson
With contributions by: Joyce Mikal-Flynn

Outcome-Based Learning Objectives

After studying this chapter, the learner will be able to:

1. Differentiate between the roles in nursing as specified by the American Nurses Association.
2. Explain the five steps of the nursing process and their relationship to each other.
3. Describe the cognitive, affective, and psychomotor skills necessary to conduct a comprehensive nursing assessment.
4. Differentiate between nursing diagnoses and collaborative problems.
5. Explain the relationship between critical thinking and the nursing process.

Research   Collaboration   Health Promotion   Nursing Process   Caring   Critical Thinking

FOR THE PAST 30 YEARS, the American Nurses Association (ANA) has published many standards of nursing practice. These standards and the social policy statement adopted by the ANA (2003) serve as national guidelines for nursing practice. A topical overview of both is shown in Chart 7–1 (p. 108).

In nursing practice, nurses' roles are defined as *independent, interdependent, and dependent* (ANA, 2004). **Independent activities** are those that nurses perform, prescribe, and or delegate based on their education and skills. Examples of independent activities are assessing, analyzing and diagnosing, planning, implementing, and evaluating. **Interdependent activities** are those activities that overlap with the activities of other health team members, physicians, social workers, pharmacists, nutritionists, and therapists (physical, speech, occupational) and require coordination and planning with these various health team members. **Dependent activities** are those prescribed by the physician and carried out by the nurse. They include implementing the physician's orders to administer medications or treatments. The nursing process, a concept coined in 1967 by Yura and Walsh (1988) and subsequently adopted by the ANA (2004), enhances each of the three roles for the patient's benefit and is the means for nurses to demonstrate accountability and responsibility to patients.

Nursing Process

The **nursing process** is defined as a variation of scientific reasoning and is used to diagnose and to treat human responses to potential and actual health problems (ANA, 2007). As the operational framework for nursing practice, the nursing process is the vehicle through which the nurse applies knowledge and skills in a systematic, goal-directed fashion to achieve the outcomes desired for the patient (ANA, 2007; King, 1971). By using the nursing process, the nurse approaches and responds to clinical situations consciously and deliberately. Such an approach avoids nursing care based on imitation ("That's how the others do it"), intuition ("This seems like a good way to do it"), or tradition ("We've always done it that way").

Nurse–Patient Relationship

The **nurse–patient relationship** is the means for applying the nursing process. This relationship is the mechanism by which the nurse works with the patient (Carpenito-Moyet, 2007; Orlando, 1961; Peplau, 1952; Rogers, 1970; Wilkinson, 2006). Three attributes are necessary to a successful nurse–patient relationship: (1) genuineness, the ability to be aware of one's own feeling, or being real; (2) respect for and acceptance of the other unconditionally;

CHART 7–1   National Guidelines for Nursing Practice

NURSING SCOPE AND STANDARDS OF PRACTICE

Scope of Nursing Practice

- Definition of Nursing
- Evolution of Nursing Practice
- Integrating the Science and Art of Nursing
- The Professional Registered Nurse
- Advanced Practice Registered Nursing
- Registered Nurses in Role Specialties
- Settings for Nursing Practice
- Continued Commitment to the Profession
- Professional Trends and Issues

Standards of Practice

- Standard 1. Assessment
- Standard 2. Diagnosis
- Standard 3. Outcomes Identification
- Standard 4. Planning
- Standard 5. Implementation
  Standard 5a. Coordination of Care
  Standard 5b. Health Teaching and Health Promotion
  Standard 5c. Consultation
  Standard 5d. Prescriptive Authority and Treatment
- Standard 6. Evaluation

Standards of Professional Performance

- Standard 7. Quality of Practice
- Standard 8. Practice Evaluation
- Standard 9. Education
- Standard 10. Collegiality
- Standard 11. Collaboration
- Standard 12. Ethics
- Standard 13. Research
- Standard 14. Resource Utilization
- Standard 15. Leadership

NURSING'S SOCIAL POLICY STATEMENT

Introduction

- The Social Context of Nursing
- Values and Assumptions of Nursing's Social Contract

Definition of Nursing

Knowledge Base for Nursing Practice

- Scope of Nursing Practice
- Specialization in Nursing
- Advanced Practice Registered Nurses
- Additional Advanced Roles

The Regulation of Nursing Practice

- Self-Regulation
- Professional Regulation
- Legal Regulation

Sources: American Nurses Association. (2004). *Standards of clinical nursing practice.* Washington, DC: Nursebooks.org; American Nurses Association. (2003). *Nursing's social policy statement* (2nd ed.). Washington, DC: Nursebooks.org.

and (3) a continuing desire to understand and empathize with the other. Effective nurse–patient relationships can be obtained when nurses are willing to look at their own values, prejudices, strengths, and limitations. Nurses must be open to the discovery of their own motivation and feelings through experience and relationships with others (Peplau, 1952; Rogers, 1970; Wilkinson, 2006).

Steps of the Nursing Process

The steps of the nursing process are progressive and successive—each step builds on previous steps and influences subsequent steps. For example, the nurse cannot develop a plan of care and select nursing interventions from that plan until valid nursing diagnoses have been formulated from an adequate database, which includes the patient's perspective and input (Carpenito-Moyet, 2007; Johnson, 1980; Orem, 1971). The nurse cannot evaluate outcomes of care unless the desired outcomes have been specified as patient goals or objectives in the care plan.

The nursing process generally consists of five successive and interrelated steps: (1) assessment, (2) diagnosis, (3) planning, (4) implementation, and (5) evaluation (Carpenito-Moyet, 2005). In 1999, however, the ANA added "outcome identification" as a discrete step of the process, although this component of the

process often is incorporated into the diagnosis phase and is presented as such in this chapter. The components of the five steps in the nursing process follow:

1. Assessment
   - Data collection
   - Analysis/synthesis of data
   - Nursing diagnosis
2. Nursing diagnosis and outcome identification
3. Planning of goals and objectives
   - Plans
   - Priorities
   - Scientific rationale
4. Implementation
5. Evaluation

These five steps and their components are depicted in more detail in Figure 7–1 ■, which illustrates the dynamic, cyclical, interdependent, and often overlapping nature of the steps of the nursing process. For example, while the nurse implements a planned intervention, such as pain relief measures, additional data may be collected that further validate and support the nurs-

FIGURE 7–1 ■ The nursing process.

ing diagnosis of pain, while also leading to the development of additional nursing diagnoses, such as a disturbance in the patient's usual sleeping patterns. Thus, during any nurse–patient interaction, the nurse is continuously collecting data that may then be helpful in planning, implementing, evaluating, or revising nursing care.

The nursing process is flexible and is, therefore, capable of being adapted to a variety of situations (Levine, 1973). It may be used in any type of clinical setting and with patients of varying ages, health status, and cultural backgrounds (Carpenito-Moyet, 2007; Leininger, 1991; Spector, 2004; Stanton, Paul, & Reeves, 1980; Wilkinson, 2006). The nursing process also can be used with families and communities as well as with individual patients. Each phase (step) of the nursing process is discussed next.

Assessment

In general terms, **assessment** is defined as the act of evaluating or appraising. Yura and Walsh (1988) provide a clear, concise, and useful definition of assessment as it relates to nursing: "The act of reviewing a situation for the purpose of diagnosing the patient's problems" (p. 110). Assessment actions include "examining the patient and identifying cues, collecting and analyzing the data, and reaching conclusions" (p. 110).

The nursing assessment begins the moment the nurse establishes initial contact with a patient. Data are collected through formal and informal interviews and a variety of other methods including observation, inspection, palpation, percussion, auscultation, and consultation with the patient and other health care providers. Data collection is a foundation of the nursing process; therefore, the nurse must strive for accuracy, completeness, and objectivity. An accurate assessment leads to identification of the patient's health status, concerns, and nursing diagnoses.

The purpose of data collection is to identify and obtain pertinent data about the patient. Nurses should consider patients in a multidimensional way; that is, the biophysical, psychological, spiritual, and sociocultural elements of the patient must be considered to ensure a comprehensive and accurate assessment (Henderson, 1966; Johnson, 1980; Watson, 1988, 2003).

Data Sources

The nurse uses two kinds of data sources: primary and secondary. The primary source of data is the patient. Secondary data sources include family, friends, other health care professionals, the patient's current health care record, and the nurse's own knowledge base. These secondary data sources should be viewed as a supplement to the data supplied by the primary source, the patient. The usefulness of information obtained from secondary sources is in clarifying, amplifying, or substantiating the data the nurse obtains from the patient.

Data Types

The nurse gathers two types of data: subjective data and objective data (Carpenito-Moyet, 2007; Wilkinson, 2006). **Subjective data** is the information that can be perceived only by the patient and not by the observer. One of the primary sources of subjective data is the nursing or health history. Because the patient is the informant, the information collected while taking a health history is subjective. **Objective data** consist of behaviors, activities, and events that can be observed or measured by another person using the five senses. Objective data are factual; they can be seen, heard, touched, smelled, or tasted. Vital signs, laboratory reports, rashes, and body posture are some examples of objective data.

Objective and subjective data are equally important in a comprehensive nursing assessment. When assessing a patient, the nurse should try to elicit objective data that correspond with the subjective data, and subjective data that correspond with objective data. By categorizing data as subjective and objective, the nurse is better able to validate data and to identify and resolve discrepancies and accurately report information to assist in communication and establishing nursing diagnoses.

Data Collection Process

Several factors influence the process of data collection: how the data are presented by the patient and how they are perceived by the nurse. The nurse and patient are influenced by their respective:

- Physical, mental, and emotional states and needs
- Cultural, social, and philosophical backgrounds
- Number and functional ability of senses
- Past experiences associated with the present situation
- Meaning of the event
- Interest, preoccupations, preconceptions, and motivational levels
- Knowledge or familiarity with the situation
- Environmental conditions and distractions
- Presence, attitudes, and reactions of others.

These factors create a situation in which both patient and nurse automatically assign personal meaning or interpretations to situations. Problems arise when the nurse's perception or interpretation is used as fact. The nursing diagnosis is the end product of the nursing assessment. The nurse analyzes the data gathered and reaches a conclusion about the health status. A patient may have one or more nursing diagnoses. Once the diagnoses have been formulated, the nurse is ready to develop a plan of care. Therefore, skill is needed in differentiating actual data from personal interpretation. The nurse's interpretation must be validated with the patient. Chart 7–2 provides examples of objective data versus personal interpretation of them.

 CRITICAL ALERT *The nurse's interpretation of the patient's problem (diagnosis) always must be validated with the patient.*

Guidelines for Data Collection

The ANA *Standards of Clinical Nursing Practice* (2004) are the guidelines for data collection. The recommended guidelines are as follows:

- Data that are collected are comprehensive and multifocal. The data need to reflect the life experiences of the patient and should consider biophysical, psychological, spiritual, socio-cultural, and socioeconomic influences. The nurse must use judgment in focusing data collection on areas that are most pertinent to the patient situation.
- A variety of sources are used for data collection. The patient is the primary source for data collection, but because perceptions of events and circumstances can vary, other sources should be used as well. Some general examples of sources are family, significant others, health care personnel, and written records.
- Appropriate tools are used for data collection. At least two data collection tools should be used to ensure the validity of the data obtained. The appropriateness of the tool used depends on the patient's age and health status.
- The data collected are objective and nonjudgmental. Data are collected through the use of observation, measurement, and interaction with the patient. Personal interpretations or perceptions of a situation may lead to further data collection, but must never be stated as data themselves.
- A systematic format is used for data collection. Theoretical and conceptual frameworks provide guides for data collection. The nurse begins data collection by assessing the patient's major concern, including multifocal influences on the concern. Then a more general assessment of the patient's health status is included as appropriate.
- The data collected reflect updating of information. Data collection is continuous in nature. The data should reflect appropriate updating of information obtained from a variety of data sources. As new data are obtained any changes in the health concerns or status of the patient must be noted.
- The data collected are recorded and communicated appropriately. Data collection is useless unless it is communicated appropriately in the patient's record. Therefore, information must be kept in a retrievable record-keeping system.

Data Collection and the Patient's Health Record

The patient's health record is a document containing (1) the medical history; (2) the findings from the physical examination; (3) the reports of laboratory tests; (4) the findings and conclusions from special examinations; (5) the findings and diagnoses of consultants; (6) the diagnoses of the responsible physician; (7) notes on treatment, including medication, surgical operations, radiation, and physical therapy; and (8) progress notes by physicians, nurses, and others. The purpose of the patient's medical record is to assist all health care providers (nurses, physicians, and others) with accurate communication and information, thus, improving the care and treatment of the patient (White, 2003). The health record also is discussed in Chapter 6 ❧.

Sequence of Components in the Health Record

The parts of the health history follow a standardized sequence, differing only in small details from one institution to another. The sequence shown in Chart 7–3 is an example used for adult patients. A different order is usually preferred by pediatricians, who set the birth history and the past history ahead of the present illness. Health history guidelines also are shown in Chapter 9 ❧.

CHART 7–2	Objective Data Versus Personal Interpretation	
Objective Data	**Personal Interpretation**
"I'd rather be left alone."	Patient is angry
Shoulder-length dark brown hair	Long, dirty brown hair
Blood pressure: 130/76	Normal blood pressure
Smiles frequently	Appears to be happy

CHART 7–3	Sequence for Taking a Health History

I. Identification and vital statistics

II. Informant, relation to the patient

III. Chief complaints (CC)

IV. Present illness (PI)

V. Medications and allergies

VI. Past history (PH)
   A. General health
   B. Infectious diseases
   C. Operations and injuries
   D. Previous hospitalizations
   E. Review of systems (ROS)
      1. Integument
      2. Lymph nodes
      3. Bones, joints, and muscles
      4. Hematopoietic system
      5. Endocrine system
      6. Allergic and immunologic history
      7. Head
      8. Eyes
      9. Ears
     10. Nose
     11. Mouth
     12. Throat
     13. Neck
     14. Breasts
     15. Respiratory system
     16. Cardiovascular system
     17. Gastrointestinal system
     18. Genitourinary system
     19. Nervous system
     20. Psychiatric history

VII. Social history (SH)

VIII. Family history (FH)

IX. Physical examination

X. Laboratory

XI. Summary

Frameworks for Data Collection

Frameworks for data collection include a health history, a physical format and functional instrument such as a growth and development chart for pediatric patients, activities of daily living (ADLs), and instrumental ADLs for older adults. Some examples of data collection tools for ADLs are provided in Charts 7–4 and 7–5 (p. 112).

Nursing Diagnosis and Outcome Identification

The assessment process is applicable to all groups of patients: individuals, families, and communities. After all data have been collected, they are sorted, organized, interpreted, and validated, and conclusions are then drawn about the patient's health status. These conclusions are called **nursing diagnoses.** Nursing diagnoses are clinical judgments about an individual, family, or community response to actual or potential health problems and life processes (North American Nursing Diagnosis Association [NANDA], 2007).

Nursing diagnoses are different from **collaborative problem**s such as medical diagnoses (diabetes, hypertension, coronary artery disease) because nurses' accountability differs for nursing diagnoses and collaborative problems. Nurses ultimately are accountable for formulating nursing diagnoses and intervening appropriately. With regard to a collaborative problem, the nurse is accountable for monitoring changes in the status of the problem and initiating the appropriate interventions, either nurse prescribed or physician prescribed. Nursing diagnoses and collaborative problems are equally important and are determined by the severity of the patient's illness at a particular point in time (Carpenito-Moyet, 2007). According to Carpenito-Moyet, there are four types of nursing diagnoses: actual, high risk, wellness, and syndrome. Each type has a specific purpose and unique components as shown in Chart 7–6 (p. 113).

Outcome Identification

Outcome identification is accomplished by analyzing the assessment data and the nursing diagnosis and deriving a desired outcome for a given problem. The **outcome** is a statement of how the patient's status will change once interventions have been successfully instituted. It is an individual measurable patient objective, or measurable criterion, that specifically indicates that the patient care objective has been met.

Planning

Once nursing diagnoses are formulated, the **planning** phase begins. The nurse is seldom able to resolve all of the patient's nursing diagnoses simultaneously; therefore, these diagnoses must be prioritized. Several factors must be considered when establishing the priority of the patient's nursing diagnoses. These include the patient's needs for biological survival and functioning, the urgency of the need, the patient's perceptions and values, and the nature of the nurse–patient relationship (Carpenito-Moyet, 2007; Wilkinson, 2006).

Certain basic human needs, such as oxygenation, fluid and electrolyte balance, temperature regulation, pain avoidance, nutrition, elimination, and protection from injury take precedence over needs such as activity, sexual needs, emotional security, attachment, and self-esteem. Basic survival needs are based on Maslow's hierarchy of needs (Maslow, 1954). For example, the needs of a patient with burn injuries for a patent airway, prevention of hypovolemic shock, and pain control must be attended to immediately. Concerns about the patient's alteration in body image and possible interferences with sexuality and self-esteem are dealt with when the patient's physiological functioning has been stabilized.

The urgency of the nursing diagnosis also must be considered. The potential threat to safety of an infant whose crib rail has been left down or to an elderly disoriented patient who tries to leave a nursing home unattended takes precedence (at least temporarily) over the infant's nutritional needs or the elderly patient's nursing diagnosis of pain resulting from arthritis.

The patient's perceptions and values are important determinants in setting priorities for nursing care—when the patient's

MyNursingKit | North American Diagnosis

CHART 7–4   Activities of Daily Living

TOILETING

_____ Cares for self at toilet completely; no incontinence (lack of bladder/bowel control).

_____ Needs to be reminded or needs help in cleaning self, or has rare (weekly at most) accidents.

_____ Soiling or wetting while asleep more than once a week.

_____ Soiling or wetting while awake more than once a week.

_____ No control of bowel or bladder.

FEEDING

_____ Eats without assistance.

_____ Eats with minor assistance at mealtimes and/or with special preparation of food; helps cleaning up after meals.

_____ Feeds self with moderate assistance for all meals.

_____ Requires extensive assistance for all meals.

_____ Does not feed self at all and resists efforts of others to feed him/her.

DRESSING

_____ Dresses, undresses, and selects clothes from own wardrobe.

_____ Dresses and undresses self with minor assistance.

_____ Needs moderate assistance in dressing or selection of clothes.

_____ Needs major assistance in dressing, but cooperates with efforts of others to help.

_____ Needs total grooming care, but can remain well groomed after help from others.

PHYSICAL WALKING

_____ Goes about grounds or city.

_____ Walks with assistance of (check one–none may apply):

     _____ Another person _____ Railing _____ Cane _____ Walker

_____ Uses a wheelchair (gets in and out without help).

_____ Uses a wheelchair (needs help getting in, out).

_____ Sits unsupported in chair or wheelchair, but cannot propel self without help.

_____ Bedridden more than half the time.

BATHING

_____ Bathes self (tub, shower, sponge bath) without help.

_____ Bathes self with help getting in and out of tub.

_____ Washes face and hands only, but cannot bathe rest of body.

_____ Does not wash self, but is cooperative with those who bathe him/her.

_____ Does not try to wash self, and resists efforts to keep himself/herself clean.

CHART 7–5   Instrumental Activities of Daily Living

ABILITY TO TELEPHONE

_____ Operates telephone on own initiative (looks up and dials numbers, etc.).

_____ Dials a few well-known numbers.

_____ Answers telephone, but does not dial.

_____ Does not use telephone at all.

SHOPPING

_____ Takes care of all shopping needs independently.

_____ Shops independently for small purchases.

_____ Needs to be accompanied on any shopping trip.

_____ Completely unable to shop.

FOOD PREPARATION

_____ Plans, prepares, and serves adequate meals independently.

_____ Prepares adequate meals if supplied with ingredients.

_____ Heats and serves prepared meals, or prepares meals but does not maintain adequate diet.

_____ Needs to have meals prepared and served.

HOUSEKEEPING

_____ Maintains house alone or with occasional assistance (i.e., heavy work done by others).

_____ Performs light daily tasks such as dish washing and bed-making.

_____ Performs light daily tasks, but cannot maintain acceptable level of cleanliness.

_____ Needs help with all home maintenance tasks.

_____ Does not participate in any housekeeping tasks.

LAUNDRY

_____ Does personal laundry completely.

_____ Launders small items: rinses socks, stockings, etc.

_____ All laundry must be done by others.

MODE OF TRANSPORTATION

_____ Travels independently on public transportation or drives own car.

_____ Arranges own travel via taxi, but does not otherwise use public transportation.

_____ Travels on public transportation when assisted or accompanied by another.

_____ Travels limited to taxi or automobile, with assistance of another.

_____ Does not travel at all.

RESPONSIBILITY FOR OWN MEDICATION

_____ Is responsible for taking medication in correct dosages at correct time.

_____ Takes responsibility if medication is prepared in advance in separate dosages.

_____ Is not capable of dispensing own medication.

ABILITY TO HANDLE FINANCES

_____ Manages financial matters independently (budgets, writes checks, pays rent and bills, goes to bank).

_____ Manages day-to-day purchases but needs help with banking, major purchases, etc.

_____ Incapable of handling money.

	Types of Nursing Diagnoses		
Actual	**High Risk**	**Wellness**	**Syndrome**
A state that has been clinically validated by identifiable major defining characteristics having four components: label, definition, defining characteristics, and related factors.	A clinical judgment that a patient is more vulnerable to develop the problem than are others in the same or similar situation having four components: label, definition, risk factors, and related factors.	A patient's clinically validated desire to move from a specific level of wellness to a higher level of wellness having only one component: the label.	A cluster of actual or high-risk nursing diagnoses that are predicted to be present because of a single event or situation having one component: the label which contains the etiology or contributing factors to the diagnosis.

CHART 7–6

perceptions of priority are ignored, the desired outcomes of care are not likely to be achieved. For example, a mother brings her toddler child in for a health checkup. The nurse observes the child drinking cola from a baby bottle and validates with the mother that the toddler consumes about three 8-ounce bottles a day. Although this is a pressing nutritional concern, the mother's chief concern is not being able to control the child's aggressive behavior. Unless the nurse focuses first on the mother's perceived priority need, success in changing the child's nutritional habits will be thwarted.

The nature of the nurse–patient relationship also will determine the order in which the nurse attempts to deal with the patient's diagnoses (Fawcett, 2005; Peplau, 1952). For example, suppose the patient's problem is interpersonal or sexual. Effective intervention will depend on a close and trusting relationship between the nurse and the patient. Such relationships take time to develop. Consequently, the nurse may assign these nursing diagnoses a lower priority until mutual rapport, trust, and respect have developed.

After nursing diagnoses have been assigned priorities, patient goals and objectives are established to clearly outline expected outcomes of care. A **goal** is a broad statement of purpose that describes the aim of nursing care; for example, "To alleviate pain and promote comfort" or "To facilitate adequate oxygenation" or "To promote acceptance of altered body image." Objectives for the individual patient should then be formulated for each goal, in terms of changes in patient behaviors that should result from nursing interventions. Objectives should include measurable criteria that provide parameters for determining whether objectives have been achieved. For example, if a hospitalized patient's nursing diagnosis is "Sleep disturbance related to environmental noise and interruptions for nursing care," the goal may be "To promote adequate rest and sleep." The objective (or outcome), then, may state, "The patient will sleep for at least two uninterrupted periods of 3 hours each during the night." It is important to formulate patient objectives that are both measurable and realistic. An objective that specifies a hospitalized patient will sleep for an 8-hour uninterrupted period is probably quite unrealistic. A realistic objective must take into account the patient's usual pattern and motivation; the health care setting; resources available to the patient and nurse; and the patient's age, cultural background, and health status. Goals and objectives that are inconsistent with the patient's cultural practices, for example, will probably not be achieved (Spector, 2004).

 CRITICAL ALERT *Goals for patient care are set based on the nurse's perspective and are differentiated from measurable objectives or outcomes, which are the patient's response to care. To assess the patient's response to care or the outcome, evaluation parameters must be identified that can be observed and measured.*

Objectives may be short term or long term. Short-term objectives can facilitate ongoing evaluation of the patient's progress toward long-term objectives. For example, a long-term objective for an obese woman might be "Patient will lose 50 pounds in 1 year." A short-term statement might be "Patient will lose approximately 1 pound per week."

Objectives are useful and effective when they are:

- Mutually acceptable to nurse, patient, and family
- Appropriate in terms of nursing and medical diagnoses and therapy
- Realistic in terms of patient's capabilities, time, energy, and resources
- Specific enough to be understood clearly by the patient and other nurses
- Measurable enough to facilitate evaluation.

Once goals and objectives have been identified, the next step is to formulate interventions for achieving the stated goals and objectives. Interventions are planned nursing actions that are likely to facilitate desired outcomes. For example, alternatives for a postoperative patient experiencing pain may include distraction and relaxation techniques, positioning for comfort, or administration of a prescribed analgesic.

After identifying nursing actions (interventions), the nurse then selects from the alternatives. In a sense, selection of nursing actions parallels the process of prioritizing the nursing diagnoses. The actions the nurse selects, and the order in which they are implemented, depend on the following factors:

- Patient preferences
- Known effectiveness of the action (based on prior knowledge, experience, and evidence)
- Time and resources available
- Possible side effects of treatments or medications.

In the case of pain relief, for example, the nurse might decide to help the patient learn conscious relaxation techniques. This action requires time, however, and if the patient is having acute, intense pain and is requesting "a pain medication" the nurse probably will choose to administer the prescribed analgesic first and then teach the patient relaxation techniques once pain relief has been achieved. This will help the patient cope with recurrence of the pain; for instance, if the pain recurs, the nurse may select distraction as the first alternative nursing action.

Implementation

Implementation is the "doing" or intervening phase of the nursing process. It involves organization and actual delivery of nursing care, which leads to achievement of stated goals and objectives. Nursing **interventions** are actions designed to facilitate achievement of positive patient outcomes. They must be purposeful and must be supported by a rationale. A sound rationale is derived from the nurse's knowledge base, prior experience, and the individualized assessment of the patient. Safe and effective nursing interventions are based on a through assessment and individualized care plan (Abdellah, Beland, Martin, & Matheney, 1960; ANA, 2007). NANDA has developed standardized nursing interventions, referred to as the Nursing Intervention Classification (NIC), that correspond with the NANDA nursing diagnoses (Ackley & Ladwig, 2007; Johnson et al., 2006; Lunney, 2001; NANDA, 2007).

Standards of care are based on research and provide an efficient method for identifying predicted problems that occur in a particular situation. Critical pathways are examples of implementation tools that anticipate and describe (in advance) the care of patients within a specified timeline (Carpenito-Moyet, 2007). The critical pathway is based on research and consists of evidence-based or benchmark practices. These practices provide rationales for care and serve to assist nurses in providing answers to the patients' questions as to why proposed interventions are the best approach to their health care. Critical pathways are discussed in Chapter 6 ∞ .

Evidence-Based Practice

Evidence-based practice (EBP) is the recommended standard in health care used by nurses (DiCenso, Guyatt, & Ciliska, 2005; Malloch & Porter-O'Grady, 2006; Melnyk & Fineout-Overholt, 2004). Omery and Williams (1999) have defined EBP as "the careful and practical use of current best evidence to guide health-care decisions" (p. 51). With this definition "current best evidence" includes clinical practice guidelines developed nationally by expert researchers, clinicians, and theorists in their areas of excellence. EBP involves the interpretation and implementation of these clinical guidelines by health care providers based on their clinical expertise, the needs and views of the patient and family, and the resources of the health care system. Thus, EBP is essential in establishing nursing interventions as part of the nursing process. As a problem-solving approach to clinical decision making, it is inherent in the nursing process and incorporates a search for the best and latest evidence, clinical expertise and assessment, and a patient's preferences and values within a context of caring (Benner & Leonard, 2005). Chapter 8 ∞ includes further discussion about EBP.

Evaluation

Evaluation focuses on a patient's behavioral changes and compares them with the criteria stated in the objectives. It consists of

both the patient's status and the effectiveness of the nursing care. Both must be evaluated continuously, with the care plan modified as needed (ANA, 2007). Thus, evaluation is ongoing through all phases of the nursing process. As the nurse works with a patient, the patient's responses to the nursing interventions are appraised to determine if the desired outcomes (objectives) have been achieved. For example, if the example states that the patient "will ambulate with assistance for 15 minutes four times a day," this intervention can easily be evaluated by confirming it with the patient and reviewing the nurses' notes. However if the objectives are not achieved, the nurse must determine:

- If the nursing diagnosis was correct
- If the goals and objectives were realistic and reasonable
- If nursing interventions were appropriate
- If any revisions and modifications in the plan are indicated.

It may be that a faulty nursing diagnosis was made from incomplete or inaccurate data or that the goals and objectives were unacceptable to the patient (unreasonable) or unrealistic in terms of the patient's usual patterns and lifestyles, and available resources (Johnson et al., 2006). Nursing interventions must be evaluated in terms of their effectiveness. If the selected intervention did not achieve the intended outcome, another should be attempted.

Patient Care Plan

The **patient care plan** is a documented record of the nursing process. Nursing diagnoses, outcomes with evaluation parameters, and interventions with supporting rationales are recorded on the care plan to communicate with the health care team and to guide patient care. The care plan also should be evaluated on the basis of information obtained from the patient evaluation. Evaluation of the patient care plan is necessary to follow a patient's increased or decreased ability to provide self-care, thus allowing for appropriate modifications. An example of how the nursing process is used with a patient care plan is shown in the Nursing Process box (p. 116). The steps of the nursing process are summarized in Chart 7–7.

■ Critical Thinking and the Nursing Process

Critical thinking and the nursing process are interrelated aspects of judgment and clinical reasoning. These processes influence and empower the nurse to demonstrate accountability to the patient through the independent, interdependent, and dependent roles inherent in nursing practice.

Critical Thinking

Critical thinking has become a popular phrase in nursing circles during the past decade. Essentially, **critical thinking** is a different way of viewing the information that one knows or learns. Critical thinking demands that one examine information in a variety of ways, exploring means of considering what is important and why some information is more important than other aspects of

CHART 7–7 **Nursing Process**

- **Assessment** is the collection of both objective and subjective data about the patient. The nurse collects physical evidence, for example, lung sounds, blood pressure, and presence or absence of peripheral pulses. The subjective data are derived from talking with the patient and family about the clinical manifestations that necessitated the need for health care. These data also include the medical history, allergies, and significant previous medical or surgical interventions. Both the subjective and objective data are then organized and documented on the patient's medical record and the patient care plan.

- **Nursing diagnoses** are derived from an analysis of the data collected during the assessment of the patient. Diagnoses include both actual and potential health problems. These diagnoses are then prioritized and categorized into those that can be managed independently by nursing and those that require a collaborative approach to management. Nurses are pivotal in coordinating the other health care professionals who contribute to positive patient outcomes.

- **Outcome identification**, often considered a part of the diagnosis step, consists of analyzing the assessment data and nursing diagnoses and deriving a desired outcome for a given problem. The outcome is a statement of how the patient's status will change once the interventions have been successfully instituted. A group of nurses from Iowa published a standardized vocabulary and classifications of nursing outcomes as they relate specifically to nursing interventions—the Nursing Outcomes Classification (NOC) (Johnson, Maas, & Moorhead, 2000).

- **Planning** is the phase of the nursing process in which interventions are planned that will achieve the identified outcomes associated with each nursing diagnosis. The interventions need to be prioritized to ensure patient safety. The planning phase may or may not be documented in the patient record. Often it is a mental process of choosing the appropriate interventions.

- **Implementation** is the carrying out of the plan identified in the previous step of the nursing process. Communication is a critical piece of the implementation process. This phase requires that the nurse identify which interventions can be accomplished independently and which require collaboration with other members of the health care team. The nurse needs to ensure that all members have received clear communication about the patient's needs. There also is a standardized classification of nursing interventions referred to as the Nursing Interventions Classifications (NIC) (Wilkinson, 2006). These standards provide a list of interventions associated with each nursing diagnosis. The final step of the implementation phase is recording the interventions on the patient record.

- **Evaluation** requires that the nurse compare the patient status to the desired outcomes. If the outcome is unmet, the care plan is revised and the process begins again until positive outcomes are achieved if at all possible.

information, and then taking what is most important and using that information to make decisions and solve problems.

Critical thinking is organized, purposeful, and disciplined. It entails the examination of elements of thought implicit in all reasoning: purpose, problem or question at issue, assumptions, concepts, reasoning leading to conclusions, implications, and consequences (Paul, 2004). Using critical thinking, the individ-

ual systematically and habitually imposes criteria and intellectual standards on the thinking process. During this process, the individual is aware of and takes charge of the thinking process, guiding his thinking to arrive at new and innovative conclusions (Paul, 2004). Critical in this respect does not mean that one is eager to find fault, but rather that one is judging carefully and competently. "Critical thinking in nursing entails purposeful, goal-directed thinking; aims to make judgments based on fact rather than guesswork; is based on principles of science and scientific method; and requires strategies that maximize human potential and compensate for problems caused by human nature" (Alfaro-LeFevre, 1995, p. 9).

At the center of critical thinking is one's ability to look at information in different ways, to question the information and assimilate it in new ways. With critical thinking comes the ability to apply new knowledge, often taken from fields outside nursing, create new options and means of implementing appropriate nursing care, and question why certain interventions give better patient outcomes. Some of the aspects of being a critical thinker are that one continually seeks new knowledge, remains open minded and receptive to new possibilities rather than merely accepting or rejecting ideas without examination, and strives to develop more innovative and effective ways to improve her decision-making capabilities. Characteristics of a critical thinker are that the individual is reflective, uses healthy, constructive skepticism, is autonomous in that he is not easily manipulated but thinks independently, is fair in his assessments, and focuses on what to do or believe.

Critical thinkers use a variety of cognitive skills in their thought processes. They are able to differentiate fact from opinion, evaluating within themselves the credibility of information sources and seeking additional sources to better evaluate the information that has been gathered. They clarify concepts, question assumptions, and ensure that the assumptions on which they base decisions and actions are accurate.

Critical thinking is essential to competent, skillful nursing care. When caring for patients, especially in stressful situations, critical thinking enables nurses to recognize important cues, respond quickly, and adapt interventions as needed. Nurses accomplish this outcome by (1) analyzing the situation to discover what issues are involved and what actions are appropriate, (2) applying standards according to established personal and professional rules, (3) discriminating by recognizing the similarities and differences among patients and diagnoses, (4) seeking additional information by searching for knowledge and gathering relevant data about the patient and her condition or diagnosis, (5) drawing conclusions that are supported by the data, (6) creating a plan of action, and (7) transforming knowledge into action. It is essential when analyzing each situation that nurses consider the ethical and legal principles involved.

Decision Making

The application of critical thinking is for decision making and effective clinical judgment. A subset of problem solving, decision making is the art of determining the best course of action to take in a given situation. In decision making, the individual selects a course of action from among two or more choices, using a variety of strategies to determine the best course of action.

NURSING PROCESS: Patient Care Plan Example

Nursing Assessment of Pain

Subjective Data:
What is your pain level at, using the 1–10 scale? A 1 is very little pain and a 10 is the worst imaginable pain.
What is your experience with pain?
Do you routinely take pain medications at home; if so, what for and what kind?
Are you allergic to any pain medication?
Do you have any cultural or religious beliefs that impact your pain control?

Objective Data:
Grimacing upon movement
Restlessness and irritability
Taut facial expression

Nursing Assessment and Diagnosis	Outcomes and Evaluation Parameters	Planning and Interventions with Rationales
Nursing Diagnosis: Acute pain related *to bilateral knee replacement therapy, physical therapy, and movement*	**Outcome:** Comfort level maintained. *Evaluation Parameters:* Able to communicate pain level and therapies that help alleviate it. On a scale of 10, reported pain will remain at 3 or less throughout hospitalization. Absence of pain behaviors such as grimacing. Nonpharmacological method of control is effective as evidenced by patient report and no pain behaviors. Reports satisfaction with pain management program.	**Interventions and *Rationales:*** Use pain scale (0–10) to quantify pain level. *Quantifying pain increases consistency.* Instruct patient to inform nurse if pain is not relieved. *Indicates need to change pain management plan.* Assess cultural and religious impact on patient's responses. *Different cultures and religions respond differently to pain.* Correct misconceptions about risk of addiction and overdose. *Decreases anxiety related to medication addiction.* Explain, prepare, and medicate patient for painful procedures (dressing change, ambulation, physical therapy) and anticipated discomforts. *Controls increased pain level related to procedure.* Provide a supportive environment in which patient is able to express pain level. *Opens communication and facilitates pain management.* Use pain control measures before it becomes severe. *Increases comfort and decreases need for medication.* Teach nonpharmacologic method of control (i.e., guided imagery, massage, and breathing exercises). *Augments pain relief.* Maintain proper positioning of affected leg. *Proper positioning reduces pain and enhances pain relief.* Provide rest periods between procedures to assist with coping with ongoing pain. *Decreases the fatigue related to long-term pain.* Revise pain management plan as wounds heal and pain decreases. *To prevent overmedication.* Plan diversional activities: relaxation, alternative sensory stimulation such as music, massage, heat/cold, movies, TV, reading, and breathing techniques. *Augments pain relief measures.*

As such, decision making is synonymous with the act of choosing, of converting information into action.

Decision making may or may not be the result of an immediate problem, but is initiated as part of an immediate problem. Elements in decision making include (1) identification of a problem, (2) establishment of criteria to evaluate potential solutions, (3) a search for alternative solutions or actions, (4) evaluation of alternative choices, and (5) selection of a course of action. The four phases of decision making are deliberation, judgment, choice, and evaluation of the effectiveness of the outcomes. Perhaps the most time-consuming phase is the deliberation phase when one determines that there is a decision to be made, begins to establish criteria for evaluating the effectiveness of potential solutions, and searches for possible solutions. The judgment phase involves a thorough understanding of the possible choices at hand and evaluation of these choices. Once these two phases have been explored, the third phase involves the selection and implementation of what has been determined to be one's best choice of action. Finally, evaluation of the effectiveness of the outcomes occurs, which may begin the process anew if desired outcomes are not attained.

A nurse can employ any of several strategies when deciding the best course of action to take. These strategies include trial-and-error methods, pilot projects, brainstorming, group input, cost–benefit analyses, cause and effect, worst-case scenarios, and the more recently endorsed EBP model (see earlier discussion). Depending on the immediacy of a needed solution and the seriousness of outcomes if an alternate course of action is taken, some of these listed strategies may not be the most appropriate strategies for decision making in different instances.

Critical Pathways

Newer forms of decision making in clinical areas include the development of critical pathways. Critical pathways identify key events of patient care and expected time frames. Their advantages include improved patient outcomes, streamlined charting, facilitation of quality assessment, improved patient education, and enhanced communication among health care providers. Again, many critical or clinical pathways are developed as a result of research and identified as one source for evidence-based practice (see Chapters 6 and 8 ⊘).

National Standards and Guidelines

National standards and guidelines also assist with decision making in clinical areas and reducing variance in professional practice patterns. National standards and guidelines have been promulgated by regulatory agencies and professional organizations. The Joint Commission promotes the use of appropriate, measurable clinical indicators in clinical settings. These measures promote quantitative measures to monitor and evaluate the quality of care. Professional organizations such as the American Association of Critical Care Nurses or the Emergency Nurses Association promote standards of care for patients served in various types of practice settings. Other standards promote care for a specialization, such as the ANA's standards of care for hospice nursing or its standards of care for ambulatory nursing care (ANA, 2004).

Clinical Judgment

Clinical judgment, sometimes referred to as reflective thinking or clinical reasoning, is the process of drawing conclusions based on a comparison of the patient's current data with specific outcome data and giving meaning to data based on that comparison. For example, clinical judgment is involved when a nurse notes that the patient's potassium level is 6.8 compared to a "normal" potassium level of 3.6 to 5.0. Thus, clinical judgment involves comparing the patient's current health status to the expected or desired status and deciding which measures are the most appropriate given that comparison. If the comparison is essentially the same, the nurse can conclude that current interventions are successful. If the comparison varies, the nurse can conclude that further interventions are required. The nurse would then use critical thinking and decision making to determine the next course of action.

Using Critical Thinking with the Nursing Process

The use of critical thinking with the nursing process enhances the validity, reliability, and effectiveness of outcomes to patients. Critical thinking is essential in nursing when the nurse is assessing, diagnosing, implementing, and evaluating the patient and developing the care plan (Wilkinson, 2006). Chart 7–8 depicts the relationship between critical thinking and the nursing process.

Critical thinking requires developing characteristics of critical thinkers as shown in Figures 7–2 ■ and 7–3 ■ (p. 118). Because critical thinking is contextual, it changes depending on circumstances. However, because the decisions nurses make affect people's lives, their judgment must be sound, precise, and disciplined. Critical thinking promotes accuracy and depth of data collection and seeks to identify the needs of the patient. This controlled thinking is essential to help people avoid illness and its complications and to help people gain optimal independence, a sense of well-being, and/or a peaceful death as appropriate.

Twelve aspects of critical thinking were initially identified by Ennis in 1962, reaffirmed in 1996, and reiterated in recent publications (Ennis, 2003, 2004). These aspects of critical thinking are shown in Chart 7–9 (p. 118) and are consistent with the definition and explanation of critical thinking as presented in Chapter 1 ⊘ of this text. In essence, critical thinking focuses on deciding what to believe or do. It is relevant not only to the formation and checking of beliefs, but also to deciding on and evaluating actions. It involves creative activities such as formulating hypotheses and plans. Critical thinking is reflective and reasonable (Ennis, 1996). As such it is a critical element in using the nursing process.

CHART 7–8   Critical Thinking, Nursing Process Actions, and Nursing Process Phases (Steps)

Critical Thinking	Nursing Process Action	Nursing Process Phase
Get a better understanding of something or someone else.	Initiate nurse–patient interaction. Collect data. Interpret and validate data.	Assessment
Identify actual and potential problems.	Formulate nursing diagnosis. Derive a desired outcome.	Nursing diagnosis and outcome identification
Make decisions about an action.	Prioritize nursing diagnosis. Formulate goals/objectives. Select planned interventions.	Planning
Reduce risk of getting undesirable results.	Organize interventions. Carry out selected nursing interventions.	Implementation
Increase likelihood of achieving beneficial results.	Determine if nursing diagnosis is correct. Determine if goals/objectives are/have been met. Make necessary revisions and modifications.	Evaluation
Find ways to improve (even when no problem exists).	Repeat the process to gain optimal independence, sense of well-being, or peaceful death.	Nursing process continues

FIGURE 7–2 ■ Critical thinking.

FIGURE 7–3 ■ Processes in critical thinking.

CHART 7–9   **Twelve Aspects of Critical Thinking**

1. Grasping the meaning of a statement
2. Judging whether there is ambiguity in the line of reasoning
3. Judging whether certain statements contradict each other
4. Judging whether a conclusion follows necessarily
5. Judging whether a statement is specific enough
6. Judging whether a statement is actually the application of a certain principle

7. Judging whether an observation statement is reliable
8. Judging whether an inductive conclusion is warranted
9. Judging whether the problem has been identified
10. Judging whether something is an assumption
11. Judging whether a definition is adequate
12. Judging whether a statement made by an alleged authority is acceptable

Sources: From Robert H. Ennis, "A Concept of Critical Thinking," *Harvard Educational Review,* 32:1 (Winter 1962), pp. 84. Copyright © by the President and Fellows of Harvard College. All rights reserved. For more information, please visit www.harvardeducationalreview.org; Ennis, R. H. (1996). *Critical thinking.* Upper Saddle River, NJ: Pearson Prentice Hall.

Summary

The nursing process is a patient-centered method for structuring the delivery of nursing care. As such, it is the common thread that unites different types of nurses who work in varied areas; it serves as the essential core of practice for the registered nurse (ANA, 2007). The nursing process is the vehicle through which the nurse applies intuitive and scientific knowledge, critical thinking, and nursing skills in a systematic, goal-directed fashion to achieve the outcomes desired for the patient. The nursing process entails gathering and analyzing data in order to identify patient strengths, potential or actual problems, and goals, and developing and evaluating a plan of nursing interventions to achieve mutually agreed-on outcomes. At every stage of the five-step process, the nurse works closely with the patient to individualize care and build a relationship of mutual respect.

REVIEW QUESTIONS

1. The nurse is conducting an independent nursing activity with a patient. Which of the following would this nurse be doing?
   1. Assessing a wound
   2. Documenting intake on a calorie count form
   3. Assisting the patient to use a walker
   4. Administering medication

2. The nurse is reviewing a patient's situation in order to diagnose the patient's problems. This nurse is conducting which phase of the nursing process?
   1. Assessment
   2. Planning
   3. Implementation
   4. Evaluation

3. The nurse does a finger stick to check a patient's current blood glucose level. The nurse is utilizing which skill for conducting this assessment?
   1. Cognitive
   2. Affective
   3. Psychomotor
   4. Psychosocial

4. At the completion of a patient's assessment, the nurse creates a clinical judgment about a potential health problem. This clinical judgment is considered:
   1. Goal setting.
   2. Planning interventions.
   3. Determining collaborative problems.
   4. Determining a nursing diagnosis.

5. The nurse is making a decision about a future action with patient care. This critical thinking activity is equated with which of the following steps of the nursing process?
   1. Assessment
   2. Planning
   3. Implementation
   4. Evaluation

Answers for review questions appear in Appendix D

KEY TERMS

assessment *p.109*
collaborative problems *p.111*
critical thinking *p.114*
dependent activities *p.107*
evaluation *p.114*
goal *p.113*

implementation *p.114*
independent activities *p.107*
interdependent activities *p.107*
intervention *p.114*
nurse–patient relationship *p.107*
nursing diagnosis *p.111*

nursing process *p.107*
objective data *p.109*
outcome *p.111*
patient care plan *p.114*
planning *p.111*
subjective data *p.109*

REFERENCES

Abdellah, F. G., Beland, K. K., Martin, A., & Matheney, R. J. (1960). *Patient centered approaches to nursing.* New York: Macmillan.

Ackley, B. J., & Ladwig, G. B. (2007). *Nursing diagnosis handbook: an evidence-based guide to planning care* (8th ed.). St Louis: Mosby.

Alfaro-LeFevre, R. (1995). *Critical thinking in nursing: A practical approach.* Philadelphia: W. B. Saunders.

American Nurses Association. (2003). *Nursing's social policy statement* (2nd ed.). Washington, DC: Author.

American Nurses Association. (2004). *Standards of clinical nursing practice.* Washington, DC: Author.

American Nurses Association. (2007). *The nursing process: A common thread amongst all nurses.* Retrieved September 16, 2007, from http://nursingworld.org/ExpeciallyForYou/StudentNurses/Thenursingprocess.aspx

Benner, P., & Leonard, V. W. (2005). Patient concerns and choices and clinical judgment in EBP. In B. Melnyk & E. Fineout-Overholt (Eds.), *Evidence-based practice in nursing and healthcare: A guide to best practices.* Philadelphia: Lippincott.

Carpenito-Moyet, L. J. (2005). *Understanding the nursing process: Concept mapping and care planning for students.* Philadelphia: Lippincott Williams & Wilkins.

Carpenito-Moyet, L. J. (2007). *Nursing diagnosis: Application to clinical practice* (12th ed.). Philadelphia: Lippincott Williams & Wilkins.

DiCenso, A., Guyatt, G., & Ciliska, D. (2005). *Evidence-based nursing: A guide to clinical practice.* Philadelphia: Elsevier.

Ennis, R. H. (1962). A concept of critical thinking. *Harvard Educational Review, 32,* 81–111.

Ennis, R. H. (2003). Critical thinking assessment. In C. Fasko (Ed.), *Critical thinking and reasoning: Current theories, research, and practice.* Cresskill, NJ: Hampton.

Ennis, R. H. (2004). Applying soundness standards to qualified reasoning. *Informal Logic, 24*(1), 23–39.

Fawcett, J. (2005). *Contemporary nursing knowledge: Analysis and evaluation of nursing models and theories* (2nd ed.). Philadelphia: F. A. Davis.

Henderson, V. (1966). *The nature of nursing.* New York: Macmillan.

Johnson, D. E. (1980). The behavioral system model for nursing. In J. P. Riehl & C. Roy (Eds.), *Conceptual models for nursing practice* (2nd ed.). New York: Appleton-Century-Crofts.

Johnson, M., Bulechek, G. M., Butcher, H., Dochterman, J. M., Maas, M., Moorhead, S., et al. (2006). *NANDA, NOC and NIC linkages: Nursing diagnoses, outcomes and interventions* (2nd ed.). Philadelphia: Elsevier.

Johnson, M., Maas, M., & Moorhead, S. (2000). *Nursing outcomes classification* (NOC) (2nd ed.). St. Louis: Mosby.

King, I. M. (1971). *Toward a theory of nursing; General concepts of human behavior.* New York: John Wiley & Sons.

Leininger, M. M. (1991). *Culture care diversity and universality: A theory of nursing.* New York: National League of Nursing Press.

Levine, M. (1973). *Introduction to clinical nursing* (2nd ed.). Philadelphia: F. A. Davis.

Lunney, M. (Ed.). (2001). *Critical thinking and nursing diagnosis: Case studies and analysis.* Philadelphia: North American Nursing Diagnosis Association.

Malloch, K., & Porter-O'Grady, T. (2006). *Introduction to evidence-based practice in nursing and health care.* Sudbury, MA: Jones and Bartlett.

Maslow, A. H. (1954). *Motivation and personality.* New York: Harper and Row Publishers.

Melnyk, B. M., & Fineout-Overholt, E. (Eds.). (2004). *Evidence-based practice nursing and healthcare: A guide to best pratice.* Philadelphia: Lippincott Williams & Wilkins.

North American Nursing Diagnosis Association. (2007). *Nursing diagnoses: Definitions & classification 2007–2008.* Philadelphia: Author.

Omery, A., & Williams, R. P. (1999). An appraisal of research utilization across the United States. *Journal of Nursing Administration, 29,* 50–56.

Orem, D. (1971). *Nursing concepts of practice.* New York: McGraw-Hill.

Orlando, I. J. (1961). *The dynamic nurse–patient relationship: Function, process, and principles.* New York: G. P. Putnam's Sons.

Paul, R. (2004). *Defining critical thinking.* Retrieved October 22, 2006, from http://www.criticalthinking.org/aboutCT/definingCT.shtml

Peplau, H. E. (1952). *Interpersonal relations in nursing.* New York: G. P. Putnam's Sons.

Rogers, M. E. (1970). *The theoretical basis of nursing.* Philadelphia: F. A. Davis.

Spector, R. E. (2004). *Cultural diversity in health & illness.* Upper Saddle River, NJ: Pearson Prentice Hall.

Stanton, J., Paul, C., & Reeves, J. S. (1980). An overview of the nursing process. In *Nursing theories: The base for professional nursing practice.* Englewood Cliffs, NJ: Prentice Hall.

Watson, J. (1988). New dimensions of human caring theory. *Nursing Science Quarterly, 1*(4), 175–181.

Watson, J. (2003). *Jean Watson and the theory of human caring.* Retrieved on February 14, 2003, from http://ww2.uchsc.edu/son/caring/content/sct.asp

White, L. (2003). *Documentation and the nursing process: A review.* Clifton Park, NY: Delmar.

Wilkinson, Judith M. (2006). *Nursing process & critical thinking* (4th ed.). Upper Saddle River, NJ: Pearson Prentice Hall.

Yura, H., & Walsh, M. B. (1988). *The nursing process* (5th ed.). New York: Appleton-Century-Crofts.

Role of Research in Nursing Practice

Annita Watson

Outcome-Based Learning Objectives

After studying this chapter, the learner will be able to:

1. Differentiate between basic and applied research.
2. Differentiate between quantitative and qualitative research.
3. Identify three types of quantitative and three types of qualitative research.
4. Describe the first step of the research process.
5. Determine how a research design is selected.
6. Differentiate between research utilization and evidence-based practice.
7. Describe the three ethical principles that guide research studies.
8. Describe the impact of HIPAA on nursing research studies.
9. Explain the four stages of completing a quantitative research critique.

Research is a formal, systematic, and organized method used to answer a question or solve a problem. It is defined as a "diligent, systemic inquiry or study that validates and redefines existing knowledge and develops new knowledge" (Burns & Grove, 2003, p. 3). Though researchers frequently attach different meanings to the term *research*, there is consensus that the term implies a formal, rigorous, and precise process intended to discover new knowledge and relationships and find solutions to problems or questions. This type of scientific inquiry provides a forum to facilitate the ongoing process of questioning and evaluating practice, informs practice based on available data, and guides new practices through research and experimental learning. As such, research is essential for defining the nursing profession, providing a mechanism for ascertaining best practices, and advancing the science of nursing practice. This chapter focuses on the process and outcomes of research and the manner in which it is used by nurses to promote clinical practice. Specific examples of research intended to change and improve medical–surgical nursing practice are discussed in the specific disorder chapters within the text.

Nursing Research

Nursing research is similar to research conducted by other professional groups or disciplines in that the same rigorous steps must be followed, and the research design and method of inves-

tigation must be appropriate to the problem or question being studied. Gillis and Jackson (2002) suggest, however, that nursing research is distinguished by the diversity of the human experience. When compared to other fields, nursing practice requires greater flexibility in the definition and interpretation of research, thereby providing for the variations that occur across professional practice settings. This has become particularly evident as globalization of the world community has highlighted the differences in nursing practice and contexts across countries.

Defining nursing research requires determining the relevant knowledge for nursing. Since Florence Nightingale's era, nurses have been expanding their professional practice foundation through research efforts designed to develop and test knowledge. In 1976, the American Nurses Association (ANA) adopted the following definition, which remains broad enough today to encompass globalization of the world community:

> Nursing research is investigation into the area of knowledge in which the physical and behavioral sciences meet and influence one another in an effort to study how health problems relate to human behavior and how behavior relates to health and illness. It addresses the human and behavioral questions that arise in the treatment of disease, in the prevention of illness, and in the promotion and maintenance of health. (ANA, 1976, p. 1)

Nursing research also may be viewed as research into phenomena that are predominantly and appropriately the responsibility of nurses in their professional practice (Gillis & Jackson, 2002). Nurses are responsible for provision of patient care, administration of nursing and health care services, and education of practitioners. Therefore, research in nursing encompasses systematic inquiry into each of these areas. With this interpretation nursing research not only adds to the knowledge base of nursing, but also influences changes for patients, their futures, and their environments. It also impacts the health care delivery system and related costs of health care.

The world is constantly changing. Much of nursing knowledge is not generated through research. Nurses typically draw on knowledge from a variety of sources, each offering something unique to holistic nursing practice. These include tradition, authority, trial and error, personal experience, intuition, and logical reasoning. However, nurses can no longer rely on the assumptions that come only from experience and trial and error. Information that is supported by data is critical to improving the clinical care provided to patients. The difficulty with non–research-based knowledge is that it has limited scientific predictability and cannot be used to justify nursing actions or provide new scientific information to direct practice.

Evidence from research must be applied to nurses' practices to assure patients that they have the best knowledge available for safe and compassionate care. In addition, research findings must be shared with others in order to broaden the current knowledge base that is available to all nurses. Increased knowledge provides opportunities to solve problems in different ways, to continually challenge the status quo of why practice is performed in a certain way, and to understand phenomena that occur in the professional sphere. In this era of rapid change it is critical for research to be used as a tool to provide caring, compassionate, and scientific care.

Basic and Applied Research

The general purpose of nursing research is to answer questions or solve problems relevant to the nursing profession. In terms of the intent of the research, a distinction can be made between basic and applied research. **Basic research,** as traditionally defined, is undertaken to extend the knowledge base in a discipline or to formulate or refine a theory. **Applied research** focuses on finding solutions to existing problems. For example, a study to determine the effectiveness of a nursing intervention to ease pain would be applied research. The specific purposes of nursing research include identification, description, exploration, explanation, prediction, and control (Polit & Beck, 2008). Practicing nurses are most apt to be involved in applied research. This, then, becomes the focus of this chapter.

Although this chapter highlights the current status of research in nursing, particularly as it relates to the development of evidence-based practice, it is necessary to understand the research process before one can participate in it. A description of the research process, the conditions under which research is undertaken, and the types of research typically used by nurses and other health care professionals provides the groundwork for the discussion of research utilization and evidence-based practice.

The Research Process

The **research process** is very similar to the nursing process in that it proceeds through discrete steps in order to answer a question. Thus, the steps of the research process should not be totally new to the learner because nurses perform similar activities every day when they engage in critical thinking, reflect on their practice, and apply the nursing process. For example, nurses engage in data collection about patients when they read the patient's chart; receive reports; and engage in dialogue with colleagues, the patient, and the family. Based on this information and observations, the nurse formulates a diagnosis of the patient's health needs. This stage is similar to naming, classifying, or identifying problems. Next, the nurse develops a plan of care specific to the patient's identified needs. This step is similar to the methodology plan that the researcher develops after the problem statement is clearly defined. The plan is based on an expectation that certain interventions produce intended outcomes for the patient. This is similar to prediction in the quantitative research process.

The nurse then evaluates the effect of the interventions on the patient's outcomes and recommends modifications to the plan as new evidence becomes available. This is similar to interpretation of findings and the recommendation stage of the research process (Gillis & Jackson, 2002). For example, a problem/question is identified, a literature search is conducted, a method or research design is selected to answer the question, data are collected and analyzed about the responses to the problem/question, and conclusions are drawn based on what the data demonstrate.

The final step is to compare outcomes of the study. The researcher asks "Do the outcomes of the study reflect current practice, is more research indicated, or does practice need to be changed from the evidence of the study?" A caution is that practices should not be changed only on the basis of one study. A research study should be replicated (repeated) in different settings, with different patients, to be sure the results are similar and that they can be generalized to other populations and settings.

A relationship between problem solving and research also can be drawn, because problem solving is the basis of the nursing process. For some, the assimilation of the research process is easier when presented in the context of problem solving and the nursing process. Chart 8–1 shows the similarities and differ-

CHART 8–1	**Problem Solving and Research: Similarities and Differences**
SIMILARITIES	**DIFFERENCES**
Critical thinking	Unique language
Complex reasoning	Rigorous application of research methods
Information is gathered	Broader focus: groups versus individuals
Observations are made	Stronger theoretical base
Problems are identified	Greater precision, rigor, and control
Plans are developed	Outcomes shared with a larger audience
Actions are taken	Research process is more complex
Effectiveness and efficiency are evaluated	
Outcomes are determined	

ences between problem solving versus research. Chart 8–2 shows a comparison of the nursing process to the problem-solving process and the research process.

Conducting Research

Discrete steps must be taken in order to conduct research. The order and progression of these steps vary depending on whether one is conducting quantitative or qualitative research. However, some of the basic elements of the process apply to both types of research approaches, including identifying the problem and purpose, conducting a literature review, collecting and analyzing data, and drawing conclusions. These steps may or may not progress in a linear way depending on the type of research being conducted, quantitative or qualitative, and are discussed under the respective topics of quantitative and qualitative research; commonalities, however, are presented next.

Research Problem and Purpose

The first step in any research process is to identify a researchable problem. A researchable problem is a situation in need of a solution, alteration, or improvement. It is an area of concern for a particular population that requires investigation and it is derived from a topical area. Not all problems are researchable. For instance, problems or questions of a moral or ethical nature are incapable of being researched because there is no right or wrong answer, only points of view that reflect one's values.

The problem concept or topical area of concern typically is very broad and generally contains numerous potential research problems. The actual research problem is a very small piece of the entire topical area. This may be thought of as a very small piece of a large puzzle or a very small slice of a very large pie. For example, pain is a general research topic/concept, and one researchable question (problem) related to pain is "Does fatigue exacerbate pain in cancer patients?" Figure 8–1 ■ (p. 124) reflects

CHART 8–2	Comparison of Steps of the Nursing Process, the Problem-Solving Process, and Stages of Nursing Research	
Nursing Process	**Problem-Solving Process**	**Stages of Nursing Research**
1. Assess to determine the degree of discrepancy between what is and what should be in relation to the optimum health of an individual patient.	1. Identify a particular problem or condition of the patient or family or a problem in the setting that requires change.	1. Identify a research problem, from clinical observations or from the literature and current theoretical thought, or from a combination of the two. Delineate the problem clearly and delimit the problem to a manageable research question or hypothesis.
2. Intervene by refining the nursing diagnoses to behavioral goals in collaboration with the patient, formulating the desired outcomes for problem resolution in the form of behavioral objectives, generating and selecting an alternate course of actions, and implementing the action alternatives.	2. Analyze the various aspects of the problem (e.g., the need for immediate or long-term change), the type of approach that is needed, the need to involve other people in the problem-solving process, and the resources that are available.	2. Collect essential facts pertaining to the problem. Review the literature, validate the significance of the problem selected, or develop the theoretical or conceptual underpinnings for the problem to explain it and its possible solution(s).
3. Evaluate to appraise the degree to which the actual outcomes match the desired outcomes (the behavioral objectives).	3. Collect data about the patient or family, the setting, related facets of the problem, and possible solutions to the problem through the use of observations, interviews, discussion with experts, and a review of the literature.	3. Create a theoretical or conceptual framework and operationalize the concepts under consideration. Develop tentative solutions to be tested in the form of hypotheses or develop the general approach that will provide the desired information in the form of research question(s).
4. Revise the plan by redesigning the behavioral objectives that have not been attained; by selecting and implementing other action alternatives; and by collecting and analyzing more data to evolve new nursing diagnoses, new behavioral objectives, and other action alternatives, all in collaboration with the patient.	4. Analyze the information collected using the analysis as a guide for appropriate actions. Establish a plan for change and a means for evaluating the success of the change.	4. Develop an appropriate design to answer the question(s) or test the hypotheses, which includes measuring instruments, setting, sample, protocol, methodology, and statistical analysis design and the rationale for each.
	5. Implement the plan of change.	5. Collect the essential data.
	6. Evaluate the effects of the change as determined by the evaluation plan developed. If the actions fail to solve the problem, begin again, looking for alternative solutions to the problem.	6. Analyze the data, interpret the findings, and generalize the results in terms of the framework, the theoretical perspective, and the sampling rationale.
		7. Disseminate the research findings.

Source: Phillips, Clinical Guide Critique and Utilization of Nursing Research, 1st, © 1986. Electronically reproduced by permission of Pearson Education, Inc. Upper Saddle River, New Jersey.

FIGURE 8–1 ■ The problem concept or topical area of concern typically is very broad, whereas the actual research problem is a very small piece of the entire topical area. This may be thought of as a very small piece of a large puzzle or a very small slice of a very large pie.

the minuteness of the research problem in relation to the problem topic. The study or **research problem** is a very specific and precise statement of the phenomenon to be studied. The study problem also may be phrased as a **research question**. Examples of research topics/concepts with related research problems are shown in Chart 8–3.

Research problems may be developed from a variety of sources, such as nursing practice, researcher and peer interactions, literature review, theory, and research priorities identified by funding agencies and specialty groups. The researcher should keep in mind that the problem selected must meet four criteria. The problems must be:

- Significant to nursing (someone must benefit from the evidence that is produced)
- Researchable (amenable to scientific inquiry)
- Feasible to address (time to complete, available study participants, cooperation of others, faculties and equipment, money, experience of the researcher, and ethically sound)
- Of interest to the researcher (genuine interest in and curiosity about the problem).

 CRITICAL ALERT

Select a research problem that:

1. *Is researchable.*
2. *Has significance to nursing practice.*
3. *Is feasible to address.*
4. *Is of genuine interest to the researcher.*

Research Purpose

The **research purpose** is generated from the problem. It identifies the goal or goals of the study and directs the development of the study. In the research process, the purpose usually is stated after the problem has been determined, because the problem identifies the gap in knowledge in a selected area and the purpose clarifies the knowledge to be generated by a study. The purpose clearly identifies the goals of the study. In quantitative research, the problem identifies an area of concern and the purpose reflects the type of study to be conducted: descriptive, correlational, quasi-experimental, or experimental. Problems formulated for qualitative studies also identify an area of concern, and the purpose indicates the focus of the investigation: a subjective concept, an event, a phenomenon, or a fact of a culture or society (Polit & Beck, 2008).

CHART 8–3 **Research Topics/Concepts and Related Research Problems/Questions**

Research Topic/Concept	Research Problem/Question
Pregnancy in teenage girls	Adaptation to pregnancy in teenage girls varies according to ethnic culture.
Quality of life among Alzheimer patients' caregivers.	Quality of life among Alzheimer patients varies according to the amount of social support received.
Testicular cancer	Instruction on testicular self-exam in adolescents is predictive of performing self-exams as an adult.
Informatics	Educational level of the registered nurse influences the use of computers in the clinical setting.
Discharge planning in acute care settings	What is the role of the staff nurse in discharge planning?
Falls in acute care setting	Fall prevention programs affect the number of falls in acute care settings.
Competence in elders	Level of competence in those over age 85 determines the ability to live independently by self.
Evidence-based practice	The use of evidence-based practice is influenced by level of education of the registered nurse.
Staffing in acute care settings	Staffing in acute care settings affects patient outcomes.
Breast cancer screening	Living in rural areas versus the city influences frequency of mammograms and other breast cancer screening mechanisms.

Literature Review

After a researchable problem has been identified and stated or posed as a research question, a **literature review** is completed. This is a critical step, and one that can be quite time consuming. It is, however, essential, and serves several purposes, one of the primary functions being to further clarify the problem identified for study. The review also helps to specify the study problem and set limits for the target population. Another function of the literature review is to verify that this is an important clinical problem, which needs answering in order to improve patient care. Thus, the literature review should be used to determine (1) if other studies similar to the one to be conducted have been done previously, (2) if prior findings would be helpful in defining the proposed study, and (3) if it would be possible to replicate a prior study. Other purposes of the literature review include finding gaps in existing knowledge that can help fill out the current study design, selecting a research design and identifying instruments to measure the central aspects of the design, and helping the researcher interpret the findings from the study.

Literature searches may be conducted by reviewing references in a library, and by conducting computer searches, which is the most common method today. Computer searches may unveil vast amounts of data, so it will be necessary to limit the search to a reasonable time period. The search also may be limited by using primary sources as the major literature source. Primary resources are those written by investigators who conducted the studies. Secondary sources are those in which a writer describes or summarizes studies done by others. Review articles are an example of secondary literature sources. They can be valuable in guiding one to primary literature. They also may be helpful in reviewing theoretical or conceptual material that assists the researcher in establishing a design and methodology.

Research Design

The third major step in the research process is selecting the type of research that will answer the question and the concomitant **research design**. The design is the overall plan or blueprint for the study and should be described in detail, including the methods used for data collection and analysis. There are a number of research design strategies that may be employed to answer the research question that has been posed. The one that will help maximize the possibilities of achieving accurate information in the results should be used. The design for the study is dictated by the research problem/question, also known as a **hypothesis**, and assumptions of the theoretical framework.

It is helpful to begin the design section by writing an overview in which the theoretical or conceptual framework is stated if one is used. The overview is an extension of the research problem. It states how and where the study will be conducted and who is going to be studied and also how the study question(s) will be evaluated (measured). Different designs would be used for describing phenomena, exploring relationships, or searching for effects of **variables**. The study design may represent qualitative or quantitative research.

Types of Research Design: Quantitative and Qualitative

There are various types of nursing research, but the most common types are quantitative and qualitative. The following descriptions provide broad distinctions between these two main types of research.

Quantitative Research **Quantitative research** is characterized by the collection of numerical values, under a controlled situation, that yield data, which can be generalized. Quantitative designs typically are descriptive, correlational, quasi-experimental, and experimental. **Descriptive research designs** often search for associations among certain variables. A **correlational research design** is aimed at examining linear relationships between two or more variables. The term **quasi-experimental** indicates a research design with an intervention, but one in which it is difficult to manipulate or control the setting, subjects, or variables as needed for a true experimental study. An **experimental research design** is used to determine the effects of an intervention, and it is highly controlled. Experimental research most often occurs in a laboratory setting, and is used to determine the effects of an intervention or of the manipulation of an independent variable. In contrast, a **nonexperimental research design,** which is not a specific type of design, consists of studies in which the researcher collects data without introducing an intervention. Quantitative research uses subjects that represent certain groups.

Research is not value free; that is, the background and biases of the researcher have an influence on study outcomes. In quantitative studies, the researcher strives to control as much bias as possible through design decisions. Understanding what biases can influence certain design decisions can be useful in the data analysis phase of the study.

In a quantitative study, the researcher moves from the beginning point of a study (posing a research question) to the end point (finding an answer). The researcher passes through five phases from the beginning to the end of the study: the conceptual phase, the design and planning phase, the empirical phase, the analytic phase, and the dissemination phase (Polit & Beck, 2008). The conceptual phase consists of thinking about the study and discussing the possibility of the study with colleagues. During this phase, the researcher calls on creativity and deductive reasoning to arrive at a researchable problem. During the second phase, the design and planning phase, the researcher develops methods to be used in conducting the study and to gather data. The third phase, the empirical phase, involves the collection of research data and the preparation of those data for analysis. During the fourth phase, the analytic phase, the data are analyzed and interpreted. Questions posed in the first phase of the study are answered. The fifth and final stage of the process is the dissemination phase. The results of the study are disseminated. This phase should include recommendations regarding how the results of the study could be incorporated into the practice of nursing. The sequential steps that occur during each phase of the research process are shown in Chart 8–4 (p. 126).

Qualitative Research **Qualitative research** describes events as they occur naturally. Qualitative research involves the use of a systematic, subjective approach to describe life experiences and give them meaning (Burns & Grove, 2005). Thus, compared to quantitative research, qualitative research uses methods that are more subjective, a smaller sample size, and fewer research controls. Qualitative research studies generally use phenomenology,

Steps in the Quantitative Research Process

PHASE 1: THE CONCEPTUAL PHASE

1. Identify a researchable problem.
2. Establish a purpose for the study.
3. Conduct a literature review.
4. Develop a theoretical/conceptual framework.
5. Formulate research objectives, questions, and hypotheses.

PHASE 2: THE DESIGN AND PLANNING PHASE

6. Select a research design.
7. Identify population to be studied.
8. Design the sampling plan.
9. Specify methods to measure the research variables.
10. Finalize and review the research plan.
11. Conduct a pilot study (if possible) and make revisions.

PHASE 3: THE EMPIRICAL PHASE

12. Collect the data.
13. Prepare the data for analysis.

PHASE 4: THE ANALYTIC PHASE

14. Analyze the data.
15. Interpret the results.

PHASE 5: THE DISSEMINATION PHASE

16. Communicate the findings.
17. Use the findings.

Activities Inherent in Qualitative Research

PHASE 1: CONCEPTUALIZING AND PLANNING THE STUDY

1. Clarify the topic area.
2. Proceed with a broad research question that may be delineated after the study is under way.
3. Conduct a literature review.
4. Identify a study site.

PHASE 2: CONDUCTING THE STUDY

5. Develop a sampling plan.[a]
6. Collect data.[a]
7. Analyze and interpret the data.[a]
8. Identify themes and categories.
9. Confirm that findings accurately reflect the feelings and experiences of participants.

PHASE 3: DISSEMINATING THE FINDINGS

10. Share findings with other nurses and health care specialists.

[a] *These activites are cyclical and may be revised as the study progresses. Analysis and interpretation are ongoing and concurrent activites, used to guide the people to sample next and the questions or observations to make. Sampling also is guided by the data.*

Qualitative studies do not follow the same linear progression of quantitative studies. The process tends to resemble a circle more than a line. The researcher is continually examining and interpreting data and making decisions about how to proceed based on what has already been discovered. There are, however, some major activities in which the researcher engages, and these too occur in phases similar to those described for quantitative research: phase 1, conceptualizing and planning the study; phase 2, conducting the study; and phase 3, disseminating the findings. These activities are discussed further in Chart 8–5.

Research Setting

The **setting** in which the study is conducted also will influence the type of research design selected. This is an important consideration when planning a study, because the setting and the dynamics within the setting can greatly influence the outcomes. Settings can be natural, in which no attempt is made to control elements of the setting; partially controlled, meaning that the setting has been modified in some way to strengthen the research design; or highly controlled, in which case a laboratory setting is usually used, such as when animal research is conducted. Many research studies use quasi-natural settings such as hospitals, clinics, or other care facilities.

Sample Selection Studies rarely gather information from an entire **population** of interest. A population is the entire aggregation of cases in which a researcher is interested, for example, all registered nurses with a master's degree in nursing who are currently practicing nursing in northern California. Instead, a sample is selected. **Sampling** is the process of selecting a portion of the population to represent the entire population. A **sample,** then, is a subset of the population.

A major concern when selecting a sample is how representative the sample is of the population; that is, how closely the sam-

grounded theory, or ethnography to explore personal meaning within a given context.

Phenomenology describes the meaning of a lived experience through the perspective of the participant. **Grounded theory** refers to the idea that conclusion of a qualitative study should be grounded in the data, that is, based on direct and careful observations of everyday life within the group. **Ethnography** focuses on the culture of a group of people, with an effort to understand the world view of those under study.

This type of research is important when little is known about a topic because it can identify factors of influence. Often the discoveries of qualitative research generate hypotheses to be used in quantitative research. Many times a combination of the two methods yields a better understanding of human phenomena as seen every day in nursing. The design of the qualitative study is not specified in advance as it is in quantitative research; instead the design tends to evolve over time during the study. Decisions about the best ways to gather data, how to schedule and record data, how many subjects will be used in the study, and so on, are all decisions made during the study. This has been called an emergent design—one that becomes clear during the study as the researcher makes decisions about what she has learned (Colling, 2003). Because qualitative studies involve researchers directly and personally, and because the design emerges during the study, the biases of the researcher must be carefully examined before the study begins.

ple mirrors the characteristics of the entire population of interest. A representative sample is one whose key characteristics closely approximate those of the population. Sampling strategies are classified as either probability sampling or nonprobability sampling (Polit & Beck, 2008). **Probability sampling** involves random selection when choosing the elements. **Nonprobability sampling** means that the elements are selected by nonrandom methods. Six common sampling strategies are explained in this chapter and are shown in Chart 8–6.

Convenience Sampling   With **convenience sampling,** the most available persons or units are selected for inclusion in the study. This also is referred to as accidental sampling (Polit & Beck, 2008). This type of sampling is easy and usually inexpensive. However, it is a weak strategy to use unless no other alternatives are possible or one is doing a **pilot study** (a small preliminary study prior to conducting a larger study). The researcher has no control over the characteristics of this sample, which may mean that the sample may be quite different from the population to which the study results are expected to be relevant. Thus, if this sampling strategy is used, it is wise to build in some limiting characteristics that the sample population must possess. Consider factors that might influence the outcome of the study, for example, socioeconomic status, gender, age, and cultural differences, and decide whether these should be included or excluded.

Quota Sampling   **Quota sampling** involves nonrandom selection of the participants in which the researcher prespecifies characteristics of the sample to increase its representation. Dividing a convenience sample into two subgroups in order to increase the potential for the sample to be representative of the total population may achieve this.

Purposive Sampling   **Purposive sampling** implies that certain people or elements are deliberately selected for the study. This type of sampling is used particularly in qualitative studies. Subjects, also called participants or informants in qualitative studies, are purposively selected for qualitative studies. They are individuals experiencing a common problem or sharing a common circumstance. Usually very few participants are needed since data collection is done through extensive interviews and observations.

Network Sampling   In **network sampling** participants refer other participants to the study. Polit and Beck (2008) also refers to network sampling as snowball sampling. This type of sampling works well for hard-to-find participant groups.

Simple Random Sampling   The **simple random sampling** strategy gives each person in a population an equal chance of being selected for the study. For example, if one were going to study a set of characteristics of breast cancer patients seen in a clinic during the past 2 years, the entire population who meet the study criteria would be listed. A sample from this population would then be randomly selected.

Random samples may be selected in a number of ways. One way is to put names or patient record numbers in a container and draw the names or numbers randomly. Another way is to flip a coin. If the toss is heads, the person is selected; if it is tails, the person is not selected. A more sophisticated method is to use a table of random numbers. Random number tables may be found in most research books. Random sampling greatly strengthens the design of the study by reducing potential selection biases.

There is a difference between random sample and random assignment that should be noted. As has been explained, a random sample means that every person within the category has an equal chance of being in the study. A **random assignment,** however, means that subjects are randomly assigned to treatment versus control groups. For example, if the category was "all cancer patients in California" and every patient in California had an equal chance of being in the study, it would be constitutive random sampling. However, in this example as in many cases this would be a too costly and time-consuming way in which to establish a random sample. Therefore, a random assignment of subjects may be done. For example, every other woman diagnosed with breast cancer in the clinic could be assigned to the treatment group for an educational intervention and every other woman assigned to the control group. Of course, random assignment would not be possible in some cases, for example, if the control group was in another location, or if ethical issues were involved.

Stratified Random Sampling   **Stratified random sampling** means that the population is first divided into two or more

CHART 8–6	**Examples of Sampling Strategies**

Type of Sampling Strategy	Explanation
Convenience sampling	The researcher uses the most conveniently available people as study participants; participants are selected because they are in the right place at the right time.
Quota sampling	The researcher identifies population strata and determines how many participants are needed from each stratum; inclusion of participants is based on predetermined characteristics; a type of convenience sampling.
Purposive sampling	Based on the belief that researchers' knowledge about the population can be used to handpick sample members; also referred to as judgmental sampling.
Network sampling	Participants are referred by other participants; also called snowball sampling.
Simple random sampling	All members of a population are enumerated and then the sample is selected from the sampling frame using random procedures; the most basic type of probability sampling design.
Stratified random sampling	The population is first divided into two or more strata, and then the sample is randomly selected from the homogeneous subsets of the sample.

strata or subpopulations, for example, participants younger than 30 years of age, those between 30 and 45, and those 46 years or older. As with quota sampling the aim is to enhance representation. Polit and Beck (2008) note that stratified sampling designs subdivide the population into homogeneous subsets from which an appropriate number of elements are selected at random. Stratification often is based on such demographic attributes as age, gender, and income level.

Regardless of the sampling strategy used, it is essential to keep a careful record of the sampling decisions and identify how many people began the study, how many completed the study, and why subjects left the study before completing it. It also is important to keep a record of those who refused to participate in the study. These records are very helpful in identifying potential biases in the study results and a clear narrative of the sampling strategy, as well as to interpret the study findings more precisely.

Sample Size Determining sample size is a major consideration in developing a research study. If subjects are hard to get or expensive to enroll in the study, it is prudent to use as few as possible to still have a credible study. However, too few subjects could result in sampling error. Studies with too few subjects to reliably "determine" an effect have low "power," meaning that tests of **statistical significance** are less likely to indicate significance even if the study has a real effect. This is particularly true if the effect is small relative to the variability of the sample. For instance, suppose that the researcher is planning a chart review study to determine if men who had prostate surgery under the age of 65 had as much postsurgery incontinence as those who were over 65. Twenty charts of those under age 65 and 20 of those over 65 are selected. From the literature review, it is expected that the incidence in older men, those over 65, will be much higher than in the younger, under age 65 men. When a test for the significance is applied, the statistic is not significant. Thus, even though there was an effect, the number of subjects was too low to be statistically significant. It is likely that with so few subjects, the variability was too homogeneous and may not have reflected the true rate of incontinence in the entire population. However, the findings from this study could lead to an examination of other factors as to why the incidence of incontinence among these men is lower than what the literature would lead one to expect.

Computing a power analysis is the gold standard in determining sample size. A **power analysis** builds on the concept of an effect size, which expresses the strength of the relationships among research variables. It increases the probability that the results are true results. Conducting a power analysis requires some knowledge of statistics, and the learner is referred to a research or statistical text for further information on power analyses.

There are no simple formulas that can advise how large a sample is needed in a given quantitative study; however, Polit and Beck (2008) suggest using the largest sample possible. The larger the sample, the more representative of the population it is likely to be. Because practical constraints such as time, subject availability, and resources often limit sample size, many nursing studies are based on relatively small samples. In many cases a small sample can lead to misleading or inconclusive results. Thus, the learner is cautioned to consider the generalizablity of

the findings based on the sample size. If there is reason to believe that the population is relatively homogeneous, a small sample may be adequate. For clinical studies that deal with biophysiological processes in which variation is limited, a small sample may adequately represent the population. However, for most nursing studies it is safer to assume a fair degree of heterogeneity, unless there is evidence from prior research to the contrary. The process of drawing a sample may vary according to the type of research design employed. Polit and Beck (2008) have, however, developed a general outline of procedures that may be employed: (1) identify the population, (2) specify the eligibility criteria, (3) specify the sample plan, and (4) recruit the sample. These steps with limited explanation are shown in Chart 8–7.

Qualitative studies almost always use small, nonrandom samples. Whereas quantitative research is concerned with measuring attributes and therefore a representative sample is needed to ensure that the measurements accurately reflect and can be generalized to the population, the aim of qualitative studies is to discover meaning and to uncover multiple realities. Thus, generalizability is not a guideline. A critical first step in qualitative sampling is selecting settings with high potential for information richness. The qualitative researcher may begin with the following types of sampling questions in mind: Who would be an information-rich data source for my study? Who should I talk to or what should I observe first, so as to maximize my understanding of the phenomenon? There are no criteria or rules for sample size in qualitative research. Sample size is largely a function of the purpose of the inquiry, the quality of the informants, and the type of sampling strategy used. Samples are usually small, probability sampling is almost never used, and final sampling decisions usually take place in the field during data collection (Polit & Beck, 2008). The main consideration for sample size is

CHART 8–7	Sampling Steps for Quantitative Studies
Identify the population.	Identify an accessible population, and then decide how best to define the target population.
Specify the eligibility criteria.	The criteria should be as specific as possible with respect to characteristics that might exclude potential subjects (e.g., inability to read Spanish).
Specify the sampling plan.	Once the accessible population has been identified, decide the method for drawing the sample and how large it will be. If possible, perform a power analysis to determine the desired number of subjects. If probability sampling is an option for selecting a sample, it should be exercised.
Recruit the sample.	Recruit prospective study participants according to the plan and after needed institutional permissions have been obtained.

Source: Polit, D.G. & Beck, C.T. (2008) *Nursing research: generating and assessing evidence for nursing practice* (8th ed.). Philadelphia: Wolters Kluwer/Lippincott Williams & Wilkins. Pages 351 and 352. http://lww.com

data saturation, which refers to sampling to the point at which no new information is obtained and redundancy is achieved (Polit & Beck, 2008). Saturation depends on a number of factors. For example, the broader the scope of the research question, the more participants will likely be needed. Data quality also affects sample size. If participants are able to reflect on their experiences and communicate effectively, saturation can be achieved with a relatively small sample. If longitudinal data are collected, few participants may be needed, because each provides a greater amount of information.

In qualitative studies, the sampling plan is evaluated in terms of adequacy and appropriateness. Adequacy refers to the sufficiency and quality of data retrieved. An appropriate sample is one in which the participants can best supply the information according to the conceptual requirements of the study. There are similarities and differences among the various qualitative approaches with regard to sampling. The similarities include the following: Sample size is generally small, probability sampling is almost never used, and final sampling decisions usually take place in the field during data collection. The differences in sampling related to qualitative approaches and tradition are shown in Chart 8–8.

Research Utilization and Evidence-Based Practice

Florence Nightingale probably was the first nursing researcher because she wrote down her observations of nursing care during the formative years of the nursing profession. In her writings, she documented her research approach. She observed what was going on, developed hypotheses, collected and analyzed the data, and then reached conclusions (Burns & Grove, 2003). Essentially, she used the research process to decrease the loss of lives from disease. Based on her skillful analyses of the factors affecting soldier mortality and morbidity during the Crimean War, she was successful in effecting some changes in nursing care and, more generally, in public health. Her landmark publication, *Notes on Nursing* (1859) described her early research interest in environmental factors that promote physical and emotional well-being, an interest of nurses that continues today, nearly 150 years later. For many years after Nightingale's work, there was little reference to research in the nursing literature. It was not until the early 1900s that nursing research began to emerge with a focus primarily on nursing education: characteristics of nurses, the supply and demand of nurses, and the amount of time required in performing certain nursing activities. A shift in focus emerged in the 1950s, accelerating the development of nursing research in the direction of clinical nursing problems. In the 1960s practice-oriented research emerged in the literature.

The advance of nursing research has continued through the last several decades, highlighted by several publications including *Advances in Nursing Science, Research in Nursing & Health, Nursing Research,* the *Western Journal of Nursing Research,* and the *Journal of Advanced Nursing.* These journals contribute to the dissemination and use of nursing research and the increased emphasis on improvement of patient care through research.

Research Utilization

The need for a systematic approach for using research to change practice was recognized in the early 1970s, leading to publication of the first model for research utilization by Stetler and Marram (Stetler, 1994). Subsequently, through the next several decades, much of the progress in using research in practice was based on that model and on work completed by the Western Interstate Commission for Higher Education's Regional Program for Nursing Research Development and the Conduct and Utilization of Research in Nursing (CURN) Project (Burns & Grove, 2005; Polit & Beck, 2008). The major emphasis of the CURN project was to increase the use of research results by direct-care nurses through facilitating organizational change. Since

MyNursingKit | National Institute of Nursing Research

CHART 8–8	Sampling Differences Related to Qualitative Approaches and Tradition
Qualitative Research Approach	**Sampling Guidelines**
Ethnography (focuses on the culture of a group of people, with an effort to understand the worldview of those under study)	Initially, researchers may contact as many members of the culture under study as possible, yet researchers rely heavily on a smaller number of key informants. Key informants are chosen purposively, as guided by the theoretical underpinnings of the study. Researchers (ethnographers) must decide on not only who to sample, but what to sample as well: observation of activities and events, examining records and artifacts, and exploring places.
Phenomenology (focuses on the lived experiences of humans)	Researchers tend to rely on a very small sample size, typically 10 or fewer. All participants must have experienced the phenomenon under study and must be able to articulate what it is like to have lived that experience. This is an example of criterion-referenced sampling.
Grounded theory (designed to develop theories and theoretical propositions grounded in real-world observations)	Theoretical sampling is done to create a sample size of 20 to 30 people. The goal is to select people who can best contribute to the evolving theory; thus, the first cases solicited may be purposive, convenient, or gained through networking. Sampling, data collection, data analysis, and theory construction occur simultaneously, so study participants are selected serially and contingently until saturation is reached (Polit & Beck, 2008).

that time there has been a growing emphasis on using research findings to improve nursing practice. This emphasis has grown in importance with the push in the United States to achieve cost-effective, high-quality patient care based on sound scientific evidence coupled with the global emphasis on quality. Though nursing has a long history of using research to make practice decisions, this process has not been well used, nor has it been well documented or labeled evidence-based practice.

The formation and adoption of the position of the National Institute of Nursing Research (NINR) in 1993 solidified the recognition of nursing research as a major component of nursing practice and moved nursing into the mainstream research path enjoyed by other health disciplines (Polit & Beck, 2008). At present, **research utilization** (RU) is perceived as the purposeful application of research findings to the clinical setting to improve patient care by using the findings from a disciplined study or set of studies in a practical, or real-world, application. Research utilization is important for the bedside nurse whose patients may benefit from implementation of research findings. Nurses in direct patient care also are the best resource for determining if a change of practice will be successful on their respective nursing unit and benefit the patients they serve. Because they are the individuals taking care of patients, nurses must use the newest research findings to keep their practice current, as well as to provide the highest standard of care to patients. Thus, research utilization is one method or source for achieving evidence-based practice.

Evidence-Based Practice

In some settings evidence-based practice and research utilization are used interchangeably; however, there are some distinct differences (Polit & Beck, 2008). **Evidence-based practice (EBP),** in contrast to research utilization, is a broader concept and relies on more than research to support and improve practice. It extends beyond research utilization and involves making clinical decisions on the basis of the best possible evidence. Though the best evidence usually comes from rigorous research, EBP also uses other sources of credible information. Some experts have differentiated between RU and EBP by explaining that RU is part of EBP and is a prescribed task of summarizing and using research findings to address a particular practice problem. In contrast, EBP is "the careful and practical use of current best evidence to guide health care decisions" (Omery & Williams, 1999, p. 51). As seen in both examples of differentiation cited earlier, EBP is broader than RU and is the interpretation chosen by most agencies adopting EBP as a practice model.

The definition of EBP posed by Omery and Williams (1999) asserts that current best evidence includes clinical practice guidelines that usually are developed nationally by expert researchers, clinicians, and theorists in their areas of excellence. EBP involves the interpretation and implementation of these clinical guidelines by health care providers based on their clinical expertise, the needs and views of the patient and family, and the resources of the health care system.

Although evidence-based practice has been emphasized in medicine for years, and expert researchers, clinicians, and theorists have developed numerous evidence-based guidelines for the prevention of illness and diagnosis and management of chronic and acute illnesses (Burns & Grove, 2005), it is in its initial stages of development in the nursing field. As the new recommended standard in health care and nursing, it is important to understand EBP and how it is used to de-emphasize ritual, isolated clinical experiences, ungrounded opinions, and tradition as a basis for nursing practice. Not only does it stress the use of research findings, it also stresses, as appropriate, the use of quality improvement data, other operational and evaluation data, the consensus of recognized experts, and affirmed experience to substantiate practice (Stetler, 1994). EBP calls for nurses to question their practice, looking to reliable evidence to improve and evaluate specific outcomes, rather than simply doing things as they have always done.

EBP is, in effect, a problem-solving approach to clinical decision making that incorporates a search for the best and latest evidence, clinical expertise and assessment, and a patient's preferences and values within a context of caring. This decision-making approach integrates clinical expertise with the best available evidence from systematic research in contrast to opinion-based health care decision making that is based primarily on values and resources. Factors that form a framework for decision making with this approach include understanding the patient's needs, concerns, and values; building on the clinical expertise or experience of the professional nurse; and seeking relevant clinical data and best practices (Malloch & Porter-O'Grady, 2006). Best practices are those proven processes that produce consistent, high-quality results.

Development of Evidence-Based Practice

Five steps are involved in developing evidence-based nursing practice: (1) defining the question, (2) collecting evidence, (3) making a critical appraisal, (4) integrating the evidence and patient factors to make and carry out the decision, and (5) evaluating the whole process (McKibbon, Eady, & Marks, 1999; Stuart, 2001). Also, five levels of evidence used in practice have been identified (Stuart, 2001). The lowest and least powerful evidence is provided by opinions of reviewers that are based on their experience and knowledge and constitute clinical practice guidelines. Somewhat stronger evidence is derived from opinions that come from well-known experts and respected authorities. Even more compelling evidence comes from the results of research studies. Three levels of evidence are derived from research. These are listed in order of increasing strength: nonrandomized controlled studies or cohort studies, small randomized controlled trials, and large randomized controlled trials. Large randomized controlled trials and meta-analyses of studies providing evidence in a specific area are considered the "gold standards" as they furnish the strongest and most powerful evidence for clinical practice.

 CRITICAL ALERT
1. *Define the question.*
2. *Collect evidence.*
3. *Make a critical appraisal.*
4. *Carry out the decision by integrating evidence and patient factors.*
5. *Evaluate the whole process.*

As a problem-solving approach to clinical decision making, EBP incorporates a search for the best and latest evidence, clinical expertise and assessment, and patient preferences and values within a context of caring. The search for evidence in an attempt to answer a burning clinical question related to the effectiveness of a clinical intervention or treatment should begin with databases that contain systematic reviews of randomized controlled trials. Critical appraisal of these reviews for validity, strength of the findings, and applicability is a necessary step in evidence-based decision making and quality patient care.

Implementation of Evidence-Based Practice

Government mandates, consumer demands for accountability, professional efforts to improve quality, and organization requirements for fiscally responsible patient care have all helped develop EBP. Alarming reports of medical errors and the consequences of poor safety practices have inspired a social and professional mandate to improve care quality. In response, a number of health care institutions are seeking to implement evidence-based nursing practice, often including it in strategic plans—with many linking it to the national accrediting body, the Joint Commission. However, two questions remain: Are health care agencies ready to provide the resources that enable nurses to participate in this promising, best-practices model, and are nurses ready to meet the challenge?

Barriers to Evidence-Based Practice

Although a laudable and critical goal, EBP within the health care setting is not easily accomplished due to human and organizational barriers. Nurses often act on experiential knowledge, rather than research evidence, in their day-to-day clinical decision making. They tend to rely most frequently on information learned about the patient, personal experience, manuals, information learned in nursing school, fellow nurses, and nonresearch nursing journals and texts. Nurses' reluctance to use research is compounded by lack of time, access, and skills (Ciliska, Pinelli, DeCenso, & Cullum, 2001; Malloch & Porter-O'Grady, 2006). Although many agencies have incorporated computer usage into the normal work environment, many nurses still have difficulty using computers to conduct database searches. The principal obstacles to nurses' progress in using computers to assist them in retrieving research data are a hectic work environment and lack of time to practice database searching. Nurses' primary responsibility rightfully remains patient care, so taking time away from the bedside to perform literature searches or participate in research projects is not only challenging, but also may be discouraged by peers and managers—especially in a time of staffing shortage.

Other types of barriers to implementing EBP may be categorized as human and institutional barriers. Nurses are attached to historical practice, for example, waking patients during the night to weigh them on standing scales versus using the hospital's newly acquired bed scales because the nurses judge them to be inaccurate. Absence of other clinicians' buy-in constitutes a barrier as does lack of manager/director support. Lack of manager support may result in the unit manager going to the hospital education session to foster staff nurses' interest in research and keeping the staff on the unit. Institutional structure and processes (i.e., red tape) are also a big obstacle. For example, a staff nurse pursuing new, evidence-based protocol on the time of an antibiotic administration must first gain approval from numerous agency committees and administrative personnel. Lack of funding for research projects constitutes another barrier in many agencies, particularly in light of attempts to reduce health care costs.

Also to be considered is the role and support of the nurse researcher, if there is one, present in the agency. The nurse researcher position often becomes one of isolation in which the researcher lacks peer and mentor support. This isolation coupled with weak, or lack of, leadership support prohibits effective use of the nurse researcher and often leads to the nurse researcher leaving the agency; thereby, absenting a role model and coordinator for nursing research. Finally, the nurse's skills, or lack thereof, may lead to the collection of unreliable data. For instance, if the unit is participating in a study on skin integrity using the Braden scale, nurses collecting the data must know how to code pressure ulcers correctly using the scale. If they do not the data are compromised.

From the barriers identified, it is obvious that research-based practice initiatives need dedicated expertise, leadership support, and grassroots enthusiasm to thrive. In many situations this means changing an organization's culture of practice.

Strategies to Promote Evidence-Based Practice

Numerous strategies to overcome the barriers of using research and clinical evidence in practice are noted in the literature. Establishing a research committee is one suggestion. A research committee could explore and adopt a research critique tool and discuss issues of concern. Another approach is to survey nurses to determine their interest in research activities. After areas of interest are established, collaborative research groups can identify research topics for investigation. A group also could be formed to look at inconsistencies in practice and varied patient outcomes, to improve patient care, and to increase the research base of practice by defining a standard protocol. Information gained from such a group could be used to develop assessments and protocols.

Other mechanisms for increasing staff participation in EBP are by forming research clubs where research studies are reviewed systematically, much like a book club. Continuing education and in-service programs also are good ways to teach nurses about research utilization. Nursing forums that focus on the research process or on research results can give nurses an increased understanding of the research utilization process. Other methods that might be useful include independent self-study packets, a newsletter, a journal club, community research groups, informal research promotion, and, of course, changes in nursing education. The main key is to stimulate interest and enthusiasm in nurses so they will want to understand and use research. It is necessary to captivate their interest and engage them in seeing the excitement of changing practice through research.

In the future, EBP should increase. Many nursing students are being taught to use research findings as a basis for interventions. Thus, the emphasis is no longer limited to research conduction. It is well known that perceptions of priority and attitudes about research influence the use of research in practice.

If the nurse does not perceive research findings to be important or relevant to his particular work setting, he will not be as likely to read research or seek out research-related outcomes to improve practice. It is absolutely necessary that nurses know that the nursing administration and the health care organization endorse the concept of EBP. Only then is it probable that the perceptions of priority will change for the nurse.

Lack of access to information is perhaps the most difficult barrier to overcome. Internet access and current literature databases must be available. Personal digital assistants can provide quick reference, but are not yet practical for most nurses, although they are becoming more useful. An on-site library is helpful, but it is not the entire solution. Information must be available and easy to access at the point of care. This will only become available when nurses start to demand it and incorporate it into their practice. Research has shown that using best practices is cost effective and reduces both complications and lengths of stay. When nurses demand tools that support their own best practice, the tools will be provided.

Practicing nurses must strive to base their practices on research in order to improve patient outcomes. Nursing manuals, policies, procedures, and protocols should reflect current research-based knowledge. It is probable that, in the future, accrediting agencies will require that nursing care interventions be research based. It follows that research utilization should be actively promoted in all health care agencies. Examples of ways in which research and clinical evidence have been used to change practice are shown in Chart 8–9.

As of December 2007, there were 15 evidence-based practice centers (EPCs) across the United States and in Canada funded by the Evidence-based Practice Program of the Agency for Healthcare Research and Quality (AHRQ). These agencies are funded to review all relevant scientific literature on clinical, behavioral, organizational, and financing topics to produce evidence reports and technology assessments. The EPCs also conduct research on methodologies to determine the effective-

ness of their implementation, to provide technical assistance in translating the reports and assessments into quality improvement tools, and to help inform coverage policies.

The 15 centers as of December 2007 are listed here:

- Blue Cross and Blue Shield Association, Technology Evaluation Center (TEC), Chicago, Illinois
- Duke University, Durham, North Carolina
- ECRI Institute, Plymouth Meeting, Pennsylvania
- Johns Hopkins University, Baltimore, Maryland
- McMaster University, Hamilton, Ontario, Canada
- Minnesota Evidence-based Practice Center, Minneapolis
- Oregon Health & Science University, Portland
- RTI International University of North Carolina at Chapel Hill
- Southern California Evidence-based Practice Center–RAND, Santa Monica
- Stanford University, Stanford, and University of California, San Francisco
- Tufts-New England Medical Center, Boston, Massachusetts
- University of Alberta
- University of Connecticut, Farmington, CT
- University of Ottawa
- Vanderbilt University, Nashville, Tennessee

Evidence-based report topics and disease category listings may be obtained via the Internet by going to www.ahrq.gov/clinic/epcindex.htm. To date, more than 80 reports have been released (AHRQ, 2007).

Research and Ethics in Health Care

The practice of ethics guides health care professionals when they are making decisions concerning life and death situations. The term *ethics* refers to the goodness and badness of human actions or to principles of what is right and wrong in conduct. The intent of ethics is to develop methods for clarifying confusing questions even if final solutions remain elusive. Ethics deals with concerns for good behavior among people and struggles to resolve ethical differences among members of society. The ethical codes and oaths of professionals do not always help, because personal feelings are often involved in each situation. Nurses and physicians often are put in a situation of conflict. Such a position may occur when participating in nursing research. A full discussion of ethical principles that guide nursing practice is given in Chapter 4.

At every stage of the research process, there are ethical considerations for nurse researchers to consider. This consideration may start with the selection of a research problem; from an ethical viewpoint, should the problem be studied or not? For example, should subjects with mental impairments who may not be able to give informed and voluntary consent be studied? As more and more nurses participate in research activities, it is imperative for the profession to operate from a sound ethical knowledge base. Because research is central to the evolution of nursing care, the avoidance of conducting nursing research might be considered unethical. Similarly, the failure to engage in

CHART 8–9 Examples of Ways in Which Research and Clinical Evidence Have Changed Practice

- Development of a heart failure center (Crowther, 2003)
- Use of saline versus heparin to maintain patency of peripheral intravenous access (DeBourgh, 2001)
- Use of Trendelenburg position for hypotension in emergencies. (DeBourgh, 2001)
- Frequency of ventilator circuit tubing change (DeBourgh, 2001)
- Use of normal saline when suctioning endotracheal tubes (DeBourgh, 2001)
- Music as an intervention in hospitals (2001)
- Maintaining oral hygiene in older people (2001)
- Assessing and managing pain in older adults (Ardery, Herr, Titler, Sorofman, & Schmittet, 2003)
- Fall risk assessment, prevention, and management (Poe, Cvach, Gartrell, Radzik, & Joy, 2005)

evidence-based practice—in other words, to base practice decisions solely on tradition or intuition rather than on empirical finding—denies patients access to the best available care and, thus, also might be considered unethical.

Nurses are involved in a variety of research efforts, including research specific to nursing, multidisciplinary research, and research of other disciplines on patients receiving nursing care. In all of these situations, nurses are expected to engage in ethical research behavior. With this expectation arises the question of how nurse researchers can make ethical decisions. What are the characteristics of ethical research? What are the rights of those participating in the study, and how does the nurse researcher guard those rights? An exploration of ethical decision making addresses these questions.

Ethical Frameworks

Two ethical frameworks have been proposed in Western society to assess the ethical acceptability of a research project. These are the utilitarian and the deontological perspectives (Gillis & Jackson, 2002). Each of these perspectives articulates ethical norms that transcend disciplinary boundaries.

Utilitarian Perspective

The utilitarian perspective suggests that ethical judgments about a research project should be made by evaluating its consequences for the participants, for society, and for the academic discipline. This view entails the belief that the good of a research project is defined by the consequences of the results. The well-known philosopher John Stewart Mill proposed that actions should be taken to promote the greatest good for the greatest number. The utilitarian perspective considers that the end justifies the means. Based on this perspective, a research project is judged ethical if it produces the greatest good for the greatest number; the problem is in determining what is good. Small-scale studies with little ability for generalization of findings to the larger society may be judged to be unethical from a utilitarian perspective. For example, research into liver transplantation that has the potential to influence quality of life for a small number of participants who receive this costly medical intervention may not be considered ethical unless it can be shown that the results will benefit a large number of people in the future. In contrast, research into the prevention of liver disease through lifestyle change is justifiable from a utilitarian perspective because lifestyle change is more likely to benefit many more people than will costly surgical procedures available to only a few. When discussing the utilitarian perspective, it is necessary to recognize that each researcher may have a different definition of what is good for the majority.

Deontological Perspective

The deontological approach to research ethics proposes absolute moral imperatives that must never be violated. In taking the deontological view, one might propose absolutes such as never using deception, never making participants' identity known, and never putting any pressure on respondents to participate in a study. Rather than assessing the consequences of a given research procedure, the deontological approach may propose, in its most extreme form, that deception in experiments is never justified,

regardless of what the positive contributions to one's knowledge might be. Immanuel Kant, a well-known deontologist, supported the categorical imperative; that is, basic laws apply without exception. For example, telling an untruth is always wrong, regardless of the consequences, or the welfare of the patient must always be placed above the integrity of the research if a conflict exists. Some deontologists take a more flexible approach, accepting more than one basic law and considering context and circumstances in determining priority. Some argue that types of harm can be distinguished: harm to a participant's interest, wrongdoing, and a moral harm. Still others argue that although harms can be compensated for, wrongs cannot be, the argument being that if doing a wrong is essential to conducting a research project, then the project should be banned (Holden, 1979).

Codes and Guidelines for Ethical Decision Making

Throughout its history, the field of nursing has been sensitive to the ethical dimension of doing nursing research. Thus, many professional organizations have developed codes of ethics to guide nurses in their research endeavors. These codes articulate the level of ethical behavior expected of nurse researchers and provide a standard for nurses working through ethical conflicts that may arise in research. They also provide guidance on ethical decision making in clinical practice, education, and administration.

During the past four decades, largely in response to human rights violations, various codes of ethics have been developed. One of the first internationally recognized efforts to establish ethical standards is referred to as the Nuremberg code, which was developed after the Nazi atrocities of World War II were made public in the Nuremberg trials. Several other international codes of ethics have been developed since then, the most notable being the Declaration of Helsinki. This declaration was adopted in 1964 by the World Medical Association and was most recently revised in 2000. Most disciplines have established their own code of ethics, as has nursing.

The American Nurses Association's Code of Ethics was adopted in 1985, and is shown in Chapter 1 . The ANA also put forth a document in 1995 entitled *Ethical Guidelines in the Conduct, Dissemination, and Implementation of Nursing Research.* This document presents nine ethical principles used to guide nursing research. These nine principles are shown in Chart 8–10 (p. 134).

In 1978, an important code of ethics was adopted in the United States that was created by the National Commission for the Protection of Human Subjects of Biomedical and Behavioral Research (1978). The commission issued a report that served as the basis for regulations affecting research sponsored by the federal government. The report, sometimes referred to as the Belmont report, also served as a model for many of the guidelines adopted by specific disciplines. The Belmont report articulated three primary ethical principles on which standards of ethical conduct in research are based: respect for persons, beneficence, and justice. Information about various codes of ethics and ethical requirements for government-sponsored research can be found in the Web links for this chapter on MyNursingkit.

CHART 8–10 **Ethical Principles in Nursing Research**

The Investigator . . .

1. Respects autonomous research participants' capacity to consent to participate in research and to determine the degree and duration of that participation without negative consequences.

2. Prevents harm, minimizes harm, and/or promotes good to all research participants, including vulnerable groups and others affected by the research.

3. Respects the personhood of research participants, their families, and significant others, valuing their diversity.

4. Ensures that the benefits and burdens of research are equitably distributed in the selection of research participants.

5. Protects the privacy of research participants to the maximum degree possible.

6. Ensures the ethical integrity of the research process by use of appropriate checks and balances throughout the conduct, dissemination, and implementation of the research.

7. Reports suspected, alleged, or known incidents of scientific misconduct in research to appropriate institutional officials for investigation.

8. Maintains competency in the subject matter and methodologies of his or her research, as well as in other professional and societal issues that affect nursing research and the public good.

9. Involved in animal research maximizes the benefits of the research with the least possible harm or suffering to the animals.

Source: From Silva, M.C. (1995). *Ethical guidelines in the conduct, dissemination, and implementation of nursing research (pp. v-vi.)* Washington, DC. American Nurses' Association. Printed in Polit & Beck, (2004). *Nursing research: Principles and methods (7th ed.).* Philadelphia: Lippincott Williams & Wilkins. http://lww.com

Principles of Ethical Research

At times ethical theories such as deontology or utilitarianism may not be adequate to guide nurses in ethical decision making. In these situations, ethical principles rather than theories may prove more helpful. The three principles from the Belmont report just discussed and elaborated on next are useful for ethical decision making.

Respect for Persons

Inherent in the principle of respect for persons are the concepts of autonomy, dignity, uniqueness, freedom, and choice. This principle forms the foundation of the participants' rights to informed consent, privacy, and confidentiality, and involves respecting people's autonomy or right to choose freely for themselves. Participants have choices based on their own values and beliefs and to be free from undue pressure or coercion by others. They must be made fully aware of any risks and benefits of the study. This principle requires that the participants' confidentiality and anonymity be safeguarded.

Beneficence

Two concepts are inherent in the principle of beneficence: nonmalfeasance, or the ability to not inflict physical or emotional harm, and beneficence, or the duty to promote or do good. To apply the concepts of beneficence, researchers must provide a standard of care. Standards of care usually are established by society and by professional role expectations. Nurses' duties to act as patient advocates require that nurses intervene if a research intervention produces more harm than benefit to a patient.

It is the researcher's responsibility to minimize risks and maximize benefits to participants; not doing so would contravene the ethical principle of beneficence. When a nurse researcher is a care provider, the potential for conflict between the duty to care and the duty to advance knowledge may be imminent. Some refer to this as the research imperative, advancement of knowledge versus the duty to care (Gillis & Jackson, 2002). Sometimes it is difficult to determine at what point the therapeutic imperative is being compromised by the research imperative. When doubt is evident, the therapeutic imperative must take precedence over the research imperative for the nurse as caregiver. This is due to the fact that the nurse must always act as the patient's advocate.

Justice

The principle of justice requires that people be treated fairly. The protection of participants from incompetence and the right to receive research treatments are expectations of the justice principle. Justice is an important principle to follow in the selection of subjects for research studies. The risks and benefits of a study should be fairly distributed among participants based on the subjects' efforts, needs, and rights. If possible, random selection of participants avoids potential sources of bias and unfairness in sample selection.

Nurses involved in any aspect of the process have a responsibility to see that research complies with the principles of respect for persons, beneficence, and justice. This is true for nurses' own research as well as for research conducted by others that affects their patients.

Methods of Protecting Human Subjects

Two methods of protecting human subjects have been developed during the past three decades. These include obtaining informed consent and the review of research proposals by an ethics committee or an institutional review board.

Informed Consent

Informed consent is based on the principle of respect for persons and incorporates the ethical concept of autonomy or the client's right to self-determination. The key elements of informed consent include disclosure of sufficient and appropriate information, understanding of information, and voluntary participation. Comprehension of information is essential to informed consent. The researcher must determine that the participants understand the information provided to them. It is incumbent on the researcher to make sure that the participants understand the risks involved as well as the benefits. They also must be fully informed about the research protocol so that they can make informed choices. Voluntary participation implies that participants agree to be part of a study of their own free will without coercion of any kind.

In obtaining informed consent, always:

- *Provide participants adequate information about the research.*
- *Make sure participants are capable of comprehending information.*
- *Make sure participants have the power of free choice.*
- *Document the informed consent.*

In qualitative investigations, the idea of process consent is suggested rather than a traditional consent. In process consent, the researcher renegotiates the consent with participants as unforeseen circumstances arise. This allows the participants to be part of the decision making as the study unfolds, and is in contrast to traditional consent, which is signed at the beginning of a study and not reconsidered.

Institutional Review Boards

Research involving humans should be submitted for approval to an ethics committee, commonly referred to as an institutional review board (IRB) or an ethics review committee. The purpose of the review is to ensure that ethical principles are appropriately applied to research involving human subjects. Most institutions, hospitals, governmental agencies, and universities in which research involving human subjects is carried out require specific information to make informed and responsible decisions regarding the ethical acceptability of a proposal. Chart 8–11 describes the type of information that should be included in a submission to an IRB (Gillis & Jackson, 2002). Additional information on IRBs is included in agency policy and also may be found in research texts.

Rules for Conducting Ethical Research

There are ethical rules that serve as guidelines for conducting research. They are organized around two themes: (1) nurse researchers' ethical responsibility to participants and (2) nurse researchers' responsibility to the discipline of nursing and society (Gillis & Jackson, 2002). These rules include the following, and are summarized in Chart 8–12 (p. 136):

1. Protect the confidentiality of participants.
2. Do not place pressure on participants.
3. Make the subjects' participation painless and free from discomfort and harm.

 Information to Be Included in Submission to an IRB

- The purpose of the study and its significance to health research
- The study design and methodology
- Potential research participants and a description of the selection process
- Risk and benefits to the participants
- Steps to ensure participant choice, confidentiality, and anonymity protection
- Areas of potential conflict of interest

Source: From Gillis, A., & Jackson, W. (2002). *Research for nurses: Methods and interpretation.* Philadelphia: F. A. Davis, page 336.

4. Identify sponsors.
5. Disclose the basis on which participants have been selected.
6. Place no hidden identification codes on questionnaires.
7. Honor promises to provide participants with research reports.
8. Informed consent is a key concern.
9. Debrief subjects.

Rules for Socially Responsible Nursing Research

Not only do nurses have ethical responsibilities to the participants but also to society at large and the nursing discipline in particular. Research-minded practitioners, educators, administrators, nursing students, and other health care professionals expect nurse researchers to do ethical research. The end result of nursing studies is to shape nurses' practice and promote excellence in nursing care. To this end, researchers should conduct unbiased studies and report results in trustworthy manners; seven rules guide this process. Researchers should:

1. Distinguish between science and advocacy.
2. Not hunt through data looking for pleasing findings.
3. Be aware of potential sources of bias.
4. Represent research literature fairly.
5. Do the best research possible.
6. Acknowledge all sources.
7. Seek advice on ethical issues.

These rules are shown and explained in Chart 8–13 (p. 136).

Privacy and the Health Insurance Portability and Accountability Act

One of the rules of conducting ethical research is that of maintaining the privacy and confidentiality of participants. Privacy is the right an individual has to determine the time, extent, and general circumstances under which personal information will be shared with or withheld from others (Burns & Grove, 2005). Such information consists of one's attitudes, beliefs, behaviors, opinions, and records. The research subject's privacy is protected if the subject is informed and consents to participate in a study and voluntarily shares private information with the researcher. An invasion of privacy occurs when private information is shared without an individual's knowledge or against her will. An invasion of privacy occurs most frequently during the data collection phase of the research process. This may occur when invasive questions are asked during an interview, an interview is taped without the subject's consent, or hidden cameras or mirrors are used to observe the subjects.

The Privacy Act of 1974 was enacted to safeguard subjects' privacy rights, and has led to scrutiny of data collection methods by an IRB or committee formed to review all research proposals. Improvements in technology also were a precipitating factor for the Privacy Act as it became so easy to collect and transmit data without the knowledge or control of the subject. With the advent of the Internet and increased access to information on individuals, including health information, the federal

CHART 8–12	**Rules for Conducting Ethical Research**

Rule	**Interpretation**
Protect the confidentiality of participants.	Confidentiality is to be treated as a sacred trust, based on the ethical principle of respect for persons. If researchers need to identify individuals' names with particular questionnaires, then number codes, rather than names, should be used. If data are released to other researchers, steps should be taken to mask the individual identities of participants.
Do not put pressure on participants.	No pressure should be put on participants to cooperate in the study. Respondents must feel free to refuse participation, to withdraw at any time, or to refuse to answer any particular question. This rule is based on the principle of respect for persons.
Make the subjects' participation painless and free from discomfort.	Researchers must not expose participants to needlessly long experimental trials or questionnaires or ask questions that pry unnecessarily into personal matters; only relevant information should be collected. Maintaining the comfort, and safety, and self-esteem of the participants should be a central concern of researchers. This is based on the principle of beneficence, which requires that one should do good and, above all, do no harm.
Identify sponsors.	Participants must be informed about who is doing the study.
Disclose the basis on which participants have been selected.	Participants have the right to know how they were selected for participation in a study. Respondents need to know if the selection was made by means of a probability sampling procedure or if it was based on special characteristics related to the research problem or phenomenon under investigation (e.g., age, health status, medical diagnosis). Selection of participants is based on the ethical principle of justice.
Place no hidden identification codes on questionnaires.	Do not place hidden identification codes on questionnaires to aid in the identification of those who have or have not returned questionnaires. If individuals are to be identified, this information should be placed directly on the questionnaire and discussed in a cover letter. The identification corresponding to participant names should be kept in a secure area to protect the identity of participants. Only the researcher should have access to this information.
Honor promises to provide participants with research reports.	When a promise to provide participants a copy of the research report is made, this promise should be fulfilled. This reinforces the idea of a reciprocal contract between the researcher and the participant.
Informed consent is a key concern.	In dealing with competent adults, participation should be based on informed consent; potential participants must be informed about the nature of the study, what kinds of issues will be explored, how participants were selected, what the risk and benefits to the participants are, and who is sponsoring the research. Prospective participants also should be informed about confidentiality and anonymity, and they should feel free to withdraw from the study at any time without prejudice if they wish to do so. Any time selective nondisclosure of information or deception is used in a research study, the researcher must question how acceptable it is to do so. With deception, the risks to the participants should be minimal and outweighed by the benefits.
Debrief subjects.	When experiments or field studies involve deception, subjects should have the study explained to them after the session. They should be told what deception was used and why it was necessary.

CHART 8–13	**Rules for Socially Responsible Nursing Research**

Rules	**Interpretation**
Researchers should distinguish between science and advocacy.	Nurses should distinguish between citizen-advocate roles and researcher roles. As a citizen-advocate, it is legitimate to comment on the evidence of others and to produce evidence that is appropriate to the issue under dispute. However, that information is being presented from the perspective of a citizen-advocate, not from that of an expert nurse scientist (Gillis & Jackson, 2002).
Do not hunt through data looking for pleasing findings.	The surest way to be guilty of misrepresentation is to search for support of one's views. To do so would be both bad science and unethical behavior.
Be aware of potential sources of bias.	Researchers have an ethical responsibility to avoid bias as much as possible.
Represent research literature fairly.	Portray the body of literature accurately. Reporting findings selectively is not acceptable.
Do the best research possible.	Always seek to do the best research possible; do research with care; strive to be competent and impartial, and report results objectively.
Acknowledge all sources.	Acknowledge people who have played a role in the research and acknowledge all literature sources that have directly influenced the study; site each literature source used.
Seek advice on ethical issues.	If ethical issues arise, seek the advice of appropriate professional bodies or institutions involved in the project.

government enacted the Health Insurance Portability and Accountability Act (HIPAA) of 1996 (Olsen, 2003). Under federal law, HIPAA's privacy requirements are intended to guarantee individuals new rights and protections against the misuse or unauthorized disclosure of their health records. Though the law does not target research, it does affect the manner in which research is conducted.

The HIPAA privacy regulations constitute an extensive reform of the way health care information is handled. Disclosures of health information for research are allowed but regulated beyond the common-rule regulations currently monitored by IRBs. HIPAA is a concern for anyone conducting or reviewing nursing research. There are three points at which the HIPAA privacy regulations will impact nursing research: (1) assessing data from a covered entity (e.g., reviewing medical records of subjects), (2) creating data (e.g., an intervention study), and (3) disclosing data (e.g., with a colleague from another institution).

- *Accessing data:* It is the covered organization's obligation not to disclose information improperly when a researcher seeks data that includes private health information. A covered organization is one that "transmits information in an electronic form, and includes health plans, health care clearing houses, and health care agencies. All covered entities are required to comply with the Privacy Rule (Connor, Smaldone, Bratts, & Stone, 2003). Researchers will be expected to work closely with clinical agencies used as research sites to ensure that both sides meet HIPAA obligations. Individually identifiable health information (IIHI) data may be accessed for research under specific conditions; the pertinent access terms and explanations for IIHI are presented in Chart 8–14.

- *Creating data:* Researchers also may be creating IIHI data. If the researcher is part of a covered entity, any protected health information obtained by any means is covered by HIPAA, and the researcher and his or her institution are bound by HIPAA regulations. When obtaining IIHI directly from the subject, the subject must authorize the use of the information. Essential elements of disclosure must be included in the authorization: who will be receiving the information, what further disclosures the researcher anticipates, and what information will be disclosed to the researcher.

- *Disclosing data:* Nurse researchers should be aware that sharing data with colleagues and students might constitute disclosures of IIHI, according to HIPAA regulations. The researcher is the holder of the IIHI and can disclose it only under appropriate conditions. When the researcher creates and holds IIHI, he must track any further disclosures made through waiver of authorization or in a review preparatory for research for 6 years and be prepared to report these to the former patient (Olsen, 2003).

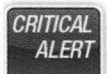 *HIPAA governs privacy in accessing data, creating data, and disclosing data.*

One may conclude that privacy of health information is widely accepted as an essential element of the researcher's obligation to respect the autonomy of subjects. To do this effectively, the nurse must understand HIPAA and its privacy provisions. They are of critical importance for current investigations as well as future research endeavors. The primary focus of HIPAA modifications in research protocols is in the areas of

CHART 8–14   Disclosure Rules for Individually Identifiable Health Information for Research Purposes

Condition of Information Disclosure	Explanation
Information pertains only to deceased persons	Information gathered about living persons from the records of the deceased, e.g., relatives, must be obtained in accordance with HIPAA.
Review preparatory to research	Allows researchers to assess the feasibility of projects by examining the information recorded in patients' records or the interventions currently in place without authorization from the potential subject or the permission of an IRB or privacy board. However, the information cannot be removed from the covered entity. The holder of the IIHI must determine how to monitor researchers' activity in this area.
Deidentification	All information that acts as an identifier as defined in the HIPAA regulations has been removed. Such information can be shared freely because it is no longer IIHI. This would include identifiers such as name, address, and date of birth. HIPAA regulations also state that IIHI can be deidentified if a person with appropriate credentials in statistics determines that the risk is very small that the information could be used to identify an individual.
Authorization	An organization, or covered agency, may disclose IIHI if the researcher presents an authorization signed by the patient. The authorization may be signed as part of the informed consent or as a separate document. Researchers also may be granted access to IIHI if an IRB or privacy board has waived the need for authorization. There are special conditions under which this waiver may be granted, and the IRB or privacy board should be contacted for this information.
Recruitment	Researchers also need to access data from the organization, or covered entity for recruitment. Under the HIPAA regulations it is inappropriate for a covered entity to disclose potential subjects for a researcher to contact. There are two alternatives. Personnel at the covered entity can make potential subjects aware of the protocol and then obtain an authorization to disclose the potential subject to the researcher, or the researcher can obtain a partial waiver of authorization from the IRB.

Source: U.S. Department of Health and Human Services, Office for Civil Rights. (2003). Standards for privacy of individually identifiable health information. *Code of Federal Regulations,* Title 45, Parts 160 & 164. Retrieved June 13, 2007 from http://www.hhs.gov/ocr/hipaa/privruletxt.txt

informed consent. Additional information on HIPAA can be obtained from the HIPAA website. HIPAA also is discussed at length in Chapter 4 .

Informatics

As has been noted, evidence-based practice is characterized by using the best available information when making clinical decisions, in lieu of intuition and unmethodical clinical experience. It is the new recommended standard in health care. Many agree that EBP has the potential to improve patient care and outcomes, yet, in order to be effective, information must be available and accessible, and practitioners must be skilled at using resources such as computers. Government mandates, consumer demands for accountability, professional efforts to improve quality, and organizational requirements for fiscally responsible patient care have all helped develop evidence-based practice. However, the questions, as previously posed, remain: "Are health care facilities ready to provide the resources that will enable nurses to participate in this promising, best-practices model? And, if so, are nurses ready to meet the challenge?" This is best answered by the acknowledgment that both health care facilities and health care providers must become skilled in informatics in order to effectively participate in evidence-based practice.

Informatics can be interpreted as a combination of computer science, information science, and health care science designed to assist in the management and delivery of health care. It is the knowledge necessary to use the computer and programs effectively to retrieve, input, and use knowledge to assist in decision making. In the case of nursing research, informatics is used to retrieve information to support an identified problem, conduct a literature review, input data for analysis, complete statistical analyses, and share findings with colleagues. The computer and specific research-oriented programs may be used to analyze both quantitative and qualitative data. Research texts typically identify computer programs that may be used for data analysis

(Burns & Grove, 2005; Gillis & Jackson, 2002; Polit & Beck, 2008). Every nurse is expected to have fundamental information management and computer literacy skills, although it is recognized that the level of skill needed may vary among nurse researchers. These levels have been defined by Staggers, Gassert, and Curran (2002) and are shown in Chart 8–15.

 CRITICAL ALERT

1. All nurses are expected to have fundamental information management and computer literacy skills.
2. All nurses must know how to use the computer to retrieve data, input data, and use knowledge for decision making.

The Research Critique

Applying research findings to practice is now recognized as essential to developing scientifically based nursing practice. A key step in this process is the ability of nurses to read nursing research studies and determine the usefulness of their findings for practice. To determine if the research is useful and applicable, the nurse must evaluate the completed research, identifying areas of adequacy and inadequacy, virtues as well as faults. This **research critique** is an intellectual process of a careful, complete examination of a study to judge its strengths, weakness, logical links, meaning, and significance. The critique involves a high level of critical thinking and analysis of each component of the study. A quality study focuses on a significant problem, demonstrates sound methodology, produces credible findings, and is easily replicated by other researchers. A critique appraisal involves judging whether or not a research study meets these quality standards and is described clearly and comprehensively enough to decide if the findings and implications are logical and believable and should be considered seriously in practice.

Generally research is critiqued to broaden understanding, summarize knowledge for use in practice, and provide a base for the conduct of a study (Polit & Beck, 2008). Research critiques are performed by nursing students, nursing instructors, practicing nurses, and nurse researchers. Each may have a different in-

Level	Competency
CHART 8–15	**Definitions for Levels of Nurses' Computer Competency Skills**
Level 1: Beginning nurses	Have fundamental information management and computer technology skills and use existing information systems and available information to manage their practice.
Level 2: Experienced nurses	Have proficiency in their domain of interest (e.g., public health, acute care, education, administration). These nurses are highly skilled in using information management and computer technology skills to support their major area of practice. Experienced nurses use current information systems, but collaborate with information specialists to suggest system improvements.
Level 3: Informatics specialists	Informatics specialists usually are registered nurses prepared at least at the baccalaureate level who possess additional knowledge and skills specific to information management and computer technology. They focus on information needs for the practice of nursing, which includes education, administration, research, and clinical practice. Informatics specialists' practices are built on the integration and application of information science, computer science, and nursing science. In their practice, informatics specialists use the tools of critical thinking, data management skills, and computer skills.
Level 4: Informatics innovators	Informatics innovators are educationally prepared to conduct informatics research and to generate informatics theory. These nurses lead the advancement of informatics practice and research.

Source: From Staggers, N., Gassert, C. A., & Curran, C. (2002). A delphi study to determine informatics competencies for nurse levels of practice. *Nursing Research, 51*(6), 383–390. http://lww.com

tent and focus; however, they all basically follow a similar process. For example, in nursing education, a critique often is seen as the first step in learning the research process. By conducting research critiques, students develop critical thinking skills, strengthen their knowledge base, and increase their use of research findings in practice. Critiques of studies by practicing nurses are essential for the implementation of evidence-based practice. These critiques tend to focus on the scientific merit of the study and on its implications for nursing practice. Educators conduct research critiques to expand their knowledge base and improve the educational process, and researchers conduct critiques to plan and implement a study. This section focuses on the general guidelines that can be used by any group to conduct a research critique.

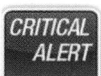

- *Applying research findings to practice is essential.*
- *Nurses must know how to read research studies and determine the usefulness of findings for practice.*

Elements of a Research Critique

Specific elements must be considered when critiquing a research study. The results of both quantitative and qualitative studies are used to improve nursing practice, so critique methods for both are discussed.

Quantitative Research Critique

Gillis and Jackson (2002) suggest the following criteria for evaluating quantitative research studies:

1. Relevant and clearly articulated statement of purpose
2. Consistency between explicitly stated purpose and problem statement or question or hypothesis
3. Comprehensive literature review identifies gaps in the research area and logically leads to the research questions under study
4. Theoretical framework provides a rationale for the study
5. Congruent match between the purpose, design, and method
6. Appropriate sample and sample selection procedures
7. Statistical procedures appropriate to the type of data collected and research questions posed
8. Adequate reliability and validity to accept findings and generalize to appropriate populations
9. Significance of study for nursing is apparent. (p. 614)

The actual review of a quantitative study uses the criteria just set forth and divides the critique into four stages of review (Gillis & Jackson, 2002; Polit & Beck, 2008):

- Stage 1 refers to a review of the purpose, problem statement, and congruency with design and methodology. The reviewer must gain a clear understanding of the meaning of the purpose and problem statement of a study, and determine if the research design and methodology are consistent with the study purpose.
- Stage 2 focuses on the conduct of the research. This refers to studying the manner in which the research was conducted

and includes determining if the methodology was applied correctly.
- Stage 3 refers to studying the findings of the research and assessing if the outcomes and conclusions are believable and supported by the findings. The focus is on the outcomes of the study.
- Stage 4 summarizes the overall quality of the study, identifying the strengths and limitations of the study, and evaluating the contributions of the study to nursing. At this point the reviewer also looks for suggestions for improving the work of the researcher.

Chart 8–16 summarizes the criteria used in each of the stages of appraising quantitative research reports. Chart 8–17 (p. 140) shows key questions that can be asked by the reviewer when critiquing quantitative designs.

Qualitative Research Critique

Critical evaluation of qualitative studies uses different standards than those of quantitative due to the nature of the study. Qualitative studies emerge from the naturalistic-inductive paradigm and as such are based on a different set of assumptions and a different worldview, and have a different purpose than quantitative studies. Qualitative research hopes to promote understanding of phenomena. A scholarly critique of qualitative studies includes a balanced evaluation of a study's strengths and weaknesses. Five

CHART 8–16	Stages of the Critiquing Process and Components of a Quantitative Research Project
Stage of Critique Process	**Review Components**
Stage 1: Purpose, problem statement, and congruency with design and methodology	• Study purpose • Problem statement • Theoretical framework • Literature review • Hypothesis or research question • Research design • Sampling procedures • Data collection procedures • Instruments • Data analysis
Stage 2: Conduct of the research	• Protection of participants' rights • Ethics of research • Consistency and integrity of procedures
Stage 3: Outcomes of the research process	• Statistical significance of results • Clinical significance of results • Discussion of findings • Implications for practice, education, and research
Stage 4: Overall quality of study	• Conclusions

Source: From Gillis, A., & Jackson, W. (2002). *Research for nurses: Methods and interpretation.* Philadelphia: F. A. Davis Co.

CHART 8-17 **Key Questions for Critiquing Quantitative Designs**

STAGE 1 QUESTIONS: CRITICAL APPRAISAL OF PURPOSE, PROBLEM STATEMENT, AND CONGRUENCE WITH DESIGN AND METHODOLOGY

Purpose or Problem Statement

- Is the study problem and purpose statement clearly articulated?
- Are the reasons for conducting the study stated?
- Is the study's potential contribution to nursing knowledge stated?
- Are the research objectives or research questions or hypotheses stated clearly and researchable (answerable through the collection of empirical data)?
- Are terms defined conceptually and operationally?

Literature Review

- Does the literature review or theoretical framework provide evidence that the researcher has synthesized the classic and current literature and placed the research question in the proper context?
- Does the literature review identify gaps in knowledge, suggest how the current study extends the knowledge base in this area, and point out contradictions in the current knowledge base?
- Does the researcher summarize the literature review, provide a rationale for the current study, and show how this study will extend previous research?

Design

- Is the study design specified, including its advantages and limitations for the research problem?
- Is there evidence that a pilot study had been conducted and the findings were used to enhance the design?
- Is the design (overall plan of research) appropriate to the research purpose and capable of answering the research question?
- How does the design control for extraneous variables?

Sample

- Was probability or nonprobability sampling used and the reason for the choice specified?
- Is the population to whom results will be generalized described?
- Are precautions taken to avoid collecting a biased sample (see Chapter 9) that would limit generalizability of the findings?
- Are the demographic characteristics of the sample described?
- Is the sample representative of the population?
- Are inclusion and exclusion criteria identified?
- Is the sample size appropriate to meet assumptions of statistical tests?

Data Collection

- Are data collection methods appropriate to meet the study purpose and answer the questions or hypotheses?
- What evidence is provided that data collection procedures are valid and reliable?
- Are adaptations to data collection tools described?
- Are data collection instruments described in sufficient detail to enable readers to ascertain method of scoring and range of values and what a particular score means?

Data Analysis

- Are data analysis procedures described?
- Are the statistical techniques appropriate for the study methodology (i.e., the type of data collected and analysis)?

- Do the statistical tests answer the research questions and specify the level of significance?
- If results are nonsignificant, is a power analysis conducted to explore nonsignificant findings?

STAGE 2 QUESTIONS: CRITICAL APPRAISAL OF THE CONDUCT OF RESEARCH

Human Rights

- How are rights of research participants protected?
- Are ethical issues anticipated and handled appropriately?

Procedures

- Are techniques used to ensure that there is consistency in the data collection process?
- What procedures were used to keep research conditions the same for all participants?
- Are there strategies to limit errors in data collection, recording, and analysis?
- Did any unplanned circumstances influence the results?
- In experimental designs, is there evidence of manipulation of independent variables, randomization in selection of sample and assignment to experimental and control groups, and control of extraneous variables?

STAGE 3 QUESTIONS: CRITICAL APPRAISAL OF RESEARCH OUTCOMES

Findings

- Are the findings presented clearly and correctly and are they related to the theoretical framework?
- Is there a clear statement of whether or not the data support the hypotheses or answer each research question?
- Are tables and graphs clearly labeled, easy to comprehend, and congruent with results presented in text form?
- Are findings presented in an unbiased manner?

Discussion

- Are alternative approaches offered for the findings?
- Does the researcher discuss both clinical and statistical significance of findings?
- Does the researcher overgeneralize the findings beyond the appropriate population?
- Are limitations of the study such as sample size, inadequate instruments, sources of bias, and so on identified and their implications discussed?

Implications and Conclusions

- Does the researcher identify important implications of the study for practice, education, or research (if appropriate)?
- How do the findings of the study advance nursing knowledge?
- Do new research questions emerge from the study?

STAGE 4 QUESTIONS: CRITICAL APPRAISAL OF THE OVERALL STUDY

Overall Quality

- What are the major strengths of the study?
- What are the major limitations of the study?
- Was the study described in sufficient detail to facilitate a replication study?
- What are the major contributions of this study to knowledge development in nursing?
- What suggestions might enhance the study and correct the limitations?

Source: From Gillis, A., & Jackson, W. (2002). *Research for nurses: Methods and interpretation.* Philadelphia: F. A. Davis Co.

standards have been proposed to evaluate qualitative studies (Burns & Grove, 2005):

- **Standard 1: descriptive vividness**—With **descriptive vividness,** the site, participants, experience of collecting data, and the thinking of the researcher are described so clearly that the reader has the sense of personally experiencing the event.
- **Standard 2: methodological congruence**—Methodological **congruence** has four dimensions: documentation rigor, procedural rigor, ethical rigor, and auditability (Burns & Grove, 2005). All elements of the study must be clearly documented, for example, the study subject, significance, purpose, research questions, assumptions, ethical implications, sampling methods, data gathering and analysis strategies, theoretical development, conclusions, and implications for practice. Documentation regarding these study elements must be clear and complete. Procedural rigor should be evident in that the researcher should clearly state the steps taken to ensure that data were accurately recorded and that the data obtained were representative of the data as a whole. Ethical rigor is reflected in the discussion by the researcher of the ethical implications related to the study, informed consent, and protection of participants' rights. Auditability refers to a decision trail. The research report should be sufficiently detailed to allow a second reader, using the original data and the decision trail, to arrive at conclusions similar to those of the original researcher.
- **Standard 3: analytical preciseness**—Analytical preciseness requires the researcher to make the effort needed to identify and record the decision-making processes through which concrete data are transformed into a theory or explanation of the phenomenon being studied.
- **Standard 4: theoretical connectedness**—Theoretical connectedness requires that the theoretical schema developed from the study be clearly expressed, logically consistent, reflective of the data, and compatible with the practice of nursing.
- **Standard 5: heuristic relevance**—The results of the study should have **heuristic relevance** for the reader. "This value is reflected in the reader's ability to recognize the phenomenon described in the study, its theoretical significance, its applicability to nursing practice, and its influence on future research" (Burns & Grove, 2003, p. 432). Dimensions of relevance include intuitive recognition, relationship to the existing body of knowledge, and applicability.

Key questions, developed by Burns and Grove (2005), can be used to critique a qualitative research report. They are grouped in four stages consistent with a review of quantitative research and are shown in Chart 8–18 (p. 142).

Future of Perspectives of Nursing Research

Research is critical to the practice of nursing, now and in the future. It is of vital importance to nursing in developing and acquiring new knowledge. This knowledge is changing practice, education, and health policy, and will continue to do so. Application of research findings to practice helps ensure the highest possible quality care that can be delivered in a cost-effective manner. This is critical to the future of nursing and health care.

Because knowledge is the foundation of professional practice, all nurses can and should develop and apply research skills in practice. As a professional nurse, the level of educational preparation will influence the role one plays in research. Though the trend is toward an expanded researcher role with advanced education, nurses at all levels of roles and responsibilities assume a role when it comes to nursing research. The ANA (1994) has defined these roles, which serve as national guidelines for education preparation, as follows:

1. **Associate degree in nursing.** Graduates of associate degree programs have several important roles to play in research. They need to develop an appreciation for research and can:
   - Help to identify clinical problems in nursing practice.
   - Assist in the collection of data within a structured format.
   - In conjunction with nurses holding more advanced credentials, appropriately use research findings in clinical practice.

2. **Baccalaureate degree in nursing.** Graduates of baccalaureate programs have an important role to play as consumers of research. This assumes that they have an intimate understanding of the research process; an ability to critically read, analyze, and critique research studies; and the judgment to interpret and evaluate research findings for application to practice. They participate in research by:
   - Identifying clinical problems
   - Assisting experienced investigators gain access to clinical sites
   - Influencing the selection of appropriate methods of data collection
   - Collecting and implementing nursing research findings.

   Baccalaureate-level nurses are prepared to understand the research protocols of other disciplines and to participate in data collection or other aspects of research.

3. **Master's degree in nursing.** Graduates of master's programs also play important roles in nursing research. They have a rich understanding of clinical practice and usually an in-depth perspective on nursing problems specific to various practice settings. This enables the researcher to identify clinically relevant problems and provide expert clinical advice on ways that services should be delivered and projects conducted. They are skilled in assisting others to use research findings appropriately. They help to create a climate in the practice setting that supports scholarly inquiry, and collaborate with others in proposal development, data collection, and data analysis and interpretation.

4. **Doctoral education.** Doctorally prepared nurses contribute to nursing knowledge through the conduct of research aimed at theory generation or theory testing. Graduates of doctoral programs are best prepared to appraise, design, and conduct research. According to the

CHART 8–18	**Key Questions for Critiquing Qualitative Designs**

STAGE 1 QUESTIONS: CRITICAL APPRAISAL OF PURPOSE, STATEMENT OF RESEARCH PHENOMENON, AND CONGRUENCE WITH DESIGN AND METHODOLOGY

Purpose or Statement of the Phenomenon of Interest

- Is the research phenomenon of interest clearly stated?
- Is rationale provided for approaching the study in an inductive, qualitative manner?
- Is the philosophy of the research tradition described?
- Is a statement of self-understanding included?
- Is there a single broad research question? Are their subquestions?
- Does the initial question become more focused as data are collected and analyzed?
- Is the study purpose clearly stated (e.g., discovery, description, theory building, and so on)?

Literature Review

- Does the qualitative method used call for a literature review before data collection?
- Does the review indicate that the researcher has expertise in the chosen area, know where gaps exist, and show how this study will eliminate such gaps?
- If a review is appropriate only after data collection, is there evidence that this is done?
- Is a framework appropriate? If so, is it presented clearly?

Design

- Is the design (i.e., overall plan for the research) appropriate to the research purpose?
- Is there congruency between the methodology and the research question?
- Is the context for the study adequately described?
- Is the researcher–participant relationship understood?

Sample

- Is purposive sampling used?
- Are informants capable of informing the study?
- Is the selection of participants appropriate to allow for saturation of data?

Data Collection

- Is data collection congruent with the study purpose, research question, and qualitative tradition selected?
- Are prolonged engagement and persistent observation in the field used to build trust with participants and ensure validity of data collection?
- Are data collection strategies and procedures described in sufficient detail?

Data Analysis

- Are data analysis procedures clearly described and appropriate to the research tradition?
- What evidence is provided that data collection and analysis are concurrent and ongoing?
- Is there evidence of decision rules for analyzing data, and does the researcher remain true to the rules?

- What evidence is there of narrowing the coding as categories are systematically discarded when they are unsupported by the data and the researcher becomes more focused on data collection and analysis?
- Is there evidence of "theoretical saturation?"

STAGE 2 QUESTIONS: CRITICAL APPRAISAL OF THE CONDUCT OF THE RESEARCH

Human Rights

- How are the rights of research participants protected?
- Are ethical issues anticipated and handled appropriately?

Procedures

- What evidence is provided that research meets the criteria of rigor (credibility: findings must be understood and viewed as credible by the informants; trustworthiness: one can believe the findings are true; and usefulness: findings shed light on an important phenomenon)?
- Creswell (1998) identifies eight procedures for testing the truth value (appropriate representation of multiple realities) and notes that researchers should use at least two of these in any given study. The critic should ask which of these the researcher uses.

  1. Prolonged engagement and persistent observation in the field to build trust with participants, learn about the culture and context, and correct distortions introduced by the researcher's presence
  2. Triangulation for purpose of corroborating evidence from different sources to shed light on a theme or perspective
  3. Peer review as an external check of the research process; this person asks hard questions about the method, meanings, and interpretations and keeps the researcher honest
  4. Negative case analysis, in which the researcher reworks the hypothesis until all cases fit it
  5. The researcher articulates researcher bias so that the reader knows what prejudices, biases, or past experiences have shaped the researcher's approach to the study
  6. Member checks to solicit informants' opinions of the accuracy and credibility of the findings and conclusions. Some methods, however, such as hermeneutic analysis, do not always conduct member checks because their emphasis is on the interpretation of meaning by the research team of the experience of the participants in the research project
  7. External audits in which a consultant examines both the process and product of the qualitative study to assess accuracy and determine if the findings, interpretations, and conclusions are supported by the data
  8. Rich, in-depth descriptions of participants and setting are provided so that the reader can make decisions regarding transferability of findings to other settings

STAGE 3 QUESTIONS: CRITICAL APPRAISAL OF THE RESEARCH OUTCOMES

Findings

- Are the findings contextualized (i.e., presented within the context of the circumstances that influence their interpretation)?
- Do readers of the report recognize the phenomenon or vicariously experience it?

| CHART 8–18 | **Key Questions for Critiquing Qualitative Designs—*Continued*** |

- Are the findings true to the data?
- Do the themes, categories, or theoretical statements present a comprehensive, plausible, and meaningful picture of the phenomenon?
- If models, diagrams, or figures are used, are they effective?
- Are the findings compatible with the field of nursing's knowledge base?
- Are reasons for incompatible findings explored by the researcher?

Discussion, Implications, and Conclusions

- Does the researcher identify implications of the study for nursing (i.e., in practice, theory building, instrument development, education, and research)?

- Is a context provided in which to use the findings?
- Do the implications and conclusions follow logically from the findings?
- Do new research questions emerge from the findings?

STAGE 4 QUESTIONS: CRITICAL APPRAISAL OF THE OVERALL QUALITY OF THE STUDY

- What are the major strengths of the study?
- What are the major limitations of the study?
- What are the major contributions of this study to knowledge development in the field of nursing?
- What suggestions might enhance the study and correct the limitations?

Source: Gillis, A., & Jackson, W. (2002). *Research for nurses: Methods and interpretation.* Philadelphia: F. A. Davis Co.

| CHART 8–19 | **Research Themes for the Future** |

1. Changing lifestyle behaviors for better health
2. Managing the effects of chronic illness to improve health and quality of life:
   - Health care practice
   - Self-management of chronic illness symptoms and treatment
   - Informal (family) caregiving.
3. Identifying effective strategies to reduce health disparities
4. Harnessing advanced technologies to serve human needs
5. Enhancing the end-of-life experience for patients and their families

Source: National Institute of Nursing Research. (2003). *Research themes for the future.* Bethesda, MD: National Institutes of Health.

ANA (1994), they develop nursing knowledge through original research and theory development. They also conduct funded independent research projects.

The vision for nursing in the 21st century is to narrow the gap between research and practice by helping nurses base their decisions and practice strategies on the best available evidence, thereby improving nursing care and patient outcomes. As the levels of sophistication and complexity in nursing increase, use of the scientific process to improve patient care and outcomes becomes more crucial, as does the educational preparation for engaging in research activities. Thus, research utilization, the process of transforming knowledge obtained from research into clinical practice, is a critical step in improving nursing care and ultimately patients' outcomes. It is, therefore, incumbent on all nurses to understand and use the research process, and to participate in the critical process of research review and utilization. This chapter has presented the basic guidelines for assisting learners to garner that knowledge, and has provided a background for interpreting research findings and future research goals presented throughout the book.

Future Research Goals

The research themes for the future as determined by the NINR are shown in Chart 8–19. Each of the five themes includes specific research goals. The themes and goals in their entirety may be found on the NINR website.

REVIEW QUESTIONS

1. The nurse is planning a study using basic research. This nurse is most likely going to be studying:
   1. The effectiveness of a type of wound dressing.
   2. The frequency of side effects from one particular medication.
   3. How Orem's theory can be applied to the nursing process.
   4. The effectiveness of teaching self-insulin administration to a patient diagnosed with diabetes mellitus.

2. The nurse researcher is conducting a quantitative research study. Which of the following will most likely be done during this study?
   1. Change the study as information is collected.
   2. Approach the process in a circular method rather than a straight line.
   3. Collect numerical values within a controlled situation.
   4. Use a small sample size.

3. The nurse researcher is planning an experimental quantitative research project. This project will most likely be conducted:

   1. On a general medical–surgical unit.
   2. In the emergency room.
   3. In the intensive care unit.
   4. In a laboratory.

4. The Quality Improvement Committee is planning to conduct a research study. Which of the following should this committee do first?

   1. Determine the patients who will participate in the study.
   2. Identify the problem to be studied.
   3. Assign data collection roles to specific committee members.
   4. Figure out how long the study will take to complete.

5. A nurse researcher is determining the best design to use for a research project. Which of the following can be used as a guide for this design?

   1. Methods used to collect data
   2. Approaches used to analyze the data
   3. Determine if the study is a quantitative or qualitative research.
   4. Write out the research problem or question.

Answers for review questions appear in Appendix D

KEY TERMS

analytical preciseness *p.141*
applied research *p.122*
basic research *p.122*
convenience sampling *p.127*
correlational research design *p.125*
data saturation *p.129*
descriptive research design *p.125*
descriptive vividness *p.141*
ethnography *p.126*
evidence-based practice (EBP) *p.130*
experimental research design *p.125*
grounded theory *p.126*
heuristic relevance *p.141*
hypothesis *p.125*
informatics *p.138*
literature review *p.125*

methodological congruence *p.141*
network sampling *p.127*
nonexperimental research design *p.125*
nonprobability sampling *p.127*
phenomenology *p.126*
pilot study *p.127*
population *p.126*
power analysis *p.128*
probability sampling *p.127*
purposive sampling *p.127*
qualitative research *p.125*
quantitative research *p.125*
quasi-experimental research design *p.125*
quota sampling *p.127*
random assignment *p.127*
research *p.121*

research critique *p.138*
research design *p.125*
research problem *p.124*
research process *p.122*
research purpose *p.124*
research question *p.124*
research utilization (RU) *p.130*
sample *p.126*
sampling *p.126*
setting *p.126*
simple random sampling *p.127*
statistical significance *p.128*
stratified random sampling *p.127*
theoretical connectedness *p.141*
variables *p.125*

PEARSON
EXPLORE **mynursingkit**™

MyNursingKit is your one stop for online chapter review materials and resources. Prepare for success with additional NCLEX®-style practice questions, interactive assignments and activities, web links, animations and videos, and more!

Register your access code from the front of your book at
www.mynursingkit.com

REFERENCES

Agency for Healthcare Research and Quality. (2007). *Evidence-based practice centers*. Retrieved December 14, 2007, from http://www.ahrq.gov/clinic/epc

American Nurses Association. (1976). *Preparation for nurses for participation research*. Kansas City, MO: Author.

American Nurses Association. (1994). *Education for participation in nursing research*. Retrieved June 10, 2007 from http://www.AmericanNursesAssociaton.org

Ardery, G., Herr, K. A., Titler, M. G., Sorofman, B. A., & Schmitt, M. G. (2003). Assessing and managing acute pain in older adults: a research base to guide practice. *MedSurg Nursing, 12*(il), 7, 13.

Burns, N., & Grove, S. K. (2003). *Understanding nursing research* (3rd ed.). Philadelphia: W. B. Saunders.

Burns, N., & Grove, S. K. (2005). *Understanding nursing research* (5th. ed.). Philadelphia: W. B. Saunders.

Ciliska, D., Pinelli, J., DeCenso, A., & Cullum, N. (2001). Resources to enhance evidence-based nursing practice. *AACN Clinial Issues, 12*(4), 520–528.

Colling, J. (2003). Desiging clinical research studies: (Demystifying clinical research studies: sample size. *Urologic Nursing, 23*(8), This article was published prior to Part 1, and was not labeled as such.

Connor, J. A., Smaldone, A. M., Bratts, T., & Stone, P. W. (2003). Ask an expert: HIPAA in 2003 and its meaning for nurse researchers. *Applied Nursing Research, 16,* 291–293.

Creswell, J. (1998). *Qualitative inquiry and research design: Choosing among five tradtions*. London: Thousand Oaks, Sage Publications.

Crowther, M. (2003). Evidence-based development of a hospital based heart failure centre. *Evidence-Based Nursing, 6,* 4–6.

DeBourgh, G. A. (2001). Champions for evidence-based practice: A critical role for advanced practice nurses. *AACN Clinical Issues, 12*(4), 491–508.

Gillis, A., & Jackson, W. (2002). *Research for nurses: Methods and interpretation*. Philadelphia: F. A. Davis.

Holden, C. (1979). Ethics in social science research. *Science, 206,* 537–540.

Malloch, K., & Porter-O'Grady, T. (2006). *Introduction to evidence-based practice in nursing and health care*. Sudbury, MA: Jones and Bartlett.

McKibbon, A., Eady, A., & Marks, S. (1999). *PDQ: Evidence-based principles and practice*. (PDQ series) Hamilton, Ont.; London: B.C. Decker.

National Commission for the Protection of Human Subjects of Biomedical and Behavioral Research (1978). *Belmont report: Ethical principles and guidelines for research involving human subjects*. Washington, DC: U.S. Government Printing Office.

Nightingale, F. (1859). *Notes on nursing: What it is and what it is not.* Philadelphia: J. B. Lippincott.

Olsen, D. P. (2003). HIPAA privacy regulations and nursing research. *Nursing Research, 52,* 344–348.

Omery, A., & Williams, R. P. (1999). An appraisal of research utilization across the United States. *Journal of Nursing Administration, 29,* 50–56.

Poe, S. S. Cvach, M. M., Gartrell, D. G., Radzik, B. R., & Joy, T. L. (2005). *Journal of Nursing Care Quality, 20*(2), 107–116.

Polit, D. F., & Beck, C. T. (2008). *Nursing research: Principles and methods* (8th ed.). Philadelphia: Lippincott Williams & Wilkins.

Staggers, N., Gassert, C. A., & Curran, C. (2002). A delphi study to determine informatics competencies for nurse levels of practice. *Nursing Research, 51*(6), 383–390.

Stetler, C. B. (1994). Refinement of the Stetler/Maram model for application of research findings into practice. *Nursing Outlook, 42,* 15–35.

Stuart, J. (2001). Evidence-based psychiatric nursing practice: Rhetoric or reality, *Journal of American Psychiatric Nurses* Association, *7,* 103–114.

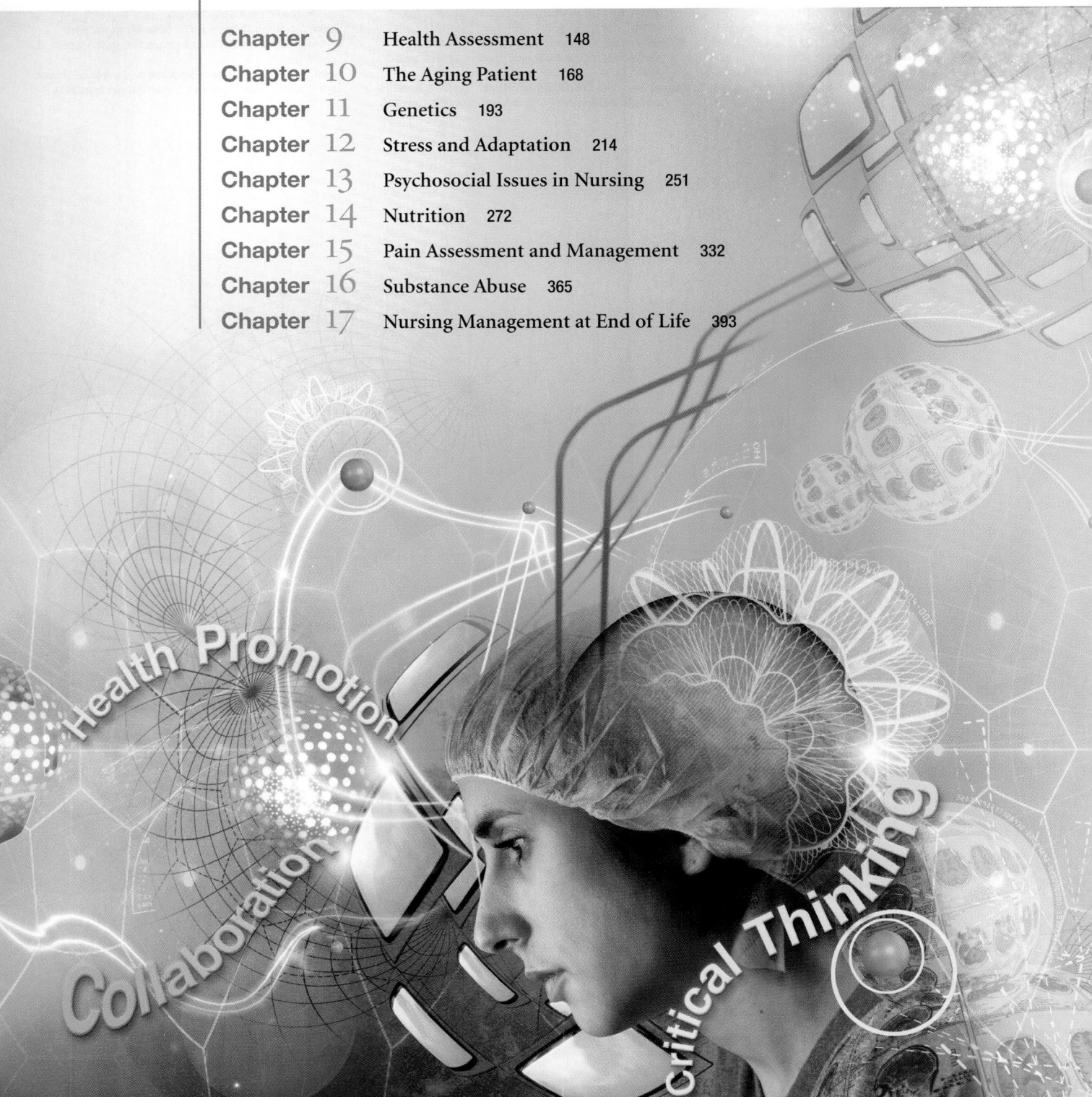

UNIT

2

General Concepts Related to Nursing Practice

Health Promotion

Collaboration

Critical Thinking

"It was this **commitment** to residents, staff, and families and a hope for innovative health care for seniors that kept me excited about going to work each day."

TERI Throughout my baccalaureate nursing program at California State University, Sacramento, I knew I wanted to work with the older population. I am sure this desire was fueled by the close relationship I had with my grandparents and the social interactions with many of their older friends as I grew up. While attending nursing school, I decided the skilled nursing facility (SNF) setting might be a good fit for me. Contrary to many negative perceptions of geriatric nursing, I saw it as a growing and challenging field. I could be at the forefront of exciting changes as the complexity and diversity of the aging population increased. I was driven by the sense that I could learn from my patients' life experiences and possibly make a difference in this last stage of their lives.

After graduation, I became a charge nurse on a 40-bed skilled nursing unit. I was responsible for the total care of 20 elderly residents, most of whom had been admitted for a short stay of 2 weeks or less for rehabilitation and others who presented with multiple diagnoses affecting their quality of life. I was responsible for administering medications, completing treatments, and documenting the patient's care regimen. I worked with the unit manager to keep the residents, their families, and the physicians apprised of all changes and to continually update the plan of care. My days were challenging, demanding, satisfying, and never boring!

After a short period of time, I was promoted to unit manager. It was in this position that my passion for geriatric nursing grew. I supervised licensed nurses and certified nursing assistants on all shifts and worked closely with the interdisciplinary team, physicians, and families to ensure that quality care was provided at all times. A sense of ownership and accomplishment was felt by all staff on the unit when our quality measures compared well to state and national averages. But more importantly, there was a sense of *family* between staff, residents, and their family members. It was easy to become emotionally attached to residents as we cared for them daily over the years, advocating for them as they negotiated the health care system. It was this **commitment** to residents, staff, and families and a hope for innovative health care for seniors that kept me excited about going to work each day.

Attending physicians in SNFs are required to see their patients within 72 hours of admission and then monthly thereafter. This lack of constant physical presence by physicians provides the SNF nurse with a great measure of autonomy in his or her practice combined with the awesome responsibility of accurate clinical assessments. The SNF nurse must be **confident** in his or her assessment and be able to demonstrate **competence** in geriatric physiology and overall assessment of the older patient in order to work with the physician in prescribing medications and treatments. I remember admitting an elderly woman, Mrs. G, following surgery for a fractured hip. Because her recovery was not as quick and complete as she had hoped, neither her interdisciplinary health team nor I could in good **conscience** recommend discharge to her home without additional help. A meeting was scheduled with the team, Mr. and Mrs. G, and the physician to discuss in an open and honest manner the team's reservations regarding a safe discharge and the resident's right and desire to go home without assistance. By demonstrating our respect for the resident's wishes and presenting a forum for open communication, Mrs. G's husband was able to express some of his own anxiety over the pending discharge. Ultimately, Mrs. G made the decision to allow home health to send a RN to her home for follow-up after discharge. Through a collaborative process and the team's professional **comportment** and **compassion**, an atmosphere of trust was built in which the resident's wishes were respected and the team was able to demonstrate their caring for the resident's continued well-being.

My experiences in skilled nursing motivated me to pursue advanced education at the master's and doctoral level in geriatrics, gerontology, and health administration. Being a geriatric nurse allows me to use a wide range of my nursing skills from medical–surgical to community health. It has led me to my current position as Director of Quality and Compliance for a large multiservice agency based in Northern California. As director, I am able to continue working with the elderly across a wide continuum of care from independent living to skilled nursing care and to become involved in making policy decisions in our community as well as statewide. I am able to influence the direction of geriatric care by precepting new nurses and gerontology students, by participating in community and government projects, and by providing input into policy development designed to improve the quality of life for this population. It is this search for the best senior care that keeps me motivated to learn more about aging and excited about my role in caring for this growing population.

Health Assessment

Rich Keegan, Cheryl Wraa, Kathleen Osborn
With contributions by: Annita Watson

Outcome-Based Learning Objectives

After studying this chapter, the learner will be able to:

1. Describe the components of the health assessment.
2. Explain the steps of the patient interview for the health history.
3. Compare and contrast verbal and nonverbal responses that enhance the collection of information.
4. Explain how the techniques of inspection, palpation, percussion, and auscultation can be applied to the physical assessment of the major body systems.
5. Differentiate between the steps of the critical thinking component as it relates to health assessment.

THE FOCUS of health care in the United States is evolving beyond treatment of illness and injury to also include prevention and promotion of wellness. This newer model requires the development of a comprehensive plan of care that will guide the patient and family toward a healthy lifestyle and away from risk factors that can increase illness and injury. The nurse takes an active role in care plan development and execution. The nursing process guides the nurse when gathering and analyzing information. It is an effective method of problem solving and provides a framework on which to make informed decisions regarding the patient's plan of care.

Assessment, the first step of the nursing process, is when the nurse gathers initial data. It is a systematic process that assists the nurse in identifying current health status, actual and potential problems, and areas that need health promotion. It also provides a baseline on which future comparisons can be made. The assessment includes data about the physical, emotional, mental, spiritual, and cultural factors that impact health. It consists of both **objective data** (collected by using the senses: observation, palpation, auscultation, percussion, and smell) and **subjective data** (information the patient or caretaker tells the nurse). Both types of data are used to formulate a nursing diagnosis. The nursing diagnosis, which evolves from the assessment data, describes conditions treated by nurses (North American Nursing Diagnosis Association, 2007). Ultimately, a thorough health assessment al-

lows the nurse to collaborate with the health care team in developing a plan that integrates personal health care with prevention efforts to reach the national goal to increase quality and years of healthy life.

As a member of the health care team, nurses must adhere to the current legislation that is in place to protect the confidentiality of the individual patient. As a nurse, it is unethical and against federal and state statutes to disclose a patient's medical information without the patient's express consent. Note, however, that in the course of providing care to a patient, health care professionals can share information in order to formulate a plan of care to meet the patient's needs. Regulatory issues are covered in detail in Chapter 3 .

■ National Guidelines: *Healthy People 2010*

Healthy People 2010: Understanding and Improving Health (U.S. Department of Health and Human Services [DHHS], 2000) is a 10-year strategy developed by the DHHS to recognize preventable threats to health and to identify and establish national goals to reduce these threats. *Healthy People 2010* has two distinct goals:

Goal 1: Increase quality and years of healthy life.

Goal 2: Eliminate health disparities.

The *Healthy People 2010* Leading Health Indicators

In addition to the two goals, 10 **leading health indicators** have been identified that reflect the major public health concerns of the 21st century for Americans: (1) physical activity, (2) overweight and obesity, (3) tobacco use, (4) substance abuse, (5) responsible sexual behaviors, (6) mental health, (7) injury and violence, (8) environmental quality, (9) immunization, and (10) access to health care. To achieve the goals and address the leading health indicators, *Healthy People 2010* is supported by specific objectives in 28 focus areas, as shown in the National Guidelines box. The nurse's role in assisting patients to achieve these goals requires an in-depth understanding of the patient's current health status. This understanding begins with a thorough health assessment.

Physical Activity

Regular physical activity helps maintain physical and psychological well-being. It also plays a significant role in reducing the incidence of many diseases including cardiovascular disease, diabetes mellitus, hypertension, colon cancer, depression, and anxiety. Physical activity is important at all ages to maintain muscle strength and decrease body fat, and it is an important component of weight control.

Physical activity is any bodily movement produced by skeletal muscles that results in an expenditure of energy. Physical fitness is defined as a set of attributes a person has with regard to a person's ability to perform physical activities that require aerobic fitness, endurance, strength, or flexibility and is determined by a combination of regular activity and genetically inherited ability. A pattern of physical activity is regular activities that are performed:

- Most days of the week, preferably daily;
- Five or more days of the week if moderate-intensity activities (in bouts of at least 10 minutes for a total of at least 30 minutes per day); or
- Three or more days of the week of vigorous-intensity activities (for at least 20 to 60 minutes per session) (Centers for Disease Control and Prevention [CDC], 2008).

One measurement of the level of exercise intensity is the **metabolic equivalent level (MET)**. The MET establishes the amount of oxygen used for physical activity, and it increases as physical activity increases. A second method of determining physical activity intensity is the Borg Rating of Perceived Exertion (RPE). Perceived exertion is how hard an individual feels like his or her body is working. It is based on the physical sensations a person experiences during physical activity, including increased heart rate, increased respiration or breathing rate, increased sweating, and muscle fatigue. Although this is a subjective measure, a person's exertion rating may provide a fairly good estimate of the actual heart rate during physical activity. The third method for measuring physical activity intensity is by determining the number of calories burned.

According to the CDC (2008), adults should strive to meet either moderate-intensity physical activity or vigorous-intensity physical activity. Moderate-intensity physical activity refers to a level of effort in which a person should experience one or more of the following:

- Some increase in breathing or heart rate
- A "perceived exertion" of 11 to 14 on the Borg RPE scale (e.g., the effort a healthy individual might expend while walking briskly, mowing the lawn, dancing, swimming, or bicycling on level terrain)
- Three to 6 METs
- Any activity that burns 3.5 to 7 Calories per minute (kcal/min).

Vigorous-intensity physical activity may be intense enough to represent a substantial challenge to an individual and refers to a level of effort in which a person should experience one or more of the following:

- A large increase in breathing or heart rate (conversation is difficult or "broken")
- A "perceived exertion" of 15 or greater on the Borg RPE scale (e.g., the effort a healthy individual might expend while jogging, mowing the lawn with a nonmotorized pushmower, participating in high-impact aerobic dancing, swimming

NATIONAL GUIDELINES for *Healthy People 2010* Focus Areas

Access to Quality Health Services	Injury and Violence Prevention
Arthritis, Osteoporosis, and Chronic Back Conditions	Maternal, Infant, and Child Health
Cancer	Medical Product Safety
Chronic Kidney Diseases	Mental Health and Mental Disorders
Diabetes	Nutrition and Overweight
Disability and Secondary Conditions	Occupational Safety and Health
Educational and Community-Based Programs	Oral Health
Environmental Health	Physical Activity and Fitness
Family Planning	Public Health Infrastructure
Food Safety	Respiratory Diseases
Health Communication	Sexually Transmitted Diseases
Heart Disease and Stroke	Substance Abuse
HIV	Tobacco Use
Immunization and Infectious Diseases	Vision and Hearing

continuous laps, bicycling uphill, carrying more than 25 lbs up a flight of stairs, standing or walking with more than 50 lbs)

- Greater than 6 METs
- Any activity that burns more than 7 kcal/ min (CDC, 2008).

Overweight and Obesity

Overweight and obese persons have a significant increased risk for heart disease, diabetes mellitus, stroke, arthritis, and serious sleep disorders. The number of obese persons has risen dramatically since the 1980s and has become a leading health problem in the United States. Obesity is more prevalent among women and proportionately higher in African American and Mexican women (D'Amico & Barbarito, 2007). Nutrition and exercise training are important factors in preventing weight gain and maintaining a healthy weight. Nutrition related to weight maintenance is discussed in detail in Chapter 14 ⚭.

Tobacco Use

Cigarette smoking is responsible for more deaths in the United States than are HIV/AIDS, drug abuse, homicide, suicide, automobile crashes, and fire combined. In addition, smoking is a risk factor associated with a number of prevalent diseases such as cardiovascular, respiratory, and cancer. Secondary smoke accounts for an increased incidence of asthma and bronchitis in children and heart and lung disease in adults (D'Amico & Barbarito, 2007). Staying away from people while they are smoking and making a choice to not smoke are two effective ways of not exacerbating these diseases.

Guidelines have been developed for professionals who are working with patients who smoke, but want to stop. For smokers who have expressed a desire to stop smoking, the guidelines include the five "A's":

- **A**sk about smoking at every visit.
- **A**dvise (that is, urge) all smokers to stop.
- **A**ssess the client's willingness to stop.
- **A**ssist or aid the patient in quitting. Work with the patient to develop a plan while providing counseling, recommending pharmacotherapy, and providing resource materials.
- **A**rrange for follow-up to determine progress or need for further assistance.

Substance Abuse

Substance abuse of alcohol and illicit drugs has been linked to many health problems, including injuries from accidents, sexually transmitted infections, cardiac and liver disease, violence, and a disruption of families. Abuse also is occurring with prescription drugs such as pain relievers, sedatives, tranquilizers, and stimulants.

Identification and diagnosis of drug abuse begins with a screening assessment. A questionnaire developed by Ewing (1984) uses the mnemonic CAGE to help professionals remember these four screening questions:

- Have you ever wanted to **C**ut down on alcohol/prescription drug use?
- Have you ever felt **A**nnoyed when remarks are made about alcohol/prescription drug use?
- Have you ever felt **G**uilty about alcohol/prescription drug use?

- Have you ever used alcohol/prescription drugs as a way to change your mood or feeling of energy?

Questions about the amount and type of alcohol/prescription drug used are included in the social history section of a health assessment (Figure 9–1 ■).

Responsible Sexual Behaviors

Unprotected sexual activity increases the risk for sexually transmitted infections (STIs) and pregnancy. According to *Healthly People 2010*, individuals must understand how STIs are transmitted in order to increase the probability that this awareness will change risky behaviors. Chapters 49 and 50 ⚭ discuss the transmission of the various STIs.

Health care providers have a pivotal role in assessing behaviors and educating individuals about prevention. Effective questions for a health assessment include the following:

- Are you sexually active?
- When was the last time you had sexual activity (oral, vaginal, anal)?
- When you had sexual activity was a condom used?
- Do you now have or have you ever had more than one sexual partner?
- Have you ever been treated for STIs?
- Have you ever had sexual activity with a partner who used intravenous drugs?

Mental Health

Mental illness affects not only individuals, but families, and even communities. According to *Healthy People 2010*, one-fifth of the people in the United States are affected by mental illness each year (D'Amico & Barbarito, 2007). Mental disorders include depression, schizophrenia, bipolar disorder, obsessive compulsive disorder, and panic disorder. Depression accounts for the majority of these cases and significantly contributes to disability and suicide. Screening for depression may be difficult because the common symptoms such as fatigue, sleep disorders, and pain are vague and can be related to many conditions. Screening for depression is accomplished through patient interviews and the use of screening questions such as these:

- Have you felt down, depressed, or hopeless in the last two weeks?
- Have you had little interest or pleasure in doing things?

When a patient answers yes to one or both of these questions, to confirm the diagnosis of depression, the nurse needs to inquire about the presence of the symptoms outlined here:

- Significant weight loss or gain
- Disturbed sleep patterns
- Agitation or slowness
- Fatigue
- Feelings of guilt or worthlessness
- Inability to concentrate or make decisions
- Thoughts of death or suicide.

If the patient answers yes to the presence of four or more of these symptoms, a diagnosis of depression is confirmed. The nurse should then assess for a family history of depression or

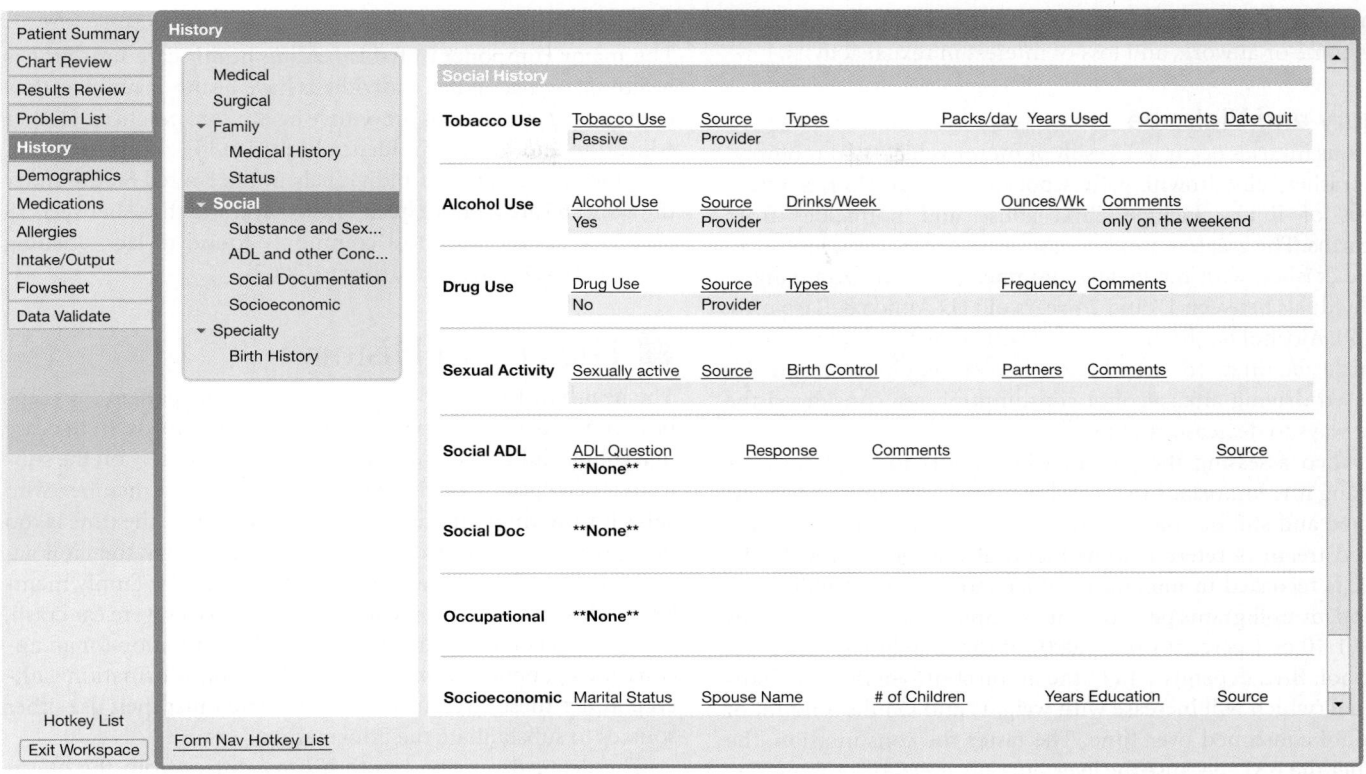

FIGURE 9–1 ■ Social history section of a health assessment.

other mental disorders, two or more chronic illnesses, stress in the home or at work, and loss of interest in sexual activity.

Injury and Violence
Serious injuries occur as a result of motor vehicle and motorcycle crashes, falls, drowning, fires, poison, guns, and knives. Other types of injury include child abuse and homicides from firearms. The greatest number of injuries occurs from motor vehicle crashes, with the greatest number of deaths occurring in individuals between 17 and 24 years old (D'Amico & Barbarito, 2007). Alcohol has been associated with almost half of all motor vehicle fatalities. Increased use of safety equipment and decreased driving after alcohol consumption are considered the best ways to decrease fatalities.

When assessing the patient who admits to drinking after driving it is important to stress how much alcohol can be consumed and still be able to drive. The amount of alcohol in the bloodstream is referred to as blood alcohol level (BAL). The BAL is recorded in milligrams of alcohol per 100 milliliters of blood, or milligrams percent. For example, a BAL of 0.10 means that 1/10 of 1 percent (or 1/1,000) of the total blood content is alcohol. BAL depends on (1) the amount of blood in the individual (which will increase with weight) and (2) the amount of alcohol consumed over time. The faster the consumption, the higher the BAL, because the liver can only metabolize about one drink per hour—the rest builds up in the bloodstream. If a person has a BAL of greater than 0.08%, most states' laws consider that person to be drunk. Disposable breathalyzers may be helpful in monitoring BAL before driving. Encourage individuals to never drive after drinking alcohol. Ask them to consider alternatives such as a taxicab or some form of public transportation.

Environmental Quality
The environment includes the physical air, water, and soil. The social environment includes housing, transportation, land use, development, and agriculture. Health risks related to the physical environment include exposure to chemical, biological, and physical agents that lead to respiratory and cardiovascular diseases and cancer. Health risks associated with the social environment include the ones in the physical environment as well as stress, injury, and violence.

Government programs and laws have been enacted that dictate standards for water treatment, food safety, and waste management. Policies vary and are more stringent in some areas such as urban settings as apposed to rural areas. When assessing patients, it is important to determine risks they may face based on their physical and social environments. *Healthy People 2010* provides information about environmental issues.

Immunization
When immunizations are consistently given to a population, they can prevent diseases, disabilities, and the spread of infection. Recommendations for childhood immunizations have been developed and when followed will reduce the incidence of many childhood illnesses. Immunizations such as pneumonia and influenza are considered an effective way to decrease death or complications from infectious diseases in older adults. Chapter 20 includes an in-depth discussion of immunizations.

Access to Health Care
The major component of this leading health care indicator is health insurance. When individuals have health insurance, they tend toward regular and preventive health care practices. Higher education and income influence health and health promotion. A significant number of individuals in the United States under the age of 65 are without health insurance, and those between 18 and 24 years old are most commonly found to lack ongoing health care (D'Amico & Barbarito, 2007).

The Health History
The health history is a detailed account of the patient's perception of his current and past health in his own words. In the case of a young child or infant, the nurse will have to rely on the subjective perceptions of the patient's adult family member who cares for the child. In the case of an adult who at the time is too ill to give an accurate account of her health history, then it is acceptable to rely on the subjective perceptions of a family member or close friend. In some instances, such as a severe car crash, total strangers may be the only source of information for an unconscious patient. To ensure the accuracy of information gathered under these circumstances, the nurse must then use other sources to substantiate the information.

The detailed nursing health history differs from the physician's medical history in that nurses are focusing on what effect the patient's current health status will have on being able to function independently in providing for activities of daily living (ADLs). For example, if an elderly patient were to be admitted for a hip fracture, the physician would be concerned with the surgical intervention needed to repair the fracture. The nurse would be focused on what the patient would need to be able to perform his ADLs while in the hospital and once cleared for discharge. The nurse would ascertain what the patient's level of functioning was before the event and apply the new limitations into a plan of care for this patient. Issues such as whether the patient requires assistive devices and whether the patient has family members or friends who are able to provide assistance once the patient goes home would all need to be assessed. The nurse must teach the caretakers all aspects of care as well as when it is appropriate to seek medical attention.

Conducting the Health Interview
When beginning the interview, nurses should address patients using their surnames and then introduce themselves and their role in the agency. They should state if they are a student. Finally, nurses should tell patients the purpose for the interview.

During the data collection phase of the interview, the nurse uses two types of questions: open ended and direct or closed. **Open-ended questions** ask for narrative information by stating the topic in general terms. This type of question is useful for introducing a subject such as "What brought you to the hospital?" A **direct question** is used to elicit specific information. Direct questions can be used to clarify specific details. For instance, if the patient stated that she is experiencing abdominal pain, a direct question would be "Is the pain sharp or dull?"

To encourage free expression, it is important for the nurse to listen carefully, not cut the patient off, and respond in a way that encourages the patient to provide more information. Responses that are helpful include the following:

- *Silence:* This allows the patient time to think and allows the nurse to observe for nonverbal cues.
- *Facilitation:* Comments such as "please continue" or nodding one's head encourages the patient to tell the nurse more.
- *Explanation:* Using factual information to explain an issue helps to clarify it for the patient. For example, telling the patient how a specific procedure is performed may decrease the patient's anxiety regarding the test.
- *Interpretation:* Interpretive responses link events or imply cause. "From what you have told me, it appears that whenever you have a meal high in fat you begin to have abdominal pain."
- *Clarification:* If patients describe an issue using ambiguous language, the nurse should ask them to clarify, such as "Please describe for me what 'feeling weird' means."
- *Empathy:* Acknowledging patients' feelings with a statement of understanding helps patients to feel accepted and more comfortable discussing the issue. An example of an empathetic response is "Not being able to do your normal activities must be frustrating for you."
- *Summary:* At the end of the interview, the nurse summarizes his perceptions of the patient's health problem from what he has learned during the interview. This acknowledges agreement between the nurse and the patient regarding the patient's health status.

Responses that are nonproductive and should be avoided by the nurse include providing false reassurance, using authoritarian language, giving unwanted advice and not allowing the patient to make decisions regarding their own solution, talking too much, using professional jargon that the patient will not understand, and using avoidance language or euphemisms to avoid reality.

An awareness of body language is an important factor during the interview. Positive nonverbal messages enhance the relationship with the patient and show attentiveness and acceptance. Examples of positive nonverbal messages are a professional appearance, a relaxed open posture, appropriate eye contact, equal-status seating, a moderate tone of voice and rate of speech, and appropriate touch. Examples of negative nonverbal messages are a tense posture, critical gestures such as pointing or finger-tapping, yawning, speaking too quickly, avoiding eye contact by focusing on notes, and inappropriate touch. Note, that it is important for the nurse to understand the different cultural norms regarding appropriate eye contact and appropriate touch as well as other related issues. Various communication norms for different cultures are discussed in the Cultural Considerations box (p. 154).

The components of the health history are consistent from one health care agency to another. The six main components of the health history include (1) biographical data; (2) present health/illness, including health patterns and beliefs; (3) past medical history, including a medication history; (4) family history; (5) psychosocial history; and (6) a review of body systems (i.e., physical assessment) (Rhodes, 2006).

Biographical Data

Biographical data, which provides baseline information about the patient, contains the following elements:

- *Name and address:* This is usually the first biographical data to be obtained. By having the patient state her name, the professional nurse is able to hear the patient speak. This assessment of whether the patient can hear and then respond appropriately helps to determine her level of consciousness.
- *Age and date of birth:* By establishing the chronological age of the patient, the nurse is then able to assess certain characteristics that occur over the age continuum. A 20-year-old male will exhibit a developed musculature and his skin will be smooth and without wrinkles, whereas a 70-year-old male will exhibit aging skin with wrinkling and will have muscle wasting secondary to inactivity.
- *Gender:* The gender of the patient in association with his or her age gives the nurse clues as to physical development and the presence of secondary sex characteristics. Adult males will typically have greater muscle mass and possess facial hair, whereas a female of the same age will not have these characteristics.
- *Birthplace:* A patient's birthplace can provide the nurse with evidence of environmental or cultural factors that may have contributed to the patient's current state of health. For example, a patient born and raised in the Central Valley of California may have signs and symptoms of reactive airway disease as a result of exposure to pesticides and dust in the region.
- *Geography:* A patient's geography refers to the country, region, section, community, or neighborhood in which he was born and raised or currently resides. Where someone was raised affects family life and general customs practiced by the individual. The availability of community resources including schools, churches, health care facilities, social systems, transportation, and support services differs depending on the region. Urban areas typically offer more services than rural areas.
- *Marital status:* By determining if the patient is single, married, widowed, or divorced, the nurse can establish whether or not there is a significant person involved in this patient's life. It is also important to ask the patient if she has ever been in a committed relationship; this encourages a response for same-gender relationships.
- *Race:* By determining the patient's race, the nurse can assess for certain characteristics that are known about certain races in the United States. Caucasians have less melanin than Hispanics or African Americans and are, therefore, more prone to skin cancers. There are also certain health-related characteristics associated with race. For example, Mexican Americans have a higher rate of adult-onset diabetes than other races (Kaushik et al., 2007).
- *Religion:* Determining the religious affiliation to which the patient ascribes is an important part of an assessment. Belonging to a religious faith can dictate whether a patient will accept the medical/nursing interventions offered. For example, a devout Jehovah's Witness will not permit blood transfusions. Persons belonging to the Jewish or Muslim faiths may not eat pork. Patients who are Roman Catholic may not eat meat on Fridays during the period of Lent.
- *Occupation:* By determining the patient's occupation, the nurse can determine if there are health-related conditions

CULTURAL CONSIDERATIONS for Communication Customs

Native American	Family may request spiritual healers. Loud voice may be associated with aggression. Avoiding eye contact is respectful.
Cambodian	It is inappropriate to touch the head without permission. Consider it impolite to disagree so may say "yes" but not mean it. Very important to speak softly and be polite.
Chinese	Eye contact with authority figures avoided as sign of respect. Chinese language is expressive and loud. Need to assess understanding of conversations because the patient or family may not ask questions as a sign of respect. Privacy very important.
Gypsies	Important to establish trust. Very respectful of elder authority, therefore will have greater respect for older health care providers and dismiss younger team members. Tone of voice is commonly loud and argumentative. Very modest; never ask personal questions in mixed company.
Hmong	Very polite and aware of disrespectful and prejudicial behavior. Prolonged eye contact considered disrespectful. Communication may be indirect; will not say "no" but may say "I will think about it." Interpreters employed by the hospital are considered to be loyal to the institution and therefore not trusted. The family may request a bilingual family member be present during discussions. Language structure is different; make sure the interpreter understands the intent of the discussion. The Hmong language has almost no medical terms. Have great respect for authority. Elders of the family will meet to make decisions regarding the patient's care. Immediate family members and female relatives may not have exclusive decision-making power.
Japanese	May not ask questions; defer to health care team to provide care. Illness not discussed outside of family. Soft voice considered polite with direct conflict avoided. Facial expressions are controlled and prolonged direct eye contact is considered disrespectful. Promptness very important. Cleanliness of body is important, as is modesty and preservation of dignity.
Mexican	Direct eye contact with authority figures is avoided. Silence may show lack of agreement with the plan of care. Touching by a stranger is considered disrespectful, although therapeutic touch is an integral part of traditional healing.
Russians	Direct eye contact is used. Respectful of elders. Tone of voice may be loud.
South Asians (India, Pakistan, Bangladesh, Sri Lanka, Nepal, Fiji, East Africa)	Touching not common; caring expressed through eyes. Prolonged direct eye contact considered rude. Modesty, humility, tolerance, and silence emphasized. Tone of voice should be soft. Loudness is considered disrespectful.
Vietnamese	Head may be considered sacred and feet profane; do not touch the feet and then the head. Avoiding eye contact is a sign of respect. Using both hands when giving a person something shows respect. Tone of voice should be soft. A loud voice or pointing of the finger is a sign of disrespect.

inherent in the type of work the patient performs. If a patient works in a factory around loud machines, there may be resultant hearing loss from repeated exposure to noise. Occupation can also be a socioeconomic indicator of the patient. Some jobs for unskilled workers often do not pay enough for the patient to have adequate housing, insurance for health care, and adequate nutrition.

- *Health insurance:* Although information about health insurance is often obtained by the registration staff, it is an important assessment of the nurse. The type of health insurance the patient has can often be a predictor of the type of health-seeking behaviors the patient may or may not have. Patients who are enrolled in a health maintenance organization (HMO) are usually aware of the preventive aspect of the insurance and the focus on healthy lifestyle and the emphasis on regular health screenings along the age continuum.

- *Source of information:* As part of the data collection process, the person providing the information must be identified. If it is the patient who is providing the health information, then this is considered the primary source. A person other than the patient who provides health information about the patient is considered a secondary source. If an interpreter is used in obtaining the health history, then that should be noted on the questionnaire. In either case, it is the responsibility of the nurse to determine the reliability of the person giving the information.

Present Health/Illness

The history of the present illness includes information about what brought the patient to the health care provider. By using open-ended questioning, the nurse can obtain the reason why the patient is seeking care. The reason is usually written verbatim in the health record and often becomes the **chief complaint**. A leading question is "Why did you come in today?" The nurse then writes down the specific responses from the patient, such as "I have lost fifteen pounds in the last two weeks." The nurse can then ask further questions to gather more subjective data from the patient, such as "How has your appetite been?"

Health Patterns

It is important for the nurse to assess the health patterns of the patient because this can be a determinant of his or her current state of health. Health patterns such as sleep can determine whether or not the patient is achieving the norm for his demographic. Open-ended questions can be used to gather this information: "How much sleep do you normally get each night?" "Is your sleep interrupted during the night?" "How many times do you have to get up to go to the bathroom during the night?" The responses that the patient provides will be a good predictor of whether or not he is getting the required 8 to 10 hours of sleep each night. Sleep patterns will usually be addressed in the neurological portion of the body system review.

Other health patterns to assess are the patient's access to preventive health maintenance. Questions such as "When was the last time you had an eye examination?" "How often do you see a dentist?" "When was your last physical exam?" "How often do you exercise?" will assist the nurse in determining the normal routine or preventive measures of the patient.

Health Beliefs and Practices

An individual's belief about health is based on knowledge, heritage, and experiences. Culture also influences these beliefs. Today with information so readily available in the mass media and on the Internet, people tend to be better informed about health issues. An increase in information about preventive medicine has made people better informed about lifestyles and habits that promote health.

The following questions and statements will assist the nurse in learning more about the patient's health care beliefs:

- What do you think it means to be healthy?
- Tell me about your own health.
- Do members of your family have the same beliefs about health as you do?

- What do you do to remain healthy?
- Do you have any behaviors that you believe are unhealthy?
- Where do you get your health information?
- Do you have a regular health care provider?
- How often do you have a complete physical examination?
- Do you have any home remedies that you use regularly?

Past Medical History

The past medical history is a timeline of the patient's health that includes childhood illnesses, immunizations, allergies, surgeries, hospitalizations, labor and deliveries, injuries, major illnesses, and any mental, emotional, or psychiatric illnesses. It is important with a chronic illness to establish when it first occurred, what has been the progression of the illness to this point, and whether there are any **sequelae** (residual problems as a result of the illness) (Zator-Estes, 2006). By determining this, the nurse can establish what effect the chronic illness has had on the patient's ability to live a "normal" life. Repeated hospitalizations, numerous doctor visits requiring invasive tests, and multiple medications can affect the patient's perception of her quality of life when living with a chronic illness such as diabetes. The past medical history is also the place to discuss whether the patient uses tobacco, alcohol, or drugs. Typical questions include these:

- Are you currently under the supervision of a health care provider for a medical condition?
- What diseases have you experienced, beginning with childhood?
- Have you ever been hospitalized? If so, tell me why, when, for how long?
- Have you been told you have any diseases that are not curable?
- Have you experienced any complications (sequelae) from diseases or injuries?
- Do you have any disabilities or special needs? If so, please describe.
- Have you ever been involved in an accident in which you were injured? If so, please describe.
- Have you ever had a blood transfusion? If so, when and where?
- Has any disease or injury affected your ability to lead a normal life?
- Have you ever suffered from any mental illnesses, such as depression?

Medications

It is necessary to obtain a complete medication history for every patient. The medication history must include both prescription and nonprescription, or over-the-counter (OTC), medications that the patient may be taking. It is important to get the name, dose, and dosage times for each medication and why the patient is taking that particular medication.

While obtaining the medication history from the patient, the nurse can determine from the responses of the patient how much he knows about the medication regime. The more complete and precise the obtained answers, the greater the indication that the patient has a comprehensive understanding of his medications. It also is important during this time to determine if the patient is taking any home remedies, vitamins, or herbs. Because many medications have the potential for reacting adversely when taken simultaneously, it is important to have a complete and accurate medication history from the patient. General questions about the safe handling of medications also are important to ascertain. Consider these sample questions:

- How long do you save unused drugs and are you aware of discard dates?
- How do you dispose of unused, outdated drugs?
- Where do you keep or store your medications?
- Do you check to see if the medication needs refrigeration?
- Do you take the entire prescription of antibiotics when prescribed?
- Do you share medications or needles with anyone?

Family History

Obtaining a detailed family history from the patient is important because this history can serve as a predictor of potential health problems that the patient may encounter later in life. If, for example, the family history reveals that the parents and all of the siblings have diabetes, the nurse could then question the patient about potential signs and symptoms of diabetes; weight loss, hunger, frequent urination.

Because many conditions occur more frequently in specific ethnic backgrounds, the family history must also include information about the ethnic background. Examples include thalassemia in Southeast Asian's and Tay-Sachs in Ashkenazi Jewish populations (Gene Clinics, 2008). Some familial illnesses do not occur in every generation; therefore, it is important to ask the patient about relatives in other generations. Typical questions that will illicit the needed information include the following:

- Please tell me about your family members and their health, including your spouse, children, siblings, parents, aunts, uncles, and grandparents.
- Do any of these individuals have medical illnesses or diseases? If so, what are they?
- Have there been any deaths in the immediate family? If so, what was the cause?
- How old were your relatives when they died and what was the cause?

Psychosocial History

Assessing behaviors of the patient during the health assessment will give the nurse *cues* to the patient's sense of self-esteem. Assessing the patient's dress, body language, and tone of voice during the interview can aid the nurse in determining the patient's emotional state at that particular time. Note, however, that the nurse must be careful not to formulate a conclusion based solely on one factor such as how the patient dressed for the interview; instead any conclusions should be based on a variety of factors. The nurse will assess for presence of eye contact during the interview and posture while seated: Was it relaxed or did the patient appear tense? Did the patient show signs of anxiety about answering the health assessment questions?

The psychosocial history includes information about the patient's occupational history, level of education, financial history, familial roles, relationships and interdependent relationships, cultural identity, and self-concept. The information gathered regarding a patient's occupational history, level of education, and financial history will alert the nurse to possible health risks both present and future. For example, a patient who is of low socioeconomic status may work in jobs that have actual or potential health hazards associated with them such as a farmworker who has worked in the fields and has been exposed to prolonged ultraviolet radiation from the sun and pesticides used on the crops.

By obtaining information regarding the patient's level of education, the nurse will gain insight into whether the patient can read and understand prescriptions or instructions given to her by a health care provider. Questions regarding the patient's financial background will give the nurse opportunities to determine the patient's health-seeking behaviors. For example, a patient who is financially secure often will have an established health care provider who is seen on a regular basis versus a patient who may be working two or more low-paying jobs and is without basic health coverage and who only seeks health care when ill.

In determining the patient's perception of role and family identity, the nurse might ask, "Is there someone significant in your life?" This "support" person may be a spouse, significant other, or a trusted friend. At this time, the nurse then can ask about siblings and other family members that the patient may be close to. Depending on the patient's chronological age, the list of significant family members may be lengthy or very short if the person is in the later stages of life. The nurse needs to inquire about the presence of family and the patient's level of participation in family life.

A patient's self-concept can be elicited by such open-ended questions as "How are you feeling about yourself?" or "Where do you see yourself in the next five years?" By gathering subjective and objective data to either support or refute a patient's perception of his self-concept, the nurse can determine if the patient has a good or a distorted view. An example would be a patient who states verbally that he has a good self-concept, yet his appearance is unkempt, he is poorly dressed, he does not maintain eye contact with the nurse, and he is slouched down in the chair during the screening interview. All of these observable signs will point toward a person who has a low self-concept. When patients have a positive self-concept, they often will have coping mechanisms in place to deal with stressors in their lives. A leading question by the nurse can be "How do you handle stress?"

Sexuality also is another component of a person's self-concept. Patients who are in a committed relationship and have a strong self-concept usually will report that their sexuality is complete or strong. The issue of sexuality is a delicate topic that patients may be reluctant to talk about, so it is important for the nurse to establish a very trusting and supportive rapport with the patient before attempting to discuss issues pertaining to sexuality. Once a level of trust and rapport has been established between the nurse and patient, such open-ended questions as "Are you dating?" or "Are you and your spouse engaging in sexual intimacy on a regular basis?" can be asked of the patient.

One final question that the nurse is required to ask of patients is whether or not they have been at risk for abuse. This may be difficult for a patient to answer if a family member or spouse is in the exam room with the patient. For this question, the nurse may need to ask the question while performing the physical exam or while alone with the patient and the patient is able to be more forthright when answering.

Stress and Coping

Stress is a physical or psychological stressor and coping is the individual's physical and emotional response to the stressor. Stress is not the event itself, but the meaning of the event to the individual. What may be a stressor for one person is not for another. The immediate physical response to acute stress is the fight-or-flight response, which is due to catecholamine release. This produces a variety of manifestations such as sweaty palms and a pounding heart. The manifestations of long-term stress are different, including habitually cold hands and suppressed immune function. Emotional reactions may include difficulty sleeping, inability to concentrate, and anxiety.

The nurse should assess the patient for the physical signs of stress including:

- Increased and pounding heart rate
- Decreased blood clotting time
- Increased rate and depth of respirations
- Dilated pupils
- Elevated glucose levels
- Dilated skeletal blood vessels
- Elevated blood pressure.

Stress in and of itself is not always bad and in fact can be a motivator to enhance performance. It is the coping skills or strategies that an individual uses that determine the impact and long-term effect. Coping is a learned behavior that develops over a person's lifetime. Chapter 12 ⊘ provides a complete discussion of stress and adaptation.

Cultural Beliefs and Practices

When inquiring about the patient's cultural identity, the nurse can open with a leading question such as "What culture do you identify with most?" Cultural identity can determine how patients view themselves and how they seek health services. Patients who identify themselves as Hispanic may have a strong sense of family and will be guided by familial desires when making health care decisions. Hispanics may also have a strong sense of spirituality and will resort to prayer for their concerns. Patients' ethnic identities might also influence their dietary habits. For example, many Asian cultures will have rice as a component with each meal.

Most Americans, when ill, seek out a health care practitioner and then comply with the traditional "Western medicine" approach to treatment. As the influx of emigrants from countries where the traditional Western model of medicine is foreign increases, it is important for the nurse to assess what health-seeking beliefs and behaviors the patient may favor. For example, when a Southeast Asian patient is ill, it is a common practice for the family to perform a "coining" ritual by rubbing a coin forcefully over the person's body in order to rid them of the spirit causing the ailment. Chinese emigrants may use herbalists to treat many ailments. Those of the Hispanic cultures may use a *curandera* (folk healer) to cast the evil from the body of the ill person.

Some leading questions that the nurse can use to determine if a patient uses alternative forms of medicine to treat illnesses are:

- Do you use any cultural or religious practices to treat illnesses?
- Do you use any home remedies to treat illnesses?
- Do you use any holistic remedies, such as meditation, yoga, or herbs, to treat illnesses?

It is then necessary to document any alternative practices that the patient may use on the health assessment (Spector, 2004).

National standards for culturally and linguistically appropriate services (CLAS) have been issued by the DHHS's Office of Minority Health. These standards are aimed at helping individuals who enter the health care system receive equitable and effective treatment in a culturally and linguistically appropriate manner.

Spiritual Beliefs

As nurses continually strive to assist patients and families with their health needs, they must also attend to their spiritual needs, because one cannot truly assess a patient/family without assessing its spirituality (Tanyi, 2006). The purpose of obtaining information about spiritual beliefs is to better understand the patient and the impact, if any, that these beliefs have on their health. As the interview is being conducted, the nurse should be alert for spiritual clues. For example, if the patient says she is a vegetarian (Hindu) or her hair has never been cut (women: Orthodox Jews), it is a good time to inquire about the basis for these practices.

While obtaining the spiritual history, the nurse should also inquire about an advance directive (living will or durable medical power of attorney). The patient's answer may involve spiritual beliefs. An example would be a patient who believes that it is up to God to decide when he dies, not anyone else.

Components of the Physical Assessment

Prior to conducting the physical assessment, the nurse should make sure that the examination area allows for privacy and the physical environment is comfortable and conducive to developing a rapport with the patient. For example, the temperature in the area should be at a comfortable level; lighting should be sufficient to see, but not glaring; distracting objects should be removed; the noise level should not be loud or distracting; and the room should be large enough to allow for 4 or 5 feet of space between the nurse and the patient.

In reviewing the body systems, a head-to-toe approach is one method used for obtaining data about each body system. Usually this is done by asking the patient a series of questions from a preprinted questionnaire regarding each body system. The assessment questionnaire will include a review of biophysical systems such as integument, head and neck, respiratory, cardiovascular, musculoskeletal, neurological, genitourinary (female/male), and reproductive (female/male).

Finally, it is important for the nurse to consider the age of the patient when performing a physical assessment. For example, aging patients' body weight will decrease during their 70s and 80s, and the distribution of fat changes with the subcutaneous

MyNursingKit | Animation: Health and Physical Assessment: Body Systems—Anatomy and Physiology fat being lost in the face and forearms and additional fat deposited in the abdomen.

Functional Assessment

The functional assessment uses observation to gather data while the patient is performing common or routine activities (D'Amico & Barbarito, 2007). As a part of the general survey, the nurse will observe such things as how patients enter the exam room; their dress, how they seat themselves and their arm movements when straightening their clothing once seated; their hand gestures while talking; and facial expressions and facial symmetry. All of the above will be interpreted by the nurse as she begins to formulate assessment data on this patient.

Physical Assessment

In conducting the physical assessment, the nurse starts with a general survey that begins at the time he first encounters the patient and then moves on to a specific examination of the body systems. The general survey is one in which the nurse observes the patient while performing the interview (described earlier) during the health assessment (Rhodes, 2006). As the nurse is asking questions, he is observing the patient and formulating a mental picture of the patient. The nurse can observe any distinguishing features such as presence or absence of facial hair in an adult male (secondary sex characteristics). During this time, the nurse will observe all that can be seen, heard, or smelled while conducting the interview. This will then set the course for the nurse when performing the physical examination. The major components of the survey are physical appearance, nutritional status, mental status, mobility, and behavior of the patient.

Physical Appearance

By looking at the patient, the nurse can formulate various facts related to the patient. If the patient looks older than her stated age, this is an important observation. The patient who appears emaciated suggests intentional or unintentional weight loss, which could be related to an underlying pathology. By looking at the patient, body symmetry can be ascertained. Does the patient's upper and lower torso have the same distance from head to pelvis as pelvis to feet? Does the patient's head appear to be in proportion to the rest of her body? By observing body shape and size, the nurse can determine whether there could be any potential disorders such as overeating or anorexia.

Nutritional Assessment

A component of the health assessment is a nutrition assessment. Such leading questions as "How many meals do you normally eat each day?" "What time do you eat your last meal of the day?" and "Do you have any dietary restrictions?" will give the nurse some insight into the patient's dietary habits. A more reliable nutrition assessment is obtained, however, by having the patient fill out a journal of the eating times and amount and type of food eaten for a 3-day period. This requires that the patient be able to write and makes the assumption that he will be honest in keeping and recording the food diary. This technique requires a subsequent visit by the patient so the diary can be added to his health assessment. Nutrition is discussed in detail in Chapter 14 .

Mental Status

The nurse can assess the patient's mental status while the patient is responding to the various questions during the health history. While asking the health questions, the nurse will be noting the patient's affect, mood, and demeanor. At this time the nurse will be able to determine if the patient is oriented to person, place, and time by virtue of how the patient responds to the questions. If the patient appears confused, the nurse can further determine the patient's mental status by asking such questions as "Do you know what day it is today?" or "What time is it?" If the patient has difficulty answering these questions, then the nurse will need to conduct a more detailed work-up.

Mobility

The nurse can observe how the patient moves when the patient enters the office area: Are the patient's movements fluid and purposeful? Is her posture erect and is she moving with a steady stride? The nurse can observe for deviations in movement and assess whether or not the patient has full range of motion in her extremities. An elderly female with advanced osteoporosis may walk with a "stooped over" posture and it may appear that the patient is having pain or is laboring to perform movements. Relative to mobility, the nurse also observes whether the patient is using any ambulatory aids such as a walker, cane, wheelchair, leg braces, or special orthotic shoes.

Behavior

The nurse can observe the patient's affect and response to questions. Is it an appropriate response, or does the patient under- or overreact to the situation. For example, if the patient is telling the nurse about the death of someone close, is there an emotional response? Lack of an appropriate response referred to as "flat affect" and should be documented in the medical record. At the other end of the spectrum, is the patient overreacting or visibly uncomfortable with unemotional queries.

Measuring Height and Weight

Height and weight are measured by the nurse as a means of obtaining baseline data about the patient. In obtaining the actual height and weight, the nurse can account for any differences in what the patient may have subjectively told the nurse during the health questioning.

The most common method of obtaining an adult patient's height and weight is with the platform scale. Once the weight is obtained, the patient turns with his back to the scale. The nurse then slides a height bar up above his head, folds out the right-angled arm and lowers it until it barely touches the patient's head, and takes the height measurement.

Many standard height and weight charts for both men and women have been developed by insurance companies and the DHHS. The nurse should make sure to use the chart that is approved by her health system. A common measure of weight to height is the body mass index (BMI). BMI is a person's weight in kilograms divided by the square of his height in meters giving a measure of kg/m^2. The BMI ranges are as follows:

- Normal range: <18.5– 24.9
- Overweight: 25.0–29.9
- Obese: >30.

Weight as it is related to cardiac risk factors is discussed in Chapter 40 .

Measuring Vital Signs

Temperature, pulse, respirations, blood pressure, and pain level are the **vital signs** that the nurse will measure during the health assessment. Temperature is often obtained with an electronic thermometer and recorded in either degrees Fahrenheit or Celsius. The most common route for obtaining a temperature is via the oral cavity. Other routes are rectal, axillary (under the arm), and tympanic (ear).

Obtaining the pulse of the adult patient is most commonly done by palpating the radial artery and counting the pulse for 15 seconds and then multiplying by 4 to arrive at a 60-second pulse rate. During the assessment the apical, bilateral radial, and bilateral pedal pulses are evaluated (Figure 9–2 ■). At the same time that the nurse is recording the pulse rate, he will also be assessing the character of the patient's pulses for such descriptors as weak, thready, bounding, regular, or irregular. If there are irregularities in the pulse rate, then the nurse should check the pulse rate for a full 60 seconds to get an accurate pulse rate. Abnormalities related to the pulse are discussed in Chapter 37 ⊘.

The respiratory rate is usually obtained while obtaining the pulse rate. Once the nurse has obtained the pulse rate, she will observe the patient's chest movement and count the number of times the patient inhales in a 15-second interval and again multiply this by 4 to achieve a 1-minute respiratory rate. The nurse should also be observing the character and movement of the patient's chest while obtaining the respiratory rate. She will be observing for a rhythmic inhalation and exhalation and for nasal flaring or use of accessory muscles in taking a breath. A more detailed examination of the patient's breathing will occur when auscultating the lungs with a stethoscope. The detailed respiratory examination is further explained in Chapter 33 ⊘.

The blood pressure is obtained by using a cuff, sphygmomanometer, and a stethoscope. The patient is placed in a sitting position. It is important for the nurse to select a cuff that is the appropriate size for the circumference of the patient's upper arm. The width of the cuff should equal 40% of the circumference of the extremity used, and the length of the cuff should equal 80% of the circumference. Using a cuff that is too narrow will give a falsely high blood pressure. The nurse must also palpate the brachial artery (Figure 9–2 ■) and align the arrows of the cuff so that they are over the artery.

Once the cuff is secure on the patient, the nurse places the bell of the stethoscope over the area where he palpated the brachial pulse. Slowly the nurse begins to inflate the cuff by squeezing the bulb and listening for the brachial pulse to be obliterated. A standard is to pump the cuff to 30 mm over the number where the pulse was first lost. The nurse then slowly releases the pressure and observes the needle of the manometer, which should be decreasing at a rate of about 2 to 3 mmHg per second. The nurse notes the manometer readings while listening. The first sound and corresponding number on the manometer will be the systolic measurement, and the last sound and corresponding number will be the diastolic measurement. Once the diastolic reading has been obtained, the nurse releases the pressure from the cuff, removes the cuff from the patient's arm, and records the findings. Abnormalities related to blood pressure are discussed in Chapters 21, 40, and 61 ⊘.

Pain

The assessment of pain, often referred to as the fifth vital sign, is essential for the nurse to obtain with each assessment of the patient (D'Amico & Barbarito, 2007). The presence of pain—whether acute or chronic, severe or mild—is a subjective experience solely unique to that individual. A pain history includes the following data:

- *Location:* The nurse asks the patient to point to the location of the pain source. Often the nurse will also use a body diagram and ask the patient to use the diagram to locate the pain. The nurse then identifies the locus of the pain using the nearest anatomic landmarks (e.g., sharp pain in right patellar region posterior and medial).
- *Intensity:* The nurse asks the patient to rate the level of pain that she is experiencing using a pain scale. For most adults, a

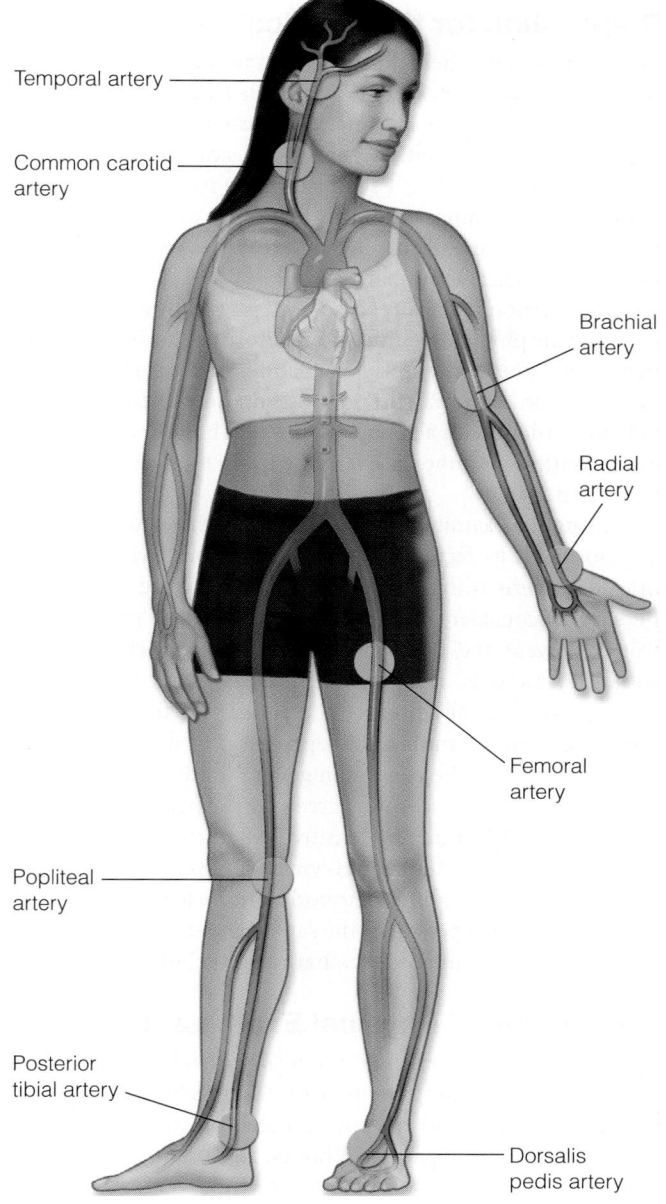

Temporal artery

Common carotid artery

Brachial artery

Radial artery

Femoral artery

Popliteal artery

Posterior tibial artery

Dorsalis pedis artery

FIGURE 9–2 ■ Apical, bilateral radial, and bilateral pedal pulse locations.
Source: From D'Amico, Barbarito, Health and Physical Assessment in Nursing (2007). Pearson Education. pp. 115 Figure 7.10

numerical pain scale of 0 to 10 can be used where 0 is no pain and 10 is the highest level of pain.

- *Quality:* Asking the patient to describe the pain as either dull, throbbing, sharp, piercing, aching, etc., gives the nurse a sense of the quality of the pain that the patient is experiencing. When using the patient's exact words to describe the quality of the pain, the nurse puts the patient's words in quotation marks.

- *Pattern:* The onset and duration of pain is noted as the pattern. The nurse assesses whether the pain is constant or intermittent. If the pain is intermittent, the nurse also asks about duration, that is, when the pain subsides and returns. Again, the nurse records the patient's response in the narrative.

- *Precipitating factors:* The nurse attempts to learn from the patient what brings on the pain. A precipitating factor could be, for example, ascending three flights of stairs (after which the patient experiences substernal chest pain).

- *Relief methods:* Along with assessing for the presence of pain, the nurse also asks the patient what she has done to attempt to relieve the pain. Here the nurse lists all prescription treatments and OTC remedies that the patient may have utilized, as well as any alternative health providers such as an herbalist, massage therapist, chiropractor, or acupuncturist. The nurse also notes which of these methods has helped in relieving the pain and for how long (duration).

- *Impact on ADLs:* By assessing how the pain is impacting the patient's ability to perform her ADLs, the nurse can obtain a clearer picture of how the pain may be affecting this particular patient and ultimately the quality of her life.

- *Coping strategies:* Coping strategies include yoga, meditation, relaxation exercises, prayer, support groups, or withdrawal. Each of these strategies is unique to the individual patient and will also be a reflection of the patient's age, culture, and belief system.

Refer to Chapter 15 👓 for a thorough discussion of pain.

Documentation of the Health History

In the acute care setting, specific forms or page screens on an electronic medical record (EMR) help guide the nurse in documentation of the health history. Figure 9–3 ■ shows examples of EMR screens for documentation of a health history in the acute care setting. Of note is the importance of documenting *who* is answering the questions. Detailed information on documentation is discussed in Chapter 6 👓.

▉ Physical Examination

There are two types of physical exams. The **comprehensive exam** (head-to-toe exam) is usually performed on new patients who will be seen on a routine basis by various clinicians. A **focused exam** is performed in emergent or urgent situations and is focused on a specific problem (Rhodes, 2006). Regardless of the type of exam to be done, an organized and systematic examination is necessary to obtain pertinent data in the shortest amount of time. An organized approach creates trust and encourages the cooperation of the patient. The information that was gathered during the health history will help to guide aspects of the physical examination. At all times during the exam, the patient's physical

and psychological comfort is taken into consideration. It is important to explain all aspects of the examination to the patient; this will enhance the patient's experience and decrease his anxiety during the examination.

Incorporating the head-to-toe examination into a nurse's routine takes practice and repeated examinations in order for the process to flow in a natural manner that is comfortable to both the nurse and the patient (Rhodes, 2006). It is important for the nurse to develop a routine that will become comfortable and will not omit any pertinent data during the examination. Expertise comes with practice, and the ability to interpret findings develops with experience. There is no one correct way to perform the head-to-toe examination. The main goal is to have a sequence that flows smoothly and allows for patient comfort and privacy. The examination of specific systems is discussed in detail throughout the book in each unit's assessment chapter.

Preparation for the Physical Examination

The environment where the physical examination is to take place must be private, quiet, and a comfortable temperature. The room needs to have adequate lighting. The nurse needs to use standard precautions throughout the entire physical examination. The equipment should all be assembled in the room prior to the beginning of the examination. It is helpful to assemble the equipment in order of use. Figure 9–4 ■ (p. 162) shows the instruments used for a physical examination.

The patient must be prepared both physically and psychologically for the physical examination. Before beginning, ask the patient if she needs to empty her bladder. If a urine specimen is needed, instruct the patient on the technique for collection. Provide the patient with a gown and instruct her to remove all necessary clothing. A drape is left in the room to be used during the examination.

During the examination the patient will have to assume various positions to facilitate the assessment and will need to be draped properly with each position change (Figure 9–5 ■, p. 163). Be sure to consider any limitations the patient may have that would prevent the usual positioning. These include arthritis, weakness, fractures, or joint deformities.

To psychologically prepare the patient for the examination, the nurse should assume a calm, professional demeanor and explain each step of the process in general understandable terms. Be sensitive to any discomfort created by exposing various parts of the body. Be culturally sensitive when dealing with people from cultures other than your own. In some cultures women are restricted from revealing their bodies to males other than their husbands. When a person of the same gender is requested for an examination, if at all possible, that request should be honored.

Techniques of Physical Examination

During the physical examination the nurse will utilize each of his senses while examining the patient. Such techniques as inspection, palpation, percussion, and auscultation are implemented to objectively assess the patient (Rhodes, 2006).

Inspection

Inspection is the deliberate, systematic examination of the patient using both sight and smell. It begins with the first encounter and continues the entire time the nurse is with the

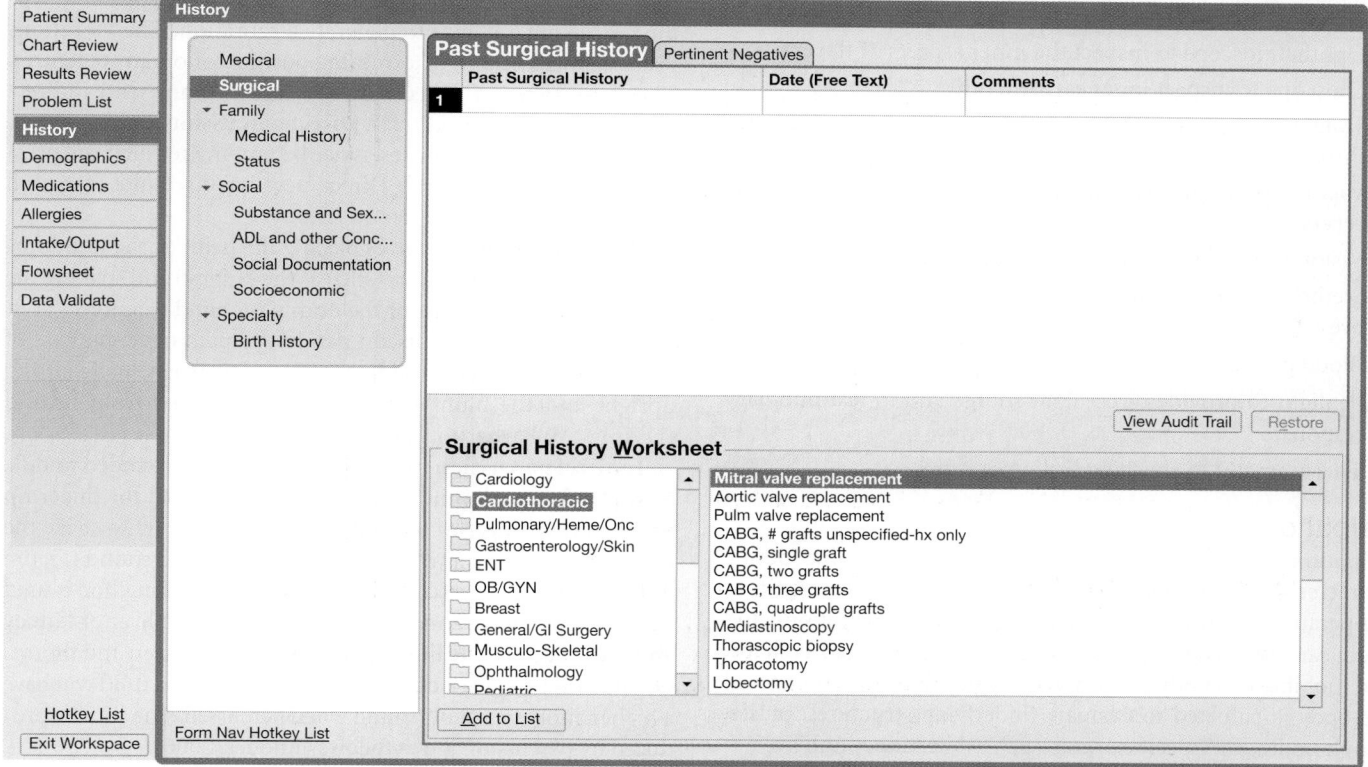

FIGURE 9–3 ■ Past medical history.

patient. The nurse observes gait, mannerisms, stature, and other physical attributes. The inspection begins by assessing the patient's appearance and comparing the right and left side of the body for symmetry. Inspection of each region of the body includes observing color, warmth, size, symmetry, contour, move-

ment, or drainage (D'Amico & Barbarito, 2007). For example, the color of the nail beds and the temperature of the fingers are assessed on each side and then a comparison of the right versus left is done. Under normal conditions the finger temperature and nail bed color are the same in both hands. A cold dusky blue

FIGURE 9–4 ■ Equipment used for physical assessment.
Source: From D'Amico, Barbarito, Health and Physical Assessment in Nursing (2007). Pearson Education. pp. 101 Table 6.1

appearance of only one hand indicates a problem with the blood supply to that area. The nurse also should note any unusual odor and determine its cause.

During most of the inspection of the patient, no instruments are needed, but some parts of the assessment require special tools that will assist the nurse. The instruments include the following:

- Ophthalmoscope to inspect the inner aspects of the eye
- Otoscope to inspect inner ear structures
- Tongue blade to inspect the inside of the mouth, tongue, and throat
- Vaginal speculum to dilate the vaginal canal and inspect the cervix
- Vision chart to test near- and farsightedness
- Stethoscope to listen to lungs, bowel sounds, and blood pressure
- Blood pressure cuff
- Penlight to provide direct light source and to test pupillary responses
- Thermometer to check body temperature

Palpation

Palpation uses touch in order to collect data to determine specific characteristics of the body (Rhodes, 2006). Such characteristics as temperature, texture, moisture, tenderness, pain, vibrations, and edema are assessed using palpation. Additionally, the size, shape, and mobility of a body part can be palpated. Each specific area of the body is palpated to evaluate underlying structures, pulses, lymph nodes, and specific organs such as the kidney and liver.

In palpating, the nurse will use the fingertips, finger pads, base of the fingers, palmar surface of the fingers, and the dorsal and ulnar surfaces of the hands (D'Amico & Barbarito, 2007) (Figure 9–6 ■, p. 164). The nurse's hand is moved slowly and intentionally and discomfort can be minimized by warming the hands, having nails cut short, and not wearing any jewelry. Gloves may be worn when there are open or exposed areas. When using latex gloves it is necessary to ask patients if they have any allergies to latex.

Palpation is characterized as being light, moderate, or deep. The nurse always begins with light palpation and culminates with deep palpation to evaluate such organ structures as the kidney and liver. The use of light palpation first will aid the nurse in assessing the texture, temperature, and any painful or reddened area on the surface of the patient's skin (Figure 9–7 ■, p. 164). Moderate palpation is used to assess major areas of the patient's anatomy especially the abdominal organs. The nurse will use the palmar aspect of the fingers and gently press down about 1 to 2 centimeters while rotating the fingers in a circular motion (D'Amico & Barbarito, 2007) (Figure 9–8 ■, p. 164). Deep palpation is used by the nurse to assess an organ that lies deep within the abdominal cavity, such as the liver and or kidneys (Figure 9–9 ■, p. 164). The level of palpation is usually 2 to 4 cm. The nurse must explain the procedure to the patient because deep palpation could cause some discomfort if the patient already experienced pain upon light to moderate palpation. It is important for the patient to be relaxed during palpation of the soft tissue areas. It is better to use the dominant hand when possible because it is more sensitive than the nondominant one.

Percussion

Percussion is the creation of sound vibrations by pushing, tapping, or using a device to generate a vibration. The vibrations produced will help in determining position of organ structures. The three types of percussion are direct, blunt, and indirect (D'Amico & Barbarito, 2007). **Direct percussion**, used to examine such areas as the sinuses, is gentle tapping to illicit the presence or absence of fluid. Direct percussion results in a dull sound (Figure 9–10 ■, p. 164).

Blunt percussion involves placing the palm of the nondominant hand over a body area (such as the kidney) and striking the palm with the closed fist of the dominant hand (Figure 9–11 ■, p. 165). This method is used to assess for pain or tenderness of the liver, gallbladder, or kidneys. The patient is usually sitting upright and the blunt percussion is performed from behind (D'Amico & Barbarito, 2007).

Indirect percussion involves using the hyperextended middle finger of the nondominant hand (pleximeter) and the finger tip of the middle finger of the dominant hand (plexor) to strike the pleximeter by using a wrist action that will elicit a sound (Figure 9–12 ■, p. 165) (D'Amico & Barbarito, 2007). This method is used to determine the location of an organ such as the liver or kidney and also to determine fluid air levels in the abdomen and thorax. Organs will produce a dull sound, whereas air and fluid will have a higher, more tympanic sound when percussed. The sounds produced by percussion are as follows (Rhodes, 2006):

- **Tympany** is a high-pitched, drum-like tone of medium duration. It is commonly heard over the air-filled intestines.
- **Resonance** is a loud hollow tone of long duration. It is commonly heard over the lungs.
- **Hyperresonance** is a loud low tone with a longer duration than resonance. It is heard when air is trapped in a space such as the lungs.

POSITION	AREAS EXAMINED	RATIONALE	CONTRAINDICATIONS
Sitting	Vital signs, head and neck, back, posterior and anterior thorax and lungs, breasts, axillae, heart, upper and lower extremities, reflexes	Sitting upright allows for full lung expansion and better visualization of upper body symmetry.	Older and weak clients may be unable to sit without support. An alternate position is supine with the head of the bed elevated.
Supine	Vital signs, head and neck, anterior thorax and lungs, breasts, axillae, heart, abdomen, extremities, peripheral pulses	This is a relaxed position for most clients. It provides access to pulse sites and prevents contracture of abdominal muscles, especially if a small pillow is placed under the knees.	Clients with cardiovascular and respiratory problems may be unable to lie flat without becoming short of breath. An alternate position is to raise the head of the bed. Clients with lower back pain may be unable to lie flat without flexing the knees.
Dorsal recumbent	Abdomen and external genitalia	Flexed knees reduce tension on lower back and abdominal muscles and increase client comfort.	Same as for supine. The client should not raise the arms over the head or clasp the hands behind the head because this increases contraction of the abdominal muscles.
Lithotomy	Female genitalia, reproductive tract, and rectum	This position maximally exposes the genitalia and facilitates the insertion of a vaginal speculum.	This position is assumed immediately before it is needed because it is embarrassing and uncomfortable. The client is kept draped. Clients with arthritis or joint deformity may be unable to assume this position. Alternate positions are dorsal recumbent and Sims'.
Sims' (posterior view)	Rectum, vagina	Flexion of the upper hip and knee improves exposure of the rectal area.	Clients with deformities of the hip or knee may be unable to assume this position. Older and obese clients may be uncomfortable.
Prone	Posterior thorax, hip movement, popliteal pulses	This position is used to assess hip extension. Sometimes popliteal pulse palpation is facilitated in this position.	This position is not well tolerated by older clients or clients with cardiovascular or respiratory problems.
Knee-chest	Rectum, prostate	This position provides maximal exposure of the anal and rectal areas and facilitates insertion of instruments into the rectum.	Poorly tolerated by clients with cardiovascular or respiratory problems. Clients with difficulty flexing hips or knees may be unable to assume this position.
Standing, bent over examining table	Rectum, prostate	This is a more comfortable position than knee-chest and allows for palpation of the prostate gland.	This position is assumed immediately before it is needed because it is embarrassing. Clients with back problems may need assistance.

FIGURE 9–5 ■ Patient positioning during physical examination.

- **Dullness** is a high-pitched tone of short duration and is soft in quality. It is heard over the large organs such as the liver and kidney.
- **Flatness** is a soft, high-pitched tone with a short duration. It is heard over muscle and bone.

Percussion sounds have characteristic features that the nurse must become familiar with through experience and practice. These features include intensity, pitch, duration, and quality. *Intensity* is the amplitude or the loudness and softness of the sound. The intensity is influenced by the amount of air and the ability of the structure to vibrate. *Pitch* refers to the frequency of vibrations of sound per second. Slow vibrations produce a low-pitched sound, whereas fast vibrations produced a high-pitched sound. The length of time that the sound can be heard is referred to as *duration*, and it can be very short to very long. *Quality* refers to the type of sound and is described as clear, hollow, muffled, or dull (D'Amico & Barbarito, 2007).

Auscultation

Auscultation is the technique of listening to body sounds (Rhodes, 2006). The nurse must use both the unassisted sense of hearing and, where needed, a stethoscope. Body sounds that can be heard unassisted include speech, coughing, respirations, and the percussion tones just described. The stethoscope (Figure 9–4 ■) is used to assess the lungs, heart, and abdomen. The stethoscope

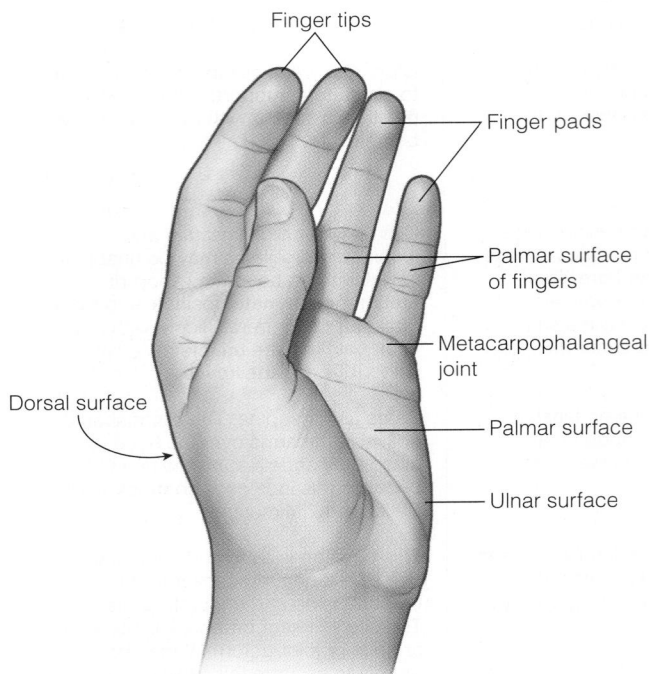

FIGURE 9–6 ■ Palpation.
Source: From D'Amico, Barbarito, Health and Physical Assessment in Nursing (2007). Pearson Education. pp. 97 Figure 6.2

FIGURE 9–7 ■ Light palpation.
Source: From D'Amico, Barbarito, Health and Physical Assessment in Nursing (2007). Pearson Education. pp. 97 Figure 6.3

FIGURE 9–8 ■ Moderate palpation.
Source: From D'Amico, Barbarito, Health and Physical Assessment in Nursing (2007). Pearson Education. pp. 98 Figure 6.4

FIGURE 9–9 ■ Deep palpation.
Source: From D'Amico, Barbarito, Health and Physical Assessment in Nursing (2007). Pearson Education. pp. 98 Figure 6.5

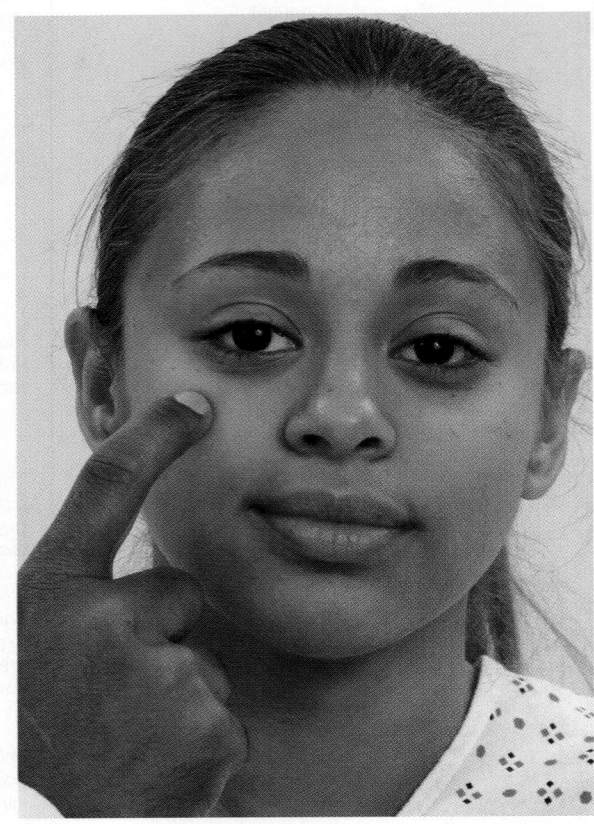

FIGURE 9–10 ■ Direct percussion.
Source: From D'Amico, Barbarito, Health and Physical Assessment in Nursing (2007). Pearson Education. pp. 99 Figure 6.6

has two end pieces, a bell, and a diaphragm. The bell has a cuplike shape and is best for hearing low-pitched sounds, such as heart murmurs. The diaphragm or flat end piece is best for high-pitched sounds such as bowel, lung, and normal heart sounds. The diaphragm should be held firmly against the patient's skin. When sounds are very soft and difficult to hear with a normal stethoscope, a Doppler ultrasound stethoscope is useful. It uses ultrasound waves to detect sounds such as fetal heart tones and peripheral pulses. Interference with the Doppler can be eliminated by applying gel to the skin.

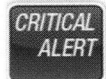 *Do not press the bell end piece of the stethoscope into the skin. This causes the skin to act as a diaphragm and will reduce audible vibratory sensations.*

When listening with the stethoscope, the environment should be as quiet as possible. Rubbing against the patient's clothing or the bed sheets or touching the stethoscope tubing will produce sounds that will interfere with body sounds. While listening, it is important to focus on only one sound at a time. Closing the eyes often assists the nurse to focus. Sounds are described in the same terms as the percussion sounds described earlier: intensity, pitch, duration, and quality.

FIGURE 9–11 ■ Blunt percussion.
Source: From D'Amico, Barbarito, Health and Physical Assessment in Nursing (2007). Pearson Education. pp. 99 Figure 6.7

FIGURE 9–12 ■ Indirect percussion.
Source: From D'Amico, Barbarito, Health and Physical Assessment in Nursing (2007). Pearson Education. pp. 99 Figure 6.8

■ Critical Thinking

Critical thinking is a cognitive skill that is needed for every aspect of a health assessment. The nursing process provides an effective framework for applying critical thinking to patient care situations. Critical thinking helps the nurse resolve problems and develop ways to manage situations. Critical thinking requires that the nurse apply logic, question the norm, and problem solve in patient care situations. The nurse must learn to recognize the relative significance of the visual, auditory, or palpable *cues* that occur during the assessment. Cues are bits of information that may hint at the possibility of a health problem. Taking advantage of the information offered by these cues necessitates the development of critical thinking skills.

The five components of critical thinking related to health assessment include collection of information, analysis of the situation, generation of alternatives, selection of alternatives, and evaluation. *Collection of information* begins with the interview and continues throughout the entire health assessment. The collection of subjective and objective data must be done in an organized manner. As the nurse is refining assessment skills, it is helpful to develop a consistent manner in which every health assessment is conducted. For example, the nurse might always use a head-to-toe approach. This helps in both the organization of data and ensures that no piece of the assessment is missed. If the patient is in acute distress, critical thinking skills will assist the nurse to alter the assessment as appropriate to maintain patient safety. For example, if the patient is in respiratory distress, it is imperative that airway management and oxygenation be assessed first.

As the nurse is collecting data, she must verify the reliability of the information. This is done by determining the ability of the patient to be a reliable historian. The nurse should look for inconsistencies and inappropriate information. This is the component where the nurse applies logic and critically assesses information. If concerned, it is sometimes helpful to ask the same question twice during the interview, and if possible check with family members for verification (D'Amico & Barbarito, 2007).

The second skill is *analysis of the situation*. During this phase the nurse must distinguish normal from abnormal. The patient's age, gender, genetic background, and culture affect the analysis. The nurse must utilize laboratory findings, diagnostic tests, charts, and measures related to development and aging. For example, some findings may be normal for an 80-year-old male but not for a 30-year-old female. When using critical thinking skills, the nurse clusters related information to assist in identifying patterns in the information. It is at this point that the nurse identifies missing information and retrieves it (D'Amico & Barbarito, 2007).

Generation of alternatives includes identifying options and establishing priorities. It begins with identification of options and then the nurse and patient work together to establish the priorities. The nurse needs to assess the patient's understanding of the situation and provide more information about the advantages and disadvantages of each option so the patient can make an informed decision.

Once informed about options, the next step is the *selection of alternatives*. The critical thinking skills needed for this step are the ability to develop outcomes and plans. The outcome is the final result of what the patient will attain, and the plan is the activities that will lead to that outcome. Some components of the plan are developed in conjunction with the health care team, whereas others are done by the patient independently.

The last step in critical thinking is *evaluation*. Evaluation requires the nurse to determine if the expected outcomes have been achieved. Each step of critical thinking is used here to determine if any omissions or misinterpretations occurred. It is essential to ensure that decisions were based on all of the facts and that reliable recourses were used (D'Amico & Barbarito, 2007).

Summary

Health assessments allow the nurse to gather information regarding the patient's past and current state of health, along with health promotion behaviors that are being utilized. This information in conjunction with the physical examination gives the nurse data to develop a plan of care to assist the patient in reaching optimum health. The development of evidence-based guidelines that assist the nurse in performing appropriate and effective health histories for specific populations is key.

NCLEX® REVIEW

1. The nurse is conducting a health assessment with a newly admitted patient. Which of the following should be included in this assessment?
   1. Subjective data only
   2. Data about the patient's physical, social, cultural, environmental, and emotional statuses
   3. Objective data only
   4. The patient's adherence to *Healthy People 2010* initiatives

2. The nurse is preparing to conduct a patient interview. Which of the following should the nurse do first?
   1. Introduce him/herself.
   2. Measure the patient's vital signs.
   3. Assist the patient into a hospital gown.
   4. Address the patient including the surname.

3. During an interview, the patient asks the nurse if she thinks he has cancer. Which of the following should the nurse make in response?
   1. Probably because your hemoglobin is low and you are exsanguinating from your rectal orifice.
   2. What makes you think that you have cancer?
   3. I'm not the doctor but I will tell you this, it's a good thing you came into the hospital while you still could because you never know what they are going to find with all of their tests and procedures.
   4. What a silly thing to say! You know, if you believe you have cancer you probably do!

4. A patient walks with two canes but is stable when ambulating and changing clothes. Which of the following assessment techniques was used to collect this data?
   1. Auscultation
   2. Palpation
   3. Inspection
   4. Percussion

5. After completing a health assessment and physical examination with a patient, the nurse begins to review the information and group similar data into clusters. Which step of the critical thinking process is this nurse functioning?
   1. Analysis of the situation
   2. Generation of alternatives
   3. Selection of alternatives
   4. Evaluation

Answers for review questions appear in Appendix D

KEY TERMS

auscultation *p.163*
blunt percussion *p.162*
chief complaint *p.155*
comprehensive exam *p.160*
direct percussion *p.162*
direct question *p.152*
dullness *p.163*
flatness *p.163*

focused exam *p.160*
hyperresonance *p.162*
indirect percussion *p.162*
inspection *p.160*
leading health indicators *p.149*
metabolic equivalent level (MET) *p.149*
objective data *p.148*

open-ended questions *p.152*
palpation *p.162*
percussion *p.162*
resonance *p.162*
sequelae *p.155*
subjective data *p.148*
tympany *p.162*
vital signs *p.159*

REFERENCES

Centers for Disease Control and Prevention. (2008). *Physical activity for everyone*. Retrieved May 6, 2008 from http://www.cdc.gov/nccdphp/dnpa/physical/everyone/recommendations/index.htm

D'Amico, D., & Barbarito C. (2007). *Health and physical assessment in nursing*. Upper Saddle River, NJ: Pearson Prentice Hall.

Ewing, J. A. (1984). Detecting alcoholism: The CAGE questionnaire. *Journal of the American Medical Association, 252,* 1905–1907.

Gene Clinics. (2008). *Gene tests*. Retrieved February 3, 2008, from http://www.geneclinics.org

Kaushik, V. P., Snih, S. A., Ray, L. A., Raji, M. A., Markides, K. S., & Goodwin, J. S. (2007). Factors associated with seven-year incidence of diabetes complications among older Mexican Americans. *International Journal of Experimental, Clinical, and Behavioral Gerontology, 53*(4).

North American Nursing Diagnosis Association. (2007). *Nursing diagnoses: Definitions and classifications 2007–2008*. Philadelphia: Author.

Rhodes, J. (2006). *Advanced health assessment and diagnostic reasoning*. New York: Lippincott Williams & Wilkins.

Spector, R. E. (2004). *Cultural diversity in health and illness*. Upper Saddle River, NJ: Pearson Prentice Hall.

Tanyi, R. A. (2006). Spirituality and family nursing: Spiritual assessment and interventions for families. *Journal of Advanced Nursing, 53*(3), 287–294.

U.S. Department of Health and Human Services http://www.cdc.gov/nccdphp/dnpa/physical/everyone/recommendations/index.htm. (2000). *Healthy people 2010: Understanding and improving health*. Retrieved February 5, 2008, from http://www.healthypeople.gov

Zator-Estes, M. (2006). *Health assessment and physical examination* (3rd ed.). Clifton Park, NY: Thompson Delmar Learning.

10

The Aging Patient

Laurie Walsh and Annita Watson

Outcome-Based Learning Objectives

After studying this chapter, the learner will be able to:

1. Identify normal age related changes of the head, neck, respiratory, cardiovascular, gastrointestinal, genitourinary, musculoskeletal, integumentary, and neurological systems when completing a nursing assessment.

2. Explain the rationale for recommended immunizations and screening exams as proposed by the U.S. Preventive Services Task Force and as stated in the chapter for the patient over 65 years of age.

3. Discuss medications contraindicated in the aging patient as identified by the Beers criteria.

4. Recognize signs and symptoms of elder mistreatment to determine appropriate referrals.

5. Differentiate between residential, assisted living, and skilled nursing care in accordance with the type of patient care services provided.

6. Provide direction and advice to the elderly by describing available innovative housing options.

7. Explain the implications of technological advancements in providing care to the elderly.

Research Collaboration Health Promotion Nursing Process Caring Critical Thinking

THIS CHAPTER focuses on nursing care of the aging patient, a cohort of individuals projected to represent 20% of the total population by 2030 (Experience CORPS, 2007). As this population grows it is incumbent on nursing and society as a whole to recognize this group's unique needs and provide special consideration to the care of these individuals. It is the intent of this chapter to present the distinctive characteristics of the aging population and to provide goals for care of the older adult. The chapter discusses the physiological and behavioral changes that occur with aging, methods of assessing for these changes, and available health care options including future innovations in caring for the elderly.

Aging is defined as the process of growing old or maturing. An individual is a composite of his chronological, physiological, and functional age. Chronological age is the number of years lived. Physiological age is the determination of age by body function, and functional age is the ability to contribute to society and to benefit self and others. An elder in some cultures is an individual who has gathered wisdom over a lifetime; an individual to be respected. The legal definition of an elder is any individual 65 years of age and older. However, many people would define an older person as "twenty years older than what I am." In other words, just because an individual has advanced in chronological age does not mean that mentally they have aged.

Theories of Aging

How a person ages largely remains a mystery in spite of frequent television infomercials offering the next new "secret" to living to a healthy old age. Factors often considered include what the person eats, where she lives, her chosen occupation, and how much she exercises. Sometimes aging is attributed to what a person inherits at birth. Although no single theory can answer all of the questions, two aging theories—biological and psychosocial—attempt to explain the physical and emotional changes that take place as an individual progresses through life.

Biological Aging Theories

Biological aging theories fall into two groups: programmed theories and error theories. The **programmed theory of aging** proposes that aging follows a biological timetable. It supports the notion that every organism is programmed to live for a certain number of years. An example of a programmed theory is the **immunologic theory of aging.** This theory asserts that the aging body is less able to distinguish its own cells from foreign cells. Alterations in B and T cells result in attacks on and eventually destruction of one's own body cells. The aging patient can boost immune function through a healthy diet and lifestyle, along with preventive health measures such as a yearly flu vaccination.

The **cross-linking theory of aging** is based on the finding that as one ages, proteins, DNA, and other molecules of the body develop inappropriate attachments to one another. These attachments cause decreased elasticity of proteins and other molecules, and prevent enzymes from breaking down proteins. As a result, damaged and unnecessary proteins are left in the system, causing problems. For example, cross-linking of collagen in the skin has been shown to be partially responsible for wrinkling. Another theory, the **rate of living theory of aging,** is based on the premise that humans possess a finite amount of a "vital substance," and when that substance is exhausted, the person dies. In other words, a human is predisposed to take only a certain number of breaths, and a human's heart is programmed to beat only a set number of times. However, this theory does not explain why some individuals live to the age of 100 and beyond (Gavrilov & Gavrilov, 2002).

Error theories of aging propose that environmental factors negatively impact the human body, causing destruction and damage. Two examples of error theories are the **free radical theory of aging** and the **wear-and-tear theory of aging.** The free radical aging theory, also called the *autoimmunity aging theory,* is based on the idea that certain chemical compounds in the body do damage that accumulates to produce aging; for example, unstable free oxygen radicals cause chromosomal changes, pigment accumulation, and collagen alteration. Cells, and eventually organs, lose function and reserve. The use of antioxidants and vitamins is thought to help slow this process. This theory, also sometimes referred to as the homeostatic theory of aging, relates to the age-related accumulation of damage produced by oxidative stress, which reduces the *homeostatic capacity of the organism* (Novoseltsev, Novoseltseva, & Yashin, 2001). The wear-and-tear aging theory compares the human body to a machine that simply wears out as a result of constant use; exposure to internal and external stressors results in the death of cells. Cellular function slows as an individual ages and becomes less efficient in responding to environmental assaults to the body (Tabloski, 2006).

Within the realm of biological theories is the genetic theory of aging, which proposes that lifespan is largely determined by the genes that one inherits. According to this theory, one's potential age is primarily determined at the moment of conception. According to Stibich (2007a), genes can explain a maximum of 35% of lifespan. The other determinants are one's behaviors, exposures, and just plain luck. Another biological theory of aging is the somatic mutation theory. The somatic mutation theory of aging purports that an important part of aging is determined by what happens to genes after they are inherited Stibich (2007b). Each time a cell divides, there is a chance that some of the genes will be copied incorrectly and result in a mutation. Additionally, exposures to toxins, radiation, or ultraviolet light can cause mutations in genes. Eventually the mutated cells accumulate, copy themselves, and cause problems in the body's functioning related to aging. The somatic mutation theory of aging is different from the genetic theory in that the genetic theory is only concerned with the genes in sperm and egg cells, whereas somatic mutations are changes in the genes that occur after they have been inherited, but they cannot be passed down to children, as can the genes in sperm and egg cells.

Psychosocial Theories of Aging

Psychosocial theories of aging describe the changes that take place emotionally and socially as one enters the later years of life. These changes tend to involve roles and social relationships. Three examples of psychosocial theories are activity theory, disengagement theory, and continuity theory. The **activity theory of aging** proposes that the more active elderly persons are, the greater their satisfaction with life; decreased activity leads to meaninglessness and life dissatisfaction. To maintain a positive sense of self, elderly persons must substitute new roles for those lost in old age, thus successful aging is achieved by staying active and extending activities enjoyed in middle age. Life care communities and senior retirement communities are designed to promote the activity theory. Such amenities as golf courses, swimming pools, and clubhouses that provide activity groups not only help support healthy aging, but also help bring individuals together to develop new relationships and interests.

The **disengagement theory of aging,** introduced in 1961, contradicts the activity theory (Tabloski, 2006). It asserts that later in life, age-related changes bring about a mutual and reciprocal withdrawal of the individual and society. In the past, mandatory retirement at age 65 with full Social Security retirement benefits may have promoted such withdrawal. With the movement toward later and more flexible retirement dates, this theory may no longer be as valid. For example, an individual born in 1937 or earlier could retire at age 65 with full benefits, whereas an individual born in 1960 or later will not be able to collect full benefits until age 67 (U.S. Social Security Administration, Office of Policy, 2007).

The **continuity theory of aging** asserts that in order to age successfully, one should substitute new roles for lost ones, and continue to maintain typical ways of adapting to the environment. One should maintain values, habits, and behaviors from his or her adult life. Older age should not be a time for major life changes, but instead one should maintain the usual activities, but at a slower pace as needed. Some older individuals would never consider a life care community or senior community because of the major changes of such a move. These adults choose to live in their established homes, along with the diversity of a neighborhood that houses both younger and older individuals, rather than living in an "all over age 65" environment (Lundell & Morris, 2004; Tabloski, 2006).

Other social theories related to aging include role theory, which maintains that role loss accompanies the aging process and could be associated with the loss of identity and esteem. Also of note are the age stratification theory, modernization theory, and the exchange theory of aging (Darkwa, 2007). Age stratification examines the movement of successive birth cohorts across time, known as *cohort flow.* Each cohort is unique in that it has its own characteristics (e.g., size, gender, and social class distribution). Each cohort experiences particular historical events that affect its members' attitudes and behaviors (Schaffer, 2006). Modernization theory argues that the role and status of the aged are inversely related to the level of societal industrialization. This tends to have a distinctly negative impact on the status of the elderly. This theory supports the premise that the more industrialized the society, the less support is given to the elderly; material family support tends to diminish (Aboderin, 2004).

Lastly, exchange theory indicates that elderly people have less power in relation to younger people because they possess fewer resources, and continued interaction with the younger population becomes more costly. Social interaction between the old and the young tends to decrease because older people have fewer resources to bring to the exchange—lower income, poorer health, and less education. Declining resources strain their possibilities for continued interaction with others (Roy & Russell, 2005).

■ Demographics of the Aging Population

In 2005, 15% of adults in the United States were over the age of 65. Elders were fairly evenly distributed throughout the United States. In Alaska, 6.5% of the population was comprised of adults age 65 and older. This was the smallest percentage for any state. Florida had the largest percentage of seniors age 65 and older, with 16.6% of the population falling into this age group. This large percentage is attributed to the many seniors who move there for the sunshine and mild climate. The percentage of adults age 65 and older fell somewhere between these two ranges for all of the other states (U.S. Census Bureau, 2005).

Women have always outlived men in the past, and the trend continues among all age groups age 65 and older. For those ages 65 to 74, there are 83 men per 100 women. For those ages 75 to 84, there are 67 men per 100 women. In the age 85 and over age group, there are 46 men per 100 women. These numbers correlate with percentages of women who are widowed. Forty one percent of women ages 65 to 84 are widowed; 79% of women age 85 and older are widowed. In the 2005 Census Bureau survey, 80% of adults ages 65 to 74 identified themselves as white; 86% of those ages 75 to 84 considered themselves white, and 87% of those ages 85 and older answered that they were white (U.S. Census Bureau, 2005).

Older Americans have attained higher levels of education than the generation before them, and this trend continues. In 1950, 17% of older adults had a high school education; only 3% had at least a bachelor's degree. By 2003, 72% were high school graduates, and at least 17% had a bachelor's degree (Administration on Aging [AOA], n.d.). Trending data indicate that advances in medicine will provide an opportunity for individuals to live a longer chronological life, however, it remains unknown as to whether a longer life will be free of disease and disability. Taking advantage of medical advances also will be influenced by educational background and finances, both of which limit one's ability to freely seek health care when it is needed. It is certain that nurses today will have a firsthand opportunity to observe how changes in medical technology affect the graying of America (Strunk, Ginsburg, & Banker, 2006).

■ Health Assessment of the Aging Patient

The nurse should view the health assessment of the aging patient as not just an opportunity to gather needed medical information, but as an opportunity to become acquainted with an individual who possesses a lifetime of experience. The health assessment includes both the health history and physical examination.

Interviewing the Older Patient to Obtain a Health History

Interviewing an older patient to collect patient health data is identified by the American Nurses Association (ANA) as a standard for clinical gerontological nursing care. See Chart 10–1 for an interpretation of the standards. The interview, as part of a comprehensive health assessment, is essential to developing a comprehensive plan of care for the aging adult (Congdon et al., 2001).

Interviewing and obtaining a health history from the aging patient can be both a challenging and rewarding experience. The experience can be challenging for a number of reasons related to complexity of the health history, as well as the impact of normal changes of aging, such as hearing and visual deficits. Eliciting a health history from an individual with memory deficits presents special challenges. The *National Health Interview Study 1989–91* revealed that 72% of the population over age 65 rated themselves in excellent or good health, yet 10% rated their health as poor (AOA, n.d.). Obtaining information from this group, who are more likely to be encountered during hospitalization, can be time consuming, yet it is essential to providing quality nursing care.

Cultural Considerations

Cultural considerations must also be taken into account when interviewing and obtaining a health history from the aging patient. Many times the nurse will become involved in the hospital setting with patients and families whose cultures are different and whose traditions seem strange and foreign. It is important for the nurse to be sensitive to the needs and customs of the patients in any health care setting. Cultural variances that nurses who work with aging patients should be aware of are discussed in the following subsections and the Cultural Considerations box.

African Americans

The family is very important in African American history and values related to the family are rooted in African traditions (Willis, 1998). The elderly are highly valued in African American families.

Asian

In Asian families family authority and structure are defined by family position, which is defined by age and gender. Older family members have higher status than younger ones, and males

---

CHART 10–1	**Scope and Standards of Gerontological Nursing Practice**

One of the responsibilities of the American Nurses Association (ANA) is to define the scope and standards of nursing practice. The *Standards of Clinical Nursing Practice* published in 1998 apply to all professional nurses. The *Scope and Standards of Gerontological Nursing Practice* contain criteria for expectations and competent care associated with the basic and advanced clinical practice of gerontological nursing. This includes nursing care demonstrated through assessment, diagnosis, outcome identification, planning, implementation, and evaluation. These processes form the foundation of clinical decision making that applies to all gerontological nurses.

Source: American Nurses Association. (2004). *Scope and standards of gerontologic nursing practice* (2nd ed.). Washington, DC: Author.

CULTURAL CONSIDERATIONS for Aging Patients

Culturally competent health care systems are those that provide culturally and linguistically appropriate services. An inability to communicate with a patient or insensitivity to cultural differences can result in a compromise in the quality of health care (Anderson, Scrimshaw, Fullilove, Fielding, & Normand, 2003). It is extremely important for the nurse to be cognizant of the cultural values of the patient and family related to aging. It is crucial that, as health care professionals, nurses understand that cultural values often are the driving forces guiding daily behavior. Cultural norms of family life and the role of elderly family members will have an impact on how the elderly are treated within society and the family. Cultural competence demands that nurses look at patients through both their own eyes and the eyes of patients and family members.

hold higher positions than females. Mutual support, cooperation, and interdependence also characterize the family, which is patriarchal in nature. Problems generally are solved within the family, and a sense of family honor and pride limits the amount and type of information to be shared with counselors or other professionals. Elders are venerated in Asia, assuming a place of great respect. As Asian immigrants grow older in the United States, they are exposed to a health care system that is very different from how they were socialized. It is a more demanding task to age in a society where their contributions are devalued, compared to a society where elders are treated with deference (Kao & Lam, 1995).

Hispanic/Latino

The Hispanic/Latino population also is a very diverse ethnic group. The family is of paramount value, which is influenced by both the Spaniards' Catholic religion as well as the values stemming from the indigenous people of the Americas. The family is an extended system that includes more than just blood relations and those related by marriage; it also includes fictive kin adopted through relationships. It is not uncommon to transfer children from one family to another during times of hardship and crises, and mutual help, protection, and caregiving are provided. In the Hispanic/Latino culture, self-sufficiency is not expected for the elderly. Children are obligated to provide care and to respect their elderly parents (Falicov, 1998).

Native American

Native Americans encompass people with many different languages, religions, organizations, and relationships with the U.S. government. The family is regarded as the cornerstone for emotional, social, and economic well-being for individuals (Red Horse, 1981). Extended family members assume very different roles. The primary relationship is not necessarily with the parents, but instead with the grandparents who assume the caregiver and disciplinarian role. Elderly family members are highly regarded. The aged are believed to be the repository of wisdom, and their role is to teach the young the traditions, customs, legends, and myths of the tribe. Consequently, in their old age they are taken care of by the tribe. Consensus often is the goal, and in decision-making processes, individuals often spend a lot of time trying to achieve consensus and harmony.

One can conclude from the brief discussion of four different cultures and the role of society in each one of them that their re-

sponse to aging and health care may be quite different. The role of the family, the environment, and manner of caring for patients vary (Mazanec & Tyler, 2003). A full discussion of cultural competence and the role of the health care provider is discussed in Chapter 1 ⊕.

People over the age of 65 in the United States account for more than one-third of all hospital stays. Most nurses will care for an aging patient on a typical medical–surgical nursing unit, necessitating the need for obtaining a health history in the hospital environment. It is useful to initially inquire about the individual's present health problem, which usually is the reason the individual has been hospitalized. It is important to determine the patient's perceptions of his health status and then obtain corroborating information from the medical record. It is important to find out how the hospitalization and illness have affected the aging patient's life, as well as the lives of family members.

Past Medical History

The next step is to interview the individual to obtain the past medical history. Collecting patient health data is essential to developing a comprehensive plan of care as identified by the ANA scope and standards of gerontological nursing care, which were shown earlier in Chart 10–1 (Congdon et al., 2001). If the patient is unable to give her medical history, the information from the medical record may be referenced and family members interviewed to fill in the "information gaps." In addition to recording medical diagnoses, obtaining information as to the length of time an individual has had a medical condition is useful. For example, the nursing management and teaching of a patient who is newly diagnosed with diabetes and has been prescribed oral medications are quite different than the management and teaching of an individual who is hospitalized with diabetic complications and has been on insulin for more than 20 years. When obtaining the past medical history, the following questions are useful to ask:

- What medical problems do you have?
- How long have you had these problems?
- What treatment have you sought in the past?
- Have you had any past surgeries? If so, when (the date), and were they successful?
- What medications are you taking?
- Do you have any history of communicable diseases such as TB, hepatitis, HIV?

Psychosocial History

Because psychosocial issues impact one's health status, a psychosocial history is an essential component of the health history. The nurse should keep in mind that education and socioeconomic status may play a role in a patient's vocabulary, self-expression, ability to comprehend, and ability to learn (Lesser, Hughes, Jemelka, & Kumar, 2005). Some questions a nurse might ask when obtaining the psychosocial history include the following:

- Where do you live? Do you live alone? Are you married?
- Do you have any history of accidents or falls?
- If you require assistance with your grooming, hygiene, or other activities of daily living (ADLs), who is available to help you?

- If you had an emergency such as falling or feeling ill, who would you contact?
- What did you do for employment when you were younger?
- Do you have children? Where do they live? Are they involved in your life/care?

Health habits must be explored as well. Questions to ask may include the following:

- Do you currently smoke tobacco? How many packs per day for how many years?
- If you have quit smoking, what was the date you quit? Have you ever had any abnormal chest x-rays?
- Do you drink alcohol? If so, how much and how often?
- Do you exercise? If so, how much and how often?
- Do you have any problems sleeping at night?
- Do you have any problems with your bowels or urinary incontinence?

Physical Assessment of the Older Patient

Nursing assessments in the elderly, as with all adults, are best carried out using a systematic approach to the physical examination. This may be done using the head-to-toe approach or by body systems. Whatever approach is chosen, it is best to stay with the same method during every assessment, so that critical elements are not overlooked and in order to identify trends in changes more clearly.

General Impression

When assessing the elderly patient, it is important to get an overall picture of the individual by looking at his general appearance:

- Is the individual clean; thin or obese?
- Is his behavior and affect appropriate?
- Does the individual seem easily angered, restless, or agitated?
- Do the facial expressions match his speech? It is known that many illnesses may affect one's facial expressions so it is important to identify a correlation, or lack thereof, of expression with speech. For example, people with Parkinson's disease often display a "masked facies," which means that their expression looks as if they are wearing a mask. People who have a long history of use of neuroleptic drugs may exhibit lip smacking, tongue thrusting, and other facial dystonias. These are irreversible side effects attributed to a history of prolonged use of this class of medications. When the medications are discontinued, these movements often remain. Such abnormal facial muscle movements also are seen in individuals with a wide variety of neurological conditions, such as Huntington's disease, Wilson's disease, head injury, and tumors (Tovey, 2007).

Assessment of the Head and Neck

When assessing the head and neck, typical changes may be found with the aging adult. Hair becomes thinner and finer with age, but the size and shape of the skull do not change. The eyes undergo many changes as the body ages. The eyelids relax, often giving the eyes a droopy appearance. When assessing the pupils for light reflex response, one may note a thin grayish-white ring at the margins of the cornea. This normal finding is called arcus senilis. The lens become less transparent and the eyelids may appear dry due to decreased lacrimal duct production. The cornea clouds with aging, and individuals lose peripheral vision. Chapter 71 ☺ describes eye disorders in detail.

Changes in the ears are related to normal age-related hearing losses. The auricle of the ear becomes less elastic; the lobes elongate and often develop linear wrinkles. Increased hair growth is seen in the auditory canals of males. The tympanic membrane may appear dull, and atrophy of the membrane itself may make the landmarks more prominent appearing. Cerumen may be harder and drier, occluding the auditory canal. A decreased sense of smell is commonly seen, along with reduced taste sensation, in advanced old age due to atrophy of papillae on the outer edges of the tongue.

Age-Related Disorders of the Head, Neck, and Mouth

Common eyelid problems seen in the elderly include ptosis, where the eyelids partially or completely cover the pupil. The lower eyelid can turn inward, called an entropion, or may turn extremely outward, called an ectropion, exposing the tissue of the conjunctiva. Because this pinkish red tissue is normally not visible, when an ectropion develops it is often misinterpreted as an eye infection. If the lower eyelid becomes excessively dry, irritated, or infected, the ectropion can be surgically repaired. Decreased tear production may cause dry eyes, which are easily treated with artificial eyedrops or lubricants. Cataracts also are common and are caused by clouding of the crystalline lens, and can be surgically repaired if they impair vision. Vision problems, even with glasses or contact lenses, affect nearly 20% of the older population (AOA, n.d.). See Chapter 71 ☺ for more information on disorders of the eye.

Relative to the ears, cerumen impaction can become a chronic problem in the aging patient if not addressed on a routine basis. Impacted cerumen can cause hearing loss as well as vertigo. Therefore, removal should be facilitated using a softening agent, such as Debrox or regular mineral oil, and irrigation by medical personnel if wax cannot be removed during showering with warm water. Accurate hearing tests cannot be conducted unless canals are free of cerumen and the tympanic membrane is readily visualized using an otoscope. Scarring and chronic perforation of the tympanic membrane resulting from years of occupational exposure to loud sounds and ear infections contribute to hearing loss as well. In 2002, almost one-half of all older men and one-third of older women reported trouble hearing without a hearing aid (AOA, n.d.). With the increase in use of personal music players with ear buds inserted into ear canals, the need for hearing aids in the next generation is expected to increase.

Dry oral mucosa along with cheilosis (dry scaling) of the mouth can be indicative of dehydration, vitamin deficiencies, poorly fitting dentures, or the result of medication side effects. Oral assessments should always include removal of dentures, because this is an area where cancerous lesions can appear.

Respiratory Assessment

Structural changes of the thoracic cavity are often seen with aging and can affect respiratory function. **Kyphosis,** which gives the patient a "stooped over" appearance, is caused by osteoporosis and collapse of vertebrae. The chest wall becomes less compliant, and changes in the breathing pattern are seen. Inspiration tends to be shallower, and expiration requires the use of accessory muscles. As a result, the measured vital capacity is decreased, and increased residual capacity will be seen if pulmonary function tests are conducted. The ciliary function of the lungs is reduced, producing a decreased cough reflex.

Age-Related Disorders of the Respiratory System

Some common disorders of the respiratory system seen in the elderly include chronic obstructive pulmonary disease (COPD), pulmonary edema due to congestive heart failure, and pulmonary emboli. Due to physiological changes, the normal PaO_2 should be corrected for age using the formula $109 - 0.43 \times$ patient's age. The PaO_2 and pH may be outside the normal range, but the response to such change is blunted. See Chapter 36 for information on complex respiratory disorders.

An increase in **sleep apnea** and sleep disorders is common. Although older adults need as much sleep as younger people, the sleep they get occurs during the lighter stages of sleep. This sleep is not as restorative as sleep that occurs during the deeper stages of sleep (Gehrman, Diana, & Impastato, 2006). The most common sleep disorder in the older adult is **insomnia,** defined as difficulty falling asleep or staying asleep with a negative impact on daytime alertness. Sleep apnea is a sleep disorder with partial or complete obstruction of airflow. The patient must awaken to resume breathing. Diagnosis is usually made after an overnight sleep study. Treatment involves wearing a nasal positive airway pressure mask at night to keep airways open and facilitate unobstructed airflow while sleeping. Sleep apnea is discussed at length in Chapter 34 .

Cardiovascular Assessment

The heart of the aging patient undergoes normal, age-related changes. A slower heart rate often is seen due to a decrease in the normal number of pacemaker cells, and may be asymptomatic. The heart valves become thicker and more rigid, along with decreased elasticity and increased rigidity of the heart muscle itself. The point of maximal impulse (PMI) may be displaced and palpated at the fifth or sixth left intercostal space at the midclavicular line. Murmurs in the older patient do not necessarily produce symptoms, and are caused by heart valves that become stiff from fibrosis and calcification. These murmurs are best heard at the base of the heart or the aortic area. The arterial walls are more irregular in size and shape, with an increase in calcium and collagen deposits. The walls themselves are thicker, less distensible, and less pliable.

Age-Related Disorders of the Cardiovascular System

Cardiovascular disorders are not specific to the elderly; however, heart disease is the number one cause of death in older people (Tabloski, 2006). Disorders commonly seen may include systolic hypertension, valvular disease (most commonly aortic stenosis), coronary artery disease with acute myocardial infarction (MI), congestive heart failure, arrhythmias, and stroke. These specific disorders are discussed at length in Unit 8 of this text.

 *Atrial fibrillation is the most common sustained arrhythmia seen in the older patient. New-onset atrial fibrillation can be caused by other illnesses such as hyperthyroidism, electrolyte disturbances, or a myocardial infarction. Any patient reporting "palpitations" or "skipped beats" while hospitalized should be reported to the health care provider for further evaluation.*

Gastrointestinal Assessment

Some of the normal age-related changes in the gastrointestinal system contribute to the perception that the elderly are fixated on their bowels. For example, the abdominal muscles of the aging patient weaken and peristalsis decreases. The liver itself becomes smaller in size and storage capacity is reduced. Alterations in insulin release often are seen as well.

Age-Related Disorders of the Gastrointestinal System

Some of the age-related disorders in digestion are caused by *dysphagia,* difficulty swallowing. Dysphagia may be caused by poorly fitted or absent dentures. Even tooth decay can cause difficulty swallowing, resulting in decreased oral intake, weight loss, and undernutrition. Dyspepsia, gastroesophageal reflux disease (GERD), and upper gastrointestinal malignancies occur more often after age 55, and affect about one in four elderly patients (Talley, 2005). GERD is caused by the backflow of gastric or duodenal contents or both into the esophagus and past the lower esophageal sphincter. The reflux causes acute epigastric pain that can radiate to the chest or arm. Pain usually occurs after meals or when the patient lies down—the increased abdominal pressure causes reflux (Moreau, 2006). Upper endoscopy is recommended for elderly patients with symptoms that trigger an alarm, new-onset GERD, or long-standing disease. Elderly patients are at risk for more severe complications from GERD. Based on safety profiles and success in general, proton pump inhibitors (PPIs) are considered to be the first-line medication treatment for GERD in the elderly (Bacak, Patel, Tweed, & Danis, 2006).

Constipation is partially caused by the decreased peristalsis mentioned earlier, but it is also caused by many other contributing factors. A decreased thirst sensation leads to decreased fluid intake, and the use of narcotics for chronic pain management leads to slowed peristalsis, all of which results in constipation. Prolonged constipation can lead to intestinal obstruction, a medical emergency due to the potential for bowel perforation. Constipation also may be caused by a tumor. The incidence of colon cancer affects men and women equally, most commonly between the ages of 60 and 80 years (Tovey, 2007).

Genitourinary Assessment

Unlike the portrayals often seen on television, not all individuals over the age of 65 are incontinent, requiring bladder pads and incontinent briefs. The incontinence product market, however, is estimated to be a billion dollar industry, some of which can be attributed to a few of the disorders seen in the aging genitourinary system. As one ages, the pubic hair thins and grays, and the bladder capacity decreases. In females, vaginal mucosa atrophies from a decrease in estrogen, which also results in a decrease in size and elasticity of the vagina and a decrease in vaginal secretions. In males, slight testicular atrophy is seen, while the prostate gland enlarges. The scrotal sac elongates as well.

Age-Related Disorders of the Genitourinary System

Common disorders of the genitourinary system seen in the aging patient include urinary tract infections (UTIs) and urinary incontinence. More frequent UTIs are thought to be caused by changes in the urinary tract. Urinary incontinence can be caused by stress incontinence, urge incontinence, overflow incontinence, or any

Management of Bowel Routines

Clinical Problem

Management of bowel routines in the acute care setting often is inadequate. Establishing bowel routines also may be complicated if the patient has dementia. Nurses need to determine that if the patient with dementia is agitated, could the agitation be related to constipation?

Research Findings

Leonard and colleagues (2006) examined the records of more than 100,000 nursing home residents living in five states in 2002. All participants were over 60 years old and diagnosed with dementia. It was found that nearly 7% of the residents had been physically aggressive in the week before the assessment, and 10.5% had been verbally aggressive in the week before assessment. It was found that physical and verbally aggressive behavior was associated with depression, delusions, and hallucinations. Physical aggression, including hitting, shoving, scratching, or engaging in sexual abuse was also associated with constipation. The study did not find significant associations with factors such as respiratory tract infections, urinary tract infections, fever, or reported pain.

Implications for Nursing Practice

Although this study took place in nursing homes, constipation is a problem often overlooked in the acute care setting as well. The nurse can play a role in intervention through advocating for preprinted bowel care orders, as well as thorough documentation and tracking of bowel movements during hospitalization. Such simple interventions may reduce the incidence of physical aggression in elderly patients with dementia.

Critical Thinking Questions

1. If a nonverbal patient with dementia who is unable to verbalize symptoms has not had a bowel movement in 3 days even with routine bowel care, what is the best way to assess for constipation?

2. What adjustments to the bowel care regimen should be considered when a nurse receives a new order to give the patient a narcotic for pain relief?

3. If a patient is having frequent small smears of liquid stool, could the patient still be constipated?

Answers to Critical Thinking Questions appear in Appendix D.

Reference

Leonard, R., Tinetti, M. E., Allore, H. G., & Drickamer, M. A. (2006). Potentially modifiable resident characteristics that are associated with physical or verbal aggression among nursing home residents with dementia. *Archives Internal Medicine, 166,* 1295–1300.

---

combination of the three. Stress incontinence, the result of weakened bladder muscles, is most commonly seen. Urge incontinence, the second most common cause, is the result of bladder spasms, a syndrome often referred to as *overactive bladder,* which can be treated with medication. Overflow incontinence is the result of a bladder that is no longer able to contract efficiently to release urine. Incontinence occurs when urine exceeds the bladder capacity. Atrophic vaginitis, the result of decreased estrogen in the vaginal tissues, can be treated with hormone replacement, although controversial. Application of estrogen vaginal cream to the labia also is sometimes helpful.

The prostate enlarges as a normal part of aging due to a decrease of androgen and increase of estrogen, resulting in an imbalance. The increased estrogen receptors trigger the androgen receptors in the prostate gland to increase. An overgrowth of normal cells begins around the urethra and can cause partial bladder neck obstruction (Moreau, 2006). The result is urinary frequency and retention. Medications in the alpha$_1$ blocker drug class work by relaxing smooth muscle in the bladder neck and prostate. The result is an improvement in urine flow. If the prostate becomes too enlarged, surgical intervention using a transurethral approach may be indicated.

Musculoskeletal Assessment

In the aging patient, one will see normal age-related changes of the musculoskeletal system. A slower reaction time, along with poorer coordination and decreased muscle strength, can all contribute to difficulties with gait. A loss of bone beginning during the fourth decade of life can affect posture and place an individual at risk for developing osteoporosis.

Age-Related Disorders of the Musculoskeletal System

Age-related disorders of the musculoskeletal system include disabilities caused by osteoarthritis, rheumatoid arthritis, gout, osteoporosis, bunions, and hammertoes. Osteoarthritis is the most common type of arthritis, affecting women more than men, with joints of the hand being the most common site affected (Figure 10–1 ■). Hip joints and knee joints also can be affected. Rheumatoid arthritis affects women and men over the age of 65 equally,

FIGURE 10–1 ■ Osteoarthritic hands.

and complications can affect mobility and one's ability to carry out ADLs, such as feeding.

Gout is a syndrome caused by deposition of urate crystals in joints and the skin. It causes acute monoarthritis and crystal deposits, called tophi, in the skin. It is more common in older people, and more common in men. Other risk factors include nonwhite ethnicity; obesity; consumption of alcohol, meat, and fish; and use of diuretics. The Mayo Clinic reported that among black men, the annual incidence of gout was 3.1/1,000 versus 1.8/1,000 in white men. Colchicine has been used for many years to treat acute gout, yet it is unknown whether this treatment is effective. The effectiveness of allopurinol in reducing the risk of recurrent attacks compared to placebo or other treatments is unknown as well (Mayo Clinic, 2007a, 2007b; Tovey, 2007).

Osteoporosis is a skeletal disorder characterized by compromised bone strength that places an individual at increased risk for fracture (National Institutes of Health Consensus Development Panel, 2001). Fractures due to osteoporosis can permanently affect function and quality of life. With the advent of bone mineral density (BMD) screening studies, health care providers are able to diagnose osteoporosis before a fracture occurs. The **U.S. Preventive Services Task Force (USPSTF),** sponsored by the Agency for Healthcare Research and Quality (AHRQ), is an independent panel of private sector experts in prevention and primary care. This panel develops recommendations about which preventive services should be incorporated routinely into primary medical care and for which populations. These are considered to be the "gold standards" for clinical preventive services based on documented evidence regarding effectiveness and outcomes of screening, counseling, and preventive medications. The USPSTF recommends bone mineral density screening at least once at age 65, with no recommendations as to how often the test should be repeated (National Guideline Clearing House, 2007). The universal recommendations for management of osteoporosis include oral calcium 1,200 mg/day, oral vitamin D 800 international units/day, fall prevention, tobacco avoidance, weight-bearing exercise, and no more than moderate alcohol consumption. Pharmacologic management should be considered based on risk factors for osteoporosis and BMD screening results. Bisphosphonates also have been shown to increase bone mineral density in the spine and hip (Reuben et al., 2007).

Bony deformities of the feet often are seen as a result of years of poorly fitting footwear and in women, years of wearing tight-fitting, high-heeled shoes. It has been said that "feet only get uglier with age." Bunions are seen in the aging patient from years of the bones in the toes being pushed to fit into tight shoes (Figure 10–2 ■). The bones of the toes take on an angled appearance, and in severe cases, the first toe of the foot will be permanently pushed over the second and third toe. These deformities can only be corrected surgically, where the bones of the feet are essentially "broken" and recast and reset into their proper alignment.

Skin Assessment
Assessment of the skin in the aging patient requires the same techniques one would use in assessing any patient, including in-

FIGURE 10–2 ■ Bunion feet.

spection of the scalp, head, neck, trunk, and limbs. The skin should be palpated to determine temperature, moisture, thickness, texture, and turgor. The amount of subcutaneous tissue present below the surface of the skin in the aging patient is decreased; thus, skin turgor may not be a reliable indicator for hydration status. Common skin changes in the aging patient include the presence of seborrheic or senile keratoses (Figure 10–3 ■), senile lentigines also known as "liver spots," cherry angiomas, and development of skin tags. Assessment of the skin is discussed more in Chapter 65 ⊙ .

Age-Related Disorders of the Integumentary System
The most common skin disorders in the elderly are skin cancers, which are the result of many years of unprotected skin exposure to the sun. Many older individuals grew up on farms or worked

FIGURE 10–3 ■ Seborrheic keratoses.

many years doing physical labor under direct exposure to the sun's rays, without the benefit of topically applied sunscreen. Thus, in their older years, many aging patients present with skin cancers, such as basal cell cancers, or precancerous lesions, such as actinic keratoses. Treatment includes surgical excision, or removal via desiccation for precancerous lesions. Herpes zoster, which produces blistering lesions along a specific dermatome, also is more commonly found in the aging patient. The USPSTF recommends a yearly skin exam in individuals aged 65 and older (AHRQ, 2007).

Dry skin is estimated to be present in approximately 75% of individuals 75 years and older (Mac-Mary, Sainthillier & Humbert, 2004). It is worse during the winter when the air is drier, and develops when the skin loses water to the air. Keratosis and pruritus are chronic problems for many aging patients, fueling an industry that sells lotions, creams, and ointments to treat dry, itchy skin.

Neurological Assessment

Contrary to common myths regarding aging, it is not routine for older people to become senile or demented. However, by age 85, the risk of developing Alzheimer's disease, a type of dementia, is nearly 50% (Alzheimer's Association, 2006). Neurological assessment is covered in detail in Chapter 28 ☞. However, there are normal changes seen in the aging patient that must be taken into consideration. The brain atrophies with age, but there are no relationships between shrinkage and change in cognition. The sense of taste and smell decrease in the aging patient. Sometimes there is a lack of awareness about food that has spoiled. This predisposes individuals to nutritional problems. Changes in reflexes include decreased deep tendon reflexes in the legs and increased reflexes in the arms, with decreased vibratory sense. There is some decrease in position sense as well. There are many medical conditions associated with pain in the older adult, but certain types of pain may be less severe than others. This may explain why a younger adult experiencing a myocardial infarction will report crushing chest pain, and the aging patient may report vague symptoms of discomfort, such as heartburn (Tabloski, 2006).

Age-Related Disorders of the Neurological System

Due to the changes just mentioned, neurological disease may be more difficult to assess in the elderly. Some abnormal neurological findings may in fact be "normal." Some disorders, such as normal pressure hydrocephalus (NPH) and dementia, may involve subtle changes in the mental status of the patient. NPH is an abnormal increase of cerebrospinal fluid (CSF) in the brain's ventricles, which occurs when the normal flow of CSF throughout the brain and spinal cord is blocked in some way. While this can occur in people of any age, it is most common in the elderly population. It may result from a subarachnoid hemorrhage, head trauma, infection, tumor, or complications of surgery. It also may occur when none of these factors is present; in these cases the cause of the disorder is unknown. Symptoms of NPH include progressive mental impairment and dementia, problems with walking, and impaired bladder control, leading to urinary frequency and/or incontinence. The person also may have a general slowing of movements, with some complaining of feeling as though her feet are stuck. This abnormal state is hard to diagnose because the symptoms often resemble other neurolog-

ical disorders, such as Alzheimer's disease, Parkinson's disease, and Creutzfeldt-Jakob disease (National Institute of Neurological Disorders and Stroke, 2007). Treatment for NPH involves surgical placement of a shunt in the brain to drain excess CSF into the abdomen where it can be absorbed. If not treated, the symptoms of NPH usually get worse over time. The success of treatment with shunts varies, but is generally favorable. Early diagnosis and treatment improves the chance of a good recovery.

The term **dementia** describes a group of symptoms that are caused by changes in brain function (destruction of brain cells) that seriously affect a person's ability to carry out daily activities (National Institute on Aging, 2006). It becomes hard for a person to remember, learn, and communicate, and the condition progresses to the point where it is hard for the person to take care of himself. Presenting symptoms include:

- Asking the same questions repeatedly
- Becoming lost in familiar places
- Being unable to follow directions
- Getting disoriented about time, people, and places
- Neglecting personal safety, hygiene, and nutrition.

Dementia also may change a person's mood and personality. At first, memory loss and trouble thinking clearly may bother the person who has dementia. Later, disruptive behavior and other problems may start, but the person who has dementia may not be aware of these problems.

People with dementia lose their abilities at different rates. It is caused by many conditions some of which are reversible and some are not. Reversible conditions can be caused by a high fever, dehydration, vitamin deficiency and poor nutrition, medication reactions, thyroid problems, or a minor head injury. Sometimes older people have emotional problems that can be mistaken for dementia. Feeling sad, lonely, worried, or bored may be more common for older people facing retirement or coping with the death of a spouse. Emotional problems and the medical problems previously noted should be professionally addressed. Family support also is critical to the care of people with dementia.

The two most common forms of dementia in older people are Alzheimer's disease (AD) and multiple-infarct dementia, sometimes referred to as vascular dementia. These types of dementia are irreversible. Alzheimer's disease is discussed in detail in Chapter 31 ☞ as a chronic neurological disease.

With multiple-infarct dementia, a series of strokes or changes in the brain's blood supply may result in the death of brain tissue. The location in the brain where the strokes occur and the severity of the strokes determine the seriousness of the problem and the symptoms that arise. Symptoms usually begin abruptly and progress in a stepwise fashion with repeated strokes. Strokes are fully discussed in Chapter 30 ☞.

Delirium is a sudden, fluctuating, and usually reversible cognitive disorder characterized by a disturbance in consciousness with decreased attention and a change in cognition or development of a perceptual disturbance that develops over a short period of time and tends to fluctuate throughout the day (American Psychiatric Association, 1994; Reuben et al., 2007). This change in cognition often manifests itself in disruptive behaviors in the hospital setting, such as disrobing, pulling out IV lines, striking out at caregivers, and resisting nursing care. Its incidence in the hospital setting is about 20%, with postoperative incidence up to 72%. It is an abnormal mental state, not a disease, and usually a sign of a newly developed disorder, which affects about one-third of hospitalized people age 70 or older.

Detection of delirium is difficult but identification is critical. The Confusion Assessment Method (CAM) is a standardized tool any clinician can use to identify delirium quickly and accurately (Inouye et al., 1990). The short version consists of four features found to have the greatest ability to distinguish delirium from other types of cognitive impairment. It identifies the presence or absence of delirium but does not assess the severity. The first two features that must be present for delirium to be diagnosed are evidence of an acute change in mental status from the patient's baseline or a fluctuation in behavior throughout the day and difficulty focusing attention. The presence of these features and either evidence of disorganized thinking, such as rambling or illogical conversation or an altered level of consciousness, must be present for diagnosis (Waszynski, 2007).

Once delirium is diagnosed, causative factors such as infection or metabolic derangement must be identified and treated. Urinary tract infections in the elderly are the most common cause of delirium, and polypharmacy is the second most common cause (Voyer, Cole, McCusker, & Belzile, 2006). Metabolic disorders such as hypo- or hypernatremia must be corrected as well. Delirium is self-limiting once the underlying problem has been corrected, and usually resolves after 5 days. In extreme cases symptoms can last 3 to 6 months (Mezey, Fulmer, Abraham, & Zwicker, 2003). If confusion and disorientation persist, other neurological disorders such as dementia must be considered. Dementia is diagnosed within 3 years in 60% of hospitalized patients with delirium (Voyer et al., 2006).

The USPSTF recommends cognitive impairment screening annually for the individual age 65 and older (AHRQ, 2007). The **Folstein Mini-Mental State Exam** is one common screening tool used by clinicians in evaluating dementia. It is easily administered after some training. The scoring ranges from 0 to 30 points, with 0 to 10 points typically scored for an individual with advanced dementia, 10 to 20 for moderate dementia, 21 to 26 points seen in mild dementia, and 27 to 30 considered normal, with adjustments made for levels of education (Folstein, Folstein, & McHugh, 1975).

Within the last 10 years, there has been increasing recognition of the elderly experiencing late-onset schizophrenia and bipolar disorders (Howard et al., 2000; Jeste, Paulsen, & Harris, 2000; Wetherell & Jeste, 2004). Late-onset schizophrenia is being diagnosed more frequently in old age and represents a sizable minority of patients diagnosed with schizophrenia (Wetherell & Jeste, 2004). This tends to be attributed to organic factors. Late-onset schizophrenia often is characterized by bizarre delusion and auditory hallucinations. Systematized delusions of physical or mental influence are seen in many of the patients, with grandiose, erotic, or somatic delusions occurring in some cases. Depressive symptoms also may be present. Persons with late-onset schizophrenia tend to have a family history of schizophrenia and have often been considered by others to be eccentric, reserved, and suspicious (Jeste et al., 2000).

Bipolor disorders in the elderly are clinically heterogeneous and present with various courses, switching from recurrent depression to mania, early onset or late bipolar disorders (Aziz, Lorberg, & Tampi, 2006). They can take on uncommon symptoms such as depressive or mixed behaviors, psychosis, mental confusion, or dementia. The prognosis of bipolar disorders in the elderly is poor due to the high prevalence of recurrences, associated somatic disorders, reduced survival, and severe handicap. As with late-onset schizophrenia, there is an immediate need for collaboration between patients, families, and clinicians to provide health care services for this population.

Parkinson's disease is a neurodegenerative disorder associated with asymmetrical bradykinesia, hypokinesia, and rigidity. More information on this disorder is presented in Chapter 31 ☺. It occurs equally in both sexes, and has a mean age onset of 65 years, with the greatest prevalence at 3.5% in the 85- to 89-year-old age group. It currently is incurable; however, dopamine agonists are used to reduce dyskinesias and motor fluctuation, and levodopa is being used to improve motor function. In patients with later onset Parkinson's disease, pallidal surgery has been associated with a high incidence of adverse effects (Tovey, 2007).

Stroke, also discussed under multiple-infarct dementia, is one of the neurological disorders affecting the elderly that can result in the greatest degree of disability. It is defined as loss of cerebral function lasting more than 24 hours or leading to death, with no apparent cause other than that of vascular origin. Ischemic stroke is caused by vascular insufficiency, often from a thromboembolism; hemorrhagic stroke is caused by a hemorrhage of a vessel. Strokes and the ramifications for nursing care are discussed in Chapter 30 ☺.

◼ Health Care Promotion and Preventive Care

The USPSTF is one of several groups that make recommendations for appropriate preventive services and screening exams in adults age 65 and older. As mentioned earlier, the USPSTF is comprised of an independent panel of experts in primary care and preventive care that systematically reviews the evidence and effectiveness of clinical preventive services and develops recommendations (AHRQ, 2007). However, such recommendations do not specifically address the appropriateness of such testing in the frail aging patient with multiple medical problems, functional decline, and a limited life expectancy. When interpreting the guidelines, it is the responsibility of the aging patient and her health care provider to discuss which recommendations are appropriate, taking all of the above factors and the individual's personal wishes into consideration.

Immunizations

Immunizations are one way the aging adult can proactively prevent potential debilitating illnesses. Hospitalization provides an opportunity for patients to update their immunizations. Many hospitals have preprinted order sheets to increase the incidence of immunization in the elderly population. Vaccines in the aging adult are about 50% to 60% effective in preventing hospitalizations from pneumonia and 80% effective in preventing death (Kaldy, 2006). Pneumococcal infections cause an estimated

40,000 deaths each year in the United States, causing more deaths than any other vaccine-preventable bacterial disease (Vlassova & Jackson, 2005). Influenza, which typically affects individuals during the winter months, has been associated with approximately 36,000 deaths per year in the United States during the time period from 1990 to 1999 (Smith et al., 2006).

Pneumococcal Vaccine

Streptococcus pneumonia is the organism responsible for pneumococcal pneumonia. All adults over 65 years old are candidates for initial vaccination, with a recommendation for revaccination for adults at age 65 who may have received the vaccination at an earlier age due to chronic health conditions. The USPSTF recommends a pneumonia vaccination once at age 65, and suggests people in that age group consider repeating the vaccine every 6 to 7 years (AHRQ, 2007). The vaccine is administered intramuscularly in the deltoid muscle or subcutaneously. It can be given with the influenza vaccine via a separate injection in the other arm without an increase in the severity of reactions or by affecting antibody response.

Influenza Vaccine

Influenza vaccines contain three virus strains: two type A and one type B. During the influenza season, selected federal "sentinel reporters" who are health care providers submit nasal swabs of individuals who present to health care institutions with influenza-type symptoms. These data are used to develop the influenza vaccine for the upcoming year. In this way, the vaccine should represent the most common viruses to which individuals will likely be exposed in the upcoming influenza season. The influenza vaccine will not always prevent the aging patient from contracting the flu; studies have shown the vaccine prevents severe illness, complications such as the development of pneumonia, and death (Kaldy, 2006). The USPSTF recommends annual influenza immunization in all individuals age 65 and older (AHRQ, 2007). The *Healthy People 2010* strategy for adult immunizations is outlined in the National Guidelines box.

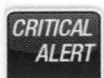 *The influenza vaccine is made from egg-grown viruses that are not infectious. Patients cannot get the flu from the vaccination; however, it is absolutely contraindicated in those who have a hypersensitivity to egg protein. The live attenuated influenza nasal vaccine should not be administered to seniors.*

Tetanus Vaccine

Many older adults are not aware that they need a tetanus immunization, and others have poor recollection of their immunization history (Fernandes, Flynn, & Masaki, 2003). Immunization against tetanus is recommended every 10 years in adults over 65 years of age (AHRQ, 2007). The vaccine is usually available in multiple-dose vials as tetanus-diphtheria toxoid (Td). The dosage for adults is 0.5 mL administered intramuscularly. The vaccine must be kept in the refrigerator to maintain potency of the vaccine.

Herpes Zoster Vaccine

Herpes zoster virus vaccine is used to prevent herpes zoster virus, also known as shingles, in people over age 60. It contains live, attenuated varicella-zoster virus in a dose 14 times greater than the varicella (chickenpox) vaccine. This larger dose is needed to boost immunity against shingles in older persons. Herpes zoster virus vaccine decreases the occurrence of herpes zoster by about half, and for those who do get herpes zoster, it reduces the severity and risk of developing postherpetic neuralgia. This is important because the pain that is associated with postherpetic neuralgia can be debilitating and persist long after the zoster rash has resolved.

About 50 million people are candidates to receive this vaccine. The cost of the vaccine is approximately $186 per dose, and is reimbursable under Medicare Part D. A single dose of zoster vaccine is recommended for adults age 60 or older whether or not they report a prior episode of herpes zoster. The Advisory Committee on Immunization Practices voted to recommend use of the vaccine for the prevention of postherpetic neuralgia in this same age group (DeYoung & Baty, 2007).

Screening Exams

Addressing screening exams in the aging patient can be a challenge for several reasons. First, unlike children who require certain exams and immunizations both to ensure normal growth and development as well as to enter school, there are no such requirements for seniors. Screening recommendations for seniors are not mandated, and must take into account the comorbidities and functional status of the individual. Second, when considering screening exams, the health care provider needs to know what will be done with the information obtained from the exam. If a patient indicates that he would not pursue treatment if cancer were found as a result of a screening test, ordering the test is most likely unnecessary. Finally, a factor that must be considered is whether the benefit of the test outweighs the burden of administering the test itself. All of these decisions require the health care provider to fully discuss the screening exam with the patient in order to make informed decisions while taking the individual's wishes into account.

Vision

The USPSTF recommends visual screening and full eye exam on an annual basis for all individuals age 65 and older (AHRQ, 2007).

NATIONAL GUIDELINES *Healthy People 2010*

Healthy People 2010 has identified an increase in adults vaccinated as one of its goals. In 1998, 64% of community-dwelling adults ages 65 and older had received the influenza vaccine, and 46% had received the pneumococcal vaccine. The 2010 targets for vaccination are as follows: 90% target for both the influenza and pneumococcal vaccine.

In the institutionalized adult (i.e., a person living in a nursing home), 59% received the influenza vaccine in 1997, and only 25% had received the pneumococcal vaccine. *Healthy People 2010's* targets for vaccination are 90% for both vaccines—the same target as for community-dwelling adults ages 65 and older.

Source: U.S. Department of Health and Human Services. (2000). Increase in adults vaccinated (Objectives 14-29a–f). In *Healthy People 2010: Understanding and improving health.* Retrieved February 11, 2007, from http://www.healthypeople.gov/document/html/objectives/14-29.htm

MyNursingKit | Medicare

MyNursingKit | Healthy People 2010 Number 14 Objective 29

Visual impairment is defined as visual acuity 20/40 or worse. Legal blindness is defined as 20/200 or worse. Such screening is important because some visual changes occur slowly over many years. The aging patient may not be aware that visual acuity has declined. Acuity testing and tonometry can identify refractive problems, cataracts, age-related macular degeneration, diabetic retinopathy, and glaucoma (Reuben et al., 2007). Mobile optometrists are available in some communities to travel to private homes, senior communities, and long-term care settings to evaluate individuals who are unable to travel to a traditional medical office. This is especially useful for evaluating individuals with dementia who may need eyeglasses but become agitated when moved from their familiar environment.

Hearing

Hearing loss is the most common sensory impairment in the older adult. The USPSTF recommends hearing impairment screening on a yearly basis for all individuals age 65 and older (AHRQ, 2007). The canals must be free of cerumen for reliable testing. Evaluation consists of screening for hearing problems (medical history, questionnaire) and audiometry, which documents the decibel loss across frequencies along with the pattern of loss. Based on the findings, augmentation with hearing aids may be considered (Reuben et al., 2007). Hearing aids can cost up to $5,000 per pair. On admission, history relating to hearing should be collected as part of the initial assessment. As the nurse develops a plan of care relating to the patient's hearing deficits, directions for the management of the patient's hearing aids must be relayed to all care providers. Developing a plan of care is one of the components of the ANA standards of clinical gerontological nursing care (Congdon et al., 2001). The ANA standards are shown earlier in the chapter in Chart 10–1 (p. 170).

Breast Exams/Breast Cancer Screening

The USPSTF recommends monthly breast self-exams and mammograms every 1 to 2 years up to the age of 70. For those over the age of 70, mammography should be continued for those who have a "reasonable life expectancy" (AHRQ, 2007). However, the term *reasonable life expectancy* has not been defined, and it is not clear as to who determines whether an individual has a reasonable life expectancy.

Pap Smears

The USPSTF recommends a Pap smear at least every 3 years in women age 65 and older. However, Pap smears may be stopped after age 65 if there is one negative Pap smear at age 65 and the woman is low risk (USPSTF, n.d.). A woman at low risk is one with an established sexual partner, history of consistent prior screening, and no history of abnormal Pap smears. Women without a cervix should not have Pap smears (Reuben et al., 2007; USPSTF, n.d.).

Prostate Exam/Prostate Cancer Screening

Prostate cancer is the most common cancer other than skin cancers that affects men. About 1 in 6 men will be diagnosed with prostate cancer during their lifetime, but only 1 in 34 will die from it (American Cancer Society, n.d.).The USPSTF recommends a yearly prostate surface antigen (PSA) test and a digital rectal exam (DRE) in males age 65 and older. However, it has been noted that men over the age of 75 with a negative DRE rarely die from prostate cancer, fueling the debate as to who should be screened in this population (Tabloski, 2006).

Prostate cancers tend to be slow growing in older patients, and for those with multiple comorbidities there is a greater chance death will occur from a disease process other than

Mammogram Screenings in Elderly Patients

Clinical Problem

When considering health promotion and disease prevention, it is debatable as to who over the age of 70 should receive screening mammograms. The recommendation for those over 70 is to only screen those with a "reasonable life expectancy," yet there is no definition of what "reasonable life expectancy" means. What criteria should be used when referring for a mammogram?

Research Findings

Schonberg and colleagues (2004) surveyed 882 women ages 80 and over to examine the relationship between health status and screening mammograms in the previous 2 years. They found that more than half of the women over age 80 in the United States receive screening mammograms. Of women likely to have life expectancies of less than 5 years due to poor health, nearly 40% received screening mammography.

Implications for Nursing Practice

When addressing the need for a mammogram, the nurse must not just consider the exam itself, but consider the aging patient's overall condition. If the patient is bedbound or unable to participate due to inability to remain still or follow instructions, a mammogram may not be appropriate. For patients with cognitive disorders or chronic

illnesses, the nurse needs to ask this question: "If an abnormality were found, would the patient seek treatment?"

Critical Thinking Questions

1. A patient refused mammograms when she was mentally alert and now has advanced dementia. Her daughter requests you schedule her for a mammogram. What should you do?

2. You are performing your usual nursing admission assessment on a medical–surgical floor on an elderly female with advanced dementia. You note a palpable golf ball–sized mass on the right breast. The patient's daughter is out in the waiting room. What should you do?

3. Your patient is only able to stand for short periods of time, but otherwise requires a wheelchair. Is she able to obtain a mammogram?

Answers to Critical Thinking Questions appear in Appendix D.

Reference

Schonberg, M. A., McCarthy, E. P., Davis, R. B., Phillips, R. S., & Hamel, M. B. (2004). Breast cancer screening in women aged 80 and older: Results from a national survey. *Journal of the American Geriatrics Society, 52,* 1688–1695.

EVIDENCE-BASED PRACTICE

prostate cancer. Older men should discuss this subject with their primary care provider. PSA levels can be falsely elevated when obtained during hospitalization due to catheterization and infection, thus they should not routinely be obtained during hospitalization.

Colon Cancer Screening

Colorectal cancer is the fourth most common cancer in the United States and the second leading cause of death from cancer (AHRQ, 2007). The USPSTF recommends colon cancer screening consisting of fecal occult blood testing (FOBT), sigmoidoscopy, and colonoscopy starting at age 50 for those at average risk for colorectal cancer. Those at high risk, for example, an individual with a first-degree relative diagnosed with colon cancer before age 60, may consider screening at an earlier age. For those age 65 and older, FOBT is recommended yearly, sigmoidoscopy every 5 years, and colonoscopy every 10 years. The appropriate age to discontinue colorectal cancer screening is not known. Most screening studies have restricted enrollees to those less than 80 years of age. The burden of screening may outweigh potential benefits in patients with advanced age and comorbid conditions that limit life expectancy. Thus, the aging patient needs to discuss benefits and potential harms associated with each screening test with a health care provider before deciding on a screening strategy (AHRQ, 2007).

◼ Pharmacology and the Aging Patient

There has been a major emphasis in the health care community on appropriate medications for the aging patient with a focus on prevention of complications from medications inappropriately prescribed (Beers, 1997; Bonk, Krown, Matuszewski, & Oinonen, 2006; Fick et al., 2003; Maio et al., 2006). This focus evolved from publication in 1991 of criteria identifying inappropriate medication use in the nursing home population. These criteria were initially developed to aid researchers in evaluating the quality of prescribing, drug utilization systems, and educational efforts in the nursing home setting. Further updates have identified medications or medication classes that should generally be avoided in persons 65 or older for two reasons. First, there are medications that are either ineffective or pose unnecessarily high risk for older persons and a safer alternative is available. Second, there are medications that should not be used in older persons known to have specific medical conditions (Fick et al., 2003). These criteria, now known as the *Beers criteria,* have been expanded to apply to older individuals living in the community, because inappropriate prescribing by health care providers has been shown to occur in both inpatient and outpatient settings (Beers, 1997; Maio et al., 2006). An adult over the age of 65 takes an average of 5.7 medications each day (American Society of Health-System Pharmacists, 2006). Often these medications may be unnecessary or inappropriately prescribed. Five percent to 15% of hospital admissions in elderly patients may be linked to drug-related problems or toxic drug effects (Mezey et al., 2003). In one study, a greater number of medications taken were associated with weight loss and impaired balance in elderly patients, after adjustment for chronic illness (Agostini, Han, & Tinetti, 2004).

Adverse drug reactions (ADRs) or **adverse drug events (ADEs)** can occur when a patient takes a medication that has been appropriately or inappropriately prescribed. An ADE is defined as "noxious and unintended patient events, such as symptoms, signs, and laboratory abnormalities caused by a drug" (Roehl, Talati, & Parks, 2006). Studies have shown that at least one inappropriate medication had been prescribed for 40% of nursing home residents and 21% of elderly living in the community (Bonk et al., 2006; Liu & Christensen, 2002; Maio et al., 2006).

Ethnic background also may place an individual at risk for ADEs. One meta-analysis of studies found this to be the case for cardiovascular medications in various ethnic groups. For example, black patients taking angiotensin converting enzyme (ACE) inhibitors are three times more likely to experience angioedema compared with nonblack patients. East Asian patients are more likely to experience cough due to ACE inhibitors compared to white patients. Black patients have a higher risk of moderate or severe bleeding following thrombolytic therapy compared to nonblack patients. Thus, ethnic background must be considered in individuals experiencing ADEs (McDowell, Coleman, & Ferner, 2006).

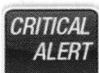 *One method to ensure that patients are not re-prescribed medications that previously caused an adverse reaction is to enter those medications in the allergy section of the patient's chart or electronic medical record, along with the reactions the patient experienced. Although not a true drug allergy, listing drug intolerances along with their adverse reaction as part of the medical record will direct providers to choose another medication for a particular condition when prescribing.*

Polypharmacy

Polypharmacy is one of the major medication issues affecting the aging patient. **Polypharmacy** is defined as the administration of many drugs together, and the administration of excessive medications (*Polypharmacy,* 2007). However, the definition itself is controversial and varies from study to study, making application of research results in the clinical setting challenging. In the clinical setting, polypharmacy occurs when an individual is using more medications than is clinically indicated. This includes prescription medications, over-the-counter (OTC) medications, and nontraditional medications. This phenomenon called polypharmacy can occur in the acute care setting, in a structured care setting such as an assisted living facility, or at home.

A thorough nursing assessment on admission to the hospital provides an opportunity to identify and eliminate polypharmacy. The following information should be collected:

- Medical diagnoses and self-diagnosed health problems
- Known drug allergies
- History of previous adverse drug reactions
- All prescribed medications taken
- All OTC medications taken
- All nontraditional medications taken
- Length of time each medication has been taken
- Actual amounts of each medication taken and how often
- Reason for taking each medication, any adverse effects
- Any problems with taking the medication in its prescribed form (*Medication Assessment,* 2005).

Medication Administration Principles for the Aging Patient

Medication administration principles for the aging patient go beyond practicing the "five rights" of medication administration. With regard to dosing, the adage to "start low, and go slow" should be followed. Often a nurse is given a choice of a range of doses for an as-needed medication. In the aging patient, the nurse should start with a lower dose than might be typically administered to a younger patient. The aging patient takes longer to metabolize and excrete medications due to decreased renal and hepatic function. Some medication reference guides list geriatric doses, which is helpful. For medications excreted renally, the nurse can calculate the estimated creatinine clearance. Serum creatinine does not accurately reflect renal function in the aging patient due to decreased lean body mass. The Cockcroft-Gault formula is used to estimate creatinine clearance (CrCl):

$$Creatinine\ clearance = \frac{(140 - age) \times weight\ (kg)}{Plasma\ creatinine\ (mg/dl) \times 2.72} (\times\ 0.85\ for\ women)$$

For drugs excreted via the kidneys, dosage adjustments may be necessary if CrCl < 60 (Roehl et al., 2006).

Many hospitalized patients have impaired swallowing or are unable to swallow medications in the traditional pill form due to altered cognition with agitation. These patients present a challenge for the nurse who must be knowledgeable about other possible methods for medication administration. For example, a patient requiring long-term pain management who is unable to swallow or take pain medications on a consistent basis may be appropriate for medication delivery via a transdermal patch (Figure 10–4 ■, p. 182). A transdermal patch delivers a continuous amount of pain medication and only requires changing every 72 hours. This method of medication delivery also may reduce caregiver burden. Chart 10-2 (p. 183) lists some of the medications with potential adverse outcomes for the aging patient.

 CRITICAL ALERT *Medications with an enteric coating as well as sustained-release medications cannot be crushed. If the patient requires her medications to be crushed or administered via nasogastric or gastrostomy tube, notify the physician or health care professional so that the equivalent short-acting medication may be ordered and crushed. Remember, if the medication is difficult to crush, there is a reason why!*

Medication Administration for Aging Patients

Clinical Problem
With all of the various mechanisms in which medications are metabolized in the elderly, how is a nurse to know which ones are not appropriate in this population? Specifically, which medications should nurses tell their aging patients to avoid?

Research Findings
The number of controlled studies on medication use in the aging patient is limited, yet the toxic effects of medications in this population can have profound consequences. The use of consensus criteria is one way to develop reliable and explicit criteria for safe medication use when precise clinical information is lacking (Fick et al., 2003). In 1991, the first research was published identifying inappropriate medication use in nursing home patients. From this original research, the Beers report update in 1997 became the accepted criteria for evaluating appropriate medication use in frail nursing home patients (Beers, 1997). By 1999, the criteria had been adopted by the Centers for Medicare & Medicaid Services for nursing home regulation. In 2003, the criteria were updated to generalize the criteria to older patients regardless of their residence. The Beers criteria identify medication or medication classes that should generally be avoided in persons 65 or older because they are ineffective or pose unnecessarily high risk for this group and safer alternatives exist.

Implications for Nursing Practice
Any nurse caring for elderly patients needs to become familiar with the Beers criteria. In addition, most medication programs that can be installed on a personal digital assistant include a section on special considerations for the elderly. In addition, any hospitalized aging patients who are exhibiting signs of delirium should have their medications reviewed to determine if adverse side effects of the medications are contributing to the delirium.

Critical Thinking Questions

1. Your 95-year-old patient had hip surgery 3 days ago and has now been admitted to your skilled nursing facility for rehabilitation. The patient is reporting aching hip pain. The x-rays are negative for any changes in the alignment of the hip. You call the on-call physician for pain medication orders and are told to give the patient "One Darvocet every four hours for moderate pain, and two Darvocet every four hours for severe pain." How would you respond to the physician?

2. An 85-year-old male on your medical floor has been receiving diphenhydramine nightly to help him sleep as was prescribed by his physician. After 3 days on your floor, he reports he is having difficulty urinating, even though he has made multiple trips to the bathroom. What do you think might be causing his problems with urination?

3. On admission to your unit, you review the admitting medication orders with your alert 90-year-old female patient. She confides in you that she has been taking diazepam 5 mg three times a day for several years that was prescribed by another physician in the community for her "nerves." Her primary care physician is not aware of her diazepam use, but she wants her medication. What should the nurse do?

Answers to Critical Thinking Questions appear in Appendix D.

References
Beers, M. H. (1997). Explicit criteria for determining potentially inappropriate medication use by the elderly. *Archives of Internal Medicine, 157,* 1531–1536.
Fick, D. M., Cooper, J. W., Wade, W. E., Waller, J. L., Maclean, J. R., & Beers, M. H. (2003). Updating the Beers criteria for potentially inappropriate medication use in older adults. *Archives of Internal Medicine, 163,* 2716–2724.

EVIDENCE-BASED PRACTICE

01/05/2007

FIGURE 10–4 ■ Fentanyl patch.

Resources for Caring for an Aging Population

When the aging patient can no longer live alone independently, all viable alternative resources should be explored. Twenty-four-hour-a-day care may be needed in a board and care facility, an assisted living facility, or a nursing home. Contrary to popular belief, Medicare does not cover private home care, board and care, assisted living, or custodial nursing home care. Custodial care residents typically live in a nursing home for an extended period of time due to their need for 24-hour-a-day supervision, nursing care, and assistance with activities of daily living. ADLs include bathing, toileting, eating, and dressing. Generally, Medicare covers skilled nursing care when an individual has been hospitalized and requires a high level of nursing care or therapy at least daily. Examples of skilled nursing care include intravenous (IV) therapy, complicated wound care, and nutrition administered via a feeding tube. Examples of therapy include daily physical, occupational, or speech therapy.

Board and care, assisted living, and many nursing homes cost between $4,000 and $7,000 per month depending on location and amenities offered. Individuals often exhaust their personal life savings paying for such care, and then rely on Medicaid to pay for their care for the remainder of their life. Some nursing homes will not accept Medicaid patients due to concerns that financial reimbursements for these patients have not kept pace with the cost of the care delivered. In fact, in many facilities, private-pay patients pay twice the amount per day that the state reimburses for Medicaid patients.

Medicare and Medicaid

A person's financial means directly affects a patient's ability to pay for housing, food, and medical care. Medical care is of special interest as funding mechanisms have changed drastically in the past 50 years. Prior to the advent of Medicare, health care was primarily a fee-for-service industry. When an individual interacted with the health care system, the provider of care was paid directly for services provided. Medicare, a federally funded health care program for individuals over the age of 65, those under the age of 65 who are disabled, and those with end-stage renal disease, was signed into law in 1965 by President Johnson. Currently Medicare pays for 54% of overall health care costs for its enrollees age 65 and over. Medicare Part A covers hospital stays, pints of blood for transfusions, home health services, hospice care, and some skilled nursing care (after a qualifying hospital stay). Most people or their spouses paid Medicare taxes while working, and will automatically receive Medicare Part A coverage without having to pay a monthly premium. Medicare Part B covers medical services such as medical care by a doctor, nurse practitioner, or physician's assistant; outpatient care; and other medical services not covered by Part A. Enrollment in Part B is optional and there is a monthly premium to pay. Part B deductible must be paid each year before Medicare begins to pay a share of Part B expenses. Some examples of services that fall under Medicare Part B are ambulance services, cardiovascular screenings, bone density measurements, mammogram screenings, and clinical laboratory services.

Individuals enrolled in Medicare can add drug coverage if they join a Medicare prescription drug plan. These plans are offered by private companies that work with Medicare to provide medication coverage. Premiums, copays, and yearly deductibles vary by plans. Each Medicare drug plan has a formulary. A formulary is a list of covered drugs. The list must include at least two drugs in all classes of drugs commonly prescribed to individuals age 65 and older. For more details review Chapter 3 ⊕ of this text.

Some individuals choose to purchase a supplemental insurance policy to cover extra health care costs not covered by Medicare. This insurance, called a "Medigap" policy, is sold by private insurance companies to fill in the gaps in Medicare coverage. Typically Medigap policies help pay a share of coinsurance, copayments, or deductibles of the costs of Medicare-covered services. Usually when one buys Medigap insurance, both Part A and Part B are covered.

For those who are low income, Medicaid provides financial coverage for health care expenses. Medicaid is a federal program enacted in 1965 at the same time President Johnson enacted Medicare. It is administered individually by each state. Eligibility is based on income and assets. Medicaid covers 10% of overall health care costs for those age 65 and over. In 2006, new rules came into effect requiring Americans to show proof of citizenship or risk losing their Medicaid benefits. This can be challenging for elderly people who lack family support systems and suffer from dementia or mental illness (Centers for Medicare & Medicaid Services [CMS], n.d.). The nurse can assist patients by identifying resources within the hospital setting that can help elderly patients submit the necessary paperwork.

Some individuals enroll in Medicare advantage plans. With these plans, their Medicare is assigned to a preferred provider organization (PPO) or health maintenance organization (HMO), which is responsible for overseeing and coordinating care. Chapter 3 ⊕ discusses these types of health plans in detail.

CHART 10–2   **Selected Medications with Potential Adverse Outcomes for the Aging Patient**

Medication Class	Medication	Rationale for Avoiding Medication in the Aging Patient
Muscle relaxants, anticholinergics, and antihistamines	Methocarbamol Carisoprodol Cyclobenzaprine Oxybutynin Chlorpheniramine Hydroxyzine Promethazine Diphenhydramine	Are very anticholinergic and produce toxic effects in the elderly such as cardiac arrhythmias, dry mouth and eyes, and urinary retention. Should be avoided in the elderly, or limited to use for 7 days or less. Diphenhydramine may cause confusion and sedation; should not be used as a sleeping agent; use smallest dose possible if needed to treat an allergic reaction.
Psychotropics and antidepressants	Amitriptyline	Has strong anticholinergic and sedating properties; better antidepressants are available such as selective serotonin reuptake inhibitors (SSRIs) other than fluoxetine.
	Fluoxetine	Has a long half-life and risk of producing excessive central nervous system (CNS) stimulation, with sleep disturbances and agitation. Other antidepressants are available for the elderly that have fewer side effects, such as other SSRIs, atypicals, or bicyclic antidepressants.
	Diazepam, flurazepam	Have a long half-life in the elderly—medications sometimes do not clear system for several days. Produce prolonged sedation, increased risk of falls and fractures. Short- and intermediate-acting benzodiazepines are preferred if needed such as low-dose lorazepam.
	Short-acting benzodiazepines at doses greater than: lorazepam, 3 mg; oxazepam, 60 mg; alprazolam, 2 mg; temazepam, 15 mg; and triazolam, 0.25 mg	Smaller doses in the elderly are effective and safer due to patients' increased sensitivity to these drugs.
Analgesics	Indomethacin	Produces the most CNS side effects of all nonsteroidal anti-inflammatory medications (NSAIDS).
	Ketorolac	Should be avoided because many elderly people have asymptomatic pathologic GI conditions.
	Long-term use of full dosage, longer half-life, non-co-oxygenase (COX) selective NSAIDS such as naproxen and piroxicam	Potential to induce GI bleeding, renal failure, high blood pressure, and heart failure.
	Meperidine	CNS effects; breakdown product can cause convulsions. Safer alternatives exist, such as acetaminophen and a short-acting opiate if necessary.
	Propoxyphene	Limited analgesic advantage over acetaminophen, but has the adverse effects of other narcotic drugs.
Cardiac medications	Digoxin > 0.125 mg/day	Doses greater than 0.125 mg should be avoided because decreased renal clearance leads to increased risk of toxic effects. Doses greater than 0.125 mg, however, can be used to treat atrial arrhythmias.
	Clonidine	Potential for hypotension and CNS effects.
	Amiodarone	Not effective in older adults; risk of torsades de pointes and QT interval problems.
	Disopyramide	Highly anticholinergic; may induce heart failure.
	Doxazosin	Can cause hypotension, dry mouth, and urinary problems.
	Methyldopa	Can cause bradycardia and exacerbate depression; alternative antihypertensives should be considered.
Miscellaneous medications	Ticlopidine	Aspirin is better in preventing clotting than ticlopidine and less toxic.
	Trimethobenzamide	Is one of the least effective antiemetic drugs; can cause extrapyramidal side effects.

Sources: Adapted from Bonk, M. E., Krown, H., Matuszewski, K., & Oinonen, M. (2006). Potentially inappropriate medications in hospitalized senior patients. *American Journal of Health System Pharmacists, 63,* 1161–1165; Beers, M. H. (1997). Explicit criteria for determining potentially inappropriate medication use by the elderly. *Archives of Internal Medicine, 157,* 1531–1536.

Medicare advantage plans provide all of the coverage of Part A and Part B and must cover medically necessary services. Medicare pays an amount every month to these private health plans, whether or not services were used in that particular month. These organizations offer benefits greater than what Medicare alone covers, thus their popularity in certain parts of the United States, such as California.

Long-Term Care Insurance

Long-term care insurance has evolved as one mechanism to ensure that individuals needing long-term care, particularly in a nursing home, will not become financially bankrupt when their time of need for care arises. Nursing home costs vary somewhat throughout the United States. The 2005 average daily rate for a private room in a nursing home was $203, and it cost an average $176 per day for a semiprivate room. Thus, the cost of living in a nursing home for a year would range from $64,240 to $74,095 (MetLife, 2005).

The aging patient has a 50% chance of spending some time in a nursing home. With more than 100 insurance companies offering long-term care insurance policies, one might think that protecting oneself from spending a lifetime of assets on nursing home care is the prudent thing to do. However, only 5% of those over 65 years of age have purchased long-term care insurance. Policies vary widely, many with restrictions, loopholes, and premiums that become unaffordable to maintain. Premiums can range from $2,000 to $10,000 per year, with annual increases. For this reason, only 5 people out of 100 who are 60 years of age or older who take out long-term care insurance policies still have the policy at age 80, when they are most likely to need it (Alexander, 2006). It is recommended that any individual considering long-term care insurance have an attorney review the policy to determine if it will indeed be useful if the time arises when care is needed.

Legal and Ethical Issues of Aging

It is often difficult and challenging for the nurse to discuss legal and ethical concerns with a patient or family member. Many nurses have little experience in this area, and bringing up issues such as elder abuse or advance directives can feel awkward and unsettling. However, such difficult conversations become easier as a nurse gains experience and becomes knowledgeable about legal and ethical issues.

Elder Mistreatment (Abuse)

Elder mistreatment or *abuse* is a broad term that describes the outcome of abuse, neglect, exploitation, or abandonment of older adults. There are three categories of elder mistreatment: domestic, institutional, and self-neglect. Domestic mistreatment occurs in the aging patient's home and involves significant others such as a child, spouse, or relatives. Institutional mistreatment occurs when an individual has a contractual agreement with a care facility such as a nursing home and is abused. Self-neglect occurs when an individual who is capable of making decisions and understanding consequences engages in behavior that threatens his or her safety or well-being (Tabloski, 2006). The seven major types of elder abuse are as follows:

- *Physical abuse* is the use of physical force that may result in injury, pain, or impairment. Some examples of physical abuse are acts of violence such as striking, slapping, kicking, or pinching. Other nonviolent examples include misuse of drugs, force feeding, or use of restraints.

- *Sexual abuse* is nonconsensual sexual contact of any kind with an elderly person. If a person is incapable of giving consent due to cognitive impairment such as dementia, sexual contact also is considered sexual abuse. Some examples include unwanted touching and all forms of sexual assault and battery, such as rape and sodomy.

- *Emotional* or *psychological abuse* involves inflicting pain or distress through verbal or nonverbal means. Insults, threats, and forced social isolation would be considered emotional/psychological abuse.

- *Neglect* is the refusal or failure to fulfill duties to an elder. Examples of neglect include failing to provide necessary personal care for a dependent adult, or failing to hire someone to provide the needed care.

- *Abandonment* is defined as desertion of an elderly person by an individual deemed responsible for the elder's care. An example is a caregiver leaving a dependent elderly person alone for a week while the caregiver takes a vacation out of town.

- *Financial* or *material exploitation* is defined as misuse of an elder's money, property, or assets. Examples of financial exploitation include tricking a dependent elder into signing checks for a caregiver's personal use and stealing money or possessions.

- *Self-neglect* is the refusal or failure of an elderly person to provide himself with adequate food, water, shelter, and health care to the point that personal health or safety is threatened. An example of self-neglect is when an individual with a cognitive impairment uses all of his money to buy cat food for 50 cats and fails to buy food for himself and becomes undernourished as a result (National Center on Elder Abuse [NCEA], 2007c).

It is important for nurses to become knowledgeable regarding elder abuse reporting laws as well as an awareness of possible signs and symptoms of elder mistreatment. Forty-four states and the District of Columbia have laws providing that individuals who care for the elderly are considered mandatory reporters and must report suspected elder abuse or mistreatment. A **mandatory reporter** is a person required by law to report allegations and/or suspicions of abuse. A nurse is a mandatory reporter. Thirty-eight state statutes specify a penalty for mandatory reporters who fail to report when they should (Daly, Jogerst, Brinig, & Dawson, 2004).

In most states, Adult Protective Services (APS) caseworkers are the first responders to reports of abuse, exploitation, and neglect. Their role for the elderly is to ensure the safety and well-being of those who are unable to take care of themselves and have no one to assist them. These caseworkers receive reports of elderly abuse, exploitation, or neglect; investigate the report; and provide case planning including emergency shelter, medical care, legal assistance, and supportive services if indicated, and monitoring and evaluation (NCEA, 2007b). On a national level, the NCEA, directed by the U.S. Administration on Aging, serves as a resource for policy makers, health care professionals, families, and others interested in ensuring that older Americans live free of abuse, neglect, and exploitation (NCEA, 2007a). Chart 10–3 lists possible signs and symptoms of elder mistreatment.

CHART 10–3	Possible Signs and Symptoms of Elder Mistreatment

Type of Mistreatment	Possible Signs and Symptoms
Physical/sexual abuse	• Multiple trips to the emergency room • A patient's report of being hit, slapped, or mistreated • Unexplained fractures or bruises in various stages of healing • Trauma or bleeding in the genital area • Unexplained veneral disease
Emotional/ psychological abuse	• Withdrawn or non-communicative patient, reluctant to answer questions with family member present • A patient who is emotionally upset or agitated • Family members who are or act irritable or refuse to allow patient to answer questions
Neglect/ abandonment	• Unexplained skin rashes, irritation, or ulcers • Family exhibits poor follow-through in obtaining needed medications and medical care for family member • Patient reports being left in unsafe situation for periods of time
Self-neglect	• Poor hygiene in an elder that impacts the individual's health • Dehydration; malnutrition; unexplained weight loss
Financial exploitation	• Discovery that patient's signature was forged • Sudden changes in a patient's financial condition • Unexplained loss of Social Security or pension checks • Visiting family members, especially previously uninvolved ones, are asking someone incapable of making decisions to sign checks or other documents, or financial activity the patient couldn't have done • Unusual interest on the part of caregivers in the patient's assets

Source: Adapted from AGS Foundation for Health in Aging. (2002). *Elder mistreatment.* Retrieved January 25, 2007, from http://www.healthinaging.org; Jaffe-Gill, E., de Benedictis, T., and Segal, J. (2008). *Elder Abuse: Types, Signs, Symptoms, Risk Factors and Prevention.* Retrieved February 8, 2009, from http://www.helpguide.org/mental/elder_abuse_physical_ emotional_sexual_neglect.htm; National Center on Elder Abuse (2007). *Major Types of Elder Abuse.* Retrieved February 6, 2009, from http://www.ncea.aoa.gov/ncearoot/Main_Site/ FAQ/Basics/Types_Of_Abuse.aspx.

Advance Directives

Advance directives provide a mechanism for individuals to place into writing their wishes regarding treatment should they become ill. Individuals typically execute such a document when they are well and able to think through the various scenarios they might experience as they age. Chapter 17 👓 describes in detail the two forms of advance directives: living wills and durable powers of attorney for health care (DPAHC). Aging patients are encouraged to draft both a living will and a DPAHC while they are healthy and able to discuss wishes re-

garding care and treatments. Once an individual is cognitively impaired and no longer has the capacity to make informed decisions, that person is not legally able to execute a living will or DPAHC. A court-appointed conservator should be pursued to allow a legally designated individual to make decisions on behalf of the patient with a cognitive impairment.

In the nursing home setting, a preferred intensity of care (PIC) or preferred intensity of treatment (PIT) form is used as an additional tool to enable patients or their designated representative to clarify treatment wishes (Figure 10–5 ■, p. 186). Depending on the facility, such forms include yes/no boxes to check to address a number of medical interventions available in the nursing home, such as CPR, nasogastric or artificial feeding methods, IV antibiotics, and transfers to the hospital.

■ Care Options for the Aging Patient

For many aging patients, hospitalization represents a sentinel event, triggering a downward spiral of health and function (Mezey et al., 2003). Social issues as well as medical issues are brought to light when a frail patient is hospitalized. However, once the crisis of hospitalization has arrived, the nurse needs to look ahead toward discharge planning. Some discussion of post-hospitalization plans should even take place at the time of admission. When the subject of post-hospitalization discharge planning is broached, many older patients oppose returning to anywhere but home. Many envision nursing homes, which in the past were referred to as "rest homes" or "convalescent homes," as dingy, dark places where people go to die. Children and family members make promises that they may not be willing or able to keep, such as "Mom will never go to a nursing home." Fortunately, a variety of housing and care options exist for the aging patient as outlined in the following subsections.

Independent Living

The aging patient has many options for independent living that go beyond remaining in one's home. Life care communities or continuing care retirement centers offer an independent living option, with an opportunity to "age in place" if the individual requires more care as time progresses. Often the independent living area offers apartment or town home living, with or without meals. Support such as housekeeping and activities are available. Such facilities also offer assisted living and skilled nursing care, usually in separate buildings, that the person can take advantage of when it is finally needed. Health plans and Medicare do not cover the expense of life care communities, unless the individual resides in the skilled nursing facility and is receiving rehabilitative services. Such facilities often require a *buy-in,* which can range from thousands to hundreds of thousands of dollars and is in addition to the monthly living expenses. The benefits of such communities are many. Most importantly, residents may move back and forth between levels of care as their health needs dictate, and couples with differing levels of health needs can be accommodated within one building.

Senior supported housing can vary from low-income apartment complexes for seniors subsidized by the government to privately paid apartments that provide some or all meals, housekeeping, and laundry services, along with social activities

ACKNOWLEDGMENT OF RECEIPT
ADVANCE DIRECTIVES/MEDICAL TREATMENT DECISIONS

This is to acknowledge that I have been informed in writing in a language that I understand of my rights and all rules and regulations to make decisions concerning medical care, including the right to accept or refuse medical or surgical treatment and the right to formulate and to issue Advance Directives to be followed should I become incapacitated.

☐ I have chosen to formulate and issue the following Advance Directives.

Initial Choices	Yes	No		Yes	No
Resuscitate	___	___	Other _____	___	___
Feeding tube(s) (N/G, G-tube)	___	___			
Antibiotic Therapy	___	___	_____	___	___
Intravenous Therapy	___	___			
Transfer to acute hospital	___	___	_____	___	___
If no, state exceptions _____					

☐ I do not choose to formulate or issue any Advance Directives at this time.
   I want efforts made to prolong my life and I want life-sustaining treatment to be provided.

Resident/Client _____   Date _____

Surrogate Decision Maker _____   Date _____

If Surrogate Decision Maker Signed, Complete the Following:

_____   _____
Print Name   Relationship to Resident

Witness _____   Date _____

— — — — — — — — — — — — — — — — — —

If Resident Unable to Sign Name, State Medical Reason:

_____

I have discussed the pertinent diagnosis (ses) and prognosis of the resident and the consequences of withdrawing or withholding life-sustaining services and other health care decisions made with: _____

FIGURE 10–5 ■ Preferred intensity of care form.

and transportation. Health plans and Medicare do not cover the expense of senior supported housing.

Adult Day Health Care and Adult Day Care

Adult day health care offers a program of health services such as nursing care and therapy, meals, social and recreational activities, and social work services in a structured daytime program. Individuals who require health services, social interaction, or supervision during the day can attend while continuing to live at home or in another care setting. Some programs offer transportation; Medicaid may pay for this program.

Adult day care, based on a social model, offers few or no health services. The emphasis of the social day care program is fostering socialization among older adults. These programs aim to keep seniors as active and healthy as possible. These programs offer respite for families and caregivers who need some time away from the caregiver role. Often these programs receive a financial subsidy and charge a daily fee. Private health plans and Medicare do not cover this program.

Residential Care Facilities

A residential care facility is the formal name for the type of facility commonly referred to as "board and care" living. Their licensing oversight varies by state, falling under the department of health. These facilities provide on-site unlicensed caregivers 24 hours a day and assistance with ADLs such as bathing, dressing, and feeding. They provide three meals a day, social activities, housekeeping, laundry services, and limited transportation. Some facilities provide medication supervision by unlicensed personnel and are not medically focused. Many are operated by individual families. Some board and care facilities are six-bed private homes; others may be larger homes designed for such clients with both private and semiprivate rooms (Kaiser Permanente, 2005).

Assisted Living Facilities

Assisted living facilities also are licensed as residential care facilities, but tend to be larger in size, often with 50 to 200 residents, and many are part of a corporation that operates assisted living facilities throughout the country. Most require individuals to be ambulatory, use a walker, or be able to propel their wheelchairs to a common dining area. Rarely are they able to accommodate special diets requiring modified food textures or special liquid consistencies. For example, rarely will an assisted living facility provide a puree diet with honey-thick liquid drinks. Some facilities will only accept an incontinent resident if that individual is able to manage their incontinence products independently.

These facilities cannot accommodate individuals who are bedbound. If an individual requires daily nursing care for problems such as pressure ulcers or an indwelling urinary catheter, the facility must apply for a special waiver to allow the person to remain in the facility. With such large variances in amenities, family members are encouraged to thoroughly examine what the assisted living facility will provide or allow in the way of services before placing a deposit. All types of residential care facilities are licensed by the department of health in the state where they are located.

Intermediate/Skilled Nursing Care

There are times when a frail aging patient has health needs that are beyond what can be provided in a home, board and care, or assisted living facility. Long-term care in an intermediate care or skilled nursing facility might be the best and, in some cases, the only option. A skilled nursing facility may also be called a nursing facility, a nursing home, a convalescent home or hospital, or occasionally a rest home.

Intermediate care facilities (ICFs) and skilled nursing facilities (SNFs) are licensed by the department of health in the state where they are located. They may also be certified to receive pay-

ETHICAL ISSUES Regarding Care of MS Patients with Urinary Retention Issues

Many patients with multiple sclerosis (MS) who are ambulatory and able to independently carry out most of their ADLs develop some degree of urinary retention due to their MS. Often, these individuals live in an assisted living settings to maximize their independence. Most assisted living facilities will not accept residents with indwelling catheters. What should the nurse do when the individual develops moderate to significant urinary retention resulting in multiple urinary tract infections and hospitalization for urosepsis?

Some options include:

- Discuss with the resident the risk/benefit of long-term catheter use; insist the resident consent to an indwelling catheter and move to a nursing home.

- Act as a patient advocate and discuss with the assisted living facility the possibility of obtaining a waiver to allow the individual with an indwelling catheter to remain living there.

- Discuss the risk/benefits of long-term urinary retention such as further damage to the bladder, antibiotic-resistant urinary tract infections, and the potential for urosepsis.

- Discuss treating the complications of urinary retention such as urinary tract infections when they occur.

- Discuss the goals of care with the patient given the progressive nature of the multiple sclerosis diagnosis, and whether the benefits of living in assisted living rather than a nursing home outweigh the risks of urinary retention and probable recurrent sepsis with hospitalization and death.

ment from Medicare and Medicaid. Approximately 1.6 million people live in the more than 16,000 nursing homes in the United States (Hamilton, 2005). ICFs care for people who are moderately independent but require 24-hour-a-day supervision and assistance, along with intermittent licensed nursing care. ICFs can provide special diets and moderate help with ADLs such as bathing and dressing. They cannot accept individuals who are nonambulatory, incontinent, or require skilled nursing care. ICFs tend to cost less than SNF care, reflecting a lower level of staffing and personal assistance.

Skilled nursing care is usually needed for a short period of time to recover from an acute illness or injury, often following hospitalization. Skilled nursing care is care that must be delivered by a licensed nurse, such as IV therapy, complicated wound care, or nasogastric or gastrostomy tube feedings. Individuals requiring daily physical, occupational, or speech therapy also would qualify for skilled therapy services. Health plans and Medicare cover skilled services and pay for nursing home days that meet established criteria.

Most residents in nursing homes receive custodial care. Custodial care residents live in a nursing home for an extended period of time, sometimes for the remainder of their lives. Some individuals recover enough to move to a less intensive level of care. For those who do not, custodial care provides a higher level of 24-hour-a-day supervision and assistance with ADLs. Licensed nursing staff are on site 24 hours a day to administer medications and deliver other nursing care. Residents who require walkers or wheelchairs for mobility and those who are bedbound or incontinent can be cared for in this setting. Some nursing homes are secured with perimeter fencing and a locked entrance/exit gate to enable those individuals with dementia who are prone to wandering to ambulate freely without becoming injured.

Medical management in the nursing home is handled on site by a physician and often a nurse practitioner who see residents at the facility. This nurse practitioner may be a **gerontological nurse practitioner (GNP),** a registered nurse with a master's degree from a nurse practitioner program specializing in the care of older adults. GNPs are educated to diagnose and manage acute and chronic diseases, using a holistic approach to address the medical, psychosocial, and functional needs of older adults. Any patient discharged from an acute care hospital to a nursing home requires the following forms: history and physical, discharge summary, and nursing home physician orders with indications or diagnoses for all medications ordered. Without these documents, the nursing home cannot admit the patient.

Home Care

Older adults who choose to live independently in their homes for as long as possible can turn to supportive services, such as home care, to provide the needed assistance. Two types of home care are available: home health care and private duty care. The main difference between the two is who pays for the service.

Traditional hospital care involving IV therapy, tube feedings, some forms of dialysis, wound vacuums for pressure ulcer management, and oxygen therapy are now administered in the home. This is partially in response to individuals' preference for care in the home and, in some cases, in response to hospitals' efforts to reign in costs (Matthews, 2006).

Home health may be covered by an individual's health plan, Medicare, or Medicaid if a physician determines the individual needs intermittent care by at least one professional, such as a registered nurse, physical therapist, occupational therapist, speech therapist, or social worker. A home health aide may be used if requested by the nurse or therapist coordinating the care.

The nurse's role as part of discharge planning during the patient's hospitalization is to determine if the patient or a willing and able caregiver is capable of administering such care in the home environment with support from the home health nurse. The ANA scope and standards of gerontological nursing practice, shown earlier in Chart 10–1 (p. 170), identify the nurse as the professional whose role it is to develop the discharge plan (Congdon et al., 2001). The nurse should begin the teaching process before the individual leaves the hospital, with home health nurses providing specialized care and reinforcement of teaching. Home health nurses typically deliver intermittent care; they may visit daily, several times a week, or weekly, depending on the individual's needs. If an individual's care needs exceed what the family can provide or a home health nurse can accomplish in a home visit, the individual may need care in a skilled nursing facility setting.

Private duty or continuous care is rendered in the home by registered nurses or nursing assistants, homemakers, or companions with the goal to provide personal care and companionship. Caregivers are hired and paid privately by the individual receiving care or through an agency. Some long-term care insurance policies cover in-home private duty care.

Hospice

Hospice services have been available in the home setting for a number of years. Hospice services have been available in nursing homes for nearly 10 years and are requested by patients and family members seeking hospice personnel's expertise in end-of-life care. Once a patient is determined to be appropriate for hospice services in a nursing home, the expectations change from cure to acceptance that a decline is inevitable and the goals change to that of promoting comfort and quality for the remainder of the patient's life. The hospice team can provide support to the family through involvement of social workers, chaplains, and a hospice nurse. Such support is above and beyond what would usually be available in a nursing home (Sattinger, 2006). See Chapter 17 🔗 for more information on hospice and end-of-life issues.

Palliative Care

There is no national consensus on the definition of palliative care. The definition proposed by the Center to Advance Palliative Care (2001) states that "Palliative care aims to relieve suffering and improve the quality of living and dying. It aims to address physical, psychological, social, spiritual and practical expectations and needs of an individual with an acute or chronic life-threatening illness." Jewish Home and Hospital Lifecare System goes on to say that "Care is a comprehensive approach to helping patients manage serious illnesses. Its main focus is to provide patients relief from pain and other distressing symptoms, along with minimizing suffering."

Palliative care programs continue to grow in the hospital setting, with 1,240 hospitals providing programs in 2005, compared to 632 programs in 2000 (*Hospitals Continue to*

Implement, 2006). Palliative care programs in the nursing home are rare, possibly due to the newness of the concept and the large amount of resources necessary to implement a program (Tuch Parrish, and Romer, 2002).

◼ Innovations in Caring for the Aging Patient

Innovations in caring for the aging patient have been slow to evolve, primarily due to lack of funding and lack of mechanisms for reimbursement under traditional Medicare and Medicaid models. Innovations currently under way include primary care in the home, the Program for All-inclusive Care of the Elderly, the Green House Project, and elder cohousing communities.

Team-Based Primary Care in the Home

The idea of health care professionals caring for an individual in the home is not new. Years ago, doctors made house calls to patients' homes. As communities grew, medical clinics emerged, and mechanisms for funding health care changed with the advent of Medicare and Medicaid, the days of house calls by a physician came to an end. The U.S. Department of Veterans Affairs (VA) has supported a program with home visits by a physician, a nurse practitioner, and an interdisciplinary team since its inception in 1972. The VA Home-Based Primary Care (HBPC) program provides comprehensive primary care in the homes of veterans with complex chronic disabling disease. Unlike home care that is focused on episodic, time-limited, and focused skilled care, HBPC provides comprehensive longitudinal care. However, this team-based care is only available for those with veterans benefits (Department of Veterans Affairs, 2007).

The concept of team-based primary care in the home is now moving to the traditional Medicare fee-for-service population through demonstration grants. A 3-year pilot project that was scheduled to end in 2008 is testing the effects of increased access and quality of care to elderly people who are chronically ill through the use of house calls by physicians. Care Level Management, the company conducting the project, utilizes a personal physician house call system of care that provides patients with direct, 24-hour access to a physician who is available to provide in-home care anytime, day or night, as needed. This level of care is designed to improve the quality of care for the most chronically ill, frail patients who represent approximately 2% of Medicare beneficiaries. Selection for the pilot project is by invitation; selection criteria include patients with two chronic illnesses and a history of at least two hospitalizations within the past 12 months. The goal is to reduce unnecessary hospitalizations and emergency department visits, thus reducing costs to the patient and the health care system (*Medicare Adds,* 2006).

Program of All-Inclusive Care for the Elderly

The Program of All-Inclusive Care for the Elderly (PACE) is based on the British day hospital model of care. PACE programs provide preventive, primary, acute, and long-term services for their enrolled members all under one roof. With a nursing focus, PACE programs are responsible for managing the health, mental, and psychosocial needs of each participant. PACE programs include the medical component of care, working from a clinic that is open 5 or 6 days a week where participants receive care from a clinic provider, either a physician or a nurse practitioner, along with specialist services such as audiology, dentistry, optometry, speech, and podiatry. These services are offered along with an adult day care program, where participants gather for socialization, recreation, and nursing care. Transportation is provided, and some PACE programs include a housing component for their participants. In their own homes, PACE participants can receive personal, home health, and respite care. If needed, PACE programs cover hospital and nursing home care (Bonifazi, 2004).

Green House Project

The Green House Project in Tupelo, Mississippi, is comprised of 10 suburban homes that have become an experiment in reinventing the nursing home. They are part of a movement to humanize the care for the aging patient with smaller, more "home-like" settings and a closer sense of community among residents and staff. The Green House model was conceptualized by Eden Alternative pioneer Bill Thomas, MD. The model was developed to address the aging patient's fears of being institutionalized, including anxieties about loss of independence and fears of abuse. In a Green House, meals are served at a communal dining table rather than on trays in a dining hall. Staff members who care for residents answer beepers to minimize the sounds of the never-ending call bells often heard in traditional nursing homes. The advantages of deinstitutionalized models are many, but potentially higher costs of operation have kept them from being widely available (Hamilton, 2005).

Elder Cohousing

Another new and innovative housing option is elder cohousing. The concept is built on a Denmark-inspired, 30-year-old community planning model typically developed for intergenerational populations. In the past few years, it has become a focus for individuals over age 55. Cohousing communities exist in California, Virginia, and Colorado and they exhibit similarities to a townhouse or condominium development run by a homeowners' association. The difference is that the residents are individuals who like living and doing things together. One community has 11 households, and all are represented on the board of directors. Members range in age from 55 to 75, with many professionals; some are retired, others are still working. Such communities are designed with the goal of encouraging aging in place through the use of universal design elements and an emphasis on home care.

As such communities develop, new questions arise. How does the community address members with dementias? How does the community address those who require around-the-clock nursing care? Only the future will tell if cohousing will take off as an option for today's aging baby boomers (*Cohousing*, 2006).

Innovations in Technology for the Aging Patient

Rapid advances in technology are beginning to have an impact on care of the aging patient in both traditional and nontraditional settings. With appropriate applications of technology,

seniors who choose to remain at home during their aging years will be able to do so successfully. New technology is making it possible for those who choose to live in board and care and assisted living to remain in those types of less restrictive environments compared to the traditional nursing home. Challenges involving telephone communication, medication administration, and overall patient monitoring can be addressed using new technology.

Telephone Communication

The challenges for the aging patient in using the telephone are numerous, due to hearing and vision difficulties. Traditional methods to address such problems include phones with higher volume and use of a text telephone (TTY) for those whose hearing renders them incapable of hearing speech over the phone. The device allows an individual to type into a TTY keyboard, which generates tones that are converted into letters by another TTY device. Newer "smart" phones provide additional options for the aging patient to communicate. For example, many individuals are moving to the Voice over Internet Protocol, which involves using the Internet rather than traditional phone lines to carry voices. The advantage is that one can communicate in several formats such as voice and text or through streaming video with multiple people at the same time (Vanderheiden, 2006).

Medication Administration Technology

Medication administration has advanced beyond the traditional pill reminder, divided up for time of day and days of the week in the home setting. Traditional methods such as pill reminders or alarm clocks that ring when a medication is due do not ensure the aging patient is taking medications when living at home. For those individuals, greater support is needed in medication administration. Newer technologies offer devices that are the size of a small TV and like an "ATM for patient medications." Such devices are wirelessly connected to software that contains an individual's medication administration record, and can be remotely adjusted by a pharmacist or health care provider. The device reminds patients when to take medications, selects the correct dose, and delivers it from the machine. Medications are loaded via blister packs. Such technology is beneficial for the home-dwelling forgetful patient, for someone with a complex drug regimen, and for someone who has difficulty understanding written directions (INRange Systems, 2006). New "closed door" pharmacies have evolved to serve this population. They deliver blister pack medications for each patient on a monthly basis.

Computer Technology

Computers continue to offer an opportunity for seniors to apply technology in their lives to simplify record keeping, even when they are no longer able to live at home. Many seniors keep track of their medical care and health history using notebooks, filing systems or, in some cases, no particular system. An innovative project at Eskaton Village Carmichael, a continuing care retirement community in Northern California, provides seniors a means to keep track of their health information via computer. The partnership between Intel Corporation and Eskaton Village in this endeavor, called the Internet Health File project, allows residents to enter health information into a secure Internet site so that it is organized and available at all times. If residents

Continuous Body Monitoring Technology

Aging patients who live at home alone may benefit from the use of technology involving continuous body monitoring. One device available is an armband, similar to a wristwatch in size, that is applied and collects continuous data on calories burned, duration and level of physical activity, and sleep–wake cycles. Using wireless transmission and software analysis, family members not living with the aging patient could be notified if, for example, the individual did not get out of bed or fell. Those who might benefit most from such technology are individuals who live alone or have an inability to call for help. Such technology might be useful in collecting accurate data for those with chronic conditions to monitor overall health and physical status over time (Matthews, 2006).

High-technology innovations such as continuous body monitoring may not be the only way to integrate technology into the aging patient's life. Simpler systems may solve the same problems at a much more reasonable cost. Miami University's Scripps Gerontology Center in Oxford, Ohio, conducted a pilot study to evaluate how electronic monitoring could alleviate caregivers' burdens of constantly keeping track of their impaired relatives. Nineteen families caring for older relatives with moderate to severe dementia were enrolled. Each home was outfitted with two video cameras with a controller, one off-the-shelf sensor for each door, a cell phone with text messaging features, and monthly broadband Internet service. The equipment cost $300 and Internet service added $50 to $60 per month. Families reported benefits of such a system, even after various system "glitches" were resolved (Piturro, 2004).

■ Summary

It is often a challenge to motivate new graduate nurses to pursue a nursing specialty in caring for the aged. Geriatrics as a field tends not to hold the same level of excitement as working in an emergency department or an intensive care unit. Helping aging patients with ADLs may not, on the surface, have the same appeal as helping deliver babies in the labor and delivery suite or taking care of children on a pediatric floor. Those nurses who grew up around an older relative or had interactions with a senior prior to becoming a nurse, however, know of the rewards of helping a group of individuals who have lived through world wars and the Depression and have gained a lifetime of wisdom. Hopefully, with some new knowledge about the aging patient, there will be renewed interest in caring for this rapidly growing population group.

NCLEX® REVIEW

1. The nurse understands that which of the following age-related changes noted during a patient's physical assessment may be expected within the elderly population:
   1. Shallow inspirations with accessory muscle use and a decreased residual capacity.
   2. Decreased taste sensation often results from hypertrophy to the tongue's papillae.
   3. Point of maximal impulse may be at the sixth left intercostal space, midclavicular line.
   4. Hyperactive bowel sounds secondary to increased peristalsis and fluid intake.

2. As it relates to recommended immunizations and screening exams by the United States Preventative Services Task Force (USPSTF) for patients over 65 years of age, the nurse understands:
   1. These guidelines strictly outline the healthcare provider recommendations for immunizations and screenings for frail elderly patients and those with functional decline.
   2. Elderly patients who are hospitalized may be immunized according to the recommendations, as this can decrease both pneumonia and its resultant death rates.
   3. The pneumococcal and influenza vaccines should be administered at different times since there is decreased antibody response and increased reaction severity when given together.
   4. Doses of the varicella virus vaccine should be 14 times greater than the vaccine for the varicella-zoster virus in order to boost immunity against shingles and its sequelae.

3. The Beers criteria were established:
   1. Because up to 25% of hospital admissions in elderly patients can be linked to adverse drug reactions or toxic effects.
   2. To provide criteria by which health care providers can assess risk for and decrease the occurrence of polypharmacy.
   3. By a panel of experts to make recommendations about preventative services to be included in primary care.
   4. As an adjunct for researchers to evaluate the quality of drug prescribing, utilization, and education in the nursing home.

4. An elderly patient presents from a nursing home, weeping and complaining of nausea. When placing the blood pressure cuff on the client's arm, the nurse notices a large hand-shaped contusion on the bicep. The nurse should:
   1. Confront the patient about what he or she did to deserve the injury.
   2. Ensure confidentiality and inquire directly about the contusion.
   3. Ignore the contusion because the patient is complaining of nausea.
   4. Call the local news to report the injury and implicate the family.

5. A patient is being discharged from the hospital after recovering from a transient ischemic attack. The patient has no residual paralysis or parasthesias and is ambulatory with a cane. They are continent, able to communicate and maintain some of their own ADLs, but do require assistance with medications. The patient and family want to consider a housing option that will meet the patient's needs and be covered by insurance. Which of the following care options is most appropriate for this patient?

1. Skilled nursing care.

2. Adult day care.

3. Residential care facility.

4. Senior supported housing.

Answers for review questions appear in Appendix D

KEY TERMS

activity theory of aging *p.169*
adverse drug event (ADE) *p.180*
adverse drug reaction (ADR) *p.180*
aging *p.168*
biological aging theory *p.168*
continuity theory of aging *p.169*
cross-linking theory of aging *p.169*
delirium *p.176*
dementia *p.176*
disengagement theory of aging *p.169*

error theories of aging *p.169*
Folstein Mini-Mental State Exam *p.171*
free radical theory of aging *p.169*
gerontological nurse practitioner (GNP) *p.187*
immunologic theory of aging *p.168*
insomnia *p.173*
kyphosis *p.172*
long-term care insurance *p.184*

mandatory reporter *p.184*
polypharmacy *p.180*
programmed theory of aging *p.168*
psychosocial theories of aging *p.169*
rate of living theory of aging *p.169*
sleep apnea *p.173*
U.S. Preventive Services Task Force (USPSTF) *p.175*
wear-and-tear theory of aging *p.169*

EXPLORE   PEARSON   **mynursingkit**™

MyNursingKit is your one stop for online chapter review materials and resources. Prepare for success with additional NCLEX®-style practice questions, interactive assignments and activities, web links, animations and videos, and more!

Register your access code from the front of your book at
www.mynursingkit.com

REFERENCES

Aboderin, I. (2004). Modernisation and ageing theory revisited: Current explanations of recent developing world and historical western shifts in material family support for older people. *Ageing and Society, 24:* 29–50.

Administration on Aging. AOA. (n.d.). *A Profile of Older Americans: 2007.* Retrieved May 19, 2008, from http://www.aoa.gov/PROF/Statistics/profile/2004/profiles2004.asp

Agency for Healthcare Research and Quality, (AHRQ). (2007). 2007 *National Healthcare Quality & Disparities Reports.* Retrieved May 19, 2008 from http://www.ahrq.gov/qual/grdr07.htm

Agostini, J. V., Han, L., & Tinetti, M. E. (2004). The relationship between number of medications and weight loss or impaired balance in older adults. *Journal of the American Geriatrics Society, 52,* 1719–1723.

Alexander, R. (Ed.). (2006). *Avoiding fraud when buying long-term care insurance.* Retrieved November 2, 2006, from http://www.consumerlawpage.com

Alzheimer's Association. (2006). *Fact sheet: Alzheimer's disease.* Retrieved January 2, 2007, from http://www.alz.org/Resources/FactSheets/FSADFacts.pdf

American Cancer Society. (n.d.). *What are the key statistics about prostate cancer?* Retrieved January 2, 2007, from http://www.cancer.org

American Psychiatric Association. (1994). *Diagnostic and statistical manual of mental disorders* (4th ed., pp. 123–133). Washington, DC: Author.

American Society of Health-System Pharmacists. (2006). Information retrieved November 1, 2006, from http://www.safemedication.com

Anderson, L. M., Scrimshaw, S. C., Fullilove, M. T., Fielding, J. E., & Normand, J. (2003). Culturally competent healthcare systems. *American Journal of Preventive Medicine, 24,* 68–79.

Aziz, R., Lorberg, B., & Tampi, R.R., (2006). Treatments for late-life bipolar disorder. *American Journal of Geriatric Pharmacotherapy,* 4(4), 347–364.

Bacak, B. S., Patel, M., Tweed, E., & Danis, P. (2006). What is the best way to manage GERD symptoms in the elderly? *Journal of Family Practice, 55,* 251–258.

Beers, M. H. (1997). Explicit criteria for determining potentially inappropriate medication use by the elderly. *Archives of Internal Medicine, 157,* 1531–1536.

Bonifazi, W. L. (2004, November 29). *Set the PACE.* Retrieved January 2, 2007, from http://www.Nursesweek.com/news/featuresNurseweek

Bonk, M. E., Krown, H., Matuszewski, K., & Oinonen, M. (2006). Potentially inappropriate medications in hospitalized senior patients. *American Journal of Health System Pharmacists, 63,* 1161–1165.

Center to Advance Palliative Care. (2001). *CAPC manual: Proposed definition of palliative care.* Retrieved May 3, 2008, from http://64.85.16.230/educate/content/elements/palliativecaredefinition.html

Centers for Medicare & Medicaid Services. (n.d.). *Proof of citizenship.* Retrieved December 30, 2006, from http://www.cms.hhs.gov/MedicaidEligibility/05_ProofofCitizenship.asp

Cohousing: The next senior housing option. Interview with Zev Paiss, Elder Cohousing network. (2006). *Nursing Homes, 55*(3), 30.

Congdon, J. G., DeCamp, J., Fletcher, K., Henningson, B., Kaplan, K., & Resnick, B. (2001). *Scope and standards of gerontological nursing practice* (2nd ed.). Silver Spring, MD: American Nurses Association.

Daly, J. M., Jogerst, G. J., Brinig, M. F., & Dawson, J. D. (2004). Mandatory reporting relationships of APS statute language on state reported elder abuse. *Journal of Elder Abuse and Neglect, 15*(2), 1–21.

Darkwa, O. (2007). *Social welfare services for the aged.* Retrieved March 16, 2008, from http://www.uic.edu/classes/socw/socw550/AGIMG/tsld001.htm

Department of Veterans Affairs. (2007). *Home-Based Primary Care Program: VHA handbook 11404.01.* Washington D.C.: Veterans Health Administration.

DeYoung, G. R., & Baty, P. J. (2007). Herpes zoster virus vaccine (Zostavax) for the prevention of shingles. *American Family Physician, 76,* 1843–1846.

Experience CORPS. (2007). *Fact Sheet on Aging in America.* Washington. DC. Experience CORPS.

Falicov, C. J. (1998). *Latino families in therapy: A guide to multicultural practice.* New York: The Guilford Press.

Fernandes, R., Flynn, B., & Masaki, K. (2003). Tetanus immunity in the elderly. *Annals of Long-Term Care, 11*(1), 21–24.

Fick, D. M., Cooper, J. W., Wade, W. E., Waller, J. L., Maclean, J. R., & Beers, M. H. (2003). Updating the Beers criteria for potentially inappropriate medication use in older adults. *Archives of Internal Medicine, 163,* 2716–2724.

Folstein, M. F., Folstein, S. E., & McHugh, P. R. (1975). Mini-Mental State: A practical method for grading the cognitive state of patients for the clinician. *Journal of Psychiatric Research, 12*(3), 189–198.

Gavrilov, L. A., & Gavrilov, N. S. (2002). Evolutionary theories of aging and longevity. *The Scientific World Journal, 2,* 339–356.

Gehrman, P., Diana, G., & Impastato, A. (2006). Wide awake in assisted living. *Assisted Living Consult, 2*(2), 26–29.

Hamilton, W. L. (2005, April 23). The new nursing home, emphasis on home. *The New York Times.* Retrieved April 24, 2005, from http://www.nytimes.com

Hospitals continue to implement palliative care programs. (2006). Retrieved January 21, 2007, from http://www.healthday.com

Howard, R., Rabins, P. V., Seeman, M. V., Jeste, D. V., & and International-Onset, Schizophrenia Group. (2000). Late-onset schizophrenia and very-late-onset schizophrenia-like psychosis: An international consensus. *American Journal of Psychiatry, 157,* 172–178.

Inouye, S., van Dyck, C., Alessi, C., Galkin, S., Siegal, A., & Horwitz, R. (1990). Clarifying confusion: the confusion assessment method. *Annals of Internal Medicine, 113*(12), 941–948.

INRange Systems. (2006). *Remote medication management systems.* Retrieved October 30, 2006, from http://www.inrangesystem.com

Intel and Eskaton team up for health. (2006). *Eskaton Connections, 8*(4), 1.

Jeste, K. V., Paulsen, J. S., & Harris, M. J. (2000). *Late-onset schizophrenia and other related psychoses.* Retrieved January 3, 2008, from http://www.acnp.org/g4GN401000138/CH135.html

Kaiser Permanente. (2005, September). *Kaiser Permanente guide to nursing facilities for members* (pp. 11–13).

Kaldy, J. (2006). Managing influenza in the assisted living facility. *Assisted Living Consult, 2*(2), 14–16.

Kao, R. S., & Lam, M. L. (1995). Asian American elderly. In E. Lee (Ed.), *Working with Asian Americans: A guide for clinicians* (pp. 208–223). New York: The Guilford Press.

Lesser, J. M., Hughes, S. V., Jemelka, J. R., & Kumar, S. (2005). Challenges and strategies for taking a comprehensive history in the elderly. *Geriatrics, 60*(11), 22–31.

Liu, G. G., & Christensen, D. B. (2002). The continuing challenge of inappropriate prescribing in the elderly: An update of the evidence. *Journal of the American Pharmaceutical Association, 42*, 847–857.

Lundell, J., & Morris, M. (2004). Tales, tours, tools, and troupes: A tiered research method to inform ubiquitous designs for the elderly. *British Computer Society Human-Computer Interaction Group, 21*, 165–178.

Mac-Mary, S., Sainthillier, J. M., & Humbert, P. (2004). Dry skin and the environment. *Exogenous Dermatology, 3*, 72–80.

Maio, V., Hartmann, C. W., Poston, S., Liu-Chen, X., Diamond, J., & Arenson, C. (2006). Potentially inappropriate prescribing for elderly patients in 2 outpatient settings. *American Journal of Medical Quality, 31*(3), 162–168.

Matthews, J. T. (2006). Existing and emerging healthcare devices for elders to use at home. *Generations, 30*(2), 13–19.

Mayo Clinic. (2007a). *Colchicine (Systemic).* Retrieved August 17, 2007, from http://222.mayoclnica.cm/health/drug-information/DR202160

Mayo Clinic. (2007b). *Probenecid and colchicine (oral route).* Retrieved August 17, 2007, from http://www.mayoclici.com/health/drug-information/DR600297

Mazanec, P. I., & Tyler, M. K. (2003). Cultural considerations in end-of-life care. *American Journal of Nursing, 103*(3), 50–58.

McDowell, S. E., Coleman, J. J., & Ferner, R. E. (2006). Systematic review and meta-analysis of ethnic differences in risks of adverse reactions to drugs used in cardiovascular medicine. *BMJ, 332*, 1177–1181.

Medicare adds nearly 14,000 beneficiaries to doctor house call project with care level management. (2006, August 24). Retrieved January 27, 2007, from http://www.carelevel.com

Medication assessment. (2005, February). Retrieved June 20, 2007 from http://www.geronurseonline.org

MetLife. (2005). *Executive summary: MetLife mature market institute market survey.* (2006). Retrieved January 2, 2007, from http://www.metlife.com

Mezey, M. D., Fulmer, T., Abraham, I., & Zwicker, D. (Eds.). (2003). *Geriatric nursing protocols for best practice* (2nd ed.). New York: Springer.

Moreau, D. (Ed.). (2006). *Pathophysiology made incredibly easy* (3rd ed.). Philadelphia: Lippincott Williams and Wilkins.

National Center on Elder Abuse. (2007a). *About NCEA.* Retrieved October 1, 2007, from http://www.ncea.aoa.gov/ncearott/Main_Site/index.aspx.

National Center on Elder Abuse. (2007b). *Adult protective services.* Retrieved October 1, 2007, from http://www.ncea.aoa.gov/ncearoot/main_site/find_help/APS/About_APS.aspx

National Center on Elder Abuse. (2007c). *Major types of elder abuse.* Retrieved October 1, 2007, from http://www.ncea.aoa.gov/ncearoot/Main_Site/FAQ/Basics/Types_of_abuse.aspx

National Guideline Clearing House. (2007). *Preventive services for adults.* Retrieved May 19, 2008 from http://www.guideline.gov/summry/summary.aspx?doc_id=11699&nbr+0060046&string=P...

National Institute of Neurological Disorders and Stroke. (2007). Normal pressure hydrocephalus information page. Retrieved January 3, 2008 from http://www.ninds.nih.gov/disorders/normal_pressure_hydrocephalus

National Institute on Aging. (2006). *Forgetfulness: It's not always what you think.* U.S. National Institutes of Health. Retrieved December 29, 2007, from http://www.niapublications.org/agepages/forgetfulness.asp

National Institutes of Health Consensus Development Panel. (2001). Osteoporosis prevention, diagnosis, and therapy. *Journal of the American Medical Association, 285*, 785–795.

Novoseltsev, V. N., Novoseltseva, J., & Yashin, A. I. (2001). A homeostatic model of oxidative damage explains paradoxes observed in earlier aging experiments: a fusion and extension of older theories of aging. *Biogerontology, 2*(2), 127–138.

Piturro, M. (2004). Assistive technology in ITC. *Caring for the Ages, 5*(12), 32–34.

Polypharmacy. (2007). Retrieved February 14, 2007, from http://www.Mercksource.com/pp/us/cns_search results.jsp

Red Horse, J. (1981). *American Indian families.* Paper presented at the Conference on American Indican Family Strengths and Stress. Elmsford, NY: Pergamon Press.

Reuben, D. B., Herr, K. A., Pacala, J. T., Pollock, B. G., Potter, J. F., & Semala, T. P. (2007). *Geriatrics at your fingertips: 2007–2008* (9th ed.). New York: American Geriatrics Society.

Roehl, B., Talati, A., & Parks, S. (2006). Medication prescribing for older adults. *Annals of Long-Term Care, 14*(6), 33–39.

Roy, H., & Russell, C. (2005). The *encyclopedia of aging & the elderly.* Iowa City, Iowa: MedRounds Publications.

Sattinger, A. M. (2006). Collaboration helps hospice work in ITC. *Caring for the Ages, 7*(3), 17–18.

Schaffer, S. (2006). "Theory and Theorizing Across Borders: Global Social Thought and Geographic Organic Intellectualism" Paper presented at the annual meeting of the American Sociological Association, Montreal Convention Center, Montreal, Quebec, Canada Online. Retrieved June 27, 2008 from http://www.allacademic.com/meta/p104982_index.html

Smith, N. M., Breese, J. S., Shay, D. K., Uyeki, T. M., Cox, N. J., & Strikas, R. A. (2006, June 28). Prevention and control of influenza. *Morbidity and Mortality Weekly Report*, pp. 1–54.

Stibich, M. (2007a). *The genetic theory of aging.* Retrieved May 15, 2008 from htt://longevity.about.com/od/reserachand medicine//p/age_genetics.htm

Stibich, M. (2007b). *Why we age–theories and effects of aging.* Retrieved May 15, 2008 from http://longevity.about.coj/od/longevity101/a/why_we_age.htm

Strunk, B. C., Ginsburg, P. B., & Banker, M. I. (2006). The effect of population aging on future hospital demand. *Health Affairs, 25*(3), 141–149.

Tabloski, P. A. (2006). *Gerontological nursing.* Upper Saddle River, NJ: Pearson Prentice Hall.

Talley, N. J. (2005). American Gastroenterological Association medical position statement: Evaluation of dyspepsia. *Gastroenterology, 129*, 1753–1780.

Tovey, D. (Ed.). (2007).*Clinical evidence handbook.* London: BMJ Publishing Group.

Tuch, H., Parrish, P., & Romer, A. L. (2002). *Integrating palliative care into nursing homes: An interview with Howard Tuch and Pam Parrish* (Vol. 4). Retrieved January 21, 2007, from http://www.edc.org/lastacts

U.S. Census Bureau. (2005). *2005 Community survey.* Retrieved February 10, 2007, from http://factfinder.census.gov

U.S. Department of Veterans Affairs. (n.d.). *What is home based primary care?* Retrieved January 21, 2007, from http://www1.va.gov/HCBC

U.S. Preventive Services Task Force. (n.d.). *Screening for colorectal cancer.* Retrieved January 1, 2007, from http://www.ahrq.gov/clinic

U.S. Social Security Administration, Office of Policy. (2007). *Fast facts & figures about social security.* Retrieved May 15, 2008 from http:www.socialsecurity.gov/p9olicy/docs/cghartbooks/fast_facts/2007/indes.html

Vanderheiden, G. (2006). Potential impact of new technologies on telecommunication for elders. *Generations, 30*(2), 9–12.

Vlassova, O., & Jackson, A. J. (2005). *December 2002 Kaiser Permanente Colorado Region adult pneumococcal vaccine recommendations.* Retrieved July 29, 2006, from http://cl.kp.org/pkc/co/cpg/cpg/immunization_toolkit/pneumovax_flyer.htm

Voyer, P., Cole, J. G., Mc Cusker, J., & Belzile, E. (2006). Prevalence and symptoms of delirium superimposed on dementia. *Clincal Nursing Research, 15*, 46–66.

Waszynski, C. M. (2007). The confusion assessment method (CAM). *Try This: Best Practices in Nursing Care to Older Adults*, 13, New York University College of Nursing: The Hartford Institute for Geriatric Nursing.

Wetherell, J. L., & Jeste, D. V. (2004). Older adults with schizophrenia. *ElderCare, 3*(2), 8–11.

Willis, W. (1998). Families with African American roots. In E. W. Lynch & M. J. Hanson (Eds.), *Developing cross-cultural competence* (pp. 165–202). Baltimore, MD: Paul H. Brookes Publishing.

Genetics

Carolyn Graff,
Ann Cashion

Outcome-Based Learning Objectives

After studying this chapter, the learner will be able to:

1. Describe the role of genetics in health care and nursing.
2. Discuss events of cell division that result in chromosomal abnormalities.
3. Describe the organization of the human genome and the DNA sequence.
4. Describe the influence of the genome on differences among patients.
5. Identify patterns of inheritance and variables influencing interpretation of inheritance patterns.
6. Discuss the role of nurses in detection, management, and care of patients with genetic disorders.
7. Describe emerging genetic technologies and therapies.

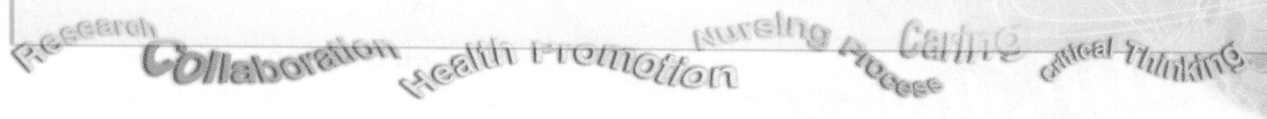

GENETICS FOCUSES on variation and heredity in all living beings. A great deal of genetics information derives from the work of many researchers, including Gregor Mendel, who is attributed with discovering the laws of genetics in 1865, and James Watson and Francis Crick, who described the double-helix structure of DNA (Watson & Crick, 1953). Fifty years after the structure of DNA was described, researchers mapped each human gene and completely sequenced the human **genome,** that is, all of the DNA in human cells. This was accomplished through an international research effort known as the **Human Genome Project (HGP).** The HGP has provided information about and insights into many diseases and development of improved methods for diagnosis and prevention.

The completion of the HGP has been described as the beginning of the genomic era (Collins, Green, Guttmacher, & Guyer, 2003). Integrating genomics into health care is critical because the use of genetic information may improve the health of individuals. **Genomics** is the field of genetics that focuses on translating the knowledge of the human genome into health benefits, including the molecular analysis of the human genome in health and illness. In addition to educating nurses and health professionals about genetic and environmental factors affecting health, findings from genetic research can be used by patients and family members to improve their own health and prevent illness. Both nurses and patients must be knowledgeable and informed so they can communicate effectively with each other and engage in discussion about the implications of genomics for health.

Foundations for Genetics

An introduction to genetics requires a foundational understanding of cells, chromosomes, and the human genome. More extensive, in-depth information can be found in genetic textbooks, such as those by Klug, Cummings, and Spencer (2005) and Lewin (2000), and appropriate websites.

Cells and Chromosomes

A typical cell has two major parts, the nucleus and the cytoplasm. The nucleus is separated from the cytoplasm by a nuclear membrane and the cytoplasm is separated from the surrounding fluids by a cellular membrane. The nucleus is the primary control center for the cell. It is within the nucleus that **chromosomes,** which house most **deoxyribonucleic acid (DNA),** are located (Figure 11–1 ■, p. 194). Each species can be characterized by its chromosome number and morphology. For example, humans have 23 pairs of chromosomes, whereas dogs have 39 pairs and tomatoes have only 12 pairs. The number of chromosomes is not associated

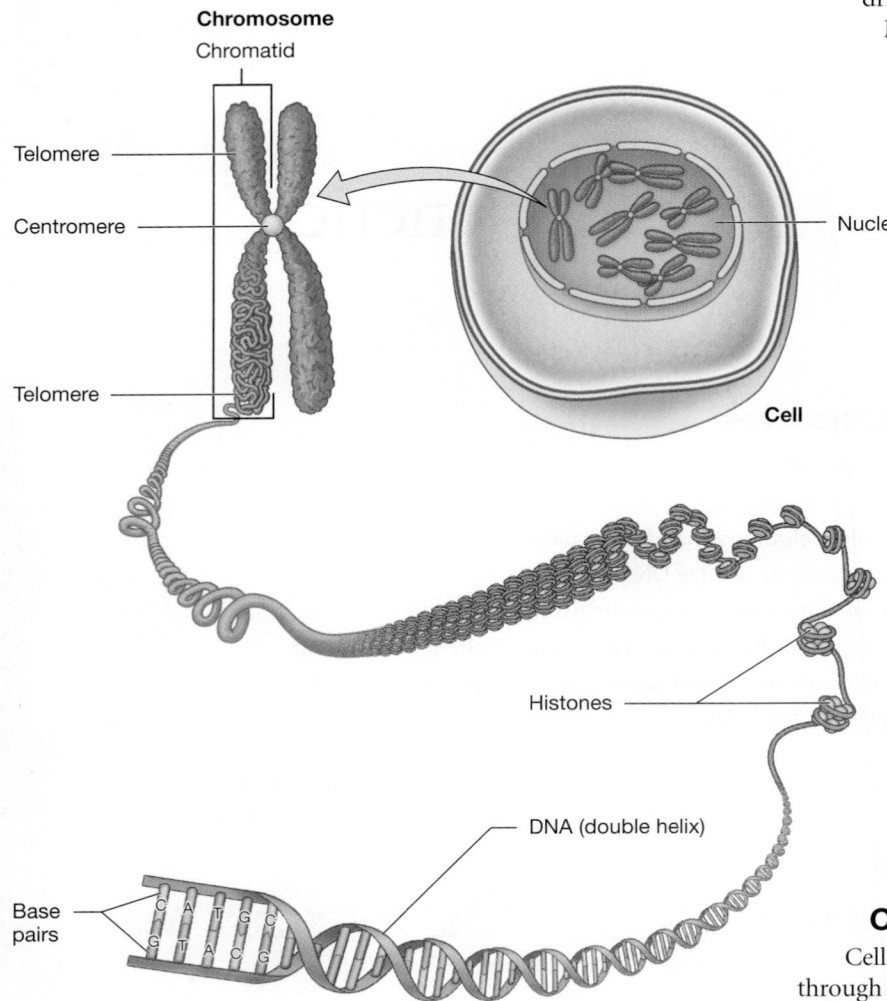

FIGURE 11–1 ■ The chromosome.

Source: Courtesy of Darryl Leja, National Human Genome Research Institute, National Institutes of Health, Bethesda, MD.

with intelligence level. The entire chromosome complement within a cell is known as the **karyotype** and is visible microscopically when cells are dividing (Figure 11–2 ■). **Cytogenetics** is the study of chromosomes, their structure, and inheritance.

Chromosomes contain genes organized into linear structural units. **Genes** are the fundamental unit of heredity that carries traits from one generation to the next. Each gene has a specific location, or locus, on the chromosome (Figure 11–3 ■). Each chromosome carries a different subset of genes; however, pairs of chromosomes carry matching genetic information in the same sequence. Because one chromosome of each pair is inherited from each parent, individuals have alternative copies of each gene, called **alleles,** one on each chromosome. For example, if an individual has type AB blood they have an A allele from one parent and a B allele from the other. Alleles are considered **homozygous** when they are the identical (i.e., type AA blood) and **heterozygous** when different (i.e., type AB blood).

Genes are found in the nucleus of almost all human cells, with a notable exception being red blood cells, which have no nucleus. Small subsets of genes are also found in the mitochon-

dria located outside the nucleus in the cytoplasm. Mitochondrial genes exclusively exhibit maternal inheritance, which means an individual can only inherit these genes from his mother.

Chromosomes are divided into two arms by the **centromere,** a constriction in the chromosome (see Figure 11–3 ■). The short or petite arm is designated *p* and the long arm is designated *q*. To identify the locus on a chromosome, both the number of the chromosome and the arm are identified. For example, the gene associated with cystic fibrosis is known as the cystic fibrosis transmembrane conductance regulator (*CFTR*) gene and is located at 7q31.2. This means that the gene is located on the long arm (q) of chromosome 7 at locus 31.2. The end of the chromosome is called the **telomere** and is thought to ensure the integrity of the chromosomes during cell division in addition to being associated with the aging process.

Of the 23 pairs of human chromosomes, 22 are classified as **autosomes** and are alike in both males and females. Only one pair is designated as the **sex chromosomes** and these differ by gender: Females have two X chromosomes (XX) and males have an X and a Y chromosome (XY).

Cell Division

Cell reproduction is controlled by DNA and occurs through one of two processes; mitosis or meiosis. Mitosis is the normal replication process used by somatic cells, which are basically all cells in the body excluding **germ line cells** (cells that give rise to egg and sperm reproductive cells). Mitosis begins in the nucleus with the duplication of all DNA in the chromosomes and ends with the formation of two new daughter cells. The daughter cells are exact copies of the parent cell.

Normal Karyotype

FIGURE 11–2 ■ Male karyotype, 46xy.

Source: © Mediscan/CORBIS All Rights Reserved

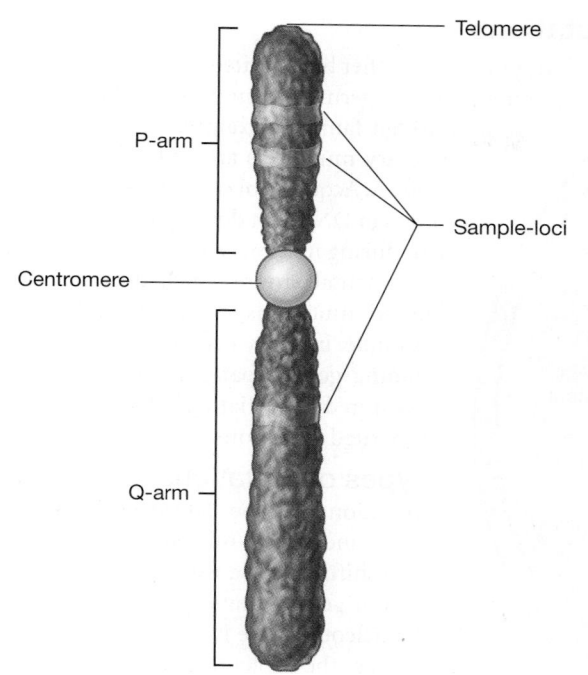

Telomere

P-arm

Centromere

Sample-loci

Q-arm

FIGURE 11–3 ■ Structure of a chromosome.

FIGURE 11–4 ■ Framework for genetic technologies.
Source: Loescher, L. J., & Merkle, C. J. (2005). The interface of genomic technologies and nursing. *Journal of Nursing Scholarship, 37*(2), 111–119.

Meiosis is the replication process that occurs in germ line cells. The product of meiosis differs from that of mitosis in that it results in the production of reproductive cells (**gametes**), which have only half the chromosomes of a somatic cell. Gametes have only one of each pair of the 23 chromosomes and are **haploid** (single chromosomes), whereas somatic cells have 46 chromosomes and are considered **diploid** (pairs of chromosomes).

The Human Genome

The **human genome** is the total set of genes carried by an individual. Genes are made of DNA.

DNA and RNA Structure

DNA is composed of four nucleotide bases, adenine (A), cytosine (C), guanine (G), and thymine (T), with the addition of sugar (deoxyribose) and phosphate (refer back to Figure 11–1 ■). The four bases, known as the building blocks of DNA, are of two types: purines and pyrimidines. The purine bases are A and G, and the pyrimidine bases are C and T. In DNA, purines and pyrimidines always pair in a complementary nature so that A always binds to T and C always binds to G. The bases align into two polynucleotide chains to create a double-helix form. Because of the complementary nature of DNA's purines and pyrimidines, the base sequence of each single strand can be deduced from that of its partner. The nature of DNA was originally identified by James Watson and Francis Crick in 1953. Together the DNA macromolecules compose the approximately 20,000 to 25,000 genes in the human genome (International Human Genome Sequencing Consortium, 2004).

The "central dogma" of molecular biology is contained in the flow of genetic information from DNA to RNA to protein (Figure 11–4 ■). More specifically, this means that DNA in the nucleus encodes ribonucleic acid (RNA), which then crosses the nuclear membrane into the cytoplasm where it attaches to ribosomes.

Once attached to ribosomes, proteins are formed using the pattern originally established by DNA. The chemical structure of RNA is similar to that of DNA, except that each nucleotide in RNA has a ribose sugar component instead of the deoxyribose sugar. In addition, uracil (U) replaces thymine as one of the pyrimidine bases.

Gene Expression

Each gene has coding regions known as **exons** and noncoding regions known as **introns.** The coding regions make up less than 10% of the human genome. A primary function of exons is to code for about 60,000 to 80,000 proteins. This is accomplished by two processes known as **transcription** and **translation** (Figure 11–5 ■, p. 196). Transcription occurs when **messenger ribonucleic acid (mRNA)** is formed using DNA as a template. In DNA, each successive section of three nucleotide base pairs forms a **codon.** The codon codes for a single amino acid. The mRNA uses DNA as a template to transfer the genetic information from the DNA to the protein-forming apparatus in the cytoplasm. Once in the cytoplasm, mRNA is decoded, or translated, to produce the protein that has been designated by the gene. Physiologically, when genes increase transcription of mRNA (sometimes known as upregulation), their expression or activity increases, resulting in the production of more proteins.

Clinical and research endeavors are targeted toward quantifying gene activity and subsequent protein formation. Although each cell contains an individual's entire genome, each gene of the genome is not actively expressed by each cell. In fact, most cells only express about 30% of the genes in the genome (Nussbaum, McInnes, & Willard, 2004). For example, neural cells only express the genes needed for normal neural function and kidney cells express genes related to renal function. To determine expression levels of a gene, the mRNA produced by the gene is measured using emerging genetic technologies such as polymerase chain reaction (PCR), real-time PCR, and microarray analysis. These genetic technologies are discussed further in a later section.

MyNursingKit | The Human Genome Project

FIGURE 11–5 ■ Transcription and translation.

■ Polymorphisms and Mutations

During the process of conception, individuals obtain one chromosome from each parent, resulting in cells having matched pairs of chromosomes. Although pairs of chromosomes carry corresponding genetic information in similar sequences, the genetic sequence for each pair of genes may not be identical. Alternative copies of each gene are known as alleles. Each individual will have two alleles (one maternal, one paternal); one on each chromosome. The most common version of an allele is considered "normal" and is called the **wild type.** Alleles that differ from the wild type are known as polymorphisms or mutations. Because molecular genetic technologies are improving, more and more specific alleles are being identified. The genetic makeup of an individual, most specifically the allelic makeup, is that individual's **genotype.**

Polymorphisms

Polymorphisms differ from mutations in that they are observed more frequently in the general population than mutations. Polymorphisms and mutations are key determinants of an individual's observable traits, or **phenotype,** and clinical status. Whether the gene variation is identified as a mutation or polymorphism has more to do with how often the allele is observed instead of whether the allele is harmful or beneficial. A **mutation** is a change in DNA sequence that has been identified in less than 1% of the population. A **polymorphism** is a change in DNA sequence that has been identified in more than 1% of the population and is, thus, more commonly observed than a mutation.

Mutations

Mutations can either be inherited or acquired. Hereditary mutations are germ line mutations that are passed down through families. Examples of diseases caused by hereditary mutations are cystic fibrosis and hemophilia A. Acquired or somatic cell mutations are changes in DNA that develop throughout the life span during normal cell mitosis or through environmental stresses such as radiation. Acquired mutations cannot be inherited, for example, in many instances of cancer. Determining genetic patterns of inheritance can assist in differentiating between somatic and inherited mutations.

Types of Mutations

Mutations can be categorized into several types including missense, nonsense, and frameshift. A **missense mutation** is the most common gene mutation. It occurs when one DNA nucleotide base is substituted for another. This changes the triplet nucleotide coding section (codon) and results in the production of an alternate amino acid. **Nonsense mutations** occur when one DNA nucleotide base is inserted for another and protein production is stopped. Both missense and nonsense mutations are also known as **point mutations** (Figure 11–6 ■). Frameshift mutations are categorized as insertion or deletion mutations. They occur when one or a sequence of nucleotide bases is either deleted or inserted into the gene. As with point mutations, frameshift mutations can alter the nucleotide bases in the coding section and thereby produce a different protein.

Disease-Causing Mutations

In general, disease-causing mutations can be categorized into four groups based on the protein outcome. They result in either (1) loss of protein function, (2) gain of protein function, (3) a new protein function, or (4) expression of the protein at the wrong time or place (Nussbaum et al., 2004). The effect of the mutation on an individual depends on what biochemical role the protein performs in the normal biology of the human body. For example, a mutation in the *HBB* gene causes sickle cell anemia, an autosomal recessive inherited blood disorder characterized by chronic anemia and periodic pain. The gene mutation produces an altered protein, resulting in changes in the structure of the hemoglobin molecule. The hemoglobin molecule functions normally except in conditions of low oxygen tension (i.e., stressful situations), at which time the hemoglobin molecule forms a sickle shape, which can produce a medical emergency.

Individual	DNA sequence		Product
Person 1	GT**T**ACC ↑		Normal protein
Person 2	GT**A**ACC ↑		Low or nonfunctioning protein

FIGURE 11–6 ■ Point mutations.

Genetic Variance and Phenotype

The associations between **genetic variance** (variations in genotypes) and phenotype are important. Knowledge of which mutation the patient has (genotype) and how that influences the clinical presentation (phenotype) affects nursing management of the patient. When considering genetic variation and its association with disease, a note of caution is required. It is important to differentiate between a gene and a mutation of a gene. It is commonly thought that if a person has the gene associated with a disease, then they are predisposed to the disease. This is not the case. All humans have essentially the same 20,000 to 25,000 genes. Therefore, it is the mutation or polymorphism in the gene, not the gene itself, which predisposes some individuals for disease. For example, each individual has a gene named the cystic fibrosis transference regulator (*CTFR*) gene. Only those who develop cystic fibrosis disease have a mutation in that gene.

 **CRITICAL ALERT** *Knowledge of which mutation the patient has (genotype) and how that influences the clinical presentation (phenotype) is essential for effective nursing management of the patient.*

■ Types of Genetic Disorders

Just about any illness is the result of some combination of genetic and environmental activity, but the role of genetics varies from small to large. The disorders caused to some extent by genetic factors are placed into three major categories: single-gene, chromosomal, and complex or multifactorial disorders.

Single-Gene Inheritance Patterns

Single-gene disorders are caused by a mutation in a single gene that may be on one or both chromosomes of a pair. A mutation is a permanent structural change in DNA. Single-gene disorders occur with a frequency of 3.6 per 1,000 by age 25 years; 16.4 per 1,000 after 25 years of age; and 20 per 1,000 over a person's lifetime (Rimoin, Connor, Pyeritz, & Korf, 2002). Commonly identified examples of single-gene disorders include cystic fibrosis, Huntington disease, and Duchenne muscular dystrophy.

Mendelian Inheritance

Single-gene characteristics are called Mendelian in recognition of Gregor Mendel's work. Mendel, an Austrian monk, is attributed with founding the principles of heredity, or Mendel's laws of inheritance. He studied the traits of garden peas and their offspring and conceived the idea of heredity units or "factors" (later called genes) in which one is recessive and the other dominant. He asserted that each individual has two factors for a trait; one factor from each parent. If two factors have identical information, the individual is called homozygous for the trait. If the two factors have different information, the individual is heterozygous.

Mendel believed that a single gene was responsible for one single trait. Today, it is known that individuals inherit genes from their parents and many genes have control over the production of traits. Genes behave as separate units and traits are the product of complex gene–gene and gene–environment interactions.

Online Mendelian Inheritance in Man (OMIM™) is an online version of Victor McKusick's (1998) listing of single-gene phenotypes. OMIM is a continuously updated catalog of human genes that includes primarily inherited genetic disorders and is considered the phenotypic companion to the Human Genome Project. It is an excellent resource for clinicians and researchers.

The patterns of single-gene disorders depend on the chromosomal location of the gene and whether the phenotype is dominant or recessive. The gene may be located on an autosome (autosomal) or the X chromosome (X-linked). The patterns of inheritance for single-gene disorders are autosomal recessive, autosomal dominant, X-linked recessive, and X-linked dominant. (Depictions of the patterns of inheritance for single-gene disorders are presented later in this chapter in Figures 11–8 ■ through 11–11 ■, p. 204.)

Autosomal Recessive Inheritance

With **autosomal recessive inheritance,** the mutant gene is located on an autosome rather than the X chromosome. The most common mechanism for transmitting a single-gene disorder with an autosomal recessive pattern of inheritance is when both parents are heterozygotes or carriers. Each heterozygous parent has one copy of the mutant gene and one copy of the wild-type or normal gene. Parents who are carriers of the mutant gene are usually asymptomatic and have no increased risk for other health problems. When each heterozygous parent gives one copy of the mutant gene to the child, however, the child is affected with a genetic disorder. Risks for the children of heterozygous carriers include the following: (1) They may be affected with the disorder, (2) they can be carriers like their parents, or (3) they can be normal without inheriting the mutant gene. The risk that a child will be affected with the autosomal recessive disorder is 1 out of 4. The risk that phenotypically normal children will be carriers is 2 out of 3. This is true for each pregnancy. Examples of autosomal recessive disorders include cystic fibrosis (CF), phenylketonuria (PKU), and Friedreich ataxia.

Autosomal Dominant Inheritance

With **autosomal dominant inheritance,** the mutant gene is on an autosome and only one copy of the dominant gene is necessary for the effects to be seen. The affected individual is heterozygous and no offspring are carriers. Homozygous individuals, or individuals who have inherited two genes for the disorder, are thought to be so severely affected that they die *in utero* or infancy. The presence of an autosomal dominant disorder in a child may indicate that one parent has the disorder also although this is not always the case. Exceptions to this may include the following: (1) The gene can be present but nonpenetrant, (2) the gene expression may be minimal and go undetected due to variable expression, (3) the disorder can be caused by a new mutation, or (4) the child is not the biological offspring of the parents. A gene is nonpenetrant when an individual carries the mutant gene but does not manifest the disorder caused by the gene.

When a child has one normal parent and one parent with the disorder, the risk for the child to inherit the gene is 50%, regardless of the child's gender. The chance of having a normal child is also 50%. This is true with each pregnancy produced by these parents. Children who are unaffected or normal have no greater risk of having an affected child than the general population, unless nonpenetrance has occurred in the child. If two individuals with the same autosomal dominant disorder have children, the risk is 25% for having a child who is an affected homozygote, 50% for having a child who is an affected heterozygote like the parents, and 25% for having a normal child without the mutant gene. These risks hold true for each pregnancy. The homozygote is usually severely affected and dies *in utero* or infancy. Examples of autosomal dominant disorders are Huntington disease and neurofibromatosis.

X-Linked Inheritance

In X-linked inheritance, the mutant gene is located on the X chromosome. Males have only one X chromosome with no counterpart for its genes. The gene is expressed when it is present in males regardless of whether it is dominant or recessive in the individual's mother. A female receives one X chromosome from each parent for a pair of sex chromosomes, XX. A male receives the X chromosome from his mother and the Y chromosome from his father for a pair of sex chromosomes, XY. Males cannot be carriers of an X-linked disorder.

In **X-linked recessive** disorders, the most common pattern of transmission is when the mother is a heterozygous carrier for the mutant gene. If the father is normal, then the parents have a 25% chance, with each pregnancy, for their child to be either (1) a female carrier like the mother, (2) a normal female without the mutant gene, (3) a normal male without the mutant gene, or (4) a male who is affected with the disorder. A mother who is a carrier usually has no obvious clinical manifestations of the mutant gene, unless X inactivation (inactivation of genes on one X chromosome in somatic cells of females, early in embryonic life) is skewed. In skewed X inactivation, the mutant allele is located on the active X and the normal allele is located on the inactive X. Variation in expression of X-linked disorders is seen commonly in heterozygotes and can range from normal to complete expression. X-linked disorders that are manifesting heterozygotes include color blindness, hemophilia A, hemophilia B, and Duchenne muscular dystrophy.

X-linked dominant disorders are seen less than the other patterns of single-gene inheritance. The mutant gene is dominant, so only one is necessary for the phenotype to manifest. Both males and females can be affected and transmit the gene. Compared to autosomal dominant disorders, in X-linked dominant disorders, an affected male usually has an affected mother because males inherit their X chromosome from their mother; some affected females may be less severely affected than males because of X inactivation; there may be an excess of female offspring in the family because some X-linked dominant genes are lethal in males; and male-to-male transmission is not seen because males transmit their X chromosome only to their daughters, not their sons.

When a female with an X-linked dominant disorder and an unaffected male have offspring, there is a 25% chance for each pregnancy to have either an affected female, an affected male, a normal female, or a normal male. There is a 50% chance that the offspring of each pregnancy will be affected regardless of the child's sex. When a male with an X-linked dominant disorder and normal female have offspring, there is a 50% chance for having an affected female and a 50% chance for having a normal male. If both the male and female had an X-linked dominant disorder, there would be a 25% chance for an affected homozygous female (probably resulting in miscarriage), a 25% chance for an affected heterozygous female, a 25% chance for an affected male, and a 25% chance for a normal male. An example of an X-linked dominant disorder is hypophosphatemic rickets or vitamin D–resistant rickets.

Atypical Patterns of Inheritance

Most patterns of inheritance follow Mendel's laws of inheritance; however, exceptions do occur. Genomic imprinting and mitochondrial mutation inheritance are examples. Originally the sex of the parent was thought to have little effect on the expression of the genes each parent transmits. For some genetic disorders, the expression of the phenotype depends on whether the mutant allele has been inherited from the father or from the mother. Differences in gene expression between the allele inherited from the mother and the allele inherited from the father result from **genomic imprinting.**

Imprinting is caused by an alteration in chromatin that affects the expression of a gene but not its DNA sequence. Examples of genomic imprinting are Prader-Willi syndrome (PWS) and Angelman syndrome. Approximately 70% of individuals with PWS have a deletion of the proximal long arm of chromosome 15 that is inherited from the individual's father only (Prader-Willi Syndrome Association, 2008). Characteristics of PWS include obesity, excessive and indiscriminant eating, small hands and feet, short stature, hypogonadism, and mental retardation. In Angelman syndrome, there is a deletion of approximately the same region on chromosome 15 inherited from the individual's mother. Angelman syndrome is characterized by unusual facial appearance, short stature, severe mental retardation, spasticity, and seizures.

The mitochondrial chromosome (mtDNA) is located in the mitochondrial organelle, not inside the nucleus. The mother's ovum or egg supplies the **zygote,** or fertilized ovum, with its mitochondria. A mother having a mutation in mtDNA passes the mutation to all of her children, and the father carrying the same mutation passes it on to none of his children. Therefore, defects in mtDNA are inherited maternally. With cell division, mtDNA replicates and sorts randomly among newly synthesized mitochondria, which are distributed randomly between the daughter cells. Each daughter cell receives different proportions of mitochondria that carry normal and mutant mtDNA. Mitochondrial function is essential to nearly all cells. The phenotypic expression of a mutation in mtDNA depends on the proportions of normal and mutant mtDNA in the cells of different tissues. Reduced penetrance, variable expression, and multiple phenotypic effects of a single gene or gene pair are typical in mitochondrial disorders. Examples of genetic disorders caused by mtDNA are Leber's hereditary optic neuropathy, Leigh disease, and progressive sensorineural deafness.

Chromosomal Genetic Disorders

Chromosomal disorders are caused by an excess or deficiency of genes contained in whole chromosomes or segments of chromosomes. There is no abnormal individual gene on the chromosome. Chromosome disorders make up a major category of genetic disorders, affect about 7 of 1,000 live-born infants, and account for almost half of all spontaneous first-trimester abortions. The frequency of chromosome disorders is 1.8 per 1,000 before age 25 years; 2 per 1,000 after age 25 years; and 3.8 per 1,000 over a lifetime (Rimoin et al., 2002).

Chromosome abnormalities are related to an abnormal chromosome number or structural rearrangements. They may involve one or more autosomes, sex chromosomes, or both. The most common and clinically significant type is aneuploidy, which occurs in 3% to 4% of all clinically recognized pregnancies. **Aneuploidy** is an abnormal chromosome number due to an extra or missing chromosome. It is usually due to an error during meiosis in which cell division results in a sperm or egg with too many or too few chromosomes.

Most individuals with aneuploidy have trisomy or monosomy, which can be associated with mental or physical developmental problems or both. **Trisomy** refers to the presence of a third or extra chromosome instead of the normal pair of a particular chromosome. **Monosomy** refers to the presence of only one chromosome instead of the normal pair of chromosomes. The most common type of trisomy in infants is trisomy 21 or Down syndrome. The chromosome number and structure seen in 95% of individuals with Down syndrome is 47, XX or 47, XY. Monosomy for an entire chromosome usually results in death, except for Turner syndrome or the monosomy for the X chromosome (45, X).

Nondisjunction

Nondisjunction, or the failure of a pair of chromosomes to separate properly during meiosis, is the most common chromosomal mechanism leading to aneuploidy. Nondisjunction can also occur in a mitotic division after formation of the zygote. A zygote with an additional chromosome 21 might lose the extra chromosome in a mitotic division, resulting in **mosaicism.** Mosaicism occurs when an individual has at least two cell lines that are different in karyotype or genotype. Mosaicism is difficult to study because an individual's karyotype is rarely done without some clinical indication to do so. Because phenotypic effects of mosaicism may not be present, clinically normal mosaic persons are seldom identified. Individuals who are mosaic for Down syndrome or Turner syndrome are usually thought to be less affected than individuals who are nonmosaic.

Deletions

Structural rearrangements of chromosomes may result from **deletions** or loss of a chromosome segment or piece. The loss of a chromosome tip is the most common deletion in humans. Occurring less commonly are two breaks in one chromosome, with rejoining of the two ends and resulting loss of the piece between the two breaks (Nussbaum et al., 2004). If the deletions occur at both ends of the chromosome, the end pieces are lost and the two broken ends unite, forming a ring chromosome. Most deletions are new or individuals with normal chromosomes have a child with a deletion. The chance that these parents will have another child who is affected similarly is probably less than 0.5%. Deletions can be large and detectable by cytogenic methods. Smaller deletions, called microdeletions, are detectable by high-resolution banding methods. Very tiny deletions are detectable only by fluorescence *in situ* hybridization (FISH) or other molecular methods, and submicroscopic ones involving the loss of a single locus are detectable only by molecular methods.

Loss of the short arm of chromosome 5 or 5p– (read "5 p minus") is a cytogenetically visible deletion. It is known as *cri du chat* syndrome or the "cat-cry syndrome" because newborns usually have a high-pitched cry like that of a kitten. Most individuals with 5p– live beyond childhood and have moderate to severe mental retardation. Other syndromes resulting from deletions include Williams syndrome (deletions in 7q) and Prader-Willi syndrome (deletions in 15q).

Translocations

Translocations occur when there are breaks in two or more chromosomes, with reattachments in new combinations. Reciprocal or balanced translocations occur when two chromosomes exchange segments and no chromosomal material is lost. Reciprocal translocations are found in approximately 1 in 600 newborns. They are generally harmless even though these translocations are more common among individuals with intellectual disabilities. Although translocations may not affect an individual's health, carriers of translocations may produce children with an unbalanced amount of chromosome material. These children are at increased risk for mental and physical disabilities, and there is increased risk of spontaneous abortions.

Robertsonian translocations involve the loss of the short arm of chromosomes 13, 14, 15, 21, or 22. Since the short arm (p) is very short on these chromosomes, this loss seems to have little or no effect. Robertsonian translocations are fairly common, occurring in 1 of 900 newborns. Robertsonian translocations between chromosomes 13 and 14 result in trisomy 13 or Patau syndrome, which is characterized by abnormalities of the brain structure and abnormalities in most of the major organ systems (Alvarez, 2006). Translocations between chromosome 14 and 21 can result in trisomy 21 or Down syndrome.

Complex or Multifactorial Disorders

Complex disorders are caused by a combination of small variations in genes that together, with environmental factors, result in or increase the susceptibility to a disorder or illness. These illnesses may be caused by single-gene mutations, yet they are not single-gene disorders. They result from complex interactions between predisposing factors to include the genotype at one or more loci and varied environmental exposures that trigger, increase, or worsen a disease process. The pattern of inheritance of the disorder or illness is not Mendelian, but follows a complex or multifactorial pattern (Nussbaum et al., 2004).

Complex disorders are considered to be disorders of adulthood. The frequency of complex disorders by age 25 years is 46.4 per 1,000; after 25 years is 600 per 1,000; and over an individual's lifetime is 646.4 per 1,000 (Rimoin et al., 2002).

A complex pattern of inheritance is the basis for conditions such as Alzheimer, cancer, cardiovascular disease, diabetes mellitus, and obesity. Although these conditions often occur in more than one member of a family, they do not follow clear Mendelian patterns of inheritance.

Alzheimer Disease

Alzheimer disease (AD) is a neurodegenerative disease characterized by chronic, progressive loss of memory and other intellectual functions. Other traits of AD include personality changes, death of neurons, development of amyloid neuritic plaques, and formation of neurofibrillary tangles within affected neurons. AD is the most common form of dementia in late life, with about 25% of AD being familial. Less than 2% of these families have early-onset familial AD (EOFAD) in which symptoms occur before age 65. Three genes have been identified as a cause of EOFAD:

1. *PSEN1,* located on chromosome 14 (a precursor for presenilin 1)
2. *AD1,* located on chromosome 21 (a precursor for amyloid beta A4 protein)
3. *AD4,* located on chromosome 1 (a precursor for presenilin-2).

EOFAD appears to follow an autosomal dominant transmission.

The majority of familial AD (FAD) occurs after age 65 or is considered to be late-onset FAD. This complex disorder is thought to involve several susceptibility genes. One of these susceptibility genes is the *APOE e4* gene on chromosome 19. Other genes located on chromosomes 2, 9, 10, 12, and 15 are being investigated for contributing to late-onset FAD. Trisomy 21 or Down syndrome appears to be related to AD because essentially all individuals with trisomy 21 will develop signs of AD after age 40. The reason for this is thought to be the lifelong overexpression of the *APP* gene on chromosome 21 (Bird, 1998).

The majority of AD (approximately 75%) is due to unknown causes. This nonfamilial or sporadic AD is thought to be multifactorial and resulting from the combination of aging, genetic predisposition, and exposure to one or more environmental influences. Factors such as head trauma, viruses, and/or toxins have been investigated for their influence on AD but have not been proven to be contributors (Cummings, Vinters, Cole, & Khachaturian, 1998).

Cancer

Cancer, a group of diseases that share common characteristics, is a disease of somatic cells. Specifically, cells experience uncontrolled growth as a result of mutations that affect a limited number of genes. Cancer cells have two characteristics that are not found in normal cells. In normal cells, cell-to-cell contact inhibits further growth and division, a process called contact inhibition. Cancer cells do not have contact inhibition; instead, they continue to grow and divide and may even pile on top of each other. If normal cells are badly damaged or starved for nutrients, they undergo apoptosis, or programmed cell death, and self-destruct. Cancer cells do not undergo apoptosis. Normal cells experience cell senescence or stop dividing in culture after about 50 divisions. Cancer cells in culture divide indefinitely. Additional information about the molecular basis of cancer and conversion of normal somatic cells to cancer cells can be found in Nussbaum et al. (2004) and Hartl and Jones (2004).

About one-third of the 565,650 cancer deaths expected to occur in the United States in 2008 will be related to nutrition, physical inactivity, and obesity or overweight. More than 170,000 cancer deaths are expected to be caused by tobacco use. Although anyone can develop cancer, risks increase as individual's age. About 77% of all cancers are diagnosed in individuals 55 years and older. Cancer researchers refer to the lifetime risk of developing cancer as the probability that an individual will, over the course of his or her lifetime, develop cancer or die from it. Relative risk is a measure of the strength of the relationship between risk factors and a particular cancer. Relative risk compares the risk of developing cancer in individuals with a certain exposure or trait to the risk in persons who do not have this exposure or trait. Male smokers are about 23 times more likely to develop lung cancer than nonsmokers, so their relative risk is 23 (American Cancer Society [ACS], 2008).

About 5% of individuals with cancer have familial cancer or cancer in which there is clear evidence that an inherited gene predisposes the individual to very high risk for a particular cancer (ACS, 2008). The remaining 95% are sporadic or cancers that occur as a result of genetic changes in somatic cells. These changes occur over the lifetime and are due to internal factors such as hormones or digestion of nutrients in cells. They may also be caused by external factors, such as tobacco, chemicals, and sunlight. Inheriting a cancer-causing gene usually does not indicate a 100% chance that cancer will develop, but it may indicate a significant risk that an individual will develop cancer at some point over his or her lifetime. Knowing this, a careful surveillance program can be instituted that will identify cancer early and decrease morbidity and mortality.

Nurses should carefully examine the family history and pedigree for clues associated with an inherited susceptibility to cancer (Chart 11–1). Cancers with a familial basis often occur at a younger age than sporadic cancers; they are usually bilateral in paired organs (e.g., breasts and kidneys), and multifocal, or occur in multiple sites in a single organ. Following analysis of the family history and pedigree, nurses should look for the presence of these clues. If a hereditary syndrome is suspected and if any of the clues are present, the patient and family should be referred to a nurse, physician, or genetic counselor with advanced professional training in cancer genetics (National Cancer Institute, 2004).

Coronary Artery Disease

Coronary artery disease (CAD) is caused by atherosclerosis or thickening and hardening of the inside walls of arteries. Some hardening of the arteries occurs normally as individuals grow older. In atherosclerosis, plaque deposits build up in the arteries. Plaque is made of fat, cholesterol, calcium, and other substances found in the blood. This buildup of plaque can narrow the arteries, resulting in less blood flowing to the heart muscle. This blockage can eventually completely block the arteries and flow of blood. Blood clots may also form and block the arteries. Risk

CHART 11–1 | **Clues Suggesting an Inherited Cancer Susceptibility Syndrome**

- Multiple cancers in close relatives
- Early age of onset; younger than 40 to 50 years for adult-onset cancers
- Multiple cancers in a single individual
- Bilateral cancer in paired organs (e.g., breast, kidney)
- Recognition of the known association between etiologically related cancers in the family
- Presence of congenital anomalies or precursor lesions that are known to be associated with increased cancer risk (e.g., presence of atypical nevi and risk of malignant melanoma)
- Recognizable Mendelian inheritance pattern

Source: National Cancer Institute. (2004, September 16). *Elements of cancer genetics risk assessment and counseling.* Last updated October 3, 2006. Retrieved November 12, 2006, from http://www.nci.nih.gov/cancertopics/pdq/genetics/risk-assessment-and-counseling.

factors for CAD include the following: age, family history of early heart disease, high blood cholesterol, high blood pressure, cigarette smoking, diabetes, obesity, and lack of physical activity. All factors except age and family history can be altered by an individual to prevent or delay onset of CAD. Individuals with a family history of early heart disease include those individuals with heart disease diagnosed before age 55 in a father or brother, and before age 65 in a mother or sister.

Single-gene disorders that cause CAD include defects in the apolipoproteins; receptor defects, such as LDL receptor disorder leading to familial hypercholesterolemia; enzyme defects, such as lipoprotein lipase deficiency; and defects in transfer proteins, such as cholesteryl ester transfer protein deficiency. Treatment with appropriate medications and lifestyle changes can reduce cholesterol levels in heterozygous individuals but may not help individuals who are homozygous for the gene contributing to CAD.

Diabetes Mellitus

The two major types of diabetes mellitus are type 1 (insulin-dependent diabetes) and type 2 (non–insulin-dependent diabetes). Of the 20.8 million individuals in the United States who have diabetes mellitus, 5% to 10% have type 1 and approximately 88% have type 2 (American Diabetes Association [ADA], 2008). Both types are complex disorders because both genetic and environmental factors are necessary for their expression.

Type 1 is an autoimmune disorder that is attributed to both an inherited risk and external triggers or factors including viruses, nutrition, and toxins. About 18 regions in the human genome are linked to influencing type 1 diabetes risk. These regions, labeled IDDM1 to IDDM18, each may contain several genes that contribute to risk. The most studied is IDDM1, which contains HLA genes, located on chromosome 6. Inheriting certain alleles of the HLA genes increases the likelihood that immune cells will attack the body's healthy cells. One of the non-HLA genes, *IDDM2,* is the insulin gene, located on chromosome 11. Inheritance of the *IDDM1* HLA genes can account for a greater than 50% genetic risk, and inheritance of the *IDDM2* gene can contribute another 10% genetic risk (Dean & McEntyre, 2004).

Type 2 diabetes has a stronger genetic basis than type 1 and is also affected by environmental factors. Risk factors include obesity and a positive family history of diabetes. Although many genes appear to be involved in the occurrence of type 2 diabetes, they have not been well defined. A rare form of diabetes called maturity-onset diabetes in the young (MODY), whose phenotype is similar to type 2 diabetes, is a single-gene disorder with autosomal dominant inheritance (ADA, 2008).

Obesity

Currently, more than 65% of U.S. adults are overweight or obese, which increases their risk for other chronic diseases such as heart disease and diabetes. In a few rare cases, gene mutations have been found to cause morbid obesity regardless of the environment. However, common forms of obesity are due to susceptibility genes acting within a receptive environment to create an obesity phenotype (Cummings & Schwartz, 2003). According to the "thrifty gene" hypothesis, evolution has favored genes that promote weight gain to protect humans against an environment that was unreliable in providing food. Unfortunately, our thrifty genes are maladaptive in today's environment of excess foods and diminished physical activity (Hill & Peters, 1998).

Studies of monozygotic and dizygotic twins have shown that estimated inheritability for obesity is 50% to 90% (Froguel & Boutin, 2001). Currently, more than 300 genes and chromosomal regions have been associated with obesity phenotypes. Genes of particular interest include leptin, leptin receptor, melanocortin 4 receptor, and single-minded 1 homologue.

Clinical studies are exploring the genetic determinants of obesity and identifying critical biologic pathways involved in maintaining energy balance. These studies could point the way toward therapeutic interventions and identify those at risk or responsive to environmental modulations.

Hemoglobinopathies

Two hemoglobinopathies, sickle cell disease and thalassemias, are good examples of disorders of hemoglobin. Both are molecular diseases in which the primary disease-causing event is an inherited or acquired mutation. A genetic disease occurs when there is an alteration in the DNA of an essential gene that changes the amount or function or both of the messenger RNA (mRNA) and protein. Single-gene disorders almost always result from mutations that change protein function.

Sickle Cell Disease

Sickle cell disease is an example of a change in the amino acid sequence that causes pathology. This is accomplished by the protein developing a new characteristic, without changing the protein's normal function. It was identified by Linus Pauling and was the first molecular disease to be recognized. The amino acid substitution in sickle cell disease changes the shape of hemoglobin from a round to a distorted sickle shape. The sickled cells' shortened life span (a few weeks compared to four months) results in anemia. Sickle cells become trapped in small blood vessels and cause tissue damage, infections, and periodic episodes of intense pain.

Sickle cell disease is an autosomal recessive disorder occurring most frequently in equatorial Africa and less commonly in the Mediterranean area and India and in countries to which people from these regions have migrated. The sickle cell gene has been described as protecting individuals against malaria, which accounts for its high frequency in areas of the world where malaria occurs. About 1 in 600 African Americans is born with sickle cell disease. Although many individuals die in early childhood, the life span of individuals with sickle cell disease is increasing (National Institutes of Health, 2006).

Thalassemias

Mutations also cause loss of protein function, the most common consequence of mutation. Although the mutations are in the same gene as the mutation that causes sickle cell disease, the red blood cells do not sickle in thalassemia. The severity of the thalassemia that results from loss-of-function mutations is generally related to the amount of function lost. When the thalassemias are grouped together, they are the most common single-gene disorder.

Thalassemia was first discovered in persons of Mediterranean origin. Both alpha- and beta-thalassemia have a high frequency in many populations, although alpha-thalassemia is more prevalent and widely distributed. Thalassemia offers protection against malaria to individuals who are carriers and is found in countries in the Mediterranean, the Middle East, and parts of Africa, India, and Asia.

Nursing Role in Detection, Management, and Care of Individuals with Genetic Disorders

The field of genetics influences all aspects of nursing, from the application of genetic principles in patient care to employing cutting-edge genetic methodologies in research protocols. As may be expected, the specific role played by the nurse depends on several factors, including the patient's needs and the nurse's expertise and knowledge of genetics. Currently, a nationwide effort is underway to increase the genetic content in all health care curricula (e.g., nursing, medicine, and pharmacy). Nurses are on the front line of patient care where the timely integration of genetic knowledge, skills, and attitudes into routine patient care is warranted to provide effective care to individuals and their families. Several organizations, including the International Society of Nurses in Genetics (2007), the National Coalition for Health Professional Education in Genetics (NCHPEG) (2000), and the Consensus Panel on Genetic/Genomic Nursing Competencies (2006), have recommended genetic core competencies and standards for nurses and other health care professionals (Chart 11–2). Principal among these are the abilities to identify who may benefit from genetic services and to make appropriate genetic referrals. As genetic content increases in nursing curricula and as more is learned about genomic determinants of common diseases, nurses will be increasingly involved in the management, interpretation, and decision making related to genetic information and services. In addition, nurses must also consider the ethical, legal, and social issues related to privacy and discrimination of genetic information. These will be discussed in a later section.

Pedigrees

Recognizing patterns of inheritance and clustering of diseases within families is a key skill needed to determine genetic risk assessment. These can be determined based on a thorough family history that is organized into a family tree, called a **pedigree.** Pedigrees enable the health care provider to visualize how diseases and characteristics are clustered within a family and through generations.

Three generational pedigrees are used by geneticists, advanced practice genetic nurses, and genetic counselors, among others, to identify disease risk and to develop a personalized prevention program for chronic conditions as well as single-gene disorders (Consensus Panel on Genetic/Genomic Nursing Competencies, 2006). Once an accurate family history has been established and genetic disorders or health care risks identified, it may be appropriate to refer the client to a geneticist or genetic counselor for follow-up.

Tools have been developed to assist health care providers in conducting a thorough family history and to draw a pedigree

(American Medical Association, 2006; Bennett et al., 1995). For each family member, the most important information to record is the current age (or age at death), ethnicity, and relevant medical conditions with onset or duration. Commonly used pedigree symbols are listed in Figure 11–7 ■ (p. 204) and used in Figures 11–8 through 11–11 ■ (p. 204) as examples of the types of inheritance patterns for single-gene disorders.

Recently, to encourage all Americans to learn more about their family health history, the U.S. Surgeon General in cooperation with other agencies, has launched a national public health campaign called the U.S. Surgeon General's Family History Initiative, My Family Health Portrait. This is a patient-friendly website designed for the general public to create a personalized family health history report from any computer with an Internet connection and an up-to-date web browser. Using the website software, the patient can create a three-generation pedigree that can be printed and shared with health care professionals.

For some disorders, cluster patterns in a pedigree do not appear to follow an autosomal dominant, recessive, or X-linked pattern of inheritance. Occasionally this is due to either incomplete penetrance or varied expressivity. These features are most commonly seen in autosomal dominant conditions. **Penetrance** is the proportion of individuals who have the genotype and actually manifest the disease or trait. It is considered an all-or-none concept. This is because an individual with a specific genotype either will, or will not, be affected with the disorder regardless of environmental or other genetic influences. Some disorders such as myotonic dystrophy, a form of muscular dystrophy characterized by generalized weakness and muscle wasting, have incomplete or reduced penetrance, meaning that some individuals with the genotype are affected and some are not.

Expressivity is the degree to which a person with a specific genotype is affected. For example, two individuals may have the same genotype, but one may have all of the symptoms of the disorder, while the second one has relatively few symptoms. This is known as variable expressivity. Marfan syndrome, an autosomal dominant disorder caused by a mutation in collagen formation, is an example of variable expressivity. Skeletal, optical, and cardiovascular abnormalities range in severity among individuals with Marfan syndrome.

Genetic Testing

The explosion in genetic knowledge and molecular technologies has led to a heightened public awareness of the genetic components of disease. Because of public access to cutting-edge research, patients are approaching their primary health care provider with requests for genetic testing for conditions ranging from rare genetic disorders to colon cancer. In the past, genetic counselors have provided guidance and counseling for genetic testing; however, there are not enough genetic counselors to meet the needs of patients referred for genetic testing. Therefore, it has become the nurses' responsibility to become knowledgeable about genetic testing and the ethical, legal, and social issues pertaining to them.

An accurate family history is a powerful initial method for determining genetic risk and this can be followed up with appropriate laboratory genetic testing. Currently, more than 1,500 diseases can be tested for using genetic tests. Genetic tests include prenatal testing, newborn screening, and carrier, diagnostic, and

Essential Nursing Competencies for Genetics and Genomics

PROFESSIONAL RESPONSIBILITIES

All registered nurses are expected to engage in professional role activities that are consistent with *Nursing: Scope and Standards of Practice* (American Nurses Association, 2004). In addition, competent nursing practice now requires the incorporation of genetic and genomic knowledge and skills in order to:

- Recognize when one's own attitudes and values related to genetic and genomic science may affect care provided to clients.
- Advocate for client's access to desired genetic/genomic services and/or resources including support groups.
- Examine competency of practice on a regular basis, identifying areas of strength, as well as areas in which professional development related to genetics and genomics would be beneficial.
- Incorporate genetic and genomic technologies and information into registered nurse practice.
- Demonstrate in practice the importance of tailoring genetic and genomic information and services to clients based on their culture, religion, knowledge level, literacy, and preferred language.
- Advocate for the rights of all clients for autonomous, informed genetic- and genomic-related decision making and voluntary action.

PROFESSIONAL PRACTICE DOMAIN

Nursing Assessment: Applying/Integrating Genetic and Genomic Knowledge

The registered nurse:

- Demonstrates an understanding of the relationship of genetics and genomics to health, prevention, screening, diagnostics, prognostics, selection of treatment, and monitoring of treatment effectiveness.
- Demonstrates the ability to elicit a minimum of a three-generation family health history information.
- Constructs a pedigree from collected family history information using standardized symbols and terminology.
- Collects personal, health, and developmental histories that consider genetic, environmental, and genomic influences and risks.
- Conducts comprehensive health and physical assessments which incorporate knowledge about genetic, environmental, and genomic influences and risk factors.
- Critically analyzes the history and physical assessment findings for genetic, environmental, and genomic influences and risk factors.
- Assesses clients' knowledge, perceptions, and responses to genetic and genomic information.
- Develops a plan of care that incorporates genetic and genomic assessment information.

Information

The registered nurse:

- Identifies clients who may benefit from specific genetic and genomic information and/or services based on assessment data.
- Identifies credible, accurate, appropriate, and current genetic and genomic information, resources, services, and/or technologies specific to given clients.
- Identifies ethical, ethnic/ancestral, cultural, religious, legal, fiscal, and societal issues related to genetic and genomic information and technologies.
- Defines issues that undermine the rights of all clients for autonomous, informed genetic- and genomic-related decision making and voluntary action.

Referral Activities

The registered nurse:

- Facilitates referrals for specialized genetic and genomic services for clients as needed.

Provision of Education, Care, and Support

The registered nurse:

- Provides clients with interpretation of selective genetic and genomic information or services.
- Provides clients with credible, accurate, appropriate, and current genetic and genomic information, resources, services, and/or technologies that facilitate decision making.
- Uses health promotion/disease prevention practices that:
  - Consider genetic and genomic influences on personal and environmental risk factors.
  - Incorporate knowledge of genetic and/or genomic risk factors (e.g., a client with a genetic predisposition for high cholesterol who can benefit from a change in lifestyle that will decrease the likelihood that the genetic risk will be expressed).
- Uses genetic- and genomic-based interventions and information to improve clients' outcomes.
- Collaborates with health care providers in providing genetic and genomic health care.
- Collaborates with insurance providers/payers to facilitate reimbursement for genetic and genomic health care services.
- Performs interventions/treatments appropriate to clients' genetic and genomic health care needs.
- Evaluates impact and effectiveness of genetic and genomic technology, information, interventions, and treatments on clients' outcome.

Source: From Consensus Panel on Genetic/Genomic Nursing Competencies. (2006). *Essential nursing competencies and curricula guidelines for genetics and genomics.* Silver Spring, MD: American Nurses Association.

□ ○	Unaffected male, female
■ ●	Affected male, female
▣ ◉	Carrier of a recessive gene
◇	Gender unknown
▨	Deceased
↗	Proband
□—○	Mating
	Siblings (2 males and 1 female) from oldest on the left to the youngest
○ ↖c	Consultand
□┤├○	Divorced/separated

FIGURE 11–7 ■ Pedigree symbols.

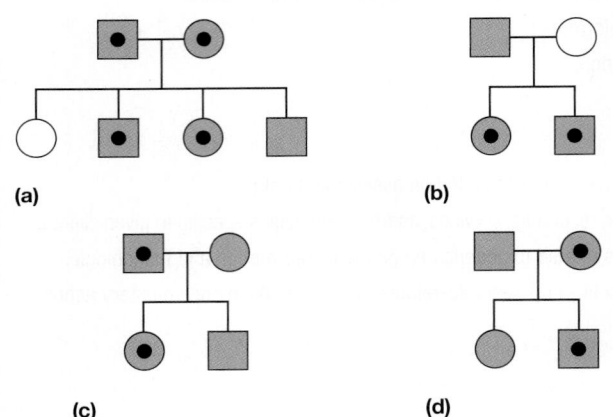

FIGURE 11–8 ■ Autosomal recessive inheritance pedigree.

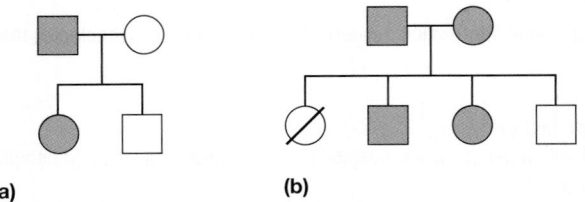

FIGURE 11–9 ■ Autosomal dominant inheritance pedigree.

predictive testing. Specimens for genetic tests include blood, urine, saliva, stool, body tissues, bone, or hair. Genetic tests include molecular analysis of DNA and RNA, linkage analysis, biochemical testing of certain proteins, and cytogenetic testing on chromosomes (University of Washington, 2006).

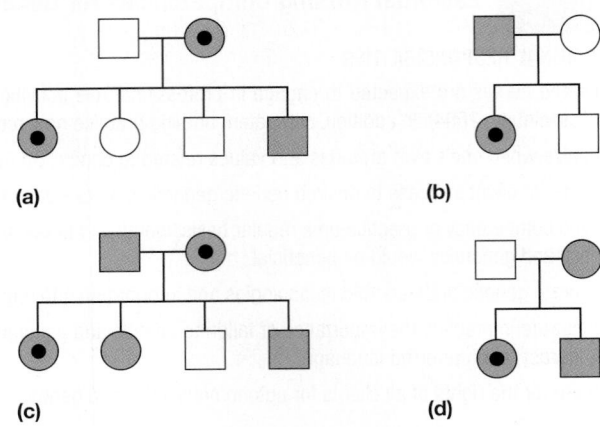

FIGURE 11–10 ■ X-linked recessive inheritance pedigree.

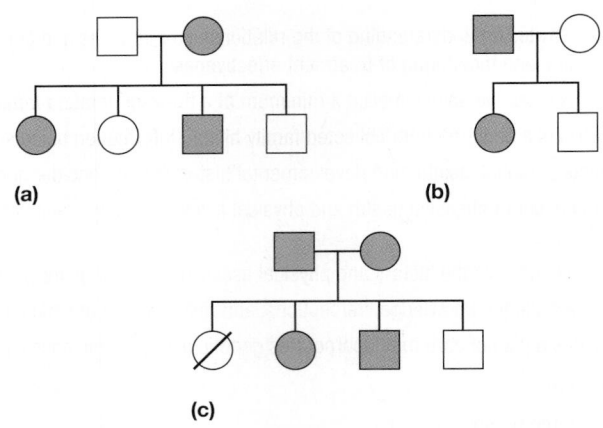

FIGURE 11–11 ■ X-linked dominant inheritance pedigree.

Prenatal Testing and Newborn Screening

Prenatal genetic testing is usually offered when there is increased risk of having a child with a genetic condition. This may be due to maternal age, family history, ethnicity, multiple marker screen, or fetal ultrasound. Biochemical, chromosomal, or molecular-based approaches are used to identify individuals with genetic disorders such as Down syndrome. Because of risks to the fetus and the mother, informed consent is required prior to conducting prenatal testing.

Each year newborns in the United States are screened using heelstick blood spots to detect genetic disorders that can be treated if found early. With the increase in new technologies such as tandem mass spectrometry, many states have expanded their newborn screening programs. The American Academy of Pediatrics Committee on Genetics (Kaye, 2006) describes the status of newborn screening for core conditions including congenital hypothyroidism, congenital adrenal hyperplasia, sickle cell disease, thalassemia, biotinidase, galactosemia, and cystic fibrosis.

Up-to-date information on what tests are required in each state can be located at the National Newborn Screening and Genetic Resource Center website.

Carrier Genetic Tests

Carrier genetic tests are conducted to determine if an unaffected, relatively healthy individual is carrying a disease-causing gene that could potentially be transmitted to offspring. This can be valuable information in common recessive disorders such as cystic fibrosis and sickle cell disease, or X-linked disorders such as hemophilia A. Knowledge of carrier status in autosomal recessive disorders is important information to use in family planning. If both parents are carriers of a recessive gene, then there is a 25% risk that each child will have the disease and a 50% chance that the child will be a carrier.

Diagnostic Genetic Tests

Diagnostic genetic tests are conducted on symptomatic individuals to identify the genetic disorder and assist with specific treatment and prognosis. For example, if a mother reports to her pediatrician that her 3-year-old son is becoming progressively weak, a DNA test can be conducted to confirm the suspected diagnosis of Duchenne muscular dystrophy. To assist with treatment or prognosis in hereditary cancers, the clinician can test for a mutation in the P53 tumor-suppressor gene. Based on the findings, a decision can be made to treat the cancer more assertively because it is more likely to grow aggressively.

As the clinical validity and utility of genetic testing is demonstrated, increasing numbers of prognostic indicators will be more closely associated with the specific mutation (i.e., BRCA1) instead of the disorder (i.e., breast cancer). Molecular approaches have largely replaced biochemical methodologies for genetic testing. In general, age is not a factor when determining whether or not to conduct a diagnostic genetic test.

Predictive Genetic Tests

Predictive genetic tests are offered to asymptomatic individuals who are at risk for a genetic disorder. The availability of predictive tests is increasing dramatically in association with the explosion in genetic technologies. Predictive tests are categorized into two groups: presymptomatic and susceptibility. Presymptomatic testing is conducted on individuals who will eventually develop the symptoms when the gene mutation is present. An example of this is an individual who has the mutation for Huntington disease, a fatal genetic disorder.

Susceptibility testing is conducted to identify individuals who are predisposed or at risk for developing the genetic disorder, but it is not certain they will develop the disorder even when the mutation is present. An example of this is hereditary nonpolyposis colorectal cancer (HNPCC), which has been associated with mutations in five genes responsible for repairing DNA. Individuals with these mutations have an 80% lifetime risk of developing colorectal cancer. Because of the ethical and psychological issues involved, many genetic laboratories conducting predictive genetic testing require documentation of patient informed consent and counseling.

An inherited gene mutation will be in the DNA of any cells in the body. Therefore, there are many sources from which to obtain samples appropriate for predictive genetic testing of an inherited disorder. DNA analysis is usually conducted using blood specimens, buccal cells (cheek cells), or skin cells because these specimens are relatively easy to obtain via noninvasive means.

Benefits and Limitations of Genetic Testing

Genetic tests differ from other medical tests because they provide genetic information about the health of individuals *and their families* and also identify asymptomatic individuals who are at risk. Benefits can include medical management that is more appropriate for the particular diagnosis and opportunities for counseling and health promotion. Activities to reduce disease risk, increase longevity, and improve quality of life may also be prescribed. Genetic testing results can be useful when making future decisions regarding children, financial planning, career choices, and lifestyle. In addition, for some individuals, knowing the test results may decrease stress and anxiety by eliminating uncertainty—even if the test is positive.

Limitations of genetic testing depend on the type of genetic test conducted. For example, a limitation of predictive testing is that it does not provide a diagnosis; instead, it identifies if the patient is "at risk." Just as a positive result does not always mean that the patient will develop a disease, a negative result does not mean the patient will not develop the disease or disorder. Diagnostic tests may provide a diagnosis, yet there may or may not be a therapeutic intervention for the genetic disorder.

Another significant limitation is that current molecular genetic tests examine for a mutation at a specific locus and do not identify mutations in other areas of the gene or the genome. For example, cystic fibrosis can be diagnosed by a mutation in the cystic fibrosis gene. However, more than 900 different mutations have been identified in that one gene. Additionally, the assay panels commonly test for only 25 of the most frequently identified mutations. Therefore, individuals with one of the other 875 mutations would not be identified and the disorder would go undiagnosed.

Concerns about the effects of information from genetic testing on the patient and family members and implications for the future should be considered. Although universal guidelines have not been developed for genetic testing, all nurses should handle information obtained from genetic testing carefully. Attention should be given to privacy, informed consent, and confidentiality. Patients have the right to privacy regarding test results to avoid future discrimination or questions about employability or insurability. Patients and health care providers should have adequate knowledge of the risks, benefits, and alternatives to genetic testing so that they understand the implications.

Ethical, Legal, and Social Issues of Genetic Information

The Ethical, Legal and Social Implications (ELSI) research program began in 1990 as an essential component of the Human Genome Project. The purpose of the program was to address the implications of the mapping and sequencing of the human genome with regard to the ethical, legal, and social consequences of the mapping and sequencing of the human genome. The intent was to stimulate discussion on these issues and develop policy options that would ensure that the information gained was used to benefit individuals and society. Funds from the National Human Genome Research Institute (NHGRI) are designated to fund ELSI research (NHGRI, 2006). There is a particular emphasis on genetic issues related to discrimination, privacy, psychological impact and stigmatization, and uncertainties associated with interpretation of predictive genetic tests. In addition, issues surrounding the availability and access to testing and treatment and their cost are being addressed.

Genetic discrimination is the concern that genetic information may be used by employers against employees, or to screen potential employees; and by insurance companies to deny or limit insurance. In May of 2008, the Genetic Information Nondiscrimination Act (GINA) was signed into law. The landmark legislation provides protection against discrimination based on an individual's genetic information in health insurance coverage and employment setting and should allow fuller use of genetic testing. In addition, the Health Information Portability and Accountability Act (HIPAA), discussed in Chapter 3 🔗, addresses privacy issues by affording genetic information increased confidentiality.

Of primary concern is the psychological impact and emotional response of the individual and family to test results. It is important to recognize that an individual's cultural background influences how she will interpret genetic information, make decisions, and adapt to genetic conditions (Greb, 1998). This cultural and ethical context should be considered when preparing the individual and family to receive genetic results. The Cultural Considerations box provides examples of this.

Careful patient assessment, counseling, and follow-up are integral to the nurse's role in the genetic testing process. Genetic information can influence future reproductive decisions and medical treatment. The results may have significant psychological ramifications. For example, it is possible for test results to inadvertently uncover a paternity or adoption issue.

Increasingly, predictive genetic testing for conditions ranging from breast cancer to cardiovascular disease is marketed directly to consumers and is available over the Internet. Because of the complexity of the interpretation of genetic tests, particularly for multifactorial diseases and predictive genetic tests, and the potential lack of counseling and follow-up, there are emerging concerns about these marketing techniques.

Emerging Genetic Technologies and Therapies

Emerging genetic technological and methodological advances are based on gene expression (the activity of the gene as measured by the amount of mRNA produced) and the complementary binding nature (A binds to T and C binds to G) of DNA bases. Loescher and Merkle (2005) have described a framework for understanding genomic technologies. Most genetic variation occurs in only 0.1% of the human genome and it is there that researchers test for an association between genetic variation (gene sequence) and disease susceptibility. These technologies allow professionals to identify disease susceptibility genes and monitor gene activity, thus bringing applied genetics to the clinical practitioner (Cashion, Driscoll, & Sabek, 2004). Chart 11–3 (p. 209) gives examples of common genetic technologies and examples of their use.

PCR and Microarrays

Although PCR has been successfully employed since 1983 to replicate, or amplify, as few as one copy of a gene into billions of copies of that gene, real-time PCR and microarrays are emerging technologies. The many exact copies of a gene made by PCR enable researchers and clinicians to identify and study that gene. Real-time PCR allows for the detection and quantification of a small fragment of replicating DNA during the amplification process. It is an improvement over PCR because it offers more rapid and sensitive quantification of the gene of interest. Clinically, real-time PCR is used to obtain viral load levels of many different viruses including cytomegalovirus and hepatitis C.

Microarray analysis is one of the emerging genetic technologies. Although primarily used in the research setting, it is transitioning into clinical practice, specifically in the area of cancer prognosis and treatment stratification. When conducting a microarray analysis, specialized equipment that uses sophisticated computer programs simultaneously evaluates up to 33,000 genes that have been placed on a small 2.5-cm (1-in.) solid support (usually glass) chip. An application of this would be to identify a genetic pattern that demonstrates which genes are most active in disease states such as leukemia. In addition, clinicians and researchers may use gene expression patterns that emerge to obtain a more specific diagnosis and to better manage patient care (Cashion & Driscoll, 2004).

Gene Therapy and Stem Cell Therapy

Since the 2001 publication of the sequencing of the human genome (Venter et al., 2001), focus has shifted from sequencing the genome to applying this knowledge to treat diseases. **Gene therapy** and stem cell therapies are two applications that are currently in clinical development. Gene therapy is the correction of a genetic mutation by the introduction of DNA into a cell as a treatment modality to improve the patient's health. Gene therapy has been used in clinical research trials to treat X-linked severe combined immune deficiency, a life-threatening disorder of the immune system. However, complications such as the short-lived nature of the treatment and significant adverse effects related to a heightened immune response have arisen in these trials. As a result of the additional research required, no human gene therapy products have been approved for commercial use. Ethical considerations such as those related to general availability of gene therapy due to excessive costs are also issues. For further information on gene therapy, refer to the Human Genome Project Information, Ethical, Legal, and Social Implications website.

In general, stem cells are unspecialized cells that have the potential to divide without limit and to develop into specialized cells. Examples of the specialized cells are nerve, muscle cells, or insulin-producing cells of the pancreas. Research is conducted on embryonic stem cells and adult stem cells. Embryonic stem cells can become all cell types of the body, whereas adult stem cells typically specialize into the cell types based on the tissue in which they originated.

Studies using human embryonic stem cells may provide information about complex aspects of human development including birth abnormalities and diseases such as cancer and Parkinson's. The focus of stem cell research is learning how undifferentiated cells become differentiated. Learning more about this process can lead to an understanding about how these conditions and diseases occur and strategies for treatment. For additional information, visit the Stem Cell Information website, an official National Institutes of Health (NIH) resource for stem cell research. Although there is hope for the treatment potential of stem cell therapies, many ethical and political issues remain to be addressed. The NIH Research Ethics and Stem Cells

CULTURAL CONSIDERATIONS for Genetics

African American	• Greeting and addressing patients should be formal, without using first names unless requested to do so by the patient or family. • Avoid imitating jargon because this may be viewed as ridicule. • Fear of admitting carrier status with sickle cell disease may be a holdover from negative experiences with mass screening in the 1970s when carriers were denied health and life insurance. • Stressing the positive, such as protection against malaria, is important when providing information about sickle cell trait. • Support systems provided by the family may be more important than support systems outside the family. • During the first counseling session, explain the session, follow up, and give suggestions related to the present. Address the future at a later time. (Telfair & Nash, 1996)
Amish	• Introductions of providers should be informal, such as "Dr. Barbara" or "Nurse David." • Decisions are made equally by husband and wife, so provide information directly to both parents. • Because of a strong belief in God, the topics of birth control, DNA storage, abortion, and artificial insemination by a donor are irrelevant. • Carrier screening may be unacceptable. Communities are aware of problems related to consanguinity and may look outside their community for a marriage partner. • Taking photographs of a patient is usually unacceptable, but may be allowed if the patient and family understand its importance in establishing a diagnosis. • Consent for autopsy is usually refused. • A lack of health insurance, which may be common in the community, can result in deciding not to proceed with extensive diagnostic testing. • Written consent may not be well understood because giving one's word is accepted in the community. • Printed visual aids may be helpful in counseling sessions. (Francomano, 1996)
Traditional Asian Indian	• Explain the importance of an in-depth family history. • Explain diagnostic tests thoroughly. Carrier testing can result in discrimination and problems if marriages are arranged. • Because decision making may be done by all family members, schedule two clinic visits so tests can be done at the second visit after family members have made a decision about the suggested tests. • Adoption is well accepted. • Autopsies may be declined by Sikhs and Hindus, whereas Muslims may consent if necessary legally. • Explain informed consent. • Visual aids may be helpful. • Surgical procedures are not readily accepted so detailed information should be given. • Results of tests that Westerners consider bad news may not be as stressful if fatalism is a strong belief. (Patil & Fisher, 1996)
Traditional Chinese	• Family members make decisions in a group and consult other family members if necessary. The oldest male has the most authority in traditional families. • Adoptions are rare. • Autopsies are viewed as irrelevant and expensive. • Carrier testing and use of other technologies may create the potential for blame, especially toward the mother. Stress the importance of "no fault." • The use of visual aids may be appropriate and helpful. • Family histories may be incomplete and mental illness may not be acknowledged or well recognized. (Jung, 1996)
Deaf	• Avoid referring to deafness as a disability because some patients do not consider it to be disabling. When this is the case, giving birth to a child who is deaf will likely not be considered a problem. • Determine how the patient prefers to be referred to (as being deaf, hard of hearing, or hearing impaired) and refer to the patient in that way. • Avoid using terms such as *abnormal* or *affected* when referring to patients who are deaf. Describe genes as altered. • Visual aids can be very helpful. Avoid communicating while the patient is looking at the pictures. • A family history form may need to be sent before clinic visits. The family history may need to be obtained through medical records or hearing family members. (Israel, Cunningham, Thumann, & Arnos, 1996)
Traditional Japanese	• Introductions should include titles with greeting of the patient and family members as Mr. or Mrs. • Adoptions, autopsies, and organ transplants are rare. • Assure the family of confidentiality and privacy. • Explain the need for consent forms. • With carrier testing and other testing, explain the importance of "no fault." • The family needs take precedence over the individual's needs. • The family members may make major decisions so allow time for the family to consult family elders if necessary. • Photographs may be refused, especially if a child has a visible disability. The disability may be viewed as shameful. (Strazaar & Fisher, 1996)

(continued)

CULTURAL CONSIDERATIONS for Genetics—*Continued*

North American Jewish	• Use of prenatal diagnosis varies widely, depending on the religious orientation. • In Orthodox families, the male is often the decision maker, but will need to consult with a rabbi. Schedule prenatal testing early enough in the pregnancy to allow for this consultation to occur. • Orthodox families may have their own internal support groups, whereas less observant Jews may use support groups outside their immediate community. • Autopsy is usually discouraged unless it is strongly recommended. Discussion with and advice from a rabbi may be necessary. (Greenstein & Bernstein, 1996)
Latino	• The eldest male is greeted first. Shake hands and ask about family to establish rapport. • Prenatal testing should be offered even though many Latinos are Catholic. • Disclosure of carrier status or a child's disability to other family members may be viewed as a loss of dignity. • Couples and patients need time to consult with other family members because family members participate in all decisions. • Loss of pregnancy is viewed as loss of a child. • Folk healers and Western physicians may be used by families and couples, so asking what other treatments are being used is important. • Visual aids may help in explaining genetic concepts. • If the patient needs to see a counselor more than once, schedule the patient with the same counselor. (Lopez-Rangel, 1996)
Native Americans of the Southwest	• Amniocentesis may be acceptable but because prenatal care may begin later in pregnancy, it is not an option. • Prenatal procedures may be more acceptable if the health provider's hands are blessed by a native healer before the procedure. • Adoption for infertile couples occurs along matrilineal lines; the couple adopts a sister's or cousin's child. • Diagnostic tests such as venipuncture, skin biopsies, and specimen samples usually present no problems. • Family planning is considered an individual's choice and may be used infrequently. • Acceptance of carrier testing is not known. • When greeting the entire family, address the maternal grandmother first. • The amount of eye contact that is comfortable for a patient may vary, so adjust accordingly. • Patients may not answer questions immediately, so allow for silence and do not consider it inattentiveness. (Hauck & Knoki-Wilson, 1996)
Countries of Southeast Asia	• If blood tests are done, avoid drawing extra blood. Use microtubes if possible. • Respect the patient's right to refuse procedures by not assuming that refusal indicates a lack of understanding. • Ask the patient or family for permission to use visual aids. (Fisher & Lew, 1996)

Source: Fisher, Nancy L., M.D., M.P.H., ed. Cultural and Ethnic Diversity: A Guide for Genetics Professionals. Pages 32–33, 55, 82–83, 96–97, 111, 127, 153–154, 193–194, 217–218, 235. © 1996 The Johns Hopkins University Press. Reprinted with permission of The Johns Hopkins University Press.

website provides links and information to explore the issues surrounding the differing views on stem cell research.

As genomic health care expands into the clinical setting, nurses will be required to understand the concepts, principles, and ethical issues underpinning emerging genetic technologies and therapies. Having a basic understanding of these concepts allows the nurse to recognize the benefits, limitations, and applications of each therapy. More importantly, the nurse can translate this knowledge for the patient, thereby improving patient care (Cashion et al., 2004).

Pharmacogenomics

Pharmacogenomics refers to the application of genomic information and methods to pharmacogenetic problems. **Pharmacogenetics** refers to the area of genetics that focuses on the variability of responses to medications due to genetic variation. These genetic variations can alter the ability of the body to absorb, transport, metabolize, or excrete medications or their metabolites. Pharmacogenetics may include any genetically determined variation in response to drugs. It is thought that many of the adverse drug reactions and some fatal adverse reactions may be "largely, if not entirely, genetically determined" (Nussbaum et al., 2004, p. 249).

The origin of polymorphisms for drug response and the mechanisms that maintain them are a challenging problem. The response to medications requires specific biochemical reactions, and the enzymes involved may participate in the metabolism of ordinary food substances. That polymorphisms for drug response may have resulted from the different diets in different populations is supported by the geographical distribution of many of these alleles. Recognizing this normal variation in response to drugs, the "potency" of a drug is defined by the dose that produces a given effect in 50% of the population. This variation is thought to be best explained by a combination of genetic and environmental factors or multifactorial inheritance.

Cytochrome P450 (CYP) enzymes are a family of liver enzymes that help break down more than 30 classes of medications. CYP polymorphisms or DNA variations in genes that code for these liver enzymes affect their ability to metabolize certain medications. When CYP enzymes are less active or inactive in terms of breaking down or eliminating medications from the patient's body, overdose can occur (Human Genome Program, 2006). CYP polymorphisms affect patients' responses to medications that are used to treat depression, psychosis, cancer, cardiovascular disorders, ulcers and gastrointestinal disorders, pain, and seizure disorders (Ingelman-Sundberg, 2004). The research findings that show strong evidence that CYP polymorphisms in genes affect the enzyme CYP2C9 and patient responsiveness to Coumadin may lead to future genotyping for P450 in patients

CHART 11–3	Commonly Used Genetic Methods		

Genetic Method	Definition	Examples of Use
Fluorescence *in situ* hybridization (FISH)	A physical mapping approach that uses a fluorescent dye to identify variations from normal in metaphase chromosomes	This technique is widely used in cytogenetics to identify deleted or transposed sections of chromosomes.
Genotype	An individual's genetic sequence at a particular locus	To diagnose genetic disease, identify paternity, and in forensic medicine.
Karyotype	A picture of the entire chromosome complement of a cell	To identify individuals with chromosomal disorders such as Down syndrome.
Microarray	Evaluates thousands of genes or gene expression levels simultaneously.	To identify subgroups of cancer to stratify for treatment therapies.
Northern blot	A technique for identifying if a gene is transcribed using electrophoresis, gels, and absorbent sheets	To examine major variations in RNA expression levels in genetic diseases such as hemoglobinopathies.
Polymerase chain reaction (PCR)	Amplifies one copy of a DNA or RNA into billions of copies	PCR has become the standard method for nucleic acid analysis.
Real-time PCR	Allows measurement of replicating DNA or RNA as the amplification process occurs	To determine viral load levels.
Southern blot	A technique for identifying if a gene is present using electrophoresis, gels, and absorbent sheets.	To diagnose genetic diseases such as cystic fibrosis.
Western blot	A technique for identifying protein using electrophoresis, gels, and absorbent sheets.	To determine if dystrophin is present in suspected cases of muscular dystrophy.

receiving Coumadin (Rettie & Tai, 2006). Clinical trials are being conducted by researchers who test for variations in CYP genes to screen and monitor patients. Pharmaceutical companies are screening the chemical compounds in medications to determine how well they are broken down by the various CYP enzymes (Hodgson & Marshall, 1998).

Malignant hyperthermia and serum cholinesterase and succinylcholine sensitivity are two genetics-related concerns that can occur during anesthesia. Malignant hyperthermia is an autosomal dominant condition that occurs in 1 out of 12,000 children and 1 out of 100,000 adults. The ratio of malignant hyperthermia in males to females is 2.5 to 1. The condition results in a dramatic adverse response to inhalational anesthetics such as halothane and muscle relaxants such as succinylcholine chloride, which can lead to death. Individuals can experience a very high temperature, sustained muscle contraction, and accompanying increased catabolism. Most cases of malignant hyperthermia are associated with mutations in a gene called *RYR1*, which maps to chromosome 19. Special precautions must be taken when individuals at risk need anesthesia. Dantrolene sodium prevents or reduces the severity of the response if an unsuspected attack occurs, and alternative anesthetics can be given to patients at risk.

The HGP has led to the understanding that genomic information can be applied successfully to pharmacogenetic problems. Two facets of pharmacogenomics include (1) the likelihood that the design of new drugs will be influenced by knowledge of all genes, and (2) that a pharmacogenetic profile of each individual who is a candidate to receive a medication can be developed, with two possible benefits. The first benefit is that it should be possible to predict those individuals who are likely to have an adverse response to a medication. This may be accomplished even without knowledge of the metabolism of the drug or of the specific alleles that modulate responses to it. A second benefit may come from the development of abbreviated pharmacogenetic profiles such that it should be possible to predict the efficacy of the medication in an individual before the drug is administered.

Overall, the role of drug metabolism in many pathophysiological processes is important. The management of patients with toxic reactions to drugs should include evaluation of the pharmacogenetic status of both the patient and members of the family, and appropriate genetic counseling about potential risks of certain drugs. The application of knowledge from the HGP to pharmacogenetics should usher in an era of "individualized medicine" in which appropriate medications and therapies consider not only the presentation and course of the disease, but also the individual's specific genetic makeup.

Health Promotion

Determining genetic patterns of inheritance can be a powerful way to establish genetic risk and to initiate health promotion activities designed to prevent the onset or lessen the severity of disease. As previously discussed, many diseases of adulthood, such as diabetes and obesity, are a result of gene–gene and gene–environment interactions. Knowing that an individual is susceptible to disease potentially provides motivation for lifestyle changes. In addition, genetic testing provides an opportunity for counseling and health promotion activities that reduce at-risk behaviors. However, for these things to occur, nurses and patients must be knowledgeable and informed so that they communicate effectively with each other and engage in discussion about the identification, monitoring, and treatment of disease using emerging genetic techniques. Refer to the Research Opportunities and Clinical Impact box (p. 210) for research ideas in the area of genetics.

RESEARCH OPPORTUNITIES AND CLINICAL IMPACT RELATED TO GENETICS

Physiological Research

- Translational research to integrate basic science and clinical research

- Pharmacogenomic research to investigate biologic pathways influencing drug metabolism

- Quantifying gene activity and subsequent protein formation in genetic disorders

- Developing animal models to investigate the interaction of genetic and environmental factors on complex disorders

Clinical Impact

- Emerging technologies and treatments would be incorporated into clinical care more rapidly.

- Medications would be individualized based on genotype, and dosage calculated based on genotypic response rather than weight and height.

- Innovative assessment and monitoring methods and treatment therapies would emerge.

- Hypotheses related to biologic pathways in complex disorders would be tested in the animal models and moved more rapidly into human testing.

Psychosocial, Ethical, and Legal Research

- Access and barriers to genetic services

- The public and policy makers use information about a genetic disorder or predisposition to a genetic disorder

- Perceptions of genetics, genetic testing, and the use of genomics by individuals and groups from varied cultural and religious backgrounds

- Strategies for providing information about the risk for complex disorders

- Patient, family, and professional communication about a genetic disorder or predisposition for a genetic disorder

Clinical Impact

- New challenges may be addressing factors such as education, economics, health care resources, values, and beliefs that facilitate or impede access to genetic services.

- Ensure policies are developed and followed that protect patients from stigmatization and discrimination.

- Awareness of the patient perceptions is essential for planning and developing appropriate nursing care with patients and their families.

- Patients should be educated about the risk for complex disorders and recommended behavior or lifestyle changes.

- Patients and their family members should be provided with up-to-date information by appropriately trained professionals to facilitate patient and family communication with themselves and others.

Nursing Management

The nursing management tips in this section were derived from the *Genetics/Genomics Nursing: Scope and Standards of Practice* (International Society of Nurses in Genetics, 2007) and the *Essential Nursing Competencies and Curricula Guidelines for Genetics and Genomics* (Consensus Panel on Genetic/Genomic Nursing Competencies, 2006). The nurse assesses the patient at risk for a genetic disorder and uses assessment data to identify diagnoses and expected outcomes. The nurse then develops interventions to achieve expected outcomes, implements interventions, and evaluates the progress made toward those outcomes. Collaboration among the nurse, patient, family, and health care providers is critical during all phases of the nursing process.

Assessment

The nurse assesses the patient and family at risk for or affected by a genetic disorder to identify risk factors and determine the patient's and family's needs for information, referral, and genetics-related services and interventions. In addition to the routine physical examination and laboratory testing, a physical examination for dysmorphology and genetic laboratory testing may be indicated. The expectations of the patient and family must be taken into consideration. These may include their cultural views, values, and beliefs; environmental risk factors; and the patient's health history. The family history is a critical element in the assessment, which can be organized in a pedigree format that includes at least three generations.

Nursing Diagnosis

The nurse analyzes data collected to identify the nursing diagnoses related to the actual or potential genetic disorder and the patient's and family's responses. Careful attention is given to the patient's knowledge of the risks for and associated with a genetic disorder; the ethical, legal, and social implications of the disorder; and the patient's decisions about managing the genetic disorder. Asking patients to communicate back to the nurse their understanding of a genetic disorder and its implications for the patient and family members can reveal gaps in knowledge, fear of the disorder, and misconceptions about the disorder.

Planning

The nurse and patient work together to develop a plan of care that may include family members, genetic nurses, genetic counselors, geneticists, other specialists, and special laboratories. Clarifying the patient's understanding of the genetic disorder can help ensure that decisions being made for treatment are made with a full understanding of the treatment and related consequences. For example, when genetic testing is pursued, results of the tests can have implications not only for the patient but also for family members.

Interventions

Implementation of interventions may include identifying those persons who have or are at risk for inheriting or transmitting genetic disorders; promoting healthy lifestyles through health teaching; coordinating services to ensure continuity of health care; promoting and maintaining the patient's health; using counseling interventions to assist patients and their family members in adjusting to and using genetic information; and using knowledge of genetic therapeutics to improve the patient's health or prevent health problems and disability.

The ability to effectively carry out interventions is directly related to a nurse's genetic and genomic knowledge. Therefore, the nurse must have current and accurate information and knowledge of resources, services, technologies, and therapeutic interventions for broad and specific genetic disorders.

The nurse considers ethical, legal, cultural, religious, and societal issues surrounding genetic and genomic information and technologies and works to define the issues that undermine the rights of each patient to make an informed decision and voluntarily take action based on that decision. The nurse refers patients as needed for routine and specialized services.

Discussion of the pedigree can lead to mutual identification of the patient's educational needs and opportunities for the nurse to share information about factors that place the patient at increased risk for genetic disorders and risk factors that are associated with the genetic disorder. The nurse considers personal and environmental risk factors, interprets information, and identifies services that are available to each patient. Genetic and genomic risk factors are incorporated into the patient's plan of care and interventions are developed with each patient to improve the patient's outcomes. The plan of care may require collaboration with other health care providers and collaboration with insurance providers/payers to facilitate reimbursement for genetic and genomic health care services.

Advanced practice nurses (APNs) use counseling interventions to promote patients' and families' understandings of the genetic disorder and promote their adjustment to the disorder. APNs who provide genetic counseling services discuss the risk for a genetic disorder, results of genetic testing, and options for genetic therapy when this is feasible. The APN may be the case manager for the patient and provide consultations to the patient and family, other nurses, and other health care providers to ensure that proper care is provided to patients and their families.

Evaluation

The nurse carefully evaluates the impact and effectiveness of genetic and genomic technology, information, interventions, and treatments on the patient's outcomes and reassesses and revises the plan of care as changes occur.

The nurse uses current genetic and genomic information to promote the patient's health, educate the patient and family, prevent illness and injury, and promote informed decision making. The patient and family who understand a genetic disorder can make better use of genetic technology and services and more actively participate in maintaining and promoting their own health. Nurses should continue to increase their knowledge and integrate research findings into practice to assure the patient and family will benefit from advances in genetics and genomics. The nurse should develop a caring relationship with the patient and family that will take into account ethical, legal, and social issues associated with the genetic disorder (International Society of Nurses in Genetics, 2007).

NCLEX® REVIEW

1. Which information best demonstrates a benefit of genetics in health care and nursing?
   1. The information gained through genetic testing can often help individuals diagnosed with the sickle cell trait to find health insurance more easily.
   2. The nurse will be able to counsel parents who are each carriers of phenylketonuria that their children have a 50% chance of being affected.
   3. After a patient has a confirmed diagnosis of Turner syndrome the nurse would be able to explain to the parents about the trisomy cause.
   4. Patients who know they are heterozygous for coronary artery disease can initiate medications and lifestyle changes to help lower cholesterol.

2. A patient asks how chromosomal abnormalities occur. The most appropriate response by the nurse would be:
   1. "With approximately 25,000 genes per chromosome things statistically go wrong."
   2. "There is always either an abundance or deficiency of genes within the chromosome."
   3. "The combination of variation in genes and environmental factors leads to changes."
   4. "There is a hereditary alteration within the DNA sequence of an individual gene."

3. Which of the following statements by the student nurse would indicate the need for further instruction regarding the human genome?
   1. "The primary function of introns is to code for proteins using transcription and translation."
   2. "When genes upregulate the mRNA, their expression also increases and forms more proteins."
   3. "A codon specifies for a single amino acid that will eventually aid in production of protein."
   4. "The alignment of purines and pyrimidines forms polynucleotide chains that form a double helix."

4. Mutations and polymorphisms within the human genome can result in a multitude of disorders. The nurse understands that an example of a condition resultant from a mutant gene located on an autosome, received from parents heterozygous for the mutation and where two mutant copies are required for expression is:

1. Marfan syndrome.
2. Cystic fibrosis.
3. Colorblindness.
4. Leigh disease.

5. When planning the care of a patient, the nurse understands the importance of obtaining the information contained in a pedigree. Which of the following statements best describes the rationale for utilizing this tool during the planning phase?

1. To help determine if unaffected or healthy individuals are carriers of disease-causing genes
2. To locate the genotypic differences among maternal and paternal alleles caused by imprinting
3. To assist in identifying disease risk and developing a customized prevention program for some conditions
4. To recognize core genetic disorders that can be treated if found early in patients with increased risk

Answers for review questions appear in Appendix D

KEY TERMS

allele *p.194*
aneuploidy *p.199*
autosomal dominant inheritance *p.197*
autosomal recessive inheritance *p.197*
autosome *p.194*
centromere *p.194*
chromosomal disorder *p.198*
chromosome *p.193*
codon *p.195*
cytogenetics *p.194*
deletions *p.199*
deoxyribonucleic acid (DNA) *p.193*
diploid *p.195*
exon *p.195*
expressivity *p.202*
gamete *p.195*
gene *p.194*
gene therapy *p.206*
genetic variance *p.197*

genome *p.193*
genomic imprinting *p.198*
genomics *p.193*
genotype *p.196*
germ line cells *p.194*
haploid *p.195*
heterozygous *p.194*
homozygous *p.194*
human genome *p.195*
Human Genome Project (HGP) *p.193*
intron *p.195*
karyotype *p.194*
missense mutation *p.196*
monosomy *p.199*
mosaicism *p.199*
messenger ribonucleic acid (mRNA) *p.195*
mutation *p.196*
nondisjunction *p.199*
nonsense mutation *p.196*

pedigree *p.202*
penetrance *p.202*
pharmacogenetics *p.208*
pharmacogenomics *p.208*
phenotype *p.196*
point mutation *p.196*
polymorphism *p.196*
sex chromosome *p.194*
single-gene disorder *p.197*
telomere *p.194*
transcription *p.195*
translation *p.195*
translocation *p.199*
trisomy *p.199*
X-linked dominant *p.198*
X-linked recessive *p.198*
wild type *p.196*
zygote *p.198*

REFERENCES

Alvarez, N. (2006). Neurology. In I. L. Rubin & A. C. Crocker (Eds.), *Medical care for children and adults with developmental disabilities* (2nd ed., pp. 249–255). Baltimore, MD: Paul H. Brookes.
American Cancer Society. (2008). *Cancer facts & figures 2008.* Atlanta, GA: Author.
American Diabetes Association. (2008). *All about diabetes.* Retrieved May 17, 2008, from http://www.diabetes.org/about-diabetes.jsp
American Medical Association. (2006, June 20). *Family history.* Retrieved November 2, 2006, from http://www.ama-assn.org/ama/pub/category/2380.html

American Nurses Association (2004). *Nursing: Scope and standards of practice.* Washington, DC: Author.
Bennett, R. L. Steinhaus, K. A. Uhrich, S. B., O'Sullivan, C. K., Resta, R. G., Lochner-Doyle, D., et at. (1995). Recommendations for standardized human pedigree nomenclature. Pedigree Standardization Task Force of the National Society of Genetic Counselors. *American Journal of Human Genetics, 56*(3), 745–752.
Bird, T. (1998, October 23). *Alzheimer disease overview.* Last updated February 2, 2005. Retrieved November 12, 2006, from http://www.geneclinics.org

Cashion, A. K., & Driscoll, C. J. (2004). Genetics and kidney dysfunction. *Nephrology Nursing Journal: Journal of the American Nephrology Nurses' Association, 31*(1), 14–18, 29.
Cashion, A. K., Driscoll, C. J., & Sabek, O. (2004). Emerging genetic technologies in clinical and research settings. *Biological Research for Nursing, 5*(3), 159–167.
Collins, F. S., Green, E. D., Guttmacher, A. E., & Guyer, M. S. (2003). A vision for the future of genomics research. *Nature, 422*(6934), 835–847.
Consensus Panel on Genetic/Genomic Nursing Competencies. (2006). *Essential nursing competencies and curricula guidelines for*

genetics and genomics. Silver Spring, MD: American Nurses Association.

Cummings, D. E., & Schwartz, M. W. (2003). Genetics and pathophysiology of human obesity. *Annual Review of Medicine, 54*, 453–471.

Cummings, J. L., Vinters, H. V., Cole, G. M., & Khachaturian, Z. S. (1998). Alzheimer's disease: Etiologies, pathophysiology, cognitive reserve, and treatment opportunities. *Neurology, 51*(1, Suppl. 1), S2–S17; discussion, S65–S17.

Dean, L., & McEntyre, J. (2004). *The genetic landscape of diabetes.* Retrieved May 22, 2008, from http://www.ncbi.nlm.nih.gov/books/bv.fcgi?rid=diabetes

Fisher, N. L., & Lew, L. (1996). Culture of the countries of Southeast Asia. In N. L. Fisher (Ed.), *Cultural and ethnic diversity: A guide for genetics professionals* (pp. 113–128). Baltimore, MD: The Johns Hopkins Unviersity Press.

Francomano, C. A. (1996). Amish culture. In N. L. Fisher (Ed.), *Cultural and ethnic diversity: A guide for genetics professionals* (pp. 176–197). Baltimore, MD: The Johns Hopkins University Press.

Froguel, P., & Boutin, P. (2001). Genetics of pathways regulating body weight in the development of obesity in humans. *Experimental Biology and Medicine, 226*(11), 991–996.

Greb, A. (1998). Multiculturalism and the practice of genetic counseling. In D. L. Baker, J. L. Schuette, & W. R. Uhlmann (Eds.), *A guide to genetic counseling* (pp. 171–198). New York: Wiley-Liss.

Greenstein, M. A., & Bernstein, B. A. (1996). Jewish culture in North America. In N. L. Fisher (Ed.), *Cultural and ethnic diversity: A guide for genetics professionals* (pp. 198–219). Baltimore, MD: The Johns Hopkins University Press.

Hartl, D. L., & Jones, E. W. (2004). *Genetics: Analysis of genes and genomes* (6th ed.). Sudbury, MA: Jones and Bartlett.

Hauck, L., & Knoki-Wilson, U. M. (1996). Culture of Native Americans of the Southwest. In N. L. Fisher (Ed.), *Cultural and ethnic diversity: A guide for genetics professionals* (pp. 60–87). Baltimore, MD: The Johns Hopkins University Press.

Hill, J. O., & Peters, J. C. (1998). Environmental contributions to the obesity epidemic. *Science, 280*(5368), 1371–1374.

Hodgson, J., & Marshall, A. (1998). Pharmacogenomics: Will the regulators approve? *Nature Biotechnology, 16*, 243–246.

Human Genome Program. (2006). *Human Genome Project information: Pharmacogenomics.* Retrieved November 12, 2006, from http://www.ornl.gov/sci/techresources/Human_Genome/medicine/pharma.shtml

Ingelman-Sundberg, M. (2004). Pharmacogenetics of cytochrome P450 and its applications in drug therapy: The past, present and future. *TRENDS in Pharmacological Sciences, 25*, 193–200.

International Human Genome Sequencing Consortium. (2004). Finishing the euchromatic sequence of the human genome. *Nature, 431*, 931–945.

International Society of Nurses in Genetics and the American Nurses Association. (2007). *Genetics/genomics nursing: Scope and standards of practice.* Silver Spring, MD: American Nurses Association.

Israel, J., Cunningham, M., Thumann, H., & Arnos, K. S. (1996). Deaf culture. In N. L. Fisher (Ed.), *Cultural and ethnic diversity: A guide for genetics professionals* (pp. 220–239). Baltimore, MD: The Johns Hopkins University Press.

Jung, J. H. (1996). Traditional Chinese culture. In N. L. Fisher (Ed.), *Cultural and ethnic diversity: A guide for genetics professionals* (pp. 86–97). Baltimore, MD: The Johns Hopkins University Press.

Kaye, C. I., & Committee on Genetics. (2006). Introduction to newborn screening fact sheets. *Pediatrics, 118*, 1304–1312.

Klug, W. S., Cummings, M. R., & Spencer, C. (2005). *Concepts of genetics and student companion website access card package* (8th ed.). Upper Saddle River, NJ: Pearson Prentice-Hall.

Lewin, B. (2000). *Genes VII.* New York: Oxford University Press.

Loescher, L. J., & Merkle, C. J. (2005). The interface of genomic technologies and nursing. *Journal of Nursing Scholarship, 37*, 111–119.

Lopez-Rangel, E. (1996). Latino culture. In N. L. Fisher (Ed.), *Cultural and ethnic diversity: A guide for genetics professionals* (pp. 19–35). Baltimore, MD: The Johns Hopkins University Press.

McKusick, V. A. (1998). *Mendelian inheritance in man.* Baltimore, MD: The Johns Hopkins University Press.

National Cancer Institute. (2004, September 16). *Elements of cancer genetics risk assessment and counseling.* Last updated October 3, 2006. Retrieved November 12, 2006, from http://www.nci.nih.gov/cancertopics/pdq/genetics/risk-assessment-and-counseling

National Coalition for Health Professional Education in Genetics. (2000). *Core competencies in genetics essential for all health care professionals,* Retrieved November 12, 2006, from http://www.nchpeg.org

National Human Genome Research Institute. (2006). *ELSI planning and evaluation history.* Retrieved November 2, 2006, from http://www.genome.gov/10001754

National Institutes of Health. (2006). *Sickle cell anemia.* Retrieved February 12, 2006, from http://www.nhlbi.nih.gov/health/dci/Diseases/Sca/SCA_WhoIsAtRisk.html

Nussbaum, R. L., McInnes, R. R., & Willard, H. F. (2004). *Thompson & Thompson genetics in medicine* (6th ed.). Philadelphia: W. B. Saunders.

Patil, S. R., & Fisher, N. L. (1996). Traditional Asian Indian culture. In N. L. Fisher (Ed.), *Cultural and ethnic diversity: A guide for genetics professionals* (pp. 142–155). Baltimore, MD: The Johns Hopkins University Press.

Prader-Willi Syndrome Association. (2008). *Research on Prader-Willi syndrome.* Retrieved March 26, 2008, from http://www.pwsausa.org/research/index.htm

Rettie, A. E., & Tai, G. (2006). The pharmacogenomics of warfarin. *Molecular Interventions, 6*, 223–227.

Rimoin, D. L., Connor, J. M., Pyeritz, R. E., & Korf, B. R. (2002). Nature and frequency of genetic disease. In D. L. Rimoin, J. M. Connor, R. E. Pyeritz, & B. R. Korf (Eds.), *Emery and Rimoin's principles and practice of medical genetics* (4th ed., pp. 55–59). Edinburgh: Churchill Livingstone.

Strazar, M. D., & Fisher, N. L. (1996). Traditional Japanese culture. In N. L. Fisher (Ed.), *Cultural and ethnic diversity: A guide for genetics professionals* (pp. 98–112). Baltimore, MD: The Johns Hopkins University Press.

Telfair, J., & Nash, K. B. (1996). African American culture. In N. L. Fisher (Ed.), *Cultural and ethnic diversity: A guide for genetics professionals* (pp. 36–59). Baltimore, MD: The Johns Hopkins University Press.

University of Washington. (2006, November 2). *Gene tests.* Retrieved November 2, 2006, from http://www.genetests.org

Venter, J. C., Adams, M. D., Myers, E. W., Li, P. W., Mural, R. J., Sutton, G. G., et al. (2001). The sequence of the human genome. *Science, 291*(5507), 1304–1351.

Watson, J. D., & Crick, F. H. (1953). Molecular structure of nucleic acids; a structure for deoxyribose nucleic acid. *Nature, 171*(4356), 737–738.

Stress and Adaptation

Annita Watson

Outcome-Based Learning Objectives

After studying this chapter, the learner will be able to:

1. Differentiate between internal and external stressors, and provide examples of each.
2. Differentiate between theories of stress as a response, a stimulus, and a transaction.
3. Explain the physiological components of the general adaptation syndrome (GAS).
4. Explain the relationship of oxidative stress to the disease process.
5. Explain ways in which a maladaptive response to stress can increase the risk of illness and cause disease.
6. Describe nursing assessment criteria for patients experiencing stress.
7. Explain the nursing management of patients with physiological stress.

Stress, a universal phenomenon, is considered to be a condition in which people respond physiologically, psychologically, and socially to life changes. These changes may be thought of as a family of related experiences, pathways, responses, and outcomes caused by a range of different events or circumstances, with different people experiencing different aspects and identifying with different definitions of stress (Manktelow, 2003). Keeping in mind that not all stress reactions are negative, the term *stress* also is used to describe a variety of feelings and reactions that accompany actual and perceived threatening or challenging situations. A certain amount of stress is actually necessary for survival. Given the various interpretations of stress, Manktelow concluded that the most commonly accepted definition of stress is that it is a condition or feeling experienced when a person perceives that demands exceed the personal and social resources the individual is able to mobilize, while recognizing that there is an intertwined instinctive stress response to unexpected events. The internal stress response is based, therefore, partly on instinct and partly on the way one thinks.

When an individual experiences an actual or perceived threat or challenge, a physiological stress response occurs. These responses are triggered when the ordinary capacity to adapt to life's demands is strained or taxed. This stress reaction maximizes the expenditure of energy, which helps prepare the body to meet the threatening or challenging situation. The individual tends to mobilize a great deal of effort in order to deal with the event, thereby

engaging both the sympathetic/adrenal and pituitary/adrenal systems to aid with the response (Bernard & Krupat, 1994). Within that context stress is viewed as a subset of the concept of adaptation, or the processes of maintaining psychobiological equilibrium during interaction with the environment.

Although a certain amount of stress is necessary for survival, prolonged stress can affect health adversely. Because stress and adaptation are interactive processes by which people respond to daily stimuli, it is important for nurses to understand the concept of stress, its effects on the total person, and how individuals respond to these phenomena.

Stress, Adaptation, and Coping

The human stress response can be viewed from several levels: the sociocultural level, the individual's psychological response (which affects the way the person presents to a health care provider), the biochemical response of the brain and central nervous system, the resulting endochronological response, and the response at the level of the human immune system and, perhaps, concomitantly at the tissue level (Haddy & Clover, 2001). Stress also can be viewed as a sequence of events that begins with a stimulus (**stressor**), which is recognized by the brain (**stress perception**), and that results in the activation of physiological fight/flight/fright systems within the body (**stress response**).

The desired outcome of stress is adaptation. **Adaptation** refers to the reaction to stress that signifies that the person is able to cope with the stressor or change. **Coping** is a compensatory process with physiological and psychological components that allows the individual to adapt to the stressor. From a functional standpoint, stressful conditions are factors that disrupt behavioral organization; distressing feelings are signals that disruption has occurred; and coping responses are efforts to restore behavioral organization and coherence (Van Egeren, 2000).

Coping is adaptive when it involves a realistic evaluation of the situation and determination of what can be done to minimize the impact of the stressor. To be adaptive, one also must deal with the emotional aspects of the situation, and develop emotional tolerance for negative life events, maintaining self-esteem, and keeping emotions in balance. Adaptive coping seeks to preserve important relationships during stressful situations. **Maladaptive coping mechanisms** are those responses to stress that are not effective. These responses generally are chronic, recurrent responses or patterns of response over time that do not promote the goals of adaptation.

The goals of adaptation are somatic or physical health; psychological health, or having a sense of well-being; and enhanced social functioning, which includes work, social life, and positive family relationships. Maladaptive coping responses frequently are cited as precursors to disease. This chapter explores the concepts of stress, adaptation, and coping as they impact the health and well-being of individuals.

Classifications of Stressors

Stress can be caused by internal or external sources (stressors) and can produce adaptive (positive) responses or maladaptive (negative) responses. The defense mechanisms of the body determine the degree to which the responses are healthy and positive or disease provoking and maladaptive. Stress also can be classified as acute or chronic, the variable being the length of time that the individual experiences stress and responds to the stressor. The third mode of classifying stress is according to the type of human response stimulated by the stressor: physical, physiological, and psychosocial. Within this mode stressors are precipitated according to developmental stages and are considered situational.

Internal and External Stressors

Internal stressors originate within a person. They include lifestyle choices, such as the use of caffeine; an overloaded schedule; negative self-talk, such as self-criticism and overanalyzing; mind traps, for example, unrealistic expectations, taking things personally, all-or-nothing thinking, exaggerating, and rigid thinking; and stressful personality traits, for example, being a perfectionist, workaholic, or pleaser. Internal stressors are precipitated by physiological or psychological stimuli, for example, cancer, stroke, depression, and anxiety, occurring within the individual.

External stressors originate outside the body and are precipitated by changes in the external environment. They can be triggered by the actual physical environment, for example, by noise, bright lights, heat, or confined spaces; the social environment, for example, by rudeness, bossiness, or aggressiveness on the part of someone else; the organizational environment, for example, rules, regulations, deadlines, and red tape; major life events, such as the birth of a baby or the sudden death of a parent; and by trauma, such as that experienced with severe burns, a motor vehicle crash, or other catastrophic events such as hurricanes, floods, and fires. Daily hassles, such as commuting long distances, misplacing keys, and experiencing mechanical breakdowns, also act as external stressors.

Acute Versus Chronic Stressors

Acute stressors are brief and involve a tangible threat that is readily identified as a stress, whereas chronic stressors have a longer duration and are not readily identified as stressors because they are often ambiguous and intangible. Chronic stressors have become such a part of modern life that they may be taken for granted and can, therefore, pose a serious health risk if they are not recognized and properly managed. Dienstbier (1989) described this phenomenon as physiological toughening. He focused on the concept that stressors vary in their duration and are intermittent in nature, alternating between periods of stress and calm. If an intermittent stressor is viewed as a challenge, it may improve one's physiological resistance to stress by causing repeated, periodic increases in sympathetic arousal, which conditions the body to better withstand subsequent stressors. Emergencies are, therefore, transformed into routine situations, decreasing the intensity of the stressful situation (Mandler, 1982).

Human Response Stressors: Developmental and Situational

Sometimes stressors are classified according to the type of human response they generate: physical, physiological, or behavioral. More often they are considered within the domains of developmental and situational, with stress developing within certain time frames of one's life and according to situations occurring in one's life.

Developmental stressors predictably occur at various points of development throughout the life span. Chart 12–1 (p. 216) depicts stressors associated with developmental stages. **Situational stressors** are precipitated by various situations; examples include illness, a new job, or the death of a child. They are unpredictable, may occur at any time during life, and, again, they may be positive or negative. The effects of the situational stressor may depend on the developmental stage of the individual experiencing the stress.

Coping

Despite the different modes by which sources of stress (stressors) are defined and classified, it is clear that stress provokes a change in the person's homeostatic or balanced state of being. Adaptive mechanisms promote adjustment to these changes, in the form of coping, in order to return the individual to a steady, or balanced, state so that the individual has the energy and resources to meet new demands.

As mentioned earlier, coping is a compensatory process with both physiological and psychological components. It has been defined by Lazarus and Folkman (1984) as constant cognitive and behavioral efforts to manage specific internal and external demands that are appraised as taxing or exceeding the resources of the person. The interpretation and treatment of stress-related

CHART 12–1	**Selected Stressors Associated with Developmental Stages**

Developmental Stage	Stressors
Child	Beginning school Establishing peer relationships Coping with peer competition
Adolescent	Accepting changing physique Developing relationships involving sexual attraction Achieving independence Choosing a career
Young adult	Getting married Leaving home Managing a home Getting started in an occupation Continuing one's education Rearing children
Middle adult	Accepting the physical changes of aging Maintaining social status and standard of living Helping teenage children to become independent Adjusting to aging parents
Older adult	Accepting decreasing physical abilities and health Accepting changes in residence Adjusting to retirement and reduced income Adjusting to death of spouse and friends

situations, both adaptive and maladaptive, are contingent on proposed stress theories. Stress theory and the concepts of stress, adaptation, and coping are explored further in this chapter as they relate to an individual's health status and to nurses' management of patients' stress in health promotion, disease prevention, and treatment via the nursing process.

Historical Development of Stress Theories

Stress theory emerged in 1865 when the French physiologist Claude Bernard developed the concept of "constancy in the internal milieu." He defined the internal milieu as the fluid that bathed the cells, and constancy was the balanced internal state maintained by physiological and biochemical processes. Bernard's principle implied a static or fixed process.

Bernard's concept was expanded on by Walter Cannon (1932) when he developed the concept of *homestasy*, physiological equilibrium or homeostasis. Cannon established the existence of the well-known "fight-or-flight" response. He also is credited with determining that the stability of the body's internal environment is coordinated by compensatory processes that respond to changes in the internal environment, thereby causing a compensatory response to minimize the change. These compensatory responses are biologic and seek physiological and chemical balance within the internal milieu. They include blood

oxygen and carbon dioxide levels, blood pressure, body temperature, blood glucose, and fluid and electrolyte balance.

Homeostasis as defined by Cannon (1932) is one of the most typical properties of highly complex open systems, such as the human body or a cell or a large organization. The structure and functions of open systems are maintained by a multiplicity of dynamic equilibriums controlled by interdependent regulation mechanisms. Open systems react to every change in the environment, or to every random disturbance, through a series of modifications of equal size and opposite direction to those that created the disturbance. The goal of these modifications is to maintain the internal balances, or to maintain homeostasis.

Dr. Hans Selye (1936), known as the father of stress theory (Gabriel, 1997), took a different approach from Cannon. Starting with the observation that many different diseases and injuries to the body seemed to cause the same symptoms in patients, he identified a general response with which the body reacts to a major stimulus, the general adaptation syndrome (GAS). While the fight-or-flight response, as identified by Cannon, works in the very short term, the GAS operates in response to longer term exposure to causes of stress.

Selye also recognized the paradox that the physiological systems activated by stress not only can protect and restore, but can damage the body. He applied his theory of stress to the "everyday stress of life" and defined a "code of behavior" to help avoid negative stress and keep an acceptable and necessary level of positive stress. Although Cannon had earlier introduced the term *stress* to medicine, it was Selye who popularized it.

In 1965, Rene Dubos provided further insight into the dynamic nature of the body's internal environment with his theory that two complementary concepts, homeostasis and adaptation, were necessary for homeostatic balance. Dubos noted that homeostatic processes occurred quickly in response to stress, making the necessary adjustments rapidly in order to maintain the internal environment. Dubos, consistent with the concepts set forth by Selye, concluded that acceptable ranges of response to stimuli existed, and these levels of acceptability varied from individual to individual. He concluded that homeostasis and adaptation are both necessary for survival in a changing world.

Contemporary Interpretations of Stress

Current theories typically portray stress in one of three ways: (1) as a stimulus, (2) as a response, and (3) as a transaction or process. As a stimulus, stress typically is generated from three sources: catastrophic events, major life events, and chronic circumstances. As a response, stress refers to how somebody responds to a particular stressor, of which there are two components, physiological and psychological. As a transaction or process, stress is an outcome of a series of interactions and adjustments between the person and the environment. Within the transaction, the person suffering stress is viewed as an active agent who can influence the impact of a stressor through behavioral, cognitive, and emotional strategies.

These three views of stress are complementary in nature and provide the framework in which stress is studied, diagnosed, and, when appropriate, treated. Nurses use these theories to identify the stressor in a particular situation and to predict the individual's responses. They can then use this knowledge to assist patients in strengthening health and coping responses and in adjusting unhealthy, unproductive responses.

Stress as a Response: The General Adaptation Syndrome

As noted earlier, stress as a response was introduced by Selye (1936) in the early 1900s. He is credited with developing the physiologically based theory of stress and adaptation. Selye's theory predicts that stressors from different sources produce a similar physical response pattern. He called these physical responses to stress the **general adaptation syndrome (GAS)**. The GAS is composed of three stages: alarm, resistance, and exhaustion. Stressors also are likely to result in a local response called the **local adaptation syndrome (LAS)**, which proceeds through the same three stages as the GAS.

Because stress is a state of the body, it can only be observed by noting the changes it produces in the body. This response of the body, the GAS, occurs with the release of certain adaptive hormones and subsequent changes in the structure and chemical composition of the body. Once the stressor or stimulus is integrated into the central nervous system (CNS), multiple responses occur because of activation of the hypothalamic–pituitary–adrenal axis and the autonomic nervous systems. It is necessary to understand these responses in the nervous, endocrine, and immune systems in order to understand the physiological and behavioral changes that occur in an individual experiencing stress.

Body organs affected by stress are the gastrointestinal tract, the adrenal glands, and the lymphatic structures. With prolonged stress, the adrenal glands enlarge considerably; the lymphatic structures, such as the thymus, spleen, and lymph nodes, atrophy; and deep rugae appear in the lining of the stomach. Also, as mentioned, the body can react locally, that is, one organ or part of the body reacts alone. An example of the LAS is inflammation. Figure 12–1 ■ depicts these three stages of adaptation to stress.

Selye also addressed the importance of conditioning factors that may affect the stress response. He coined the term **eustress** to refer to stress associated with positive events such as winning a race or a tennis match. The health consequences of eustress were never fully explained, but the concept is similar to that discussed under the "uplifts" concept proposed by Lazarus when he described stress as a stimulus (see the Hassles and Uplifts section later in this chapter).

Alarm Stage

The first stage of the stress response is the alarm reaction of the GAS, in which the individual experiences a stressor physically or mentally, and the fight-or-flight response is initiated. When the stressor is of sufficient intensity to threaten the steady state of the individual, a reallocation of energy is required so that adaptation can occur. This temporarily decreases an individual's resistance and may even result in disease or death if the stress is

FIGURE 12–1 ■ The three stages of Selye's adaptation to stress model.

prolonged and severe (as in the case of burns or extreme temperature changes). The body has a limited amount of energy available for adapting to a stressor in this acute stage.

The alarm stage can be divided into two parts: the shock phase and the countershock phase (see Figure 12–1 ■) (Selye, 1976). During the shock phase, the stressor may or may not be perceived by the person. The autonomic nervous system reacts, and large amounts of epinephrine (adrenaline) and cortisone are released into the body, accounting for the fight-or-flight syndrome. This primary response is short lived, lasting from 1 minute to 24 hours. During the countershock phase, the changes produced in the body during the shock phase are reversed. Thus, a person is best prepared to react during the shock phase of the alarm reaction.

Physical Signs and Symptoms

Physical signs and symptoms of the alarm reaction generally are those of the sympathetic nervous system stimulation. They include increased blood pressure, increased heart and respiratory rate, decreased gastrointestinal motility, pupil dilation, and increased perspiration. The patient also may complain of such symptoms as increased anxiety, nausea, fatigue, anorexia, and weight loss.

Resistance Stage

The resistance stage reflects the individual's adaptation to the stressor. Ideally the individual moves from the alarm stage to the resistance stage quickly so that physiological forces are used to increase the resistance to stress. At this time, adaptation may occur, involving mediation of the external and internal environments. Resistance is high at this time compared with the normal state. The body attempts to cope with the stressor and to limit the stressor to the smallest area of the body that can deal with it. The amount of resistance varies among individuals, depending on the level of physical functioning, coping abilities, and total number and intensity of stressors experienced.

Physical Signs and Symptoms

There are fewer signs and symptoms at this stage compared to the alarm or acute stage; however, the bodily symptoms of the alarm reaction disappear, and resistance rises above normal. For example, instead of continuing to lose weight, such as occurred in the alarm stage, the person returns to a "normal" weight. Throughout the resistance stage, the person is expanding energy in an attempt to adapt. This adaptive response is limited by the resources of the individual. When resources are adequate, the individual may successfully recover from a stressor such as surgery and return to a normal coping state. If adaptation does not occur, the person may move to the next stage of the GAS, the stage of exhaustion.

Exhaustion Stage

The stage of exhaustion is the final stage of the GAS. The adaptation that the body made during the second stage cannot be maintained, meaning that the means used to cope with the stressor have been exhausted. This stage occurs only if the stress becomes overwhelming or is not removed, or if the individual is ineffective in dealing with it. If adaptation has not overcome the stressor, the stress effects may either rest and return to normal, or death may be the ultimate consequence.

Physical Signs and Symptoms

Physical symptoms of the alarm reaction may reappear briefly as the body makes a final attempt to survive. This is exemplified by a terminally ill person whose vital signs become stronger just before death. The individual in the stage of exhaustion usually becomes ill and may die if assistance from outside sources is not available. Often this stage can be reversed by external sources of adaptive energy such as medication, blood transfusion, and/or psychotherapy. The end of this stage largely depends on the adaptive energy resources of the individual, the severity of the stressor, and the external adaptive resources that are provided.

Interruption Theory as a Response Theory

Mandler (1982) defined stress as an emergency that signals interruption, the basic premise being that autonomic activity results when some organized action or thought process is interrupted. The term *interruption* is used in the sense that any event, whether external or internal to the individual, prevents completion of some action, thought sequence, or plan, and is considered to be interrupted. Interruption can occur in the perceptual, cognitive, behavioral, or problem-solving domains. The consequences of the interruption will always be autonomic activity and will be interpreted emotionally in any number of ways, ranging from the most joyful to the most noxious.

Stress as a Stimulus

According to the stimulus-based theory of stress, stress is defined as a stimulus, a life event, or a set of circumstances that arouses physiological and/or psychological reactions that result in a disrupted response that may increase the individual's vulnerability to illness. Historically, this theory evolved from attempts to develop questionnaires to measure stress in terms of life changes or life events (Holmes & Masuda, 1966; Holmes & Rahe, 1967; Horowitz, Schaefer, Hiroto, Wilner, & Levin, 1977). Two such scales have been developed and are used as the classic foundation for development of this theory: the Social Readjustment Rating Scale (SRRS) and the Schedule of Recent Experiences (SRE). These scales were developed in an attempt to numerically weigh the impact (stress) of various life changes, for example, death of a spouse, divorce, trouble with the boss. In their classic work, *The Social Readjustment Rating Scale*, Holmes and Rahe, with reliability reestablished in 1977 by Horowitz and colleagues, assigned a numerical value to 43 life changes or events. The SRRS is used to document a person's relatively recent experiences. In this view, both positive and negative events are considered stressful.

The Holms and Rahe scale was assigned numerical values by volunteers according to the amount of adjustment required by each event. The highest rated event on the scale was the death of a spouse. Other events were marriage, loss of a job, starting school, bankruptcy, and many others. These researchers placed the items in a questionnaire and scored each according to the rating they got from the first set of volunteers. They gave the questionnaire to people in an emergency room, both to the patients who were sick and to the people who accompanied them; then they compared the scores. The result astounded the world of psychology and medicine: sick people had experienced far more of these life events in the year prior to their illness than the healthy people who brought them to the hospital emergency room. The 43 items included in the Holmes and Rahe Social Readjustment Rating Scale, with assigned numerical values, is shown in Chart 12–2.

It was originally theorized that the greater the number of stressful life events occurring throughout a specific period of time, the greater the vulnerability to illness. Research has demonstrated a significant relationship between number and intensity of life events and the resulting probability of physical and emotional illness following the events (Holmes & Masuda, 1966). However, the relationships often are weak, and findings contrary to these studies also have been reported. Thus, methodological issues regarding additional factors (age, perception, health, previous experiences) must be taken into account when considering life events.

Note also that other factors influence an individual's response to life events. These include cultural influences, personality, clustering of events, biologic variables, socioeconomic status, timing, and interpersonal support systems. Outcomes are another important factor to consider. Disease outcomes often are confused with illness outcomes (total effect of the disease on an individual), leading to inconclusive results. These factors highlight the need to use a holistic approach when assessing the patient.

CHART 12–2	Holmes and Rahe Social Readjustment Rating Scale

LIFE EVENTS SCORE

1. Death of spouse 100
2. Divorce 73
3. Marital separation from mate 65
4. Detention in jail, other institution 63
5. Death of a close family member 63
6. Major personal injury or illness 53
7. Marriage 50
8. Fired from work 47
9. Marital reconciliation 45
10. Retirement 45
11. Major change in the health or behavior of a family member 44
12. Pregnancy 40
13. Sexual difficulties 39
14. Gaining a new family member (e.g., through birth, adoption, oldster moving, etc.) 39
15. Major business readjustment (e.g., merger, reorganization, bankruptcy) 39
16. Major change in financial status 38
17. Death of close friend 37
18. Change to different line of work 36
19. Major change in the number of arguments with spouse 35
20. Taking out a mortgage or loan for a major purchase 31
21. Foreclosure on a mortgage or loan 30
22. Major change in responsibilities at work 29
23. Son or daughter leaving home (e.g., marriage, attending college) 29
24. Trouble with in-laws 29
25. Outstanding personal achievement 28
26. Spouse beginning or ceasing to work outside the home 26
27. Beginning or ceasing formal schooling 26
28. Major change in living conditions 25
29. Revision of personal habits (dress, manners, associations, etc.) 24
30. Trouble with boss 23
31. Major change in working hours or conditions 20
32. Change in residence 20
33. Change to a new school 20
34. Major change in usual type and/or amount of recreation 19
35. Major change in church activities (a lot more or less than usual) 19
36. Major change in social activities (clubs, dancing, movies, visiting) 18
37. Taking out a mortgage or loan for a lesser purchase (e.g., for a car, TV, freezer) 17
38. Major change in sleeping habits 16
39. Major change in the number of family get-togethers 15
40. Major change in eating habits 15
41. Vacation 13
42. Christmas season 12
43. Minor violations of the law (e.g., traffic tickets) 11

SCORING

Less than 150 life change units = 30% chance of developing a stress-related illness

150–299 life change units = 50% chance of illness

More than 300 life change units = 80% chance of illness

Hardiness and Sense of Coherence

Research has demonstrated that some individuals who experience high scores in terms of changing life events do not experience illness. A mediating factor in this process, that may act as a predictor of illness is the condition termed **hardiness** (Kobasa, Maddi, & Zoda, 1983). The hardy person has (1) a clear sense of personal values and goals, (2) a strong tendency toward interaction with the environment, (3) a sense of meaningfulness, and (4) an internal rather than an external locus of control.

Sense of coherence (SOC) is a closely related concept to hardiness and has been defined and developed by Antonovsky (1987). SOC refers to how an individual sees the world and one's life in it. It is a personality characteristic or coping style rather than a response to a specific situation. The three components of SOC are comprehensibility, manageability, and meaningfulness. Comprehensibility means that stimuli derived from one's internal and external environments are structured, predictable, and explicable. Manageability implies that resources are available to meet the demands posed by these stimuli. Meaningfulness suggests that the demands are challenges worthy of investment and engagement. An individual with a strong SOC has an enduring tendency to see one's life as ordered, predictable, and manageable.

Stress as a Transaction

Transactional theories of stress are based on the work of Lazarus (1966). Lazarus purports that the stimulus and response theories do not consider individual differences. He asserts that neither theoretical approach explains which factors lead some people and not others to respond effectively, nor interprets why some people are able to adapt for longer periods of time than are others. Consequently, Lazarus focused on the person–environment transaction and the cognitive appraisals of demands and coping options (Lazarus & Folkman, 1984). In other words, the way in which a person appraises or interprets (cognition) his relationship with the environment (objects, persons, and situations in the surroundings) determines whether or not the individual perceives the situation as stressful (Lazarus & Folkman, 1984).

According to Lazarus (1966), psychological stress consists of the demands that tax or exceed available resources (internal and external) as perceived by the individual involved. Whether positive or negative (an opportunity for growth or gain versus a damaging or injurious situation), psychological stress does not reside exclusively in either the environment or the person. Instead, stress is generated from the transaction, the mutual influence that occurs between the person and the environment one interacts with during the course of an encounter. Thus, the emphasis is on the process, or dynamics, of what is happening in any given stressful event and how changes are occurring during the event. The transaction is not a static process, but a dynamic one.

Although Lazarus recognized that certain environmental demands and pressures produce stress in substantial numbers of people, he emphasized that people and groups differ in their sensitivity and vulnerability to certain types of events, as well as in their interpretations and reactions. Thus, the Lazarus model takes into account cognitive processes that intervene between the encounter and the reaction and the factors that affect the nature of this process. In contrast to Selye, who focused on physiological responses, Lazarus includes mental and psychological components or responses as part of the concept of stress. His theory encompasses a set of cognitive, affective, and adaptive (coping) responses that arise out of person–environment transactions.

Lazarus proposed that multitudes of internal and external data are received at the neurocognitive level, and that these data are interpreted during the process of cognitive appraisal. Appraisal is a judgment process that includes recognizing the degree of demands, or stressors, placed on the individual. This process also involves the recognition of available resources or options that help when dealing with potential or actual demands. The two major forms of cognitive appraisal are primary and secondary appraisals.

Primary Appraisal

Primary appraisal is the process of evaluating the significance of the transaction as it relates to a person's well-being. During the initial appraisal, a person seeks answers as to the meaning of the situation with regard to his well-being. One of three types of appraisals could be made: (1) It is irrelevant; (2) it is good, or benign-positive; or (3) it is stressful. If demands are appraised as stressful, they can be classified as representing harm or loss, threat, or challenge. Harm or loss demands involve actual damage, and threat demands involve anticipated harm or loss. Challenge demands differ from threat and harm or loss demands because they are viewed as a potential for personal gain or growth. The stress transaction also can be vivacious, such as empathizing with others who are in stress. Therefore, stress is a situation in which demands exceed the individual's adaptive resources. If an adaptive response to those demands does not occur, negative consequences will result (Lazarus & Launier, 1976).

Secondary Appraisal

Secondary appraisal is the process of evaluating the significance of the transaction between the person and her environment as it relates to available coping resources and options. Primary and secondary appraisals often occur simultaneously

and interact with each other in determining stress. They are equally important in the person's cognitive assessment of an event. Figure 12–2 ■ shows a diagram of stress as a transaction. A secondary appraisal can actually cause a primary appraisal. Secondary appraisals include feelings of not being able to deal with the problem.

Cognitive Reappraisal

In addition to primary and secondary appraisal, the act of reappraisal also occurs. **Cognitive reappraisal** develops from the feedback of changes in the person–environment relationship and from reflection about the coping process. Reappraisal allows for changes in the person's evaluation of the event, or a relabeling of the cognitive appraisal. Certain factors influence the labeling of appraisals. Situational factors include the intensity of the external demands, the immediacy of the expected impact, and ambiguity. Person-related factors include motivational characteristics, belief systems, and intellectual resources and skills.

The event may be reappraised and evaluated as nonstressful due to changes in the relationship between the person and the environment. For example, a hospitalization initially may be deemed stressful by the individual, based on primary and secondary appraisal. The event may be reappraised and evaluated as nonstressful, however, because of changes in the relationship between the person and the environment, such as a positive outcome of improved health from the hospitalization.

Hassles and Uplifts

Daily hassle scores have been found to be an important supplement to the life-events approach in predicting health and illness outcomes related to the impact of a stressor. Daily **hassles** are experiences and conditions of daily living that have been appraised as relevant and harmful or threatening to an individual's well-being (Lazarus & Folkman, 1984). The frequency and intensity of daily hassles have a stronger relationship with somatic

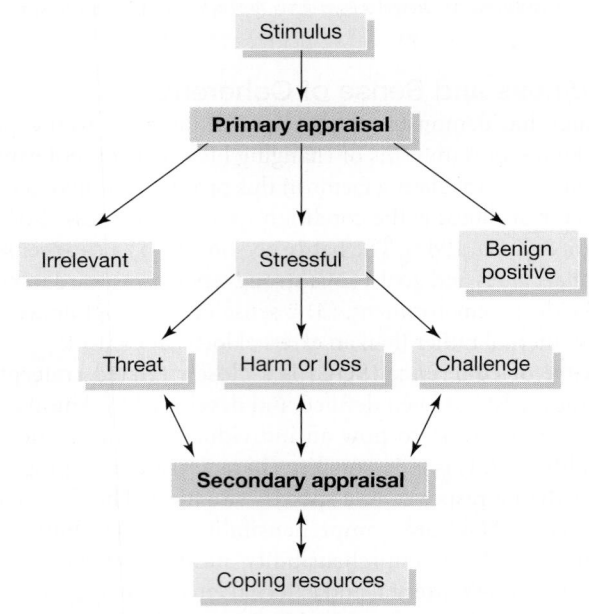

FIGURE 12–2 ■ Stress as a transaction.

illness than with the life-events scale (Lazarus & Folkman, 1984). Items shown on the daily hassles scale reflect work, family, social activities, environment, practical considerations, finances, and health (Lazarus & Folkman, 1984). Examples of daily hassles are shown in Chart 12–3.

Uplifts, the counterpart to hassles, are defined as positive experiences that are likely to occur in everyday life (Lazarus & Folkman, 1984). This concept seems comparable to the eustress described earlier by Selye. Little evaluation has been completed to determine the effects of positive experiences on health outcomes.

Factors That Lead to Stressful Appraisals

Personal factors that lead to stressful appraisals include intellectual, motivational, and personality characteristics. People who have high self-esteem are likely to believe that they have the resources to meet demands. Stressful events are seen as challenging rather than as threatening (Lazarus and Cohen, 1977). In regard to motivation, the more important the threatened goal is, the more stress the person is likely to perceive. Events that involve very strong demands and are imminent tend to be seen as stressful. Life transitions also can be stressful: starting school, moving a household, reaching puberty, starting or changing a career, becoming a parent, losing a spouse, and retiring.

Ambiguity, such as role and harm ambiguity, also can cause stress. Role ambiguity can occur in the workplace, for instance, when people are working without clear guidelines, no standards for performance, and no clear consequences. This is stressful because people are uncertain about what actions and decisions to make. Harm ambiguity occurs when people are not sure what to do to avoid harm. Stress depends on the person's personality, beliefs, and general experience (Lazarus & Folkman, 1984). A person who is seriously ill and does not have clear information might draw hope from this ambiguity, believing that he will get well. Another person in the same situation may believe that people are deliberately giving ambiguous information because the prognosis is poor.

The desirability and controllability of the situation also are important factors. Many of life's events, whether desirable or undesirable, can produce stress. Generally, undesirable events are more likely to be appraised as stressful. People also tend to appraise uncontrollable events as being more stressful than controllable events (Litt, 1988). There are two types of control: behavioral and cognitive. Behavioral control means performing some action, for example, taking a pain control tablet for a headache to make experiencing a headache less stressful. In the case of cognitive control, one can affect the impact of events by using some mental strategy, such as distraction, or by developing a plan to overcome the problem.

Cognition, Emotions, and Stress

A high level of stress impairs people's memory and attention during cognitive activities such as when taking examinations. Disturbing or worrying thoughts can perpetuate stress and make it chronic. Cognitive appraisal processes can influence both the stress and the emotional experience. For example, something that frightens one person, such as running into a black bear on a hike, may make another person feel excited. Fear is a common emotional reaction that can be classified into two categories: phobias and anxiety.

Phobias are intense and irrational fears that are associated with specific events and situations. An example of this would be claustrophobia, a fear of being enclosed in small rooms or crowded conditions. Anxiety is a vague feeling of uneasiness or apprehension. This may be typified by anticipation of impending doom caused by a relatively uncertain or unspecified threat. People may not be aware of situations that seem to arouse anxiety or to know how the "doom" will be manifested. Anxiety also may result from appraisals of low self-worth and the anticipation of a loss of self-esteem.

Another emotional reaction to stress is anger. This often occurs when the person perceives the situation as harmful or frustrating. When stress is accompanied by anger, negative social behaviors tend to increase. Stress-produced anger increases aggressive behavior, and these negative effects tend to continue after the stressful event is over (Helfer & Kempe, 1976). As an example, child abuse often is related to parental stress. Stress may also affect helping behavior. Those experiencing a high level of stress tend not to help others who are experiencing some stressful incident, whereas those experiencing a less stressful event may do so.

Theoretic Summary

Perception is the key to understanding and differentiating between the three major types of stress theories presented. In stress response theory, all demands are stressors with the capacity to elicit a physiological response. Individuals' conditioning factors influence the stress response. In the life-change theory, the perceived stressfulness of the event is not a consideration because all individuals receive the same score on the event scale for a certain stressor. In the transaction theory, the cognitive appraisal process determines whether the demands will be assessed as stressful. Through cognitive appraisal, individuals experience different outcomes in dealing with demands, not only because of conditioning factors, but also as a result of how the demand is perceived and labeled during the person–environment interaction. An event that is stressful to one individual is not necessarily stressful to another individual.

Despite the differentiation made in the types of stress theory, nurses should recognize that stress is ever present, is inevitable,

| CHART 12–3 | **Examples of Daily Hassles** |

Concerns about job security
Problems with coworkers
Chronic pain
Difficulties with friends
Marital problems
Inadequate financial resources
Traffic to and from work
Caring for parents
Deadlines
Misplacing or losing things
House repairs

and is a familiar aspect of life as are the stressors that precipitate the stress response. The stressors may, however, originate from different sources, and for some may precipitate stress as a stimulant, whereas for others it becomes a burden. Thus, it is recognized that an integrated stress response consists of the fight-or-flight response, the general adaptation syndrome, and one's mental response to stress as separate mechanisms that fit together in one response.

Stress Research

Traditionally, stress research has been oriented toward studies involving the body's reaction to stressors (biophysiological perspective) and the cognitive processes and transactional processes that appraise the event or interaction/situation as a stressor. However, current social perspectives of the stress response have noted that different people experiencing similar life conditions are not necessarily affected in the same manner. There continues to be a growing interest in the epidemiology of disease thought to result from stress. It has been noted that the incidence of hypertension, cardiovascular ailments, and depression varies with such factors as race, sex, marital status, and income. This kind of socioeconomic variation for disease indicates that the stressors that presumably dispose people toward these illnesses are somehow linked to the conditions that people confront as they occupy their various positions and status in society.

The concept of stress, as recently defined, views the human in an interactive relationship with the environment, with an increasing awareness and emphasis on the social and cultural contexts involved in stress and coping. The biopsychosocial model of stress incorporates a variety of social factors that influence stress reaction and perception. Culture and society may shape what events are perceived as stressful and what coping strategies are acceptable to use in a particular society. As research progresses on a sociocultural perspective of stress, stress may be redefined to reflect both social and cultural differences. The definition of stress may then evolve to be that stress is a set of neurological and physiological reactions that serve an adaptive function in the environmental, social, and cultural values and structures upon which the individual acts. This concept also is used to form the basis for nursing theories that guide nursing practice.

Nursing Theories Based on Systems and Adaptation

Several nursing theories are based on the concepts of stress and adaptation, and are derived from systems theory. Notable among them are those theories credited to Florence Nightingale, Imogene King, Martha Rogers, Betty Neuman, and Sister Callista Roy:

- Florence Nightingale sought to improve nursing by improving the environment. Her *Notes on Nursing* emphasized that a clean environment, warmth, ventilation, and a quiet environment led to good health (Lobo, 2002; Nightingale, 1957).
- Imogene King developed a conceptual model for nursing in the mid-1960s with the idea that human beings are open systems interacting with their environment (Fawcett, 2005;

King, 1971). She based her framework on the premise that there are three interacting systems, with each system having its own distinct group of concepts and characteristics. These systems include personal, interpersonal, and social systems.

- In the 1970s Martha Rogers advanced the theory of the "science of unitary human beings," also known as Rogerian (Fawcett, 2005; Marriner-Tomey & Alligood, 2006; Rogers, 1970). Rogers' model identifies the individual as a unified whole in constant interaction with the environment. Rogers and her colleagues saw human beings as the central phenomenon of interest to nursing, and her model is designed to explain the nature of human beings (Malinski, 2006). In so doing Rogers drew on a vast array of subjects that formed the theoretical underpinning of her framework, including anthropology, astronomy, and mathematics. She focused on treating the whole patient—not just the illness—with the assumption that individuals achieve maximum well-being within their potential.
- Betty Neuman's health care systems model (2002) focuses on the person as a complete system, the subparts being interrelated physiological, psychological, sociocultural, spiritual, and developmental factors (Fawcett, 2005; Polit & Beck, 2008). She defines health as "expanding consciousness," or increasing complexity. The nurse's role is to recognize the person's unique pattern of life and to work within that pattern with the person to achieve the person's goals (George, 2002; Tomey & Alligood, 2005).
- In Sister Callista Roy's adaptation model, humans are purported to be adaptive systems that cope with change through adaptation. Nursing helps to promote client adaptation during health and illness (Fawcett, 2005; Roy, 1990). Both Selye and Lazarus influenced Roy's development of this model. Although the original model was developed in the early 1960s and 1970s, Roy redefined adaptation for the 21st century in 1990. In the latest version of her model, Roy included expanding the adaptive model to include relational persons as well as the individual person, and describing adaptation on three levels of integrated life processes, compensatory processes, and compromised processes (Fawcett, 2005; Roy & Andrews, 2005; Marrner-Tomey & Alligood, 2006).

Nursing theories, such as those just discussed, often form the framework for implementing the nursing process in service settings. Both Neuman and Roy have been used extensively in nursing practice and nursing education as a framework for defining nursing and implementing the nursing process (Parker, 2006).

Physiological Responses to Stress

Physiological responses to stress should be considered within the context of the body as an open living system with an internal and external environment, with information and matter being exchanged continuously between these two environments. Within the internal environment each organ, tissue, and cell is a system unto itself and a subsystem of the whole, with each system exchanging information and matter. Each subsystem also exchanges information and matter in an attempt to maintain a dynamic balance, or a **steady state**, even in the presence of change, so as to maintain harmony with each other; in other words, homeostasis.

When stress occurs that causes a body function to deviate from its stable range, processes are initiated to restore and maintain the dynamic balance. When these compensatory processes are not adequate, the steady state is threatened, function becomes disordered, and pathophysiological mechanisms occur. The pathophysiological mechanisms can lead to disease, thus, becoming a threat to the steady state. Disease is an abnormal variation in the structure or function of any part of the body that occurs within a living system when the sum of stressors acting on that living system exceeds the system's ability to adapt. It disrupts function and therefore limits the person's freedom of action. Because disease may be localized or generalized, it can affect part of the living system or the entire living system (Wilkin, 2005).

The physiological components involved in the stress response include the CNS, the hypothalamus, the sympathetic nervous system, the anterior and posterior pituitary glands, the adrenal medulla, and the adrenal cortex. The physiological components and their secretions (hormones and catecholamines) are responsible for the neuroendocrine response to stressors. The neuroendocrine response involves the nervous system, the endocrine system, and the immune system. Because these three systems are interrelated, the ultimate responses of the person to stress reflect the integration of the three systems. Figure 12–3 ■ depicts the physiological responses to stress.

Nervous System

The body responds physiologically to both actual and symbolic stressors. The hypothalamus participates in both the emotional and physical response to stressors. In addition to the hypothalamus, other parts of the CNS, including the cerebral cortex, limbic system, and reticular formation, are involved in the neural control of emotions and the physiological responses to stress. The functions of these structures are interrelated.

FIGURE 12–3 ■ Neurochemical links among the nervous, endocrine, and immune systems. The communication is bidirectional among the three systems.

Cerebral Cortex

Following an external event, afferent input is sent to the cerebral cortex via sensory impulses from the peripheral nervous system including the eyes and ears. Afferent impulses that travel to the cortex from the periphery via the spinal cord (spinothalamic pathways) also activate the reticular formation in the area of the brainstem. The reticular formation relays input to the thalamus and from the thalamus to the cerebral cortex. This network of neurons, which is involved with arousal and consciousness, is called the **reticular activating system (RAS)**. The RAS functions to maintain wakefulness and alertness.

The somatic, auditory, and visual associative areas of the cerebral cortex receive input from the peripheral sensory fibers, and then interpret them. The prefrontal area serves to reduce the speed of the associative functions so that the person has time to evaluate the information in light of past experiences and future consequences (primary and secondary appraisal) and to plan a course of action. All of these functions are involved in the perception of a stressor. The temporal lobes of the cerebral cortex contain the auditory association areas, which when stimulated produce the sensation of fear. Stimulation of the temporal lobes can result in sounds that seem louder or softer, visual displays that seem nearer or further, and experiences that seem familiar or strange. These effects modify the perception of stress.

Limbic System

The limbic system, lying in the inner midportion of the brain near the base, includes the septum, cingulated gyrus, amygdala hippocampus, and anterior nuclei of the thalamus. It is thought to be primarily responsible for emotions and behaviors. When stimulated, emotions, feelings, and behaviors can occur that ensure survival and self-preservation, such as feeding, sociality, and sexuality. Endorphins are found in structures of the limbic system and are known to reduce the perception of painful stimuli.

Reticular Formation

The reticular formation is located between the lower end of the brainstem and the thalamus. It contains the RAS, which sends impulses contributing to alertness to the limbic system and to the cerebral cortex and thalamus. The RAS also receives impulses from the hypothalamus. When stimulated the RAS increases its output of impulses, leading to wakefulness. Both physiological and perceived stress usually increase the degree of wakefulness.

Hypothalamus

The hypothalamus, which lies just above the pituitary gland, integrates autonomic nervous system mechanisms that maintain the chemical constancy of the internal environment of the body. Together with the limbic system, it regulates emotions and many visceral behaviors necessary for survival, such as eating, drinking, temperature control, reproduction, defense, and aggression. The hypothalamus receives information regarding traumatic stimuli via the spinothalamic pathway, pressure-sensitive input from the baroreceptors via the brainstem, and emotional stimuli via the limbic system.

Because the hypothalamus secretes peptide hormones and factors that regulate the release of hormones by the anterior pituitary, it is central to the connection between the nervous and endocrine systems in responding to stress. Additionally, the hypothalamus regulates the function of both the sympathetic and parasympathetic branches of the autonomic nervous system. Thus, when an individual perceives the presence of a stressor, the hypothalamus mediates both the neural and endocrine responses. It does this by activating the sympathetic nervous system and by releasing corticotropin-releasing hormone (CRH), which stimulates the pituitary to release adrenocorticotropic hormone (ACTH). In response to certain stress conditions, the parasympathetic nervous system is stimulated. This may be manifested as increased gastrointestinal motility, flushing, or bronchial constriction.

Sympathetic Nervous System Response

The sympathetic nervous system response is rapid and short lived, a response to acute stress. Norepinephrine is released at nerve endings that are in direct contact with the respective end organs to cause an increase in function of the vital organs and a state of general body arousal. Heart rate is increased and peripheral vasoconstriction occurs, raising the blood pressure. Blood also is shunted away from abdominal organs in order to provide better blood supply to the vital organs, brain, heart, and skeletal muscles. Blood glucose is increased, supplying a more readily available energy. Pupils are dilated, mental activity is increased, and a greater sense of awareness exists.

Constriction of the blood vessels of the skin limits bleeding in the event of trauma. The person is likely to experience cold feet, clammy skin and hands, chills, palpitations, and a knot in the stomach. Typically, the person appears tense, with the muscles of the neck, upper back, and shoulders tightened, and respirations may be rapid and shallow, with a tense diaphragm. Figure 12–4 ■ depicts the increased sympathetic activity present in a stress response.

Endocrine System

Once the hypothalamus is activated in response to stress, the endocrine system becomes involved. The sympathetic nervous system also stimulates the medulla of the adrenal gland to release the hormones epinephrine and norepinephrine (catecholamines) into the bloodstream. The effect of catecholamines and the sympathetic nervous system, including the adrenal medulla, is referred to as the sympathoadrenal response. These hormones prepare the body for the fight-or-flight response, which is depicted in Figure 12–4 ■. This response is activated by physical stressors such as hypovolemia and hypoxia and emotional states such as anger, excitement, and fear. Catecholamines can be measured in the blood and urine.

The Hypothalamic–Pituitary–Adrenal Response

The hypothalamus releases CHF, which stimulates the anterior pituitary to produce ACTH. ACTH, in turn, stimulates the adrenal cortex to produce glucocorticoids, primarily cortisol. Glucocorticoids, particularly cortisol, are essential for the stress response. Cortisol stimulates protein catabolism, releasing amino acids; stimulates liver uptake of amino acids and their conversion to glucose; and inhibits glucose uptake (anti-insulin action) by many body cells, but not those of the brain or heart. Cortisol also potentiates the action of catecholamines on blood vessels and inhibits the inflammatory response. These cortisol-induced metabolic effects provide the body with a ready source of energy during a stressful situation. These effects are important to consider in relation to people experiencing stress. Any patient who is under stress (perhaps caused by surgery, illness, trauma, or prolonged psychological stress) catabolizes body protein and needs supplements.

In addition to the catecholamines, epinephrine and norepinephrine, and cortisol, other hormones also are released. These are the antidiuretic hormone (ADH) from the posterior pituitary and aldosterone from the adrenal cortex. ADH promotes water reabsorption by the distal and collecting tubules of the kidneys, and aldosterone acts to increase sodium reabsorption in the kidney tubules. As a result, both ADH and aldosterone in-

FIGURE 12–4 ■ Alarm reactions resulting from increased sympathetic activity. These responses commonly are referred to as the "fight-or-flight" reaction.

crease extracellular fluid (ECF) by promoting water and sodium retention. This is an adaptive mechanism in the event of hemorrhage or loss of fluids through excessive perspiration.

Stimulation of both the adrenal medulla and cortex results in an increased blood glucose level. This elevation provides the additional fuel for the increased metabolism needed for fighting or fleeing. The increased cardiac output (resulting from the increased heart rate and increased ECF), increased blood glucose levels, and increased metabolic rate make the physical responses possible. Also, the dilation of skeletal muscle blood vessels and resulting increased blood supply to the large muscles and the brain provide for quick movement and increased alertness. The increased blood volume (from ECF and the shunting of blood from the GI system) and increased clotting time function to help maintain adequate circulation to vital organs in case of traumatic blood loss. These responses to stress illustrate the complexity and interrelated nature of the processes involved.

Immune System

The immune system is the body's surveillance system. It detects and battles foreign invaders, such as bacteria, viruses, and tumor cells. The immune system comprises several organs, including bone marrow, spleen, thymus, and the lymph nodes. The most important elements of the immune system are lymphocytes, which are specialized white blood cells that fight bacteria, viruses, and other foreign invaders. Lymphocytes are originally manufactured in the bone marrow and then migrate to the other immune system organs, where they develop and are stored until needed.

Research has demonstrated the connection of the immune system to the neuroendocrine and autonomic systems. Negative stressors lead to alterations in immune function in humans through processes involving the hypothalamic–pituitary–adrenal (HPA) axis and the autonomic nervous system that affect immune function. In return, the immune system also affects endocrine and CNS responses. Both corticosteroids and catecholamines are known to suppress immune function. Figure 12–5 ■ demonstrates the physiological response to stress stimuli originating in the cerebral cortex and ending with the inhibition of the immune system.

Physiological Responses of Acute Versus Chronic Stress

With **acute stress**, as defined under the description of the HPA system or axis, catecholamines suppress activity in areas at the front of the brain concerned with short-term memory, concentration inhibition, and rational thought. This sequence of mental events allows a person to react quickly to the stressful event, to either fight or flee. It also hinders the ability of the person to handle the complex social or intellectual tasks and behaviors associated with the event.

The body actually responds to the stressful event by demonstrated changes in the heart rate, breathing, and blood pressure; the immune system; the skin; and metabolism.

- Breathing becomes rapid and the lungs take in more oxygen. Blood flow increases, sometimes up to 300% to 400%, priming the muscles, lungs, and the brain for added demands, and the spleen discharges red and white blood cells, allowing the blood to transport more oxygen.

FIGURE 12–5 ■ System progression of the stress response.

- The immune system responds by marshalling a defense to the stress invaders. The steroid hormones diminish parts of the immune system so that infection or other immune molecules can be redistributed. These immune-boosting cells are sent to the injured or infected part of the body (e.g., the skin, the bone marrow, and the lymph nodes).
- The stress effect diverts blood flow away from the skin to support the heart and muscle tissues. The physical effect is cool, clammy, sweaty skin. The scalp also tightens so that the hair seems to stand up.
- Stress shuts down digestive activity, which is considered a nonessential body function during short-term periods of physical exertion or crisis.

Once the threat has passed and the effect has not been harmful, the stress hormones return to normal. This phenomenon is known as the relaxation response.

In contrast, and as previously defined, **chronic stress** is that which occurs on a daily basis and is a result of an ongoing situation. With chronic stress the urge to act (fight or flee) must be suppressed. Chronic stressors include ongoing highly pressured work situations, long-term relationship problems, loneliness, and persistent financial worries. The entire concept of the body's physiological response to stress is shown in Figure 12–6 ■ (p. 226).

Stress at the Cellular Level

Stress also affects the internal milieu of the body at the cellular level, with alterations in cellular structure and function contributing to changes in the steady state. Thus, the processes of

FIGURE 12–6 ■ Current concepts regarding the body's response to stress syndrome. *ACTH,* Adrenocorticotropic hormone; *ADH,* antidiuretic hormone; *CRH,* corticotrophin-releasing hormone.

health and disease or adaptation and maladaptation all can oc-cur at the cellular level.

Cells are complex units that dynamically respond to the changing demands and stresses of daily life. They exist on a con-tinuum of structure and function, ranging from the normal cell, to the adapted cell, to the injured or diseased cell, to the dead cell. Changes from one state to another can occur rapidly and may not be easily discernible.

Cells possess a maintenance function and a specialized func-tion; Goodyear-Bruch & Pierce, 2002; Porth, 2007). The main-tenance function refers to activities that the cell must perform with respect to itself; specialized functions are those that the cell performs in relation to the tissues and organs of which it is a part. Individual cells may cease to function without negatively

affecting the organism; however, if the specialized functions of the tissue are altered, the individual's health is threatened.

Cells adapt to environmental stress through structural and functional changes. Some of these adaptations are hypertrophy, atrophy, hyperplasia, dysplasia, and metaplasia:

- **Hypertrophy** and atrophy lead to changes in the size of cells and hence the size of the organs they form. Compensatory hy-pertrophy is the result of an enlarged muscle mass and com-monly occurs in skeletal and cardiac muscles that experience a prolonged, increased workload.

- **Atrophy,** a reduction in size of the cell, can be the conse-quence of a disease or of decreased use, decreased blood sup-ply, loss of nerve supply, or inadequate nutrition. Disuse of a body part often is associated with aging. Structures primarily affected by the decrease in cell and organ size are the skeletal muscles, the secondary sex organs, the heart, and the brain.

- **Hyperplasia** is the increase in the number of new cells in an organ or tissue. Hyperplasia results when cells multiply and are subjected to increased stimulation; the tissue mass enlarges. This represents a mitotic response to change, but is reversible when the stimulus is withdrawn, thereby distinguishing it from a malignant growth, which continues after the stimulus is removed.

- **Dysplasia** is the change in the appearance of cells after they have been subjected to chronic irritation. Dysplastic cells have a tendency to become malignant. They commonly are seen in epithelial cells in the bronchi of smokers.

- **Metaplasia** is a cell transformation in which a highly specialized cell changes to a less specialized cell. This serves as a protective mechanism because the less specialized cell is more resistant to the stress that stimulated the change.

Examples of these cellular changes are shown in Chart 12–4. These adaptations allow the survival of the organism, and they reflect the changes of the cell in response to stress. If the stress is unremitting, the function of the adapted cell may succumb, and cell injury will occur.

Cellular Injury

Any stressor that alters the ability of the cell or system to maintain optimal balance of its adjustment processes will lead to injury. Structural and functional damage then occurs. This may be reversible, permitting recovery, or irreversible, leading to disability or death. With adaptive changes, compensation occurs and a steady state is achieved, although it may be at new levels. With injury, steady-state regulation is lost, and changes in functioning follow.

Causes of changes in the system (cell, tissue, organ, body) may arise from the internal/external environment and include hypoxia, nutritional imbalance, physical agents, chemical agents, infectious agents, immune mechanisms, genetic defects, and psychogenic factors. The most common are infectious agents, hypoxia, and chemical agents. The presence of one injury

may precipitate another, and it may become a ripple effect. For example, the inadequate oxygenation and nutritional deficiencies make the system vulnerable to infection. These agents act at the cellular level by damaging or destroying the integrity of the cell membrane necessary for ionic balance and the ability of the cell to transform energy, synthesize enzymes and other necessary proteins, and to grow and reproduce.

Hypoxia

Inadequate cellular oxygenation interferes with the cell's ability to transform energy. Hypoxia may be caused by several factors including a decrease in blood supply, decreased hemoglobin, a ventilation/perfusion or respiratory problem, and a problem in the cell's enzyme system that makes it unable to use the oxygen delivered to it. Ischemia is the usual cause. This commonly is seen in myocardial cell injury in which arterial blood flow is decreased because of atherosclerotic narrowing of blood vessels. Ischemia also results from intravascular thrombi or emboli that may form and interfere with blood supply. These commonly result in cerebrovascular accidents (strokes). The amount of time tissues can survive without oxygen varies; however, if the hypoxia is slow and progressive, collateral circulation may develop, whereby blood is supplied to the tissues by other blood vessels. This does not guarantee resolution of the problem. See Chapter 29 for more information on strokes.

Nutritional Imbalance

Nutritional imbalance refers to a deficiency or excess of one or more essential nutrients. This imbalance results from inadequate nutrition (calories) or too much nutrition (calories). Caloric excess leads to obesity and overloads the cells in the body with lipids. Obesity places a strain on the body because it requires more energy to maintain the extra tissue, and obesity has been associated with the development of disease, especially cardiovascular and pulmonary disease.

Specific diseases can result when an essential nutrient is absent or when there is an imbalance of nutrients. For example, an energy deficit leading to cell injury can occur if there is insufficient glucose or insufficient oxygen to transform the glucose

CHART 12–4 Cellular Adaptation to Stressors

Stressor	Adaptation	Example
Increased use (workload)	Hypertrophy—increase in size of cells leading to increase in organ size	Leg muscles of runner Arm muscles in tennis player Cardiac muscle in person with hypertension
Decreased use resulting in decreased blood supply, nutrition, and innervation	Atrophy—reduction in size of cell leading to decreased organ size	Extremity immobilized in cast Secondary sex organ in older adult
Hormonal change	Hyperplasia—increase in number of new cells	Breast changes of a girl in puberty or of a pregnant woman Regeneration of liver cells New red blood cells in blood loss
Reproduction of cells with alteration of size and shape	Dysplasia—change in the appearance of cells subject to chronic irritation	Alterations in epithelial cells of the skin or the cervix could be precursors of a malignancy
Stress applied to highly specialized cells	Reversible transformation of one adult cell type to another	Changes in epithelial cells lining bronchi in response to tobacco irritation (cells become less specialized)

Source: Matthews, B. D., Overby, D. R., Mannix, R., & Ingber, D. E. (2006). Cellular adaptation in mechanical stress: Role of integrins, Rho, cytoskeletal tension and mechanosensitive ion channels. Journal of Cell Science, 119, 509–518.

into energy. Conversely, a lack of insulin, or the inability to use insulin, also may prevent insulin from entering the cell from the blood. This occurs in diabetes mellitus. See Chapters 14 and 53 , respectively, for more information on nutrition and diabetes.

Physical Agents

Physical agents that can cause injury to the cells include temperature extremes, radiation and electrical shock, and mechanical trauma. Extremely high temperatures precipitate hypermetabolism as manifested by an increase in respiratory rate, heart rate, and basal metabolic rate. With fever induced by infections, the hypothalamic thermostat may be reset at a higher temperature, then returns to normal when the fever goes down. Body temperatures greater than 41°C (106°F) suggest hyperthermia; the physiological function of the thermoregulatory center breaks down and the temperature soars. Eventually, the cell proteins coagulate and the cells die. The local response to thermal or burn injury is similar. There is an increase in metabolic activity and as heat increases, protein coagulates, enzyme systems are destroyed, and, in the extreme, charring or carbonization occurs. See Chapter 68 for information on burn injuries.

Low temperature extremes, or cold, cause vasoconstriction. Blood flow becomes sluggish and clots form, leading to ischemic damage in the involved tissues. With still lower temperatures, ice crystals may form and the cells may rupture.

> **CRITICAL ALERT**
> *Extremely high temperatures of 41°C (106°F) cause hyperthermia, which results in cell protein coagulation and cell death. Extremely low temperatures cause vasoconstriction leading to ischemia in involved tissues.*

Radiation and electrical shock, though used for diagnosis and disease treatment, also may cause injury by their destructive action. Radiation decreases the protective inflammatory response of the cell, creating a favorable environment for opportunistic infections. Electrical shock produces burns as a result of the heat generated when electrical current travels through the body. It also may stimulate nerves abnormally, as in cardiac fibrillation.

Mechanical trauma can result in wounds that disturb the cells and tissues. The outcome of mechanical trauma is dependent on the severity of the wound, the amount of blood lost, and the extent of nerve damage.

Chemical Agents

Chemical injuries are caused by poisons that have a corrosive action on epithelial tissues, such as lye, or by heavy metals, such as mercury, arsenic, and lead. Many other chemicals are toxic in specific amounts, in certain people, and in certain tissues. An example of such is excessive amounts of hydrochloric acid, which can damage the stomach lining. Large amounts of glucose can cause osmotic shifts, which affect the fluid and electrolyte balance, and too much insulin can cause subnormal levels of blood glucose and lead to coma.

Drugs also can cause chemical poisoning as can alcohol. The individual's drug tolerance must be carefully assessed when prescribing medications to prevent toxic reactions to the usual or customary dosages. Aging tends to decrease tolerance to medications. Polypharmacy also frequently occurs in the aging pop-

ulation and is a problem due to the unpredictability of medication interactions. Alcohol is a chemical irritant. Alcohol breaks down into acetaldehyde in the body, which has a direct toxic effect on liver cells that leads to a variety of liver abnormalities, including cirrhosis in susceptible individuals. Disordered liver cell function leads to complications in other body organs.

> **CRITICAL ALERT**
> *The elderly are susceptible to polypharmacy. This potentially is harmful because drug interactions are common with polypharmacy.*

Infectious Agents

Infectious agents known to cause disease in humans are viruses, bacteria, rickettsiae, mycoplasmas, fungi, protozoa, and nematodes. The severity of the infectious disease depends on the number of microorganisms entering the body, their virulence, and the host's defenses (e.g., health, age, immune defenses). Typically, an inflammatory response and immune reaction are the physiological responses of the body to the presence of infection. These processes are discussed at length in Chapters 59, 60, and 61 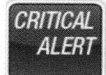.

Cellular Response to Injury

Cells may be injured or killed from the many agents just discussed. When this happens an inflammatory response naturally occurs in the tissues surrounding the injury. **Inflammation** is a defensive mechanism intended to neutralize, control, or eliminate the offending agent to prepare the site for repair. It is a nonspecific response that is meant to serve a protective function. Thus, the mechanism of inflammation basically is the same regardless of the injuring agent. The intensity of the response depends on the extent and severity of injury and on the reactive capacity of the injured person.

Contrary to a popular misconception, inflammation is not the same as infection. Inflammation always is present with infection, but infection is not always present with inflammation. An infection involves invasion of tissues or cells by microorganisms such as bacteria, fungi, and viruses. In contrast, inflammation also can be caused by nonliving agents such as heat, radiation trauma, and allergens. If infection is present, it is from a superimposed invasion of microorganisms. An infectious agent is only one of several agents that may trigger an inflammatory response. An infection exists when the infectious agent is living, growing, and multiplying in the tissues and is able to overcome the body's normal defenses.

> **CRITICAL ALERT**
> *Inflammation and infection are not the same thing. Whereas inflammation is always present with infection, infection is not always present with inflammation. Infection is caused by invasion of cells and tissues by an organism (bacteria, fungi, virus). Inflammation also can be caused by heat, radiation, trauma, and allergens. An infection exists when the invading agent is living, growing, and multiplying in the tissues, thereby overcoming the body's defense system.*

The mechanism of inflammation basically is the same regardless of the injuring agent. The intensity of the response depends on the extent and severity of injury and on the reactive capacity of the injured person. The inflammatory response involves changes in the microcirculation, including vasodilation, increased vascular permeability, and leukocytic cellular infiltration. As these changes take place, five cardinal signs of inflammation are produced: redness, heat, swelling, pain, and loss of function. Initially transient vasodilation results in hyperemia, which raises filtration pressure. Vasodilation and chemical mediators cause endothelial cell retraction, which increases capillary permeability. The pain produced is attributed to the pressure of fluids or swelling on nerve endings and to the irritation of nerve endings by chemical mediators released at the site. Bradykinin is one of the chemical mediators suspected of causing pain. Loss of function is most likely related to the pain and swelling; however, the exact mechanism is not known.

 Five cardinal signs of inflammation are:

- *Redness*
- *Heat*
- *Swelling*
- *Pain*
- *Loss of function.*

As blood flow increases and fluid leaks into the surrounding tissues, the formed elements (red blood cells, white blood cells, and platelets) remain in the blood, causing it to become more viscous. Leukocytes (white blood cells) collect in the vessels, exit, and migrate to the site of injury to engulf offending organisms and to remove cellular debris in a process called phagocytosis. Fibrinogen in the leaked plasma fluid coagulates, forming fibrin for clot formation, which serves to wall off the injured area and prevent the spread of infection.

Injury initiates the inflammatory response, but chemical substances released at the site induce the vascular changes. Histamine and kinins are foremost among these chemicals. Histamine is responsible for the early stages of vasodilation and vascular permeability. Kinins increase vasodilation and vascular permeability. They also attract neutrophils to the area. Prostaglandins, another group of chemical substances, also are suspected of causing increased permeability.

The inflammatory response often is confined to the site, causing only local signs and symptoms. However, systemic responses also can occur. Fever is the most common sign of a systemic response to injury, and it is most likely caused by endogenous pyrogens released from neutrophils and macrophages. The systemic inflammatory response is discussed fully in Chapter 61 ⊕ .

 Fever should not be ignored, because it signifies a systemic response to an infectious agent.

Cellular Healing

The reparative process of cellular injury begins at approximately the same time as the injury and is linked with inflammation. Healing progresses after the inflammatory debris has been removed. Healing may occur by regeneration or by replacement. In regeneration, gradual repairs of the defect occur by proliferation of cells of the same type as those destroyed. During replacement, cells of another type, usually connective tissue, fill in the tissue defect and result in scar formation.

The ability of cells to regenerate depends on whether they are labile, permanent, or stable. Labile cells multiply constantly to replace cells worn out by physiological processes, such as the epithelial cells of the skins. Permanent cells include neurons, the nerve cell bodies, not their axons. If normal activity is to return, tissue regeneration must occur in a functional pattern, especially in the growth of several axons. Stable cells have a latent ability to regenerate. If they are damaged or destroyed, they are able to regenerate. These include cells of the kidney, liver, and pancreas.

Healing by replacement may occur through primary intention and/or secondary intention. In primary intention healing, the wound is clean and dry and the edges are approximated, as in a surgical wound. There is little scar formation. In secondary intention, the wound or defect is larger and gaping, and has necrotic or dead material. The wound fills from the bottom upward with granulation tissue. This repair process takes longer and results in more scar formation, with loss of specialized function. For information on wound healing, see Chapter 67 ⊕ . This is seen in the case of myocardial infarction and is detected on electrocardiographic (ECG) tracings because the electrical signal cannot be conducted through the connective tissue that has replaced the infarcted area. For information on ECGs, see Chapter 38 ⊕ .

The condition of the host, the environment, and the nature and severity of the injury affect the processes of inflammation and cell repair. Any of the injuries previously discussed can lead to death of the cell. The cell membrane becomes impaired, resulting in a nonrestricted flow of ions. Sodium and calcium enter the cell, followed by water, which leads to edema, and energy transformation ceases. Nerve impulses no longer are transmitted; muscles no longer contract. The cells rupture, lysosomal enzymes that destroy tissues escape, and cell death and necrosis occur. See Chapter 18 ⊕ for information on fluid and electrolytes.

Oxidative Stress (OS)

Oxidative stress is rapidly becoming the nutritional and medical buzzword for the 21st century. It is receiving much attention as a way of interpreting the body's physiological response to stress, and it is implicated in a growing list of diseases, from cataracts to cancer. Health conscious people, taking heed of the news about oxygen free radicals, also are taking steps to protect themselves from these active "criminals" that are sabotaging health.

Oxidative stress (OS) is a physiological response to both internal and external stressors. Though in and of itself, it is not a disease, it is a condition that can lead to or accelerate disease development. OS occurs when the available supply of the body's antioxidants is insufficient to handle and neutralize free radicals of different types. The result is massive cell damage, which can result in cellular mutations, tissue breakdown, and immune compromise. The increasing focus on OS makes it increasingly important that nurses understand and appreciate the concept of oxidative stress, both from a treatment perspective and a preventive/educational perspective. The process that allows oxidative stress to occur is discussed next and is related to the physiological development of oxygen-derived free radicals.

Oxygen is necessary for the metabolic production of energy. Mitochondria, through the electron transport chain, use oxygen to oxidize other molecules and generate energy in the form of adenosine triphosphate. During this process oxygen is reduced to water, producing several intermediary **reactive oxygen species** (**ROS**). These species are a major contributing factor in diseases in patients who are critically ill. ROSs are controlled by a defense system that depends on the activity of enzymes and other nonenzyme substances. The imbalance between ROSs and the body's defense system is called oxidative stress.

Formation of ROS

During chemical processes, molecules can be reduced or oxidized. A molecule with an unpaired electron can combine with a molecule capable of donating an electron. The donation of an electron is called *oxidation*. The gain of an electron is called *reduction*. During these reactions, the molecule that donates the electron is oxidized and the molecule that accepts the electron is reduced. Reduction and oxidation can leave the reduced molecule unstable and free to react with other molecules to cause damage to cell membranes, proteins, and DNA. These reduced substances are called *free radicals* (Pugliese, 1995).

In homeostasis, the rates of reduction and oxidation are equal. The reduction–oxidation (redox) balance is maintained by physiological defenses such as specialized enzymes and antioxidants. These antioxidants and enzymes remove or inactivate the free radicals. The enzymes and antioxidants can become overwhelmed by an increase in reduced molecules or by a decrease in the defense system, allowing the accumulation of free radicals (Espat & Helton, 2000).

Free radicals are involved in many cellular functions and are a normal part of living. For example, mitochondria within a cell burn glucose for fuel. This process oxidizes the glucose and in so doing generates free radicals. White blood cells also use free radicals to attach and destroy bacteria, viruses, and virus-infected cells. The detoxifying actions of the liver also require free radicals. Although free radicals have useful functions in the body under controlled conditions, they are extremely unstable molecules that can damage cells if left uncontrolled.

Normally, oxygen free radicals are neutralized by antioxidants such as vitamin E or enzymes such as superoxide dismutase. However, in some patients, oxygen free radicals become a problem when either a decrease in the removal of or an overproduction of the radicals occurs. When the body is overwhelmed by increased production of oxidative agents and defense against these agents is decreased, the ensuing damage contributes to cellular derangements, cell injury, and death. The free radicals tend to accelerate aging and contribute to the development of many diseases, such as cancer, ischemia-reperfusion injury, and systemic inflammatory response (Byrnes, 2003).

Evidence-based research confirms the link between oxidative stress and pathophysiological syndromes and diseases, including those mentioned earlier as well as cardiogenic shock, sepsis, acute respiratory distress syndrome (ARDS), diaphragm fatigue, and burns (Goodyear-Bruch & Pierce, 2002). A relationship also has been determined between oxidative stress and septic shock, disseminated intravascular coagulation, multiple organ dysfunction, cardiovascular disease, diabetes mellitus, and trauma, as well as nonhereditary degenerative diseases such as Parkinson's and Alzheimer's (Byrnes, 2003; Emory University Health Sciences Center, 2006).

Poor nutrition in general also contributes to OS. When the body is fed poorly, it slowly starves and all of its systems suffer.

Weak organ systems are prime targets for free radical attack. Even psychological and emotional stress can contribute to OS. When the body is under stress, it produces certain hormones that generate free radicals. Moreover, the liver must eventually detoxify them in a process that also generates free radicals.

Everyone is exposed to free radicals from a variety of sources. Because oxidative stress is associated with a variety and severity of illnesses, the care of patients depends on preventing and controlling production of ROS. Within this realm, collaborative care, which includes nutritional counseling, is an essential component of the patient's care and is focused on removing as many related stressors as possible.

Negative (Maladaptive) Effects of Stress

In prehistoric times, the physical changes in response to stress were an essential adaptation for meeting natural threats. Even now in the modern world the stress response can be an asset for raising levels of performance during critical events such as sports activities, an important meeting, or in situations of actual danger or crisis. However, if stress becomes persistent and low level, all parts of the body's stress apparatus (the brain, heart, lungs, vessels, and muscles) become chronically over- or underactivated. This may produce psychological or physical damage over time. Acute stress also can be harmful in certain situations.

Stress-related conditions that are most likely to produce negative physical effects include:

- An accumulation of persistent stressful situations, particularly those that a person cannot easily control (e.g., high-pressure work plus an unhappy relationship)
- Persistent stress following a severe acute response to a traumatic event, such as an automobile crash
- An inefficient or insufficient relaxation response
- Acute stress in people with serious illness, such as heart disease or cancer.

Psychological Effects of Stress

Studies suggest that the inability to adapt to stress is associated with the onset of depression or anxiety (Manktelow, 2003). Some evidence suggests that repeated release of stress hormones produces hyperactivity in the HPA axis and disrupts normal levels of serotonin, the nerve chemical that is critical for feelings of well-being. On a more obvious level, stress diminishes the quality of life by reducing feelings of pleasure and accomplishment, and relationships often are threatened.

Stress and Illness

Stress may increase vulnerability to almost any illness. It has long been suspected to play a role in the etiology of many diseases. (Refer back to the discussion on oxidative stress.) How a stress-provoking event is perceived and how one reacts to it determines its impact on health. When something happens to an individual, she automatically evaluates the situation mentally and decides if it is threatening. She then decides how to deal with the situation and what skills she can use. If she decides that the demands of the situation outweigh the skills she has, the situation is labeled "stressful" and the classic stress response begins. If the individual decides that her coping skills outweigh the demands of the situation, then it is not viewed as stressful.

A threat to one's life or safety is considered stressful and triggers a primal physical response by the body. From deep within the brain, a chemical signal speeds stress hormones through the bloodstream, priming the body to be alert and ready to escape danger. Concentration becomes more focused, reaction time faster, and strength and agility increase. When the stressful situation ends, hormonal signals switch off the stress response and the body returns to normal. But in modern society, fraught with stressful daily events, hassles, and relationships, and also contingent on the individual's hormonal response, stress does not always let up. The stress hormones continue to wash through the system at high levels, never leaving the blood and tissues. Research now shows that long-term activation of the stress system can have a hazardous, even lethal effect on the body, increasing the risk of obesity, heart disease, depression, and a variety of other illnesses. Dr. Gabor Maté (2003) theorized in his treatise *When the Body Says No: Understanding the Stress–Disease Connection* that repressed stressful emotions can interfere with the psychoneuroimmune axis and predispose a person to a variety of diseases—from rheumatoid arthritis to cancer. Manktelow (2003) also has commented on the relationship of stress to disease.

Stress Circuit

The stress response results from the complex interplay between the nervous system and stress hormones, or the hormonal systems known as the **hypothalamic–pituitary–adrenal (HPA) axis** (Figure 12–7 ■). As described earlier, the HPA axis is a feedback loop by which signals from the brain trigger the release of hormones needed to respond to stress. Because of its function the HPA axis also is referred to as the *stress circuit*.

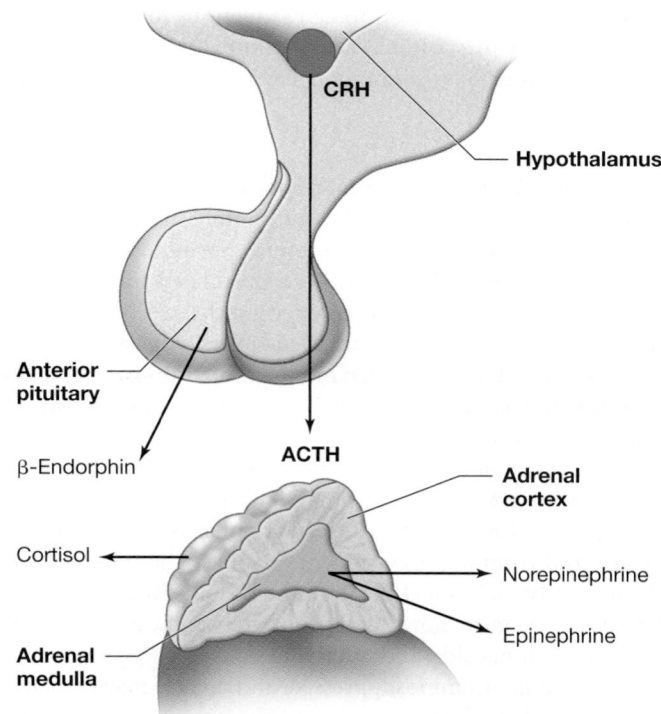

FIGURE 12–7 ■ The hypothalmic–pituitary–adrenal axis (HPA). *ACTH,* Adrenocorticotropic hormone; *CRH,* corticotrophin-releasing hormone.

The stress circuit, or HPA axis, affects systems throughout the body, the autonomic nervous system, regions of the brain, and glandular systems. Short-term response to the stress may be helpful, allowing biochemical resources to be diverted to deal with the threat. Long-term response can result in exacerbations of chronic conditions or major disorders.

The HPA axis also can alter its functioning in response to environmental influences. It may be permanently altered in response to extreme stress during the life cycle—adulthood, adolescence, early childhood, or even in the womb. If a person experiences major stresses in early childhood, the HPA feedback loop becomes stronger and stronger with each new stressful period. This usually results in an adult individual who overreacts hormonally to comparatively minor situations. Thus, from a physiological perspective, it is understandable that chronic and acute events are linked closely to stress. Certain chronic conditions, many of them difficult to treat, have a particularly close link to stress. These include pain and fatigue, mood and anxiety, and addiction and substance abuse. Research also has shown that stress plays an integral part in many disease processes that affect specific organs, body systems, and or behavioral phenomena. Some of these are discussed in the following subsections (Wein, 2000). Figure 12–8 ■ (p. 232) illustrates some disorders that may be caused or aggravated by stress.

Cardiovascular System

An impaired ability to adapt to physiological and psychological stress may contribute to the pathogenesis of cardiovascular disease (Pickering, 2001), because the cardiovascular system is particularly vulnerable to stress (Manktelow, 2003; Schwaertz et al., 2003; Wan, Camandolal, & Mattson, 2003). Excessive exposure to uncontrollable stressors and/or the inability to adapt to stress are implicated in the pathogenesis of several different disorders including hypertension and atherosclerotic vascular disease. Moreover, acute stressors can trigger myocardial infarctions and strokes (Kop, 1999; Manktelow, 2003). Stress is a major trigger for angina as physical stress. Incidents of acute stress have been associated with a higher risk for serious cardiac events, such as heart dysrhythmias and heart attacks, and even death from such events in people with heart disease.

The sympathetic nervous system regulates a broad range of visceral functions and, during extreme emotional or physical states, activates both the cardiovascular and adrenal catecholamine systems for homeostatic adjustments. The CNS neurons responsible for coactivation of these autonomic changes are thought to be governed by a common set of central command neurons that provides dual projections to the sympathetic outflow systems that control the heart and adrenal gland. Stress activates the sympathetic nervous system (the autonomic part of the nervous system that affects many organs, including the heart). The heart may be negatively affected in several ways:

- Sudden stress increases the pumping action and rate of the heart and causes the arteries to constrict, thereby posing a risk for blocking blood flow to the heart.
- The emotional effects of stress alter the heart rhythms and pose a risk for serious arrhythmias in people with existing heart rhythm disturbances.
- Stress causes blood to become stickier (possibly in preparation for potential injury), increasing the likelihood of an artery-clogging blood clot.

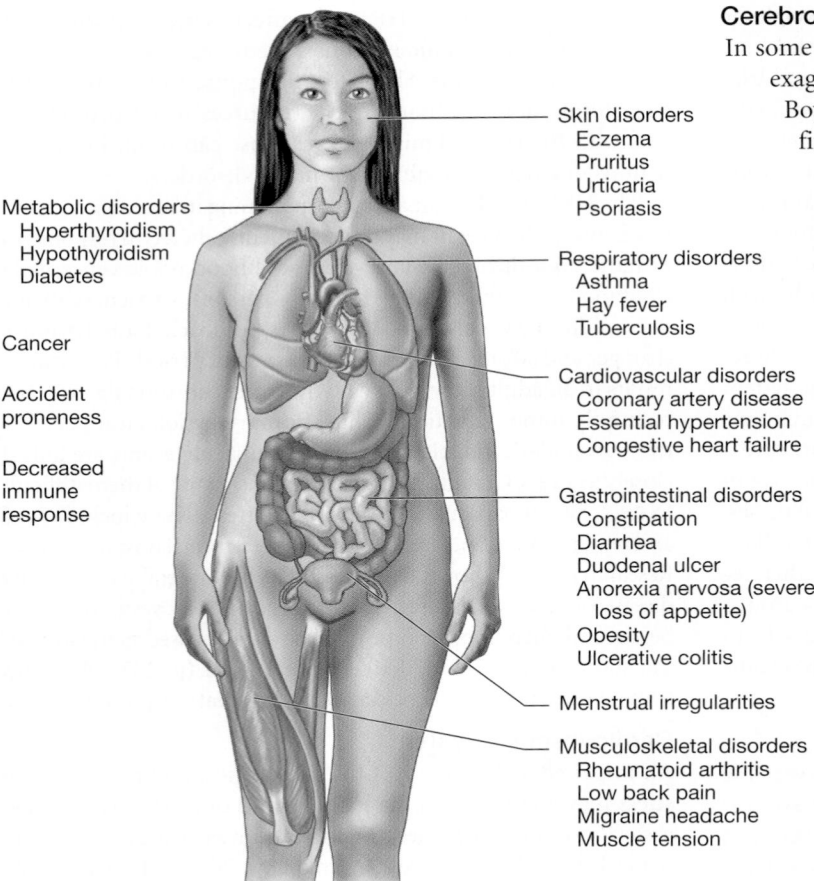

Metabolic disorders
  Hyperthyroidism
  Hypothyroidism
  Diabetes

Cancer

Accident
proneness

Decreased
immune
response

Skin disorders
  Eczema
  Pruritus
  Urticaria
  Psoriasis

Respiratory disorders
  Asthma
  Hay fever
  Tuberculosis

Cardiovascular disorders
  Coronary artery disease
  Essential hypertension
  Congestive heart failure

Gastrointestinal disorders
  Constipation
  Diarrhea
  Duodenal ulcer
  Anorexia nervosa (severe
    loss of appetite)
  Obesity
  Ulcerative colitis

Menstrual irregularities

Musculoskeletal disorders
  Rheumatoid arthritis
  Low back pain
  Migraine headache
  Muscle tension

FIGURE 12–8 ■ Disorders caused or aggravated by stress.

- Stress may signal the body to release fat into the blood-stream, raising blood cholesterol levels, at least temporarily.
- In women, chronic stress may reduce estrogen levels, which are important for cardiac health.
- Stressful events may cause men and women who have relatively low levels of the neurotransmitter serotonin (and, therefore, a higher risk for depression or anger) to produce more of certain immune system proteins, called cytokines, which in high amounts cause inflammation and damage to cells, including possibly heart cells.
- Recent evidence confirms the association between stress and hypertension. People who regularly experience sudden increases in blood pressure caused by mental stress may, over time, develop injuries in the inner lining of their blood vessels.

More research is needed to confirm the actual harm of stress on the heart, although it has been scientifically demonstrated that mentally stressful tasks in patients with coronary artery disease (CAD) can produce acute cardiac effects that are consistent with ischemia, including reductions in left ventricular function, and relative myocardial perfusion (Arrighi et al., 2000). It also is possible that people who work under high-stress conditions try to cope with the situation by resorting to unhealthy habits including high-fat and high-salt diets, tobacco use, alcohol abuse, and a sedentary lifestyle, thereby, contributing to cardiovascular disorders.

Cerebrovascular System

In some people prolonged or frequent mental stress causes an exaggerated increase in blood pressure (Truelsen, Nielsen, Boysen, & Gronbaeck, 2003). A 2001 study linked for the first time a higher risk for stroke in adult Caucasian men and elevated blood pressure during times of stress (Everson et al., 2001).

Gastrointestinal System

Many of the same hormones stimulate the brain and the intestine. Although stress does not cause gastrointestinal problems directly, it can be a trigger (Grumman, 1998; Mayer, Naliboff, & Craig, 2006). The stress circuit influences the stomach and intestines in several ways. The CRH directly hinders the release of stomach acid and emptying of the stomach. The CRH also directly stimulates the colon, speeding up the emptying of its contents. In addition to the direct effects on the stomach, the entire HPA axis, through the autonomic nervous system, also hinders stomach acid secretion and emptying and increases the movement of the colon. Thus, prolonged stress can disrupt the digestive system, irritating the large intestine and causing diarrhea, constipation, cramping, and bloating. Excessive production of digestive acids in the stomach may cause a painful burning. Conditions of the digestive systems strongly related to stress are irritable bowel syndrome, peptic ulcers, and inflammatory bowel disease. According to Levenstein (1998), there is solid evidence that psychological stress triggers many ulcers and impairs responses to treatment. Levenstein (2003) also draws a relationship between stress and ulcerative colitis. Psychological stress probably functions most often as a cofactor with *H. pylori*. It may act by stimulating the production of gastric acid or by promoting behavior that causes a risk to health.

Immune System

As has been noted, physiological responses to stress involve the pituitary–adrenal axis and the autonomic nervous system through the release of corticosteroid hormones and catecholamines, respectively. It has been postulated that the relationship between the immune system and the CNS provides confirmation that the autonomic and physiological pathways through which stress passes can modulate an immune response. According to Glaser and Kiecolt-Glaser (1994) and Segerstrom and Miller (2004), the field of psychoneuroimmunology proposes that a relationship exists between stress, immunological impairment, and health outcomes. The ramifications of this finding are that intense stressors, such as death of a loved one, divorce, and commonplace stressors such as school exams and job stress, adversely affect the immune system. Stress can cause wounds to heal more slowly and people to become more susceptible to infection, colds, and other illness.

Stress can be immunosuppressive and, hence, may be detrimental to health. Glucocorticoid stress hormones are widely regarded as being immunosuppressive and are used clinically as anti-inflammatory agents. The HPA axis interacts with the immune system, increasing vulnerability to colds, flu, fatigue, and infections. In response to an infection or an inflammatory disorder such as arthritis, cells of the immune system produce three substances that cause inflammation: interleukin 1 (IL-1), interleukin 6 (IL-6), and tumor necrosis factor (TNF), working either singularly or in combination to cause the release of CRH. IL-6 also promotes the release of ACTH and cortisol. Cortisol and other compounds then suppress the release of IL-1, IL-6, and TNF, thereby switching off the inflammatory response. Ideally, stress hormones switch off, or dampen, the immune response when it has run its course. However, if the HPA axis is continually running at a high level, the damping down can have a down side, leading to decreased ability to release the interleukins and fight infection.

In some cases, stress can have the opposite effect, making the immune system overreactive. The result is an increased risk of autoimmune diseases, in which the immune system attacks the body's own cells. Stress also can worsen the symptoms of autoimmune disease. For example, stress is one of the triggers for the sporadic flare-ups of symptoms in lupus.

Additionally, the high cortisol levels resulting from prolonged stress could serve to make the body more susceptible to disease by switching off disease-fighting white blood cells. It also has been hypothesized that this same deactivation of white blood cells also might increase the risk for certain types of cancer (National Institutes of Health [NIH], 2004). Conversely, there is evidence to suggest that a depressed HPA axis can result in too little corticosteroid, leading to a hyperactive immune system and increased risk of developing autoimmune diseases (diseases in which the immune system attacks the body's own cells).

The phenomenon of stress has been shown to adversely affect a variety of natural-resistance responses and specific immunological modifications in both animals and men. Although consensus has not been reached on the effects of stress on the immune system, some responses have been validated (Norman, 2003). Stress can have mixed effects on autoimmune diseases (those which are caused by inflammation and damage from immune attacks on the body). It has been shown, for example, that eczema, lupus, and rheumatoid arthritis may demonstrate changes ranging from improvement to deterioration in response to stress. It also has been shown that short-term stress appears to have no negative effect on multiple sclerosis, but chronic stress is a major risk factor for flare-ups.

Susceptibility to Infection Stress also has been found to impair the immune system. Chronic stress appears to blunt the immune response and increase the risk for infections and may even impair a person's response to immunizations. Studies have shown that subjects experiencing chronic stress have low white blood cell counts and are vulnerable to colds. People who harbor herpes or HIV viruses may be more susceptible to viral activation following exposure to stress. Some research has found that HIV-infected men with high stress levels progress more rapidly to AIDS when compared to those with lower stress levels (Green & Smith, 2004). Stressful events most linked with a higher incidence of infections seem to be interpersonal conflicts, such as those at work or in a relationship (Thomas, Nelesen, Ziegler, Bardwell, & Dimsdale, 2004).

Endocrine System

The endocrine system also has been found to be affected by stress. Chronic stress has been associated with the development of insulin resistance, a condition in which the body is unable to use insulin effectively to regulate glucose (blood sugar). Insulin resistance is a primary factor in diabetes. Stress also can exacerbate existing diabetes by impairing the patient's ability to manage the disease effectively.

Stress and Growth The hormones of the HPA axis also influence hormones needed for growth. Prolonged HPA activation hinders the release of growth hormone and insulin-like growth factor 1, (IGF-1), both of which are essential for normal growth. According to the NIH (2004), old research also has shown that the stress from emotional deprivation or psychological harassment may result in the short stature and delayed physical maturity of the condition known as psychological short stature (PSS).

Reproductive System

Stress suppresses the reproductive system at various levels. CRH prevents the release of gonadotropin releasing hormone (GnRH), the master hormone that signals a cascade of hormones that direct reproduction and sexual behavior. Similarly, cortisol and related glucocorticoid hormones not only inhibit the release of GnRH, but also inhibit the release of luteinizing hormone, which prompts ovulation and sperm release.

Glucocorticoids also inhibit the testes and ovaries directly, hindering production of the male and female sex hormones testosterone, estrogen, and progesterone. Thus, it has been shown that stress can lead to diminished sexual desire and an inability to achieve orgasm in women. Stress response also can cause temporary impotence in men. Part of the stress response involves the release of brain chemicals that constrict the smooth muscles of the penis and its arteries. This constriction reduces the blood flow into and increases the blood flow out of the penis, which can prevent erection.

Other reactions to stress may manifest as decreased fertility and a higher risk for miscarriage in pregnant women. Stress also has been associated with lower birth weights and an increased incidence of premature births, both of which are risk factors for infant mortality. Stress may cause physiological alterations, such as increased adrenal hormone levels or resistance in the arteries that may interfere with normal blood flow to the placenta.

Conversely, the interaction between the HPA axis and the reproductive system is a two-way reciprocal process. The female hormone estrogen exerts partial control of the gene that stimulates CRH production. This may explain why women, on average, have slightly elevated cortisol levels. In turn, higher cortisol levels, in combination with other, as yet unknown, factors, may be the reason why women are more vulnerable than men to depression, anorexia nervosa, panic disorder, obsessive compulsive disorder, and autoimmune diseases such as lupus and rheumatoid arthritis (Kalantaridou, Makrigiannakis, Zoumakis, & Chrousos, 2004).

It also has been scientifically demonstrated that females under "attack" are less likely to fight or flee and are more apt to attempt to protect their children and seek help from others, particularly other females (Taylor & Klein, et. al, 2000). Taylor and Klein call this pattern of behavior the "tend-and-befriend" response. They suggested an evolutionary explanation for the difference. In many situations it could be disastrous for a woman who is pregnant, nursing, or caring for young children to fight or flee. Befriending, on the other hand, establishes a support system for the mother and child and also helps to defend women against male violence. Taylor and Klein believed that hormones, especially sex hormones and the pituitary hormone oxytocin, are one reason for the difference in response to stress between men and women. Oxytocin, which induces relaxation and lowers anxiety, is released in response to stress by both males and females, but its effects are enhanced by female hormones and reduced by male hormones. In contrast, the fight-or-flight response activates the nervous system and causes the secretion of the stress hormones adrenaline and cortisol. Both sexes release these hormones under stress, but men also release testosterone, which tends to increase hostility and aggression. Because female aggression is less closely linked to nervous system arousal, it has been suggested that their stress is more easily moderated by learning and culture, whereas men tend to do this less easily. Studies on the relationship between oxytocin and stress have concentrated on men, and more research needs to be conducted that also focuses on women.

Cancer

To date, there is no current evidence to support the idea that stress causes cancer. However, Dr. David Spiegel of Stanford University purports that the link between postdiagnosis stress and cancer survival is gaining momentum (Senior, 2001). He has reported that four recent studies have indicated that higher levels of stress hormones lead to more rapid cancer progress. Cortisol concentrations have been found to be a reliable indicator of chronic and severe stress. In one of Dr. Spiegel's most recent studies, he found that patients with abnormally flat cortisol measurements had significantly lower numbers of natural killer cells, which suggests a link between the immune system, stress, and the body's ability to fight breast cancer.

It also has been demonstrated that lack of control over stress (not simply stress itself) has had negative effects on immune function and has contributed to tumor growth in animals. Two small studies on melanoma and breast cancer patients reported improved survival with therapies that offered emotional support (Reuters Health, 2004). More information on cancer can be found in Chapter 64 ☺.

Pain

Pain and agitation are common in patients who are critically ill. The stress response causes tremendous neurohumoral elevations of plasma catecholamine, cortisol, glucose, ADH, and acute-stage protein levels. These elevations can result in tachycardia, hypertension, vasoconstriction, increased oxygen consumption, salt and water retention, and blunting of the immune response.

The primary goals of sedation and analgesia are to relieve pain and anxiety, attenuate the stress response, and improve compliance with care. In certain situations neuromuscular blocking agents are necessary. Appropriate use of these medications requires a thorough understanding of drug indications, metabolism, side effects, and monitoring techniques. Sedation needs may vary over the course of a patient's stay. In the acute phase, a profound stress response may require deeper sedation and higher doses of analgesics. When a plateau is reached, sedative and analgesic requirements may decrease, but delirium may

emerge. In the recovery phase, sedation and analgesics are tapered and discontinued. Use of agents needs to be tailored to the needs of individual patients; indications, anticipated length of need, and underlying organ system derangements are important considerations (Blanchard, 2002).

Chronic pain caused by arthritis and other conditions may be intensified by stress. Psychological distress also plays a significant role in the severity of back pain. Tension-type headaches are highly associated with stress and stressful events. Some research suggests that tension-type headache sufferers may actually have some biological predisposition for translating stress into muscle contraction. Emotional stress is among the wide range of possible migraine triggers.

Eating Problems

Stress can have varying effects on eating problems and weight. Stress often is related to weight gain and obesity. Many people develop cravings for salt, fat, and sugar to counteract tension and, thus, gain weight. Scientists at the University of California found that comfort foods such as chocolate cake and ice cream literally blunt the body's response to chronic stress (Manisses Communications Group, 2003; SixWise.com, 2006). Eating calorie-rich food seems to calm the nerves, but eating too much can lead to obesity, depression, and more stress.

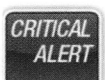 *Comfort foods, those rich in calories (e.g., chocolate cake and ice cream), may act as a stress blocker. Too much comfort food, however, leads to obesity, depression, and more stress. Obesity may be a predictor of diabetes and heart problems.*

The weight gained is often abdominal fat, a predictor of diabetes and heart problems. The release of cortisol, a major stress hormone, appears to promote abdominal fat and may be the primary connection between stress and weight gain in people. Rivas (2003) has demonstrated that a hormonal cascade causes hunger. When a stress response is activated, the brain releases CRH, which suppresses the appetite. The adrenal glands then secrete their powerful fight-or-flight stress hormones, adrenaline, and cortisol, which propel sugar into the bloodstream for a short-term energy rush. After that rush, cortisol sparks ravenous hunger for carbohydrates and fat.

If under continuous stress, the result is prolonged, thus elevating cortisol levels that spur the release of insulin, the hormone directs the body to hang on to the fat it has and store more. If one has many stressors, one has many periods of rebound insulin secretion. The cumulative effect is a push toward obesity. Also noted is the fact that the brain's complex appetitive and satiety control system can go haywire under stress. Rivas (2003) contends that most people who overeat when stressed are genetically prone to an imbalance among at least three of the brain's neurotransmitters (serotonins, dopamine, and norepinephrine), which help the body regulate both appetite and mood. When an already short supply of serotonin dwindles further under stress, overeaters launch into desperate forays for sweets because carbohydrates raise serotonin levels (SixWise.com, 2006).

Conversely, some people experiencing stress suffer a loss of appetite and lose weight. In rare cases, stress may trigger hyperactivity of the thyroid gland, stimulating appetite but causing the body to burn up calories at a faster than normal rate. Several eating disorders, such as anorexia nervosa and bulimia, are highly associated with adjustment problems in response to stress and emotional issues.

Sleep Disturbances

The tensions of unresolved stress frequently cause insomnia, generally keeping the stressed person awake or causing awakening in the middle of the night or early morning. Researchers also have theorized that persistent insomnia may result from a disorder of the stress system (NIH, 2004). They found that, when compared to a group of people who did not have difficulty falling asleep, the insomniacs had higher ACTH and cortisol levels, both in the evening and in the first half of the night. The insomniacs with the highest cortisol levels tended to have the greatest difficulty falling asleep. Their ACTH and cortisol levels indicated that the insomniacs had nervous systems that were on overdrive, alert, and ready to deal with a threat, when they should otherwise be quieting down. Thus, the researchers suggested that, rather than prescribing hypnotics to regulate sleep system, the physicians might have more success in prescribing antidepressants to help calm an overactive stress system. Behavior therapy also was recommended.

Memory, Concentration, and Learning

Cognitive changes occur in response to acute, uncontrollable stress. One can become distracted and disorganized, and the working memory abilities worsen, leaving habitual response to control behavior. Neurological research now can begin to explain many of these cognitive changes in response to stress. The neuromodulators called catecholamines (dopamine, norepinephrine, and epinephrine) are released through the peripheral and central nervous systems during stress. Just as catecholamines "turn on" the heart and muscles and "turn off" the stomach to prepare for fight-or-flight responses during stress, similar opposing actions in the brain may turn on a structure called the amygdala and turn off the prefrontal cortex (a higher cognitive center), allowing posterior cortical and subcortical structures to control behavior (Arnsten, 1998). The amygdala is a phylogenetically older structure in the medial temporal lobe, long known to be essential for the expression of emotion and the formation of associations between stimuli and emotions (Aggleton, 1992). In contrast, the prefrontal cortex expands greatly and permits working memory to guide behavior, inhibiting inappropriate responses or distractions and allowing one to plan and organize effectively. High levels of catecholamines exert opposite actions on these brain regions (Arnsten, 1998).

Thus, it can be concluded that stress has substantial effects on the brain, particularly on memory. Typically, one who is experiencing severe stress suffers loss of concentration and may become inefficient at work and home and accident prone. It also has been shown that the immediate effect of acute stress impairs short-term memory, particularly verbal memory. Prolonged exposure to cortisol, the major stress hormone, causes shrinkage in the hippocampus, the center of memory.

Other Disorders

Other disorders precipitated by stress include allergies, skin disorders, hair loss, and periodontal disease, along with depression. Research suggests that stress may actually be a cause of the so-called "sick-building syndrome," which produces allergy-like symptoms, such as eczema, headaches, asthma, and sinus prob-

lems (NIH, 2004). Stress also plays a role in exacerbating some skin conditions including hives, psoriasis, acne, rosacea, and eczema. Unexplained itching also may be caused by stress as can unexplained hair loss (alopecia areata). This is hair loss that occurs in localized patches. The exact cause is unknown, but stress is suspected as a player in this condition, for it has been noted that hair loss often occurs during periods of intense stress, such as mourning. Stress also has been implicated in increasing the risk for periodontal disease.

Depression

Evidence suggests that early adverse experiences play a preeminent role in development of mood and anxiety disorders and that a corticotropin-releasing factor (CRF) systems may mediate this association (Heim et al., 2000; Mayer, Naliboff, & Craig, 2006). Melancholic depression has been found to be a major disorder characteristic of an overactive HPA axis. Research has shown that people with depression have a blunted ability to "counterregulate," or adapt, to the negative feedback of increases in cortisol. The body turns on the fight-or-flight response, but cannot turn it off again, thereby, producing anxiety and overreaction to stimulation. This is followed by the paradoxical response called "learned helplessness," in which victims apparently lose all motivation. This form of depression manifests itself as anxiety, loss of appetite, loss of sex drive, rapid heart beat, high blood pressure, and high cholesterol and triglyceride levels. Individuals with this condition tend to produce higher-than-normal levels of CRH, which is probably due to a combination of environmental and hereditary causes, depending on the person affected. However, rather than producing higher amounts of ACTH in response to CRH, depressed people produce smaller amounts of this substance, presumably because their hippocampi have become less sensitive to the higher amounts of CRH.

In an apparent attempt to switch off excess CRH production, the systems of people with melancholic depression also produce high levels of cortisol, the by-products of which are produced in response to high levels of the substance. Thus, these by-products of the cortisol serve as sedatives and perhaps contribute to the overall feeling of depression.

Other conditions also are associated with high levels of CRH and cortisol. These include anorexia nervosa, malnutrition, obsessive-compulsive disorder, anxiety disorder, alcoholism, alcohol and narcotic withdrawal, poorly controlled diabetes, childhood sexual abuse, and hyperthyroidism (NIH, 2004). The excessive amount of the stress hormone cortisol produced in patients with any of these conditions is responsible for many of the observed symptoms. Most of these patients share psychological symptoms including sleep disturbances, loss of libido, and loss of appetite as well as physical problems such as an increased risk for accumulating abdominal fat and hardening of the arteries and other forms of cardiovascular disease. They also may experience suppression of thyroid hormones and of the immune system. Such patients are likely to have their life spans shortened by 15 to 20 years if they remain untreated due to their risk for health problems.

Self-Medication with Unhealthy Lifestyles

People under chronic stress often seek unhealthy means to relieve the stress: drug or alcohol abuse, tobacco use, abnormal eating patterns, or passive activities, such as watching television. The damage caused by these self-destructive habits under ordinary circumstances is exacerbated by the physiological effects of stress itself. The cycle becomes self-perpetuating. A sedentary routine, an unhealthy diet, alcohol abuse, and smoking promote heart disease, interfere with sleep patterns, and lead to increased rather than reduced tension levels.

 *Unhealthy lifestyle practices used to reduce stress include alcohol use, tobacco use, abnormal eating patterns, and passive activities.*

Although many disorders result from an overactive stress system, some result from an underactive stress system. This occurs in the case of Addison's disease due to the lack of cortisol. Lack of the hormone CRH also results in the feelings of extreme tiredness common to people suffering from chronic fatigue syndrome. CRH also is central to seasonal affective disorder (SAD), the feelings of fatigue and depression that plague some patients during winter months.

Risk Factors for Stress

At some point in everyone's life, stressful events or conditions develop that overwhelm natural coping mechanisms. Many factors influence susceptibility to stress. People respond differently depending on different factors. These factors have been mentioned before and include early nurturing, personality traits, genetic factors, immune-regulated diseases, and the length and quality of the stressors. Some people are more vulnerable than others to the effects of stress. People who are less emotionally stable or have high anxiety levels tend to experience specific events as more stressful than others. It also has been demonstrated that the lack of an established network of family and friends predisposes one to stress disorders and stress-related health problems, including heart disease and infections (Mayo Clinic, 2006).

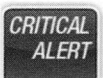 *Stress responses may be influenced by early nurturing or lack thereof, personality traits, genetic factors, immune-related diseases, and length and quality of stressors.*

Work risk factors also must be considered when discussing stress. Job-related stress is particularly likely to become chronic because it is such a large part of daily life (MacDonald, Karasek Punnett, & Scharf, 2001; Parikh, 2004). Stress, in turn, reduces a worker's effectiveness by impairing concentration, causing sleeplessness, and increasing the risk for illness, back problems, accidents, and lost time. Extreme stress, such as harassment or violence on the job, places a burden on the heart and the cardiovascular system.

From a biological perspective, some people exhibit an absent or inadequate relaxation response to stress. Stress hormones remain elevated instead of returning to normal levels. This may occur in highly competitive athletes or people with a history of depression. Scientists also have reported the discovery of a small protein in the brain (orphaninFQ/nocicptin) that plays an important role in the stress response. Animals with a genetic deficiency in this protein are unable to manage stress response and exhibit overanxious behavior in response to new situations. Future research may reveal similar findings in humans (Reuters

Health, 2004). The types of individuals at higher risk for stress are listed in the Risk Factors box.

Coping Strategies for Stress

It has long been understood that how a person adjusts to life stresses is a major component of his ability to lead a fulfilling life. Yet, it was not until the 1980s that coping became a discrete topic of psychological inquiry. Since then, coping has risen to a position of prominence in the modern psychological discourse, especially within the personality, cognitive, and behavioral spheres. As previously discussed the concept of coping has been defined as a compensatory mechanism wherein cognitive and behavioral efforts change constantly to manage specific external or internal demands that are appraised as taxing or exceeding the resources of the person (Lazarus & Folkman, 1984).

RISK FACTORS for Stress

Younger adults	Stress may go unnoticed in the very young and old.
Women in general	Women may be at higher risk than men for stress-related chest pain, but men's hearts may be more vulnerable to adverse effects from long-term stress.
Working mothers	Working mothers face higher stress levels and possibly adverse health effects, most likely because they bear a greater and more diffuse workload than men or other women.
Caregivers of family members	Caregivers of family members with physical or mental disabilities are at risk for chronic stress. They are particularly vulnerable to stress-related health threats such as influenza, depression, and heart disease.
Less educated individuals	Less educated individuals may be at higher risk because they may not be able to differentiate the causes of stress.
Divorced or widowed individuals	Unmarried people generally do not live as long as their married contemporaries.
The unemployed	Being unemployed is an environmental stressor that threatens security.
Isolated individuals	Such individuals usually lack support systems.
People who are targets of racial or sexual discrimination	Discrimination is an environmental stressor that is beyond individual control.
Those without health insurance	This is a threat to one's health that can lead to stress.
People who live in cities	City dwellers may be more stressed as a result of external stressors beyond their control.

Stress and Premature Aging

Clinical Problem

It is well known that stress has a physiological impact on the body and may advance disease and the aging process. Although there has been a deeply held belief that stress leads to premature aging, there has been no hard evidence as to how this might happen until recently. It has now been scientifically demonstrated that prolonged psychological stress affects molecules believed to play a key role in biological aging and, possibly, disease development (Epel et al., 2004; Sapolsky, 2004).

A recent study conducted by Epel and her colleagues (2004) concluded that psychological stress appears to cause cellular damage and premature aging, thereby explaining why intense, long-term emotional strain can make people get sick and grow old before their time. Perceived long-term stress negatively impacts cellular molecules, resulting in increased oxidative stress, lower telomerase activity, and shorter telomere length, all of which are related to cell longevity and disease.

Telomeres are the protective structures (caps) at the end of chromosomes that prevent the DNA strands from unraveling. They also promote genetic stability. Each time a cell divides, the telomeres shorten so that daughter cells have slightly shorter telomeres than their parents and a portion of telomeric DNA dwindles away by a few base parts. After many rounds of cell division, so much DNA has diminished that the aged cell stops dividing. At this point, when the cell stops dividing, it no longer performs its vital functions, and is close to dying. Thus, telomeres play a critical role in determining the health and life span of cells, as well as whatever tissues those particular cells may form.

In effect, chronic stress appears to hasten the shriveling of the tips of the bundles of genes inside cells (the DNA), which threatens their life span and the body's deterioration. The cellular enzyme telomerase acts to replenish a portion of telomeres with each round of cell division, thus protecting these structures. In young people the telomerase is effective in protecting and correcting the cell division process by regenerating the ends. However, as people age, the telomeres shorten significantly and eventually their replication stops all together. Oxidative stress is related to an overabundance of free radical toxins in the body. Free radicals damage lipids, proteins, and DNA, including the DNA of telomeres. Nurses need to understand this degenerative physiological process because it is directly correlated to the perception of high psychological stress. Through assessment and intervention, nurses may be able to help patients cope with stress and mitigate the maladaptive physiological response to stressors, thus, reducing the aging and disease processes.

Research Findings

In 2004 Epel and colleagues at the University of California, San Francisco, conducted a landmark research study in which they found evidence to support the long-suspected association between stress and cellular aging. In a comparison correlational study, they investigated the hypothesis that stress impacts health by modulating the rate of cellular aging through an increase in oxidative stress, lower telomerase activity, and shorter telomere length. They studied both objective (event- or environment-based phenomenon) and subjective (perception-based) stress in 58 healthy premenopausal women who were biological mothers of either a healthy child (*n* = 19, control mothers), or mothers of a child with a chronic illness (*n* = 39, women called caregivers). The latter were predicted to have, on average, environmental exposure to stress. Women in both groups completed a standardized 10-item

questionnaire assessing their levels of perceived stress during the past month. This design allowed the researchers to examine the importance of perceived stress and measures of objective stress (caregiving status and chronicity of caregiving stress based on the number of years since a child's diagnosis). They also looked at the chromosomes in the white blood cells of the study participants. Mean telomere length and telomerase activity were measured quantitatively as was oxidative stress.

The research findings did substantiate the proposed hypothesis of the study. As expected, the average perceived stress level was significantly higher in caregivers than in the control group. As a group, caregivers did not differ from controls in telomere length, telomerase activity, or oxidative stress index, but the duration of their chronic stress (number of years spent as a caregiver) varied greatly, from 1 to 12 years. The more years of caregiving, the shorter the length of the telomeres, the lower the telomerase activity, and the greater the oxidative stress level.

The researchers also found significant correlations between perceived stress and all three markers of cellular aging across the entire sample of caregivers and noncaregivers. Notably, telomere length was related to perceived stress in both the control group and the caregiving group. Hence, the relationship between perceived stress and shorter telomeres is not simply because of the severe stress experience by many of the caregivers or because of some biological vulnerability that predisposed their child to have a chronic condition, but rather existed across the continuum of normative stress levels. Although being a caregiver per se was not related to telomere length, the chronicity of caregiving stress was related to telomere length. This finding supported the premise that the perception of being stressed correlated in both the care and control groups with the biological markers.

This correlation held true for oxidative stress as well: The worse the perceived psychological stress, the greater the oxidative stress. In fact, in the most stunning result, the telomeres of women with the highest perceived psychological stress—across both groups—had undergone the equivalent of approximately 10 years of additional aging compared with women across both groups who had lower perceptions of being stressed. The highest stress group also had significantly decreased telomerase activity and higher oxidative stress that the lowest stress group. This was the fist evidence that psychological stress, and how a person perceives stress, may modulate the rate of cellular aging. Further research will explore the relationship of how elevated levels of stress affect the telomeres and telomerase levels by asking the question "Do the chronically elevated levels of stress hormones such as cortisol damage the telomeres and other genes in the body and lower telomerase levels, inhibiting the cells' ability to respond?"

In summary, the study provided evidence that psychological stress, both perceived and chronic, significantly affects cellular integrity and longevity. These findings have implications for understanding how, at the cellular level, stress may promote earlier onset of age-related diseases. This work quantifies a physiological price to feeing highly stressed, drawing on the relationship of mind and body interaction. The researchers concluded that stress is a risk factor—rather than a direct marker—of cell aging. Cell aging, in turn, is a risk factor for later disease. The study also suggests that health care professionals can use these cell markers as a way to monitor health, with very low telomerase or very short telomeres serving as a red flag and indicating the need for professional intervention. Thus,

EVIDENCE-BASED PRACTICE

(continued)

EVIDENCE-BASED PRACTICE

Stress and Premature Aging—*Continued*

the study emphasizes the importance of managing feelings of stress as much as possible in order to give the body a break from the degenerative process. This often means that one has to make life changes that promote a greater sense of well-being.

Implications for Nursing Practice

This study clearly indicates a need for nurses to be aware of the physiological response to chronic stress at the cellular level, which can precipitate or augment disease and aging, particularly in women. Implications for nursing practice begin with the nursing assessment. It is important to specifically question the individual's history and duration of chronic stress. The study emphasizes the importance of having some respite from perceived long-term chronic stress.

It is an inherent responsibility of nurses to determine if the patient perceives chronic stress, to what it is attributable, and how long the perception of high stress has lasted. Following assessment and diagnosis of such, the nurse must be prepared to intervene by providing resources and education to the patient on ways of coping or managing the situation in order to reduce the stress. Most probably this will involve collaborative efforts with the entire health team.

Critical Thinking Questions

1. Explain the relationship of chronic stress to the aging process.

2. Differentiate between the response of young adults and older adults to psychological stress from a physiological and cellular perspective, and explain the relevance of this information to nursing.

3. Classify stress reduction measures that nurses may advise individuals to use when experiencing high psychological stress.

Answers to Critical Thinking Questions appear in Appendix D.

References

Epel, E., & Blackburn, E. H., Lin, J., Dhabhar, F. S., Adler, N. E., Morrow, J. D., et al. (2004). Accelerated telomere shortening in response to life stress. *Proceedings of the National Academy of Sciences of the United States of America, 101*(49), 17312–17315.

Sapolsky, R. M. (2004). Organismal stress and telomeric aging: An unexpected connection. *Proceedings of the National Academy of Sciences of the United States of America, 101*(50), 17323–17324.

CRITICAL ALERT *Coping is influenced by control over the situation. The more control a person has over a situation, the better the person copes. Control is perceived when the stress is internal, transient, and specific. Lack of control stems from stressors that are external, stable, and global.*

Cognitive appraisal and coping are affected by internal characteristics such as health, energy, personal belief systems, commitments or life goals, self-esteem, control, mastery, knowledge, problem-solving skills, and social skills. To date, nursing research has focused on health promotion and hardiness. In many circumstances, it has been found to be more feasible to promote a healthy lifestyle than to alter the stressors. The research often is guided by the transactional model of stress and coping as developed by Glanz, Rimer, & Lewis, 2002. This model provides a framework for evaluating the processes of coping with stressful events. Within this framework stressful experiences are construed as person-environment transactions; these transactions depend on the impact of the external stressor. The impact is mediated by the person's appraisal or perception of the stressor and the individual's availability of social and cultural resources with which to deal with the stressor. Chart 12–5 depicts the key concepts of the Transaction Model of Stress and Coping (Glanz, Rimer, & Lewis, 2002).

Coping strategies, also referred to as stress management, refer to the specific efforts, both behavioral and psychological, that people employ to master, tolerate, reduce, or minimize stressful events (Edelman & Rémond, 2004; MacArthur & MacArthur, 1998; Manktelow, 2003). A distinction that often is made in the coping literature is between active and avoidant coping strategies. Active coping strategies are either behavioral or psychological responses designed to change the nature of the stressor itself or how one

CHART 12–5 **Key Constructs of the Transaction Model of Stress and Coping**

Concept	Definition
Primary appraisal	Evaluation of the significance of a stressful event
Secondary appraisal	Evaluation of the controllability of the stress; a person's coping resources
Coping efforts	Actual strategies used to mediate primary appraisals Strategies directed at changing a stressor.
Problem management, emotional regulation	Strategies aimed at changing the way one feels about a stressful situation
Outcomes of coping	Emotional well-being; functional status

thinks about it, whereas avoidant coping strategies lead people into activities that are considered nonhealthy, for example, alcohol abuse. Generally speaking, active coping strategies, whether behavioral or emotional, are thought to be better ways to deal with stressful events. Avoidant coping strategies appear to a psychological risk factor or marker for adverse responses to stressful life stimuli (Holahan & Moos, 1987) and may become maladaptive. Defense processes, such as denial, also may be included as coping processes, because both defensive and coping processes intertwine and are intrinsic to the psychological integrity of the individual.

Coping resources are defined as characteristics or actions drawn on to manage stress. They include factors in the person or environment that encompass categories such as (1) health, energy, and morale; (2) positive beliefs; (3) problem-solving skills; (4) social skills; (5) social networks; and (6) material networks. According to Lazarus and Folkman (1984), coping mechanisms function in two ways, as problem solving and emotion regulating, being problem focused and emotionally focused. As an individual attempts to deal with demands, internal or environmental, or confront obstacles that create the demands, the person is using the problem-solving method. If, however, the person is concentrating on methods of regulating the emotional response to the problem, the person is using the emotion-focused response to the problem. Coping that is emotion focused seeks to make the person feel better by reducing the emotional distress felt, whereas problem-focused coping aims to make direct changes in the environment so that the situation can be managed more effectively. Oftentimes a combination of problem-focused and emotional-focused coping is used (MacArthur & MacArthur, 1998).

Manktelow's interpretation of stress management is similar to that posed by Lazarus and Folkman, and also can be used as a framework for developing coping strategies. According to Manktelow (2003), three major approaches can be used to manage stress:

- *Action oriented:* in which one seeks to confront the problem causing the stress, often changing the environment or the situation
- *Emotionally oriented:* in which one does not have the power to change the situation, but can manage stress by changing the interpretation of the situation and the way one feels about it
- *Acceptance oriented:* in which something has happened over which one has no power and no emotional control, and where the focus is on surviving the stress.

To be able to take an action-oriented approach, the person must have some power in the situation. If a person does not have the power to change a situation, the situation can be changed by the way the person views it and feels about it. These three approaches to stress management help people to manage the demands placed on them, help people to adjust to perceptions of the situation, and help people survive the situations that they genuinely cannot change.

As a person begins to deal with a stressor, modes of coping may include the following:

- Information seeking (gathering data about the problem and possible solutions to the problem)
- Direct actions (performing concrete acts to alter self or environment)
- Inhibition of action (refraining from an action)
- Intrapsychic processes (reappraising the situation; initiating cognitive activity aimed at improving feelings)
- Obtaining emotional support by turning to others
- Escaping or avoiding.

The choice of coping strategies depends on various factors, such as degrees of uncertainty, threat, or helplessness, and the presence of conflict (Seaward, 2006). If the person is experiencing high uncertainty, direct action is less likely to be selected as a coping strategy. If the degree of threat is severe, more primitive coping modes such as panic are more likely to

occur. In the presence of conflict, an individual may not be able to take direct actions. Helplessness promotes immobilization. The strategy chosen also may be influenced by the outcome of the cognitive appraisal that categorizes the stressor as harm or loss, threat, or challenge. Examples of stress demands and the coping mechanisms people use to handle the stress are shown in Chart 12–6, along with indications of which examples are problem-solving strategies and which are emotion-regulating efforts.

Cultural Considerations

Culture plays a very important role in the choice of a person's coping strategies. Cultures and societies have their own set of rules about what they perceive to be stressful or not. For example, educational systems vary from culture to culture, with some cultures placing greater emphasis on how students do in schools. Access to higher education—and ultimately the better jobs—is determined solely through academic performance. Thus, the stress that the students experience due to this cultural expectation is very high.

People in a monogamous culture will have different responses than those from a polygamous culture. Stressful life events, as described by Holmes and Rahe (1967), will vary among cultures due to different norms and values. Cultural and societal norms must be considered when assisting those from different cultures to identify stressors, stressor resources, and strategies to reduce the stress (Noh & Kaspar, 2003; Wong & Wong, 2006). The Cultural Considerations box (p. 240) discusses two types of cultures, individualist and collectivist, and how they respond to stress.

 Cultural assessment is instrumental in identifying stressors, stress resources, and coping strategies. Perceptions of stressful life events vary among cultures and are dependent on different norms and values. Nursing interventions must consider cultural norms in order to meet desired outcomes.

Workplace Culture

Cultural influence also is applicable when discussing work-related stress. Culture has been described as a "defining force" in understanding work habits (Frey-Ridgway, 1997; Parikh, 2004).

CHART 12–6   Examples of Demands and Coping

Demands	Coping
Failing an examination, such as the state board test for nursing	Taking a review course (PS) Studying with friends (PS)
Giving an oral presentation in class for the first time	Practicing in front of a mirror (PS) Taking a walk before class (ER)
Being diagnosed with cancer	Seeking information from a resource library (PS) Discussing with family and friends (ER)
Finding self with insufficient funds to pay monthly bills	Seeking the advice of a financial planner (PS) Exercising daily at the gym (ER)

PS = problem-solving strategy, ER = emotion-regulating strategy.

CULTURAL CONSIDERATIONS Responses by Individualist and Collectivist Cultures to Stress

Individualist cultures (most Western cultures) tend to emphasize personal autonomy and personal responsibility when dealing with problems. They tend to emphasize the importance and value of exerting control over stressful situations. Therefore, members of this type of culture are less likely to seek social support in stressful situations than are people from collectivist cultures (generally Asian and other Eastern countries). Collectivist cultures tend to be more oriented toward their social group, family, or community and toward seeking help with their problems. However, in collectivist cultures, a greater emphasis is placed on controlling one's personal reactions to a stressful situation rather than trying to control the situation itself. It stands to reason then that the learned component of coping, which is arrived at through experiential and reinforcement situations, may stem from cultural and societal values and beliefs.

Each organization or work setting has a unique culture. When there is discord in the work setting or when a person's values and beliefs are at odds with the culture of the setting, stress develops. In fact, work stressors can be identified in almost all aspects of a person's job. Chart 12–7 describes categories and specific components of work-related stressors. The feelings or stressors identified in this chart also can be used as a guided inventory to identify one's own work-related stressors. Difficult interpersonal relationships, discourse with management, and untoward incidents also must be considered as attempts are made to reduce work-related stress.

In most work situations, stress responses cause performance to suffer. As workers become uncomfortably stressed, distractions, difficulties, anxieties, and negative thinking begin to crowd their minds. These thoughts tend to compete with performance of the task for attentional capacity. Concentration suffers, and focus narrows as the brain becomes overloaded. The more overloaded the brain becomes, the more performance can suffer. The more performance suffers, the more new distractions, difficulties, anxieties, and negative thoughts develop.

Research also has shown that stress reduces people's ability to deal with large amounts of information. Both decision making and creativity are impaired because people are unable to take account of all of the information available. This inability accounts for the frequent observation that highly stressed people will persist in a course of action even when better alternatives are available. It also explains why anxious people perform best when they are not put under a lot of additional stress, whereas calm people may need additional pressure to produce a good performance. People perform at their best when they are normally able to concentrate, and focus all of their attention on the important task at hand. It is then that people are sufficiently motivated to resist competing temptations, and anxieties and distractions do not interfere with clear thought (Manktelow, 2003).

Acculturative Stress

In the fast-paced world of today, job-related stress is becoming increasingly recognized as a nontrivial malady that impacts the well-being of both the employees and the organization. Globalization, an irreversible trend of the 21st century, has been widely

acknowledged as having a stress-producing impact on the work setting. The increasing permeability of international borders, cross-border transfers of people and technology, and international mergers and partnerships that fuel globalization are influencing the culture of work settings.

When diverse cultures come together for collective effort in an organization, culture shock could be experienced. This also is known as **acculturative stress**, which can be defined as job-related stress that is exacerbated by cultural differences such as diverse assumptions, values, and beliefs among the participants (Sohmen, 2005). Acculturative stress as a distinct subset of general job-related stress is suggested as a key impediment to personal satisfaction, team morale, and organizational success. Thus, acculturative stress involves multicultural players with more complex, culture-based causes, but with similar symptoms as in job-related stress such as depression, absenteeism, psychosomatic illnesses, low morale, and high turnover (Friedman, Tidd, Currall, & Tsai, 2000).

Gerontological Considerations

It has been found that the ability to achieve a relaxation response after a stressful event becomes more difficult as people age. Elderly people appear to have an impaired resiliency of the HPA axis response to the acute effects of stress (Spencer & Hutchinson, 1999). Conversely, chronic stress may accelerate the aging process by causing overactivity of the HPA axis. Aging may simply wear out the systems in the brain that respond to stress, so that they become inefficient.

Other physiological responses also vary as one ages. It has been scientifically demonstrated that the cardiovascular response to stress is increased in the elderly including such factors as the heart rate, systolic and mean arterial pressure, peripheral resistance and rate pressure product, and lower cardiac output and stroke volumes (Boutcher & Stocker, 1996). In assessing stress among the elderly, the nurse must consider that the elderly very often are exposed to major stressors such as medical problems, the loss of a spouse and friends, a change in a living situation, and financial worries.

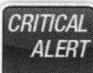 *The elderly are affected uniquely by stress. Cardiovascular responses to stress are reflected in changes in:*

- *Heart rate*
- *Systolic and mean arterial pressures*
- *Peripheral resistance*
- *Rate pressure product*
- *Lower cardiac output and stroke volume.*

Stress responses also are influenced by lack of coping resources:

- *Social support*
- *Problem-solving skills*
- *Material resources*
- *Medical problems.*

The proposed physiological changes that appear in the elderly also impact their coping responses to stress. Situations perceived as potentially menacing vary throughout life, and consequently, coping styles change. It has been found that coping styles probably vary with age, and that when people age they

CHART 12–7 Work-Related Stressor Categories and Their Specific Components

Stressor Category	Specific Components of Category
Disagreement and indecision	Unsure of coworkers' expectations. Unfriendly attitude in coworkers. Job responsibilities go against your better judgment. Cannot satisfy conflicting demands from superiors. Trouble refusing overtime.
Pressure on the job	Overloaded at work, unable to complete tasks during an average day. Too much supervision. Job requirements are taking their toll on your private life. Rushed to complete work or short on time. Too much red tape.
Job description conflict	Uncertainty about your exact job responsibilities. Too much teamwork. Poor flow of information, which makes it difficult to carry out the job. Not enough authority for you to properly do the job. Discomfort in handling unethical assignments.
Communications and comfort with supervisor	Ideas differ from those of the supervisor. Trouble talking to boss. Unable to predict supervisor's reactions. Boss gives little feedback about the work done. Boss is overly critical of the work.
Job-related health concerns	Work conditions are unhealthy. Physical danger exists at workplace. Heavy physical tasks to complete. Hostile threats from coworkers. Sick days are discouraged.
Work overload stress	Cannot consult with others on projects. Coworkers are inefficient. Often take work home to complete. Responsible for too many people/projects. Shortage of help at work.
Work underload stress	Too little responsibility at work. Overqualified for the job. Little chance for growth exists. Trying to "look" busy on job. Feeling unstimulated.
Boredom-induced stress	Performing a repetitive, highly specialized routine. Not learning anything new. Cannot see final outcome of your efforts. Job is too easy. Frequent daydreaming.
Problem of job security	Fear of being laid off or fired. Worry about poor pension. Concern about low wages. Need "pull" to get ahead. Could be fired without cause.
Time pressure	Constant reminders that "time is money." Starting and ending times are rigid. Monotonous pace of work. Not enough break or mealtime. Work pace is too fast.
Job barrier stress	Hope for advancement or raise is limited. Sex/age discrimination exists at job. Not suited to job. Work has no personal meaning. Work goes unrecognized.

Source: American Institute for Preventive Medicine. (2005) Systematic Stress Management Program. www.HealthyLife.com

shift from an active coping style to a more passive one. In addition to the physiological responses to stressors that change, so do some of the cognitive and behavioral responses. Many elderly live alone and many do not have a social support system in place to help them cope. Cognitive problem-solving skills also may be diminished.

Ongoing research in gerontology seeks to examine those situations that elderly adults perceive as potentially menacing, the physical psychosocial implications, and what material resources they have available to face daily demands and establish coping strategies used to diminish the perceived menace. It is critically important for nurses to take these factors into account when assessing the elderly patient and to assist them to evaluate their coping resources and options and to develop effective coping strategies.

Nursing Management

Knowledge of stress, adaptation, and coping theories provides a framework for practice that is applicable to every stage of the nursing process. In caring for patients, the nurse needs to be aware of situations that are likely to be stressful and also to assess and determine the patient's appraisal of the situation and response to the stressor. The nurse also needs to determine the patient's coping resources and strategies as these too impact the patient's physiological and psychosocial response to stressors.

Assessment

Three major areas, previously discussed, serve as a useful guide in the assessment process. These are demands (stressors), the human response to stress, and coping. Although the manifestations of stress vary among individuals, the nurse should assess the patient for the signs and symptoms of the stress that occur as a result of changes in the nervous, endocrine, and immune systems. Also the age of the patient should be considered because many developmental stressors occur at predictable times throughout an individual's life.

Stressors on the patient may include major life changes, events, or situations such as changes in family constellations or daily hassles that the patient is experiencing. The stressors also may be classified as internal and external. Internal demands, aside from perceived tasks and goals, may include physical demands resulting from disease or injury. Additionally, the number of simultaneous demands, the duration of those demands, and previous experience with similar demands should be assessed. It is essential to determine the patient's primary appraisal or perception of the demands to determine if they represent harm or loss, threat, or challenge. Family responses to the patent's demands also should be assessed.

The physiological effects of demands (stressors) that are appraised as stressful are mediated primarily by the sympathetic nervous system and the HPA system. This results in responses such as an increased heart rate, increased blood pressure, loss of appetite, sweating, and dilated pupils. Additionally, the patient may exhibit signs and symptoms related to maladaptation of the immune system or other disorders. Chart 12–8 lists some physiological indicators of stress.

CHART 12–8   **Physiological Indicators of Stress**

- Pupils dilate to increase visual perception when serious threats to the body arise.
- Diaphoresis increases to control elevated body heat due to increased metabolism.
- Heart rate and cardiac output increase to transport nutrients and by-products of metabolism.
- Skin pales due to constriction of peripheral blood vessels, an effect of norepinephrine.
- Sodium and water retention increase due to release of mineralocorticoids, resulting in increased blood volume.
- Rate and depth of respirations increase because of dilated bronchioles, promotion of hyperventilation.
- Urinary output decreases.
- Mouth may be dry.
- Peristalsis of intestines decreases, resulting in possible constipation and flatus.
- Muscle tension increases in preparation for the fight-or-flight response.
- Blood sugar increases due to the release of glucocorticoids and gluconeogenesis.
- Mental alertness improves with serious threats.

Source: From Kozier, Barbara J.; Erb, Glenora; Berman, Audrey J.; & Snyder, Shirlee J. Fundamentals of Nursing: Concepts, Procedures, & Practices, 7th, © 2004. Electronically reproduced by permission of Pearson Education, Inc., Upper Saddle River, New Jersey.

Behavioral responses include observable actions and cognition of the patient. These may include such behaviors as accident proneness, impaired speech, and anxiety, crying, and shouting. Work-related demands may be manifested in responses such as absenteeism, tardiness, reduced productivity, and job dissatisfaction. Observable cognitive responses include self-reports of excessive demands, inability to make decisions, and forgetfulness. Signs and symptoms of stress are shown in Chart 12–9.

Evaluation of the adequacy and effectiveness of a patient's coping strategies and resources should be assessed. It also is necessary to assess whether or not a certain coping strategy will bring about the desired result. Positive resources might include supportive family members, adequate finances, and the ability to solve problems.

In assessing the individual who seeks health care, it is critical to remember that objective signs and subjective symptoms are the primary indicators of the physiological processes that are occurring. Further signs of change are indicated in diagnostic studies such as computed tomography (CT) and magnetic resonance imaging (MRI). Objective data also may be obtained from laboratory data (e.g., blood glucose, electrolytes, and urinalysis). In making a diagnosis the nurse must relate the symptoms or complaints expressed by the patient to the physical and behavioral signs that are present.

Nursing Diagnoses

Many nursing diagnoses are possible for patients suffering from stress. Anxiety, frustration, anger, and feelings of inadequacy, helplessness, or powerlessness often are emotions associated

CHART 12–9 Signs and Symptoms of Stress

General irritability, hyperexcitation, or depression

Dryness of throat and mouth

Urge to cry, scream, or run and hide

Easily fatigued, constantly tired

Floating anxiety

Easily startled

Stuttering

Pacing, moving about, cannot sit still

Gastrointestinal signs and symptoms: "butterflies" in the stomach, diarrhea, vomiting

Changes in menstrual cycle

Loss of or excessive appetite

Increased use of legally prescribed drugs

Injury prone

Disturbed behavior

Pounding of the heart

Emotional instability, impulsive behavior

Inability to concentrate

Feelings of unreality, weakness, or dizziness

Tension

Trembling, nervous tics

Nervous laughter

Grinding of teeth

Insomnia, nightmares, or other sleep difficulties

Excessive perspiration

Frequent urination

Muscle tension and headaches

Pain in the neck or lower back

Increased smoking

Alcohol and drug addiction

Source: This article was published in Stress in health and disease. Selye, H. (1976). Stoneham, MA: Butterworth-Heinemann. Copyright Elsevier, 1976.

with stress. In the presence of these emotions, the customary activities of daily living may be disrupted. For example, a sleep disturbance may be present, activity and eating patterns may be altered, and family processes and roles may be changed.

According to Carpenito (2007), a coping–stress–tolerance pattern has been identified as 1 of 11 functional health patterns. Assessment of the health pattern elicits a description of the coping–stress–tolerance level of a patient, and enables the nurse to identify stressors at the individual or family level. Two overriding diagnoses related to stress have been identified: *Ineffective Coping* and *Compromised, Family Coping*. **Ineffective Coping** is defined as an inability to manage internal or environmental stressors appropriately as a result of inadequate resources (physical, psychological, behavioral, or cognitive). Potential etiologies include disruption of emotional bonds, unsatisfactory support system, sensory overload, and inadequate psychological and physical resources (Carpenito, 2007). **Compromised Family**

CHART 12–10 Nursing Diagnoses in Coping–Stress–Tolerance Pattern

Risk Prone Health Behavior

Caregiver Role Strain

Ineffective individual coping:
   Defensive Coping
   Ineffective Denial

Ineffective family coping:
   Coping: Family, Compromised
   Coping: Family, Disabled

Risk for Self-Mutilation

Risk for Other-Directed Violence

Post-Trauma Syndrome

Relocation Stress Syndrome

Coping: Compromised refers to the usually supportive primary person (family member or friend) providing insufficient, ineffective, or compromised support, comfort, assistance, or encouragement that may be needed by the patient to manage the adaptive strategies related to the health challenge (Carpenito, 2007). Specific nursing diagnoses that are derived from the coping–stress–tolerance pattern are shown in Chart 12–10.

NANDA International (formerly the North American Nursing Diagnosis Association) has identified nursing diagnoses related to stress, adaptation, and coping (NANDA, 2007). These are listed below in alphabetical order:

- *Anxiety*: A vague, uneasy feeling of discomfort or dread, the source of which may not be known. It is an alerting signal that warns of impending danger and enables the individual to take measures to deal with a threat.

- *Caregiver Role Strain*: Difficulty in performing the role of caregiver.

- *Compromised Family Coping*: Primary supportive person provides insufficient, ineffective, or compromised support, comfort, or assistance that may be needed by the patient to manage adaptive tasks.

- *Decisional Conflict (Specify)*: Uncertainty about course of action to take when the choice involves risk, loss, or challenge to personal life values.

- *Defensive Coping*: Repeated projection of falsely positive self-evaluation based on a self-protective pattern that defends against underlying perceived threats to positive self-regard.

- *Disabled Family Coping*: Behavior of significant person that disables his or her capacities and the patient's capacities to effectively address tasks essential to adaptation to the health challenge.

- *Fear*: Response to perceived threat that is consciously recognized as a danger.

- *Risk Prone Health Behavior*: Inability to modify lifestyle/behavior in a manner consistent with a change in health behavior.

- *Ineffective Coping*: Inability to form a valid appraisal of the stressors, inadequate choices of practiced responses, and/or inability to use available resources.

- *Ineffective Denial:* Conscious or unconscious attempt to disavow the knowledge or meaning of an event to reduce anxiety/fear, but leading to the detriment of health.
- *Post-Trauma Syndrome:* Sustained maladaptive responses to a traumatic, overwhelming event.
- *Relocation Stress Syndrome:* Physiological and/or psychosocial disturbance following transfer from one environment to another.

Other Nursing Diagnoses

In addition to the examples of nursing diagnoses provided in the preceding section, other applicable diagnoses dealing with stress also include *Social Isolation, Risk for Impaired Parenting, Spiritual Distress, Readiness for Enhanced Family Coping, Situational Low Self-Esteem,* and *Powerlessness.* Because human responses to stress are so varied, as are the sources of stress, arriving at an accurate diagnosis allows interventions and goals to be more specific and leads to improved outcomes.

Outcomes and Evaluation Parameters

Stress management is directed toward reducing and controlling stress and improving coping. The desired patient outcomes of nursing interventions are: illness prevention, improved quality of life as defined by patient, and fewer maladaptive responses to stress. Specific parameters of success in meeting these goals include identification of stressors, identification of stress resources, and use of coping strategies. These serve as measurable parameters on which to evaluate the patient's responses to nursing interventions.

Interventions

Interventions are based on the plans developed in collaboration with the patient, significant support people if possible, and other members of the health care team. They are dependent on the patient's state of health, level of anxiety, support resources, coping mechanisms, and sociocultural and religious affiliation. The nurse and patient need to set goals to change the existing responses to the stressor or stressors.

Although stress is commonplace and occurs daily in one form or another, it also is highly individual. It is, therefore, important to tailor the stress reduction approaches to the individual patient. Interventions that seem to be universal in reducing stress include adequate rest and sleep, time management, optimal nutrition, and physical exercise.

Specific nursing interventions that assist in meeting the goals of stress reduction include the following: promoting a healthy lifestyle, providing stress management education, and recommending support and therapy groups, all of which are discussed next.

Health Promotion

Health and energy aid individuals with their coping strategies; thus, a health-promoting lifestyle provides resources and buffers the impact of stressors. A health risk appraisal may identify lifestyles or habits that place the patient at risk for illness. A health risk appraisal is an assessment method that is designed to promote health by examining an individual's personal habits and recommending changes when a health risk is evident.

Health risk questionnaires estimate the likelihood that a person with a given set of characteristics will become ill. Hopefully, if provided this information, individuals will alter their activities to improve their health. However, research so far has not demonstrated that providing people with such information motivates them to change their behavior. It has been found that the single most important factor for determining health status is social class, and within social class the major factor influencing health is education (Mickler, 1997).

Factors that have been found to be successful in reducing stress include exercise, nutrition, rest and sleep, and time management. Regular exercise promotes both physical and emotional health. Physiological benefits include improved muscle tone, improved cardiopulmonary function, and weight control. Psychological benefits include relief of tension, a feeling of well-being, and relaxation. Good nutrition is essential in increasing the body's resistance to stress. Reducing caffeine, salt, sugar, and fat intake and increasing vitamin and mineral intake will minimize the negative effects of stress, irritability, hyperactivity, and anxiety. Rest and sleep restore the body's energy levels and are an essential element of stress management. Patients may need help in achieving this goal if in pain and they also may need to learn relaxation techniques. People who manage their time effectively usually experience less stress because they feel more in control of their situation. Thus, the nurse may need to help patients prioritize tasks and to consider whether modifications can be made to decrease role demands. This is an important consideration in both inpatient and outpatient settings, particularly as nurses help patients prepare for discharge from acute care to a home environment.

Minimizing anxiety and mediating anger are helpful and appropriate nursing interventions. Nurses carry out measures to reduce patients' anxiety on a daily basis and these activities should be reinforced. These include such measures as explaining procedures before they are performed, administering a massage to help the patient relax, controlling the environment to make it less stressful, providing emotional support to the patient and family, providing an atmosphere of caring and trust, and listening to and validating the patient's perceptions of what is happening and how she is feeling. Mediating anger also is important. Many nurses become upset with the angry patient, who seems irrational, refuses treatment, or becomes verbally abusive. Nurses tend to respond in ways that reduce their own stress, not that of the patient. Fontaine and Fletcher (2003) recommend the following strategies for dealing with patients' anger:

- Know and understand your own response to the feelings and expressions of anger.
- Accept the patient's right to be angry; feelings are real and cannot be discounted or ignored.
- Try to understand the meaning of the patient's anger.
- Ask the patient what contributed to the anger.
- Help the patient "own" the anger; do not assume responsibility for his feelings.
- Let the patient talk about his anger.
- Listen to the patient, and act as calmly as possible.
- After the interaction is completed, take time to process your feelings and your responses to the client with your colleagues.

Always ensure the safety of the patient and others. Do not hesitate to seek help if needed from other staff or security personnel.

 CRITICAL ALERT *Patients may react to stress through anger. The nurse should respond to the angry patient in a constructive manner, not through anger. Always seek help to manage the angry patient when appropriate.*

Using and teaching relaxation techniques are useful mechanisms for stress reduction. Commonly used relaxation techniques include progressive muscle relaxation, meditation, and guided imagery. Specific relaxation techniques that a nurse can teach a patient to help quiet the mind include breathing exercises, massage, biofeedback, yoga, therapeutic touch, music therapy, and humor and laughter. Many agencies have relaxation tapes available for patient use.

Crisis intervention is a short-term helping process of assisting patients to (1) work through a crisis to its resolution, and (2) to restore their precrisis level of functioning. Those in crisis are experiencing an acute, time-limited state of disequilibrium resulting from situational, developmental, or societal sources of stress. They are incapable of coping with or adapting to the stressor by using previous methods of problem solving. They generally have a distorted perception of the event and do not have adequate situational support of coping mechanisms. This is a temporary situation requiring intervention from a professional individual, such as a nurse, physician, psychologist, clergy, or social worker.

The traditional steps of the nursing process closely correspond to the steps of crisis intervention. In the assessment phase, the nurse must focus on the person and the problem, collecting data about the patient, the patient's coping style, the precipitating event, the situational supports, the client's perception of the crisis, and the person's ability to handle the problem. This information provides a basis for future decisions about how and when to intervene and whom to call. An individual's perception of the event and personal response will determine the nursing diagnoses. Diagnoses previously described also are common for people in crisis. Additionally, diagnoses such as *Risk for Self-Directed Violence, Risk for Other-Directed Violence, Rape-Trauma Syndrome,* and *Hopelessness* may be appropriate. Effective planning for crisis intervention must be based on careful assessment and developed in active collaboration with the person in crisis and the significant people in that person's life. Implementation involves crisis counseling and crisis home visits. Crisis counseling focuses on solving immediate problems and it involves individuals, groups, or families. Crisis home visits may be made when telephone counseling does not suffice or when the crisis workers need to obtain additional information by direct observation or to reach a patient who is unobtainable by telephone.

Educating About Stress Management

The goals of nursing educational interventions are to reduce stress and improve the patient's coping ability. These generally are met by providing sensory information and providing procedural information (e.g., preoperative teaching). Teaching structure content, such as a review of cardiovascular anatomy for the cardiac patient or a description of sensations the patient will experience during cardiac catheterization, is one type of preparatory education. This type of education may alter the person–environment relationship such that something that might have been viewed as threatening becomes perceived more positively. Providing patients with information also tends to reduce the emotional response so patients can concentrate and problem solve more effectively.

Enhancing Social Support

As noted, social support has been demonstrated to be effective in mediating life stress. Typically, social support tends to make people feel loved, appreciated, esteemed, and valued. In turn, this tends to elevate the person's sense of self-worth. Those who belong to a social support network share information and make goods and services available to the members on demand. The critical qualities within a social network are the exchange of intimate communications and the presence of solidarity and trust. These social support qualities facilitate an individual's coping behaviors, and create a sense of sharing the stress burden with the individual. The emotions that accompany stress are unpleasant and often increase in a spiraling fashion if relief is not provided. Being able to talk with someone and express feelings openly may help the person gain control of the situation. Nurses can provide this support; however, it is important to identify the person's social support system and encourage its use. Persons who are loners, who are isolated, or who withdraw in times of stress have a high risk of coping failure.

Anxiety also can alter a person's ability to process information, thus, it helps to seek information and advice from others who can assist with analyzing the threat and developing a strategy to manage it. This assists the person in maintaining control and retaining self-esteem. Social networks assist with management of stress by providing the individual with:

- A positive social identity
- Emotional support
- Material aid and tangible services
- Access to information
- Access to new social contacts and new social roles.

Support and Therapy Groups

Support groups are formed for people in similar stressful situations: cancer survivors, people with ostomies, mastectomy patients, parents of autistic children, and those with chronic illnesses and disabilities. There also are groups for drug abusers and alcoholics. Being a member of a group with similar problems or goals generates a releasing effect on a person that promotes freedom of expression and an exchange of ideas. Although not all individuals benefit from membership in such groups, many do. It is the nurse's responsibility, when assessing an individual's stressors and coping resources and strategies, to determine if such an intervention might be helpful to the individual.

Intervention Summary

As noted, a person's psychological and biologic health, internal and external sources of stress management, and relationships with the environment are predictors of health outcomes. These factors are related directly to the individual's health patterns. The nurse plays a significant role in identifying the health patterns of the individual receiving care. If the patient's health patterns are not achieving physiological, psychological, and social balance, the nurse is obligated, with the consent and assistance of the patient, to seek ways to promote balance through nursing interventions. Many examples of stress reduction techniques, are shown in Chart 12–11. Interventions designed to mediate physiological stress and its effect on the body systems are addressed in greater depth in other chapters of this book.

Evaluation

Desired outcomes provide a guide for evaluating the patient's response to nursing interventions. They serve as indicators of accomplishment or lack of accomplishment in helping the patient reduce the stressors or manage the stressful situation. If outcomes are not achieved, the nurse, patient, support resources, and the health care team need to explore the reasons and revise the interventions as appropriate. Questions such as the following need to be considered:

- How does the patient perceive the problem?
- Is there an underlying problem that has not been identified?
- Were existing coping strategies sufficient to meet intended outcomes?
- How does the patient perceive the effectiveness of new coping strategies?
- Did the patient implement new coping strategies properly?
- Did the patient access and use available resources?
- Have the family and significant others provided effective support?

Additionally, the health care provider should assess physiological values that are indicators of stress. These include vital signs, heart rate, blood pressure, and respiratory rate measurements; level of pain; sleep and rest patterns; and dietary habits.

Collaborative Management

Humans experience stress as an intrinsic part of life and in conjunction with many standard diagnostic, clinical, and experimental manipulations. Unintended stressors, as well as those intended, may significantly affect diagnostic and clinical measures and overall health outcomes. Thus, when conducting clinical, diagnostic, or experimental manipulations, it may be prudent to account for the effects of stress on the specific physiological parameter or health outcome being measured.

Responding to stress signs and symptoms and creating a plan of care require collaboration with all members of the health care team. Depending on the signs and symptoms, the nurse will work with a physician, dietician, physical therapist, respiratory therapist, social worker, and/or home care coordinator. Acute physiological responses to stress in which the patient is experiencing signs and symptoms of critical illness will require close collaboration with the physician in planning, treating, and monitoring care. Other members of the health care team will play an active part in treating respiratory problems, cardiovascular problems, pain, and nutritional imbalances. If stress manifestations are psychological and/or behavioral, it would be prudent for the nurse to collaborate with a psychologist or social worker. The same would hold true for a patient with a nutritional imbalance, or eating habit problems, where the nutritionist or dietician would become a key player.

CHART 12–11 Stress Reduction Techniques

Maintain a healthy lifestyle by looking after your body.	Maintain regular exercise and a healthy diet rich in a variety of whole grains, vegetables, and fruits, and avoid excessive alcohol, caffeine, and tobacco. Exercise helps by creating a distraction from stressful events and releasing nervous energy.
Discover how to relax.	Relaxation is the polar opposite of the stress response. Deep-breathing exercises may help. If persistently unable to relax, try yoga or t'ai chi. Therapeutic massage also may loosen taut muscles and calm frazzled nerves.
Reduce stress through cognitive-behavioral methods.	Identify sources of stress and question those sources. Whose goals do the stressful activities meet? Can the assumed tasks be reasonably accomplished?
Restructure priorities; add stress-reducing activities.	Shift the balance from stress-producing to stress-reducing activities. Consider as many relief options as possible (e.g., walks, recreation).
Discuss feelings.	Explain your feelings and needs to a trusted individual, in a positive way, or use a journal or letter to express feelings. In return, listen to others.
Keep perspective and look for the positive; shift your outlook.	Focus on positive outcomes; this helps reduce tension and achieve goals. Choose to look at a situation in a more positive way. Step back from the conflict or worry that has put you in knots and ask what part of it is troubling you most. Are you afraid of losing face, or are you so angry that you are in danger of losing self-control. Is your reaction out of proportion? Take a break, talk to someone close and get a different perspective on your troubles.
Use humor.	Use humor and laughter to release pent-up feelings and keep perspective. Laughter also appears to have physical effects that reduce stress hormone levels.
Get help.	Seek professional help from psychiatrists, psychologists, or licensed clinical social workers if unable to change your habitual patterns of thought and behavior that trigger your stress response. Professionals are trained to help you break free of these patterns.

In preparing a patient for discharge from an acute care hospital, the nurse would need to coordinate with, and rely on, the expertise of many other members of the health care team in order to provide a comfortable transition from acute care to the home or extended care environment. And, perhaps most important of all, is the need for the nurse to coordinate with the patient and the patient's family or significant others. As noted throughout the chapter, these people play a key role in providing coping resources and in developing coping strategies. The nurse uses these resources as key elements in implementing the nursing process and developing the plan of care for patients.

Health Promotion

Stress can be a factor in a variety of physical and emotional illnesses, which should be professionally treated. However, many stress symptoms can be managed with over-the-counter medications, for example, aspirin, acetaminophen, or ibuprofen for tension headache, and antacids and antidiarrhea medications for mild stomach distress. However, a physician should be consulted for physical symptoms that are out of the ordinary, particularly those which progress in severity or awaken the patient at night. A mental health professional should be consulted for unmanageable acute stress or for severe anxiety or depression.

In choosing specific strategies for treating stress, several factors should be considered:

- No single method is uniformly successful.
- What works for one person does not necessarily work for someone else.
- Stress can be positive as well as negative. Appropriate and controllable stress can enhance an individual's interest and excitement and motivate the individual to greater achievement. A lack of stress may lead to boredom and depression.
- Stress may play a part in making people vulnerable to illness. A physician or psychologist should be consulted if there are any indications for accompanying medical or psychological conditions, such as cardiac symptoms, significant pain, anxiety, or depression.

Stress Reduction and Impact on Health

An individual's reaction to a specific stressor is different from anyone else's. Some people are naturally laid-back about almost everything, whereas others react strongly at the slightest hint of stress, and most fall somewhere between those extremes. Genetic variations may partly explain the differences. The genes that control the stress response keep most people on a fairly even keel, only occasionally priming the body for fighting or fleeing. Overactive or underactive stress responses may stem from slight differences in these genes. The availability of genetic information and technology enables health care providers to perform screening, testing, and counseling for patients with genetic concerns. Knowledge obtained from the Human Genome Project also has created opportunities for assessing a person's genetic profile and preventing or treating disease.

Life experiences may increase the individual's sensitivity to stress as well. Strong stress reactions sometimes can be traced to early environmental factors. People who were exposed to extreme stress as children tend to be particularly vulnerable to stress as adults.

As explained, stressors develop when the demands of life exceed the ability to cope with them. It follows, then, that stress can be managed by:

- Changing one's environment so that the demands are not so high
- Learning how to better cope with the demands in the environment
- Doing both.

Helpful techniques to accomplish these goals were shown earlier in Chart 12–11.

It is emphasized that treating stress cannot cure medical problems. Stress management is not, therefore, a substitute for standard medical treatments, but it can be an important component in a medical regimen. It has been reported that treatments that reduce psychological distress after a heart attack appear to improve patients' long-term outlooks. It also has been reported that stress management programs may reduce the risk of heart events. Stress management has been found to be effective in coping with anger associated with lowering blood pressure. It also has been found to be effective when used with medications, such as tricyclics, in reducing headaches.

Stress management requires continuous practice as one goes through life and deals with change, often unexpected change. Even if frustrations are taken in stride, the stress response can surge up when dealing with something big, such as illness, job loss, or bereavement. The body's fight-or-flight reaction has strong biological roots. It is there for self-preservation, even if not much help in a demanding job or a difficult relationship. If stress becomes difficult and is potentially causing long-term effects, it is necessary to take action by learning how to recognize the symptoms and by seeking help to mediate the effects of the stress.

Summary

Just as stress is universal, it is a constant factor in caring for patients. The nurse must be able to recognize and treat the physical, psychological, and social manifestations of stress. It is important that nurses recognize the signs and symptoms of stress, both within patients and within themselves, and promote positive adaptive outcomes. To do so, nurses must become familiar with stress theories, understand the physiological, behavioral, and psychosocial responses to stress, and engage in evidence-based practice. Collaborative health care practices are integral to achieving these outcomes and to applying research findings to practices designed to foster improved patient outcomes. Future research opportunities and their impact on clinical practice are shown in the Research Opportunities and Clinical Impact box (p. 248).

RESEARCH OPPORTUNITIES AND CLINICAL IMPACT RELATED TO STRESS

Research	Clinical Impact
Physiological	
Determine types of sedation and analgesics that can best alleviate the stress response and attenuate pain and anxiety.	Provide for appropriate use of sedation and analgesic to improve compliance with care.
Identify the effect of repressed stressful emotions on the psychoneuroimmune axis and the predisposition to illnesses.	Develop treatments specific to the stress-related illnesses. Educate patients about themselves and the body's response to stress.
Determine the effect of stress on wound healing.	Develop wound-healing protocols.
Distinguish between the effects of physical and psychosocial workplace stressors on the etiology of work-related musculoskeletal disorders.	Develop insight into the nature of risk for work-related musculoskeletal disorders.
Identify the possible potentiation of oxidative stress by nursing care activities.	Develop guidelines for care of patients who are critically ill that minimize oxidative stress.
Determine the relationship, if any, between an impaired HPA and axis resiliency during aging.	Realize the affect of stress on aging, and whether or not the HPA axis returns to basal levels after acute stress or to habituate after repeated stress in the elderly.
Explore relationship between postdiagnostic stress and cancer survival.	Provide psychological intervention during the treatment of breast cancer to promote and foster survival.
Explore the relationship between different kinds of abuse at different development stages and potential reversibility of the biological stress vulnerability after psychotherapeutic and psychopharmacological interventions.	Identify implications for the prevention and treatment of mood and anxiety disorders in survivors of early trauma.
Determine if there is a relationship between the clustering of stress indicators and *H. pylori* in the general population.	Treat stress effects on the gastrointestinal system more effectively.
Psychosocial	
Examine social support and its relationship to personality, health, and adjustment	Evaluate the role of social support as a coping resource.
Explore the role that psychosocial factors play in the development of peptic ulcers.	Develop a new paradigm for applying the integrated psychosocial model to medical disorders.
Develop coping measurements.	Expand availability of measurement tools to assess coping.

NCLEX® REVIEW

1. During a focused health interview, a patient identifies a number of external stressors. Which of the following would be considered an external source of stress?
   1. Smoking
   2. Negative self-image
   3. Long commute to work each day
   4. Personal need to work 16 hours each day

2. During a routine health assessment, a patient reports a recent loss of job and divorce however has no health issues to report or discuss. The nurse attributes this patient's ability to handle stress as being:
   1. Disrupted.
   2. Attributed to hardiness.
   3. Able to handle daily hassles.
   4. Situational uplifts.

3. During an assessment, the patient demonstrates physical signs of the alarm phase within the General Adaptation Syndrome. Which of the following is a sign of this phase?
   1. Elevated blood pressure
   2. Normal heart rate
   3. Maintenance of normal weight
   4. Constricted pupils

4. A patient tells the nurse that she needs to be discharged from the hospital soon because she has a job to go to and a family who needs her. The nurse realizes this patient is at risk for additional illnesses because:
   1. She hasn't fully recovered from her current hospitalization.
   2. She shouldn't return to work yet.
   3. The additional stresses of daily life add more stress hormones to the body which can lead to disease.
   4. She isn't focused on her own health.

5. Which of the following would be beneficial to instruct a patient demonstrating signs of oxidative stress?
   1. Strive to remove all free radicals from the body.
   2. Limit the ingestion of water-based foods.
   3. Ingest high doses of vitamin C.
   4. Improve nutritional intake including foods containing vitamin E.

6. A patient is demonstrating signs of increasing stress. Which of the following would the nurse assess in this patient?
   1. Increased heart rate and blood pressure
   2. Cool skin
   3. Respiration rate of 12 per minute and regular
   4. Bowel sounds present in all quadrants

Answers for review questions appear in Appendix D

KEY TERMS

acculturative stress *p.240*
acute stress *p.225*
acute stressor *p.215*
adaptation *p.215*
atrophy *p.226*
chronic stress *p.225*
cognitive reappraisal *p.220*
Compromised Family Coping p.243
coping *p.215*
developmental stressor *p.215*
dysplasia *p.217*
eustress *p.217*
external stressor *p.215*
general adaptation syndrome (GAS) *p.217*

hardiness *p.219*
hassles *p.220*
homeostasis *p.216*
hyperplasia *p.227*
hypertrophy *p.226*
hypothalamic–pituitary–adrenal (HPA) axis *p.231*
Ineffective Coping p.243
inflammation *p.228*
internal stressor *p.215*
local adaptation syndrome (LAS) *p.217*
maladaptive coping mechanisms *p.215*
metaplasia *p.227*
nutritional imbalance *p.227*

oxidative stress *p.229*
primary appraisal *p.220*
reactive oxygen species (ROS) *p.230*
reticular activating system (RAS) *p.223*
secondary appraisal *p.220*
sense of coherence (SOC) *p.219*
situational stressor *p.215*
steady state *p.222*
stress *p.214*
stress perception *p.214*
stress response *p.214*
stressor *p.214*
uplifts *p.221*

EXPLORE **PEARSON mynursingkit™**

MyNursingKit is your one stop for online chapter review materials and resources. Prepare for success with additional NCLEX®-style practice questions, interactive assignments and activities, web links, animations and videos, and more!

Register your access code from the front of your book at
www.mynursingkit.com

REFERENCES

Aggleton, J. P. (1992). *The amygdatale*. New York: Wiley-Liss.

Antonovsky, A. (1987). *Unravelling the mystery of health: How people manage stress and stay well*. San Francisco: Jossey-Bass.

Arnsten, A. F. T. (1998). The biology of being frazzled. *Science, 280*(5370), 1711–1712.

Arrighi, J. A., Burg, M., Cohen, I. S., Kao, A. H., Pfau, S., Caulin-Glaser, T., et al. (2000). Myocardial blood-flow response during mental stress in patients with coronary artery disease. *Lancet, 356*(9226), 310–311.

Bernard, L. C., & Krupat, E. (1994). *Health psychology: Biopsychosocial factors in health and illness*. New York: Harcourt Brace.

Blanchard, A. R. (2002). Sedation and analgesia in intensive care: Medications attenuate stress response in critical illness. *Postgraduate Medicine, 3*(2), 59.

Boutcher, S. H., & Stocker, D. (1996). Cardiovascular response of young and older males to mental challenge. *Journals of Gerontology Series B: Psychological Sciences and Social Sciences, 51*(5), P261-P267.

Byrnes, S. (2003). Staying on top of oxidative stress. *The Weston A. Price Foundation modern diseases*. Retrieved January 4, 2007, from http://www.westonaprice.org/moderndiseases/oxidativesterss.html

Cannon, W. B. (1932). *The wisdom of the body*. New York: Norton.

Carpenito, L. J. (2007). *Nursing care plans and documentation: Nursing diagnosis and collaborative problems* (4th ed.). Philadelphia: Lippincott Williams & Wilkins.

Dienstbier, R. A. (1989). Arousal and physiological toughness: Implications for mental and physical health. *Psychological Review, 96*, 84–100.

Edelman, S., Rémond, L. (2004). *Taking charge: A guide for teenagers*. St. Leonards: Foundation for Life Sciences.

Emory University Health Sciences Center. (2006). *Scientists discover possible link between oxidative stress and non-hereditary degenerative disease*. Retrieved January 4, 2007, from http://eurekalert.org/pub_releases/2006-04/euhs-sdp0427-6.php

Espat, N. J., & Helton, W. S. (2000). Oxygen free radicals, oxidative stress, and antioxidants in critical illness. *Support Line, 22*, 11–20.

Everson, S. A., Lynch, J. W., Kaplan, G. A., Lakka, T., Sivenius, J., & Salonen, J. T. (2001). Stress-induced blood pressure reactivity and incident stroke in middle-aged men. *Stroke, 32*, 1263–1270.

Fawcett, J. (2005). *Contemporary nursing knowledge: Analysis and evaluation of nursing models and theories* (2nd ed.). Philadelphia: F. A. Davis.

Fontaine, K. L., & Fletcher, J. S. (2003). *Mental health nursing* (5th ed.). Upper Saddle River, NJ: Pearson Prentice Hall.

Frey-Ridgway, S. (1997). The cultural dimensions of international business. *Collection Building, 16*(1), 12–23.

Friedman, R. A., Tidd, S. T., Currall, S. C., & Tsai, J. C. (2000). What goes around comes around: The impact of personal conflict style on work conflict and stress. *International Journal of Conflict Management, 11*(1), 32–55.

Gabriel, G. (1997). Hans Selye: The discovery of stress. In *Brain Connection*. Oakland, CA: Scientific Learning Corporation. Retrieved December 9, 2006, from http://www.brainconnection.com/topics/printindex.php3?main=fa/Selye

George, J. (Ed.). (2002). *Nursing theories: The base for professional nursing practice*. (5th ed.). Norwalk, CT: Appleton and Lange.

Glanz, K., Rimer, B. K., & Lewis, F. M. (2002). *Health behavior and health education: Theory, research and practice*. San Francisco: Wiley & Sons.

Glaser, G., & Kiecolt-Glaser, J. K. (1994). *Handbook of human stress and immunity*. San Diego: Academic Press.

Goodyear-Bruch, C. & Pierce, J. D. (2002). Oxidative stress in critically ill patients. *American Journal of Critical Care, 11*(6), 543–653.

Green, G., & Smith, R. (2004). The psychosocial and health care needs of HIV-positive people in the United Kingdom: A review. *HIV Medicine, 5*(1), 4.

Grumman, R. (1998). Stomach, digestive system, ulcers, stress. *New Woman, 28*(12), 46–47.

Haddy, R. I., & Clover, R. D. (2001). The biological processes in psychological stress. *Families, System, & Health, 19*(3), 291–302.

Heim, C., Newport, D. J., Heit, S., Graham, V. P., Wilcox, M., Bonsall, R., et al. (2000). Pituitary-adrenal and autonomic responses to stress in women after sexual and physical abuse in childhood. *Journal of American Medical Association, 284*(5), 592–597.

Helfer, R. E., & Kempe, C. H. (1976). *The Abused Child.* Cambridge, MA: Ballinger Publishing Company.

Holahan, C. J., & Moos, R. H. (1987). Risk, resistance, and psychological distress: A longitudinal analysis with adults and children. *Journal of Abnormal Psychology, 96,* 3–13.

Holmes, T. A., Masuda, M. (1966). Magnitude estimations of social readjustments. *Journal of Psychosomatic Research, 11,* 219–225.

Holmes, D., & Rahe, R. (1967). The social readjustment rating scale. *Journal of Psychosomatic Research, 11,* 213–218.

Horowitz, M., Schaefer, C., Hiroto, D., Wilner, N., & Levin, B. (1977). Life event questionnaires for measuring presumptive stress. *Psychosomatic Medicine, 39*(6), 413–431.

Kalantaridou, S. N., Makrigiannakis, A., Zoumakis, E., & Chrousos, G. P. (2004). Stress and the female reproductive system. *Journal of Reproductive Immunology, 62*(1), 61–68.

King, I. (1971). *Toward a theory of nursing: General concepts of human behavior.* New York: John Wiley & Sons, Inc.

Kobasa, S. C., Maddi, S. R., & Zoda, M. A. (1983). Type A and hardiness. *Journal of Behavioral Medicine, 6*(1), 41–51.

Kop, J. J. (1999). Chronic and acute psychological risk factors for clinical manifestations of coronary artery disease. *Psychosomatic Medicine, 61,* 476–487.

Lazarus, R. S. (1966). *Psychological stress and the coping process.* New York: McGraw-Hill.

Lazarus, R. S., & Cohen K. B. (1977). Environmental stress. In I. Altman & J. F. Wohlwill (Eds.), *Human behavior and environment* (Vol. 2). New York: Plenum Press.

Lazarus, R. S., & Folkman, S. (1984). *Stress, appraisal, and coping.* New York: Springer Publishing.

Lazarus, R. S., & Launier, R. (1976). Stress related transactions between person and environment. In L. A. Pervin & M. Lewis (Eds.), *Perspectives in international psychology* (pp. 87–327). New York: Plenum Press.

Levenstein, S. (1998). Stress and peptic ulcer: Life beyond *Helicobacter. British Medical Journal, 316,* 538–541.

Levenstein, S. (2003). Stress and ulcerative colitis: Convincing the doubting Thomases. *American Journal of Gastroenterology, 98*(10), 2203–2208.

Litt, M. D. (1988). Cognitive mediators of stressful experience: self-efficacy and perceived control. *Cognitive Therapy and Research, 12*(3), 241–260.

Lobo, M. L. (2002). Environmental model: Florence Nightingale. In J. B. George (Ed.), *Nursing theories: The base for professional nursing practice* (5th ed., pp. 43–60). Upper Saddle River, NJ: Pearson Prentice Hall.

MacArthur, J. D., & MacArthur, C. T. (1998). *Coping strategies.* Research Network on Socioeconomic Status and Health. Retrieved March 2, 2005, from http://www.maces.ucsf.edu/Reserach/Psychosocial/notebook/coping.html

MacDonald, L. A., Karasek, R. A., Punnett, L., & Scharf, T. (2001). Covariation between workplace physical and psychosocial stressors: Evidence and implications for occupational health research and prevention. *Economics, 44*(7), 696–718.

Malinski, V. M. (2006). Rogerian science-based nursing theories. *Nursing Science Quarterly, 19,* 7–12.

Mandler, G. (1982). Stress and thought processes. In L. Goldgerger and S. Breznitz (Eds.), *Handbook of stress: Theoretical and clinical aspects.* New York: The Free Press.

Manisses Communications Group. (2003). In case you haven't heard. *Mental Health Weekly, 13*(36), 8.

Manktelow, J. (2003). *Stress management techniques from mind tools: Introduction to stress management.* Retrieved December 14, 2006, from http://www.mindtools.com/stress/UnderstandStress/StressIntro.htm

Marriner-Tomey, A., & Alligood, M. R. (2006). *Nursing theorists and their work,* (6th ed.). St. Louis: Mosby.

Maté, G. (2003). *When the body says no: Understanding the stress–disease connection.* Hoboken, New Jersey: Wiley & Sons.

Mayer E. A., Naliboff, B. D., Craig, A. D. (2006). Neuroimaging of the brain-gut axis: from basic understanding to treatment of functional GI disorders. *Gastroenterology,131,* 1925–42.

Mayo Clinic. (2006). *Reduce stress with a strong social support network.* Retrieved January 5, 2007, from http://www.mayoclinic.com/health/social-support/SR00033

Mickler, M. (1997). *Community organizing and community building for health.* New Brunswick, NJ: Rutgers University Press.

NANDA International. (2007). *NANDA nursing diagnoses: Definitions and classification 2007–2008.* Philadelphia: Author.

National Institutes of Health. (2004). *Stress system malfunction could lead to serious, life threatening disease.* Retrieved November 12, 2004, from http://www.mayoclinic.com/findinformation/condiotncenters/subcenters/cfm

Neuman, B., & Fawcett, J. (2002). *The Neuman systems model* (4th ed.). Upper Saddle River, NJ: Pearson Prentice Hall.

Nightingale, F. (1957). *Notes on nursing.* Philadelphia: J. B. Lippincott. (Original publication in 1859).

Noh, S., & Kaspar, V. (2003). Perceived discrimination and depression: Moderating effects of coping, acculturation, and ethnic support. *American Journal of Public Health, 93*(2), 232–238.

Norman, D. (2003). The effects of stress on wound healing and leg ulceration. *British Journal of Nursing, 12*(21), 1256–1263.

Parikh, P. (2004). Occupational stress and coping in nurses. *Journal of Health Management, 6*(2), 115–127.

Parker, M. E. (2006). *Nursing theories and practice.* Sudbury, MA: Jones and Bartlett.

Pickering, T. G. (2001). Mental stress as a causal factor in the development of hypertension and cardiovascular disease. *Current Hypertension, 3,* 249–254.

Polit, D., & Beck, C.T. (2008). *Nursing research: Generating and assessing evidence for nursing practice* (8th ed.). Philadelphia: Lippincott Williams & Wilkins.

Porth, C. M. (2007). *Essentials of pathophysiology: Concepts of altered health states.* Philadelphia: Lippincott Williams & Wilkins.

Pugliese, P. (1995). The skin, free radicals, and oxidative stress. *Dermatology Nursing, 7,* 316–369.

Reuters Health. (2004). Retrieved January 20, 2004, from http://www.reutershealth.com/wellconnected/doc31.html

Rivas, P. (2003). *Turn off the hunger switch naturally.* Ferndale, WA: Appleton Publishing.

Rogers, M. (1970). *The theoretical basis of nursing.* Philadelphia: F. A. Davis Co.

Roy, C. (1990). Response: conceptual clarification. *Nursing Science Quarterly, 3,* 64–66.

Roy, C., & Andrews, H. A. (2005). *The Roy adaptation model* (3rd ed.). Upper Saddle River, NJ: Pearson Prentice Hall.

Schwaertz, A. R., Gerin, W., Davidson, K. W., Pickering, T. G., Brosschot, J. F., Thayer, J. F., et al. (2003). Toward a causal model of cardiovascular responses to stress and the development of cardiovascular disease. *Psychosomatic Medicine, 65*(1), 22–35.

Seaward, B. L. (2006). *Managing stress: Principles and strategies for health and well-being* (4th ed.). Sudbury, MA: Jones and Bartlett.

Segerstrom, S. C., & Miller, G. E. (2004). Psychological stress and the human immune system: A meta-analytic study of 30 years of inquiry. *Psychological Bulletin, 104,* 601–630.

Selye, H. A. (1936). Syndrome produced by diverse nocuous agents. *Nature, 138,* 32.

Selye, H. (1976). *The stress of life* (rev. ed.). New York: McGraw-Hill.

Senior, K. (2001). Should stress carry a health warning? *Lancet, 357*(9250), 126.

SixWise.com. (2006). *Stress now proven to cause weight gain in women: Five key stress-reduction tips.* Retrieved January 4, 2007, from http://www.sixwise.com/newsletters/05/03/15/stress_now_proven_to_cause_weight_gain_i...

Sohmen, V. (2005). *Acculturative project stress.* Umed School of Business & Economics, Umed University, Sweden. Retrieved December 28, 2006, from http://www.fek.umu.se/~VS

Spencer, R. L., & Hutchinson, K. E. (1999). Alcohol, aging, and the stress response. *Alcohol Research & Health, 23*(4), 272–283.

Taylor, S. E., Klein, L. C., Lewis, B. P., Gruenewald, T. L., Gurung, R. A. R., & Updegraff, J. A. (2000). Biobehavioral responses to stress in females: Tend-and-befriend, not fight-or-flight. *Psychological Review, 107,* 411–429.

Thomas, K. S., Nelesen, R. A., Ziegler, M. G., Bardwell, W. A., & Dimsdale, J. E. (2004). Job strain, ethnicity, and sympathetic nervous system activity. *Hypertension, 44*(6), 891–896.

Tomey, A. M., & Alligoud, M. R. (2005). *Nurse theorists and their work* (6th ed.). Philadelphia: Mosby.

Truelsen, T., Nielsen, N., Boysen, G., & Gronbaeck, M. (2003). Self-reported stress and risk of stroke. *Stroke, 34,* 856–866.

Van Egeren, L. V. (2000). Stress and coping and behavioral organization. *Psychosomatic Medicine, 62,* 451–460.

Wan, R., Camandolal, S., & Mattson, M. P. (2003). Intermittent food deprivation improves cardiovascular and neuroendocrine responses to stress in rats. *The Journal of Nutrition, 133,* 1921–1930.

Wein, H. (2000). *Stress and disease: New perspectives. The NIH Word on Health.* Retrieved March 9, 2006, from http://www.nih.gov/news/WordonHealth/soryol.htm

Wilkin, T. (2005). A definition of disease. *Future Positive.* Retrieved January 4, 2007, from http://futurepositive.synearth.net/eoo5/12/05?print-friendly=true

Wong, P. T. P. , & Wong, L. C. J. (Eds.). (2006). *Cross cultural psychology.* New York: Springer Publishing.

Psychosocial Issues in Nursing

Leslie Rittenmeyer

Outcome-Based Learning Objectives

After studying this chapter, the learner will be able to:

1. Discuss conceptual foundations that inform psychosocial nursing.
2. Define the characteristics of a therapeutic nurse–patient relationship.
3. Utilize culturally competent principles of therapeutic communication for the care of patients and significant others.
4. Apply the principles of teaching and learning to the care of patients and significant others.
5. Identify the dimensions of crisis and the nursing actions that promote adaptive coping.
6. Discuss the impact of illness and hospitalization on patients and significant others.
7. Compare and contrast the psychodynamics of anxiety, frustration, anger, depression, and loss and grief.
8. Utilize the nursing process for patients experiencing loss and grief, anxiety, depression, and anger.

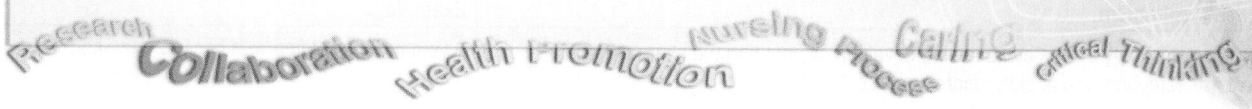

Research   Collaboration   Health Promotion   Nursing Process   Caring   Critical Thinking

NURSING IS about caring for persons throughout their life span. Nurses are privileged to share some of the most intimate moments in people's lives. They are present for joyful events, like the birth of a child or the successful outcome of a health care crisis, and heartrending events, like the death of a loved one or being presented with a grave prognosis. When nurses care for the whole person, they learn about the rich fabric of their patient's life.

During a person's life span, experiencing periods of both health and illness is inevitable. These experiences influence how people perceive themselves in relation to their own health belief model as well as the health care delivery system. Nurses play a pivotal role in shaping these experiences, and it is often through their influence that patients are able to give meaning to their experiences. In the process patients are empowered to assume more autonomy for their health care decisions. To achieve a positive health care outcome, nurses need to monitor and respond to the holistic needs of patients and their families. This means acknowledging patients as biopsychosocial spiritual beings who are more than the sum of their parts. Developing a knowledge base in the principles of psychosocial nursing helps the nurse apply the nursing process to psychosocial concerns in a holistic way.

◼ Theoretical Foundations

An array of theoretical perspectives informs the practice of psychosocial nursing. Theories provide a scientific basis for practice

and further aid in conceptualizing practice situations. Theories also offer a road map for predicting what may happen in a particular practice situation and often provide guidance about what has been effective in the past. A wide variety of theories are applicable to psychosocial nursing. Some of these theories have been borrowed from other disciplines; others are shared theories and have been modified for nursing practice; and yet others are theories specific to the discipline of nursing. This chapter introduces the reader to some of the theories that are most relevant to the practice of psychosocial nursing.

Psychoanalytical Perspective

The psychoanalytical perspective is attributed to the work of Sigmund Freud (1935). The work of Freud was revolutionary for the time, and he was one of the first scientists to suggest a mind–body interaction. He was also one of the first to suggest the importance of the unconscious in mental functioning. He divided aspects of the conscious into three categories. The first category he called the **conscious**, which includes all things that are easily remembered, such as one's mother's name, one's address, or one's favorite food. The second category was termed the **subconscious** and includes those things that have been forgotten but can easily be brought to consciousness, such as an old address, the feelings a man had on his wedding day, or the feeling of wonder at the birth of a first child. The third category was termed **unconscious** and encompasses all of those things that cannot be remembered or brought to conscious thought.

Freud also conceptualized three components of personality. He called these the id, ego, and superego. The **id** represents all of a person's biological and psychological drives. Drives are inborn psychological tensions that call for mental action in order to obtain instant gratification of needs. The id is primitive and instinctual and is often associated with sexual and aggressive impulses. The id does not consider reality or morality as it attempts to reduce psychic tension. The principle of tension reduction is called the **pleasure principle.**

The purpose of the **ego** is to mediate the urges of the id with a dose of reality. It helps individuals make a connection between the realities of the real world and the demands of the id in a way that promotes well-being and survival. An additional function of the ego is to protect the mind against conflict-laden impulses coming from the id. The ego obeys a reality principle.

The ego does not concern itself with morality or social norms. This role is reserved for the **superego.** The superego is really an extension of the ego and represents individuals' early moral training and ideal values imparted by societal norms. The emphasis of superego functioning is not reality but the ideal. To put it simply, the superego tells a person what is right and what is wrong and acts as a control system to help the ego assist the id in choosing objects of gratification that are not immoral.

The concept of anxiety is a thread that runs through the psychoanalytical perspective. Anxiety is conceptualized by Freud as a feeling of discomfort and tension that alerts the ego to a perceived threat or loss of inner control. Once warned, the ego can then undertake a wide variety of rationale defenses to decrease the feelings of discomfort and tension. If, however, the anxiety is overwhelming and the ego is unable to cope, the ego resorts to less rationale coping mechanisms. These processes are called the **ego defense mechanism** and are utilized to alleviate anxiety by denying, distorting, and misinterpreting reality. Although the ego defense mechanisms are helpful for a time, their overuse does not constitute healthy coping. For the most part the ego defense mechanisms operate at an unconscious level. Chart 13–1 provides an explanation of the ego defense mechanisms.

Developmental Perspective

Erik Erikson (1963) is best known for his theory on how humans develop across the life span. He embraced some of Freud's conceptualizations but expanded them to include the influence of culture and society on human development. He felt that the determinants of personality development were not

---

CHART 13–1 **Ego Defense Mechanisms**

Defense Mechanism	Example
Identification: Helps people avoid feeling devalued by adopting the characteristics or behavior of someone who is either feared or respected.	A young girl identifies with her teacher whom she admires.
Introjection: Helps people gain social acceptance by accepting the norms and values of others even if contrary to own beliefs.	A teen who uses drugs tells her brother that it is wrong to use drugs.
Projection: Allows people to avoid acknowledging their own shortcomings by blaming others or the environment for their own unacceptable motives.	A employee who does not do his job blames the incompetence of his boss.
Displacement: Allows people to discharge their emotions on a safer object or person by substituting a less threatening target or person for the recipient of their emotions.	A teenager has a very bad day at school and comes home and fights with her sister.
Rationalization: Allows people to cope with their inability to meet certain goals or standards by justifying behavior that is unacceptable as a socially acceptable rationale.	A man who verbally abuses his wife says "At least I don't hit her."
Denial: Allows people to avoid the full impact of a threatening situation by ignoring or screening the realities of the situation.	A patient who has been told she has a terminal illness is heard making plans for an extended trip abroad.
Repression: Helps people avoid trauma until they have the resources to do so by keeping a threatening thought out of awareness. The repressed material is denied entry into consciousness.	A person who was present at a terrorist attack cannot remember any of the details.
Regression: Helps people to return to a more comfortable time by allowing them to return to a level of functioning that is less demanding.	A very ill patient allows his nurse to nurture and care for him.
Reaction formation: A mechanism that allows people to act the opposite to the way they really feel.	A person who privately likes pornography becomes an advocate of censorship.
Intellectualization: Allows people to protect themselves from hurt by using a rational explanation to remove the personal significance of an incident.	A man's ill father dies and the son says "He wouldn't have wanted to live like that."
Undoing: Allows people to relieve guilty feelings or make amends by acting to annul some act or thought.	A teacher who makes a test too hard curves it so almost everyone passes.
Compensation: Allows people to overcome deficits by emphasizing a more desirable trait or by overachieving in a more comfortable area.	A nonathletic person becomes a sports announcer.
Sublimation: Allows people to avoid acting in socially unacceptable ways by substituting acceptable behavior.	A person with uninhibited sexual drives becomes morally religious.
Substitution: Allows people to keep frustrations to a minimum by replacing a highly valued or nonattainable object with an acceptable or attainable object.	A person wants to write for the *New York Times* but settles for working for her hometown newspaper.

just instinctual and biological as Freud theorized, but social and cultural as well.

Erikson conceptualized eight developmental stages, starting at birth and ending at death. Each of these stages is characterized by a developmental task that must be achieved in order for the person to develop in a healthy manner. Erikson did believe that if a task was not met at an earlier developmental stage, a person could later go backwards and meet the task of that stage successfully. Chart 13–2 provides an explanation of Erikson's developmental stages and tasks and their defining characteristics.

Another developmental theorist who has gained attention is Urie Bronfenbrenner (1979). In his work Bronfenbrenner emphasizes the social contexts in which children develop. A major thesis of his work is that "human abilities and their realization depend in significant degree on the larger social and institutional context of individual activity" (p. 23). His theory of ecological development calls attention to the importance of considering the influences of multiple settings on development. Chart 13–3 (p. 254) provides a summary of Bronfenbrenner's ecological theory.

CHART 13–2 Erikson's Stages of Growth and Development

Stage	Developmental Period	Explanation
Trust vs. mistrust	Infancy (first year)	Occurs in the first year of life. The development of trust requires consistent, nurturant caregiving. A positive outcome is the development of feelings of comfort and security attained from having needs met. A sense of mistrust develops when a child is treated negatively and/or is neglected and cannot consistently get her needs met.
Autonomy vs. shame and doubt	Infancy (second year)	Occurs in late infancy and early toddler years. After gaining trust in their caregivers, infants begin to realize that their behavior is their own. It is natural for them to assert their independence and realize that they have a mind of their own. This is how they gain a sense of their own autonomy. If infants are restrained too much (overprotected) or punished too harshly, a sense of shame and doubt occurs.
Initiative vs. guilt	Early childhood (preschool years, ages 3–5)	As young children experience a widening social circle, they are challenged more than they were as infants. To cope with these changes, they need to engage in active, purposeful behavior. In this stage adults expect children to become more responsible and require them to assume more responsibility for taking care of their bodies and belongings. Developing a sense of responsibility increases the child's sense of initiative. Children develop an uncomfortable guilt feeling if they are irresponsible or made to feel too anxious.
Industry vs. inferiority	Middle and late childhood (elementary school years, age 6 to puberty)	The development of initiative in the previous stage brings children into contact with a wealth of new experiences. As they move into the elementary school years, they direct their energy toward mastering knowledge and intellectual skills. At no time are children more enthusiastic about learning than at the end of their childhood, when this imagination is expansive. The danger of this developmental stage is developing a sense of inferiority, unproductiveness, and incompetence.
Identity vs. identity confusion	Adolescence (ages 10–20)	Adolescents try to figure out who they are, what they are about, and where they are going in life. They are confronted with many new roles, some of them adult roles (such as vocational and romantic). Adolescents need to be allowed to explore different paths to attain a healthy identity. It is a time for them to practice the skills they need to become adults. If adolescents do not adequately explore different roles and are not allowed to practice for their adult roles, they develop confusion about their own independence and identity.
Intimacy vs. isolation	Early adulthood (20s and 30s)	The developmental task is to form positive close relationships with others. Erikson describes intimacy as finding one's self but losing one's self in another person. The hazard of this stage is that one will fail to form an intimate relationship with either a romantic partner or through friendship and thus become socially isolated. For such individuals loneliness becomes a looming problem.
Generativity vs. stagnation	Middle adulthood (40s and 50s; later for some)	Generativity means transmitting something positive to the next generation. This can be done through roles of parenting, teaching, or through social activism. Generativity is about leaving a legacy to the next generation. Stagnation is the feeling of having done nothing to help the next generation or failure to leave a legacy.
Integrity vs. despair	Late adulthood	Older adults review their lives, reflecting on what they have done and accomplished. If the retrospective evaluations are positive, a sense of integrity is felt. That is, they can say to themselves "My life was worth living." In contrast, older adults become despairing if, when they look backward, their evaluations are predominantly negative.

Source: Ball, J. W., & Bindler, R. C. (2006) *Child health nursing: Partnering with children & families.* Upper Saddle River, NJ: Pearson Prentice Hall.

MyNursingKit | Erikson Institute

CHART 13–3	**Bronfenbrenner's Ecological Theory**
System	**Description**
Microsystem	A setting in which the individual spends a lot of time. Most immediate influence on the person. Focus is on face-to-face interactions. Developmental influences include family, peers, school and neighborhood, and religious institutions. Within these microsystems the individual has interaction with parents, teachers, peers, and others. The individual is not a passive recipient of experiences in these settings, but someone who reciprocally interacts with others and helps to construct the setting.
Mesosystem	Links microsystems together. Examples are the connections between family experiences and school experiences, for example, parent–teacher conferences. Experience in one microsystem can affect experiences in another microsystem. For example, an abused child may have difficulty being successful in school.
Exosystem	Setting in which a person does not actually participate but nonetheless exerts an influence. For example, a major layoff by a city's largest employer can affect families. The raising of property taxes by a city council can affects city schools, which in turn affects the individual.
Macrosystem	International and global influences, including the attitudes and ideologies of the culture. Involves the broader culture in which the individual lives, including the society's values and customs. Culture is a broad concept and affects the development of individuals in different ways. For instance, gender roles in one culture are transmitted differently in another culture. Culture includes the roles of ethnicity and socioeconomic factors in development.
Chronosystem	The sociohistorical conditions of an individual's development. For example, children today are living a childhood of firsts: the first day care generation, the first technological generation, the first post–sexual revolution generation. All of these sociohistorical contexts affect the development of individuals.

Source: Paquette, D., & Ryan, J. (2008). Brofenbrenner's ecological theory. National-Louis University. Accessed 5/24/2008 at http://pt3.no.edu/paquetteryanwebquest.pdf

Humanistic Perspective

The work of Abraham Maslow represents what is known as the "third force" in the field of psychology. He wished to provide an alternative to the somewhat mechanistic view of the psychoanalytical and behaviorist perspectives. The humanistic perspective believes that behavior is shaped by people's own perceptions of themselves, their subjective views of the world, and the need of all human beings to experience growth.

Maslow theorized a hierarchy of human needs in which some needs are perceived as more prevailing than other needs. The physiologic needs, such as air, water, and food, are placed on the

bottom rung of the hierarchy. The next rung is the need of individuals to feel safe and secure, followed by the need for love and belonging. Further toward the top of the hierarchy is the need for self-esteem. Needs on the first four rungs of the hierarchy are labeled **basic human needs**. Maslow labeled these lower rung needs as *deficit needs*. The next group on the hierarchy is the group of **growth needs**. Maslow identified these as the need to know and understand, aesthetic needs, and self-actualization and transcendence needs. He believed that the higher needs are met only after the lower needs have been satisfied. For example, if a person is without food, it is unlikely that the person will be concerned about her aesthetic needs. Figure 13–1 ■ illustrates Maslow's hierarchy of basic human needs.

Cognitive Development

Jean Piaget (1969) was interested in the cognitive development of children. He theorized that children develop cognitively through their exposure to the world around them. The basic mental structure of Piaget's theory is called a **schema**. Schemas are coordinated patterns of recurring action and are created for the purpose of organizing and interpreting information. As such, children's ability to think matures through two processes, assimilation and accommodation. **Assimilation** occurs when a child incorporates new knowledge into an already existing schema. **Accommodation** occurs when a child must modify an existing schema because the incorporation of new knowledge does not fit into his existing schema (Ball & Bindler, 2006). For example, a child is given a broom to sweep the floor. He has never really swept a floor before, but has watched his father do it and knows that to sweep one has to move the broom back and forth over the floor. He assimilates his behavior into what schemas he already has. But the broom is too big for him and he is holding it up close to the top, so he adjusts his hands lower on the broom handle in order to get a better sweeping action, therefore accommodating adjustments to his existing schema.

Piaget further theorized that children move through stages of cognitive development. The speed at which a child develops cognitively is variable and often depends on a multitude of factors such as genetics and the environment. This information is important to the nurse when considering developmentally appropriate teaching–learning strategies. Chart 13–4 summarizes Piaget's stages of cognitive development.

Cognitive Theory

Cognitive theory has impacted the treatment of a broad range of emotional and mental health disorders. It is based on the premise that mental health symptoms are related to how individuals view themselves and the world around them. Cognitive theory posits that individuals develop a set of core beliefs as a result of interacting with the environment. These beliefs or schemas can be positive or negative. A positive example could be the belief that women are strong and powerful. A negative belief could be the belief that women are weak and helpless. Schemas influence how individuals interpret and evaluate experiences, and behaviors are often the result of these interpretations.

Another construct in cognitive theory is that of the cognitive triad. The cognitive triad is influenced by negative schemas that influence people to (1) see themselves as inadequate, (2) negatively misinterpret an experience, and (3) view the future in a

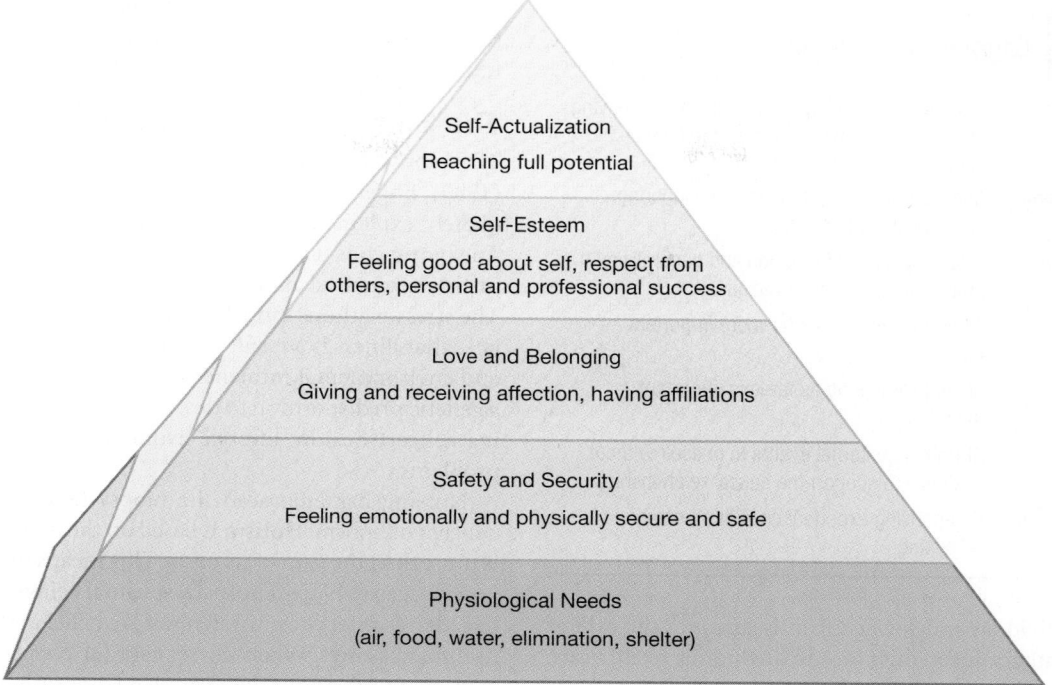

FIGURE 13–1 ■ Maslow's hierarchy of needs.

CHART 13–4	Piaget's Stages of Cognitive Development
Stage	**Typical Achievements and Behaviors**
Sensorimotor (birth–1½ or 2 years)	Thought is based on action. Infants suck, grasp, look, reach. A child learns about objects through sensory input. These responses become organized into complex activities such as eye–hand coordination and are applied to the environment to solve problems such as reaching for and manipulating objects.
Preoperational (1½–7 years)	Children begin to acquire language and mental imagery. They learn to do symbolic play. They may have difficulty understanding that another person sees, feels, or thinks differently from themselves (egocentrism). Thinking is unidimensionally focused on a single concept. They exhibit precausal (transductive) reasoning, having an incomplete understanding of cause and effect. One manifestation of precausal reasoning is magical thinking, that is, thinking that they can make things happen. Another manifestation is animism, the tendency to attribute human characteristics to inanimate objects. Ability to reason is inconsistent.
Concrete operational (7–11 years)	Children in this stage are capable of mental operations, which follow logical rules for transforming and manipulating information. They develop the ability to classify things. They are no longer fooled by appearances. They can reason effectively about classes of objects and their relationships.
Formal operational (11 years and older)	Adolescents are able not only to imagine but to reason about hypothetical situations. Abstract issues (for example, religion, morality, alternative life styles) can be considered and systematically evaluated. Adolescents are able to think about their own thinking (metacognition). There is a renewed egocentrism, a belief that one is unique and the center of others' attention.

Source: Ball, J. W., & Bindler, R. C. (2006) *Child health nursing: partnering with children & families.* Upper Saddle River, NJ: Pearson Prentice Hall.

negative way. Beck and Freeman (1990) suggest that being stuck in the cognitive triad leads to the development of cognitive distortions, which in return may result in the development of mental health symptoms. See Chart 13–5 (p. 256) for examples of cognitive distortions.

Assessing the cognitive distortions of patients and identifying how their cognitive triads influence the ways in which they are evaluating their health care situation can help the nurse design more effective interventions. One way to challenge cognitive distortions is to provide education that assists patients and

families in examining all available evidence about a situation so that they are informed about options and alternatives. This helps them develop problem-solving strategies that focus away from the most negative extremes of the situation.

Family Systems

In the practice of nursing, it is inevitable that the care of patients will call for inclusion of the family. In today's culture, "family" includes all of those significant others in a person's life such as life partners, friends, or roommates. The family is the mediator

CHART 13–5 **Cognitive Distortions**

Arbitrary inference	Coming to a specific conclusion without having any supporting evidence or in the face of contradictory evidence.
Selective abstraction	Conceptualizing a situation while ignoring contradictory information.
Overgeneralization	Taking specific information and generalizing it broadly to unrelated situations.
Magnification	Seeing something as far more important than it is.
Minimization	Seeing something as far less important than it is.
Personalization	Attributing external events to oneself without evidence to support the causal relationship.
Dichotomous thinking	Categorizing experiences with all-or-none reasoning.

between the individual and society. Family assumes the role of helping its members meet their needs, including health care needs. The family often wishes to be involved in all aspects of health care delivery to its individual members. It is important that nurses acknowledge the importance of patients' families in achieving desirable health care outcomes.

Hospital policies often apply traditional definitions of family to include only those individuals who are related by marriage, blood, or adoption. Although this definition applies to many families, it also serves to exclude those families that have chosen variant family forms. Friedman (1998) provided a broader definition of family that is more inclusive. She defined family as "two or more persons who are joined together by bonds of sharing and emotional closeness and who identify themselves as being part of the family" (p. 9). A more contemporary belief is that family is anyone who the patient says is a family member.

One theoretical approach that has influenced how to look at families is systems theory. Systems theory examines a unit and describes its relationship to a greater whole. Systems theory is concerned with how things interrelate and it creates an umbrella under which other theories may be applied. The major assumption of systems theory is that all matter forms a system that is capable of being studied. Families are considered to be open social systems because they interact with the environment around them. Families also have discrete boundaries that separate them from the environment. These boundaries are porous and serve to allow the family to control how much input the family receives from the environment. For example, if a family member has a major illness, the family may curtail some of its activities in order to better deal with the health care crisis. Families must continually adapt in order to maintain equilibrium. When families are faced with stress, they must mobilize their adaptive resources in order to maintain a steady state. Stress places more strain on the family unit and creates a situation in which they may need help from outside resources in order to maintain equilibrium. Health care problems are stressful for families and the nurse is in a particularly good position in which to offer assistance to encourage healthy adaptations. Systems theory helps

nurses realize that patients and their families are connected to the outside world and what happens to one member has an effect on the whole.

The Biopsychosocial Model

The biopsychosocial model was formalized by George Engel (1980). Engel believed that mental disorders could not be adequately explained by reducing them to biological causations. The biopsychosocial model offered an alternative to the mechanistic, biomedical model and provided a holistic perspective. The stress diathesis model takes this concept further and postulates that illness is a result of both genetic and biological factors and environmental influences. For example, a person may have a genetic predisposition to develop heart disease, but by embracing a heart-healthy lifestyle avoids the development of heart problems.

Nursing has embraced the biopsychosocial model and the concept of holism. **Holism** is based on the premise that the whole is more than the sum of its parts. This means that patients are acknowledged as biopsychosocial spiritual beings that cannot be reduced to a variety of subsystems. It is a belief in the unitary nature of human beings. When nurses care for people holistically, they consider all aspects of their care. The biopsychosocial model and holism are compatible with systems theory. Individuals as open systems are in constant interaction with their environment; therefore, change in one area of their life affects the total system. There is recognition of health as more than the absence of disease and in providing care, nurses should consider not only the individual, but family and social support systems as well. All of this serves to promote the provision of patient-centered care.

The theories just discussed provide a framework within which psychosocial nursing care can be conceptualized. They provide a rationale for the way to frame nursing problems and apply the nursing process for effective patient-centered care. All nursing care takes place in the context of interpersonal relationships and effective communication. It is through the nurse–patient relationship, therapeutic communication, and patient education that persons are empowered to take an active role in their own health care decisions. The following sections provide an overview of the therapeutic nurse–patient relationship, therapeutic communication, and principles of patient education.

The Therapeutic Nurse–Patient Relationship

The word *relationship* suggests human interaction in which the persons involved affect each other in some way. There are differences between social relationships and professional relationships. Professional relationships are meant to be therapeutic. To enter into a professional relationship, specific skills and knowledge are required. The professional or therapeutic nurse–patient relationship sets the stage for application of the nursing process in which assessment, diagnosis, planning, goal setting, intervention, and evaluation are carried out. There is also an emphasis on problem solving and a mandatory duty to accountability, responsibility, and confidentiality. Integral to the nurse–patient relationship is the concept of empowerment. When people are empowered, they are more able to develop the resources needed to make informed decisions about their health care based on their own priorities.

Certain actions foster the nurse–patient relationship. Conveying respect for a person's uniqueness, being nonjudgmental, showing attentiveness, and being empathetic all create the building blocks of a therapeutic nurse–patient relationship. Patients need to feel safe, secure, and understood. Also pivotal is that the nurse is perceived as knowledgeable, trustworthy, sensitive, and unambiguous.

Hildegard Peplau (1952), a nurse theorist, conceptualized the nurse–patient relationship as moving through three phases: introductory (orientation), working, and termination. During each of the phases, particular goals are achieved and particular events take place. The phases, which are often overlapping, are discussed next.

Introductory (Orientation) Phase

The introductory phase begins when the therapeutic relationship is initiated. Introductions take place and the patient is given initial information pertinent to her circumstances. The nurse starts to develop a trusting relationship. It is during this phase that the nurse and the patient establish an agreement—and in some cases a contract—about the purposes and direction of the relationship. This agreement or contract is usually verbal in nature, and in some settings it will be informal and in others more formalized. It is also during this phase that mutual goal setting is initiated. It is important for the goals of the nurse and the goals of the patient to be in alignment.

Another important activity that takes place during this phase is initial assessment. Although assessment takes place throughout the therapeutic relationship, it is essential during the introductory phase because it leads to the initial identification of nursing diagnoses and leads to mutual goal setting. The activities of this stage are built on a foundation of beginning trust and rapport.

Working Phase

The second phase is called the working phase. It is during this phase that a **therapeutic alliance** is established. A therapeutic alliance is one in which the nurse and the patient consciously work together to reach mutually agreed-on goals. Application of the nursing process is continuous during this stage and it is sometimes necessary to seek additional assessment data, realign goals, try new interventions, and reevaluate outcomes. Because new information and unanticipated events sometimes occur, problem solving is also continuous during this phase. Most patient education takes place during the working phase. Trust and rapport continue to grow during this stage. Patients begin to reach clarity and learn to exploit all of the resources that are available to them. Some refer to this as the exploitation phase.

Termination

The third phase of the therapeutic nurse–patient relationship is termination. Depending on the nature, length, and intensity of the therapeutic relationship, the termination phase can be difficult for patients. For this reason termination is introduced during the initial phase and often discussed during the working phase. During this phase the nurse and patient review what occurred during the working phase and what goals have been met and what progress was made. It is important for the nurse to understand that patients often feel a sense of loss and insecurity during this phase. These feelings on the part of the patient might cause them to present some self-protective behaviors such as displays of hostility or regressing backward in their treatment. This is considered normal during this stage and needs to be worked through. Termination should begin during the introductory phase.

Self-Awareness in the Nurse–Patient Relationship

Hildegard Peplau expressed the importance of each nurse taking on the responsibility of expanding his or her own insight. She believed that the nurse's personality was an important factor in the development of an interpersonal relationship. According to Peplau, a basic task of nursing education should be the development of each nurse as a person who wants to nurse patients in a helpful way with the direction of this development being maturity (Vandemark, 2006).

Caring

The nurse–patient relationship also takes place in a context of caring. Watson (1985) feels that caring is one of the most fundamental attributes in nursing. She believes in general that caring serves to advance health in individual and families and allows for the development of human potential and health autonomy. She has identified 10 carative factors, as listed in Chart 13–6.

Interpersonal relationships between patients and nurses are strengthened when patients perceive the nurse as interpersonally competent. Foshbinder (1994), in a study that analyzed patient perceptions of nursing care, identified four themes that strengthened the perception on the part of patients that the nurse was interpersonally competent. The themes were identified as translating, getting to know you, establishing trust, and going the extra mile. The nursing behaviors that illuminated these themes were when nurses were forthcoming, gave needed information, provided patient teaching, were friendly and interested, took

CHART 13–6	Watson's Carative Factors

1. Forming a humanistic-altruistic value system
2. Instilling faith and hope
3. Cultivating sensitivity to oneself and to others
4. Developing a helping, trusting relationship
5. Promoting expression of positive and negative feelings
6. Systematically using the scientific problem-solving method for decision making
7. Promoting interpersonal teaching–learning
8. Providing support of a protective or corrective mental, physical, sociocultural, and spiritual environment
9. Assisting with gratification of human needs
10. Allowing for existential phenomenological forces

Source: Watson, J. (1999). *Nursing: Human science and human care.* Boston: Jones and Bartlett.

charge, appeared to enjoy their work, and provided care beyond expectations. In a study focusing on emotional support provided by nurses to patients with breast cancer, Paisson and Norberg (1995) found that supportive emotional support improved the women's sense of control and, therefore, their sense of well-being.

As nurses enter into therapeutic relationships, they do so with persons of diverse beliefs and values. These beliefs and values are born from cultural and subcultural socialization. Paying attention to cultural influences that may affect the nurse–patient relationship is very important. Providing culturally sensitive care requires a responsible relationship between health care providers and patients, their families, and communities that is based on trust and respect. Nurses are expected to be culturally sensitive and competent. Cultural competence is defined by Camphina-Bacote (1999) as the continual striving by the nurse to provide culturally appropriate care to patients and families. Camphina-Bacote and Munoz (2001) identify five components in their cultural competence model: (1) cultural awareness, (2) adequate cultural knowledge, (3) skill to carry out a cultural assessment, (4) experience with cultural encounters, and (5) the desire to be culturally competent. In a study that looked at culturally diverse nurse–patient interactions, Cioffi (2006) found that relationships between nurses and culturally diverse patients are often tense.

Recommendations from the study suggested better education of nurses and more research in order to develop better models of culturally diverse interaction.

The Office of Minority Health (2001) has developed the *National Standards on Culturally and Linguistically Appropriate Services in Health Care*. These are referred to as the CLAS standards and they are listed in the National Guidelines box. These standards have been cross-referenced to the Joint Commission standards for accreditation of hospitals.

■ Therapeutic Communication

Having the ability to communicate skillfully is essential to good nursing care. Communication involves both a sender and receiver. It entails a two-way interaction in which a message is sent by the sender, heard and interpreted by the receiver, and a response given. Effective communication calls for active listening skills and allows for feedback and clarification.

Communication also involves nonverbal messages. Nonverbal messages can be delivered through voice tone, rate and volume of speech, the use of silence, the use of touch, and body language. For instance, patients may verbally relate that they feel fine, but they may appear to be very sad. If a verbal and the non-

---

NATIONAL GUIDELINES The CLAS Standards

Standard 1: Health care organizations should ensure that patients/consumers receive from all staff members effective, understandable, and respectful care that is provided in a manner compatible with their cultural health beliefs and practices and preferred language.

Standard 2: Health care organizations should implement strategies to recruit, retain, and promote at all levels of the organization a diverse staff and leadership that are representative of the demographic characteristics of the service area.

Standard 3: Health care organizations should ensure that staff at all levels and across all disciplines receive ongoing education and training in culturally and linguistically appropriate service delivery.

Standard 4: Health care organizations must offer and provide language assistance services, including bilingual staff and interpreter services, at no cost to each patient/consumer with limited English proficiency at all points of contact, in a timely manner during all hours of operation.

Standard 5: Health care organizations must provide to patients/consumers in their preferred language both verbal offers and written notices informing them of their right to receive language assistance services.

Standard 6: Health care organizations must assure the competence of language assistance provided to limited English proficient patients/consumers by interpreters and bilingual staff. Family and friends should not be used to provide interpretation services (except on request by the patient/consumer).

Standard 7: Health care organizations must make available easily understood patient-related materials and post signage in the languages of the commonly encountered groups represented in the service area.

Standard 8: Health care organizations should develop, implement, and promote a written strategic plan that outlines clear goals, policies,

operational plans, and management accountability/oversight mechanisms to provide culturally and linguistically appropriate services.

Standard 9: Health care organizations should conduct initial and ongoing organizational self-assessments of CLAS-related activities and are encouraged to integrate cultural and linguistic competence-related measures into their internal audits, performance improvement programs, patient satisfaction assessments, and outcomes-based evaluations.

Standard 10: Health care organizations should ensure that data on the individual patient's/consumer's race, ethnicity, and spoken and written language are collected in health records, integrated into the organization's management information systems, and periodically updated.

Standard 11: Health care organizations should maintain a current demographic, cultural, and epidemiological profile of the community as well as a needs assessment to accurately plan for and implement services that respond to the cultural and linguistic characteristics of the service area.

Standard 12: Health care organizations should develop participatory, collaborative partnerships with communities and utilize a variety of formal and informal mechanisms to facilitate community and patient/consumer involvement in designing and implementing CLAS-related activities.

Standard 13: Health care organizations should ensure that conflict and grievance resolution processes are culturally and linguistically sensitive and capable of identifying, preventing, and resolving cross-cultural conflicts or complaints by patients/consumers.

Standard 14: Health care organizations are encouraged to regularly make available to the public information about their progress and successful innovations in implementing the CLAS standards and to provide public notice in their communities about the availability of this information.

Source: Office of Minority Health. (2001). *National standards for culturally and linguistically appropriate services in health care. Final report.* Rockville, MD: Author.

verbal message do not match in emotional tone, then the message is said to be incongruent. Incongruent messages are confusing for the receiver and leave interpretation to the imagination.

Therapeutic communication is purposeful communication and is designed to convey openness and caring. Skillful use of therapeutic communication requires the nurse to have an awareness of the feeling environment of the patient. It consists of those words and actions that enhance the nurse–patient relationship and empower patients to make informed choices about their health care. At times, without realizing it, nurses communicate in such ways that create barriers to effective communication. Developing an understanding of therapeutic and nontherapeutic communication techniques helps the nurse avoid communication pitfalls. Chart 13–7 (p. 260) provides a summary of therapeutic and nontherapeutic communication techniques.

Culture also plays a role in therapeutic communication, as discussed in the Cultural Considerations box.

The Teaching–Learning Process

Nurses fulfill many roles as members of the health care delivery team. The nurse as teacher or patient educator is one of those roles. It is often nurses who assume the primary responsibility for patient education. The reality of shorter hospital stays and the fact that many medical problems are treated in outpatient settings create circumstances in which it is essential that patients and families be provided with the necessary patient education. In a meta-analysis study that sampled 116 intervention studies that measured the effects of psychoeducational care provided to adults with cancer, Devine and Westlake (1995) found that psychoeducational care benefited adults with cancer with regard to reducing anxiety, depression, nausea, vomiting, pain, and perceived knowledge.

CULTURAL CONSIDERATIONS for Therapeutic Communications

Munoz and Luckmann (2005) provide a rationale for the growing need for transcultural communication. They cite the increasing ethnic, racial, and cultural diversity of the United States; the increase in the number of patients who represent different culturally influenced patterns of health behavior; the different cultural meanings of health care; the different ways in which patients and families respond to health care; the multicultural nature of health care settings; and the nursing profession's commitment to culturally competent humanistic care. They further contend that talking to strangers about deeply personal issues is often difficult and may be particularly so for patients who are from different cultural backgrounds. They identify several behaviors on the part of nurses that are necessary to encourage patents to talk about themselves. Nurses must convey empathy, show respect, build trust, establish rapport, listen actively, provide appropriate feedback, and demonstrate genuine interest (p. 148). They also identify barriers to effective transcultural communication as follows: nurses' lack of knowledge, bias, ethnocentrism, prejudice, and stereotyping. Further, language differences, differences in the understanding of terminology, and differences in perceptions and expectations also create barriers (p. 162).

Teaching is defined as any deliberate act that involves the planning, implementation, and evaluation of instructional strategies that meet expected learner outcomes. It is a planned method or series of methods used to help someone learn. Learning has occurred when there is a change in behavior (cognitive, affective, or psychomotor) as a result of being exposed to environmental stimuli. It is an internal experience that represents an integration of thoughts, ideas, theory, and experience. Learning is divided into three domains; cognitive, affective, and psychomotor. Cognitive learning involves the storing and recalling of new knowledge and information in the brain. **Affective learning** involves changes in attitudes, values, and feelings. **Psychomotor learning** involves learning that occurs when a physical skill has been acquired.

The teaching–learning process is facilitated by the existence of a therapeutic nurse–patient relationship. The nurse as teacher needs to be able to communicate effectively with individuals, families, and groups. The teaching–learning process can be conceptualized into four steps: assessment of learning needs, developing a teaching plan, implementation of a teaching plan, and evaluation of the teaching plan.

Assessment of Learning Needs

When nurses assess the learning needs of an individual, group, or family, they should use all appropriate information available to them. Patients and families can provide the most accurate information. Unfortunately, there are times when for one reason or another a patient or family member is not a good historian. In such cases, it is necessary to get information from additional sources such as other family members or old medical records. During the assessment process, it is important for the nurse to identify the particular knowledge, skills, and attitudes that are needed by the patient or family. Once this is accomplished the nurse must then assess the emotional and experiential readiness of the patient or family to learn. The following factors should be considered when assessing emotional and experiential readiness to learn:

- The level of emotional health
- Motivation to learn
- Self-concept and body image
- Social and economic stability
- Past experiences with learning
- Attitude toward learning.

Assessing the patient's ability to learn is necessary so an appropriate teaching plan can be designed. The following factors need to be considered:

- Physical condition of the patient and acuity of the illness
- Acuity of the patient's senses
- Developmental considerations
- Level of education
- Literacy
- Communication skills
- Primary language
- Pain level
- Prognosis.

CHART 13–7	**Therapeutic and Nontherapeutic Communication Techniques**	

Techniques	Rationale	Examples
Therapeutic Techniques		
Using silence	Gives the patient the opportunity to collect and organize thoughts, to think through a point, or to consider introducing a topic of greater concern than the one being discussed.	When discussing difficult subjects, such as sexual history, or possible abusive situations.
Accepting	Conveys an attitude of reception and regard.	"Yes, I understand what you said." Eye contact, nodding.
Giving recognition	Acknowledging; indicating awareness. Better than complimenting, which reflects the nurse's judgment.	"I see you attended therapy today" or "I see you made your bed."
Offering self	Making oneself available on an unconditional basis increases patient feelings of worth.	"I'll stay with you for awhile," "Let me sit with you awhile," or "I'll be here with you."
Giving a broad opening	Allows the patient to take the initiative in introducing the topic. Emphasizes the importance of the patient's role in the interaction.	"What would you like to talk about today?" or "Tell me what you are thinking."
Offering general leads	Offers the patient encouragement to continue.	"Go on," "Yes, I see," or "And after that?"
Placing the event in time or sequence	Clarifies the relationship of events in time so that the nurse and patient can view them in perspective.	"What seemed to lead up to this," "Was that before or after?" or "When did that happen?"
Making observations	Verbalizing what is observed or perceived. This encourages the patient to recognize specific behaviors and compare perceptions with the nurse.	"You seem tense," "I notice you are pacing a lot," or "You seem uncomfortable."
Encouraging description of perceptions	Asking the patient to verbalize what is being perceived. Often used when a patient is experiencing hallucinations.	"Tell me what is happening now," "Are you hearing the voices now?" or "What do the voices seem to be saying?"
Encouraging comparison	Asking the patient to compare similarities and differences in ideas, experiences, or interpersonal relationships. Helps the patient recognize life experiences that tend to recur as well as aspects of life that are changeable.	"Was this something like. . .," "How does this compare to the time when. . .," or "What was your response the last time this situation occurred?"
Restating	The main idea of what the patient has said is repeated. Lets the patient know whether or not an expressed statement has been understood and gives him or her the chance to continue or clarify.	Pt: "I can't study. My mind seems to wander." Nurse: "You have difficulty concentrating." Pt: "I can't take a new job. What if I fail?" Nurse: "You are afraid you will fail in this new position?"
Reflecting	Questions and feelings are referred back to the patient so they may be recognized and accepted, and so the patient may recognize that his or her point of view has value. A good technique to use when a patient asks the nurse for advice.	Pt: "What do you think I should do about. . .?" Nurse: "It sounds as if you are having difficulty deciding what to do." Pt: "My sister won't help a bit towards my mother's care. I have to do it all." Nurse: "You feel angry when she doesn't help."
Focusing	Taking notice of a single idea or even a single word. Works well with a patient who is moving rapidly from one thought to another. This technique is not therapeutic for someone who is very anxious. Focusing should not be pursued until the anxiety abates.	"This point seems worth looking at more closely. Perhaps you and I can discuss it together."
Exploring	Delving further into a subject, idea, experience, or relationship. Especially helpful with patients who tend to remain on a superficial level. However, if the patient chooses not to disclose further information, the nurse should refrain from pushing or probing in an area that obviously creates discomfort.	"Please help me understand that situation in more detail" or "Tell me more about that."
Seeking clarification and validation	Striving to explain that which is vague or incomprehensible and searching for mutual understanding. Clarifying the meaning of what has been said facilitates and increases understanding.	"Tell me if my understanding agrees with yours" or "Do I understand correctly that you said. . .?"

(continued)

CHART 13–7	Therapeutic and Nontherapeutic Communication Techniques—*Continued*	
Techniques	**Rationale**	**Examples**
Presenting reality	When a patient has a misperception of the environment, the nurse defines reality or indicates his or her perception of the situation for the patient.	"I understand that the voices seem real to you, but I do not hear any voices," or "I can only see you and me in the room right now."
Voicing doubt	Expressing uncertainty as to the reality of the patient's perceptions. Often used with patient's who are experiencing delusional thinking.	"I find that unusual" or "That seems rather doubtful to me."
Verbalizing the implied	Putting into words what the patient has only implied or said indirectly. Can also be used with the patient who is mute or is otherwise experiencing impaired verbal communication. Clarifies what is implicit rather than what is explicit.	*Pt:* "It's a waste of time to be here, I can't talk to you anymore." *Nurse:* "Are you feeling that no one understands?" *Pt:* (Refuses to speak.) *Nurse:* "I'm wondering if you are feeling angry right now."
Attempting to translate words into feelings	When feelings are expressed only indirectly, the nurse tries to "desymbolize" what has been said and find clues to the underlying meaning.	*Pt:* "I feel like I'm adrift in the ocean." *Nurse:* "You must be feeling lonely right now."
Formulating a plan of action	Helping the patient design a plan to deal with an uncomfortable stressful situation using effective coping strategies.	"What could you do to express your anger harmlessly?" or "Next time this comes up what might you do to handle it differently?"
Nontherapeutic Techniques		
Giving reassurance	Indicates to the patient that there is no cause for anxiety, thereby devaluing the patient's feelings. May discourage the patient from further expressions of feelings if he or she believes that they will only be downplayed.	"I wouldn't worry about that" or "Everything will be all right." Better to say: "We will work on that together."
Rejecting	Refusing to consider or showing contempt for the patient's ideas or behavior. This may cause the patient to discontinue interaction with the nurse for fear of further rejection.	"Let's not discuss. . ." or "Let's not talk about that now." Better to say: "Let's look at that a little closer."
Giving approval or disapproval	Sanctioning or denouncing the patient's ideas or behavior. Implies that the nurse has the right to pass judgment on whether the ideas or behaviors are good or bad, and the patient is expected to please the nurse. The nurse's acceptance of the patient is then seen as conditional depending on the patient's behavior.	"That's good, I'm glad that you. . ." or "That's bad. I'd rather you wouldn't." Better to say: "Let's talk about how your behavior at dinner invoked anger in the other patients."
Agreeing or disagreeing	Indicating accord with or opposition to the patient's ideas or opinions. Implies that the nurse has the right to pass judgment on whether the patient's ideas or opinions are "right" or "wrong." Agreement prevents the patient from later modifying his or her point of view without admitting error. Disagreement implies inaccuracy, provoking the need for defensiveness on the part of the patient.	"That's right, I agree," "I don't believe that," or "I wouldn't do it like that." Better to say: "Let's discuss what you feel is unfair about the new rules."
Giving advice	Telling the patient what to do and how to behave implies that the nurse knows what is best and the patient is incapable of self-direction. Nurtures the patient in the dependent role and discourages independent thinking.	"I think you should" or "I wouldn't do it like that." Better to say: "What do you think you should do."
Probing	Persistent questioning of the patient. Pushing for answers to issues the patient does not wish to discuss. Causes the patient to feel used and valued for only what he or she shares. Causes patient to feel defensive.	"Tell me about your abuse" or "How come you were drinking and driving?"
Defending	Attempting to protect someone or something from verbal attack. To defend what the patient has criticized is to imply that she or he has no right to express ideas, opinions, or feelings. Defending does not change the patient's feelings and may cause the patient to think the nurse is taking sides with those being criticized.	"No one here would lie to you" or "You have a very capable doctor, I'm sure he has your best interest at heart." Better to say: "I will try to answer your questions and clarify some issues regarding your treatment."

(continued)

CHART 13–7	Therapeutic and Nontherapeutic Communication Techniques—*Continued*	
Techniques	**Rationale**	**Examples**
Requesting an explanation	Asking the patient to provide explanations for thoughts, feelings, behavior, and events. Asking "why" a patient did something or feels a certain way can be very intimidating and implies that the patient must defend his or her behavior or feelings.	"Why do you think that?" "Why do you feel that way?" or "Why did you do that?" Better to say: "Describe what you were feeling just prior to this occurrence."
Belittling feelings	When the nurse misjudges the degree of the patient's discomfort, a lack of empathy and understanding may be conveyed. This causes the patient to feel insignificant or foolish. It is no relief to a patient to hear that others are or have been in similar situations.	*Pt:* "I'm so down today." *Nurse:* "Cheer up." *Pt:* "I'm always unhappy." *Nurse:* "Most people are unhappy sometimes." Better to say: "You sound upset. Tell me what you are feeling right now."
Making stereotyped comments	Clichés and trite expressions are meaningless in the nurse–patient relationship. For the nurse to make empty conversation is to encourage a like response from the patient.	"Hang in there," "Keep your chin up," or "It's good for you." Better to say: "Let's talk about your feelings."
Using denial	When the nurse is uncomfortable with a patient's problem and blocks discussion with the patient and avoids helping the patient identify and explore areas of difficulty.	*Pt:* "I've amounted to nothing in my life." *Nurse:* "Everyone has some accomplishments." Better to say: "Let's talk about how you have come to that conclusion."
Interpreting	The nurse attempts to tell the patient the meaning of her or his experience.	"What you really mean is. . ." or "Unconsciously you feel. . . ."
Changing the subject	Changing the subject causes the nurse to take over the discussion. The nurse may do this in order to meet his own agenda or to avoid talking about something he wishes to avoid.	*Pt:* "I think I'm going to die." *Nurse:* "Did you have visitors this weekend?"

Developing a Teaching Plan

The teaching–learning process is more effective when mutual goal setting takes place. Unless the patient values the learning objectives, it is unlikely that much learning will occur. It is also important for all learning goals to be realistic and appropriate for the patient and situation. The following are important steps when designing a teaching plan:

- Identify short- and long-term goals.
- Prioritize the goals.
- Determine who should be included in the teaching.
- Match content with appropriate teaching strategies and learner activities.
- Relate teaching content to the patient's interests, resources, and patterns of everyday living.
- Decide on group versus individual teaching and formal versus informal teaching.
- Design a plan that is realistic for time constraints.

Implementing a Teaching Plan

The implementation of the teaching plan should include varied teaching strategies delivered in an organized manner. The strategies should be appropriate for the type of learning that is desired. Chart 13–8 lists some teaching strategies that might be considered.

CHART 13–8	Suggested Teaching Strategies	
Cognitive Learning	**Affective Learning**	**Psychomotor Learning**
Lecture	Role modeling	Demonstration
Panel discussion	Panel discussion	Self-discovery
Printed materials	Printed materials	Printed materials
AV materials	AV materials	AV materials
Program instruction	Role playing	Practice
Computer instruction	Peer counseling	

Evaluating a Teaching Plan

The mutually set learning goals provide the basis for evaluating whether learning has occurred. This can be accomplished by:

- Direct questioning of the patient
- Observation of behavior
- Return demonstrations
- Paper-and-pencil tests
- Pretests and post-tests
- Patient questionnaires
- Self-evaluation
- Postdischarge follow-up

If the learning objectives have not been met, the learning content and teaching strategies may need to be altered. Further assessment may be needed, new goals agreed on, and the teaching repeated.

■ Psychodynamics of Illness and Hospitalization

Many complex factors can influence a patient's perception of a serious illness or hospitalization. Understanding these different factors and providing appropriate nursing care will improve a patient and family's outlook on health and illness and possibly improve patient outcomes.

Crisis

For many people a serious illness and hospitalization constitute a crisis. A **crisis** can develop when an event or series of events occurs that creates a situation that is perceived as threatening. These events can be personal such as illness or death of a loved one, or more global such as experiencing a terrorist attack. A crisis is said to be maturational when the stressors are related to developmental events. An example of this would be an adolescent who develops an identity crisis. A situational crisis occurs when the stress stems from an unexpected event, such as the development of an acute illness. An adventitious crisis is one that is the result of unexpected natural disasters such as tornadoes or plane crashes.

A crisis develops in response to a series of events. It is not the situation itself that leads to the development of a crisis state, but rather the individual's perception and response to the event. The development stages of a crisis are as follows:

- The individual or family is in a state of homeostasis.
- A stressful event or events occur.
- The event is perceived as a threat.
- Well-known coping skills are applied but fail to reduce the threat.
- A period of disequilibrium occurs with a decrease in problem-solving ability and an increase in feelings of anxiety and depression.
- The problem is either resolved or personal disintegration occurs.

A crisis is also self-limiting. Caplan (1964) found that in a typical crisis state, equilibrium is restored in approximately 4 to 6 weeks. Because of the extreme feelings of disorganization during an active crisis, individuals often need to turn to outside resources in order to return to a state of equilibrium. Nurses are often in contact with individuals and families when they are vulnerable to crisis or already in crisis and therefore become a valuable resource. Early intervention is essential to reduce the effects of the crisis. Providing information and resources sometimes serves to prevent a full-blown crisis from occurring. Intervention should meet the level of disorganization that is felt and should be done as quickly as possible.

Rapport needs to be established quickly. Initially, an assessment should be done to define the problem. Because crisis is about perception of the problem, it is essential that information be described from the patient's perspective. It is important to understand the meaning the event has for the patient. Further, allowing for free expression of feelings can be cathartic in itself. Once these things are accomplished, the nurse can then help the patient clarify the series of events that led to the crisis.

Once the problems have been defined, the nurse and the patient develop an initial plan of action. If the patient is very disoriented, the nurse may need to take a directive role while still allowing for as much input as possible. During this time the nurse can provide practical, concrete help to the patient. The nurse may have to do some things for the patient that under different circumstances the patient would do for himself. It is sometimes helpful to have the patient make a list of his needs and concerns from most important to least important. This can help the nurse plan interventions that will decrease the sense of disequilibrium, reduce feelings of anxiety and depression, and mobilize supportive resources. If there is a concern about self-harm, the patient should be protected and an immediate referral made.

Once the crisis has been stabilized, the nurse can help the patient problem solve and explore alternatives. It is here that new coping skills can be taught. Teaching new coping skills empowers patients to better handle future crisis events. It is for this reason that a crisis is often seen as an opportunity for growth. The nurse provides continual emotional support through this process because the change can be very anxiety producing.

Sick Role Behavior

Illness and hospitalization are often perceived as stressful and make patients more vulnerable to experiencing a crisis. When individuals become ill and must be hospitalized, they are expected to behave in certain ways and assume a sick role. A **sick role** is a set of expectations that people who are ill must meet and which society including caregivers expects of them. When a person enters the hospital, that person is immediately oriented to hospital rules, regulations, policies, and procedures. It is expected that patients and their families will adhere to these rules. The patient is expected to be cooperative, dependent, and non-demanding. Wilson (1963) explains this well:

> The patient comes unbidden to a large organization which awes and irritates him, even as it also nurtures and cares. As he strips off his clothing so he strips off, too, his favored costume of social roles, his favorite style, and his customary identity in the world. He becomes subject to a time schedule and a pattern of activity not of his own making. (p. 70)

Hospitals are bureaucratic entities and services are often fragmented. The hospital is frequently organized for the convenience of the staff and not the patient. Patients are repeatedly the victims of this fragmentation and frequently perceive that they are losing control. This feeling of losing one's autonomy is more disturbing to some patients than to others. The term **locus of control** refers to the perception people have about how much control they exert over the events that happen in their lives. People with an **internal locus of control** orientation believe that events in their lives are controlled by their own actions and decisions. People with an **external locus of control** orientation believe that events in their lives are controlled more by fate, luck, and external circumstances.

Even though health professionals are literally strangers, health care professionals continually ask patients to entrust themselves to their care. Nurses may ask patents to trust their competence, motives, and decision making. Because of a strong need to control their own autonomy, patients with an internal locus of control orientation will find this paternalism in health care bureaucracies frustrating. Patients with an external locus of control orientation will most likely not feel as uncomfortable and actually might need assistance in being more involved in their own health care decision making. Shattel (2004) found that issues such as power, social and cultural contexts, and interpersonal competence influence the nurse–patient relationship. Russell, Daly, Hughes, and op't Hoog (2003) concluded that to provide patient-centered care, power and authority need to be transferred away from health care professionals and to patients. The following are ways in which nurses can demonstrate interpersonal competence and therefore empower patients to be more involved in their health care decisions:

- Answer questions honestly and knowledgeably.
- Do mutual goal setting.
- Inform patients in advance of procedures.
- Prepare the patient for procedures.
- Let patients know what to expect.
- Listen patiently to expressions of concern.
- Do not treat patients as children.

It is important to encourage patients to share their experiences and perceptions with the nurse. Venke, Torjuul, Ross, and Kihigren (2006), in a study that attempted to illuminate the experience of being a "patient," found that patients, even when generally satisfied with their care, made compromises about the things they found as less than optimal. The patients considered this as a necessary part of their experience and did not share their perceptions, therefore making them more vulnerable. Clinical recommendations from the study suggested that nurses need to be aware of the content of their patient's vulnerabilities and act as patient advocates.

Loss and Grief

When patients and significant others are confronted with a serious illness, they often experience feelings of loss and grief. The amount of loss that is perceived by the patient and significant others is individual and should be assessed accordingly. The grieving process can be initiated by any loss. Although impending death represents a major loss, other types of losses can be extremely significant for patients and their significant others and therefore trigger the grieving process. Illness can cause loss of physiological functioning, loss of familiar roles, loss of relationships, loss of financial security, loss of self-esteem, loss of autonomy, and many more losses individual to each situation. How each patient and significant other adapts to their losses depends on their perception of the significance of the loss, their coping skills, their support systems, and the replaceability of the loss. Although each patient and significant others will cope with their losses in an individualized way, each will also go through a grief response process. Chart 13–9 presents the stages of grief response as identified by Kübler-Ross & Kessler (2005).

CHART 13–9	**Kübler-Ross's Stages of Grief and Mourning**
Denial	Individuals react with a shocked "No, not me." This is healthy and allows individuals and significant others time to gather coping resources.
Anger	Individuals say "Why me?" or "Why us?" During this stage people sometimes blame others, including God.
Bargaining	Individuals say "Yes me, but. . . ." or "If you just give me enough time to see my daughter married, I'll be ready."
Depression	Individuals say "Yes me." With this acknowledgment of the reality of the situation comes feelings of depression.
Acceptance	Facing the loss or death peacefully. In the case of death, individuals tend to withdraw into themselves.

Source: Kübler-Ross, E., & Kessler, D. (2005). *On grief and grieving: Finding the meaning of grief through the five stage of loss.* New York: Scribner.

◼ Nursing Management

Nurses are often in the best position to offer support to patients and significant others as they move through the grieving process. It is most important to provide a safe environment for grieving to be expressed. Nurses need to be sensitive to individual differences in expressing grief. Some differences in grieving rituals are culturally influenced. Some people grieve quietly, some loudly, some verbalize a great deal, some not at all, and some are very stoic. Others are very emotional. Nurses provide a quiet acceptance of all grieving practices.

In a systematic review of the effectiveness of palliative care teams in improving the health outcomes of cancer patients, Hearn and Higginson (1998) found that when compared to conventional care, palliative care teams were better able to meet the needs of cancer patients and their families, possibly reducing the overall cost of care.

Assessment

The nurse should answer the following questions when assessing a patient experiencing grief and loss:

- What is the perceived or observable loss as experienced by the individual and/or significant others?
- How does the individual and/or significant others explain or describe the loss?
- Is the individual or significant others able to identify their own feelings about the loss?
- Is the individual or significant others in denial about the loss?
- Is the individual or significant others expressing feelings of helplessness or hopelessness?
- Are there outward expressions of grief such as crying?
- Are there observable symptoms of depression?
- In what stage of the grieving process is the individual or significant others?

Nursing Diagnosis

Possible nursing diagnosis for patients experiencing grief and loss include:

- *Grieving*
- *Coping Ineffective*
- *Spiritual Distress*
- *Knowledge Deficit* related to feelings of loss and grief
- *Hopelessness.*

Planning

The plan of care should facilitate a healthy grieving process.

Outcomes and Evaluation Parameters

An outcome for the grieving patient is the ability to work through the grieving process. This is evaluated by the patient's ability to:

- Verbalize an awareness of the loss.
- Verbalize the significance of the loss.
- Verbalize an awareness of the grieving process.
- Accept support while moving through the grieving process.
- Move toward acceptance of the loss.

Interventions and Rationales

The following interventions and rationales would be appropriate for the patient experiencing loss and grief:

- Assess the individual's and/or significant others' stage in the grief and loss process. *Identifying any issues that may be unresolved facilitates the grieving process. The patient and family members are frequently at different phases of grieving and should be treated appropriately.*
- Provide nonjudgmental support. *Allowing patients to express feelings openly may allow them to move through the phases of grieving more easily. Nonjudgmental listening allows patients to express their feelings without the fear of rejection.*
- Provide a safe environment in which the individual and/or significant others can express all feelings. *When the nurse spends time with the patient and family it may assist with the necessary review and processing of the loss. Being with the patient can decrease feelings of loneliness and reassure them that caregivers perceive the loss as significant.*
- Educate the individual and/or significant others about the grieving process. *Understanding of the grief process allows the patient and significant others to move through the process more easily.*
- Help individuals and/or significant others to identify and reach out to additional support systems. *Assist the patient to identify resources. Referrals to appropriate support groups will help to meet emotional needs.*
- Help individuals and/or significant others problem solve. *Providing the patient and significant others with accurate information prevents misconceptions and may decrease their fears. Allowing patients to make decisions whenever possible enables them to maintain control.*

Evaluation

The patient will be able to move through the grief process in a healthy manner and exhibit effective coping mechanisms.

Depression

Experiencing feelings of depression is a predictable response to illness and hospitalization and often accompanies loss and grief. The DSM-IV-TR (American Psychiatric Association [APA], 2000) provides diagnostic criteria for all of the affective disorders, for example, Major Depressive Disorder, Bipolar Disorder, and Dysthymic Disorder. Specific exploration of these disorders is beyond the scope of this chapter. The focus for this discussion is on depression as a psychological response to the losses associated with illness and hospitalization.

Patients are more vulnerable to developing depressive symptoms when they are experiencing severe, prolonged stress or crisis. The depression can act as a protective mechanism when people exhaust their coping abilities. The ability to adapt to stressors is dependent on the effectiveness of the individuals' coping mechanisms and the amount of perceived stress. Even individuals with excellent coping skills can become overwhelmed when the amount of stressors transcends their ability to cope with them.

Depression is also prevalent with certain diseases. Hackett, Yapa, Parag and Anderson (2005) did a systematic review of the frequency of depression after stroke. Their conclusions were that depression is common among stroke patients and that this needs to be addressed in clinical practice. A study on depression and anxiety as predictors of health outcomes after myocardial infarction found that patients who are worried and unhappy in the hospital are at higher risk for negative psychological and quality-of-life outcomes (Mayou, Gill, and Thompson, 2000). In their conclusions they argue for in-hospital identification and treatment of depression and anxiety.

Sherbourne and colleagues (2000) studied the impact of psychiatric conditions on health-related quality-of-life issues in persons with HIV infection. The results of this study found that comorbid psychiatric conditions predispose patients to impaired functioning and loss of a sense of well-being. Barsevick, Dudley, and Beck (2006) researched cancer-related fatigue, depressive symptoms, and functional status. They found that when fatigue caused patients to have difficulty carrying out routine activities they tended to experience more depressive symptoms. They suggest that interventions should be aimed at reducing the likelihood of impaired functioning that could result in increased depressive symptoms.

■ Nursing Management

It is often nurses who provide the frontline care for individuals who are experiencing feelings of depression. Intervening with patients who are depressed can sometimes be difficult because dealing with others' pain can be depressing in itself. Because of this, at times there is the tendency to want to avoid depressed patients. It can be hard to find the time to properly intervene, and the fast pace of the hospital environment is counterproductive to the slowed pace of the depressed patient. Sometimes other people view depressed individuals as not doing enough to help themselves. They feel that if depressed people would just try harder, they could pull themselves out of their depressed mood. It is important to understand that depression is a clinical diagnosis and needs to be assessed and treated just like any other disease.

Assessment

Depression is an uncomfortable psychological and physical experience of sadness. To a degree ranging from mild to severe, individuals experience behavioral, physical, affective, and cognitive changes as follows:

Behavioral Changes

- Loss of interest in usually enjoyed activities
- Body posture slumped, dejected looking
- Difficulty making eye contact
- Difficulty carrying out activities of daily living
- Crying.

Physical Changes

- Weight loss or weight gain
- Appetite changes
- Loss of sexual desire
- Somatic symptoms
- Sleep disturbances
- Fatigue
- Lack of energy
- Change in bowel habits.

Affective Changes

- Feelings of emotional sadness
- Low self-esteem
- Labile mood
- Feelings of helplessness or hopelessness
- Pessimistic outlook
- Ambivalence.

Cognitive Changes

- Cognitive distortions
- Slowing of thought processes
- Inability to concentrate
- Indecisiveness
- Loss of memory
- Difficulty problem solving
- Feelings of guilt
- Possible suicidal ideation
- Difficulty looking into the future.

Nursing Diagnosis

Possible nursing diagnoses for a person with depression include:

- *Coping, Ineffective*
- *Impaired Verbal Communication*

- *Social Isolation*
- *Ineffective Health Maintenance*
- *Self-Care Deficits*
- *Sleep Deprivation*
- *Self-Esteem Disturbance*
- *Ineffective Role Performance*
- *Knowledge Deficit*
- *Spiritual Distress*
- *Risk for Self-Directed Violence.*

Planning

Nursing priorities for the patient with depression include establishing rapport and trust, indentifying threat and coping resources, providing interventions to optimize coping skills, and evaluating the effectiveness of interventions.

Outcomes and Evaluation Parameters

Outcomes for the patient with depression include identification of ineffective coping and the ability to participate in developing a plan of care. This will be exhibited by the patient's ability to:

- Identify significant losses.
- Verbalize the significance of losses.
- Verbalize factors that he or she can control.
- Participate in own health care decision making.
- Exhibit reduced symptoms of depression.
- Remain free from self-harm.

Interventions and Rationales

The following interventions and rationales would be appropriate for the patient experiencing depression:

- Validate the presence of the depression. *Acceptance by the nurse allows the patient to feel positive about the therapeutic relationship. This helps with healing, decreases isolation, and increases coping ability.*
- Provide emotional support through empathetic listening. *Empathetic listening helps to build trust and strengthens the therapeutic relationship.*
- Encourage the expression of feelings both positive and negative. *Patients may not fully understand what is happening to them. If they can express feelings freely, the nurse can plan specific actions to assist the patient to see the situation clearly.*
- Avoid excessive cheerfulness and false reassurance. *This will not help patients to work through their problems.*
- Encourage patient to be involved in his or her care. *The ability to control aspects of one's life helps to allay feelings of helplessness.*
- Assist the patient in goal setting and problem solving. *Patients may be overwhelmed by their situation. Assisting them to view the problem in its component parts will reduce anxiety and assist with effective coping behaviors.*
- Assess for suicidal ideation and if present ensure safety and make a referral. *Involve the healthcare team if you suspect that the patient is suicidal.*

- If necessary, refer for psychotherapy and pharmacological intervention. *It is important to ensure safety and prevent patients from harming themselves.*

Evaluation

The nurse should frequently reevaluate the patient's coping mechanism. The patient should be able to describe his or her emotional state, participate in developing a plan of care, and use support offered by caregivers.

Anxiety

Anxiety is a universal psychological response. Without some amount of anxiety, individuals would not be able to accomplish their goals or meet their challenges. When faced with illness and possible hospitalization, most people will experience increased feelings of anxiety. They often become worried about their diagnosis, prognosis, and ability to cope with their illness. Anxiety is a primary emotion from which other emotions such as anger stem. As with depression the DSM-IV-TR (APA, 2000) provides diagnostic criteria for an array of anxiety disorders, for example, Panic Disorder, Generalized Anxiety Disorder, and Posttraumatic Stress Disorder. An explanation of these specific anxiety disorders is beyond the scope of this chapter. The focus for this discussion is on anxiety as a predictable psychological response to the stress of illness and hospitalization.

Anxiety is an uncomfortable feeling of discomfort, dread, apprehension, and unease, the cause of which can be specific or nonspecific. Oftentimes individuals are unable to identify what is making them feel anxious. The symptoms of anxiety are physiological, psychological, and behavioral. Several factors affect the severity of the anxiety: the strength and intensity of the stressors, the duration of the stressors, the individual's coping abilities, and the individual's perceived sense of helplessness. Variables such as culture, religion, education, and past experiences can also influence how well individuals cope with a particular situation. Many variables affect the development of anxiety, including perceived threats to biological integrity, perceived threats to self-esteem, frustration of needs or motives, the inability to control or influence meaningful events, or mental association with previously anxiety-producing events. When patients are exposed to the health care system, events such as hospitalization, waiting for test results, waiting for a diagnosis, needing surgery, and losing time from work, anticipating the outcome of treatment, and experiencing lifestyle changes can all lead to increased anxiety.

Anxiety is both physiological and psychological. This is a very important fact because the mind will perceive a stressor as a threat, but it is the physiological response that causes the feelings of tension and discomfort. This is because the anxiety response is a sympathetic nervous system response, causing symptoms such as increased heart rate, increased respirations, increased blood pressure, and increased glucose. When this occurs individuals want to feel relief from the uncomfortable feelings that the anxiety produces, and if they are unable to apply anxiety-reducing interventions that decrease the physiological arousal the anxiety tends to increase in severity. In the case of chronic anxiety, the increased arousal of the sympathetic nervous system causes danger-

ous wear and tear on the body. This is why early assessment and intervention to decrease the anxious symptoms is vital.

Anxiety can be conceptualized on a continuum moving from mild to moderate to severe to panic. The higher the level of anxiety the more uncomfortable the symptoms will feel. Immediate interventions that are designed to decrease the physiologic arousal are of utmost importance. The longer the symptoms go unchecked the more anxious the person will feel.

Nursing Management

Nursing interventions to reduce anxiety are variable. Jung-Soon and Kyung-Sook (2001) studied the effects of handholding on anxiety in cataract surgery patients under local anesthesia and found that this cheap noninvasive intervention had potential for reducing anxiety in this group of patients. Vingerhoets (1998) found that patients who go into open heart surgery with high levels of anxiety tend to remain highly anxious after their open heart surgery. In a 1997 study that looked at the effects of relaxation exercises on anxiety and other symptoms of chemotherapy, Arakawa found that patients who received the intervention of relaxation reported less subjective feelings of anxiety. In a systematic review of implementing music in hospitals, Evans (2001) found that the evidence suggests the use of music can reduce anxiety in hospitalized patients. Badger, Segrin, Dorros, Meek, and Lopez (2007) found that phone-delivered psychosocial interventions decreased anxiety and depression in women with breast cancer and their partners.

Assessment

The nurse should assess for the following types of anxiety:

Mild Anxiety
- Alert, attentive, confident
- Open to new experiences
- Good problem-solving abilities
- Perceptual fields open, can deal with more than one thing at a time
- Can apply coping mechanisms.

Moderate Anxiety
- Signs and symptoms are beginning to become noticeable
- Ability to pay attention is narrowed
- Perceptual fields begin to narrow
- Verbalization is increasing
- Problem solving is more rigid
- Increased respiratory rate, heart rate, and muscle tension
- Dry mouth, clammy palms, and sometime palpitations
- General feeling of restlessness.

Severe Anxiety
- Anxiety is obvious
- Cognitive functioning is impaired
- Perceptual fields extremely narrowed
- Can only focus on one detail at a time
- Ability to concentrate decreased significantly

- Learning cannot occur
- Pacing, need for motor activity
- Sweating
- Hyperventilation, tachycardia
- Tremors, numbness, tingling
- Nausea, headache, dizziness.

Panic

- Chest pain, breathlessness, tachycardia
- Feelings of impending death
- Extreme discomfort
- Perceptual fields closed
- Unrealistic distorted perceptions
- Inability to communicate clearly
- Must be resolved quickly.

Planning

Priorities for nursing management for the patient with anxiety should include providing appropriate health information, assisting the patient with applying the information to his or her current health situation, and promoting identification of methods to cope with anxiety. The plan should also identify ways to minimize or prevent the escalation of the patient's anxiety and promote the overall well-being of the patient.

Nursing Diagnosis

Possible nursing diagnoses for the patient experiencing anxiety include:

- Anxiety
- Coping Ineffective
- Social Isolation
- Sleep Deprivation
- Hopelessness
- Powerlessness
- Knowledge Deficit.

Outcomes and Evaluation Parameters

The patient will be able to recognize the symptoms of anxiety resulting from identified fears by:

- Acknowledging to the nurse the presence of the anxiety.
- Demonstrating the appropriate use of coping mechanisms.
- Demonstrating increased problem solving.
- Verbalizing feeling less anxious.
- Exhibiting a decrease in the symptoms of anxiety.

Interventions and Rationales

The following interventions and rationales would be appropriate for the patient experiencing anxiety:

- Acknowledge the presence of the anxiety. *Recognition of the anxiety helps the patient to feel accepted and strengthens the therapeutic relationship.*
- Ask the patient to perform deep-breathing exercises. *Deep breathing assists the body to relax and the mind to be focused.*

Learning new techniques allows the patient to participate in promoting personal well-being.

- Offer music. *Music can distract the patient and help to focus his or her thoughts.*
- If possible, identify the stimulus for the anxiety. *Identifying the stimulus helps the patient to clarify realistic and unrealistic perceptions and develop appropriate ways of handling the distress.*
- Provide the patient with needed information. *Written materials give the patient information for discussion with the health care team and significant others. The materials can also be used as a reference when questions arise.*
- Remove anxiety-producing environmental stimuli. *When anxious, the patient may have increased sensitivity to environmental stimuli.*
- Stay with the patient and provide support. *Acceptance by the nurse allows the patient to feel positive about the therapeutic relationship. This helps with healing, decreases isolation, and increases coping ability.*
- Encourage the expression of feelings. *Patients may not fully understand what is happening to them. If they can express feelings freely, the nurse can plan specific actions to assist the patient to see the situation clearly.*
- Explore with the patient usual coping mechanisms. *Understanding the patient's baseline ability starts interventions from the place where the patient is comfortable. It also identifies unhealthy coping skills that need to be changed.*
- Acknowledge to the patient the effective use of coping mechanisms. *Positive reinforcement.*
- Assist the patient in problem solving. *The patient may be overwhelmed by his or her situation. Assisting the patient to view the problem in its component parts will reduce anxiety and assist with effective coping behaviors.*
- Provide opportunities to give the patient more control. *The ability to control aspects of one's life helps to allay feelings of helplessness.*
- Teach the patient relaxation techniques. *Helps the patient to focus.*
- In panic levels of anxiety:
  - Do not leave the patient.
  - Do not ask the patient for explanations.
  - Assure patient you will stay with him or her.
  - Allow patient to rest after attack is over.
  - Refer patient for further evaluation.

Evaluation

It is important for the nurse to assess the effectiveness of the patient's coping strategies. As the patient improves he or she will be able to identify effects of increasing anxiety, understand the sources of his or her anxiety, learn useful coping skills, and differentiate between healthy and unhealthy coping strategies.

Anger

Anger and anxiety are two emotions that are often related. When individuals feel anxious, they also experience accompanying feelings of frustration and helplessness. These feelings can in turn cause individuals to feel powerless to control their own autonomy. Anger develops to a greater or lesser degree as a response to the feelings of powerlessness and helplessness. At least temporarily, anger is a powerful feeling that helps individuals feel more in control. For some people the intolerable feeling of anxiety is replaced with the more powerful feeling of anger. This is effective as a temporary coping mechanism, but not meant to be the only coping strategy. Long-standing anger feelings do not promote health. In fact, Matthews, Gump, Harris, Haney, and Barefoot, (2004) found that long-standing hostility may place people at higher risk for cardiovascular mortality.

In society the open expression of anger is sometimes discouraged and causes others to feel uncomfortable. It is important to recognize that anger is a natural emotion and that the rational expression of angry feelings can be appropriate for some situations. For example, a patient whose diagnostic test results are lost and has to repeat the test would be justified in feeling angry.

Nurses are often the recipients of angry feelings and it is sometimes difficult for them not to personalize their response to these expressions of anger. When patients are angry, nurses can experience feelings of powerlessness and anxiety and respond to the patients' anger with anger of their own. This, of course, only serves to escalate the angry feelings. When anger is conceptualized as anxiety, nurses feel more in control and are able to intervene professionally and rationally.

Nursing Management

The expression of anger can be blatant, for example, when someone yells or throws something, or subtle, such as when someone is a little sarcastic or refuses to speak much. It is important to pick up the early signs of anger because angry feelings tend to increase if the cause for the anger is not dealt with. The earlier the nurse intervenes to reduce the anger and accompanying anxiety, the better the chance for a positive outcome. If a patient's expression of anger is not rationale, the nurse will need to set clear limits. Sometimes patients need to be informed about the types of behaviors that are acceptable and those that are not.

Assessment

Anger can be conceptualized on a continuum ranging from mild, to moderate, to severe, to rage.

Mild Anger
- Feeling tense
- Feeling irritable
- Argumentative
- Difficult to please
- Scowling facial expression
- Sarcasm.

Moderate Anger
- Increasing rumination
- Angry behavior more obvious
- Motor agitation
- Voice pitch increases
- Potential for acting out behavior.

Severe Anger
- Signs of acting-out behavior
- Cursing
- Distinct danger of becoming out of control.

Rage Anger
- Rage is an out-of-control situation and appropriate interventions to protect the safety of the patient and staff must be implemented immediately.

Nursing Diagnosis
Possible nursing diagnoses for an angry person include:
- *Coping Ineffective*
- *Noncompliance* with treatment
- *Social Isolation*
- *Powerlessness*
- *Risk for Other-Directed Violence.*

Planning
Nursing planning begins with establishing rapport and trust with the patient. Following is the identification of the cause of the anger, intervene and identify coping strategies, and evaluate the effectiveness of the interventions.

Outcomes and Evaluation Parameters
The patient will be able to recognize the cause of the anger and use effective coping strategies as evidenced by the ability to:
- Verbalize the presence of anger.
- Demonstrate decreased symptoms of anger.
- Demonstrate decreased symptoms of anxiety.
- Verbalize that he or she feels less angry.

Interventions and Rationales
- Prevention and anger reduction techniques, as listed next, can be useful. *Acceptance by the nurse allows the patient to feel positive about the therapeutic relationship. This helps with healing, decreases isolation, and increases coping ability.*

Prevention
- Listen when patients talk to you.
- Do not dismiss people's concerns.
- Treat each patient as an individual.
- Talk to patients not at them.
- Respect patients' privacy.
- Do not make rules that treat adults as children.
- Recognize when patients are feeling anxious and intervene to reduce the anxiety.

Anger Reduction
- Help patient verbalize angry feelings.
- Validate the patient's anger.
- Avoid defensive responses.
- Use therapeutic communication skills.
- Assist patient to identify the source of anger.

- Allow patient an outlet for angry feelings.
- Do mutual problem solving.
- Allow patient more control over health care decisions.
- Teach patient techniques such as deep breathing and relaxation.

Evaluation

As the patient develops healthy coping strategies he or she should exhibit the ability to describe his or her emotional state to the nurse, articulate an accurate understanding of the current situation, and accept support offered by caregivers.

Summary

This chapter discussed the basic principles and concepts of psychosocial nursing care. They are the concepts that nurses often forget when the pressures exerted by the health care delivery system take precedence. They are also the aspects of nursing care that make nursing a patient-centered and holistic profession.

Several topics for future research are listed in the Research Opportunities and Clinical Impact box.

RESEARCH OPPORTUNITIES AND CLINICAL IMPACT RELATED TO PSYCHOSOCIAL NURSING

Research	Clinical Impact
What interventions will help to relieve the "compassion fatigue" described by nurses?	Developing interventions to relieve the discomfort surrounding care of patients and families will improve the care given to the patients.
What is the best teaching methodology for therapeutic communication?	Best teaching practices would enhance relationship-based care.
What interventions can be done to support culturally appropriate care?	The promotion of cultural customs and rituals surrounding illness can enhance patient care.

NCLEX® REVIEW

1. A patient tells the nurse "I don't have diabetes; just a touch of sugar." The nurse realizes this patient is demonstrating a concept from which of the following theories?
   1. Erikson
   2. Freud
   3. Maslow
   4. Piaget

2. A patient is ambivalent about the types of treatment available for a disease process. Which of the following actions would support a therapeutic nurse–patient relationship?
   1. Encouraging the patient to follow the doctor's orders, without question
   2. Instructing the patient to figure it out and then let the nurse know the decision
   3. Asking the patient if more information is needed to help in the decision-making process
   4. Telling the patient that he has more information about the disease than the nurse

3. A foreign-born patient is trying to explain his current health status. Which of the following would demonstrate culturally sensitive therapeutic communication by the nurse?
   1. Leave the patient alone until he's ready to explain his current health issue.
   2. Sit with the patient and encourage him to explain to the best of his ability.
   3. Stand at the bedside and write down whatever the patient says being careful to avoid eye contact.
   4. Tell the patient he can explain his health problem to the doctor.

4. The nurse is planning to instruct a patient newly diagnosed with diabetes mellitus how to self-inject insulin. Which of the following responses indicates the patient is ready to learn the information?
   1. I will do my best to learn how to do this. I have to.
   2. I don't know why you are doing this. I don't have diabetes.
   3. Wait until my wife comes in. She's the one who will do it.
   4. Can't you do this for me? I don't want to worry about this every day.

5. A patient just learns he has prostate cancer. Which of the following should the nurse do to assist this patient?
   1. Sit with the patient and be prepared to answer any questions.
   2. Leave the patient alone to handle his emotions privately.
   3. Ask the physician to sit with the patient.
   4. Call a social worker to help the patient understand the implications of the diagnosis.

Answers for review questions appear in Appendix D

KEY TERMS

accommodation *p.254*
affective learning *p.259*
assimilation *p.254*
basic human needs *p.254*
conscious *p.251*
crisis *p.263*
ego *p.252*
ego defense mechanisms *p.252*

external locus of control *p.263*
growth needs *p.254*
holism *p.256*
id *p.252*
internal locus of control *p.263*
locus of control *p.263*
pleasure principle *p.252*
psychomotor learning *p.259*

schema *p.254*
sick role *p.263*
subconscious *p.251*
superego *p.252*
teaching *p.259*
therapeutic alliance *p.257*
therapeutic communication *p.259*
unconscious *p.252*

EXPLORE   PEARSON mynursingkit™

MyNursingKit is your one stop for online chapter review materials and resources. Prepare for success with additional NCLEX®-style practice questions, interactive assignments and activities, web links, animations and videos, and more!

Register your access code from the front of your book at
www.mynursingkit.com

REFERENCES

American Psychiatric Association. (2000). *Diagnostic and statistical manual of mental disorders, text revision* (4th ed.). Washington, DC: Author.

Badger, T., Segrin, C., Dorros, S. M., Meek, P., & Lopez, A. M. (2007). Depression and anxiety in women with breast cancer and their partners. *Nursing Research, 56*(1), 44–53.

Ball, J. W., & Bindler, R. C. (2006). *Child health nursing: Partnering with children & families.* Upper Saddle River: Pearson Prentice Hall.

Barsevick, A. M., Dudley, W. N., & Beck, S. L. (2006). Cancer-related fatigue, depressive symptoms, and functional status. *Nursing Research, 55*(5), 366–372.

Beck, A. T., & Freeman, A. (1990). *Cognitive theory of personality disorders.* New York: Guilford Press.

Bronfenbrenner, U. (1979). *The ecology of human development: Experiments by nature and design.* Cambridge, MA: Harvard University Press.

Camphina-Bacote, J. (1999). A model and instrument for addressing cultural competence in health care. *Journal of Nursing Education, 38*(5), 203–207.

Camphina-Bacote, J., & Munoz, C. (2001). A guiding framework for delivering culturally competent services in case management. *The Case Manager, 12,* 48–52.

Caplan, G. L. (Ed.). (1964). *Principles of Preventive Psychiatry.* New York: Basic Books.

Cioffi, J. (2006). Culturally diverse patient–nurse interactions on acute care wards. *International Journal of Nursing Practice, 12,* 319–325.

Devine, E. C., & Westlake, S. K. (1995).The effects of psychoeducational care provided to adults with cancer: Meta-analysis of 116 studies. *Oncology Nursing Forum 22*(9), 1369–1381.

Engel, G. L. (1980). The clinical application of the biopsychosocial model. *American Journal of Psychiatry, 137,* 535–544.

Erikson, E. (1963). *Childhood and society* (2nd ed.). New York: Norton.

Evans, D. (2001). *Music as an intervention for hospital patients: A systematic review.* Adelaide, Australia: Joanna Briggs Institute for Evidence Based Nursing and Midwifery.

Foshbinder, D. (1994). Patient perceptions of nursing care: An emerging theory of interpersonal competence. *Journal of Advance Nursing, 20*(6), 1085–1093.

Freud, S. (1935). *A general introduction to psychoanalysis.* New York: Simon and Schuster.

Friedman, M. (1998). *Family nursing: Research, theory and practice* (4th ed.). Stamford, CT: Appleton and Lange.

Hackett, M. L., Yapa, C., Parag, V., Anderson, C. S. (2005). Frequency of depression after stroke: A systematic review of observational studies. *Stroke, 36*(6):1330–40.

Hearn, J., & Higginson, I. (1998). Do specialist palliative care teams improve outcomes for cancer patients?: A systematic review. *Palliative Medicine, 12*(5), 317–332.

Jung-Soon, M., & Kyung-Sook, C. (2001). The effects of handholding on anxiety in cataract patients under local anesthesia. *Journal of Advanced Nursing, 353*(3), 407–415.

Kübler-Ross, E., & Kessler, D. (2005). *On grief and grieving: Finding the meaning of grief through the five stages of loss.* New York: Scribner.

Mayou, R., Gill, D., & Thompson, D. R. (2000). Depression and anxiety as predictors of outcome after myocardial infarction. *Psychosomatic Medicine, 62,* 212–219.

Matthews, K. A., Gump, B. B., Harris, K. F., Haney, T. L., & Barefoot, J. C. (2004). Hostile behaviors predict cardiovascular mortality among men enrolled in the multiple risk factor intervention trial. *Circulation, 109,* 66–70.

Munoz, C., & Luckmann, J. (2005). *Transcultural communication in nursing.* Clifton Park, NY: Thomson/Delmar Learning.

Office of Minority Health. (2001). *National standards for culturally and linguistically appropriate services in health care. Final report.* Rockville, MD: Author.

Paisson, M. B., & Norberg, A. (1995). Breast cancer patients' experiences of nursing care with the focus on emotional support: The implementation of a nursing intervention. *Journal of Advanced Nursing, 21*(2), 277–285.

Peplau, H. E. (1952). *Interpersonal relations in nursing.* New York: Putnam.

Piaget, J., & Inhelder, B. (1969). *Psychology of the child.* New York: Basic Books.

Russell, S., Daly, J., Hughes, E., & op't Hoog, C. (2003). Nurses and "difficult" patients: Negotiating non-compliance. *Journal of Advanced Nursing, 43*(3), 281–287.

Shatell, M. (2004). Nurse–patient interaction: A review of the literature. *Journal of Clinical Nursing, 13*(6), 714–722.

Sherbourne, C., Hays, R. D., Fleishman, J. A., Benedetto, V., Magruder, K. M., Bing, E. G., et al. (2000). Impact of psychiatric conditions on health related quality of life in persons with HIV infection. *American Journal of Psychiatry, 157,* 248–254.

Vandemark, L. M. (2006). Awareness of self and expanding consciousness: Using nursing theories to prepare nurse-therapists. *Issues in Mental Health Nursing, 27,* 605–615.

Venke, S., Torjuul, K., Ross, A., & Kihigren, M. (2006). Satisfied patients are also vulnerable patients—Narrative from a acute care ward. *Journal of Clinical Nursing, 15*(10), 1240–1244.

Vingerhoets, G. (1998). Perioperative anxiety and depression on open heart surgery. *Psychosomatics, 39,* 30–37.

Watson, J. (1985). Nursing: Human science and human care. Norwalk, CT: Appleton-Century-Crofts.

Watson, J. (2004). *Caring science as sacred science.* Philadelphia: F. A. Davis Company.

Wilson, R. (1963). The social structure of a general hospital. *Annals of the American Academy of Political and Social Sciences, 346,* 67–76.

Nutrition

Sheila Tucker

Outcome-Based Learning Objectives

After studying this chapter, the learner will be able to:

1. Explain components of a comprehensive nutrition assessment as part of the nursing care process.
2. Apply the nutritional component of national standards for disease prevention and treatment.
3. Discuss the metabolic effects of physiological stress and the potential impact on nutrition status.
4. Outline the nutrition therapy guidelines for patients with physiological stress, such as postoperative wound healing and burn injury.
5. Differentiate among the principles of medical nutrition therapy in treating general medical conditions.
6. Explain the indications and nursing interventions associated with enteral and parenteral nutrition support.
7. Defend the important role of nursing care in successful medical nutrition therapy.

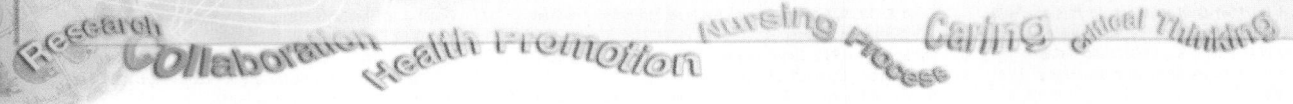

Research   Collaboration   Health Promotion   Nursing Process   Caring   Critical Thinking

NUTRITION PLAYS a crucial role in both the prevention and treatment of disease. Both overnutrition and undernutrition can lead to negative health outcomes. For example, **overnutrition** from excess intake of calories and fat can result in weight gain, elevated blood lipids, and risk of hypertension, diabetes, and some cancers. **Undernutrition,** in which dietary intake is less than the body's requirement, can result in impaired wound healing, poor response to medical treatment, and loss of functional capacity.

Medical nutrition therapy is an integral part of the health care process. Proper nutrition, whether accomplished through a therapeutic diet, nutrition support, or general healthy eating, is associated with positive outcomes. The nurse is uniquely positioned to take an active role in the nutrition care process of medical and surgical patients. The nutrition care process involves assessment, evaluation, and setting of patient goals and objectives in a fashion that can be easily dovetailed into the nursing care process. The registered dietitian is the health care professional with the primary responsibility for overseeing medical nutrition therapy in most settings. However, the nurse's active position on the front line of patient care presents an important opportunity for improving nutritional care with efficient screening and assessment of nutrition status, appropriate and timely referrals, reinforcement of patient education, and close monitoring of nutrition intervention.

▮ Nutrition Assessment

The cornerstone of all nutritional care is based on the foundation of a well-done nutrition assessment. Objective and subjective data gathered as part of the nursing assessment can be evaluated to determine a patient's existing or potential risk for undernutrition or overnutrition. Appropriate nursing diagnoses and interventions can then be developed based on findings from the nutrition assessment.

Nutrition Assessment Parameters

No one parameter or single piece of data should be used as an indicator of nutrition status. Data gathered during the physical exam and laboratory assays together with subjective data from the focused interview provide a comprehensive set of information on which to base a nutritional assessment. A nutrition assessment based on limited data has limited clinical value since many parameters used in a nutrition assessment can be influenced by nonnutritional factors. When compiling a nutrition assessment, the nurse should use as many sources of data as are available along with sharp clinical judgment.

Physical Assessment

The physical assessment portion of a nutrition assessment includes the clinical exam along with anthropometric measurements. Pertinent data from the medical history and treatment plan should be considered for any influence on nutrition status because of alterations in physical health. The presence of pain, gastrointestinal symptoms, medication side effects, and impaired cognition or mobility are examples of physical factors that can have negative effects on nutrition status. The Risk Factors chart outlines the potential influences of physical symptoms and health on nutrition status.

Observations from the clinical examination can be incorporated into the nutrition assessment. Nutritional deficiencies can have few, if any, clinical symptoms until nutrient status is compromised for a length of time. The nurse should not dismiss suspicion of poor nutrition health simply because no physical findings are apparent. Physical changes associated with altered nutrition status can also occur for medical or environmental reasons and so deserve further investigation when discovered. Chart 14–1 (p. 274) outlines physical findings that can be indicative of altered nutrition health.

Anthropometric measurements are an important component of the assessment and include any scientific measurement of the body. Measured current weight and height should be obtained during an initial assessment. Weight should be measured at regular intervals thereafter. Self-reported height and weight are not considered accurate and are subject to overreporting and underreporting bias by adults of all ages (Brown, Feng, & Knapp, 2002; Kuczmarski, Kuczmarski, & Najjar, 2001). Use of self-reported weight in a patient with undetected weight loss

will result in an unaddressed clinical change and subsequent delayed intervention. A patient should be weighed with a minimal of clothing and after voiding. Presence of edema or ascites and any unremoved casts or appliances should be noted. Additionally, adjustments in weight should be made for missing limbs following established guidelines (Osterkamp, 1995).

A weight history should also be obtained and confirmed by checking medical records. An unplanned weight loss of >5% in 1 month or >10% in 6 months is clinically significant and warrants attention. Patients who cannot stand to be measured or weighed can be measured using alternative methods. Chair and bed scales can be used to obtain current weight while arm span, knee height, or recumbent measures will provide estimates of height. Recumbent height will yield an overestimation of height by approximately 4 cm (1.5 in.) from changes in spinal compression when standing (American Medical Directors Association, 2001).

Body mass index (BMI) is used to calculate appropriate weight for height using the formula weight (kg)/height^2 (m). Morbidity and mortality statistics have been employed to determine cutoff points to define overweight, obesity, underweight, and healthy weight. Figure 14–1 ■ (p. 275) depicts a table from the National Institute of Health (NIH) that can be used as a tool to determine BMI. Because BMI calculations use simple height and weight measurements, its use does not take into account body composition. Individuals with large bone structure or ample muscle mass can be categorized erroneously as overweight using this single assessment tool. The nurse should discover this discrepancy when conducting a physical exam.

Waist circumference can be used in a nutrition assessment, especially when cardiovascular disease risk is suspected or known. Deposition of excess abdominal fat is considered to be an independent risk factor for heart disease in adults (National Heart Lung, and Blood Institute [NHLBI], 2002). A waist circumference of >102 cm (40 in.) in men or >88 cm (35 in.) in women is associated with risk. Measurement should be made following proper technique with use of bony landmarks. Simply measuring waist circumference just below the umbilicus is not accurate in the obese patient in whom the position of the umbilicus has changed with weight gain (Lean & Han, 2002). Waist circumference measurements are not of nutritional value in patients who are pregnant or have ascites or other fat-free mass increases in abdominal girth because of disease.

Body composition can be tested using a variety of techniques. Skinfold measurements, bioelectrical impedance analysis, near-infrared, and dual x-ray absorptiometry (DEXA) are utilized in different clinical settings to estimate body fat and muscle mass. Bone mineral content and fluid composition can be estimated with more sophisticated technology. Care must be taken to ensure that the most accurate measurements are performed, realizing even then that most methods have a margin of error associated with them. Skinfold measurements are best performed by a practiced clinician, because repeated accurate measurement is difficult. The presence of edema at the measurement site invalidates the findings. Bioelectrical impedance is subject to error caused by changes in hydration. Near-infrared measurements have an increased margin of error when performed on obese subjects (Wagner & Heyward, 1999).

RISK FACTORS for Poor Nutrition Health

Condition	Contributing Symptoms
Chronic disease, acute illness, injury	Disease symptoms (including pain) or treatment can ↓ appetite, ↓ intake, cause malabsorption, or change nutritional requirements
Multiple medications	Gastrointestinal side effects, altered taste, decreased saliva, nutrient interactions
Restrictive eating	Chronic dieting, disordered eating, food beliefs, or faddism can lead to poor intake
Poor oral health	Loose, missing teeth, ill-fitting dentures, gum disease, and mouth sores can ↓ intake
Alcohol abuse	Poor dietary intake and nutrient absorption
Psychosocial issues	Depression, bereavement, social isolation can lead to ↓ intake. Lack of finances or access to adequate food impairs intake. Lack of nutrition knowledge or food preparation skills can yield poor-quality intake
Altered functional status	Immobility, altered cognition can ↓ intake
Sensory changes	Vision, hearing, taste alterations alter ability to prepare or enjoy food or dining

CHART 14–1   Physical Findings Associated with Altered Nutrition

	Finding	Potential Altered Nutrient
Hair	Dull, sparse, brittle, dyspigmented	Protein, zinc, biotin
Face	Puffy/moon face, temporal wasting	Protein
	Pallor	Iron
Eyes	Sunken	Water
	Dry mucosa, night blindness	Vitamin A
	Pale conjunctiva	Iron
	Fatty deposits around lids	Elevated serum cholesterol
Mouth	Long tongue furrows	Water
	Cracked corners, lips, magenta tongue	Niacin, vitamin B_6, riboflavin
	Atrophic papillae	Iron
	Spongy, bleeding gums	Vitamin C
	Lack of taste (hypogeusia)	Zinc
Glands	Enlarged thyroid (goiter)	Iodine
Skin	Poor wound healing	Protein, zinc, vitamin C
	Dry, scaly	Vitamin A, zinc, fat
	Bruising	Vitamins C and K
	Pinpoint hemorrhages (petechiae)	Vitamin C
	Photosensitive symmetric rash	Niacin
	Tenting, dry mucous membranes or axillae	Water
Skeleton/trunk	Ascites	Protein
	Beading on ribs, bowed legs	Vitamin D
	Loss of fat, muscle wasting	Protein and calories
Limbs	Edema, loss of muscle, fat	Protein and calories
Nails	Spoon shaped, ridges	Iron
Central nervous system	Confusion, headache, lethargy	Water
	Confabulation, hyporeflexia	Thiamine
	Dementia, ataxia, neuropathy	Vitamin B_{12}
Cardiac	Arrhythmias	Magnesium, potassium

Reference values for all body composition measurements should be current and age and gender specific. The best use of composition measurements is in the serial monitoring of a patient, with the patient's own baseline measures serving as the initial point of reference.

Laboratory Measurements

Laboratory values can be a useful adjunct to other parameters used in a nutritional assessment. No single laboratory value is uniquely indicative of current nutritional status because confounding variables exist for each. Disease, infection, and the inflammatory process can alter laboratory values used in an assessment. Varying half-lives and the body's pool size of plasma proteins will yield differences in the snapshot of nutrition status reflected by their values. Albumin, with its long half-life, provides an older picture of nutrition status than prealbumin with its shorter half-life. Chart 14–2 outlines laboratory testing used in a nutrition assessment.

Nutrition History

A nutrition history can conveniently be incorporated into the focused interview done during a nursing assessment. The nutrition history can include a 24-hour diet recall and a food frequency questionnaire. In the clinical setting where patients receive subsequent monitoring, a food record or diary can be a useful adjunctive tool to evaluate nutrition intervention.

A 24-hour diet recall provides a 1-day snapshot of the patient's intake on which to base an assessment. All meals, snacks, liquids, and nutrition supplements should be recorded with estimates of preparation method and portion size. Because no single day usually illustrates all dietary habits, it is best to ask the patient about other general nutrition habits. A second recall can be performed to improve the type of data, for example, the nurse could query the patient about intake on a workday and a nonworkday. Chart 14–3 (p. 276) outlines data to be considered when conducting a nutrition history.

A food frequency questionnaire can be used to supplement the limited data of a 24-hour recall. The patient can provide information on the frequency of consumption of different food groups by filling out a questionnaire or answering questions during the nutrition history. For example, a nurse may find no fruit intake on the limited recall, but a food frequency questionnaire might reveal that 10 pieces of fruit are eaten a week.

During the nutrition history, the nurse should ask open-ended questions and make no assumptions about types and patterns of intake. Asking a question such as "What did you have for breakfast?" assumes the patient had breakfast or appears to

Body Mass Index Table

	Normal						Overweight					Obese										Extreme Obesity																
BMI	19	20	21	22	23	24	25	26	27	28	29	30	31	32	33	34	35	36	37	38	39	40	41	42	43	44	45	46	47	48	49	50	51	52	53	54
Height (inches)																**Body Weight (pounds)**																				
58	91	96	100	105	110	115	119	124	129	134	138	143	148	153	158	162	167	172	177	181	186	191	196	201	205	210	215	220	224	229	234	239	244	248	253	258
59	94	99	104	109	114	119	124	128	133	138	143	148	153	158	163	168	173	178	183	188	193	198	203	208	212	217	222	227	232	237	242	247	252	257	262	267
60	97	102	107	112	118	123	128	133	138	143	148	153	158	163	168	174	179	184	189	194	199	204	209	215	220	225	230	235	240	245	250	255	261	266	277	276
61	100	106	111	116	122	127	132	137	143	148	153	158	164	169	174	180	185	190	195	201	206	211	217	222	227	232	238	243	248	254	259	264	269	275	280	285
62	104	109	115	120	126	131	136	142	147	153	158	164	169	175	180	186	191	196	202	207	213	218	224	229	235	240	246	251	256	262	267	273	278	284	289	295
63	107	113	118	124	130	135	141	146	152	158	163	169	175	180	186	191	197	203	208	214	220	225	231	237	242	248	254	259	265	270	278	282	287	293	299	304
64	110	116	122	128	134	140	145	151	157	163	169	174	180	186	192	197	204	209	215	221	227	232	238	244	250	256	262	267	273	279	285	291	296	302	308	314
65	114	120	126	132	138	144	150	156	162	168	174	180	186	192	198	204	210	216	222	228	234	240	246	252	258	264	270	276	282	288	294	300	306	312	318	324
66	118	124	130	136	142	148	155	161	167	173	179	186	192	198	204	210	216	223	229	235	241	247	253	260	266	272	278	284	291	297	303	309	315	322	328	334
67	121	127	134	140	146	153	159	166	172	178	185	191	198	204	211	217	223	230	236	242	249	255	261	268	274	280	287	293	299	306	312	319	325	331	338	344
68	125	131	138	144	151	158	164	171	177	184	190	197	203	210	216	223	230	236	243	249	256	262	269	276	282	289	295	302	308	315	322	328	335	341	348	354
69	128	135	142	149	155	162	169	176	182	189	196	203	209	216	223	230	236	243	250	257	263	270	277	284	291	297	304	311	318	324	331	338	344	351	358	365
70	132	139	146	153	160	167	174	181	188	195	202	209	216	222	229	236	243	250	257	264	271	278	285	292	299	306	313	320	327	334	341	348	355	362	369	376
71	136	143	150	157	165	172	179	186	193	200	208	215	222	229	236	243	250	257	265	272	279	286	293	301	308	315	322	329	338	343	351	358	365	372	379	386
72	140	147	154	162	169	177	184	191	199	206	213	221	228	235	242	250	258	265	272	279	287	294	302	309	316	324	331	338	346	353	361	368	375	383	390	397
73	144	151	159	166	174	182	189	197	204	212	219	227	235	242	250	257	265	272	280	288	295	302	310	318	325	333	340	348	355	363	371	378	386	393	401	408
74	148	155	163	171	179	186	194	202	210	218	225	233	241	249	256	264	272	280	287	295	303	311	319	326	334	342	350	358	365	373	381	389	396	404	412	420
75	152	160	168	176	184	192	200	208	216	224	232	240	248	256	264	272	279	287	295	303	311	319	327	335	343	351	359	367	375	383	391	399	407	415	423	431
76	156	164	172	180	189	197	205	213	221	230	238	246	254	263	271	279	287	295	304	312	320	328	336	344	353	361	369	377	385	394	402	410	418	426	435	443

FIGURE 14–1 ■ BMI table.
Source: From National Institutes of Health website: http://www.nhlbi.nih.gov/guidelines/obesity/bmi_tbl.htm

CHART 14–2 Laboratory Tests Used in Nutrition Assessment

Laboratory Test Normal Finding	Half-life (days)	Expected Abnormality with Mild Malnutrition	Expected Abnormality with Moderate Malnutrition	Expected Abnormality with Severe Malnutrition	Rationale
Albumin 3.5–5 g/L	14–20	2.8–3.4 g/L	2.1–2.7 g/L	<2.1 g/L	↓ w/liver disease, inflammation, infection, renal losses
Transferrin >200 mg/L	8–10	180–200 mg/L	160–180 mg/L	<160 mg/L	↓ w/renal losses, liver disease; ↑ w/infection, inflammation, iron deficiency
Prealbumin 150–350 mg/L	2–3	110–150 mg/L	50–109 mg/L	<50 mg/L	↓ w/liver disease, inflammation, infection, renal losses
Total lymphocytes 2,000–3,500 cells/m³	NA	1,200–1,500 cells/m³	800–1,200 cells/m³	<800 cells/m³	↓ w/steroid, immunosuppression, cancer treatment

Sources: Beck, F. K., & Rosenthal, T. C. (2002). Prealbumin: A marker for nutritional evaluation. *American Family Physician, 65,* 1575–1578; Omran, M. L., & Morley, J. E. (2000). Assessment of protein-energy malnutrition in older persons, part II: Laboratory evaluation. *Nutrition, 16,* 131–140; Shenkin, A., Cederblad, G., Elia, M., & Isaksson, B. (1996). Laboratory assessment of protein energy status. *Clin Chim Acta, 253,* S5–S59.

CHART 14-3	Nutrition History Data

DIET RECALL AND FOOD FREQUENCY
- All meals and snacks
- All liquids, including alcohol, water, and caffeinated beverages
- Location of meals (home, school, restaurant, car, work, etc.)
- Preparation methods (convenience food, added fat, salt, etc.)
- Portion size
- Meal patterns: number of meals, missed meals

SUPPLEMENT AND MEDICATION USE
- Vitamin and mineral use; include dose, frequency, and ingredients
- Herbal supplement use; include dose, frequency, and ingredients
- Weight loss and sports supplements; include dose, frequency, and ingredients
- Assess over-the-counter and prescription medications for drug–nutrient interactions

FOOD BELIEFS AND PRACTICES
- Use of therapeutic diet for allergy, food intolerance, or medical nutrition therapy
- Lifestyle nutrition choices and food faddism; avoidance of certain foods or food groups, trendy nutrition practices, vegetarianism or vegan diet
- Cultural or religious dietary influences
- Pica: consumption of nonfood items or unusual intake of single foods

OTHER INFLUENCES ON NUTRITION
- Education and literacy as it relates to nutrition knowledge and cooking skills
- Social environment: isolation, food security, access to cooking facilities and refrigeration, presence of substance abuse
- Economics: adequate funds for food
- Functional capacity related to ADLs and I-ADLs: cooking, shopping, self-feeding, meal preparation, general activity level

CULTURAL CONSIDERATIONS in Nutrition Assessment

- Cultural and religious beliefs and traditions can affect dietary habits and practices in many ways. Preparation methods, food choices, and patterns of intake can be based on beliefs of a group or individual interpretation.
- Explore the influence of cultural interpretations and religious beliefs on individual nutrition habits and beliefs. Diversity exists within groups and it is best to discuss an individual's personal practices rather than make assumptions based on generalities.
- Ask about religious dietary laws, food preparation methods, food practices for special occasions (including whether fasting is practiced), and beliefs related to food and health. Medicinal herb use varies among cultures and can play an important role.

the gold standard for evaluating nutrition status in adults. Thus, many tools exist and will continue to be developed. When choosing a tool, it must be validated for use in the intended population. Most assessment tools have cutoff points as part of a scoring system. Because poor nutrition health occurs along a continuum, sharp clinical judgment is a needed accessory to any nutrition assessment tool in order to avoid missed opportunities for intervention and improved outcome.

REAP and WAVE

The Rapid Eating and Activity of Patients (REAP) and Weight, Activity, Variety and Excess (WAVE) validated tools were developed for use by health care providers to improve nutrition assessment and education during clinical encounters (Gans et al., 2003). The tools can be used alone or together to provide assessment and education in less than 9 minutes. The WAVE tool uses the Food Guide Pyramid as a foundation to evaluate a diet recall and the BMI to assess weight and also includes an assessment for risks of overnutrition. The REAP questionnaire can be completed by the patient before the assessment and is meant to supplement the overall assessment. Chart 14–4 (p. 278) depicts the REAP and WAVE tools.

Mini Nutrition Assessment and Subjective Global Assessment

The Mini Nutrition Assessment (MNA) and Subjective Global Assessment (SGA) have both been validated as nutrition assessment tools (Persson, Brismar, Katzarski, Nordenstrom, & Cederholm, 2002). The SGA was developed more than 20 years ago and had been validated in several adult populations since then. The MNA is a newer tool and is specific to older adults (Vellas et al., 1999). The MNA can be incorporated into the nursing assessment or used alone.

■ Special Considerations Affecting Nutrition Care

Both malnutrition and physiological stress place additional nutritional requirements on the medical–surgical patient. Existing malnutrition can compromise medical treatment and contribute to adverse medical and surgical outcomes. The presence of physiological stress increases nutritional requirements in the patient who may already be at nutritional risk because of a medical condition or disease.

judge that breakfast consumption is expected. This type of questioning can lead the patient to craft an answer to meet the perceived expectations of the nurse rather than answer factually. A better choice to begin the recall would be "What was the first thing you had to drink or eat yesterday? When/what was that?" followed by "When was the next time that you had something?"

Underreporting bias exists in giving a nutrition history. Patients who are seeking the social approval of the interviewer or want to avoid disapproval tend to underreport intake (Novotny et al., 2003). Patients who smoke, are obese, or are of lower socioeconomic or educational level underreport intake more than others. In addition, alcohol intake can be underreported. Cultural influences on the nutrition assessment are outlined in the Cultural Considerations box, and gerontological influences are outlined in the Gerontological Considerations box.

Nutrition Assessment Tools

Data from a nutrition assessment can be gathered following a protocol, the nursing care process, or by using a validated tool. No one screening or assessment tool is universally accepted as

GERONTOLOGICAL CONSIDERATIONS for Nutrition Assessment

Nutrition assessment of the older adult should utilize the same parameters outlined for the general population. However, because of the prevalence of malnutrition in the elderly, specific attention should be paid to assessment of contributing factors to unintentional weight loss and malnutrition.

Physical Exam and Focused Interview
Assess:

- Signs of malnutrition during clinical exam as outlined in Chart 14–1 (p. 274)
- Signs of dysphagia or chewing difficulties; note pocketed food, drooling, mouth sores, dental health, fit of dentures, xerostomia (lack of saliva)
- Cognitive impairment or dependency on others for feeding or meal preparation
- Altered functional status: immobility, loss of strength, fatigue
- Gastrointestinal, appetite, or oral complaints from disease or medication side effects
- Pain
- Psychosocial health: depression, bereavement, isolation, dependency, food security
- Sensory losses and neurological symptoms: vision, hearing, taste, neuropathy, tremors
- Medical conditions or treatment that alter intake, absorption, or nutritional requirements

- Hypermetabolic conditions: fever, infection, sepsis, fracture, wounds, cachexia, burns.

Anthropometric Measurements
Assess:

- Measured height and weight
- Serial weights; check medical record for weight history to confirm
- Body composition measurements must use age and gender-specific references because alterations in skin elasticity, muscle mass, fat distribution, bone density and water content can change with age.

Nutrition History
Assess:

- Nutrition data as outlined in Chart 14–3
- Whether use of therapeutic diet is appropriate
- Use of alcohol
- Access to personal, cultural, or religious food preferences (especially hospitalized or dependent elderly)
- Iatrogenic malnutrition risk: assess days NPO, on clear liquid, or other insufficient diet; inadequate delivery of supplements or tube feedings; overuse of restricted diet resulting in poor intake; insufficient feeding assistance; missed meals for testing.

Malnutrition

Malnutrition can be defined as a deficiency of one or more nutrients. The terms *undernutrition* and *malnutrition* are used interchangeably. A deficiency of macronutrients (carbohydrate, protein, and fat) can result in weight loss from insufficient energy and muscle wasting. Often the general term *malnutrition* is synonymous with the specific term **protein-calorie malnutrition.** Deficiency of any micronutrient may initially be less physically evident than with macronutrient deficiency because a lack of vitamins and minerals can take many weeks or months to manifest clinical symptoms.

Malnutrition occurs because of decreased intake, increased losses, or unmet increased needs for energy or any nutrient. Patients have decreased intake for a number of medical and psychosocial reasons. Nutrient losses can occur from malabsorptive disease or drug interactions. Hypermetabolism during physiological stress, or increased energy needs because of growth, development, and physical activity can cause increased nutritional needs that must be met or malnutrition will develop. The accompanying Risk Factors box (p. 278) outlines the many contributing risk factors to malnutrition.

Malnutrition has adverse consequences such as poor wound healing, risk of decubitus ulcer development, loss of muscle mass (including respiratory and heart) with subsequent loss of strength and functional decline, diminished immunocompetence, and altered pharmacokinetics (Covinsky, 2002; Hoffer, 2001; Holmes, 2003; Sullivan, Bopp, & Roberson, 2002). Weight loss exceeding 40% of body weight is associated with mortality (Hoffer, 2001). Successful treatment of malnutrition is contingent on discovery of the underlying etiology. Provision of adequate nutrition in a well-tolerated form is best

based on the recommendations of a registered dietitian who is trained to assess the impact of physiological stress, disease, and alterations in metabolism on baseline nutritional requirements across the life span. Specific nutrition interventions are presented in later discussions in this chapter of medical nutrition therapy.

Physiological Stress

A hypermetabolic response to injury or disease can have significant nutritional ramifications. Major surgery, thermal injury, sepsis, and trauma are examples of **physiological stress**. Unlike periods of inadequate energy intake that result in weight loss and some muscle wasting, a hypermetabolic response because of physiological stress can lead to rapid protein catabolism even when it seems energy and protein intake are sufficient (Hoffer, 2001). The body's response to this metabolic stress leads to a cascade that includes release of catecholamines and cortisol, and a systemic inflammatory response (Hoffer, 2001; Holmes, 2003; Kotler, 2000). Systemic inflammatory response is described in detail in Chapter 61 . The result can be catabolization of skeletal muscle to provide substrate for gluconeogenesis and a degradation of plasma proteins, such as albumin, that are considered acute-phase reactant proteins. Resting energy needs are elevated, which is referred to as **hypermetabolism**. Thus, physiological stress results in hypermetabolism and hypercatabolism. **Hypercatabolism** occurs when catabolism exceeds normal physiological rates. Each of these represents a nutritional challenge that is compounded when present together. The patient who is already malnourished before surgery, injury, or disease will have less available body stores to draw on during a metabolically challenging circumstance. In severe circumstances the rate

CHART 14–4 **REAP and WAVE Tools**

WEIGHT

Assess patient's Body Mass Index.*
Patient is overweight if BMI>25.

Height	Body Weight lbs	Height	Body Weight lbs
4'10"	>119	5'8"	>161
4'11"	>124	5'9"	>169
5'0"	>128	5'10"	>174
5'1"	>132	5'11"	>179
5'2"	>136	6'0"	>184
5'3"	>141	6'1"	>189
5'4"	>145	6'2"	>194
5'5"	>150	6'3"	>200
5'6"	>155	6'4"	>305
5'7"	>159		

*Certain pts may require assessment for underweight and/or unintentional weight loss

VARIETY

Is patient eating a variety of foods from important sections of the food pyramid?

Grains (6–11 servings)

Fruits (2–4 servings)

Vegetables (3–5 servings)

Protein (2–3 servings)

Dairy (2–3 servings)

Determine Variety and Excess using one of the following methods:

- Do a quick one-day recall.
- Ask patient to complete a self-administered eating pattern questionnaire.

ACTIVITY

Ask patient about any physical activity in the past week: walking briskly, jogging, gardening, swimming, biking, dancing, golf, etc.

1. Does patient do 30 minutes of moderate activity on most days/wk?
2. Does pt do "lifestyle" activity like taking the stairs instead of elevators, etc.?
3. Does patient usually watch less than 2 hours of TV or videos/day?

If patient answers NO to above questions, assess whether patient is willing to increase physical activity.

EXCESS

Is patient eating too much:

Fat? Saturated fat?

Calories?

Salt?

Sugar?

Alcohol?

- Ask about serving/portion sizes, preparation methods and added fats like butter, mayonnaise, sour cream, salad dressing, etc.
- Does patient eat 4 or more meals from sit-down or take-out restaurants per week?
- Does patient indulge on the weekends?
- *What does patient think are pros/cons of his/her eating pattern?*
- *If patient needs to improve eating habits, assess willingness to make changes.*

Source: Gans, K. M., Ross, E., Barner, C. W., Wylie-Rosett, J., McMurray, J., & Eaton, C. (2003). REAP and WAVE: New tools to rapidly assess/discuss nutrition with patients. *Journal of Nutrition, 133,* 556S–562S.

RISK FACTORS for Malnutrition

Decreased Intake

- Anorexia
- Gastrointestinal symptoms: nausea, vomiting, diarrhea
- Medication side effects
- Pain
- Dysphagia
- Poor dental health or chewing difficulties
- Sensory changes: loss of vision, taste, neuropathy
- Depression, anxiety, cognitive impairment, or other neuropsychological symptoms
- Socioeconomic issues: lack of finances, food insecurity, social isolation, bereavement, dependency on others for food or feeding
- Alcoholism.

Increased Nutrient Losses

- Malabsorptive disease
- Short bowel syndrome
- Alcoholism
- Drug–nutrient interactions.

Increased Nutrient Requirements

- Fever
- Infection or sepsis
- Wounds
- Fracture
- Hypermetabolic disease
- Increased energy expenditure from increased physical activity.

of protein degradation exceeds the body's ability to replenish muscle and plasma stores and, thus, physical and biochemical evidence of malnutrition ensues.

The severe muscle wasting seen with physiological stress is referred to as **cachexia** (Kotler, 2000). When cachexia becomes evident, nutritional repletion is difficult because of the confounding chronic systemic inflammatory response. High energy and protein intake alone often does not overcome the effects. Considerable research has focused on supplementation with so-called "conditionally essential" amino acids, such as glutamine and arginine. Researchers believe that these nonessential amino acids become essential during extreme metabolic stress, such as with trauma or burns (Wilmore, 2001). Amino acid–enhanced nutritional products are available (and prescribed), but their use remains controversial (Buchman, 2001). More recently, resistance training, pharmacological intervention with anabolic agents, cytokine inhibitors, and other metabolic regulators have all been under investigation for a potential role in cachexia treatment (Kotler, 2000; Nerad et al., 2003). Further discussion of the nutritional effects of physiological stress under specific circumstances is provided later in this chapter. The effects of malnutrition on the elderly is presented in the Gerontological Considerations box.

Health Promotion

Health promotion includes nutrition education on both preservation of wellness and disease prevention through diet. The nurse can assist the patient in the development of strategies for lifestyle modifications aimed at improving nutrition health. Several national standards exist with supporting educational tools to guide the nurse in nutrition health promotion.

The *Dietary Guidelines for Americans, 2005 Edition* (U.S. Department of Health and Human Services [DHHS], 2005) are national standards that can be used when advising patients about health maintenance and disease prevention. These science-based general recommendations are targeted to the general population age 2 years and older and serve as the foundation for other federal nutrition guidelines and information, such as the development of the *Healthy People* objectives for the nation (DHHS, 2000). These guidelines are translated for the public into key messages providing diet and physical activity guidance. These messages can become a template for general nutrition education as well as more specific advice about disease prevention. The National Guidelines box outlines the

GERONTOLOGICAL CONSIDERATIONS
Malnutrition

The prevalence of malnutrition among older adults is disproportionately high compared to younger adults. Up to 60% of hospitalized elderly or those under dependent care are malnourished (Singh, Watt, Veitch, Cantor, & Duerksen, 2006; Sullivan, Sun, & Walls, 1999; Thomas et al., 2002). Hospitalized malnourished older adults have twice the 1-year mortality rate after discharge compared to well-nourished older adults (Persson et al., 2002).

Alterations in pharmacokinetics from malnutrition are especially pertinent in the elderly because of the probability of polypharmacy. Low plasma protein levels affect drug binding for certain classes of medications, leaving an increased circulating free fraction of those drugs. Polypharmacy further complicates this when multiple drugs compete for diminished protein binding sites, increasing the likelihood of an adverse drug reaction. Enzymes required for drug metabolism can be affected by inadequate protein and micronutrient status (Holmes, 2003). Malnutrition can affect pharmacokinetics at both the absorptive and cell level for drug and herb metabolism. Unintentional weight loss and signs of malnutrition among the elderly should not be considered a normal part of the aging process and always deserve full consideration and attention to determine the etiology and provide appropriate intervention.

nine major messages of the *Dietary Guidelines for Americans, 2005 Edition*.

Nutrition health promotion also includes the elimination of health disparities that affect nutrition status. The DHHS along with the U.S. Department of Agriculture developed the *Healthy People 2010* document to establish goals and objectives for the nation aimed at improving quality and years of life as well as reducing health disparities (DHHS, 2000). The *Healthy People 2010* objectives can help the nurse to target appropriate interventions for specific population groups. Another National Guidelines box (p. 280) outlines the objectives from *Healthy People 2010* that relate to nutrition health.

Medical Nutrition Therapy for Medical–Surgical Patients

Medical nutrition therapy (MNT) plays a central role in the care of the medical or surgical patient. MNT includes the use of specific nutrition guidelines, nutrients, or therapeutic diets to treat an illness or medical condition. Therapeutic diets are used in the

---

NATIONAL GUIDELINES *Dietary Guidelines for Americans, 2005 Edition*

- Consume a variety of foods within and among the basic food groups while staying within energy needs.
- Control calorie intake to manage body weight.
- Be physically active every day.
- Increase daily intake of fruits and vegetables, whole grains, and nonfat or low-fat milk and milk products.

- Choose fats wisely for good health.
- Choose carbohydrates wisely for good health.
- Choose and prepare foods with little salt.
- If you drink alcoholic beverages, do so in moderation.
- Keep food safe to eat.

Source: U.S. Department of Health and Human Services. (2005). *Dietary guidelines for Americans, 2005 edition.* Retrieved May 17, 2008, from http://www.health.gov/DietaryGuidelines/dga2005/document.

NATIONAL GUIDELINES *Healthy People 2010* Nutrition Objectives

- Increase the proportion of adults who are at a healthy weight.
- Reduce the proportion of adults who are obese.
- Reduce the proportion of children and adolescents who are overweight or obese.
- Reduce growth retardation among low-income children under age 5 years.
- Increase the proportion of persons age 2 years and older who consume at least:
  - Two daily servings of fruit
  - Three daily servings of vegetables, with at least one green or dark orange
  - Six daily servings of grain products, with at least three whole-grain choices
  - And who meet the dietary recommendations for calcium.

- Increase the proportion of people age 2 years and older who consume less than:
  - 10% of calories from saturated fat
  - 30% of calories from total fat
  - 2,400 mg of sodium.
- Reduce iron deficiency anemia among young children and females of childbearing age.
- Reduce low birth weight and very low birth weight.
- Increase the proportion of pregnancies begun with optimum folic acid level.

Source: U.S. Department of Health and Human Services. (2000). *Healthy people 2010: Understanding and improving health.* Retrieved February 5, 2008, from http://www.healthypeople.gov

---

treatment of many diseases and conditions. Descriptions of specific diets are contained within the discussion of each disease state outlined in this chapter. Nutrition support in the form of tube feedings or intravenous nutrition is a type of MNT and is also discussed. Both hospitals and long-term care institutions are required by accrediting agencies to have a diet manual specific to their organization available in each medical unit. Diet manuals describe the specifics of all therapeutic diets and texture-modified diets offered at the institution. The nurse should refer to this manual to become familiar with the modified diets available for patients.

Many patients may not require a therapeutic diet while hospitalized. A house or regular diet is ordered for such patients. Some patients have a temporary or permanent need for a texture-modified or liquid diet while hospitalized. Clear liquid diets can be used postoperatively or as part of preparation for diagnostic testing. A clear liquid diet contains little in the way of adequate nutrition for the patient and should not be used for more than a day or two without consideration given to additional nutrition intervention. Many institutions require daily renewable prescriptions for a clear liquid diet in the hope it fosters regular reevaluation of the need for the diet. A registered dietitian should be consulted when patients remain on a clear liquid diet as the sole form of nutrition for more than a few days. Difficulties with either chewing or swallowing warrant a nutrition evaluation for the appropriateness of a texture-modified diet. Chart 14–5 outlines various hospital diets prescribed for transitional and texture-modified diets.

Weight Management

Care of the patient who is either overweight or underweight requires a central nutrition component. The approach to medical nutrition therapy in the area of weight management is constantly evolving and requires the need to keep a current knowledge base. Both overweight and underweight states can lead to additional health risks in the medical–surgical patient.

Overweight and Obesity

Overweight and obesity are linked with a multitude of comorbidities, including cardiovascular disease, hypertension, type 2 diabetes, degenerative joint disease, some pulmonary disease, and cancers (NHLBI, 1998). Obesity has been reported to lessen life expectancy, especially in younger adults (Fontaine, Redden, Wang, Westfall, & Allison, 2003). The prevalence of overweight and obesity is increasing among all population groups in the United States, where 63% of all men and 55% of women 20 to 74 years of age are considered overweight or obese (Hedley et al., 2004). Further parental obesity has been reported to more than double the risk of adult obesity among children less than 10 years of age (Whitaker, Wright, Pepe, Seidel, & Dietz, 1997). This worrisome association could lead to future increases in obesity prevalence.

Many factors are postulated as contributing to the prevalence of overweight and obesity. Genetic, metabolic, psychological, and environmental causes have been cited (American Dietetic Association, 2002b; NHLBI, 1998). Hormones, such as leptin, have been hypothesized to have a potential role in the metabolic link to obesity (American Dietetic Association, 2002b). Certain medications, such as psychotropics, can foster weight gain. Medications that block receptors for histamine, serotonin 5-5HT, and dopamine are examples in this category (Devlin, Yanovski, & Wilson, 2000). Although genetic and metabolic contributors to obesity are important, most researchers agree that energy imbalance is a more significant contributor (American Dietetic Association, 2002b). Increased dietary intake, decreased physical activity, or a combination of both can lead to an imbalance in which energy expenditure is less than energy consumption and weight gain follows.

Increased energy consumption occurs for many reasons. One reason is that Americans consume more food outside the home than in the past. Foods prepared outside the home are calorically dense and come in larger portions than in previous years (Harnack & French, 2003; Young & Nestle, 2003). Larger portions are often marketed as a value to the cost-conscious consumer. The consumer may have lost sight of standard food portions with the expansion of market portions between two- and eightfold in the past decades (Young & Nestle, 2003). A sedentary lifestyle can further tip the energy balance equation and contribute to weight gain. More than 25% of U.S. adults are considered sedentary

CHART 14–5	Transitional and Texture-Modified Diets			
Diet	**Definition**	**Sample Contents**	**Indications**	**Special Concerns**
Clear liquids	Liquid at room or body temperature and able to be seen through clearly	Clear juices like apple and cranberry, popsicles, gelatin, clear broth, tea	Preparation for diagnostic testing, transition from NPO to reintroduction of oral intake such as after an acute gastrointestinal (GI) event or postoperatively	Provides hydration and some electrolytes and carbohydrate, but nutritionally inadequate. Limit duration of use.
Full liquids	Pourable consistency at room or body temperature	All liquids, including milk and nutrition supplement drinks, ice cream, cooked cereal	Fractured mandible, difficulty chewing or swallowing other consistencies	Ensure safety of this consistency in patients at risk for aspiration, avoid overmodifying texture unnecessarily. Can be modified to exclude lactose-containing foods.
Mechanical soft	Soft or chopped foods without connective tissue, casings, tough skins	Full range of soft foods; can be chopped or mashed	Chewing or swallowing difficulties	Vary texture to patient tolerance. Avoid overly chopped or mashed consistency when not necessary.
Puree	Mechanically blenderized foods to spoon-thick consistency	Mashed potato, pureed hamburger, pureed peas, pudding	Chewing or swallowing difficulties	Avoid more texture modification than is needed. Ensure attractive eating environment to improve visual appeal of diet.
House or regular	All foods	Full choice of available menu items in all food groups	No condition requiring diet modification	Provides complete nutrition. Monitor tolerance and intake.

(Centers for Disease Control and Prevention [CDC], 2001). Reliance on technology, the automobile, and energy-saving devices has made it easier to expend less energy to do work and leisure activities (Nestle & Jacobson, 2000). "Screen time" watching television, videos, or computer games has been linked to obesity in adults and children (Hu et al., 2001; Hu, Li, Colditz, Willett, & Manson, 2003; Shields, 2006).

A nutrition assessment focusing on parameters to measure weight status is an intuitive step before determining treatment interventions for the overweight patient. Overweight is defined as a BMI of 25 to 29.9. Obesity is defined as a BMI greater than 30. Additional stratification exists to denote different classes of obesity. Chart 14–6 lists BMI classifications. Figure 14–1 ■ (p. 275) illustrates BMI calculations and classifications. In the

CHART 14–6	BMI Classifications	
BMI	**Classification**	
18.5–24.9	Normal	
25–29.9	Overweight	
30–34.9	Obese class 1	
35–39.9	Obese class 2	
≥40	Obese class 3	

Source: National Heart, Lung, and Blood Institute. (1998). *Clinical guidelines on the identification, evaluation, and treatment of overweight and obesity in adults—the evidence report.* Retrieved February 5, 2004, from www.nhlbi.nih.gov/guidelines/obesity/ob_gdlns.pdf

past, height–weight tables were used to determine appropriate weight and to diagnose overweight. These tables have been replaced by the BMI table in the clinical setting.

Other considerations to include in the assessment process are the presence of obesity risk factors, weight and dieting history (including failures and successes), and patient readiness to attempt weight loss. The nurse needs to assess the patient's readiness for weight loss based on the Stages of Change model. This model can be used to assess readiness for any behavior change and categorizes individuals according to where they are on a spectrum of thinking or action about new behavior using the terms precontemplation, contemplation, action, and maintenance (Kushner, 2003). Patients not ready or unwilling to attempt weight loss should be encouraged to prevent further weight gain (NHLBI, 1998; Serdula, Kettel Khan, & Dietz, 2003). Figure 14–2 ■ (p. 283) shows an algorithm developed by the NIH for weight loss treatment. Chart 14–7 (p. 282) outlines important factors to consider when assessing a patient before weight loss intervention.

The nurse can guide the patient in establishing a reasonable weight loss goal. Generally a goal of 5% to 10% loss of weight is recommended over a 6-month period and is associated with a reduction in health risks associated with obesity (NHLBI, 1998). Many patients wish to attempt a larger weight loss, but this should be discouraged because weight loss maintenance of larger losses can prove frustrating and difficult and lead to weight regain (American Dietetic Association, 2002b; Serdula et al., 2003). The nurse should encourage the patient to attempt weight loss by stressing the associated health benefits with even

CHART 14–7 **Assessment of Patients Who Are Overweight or Obese for Weight Loss Intervention**

Assess for obesity comorbidities.

Assess anthropometrics:
- Weight, weight history, maximum and minimum adult weights
- BMI and waist circumference.

Assess dieting history:
- Amount, frequency, duration, and types of diets
- Use of supplements, devices, or medications for weight loss
- Contributors to weight gain or regain
- Barriers to weight loss or maintenance in past and currently
- Source of information on dieting and nutrition.

Assess current eating according to Chart 14–3.

Assess for symptoms of disordered eating or binge eating.

Assess psychosocial influences:
- Social support
- Financial implications of weight loss treatment
- Readiness, motivation to change.

Assess physical activity frequency, intensity, and duration.

Sources: Kushner, R. F. (2003). *Roadmaps for clinical practice—Case studies in disease prevention and health promotion: Assessment and management of adult obesity—A primer for physicians.* Chicago, IL: American Medical Association. Retrieved December 18, 2003, from http://www.ama-assn.org/ama/pub/category/10931.html; American Dietetic Association 2002; National Institute of Health, National Heart, Lung, and Blood Institute. (NHLBI). (1998). *Clinical guidelines on the identification, evaluation, and treatment of overweight and obesity in adults—The evidence report.* Retrieved February 5, 2004, from http://www.nhlbi.nih.gov/guidelines/obesity/ob_gdlns.pdf; Serdula, M. K., Kettel Khan, L., & Dietz, W. H. (2003). Weight loss counseling revisited. *Journal of the American Medical Association, 289,* 1747–1750.

modest loss. Less than half of obese patients surveyed reported being advised by a health care provider to lose weight (Jackson, Doescher, Saver, & Hart, 2005).

An energy deficit of 500 to 1,000 kilocalories per day can result in weight loss of between 1 to 2 pounds per week. This deficit is best accomplished with a combination of decreased intake and increased energy expenditure (NHLBI, 1998). Any diet with a lower calorie intake than at baseline will produce weight loss. Most current research supports the idea than macronutrient composition (amount of carbohydrate, protein, or fat) does not play a major role, but rather overall calorie deficit does (Freedman, King, & Kennedy, 2001). In published reports of popular low-carbohydrate diets, subjects indeed lost weight but this was reportedly because of an overall reduction in calorie intake and not the carbohydrate content alone (Bravata et al., 2003; Foster et al., 2003; Samaha et al., 2003). Fad and fringe diets may target macronutrient composition or the "magical" combining powers of foods. Those that lead to successful weight loss do so because of calorie reduction and the self-limiting nature of their diet restrictions.

Low-calorie diets occur along a continuum from starvation or fasting to the recommended modest calorie reduction of 500 to 1,000 kilocalories per day. Extreme calorie reduction can lead to unhealthy loss of muscle mass, minerals, electrolytes, and water. In select obese patients, extremely low calorie diets (those with <1,000 kilocalories per day) are used, but with close medical supervision to monitor fluid and electrolyte status as well as general health. Such diets are not recommended for long-term

success (American Dietetic Association, 2002b). Targeting high-fat foods and empty calorie foods with little nutritional content can accomplish a 500- to 1,000-kilocalorie daily reduction in intake. Foods can be replaced with lower calorie foods or omitted. The choices should be realistic and sensible and not contribute to an overall sense of deprivation. Chart 14–8 (p. 284) outlines some examples of lower calorie food swaps.

Some patients want or need the structure of a more formal diet when attempting weight loss. The nurse can educate patients about the components of a healthy diet and guide them in an evaluation of any popular diet they are considering. Chart 14–9 (p. 284) outlines the components of a healthy weight loss diet. Patients who need extensive nutrition guidance and education should be referred to a registered dietitian. Commercial programs are also available for the patient who may benefit from the weekly social support. The nurse can guide the patient to an appropriate individual treatment choice.

Physical activity and a reduction in sedentary activity should be encouraged. Adults with long-term success at weigh loss report ongoing physical activity as a major contributing factor (McInnis, Franklin, & Rippe, 2003). Physical activity has a positive effect on energy balance and can improve body composition and cardiovascular fitness. Weight loss without a physical activity component can lead to loss of lean body mass and a reduced metabolic rate; in contrast, including exercise helps to preserve lean mass (McInnis et al., 2003). The nurse should emphasize the importance of physical activity in preventing weight regain. Exercise can be initiated slowly to eventually accumulate at least 30 minutes of moderate intensity exercise on most days (NHLBI, 1998). Even activities such as walking can replace sedentary activities such as riding an elevator or driving. The nurse can explore any barriers to increasing activity with the patient and offer suggestions tailored to the patient.

Behavior modification is essential for long-term weight loss maintenance and relapse prevention. Weight loss maintenance is a bigger challenge than the initial weight loss for many patients. A lifestyle approach to weight maintenance and healthy social support and coping mechanisms are important. Chart 14–10 (p. 284) outlines behavior modification use in weight loss.

Approved pharmacological treatment for obesity is reserved for patients with a BMI ≥ 30 with no obesity comorbidities or a BMI ≥27 if comorbidities exist. Lifestyle diet and exercise modifications should first be attempted for at least 6 months before considering adjunctive medication (NHLBI, 1998; Yanovski & Yanovski, 2002). Pharmacological treatment is not appropriate for cosmetic weight loss attempts.

Bariatric surgery is a treatment option for select clinically severe obese patients (BMI ≥ 40 or >35 with comorbidities). Gastric reduction surgery, including vertical banded gastroplasty, and gastric bypass surgery, such as the Roux-en-Y procedure, are types of bariatric surgery. Weight loss occurs over many months postoperatively. Bypass procedures produce greater weight loss than simpler gastric reduction surgery (American Society for Metabolic and Bariatric Surgery, 2005). Patients undergoing bariatric surgery require intensive presurgical screening and lifelong medical monitoring because of possible short- and long-term health complications (Garza, 2003). Nutrition guidelines following bariatric surgery are discussed later in this chapter.

FIGURE 14–2 ■ Obesity treatment algorithm.

Source: From National Institutes of Health website: http://www.nhlbi.nih.gov/guidelines/obesity/ob_gdlns.pdf

The nurse should be aware of the many alternative approaches to weight loss that a patient may pursue. Nutrition and herbal supplements, fad diets, and various devices are marketed to the patient as alternative and often "no effort" methods to lose weight. Federal regulation of supplements is minimal because these products are regulated as food and not medicine by the Food and Drug Administration (FDA). The Federal Trade Commission regulates the advertising of such products, however, and

CHART 14–8 Calorie-Saving Examples for Weight Loss Intervention

Original Food	Alternative Food Suggestion	Approximate Calories Saved
1 C whole milk	1 C skim milk	65
1 C premium ice cream, vanilla	1 C low-fat soft-serve frozen yogurt, vanilla	300
2 TBSP cream cheese	2 TBSP fat-free cream cheese	70
2 TBSP half-and-half coffee creamer	2 TBSP fat-free half-and-half creamer	30
3 oz chicken thigh w/skin, roasted	3 oz chicken breast, skinless, roasted	90
4 oz pork sparerib, braised	4 oz pork tenderloin, trimmed, braised	233
Bagel, 4-1/2-in. diameter	2 English muffin halves	100
Yellow cake, no frosting, 1/12 of 8-in. cake	Angelfood cake, no frosting, 1/12 of 10-in. cake	115
Vanilla crème cookie, 1-3/4 in.	Vanilla wafers, 1 medium	30
1 TBSP oil for sautéing	Cooking spray for sautéing	100
2 TBSP mayonnaise	2 TBSP reduced-calorie mayonnaise	100
2 TBSP Ranch salad dressing	2 TBSP fat-free Ranch salad dressing	100

Note: Not all fat-free or reduced fat foods are lower in calories than the original version. The nurse should instruct patients to compare labels.

Source: USDA Nutrient Data Laboratory http://www.nal.usda.gov/fnic/foodcomp/search

CHART 14–9 Components of a Healthy Weight Loss Diet

- Contains foods from all the major food groups.
- Diet is practical and realistic; can be adhered to without social interruption.
- Fosters no more than a 2 lb per week weight loss on average; higher losses can yield loss of muscle, fluid and electrolytes.
- Emphasis on lean sources of protein: skinless poultry, fish, lean meats, legumes.
- Fruits, vegetables, and whole grains emphasized.
- Intake of 20 to 35 g fiber daily encouraged.
- Adequate low-fat sources of calcium included: nonfat or low-fat milk, yogurt, cheese, or dairy alternatives such as fortified soy milk.
- Adequate water intake of at least 64 oz daily.
- Limited alcohol, if any.
- Minimizes intake of saturated fat, total fat, cholesterol, and sodium.
- Place emphasis on portion sizes.
- No skipped meals; avoids becoming overhungry and overeating as result. Some protein with each meal may satiate longer than an all-carbohydrate meal.
- Physical activity is encouraged.

Sources: Kushner, R. F. (2003). *Roadmaps for clinical practice—Case studies in disease prevention and health promotion: Assessment and management of adult obesity—A primer for physicians.* Chicago, IL: American Medical Association. Retrieved December 18, 2003, from http://www.ama-assn.org/ama/pub/category/10931.html; Jackic, J. M., Clark, K., Coleman, E., et al. (2001). American College of Sports Medicine position stand on the appropriate intervention strategies for weight loss and prevention of weight regain in adults. *Medicine, Science, Sports and Exercise, 33,* 2145–2156; National Institute of Health, National Heart, Lung, and Blood Institute. (2000). *The practical guide: Identification, evaluation and treatment of overweight and obesity in adults.* Retrieved February 5, 2004, from http://www.nhlbi.nih.gov/guidelines/obesity/practgde.htm

CHART 14–10 Behavior Modification in Weight Management

- Allow patient to set goals.
- Encourage self-monitoring of goals; e.g., food diaries and activity logs.
- Identify small steps to take toward daily lifestyle changes.
- Identify environmental cues and contributors to old eating habits. Develop ideas for new cues for exercise and eating habits.
- Discuss and brainstorm coping strategies for relapse prevention: stress management, social support, dealing with boredom or emotions.
- Cognitive restructuring; change self-talk that undermines weight loss or exercise.
- Encourage self-reinforcement; give nonfood rewards when milestones are reached.

Sources: Poston, W. S. C., & Foreyt, J. P. (2000). Successful management of the obese patient. *American Family Physician, 61,* 3615–3622; McInnis, K. J., Franklin, B. A., & Rippe, J. M. (2003). Counseling for physical activity in overweight and obese patients. *American Family Physician, 67,* 1266–1268; National Heart, Lung, and Blood Institute. (1998). *Clinical guidelines on the identification, evaluation, and treatment of overweight and obesity in adults—The evidence report.* Retrieved February 5, 2004, from http://www.nhlbi.nih.gov/guidelines/obesity/ob_gdlns.pdf; National Heart, Lung, and Blood Institute. (2000). *The practical guide: Identification, evaluation and treatment of overweight and obesity in adults.* Retrieved February 5, 2004, from http://www.nhlbi.nih.gov/guidelines/obesity/practgde.htm

Weight management for elderly adults is presented in the Gerontological Considerations box and a patient care plan for obesity is presented in the Nursing Process feature (p. 286).

Disordered Eating

Disordered eating consists of behavioral, psychological, and physical symptoms that surround abnormal perceptions regarding food and body weight. Disordered eating patterns occur along a continuum from minor alterations in food-related behaviors to a clinical eating disorder that meets all established diagnostic criteria. Clinical eating disorders include anorexia nervosa, bulimia nervosa, and eating-disorders-not-otherwise-specified (ED-NOS), which includes binge-eating disorder and disordered eat-

can pursue a manufacturer for flagrantly misleading advertising. Patients need to be educated to view such products with a critical eye. Chart 14–11 outlines examples of alternative products marketed for weight loss, and Chart 14–12 provides educational pointers for evaluating alternative products.

Sample Alternative Diet Products (Found Alone or in Combination Products)

Product	Purported Action	Clinical Evidence or Alert
Chitosan	Weight loss from fat "trapping"	Lack of sufficient research. Caution if shellfish allergy. Can alter medication absorption.
Chromium	Lose fat and gain muscle	Deficiency of mineral uncommon. Little evidence products available alter body composition.
Ephedra	Weight loss stimulant	FDA banned the sale of ephedra because of risk of morbidity and mortality from vascular events.
Ginseng	Energy booster	Limited research, little evidence it ↑ energy. Can interact with medication, coagulation.
Hydroxycitric acid or garcinia	Inhibits enzymes of fat metabolism	Controlled trials do not support benefit.
Vanadium	Increase muscle	Limited research showing little to no effect on muscle. Can interact with coagulation.
Mate, guarana, kola nut, green tea	Caffeine-like stimulants of metabolism	Exert caffeine-like effect on central nervous system. Can potentiate other stimulant ingredients. Side effects on blood pressure (BP) and heart rate mimic those of excess caffeine. Labels do not list cumulative "caffeine" equivalent.

Sources: Food and Drug Administration. (2004). *FDA issues regulation prohibiting sale of dietary supplements containing ephedrine alkaloids and reiterates its advice that consumers stop using these products.* News release, retrieved February 6, 2004, from http://www.cfsan.fda.gov/~lrd/fpephed6.html; Morelli, V., & Zoorob, R. J. (2000). Alternative therapies: Part 1. Depression, diabetes, obesity. *American Family Physician, 62,* 1051–1060; Roerig, J. L., Mitchell, J. E., deZwaan, M., Wonderlich, S. A., et al. (2003). The eating disorders medicine cabinet revisited: A clinician's guide to appetite suppressants and diuretics. *International Journal of Eating Disorders, 33,* 443–457; Sarubin Fragakis, A. (2003). *The Health Professional's Guide to Popular Dietary Supplements* (2nd ed.). Chicago, IL: American Dietetic Association.

CHART 14–12   Spotting Quackery in Weight Loss Products

- Weight loss claim is "too good to be true."
- Quick dramatic results are promised with little or no effort.
- Miracle blocking or trapping of fat or carbohydrates is claimed.
- Weight loss occurs while you can eat all you want.
- The product is worn or rubbed on skin and causes weight loss without diet or exercise.
- Pseudomedical jargon is used to infer scientific expertise.
- Anecdotes and testimonials are touted instead of peer-reviewed controlled studies.
- Advertising is condescending to established medical treatment. Claims of hidden medical secret are made.
- Food or groups of foods are labeled as toxic or "poisonous to the system."
- Special powers or attributes are assigned to certain foods (e.g., grapefruit burns fat).

Federal Trade Commission (2003). *Red flag bogus weight loss claims.* Retrieved May 30, 2008 from http://www.ftc.gov/bcp/conline/pubs/buspubs/redflag.pdf

 GERONTOLOGICAL CONSIDERATIONS
Weight Management

Adults over age 65 years can benefit from weight management with improved day-to-day functioning and reduced cardiovascular risk. Before weight loss is recommended or attempted, however, a thorough nutrition assessment should be considered because of the high prevalence of malnutrition among older adults. Improper dieting attempts could unwittingly contribute to increased risk of malnutrition. Patients should be evaluated for their individual risks and benefits associated with potential weight loss. Specific attention should be given to preservation of muscle mass with physical activity. Appropriate referrals should be made for monitoring nutrition and exercise in the elderly.

ing not meeting the strict criteria for anorexia or bulimia. Criteria for clinical diagnoses are outlined in the *Diagnostic and Statistical Manual of Mental Disorders, Fourth Edition, Text Revision* (DSM-IV) (American Psychiatric Association [APA], 2000a).

Eating disorders are prevalent in up to 5% of the U.S. population (American Dietetic Association, 2001). Much debate surrounds the etiology of these complex disorders. Biology (including genetics), psychology, and sociocultural influences have all received attention as contributors (Fairburn & Harrison, 2003). More than half of patients with bulimia and almost half of patients with binge-eating disorder have substance abuse disorder. Obsessive-compulsive disorder, anxiety, depression, and other mood disorders are prevalent in all forms of eating disorders (APA, 2000b; American Dietetic Association, 2001; Pritts & Susman, 2003). Chart 14–13 (p. 286) lists population groups felt to be at higher risk for an eating disorder. When conducting a nursing assessment, these groups should be screened for eating disorder signs and symptoms.

Although eating disorders are considered a psychiatric diagnosis, medical and nutritional complications often place the patient in the medical care setting. It is important for the nurse to recognize the physical symptoms when assessing patients and to be involved in the medical and nutritional interventions of any treatment.

Anorexia Nervosa

Patients with anorexia nervosa are at 85% or less of expected body weight yet have an intense fear of gaining weight and a disturbed

MyNursingKit | Video: Nutrition: Eating Disorders—Anorexia

Populations at Risk for Eating Disorders

Athletes in sports with

- Subjective scoring (e.g., figure skating, gymnastics)
- Performance thinness philosophy (e.g., dance, distance running)
- Contour-revealing clothing (e.g., cheer leading, swim, dance)
- Emphasis on prepubescent body (e.g., gymnastics, figure skating)
- Weight categories (e.g., rowing, wrestling).

Fashion models

People who are obese

Young people with limited diets because of disease (e.g., diabetes)

Family history of mood, anxiety disorder, substance abuse

Family environment of adverse, critical, controlling, or distance parenting; family dieting; comments on physical appearance

Sources: American Dietetic Association. (2001). Position of the American Dietetic Association: Nutrition intervention in the treatment of anorexia nervosa, bulimia nervosa, and eating disorders not otherwise specified (EDNOS). *Journal of the American Dietetic Association, 101,* 810–819; Fairburn, C. G., & Harrison, P. J. (2003). Eating disorders. *Lancet, 361,* 407–416; McNulty, K. Y., Adams, C. H., Anderson, J. M., & Affenito, S. G. (2001). Development and validation of a screening tool to identify eating disorders in female athletes. *Journal of the American Dietetic Association, 101,* 886–892; Rubenstein, S., & Caballero, B. (2000). Is Miss America an undernourished role model? *Journal of the American Medical Association, 283,* 1569.

body image. Weight loss can have occurred as a result of restrictive dieting, excessive exercise, or a combination of both. A BMI ≤17.5 is considered indicative of anorexia (American Dietetic Association, 2001; Becker, Grinspoon, Kilbanski, & Herzog, 1999). Other physical symptoms that may be present on a physical exam are listed in Chart 14–14 (p. 289). During the focused interview, the nurse can use established screening tools to assess for disordered eating or simply rely on informal questions on eating and exercise patterns, dieting behaviors, perception of body weight, and proper nutrition. A vegetarian diet is used by some as a method of masking restrictive eating (Klopp, Heiss, & Smith, 2003). Suspicion of disordered eating accompanied by a new vegetarian lifestyle should be investigated further.

Comprehensive evaluation tools exist but are cumbersome in the primary care setting and best intended for use by mental health professionals (Pritts & Susman, 2003). A quick screening tool appropriate in the medical setting is the SCOFF screening instrument outlined in Chart 14–15 (p. 289) (Morgan, Reid, & Lacy, 1999; Perry et al., 2002). Some patients do not present with symptoms that meet the strict DSM-IV criteria but have abnormal eating or exercise patterns and a significant weight loss history. The nurse should use sound judgment in determining

NURSING PROCESS: Patient Care Plan for Obesity

Assessment of Current Nutritional Status

Subjective Data:

Have you recently gained or lost weight?

Do you prepare your own meals?

How often do you eat in restaurants?

Do you live/eat alone?

Do you have a regular meal schedule? What is it?

Do you eat during the night?

Objective Data:

Current measured weight in pounds/height with minimal clothing and after urination

Serial weights from medical records

Presence of abdominal adiposity

Nursing Assessment and Diagnoses	Outcomes and Evaluation Parameters	Planning and Interventions with *Rationales*
Nursing Diagnosis: *Imbalanced Nutrition: More than Body Requirements* related to imbalance in dietary requirements and energy requirements	**Outcome:** Balanced nutrition ***Evaluation Parameters:*** Maintaining BMI within normal range.	**Interventions and *Rationales:*** Perform a complete physical assessment and nutritional history on admission *to assess current nutritional status and to provide a nutritional baseline of data.* Calculate BMI to determine overweight/obesity status. Current weight is compared to BMI charts, height weight charts, and waist measurement *to determine degree of overweight status, overweight, obese, or morbidly obese.* Measure waist circumference *to determine cardiovascular disease risk.* Differentiate weight gain of obesity from weight gain of edema, and other nonadiposity causes *to determine cause of weight gain.*

Assessment of Current Nutritional and Dietary Intake

Subjective Data:

24-hour and possibly 3-day recall of all meals, snacks, liquids

Location of meals

Method of food preparation

Portion size

Meals missed

Other factors that may influence intake, such as recent acute illness or cultural or religious influences on food intake patterns.

Alcohol intake

Objective Data:

Ask spouse or significant other to validate data if patient agrees

NURSING PROCESS: Patient Care Plan for Obesity—*Continued*

Nursing Assessment and Diagnoses	Outcomes and Evaluation Parameters	Planning and Interventions with *Rationales*
Nursing Diagnosis: *Imbalanced Nutrition: More Than Body Requirements* related to individual factors and patterns in food preparation and eating styles	**Outcome:** Patient lists all foods honestly so that a true intake record is gathered. ***Evaluation Parameters:*** Patient aware of sources of intake and eating habits. Patient states motivation to change unhealthy habits.	**Interventions and *Rationales:*** List food intake for the past 24 hours and the past 3 days *to determine patterns, frequency of certain foods, location of meals, and intake patterns that place patient at high risk for increased nutritional intake.* Observe and identify possible patterns of food intake such as nighttime eating, eating while driving, eating while watching television *to determine total calorie intake and patient's awareness, or lack there of, about the amount of intake.* Keeps a food diary of frequency of intake of high-calorie items *to determine calorie intake.*

Assessment of Disease Risk Factors Influenced by Overweight Status

Subjective Data:

Do you have diabetes?
Is there a history of diabetes in your family?
When was the last time you had your blood sugar tested and what were the results?
Do you have high blood pressure?
When was the last time you had your blood pressure checked and what was the reading?
Do you have any problems with your heart?
When was your last physical examination?
What medications do you take?

Objective Data:

Cholesterol level
Triglyceride level
Blood glucose level
Blood pressure
Medication evaluation

Nursing Assessment and Diagnoses	Outcomes and Evaluation Parameters	Planning and Interventions with *Rationales*
Nursing Diagnosis: Health Maintenance Ineffective risk related to known risk factors for chronic diseases based on overweight status	**Outcomes:** Patient is able to verbalize risk for cardiac disease. Patient establishes a short-term and a long-term weight loss goal that is realistic. ***Evaluation Parameters:*** Verbalization allows the patient to admit that weight is problematic in terms of health status. Verbalizes understanding of impact of excess weight on health status.	**Interventions and *Rationales:*** Ask patient what disease risk factors are related to overweight status. *This question elicits the patient's understanding of how overweight status may affect health status.* Establish a weight goal that is reasonable and achievable *to reduce disease risks.*

Assessment of Changes That Can Be Made in Food Intake to Lower Caloric Intake, Including Patient Readiness to Change Food Intake

Subjective Data:

List the foods you typically eat daily.
Is there a particular food that you eat in excess when you are stressed, sick, or disturbed about something?
What activities do you do when you are stressed?
Do you increase your food intake when stressed?
Do you feel a need to change your dietary habits?
Are you motivated to learn new habits and try instituting them?
Do you have an exercise program?
Are you interested in starting an exercise program?

Objective Data:

Caloric intake per 24 hours based on above food diary
Cholesterol and fat grams in food
Carbohydrate counting
BMI
Daily, weekly, and/or monthly weigh-ins

(continued)

NURSING PROCESS: Patient Care Plan for Obesity—*Continued*

Nursing Assessment and Diagnoses	Outcomes and Evaluation Parameters	Planning and Interventions with *Rationales*
Nursing Diagnosis: *Impaired Home Maintenance* related to changes in eating patterns that may affect lifestyle, planning, and financial matters	**Outcomes:** Begins and maintains a change in eating habits. Develops healthy choices to deal with stress. ***Evaluation Parameters:*** Patient can write down changes in food intake that he/she is willing to do in order to lose weight. Keeps weight loss records, measure body circumference area, for progress toward goal. Writes daily weight in a weight loss calendar/diary. Loses 1–2 lb of weight per week.	**Interventions and *Rationales:*** Determine caloric intake for 24-hour period based on patient's size and weight goals. *Weight loss of 7%–10% has been recommended to be a manageable level to achieve and maintain and will also provide a benefit in glucose levels for those who have prediabetes or overt diabetes.* Provide some simple ways to lower caloric counts (e.g., removing skin from chicken, avoiding fried foods, avoiding extra fat and caloric intake such as butter and jelly). *Most nutritious foods can be reduced in terms of calories by the method of preparation and the patient will not feel deprived.* Recommend using a support group *to provide emotional support while losing weight.* Teach patient to eat nutritious foods when hungry at regular times. *This strategy will help patient avoid food items with high caloric value and little to no nutritional value (e.g., cake, donuts, chips, etc.).* Teach the patient who wants a structured diet to count calories, carbohydrates, and/or fat grams in food. *Some patients benefit more from a structured weight loss plan, whereas others prefer less structure.* Teach patient recommendations regarding cholesterol and saturated fat intake. Discuss an exercise program and set realistic goals *to increase calorie burning and promote a healthy lifestyle.* Encourage cues to weight loss action, such as keeping a food diary and putting reminders on the refrigerator regarding physical activity. *Cues to action serve as reminders for health promotion behaviors.* Teach patient to avoid triggers to overeating *to prevent weight gain.* Increase activities that are enjoyable other than eating *to minimize food intake.*

Assessment of Activity Level

Subjective Data:
Do you exercise; if so, what type?
How many times per week do you exercise?
Do you take your pulse during and after exercise?

Objective Data:
Pedometer readings
Documented visits to personal health trainer

Nursing Assessment and Diagnoses	Outcomes and Evaluation Parameters	Planning and Interventions with *Rationales*
Nursing Diagnosis: *Activity intolerance* related to lack of motivation and current health status	**Outcome:** Patient walks at least 30 minutes per day at least four times per week. ***Evaluation Parameters:*** Activity log shows daily entries of time engaged in activity. Activity levels show a steady increase in time and distance achieved.	**Interventions and *Rationales:*** Encourage 30 minutes of physical activity most days of the week, *which will tone the body and assist in weight loss.* If patient has been physically inactive previously, activity levels should gradually increase *to prevent activity intolerance and cardiac stress.*

Assessment of Knowledge Regarding Surgical Methods of Weight Loss

Subjective Data:
What are your thoughts on surgical intervention for weight loss?
Do you have questions about the various procedures?

Objective Data:
Patient inquires of health provider about suitability of these methods for himself.
Patient attends a surgical information session.

NURSING PROCESS: Patient Care Plan for Obesity—*Continued*

Nursing Assessment and Diagnoses	Outcomes and Evaluation Parameters	Planning and Interventions with *Rationales*
Nursing Diagnosis: *Deficient Knowledge* regarding surgical weight loss methods	**Outcome:** Patient verbalizes knowledge regarding various surgical techniques. *Evaluation Parameters:* Patient states will continue to consider surgical means if weight loss is unsuccessful.	**Interventions and *Rationales:*** Discuss the surgical means of weight loss, including lap band surgery and intestinal bypass *to help patient understand the new concepts of surgical intervention.* Discuss the pros and cons of weight loss surgery *to assist the patient in being well informed.* Emphasize the importance of using medical means of weight loss until a decision is reached about the appropriateness of surgery for the patient. *The patient needs to understand that surgical interventions take time to consider and that surgery is more successful with fewer complications if about 10% of body weight has been lost prior to surgery by conventional means.*

CHART 14–14   Symptoms of Eating Disorders

Disorder	Potential Physical Findings
Anorexia/restrictive eating	Alopecia Lanugo (soft light hair growth on body) Dry skin Cold intolerance, loss of subcutaneous fat Hypotension Bradycardia Amenorrhea in nonpregnant women Muscle mass and strength loss Fatigue Pedal edema GI complaints: bloating, constipation
Bulimia/binge–purge behavior	Swollen parotid glands Dental enamel erosion Poor or absent gag reflex Bloodshot eyes, broken blood vessels on face Hoarse voice Scarred knuckle calluses on dorsal surface of hand Weight fluctuations GI complaints: reflux, bloating, constipation

CHART 14–15   SCOFF Tool for Screening for Eating Disorders

Do you make yourself **S**ick (induce vomiting) because you feel uncomfortably full?

Do you worry you have lost **C**ontrol over how much you eat?

Have you recently lost more than **O**ne stone (14 lb) in a 3-month period?

Do you feel yourself to be **F**at when others say you are too thin?

Would you say that **F**ood dominates your life?

Scoring: One point for every yes. A score $\geq$ 2 indicates a likely case of anorexia or bulimia.

British Medical Journal, 1999, 319:1467–1468. Morgan J. F. Reid F, Lacey J. H. (1999) The SCOFF questionnaire: Assessment of a new screening tool for eating disorders. Reproduced with permission from the BMJ Publishing Group.

whether the patient is at risk for an eating disorder or in need of further evaluation for psychiatric, medical, or nutritional issues.

Anorexia nervosa is treated either in the inpatient or outpatient setting depending on the severity of symptoms. Outpatient care is preferred unless the patient is refractory to treatment with a weight of less than 75% expected or has an emergent mental health event or severe cardiovascular risk, such as bradycardia (<40 beats/min), hypotension (<60 systolic) or hypokalemia (<3 mg/dL). Hypothermia (36°C [<97°F]) is also indicative of need for inpatient treatment (APA, 2000b). A team approach to treatment is recommended because of the complex medical, psychiatric, and nutritional issues; no one clinician or profession is solely able to provide the scope of care required. Goals for treatment include cessation of weight reduction and weight reduction behaviors, weight restoration, improved behaviors related to food and eating, and improvement of any medical or psychiatric conditions (American Dietetic Association, 2001; APA, 2000b).

Nutrition intervention in anorexia initially focuses on cessation of weight loss and then restoration of body weight. Outpatient weight restoration is recommended at 1 to 2 pounds per week; inpatient restoration of 2 to 3 pounds per week can be safely monitored (American Dietetic Association, 2001). Determination of the appropriate meal plan and its progression is the responsibility of the dietitian (American Dietetic Association, 2001; APA, 2000b). The nurse plays an important role in educating the patient on the physiological symptoms and consequences of starvation, reinforcing and monitoring the nutrition plan (including assessing for excessive exercise or squirreling away of uneaten food in the inpatient setting), monitoring for changes in vital signs and body weight, and assessing for symptoms of refeeding syndrome. **Refeeding syndrome** can occur following starvation and reintroduction of fuel in any medical or surgical situation, including eating disorders. As fuel substrate is reintroduced to the body and metabolism increases, fluid and electrolyte shifts can occur. Serum phosphorous levels can become dangerously low as new ATP is generated. The Critical Alert outlines essential assessment data when refeeding begins. The Nursing Process Patient Care Plan (p. 291) outlines nursing management of the weight loss patient.

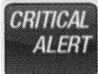 *Patients with refeeding syndrome are at risk for cardiac dysrhythmia and sudden death. The nurse needs to assess the patient for the following symptoms (American Dietetic Association, 2001; APA, 2000b; Crook et al., 2001; Ornstein et al., 2003):*

- *Hypophosphatemia*
- *Hypokalemia*
- *Hypomagnesemia*
- *Cardiac dysrhythmia, specifically prolonged QT interval*
- *Edema (can be normal part of refeeding; monitor for presence with other symptoms)*
- *Heart failure.*

Food intake is increased gradually in both the inpatient and outpatient setting to avoid refeeding syndrome and to allow the patient to become comfortable physically and emotionally with increased intake. Use of food, and not tube feedings or parenteral nutrition, is the recommended route for nutrition intervention unless the patient is acutely refusing food (APA, 2000b). This allows for addressing food phobias and assists with eating behavior change. Prescriptive limits or avoidance of exercise is included in the treatment of those patients who exercise excessively. As the patient's condition improves, exercise limitations can slowly be lifted.

The treatment team determines which clinician is most appropriate for monitoring ongoing weight and whether the patient will learn weight measurements or be "blinded" (weighed while standing backwards on the scale). These determinations are made individually. When weighing patients, the nurse should ensure that weights are done in a private setting and not in a common area. The patient should wear minimal clothing and void before the weight measure. Some patients will drink excessive amounts of liquids before being weighed. The voided urine can be assessed for specific gravity to determine if this is happening. An assessment should be done for any hidden weights in or under clothing or undergarments. Weight alone should not be the sole parameter used to determine recovery.

Bulimia Nervosa

Bulimia nervosa is prevalent in 5% of the U.S. population and is characterized by chaotic eating patterns such as binge eating and compensatory purging, and is accompanied by a sense of loss of control as a result (American Dietetic Association, 2001). Patients with bulimia often have a personal set of "rules" governing "good" and "bad" foods and amounts of food. It is not uncommon for patients with bulimia to be restrictive eaters when not bingeing. Binges can be triggered by a perception of breaking such a "rule," hunger from restrictive eating, perceived fullness, or an emotional cause. Compensatory action can be purging with self-induced vomiting, laxative use, diuretic use, or excessive exercise. At-risk patients should be assessed for use of over-the-counter, prescription, and alternative medicine versions of laxatives and diuretics. Assessment should also include whether syrup of ipecac is used because it has negative cardiovascular effects such as cardiomyopathy (Mehler, 2003). Type, duration, and frequency of exercise should be ascertained as well.

DSM-IV criteria call for binge–purge behavior at least twice a week for 6 months. The nurse may find on assessment that patients engage in this behavior more frequently but not for 6 months duration. Some patients purge up to 10 times in a day (Mehler, 2003). Any binge–purge behavior is deserving of further evaluation. Symptoms of bulimia are subtler than with anorexia. Patients with bulimia are often of normal weight or slightly overweight, making assessment more difficult. Symptomology depends on mode and duration of compensatory purging (Mehler, 2003). Signs and symptoms of bulimia nervosa are listed in Chart 14–14 (p. 289).

Nutrition intervention for bulimia centers on normalizing eating patterns to interrupt the binge–purge cycle. This includes avoidance of hunger and chaotic eating patterns and slow reintroduction of forbidden foods. Generally a more structured eating pattern is prescribed by the dietitian to meet this goal. Finger foods are avoided because portion control is difficult. When excessive exercise is used as a compensatory purging method, prescriptive limits are generally placed on activity. The nurse can be instrumental in reinforcing the meal pattern to encourage avoidance of long time spans between eating. A food record can be helpful to assess this.

Corrections of misconceptions about weight and nutrition are also important. The nurse can educate the patient about normal transient symptoms to expect with the normalization of eating patterns. These include water retention (which will worsen if fluid is restricted or diuretics or laxatives abused) and bloating from delayed gastric emptying or from constipation with laxative reliance. Additionally, the nurse can be effective in counseling the patient who abuses laxatives or diuretics as to the ineffectiveness of those treatments in eliminating calories or fat from the body, in addition to their medical dangers. A high-fiber and high-fluid diet should be encouraged for the patient who is weaning from laxative abuse.

Binge-Eating Disorder

Binge-eating disorder (BED) is prevalent in up to 2% of the U.S. population (American Dietetic Association, 2001). BED is characterized by the same type of binge eating as bulimia nervosa but without the compensatory purging. Most patients with binge-eating disorder are overweight (American Dietetic Association, 2001). Increased focus is pointing to the effects of chronic restrained eating, increased prevalence in some families, and depression and other psychiatric diagnoses as contributing to binge eating (Hudson et al., 2006; Meno, Hannum, Espelage, & Douglas Low, 2008). The nurse should screen obese patients who may be at risk for binge-eating disorder (Striegel-Moore et al., 2003).

Treatment of binge-eating disorder involves medical treatment of any complications of obesity, psychological treatment of any underlying mental health issues, and nutrition treatment to normalize eating patterns. It is under debate whether any attempt at weight loss should occur during binge-eating treatment or be delayed until behaviors are stabilized (American

NURSING PROCESS: Patient Care Plan for Malnutrition (Undernutrition)

Assessment of Current Nutritional Status

Subjective Data:
Have you lost weight in the last 3 months, if so how much?
Have you changed your eating habits in the last 3 months?
Do you have any discomfort such as pain or bloating after you eat? Does it occur with any particular type of food?
Ask patient or family how long nutritional intake has been reduced to help determine severity of malnutrition.

Objective Data:
Patient has experienced an unintentional weight loss of >5% or more in 1 month or >10% in 3 months
Current measured weight and height compared to standardized tables of measurement
BMI < 18.5 kg/m^2
Gastrointestinal symptoms including constipation, diarrhea, pain or cramping
List of current medications that can cause nutritional side effects (diarrhea, loss of appetite, etc.)

Nursing Assessment and Diagnoses	Outcomes and Evaluation Parameters	Planning and Interventions with *Rationales*
Nursing Diagnosis: *Imbalanced Nutrition: Less Than Body Requirements* related to inability to eat adequate amounts of food to maintain weight	**Outcome:** Normal intake of a balanced diet without side effects. *Evaluation Parameters:* Weight is at recommended level for the height and musculature for the patient. Treatment of gastrointestinal clinical manifestations is effective.	**Interventions and *Rationales*:** Perform a complete physical assessment and nutritional history on admission *to assess current nutritional status and to provide a nutritional baseline of data for plan development.* Instruct patient to weigh daily before breakfast, after urination, using the same scale *to monitor weight gain.* Consult registered dietician *for detailed nutritional analysis and specialized planning.*

Assessment of Current Nutritional and Dietary Intake

Subjective Data:
What is your normal daily dietary intake?
How much alcohol do you drink weekly?
What types of food do you use for snacks?
How many meals a day do you eat and at what time?
Do you use vitamin, herbal, and over the counter (OTC) medications?
Have you taken any weight loss medications or used laxatives for weight loss?
Do you have any difficulty with swallowing or chewing?

Objective Data:
Serial weights from medical records.
Assess muscle wasting.
Assess for acute and/or chronic disease states, e.g., kidney, liver, diabetes, anorexia, cancer.
Test serum albumin level, serum prealbumin level, serum creatinine level, total lymphocyte count, and transferrin level.

Nursing Assessment and Diagnoses	Outcomes and Evaluation Parameters	Planning and Interventions with *Rationales*
Nursing Diagnosis: *Imbalanced Nutrition: Less Than Body Requirements* related to factors inhibiting successful eating patterns to maintain weight	**Outcomes:** Maintain normal nutrition. BMI within normal limits *Evaluation Parameters:* Current weight is compared to BMI charts and height–weight charts to determine level of malnutrition (mild, moderate, or severe). The nurse must use the evaluation parameters that correlate with the etiology of the nutritional deficit. See charts in this chapter for specific deficits in specific disease processes. Food intake is less than energy expenditure.	**Interventions and *Rationales*:** Ask patient/family to list the foods and portion sizes consumed for the last 24 hours and the past 3 days *to assess adequacy of calorie intake.* Explore nutritional beliefs, cultural and religious attitudes toward food, food taboos, use of alcohol, medication and OTC use, and problems with dentition or self-feeding difficulties *to determine factors that impact food intake.* List the calorie count for each food consumed *to determine adequacy of calorie intake.* Measure triceps skinfold, midarm muscle circumference in the younger but not the older patient *to determine baseline for muscle wasting.*

Assessment of Disease Risk Factors That Are Influenced by Underweight Status

Subjective Data:
Do you have any acute or chronic diseases?
When was the last time you had a complete physical examination?

Objective Data:
Assess for cachexia, renal dysfunction, fever, infection, wounds, diabetes mellitus, gastrointestinal pain, and bloating.

(continued)

NURSING PROCESS: Patient Care Plan for Malnutrition (Undernutrition)—*Continued*

Nursing Assessment and Diagnoses	Outcomes and Evaluation Parameters	Planning and Interventions with *Rationales*
Nursing Diagnosis: *Ineffective Health Maintenance* related to disease factors that can result in loss of weight	**Outcome:** Identification and management of disease/s that caused weight loss. ***Evaluation Parameters:*** Prealbumin levels within normal limits. BMI within normal limits.	**Interventions and *Rationales:*** Assess patient for risk factors for malnutrition *to determine problem priority.* Risk factors include acute and chronic illness, depression in the elderly, functional status, polypharmacy, and frailty. Assess patient for signs of impaired wound healing (e.g., pressure ulcers, fistulas), burns, muscle wasting, muscle weakness, loss of calcium, increased risk for falls leading to increased risk for fractures. *These factors indicate patient has high risk for malnutrition.* In oncology patients, assess for weight loss >5%, *which can result in increased mortality, poor response to chemotherapy, and treatment complications.*

Assessment of Changes That Can Be Made in Food Intake to Increase Caloric Intake, Including Readiness to Change Food Intake

Subjective Data:
List the foods you enjoy eating and eat frequently.

Objective Data:
Caloric intake per 24 hr based on above food diary.
Write down each food consumed along with portion size for calculation of food intake by dietician.

Nursing Assessment and Diagnoses	Outcomes and Evaluation Parameters	Planning and Interventions with *Rationales*
Nursing Diagnosis: *Imbalanced Nutrition: Less Than Body Requirements* related to need to increase caloric intake	**Outcomes:** Patient verbalizes changes to increase food intake. ***Evaluation Parameters:*** Weight gain of 1–2 lb per month for 6 months.	**Interventions and *Rationales:*** Reassess hospitalized patients weekly for nutritional status. Encourage balanced nutrition. *To assess progress toward normal BMI.* Measure upper arm and thigh monthly *to assess growth in muscle mass.* Encourage small, frequent meals of foods that patient enjoys. *Potentially increases calorie intake.* *For hospitalized patients:* Monitor tolerance for prescribed tube feedings, total parenteral nutrition (TPN), and other nutritional support as needed including electrolytes and vitamins *to prevent malnutrition.* Provide feeding assistance if needed; if assistance is provided, do not hurry the patient and sit down while feeding *so patient doesn't feel rushed to eat.* Place patient in an upright position while eating and for 30 minutes afterward *to prevent regurgitation.* Provide a pleasant environment for mealtime *to encourage the appetite.* Encourage communal environment for mealtime *to encourage social milieu and appetite.* Avoid prolonged NPO status while inpatient *because this contributes to further loss of intake.*

Dietetic Association, 2001; Goldfein, Devlin, & Spitzer, 2000). The Genetic Considerations box discusses speculation about the roles genetics may play in weight management.

Nutrition and Cardiovascular Disease

Nutrition intervention can have a significant impact on risk reduction with cardiovascular disease. Following lifestyle modifica-

tions, including nutrition recommendations, can help prevent or manage hypertension and coronary artery disease. Medical nutrition therapy is also indicated in the treatment of heart failure.

Hypertension

Lifestyle modifications, including diet, have been shown to have both clinical and public health significance in reduction of blood

GENETIC CONSIDERATIONS Implications for Weight Management

Speculation about the genetic implications in weight management has existed for some time. The specific roles of genetics as related to risk of obesity and eating disorders are being investigated. Risk factors for the development of eating disorders have been linked to genetic phenotypes for other disorders, such as the traits for obsessive-compulsive disorder and disturbances of dopamine systems (Kaye et al., 2004; Shinohara et al., 2004).

The role of genetics and the possibility of genetic manipulation have been heavily researched in the hope of identifying obesity risk factors and treatment options. Substances involved in appetite regulation, such as neuropeptide Y and ghrelin, proteins involved in thermogenesis, and leptin, and their relation to obesity are among the areas of research (Campion, Milagro, & Martinez, 2004; Marti, Moreno-Aliaga, Hebebrand, & Martinez, 2004). Although the topic of genetic influence on the development of both eating disorders and obesity is intriguing, it is difficult to draw firm conclusions without further research into these areas (Bulik, Sullivan, Wade, & Kendler, 2000; Kaye et al., 2004).

CHART 14–16 Lifestyle Modifications for Hypertension

Lifestyle Component	Recommendation
Weight management	Practice weight reduction or management of normal weight.
Diet	Eat a diet rich in fruits, vegetables, and low-fat dairy foods and low in saturated and total fat.
	Reduce sodium intake to not more than 2,400 mg or 6 g NaCl daily.
	Limit alcohol to not more than 2 drinks a day for men and not more than 1 drink a day for women and small men. One drink is 12 oz beer, 5 oz wine, or 1-1/2 oz 80-proof spirits.
Physical activity	Engage in physical activity at least 30 minutes most days.

Sources: Chobanian, A. V., Bakris, G. L., Black, H. R., Cushman, W. C., et al. (2003). The seventh report of the Joint National Committee on Prevention, Detection, Evaluation and Treatment of High Blood Pressure. *Journal of the American Medical Association, 289,* 2560–2572; National Heart, Lung, and Blood Institute. (2004). *The seventh report of the Joint National Committee on Prevention, Detection, Evaluation and Treatment of High Blood Pressure (JNC7).* Retrieved February 5, 2004, from http://www.nhlbi.nih.gov/guidelines/hypertension/express.pdf; Whelton, P. K., He, J., Appel, L. J., Cutler, J. A., Havas, S., Kotchen, T. A., et al. (2002). Primary prevention of hypertension: Clinical and public health advisory from the National High Blood Pressure Education Program. *Journal of the American Medical Association, 288,* 1882–1888.

---

pressure in people with hypertension and those with high normal blood pressure, or prehypertension (Chobanian et al., 2003; Khan et al., 2006; Writing Group of the PREMIER Collaborative Research Group, 2003). The prevalence of hypertension in America is increasing, with almost 29% of all adults exhibiting elevated blood pressure. Of those diagnosed with hypertension and on antihypertensive medication, only 53% had measured blood pressure within the recommended target (Hijjar & Kotchen, 2003). Clearly, improved primary prevention and treatment of hypertension are needed to avoid the negative effects of elevated blood pressure on cardiovascular risk across the life span.

Lifestyle modifications recommended for prevention and management of high blood pressure include several nutrition-centered modifications as well as engaging in regular physical activity. Decades of research have shown the individual and additive effects on blood pressure reduction with weight reduction in overweight people, limiting sodium, alcohol, and total and saturated fat while consuming a diet rich in fruits, vegetables, and low-fat dairy products (Chobanian et al., 2003; Whelton et al., 2002; Writing Group of the PREMIER Collaborative Research Group, 2003). Current national guidelines recommend lifestyle modifications for all people for the primary prevention and management of high blood pressure (Chobanian et al., 2003; NHLBI, 2004; Whelton et al., 2002). Specific guidelines are outlined in Chart 14–16.

The nurse is uniquely positioned to be instrumental in detecting elevated blood pressure and educating patients on prevention and management of hypertension. In addition to weight management methods discussed in this chapter, the nurse can be involved in patient education and monitoring of other nutrition-related lifestyle modifications.

Reduction of dietary sodium intake has been reported to lower systolic blood pressure as a single intervention or in conjunction with other lifestyle modifications or pharmacology (Chobanian et al., 2003; Khan et al., 2006). Further, a low sodium intake compared with usual sodium intake has been reported to reduce the amount of antihypertensive medication needed in some patients (Mulrow, 2001). The primary source of sodium in the American diet is from packaged, processed, and ready-to-eat food prepared outside the home. Discretionary added sodium in the form of table salt used in the home only accounts for 20% to 30% of sodium consumption (Mulrow, 2001). The nurse should question the patient about eating patterns and preparation methods during the nutrition portion of a nursing assessment. Specifically asking about frequency of restaurant meals and use of convenience products is important to estimate sodium intake. Chart 14–17 lists sources of high-sodium foods.

The NIH's Dietary Approaches to Stopping Hypertension (DASH) diet has taken nutrition intervention for high blood

---

CHART 14–17 Dietary Sources of High Sodium

- In general, processed, preserved, and convenience foods are high in sodium. Terms such as *pickled, cured, dehydrated, smoked, seasoned, ready-to-eat,* and *added sauce* hint at a high sodium content.

- Plain forms of most food have low or moderate sodium content. Fresh fruit, juice, fresh or plain frozen vegetables, plain grains and breads, milk, plain meat, poultry, fish, and dried beans, peas, and lentils are not naturally high in sodium.

- Canned vegetables, frozen vegetables with sauce, canned tomato products, grain mixes, cured or luncheon meats, cheeses, canned meat, fish, beans and poultry, and boxed or frozen meals are higher in sodium than their fresh or plain counterparts.

- Foods labeled "reduced sodium" have 25% less sodium than the original, but may not be low in sodium. Foods labeled "low sodium" have 140 mg sodium or less per serving.

pressure beyond the single low-sodium diet approach. The DASH diet emphasizes fruits, vegetables, nuts, and low-fat dairy while also containing reduced fat and saturated fat levels. The diet is rich in potassium, which has been associated with independent reductions in blood pressure and risk of stroke (Khan et al., 2006). Magnesium and calcium sources are also plentiful in the DASH diet, but results from research on their effects independently or in supplemental form are unclear. Supplemental calcium in amounts of 1,000 to 1,500 mg has had small, inconsistent effects on blood pressure reduction in hypertensive individuals, but this amount is already within recommended levels for intake in the general population (Whelton et al., 2002). The DASH diet recommends the use of foods to attain its goals and remains silent on the use of supplements. Chart 14–18 outlines the DASH diet. The nurse should note that the DASH diet contains various calorie levels that can be used or modified as a weight reduction plan for the overweight patient (NHLBI, 2004).

Alcohol intake above one drink a day for women and lighter weight men or two drinks a day for men has been shown to have a direct negative effect on blood pressure (Chobanian et al., 2003; Khan et al., 2006; Whelton et al., 2002). Although some patients tout the reputed cardioprotective effects of alcohol consumption, intake beyond the recommended limit is not conferring additional benefit. Overweight or obese patients trying to lose weight should be made aware of the significant calorie content that alcoholic beverages can contribute to the diet.

Chapter 21 ☞ includes a complete description of hypertension.

Coronary Heart Disease

Aggressive management of serum lipids is recommended as a primary strategy in the prevention and treatment of cardiovascular disease. Management of elevated serum low-density lipoprotein (LDL) cholesterol should receive priority attention because of its established association with increased risk of coronary heart disease (NHLBI, 2002). Total cholesterol and high-density lipoprotein (HDL) cholesterol levels are also important predictors of cardiac risk. Target values for serum lipid

levels based on the NHLBI's National Cholesterol Education Program (NCEP) are discussed in Chapter 37 ☞.

The general population as well as those patients with established coronary heart disease can benefit from dietary approaches aimed at reducing serum lipids, controlling blood pressure, and managing body weight in an effort to reduce cardiac risk (Lichtenstein et al., 2006). Diet modifications, called **therapeutic lifestyle changes (TLC)**, are recommended as an initial strategy for treating elevated LDL cholesterol or in conjunction with pharmacologic intervention when indicated. Medical nutrition therapy for hyperlipidemia and coronary heart disease targets reduction of both lipid and nonlipid cardiac risk factors. A fat-controlled diet coupled with weight management and increased physical activity comprises the foundation of the therapeutic lifestyle changes. Therapeutic lifestyle changes are outlined in Chart 14–19.

Saturated Fats and Cholesterol

The NCEP guidelines focus on reducing dietary saturated fat and cholesterol. A dose response exists between saturated fat intake and serum LDL cholesterol (NHLBI, 2002). Saturated fats exist primarily in fats from animal-based foods such as fatty meats or whole-milk dairy products. Tropical fats are also saturated fats and include palm oil, coconut oil, and cocoa butter. Hydrogenated and *trans* fats are included in the recommendation to reduce saturated fat intake. These fats originate as *un*saturated oils, but become saturated during food processing when the manufacturer removes hydrogen molecules to make a fat that is more solid at room temperature. Examples include fats used in shortening, stick margarine, and many baked goods and snacks. High intake of dietary cholesterol is associated with increased LDL cholesterol. Dietary cholesterol is present only in foods of animal origin. Fatty and organ meats, egg yolks, and shellfish are among the higher sources of dietary cholesterol.

Unsaturated Fats

Unsaturated fats, which are liquid at room temperature, are not associated with elevated LDL cholesterol. The monounsaturated fats present in olive, peanut, and canola oils and most nuts and

---

| CHART 14–18 | DASH Eating Plan: Number of Daily Servings for Other Calorie Levels |

Food Groups	Servings/Day		
	1,600 Calories/Day	2,600 Calories/Day	3,100 Calories/Day
Grains*	6	10–11	12–13
Vegetables	3–4	5–6	6
Fruits	4	5–6	6
Fat-free or low-fat milk and milk products	2–3	3	3–4
Lean meats, poultry, and fish	3–6	6	6–9
Nuts, seeds, and legumes	3/week	1	1
Fats and oils	2	3	4
Sweets and added sugars	0	≤2	≤2

*Whole grains are recommended for most grain servings as a good source of fiber and nutrients.

Source: National Heart, Lung, and Blood Insitute. (2006). *Your guide to lowering your blood pressure with DASH*. Retrieved May 30, 2008 from http://www.nhlbi.nih.gov/health/public/heart/hbp/dash/new_dash.pdf

CHART 14–19 Therapeutic Lifestyle Changes for Cardiovascular Disease

Lifestyle Component	Recommendation
Diet	Saturated fat: <7% total daily calorie intake. *Trans* fatty acids should also be limited.
	Monounsaturated fat: up to 20% total daily calorie intake.
	Polyunsaturated fat: up to 10% total daily calorie intake.
	Total fat: 25%–35% total daily calorie intake.
	Cholesterol: <200 mg/day.
	Fiber: 20–30 g/day with consideration given to include 10–25 g soluble fiber daily.
	Carbohydrate: 50%–60% of total daily calorie intake. Emphasize whole grains, fruits, and vegetable sources.
	Protein: approximately 15% of total daily calorie intake.
	Energy intake to maintain desirable weight and prevent weight gain.
Weight management	Maintain desirable weight, avoid weight gain, lose weight if indicated.
Physical activity	Increase physical activity. Energy balance to include at least 200 calories of energy expenditure from moderately intense activity most days.

Source: National Heart Lung and Blood Institute. (2002). *Third report of the National Cholesterol Education Program expert panel on detection, evaluation, and treatment of high blood cholesterol in adults (Adult treatment panel III).* Retrieved February 5, 2004, from http://www.nhlbi.nih.gov/guidelines/cholesterol/atp3full.pdf

avocado have been shown to lower LDL cholesterol when substituted for saturated fats in the diet (NHLBI, 2002). Polyunsaturated fats also can foster a decrease in saturated fats when substituted for saturated fats but can adversely contribute to a small decrease in beneficial HDL cholesterol as well (NHLBI, 2002). Sources of polyunsaturated fats include corn, safflower, sunflower, and soybean oils and are included on Chart 14–20 (p. 296), which lists practical interventions that can be used to make therapeutic lifestyle changes.

Carbohydrate and Fiber

Carbohydrate can be substituted for saturated fat as a strategy for decreasing LDL cholesterol (NHLBI, 2002). However, high carbohydrate intake exceeding 60% of the diet's energy value has been associated with a decrease in HDL cholesterol and an increase in serum triglycerides, neither of which is beneficial to cardiac risk (NHLBI, 2002). Carbohydrate-containing plant foods that contain fiber, specifically soluble fiber, are recommended for their cholesterol-lowering capabilities (Shamliyan, Jacobs, Raatz, Nordstrom, & Keenan, 2006). Soluble fiber is associated with a 3% to 5% reduction of LDL cholesterol when 5 to 10 grams are consumed daily (NHLBI, 2002). Soluble fiber is present in several plant foods such as oats, oat bran,

legumes, and barley. Chart 14–20 (p. 296) lists additional sources of soluble fiber.

Plant Sterol and Stanol Esters

Plant sterol and stanol esters are poorly absorbed derivatives of soybean and wood oils that have been reported to lower total and LDL cholesterol up to 20% with maximum effective intake of 2 g/daily (Lichtenstein et al., 2006). Several brands of margarine and salad dressings exist that have sterol or stanol esters listed as ingredients on the label.

Soy Protein

Soy protein in the diet has been reported to lower plasma LDL cholesterol, especially when consumed with soluble fibers and used to replace animal proteins (Jenkins et al., 2006; Lichtenstein et al., 2006). The mechanism by which soy affects cholesterol and cardiac risk is complex and not fully understood. It may involve both lipid-lowering effects and changes in platelet aggregation and vascular inflammation (Anderson, 2003; Morelli & Zoorob, 2000). Soy protein can be found in soybeans, tofu, soy milk, and many soy "meat" alternatives.

Omega-3 Fatty Acids

Omega-3 fats are associated with decreased risk of cardiac events, specifically cardiac death in people with established coronary heart disease (Gebauer, Psota, Harris, & Kris-Etherton, 2006). Reduction of plasma triglycerides, decreased platelet aggregability, reduction in cardiac dysrhythmias, and improvement in endothelial dysfunction all play a role in the mechanism (Gebauer et al., 2006). The American Heart Association recommends intake of oily fish twice a week for the general adult population and 1 g/day of omega-3 fats from fish or a fish supplement in those with existing atherosclerosis (Lichtenstein et al., 2006). One serving of a fatty fish such as salmon or bluefish has 900 mg of omega-3 fat. Plant sources of omega-3 fats contain smaller amounts of these fats in a serving and include flaxseed and canola oil. The nurse should caution patients who choose to take supplemental forms of omega-3 fats about negative side effects as outlined in the Critical Alert.

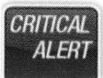 *Omega-3 supplements decrease platelet aggregability. Take care to assess patients for any interaction with medications such as Coumadin or aspirin therapy that potentiate this effect. Additionally, assess for other dietary supplements and herbs with antiplatelet action, such as garlic, feverfew, ginkgo biloba, and vitamin E. Make sure the patient respects proper dosage recommendations of any omega-3 fat supplements.*

Alcohol

A moderate intake of alcohol can reduce the risk of coronary heart disease in adults (Lichtenstein et al., 2006). Moderation is described as no more than one drink per day for a woman and two per day for a man. Wine, specifically red wine, has received great focus when researching the potential cardioprotective effects of alcohol, yet most studies do not support reduced cardiac risk with a specific type of alcohol (Lichtenstein et al., 2006). Red wine is singled out by some because of its antithrombolytic action and antioxidant content perhaps contributing additional benefits over other types of alcohol. Higher intake of alcohol does not confer additional cardioprotection, can be the source of

CHART 14–20	Practical Interventions to Achieve Therapeutic Lifestyle Changes (TLC)

Choose	Limit
Monounsaturated and polyunsaturated fats, oils, and margarines to replace saturated fat ingredients:	Saturated fat and cholesterol sources.
	Fats that are hard at room temperature tend to be saturated fats:
• Olive oil, canola oil, peanut oil = mono	• Fatty meats, luncheon meats, organ meats
• Sunflower, soybean, safflower, corn, sesame = poly.	• Poultry w/skin
Lower fat and saturated fat protein foods:	• Whole-fat dairy products
• Dried beans, peas, lentils, soy (these also contain soluble fiber)	• Commercial baked goods made with *trans* and hydrogenated fats or lard
• Skinless poultry	• Tropical oils found in processed foods: palm oil, cocoa butter, coconut oil
• Fish	• Stick margarine, shortening, lard.
• Lean, trimmed cuts of meat (round/loin)	High-fat food preparation methods:
• Fat-free and low-fat dairy foods.	• Deep-fat or pan frying
Omega-3 polyunsaturated fat sources:	• Adding sauces, gravies, creams, creamy dressings, or mayonnaise to foods
• Fish: deep, cold-water fish such as salmon, tuna, bluefish, mackerel	• Leaving on poultry skin or visible meat fat on during cooking
• Flaxseed	• Recipes with high oil, butter, margarine, lard, cream, or full-fat cheese content.
• Canola oil	
• Nuts	
• Soy.	
Low-fat food preparation methods:	
• Bake, grill, sauté w/ broth or cooking spray	
• Remove fat/skin from proteins before cooking	
• Use low-fat marinades	
• Substitute low fat ingredients in recipes for high fat version.	
Five or more fruits and vegetables daily. Soluble fiber sources include fruit and vegetables w/edible skins.	
Whole grains, including soluble fiber sources such as oats, oat bran, barley.	

Source: Adapted from National Heart Lung and Blood Institute. (2002). *Third report of the National Cholesterol Education Program expert panel on detection, evaluation, and treatment of high blood cholesterol in adults (Adult treatment panel III)*. Retrieved February 5, 2004, from http://www.nhlbi.nih.gov/guidelines/cholesterol/atp3full.pdf

excess calorie intake, and can contribute to an elevated triglyceride level in addition to other medical risks (Lichtenstein et al., 2006). There is little justification to recommend drinking alcohol to patients who do not already do so.

Homocysteine and B-Vitamins

Elevated plasma homocysteine has emerged as a risk factor of cardiovascular disease. It is unclear whether homocysteine is simply a marker of disease or causative in nature (Hackam & Anand, 2003). Homocysteine is an amino acid that is metabolized in the body with the help of folic acid, pyridoxine (vitamin B_6), and vitamin B_{12}. Diets high in folic acid or all three vitamins have been reported to lower plasma homocysteine levels. Whether a reduction of homocysteine levels will lead to a reduction in coronary heart disease remains a matter of debate (Lichtenstein et al., 2006).

Other Supplements and Botanicals

Antioxidant vitamins such as vitamins E and C have been investigated for a possible role in reducing coronary heart disease. To date, observations made in epidemiologic studies regarding these antioxidants have not illustrated a reduction in cardiac risk when investigated in controlled clinical trials (Morris &

Carson, 2003). In several studies of patients with existing cardiovascular disease, antioxidant therapy failed to decrease the risk of future cardiac events or disease. Additionally, antioxidant therapy lessened the interventional effects of a HMG CoA reductase inhibitor (a cholesterol-lowering drug) and nicotinic acid regimen (niacin) (Brown et al., 2001; Waters et al., 2002). The American Heart Association stresses that studies have pointed to the health benefits of diets rich in fruits and vegetables, food sources of antioxidants, but therapeutic use of antioxidant supplements is not recommended because of negative outcomes in research trials (Lichtenstein et al., 2006).

Many other dietary supplements, including herbs, have received attention for possible roles in the reduction of cholesterol or other cardiac risk factors. To date, none has withstood the test of a long-term clinical trial to prove a benefit. Supplemental garlic has been investigated for a mild cholesterol-lowering effect compared to placebo in some trials, but not others (Morelli & Zoorob, 2000; Rahman, 2001; Stevinson, Pittler, & Ernst, 2000). Gugulipid, or guggul gum, has received attention for reported cholesterol-lowering power in clinical trials in India but more recent reports find little effect (Morelli & Zoorob, 2000). Both of these examples serve as a reminder of the uncertainty of using dietary supplements without clinical evidence of efficacy. Controlled research on such supplements is limited, making it difficult to make a good clinical recommendation when queried by patients seeking to avoid or augment the use of pharmacologic therapies. Current lack of research and limited knowledge regarding safety does not support the use of these products in treating coronary heart disease. Additionally, standardization of supplement dosing and ingredients is lacking in the United States, making it a game of roulette when choosing underresearched products. Despite the lack of standardization and research, many consumers are willing to try these supplements and may not volunteer this information to their health care providers. The nurse should assess patients for use of supplements and discuss the lack of clinical studies, any safety concerns, and the potential for drug–supplement interactions.

Weight Management

Overweight and obesity are associated with an increased risk of coronary heart disease, among other comorbid conditions (NHLBI, 2002). Weight management is included in the TLC recommendations for targeting LDL cholesterol reduction. Weight loss of even a few pounds has been reported to reduce LDL cholesterol (NHLBI, 2002). The NCEP and the American Heart Association encourage weight loss through decreased energy intake and increased physical activity. Prevention of weight gain is emphasized (Lichtenstein et al., 2006; NHLBI, 2002). A balanced low-fat diet containing all food groups is stressed for long-term benefit and overall health. A reduction in sedentary time and the addition of moderate physical activity on most days is also encouraged (Lichtenstein et al., 2006). Weight reduction was discussed earlier in the chapter.

Metabolic Syndrome

Recently a cluster of cardiovascular risk factors, referred to as *metabolic syndrome,* has been defined as having three out of the five following conditions: (1) abdominal obesity, (2) high triglycerides, (3) low HDL-C, (4) high blood pressure, and (5) fasting glucose ($\geq$110 mg/dL). The presence of metabolic syndrome can place the overweight patient at additional cardiac risk. Overweight patients with abdominal obesity (apple shape), elevated triglycerides, low HDL cholesterol levels, high blood pressure, or elevated fasting glucose should be assessed for the metabolic syndrome as discussed in Chapters 37 and 40 🔗. Treatment recommendations begin with a 3-month trial of standard TLCs (see Chart 14–19, p. 295) emphasizing LDL cholesterol reduction and weight loss. If parameters of metabolic syndrome are still present after 3 months, intensified weight loss efforts are indicated. Elevated triglycerides of $\geq$500 mg/dL should be attended to urgently because of an associated risk of pancreatitis (NHLBI, 2002). A very low fat diet ($\leq$15% of daily calorie needs from fat), weight loss, physical activity, and possible pharmacologic intervention are indicated with this level of hypertriglyceridemia (NHLBI, 2002).

Much attention has been given to the concept of carbohydrate-containing foods and elevated postprandial plasma glucose levels, especially in individuals with insulin resistance at risk for metabolic syndrome. Diets that are high in carbohydrate (>60%) are associated with elevated triglyc-

erides and lowered HDL cholesterol. Individuals with metabolic syndrome or insulin resistance can benefit from replacement of dietary saturated fat with unsaturated fats, specifically monounsaturates, as an alternative to adding carbohydrate food sources to replace needed calories (Lichtenstein et al., 2006).

Additionally, the nurse should encourage high-fiber fruits, vegetables, and whole grains as choices for needed carbohydrate sources, nutrient composition, and to promote satiety. Fiber intake has been shown to have benefit in postprandial glycemic control and improvement of blood lipid levels in diabetic patients (American Diabetes Association [ADA], 2003a; Lichtenstein et al., 2006). Some refer to a tool called the glycemic index (GI) that predicts postprandial glucose response to varying foods. The content of individual food constituents such as fiber and fat and the preparation method affect the glycemic response (ADA, 2003a). The GI may prove useful in the future for providing advice to patients with metabolic syndrome and diabetes mellitus. Currently, the tool considers only the glycemic effect of the food when eaten singly and not its consumption in a mixed meal, as would be the usual pattern, making it too cumbersome for practical clinical use (Franz, 2003). The patient who inquires about use of the GI should be encouraged to consume carbohydrates that are unprocessed and retain their original fiber content such as fruits, vegetables, and whole grains. Fruits and vegetables with edible skin or seeds, whole-grain cereals and breads, brown rice, barley, and dried beans are examples.

Heart Failure

A low-sodium diet is prescribed as medical nutrition therapy for cardiac failure. Reduction of dietary sodium along with pharmacologic intervention can help reduce extracellular fluid burden and reduce cardiac workload. Commonly, a 2-g sodium restriction is recommended (see Chart 14–17 (p. 293) for a list of high-sodium foods). A 2-g sodium restriction requires the elimination of table salt use and replacement of high-sodium processed foods with unprocessed versions. The use of low-sodium specialty foods is not necessary to comply with the diet unless the patient's situation requires ongoing use of processed foods.

Advanced cardiac failure can place increased metabolic needs on the patient when lung function becomes compromised and respiration is altered. Increased respiratory rate and use of auxiliary muscles for labored breathing can increase the body's caloric requirement. Fatigue, early satiety, restrictive diet, and medication side effects can hamper appetite and put the patient at further risk for malnutrition. The term *cardiac cachexia* describes the consequences and physical symptoms seen in advanced cardiac failure when nutritional needs go unmet and muscle and fat wasting ensue.

The nurse should monitor patients for signs of weight loss that can be masked by edema. Temporal wasting, loss of adipose muscle, and lack of strength can be indicative of malnutrition. The patient should be encouraged to consume small, frequent meals to minimize early satiety and difficulty with breathing. Nutrient-dense foods high in protein and calories should be encouraged to maximize intake and "make every bite count." In patients consuming insufficient calories, it is prudent to evaluate intake of sodium. Sodium intake may be extremely low because of lack of general intake. Appropriate consideration can be given to allowing intake of some higher sodium foods to promote intake while remaining within the parameters of an overall sodium-restricted diet. Chart 14–21 lists food suggestions for improving intake in patients at risk for cardiac cachexia.

Diabetes Mellitus

Medical nutrition therapy is an essential lifestyle component in the management of diabetes. Nutrition choices and habits following recommended guidelines can improve glycemic control and reduce the risk of diabetic complications such as macrovascular disease in patients with existing disease (Franz et al., 2002). Additionally, lifestyle modifications, including diet, have a positive effect on disease reduction in those with impaired glucose tolerance and at risk for type II diabetes (Diabetes Prevention Program Research Group, 2002). Goals of medical nutrition therapy for diabetes are outlined in Chart 14–22.

The nutrition recommendations for diabetic patients has evolved beyond the old-school "ADA" diet (named for the American Diabetes Association), in which a specific calorie level was prescribed by the health care provider based on an exchange list of foods according to carbohydrate, protein, and fat content. The ADA (2003b) no longer recommends any single type of meal plan for all type I or type II diabetic individuals and urges that this terminology no longer be used.

Current recommendations call for attention to a healthy diet that is mindful of carbohydrate content, matching food choices and consistency of intake to individual needs. The overall diet also should incorporate TLCs known to reduce risk of coronary heart disease through the prevention of dyslipidemia, overweight, and high blood pressure. Rather than provide a blanket recommendation of a specific diet, the focus is now on individual management decisions. The patient is to be included in decision making along with the treatment team. The ADA (2003a)

CHART 14–21	Suggested Nutrition Interventions for Cardiac Cachexia
Add "more calories per bite"	Add calorie sources to existing foods: • Butter, gravy,* sauces,* dressings* • Grated cheese* • Powdered milk mixed into regular milk • "Double milk" in baking recipes, desserts, soups,* milkshakes.
Increase intake of nutrient-dense foods	• Encourage more intake at the start of the day or start of the meal when intake is best • Limit mealtime liquids to avoid fullness • High-protein desserts made w/egg or milk such as pudding, custard, ice cream • Frequent snacks of high energy, protein foods like yogurt, peanut butter on crackers,* cheese* • Cream soup* vs. clear soup, juice vs. water.

Monitor overall sodium intake and urge lower sodium versions if intake is high.

CHART 14–22	Medical Nutrition Therapy Goals for Diabetes

Attain and maintain optimal metabolic outcomes including:
- Blood glucose levels in the normal range or close to normal to prevent or reduce risk of complications of diabetes.
- A lipid profile that reduces risk of macrovascular disease.
- Blood pressure levels that reduce the risk of vascular disease.
- Prevent and treat chronic complications of diabetes. Modify nutritional intake and lifestyle as appropriate for prevention and treatment of obesity, dyslipidemia, cardiovascular disease, hypertension, and nephropathy.
- Improve health through healthy food choices and physical activity.
- Address individual nutritional needs taking into consideration personal and cultural preferences and lifestyle.

Franz, M. J., Bantle, J. P., Beebe, C. A., Brunzelli, J. D., Chiasson, J., Garg., et al. (2002). Technical review: Evidence-based nutrition principles and recommendations for the treatment and prevention of diabetes and related complications. *Diabetes Care 25,* 148–198. Copyright © 2002 American Diabetes Association From Diabetes Care, Vol. 25, 2002; 148–198. Reprinted with permission from *The American Diabetes Association.*

recommends that the registered dietitian be the treatment team member who provides the medical nutrition therapy, but that all team members are knowledgable about its parameters.

Carbohydrate Recommendations

Carbohydrates are an essential component of a healthy diet. Diabetic patients are urged to include carbohydrates in the form of whole grains, fruits, vegetables, and low-fat milk products. Together with monounsaturated fats, combined intake of carbohydrate and monounsaturated fats should be 60% to 70% of total energy intake (ADA, 2003a). No individual recommendation is given for just carbohydrate intake. The carbohydrate content of the diet and any given meal is determined individually. Some patients with type I diabetes adjust premeal insulin based on the meal's carbohydrate content, whereas others who are on a fixed dose of insulin keep a consistent pattern of day-to-day carbohydrate intake (ADA, 2003a; Franz et al., 2002). Additionally, physical activity can require an adjustment of insulin or carbohydrate intake by some individuals because of increased uptake of plasma glucose by exercising muscle (Franz et al., 2002). The treatment team and patient determine initial parameters for carbohydrate intake based on the registered dietitian's assessment of nutritional needs. Adjustments are made over time to further individualize intake. Patients are educated to read carbohydrate content on food labels and to use a basic system of carbohydrate counting based on a food exchange system. Chart 14–23 provides an example of this system.

It is recommended that patients be educated to recognize their individual glycemic responses to varying foods, levels of activity, and any hypoglycemic agents and to incorporate this into the advice given by the treatment team. The nurse is instrumental is this educational effort.

The ADA (2003a) does not currently support the use of the glycemic index (discussed earlier in this chapter in the Metabolic Syndrome section) in the management of diabetes, citing lack of overall definitive conclusions among limited clinical trials as well as study design criticisms. Much debate has surrounded this topic and varying clinical trials support all sides of the discussion (Brand-Miller, Hayne, Petocz, & Colagiuri, 2003). Glycemic index use is supported by national recommendations in other

CHART 14-23 Sample Carbohydrate Counting for Diabetes Management

Food Group	Serving Size Examples	Grams of Carbohydrate
Starches (grains, breads, cereals, legumes, starchy vegetables)	1/2 cup cooked grain, 1-oz slice equivalent (bread, rolls, and buns), 3/4 cup cold cereal	15
Fruit	1 medium peach, 1/2 cup apple juice, 1/2 cup melon	15
Vegetables	1 cup raw or 1/2 cup cooked greens	5
Dairy	1 cup milk or yogurt	12
Miscellaneous foods w/carbohydrate (snack foods, desserts, etc.)	Read label for portion	15

Note: An RD would help determine an individual carbohydrate recommendation for a patient. Patients monitor grams of carbohydrate in their diet or use a system of "carbohydrate choices." One carbohydrate choice is the serving of a food with ≅15 g of carbohydrate. Portions are important to accurately judge intake. Patients learn to manage the diet by reading labels and utilizing the generic exchange system in this chart for carbohydrate-containing foods. Foods not containing carbohydrate (meats, fish, poultry, cheese, fats) must be monitored to avoid cardiovascular risk, but are not part of the carbohydrate-counting system.

Sources: American Diabetes Association & American Dietetic Association. (1995a). *Carbohydrate counting: getting started.* Alexandria, VA, and Chicago, IL: Authors; American Diabetes Association & American Dietetic Association. (1995b). *Exchange lists for meal planning.* Alexandria, VA, and Chicago, IL: Authors; Wheeler, M. L. (2003). Nutrient database for the 2003 exchange lists for meal planning. *Journal of the American Dietetic Association, 103,* 894–920.

countries (Ludwig, 2002). The ADA (2003a) does acknowledge that foods have individual effects on glycemic response, but, given *equal* amounts of carbohydrate, *total amount* of carbohydrate at meals and snacks is more important than *source or type* when considering glycemic response (Franz et al., 2002). Consistent with this message, no type of carbohydrate is prohibited from the diet. Sucrose (table sugar) and other traditionally taboo, empty-calorie "sweets" sources of carbohydrate are allowed, but within the context of an overall healthy diet. The carbohydrate content of these foods should be calculated and considered as is done with all other carbohydrates in the diet. When asked for glycemic index advice by patients, the nurse can encourage intake of recommended plant sources of carbohydrate such as high-fiber fruits, vegetables, and whole grains. High-fiber carbohydrates, especially soluble fiber sources, have been shown to benefit glycemia and a high-fiber diet may be a de facto form of a low-glycemic index diet (Brand-Miller et al., 2003).

Fat Recommendations

Aggressive lipid management and prevention of coronary heart disease are important goals for diabetics (ADA, 2004). Saturated fat and cholesterol intake should be limited to assist with management of LDL cholesterol levels. Guidelines outlined under medical nutrition therapy for coronary heart disease in this chapter should be followed for the patient with diabetes as well. Monounsaturated fats or carbohydrates should be encouraged as calorie replacements for displaced saturated fat in patients seeking to maintain energy balance and body weight. Patients attempting weight loss doubly benefit from reduced saturated fat intake by not replacing saturated fat with equivocal calorie sources and therefore foster a deficit of energy intake. Substitution of monounsaturated fats over carbohydrates is preferred for individuals with elevated triglycerides, elevated postprandial glucose, or low HDL cholesterol. However, this recommendation should be assessed on an individual basis because excess calorie intake from fats and weight gain can ensue if fat is taken *ad libitum* (ADA, 2003a; Franz et al., 2002). Consumption of fatty fish is encouraged for the cardiovascular disease benefits associated with omega-3 fats as discussed earlier.

Vitamin and Mineral Recommendations

The position of the ADA is that no clear evidence exists to support any different advice on vitamin and mineral intake specific to people with diabetes than already exists for the general population. Antioxidants have been researched for their potential effects on clinical outcome with no conclusion specific to people with diabetes. Minerals such as chromium have also been investigated for a role in blood glucose control, but results are limited and seem to apply only to those who have a chromium deficiency, which is uncommon. Thiamine, pyridoxine (B_6), and vitamin B_{12} are used by some to treat diabetic neuropathy, but the efficacy of this is not clear and the ADA does not support this practice (ADA, 2003a; Franz et al., 2002).

Alcohol Recommendations

Like much of the nutritional advice for people with diabetes, alcohol recommendations coincide closely with those for the general adult population. People with diabetes must be aware of the potential hypoglycemic and hyperglycemic effects of alcohol and consume any intake along with food (Franz et al., 2002). Moderate intake is stressed in those who do choose to consume alcohol.

Special Considerations

Additional dietary considerations need to be made for the patient with diabetes who is acutely ill or experiencing other specific circumstances. Changes in diet and insulin needs occur under special circumstances. It is imperative for the nurse to teach the patient and family how to adjust insulin dosages depending on the given circumstance. The most common special considerations are discussed next.

Overweight and Obesity

Patients with diabetes who are also overweight or obese can benefit from weight management. Weight loss specifically in people with type II diabetes can lessen insulin resistance and decrease the risk of coronary heart disease (NHLBI, 2002). The nurse can encourage and support even small amounts of weight loss in these patients. Lifestyle changes for weight reduction outlined earlier in the chapter coincide with recommendations for the patient with diabetes (ADA, 2003a). The use of high-protein, low-carbohydrate diets for weight loss in patients with diabetes is not supported. Long-term effects of high levels of protein intake on the risk of nephropathy development deserve further study. Concern also exists regarding long-term effects of these diets on LDL cholesterol.

Exercise and Type I Diabetes

Glucose uptake is increased by exercising muscle. After consultation with the treatment team, a patient can compensate for this effect by reducing insulin before planned exercise or with consumption of carbohydrate. A registered dietitian could advise the patient on suitable food or beverage choices to fit the intensity, type, and duration of exercise given these parameters for glucose uptake.

Hypoglycemia

Blood glucose levels of ≤50 mg/dL require immediate treatment, whereas those in the range of 60 to 80 mg/dL can follow a decision-making process determined by the health care team (ADA, 2003a). Glucose is the preferred form of carbohydrate replacement to treat hypoglycemia because of its quicker glycemic response compared with other sources, but any carbohydrate source can be used (Franz et al., 2002). Guidelines call for an initial 15- to 20-g ingestion of carbohydrate followed by a reevaluation of blood glucose approximately 60 minutes later (ADA, 2003a). The nurse can guide the patient in pinpointing potential contributors to low blood sugar and suggest interventions to avoid future episodes.

Acute Illness

Symptoms from some acute illnesses can cause eating and diet tolerance to be jeopardized. The need for insulin can persist or be increased despite reduced intake because of the effects of illness on hormone secretion (Franz et al., 2002). Patients with type I diabetes in whom intake is compromised should be encouraged to maintain a carbohydrate intake of 150 to 200 g divided over the day (Franz et al., 2002). Easy-to-tolerate and liquid carbohydrates should be stressed for improved intake and hydration. Clear liquid and full liquid diets should *not* be sugar free (ADA, 2002b). Chart 14–24 outlines examples of appropriate carbohydrate sources to offer a person with diabetes who is ill.

CHART 14–24   **Sick Day Nutrition Suggestions for Diabetes**

The following foods are approximately 15 g of carbohydrate each or one "carbohydrate choice." Patients should try to approximate normal amount of carbohydrate intake.

Ginger ale, 5 oz	Apple juice, 1/2 cup
Cranberry juice cocktail, 1/3 cup	Fruit juice, frozen bar, 3oz
Sports drink, 1 cup (check labels)	Chicken noodle soup, 1 cup
Gelatin, 1/2 cup	Pudding, 1/4 cup
Sherbert, 1/4 cup	Breakfast bar, 1/2 of a 1-oz bar (check labels)
Canned fruit cocktail in juice, 1/2 cup	Jam, jelly, 1 TBSP
Toast, plain, 1 slice	Rice, plain, 1/3 cup
Noodles, plain, 1/3 cup	

Source: USDA Nutrient Data Laboratory http://www.nal.usda.gov/fnic/foodcomp/search

---

Hospitalized patients with diabetes who require enteral tube feedings or parenteral nutrition support can receive a standard or slightly lower carbohydrate feeding (40% of energy) with close attention paid to glycemic control and hydration. Care must be taken to avoid overfeeding because glycemic control will be adversely affected (Franz et al., 2002). Other parameters used in providing nutrition support also apply to the patient with diabetes.

Special considerations for elderly patients with diabetes are discussed in the Gerontological Considerations box.

Disorders of the Gastrointestinal Tract

Disorders of the gastrointestinal (GI) tract can affect overall health by altering digestion or absorption of food and nutrients. Minor GI complaints are commonplace and may have little impact on nutrition health if short term. Chronic GI conditions or disease can lead to altered intake of food or compromised absorption. Medical nutrition therapy plays a central role in the treatment of most GI diseases.

Swallowing Dysfunction

Dysphagia, or difficulty swallowing, can occur for a number of reasons. Dysphagia is associated with head and neck trauma or disease, neuromuscular disease, stroke, and dementia. Sedation and other medication side effects can impact swallowing directly or indirectly because of diminished saliva production. The patient who experiences dysphagia is at risk for "starvation, dehydration and aspiration" (Palmer, Drennan, & Baba, 2000). Difficulty swallowing can lead to inability to handle oral liquid boluses. Aspiration or loss of fluid volume from drooling or spitting liquids can also lead to dehydration because of diminished intake. Patients can become fearful of drinking liquids and voluntarily self-restrict fluid. Similarly, chewing and swallowing more solid foods can be risky or difficult, so patients may be unable to safely consume adequate nutrition orally.

The nurse should conduct a bedside evaluation to screen for dysphagia. The presence or absence of a gag reflex is not considered an accurate assessment tool (Palmer et al., 2000; Perry, 2001). Screening tools exist that have been validated for use by nurses (Perry, 2001). Warning signs of dysphagia during feeding include drooling or food spilling from the mouth; pocketing of food in the cheek, under the tongue or palate; repeated attempts to swallow a single food bolus; complaint of food sticking or heartburn while eating; frequent throat clearing or coughing while eating (Finestone & Greene-Finestone, 2003; Palmer et al., 2000).

 GERONTOLOGICAL CONSIDERATIONS
Nutrition for Elderly Patients with Diabetes

There is no evidence to support the use of any dietary restrictions in elderly patients with diabetes who reside in long-term care (ADA, 2003b). Long-term care elderly should receive a standard diet individualized to promote adequate intake and prevention of undernutrition, a common risk in older adults (American Dietetic Association, 2002a). In institutionalized elderly, a restricted diet does not provide superior blood glucose control and can lead to diminished intake. The use of "no concentrated sweets" or "no added sugar" diets is generally contraindicated in this population.

Patients with symptoms of dysphagia should be referred to the interdisciplinary team for a thorough evaluation. Speech/language pathologists (SLPs) and advanced practice nurses are the experts in management of swallowing problems and would guide the team in treatment. A dietitian works closely with the team to accommodate appropriate texture modifications to the diet to ensure safe swallowing and provision of adequate fluid and nutrition. The goals of medical nutrition therapy are to reduce choking risk, facilitate independent eating, and enhance enjoyment of eating (Dorner, 2002).

Often, texture modification to the diet can be presented in an unattractive fashion if attention is not given to preparation. Pureed or chopped meals can be made more attractive with sauces, gravies, colorful garnishes, and casseroles rather than being served in lumpy mounds with an ice cream scoop. The nurse should help the patient to have meals in as attractive a surrounding as possible to improve the eating environment. To improve nutrition, whenever possible, the patient should not be interrupted during mealtime for tests or procedures.

When patients with dysphagia are evaluated and transition through various diet modifications, the nurse should monitor the patient for tolerance to texture changes. Foods that form a cohesive bolus are most easily handled and are often attempted first; thin liquids are generally most easily aspirated (Dorner, 2002). The nurse should become familiar with hospital protocol for the dysphagia diet, and learn which foods are permitted with each transitional stage. *Pureed, mechanically altered,* or *mechanical soft* are common terms for food consistency. *Spoon-thick, honey-like, nectar-like,* and *thin* are liquid diet prescriptions (McCallum, 2003). Each patient should have an individualized prescription based on the hospital's dysphagia protocol. An inadvertent mistake in meal delivery could lead to aspiration. The patient should be watched closely for signs of aspiration, food pocketing, or other dysphagia symptoms. Fluid status should be monitored to ensure adequate intake. Commercial products are available to thicken liquids or foods as appropriate. The nurse can also assist the patient with compensatory swallowing techniques or exercises prescribed by the SLP.

Some patients are not able to safely consume adequate food or fluid. Enteral nutrition support with a feeding tube is then indicated. It is important to note that risk of aspiration still exists as do the possibility of gastroesophageal reflux. Nursing interventions to minimize aspiration risk are outlined later in this chapter in the discussion on enteral nutrition support.

Gastroesophageal Reflux Disease, Hiatal Hernia, Esophagitis, and Ulcer Disease

Lifestyle modifications, including dietary manipulation, are used as an adjunct to other treatment throughout the course of therapy for disorders of the upper GI tract. Nutrition therapy is targeted at relief of symptoms from gastroesophageal reflux and mucosal irritation by gastric acid. Additionally, certain foods can precipitate reflux from specific effects on reducing lower esophageal sphincter (LES) pressure in some patients (DeVault, Castell, & Practice Parameters Committee, 1999; Katz, 2003). The nurse should assess the patient for intake of foods or habits that affect LES pressure or intra-abdominal pressure. Chart 14–25

CHART 14–25 Nutrition Therapy for GERD

Limit foods that predispose to ↓ lower esophageal sphincter pressure:
- Fat
- Alcohol
- Coffee, tea, cola
- Chocolate
- Carminatives (mint).

Limit foods that irritate esophagus:
- Citrus
- Tomato
- Spicy.

Limit gastric pressure:
- Avoid tight clothing, belts.
- Avoid large meals and excessive carbonated drinks.
- Avoid recumbency after meals.
- Lose weight if indicated.

Sources: DeVault, K. R., Castell, D. O., & Practice Parameters Committee. (1999). Practice guidelines: Updated guidelines for the diagnosis and treatment of gastroesophageal reflux disease. *The American Journal of Gastroenterology, 94,* 1434–1442; Katz, P. O. (2003). Optimizing medical therapy for gastroesophageal reflux disease: State of the art. *Reviews in Gastroenterological Disorders, 3,* 59–69; National Institute of Diabetes and Digestive and Kidney Diseases. (2003a). *Gastroesophageal reflux.* Retrieved January 13, 2004, from http://digestive.niddk.nih.gov/ddiseases/pubs/gerd/index.htm#4

provides general guidelines for adjunctive dietary treatment for gastro-esophageal reflux disease (GERD). Individual patient food intolerances should be added to these guidelines. The nurse should assess the nutritional adequacy of the diet of patients who seem intolerant to many foods or those who have broadly eliminated any major food group assuming intolerance to all of its constituents. An example of this would be the patient who consumes no fruits after poor tolerance of a citrus juice. Such patients need encouragement to try other foods within the food group to ensure adequate intake.

Dumping Syndrome

Dumping syndrome is a condition often resulting from full or partial gastric resection or the removal of the pyloric sphincter. Symptoms include abdominal cramping, diarrhea, sweating, and shakiness following a meal because of rapid emptying of gastric contents into the small intestine. Dumping syndrome can also result following bariatric surgery for morbid obesity. Postoperative nutrition guidelines for bariatric surgical patients are discussed later in this chapter.

The goals of nutrition treatment of dumping syndrome include the prevention of rapid gastric emptying and the reduction of hyperosmolar intestinal contents. Foods high in simple sugars have a concentrated, or hyperosmolar, content that will draw fluid into the gut because of a concentration gradient between plasma and the intestine. This rapid entry of fluid into the gut can contribute to the symptoms of dumping syndrome (NIDDK, 2003). Large meals, fluids with meals, and extreme food temperatures (very hot or very cold) can promote more rapid gastric emptying than usual. Eating smaller meals, avoiding liquids at mealtime, and lying down following a meal can be helpful. Chart 14–26 (p. 302) outlines the guidelines for treatment of dumping syndrome.

CHART 14–26	Nutrition Guidelines for Dumping Syndrome

- Limit consumption of simple sugars and carbonated drinks.
- Avoid extremes of hot or cold foods.
- Eat small meals.
- Save liquid for between meals.
- Lie down if needed after eating.

Source: National Heart Lung and Blood Institute. (2002). *Third report of the National Cholesterol Education Program expert panel on detection, evaluation, and treatment of high blood cholesterol in adults (Adult treatment panel III).* Retrieved February 5, 2004, from http://www.nhlbi.nih.gov/guidelines/cholesterol/atp3full.pdf

Lactose Intolerance

Lactose is the principal disaccharide present in milk products that requires the small intestine enzyme lactase for digestion. Insufficient production of lactase can foster maldigestion of lactose-containing foods with resultant intestinal complaints, which can include bloating, cramping, and diarrhea. The nurse should help educate the patient that a lactose intolerance is not an allergy to milk. Lactose maldigestion or intolerance is a common complaint among people with gastrointestinal symptoms. The prevalence of lactose-intolerance symptoms is high among many ethnic groups with the exception of those of Northern European descent (Swagerty, Walling, & Klein, 2002). Several researchers have found that people mistakenly claim they have lactose intolerance when in fact breath hydrogen tests show normal findings, leading some to conclude that the prevalence statistics are overstated (Saltzman et al., 1999). Insufficient lactase production can occur from birth, which is uncommon, or later in life. Secondary lactose intolerance can occur from damage to the small intestine mucosa, such as with infection, small bowel disease, chemotherapy, or intestinal radiation, and may be temporary (Montalto et al., 2006). The degree of lactose intolerance varies among individuals and can be dose dependent (Montalto et al., 2006). Nutrition treatment of lactose intolerance is largely not dependent on the etiology of the intolerance.

A general consensus exists that most people who complain of lactose intolerance are capable of tolerating some lactose in their diets. Additionally, it is believed that tolerance to lactose can be improved with the continual consumption of some lactose-containing foods. Some milk-based foods, such as aged cheeses, naturally contain less lactose than others do. Many yogurts and other fermented dairy products have reduced lactose content and advantageous probiotic bacteria that have a lactase-producing ability that benefits digestion of lactose content (Kopp-Hoolihan, 2001; Montalto et al., 2006; Swagerty et al., 2002).

Because each patient with lactose intolerance has a different ability to produce lactose, medical nutrition therapy occurs along a continuum. The nurse should assess the patient for lactose tolerance among different milk-based foods and under different patterns of consumption. Lactose-containing foods tend to be better tolerated with a meal than when consumed alone (Montalto et al., 2006). The patient's diet should be assessed for adequate calcium and vitamin D sources, especially for those who have broadly eliminated dairy foods from their diets. Chart 14–27 lists suggestions for improving tolerance to lactose and adequate intake of calcium and vitamin D.

CHART 14–27	Nutrition Guidelines for Lactose Intolerance

- Try 1/2 to 1 cup milk with meals.
- Gradually increase milk intake in small increments.
- Try cultured and fermented dairy products: yogurt with active cultures, buttermilk, aged cheese.
- Use digestive aides as needed: oral lactase enzyme products or enzyme-incubated milk.
- Monitor diet for adequate calcium and vitamin D intake.
- Be mindful of hidden lactose in baking mixes, processed foods, instant soups, mashed potato mix, cold cuts, commercial sauces, and medicines.
- Read labels for "nonfat milk solids" or "milk by-products" because lactose may be present.

Sources: Montalto, M., Curigliano, C., Santoro, L., Vastola, M., Cammarota, G., & Manna, R. (2006). Management and treatment of lactose malabsorption. *World Journal of Gastroenterology, 12,* 187–191; National Institute of Diabetes, and Digestive Disorders and Kidney Diseases. (2003b). *Lactose intolerance.* Retrieved January 13, 2004, from http://digestive.niddk.nih.gov/ddiseases/pubs/lactoseintolerance; Swagerty, D. L., Walling, A. D., & Klein, R. M. (2002). Lactose intolerance. *American Family Physician, 65,* 1845–1850.

Inflammatory Bowel Disease

A diagnosis of either Crohn's disease or ulcerative colitis can place a patient at risk for malnutrition. Chapter 45 ⊕ provides a complete description of Crohn's disease. Crohn's patients generally tend to have more extensive nutritional risk factors than do patients with ulcerative colitis because of potential small bowel disease location, severity of symptoms, and fistula formation (Goh & O'Morain, 2003; Jeejeebhoy, 2002a). Active inflammatory bowel disease can cause diminished nutrient intake, increased gut nutritional losses and additional metabolic requirements (Goh & O'Morain, 2003; Jeejeebhoy, 2002a). Together, or singly, these disease consequences present nutritional challenges to the patient and the clinician. Pain, anorexia, fever, and medication side effects can lead to poor intake in the face of the increased metabolic needs required for tissue healing and to compensate for malabsorptive losses. Patients with inflammatory bowel disease require a comprehensive nutrition assessment on which to base the foundation of nutrition therapy. The Risk Factors box lists common nutrition problems association with Crohn's disease.

RISK FACTORS for Malnutrition in Inflammatory Bowel Disease

Risk Factor	Etiology of Malnutrition Risk
Decreased intake	• Nausea, vomiting, diarrhea • Pain or fear of pain • Discomfort associated w/certain foods • Anorexia
Increased nutrient losses	• Malabsorption; depends on disease site • Drug–nutrient interactions (sulfasalazine and folic acid, steroids and calcium, vitamin D) • Iron losses w/bleeding
Increased nutrient needs	• Hypermetabolism from inflammation • Fistula healing requirements

Physical symptoms and disease severity will dictate the nutrition care plan. Small bowel disease in Crohn's can lead to malabsorption of multiple nutrients, depending on the specific location of the disease. Calcium, magnesium, iron, and other minerals are generally absorbed in the proximal small intestine, whereas vitamin B_{12}, fat, and fat-soluble vitamin absorption occur in the ileum. Fat malabsorption can lead to a cascade of other nutritional problems such as vitamin A, D, E, and K and calcium malabsorption, increased absorption of oxalates (with subsequent increased risk of oxalate kidney stones), and loss of the valuable energy derived from fat. Fluid and electrolyte status can also become compromised because of losses from diarrhea. Inadequate absorption of calcium and vitamin D can lead to bone disease and further complicate the nutritional consequences of the steroid therapy often used in these patients (Jeejeebhoy, 2002a).

Anemia from blood losses and poor iron, folate, and vitamin B_{12} absorption can contribute further to the fatigue experienced from inadequate intake and the disease process. Enteric fistula formation can cause intestinal losses of crucial nutrients, as well as fluid and electrolytes. Surgical resection of diseased intestine can result in the loss of crucial absorptive surface and further place the patient at nutritional risk. Short bowel syndrome can be the result and is discussed in a later section. Knowledge of the extent and location of disease, along with a complete nutrition history, is essential to identify nutrition risk and goals.

Nutrition treatment of inflammatory bowel disease focuses on correction of malnutrition and provision of adequate nutrients and energy to promote disease remission. Nutrition plays a central role in disease management and remission but is not the primary treatment (American Gastroenterological Association [AGA] 2001a; Ireton-Jones, 2000; Jeejeebhoy, 2002a). Patients with severe fulminant disease can require nutrition support in the form of a low-fat elemental or polymeric enteral nutrition formula, which is discussed later. These formulas can be taken orally or delivered via a feeding tube. Such formulas require minimal digestion for absorption and can be a better tolerated mode of providing nutrition than a usual diet, though palatability of some formulas is low. A registered dietitian would determine the appropriate type and amount of enteral nutrition support and make a recommendation for treatment.

The nurse should monitor intake and tolerance as described in Chart 14–28 (p. 304). Unless a patient has developed a bowel obstruction, perforation, or severe short bowel syndrome, there is no specific need for parenteral nutrition in disease treatment as compared with enteral support. Achievement of disease remission does not require bowel rest (AGA, 2001a). It is postulated that use of the gut with enteral nutrition provides an additional beneficial effect toward recovery, besides just nutrient content, by preventing intestinal bacterial translocation that can occur when the gut is not used (Goh & O'Morain, 2003; Jeejeebhoy, 2002a).

A low-residue diet with adequate energy and protein is indicated as patients are recovering from a disease flare and transitioning a return to their usual diet (George, Day, & Zeiter, 2000; Ireton-Jones, 2000). Fibrous fruits and vegetables, whole grains, seeds, and nuts are avoided to decrease fecal residue and stool frequency. Patients with stricture should avoid a high-fiber diet to decrease the risk of intestinal obstruction (Jeejeebhoy, 2002a).

Lactose-containing foods may need to be limited in patients for whom secondary lactose intolerance has developed. Due to lack of small bowel involvement, patients with ulcerative colitis are not likely to benefit from altering lactose intake. As the patient improves, the diet can be liberalized as tolerated.

Nutrient supplementation is often indicated for patients unable to tolerate adequate variety in the diet or with active disease. Anemia should be treated with the appropriate dose of iron, folic acid, or vitamin B_{12} depending on anemia type. (Anemia is discussed later in this chapter.) Calcium supplementation to meet the federal Recommended Dietary Allowance (RDA) of 1,000 to 1,200 mg are indicated for patients with a limited diet, steroid therapy, or malabsorption. Adequate vitamin D is needed as well. Zinc is lost when there is high-volume intestinal output as with diarrhea or an enteric fistula. Wound healing, including fistula repair, requires zinc. Zinc replacement of 12 to 15 mg/day per liter of stool output or 20 to 40 mg/day zinc gluconate is recommended (Ireton-Jones, 2000; Jeejeebhoy, 2002b). Magnesium replacement therapy may also be necessary, but care must be used to avoid magnesium salts known to precipitate diarrhea (Jeejeebhoy, 2002b). The nurse should routinely assess patients with inflammatory bowel disease for inadequate or overly restrictive intake and refer appropriate patients for nutritional counseling.

Celiac Sprue

Celiac sprue, or gluten-sensitive enteropathy, is a lifelong condition affecting the small intestine in which the villi morphology is damaged from the presence of gluten in the diet. Gluten is a protein found in grain products, specifically wheat, rye, and barley. The presence of gluten in the intestine leads to villi atrophy and loss of absorptive surface. Diarrhea with malabsorption of most nutrients can follow with risk of weight loss and malnutrition. Individuals vary in their degree of presenting malabsorptive symptoms (AGA, 2001b).

Medical nutrition therapy is essential for resolution of symptoms and return of normal villi morphology (AGA, 2001b). Gluten-containing foods must be avoided to eliminate disease symptoms (NIDDK, 2005a). There is agreement that foods made from wheat, rye, and barley should be eliminated, but considerable debate exists about several other grains. Oats have traditionally been excluded in the diet as well, but more recently evidence exists that oats do not exhibit toxicity and can be well tolerated (NIDDK, 2005a). The AGA permits oat products as part of a gluten-free diet, but warns of the possibility of wheat contamination of oat flour (AGA, 2001b). The chance of wheat contamination has led some to recommend avoidance of oats until disease remission and then only consumption of oat products from a trustworthy source (Farrell & Kelly, 2002). Buckwheat, quinoa, and amaranth are grains recommended by some clinicians and celiac sprue organizations citing different plant taxonomy than offending grains, but they are banned by others because of insufficient information on toxicity (Thompson, 2000b, 2001a). No consensus exists on advice to give patients regarding these three grains. The recommendation regarding wheat-starch faces a similar dilemma in that some recognize it as gluten free, whereas others contend it still has offending protein components (Thompson, 2001b). Distilled vinegar, millet, and wild rice are also debated. Chart 14–29 (p. 305) outlines common dietary sources of gluten.

| CHART 14–28 | **Nursing Interventions in Enteral Nutrition Support** |

Problem	Intervention
Potential for foodborne illness	• Wash hands before handling formula and equipment. • Wipe off top of formula container before opening. • Label, cover, and store open formula in refrigerator for not >24 hours. • Limit "hang time" to 4 hours if water or other additions made to formula. Otherwise 8- to 12-hour hang time allowed if canned formula w/no additives is being used.
Aspiration	• Check gastric residuals. Hold feeding for large volume (>150 mL but treat individually and according to physician's order). • Elevate head of bed to at least a 30-degree angle. • Avoid bolus feedings. • Consider smaller bore or longer tube if nasally intubated. Routinely confirm tube placement. • Consider G-tube or J-tube if long-term feeding is required.

Clogged tube	• Administer feeding with pump vs. gravity drip.
	• Administer room temperature feeding. High-temperature storage or heating of formula will cause protein content to coagulate.
	• Follow guidelines for medication administration:
	  1. Flush tube with 20 to 30 mL water before, between, and after each single medication.
	  2. Consult pharmacist regarding suitability of crushing medication with a small amount of water and availability of medication elixirs.
	
	Note: If using longer feeding tubes, ensure medication absorption site is not bypassed by tube.

Diarrhea	• Administer feeding at room temperature. Cold feeding increases gut peristalsis. • Consider lactose-free formula. • Consider formula with fiber. • Consider medications w/cathartic effect: antibiotics, magnesium, potassium, digoxin, theophylline, acetaminophen elixir, and others. • Administer continuous drip vs. bolus. • Consult registered dietitian regarding temporarily altering formula concentration or rate of delivery. • Rule out infection, *Clostridium difficile,* medical etiology.
Constipation	• Consider formula with added fiber. • Monitor hydration; ensure adequate intake. • Encourage ambulation as indicated. • Assess for contributing medications (e.g., narcotics, some antacids). • Consider obstruction or medical causes.
Dehydration	• Monitor hydration: weight, intake & output, physical signs. • Ensure adequate free water intake. Need 1 mL water per 1 kcal of intake. Most formulas are 50%–75% free water (formula with >1 kcal/mL or high protein content have less free water).

Sources: Rees Parrish, C., & Falls McCray, S. (2003). Nutrition support for the mechanically ventilated patient. *Critical Care Nurse, 23,* 77–80.; Dobson, K., & Scott, A. (2007). Review of ICU nutrition support practices: Implementing the nurse-led enteral feeding algorithm. *Nursing in Critical Care, 12,* 114–123; Swanson, R. W., & Winkelman, C. (2002). Exploring the benefits and myths of enteral feeding in the critically ill. *Critical Care Nursing Quarterly, 24,* 67–75.

The patient with celiac sprue has to be dedicated to label reading and attentive to the diet at all times. Wheat, rye, and barley are present in both obvious and hidden sources in the diet. Some patients with celiac sprue also have secondary lactose intolerance and must adhere to guidelines for that treatment as well. Product reformulation can lead to changes that add or delete ingredients so continued label reading is essential. The nurse should warn patients to be suspect of labels touting "new and improved" versions because ingredients could be altered. The nurse can be empathetic about the need for restrictions and stress the role of diet in avoiding ill health and correcting existing deficiencies.

Gluten-free versions of grain foods can replace the displaced wheat, rye, and barley products. Corn, potato, rice, and soy flours can be used to make alternative breads, pasta, and baked goods. Many stores and online sources sell these products. A local or online celiac sprue support group and a knowledgeable dietitian can provide patients with lists of available products. Wheat flour products are commonly fortified with iron, folic acid, and other B-complex vitamins. Alternative gluten-free products often are not routinely fortified with these nutrients. Alternative sources of iron and B-complex vitamins should be encouraged. The limited diet warrants a recommendation of a gluten-free multivitamin supplement (Thompson, 1999, 2000a).

CHART 14–29 Dietary Sources of Gluten

Label reading is essential. In addition to more obvious sources of barley, rye, and wheat, fillers and additives contain hidden sources of gluten that can be discovered by reading ingredient panels. Dietary sources of gluten include:

- Barley including beer, malt beverages, and cereal
- Rye
- Wheat including all wheat flour products (pastas, cereals, baked goods, pizza crust, etc.), wheat or food starch, couscous, spelt, triticale, semolina, distilled vinegar, soy sauce, caramel coloring. Wheat or food starch can be a filler in many products, including instant mixes, sauces, condiments, hot dogs, sausage.

It is under debate whether or not the following grains should be restricted. Patients should be assessed individually and given personal advice:

- Oats
- Buckwheat
- Amaranth
- Quinoa
- Millet
- Sorghum.

Sources: American Gastroenterological Association (AGA). (2001a). Medical position statement: Celiac sprue. Gastroenterology, 120, 1761–1778; Farrell, R. J., & Kelly, C. (2002). Celiac sprue. New England Journal of Medicine, 346, 180–188; National Institute of Diabetes and Digestive and Kidney Diseases. (2005a). Celiac disease. Retrieved November 13, 2006, from http://www.digestive.niddk.nih.gov/ddiseases/pubs/celiac/index.htm; Thompson, T. (2001a). Case problem: Questions regarding the acceptability of buckwheat, amaranth, quinoa, and oats from a patient with celiac disease. Journal of the American Dietetic Association, 101, 586–587; Thompson, T. (2001b). Wheat starch, gliadin, and the gluten-free diet. Journal of the American Dietetic Association, 101, 1456–1459.

Short Bowel Syndrome

Short bowel syndrome (SBS) describes a set of symptoms that can result from a large surgical resection of any combination of small intestine and colon. Most commonly, the resection is a result of a single or several surgical interventions for inflammatory bowel disease. Bowel infarct, gastric bypass surgery, neoplastic disease treatment, and congenital abnormalities are among other etiology of SBS. In some forms of gastric bypass surgery for morbid obesity, the loss of small intestine absorptive surface is a deliberate attempt to have malabsorption contribute to weight loss efforts. Such surgery and its nutrition intervention are discussed later in the surgical nutrition section of this chapter. Symptoms of SBS can include rapid gut transit time, diarrhea, altered fluid and electrolyte status, malabsorption, and subsequent weight loss and malnutrition (AGA, 2003; Atalay et al., 2003; Jeejeebhoy, 2002b). Loss of absorptive surface and the presence of unabsorbed substrate in the colon are responsible for the symptoms.

A patient with <200 cm (6.5 ft) of small intestine is at risk for short bowel syndrome. Patients with <100 cm (3.3 ft) of remaining small intestine most likely will have some symptoms of this syndrome, especially if losses include the terminal ileum or remaining bowel has disease (AGA, 2003). The terminal ileum is the site of reabsorption of bile salts that are responsible for fat and fat-soluble vitamin absorption. Additionally, vitamin B_{12} and some water and electrolyte absorption occur here. When all of these substances remain unabsorbed and pass into the colon,

their hyperosmolar content draws fluid from the plasma that leads to diarrhea, malabsorption, and altered hydration. If both ileum and colon have been resected, an end jejunostomy is the result and has compromised absorptive ability (AGA, 2003; Jeejeebhoy, 2002b). Postsurgical intestinal adaptation can occur over the course of 1 to 2 years and improve absorptive capability. The ileum can adapt to compensate for the absorptive needs previously met by a resected jejunum, but conversely, the jejunum is less able to compensate for a resected ileum (Jeejeebhoy, 2002b).

Medical nutrition therapy for SBS is essential. Patients must receive adequate nutrition to promote wound healing and prevent malnutrition in the postoperative period. Initially, patients will require at least a 7- to 10-day course of parenteral nutrition to meet fluid, electrolyte, and nutritional demands while potential bowel function begins to return (AGA, 2003). Gradual conversion to enteral nutrition occurs according to patient tolerance. Those patients with more than 100 cm (3.3 ft) of remaining small intestine, especially those with an intact ileum and colon, typically are able to progress to a standard diet, often with few restrictions (Atalay et al., 2003). In contrast, patients with 35 to 100 cm (about 1 to 3.3 ft) of intestinal remnant may progress more slowly from parenteral nutrition to an enteral formula and then to trials of a modified diet over the course of several months to years (AGA, 2003; Atalay et al., 2003). Intestinal absorptive adaptation takes time and requires enteral nutrition in order to occur. Patients with <50 cm (1.6 ft) of remaining intestine present a unique medical challenge because of severely altered absorption and the potential for ongoing disturbances in hydration and electrolyte status and acid–base balance (AGA, 2003; Atalay et al., 2003; Jeejeebhoy, 2002b). Most often these patients require permanent parenteral nutrition to meet their nutritional and fluid and electrolyte requirements, because adaptation is less likely to occur than in cases with larger bowel remnants.

When the patient is hemodynamically stable and bowel sounds return, sips of isotonic liquids can be attempted. Isotonic enteral formula and rehydration solutions are recommended (AGA, 2003). Hypertonic liquids, such as elemental nutrition formula and sugary drinks, or hypotonic liquids (water or overly diluted drinks) are not recommended initially because of potential intestinal fluid and electrolyte shifts compensating for a concentration gradient (AGA, 2003). Sorbitol should be avoided in sugar-free beverages because of its laxative effect. The nurse should monitor fluid intake and tolerance with a careful comparison to measured fluid output. Laboratory values should also be monitored for assessing hydration and electrolyte status, that is, sodium, chloride, potassium, hemoglobin, and hematocrit. Sodium, potassium, magnesium, and zinc losses can be substantial and require replacement (Jeejeebhoy, 2002b). Patients will vary in their ability to successfully attempt this stage of diet transition. Some may require months of parenteral support first.

After several months of tolerance to enteral formula, the patient with SBS can begin the challenging process of further intestinal adaptation with a more solid diet. Patients with <100 cm (3.3 ft) of bowel remnant can require intake of twice their estimated nutrition needs in order to absorb adequate macro- and micronutrients. Protein absorption occurs in the duodenum and generally is not compromised as severely as other nutrients

(Jeejeebhoy, 2002b). A modified diet is encouraged as tolerated following the parameters outlined in Chart 14–30. The diet may be modified to include less lactose and low oxalate content, but not low fat. Altering fat has little effect on symptoms and deprives the patient of needed calories. A lactose-modified diet is recommended only if lactose maldigestion in known. Patients with SBS and an existing colon are at risk for increased absorption of oxalate (AGA, 2003). Oxalate is a substance found in foods such as spinach, chocolate, tea, and rhubarb and normally is bound with calcium and poorly absorbed. However, during fat malabsorption, calcium binds with free fats, leaving oxalates unbound and more apt to be absorbed by the intestine. Eventually such elevated oxalate absorption can lead to calcium oxalate kidney stones (Morton, Iliescu, & Wilson, 2002).

Nutrient supplementation is often necessary if the ileum has been resected. Fat-soluble vitamins A, D, E, and K are needed in a liquid form if **steatorrhea,** or diarrhea from fat malabsorption, is present. This can be confirmed with a Sudan stain of a stool sample. Zinc replacement should correspond with intestinal output. Calcium supplements are needed if a lactose modification is needed or fat malabsorption is present. Calcium supplements can advantageously assist with lessening oxalate absorption. The need for magnesium replacement should also be assessed. Vitamin B_{12} injections are needed in patients without an ileum (AGA, 2003; Jeejeebhoy, 2002b). Patients who experience SBS require long-term monitoring by an experienced health care team to prevent malnutrition, dehydration, and altered electrolyte status.

Constipation

A high-fiber diet is recommended for the treatment of most types of constipation (AGA, 2000). A low-fiber diet and sedentary lifestyle contribute to the occurrence of constipation in adults (Arce, Ermocilla, & Costa, 2002). Fiber is present only in plant foods and can be removed during processing. Adequate fiber intake benefits intestinal motility by contributing to stool bulk and shortening intestinal transit time. The National Academy of Science has set the daily recommendation for fiber at 38 g for men and 25 g for women up to age 50 years. After age 50, the recommendation drops to 30 g and 21 g, respectively (Institute of Medicine [IOM], 2002). The nurse should advise the patient to gradually add fiber to the diet in order to minimize intestinal bloating. Adequate fluid intake is also recommended to both prevent and treat constipation. The established daily adequate intake (AI) of water for men and women is 3.7 and 2.7 liters, respectively (IOM, 2004). Chart 14–31 outlines sources of fiber to recommend.

Diverticular Disease

Patients with uncomplicated diverticulosis should be encouraged to consume adequate fiber to lessen potential symptoms and potentially avoid diverticulitis. Although there is no evidence that a high-fiber diet will decrease intraluminal pressure and subsequent development of diverticula, the recommendation to consume sufficient fiber is felt to be a reasonable approach to amelioration of symptoms of this condition (NIDDK, 2005b; Stollman, Raskin, & Practice Parameters Committee, 1999). Traditionally most fiber sources have been recommended with the exception of seeds and nuts feared to foster diverticulitis when trapped in diverticulum. The AGA does not find sub-

---

CHART 14–30	Nutrition Therapy for Short Bowel Syndrome
Early diet	• Use isotonic feedings to minimize diarrhea.
	• Replace fluid and electrolyte losses.
	• Determine nutrients at risk for malabsorption based on resection site.
Adaptation	• Maximize intake of energy (including fat) and protein, adjust to tolerance.
	• Give frequent meals w/liquids separately.
	• Dilute sugary drinks.
General recommendations	• Limit caffeine, oxalates, lactose, sugar alcohols (such as sorbitol, mannitol).
	• Monitor and replace electrolytes/minerals, including zinc, potassium, and magnesium.
	• Replace fat-soluble vitamins and B_{12} if ileum resected/fat malabsorbing.

Sources: Atalay, F., Ozcay, N., Gundogdu, H., Orug, T., et al. (2003). Evaluation of the outcomes of short bowel syndrome and indications for intestinal transplantation. *Transplant Proceedings, 35,* 3054–3056; Jeejeebhoy, K. N. (2002b). Short bowel syndrome. *Canadian Medical Association Journal, 166,* 1297–1302; Stahl, P. (2000). Nutrition protocols for small-bowel transplant patients. *Journal of the American Dietetic Association, 100,* 689.

CHART 14–31	Fiber Content of Selected Foods*			
≤1 g Fiber	**2 g Fiber**	**3 g Fiber**	**4 g Fiber**	**≥5 g Fiber**
1-oz white bread	1-oz whole-wheat bread	1 med banana	1 C brown rice	1 C bran flake cereal
1 dinner roll, average	2 C popcorn	1 C corn	1/2 C cooked barley	1/2 C dried fruit
1 boiled potato without skin	1 C couscous	1/2 C winter squash	1 C cooked oatmeal	1/2 C cooked beans, peas, or
1 C iceberg lettuce	1 medium peach	1/4 cup soy nuts	1 med apple or pear with skin	lentils
1 C mushrooms	1/2 cup cooked carrots		1 med baked potato with skin	1 C cooked collards
			1 C cooked spinach	1 kiwi
			2 TBSP almonds	

*The nurse should advise the patient that fiber content is listed on "Nutrition Facts" food labels.

Source: USDA Nutrient Data Laboratory http://www.nal.usda.gov/fnic/foodcomp/search

stantial clinical evidence to support this seed and nut restriction (Stollman et al., 1999). The NIH and others still advise against consumption of nuts, popcorn hulls, and seeds (Cunningham & Marcason, 2002; NIDDK, 2005b).

Nutritional management of an episode of diverticulitis requires a short course of a clear liquid diet while medical treatment is given and symptoms abate within a few days (Stollman et al., 1999). Patients who require surgical intervention, an extended course of nil per os (NPO), or more prolonged intake of clear liquids need close nutritional assessment and monitoring with appropriate referral to the registered dietitian as needed. Once diverticulitis is resolved and the patient is free of symptoms, the high-fiber diet should be resumed.

Chronic Diarrhea

Chronic diarrhea can occur for many reasons. Appropriate nutrition intervention is determined by the etiology of the diarrhea, if known. Patients in whom pancreatic exocrine function is compromised may require a low-fat diet as outlined in the nutrition treatment of pancreatic disease. Small bowel disease and lactose intolerance can also result in chronic diarrhea if not adequately treated. (Nutrition therapy for each of these causes was discussed in an earlier section.) The nurse can assess the patient for excessive intake of sugar alcohols, such as sorbitol, which can contribute to diarrhea. The presence of eating disorder symptoms can also be cause to suspect laxative abuse, which can lead to chronic diarrhea. Patients with chronic diarrhea should be routinely assessed for fluid, electrolyte, weight loss, and nutrition depletion. Parenteral nutrition may be required in cases where intestinal losses from the condition exceed enteral ability to compensate and maintain adequate nutrition or fluid balance (AGA, 1999).

Irritable Bowel Syndrome

Irritable bowel syndrome (IBS) is characterized by abdominal pain, constipation, or diarrhea that has no known coexisting organic cause. Nutrition treatment is largely trial and error according to the individual patient's situation. Often a symptom diary is helpful to guide the patient in finding any lifestyle factors, including offending foods, that trigger symptoms (AGA, 2002a). No single food or food group has proven to universally contribute to symptoms though a significant placebo effect was noticed in many research trials. Caffeine, alcohol, fat, and sorbitol are the most commonly mentioned trigger foods. Sorbitol is a sugar alcohol present in dietetic candies and foods that has a laxative effect (Burden, 2001; Viera, Hoag, & Shaughnessy, 2002).

Many patients with IBS can benefit from a psychosocial assessment and appropriate intervention because coexisting stress, coping difficulties, depression, and anxiety occur in these patients (Viera et al., 2002). The nurse can guide the patient in recognizing any individual foods that trigger symptoms and suggest experimenting with limiting caffeine, alcohol, sorbitol, and fat in the diet. Lactose intolerance is often a complaint because of similar symptoms, but can be unfounded. Lactose should be managed only in patients known to have lactase deficiency (Viera et al., 2002).

Liver Disease

The liver performs various functions related to the storage, metabolism, or excretion of most nutrients. Liver disease impacts nutrition status by decreasing nutrient storage and interfering with efficient metabolism. The body's ability to maintain nutritional health is altered when any aspect of nutrient metabolism is compromised by liver disease.

Fatty Liver

Deposition of fatty deposits in the liver can occur from excessive alcohol intake but can also be associated with nonalcoholic etiology. Many cases of fatty liver, or steatosis, are associated with nutritional contributors. Daily intake of more than 20 to 30 g of alcohol, obesity, severe weight loss (as in starvation or following gastric bypass surgery for obesity), total parenteral nutrition, elevated blood triglyceride levels found in type 2 diabetes, and metabolic syndrome are associated with steatosis (AGA, 2002b). Nutrition therapy for fatty liver requires knowledge of the pathogenesis of the condition. Abstinence from alcohol, weight loss if overweight, and control of plasma glucose and lipids are the primary therapies for uncomplicated fatty liver.

Alcohol and Nutrition Status

Malnutrition can be a complication of excessive alcohol intake and is associated with a more dismal prognosis than observed in better nourished people with alcoholic liver disease (Stickel et al., 2003). It is important for the nurse to understand the overall potential impact of alcohol on nutrition status when assessing patients with any type of alcoholic liver disease. Both primary and secondary malnutrition can occur from excessive alcohol intake. Poor-quality food, infrequent food intake, and anorexia are examples of risk factors for primary malnutrition. Secondary malnutrition can occur because of indirect effects such as nutrient malabsorption and altered metabolism. Alcohol contains significant calories (7.1 per gram), which can be a concern in the casual drinker trying to maintain or lose weight. However, when intake of alcohol is excessive, altered and inefficient metabolism of alcohol occurs, resulting in weight loss when significant food calories are replaced by alcohol calories (Santolaria et al., 2000; Stickel et al., 2003). Chart 14–32 (p. 308) lists the contributing causes of both primary and secondary malnutrition with excessive alcohol intake.

A careful assessment of nutrition status should be done when excessive alcohol intake is suspected. Unfortunately, an accurate diet history is difficult to obtain if the patient has suffered periods of altered consciousness. Irregular feeding habits and transient diet quality further make generalizations from a diet recall difficult (Santolaria et al., 2000).

Patients in whom alcohol comprises more than 30% of total calorie intake have been shown to have decreased intake of protein, fat, vitamins A and C, thiamin, calcium, and iron (Lieber, 2000). The altered absorption and metabolism of those nutrients from alcohol can further worsen nutrition health. Physical assessment of the patient should focus on skin integrity, presence of muscle or fat wasting, and edema or ascites. Chapter 46 ⊙ has a complete description of ascites due to liver disease. Altered fluid status can mask changes in body weight, making weight or BMI unreliable assessment tools for nutrition status. If liver disease is present, plasma protein production can be diminished unrelated to nutrition. Malnutrition can also lower serum albumin, prealbumin, or transferrin levels, but it is impossible to differentiate the major cause with the compounded effects of liver disease and poor nutrition status.

CHART 14–32	Effect of Alcohol on Nutrition Status
Primary malnutrition	Replaces nutrient and food intake with alcohol. Appetite can be suppressed.
Secondary malnutrition	Decreased nutrient absorption: • Thiamine • Folate • Vitamin B$_{12}$ • Protein. Increased urinary losses of nutrients: • Folate • Magnesium • Zinc • Nitrogen. Decreased nutrient storage: • Folate • Riboflavin • Vitamin B$_6$.

Sources: Lieber, C. S. (2000). Alcohol: Its metabolism and interaction with nutrients. *Annual Review Nutrition, 20,* 395–430; Stickel, F., Hoehn, B., & Seitz, H. K. (2003). Nutrition therapy in alcoholic liver disease. *Alimentary Pharmacology Therapy, 18,* 357–373.

Nutrition supplementation is recommended for several nutrients when excessive alcohol intake is suspected or known and nutrition intake is poor. A multivitamin supplement with ample water-soluble vitamins is reasonable, with special attention given to thiamine and folic acid (Stickel et al., 2003). Both nutrients are poorly absorbed in the presence of alcohol. Thiamine supplementation in the alcoholic patient is crucial in order to avoid development of Wernicke-Korsakoff syndrome (Thiamine, 2003). Thiamine is routinely administered on admission to patients suspected or known to abuse alcohol. Trace mineral status should be assessed and deficiencies replaced accordingly. Zinc levels are often diminished from low intake and increased urinary zinc excretion in people with alcoholic liver disease (Lieber, 2000). Abstinence from alcohol is the primary goal.

Hepatitis

Anorexia, fatigue, and gastrointestinal complaints are common symptoms with hepatitis that can place a patient at increased risk for malnutrition. Fever and hypermetabolism require closer than usual attention to energy intake and hydration. Nutrition care of a patient with hepatitis should stress the need for calories and protein to enhance hepatocyte regeneration and prevent weight loss. Patients can require an additional 10% to 40% more calories above normal and up to 1.5 g of protein per kilogram ideal weight (Dietitians of Canada, 2003). Lack of appetite and nausea make meal consumption difficult. Small, more frequent nutrient-dense meals can promote overall increased intake and help with nausea, which is often worsened by an empty stomach. A multivitamin supplement should be considered in patients with poor intake. Importantly, high doses of some vitamins, such as vitamin A and niacin, are hepatotoxic and should be avoided (Riley & Bhatti, 2001).

The nurse should assess the patient for self-prescribed use of supplements and provide education about consuming excesses. Additionally, the patient should be assessed for use of alternative medicine supplements. Many herbal supplements are hepatotoxic. Chaparral, comfrey, and mistletoe are examples of hepatotoxic herbs. Others, like milk thistle, are touted by some for their ability to improve liver function (Riley & Bhatti, 2001). The nurse should consult with a pharmacist knowledgeable about herb safety and review the latest medical research when questions arise. Few recommendations exist on herbal remedies for liver disease and this should not be misinterpreted to mean untested herbs are efficacious or safe.

Cirrhosis

Malnutrition can be a common complication in patients with cirrhosis. Poor nutrition is more likely to occur in cirrhosis from alcoholic liver disease than nonalcoholic liver disease. Nutrition status is related to the etiology of the liver disease as well as its severity. An accurate nutrition assessment is often complicated by the presence of edema and ascites, as well as decreased production of plasma proteins—all secondary to liver disease. Digestion, absorption, metabolism, and storage of nutrients are all negatively affected by cirrhosis. Poor glycogen storage with enhanced breakdown of fat and protein occurs and resembles metabolic alterations seen in short-term starvation. Decreased production of bile salts by the liver can cause energy loss from fat because of steatorrhea. Pancreatic exocrine insufficiency is found in alcoholic liver disease and can impact fat absorption as well (Stickel et al., 2003). Ascites can cause the sensation of early satiety because of abdominal pressure and lead to diminished intake at meals.

Nutrition therapy in cirrhosis should include adequate protein to foster potential hepatic regeneration (Blei, Cordoba, & Practice Parameters Committee, 2001). Frequent meals and snacks should be offered to compensate for hypermetabolism and poor glycogen storage. Hypermetabolism has been reported in some, but not all, patients with cirrhosis. The reason for this increase is not fully understood but can contribute to malnutrition if energy needs go unmet. Energy needs vary individually and are estimated to be between 35 and 40 calories per kilogram dry weight (Kondrup, 2006). Smaller, more frequent meals help if early satiety is an issue. A low-sodium diet (2 g) is indicated in decompensated cirrhosis when ascites or edema is present (Riley & Bhatti, 2001). The nurse should monitor and encourage intake, stressing the importance of the dietary intake to avoid further nutrition risk and compromised health. Malnutrition has been shown to be an independent predictor of survival in patients with cirrhosis (Alberino et al., 2001). Patients with cirrhosis and malnutrition who require liver transplantation or other surgery are considered to be a higher surgical risk than those who are better nourished (Kondrup, 2006).

Hepatic Encephalopathy

Many theories exist as to the pathogenesis of hepatic encephalopathy, but it is agreed that unmetabolized ammonia in the intestinal tract is the major precipitating factor (Blei et al., 2001). Ammonia is normally metabolized by the liver and skeletal muscle, but this can be compromised with liver damage. Elevated ammonia blood levels then lead to sequelae that include altered neurotransmission and encephalopathy. Medical nutrition therapy targeting a reduction in blood ammonia plays a central role in treatment. Ammonia is produced in response to excessive protein from the diet and from metabolism of protein compounds found in the intestine. Intestinal bacteria contribute to this metabolic effect. Constipation, gastrointestinal bleeding, and infection can also increase ammonia production by providing a favorable environment or substrate for intestinal bacteria to produce ammonia. Traditionally, a low-protein diet has been used to treat hepatic encephalopathy, but this approach is now considered to contribute to encephalopathic symptoms when maintained over time (Blei et al., 2001). Protracted restriction of protein can lead to skeletal muscle catabolism and availability of substrate for ammonia production. Additionally, ammonia is normally taken up by skeletal muscle. Catabolism of skeletal muscle can diminish the amount of ammonia that can be taken up by muscle.

Current recommendations for medical nutrition therapy of hepatic encephalopathy call for an initial, short-term protein restriction of 0.5 g/kg ideal weight per day (Blei et al., 2001). This restriction should be prescribed for 1 to 2 days while monitoring the patient for signs of improvement. Depending on the patient's level of consciousness, nutrition can be administered as an oral diet or tube feeding. Enteral feeding is contraindicated in patients with active gastrointestinal bleeding. The diet should then be advanced in small increments to include increasing amounts of protein while monitoring patient tolerance. Ultimate protein intake should reach 1.0 to 1.5 g/kg ideal weight per day (Blei et al., 2001). A 70-kg (about 150-lb) ideal weight patient would need 70 to 105 g of protein. Examples of foods containing protein to meet incremental protein increases are listed in Chart 14–33. Some patients have improved protein tolerance when a portion of their intake is derived from plant protein sources. From 30 to 40 g of plant protein is tolerated without the intestinal side effect of bloating. It is believed that the fiber content of these foods quickens gut transit time and alters the intestinal pH environment by providing substrate for beneficial bacteria action (Blei et al., 2001).

As a last resort in the patient who seems chronically intolerant of protein, enteral formula with enhanced branch chain amino acid (BCAA) content may be tried. BCAA may be better tolerated than other protein sources in some patients. These formulas are expensive and do not contain complete nutrition, but

CHART 14–33   Incremental Protein in Treatment of Hepatic Encephalopathy

The following foods contain approximately 7 to 10 g of protein per serving listed:

1 egg, whole

1 oz meat, fish, poultry, cheese

1 cup milk or yogurt

1 oz firm tofu

1/2 cup cooked beans, peas, lentils

2 TBSP peanut butter

2 oz nuts, average.

Source: USDA Nutrient Data Laboratory http://www.nal.usda.gov/fnic/foodcomp/search

may be of some benefit in this limited population (Blei et al., 2001). These nutrition-based treatments are used to augment pharmacologic management aimed at lowering ammonia production in the lower GI tract, such as with lactulose or neomycin.

Adequate calorie intake is an essential component of the diet to ensure that energy needs are met. Inadequate energy intake can lead to catabolism of skeletal tissue to provide protein substrate for gluconeogenesis. Altered metabolism of glucose and lipids or overall hypermetabolism compound the difficulty of providing adequate nutrition. Ensuring the delivery of proper nutrition to patients with hepatic encephalopathy can be a challenge for the nurse. Patients have varying levels of somnolence, restlessness, disorientation, agitation, and tremor that can affect their ability to take an oral diet safely. Aggressive or inappropriate behavior in advanced stages of encephalopathy can lead to removal of any feeding tube in place. Family and other visitors who bring gifts of food need to be educated about the incremental protein prescription in order to avoid inadvertent dietary noncompliance that can affect the assessment of protein tolerance. Chapter 46 ◯ provides a complete description of hepatic encephalopathy.

Pancreatitis

Most patients who present with acute pancreatitis experience resolution of their symptoms within 5 to 7 days, and do not require aggressive nutritional intervention. However, 20% to 30% of patients exhibit severe disease (≥3 Ranson criteria as described in Chapter 46 ◯) and will need multidisciplinary intervention, including nutritional support (Abou-Assi & O'Keefe, 2002). Symptoms of acute pancreatitis such as pain, nausea, and vomiting can preclude oral intake by patients before they seek medical attention. Hypermetabolism and an 80% increase in catabolic rate occur with severe disease because of the local and systemic inflammatory responses by the body (Abou-Assi & O'Keefe, 2002; Alsolaiman, Green, & Barkin, 2003). The combination of inability to consume adequate oral nutrition in the face of a hypermetabolic and hypercatabolic state places these patients at high risk for malnutrition and related complications. The patient who goes on to develop further infection, sepsis, abscess, or pancreatic fistula—all complications of acute pancreatitis—will be at even greater risk.

Medical nutrition therapy for acute pancreatitis centers on the widely held belief that stimulation of the exocrine pancreas needs to be avoided in order to minimize pain and enzyme secretion. Pancreatic rest through bowel rest and provision of nutrition via the parenteral route were treatments of choice for decades. More recently, debate has arisen about the use of enteral versus parenteral nutrition in achieving pancreatic rest, and providing adequate nutrition while minimizing complications. This debate holds only for patients with a functioning gut and not for those in whom an ileus precludes enteral support. It has been demonstrated that most patients with acute pancreatitis tolerate an enteral nutrition formula infused into the jejunum distal to the ligament of Treitz (Abou-Assi & O'Keefe, 2002; McClave, 2004; Olah et al., 2002). Elemental or semielemental small peptide formulas are used that have negligible fat and free amino acids or di- and tripeptides versus intact whole proteins. Such formulas require no pancreatic enzyme secretion for absorption and do little to stimulate the exocrine pancreas (Abou-Assi & O'Keefe, 2002; Alsolaiman et al., 2003; McClave, 2004; Olah et al., 2002).

Parenteral nutrition also is effective in achieving nutrition goals and pancreatic rest, but it has coincidental risks not associated with enteral nutrition. Studies comparing distal jejunal feeding with parenteral nutrition have illustrated equivocal provision of nutrition, achievement of pancreatic rest, and overall mortality. However, in some studies, but not all, parenteral nutrition was associated with more frequent hyperglycemia, a longer hospital stay, and infection (Abou-Assi, Craig, & O'Keefe, 2002; Jeejeebhoy, 2001). Acute pancreatitis can already cause glucose intolerance because of endocrine pancreas involvement. High glucose parenteral formula can cause greater blood glucose elevations. Catheter-related problems include both local and systemic infections. Those ascribing to the preferential use of the gut for feeding believe that prevention of gut atrophy, maintenance of beneficial gut microflora, and prevention of bacterial translocation are crucial. The theory exists that all of these factors play an important part in preventing changes in gut permeability associated with more advanced complications of pancreatitis (Abou-Assi & O'Keefe, 2002; Olah et al., 2002). Other researchers report that there are insufficient clinical trials supporting either route of nutrition as being superior or preferable, but they are in agreement that nutrition support is a cornerstone of treatment (Jeejeebhoy, 2001).

A reasonable approach to providing nutrition care to the patient with acute pancreatitis is to begin with a jejunal feeding early in the course of severe disease. Patients with evidence of severe disease are most likely to require nutrition support. A small-bore jejunal tube should be placed distal to the ligament of Trietz. After confirmation of tube placement, an elemental or small peptide enteral formula can begin. A registered dietitian should be consulted to recommend the needed volume of feeding and a protocol for advancing the rate and concentration of the formula. Such formulas are hyperosmolar and should not be started at a full-strength concentration or full volume. The nurse should monitor the patient closely for tolerance to the formula and rate changes. An increase in pain, nausea, vomiting, or diarrhea can indicate intolerance and deserves evaluation. Further elevation of the serum pancreatic enzymes, amylase or lipase, indicates intolerance to enteral nutrition. The patient should also be monitored at the bedside with a stethoscope for signs of tube migration. Movement of the tube into the proximal jejunum or duodenum may precipitate pancreatic stimulation and feeding intolerance. A pharmacist should be consulted relative to the administration of medications via a jejunal tube because the site may bypass the point of absorption of many drugs. Additionally, small-bore tubes are prone to clogging and a precipitate from medications could form. Therefore, when administering medication the nurse needs to ensure adequate flushing of the system to maintain patency.

Parenteral nutrition support is indicated when the patient is unable to tolerate enteral support or has an ileus. The nutrition support team will recommend an appropriate parenteral formula to meet the patient's nutritional and fluid and electrolyte needs. The patient should be monitored for hyperglycemia and hypertriglyceridemia because both can occur with pancreatitis and be exacerbated by total parenteral nutrition.

Patients with mild pancreatitis may only require a short period of time NPO and no aggressive nutritional support before resumption of a low-fat oral diet. Fat is minimized to reduce stimulation of the pancreas. Patients transitioning from nutrition support should also receive a low-fat diet.

Chronic pancreatitis can lead to longer term weight loss and malabsorption when the disease affects the majority of the pancreas. Permanent glucose intolerance can also occur. In addition to oral enzyme replacement therapy, many patients will require a modified fat diet and supplementation with a water-miscible, fat-soluble vitamin. Bone disease and clotting abnormalities have been noted from malabsorption of fat-soluble vitamins D and K, respectively. Vitamin B_{12} may also need to be supplemented if insufficient protease production prohibits the cleaving of vitamin B_{12} from its protein. Medium-chain triglycerides do not require pancreatic lipase for absorption and can be prescribed to provide needed calories for patients who have poor intake. Patients with endocrine pancreas dysfunction will also require modification of the carbohydrate content as outlined in the medical nutrition therapy of diabetes. Chapter 45 ⊘ provides a complete description of pancreatitis.

Renal Disease

The kidney plays an important role in maintaining homeostasis in the body. Regulating nutrition processes and excreting nutrient by-products of metabolism, such as nitrogen, are among the crucial functions performed by the kidney. Kidneys also regulate fluid and electrolyte balance. Additionally, the kidneys are responsible for orchestrating the delicate balance between calcium, phosphorus, and vitamin D in the body. Vitamin D reaches its metabolically active form after being hydroxylated in the kidney.

A complete description of renal disease is provided in Chapter 47 ⊘.

Nephrotic Syndrome

Damage to the capillary walls of the glomeruli can cause significant losses of protein in the urine. Following significant proteinuria, decreases in plasma albumin can result with subsequent edema formation. Medical nutrition therapy for nephrotic syndrome focuses on replacement of protein losses to prevent malnutrition, slow the disease progression, and minimize edema. Dietary sodium is limited to control edema (Appel, 2006).

The nurse can educate the patient and reinforce the importance of a low-sodium diet in reducing edema. (A list of high-sodium foods can be found in Chart 14–17 (p. 293) earlier in this chapter). Adequate, but not high, protein is recommended to provide needed protein without contributing to disease progression. A patient should have a 24-hour urine protein assessment to determine the amount of protein replacement needed in addition to the RDA for protein baseline requirement. A registered dietitian would calculate this recommendation for the patient and outline suitable food choices. Adequate nonprotein sources of calories are needed to provide energy and prevent malnutrition because of catabolism of skeletal muscle for gluconeogenesis. If inadequate energy intake occurs, the protein intake will be sacrificed by the body for use as energy instead of as a substrate for anabolic functions.

Renal Failure

Medical nutrition therapy for both acute and chronic renal failure is determined by whether or not dialysis is part of the treatment strategy for the patient. Additionally, current laboratory values, amount of urine production, and any underlying disease will dictate an individualized diet prescription. Uremia results from the buildup of metabolic by-products in the body that is normally excreted via the kidneys. Nitrogenous waste products and inorganic ions are responsible for the clinical manifestations of uremia (National Kidney Foundation [NKF], 2000).Uremia can predispose the patient with renal failure to malnutrition. Anorexia, nausea, and altered taste perception can lead to decreased intake. Medication side effects and a restricted diet can further the potential for nutrition risk.

The short-term goals of medical nutrition therapy are to minimize uremia, manage fluid status, and provide adequate nutrition. Long-term nutrition care is focused on prevention of disease progression and malnutrition. Patients who also have comorbid conditions, such as diabetes or hypertension, must also receive appropriate nutrition intervention for those diseases. Overall, the resultant diet prescription can be quite stringent and patients require close monitoring. The National Kidney Foundation (2000) recommends reassessment and updating of the patient's care plan every 3 to 4 months.

Nutrition assessment is essential before an individualized diet prescription can be tailored to fit established guidelines. Parameters normally used to assess nutrition status can require adjustment in this population. Fluid shifts and resultant weight gain call for use of either a calculated ideal weight or postdialysis edema free body weight in calculating nutritional needs (Wells, 2003).The dietitian will rely on nursing expertise to make a determination of dry weight. Blood pressure monitoring, heart rate, postdialysis symptoms, presence of any hemoconcentration, edema, or increased gastrointestinal losses will all factor into dry weight estimations (Reams & Elder, 2003). Plasma samples obtained to assess albumin or other proteins should be taken before dialysis to avoid the effect of interdialytic protein losses (NKF, 2000). Creatinine index and serum creatinine can be employed to assess for loss of muscle mass or poor protein intake (NKF, 2000; Wells, 2003).

Dietary protein is responsible for the development of nitrogenous by-products during metabolism that contribute to uremia.

Thus, a controlled protein diet is recommended to control uremia. The contribution of a high-protein diet to renal disease progression or, conversely, whether a low-protein diet slows progression is the subject of debate. Following a protein-modified diet is associated with a decreased risk of death associated with renal disease in patients with existing kidney failure (Foque, Laville, & Boissel, 2006). Patients *not* receiving dialysis treatment and with a GFR of <25 mL/min are advised to follow a daily protein restriction of 0.6 g/kg ideal weight (Beto & Bansal, 2004). Some patients are unable to consume this low level of protein without becoming at risk for malnutrition. In such patients, the diet may be liberalized to 0.75 g protein/kg ideal weight (NKF, 2000). Because of protein losses during dialysis, patients receiving hemodialysis or peritoneal dialysis as part of treatment can consume more protein than those not dialyzed. Chart 14–34 outlines recommended protein levels for renal failure.

To achieve the most efficient metabolism, the majority of protein consumed should be of high biological value, having all essential amino acids, such as animal proteins (meats, poultry, fish, dairy) and soy. Use of high biological value proteins is most important for patients consuming low amounts of protein (Beto & Bansal, 2004). Adequate nonprotein calorie intake is essential to support energy needs and not have protein wasted as an energy source. The majority of patients will require 35 calories/kg per day (Beto & Bansal, 2004). The dietitian can recommend appropriate individual adjustments to this recommendation for patients who are sedentary, obese, or hypermetabolic. Additionally, patients receiving peritoneal dialysis can require modification of calorie intake because of the dextrose calories absorbed from the dialysate (Beto & Bansal, 2004).

Nutrition management of altered fluid status and plasma electrolyte and mineral abnormalities also is recommended with renal failure. General guidelines are presented in Chart 14–34, but it should be understood that each patient should have a customized diet prescription that fits his or her individual needs and laboratory parameters (NKF, 2000). A registered dietitian provides this individualized assessment and diet recommendation. Potassium restrictions vary according to treatment mode and laboratory values. Intake of minerals should be matched with excretion (Wells, 2003). The nurse can be instrumental in reinforcing the immediate importance of low-potassium food choices in this

---

CHART 14–34	**Medical Nutrition Therapy for Chronic Renal Disease**			
	Hemodialysis	**Peritoneal Dialysis**	**No Dialysis**	**Nephrotic Syndrome**
Protein (g/kg dry weight)	1.2 g	1.2–1.3 g	0.6–0.75	0.8
Sodium (g)	2–4*	2–4*	2–4*	2–3*
Potassium (g)	2–3*	3–4*	2*	No restriction
Fluid (mL)	500–1,000 + UOP volume	Assess individually	500–1,000 + UOP volume	No restriction
Calories* (kcal/kg)	35 in those < age 65 30–35 in those > age 65	35 in those < age 65 30–35 in those > age 65	35 in those < age 65 30–35 in those > age 65	Assess individually

Note: Emphasis should be placed on individual diet recommendations based on overall renal function, nutrition status, and general health. All parameters outlined in this chart are general and should be adapted to meet patient requirements.

Sources: Beto, J. A., & Bansal, V. K. (2004). Medical nutrition therapy in chronic kidney failure: Integrating clinical practice guidelines. *Journal of the American Dietetic Association, 104,* 404–409; National Kidney Foundation. (2000). *Kidney disease outcomes quality initiative (K/DOQI). Clinical practice guidelines for nutrition in chronic kidney disease.* Retrieved November 16, 2006, from http://www.kidney.org/professionals.doqi/index/cfm; Wells, C. (2003). Optimizing nutrition in patients with chronic kidney disease. *Nephrology Nursing Journal, 30,* 637–646.

population. Noncompliance with a potassium restriction can result in quick deleterious consequences with elevated blood potassium leading to lethal cardiac dysrhythmias and cardiac arrest. Chart 14–35 outlines high potassium foods. Sodium and fluid restrictions correspond to amount of urine production and accumulation of fluid between dialysis treatments. Generally, fluid intake is 500 to 1,000 mL plus volume of 24-hour urine output (Wells, 2003). Patients with acute renal failure who are in the diuretic phase need to have fluid intake reevaluated to match changes in output (see Chapter 47). For patients receiving dialysis, large interdialytic fluid gains present medical risk and dialysis difficulties and should be avoided. Interdialytic weight gain should be limited to 2% to 5% of dry weight (Wells, 2003). Compliance with the fluid restriction can be difficult for many patients. The nurse can offer suggestions for helping with thirst, such as mouth care or rinses and sucking on hard candy, and suggest low-potassium fluid choices within restriction parameters.

Chronic renal failure and ongoing dialysis treatment can result in additional nutritional concerns. Water-soluble vitamins are lost in the dialysate and require replacement. Dietary restrictions and poor intake also contribute to poor vitamin status. Formulations are available specifically for renal failure use. Kidney endocrine function becomes compromised and final synthesis of active vitamin D is diminished. Calcitriol, an oral supplement of active vitamin D, is given. Without adequate vitamin D, calcium absorption is lowered, predisposing the patient to bone disease. Plasma phosphorous levels are often elevated and complicate the intricate feedback mechanisms among vitamin D, calcium, and parathyroid hormone. Dietary restriction of phosphorus is indicated but only to the level achieved by the simultaneous protein restriction. Phosphorus is found primarily in milk products, nuts, and legumes. Overreliance on dietary restriction of phosphorus could result in insufficient intake of high-quality protein. Further reduction in plasma phosphorus is achieved with binding medications such as calcium carbonate. These are consumed along with a meal. Erythropoietin production is diminished with resultant anemia because of lowered red blood cell production by the bone marrow (see Chapter 47). An erythropoiesis-stimulating agent is given. Additional contributors to anemia should be investigated. Transferrin saturation and ferritin are assessed to determine appropriate intervention for iron deficiency. Intravenous iron replacement is the preferred route of administration in this anemic population (NKF, 2006).

The patient with end-stage renal disease has unique dietary restrictions that make consumption of adequate nutrition a challenge. Patients on low-protein diets without dialysis treatment are at higher risk of malnutrition than those who receive dialysis because of the nature of the diet and disease symptoms (Beto & Bansal, 2004). Restrictions accompanying comorbid conditions such as diabetes present additional considerations. The nurse can provide much needed reinforcement of the importance of dietary compliance in both short-term well-being and long-term disease management.

Renal Stones

Supersaturation of urine favors nucleation and growth of crystals that can cause nephrolithiasis (Bushinski, 2002). Medical nutrition therapy of kidney stones focuses first on adequate fluid intake to promote ample urine volume and flow. Consumption of enough fluid to produce between 2 and 3 L of urine daily is recommended (Morton et al., 2002). Tailoring intake is required with changes in climate when insensible fluid losses increase and urine output is lessened if fluid intake is not adjusted.

Calcium oxalate stones are the predominant type of kidney stone, comprising up to 70% of all stones (Bushinski, 2002; Morton et al., 2002). In the past, a low-calcium diet was recommended in an attempt to decrease hypercalciuria and the likelihood of stone precipitation. However, although this advice resulted in decreased urinary excretion of calcium, it also fostered increased absorption of oxalate from the intestine and increased oxalate in urine. The result was no improvement in relative risk of stone formation and an increased risk of bone disease with insufficient calcium intake (Bushinski, 2002). Current recommendations advise adequate calcium intake, avoidance of excess oxalate intake (spinach, rhubarb, nuts, beets, chocolate, tea, and wheat bran are significant absorbable sources) (Morton et al., 2002). Additionally, excess intake of nondairy animal proteins and sodium has been shown to contribute to stone formation. Excessive animal protein promotes an acid environment in the body to which the body responds by buffering with calcium release from bone. Sodium excretion is associated with calcium excretion in the urine and thus is a target for control of calciuria. A long-term trial of a normal calcium diet that avoided excess sodium and animal protein resulted in a decreased relative risk of stone recurrence when compared with the old calcium-restricted approach (Borghi et al., 2002). Patients at risk for calcium stones should be educated to avoid excess vitamin D and C supplements. Vitamin D causes calcium absorption. Vitamin C promotes increased oxalate, an end product of the metabolism of ascorbate (Massey, Liebman, & Kynast-Gales, 2005; Morton et al., 2002).

Less common uric acid, cystine, and struvite kidney stones require medical management and ample fluid intake to avoid urine supersaturation. Additional dietary manipulations are not common modes of treatment in the prevention of these stones. Purines in meats and organ meats contribute to uric acid formation if consumed in significant quantities on a regular basis. However, management generally involves manipulation of urine pH rather than changes in diet for uric acid nephrolithiasis (Morton et al., 2002).

CHART 14–35 **High Potassium Food Sources**

- Banana
- Dried fruit: apricots, raisins, prunes, dates, figs
- Green leafy vegetables: Swiss chard, spinach, mustard greens
- Legumes: dried beans, peas, lentils
- Melon: cantaloupe, honeydew
- Oranges, orange juice
- Potato
- Tomato
- Whole grains, bran.

Note: Check labels on salt substitutes. Many contain potassium.

Patients at risk for kidney stones should have a nutrition history done to assess for fluid intake and urine output, use of vitamin supplements (vitamins C and D, calcium), and excessive intake of protein and sodium. The nurse should educate the patient to consume adequate fluid to produce between 2 and 3 L of urine daily. Patients who exercise or live in climates where insensible losses are increased should be educated to tailor fluid intake accordingly. Nonnutritional risk factors for kidney stone formation are discussed in Chapter 47 ⊘.

Anemias

Nutrition therapy for anemia first requires an established etiology for the hematologic changes. Indiscriminate treatment with vitamin or mineral supplements can mask underlying causes and result in additional negative consequences. This is especially illustrated with macrocytic anemia treatment using folic acid alone, without screening for potential vitamin B_{12} deficiency (Little, 1999). Folic acid therapy can result in improved hematologic indices while masking neurological damage from ongoing deficiency of vitamin B_{12}. Full discussion of anemia testing and treatment is presented in Chapter 63 ⊘.

Iron Deficiency

Iron deficiency anemia is the most common nutritional anemia worldwide (CDC, 2002). In addition to the medical etiology of iron deficiency, inadequate diet or poor iron absorption can contribute to the prevalence of this condition. Correction of iron deficiency anemia requires use of iron salt supplementation, but improved iron intake and absorption can facilitate repletion and prevent recurrence once the etiology has been treated. Repletion can take 4 to 6 months unless the patient is experiencing continued abnormal blood loss (Little, 1999).

The nurse can assess the patient for adequacy of iron intake and presence of inhibitors of absorption to facilitate improved iron repletion. Iron is present in animal protein foods such as meats and poultry as well as plant sources. Iron obtained from a "blood source" of iron is called heme iron, and is better absorbed than nonheme sources. Nonheme iron is present in plant sources of iron such as legumes (beans, soy), dried fruit, and iron-fortified products (cereals and pasta, for example). Absorption of iron, especially nonheme iron, can be affected by other dietary substances. Vitamin C sources with a meal enhance iron absorption, whereas consumption of tea, coffee, and calcium during a meal inhibit absorption (Nelson & Poulter, 2004). In patients at risk for iron deficiency, it is recommended that tea consumption in particular be limited to 1 hour outside the mealtime because tea can decrease iron absorption by up to 85%, depending on meal content (Nelson & Poulter, 2004). Chart 14–36 outlines iron content of foods and potential inhibitors and enhancers of iron absorption.

Vitamin B_{12} Deficiency

Adequate stores of vitamin B_{12} can meet nutritional requirements for up to 5 years. Thus, a deficiency of vitamin B_{12} generally occurs following prolonged inadequate intake or absorption (Oh & Brown, 2003). Vitamin B_{12} is present in only foods of animal origin. Any patient following a vegan diet (which contains no animal products) who does not take synthetic vitamin B_{12} to supplement his diet is at risk for deficiency. Plant-based supple-

---

| CHART 14–36 | **Iron Sources and Absorption** |

FOOD SOURCES OF IRON

- Meat, shellfish, dark poultry, dried beans, peas, and lentils
- Green leafy vegetables
- Dried fruit
- Whole grains, fortified cereals, and grain products.

IRON ABSORPTION ENHANCERS

- Vitamin C
- Meat, seafood, poultry.

IRON ABSORPTION INHIBITORS

- Tea
- Coffee
- Binders: oxalates and phytates (e.g., in green leafy vegetables)
- Calcium
- Antacids and other acid reduction medications.

Sources: Hallberg L. & Hulthen, L., (2000). Prediction of dietary iron absorption: An algorithm for calculating absorption and bioavailability of dietary iron. *American Journal of Clinical Nutrition, 71,* 1147–1160.; Little, D. R. (1999). Ambulatory management of common forms of anemia. *American Family Physician, 59,* 1598–1604; Nelson, M., & Poulter, J. (2004). Impact of tea drinking on iron status in the UK: A review. *Journal Human Nutrition Dietetics, 17,* 43–54.

ments available on the market are not bioavailable and therefore not recommended (American Dietetic Association & Dietitians of Canada, 2004). Alcoholics or elderly also are at potential risk because of poor intake (Oh & Brown, 2003).

Decreased absorption of vitamin B_{12} can occur for two main reasons. First, an acid environment is required in the stomach to cleave vitamin B_{12} from its protein. Patients with gastric resection, long-term acid suppression treatment, or achlorhydria are at risk of vitamin B_{12} malabsorption because of diminished acid production (Oh & Brown, 2003). Second, intrinsic factor (IF) is required to bind with B_{12} and then be absorbed in the terminal ileum. Lack of IF production by parietal cells, poor binding of IF in the duodenum, and ileal disease or resection all place the patient at risk for malabsorption (Oh & Brown, 2003). Traditionally, an oral supplement of vitamin B_{12} was given to patients with poor acid environment while vitamin B_{12} injections were administered for IF and small bowel related problems (Oh & Brown, 2003). Now, a second passive route of absorption has been recognized and high-dose oral supplementation can be used for many patients to good effect (Nyholm et al., 2003). The nurse can assess patients for risk of vitamin B_{12} deficiency through a diet history and screening for potential factors associated with poor absorption. Patients consuming inadequate vitamin B_{12} need to be advised of important nutritional sources. Animal products, vitamin B_{12}–fortified cereals or milk alternatives, and synthetic supplements are emphasized. Deficiency should resolve within 3 to 4 weeks of treatment unless neurological manifestations have occurred; 6 months or more can pass before any possible neurological improvement is evident (Little, 1999). The risk of vitamin B_{12} deficiency faced by the elderly is discussed in the Gerontological Considerations box (p. 314).

GERONTOLOGICAL CONSIDERATIONS
Associated with Vitamin B₁₂ Deficiency

The elderly are at particular risk of vitamin B_{12} deficiency because of age-related atrophic changes in the stomach with resultant achlorhydria. Production of intrinsic factor can also be affected. This alteration in gastric pH and diminished IF production result in decreased absorption of vitamin B_{12}. Consideration of routine vitamin B_{12} supplementation is uniquely recommended for adults older than 70 years of age for this reason (IOM, 1998; Russell, Rasmussen, & Lichtenstein, 1999). Adults older than 65 years of age already at risk for poor vitamin absorption who are receiving prolonged acid suppression medication should be assessed for vitamin B_{12} deficiency (Oh & Brown, 2003).

Folate Deficiency

Folate deficiency can occur from decreased intake or absorption, unmet increased needs, or a combination. People with alcoholic liver disease and others with poor-quality diets are at risk for poor folate status. Several medications are folate antagonists or alter absorption; examples include methotrexate, triamterene, phenytoin, sulfasalazine, and corticosteroids (Little, 1999; White & Ashworth, 2000). Folate, which is the name of this B vitamin when found in foods, is present in orange juice, green leafy vegetables, and legumes. It is also present in white flour products as a result of government-mandated folic acid fortification begun in 1996 in the United States. Folic acid is the name used by some to denote supplemental forms of the vitamin.

Generally, a 1-mg dose per day of folic acid is prescribed for deficiency. This is the tolerable upper limit of the vitamin (IOM, 1998). Careful screening to rule out deficiency of vitamin B_{12} is first essential because this level of folic acid repletion can mask a vitamin B_{12} deficiency. Many recommend that unopposed folic acid supplementation at or near the 1-mg dose not be given, but rather complementary vitamin B_{12} also be administered (Fletcher & Fairfield, 2002). The nurse can screen patients for folate intake and the presence of any inhibitory medications. Consumption of good sources of folate should be encouraged. Women of childbearing age should be especially encouraged to consume adequate folate or take a multivitamin supplement with the RDA of 400 mcg folic acid. Adequate maternal folate status is associated with decreased risk of development of neural tube defects in a developing fetus (IOM, 1998).

Acquired Immunodeficiency Syndrome (AIDS)

Nutritional problems, from malnutrition to dyslipidemia, can occur in human immunodeficiency virus (HIV) infection. Malnutrition can occur for a variety of reasons such as opportunistic infection. For example, oral candidiasis can lead to inadequate intake because of pain and dysphagia accompanying inflammation. Other infections can lead to anorexia, fatigue, malabsorption, hypermetabolism from fever and inflammation, nausea and vomiting, or altered cognition and functional status (Nerad et al., 2003).

Pharmacologic treatment of infection can cause gastrointestinal side effects and food and drug interactions. Often, complicated medication schedules and food interactions can make adequate intake a challenge (Nerad et al., 2003). Chemical dependency and socioeconomic issues present additional challenges to nutrition status. These factors in combination or alone can predispose patients with HIV infection to malnutrition. Development of malnutrition can diminish immunocompetence and leave the patient at further risk of opportunistic infection (American Dietetic Association & Dietitians of Canada, 2004). The effectiveness of pharmacologic interventions can be reduced with malnutrition because many medications require critical levels of protein stores or body cell mass for metabolism (American Dietetic Association & Dietitians of Canada, 2004). Many medications require specific food recommendations without which serum drug levels are affected (Gagnon & Therrien, 2006; Nerad et al., 2003). Some patients are unable to tolerate adequate intake, resulting in impaired drug treatment along with poor nutrition status. Thus, a vicious cycle of malnutrition and infection can follow. Weight loss, loss of muscle, adipose, and nutrient deficiencies lead to further negative consequences. Malnutrition in HIV infection is associated with adverse outcomes, such as disease progression and mortality (Grinspoon & Mulligan, 2003; Knox et al., 2003).

Some wasting occurs despite a clear single etiology. In addition to suspected contributors to malnutrition such as inadequate intake and malabsorption, wasting occurs because of changes in metabolism, hypogonadism, and excessive cytokine production associated with HIV (Grinspoon & Mulligan, 2003). No matter what the etiology, the health impact resulting from loss of lean muscle and total body weight is significant.

Current medical treatment of patients with HIV infection using highly active antiretroviral treatment (HAART) has presented clinicians with additional sequelae of potential nutritional problems. Hyperlipidemia, insulin resistance, and body fat redistribution have been associated with the use of protease inhibitors (Dube et al., 2003; Graber, 2001; Nerad et al., 2003). Additionally, length of HIV infection, age, and gender may play a role (Chen, Misra, & Carg, 2002). Limited literature is available to assess the influence of diet on this complication. Patients may present with elevated plasma cholesterol, triglyceride, glucose intolerance, and unique **lipodystrophy**. Lipodystrophy is characterized by adipose loss in the face and extremities and excess fat deposition in the abdomen and over the dorsocervical spine (Chen et al., 2002; Graber, 2001). Such alterations in morphology may lead some patients to alter their diet or medication strategies in an attempt to deal with body image conflicts. This, in turn, may place these patients at risk for poor nutrition or ineffective medication concentration (Nerad et al., 2003). Some patients may experiment with alternative medicine in place of, or in addition to, HAART to counteract the metabolic effects. Not all nutritional and herbal supplements can be safely used by patients with HIV infection and some may compromise effective treatment.

Medical nutrition therapy for HIV infection is based on an up-to-date comprehensive nutrition assessment. It is recommended that a thorough assessment be completed at the time of diagnosis to establish a baseline for later comparison *and* that reevaluation take place up to twice a year in the asymptomatic patient and up to six times a year in patients experiencing HIV-related symptoms (Knox et al., 2003). No nutritional evaluation tool has been validated for exclusive use in assessment of patients with HIV infection. Standard nutrition assessment parameters should all be used, but tailored for specificity with this population. Anthropometric measurements are important to obtain at baseline for potential future estimations of any lipodystrophy. Serial weights should be monitored. Skinfold measurements and waist and hip circumferences are recommended to assess for changes in adipose deposition (Gerrior, Kantaros, Coakley, Labrecht, & Wanke, 2001; Knox et al., 2003).

Weight alone will not suffice for such comparisons because muscle loss and fat gains can mask weight change. Weight alone may also underestimate the presence of malnutrition (Mangili, Murman, Zampini, & Wanke, 2006). Laboratory parameters such as plasma proteins may be reflective of nutrition status or infection-related inflammation and cannot be solely relied on to assess nutrition (American Dietetic Association & Dietitians of Canada, 2004). Serum vitamin B_{12} and zinc levels, among other micronutrients, are often diminished and this has been associated with increased risk of disease progression (American Dietetic Association & Dietitians of Canada, 2004; Baum, Campa, Lai, Lai, & Page, 2003; Fawzi, 2003; Woods et al., 2003).

During the focused interview and the physical examination, the nurse should closely assess the patient for presence of any factor known to influence nutrition health. Knowledge regarding HIV-related nutrition risk factors is important for nurses because the nurse is often first in line to assess a patient. Existing opportunistic infections, oral and digestive symptoms, medication, use of alternative medicines and supplements, and functional status are among the many parameters that are essential to the assessment. Chart 14–37 outlines essential components of the nutritional assessment of patients with HIV infection.

The findings from the nutritional assessment will determine the extent of needed nutrition intervention. Nutrition care and education are central to management of HIV infection. Asymptomatic patients may benefit from general nutrition education about a healthy diet to maintain important muscle mass and body weight. It is important for the nurse to discuss the use of herbal and nutritional supplements that may impact medical management. For example, it has been shown that St. John's wort may decrease crucial therapeutic plasma levels of protease inhibitors (American Dietetic Association & Dietitians of Canada, 2004). Education about the importance of food and water safety is also important to prevent or lessen the risk of foodborne illness. Improperly handled foods and water from unsafe sources each pose a risk to patients who are immunocompromised. Many pathogens identified in patients with opportunistic infection are recognizable as having potentially originated in a food or water source. Salmonella, listeria, cryptosporidia, and *Vibrio vulnificus* are examples (Hayes, Elliot, Krales, & Downer, 2003). Chart 14–38 (p. 316) outlines important aspects of food and water sanitation.

Patients with malnutrition or at risk for malnutrition require quick intervention to prevent further deterioration of nutrition health. Underlying factors responsible for malnutrition must be identified and treated or controlled. Nutrition intervention should be tailored to maximize nutrient repletion while minimizing side effects and symptoms. Chart 14–39 (p. 316) outlines

---

CHART 14–37 Nutrition Assessment in HIV Infection

Physical exam/interview
Assess weight, serial weights.
Assess baseline body composition and waist-to-hip ratio and monitor serially for muscle wasting or fat redistribution.
Assess for risk of ↓ intake:

- Oral pain, dysphagia, thrush, oral health
- Nausea, vomiting, diarrhea
- Food intolerances
- Altered cognition
- Medication side effects
- Complicated food/medicine schedule
- Depression, anxiety
- Fatigue, shortness of breath
- Chemical dependency
- Lack of economic resources
- Impaired functional status.

Assess for risk of ↑ nutrient losses:

- Malabsorption because of infection
- Enteropathy
- Medication interactions.

Assess for risk of ↑ nutrient needs:

- Active infection/viral load
- Fever
- Wounds
- Other disease.

Laboratory tests
Plasma proteins
Lipids
Vitamin B_{12}
Zinc

Nutrition history
Assess nutrition history data in Chart 14–3 (p. 276).
Note use of alternative nutrition therapy, vitamins/minerals, and herbal or other supplements.
Assess food and water safety practices.

Sources: American Dietetic Association & Dietitians of Canada. (2004). Position of the American Dietetic Association and Dietitians of Canada: Nutrition intervention in the care of persons with human immunodeficiency virus. *Journal of the American Dietetic Association, 104,* 1425–1441; Knox, T. A., Zafonte-Sanders, M., Fields-Gardner, C., Moen, K., Johansen, D., & Paton, N. (2003). Assessment of nutritional status, body composition, and human immunodeficiency virus-associated morphologic changes. *Clinical Infectious Diseases, 36,* S63–S68; Nerad, J., Romeyn, M., Silverman, E., Allen-Reid, J., Dietrich, D., Merchant, J., et al. (2003). General nutrition management in patients infected with HIV. *Clinical Infectious Diseases, 36,* S52–S62.

---

common causes of malnutrition in HIV infection and sample nutrition strategies the nurse can suggest.

Patients in whom lipodystrophy is evident may require nutrition intervention for any glucose intolerance or hyperlipidemia. Current recommendations advise the prescription of the same diet treatment as for any patient with hyperlipidemia or hyperglycemia (Dube et al., 2003). This area requires more research to determine the efficacy of nutrition therapy in treating these metabolic changes when they occur in this population. Current

CHART 14–38	Guidelines for Safe Food and Water Handling

Prepare foods safely:
- Clean surfaces and utensils.
- Wash hands before preparing food and after handling raw meats, poultry, or fish.
- Wash surfaces and utensils after preparing raw meat, poultry, and fish. Use separate cutting board if possible for raw products.
- Cook foods until done and proper temperature; meats, poultry > 165°F internally; fish should be opaque and flaky. Reheat leftovers to 165°F. Bring leftover soup, gravy, or sauce to a boil. Only keep leftovers for 3 to 4 days in refrigerator.

Do not consume raw or undercooked eggs, meat, fish, or poultry:
- Avoid sushi or raw bars, real eggnog, dressings made with raw egg, runny eggs.
- Do not taste test marinades used for tenderizing proteins.

Consume pasteurized juices, milk, and dairy foods.

Wash and peel fruits and vegetables.

Do not drink water from streams, lakes, springs, rivers.

Boil tap water if advised by local health department.

Store foods safely:
- Place raw meat, poultry, and fish in lower shelf of refrigerator to avoid drips onto other food.
- Separate raw products in grocery cart and when bagged in store.
- Keep stored perishable foods out of the 40°–140°F danger zone. Cool hot foods quickly in shallow dish. Keep foods properly refrigerated or frozen.

Sources: Centers for Disease Control. (2007). *Safe food and water.* Retrieved May 30, 2008 from http://www.cdc.gov/hiv/resources/brochures/food.htm; Food and Drug Administration. (2001). *Food safety for you!* Retrieved January 27, 2004, from http://www.cfsan.fda.gov/~dms/fttclean.html; Hayes, C., Elliot, E., Krales, E., & Downer, G. (2003). Food and water safety for persons infected with HIV. *Clinical Infectious Diseases, 36,* S106–S109.

nutrition recommendations are made largely in the absence of data on their use in patients with HIV. Nutrition intervention to alter the effects of fat redistribution or to specifically increase muscle mass in wasting has little reported effect. Strength training and use of pharmacologic interventions are current strategies being suggested (Grinspoon & Mulligan, 2003). A complete description of HIV/AIDS is in Chapter 60 .

Cancer

Patients diagnosed with cancer are at risk for poor nutrition status because of the effects of the disease as well as the treatment. Anorexia, nausea, and vomiting, changes in taste perception, dysphagia, mucositis, diarrhea, and fatigue can predispose a patient to malnutrition whether the symptoms are caused by tumor effects, radiation, or chemotherapy. Malnutrition that may begin from disease alone may be worsened with treatment side effects. A baseline nutrition assessment at diagnosis followed by reassessment periodically through treatment will allow for early intervention when nutrition risk is evident. The nurse who is part of the treatment team during chemotherapy, radiation, or surgery can be instrumental in identifying symptom changes that prevent adequate intake and planning appropriate intervention. Chart 14–40 lists nutrition interventions that the nurse can recommend to patients and caregivers.

CHART 14–39	Nutrition Strategies for Common Problems with HIV Infection

Problem	Nutrition Intervention
Anorexia	Eat small, frequent meals. Choose nutrient dense foods: peanut butter, cheese, meal replacement or breakfast-type drinks, smoothies. See Chart 14–21 (p. 298) for "more calories per bite" food recommendations.
Nausea and vomiting	Nibble on dry carbohydrates: toast, crackers, dry cereal. Eat small meals to avoid empty stomach or feeling too full. Avoid greasy foods, strong odors. Sip flat ginger ale, weak ginger, or mint tea.
Diarrhea	Limit fat, caffeine, and fiber. Assess for lactose intolerance. Replace fluids.
Oral pain or dysphagia	Eat smooth, cool foods: pudding, ice cream, cooled soup, liquid supplement drinks. Avoid citrus, tomato, and hot foods. Use a straw to bypass mouth.
Fatigue	Keep ready-to-eat and convenience foods in stock: microwave or toaster oven items, single-serve pudding, yogurt, hearty soups. Eat nutrient-dense foods early in day and meal when energy level is best.

Patients undergoing treatment with a hematopoietic stem cell transplant require highly specialized nutrition care. Parenteral nutrition is required post-transplant because of treatment-induced mucositis. Nutrition risk is heightened by multiple medications, side effects, and potential graft-versus-host disease (GVHD). GVHD may lead to malabsorptive and liver problems, which in turn alter nutrition requirements and medical nutrition therapy. Treatment of GVHD requires use of medications, such as glucocorticoids, that present additional challenges to maintenance of nutrition health (Roberts & Thompson, 2005). A multidisciplinary care team closely manages medical and nutrition treatment in this population. A complete description of hematopoietic stem cell transplant is included in Chapter 63 . A description of GVHD is presented in Chapter 59 .

The nurse should be knowledgeable of current recommendations regarding use of nutritional supplements during active treatment with chemotherapy or radiation. Limited research to date has provided little on which to build the foundation of evidence-based clinical advice. Few studies have investigated the variability in response to conventional treatment when accompanied by use of supplements (Bruemmer, Patterson, Cheney, Aker, & Witherspoon, 2003). A theoretical concern exists that the use of antioxidants during radiation or with certain types of chemotherapy may interfere with the intended cytotoxic effects of those therapies (Norman et al., 2003; Weiger et al., 2002). Antioxidants have been investigated for their potential in minimizing oxidative damage to cells and therefore preventing or slowing cancer. Examples of antioxidant nutrients include beta-carotene (vitamin A precursor), vitamins C and E, and selenium. Patients may take these supplements hoping to minimize disease and spare healthy cells the effects

CHART 14-40   Suggested Nutrition Interventions in Cancer Care

Symptom	Nutrition Intervention
Anorexia or early satiety	Eat small, frequent meals. Eat nutrient-dense foods first. See Chart 14-21 (p. 298) for "more calories per bite" food recommendations.
Nausea	Nibble on dry carbohydrates: toast, crackers, dry cereal. Eat small meals to avoid empty stomach or feeling too full. Avoid greasy foods, strong odors. Sip flat ginger ale. Minimize physical movement before mealtime.
Altered taste	Eat tart candy, juice, or seasonings. Practice good oral care. Eat room temperature or cool foods, especially proteins.
Painful mouth or swallowing	Eat smooth, cool foods: pudding, ice cream, cooled soup, liquid supplement drinks. Avoid citrus, tomato, and hot foods. Use a straw to bypass mouth.
Xerostomia (lack of saliva)	Eat moist foods. Add sauces, gravies, butter, and liquids to foods. Avoid hot foods, alcohol, and dry foods.
Food aversions	To minimize "learned" food aversions from association, avoid favorite foods following treatment when side effects are more likely.

of treatment. The controversy arises in that antioxidants may also theoretically spare diseased tissue from the cytotoxic effects of treatment, thereby diminishing treatment efficacy. Current recommendations are to take only moderate doses of antioxidants, such as in a multivitamin, during treatment until more definitive evidence is available (Norman et al., 2003; Weiger et al., 2002).

Soy supplements are also popular choices of adjuvant therapy in patients who have heard about their natural phytoestrogen content. Phytoestrogens are weak plant estrogens that may possibly have some effect on reproductive cancer risk (Weiger et al., 2002). Until more definitive evidence is available, it is recommended that patients with breast cancer or receiving tamoxifen avoid phytoestrogen supplements (Weiger et al., 2002). Soy isoflavonoids and red clover are examples of phytoestrogens. Essiac tea is often used by patients seeking alternative therapies and can contain red clover (Weiger et al., 2002). Research on soy-based supplementation in prostate cancer is ongoing. The current recommendation is to accept the use of soy supplements by patients with prostate cancer who have chosen to use them (Weiger et al., 2002).

Patients may also choose to use herbal remedies for treatment side effects such as ginger for nausea. The nurse should query the patient for use of all supplements and educate the patient about any known interactions with treatment or medications, possible anticoagulant effects, or other contraindications to use. The safety and efficacy of nutrition and herbal supplement use before, during, and after cancer treatment are areas deserving future research.

Chronic Obstructive Pulmonary Disease and Mechanical Ventilation

Chronic obstructive pulmonary disease (COPD) symptoms such as dyspnea and fatigue can predispose patients to malnutrition by altering diet consumption. Patients may experience shortness of breath that precludes sufficient intake if chewing and swallowing alter breathing patterns and potentially affect arterial oxygen saturation. Early satiety can occur if gastric filling affects perceived or real breathing capacity. **Aerophagia**, or swallowing of air, may occur while eating and lead to bloating and early satiety as well. Fatigue can impair adequate intake when meal preparation and even simple tasks like cutting meats or opening lids prove too exhausting. Medications such as glucocorticoids may cause appetite stimulation but also gastrointestinal upset and altered intake.

COPD may also lead to an increase in energy expenditure due in part to inefficient respiratory mechanics and the increased work of the respiratory muscles. This effect is noted at rest and increases further during activity or exacerbation of respiratory symptoms (Gronberg, Slinde, Engstrom, Hulthen, & Larsson, 2005). Acute treatment with beta-2 agonists and theophylline may elevate energy expenditure (Mallampali, 2004). If the increased need for calories goes unmet, weight loss will occur. Weight loss may occur slowly or be exacerbated during acute disease or infection when nutritional needs are further increased.

Patients with elevated resting energy needs have also been reported to have increased protein turnover in the body, resulting in disproportionate loss of muscle mass or "wasting." Loss of muscle does not spare respiratory muscle; diaphragmatic and auxiliary respiratory muscle can be lost. In some patients this loss of muscle occurs even with maintenance of body weight. The muscle wasting seen in this subpopulation is referred to as pulmonary cachexia (Schols, 2002). Patients with pulmonary cachexia may suffer from loss of respiratory strength and endurance as well as functional capacity. A vicious downward spiral can occur when this in turn leads to further decreased intake and malnutrition. Malnutrition can alter immunocompetence, leaving the patient more susceptible to infection (Cai et al., 2003). A reduced BMI in COPD is associated with reduced survival (Mallampali, 2004).

The goal of medical nutrition therapy for COPD is to prevent malnutrition and weight loss that may occur with advanced disease. In patients who have hypercapnia, nutrition therapy should also focus on minimizing CO_2 production from nutrient metabolism. Each macronutrient produces a given amount of CO_2 for each molecule of O_2 consumed. This is called its **respiratory quotient (RQ)**. Carbohydrates have a higher RQ than do protein and fat and thus have the potential to produce more CO_2 at a given intake. Overfeeding a patient in total calories will also produce more CO_2 than feeding adequate calories (Cai et al., 2003). Providing excess calories or a high carbohydrate load is not recommended for patients with hypercapnia (Cai et al., 2003; Mallampali, 2004).

Nutrition intervention should focus on providing optimal nutrition in a well-tolerated form. For patients with dyspnea, nutrient-dense foods with "more calorie per bite" should be encouraged. When fatigue is a problem, the nurse can encourage intake of higher calorie sources first in the meal (and also earlier in the day) to optimize intake before the patient becomes too tired to eat. The patient should be offered assistance with opening cartons or other tasks when in hospital to conserve energy for eating. Patients experiencing early satiety can be advised to consume many small meals and to minimize filling up on empty-calorie liquids. Supplementation with an oral liquid nutrition supplement may be helpful between meals, but has been found to just replace intake in many studies, resulting in no nutritional improvements (Mallampali, 2004). Chart 14–41 outlines nutrition interventions for the patient with COPD. The patient should be monitored for overall intake and routinely screened for weight loss and muscle wasting. When risk factors exist for malnutrition, the nurse can make suggestions as outlined in Chart 14–41.

Any patient requiring mechanical ventilation and with a functioning gut will require enteral nutrition support. Parenteral nutrition is indicated for patients in whom gut function contraindicates enteral support. Nutrition support of patients on mechanical ventilation should focus on preservation of body weight and muscle, including crucial respiratory muscles essential for weaning from the ventilator. A registered dietitian should assess the patient and determine required nutrition needs and appropriate formula. Generally, standard enteral or parenteral nutrition formulas are used with a focus on not contributing to excess CO_2 production. Overfeeding ventilator patients or prescribing excess carbohydrates is not recommended (Parrish & McCray, 2003). Enteral formulas exist that are higher in fat than standard versions and are marketed for pulmonary use. Current clinical trials do not find that these formulas possess any advantage in duration on ventilation or weaning over standard formulas when overfeeding is avoided (Cook et al., 2001; Parrish & McCray, 2003).

Nutrition and Wound Healing

The presence of a cutaneous wound places metabolic demands on the body that must be met in order for healing to progress. Each stage of wound healing requires adequate nutritional substrate and is contingent on successful outcome of the prior healing phase. Healing phases are described in Chapter 67 . As a result, delayed wound healing may occur in patients with malnutrition (Casey, 2003). Poor baseline nutrition status prior to wound development or subsequent inadequate intake may predispose a patient to weight loss and poor vitamin, mineral, and protein status that can impact healing and increase the risk for

---

CHART 14–41 **Suggested Nutrition Interventions for COPD**

Dyspnea, early satiety, bloating, and fatigue all contribute to poor intake. Suggested interventions include the following:

- Consume higher calorie, higher protein foods first.
- Get more "calories per bite," especially by adding fat to foods with butter, margarine, mayonnaise, sauces, cream, dressings, and gravy.
- Consume frequent small meals.
- Save liquids for between meals.
- Limit intake of carbonated beverages.
- Keep convenient and ready-to-eat nutrient dense foods available for when fatigued.

---

infection. Inadequate fluid intake offset further by wound exudative fluid losses, fever, diarrhea, or excessive insensible losses can lead to dehydration. Decreased blood volume will not only impair needed oxygen delivery to the wound but also essential nutrients required for tissue repair (Leninger, 2002).

Knowledge of the role of nutrition in wound healing is beneficial to the nurse when completing an assessment of patients with existing wounds or those at risk of pressure ulcers. The early stages of wound healing require adequate protein stores to provide substrate for the inflammatory process. Diminished plasma protein levels before injury may worsen during this acute reaction (Leninger, 2002). Edema can result with decreased plasma proteins and this can impact healing. Collagen synthesis and tissue repair require adequate protein, vitamins C and A, and zinc, among other nutrients (Casey, 2003; Leninger, 2002). Protein is also essential for maintenance of immune function and avoidance of infection risk. Sufficient calorie intake is needed to prevent the use of crucial protein as energy instead of as a building block for tissue repair. Inadequate calorie intake can delay healing and also lead to skeletal muscle catabolism. The dietitian should be consulted to assess calorie, protein, and general nutrition needs. The size of the wound, amount of exudate (which can contribute to protein losses), presence of fever, coexisting injuries or disease, and the patient's baseline nutrition status will all affect nutritional recommendations.

The nurse should assess the patient for baseline nutrition status, paying close attention to protein status, physical signs of malnutrition including overall skin integrity, and diet history. The patient should be monitored for adequate intake of calories, protein, and fluid. The routine use of vitamin supplementation in wound healing is a common practice, yet benefits to this practice have only been reported for those patients who have existing nutritional deficiencies (Casey, 2003; Leninger, 2002). Vitamin C is necessary for collagen formation and is found in many fruits and vegetables, especially citrus or tropical fruit and green leafy vegetables. Zinc supplements are also commonly prescribed based on research that patients who are deficient have delayed reepithelialization of the wound and decreased wound strength (Casey, 2003). Long-term or excessive zinc supplementation can precipitate an imbalance in copper status and gastrointestinal upset (IOM, 2001). Zinc is found in most foods that contain protein, such as meats, poultry, legumes, and nuts. Fluid status should be monitored to provide at least the recommended AI of 2.7 or 3.7 liters of water daily for women and men, respectively (IOM, 2004). Adjustments should be made for excessive fluid losses from the gastrointestinal tract or the wound. Patients managed with an air-fluidized bed should receive an extra 10 to 15mL/kg fluid because of the associated increased insensible fluid losses (Leninger, 2002).

Pressure Ulcers

Malnutrition is among the many potential risk factors for development of a pressure ulcer (Langemo et al., 2006). As with the presence of any wound, adequate nutrition can benefit the healing process by providing necessary nutrients for each phase of tissue repair. Elderly and malnourished patients with a decubitus ulcer require close monitoring to ensure that nutritional needs are met. Individual consideration should be given to the liberalization of any dietary restrictions in these populations to encourage intake. Supplementation with oral nutrition formula may be beneficial if it does not replace normal intake. Multivitamin use is reasonable with consideration given to extra vitamin C and zinc in those found to be deficient (Langemo et al., 2006). Pressure ulcers are discussed in detail in Chapter 67 .

Burns

Medical nutrition therapy for the patient with a thermal injury focuses on two important management aspects. Both the metabolic response to a burn as well as the healing process require special attention with aggressive nutrition support. Severe burns cause a catabolic response by the body whereby hormonal and inflammatory responses to the injury precipitate tissue losses that compound the burn itself (Andel, Kamolz, Horauf, & Zimpfer, 2003). Patients are also in a hypermetabolic state because of the injury (Demling, DeSanti, & Orgill, 2004). The nutritional requirements for tissue repair must be met in addition to those that result from catabolism and hypermetabolism. With a severe burn, the result is a daily requirement for high levels of calorie and protein intake.

Early enteral feeding is most often recommended for the burn patient (Andel et al., 2003; Demling et al., 2004). Oral nutrition, continuous tube feedings, or supplemental nocturnal tube feedings can be utilized to deliver adequate nutrition in the patient who has a functioning gastrointestinal tract. Patients with gastric stasis may tolerate postpyloric enteral feeding in the duodenum or jejunum rather than via a basic nasogastric tube, because the latter could result in high residual gastric feeding volumes and increase aspiration risk (Andel et al., 2003; Sefton, Boulton-Jones, Anderton, Teahon, & Knights, 2002). Parenteral nutrition may be necessary in patients with ileus or intolerance to sufficient volume of enteral nutrition support. The large dextrose content of parenteral nutrition can supply fodder for bacterial growth; thus, strict aseptic technique is required for the parenteral nutrition intravenous site in order to avoid a disastrous infection.

Nutritional recommendations focus on modulating tissue catabolism and providing sufficient nutrition for tissue repair. Many different equations exist to estimate calorie and protein needs in a burn patient. None is universally accepted due to differences such as technique for factoring the effects of varying degree and percentage of body surface area burned. Typically 35 to 40 calories/kg per day are required for adults; this can be adjusted if **indirect calorimetry** technology is available to estimate energy needs based on oxygen consumption and carbon dioxide production. Up to 2 g protein/kg per day is suggested (Demling et al., 2004). Adjustments can be made based on wound healing progress. Supplemental amino acids in the form of glutamine and arginine may play a role in mediating catabolism post-burn. There have been hopeful research reports resulting in their use by some, but the supplements remain controversial as a standard of care in thermal injury (Andel et al., 2003; Buchman, 2001; Demling et al., 2004; Wilmore, 2001). Supplemental vitamins and minerals are prescribed to support tissue synthesis and the needs of a hypermetabolic state.

The nurse should monitor the patient's tolerance to enteral or parenteral nutrition. Close attention should be given to the amount and type of intake and fluid balance. Serial weights should be monitored to assess for weight loss. Loss of >10% body weight will impair healing. Larger losses of lean muscle mass are associated with increased mortality (Andel et al., 2003). Some patients are able to tolerate adequate oral intake, whereas others require nocturnal supplementation with a tube feeding. The nurse can help optimize intake by facilitating a comfortable eating environment. Dressing and wound care, venipuncture, and any major repositioning are best avoided near mealtime to minimize discomfort. Optimal pain management during meals is also helpful. Depression, pain, and medication side effects, including sedation, can lead to diminished intake. The patient with a thermal injury requires close monitoring and reevaluation of nutrition status throughout the course of injury and recovery. Chapter 68 describes the complete care of the burn patient.

Nutrition and the Surgical Patient

Malnutrition is associated with poor surgical outcome and increased postoperative mortality (Howard & Ashley 2003). Impaired wound healing, infection, and reduced strength for postoperative rehabilitation can result because of poor baseline nutrition status. Every effort should be made to ensure that a patient is in good nutritional health preoperatively. Lengthy hospitalization with multiple diagnostic tests requiring withheld or clear liquid feeding can contribute to iatrogenic deterioration of nutrition status. Trauma as a precursor to surgery leads to preoperative metabolic stress with characteristic hypercatabolism and hypermetabolism compromising nutrition status (McKibbin, Cresci, & Hawkins, 2003). Chronic disease existing before surgery, such as organ failure requiring transplantation, can place a patient at risk for malnutrition because of the need for a restrictive diet, medication side effects, and depression and anxiety, as well as a host of other medical symptoms. A nutrition assessment should be routinely included in the preoperative work-up of any patient when possible. Patients found to be at risk for poor nutrition status should receive appropriate referral for further evaluation and intervention. Although it seems intuitive that preoperative improvement in nutrition status will benefit the malnourished patient, it is controversial whether a short course of nutrition support prior to surgery improves operative outcome in this population (Howard & Ashley, 2003).

An assessment of preoperative nutrition and medication use is essential. The nurse should inquire about use of nutrition and herbal supplements during the preoperative nutrition assessment. In one study, up to 34% of patients surveyed reporting using a nutrition or herbal supplement that could interfere with anesthesia or inhibit coagulation (Norred, 2002). Women, people with higher education, and people practicing preventive health measures such as regular exercise, a low-fat diet, and not smoking are more likely to use herbal or nutrition supplements (Gunther, Patterson, Kristal, Stratton, & White, 2004). The Critical Alert outlines herbal and nutritional supplements that should be noted during preoperative screening.

CRITICAL ALERT   *The following supplements can alter coagulopathy or sedation (Fugh-Berman, 2000; Hodges & Kam, 2002; Norred, 2002):*

Borage	Bromelain	Danshen
Devils claw	Dong quai	Evening primrose
Feverfew	Fish oil	Garlic
Ginger	Ginkgo	Ginseng
Kava kava	Papaya	Red clover
St. John's wort	Vitamin E	

Adequate nutrition in the postoperative period is essential to contend with the increased metabolic demands caused by the physiological stress of the surgery. Additionally, wound healing, preservation of nutritional stores, and immunocompetence require sufficient energy, protein, and micronutrient intake. Patients should be transitioned to diet or enteral feeding as quickly as possible. Parenteral nutrition support may be indicated following some surgeries. Prolonged NPO status, reliance on only peripheral dextrose intravenous fluid, or extended use of a clear liquid diet postoperatively will not provide sufficient energy to meet even baseline needs and nutrition health can become compromised beginning with weight loss. The nurse should know that 2 L of a 5% dextrose solution provides only 340 calories! Nurses are uniquely positioned to closely monitor patients for lack of intake or poor intake and to ensure communication of prolonged NPO, clear liquid, and other forms of inadequate intake to the health care provider and nutrition staff. It is not uncommon for hospitalized patients to have periods of continuous or significantly cumulative NPO or poor quality intake to slip by without intervention when good communication patterns have not taken place. Such iatrogenic contribution to malnutrition was reported in one study where hospitalized elderly patients with already poor intake were ordered NPO for 38% of their meals (Sullivan et al., 1999). The reason for the NPO order was not clinically apparent 17% of the time and related to unnecessary delay in returning to a normal diet 20% of the time.

Some specific surgeries require additional postoperative nutrition intervention. Generally a registered dietitian with specialized training in the care of these patients is an active member of the treatment care team. It is important for the nurse to understand the nutrition protocol prescribed and participate in the team effort to ensure adequate nutrition contributes to good surgical outcome.

Bariatric Surgery for Morbid Obesity

Gastroplasty or gastric bypass surgery is indicated for weight loss treatment in some patients with morbid obesity. Gastroplasty is called a gastric restrictive procedure because the goal is to simply reduce gastric volume and therefore limit the amount (and energy content) of intake without causing malabsorption. In contrast, gastric bypass surgery involves reduction of the gastric volume but also causes deliberate malabsorption by bypassing absorptive surface in the small intestine. A Roux-en-Y procedure is the most commonly used bypass configuration; it bypasses the gastric fundus, duodenum, and proximal jejunum (Figure 14–3 ■) (Elliott, 2003). Postoperative care of patients who have undergone bariatric surgery follows careful steps in reintroduction of nutrition. Patients must learn to accommodate the reduction in gastric volume without precipitating nausea, vomiting, or dumping syndrome. Diets are advanced slowly over weeks and months from just liquids to texture modified foods until tolerance improves.

Patients with malabsorptive procedures or protracted vomiting must be closely monitored for nutrition risk. Commonly, supplemental vitamin B_{12}, folic acid, and calcium are prescribed (Elliott, 2003). Individual assessment of iron status may dictate an iron supplement as well since iron may be malabsorbed because of diminished acid production (Elliott, 2003). A chewable multivitamin is often generically recommended (Cunningham & Mar-

Vertical banded gastroplasty

Roux-en-Y gastric bypass

FIGURE 14–3 ■ Gastric bypass line drawing.
Source: National Institutes of Health. (2000). *The Practical Guide: Identification, Evaluation, and Treatment of Overweight and Obesity in Adults.* Retrieved December 10, 2008 from, http://www.nhlbi.nih.gov/guidelines/obesity/prctgd_c.pdf

cason, 2000). Chart 14–42 provides a sample diet recommendation and discharge instructions following bariatric surgery.

Transplant Surgery

Patients presenting for organ, intestinal, or bone marrow transplant are often already nutritionally at risk because of preexisting disease (Weimann et al., 2006). Most will have been closely monitored and have received appropriate nutrition intervention despite the presence of malnutrition. Postoperative recovery requires adequate nutrition for wound healing, repletion of nutrition stores, and support for the hypermetabolic demands of surgery. Patients undergoing renal or hepatic transplantation may have been on a restrictive diet that potentially may be liberalized following surgery when organ function improves. These recommendations are made on an individualized basis according to metabolic changes following surgery (Anbar, Lipa, Zinger, & Mor, 2003). Therapeutic use of immunosuppressive medications requires careful attention to risk factors for infection, including foodborne illness. The patient and family should be instructed about safe food handling (see Chart 14–38, p. 316).

 Educate patients about the deleterious effects of combining some nutritional and herbal supplements with medications. St. John's wort has been reported to decrease crucial plasma levels of cyclosporine therapy, leading to graft rejection (Henderson et al., 2002).

Patients undergoing intestinal transplant most commonly have been on some parenteral nutrition support preoperatively because of short bowel syndrome. The postoperative goal is to support the patient with enteral nutrition (Silver & Castellanos, 2000). Patients are closely monitored for return of intestinal motility and function. Enteral nutrition progresses according to patient tolerance and may consist of an oral diet, enteral formula, or a combination of both.

Following allogenic bone marrow transplant, patients routinely receive parenteral nutrition because of treatment-induced mucositis. The ability to take adequate enteral nutrition may not occur for several weeks and requires close monitoring by the team. Better nourished patients have been reported to have a shortened time to engraftment than malnourished patients (Muscaritoli, Grieco, Capria, Iori, & Fanelli, 2002). GVHD can place these patients at higher nutrition risk if malabsorption occurs. Parenteral or enteral supplementation with the amino acid

CHART 14–42 **Diet Progression and Discharge Planning Following Bariatric Surgery for Weight Loss**

DIETARY CHANGES

Liquids for 1–2 weeks postoperatively:
- Begin with clear liquids and add full liquids as tolerated.
- Avoid sugary beverages.
- Avoid carbonation.
- Slowly work toward intake of 64 oz daily.

Progress to pureed and soft foods 1 month postoperatively:
- Start with 2 TBSP and increase as tolerated per meal.
- Consume many small meals.
- Eat slowly. Eating too much or too fast will cause nausea and vomiting.

Follow guidelines for dumping syndrome if present. Dumping syndrome refers to abdominal pain, nausea, and bloating that occur after eating foods high in sugar, such as ice cream and milkshakes, following a bariatric procedure. Diarrhea, sweating, and fainting can also occur. Avoid foods that could cause this.

Eat slowly and chew well.

Save liquids for between meals.

Drink liquids in smaller amounts than prior to surgery. Continue to drink liquids to prevent dehydration. Signs of dehydration include dry mouth and dark urine.

Use a chewable or liquid multivitamin. Bypass patients require Vitamin B_{12}, iron, folic acid, and fluid and electrolyte monitoring.

ACTIVITY

Keep in mind that recovery takes several weeks.

It is normal to feel tired. Rest as needed.

Walk as often as able. Increase activity slowly.

Do not lift anything heavier than 10 pounds.

Avoid strenuous chores, such as vacuuming or lifting full bags of garbage, until the surgeon says it is safe to do so.

Climb stairs slowly and pause after every few steps.

Start an exercise program 1 week after discharge. You can benefit from simple activities such as walking or gardening. Ask your surgeon how to get started.

Ask your surgeon when you can expect to return to work.

HOME CARE

Continue the coughing and deep-breathing exercises you learned in the hospital.

Shower as needed. But avoid baths, swimming pools, and hot tubs for 2 weeks after going home. This helps prevent infection of the incision site.

Keep the incision clean and dry. Wash the incision gently with mild soap and warm water. Then gently pat the incision dry with a towel.

Follow your surgeon's instructions about caring for the dressing covering your incisions.

If Steri-Strips (small white adhesive strips) were used to close the incision, do not remove them. Let the strips fall off on their own. If they do not come off within 2 weeks after you were sent home, call your surgeon.

Take medications in crushed or liquid form for 3 weeks after surgery and as instructed.

Keep in mind that medications and dosages may need to be adjusted with weight loss.

Do not drive for 2 weeks after surgery.

WHEN TO CALL THE SURGEON

Call the surgeon if these following are present:
- Cloudy or smelly drainage from the incision site
- Fever of 100.4°F or higher, or shaking chills
- Fast pulse
- Night sweats
- Persistent pain, nausea, or vomiting after eating
- Diarrhea beyond the first week after discharge
- Pain in your upper back, chest, or left shoulder
- Persistent hiccups
- Confusion, depression, or unusual fatigue
- Signs of bladder infection (urinating more often than usual; burning, pain, bleeding, or hesitancy when urinating).

Sources: American Society for Metabolic and Bariatric Surgery. (ASBS). (2005). *Rationale for the surgical treatment of morbid obesity.* Retrieved November 21, 2006, from http://www.asbs.org/html/patients/rationale; Cunningham, E., & Marcason, W. (2000). Surgical treatment for obesity. *Journal of the American Dietetic Association, 100,* 1056; University of California, Davis Medical Center. (2007). Discharge instructions for bariatric (obesity) surgery. Davis, CA: Author.

glutamine has been reported to have beneficial effects on mitigating treatment toxicity effects on the GI tract because it is a primary fuel for the enterocyte. This area is deserving of further research (Muscaritoli et al., 2002; Weimann et al., 2006).

Trauma

Patients who sustain major trauma are at nutritional risk because of the hypermetabolic and hypercatabolic metabolic response that follows injury. Blunt or penetrating trauma and head injuries are examples of trauma associated with high nutritional risk. Early and aggressive nutrition support is indicated once the patient is generally hemodynamically stable (McKibbin et al., 2003). Enteral nutrition support is the preferred route unless bowel obstruction or other contraindication exists. The preservation of gut function and potential reduction of bacterial

translocation and septic complications are cited as benefits of enteral over parenteral nutrition support in trauma patients (Swanson & Winkelman, 2002). Longer length feeding tubes, such as those used with a jejunostomy, may be required to deliver nutrition in the distal intestine following abdominal surgery or because of altered gastric emptying associated with stress.

■ Nutrition Support

Nutrition support with enteral or parenteral feeding is indicated when a patient cannot or will not take adequate nutrition to meet their individual needs. Enteral nutrition utilizes the intestinal tract for feeding. Parenteral nutrition is delivered intravenously and is generally reserved for situations where intestinal function is grossly compromised (Weimann et al., 2006).

Enteral Nutrition

Enteral nutrition is the preferred route of delivery for nutrition support. Much has been written on the beneficial effects of maintaining gut integrity and function by continued use of the gastrointestinal tract, even when only small amounts of enteral feeding supplement parenteral nutrition. Increased intestinal permeability and atrophy of intestinal villi occur when the gut is not used (Sun, Spencer, Yang, Haxhija, & Teitelbaum, 2006). Risk of bacterial translocation and sepsis may be reduced when patients receive enteral nutrition support compared to parenteral support or no nutrition support (Olah et al., 2002). Enteral nutrition support is also less costly than parenteral support. Although in the past, many clinicians were quick to institute parenteral nutrition for many gastrointestinal or abdominal conditions, it is now realized that enteral nutrition may be tolerated and beneficial to these patients. Acute pancreatitis, postoperative bowel surgery, and active inflammatory bowel disease are examples of situations where enteral nutrition may be used effectively in most patients, replacing the older practice of using parenteral nutrition. Other indications for enteral nutrition include situations where a patient cannot or will not take an adequate oral diet, but has a functioning GI tract. Anorexia, dysphagia, head and neck surgery or tumor, and mechanical ventilation are examples of conditions that may prevent adequate oral intake. Chapter 45 ☞ describes GI disorders.

Types of Enteral Formulas

A wide variety of enteral nutrition formulas exist. Most fall into the category of a complete formula, which is one that contains all essential nutrients. Modular feedings are also available that can be used to supplement a complete formula with a single nutrient (for example, fat or protein) or to build a customized formula comprised of all modular components. The latter use is less common.

Complete formulas are further categorized by nutrient composition, density, and form. Some are marketed specifically for a certain disease state, but whether they are superior to generic formulas of similar composition is unknown. Standard complete formulas contain intact nutrients and require full digestive and absorptive ability by the patient. For example, protein is present in its intact form as found in foods, such as soy protein or casein from milk. Some standard formulas contain lactose or added fiber. Fiber in enteral feedings may be beneficial for normal bowel function, especially in patients on long-term feeding. Elemental formulas contain nutrients in a hydrolyzed form such that the patient does not need full digestive or absorptive ability to benefit from the feeding. Instead of whole proteins, an elemental formula may have protein already broken down to amino acids or di- and tripeptides. Generally these formulas have a minimal fat content as well. An elemental formula may be used with a patient with malabsorptive disease, bowel resection, or impaired pancreatic enzyme function. Both standard and elemental formulas contain between 1 and 2 kilocalories/mL. Many are also available in a high-protein version. Higher and lower calorie and protein contents allow for patients with increased or decreased fluid and/or nutritional needs.

When the composition of a 1 kilocalorie/mL formula is made of intact nutrients, the formula is usually isotonic in concentration. An **isotonic formula** has a concentration similar to that of the plasma and therefore should not contribute to an osmotic draw of fluid into the gut. When fluid is drawn into the gut to dilute a concentrated solution, cramping, bloating, and diarrhea can occur. Other types of formula can be **hypertonic** because they have a higher concentration of electronically active particles, as in the case of elemental formulas that have many small amino acids instead of large protein molecules. Higher calorie or higher protein formulas are also hypertonic because of their increased concentration. Hypertonic formulas may cause an osmotic draw of fluid into the gut in some patients and are often begun at a diluted strength to avoid this consequence initially. The choice of appropriate formula will be driven by whether the patient has full or compromised digestive and absorptive ability and their overall nutrition and fluid requirements.

Routes of Delivery

Enteral nutrition formula may be taken orally or delivered via a small-bore feeding tube of varying lengths. The oral route is used when the patient is able to tolerate liquid intake safely and requires a supplement to the diet, a liquid diet, or an elemental diet. For example, patients with short bowel syndrome may take minimal food and instead consume an elemental formula because of altered absorption. When a tube feeding is indicated, nasogastric, nasoduodenal, or nasojejunal tubes are available. The longer length tubes are used when the upper GI tract is dysfunctional or to reduce risk of aspiration compared with a nasogastric tube. Longer tubes do not remove risk of aspiration, but may lessen risk. The Evidence-Based Practice guidelines discuss the reduction of aspiration risk during tube feeding administration.

Surgical placement of a gastrostomy or jejunostomy feeding tube is used when long-term enteral support is anticipated. Permanent tubes have the advantage of avoiding the irritation and discomfort of a nasal tube. Permanent tubes do not hold open the lower esophageal sphincter or pylorus, which potentially lessens the risk of aspiration. When a feeding tube is placed in the jejunum, an elemental formula must be used because the site of the tube has bypassed the natural sites for digestion of intact nutrients and enzyme secretion. Figure 14–4 ■ demonstrates the various placements and lengths of feeding tubes.

Administration of Feedings

Enteral feedings may be administered in a variety of ways. Bolus feedings can be given several times during the day, mimicking normal food or fluid intake, when the patient is alert and not at risk of aspiration. This would not be unlike a patient consuming an oral diet who consumes a 240-mL cup of a beverage at one sitting. An example of this is a patient with a G-tube secondary to a resected head and neck tumor who is otherwise well and now receiving long-term enteral feedings.

Patients with longer feeding tubes reaching the small bowel will not tolerate bolus feedings because of the osmotic load of the formula. Intermittent or continuous feedings are more common in the acute care setting. Intermittent feedings are delivered at a set rate for intermittent periods of time (for example, all night), whereas continuous feedings are delivered around the clock. Intermittent feedings may be the sole nutrition provided or they may be used to augment oral intake or parenteral nutrition. For example, a patient recovering from burns or a head injury may take an oral diet during the day with no tube feedings to impede appetite, and then receive intermittent feeding during the night in order to meet her high nutritional needs. Slower de-

Reducing Aspiration Risk During Tube Feeding Administration

Clinical Problem

Tube feedings are often stopped or held in patients at high risk of aspiration if gastric residuals are elevated. As a result, the patient does not receive the goal volume of feeding needed to obtain nutritional requirements.

Research Findings

Tube feedings are stopped or held for gastric residual volumes of 150 mL or more out of fear of aspiration. McClave and Snider (2002) report that a cutoff volume for holding feedings can be closer to 400 mL without negative effect on aspiration risk in low-risk patients, or 250 mL in patients at higher risk of aspiration. Saliva and gastric secretions alone amount to almost 190 mL/hr, a factor that deserves consideration when evaluating gastric emptying (McClave & Snider, 2002). An evidence-based review of gastric residual volume urges acceptance of an isolated residual of 250 mL followed by clinical evaluation when two or more consecutive volumes exceed 250 mL (Kattlemann et al., 2006). They report that when single residuals of 250 mL are accepted, greater formula delivery results without altered aspiration risk.

Postpyloric placement of the feeding tube tip has been shown in multiple studies to decrease gastric residual volume and gastric reflux of formula, both risk factors for aspiration (Kattelmann et al., 2006). In turn, patients with postpyloric feeding tube placement are reported to receive formula volume that more closely approximates estimated goals than individuals with gastric placement (Morgan, Dickerson, Alexander, Brown, & Minard, 2004).

Aspiration risk is diminished with proper patient positioning. When possible, elevating the head of the bed to a 45-degree angle during feedings will lessen the risk of reflux of gastric contents (Kattlemann et al., 2006). Positioning patients in this fashion is reported to decrease risk of aspiration pneumonia compared with patients in the supine position during feedings (Collard, Saint, & Mathay, 2003).

Nursing Implications

Critically ill patients are often at high risk of malnutrition. Promoting improved tube feeding tolerance and reduction in risk of aspiration pneumonia through patient positioning and feeding tube placement may offer an additional benefit of increased delivery of crucial nutrition.

Critical Thinking Questions

1. A patient who is sedated and in the supine position has not received any nutrition support because of aspiration risk. What suggestions can the nurse make regarding delivery of nutrition?

2. Sedatives can slow gastric emptying. What parameters should be used for holding any enteral feeding?

Answers to Critical Thinking Questions appear in Appendix D.

References

Collard, H. R., Saint, S., & Mathay, M. A. (2003). Prevention of ventilator-associated pneumonia: An evidence-based systematic review. *Annals of Internal Medicine, 138*, 494–501.

Kattlemann, K. K., Hise, M., Russell, M., Charney, P., Stokes, M., & Compher, C. (2006). Preliminary evidence for a medical nutrition therapy protocol: Enteral feedings for critically ill patients. *Journal of the American Dietetic Association, 106*, 1226–1241.

McClave, S. A., & Snider, H. L. (2002). Clinical use of gastric residual volumes as a monitor for patients on enteral tube feedings. *Journal of Parenteral and Enteral Nutrition, 26*, S43–S48.

Morgan, L. M., Dickerson, R. N., Alexander, K. H., Brown, R. O., & Minard, G. (2004). Factors causing interrupted delivery of enteral nutrition in trauma intensive care unit patients. *Nutrition in Clinical Practice, 19*, 511–517.

EVIDENCE-BASED PRACTICE

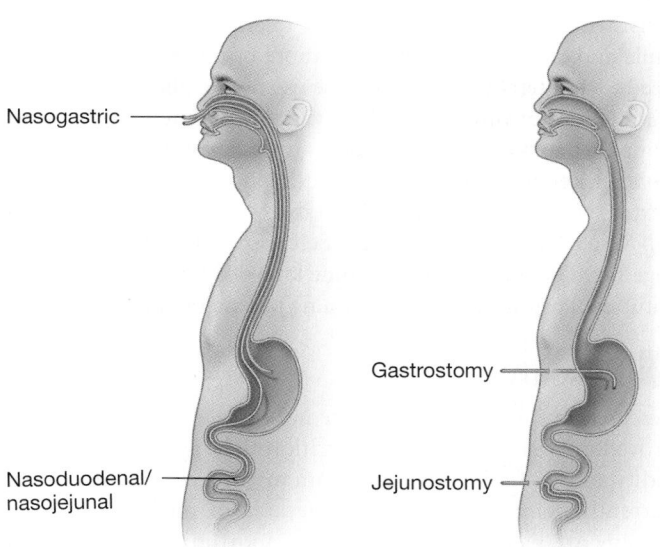

Nasogastric

Nasoduodenal/
nasojejunal

Gastrostomy

Jejunostomy

FIGURE 14–4 ■ Feeding tube placement.

livery of the formula results in avoidance of large gastric or intestinal volumes, minimizing the effect on aspiration risk and intolerance to hypertonic concentration. Feedings may be administered via gravity drip or with a feeding pump. Gravity drip delivery runs the risk of an accidental bolus occurring and should be avoided in patients at risk of aspiration.

The registered dietitian generally will recommend the appropriate formula and volume to meet the patient's needs. Depending on the formula content, the location of the feeding tube, and the patient's medical condition, feedings may be initiated at a diluted concentration or full strength. Isotonic feedings may be initiated at full-strength concentration is some patients, but hypertonic formula routinely are initiated at one-quarter to one-half strength. The concentration is gradually increased to full strength over one or more days depending on patient tolerance. The rate of formula delivery begins at about 50 mL/hr and is also increased as tolerated until recommended volume is achieved. Individual rate and concentration recommendations should be made for each patient.

Nutrition support requires close monitoring by the nurse. Tolerance to formula, amount delivered, and the fluid balance are crucial factors in determining effectiveness of treatment. Starting and stopping feedings for various interventions and repositioning can result in inadequate delivery of feeding and should be monitored for cumulative effect. The nurse must monitor the patient for symptoms such as high gastric residuals of formula, diarrhea, nausea, or vomiting. Severe vomiting or coughing can cause nasal tube displacement and warrants reassessment of placement. Diarrhea is commonly blamed on enteral formula even when other factors contribute more significantly (Parrish & McCray, 2003). Medications including antibiotics, infection, or bowel edema from hypoalbuminemia may be to blame and deserve investigation. Loose stools are to be expected with tube feeding and can be erroneously diagnosed as diarrhea. Formulas with added fiber are helpful in normalizing bowel function in appropriate patients (Swanson & Winkelman, 2002). To minimize risk of aspiration, patients should be fed with the head of the bed up at a 45-degree angle (Kattlemann et al., 2006).

Some medications can be administered through the feeding tube, but not all. Longer tubes may bypass drug absorption sites. Liquid suspension of some medications is not available and crushing medication can alter its action. A pharmacist should be consulted to determine compatibility of medication with tube feeding delivery. Tubes should be flushed before, between, and after medication delivery to avoid formation of precipitates that will clog the tube. A clogged tube or the need to replace a tube will inconvenience both the nurse and the patient. Taking the time to ensure that medication delivery does not lead to tube obstruction is time well spent. Handling of the equipment and formula requires fastidious sanitation to avoid the risk of feeding contamination. Chart 14–28 (p. 304) earlier in the chapter outlines nursing interventions for common problems related to tube feedings.

Parenteral Nutrition

Parenteral nutrition support is indicated in the patient who is unable to tolerate adequate enteral nutrition for more than 1 week (AGA, 2001a). Bowel obstruction, severe intolerance to enteral feeding (such as can occur with short bowel syndrome), and with bone marrow transplant are situations where parenteral nutrition is used. Parenteral formula delivered via a central line is referred to as **total parenteral nutrition (TPN)**. This is indicated in patients requiring support for at least 10 days. Formula delivered via a peripheral vein is called **peripheral parenteral nutrition (PPN)** and must be isotonic. PPN is used as short-term nutrition intervention to offset nutritional requirements until transition to alternative enteral nutrition is initiated. TPN is able to meet most patients' complete nutritional requirements. PPN is limited by the volume of fluid that can be tolerated peripherally and the lower concentration of nutrients that is required to maintain an isotonic concentration. Thus, it may not provide complete nutrition for some patients and is only a short-term solution.

Formula Composition

Parenteral formulas consist of a mix of carbohydrate, protein, fat, micronutrients, and electrolytes in amounts that are individually determined for each patient. Carbohydrate is in the form of dextrose and can be a 5% to 70% solution. Solutions that are more than 10% dextrose are hypertonic and cannot be delivered peripherally. Protein is in the form of amino acids and

begins at concentrations of 5%. A 5% amino acid solution, but not greater, can be tolerated peripherally. Fat can be administered centrally or peripherally and is an important calorie-dense component, a useful benefit when fluid volume is an issue. Both 10% and 20% solutions are available. Vitamins, minerals, and electrolytes are also administered with the formula admixture and can be customized to meet patient needs.

The nutrition support team makes recommendations on formula choice after a thorough assessment of the patient's nutritional, metabolic, and medical needs. Parenteral support is initiated at a low rate (about 50 mL/hr) and increased gradually to reach recommended volume. Maximum rates and volumes for both dextrose and fat administration are individually adjusted to avoid hyperglycemia, poor lipid clearance, and fatty liver. Blood glucose and triglyceride levels are monitored to assess tolerance to formula composition of dextrose and lipid loads, respectively.

The nurse is involved in the close monitoring of parenteral nutrition whether as a member of the nutrition support team or as a staff nurse. Most hospitals or institutions have clinical pathways or protocols that dictate frequency and type of nursing interventions in the care of patients on parenteral support. The nurse should become familiar with the specific protocol. Meticulous care of the access site for parenteral nutrition is imperative to avoid local or systemic infection risk because the high dextrose load of the feeding is fuel for bacteria. Accurate fluid balance calculations along with daily weights are essential. A short-term weight gain of >1 kg is more likely associated with fluid gain than accumulation of lean or adipose tissue. Clinical protocols will also outline metabolic monitoring for hyperglycemia and frequency of required laboratory assays. Close attention is paid to overall fluid and electrolyte status and formula adjustments can be made accordingly.

Patients continuing parenteral nutrition to the home care setting will require regular nursing care and monitoring following modifications of the in-hospital monitoring parameters. Before parenteral nutrition is discontinued, it should be documented consistently that the patient is able to tolerate a diet or enteral formula and consume two-thirds or more of estimated nutritional needs. Parenteral nutrition may be weaned to allow for appetite stimulation. Institutional policy will also outline guidelines for stopping parenteral support. Some advocate substitution of a peripheral dextrose solution to avoid hypoglycemia once a high-dextrose central solution has been discontinued, whereas others call for a reduced rate of delivery before stopping the solution altogether. The nurse should become knowledgeable about the institutional protocol for discontinuing parenteral nutrition.

Research

Research in the area of nutrition and disease can facilitate improved provision of medical nutrition therapy as well as morbidity and mortality outcomes from medical conditions. Topics currently being investigated in the area of medical nutrition therapy are listed in the Research Opportunities and Clinical Impact box. Results of this research can be monitored by reviewing the medical literature referenced through the National Library of Medicine.

RESEARCH OPPORTUNITIES AND CLINICAL IMPACT RELATED TO MEDICAL NUTRITION THERAPY

Research Area	Clinical Impact
Weight Management and Nutrition	
• Specific alterations in dietary carbohydrate, protein, and fat and weight loss efficacy	Improved advice on most effective diet for healthy weight loss
• Effects of significant restricted eating on short- and long-term alterations in brain chemistry and ability of diet to normalize changes.	Better understanding of treatment outcomes in disordered eating management
Coronary Artery Disease and Nutrition	
• Effect of lowering plasma homocysteine levels with diet on disease risk reduction	Potential reduction of disease risk factors
• Effect of antioxidants on disease risk	
• Effect of herbal dietary supplements on disease risk.	
Diabetes Mellitus and Nutrition	
• Use of the glycemic index to improve blood sugar control.	Improved short- and long-term glycemic control
Nutrition and Physiological Stress	
• Use of amino acid supplements, such as glutamine or arginine, in lessening catabolism in burns, trauma, bone marrow transplant, and other conditions	Lessened catabolic response to certain conditions and illnesses
• Use of early enteral nutrition support to prevent bacterial translocation.	
HIV and Nutrition	
• Effect of diet on occurrence and treatment of wasting and lipodystrophy.	Improved maintenance of nutrition status or nutrition repletion in acute care
Nutrition and Cancer	
• Effect of antioxidants on cancer prevention	Decreased incidence and improved treatment of alterations in body composition in HIV patients
• Effect of antioxidants on cancer treatment, including negative effects of antioxidants on chemotherapy or radiation efficacy.	Decreased disease risk
Nutrition and Renal Disease	
• Effect of limiting dietary protein on disease progression in renal failure	Improved treatment response to chemotherapy and radiation
• Effect of high-protein intake on risk of renal disease.	Limited disease progression
	Avoidance of disease risk from excess

Clinical Preparation

Read

- History of Current Illness
- Past Medical History
- Physical Exam
- Admitting Medical Orders
- Laboratory Study Results

Document

- Summary of Hospitalization
- Pathophysiology Form
- Laboratory Values
- Laboratory Results Explanation

Apply

- List of Potential Nursing Diagnoses
- Concept Map
- Critical Thinking Questions

Log on to MyNursingKit.com to download forms you will need and to complete further steps in the Clinical Preparation assignment.

HISTORY OF PRESENT ILLNESS

A 57-year-old unmarried female office worker was admitted to the telemetry unit through the emergency department (ED) after presenting in the early hours of the morning with a complaint of several hours of severe chest pain. On interview, the patient, Ms. Nance, reports that she was experiencing intermittent, nonradiating chest pain during the late evening after returning home from an elaborate dinner party. She relates that she has had this type of pain in the evening multiple times before during the last year and it eventually goes away on its own; for this reason she tolerated this episode of pain for several hours and it eventually became constant in nature. She then waited several more hours before calling a friend who urged her to seek medical help and drove her to the hospital.

On admission to the ED, she was found to be in sinus tachycardia with no ST segment changes. Initial serial cardiac enzymes were within normal limits (WNL). Nonfasting laboratory values were WNL with the exception of serum cholesterol of 215 mg/dL and blood glucose of 162 mg/dL. Ms. Nance's blood pressure was found to be elevated at 175/110 mmHg and she was begun on antihypertensive medication. The admitting health care provider assessed that her chest pain might be related to gastroesophageal reflux and treated her with a proton pump inhibitor. She was admitted for overnight observation with a diagnosis of acute coronary syndrome due to continued, though milder, chest pain with midepigastric tenderness.

Medical–Surgical History

Her medical history is unavailable because Ms. Nance has not had a physical examination or other health care intervention in more than 20 years. Ms. Nance reports no prior physical complaints. She reports NKA, no prescribed or OTC medications, and no surgical history. Both of her parents died in their mid-70s of CAD.

Physical Exam

On physical examination, significant findings include a blood pressure of 170/105 mmHg and a complaint of moderate midepigastric tenderness. Ms. Nance is 5'5" in height and weighs 198 pounds. Fasting laboratory values reveal serum cholesterol of 209 mg/dL with LDL cholesterol of 151 mg/dL and HDL cholesterol of 35 mg/dL. Her fasting blood glucose is 130 mg/dL. Cardiac enzymes remain normal. You find the following after eliciting her history:

- Ms. Nance is unable to give a good weight history because she does not own a scale, but you discover that her dress size has climbed by one or two sizes a year for the last 5 years.
- Ms. Nance attempted to lose weight 1 year ago before a nephew's wedding by following a high-protein, very-low-carbohydrate diet. She was able to fit into a dress two sizes smaller after dieting for 6 weeks, but also reported that her chest pain symptoms began while on the diet, leading her to stop adhering to it.
- Her nutrition history reveals that she eats two meals per day, lunch and dinner plus frequent snacks. She has her first meal at work at noon, but does drink several cups of coffee with cream in the morning. She has four or five cups of coffee a day. She buys her lunch at the office, choosing a meat with gravy or other sauce or a stir-fried dish and a potato or fried rice. She does not eat vegetables because she does not like how they are prepared by the office restaurant. Ms. Nance eats dinner out in a restaurant about four times a week with a preference for steak house establishments. Again, she tends to order red meat or chicken and a potato, plus dessert. When home for dinner, she heats a ready-made meal in her microwave or has instant soup. She always has at least one glass of wine with dinner, two if she is at a restaurant. Her snacks consist of chips or pretzels and crackers and cheese. A food frequency assessment reveals that her only fruit intake is orange juice on occasion when she feels she is getting a cold. Her only dairy intake is cream in her coffee. She takes no dietary supplements of any sort.
- Ms. Nance walks to and from her car in the office parking lot five days a week. This is her only exercise and takes approximately 5 minutes each way. On weekends, she remains indoors doing sedentary activities around her apartment and dining out in the evening with friends.

Allergies:	NKA
Medications:	none
Illness:	none reported
Surgeries:	none

Social History

Both parents died in their 70s of CAD. No siblings. Single, never married, lives alone, sedentary office worker. Active social life revolving around dining out with friends.

Physical Exam

Oxygen saturation 94% on RA

BP: 170/105 HR: 90 RR: 20 Temp: 37.1°C (98.9°F)

HEENT: nearsighted, glasses

Skin color: ruddy

Mucous membranes: pink

Sclera: white, no masses

Teeth: partial bridge, no obvious decay

Heart: regular rhythm, with no murmurs/rub, tachycardia

Lungs: clear, reports mild DOE

Abdomen: obese, soft, +BS, mild midepigastric tenderness

Pulses: −1 + radial and pedal

Extremities: no edema, warm and dry, no clubbing of fingers

Neuro exam 1: alert and oriented ×4; speech clear and coherent

Skin: good skin turgor, no rashes, no bruising

ECG: NSR, mild tachycardia, no elevated ST segments

Admitting Medical Orders

Admit to cardiology service

Type of floor: telemetry

Condition: good

Admitting diagnosis: acute coronary syndrome, GERD

Final diagnosis: GERD, HTN, obesity, hypercholesterolemia

No known allergies

Vital signs and oxygen saturation q2h

Activity bed rest, with bathroom privileges

Diet: low fat, saturated fat and cholesterol, 2 g sodium, no caffeine; nutrition consult

Call house officer: Pulse < 60 & > 130/minute; BP < 90 & > 160 systolic; temperature > 38.5°C (101.3°F); urine output < 30 mL/hr for 2 hours; respiratory rate > 30/minute; oxygen saturation < 92%

IV: saline lock; flush with NS q8h

Strict in/out

Sequential compression devices (SCD) to lower extremities

Oxygen 2 L nasal cannula

ECG continuous monitoring

12-lead ECG daily

Daily weight

Scheduled Medications

Omeprazole 20 mg po daily

Vasotec 10 mg po daily

PRN Medications

Phenergan 25 mg IV q6h prn nausea

Triazolam 0.125–0.25 mg q noc, prn sleep

Ativan 0.5–2 mg IV q6–8h prn anxiety (not to exceed 10 mg/24 hours)

Tylenol 650 mg po/pr q4h for pain

Ordered Laboratory Studies

Troponin I q3h × 3

CPK–MB q8h × 3

Chemistry 20 and PO$_4$ on admission and chemistry 7 q12h for first 2 days, then daily

CBC q a.m.

Mg^{2+} q a.m.

UA

Ordered Diagnostic Studies

Chest x-ray on admission and with adverse changes in O$_2$ saturation, increased shortness of breath, and/or increasing rales

GI consult for endoscopy

LABORATORY STUDY RESULTS

Test	Day 1	Day 2	Day 3
Sodium	142 mEq/L	137 mEq/L	140 mEq/L
Potassium	4.0 mEq/L	3.5 mEq/L	3.4 mEq/L
Chloride	106 mEq/L	100 mEq/L	102 mEq/L
Calcium	9.5 mg/dL		
Venous carbon dioxide	24 mEq/L	29 mEq/L	29 mEq/L
Blood urea nitrogen (BUN)	15 mg/dL	10 mg/dL	12 mg/dL
Creatinine	1.1 mg/dL	0.6 mg/dL	0.8 mg/dL
Blood glucose	162 mg/dL	130 mg/dL	129 mg/dL
Total proteins	5.2 g/dL		
Magnesium	2.1 mEq/L	2.0 mEq/L	2.1 mEq/L
Phosphorus	3.2 mg/dL		
Troponin I	0.26/0.23/ 0.28 ng/mL		
Myoglobin	0.5 µg/L		
Albumin	4.5 g/dL		
GOT	15 units/L	20 units/L	19 units/L
T. bilirubin	0.5 mg/dL		
CPK total	10 units/L	15 units/L	7 units/L
CPK MB	1.8%		
LDH	80 units/L	90 units/L	87 units/L
WBC	6,000/mm^3	5,200/mm^3	5,400/mm^3
Hemoglobin	16 g/dL	12 g/dL	14 g/dL
Hematocrit	45%	38%	40%
RBC	5/mm^3		
Platelets	395/mm^3	325/mm^3	250/mm^3
ABGs			
PO$_2$	80 mmHg	90 mmHg	91 mmHg
O$_2$ saturation	94%	97%	97%
pH	7.32	7.40	7.39
PCO$_2$	35 mmHg	40 mmHg	41 mmHg
HCO$_3$	22 mEq/L	26 mEq/L	24 mEq/L

CRITICAL THINKING QUESTIONS

1. What are this patient's risk factors for hypertension? Coronary artery disease?

2. What nutrition advice would you give to improve her blood pressure control and decrease her risk of coronary artery disease?

3. What components of the patient's diet may contribute to her symptoms of gastroesophageal reflux?

4. What nutrition advice for cardiac risk reduction should also help with management of reflux symptoms?

Answers to Critical Thinking Questions appear in Appendix D.

NCLEX® REVIEW

1. The nurse should plan to include the following anthropometric measurements when assessing a patient's nutritional status.
   1. Body Mass Index (BMI), weight and waist circumference
   2. Body Mass Index (BMI), blood pressure and pulse
   3. A weight diary and food frequency diary
   4. A twenty-four-hour food recall and blood pressure

2. The nurse should include which nursing intervention when caring for a patient with bulimia?
   1. Offer the patient frequent small servings of finger foods.
   2. Instruct patient to avoid eating unless hungry.
   3. Encourage frequent periods of vigorous exercise.
   4. Explain importance of adhering to scheduled mealtimes.

3. A patient with type I diabetes calls the clinic and reports having nausea and diarrhea secondary to the flu. Which instruction should the nurse provide?
   1. Restrict your intake of proteins and carbohydrates.
   2. Try to eat a lot of sugar-free jello and pudding.
   3. Maintain your carbohydrate intake by eating noodles, toast, and sports drinks.
   4. Do not take your insulin injection until you can eat solid foods.

4. A patient with a large abdominal wound has low albumin levels. The nurse identifies the following condition in the patient will contribute to further protein losses.
   1. The patient is receiving two different antibiotics.
   2. The wound drains large amounts of exudates.
   3. The patient eats a lot of dairy products.
   4. The wound needs surgical debridement.

5. The nurse recognizes the need for intermittent enteral tube feedings may be indicated in the patient recovering from which condition?
   1. Burn injuries
   2. Cholecystitis
   3. Renal transplant
   4. Bulimia

Answers for review questions appear in Appendix D

KEY TERMS

aerophagia *p.317*
anthropometric measurements *p.273*
binge-eating disorder (BED) *p.290*
cachexia *p.279*
celiac sprue *p.303*
dysphagia *p.300*
enteral nutrition *p.322*
hypercatabolism *p.277*
hypermetabolism *p.277*

hypertonic formula *p.322*
indirect calorimetry *p.319*
isotonic formula *p.322*
lipodystrophy *p.314*
malnutrition *p.277*
overnutrition *p.272*
parenteral nutrition *p.324*
peripheral parenteral nutrition (PPN) *p.324*

physiological stress *p.277*
protein-calorie malnutrition *p.277*
refeeding syndrome *p.289*
respiratory quotient (RQ) *p.317*
steatorrhea *p.306*
therapeutic lifestyle changes (TLC) *p.294*
total parenteral nutrition (TPN) *p.324*
undernutrition *p.272*

REFERENCES

Abou-Assi, S., & O'Keefe, S. J. D. (2002). Nutrition support during acute pancreatitis. *Nutrition, 18,* 938–943.

Abou-Assi, S., Craig, K., & O'Keefe, S. J. D. (2002). Hypocaloric jejunal feeding is better than total parenteral nutrition in acute pancreatitis: results of a randomized, comparative study. *American Journal of Gastroenterology, 97,* 2255–2262.

Alberino, F., Gatta, A., Amodio, P., Merkel, C., et al. (2001). Nutrition and survival in patients with liver cirrhosis. *Nutrition, 17,* 445–450.

Alsolaiman, M. M., Green, J. A., & Barkin, J. S. (2003). Should enteral feeding be the standard of care for acute pancreatitis? *American Journal of Gastroenterology, 98,* 2565–2567.

American Diabetes Association. (2003a). Evidence-based nutrition principles and recommendations for the treatment and prevention of diabetes and related complications. *Diabetes Care, 26,* S51–S61.

American Diabetes Association. (2003b). Translation of the diabetes nutrition recommendations for healthcare institutions. *Diabetes Care, 26,* S70–S72.

American Diabetes Association. (2004). Dyslipidemia management in adults with diabetes. *Diabetes Care, 27,* S68–S70.

American Dietetic Association. (2001). Position of the American Dietetic Association: Nutrition intervention in the treatment of anorexia nervosa, bulimia nervosa, and eating disorders not otherwise specified (EDNOS). *Journal of the American Dietetic Association, 101,* 810–819.

American Dietetic Association. (2002a). Position of the American Dietetic Association: Liberalized diets for older adults in long-term care. *Journal of theA merican Dietetic Association, 98,* 201–204.

American Dietetic Association. (2002b). Position of the American Dietetic Association: Weight management. *Journal of the American Dietetic Association, 102,* 1145–1155.

American Dietetic Association & Dietitians of Canada. (2004). Position of the American Dietetic Association and Dietitians of Canada: Nutrition intervention in the care of persons with human immunodeficiency virus. *Journal of the American Dietetic Association, 104,* 1425–1441.

American Gastroenterological Association (AGA). (1999). Medical position statement: Guidelines for the evaluation and management of chronic diarrhea. *Gastroenterology, 116,* 1461–1463.

American Gastroenterological Association (AGA). (2000). Medical position statement: Guidelines on constipation. *Gastroenterology, 119,* 1522–1525.

American Gastroenterological Association (AGA). (2001a). Medical position statement: Celiac sprue. *Gastroenterology, 120,* 1761–1778.

American Gastroenterological Association (AGA). (2001b). Medical position statement: Parenteral nutrition. *Gastroenterology, 121,* 966–969.

American Gastroenterological Association (AGA). (2002a). Medical position statement: Irritable bowel syndrome. *Gastroenterology, 123,* 2105–2107.

American Gastroenterological Association (AGA). (2002b). Medical position statement: Nonalcoholic fatty liver disease. *Gastroenterology, 123,* 1702–1704.

American Gastroenterological Association (AGA). (2003). Medical position statement: Short bowel syndrome and intestinal transplantation. *Gastroenterology, 124,* 1105–1110.

American Medical Directors Association (AMDA). (2001). *Altered nutritional status: Clinical practice guideline.* Columbia, MD: Author.

American Psychiatric Association (APA). (2000a). *Diagnostic and Statistical Manual of Mental Disorders* (4th ed., text revision). Washington, DC: Author.

American Psychiatric Association (APA). (2000b). Practice guidelines for the treatment of patients with eating disorders. *American Journal of Psychiatry, 157*(s), 1–39.

American Society for Metabolic and Bariatric Surgery. (2005). *Rationale for the surgical treatment of morbid obesity.* Retrieved November 21, 2006, from http://www.asbs.org/html/patients/rationale

Anbar, R., Lipa, R., Zinger, P., & Mor, E. (2003). The role of nutrition support in transplant recipients: Two case reports. *Transplant Proceedings, 35,* 614–616.

Andel, H., Kamolz, L., Horauf, K., & Zimpfer, M. (2003). Nutrition and anabolic agents in burned patients. *Burns, 29,* 592–595.

Anderson, J. W. (2003). Diet first, then medication for hypercholesterolemia. *Journal of the American Medical Association, 290,* 531–533.

Appel, G. B. (2006). Improved outcomes in nephrotic syndrome. *Cleveland Clinic Journal of Medicine, 73,* 161–167.

Arce, D. A., Ermocilla, C. A., & Costa, H. (2002). Evaluation of constipation. *American Family Physician, 65,* 2283–2290.

Atalay, F., Ozcay, N., Gundogdu, H., Orug, T., et al. (2003). Evaluation of the outcomes of short bowel syndrome and indications for intestinal transplantation. *Transplant Proceedings, 35,* 3054–3056.

Baum, M. K., Campa, A., Lai, S., Lai, H., & Page, J. B. (2003). Zinc status in HIV type1 infection and illicit drug use. *Clinical Infectious Diseases, 37,* S117–S123.

Becker, A. E., Grinspoon, S. K., Kilbanski, A., & Herzog, D. B. (1999). Eating disorders. *New England Journal of Medicine, 340,* 1092–1098.

Beto, J. A., & Bansal, V. K. (2004). Medical nutrition therapy in chronic kidney failure: Integrating clinical practice guidelines. *Journal of the American Dietetic Association, 104,* 404–409.

Blei, A. T., Cordoba, J., & Practice Parameters Committee. (2001). Practice guidelines: Hepatic encephalopathy. *The American Journal of Gastroenterology, 96,* 1968–1976.

Borghi, L., Schianchi, T., Meschi, T., Guerra, A., et al. (2002). Comparison of two diets for the prevention of recurrent stones in idiopathic hypercalciuria. *New England Journal of Medicine, 346,* 77–84.

Brand-Miller, J., Hayne, S., Petocz, P., & Colagiuri, S. (2003). Low-glycemic index diets in the management of diabetes. *Diabetes Care, 26,* 2261–2267.

Bravata, D. M., Sanders, L., Huang, J., Krumholz, H. M., Olkin, I., et al. (2003). Efficacy and safety of low-carbohydrate diets: A systemic review. *Journal of the American Medical Association, 289,* 1837–1850.

Brown, J. K., Feng, J., & Knapp, T. R. (2002). Is self-reported height or arm span a more accurate alternative measure of height? *Clinical Nursing Research, 11,* 417–432.

Brown, B. G., Zhao, X., Chait, A., Fisher, L. D., et al. (2001). Simvastatin and niacin, antioxidant vitamins, or the combination for the prevention of coronary disease. *New England Journal of Medicine, 345,* 1583–1592.

Bruemmer, B., Patterson, R. E., Cheney, C., Aker, S., & Witherspoon, R. P. (2003). The association between vitamin C and vitamin E supplement use before hematopoietic stem cell transplant and outcome to two years. *Journal of the American Dietetic Association, 103,* 982–990.

Buchman, A. L. (2001). Glutamine: Commercially essential or conditionally essential? A critical appraisal of the human data. *American Journal of Clinical Nutrition, 74,* 25–32.

Bulik, C. M., Sullivan, P. F., Wade, T. D., & Kendler, K. S. (2000). Twin studies of eating disorders: A review. *International Journal of Eating Disorders, 27,* 1–20.

Burden, S. (2001). Dietary treatment of irritable bowel syndrome: Current evidence and guidelines for future practice. *Journal Human Nutrition Dietetics, 14,* 231–241.

Bushinski, D. A. (2002). Recurrent hypercalciuric nephrolithiasis—Does diet help? *New England Journal of Medicine, 346,* 124–125.

Cai, B., Zhu, Y., Ma, Y., Xu, Z., et al. (2003). Effect of supplementing a high-fat, low-carbohydrate enteral formula in COPD patients. *Nutrition, 19,* 229–232.

Campion, J., Milagro, F. I., & Martinez, A. (2004). Genetic manipulation in nutrition, metabolism and obesity. *Nutrition Reviews, 62,* 321–330.

Casey, G. (2003). Nutrition support in wound healing. *Nursing Standard, 17,* 55–58.

Centers for Disease Control (CDC). (2001). Physical activity trends in the US 1990–1998. *Morbidity and Mortality Weekly Review, 50,* 166–169.

Centers for Disease Control (CDC). (2002). Iron deficiency—United States, 1999–2000. *Morbidity and Mortality Weekly Report, 51,* 897–899.

Chen, D., Misra, A., & Carg, A. (2002). Lipodystrophy in HIV-infected patients. *Journal Clinical Endocrinology Metabolism, 87,* 4845–4856.

Chobanian, A. V., Bakris, G. L., Black, H. R., Cushman, W. C., et al. (2003). The seventh report of the Joint National Committee on Prevention, Detection, Evaluation and Treatment of High Blood Pressure. *Journal of the American Medical Association, 289,* 2560–2572.

Cook, D., Meade, M., Guyatt, G., Butler, R., Aldawood, A., & Epstein, S. (2001). Trials of miscellaneous interventions to wean from mechanical ventilation. *Chest, 120,* 438S–444S.

Covinsky, K. E. (2002). Malnutrition and bad outcomes. *Journal of General Internal Medicine, 17,* 956–957.

Crook, M. A., Hally, V., & Panteli, J. V. (2001). The importance of the refeeding syndrome. *Nutrition, 17,* 632–637.

Cunningham, E., & Marcason, W. (2000). Surgical treatment for obesity. *Journal of the American Dietetic Association, 100,* 1056.

Cunningham, E., & Marcason, W. (2002). What role does fiber play in diverticular disease? *Journal of the American Dietetic Association, 102,* 225.

Demling, R. H., DeSanti, L., & Orgill, D. R. (2004). *Metabolism & nutrition.* Retrieved November 30, 2004, from http://www.burnsurgery.org/index_4x.htm

DeVault, K. R., Castell, D. O., & Practice Parameters Committee. (1999). Practice guidelines: Updated guidelines for the diagnosis and treatment of gastroesophageal reflux disease. *The American Journal of Gastroenterology, 94,* 1434–1442.

Devlin, M. J., Yanovski, S. Z., & Wilson, G. T. (2000). Obesity: What mental health professionals need to know. *American Journal of Psychiatry, 157,* 854–866.

Diabetes Prevention Program Research Group. (2002). Reduction in the incidence of type 2 diabetes with lifestyle intervention or metformin. *New England Journal of Medicine, 346,* 393–403.

Dietitians of Canada. (2003). *Hepatitis C: Nutrition care—Canadian guidelines for healthcare providers.* Retrieved December 18, 2003, from http://www.dietitians.ca/resources/HepatitisC_Guidelines.htm

Dorner, B. (2002). Tough to swallow. *Today's Dietitian,* August, 28–31.

Dube, M. P., Stein, J. H., Aberg, J. A., Fichtenbaum, C. J., Gerber, J. G., Tashima, K. T., et al. (2003). Guidelines for the evaluation and management of dyslipidemia in HIV-infected adults receiving antiretroviral therapy: Recommendations of the HIV Medicine Association and the Infectious Disease Society of America and the Adult AIDS Clinical Trials Group. *Clinical Infectious Diseases, 37,* 613–627.

Elliot, K. (2003). Nutritional considerations after bariatric surgery. *Critical Care Nursing Quarterly, 26,* 135–138.

Fairburn, C. G., & Harrison, P. J. (2003). Eating disorders. *Lancet, 361,* 407–416.

Farrell, R. J., & Kelly, C. (2002). Celiac sprue. *New England Journal of Medicine, 346,* 180–188.

Fawzi, W. (2003). Micronutrients and HIV type 1 disease progression among adults and children. *Clinical Infectious Diseases, 37,* S112–S116.

Finestone, H., & Greene-Finestone, L. S. (2003). Rehabilitation medicine: 2. Diagnosis of dysphagia and its nutritional management for stroke patients. *Canadian Medical Association Journal, 169,* 1041–1044.

Fletcher, R. H., & Fairfield, K. M. (2002). Vitamins for chronic disease prevention in adults: Clinical applications. *Journal of the American Medical Association, 287,* 3127–3129.

Fontaine, K. R., Redden, D. T., Wang, C., Westfall, A. O., & Allison, D. B. (2003). Years of life lost due to obesity. *Journal of the American Medical Association, 289,* 187–193.

Foque, D., Laville, M., & Boissel, J. P. (2006). Low protein diets for chronic kidney disease in nondiabetic adults. *Cochrane Database Review, 19,* CD 001892.

Foster, G. D., Wyatt, H. R., Hill, J. O., McGuckin, B. G., Brill, C., Mohammed, B. S., et al. (2003). A randomized trial of a low-carbohydrate diet for obesity. *New England Journal of Medicine, 348,* 2082–2090.

Franz, M. J., Bantle, J. P., Beebe, C. A., Brunzelli, J. D., Chiasson, J., Garg., et al. (2002). Technical review: Evidence-based nutrition principles and recommendations for the treatment and prevention of diabetes and related complications. *Diabetes Care 25,* 148–198.

Franz, M. J. (2003). The glycemic index: Not the most effective nutrition therapy intervention. *Diabetes Care, 26,* 2466–2468.

Freedman, M. R., King, J., & Kennedy, E. (2001). Popular diets: A scientific review. *Obesity Research 9,* 1S–40S.

Fugh-Berman, A. (2000). Herb-drug interactions. *Lancet, 355,* 134–138.

Gagnon, A. J., & Therrien, R. (Eds.). (2006). *HIV Medication Guide V2.05.* Retrieved January 15, 2004, from http://www.hivmedicationguide.com

Gans, K. M., Ross, E., Barner, C. W., Wylie-Rosett, J., McMurray, J., & Eaton, C. (2003). REAP and WAVE: New tools to rapidly assess/discuss nutrition with patients. *Journal of Nutrition, 133,* 556S–562S.

Garza, S. F. (2003). Bariatric weight loss surgery: Patient education, preparation and follow-up. *Critical Care Nursing Quarterly, 26,* 101–104.

Gebauer, S. K., Psota, T. L., Harris, W. S., & Kris-Etherton, P. M. (2006). N-3 fatty acid dietary recommendations and food sources to achieve essentiality and cardiovascular benefits. *American Journal of Clinical Nutrition, 83,* 1526S–1535S.

George, M. B., Day, L., & Zeiter, T. (2000). Case problem: Medical nutrition therapy for a patient with Crohn's disease. *Journal of the American Dietetic Association, 100,* 474–475.

Gerrior, J., Kantaros, J., Coakley, E., Labrecht, M., & Wanke, C. (2001). The fat redistribution syndrome in patients infected with HIV: Measurements of body shape abnormalities. *Journal of the American Dietetic Association, 101,* 1175–1180.

Goh, J., & O'Morain, C. A. (2003). Nutrition and adult inflammatory bowel disease. *Alimentary Pharmacology Therapy, 17,* 307–320.

Goldfein, J. A., Devlin, J. H., & Spitzer, R. L. (2000). Cognitive behavior therapy for the treatment of binge eating disorder: What constitutes success? *American Journal of Psychiatry, 157,* 1051–1056.

Graber, A. L. (2001). Syndrome of lipodystrophy, hyperlipidemia, insulin resistance and diabetes in treated patients with HIV infection. *Endocrine Practice 7,* 430–437.

Grinspoon, S., & Mulligan, K. (2003). Weight loss and wasting in patients infected with HIV. *Clinical Infectious Diseases, 36,* S69–S78.

Gronberg, A. M., Slinde, F., Engstrom, C. P., Hulthen, L., & Larsson, S. (2005). Dietary problems in patients with severe chronic obstructive pulmonary disease. *Journal of Human Nutrition & Dietetics, 18,* 445–452.

Gunther, S., Patterson, R. E., Kristal, A. R., Stratton, K. L., & White, E. (2004). Demographic and health-related correlates of herbal and specialty supplement use. *Journal of the American Dietetic Association, 104,* 27–34.

Hackam, D. G., & Anand, S. S. (2003). Emerging risk factors for atherosclerotic disease: A critical review of the evidence. *Journal of the American Medical Association, 290,* 932–940.

Harnack, L., & French, S. (2003). Fattening up on fast food. *Journal of the American Dietetic Association, 103,* 1296–1297.

Hayes, C., Elliot, E., Krales, E., & Downer, G. (2003). Food and water safety for persons infected with HIV. *Clinical Infectious Diseases, 36,* S106–S109.

Hedley, A. A., Ogden, C. L., Johnson, C. L., Carroll, M. D., Curtin, L. R., & Flegal, K. M. (2004). Prevalence of overweight and obesity among US children, adolescents and adults. *Journal of the American Medical Association, 291,* 2847–2850.

Henderson, L., Yue, Q. Y., Gerden, B., & Arlet, P. (2002). St. John's wort: Drug interactions and clinical outcomes. *Journal Clinical Pharmacology, 54,* 349–356.

Hijjar, I., & Kotchen, T. A. (2003). Trends in prevalence, awareness, treatment, and control of hypertension in the United States, 1988–2000. *Journal of the American Medical Association, 290,* 199–206.

Hodges, P. J., & Kam, P. C. A. (2002). The perioperative implications of herbal medicines. *Anaesthesia, 57,* 889–899.

Hoffer, L. J. (2001). Clinical nutrition: 1. Protein-energy malnutrition in the inpatient. *Canadian Medical Association Journal, 165,* 1345–1349.

Holmes, S. (2003). Undernutrition in hospital patients. *Nursing Standard, 17,* 45–52.

Howard, C., & Ashley, C. (2003). Nutrition in the perioperative patient. *Annual Review of Nutrition, 23,* 63–82.

Hu, F. B., Leitzmann, M. F., Stampfer, M. J., Colditz, G. A., Willett, W. C., & Rimm, E. B. (2001). Physical activity and television watching in relation to risk for type 2 diabetes mellitus in men. *Archives of Internal Medicine, 161,* 1542–1548.

Hu, F. B., Li, T. Y., Colditz, G. A., Willett, W. C., & Manson, J. E. (2003). Television watching and other sedentary behaviors in relation to risk of obesity and type 2 diabetes mellitus in women. *Journal of the American Medical Association, 289,* 1785–1791.

Hudson, J. I., Lalonde, J. K., Berry, J. M., Pindyck, J. L., Bulik, C. C., Crow, S. J., et al. (2006). Binge-eating disorder as a distinct familial phenotype in obese individuals. *Archives of General Psychiatry, 63,* 313–319.

Institute of Medicine. (1998). *Dietary reference intakes for thiamine, riboflavin, niacin, vitamin B-6, folate, vitamin B-12, pantothenic acid, biotin and choline.* Washington, DC: National Academy Press.

Institute of Medicine. (2001). *Dietary reference intakes for vitamin A, vitamin K, arsenic, boron, chromium, copper, iodine, iron, manganese, molybdenum, nickel, silicon, vanadium and zinc.* Washington, DC: National Academy Press.

Institute of Medicine. (2002). *Dietary reference intakes for energy, carbohydrate, fiber, fatty acids, cholesterol, protein and amino acids.* Washington, DC: National Academy Press.

Institute of Medicine. (2004). *Dietary reference intakes for water, potassium, sodium, chloride and sulfate.* Washington, DC: National Academy Press.

Ireton-Jones, C. (2000). Case problem: Medical nutrition therapy for a patient with Crohn's disease. *Journal of the American Dietetic Association, 100,* 472–474.

Jackson, J. E., Doescher, M. P., Saver, B. G., & Hart, L. G. (2005). Trends in professional advice to lose weight among obese individuals, 1994–2000. *Journal of General Internal Medicine, 20,* 814–818.

Jeejeebhoy, K. N. (2001). Total parenteral nutrition: Potion or poison? *American Journal of Clinical Nutrition, 74,* 160–163.

Jeejeebhoy, K. N. (2002a). Clinical nutrition: 6. Management of nutritional problems of patients with Crohn's disease. *Canadian Medical Association Journal, 166,* 913–918.

Jeejeebhoy, K. N. (2002b). Short bowel syndrome. *Canadian Medical Association Journal, 166,* 1297–1302.

Jenkins, D. J., Kendall, C. W., Faulkner, D. A., Nguyen, T., Kemp, T., Marchie, A., et al. (2006). Assessment of the longer term effects of a dietary portfolio of cholesterol-lowering foods in hypercholesterolemia. *American Journal of Clinical Nutrition, 83,* 582–591.

Kattlemann, K. K., Hise, M., Russell, M., Charney, P., Stokes, M., & Compher, C. (2006). Preliminary evidence for a medical nutrition therapy protocol: Enteral feedings for critically ill patients. *Journal of the American Dietetic Association, 106,* 1226–1241.

Katz, P. O. (2003). Optimizing medical therapy for gastroesophageal reflux disease: State of the art. *Reviews in Gastroenterological Disorders, 3,* 59–69.

Kaye, W. H., Devlin, B., Barabarich, N., Bulik, C. M., Thornton, L., Bacarus, S., et al. (2004). Genetic analysis of bulimia nervosa. *International Journal of Eating Disorders, 35,* 556–570.

Khan, N. A., McAlister, F. A., Rabkin, S. W., Padwal, R., Feldman, R. D., Campbell, N. R., et al. (2006). The 2006 Canadian Hypertension Education Program recommendations for the management of hypertension: Part II—Therapy. *Canadian Journal of Cardiology, 22,* 583–593.

Klopp, S. A., Heiss, C. J., & Smith, H. S. (2003). Self-reported vegetarianism may be a marker for college women at risk for disordered eating. *Journal of the American Dietetic Association, 103,* 745–747.

Knox, T. A., Zafonte-Sanders, M., Fields-Gardner, C., Moen, K., Johansen, D., & Paton, N. (2003). Assessment of nutritional status, body composition, and human immunodeficiency virus-associated morphologic changes. *Clinical Infectious Diseases, 36,* S63–S68.

Kondrup, J. (2006). Nutrition in end stage liver disease. *Best Practice and Research: Clinical Gastroenterology, 20,* 547–560.

Kopp-Hoolihan, L. (2001). Prophylactic and therapeutic uses of probiotics: A review. *Journal of the American Dietetic Association, 101,* 229–238.

Kotler, D. P. (2000). Cachexia. *Annals of Internal Medicine, 133,* 622–634.

Kuczmarski, M. F., Kuczmarski, R. J., & Najjar, M. (2001). Effects of age on validity of self-reported height, weight, and body mass index: Findings from the third National Health and Nutrition Examination Survey 1988–1994. *Journal of the American Dietetic Association, 101,* 28–34.

Kushner, R. F. (2001). *Roadmaps for clinical practice—Case studies in disease prevention and health promotion: Assessment and*

management of adult obesity—A primer for physicians. Chicago, IL: American Medical Association. Retrieved December 18, 2003, from http://www.ama-assn.org/ama/pub/category/10931.html

Langemo, D., Anderson, J., Hanson, D., Hunter, S., Thompson, P., & Posthauer, M. E. (2006). Nutritional considerations in wound care. *Advances in Skin and Wound Care, 19,* 297–298, 300, 303.

Lean, M. J., & Han, T. S. (2002). Waist worries. *American Journal of Clinical Nutrition, 76,* 699–700.

Leninger, S. M. (2002). The role of nutrition in wound healing. *Critical Care Nursing Quarterly, 25,* 13–21.

Lichtenstein, A. H., Appel, L. J., Brands, M., Carnethon, M., Daniels, S., Franch, H. A., et al. (2006). Diet and lifestyle recommendations revision 2006: A scientific statement from the American Heart Association. *Circulation, 114,* 82–96.

Lieber, C. S. (2000). Alcohol: Its metabolism and interaction with nutrients. *Annual Review Nutrition, 20,* 395–430.

Little, D. R. (1999). Ambulatory management of common forms of anemia. *American Family Physician, 59,* 1598–1604.

Ludwig, D. S. (2002). The glycemic index: Physiological mechanisms relating to obesity, diabetes and cardiovascular disease. *Journal of the American Medical Association, 287,* 2414–2423.

Mallampali, A. (2004). Nutritional management of the patient with chronic obstructive pulmonary disease. *Nutrition in Clinical Practice, 19,* 550–556.

Mangili, A., Murman, D. H., Zampini, A. M., & Wanke, C. A. (2006). Nutrition and HIV: Review of weight loss and wasting in the era of highly active antiretroviral therapy from the Nutrition for Healthy Living cohort. *Clinical Infectious Diseases, 42,* 836–842.

Marti, A., Moreno-Aliaga, M. J., Hebebrand, J., & Martinez, J. A. (2004). Genetics, lifestyles and obesity. *International Journal of Obesity and Related Metabolic Disorders, 3,* 529–536.

Massey, L. K., Liebman, L. M., & Kynast-Gales, S. A. (2005). Ascorbate increases human oxaluria and kidney stone risk. *Journal of Nutrition, 135,* 1673.

McCallum, S. L. (2003). The national dysphagia diet: Implementation at a regional rehabilitation center and hospital system. *Journal of the American Dietetic Association, 103,* 381–384.

McClave, S. A. (2004). Defining the new gold standard for nutrition support in acute pancreatitis. *Nutrition in Clinical Practice, 19,* 1–4.

McInnis, K. J., Franklin, B. A., & Rippe, J. M. (2003). Counseling for physical activity in overweight and obese patients. *American Family Physician, 67,* 1266–1268.

McKibbin, B., Cresci, G., & Hawkins, M. (2003). Nutrition support for the patient with an open abdomen after major abdominal trauma. *Nutrition, 19,* 563–566.

Mehler, P. S. (2003). Bulimia nervosa. *New England Journal of Medicine, 349,* 875–881.

Meno, C. A., Hannum, J. W., Espelage, D. E., & Douglas Low, K. S. (2008). Familial and individual variables as predictors of dieting concerns and binge eating in college females. *Eating Beahviors, 9,* 91–101.

Montalto, M., Curigliano, C., Santoro, L., Vastola, M., Cammarota, G., & Manna, R. (2006). Management and treatment of lactose malabsorption. *World Journal of Gastroenterology, 12,* 187–191.

Morelli, V., & Zoorob, R. J. (2000). Alternative therapies: Part 1. Depression, diabetes, obesity. *American Family Physician, 62,* 1051–1060.

Morgan, J. F., Reid, F., & Lacey, J. H. (1999). The SCOFF questionnaire: Assessment of a new screening tool for eating disorders. *British Medical Journal, 319,* 1467–1468.

Morgan, L. M., Dickerson, R. N., Alexander, K. H., Brown, R. O., & Minard, G. (2004). Factors causing interrupted delivery of enteral nutrition in trauma intensive care unit patients. *Nutrition in Clinical Practice, 19,* 511–517.

Morris, C. D., & Carson, S. (2003). Routine vitamin supplementation to prevent cardiovascular disease: A summary of the evidence for the US Preventative Services Task Force. *Annals of Internal Medicine, 139,* 56–70.

Morton, A. R., Iliescu, E. A., & Wilson, J. W. L. (2002). Nephrology: 1. Investigation and treatment of recurrent kidney stones. *Canadian Medical Association Journal, 166,* 213–218.

Mulrow, C. (2001). Sound clinical advice for hypertension patients. *Annals of Internal Medicine, 135,* 1084–1086.

Muscaritoli, M., Grieco, G., Capria, S., Iori, A. P., & Fanelli, F. R. (2002). Nutritional and metabolic support in patients undergoing bone marrow tranplantation. *American Journal of Clinical Nutrition, 75,* 183–190.

National Heart, Lung, and Blood Institute. (1998). *Clinical guidelines on the identification, evaluation, and treatment of overweight and obesity in adults—The evidence report.* Retrieved February 5, 2004, from http://www.nhlbi.nih.gov/guidelines/obesity/ob_gdlns.pdf

National Heart, Lung, and Blood Institute. (2002). *Third report of the National Cholesterol Education Program Expert Panel on Detection, Evaluation, and Treatment of High Blood Cholesterol in Adults [Adult Treatment Panel III (ATPIII)].* Retrieved February 5, 2004, from http://www.nhlbi.nih.gov/guidelines/cholesterol/atp3full.pdf

National Heart, Lung, and Blood Institute. (2004). *The seventh report of the Joint National Committee on Prevention, Detection, Evaluation and Treatment of High Blood Pressure (JNC7).* Retrieved February 5, 2004, from http://www.nhlbi.nih.gov/guidelines/hypertension/express.pdf

National Institute of Diabetes and Digestive and Kidney Diseases (2003). *Gastroesophageal reflux.* Retrieved January 13, 2004, from http://digestive.niddk.nih.gov/ddiseases/pubs/gerd/index.htm#4.

National Institute of Diabetes and Digestive and Kidney Diseases. (2005a). *Celiac disease.* Retrieved November 13, 2006, from http://www.digestive.niddk.nih.gov/ddiseases/pubs/celiac/index.htm

National Institute of Diabetes and Digestive and Kidney Diseases. (2005b). *Diverticulosis and diverticulitis.* Retrieved November 13, 2006, from http://www.digestive.niddk.nih.gov

National Kidney Foundation. (2000). *Kidney disease outcomes quality initiative (K/DOQI). Clinical practice guidelines for nutrition in chronic kidney disease.* Retrieved November 16, 2006, from http://www.kidney.org/professionals.doqi/index/cfm

National Kidney Foundation. (2006). *Kidney disease outcomes quality initiative (K/DOQI). Clinical practice guidelines and clinical practice recommendations for anemia in chronic kidney disease.* Retrieved November 16, 2006, from http://www.kidney.org/professionals/kdoqi/guidelines_anemia/index.htm

Nelson, M., & Poulter, J. (2004). Impact of tea drinking on iron status in the UK: A review. *Journal Human Nutrition Dietetics, 17,* 43–54.

Nerad, J., Romeyn, M., Silverman, E., Allen-Reid, J., Dietrich, D., Merchant, J., et al. (2003). General nutrition management in patients infected with HIV. *Clinical Infectious Diseases, 36,* S52–S62.

Nestle, M., & Jacobson, M. F. (2000). Halting the obesity epidemic: A public health policy approach. *Public Health Reports, 115,* 12–24.

Norman, H. A., Butrum, R. R., Feldman, E., Heber, D., et al. (2003). The role of dietary supplements during cancer therapy. *Journal of Nutrition, 133,* 3794S–3799S.

Norred, C. L. (2002). Complementary and alternative medicine use by surgical patients. *AORN, 76,* 1013–1021.

Novotny, J. A., Rumpler, W. V., Riddick, H., Hebert, H., Rhodes, D., Judd, J. T., et al. (2003). Personality characteristics as predictors of underreporting of energy intake on a 24-hour dietary recall interview. *Journal of the American Dietetic Association, 102,* 1146–1151.

Nyholm, E., Turpin, P., Swain, B., Daly, S., et al. (2003). Oral vitamin B-12 can change our practice. *Postgraduate Medical Journal, 79,* 218–221.

Oh, R. C., & Brown, D. L. (2003). Vitamin B-12 deficiency. *American Family Physician, 67,* 979–986.

Olah, A., Pardavi, G., Belagyi, T., Nagy, A., et al. (2002). Early nasojejunal feeding in acute pancreatitis is associated with a lower complication rate. *Nutrition, 18,* 259–262.

Ornstein, R. M., Golden, N. H., Jacobson, M. S., & Shenker, I. R. (2003). Hypophosphatemia during nutritional rehabilitation in anorexia nervosa: Implications for refeeding and monitoring. *Journal of Adolescent Health, 32,* 83–88.

Osterkamp, L. K. (1995). Current perspective on assessment of human body proportions of relevance to amputees. *Journal of the American Dietetic Association, 95,* 215–218.

Palmer, J. B., Drennan, J. C., & Baba, M. (2000). Evaluation and treatment of swallowing impairments. *American Family Physician, 61,* 2453–2462.

Parrish, C. R., & McCray, S. F. (2003). Nutrition support for the mechanically ventilated patient. *Critical Care Nurse, 23,* 77–80.

Perry, L. (2001). Screening swallowing function of patients with acute stroke. Part 1: Identification, implementation and initial evaluation of a screening tool for use by nurses. *Journal of Clinical Nursing, 10,* 463–473.

Perry, L., Morgan, J., Reid, F., O'Brien, A., Luck, A., & Lacey, H. (2002). Screening for symptoms of eating disorders: Reliability of the SCOFF screening tool with written compared to oral delivery. *International Journal of Eating Disorders, 32,* 466–472.

Persson, M. D., Brismar, K. E., Katzarski, K. S., Nordenstrom, J., & Cederholm, T. E. (2002). Nutritional status using Mini Nutritional Assessment and Subjective Global Assessment predict mortality in geriatric patients. *Journal of the American Geriatric Society, 50,* 1996–2002.

Pritts, S. D., & Susman, J. (2003). Diagnosis of eating disorders in primary care. *American Family Physician, 67,* 297–304.

Rahman, K. (2001). Historical perspective on garlic and cardiovascular disease. *Journal of Nutrition, 131,* 977S–979S.

Reams, A. M., & Elder, V. (2003). Dry weight: To be set or not to be. *Nephrology Nursing Journal, 30,* 236.

Riley, T. R., & Bhatti, A. M. (2001). Preventative strategies in chronic liver disease. Part 1: Alcohol, vaccines, toxic medications and supplements, diet and exercise. *American Family Physician, 64,* 1555–1560.

Roberts, S., & Thompson, J. (2005). Graft-vs.-host disease: Nutrition therapy in a challenging condition. *Nutrition in Clinical Practice, 20,* 440–450.

Russell, R. M., Rasmussen, H., & Lichtenstein, A. H. (1999). Modified food guide pyramid for people over 70 years of age. *Journal of Nutrition, 129,* 751–753.

Saltzman, J. R., Russell, R. M., Golner, B., Barakat, S., et al. (1999). A randomized trial of lactobacillus acidophilus to treat lactose intolerance. *American Journal of Clinical Nutrition, 69,* 140–146.

Samaha, F. F., Iqbal, N., Seshadri, P., Chicano, K. L., Daily, D. A., McGrory, J., et al. (2003). A low-carbohydrate as compared with a low-fat diet in severe obesity. *New England Journal of Medicine, 348,* 2074–2081.

Santolaria, F., Perez-Manzano, J. L., Milena, A., Gonzalez-Reimers, E., et al. (2000). Nutrition assessment in alcoholic patients. *Drug and Alcohol Dependence, 59,* 295–304.

Schols, A. M. W. J. (2002). Pulmonary cachexia. *International Journal of Cardiology, 85,* 101–110.

Sefton, E. J., Boulton-Jones, J. R., Anderton, D., Teahon, K., & Knights, D. T. (2002). Enteral feeding in patients with major burn injury: The use of nasojejunal feeding after the failure of nasogastric feeding. *Burns, 28,* 386–390.

Serdula, M. K., Kettel Khan, L., & Dietz, W. H. (2003). Weight loss counseling revisited. *Journal of the American Medical Association, 289,* 1747–1750.

Shamliyan, T. A., Jacobs, D. R., Raatz, S. K., Nordstrom, D. L., & Keenan, J. M. (2006). Are your patients with risk of CVD getting the viscous soluble fiber they need? *Journal of Family Practice, 55,* 761–769.

Shields, M. (2006). Overweight and obesity among children and youth. *Health Reports, 17,* 27–42.

Shinohara, M., Mizushima, H., Hirano, M., Shioe, K., Nakazawa, M., Hiejma, Y., et al. (2004). Eating disorders with binge eating behaviours are associated with the s allele of the 3'-UTR VNTR polymorphism of the dopamine transported gene. *Journal of Psychiatry Neuroscience, 29,* 134–137.

Silver, H. J., & Castellanos, V. H. (2000). Nutritional complications and management of intestinal transplantation. *Journal of the American Dietetic Association, 100,* 680–684.

Singh, H., Watt, K., Veitch, R., Cantor, M., & Duerksen, D. R. (2006). Malnutrition is prevalent in hospitalized medical patients: Are housestaff identifying the malnourished patient? *Nutrition, 22,* 350–354.

Stevinson, C., Pittler, M. H., & Ernst, E. (2000). Garlic for treating hypercholesterolemia: A meta-analysis of randomised clinical trials. *Annals of Internal Medicine, 135,* 420–429.

Stickel, F., Hoehn, B., & Seitz, H. K. (2003). Nutrition therapy in alcoholic liver disease. *Alimentary Pharmacology Therapy, 18,* 357–373.

Stollman, N. H., Raskin, J. B., & Practice Parameters Committee. (1999). Practice guidelines: Diagnosis and management of diverticular disease of the colon in adults. *The American Journal of Gastroenterology, 94,* 3110.

Striegel-Moore, R. H., Dohm, F. A., Kraemer, H. C., Taylor, C. B., Daniels, S., Crawford, B. P., et al. (2003). Eating disorders in white and black women. *American Journal of Psychiatry, 160,* 1326–1331.

Sullivan, D. H., Bopp, M. M., & Roberson, P. K. (2002). Protein-energy undernutrition and life-threatening complications among the hospitalized elderly. *Journal of General Internal Medicine, 17,* 923–932.

Sullivan, D. H., Sun, S., & Walls, R. C. (1999). Protein-energy undernutrition among elderly hospitalized patients. *Journal of the American Medical Association, 281,* 2013–2019.

Sun, X., Spencer, A. U., Yang, H., Haxhija, E. Q., & Teitelbaum, D. H. (2006). Impact of caloric intake on parenteral nutrition-associated intestinal morphology and mucosal barrier function. *Journal of Parenteral and Enteral Nutrition, 30,* 474–479.

Swagerty, D. L., Walling, A. D., & Klein, R. M. (2002). Lactose intolerance. *American Family Physician, 65,* 1845–1850.

Swanson, R. W., & Winkelman, C. (2002). Exploring the benefits and myths of enteral feeding in the critically ill. *Critical Care Nursing Quarterly, 24,* 67–75.

Thiamine. (2003). *Alternative Medicine Reviews, 8,* 59–62.

Thomas, D. R., Zdrowski, C. D., Wilson, M. M., Conright, K. C., Lewis, C., Tariq, S., et al. (2002). Malnutrition in subacute care. *American Journal of Clinical Nutrition, 75,* 308–313.

Thompson, T. (1999). Thiamin, riboflavin and niacin content of the gluten-free diet: Is there cause for concern? *Journal of the American Dietetic Association, 99,* 858–862.

Thompson, T. (2000a). Folate, iron and dietary fiber contents of the gluten-free diet. *Journal of the American Dietetic Association, 100,* 1389–1393.

Thompson, T. (2000b). Questionable foods and the gluten-free diet: Survey of current recommendations. *Journal of the American Dietetic Association, 100,* 463–465.

Thompson, T. (2001a). Case problem: Questions regarding the acceptability of buckwheat, amaranth, quinoa, and oats from a patient with celiac disease. *Journal of the American Dietetic Association, 101,* 586–587.

Thompson, T. (2001b). Wheat starch, gliadin, and the gluten-free diet. *Journal of the American Dietetic Association, 101,* 1456–1459.

U.S. Department of Health and Human Services. (2000). *Healthy people 2010: Understanding and improving health.* Retrieved February 5, 2008, from http://www.healthypeople.gov

U.S. Department of Health and Human Services. (2005). *Dietary guidelines for Americans, 2005 edition.* Retrieved May 17, 2008, from http://www.health.gov/DietaryGuidelines/dga2005/document

Vellas, B., Guigoz, Y., Garry, P. J., Nourhashemi, F., Bennahum, D., Lauque, S., et al. (1999). The Mini Nutritional Assessment and its use in grading the nutritional state of elderly patients. *Nutrition, 15,* 116–122.

Viera, A. J., Hoag, S., & Shaughnessy, J. (2002). Management of irritable bowel syndrome. *American Family Physician, 66,* 1867–1874.

Wagner, D. R., & Heyward, V. H. (1999). Techniques of body composition assessment: A review of laboratory and field methods. *Research Quarterly for Exercise and Sport, 70,* 1–17.

Waters, D. D., Alderman, E. L., Hsia, J., Howard, B. V., et al. (2002). Effects of hormone replacement therapy and antioxidant vitamin supplements on coronary atherosclerosis in postmenopausal women. *Journal of the American Medical Association, 288,* 2432–2440.

Weiger, W. A., Smith, M., Boon, H., Richardson, M. A., et al. (2002). Advising patients who seek complementary and alternative medical therapies with cancer. *Annals of Internal Medicine, 137,* 889–903.

Weimann, A., Braga, M., Harsanyi, L., Laviano, A., Ljungqvist, O., Soeters, P., et al. (2006). ESPEN guidelines on enteral nutrition: Surgery including organ transplantation. *Clinical Nutrition, 25,* 224–244.

Wells, C. (2003). Optimizing nutrition in patients with chronic kidney disease. *Nephrology Nursing Journal, 30,* 637–646.

Whelton, P. K., He, J., Appel, L. J., Cutler, J. A., Havas, S., Kotchen, T. A., et al. (2002). Primary prevention of hypertension: Clinical and public health advisory from the National High Blood Pressure Education Program. *Journal of the American Medical Association, 288,* 1882–1888.

Whitaker, R. C., Wright, J. A., Pepe, M. S., Seidel, K. D., & Dietz, W. H. (1997). Predicting obesity in young adulthood from childhood and parental obesity. *New England Journal of Medicine, 337,* 869–873.

White, R., & Ashworth, A. (2000). How drug therapy can affect, threaten and compromise nutritional status. *Journal Human Nutrition Dietetics, 13,* 119–129.

Wilmore, D. (2001). The effect of glutamine supplementation in patients following elective surgery and accidental injury. *Journal of Nutrition, 131,* 2543S–2549S.

Woods, M. N., Tang, A. M., Jones, C., Hendricks, K., et al. (2003). Effect of dietary intake and protease inhibitors on serum vitamin B-12 levels in a cohort of HIV-positive patients. *Clinical Infectious Diseases, 37,* S124–S131.

Writing group of the PREMIER Collaborative Research Group. (2003). Effects of comprehensive lifestyle modification on blood pressure control. *Journal of the American Medical Association, 289,* 2083–2093.

Yanovski, S., & Yanovski, J. A. (2002). Drug therapy: Obesity. *New England Journal of Medicine, 346,* 591–602.

Young, L. R., & Nestle, M. (2003). Expanding portions sizes in the US marketplace: Implications for nutrition counseling. *Journal of the American Dietetic Association, 103,* 231–234.

15

Pain Assessment and Management

Claudia E. Campbell, Kathleen Osborn

Outcome-Based Learning Objectives

After studying this chapter, the learner will be able to:

1. Recognize pain as a distinct and frequently encountered human problem in the health care field.
2. Compare and contrast the ethical and legal issues related to pain and pain management.
3. Distinguish the sensory, cognitive, affective, and behavioral components of pain.
4. Apply common pain assessment tools and strategies to elicit details of the multidimensional pain experience.
5. Differentiate between acute, chronic, and cancer-related pain.
6. Describe and give examples of basic pharmacodynamic and pharmacokinetic properties of commonly used pharmacologic therapies, including the role of balanced analgesia in pain management.
7. Examine the usefulness of nonmedication interventions to alleviate pain in clinical practice.
8. Apply nursing pain management techniques in relation to established theories and current research.
9. Specify the major patient-related barriers to adequate pain management and demonstrate effective collaboration as a nurse-member of a multidisciplinary team in the management of pain.

Research   Collaboration   Health Promotion   Nursing Process   Caring   Critical Thinking

PAIN IS a symptom common to almost every illness, disease, or traumatic injury regardless of a person's age, gender, or socio-economic status. All cultures recognize the experience of pain although it may be expressed and responded to differently. It is pain that alerts an individual to an injury and encourages guarding of the injury to prevent further damage. To most, pain is a transient and unpleasant experience that persists for only moments before becoming an annoyance and then a memory. Pain is a reminder to avoid the activity that caused pain. For most people, the experience of pain leads to a diagnosis of the source of pain, successful treatment, and resolution of pain within a relatively short period of time. For others, pain becomes a complex experience that may not lead to a diagnosis or successful treatment. For some, pain is a disease. These patients are left to live with pain that persists for years and in many cases for the rest of their lives.

Pain is a major health problem of epidemic proportions. Millions of patients are unable to find health care providers who are knowledgeable and willing to treat pain. Pain management specialists are relatively few in number, clinics are generally located only in metropolitan areas, and health care coverage for pain treatment is often limited. Health care professionals, patients, and their family members are oftentimes misinformed so that misconceptions and myths regarding pain and pain treatments abound, creating conflict as patients seek relief from their pain.

In this challenging environment, patients are burdened with navigating an unfriendly health care system at a time when they are in pain, unable to or have a limited ability to self-advocate, and left vulnerable to accepting whatever health care they can easily access. When pain is chronic, patients are likely to experience personal distress from strained relationships, loss of independence, and depression. Patients are often unable to consistently participate in work-related activities, leading to loss of income and financial instability. A survey of chronic pain in America estimated that the annual costs associated with medical care, loss of income, and reduced work productivity are approximately $100 billion (American Pain Society [APS], 2000).

Epidemiology

A national health survey estimates that one-third of the people in the United States experience some type of pain (Lethridge-Cejku & Vickerie, 2005). Although pain management has improved during the past decade, the literature supports the consensus that many patients will experience severe postoperative or post-traumatic pain that is unrelieved (Ferrell et al., 2001). Of those patients experiencing chronic pain, one-half to two-thirds are partially or totally disabled for days, months, years, or even permanently (Bonica & Loeser, 2001). In evaluating the cost of treating pain, both the direct cost (office visits and medications) and the indirect cost (time away from work, reduced productivity, and/or tax revenue) must be considered (Turk, 2006).

Pain is associated with significant personal, economic, and social distress. Research indicates that hospitalized patients suffering unrelieved pain are more likely to experience delayed wound healing, pneumonia, and other postoperative complications (Shea, Brooks, Dayhoff, & Keck, 2002). Pain also is associated with decreased mobility, agitation, sleep deprivation, and postoperative delirium (Pasero & McCaffery, 2001b; Swarm, Karanikolas, & Kalauokalani, 2001). Scientific studies in recent years have just begun to uncover the connection between persistently unrelieved acute pain, subsequent hypersensitivity, and the transition to chronic pain syndromes (APS, 2003; Brookhoff, 2000; Byers & Bonica, 2001). These consequences of unrelieved pain are commonly associated with increased costs of providing health care. They also create financial and personal burdens for patients and underscore the need to make every effort possible to relieve pain in acute stages.

Pain management is associated with legal, ethical, and political concerns. The Joint Commission released pain management standards in 2000 that require accredited health care organizations to educate patients regarding their right to receive appropriate assessment and management of pain (Pasero & McCaffery, 2005). As a result patients are becoming better informed health care consumers who have expectations that their pain will be assessed and managed appropriately. Increased consumer awareness has improved patients' self-advocacy skills so that failure to manage pain is now resulting in increased legal liability for health care institutions, health care providers, and nurses (Pasero & McCaffery, 2001c). More than ever before, nurses must be aware of the importance of statutes and regulations that address the appropriate treatment of pain. Administering excessive amounts of pain medication can lead to sanctions and even criminal penalties for nurses. Now, nurses who do not appropriately treat pain can be investigated and disciplined as well (Frank-Stromborg & Christensen, 2001).

In addition to legal responsibilities, nurses have an ethical obligation to relieve pain. Nurses' ethical responsibilities when caring for patients are outlined in the American Nurses Association (ANA) *Code of Ethics* (ANA, 2001). Additionally, *The ICN Code of Ethics for Nurses* preamble states that nurses have the fundamental responsibility to alleviate suffering (International Council of Nurses [ICN], 2006). The use of placebos in the treatment of pain, treating the patient who has an addiction and pain, and treatment of pain at the end of life are examples of ethical challenges that nurses face in everyday practice. The American Society for Pain Management Nursing (ASPMN) has issued position statements, such as those listed in Chart 15–1, that are useful guides to nurses when they are confronted with difficult ethical situations in the course of managing pain (ASPMN, 2007). The Ethical Issues box discusses additional ethical issues related to pain management.

The science of pain is expanding at an unprecedented pace. The U.S. Congress publicly recognized the need for increased pain research by designating the period beginning January 1, 2001, to December 31, 2010, as the "Decade of Pain Control and Research." With this declaration, Congress recognized that much is still unknown regarding the complexity of pain and that to respond fully to those suffering with unrelenting pain time

---

| CHART 15–1 | **American Society for Pain Management Nursing Position Statements** |

- *Use of Placebos for Pain Management* (Coggins, Arnstein, & Leahy, 2004)
- *Pain Management at the End of Life* (Brown, Phillips, Cusimano, & Osteyee, 2003)
- *Assisted Suicide* (ASPMN, 2007)
- *Pain Management in Patients with Addictive Disease* (Coggins, McCaffery, Pasero, St. Marie, & Nichols, 2002)
- *Authorized and Unauthorized ("PCA by Proxy") Dosing of Analgesic Infusion Pumps* (Wuhrman et al., 2006)
- *The Use of "As-Needed" Range Orders for Opioid Analgesics in the Management of Acute Pain* (Phillips, Gordon, & Frandsen, 2006)
- *Registered Nurse Management and Monitoring of Analgesia by Catheter Techniques* (Primeau, Cowley, Eksterowicz, & Pasero, 2007)

Note: The full position statements are available at www.aspmn.org.

ETHICAL ISSUES in Nonmalignant Pain Management

Chronic nonmalignant pain is not usually proportional to objective disease severity; therefore, confusion about treatment goals and confusion about the reality of pain entangle therapeutic efforts. Doubts about the reality of the pain raise concerns about the issue of medication addiction and often cloud the efforts for relief. The ethical question is not whether chronic nonmalignant pain is real or proportional to objective disease severity, but how it should be managed to optimize the patient's quality of life. Sullivan and Ferrell (2005) proposed patient-centered principles to guide efforts to relieve chronic nonmalignant pain, including these:

- Accept all patient pain reports as valid, but negotiate treatment goals early in care.
- Avoid harming patients.
- Incorporate chronic opioids as one part of the treatment plan if they improve the patient's overall health-related quality of life.

The ban on opioid use in chronic nonmalignant pain is no longer ethically acceptable. Note, however, that ensuring opioids provide overall benefit to patients requires that patients with nonmalignant pain should be assessed and treated for concurrent psychiatric disorders. The presence of a psychiatric diagnosis does not mean that these patients are not entitled to equivalent efforts at pain relief. See the Pharmacology Summary (p. 344) regarding the use of antidepressant medications in the pain management treatment plan.

---

and resources must be dedicated to finding answers. Federal and state legislators are beginning to recognize the importance of pain management in the lives of their constituents. Legislation about issues such as regulatory barriers to appropriate pain management, the use of electronic prescription monitoring programs to monitor for diversion and abuse, establishing intractable pain treatment acts, and mandating pain education for health care professionals is only beginning to address some of the barriers to appropriate pain management (Dahl, 2002). The National Institutes of Health publishes guidelines about pain management, as noted in the National Guidelines box (p. 334).

NATIONAL GUIDELINES for Pain Management

The National Institutes of Health provides a web page with a plan for comprehensive pain management that spans all age groups. Topics covered include:

- Diagnosis/symptoms
- Treatment
- Health check tools
- Alternative therapy
- Coping
- Disease management
- Specific conditions
- Financial issues.

Source: National Institutes of Health. (2008). Retrieved May 28, 2008, from http://medlineplus.nlm.nih.gov/medlineplus/pain.html#fromthenationalinstitutesofhealth

In spite of positive strides, significant barriers prevent the provision of appropriate pain management for many patients. Patients and family members continue to be fearful that the use of opioids to treat pain will, as a singular event, result in addiction. Health care professionals confuse physical dependence and tolerance to opioids as addiction, and consumers are bombarded with inaccurate data and information regarding opioid abuse and diversion. Health care provider, nursing, and pharmacy educational curricula lack evidence-based information regarding pain and pain management, and health care professionals enter their practice without adequate knowledge of pain management principles. Health care institutions and insurance providers continue to provide financial incentives for major procedures or surgeries but fail to provide access to appropriate pain medications, treatments, and health care providers specializing in pain management. See examples of common barriers to appropriate pain management in Chart 15–2.

◼ Definitions of Pain

Discussion of pain is difficult without initially defining the terms commonly used to describe pain. The lack of consistent language is confusing to patients and family members as well as

CHART 15–2 Barriers to Appropriate Pain Management

- Inaccurate consumer education and consumer fears related to addictive disease
- Professional educational curriculums that do not include evidence-based instruction regarding principles of pain management
- Prescribing providers' fears of abuse, diversion, and regulatory scrutiny
- Federal and state laws, policies, and regulations that restrict appropriate access to pain medications and pain management specialists
- Inaccurate media coverage of abuse and diversion of prescription opioids
- Inadequate provider reimbursement for pain management treatments and therapies.

health care providers. Is pain the same as suffering? What is the difference between acute pain and chronic pain? Improved understanding of the principles of pain management begins with learning the terms that are commonly used and then using consistent language in discussions with professional colleagues and when educating patients and families.

Pain is defined as an unpleasant sensory and emotional experience associated with actual or potential tissue damage, or described in terms of such damage (International Association for the Study of Pain [IASP], 1993; Mersky, 1994; Wittbrodt & Tietze, 2004). Pain is always a subjective experience (APS, 2003). It is the subjective nature of pain that creates difficulty for the clinician who feels compelled to prove whether pain is present. Nurses must recognize that the physical assessment is incomplete without assessing patients' understanding of their illness including their pain. In 1968, Margo McCaffery's definition, "Pain is whatever the experiencing person says it is, existing whenever he says it does," described the need to appreciate that behaviors may not be consistent with the experience of pain and the most reliable indicator of the presence of pain is the patient's self-report (McCaffery, 1968; National Institutes of Health [NIH], 1987).

Pain Descriptors

Acute pain is considered to be of relatively short duration and coincides with injury, surgery, or illness. When healing occurs, acute pain decreases and resolves within a relatively predictable period of time (APS, 2003; Pasero, Paice, & McCaffery, 1999). However, it is difficult to classify pain based only on the criterion of duration. Acute pain may persist but still coincide with a high degree of pathology that does not meet the criteria expected for chronic pain. It has been suggested that it may be appropriate to consider pain that is associated with high levels of pathology that can usually be linked to the injury, surgery, or illness as acute regardless of the duration (Turk & Okifuji, 2001).

Acute pain episodes that are relatively short in duration and then completely resolve, leaving the patient pain free for a period of time before pain reoccurs, is defined as **recurrent pain**. This type of pain is usually associated with a chronic disease process that is painless except for episodes of acute pain (e.g., sickle cell disease, pancreatitis, or Crohn's disease). However, recurrent pain also is an appropriate designation when a patient has had multiple surgeries where pain has completely resolved between surgeries that are sequential (Turk & Okifuji, 2001).

When resolution of pain does not occur within the expected time frame, and is persistent beyond 3 to 6 months, it is considered to be **chronic pain**. Chronic pain is sometimes difficult to connect to an injury or illness and may persist for months, years, or even the lifetime of the patient. Chronic pain is associated with low or absent levels of pathology that can be linked to injury, surgery, or illness. The intensity of pain perceived by the patient may appear to be inconsistent with the existing pathology (Sullivan & Ferrell, 2005; Turk & Okifuji, 2001). Common types of chronic pain complaints include headache, low back pain, arthritis pain, or pain resulting from damage to the peripheral nerves or to the central nervous system (CNS) itself. A less common example of chronic pain is when pain is not due to past disease or injury or any visible sign of damage inside or outside the nervous system (psychogenic pain) (National Institute of Neurological Disorders and Stroke [NINDS], 2007a). Untreated chronic pain is currently being recognized as a major health problem in the United States (Sullivan & Ferrell, 2005).

Transient pain is acute pain that is brief and then resolves completely such as the pain associated with a needlestick for phlebotomy or an intramuscular injection. Transient pain is associated with minor tissue damage rather than disease or significant tissue damage.

Breakthrough pain is defined as a "transitory exacerbation of pain that occurs on a background of otherwise stable pain in a patient receiving chronic opioid therapy" (Portenoy & Hagen, 1990). It is referred to as breakthrough pain because the pain "breaks through" the patient's regular pain medication. Breakthrough pain is commonly associated with cancer pain although it can occur with chronic pain as well. Breakthrough pain may be easily confused with the pain caused by a painful procedure (acute pain) or the pain experienced as the effects of analgesic medications decline (end-of-dose failure).

Cancer pain is associated with malignancy and can be acute and chronic in nature. Acute cancer pain is generally caused by disease progression, surgery or procedures, and medications or therapies used in the treatment of cancer. Chronic cancer pain can also occur as a result of nerve injury leading to painful neuropathies (APS, 2005; Turk & Okifuji, 2001). Cancer pain is discussed in detail in Chapter 64 ☺.

Evolution of Pain Theories

Theories on pain have been recorded since ancient times when some believed that pain was punishment as a result of wrongdoing or an expression of mental instability. There are a number of theories to explain the physiological basis of pain (Porth, 2005). The **specificity theory** asserts that pain is directly related to the degree of injury. Once a noxious stimulus has occurred, the message is carried directly to the pain centers in the brain. In 1664, Descartes first described pain as a physical experience using the example of the automatic withdrawal of the injured foot from the fire that burned it (Melzack & Wall, 1983). The **pattern theory** is a group of theories which assert that pain receptors share nerve pathways with other sensory pathways and that the intensity of the stimulus determines the frequency of firing of the receptor (Porth, 2005). Light touch would produce low-frequency firing, whereas intense or painful pressure would produce high-frequency firing of the same receptor, signaling pain. These theories do not account for emotional or learned responses to pain.

The **gate control theory** proposes that the spinal cord has a gating mechanism that either permits or inhibits the transmission of pain information to the brain. The pain is modulated at the substantia gelatinosa in the dorsal horn where there are "gates" that either inhibit or transmit noxious stimuli. Messages are transmitted via either small, nociceptive neurons or by large nonnociceptive neurons. The large neurons transmit nonnoxious stimuli such as massage or electrical stimulation, whereas the small nociceptive neurons transmit painful stimuli. The large nonnociceptive transmissions can inhibit the small transmissions, thereby interrupting the pain transmission. For example, when sudden pain occurs due to a fall, if the area is briskly rubbed the pain diminishes.

The more recent **neuromatrix theory** addresses the brain's role in pain perception as well as other determinants (Melzack, 1999; Porth, 2005). This theory proposes that the brain contains a widely distributed neural network referred to as the *body-self neuromatrix*. This matrix contains somatosensory, limbic, and thalamocortical components whose synaptic architecture is determined by genetics and sensory influences. An individual's matrix integrates multiple sources of input, which results in a multifaceted pain response. This theory is used to explain chronic pain or phantom limb pain where there is no direct relationship. **Phantom limb pain** is felt in the amputated part of the body as a result of the brain misinterpreting the nerve signals as coming from the site of the amputation (Merck, 2007). This theory also helps to explain the highly variable individual perception of painful stimuli (Porth, 2005).

◼ Pain as a Multidimensional Phenomenon

The currently accepted definition of pain and the evolving pain theories of the 20th century all support the rationale that pain is much more than the physical response to tissue damage. Pain is multidimensional and includes the patient's emotions, behaviors, and functionality both physically and mentally in response to the pain. Just as a singular description of pain is not accurate, consideration of all of the dimensions of pain is necessary to fully appreciate the individuality and complexity of the experience of pain. The multiple dimensions of pain discussed in the following subsections are physiological, sensory, affective, cognitive, and behavioral.

Physiological Dimension

Both the peripheral and central nervous systems are involved in processing the perception of pain. The origin of pain can be either nociceptive (tissue) or neuropathic (nerves). Three pathways transmit nociceptive painful stimuli: first-order, second-order, and third-order neurons. First-order neurons, or nociceptors, are nerve endings found in the skin, dental pulp, periosteum, meninges, and some internal organs that exclusively respond to chemical, thermal, and mechanical noxious stimuli. **Nociception**, which means "pain sense," is the process by which **noxious stimuli** (tissue damage) activate sensory neurons to send the message to the CNS, resulting in a **nociceptive pain** response (Porth, 2005).

Nociceptors branch from the skin, sending fibers to local blood vessels, mast cells, hair follicles, and sweat glands. The transmission of pain from these peripheral fibers to the CNS is referred to as **transduction**. Transmission of pain impulses occurs via two types of nerve fibers, fast-conducting A-delta fibers and slower conducting C-fibers. Localized sharp pain is conducted by A-delta fibers, and dull, aching pain is conducted by C-fibers. When noxious stimuli stimulate the nociceptors, histamine is released from the mast cells, causing vasodilation at the injury site. Nociceptors transfer the noxious stimuli into electrical activity, known as action potentials. Once nociception is initiated, the action potentials are transmitted through the peripheral nervous system to the internal organs and the spinal cord (Porth, 2005; Wittbrodt & Tietze, 2004). These action potentials are transmitted via the sensory neurons and converge onto common second-order neurons in the dorsal horn of the spinal cord, where they are processed (Porth, 2005).

The substantia gelatinosa in the dorsal horn is the major site for pain modulation, an individual's perception of the experience.

From the dorsal horn, pain messages are transmitted through the third-order neurons to the thalamus and cerebral cortex where pain is integrated and modulated. The ascending tracts send information about the quality, intensity, and the affective meaning of pain, and will activate the descending pathways. **Endorphins** and **enkephalins** are endogenous morphine-like substances that reduce or suppress the pain perception in the descending pathways. These descending spinal pathways conduct inhibitory impulses by releasing serotonin, norepinephrine, and endorphins, which reduce nociceptive transmission in the CNS. This process modulates the pain, making it highly personal and individualized (Porth, 2005). Response to pain is dependent on past experience with pain, the concept of the cause of the pain, learned cultural responses, fear, anxiety, age, and individual beliefs.

The second type of pain, neuropathic pain, occurs when there is direct damage to the nerves (Porth, 2005). **Neuropathic pain** is a result of injury or dysfunction in the peripheral nervous system and can progress to the CNS, altering its function and resulting in a chronic painful disease (Backonja, 2001; NINDS, 2007a). Instead of loss of sensation, as would be expected with nerve damage, some injuries are associated with abnormal pain. Normal stimuli such as light pressure may result in significant pain, and normal noxious stimulation such as bumping the affected area produces a supernormal pain response. Traumatic nerve injury, certain diseases (especially shingles and diabetes), and certain toxins (anticancer medications) can cause these painful neuropathies.

The type of injury or disease dictates the origin of the pain. Pain that originates in the skin and subcutaneous tissue is referred to as *superficial*, whereas pain from muscles and bones is *somatic* and pain originating in the organs is *visceral*. Somatic pain is typically described as dull or sharp, and aching, and is most commonly caused by a cut, heat such as a burn injury, ischemia, and bone displacement. Visceral pain typically is described as dull or sharp, aching, and cramping and is caused by distention, ischemia, spasms, and chemical irritants such as medications or spicy food.

Physiological and Pathological Consequences of Unrelieved Pain

Undertreated pain can produce serious adverse physiological, psychological, and immunological effects. Inadequate pain control can stimulate a stress response that involves the cardiovascular, pulmonary, gastrointestinal, metabolic, and neuroendocrine systems (Pasero et al., 1999; Rothley & Therrien, 2002). Pain causes catabolism, which leads to poor wound healing, weakness, and muscle breakdown. Increased heart rate and blood pressure increases the risk of thromboembolic events due to stress hormone effects and decreased mobility. Chapter 12 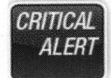 describes the relationship of the stress response and pain. Effective respiratory effort is impaired, increasing the risk of infection and hypoxemia. Pain increases salt and water retention, resulting in fluid overload and hypokalemia. Pain also causes decreased gastrointestinal motility and increased blood pressure. Anxiety, depression, and sleep deprivation are commonly associated with pain. Immunologically, pain is associated with reduced natural killer cell counts indicating impaired immune response (APS, 2003; Pasero et al., 1999). Increasing evidence suggests that un-dertreated acute pain may predispose patients to chronic pain syndromes due to neuronal plasticity (APS, 2003).

Sensory Dimension

The **sensory dimension of pain** includes consideration of the location, intensity, quality, and temporal patterns. An understanding of these factors will influence the diagnosis and ultimately the treatment. Many patients will experience more than one location of pain, and each location may be associated with a different intensity, quality, and pattern. Neuropathic pain, for example, is generally located along the anatomic distribution of the nerve or where the spinal cord is affected. Nociceptive pain may be localized to the injury and the immediate surrounding area. Pain intensity may be described in a variety of ways. Patients can be instructed to use numbers from a scale, select a drawing of a face that best illustrates their pain, or select descriptive words such as *mild* or *severe* (Chart 15–3). If encouraged to describe the quality of their pain, most patients can provide a fairly graphic description using one or two words without coaching. The temporal pattern of pain is generally described in terms of the onset and duration using terms such as *constant* or *steady*, *intermittent*, and *episodic*.

Affective Dimension

The **affective dimension of pain** describes the emotions patients assign to their pain. Patients' emotions can impact the experience of pain both positively and negatively. Postoperative pain for a patient recovering from surgery to remove a mass that was found to be benign would possibly assign different emotions to their pain than another patient would whose tumor was found to be malignant. In addition to the patient's own emotions related to her pain, the emotions and support of friends and family will impact the pain experience. Feeling loved and supported by those who are meaningful in the patient's life can reduce the intensity of pain (Price, Riley, & Wade, 2001). Conversely, patients who do not have a good support system will report greater discomfort. Nurses have long noted that fear, frustration, anger, stress, and anxiety are all associated with increased pain intensity. Descriptive words such as *unbearable*, *punishing*, and *terrifying* convey a different meaning than do *annoying*, *tiring*, and *exhausting*. When negative emotions overwhelm the patient, the term *suffering* is used to describe the unpleasant physical and emotional components of pain. Suffering is hallmarked by feelings of uncontrollability, hopelessness, helplessness, and intolerability that undermine the patient's self-identity and integrity (Turk & Okifuji, 2001).

CRITICAL ALERT *Evaluation of the affective dimension of pain requires the nurse to be attentive to the verbal and nonverbal cues that indicate that the patient's emotions may be negatively impacting his pain.*

Cognitive and Cultural Dimensions

The **cognitive dimension of pain** includes the impact of personal beliefs, attitudes, and meanings attached to pain. Factors such as self-efficacy, self-control, and the locus of control can be beneficial or negative in the experience of pain. Patients who have a history of psychological problems generally report pain

CHART 15–3 Unidimensional Pain Intensity Measurement Tools

Numeric Pain Rating Scale (NRS)

0	1	2	3	4	5	6	7	8	9	10

No Pain   Moderate Pain   Worst Pain

Visual Analog Scale (VAS)

No Pain   Pain as bad as it
                                                                could possibly be

Simple Verbal Descriptive Scale (SVDS)

No pain (None)	Mild pain (Mild)	Moderate pain (Discomforting)	Severe pain (Distressing)	Very severe (Horrible)	Worst possible (Excruciating)

that is out of proportion to their physical disability and are prone to a greater degree of disability and depression when pain is chronic (Merck, 2007). Successful treatment of chronic pain often includes assisting the patient to convert unrealistic expectations into willingness to acknowledge and then accept pain as a part of his life. Acceptance enhances the patient's ability to cope and results in improved outcomes and satisfaction with the quality of life (Arnstein, Wells-Federman, & Caudill-Slosberg, 2002). Patients need to be encouraged to develop cognitive control by reducing their focus on pain-related thoughts and shifting to acceptance that meaningful life is possible despite pain. The Cultural Considerations box discusses how spiritual beliefs and culture affect patients' cognitive responses to pain.

Behavioral Dimension

The **behavioral dimension of pain** includes responses to pain that may be situational, developmental, or learned. Behaviors commonly associated with the expression of pain are both verbal and nonverbal. Grimacing or furrowed brow, guarding, agitation, and avoiding required activities are examples of nonverbal expressions of pain. Verbal expressions of pain include crying, moaning, and verbalization. It is appropriate to expect a patient to demonstrate anxiety in situations that are not familiar to him such as treatment in an emergency depart-

CULTURAL CONSIDERATIONS Related to Patient Responses to Pain

Spiritual beliefs, culture, and family affect patients' cognitive responses to pain. A child learns from an early age how to respond to and express pain from observation of her family members. Acceptable responses vary among different cultures. Some cultures believe pain is a punishment for wrongdoing, whereas others feel it is a direct result of a past or future event. Spiritual rituals such as prayer may play an important comforting role in some cultures, whereas other cultures use food rituals to restore balance in the body. Patients may be stoic, remaining silent about their pain, or they may be verbally expressive and prone to pain behaviors such as moaning or crying. In some cultures the patient may remain silent while the head of the family speaks for the patient. Each of these situations and responses plays an important role in the individual's cognitive responses to pain.

ment or hospitalization. Patients who have developmental delays will demonstrate behaviors consistent with the situation and their developmental age. When pain is well controlled, pain behaviors alleviate or resolve and patients appear relaxed, calmer, and are able to participate in daily activities. Participation in required activities of recovery is facilitated.

Failure to respond to a patient's self-report of pain may encourage the development of learned pain behaviors. Patients who come to understand that unless they appear to be uncomfortable their reports of pain will not be believed may purposefully demonstrate behaviors consistent with pain when clinicians are present (McCaffery & Pasero, 1999).

Pain Measurement and Assessment

Failure to measure and assess pain has long been recognized as a barrier to appropriate pain management. It is essential for nurses and all health care team members to understand the significance of assessing and providing effective pain management. To emphasize this point, the American Pain Society launched a campaign in the late 1990s to increase awareness of the importance of the assessment of pain intensity. The statement "Pain is the fifth vital sign" was designed to encourage health care providers and organizations to consider the assessment of pain just as essential as the assessment of the patient's temperature, pulse, blood pressure, and respiratory rate. Pain assessment should be incorporated into routine vital sign assessments (Campbell, 1995).

Not only is it important to regularly assess pain, it is important to assess it correctly and thoroughly to create a pain management plan tailored to meet the individual needs of the patient. Those needs must be based on a unidimensional measurement of pain intensity in addition to the complete assessment of the multidimensional experience of pain.

Assessment and measurement tools have evolved during the past decade such that multiple tools are now available to meet the specific needs of patients with different disease states, ages and developmental stages, and cognitive abilities. Depending on the patient's needs, any one of the tools may be appropriate in a given situation. Regardless of the tool selected, patients should be educated in its use, and the same tool should be used consistently to encourage accurate trending of changes, to facilitate familiarity with the tool, and to ultimately increase the ease of use. Because these tools rely on the patient's ability to understand how to use them properly, patients who speak a language other than that of the health care team should be provided a tool with numbers and descriptors written in their own language to prevent misunderstandings due to language barriers. Whether patients have unique needs or not, assessment tools should always be validated by research and found reliable in the patient population where they will be used. Additionally, tools that are easy for the nurse and the patient to use and document will be more likely to be used routinely.

At times, nurses express frustration over the inability to verify the accuracy of the patient's self-report of pain intensity. Although most patients with pain will not attempt to lie or deceive, some patients will. Regardless, clinicians are required to accept the patient's report of pain (APS, 2003). However, accepting does not require believing. When there is doubt regarding the truthfulness of a patient's response, it is important to recognize that potential of accepting a false report of pain, and responding to that report with an appropriate intervention is justified by the importance of accepting the many reports of pain that are valid and truthful (Pasero & McCaffery, 2001b). Nurses must value the fact that the patient is the only one who

can identify the intensity of pain. Examples of unidimensional tools used to measure pain intensity include the numeric rating scale, the simple verbal descriptive scale, and the visual analog scale (see Chart 15–3, p. 337).

Unidimensional Measurement Tools

Unidimensional measurement tools are used to measure only one component of the pain assessment. The unidimensional measurement of pain is an incomplete assessment if the remaining multidimensional aspects of pain are not evaluated. In most cases, unidimensional tools are used to determine the patient's self-report of the intensity or severity of pain.

Numeric Rating Scale

The **numeric rating scale (NRS)** is a horizontal line with numbers from 0 to 10 ranging from left to right (see Chart 15–3, p. 337). Three interval descriptors of pain are located along the scale: "No Pain," "Moderate Pain," and "Worst Pain." Once a patient is instructed on how to use the scale, it is relatively easy to use and assessment can be completed within a few minutes, making it easy for the both the patient and the clinician to use, document, and trend.

Simple Verbal Descriptive Scale

The **simple verbal descriptive scale (SVDS)** also uses a horizontal line with numbers 0 to 10 ranging from left to right. However, interval descriptors of "No Pain," "Mild," "Discomforting," "Distressing," "Horrible," or "Excruciating" pain provide the patient with a few more descriptive options. As with the NRS, this scale is relatively quick and easy for both the patient and the clinician to use.

Visual Analog Scale

The **visual analog scale (VAS)** does not have numeric intervals; rather it uses "No Pain" and "Pain as Bad as It Can Possibly Be" as descriptors at either end of a horizontal line measuring 10 centimeters in length. Each centimeter on the scale corresponds to a number from 0 to 10. The patient is instructed to draw a vertical line through the scale to indicate the intensity of their pain. Although this scale is relatively easy for the patient to use, it requires measurement from the start of the scale to the point where the vertical line is drawn to determine the 0 to 10 score. This makes the scale less useful to a busy clinician.

Behavioral Assessment

When patients are unable to provide a self-report of pain intensity, behavioral assessment tools can be used to guide observation for pain-related behaviors. This type of unidimensional tool, often validated for use with preverbal pediatric patients, should be used with caution in adults since pain-related behaviors may be inconsistent (either over- or underemphasized) with actual pain. With the behavioral assessment, the nurse must make an observational judgment that may lead to undermanagement of pain (AHCPR, 1992; APS, 2003).

Patients who are critically ill represent a large population of nonverbal patients. This puts this population at considerable risk for unrelieved pain. One of the primary reasons for inadequate pain relief is the lack of an appropriate pain relief assessment for nonverbal patients (Puntillo, 2007). Nursing researchers are currently studying ways to measure pain in this population (Gelinas, Fortier, Viens, Fillion, & Puntillo, 2004; Puntillo et al., 2004). Pain behaviors in the acutely/critically ill population noted during common painful procedures such as dressing changes included grimacing, rigidity, wincing, shutting of eyes, moaning, verbalization, and clenching of fists.

To date no valid standardized assessment tool exists for use in all populations of critically ill patients. A Critical-Care Pain Observation Tool (CPOT) has been researched and validated in cardiac patients who are critically ill, and it is hoped that this tool and other tools can be further validated in other critically ill populations in the future (Gelinas, Fillion, Puntillo, Viens, & Fortier, 2006). For now, though, nurses need to be aware of the common manifestations of pain in this population in order to assess a patient's specific response. Pasero & McCaffery (2005) recommend the following guidelines for individual nonverbal patient assessment:

- On admission, document reason self-report cannot be used for pain assessment.
- Document underlying conditions, such as chronic pain condition or trauma, as well as any painful activities such as physical therapy and turning.
- Look for individual behaviors that indicate pain.
- Ask caregivers, family, and significant others about behaviors that indicate pain.
- Draw a conclusion about the patient's pain based on the preceding information.
- Devise a pain management plan.
- Initiate an analgesic trial.
- Evaluate response to analgesics.
- Make appropriate adjustments.

Multidimensional Assessment and Measurement Tools

Multidimensional assessment and measurement tools such as the patient interview, the **McGill Pain Questionnaire (MPQ)**, and the **Brief Pain Inventory (BPI)** assess more than one dimension of pain. The MPQ provides 20 sets of words patients can use to describe pain, and scores the responses. Each set of words varies in intensity and measures either the sensory or affective dimension of pain. One set scores the intensity of pain. Patients document the location of pain on a body diagram provided as part of the questionnaire.

The BPI asks multiple questions regarding pain and its impact on patient function and addresses the multidimensionality of the pain experience. Depending on the situation, these tools have advantages and disadvantages that may make them more useful or inappropriate. Most of these tools require the patient to have the cognitive ability to complete the tool, not to mention the time. These two requirements make some of the tools difficult for both the patient and busy nurses to use routinely. However, when pain management is complex, the time spent completing a multidimensional tool can be invaluable.

Patient Interview

The patient interview is the most commonly used multidimensional tool in nursing practice. A unidimensional tool is usually used in addition to the interview questions to determine pain intensity. However, the patient interview can also be combined with any multidimensional tool when appropriate. Prior to conducting an interview, the nurse should review the patient's medical history. Components of the patient's history that are specifically useful in the assessment of pain include:

- Previous experiences with pain including trauma, surgery, or chronic pain
- Medications taken previously or currently to relieve pain
- Significant social history including drug, alcohol, or tobacco abuse
- Comorbid conditions, such as renal insufficiency, pulmonary disease, or hepatic dysfunction, that should be considered when administering analgesics.

During the patient interview, the nurse's demeanor should be supportive and interested. Allow sufficient time for the patient to answer the questions. Patients experiencing moderate to severe pain may have difficulty answering questions. Every effort should be made to make the patient as comfortable as possible before the interview takes place. Interview questions may include the following:

- Where are you having pain?
- Are you having pain anywhere else?
- How intense is the pain?
- What does the pain feel like?
- When did the pain begin?
- How long does the pain last?
- What makes the pain worse?
- Have you had this type of pain before?
- How does your pain affect your daily activities, sleep, mood, and relationships?
- What do you do to reduce the pain?

When asking questions that require the use of an assessment tool, the nurse should first assess the patient's ability to use and understand the tool. Once an appropriate tool has been selected, all members of the health care team should use that same tool consistently to improve the patient's ability to provide self-reports of the details concerning her pain experience.

Location of Pain

Patients may have pain in more than one location due to radiation of the pain, metastases of carcinoma, or multiple injuries, as is often the case with traumatic injuries. Each location of pain may have different characteristics. Unless encouraged to discuss all locations, the patient may not offer this information.

Assist the patient to identify each location of pain. The nurse should then ask all of the interview questions about each location. This will encourage patients to identify sources of pain that may be impacting their level of comfort, but that may be unrelated to the reason they are seeking medical assistance. Locations of pain can be reported verbally or by using a pain assessment tool such as the MPQ as described earlier.

Duration and Pattern of Pain

Pain can be persistent or intermittent. It can occur in a sudden flare of breakthrough pain that resolves quickly, or it may flare and linger, resolving after a period of time, as is the case with recurrent pain. Analgesic medication formulations are becoming more sophisticated and are designed to address the specific durations and patterns of pain. Complementary or alternative treatments may be better suited to relieving pain that is mild in intensity and short in duration. An appropriate treatment plan requires that a thorough assessment of the duration and pattern of the pain be elicited. The nurse can help the patient provide this information by asking the following questions:

- Do you have pain for most of the day and night?
- Does the pain come and go or is it constant?
- Do you have sudden episodes of severe pain that occur without warning or that happen with certain activities?

Pain Intensity

The patient should be instructed in the use of the pain intensity tool. The tool that is used in the assessment should be one that the patient understands and can easily use. The intensity of pain is not generally static regardless of whether the pain is acute or chronic, so a score should be obtained for the least intense pain (usually at rest), the most intense pain (usually with activity), and with sudden flares of breakthrough pain. The nurse can elicit this information with the following questions:

- What is your pain score when you are having the least amount of pain?
- What is your pain score when you are having the most pain?
- Do you have sudden episodes of moderate to severe pain?
- If so, what is your pain score during these episodes?

This level of detail discourages patients from averaging their pain intensity scores to achieve one score that will not provide the information necessary to individualize the treatment plan. More aggressive treatment should be provided during times when pain is the most intense and in anticipation of breakthrough pain episodes. The assessment and reassessment of pain intensity needs to be documented before and after pain interventions to evaluate the effectiveness of pain treatments and to provide trends that will direct adjustments to the pain treatment plan.

Character of Pain

The character of the pain provides clues as to the source of the pain and may indicate which analgesic medication should be used to provide relief. When asked to describe their pain, patients generally use similar terms such as *aching, dull, sharp, stabbing, knife-like, electrical, shooting,* and *burning.* Neuropathic pain is often described as *tingling, shooting, electric,* or *shock-like* and requires different treatments than nociceptive pain, which may be reported as *sharp, stabbing, cutting,* or *throbbing.* As mentioned, the character of the pain may give a clue to its cause. For example, the pain of angina is rarely described as sharp; instead it is described as crushing, pressure, like "an elephant is sitting on my chest." Therefore, if a patient complains of sharp chest pain, the nurse knows to assess for causes other than cardiac ischemia.

Occasionally patients have difficulty describing their pain. They may say "It just hurts." If patients are reluctant to report the characteristic of their pain, the nurse should explain the importance of this information in selecting the medications to be used to treat the pain. For example, incisional pain, cardiac-related chest pain, and neuropathic pain are different in etiology and in treatment. Patients who understand that only *they* can provide this information and that it will be used when determining their treatment are often more willing to try to provide a description of their pain. Provide a few descriptors to give the patient an example of what is needed: Is it sharp, stabbing, burning, sharp-shooting, tight, or pressure pain? Be sure to select a variety of descriptors so that patients can choose one that best represents their pain or can think of one of their own.

Exacerbation of Pain

Assist the patient to identify circumstances when the pain is more intense. Common recovery activities after surgery such as getting in and out of bed, coughing, and walking in the halls may be mentioned. Patients with chronic pain may experience exacerbation of pain with activities of daily living (ADLs). The nurse may help the patient provide information about exacerbation of pain by asking the following questions:

- What do you do that makes your pain more intense?
- What do your doctors and nurses do to you that increases your pain?

When it is known that specific activities or procedures exacerbate pain, the nurse should provide pain treatments prior to the painful event to facilitate the ability to do ADLs, participate in physical therapy, and tolerate medical procedures. If the exacerbation of pain is associated with new pain of a different intensity, location, or character, it may indicate that there is a complication such as infection, that disease is progressing, or that there is a surgical complication. Sudden onset of new pain should be considered an emergency, evaluated, and reported to the health care provider or independent licensed practitioner.

Pain Relief

Encourage the patient to report all nonmedication and medication methods they currently or previously used to relieve the pain. The pain treatment plan should include the patient's preferred methods and medications, whenever it is appropriate. This is especially true when the patient has chronic pain and has a well-established pain management plan that has been effective in relieving their pain. It is important to be specific when questioning the patient to ensure that information about prescription and nonprescription medications is elicited. In addition, the patient should be asked specifically about herbal or dietary supplements so that potential medication interactions can be identified. Sensitive subjects such as abuse of alcohol, prescription medications, or illicit drugs should be approached after developing a rapport with the patient; thus, questions about medications are usually saved until the end of the interview. The nurse should use a nonjudgmental and direct approach and reassure the patient and family that the information they provide will be considered when selecting medications and dosages for the pain treatment plan. The following are examples of questions that can be used to encourage the patient to discuss these sensitive subjects:

- Do you take any pain medications that you can buy without a prescription (e.g., acetaminophen, nonsteroidal anti-inflammatory drugs [NSAIDS])?

- Do you take any pain medications that you buy from the pharmacy with a prescription?

- Do you take any herbal or dietary supplements to relieve your pain?

- Do you drink alcohol daily, weekly, monthly? Do you ever take your pain medications when you are drinking alcohol?

- Have you ever or are you now taking illegal drugs to relieve your pain?

- Have you ever been involved in a drug treatment or methadone program?

- Do you have any concerns regarding addiction?

Impact on Quality of Life and Function

During the interview, observation of the patient and attention to the patient's responses provide information regarding the affective, cognitive, and behavioral dimensions of pain. Observe for expressions of hope or optimism that the pain can be relieved as opposed to hopelessness, helplessness, or even expression of suicidal ideations. Patients may be calm and cooperative or angry, frustrated, anxious, and focused on placing blame. Be watchful for information to be gained from the responses of family members regarding the impact of pain in their personal relationships and the patient's quality of life. Use interviewing techniques such as open-ended questions to encourage the patient and family members to share details about pain and the role it plays in their lives. Patients and family members are observant of the general demeanor of the interviewer and will respond based on the perception that the interviewer is caring and concerned and has time to listen or that time is limited and questions are asked for the purpose of documentation rather than for use in determining a plan for care.

Multidimensional Assessment of At-Risk Patients

Factors such as developmental delays, cognitive impairment, severe emotional disturbance, and critical illness may render patients incapable of providing an accurate report of pain intensity and preclude participation in the patient interview (Puntillo, 2007). Patients who are unable to provide a self-report of pain intensity are at risk for undermanagement of pain (APS, 2003; Herr et al., 2006; Puntillo, 2007). Nurses should take care to avoid erroneously concluding that a patient cannot provide a self-report. Studies have demonstrated that patients with mild to moderate cognitive impairment are able to provide a self-report using unidimensional measurement tools and short versions of some multidimensional assessment tools (Soscia, 2003). Pasero and McCaffery (2000) suggest that five factors be considered to ensure that the patients who are at risk of poor pain management are appropriately managed and plans for pain management care reflect the individual patient's special needs. Chart 15–4 provides steps for assessing patients at risk.

Documentation of Pain Assessment

As the health care team member most likely to spend the greatest amount of time with the patient and family, nurses are pivotal in the appropriate management of pain (McCaffery, Ferrell, & Pasero, 2000). Documentation of assessment findings is a vital part of the patient's medical record. Nurse documentation is

---

CHART 15–4 | **Five Assessment Steps for At-Risk Patients**

1. Be sure that the patient is unable to self-report pain.
2. Consider pathologic conditions and procedures known to be painful.
3. Observe for behaviors consistent with pain.
4. Use a proxy pain rating from close family members or caregivers.
5. Consider physiological measures as a last resort.

Source: Pasero, C., & McCaffery, M. (2000). When patients can't report pain. *American Journal of Nursing, 100,* 22–23.

reviewed by many members of the multidisciplinary team and provides detail that team members may not have had an opportunity to elicit. It is important that details about the pain assessment, treatments, and the patient's response to treatments are accurately and completely documented on the medical record so that decisions regarding the plan of care are made with consideration of the information the nurse has compiled.

Whether recorded on a paper flow sheet, in an electronic medical record (EMR), or written in narrative, the nurse's documentation of pain assessment and measurement creates a baseline by which improvement or negative trends are measured (Campbell, 2006). The Joint Commission standards on pain management require that health care organizations have policies regarding the assessment and management of pain. The nurse must know and understand the contents of policies specific to their workplace, and the nursing documentation should reflect that nursing care was given according to institutional policy.

 *Nursing documentation in the legal medical record should reflect topics such as these:*

1. *Pain management that was delivered following institutional policy, with consideration of the patient assessment and responses to treatments, and utilizing ordered interventions*
2. *Responses to unrelieved pain, including administration of additional analgesic medications; use of nonmedication treatments; and health care provider or licensed independent practitioner contact and subsequent changes to the patient's pain management plan of care*
3. *The avoidance of labels such as psychotic, whiner, drug seeking, or addict.*

◼ Pain Management

In 1992, the Agency for Health Care Policy and Research (AHCPR) published the first edition of the *Clinical Practice Guideline for Acute Pain Management: Operative or Medical Procedures and Trauma.* A panel of experts completed an exhaustive literature review to establish evidence-based guidelines, and where no evidence was available, best practices were determined (AHCPR, 1992). In 1994, AHCPR published the first edition of the *Clinical Practice Guideline for Management of Cancer Pain* using the same model and goals (Jacox et al., 1994). Nearly a decade later, pain management had not improved significantly. In response, the Joint Commission released new standards on pain management in 1999. These standards are based on the same valid recommendations published in the AHCPR guidelines of 1992 and 1994 and require health care organizations to implement a multidisciplinary team and create an institutional commitment to pain management (Joint Commission, 2002).

Rather than becoming discouraged by the lack of improvement in pain management over the years, nurses are beginning to embrace the potential for improvement by researching the knowledge of student nurses and the relationship between nurses' knowledge and patient outcomes, determining appropriate curriculum components for pain management education in nursing schools, and outlining competency guidelines (Chiu, Trinca, Lim, & Tuazon, 2003; IASP, 1993; Watt-Watson, Stevens, Garfinkel, Streiner, & Gallop, 2001; Wisconsin Cancer Pain Initiative Nursing Education Committee, 1995). However, in spite of these efforts, nursing knowledge and the reported comfort and amount of medication their patients receive continue to be at odds (Watt-Watson et al., 2001). Now is the time for nurses to take the lead professionally by demanding that comprehensive pain management education be provided during professional preparation. Nurses are necessary to the successful implementation of evidence-based pain management practices. In addition, until nurses begin to support improved competency of all health care team members, patients will continue to experience unrelieved pain in spite of the fact that pain can be relieved. Patients with pain must be able to rely on nurses to be knowledgeable regarding pain management principles and practices, professional in the application of pain-relieving treatments, and to advocate on behalf of their patients. No patient should look to the nurse as one of the reasons for his or her unrelieved pain. Management of pain at the end of life is discussed in depth in Chapter 17 🔗.

Acute Pain Management Therapeutic Goals

Acute pain is often the result of surgical procedures, trauma, or burns. Acute pain problems are the most common reason why patients seek medical assistance, and nurses spend a significant portion of their time at the bedside providing pain-relieving treatments and medications (Coda & Bonica, 2001). The plan for pain management provides for organized and rational treatment appropriate to all phases of recovery including the critical or emergent phase, subsequent healing and recovery, and finally rehabilitation.

Management of acute pain is focused on (1) reducing the sympathetic stress response, (2) safely optimizing comfort during treatment and recovery, (3) facilitating participation in recovery and rehabilitation activities, and (4) improving patient outcomes. Nurses educate patients and family members with the goal of improving their understanding of (1) the importance of pain management in the patient's recovery, (2) the role of medications and nonmedication treatment, and (3) the differences between physical dependence, tolerance, and addiction to opioid medications. Establishing comfort and function goals encourages the patient and health care team to work toward meeting a defined pain intensity score and a specific functional goal rather than an elusive or poorly defined therapeutic goal. For example, the patient with acute pain might select a pain intensity score of 3 from the 0–10 NRS and the goal of ambulating three times daily as a postoperative recovery activity.

Chronic Pain Management Therapeutic Goals

The long-term, persistent nature of chronic pain increases the likelihood that psychosocial and environmental factors will contribute to the emotional distress and physical disability that is frequently seen with pain that has limited ongoing pathology. Management of chronic pain is focused on (1) reducing the focus on pain; (2) safely optimizing comfort through appropriate use of analgesic treatments and complementary or alternative strategies; (3) increasing active participation in ADLs, work, and relationships; and (4) restoration of joy and a sense of purpose despite persistent pain (Arnstein, 2003). Nurses educate patients and family members with the goal of improving understanding of (1) the role anxiety, depression, and anger can have in escalation of pain; (2) the role of medications and complementary or alternative treatments in improving function; and (3) the differences between physical dependence, tolerance, and addiction to opioid medications.

When encouraging the patient with chronic pain to establish comfort and function goals, the process is the same as with acute pain, but the scores and functional goals are likely to be very different. Patients who experience moderate to severe pain on a daily basis may consider even a very small reduction in pain intensity as a success. Often functional goals are focused around achieving or maintaining independence in ADLs, work, or relationships and leisure activities. It may be necessary to encourage the patient to identify realistically achievable goals as an intermediate step to his ultimate goals to avoid discouragement.

Cancer Pain Management Therapeutic Goals

The management of cancer pain is a combination of the acute and chronic pain therapeutic goals mentioned previously. Given the dual nature of cancer pain, it is appropriate to have goals that address healing, recovery, and finally rehabilitation for the acute pain associated with surgery and cancer treatments. However, it is also appropriate to consider the role that a potentially lethal diagnosis has on increasing the likelihood of emotional distress and physical disability that is frequently seen with the pain of malignancy. Management of cancer pain is focused on (1) reducing the sympathetic stress response following surgeries or treatments; (2) safely optimizing comfort through appropriate use of analgesic treatments and complementary or alternative strategies; (3) facilitating participation in recovery and rehabilitation activities; (4) increasing active participation in ADLs, work, and relationships; and (5) preservation of a sense of purpose despite a potentially lethal diagnosis.

Nurses educate patients and family members with the goal of improving understanding of (1) the role that anxiety, depression, and anger can have in escalation of pain; (2) the role of medications and complementary or alternative treatments in improving function; and (3) the differences between physical dependence, tolerance, and addiction to opioid medications. When encouraging the patient with cancer pain to establish a comfort and function goal, the process is the same as with acute and chronic pain. Often functional goals are focused around achieving or maintaining independence in daily activities. As with acute and chronic pain, the comfort and function goals should guide the treatment plan. An in-depth discussion of the diagnosis and treatment of cancer is included in Chapter 64 🌐 .

Pharmacologic Strategies

In pain management pharmacology, the multidisciplinary team focus is on establishing a regimen that includes a balance of nonopioid, nonsteroidal anti-inflammatory, adjuvant, and opioid medications whenever possible to optimize the quality of analgesia with minimal medication side effects. This method of managing pain is often referred to as *balanced* or *multimodal analgesia*. The pharmacologic pain management plan is accomplished through the combined efforts of multiple disciplines. The selection of medications requires that the health care provider consider the patient's medical history, including previous and current pain, and the findings of the patient interview and pain assessment as previously discussed. Treatment plans crafted in the absence of this information are often unsuccessful in relieving pain or alternatively more likely to cause adverse effects and potentially patient harm.

Nurses are central to the effectiveness and safety of medication administration with multiple responsibilities at every stage of the prescription process. Prescriptions must be reviewed on the medical record and considered for their appropriateness based on the patient assessment and relevant laboratory studies. If there are questions regarding the prescription, the prescribing health care provider must be contacted for clarification. When it is time to administer the medication, rigorous double checks are completed to ensure the correct prescription is administered to the patient.

Pharmacologic Interventions

When discussing pharmacologic interventions, it is necessary to consider the patient's physiological status in relationship to the pharmacology of each medication that is selected including how it is absorbed, distributed, metabolized or biotransformed, and eventually excreted. In addition, the mechanism of action and therapeutic and adverse effects of each medication should guide the medication selection and monitoring that will be necessary to ensure the patient's safety.

Absorption describes the process by which the medication leaves the site of administration to cross membranes as it journeys to the site of action (Youngkin, Sawin, Kissinger, & Israel, 2005). For example, medications that are administered into the gastrointestinal system absorb from the stomach, small intestine, large intestine, colon, and even the rectum into the systemic circulation for distribution. In contrast, medications that are administered directly into the systemic circulation bypass the absorptive process and are immediately distributed (Youngkin et al., 2005).

Distribution refers to the process of moving the medication into the bloodstream, the extracellular, and the intracellular compartments, as well as in the compartment that is the site of absorption and storage (Youngkin, Sawin, Kissinger, & Israel et al., 2005). Factors that will effect the distribution of a medication are the size of the molecule, the degree to which it binds to protein, and the solubility of the medication. Large molecules and those that bind to protein usually stay in the bloodstream. Hydrophilic drugs, like morphine, are more slowly distributed

in both the bloodstream and the extracellular compartments. Lipid-soluble medications, like fentanyl, are more rapidly absorbed and distributed throughout all three compartments (Miyoshi & Leckband, 2001).

Biotransformation or **metabolism** describes the process of changing a medication's structure in preparation for elimination (Youngkin et al., 2005). Metabolism occurs primarily in the liver, but also the kidneys, and to a very small degree in other organ systems. Once a medication has metabolized, it is no longer the same and effectively discontinues its pharmacologic activity. **Hepatic first-pass metabolism** refers to the reduction of the medication's effect due to partial metabolism in the liver prior to distribution to the ultimate site of action. Medications may produce active metabolites that then exert a pharmacologic action of their own. This is of particular concern when the metabolite has significant adverse effects.

Elimination is the process of excretion from the body and is generally accomplished in the renal system (Youngkin et al., 2005). Elimination can occur after a medication has metabolized or the medication may be eliminated in its primary form. Alterations in the renal system that impair elimination result in prolonging the effects of the primary medication and any metabolites that have been formed, potentially increasing the risks of adverse effects.

Classifying Analgesics

The three-step analgesic ladder designed by the World Health Organization (WHO) outlines recommendations for classes of analgesic medications that would be appropriate for treating mild, moderate, and severe pain (Bajwa, Warfield, & Wootton, 2006; Jacox et al., 1994). Figure 15–1 ■ illustrates the WHO three-step analgesic ladder. This ladder provides a stepped approach based on pain severity. For example, step 1 analgesics include acetaminophen or an NSAID. If the pain persists or worsens despite appropriate dose increases of step 1 drugs, a change to a step 2 or step 3 analgesic is indicated. If the patient presents with moderate to severe pain, step 1 can be skipped (National Cancer Institute, 2007).

It is reasonable to choose the step that most closely describes the patient's pain intensity as a guide in determining a pain

FIGURE 15–1 ■ World Health Organization three-step analgesic ladder.

treatment plan that would provide the best level of analgesia with the fewest potential adverse effects. The steps on the analgesic ladder are additive, meaning as one progresses up the ladder, more medications are added to those already in use to achieve improved analgesia than would be possible with a single medication for a balanced or multimodal approach to pain management. It is important to recognize that when pain is severe, the appropriate step on the analgesic ladder would be at the top and movement through each step to reach the top is not necessary. This method of medication selection has been proven effective in acute, chronic, and cancer pain management. Nurses are vital to the medication administration and monitoring process and so must understand the basic mechanism of action, pharmacology, and adverse effects of each group of medications to function effectively in their role.

Acetaminophen

Acetaminophen is one of the most widely used analgesic medications and is considered a first-line analgesic for treating mild acute and chronic pain (Smith, 2003). It is the first step in the

WHO three-step approach to pain management (APS, 2003; Jacox et al., 1994; Smith, 2003). It is also included as an important medication in steps 2 and 3. The Pharmacology Summary feature includes an in-depth discussion of acetaminophen.

Nonsteroidal Anti-Inflammatory Drugs

NSAIDS effectively reduce inflammation, pain, and fever. More than 20 different NSAIDS are currently available in the United States, and they are one of the most commonly used classes of drugs in the world (Simon, 2003). At equal doses all NSAIDS are equally effective in relieving pain. However, there is an intrapatient variability in response that warrants trying a different NSAID if the desired effect is not achieved on the current NSAID at the maximum recommended dosage (APS, 2003). NSAIDS, along with acetaminophen, are the first step in the WHO analgesic ladder (see Figure 15–1 ■, p. 343) for mild to moderate pain and should be used in conjunction with acetaminophen and opioids on the second and third steps for moderate to severe pain. The Pharmacology Summary includes an in-depth discussion of NSAIDS.

PHARMACOLOGY Summary of Medications Used for Pain Relief

Medication Category	Action	Application/Indication	Nursing Responsibility
Acetaminophen			
First-line analgesic for treating mild acute and chronic pain. Available over the counter in a variety of formulations including liquid, tablets, capsules, caplets, and rectal suppository. Is found in combination with many medications such as the opioids Lortab and Percocet.	Specific action is unclear; thought to be inhibition of the third isoform of the cyclooxygenase (COX-3) pathway only found in the CNS. Absorbed rapidly from the gastrointestinal tract, and its low molecular weight permits easy penetration of the spinal tissues (Smith, 2003).	The first step in the WHO three-step analgesic ladder approach to pain management and included in steps 2 and 3 (see Figure 15–1 ■, p. 343). Used in addition to anti-inflammatory medications, opioids, and adjuvants in the analgesic treatment plan unless contraindicated.	Used with caution in patients who have been fasting for prolonged periods of time or who drink more that three alcoholic beverages per day. The Food and Drug Administration (FDA) now requires acetaminophen to be labeled with warnings for the patient who consumes alcohol on a daily basis and includes cautions for all patients to avoid exceeding eight tablets of 500 mg or a total of 4,000 mg total in 24 hours (Karch & Karch, 2003). Monitor liver function studies. Patients must be educated about potential side effects of overdose to prevent overdose and liver damage.
Nonsteroidal Anti-Inflammatory Drugs (NSAIDS)			
Aspirin Ibuprofen Naproxen Ketoprofen Advil Feldene Celebrex Indocin Motrin Relafen Toradol (only injectable NSAID)	Inhibit prostaglandin production, primarily the prostaglandin E series, via inhibition of the COX enzymes. Absorbed from the gastrointestinal tract and are, in general, highly protein bound.	First step in the WHO three-step analgesic ladder approach to pain (see Figure 15–1). Used alone for mild to moderate pain. Used in conjunction with acetaminophen and opioids on the second and third steps for moderate to severe pain. Aspirin inhibits platelet aggregation for the life of the platelet, therefore, making it useful for preventing thromboembolic events.	Assess character, duration, and intensity of pain prior to administration to determine baseline for effectiveness. Monitor for gastric pain, bleeding, and acute renal failure. Monitor BUN, ALT, AST, creatinine, and hemoglobin before and during continued use. Should be discontinued for several days to 1–2 weeks, if taking aspirin, before surgery or invasive procedures to reduce the risk of bleeding. When using NSAIDS in combination with opioids, frequently the dose of the opioid can be reduced (Bajwa et al., 2006).

PHARMACOLOGY Summary of Medications Used for Pain Relief—*Continued*

Medication Category	Action	Application/Indication	Nursing Responsibility
Opioids			
Codeine Dihydrocodeine Hydrocodone Propoxyphene Oxycodone Morphine Methadone Levorphanol Fentanyl Hydromorphone Meperidine	A natural or synthetic morphine-like substance. Produce their pharmacologic effects and side effects by binding to opioid receptor cells throughout the CNS and peripheral tissues. There are three types of opioid receptors: mu, kappa, and delta. When the mu receptor is stimulated, analgesia, euphoria, reduced gastric motility, sedation, nausea, tolerance, and physical dependence occur.	Third step in the WHO three-step analgesic ladder (see Figure 15–1 ■, p. 343). Symptomatic control of moderate to severe pain and as preanesthetic medication.	Assess character, duration, and intensity of pain prior to administration to determine baseline for effectiveness. Monitor vital signs before and during treatment. Do not administer opioids if the respiratory rate is less than 12 per minute. Monitor level of consciousness and respiratory rate and depth after administration. Obtain allergy history and current and prior drug use. Monitor liver function tests. Document bowel movements. Administer antihistamines (pruritus) and antiemetics (nausea) as ordered. Have a narcotic antagonist (Narcan) readily available if respirations fall below 10 per minute. Monitor urinary output for urinary retention.
Anticonvulsants			
Gabapentin Carbamazepine Phenytoin Diazepam	Limits aberrant nerve firing, leading to neural membrane stabilization.	Neuropathic pain syndrome that is shooting or electrical in nature.	Assess character, duration, and intensity of pain prior to administration to determine baseline for effectiveness. Assess for alteration in vision, concentration, and coordination.
Antidepressants			
Elavil Asendin Tofranil Pamelor Venlafaxine Trazodone Doxepin Amitriptyline Imipramine Venlafaxine	Precise mechanism of analgesic effect unknown. Thought to inhibit the reuptake of serotonin and norepinephrine involved in the descending inhibitory pain pathway. Enhanced endorphin secretion, sodium channel blockade inhibition of substance P, a neuropeptide involved in both pain and depression. Doses for pain relief are lower than doses for depression.	Chronic pain, cancer pain, fibromyalgia, tension migraine headaches, postherpetic neuralgia, diabetic neuropathy, arthritis, low back pain. Most effective in treating burning neuropathic pain.	Assess character, duration, and intensity of pain prior to administration to determine baseline for effectiveness. Monitor for nausea and dry mouth. Gum will help with the dry mouth. Patient education includes time of onset (tricyclics take several weeks to achieve therapeutic effect). Monitor patient for oversedation and insomnia. Educate patient not to discontinue use abruptly. Monitor for orthostatic hypotension. Instruct patient not to rise suddenly from a lying position.
Glucocorticoids			
	Exert anti-inflammatory properties through inhibiting leukotriene and prostaglandin synthesis.	Nerve compression pain, chronic pain.	Assess character, duration, and intensity of pain prior to administration to determine baseline for effectiveness. Due to the impact on certain conditions, prior to therapy the patient needs to be assessed for infection, osteoporosis, diabetes, heart failure, hypertension, and renal disease. Instruct patient to take medication with food and water to prevent gastric irritation. Do not discontinue drug abruptly; therapy needs to be tapered off.

Sources: Adams, M. P., Josephson, D. L., & Holland, L. N. (2005). *Pharmacology for nurses: A pathophysiological approach.* Upper Saddle River, NJ: Pearson Prentice Hall; American Pain Society (APS). (2003). *Principles of analgesic use in the treatment of acute pain and cancer pain* (5th ed.). Glenview, IL: Author; Chandrasekharan, N., Dai, H., Roos, K., Evanson, N., Tomsik, J., Elton, T., et al. (2002). Cox-3, a cyclooxygenase-1 variant inhibited by acetaminophen and other analgesic/antipyretic drugs: Cloning, structure, and expression. *Proceedings of the National Academy of Sciences, 99,* 13926–13931; MacDonald, T., & Wei, L. (2003). Effect of ibuprofen on cardioprotective effect of aspirin. *Lancet, 36,* 542–544; McCaffery, M., & Portenoy, R. K. (1999). Nonopioids. In M. McCaffery & C. Pasero (Eds.), *Pain: Clinical manual* (2nd ed., pp. 129–160). St. Louis, MO: Mosby; Simon, L. S. (2003). Nonsteroidal anti-inflammatory drugs and cyclooxygenase-2 selective inhibitors. In H. S. Smith (Ed.), *Drugs for pain* (pp. 41–54). Philadelphia: Hanley & Belfus; Youngkin, E. Q., Sawin, K. J., Kissinger, J. F., & Israel, D. S. (2005). *Pharmacotherapeutics: A primary care guide* (2nd ed.). Upper Saddle River, NJ: Pearson Prentice Hall.

Opioids

Opioids have long been recognized for their role in relieving pain (Bajwa et al., 2006). The earliest accounts of opioid use date back to the ancient Mesopotamia in Asia Minor in 3500 B.C., where opium was referred to as the *hul gil* or the *joy plant* (Maher & Chaiyakul, 2003). In 1806, Serturner, a German pharmacist, first isolated morphine from the opium extract and named it *morphine* after the god of dreams, Morpheus (Maher & Chaiyakul, 2003). Opioids, morphine-like medications, play a major role in current-day management of moderate to severe pain for acute, cancer, and in certain situations chronic pain. As with all of the analgesic medications, opioids should only be initiated after an assessment of the patient's pain in conjunction with the significant findings of the medical history and physical exam (APS, 2003).

Opioids should be added to nonopioids, NSAIDS, and adjuvants for pain that is not responsive to these analgesics alone (APS, 2003). Unlike acetaminophen and NSAIDS, opioids do not have a ceiling effect and unless combined with acetaminophen or an NSAID (e.g., Lortab, Percocet, Vicoprofen), an opioid dosage can be escalated as needed to relieve pain. The analgesia achieved by opioid administration is dose dependant and with the appropriate dosing, opioids can usually relieve all intensities of pain (Miyoshi & Leckband, 2001). There is, however, a wide variation in the dosages required by individual patients to achieve pain relief. It is unrealistic to expect the same dose of opioid to be safe and effective for all patients. Opioid dosages should be increased or decreased incrementally to achieve the best level of pain relief with the lowest incidence of opioid-induced side effects.

Major barriers to the effective use of opioid medications are usually centered on misunderstandings regarding tolerance and physical dependence and on unfounded concerns that addiction is inevitable. Opioids require a prescription and are regulated by the Drug Enforcement Administration (DEA) to reduce the risk of abuse and diversion. The challenge of finding a balance between this risk and the need for appropriate management of pain with opioids is an additional barrier. It is of concern that the most significant barriers to effective pain relief using opioid analgesics are not complicated pharmacology or lack of good medications, but bias, regulatory scrutiny, and lack of education (Miyoshi & Leckband, 2001). Discussion of opioid tolerance, physical dependence, addiction, and pseudoaddiction is provided in Chart 15–5.

MyNursingKit | American Academy of Pain Management

MyNursingKit | American Society of Addiction Medicine

CHART 15–5   **Opioid Tolerance, Dependence, and Addiction**

One of the most significant barriers to pain management is the concern that opioid analgesics will cause addiction. *Opiophobia* (Morgan, 1985) is the term that is frequently used to describe the fears that health care providers and patients share: that exposure to opioids will cause addictive disease.

When nurses have insufficient knowledge of the risks and realities of addictive disease, unethical clinical practices such as withholding opioids, administering subtherapeutic dosages when therapeutic dosages are prescribed, administering placebos, and withholding compassionate nursing care may become the hallmark of their professional practice. Nurses play a pivotal role in pain management and are recognized as patient advocates whose professional practice should be based on scientific understanding of addictive disease. They must recognize the important role of opioid therapy in pain management and develop the skills necessary to appropriately provide nursing care and education to patients who have fears regarding opioids, who are recovering from opioid addiction, or who have active addictive disease.

Confusion regarding opioid tolerance, physical dependence, and addiction is common. Defining these conditions and then using these definitions consistently in professional and well as patient interactions is the first step.

- *Tolerance* is "a state of adaptation in which exposure to a drug induces changes that result in a diminution of one or more of the drug's effects over time" (American Academy of Pain Medicine [AAPM], American Pain Society [APS], & American Society of Addiction Medicine [ASAM], (2001).

- *Physical dependence* is "adaptation that is manifested by a drug class specific withdrawal syndrome that can be produced by abrupt cessation, rapid dose reduction, decreasing blood level of the drug, and/or administration of an antagonist" (AAPM/APS/ASAM, 2001).

- *Addiction* is "a primary, chronic, neurobiological disease with genetic, psychosocial, and environmental factors influencing its development and manifestations. It is characterized by behaviors that include one or more of the following: impaired control over drug use, compulsive use, continued use despite harm and craving" (AAPM/APS/ASAM, 2001).

Tolerance, physical dependence, and addiction are individual conditions, but they are often found in combination. *Pseudoaddiction* is a term used to describe the behaviors that can result from undertreatment of pain such as watching the clock, requesting medications more frequently than allowed or in larger doses (drug seeking), and expressing anger or feelings of being unfairly judged. Pseudoaddiction is commonly mistaken for addiction, but unlike addiction, behaviors will resolve when pain is appropriately relieved (Weissman & Haddox, 1989).

The following are suggestions for the nurse to consider when administering opioids for pain management:

- Assume the patient and family members have concerns regarding the risk of addiction and provide education based on scientific evidence to refute misconceptions.

- Manage pain appropriately and advocate for improvement when pain is unrelieved.

- Recognize that an opioid-tolerant patient will require higher dosages of opioid to achieve pain relief and that this does not equal addiction.

- Respond promptly, with respect and compassion, to requests for pain medications for all patients including those with opioid tolerance, dependence, or addiction.

- Avoid personal biases, labeling of patients, or unethical practices.

Opioids that have modified release formulations to make them long acting are not appropriate for prn dosing (APS, 2003). Controlled-release or sustained-release opioids are designed to provide 12 to 24 hours of analgesia (up to 72 hours of analgesia in the case of transdermal fentanyl patches). Many of these opioids take as long as 4 hours to achieve peak effects and last much longer than short-acting opioids, increasing the risk of oversedation and respiratory depression with prn use.

Sources: Bajwa, Z. H., Warfield, C. A., & Wootton, R. J. (2006). *Overview of treatment for chronic pain,* and Passik, S. D., & Kirsh, K. L. (2003). *Pain management and addiction.* Both retrieved February 25, 2007, from UpToDate website: http://utdol.com/utd/store/index.do.

Opioids are available in two major groups, agonists and agonist-antagonists. **Agonist** opioids are often referred to as morphine-like, or mu, agonists because they bind to the mu, kappa, and delta receptors of the cell, which are located in the CNS, peripheral nervous system, and gastrointestinal tract. Agonist opioids include opioids such as morphine, codeine, meperidine, dihydromorphinone, and methadone. **Agonist-antagonist** opioids are kappa and mu receptor partial agonists and are generally considered to be less efficacious than the pure mu agonists. Of note, a ceiling effect on analgesia has been identified with this group of opioids (Miyoshi & Leckband, 2001). Agonist-antagonist opioids include opioids such as buprenorphine, butorphanol, pentazocine, nalbuphine, and dezocine.

Both agonist and agonist-antagonist effects are reversible with the administration of a pure antagonist such as naloxone. **Antagonists** displace and replace the opioid at the receptor reversing the opioid's pharmacologic effect and side effects such as respiratory depression. The Pharmacology Summary (p. 344) and Chart 15–6 outline essential information about the mechanism of action and side effects of opioids.

Adjuvant Medications

Medications that are traditionally prescribed and administered for reasons other than pain relief are often used in pharmacologic treatment plans for chronic and cancer pain. Although less commonly used in acute pain, these medications may be of benefit in cases of trauma, burns, and some complex acute pain situations. These medications may enhance the effects of the opioids or NSAIDS, provide analgesia on their own, or reduce the side effects of other analgesic medications (APS, 2003). **Adjuvant medications** by definition are not primarily indicated for treatment of pain (Portenoy & McCaffery, 1999), so the

CHART 15–6 Side Effects of Opioids

Side Effect	Rationale	Nursing Action/Responsibility
Nausea and vomiting	Very common adverse effect of opioid therapy. Often related to dosages that exceed the patient's individual requirement for pain relief. Physiological explanation for this adverse effect is the stimulation of the chemoreceptor trigger zone in the medulla and vestibular stimulation, which explains the increased nausea associated with the upright position (Miyoshi & Leckband, 2001).	Assess for nausea and vomiting. Reduce the dosage of opioid by 25–50% if patient is comfortable. Consider advocating for an alternative opioid if vomiting persists. Monitor intake and output if vomiting persists. Obtain order for a nonsedating antinausea medication. Use extreme caution when administering a sedating antiemetic such as prochlorperazine. Co-sedation is likely to occur, increasing the risk of respiratory depression. A patient who is compromised by sedation is at risk for aspiration pneumonia, especially after anesthesia. If unable to tolerate food and drink, hold diet and advocate for another route of opioid administration (e.g., IV).
Pruritus	Pruritus, itching without a rash, is most commonly associated with administration of spinal opioids, but may also occur with any route of administration. More likely to occur with dosages that exceed the patient's requirements for pain relief. Usually limited to the face and torso. Increased tolerance to opioids will reduce the incidence of this adverse effect.	Report to health care provider to obtain orders for a nonsedating antipruritic medication. Reduce the dosage of opioid by 25–50% if patient is comfortable. Consider advocating for an alternative opioid if pruritus persists. Antihistamines are used to treat pruritus, however, these medications can be sedating and combined with opioids often lead to significant sedation and respiratory compromise. Assess for skin breakdown. Apply gloves to patient if scratching is causing a loss of skin integrity.
Constipation	Results from the generalized depressant effect of the opioid on the gastrointestinal motility. Slows emptying of gastrointestinal track by reducing peristalsis. This leads to increased absorption of water and drying and compacting of the intestinal contents (Miyoshi & Leckband, 2001). Constipation increases with larger dosages.	Administer a stimulating laxative and stool softener routinely while opioids are administered. Encourage fluid intake. Encourage ambulation if possible. Administer as low a dose of opioid as possible to provide pain relief and ensure patient is receiving acetaminophen and an NSAID if possible to augment pain relief.
Urinary retention	Occurs as a result of increased sphincter tone, making urination difficult or impossible, requiring catheterization of the bladder. This adverse effect decreases as tolerance to opioids develops.	Assess intake and output. Scan bladder to assess retention after urination. Notify health care provider and obtain order for urinary catheter as necessary to prevent retention.

(continued)

CHART 15–6	Side Effects of Opioids—*Continued*		
Side Effect	**Rationale**		**Nursing Action/Responsibility**
Sedation	Opioid-induced sedation is more likely to occur when patients are not tolerant to opioids or when opioids are given in doses that exceed the patient's individual requirements. First clinical manifestation is slowed cognition while remaining oriented. May experience drowsiness, drifting into sleep unless stimulated with conversation. Excessive sedation can result in confusion, dizziness, and increased risk for falling. If not treated, may lead to respiratory depression.		Assess for cosedating medications the patient is receiving and eliminate whenever possible. These medications will limit the amount of opioid the patient is able to safely use to relieve pain. Assess level of sedation. Assess breathing and oxygen saturation. If sedation is noted, notify the prescribing health care provider, decrease opioid dosage by 25–50%, and increase the frequency of monitoring until sedation resolves. Provide for patient safety with side rails and close observation. It may be necessary to use an antagonist (naloxone) to reverse significant sedation. Unresponsiveness that is not accompanied by respiratory depression is likely of another etiology and needs to be explored (e.g., cosedating medications, sepsis, and stroke).
Respiratory depression	Opioids reduce the responsiveness of the respiratory center in the pontine and bulbar brainstem to rising carbon dioxide (CO_2) tension, thus depressing the respiratory drive (Maher & Chaiyakul, 2003; Miyoshi & Leckband, 2001). Normally when CO_2 levels increase, the respiratory center responds by stimulating increased respiratory rate to rid the body of the excessive CO_2. Opioids defeat this response and can cause respirations to slow, become irregular, and eventually progress to apnea. Often the cause of undertreatment of pain that could easily be relieved.		Assess rate and depth of respirations and oxygen saturation. Administer oxygen as necessary. Stimulate the patient. Stop opioid administration. Report respiratory depression to the health care provider to obtain further orders. Resume opioid administration at 50% of the previous dosage once sedation and respiratory depression have resolved. Risk of respiratory depression increases when dosages exceed the requirements to achieve adequate pain relief.
Other adverse effects	Opioids impact in the limbic system resulting in euphoria, tranquility, or alternatively dysphoria through mechanisms that are not entirely clear (Miyoshi & Leckband, 2001). Cough suppression may be a desired effect or a potentially harmful adverse effect. Too rapid IV injection can cause chest wall rigidity. Accumulation of opioid and opioid metabolites occurs when renal function is impaired. The development of tolerance to opioids can be considered a benefit or an adverse effect. See discussion of tolerance, physical dependence, and addiction in Chart 15–5 (p. 346). Two very commonly prescribed opioids, meperidine and propoxyphene, both metabolize into active metabolites (normeperidine and norpropoxyphene, respectively) that have long half-lives. Accumulation is a concern with repeated dosing and if excretion is impaired through renal insufficiency (APS, 2003; Maher & Chaiyakul, 2003). As with normeperidine, norpropoxyphene can cause seizures (APS, 2003; Maher & Chaiyakul, 2003). The CNS excitatory effects of normeperidine can cause dysphoria, agitation, and seizures, making meperidine less useful for pain management (APS, 2003; Jacox et al., 1994).		The nurse must consult with the pharmacist as a collaborative resource especially when the patient has multiple disease states, making opioid therapy potentially more likely to result in an adverse effect. Provide patient safety with use of side rails and close observation. Assess oxygen status and lung sounds. Conduct ongoing assessments of renal function studies and report to the health care provider any increase in values. When giving IV, administer slowly and observe for chest rigidity. Assess drug effectiveness and need for increased dosage. Meperidine continues to be useful in small dosages appropriate for treating postanesthetic shivering and rigors. Norpropoxyphene should be limited in its use, especially in the older adult as discussed in this chapter. It is recommended that the use of meperidine be limited to situations where use of an alternative opioid is not possible (e.g., patients who have intolerable side effects with other opioids).

nurse must be aware of the rationale for the specific medication within the context of pain management and be prepared to offer education regarding its use to patients and family members to avoid confusion. Adjuvants may include tricyclic antidepressants, antiepileptic medications, local anesthetics, glucocorticoids, skeletal muscle relaxants, antispasmodic agents, antihistamines, benzodiazepines, caffeine, topical agents, and dextroamphetamine. Bisphosphonates and radionuclides are also useful in the treatment of metastatic bone pain (APS, 2003; Maher & Chaiyakul, 2003).

Routes of Administration

Pain medications are available in a variety of formulations that can be administered via many different routes. This allows the prescribing provider to select a route of medication administration based on the individual needs of the patient given the specific situation. Routes of medication administration provide for a range of absorption times from rapid onset (e.g., transmucosal, intravenous) to delayed onset (e.g., transdermal). Each route of administration has advantages and disadvantages that should be considered. It is appropriate to deliver medications by the least invasive route when possible (APS, 2003).

Oral Route

The oral route of administration is generally preferred because it is the least invasive, most convenient, and often most cost effective. Most analgesic medications come in tablets, capsules, or in a liquid formulation that allow for ease of oral administration. The oral route of administration is preferred in the treatment of chronic and cancer pain because it reduces the need for frequent analgesic administration thus reducing the burden on the patient and caregiver, and it reduces the focus on pain and the "sick role" (APS, 2003). When treating acute pain, the oral route of administration may not be available initially after surgery due to nausea, vomiting, and postoperative ileus. As soon as bowel function is reestablished, transition to the oral route of administration is recommended. The oral route of administration has the disadvantage of slower onset and delayed peak effect. The rate of gastric emptying and intestinal motility can increase or decrease medication absorption (Glen & St. Marie, 2002). Once absorbed, oral analgesics undergo first-pass metabolism in the small intestine and the liver. Gastrectomy and major bowel resection may reduce adequate medication absorption.

Oral Transmucosal Route

The oral cavity provides several locations for medication administration via the vascular mucosal membranes including sublingual, buccal, and gingival. When administering a medication sublingually, the medication is placed under the tongue and held there until it is completely dissolved and absorbed. Buccal administration requires the medication to be placed between the gums of the upper molars and the cheek. Gingival drugs are placed between the gums of the upper incisors and the upper lip (McCaffery & Portenoy, 1999).

Absorption from the oral mucosa is optimal if the medications are lipid soluble and designed specifically for transmucosal delivery. An example is oral transmucosal fentanyl citrate (Actiq). Medications that are less lipid soluble, such as morphine, are not well absorbed by the mucosal membrane. An advantage of transmucosal administration is that the drug is absorbed directly into the venous blood flow going to the superior vena cava with minimal first-pass metabolism by the liver (Glen & St. Marie, 2002).

The nurse should assess the patient's ability to hold the medication under the tongue until completely absorbed. Many patients are unable to either understand or tolerate sublingual administration and instead swallow the medication, resulting in gastric absorption and hepatic metabolism, which reduces the effectiveness of the medication dramatically.

All of the oral transmucosal locations can become irritated with repeated application of a medication. Assessment of the integrity of the mucosa and rotating the site of application from side to side will help reduce this irritation.

Rectal Route

The rectal route of medication administration is generally reserved for use when nausea or vomiting precludes oral administration and in situations where the additional expertise of intravenous administration is not available or desirable. Most medications that can be taken orally may be given rectally with similar dissolution, absorption, and effectiveness. Medications administered into the rectum are absorbed into the superior, middle, and inferior rectal veins through contact with a relatively small area of the rectal wall and without the assistance of digestive enzymes (Glen & St. Marie, 2002; McCaffery & Portenoy, 1999). Relatively rapid systemic absorption and avoidance of hepatic metabolism are possible if the medication is inserted just past the rectal sphincter (Davis, Walsh, LeGrand, & Naughton, 2002). Medications that are formulated or coated so that absorption occurs in the intestine (e.g., enteric coated) are not effective when administered using the rectal route. The pH of the colon is alkaline and enteric-coated medications require the acidic environment of the intestines (McCaffery & Portenoy, 1999). An important disadvantage of the rectal route of administration is the actual placement, which most patients find unpleasant and embarrassing. If medications must be administered frequently, rectal irritation can occur.

Intravenous Route

Intravenous (IV) administration of medications allows for the most rapid onset of effect because medications are delivered directly into the systemic circulation. First-pass hepatic metabolism is avoided. When administering opioids to treat severe pain, IV boluses can be administered by titration (frequent administration of small doses) for rapid control of escalating pain (APS, 2003; McCaffery & Portenoy, 1999; Miyoshi & Leckband, 2001). Because of the rapid onset of effect, the IV route of administration is also associated with the highest level of toxicity. Care must be taken to administer medications slowly or in small doses in order to reduce adverse effects (McCaffery & Portenoy, 1999). Other disadvantages of the IV route of administration include increased risk of infection with vascular access and the expertise required to administer medications aseptically.

The IV route of administration is commonly reserved for acute pain management or in cases of chronic and cancer pain where patients are experiencing severe pain that requires rapid relief or are unable to take oral analgesics due to adverse effects or situations such as disease that impairs gastrointestinal function.

Intramuscular Route

Intramuscular (IM) injection of analgesics should be avoided. The IM route of administration has significant disadvantages. The IM absorption is unreliable with a 30- to 60-minute lag time to peak effect with a rapid falloff of action as compared with oral analgesic administration (APS, 2003; McCaffery & Portenoy, 1999). If the IM route of administration must be used, the deltoid muscles and vastus lateralis muscles have better perfusion, and absorption may be more rapid than with the gluteal muscle (APS, 2003; Glen & St. Marie, 2002). Although hepatic first-pass metabolism is avoided using this route of analgesic administration, the risk of tissue injuries such as sterile abscesses and fibrosis of the muscle and soft tissue as well a nerve injury resulting in persistent neuropathic pain make IM injection a poor choice in pain management situations (APS, 2003; McCaffery & Portenoy, 1999).

Subcutaneous Route

The subcutaneous route of administration is similar to the IM route of administration with the disadvantage of painful injection and variability of absorption based on the location of injection. Hepatic first-pass metabolism is avoided. However, in situations where oral and IV routes of delivery are not available, subcutaneous offers an alternative for administering analgesics. When treating pain in palliative care or end-of-life settings, subcutaneous administration may be an effective option when IV access if difficult. If subcutaneous medications are delivered by continuous infusion, the volume of the medication should be limited to 2 or 3 mL/hour to optimize absorption (APS, 2003; McCaffery & Portenoy, 1999). If higher infusion rates are necessary, the total volume to be infused can be split between two sites to prevent irritation, pain, necrosis, and sloughing at the site (McCaffery & Portenoy, 1999).

Transdermal Route

Transdermal administration of analgesic medications relies on absorption of lipid-soluble medications through the barrier of the intact skin into the local tissues and the systemic circulation. These medications are generally formulated in transdermal patches or topical creams, ointments, or gels. Absorption of the medication can be unintentionally increased with the application of heat or by massaging the skin to increase the blood flow to the area, resulting in rapid absorption and potential overdose (Glen & St. Marie, 2002). Fentanyl, lidocaine, and clonidine are examples of transdermal medications that are commonly used in pain management.

Spinal (Epidural and Intrathecal) Route

Epidural and intrathecal routes of administration are useful for acute pain management for postoperative and trauma pain and also for specific cancer and chronic pain management situations. These routes of medication administration bypass metabolism in the liver and systemic circulation. For this reason, the dosage of medication used to achieve adequate analgesia is very small compared to those administered by other routes.

The epidural space is separated from the spinal cord by the spinal meninges. When opioids, anesthetics, or other medications are administered by the epidural route, they must diffuse across the meninges, into the cerebrospinal fluid (CSF), and subsequently penetrate the spinal cord tissues. Medications injected directly into the intrathecal space have immediate access to the spinal cord tissues without diffusion across the meninges.

Both epidural and intrathecal administration of medications requires access to the spinal tissues through an invasive procedure, either injection through a spinal needle alone or in combination with placement of an indwelling catheter. The epidural or intrathecal catheter is usually temporarily indwelling and can be a potential source of infection. If the intention is to use the epidural or intrathecal route for longer durations, a permanent catheter is tunneled under the subcutaneous tissue to reduce the risk of infection or a fully implanted infusion pump with catheter is placed during a surgical procedure.

Regional Nerve Route

Injection of anesthetic medications into or near a nerve is commonly referred to as regional anesthesia or a nerve block. A variety of regional anesthetic blocks are performed to diagnose nerve pain, as a prognostic prior to a more invasive procedure, or to relieve chronic and cancer pain. When the anesthetic is injected, it is delivered directly to the nerve tissue. The anesthetic blocks the conduction of both afferent and efferent neural fibers (Buckley, 2001).

Regional anesthetic techniques are often used to diagnose whether pain originates from a peripheral nerve or from the CNS, a technique that is valuable in chronic pain of unknown etiology. Continuous infusion of anesthetics to regional nerves is becoming a very popular option for acute pain management and in situations where it is desirable to reduce the amount of opioid a patient receives throughout the operative and postoperative course (e.g., multiple comorbidities). The nerve block is generally established prior to surgery as a single dose. In some cases a catheter is placed to allow for continuous infusion of anesthetic so that the medication effects continue throughout the operative course and into the postoperative period, improving the quality of pain relief.

Methods of Medication Delivery

Clinical decisions regarding the dosing intervals for the various analgesic medications are based on multiple factors, including the type and intensity of the pain, the pharmacologic attributes of the medication, and the clinical setting. Consideration of the patient's preferences and need for simple dosing schedules is essential. Analgesics may be given as a single dose, multiple intermittent doses, by continuous dosing, or at the patient's request. As with many aspects of pain management, the dosing schedule should be customized to meet the individual needs of the patient to achieve the best results.

Single Dose

Single dosing of analgesic medications is generally a strategy used to treat pain caused by a painful procedure or in some circumstances injury. When premedicating a patient for a painful procedure, the analgesic should be administered so that the peak effects occur just prior to the start of the procedure. For example, a single dose of IV fentanyl administered to the patient just prior to beginning a colonoscopy allows time for the fentanyl to peak and adequately relieve the pain caused by this relatively brief procedure. A single dose of steroid administered into the epidural space may be sufficient to relieve the pain and inflammation associated with an acute low back injury. Single doses of analgesics are sometimes administered as a loading dose in order to rapidly achieve therapeutic blood levels.

Pro re Nata (prn)

Pro re nata (prn), or "as needed," is a common dosing strategy that allows for flexibility in the dosing schedule when pain is intermittent and the analgesic medication is appropriate for intermittent dosing. It is most commonly used for acute pain when pain is not consistent or is expected to decline rapidly as healing occurs. For example, a patient may have a prescription for a short-acting opioid analgesic that can be taken every 4 hours prn, allowing her to take the ordered medication as often as every 4 hours and as infrequently as her pain allows. Disadvantages of the prn dosing schedule are evident when a patient waits too long between doses of medication, allowing the pain to become severe, or when she is experiencing continuous pain that would be best managed with a continuous dosing pattern.

If continuous pain is managed with prn dosing, the patient can be taught to determine the duration of pain relief he experiences with a dose of medication and to then schedule the prn doses at that frequency to be taken routinely. This is an effective strategy for severe acute pain and for chronic or cancer pain. For example, the patient takes the ordered dose of oxycodone and begins to experience the onset of pain after 5 hours of good pain relief. Another dose of medication is taken to avoid the escalation of pain intensity and good pain relief is achieved for another 6 hours. Based on this information, the patient should adjust his prn schedule to a continuous dosing schedule with intervals of every 5 to 6 hours around the clock (ATC).

The use of prn dosing is appropriate when treating breakthrough pain episodes that occur in spite of well-controlled persistent pain. Breakthrough pain is generally unpredictable and severe, requiring the flexibility of a short- or rapid-acting analgesic that can be administered as soon as the breakthrough pain begins. For example, the patient is using a fentanyl transdermal patch once every 72 hours and treats breakthrough pain episodes two to three times daily with oral transmucosal fentanyl citrate (Actiq) units prn.

When the nurse manages prn dosing, the potential for undertreatment of pain becomes a very real concern. Patients often rely on their nurse to know what dosing schedule is best for them, and nurses frequently feel that the patient should ask for medication when they begin to experience the onset of pain. The result is a roller-coaster of severe pain alternating with pain relief. This common scenario is dissatisfying, instills a lack of trust, encourages "clock watching," and increases the risk for undertreatment of pain. Nurses should determine the optimal dosing schedule based on the patient's response to the medication and then offer doses routinely and prior to the onset of severe pain.

At times, the ordered interval for prn dosing is not frequent enough to allow dosing prior to the onset of pain, resulting in undertreated pain if the dosing schedule is followed. The nurse is responsible for conveying this information to the prescribing clinician and advocating for an appropriate dosing interval or an increase in dosage based on assessment findings. Likewise, if the prescribed dosing interval is too frequent to be realistically implemented, it is appropriate for the nurse to contact the prescribing clinician and advocate for an alternative dosing schedule or method. For example, boluses of IV fentanyl every 30 minutes prn for postoperative pain management may be optimally delivered using a continuous infusion or patient-controlled analgesia to avoid missed doses and subsequent undertreatment of pain.

Continuous

When pain is consistently present, analgesic medications should be administered continuously. This dosing strategy is most commonly used for severe pain. The goal of continuous dosing is to maintain a therapeutic level of the medication that provides optimal pain relief without adverse effects. To accomplish continuous dosing, short-acting analgesics may be administered ATC as mentioned or infusion pumps can be used to deliver IV analgesics continuously.

Other analgesic medication formulations have long half-lives or modified delivery to make them long acting and designed specifically for continuous dosing. These medications should be prescribed with a routine dosing interval based on the pharmacology of the medication. For example, controlled-release morphine that is designed so that the medication is released over a period of 24 hours should be prescribed for once-a-day dosing. When the frequency of analgesic dosing is reduced, patients with chronic and cancer pain benefit from the consistent pain relief and a reduced focus on medication administration and the sick role, and they generally experience improved quality of life. Continuous dosing of opioid analgesics should be used with extreme caution when patients are opioid naïve due to increased risk of adverse effects (APS, 2003).

Patient-Controlled Analgesia

Patient-controlled analgesia (PCA) is a dosing strategy that allows patients to request a small dose of analgesic medication when they begin to feel pain. PCA infusion pumps are designed with a patient dose button that the patient can press to activate medication delivery. The prescription includes a dosage and dosing interval that are programmed into the pump so that the patient receives the prescribed dosage no more often than allowed by prescription in spite of the possibility of more frequent button presses to request doses. The PCA can be used successfully to administer analgesic medications by a variety of routes including IV, subcutaneous, epidural, intrathecal, and peripheral nerve. The PCA may be used alone as a prn dose or in combination with a continuous infusion. PCA dosing is generally used in moderate to severe acute pain or in cases of chronic pain where alternate routes of analgesic administration are not available or effective.

The benefits of PCA include increased patient control and participation in pain management. PCA is very effective for acute pain management postoperatively or post-trauma when patients are unable to take oral analgesics and the severity of pain would require an unrealistic frequency of IV medication administration given the nurse's other responsibilities. Reduced time waiting for the nurse to deliver a requested analgesic is another benefit that often makes patients reluctant to relinquish control even when they are able to transition to oral analgesics prn. As mentioned previously, use of continuous dosing of opioids should be used with extreme caution for opioid naïve patients. This is especially true when continuous dosing is combined with PCA dosing.

Complementary and Alternative Therapies

A balanced analgesic medication treatment plan is the foundation of acute and cancer pain management. This is rapidly becoming the case in chronic pain management as well. However, the integration of appropriate complementary therapies is often used to fully treat the multidimensional experience of pain. In spite of the lack of scientific evidence that these therapies are effective in pain relief, the underlying principle of the mind, body, and spirit connection in promoting balance, harmony, and healing is a strong argument for their use (Snyder & Wieland, 2003). Generally, patients use complementary therapies as an additional strategy along with their pharmacologic treatments. However, some patients prefer to use only alternative therapies. Alternative therapies may be attractive to patients who desire to avoid medications and their potential adverse effects or to those who simply have not found medications to be effective in relieving their pain.

The nurse should have a basic understanding of common complementary therapies and include an assessment of the patient's use of complementary therapies in the overall assessment of pain. Patients may be reluctant to discuss their decision to use a complementary or alternative therapy for fear of ridicule or concern that the nurse will attempt to dissuade them from its use (Snyder & Wieland, 2003). The following questions may be used to encourage discussion regarding complementary therapies the patient might be using or desire to learn more about:

- Do you do anything to treat your pain besides taking medications?
- Have you ever used music, massage, or meditation to distract you when you are in pain?

The Complementary and Alternative Therapies feature discusses the use of art in managing pain.

Nursing Management

The nurse's knowledge of the multidimensions of pain management, effective assessment techniques, and common pharmacologic and complementary or alternative strategies is the foundation necessary to provide safe and appropriate nursing care. Consistent with the nursing process, data gathered from the pain assessment is analyzed along with the data gathered from all other aspects of the physical assessment and used in the planning of interventions.

Assessment

The assessment findings related to the physiological dimension should prompt the nurse to recognize the potential harm that unrelieved pain could cause to the patient, especially those who

are acutely or critically ill, who are frail or debilitated, or those with multiple disease states that would likely be impacted by a significant stress response.

Specific assessment data includes:

- Type (sharp, dull, burning, pressure)
- Location: including transmission patterns
- Duration
- What brings it on
- What relieves it
- When did it start
- Is it getting worse or better
- Intensity (using a pain scale)

Analysis of the data gathered regarding the sensory dimension of pain provides a baseline that future data may be compared against to determine if the treatment plan is resulting in a positive trend toward adequate pain relief. The quality of the pain will provide some direction in the selection of medications suited to nociceptive or neuropathic pain. The temporal pattern of the pain is important to the selection of formulations and timing of the administration of medications. Sustained-release, modified release, or continuous infusions of analgesics are particularly suited to pain that is constant and persistent and may potentially cause harm when administered for pain that is intermittent or transient. The sudden onset of severe breakthrough pain may require the use of a rapid-acting transmucosal or IV opioid.

COMPLEMENTARY & ALTERNATIVE THERAPIES — Art

Description:
Art therapy is a creative process that uses psychotherapy and visual art to further self-understanding. In the process of art therapy, the patient's created work becomes a reflection of his or her personality, development, abilities, pain, and conflict. This type of therapy includes a range of modalities that include, but are not limited to:

- Painting with oil, acrylic, or water color on canvas or finger painting.
- Basket or loom weaving.
- Sculpturing with wood, metal, marble, or other materials.
- Creating pottery and working with clay.

Research Support:
It is thought that visual creativity consists of not only originality and a special talent, but also sensitivity and even deeper dynamics of the human personality, such as sublimation, reparative-compensating mechanisms, and mental well-being. Art therapy combines all of these capacities and utilizes them in self-healing (Hardi, 2006). Individuals and families use a process of meaning construction to make sense of the world and their experiences. When an individual receives a life-threatening or life-altering illness diagnosis, it often forces the individual to revise his or her "life narrative" and to reconstruct meaning in his or her life. Expressive arts and ritual provide the means by which the individual can create meaning and connection. It is vital for each member of the health care team to help patients and their families express their feelings about their illness and find meaning and purpose at the end of life. Art therapy can allow the relationship among patient, family, and practitioner to be powerfully therapeutic and potentially transformative for all involved (Romanoff & Thompson, 2006).

The goal in art therapy is to facilitate positive change in an individual by engaging with the therapist and the art materials in a safe environment. Art therapy is used with success among all age populations. The therapeutic change occurs during the process of physical involvement with the art materials, such as the process of making of a significant art object, the process of expressing feelings through the created images, and the process of communication with the therapist by means of the art object (Waller, 2006).

Several art therapy programs have been created for use with the elderly population and serve as models for instituting art therapy into nursing practice. For example, The University of Pennsylvania's School of Nursing created a Living Independently for Elderly (LIFE) Program. At a Program of All-Inclusive Care for the Elderly (PACE) site in an urban African American community, art therapy practitioners offer the choice of art media and options for working with elderly clients (Johnson & Sullivan-Marx, 2006).

References
Hardi, I. (2006). Creativity and visual expression. *Psychiatria Hungarica, 21*(4), 268–278.
Johnson, C. M., & Sullivan-Marx, E. M. (2006). Art therapy: Using the creative process for healing and hope among African American older adults. *Geriatric Nursing, 27*(5), 309–316.
Romanoff, B. D., & Thompson, B. E. (2006). Meaning construction in palliative care: The use of narrative, ritual, and the expressive arts. *American Journal of Hospice Palliative Care, 23*(4), 309–316.
Waller, D. (2006). Art therapy for children: How it leads to change. *Clinical Child Psychology and Psychiatry, 11*(2), 271–282.

The affective dimension of pain will yield assessment data that has the potential to undermine even the most carefully planned treatments. The patient's emotions and assignment of meaning to the pain should be considered when prioritizing time spent with the patient. Education and emotional support should be tailored to meet the specific needs of patients who are suffering or have a negative perception of their pain. Involvement of a psychiatric specialist, psychologist, or social worker may be indicated, and based on the analysis of the affective dimension findings, the nurse is in an excellent position to advocate for this on behalf of the patient who may not be able to recognize that this is a concern.

Consideration of assessment findings in the cognitive dimension will assist the nurse in providing for specific religious and cultural needs. In addition, understanding the culturally appropriate response to pain assists the nurse in interpreting pain-related behaviors more accurately. For example, when a patient who is culturally inclined to be quite stoic in the expression of pain becomes more vocal, it should prompt the nurse to consider that pain might be severe in spite of the patient's subdued response. Patients who feel a loss of control might be comforted by having choices in their pain treatment whenever possible. For example, opioids that are ordered to be administered IV prn might be administered using a PCA infusion device, allowing postoperative patients significant control and increasing self-efficacy in their acute pain management.

Assessment of the behavioral dimension of pain is a necessary baseline to determine whether pain-related behaviors are reduced following the implementation of the pain treatment plan for patients who are unable to provide a self-report of pain. The nurse who finds that the patient has developed some unfortunate learned pain behaviors has the opportunity to reduce the use of these behaviors by establishing a trusting relationship, providing pain treatments appropriately as needed rather than waiting until pain behaviors are demonstrated, and reassuring the patient that the health care team is committed to relieving pain and will do everything possible to accomplish that goal. In addition, these findings should prompt the nurse to consider encouraging and assisting patients to develop their skills in using cognitive-behavioral strategies such as meditation, journaling, or redirecting thoughts into a more positive pattern.

Planning

The analysis of assessment findings and planning of interventions should be focused around the therapeutic goals described in this chapter. The baseline assessment of pain intensity and functional ability is matched with the comfort and function goal to establish the means by which progress may be measured. Interventions are defined and initiated using the goals established in the planning phase. Evaluation will determine whether the goals and patient outcomes have been accomplished and redirect the plan if they have not.

Nursing Diagnosis

Nursing diagnoses that may apply to the patient experiencing pain include:

1. Pain, acute
2. Pain, chronic
3. Fatigue

4. Coping ineffective
5. Hopelessness
6. Mobility impaired
7. Powerlessness

Interventions and Rationales

Implementation of interventions, particularly pharmacologic interventions, is multifaceted and focused on patient safety as well as optimizing the potential efficacy of the treatment plan. The nurse uses the knowledge of pharmacologic interventions to review the medications that have been prescribed for the patient. The following questions might be considered:

- Could this medication or dosage cause the patient to experience adverse effects given her physiological status or allergies?
- Is the medication appropriate to treat this patient's source of pain (e.g., neuropathic, nociceptive)?
- Is it likely that this medication and dosage will be able to relieve the intensity of pain this patient is experiencing?
- Is this medication ordered with an appropriate frequency for administration?
- Is the formulation (long-acting, short-acting, etc.) and route of administration appropriate to treat this patient's pattern of pain?
- Does the patient have adequate understanding of how to use the medication to prevent harm through inadvertent misuse?
- Are there other medications that might be appropriate to add to this treatment plan to optimize the effectiveness and safety of pain relief for this patient?

The nurse is the "guardian of patient safety" at the patient's bedside to ensure that when medications are administered they will not cause harm (Campbell, 2006). If there is any concern that the prescribed medication may not be appropriate or ordered in an appropriate dosage or frequency of administration, it is the nurse's responsibility to notify the prescribing clinician and request clarification of the order. The patient's physical condition must be considered when implementing pharmacologic strategies to avoid administration of a medication that has the potential to cause adverse effects or that could result in patient harm and when selecting or implementing complementary or alternative strategies. Because pain medications, particularly opioids, have the potential to cause serious adverse effects, this important nursing role cannot be stressed enough.

Successful implementation of complementary or alternative intervention is based on the selection of a strategy that is embraced by the patient and his family. Some interventions are less demanding of the patient's time and energy (e.g., music, massage), whereas others require the patient to be actively engaged (e.g., meditation, journaling). It is important to consider the selected strategies given the patient's specific needs and to consider alternative strategies if necessary.

Prior to initiating interventions, the patient and family must be educated regarding the goals, rationale, expected outcomes, and potential adverse effects associated with the intervention. Some patients will only be able to understand or desire to learn the most basic concepts regarding their treatments. For these patients, a base of knowledge should be established and then built on with subsequent educational opportunities. Ensure that the patient does not have a cultural barrier to learning such as speaking a language other that of the health care team or having a cognitive impairment (e.g., confusion, sedation). It is important to remember that the presence of severe pain is a barrier to learning and should be relieved as quickly as possible to facilitate the patient's participation in their care. Other patients will want detailed information, and education may have to be provided on multiple occasions to fully answer all of their questions. Educational tools such as diagrams, diaries, audiovisual programs, and demonstrations may provide another avenue of learning for patients who learn more effectively from visual instruction. The education provided must be tailored to meet the specific needs of each patient and their family members.

Equianalgesia

Early studies of the relative potency of various opioids were accomplished by comparing single doses of oral and IV/IM opioids to 10 mg of IV morphine in patients with postoperative and cancer pain (Houde, Wallenstein, & Beaver, 1996). The term *equianalgesia* refers to the ratio derived from these studies that allows selection of a dosage of an opioid that is relatively the same in potency to an opioid that is already in use. For example, a patient receiving IV morphine for postoperative pain can be transitioned to an oral opioid with the goal of providing approximately the same level of pain relief by calculating the equianalgesic dose (Kaplow & Hardin, 2007). An understanding of basic equianalgesia gives the nurse the information necessary to respond appropriately to patients who are rotating to a new opioid and/or new route of administration.

To perform an equianalgesic calculation, the nurse must have access to an equianalgesic chart. Although equianalgesic charts may be published in different formats and with different associated information, the equianalgesic doses are consistent. The nurse should obtain an approved equianalgesic chart from the pharmacy. The opioids listed on the chart will have equianalgesic dosages listed for the IV/IM route of administration and the oral route. A simple calculation allows the nurse to determine the equianalgesic dose:

- First determine the amount of opioid the patient has received in the past 24 hours, being careful to add up all doses given.
- Locate the opioid that has been given in the past 24 hours on the equianalgesic chart and locate the equianalgesic dose under the correct route of administration.
- Divide the 24-hour total dose of opioid by the equianalgesic dose.
- Identify the new opioid's equianalgesic dose on the equianalgesic chart using the new route of administration.
- Multiply the 24-hour total equianalgesic dose by the new opioid equianalgesic dose.
- The answer represents the 24-hour total amount of the new opioid that is relatively equal in potency to the 24-hour total dose of the opioid currently being administered.
- Divide the total 24-hour dose of the new opioid into administration intervals by dividing by the number of doses desired within 24 hours (APS, 2003).

For example, a patient has received IV morphine 1 mg/hr for postoperative pain equaling 24 mg for the past 24 hours. The equianalgesic dose for IV morphine is located on the chart and

is 10. The nurse divides 24 mg by 10 to equal 2.4 equianalgesic dose units. The order for oxycodone (Percocet) has been written and so the nurse locates the equianalgesic dose of 20 for oral oxycodone on the chart. The nurse then multiples the equianalgesic dose units of 2.4 by 20 to equal 48 mg, which is the 24-hour total amount of oxycodone that would be required to provide the same pain relief as 24 mg of IV morphine. As a final step, the nurse then divides 48 mg into 6 equal doses for a q4h administration interval. The 8-mg dose of oxycodone is within the range of the health care provider's order for one to two Percocet (5 mg each tablet) q4h prn. Additionally, the nurse also knows that the patient is likely to need two tablets rather than one tablet given the equialangesic dose.

The nurse should note the following when doing equianalgesic dose calculations:

- If several different opioids or routes of administration are used, the equianalgesic dose units should be determined for each different opioid/route and then added before multiplying by the new opioid equianalgesic dose.
- Patients may have different responses to different opioids and/or routes of administration, so a degree of variability should be expected and monitoring for opioid side effects and pain relief should be increased until the patient is safely transitioned to the new opioid.
- If an order for a new opioid is either too large or too small given the equianalgesic dose calculation, the nurse should request clarification with the prescribing health care provider.
- As a colleague, the pharmacist is generally an excellent resource for assistance with equianalgesic dose calculations.

Management of Unrelieved Pain

As an advocate for change, it falls to the nurse to accurately and concisely communicate the details of the pain assessment, interventions that have been implemented, and the evaluation of the patient's response. Chart 15–7 provides suggestions for using collaborative communication to improve pain management.

Evaluation

Evaluation data is aimed at determining whether pain relief has been achieved. The nurse needs to evaluate each tenant of the plan to determine the most effective interventions. It may not always be realistic to achieve total relief, especially with chronic diseases such as arthritis. The realistic goal may need to be a level of comfort that allows the patient to perform activities of daily living and maintain some quality of life. It is essential that the nurse helps the patient and family identify behaviors that increase the pain and how to avoid these activities.

Reassessment of pain and assessment of the patient's response to interventions is necessary to successfully measure improvement in the quality of pain management as compared to baseline assessments. The reassessment of pain should follow the same pattern used at baseline, including using the same tools to reinforce concepts that were taught during the assessment. Some minor alterations should be made to elicit the details needed to determine if there has been a change after intervention. For example:

- How would you rate your pain intensity on the 0 to 10 scale at rest? With activity? During _____ (the patient's previously identified most painful time)?

CHART 15–7   Collaborative Communication to Improve Pain Management

When collaborating with other members of the health care team to improve pain management, it is vital that the nurse be prepared to concisely, accurately, and knowledgeably convey the details necessary for the health care provider to make a logical and appropriate decision regarding the patient's care. Poorly prepared nurses may actually indirectly cause harm if they communicate inaccurate or incomplete information. Nurses are the eyes, ears, and hands of the other members of the health care team when those members must make decisions away from the patient's bedside (Griffie, 2003). An effective nurse who has the best interests of the patient and the health care team in mind during communications will command a level of trust that encourages support from colleagues and discourages arguments and denial of requests.

Prepare to provide the following:

- Patient name, location, age, and diagnosis or surgery
- Patient's primary health care provider (if speaking with another member of the team)
- Pertinent details of the pain assessment (e.g., pain intensity, location, character)
- Impact of the pain on the patient's function
- Interventions that have been implemented (e.g., medications, therapies)
- The appropriate next step to improve the situation.

The following hypothetical patient scenario provides an example script and rationale for steps that a nurse could follow to improve communication when discussing postoperative pain management with an orthopedic surgeon who is covering for her colleague.

INTRODUCE YOURSELF AND THE PATIENT

"Dr. Smith this is (state your name), I am a nurse here on the medical–surgical unit." Introduce yourself professionally avoiding meaningless chatter. This is an important step that helps the health care provider, in this case, to know whom she is speaking with and their credentials.

"I am caring for Mrs. Jones in Room 246. She is a 78-year-old female who has degenerative arthritis and underwent a total knee arthroplasty yesterday by Dr. Black." This information alerts the health care provider to the fact that this patient is an older adult, recently postanesthetic, and expected to have a significant amount of pain. These are all considerations that will be used in medical decision making. Additionally, this information allows the health care provider time to focus on any information her health care provider colleague may have reported to her and to visualize this patient if she has seen her before.

BRIEFLY REVIEW THE GOALS OF THE PAIN TREATMENT PLAN

"Mrs. Jones' comfort and function goals are a pain score of 4/10 and to be able to participate in her physical therapy two times today." This gives the health care provider a direction and makes the patient's report of pain meaningful in the context of an outcome.

COMMUNICATE THE PERTINENT DETAILS OF THE PAIN ASSESSMENT

"She has reported a pain score of 8/10 for the past 2 hours, and describes the pain as constant, sharp, and throbbing and localized to her left knee.

She has been coping fairly well, but is beginning to express some frustration and anxiety. Her husband is supportive and in the room with her. She grimaces and stiffens up when the continuous passive motion machine reaches its highest and lowest points." This is a concise summary of the sensory assessment (pattern, character, location, and intensity) and the affective and cognitive assessments (emotions and coping), as well as the behavioral assessment (grimacing, stiffening).

DISCUSS THE IMPACT OF THE UNRELIEVED PAIN

"The physical therapist came to take Mrs. Jones to the joint therapy class, but felt she would be unable to participate until her pain was more appropriately relieved." This is strong outcome-based evidence that a change is warranted and validated by two members of the health care team.

REVIEW THE PAIN TREATMENT PLAN AND EVALUATION OF THE PATIENT'S RESPONSE

"Mrs. Jones has IV PCA morphine ordered with settings of zero continuous infusion, 1 mg PCA demand dose, a 15-minute lock-out time, and the hourly limit is set at 4 mg. She has requested an average of three doses to each of the three or four doses she has received since her surgery. She has an ice wrap on her knee. She is alert and oriented. Her respiratory status is stable with good oxygen saturations. She doesn't have any opioid-induced adverse effects." At this point, the health care provider has a very clear direction that is reasonable and based on good physical evidence that a change is not only necessary but will be well tolerated and is prepared to listen to the nurse's request respectfully. In addition, the nurse has established a base of trust through professional communication that will most likely be remembered in future opportunities for collaboration.

MAKE A RECOMMENDATION

"I would like an order to give a bolus of IV morphine 2 mg now and I think it would be helpful to have it available for prn use 10 minutes prior to physical therapy. I think we should decrease the PCA lock-out time to 10 minutes, and increase the hourly limit to 6 mg. As soon as Mrs. Jones is eating, I recommend we start acetaminophen 500 mg PO every 6 hours ATC and celecoxib (Celebrex) 100 mgs PO bid." In approximately 2 to 3 minutes the nurse has conveyed a clear, strong, and appropriate request for a balanced or multimodal approach to acute pain management. The dosages requested reflect an understanding of the patient's potential sensitivity to medication adverse effects due to her age and renal and hepatic function. However, the nurse should be prepared to discuss hepatic and renal function lab results when requesting these medications.

KNOWLEDGEABLY DISCUSS OTHER OPTIONS

"Is there something else you would like for me to try?" Once the nurse's request has been presented, it is important to acknowledge that there may be another equally appropriate change that the health care provider may have in mind or that the health care provider may have information that would make another option more appropriate.

- Is your pain in the same place?
- Do you have any new pain?
- Does your pain feel the same (e.g., aching, burning)?
- Do you feel like the pain treatments are helping to relieve your pain?
- Are you having any nausea, vomiting, itching, or constipation?
- Are you able to urinate? (If opioid analgesics have been administered)
- Do you feel alert and able to keep up with conversations around you when you are not resting?
- Are you able to do _____ (the patient's previously identified goal for function)?

In addition to these assessment questions, the patient's vital signs should be checked with specific attention to respiratory status including depth, quality, and rate of respirations when opioid analgesics have been administered.

If the analgesic treatment plan includes delivery of medications using infusion devices such as a PCA pump, analysis of the data provided by the device becomes an important component of the evaluation process. Review of the pump settings to ensure appropriate programming will prevent errors or encourage rapid identification of an error should one occur. PCA pumps track the number of milligrams, micrograms, or milliliters of medication that is administered to the patient. The PCA pump also tracks the number of times the patient pushes the PCA button to request a dose and the number of times they actually receive a dose. Evaluation of this data can provide important trending information and provide a prompt to initiate a change when necessary.

The frequency of evaluation or reassessment is determined by institutional policies and procedures. However, it is the nurse's obligation to increase the frequency of reassessment if the patient's condition warrants. For example, a patient who is found to be slightly drowsy with a marginal respiratory rate of 10 breaths per minute is scheduled to be reassessed again in 2 hours. Instead, the nurse should identify the potential for significant respiratory depression and reassess the patient more frequently until her respiratory status is stable.

Collaborative Management

A successful pain management plan requires the focused attention of the multidisciplinary team. Nurses are recognized as the team members most likely to spend significant amounts of time with the patient; hence, they play a vital role in the coordination of the care of the multidisciplinary team. It is the nurse's responsibility to assess the ongoing effects and intensity of pain, administer medications and nonmedication treatments, communicate changes in the patient's condition to the other members of the team, and advocate for change. Members of the health care team depend on the knowledge and skill of the nurse to manage the patient's pain adequately facilitating participation in necessary therapies and procedures.

To meet the goals of pain management, the multidisciplinary team draws on the additional support of services such as pain management services, chaplain services, psychologists/psychiatrists, financial assistance, social services, and specific support groups for patients and family members. Pain management services provide expert assistance with complex pain management problems and are skilled in the management of high-technology modalities such as IV PCA, epidural or intrathecal infusion of opioids and anesthetics, and regional anesthetic techniques. Chaplin services, psychologist/psychiatrist, and social services assist with identification and management of concerns in the affective, cognitive, and behavioral dimensions of pain. Financial services assist the patient in meeting immediate needs such as purchasing medications and obtaining specialty pain management care, and providing counseling regarding long-term needs if the patient is unable to return to gainful employment. Finally, specific support groups may be especially beneficial to patients with chronic and cancer pain. Meeting with others who are living with similar challenges allows the patient and family to openly discuss their concerns, exchange ideas, and receive encouragement.

Discharge Planning

Transitioning from one care setting to another can cause a patient and family members to feel anxious, frightened, confused, and even frustrated as they try to understand their pain management plan. Patients and family members should be prepared for discharge throughout the entire course of the admission through the coordinated efforts of all members of the multidisciplinary team. Nurses play a significant role in assessing the needs of the patient and family for discharge.

Initial Discharge Planning

Planning for the pain management regimen should be initiated with consideration of the patent's ability to appropriately use the medications and complementary or alternative strategies. Complex medication plans, although they may provide superior pain relief, may not be appropriate if the patient will not be able to manage the complexity of the plan independently after discharge. Likewise, nonmedication strategies that are difficult to perform without expert skills are less likely to be used after discharge.

Financial considerations such as prescription coverage or ability to pay for prescription medications, if considered during the planning stages, will enhance the patient's willingness and ability to adhere to the medication regimen after discharge. Many patients do not have adequate health care insurance or prescription coverage and the cost of pain medications may be a financial burden. Although it is not always possible, medications should be selected based on the lowest appropriate cost in addition to most appropriately meeting the needs of the patient. However, care must be taken to avoid selecting a less costly medication based on cost alone. A medication that causes side effects that must then be treated with yet another medication will negate any cost savings to the patient.

Some patients have complex pain management needs and the care of a pain management specialist after discharge may be determined to be necessary. In these cases, it is appropriate to begin the process of referral early to facilitate a smooth transition of care after discharge. If a pain management specialist is not available in the patient's community, appropriate follow-up care may be available from a health care provider or licensed independent practitioner in the community. Time will be needed to select a provider and secure an appointment for follow-up care.

Ongoing Discharge Planning

Once a pain management plan is determined, it should be implemented and modified until the best level of pain relief and functionality are achieved with minimal side effects. When pain medications are administered, the patient and family members should be instructed regarding expected onset of relief, side effects that may be experienced, and when additional medication will be provided or should be requested. Treatments of medication side effects should also be reviewed with the patient and family. When assisting a patient with the use of a complementary or alternative strategy, it is imperative to provide adequate opportunity to practice the technique to facilitate the skillful use of the strategy after discharge. Repeated administration of medications and use of nonmedication strategies will allow the patient and family members the opportunity to hear instructions many times before discharge. This approach reduces the stress of having to learn everything on the day of discharge.

Health Promotion

Patient teaching prior to discharge should be a review of the teaching that has been provided during the patient's stay. New information will be very difficult for the patient and family to incorporate this late in their care. Every effort should be made to ensure that the plan for pain management is providing adequate relief of pain and optimal function with minimal side effects so that last minute changes are avoided when possible.

The nurse is the patient's final contact before discharge in most settings. Discharge responsibilities include presenting information in a calm and reassuring manner that will support the patient's need to be confident that he will be able to efficiently continue the plan independent of the support of the health care team.

Determining when to take pain medications can be confusing and requires a thought process that is similar to managing diabetes with insulin injections. Patients must "measure" their pain and its impact on function to determine if additional pain medication is needed and how much. To facilitate optimal understanding, it is important to provide clear and accurate written discharge instructions (AHCPR, 1992; Jacox et al., 1994). Supportive graphics to illustrate the use of each medication may be useful when discussing more complex pain management concepts such as persistent pain and breakthrough pain. Written instructions should include the times that medication was given to the patient while the patient was admitted including when the last dose was taken and when the next dose is due. The nurse should explain how medication administration is recorded to reduce reliance on memory and the chance for errors. Encourage patients to use a similar system to track their own medications after discharge. Patients may find it helpful to use a notebook to document their pain scores, daily function, side effects, and when medications are taken. A written record may provide additional understanding of how much medication they are taking and the impact that pain has on their lives. Patients' and family members' perceptions regarding pain management are occasionally different and a written record may help each to gain an appreciation of the other's perspective.

If the patient participated in a complementary or alternative strategy as part of the pain management plan, written instructions should be provided including when the strategy was used and how it was most effectively executed (e.g., which music was most relaxing). Appropriate referral information should be provided in cases where the strategy requires a specialist (e.g., acupuncture).

The patient and family should be given the opportunity to voice any concerns or questions they may have prior to discharge. In addition, the nurse should review the following concepts:

- Pain management plays an important role in the recovery process.
- Several different pain medications may be prescribed together to relieve pain through different mechanisms.
- When pain is persistent pain medications should be taken routinely.
- Physical dependence and tolerance to opioid pain medications are not addiction.

Many times patients and families are overwhelmed and are not sure what to ask. The nurse should provide the patient and family members with the name of their provider and phone number to contact if they have questions after discharge. Discharge instructions are outlined in the Patient Teaching & Discharge Priorities box (p. 358).

◼ Gerontological Considerations

The older adult patient is at risk for undermanagement of pain due to many barriers unique to the aging population. Myths such as pain is a natural part of aging, older adults are less sensitive to pain, and opioids should be avoided when treating pain are often believed by health care professionals, patients, and their family members. Barriers to appropriate pain management in older adults may include the patient's own reluctance to report pain due to the belief that pain is an expected consequence of aging and disease (Pautex & Gold, 2006). They may have fears about the meaning of pain in terms of disease and the potential impact that it may have on their ability to remain independent. In addition, many patients have fixed incomes and very minimal or no health care benefits. Financial concerns may cause them to delay seeking health care or to choose not to purchase prescribed medications. In addition to these and other age-specific barriers, many patients have multiple medical diagnoses and increased sensitivity to analgesic medications due to altered hepatic and renal function.

Consequences of Unrelieved Pain

The impact of undertreated pain in the older adult is costly on many levels. Older adults with pain may be less active, leading to deconditioning, gait disturbances, and increased risk of falling. Sleep disturbances are common for patients with pain, but have an even greater impact on the older adult, causing decreased energy, depression, and cognitive impairment (Jakcobsson, Klevsgard, Westergren, & Rahm Hallberg, 2003; Pautex & Gold, 2006). As the ability to independently perform daily activities declines, burdens on the health care system, dependence on caregivers, and social isolation increase and exert a negative impact on the quality of life (Weiner & Hanlon, 2001).

Pain Assessment and Measurement

Assessing and measuring the multiple dimensions of pain in the older adult can be accomplished in the same manner as with any adult patient in most cases. The American Geriatrics Society (AGS) has published *The Management of Persistent Pain in Older Persons* as a guide to appropriate pain management (AGS, 2002). It should not be assumed that the older adult would have difficulty with the pain assessment. Instead, the nurse should pay special attention to preparing for the interview so that the best outcomes are possible. The location of the interview should be quiet and free of interruptions. Plan for sufficient time so that the patient is able to take the time needed to answer the questions. Speak clearly while facing the patient and use body language to convey the meaning of the question. Ensure that patients with hearing impairments are wearing their hearing aids if possible. Likewise, ensure that patients are wearing their eyeglasses if vision is impaired. Assessment tools should be enlarged so that the pictures and font of the type are easily visualized.

PATIENT TEACHING & DISCHARGE PRIORITIES for Pain Management

Need	Teaching
PRESCRIPTION MANAGEMENT Patient/family	Prescriptions for pain medications should be filled as soon as possible so that the next dosage can be taken on time.
	Secure prescription pain medications to prevent loss or theft.
	Avoid opening medication bottles over the sink or toilet.
	Follow your prescribed pain medication taper plan. • Contact your prescribing health care provider prior to taking extra doses of medication or if dosage needs to be reduced.
	Report unrelieved or new pain to your health care provider.
	If an additional prescription is necessary, notify your prescribing health care provider 2 to 3 days before it is needed.
	Assess pain intensity and ability to perform necessary activities prior to taking pain medications. • Take routine medications on schedule without skipping dosages. • Take "as-needed" medications prior to the onset of severe pain. • Use a notebook or journal to record the pain score, activity at the time of medication, the time and dosage of medication, and notes describing your concerns.
	Assess for pain medication side effects. • Take pain medications with food to prevent nausea. • Take stool softeners and stimulating laxatives routinely if taking opioid pain medications to prevent constipation. • Contact your prescribing health care provider if your opioid pain medication causes excessive sleepiness or heavy snoring.
	Assess knowledge of pain medications and pain management plan.
Family/support system	• Assess knowledge of pain medication side effects and treatments. • Assess knowledge of physical dependence, tolerance, and addiction. • Assess financial needs and resources for prescription coverage. • Provide example of journal or notebook for patient use.
Setting	• Assess discharge referral needs: Pain management specialist/clinic, psychiatrist or psychologist, primary care provider. • Assess need for follow-up appointments.
NONMEDICATION STRATEGY MANAGEMENT Patient/family	Nonmedication strategies that were helpful during admission should continue to be used in addition to pain medications.
	Assess pain intensity and ability to perform necessary activities prior to performing nonmedication strategies. • Record the pain score, activity at the time of the nonmedication strategies, the time, and notes describing your feelings or concerns in the journal or notebook.
Family/support system	Assess knowledge of selected nonmedication strategies role in the pain management plan.
Setting	Assess discharge referral needs: physical therapist, massage therapist, acupuncture practitioner.
	Assess for need for follow-up appointments.
PAINFUL PROCEDURE MANAGEMENT Patient/family Family/support system Setting	Medications that are prescribed for use prior to painful procedures should be taken allowing sufficient time for onset of pain relief prior to beginning procedure.
	Assess pain score prior to, during, and after procedure. • Utilize nonmedication strategies to encourage relaxation or distraction. • Report unrelieved pain during procedures to your prescribing health care provider.
	Assess understanding of the role of premedication in successful procedural pain management.
	Assess knowledge of pain medications and nonmedication strategies to be used prior to and during painful procedures.
	Assess for need for professional home health assistance with procedural pain management.

Many of the common pain intensity measurement tools are valid and acceptable to use when assessing the older adult (AGS, 2002; McDonald, 2006; Pautex & Gold, 2006). It is suggested that the 0–10 numeric rating scale is a good first choice. If the patient has difficulty with the NSR, the nurse should try the simple verbal descriptor scale next, followed by the pain thermometer (a diagram of a thermometer with descriptions that show increasing pain intensity), and then finally the faces pain scale (Herr, 2002). When older adult patients have cognitive impairment (e.g., dementia, Alzheimer's disease, or stroke) assessment of pain can be challenging, as discussed next.

Pain Assessment in Older Adults with Cognitive Impairments

Assessment of pain in an older adult who is cognitively impaired presents a significant nursing challenge. Impairments may range from minor deficits in memory to the advanced stages of Alzheimer's disease. In spite of the difficulty that cognitive impairment presents, studies support the validity of specific pain assessment tools for use in this population and demonstrate that a surprising number of older adults with cognitive impairments are able to use these tools effectively (Soscia, 2003). Just as with cognitively intact patients, the nurse should select a pain assessment tool that specifically meets the needs of the patient. Research findings suggest that the McGill Pain Questionnaire short form is the most reliable and valid for use in the mildly or moderately cognitively impaired older adult patient in the nursing home with only 27% of older cognitively impaired adults being unable to complete the tool (Wynne, Ling, & Remsburg, 2000). Other assessment tools studied were the visual descriptor scale (49% unable to use), the visual analog scale (43% unable to use), and the faces pain scale (39% unable to use) (Wynne et al., 2000). Additional studies suggest that the visual analog scale may be more useful if presented in a vertical form like a thermometer so that patients can relate more intense pain to the rising of the temperature (Herr & Garand, 2001; Herr & Mobily, 1991).

Careful assessment of the behavioral dimension of pain is helpful when the use of most other assessments is not possible. Common pain-related behaviors demonstrated by older adults with cognitive impairment include:

- Aggressiveness
- Restlessness
- Agitation
- Increased or decreased verbalization or vocalization
- Changes in appearance, facial expressions, or body language (AGS, 2002; Parke, 1998).

To fully appreciate the subtle changes that indicate a patient with cognitive impairment is experiencing pain, the nurse must become familiar with the patient's everyday personality, habits, and activities (AGS, 2002; Soscia, 2003). Family members and caregivers can be very helpful in establishing a baseline for the patient's behavior, as well as assisting with identification of changes from baseline (AGS, 2002).

Pain assessment is possible in older adults with cognitive impairments if the nurse recognizes the special assessment needs of this population by selecting the correct assessment tools, utilizing the behavioral assessment, and establishing the patient's normal baseline with the patient's family members or caregiver.

Pharmacologic Considerations

When selecting analgesic medications for the treatment of pain in the older adult, the changes that occur with aging must be considered to reduce the risk of medication side effects. Changes in gastric pH, increased gastric emptying, and decreased intestinal blood flow are common changes that will slow the absorption of medications. When the older adult has decreased lean body mass, increased body fat, decreased body water, and increased plasma protein, the distribution of medications is altered (Smith, 2003; St. Marie & Loeb, 2002). Medications are stored in the tissue longer extending their effects. When hepatic changes such as decreased hepatic mass and blood flow are present, metabolism is impacted, increasing the half-life of medications and reducing clearance or elimination as a result. Older adults also may experience decreased clearance or elimination of medications as a result of decreased glomerular filtration rate, decreased creatinine clearance, and decreased renal blood flow.

The physiological changes that occur with advancing age often result in a more potent effect and longer half-life of medications commonly used to treat pain. Generally those adults who are older than 70, who also have altered absorption, distribution, metabolism, and excretion, should be started on 25% to 50% of the recommended adult starting doses (AHCPR, 1992; APS, 2003). Once the patient's response to the medication is determined, dosages should be slowly increased or decreased as indicated until the desired effects are achieved. Specific medication cautions for the older adult are listed in Chart 15–8.

CHART 15–8 Medication Cautions for the Older Adult

NSAIDS	Highly protein bound NSAIDS, such as aspirin, diflunisal, ibuprofen, naproxen, indomethacin, meclofenamate, and piroxicam are more likely than the younger population to cause toxicities.
Meperidine (Demerol)	The active metabolite normeperidine can cause CNS irritability leading to seizures. Delirium and agitation are more likely when used to treat the postoperative older adult. Metabolite accumulation and toxicity occur when renal function is impaired.
Propoxyphene (Darvon, Darvocet)	The active metabolite norpropoxyphene can make seizures and cardiac arrhythmias more likely to occur. Accumulation and toxicity occur when renal function is impaired.
Pentazocine (Talwin)	More likely to cause seizures, cardiac arrhythmias, and agitation. Analgesia is similar to aspirin.
Tricyclic antidepressants	Anticholinergic effects are often intolerable.
Sedatives, hypnotics, and antiemetics	Long duration of action and sedation side effects make the older adult more prone to delirium, and unstable gait leads to increased risk of falls. Can cause respiratory depression especially when given with opioids.
Antihistamines	Anticholinergic effects are often intolerable. Use should be limited to less than 12 weeks, and in lower dosage ranges.

Sources: American Geriatric Society, Panel on Chronic Pain in Older Persons. (2002). The management of persistent pain in older persons: AGS panel on persistent pain in older persons. *Journal of the American Geriatrics Society, 6*(50), 205–224; St. Marie, B. (2002). Gerontologic pain management. In B. St. Marie (Ed.), *Core curriculum for pain management nursing* (pp. 417–426). Philadelphia: W. B. Saunders; Pasero, C., & McCaffery, M. (2000). When patients can't report pain. *American Journal of Nursing, 100,* 22–23.

RESEARCH OPPORTUNITIES AND CLINICAL IMPACT RELATED TO PAIN MANAGEMENT

Research Area	Clinical Impact
Assessment tools that are culturally sensitive for ethnic minorities who speak English dialects and have low literacy levels	Improved ability to assess pain in this at-risk population of patients
Assessment tools that are disease specific	Improved ability to capture the unique components of pain in diseases such as sickle cell, HIV, or cancer
Outcomes related to high-technology implanted modalities	Improved understanding of when high technology will improve outcomes to facilitate development of clinical guidelines outlining best practices
Neural remodeling as a mechanism of chronic pain	Identification of preventive, management, and restorative treatment possibilities
Use of opioids for the treatment of chronic pain	Improved understanding of the impact of opioids on long-term health to facilitate development of clinical guidelines and consensus on best practice
Gender differences in chronic pain	Improved understanding of sex-related factors and mechanisms that could lead to the development of new medications and management strategies
Clinical trials of complementary and alternative therapies	Establishment of a base of scientific evidence to validate the use of these therapies in specific pain states
Genes that are relevant to pain and inhibitory mechanisms	Development of gene therapy models targeting specific structures within the central nervous system
The role of sleep and circadian variations in perception and modulation of pain	Understand the differences in pain perception and modulation for patients who have unusual sleep/rest/activity needs (e.g., night shift workers, people with insomnia)
Barriers to patient compliance with pain treatment plan	Development of assessments, tools, educational materials, or specific helps that are demonstrated to improve compliance

EVIDENCE-BASED PRACTICE

Pain Management

Clinical Problem

Management of patients' pain is an ongoing nursing challenge. Due to patients' individual perceptions and responses, it can be difficult to quantify the pain. Typically, health care providers order a variety of medications and dosages that can be administered based on the level of pain. Therefore, it is essential that nurses make an accurate assessment of the pain in order to make a decision regarding choice of medication. A number of pain intensity scales, as described earlier in this chapter, have been developed to assist in standardizing pain levels and subsequent management, but the controversy continues about the best method to quantify pain (Pasero & McCaffery, 2005).

Research Findings

McDonald, LaPorta, and Meadows-Olive (2007) conducted a study to determine nurses' responses to patients' reports of pain. The study evaluated three different methods patients used to describe their pain:

Personal description along with a numeric scale

Personal description only

Numeric scale only.

Nurses were randomly assigned to three groups and all were given a vignette about a trauma patient with moderate to severe pain. The vignettes were identical except for the three different methods used by the patients to describe their pain and the patient's age. The results showed that there was no difference in the nurses' responses to the pain management between the three modes. The authors further noted that a relatively small number of pain management strategies were identified by the sample nurses in response to moderately severe pain.

Implications for Nursing Practice

Knowledge of effective pain management is still an evolving area of health care. It is a multifaceted area with issues of effective relief, addiction, and legal ramifications woven into the management decisions. Nurses are in a pivotal position in the pain management arena and therefore must have knowledge of and an appreciation for these issues. Nurses' approach to pain management also requires sensitivity to individual responses to pain. When using the numeric scores it is important to use the appropriate terminology and to further inquire about the reason for the score on the pain scale (Thompson American Health Consultants, 2004). For example, some patients report a pain number and then state they are comfortable with a certain pain level as it relates to their diagnosis and do not require medication, whereas other patients report the same score and are not comfortable and therefore require treatment.

Prior use of both legal and illegal medications also may impact pain scores. Occasionally, patients with illicit drug histories demonstrate "drug-seeking" behaviors such as fabricating pain levels in order to receive medication. Nurses must come to understand individual nuances to effectively manage pain. Use of both personal account and numeric scales provides the nurse with more data when making treatment decisions.

Critical Thinking Questions

1. When a patient reports a pain score what further information is needed to determine the appropriate pain intervention?

2. How would a nurse assess the pain level in a nonverbal patient?

Answers to Critical Thinking Questions appear in Appendix D.

References

Pasero, C., & McCaffery, M. (2005). Pain control: No self-report means no pain-intensity rating: Assessing pain in patients who cannot provide a report. *American Journal of Nursing, 105*(10), 50–53.

Thompson American Health Consultants. (2004). *Managing pain and end of life issues* (Vol. 2). Atlanta: Author.

Research

The science of pain management is expanding with astonishing speed due to the ongoing efforts of scientists, nurses, and other health care providers who have dedicated time and energy to discovery. The "Decade of Pain Research" provides an opportunity to accomplish even more. The Research Opportunities and Clinical Impact feature provides a list of both medical and nursing research topics still under investigation.

Clinical Preparation

Read

- History of Current Illness
- Past Medical History
- Physical Exam
- Admitting Medical Orders
- Laboratory Study Results

Document

- Summary of Hospitalization
- Pathophysiology Form
- Laboratory Values
- Laboratory Results Explanation

Apply

- List of Potential Nursing Diagnoses
- Concept Map
- Critical Thinking Questions

Log on to MyNursingKit.com to download forms you will need and to complete further steps in the Clinical Preparation assignment.

HISTORY OF PRESENT ILLNESS

As the on-coming nurse on the orthopedic nursing unit in a major trauma hospital, you are receiving report about Mr. X, a 27-year-old male who was admitted to the hospital following a motor vehicle collision in which he was the unrestrained driver. Mr. X was ejected from the vehicle, but did not lose consciousness and was able to provide a brief medical history to paramedics at the scene. In the report, the night nurse stated that the patient was now 24 hours post-op following stabilization of an open book pelvic fracture with external fixation. He has multiple lacerations over his arms and legs and a large laceration on his head that the plastic surgeon repaired during surgery.

Medical–Surgical History

His past medical history includes asthma and multiple knee arthroscopies for sports-related injuries.

Social History

Mr. X is married and the father of two children ages 1 and 3. Mr. X's wife and parents are at his bedside. He denies medication allergies, alcohol, smoking, or drug abuse.

Physical Exam

Mr. X is alert, oriented, with no sedation. His respiratory status includes deep, even, respirations at a rate of 14 breaths per minute. He is able to maintain oxygen saturations of 93% to 97% on room air. He has clear breath sounds.

His pulse is regular and strong with an apical heart rate of 68 beats per minute with no extra heart sounds. He has 3+ peripheral pulses with capillary refill < 3 seconds in all extremities. Blood pressure is measured at 132/56.

Bowel sounds are present in all four quadrants of the abdomen and he denies nausea. He has passed flatus and his surgeon has prescribed advancement of diet as tolerated. He has not had a bowel movement since surgery.

A urinary catheter has been placed and is draining approximately 30 mL of dark yellow-brown urine per hour.

Current Pain Assessment

Mr. X reports pain in his lower abdomen bilaterally, right groin, and right shoulder. He rates his pain intensity using the numeric rating scale of 0 to 10 as 7/10 in his abdomen, 9/10 in his right groin, and 5/10 in his right knee. Mr. X describes the pain in his abdomen and right groin as constant, sharp, stabbing with occasional spasms, and the right knee pain as a constant, aching, throbbing pain. He reports his pain is unbearable when he is turned in bed to change the linens.

Mr. X expresses frustration and anger that his pain is unrelieved and that his life is ruined because of the injuries he has sustained. His wife expresses concern that he is not coping as he usually does when faced with difficult circumstances. The hospital chaplain has attempted to visit with Mr. X and his wife on two separate occasions, but each time Mr. X declines the visit stating that he is in too much pain. When Mr. X's wife leaves the room he is calm and watches the sports channel on the TV.

Admitting Medical Orders
Admit to trauma service
Diagnosis: multiple lacerations over arms, legs, and head; rule out internal injuries; open book pelvic fracture
No known allergies
Vital signs every 4 hours
Bed rest
Sequential compression devices (SCD) to lower extremities
Peroxide ½ strength to clean pin sites q12h
Foley catheter
Intake and output
IV: D5½NS plus KCl 20 mEq at 125 hour
NPO
Incentive spirometer q1h while awake and q4h at night
Clean lacerations with ½ strength hydrogen peroxide q8h
Call house officer: Pulse < 60 & > 110/minute; BP < 90 & > 160 systolic; temperature > 38.5; urine output < 30 mL/hr for 2 hours; respiratory rate > 30/minute

Scheduled Medications
IV PCA morphine 1 mg/mL; no continuous infusion, 1 mg PCA demand dose, a 6-minute lockout time, and a 12-mg hourly limit; may bolus with 2 mg every hour prn severe pain

PRN Medications
Phenergan 25 mg IV q6h prn nausea
Ativan 0.5–2 mg IV q6–8h prn anxiety (not to exceed 10 mg/24 hours)
Tylenol 650 mg PR q4h for pain
Benadryl 25–50 mg IV qhs

Ordered Laboratory Studies
CBC q6h times 24 hours, then daily; basic metabolic panel daily, UA ×1 now

Ordered Diagnostic Studies
12-lead ECG
PA and lateral chest x-ray
X-ray of right knee and pelvis post-fixation

LABORATORY STUDY RESULTS

Test	Day 1	Day 2	Day 3
Potassium	4.4 mEq/L	3.8 mEq/L	3.7 mEq/L
Chloride	106 mEq/L	106 mEq/L	111 mEq/L
Sodium	142 mEq/L	141 mEq/L	144 mEq/L
Carbon dioxide (CO_2)	24 mEq/L	24 mEq/L	27 mEq/L
Anion gap	12.4 mEq/L	11.8 mEq/L	7.1 mEq/L
Glucose	97 mg/dL	99 mg/dL	119 mg/dL
Blood urea nitrogen (BUN)	22 mg/dL	22 mg/dL	20 mg/dL
Creatinine	0.8 mg/dL	0.8 mg/dL	1.4 mg/dL
Calcium	8.2 mg/dL	8.2 mg/dL	7.7 mg/dL
Hemoglobin	10/10.2/9.8/10/9.9/10.1 g/dL	10.1 g/dL	10.4 g/dL
Hematocrit	33/33.4/34/32.3/33/34/33/%	33.6 %	34%
Urinalysis			
Appearance and color	Dark amber and clear		
pH	6.2		
Protein	6 mg/dL		
Specific gravity	1.025		
Leukocytes, nitrates, ketones, and bilirubin	All negative		
Urobilinogen	0.02 units/mL		
Crystals and casts	None		
Glucose	None		
WBC and RBC	None		

CRITICAL THINKING QUESTIONS

1. Which dimensions of pain would you consider significant when reviewing your assessment of Mr. X's pain?

2. Which nursing intervention would be appropriate for the change in behavior when Mr. X's wife leaves the room?

3. What additional assessments would be important to consider prior to contacting the prescribing health care provider to advocate for changes to Mr. X's pain medications?

Answers to Critical Thinking Questions appear in Appendix D.

NCLEX® REVIEW

1. After attending a symposium on pain assessment and management, the well-informed nurse understands that pain:
   1. Is a common symptom to most illnesses, disease processes, and traumatic injuries.
   2. Is recognized, expressed, and responded to similarly among all cultures.
   3. Is addressed by a friendly health care system that is willing and able to manage pain.
   4. Is rarely associated with significant personal, social, or economic distress.

2. Confusion about treatment goals and the reality of pain abound, requiring nurses to make many legal and ethical decisions regarding pain and pain management. The nurse implementing a plan of care for the patient with chronic nonmalignant pain should:
   1. Identify that chronic nonmalignant pain is usually directly proportional to objective disease severity.
   2. Exclude the use of chronic opiates when the patient also requires treatment for concurrent psychiatric disorders.
   3. Recognize the fundamental responsibility of all nurses to help alleviate patient suffering and relieve pain.
   4. Acknowledge the patient's own fears of facing criminal penalties for receiving excessive amounts of opiates.

3. The nurse is educating the patient with chronic pain about his condition. The nurse knows the patient has a clear understanding of chronic pain with verbalization of the statement:
   1. "My pain should be brief and then resolve completely."
   2. "The pain I am having coincides with my recent surgery."
   3. "This pain will not last long, but will come back soon."
   4. "My pain may last for months, years, or for my whole life."

4. The nurse recognizes that two of the most accurate multidimensional evaluation methods when assessing a patient's pain would be:
   1. A patient's pain intensity self-report and behavioral assessment.
   2. The McGill Pain Questionnaire and the patient interview.
   3. The numeric rating scale and simple verbal descriptive scale.
   4. A Critical-Care Pain Observation Tool and visual analog scale.

Answers for review questions appear in Appendix D

KEY TERMS

absorption *p.343*
acute pain *p.334*
adjuvant medications *p.347*
affective dimension of pain *p.336*
agonist *p.341*
agonist-antagonist *p.347*
antagonist *p.347*
behavioral dimension of pain *p.337*
biotransformation *p.343*
breakthrough pain *p.335*
Brief Pain Inventory (BPI) *p.339*
cancer pain *p.335*
chronic pain *p.334*

cognitive dimension of pain *p.336*
distribution *p.343*
elimination *p.343*
endorphins *p.336*
enkephalins *p.336*
gate control theory *p.335*
hepatic first-pass metabolism *p.343*
McGill Pain Questionnaire (MPQ) *p.339*
metabolism *p.343*
neuromatrix theory *p.335*
neuropathic pain *p.336*
nociception *p.335*
nociceptive pain *p.335*

noxious stimuli *p.335*
numeric rating scale (NRS) *p.338*
pain *p.334*
pattern theory *p.335*
phantom limb pain *p.335*
recurrent pain *p.334*
sensory dimension of pain *p.336*
simple verbal descriptive scale (SVDS) *p.338*
specificity theory *p.335*
transduction *p.335*
transient pain *p.335*
visual analog scale (VAS) *p.338*

EXPLORE PEARSON mynursingkit™

MyNursingKit is your one stop for online chapter review materials and resources. Prepare for success with additional NCLEX®-style practice questions, interactive assignments and activities, web links, animations and videos, and more!

Register your access code from the front of your book at
www.mynursingkit.com

REFERENCES

Agency for Health Care Policy and Research, Acute Pain Management Guideline Panel. (1992, February). *Acute pain management: Operative or medical procedures and trauma* (Clinical Practice Guideline, AHCPR Pub. No. 92-0032). Rockville, MD: Author.

American Academy of Pain Medicine, American Pain Society, & American Society of Addiction Medicine. (2001). *Definitions related to the use of opioids for the treatment of pain.* Glenview, IL: American Pain Society.

American Geriatric Society, Panel on Chronic Pain in Older Persons. (2002). The management of persistent pain in older persons: AGS panel on persistent pain in older persons. *Journal of the American Geriatrics Society, 6*(50), 205–224.

American Nurses Association. (2001). *Code for nurses with interpretive statements.* Kansas City, MO: Author.

American Pain Society. (2000). *Principles of analgesic use in the treatment of acute pain and cancer pain* (4th ed.). Glenview, IL: Author.

American Pain Society. (2003). *Principles of analgesic use in the treatment of acute pain and cancer pain* (5th ed.). Glenview, IL: Author.

American Pain Society. (2005). *Guideline for the management of cancer pain in adults and children.* Glenview, IL: Author.

American Society for Pain Management Nursing. (2007). *ASPMN position statement: Assisted suicide.* Retrieved February 12, 2007, from http://www.aspmn.org/pdfs/Assisted%20Suicide.pdf

Arnstein, P. M. (2003). Comprehensive analysis and management of chronic pain. *The Nursing Clinics of North America, 38*(3), 403–417.

Arnstein, P. M., Wells-Federman, C. L., & Caudill-Slosberg, M. A. (2002, August). *Change in self efficacy as a predictor of clinical outcomes and coping skill use at 1 year following participation in a cognitive behavioral pain treatment program.* Paper presented at the 10th World Congress on Pain, San Diego, CA.

Backonja, M. (2001). Painful neuropathies. In J. D. Loeser, S. H. Butler, C. R. Chapman, & D. C. Turk (Eds.), *Bonica's management of pain* (3rd ed., pp. 371–387). Philadelphia: Lippincott Williams & Wilkins.

Bajwa, Z. H., Warfield, C. A., & Wootton, R. J. (2006). *Overview of treatment for chronic pain.* Retrieved February 25, 2007, from UpToDate website: http://utdol.com/utd/store/index.do

Bonica, J. J., & Loeser, J. D. (2001). History of pain concepts and therapies. In J. D. Loeser, S. H. Butler, C. R. Chapman, & D. C. Turk (Eds.), *Bonica's management of pain* (3rd ed., pp. 3–16). Philadelphia: Lippincott Williams & Wilkins.

Brookhoff, D. (2000). Chronic pain: A new disease? *Hospital Practice,* 23–50.

Brown, J., Phillips, P. Cusimano, C., & Osteyee, J. (2003). *ASPMN position statement: Pain management at the end of life.* Retrieved from American Society for Pain Management Nursing website: http://www.aspmn.org

Buckley, P. F. (2001). Regional anesthesia with local anesthetics. In J. D. Loeser, S. H. Butler, C. R. Chapman, & D. C. Turk (Eds.), *Bonica's management of pain* (3rd ed., pp. 1893–1966). Philadelphia: Lippincott Williams & Wilkins.

Byers, M. R., & Bonica, J. J. (2001). Peripheral pain mechanisms and nociceptor plasticity. In J. D. Loeser, S. H. Butler, C. R. Chapman, & D. C. Turk (Eds.), *Bonica's management of pain* (3rd ed., pp. 26–72). Philadelphia: Lippincott Williams & Wilkins.

Campbell, C. E. (2006). The role of nursing in pain management. In M. V. Boswell & B. E. Cole (Eds.), *Weiner's pain management: A practical guide for clinicians* (7th ed., pp. 165–175). Boca Raton, FL: Taylor & Francis Group.

Campbell, J. (1995, November 11). *Pain: The fifth vital sign.* Presidential address presented at the meeting of the American Pain Society, Los Angeles.

Chiu, L. H., Trinca, J., Lim, L. M., & Tuazon, J. A. (2003). A study to evaluate the pain knowledge of two sub-populations of final year nursing students: Australia and Philippines. *Journal of Advanced Nursing, 41,* 99–108.

Coda, B. A., & Bonica, J. J. (2001). General considerations in acute pain. In J. D. Loeser, S. H. Butler, C. R. Chapman, & D. C. Turk (Eds.), *Bonica's management of pain* (3rd ed., pp. 222–254). Philadelphia: Lippincott Williams & Wilkins.

Coggins, C., Arnstein, P., & Leahy, S. (2004). *ASPMN position statement: Use of placebos for pain management.* Retrieved from American Society for Pain Management Nursing website: http://www.aspmn.org

Coggins, C., McCaffery, M., Pasero, C., St. Marie, B., & Nichols, R. (2003). *ASPMN position statement: Pain management in patients with addictive disease.* Retrieved from American Society for Pain Management Nursing website: http://www.aspmn.org

Dahl, J. L. (2002). Working with regulators to improve the standard of care in pain management: The U.S. experience. *Journal of Pain and Symptom Management, 24,* 136–157.

Davis, M. P., Walsh, D., LeGrand, S. B., & Naughton, M. (2002). Symptom control in cancer patients: The clinical pharmacology and therapeutic role of suppositories and rectal suspensions. *Support Care Cancer, 10,* 117–138.

Ferrell, B. R., Novy, D., Sullivan, M. D., Banja, J., Dubois, M. Y., Gitlin, M., et al. (2001). Ethical dilemmas in pain management. *Journal of Pain, 2*(3), 171–180.

Frank-Stromborg, M., & Christensen, A. (2001). A serious look at the undertreatment of pain: Part I. *Clinical Journal of Oncology Nursing, 5*(5), 235–236.

Gelinas, C., Fillion, L., Puntillo, K. A., Viens, C., & Fortier, M. (2006). Validation of the Critical-Care Pain Observation Tool in adult patients. *American Journal of Critical Care, 15*(4), 420–427.

Gelinas, C., Fortier, M., Viens, C., Fillion, L., & Puntillo, K. A. (2004). Pain assessment and management in critically-ill intubated patients: A retrospective study. *American Journal of Critical Care, 13*(2), 126–135.

Glen, V. L., & St. Marie, B. (2002). Overview of pharmacology. In B. St. Marie (Ed.), *Core curriculum for pain management nursing* (pp. 181–202). Philadelphia: W. B. Saunders.

Griffie, J. (2003). Addressing inadequate pain relief. *American Journal of Nursing, 103*(8), 61–63.

Herr, K. (2002). Pain assessment in cognitively impaired older adults. *American Journal of Nursing,102,* 65–67.

Herr, K., Coyne, P. J., Key, T., Manworren, R., McCaffery, M., Merkel, S., et al. (2006). Pain assessment in the nonverbal patient: Position statement with clinical practice recommendations. *Pain Management Nursing, 7*(2), 44–52.

Houde, R., Wallenstein, S., & Beaver, W. (1996). Evaluation of analgesics in patients with cancer pain. In L. Lasagna (Ed.), *International Encyclopedia of Pharmacology and Therapeutics. Section 6, Clinical Pharmacology* (Vol. 1, pp. 59–98). Oxford: Pergamon Press.

International Association for the Study of Pain. (1993). *Outline curriculum on pain for schools of nursing.* Retrieved February 23, 2007, from http://www.iasp-pain.org/nursing_toc.html

International Council of Nurses. (2006). *The ICN code of ethics for nurses.* Geneva, Switzerland: Author.

Jacox, A., Carr, D. B., Payne, R., et al. (1994, March). *Management of cancer pain* (Clinical Practice Guideline No. 9, AHCPR Pub. No. 94-0592). Rockville, MD: Agency for Health Care Policy and Research.

Jakobsson, U., Klevsgard, R., Westergren, A., & Rahm Hallberg, I. (2003). Old people in pain: A comparative study. *Journal of Pain and Symptom Management, 26,* 625–636.

Joint Commission on Accreditation of Healthcare Organizations. (2002). *Pain assessment and management: An organizational approach.* Retrieved February 26, 2007, from http://www.jointcommission.org

Kaplow, R., & Hardin, S. R. (2007). *Critical care nursing: Synergy for optimal outcomes* (pp. 41–51). Sudbury, MA: Jones and Bartlett.

Karch, A. M, & Karch, F. E. (2003). Acetaminophen's hidden dangers. *American Journal of Nursing, 103,* 101.

Lethridge-Cejku, M., & Vickerie, J. (2005). Summary health for U.S. adults: National health interview survey, 2003. *National Center for Health Statistics, 10,* 225.

Maher, T. J., & Chaiyakul, P. (2003). Opioids (Bench). In H.S. Smith, *Drugs for pain* (pp. 83–96). Philadelphia, PA: Hanley & Belfus, Inc.

McCaffery, M. (1968). *Nursing practice theories related to cognition, bodily pain, and man–environment interactions.* Los Angeles: University of California at Los Angeles Students' Store.

McCaffery, M., & Pasero, C. (1999). Assessment: Underlying complexities, misconceptions, and practical tools. In M. McCaffery & C. Pasero (Eds.), *Pain: Clinical manual* (2nd ed., pp. 35–102). St. Louis, MO: Mosby.

McCaffery, M., & Portenoy, R. K. (1999). Nonopioids. In M. McCaffery & C. Pasero (Eds.), *Pain: Clinical manual* (2nd ed., pp. 129–160). St. Louis, MO: Mosby.

McCaffery, M., Ferrell, B. R., & Pasero, C. (2000). Nurses' personal opinions about patients' pain and their effect on recorded assessments and titration of opioid doses. *Pain Management Nursing, 1*(3), 70–87.

McDonald, D. D. (2006). Postoperative pain management for the aging patient. *Geriatrics Aging, 9*(6), 395–398.

Melzack, R., & Wall, P. D. (1983). *The challenge of pain.* New York: Basic Books.

Melzack, R. (1999). From gate to neuromatrix. *Pain, 6*(Suppl.), S121–S126.

Merck. (2007). Types: Pain. In *The Merck Manual of Medical Information—Home Edition.* Retrieved May 27, 2008, from http://www.merck.com/mmhe/sec06/ch078/ch078b.html?qt=types:%20pain&alt=sh

Mersky, H. (1994). Classification of chronic pain: Descriptions of chronic pain syndromes and definitions of pain terms. *Pain* (Suppl. 3), S215–S221.

Miyoshi, H. R., & Leckband, S. G. (2001). Systemic opioid analgesics. In J. D. Loeser, S. H. Butler, C. R. Chapman, & D. C. Turk (Eds.), *Bonica's management of pain* (3rd ed., pp. 1682–1709). Philadelphia: Lippincott Williams & Wilkins.

Morgan, J. P. (1985). American opiophobia: Customary underutilization of opioid analgesics. *Advances in Alcohol and Substance Abuse, 86*(5), 163–173.

National Cancer Institute. (2007). *Pain PDQ: Pharmacologic management.* Retrieved February 19, 2007, from http://www.cancer.gov/cancertopics/pdq/supportivecare/pain/HealthProfessional/Page3

National Institutes of Health. (1987). The integrated approach to the management of pain. *Journal of Pain and Symptom Management, 2,* 35–44.

National Institute of Neurological Disorders and Stroke. (2007a). *Chronic pain information page.* Retrieved February 19, 2007, from http://www.ninds.nih.gov/disorders/chronic_pain/chronic_pain.htm

National Institute of Neurological Disorders and Stroke. (2007b). *Gene therapy relieves neuropathic pain.* Retrieved February 19, 2007, from http://www.ninds.nih.gov/news_and_events/news_articles/news_article_pain_gene_therapy.htm

Parke, B. (1998). Gerontological nurses' ways of knowing. Realizing the presence of pain in cognitively impaired older adults. *Journal of Gerontological Nursing, 24*(6), 21–28.

Pasero, C., & McCaffery, M. (2000). When patients can't report pain. *American Journal of Nursing, 100,* 22–23.

Pasero, C., & McCaffery, M. (2001b). The patient's report of pain: Believing vs. accepting. There's a big difference. *American Journal of Nursing, 101,* 73–74.

Pasero, C., & McCaffery, M. (2001c). The undertreatment of pain: Are providers accountable for it? *American Journal of Nursing, 101,* 62–65.

Pasero, C., & McCaffery, M. (2005). Pain control: No self-report means no pain-intensity rating: Assessing pain in patients who cannot provide a report. *American Journal of Nursing, 105*(10), 50–53.

Pasero, C., Paice, J. A., & McCaffery, M. (1999). Basic mechanisms underlying the causes and effects of pain. In M. McCaffery &

C. Pasero (Eds.), *Pain: Clinical manual* (2nd ed., pp. 15–34). St. Louis, MO: Mosby.

Pautex, S., & Gold, G. (2006) Assessing pain intensity in older adults. *Geriatrics Aging. 9*(6), 399–402.

Phillips, P., Gordon, D., & Frandsen, J. (2006). *ASPMN position statement: The use of "as-needed" range orders for opioid analgesics in the management of acute pain.* Retrieved from American Society for Pain Management Nursing website: http://www.aspmn.org

Portenoy, R. K., & Hagen, N. A. (1990). Breakthrough pain: Definition, prevalence and characteristics. *Pain, 41,* 273–281.

Portenoy, R. K., & McCaffery, M. (1999). Adjuvant Analgesics. In M. McCaffery & C. Pasero (Eds.), *Pain: Clinical manual* (2nd ed., pp. 302). St. Louis, MO: Mosby.

Porth, C. M. (2005). *Pathophysiology: Concepts of altered health states* (7th ed.). Philadelphia: Lippincott Williams & Wilkins.

Price, D. D., Riley, J. L., & Wade, J. B. (2001). Psychological approaches to measurement of the dimensions and stages of pain. In D. C. Turk & R. Melzack (Eds.), *Handbook of pain assessment* (2nd ed., pp. 53–75). New York: Guilford Press.

Primeau, M., Cowley, C., Eksterowicz, N., & Pasero, C. (2007). *ASPMN position statement: Registered nurse management and monitoring of analgesia by catheter techniques.* Retrieved from the American Society for Pain Management Nursing website: http://www.aspmn. org

Puntillo, K. A. (2007). Managing pain, delirium, and sedation. *Critical care nurse* (Suppl.), 8–10.

Puntillo, K. A., Morris, A. B., Thompson, C. L., Stanik-Hutt, J. A., White, L., & Wild, L. J. (2004). Behaviors observed during six common procedures: Results from thunder project II. *Critical Care Medicine, 32*(2), 412–427.

Rothley, B. B., & Therrien, S. R. (2002). Acute pain management. In B. St. Marie (Ed.), *Core curriculum for pain management nursing* (pp. 239–272). Philadelphia: W. B. Saunders.

Shea, R. A., Brooks, J. A., Dayhoff, N. E., & Keck, J. (2002). Pain intensity and postoperative pulmonary complications among the elderly after abdominal surgery. *Heart & Lung, 31,* 440–449.

Simon, L. S. (2003). Nonsteroidal anti-inflammatory drugs and cyclooxygenase-2 selective inhibitors. In H. S. Smith (Ed.), *Drugs for pain* (pp. 41–54). Philadelphia: Hanley & Belfus.

Smith, H. S. (2003). Acetaminophen (bedside). In H. S. Smith (Ed.), *Drugs for pain* (pp. 33–40). Philadelphia: Hanley & Belfus.

Snyder, M., & Wieland, J. (2003). Complimentary and alternative therapies: What is their place in management of chronic pain? *The Nursing Clinics of North America, 38*(3), 495–508.

Soscia, J. (2003). Assessing pain in cognitively impaired older adults with cancer. *Clinical Journal of Oncology Nursing, 7*(2), 174–177.

St. Marie, B., & Loeb, J. L. (2002). Gerontologic pain management. In B. St. Marie (Ed.), *Core curriculum for pain management nursing* (pp. 417–426). Philadelphia: W. B. Saunders.

Sullivan, M., & Ferrell, B. (2005). *Ethical challenges in the management of chronic nonmalignant pain: Negotiating through the cloud of doubt.* Retrieved February 25, 2007, from American Pain Society, http://www.ampainsoc.org/press/2005_jop/0105.html

Swarm, R. A., Karanikolas, M., & Kalauokalani, D. (2001). Pain treatment in the perioperative period. *Current Problems in Surgery, 38,* 835–920.

Turk, D. C. (2006). Pain hurts—Individuals, significant others, and society. *American Pain Society Bulletin, 16*(1).

Turk, D. C., & Okifuji, A. (2001). Pain terms and taxonomies of pain. In J. D. Loeser, S. H. Butler, C. R. Chapman, & D. C. Turk (Eds.), *Bonica's management of pain* (3rd ed., pp. 17–25). Philadelphia: Lippincott Williams & Wilkins.

Watt-Watson, J., Stevens, B., Garfinkel, P., Streiner, D., & Gallop, R. (2001). Relationship between nurses' pain knowledge and pain management outcomes for their postoperative cardiac patients. *Journal of Advanced Nursing, 36,* 535–545.

Weiner, D. K., & Hanlon, J. T. (2001). Pain in nursing home residents: Management strategies. *Drugs and Aging, 18*(1), 13–19.

Weissman, D. E., & Haddox, J. D. (1989). Opioid pseudoaddiction—An iatrogenic syndrome. *Pain, 36,* 363–366.

Wisconsin Cancer Pain Initiative Nursing Education Committee. (1995). Competency guidelines for cancer pain in nursing education and practice. Retrieved May 27, 2008, from http://www.cityofhope.org/prc/pdf/Competency_Guidelines_ WCPI.pdf

Wittbrodt, E. T., & Tietze, K. J. (2004). *Pain control in the intensive care unit.* Retrieved February 25, 2007, from UpToDate website: http://utdol.com/utd/store/index.do

Wuhrman, E., Cooney, M. F., Dunwoody, C. J., Eksterowicz, N., Merkel, S., & Oakes, L. L. (2006). *ASPMN position statement: Authorized and unauthorized ("PCA by proxy") dosing of analgesic infusion pumps.* Retrieved from American Society for Pain Management Nursing website: http://www.aspmn.org

Wynne, C. F., Ling, S. M., Remsburg, R. (2000). Comparison of pain assessment instruments in cognitively intact and cognitively impaired nursing home residents. *Geriatric Nursing, 21,* 20–23.

Youngkin, E. Q., Sawin, K. J., Kissinger, J. F., & Israel, D. S. (2005). *Pharmacotherapeutics: A primary care guide* (2nd ed.). Upper Saddle River, NJ: Pearson Prentice Hall.

Substance Abuse

Eileen Trigoboff

Outcome-Based Learning Objectives

After studying this chapter, the learner will be able to:

1. Explain the major theories about substance-related disorders.
2. List why some groups are at risk for substance-related disorders.
3. Discuss how the physical, psychological, and withdrawal effects of the major categories of substances manifest themselves.
4. Incorporate nursing assessment components to detect patients who have substance-related disorders.
5. Demonstrate knowledge of a variety of short-term and long-term nursing intervention strategies for clients who have substance-related disorders.
6. Develop outcome criteria for clients who have substance-related disorders.
7. Establish what impact your own feelings and attitudes about clients with substance-related disorders have in your nursing care.

SUBSTANCE ABUSE is the clinical term for people who use or abuse prescription or recreational substances in order to experience one of the following: escape, relief, get a buzz, get away, get in touch, get cushioned, deserve a break, feel high, feel happy, feel numb, feel something, feel normal, feel distant, leave this realm of existence, or any other phrase describing the urge behind the behavior. This behavior is a way for people to cope or escape stress through substance abuse.

Substance abuse affects society as a whole by robbing it of valuable members. It increases the crime rate, automobile crash deaths, number of teenage pregnancies, and the suicide rate, while decreasing the quality of life for individuals and families (National Drug Intelligence Center [NDIC], 2006). There is not a single aspect of a substance abuser's life—social life, family life, community involvement, work productivity, coworker relationships, physical health—that escapes being affected.

The American Nurses Association (ANA) Standards of Addictions Nursing Practice demonstrate how important it is for nurses to understand the implications of addiction. There is an ongoing need for thorough assessment and collaborative treatment with other health care providers. The high incidence of substance abuse in society demands that nurses exhibit competence when treating patients with addictions. See the National Guidelines box for a list of the ANA standards (p. 366).

Definitions and Terminology

Nurses must know the language for this particular area of health care. The terms used to describe substance use and abuse include the names of the various stages of substance use as well as characteristics of behavior within that stage. Accurate nursing assessment is based on a good understanding of these terms.

Substance-Related Disorders

According to the *Diagnostic and Statistical Manual of Mental Disorders*, Fourth Edition, Text Revision (DSM-IV-TR) (American Psychiatric Association [APA], 2000), substance-related disorders are disorders that are (1) a consequence of abusing a drug (such as alcohol), (2) the side effects of a medication (antihistamines, for example), or (3) related to exposure to a toxin (fuel, paint, or other inhalants). Substance-related disorders are divided into two groups:

1. Substance use disorders that include substance dependence and substance abuse
2. Substance-induced disorders (including substance intoxication, substance withdrawal, and substance-induced cognitive disorders and mood disorders).

This chapter focuses on substance abuse. Material in this chapter refers to intoxication and withdrawal issues for some

NATIONAL GUIDELINES ANA Standards of Addictions Nursing Practice

Standard 1: Assessment

The addictions nurse collects patient health data.

Standard 2: Diagnosis

The addictions nurse analyzes the assessment data in determining diagnoses.

Standard 3: Outcome Identification

The addictions nurse identifies expected outcomes individualized to the patient.

Standard 4: Planning

The addictions nurse develops an individualized plan of care that prescribes interventions to attain expected outcomes.

Standard 5: Implementation

The addictions nurse implements the interventions identified in the plan of care.

Standard 5a: Therapeutic Alliance: The addictions nurse uses the "therapeutic self" to establish a therapeutic alliance with the patient and to structure nursing interventions to promote development of insight, coping skills, and motivation for change in behavior that promotes health.

Standard 5b: Health Teaching: The addictions nurse, through health teaching, assists individuals, families, groups, and communities in achieving satisfying, productive, and healthy patterns of living.

Standard 5c: Self-Care and Self-Management: The addictions nurse uses the knowledge and philosophy of self-care and self-management to assist the patient in learning new ways to address stress, maintain self-control, accept personal responsibility, and integrate healthy coping behaviors into lifestyle choices.

Standard 5d: Pharmacological, Biological, and Complementary Therapies: The addictions nurse applies knowledge of pharmacological, biological, and complementary therapies and uses clinical skills to restore the patient's health and prevent consequences from addiction.

Standard 5e: Therapeutic Milieu: The addictions nurse structures, provides, and maintains a therapeutic environment in collaboration with the patient and other health care providers.

Standard 5f: Counseling: The addictions nurse uses counseling interventions to assist patients in promoting healthy coping abilities, preventing addiction, and addressing issues related to patterns of abuse and addiction.

Standard 6: Evaluation

The addictions nurse evaluates the patient's progress toward attainment of expected outcomes.

Reprinted with permission from American Nurses Association and International Nurses Society on Addictions, Scope and Standards of Addictions Nursing Practice, © 2004 Nursesbooks.org, Silver Spring, MD.

classes of substances that have traditionally been called psychoactive drugs. Some of the often-abused drugs are listed in the Pharmacology Summary box.

Substance Dependence

Substance dependence is defined as a maladaptive pattern of substance use leading to clinically significant impairment or distress. The hallmarks of this pattern are:

- **Tolerance**, or needing increased amounts of a substance to achieve the desired effect
- **Withdrawal**, or the uncomfortable and maladaptive physiological and cognitive behavioral changes that are associated with lowered blood or tissue concentrations of a substance after an individual has been engaged in heavy use
- Compulsive use
- Needing larger amounts of the substance than intended
- Making unsuccessful efforts to cut down or regulate substance use
- Devoting a great deal of time trying to obtain the substance
- Using the substance or recovering from the effects of the substance
- Continuing to use the substance despite the recognition of associated adverse effects and difficulties (APA, 2000).

This diagnosis can be made for every class of substance except caffeine.

Substance Abuse

Substance abuse is characterized by a pattern of repeated consumption of substances that are used despite harm. Examples of the harm that can result include the failure to fulfill major role obligations (such as parenting), using substances in physically hazardous situations (such as crack houses), and repeated social and relationship problems (domestic violence) (Libby et al., 2006).

Substance Intoxication

Substance intoxication refers to a reversible syndrome of maladaptive physiological and behavioral changes that are due to the effects of a substance on a person's central nervous system (CNS). The syndrome includes disturbances of mood (such as belligerence or mood lability), perception, the sleep–wake cycle, attention, thinking, judgment, and psychomotor as well as interpersonal behavior (Doweiko, 2006).

Substance Withdrawal

Substance withdrawal refers to the development of maladaptive physiological, behavioral, and cognitive changes that are due to reducing or stopping the heavy and regular use of a substance. Some examples include muscle aches, nausea, diarrhea, and increased blood pressure. **Substance withdrawal syndrome** is associated with distress and/or impairment in important areas of social functioning.

Postacute Withdrawal Syndrome

Postacute withdrawal syndrome (PAWS) occurs well after the usual withdrawal symptoms have resolved. It is a physiological state stimulated or stamped on the individual's metabolism and physical responses through drug use. The syndrome is seen as enduring physical remnants of neurotransmitter production and/or receptor site damage. Neurotransmitter production problems, either overproduction or underproduction, affect

PHARMACOLOGY Summary of Medications to Treat Substance-Related Disorders

Medication Category	Action	Application/Indication	Nursing Responsibilities
Replacement Agent/ Anticonvulsant Magnesium sulfate	Anticonvulsant Activities Produced by CNS depression	Magnesium deficiency Seizure treatment and prevention	• Monitor for adverse effects: hypotension, hypothermia, stupor, respiratory depression. • Observe for signs of magnesium toxicity: cathartic effect, profound thirst, sedation, confusion, muscle weakness. Have calcium gluconate available as antidote. • Monitor EKG and vital signs when given IV. • Monitor renal function, magnesium, calcium, and phosphorous levels.
Anxiolytic/Anticonvulsant Diazepam (Valium) Chlordiazepoxide (Librium)	Reduces withdrawal symptoms by action on limbic and subcortical levels of CNS	Symptoms of acute alcohol withdrawal, prophylaxis and treatment of seizures, delirium tremens	• Monitor for adverse effects: drowsiness, fatigue, weakness, ataxia. • Monitor vital signs closely if given parenterally. • Be aware of drug interactions (phenytoin, cimetidine, CNS depressants and others). • Be aware of multiple IV incompatibilities (furosemide, heparin, potassium chloride, and others). • Monitor CBC and liver function if used long term. • Warn patient not to abruptly stop drug.
Antialcohol Agent Disulfiram (Antabuse)	Produces undesirable symptoms as a deterrent to alcohol ingestion by inhibiting acetaldehyde dehydrogenase which normally detoxifies and metabolizes alcohol	Alcohol cessation aid	• Monitor liver function, CBC. • Do not administer unless patient has been alcohol free for a minimum of 12 hours. • Be aware of drug interactions (warfarin, phenytoin, barbiturate, and others). • Warn patient not to consume alcohol in any form including cough and cold preparations, mouthwash, sauces, etc. • Warn patient of potential severe reactions if alcohol ingested while on medication (myocardial infarction, convulsions, respiratory depression, sudden death).
Opiate Antagonist Naltrexone (ReVia)	Reduces euphoria and drug craving by binding with opioid receptors	Adjunct to treatment of narcotic addiction and alcohol dependence	• Give naloxone challenge test before starting naltrexone. • Monitor for adverse effects: nausea, vomiting, abdominal cramps, muscle pain, insomnia, anxiety. • Monitor liver function. • Warn patient to check with physician before using OTC drugs. • Warn patient of risk of overdosing if opiates used.

mood, interpersonal interactions, and cognitive skills. Receptor site damage means that naturally produced neurotransmitters cannot be normally recognized, absorbed, or provide feedback. Therefore, normal functioning is impaired.

Evidence of PAWS is seen as unusual or flattened interpersonal styles, disabilities in functioning within demanding zones such as personal finances and stress, poor occupational/vocational functioning, and difficulties establishing and maintaining relationships. Typical symptoms of PAWS include inability to think clearly, memory problems, emotional overreactions or numbness, sleep disturbances, difficulty with physical coordination, and stress sensitivity. A common reaction from others is to believe that the person who was dependent on a substance and has been abstaining is now using again. This creates social stressors in addition to the physiological and cognitive problems.

Clinicians reporting on their work with alcohol- and substance-dependent individuals anecdotally reported these problems. For a period of time in the 1990s attempts were made to codify these reports in the hope of establishing a verifiable postacute withdrawal syndrome. However, since about 2000 it appears that efforts to accomplish this have been discontinued. It seems likely that the reported aftereffects may be variable enough such that they do not cohere to form a true medical syndrome.

Etiology

The etiology of substance abuse, or what the causative factor or factors may be, describes how the problem of using substances inappropriately came into being. It is important to determine where and why the problem started in order to develop interventions to address the source.

Biological Theories

The biological explanation of substance abuse has had a great deal of support from recent developments in technology. With the use of magnetic resonance imaging (MRI) and positron emission tomograph (PET) scans, more details about the brain's function can be seen than ever before. Advances in neuroimaging and anatomic discoveries help explain substance abuse in terms of changes in the limbic area of the brain (Heimer & Van Hoesen, 2006). Other studies show biologic explanations of substance abuse and how genes affect the functioning of differential biochemical systems (Serretti et al., 2006), genotypes consistently indicating a relationship with substance abuse problems (Prescott et al., 2006), and the role of family genetics in the development of substance use disorders (Vieten, Seaton, Feiler, & Wilhelmsen, 2004).

Substance abuse prior to conception and pregnancy has such a strong biologic impact that in both males and females it has been validated as damaging to the genetic makeup of the child (Muthen, Asparouhov, & Rebollo, 2006). Research demonstrates that children of people who abuse alcohol have a fourfold risk of becoming alcohol abusers themselves. Even if different families adopt them at birth, identical twins of alcoholic parents have more than a 60% chance of becoming alcoholics; fraternal twins have just under a 30% chance.

Neurobiologic studies clearly support the fact that biologic factors such as genetics shape vulnerability to substance-related disorders and also result from them. Additional biologic foundations can be seen in the treatment of substance abuse. The body's responses to medications with anxiolytic and antidepressant effects used in detoxification and relapse-prevention treatment further support a biologic framework for substance abuse. Genetics may also be involved, as discussed in the Genetic Considerations box.

Psychological Theories

Psychological theories about substance abuse indicate that the psychological underpinnings of experiences and behaviors come together to form the motivations for using substances in a destructive manner. People respond to environmental influences through their underlying neurobiologic system. The remarkable frequency of some disorders—such as bipolar disorder—along with substance abuse further supports how psychological experiences and symptoms affect subsequent maladaptive coping (Albanese, 2005).

Dimensions of a person's personality, up to and including a characterological or personality disorder, can be detected in drug abusers. Routinely identified characteristics include inner dishonesty and self-centeredness, although self-centeredness could be related to the addiction itself. When someone is addicted to a substance, nothing is as important as the drug and the acquiring of it. A number of personality traits, as listed in Chart 16–1, are often associated with disruptive substance abuse.

GENETIC CONSIDERATIONS Related to Substance Abuse

We now have an understanding that a genetic predisposition can provide the base for vulnerabilities to substance abuse, but environment and experiences have an enormous influence on whether those genetics are expressed (Dick & Bierut, 2006). Questions such as whether genes have a substantial influence on adolescent substance abuse are answered considering the variety of contributions to adolescent behavior. Substance use and abuse is not a simple formula with two ingredients but a complex layering and melding of experiences and susceptibilities.

Drug use affects human development on the genetic level because drug use impacts sperm and egg health. Each partner contributes, such as when a male uses a substance and subsequently impregnates a woman, when a woman uses drugs prior to pregnancy, or when a woman uses substances during pregnancy. Birth defects are more commonly linked with paternal DNA damage than with maternal DNA damage (NDIC, 2006). The substance abuse genetics equation is a formula where the preceding circumstances combine to equal a number of physiological consequences for the offspring in addition to an increased risk for the offspring to have substance abuse issues.

Adult alcoholism develops as a result of the considerable role genetics plays when the gene pool has alcohol abusers in it. However, it is acknowledged that family environmental factors do supply a significant platform in terms of how the addiction is allowed to be asserted (Doweiko, 2006). Similarly, adult substance abuse has been examined in those who were adopted and had birth parents who were substance abusers. Again it is supported that having the genes for substance abuse does not, in and of itself, guarantee an addicted adult. The environment must interact with the genetics to create the development of highest risk (Dick & Bierut, 2006).

CHART 16–1 Personality Traits Associated with Substance Abuse

It has been hypothesized that people who have substance abuse problems also share certain personality traits. Given that people and adaptive responses, as well as maladaptive responses such as substance abuse, can vary tremendously, this can be a contradictory set of characteristics. Listed below are some personality traits that may be seen in substance abusers:

- Anxiety and tension
- Social conformist
- Impulsive
- Irritable
- More easily fatigued than those without substance abuse
- Less satisfaction with present life situation
- Reports dissatisfaction with childhood experiences
- A tendency to act rashly when distressed
- Extroversion
- A prominence of Cluster B (dramatic, emotional, or erratic) personality patterns
- Choosing a substance when seeking comfort from stress
- Denial of a problem or minimizing the problem
- Projection of feelings onto another person
- Conning, bargaining, feigning
- Rationalization
- A routine of sensation seeking.

Comprehending the psychological infrastructure of substance abuse includes the possible contribution of attachment theory (Shorey & Snyder, 2006). The substance abuser may develop an attachment to the drug much like he would an attachment to another person. The drug becomes the partner in the relationship. The interaction between the person and the drug becomes the primary relationship with experiences and attitudes not unlike any other close bond. This theoretical framework may assist in treatment for this group of patients using support and exploration.

Sociocultural Theories

A sociocultural theoretical framework holds that both the social influences on an individual as well as the culture within that social structure define what has happened to create substance abuse. Poverty and wealth along with youth and age can contribute to the problems that compel some to abuse substances. Some of the sociocultural reasons people may use substances include the following:

- It was learned from the family.
- It was learned from friends.
- It results from a lack of alternative coping skills.
- It helps with anger.
- It helps deal with the side effects of medications.
- It makes them feel better (smarter, interesting, creative, powerful, etc.).

- They think it is normal and usual.
- It helps them cope with the difficulties of life.
- It numbs sexual, physical, emotional trauma.

Neaigus et al. (2006) and Vieten et al. (2004) explored the context of substance abuse and the typical groups at risk for it. After numerous surveys of the population, study summaries maintain that the component parts are the economics of drug use, what place those who are addicted hold in society, how the drug is produced, and what links the sociocultural network together. Learning about the context has been helpful in understanding how epidemics of drug use, such as heroin and methamphetamine, occur.

In a sociocultural framework, the roles different family members play and the importance of family rituals contribute to the problem of substance abuse and its treatment. For example, the family of a person who abuses alcohol may see the annual family reunion as a time when excessive drinking is not only allowed but expected and part of the event's relaxation. Entering a substance abuse treatment program prior to the reunion would be rejected. Similarly, the family of a young man abusing a methamphetamine with cardiac implications may nurse him back to health with each setback. The roles of caretaker may be more important to the family than any other role. Involving the community in substance abuse treatment can take shape in a variety of ways. The National Institute on Alcohol Abuse and Alcoholism has developed several guidelines for effective interventions in dealing with college campus drinking incidents (LaBrie, Pedersen, Lamb, & Bove, 2006). Projects like this target high-risk populations on campus and help students make responsible drinking decisions.

Substance abuse is thought to be created within social and cultural systems, so culture-specific approaches to the treatment of drug addiction would, therefore, be most effective. Treatment approaches that exist vary greatly and exceed the scope of this chapter. However, it is interesting to note that tradition-imbedded practices exist for substance abuse such as the Buddhist temple cure in Thailand, the San Pedro drink therapy (mescaline) for alcoholism in the northern coast of Peru, or the Danshukai groups and the Naikan treatment methods used in Japan.

■ Management of Patients Who Are Substance Abusers

Competent nursing care involves an understanding of the substance of abuse and how to most effectively treat the prioritized problems. This chapter focuses on the main substances of abuse.

Alcohol

Alcohol is a common substance that has just as much destructive power as any other substance of abuse. It is a legal, liquid, recreational drug. Characteristic features seen with abuse of this drug include slurred speech, ataxia, slowed reaction times, disinhibition, and interactions including repetitive argumentativeness or profuse apologizing for drinking. The nurse needs to know how this drug impacts on the patient's physiology. The range of physiological impacts on a patient with blood alcohol levels (BALs) ranging from 0.05 to 0.5 g/dL are presented in Chart 16–2 (p. 370).

CHART 16–2 Escalating Physiological Impacts of Alcohol

CNS

- Disinhibition (behaviorally and sexually)
- Memory, concentration degradation
- Decrease in reasoning abilities
- Blackouts
- Motor skill degradation
- Labored breathing, severe respiratory depression
- Drowsiness, stupor, unconsciousness, coma, death

MOOD

- Euphoria
- Depression
- Mood lability

BEHAVIOR

- Outbursts
- Ataxia
- Slurred speech
- Incoherent speech
- Vomiting
- Violence

SENSES

- Diplopia

Public figures and famous people are often involved in alcohol-related incidents that the public does not view as being significantly problematic. The same casual attitude seeps into the overall perception of alcoholism in communities; that is, there is a certain level of acceptance about the use of alcohol and alcoholism. Alcohol-related disasters occur in which both the amount of alcohol and the resulting disaster are minimized by those involved: "I only had a couple drinks, of course I could drive." It is not wise to leave the decision to function competently to the person whose judgment is tainted. When those charged with maintaining social order focus on the dangerous combination of alcohol consumption and participation in activities that require judgment and motor skill, the result is a community that is slightly more aware of the problems alcohol consumption creates.

Alcoholism has been, and often still is, viewed as a sign of weakness by those who are unenlightened; note, however, that clinical investigation has redefined alcoholism as a disease. As research about its biochemical aspects has become known, the social stigma attached to alcoholism has decreased and more people have sought help. Professionals, laypeople, students, alcoholics, and nonalcoholics are attending seminars and college courses on alcoholism. Recovery programs are reported widely in the popular media and rehabilitation programs have become common knowledge. Information about alcohol recovery programs is easily accessible on the Internet and in print materials.

It is hard for the person imbibing to see what is happening to her body and quality of life. The devastation is usually seen and felt by others first. Some of the effects of alcoholism include depression; loss of self-respect; alienation from family, friends, and coworkers; malnutrition; decreased competence in self-care; infections; and damaging physiological effects to most body systems. A structured conversation by family and friends with the person who is abusing alcohol may be the first time all of the problems of a person's alcoholism are aired in a matter-of-fact manner.

The patterns of alcohol use vary and include regular daily intake of large amounts of alcohol, regular heavy drinking limited to weekends, or long periods of sobriety interspersed with binges of heavy drinking that last for weeks or months. The pattern does not change the physiological effects or the designation "alcoholic."

The Effects of Alcohol

A sedative anesthetic (CNS depressant), alcohol begins to be absorbed in the mouth, with absorption completed in the stomach and small intestine. Approximately 95% of alcohol is broken down by the liver; the rest is excreted through the lungs, kidneys, and skin. Generally, a person can metabolize 30 mL of alcohol (1 oz of whiskey) every 90 minutes. The rate of absorption varies based on weight, intake of food, liver function, and many other factors. If taken in exceedingly high doses, alcohol can depress respiration and cause death. Intoxication occurs when a person's BAL is 0.10% or more. This blood alcohol level is the legal definition of inebriation in most states, although there is a vigorous trend toward lowering the level to 0.08.

Assessment Aides

Useful, structured assessments around alcohol abuse include the CAGE questionnaire (Chart 16–3). CAGE is an acronym for the main words in the four specific questions about alcohol use. It is quick and direct, and allows professionals in other specialties and nonprofessionals the opportunity to screen for alcohol abuse. Because of its brevity, one of its disadvantages is that it may result in missed opportunities to obtain information. In addition, those particular questions could be offensive and impair communications about substance abuse.

Another quick assessment aid is the World Health Organization's Alcohol Use Disorders Identification Test (AUDIT) test. This is a 10-question assessment developed in 1992 that some consider to be less confrontational than the CAGE. The BEAST acronym (Chart 16–4), described in detail later in this chapter, is used to help addicts avoid taking another drink or drug.

CHART 16–3 CAGE Questions

The CAGE questionnaire is most frequently used for the detection of alcoholism in clinical settings. CAGE is a mnemonic for these four questions:

1. Have you ever felt like you should **C**ut down on your drinking?
2. Have people **A**nnoyed you by criticizing your drinking?
3. Have you ever felt bad or **G**uilty about your drinking?
4. Have you ever had a drink in the morning as an **E**ye-opener to get rid of a hangover?

BEAST Acronym

- **B** is for Boozing Opportunities (weddings, parties, trips, and so on). RR says to be aware of the pitfalls but do not necessarily avoid them. You are not powerless in the face of temptations, and you can choose not to succumb.
- **E** is for Enemy Recognition. Distinguish those thoughts from the Enemy (Beast) that are positive about booze or drugs.
- **A** is for Accuse the Beast of Malice. You can be angry at the Beast for its evil deeds (trying to tempt you), or you can laugh at it. Either way, make clear to the Beast that you have the upper hand and you won't relinquish it.
- **S** is for Self-Control and Self-Worth Reminders. Find ways of showing the Beast you have self-control (like moving your hands in front of your face and holding them there, totally in your control, until the Beast backs down). Find ways of telling yourself that you are a worthwhile person. Choose not to drink for the same reason you drank: to feel good about yourself.
- **T** is for Treasuring Your Sobriety. Focus on the pleasures of life that are attainable only in sobriety (a concept similar to that in AA).

Alcohol Withdrawal Syndrome

Alcohol withdrawal often includes the symptoms described in the following subsections and in Chart 16–5.

Hangover

The term *hangover* is used to describe the unpleasant symptoms of mild alcohol withdrawal occurring approximately 4 to 6 hours after the last alcohol ingestion. These symptoms include:

- Nausea and vomiting
- Gastritis
- Headache
- Fatigue
- Sweating and thirst
- Restlessness
- Irritability
- The "shakes"
- Vasomotor instability.

Chemicals known as congeners are formed during alcohol processing and maturation and increase the likelihood and severity of a hangover. The darker the liquor, the more congeners it contains. The toxins in congeners are distributed throughout the body as the liver breaks down the alcohol. Hangovers change various blood hormone levels that in turn create more symptoms. Alcohol inhibits the antidiuretic hormone, which leads to excessive urination and dehydration. Blood aldosterone and rennin levels increase with a hangover, but how this affects symptoms is unclear. A person is more prone to a hangover if the following circumstances apply:

- Drinks alcohol rapidly
- Mixes different types of alcoholic drinks
- Does not dilute the absorption of liquor with food and non-alcoholic beverages.

Alcohol Withdrawal Symptoms

Symptom	Occurrence Time Frame after Last Drink	Duration Time Frame
Slight at-rest tremors/pronounced and irregular during activities	24 hours	1 week
Diaphoresis	24 hours	3–4 days
Nausea, vomiting, anorexia	24 hours	3–4 days
Increased vital signs	24 hours	3–4 days
Agitation, inner shakiness	24 hours	2 weeks
Insomnia, vivid nightmares	24 hours	At least 2 weeks
Visual hallucinations (usually of disasters during everyday events)	24 hours	3 days
Auditory hallucinations, feeling persecuted, agitation, increased risk for lethality (self and others)	24 hours	3 days to 2 weeks
Delirium tremens (delirium, generalized seizures, disorientation for time and place, visual hallucinations, agitation, panic)	24–48 hours	3–5 days
Rum fits (2–6 generalized seizures)	24–48 hours	3–5 days

The following can help lessen the distressing symptoms of a hangover:

- Sugar and fluids help overcome hypoglycemia and dehydration.
- Anti-inflammatory drugs can reduce headache (aspirin may irritate the stomach; alcohol amplifies the toxic effects of acetaminophen on the liver).

Delirium Tremens

Delirium tremens (DTs), one symptom of withdrawal, is a condition of severe memory disturbance, agitation, anorexia, and hallucinations. Generally, DTs begin a few days after drinking stops and end within 1 to 5 days. They may, however, appear as late as the second week of abstinence from alcohol, especially when there is cross-addiction to other drugs. Additional medical illnesses may be present, such as pneumonia, pancreatitis, and hepatic decompensation.

Medical Detoxification

Medical treatment of alcoholism involves the management of withdrawal symptoms and the use of medication to deter the addicted individual from drinking. Alcohol withdrawal occurs after the individual stops drinking. This syndrome is composed of a constellation of physiological and behavioral symptoms that occur when the alcohol level drops.

Minor Withdrawal

A minor withdrawal from alcohol can occur within 6 to 12 hours after the alcoholic's last drink. Early symptoms include anxiety, agitation, and irritability. As the syndrome progresses other symptoms occur. These include tremor, tachycardia, hypertension, diaphoresis, and hallucinations. Gastrointestinal symptoms of nausea, vomiting, diarrhea, and anorexia may also be present. The appearance of hallucinations (visual, auditory, olfactory, or tactile) and seizures marks the onset of a major withdrawal.

Major Withdrawal

A major withdrawal is the most advanced, potentially life-threatening stage of alcohol withdrawal. Symptoms associated with DTs usually develop 72 hours after the last drink. Physical symptoms of impending DTs include elevated temperature, severe diaphoresis, hypertension, and tachycardia. Behavioral symptoms include confusion and disorientation, agitation, tremors, and alterations in sensory perception (auditory and visual hallucinations). The best treatment for major alcohol withdrawal involves early detection. Medical treatment for withdrawal includes:

1. Monitoring the patient's fluid status. Although some patients are overhydrated, many are dehydrated or have the potential to develop a fluid volume deficit. Fluids should be encouraged, up to 3000 mL/day, if no evidence exists to contraindicate this. Intravenous fluids are indicated if the patient is unable to take fluids by mouth.

2. Many people who abuse alcohol suffer from a magnesium deficiency. Administering magnesium sulfate decreases irritability caused by low magnesium levels and prevents seizures.

3. Administering vitamins, especially thiamine (vitamin B_1), because alcohol interferes with the absorption of B vitamins.

4. Prescribing benzodiazepines, such as diazepam (Valium) or chlordiazepoxide (Librium), to help prevent DTs. Seizures may be treated with IV diazepam, and the patient may be placed on an anticonvulsant.

5. Prescribing disulfiram (Antabuse, an agonist medication). The use of disulfiram may be prescribed in the treatment of patients with alcoholism. Disulfiram inhibits acetaldehyde dehydrogenase, which normally metabolizes acetaldehyde. The mechanism causes acetaldehyde to accumulate if alcohol is consumed. Acetaldehyde is highly toxic, producing nausea and hypotension. Hypotension leads to shock and may be fatal. If the patient uses alcohol, a powerful disulfiram reaction may occur and last for up to 2 weeks. Reaction symptoms include nausea, vomiting, flushing, dizziness, and tachycardia. Because of the potential danger of disulfiram, instruct the patient, orally and in writing, not to use alcohol in any form including alcohol-based cough syrups, cold remedies, or oral hygiene products.

6. Prescribing naltrexone (ReVia, Trexan). Developed in 1984 for treatment of heroin abuse, this drug was approved in January 1994 for blocking the craving for alcohol and the pleasure derived from drinking it. Rather than making the patient sick, it blocks the need to ingest alcohol and the pleasure derived from it, and thus may help prevent relapse when it is combined with long-term support groups and individual counseling. It has had more success as an active treatment mode than the punitive pharmacologic agent disulfiram.

Blackouts

Having **blackouts** is frequently confused with passing out. In fact, passing out refers to unconsciousness, whereas a blackout is anterograde amnesia: loss of short-term memories with retention of remote memories. A person can be fully functional for up to several days—working, talking on the telephone, and driving—yet have absolutely no memory of doing so. To others, the person abusing alcohol may appear normal or "high." Interestingly, alcohol abusers appear unconcerned by the blackouts and eventually learn effective coverups. This appearance of unconcern may be due, in part, to euphoric recall: The alcoholic recalls the feeling that fun or interesting events occurred, but does not recall specific behaviors. Reality is distorted. Some patients find blackouts very disturbing and seek treatment after the first blackout.

Blackouts appearing later in the disease process may indicate physical dependence and are not related to the amount of alcohol consumed. They are unpredictable, and exactly how or why they occur is not clear. One theory holds that blackouts are an acute syndrome caused by dehydration of brain tissue. When assessing a patient who abuses alcohol, determine whether blackouts have occurred.

Fetal Alcohol Syndrome

Fetal alcohol syndrome (FAS) is found in children of women who engage in alcohol consumption during pregnancy. Nurses need to be aware of the harmful effects of alcohol on pregnant women and unborn children. As many as 12,000 infants are born each year in the United States with FAS and three times as many with alcohol-related neurodevelopmental disorder (ARND) and alcohol-related birth defects (ARBD) according to the National Organization on Fetal Alcohol Syndrome. All will suffer varying degrees of effects, ranging from mild learning disabilities to major physical, mental, and intellectual impairment. Physical and mental defects include severe growth deficiency, heart defects, malformed facial features, mental retardation, low birth weight, learning problems, and hyperactivity. If a child has one or two of these characteristics, the condition is called fetal alcohol effects (FAE). Of individuals with FAE between the ages of 12 and 51, many will have mental health problems and disrupted school experiences, as well as trouble with the law and confinement in prison, drug or alcohol treatment centers, or mental institutions. A baby born to an alcoholic mother may need to be withdrawn gradually from alcohol immediately after birth. O'Connor et al. (2006) demonstrated evidence of improvement in the social skills deficits and behavioral problems seen in this population following training involving friendship behavior.

Amphetamines

Amphetamines, also known as "speed," belong to a group of compounds called the sympathomimetics. This group of compounds is comprised of synthetic drugs derived from ephedrine that stimulate the release of adrenaline and do speed up someone's system, thus the common name.

Amphetamines were first synthesized in 1887 and experimental medical use began in the 1920s (McGuinness, 2006). In the 1950s and 1960s, amphetamines were heralded as wonder drugs for depression, management of obesity, and exhaustion. By the 1970s their dangers became known and today they are

CHAPTER 16 Substance Abuse **373**

prescribed less frequently because alternative compounds are available to effectively and safely treat those symptoms. Amphetamines are still used to control appetite and treat depression, narcolepsy, and minimal brain dysfunctions, along with attention deficit hyperactivity disorders in children. Amphetamine abusers are usually teenagers or young adults who are looking for a good time. The uninformed hope for alertness and improved performance through use of these substances, which can lure truck drivers working on long road trips, students during exams, and athletes, among others, into the speed trap.

In small doses, amphetamines cause people to feel energetic, euphoric, and in touch with their surroundings. Users take these CNS stimulants to feel good. A growing number of people who do uppers and downers in a cyclic fashion take amphetamines (the upper) to balance the effects of barbiturates (the downer). Amphetamines are dangerous because they alter judgment and obscure sensations. Taken in high doses or intravenously, amphetamines can have dangerous effects.

Amphetamines act by mimicking two of the brain's most important neurotransmitters, dopamine and norepinephrine. A drug must be able to act on a receptor site or on a number of receptor sites to have an impact. The body may not have a specific amphetamine or cocaine receptor site, so amphetamine and cocaine will take what is called illegal control at the existing receptor sites. Dopamine and dopamine receptor sites are intricately involved in the effects substances of abuse have on the nervous systems of patients. Chronic use of methamphetamines changes the way a person thinks and behaves, because the brain's cortex is no longer activated during decision making. This change in the ability of the brain to transport dopamine to any significant degree creates the clinical characteristics of severe psychiatric symptoms (Kim et al. 2006).

Tolerance develops rapidly, and chronic abusers may suffer a toxic psychosis presenting with the symptoms of paranoid schizophrenia. Argumentativeness, delusions, hallucinations, stereotypic compulsive behavior, increased libido, interpersonal sensitivity, panic, and violence may occur (APA, 2000). Substance abuse with amphetamines means a craving for these drugs and requiring higher and higher dosages. Abusers are rowdy, paranoid, and irritable. A "crash" (depression), often with suicidal symptoms, may last for several weeks. This is so uncomfortable that the user ingests more of the drug in an attempt to feel better and develops a cyclical pattern of abuse and crashing.

Physiologically, the overuse of speed has been tied to stroke and death. Depression, anxiety, and increased stress symptoms are the most common psychological pitfalls in recovering from the use of speed. Changes in neurotransmitter activity increase the patient's sensitivity to stress and may contribute to the spontaneous recurrence of amphetamine and methamphetamine psychosis, called flashbacks. Recurrent flashbacks contribute to recurrent major mood disorders (Barr et al., 2006).

Methamphetamine

The most hypercharged form of speed is methamphetamine (MA). It is less expensive than cocaine and has similar CNS stimulant characteristics. Recently MA has become an enormous public health/substance abuse issue. Recipes to manufacture MA in home drug labs using everyday ingredients (over-the-counter

pseudoephedrine, starter fluids, and drain cleaner) are widely available and have impacted how these products are sold (see the Combat Methamphetamine Epidemic Act of 2005). Lower quality MA is called "speed" or "crank"; higher quality MA is sold in small chunks as "glass" or "ice" because of its crystalline appearance. It is a maximum stimulant with maximum risks.

Exposure to MA is neurotoxic and long-term use leads to extensive neural damage. Physiological changes include cognitive impairments, MA-induced psychosis, inadequate perfusion, and ischemic lesions of the brain. What nurses will see is an inability to competently perform activities of daily living (brush teeth, wash face, etc.), difficulty remembering or problem solving, and delusional accusations or reactions with strong emotional content to something the patient is experiencing (seeing, hearing, feeling). MA morphologically changes the corpus callosum and causes skin lesions, perinatal complications, and hypertension (Arria et al., 2006; Barr et al., 2006; McGuinness, 2006). Each of these impacts has consequences that are far reaching for a person's health and functioning. Before and after photographs of people who use methamphetamine are striking in the differences from weight loss, skin integrity problems, and general poor state of health.

Caffeine

Trimethylxanthine is a drug that keeps one awake and alert with a feeling of goodwill. The drug is caffeine. It is one of the most popular drugs in North America. On average, 90% of adults consume 300 mg of caffeine every day. Chart 16–6 lists the caffeine content of certain beverages and foods.

Caffeine is able to accomplish the physiological effect of stimulation through binding to adenosine receptors; adenosine is a chemical that gives instructions about going to sleep. When adenosine is bound to its receptors, it causes drowsiness by slowing down nerve cell activity in the brain. Caffeine takes illegal control of that receptor so adenosine cannot do its job. When the

CHART 16–6	Caffeine Content of Selected Beverages and Foods
Source	**Approximate Caffeine Content per Average Serving**
Cup of instant coffee	65–100 mg
Mug of drip coffee	115–175 mg
Cup of brewed coffee	80–135 mg
Espresso coffee, 2 oz	100 mg
Decaf coffee, brewed	3–4 mg
Decaf coffee, instant	2–3 mg
Cup of tea	30–60 mg
Green tea	15 mg
Cola drink	Up to 40 mg
Certain carbonated sodas	34–80 mg
Energy drink	Up to 80 mg
Hot cocoa	14 mg
Bar of chocolate	Up to 50 mg

receptors are occupied and controlled by caffeine, the nerve cannot respond to the adenosine. Nerve cell activity speeds up and the patient is not able to relax.

This increased neural firing has an impact on the pituitary gland. Increased neural activity usually accompanies a crisis or stressor and the pituitary gland acts in stressful situations by communicating with the adrenal gland to add adrenaline to the system. This is a survival mechanism to help maintain alertness. Adrenaline causes pupils to dilate, increases the heart rate, and readies skeletal muscles for action. As adrenaline wears off, feelings of fatigue and depression appear. Peak concentrations of caffeine are achieved 30 to 60 minutes after ingestion. The half-life of caffeine is about 6 hours. If a patient drinks caffeine first thing in the morning, another dose would be needed in the afternoon to fight off the fatigue and depression.

Caffeine also increases dopamine levels in the brain. Dopamine is a neurotransmitter that, as discussed later in this chapter, impacts mood and a sense of well-being. The dopamine response is partly responsible for caffeine addiction. Moderate caffeine use is typically defined as up to 300 to 400 milligrams a day; while greater amounts are considered heavy consumption. People who use caffeine use it for its stimulant properties. Typical use is seen upon awakening, during times of low energy or fatigue, and when an external source of comfort is required. Once a pattern of use has been established, individuals continue to use so that they do not suffer withdrawal symptoms (Jones & Lejuez, 2005).

Caffeine is a common substance that is intrinsic to a number of plant products. It is encountered in coffee, tea, chocolate, carbonated beverages, and some pain relievers. The color of a substance is not indicative of its caffeine content—some of the highest caffeine content is found in clear carbonated beverages. Caffeine use—and abuse—has only recently become a health concern. In the United States more than half of the population over the age of 10 drinks coffee. Individuals may have a sensitivity to caffeine that causes physical distress (muscle cramping, cardiac effects, diarrhea). There is evidence that combining alcohol with caffeine, as in popular cocktails, impacts cognition, particularly of those making self-assessments of intoxication (Marczinski & Fillmore, 2006).

The amount of caffeine in tea varies according to the plant variety it is made from and how long it is brewed: The longer it is brewed, the higher the caffeine levels. Coffee also has variable amounts of caffeine depending on its preparation method. For instance, brewed coffee has substantially more caffeine than instant coffee.

If coffee is withdrawn suddenly from people who drink large quantities of brewed coffee (six or more cups a day), they might become irritable and suffer from headaches. Given the stimulant effect of caffeine, it makes sense to advise those who complain of insomnia to switch to decaffeinated coffee or to have their last cup of coffee at least 3 hours before going to bed. Remember, "decaffeinated" does not mean there is no caffeine in the coffee or tea; it means the caffeine content is much reduced but still present. Because tea has much less caffeine per cup than coffee, it does not have as strong a stimulating effect. But if there is a complaint of insomnia, good sleep hygiene demands not drinking large quantities of caffeinated tea just before going to bed in an attempt to minimize stimulation.

A successful strategy for lowering the negative physiological impacts of caffeine is to reduce the harm mode. The individual would decrease overall intake of the substance vehicle (such as coffee or tea), start using decaffeinated mixtures in increasing proportions, then complete the effort with cessation of caffeine ingestion. This process weans the individual from the substance without causing, or at least by minimizing, abrupt and uncomfortable withdrawal symptoms. Health care facilities frequently limit or restrict access to caffeinated beverages so that interference from the stimulating impacts does not complicate health care treatments. Advance planning for alternative behaviors in social and occupational situations is helpful for the patient working on discontinuing this particular form of substance abuse.

Cannabis

Marijuana has been illegal in the United States since 1937, although it has been fairly easy to obtain since the early 1900s. As of this writing, despite a U.S. Supreme Court ruling to the contrary, the federal Drug Enforcement Administration considers it illegal and opposes its use for medical purposes. Legal conflicts remain regarding medical marijuana. A 1996 California law legalized some medical use of it, a federal law prohibits distribution or use of marijuana regardless of state law, and health care providers in seven states are allowed to discuss medical marijuana for pain relief without risking loss of license. But this is a topic, and a treatment, in flux.

Marijuana is the most used illicit drug. It is derived from an Indian hemp plant (*Cannabis sativa*) and contains the psychoactive substance delta 6-3,4-tetrahydrocannabinol (THC). THC is found in the sticky yellow resin secreted by the tops and leaves of the ripe plants.

THC is transformed into metabolites in the body. Unlike alcohol, which is water soluble and leaves the body through urine, breath, and perspiration, THC is stored in the fatty tissues (especially the brain and reproductive system). Consequently, it can be detected in the body for up to 6 weeks. The potency of marijuana has steadily increased over the years. Although marijuana contains more than 400 chemicals, the THC content determines the potency. With an increase in potency comes an increase in health problems. There is compelling evidence that underlying neurochemical mechanisms are at work reinforcing the reward and dependence features of this drug and contributing to addiction (Fride, Perchuk, Hall, Uhl, & Onaivi, 2006).

Researchers have found that marijuana produces a significant analgesic effect and is modestly effective against the nausea and vomiting associated with chemotherapy. Medicinal applications of both THC and cannabidiol for pain have been examined and show significant pain relief (Trossman, 2006). Dronabinol is a synthetic delta-9-tetrahydrocannabinol or delta-9-THC that contains standardized THC content in an FDA-approved pharmaceutical. It is mainly used to treat the weight loss, nausea, and vomiting associated with a number of medical conditions.

Although marijuana does decrease intraocular pressure, it requires high doses and has a short-lived effect, making it inappropriate for the treatment of glaucoma. The cannabinoids of marijuana cross the placental barrier and are distributed to fetal tissues. The risk of fetal death and abnormalities—CNS disturbances, low birth weight, decreased length, and smaller head circumference—increases when the mother uses marijuana. Long-term marijuana smoking is associated with lung damage, increased risk of respiratory cancer, and poorer pregnancy outcomes.

Cocaine

Cocaine is a stimulant extracted from the leaves of the coca plant found in Bolivia and Peru. South Americans chewed coca leaves, enjoying the effects of decreased appetite and increased ability to work at high altitudes, for hundreds of years. Common knowledge held that slaves became more productive when given cocaine. It was an ingredient in the popular soft drink Coca Cola—thus the name—before federal regulations prohibited it in 1903. Today, cocaine is used as a local anesthetic in ear, nose, and throat surgery. When inhaled or injected, cocaine produces alertness and energy and makes users feel sociable and confident. The drug blocks appetite and erases fatigue, which makes it appear to be an ideal performance booster although that is an illusion. Cocaine addicts develop a tolerance to the drug and use amounts that would have been lethal to them earlier.

An estimated 5.7 million Americans chronically use cocaine according to the National Institute on Drug Abuse. Because cocaine abuse has been recognized as a widespread problem, the government invests resources to limit access. Cocaine is purer today than ever before. It is available to all cultural and socioeconomic groups and is used equally by women and men. The cocaine industry is a multibillion dollar illegal drug enterprise that affects every aspect of civilization.

Cocaine's impact is both behavioral and biochemical. It produces a euphoria that diminishes after approximately 5 to 10 minutes. The euphoria, or high, is followed by a terrible letdown called the "postcoke blues" or cocaine abstinence syndrome. Anxiety, depression, and fatigue are part of this syndrome. Cocaine initially increases dopamine (DA) neurotransmission. The cocaine crash, lasting for approximately 30 to 60 minutes, results from depletion of DA, the neurotransmitter responsible for feelings of pleasure and well-being. The development of new dendrites (branches of the nerve cells) to aid in the uptake of the increased amount of DA accounts for the tolerance. Over time, however, cocaine abuse depletes DA in the brain and this depletion may be the basis for the supremely compelling cravings associated with its use (Meyers, Zavala, Speer, & Neisewander, 2006).

Ultimately, cocaine no longer produces pleasure, but not taking it feels even worse. As the DA eventually becomes depleted, the user becomes chronically fatigued, irritable, and anxious. Psychiatric symptoms such as confusion and paranoia emerge. Suicide attempts, accidents, and overdoses are common. The only effect of cocaine that is increased as tolerance develops is its ability to induce a convulsion or seizure. Research with cocaine users indicates that the drug bromocriptine mesylate (Parlodel), a DA receptor agonist, eliminates the craving that users feel after they stop using cocaine.

Although the brain needs to synthesize more DA as a result of the chemical misprogramming from the addiction, it craves more cocaine, which offers immediate relief. The crash intensity appears related to the amount of cocaine used. Addicts often use other drugs, such as alcohol, marijuana, or sleeping pills, during the crash.

When someone is intoxicated with cocaine, the person will be sweating and exhibit dilated pupils, psychomotor agitation, and increased blood pressure and heart rate. Higher doses of cocaine produce high fever, cardiac arrhythmia, seizures, hallucinations, and a paranoid schizophrenic syndrome. Hallucinations typically involve "cocaine bugs," described as feeling like bugs are crawling under the person's skin. The patient may scratch and dig in an attempt to get rid of them. Antipsychotics are used to combat the psychotic symptoms, but the use of those that can further decrease the seizure threshold is avoided.

Detoxification for cocaine abusers depends on the patient's symptoms. Some hospitals use nothing; others administer diazepam (Valium) intravenously 1 to 20 mg at a slow rate (not more than 5 mg/min). Some Valium protocols last approximately 4 days; Valium is decreased from 10 mg q4h PO/IM to 5 mg q8h PO/IM, with additional doses as needed if the patient has withdrawal symptoms. Other hospitals have prn Valium orders only. Another protocol involves the use of phenobarbital in decreasing doses and imipramine hydrochloride (Tofranil).

Because the depression associated with cocaine detoxification is significant, Tofranil or other tricyclic antidepressants may be given for several weeks after the acute detoxification. Tricyclics build up existing levels of neurotransmitters and make them available for transmission.

 Beta-adrenergic blockers such as propranolol (Inderal) may be used to counteract the tachycardia and hypertension that accompany acute cocaine intoxication. Their use may result in paroxysmal hypertension due to unopposed alpha-adrenergic stimulation. Use cautiously and with constant blood pressure monitoring.

Synaptic treatment uses tricyclic antidepressants to increase the number of neurotransmitters in the synapse. Postsynaptic treatment for cocaine withdrawal and dependence includes the use of drugs such as bromocriptine (Parlodel) or amantadine (Symmetrel), which increase dopaminergic activity in the synapse and enhance the effects of DA on the postsynaptic receptors. Other medications such as buprenorphine can promote abstinence and there has been success with agonist substitution treatments (Gross, Marsch, Badger, & Bickel, 2006; Lile, 2006). Historically, presynaptic treatment was employed using amino acids such as tryptophan. This was used until 1989, when tryptophan was removed from the market because of several deaths associated with its use. The rationale for instituting presynaptic treatment was based on the body's conversion of amino acids to neurotransmitters. Cocaine abuse depleted neurotransmitters and the tryptophan was thought to replace it to some extent.

Auricular acupuncture for cocaine dependence is widely used (Gates, Smith, & Foxcroft, 2006), but research has not supported its effectiveness. Placing acupuncture needles into specific sites in the ear can promote relaxation and be a stress management technique. This nonpharmacologic intervention requires more robust and reliable research to determine whether it contributes to helping the dependent individual abstain from cocaine use.

Crack

Crack, or "rock" cocaine, recently labeled "the most addictive drug known to man," is a potent form of hydrochloride cocaine that is mixed with baking soda and water, heated, allowed to harden, and then broken or "cracked" into little pieces and smoked in cigarettes or glass water pipes. Smokable forms of cocaine have effects similar to those of the injectable drug. Crack is more insidious, addictive, and toxic than cocaine. It is not unusual for someone to become addicted after using crack twice.

Crack is cheap and easily acquired. A crack high has a rapid onset and is intensely euphoric, followed by a dramatic crash. Within seconds after the crash, users feel compelled to smoke more crack. Repeatedly smoking cocaine affects the central serotonergic and dopaminergic functions of the brain. The long-lasting and selective disruptions in serotonin pathways following chronic cocaine use may provide a neurochemical basis for the mood changes commonly reported during cocaine withdrawal (Meyers et al., 2006).

Symptoms of crack use include irritability, paranoia, depression, and physical symptoms that go along with the smoking of a toxic chemical, such as wheezing and coughing blood, and black phlegm. Cardiac arrhythmias caused by crack use may lead to death. There is an increase in the number of babies being born to mothers who use crack. These babies are more likely to be premature, have microcephaly, or have low birth weights. They are irritable, and have tremors and muscle rigidity. The children have adjustment problems and are quick to express frustration and have generally disruptive styles of interacting (Dennis, Bendersky, Ramsay, & Lewis, 2006).

Treatment for this addiction is very difficult. Many people seek help only when they can no longer support their habit. That point is much further along than it would be with a more expensive drug, so patients are very debilitated by the time they seek treatment and have usually been coerced by others to do so. It is an extremely problematical drug to stop using. Recidivism is estimated at more than 90%.

Freebase

Freebase is a purified form of cocaine made by applying solvents to ordinary cocaine. Melting the cocaine with a small butane torch helps in the purifying and delivery process. This action alone is dangerous due to the hazard of the solvent exploding. The effects of the freebase are brief but intense, and the short euphoria (3 to 5 minutes) immediately becomes a restless desire for more "base." This sequential abuse of the substance has caused the death of a number of public figures in recent decades.

Hallucinogens

Hallucinogens are synthetic and natural drugs that cause hallucinations and unusual sensory experiences. A variety of plant species have impacts on the CNS that can be exploited as drugs of abuse. Peyote, the active hallucinogen in cactus buttons, is still an integral part of religious rituals of Native Americans in the southwestern United States and Mexico. Psilocybin is the active hallucinogen in certain mushrooms. Recipes using psilocybin mushrooms encompass everyday foods, tea, and honey concoctions. There continues to be controversy around whether psilocybin-containing mushrooms can be smoked to produce a psychoactive effect. People around the world continue to use many species of hallucinogenic plants to achieve distortions in their state of mind (Vaitl et al., 2005). Developed in 1938 for scientific research, LSD (an abbreviation of the German words for lysergic acid diethylamide) is the drug most commonly identified with the term *hallucinogen* and the most widely used in this class of drugs. It is considered the typical hallucinogen, and characteristics of its action and effects apply to other hallucinogens, including mescaline, psilocybin, and ibogaine.

In the 1960s and 1970s, the U.S. Army experimented with LSD by giving it without informed consent to unsuspecting army employees. One dramatic and much publicized event concerned the army officer who leapt to his death from a window after unknowingly ingesting LSD. At this time the danger of LSD became publicized, as did the unethical research. Physician researchers also were interested in experimenting with the uses of LSD in the treatment of a variety of diseases; however, in 1966 LSD became illegal and could no longer be used in human research.

After a lull in use, LSD ("acid") is again being used because it is cheap ($2 to $5 a "hit") and causes an intense high that lasts 6 to 12 hours. Users today are unacquainted with the horror stories of the 1960s, typically because they are teenagers and young adults. Psychological and physical dependence are unlikely because each experience with a hallucinogen is different. Visual hallucinations, a sense of increased creativity, and revelations regarding the essential meaning of life are the presumed effects of the drugs. If these occur, they are short-lived excursions.

The dangers of hallucinogens include "bad trips" and flashbacks. Users who experience bad trips may appear psychotic and extremely fearful. Reassuring the person and pointing out reality are helpful; occasionally tranquilizers or antipsychotics are given. The symptoms usually disappear within 12 hours but may persist for months.

Flashbacks are a spontaneous reliving of the experiences the person felt while under the influence of the drug, even though the person is currently drug free. The experience may involve perceptual distortions, a variety of physical feelings, and strong emotions such as fear and pleasure. Flashbacks are generally brief, and they occur less frequently over time. Flashbacks may be induced by stress, fatigue, and drug or alcohol ingestion (Vaitl et al., 2005). There exists a clinical concern that hallucinogens pose a particular danger to adolescents in that they may precipitate psychosis. Because teenagers' egos and defenses are weak, they may be especially susceptible to the effects of hallucinogens.

Inhalants

Inhalants are popular among teenagers and school-age children because they are inexpensive, easy to obtain, and are generally typical household items—such as glue, fuels, paints, aerosols, air fresheners, the substance used to resole shoes, and the propellants in canned whipped cream—with the exception of one unusual source: embalming fluid. The abuse of inhalants is increasing at a frightening rate. Their use causes euphoria, light-headedness, and excitement. Children are the most frequent users. Adult users often have a long history of polydrug abuse.

Inhalants are sniffed or inhaled (called "huffing") in a variety of ways. Huffing a rag soaked with the inhalant and placed in a plastic bag or inhaling the gas directly from a tank are the two most common behaviors. Amyl and butyl nitrate (called "poppers") can be easily concealed and passed around a classroom, and paint thinner can be concealed in a soft drink can. Use of these inhalants and solvents can cause ventricular fibrillation, decreased cardiac output, serious brain damage, and sudden death.

Although withdrawal must be managed as with the other substances covered in this chapter, careful assessment, early identification, detoxification, education, and prevention are particularly critical because so many inhalant abusers are children under the age of 12. The appalling consequences of young children's abuse of inhalants cannot be understated (Eaton et al., 2006). Nurses need to be aware of the programs and resources available and should support legislation to make it more difficult for minors to obtain glue and paint products.

Nicotine

Nicotine is the psychoactive stimulating substance found in tobacco. The behavioral and physiological effects of nicotine frequently lead to addiction, and access to this legal drug for adults endangers those under the legal smoking age. Populations with psychiatric conditions and substance abuse problems have higher rates of smoking and show a lack of responsiveness to smoking cessation treatments (Ranney et al., 2006).

Nicotine is a stimulant that acts in the central and peripheral nervous systems on cells that are normally acted on by the neurotransmitter acetylcholine. In the CNS nicotine occupies the receptors for acetylcholine in both dopamine and serotonin neural pathways. This causes the release of both dopamine and norepinephrine. The stimulant nicotine initially increases alertness and cognitive ability, and then has a depressant effect.

Research suggests a role for dopaminergic processes regulating the reinforcing effects of nicotine, making cessation of use more difficult. Dopamine blockers can alter smoking behavior for a limited time, but people compensate for this by then increasing their amount of smoking (Glover, 2006). The usual impact of dopamine being turned over in the system at an increased rate is the reduction of hunger impulses. Once someone tries to quit smoking, hunger impulses return and the person may gain weight.

Smoking rates of the general population have fallen during the past 25 years from 34% in 1980 to close to 22% in 2005 (Hoeppner et al., 2006; Ranney et al., 2006), but are still of concern given the negative physiological impacts of the addiction. Nicotine use is associated with cancer, heart disease, emphysema, hypertension, and death. Smoking cigarettes is an extremely common addiction and is seen routinely despite smoke-free environments and restrictions on cigarette access. Evidence indicates that smoke-free environments protect people from the force of secondhand smoke but do not reduce actual smoking. Instead, smokers will practice anticipatory smoking to ensure their desired level of nicotine is maintained (Doweiko, 2006). There are also socioeconomic differences in smoking rates. The prevalence of smoking in Medicaid recipients is 44% compared to the general population.

Typically, people begin smoking at young ages, during peer pressure contacts, or during times of stress and thereafter find it very difficult to quit successfully. Use of tobacco products can be interrupted briefly during respiratory illnesses, hospitalizations, pregnancy, and following health care provider advice on smoking cessation. Return to tobacco use after a brief time is all too usual. Long-term quit rates range from 10% to 25% including pharmacologic cessation support (nicotine replacement systems, psychopharmacology) (Evans, Blank, Sams, Weaver, & Eissenberg, 2006; Killen et al., 2006).

The most commonly used approach for treating nicotine dependence is nicotine replacement therapy (patch, inhaler, lozenge, gum), which reduces cravings by maintaining the blood level of nicotine. Bupropion (Zyban), an antidepressant, has demonstrated effectiveness in short-term abstinence. Support in a variety of forms is also useful in assisting patients with this difficult addiction. Educational programs targeting the smoking cessation knowledge base of health care providers in prenatal, pediatric, and community health are needed to promote effective treatment of nicotine dependence (Klesges et al., 2006).

Every person trying to make a change in behavior must go through stages before, during, and after the change is made. The transtheoretical model of behavior change (TTM) has been applied successfully to substance abuse as well as co-occurring disorders (Finnell & Osborne, 2006). TTM describes a continuum of five stages of behavior change (see Chart 16–7) and the underpinnings of movement from stage to stage. The beginning of this process is called assessing readiness to change. The entire model describes each of the stages in the process. There is a great deal within the TTM that can be useful to nurses throughout their careers.

CHART 16–7 **The Transtheoretical Model of Behavior Change**

Any desired change in health care behavior is best understood with a model that explains human behavior. TTM explains the stages of change and the processes of change. Features of change that occur throughout the stages, such as how decisional balance affects the change process, an individual's vision of how effective efforts will be, and how temptation will likely be handled, make this perspective a useful one for promoting change.

Stage	Processes and Principles
Precontemplation	The patient does not intend to change the health behavior in the near future. This stage usually lasts approximately 6 months. What the nurse sees is an avoidance of communications designed to help change occur.
Contemplation	The patient does intend to change the health behavior in the next 6 months. There is awareness of the benefits of change, but the barriers and ambivalence are potent and interfere.
Preparation	The patient intends to make the change within the next month. The patient develops a plan of action with small, important steps taken toward change.
Action	The patient demonstrates modified risky behavior and makes the change. There is significant risk of reverting to previous problematic health behaviors. Healthy action requires considerable time and energy.
Maintenance	Work to prevent relapse occurs in this stage. Temptation gradually diminishes over 6 months to 5 years. This stage is meant to extend through the patient's life.

Source: Reprinted from Addictive Behaviors. Vol 31(8), Hoeppner, B. B., Velicer, W. F., Redding, C. A., Rossi, J. S., Prochaska, J. O., Pallonen, U. E., & Meier, K. S. Psychometric evaluation of the smoking cessation Processes of Change scale in an adolescent sample. Addictive Behaviors, pp. 1363–1372, Copyright 2006, with permission from Elsevier.

Opiates

Opiates as a category of drugs of abuse include heroin and morphine (which are derived from the poppy plant) and synthetic drugs (such as oxycodone, meperidine, codeine, and methadone). Opiates have analgesic qualities and are usually prescribed after a surgical procedure or for chronic pain. They are quite potent and have the ability to decrease awareness of painful stimuli. Depending on the person, the drugs may produce a euphoric high, as it does in drug addicts, but opiates generally cause people to feel drowsy and out of touch with the world (Martin, Loder, Taylor, Almas, & Hilliard, 2005). For information on chronic pain conditions, see Chapter 15 .

Heroin as a drug is not inherently dangerous. Unless there is an accidental overdose, the heroin alone as a substance will not harm the individual. But addiction to heroin exposes the patient to the dangerous and deadly ancillary issues of:

- Diluting agents (which are likely contaminated)
- Needle cleanliness
- Exposure to transmissible diseases such as hepatitis, TB, and HIV
- Overdose
- Malnutrition
- Poisoning by impurities
- Criminal behaviors necessary to support the addiction, which can put the individual at great risk.

These issues and others make the addicted individual of concern to others. The Harrison Narcotics Act of 1914 restricted use of opiates in the United States due to their dangerous impacts. Drugs such as heroin are used for clinical purposes in Europe and the United Kingdom; heroin in particular is used to control pain because it is relatively inexpensive.

Constricted pupils, euphoria, psychomotor retardation, slurred speech, and/or drowsiness indicate opiate intoxication. If a client overdoses, naloxone (Narcan) can be used if it is immediately administered. Abdominal cramps, rhinorrhea, and lacrimation may be treated with belladonna alkaloids or with phenobarbital.

> **CRITICAL ALERT** *Heroin overdoses, if identified quickly, can be treated with naloxone (Narcan). Naloxone is a fast-acting narcotic antagonist that counteracts respiratory depression. The dose is usually 0.4 to 0.8 mg IV repeated in 5 to 15 minutes.*

Because opiates are physically addictive, withdrawal is a physiological threat. People who use high doses of a drug and who use the drug intravenously are at high risk for severe withdrawal symptoms. Withdrawal symptoms are usually evident within 12 hours after the last dose. The person experiences the most severe withdrawal within 36 to 48 hours with the symptoms decreasing gradually over 2 weeks. Clonidine has been useful in this process. Clonidine blocks the withdrawal symptoms, making the detoxification process less painful. Psychologically, the patient feels less anxious and depressed.

During this stressful withdrawal, the person craves the drug. Babies who are born to addicted mothers must be treated for opiate withdrawal. These babies are irritable, have high-pitched crying, increased respirations, fever, sneezing, yawning, and tremors.

In 1964, methadone was introduced to treat opiate addiction. By the late 1960s and early 1970s, when federal governments allocated money for treatment, methadone maintenance programs mushroomed all over North America. Methadone, a synthetic narcotic, was dispensed daily at clinics to narcotic addicts by prescribers with special licensure to do so. Although addictive, methadone does not produce the ecstatic feeling associated with heroin. Methadone alleviates the addict's craving for narcotics and, therefore, was expected to decrease the illicit drug trafficking, theft, prostitution, and crime necessary to obtain money for the drugs. It was thought that dwindling drug trafficking would allow addicts to lead productive lives. Also, methadone therapy is far less expensive than residential programs or jail. Methadone as a treatment option for these patients has been successful to a certain extent, but has had controversial aspects. The ethics of methadone treatment, as well as the economic aspects of the treatment, are viewed as public health concerns.

Federally controlled substances, including buprenorphine, are alternatives to methadone. Buprenorphine is an opioid mixed agonist and potent analgesic. Buprenorphine, a potential treatment for opiate addiction, is administered under the tongue via a small syringe by specially licensed professionals. Patients do not swallow the medication but allow it to be absorbed through the mucous membranes that line the inside of the mouth (Gross et al., 2006). This medication will not replace methadone therapy that is provided through special methadone treatment facilities, but will provide the office-based prescriber an opportunity to treat patients for addiction to heroin or other opiates, including prescription painkillers. In 1993, LAAM (1-alpha-acetylmethadol) was approved for the management of opiate dependence. Buprenorphine joins methadone, naltrexone, and LAAM as the fourth medication available for treating heroin and other opiate addictions. With most opioid substitution treatment, the patient continues some level of illicit drug use (Carroll, Walsh, Bigelow, Strain, & Preston, 2006).

Phencyclidine

Drugs such as phencyclidine (PCP) and ketamine, which were initially developed as general anesthetics for surgery, distort perceptions of sight and sound and produce feelings of detachment—dissociation—from the environment and self. But these mind-altering effects are not hallucinations. PCP and ketamine are therefore more properly known as "dissociative anesthetics." Dextromethorphan, a widely available cough suppressant, when taken in high doses can produce effects similar to those of PCP and ketamine. The dissociative drugs act by altering distribution of the neurotransmitter glutamate throughout the brain. Glutamate is involved in the perception of pain, responses to the environment, and memory. PCP is considered the typical dissociative drug, and the descriptions of PCP's actions and effects largely apply to ketamine and dextromethorphan as well (Lofwall, Griffiths, & Mintzer, 2006).

PCP was originally used as an anesthetic for humans and as a tranquilizer for animals. Because of its dangerous side effects, it was removed from the market except for veterinary use. However, by the mid-1960s PCP was readily available as a street drug. PCP is inexpensive and easily synthesized by home chemists, making a supply always available.

People who use PCP frequently arrive at the emergency room in a psychotic, violent, and agitated state. The agitation and the sensations experienced by the user generate incredible power and strength. Even a small, slight person can break heavy glass doors or fight several people at once. Some users fluctuate between coma and violence. Hallucinations are common. A differential diagnosis is important but difficult because the symptoms are similar to those of schizophrenia.

A PCP high sets in about 5 minutes after a person takes the drug and lasts 4 to 6 hours. Effects may last up to 48 hours. PCP may be recovered from the blood and urine for 7 to 10 days. While using PCP, a person experiences a wide variety of feelings ranging from euphoria and utter peace to violence, confusion, and disorganization. Distorted sensory perceptions are common. During a "bad trip," anxiety, fear, and paranoia predominate. The dramatic physical and emotional effects of PCP may last for several weeks. Users may suffer from poor impulse control, depression, fatigue, memory loss, and concentration difficulties.

Variable concentrations and questionable purity are vital problems with PCP. Because it is generally manufactured illegally, users never really know what they are buying. Contaminants are often toxic to humans, causing a wide variety of physiological responses including death. PCP is recognized for its potential to cause violence, especially when the drug is taken in high dosages.

Treatment of acute PCP intoxication may include the use of diazepam for muscle spasms, seizures, and agitation. Risperidone or haloperidol may be used for severe psychotic behavior, but phenothiazines should not be used because PCP is anticholinergic. Calcium channel blockers such as verapamil may be given. These drugs are thought to prevent or reverse PCP-induced vasospasms, thereby decreasing the hallucinogenic effects of PCP. This treatment is controversial, however, because some clinicians feel that the use of verapamil may potentiate the effects of PCP. Nursing care during this period should focus on protecting the patient and others from injury and reorienting the person to reality. Providing a quiet, safe environment and addressing the person in a calm, reassuring manner are important.

A substance very similar to PCP is ketamine, a veterinary anesthesia agent also known as Special K, K, Vitamin K, and Cat Valium. It has a much shorter duration of action than PCP and is used recreationally because of its sedative and hallucinogenic properties (Lofwall et al., 2006). It can cause delirium, amnesia, tachycardia, anxiety, and high blood pressure. Ketamine is also used for pediatric conscious sedation.

Sedatives, Hypnotics, and Anxiolytics

Barbiturates are highly addictive sedatives that cause people to feel euphoric, yet relaxed. They are frequently prescribed to reduce anxiety, prevent or relieve pain, and induce sleep but have inherent dangers because of their ability to cause significant CNS depression and lethality if used to overdose. Migraine overuse headache (MOH) can occur when these medications are used too often and requires a withdrawal strategy (Rossi, Di Lorenzo, Faroni, Cesarino, & Nappi, 2006). Overprescribing may be due to health care providers treating the symptoms of anxiety, stress, or insomnia without determining, and then appropriately eradicating, the cause.

Anxiolytic drugs, typically the benzodiazepines (BZDs) and nonbenzodiazepines, began to be widely used because of their ability to reduce anxiety without causing significant CNS depression. These drugs are thought to modify anxiety by altering the balance of neurotransmitters, especially norepinephrine and gamma-aminobutyric acid (GABA) in the brain's limbic system. The limbic system is involved in the regulation of emotion.

BZDs include diazepam (Valium), clorazepate (Tranxene), lorazepam (Ativan), and alprazolam (Xanax). These, and others, are known to produce dependence and withdrawal syndromes. They have a high risk for abuse and physical dependence. When the drug stops working and tolerance builds up, people tend to increase the dosage just "to cope." Even the nonbenzodiazepines such as zolpidem (Ambien) and zaleplon (Sonata) can be used to excess and have dependence issues associated with use.

One type of abuse of these substances involves taking high doses of barbiturates, often in combination with alcohol, to get the "high." The resultant CNS depression makes this practice especially dangerous. "Speed freaks" (amphetamine abusers) use barbiturates to "come down" from a high. Dependence, tolerance, and cross-tolerance to other depressant drugs develop rapidly.

The liver conducts a staged metabolism of barbiturates. Oral ingestion is followed by initial absorption and partial metabolism. The unmetabolized parts of the drug become active metabolites that are stored in the patient's fatty tissues. Taking these drugs over a period of time results in a cumulative effect, unsuspected dependence, and possible overdose. Death from barbiturate overdose commonly occurs when people take alcohol and barbiturates together. While judgment is impaired, they take more pills, thereby unintentionally overdosing. Because alcohol and barbiturates are synergistic, an overdose can occur quickly. Barbiturates are often used in suicide attempts. A deep sleep is followed by decreased respiration, coma, and sometimes death.

Barbiturate withdrawal is unpleasant and life threatening. Babies born to mothers addicted to barbiturates are physically dependent and need to be helped through withdrawal. Withdrawal from BZDs may produce symptoms similar to those of barbiturate withdrawal. The onset of withdrawal symptoms begins within 24 to 72 hours of the last dose, depending on the half-life of the drug used. Symptoms include autonomic hyperactivity (alterations in vital signs and diaphoresis), marked anxiety, agitation, insomnia, depression, and seizures. Medical detoxification can prevent a potentially serious emergency during withdrawal.

Gerontological Considerations

A number of reasons make geriatric substance abuse a major medical concern. People over the age of 65 consume more prescription medications than all other age groups combined. This alone puts this group at risk for deliberate or inadvertent prescription drug abuse. Misunderstandings about what the medication is supposed to accomplish and how exactly it is supposed to be taken combine with poor or slow responses to encourage inaccurate or abusive ingestion. In addition, the medical health of this group is compromised. Overuse or abuse of prescription substances is more dangerous in older people because less-than-optimal liver functioning and other system frailties can potentiate physiological consequences (Oslin, 2005).

The onset of substance abuse late in life may not be the norm for geriatric substance abuse. Lifelong substance abuse that continues into geriatric years occurs frequently and is evident in chronic damage to body systems and concomitant health problems. Typical to substance abuse is the presence of violence that further complicates treatment as support systems are compromised. Addiction to a substance throughout adult milestones has had psychosocial impacts on the patient in profound ways. Wrestling an addiction is not easy at any stage in life; trying to conquer substance abuse after decades is daunting. Specific treatment incorporating gerontology and substance abuse considerations must be put into practice (Mansell, 2005).

Alcohol is the drug of choice in the geriatric patient population. Identifying late-life alcoholism, either sustained from earlier years or as a new addiction, requires a significant knowledge base about alcoholism and aging. Recognizing the effects of alcoholism on the body and developing evidence-based practice and treatments for those effects is vital.

Impaired Health Care Professional

The health care provider with a chemical dependency is not an unusual scenario. Health care workers, in general, work under a great deal of stress, may have physical injuries leading to pain syndromes, and have easy access to drugs. In the midst of daily pain-relieving functions with patients such as administering pain medications, the professional may consider self-medicating. If the professional has a chronic pain condition, it needs to be managed in an effective manner. Performing professional functions is difficult when chronic pain interferes and being able to function and work while being treated for chronic pain (with pain medications) is a proven positive treatment strategy (Turk & McCarberg, 2005). Effective treatment reduces the abusive use of medications in the workplace as a route to pain relief.

Health care providers become substance abusers for the same reasons anyone becomes dependent on or addicted to a substance. And when the substance is abused, the substance becomes more important than anything else in that person's life. Such behavior is dangerous in a health care environment, is a violation of state practice acts and ethical standards of practice, and, depending on the drug and method of obtaining it, may be a criminal offense.

Colleagues of chemically dependent health care workers need to be alert to behavior that suggests a substance abuse problem. They should assess the safety of attempting to talk with the professional who is having difficulty, and if deemed appropriate use the contact to clarify impressions and gather facts. Typical behaviors of impaired health care professionals are listed in Chart 16–8. The nurse's concerns about a colleague should be reported to a supervisor. A coworker relationship, a friendship, family ties, and the nurse's feelings of guilt or fear are not sufficient to neglect protecting patients from exposure to an impaired health care provider.

It is very common to cover up the addicted behavior. Shielding such a health care provider, whatever the professional discipline, puts patients, the health care provider, and the profession at risk and violates professional practice, the code of ethics, and the law in many states. Nurses, however, need to understand that their chemically dependent colleagues have a disease, not a moral problem. This understanding empowers nurses to work together to help each other. Most states have drug treatment or

---

CHART 16–8 | **Typical Behaviors Exhibited by Substance-Abusing Health Care Providers**

- Frequent absenteeism (usually before or after scheduled days off)
- Always working (in order to obtain supply)
- Abrupt mood changes; inappropriate affect
- Sloppy charting and patient care
- On duty when drugs are missing
- Frequent "wasting" of drugs or inaccurate control drug records
- Frequent disappearance from assigned work area
- Offering to give medication to patients not assigned to them
- Patients receiving medications from the health care provider complain of little or no pain relief.

---

support groups affiliated with the state nurses' association to address the impaired nurse. Disciplinary action, mandated treatment, and determination of suitability to practice all work well in a holistic approach (McKeon, Fogarty, & Hegney, 2006). A humane and rehabilitative approach such as treatment returns competent nursing colleagues to the work force.

Taylor (2004) suggested the following steps to take in supporting a colleague who is in recovery:

- Do not be judgmental or condescending.
- Let your colleague know you will be there for him and be supportive.
- Be available to step in when recovery is in jeopardy.
- Be honest about mentioning troubling behaviors.
- Be ready to intervene if evidence of relapse appears.
- Promote collaborativeness, not an us-against-you attitude.
- Step in and take a stand when others are intolerant.
- If intolerant behavior continues, report it to management.
- Ask questions about recovery, addiction, and relapse.
- Treat the colleague as you would want to be treated.

Remember, a physical injury and a painful rehabilitation can leave any nurse dependent on pain medications and subject to the physical, emotional, and professional problems just discussed (Sinuk & Taylor, 2004).

Nursing Management

Admission to hospitals and clinics for help with intoxication and withdrawal defines the majority of medical–surgical nursing intervention venues for substance abuse. This tends to be a cyclic process; one in which the patient has a negative physiological consequence of the substance abuse, realizes treatment is needed or is forced to participate in treatment, followed by eventual slippage of the drive to abstain and abuse of the substance recurs. Recognizing and accepting that substance abuse problems are chronic, often with remissions and exacerbations, should keep the nurse from succumbing to the frustration felt by many who treat substance abusers who relapse. At stressful times in life, anyone may develop a dependence on drugs or alcohol; however, certain people seem to be predisposed to the illness. The nurse's focus in performing the nursing process with these patients should be on promoting self-awareness, good health, and good interpersonal relationships so that patients can lead healthier, more constructive lives.

Medical–surgical nurses must be prepared to manage patients who have a substance abuse problem in addition to a medical or surgical issue. For example, management of a patient admitted for an extraordinarily painful acute pancreatitis would involve use of the nurse's physical assessment skills, history taking to pinpoint potential contributing factors such as drug abuse, the design and completion of competent pain assessments, provision of pain medications, and incorporation of ongoing assessment of behaviors around pain and its relief.

Assessment

The major approaches to assessing for substance abuse include interviews, questionnaires, and biological measures of biochemical and hematological markers. Nurses must keep up with current trends in drug use to assess and treat competently patients who are substance abusers. This can be accomplished with the knowledge acquired from reading, continuing education programs, and seminars as well as recognition of the realities of drug use in the local community.

The nurse must make an accurate assessment of the substances used and abused to anticipate potential toxic and withdrawal effects. Different substances require different modes of treatment.

Nursing care plans for a patient with chronic alcoholism who is malnourished, exhausted, and depressed include immediate diet regulation, rest, and gradual involvement in a treatment program. The nursing care also involves incorporating the psychosocial and physiological aspects of the disease. The nursing process organizes care from assessment through interventions. The Nursing Process: Patient Care Plan for Chronic Alcoholism box (p. 382) details the assessment of the patient with chronic alcoholism and gives examples of the expected nursing diagnoses. The outcomes of the care as well as the evaluation of the interventions are delineated in addition to the plan for care and the interventions.

People who abuse cocaine or crack are likely to be resistant to treatment and need active staff intervention and a structured program to involve them in treatment. They should not be left alone or purposefully isolated, as might be done with someone who abuses alcohol. The nursing care for a patient with cocaine intoxication focuses on the immediate needs of the patient and the plan for the longer term. As with the chronic alcoholism nursing process care plan, the Nursing Process: Patient Care Plan for Cocaine Intoxication (p. 382) details the assessment of the patient who is intoxicated from cocaine and gives examples of the expected nursing diagnoses, outcomes of the care, and evaluations and rationales. Notice how the focus of one care plan differs from the other.

The nurse should conduct a thorough, nonjudgmental substance use assessment. Some of the interview questions found in Chart 16–9 may be useful. Simply asking "How many drinks do you have at a time?" is insufficient and can minimize the problem if each drink exceeds standard bar amounts of about 2 oz. The CAGE questions discussed earlier in Chart 16–3 (p. 370) are also helpful. Accurate responses to these questions are most

| CHART 16–9 | **Substance Abuse Interview Questions** |

- How many packs of cigarettes do you smoke daily?
- Do you take any prescription drugs now?
- Do you drink alcohol each day? If yes, do you drink a pint or about a quart? (Let the patient correct an overstatement.)
- Do you drink a pint or quart of alcohol or more on occasion?
- When was your last drink?
- Do you have a drug habit?
- What drugs do you use?
- What is your daily cost?
- When did you last drink more than you wanted to?

likely when they are part of an interview that includes general lifestyle inquiries about cigarette smoking, coffee consumption, and exercise habits. Experts agree that skillful assessment interviewing of patients and their family members remains the best source of data.

In an emergency situation the patient may be unable to answer key questions such as these:

- What did you take?
- How much did you take?
- When did you take it?
- What have you taken in the last 24 hours? In the last week?

When this happens, the nurse must rely on family or friends as data sources, and then corroborate what is learned with the patient once she is alert.

People who abuse alcohol and other drugs tend to deny they have a problem or minimize the problem by making it appear perfectly normal: "I drink/use every day, but it rarely interferes with my work." Rationalization is common: "I know I shouldn't use, and I'll stop as soon as I get through this problem. It keeps me calm so I can do what I need to do." A detailed assessment generally reveals that the problem is worse than the patient says. Cocaine users tend to project and blame their difficulties on others, often a family member. "I don't need help. My boyfriend's marijuana smoking is the real problem. He can't remember to do anything so I have to stay on the ball to make up for it."

Substance abusers manipulate people and situations to get drugs. The term *drug-seeking behaviors* (DSBs) refers to these manipulations. Examples include feigning illness or an injury to get a drug. It becomes more important to obtain the substance of choice than to function with integrity, honesty, love, or reliability.

An assessment of behavioral changes can cue the nurse to drug use. Less dramatic physical findings that aid in detection may include dry skin, hangnails, malnutrition, ascites, elevated blood pressure, and the smell of alcohol or an inhalant on the patient's breath. As alcoholism progresses, the nurse should be alert to signs and symptoms of liver cirrhosis.

Laboratory Tests

For years, researchers and clinicians have been searching for an objective biologic marker that will reflect problem drinking and make assessment less challenging. Common laboratory tests in

Assessment of Coping Style and Effectiveness

Subjective Data:
What kinds of experiences do you have before you drink alcohol?
What do you consider stressful?
Does stress seem easier to manage when you drink?
How many hours do you sleep at night?
What do you do to promote sleep for yourself?
What do you usually eat throughout the day?

Objective Data:
Inability to manage stress without resorting to substance use
Limited coping skills
Compromised liver function
Insomnia
Poor metabolic health
Malnutrition

Nursing Assessment and Diagnoses	Outcomes and Evaluation Parameters	Planning and Interventions with *Rationales*
Nursing Diagnoses: *Coping, Ineffective* related to alcohol abuse *Sleep Deprivation* related to alcohol abuse *Nutrition, Imbalanced: Less than Body Requirements* related to alcohol abuse	**Outcomes:** Reduction of ineffective and self-destructive coping through alcohol abuse and regular use of more effective coping styles. Sleeping a total of a reasonable number of hours/night indicates successful resolution of sleep deprivation. Patient eats 3 meals every day plus snacks and takes multivitamin as recommended. ***Evaluation Parameters:*** Has begun to substitute effective coping for alcohol use when stressed. Uses sleep-inducing strategies nightly and reports satisfaction with quality of sleep. Reestablishes a consistently healthy sleep routine. Patient identifies and understands relationship between alcoholism and malnutrition. Patient gains weight through a balanced diet.	**Interventions and *Rationales:*** Identify two effective coping mechanisms. *Patients need to have ready choices on how to cope with stress without their addictive substance.* Inventory those situations that challenge patient's abilities to cope. *This prepares the patient for difficulties so rehearsal and skill building can take place.* Rehearse various coping strategies to prepare and select two for regular use. *Rehearsal allows the patient to get familiar with the skill and to learn how to use it.* Teach alternative, healthy coping mechanisms. *Revision of coping styles requires identification of the situations placing the patient at risk, typical problematic responses, and acknowledgment of a need to learn.* Assess for cirrhosis of the liver. *Years of substance abuse may result in cirrhosis.* Assess for depression and feelings of self-reproach and guilt for years of drinking and the effect on others. *Alcohol is a depressant and contributes to deepening existing depressions.* Promote recognition of automatic mechanisms involved in habitually responding to stress with alcohol. *How to cope with stress in adaptive ways will be a new skill.* Consider AA groups, psychiatric treatment, hospitalization, 28-day alcohol treatment programs. *These specialized interventions may be necessary to treat the acute problem.* Evaluate suicide or violence potential. *Alcohol as a depressant certainly raises risk of lethality, plus abstinence may highlight the deep and various life problems the patient has where problem solving sober may seem too big a burden to bear.* Assess for history of insomnia. *Alcohol initially causes somnolence, but chronic use causes insomnia.* Assess current sleep pattern and effective strategies. *Teach and promote healthy sleep hygiene such as warm milk, reading, and other relaxation strategies that counteract ineffective sleep hygiene routines.* Employ effective sleep strategies regularly. *To counteract the alcoholism-disturbed sleep pattern, retraining must take place.* Assess malnourishment from chronic alcoholism. *Vitamins, especially vitamin B, are not metabolized well in an alcoholic's body.* Long-term alcoholism interferes with self-care abilities such as proper nourishment. *Malnutrition from chronic alcoholism can be addressed with a comprehensive nutrition program.* Monitor intake of meals and snacks *to ensure proper intake.* Initiate dietary consult *to explore depth of nutrition problem and educate patient about healthy eating.* Investigate dietary preferences to maximize patient's abilities to expand intake appropriately. *It is easier to reshape a patient's diet when preferences are incorporated.* Educate patient regarding the impact of chronic alcohol ingestion on the digestive tract, metabolism, and overall health. *Alcohol impacts are not commonly known or understood.* Offer frequent food and fluids throughout contacts *to reestablish proper electrolyte, protein, and carbohydrate levels.*

NURSING PROCESS: Patient Care Plan for Cocaine Intoxication

Assessment of Coping Style and Effectiveness

Subjective Data:
What kinds of experiences do you have before you use cocaine?
What do you consider stressful?
Does stress seem easier to manage when you use cocaine?
How are your relationships affected by your cocaine use?

Objective Data:
Inability to manage stress without resorting to substance use
Limited coping skills
Poor social and occupational functioning

Nursing Assessment and Diagnoses	Outcomes and Evaluation Parameters	Planning and Interventions with *Rationales*
Nursing Diagnosis: *Ineffective Coping* related to cocaine abuse	**Outcomes:** Reduction of ineffective and self-destructive coping through cocaine abuse and regular use of more effective coping styles. **Evaluation Parameters:** Has begun to substitute effective coping for cocaine use when stressed. Patient will complete a cocaine detoxification program and will remain free of cocaine. "Clean" urine 72 hours after last use. Replacement of destructive coping with two effective individual coping options.	**Interventions and *Rationales:*** Conduct individual meetings with patient regarding consequences of drug use in work, home, social, and physical arenas. *Defense mechanisms solidly in place throughout the substance abuse period make recognition of self-imposed difficulties difficult.* Discuss prioritization of the work on problem areas. *Immediate medical–surgical concerns take priority over the longer term issues of substance abuse treatment and therapy.* There will be treatment offered for cocaine withdrawal. Arrange access to individual and group therapy. *Team discussions will shape the treatment for the problem in the forefront.* Observe every 1/2 hour. *Withdrawal from cocaine can be a difficult and dangerous time. Lethality risk exists.* Monitor drug-seeking behaviors as an inevitable aspect of this problem. *Long-standing interpersonal styles are not immediately resolved.* When drug-seeking behavior (DSB) commences, interact about patient's feelings and educate about cravings and time frames for resolution. *DSB may be out of patient's awareness and needs to be labeled and addressed.* Help patient recognize the automatic mechanisms involved in turning to cocaine. *Over time the patient sees the connection between stress and demands and the urge to escape through cocaine use.* Identify two effective coping mechanisms. *Patients need to have ready choices on how to cope with stress without their substance.* Help patient rehearse various coping strategies to prepare and select two for regular use. *Revision of coping styles requires learning and practice. Options for coping are more effective and promote resiliency.* Patient begins to substitute effective coping for cocaine use. *Once substitution occurs, there is still the risk of returning to familiar, if maladaptive, responses to stress.* Improve patient's awareness of behaviors, reduce denial, and educate about the addiction. *This intervention serves to supply an educative process that was missing or ineffective before addiction was established.*

which elevated values are associated with excessive alcohol intake are:

- Blood alcohol concentration
- Gamma-glutamyl transferase (GGT)
- Alanine aminotransferase (ALT, formerly SGPT)
- Aspartate aminotransferase (AST, formerly SGOT)
- Lactate dehydrogenase
- Alkaline phosphatase
- Total bilirubin
- Cholesterol
- Triglycerides
- Uric acid
- Mean corpuscular volume (MCV).

These elevated laboratory test values are only one of the alerting factors for problem drinking. (The Diagnostic Tests box provides an overview of the rationale for these tests.) No single test or combination of tests alone to date is appropriate for clinical screening. Confirmation of the excessive use of alcohol in a sensitively conducted assessment interview remains the preferred assessment approach and is considered a prerequisite for successful intervention.

Nursing Diagnosis

Because substance-related disorders are associated with physiological, psychosocial, and spiritual distress, a wide variety of nursing diagnoses are likely to be fundamental to planning comprehensive care. Applicable diagnoses include:

- *Coping, Ineffective*
- *Family Processes, Dysfunctional: Alcoholism*
- *Anxiety*
- *Nutrition Imbalanced: Less than Body Requirements*
- *Decisional Conflict*
- *Pain*
- *Sensory Perception, Disturbed*
- *Social Interaction, Impaired*
- *Thought Processes, Disturbed.*

Outcomes and Evaluation Parameters

When designing care for substance abusers, outcomes must be specifically stated. Although the outcome of total and permanent abstinence may be achievable for some patients with some abuse disorders, for others it may be an unattainable goal. Each situation must be assessed individually. Make sure outcomes can be measured so the treatment team is aware of progress and relapse. Outcome criteria for substance abusers include:

- Coping *as exhibited by goal-directed behavior with resolution of problems.*
- Decision making *as exhibiting patterns of choosing courses of action that meet short- and long-term health-related goals.*
- Impulse control *as exhibited by abstinence.*

See the Patient Teaching & Discharge Priorities box for general guidelines on planning the discharge for these patients.

All of these outcomes impact on sobriety, abstinence from drugs and alcohol, and "getting straight." Further outcomes include risk reduction; improvement of work, family, and social relationships; and lifestyle changes that may include a growing sense of spirituality. No addiction or abuse situation is going to be easy to abandon as a lifestyle. Interventions promote more effectiveness in using new attitudes and behaviors. Although the fear of relapse is always present, over time the craving for chemicals diminishes, and the patient establishes a healthier lifestyle.

Planning and Interventions

Treatment for substance abuse includes promoting adaptive mechanisms and healthy perspectives on self-care and addressing the psychodynamics of drug addiction (Killen et al., 2006; Lile, 2006; Mathias & National Institute on Drug Abuse, 2006). Treatment interventions range from traditional medical interventions and psychiatric care through shamanistic practices. In general, planning care focuses on reducing the harmful use pattern.

Coerced treatment by family, friends, physicians, or the police—a frequent eventuality—inevitably causes the patient to feel anger and resentment. These patients may lash out at people (including the nurse), blame them, and demonstrate resistant or arrogant behavior. In these difficult situations, the nurse must remain detached and nonjudgmental to avoid both power

---

DIAGNOSTIC TESTS for Substance Abuse

Test	Expected Abnormality	Rationale for Abnormality
Liver function profiles	Indications that the liver enzymes are not effective or that the liver would not be able to competently metabolize medications	Alcohol interferes with the liver's abilities to function adequately. Long-standing problems with alcohol cause cirrhosis.
Drug screens (blood and urine)	Evidence of drug in blood or urine	Patient may deny use of substances, but drug screens are able to detect presence.
Breathalyzer	Evidence of alcohol, and the extent of the alcohol, in the expired breath of the patient	Determines the BAL following ingestion of an amount of alcohol.

Sources: Albanese, M. J. (2005). Assessing and treating the bipolar patient with comorbid substance use disorder. *Directions in Psychiatry, 25*(4), 281–290; Kasper, D. L., Braunwald, E., Fauci, A., Hauser, S., Longo, D., & Jameson, J. L. (2007). *Harrison's principles of internal medicine* (16th ed.). New York: McGraw-Hill.

PATIENT TEACHING & DISCHARGE PRIORITIES for Substance Abuse

Need	Teaching
Stabilization of the physiological condition	Patient will be able to demonstrate the need for attention to the physiological demands placed on him as a result of substance abuse.
Involvement in substance abuse treatment	Patient will initiate and continue involvement with substance abuse treatment framework.
Awareness of the substance abuse problem and the necessary treatment	Family members are able to list the signs of substance abuse evident in their relative and the appropriate interventions applicable to the situation.
Contact and linkage with the treatment venue associated with the substance of abuse	The setting of the substance abuse treatment varies depending on the drug of abuse. Alcoholism can be treated via inpatient programs such as a detoxification unit, in a 28-day program, in a halfway house, through self-help such as AA, or as an outpatient. Other substances offer a similar array of treatment choices with heroin addiction having an extra component of the methadone clinic as a treatment avenue.

struggles and taking the role of persecutor or rescuer. Interactions are matter of fact: "I know you are [uncomfortable, anxious, afraid, angry] right now. To help you feel better, I need to ask you some questions about your drug use."

General Hospital Care

Substance abusers who are suicidal or acutely ill with DTs, hepatic coma, respiratory depression, or cardiac arrhythmias are often treated in the medical–surgical unit of a general hospital. Life-threatening physiological symptoms are prioritized. When the client is out of danger, the alcoholism or drug addiction issues can be addressed. In this setting, nurses:

- Monitor vital signs and respiratory and cardiovascular support.
- Administer prescribed medications.
- Apply ice packs for fever, such as fever caused by amphetamine intoxication or following cocaine use.
- Decrease stimulation; provide a darkened quiet room.
- Point out reality: "I know you are seeing things, and I know you are frightened. You are in the hospital, and we are caring for you. There are no bugs or monsters here. You are safe and will feel better soon."
- Make sure clients get adequate nutrition and fluids (they are disoriented and generally forget to eat and drink).
- Assess changes in level of consciousness.
- Monitor fluid intake and output.
- Protect skin integrity.
- Offer emotional support and encouragement to the patient and his family.
- Refer patients to community resources for recovery programs.

Other Treatment Settings

Specialized care is given in inpatient hospital units that are geared specifically for the treatment of substance abuse. If the hospital is equipped with trained personnel and appropriate resources, acutely ill patients, including those who are intoxicated, may be admitted. The physical environment is modified to handle problems with substance abusers. For example, rooms devoid of furniture and potentially harmful materials offer a quiet, unstimulating environment that prevents convulsions and decreases anxiety. A primary nurse may be assigned to decrease confusion and stimulation. Members of the staff are experts in detoxification, education, and treatment. Patients also receive treatment for coexisting medical and psychiatric problems. Staff efforts are geared toward stabilization.

Residential rehabilitation facilities offer inpatients expert care for substance abuse, but in some cases staff members are not skilled in treating medical or psychiatric problems. Extended care facilities provide services for people with physical impairments and a home for recovering alcoholics or drug addicts who have been rejected by their families. Apartments for independent living are useful when available. The nurse working in one of these settings would be aware of each patient's history and propensities around substance use and abuse and be alert to signs and symptoms of relapse to the drug of choice. Impacts on the individual's ability to remain in that health care setting would be a foremost consideration in nursing care.

Outpatient care may consist of daily, weekly, or monthly individual, group, or family therapy in a variety of treatment centers. Daily care is usually given only in intensive programs of limited duration, usually 1 month. Employee assistance programs (EAPs) are now common in many industries and are one example of outpatient care given not in a clinic but in the workplace. Substance abuse outreach counselors work with employees who are chemically dependent.

Self-Help Groups

Self-help groups for addictions have similar goals as other self-help groups: to be a source of mutual aid to individuals who have addictions. Further goals may include serving as a resource to addicts and loved ones as well as increasing awareness of the addiction in the community and its treatment among clinical professionals. Self-help groups may have a specific focus within the support they provide, such as promoting spirituality or helping with a particular addiction. But because longitudinal studies associate self-help group involvement with reduced substance use, improved psychosocial functioning, and lessened health care costs (Guha, 2006), nurses involved in treating addictive processes need to be aware of the benefits of peer groups.

Twelve-Step Programs

In contrast to the previously described treatment programs, Alcoholics Anonymous (AA) and Narcotics Anonymous (NA) are not professionally designed treatment programs. They are spiritual programs based on fellowship among its members. Both are successful self-help groups that meet daily, or more often, in different parts of large cities and weekly in smaller towns in places of worship, schools, town halls, and various mental health treatment facilities. Anyone who has a desire to stop drinking or taking drugs is welcome. This belief pervades both organizations: "Once an alcoholic/addict, always an alcoholic/addict." Members admit they are powerless over chemicals, live "one day at a time," recite the serenity prayer, and believe in "a power greater than man." Members learn to turn their problems over to "the God of my understanding." Their philosophy is revealed in part through their key slogans: "First things first," "Easy does it," and "Let go and let God." Alcoholics learn the "Twelve Steps of AA" (see Chart 16–10).

CHART 16–10 **Twelve Steps of Alcoholics Anonymous**

1. We admitted we were powerless over alcohol—that our lives had become unmanageable.
2. Came to believe that a Power greater than ourselves could restore us to sanity.
3. Made a decision to turn our will and our lives over to the care of God, as we understand Him.
4. Made a searching and fearless moral inventory of ourselves.
5. Admitted to God, to ourselves, and to another human being the exact nature of our wrongs.
6. Were entirely ready to have God remove all these defects of character.
7. Humbly asked Him to remove our shortcomings.
8. Made a list of all people we had harmed, and became willing to make amends to them all.
9. Made direct amends to such people wherever possible, except when to do so would injure them or others.
10. Continued to take personal inventory and when we were wrong, promptly admitted it.
11. Sought through prayer and meditation to improve our conscious contact with God, as we understand Him, praying only for knowledge of His will for us and the power to carry that out.
12. Having had a spiritual awakening as the result of these steps, we tried to carry this message to alcoholics, and to practice these principles in all our affairs.

Source: The Twelve Steps are reprinted with permission of Alcoholics Anonymous World Services, Inc. (AAWS). Permission to reprint the Twelve Steps does not mean that AAWS necessarily agrees with the views expressed herein. AA is a program of recovery from alcoholism only—use of the Twelve Steps in connection with programs and activities, which are patterned after AA but which address other problems, or in any other non-AA context, does not imply otherwise.

Through AA/NA, people learn to change negative attitudes and behaviors into positive ones. A key concept of AA/NA is that total abstinence is essential to recovery. As members become sober or drug free, they begin "sponsoring" (helping) other substance abusers. This offering of support is believed to be vital to recovery, as is regular attendance at AA/NA meetings. Twelve-step recovery programs also emphasize spirituality through meditation and prayer rather than willpower as the means to recovery. Recognizing that AA's 12 steps were written in the 1930s by and for white Christian males may require that the nurse adapt some of the language to a less patriarchal, less religious, and more generally spiritual and culturally relevant usage.

Women for Sobriety

Women for Sobriety (WFS) is another self-help group. Unlike AA/NA, WFS is not based on a spiritual philosophy; instead, the program is based on abstinence. WFS's 13 acceptance statements focus members on new ways of thinking. Women learn to cope and, over time, to change their daily lives. The group recognizes the differences of alcoholism in males and females.

Rational Recovery

Alcoholics and addicts who were not comfortable in AA but were nevertheless determined to become sober have founded Rational Recovery (RR), a self-help approach that rejects the spiritual approach of AA. RR also rejects the notion that alcoholics and addicts are powerless to stop their addictions, suggesting instead that until now they simply have not chosen to do so. Instead of reliance on a higher power (which RR considers another form of dependence), RR members are urged to build on strengths within themselves; the movement inspires independence whenever humanly possible. A constant theme is "Think yourself sober."

In RR, there are no steps, sponsors, moral inventories, making amends to others, or even caring about what others think of you. According to rational emotive therapy, on which RR is based, human beings should love themselves because they are human beings and not because others think well of them. The concept of staying sober one day at a time is rejected in favor of a decision to never drink or use again, period. Sobriety is not supposed to become the cornerstone of one's life. The goal is for members to wean themselves from dependence on alcohol, then from dependence on people, and finally from dependence on the group.

Meetings take place only twice a week, and most people attend for only 1 year, after which they may be pronounced "recovered." They can, however, return to meetings whenever the need arises. Discussions at meetings focus on the here and now rather than past history, and interactive discussion is encouraged.

Whereas AA relies totally on nonprofessionals helping one another, professional coordinators run RR, and each group has volunteer professional advisers available for advice and input. This is necessary because, unlike AA, there are no old-timers around to help newcomers. Advisers attend meetings only occasionally. RR, like AA, offers written materials, the core of which is *Rational Recovery from Alcoholism: The Small Book* (meant to contrast with the Big Book of AA).

RR suggests looking within oneself for strength and direction. Everyone has an inner voice, says RR, that challenges one to go wrong. It is this voice, nicknamed "Beast," that urges one to drink or use drugs, takes over during blackouts, gets one to do terrible things, and speaks louder than one's rational self. It's the voice that tells one things like "You can stop anytime (but not now)" or "You're not really addicted (you just like the taste)" and that tears angrily into those who criticize or try to help. BEAST is an acronym used to help RR members avoid taking another drink or drug. See Chart 16–4 (p. 371) for specifics about the BEAST acronym.

Relapse

Relapse is common among substance abusers, and it seriously complicates treatment. Authorities in the field of alcoholism estimate that 60% to 75% of those who complete treatment programs drink again within the first 90 days. Data suggest that only 10% to 20% of alcoholics remain abstinent for 1 year following treatment, and that only 35% of these are abstinent 5 years later. In fact, recidivism rates are notoriously high across the spectrum of addictive behaviors (Doweiko, 2006; Finnell & Osborne, 2006).

After a successful initial change, the patient experiences perceived control while remaining abstinent. This feeling of perceived control continues until the patient encounters a high-risk situation involving negative emotional states, interpersonal conflict, or social pressure. The patient can avoid relapse by using effective coping responses in the high-risk situation. If, however, the patient cannot cope successfully, an initial "lapse" occurs in which she resorts to the use of a chemical to control stress. The patient then feels less able to exert control and develops a tendency to "give in" to the situation ("It's no use, I can't handle this"). In subsequent high-risk situations, the patient again resorts to the use of chemicals to relieve stress. Repeated lapses set the stage for a return to uncontrolled use (relapse).

Many treatment centers are now incorporating the concept of relapse prevention into their treatment programs. This concept is designed to teach patients how to anticipate relapse. By learning skills to use in high-risk situations, patients gain confidence and the expectation of being able to cope successfully, thus decreasing the probability of relapse.

Research indicates that participation in a 12-step program can help prevent relapse. These programs focus on the patient being "in recovery" and maintaining sobriety, as opposed to having recovered or being cured.

Other Treatment Approaches

Substance abuse is a complex problem, so a single treatment approach is not likely to address the majority of needs. Therefore, a variety of treatments are typically engaged, as discussed in the following subsections.

Complementary and Alternative Therapies

Interest in alternative and complementary treatments has increased and is useful to explore with regard to substance abuse. Treatment for substance abuse is a difficult process prone to failure. The addict must fight the physiological demands of the addiction as well as the psychological repercussions of being in the world without the relief or escape of the drug of choice. Short-lived abstinence can be viewed as a partial success.

Complementary and alternative treatments for substance abuse take on a different form than for other health problems in that an herbal or food supplement substance is not substituted

for the pharmaceutical or illicit drug of abuse. As a matter of fact, there are a number of complementary and alternative substances that can be abused for their escapist and stimulating qualities, so suggesting those as a mode of treatment would be counterproductive. Consider the therapeutic impact and the holistic functioning of the person when integrating these aspects of care.

For substance abuse, alternative treatments may include more ethnomedical treatments or those discovered through research on cross-cultural styles rather than substituting a benign botanical for the abused drug. Interventions based on behaviors and beliefs would be alternative to the medical model of drug treatment. Treatments that attend to the cultural aspects of human existence include encouraging traditional values that discourage deviant behaviors such as drug abuse (Gates et al., 2006; Peterson, Mitchell, Hong, Agar, & Latkin, 2006), inducing a relaxation response and thus providing a healthy coping mechanism, or using a nondrug reward for abstinence through the traditional operant behavior analysis style (Turk & McCarberg, 2005).

The use of acupuncture for treating substance abuse is discussed in the Complementary and Alternative Therapies box (p. 388).

Using Confrontation Strategies

Interventions for substance abuse can occur as soon as the problem is identified. Group intervention/confrontation is one strategy that aims to break down the substance abuser's denial. Nurses are often "intervention specialists" and leaders in this process.

Several family members, friends, employers, coworkers, and an alcohol/drug intervention specialist confront the substance abuser in a private meeting. They list the evidence by going around the group, one by one. The family, friends, employer, and so on, following the leader's cues, speak calmly and slowly with minimal emotion. They are presenting the facts, the objective evidence, to the alcoholic/drug abuser. Yelling, blaming, and haranguing are avoided because the alcoholic/drug abuser will inevitably respond by denying the behavior or making excuses. However, confrontation by several people who really care and who persistently present the facts breaks through the denial.

The next step in group intervention/confrontation requires the family, friends, employer, etc., to make clear and direct statements to the alcoholic/drug abuser about the consequences of his behavior:

- "Either you get help now or we will take you off the job."
- "Either you enter a treatment program now or I will move out with the kids."

If the patient agrees to treatment, the caring people agree to remain involved.

Education

Videotapes and talks by recovered substance abusers or experts in the effects of substance abuse are helpful. Education may take place in or out of the hospital, in one comprehensive session or several sessions over time. Nurse-educators should focus on the types of abused substances and their physical, psychological, and social effects. Families are often involved in these sessions because substance abuse is a family problem. The belief underlying such education is that knowledge and awareness may be useful in decreasing self-destructive behavior. But knowledge alone is never enough. Culturally sensitive and relevant educational resources should be used.

Referral and Self-Help Groups

Support and self-help groups are extremely useful in helping patients feel better about themselves and acquire new attitudes and behaviors. Merely being with many people who are suffering in similar ways is beneficial. By observing people who have been sober or drug free for long periods, patients can begin to learn similar behaviors. They can see that there is hope and that recovery is possible. Self-help groups also provide new friends, generally with healthy lifestyles. Patients may choose to attend support groups for the rest of their lives. Some patients who experiment with drugs or alcohol during one period of their lives and who succeed in stopping may attend only during the crisis.

Lifestyle Change

An emphasis on the requirement for a total lifestyle change is necessary. Nurses can help patients discuss ways to alter their destructive habits by suggesting different coping strategies and by encouraging them to discover new interests and capabilities within themselves. Nurses and patients can role-play new responses to old situations. Recognizing that relapse is always a threat, nurses may set up behavioral contracts. For example, there may be an agreement to contact the nurse or an AA/NA sponsor if and when they feel the urge to drink or do drugs. This agreement represents new behaviors that are necessary for a lifestyle change.

Part of a total lifestyle change includes the patients' realization that it is no longer possible to remain abstinent while spending time with friends who are substance abusers or hanging out at places where they used to take drugs or alcohol. The mere sight or smell of paraphernalia or the desired substance is often enough to trigger a relapse. Old ties must be broken; new friends and activities must be pursued. See the Nursing Process: Patient Care Plan (p. 382) earlier in this chapter for specifics on lifestyle changes with cocaine use.

COMPLEMENTARY & ALTERNATIVE THERAPIES — Acupuncture/Acupressure

Description:

Acupuncture is based on the philosophy that Qi (pronounced "chee"), or a person's vital energy, flows through specific energy meridians throughout the body. An acupuncturist inserts very fine needles into the skin to stimulate these energy meridians in order to influence physiological, emotional, and psychological functions of the mind and body. A related CAM therapy, acupressure, uses finger pressure rather than needles along these energy meridians to exert the same influence on the flow of energy. Most acupuncture and acupressure practitioners are health care providers who have chosen to add these therapies to their current practice. These practitioners may choose one or both of the therapies, then pursue certification programs.

Research Support:

A placebo-controlled pilot study was carried out in a community mental health center in a United States–Mexico border city. Most participants were Hispanic males with an average age of 32.8 years. The goal of the study was to examine the effectiveness of acupressure on cravings in drug-addicted individuals. Participants reported an average lifetime use of drug of choice of 14 years. In addition to conventional medical care, participants received specific acupressure treatment once a week for 6 consecutive weeks, and placebo acupressure treatment. Researchers administered the Hopkins Symptom Checklist (SCL-20) Depression Scale to assess changes in emotional distress before and after 6 weeks of treatment. In order to assess changes in craving, researchers used the Brief Substance Craving Scale at baseline and weekly for 6 weeks. The results showed that both specific and placebo acupressure groups experienced a significant reduction in craving at the end of treatment. The specific acupressure group had a greater and more steady reduction in craving. Both specific acupressure and conventional-care-only groups demonstrated a significant reduction in emotional stress (Tian & Krishnan, 2006).

In another study, the effects of acupuncture on 40 HIV-seropositive, cocaine-abusing, methadone-maintained drug users were studied. These participants were randomized to one of two protocols: the standard five-needle National Acupuncture Detoxification Association (NADA) protocol or a reduced, escalating dose (one- to three-needle) protocol. The last 15 of the participants also received a spirituality-focused group therapy intervention in addition to their assigned acupuncture treatments that were offered 5 days per week for 8 weeks. Urine samples from each participant were collected twice weekly and were analyzed for the presence of both cocaine and heroin. Participants' levels of depression and anxiety were assessed both pre- and post-treatment. Results showed that there was no difference in the number of weeks in which urine samples tested negative for heroin and cocaine use between the two acupuncture protocols. However, patients who received the spirituality-focused group therapy in addition to acupuncture treatment showed significantly longer abstinence from heroin and cocaine and greater reductions in depression and anxiety than the patients who did not receive spirituality-focused psychotherapy (Margolin, Avants, & Arnold, 2005).

The goal of another study was to develop an Internet-assisted smoking cessation program accompanied by auricular acupressure. Researchers aimed to compare the abstinence rate and self-efficacy of youth smokers receiving auricular acupressure with and without the Internet-assisted smoking cessation program. Participants were assigned nonrandomly to two groups. Group 1 received auricular acupressure plus the Internet-assisted smoking cessation program, while group 2 received auricular acupressure only. Researchers collected demographic factors, serum nicotine, quitting rate, nicotine dependence, and self-efficacy data before and after a 4-week intervention. The results showed that after intervention, the abstinence rate was 15.78% in group 1 and 2.56% in group 2. Group 1 showed significantly lower nicotine dependence, nicotine dependence remained unchanged in group 2. Self-efficacy improvement between groups 1 and 2 was significantly different. The combination of auricular acupressure and Internet-assisted smoking cessation program was more effective than auricular acupressure alone in terms of the abstinence rate (Chen, Yeh, & Chao, 2006).

References

Chen, H. H., Yeh, M. L., & Chao, Y. H. (2006). Comparing effects of auricular acupressure with and without an internet-assisted program on smoking cessation and self-efficacy of adolescents. *Journal of Alternative and Complementary Medicine, 12*(2), 147–152.

Margolin, A., Avants, S. K., & Arnold, R. (2005). Acupuncture and spirituality-focused group therapy for the treatment of HIV-positive drug users: A preliminary study. *Journal of Psychoactive Drugs, 37*(4), 385–390.

Tian, X., & Krishnan, S. (2006). Efficacy of auricular acupressure as an adjuvant therapy in substance abuse treatment: A pilot study. *Alternative Therapies in Health and Medicine, 12*(1), 66–69.

Helping the Family

Substance abuse affects the entire family system. Family members often engage in behaviors that enable substance abusers to continue with their substance abuse by protecting them from the consequences of their behavior. Helping family members to be healthier includes clarifying the problem and presenting possible solutions (treatment) and creating a support system for family members. Referring family members to Al-Anon can be a very helpful strategy. Al-Anon is a program for family members and friends whose lives have been affected by a person who abuses alcohol. The program helps them to understand the addiction, the psychological affects of being near someone who abuses alcohol, and to learn coping mechanisms.

In dysfunctional families, the substance abuser often becomes the "identified patient," focusing attention on that individual and away from the other problems in the family. Treatment for the substance abuser may require including some type of family therapy. Family members may need treatment for codependence through group or individual therapy or involvement in a 12-step program such as Al-Anon or Codependents Anonymous (CODA). The Adult Children of Alcoholics (ACOA) support groups could be helpful for those who respond to 12-step self-help groups (Timko, Billow, & DeBenedetti, 2006).

Evaluation

Evaluating nursing interventions for patients who are substance abusers hinges on an evaluation of the patient's abilities to change. Is there evidence of patient honesty, openness, and willingness to take responsibility for his own actions? Regardless of the substance of abuse, once a patient stops blaming others for her use/abuse, treatment has made a positive impact. Another criterion is the amount of substance the patient is placing in his body. Has it decreased? Other indications of positive treatment outcome are increased job stability, improvement in interpersonal relationships with others, and improved problem-solving techniques. Evaluating implementation of the necessary changes in people, places, and things is critical for victory over substance dependence.

Collaborative Management

Treating chronic alcoholism in an effective manner involves nurses, physicians, rehabilitation therapists, and psychotherapists (such as clinical nurse specialists, psychologists, and psychiatrists), social workers, dieticians, and peer advocacy/support. This disease process is a composite of genetic predisposition, a variety of underlying psychological dynamics, exposure and reactions to stress, and the physiological consequences of the behavior of using alcohol as a coping mechanism.

Each team member will address, in a planned manner, how the patient will move toward recovery from chronic alcoholism. The psychologist can provide psychological testing when there are questions about coexisting psychological problems, and can provide psychotherapy (individual or group) for patients who abuse alcohol whose problems require multifaceted clinical interventions. The dietician will help increase the nutritional status of the patient that has been compromised by malnutrition and the interference of alcohol in metabolizing necessary vitamins and nutrients. The peer support approach of AA has had a significant impact on people addicted to alcohol. The self-help component of this contact is an important factor in the overall success and recovery of an alcoholic. The collaborative team approach offers the best response to the treatment needs of this patient from the day of admission to the ongoing, sustained approach that will help this patient maintain a healthier lifestyle.

Effective treatment of a patient who is intoxicated by cocaine usually involves the same team members used for treating patients with alcoholism. Teams intervene during the intoxication stage and beyond, providing services to enhance the patient's abilities to choose a healthier lifestyle. The rehabilitation counselor provides additional information about the use of cocaine and develops, with the rest of the team, a plan for the patient to maintain cocaine abstinence. As with alcoholism, peer support through Narcotics Anonymous has been proven to be an effective mechanism for recovery. The collaborative team approach offers the best response to the treatment needs of this patient from the day of admission to the ongoing, sustained approach that will help this patient maintain a healthier lifestyle.

Summary

Substance abuse knows no social boundaries. It is important nurses educate themselves and others about the effects of substance abuse. Through the understanding of addiction, the nurse will be able to observe the patient for behaviors or physical symptoms of abuse and report him or her to the health care team. Caring for patients who are substance abusers requires knowledgeable and skilled nursing to develop and implement effective multidisciplinary plans of care.

RESEARCH OPPORTUNITIES AND CLINICAL IMPACT RELATED TO SUBSTANCE ABUSE

Research Area	Clinical Impact
Standards of Addictions Nursing Practice, Standard XII: Research. This standard states that the nurse contributes to the nursing care of patients with addictions and to the addictions area of practice through innovations in theory and practice and participation in research, and communicates these contributions.	The clinical impact of research in this area of nursing care provides evidence-based practices for addictions and substance abuse treatment providers and deepens one's knowledge base within nursing. When research results are shared throughout the nursing community, patient care is enhanced.
Research demonstrates that children of alcoholics are at higher risk of becoming alcoholics. Even if different families adopt them at birth, identical twins of alcoholic parents have more than a significant chance of becoming alcoholics; fraternal twins have a smaller but still elevated chance (Dick & Bierut, 2006).	Research into addressing the environments vulnerable children are raised in could ultimately lower the risk factors associated with having genetic predispositions to substance abuse.
Alcoholism clinical investigations have redefined alcoholism as a disease. As research about its biochemical aspects became known, the social stigma attached to alcoholism decreased and more people sought help. Professionals, laypeople, students, alcoholics, and nonalcoholics are attending seminars and college courses on alcoholism. Recovery programs are reported widely in the popular media and rehabilitation programs have become common knowledge. Information about alcohol recovery programs is easily accessible on the Internet and in print materials.	Further research into alcoholism would drive the stigma and lack of knowledge into retreat and provide a better venue for the definitions of the illness, effective treatment frameworks, and acceptance of people with alcoholism.
Researchers have found that marijuana produces a significant analgesic effect and is modestly effective against the nausea and vomiting associated with chemotherapy (Trossman, 2006). Dronabinol is a synthetic delta-9-tetrahydrocannabinol or delta-9-THC that contains standardized THC content in an FDA-approved pharmaceutical.	Examination of substances for their beneficial actions contributes to opportunities to capitalize on available treatment and encourage the development of additional compounds to treat clinical problems.
Use of an atypical antipsychotic for the treatment of stimulant abuse and dependence (Stoops et al., 2006) was found to be effective and directs future research for combinations specifically with methamphetamine and cocaine.	Thorough clinical trials of the biochemistry of substance abuse helps assess the process of abuse, identifies the pathways involved, and can direct clinical interventions more accurately.
Research suggests a role for nicotine replacement in smoking cessation. In time this management option and the only nonnicotine smoking management option approved by the FDA (bupropion SL) may be joined by investigational drugs in the near future (Glover, 2006).	Understanding how, when, and why neurochemicals act as they do and how those actions can be translated into human behavior gives treatment providers a scientific basis for care.
For years, researchers and clinicians have been searching for an objective biologic marker that will reflect problem drinking and make assessment less challenging (Muthen et al., 2006; Prescott et al., 2006; Vieten et al., 2004).	Finding an objective biologic marker for alcoholism can be formulated as prevention as well as enhancing treatment.
Research indicates that participation in a 12-step program can help prevent relapse. These programs focus on the patient maintaining sobriety, as opposed to having recovered or being cured (Timko et al., 2006).	Clinical research debunked the formerly held view that alcoholics could imbibe moderately as long as they were in control of their consumption. Science showed that the vast majority of alcoholics relapsed quickly with negative consequences if they drank alcohol. Continued research keeps treatment accurately focused.

NCLEX® REVIEW

1. A pregnant patient seen in the clinic informs the nurse she does not consume alcohol or use illicit drugs, but her husband has been abusing cocaine for a few years. When the patient asks, "Will my baby be okay" the nurse explains:

   1. "Since you have abstained from alcohol and drugs, the baby should be fine."
   2. "There is a potential for the baby to have birth defects."
   3. "You should use some form of barrier contraception for the remainder of the pregnancy."
   4. "Sociocultural and environmental factors have a greater influence on substance abuse."

2. The nurse identifies the patient with the following personality traits to be most at risk for disruptive substance abuse:

   1. Outgoing and gregarious
   2. Quiet and studious
   3. Independent and loyal
   4. Impulsive and extroverted

3. The nurse is caring for a patient with a history of alcoholism who has been hospitalized for 48 hours. The nurse suspects the patient is beginning major alcohol withdrawal when the following symptoms are displayed.

   1. Hypothermia
   2. Bradycardia
   3. Diaphoresis
   4. Abdominal pain

4. The nurse caring for a patient in the emergency department who has been sniffing paint solvents places priority on monitoring the patient for:

   1. Cardiac arrhythmias
   2. Suicidal tendencies
   3. Outbursts of rage
   4. Visual hallucinations

5. A patient admitted to the emergency department is displaying symptoms of PCP intoxication. The nurse prepares to administer which drug?

   1. Naloxone, Narcan
   2. Prochloperazine, Phenergan
   3. Diazepam, Valium
   4. Amitriptyline, Elavil

Answers for review questions appear in Appendix D

KEY TERMS

blackouts *p.372*
delirium tremens (DTs) *p.371*
fetal alcohol syndrome (FAS) *p.372*
postacute withdrawal syndrome
  (PAWS) *p.366*

substance abuse *p.366*
substance dependence *p.366*
substance intoxication *p.366*
substance withdrawal *p.366*

substance withdrawal syndrome *p.366*
tolerance *p.366*
withdrawal *p.366*

REFERENCES

Albanese, M. J. (2005). Assessing and treating the bipolar patient with comorbid substance use disorder. *Directions in Psychiatry, 25*(4), 281–290.

American Psychiatric Association. (2000). *Diagnostic and statistical manual of mental disorders* (4th ed., text revision). Washington, DC: Author.

Arria, A. M., Derauf, C., LaGasse, L. L., Grant, P., Shah, R., Smith, L., et al. (2006). Methamphetamine and other substance use during pregnancy: Preliminary estimates from the Infant Development, Environment, and Lifestyle (IDEAL) study. *Maternal and Child Health Journal, 10*(3), 293–302.

Barr, A. M., Panenka, W. J., MacEwan, G. W., Thornton, A. E., Lang, D. J., Honer, W. G., et al. (2006). The need for speed: An update on methamphetamine addiction. *Journal of Psychiatry and Neuroscience, 31*(5), 301–313.

Carroll, C. P., Walsh, S. L., Bigelow, G. E., Strain, E. C., & Preston, K. L. (2006). Assessment of agonist and antagonist effects of tramadol in opioid-dependent humans. *Experimental and Clinical Psychopharmacology, 14*(2), 109–120.

Dennis, T., Bendersky, M., Ramsay, D., & Lewis, M. (2006). Reactivity and regulation in children prenatally exposed to cocaine. *Developmental Psychology, 42*(4), 688–697.

Dick, D. M., & Bierut, L. J. (2006). The genetics of alcohol dependence. *Current Psychiatry Reports, 8*(2) 151–157.

Doweiko, H. F. (2006). *Concepts of Chemical Dependency* (2nd ed.). Washington, DC: American Psychological Association.

Eaton, D. K., Kann, L., Kinchen, S., Ross, J., Hawkins, J., Harris, W. A., et al. (2006). Youth risk behavior surveillance—United States, 2005. *Morbidity and Mortaility Weekly Report 9, 55*(Suppl. SS-5), 1–107.

Evans, S. E., Blank, M., Sams, C., Weaver, M. F., & Eissenberg, T. (2006). Transdermal nicotine-induced tobacco abstinence symptom suppression: Nicotine dose and smokers' gender. *Experimental and Clinical Psychopharmacology, 14*(2), 121–135.

Finnell, D. S., & Osborne, F. H. (2006). Support for psychotropic medication adherence and substance cessation. *Archives of Psychiatric Nursing, 20*(4), 166–174.

Fride, E., Perchuk, A., Hall, F. S., Uhl, G. R., & Onaivi, E. S. (2006). Behavioral methods in cannabinoid research. *Methods in Molecular Medicine, 123,* 269–290.

Gates, S., Smith, L. A., & Foxcroft, D. R. (2006). Auricular acupuncture for cocaine dependence. *Cochrane Database of Systematic Reviews,* Issue 1, CD005192. Retrieved from http://www.cinahl.com/cgi-bin/refsvc?jid=s3053&accno=2009359326

Glover, E. D. (2006). Successfully treating nicotine dependence. *American Journal of Health Education, 37*(1), 6–14.

Gross, A., Marsch, L. A., Badger, G. J., & Bickel, W. K. (2006). A comparison between low-magnitude voucher and buprenorphine medication contingencies in promoting abstinence from opioids and cocaine. *Experimental and Clinical Psychopharmacology, 14*(2), 148–156.

Guha, M. (2006). Book reviews (*Review of fleeting pleasures: A history of intoxicants; Cannabis and young people: Reviewing the evidence; Overcoming problem drinking: A self-help guide using cognitive behavioral techniques; Alcohol, gender and drinking problems: Perspectives from low and middle income countries; Substance use among young people in urban environments;* and *Adolescent risk behaviors: Why teens experiment and strategies to keep them safe). Journal of Mental Health, 15*(6), 713–716.

Heimer, L., & Van Hoesen, G. W. (2006). The limbic lobe and its output channels: Implications for emotional functions and adaptive behavior. *Neuroscience & Biobehavioral Reviews, 30*(2), 126–147.

Hoeppner, B. B., Velicer, W. F., Redding, C. A., Rossi, J. S., Prochaska, J. O., Pallonen, U. E., et al. (2006). Psychometric evaluation of the smoking cessation Processes of Change scale in an adolescent sample. *Addictive Behaviors, 31*(8), 1363–1372.

Jones, H. A., & Lejuez, C. W. (2005). Personality correlates of caffeine dependence: The role of sensation seeking, impulsivity, and risk taking. *Experimental and Clinical Psychopharmacology, 13*(3), 259–266.

Killen, J. D., Fortmann, S. P., Murphy, G. M., Jr., Hayward, C., Arredondo, C., Cromp, D., et al. (2006). Extended treatment with bupropion SR for cigarette smoking cessation. *Journal of Consulting and Clinical Psychology, 74*(2), 286–294.

Kim, S. J., Lyoo, I. K., Hwang, J., Chung, A., Hoon Sung, Y., Kim, J., et al. (2006). Prefrontal grey matter changes in short-term and long-term abstinent methamphetamine abusers. *International Journal of Neuropsychopharmacology, 9*(2), 221–228.

Klesges, R. C., DeBon, M., Vander Weg, M. W., Haddock, C. K., Lando, H. A., Relyea, G. E., et al. (2006). Efficacy of a tailored tobacco control program on long-term use in a population of U.S. military troops. *Journal of Consulting and Clinical Psychology, 74*(2), 295–306.

LaBrie, J. W., Pedersen, E. R., Lamb, T. F., & Bove, L. (2006). Heads up! A nested intervention with freshmen male college students and the broader campus community to promote responsible drinking. *Journal of American College Health, 54*(5), 301–304.

Libby, A. M., Orton, H. D., Heather, D., Barth, R. P., Webb, M. B., Burns, B. J., et al. (2006). Alcohol, drug, and mental-health specialty treatment services and race/ethnicity: A national study of children and families involved with child welfare. *American Journal of Public Health, 96*(4), 628–631.

Lile, J. A. (2006). Pharmacological determinants of the reinforcing effects of psychostimulants: Relation to agonist substitution treatment. *Experimental and Clinical Psychopharmacology, 14*(1), 20–33.

Lofwall, M. R., Griffiths, R. R., & Mintzer, M. Z. (2006). Cognitive and subjective acute dose effects of intramuscular ketamine in healthy adults. *Experimental and Clinical Psychopharmacology, 14*(4), 439–449.

Mansell, D. (2005). Geriatric substance abuse: An opportunity to improve care. *Substance Abuse, 26*(2), 48.

Marczinski, C. A., & Fillmore, M. T. (2006). Clubgoers and their trendy cocktails: Implications of mixing caffeine into alcohol on information processing and subjective reports of intoxication. *Experimental and Clinical Psychopharmacology, 14*(4), 450–458.

Martin, V. T., Loder, E., Taylor, K., Almas, M., & Hilliard, B. (2005). Eletriptan treatment of migraine in patients switching from barbiturate-containing analgesics: Results from a multiple-attack study. *Cephalalgia, 25*(9), 726–734.

Mathias, M., & National Institute on Drug Abuse. (2006). Alcohol-treatment medication may help reduce cocaine abuse among heroin treatment patients. *NIDA Notes Research Findings, 16*(1), 1–4.

McGuinness, T. M. (2006). Nothing to sniff at: Inhalant abuse & youth. *Journal of Psychosocial Nursing and Mental Health Services 44*(8), 15–18.

McKeon, C. M., Fogarty, G. J., & Hegney, D. G. (2006). Organizational factors: Impact on administration violations in rural nursing. *Journal of Advanced Nursing, 55*(1), 115–123.

Meyers, R. A., Zavala, A. R., Speer, C. M., & Neisewander, J. L. (2006). Dorsal hippocampus inhibition disrupts acquisition and expression, but not consolidation, of cocaine conditioned place preference. *Behavioral Neuroscience, 120*(2), 401–412.

Muthen, B., Asparouhov, T., & Rebollo, I. (2006). Advances in behavioral genetics modeling using Mplus: Applications of factor mixture modeling to twin data. *Twin Research and Human Genetics: The Official Journal of the International Society for Twin Studies, 9*(3), 313–324.

National Drug Intelligence Center. (2006). National drug threat assessment 2006: Product No. 2006-Q0317-001. Johnstown, PA: U.S. Department of Justice. Retrieved from http://www.usdoj.gov/ndic/topics/titles2.htm

Neaigus, A., Gyarmathy, V. A., Miller, M., Frajzyngie, V. M., Friedman, S. R., & Des Jarlais, D. C. (2006). Transitions to injecting drug use among noninjecting heroin users: Social network influence and individual susceptibility. *Journal of Acquired Immune Deficiency Syndromes, 41*(4), 493–503.

O'Connor, M. J., Frankel, F., Paley, B., Schonfeld, A. M., Carpenter, E., Laugeson, E. A., et al. (2006). A controlled social skills training for children with fetal alcohol spectrum disorders. *Journal of Consulting and Clinical Psychology, 74*(4), 639–648.

Oslin, D. W. (2005). Evidence-based treatment of geriatric substance abuse. *Psychiatric Clinics of North America, 28*(2), 897–911.

Peterson, J., Mitchell, S. G., Hong, Y., Agar, M., & Latkin, C. (2006). Getting clean and harm reduction: Adversarial or complementary issues for injection drug users. *Cadernos de Saude Publica, 22*(4), 733–740.

Prescott, C. A., Sullivan, P. F., Kuo, P. H., Webb, B. T., Vittum, J., Patterson, D. G., et al. (2006). Genomewide linkage study in the Irish affected sib pair study of alcohol dependence: Evidence for a susceptibility region for symptoms of alcohol dependence on chromosome 4. *Molecular Psychiatry, 11*(6), 603–611.

Ranney, L., Melvin, C., Lux, L., McClain, E., Morgan, L., & Lohr, K. (2006). *Evidence report on tobacco use: Prevention, cessation, and control* (Evidence Report/Technology Assessment 140, AHRQ Publication 06-E 015). Rockville MD: Agency for Healthcare Research and Quality.

Rossi, P., Di Lorenzo, C., Faroni, J., Cesarino, F., & Nappi, G. (2006). Advice alone vs. structured detoxification programmes for medication overuse headache: A prospective, randomized, open-label trial in transformed migraine patients with low medical needs. *Cephalalgia, 26*(9), 1097–1105.

Serretti, A., Liappas, I., Mandelli, L., Albani, D., Forloni, G., Malitas, P., et al. (2006). Interleukin-1 alpha and beta, TNF-alpha and HTTLPR gene variants study on alcohol toxicity and detoxification outcome. *Neuroscience Letters, 406*(1–2), 107–112.

Shorey, H. S., & Snyder, C. R. (2006). The role of adult attachment styles in psychopathology and psychotherapy outcomes. *Review of General Psychology, 10*(1), 1–20.

Sinuk, P., & Taylor, A. (2004). Nurses' addictions. *American Journal of Nursing, 104*(6), 13.

Stoops, W. W., Lile, J. A. Glaser, P. E. A., & Rush, C. R. (2006). A low dose of aripiprazole attenuates the subject-rated effects of d-amphetamine. *Drug and Alcohol Dependence, 84*(2), 206–209.

Timko, C., Billow, R., & DeBenedetti, A. (2006). Determinants of 12-step group affiliation and moderators of the affiliation-abstinence relationship. *Drug and Alcohol Dependence, 83*(1), 111–121.

Trossman, S. (2006). Issues update. Rx for medical marijuana? Promoting research on and acceptance of this treatment option for patients. *American Journal of Nursing, 106*(4), 77–79.

Turk, D. C., & McCarberg, B. (2005). Non-pharmacological treatments for chronic pain: A disease management context. *Disease Management and Health Outcomes, 13*(1), 19–30.

Vaitl, D., Birbaumer, N., Gruzelier, J., Jamieson, G., Kotchoubey, B., Kübler, A., et al. (2005). Psychobiology of altered states of consciousness. *Psychological Bulletin, 131*(1), 98–127.

Vieten, C., Seaton, K. L., Feiler, H. S., & Wilhelmsen, K. C. (2004). The University of California, San Francisco, family alcoholism study. I. Design, methods, and demographics. *Alcoholism: Clinical and Experimental Research, 28*(10), 1509–1516.

CHAPTER

17

Nursing Management at End of Life

Cheryl Wraa, Pamela Coulter, Linda Kelly

Outcome-Based Learning Objectives

After studying this chapter, the learner will be able to:

1. Review ethical theories that influence decisions in end-of-life care.
2. Define advanced directives and their role in end-of-life care.
3. Compare and contrast pharmacological and nonpharmacological therapies used for relief of pain at end of life.
4. Discuss beliefs surrounding death held by various cultures and religions.
5. Identify the need for interdisciplinary collaboration in planning end-of-life care.
6. Identify the role of hospice during end-of-life care.
7. Review the principles of palliative care.

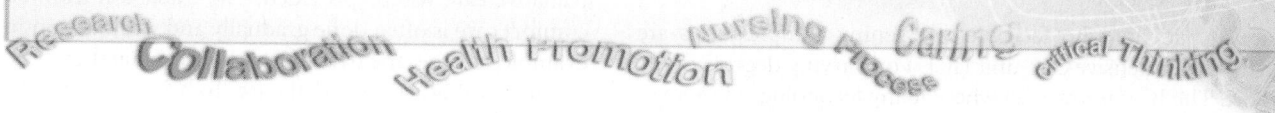

DEALING WITH end-of-life decisions can be an extremely difficult and complex situation for caregivers. This is particularly true in the acute care setting because often the critical nature of the illness or injury is sudden and unexpected. Recent studies report on the dissatisfaction expressed by families with the quality of care their family member received when they died while in the hospital (Heyland et al., 2005; Teno et al., 2004). Family satisfaction depends largely on the information the family receives and the way it is provided.

End of Life in the Acute Care Setting

Palliative care, comprehensive care focused on alleviating suffering and promoting the quality of remaining life of patients living with a chronic, life-threatening, or terminal illness, allows patients and families to guide treatment and set goals for care (National Consensus Project for Quality Palliative Care, 2004). Although palliative care is well defined for patients who are terminally ill, it has not been well defined for patients in the acute care setting who are critically ill.

For health care providers, the transition from providing "curative care" to "comfort care" can be difficult. There are several reasons why making this transition is difficult. First, ethical dilemmas may arise on a daily basis as the choice of extending

life versus postponing death occurs. Second, nurses are influenced by their own values, culture, religion, education, and life experiences. Third, the role of the nurse is to participate as a member of the health care team to assist the patient and families to make fully informed decisions with full knowledge of their options. Finally, it is critical that everyone involved with the patient's care communicate with one another and have consensus prior to discussions with the family. In addition to the normal nursing interventions needed to provide clinical care, there are additional key nursing interventions discussed throughout the chapter that are helpful at end of life. These key nursing interventions include:

- Recognition of autonomy
- Honesty
- Expert communication
- Presence
- Compassion
- Touch
- Assisting in transcendence or developing a sense of meaning and peace with death (Saunders, 2007).

Advances in technology, changes in managed care, and changes in social and family structures have also added to the complexity of end-of-life care (Bednash & Ferrell 2002b). Advances in technology in critical care medicine have added therapeutic options never before available. Today patients who were considered physiologically brittle, including those who are elderly or chronically ill, are receiving operations and complex procedures. Most will survive the operation and recover with few or no complications. Issues arise, however, when complications occur and despite massive resuscitative efforts, the patient continues to deteriorate and further care is deemed futile. The transition from curative to noncurative is particularly difficult for surgeons, due in part to their training (Buchman, Cassell, Ray, & Wax, 2002). An ethnographic study of surgical services completed by C. Bosk at the University of Chicago revealed that one characteristic that sets surgeons apart from their medical colleagues is their sense of accountability for the patient's outcome (Buchman et al., 2002). Surgeons are trained to be heroic, because surgical patients often require immediate decision making and actions. Surgeons' personalities tend to exude confidence and commitment to successful outcomes. This heroic optimism may be a barrier to discussions with families when offering comfort, as opposed to curative care, because the surgeon may view this as a failure on his part. The nurse working in a surgical area may need to assist the family in approaching the surgeon for discussions regarding end-of-life issues.

End of Life in the Intensive Care Unit

Typically, patients who face life-threatening complications are placed in the intensive care unit (ICU) on varying degrees of life support. The ICU is one area where many technological innovations have been developed to prevent death. Therefore, decisions regarding withholding or withdrawing life-sustaining treatment are more consequential than in many other settings. Monitoring in the ICU provides an enormous amount of data regarding the patient's condition—pulse, blood pressure, cardiac output, and oxygen saturation, to name a few. The data may be confusing to the family because one bit of information could bode well at the same time that another bodes poorly. These discordant data make it difficult for a family to comprehend the situation and know how to respond. The Institute of Medicine believes this is especially true because society places a great deal of faith in technology (Buchman et al., 2002). The Institute of Medicine recently asked:

> Are ICU staff, specialty services, and other personnel trained to recognize patients (and families) for whom the goals of curative or life-prolonging care should be reconsidered with particular attention to the goals of physical and emotional comfort and symptom relief? Are procedures in place for arranging appropriate care and consultations? Are the important roles of nurses, social workers, and others recognized and supported? (Buchman et al., 2002, p. 666)

The answer to these questions depends on all members of the health care team being able to acknowledge when rescue attempts are failing.

Nurses spend most of their time at the bedside and are integral to relaying and reinforcing information to patients' families and other members of the health care team. Families in crisis need information repeated or at times explained in a different way. Stud-

ies have demonstrated a significant difference between what clinicians think they said and what patients and families understood (Chaitin & Arnold, 2005). Therefore it is essential that every member of the health care team, especially nurses because of their close and frequent contact with the patient and family, be aware of discussions that are held with the family and the plan of care for the patient. Nurses are instrumental in helping the family not feel abandoned at the end of life. A core nursing function at end of life is to be present and bear witness during the dying process and to help the patient and family find meaning in the experience.

The Study to Understand Prognoses and Preferences for Outcomes and Risks of Treatments (SUPPORT) in 1995 revealed that some physicians have difficulty listening to nurses unless the nurse is responding to a posed question (Buchman et al., 2002). Although physicians in the ICUs believed that their relationships with nurses was collaborative and believed that the information received from nurses was valuable, they tended not to involve them in end-of-life decision-making processes (Buchman et al., 2002). Studies have shown that for families, communication with caregivers is identified as the single most important factor for them during end-of-life care (Chaitin & Arnold, 2005; Heyland et al., 2006). Families, when surveyed, revealed that not just communication but continuity of communication is an essential ingredient (Heyland et al., 2006). As the plan of care shifts from cure to comfort, it is important to repeatedly reassure the family through words and actions that the patient and they will not be ignored or abandoned and that attentive palliative care will be provided. The transition from curative to comfort care is often done gradually and without continuity. For example, at times the patient may be receiving therapies aimed at comfort and others aimed at cure. To bring continuity to the situation, the health care team needs to change to a model focused primarily on symptomatology. In this new model the criteria for an intervention is based on improvement of symptom relief, functional status, or amelioration of emotional, psychological, or spiritual concerns (Chaitin & Arnold, 2005).

Research has shown that nurses in the ICU feel immense frustration about the lack of consensus concerning end-of-life care and that ICUs do not deliver compassionate end-of-life care (Buchman et al., 2002). One way to alleviate this type of frustration is to develop guidelines for end-of-life care in the ICU. Evidenced-based guidelines will assist with health care team continuity and will assist in facilitating discussion regarding a shift from curative to comfort care. Open communication among all members of the health care team will also assist with the psychological and emotional stress incurred by ICU staff when involved in palliating a patient who is dying, as discussed further in the Evidence-Based Practice box.

Oncology nurses who frequently care for patients who are terminally ill are more comfortable with and better understand palliative care (Davidson et al., 2003). Unfortunately, nurses who do not care for patients who are terminally ill on a daily basis usually do not have this knowledge of and familiarity with end-of-life care. A recent exploratory study of the perceptions of palliative care among cardiorespiratory nurses revealed several themes (Davidson et al., 2003). First, nurses felt there was philosophical and cognitive dissonance between acute care and palliative care philosophies. Second, there is a lack of continuity in planning and negotiating with the patient or the family. Often decisions are left

For End-of-Life Care

Clinical Problem

In the hospital setting, conflicts between families and health care providers regarding end-of-life decisions are common. Decisions should be a cooperative effort to achieve treatment goals. When discussions are perceived as conflicts, families often feel misunderstood or isolated, and may doubt the health care providers' commitment to the patient's well-being.

Research Findings

In a study by Breen, Abernethy, Abbott, and Tulsky (2001), health care providers reported that 63% of conflicts with families involved decision making at the end of life. The Center for Gerontology and Health Care Research at Brown Medical School found that many patients and family members of people dying in institutions reported having unmet needs for symptom amelioration, physician communication, emotional support, and being treated with respect (Teno et al., 2004). In Canada, Heyland et al. (2006) conducted a study to describe what seriously ill patients in the hospital and their family members considered to be the key elements of quality end-of-life care. In their results, elements rated as "extremely important" included trust and confidence in their doctors; not to be kept alive when there is little hope for recovery; information regarding their disease being communicated in an honest manner; and preparing for end of life, that is, resolving conflicts, saying good-bye, and life review.

Implications for Nursing Practice

Supportive communication involves active listening and letting the family know that providers are present and are accepting of their strong emotions. For the family, knowing that caregivers listen to and understand what they are going through is therapeutic. The acronym NURSE is a useful tool for how one can be empathetic to families' strong emotions:

Acronym	Request	Example
N	Name *Help the patient or family member understand and give their feelings a name.*	It sounds like you are frustrated.
U	Understanding *Let the family know that you are aware and empathetic of their situation.*	It is hard for me to imagine what it is like to be in this situation.
R	Respect *When a family makes an end-of-life decision, acknowledge how difficult it can be.*	I respect how hard you have tried to follow your loved one's wishes.
S	Support *Let the family know that you are available.*	I am here if you have any questions.
E	Explore *Take time to listen to the family. Help them sort out their feelings.*	Tell me more about what you are thinking.

Critical Thinking Questions

1. After a family meeting with the health care team, you notice that a family member looks confused. How would you approach this person?

2. How will you show support to the patient and family?

Answers to Critical Thinking Questions appear in Appendix D.

References

Breen, C. M., Abernethy, A. P., Abbott, K. H., & Tulsky, J. A. (2001). Conflict associated with decisions to limit life-sustaining treatment in intensive care units. *Journal of General Internal Medicine, 16*, 283.

Heyland, D. K., Dodek, P., Rocker, G., Groll, D., Gafni, A., Pichora, D., et al. (2006). What matters most in end of life care: Perceptions of seriously ill patients and their family members. *Canadian Medical Association Journal, 184*(5), 627–633.

Teno, J. M., Clarridge, B. R., Casey, V., Welch, L. C., Wetle, T., Shield, R., et al. (2004). Family perspectives on end of life care at the last place of care. *Journal of the American Medical Association, 291*(1), 88–103.

EVIDENCE-BASED PRACTICE

to a crisis point and there is poor communication between clinical teams about end-of-life issues. Third, there is discomfort in dealing with death and dying. Fourth, there is a lack of consistency of messages among the health care team. Nurses felt that if the death of the patient had not been managed optimally that it became a critical incident for them. Finally, Davidson and colleagues found that there is a lack of awareness of palliative care philosophies and resources and a need for education on palliative care principles.

◼ Ethical Issues

The transition to end-of-life care in the acute care setting begins with the process of shared decision making to change the focus from care aimed at cure to care aimed at comfort and freedom from pain. When the health care team begins to discuss decisions regarding life-sustaining versus end-of-life interventions, ethical issues and dilemmas are inherent in the discussions. Ethical decision making involves a systematic appraisal of a situation using moral principles and ethical theories to justify the resolution (Gillick, 2004; Jackson & Abrahm, 2005).

Respect for Persons

Fundamental to nursing practice is the respect for the worth, dignity, and rights of every individual. It requires that people be treated as individuals with respect for their human dignity. It is this principle that prevents interference with the plans, privacy, or decisions made by capable adults (Bednash & Ferrell, 2002a).

Privacy

Individuals have a right to privacy and caregivers have a duty to respect the confidentiality of patient information (Saunders, 2007). Any discussion regarding the patient's diagnoses, consultation, examination, and treatment should be conducted discreetly.

Autonomy

Capable adults have the moral and legal right to determine what will be done with their own person. They have the right and ability to determine how they wish to live and to determine what therapies to accept or reject, even if the health care team does not agree. The principle of autonomy is referred to as the right to self-determination (Bednash & Ferrell, 2002a; Gillick, 2004).

 Caregivers are duty bound to respect patients' choices in all situations unless a choice is overridden by another moral principle of greater weight.

Veracity

Caregivers have a duty to be truthful. When information is withheld from patients and family or they are not told the truth, they can no longer make informed choices. It is important for the nurse to find out how much and the type of information the patient wants so her goals can be adjusted to fit the time she has left (Bednash & Ferrell, 2002a; Saunders, 2007).

Beneficence

This principle means to do or promote good. It is different from nonmaleficence, or the duty to not inflict harm. It is sometimes difficult when caring for patients to distinguish between preventing harm and providing benefit. When the duty not to inflict harm conflicts with the duty to provide benefit, there is support for the view that the obligation not to injure others is greater than the obligation to benefit them (Bednash & Ferrell, 2002a). Therefore, care given in the acute care setting is focused primarily on the curative model of care. Decisions regarding invasive monitoring, diagnostic tests, or therapeutic interventions are based on whether doing this procedure will contribute to the patient's recovery from the illness. In palliative care, the decision about whether to do an intervention should be based on whether it will improve symptom relief, functional status, or ameliorate emotional, psychological, or spiritual concerns (Peterman & Cella, 2005). Bednash and Ferrell (2002a) state, "Patients at the end of their lives may be particularly vulnerable to harm. They are harmed when they receive unwanted or unnecessary interventions, when they are overtreated with burdensome technological interventions that serve only to prolong dying and when treatments are withdrawn without their consent or agreement. They are most certainly harmed when their pain is not adequately managed due to the nurse's fear that the patient's death might be hastened as a result of pain management with high dose opiates" (p. 4).

The American Nurses Association's Code of Ethics for nurses states "the nurse may provide interventions to relieve symptoms in the dying client even when the interventions entail substantial risks of hastening death" (Bednash & Ferrell, 2002c, p. 75). So at the end of life, not titrating a drug to relieve symptoms because it may hasten death would be viewed as causing the patient harm because it would increase suffering.

Nonmaleficence

Caregivers are required to avoid intentionally causing patients unnecessary harm or pain, both physical and mental (Bednash & Ferrell, 2002a). Health care teams often do procedures that may harm patients in order to benefit them or to prevent a greater harm from occurring. Morally they must decide whether causing the harm is justified.

Justice

This principle is understood as fairness. It involves the determination of what is owed a person or a group. Justice also takes into consideration cultural and religious preferences. Incorporating justice into medical decisions includes the likelihood of medical benefit as well as present and future quality-of-life criteria. Most believe that if a treatment will not benefit a patient, then it is considered futile and, as such, its use is morally and professionally unwarranted. Therefore treatments that are futile should not be suggested or offered to patients or families (Gillick, 2004).

◼ Ethical Issues and Dilemmas at End of life

As stated before, the change from "curative care" to "comfort care" can be a difficult transition. Communication among the health care team and family is of great importance during this transition time because a number of ethical issues and dilemmas may arise at the end of life.

Advanced Care Planning

Patients must have the capacity to comprehend information in order to make informed consent. For the patient who is unable to consent for himself, it is important to determine whether he has done any advanced care planning.

Advance Directives

Advance directives lay the groundwork for decision making at the time of acute illness. They are a significant part of the Patient Self-Determination Act and include the living will, the durable power of attorney for health care, and the directive for organ donation (Saunders, 2007). Advance directives give patients peace of mind that their wishes will be followed even if they cannot communicate. The directives give clear directions for significant others and the health care team regarding the patients' wishes. All advance directive statutes contain provisions that grant immunity to health care professionals when they act in good faith and in accordance with state statutes in regard to advance directives.

 It is the nurse's responsibility to be aware of a patient's advance directive and to advocate for respecting the patient's wishes.

Living Wills

Living wills, a form of an advance directive, describe the patient's preferences in case she becomes incapacitated. They usually describe what level of life-prolonging interventions the patient would or would not want and under what circumstances they should be completed, withheld, or withdrawn. Living wills require the signature of two witnesses (Bednash & Ferrell, 2002a; Gillick, 2004).

Durable Power of Attorney

A **durable power of attorney for health care (DPAHC)**, **medical durable power of attorney (MDPA)**, or health care proxy allows the patient to appoint a decision maker in the case of future incapacity. The DPAHC or MDPA specifically states which powers the patient gives to the surrogate. The appointed person responsible for making medical decisions does not need consent from other family members or friends (Bednash & Ferrell, 2002a; Gillick, 2004).

In the ICU setting where initially aggressive lifesaving technology is used, when it is apparent that the patient will not return to his former health, it is often difficult to choose to reject that support. Patients and families may continue to opt for invasive or high-technology therapy out of fear of a painful death or of giving up too soon. When caregivers discuss specific treatments with the patient and family, it is important to explain the potential benefits versus the potential burdens. For the family, it can be emotionally more difficult to withdraw life-sustaining treatments that have been initiated than to withhold them (Gillick, 2004). Health care teams must remember that ethically based medical decisions are a shared process and are based on open communication and a relationship with the patient that respects the patient's privacy and autonomy. Decisions must be made with regard to providing the best recommendation for the patient and not to relieve the stress of any individual in the family or health care team caused by having to make the decision.

Communication During End-of Life Care

Patients and their families have expressed that communication with caregivers is an extremely important factor during end-of-life care (Heyland et al., 2006). Even though health care providers feel overburdened with time constraints, it is important to take the time to sit with the patient and family and communicate with them in an open, genuine manner regarding the patient's illness.

Many critical care clinicians have difficulty initiating a straightforward discussion about death with a patient and/or family because they have been trained to restore health. If the primary goal is to make patients well, then death is often viewed as failure. Adding to the conflict is the question of how certain the health care team is about the patient's prognosis. The team may decide that any further care is futile and suggest withdrawing all life-sustaining treatment and giving comfort care only. On the other hand, it may be decided that there is some chance of survival, but that additional interventions would be burdensome. In this case, conversations would be held regarding continuing the current level of life support, but forgoing additional support in the event of further complications. Another option is a plan that considers each new problem or complication as it arises and weighs the potential burdens and benefits of the treatment that might be administered.

Caring for the acutely ill patient may require that decisions and interventions be made quickly, although the appropriateness of some of these decisions becomes clearer as time passes and as the illness takes its course (Chaitin & Arnold, 2005). If the patient is in a teaching hospital, the family may receive conflicting messages from the multiple teams of physicians caring for the patient. It is better to have a representative from each team present during a family meeting and to ask open-ended questions of the family to ascertain if they clearly understood what was presented. Recom-

mendations are to give information at a ninth-grade level with as little medical jargon as possible. Family members are under stress and their ability to understand large amounts of information is difficult. Experts suggest not giving more than three pieces of information without stopping to check the family members' understanding (Chaitin & Arnold, 2005).

Formal training in end-of-life care skills is not included in most caregivers' education. Most caregivers learn these skills through experience and on-the-job exposure. In Canada, Stevens et al. (2002) completed a study of the perceptions of the limitations of ethics education in end-of-life care for residents. Prior to their ICU rotation, the residents felt that out of 19 determinants considered in the decision for withdrawal of life support, the three factors most important to the decision were patient advance directives, the likelihood of surviving the current illness, and family directives. After completing their ICU rotation, the three most important factors were patient advance directives, the likelihood of surviving the current illness, and the likelihood of long-term survival. Of the 19 determinants, the two that increased the most in importance for the decision to withdraw life support were likelihood of long-term survival and preferences of the attending physicians. From this study, the participating residents recommended more formal and informal education and practical experience in end-of-life issues in the ICU. Specifically they suggested more opportunities to observe senior clinicians during family meetings, discussions on approaches to withdrawal of life support, more patient-centered discussions, and opportunities to lead family meetings to improve their communication skills. The residents felt that formal lectures and grand rounds on the ethical aspects of end-of-life care in the ICU were not of much benefit.

Many clinicians do not feel comfortable with death and are not trained in good communication skills. This combination creates difficult situations for dying patients and their families. The ability to give compassionate, nurturing, end-of-life care is based on the caregiver's ability to be comfortable with death. The structure of tightly organized rounds that occurs in teaching hospitals in the ICU is a wonderful opportunity to include detailed discussion of the goals for care in light of the patient's needs and values. A particular principle that should be taught is that the goals of care should drive the use of technology, not the other way around. These discussions will help caregivers to learn to ask questions such as these: Are the patient's goals and values known? If so, are the treatments the patient is receiving consistent with these goals? If not, why not and what needs to change? Although it is important to be sensitive to the family's wishes, discussions should be guided by respect for what the patient's goals and wishes were.

Additionally, these discussions and having students and nurses accompany the physician team during family meetings give them the opportunity to recognize and deal with the suffering that the family may be experiencing. The ICU also gives caregivers the opportunity to learn the multidisciplinary nature of critical care, collaborative decision making, and effective teamwork.

■ Ensuring the Patient's Comfort

The transition from curative care to comfort care can be inconsistent with some therapies aimed at comfort and some at cure. In a study done by Heyland et al. (2006), patients and their families identified four issues that were considered extremely important in end-of-life care: (1) trust and confidence in the physicians caring for them, (2) avoiding inappropriate prolongation of death, (3) information about their illness being communicated in an honest manner, and (4) completing things and preparing for life's end.

One suggestion for making the transition from curative to comfort care is to completely rewrite the patient's orders and review the plan of care as if the patient were just now being admitted. Each test or intervention should be reviewed for its need and how it will further the patient's wishes, improve symptom relief, and ameliorate emotional or spiritual concerns. The treatment orders should be organized by symptoms rather than by organ system or disease. The symptom list should be actual and potential and each symptom should be managed separately.

Pain

If the patient is unable to communicate, assessment of pain at the end of life may rely on evaluation of physical signs such as consciousness, breathing pattern, change in blood pressure and heart rate, and facial grimaces.

At the end of life, allowing hypoxia in the face of normocarbia is the fastest path to unconsciousness with the least amount of agitation. Decreased cardiac activity leads to hypoperfusion and decreased cerebral function. Also, lack of oral intake will lead to dehydration, which also decreases cerebral function. This phenomenon has been referred to as *starvation euphoria* and is thought to be related to endogenous opioid production or the analgesic effects of ketosis. So the withdrawal of some treatments may actually assist the patient to be more comfortable.

Environment also plays a factor in the patient's comfort. The hospital is rarely considered a peaceful environment although measures can be taken to enhance the patient's comfort, such as reducing lighting and noise, eliminating unnecessary monitors and machines, removing restraints, and providing room for the patient's significant others. Cultural and spiritual factors such as prayer, ritual, and music can also increase the patient's comfort.

Pharmacologic Therapies

The use of pharmacologic therapies, with attention paid to the pharmacokinetics and pharmacodynamics of the drugs used, can ease many or all of the symptoms the dying patient may experience. The symptoms most often experienced by dying patients are pain, fatigue, dyspnea, excessive respiratory secretions, nausea and vomiting, constipation, and diarrhea (Saunders, 2007). In addition to the specifics discussed in the following subsections, the Pharmacology Summary feature provides more information about the use of medications for a patient who is at the end of life.

Opioids

Opioids are the most common class of drug used for the treatment of pain and suffering in the dying patient. Opioids instill analgesia, sedation, and euphoria by binding to receptor sites in the brain and spinal cord to prevent the release of neurotransmitters involved in pain transmission. The most frequently used opioids are morphine, hydromorphone, and fentanyl. Meperidine is not recommended because its metabolite, normeperidine, produces signs of central nervous system (CNS) excitation such as tremors, and if not excreted, as in the patient with renal insufficiency, is toxic to the CNS and places the patient at risk for seizures (Bednash & Ferrell, 2002c; Jackson & Abrahm, 2005).

Most patients in the acute care setting are already receiving analgesics and may have already developed some tolerance to their effects. For this reason, there is no set dosage for opioids at the end of life. Analgesic drips should be titrated to effect and should not be limited by recommended maximal doses. As stated previously, the increasing of the titration of the opioid is intended to relieve pain and suffering, not to directly cause death (Bednash & Ferrell, 2002c; Jackson & Abrahm, 2005).

 CRITICAL ALERT *It is important to document the indication for increasing the dose clearly.*

It is also appropriate to use anticipatory dosing. When withdrawing mechanical ventilation, an increase in dyspnea can be an-

PHARMACOLOGY Summary of Drugs Used in End-of-Life Care

Medication Category	Action	Application/Indication	Nursing Responsibility
Opioid analgesics	Bind with and activate opioid receptors in brain and spinal cord to produce analgesia and euphoria	Treatment of pain and nonpain symptoms associated with dying.	Conduct regular, frequent assessment of pain and nonpain symptoms (e.g., shortness of breath, anxiety). Ensure safe and timely reduction of pain and symptom levels. Address barriers to effective pain management, including inappropriate fears of risk of side effects, addiction, respiratory depressions, or hastening of death.
Benzodiazepines	Produce a calming effect and relax skeletal muscles by increasing the activity of gamma-aminobutyric acid, a major inhibitory neurotransmitter in the brain.	Synergistic sedative effect with opioids. May help prevent development of premorbid seizures.	Same as for opioids.

ticipated. It would not be sufficient to wait for the distress to respond, so adequate medication should be given prior to the withdrawal (Jackson & Abrahm, 2005). Lynn, Lynch Schuster, and Kabcenell (2000) describe a prospective study done by Campbell et al. in 1999 of patient responses during terminal weaning of unconscious patients. The investigators reported that 35% of the patients required no analgesia or sedation at any time during the procedure. Also, there were no significant correlations between the amount of morphine used and the duration of survival after removal from the ventilator. Additionally, when comparing the patients who received morphine and those who did not, there was no difference in length of survival. During this study, the average dose of morphine used was 5.5 mg/hr.

Benzodiazepines

Benzodiazepines have a synergistic sedative effect with opioids, are anticonvulsants, and may help prevent the development of premorbid seizures (Truog et al., 2001). Midazolam, when administered intravenously, changes to a lipophilic (i.e., having an affinity for fat) compound that rapidly penetrates the CNS. The drug is short acting but will have a sustained effect when given by continuous infusion. Starting doses for adult continuous infusion is 1 to 5 mg/hr. Lorazepam is an intermediate-acting benzodiazepine and reaches a peak effect approximately 30 minutes after intravenous infusion. The starting dose for adult continuous infusion is 1 to 8 mg/hr. Further discussion about the use of opioids and benzodiazepines at the end of life is provided in the Ethical Issues box.

Neuroleptics

Neuroleptics, such as haloperidol, may be helpful for patients exhibiting delirium. It is important to try to distinguish between anxiety and delirium, an acute confusional state. The distinction is important because the use of opioids or benzodiazepines can worsen the symptoms of delirium. It has been shown that patients who are given haloperidol for acute delirium require less sedation than with other medications (Truog et al., 2001). Starting doses of haloperidol in adults range from 0.5 to 20 mg. Recommendations are to titrate additional doses at 30-minute intervals until symp-

ETHICAL ISSUES for Pain Management at End of Life

Management of pain at the end of life is the right of the patient and the duty of the caregiver. Many families state that their loved ones suffered from untreated pain at the end of their life (Jackson & Abrahm, 2005). Failure to treat the pain adequately can arise from the caregiver's fear of violating ethical and moral tenets in the administration of pain medication to the dying patient.

At the end of life, the use of opioids, benzodiazepines, and other medications in doses high enough to control the patient's symptoms may unintentionally hasten death. This is referred to as double effect, where an action may have two possible effects, one good and one bad. The action is not considered immoral if it is undertaken with the intention of achieving the good effect without intending the bad effect, even though it may be foreseen. At the end of life not administering a drug to relieve symptoms because it may hasten death would be viewed as causing the patient harm and increased suffering.

toms are controlled. The drug can also be given by continuous infusion ranging from 3 to 25 mg/hr. The use of restraints should be avoided when possible (Truog et al., 2001).

Complementary and Alternative Therapy

Complementary therapies may be helpful to patients who are at the end of life, as discussed in the accompanying Complementary and Alternative Therapies box (p. 400).

Dyspnea

Dyspnea is shortness of breath and can be extremely distressing and frightening. The neuropathways responsible for the sensation are poorly understood (Kuebler, Heidrich, & Esper, 2007). Many patients may be unable to report dyspnea due to their level of consciousness. Physical symptoms that should be considered signs of dyspnea are tachypnea, restlessness, accessory muscle use, grunting at the end of each breath, and nasal flaring. Nonpharmacologic techniques that may lessen the sensation of dyspnea are to elevate the head of the bed to reduce choking sensations and promote expansion of the lungs, and the use of fans that circulate air. Cool air directed gently on the face may reduce the perception of breathlessness (Bednash & Ferrell, 2002c; Truog et al., 2001). The use of oxygen may be effective if the patient is hypoxic, but the use of a face mask may increase the sensation of dyspnea if it makes the patient feel claustrophobic (Truog et al., 2001). Opioids are highly effective in relieving dyspnea by depressing respiratory drive; causing vasodilation, which can reduce pulmonary vascular congestion; and producing sedation and euphoria. The use of opioids for relief of dyspnea in a patient who is near death is considered the standard treatment (Kuebler et al., 2007).

Dyspnea is reported in up to half of dying patients. It is important to educate the family and the patient, if the patient is conscious, regarding the specific symptoms of dyspnea and ways to relieve the sensation and make the patient comfortable (Bednash & Ferrell, 2002c).

Fever

Fevers and infections occur frequently in the acute care setting. For the dying patient, fever can be uncomfortable and antipyretics should be given. Any measure that would cause the patient more discomfort, such as a cooling blanket or alcohol bath, should not be used.

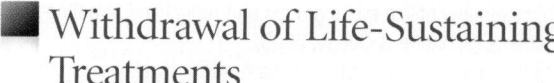 Withdrawal of Life-Sustaining Treatments

The goal of palliative and end-of-life care is to achieve the best quality of life for the patient and her family, consistent with their goals and values, regardless of the location of the patient. Components of palliative care should be offered, discussed, and incorporated into the plan of care at the time of diagnosis of a life-threatening illness. As the disease progresses, the patient or family may decide to forgo or withdraw life-sustaining treatments. When discussing with the family the decision not to initiate cardiopulmonary resuscitation, providing survival statistics to the family can facilitate decision making. Chances of survival to discharge for patients who have suffered an arrest in the hospital range from 6% to 15%, with 30% of survivors suffering a significant decrease in quality of life and the ability to be independent (Carney & Meier, 2000).

Discontinuation of mechanical ventilation usually occurs when the burdens of continuing life-prolonging interventions outweigh their benefits. Withdrawal of mechanical ventilation should be planned carefully, ensuring the patient's comfort and allowing the family to be present at the bedside if they wish. Unfortunately, death can be viewed as a failure by the health care team and the antithesis of everything in which they believe. For this reason, the dying patient can become the object of intense effort where death occurs in an arena of machines, tubes, and technicians (Bednash & Ferrell, 2002b). Because the attitudes of both society and members of the health care team can greatly influence the process of dying, it is important to educate all members of the team on the ways in which life-sustaining treatments can be withdrawn (Bednash & Ferrell, 2002a).

Terminal Wean

In 1983 A. Grenvik was the first to describe a systematic approach to ventilator withdrawal by a gradual reduction in the ventilator settings over several hours. The process is a gradual reduction of the fractionated inspired oxygen (FIO_2) and pressure support or control, leading to development of hypoxia and hypercarbia. It is important to remember that in the ICU setting, the sedation and

analgesia adequate for the patient who is currently receiving mechanical ventilation are inadequate to treat his symptoms during terminal weaning. A study done at two San Francisco teaching hospitals by Wilson et al. found that 75% of adult patients from whom life support was withheld or withdrawn received nearly a threefold increase in sedatives, analgesics, or both during the process (Burns et al., 2000). An advantage to terminal weaning is that the patient does not develop any signs of upper airway obstruction and, with the proper administration of sedatives and analgesics, the patient does not develop symptoms of acute air hunger. These advantages promote the comfort of the patient and reduce the anxiety of the family. The disadvantage of terminal weaning is that it may prolong the death by several days and some family members may perceive it as an attempt to have the patient successfully survive separation from the ventilator.

Terminal Extubation

The obvious advantage to terminal extubation is that it does not prolong the dying process and allows the patient to be free from an unnatural tube. It is important to be anticipatory of the distress a patient may experience during terminal extubation. Therefore, the patient should receive anticipatory doses of analgesics and sedatives that are then titrated as necessary to the observed level of the patient's distress.

COMPLEMENTARY & ALTERNATIVE THERAPIES   Journaling

Description:

Many people have found that recording thoughts in a journal helps to relieve pain and emotional suffering. People who are at the end of life, and who create a historical record that lives on after their death often reduce their perception of stress. A diary is the most common form of journaling.

Research Support:

Nursing literature and educational literature frequently discuss journaling as an active technique that can enhance a nurse's reflective practice, which is a means of self-examination. Reflective practice involves looking back over what has happened in practice in an effort to improve, or encourage, professional growth. Some of its benefits include discovering meaning, making connections between clinical experiences and the classroom, instilling values, learning others' perspectives, and developing critical thinking (Blake, 2005). Reflective journaling is also used in the hospice setting, and many hospices now utilize focus groups and reflective journaling with their dying patients (Schaefer & Curley, 2005).

Journaling is reported to have therapeutic benefits by allowing patients a way of making sense of dying in addition to having a strong sense of purpose in sharing their story. This was confirmed when Bingley et al. (2006), a team of English investigators, reviewed samples of narratives written since 1950 by people who were facing death from cancer and other diseases. The investigators' goal was to compare experiences and identify how these experiences relate to broad changes in practice in end-of-life care. The investigators conducted a bibliographic search of libraries, archives, journals, and Internet-based sources. They located English spoken literature, including books, poems, newspapers, journal articles, diaries, and Internet postings of writings by people facing terminal disease. They conducted bibliometric and qualitative content analysis that explored changing authorship, experiences, purpose in writing, and the impact on readers. They applied inclusion/exclusion criteria to the initial search that located a wide range of published and unpublished narratives, which yielded 148 narratives by different au-

thors since 1950. They reviewed a subsample of 63 of these narratives. The investigators found that, over the last 56 years, there have been changes in both the volume of available literature and patterns of writing about the end-of-life experience. The results showed that patients have a clear awareness of social needs when dying. Patients also express issues of communication with medical staff, symptom control, realities of suffering, and spiritual aspects of dying (Bingley et al., 2006).

One component of journaling (or narrative therapy) has been well defined: It allows the patient to externalize problems. One study by Keeling and Bermudez (2006) examined an innovative externalization exercise that combined sculpture and journaling over a period of 4 weeks. Researchers studied the voices and experiences of 17 participants. The principal investigator also engaged in the exercise in an attempt to better understand the participants' experience. The findings were positive: The intervention helped participants express emotions, increase their awareness of personal resources and agency, separate problems from self-decreased symptoms and problem behaviors, and foster a sense of empowerment. This study reveals that physically externalizing problems and interacting with them deliberately over time have potential usefulness as a CAM therapy (Keeling & Bermudez, 2006).

References

Bingley, A. F., McDermott, E., Thomas, C., Payne, S., Seymour, J. E., & Clark, D. (2006). Making sense of dying: A review of narratives written since 1950 by people facing death from cancer and other diseases. *Palliative Medicine, 20*(3), 183–195.

Blake, T.K. (2005). Journaling: An active learning technique. *International Journal of Nursing Education Scholarship, 2*, 7.

Keeling, M. L., & Bermudez, M. (2006). Externalizing problems through art and writing: Experiences of process and helpfulness. *Journal of Marital and Family Therapy, 32*(4), 405–419.

Schaefer, K. M., & Curley, C. (2005). Use of focus groups and reflective journaling in a hospice experience. *Nurse Educator, 30*(3), 93–94.

An issue that may arise during both terminal weaning and terminal extubation is with the patient who is receiving neuromuscular blocking agents. An effort should be made to allow restoration of neuromuscular function before withdrawal of mechanical ventilation. Unfortunately, in some patients with multisystem organ failure, the clearance of the drug may become prolonged and restoration of full neuromuscular function could take days or weeks. Therefore, it may be morally justified to withdraw mechanical ventilation from a patient who is still experiencing the effects of residual blocking agents that were started prior to the decision to forgo life-sustaining measures. This decision must be balanced between the reasons to wait for restoration of neuromuscular function versus the added suffering of continued use of life-sustaining interventions.

Environment

When a patient is dying, it is important to create an environment that facilitates family presence. Discussions with family members regarding end-of-life decisions should not be held in a hallway or in the busy ICU. It is important to schedule a time and find a quiet place where family members can listen and feel comfortable asking questions. Once the decision is made for comfort care only, the patient care area should facilitate comfort for the patient and their family and friends. Rules regarding visiting hours and numbers of persons allowed in the room should be adjusted. Carney and Meier (2000, p. 204) describe a 10-step protocol for patients who are to be withdrawn from the ventilator:

1. Shut off and remove all monitors and alarms from the patient's room.
2. Remove equipment impeding access to hands. Hands are for holding.
3. Remove encumbering, disfiguring devices from the bedside.
4. Invite family to be with patient.
5. Quietly and personally request that vasopressors be turned off and that intravenous lines be set to keep open.
6. Watch for symptoms to develop and treat appropriately.
7. Turn FIO_2 down to 21% and observe patient for respiratory distress.
8. If patient and scene appear comfortable, remove endotracheal tube with clean towel in hand.
9. Educate and debrief house staff and nursing staff about process.
10. Consider contacting family during bereavement period whether by letter or visit.

The goal is to provide a peaceful, pain-free death for the patient and to create a supportive environment for the family.

Cultural Considerations

The manner in which individuals handle death is influenced by their culture, religion, family traditions, and individual preferences (Kuebler et al., 2007). When caring for a patient who is dying, it is important to discuss with the patient and family their cultural beliefs. Cultural practices bring security, integrity, and belonging to the individual. In some cultural groups, the family or a religious representative traditionally prepares the body af-

ter death (Andrews & Boyle, 2003). Most acute care facilities have a standardized procedure for preparation of the body following death. Family members, however, may view this as the facility performing a task that should be done by them. It is important to ask the family about their preferences and to facilitate any ritual that may be important to the patient and to them. Chart 17–1 (p. 402) discusses religious beliefs and traditions relating to end-of-life care.

In addition to religious beliefs, some cultures have specific customs with regard to end-of-life care. Cultural customs may come into play during communication with the patient and their family. Things to be aware of are conversational style and pace, eye contact, personal space, touch, and time orientation (Lipson & Dibble, 2007). The Cultural Considerations box (p. 404) lists known death rituals and communication customs for different cultures.

Grief

At the end of life, loss, grief, and bereavement can affect the family and members of the health care team. Part of the nurse's role at the end of life includes facilitating the grieving process. What is important to understand is that grief is a process an individual must experience to finally accept the reality of the loss (Bednash & Ferrell, 2002a). The grieving process includes a series of stages that the individual must move through to help resolve the grief. The process is not predictable, but fluid and unique to each individual.

There are several theories describing the stages of grief. The stages of grief described by Elizabeth Kubler-Ross are the most well known and are applied to those facing a death as well as those who have experienced a loss. Kubler-Ross identified five stages of grief: denial and isolation, anger, bargaining, depression, and acceptance. The loss of a loved one usually brings with it an intense grief response and may develop into a complicated grief response. Normal grief affects all aspects of a person's being—physical, emotional, cognitive, behavioral, and spiritual.

After a death, the bereaved person is at risk for new illness or worsening of an existing illness during the first year after the loss. Emotional acceptance takes time as the bereaved person feels the pain of the loss. Sadness may lessen at times but returns with reminders of the loved one, such as an anniversary or a photograph. Even if the death was expected at the time, cognitively it will still be a shock. The loss is so intense that the person can hardly believe that the patient is really dead. Behaviorally, the bereaved person gradually returns to daily functioning after the funeral or burial. Maladaptive behaviors may arise such as substance abuse. Spiritual beliefs will affect the way a person grieves. The patient may have held certain religious or cultural beliefs that prescribe certain acts and behaviors after death, but not all significant others may hold those beliefs.

Complicated or abnormal grief response may occur and arises from various internal and external factors. One of these factors is the bereaved person's relationship with the deceased before the death. If the bereaved person still holds unexpressed hostility toward the deceased, then that person is likely to feel anger and guilt, which inhibits the grief process. Chart 17–2 (p. 405) lists characteristics of complicated grief. Nursing care for significant others during end of life includes providing information with sensitivity to what significant others want to know,

CHART 17–1	**Religion and End-of-Life Care**

Religion	Beliefs	Traditions/Rituals
Christianity • Catholic • Orthodox • Protestant • Amish • Other	Christians believe that Jesus is the messiah.	**Catholic** • Anointing of the sick is done by a priest before the person's death. • Belief in preservation of life but not obligated to take extraordinary means. • Donation of organs is acceptable. • Funerals are generally held 2–3 days after death. **Orthodox** • Last anointing may be conducted before or after death. • Confession and holy communion are important rituals and are conducted by priests. • A memorial service is held on the closest Sunday to the 40th day after death. **Protestant** • There are no last rites. Prayers are given to offer comfort and support. • Some Pentecostal and neocharismatic churches believe in faith healing. **Amish** • Use of narcotic drugs is prohibited. • Prolongation of life and euthanasia are personal matters that may be discussed with the bishop and/or family members. • Autopsy is acceptable in the case of medical necessity or legal requirement. • Prefer to bury the body intact so generally do not donate organs. **Others** • Mormons will administer a sacrament if the patient requests. • Important to Mormons that death be peaceful and dignified. • Jehovah's Witnesses do not believe in sacraments. • Jehovah's Witnesses will be excommunicated if they receive a blood transfusion. • Jehovah's Witnesses do not believe in organ donation. • Christian Scientists rely mostly on spiritual healing. It is unlikely they will seek medical help to prolong life.

Islam	The founder of Islam, Mohammed, received a vision while meditating. This vision later became the Qur'an or Koran. *Allah* is the Arabic word for "God." A follower of Islam is called Moslem or Muslim.	• Second-degree male relatives (cousins or uncles) should be the contact person. They will determine whether the patient and/or family should be told about diagnoses, prognoses, etc.
		• Patients may choose to face Mecca (west or southwest in the United States). The head should be elevated above the body.
		• Discussions about death are not usually welcomed.
		• Stopping medical treatment is viewed as against Allah's will.
		• Grief may be expressed through slapping or hitting the body. Counseling is not well accepted.
		• It is important in Islam to follow prescribed burial procedures:
		  1. Washing of the dead body according to Muslim tradition. Muslim women cleanse a woman's body. Muslim men cleanse a man's body.
		  2. The body is washed three times and then wrapped in three pieces of clean white cloth.
		  3. Special prayers for the dead are required.
		  4. The body should be buried as soon as possible and should be positioned so that the head faces toward Mecca.
		  5. These burial practices are followed for fetuses after a gestational age of 130 days.

CHART 17–1	Religion and End-of-Life Care—*Continued*	
Religion	**Beliefs**	**Traditions/Rituals**
Judaism	The Sabbath is celebrated from sunset on Friday to sunset Saturday evening. Sabbath is a day of rest.	• No actions to hasten death are permitted but if a physician states that death is inevitable, no new therapeutic measures that would artificially extend life should be initiated. • A dying person should not be left alone. The exact time of death is noted for the purpose of honoring the deceased the first year after death. • Autopsy and cremation are forbidden. If an autopsy is required, it should be limited to essential organs or systems. All body parts must be returned for burial. • The funeral is usually held the day after death. The body is ritually washed and then clothed in a simple white burial shroud. Embalming and cosmetic treatment of the body are forbidden. • The family mourns for 7 days.
Hinduism	Hindus believe in multiple gods and goddesses, with one great spirit, Brahman. Karma is the working out in this life of events that occurred in a previous life. Reincarnation is a strong belief.	• Life is a perpetual cycle, so death is seen as just one more step toward nirvana. • Rituals include tying a thread around the neck or wrist of the dying person, sprinkling them with water from the Ganges River, or placing a leaf of basil on their tongue. • After death, do not remove sacred threads or wash the body.
Buddhism	The teachings of Buddha included the Four Noble Truths that expound on suffering: the truth of suffering, the truth of the origin of suffering, the truth that suffering can be destroyed, and the way that leads to the cessation of pain. The original teachings also included the Noble Eightfold Way: right views, right intention, right speech, right action, right livelihood, right effort, right mindfulness, and right concentration. Buddhism does not dictate any specific practices so individual differences can be expected and should be respected.	• Buddhist monks should be consulted to offer spiritual support. • A shrine to Buddha may be placed in the patient's room. • "Mindfulness" is an important state of being. Patients may refuse medications because they may alter alertness. • Buddhists generally accept death. • After death, a monk may recite prayers for 1 hour. The prayers need not be said in the presence of the body because it is considered but a shell. • Organ donation is encouraged. • Cremations are common.
Baha'i Faith	Belief is to know and worship God and carry forward an ever-advancing civilization. They believe that all the great religions of the world are divine in origin.	• Baha'is believe that life is unique and precious, so destruction of a human life is not permitted. When natural death has occurred, it is considered in the light of current medical science and legal rulings. • Baha'i law states that the body is not to be embalmed or cremated. • The place of burial must be within 1 hour's travel from the place of death; exceptions are possible.

Sources: Andrews, M., & Boyle, J. (2003). *Transcultural concepts in nursing care* (4th ed.). New York: Lippincott Williams & Wilkins; Bednash, G., & Ferrell, B. (2002a). Ethical and legal issues in end of life care. In *Continuing Education for Nurses* (pp. 21–65). Roseville, CA: CME Resource; Spector, R. (2009). *Cultural diversity in health and illness* (7th ed.). Upper Saddle River, NJ: Pearson Prentice Hall.

providing emotional support, suggesting appropriate referrals to mental health resources, recognizing abnormal grief reactions, and legitimizing the death (Saunders, 2007).

Interventions are designed to help an individual accept the reality of the loss. Interventions may include:

- Presence, active listening, touch
- Providing emotional support
- Encouraging verbalization
- Identifying support systems
- Normalizing the grief process and allowing for individual differences
- Identifying need for additional assistance and making referrals.

To be effective caregivers at end of life, nurses must come to terms with their own views on death and dying. As with patients and their families, nurses' comfort with death is affected by their personality, culture, spiritual belief system, and life experiences. Encouraging nurses to verbalize their feelings and express emotions will help them to process grief and loss and provide quality care at the end of life.

End-of-Life Care for Patients Who Are Terminally Ill

End-of-life care for patients who are terminally ill follows the same principles as those used for patients and families faced

CULTURAL CONSIDERATIONS Communication Customs and Death Rituals

American Indians	• Most embrace the present and avoid contact with the dying. If they feel comfortable being present, they will include immediate and extended family with children. The family will remain positive and even jovial because sadness and mourning are to be done in private. • Family may request spiritual healers. • Loud voice may be associated with aggression. Avoiding eye contact is respectful.
Cambodians	• The family may be quiet and passive. Monks and *aacha* are called to recite prayers, especially on the night of death. • It is inappropriate to touch their heads without permission. • They consider it impolite to disagree so they may say yes but not mean it. • Very important to speak softly and be polite. • After death, the family or monks may wash the body and then shroud it in a white cloth.
Central Americans • Guatemala • Nicaragua • El Salvador	• Spanish language is rich and full of intonations and meanings. It is important to closely observe body language. Loud, boisterous voices are acceptable. • Women are very modest around strangers. • Crosses, rosary beads, or figures of saints may be important. Female children may be protected by wearing red earrings because red is a strong color. Male babies may wear red knitted caps. Both may wear a little red bag (bolsita) of herbs around the neck to protect them from harm. Always check with parents before removing any red item. • If a young person dies it is believed to be a greater loss because of the unfulfilled life. • If the patient can be kept comfortable, they consider prolonged death a relief because it enables more relatives to say their good-byes. • The eldest male in the family should be informed of impending death. • Traditionally family members prepare the body for burial. Nurses should ask if the family wants to prepare the body for the mortuary. • They consider death a spiritual event, so family members need time to say good-bye to the deceased.
Chinese	• Eye contact with authority figures is avoided as a sign of respect. • Chinese language is expressive and loud. • Need to assess understanding of conversations because the patient or family may not ask questions as a sign of respect. • Privacy is very important. • Special amulets and cloths may be placed on the body.
Roma (Gypsies)	• Important to establish trust. • Very respectful of elder authority, therefore will have greater respect for older health care providers and dismiss younger team members. • Tone of voice is commonly loud and argumentative. • Very modest; they never ask personal questions in mixed company. • Moment of death is very significant because the feelings of the dying person at that moment give the family a sense of what will happen in the year after death. The last words of the dying patient are very important and the family will want to hear them.
Hmong	• Very polite and aware of disrespectful and prejudicial behavior. • Prolonged eye contact is considered disrespectful. • Communication may be indirect. Will not say "no" but may say "I will think about it." • Interpreters employed by the hospital are considered to be loyal to the institution and therefore not trusted. The family may request a bilingual family member be present during discussions. • Language structure is different; make sure the interpreter understands the intent of the discussion. The Hmong language has almost no medical terms. • Have great respect for authority. • Elders of the family will meet to make decisions regarding the patient's care. Immediate family members and female relatives may not have exclusive decision-making power. • Traditional beliefs say that at the time of death, the person goes to the next world in the same appearance. It is considered shameful to enter the next world poorly dressed or unclothed. If possible, allow the family to dress the patient in traditional clothing near the time of death. • Do not remove amulets from the dying patient's body.
Japanese	• May not ask questions, deferring to health care team to provide care. • Illness is not discussed outside of the family. • Soft voice is considered polite with direct conflict avoided. • Facial expressions are controlled and prolonged direct eye contact is considered disrespectful. • Promptness is very important. • Family and patient may avoid discussing illness or impending death. The decision not to resuscitate is a difficult one and is decided by the entire family. • Cleanliness of body is important, as is modesty and preservation of dignity.

CULTURAL CONSIDERATIONS Communication Customs and Death Rituals—*Continued*

Mexicans	• Direct eye contact with authority figures is avoided. • Silence may show lack of agreement with the plan of care. • Touching by a stranger is considered disrespectful although therapeutic touch is an integral part of traditional healing. • Family may hang spiritual amulets, religious medallions, or rosary beads near the patient. • After the patient dies, the family will request some time to say good-bye.
Russians	• Direct eye contact is used. • Respectful of elders. • Tone of voice may be loud. • Family members decide whether patients should be told about their condition and prognosis to not burden them. • Tend to use DNR orders for an elderly patient to allow him or her to die comfortably and not on life support. • After death the body is respected and considered sacred.
Asians and Africans • India • Pakistan • Bangladesh • Sri Lanka • Nepal • Fiji • East Africa	• Touching not common; caring is expressed through the eyes. • Prolonged direct eye contact is considered rude. • Modesty, humility, tolerance, and silence are emphasized. • Tone of voice should be soft. Loudness is considered disrespectful. • Family decides whether the patient should be told about his or her condition and prognosis. • Family members will want to be at the bedside at the time of death. Grief will be expressed openly.
Vietnamese	• Head may be considered sacred and feet profane; do not touch the feet and then the head. • Avoiding eye contact is a sign of respect. • Using both hands when giving a person something shows respect. • Tone of voice should be soft. • A loud voice or pointing of the finger is a sign of disrespect. • Family may want to wash the body themselves as the body is highly respected.

Source: Adapted from Lipson, J., & Dibble, S. (Eds.). (2005). *Culture and clinical care.* San Francisco: UCSF Nursing Press.

CHART 17–2   Characteristics of Complicated Grief

Complicated Grief Type	Characteristics
Exaggerated	• Response is out of proportion. • Response is more intense than expected. • The person is disabled with clinical depression or other psychiatric disorders.
Masked	• Feelings are expressed as physical symptoms. • Feelings are expressed as maladaptive behavior. • Feelings are not expressed at all. • The person may not realize that symptoms or behaviors are related to the loss.
Delayed	• Feelings may not arise until another person is lost. • Feelings surrounding the loss are not expressed until the person suffers another loss.
Chronic	• The person never reaches resolution with regard to the loss. • The reaction to the loss is unusually long.

Source: Adapted from Saunders, C. A. (Ed.). (2007). *End of life: A nurse's guide to compassionate care.* Philadelphia: Lippincott Williams & Wilkins, page 235.

with an unexpected death. The main difference is that the patient with a terminal illness has the opportunity to participate in the planning for his death.

Hospice

Hospice is the provision of care at the end of life aimed at comfort instead of cure. It is based on a model that is interdisciplinary and tailored to meet the values and goals of the patient and family. The care is aimed at relieving physical, psychosocial, and spiritual suffering for the patient and to facilitate the grieving and coping strategies of families and caregivers.

Death is an inevitable aspect of the human condition; dying badly is not. (Jennings, Ryndes, D'Onofrio, & Baily, 2003). As the aging of the population continues, more and more individuals will face decisions regarding their end-of-life care. The challenge of end-of-life care will grow during the next three decades because the population of seniors in the United States is projected to more than double during the next 30 years, rising from 34 million in 1997 to more than 69 million by 2030. Despite significant advances in preventive care and treatment modalities that prolong health and life, all but those who die suddenly and unexpectedly will have to make decisions about serious or life-threatening illness.

The History of Hospice

The root word *hospitality* led to the term *hospice*. As far back as medieval times, it originally meant a place for travelers to rest. The first modern hospice established to care for dying patients was founded by Dame Cicely Saunders in 1967 in London. Soon she was lecturing at Yale to medical students and nurses regarding hospice care. This heralded the start of the modern hospice movement.

In 1969, Elizabeth Kubler-Ross published her book *On Death and Dying*, which describes the phases of the dying process and pioneered the concepts of patient choice and self-direction. In 1972 she testified at Senate hearings on aging, which led to an unsuccessful attempt to establish legislation for federal funding of hospice care. In 1979, the Healthcare Financing Administration authorized 26 hospice demonstration projects across America. In 1980, the W. K. Kellogg Foundation awarded a grant to the Joint Commission to develop hospice standards. In 1986 Congress enacted the Medicare Hospice Benefit, which established a reimbursement mechanism for Medicare-eligible beneficiaries. Over the years, Congress has granted several increases and has recommended the incorporation of hospice care into the care of military veterans and Native Americans.

Terminology

Nurses need to have a clear understanding of hospice care, beginning with the customary terminology used. Nurses play a crucial role in assisting patients and families in increasing their knowledge of hospice care and dispelling myths and fears. Hospice care focuses on comfort care versus curative care. An interdisciplinary team of health care providers including physicians, nurses, social workers, spiritual counselors, dieticians, home health aides, and volunteers provides hospice. The care plan encompasses both the patient and family/caregiver as the unit of care, and the care plan is individualized to meet their values and goals. Patients receiving hospice care are generally defined as those patients who have a prognosis of 6 months or less if their terminal disease runs a normal course.

One of the core operating principles of hospice is the ongoing collaboration of the interdisciplinary team to ensure holistic, comprehensive care to meet not only physical needs but psychosocial and spiritual needs. Hospice care is provided to the patient in various settings, although most often this is the patient's home or living facility. According to the National Hospice and Palliative Care Organization (NHPCO, 2006), in 2004, 95.8% of the days of hospice services provided by the nation's hospices were at the home care level. Hospice care is also provided in the inpatient setting. In fact, many hospice programs have dedicated beds or inpatient units to provide hospice care. Inpatient care is generally provided for management of symptoms and periods of caregiver crisis. NHPCO states that, in 2004, 3% of hospice care was provided in an inpatient setting.

Hospices also provide respite care. Respite is care given to a hospice patient by another caregiver so the usual caregiver can rest. Respite care is provided in a hospice facility, hospital, or a skilled nursing facility. Hospices may also provide short-term continuous nursing care in a patient's home to prevent a hospitalization during a period of medical crisis. This allows patients to remain in the comfort of their own home and attain symptom control.

Hospice care also encompasses bereavement services after the death of the patient. These services are available for a minimum of 1 year after the death of the patient and provide support for families and caregivers during the grieving process. Bereavement is provided by telephone and in person, and on an individual or group basis. Most hospice programs also have groups that are available to the community to deal with grief and coping issues.

The term *palliative care* has risen to the forefront in recent years. The World Health Organization's (WHO's) definition of palliative care makes it virtually identical with hospice: "Palliative care is an approach that improves the quality of life of patients and their families facing the problem associated with life-threatening illness, through the prevention and relief of suffering by means of early identification and impeccable assessment and treatment of pain and other problems, physical, psychosocial and spiritual" (2006). From another perspective, however, the two terms are often taken to refer to different caregiving orientations, time frames, and institutional settings. WHO's definition goes on to add "Many aspects of palliative care are also applicable earlier in the course of the illness, in conjunction with anti-cancer treatment." From a medical perspective, then, palliative care may be taken as the broader term, covering all forms of the prevention and treatment of suffering (Jennings et al., 2003).

The concept of comfort care versus curative care is important for nurses who are caring for patients with cancer to fully understand. Comfort care is aimed at improving the quality of life, not necessarily aimed at prolonging the quantity of life. Effective symptom relief may not only improve the quality of life but occasionally will demonstrate some secondary gain in quantity of life. The key to understanding comfort care versus curative care is to ask "What is the primary intent of the treatment intervention?" There are instances where modalities such as chemotherapy and radiation are curative in nature. For example, providing radiotherapy to decrease tumor size may result in less pain. This is different than choosing these therapies in the setting of a more aggressive approach, with the goal being cure.

Most people will progress through the dying process in much the same way that they lived, with a set of values and beliefs that are important to them. The very decision to choose hospice care is rooted in these values and beliefs. For some individuals the concept of hospice means "giving up" and may be in conflict with their core belief system. For those patients who choose hospice, the hospice team individualizes the care plan in collaboration with the patient and family to be sure that the hospice care provided is what they desire. This individualized values-based care allows patients to maintain their independence and have their personal values and preferences respected as they are dying. The majority of Americans have an affinity for as much independence in their lives as possible, even during their final days. Nurses play a pivotal role in providing patients and their families with information about what is happening to them and what options are available to them (Kuebler et al., 2007).

Interdisciplinary care involves interdisciplinary teamwork, which is a hallmark of hospice care. Utilizing the knowledge and expertise of physicians, nurses, social workers, spiritual counselors, dietitians, aides and volunteers, the care is designed to be comprehensive and constantly updated to meet the patient and family needs. Team meetings should be held at regular intervals to discuss all aspects of a patient's care including symptom management, patient and family psychosocial needs, spiritual needs, and the ability to maintain or receive assistance in activities of daily living. All members of the team bring their individual perspectives to the care and have input into care decisions.

Suffering is unrelieved physical, psychological, or spiritual distress. Hospice recognizes the interdependence of all of these factors and relieving these is critical in truly achieving a "good death." An example of *relief of suffering* is resolving psychological or spiritual needs that may be impeding the success of pharmacologic pain control measures. Suffering can also be existential in nature. Existential suffering differs from physical, psychosocial, or spiritual symptoms that may respond to intervention. Existential suffering includes hopelessness, disappointment, remorse, death anxiety, disruption of personal identity, and the meaninglessness of continued life. The goal of hospice is to address all of these needs in an integrated and holistic manner.

Payer Sources

In the United States, hospice care provided at home for patients over the age of 65 or for patients who have been disabled for more than 2 years is covered through Medicare. Most private insurance and health maintenance organizations provide hospice benefits. Hospice care covers physician services, nursing services, social work counseling, dietary instruction, aides and homemakers, volunteers, medical equipment, and drugs prescribed for the terminal illness. Additionally, hospice programs also receive donated funds, most often in memory of one of their patients who has died. These funds may be used to care for patients who do not have medical coverage for hospice care.

Medicare is the largest payer source in America for hospice care. In 1982 the Hospice Benefit was created as part of Medicare. To be eligible for Medicare hospice care, the patient must have Medicare Part A, and the attending physician and the hospice medical director must certify that the patient has a prognosis of 6 months or less if the disease runs its normal course. Patients are reevaluated on an ongoing basis and at intervals defined by Medicare for continued appropriateness for hospice. If the patient's disease does not progress and the patient's condition stabilizes, the patient may be taken off the hospice benefit. Likewise, if a patient changes her mind and wishes to pursue aggressive therapy, the patient may revoke the hospice benefit. However, the patient, in either of these two scenarios, can return to the hospice benefit if disease progression returns and the physician certifies that the patient has a 6-month prognosis. Despite the payer source, most hospice programs model their care under the federal regulations for participation in the Medicare Hospice Program, entitled the Medicare Conditions of Participation.

Access to Hospice Care

NHPCO (2006) estimates that in the year 2004, approximately 3,650 established hospice programs served 1,060,000 patients. Hospice care is provided to patients of all ages; however, the majority of care is provided to those 65 years of age or older.

Hospice care has expanded over the years to include serving patients other than those with cancer diagnoses. Hospices are now caring for patients with other life-threatening, chronic illnesses such as heart disease, respiratory disease, and HIV/AIDS. In 2006, NHPCO reported that in 2004, 46% of hospice patients had a cancer diagnosis. NHPCO reports the top five noncancer causes of death in hospice patients in 2004 as follows: 12.2%, end-stage cardiac disease; 8.9%, dementia; 8.2%, debility; 7.1%, lung disease; and 3.1%, end-stage kidney disease.

Barriers to Hospice Care

With only one in four Americans receiving hospice care at the time of death, it is clear that barriers to hospice care exist. By the year 2030, 20% of Americans will be age 65 or older. One in nine baby boomers is expected to live to age 90, and by 2040, the number of Americans over age 85 will be nearly four times greater than today. The United States already struggles to provide basic primary care to its population; more than 40 million Americans are without consistent, adequate health insurance coverage. Geography plays a significant role in preventing access to services provided by hospice. Patients in inner city, rural, and remote inaccessible areas are likely to be underserved (Jennings et al., 2003).

Physician reluctance to refer to hospice has remained a barrier. Patients depend on their physicians for health care information and guidance; however, many individuals are never introduced to the concept of hospice care by their physicians or health care providers. In a recent study, a significant subgroup of physicians had reservations about the physician being the most appropriate person to introduce the concept of hospice to the patient and was also concerned that discussion of hospice would lead to a sense of hopelessness (Ogle, Mavis, & Wang, 2003).

Information technology has heightened the awareness of patients and their families to promising new treatments and disease-fighting drugs. Consumers are enticed by the media and the Internet to investigate the use of these modalities without much discussion of the associated burden or risk. Patients and families often do not want to hear about hospice, but rather want to avail themselves of every option. Some feel that the regulatory and policy issues represent a barrier to hospice care. As technological options increase for consumers, it is hoped that regulations regarding the requirement that the patient forgo curative treatment will be reevaluated. The ability to expand the types of hospice care provided would benefit patients and families and promote receiving hospice services earlier in their illness.

Nurses will no doubt experience the challenge of end-of-life care more significantly during the next three decades. The lack of available qualified nurses is impacting the ability to provide hospice care in some hospices. The challenge of the shortage will be multiplied by the projected aging of the population.

With the tendency of Americans to deny their mortality, along with physician reluctance and access to increased information regarding new treatments, patients and families are either not referred to or refuse hospice services until very late in their disease course. NHPCO (2006) states the average length of service in 2002 was 51 days, and the median length of stay was 26 days. These short stays do not allow the hospice team to maximize symptom control, to provide psychological and spiritual support, and to begin work on anticipatory grieving. The crucial development of a trusting therapeutic relationship between the patient/family and the hospice team is difficult to achieve in such a limited amount of time.

Diversity

Culture is not the same as race. Culture includes traditions, customs, religious beliefs, and attitudes that occur at a variable pace (Lipson & Dibble, 2007). Language and immigration history also influence cultures. Hospice must work within the culture of each patient and family unit. The hospice team must seek input from the patient and family to develop a plan that is realistic and not in opposition to strongly held cultural beliefs. The Cultural Considerations box (p. 404) discusses details of end-of-life care as it relates to cultural variations.

NHPCO (2006) reports that in 2004, 77.3% of all hospice patients identified themselves as white or Caucasian, 8.1% as black or African American, 6.2% as Hispanic or Latino, 6.4% as multiracial, and 1.7% as Asian or Pacific Islander. The results of a recent study (Colon & Lyke, 2003) indicate that there are significant differences between ethnic groups who use hospice care. Most importantly, the study also determined that African Americans and Latinos are clearly underusing hospice services relevant to their prevalence in the general population.

Identified differences between ethnic groups include age, cultural adaptation, high-risk behaviors, caregivers, and payment method. Hospice programs need to focus on increasing awareness of services within minority communities as well as making the treatment itself more culturally sensitive.

Sexual diversity applies to groups such as lesbians, gays, bisexuals, and transgendered individuals. These groups require special consideration in hospice care due to the fact that, despite advances, social stigmas still exist within certain groups and locales. This may discourage access to hospice care, especially if the terminal illness is associated with lifestyle choices.

The Role of Nursing in Hospice

The professional nurse plays a number of key roles in hospice care. The nurse is critical in not only directing the provision of high-quality, competent care, but also in promoting the hospice concept and advocating for patients and families. Most hospice programs identify the registered nurse as the case manager for a panel of hospice patients. The nurse is accountable for the interdisciplinary collaboration and oversight of the care of the patient and family.

The nurse can play a role in influencing physicians and other health care providers to consider the hospice option for their patients. The nurse can provide knowledge and information, correct myths, and influence the effort for earlier referrals to hospice. The nurse also plays a key role in the education of patients and families about hospice, exploring their concerns and fears, and assisting them in navigating the numerous care options. The nurse is always the patient advocate, ensuring that whatever course is chosen is in alignment with the patient's and family members' values and goals, done with their full knowledge about the options, and the implications of their choices.

Hospice programs have grown tremendously during the past 10 years. NHPCO (2006) reports that in 1992 there were 1,935 hospice programs, growing to 3,650 in 2004. More patients and families are choosing hospice care, up from 246,000 in 1992 to 1,060,000 in 2004. Despite this growth there are challenges. Access issues and barriers to care continue. Hospices are faced with an increasingly diverse population. Physician willingness to refer remains an issue. These challenges exist in a health care system faced with an increasing number of aged Americans, the issues of payer reimbursement, and complex regulations from payers, government agencies, and accrediting organizations. However, there is reason to be optimistic. The hospice movement and the palliative care movements can exist in collaboration to improve

the overall quality of end-of-life care. Structured end-of-life education is being provided to physicians during training and later as continuing education. Education in end-of-life care is being presented to nurses, and increasing numbers of hospice nurses are receiving certification in the specialty of hospice and palliative care. Professional organizations such as NHPCO and state hospice organizations are advocating legislative reforms to increase access to hospice programs, decrease barriers especially with regard to eligibility, and promote increasing the lengths of stay in hospice programs. To provide the impetus for policy and practice changes that will increase access to hospice care, hospice must be re-envisioned as a concept of health care—a new way of thinking about the nature and goals of health care itself, rather than an end-stage form of care (Jennings et al., 2003).

Palliative Care

Palliative care is a relatively new field in nursing. Nurses have traditionally contributed their resources to a health care system that has focused primarily on attempts at curing diseases. Yet, many diseases are incurable including congestive heart failure (CHF), chronic obstructive pulmonary disease (COPD), some cancers, stroke, and dementias, to name a few. Modern medicine continues to overtreat by attempting to cure when cure is no longer possible. Perhaps it is more appropriate to treat death as a natural process rather than an enemy, particularly when the patient's end of life is near.

Palliative care nurses serve patients with incurable illnesses, and their family members, by assisting in the management of their multifaceted symptoms, ultimately enabling them to live within the confines of their illnesses. Traditional disease-centered focus should be aligned with the caring model of nursing, one that focuses on the whole patient, embracing a model that includes the art of caring for ill patients, as well as the science.

Palliative care was recognized as its own field of medicine in 1987, with its roots stemming from hospice, being viewed as active care versus total care (Kuebler et al., 2007). In 1990 the WHO introduced their definition of palliative care as "the active total care of a patient whose disease is manageable but not curable." This includes interventions that:

1. Affirm life and regard dying as a normal process.
2. Neither hasten nor postpone death.
3. Provide relief from pain and other distressing symptoms.
4. Integrate the psychological and spiritual aspects of patient care.
5. Offer a support system to help patients live as actively as possible until death.
6. Offer a support system to help the family cope during the patient's illness and in their own bereavement.

Nurses should be familiar with how palliative care emerged and the types of programs and activities available to patients and their families. It is also important to recognize the barriers those providing palliative care face.

Emergence of Palliative Care

There is a rapidly growing nation movement to improve end-of-life education and the delivery of palliative care. Forces behind the

MyNursingKit | Center to Advance Palliative Care

MyNursingKit | Last Acts Campaign

motivation to change have been changes in the delivery of health care in the last century, results of research studies, and the development of programs and projects by renowned organizations.

Changes in the last century in medical science have led to unparalleled progress in the effective treatment of disease, which has, for many, led to prolonged periods of illness, decline, and suffering. Chart 17–3 compares care in the early 20th century to care early in the 21st century, which has been changed tremendously by the advances of modern medicine.

Most people die in the hospital, although surveys indicate that more than 70% of people would prefer to die at home (Solloway, Lafrance, Bakitas, & Gerken, 2005). In a chart review of 782 deaths in hospitals, nursing homes, and hospice/home care in one state, significant differences were found among symptom assessment and provision of emotional and spiritual support for patients and families. Within the hospitals, 56% of deaths were in acute care beds, 30% were in ICUs, and only 4% were in palliative care beds. Nineteen percent of decedents received interventions such as being placed on a ventilator or surgery in the 48 hours preceding death. More than 80% had a do-not-resuscitate (DNR) order, 45% had a DPAHC, and 37% had a living will. Age and setting were significant factors in the presence of advance directives (Solloway et al., 2005). How unfortunate that many Americans die after suffering miserably. Fear of the dying process is a very real emotion for many adults. Many fear the care they will receive during and before end of life, the loss of control they will experience, being attached to machines, dying away from home, and being separated from loved ones.

End-of-life education for health care professionals has been scarce at best. Both medical schools and residency programs devote inadequate efforts to end-of-life care instruction (McPhee, Rabow, Pantilat, Markowitz, & Winker, 2000). Up until recently, nursing textbooks devoted only 2% of the total content to end-of-life care. However, much of the information was found to be inaccurate (Ferrell & Coyle, 2002).

Several organizations are aspiring to better the end-of-life care provided around the country. They are committed to the vision of ensuring a "good death" for patients and their families, where the period prior to death is dignified and comfortable. Included are the Last Acts Campaign of the Robert Wood Johnson (RWJ) Foundation, the Education for Physicians on End of Life Care of the American Medical Association, the Center to Advance Palliative Care, and Americans for Better Care of the Dying. Also, of special mention, are the hospice programs that improve the quality of life for those who are dying and their families (Ditillo, 2002).

The End-of-Life Nursing Education Consortium of the American Association of Colleges of Nursing and the City of Hope National Medical Center is a program funded by the RWJ foundation. It is a 3-day course designed to train nurses who provide continuing education courses and equip them with the resources to integrate end-of-life care into their courses. Renowned researchers, educators, authors, and leaders facilitate the training in the specialty of palliative care. Modules include nursing care at the end of life, pain and other symptom management, cultural issues, ethical/legal considerations, communication, bereavement, and care and preparation for death.

Provision of Palliative Care

As the specialty of palliative care is emerging, so is the evolution of the provision of care. Types of programs are varied, yet many of the activities are common. And, as with all programs, come the inevitable barriers to providing effective care.

Determining the type of palliative care program that would be most effective is very challenging. Many elements need to be considered, and range from selecting the patient population to funding reimbursement. Palliative care units and services can be useful approaches to caring for people who are terminally ill, and include those patients who are chronically ill and may live for years in their disease state.

A palliative care service may include either inpatient and/or outpatient consultations, ranging from comprehensive case management or care coordination to a one-time visit. Types of patients to be seen may include those with chronic illnesses that are incurable and decline over time, such as CHF, COPD, dementia, cancers, and strokes. No single health care provider can successfully meet all of the palliative care needs of patients who have incurable illnesses and the needs of their families. The interdisciplinary team approach is essential because it is comprised of a variety of disciplines that pool their data to reach a consensus about goal setting, and the development of a comprehensive plan of care. Team members may include, but are not limited to, physicians, nurses, social workers, and chaplains. Other ancillary support may be needed depending on the needs of the patient, and include experts in the fields of mental health, physical therapy, nutrition, pharmacy, respiratory therapy, and ethics.

Nurses working in a palliative care program should understand that targeted interventions are common regardless of the program design, and include pain and symptom management, end-of-life care planning, and support that encompasses psychosocial and spiritual needs. The National Guidelines box (p. 410) discusses standards and guidelines for palliative care.

Symptoms will vary according to the disease state and should be monitored and controlled regardless of the proximity to end of life. For patients close to the end of life, symptoms experienced are often distressing and include pain, dyspnea, nausea, constipation, anxiety, restlessness, delirium, fatigue, dehydration, and "death rattles." Palliative care nurses play a pivotal role in accurately assessing, reporting, and ensuring that symptoms are appropriately managed. A patient's quality of life is contingent on an astute, competent nurse who has received thorough education in pain and symptom management and is assertive

CHART 17–3	Effects of Changes in Care: Now and Then	
	1900	**2000**
Average age at death	46 years	78 years
Cause of death	• Infection	• Cancer
	• Accidents	• Heart disease
	• Childbearing	• Stroke
		• Dementias
Location where death occurred	• Home	• Hospital
Prevalence of disability	• Rare	• Average 4 years

MyNursingKit | End of Life Nursing Education Consortium

NATIONAL GUIDELINES for Quality Palliative Care

In 2002, the Hospice and Palliative Nurses Association and the American Nurses Association developed the *Scope and Standards of Hospice and Palliative Nursing Practice*. Part of the standards follow the nursing process (Saunders, 2007):

Assessment	Collect Patient and Family Data
Diagnosis	Analyze the assessment data and develop diagnoses using an accepted framework that supports hospice and palliative nursing knowledge.
Outcomes	In partnership with a multidisciplinary team, identify expected outcomes relevant to the patient and family.
Planning	In partnership with the patient, family, and multidisciplinary team, develop a plan of care that includes interventions and treatments to attain expected outcomes.
Implementation	Implement the plan of care.
Evaluation	Evaluate the patient's and family's progress in attaining the expected outcomes.

In 2004, the National Consensus Project for Quality Palliative Care, the Center to Advance Palliative Care, and the Last Acts Partnership created the *Clinical Practice Guidelines for Quality Palliative Care* (National Consensus Project for Quality Palliative Care, 2004). More than 100 experts contributed to the evidence-based guidelines. The framework for the clinical practice guidelines include:

- Structure and processes of care
- Physical aspects of care
- Psychological and psychiatric aspects of care
- Social aspects of care
- Spiritual, religious, and existential aspects of care
- Cultural aspects of care
- Care of the imminently dying patient
- Ethical and legal aspects of care.

Source: National Consensus Project for Quality Palliative Care (2004). Clinical practice guidelines for quality palliative care. http://www.nationalconsensusproject.org

enough to advocate for patients in an environment where the proper use of analgesics and adjunct medications may not be understood. Doses often need to be titrated and tailored to a level particular to the individual. Nurses need to recognize that many health care providers lack the expertise to appropriately manage the common and complex symptoms that occur at or near death.

Another key function of the palliative care team is to assist the patient who has an incurable illness to develop a plan of care prior to advancement of his disease process. The plan should be rational and customized to the individualized patient's goals and values. This can be accomplished in an interdisciplinary team setting and should include the patient and key people in his life. A systematic or methodical approach may be very beneficial. It would include a discussion regarding what the patient knows or wants to know about his disease state, and whether or not he is ready to engage in this type of discussion. The provider may then educate the patient regarding the potential trajectory of the illness, and the risk, benefit, and burden measure of each treatment option. Next, the patient would be assisted to set goals of care based on the individual's values.

Remember that any expression of a patient's wishes should be considered valid and binding, whether it is written or oral. Even though it is beneficial for potential agents to witness the patient's statements about what may or may not give meaning and value to one's life, a formal written document signed by the patient helps to avoid ambiguity. The patient should choose a health care agent whom she trusts and is confident would carry out previously discussed wishes, in the event that she cannot speak for herself. The document should be readily available when decisions need to be made. Statute requirements for the state where the patient resides can be determined by contacting the local hospital, state attorney general's office, public health office, local medical society, or state board of nursing.

Paramount to providing good palliative care is the ability of the provider to be absolutely honest with the patient. The concept of truth-telling urges practitioners to overcome the tendency to avoid accurate disclosure when talking to dying patients so they may begin planning for their end-of-life journey (Saunders, 2007). When a curative model of care is offered to a dying patient, it becomes more difficult to allow discussions that are completely truthful in nature. Nurses build relationships with dying patients that allow for discussions centered on shifting the focus of care from curative to more of a palliative model. Staying focused on a curative model fosters false hope and may rob a patient of intimacy and closure at the end of life.

To be effective in providing palliative care for those with terminal illnesses, providers need to be tuned in to the various psychosocial needs of the patient and family. Nurses need to be able to recognize grief and assist with the appropriate interventions to cope, whether that is by nursing actions or consultation with the palliative care team for appropriate referral to psychiatrists, grief counselors, social services, or spiritual counselors. Patients facing incurable and life-threatening illnesses experience losses of function, control, independence, body image, dignity, and of a future.

Spirituality is an inherent and pervasive dimension for persons, particularly those faced with the closure of their lives. Effective palliative care nurses must become comfortable and competent in performing a spiritual assessment. When the nurse queries a patient about spiritual issues, the patient is assisted to reflect on his own humanity. In doing so, the nurse is offering support for patients who naturally grapple with spiritual issues surrounding illness and impending end of life. Last, it is an opportunity for the nurse to be present and witness the sacredness of this life event. Nurses who assist patients may find this involvement in the intimate stories of patients' lives to be an honor, a gift, and a tremendous opportunity for growth as a person.

Barriers to the provision of palliative care are multifaceted. Financial reimbursement to fund palliative care programs is a challenge. Providers have a fear of prescribing controlled substances due to the regulation of narcotics and other medications. There is a general lack of understanding of the services offered by a palliative care team. Providers must overcome the natural tendency to participate in the conspiracy to withhold the facts about prognoses for fear of erasing the patient's hope.

The health care system has the unique opportunity to improve on the services provided to those who are facing chronic, terminal, incurable illnesses. Palliative care programs will no doubt develop and evolve over time, basing changes on the experiences of current-day programs.

Palliative care nurses have been given the honor of assisting patients and their families through a momentous time by alleviating suffering, both physically and emotionally. Caring for those who are preparing the closure of their life provides nurses with a unique challenge—that of being put at a vantage point where one comes face to face with the obviousness of one's own human mortality. In turn, this perspective provides an opportunity to look at the great gift of life, how one might choose to appreciate it and live it well, and how nurses can make an everlasting difference in the death of one and the lives of the remaining.

Nursing Management

Variation in the delivery of care to patients is a leading cause of inadequate care. The number of patients who have died in the ICU following a decision to withdraw life support or limit therapy is increasing. Even so, evidence indicates that patients and families are dissatisfied with the care given during end of life (Heyland et al., 2006; Teno et al., 2004). Educating health care professionals in end-of-life care is an important aspect of improving their ability to properly care for dying patients and their families. The goal is to add life to the patient's time, not simply time to the patient's life. A detailed patient care plan for end-of-life care is provided in the Nursing Process box.

Collaborative Management

Achievement of a pain-free and meaningful death experience for the patient and family requires a multidisciplinary approach. The nurse is in a pivotal role to bring together the members of

NURSING PROCESS: Patient Care Plan for End-of-Life Care

Assessment of Therapeutic Regimen
Subjective Data:
Are all members of the health care team clear on the plan of care and goals and expected outcomes?
What did the doctor tell you about your family member's prognosis?
Do you know your family member's resuscitation wishes and are you in agreement?
Is there a written advance directive?

Objective Data:
Family and significant others are calm and do not appear surprised by treatment regimen.

Nursing Assessment and Diagnoses	Outcomes and Evaluation Parameters	Planning and Interventions with *Rationales*
Nursing Diagnosis: *Ineffective Therapeutic Regimen Management* related to the acceleration (expected or unexpected) of illness symptoms	**Outcome:** The health care team has a clear understanding of the plan of care. *Evaluation Parameters:* All members of the health care team express understanding regarding: Disease process, Rationale for treatment regimen, Expectations of regimen, Methods to monitor condition, Signs or symptoms of complications, Honoring the patient's wishes. **Outcome:** The patient and/or family verbalize understanding of the seriousness of the patient's preferences and prognosis. *Evaluation Parameters:* The patient and/or family will verbalize an understanding of the seriousness of the patient's condition. The patient and/or family will be able to verbalize patient's preferences for quality-of-life issues.	**Interventions and *Rationales:*** Request a multidisciplinary meeting with the health care team *to identify concerns and clarify goals and expected outcomes for the patient.* Facilitate multidisciplinary family conference. Be respectful of cultural conversational norms. Listen to identify concerns. Attempt to match expressed needs with services the nurse can provide or facilitate. Demonstrate honesty, consistency, and stability. Maintain preestablished contacts in person or by phone. *To build trust and strength.* Discuss with patient and/or family their understanding of the prognosis; perception of seriousness; perceived level of anxiety; support system; emotional status; and cognitive ability *to identify factors that influence understanding.* Solicit expressions of feelings and questions. Identify if any advance directives were done and/or who will be responsible for care decisions. Encourage patient and family to seek information and make informed decisions. *To promote active participation of the patient and family.*

(continued)

NURSING PROCESS: Patient Care Plan for End-of-Life Care—*Continued*

Assessment of Grieving

Subjective Data:
What is your past experience with loss?
Do you have a support system?
Are there any cultural or religious practices that I can assist you with?

Objective Data:
Observe family interaction with staff and significant others.
Observe the family members' comfort level while in the patient room.
Observe family's ability to cope with the situation.

Nursing Assessment and Diagnoses	Outcomes and Evaluation Parameters	Planning and Interventions with *Rationales*
Nursing Diagnosis: *Grieving*	**Outcome:** Patient/family will demonstrate the ability to make mutual decisions regarding the anticipated death. ***Evaluation Parameters:*** Expresses thoughts, feelings, and spiritual beliefs about the loss. Verbalizes fears/concerns regarding the impending death. Exhibits no somatic distress.	**Interventions and *Rationales:*** When assisting with family discussions, use clear words, such as *death* or *died*, rather than euphemisms. Assist patient/family to verbalize fears/concerns regarding impending loss, including impact on the family unit. *To assist the patient/family to share mutual fears, plans, and concerns with each other.* Teach the patient/family about the normal events of the dying process. Encourage patient/family to implement cultural, religious, and social customs associated with death. Teach the patient/family characteristics of normal and abnormal grieving. *To help the patient and family move through the grieving process.* Arrange equipment and furniture in the patient's room to facilitate family presence and interaction with the patient. Remove as much monitoring equipment and intravenous lines from the patient as possible. Facilitate privacy for the family. Facilitate cultural/religious rituals. *To provide a peaceful, pain-free death for the patient and to create a supportive environment for the family.* Refer to appropriate resources: support groups, legal assistance, financial assistance, social services, and chaplain. *To assist the patient and family with putting the patient's legal affairs in order and to create an environment for emotional closure.*

Assessment of Pain

Subjective Data:
On a scale of 1–10 with one being a little pain and 10 being the worst pain you have ever felt, at what level is your pain?
Do you routinely take pain medication at home? If yes, what is the name of the medication and why do you take it?
Are you allergic to any medications?

Objective Data:
Monitor:
Facial grimacing
Change in breathing pattern
Change in blood pressure and/or pulse rate
Diaphoresis
Agitation

Nursing Assessment and Diagnoses	Outcomes and Evaluation Parameters	Planning and Interventions with *Rationales*
Nursing Diagnosis: *Pain*	**Outcome:** Pain level will be tolerable and the patient will not suffer. ***Evaluation Parameters:*** Patient will not exhibit symptoms of pain or suffering.	**Interventions and *Rationales:*** *Nonpharmacologic:* Reduce lighting and noise, eliminate unnecessary monitors and machines, remove restraints, and provide room for the patient's significant others. Cultural and spiritual factors such as prayer, ritual, and music can also increase the patient's comfort. *Promotes relaxation and comfort.* *Pharmacologic:* Morphine drip: titrate for symptom relief. At end of life, there is no recommended maximal dose. *Titration is intended to relieve pain and suffering.* Benzodiazepines: Midazolam drip: starting dose for adult continuous infusion: 1–5 mg/hr. Titrate for symptom relief. Lorazepam drip: starting dose for adult continuous infusion: 1–8 mg/hr. Titrate for symptom relief. *Benzodiazepines have a synergistic sedative effect with opioids, are anticonvulsants, and may help prevent the development of premorbid seizures.*

NURSING PROCESS: Patient Care Plan for End-of-Life Care—*Continued*

Assessment of Respiratory Distress

Subjective Data:
If patient is responsive ask if he/she is feeling short of breath.

Objective Data:
Observe nonintubated patient for:
Tachypnea
Restlessness

Accessory muscle use
Grunting at the end of each breath
Nasal flaring

Nursing Assessment and Diagnoses	Outcomes and Evaluation Parameters	Planning and Interventions with *Rationales*
Nursing Diagnosis: *Ineffective Breathing Pattern*	**Outcome:** Breathing pattern will be effective. **Evaluation Parameter:** Patient will not exhibit symptoms of respiratory distress.	**Interventions and *Rationales:*** *Nonpharmacologic:* Elevate the head of the bed. Place a fan in the room that blows gently on the patient's face. *To promote comfort.* *Pharmacologic:* Morphine drip: titrate for symptom relief. At end of life there is no recommended maximal dose. *Titration is intended to relieve pain and suffering.*

Assessment of Body Temperature

Objective Data:
Assess:
Skin temperature
Tachypnea

Tachycardia
Shivering

Nursing Assessment and Diagnoses	Outcomes and Evaluation Parameters	Planning and Interventions with *Rationales*
Nursing Diagnosis: *Imbalanced Body Temperature*	**Outcome:** The patient will not exhibit signs of physical discomfort from a fever. **Evaluation Parameters:** Normal body temperature Free from shivering	**Interventions and *Rationales:*** *Pharmacologic:* Administer an antipyretic *to decrease body temperature. Any measure that would cause the patient more discomfort, such as a cooling blanket, should not be used.*

the team necessary to achieve this objective. It is the nurse's responsibility to ensure that all members of the team are notified regarding the patient and family needs. Additionally, the health care team requires support and assistance to optimally assist the patient and family with this process. Services that may be used include hospital ethics committee, chaplain services, psychologist/psychiatrist, legal services, financial assistance, social services, hospice, and specific support groups for family members.

The ethics committee intervenes when there is conflict among the health care team and/or family regarding the prognosis and continuation of curative care for the patient. Once the decision is made to place the patient on palliative care, the family may need help regarding legal and financial assistance to ensure the patient's affairs are in order. The chaplain, social services, or a psychologist/psychiatrist assists the family to work through the grieving process and bring closure to the situation. If the patient is able to return home to die, hospice services aid the patient and family to facilitate this process in the home setting. Finally, specific support groups will help the family to work through the grieving process both before and after death.

Research Opportunities

There is an abundance of literature and research regarding hospice care for the terminally ill. Unfortunately, little research has been done with regard to end-of-life care when the death is un-

expected. See the Research Opportunities and Clinical Impact box (p. 414) for research topics in this area.

Many hospitals and organizations are working to improve end-of-life care and are committed to ensuring that all patients and families experience a "good death." Unfortunately, though, deciding who is "dying" in the acute care setting can be subjective or more a matter of perspective. Caregivers feel comfortable when pursuing a cure, but once the decision is made that any further care would be futile, caregivers often feel uncomfortable because this is not the "norm." Today's health care system is tailored to handle emergencies and injuries, diagnostic tests, and the most technologically advanced care in the world. It is not designed to accommodate the diverse needs of patients who are dying. Education and care guidelines will help to alleviate the discomfort of caregivers when they end up doing something that is perceived as the opposite of their normal goals.

Summary

As a nurse, one of the most rewarding experiences will be to allow natural death for a patient and to support him or her during this time. Helping the patient and significant others to meet their goals at end of life is challenging and rewarding. We ourselves will come to die and that alone should be reason enough to advocate for a system of care for people at the end of life.

RESEARCH OPPORTUNITIES AND CLINICAL IMPACT RELATED TO END-OF-LIFE CARE

Research Area	Clinical Impact
What interventions will help to relieve the discomfort felt by critical care nurses caring for end-of-life patients?	Developing interventions to relieve the discomfort surrounding end-of-life care will improve the care given to patients at end of life.
Is there a way to measure quality of life as an end point of treatment?	A tool that could accurately measure quality of life would assist in decisions for the end point of treatment.
What interventions can be done to support culturally appropriate end-of-life care?	To promote cultural customs and rituals surrounding end of life.
Compare the efficacy of terminal weaning versus terminal extubation during withdrawal of care.	This research could determine the best approach to withdrawal of ventilatory life support.

NCLEX® REVIEW

1. A family member inquires about the numbers and variety of different health care personnel attending to the patient receiving palliative care. The nurse should inform the patient and family that:
   1. Integrating the goals and expertise of many different disciplines encourages the development of the most comprehensive plan of care.
   2. Increased numbers of health care teams can help to ensure continuity in communication with the patient and family members.
   3. The utilization of an interdisciplinary team decreases the likelihood of civil or criminal liability following new treatment decisions.
   4. A multidisciplinary approach to end-of-life care guarantees that the latest in palliative care technology will guide patient care goals.

2. Which statement made by the student nurse would indicate the need for further instruction regarding end-of-life care?
   1. "The focus of the plan of care should be changed from curative processes to comfort advances."
   2. "The rights of self-determination and confidentiality are essential for all palliative care patients."
   3. "The patient has the right to conclude what treatments or lack of treatments affect his own body."
   4. "The family usually finds it easier to withdraw life-sustaining treatments than to withhold them."

3. The nurse has just completed educating a patient about advanced directives. Which statement made by the patient would indicate the need for further instruction?
   1. "Advance directives will guide the health care team as to my wishes regarding medical treatments should I become incapacitated."
   2. "By signing the advance directive my appointed family member will have the ability to make health care decisions for me if I become ill."
   3. "The advanced directive is supposed to help direct the decision-making process about my intentions for life-sustaining treatments."
   4. "My living will is a type of advanced directive that describes what level of life-prolonging care I desire in the event I become incapacitated."

4. The patient is being admitted for inpatient hospice care. Which instructions should be provided to the patient and his or her family regarding pain control?
   1. "We will continue to increase the pain medication until the symptoms are relieved."
   2. "We are going to limit family visits because the excess stimulation can be detrimental."
   3. "We are planning on reducing the amount of anxiety medication for fear of dependence."
   4. "We feel all the excess lights and noise will help the patient forget all about the pain."

5. A new nurse is being oriented to a hospice position in a culturally diverse area. Which statement made by this new employee would reflect a thorough understanding of cultural diversity as it relates to end-of-life care?
   1. "Many followers of Judaism believe that death is a private matter, and therefore, the dying person should be left alone."
   2. "Some Russians may make their elderly family members a DNR so they will die comfortably and without life-sustaining treatments."
   3. "Believers in the Baha'i faith consider the body as just a shell, so cremations are common and organ donation is encouraged."
   4. "Persons from South Asia may remain positive and upbeat when around the health care team but then mourn in private."

Answers for review questions appear in Appendix D

KEY TERMS

durable power of attorney for health care
    (DPAHC) *p.397*
hospice *p.405*

living wills *p.396*
medical durable power of attorney
    (MDPA) *p.397*

palliative care *p.393*

REFERENCES

Andrews, M., & Boyle, J. (2003). *Transcultural concepts in nursing care* (4th ed.). New York: Lippincott Williams & Wilkins.

Bednash, G., & Ferrell, B. (2002a). Ethical and legal issues in end of life care. In *Continuing Education for Nurses* (pp. 21–65). Roseville, CA: CME Resource.

Bednash, G., & Ferrell, B. (2002b). Nursing care at the end of life. In *Continuing Education for Nurses* (pp. 2–18). Roseville, CA: CME Resource.

Bednash, G., & Ferrell, B. (2002c). Pain and symptom management in end of life care. *Continuing Education for Nurses* (pp. 21–65). Roseville, CA: CME Resource.

Buchman, T., Cassell, J., Ray, S., & Wax, M. (2002). Who should manage the dying patient? Rescue, shame, and the surgical ICU dilemma. *Journal of the American College of Surgeons, 194*(5), 664–673.

Burns, J., Mitchell, C., Outwater, K., Geller, M., Griffith, J., Todres, I., et al. (2000). End of life in the pediatric intensive care unit after the forgoing of life-sustaining treatment. *Critical Care Medicine, 28*(8), 3060–3066.

Carney, M., & Meier, D. (2000). Palliative care and end of life issues. *Anesthesiology Clinics of North America, 18*(1), 183–209.

Chaitin, E., & Arnold, R. (2005). *Communication in the ICU: Holding a family meeting*. Retrieved May 2, 2006, from UpToDate website: http://www.uptodate.com

Colon, M., & Lyke, J. (2003). Comparison of hospice use and demographics among European Americans, African Americans, and Latinos. *American Journal of Hospice and Palliative Care, 20*(3).

Davidson, P., Introna, K., Daly, J., Paull, G., Jarvis, R., Angus, J., et al. (2003). Cardiorespiratory nurses' perceptions of palliative care in nonmalignant disease: Data for the development of clinical practice. *American Journal of Critical Care, 12*(1), 47–53.

Ditilio, B. (2002). The emergence of palliative care: A new specialized field of medicine requiring an interdisciplinary approach. *Critical Care Nursing Clinics of North America,14*, 127–132.

Ferrell, B. R., & Coyle, N. (2002). An overview of palliative nursing care. *American Journal of Nursing 102*(5), 26–31.

Gillick, M. (2004). *Ethical issues near the end of life*. Retrieved April 24, 2006, from UpToDate website: http://www.uptodate.com

Heyland, D. K., Dodek, P., Rocker, G., Groll, D., Gafni, A., Pichora, D., et al. (2006). What matters most in end of life care: Perceptions of seriously ill patients and their family members. *Canadian Medical Association Journal, 184*(5), 627–633.

Heyland, D. K., Groll, D., Rocker, G., Dodek, P., Gafni, A., Tranmer, J., et al. (2005). End-of-life care in acute care hospitals in Canada: A quality finish? *Journal of Palliative Care, 21*(3), 142–150.

Jackson, V., & Abrahm, J. (2005). *Ethical considerations in effective pain management at the end of life*. Retrieved May 2, 2006, from UpToDate website: http://www.uptodate.com

Jennings, B., Ryndes, T., D'Onofrio, C., & Baily, M. (2003). Access to hospice care: Expanding boundaries, overcoming barriers. *The Hastings Center Report, 33*.

Kuebler, K. K., Heidrich, D. E., & Esper, P. (Eds.). (2007). *Palliative and end of life care*. St. Louis, MO: Saunders.

Lipson, J., & Dibble, S. (Eds.). (2007). *Culture and clinical care*. San Francisco: UCSF Nursing Press.

Lynn, J., Lynch Schuster, J., & Kabcenell, A. (2000). *Improving care for the end of life*. New York: Oxford University Press.

McPhee, S. J., Rabow, M. W., Pantilat, S. Z., Markowitz, A. J., & Winker, M. A. (2000). Finding our way —perspectives on care at the close of life. *JAMA 284*(19), 2502–2507.

National Consensus Project for Quality Palliative Care. (2004). *Clinical practice guidelines for quality palliative care*. Pennsylvania: Author. Retrieved May 31, 2008, from http://www.nationalconsensusproject .org

National Hospice and Palliative Care Organization. (2006). *Facts and figures*. Retrieved August 8, 2006, from http://www.nhpco.org/ files/public/Facts_Figures_for2004data.pdf

Ogle, K., Mavis, B., & Wang, T. (2003). Hospice and primary care physicians: Attitudes, knowledge and barriers. *American Journal of Hospice and Palliative Care, 20*(1).

Peterman, A., & Cella, D. (2005). *Evaluation of quality of life*. Retrieved April 24, 2006, from UpToDate website: http://www.uptodate.com

Saunders, C. A. (Ed.). (2007). *End of life: A nurse's guide to compassionate care*. Philadelphia: Lippincott Williams & Wilkins.

Solloway, M., Lafrance, S., Bakitas, M., & Gerken, M. (2005). A chart review of seven hundred eighty-two deaths in hospitals, nursing homes, and hospice/home care. *Journal of Palliative Medicine, 8*(4), 789–796.

Stevens, L., Cook, D., Guyatt, G., Friffith, L., Walter, S., & McMullin, J. (2002). Education, ethics, and end of life decisions in the intensive care unit. *Critical Care Medicine, 30*(2).

Teno, J. M., Clarridge, B. R., Casey, V., Welch, L. C., Wetle, T., Shield, R., et al. (2004). Family perspectives on end of life care at the last place of care. *Journal of the American Medical Association, 291*(1), 88–103.

Truog, R., Cist, A., Brackett, S., Burns, J., Curley, M., Danis, M., et al. (2001). Recommendations for end of life care in the intensive care unit: The Ethics Committee of the Society of Critical Care Medicine. *Critical Care Medicine, 29*(12) 2332–2348.

World Health Organization. (2006). *WHO definition of palliative care*. Retrieved August 8, 2006, from http://www.who.int/cancer/ palliative/definition/en

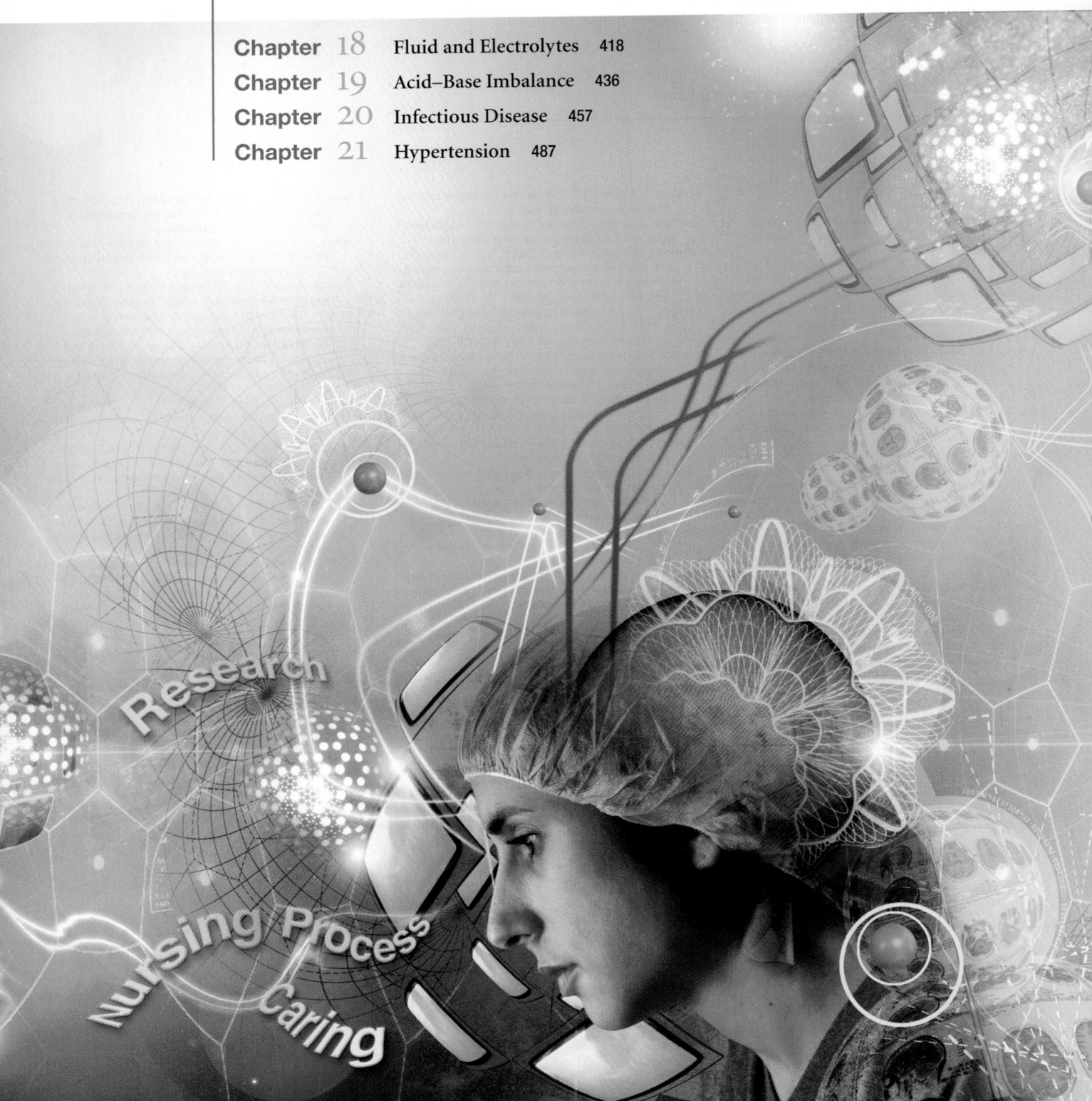

UNIT

3

Physiological Concepts
Related to Nursing Practice

Research

Nursing Process

Caring

SHERRI   My name is Sherri and I am the critical care epidemiologist at a teaching hospital in Northern California. This hospital is a Level 1 trauma center with a Level 3 neonatal intensive care unit (ICU), a burn ICU, and seven other critical care units. I am certified in infection control and my job is to monitor infectious diseases. Much of my time is spent in surveillance for hospital-acquired infections within the critical care units. This surveillance is part of our Infection Control Program and is mandated by the Joint Commission. I perform this surveillance by doing detailed chart reviews monthly. My reports are then sent to the Infection Control Committee and to unit managers as well as unit medical directors. I also make rounds in the ICUs giving the staff an opportunity to ask infection control–related questions. I discuss issues such as patient placement and isolation for those with resistant organisms. At times, I must also interact with the county and state health departments with regard to reporting communicable diseases.

I receive calls from every area of the hospital and clinics requesting information on a variety of subjects related to infection control. I am also called on to collaborate on construction projects that impact critical care especially with regard to dust control and other environmental safety hazards that may pose an infectious disease risk to our patient populations.

In addition, I am involved in studies and interventions designed to reduce or eliminate infections. The most recent initiative is one to eliminate catheter-associated bloodstream infections. The team leading this initiative designed a "Six Step Program to a Cleaner Line" and we have seen the rate of these types of infections decrease dramatically. Daily I review reports showing all microbiology results in order to find potential cases of hospital-acquired infection. I determine which patients have significant culture results and then review the medical record looking for the cause. After reviewing all potential cases, I generate device-related infection rates and present the data at Infection Control Committee meetings to help identify trends and infection control–related problems and to provide evidence of the success or failure of infection control interventions.

Controlling outbreak of infections is another aspect of my position. We monitor microbiology reports for sentinel organisms or for the emergence of the same organism in the cultures of many patients in a single unit. For example, the neonatal ICU had several babies who were positive for *Clostridium difficile* toxin. I worked with the unit manager, the nursing and ancillary staff, physicians, and environmental services to bring the situation to an end. Doing so required isolating and cohorting patients positive for *C. difficile* toxin, repeated cleaning of the environment with a diluted bleach solution, removal of alcohol-based hand rubs from the unit during the outbreak, limiting the movement of patients as much as possible, and touring the unit to look for possible areas of cross contamination. After approximately 15 cases, the outbreak came to an end.

My hospital has participated in the National Nosocomial Infection Surveillance study with the Centers for Disease Control and Prevention, which produced a new data collection system and became the National Health and Safety Network. The system provides specific criteria to help identify hospital-acquired infections.

There are occasions when I am called to help patients and their families in infection control–related situations both via telephone consultation and in person. In one case, a primary care physician called our office and needed help with a patient diagnosed with a pneumonia caused by *Neisseria meningitidis*, the causative organism for meningococcal meningitis. The physician referred him to our department for additional information. In talking with and teaching him about the organism, he was much calmer and felt he could speak intelligently with his close contacts about his situation now that he was armed with information.

Sometimes, the telephone consultation is not enough and intervention in the patient care environment is required. One such case was that of a 2-year-old patient in the pediatric ICU who had trisomy 21 and was currently hospitalized with leukemia. Her microbial flora were changing as she was exposed to antimicrobial therapy, which resulted in the growth of very resistant *Stenotrophomonas maltophilia*. The toddler was appropriately placed in Contact Precautions. I received a call from the unit staff telling me that the patient's family was not complying with the isolation precautions despite multiple reminders. I offered to talk with them in order to take the direct patient caregivers out of the situation so they could concentrate on the care the child required. I approached the family to discuss the resistant organisms and the isolation requirement. They wanted to be able to touch their child without gloves. We discussed options and came to a compromise that worked for everyone. They understood the concepts and I felt sure they would be very careful in their efforts to prevent transmission of the organisms. I gave them my contact numbers and over the subsequent days, I stopped in to chat with the family.

> "Sometimes, the telephone consultation is not enough and intervention in the patient care environment is required."

Fluid and Electrolytes

Darlene Gilcreast

Outcome-Based Learning Objectives

After studying this chapter, the learner will be able to:

1. Explain the normal composition of fluids and electrolytes in the body.
2. Describe the normal osmolality of the blood and urine.
3. Define the normal ranges of electrolytes in the body.
4. Discuss various circumstances that place the patient at risk for fluid and electrolyte imbalances.
5. Evaluate fluid status of an adult according to normal fluid and electrolyte values.
6. Identify nursing interventions to restore fluid and electrolyte balance.
7. Explain discharge teaching implications to assist patients to maintain fluid and electrolyte balance.

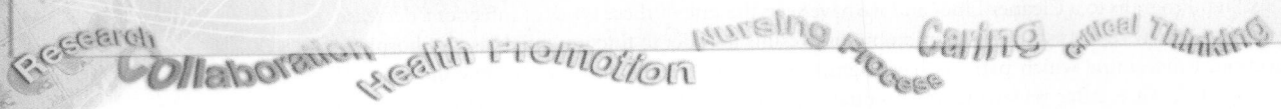

Research · Collaboration · Health Promotion · Nursing Process · Caring · Critical Thinking

FLUIDS and electrolytes are the basic elements of life. All chemical reactions within the body take place in fluids. The causes of the reactions are electrolytes because they have an electrical charge, negative or positive. The primary fluid of the body is water. Water comprises 70% of living cells, 60% of an average adult's total body weight, and 70% to 80% of body weight in infants (Goyne, 2003). An average healthy person needs about 2 to 2.5 liters of water per day to meet the body's fluid requirements. This is based on the fact that healthy individuals need about 1 to 1.5 ounces of water per kilogram of body weight per day to dissolve and metabolize wastes (Grandjean, Reimers, & Buyck, 2003). Fluids are continually lost through respiration, formation of urine and feces, and perspiration. Most adults produce about 1,500 mL of urine per day (Whitmire, 2003). Additional fluids are lost during illness through **insensible fluid loss**, water that passes through the skin and from the respiratory tract and is lost by evaporation or with fever, wound drainage, vomitus, or diarrhea.

Body Fluid Composition and Function

Basically, there are two body fluid compartments: the **intracellular fluid (ICF)** and the **extracellular fluid (ECF)**. The ICF is all fluids that exist within the cell cytoplasm and nucleus. The ECF is all fluids that exist outside the cell, such as **interstitial fluid** between cells, fluid in the bloodstream (serum), cere- brospinal fluid (CSF) in the central nervous system, gastrointestinal secretions, sweat, and urine. Two-thirds of the body's water is ICF and one-third is ECF (Felver, 2000). Only 5% of body fluid is normally in the blood (Johnson, 2007; Porth, 2007).

The functions of body fluids are many. Enzymes in saliva and mucus assist the passage of food into the gut and provide mechanisms for hydrolyzing food into elements the body can absorb. ECF in blood and CSF serves as a transport mechanism to deliver electrolytes, oxygen, nutrients, and hormones to tissues. Body fluids also carry immune cells to injury sites for the body's defense. ECF eliminates the body's waste products through the kidneys, bowels, and perspiration. Body functions depend on fluids facilitating the movement of electrolytes from one body compartment to another, often multiple times per minute, to effect an electrochemical action (i.e., the heartbeat, the secretion of a hormone, or a neuromuscular transmission). Another vital function of ECF is the regulation of body temperature through perspiration and capillary dilation to give off excess heat or conserve heat through the skin.

Osmolality

Osmolality is the number of molecules of solute per kilogram of water (Felver, 2000; Hogan, et al., 2006; Mushnick, 2007). The normal osmolality of blood is 275 to 295 milliosmoles per kilogram (mOsm/kg) of body weight. Fluids having osmolalities within this range are known as **isotonic** fluids (Goyne, 2003).

Fluids with osmolalities above 295 mOsm/kg are known as **hypertonic** fluids and fluids with osmolality below 275 mOsm/kg are **hypotonic**.

Electrolytes

Electrolytes are ionized minerals (calcium, chloride, magnesium, phosphorus, potassium, and sodium) that serve as energy transfer mechanisms to cause normal bodily functions by attractions, repulsions, and combinations. Ions either have a positive charge (cations), such as sodium (Na^+), or a negative charge (anions), such as chloride (Cl^-). Electrolytes move from one body compartment to another via the fluids and cause movement of various elements of the body by electrochemical interactions (see Chapter 38 ⊚).

Fluids and electrolytes each have normal ranges in which the body functions well. When elements or fluids are outside normal ranges, dysfunction or decreased performance occurs (Goyne, 2003).

Regulation of Body Fluid

Body fluids are regulated by osmosis, diffusion, and filtration (Goyne, 2003). In **osmosis**, water moves through a semipermeable membrane from an area of lower particle concentration toward one of higher particle concentration. Osmosis is based on the relationship of the molecules of solute (i.e., electrolytes) to water molecules (Goyne, 2003).

Diffusion occurs by movement of molecules from an area of higher concentration to an area of lower concentration. Diffusion depends on the size of the molecules, electrical charges, and pressure gradients. An elevated pressure gradient resists the transfer of elements into the high-pressure area and filters ions from the high-pressure area into a lower pressure area. An example of this process is the filtration done by the kidneys (Goyne, 2003). Pressure gradients are determined by conditions such as blood pressure within arterioles and the surrounding tissues. For example, the kidney juxtaglomerular apparatus exhibits higher pressure in the arterioles than in the renal collecting tubules, thus favoring transfer of fluids and solutes into the renal collecting tubules. Molecules must be small enough to pass through semipermeable membranes. Thus, in the kidney, large protein molecules are not normally filtered. Electrical charges must balance negative and positive ions or move from an area of higher concentration to an area of lower concentration.

Diffusion may be simple or facilitated. An example of simple diffusion is when lipid-soluble molecules pass through the phospholipid bilayers of cellular membranes and through protein channels for lipid-insoluble molecules. Facilitated diffusion requires carrier proteins to carry the substance through the cellular membrane (Porth, 2007). The movement of an ion against an electrochemical gradient is called *active transport* because energy must be used to transfer the molecule (Bond, 2000).

Filtration takes place when molecules from an area of higher concentration move through permeable membranes to an area of lower concentration as a result of hydrostatic pressure (Metheny, 2000). Hydrostatic pressure is the pressure exerted on the surrounding tissues due to the presence of water. Filtration occurs in the body because of hydrostatic pressure generated by the pumping action of the heart. On the arterial side of the capillary, the hydrostatic pressure is 32 millimeters of mercury (mmHg). On the venous side of the capillary, the hydrostatic pressure is about 15 mmHg. This favors movement of fluids from the bloodstream into the tissues on the arterial side of the capillary and back into the bloodstream on the venous side of the capillary after filtering through the tissues and bathing the cells in interstitial fluid (Metheny, 2000).

Filtration is directly opposed by the oncotic pressure of plasma proteins, especially albumin in the bloodstream (Metheny, 2000). **Oncotic pressure** is the influence of plasma proteins on the movement of water into and out of the blood stream based on the fact that plasma proteins maintain a negative ionic charge. Plasma oncotic pressure is about 22 mmHg. In a steady state, the ECF and ICF pressures are equal (Porth, 2007). To maintain homeostasis, fluid loss must equal fluid intake.

Tests for Evaluating Fluid Status

Laboratories routinely test the osmolality of blood. The Diagnostic Tests box (p. 420) lists normal and low and high values for use when evaluating fluid status. The normal range is 275 to 295 mOsm/kg of water (Goyne, 2003). Values above 295 indicate that there are too many molecules of solute per molecule of water, or a water deficit. Values below 275 indicate that there are too few molecules of solute per molecule of water, or a water excess (Goyne, 2003). Both conditions can result in bodily dysfunction. Serum osmolality may be roughly calculated by doubling the serum sodium value (Goyne, 2003; Hogan, et al., 2006).

Another test to evaluate hydration is the serum hematocrit measurement, which is the percentage of blood cells in a given volume of blood. A normal value is ~ 40% to 50%, with males at 42% to 52% and females at 37% to 47%. If the serum is dilute (symbolic of overhydration), the hematocrit will be low with decreased values for sodium, chloride, potassium, and bicarbonate. If the serum is concentrated, the hematocrit, sodium, potassium, chloride, and bicarbonate values will be high. Normal laboratory values for measuring electrolyte and fluid balance are presented in the Diagnostic Tests box (p. 420). Serum concentration can be measured indirectly by measuring the osmolality (**specific gravity** or **SG**) of urine. Normal SG is 1.016 to 1.022. SG will be low when the blood is dilute, and high when the blood is concentrated (Goyne, 2003; Hogan, Gingrich, Ricci, & Overby, 2006) unless other physiological abnormalities are present.

Clinical Manifestations of Overhydration and Dehydration

The body normally does not have excess fluid in the absence of diseases, such as renal failure, congestive heart failure (CHF), or syndrome of inappropriate antidiuretic hormone (Goyne, 2003; Hogan et al., 2006). However, if the blood is dilute, water is redistributed by osmosis from the blood to the ECF and ICF spaces. As a result, cellular edema occurs. Edema between the cells will follow gravity and will be reflected by lower extremity edema in people who are upright and sacral edema in people who are confined to bed. When cells are swollen with water, normal function is slowed or interrupted. Excess fluid volume is common in individuals with reduced renal sodium and water excretion and in patients with liver cirrhosis or CHF (Joy & Hladik, 2007).

DIAGNOSTIC TESTS for Evaluating Fluid Status (Adult Values)

Test and Normal Values	Expected Normal Values	Low (Overhydration)	High (Dehydration)
Urinalysis			
Specific gravity	1.005–1.030	<1.005	>1.030
Urine osmolality	50–1200 mOsm/kg water	<50 mOsm/kg	>1,200 mOsm/kg
Urine electrolytes			
Sodium	40–220 mEq/day	<40 mEq/d	>220 mEq/d
Potassium	25–100 mEq/day	<25 mEq/d	>100 mEq/d
Serum osmolality	285–295 mOsm/kg water	<285 mOsm/kg	>295 mOsm/kg
Hematocrit	Male: 42–52%	Male: <42%	Male: >52%
	Female: 37–47%	Female: <37%	Female: >47%
Serum electrolytes			
Sodium	136–145 mEq/L	<135 mEq/L	>146 mEq/L
Potassium	3.5–5.0 mEq/L	<3.5 mEq/L	>5.0 mEq/L
Chloride	98–106 mEq/L	<98 mEq/L	>106 mEq/L
Bicarbonate	22–26 mEq/L	<22 mEq/L	>26 mEq/L

Sources: Cavanaugh, B. M. (2001). *Nurse's manual of laboratory and diagnostic tests* (3rd ed.). Philadelphia: EA; Davis Company. Ehmann, W.C. (1). ...; Kee, J.L. (2005). *Laboratory and diagnostic tests with nursing implications* (7th ed.). Upper Saddle River, New Jersey: Prentice Hall.

Excess fluid may build up in the lung capillaries and pool in the lung alveoli (air sacs). The fluid can be detected by auscultating the lung bases and hearing "crackles," a sound similar to rubbing the hair between your fingers just in front of your ear. The nurse may also hear an extra heart sound (S_3, just following the S_2). This sounds like "lub-dub-dee" instead of the normal "lub-dub" of the heart. Many use the mnemonic "Kentucky" to distinguish this rhythm from the S_4, a "dee-lub-dub" or "Tennessee." The S_3 sound results from the atria of the heart being overly distended by fluid backup in the central venous system and the forcible contraction of the atria (O'Gara & Braunwald, 2001).

The S_3 heart sound is common in children, but not in people over the age of 40 years. The fluid in the alveoli increases the oxygen–carbon dioxide diffusion distance in the pulmonary capillaries and results in less efficient gas exchange. This is exhibited in patients by perceived shortness of breath, reduced blood oxygen levels, higher blood carbon dioxide levels, and a condition known as respiratory acidosis, in which the serum pH is less than 7.35, caused by a buildup of carbonic acid and dissolved carbon dioxide in the blood (O'Gara & Braunwald, 2001). Patients will increase respiratory rates above 24 breaths per minute in an attempt to compensate for reduced gas exchange. Hypervolemia is usually treated with large doses of loop diuretics, such as furosemide, that are efficient in removing free water from the blood via the distal tubules (Joy & Hladik, 2007).

The most common cause of dehydration (pure water deficit) is the excessive loss of free water through urine, such as in people with diabetes insipidus (a condition in which antidiuretic hormone from the pituitary gland is lacking), hyperglycemia (serum glucose above 200 mg/dL and usually above 300 mg/dL) in diabetes mellitus, failure to drink replacement fluids (as may happen in people with altered mental status), or overuse of diuretics (Goyne, 2003; Johnson, 2007). Elderly individuals have decreased perception of thirst due to aging and may not replace fluids appropriately. The elderly are particularly vulnerable to

dehydration because many are taking prescription diuretics for high blood pressure. Other causes of fluid deficit may be nausea, vomiting, and diarrhea resulting from gastrointestinal flu, food poisoning, or hyperemesis gravidarum (vomiting related to pregnancy). The elderly are very vulnerable to influenza and contagious diseases because the immune system becomes less effective as the body ages.

Clinical manifestations of dehydration include severe thirst (may be absent in the elderly), dry mouth and tongue, possible cracked and peeling lips, dry skin that "tents" when it is lightly lifted (the skin creates an upward fold that does not return quickly to its original position), and body temperature that may rise one or two degrees (Goyne, 2003; Hogan et al., 2006). Patients will have orthostatic hypotension. Orthostatic hypotension is determined by an increase in pulse of 20 beats/min or blood pressure drop of 20 mmHg or more in the systolic blood pressure or 10 mmHg in the diastolic blood pressure upon changing from the supine to the standing position (Saseen & Carter, 2005). Patients will have tachycardia and weak pulses because of decreased circulating blood volume in dehydration. The extremities may take on a "mottled" (patches of purple and white) appearance due to decreased perfusion (O'Gara & Braunwald, 2001).

◼ Nursing Management

Assessing the hydration of patients is part of the initial and ongoing nursing assessments. Assessments, as defined in Chapter 9 ☺, include both the oral history and physical assessments. Many symptoms, such as headache, dizziness, or syncope (faintness), can be reduced with attention to adequate hydration. In the patient with heart failure, overhydration may lead to symptoms of dyspnea, shortness of breath, and intolerance for walking and other activities of daily living (ADLs). Overhydration can lead to orthopnea (difficulty breathing when lying flat), which may necessitate propping up the patient in bed with several pillows or having the patient sit in a recliner chair to sleep (O'Gara & Braunwald, 2001). Sample hydration assessment questions are included in the Nursing Process: Patient Care Plan boxes for dehydration and overhydration (p. 422). The care plans apply the nursing process to relevant nursing diagnoses and provide outcomes and interventions for patients with alterations in hydration.

Collaborative Management

To achieve the optimal balance of fluid and electrolytes, patients need a multidisciplinary health care team. The team includes nurses, nursing assistants, physicians, laboratory personnel, dietitians, and dietary assistants. Nurses and physicians assess the patient for alterations in fluids and electrolytes by conducting a thorough history and physical and by maintaining accurate intake and output (I&O) documentation. Nursing assistants often are responsible for maintaining I&O charts, particularly in inpatient settings. However, the nurse, as the supervisor for the nursing assistants, is responsible for the accuracy of the I&O data. Laboratory personnel assist by performing laboratory tests that provide more specific data about the fluid and electrolyte balances of patients. Dietitians and dietary assistants provide appropriate medical nutrition therapy for patients, including appropriate fluids in the right amounts (Goldstein-Fuchs & McQuiston, 2003).

Often, patients need to monitor their fluid status at home. Therefore, a plan for appropriate hydration (avoiding excesses and deficits) may be part of discharge planning. Daily weights may be part of the fluid assessment if patients have a tendency toward overhydration. Daily weights need to be repeated under the same conditions, on the same scale, at the same time of day, dressed in the same clothing (i.e., gown or pajamas), with all drainage tubes empty, for consistency of weighing conditions (Indiana State University, 2007). A weight gain of more than 5 pounds per day indicates that the health care provider should be notified because the retention of 1 pint of fluid results in a gain of 1 pound (Johnson, 2007). Because patients may not prepare their own meals, the person who prepares the meals for the patient must be included in the planning and teaching.

Assessing the frequency and consistency of stools also is a layperson's way of determining the adequacy of hydration. In dehydration, constipation occurs and stools become hard and difficult to pass. When stools are of a normal frequency for the individual, are soft, and easy to pass, it may be assumed that hydration is adequate (Grandjean et al., 2003). Although this may seem a mundane task, monitoring the frequency and quality of patients' bowel movements is important to fluid intake monitoring. If stools become too hard and difficult to pass, patients can induce cardiac dysrhythmias due to excessive internal pressure generated with the Valsalva maneuver, closing the glottis of the throat, and bearing down to pass stools (Ahlquist & Camilleri, 2001). The elderly are more likely to suffer from constipation secondary to decreased physical activity and slowing of bowel activity with aging.

Homeostatic Mechanisms

Serum osmolality is regulated by the osmoreceptors of the hypothalamus. When body water loss is 2% of normal body

NURSING PROCESS: Patient Care Plan for Dehydration

Assessment of Dehydration

Subjective Data:
Are you feeling thirsty?
Have you had difficulty drinking fluids and keeping them down?
Have you had any nausea, vomiting, diarrhea, or fever lately?
Have you experienced any dizziness on standing?

Objective Data:
Weigh patient and compare weight to usual weight (loss of >2 lb/day indicates dehydration).
Measure temperature (>99°F or 37°C compatible with dehydration), pulse (greater than 100 beats/min), blood pressure (lower than normal, take lying, sitting, standing), and respirations.
Examine mouth for, cracked lips, dried tongue and mucous membranes.
Lift the skin on the back of the hands to assess for "tenting" (skin is slow to return to its normal position).
Obtain urinalysis with specific gravity and serum electrolytes.

Nursing Assessment and Diagnoses	Outcomes and Evaluation Parameters	Planning and Interventions with *Rationales*
Nursing Diagnosis: *Risk for Imbalanced Fluid Volume* related to excessive fluid loss/inability to take fluids as evidenced by low blood pressure, rapid pulse, increased body temperature, and dizziness on standing.	**Outcome:** Adequate fluid balance *Evaluation Parameters:* Temperature, pulse, and blood pressures within normal limits. No evidence of dizziness on standing. Able to drink and retain 8 glasses of water per day.	**Interventions and *Rationales:*** Provide a source of fluids that the patient can retain (oral or parenteral). If nausea and vomiting are the source of dehydration, parenteral fluids will be needed. *Inadequate hydration requires restoration of normal circulating volume in order to maintain blood pressure and provide sufficient cardiac output to circulate nutrients to the body. When the fluids cannot be taken and retained orally, a parenteral source of fluids will need to be provided to restore balance.*

NURSING PROCESS: Patient Care Plan for Overhydration

Assessment of Overhydration

Subjective Data:
Have you had any difficulty urinating lately?
How much fluid have you ingested in the last 24 hours?
Have you eaten a lot of salt or soy sauce?
Have you experienced any shortness of breath with walking or exercise?
Are you able to sleep lying flat? If not, how many pillows do you need for your head?
Do you sleep sitting in a recliner chair?

Objective Data:
Weigh patient and compare weight to usual weight (an increase in weight greater than 2 lb/day indicates fluid retention).
Measure temperature, pulse, blood pressure (higher than normal), and respirations (will be more rapid than normal).
Assess skin on the legs and ankles for dependent edema. If the patient is confined to bed, this will be in the sacral area.
Obtain urinalysis and serum electrolytes.

Nursing Assessment and Diagnoses	Outcomes and Evaluation Parameters	Planning and Interventions with *Rationales*
Nursing Diagnosis: *Risk for Imbalanced Fluid Volume* related to excessive fluid intake/decreased urination as evidenced by high blood pressure, rapid breathing, shortness of breath, and dependent edema.	**Outcome:** Adequate fluid balance *Evaluation Parameters:* Temperature, pulse, and blood pressures within normal limits. No evidence of dependent edema. Voiding at least 240 mL/8 hr.	**Interventions and *Rationales*:** Reduce oral fluid and sodium intake as directed by health care provider (about 1 L/day with most taken in the waking hours and <2,000 mg of sodium/day). A fluid-intake schedule is arranged and the patient instructed in fluid restriction. Administer diuretics as prescribed, monitoring serum potassium levels. *Overhydration requires restoration of normal circulating volume to decrease blood pressure and reduce the workload on the heart. When the fluids are excessive, fluids will cross the alveolar capillary barrier and pool fluids in the lungs (pulmonary edema), interfering with oxygen–carbon dioxide diffusion. This reduces blood oxygen levels. When dependent edema is present, it interferes with normal circulation in the tissues resulting in lower tissue oxygen. The patient's cooperation will have to be obtained in order to succeed at fluid restriction. Rapid diuresis will often result in low serum potassium. Serum potassium within the normal range is essential for normal cardiac function.* If the patient is not able to urinate due to renal failure, hemofiltration or dialysis may need to be arranged *to assist in restoration of normal fluid balance.* Additionally, potassium levels will need to be monitored *to ensure the patient is not retaining too much potassium.* Reposition patient every 2 hours *to decrease risk to skin.*

weight, the hypothalamus stimulates the posterior pituitary to secrete **antidiuretic hormone (ADH)**. ADH signals the kidneys to conserve water by reabsorbing water from the distal renal tubules. Additionally, the perception of thirst is stimulated to promote drinking of water to restore normal serum osmolality (Goyne, 2003; Mushnick, 2007).

In the presence of severe dehydration, such as results from vomiting, baroreceptors (pressure-sensitive cells) in the carotid artery sinuses and aorta stimulate the secretion of ADH. Baroreceptors in the afferent glomerular arterioles of the kidneys detect reduced perfusion and secrete renin. Renin causes the conversion of angiotensinogen to angiotensin I, which is converted to angiotensin II in the lungs by angiotensin converting enzyme. Angiotensin II stimulates aldosterone release from the adrenal glands, which promotes retention of sodium (Goldstein-Fuchs & McQuiston, 2003). This mechanism becomes a problem in the elderly. Atherosclerosis narrows the renal arteries in the same fashion as it does the coronary arteries. In response to decreased blood through the kidneys, renin is released stimulating the cascade of sodium and fluid retention. Health care providers address this problem by prescribing angiotensin converting enzyme inhibitors (ACEI) and angiotensin-receptor blocking (ARB) medications (Bomback & Klemmer, 2007).

Electrolyte Balance

Electrolyte balance is the sum of electrolyte intake, absorption, distribution, and electrolyte loss through normal and abnormal routes. Intake is primarily oral, but may include the rectal route if patients use enemas. In the hospital, intravenous fluids are another source of electrolytes for patients (Felver, 2000). Once absorbed, electrolytes are distributed in different ways in the body. For example, the reservoirs for calcium are the teeth and bones, the reservoir for potassium is inside the cells of the body, and sodium and chloride are found primarily in blood. Most electrolytes are lost via the gastrointestinal (GI) tract, urinary tract, and sweat. Other sources of loss may be vomitus, nasogastric suction, wound drainage, or hemorrhage (Felver, 2000).

Electrolyte Imbalances

Because every bodily function is dependent on the electromotive force (the exchange of electrons between molecules), electrolyte imbalances decrease the body's ability to conduct normal activities. These activities include transmission of neural signals, contraction of muscles including the heart, secretion of hormones by secretory glands, and regulation of normal bodily functions, such as oxygenation and metabolization of wastes. The nature of the imbalance is reflected by which electrolyte is out of balance. Often, the complementary electrolyte with which the primary electrolyte combines also is affected. The following sections provide details regarding specific electrolyte imbalances.

Sodium

Sodium is the most numerous cation in the ECF. It maintains ECF volume through osmotic pressure, regulates acid–base balance by combining with chloride or bicarbonate ions, and conducts nerve impulses via the sodium channels of cells. Normal values for sodium are 135 to 145 milliequivalents/liter (mEq/L) (Johnson, 2007). Acid–base balance is discussed thoroughly in Chapter 19 🔗.

Three hormones are responsible for regulating the sodium level in the ECF: (1) **aldosterone**, a hormone secreted by the adrenal cortex; (2) ADH, secreted by the posterior pituitary gland; and (3) **atrial natriuretic peptide (ANP)**, secreted by the atrium of the heart. Aldosterone is secreted in response to low ECF sodium levels, an increase in ICF potassium, low cardiac output, and stress. Aldosterone causes increased retrieval of sodium from the kidney filtrate. Water follows the osmotic attraction of sodium; thus, body ECF is increased. ADH is secreted in response to increased ECF osmolality detected by the osmoreceptors (receptors that detect the osmolality of the serum) in the hypothalamus and causes the reabsorption of water from the kidney distal tubules (Goyne, 2003). When the atria are excessively stretched due to excessive ECF volume in the blood, ANP is secreted as an antagonist to aldosterone to cause increased sodium excretion through the kidneys. As a result, water is also lost into the urine, reducing blood volume and increasing water loss (Porth, 2007).

Hypernatremia (Sodium Excess)

Hypernatremia (sodium above 145 mEq/L) represents a deficit of water in relation to the body's sodium levels. It occurs when there is an excess loss of body fluids that have a lower than normal concentration of sodium so that water is lost in excess of sodium. For example, Cushing's syndrome (aldosterone excess) causes excess sodium retention, or diabetes insipidus causes excessive fluid loss. Initially, fluid moves from the cells into the serum via osmosis to maintain osmolality within the normal parameters (below 295 mOsm/kg) and reduce serum sodium (to 145 mEq/L or below). Thirst is increased due to the increase in serum sodium and osmolality (Johnson, 2003; Porth, 2007).

Clinical symptoms resulting from hypernatremia caused by water loss are largely those of ECG fluid loss and cellular dehydration: thirst, low-grade fever, peripheral and pulmonary edema, and postural hypotension with excess fluid loss (Grogan, 2006; Porth, 2007). A simple test for hypernatremia is whether patients' rings have suddenly become tight on their fingers. This must be closely monitored to make sure that swollen fingers with rings do not threaten the tissue integrity of the fingers. Patients rings should be removed with permission, if they threaten the circulation in the finger. Laboratory values will show increased serum osmolality, elevated serum sodium, and a possible increase in urine specific gravity because of the effect of ADH to conserve water.

Pathophysiologic symptoms of hypernatremia are most likely to occur with sudden onset (Singer & Brenner, 2001). Brain symptoms resulting from hypernatremia are altered mental status, neuromuscular irritability, and occasionally coma or seizures (Singer & Brenner, 2001). One cause of this type of hypernatremia is excess sweating without fluid replacement, such as in heat stroke. Mortality associated with serum sodium levels above 180 mEq/L is very high (Singer & Brenner, 2001).

The brain cells adjust to ECF hypertonicity after 24 hours by moving the excess ions into brain cells. The resulting hyperosmolality inside the cells results in increased hydration inside brain cells to correct cellular dehydration. A potential danger of administering intravenous fluids too aggressively to reduce the osmolality of the blood is that of excess fluids moving into cerebral cells, resulting in cerebral edema (Singer & Brenner, 2001). This can lead to cellular dysfunction in the brain and increased intracranial pressure. Seizures or permanent brain damage could result (Singer & Brenner, 2001). Therefore, the water deficit should be replaced slowly over 48 to 72 hours with oral fluids being the preferred route (Singer & Brenner, 2001).

As mentioned earlier, one possible cause of hypernatremia is Cushing's syndrome. Cushing's syndrome is overactivity of the adrenal glands releasing excess aldosterone, which causes sodium retention. Symptoms of Cushing's syndrome are excess adrenal hormones that include cortisone, aldosterone, and androgens. The person will exhibit truncal obesity (large waist compared to the rest of the body, "apple" figure type) and may have a "buffalo hump" on the nape of the neck, a rounded "moon-shaped" face, fragile skin that bruises easily, muscle wasting of the arms and legs, osteoporosis with possible forward curvature of the spine (kyphosis), mood changes, and increased susceptibility to infections. Females may have excessive facial hair due to excess androgen (male) hormones. Fluid retention secondary to sodium retention results in expanded blood volume with hypertension and subsequent weight gain.

Nursing Management

Treatment requires diagnosis of Cushing's syndrome, possible surgery for tumors of the adrenal or pituitary glands, or drugs to decrease the activity of the adrenal glands (ketoconazole, metyrapone, aminoglutethimide, or mitotane) (Gums & Tovar, 2007). Ketoconazole reduces cortisol in Cushing's syndrome. Ketoconazole, however, can cause gynecomastia and lower testosterone levels. Metyrapone inhibits cortisol synthesis and patients may show an increase in plasma adrenocorticotropic hormone (ACTH). Side effects of metyrapone are nausea, vomiting, vertigo, headache, dizziness, abdominal discomfort, and an allergic rash. Aminoglutethimide inhibits cortisol production and is indicated for short-term use in inoperable Cushing's syndrome with ectopic ACTH production. Mitotane is a cytotoxic drug that reduces the synthesis of cortisol and corticosterone. It selectively inhibits adrenocortical function without causing cellular destruction. Because mitotane can severely inhibit cortisol production, the patient should be hospitalized to initiate therapy (Gums & Tovar, 2007, pp. 1396–1397).

Diabetes insipidus (uncontrolled loss of water in the urine) is due to an absence of ADH related to pituitary damage. This loss of ADH could be due to tumors or possible head injury by accident or as a result of surgery. Because the body lacks ADH, there is decreased water resorption in the distal tubules of the kidneys, resulting in marked increased urinary output with cellular dehydration. Volumes of 5 to 20 L of urine per day are common, with the urine having the appearance of water. The urine specific gravity will be <1.005. The person with diabetes insipidus will have an unquenchable thirst and will drink between 4 and 40 L of fluids per day. The blood osmolality will be high (about 295 mOsm) and serum sodium will be greater than 145 mEq/L because the blood becomes very concentrated due to water deficit (Guin, 2006). Management of diabetes insipidus is the administration of ADH in the form of a drug known as desmopressin acetate, which is administered as a nasal spray (Guin, 2006).

The nursing care of patients with hypernatremia, as outlined in the Nursing Process: Patient Care Plan box, is very important because of the risk for cerebral edema if the serum sodium level is lowered too rapidly. The rate at which sodium is lowered should not exceed 0.5 to 1 mEq/hr (Porth, 2007). To lower it more quickly risks brain dysfunction with neurological problems, such as seizures.

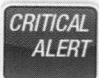 *Excess sodium is stored in brain cells during hypernatremia to reduce serum sodium. When IV fluids are administered too aggressively, excess fluid may move into cerebral cells, resulting in edema and life-threatening brain dysfunction. Serum sodium should be lowered no faster than 0.5 to 1 mEq/L per hour (Johnson, 2007; Joy & Hladik, 2007).*

Hyponatremia (Low Serum Sodium)

Hyponatremia (serum values below 135 mEq/L) develops with excessive retention of water, inadequate sodium intake, or loss of sodium-rich fluids that are replaced with water. Diuretics, vomiting, diarrhea, GI suctioning, or loss of wound fluids from very large wounds (e.g., burn wounds) may cause sodium deficiency (Johnson, 2007). Excessive use of dextrose 5% intravenous (IV) fluid can result in hyponatremia due to free water being created when glucose is metabolized. In fact, about 2.5% of hospitalized patients experience hyponatremia largely due to IV fluids (Johnson, 2007). Diuretic-induced hyponatremia can result from the administration of thiazide diuretics by the blocking of sodium resorption in the distal tubules. Thus, water is retained in excess of sodium (Joy & Hladik, 2007).

Symptoms of sodium deficit are reduced ability of cells to depolarize and repolarize. Often patients are asymptomatic because both the relative sodium deficit and the rapidity of onset determines symptoms. As sodium levels drop below 120 mEq/L, neurological changes such as lethargy, headache, confusion, personality changes, apprehension, seizures, and even coma could result (Johnson, 2007). Symptoms of hypotension may reduce osmotic pressure in the blood to retain circulating fluid volume. Tissue edema may accompany dilutional hyponatremia caused by inappropriate intravenous fluids. In a syndrome of inappropriate antidiuretic hormone (SIADH), the urine will be concentrated in spite of hyponatremia due to the lack of ADH. Permanent brain damage, such as central nervous system demyelination, may occur if the serum sodium level drops below 115 mEq/L or is corrected too rapidly (Singer & Brenner, 2001). Symptoms of osmotic demyelination syndrome are flaccid paralysis, dysarthria, and dysphagia. Mortality is high with this syndrome, even in the hospital. People who are most likely to suffer this syndrome are those with chronic hyponatremia (Singer & Brenner, 2001).

SIADH usually occurs as a result of brain trauma that causes increased secretion of ADH despite a normal fluid volume or it may be caused as a side effect of lithium, diuretics, or anticancer drugs (Johnson, 2007). Fluid overload and, hence, delusional hyponatremia are the result. The serum sodium will be less than 135 mEq/L and urine will be concentrated due to fluid retention. Symptoms are bounding pulse, hypertension, pale dry skin, weight gain and edema, renal failure, weakness, confusion, and possible seizures. The cause must be identified and treated to restore fluid and sodium volumes to normal (Johnson, 2007).

◼ Nursing Management

The nursing care for a patient with hyponatremia is dependent on the cause. Therapeutic goals are to return serum sodium to near normal (135 mEq/L). Restriction of water intake to 1,000 mL/day is usually implemented to assist sodium increase and to prevent the sodium level from dropping further due to dilution (Johnson, 2007). Foods high in sodium (highly processed foods, such as chips) will be given, unless the patient is NPO (nothing by mouth). Correction of sodium levels may require adjusting other electrolytes to establish balance. Hypertonic saline intravenous fluids are used only in severe cases where seizures have occurred (Johnson, 2007). Overly aggressive correction of chronic hyponatremia could result in permanent brain damage. When hypertonic saline intravenous fluid is given, only sufficient 3% sodium chloride is given to correct symptoms—not to return the sodium to 135 mEq/L (Porth, 2007). See the Nursing Process: Patient Care Plan for hyponatremia (p. 426).

 In hyponatremia, when the sodium level drops to 120 mEq/L, neurological changes occur: lethargy, confusion, personality changes, apprehension, seizures, and coma. Permanent brain damage may occur if the serum sodium level drops below 115 mEq/L or if correction of chronic hyponatremia is overly aggressive due to destruction of myelin (Johnson, 2007; Joy & Hladik, 2007). Hypertonic saline IV fluids are used only in severe cases after seizures have occurred (Johnson, 2007).

Potassium

Potassium (K⁺) is an intracellular cation primarily. Ninety-eight percent of potassium is found within cells (Rhyne, 2003b). Small amounts are found in blood (3.5 to 5.0 mEq/L) and bone (Rhyne, 2003b). The function of potassium is to maintain intracellular osmolality and participate in the sodium-potassium exchange that causes cellular depolarization and repolarization. The sodium-potassium-ATPase pump in cellular membranes uses active transport to transport sodium out of the cell and potassium into the cell at a ratio of 3:2 to maintain the appropriate balance (Brophy

NURSING PROCESS: Patient Care Plan for Hypernatremia (Sodium Excess)

Assessment of Hypernatremia

Subjective Data:
How thirsty have you been lately?
Have you been able to drink water and keep it down?
How much salt or soy sauce have you taken lately?

Objective Data:
Excessive thirst
Low-grade fever (99°F or 38°C)
Peripheral edema
Pulmonary edema (auscultation of S_3 heart sound at left apex and "crackles" in lungs)
Postural hypotension (with large fluid loss)
Cushing's syndrome
Diabetes insipidus
Decreased fluid intake or excessive sodium intake
Laboratory values: increased serum osmolality, sodium, increased urine specific gravity

Nursing Assessment and Diagnoses	Outcomes and Evaluation Parameters	Planning and Interventions with *Rationales*
Nursing Diagnosis: Risk for imbalanced fluid volume with potential for life-threatening cerebral edema related to excess fluid loss or excess sodium retention as evidenced by serum sodium >148 mEq/L	**Outcomes:** Fluid and electrolyte balance Acid–base balance Adequate hydration ***Evaluation Parameters:*** Normal sensorium for patient Serum sodium 135–145 mEq/L Hematocrit: 37–47% for women, 40–50% for men Serum pH 7.35–7.45	**Interventions and *Rationales:*** Monitor fluids and electrolytes, acid–base balance, blood pressure, pulse, temperature *to guide treatment decisions to ensure patient safety.* Administer IV fluids to lower serum sodium slowly at a rate of 0.5–1.0 mEq/L until it reaches 147 mEq/L *to avoid cerebral edema. Chloride follows sodium and chloride is involved in acid–base balance.* Assess level of consciousness every 4 hours. Observe for lethargy, headache, nausea, vomiting, increased blood pressure, or altered sensorium. Notify health care provider of changes. *To recognize the symptoms of cerebral edema early.* Pad bed rails with blankets if seizures are likely *to prevent injury in the event of a grand mal seizure.*

Assessment of Patient's/Family's Knowledge Regarding Cause of Hypernatremia

Subjective Data:
Do you understand how your/the patient's blood levels became out of balance?
What will you be able to do in the future to keep this from happening again?
Do you understand the risks involved with high salt in your blood?

Objective Data:
Patient's/family's answers to above questions and whether they reflect understanding
Rehospitalizations for similar conditions

Nursing Assessment and Diagnoses	Outcomes and Evaluation Parameters	Planning and Interventions with *Rationales*
Nursing Diagnosis: *Deficient Knowledge* on part of patient and family related to cause and treatment of hypernatremia	**Outcomes:** Appropriate knowledge of the definition, causes, and clinical manifestations of hypernatreumia. ***Evaluation Parameters:*** Patient and family member verbalize understanding of causes and treatment of high serum sodium *to reduce likelihood of recurrence* Patient adheres to treatment regimen *to reduce future threats to patient's health and need for hospitalization*	**Interventions and *Rationales:*** Provide discharge instructions to patient and family member on causes and treatment of hypernatremia at an appropriate educational, cultural level *to inform patient/family why hypernatremia occurred, to promote adherence to treatment, and to prevent recurrence.* Provide reminders of adequate fluid intake and treatment adherence for Cushing's syndrome or diabetes insipidus *to prevent future occurrences of hypernatremia.*

NURSING PROCESS: Patient Care Plan for Hyponatremia (Sodium Deficit)

Assessment of Sodium Deficit

Subjective Data:

How thirsty have you been lately?

Have much water have you been drinking?

How much salt or soy sauce have you taken lately?

Are you having any headaches?

Are you having any difficulty thinking or remembering things?

Objective Data:

Is the patient receiving IV fluids?

Does the patient have psychological problems leading to water intoxication?

Is the patient taking diuretics that may have caused electrolyte imbalance?

Does the patient exhibit neurological changes?

Laboratory values: increased serum osmolality, sodium increased, decreased urine specific gravity

Nursing Assessment and Diagnosis	Outcome and Evaluation Parameters	Planning and Interventions with *Rationales*
Nursing Diagnosis: *Risk for imbalanced body fluids with* potential for life-threatening cerebral edema related to excess fluid retention or sodium deficit as evidenced by serum sodium <135 mEq/L	**Outcomes:** Fluid and electrolyte balance Acid–base balance Adequate hydration **Evaluation Parameters:** Patient free from injury with normal sensorium Serum sodium 135–145 mEq/L Hematocrit 38–47% (women), 40–50% (men) Serum pH 7.35–7.45	**Interventions and *Rationales:*** Monitor neurological status (orientation to person, place, time), fluid and electrolytes, and acid–base balance *to determine whether the patient's condition is worsening, improving, or staying constant.* Restrict fluids to <1,000 mL/day *to prevent further dilution of sodium.* Assess blood pressure, dizziness, sensorium *to allow early intervention and maintain normal blood pressure.* Assist patient with ambulation. Maintain bed in lowest position with bed rails up and brakes on *to prevent falls and injury.* Explain to patient and family that disorientation is temporary *to decrease fear.* Use clocks, calendars, and familiar personal items *to reorient the patient and reduce confusion.* Pad the bed rails with blankets if seizures are likely *to prevent injury in the event of a seizure.* If seizures occur, administer hypertonic IV fluids (3% sodium) as ordered *to raise sodium to 135 mEq/L and prevent injury.*

Assessment of Patient's/Family's Knowledge Regarding Cause of Hyponatremia

Subjective Data:

Do you understand how your/the patient's blood levels became out of balance?

What will you do in the future to keep this from happening again?

Do you understand the risks involved with low salt in your blood?

Objective Data:

Patient's/family's answers to above questions reflect whether they understand

Rehospitalizations for similar conditions

Nursing Assessment and Diagnosis	Outcome and Evaluation Parameters	Planning and Interventions with *Rationales*
Nursing Diagnosis: *Deficient Knowledge* on the part of the patient and family related to cause and treatment of hyponatremia	**Outcome:** No future recurrence of low serum sodium **Evaluation Parameters:** Patient and family member identify the correct cause of the problem and identify proper treatment *to prevent recurrence*	**Interventions and *Rationales:*** Provide discharge instructions *to identify cause, to teach adherence to treatment, and to prevent future occurrences of hyponatremia.*

& Gehr, 2007). About 70% of intracellular potassium is located in muscle, thus when a person eats meat, potassium is gained. The remaining 30% is in the liver and red blood cells (Brophy & Gehr, 2007). Potassium is essential for cellular integrity, transmission of neuromuscular impulses, acid–base balance, conversion of carbohydrates into energy, and the formation of amino acids into proteins (Rhyne, 2003b). Serum potassium affects the strength and rate of cardiac contraction. Both hypokalemia and hyperkalemia can result in potentially fatal cardiac dysrhythmias because of potassium's essential role in cardiac cell polarization and depolarization (Brophy & Gehr, 2007) (see Chapter 19).

Potassium is gained by eating meat, potatoes, bananas, and other foods (Rhyne, 2003b). (See Chapter 14 for information on nutrition.) Most people consume about 100 mmol/day. Because some potassium is found in most foods, when caloric intake increases, so does the intake of potassium. When the body is in an anabolic state (building new tissue), potassium is stored in the cells. Movement of potassium into the blood occurs (1) with tissue injury or catabolism, when cells are broken down for energy during starvation, or (2) during periods of acidosis, when potassium moves from inside the cell into the blood to allow hydrogen ions to move into the cells to decrease the acidity of the blood (Rhyne, 2003b). Potassium is lost from the body via the kidneys where it is exchanged for sodium and via the GI tract where it is used to buffer hydrochloric acid.

Hyperkalemia

Hyperkalemia (serum potassium greater than 5.0 mEq/L) may occur because of increased potassium intake, decreased urinary excretion, or cellular damage that releases a lot of potassium into the blood (Hogan et al., 2006; Rhyne, 2003b). It may be the result of inappropriate potassium supplementation in IV fluids during hospitalizations or potassium supplementation medication. Decreased potassium excretion, causing hyperkalemia, may be the result of acute or chronic renal failure (urine output less than 30 mL/hr) or potassium-sparing diuretics (amiloride, spironolactone, triamterene) (Brophy & Gehr, 2007). Severe acidosis may greatly increase serum potassium by movement of potassium out of the cells to allow the intracellular storage of hydrogen ion to the buffer blood pH. Cellular release of potassium can occur with surgery, fever, sepsis, or trauma (Rhyne, 2003b). Decreases in the secretion of aldosterone can cause secretion of potassium in exchange for sodium and increase serum potassium levels (Rhyne, 2003b).

Clinical symptoms of hyperkalemia differ based on the degree of potassium elevation. Some common manifestations are muscular weakness and changes in the electrocardiogram (ECG) tracings with progressively widening PR and QRS intervals (Brophy & Gehr, 2007). Because of the increase of potassium inside the cell, potassium cellular repolarization is heightened, resulting in an enlarged or "tented" T wave during repolarization (Brophy & Gehr, 2007). Severe hyperkalemia (>6.0 mEq/L) results in prolonged PR intervals with loss of the P wave at levels above 7.0 mEq/L (complete heart block), wide QRS to a bizarre W configuration, and merging of the QRS and T wave (Brophy & Gehr, 2007) (see Chapter 38 😊). Calcium affects the cellular threshold potential and may compensate for some degrees of hyperkalemia (Brophy & Gehr, 2007; Rhyne, 2003b).

◼ Nursing Management

Nursing management of patients with hyperkalemia includes assessing, planning of interventions, and evaluation.

Assessment

A thorough nursing assessment is essential to identify risks for and symptoms of hyperkalemia. Hyperkalemia is likely in cases of severe cellular injury such as crush injuries or burns, renal disease, insulin deficiency (diabetic ketoacidosis or hyperosmolar hyperglycemic nonketotic syndrome), Addison's disease (hypoaldosteronism), or the use of potassium supplements (Rhyne, 2003b). Symptoms may include irregular pulse, irritability, abdominal distention, cramping, muscle weakness, paresthesia, and diarrhea (Hogan et al., 2006; Rhyne, 2003b). Arterial blood gases (ABGs) may show metabolic acidosis (Brophy & Gehr, 2007).

Outcomes and Evaluation Parameters

Nursing goals are to reduce cardiac risk within 6 hours of admission (Porth, 2007). Positive results are a heart rate within the normal range of 60 to 120 beats/min and an ECG that is reflective of normal rhythm (contains a P wave, QRS is within 0.12 second with normal amplitude, ST segment is no longer depressed, and the T wave is less "tented" in its appearance). See Chapter 38 😊 for more about ECGs.

Planning, Interventions, and Rationales

Treatment for hyperkalemia includes reducing oral or IV intake of potassium while treating the underlying cause of the hyperkalemia by administering potassium reducing agents: Kayexalate enemas (retained for 30 minutes) to exchange potassium for sodium in the gut or oral Kayexalate combined with sorbitol to rapidly remove potassium from the gut via diarrhea (Rhyne, 2003b). Some drugs will temporarily reduce potassium to allow more time for correcting the underlying cause: (1) 1 ampule of 10% calcium gluconate is administered IV, (2) combining administration of IV glucose (dextrose 50%) and IV insulin, (3) beta-adrenergic agonists such as albuterol, or (4) sodium bicarbonate (if the hyperkalemia is due to metabolic acidosis) (Brophy & Gehr, 2007). When these measures are insufficient to reduce the risks associated with hyperkalemia, patients may receive dialysis to remove the potassium (Hogan et al., 2006; Rhyne, 2003b).

When correcting hyperkalemia, the nurse should observe for possible symptoms of hypokalemia due to overcorrection.

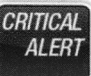 *In hyperkalemia, serum potassium levels greater than 6.0 mEq/L can be life threatening due to decreased ability of the heart to repolarize as evidenced by a "tented" T wave, loss of the P wave, and a wide, bizarre QRS with a depressed ST segment (Brophy & Gehr, 2007; Rhyne, 2003b). Should this occur, stop any potassium supplementation and take measures to reduce serum potassium before life-threatening dysrhythmias occur (Brophy & Gehr, 2007). Measures to reduce serum potassium are Kayexalate enemas, oral Kayexalate given with sorbitol, temporarily moving potassium into cells with the administration of IV glucose and insulin, and beta-adrenergic medications (albuterol). Renal dialysis may be needed (Brophy & Gehr, 2007; Rhyne, 2003b).*

Hypokalemia

Hypokalemia occurs when the serum potassium level is less than 3.5 mEq/L. Average daily losses of potassium are 5 to 10 mEq/L in feces, 0 to 20 mEq/L in sweat, and 40 to 120 mEq/L in urine (Rhyne, 2003b). Lowered serum potassium may or may not be reflective of total body loss of potassium due to the fact that potassium primarily is an intracellular cation. Generally, hypokalemia is not a problem unless people are receiving non–potassium-sparing diuretics, such as furosemide, bumetanide, or ethacrynic acid. Hypomagnesemia also is associated with hypokalemia. In fact, hypomagnesemia should be corrected before potassium is corrected because low magnesium promotes the loss of potassium from the kidneys (Brophy & Gehr, 2007).

Other common causes of low serum potassium are decreased potassium intake, GI and renal disorders, Cushing's disease, potassium-wasting diuretics, and elevated serum insulin (Rhyne, 2003b). Diarrhea may increase excretion of potassium to 200 mEq/day (Rhyne, 2003b). Vomiting or nasogastric suction can increase loss through GI fluids removed. Stress may predispose the body to hypokalemia because of increased aldosterone secretion in response to elevated ADH. This would result in increased sodium retention and increased potassium excretion in the urine. In acidosis serum potassium moves out of the cell to allow hydrogen ions to move intracellular to buffer pH. Hypokalemia can occur when the potassium returns to the ICF and hydrogen ions return to the serum. During the temporary movement of potassium into the ECF to buffer hydrogen ion, potassium may have been lost in the urine, resulting in hypokalemia when the acidosis is corrected (Brophy & Gehr, 2007).

Nursing Management

Nursing management of patients with hypokalemia includes assessing, planning of interventions, and evaluation.

Assessment

Clinical symptoms of hypokalemia are muscle weakness, cramps, nausea, vomiting, decreased bowel sounds with possible ileus (paralysis of the bowels), and paresthesias (Porth, 2007; Rhyne, 2003b). Cardiac manifestations of low serum potassium are a weak, irregular pulse. The ECG shows a flattened T wave followed by a U wave, which is an extra cardiac negative-deflection that is not normally present. Ventricular ectopy may be common due to slow repolarization of the myocardium and could progress to dangerous dysrhythmias, for example, ventricular tachycardia with hemodynamic changes (Rhyne, 2003b).

Planning, Interventions, and Rationales

Nursing interventions are directed at treating the underlying cause and replacing serum potassium as ordered without overcorrecting it (Brophy & Gehr, 2007). A diet containing about 50 to 100 mEq of potassium daily should be provided. Vegetables such as spinach, broccoli, carrots, green beans, tomato juice, acorn squash, and potatoes are good sources of potassium (Hogan et al., 2006; Rhyne, 2003b). The usual dosage of intravenous potassium supplementation is 20 to 40 mEq/hr (Rhyne, 2003b). Intravenous potassium is essential if hypokalemia is severe or if the patient is unable to take oral potassium. Potassium is **never** administered IV push! Too rapid administration of potassium can result in hyperkalemia with life-threatening dysrhythmias and death.

 CRITICAL ALERT *Potassium is **never** administered IV push! Too rapid administration of potassium can result in life-threatening dysrhythmias. If potassium is replaced too quickly, hyperkalemia may result (Brophy & Gehr, 2007; Rhyne, 2003b).*

The IV fluid of choice for replacing potassium is normal saline because dextrose 5% will result in free water once the glucose is utilized. This, in turn, will increase the dilution of potassium in the serum, consequently decreasing the rate of correction (Rhyne, 2003b). IV supplementation usually is reserved for severe cases of hypokalemia (<2.5 mEq/L) and for patients exhibiting cardiac symptoms of hypokalemia via ECG, patients with muscle spasms, or patients unable to take oral therapy (Brophy & Gehr, 2007). "In cases of severe potassium depletion, patients may require as much as 300–400 mEq/day. It is common practice to dilute 40–60 mEq in 1,000 mL of 0.45%

normal saline and infuse at a rate not exceeding 40 mEq/hour" (Brophy & Gehr, 2007, p. 971). It is preferable for this administration to take place under continuous ECG monitoring.

Evaluation

Supplementation of potassium should not be given unless the patient has adequate urinary output (15 to 20 mL/hr). The patient should be monitored for adequate respirations (above 12 per minute) and a peripheral oxygen saturation of >90%. Respirations may be weak due to the weakened muscle contractions present with hypokalemia (Rhyne, 2003b).

Calcium

Calcium (Ca^{2+}) is important for neuromuscular transmission, contraction of muscles, blood clotting, bone and tooth construction, cellular membrane function, and energy conversion (Hogan et al., 2006; Nielson, 2003). Cellular membrane stability relies on calcium. Calcium exerts a sedative effect on nerves (Nielson, 2003). Ninety-eight percent of calcium in the body is found in the bones and teeth. Two percent is in the blood serum (8.5 to 10.5 mg/dL, 50% ionized and 45% bound to albumin) (Nielson, 2003). Ionized calcium, 4.0 to 5.0 mg/dL, is responsible for the physiological actions of calcium, such as blood clotting and muscle contraction. Serum pH greatly affects the level of ionized calcium (Nielson, 2003). Metabolic acidosis decreases calcium binding to albumin, its carrier protein, and causes increased ionized calcium. Metabolic alkalosis has the opposite effect (Joy & Hladik, 2007). Tetany and muscle cramping occur with decreased ionized calcium levels. In the bone, calcium combines with phosphorus to form **hydroxyapatite**, the inorganic hexagonal matrix of bone (Nielson, 2003).

Regulation of calcium serum levels is controlled by vitamin D, calcitonin from the thyroid gland, and parathyroid hormone (PTH) from the parathyroid glands. PTH mobilizes calcium from the bones and causes increased reabsorption of calcium by the kidneys to increase serum calcium levels. Calcitonin inhibits calcium resorption, causes deposition of calcium in the bones and teeth, and increases renal excretion of calcium to lower serum calcium levels (Nielson, 2003). Vitamin D (cholecalciferol), a fat-soluble vitamin, is essential for the absorption of calcium and phosphorus from the gut (Joy & Hladik, 2007). It may be consumed in the diet or manufactured in the skin by ultraviolet light (Nielson, 2003). The kidneys must activate 1,25-dihydroxyvitamin D3 to vitamin D before it is physiologically active (Joy & Hladik, 2007).

Hypercalcemia

Hypercalcemia occurs when serum calcium is greater than 10.5 mg/dL or ionized calcium is greater than 5.5 mg/dL (Nielson, 2003). Symptoms may occur with an increase in total calcium or an increase in ionized calcium because it is the ionized calcium that is active. The latter may occur with acidosis (Nielson, 2003).

Three causes account for 80% of hypercalcemia: primary hyperparathyroidism (dysfunction of the parathyroid gland), bone malignancy, and drug toxicity (from thiazide-related drugs, i.e., thiazide diuretics, lithium carbonate, and vitamins A and D) (Guin, 2006). PTH mobilizes calcium from the bones and causes increased reabsorption of calcium by the kidneys, thus increasing serum calcium levels. Malignancy may involve metastases resulting in bone destruction and the liberation of calcium. Thiazide diuretics can cause renal tubule dysfunction and prevent the excretion of calcium. Vitamins A and D promote the absorption of calcium from the GI tract. Other causes of hypercalcemia are prolonged bed rest causing mobilization of bone calcium, adrenal insufficiency, hyperthyroidism, and rhabdomyolysis (massive muscle destruction resulting in release of myoglobin into the blood with subsequent clogging of the renal glomeruli) (Guin, 2006).

Clinical symptoms of hypercalcemia affect most systems/organs of the body as follows:

1. **Central nervous system**—fatigue, weakness, decreased deep tendon reflexes, headache, impaired concentration, memory defects, personality changes, confusion, lethargy, and depression (Guin, 2006; Joy & Hladik, 2007).

2. **Renal system**—polyuria, kidney stones, acute or chronic renal failure with decreasing urine concentrating ability (Joy & Hladik, 2007).

3. **Gastrointestinal system**—anorexia, nausea, vomiting, pain, constipation; in severe cases, pancreatitis (Joy & Hladik, 2007).

4. **Cardiovascular system**—cardiac dysrhythmias with shortening of the ST segment and QT interval and a prolonged PR interval that can lead to heart block and possible cardiac arrest (Guin, 2006). Hypertension usually is present. "Calcium or calcium-phosphorus complex deposition in blood vessels and multiple organs is a complication of chronic hypercalcemia and/or concomitant hyperphosphatemia and hyperparathyroidism" (Joy & Hladik, 2007, p. 951). These atherosclerotic lesions contribute to heart and vascular disease.

5. **Musculoskeletal system**—muscle weakness, acute arthritis, painful joints, itching, and bony cysts.

6. **Eyes and skin**—conjunctival calcifications leading to conjunctivitis. The severity of the symptoms is proportionate to the level of hypercalcemia. Soft tissue calcifications may occur throughout the body if calcium and phosphorus are elevated simultaneously (Porth, 2007). When excess calcium deposits in the skin, it can cause **calciphylaxis** (Beitz, 2004). Lesions occur primarily in the lower extremities as irregular violet plaques or nodules. They are painful and pruritic and may progress to necrosis and gangrene.

■ Nursing Management

Treatment of hypercalcemia basically is treatment of the underlying cause, that is, partial parathyroidectomy for excess PTH, chemotherapy for malignancy, discontinuation of vitamins A and D and calcium supplementation with a low calcium diet, and discontinuation of thiazide diuretics.

Assessment

As with all electrolyte imbalances, assessment of the patient is critical. Key factors include monitoring the patient's intake and output to prevent fluid overload and ensure adequate kidney function. The patient should be turned carefully to avoid possible pathologic fractures secondary to calcium mobilization from the bones. The nurse also should auscultate breath sounds for "crackles" and rhonchi and heart sounds for the development of an S_3 heart sound with vital signs to detect fluid overload at earliest onset (O'Gara & Braunwald, 2001). In the event that the patient is on digitalis, digitalis toxicity must be considered.

Planning, Interventions, and Rationales

Frequently, normal saline is administered rapidly concurrently with furosemide to dilute the blood and result in increased calcium secretion. Cortisone may be given to compete with vitamin D and decrease calcium absorption (Nielson, 2003). Bisphosphonates can be given to reduce decalcification of the bone in the presence of malignancy. Weight-bearing activity will reduce bone resorption. Calcitonin can be given to promote calcium deposition in the bone and increase calcium excretion. Gallium nitrate may be given to inhibit malignancy-related bone resorption.

 When treating hypercalcemia, if the patient is also receiving digitalis, monitor for digitalis toxicity (visual green halo around objects, serum level > 2 ng/mL) to avoid the occurrence of lethal dysrhythmias (Joy & Hladik, 2007; Nielson, 2003).

Hypocalcemia

Hypocalcemia occurs when the serum calcium level is less than 8.5 mg/dL and ionized levels are less than 4.0 mg/dL (Nielson, 2003). Because physiological effects are dependent on ionized calcium, symptoms of hypocalcemia may occur at higher serum levels, especially with a rise in serum pH (Nielson, 2003). Hypocalcemia can occur if the patient receives a large volume of citrated blood because the citrate combines with calcium, thus deactivating it.

Causes of hypocalcemia are reduced calcium intake or absorption (vitamin D deficiency or excessive phosphorous intake), decreased PTH, elevated serum phosphorus, decreased magnesium levels, hypoalbuminemia, and alkalosis. Often, the parathyroid glands are disrupted following thyroid surgery and PTH is reduced. Unless the parathyroid glands were accidentally removed with the thyroid gland, this condition will be temporary (Joy & Hladik, 2007). To monitor this condition, serum calcium concentrations should be checked every 6 hours for 1 to 2 days following thyroid surgery (Joy & Hladik, 2007). On a worldwide basis, vitamin D deficiency is the most common cause of hypocalcemia. Rickets and osteomalacia result (Joy & Hladik, 2007).

Phosphorus and calcium combine in the GI tract under the influence of vitamin D and are exchanged for one another in the kidney. Gastrointestinal surgery, chronic pancreatitis, and small-bowel disease can result in decreased levels of vitamin D and, thus, decrease calcium and phosphorous absorption. Vitamin D supplementation may be needed by an intravenous route (Joy & Hladik, 2007). Renal failure may decrease phosphorous excretion and result in excessive calcium loss. Large calcium losses may occur if the patient is taking loop diuretics (Nielson, 2003). Pancreatitis may cause decreased levels of ionized calcium because of free fatty acids binding calcium (Nielson,

2003). Severe hypomagnesemia also may be associated with severe symptomatic hypocalcemia (Joy & Hladik, 2007).

The faster the drop in serum calcium, the more acute the symptoms become. Symptoms of hypocalcemia are changes in the ECG showing prolonged QT intervals and cardiac contractility that could progress to congestive heart failure (Joy & Hladik, 2007). Dysrhythmias, bradycardia, and hypotension could occur (Joy & Hladik, 2007). Patients with low calcium experience numbness and tingling of the fingers and circumoral area, hyperactive reflexes, muscle cramps, laryngeal spasm, bronchospasm, muscle tetany, confusion, hallucinations, and possible tonic-clonic seizures (Joy & Hladik, 2007; Nielson, 2003). Mental changes can include anxiety, depression, or even psychosis. Pathologic fractures may occur due to calcium-poor bones. Trousseau's sign (carpopedal spasm) or Chvostek's sign may be present. Trousseau's sign is induced by inflating a blood pressure cuff on the upper arm 20 mm above the systolic blood pressure and maintaining the inflation for 3 minutes, resulting in wrist and fingers contracting inward (Nielson, 2003). Chvostek's sign is twitching of the facial muscles obtained by tapping the facial nerve just below the temple on the zygomatic arch. Laryngeal spasm can occur with severe hypocalcemia, resulting in asphyxiation (Nielson, 2003).

■ Nursing Management

Treatment of hypocalcemia includes oral or IV administration of calcium.

Planning, Interventions, and Rationales

Phosphorous levels should be checked to ensure that hyperphosphatemia is not the cause of the hypocalcemia (Joy & Hladik, 2007). "The elevated levels of calcium and phosphorus product result in precipitation in the arteries, joints, soft tissues and viscera and can result in tissue ischemia termed, calciphylaxis" (Joy & Hladik, 2007, p. 959). For tetany, 10 to 20 mL of 10% calcium gluconate is given IV push at a rate of 0.5 mL/min or by piggyback infusion in 100 mL of 10% calcium gluconate in a 1-L bag of D5W over at least 4 hours (Guin, 2006).

Too rapid administration of calcium can result in cardiac arrest or hypotension. Calcium gluconate is usually preferred over calcium chloride because calcium gluconate is less irritating to veins. "Calcium should not be infused at a rate greater than 60 mg of elemental calcium per minute because severe cardiac dysfunction may result" (Joy & Hladik, 2007, p. 957). Intravenous calcium should be administered with caution in patients taking digitalis glycosides because cardiac dysrhythmias could result. Calcium should not be administered in the same IV line as sodium bicarbonate because a precipitation could result, causing adverse effects (Joy & Hladik, 2007). "The bolus of calcium is usually only effective for one to two hours and should be followed by a continuous infusion of elemental calcium at a rate of 0.5 to 2 mg/kg per hour. Serum calcium concentrations should be monitored every four to six hours during the intravenous infusion" (Joy & Hladik, 2007, p. 958).

Replacement of magnesium should be considered because hypomagnesemia-induced hypocalcemia may recur if calcium is administered alone. Vitamin D should be administered to facili-

tate calcium absorption from the GI tract. Phosphate-binding antacids may be given to reduce phosphorous levels to promote calcium absorption (Nielson, 2003). Oral calcium and vitamin D supplements will be prescribed for patients with chronic hypocalcemia. Discharge instructions include that oral calcium should be taken 30 minutes before meals or at bedtime for maximum absorption. Phosphorous-binding antacids should be taken with meals (Nielson, 2003).

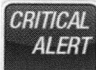 *With hypocalcemia, sudden drops in blood pressure may occur because of vasodilation and decreased cardiac contractility with rapid administration of IV calcium. Infuse calcium at a rate less than 0.5 to 1 mL/min to avoid hypotension (Joy & Hladik, 2007; Nielson, 2003). Observe closely the type of calcium that is administered because of similarity in packaging. Calcium chloride contains 13.6 mEq of calcium and calcium gluconate contains 4.5 mEq of calcium (both come in 10-mL ampules). To relieve tetany, 10 to 20 mL of 10% calcium gluconate is given IV push or piggyback infusion over at least 4 hours (Joy & Hladik, 2007; Nielson, 2003).*

Magnesium

Magnesium (Mg^{2+}) is an intracellular cation. More than 50% of body magnesium is stored in muscle and bone and only 1% is in the blood (1.4 to 2.1 mg/dL) (Adkins, 2003). Two-thirds of serum magnesium exists in ionized form and one-third is bound to plasma proteins. Forty-five percent of magnesium in the body is intracellular with most of it in the mitochondria where it is a cofactor in enzymatic activities and contributes to neuromuscular interactions, neurotransmission, and cardiac contraction (Adkins, 2003). Magnesium is involved in energy conversion of adenosine triphosphate, carbohydrate metabolism, protein synthesis, and muscular contraction (Adkins, 2003).

Magnesium is absorbed from the diet and excreted by the kidney. The body's requirement for magnesium is 4.5 mg/kg of body weight. In the average diet, 168 to 720 mg of magnesium are consumed each day (Adkins, 2003). The proportion absorbed by the GI tract varies with the amount consumed. Sources of magnesium in the diet are green leafy vegetables, nuts, legumes, seafood, whole grains, bananas, oranges, and chocolate. Magnesium absorption decreases in kidney disease because vitamin D is not activated. Phytates, oxalates, and fat in the diet decrease magnesium absorption. In magnesium-depleted states, absorption of magnesium competes with calcium absorption. When calcium absorption goes up, magnesium absorption goes down (Adkins, 2003). Average daily urinary excretion of magnesium is 100 mg/dL in men and 90 mg/dL in women. The kidney reabsorbs 20% to 30% of filtered magnesium. Excessive magnesium losses occur with diuresis (Adkins, 2003). Alcohol ingestion decreases renal magnesium reabsorption.

Hypermagnesemia

Hypermagnesemia (serum levels greater than 2.1 mg/dL) may occur due to renal failure (Adkins, 2003). It can occur in people with adrenal insufficiency or in obstetrical settings where women receive intravenous magnesium to decrease symptoms of pregnancy-induced hypertension (Adkins, 2003).

Clinical manifestations are related to decreased neuromuscular activity, such as those seen in hyperkalemia. Cardiovascular symptoms are hypotension, bradycardia, flushing and sense of warmth, and possible respiratory or cardiac arrest (Adkins, 2003). Gastrointestinal symptoms are nausea and vomiting; neurological symptoms are mental changes (drowsiness), respiratory depression, and decreased deep tendon reflex (Adkins, 2003). Deep tendon reflexes are usually lost at 8 mg/dL and respiratory failure is likely if the serum level exceeds 10 mg/dL. Coma can occur at a level of 10 mg/dL, and cardiac arrest is possible at levels >15 mg/dL (Porth, 2007).

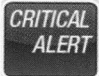 Nursing Management

Assessment

Nursing assessments should include tendon reflex as well as respiratory status. Both can be compromised with an increased magnesium serum level. The IV site should be monitored closely because extravasated calcium can result in tissue sloughing (Adkins, 2003).

Planning, Interventions, and Rationales

Treatment for serious hypermagnesemia includes immediate cessation of magnesium-containing products, IV push administration of 10 mL of 10% calcium gluconate, or dialysis. If the kidneys are intact, 0.45% normal saline may be given intravenously with diuretics to promote the renal excretion of magnesium (Adkins, 2003).

> **CRITICAL ALERT**
> In hypermagnesemia, the deep tendon reflex is lost at 8 mEq/L and respiratory failure is likely if the serum level exceeds 10 mEq/L (Adkins, 2003; Brophy & Gehr, 2007).
> Complete heart block may occur at levels of more than 15 mEq/L (Adkins, 2003). If this occurs stop magnesium-containing products and provide IV push administration of 10 mL of 10% calcium gluconate or dialysis.

Hypomagnesemia

Hypomagnesemia (serum magnesium of <1.4 mg/dL) occurs because of malnutrition (inadequate intake of magnesium-containing foods) or increased urinary excretion of magnesium due to alcoholism, osmotic diuresis in diabetes, and loop diuretics. It may occur by GI loss with vomiting, diarrhea, or malabsorption syndromes (Adkins, 2003). The most common cause is a combination of factors. Hypomagnesemia, in turn, is a cause of hypertension, cardiac dysrhythmias, and sudden cardiac death (Adkins, 2003; Brophy & Gehr, 2007).

Symptoms of hypomagnesemia are most common when the serum level is ≤1 mg/dL (Adkins, 2003). Severe deficiency may cause confusion, lethargy, seizures, hyperreflexia of deep tendon reflexes, tetany, hallucinations, nausea and vomiting, hypertension, cardiac dysrhythmias, and death (Adkins, 2003). Cardiac symptoms include supraventricular tachycardia, possible coronary artery spasms, and paresthesia (Adkins, 2003). Digitalis toxicity occurs more frequently with low serum magnesium (Adkins, 2003).

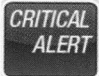 Nursing Management

Treatment for hypomagnesemia is parenteral and oral administration of magnesium supplements.

Planning, Interventions, and Rationales

Severe hypomagnesemia is treated with the IV route. IV magnesium must be administered carefully with close observation because of the possibility of developing hypermagnesemia due to overcorrection. Chronic, less severe hypomagnesemia is treated with oral magnesium salts, magnesium-containing antacids, and foods high in magnesium.

> **CRITICAL ALERT**
> When treating hypomagnesemia, IV magnesium must be administered carefully with close observations because of the possibility of developing hypermagnesemia.

Phosphorus

Eighty-five percent of phosphorus is in a structural matrix with calcium and collagen forming teeth and bones (Rawls & Hogan, 2003). The remainder is found intracellularly and in blood (2.5 to 4.5 mg/dL) (Rawls & Hogan, 2003). **Phosphorus** is essential to carbohydrate, lipid, and protein metabolism and to nerve and muscle function (Rawls & Hogan, 2003). It is part of the basic energy units of the body, adenosine triphosphate (ATP), adenosine diphosphate (ADP), and adenosine monophosphate (AMP). Phosphorus is in phospholipids, which make up the cellular and organelle membranes. It is found in red blood cells in 2,3-diphosphoglycerate, which is a hormone that increases the amount of oxygen carried in red blood cells (Rawls & Hogan, 2003).

About 800 to 1,600 mg of phosphorus is consumed per day and absorbed with the help of vitamin D. Phosphate levels are regulated by calcitonin, parathyroid hormone, and vitamin D in conjunction with calcium regulation (Rawls & Hogan, 2003). PTH blocks the reabsorption of phosphorus. When calcium is reabsorbed from the kidney tubules, phosphate is excreted (Rawls & Hogan, 2003). However, normally 80% to 90% of phosphorus is reabsorbed. Plasma phosphorous levels vary with acid–base balance. The consumption of glucose, insulin, or sugar-containing foods temporarily shifts phosphorus into the cells.

Hyperphosphatemia

Phosphorous balance is regulated primarily by the kidneys (Rawls & Hogan, 2003). Hyperphosphatemia (serum levels greater than 4.5 mg/dL) is due chiefly to renal disease and decreased excretion of phosphorus (Rawls & Hogan, 2003). Other causes may be excessive phosphate replacement or the overuse of phosphate-based enemas (Rawls & Hogan, 2003). Acidosis may cause an extracellular shift of phosphorus because phosphate serves as a buffering anion in acidosis. Cellular destruction, such as with malignancy, chemotherapy, radiation therapy, or rhabdomyolysis, may release large amounts of phosphate because it is mostly an intracellular anion (Rawls & Hogan, 2003). As serum phosphorous levels increase, serum calcium decreases, which may result in hypocalcemia.

The most common complication of hyperphosphatemia is the deposition of calcium phosphate in soft tissues. This occurs when the product of the serum calcium level and serum phosphorous level exceeds 70 mg/dL (Rawls & Hogan, 2003). Deposition of calcium phosphate in the heart muscle could result in cardiac dysrhythmias. Symptoms directly due to hyperphosphatemia are few. Most adverse symptoms relate to the resulting hypocalcemia.

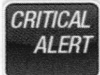 Nursing Management

Planning, Interventions, and Rationales

Treatment for hyperphosphatemia is administration of phosphorous-binding antacids, such as calcium carbonate or calcium acetate (Rawls & Hogan, 2003). Phosphorous absorption is reduced and excretion of phosphorus in the feces is increased. Calcium-based antacids are preferred in renal failure because of the potential for hypermagnesemia (Rawls & Hogan, 2003). If hyperphosphatemia is accompanied by hypocalcemia, the correction of the calcium level may reduce the phosphate level (Joy & Hladik, 2007).

> **CRITICAL ALERT**
> *Deposition of calcium phosphate in soft tissues can occur as a result of hyperphosphatemia when the product of serum calcium and phosphorous levels exceeds 70 mg/dL. In heart muscle, this could result in cardiac dysrhythmias (Joy & Hladik, 2007; Rawls & Hogan, 2003). This phenomenon occurs primarily with renal failure. As serum phosphorus levels increase, there is a simultaneous drop in calcium, resulting in symptoms of hypocalcemia (Joy & Hladik, 2007; Rawls & Hogan, 2003).*

Hypophosphatemia

Hypophosphatemia occurs when the serum phosphate level is less than 2.0 mg/dL (Medline Plus, 2006; Rawls & Hogan, 2003). Common causes are vitamin D deficiency, bowel disorders that lead to malabsorption, excessive use of phosphate-binding antacids (aluminum hydroxide or magnesium hydroxide), alcoholism, or diabetic ketoacidosis. Prolonged respiratory alkalosis can contribute significantly to hypophosphatemia (Joy & Hladik, 2007; Rawls & Hogan, 2003). In acidosis, such as diabetic ketoacidosis, phosphate is consumed as an acid buffer (Rawls & Hogan, 2003). The kidney may fail to reabsorb phosphorus in the presence of elevated PTH. Rhabdomyolysis (breakdown of striated muscle) also may be a source due to heat stroke, viral infections, or catabolic states (Rawls & Hogan, 2003).

Phosphate deficiency commonly impairs neurological function, which may be manifested by confusion, seizures, and coma. Peripheral neuropathy and ascending motor paralysis, similar to Guillain-Barré syndrome, may occur. Extrapontine myelinolysis has been reported (Mailhot, Richard, & Hemphill, 2006).

Hematologic function also may be impaired. The hemolytic anemia associated with severe hypophosphatemia has been attributed to the inability of erythrocytes to maintain integrity of cell membranes in the face of ATP depletion, leading to their destruction in the spleen. Phosphate deficiency also compromises oxygen delivery to the tissues due to decreases in erythrocyte 2,3-DPG and the resulting leftward shift in the oxygen–hemoglobin dissociation curve. Diminished oxygen delivery to the brain may be the cause of some of the neurologic manifestations mentioned earlier (Mailhot et al., 2006).

■ Nursing Management

Assessment

Clinical symptoms of hypophosphatemia are decreased availability of ADP and reduced oxygen-carrying capacity of red blood cells because of 2,3-diphosphoglycerate deficiency with a shift of the oxygen–hemoglobin dissociation curve to the left (greater resistance of oxygen release to the tissues) (Joy & Hladik, 2007; Rawls & Hogan, 2003). Tissue hypoxia can cause dysrhythmias and heart block. If the deficiency is severe, it can result in metabolic encephalopathy syndrome, in which the patient may be irritable, confused and have seizures or chest pain. Respiratory failure is possible due to muscular weakness and diaphragmatic contractile dysfunction (Joy & Hladik, 2007). Thus, phosphate serum monitoring is indicated for patients with respiratory weakness. Neurological symptoms may include apathy, delirium, hallucinations, and paranoia (Joy & Hladik, 2007). Bones may be weakened due to resorption of the bone matrix to salvage phosphate (Rawls & Hogan, 2003). Bone pain and pathologic fractures may occur due to mobilization of phosphate to replace serum losses (Joy & Hladik, 2007).

Planning, Interventions, and Rationales

Treatment of hypophosphatemia is by treating the underlying cause and promoting a high phosphate diet, especially milk, if it is tolerated. Other foods high in phosphate are dried beans and peas, eggs, fish, organ meats (brain, liver, kidney), Brazil nuts and peanuts, poultry, seeds (pumpkin, sesame, sunflower), and whole grains (oats, barley, bran) (Rawls & Hogan, 2003) (see Chapter 14). Phosphate-binding antacids should be avoided. Mild hypophosphatemia may be corrected by oral supplements, such as Neutra-Phos liquid (sodium and potassium phosphate) or Phospho-Soda (sodium phosphate) (Rawls & Hogan, 2003). Intravenous phosphate salts are not commonly administered to correct hypophosphatemia because of the danger of hyperphosphatemia causing hypocalcemia followed by tetany (Rawls & Hogan, 2003). The IV route is reserved for cases of severe hypophosphatemia or in situations where the bowel is not functioning (Mailhot et al., 2006; Rawls & Hogan, 2003). When intravenous hyperalimentation solutions are administered, 12 to 15 mmol/L of phosphorus should be added (Joy & Hladik, 2007). Acidosis should be corrected, whether metabolic or respiratory.

> **CRITICAL ALERT**
> *The IV route of phosphate is reserved for cases of severe hypophosphatemia or in situations where the bowel is not functioning because of the danger of hyperphosphatemia (Joy & Hladik, 2007; Rawls & Hogan, 2003). Acidosis should be corrected, whether metabolic or respiratory. Respiratory alkalosis causes serum phosphorus to move into the cells, thereby aggravating hypophosphatemia (Joy & Hladik, 2007; Rawls & Hogan, 2003).*

Chloride

Chloride (Cl^-) is the primary anion in the ECF (blood level: 95 to 108 mEq/L) (Covington, 2003). Chloride combines with sodium to create electrical neutrality in the body; therefore, it usually is found in combination with sodium (Covington, 2003). It assists in the reabsorption of sodium in the kidneys (Covington, 2003). Another major function of chloride is to combine with hydrogen ion (H^+) to form hydrochloric acid for digestion and hydrolyzing nutrients for absorption in the GI tract. An ample amount of chloride ion is essential for reabsorbing hydrogen ion in the kidneys to buffer alkalosis. Bicarbonate is another major anion in the ECF, and chloride tends to vary inversely with the changes in bicarbonate (Covington, 2003).

When carbon dioxide increases in the blood, chloride moves to the intracellular space to allow bicarbonate into the blood to buffer the carbonic acid. The range of variation of chloride in response to bicarbonate is 10 to 20 mEq/L (Rhyne, 2003a).

Chloride is consumed with sodium in the diet in the form of salt with the recommended daily allowance being 750mg/day. Normal excretion of acid by the kidneys includes the excretion of chloride. Chloride is lost through vomiting, excessive sweating, and in the urine, especially with diuretics (Covington, 2003). Because the serum chloride level usually remains so stable, it is used to calculate the "anion gap" (Rhyne, 2003a). The anion gap is calculated by adding the chloride and bicarbonate levels together and deducting it from the sum of the sodium and potassium levels (Rhyne, 2003a). A normal anion gap is 15 to 30. Anion gaps above 30 indicate excess organic acids, such as lactic acid or ketone acids (Rhyne, 2003a).

Hyperchloremia

Hyperchloremia (serum chloride > 108 mEq/L) may result from metabolic acidosis (arterial pH < 7.35). Common causes are hyperparathyroidism, dehydration, and respiratory alkalosis. Symptoms are increased depth and rate of respiration, lethargy, stupor, disorientation, and coma if the acidosis is not treated (Covington, 2003).

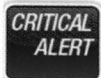 *Hyperchloremic acidosis occurs when serum Cl⁻ ion levels are increased, and can develop as the result of abnormal absorption of Cl⁻ by the kidneys or as a result of treatment with chloride-containing medications (i.e., sodium chloride, amino acid-chloride hyperalimenation solutions, and ammonium chloride). Metabolic acidosis is characterized by a decrease in pH (<7.35) and a decrease in serum HCO₃ levels (<24mEq/L). Though metabolic acidosis seldom is a primary disorder, the nurse should be aware of signs and symptoms of metabolic acidosis that typically begin to appear when plasma HCO₃⁻ falls to 20mEq/L or less. Acidosis typically produces a compensatory increase in respiratory rate with a decrease in PCO₂. Additional compensatory mechanisms of hyperchloremic acidosis are: hyperkalemia, acid urine, and increased ammonia in urine. Symptomatic manifestations of hyperchloremic acidosis include disorders of the gastrointestinal, nervous, and cardiovascular systems, including anorexia, nausea and vomiting, abdominal pain, weakness, lethargy, confusion, peripheral vasodilation, increased heart rate, and cardiac arrhythmias. The skin also may be warm and flushed (Porth, 2007).*

Hypochloremia

Hypochloremia (95 mEq/L) occurs due to loss of gastric fluids in the form of hydrochloric acid with nasogastric suctioning and severe vomiting (Covington, 2003). Serum chloride will be reduced and bicarbonate significantly elevated (30 to 40 mEq/L). One cause is stomach pyloric obstruction due to duodenal ulcer or prolonged vomiting, possibly due to bowel obstruction (Covington, 2003). Diabetic ketoacidosis may result in chloride loss because of the osmotic diuresis and elevated bicarbonate. A rare condition is Bartter's syndrome, a congenital defect that prevents renal chloride reabsorption (Devarajan, 2006)

Hypochloremia may cause hypochloremic alkalosis with chloride levels < 95 mEq/L and arterial serum pH > 7.45. Bicarbonate will be excessively retained to maintain electrical neutrality and buffer acid–base imbalances (Rhyne, 2003a).

Symptoms of alkalosis are paresthesias of the face and extremities, muscle spasms and tetany, slow and shallow respirations, and dehydration.

 Hypochloremia results when there is an abnormal depleted level of the chloride into in the blood. It rarely occurs in isolation, but is usually seen in combination with other disorders. Extra renal courses included inadequate sodium chloride intake, loses of certain gastrointestinal fluids (e.g., vomiting and nasogastric suction, or diarrhea as a result of abnormalities in small bowel transport), and loss of fluids through the skin occurring as a result of trauma, e.g., burns. Metabolic alkalosis may result in which case signs of compensation include decreased respirations (rate and depth) with various degrees of hypoxia and respiratory acidosis. Nervous system effects may include: hyperactive reflexes, tetany, confusion, and seizures. Cardiovascular system effects may include hypertension and cardiac arrhythmias (Porth, 2007).

Collaborative Management

Care of the patient with electrolyte imbalances involves collaboration with a multidisciplinary team. The health care provider directs the patient's care and writes medication, fluid replacement, and laboratory test orders to ascertain the electrolyte status and the outcomes of directed therapies. Pharmacists ensure that the IV fluids and medications administered will bring about the desired change in the patient. Nurses are vigilant at the bedside to notify the health care provider of changes in the patient's clinical condition. Dietitians provide specified diets and nutritional teaching when patients are allowed to eat and are ready for discharge. The team collaboration aspect of care is reflected in the patient care plans included in this chapter.

Research

Opportunities for nursing research related to fluid and electrolyte imbalances are investigations into ways of promoting patient awareness of problems with electrolyte abnormalities and corrective actions to be taken. Because of emphasis on prevention of osteoporosis, nutritional research might address overuse of antacids in combination with high milk ingestion or calcium-supplement therapy. The Research Opportunities and Clinical Impact box (p. 434) outlines research topics on the area of fluid and electrolyte imblances.

Summary

The human body has a complex internal environment that requires cations and anions to balance in the proper fluid volume and space (ICF or ECF). Sodium, potassium, chloride, bicarbonate, calcium, magnesium, and phosphorus have separate roles and precise levels. Cellular life cannot exist outside these boundaries; cellular swelling or shrinkage is fatal. Proper maintenance of electrochemical and neuromuscular activity is dependent on each electrolyte being present in the proper ECF or ICF compartment when it is needed.

When the complexity of the body and human nature is examined, one is amazed by the intricacies of balance that are required to keep bodily systems functioning in normal conditions. Nurses can assist patients by educating them on electrolyte abnormalities that may occur as a result of disease processes and how to avoid health problems.

RESEARCH OPPORTUNITIES AND CLINICAL IMPACT RELATED TO FLUID AND ELECTROLYTE IMBALANCES

Research Area	Clinical Impact
Overuse of antacids in combination with high milk ingestion or calcium-supplement therapy	Prevention of osteoporosis
Low serum magnesium in diabetics due to the diuresis associated with hyperglycemia	Determining what role, if any, this electrolyte abnormality plays in cardiac symptoms in the diabetic population
Assessing the accuracy of bedside monitoring of intake and output reports	Improving the quality of data on patients' intakes and outputs of fluids

NCLEX® REVIEW

1. A patient is experiencing nausea with severe vomiting. The nurse realizes that this patient is at risk for which of the following?
   1. Interstitial fluid volume overload
   2. Intracellular fluid volume deficit
   3. Extracellular fluid volume deficit
   4. Interstitial fluid volume deficit

2. A male patient's hematocrit is 56% with serum sodium of 150 mEq/L and potassium of 5.8 mEq/L. Which of the following would be indicated for this patient?
   1. Prepare to administer a hypertonic intravenous solution.
   2. Prepare to administer a hypotonic intravenous solution.
   3. Prepare to administer an isotonic intravenous solution.
   4. Implement a fluid and sodium restriction for the patient.

3. The nurse is caring for a patient and has just received the laboratory data report. Which of the following results would cause the most concern to the nurse?
   1. Na+: 115 mEq/L
   2. K+: 4.0 mEq/L
   3. Ca+: 9 mg/dL
   4. Mg+: 2.0 mg/dL

4. The nurse is caring for a patient with severe vomiting and diarrhea and a nasogastric tube to low wall suction. The nurse realizes that this patient is at risk for which of the following electrolyte imbalances?
   1. Hypokalemia
   2. Hypercalcemia
   3. Hypermagnesemia
   4. Hypophosphatemia

5. A patient is admitted to the hospital with a fluid volume excess. Which of the following will the nurse most likely assess for this patient?
   1. Dependent edema
   2. Blood pressure: 92/55 mmHg
   3. Respiratory rate 14 breaths/minute and unlabored
   4. Heart rate 86 beats per minute without ectopy

6. The nurse is caring for a patient in renal failure with a serum potassium level of 7.1 mEq/L. Which of the following should the nurse do first to assist this patient?
   1. Assess level of consciousness
   2. Measure urine output hourly
   2. Have arterial blood gases drawn
   4. Obtain an electrocardiogram

7. The nurse is providing discharge instructions to a patient with hypokalemia. Which of the following should the nurse include in these instructions?
   1. Take oral Kaexylate as prescribed.
   2. Limit the intake of spinach and carrots, and green, leafy vegetables.
   3. Eat a balanced diet including tomato juice and potatoes.
   4. Expect muscle cramps and weakness for at least six weeks.

Answers for review questions appear in Appendix D

KEY TERMS

aldosterone *p.423*
antidiuretic hormone (ADH) *p.422*
atrial natriuretic peptide (ANP) *p.423*
calciphylaxis *p.429*
calcium *p.428*
chloride *p.432*
diffusion *p.419*
electrolytes *p.419*
extracellular fluid (ECF) *p.418*

filtration *p.419*
hydroxyapatite *p.428*
hypertonic *p.419*
hypotonic *p.419*
insensible fluid loss *p.418*
interstitial fluid *p.418*
intracellular fluid (ICF) *p.418*
isotonic *p.418*

magnesium *p.430*
oncotic pressure *p.419*
osmolality *p.418*
osmosis *p.419*
phosphorus *p.431*
potassium *p.424*
sodium *p.423*
specific gravity (SG) *p.419*

EXPLORE   PEARSON   **mynursingkit**™

MyNursingKit is your one stop for online chapter review materials and resources. Prepare for success with additional NCLEX®-style practice questions, interactive assignments and activities, web links, animations and videos, and more!

Register your access code from the front of your book at
www.mynursingkit.com

REFERENCES

Adkins, J. A. (2003). Magnesium balance and imbalances. In M. A. Hogan & D. Wane (Eds.), *Fluids, electrolytes, and acid–base balance: Reviews and rationales* (pp. 113–126). Upper Saddle River, NJ: Pearson Prentice Hall.

Ahlquist, D. A., & Camilleri, M. (2001). Diarrhea and constipation. In E. Braunwald, A. S. Fauci, D. L. Kasper, S. L. Hauser, D. L. Longo, & J. L. Jameson (Eds.), *Harrison's principles of internal medicine* (15th ed., pp. 241–249). New York: McGraw-Hill.

Beitz, J. M. (2004). Wound wise: Calciphylaxis. *American Journal of Nursing, 104,* 36–37.

Bomback, A. S., & Klemmer, P. J. (2007). The incidence and implications of aldosterone breakthrough. *Nature Clinical Practice of Nephrology, 3*(9), 486–492.

Bond, E. F. (2000). Cardiac anatomy and physiology. In S. L. Woods, E. S. Sivarajan Froelicher, & S. A. Underhill Motzer (Eds.), *Cardiac nursing* (4th ed.). Philadelphia: Lippincott Williams & Wilkins.

Brophy, D. F., & Gehr, T. W. B. (2007). Disorders of potassium and magnesium homeostasis. In J. T. DiPiro, R. L. Talbert, G. C. Yee, G. R. Matzke, B. G. Wells, & L. M. Posey (Eds.), *Pharmacotherapy: A pathophysiologic approach* (6th ed., pp. 967–981). New York: McGraw-Hill.

Covington, L. W. (2003). Chloride balance and imbalances. In M. A. Hogan & D. Wane (Eds.), *Fluids, electrolytes, and acid–base balance: Reviews and rationales* (pp. 127–144). Upper Saddle River, NJ: Pearson Prentice Hall.

Devarajan, S. (2006). Bartter Syndrome. *Emedicine.* Retrieved June 14, 2006 from http://www.emedicine.com/PED/topic210.htm

Felver, L. (2000). Fluids and electrolytes balance and imbalance. In S. L. Woods, E. S. Sivarajan Froelicher, & S. A. Underhill Motzer (Eds.), *Cardiac nursing* (4th ed., pp. 132–148). Philadelphia: Lippincott Williams & Wilkins.

Goldstein-Fuchs, D. J., & McQuiston, B. (2003). Renal failure. In L. E. Matarese & M. M. Gottschlich (Eds.), *Contemporary nutrition support practice: A clinical guide* (2nd ed., pp. 460–483). Philadelphia: W. B. Saunders.

Goyne, J. S. (2003). Fluid balances and imbalances. In M. A. Hogan & D. Wane (Eds.), *Fluids, electrolytes, and acid–base balance:*

Reviews and rationales (pp. 1–36). Upper Saddle River, NJ: Pearson Prentice Hall.

Grandjean, A. C., Reimers, K. J., & Buyck, M. E. (2003). Hydration: Issues for the 21st century. *Nutrition Reviews, 61*(8), 261–271.

Guin, P. R. (2006). Endocrine disorders. In *Lippincott manual of nursing practice* (8th ed., pp. 873–909). Philadelphia: Lippincott Williams & Wilkins.

Gums, J. G., & Tovar, J. M. (2007). Adrenal gland disorders. In J. T. DiPiro, R. L. Talbert, G. C. Yee, G. R. Matzke, B. G. Wells, & L. M. Posey (Eds.), *Pharmacotherapy: A pathophysiologic approach* (6th ed., pp. 1391–1406). New York: McGraw-Hill.

Hogan, M. A., Gingrich, M. M., Ricci, M. J., & Overby, P. (2006). *Fluids, electrolytes, and acid–base balance* (2nd ed.). Upper Saddle River, NJ: Pearson Prentice Hall.

Indiana State University. (2007). *Nursing management of fluids and electrolytes: Daily weights.* Retrieved November 25, 2007, from http://www.indstate.edu/mary/Fluidlytecf/slide13.htm

Johnson, A. P. (2007). Sodium balance and imbalances. In M. A. Hogan & D. Wane (Eds.), *Fluids, electrolytes, and acid–base balance: Reviews and rationales* (pp. 37–59). Upper Saddle River, NJ: Pearson Prentice Hall.

Joy, M. S., & Hladik, G. A. (2007). Disorders of sodium, water, calcium and phosphorus homeostasis. In J. T. DiPiro, R. L. Talbert, G. C. Yee, G. R. Matzke, B. G. Wells, & L. M. Posey (Eds.), *Pharmacotherapy: A pathophysiologic approach* (6th ed., pp. 937–966). New York: McGraw-Hill.

Mailhot, T., Richard, A. J., & Hemphill, R. R. (2006). *Hypophosphatemia.* Retrieved February 16, 2008, from eMedicine website: http://www.emedicine.com/emerg/topic278.htm

Medline Plus. (2006). *Serum phosphorus.* Retrieved February 16, 2008, from http://www.nlm.nih.gov/medlineplus/ency/article/003478.htm

Metheny, N. M. (2000). *Fluid and electrolyte balance* (4th ed.). Philadelphia: Lippincott Williams & Wilkins.

Mushnick, R. (2007). Osmolality. *Medline Plus.* Retrieved June 14, 2008 from http://www.nlm.nih.gov/medlinieplus/ency/article/003463.htm

Nielson, K. A. (2003). Calcium balance and imbalances. In M. A. Hogan & D. Wane (Eds.), *Fluids, electrolytes, and acid–base balance: Reviews and rationales* (pp. 85–112). Upper Saddle River, NJ: Pearson Prentice Hall.

O'Gara, P. T., & Braunwald, E. (2001). Approach to a patient with a heart murmur. In E. Braunwald, A. S. Fauci, D. L. Kasper, S. L. Hauser, D. L. Longo, &, J. L. Jameson (Eds.), *Harrison's principles of internal medicine* (15th ed., pp. 207–210). New York: McGraw-Hill.

Porth, C.M. (2007). Essentials *of pathophysiology: Concepts of altered health states.* Philadelphia: Lippincott Williams & Wilkins.

Rawls, M. C., & Hogan, M. A. (2003). Phosphorus balance and imbalances. In M. A. Hogan & D. Wane (Eds.), *Fluids, electrolytes, and acid–base balance: Reviews and rationales* (pp. 145–163). Upper Saddle River, NJ: Pearson Prentice Hall.

Rhyne, L. (2003a). Acid–base balance and imbalances. In M. A. Hogan & D. Wane (Eds.), *Fluids, electrolytes, and acid–base balance: Reviews and rationales* (pp. 165–192). Upper Saddle River, NJ: Pearson Prentice Hall.

Rhyne, L. (2003b). Potassium balance and imbalances. In M. A. Hogan & D. Wane (Eds.), *Fluids, electrolytes, and acid–base balance: Reviews and rationales* (pp. 61–83). Upper Saddle River, NJ: Pearson Prentice Hall.

Saseen, J. J., & Carter, B. L. (2005). Hypertension. In J. T. DiPiro, R. L. Talbert, G. C. Yee, G. R. Matzke, B. G. Wells, & L. M. Posey (Eds.), *Pharmacotherapy: A pathophysiologic approach* (6th ed., pp. 185–218). New York: McGraw-Hill.

Singer, G. G., & Brenner, B. M. (2001). Fluid and electrolyte disturbances. In E. Braunwald, A. S. Fauci, D. L. Kasper, S. L. Hauser, D. L. Longo, &, J. L. Jameson (Eds.), *Harrison's principles of internal medicine* (15th ed., pp. 271–282). New York: McGraw-Hill.

Whitmire, S. J. (2003). Fluid, electrolytes, and acid–base balance. In L. E. Matarese & M. M. Gottschlich (Eds.), *Contemporary nutrition support practice: A clinical guide* (2nd ed., pp. 122–144). Philadelphia: W. B. Saunders.

Acid–Base Imbalance

Gail Thurkauf

Outcome-Based Learning Objectives

After studying this chapter, the learner will be able to:

1. Describe the role of hydrogen ions in the determination of plasma pH.
2. Compare and contrast the processes that produce respiratory and metabolic acids in the body and the processes by which they are eliminated.
3. Calculate minute ventilation and explain the effect of minute alveolar ventilation on acid–base balance.
4. Evaluate the process of respiratory compensation for a metabolic abnormality.
5. Discuss the renal handling of hydrogen ion and bicarbonate.
6. Discuss a systematic stepwise process for the interpretation of the arterial blood gas values related to acid–base balance.
7. Relate the major causes, pathophysiology, signs, symptoms, consequences, and medical management for respiratory acidosis and alkalosis and metabolic acidosis and alkalosis.
8. Describe the nursing assessment used in the assessment of acid–base abnormalities.
9. Describe nursing actions to alleviate the symptoms of acid–base abnormalities.

Research Collaboration Health Promotion Nursing Process Caring Critical Thinking

DISORDERS OF THE balance between the acids and the alkali or bases in the body are common clinical problems that result from or accompany a wide variety of pathologic conditions and diseases. A basic understanding of the effect of these imbalances on organ systems is important for nurses when assessing and caring for patients in all clinical settings.

Acid–Base Homeostasis

A **hydrogen ion** is a single charged particle (proton) that is not orbited by any electrons. The hydrogen ion (H^+) is the smallest ionic particle and it is extremely reactive. Because of this reactivity, the hydrogen ion has a significant effect on physiological functions despite the fact that it is present in very low concentrations. The hydrogen ion combines with alkali/bases or other negatively charged ions at low concentrations. Proteins contain many negatively charged and positively charged groups within their structure. Therefore, even small changes in hydrogen ion concentration can alter protein and enzyme functioning. More extreme changes may totally disrupt the protein's structure, a process referred to as *denaturing* them. Disturbances in hydrogen ion concentration may result in abnormalities of function in many organs such as the pulmonary, renal, or cardiac systems and can also alter such processes as blood clotting and the metabolism of drugs (Schlichtig, 2005).

Plasma **pH** is an indicator of hydrogen ion concentration. It is the negative logarithm of the hydrogen ion concentration measured in nanomoles per liter (nmol/L). A normal pH of 7.40 is equivalent to 40 nmol/L of hydrogen ion. In terms more commonly used, this would be equal to 0.0004 mEq/L. Contrast that with a normal serum potassium level of 4 mEq/L or normal serum sodium of 140 mEq/L. Because it is a *negative* log, as the hydrogen ion concentration increases, the pH decreases. Conversely, as the hydrogen ion concentration goes down, pH goes up. Homeostatic mechanisms work to keep pH within a relatively narrow range of 7.35 to 7.45 for optimal cell functioning. As the pH changes either higher or lower, enzymes may stop functioning, nerve and muscle activity weaken, and, if the change is extreme, all metabolic activity may become deranged. The pH range that is usually considered compatible with life is 6.8 to 7.8.

Acids are compounds that form hydrogen ion in solution. Because of this, they are referred to as proton *donors*. As an example, hydrochloric acid (HCl) gives up H^+ when added to blood. Strong acids hold their hydrogen ion weakly, so the ion dissociates easily and can then act on other substances. Weak acids hold onto their hydrogen ion more tightly so they do not contribute as much to the free hydrogen ion concentration. Because of this, the solution will have a higher (less acid) pH (Argyle, 2002).

Bases or **alkalis** are compounds that combine with hydrogen ion in solution; they are proton *acceptors*. **Sodium bicarbonate**

(NaHCO$_3^-$) removes hydrogen ion when added to the blood. Acids and bases constantly react with one another to neutralize changes in hydrogen ion concentration.

Carbon dioxide (CO$_2$) can be thought of as a potential acid. When it is dissolved in water, it becomes **carbonic acid**:

$$CO_2 + H_2O \rightarrow H_2CO_3 \text{ (carbonic acid)}$$

Carbonic acid then dissociates into hydrogen ion and bicarbonate:

$$H_2CO_3 \rightarrow H^+ + HCO_3^-$$

In plasma, under normal circumstances, there are 20 parts of bicarbonate to 1 part carbonic acid, a ratio of 20:1. If this 20:1 ratio is altered in either direction, the plasma pH will change (Schlichtig, 2005).

Body metabolism continually produces CO$_2$ (the respiratory acid) and other nonrespiratory acids, called metabolic acids. These acids are released into capillary blood, lowering the pH. Under normal conditions, this pH change is quite small. Blood arrives in the arterioles with a pH of 7.4 (which is equivalent to 40 nmol/L of hydrogen ion) and leaves the venules with a pH of 7.36 (equal to 44 nmol/L of hydrogen ion). Hydrogen ions have been added to the blood from the cell interior, which has a pH of about 7.0, equivalent to 100 nmol/L of hydrogen ion (Grogono, 2006).

The amount of respiratory acid produced is about 288 L/day (Grogono, 2006). This large amount is matched to the lung ventilation, which is its means of excretion. By comparison, very little metabolic acid is produced on a daily basis: about 0.1 mol (100 mEq). The main metabolic acids are lactic acid, pyruvic acid, ketoacids seen in diabetic acidosis, acetoacetic acid, and beta-hydroxybutyric acid. These acids are eliminated by the kidneys or they are metabolized by the liver. The capacity for elimination of these metabolic acids is much less than that of the lungs.

Abnormalities in the balance of acid to base can be grouped into four basic categories:

- **Respiratory acidosis**—excess of carbon dioxide leading to an acid pH
- **Respiratory alkalosis**—lower than normal level of carbon dioxide leading to an alkaline pH
- **Metabolic acidosis**—excess of hydrogen ion or a deficiency in bicarbonate leading to an acid pH
- **Metabolic alkalosis**—excess of bicarbonate leading to an alkaline pH.

Chart 19–1 provides a summary of acid–base terminology. The body's response to changes in acid–base status has three components:

1. **The first defense**—buffering
2. **The second defense**—changing the level of CO$_2$
3. **The third defense**—changing the level of HCO$_3^-$.

Buffer Systems

A **buffer** is a compound that minimizes the change in hydrogen ion concentration and, thus, the change in pH when these ions are added or removed from solution. A buffer acts like a sponge:

CHART 19–1 **Acid and Base Terminology**

Acidemia/Acidosis	Alkalemia/Alkalosis
Blood pH <7.40	Blood pH > 7.40
Caused by loss of base/alkali; increase of acid	Caused by increase of base/alkali; loss of acid
Lowers the 20:1 bicarbonate-to-carbonic acid ratio	Raises the 20:1 bicarbonate-to-carbonic acid ratio
Less base/more acid	More base/less acid

When there is an excess of hydrogen ion, the sponge soaks up the extra ions. When the level of hydrogen ion is decreased, the sponge can be squeezed out to release hydrogen ions back into the blood. Buffer systems act quickly to prevent excess changes in the pH.

There are buffers within body cells and in the extracellular fluid (ECF). The primary buffers of the extracellular system are carbonic acid and bicarbonate. The concentrations of these two substances are regulated by two independent systems. Carbonic acid is controlled by respiration via the lungs, and bicarbonate is controlled by excretion via the kidneys. Oxidative (aerobic) metabolism of amino acids and the anaerobic metabolism of glucose to lactate and pyruvic acid produce CO$_2$, which, again, can be thought of as a potential acid. Although CO$_2$ does not contain hydrogen ions, it reacts rapidly with water to form carbonic acid, which then dissociates into hydrogen and bicarbonate ions, as noted previously. This reaction can be written:

$$CO_2 + H_2O \rightarrow H_2CO_3^- \leftrightarrow HCO_3^- + H^+$$

This reaction occurs throughout the body and, in certain circumstances such as within red blood cells, can be sped up by the enzyme carbonic anhydrase.

Excess carbon dioxide is exhaled by the lungs as carbon dioxide gas. The concentration of bicarbonate ions is controlled by the kidneys. Under normal circumstances, the kidneys reabsorb and retain all of the bicarbonate presented to them by glomerular filtration. The kidneys also excrete small amounts of acid in the renal tubule. In alkalosis, either respiratory or metabolic, the kidneys retain hydrogen ion and excrete bicarbonate. In contrast, in respiratory acidosis and most cases of metabolic acidosis, the kidneys excrete hydrogen ion and conserve bicarbonate to correct the pH.

The intracellular buffer system is the phosphate buffer system. This system consists of dihydrogen phosphate ion (H$_2$PO$_4$) as the hydrogen ion donor (the acid) and hydrogen phosphate (HPO$_4$) as the hydrogen ion acceptor, the base. These two compounds are in equilibrium with one another inside the cell. When there is excess hydrogen ion in blood plasma, the hydrogen ions cross the cell membrane, enter the intracellular fluid (ICF), and are consumed by reacting with HPO$_4$. If there is extra hydroxide, or base, these compounds enter the intracellular fluid where they react with the H$_2$PO$_4$.

Protein buffers in the blood include plasma proteins and hemoglobin. Hemoglobin (Hgb) is the more important of these because it can bind to both CO$_2$ and H$^+$. Hemoglobin exists in two forms. It leaves the left side of the heart carrying its load of oxygen as oxyhemoglobin. After delivering the oxygen to the

MyNursingKit Animation: Fluids and Electrolytes: Acid–Base and pH: Anatomy and Physiology cell, the oxygen content is depleted and it has now become de-oxygenated Hgb. Deoxygenated Hgb is a better buffer than oxygenated Hgb because it has a stronger affinity for both the CO_2 and the hydrogen ion. Oxygen unloading at the tissues increases the amount of deoxygenated Hgb, thus producing the superior buffer exactly where it is needed to buffer the additional hydrogen ion being produced by metabolism (Breen, 2001).

At the tissue level, dissolved CO_2 enters the red blood cells (RBCs) where it combines with water to form carbonic acid. Carbonic anhydrase, present in the RBCs, is the enzyme that catalyzes this reaction. The carbonic acid then dissociates into bicarbonate and hydrogen ions. The hydrogen ions then bind to deoxygenated Hgb when they are soaked up by the buffer "sponge." Hemoglobin's buffering capacity is due to a chain within its structure, the imidazole chain. Imidazole can accept an extra proton, the hydrogen ion, or donate it back when the body pH is corrected (Argyle, 2002). The bicarbonate ions formed by the dissociation pass through RBC membranes back into the plasma in exchange for chloride ions (Cl^-). This ensures that there is no gain or loss of negative ions within the RBCs.

When the RBCs reach the lungs, this process is reversed. Hydrogen ions that were bound to the hemoglobin recombine with the bicarbonate to form CO_2, which passes through the RBC membranes into the alveoli so it can be expired. The deoxygenated Hgb combines with oxygen to prepare to return to the tissues. This process is illustrated in Figure 19–1 ■.

In addition to the buffer systems just described, bones also act as a buffer. The carbonate and phosphate salts in bone provide a long-term supply of buffer. They act as a reserve for alkalis. In acute metabolic acidosis, bone can take up hydrogen ion in exchange for calcium (Ca^{2+}), sodium (Na^+), and potassium (K^+). In chronic metabolic acidosis, calcium carbonate is released from bone as bone crystals dissolve. This situation can lead to the osteodystrophy often seen in chronic renal failure, which is a cause of chronic metabolic acidosis (Androgue & Androgue, 2001).

■ The Role of the Lungs

The lungs help to regulate plasma pH on a minute-to-minute basis by regulating the level of carbon dioxide, the respiratory acid. Carbon dioxide is measured as the partial pressure of carbon dioxide in arterial blood, the $PaCO_2$. This level is tightly controlled under normal conditions and kept within a narrow range of 35 to 45 mmHg at sea level. The lungs can either retain or excrete CO_2 by altering the rate and depth of ventilation. The amount of ventilation is generally quantified by how much air the lungs move in 1 minute, referred to as the **minute ventilation**. Minute ventilation is the product of respiratory *rate* and *depth*, referred to as the tidal volume (V_t). Normal resting respiratory rate is about 12 breaths per minute. Normal resting depth tidal volume is about 500 mL. This yields a normal minute ventilation of 6 L/min:

$$12 \; breaths/min \times 500 \; mL \; V_t = 6,000 \; mL \; or \; 6 \; L$$

The tidal volume refers to the total amount of air inhaled and exhaled with each breath. A portion of that volume, however, is in the large conducting airways such as the trachea and bronchi. That volume, referred to as **anatomic dead space**, does not reach the alveolar airspaces to take part in the exchange of oxygen and carbon dioxide with the blood. The amount of anatomic dead space can be estimated as 1 mL/lb of ideal body weight. Thus, a person with an ideal body weight of 150 pounds has about 150 mL of anatomic dead space.

The remainder of the tidal volume, that portion which *does* reach the alveoli and participates in gas exchange with capillary blood, is termed *alveolar volume*. Minute alveolar ventilation is the volume of alveolar air per minute that takes part in gas exchange, transferring oxygen to the blood and removing carbon dioxide from the blood. It is actually this minute alveolar ventilation that determines the $PaCO_2$. Normal minute alveolar ventilation can be calculated as follows:

$$Tidal \; volume - anatomic \; dead \; space = alveolar \; volume$$
$$500 \; mL - 150 \; mL = 350 \; mL$$
$$Respiratory \; rate \times alveolar \; volume =$$
$$minute \; alveolar \; ventilation$$
$$12 \; breaths/min \times 350 \; mL = 4,200 \; mL \; or \; 4.2 \; L/min$$

This normal minute alveolar ventilation should yield a normal $PaCO_2$. In clinical practice, the terms *hyperventilation* and *hypoventilation* apply only to alveolar ventilation and its effect on the $PaCO_2$.

Dead space ventilation is that part of the minute ventilation which does not take part in gas exchange; it is actually "wasted ventilation." Dead space ventilation includes the air in the conducting airways, the anatomic dead space as discussed earlier, and the air that *does* reach the alveoli but doesn't take part in gas exchange, typically referred to as **pathologic dead space**. Different disease states such as emphysema can alter this pathologic dead space and affect the ability of the lungs to oxygenate and ventilate.

The respiratory center located in the medulla in the brainstem controls the rate and depth of ventilation in response to the level of arterial CO_2, denoted as $PaCO_2$. Chemoreceptors located on the surface of the medulla are in contact with cerebrospinal fluid (CSF). These receptors are termed "central" because they are located within the central nervous system (CNS). As the level of $PaCO_2$ rises, the arterial $PaCO_2$ reaches equilibrium with the CO_2 in the CSF. That CO_2 in the CSF combines with water to form carbonic acid, as previously described. The carbonic acid dissociates into hydrogen ion and bicarbonate. The CSF hydrogen ion diffuses into the medullary tissue and stimulates the chemorecep-

Red blood cell

FIGURE 19–1 ■ Red blood cell.

tors. They, in turn, stimulate the diaphragm and intercostal muscles to increase the rate and depth of ventilation. This increase in minute ventilation will "blow off" excess CO_2, returning it back toward normal, thereby correcting the pH.

The reverse happens when there are abnormally low levels of CO_2. In this state of hyperventilation, the medullary centers slow the rate and depth of ventilation to allow accumulation of CO_2 back toward normal, thereby correcting the pH.

The level of $PaCO_2$, acting on the central chemoreceptors by altering the pH of the CSF, is the most important single determent of ventilation, and is referred to as the **hypercarbic drive**. There are also peripheral chemoreceptors that are responsive to the level of oxygen in the blood and hydrogen ion as well as the $PaCO_2$. These peripheral receptors are located in the carotid arteries at the bifurcation of the common carotid and in the arch of the aorta. The carotid receptors are sensitive to PaO_2, $PaCO_2$, and pH. The aortic receptors are sensitive to PaO_2 and $PaCO_2$ but not pH. Neural impulses from the carotid bodies increase as the PaO_2 falls below about 60 mmHg and stimulate the respiratory centers to increase both rate and depth of ventilation in an attempt to increase the body's oxygen supply. This responsiveness to low oxygen tension, referred to as the **hypoxic drive**, is potentiated by acidosis and hypercapnia.

The hypercarbic drive is a response to *acute* respiratory acidosis. If a person suffers from chronic ventilatory failure, such as a patient with end-stage emphysema that leads to chronically high $PaCO_2$ levels (chronic respiratory acidosis), bicarbonate will cross the blood–brain barrier to buffer the CSF hydrogen ion changes. It takes hours to days for this adaptation to occur. Due to this increased bicarbonate on the brain side of the blood–brain barrier, the central chemoreceptors become less sensitive to changes in the level of CO_2, which results in a decrease in the strength of the ventilatory drive moderated by these central receptors. When this occurs, the only remaining drive to breathe is the stimulation of the peripheral receptors by a low PaO_2, the hypoxic drive.

The terms *hyperventilation* and *hypoventilation* are defined by the $PaCO_2$. Low $PaCO_2$, or hypocapnia, defines the state of **hyperventilation**. A high $PaCO_2$, hypercapnia, defines the state of **hypoventilation**. There is a tendency to describe someone who is breathing rapidly and deeply as "hyperventilating," but this cannot actually be determined without obtaining an arterial blood gas and looking at the $PaCO_2$.

In addition to the level of CO_2, an increase in the arterial hydrogen ion concentration will also stimulate the central chemoreceptors of the respiratory control center, but to a lesser degree because hydrogen ions do not diffuse into the CSF as easily as the lipid-soluble CO_2, so the response is slower. But in a state of metabolic acidosis, such as that which exists during diabetic ketoacidosis, the medullary centers will stimulate the lungs to increase the minute ventilation to blow off CO_2, even if that level is normal. These rapid, deep respirations, referred to as Kussmaul's respirations, are an attempt to correct the arterial pH by decreasing respiratory acid. This process is referred to as **compensation**.

The Role of the Kidneys

The kidneys perform two basic functions to maintain acid–base balance: They secrete hydrogen ions and they restore or reclaim bicarbonate. Bicarbonate ions are freely filtered in the kidneys by glomerular filtration. The level of bicarbonate in the renal tubular fluid is the same as that of plasma. To help make this clear, think of tubular fluid as being outside of the body. During glomerular filtration, plasma, water, and solutes are forced by hydrostatic pressure across the membrane of the glomerular capillaries into the lumen of the tubule. If substances remain in the tubular fluid or other substances are secreted into that fluid, they will eventually leave the body in urine. **Secretion** is the active process of moving substances, such as hydrogen ion, from the blood into the tubular fluid against the concentration gradient. If substances are reabsorbed from the tubular fluid back across the membrane and into the blood, they are being reclaimed back into the body.

The reabsorption of bicarbonate that has been filtered into the tubular fluid occurs primarily in the proximal convoluted tubule of the nephron. Filtered bicarbonate combines with the secreted hydrogen ions to form carbonic acid, which then dissociates into CO_2 and water.

$$HCO_3^- + H^+ \leftrightarrow H_2CO_3 \leftrightarrow CO_2 + H_2O$$

This reaction is catalyzed by carbonic anhydrase, the same enzyme contained in the red blood cells. The CO_2 crosses from the tubular fluid into the cells lining the tubule. Here, the CO_2 recombines with water to again form carbonic acid, which then dissociates to hydrogen ion and bicarbonate. This is the reverse of the preceding equation:

$$CO_2 + H_2O \rightarrow H_2CO_3^- \leftrightarrow HCO_3^- + H^+$$

The bicarbonate passes from the cell back across the membrane into the blood while the hydrogen ion passes back into the tubular fluid. This hydrogen ion is exchanged for sodium ion, another positive ion.

In the face of a high load of metabolic acids, the kidneys also increase their production of the urinary buffer, ammonia (NH_4). Under normal circumstances, NH_4 excretion is about 30 mmol/day, or about 0.5 mmol/kg. This excretion can increase to about 280 mmol/day but this response takes several days to be completed (DuBose, 2004).

In the event of respiratory acidosis, where there is an excess of plasma CO_2, and in most cases of metabolic acidosis, the kidneys excrete hydrogen ion and conserve bicarbonate to help restore acid–base balance and return the pH toward normal. In respiratory and metabolic alkalosis, the kidneys retain hydrogen ion and excrete bicarbonate. This metabolic compensation is slow compared to respiratory compensation. It can take hours to days to occur. Note that the average ventilation rate is about 6 L/*minute*, whereas the renal excretion rate is only about 2 L/*day* (Schlichtig, 2005).

Assessment of Acid–Base Balance

Arterial blood gas (ABG) values are most often used to assess acid–base balance, although serum electrolytes will help fine-tune the analysis. The Diagnostic Test box (p. 440) outlines the commonly assessed laboratory values.

Normal ABG values are:

$$pH = 7.40 \, (range: 7.35 - 7.45)$$

$$PaCO_2 = 40 \, mEq/L \, (range: 35 - 45)$$

$$HCO_3^- = 22 - 28 \, mEq/L$$

DIAGNOSTIC TESTS for Acid–Base Imbalances

Test	Expected Abnormality	Rationale for Abnormality
pH	↓ 'd < 7.35 in uncompensated respiratory or metabolic acidosis ↑ 'd > 7.45 in uncompensated respiratory or metabolic alkalosis	
$PaCO_2$	>45 mmHg in respiratory acidosis <35 mmHg in respiratory alkalosis	CO_2 is a respiratory acid. An excess will lead to acidosis; a deficiency will lead to alkalosis.
HCO_3^-	<22 mEq/L in metabolic acidosis >28 mEq/L in metabolic alkalosis	HCO_3^- is a base. A deficiency will lead to acidosis; an excess will lead to alkalosis.
Base excess (BE)	> −3 in metabolic acidosis > +3 in metabolic alkalosis	Quantifies the milliequivalents of bicarbonate that are deficient/in excess per liter of ECF.
Serum potassium	↑ 'd with acidosis	Excess hydrogen ion moves into cells and displaces K^+ out of the cell and into the serum.
Ionized calcium	↓ 'd in alkalosis	Alkalosis ↑ 's the binding of calcium to albumin, resulting in a decrease in free, ionized calcium in the serum.
Anion gap	↑ 'd above 10–14 in high anion gap acidosis Normal in nonanion gap metabolic acidosis	Indicates an increased anion load (lactic acidosis, ketoacidosis, ingestion of acids, rhabdomyolysis). Loss of bicarbonate (diarrhea, fistula, renal dysfunction) or ingestion of base.

Along with these values, most ABGs also report the **base excess**. This is a calculated value that is based on the bicarbonate level, the $PaCO_2$, and the hematocrit. The base excess refers to the number of milliequivalents of bicarbonate per liter of ECF that one has too much of (base excess) or too little of (base deficit). As an example, a patient has a base excess of +6. This indicates a metabolic alkalosis and quantifies it. Every liter of the patient's ECF has 6 mEq too much bicarbonate or other base. In an opposite example, a patient has a base excess of −10. This indicates a metabolic acidosis and every liter of ECF is deficient in bicarbonate by 10 mEq. This number can help guide clinicians when they are considering how much bicarbonate to administer to a patient with severe metabolic acidosis. (*Note:* Although a positive number indicates a base excess and a negative number indicates a base deficit, in clinical practice, only the term *base excess* is commonly used.) A negative number is referred to as a "base excess of minus *x*." A normal base excess, then, is zero; not too little or too much bicarbonate. The normal range is usually considered to be ±3 mEq. Outlined here is the recommended stepwise approach for the interpretation of ABGs, which is also illustrated in Figure 19–2 ■:

1. **Assess the pH**—is it normal, low, or high? This first step is crucial because it guides the approach to the rest of the values. If the pH is less than 7.35, there is an acidosis. If the pH is greater than 7.45, there is an alkalosis.

2. **Assess the respiratory component**—Is the $PaCO_2$ normal, low, or high? If the cause of an abnormality is a respiratory problem, the $PaCO_2$ and the pH move in opposite direc-

FIGURE 19–2 ■ Stepwise approach to ABG interpretation.

tions. In ventilatory failure, the $PaCO_2$ rises and causes a lowered acid pH. If both the pH and the $PaCO_2$ have moved in the same direction (i.e., both are increased or both are decreased), then the cause of the abnormality is a metabolic one. Refer to the examples in Chart 19–2.

3. **Assess the metabolic component**—Are the bicarbonate and the base excess (BE) normal, low, or high? In a metabolic abnormality, the pH and the bicarbonate move in the same direction. If the bicarbonate is increased, pH will be increased. If the bicarbonate is decreased, the pH will also be lower. Refer to the examples in Chart 19–3.

Steps 2 and 3 will identify the primary problem if there is one. Next, evaluate compensation. Any change in the acid–base equilibrium will cause the system that is *not* the primary cause of the abnormality to respond to attempt to restore the 20:1 ratio of

CHART 19–2 Examples of Abnormalities of the Respiratory Component

Example 1: Mrs. A has a $PaCO_2 = 56$ and a pH = 7.27.
The $PaCO_2$ is increased (16 mmHg above normal). The pH is decreased by 0.13.
In respiratory acidosis, the $PaCO_2$ and the pH move in opposite directions, so:
Mrs. A has a respiratory acidosis.

Example 2: Mr. B has a $PaCO_2 = 28$ and a pH = 7.52.
The $PaCO_2$ is decreased by 12 mmHg. The pH is increased by 0.12.
In respiratory alkalosis, the $PaCO_2$ and the pH move in opposite directions, so:
Mr. B has a respiratory alkalosis.

Example 3: Ms. C has a $PaCO_2 = 52$ and a pH = 7.48.
The $PaCO_2$ is increased. The pH is also increased.
Because both the $PaCO_2$ and the pH are elevated (moving in the same direction), it cannot be a respiratory problem. If it isn't a respiratory problem, then it has to be a *metabolic derangement*. (This is known even though a value for bicarbonate hasn't been given.)

CHART 19–3 Examples of Abnormalities of the Metabolic Component

Example 1: Mr. E has a HCO_3^- of 16 and a pH of 7.24.
Base excess = −6.
The bicarbonate and the pH are both decreased. In a metabolic acidosis, the bicarbonate and the pH move in the same direction.
This is a metabolic acidosis. The base excess of −6 indicates that every liter of Mr. E's extracellular fluid needs 6 mEq of additional bicarbonate to normalize the pH.

Example 2: Mr. F has a HCO_3^- of 34 mEq and a pH of 7.50.
Base excess = +5.
The bicarbonate and the pH are both elevated. In metabolic alkalosis, the bicarbonate and the pH move in the same direction.
This is a metabolic alkalosis. The base excess of +5 indicates that every liter of Mr. F's extracellular fluid has 5 mEq too much bicarbonate or other anion.
(A base excess is not as clinically helpful as a base deficit. A specific number of milliequivalents of bicarbonate cannot be dialyzed or otherwise removed and acids are rarely administered to patients to correct a metabolic alkalosis.)

bicarbonate-to-carbonic acid and bring the pH back toward normal. If the primary problem is a metabolic abnormality, the lungs will increase or decrease total minute ventilation to attempt to bring the pH back toward normal. If the cause of the problem is respiratory, the kidneys will retain or secrete hydrogen ion and/or bicarbonate to restore balance.

Because renal/metabolic compensation is slower, taking hours to days, one can infer whether a respiratory abnormality is an acute problem or a chronic one. If the kidneys have not had enough time to compensate, the problem is acute. If metabolic compensation has taken place, the problem is likely to be a chronic one. Once the primary cause has been identified (CO_2 or HCO_3^-), look at the other value. If that parameter is abnormal, but is moving in a direction that would bring the pH back toward normal, then compensation is occurring. If the pH is in the normal range, then complete compensation has occurred. If the pH is not within the normal range, but moving in the right direction, then partial compensation has occurred. See Chart 19–4 for a summary of the blood gas changes seen in respiratory and metabolic disturbances.

Complex Acid–Base Disorders

Sometimes patients will have combined disorders. For example, a critically ill patient who has recently suffered a cardiac arrest

may have both a respiratory and a metabolic acidosis. It can be helpful, sometimes, to look at the magnitude of the change in the CO_2 or HCO_3^- and compare it to the expected change in the pH. A simple rule of thumb to use is this: For every 10 mmHg change in the $PaCO_2$, there should be a corresponding pH change of 0.08 to 0.1 in the opposite direction. Using the 0.1 is easiest to calculate:

$$Normal\ PaCO_2 = 40;\ normal\ pH = 7.40$$

If the $PaCO_2$ increases to 50 (a change of 10 mmHg from normal), the pH should decrease by 0.10 to 7.30 if there is only a respiratory acidosis. Conversely, if the $PaCO_2$ decreases to 22 (a change of 18 mmHg from normal), the pH should increase to 7.58, a 0.18 increase, if there is only a respiratory alkalosis. However, if the $PaCO_2$ increases to 50 (a change of 10 mmHg), but the pH is 7.15 (a change of 0.25), this change in the pH is much greater than it would be if there was a respiratory acidosis alone. In this case, a concurrent metabolic acidosis must be causing the large drop in pH with a rather moderate increase in the $PaCO_2$.

Acid–Base Imbalances

Imbalances between acids and bases almost always occur as a result of diseases, organ dysfunction, or other pathologic conditions. The following descriptions of the four imbalances

CHART 19–4 Blood Gas Changes in Acid–Base Imbalances

Acid–Base Disorder	pH Normal = 7.35–7.45	$PaCO_2$ Normal = 35–45 mmHg	HCO_3^- Normal = 22–28 mEq/L
Respiratory acidosis	↓	↑	Normal (↑'d if compensating)
Respiratory alkalosis	↑	↓	Normal (↓'d if compensating)
Metabolic acidosis	↓	Normal (↓'d if compensating)	↓
Metabolic alkalosis	↑	Normal (↑'d if compensating)	↑

Note: $PaCO_2$ and pH move in *opposite* directions. HCO_3^- and pH move in the *same* direction.

describe them as distinct abnormalities, but they must be evaluated in the context of the patient's underlying pathology when caring for patients in the clinical setting. Chart 19–5 summarizes the causes of acid–base imbalances.

Respiratory Acidosis

Also referred to as primary hypercapnia, the primary derangement of acid–base balance in this situation is an excess of arterial CO_2 accompanied by a decrease in the pH. The CO_2 is regulated in part by the respiratory rate. When respirations increase, the CO_2 decreases and vice versa with a decreased respiratory rate, thereby increasing the CO_2.

Etiology and Pathophysiology

Whenever excretion of CO_2 via the lungs fails to keep up with the body's CO_2 production, respiratory acidosis will occur. This respiratory system failure may be *acute*, occurring rapidly due to a sudden event. In this situation, the elevation in the $PaCO_2$ results in acidemia and a low pH. Respiratory acidosis may also be *chronic*, where there has been a sustained increase in the $PaCO_2$ that leads to renal compensation and elevated serum bicarbonate. Causes of acute and chronic ventilatory failure are noted in Chart 19–6.

Most of these conditions impair the lung's ability to eliminate CO_2 by impairing ventilation. Conditions that cause alveolar hypoventilation can be categorized as being due to a decreased respiratory drive (patients who "won't breathe") or a decrease in respiratory muscle or chest wall function (patients who "can't breathe"). Normally, an increase in the $PaCO_2$ leads to a marked increase in the ventilatory drive. If there is an abnormality of ventilatory control, there will be an inappropriately low to absent ventilatory drive despite elevations in the $PaCO_2$. This can occur with a neurological event such as cerebral anoxia or from depression of the respiratory centers by drugs such as narcotics.

Another influence on the respiratory drive is the level of CNS arousal. During non–rapid eye movement (NREM) sleep, the ventilatory response to $PaCO_2$ is blunted and the minute ventilation decreases, primarily secondary to a lower tidal volume. The $PaCO_2$ can increase by about 3 to 10 mmHg. This is not clinically a problem unless the person suffers from preexisting hypercapnia, in which case respiratory acidosis may worsen.

Chest wall or respiratory muscle abnormalities can be the result of CNS disorders, neuromuscular disorders, or restrictive lung conditions such as pulmonary fibrosis. These conditions can lead to acute or chronic hypoventilation. A condition worth noting in this category is obesity hypoventilation syndrome. Some people who are morbidly obese, which is defined as having a body mass index (BMI) > 40, have a syndrome that is characterized by chronic hypoventilation and chronic respiratory failure. Chronic respiratory failure develops over a longer period of time, allowing for renal compensation by the retention of bicarbonate. Chapter 36 👁 discusses the diagnosis and treatment of respiratory failure. These patients have a decreased ventilatory drive and an increased work of breathing. This work of breathing increase is due to a reduction in lung compliance ("stretchiness") and abdominal influences. These persons are prone to the development of obstructive sleep apnea, which causes both hypoventilation and hypoxemia. Chapter 34 👁 describes obstructive sleep apnea.

CHART 19–5 | **Causes of Acid–Base Disorders**

Acute Respiratory Acidosis	Metabolic Acidosis
CNS Depression Drug overdose Head trauma Encephalitis Stroke	**Excess H+ Production** Lactic acidosis due to tissue hypoxia Ketoacidosis: diabetic, alcoholic, starvation
Neuromuscular Disease Guillain-Barré syndrome Myasthenic crisis Spinal cord injury	**Ingestion of Acids** Poisoning with agents such as ethylene glycol (antifreeze) or aspirin
Airway Disease Status asthmaticus Upper airway obstruction	**Inadequate Acid Excretion** Renal dysfunction Endocrine disturbances (e.g., hypoaldosteronism)
Pleural or Chest Wall Abnormalities Pneumothorax Large pleural effusion	**Excessive Loss of Bicarbonate** Excessive diarrhea Acetazolamide

Chronic Respiratory Acidosis

Impaired Central Ventilatory Drive
Central sleep apnea
Obesity hypoventilation

Neuromuscular Disease
Amyotrophic lateral sclerosis
Muscular dystrophy
Poliomyelitis
Multiple sclerosis
Spinal cord injury

Airway and Lung Parenchyma Disease
Emphysema
Chronic bronchitis
Interstitial lung disease

Other:
Kyphoscoliosis
Diaphragmatic paralysis

Respiratory Alkalosis	Metabolic Alkalosis
Central Nervous System Pain Anxiety Psychosis Fever Stroke Meningitis, encephalitis Tumor Trauma Hypoxemia	**Excessive Loss of H+** Protracted vomiting Nasogastric suction **Acid Shifts into Cells** Potassium deficiency **Excessive Reabsorption of Bicarbonate** Hypochloremia Thiazide and loop diuretics
Drugs Salicylates, nicotine, progesterone Pregnancy Sepsis Hepatic failure Iatrogenic on mechanical ventilation	

CHART 19–6 **Causes of Hypercapnic Ventilatory Failure**

Site of Disturbance	Acute	Chronic
Respiratory center	Drug overdose Trauma Stroke	Tumor
Neuromuscular disease	Guillain-Barré syndrome Myasthenia gravis	Polio Spinal cord injury Amyotrophic lateral sclerosis
Chest wall	Trauma Pleural effusion (large) Pneumothorax	Kyphoscoliosis
Upper airway obstruction	Tumor Laryngeal edema Foreign body	
Peripheral airway obstruction	Asthma (severe)	Emphysema Chronic bronchitis Obesity Hypoventilation

Aside from conditions that cause alveolar hypoventilation, respiratory acidosis can result from an increase in pathologic dead space. The matching of alveolar ventilation to the perfusion of the pulmonary capillaries is most important to the maintenance of normal oxygenation, but it is also important to the maintenance of CO_2 balance. The CO_2 must be delivered from the tissues via the blood to the lungs so it can be excreted. The elimination of CO_2 decreases when perfusion to a segment of the lungs is reduced, such as occurs with a pulmonary embolism or pulmonary vascular disease. This is usually not clinically a problem because the ventilatory centers will increase the rate and depth of ventilation to compensate.

As discussed earlier, anatomic dead space is that portion of the inhaled volume that remains in the large conducting airways and does not take part in the exchange of oxygen and CO_2. The anatomic dead space is a fixed volume, so increase in the tidal volume will increase the alveolar ventilation. Conversely, a decreased tidal volume will result in less air reaching the alveoli and can result in hypercapnia and respiratory acidosis. In acute respiratory failure, patients often resort to a pattern of rapid, shallow breathing that can lead to a higher proportion of dead space to tidal volume. This also is the pattern of breathing seen with neuromuscular disease such as Guillain-Barré syndrome and amyotrophic lateral sclerosis (Priestley & Levine, 2006). Other causes of increased dead space include decreased lung perfusion as noted previously and destruction of pulmonary parenchyma by diseases such as emphysema and pulmonary fibrosis.

In chronic obstructive pulmonary diseases such as emphysema or chronic bronchitis, elevations in the $PaCO_2$ are thought to be a poor prognostic sign. With emphysema, there is decreased surface area for gas exchange that first leads to a decrease in arterial oxygenation, but, in the most severe cases, also leads to chronic hypercapnia. Air trapping in the alveolar airspaces also leads to lung hyperinflation. This hyperinflation flattens out the diaphragm, which, in the relaxed position, is shaped like an upside-down bowl. When the lungs are permanently inflated, this flattened diaphragm impairs the person's ability to generate negative inspiratory pressure, which is needed to pull air into the lungs. This leads to impaired ventilation and greatly contributes to the sensation of breathlessness from which these patients suffer. (Try this yourself: Take a deep breath in and hold it. Now take in more air. Hard, isn't it? And very uncomfortable.)

In some conditions the major problem is increased production of CO_2, rather than impaired elimination. These conditions include exercise, fever, burns, and thyrotoxicosis and catabolic states such as are seen with multiple-organ failure. Using fever as an example, for every degree of temperature elevation, CO_2 production increases by about 13%. Thus, a patient with a fever of 40°C (104°F) must increase alveolar ventilation by about 40% to maintain a normal $PaCO_2$. Increased CO_2 production rarely leads to hypercapnia in otherwise healthy persons because increased production leads to increased ventilation and subsequent CO_2 excretion. Patients with preexisting pulmonary diseases, however, may not be able to increase their ventilation enough to handle the excess CO_2 and their levels will rise.

In acute respiratory acidosis, cellular buffering occurs over minutes to hours. Renal compensation occurs over several days. The kidneys reabsorb bicarbonate and excrete acid. The plasma bicarbonate increases about 3.5 mEq/L for each increase of 10 mmHg in the $PaCO_2$. In acidemia, hydrogen ion moves into cells and displaces K^+ out of the cell into the serum, although respiratory acidosis does not usually cause clinically significant hyperkalemia.

Signs, Symptoms, and Consequences

Acute hypercapnia can be life threatening when it causes severe respiratory acidosis. This usually occurs in conjunction with hypoxemia. Carbon dioxide crosses cell membranes rapidly and leads to a low intracellular pH, which can affect many body systems. CNS symptoms dominate and their severity depends on the magnitude of the increase, the speed with which it occurs, and the accompanying degree of hypoxemia. Carbon dioxide rapidly crosses the blood–brain barrier and lowers CSF pH. The acute effects are cerebral vessel dilation, increased cerebral blood flow, and increased intracranial pressure. Clinical manifestations of these changes include anxiety, irritability, headache, confusion, disorientation, somnolence, and lethargy. Patients may complain of dyspnea. More serious alterations of consciousness such as stupor or coma are rare but are seen when the $PaCO_2$ is markedly elevated, typically more than 70 to 100 mmHg (Priestley & Levine, 2006).

The other major organ system that may be affected in respiratory acidosis is the cardiovascular system. Mild to moderate hypercapnia causes release of the catecholamines epinephrine and norepinephrine and peripheral vasodilation. Catecholamines usually cause peripheral vasoconstriction, but the elevated CO_2 has an inhibitory effect on vascular smooth muscle, which leads to vasodilation. These changes results in an increase in heart rate with normal or elevated blood pressure. Because of the peripheral vasodilation, the patient's skin is often warm, flushed, and diaphoretic.

In chronic hypercapnia, the effects are not as dramatic because organ systems have a chance to adapt and renal compensation has time to occur. The cerebral blood flow returns to normal and the only symptom may be a morning headache, mild irritability, and lethargy. It is important to remember that patients with chronic respiratory failure may develop acute respiratory failure as well. If a patient with a chronically high level of CO_2 presents with an acid pH, he is suffering from acute respiratory failure. See examples in Chart 19–7.

Medical Management

Acid–base disturbances are rarely isolated conditions; they usually accompany other pathophysiologic processes. The main treatment for respiratory acidosis is correction of the underlying disorder that led to its development. This might include a reversal of a drug overdose to counteract respiratory depression, the use of inhaled bronchodilators and steroids to treat the bronchospasm that accompanies acute asthma, or the use of antibiotics to treat pneumonia and improve ventilation, thus correcting the acidosis. Administration of sodium bicarbonate is almost never indicated in the treatment of respiratory acidosis because the bicarbonate will eventually be converted to CO_2. Thus, in the long run, it can actually worsen a respiratory acidosis although, its use may be considered in the situation of cardiac arrest with extremely low pH (<7.0 to 7.1). In this situation, metabolic acidosis is usually combined with respiratory acidosis (Priestley & Levine, 2006). The metabolic acidosis is a lactic acidosis that results from anaerobic metabolism that occurs because of the lack of tissue perfusion during cardiac arrest.

Treatment also is aimed at assisting or increasing ventilation. This can be accomplished invasively through endotracheal intubation and the use of mechanical ventilation or noninvasively through the use of nasal continuous positive airway pressure (CPAP) or nasal bilevel ventilation (BiPAP).

Bilevel Positive Airway Pressure

BiPAP is a noninvasive method of assisting ventilation in children and adults with chronic hypoventilation. The system consists of a blower or compressor attached via tubing to a cushioned nose mask that is held to the face with an elastic headband or a specially designed cap. Patients with sleep-related hypoventilation disorders may only need to use the device at bedtime, whereas others may need the system for longer periods of time. Chapter 36 ⊘ discusses BiPAP. When positive pressure is applied to the nasopharynx, the soft palate comes in contact with the tongue. These structures are held together and

pushed forward away from the posterior wall of the pharynx, effectively sealing off the oral cavity from the wall of the oropharynx. This prevents air from leaking out through the patient's mouth.

In BiPAP, one level of positive pressure is applied during inspiration and another (lower) level is applied during expiration. In the system, the clinician sets:

- Inspiratory positive airway pressure (IPAP): between 2 and 25 cmH_2O
- Expiratory positive airway pressure (EPAP): between 2 and 20 cmH_2O
- The frequency of the cycling: usually between 6 and 30 cycle/min
- The percentage of IPAP-to-EPAP: set between 10% and 90%, but is usually around 40%. This means that for 40% of the time of each respiratory cycle, the pressure delivered is the IPAP and 60% of the time it is the EPAP. This percentage of IPAP to EPAP is titrated to achieve the optimum tidal volume with each breath.

The difference between the two pressures is referred to as the *pressure boost* (PB). If the IPAP is 20 cmH_2O and the EPAP is 5 cmH_2O, then the PB would be 15 cmH_2O.

The system does have a backup mode that will kick in if the patient ceases to breathe.

The side effects are few although patients may complain of drying of the nasal mucosa, which can lead to nosebleeds. Pressure through the eustachian tubes can cause "ear popping" discomfort. If the mask is too tight or is not fitted properly, skin breakdown can occur at the bridge of the nose.

Intubation

There are no absolute criteria for deciding when to intubate someone in respiratory distress, but the general rule is that intubation is indicated if the patient has a $PaCO_2$ in the 80- to 90-mmHg range and a pH of less than 7.10 to 7.25. It is often a clinical decision based on the medical team's estimation of whether the patient will be able to keep on or will approach exhaustion. Once the patient is on mechanical ventilation, the patient can be supported while health care clinicians work to correct the underlying pathology. After treating the problem the patient can gradually be weaned off of the ventilatory support.

For patients with chronic hypercarbia, care must be taken when they are placed on mechanical ventilation to correct them slowly. Too efficient ventilation of the patient will correct the $PaCO_2$ too rapidly, and the patient will develop a metabolic alkalosis because of the excess retained bicarbonate. This can alkalinize the CSF and may cause seizures (Priestley & Levine, 2006). Chapter 36 ⊘ includes a discussion of the various modes of mechanical ventilation.

Supplemental Oxygen

Many patients with hypercapnea are also hypoxemic, so the use of supplemental oxygen may be indicated. It has been shown to decrease mortality and leads to better outcomes. The use of supplemental oxygen in patients with chronic respiratory acidosis, however, must be approached with caution. Because chronic hypercapnea blunts the central hypercarbic drive, these patients'

CHART 19–7 | **Acute Ventilatory Failure in the Patient Who Has Chronic Ventilatory Failure**

Example 1: Mr. T has $PaCO_2 = 60$, pH = 7.37, $HCO_3^- = 35$ mEq/L.
Despite the elevated $PaCO_2$, the pH is normal because the kidneys have retained bicarbonate.
In this patient's case, *Mr. T is at or near his baseline $PaCO_2$.*

Example 2: Ms. Y has $PaCO_2 = 73$, pH = 7.28, $HCO_3^- = 35$ mEq/L.
The $PaCO_2$ is elevated but the pH is acidic despite the elevated bicarbonate.
This $PaCO_2$ of 73 is higher than the patient's baseline. If it was her baseline, her pH would be at/close to the normal range.
This patient has an *acute respiratory failure superimposed on chronic respiratory failure.*

main stimulus to ventilation is the peripheral hypoxic drive. These patients breathe because their level of PaO_2 goes down. High levels of supplemental oxygen may blunt this hypoxic drive, leading to a further decrease in ventilation and a worsening of hypercapnea. Oxygen should be carefully administered to keep the oxygen saturation level in the low 90% range with a PaO_2 of 60 to 65 mmHg.

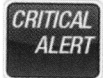 *Patients with chronic obstructive pulmonary disease who have chronically elevated levels of $PaCO_2$ may have a blunted hypercarbic drive. Their main stimulus of ventilation is the hypoxic drive. If a person who is a chronic CO_2 retainer receives a high concentration of supplemental oxygen that raises his PaO_2 above the stimulus level, respirations may be depressed. This does not mean that these patients should not receive oxygen if they are hypoxemic. It means clinicians have to be careful and monitor them more closely. (Note: This applies only to persons who are chronic CO_2 retainers. Not all patients who have chronic lung disease retain CO_2.)*

Respiratory Alkalosis

This acid–base derangement is characterized by a lower than normal $PaCO_2$ accompanied by an elevated pH. Respiratory rate is a major determinant of the $PaCO_2$ level. Excessively fast or deep ventilation "blows off" the carbon dioxide, decreasing the level and increasing the pH, causing alkalosis.

Etiology and Pathophysiology

Respiratory alkalosis is an acid–base disturbance caused by alveolar overventilation. The overventilation leads to a decreased $PaCO_2$, altering the 20:1 bicarbonate-to-carbonic acid ratio and causing an increased pH. The lungs are removing carbon dioxide faster than the tissues are producing it. This can be an acute or chronic problem. In acute respiratory alkalosis, the pH will be higher than normal. In chronic respiratory alkalosis, the $PaCO_2$ is lower than normal, but the pH is within normal limits because the kidneys have had time to eliminate bicarbonate and normalize the pH. This is renal compensation and it takes about 2 to 4 days to be completed.

Under normal circumstances, a drop in the $PaCO_2$ has an inhibitory effect on the central respiratory centers, but certain disease processes or psychological conditions can stimulate ventilation and lead to hypocapnia. Acute respiratory alkalosis leads to changes in serum electrolytes. Hydrogen ions shift from the intracellular compartment to the plasma. The positively charged hydrogen ions move out of cells in exchange for other positively charged ions, specifically potassium and phosphate, which move into the cells, resulting in hypokalemia and hypophosphatemia. There is also a reduction in free serum calcium because in alkalemia, there is increased binding of Ca^{2+} to serum albumin. Because the only calcium that is physiologically active is the free, nonionized calcium, the patient can develop symptoms of hypocalcemia.

Respiratory alkalosis is often caused by hypoxemia. When the PaO_2 drops, the peripheral chemoreceptors send impulses to the central respiratory control centers. They, in turn, increase ventilation in an attempt to raise the PaO_2. This increased ventilation, however, causes the patient to excrete too much CO_2. This same process occurs in the presence of a metabolic acidosis; the lungs increase ventilation to eliminate CO_2 and normalize the pH.

Neurological conditions such as a stroke, meningitis, encephalitis, head trauma, or tumor can lead to excessive ventilation. Psychological conditions such as anxiety and panic or severe pain can also cause overventilation. During pregnancy, progesterone levels are increased. This situation stimulates the respiratory center and can lead to respiratory alkalosis (Hayes, 2005). It also can be an iatrogenic problem resulting from inappropriate machine settings when the patient is on mechanical ventilation.

Signs, Symptoms, and Consequences

The signs and symptoms of respiratory alkalosis are nonspecific, and often vary according to the underlying illness or cause. Patients may appear anxious; tachycardia and tachypnea are common. CNS effects are due to the cerebral vessel vasoconstriction that occurs with alkalosis. This vasoconstriction causes a significant decrease in cerebral blood flow. Vertigo, anxiety, clumsiness, and forgetfulness are often seen. The cardiovascular effects are nonspecific, but may include tachycardia and atrial and/or ventricular arrhythmias (Hayes, 2005).

Alkalosis of any origin favors the binding of calcium to albumin. When there is increased binding of calcium, there is less free, ionized calcium in the serum. Because only free, ionized calcium is biologically active, any time there is less of it circulating, patients will exhibit signs and symptoms of hypocalcemia. Some of the symptoms seen with respiratory alkalosis symptoms may be the result of hypocalcemia and can include numbness and/or tingling around the mouth or in the hands and fingers. A positive Chvostek's sign or carpopedal (Trousseau's sign) spasm may be seen. Both Chvostek's sign and carpopedal spasm are discussed in Chapter 18 . Muscle cramps also may be experienced.

Medical Management

Treatment is primarily directed at correcting the underlying disorder. This is rarely a life-threatening abnormality and treatment is usually not indicated unless the pH is > 7.50 (DuBose, 2004). If the hypocapnia is secondary to a hypoxemia, supplemental oxygen should be administered. If the patient is on mechanical ventilation, the tidal volume and/or respiratory rate settings should be adjusted to decrease the minute ventilation to the point where the $PaCO_2$ is in the normal range. Chapter 36 includes a discussion of ventilator settings and their impact on the acid–base balance.

Patients with psychological hyperventilation syndromes should benefit from reassurance and methods to decrease stress. During acute episodes, it may be necessary to have them breathe into a paper bag, which causes people to "rebreathe" their CO_2 and minimize loss by ventilation. The nurse plays an important role by maintaining a calm, reassuring demeanor and explaining the reason for the rebreathing. Sedatives should be reserved for patients who do not respond to conservative treatment (Hayes, 2005).

Metabolic Acidosis

This disturbance is characterized by an increase in total body acid, leading to a decreased pH. Any disorder that alters metabolism in the body can contribute to the development of metabolic acidosis.

Etiology and Pathophysiology

Metabolic acidosis is a sign of some underlying disease process. It can be induced in two ways:

- An addition of hydrogen ions or an inability to excrete the H^+ load from dietary metabolism
- A primary decrease in plasma bicarbonate to < 22 mEq/L.

The increased hydrogen ion load can come from numerous sources; lactic acidosis is believed to be the most common cause of metabolic acidosis in the hospitalized patient (Casaletto, 2005). It represents an imbalance between lactate production and utilization. Tissue hypoxia is the most common cause of clinically significant lactic acidosis. The tissue hypoxia is the result of increased oxygen demand or decreased oxygen delivery to body tissues. Without oxygen, tissues resort to anaerobic metabolism. In the face of anaerobic metabolism, body tissues are unable to completely oxidize sugar to CO_2; instead, sugars are partially oxidized to lactic acid. This acid cannot be excreted via the lungs; therefore, it remains in the circulation and causes a metabolic acidosis.

Ketoacidosis from uncontrolled diabetes mellitus, alcoholism, or prolonged starvation can also cause an accumulation of the ketone bodies acetoacetic acid and beta-hydroxybutyric acid. Ingestion of toxins such as a salicylate (aspirin) overdose, methanol, and ethylene glycol (antifreeze) will also cause metabolic acidosis.

A certain amount of acid is produced when dietary proteins are metabolized. These proteins contain sulfate and phosphate groups that, after metabolism, form sulfuric and phosphoric acid. These acids normally amount to about 150 mEq/day and they must be excreted through kidney filtration. If the kidneys fail, acidosis will occur in several days (Casaletto, 2005).

A failure to excrete the hydrogen ion load may be due to renal damage at several sections of the nephron. The term *renal tubular acidosis* refers to a group of renal pathologies that result in diminished hydrogen ion excretion or excess renal loss of bicarbonate. Type 1 renal tubular acidosis (RTA) is referred to as classic RTA or distal RTA because the malfunction is at the level of the distal convoluted tubule. The problem here is an inability to maximally acidify urine. This can be due to an inability of the H^+ pump to work against the osmotic gradient, back-diffusion of the hydrogen ion through leaky tubules, or an insufficient hydrogen ion pumping capacity due to tubular damage. There is low acid secretion and continued excretion of bicarbonate at a time when it should be retained. There is also loss of sodium and potassium in the urine (DuBose, 2004).

Type 2 RTA is also called proximal renal tubular acidosis because the site of damage is the proximal convoluted tubule. The pathology here results in impaired reabsorption of bicarbonate in the proximal tubule. The result is a high urinary bicarbonate loss, a systemic acidosis, and an inappropriately alkaline urine pH. There is accompanying renal loss of potassium that can lead to systemic hypokalemia.

Type 4 RTA is associated with a number of different conditions, but most patients with this pathology have renal failure that results in damage to the renal interstitium and tubules. Here, the defect causes impaired exchange of cations in the distal tubules. This results in reduced secretion of both hydrogen ion and potassium, which may result in hyperkalemia as well as

acidosis (DuBose, 2004). (*Note:* There is a Type 3 RTA, but it is a rare variant of Type I RTA seen exclusively in children and not clinically relevant to the discussion here.)

When assessing a patient with metabolic acidosis, it is helpful to calculate the **anion gap**. The anion gap concept is based on the principle of **electroneutrality**. The sum of all of the cationic (positive) charges in the plasma must always be equal to the sum of all of the anionic (negative) charges. However, not all ions are measured and reported by the laboratory. The primary cations that are measured in venous plasma are sodium and potassium; the main anions are chloride and bicarbonate or serum CO_2. Typically, there are more unmeasured anions than cations. This difference is referred to as the anion gap. Several other anions that are not normally measured include phosphates, sulfates, organic ions, and proteins (Bartlett, 2005). Those anions make up the anion gap, which is calculated in one of two ways:

$$(Na^+ + K^+) - (Cl^- + HCO_3^-)$$

or

$$Na^+ - (Cl^- + HCO_3^-)$$

Because the value of potassium is so small, 4 mEq/L, it is sometimes ignored when calculating the anion gap. A normal anion gap is 10 ± 4 when K^+ is not included in the equation, although different sources cite different values for this "normal":

$$(Na^+) - (Cl^- + HCO_3^-)$$
$$140 - (105 + 22) = 13$$

Figure 19–3 ■ graphically depicts the anion gap.

If the anion gap is abnormally large, there are more negative ions than can be explained by the usual unmeasured substances. These extra negative substances are often lactate or the ketone bodies seen with diabetic ketoacidosis: acetoacetic acid and/or

Na⁺ 140 mEq	Cl⁻ 105 mEq
K⁺ 4 mEq	HCO₃⁻ 22 mEq
	Anion Gap

OR

Anions and Cations in Serum

The equivalents of cations in a solution always balances the equivalents of anions

Cations	Anions	
Sodium 140	Chloride 105	
Potassium 4.5	Bicarbonate 24	
Calcium 5	Other = 22	⎤ Anion gap
Magnesium 1.5		
Total = 151	Total = 151	

FIGURE 19–3 ■ Anion gap.

beta-hydroxybutyric acid. In this situation, termed *high anion gap acidosis,* the acid dissociates into hydrogen ion and unmeasured anion. The hydrogen ion is buffered by bicarbonate while the unmeasured ion accumulates in the serum. For example:

$$pH = 7.1 \ Na^+ = 145 \ K^+ = 5 \ Cl^- = 97 \ HCO_3^- = 12$$

$$Gap \ = \ 145 \ - \ (97 \ + \ 12)$$

$$Gap \ = \ 36$$

This significant elevation indicates high anion gap acidosis. Sometimes, calculating the anion gap will help identify a metabolic acidosis even when the pH is normal. High anion gap acidosis can also be caused by ingestion of salicylate, methanol, ethylene glycol (antifreeze), or other substances (DuBose, 2004).

If the patient has metabolic acidosis, but the anion gap is within normal limits, the problem is likely to be a loss of bicarbonate rather than an excess of acid. This occurs with gastrointestinal losses of bicarbonate such as that seen with extensive diarrhea or bowel fistulae that cause high output of lower GI fluids. The intestinal fluids beyond the stomach, including pancreatic and biliary secretions, are alkaline and consist of both bicarbonate and other organic anions. When these fluids are absorbed through the intestine, they are converted to bicarbonate in normal metabolism. If these fluids are lost through diarrhea or fistula output, the bicarbonate cannot be reclaimed and pH falls. This scenario also is typically associated with an increase in plasma chloride concentrations. The chloride ions replace plasma bicarbonate. Urinary diversions, such as a ureterosigmoidostomy, can cause hyperchloremic metabolic acidosis in as many as 80% of patients. The colon has an anion exchanger that exchanges HCO_3^- for the high chloride usually found in urine. So, when the urine is diverted to the colon, the urinary chloride is exchanged for bicarbonate, which is then lost in urine. In addition, the colon can directly absorb ammonia (NH_4), which is derived from urine and colonic bacteria. The absorbed NH_4 is converted into NH_3 and hydrogen ion in the liver, leading to hydrogen ion excess (Thomas & Kahled, 2007).

Signs, Symptoms, and Consequences

Patients with metabolic acidosis often complain of dyspnea because of the Kussmaul respirations that occur as the respiratory system tries to compensate. Tachypnea and hyperpnea (deeper than normal respirations) are usually prominent. If the acidosis is severe with a pH < 7.10, patients may develop potentially serious or fatal cardiac dysrhythmias such as ventricular tachycardia. This abnormality may also reduce cardiac contractility and lead to hypotension and heart failure.

Neurological symptoms are nonspecific, but may be manifestations of the underlying cause of the metabolic acidosis, particularly if it is associated with the ingestion of toxic substances such as ethylene glycol or methanol. Patients may complain of headache, visual changes, or mental confusion. Gastrointestinal symptoms include nausea and vomiting, abdominal pain, diarrhea, anorexia, and weight loss (Stavile et al., 2005). Chronic metabolic acidosis such as that associated with uremia or renal tubular acidosis is associated with bone disease due to the buffering of calcium carbonate and increases the risk of fractures in adults.

Laboratory studies used in the evaluation of metabolic acidosis include an ABG, which shows a low pH and low HCO_3^- as well as a base deficit more negative than −3. (Remember that bicarbonate and pH move in the *same* direction.) If the lungs have increased their alveolar ventilation to attempt to compensate for the acidosis, the $PaCO_2$ may also be lower than normal.

A metabolic panel with electrolyte assay is required when assessing patients in metabolic acidosis. The serum sodium, potassium, chloride, and bicarbonate levels are useful when calculating the anion gap. Hyperkalemia often complicates a metabolic acidosis. The excess hydrogen ions cross cell membranes and enter the intracellular space. They, in turn, "bump out" potassium ions, which are in high concentrations inside the cell. Glucose levels will be elevated in the presence of diabetic ketoacidosis; the blood urea nitrogen (BUN) and creatinine will be elevated in uremic acidosis.

Medical Management

The treatment of metabolic acidosis is directed at the correction or treatment of the underlying disorder or cause. The use of alkalinizing therapy is rarely indicated except in the most severe, life-threatening instances. In many cases, the treatment of the underlying cause and the restoration of intravascular volume and arterial oxygenation will be enough to allow for the metabolism of the organic acids (lactate and ketoacids) back to bicarbonate or for the kidney to regenerate new bicarbonate to replace the losses (Black, 2003).

The administration of sodium bicarbonate in acute metabolic acidosis is controversial. Recent studies have shown that giving bicarbonate is ineffective and may actually be detrimental to the patient's welfare (Stavile et al., 2005). The problem is that, when exogenous bicarbonate is administered to a patient who is acidemic, the bicarbonate reacts with hydrogen ions to form carbonic acid. The carbonic acid then dissociates into CO_2 and water, so the $PaCO_2$ rises. When the CO_2 cannot be eliminated, the pH correction will be very slight, or it may become more acidotic.

Metabolic Alkalosis

Metabolic alkalosis is characterized by a primary elevation in the plasma bicarbonate accompanied by an elevated pH. In metabolic imbalances, bicarbonate and pH move in the *same* direction. If bicarbonate is elevated, the pH will be elevated. If bicarbonate is decreased, the pH will decrease. The mortality of severe metabolic alkalosis is quite high, 45% in patients with an arterial pH of 7.55 and 80% when the pH is greater than 7.65 (Yaseen & Thomas, 2006).

Etiology and Pathophysiology

Metabolic alkalosis is caused by pathologic processes that lead to an accumulation of base or a loss of acid in the extracellular fluid. The increase in arterial pH usually causes a depression of the rate and depth of ventilation. This results in an increase in the $PaCO_2$ and a buffering of the alkalemia, which is the respiratory compensation component. Respiratory compensation for metabolic alkalosis is limited, however, because the respiratory center will not depress respiration to the point where oxygenation begins to suffer.

Metabolic alkalosis is a relatively common disorder that is seen with diuretic use or the loss of gastric secretions due to excessive vomiting or nasogastric suction. It also can be caused by alkali administration, loss of hydrogen from extracellular fluid, or depletion of electrolytes such as chloride or potassium, or from intravascular volume depletion.

In addition to the primary pathology, factors must be present that increase the reabsorption of bicarbonate from the kidneys. An excess of bicarbonate or "base loading" is rarely a sole cause of significant persistent metabolic alkalosis because the normal kidney is very efficient at excreting bicarbonate (Yaseen & Thomas, 2006). Transient alkalosis may occur after a patient has received oral or intravenous $NaHCO_3^-$ or a basic/alkaline equivalent such as citrate. Citrate is used as the anticoagulant in transfused blood and fresh frozen plasma. When patients receive multiple blood or plasma transfusions, they receive a significant amount of citrate and this can lead to a metabolic alkalosis. Metabolic alkalosis also may occur temporarily in patients with a chronic respiratory acidosis who have been placed on mechanical ventilation and whose $PaCO_2$ has been corrected too rapidly, before their kidneys have had a chance to excrete the excess bicarbonate.

Loss of hydrogen can occur from the GI tract or in urine. Gastric contents have high concentrations of hydrochloric acid (HCl^-) and a smaller amount of potassium chloride (KCl^-). Gastric hydrogen secretion stimulates, and is matched by, pancreatic bicarbonate secretion. When the acid contents of the stomach pass through the pylorus into the duodenum, they stimulate the pancreas to secrete lytic enzymes and bicarbonate. This bicarbonate neutralizes the acidity of the stomach contents. If the patient suffers excessive vomiting or the gastric secretions are removed by nasogastric suction before they can pass into the duodenum, there is no stimulus to the secretion of bicarbonate and it accumulates.

An excess loss of hydrogen in urine can be caused by a number of pathologic conditions or as a side effect of therapies. An increase in the secretion of the mineralocorticoid aldosterone causes an increased reabsorption of sodium from the kidney tubule back into the kidney interstitium. Under normal conditions, when a person has abnormally low blood pressure, the renin-angiotensin system is stimulated. Angiotensin release stimulates the release of aldosterone, which, in turn, promotes the reabsorption of sodium from kidney tubules. As the sodium is reabsorbed, water follows with it and the intravascular fluid volume increases, thus helping to increase blood pressure. This reabsorption of Na^+, a positive ion, renders the lumen of the tubule more electronegative. Because the lumen is now more negative, hydrogen ion stays in the tubule (again, think of the interior of the kidney tubule as being outside the body). When hydrogen ion reabsorption is inhibited, more of it is lost in the urine. An excess of mineralocorticoids (so named because they affect mineral metabolism) can be seen with primary conditions such as primary aldosteronism or as a secondary problem of many conditions including malignant hypertension or renal cell carcinoma (Black, 2003). Certain classes of diuretics, the loop (so named because they act on the nephron of the kidney at the site of the loop of Henle) or thiazide diuretics, can cause an increased secretion of aldosterone and lead to increased urinary hydrogen secretion as well as decreased intravascular volume.

Chloride helps to maintain the balance of cations to anions in the extracellular fluid to maintain electroneutrality. It does this through its inverse relationship with bicarbonate. If excessive amounts of bicarbonate ions (anions) accumulate, the number of chloride ions (also anions) decreases to maintain the number of negative charges. If sodium ions (cations) increase,

the number of chloride ions increases as well, to maintain the balance of positive to negative charges. Chloride and sodium work together; sodium and bicarbonate have an inverse relationship. If serum sodium goes down, chloride also decreases. Chloride losses result in an increase in bicarbonate. Chloride depletion may occur through the loss of gastric secretions, which are rich in chloride ions, or through the kidneys with the loop or thiazide diuretics.

Hypokalemia participates in perpetuating metabolic alkalosis in several ways. When there is a decrease of K^+ in the extracellular fluid, hydrogen ions shift to the intracellular compartment to keep the electrical charge balanced. This makes the inside of the cells acidic. This intracellular acidosis stimulates reabsorption of bicarbonate from the collecting of the kidney. Hypokalemia stimulates an enzyme that promotes potassium ion reabsorption, but the potassium is exchanged for hydrogen ion, the loss of which leads to alkalosis (DuBose, 2004).

When a patient is hypovolemic and has lost relatively large volumes of bicarbonate-free fluid, this can lead to contraction alkalosis. The plasma bicarbonate concentration rises because there is a contraction of the extracellular volume around a relatively constant quantity of bicarbonate. This can occur when a loop diuretic is given to induce rapid fluid removal from a very edematous patient (Rose, 2005). To simplify this, think of a cup of water containing 4 tablespoons of sugar. If one-third cup of the water is poured off, leaving the same 4 tablespoons of sugar, the water will be much sweeter because it has a higher concentration of sugar.

Signs, Symptoms, and Consequences

The symptoms of metabolic alkalosis are difficult to separate from the symptoms of the chloride volume or potassium depletion. The effect on the CNS is the same as with respiratory alkalosis. Cerebral vessels constrict and cerebral blood flow is decreased. This can lead to lethargy, confusion, and/or apathy. If the alkalemia is very severe, coma or seizures may result (Yaseen & Thomas, 2006). The respiratory centers are depressed to attempt compensation, decreasing alveolar ventilation. This decrease in tidal volume can lead to problems with atelectasis and may contribute to the development of pulmonary infection in very ill or immunocompromised patients.

The increased binding of calcium to albumin described in the earlier section about respiratory alkalosis also occurs with metabolic alkalosis. This may lead to neuromuscular irritability resulting in muscle twitching, muscle spasm, and tetany. Positive Chvostek and Trousseau's signs may be present.

Metabolic alkalosis has effects on cardiac function. Myocardial contractility is depressed. Electrocardiogram (ECG) changes include prolongation of the QT interval as well as atrial and ventricular arrhythmias. Hypokalemia and hypomagnesemia often coexist with metabolic alkalosis and these electrolyte imbalances may exacerbate the effect of the alkalosis on cardiac function and rhythm (Yaseen & Thomas, 2006).

The diagnosis of the cause of metabolic alkalosis is usually discerned from the patient's history. A history of vomiting or the use of nasogastric suction or diuretic therapy is easily uncovered during a careful patient history. Sometimes, however, no obvious cause can be found. This may be due to a patient's surreptitious use of diuretics or self-induced vomiting, or to conditions that cause excess mineralocorticoids, usually aldosterone. With vomiting or diuretic use, intravascular volume depletion generally occurs; with hyperaldosteronism, mild volume expansion is usually present.

Medical Management

Once the origin of the metabolic alkalosis is determined, the treatment is quite obvious. Treatment is aimed at correcting the volume depletion, the potassium depletion, or the chloride depletion. In patients with low intravascular volume due to vomiting, gastric suction, or diuretic use, the administration of sodium chloride can correct the dehydration and replete the chloride. Any other electrolyte deficits should be corrected by replacing them. The administration of potassium chloride is important in the correction of metabolic alkalosis. This exogenous (from the outside the body) potassium moves into body cells in exchange for hydrogen ion to maintain electroneutrality. This hydrogen ion buffers excess extracellular bicarbonate in the serum, bringing pH down toward normal. In addition, the correction of intracellular acidosis in renal tubular cells reduces the secretion of hydrogen ion and the reabsorption of bicarbonate (Yaseen & Thomas, 2006).

If the primary cause is an excess of mineralocorticoid, steroids may be used to suppress hormone secretion or the patient may be given the drug spironolactone. Spironolactone is a synthetic steroid with a structure much like that of aldosterone. It acts as a competitive antagonist at the aldosterone receptors in the kidney. This drug is administered until definitive therapy is undertaken to treat the primary disorder (Black, 2003). If the patient is on hemodialysis, the bath solution used for dialysis can be made more acidic. If the patient has posthypercapnic alkalosis, the administration of the drug acetazolamide can speed up the renal elimination of excess bicarbonate.

In very rare cases of severe alkalosis, the administration of intravenous hydrochloric acid may be indicated. This intravenous HCl will buffer excess bicarbonate. This is usually administered over a period of about 24 hours and must be given into a major central vein due to its corrosive nature.

Nursing Management

Disorders of acid–base balance do not exist in a vacuum; instead they are a product of other underlying pathology. The nurse must be aware of patients who are at risk for acid–base disorders. The risk may be from the disorder itself or from a clinical manifestation such as fever, vomiting, diarrhea, age, and sepsis. The risk may be due to a treatment such as diuretics, mechanical ventilation, and total parental nutrition or enteral nutrition that is high in carbohydrates. Finally, the risk could be due to comorbid conditions such as respiratory or cardiac disorders or diabetes. The older adult may have multiple risk factors present from all three categories. The nursing care outlined in Nursing Process: Patient Care Plan for Acid–Base Imbalances (p. 450) must be incorporated into a larger plan of care that addresses the primary pathology or disorder. The Nursing Process: Patient Care Plan box (p. 450) outlines the nursing care required for patients experiencing acid–base disorders. Caring for elderly patients who may have acid–base imbalances is discussed in the Gerontological Considerations box.

GERONTOLOGICAL CONSIDERATIONS: Related to Acid–Base Imbalances in the Elderly

The normal pH range of extra cellular fluid (ECF) is not affected by advanced age. Some changes in respiratory and renal function, however, may affect acid–base balance. These lung and kidney changes are more likely to affect the body's ability to respond to a physiological challenge with compensation may be blunted.

In the lungs, there is uneven ventilation of the alveoli that leads to an altered ventilation/perfusion balance. This causes a drop in arterial oxygen tension, but the $PaCO_2$ remains unchanged. This may be partly due to a drop in the production of CO_2 due to a decrease in the basal metabolic rate that happens during the aging process (Rosenthal & Kavic, 2004). The ability to hyperventilate in response to an acute metabolic acidosis may be blunted and lead to a persistent acidosis.

Renal tubular function is also affected by aging. The ability to conserve sodium and excrete hydrogen ion falls, so the aging kidney may be slower to respond to an acid load (either respiratory or metabolic) and blood pH may take longer to normalize (Marik, 2006). Dehydration is a particular problem because the aging kidney does not respond to fluid and sodium loss by its usual mechanism of increasing sodium retention, thus conserving water (Rosenthal & Kavic, 2004). In addition, many drugs commonly used by elderly people such as salicylates, diuretics, and laxatives may precipitate acid–base disturbances.

Collaborative Care

The care of a patient with a disorder that produces an imbalance of acid–base homeostasis involves nurses and physicians, but may also require respiratory therapy for assistance with bronchodilator therapy or assisted ventilation when treating respiratory causes of imbalance. Other nursing specialists such as dialysis nurses may also be called on for the expertise. Pharmacists may be used as consultants when electrolytes are being administered or when the absorption or action of medications may be altered in the presence of an abnormal pH.

Case managers and discharge planners evaluate placement and discharge needs. They can provide assistance in the arrangement of home nursing and/or respiratory therapy and durable medical equipment such as nebulizers or CPAP or BiPAP machines.

Health Promotion

Many patients with disturbances of acid–base balance suffer from chronic conditions that are the underlying causes of imbalances. Nurses are in a unique position to promote healthy behaviors in the face of chronic illness. These interventions can decrease symptoms and improve quality of life. Several examples are presented here.

Patients with chronic ventilatory failure often experience disabling symptoms such as chronic dyspnea. This can lead to malnutrition because the patient is too short of breath to eat. The nurse can explore the patient's daily routines and make suggestions about switching to five to six small meals per day and limiting mealtime conversation to conserve energy. Dietitians can suggest the best types of foods to conserve energy while supplying adequate nutrition. Subjective feelings of breathlessness can be eased by keeping the environment relatively cool and using fans to create air movement. Positioning for optimal lung expansion may involve the use of a recliner for sleeping and supporting

NURSING PROCESS: Patient Care Plan for Acid–Base Imbalances

Assessment of Respiratory Acidosis

Subjective Data:
Do you have a history of shortness of breath or exercise-limiting symptoms?
Do you have a cough? Is it productive? Sputum description?
Any history of sleep-disordered breathing? (Sleeping partner may be aware of excessive snoring.)

Objective Data:
Auscultate breath sounds; be alert for decreases in intensity, diffuse wheezing, stridor
Respiratory rate
Examine fingers for signs of clubbing
Observe for presence of a barrel chest
Laboratory evaluation: ABGs, complete blood count, serum electrolytes, drug screen (if there is suspicion of respiratory depression by drugs)

Nursing Assessment and Diagnoses	Outcomes and Evaluation Parameters	Planning and Interventions with *Rationales*
Nursing Diagnoses: *Impaired Gas Exchange* *Ineffective Airway Clearance*	**Outcomes:** Airway patency will be maintained. Gas exchange will be optimized **Evaluation Parameters:** $PaCO_2$ will return to patient's baseline with a pH in the normal range. Any dyspnea will be relieved as reported by the patient. Patient will return to baseline level of physical activity.	**Interventions and *Rationales*:** Position the patient sitting upright with arms supported on an overbed table. (Positioning in a chair may be preferable to the bed.) *This position helps maximize lung inflation.* Administer any bronchodilators that are ordered. Ensure that the patient is using proper technique if self-administering. *Patients who self-administer metered-dose inhalers (MDI) at home often prefer to continue self-administration while in the hospital as a way to retain control. However, improper technique is a frequent problem in the use of metered-dose inhalers (MDI). Enlist the help of a respiratory therapist.* Encourage the use of an incentive spirometer. Use should be at least every 4 hours while awake. *This is one way to encourage the patient to take deep breaths to help prevent atelectasis.* Encourage early ambulation. Set increasing distance goals with the patient each time. *Helps the patient to avoid complications of immobility.*

Assessment of Respiratory Alkalosis

Subjective Data:
Do you have any shortness of breath, numbness around the mouth, or paresthesias?
Do you have any history of anxiety or acute pain?

Objective Data:
Assess respiratory rate
Laboratory evaluation: ABGs, serum electrolytes, complete blood count

Nursing Assessment and Diagnoses	Outcomes and Evaluation Parameters	Planning and Interventions with *Rationales*
Nursing Diagnosis: *Ineffective Breathing Pattern*	**Outcomes:** Gas exchange will be optimized. Any excess anxiety or pain will be relieved. **Evaluation Parameters:** $PaCO_2$ will return to patient's baseline with a pH in the normal range. Respiratory rate and depth will be within normal parameters.	**Interventions and *Rationales*:** Encourage slow, deep respirations. In the acute stage, this may require the constant presence of the nurse. *A calm, reassuring nurse will help promote relaxation in the patient.* If that is difficult for the patient, the use of a rebreather mask or having the patient breathe into a simple paper bag may be required. *Promotes the rebreathing of exhaled CO_2 to help return levels to normal. Explain the reason for the rebreathing to the patient.* Evaluate for the presence of pain using objective criteria such as the visual analog scale. Medicate the patient to a level of pain that is acceptable to the patient. Reassess pain levels 30 minutes after IV medication and 1 hour after oral medication. *Pain can cause an increased respiratory rate. Relief of pain should help return the rate toward normal.* If the cause of the hyperventilation was anxiety or fear, help the patient explore the cause to help identify strategies to avoid future episodes. *Patients may need guidance in stress relief or anticipatory guidance about how to avoid such stress in the future.*

Assessment of Metabolic Acidosis

Subjective Data:

Ask about symptoms that may help determine cause: history of diabetes, renal insufficiency/failure, diarrhea or other loss of intestinal fluids. Ask about dyspnea; count respiratory rate. Observe for Kussmaul respirations.

Objective Data:

Laboratory evaluation:

- ABGs; evaluate pH and HCO_3^-; also examine PaO_2 to evaluate for hypoxemia as a cause of lactic acidosis
- Serum electrolytes; calculate anion gap
- Urine electrolytes, osmolarity
- Blood glucose (to evaluate for uncontrolled diabetes mellitus)
- BUN and creatinine (to evaluate renal function)

Evaluate for physical signs of malnutrition or dehydration

Nursing Assessment and Diagnoses	Outcomes and Evaluation Parameters	Planning and Interventions with *Rationales*
Nursing Diagnoses: *Imbalanced Nutrition: More than body requirements Deficient Fluid Volume*	**Outcomes:** Acid–base balance will be restored. The underlying cause of the acidosis will be identified and treated. Recurrence will be avoided. ***Evaluation Parameters:*** Serum bicarbonate will return to normal levels with a pH within the normal range. Fluid balance will be optimized.	**Interventions and *Rationales:*** *Note:* Much of the nursing care will be directed by the underlying cause of the acidosis. Obtain a baseline weight and weigh the patient frequently during rehydration, if applicable. *An accurate patient weight is a better parameter to measure than is the intake and output measurement. This is particularly true in cases where the cause of any dehydration is excessive diarrhea or fistula output. The patient should be weighed with the same amount of clothing each time.* If the cause of the acidosis is an exacerbation of diabetes or renal failure, it is important to explore the reasons with the patient and family. The problem may be a failure to comply with recommended treatment or may be caused by a concurrent event such as an infection. *An assessment of the patient's knowledge of any underlying disease and its management may help uncover causes of noncompliance or condition exacerbation. Extensive patient and family education or reeducation may be required to help prevent episodes in the future. This may be beyond the scope of the inpatient nurse when hospital stays continue to shorten. Referral to an outpatient facility or consultant such as a diabetes educator may be required.*

Assessment of Metabolic Alkalosis

Subjective Data:

Ask about history that may help identify a cause: vomiting, diarrhea, use of diuretics.
Ask about symptoms of hypokalemia: weakness, muscle aches.
Ask about symptoms of hypocalcemia: tingling around the mouth, muscles cramps.

Objective Data:

Evaluate fluid volume status
Evaluate for signs of hypocalcemia: tetany, Chvostek's sign
Laboratory evaluation:
ABGs; serum electrolytes and calcium, osmolarity; urine electrolytes

Nursing Assessment and Diagnoses	Outcomes and Evaluation Parameters	Planning and Interventions with *Rationales*
Nursing Diagnosis: *Deficient Fluid Volume*	**Outcomes:** Acid–base balance will be restored. The underlying cause of the alkalosis will be identified and treated. Recurrence will be avoided. ***Evaluation Parameters:*** Serum bicarbonate will return to normal levels with a pH within the normal range. Fluid balance will be optimized. Any excess vomiting or gastric suction will be corrected. Any chloride or potassium depletion will be corrected.	**Interventions and *Rationales:*** *Note:* Much of the nursing care will be directed by the underlying cause of the acidosis. Obtain a baseline weight and weigh the patient frequently during rehydration, if applicable. *An accurate patient weight is a better parameter to measure than is the intake and output measurement. This is particularly true in cases where the cause of any dehydration is excessive vomiting. The patient should be weighed with the same amount of clothing each time.* Control any vomiting with antiemetics. If the patient must be on continuous gastric suction, the use of a histamine-2 receptor blocker or a proton pump inhibitor may be indicated. *The goal is to stop the loss of hydrochloric acid from the stomach. The drugs decrease the secretion of acid into the stomach and, hence, stop its loss.* If the alkalemia is severe and the patient's respirations are depressed, encourage frequent deep breathing and the use of an incentive spirometer. *The decrease in tidal volume can lead to atelectasis and may contribute to the development of a pulmonary infection.* If there is no obvious cause for the alkalosis, a sensitive exploration into the possibility of self-induced vomiting or the use of diuretics may be required. *These may be attempts at weight loss or may be symptoms of a disorder such as bulimia.*

the arms on pillows. Patient and family education about the precautions to be taken when oxygen is in use in the home can help to decrease the risk of fire or excess oxygen administration. If the patient uses an oxygen concentrator, a plan about what to do in case of an emergency such as a power outage should be formulated by the patient and the nurse.

Patients with obstructive sleep apnea that leads to respiratory acidosis must be counseled about the dangers of excessive daytime sleepiness. When possible, patients should undergo an outpatient sleep study and evaluation for the use of nasal CPAP to decrease apneic arousal episodes at night and to promote better REM sleep. Patients are often reluctant to use home CPAP machines, and the nurse is in a position to provide encouragement about their use for patient safety. Patients who frequently fall asleep during the day should be counseled about the risks associated with driving because they are prone to accidents.

When patients with diabetes experience an episode of ketoacidosis, the nurse should explore with the patient and family what may have led to the episode. If it is a stressor such as infection, diabetic teaching should be begun or reinforced and the patient counseled to have a "sick day" plan to decrease the chance that blood sugar levels will get out of control. If there is any suspicion that the patient is not following her diabetes management regimen adequately, the nurse will be able to explore the reasons for noncompliance. If the problem is a lack of knowledge, intensive diabetic teaching and reinforcement of previous teaching should be started in the inpatient setting and continued in the outpatient or home care setting.

 Research

Current and future research needs to focus on control of symptoms with chronic conditions such as dyspnea and enhancing the quality of life of patients with chronic illnesses. Additionally, improved monitoring systems and treatment measures need to detect and treat symptoms before they progress to cause a debilitating state. The Research Opportunities and Clinical Impact box outlines research topics in the area of acid–base imbalances.

 Summary

Acid–base imbalances almost always occur in conjunction with diseases or pathologic conditions that are the primary focus for the nurse caring for the patient. A basic understanding of how these imbalances affect organ systems and blood chemistries will enable nurses to provide focused assessments of the patients in their care and plan nursing interventions accordingly.

RESEARCH OPPORTUNITIES AND CLINICAL IMPACT RELATED TO ACID–BASE IMBALANCES

Research Area	Clinical Impact
Patient Assessment	
• Assessing the severity of dyspnea	Establish a standard measure of dyspnea to measure severity and to gauge the effectiveness of interventions and relief strategies.
• Exploration of ethnic/cultural differences in the description of symptoms such as dyspnea	Enhance cultural sensitivity and ensure that symptoms are recognized and that strategies are undertaken to relieve symptoms.
• Assess accuracy of noninvasive methods of measuring $PaCO_2$	To promote noninvasive methods of assessing the adequacy of ventilation.
• Compare the accuracy of the recording of intake and output vs. accurate patient weight in the assessment of fluid loss/gain	Intake and output recording is time consuming and often inaccurate. Explore more accurate methods of assessment of fluid volume status.
Nursing Intervention Research	
• Effectiveness of interventions to relieve dyspnea	Dyspnea is a strong, subjective experience of physiological distress. Relief of this symptom can enhance quality of life and improve end-of-life care.
• Enhancing quality of life in patients with chronic illness	
• Examine the most effective methods of patient education during short hospital stays	Shorter inpatient hospitalization reduces the time available for patient and family education about disease processes and their management. Evaluation of the most effective methods that can be undertaken in a short time period has a goal of improving comprehension and retention of information.

Clinical Preparation

 Read

- History of Current Illness
- Past Medical History
- Physical Exam
- Admitting Medical Orders
- Laboratory Study Results

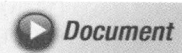 **Document**

- Summary of Hospitalization
- Pathophysiology Form
- Laboratory Values
- Laboratory Results Explanation

 Apply

- List of Potential Nursing Diagnoses
- Concept Map
- Critical Thinking Questions

Log on to MyNursingKit.com to download forms you will need and to complete further steps in the Clinical Preparation assignment.

HISTORY OF PRESENT ILLNESS

A.B. is an 82-year-old male who began to feel unwell 2 days prior to presenting to the emergency department (ED). He complained of feeling "achy all over" and developed a cough that was productive of yellowish sputum. He was unable to sleep flat in bed and had begun to try to sleep sitting up in his recliner. The coughing left him short of breath and unable to sleep. He was unable to walk farther than a few steps without becoming increasingly short of breath. Consequently, his wife drove him to the ED. He presented with a complaint of increasing shortness of breath and a productive cough. He had a temperature of 38.2°C and a respiratory rate of 24 breaths/minute with an oxygen saturation of 93% on room air. Chest radiograph showed evidence of pneumonia.

Medical–Surgical History

History of coronary artery disease; two coronary stents placed 1 year prior to admission
Emphysema
No other significant medical history
Allergies: none known
Drug intolerance: none known

Social History

A.B. lives with his wife independently. He has two sons who live in other states. He depends on friends and neighbors when he needs assistance. He has a 50 pack/year smoking history although the patient stopped smoking 8 years ago after he was told that he had emphysema. Denies use of alcohol.

Physical Exam

The patient appears ill. Vital signs reveal: temperature: 38.2°C; pulse: 112 beats/minute; BP: 156/92; respirations: 24 breaths/minute.

The patient is moderately obese with a barrel chest. On auscultation, coarse rhonchi can be heard throughout. Breath sounds are decreased in the bases and there is a slight expiratory wheeze.

HEENT: PERRLA, ears appear normal; pharynx pink with exudate
Neck: no cervical lymphadenopathy; thyroid nonpalpable
Heart: regular rate and rhythm; no extra heart sounds
Abdomen: bowel sounds present × 4 quadrants; soft and nondistended; no tenderness or masses; no hepatomegaly
Pulses: apical, radial, and pedal pulses present and regular
Arterial blood gas: PaO_2: 88 mmHg; $PaCO_2$: 66 mmHg; pH: 7.28; HCO_3^-: 34 mEq/L; BE: +5; saturation: 92% on room air

White blood cell count: $14.1 \times 10^3/\mu L$
Chest radiograph revealed a consolidation in the right lower lobe but no effusion.
Sputum gram stain showed a few gram-positive cocci in pairs and 12 to 20 white cells. The culture later grew out *Streptococcus pneumoniae*.

Admitting Medical Orders

Admit to medicine
No known allergies
Diagnosis: exacerbation of COPD and community-acquired pneumonia
Vital signs, oxygen saturation every 4 hours
Call house officer: pulse < 60 or > 120/minute; BP < 90 or > 160 systolic; temperature > 38.5; RR < 10 or > 30; oxygen saturation < 92% or patient complaint of increased dyspnea
Activity: bed rest with bathroom privileges tonight. Up ad lib tomorrow morning
Diet: AHA (2 g sodium)
Bronchodilator protocol: levalbuterol nebulizer q6h
Oxygen: place patient on least amount of oxygen needed to maintain saturation > 92%
Sequential compression devices (SCD) to lower extremities
IV fluids: D5½NS 100 mL/hr
Incentive spirometer q2h while awake
Patient education: obtain spacer; educate patient in use of metered-dose inhaler (MDI) and spacer
Case management for discharge planning: possible home oxygen, home nebulizer, referral to community pulmonary rehab program

Scheduled Medications

Methylprednisolone sodium succinate (Solu-Medrol) 60 mg IV push q6h
Lasix 40 mg po bid
Ceftazidime 1 g q8h IV
Aspirin 81 mg po/day
Clopidogrel 75 mg po/day
DVT prophylaxis: enoxaparin 30 mg subcutaneously twice a day

PRN Medications

Tylenol 325 mg × 2 po q4h for fever > 38.5°C
Morphine 0.3–5 mg IV q4h prn pain

Temazepam 15-30mg po HS prn insomnia
Droperidol 1.25–2.5mg IV q6h prn nausea

Ordered Laboratory Studies

Chemistry 20 on admission; Chemistry 7 q a.m.
Blood cultures now
CBC w/diff every a.m.
PTT, PT, INR every a.m.
Sputum culture

Ordered Diagnostic Studies

Chest x-ray PA and lateral in a.m.

LABORATORY STUDY RESULTS

TEST	Day 1	Day 2	Day 3
Chemistry			
Sodium	135 mEq/L	137 mEq/L	141 mEq/L
Potassium	4.8 mEq/L	4.0 mEq/L	3.9 mEq/L
Chloride	103 mEq/L	107 mEq/L	105 mEq/L
Carbon dioxide (CO_2)	34 mEq/L	34.5 mEq/L	34.4 mEq/L
Blood urea nitrogen	32 mg/dL	28.8 mg/dL	26 mg/dL
Creatinine	1.7 mg/dL	1.5 mg/dL	1.3 mg/dL
Blood glucose	120 mg/dL	126 mg/dL	118 mg/dL
Calcium	8.8 mg/dL	9.0 mg/dL	9.2 mg/dL
Amylase	110 units/L		
Magnesium	2 mEq/L	2.1 mEq/L	1.8 mEq/L
Phosphorus	3.3 mg/dL		
Alkaline phosphatase	174 units/L		
T. bilirubin	1.0 mg/dL		
CPK total	220 units/L		
LDH	188 units/L		
AST	16 units/L		
ALT	17 units/L		
Hematology			
WBC	14.1/mm³	13.9/mm³	12.8/mm³
Hemoglobin	17.2 g/dL	16.4 g/dL	16.5 g/dL

TEST	Day 1	Day 2	Day 3
Hematocrit	53.5%	50.2%	51.1%
RBC	5.2/mm³	5.0/mm³	5.0/mm³
Platelets	356/mm³		
PTT	29 seconds	31 seconds	28 seconds
PT	11.8 seconds	12.6 econds	14.3 seconds
INR	1.0	1.10	1.14
ABGs			
%O_2	21%	28%	28%
PO_2	88	90	89
O_2 Sat	92%	96%	95%
pH	7.28	7.32	7.33
PCO_2	66	58	56
HCO_3	34	34	31
Miscellaneous			
Digoxin level	Negative		
Toxicology screen	Negative		
Blood alcohol level	Negative		
Sputum culture	*Streptococcus pneumoniae*		
Blood culture	Negative		

CRITICAL THINKING QUESTIONS

1. What does the blood gas indicate in terms of acid–base balance?
2. What were this patient's risk factors for developing pneumonia?
3. What factor(s) contributed to the $PaCO_2$ of 66 mmHg?
4. What nursing measures would help bring the $PaCO_2$ back into normal range?

Answers to Critical Thinking Questions appear in Appendix D.

NCLEX® REVIEW

1. A patient's blood pH is decreasing. The nurse realizes that this patient's hydrogen ion concentration is:
   1. Increasing.
   2. Decreasing.
   3. Being affected by oxygen concentration.
   4. Stabilizing.

2. A patient is admitted with the diagnosis of diabetic ketoacidosis. The nurse realizes that this patient's body will attempt to attain acid–base balance by:
   1. Decreasing the respiratory rate.
   2. Increasing the reabsorption of hydrogen ions.
   3. Increasing the secretion of hydrogen ions.
   4. Decreasing the reabsorption of bicarbonate.

3. A patient has a respiratory rate of 20. The nurse calculates this patient's minute ventilation to be:
   1. 1 L/min.
   2. 2 L/min.
   3. 5 L/min.
   4. 10 L/min.

4. The nurse, admitting a patient with diabetes, believes the patient is attempting to correct an acidotic condition. Which of the following did this nurse most likely observe while assessing this patient?
   1. Slow methodical respirations
   2. Deep rapid respirations
   3. Change in level of consciousness
   4. Intact extraoccular movements

5. The nurse is caring for a patient with metabolic acidosis. The nurse realizes that which of the following laboratory values might be altered for this patient?
   1. Ammonia
   2. Blood-urea-nitrogen
   3. Creatinine
   4. Prothrombin

6. The nurse is reviewing a patient's arterial blood gas results. Which of the following values should the nurse study first?
   1. $PaCO_2$
   2. HCO_3
   3. Compensation
   4. pH

7. The nurse is caring for a patient with pneumonia who has arterial blood gas values of: pH 7.20, $PaCO_2$ 75, HCO_3^- 28, PaO_2 44. Which of the following would be a priority for this patient?
   1. Assist the patient to breathe into a paper bag.
   2. Prepare to administer sodium bicarbonate IV.
   3. Place the patient in high Fowler's position.
   4. Administer the prn sedative available.

8. A patient is admitted in respiratory acidosis secondary to barbiturate overdose. Which of the following will the nurse most likely assess in this patient?
   1. Kussmaul's respirations
   2. Seizures
   3. Slow, shallow respirations
   4. Increased deep tendon reflexes

9. The nurse is providing discharge instructions to a patient with respiratory alkalosis. Which of the following statements indicates the patient understands the instructions?
   1. "I will not take my Lasix without a potassium supplement."
   2. "I will not use Mylanta 5–6 times a day like I used to."
   3. "I will take a stress management class or seek counseling."
   4. "I will call my MD the next time I have diarrhea for a few days."

Answers for review questions appear in Appendix D

KEY TERMS

acids *p.436*
alkalis *p.436*
anatomic dead space *p.438*
anion gap *p.446*
base excess *p.440*
bases *p.436*
buffer *p.437*
carbon dioxide *p.437*

carbonic acid *p.437*
compensation *p.439*
dead space *p.438*
electroneutrality *p.446*
hydrogen ion *p.436*
hypercarbic drive *p.439*
hyperventilation *p.439*

hypoventilation *p.439*
hypoxic drive *p.439*
minute ventilation *p.438*
pathologic dead space *p.438*
pH *p.436*
secretion *p.439*
sodium bicarbonate *p.436*

EXPLORE PEARSON **mynursingkit**

MyNursingKit is your one stop for online chapter review materials and resources. Prepare for success with additional NCLEX®-style practice questions, interactive assignments and activities, web links, animations and videos, and more!

Register your access code from the front of your book at
www.mynursingkit.com

REFERENCES

Androgue, H. E., & Androgue, H. J. (2001). Acid–base physiology. *Respiratory Care, 46*(4), 328–341.

Argyle, B. (2002). *Blood gas computer program manual.* Retrieved March 10, 2004, from Mad Scientists Software website: http://www.madscientistsoftware.com

Bartlett, D. (2005). Understanding the anion and osmolal gap lab values. *Journal of Emergency Nursing, 31*(1), 109–111.

Black, R. M. (2003). Metabolic acidosis and metabolic alkalosis. In R. Irwin & J. Rippe, *Intensive care medicine* (5th ed., pp. 854–864). Philadelphia: Lippincott Williams & Wilkins.

Breen, P. (2001). ABG and pH analysis. *Anesthesia Clinics of North America, 19*(4), 885–906.

Casaletto, J. (2005). Differential diagnosis of metabolic acidosis. *Emergency Medicine Clinics of North America, 23*(3), 1–12.

DuBose, T. (2004). Acid–base disorders. In B. M. Brenner, *The Kidney* (7th ed.). Philadelphia, Elsevier, Inc.

Grogono, A. (2006). *Acid–base tutorial.* Retrieved April 1, 2007, from http://www.acid-base.com

Hayes, J. A. (2005, June 30). *Respiratory alkalosis.* Retrieved April 6, 2007, from http://www.emedicine.com/topic2009

Marik, P. (2006). Management of the critically ill geriatric patient. *Critical Care Medicine, 34*(9 Suppl.), S176–S182.

Priestley, M., & Levine, G. (2006). *Respiratory acidosis.* Retrieved April 6, 2007, from http://www.emedicine.com/ped/topic16.html

Rose, B. (2005, September 3). *Urine electrolytes in diagnosis of metabolic acidosis.* Retrieved April 1, 2007, from UpToDate website: http://www.utdol.com/application/topic/topicTest.asp?fil.../18016&type=A&selectedTitle=4~4

Rosenthal, R., & Kavic, S. (2004). Assessment and management of the geriatric patient. *Critical Care Medicine, 32*(4 Suppl.), S92–S105.

Shlichtig, R. (2005). Acid–base balance. In *Textbook of critical care* (5th ed., pp. 829–838). Philadelphia: W. B. Saunders.

Stavile, K. L., et al. (2005). *Metabolic acidosis.* Retrieved April 1, 2007, from http://www.emedicine.com/emerg/topic31.2

Thomas, C., & Khaled, H. (2007, February 1). *Metabolic acidosis.* Retrieved April 6, 2007, from http:///www.emedicine.com/med/topic1458.htm

Yaseen, S., & Thomas, C. (2006). *Metabolic alkalosis.* Retrieved March 21, 2007, from http://emedicine.com/med/topic1459

Infectious Disease

Teri Murray
Peggy Ellis

Outcome-Based Learning Objectives

After studying this chapter, the learner will be able to:

1. Describe the infectious process and its effects on the body.
2. Identify risk factors for infection.
3. Describe the chain of infection.
4. Describe measures to prevent and control infection.
5. Identify common pathogens causing infection.
6. Differentiate between active and passive immunity.
7. Describe *Healthy People 2010* guidelines for prevention of infection.
8. Identify the assessment and interventions required by a patient with an infection.

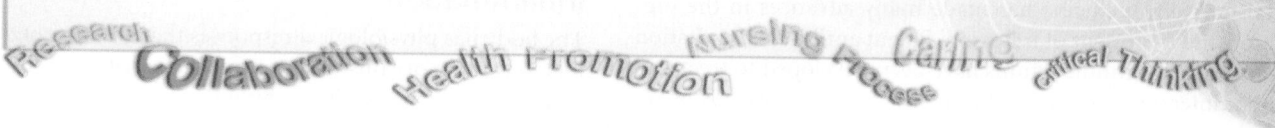

Research Collaboration Health Promotion Nursing Process Caring Critical Thinking

INFECTIOUS DISEASE is a major health problem. Infection occurs when a microorganism enters the body and is able to colonize and multiply, leading to an infection and subsequent immune response. A microorganism is a microscopic body such as a bacterium, virus, fungus, or parasite. Some microorganisms live on the human body normally and are beneficial. For example, certain microorganisms live in the intestines and produce enzymes that facilitate digestion. If the immune and inflammatory systems are compromised, as can occur when an individual has a decreased immunity, organisms that usually benefit the body will leave their normal sites and travel to other areas of the body and cause an infection. A microorganism that produces disease is called a pathogen. True pathogens are able to cause disease regardless of the body's normal defenses.

When an infection is acquired outside a health care facility it is considered a **community-acquired infection**. When an infection occurs in a hospitalized patient, it is known as a **nosocomial infection.** Nosocomial infections have been blamed for numerous complications in the hospitalized patient leading to a cost of many lives and billions of health care dollars. Many infections in the hospital are related to the use of invasive devices such as urinary catheters, intravenous catheters, surgical drains, nasogastric tubes, and endotracheal tubes. Because of the increased susceptibility to infection, invasive devices should only be used when necessary for patient care and should be discontinued as quickly as possible. Clean or sterile technique should be used when caring for anyone with invasive devices in order to avoid infection. Patients who develop nosocomial infections are often critically ill with an increased susceptibility to infection.

Nosocomial infections may also occur because the overuse of broad-spectrum antibiotics alters the body's natural defenses and leads to antibiotic resistance in harmful bacteria. Many nosocomial infections are caused by multidrug-resistant organisms (MDROs). The National Nosocomial Infections Surveillance (NNIS) system was formed by the Centers for Disease Control and Prevention (CDC) to create a national database of nosocomial infections. It began in 1970 and is a voluntary, hospital-based reporting system to monitor and accurately describe hospital-acquired infections and provide statistical analysis of those infections. This information aids the infection control practitioner and hospital epidemiologist to develop strategies to reduce nosocomial infection rates. The goals of NNIS are to:

- Collect surveillance data from a sample of acute care hospitals in the United States to permit valid estimation of the magnitude of nosocomial infections (NI) in hospitalized patients.

- Analyze and report NI surveillance data to permit recognition of trends in infection rates, antimicrobial resistance, and nosocomial pathogens.

- Provide hospitals with risk-adjusted NI data that can be used for comparison.
- Assist hospitals in developing surveillance and analysis methods that permit timely recognition of NI problems and prompt intervention with appropriate infection control measures.
- Conduct collaborative research studies with NNIS hospitals (e.g., describe the epidemiology of emerging infections and pathogens, assess the importance of potential risk factors, further characterize nosocomial pathogens and mechanisms of resistance, and evaluate alternative surveillance and prevention strategies).

The NNIS produces a national nosocomial infection database that is used to (1) describe the epidemiology of nosocomial infections, (2) describe antimicrobial resistance trends, and (3) produce NI rates to use for comparison purposes. This information is used to help infection control practitioners and hospital epidemiologists develop guidelines for prevention, timely recognition, and prompt intervention with appropriate infection control measures. The data show that surgical site infections are the leading type of infection in hospitalized patients. The respiratory tract, urinary tract, bloodstream, and surgical wounds are the most common sites and are the most frequently monitored for the occurrence of infection. Although, the rates of infection have decreased during the last 10 years, the prevention of infection in hospitalized patients remains part of the national health objectives for 2010 (U.S. Department of Health and Human Services [DHHS], 2000).

Historically, medicine has made many advances in the prevention and treatment of infection. Potent antibiotics, sanitation programs, and immunizations have been developed to treat and prevent infection. In spite of this, many infectious organisms remain and new varieties and strains are developing. Some of these strains are resistant to antibiotics, making treatment more difficult due to increased susceptibility to infection, which then increases morbidity and mortality and length of hospital stay.

Antimicrobial resistance is becoming an increasingly important problem in health care. It is primarily due to the prolonged or inappropriate use of antibiotics. Bacteria sometimes survive after the use of antibiotics and become able to change their genetic makeup so that the antibiotic is no longer effective. Currently, the most well-known resistant organisms are methicillin-resistant *Staphylococcus aureus* (MRSA), multidrug-resistant tuberculosis (MDR-TB), penicillin-resistant *Streptococcus pneumoniae* (PRSP), vancomycin-resistant enterococci (VRE), vancomycin intermediate-resistant *S. aureus* (VISA), and vancomycin-resistant *S. aureus* (VRSA) (CDC, 2004). Antimicrobial resistance has occurred for a variety of reasons, including but not limited to inappropriate prescribing practices, inconsistent infection control techniques, promotion of antibiotic use by pharmaceutical companies, lack of public knowledge about appropriate antibiotic use, availability of antibiotics without prescription in some parts of the world, and use of antibiotics in agriculture on crops and livestock. Chart 20–1 lists various actions that can be taken to address this problem.

■ Defense Mechanisms

Most human beings have defenses for prevention of infectious disease including physical, chemical, and immune mechanisms.

| CHART 20–1 | **Actions to Address Antimicrobial Resistance** |

- Use antibiotics judiciously. Obtain cultures and do not use antibiotics for prophylactic purposes when the likelihood of infection is low.
- Use the most appropriate narrow-spectrum antibiotic possible. Use a full dose of the antibiotic for the shortest course needed to kill the microorganism.
- Use standard, approved infection control measures. Proper hand hygiene as outlined in Charts 20–3, 20–4, and 20–5 (pp. 462, 463) is essential. Wear gloves when necessary and follow standard precautions for all patients.
- Teach patients the importance of practicing infection control, and when antibiotics are necessary and when they are not.

Whether or not an organism causes disease depends, in part, on the success or failure of these mechanisms. These defense mechanisms include the skin, enzymes that kill microorganisms, structures such as cilia that trap microorganisms and sweep them out of the bronchial tubes, membranes that secrete mucus to prevent the adherence of the organisms, chemical secretions such as hydrochloric acid in the stomach, and the immune system. The immune system produces enzymes, and uses other factors and cells to trap and kill microorganisms. Chart 20–2 depicts human defenses against infection. Chapters 59 and 60 address immune assessment and immune response.

Inflammation

The body has physiological responses that are designed to eliminate invading organisms and protect against infection. The inflammatory response is a physiological process that attacks, confines, and kills invading organisms. It also allows for tissue repair after damage from an invading organism or from tissue injury and death. The steps in the inflammatory process are di-

---

| CHART 20–2 | **Defense Mechanisms Against Infection** |

Mechanism	Purpose
Skin	Offers a protective barrier of five to seven layers with the top layer being shed constantly.
Mucous membranes	Line orifices of body open to the environment, trap microorganisms, contain bacteriostatic agents, secrete IgA, an immunoglobulin that fights infection. Wash out microorganisms and prevent them from adhering to mucosal surfaces.
Respiratory cilia	Trap microorganisms and push them out of the body.
Secretions of oil and moisture from glands	Inhibit penetration of pathogens; inhibit pathogen growth.
Normal flora	Flora that normally exist in the gastrointestinal tract and vagina compete with pathogens for placement.
Chemical secretions	Gastric acid and acidic urine create an atmosphere not conducive to the growth of microorganisms.

agramed in Figure 20–1 ■. The inflammatory process involves a vascular phase and a cellular phase. The vascular phase consists of the following processes, which occur almost simultaneously:

- Temporary vasoconstriction to avoid blood loss after injury
- Vasodilation to increase blood supply to the area, leading to redness and increased warmth of the area
- Increased hydrostatic pressure related to the increase in blood flow
- Increased permeability of blood vessel walls caused by chemical mediators
- Leakage of fluid and cells out of capillaries into interstitial spaces so that toxins are diluted. This leakage of fluid and eventually protein leads to increased osmotic pressure in the interstitial spaces and edema.

The cellular phase involves the response of white blood cells (WBCs) to the cellular injury. It begins as chemotactic substances are released from the tissues by cellular injury and complement is activated. Neutrophils are the first WBCs to arrive at the site and are the main phagocytic cell. The processes involved in the cellular phase are as follows:

- An increased number of WBCs are attracted to the site of injury by chemotactic factors.

- WBCs adhere to the vessel wall during a process called margination.
- WBCs migrate through the vessel wall into the interstitial tissue during a process called diapedesis or emigration.
- WBCs are attracted to the inflamed site by chemotactic factors.
- Neutrophils ingest the bacteria and dead cells through a process of coating microorganisms called opsonization.
- This coating allows the bacteria and dead cells to be easily engulfed and killed by WBCs.
- Neutrophils then die, releasing proteolytic enzymes that liquefy the dead cells and bacteria, resulting in the formation of pus.
- Fibrin is secreted by fibroblasts and serves to wall off the area to prevent the spread of bacteria and lay the groundwork for tissue rebuilding.

The inflammatory phase of wound healing is discussed in Chapter 67 .

Manifestations of Inflammation

The signs and symptoms related to inflammation can be local and/or systemic depending on the location and severity of the inflammatory response. There are five cardinal local symptoms of inflammation: (1) redness from increased blood flow to the area, (2) heat due to increased blood flow to the area, (3) swelling due

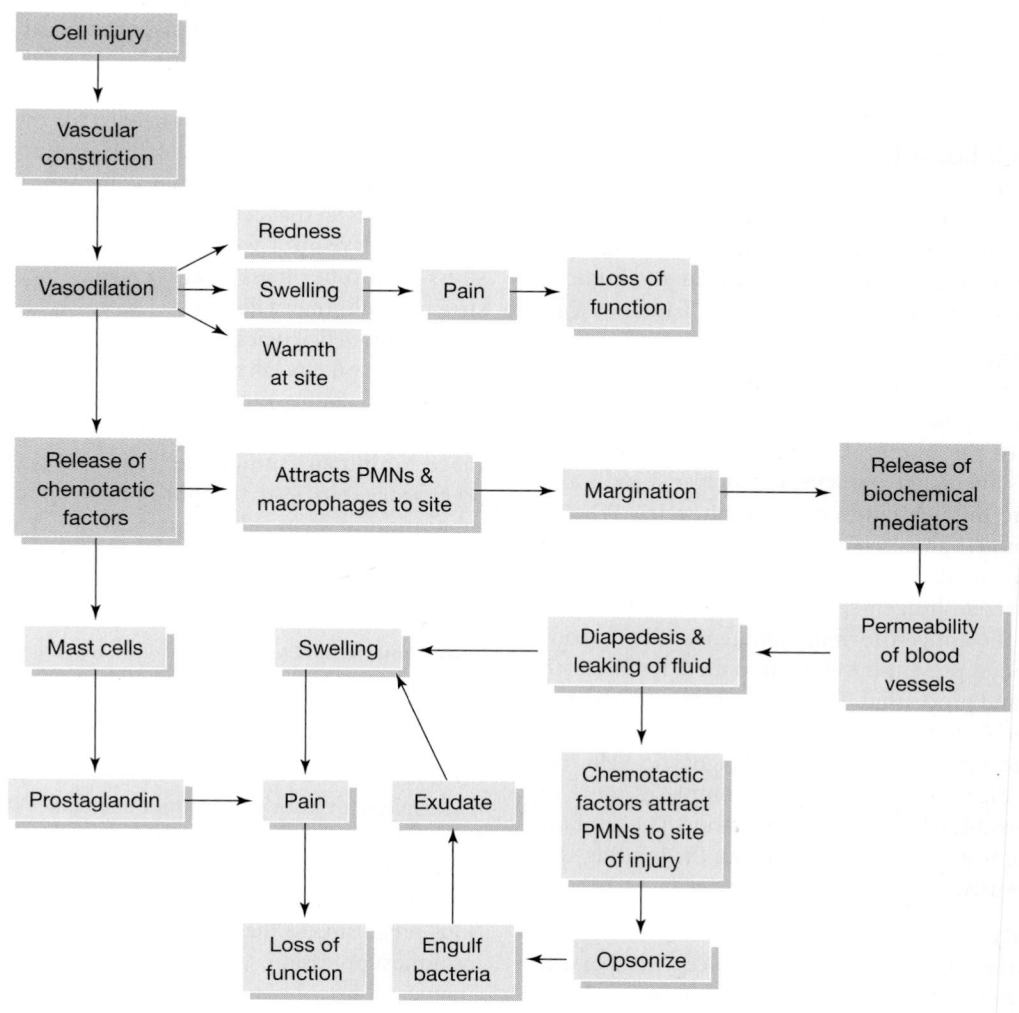

FIGURE 20–1 ■ Steps in the inflammatory process.

to the fluid exudates that form in the interstitial tissue, (4) pain caused by the pressure of the exudates and release of chemicals that irritate nerve endings, and (5) loss of function related to the pain and swelling.

The major systemic symptoms are fever and leukocytosis. Fever occurs because of the release of endogenous pyrogens at the site of inflammation. These endogenous pyrogens consist of substances such as prostaglandins and leukotrienes from injured cells and WBCs that accumulate at the site. These substances are carried to the temperature-regulating center in the hypothalamus where an increased temperature is stimulated. Fever is part of the body's defense mechanism and helps to fight infections.

Leukocytosis is a systemic sign of inflammation that is stimulated by the release of leukopoietins from damaged cells. Leukopoietins stimulate the increased production of WBCs and the release of mature neutrophils by the bone marrow. As inflammation continues the bone marrow releases immature neutrophils known as bands to help meet the body's needs. An increase in the number of bands on a differential WBC count is known as a "shift to the left" and indicates an ongoing acute inflammation. WBC response to infection and inflammation is discussed further in Chapter 61 ☁.

Immune Responses

The immune responses are specific reactions of the body to invading foreign materials. The body's immune responses are complex and not completely understood. However, it is known that the immune responses work to defend the body against agents that are able to produce infection.

Humoral and Cellular Immunity

The immune responses can be divided into two types: humoral immunity and cellular immunity. The humoral response involves the antigen–antibody reactions, whereas the cellular response involves the reaction of the WBCs. Cellular and humoral defenses against infection also are discussed in Chapter 61 ☁.

Humoral Immunity

Foreign materials are called antigens and the body responds to antigens by producing antibodies. These antigen–antibody responses are part of the humoral immune response. The humoral response is mediated by activated helper T cells that induce growth and differentiation of B lymphocytes. When B lymphocytes encounter an antigen such as a pathogen, they are stimulated to differentiate into antibody-producing cells called plasma cells that secrete antigen-specific antibodies. These antibodies bind with the antigen-forming antigen–antibody complexes. The antibodies present the antigen to the T lymphocytes for identification and processing. These complexes serve to neutralize the bacterial toxins and viruses, lyse and destroy pathogens, and facilitate phagocytosis. Phagocytic cells can bind, engulf, and digest antigen–antibody complexes more effectively than is possible when the antigen is alone. The antibodies also serve to neutralize a virus by blocking the binding sites on a virus that are used to bind to and infect a cell.

Cellular Immunity

The cellular immune response is a complex process involving an increase in the number of lymphocytes and macrophages in response to the invading organism. T cells mature in the thymus and in the process of growing become able to recognize specific antigens through the growth of antigen-specific receptors. After exposure to the antigens, the production of helper T cells is stimulated. This in turn, increases the production of cytotoxic T cells and natural killer cells that enhance the engulfment and killing of the antigen directly by macrophages.

Increased Susceptibility to Infection

Some known factors make an individual more susceptible to infection. For instance, individuals who are very old or very young have an increased susceptibility to infection. For the very young, the immune system is not fully developed until about the age of 6 months. Susceptibility to childhood infections increases as children are exposed to pathogens at day care facilities and schools. In the elderly, the immune system weakens as a result of decreasing thymus gland function. Changes in lymphocytes may occur as people age, contributing to decreased defenses. It is known that some of the lymphocytes important to immunity become less responsive in the elderly, whereas others function normally.

Defense mechanisms can be improved through lifestyle changes. Good hygiene is important in maintaining strong defense mechanisms. Skin that is unclean serves as a medium for bacterial growth and is more likely to allow invasion of microorganisms. Dust in the environment can serve as a reservoir for pathogens and helps with transportation of pathogens into the body. A balanced diet helps the body maintain an effective immune system by providing the nutrients needed for growth of new, healthy tissue. Protein is needed for the production of antibodies and the functioning of the immune system. Vitamins and minerals are also important to help the body digest and utilize nutrients so that cells can grow and remain strong. Individuals may develop a weakened immune system from chronic stress or chronic illness such as diabetes mellitus or chronic obstructive pulmonary disease.

Immunodeficiencies involve impaired functioning of one or more components of the immune response or inflammatory process. The failure of these defense mechanisms can be caused by a genetic abnormality or by an acquired abnormality such as cancer or human immunodeficiency virus (HIV). An immunodeficiency can lead to abnormal lymphocyte development, prevention of stem cell maturation into T or B cells, or a decrease in the production of a specific class of immunoglobulin. Regardless of the cause, a failure in the immune system will lead to a tendency to develop unusual or recurrent, severe infections. Immunodeficiency should be considered when an individual has frequent severe, documented infections such as otitis media, pneumonia, candidiasis, or meningitis. It should also be suggested when the infections are unusual such as *Pneumocystis carinii*.

People with known immunodeficiencies should be protected from infection. It may be unsafe or even fatal to administer immunizations or perform even simple procedures such as drawing blood. Care should be taken by nurses to avoid transmitting infectious organisms to these individuals. An in-depth discussion of immunosuppression and immunodeficiency is included in Chapter 60 ☁.

Infectious Process

Infections can range from mild to debilitating or death producing. The severity of the infection depends on the **pathogenicity** or disease-causing potential of the microorganism, the number of invading microorganisms, and the host defenses. The common sequence of events is known as the chain of infection. All links of the chain must be present for infection to occur. The **chain of infection** consists of a causative agent, reservoir, portal of exit, mode of transmission, portal of entry, and a susceptible host (Figure 20–2 ■).

Chain of Infection

A causative agent or microorganism must exist in order for infection to occur. This can be any organism capable of causing disease. This organism must have a **reservoir** or a place where it can survive and may or may not multiply. Humans can serve as reservoirs as can inanimate objects such as soil, water, or equipment. Human reservoirs can be **carriers** or people or animals that do not have symptoms of infection but carry an active pathogenic microorganism. These individuals can be (1) in a period of incubation or before the onset of symptoms, (2) have a subclinical infection, (3) be recovering from an infection, or (4) be chronic carriers of the pathogen.

There must be a **portal of exit** or a path that allows the causative agent to escape from the reservoir. The portal of exit is usually associated with the site where the organism grows. Common human portals of exit include the respiratory system, the gastrointestinal system, the genitourinary (GU) system, and the skin and mucous membranes. Causative agents can be found in blood, sputum, emesis, stool, urine, wound drainage, and genital secretions. The portal of exit will vary depending on the microorganism.

In order for the organism to leave the reservoir, it needs a **mode of transmission,** which is the means by which it travels from the reservoir to a susceptible host. Transmission occurs through one of four modes: *contact, airborne, vehicle,* and *vector-borne.* Contact transmission can occur by direct contact, indirect contact, or droplets. Direct contact occurs when there is actual person-to-person or person-to-source physical contact, such as occurs when a sexually transmitted infection is obtained through sexual activity. Indirect contact involves the susceptible person being exposed to the organism through a contaminated object. An example of indirect contact is exposure to a contaminated dressing or surgical instrument. Droplet transmission occurs when the organism is expelled from its reservoir through the respiratory system in droplets, for instance, when someone sneezes or coughs. These large particles can travel up to 3 feet and can be inhaled by another susceptible person within a 3-foot radius around the person generating the droplets. They set up infection in a new susceptible host by being inhaled.

Airborne transmission occurs when the organism is expelled from the infected person and remains suspended in the air in tiny droplets no larger than 5 microns. These droplets are carried by air currents or on dust and inhaled by the susceptible host. They differ from droplet transmission in that these droplets are small enough to remain suspended in the air for prolonged periods of time. Tuberculosis (TB) is spread by airborne transmission.

Vehicle transmission occurs when the organism's life is maintained on something outside the reservoir until it is passed to the susceptible host. The vehicle is a nonliving object that is not normally harmful but acts as an intermediary for the infectious agent. Pathogenic organisms are contained in contaminated water or food, blood, or other items and transmitted to a susceptible host. This is the method of transmission for hepatitis B, which is transmitted through contaminated blood or blood products or through the salmonella infection.

Vector-borne transmission occurs when a disease-producing organism is carried by a living intermediate host that transfers the organism to a susceptible host. Examples of vectors include mosquitoes that carry West Nile virus and ticks that carry Lyme disease.

A portal of entry is needed to continue the chain of infection. A **portal of entry** is the path by which the infective organism enters the new susceptible host. These sites are usually the same as those for the portal of exit. Once the organism enters a host, the host must be susceptible to infection before an infection will occur. As long as the body's defenses against infection function normally, no infection will occur, but if the body has weakened defenses and is at increased risk, infection can occur.

Stages of the Infectious Process

Once the organism enters the susceptible host, the infectious disease develops in four stages. The first stage is the incubation period. During the incubation period the organism is establishing itself. It is replicating and spreading to other organs or tissues in the body but not yet causing symptoms. This stage can

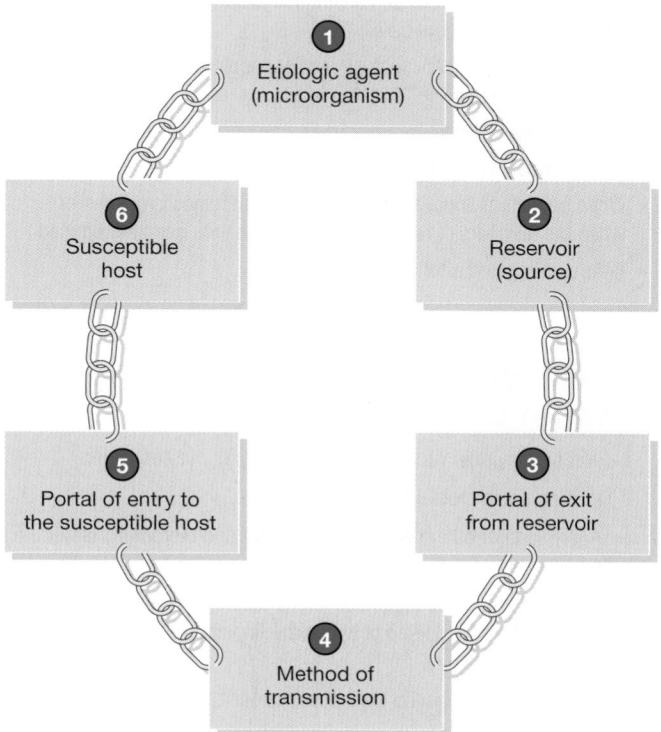

FIGURE 20–2 ■ Chain of infection.

pass by quickly or last for years, but during this time the infected person is contagious. The second stage is the prodromal phase. During the prodromal stage, the symptoms begin to appear. At this point, the symptoms are usually nonspecific such as general malaise, fever, myalgia, and fatigue.

Acute illness occurs during the third stage. During this stage the infective organism is growing and spreading rapidly in the body. The microorganisms produce toxins leading to cell lysis and death. An inflammatory response and immune reaction occur, leading to tissue damage. Along with the vague symptoms, the patient develops more specific symptoms. These include the classic signs of inflammation: swelling, redness, pain, and warmth at the site of infection, along with tachycardia and tachypnea from increased metabolic demands. There are usually other more specific symptoms related to the site of infection and the virulence of the pathogen. As the infection is contained and the pathogen confined by the body's defenses, the individual enters the convalescent stage. During this stage, the damaged tissues begin to heal and symptoms resolve.

An infection can be localized or generalized, acute or chronic. A localized infection affects the host in a small, focal area. Proper care can control the spread of the infection and minimize the illness. Symptoms are localized and may include pain and tenderness at the wound site. A generalized or systemic infection indicates involvement of a large part of the body instead of a single organ or part.

Infections are usually acute, which means that symptoms develop quickly and the body's response is temporary. However, infections can become chronic. In a chronic infection the associated inflammation is covert with the body trying to heal, but with the inflammation flaring up intermittently. It is almost like a battle without either the organism or the body's defenses ever gaining the upper hand.

■ Infection Control and Prevention

Many actions can be taken to control and prevent infection. Health care facilities are prime targets for the development and transfer of infectious organisms. As discussed earlier, patients in health care facilities generally have weakened defenses and are easy targets for bacteria and other types of infectious organisms. Hospital-acquired infections are as high as 30% in intensive care units (Creedon, 2005).

Hand Hygiene

The single most important action in the control and prevention of infection is hand hygiene. Inadequate hand hygiene is considered the leading cause of health care–associated infections and the spread of multidrug-resistant organisms. Infection associated with the delivery of health care is a topic being addressed by the first Global Patient Safety Challenge. Within that effort is a campaign to promote hand hygiene titled "Clean Hands Are Safer Hands." The simple act of hand washing can decrease the occurrence of infections associated with the delivery of health care (Larson et al., 2006).

The purpose of performing hand hygiene is to remove dirt, organic material, and transient microorganisms, and to prevent the spread of organisms leading to infection. Hands are contaminated daily simply through exposure to skin, patient gowns, bed

linen, bedside furniture, and other objects in the patient's immediate environment that are contaminated with the patient's flora. Simple activities such as lifting a patient, taking a patient's pulse, or touching a hand or shoulder can result in contamination of the hands enough to spread infection to others. It is important to perform hand hygiene before and after patient contact, but there are other indications for hand hygiene as well, as listed in Chart 20–3.

Although hand washing with soap and water may seem like a simple procedure, there are many things to consider when washing hands to prevent spread of infection. It is important to perform the procedure properly in order for it to be effective (Chart 20–4). The compliance of health care workers with hand hygiene recommendations is only about 40% or less (Widmer, Conzelmann, Tomic, Frei, & Stranden, 2007). Health care workers often wash their hands incorrectly and not frequently enough. When using soap and water, the hands should be washed for at least 15 seconds, covering all surfaces of the hands and fingers so that nothing is missed. This allows time for the antimicrobial products to work. The area around and under the fingernails contains higher microbial counts and should be washed thoroughly with debris removed from under the fingernails. The hands are then thoroughly rinsed to remove soap

---

CHART 20–3 **Hand Hygiene Requirements**

Hand hygiene procedures should be followed in these circumstances:

- When hands are visibly soiled.
- Before and after patient contact.
- After contact with body fluids or excretions, mucous membranes, and wound dressings.
- When hands are moved from a contaminated body site to a clean body site during patient care.
- After contacting objects such as medical equipment in the immediate vicinity of the patient.
- After removing gloves.
- Before invasive procedures are performed.
- When persistent antimicrobial activity on the hands is desired or when the numbers of resident flora on the hands must be reduced.
- Before eating and after using a restroom.

CHART 20–4 **Steps in Proper Hand Washing When Using Soap and Water**

1. Wet hands under running water using tepid, *not hot,* water.
2. If using antimicrobial soap, use 3 to 5 mL.
3. Apply soap or other hand-washing agent and thoroughly distribute over hands.
4. Vigorously rub hands together for 15 seconds, generating friction on all surfaces including between the fingers and under fingernails.
5. Thoroughly rinse hands to remove residue soap.
6. Dry hands thoroughly using paper towels.
7. Use foot controls or a paper towel to shut off faucet.

residue and then thoroughly dried as well. Microorganisms can be transferred more easily on wet hands than on hands that have been completely dried.

Even when hands are washed and dried correctly, recontamination can occur with the touching of faucet handles that are likely to be contaminated. If the hands are washed correctly and then the faucets are touched to turn them off, the washing is negated. Therefore, faucets should be automatic or controlled by foot, or paper towels should be used for turning them off. When washing the hands for surgical asepsis, the procedure is different, as outlined in Chart 20–5.

Many agents have been tested for use in hand hygiene. The use of plain soap for hand washing is effective in removing dirt, soil, and organic substances; however, plain soap has little antimicrobial activity. The use of antimicrobial hand hygiene products is recommended in any setting where there is a high risk of infection. A 70% ethanol agent effectively reduces microbial counts in less time than other cleansing agents. Alcohol-based agents have been shown to be effective against microorganisms and some viruses and can be more effective than soap in preventing pathogen transmission. The use of an alcohol-based agent results in better adherence to hand hygiene guidelines and saves time for nurses (Somner, Scott, & Gibb, 2007). If using an alcohol-based rub, the product should be applied to the palm of one hand, the hands should be rubbed together, covering all surfaces of the hands and fingers, until the hands are dry.

Some health care facilities have made alcohol-based hand rubs readily available by providing containers to be carried in the nurses' pockets for use at the patient's bedside or close to areas of patient care. Alcohol is not adequate, however, when there is visible dirt or contamination with protein-type materials. Other antiseptic agents used for hand hygiene include chlorhexidine gluconate (CHG), hexachlorophene, and chloroxylenol. These agents work more slowly than alcohol, but have effective residual effects. In addition, agents such as CHG build up an antimicrobial residual, unlike alcohol products.

The wearing of rings and artificial nails can contribute to the spread of infectious organisms (Trick et al., 2003). Rings increase the pathogen counts on the skin, and the more rings that are worn, the greater the contamination (Trick et al., 2003). Therefore, rings should be avoided. Artificial nails are more likely to encourage the growth of microorganisms than are natural nails and should not be used when caring for patients at high risk for infection. Natural nails should be short enough to allow for thorough cleaning underneath the nail and to prevent tears in gloves. Microorganisms can be found in higher concentrations in subungual areas. Nail polish does not increase the microorganism count, however, chipped nail polish does support the growth of microorganisms on the hands.

Hand hygiene is important regardless of whether gloves are used. However, gloves do provide a protective barrier to the transmission of microbes and prevent heavy contamination of the hands. Some transmission can still occur because gloves may have small defects or be torn during use. The hands can also be contaminated during glove removal. Therefore, hand washing with soap and water or the use of an antiseptic hand rub is recommended after glove removal. Gloves should be changed between patients and between contaminated body sites. Single-use disposable gloves should *not* be reused.

Hand washing can lead to dermatitis from the frequent contact with water and cleansing agents. The cracked, dry skin associated with dermatitis is more readily colonized with pathogens. The tenderness of dry, cracked skin can also lead to the avoidance of hand washing. Therefore, it is important to prevent or correct hand dermatitis. Currently the Occupational Safety and Health Administration (OSHA) recommends avoiding the use of petroleum-based moisturizers because they can lead to a deterioration of latex gloves. The use of an appropriate moisturizer that contains humectants along with fats and oils can increase skin hydration, providing a protective skin barrier without interfering with gloves or antibacterial agents (Larson et al., 2006). The use of tepid water rather than hot water is also recommended to help prevent hand dermatitis and the spread of pathogens.

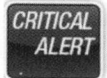 *Hand washing done using the correct procedure and frequency has been shown to be the most important single action in preventing the spread of infection.*

Patient Placement

Placement of a patient with an infection in the hospital setting can be a significant factor in preventing the spread of infection. A private room is the best solution, especially if the infected patient has poor hygiene or cannot assist in implementing precautions to avoid transmission of the microorganisms. If a private room is not available, the infected patient should be placed in a room with the proper roommate. First, consider another patient with the same microorganism as a roommate. If this is not possible, consider the epidemiology and mode of transmission of the infecting pathogen.

Protective Equipment

The use of personal protective equipment (PPE) such as gloves, gowns, and masks plays an important role in the prevention of the spread of pathogens. Protective gowns help prevent the contamination of clothing and protect the skin and clothing of personnel from exposure to blood and body fluids. Gowns can help prevent the transmission of pathogens from patients or equipment in the environment to other patients or equipment. The Healthcare Infection Control Practices Advisory Committee (HICPAC) of the CDC recommends the use of gowns and gloves

---

CHART 20–5 **Surgical Hand Antisepsis**

1. Hands should be scrubbed before putting on gloves.

2. Remove rings, watches, and bracelets before beginning the scrub.

3. Remove debris from underneath fingernails using a nail cleaner under running water.

4. Using antimicrobial soap or alcohol-based rub, scrub hands and forearms the length of time recommended by the manufacturer, usually 2 to 6 minutes.

5. When using an alcohol-based surgical hand scrub, follow the manufacturer's instructions. Wash hands with non-antimicrobial soap, and dry hands thoroughly before using the alcohol-based scrub.

---

to prevent nosocomial infections. Gowns need to be impervious to fluids for procedures that may involve fluids. Gowns should *always* be removed before leaving patients' rooms and hand hygiene should be performed.

Masks and face shields or eye shields should be worn by health care personnel when performing procedures that are likely to cause splashing of blood or body fluids. These activities protect the mucous membranes of the eyes, nose, and mouth from exposure to pathogens. When an infected patient leaves his room, a mask is required.

Housekeeping practices should be observed to decrease dust and environmental reservoirs of pathogens. Spills of blood and body fluids must be cleaned up immediately with hospital disinfectant or household bleach and water. Reusable equipment such as blood pressure cuffs and stethoscopes can carry pathogens from patient to patient. Stethoscopes can be disinfected with isopropyl alcohol or disposable covers can be used between patients. Before and after each shift, the bell, diaphragm, and earpieces of stethoscopes need to be wiped down with alcohol. All equipment used on patients in isolation should be left in the room for use only with that patient. If this is not possible, any equipment removed from the room must be disinfected with hospital-grade disinfectant before being used with another patient.

It is important to note that *Clostridium difficile* is a frequent colonizer of the hospital environment. It is a spore former that can live in the environment for very long periods and is able to withstand many normal cleaning procedures.

Disposal of Soiled Equipment

Appropriate disposal of used and/or contaminated equipment is essential in order to protect both health care workers and prevent the spread of disease (Kozier, Erb, Berman, & Snyder, 2004). Linens should be changed so that there is little contact between the dirty linens and the nurse's uniform. Linens are to be carried away from the nurse's body and placed in an appropriate hamper. Throwing dirty linen on the floor or laying it in a chair should be avoided because it could lead to further contamination of the environment. Linens should never be shaken in the air because that creates air currents that spread pathogens. Needles and syringes should be disposed of in a container specifically made for disposal of sharp objects (Figure 20–3 ■). Inadvertent sticks with used sharps can lead to exposure to pathogens.

Contaminated materials need to be placed in plastic bags that are impervious to microorganisms before removing them from an isolated area. The CDC recommends a single bag unless the outside becomes contaminated. The single bag needs to be placed in a second bag if outside contamination occurs (CDC, 1997).

Pathogens Causing Infectious Disease

Pathogens must be present in the right quantity in a susceptible host in order to cause infection. The number needed is variable depending on the pathogen and the susceptibility of the host. The severity of the illness depends on the pathogen's pathogenicity or its ability to induce disease. Several factors influence the pathogenicity of an organism, including the pathogen's infectivity or in-

FIGURE 20–3 ■ Sharps container.

vasiveness, virulence, antigenicity, and viability. These terms are defined as follows:

- **Infectivity** or **invasiveness** is the ability of a pathogen to enter the host and then live and grow. Some pathogens are capable of producing toxins or enzymes that help them to invade the host and increase their resistance to the host's defenses.
- **Virulence** is related to the severity of disease a pathogen is capable of causing. Virulence can vary depending on the ability of the host to mount an immune response. It is expressed as the number of cases of infection that are serious or produce a disability in all those infected.
- **Antigenicity** is the ability of the pathogen to elicit an immune defense in the host. It affects the ability of the host to develop long-term immunity.
- **Viability** is the ability of the pathogen to survive outside of the host. Most pathogens cannot live and grow outside the host.

Human pathogens are divided into different categories of disease-causing agents. These include bacteria, viruses, *Mycoplasma*, rickettsiae, fungi, and parasites.

Bacteria

Bacteria are single-celled microorganisms that have a cell membrane that can be penetrated by antibiotics. They are classified in many different ways. They can be round or oval cocci, rod shaped, or spirochetes. Cocci can appear in pairs, called diplococci; or chains, like streptococci; or in clusters, like staphylococci. They can be rod-shaped bacilli, spiral shaped as seen in spirochetes, or curved. Bacteria can be intracellular like *Neisseriae gonorrhoeae* or extracellular like *Staphylococcus*.

Bacteria can be classified according to their need for oxygen. Aerobic bacteria must have oxygen for survival, whereas anaerobic bacteria can survive without oxygen. Bacteria are also classified according to their ability to be stained with crystal violet. Some bacteria have a substance in their outer cell wall that absorbs dye. Gram-positive bacteria stain blue when subjected to crystal violet stain; gram-negative bacteria remain colorless. Yet another classification for bacteria is according to their ability to form protective capsules and spores. See Chart 20–6 for classifications of common bacterial diseases.

Bacteria can cause disease in several ways. Gram-negative bacteria have endotoxins in their outer cell wall. These **endotoxins** are produced by live bacteria and are released when the bacteria are killed. Endotoxins stimulate the immune response, which can lead to changes in coagulation of blood and functions of vital body systems. Endotoxins can stimulate regulatory systems in humans, leading to inflammation, bleeding, hypotension, and fever. **Exotoxins** are proteins released by the bacterial cell during growth and have very specific actions. Exotoxins modify cell enzymes and functions leading to cell death or dysfunction. They are usually named for the site they affect. For example, enterotoxins affect the gastrointestinal tract. Some toxins disrupt cell membranes causing them to lyse, leading to cell death. Examples of bacteria include *Streptococcus, Staphylococcus, Neisseriae gonorrhoeae, Enterococcus,* and *Pseudomonas aeruginosa.*

Viruses

Viruses are the smallest of human pathogens. They occupy the body intracellularly because they require the genetic material of the host cell to replicate. Viruses contain a core made up of either RNA or DNA surrounded by a protein coat that helps the virus attach to the host cell. They cannot live and grow outside of a host cell. Viruses are classified according to the type of genetic material (RNA or DNA), the type of disease they cause (hepatitis, herpes), and how they reproduce (retrovirus) or how they are transmitted (as an enterovirus or sexually).

Viruses attach to receptors on the host cell membrane and penetrate the cell. Once inside the cell, the virus uses the cell's genetic material to replicate itself. The virus then matures and exits the cell ready to invade another host cell. The virus causes disease through the process of entering the cell and replicating, which leads to disruption of the cell's normal functions. The virus evokes an immune response against the host cell as it spreads from cell to cell. Most viruses are self-limiting, but viruses can also cause irreversible and lethal injury in a susceptible host. Examples of diseases caused by a virus include the common cold, acquired immunodeficiency syndrome (AIDS), hepatitis, mononucleosis, and herpes simplex.

CHART 20–6 | **Common Classifications of Bacterial Disease**

Organism	Area of the Body	Antibiotic Treatment
Gram-Positive Cocci		
Staphylococcus aureus	Found in nasopharynx, skin, clothing. Common in subcutaneous and cutaneous abscesses, and foreign devices such as IVs. Frequent cause of osteomyelitis, pneumonia.	Penicillin, first-generation cephalosporins, vancomycin, erythromycin
Staphylococcus epidermidis	Found commonly on the skin, nasopharynx, and lower GU tract. Infection occurs with indwelling devices that are inserted through the skin, such as catheters. Can be a contaminant of cultures if area not properly disinfected prior to obtaining the culture.	Penicillins, first-generation cephalosporins, vancomycin
Group A beta-hemolytic streptococci	Found in nose and throat, respiratory secretions, hands. Cause of acute pharyngitis, cutaneous impetigo, and systemic infection.	Penicillin, erythromycin, first-generation cephalosporins, vancomycin
Gram-Positive Bacilli		
Corynebacterium diphtheriae	Present in nasopharyngeal secretions, respiratory infections, and skin infections. Transmitted by airborne droplets and direct contact with exudates from infected lesions.	Erythromycin, penicillin
Gram-Negative Diplococci		
Neisseria meningitidis	Found in the nasopharynx and transported through respiratory tract. Causes meningitis.	Penicillin, third-generation cephalosporins
Gram-Negative Bacilli		
Enterobacteriaceae	Important in nosocomial infections. Can be found in the intestinal tract. Causes lower respiratory tract infections, urinary tract infections, and traveler's diarrhea.	Third-generation cephalosporins, penicillins, imipenem
Pseudomonas	Found in the soil, water, raw fruits and vegetables, plants, animals and man. Causes nosocomial infections. Can affect any body system but frequently seen in moist wounds and upper airways.	Penicillins, aminoglycosides, ciprofloxacin, ceftazidime, imipenem
Anaerobic Bacteria		
Clostridium difficile	Occurs as an overgrowth in the gut of patients during or after antibiotic therapy. Also transmitted on the hands and unsterilized equipment and is a frequent colonizer of the hospital environment. It can live in the environment for long periods and is able to withstand normal cleaning procedures.	Discontinue antibiotics, vancomycin, metronidazole

Mycoplasma

Mycoplasma is a small pathogen that is neither bacteria nor virus. It lives independently and does not require a host cell. It does not have a cell wall but does have a lipid outer membrane (Porth, 2007). This characteristic makes *Mycoplasma* resistant to antibiotics that usually attack cell walls. *Mycoplasma* has the ability to kill cells directly and leads to an autoimmune, antigen–antibody response and inflammation. It usually infects the respiratory tract and leads to many serious respiratory problems such as pneumonia. It also is responsible for pharyngitis, urethritis, and pelvic inflammatory disease (Porth, 2007).

Rickettsiae

Rickettsiae are small, intracellular, gram-negative organisms. They have no cell wall and, therefore, require a host cell to live and multiply. Rickettsiae are transmitted through the bites of arthropods such as ticks, lice, fleas, or mites or through exposure to their waste products. They primarily attack vascular epithelial cells causing vasculitis. Infections related to rickettsiae include Rocky Mountain spotted fever, typhus, and Q fever.

Fungi

Fungi have a nuclear membrane and a nucleus with several chromosomes. They can reproduce sexually or asexually. They are classified as either molds or yeasts. Molds are organisms with hyphae that produce spores for reproduction. Yeasts are single-celled, oval-shaped organisms that reproduce by budding. Fungal disease is also known as mycosis.

Fungi are found most everywhere on earth. They can live in a wide variety of environments and do not necessarily need a host. Temperature is important to the survival of fungi. Some can grow only on cooler surfaces like the skin, whereas others require warmer core body temperatures. Cutaneous mycosis is caused by skin contact. Systemic disease is due to inhalation of the fungi, which is then spread through the lymphatic system. Examples of cutaneous myosis include candidiasis, *tinea pedis,* and *tinea capitis.* Examples of systemic mycosis include cryptococcosis, histoplasmosis, and aspergillosis.

Parasites

Parasites are pathogens that infect and cause disease in other animals. Protozoa and helminths belong to this classification. Protozoa are small, single-celled animals that can be transmitted to the host by direct or indirect contact. They are mainly transmitted through ingested food or water or through an arthropod vector. They reproduce inside the host and are easily mobile in the body. Once inside, they stimulate an inflammatory response or cause disease by ingesting and/or invading human tissue.

Helminths are multicellular parasites. They require intermediate hosts and cannot reproduce inside the human host. Therefore, many exposures are required before a human can be infected. Helminths are transmitted by ingestion of eggs, breaks in the skin, or arthropod vectors. Like protozoa, helminths stimulate an inflammatory response. Infestation by helminths can lead to malnutrition and anemia in the host because they compete with the host for nutrients in the gastrointestinal tract.

New or Reemerging Infection

Infectious diseases are constantly emerging and reemerging. Since 1973, 30 new infections have been identified such as Lyme disease, Ebola virus, West Nile virus, severe acute respiratory syndrome (SARS), and AIDS (CDC, 2004). Diseases that were thought to be under control have reemerged due to antibiotic resistance and the development of new strains of pathogens. Tuberculosis is an example of a reemerging disease.

Biological Warfare

Biological warfare has become a concern since the terrorist attacks of September 11, 2001. The most likely pathogens to be used in biological warfare are the smallpox virus, *Bacillus anthracis* (anthrax), *Clostridium botulinum* (botulism), and viruses that cause hemorrhagic fevers. Smallpox immunizations were stopped in 1972 because the World Health Organization believed the disease had been eradicated. Smallpox is caused by the poxvirus *Variola* and spreads by direct contact or inhalation of respiratory droplets. Symptoms include high fever, headache, malaise, and a vesicular/pustular rash on the face and extremities. It is highly contagious and has a high mortality in unvaccinated people. Anthrax is an acute bacterial infection caused by a gram-positive, spore-producing organism that occurs in inhaled, cutaneous, and gastrointestinal forms. The inhaled form has the highest mortality rate (CDC, 2003). The symptoms are flu-like and include fever, nonproductive cough, headache, and malaise. Eventually the patient develops respiratory failure and hemodynamic collapse that can lead to death in 2 to 3 days.

Health care workers need to be alert to unusual illness patterns that indicate unusual infections. Signs to watch for include an increased incidence in the same geographic area, a disease pattern that is inconsistent with the patient's age, or patient presentation with symptoms of a rare disease. The presence of these indicators should be reported to the public health authorities. Biological warfare is covered in detail in Chapter 72 ∞.

Isolation Precautions

In 1996, HICPAC developed isolation precautions that were then updated in 2007 (Siegel, Rhinehart, Jackson, Chiarello, & HICPAC, 2007). HICPAC's guidelines follow a two-tiered program. The first tier involves standard precautions. Standard precautions are designed to reduce the risk of transmission of pathogens from blood and body fluids containing blood. Patients with HIV or hepatitis B often have no apparent symptoms but can transmit the disease to others. Therefore, standard precautions apply to all hospitalized patients regardless of their diagnosis. The HICPAC guidelines are designed to control the spread of these diseases, as well as other nosocomial infections. The HICPAC guidelines should be used by all health care workers who have direct or indirect contact with patients or with their body fluids. This includes not only nurses and physicians, but those who empty trash, change linens, or clean the room. Standard precautions apply to blood, body fluids and secretions, nonintact skin, and mucous membranes. The National Guidelines box lists the HICPAC standard precautions.

The second tier is the transmission-based precautions, also outlined in the National Guidelines box. These precautions are

NATIONAL GUIDELINES for Standard and Transmission-Based Precautions

Category	Precaution
Standard Precautions	
Hand hygiene	Perform hand hygiene after touching blood, body fluids, secretions, excretions, and contaminated items whether or not gloves are worn.
Gloves	Wear clean, nonsterile gloves when touching blood, body fluids, secretions, excretions, and contaminated items. Put on clean gloves just before touching mucous membranes and nonintact skin.
Mask, eye protection, face shield	Worn to protect mucous membranes of the eyes, nose, and mouth during procedures and patient care activities that generate splashes or sprays of blood, body fluids, secretions, or excretions.
Gown	Wear a clean, nonsterile gown to protect skin and prevent soiling of clothing during procedures and patient care activities that may generate splashes or sprays of blood, body fluids, secretions, or excretions. Gowns should be impervious to fluids.
Patient care equipment	Handle used patient care equipment soiled with blood, body fluids, secretions, or excretions in a manner that prevents skin and mucous membrane exposure and contamination of clothing, and transfer of microorganisms to other patients and environments.
Environmental control	Adequate procedures should be in place for routine care, cleaning, and disinfection of environmental surfaces.
Linen	Handle soiled linen in a manner that prevents skin and mucous membrane exposure and contamination of clothing.
Occupational health and bloodborne pathogens	Prevent injuries when using and disposing of needles, scalpels, and other sharp instruments or devices. Never recap needles or use any technique that involves pointing the sharp end toward part of the body. Use mouthpieces, resuscitation bags, or other ventilation devices as an alternative to mouth-to-mouth resuscitation.
Patient placement	Place a patient who contaminates the environment in a private room if possible. If not possible, place patients with the same diagnosis in the same room.
Transmission-Based Precautions	
Airborne precautions	1. Place patient in private room with N95 respirator, monitored negative air pressure, 6 to 12 air changes per hour, and appropriate discharge of air outdoors. Keep room door closed and patient in room. 2. Wear respiratory protection when entering room. 3. If leaving the room, the patient should wear a mask. 4. Limit the movement and transport of the patient from the room.
Droplet precautions	1. Place patient in private room or in a room with cohort patients with the same disease. 2. Wear a mask when working within 3 feet of patient. 3. If leaving the room, the patient should wear a mask. 4. Limit movement and transport of patient from room.
Contact precautions	1. Place patient in private room or with a very low risk roommate. 2. Wear gloves when entering room and remove gloves before leaving room. Then perform hand hygiene. 3. Wear a gown when entering the room and remove gown before leaving room. 4. Limit the movement and transport of the patient from the room. 5. Dedicate the use of noncritical patient care equipment to a single patient.

Source: Siegel, J. D., Rhinehart, E., Jackson, M., Chiarello, L., & the Healthcare Infection Control Practices Advisory Committee. (2007, June). *Guideline for isolation precautions: Preventing transmission of infectious agents in healthcare settings 2007.* Retrieved June 6, 2008, from http://www.cdc.gov/ncidod/dhqp/pdf/guidelines/Isolation2007.pdf.

for patients "known or suspected to be infected by highly transmissible or epidemiologically important pathogens" (Siegel et al., 2007). They are used in addition to standard precautions. They are classified into three types: airborne precautions, droplet precautions, and contact precautions (Garner, 1996). These precautions can be used either singularly or in combination for diseases that have multiple routes of transmission.

Airborne precautions are designed to protect against infectious agents that are transmitted through particles that remain suspended in the air and can become inhaled or deposited on a host. These precautions require the use of special ventilation and air handling, such as a room with negative air pressure and an increased number of air changes with the air discharged to the outside and no recirculation of the air in the room. If the air is recirculated, the return air must be filter through a high-efficiency particulate air (HEPA) filter (Schulster & Chinn, 2003). Personal respiratory protection or a mask is indicated for persons entering the room when caring for the patient. Precautions include the use of a National Institute for Occupational Safety and Health (NIOSH)-approved N95 particulate respirator with qualitative fit testing of the respirator required. Use of these engineering controls is needed for TB, varicella (and disseminated varicella-zoster), measles, and smallpox.

Droplet precautions protect against the risk of transmission of infection through droplets in the air. Infected droplets can make contact with the conjunctivae or the mucous membranes of the nose or mouth. They are generated primarily during talking, coughing, or sneezing by someone who is infected with the organism. These droplets do not remain suspended in the air and travel only short distances (usually 3 feet or less), therefore, special air handling is not required. The wearing of masks is important if working closely with a patient, when doing procedures such as suctioning. Droplet precautions may be necessary to use when caring for a patient with meningitis or diphtheria.

Contact precautions reduce the risk of organism transmission by direct or indirect contact. Direct contact occurs when there is skin-to-skin contact such as might occur when turning or bathing a patient or even touching an infected patient's hand. Transmission could also occur from an infected patient to a susceptible patient if the patients shake hands or touch in some way. Indirect contact involves contact of a host with a contaminated intermediate object in the patient's environment. Contact precautions involve wearing gloves and gowns and dedicating the use of equipment to a single patient. This type of precaution would be necessary when caring for a patient with *Clostridium difficile* infection or a major abscess.

Patients who are immunocompromised may be at high risk of developing infections, especially is they are severely neutropenic with an absolute neutrophil count of less than 500 cells/mm³ (cubic millimeter) (Porth, 2007). This may occur in patients who have had a transplant or have leukemia. These patients must be in a protective environment that minimizes exposures to pathogens. Of course, the standard isolation precautions are observed. The length of time this patient is outside the room for diagnostic procedures or other activities must be limited. If the patient must be outside the room, respiratory protection should be provided. The room should be kept very clean without dust. All visitors and health care workers should perform hand hygiene carefully before entering the room or touching the patient. No one with any type of infection should be allowed to enter the room.

The 2007 expanded and revised isolation guidelines (Siegel et al., 2007) include specific diseases and new terminology and equipment. The National Guidelines box summarizes these 2007 revisions of the 1996 guidelines.

Immunization Programs

Prevention of infection is the best approach, and immunizations help protect children and adults against infections. Infection can be prevented anywhere along the chain of infection. Efforts to prevent infection include anything from eradication of infectious agents, to eliminating the reservoirs for infection, to eliminating a vector that carries the disease. One method used to eliminate the risk for some infections is immunization. Active or passive immunization improves the host's defenses. **Active immunization** involves the introduction of a live, killed, or attenuated toxin of a disease organism into the body. The immune system responds by producing antibodies. Active immunization provides long-term and possibly lifelong immunity. Some vaccines require boosters to maintain the immunity. Examples of active immunizations include those for measles, mumps, hepatitis B, and hepatitis A.

Passive immunization provides immunity for a short period of time, usually around 6 to 12 weeks. This involves the injection of already formed antibodies into the body. The individual may still have the disease, but it will be a less severe case. An example of this type of immunity is immunoglobin injections given to people exposed to hepatitis A. The recommendations regarding immunizations are based on scientific knowledge regarding the principles of active and passive immunization, the epidemiology and burden of disease, the safety of vaccines, and the cost analysis of preventive measures.

Certain benefits and risks are associated with immunizations. No vaccine is completely safe or 100% effective. Benefits include protection against the consequences of disease to the individual and to society as a whole. This protection includes not having to experience the symptoms of the illness, improved quality of life and productivity, and prevention of death. The risks of immunization include common, minor, and local adverse effects and rare, severe, and life-threatening conditions. The recommendations for immunizations represent a balance of the benefits for each person and society against the potential risks and problems associated with vaccinations. A vaccination schedule has been developed based on age-specific risks for disease, age-specific risks for complications, ability of an individual to respond to the vaccine, and potential interference with the immune response by passively transferred maternal antibodies. Studies have demonstrated that recommended ages and intervals between doses of multiple-dose antigens provide optimal protection or have the best evidence of efficacy. The immunization schedule for children is revised annually and published each year in January by the Centers for Disease Control and Prevention (2008). The schedule for adolescents and adults is revised less frequently, except for the influenza vaccine recommendations that are published annually.

Although immunizations are relatively safe, there are some contraindications and certain precautions should be followed. Most are adverse reactions are temporary and the vaccination can be given at a later time. A contraindication is any condition that increases the risk for a serious adverse reaction. The only true contraindication applicable to all vaccines is a history of a severe allergic reaction after a prior dose of vaccine or to a vaccine constituent. For example, a person who has an anaphylactic allergy to egg protein should not receive the influenza vaccine because it could cause serious illness or death in the recipient. A precaution is a condition in a recipient that might increase the risk for a serious adverse reaction or might compromise the ability of the vaccine to produce immunity. Those individuals with mild, acute illness such as diarrhea or upper respiratory tract infection can be safely vaccinated. Individuals with moderate or severe illness should be vaccinated as soon as possible after they have recovered from the acute illness. All vaccines may cause adverse reactions that are local, systemic, or allergic. Local reactions are least severe and mainly involve redness or soreness at the site. Systemic reactions such as fever occur less frequently. Serious allergic reactions such as anaphylaxis are rare.

NATIONAL GUIDELINES Summary of 2007 Revisions to the HICPAC Isolation Guidelines

Standard Precautions: New Elements

Respiratory hygiene/cough etiquette

Use of masks: to insert catheters for injections into spinal or epidural spaces, via lumbar puncture (e.g., myelogram, spinal or epidural anesthesia)

Safe injection practice

Safe Injection Practice: Defined

Use sterile, single-use needles and syringes for each injection given.

Prevent contamination of injection equipment, medication, and spaces used to prepare the injections.

Use single-dose vials whenever possible.

Include these practices in policies and training programs and monitor for adherence.

Empiric Transmission-Based Precautions

These precautions are to be observed in addition to standard precautions, pending confirmation of diagnosis. More than one transmission-based precaution may be used for diseases that have multiple routes of transmission. Some examples follow:

Meningitis

Neisseria meningitides: Use droplet precautions for the first 24 hours of antimicrobial therapy; mask and face protection for intubation. (*Note:* This is the *only type of meningitis* that requires transmission-based precautions.)

Enteroviruses: Use contact precautions for infants and children.

Mycobacterium tuberculosis: Use airborne precautions if pulmonary infiltrate; use airborne plus contact precautions if potentially infectious draining body fluid is present.

Respiratory Infections

In infants and young children, especially bronchiolitis and pneumonia (RSV, parainfluenza, adenovirus, influenza virus, human metapneumonia virus): Use contact plus droplet precautions; droplet may be discontinued when influenza and adenovirus have been ruled out.

Cough/ fever/ upper lobe pulmonary infiltrate (M. tuberculosis, respiratory viruses, Staphylococcus pneumoniae and/or S. aureus (MSSA or MRSA): Use airborne plus contact precautions, or resistant organism (RO) precautions for MRSA.

For HIV-positive patients (or patients at high risk for HIV infection): Use eye/face protection if aerosol-generating procedure performed or contact with respiratory secretions anticipated. Tuberculosis is more likely in an HIV-infected individual than in an HIV-negative individual. If tuberculosis is unlikely and there is no airborne infection isolation room or respirator available, use droplet instead of airborne precautions.

For patients with history of recent travel (10 to 21 days) to countries with active outbreaks of SARS (avian influenza): Use airborne plus contact precautions plus eye protection. If SARS and/or TB are unlikely, use droplet only instead of airborne.

Ambulatory Care

Patient-to-patient transmission of *Burkholderia* species and *Pseudomonas aeruginosa* can occur in outpatient clinics for adults and children with cystic fibrosis. Implement transmission-based precautions. Segregate patients in the waiting room and decontaminate surfaces.

New Terminology

Airborne infection isolation room (AIIR) replaces *negative pressure room.*

Transmission-based precautions replaces *isolation categories.*

New Equipment: Purified Air Particulate Respirator

The purified air particulate respirator (PAPR) is a type of respiratory protection used for rule-out and confirmed TB, SARS, and avian influenza.

The N95 respirators will continue to be used. Annual fit-testing is required for the N95 respirators. N95 respirators have different shapes, sizes, and colors.

Please continue to use surgical masks for standard, droplet, and contact transmission-based precautions.

Source: Centers for Disease Control. (2007a). *Guidelines and recommendations: Infection control guidance for the prevention and control of influenza in acute-care facilities.* Retrieved June 20, 2007, from http://www.cdc.gov.

Healthy People 2010 Guidelines

The *Healthy People 2010* guidelines (DHHS, 2000) are a set of national health objectives designed to serve as a basis for the development of state and community health plans. It allows for diverse groups to work together as teams to improve health for everyone. These objectives were developed by leading federal agencies based on the best scientific knowledge available and designed to measure program outcomes over time. One of the objectives included in the *Healthy People 2010* report is to "[p]revent disease, disability, and death from infectious diseases, including vaccine-preventable diseases" (DHHS, 2000). Infectious diseases remain a major cause of illness, disability, and death in this country and worldwide. Pneumonia, influenza, and septicemia were among the top 10 causes of death in the United States in 2003. Infectious diseases are an economic drain on society, not only in terms of financial costs but also in terms of time lost from work and treatment of disabilities.

Immunizations can prevent infectious diseases and the disabilities caused by the diseases. The vaccines not only protect the person who is vaccinated but also protect society. When the vaccination levels in the community are high, those who have not been vaccinated due to contraindications are not likely to get the disease. Significant progress has been made, with vaccine-preventable diseases at or near record-low levels; however, these efforts need to be continued. The organisms responsible for these diseases have not disappeared—they have merely receded. Therefore, the major strategies identified by *Health People 2010* to protect people from vaccine preventable diseases are as follows:

- Improve the quality and quantity of vaccinated delivery services.
- Minimize financial burdens for needy persons.
- Increase community participation, education, and partnership.

- Improve monitoring of disease and vaccination coverage.
- Develop new or improved vaccines and improve vaccine use.

The National Guidelines box summarizes the *Healthy People 2010* objectives related to immunizations and infectious diseases.

■ Nursing Management

The nursing management of a patient with an infection requires the assessment of the patient and the development of a specific plan to meet the individual patient's needs. Nursing care should be well planned and adapted as necessary so that the patient receives quality care, further infection is prevented, and infections are not transmitted to others. Nursing assessment is essential to identify potential complications and responses to treatment.

Assessment

When assessing the patient with an infection, the nurse should take into account the signs and symptoms of the infection, the site of the infection, the pathogenicity of the organism, and the body's immune response. A thorough assessment will help identify the infection and/or its complications so that appropriate therapy can be implemented.

Fever

One feature common to most infections is a fever. Fever is defined as a body temperature of more than 38°C (100°F). Fever is an indication of the severity of the inflammatory response in the patient with an intact immune response. As stated earlier in this chapter, fever is induced by mediators known as endogenous pyrogens that act directly on the hypothalamic regulating center that controls the body's temperature. Fever can be beneficial because some microorganisms are very sensitive to changes in temperature and cannot survive when temperatures go up. Fever can also be present when no infectious process is occurring, such as with malignancy or myocardial infarction. In these cases, the injured cells produce endogenous pyrogens, resulting in a fever.

Although a fever can have beneficial effects, a fever of 40°C (104°F) can be harmful. *Hyperpyrexia,* an elevated body temperature, leads to an increased metabolic rate, which increases the demand for oxygen and the need for calories. This is associated with tachycardia and tachypnea. These conditions put an increased workload on the heart and lungs and can lead to impaired cardiac and pulmonary function. The increased need for calories can lead to protein breakdown for energy. With the increase in temperature, diaphoresis increases, which can lead to dehydration. High fevers can also lead to febrile seizures.

NATIONAL GUIDELINES *Healthy People 2010* Objectives Related to Immunization and Infectious Disease

Diseases Preventable Through Universal Vaccination
Reduce or eliminate indigenous cases of vaccine-preventable diseases.

Reduce chronic hepatitis B virus infections in infants and young children.

Reduce hepatitis B.

Reduce bacterial meningitis in young children.

Reduce invasive pneumococcal infections.

Diseases Preventable Through Targeted Vaccination
Reduce hepatitis A.

Reduce meningococcal disease.

Reduce Lyme disease.

Infectious Diseases and Emerging Antimicrobial Resistance
Reduce hepatitis C.

Increase the proportion of persons with chronic hepatitis C infection identified by state and local health departments.

Reduce tuberculosis.

Increase the proportion of all tuberculosis patients who complete curative therapy within 12 months.

Increase the proportion of contacts and other high-risk persons with latent tuberculosis infection who complete a course of treatment.

Reduce the average time for a laboratory to confirm and report tuberculosis cases.

Increase the proportion of international travelers who receive recommended preventive services when traveling in areas of risk for select infectious diseases: hepatitis A, malaria, and typhoid.

Reduce invasive early-onset group B streptococcal disease.

Reduce hospitalizations caused by peptic ulcer disease in the United States.

Reduce the number of courses of antibiotics for ear infections in young children.

Reduce the number of courses of antibiotics prescribed for the sole diagnosis of the common cold.

Reduce hospital-acquired infections in intensive care unit patients.

Reduce antimicrobial use among intensive care unit patients.

Vaccination Coverage and Strategies
Achieve and maintain effective vaccination coverage levels for universally recommended vaccines among young children.

Maintain vaccination coverage levels for children in licensed day care facilities and children in kindergarten through the first grade.

Increase the proportion of young children and adolescents who receive all vaccines that have been recommended for universal administration for at least 5 years.

Increase the proportion of providers who have measured the vaccination coverage levels among children in their practice population within the past 2 years.

Increase the proportion of children who participate in fully operational population-based immunization registries.

Increase routine vaccination coverage levels for adolescents.

Increase hepatitis B vaccine coverage among high-risk groups.

Increase the proportion of adults who are vaccinated annually against influenza and ever vaccinated against pneumococcal disease.

Vaccine Safety
Reduce vaccine-associated adverse events.

Increase the number of persons under active surveillance for vaccine safety via large linked databases.

Source: U.S. Department of Health and Human Services. (2000). *Healthy people 2010: Understanding and improving health.* Retrieved June 5, 2008, from http://www.healthypeople.gov.

The assessment of fever can provide information about the possible cause of the infection. The pattern of fever occurrence should be observed. Fever can be described as intermittent, remittent, sustained, or relapsing. An intermittent fever is defined as a fever that is cyclical. The temperature goes up and then returns to normal at least once in 24 hours. The remittent fever is one in which the fever stays elevated throughout the day but can vary a few degrees. Sustained fever is a continuous fever that has very little variation. A relapsing fever resolves but returns after a period of time in which the infection was thought to be resolved. A fever that lasts 2 weeks or more without identification of the cause is known as a **fever of unknown origin (FUO).**

 A fever of 40.5°C (105°F) can cause or worsen cardiac and pulmonary problems and also cause febrile seizures.

Patient History

When assessing the patient for a risk for infection or the presence of an infection or fever, the first step is to take a history. A thorough history can help identify the cause of the infection and can direct the focus for the physical examination and diagnostic tests. The first part of a patient history is the *history of present illness*. This section should provide an in-depth view of the patient's problem. One way to remember what should be included in the history of present illness is the mnemonic OLD CARTS (Chart 20–7). It is usually beneficial to begin with a general question such as "What brought you here?" Then direct the patient—without putting words in the patient's mouth—so that pertinent information is obtained.

Information pertaining to past medical history is gathered next. This should include information on any previous infectious diseases such as hepatitis, sexually transmitted infections, or TB. History of childhood infections and vaccinations should be included in the inquiry. The patient should be asked about any preexisting conditions that might affect the immune system such as the use of steroids, chemotherapy, transplants, or other chronic illnesses. A travel history should be included. Where has the patient traveled, how long, and what were the living circumstances? Hiking, camping, and caving can increase the risk of infection as well as travel to countries where sanitation is poor. It is important to note what foods were eaten and whether the foods were cooked or raw.

CHART 20–7 **History of Present Illness: OLD CARTS**

The OLD CARTS mnemonic can be used to elicit information about a patient's current illness:

Onset

Location

Duration

Character

Aggravating/alleviating factors

Relieving factors

Temporal factors

Severity

Has the patient been exposed to any infected animals? If the patient has pets, how are the animal feces handled? Has the patient recently experienced any insect bites or been exposed to rodents in the home? Exposure to infected people is also important. The nurse should inquire about sexual history. It is important to know about all sexual partners and whether the sexual activity is high risk. Ask the patient about drug, tobacco, and alcohol use. Drugs and alcohol can lead to exposure to bloodborne pathogens via needles and sexual contact. Smoking increases the risk of respiratory infections due to effects of smoke on cilia that normally protect the airway. Sharing tobacco products, drinks, lip balm, and so forth has been implicated in the transmission of gram-negative diplococci *Neisseria meningitidis,* which may lead to meningococcal disease. Diet history should be obtained related to what is eaten, as well as the sanitation of food, dining out, how food is cooked, and where it is obtained.

Physical Examination

Once the history is completed, the physical examination should focus on the areas identified in the history as being the potential source of infection. A focused physical exam aimed at assessing for an infection should include the following:

- *Vital signs:* Record height and weight, temperature, respiratory rate, pulse rate, and blood pressure.
- *Skin and mucous membranes:* Inspect for breaks in skin integrity, redness, warmth, rash, jaundice, signs of insect bites; check skin turgor and hydration status, drainage from lesions or wounds. Inspect skin folds for candidal skin infections and scabies.
- *Head and neck:* Examine eyes, nose, and ears for redness, drainage, or swelling. Assess visual acuity. Assess pharynx for redness, swelling, the presence of masses, and the presence of discharge or exudates. Inspect the oral mucosa for lesions and the teeth for caries, swelling of the gums, foul smell, or drainage. Palpate over the sinuses for pain or swelling.
- *Lymph nodes:* Palpate all superficial lymph nodes. Check for enlargement and pain. Also note the size of the lymph nodes and whether they are movable or very firm.
- *Lungs:* Auscultate lungs for abnormal breath sounds. Note decreases in breath sounds, the presence of crackles, rhonchi, friction rubs, or wheezes. Note the presence of a cough. Note color and consistency of sputum.
- *Heart:* Auscultate the heart for the rate and rhythm of the heart sounds. Note any abnormal sounds such as murmurs or friction rubs.
- *Abdomen:* Auscultate for the presence of bowel sounds. Palpate for masses, tenderness, and enlarged liver or spleen. If diarrhea is present, note amount, frequency, color, and consistency. Note presence of vomiting including the consistency, color, and amount.
- *Genitourinary tract:* Assess for costovertebral angle tenderness, suprapubic tenderness, fullness over the bladder. Inspect the perineum for redness or drainage.
- *Reproductive system:* Pelvic examination should be completed on women as indicated by the history. Check for discharge, cervical motion tenderness, or masses. The prostate gland should be assessed on men when indicated by history.

Check for size, tenderness, and discharge. Note color, odor, and amount of urine.

- *Nervous system:* Assess for changes in mental status. Note any changes in neurological signs such as weakness, tremors, seizures, or parenthesis.

 Frequently assess areas where tubes enter or leave the body for signs of infection such as increasing redness or drainage around the tube.

Diagnostic Tests

Diagnostic tests are used to confirm the diagnosis, to decide on or see the response to treatment options, or to pinpoint the location and severity of the infection. The Diagnostic Tests box summarizes the tests related to infection. One of the most important diagnostic tests is the complete blood count. The number and variety of leukocytes, or WBCs, can give the nurse some insight into the presence and severity of an infection. The normal count is 5,000 to 10,000 WBC/mm³. A WBC of more than 10,000

DIAGNOSTIC TESTS Related to Infection

Test and Normal Values	Expected Abnormality	Rationale for Abnormality
WBC count, n = 5,000–10,000 cells/mm³	Elevated in acute infections, tissue injury, tissue necrosis. Decreased in viral infections, some bacterial infections, bone marrow depression.	WBC count increases in order to phagocytize or kill bacteria or cell debris.
• Neutrophils, n = 50–70% of the total WBC count; band, n = 3–6%	Neutrophils and bands are elevated in acute infections.	Neutrophils are the first WBCs to arrive at the site of infection. They have a short life span and must be continually produced when needed. So the immature neutrophil or band will be elevated quickly.
• Basophils, n = 0.5–1.0% of total WBC count	Elevated with allergic and parasitic responses. Do not respond to bacterial or viral infections.	Involved in phagocytosis of antigen–antibody complexes.
• Eosinophils, n = 1–4% of total WBC count	Elevated in allergic and parasitic reactions.	Respond later in inflammation and help control the inflammatory process.
• Monocytes, n = 2–8% of total WBC count	Elevated with infection, tuberculosis, bacterial endocarditis.	Phagocytic cells that perform like neutrophils but start later and stay longer in the bloodstream.
• Lymphocytes, n = 20–40% of total WBC count	Elevated with some bacterial diseases, infectious mononucleosis, leukemia, some viral diseases.	Function to fight chronic bacterial infection and acute viral infections. Responsible for immune reactions.
Erythrocyte sedimentation rate (ESR): *Males:* up to 15 mm/hr *Females:* up to 20 mm/hr	Elevated with acute and chronic infection, inflammation, cancer, tissue necrosis.	Nonspecific test that measures the rapidity at which red blood cells (RBCs) clump together. This process occurs more rapidly when there is an alteration in blood proteins due to inflammation. Therefore, an elevation indicates the presence of an inflammatory process.
Culture and sensitivity: Normally negative	Positive if pathogens are present in the specimen. The culture will identify the organism and the sensitivity will identify what antibiotic will work best.	If pathogens are present on the substance being tested, they will grow on a special culture medium and can be identified.
Gram stain: None with no organisms present	Differentiates between gram-negative and gram-positive organisms.	Useful for identifying the microorganisms so proper treatment can occur.
Febrile agglutinins: No agglutinins in titers ≤1:80	Increased in infectious diseases such as rickettsial disease, salmonellosis, brucellosis, and tularemia.	A group of tests that helps identify the type of organism responsible for an infection based on antibodies.
Viral antibody tests: None with no organisms present	This is a group of tests for specific viruses. Will be elevated with viral infections.	Used to determine exposure to or existing viral infections that are difficult to culture. Includes several tests, each specific to an organism and antibody reaction. They must be specifically ordered.
Fungal infection: Antibody tests negative	Elevated in the presence of a fungal-induced infection.	Looks for the presence of antibodies related to fungal infections or the presence of parasitic organisms.

WBC/mm³ usually indicates the presence of inflammation and/or infection. The higher the WBC count, the more serious the infection is thought to be. A viral infection can often cause the WBC count to decrease. The differential count of WBCs should also be assessed. There are five types of WBCs; neutrophils, eosinophils, basophils, lymphocytes, and monocytes. Neutrophils are the first type of WBC to arrive at the site of inflammation or infection and their job is to phagocytize or ingest bacteria. This process is described in Chapters 62 and 63 .

Cultures are also very important in diagnosing and treating infections. The nurse is often responsible for collecting the specimen to be cultured. Each institution has its own policy for collecting specimens, however, it is very important to collect the specimen correctly so that the results of the culture are useful. The following guidelines should be followed:

- Sufficient material must be collected to ensure an accurate examination.
- The specimen should be collected where the suspected organism is most likely to be found.
- Observe standard precautions when collecting the specimen.
- Culture only for a specific pathogen and not where there are areas of normal flora.
- Collect the specimen in a sterile container with a tight-fitting lid. Polyester-tipped swabs in a collection system with a transport medium ensure the adequacy of the specimen for 72 hours.
- Place the specimen in a biohazard bag.
- Label the specimen correctly with patient information, the source of the specimen, and the time of collection.
- Make sure the specimen gets to the laboratory as soon as possible. Most specimens can be refrigerated for a few hours if necessary.

CRITICAL ALERT *Remember to collect specimens for culture before beginning treatment with an antibiotic. This gives a more accurate picture of the original infection.*

Emotional care of the patient is very important. Patients and their families may not know the origin of the infection, and may therefore be apprehensive about the effectiveness of treatments. The use of standard precautions or transmission-based precautions makes visits with family and friends difficult. Hugs and touching are hindered by gloves and masks. The necessary use of protective masks, gloves, and gowns may make the patient feel isolated and rejected. Education about the necessity of isolation procedures is important for the patient and family. The nurse needs to allow the patient to verbalize feelings about the isolation and the concerns about being ostracized.

Nursing Diagnosis

Nursing diagnoses are determined based on an in-depth analysis of the data from the patient history and physical examination. Nursing diagnoses will vary depending on the type and location of the infection or an increased risk for infection. For example, the patient with pneumonia may also be given the nursing diagnosis of *Ineffective Airway Clearance*. Another example might be the patient with a wound infection who has a nursing diagnosis of *Impaired Tissue Integrity*.

When the patient is at risk for an infection the nursing diagnosis is *Risk for Infection*. The etiology or cause may be a break in the body's defense mechanisms, an alteration in secondary defenses such as a low hemoglobin or suppressed inflammatory response, the presence of a chronic disease, malnutrition, or increased environmental exposure. The Nursing Process: Patient Care Plan (p. 474) outlines the nursing management for a patient with an infectious communicable disease.

Health Promotion

Prevention and control of infection is the number one goal of health care no matter what the setting. Health care–associated infections are an increasing problem. The best way to address infection is to prevent it. Prevention requires education of health care professionals and the general public. An educational program related to the prevention of infection has several facets. Everyone should be educated on the importance of proper hand hygiene. Understanding the importance of immunization is an important part of educating the public. Family members must be instructed to check all immunization records and keep them up to date. Community members should understand the disease they are being protected against, why the immunization is necessary, the relative safety of immunizations, and when booster doses are due.

It is important to educate the public on the use of antibiotics. Antibiotics are not effective for all organisms. Many infections will resolve completely without the use of antibiotics. Antibiotic resistance is occurring, in part, because of the misuse of antibiotics. Patients need to have an understanding of when antibiotics are effective and when alternatives may be appropriate. It is important to stress that it is necessary to take all of the medication prescribed. If the full treatment is not taken, this could result in a worse infection due to the development of resistant organisms. The Pharmacology Summary (p. 477) lists medications used to treat infectious disease.

A healthy lifestyle is a deterrent to infection. An individual, who practices good hygiene, eats a well-balanced diet, exercises regularly, and gets an adequate amount of sleep will have a stronger immune system and be better able to resist infection. Although exposure will occur no matter how careful an individual is, it is important to prevent transmission of the organism. To decrease exposure, an individual should do the following:

- Avoid crowds and contact with susceptible persons.
- Use disposable tissues when coughing or sneezing.
- Use appropriate food-handling precautions.
- Practice frequent hand hygiene.
- Clean equipment and eating utensils.
- Avoid contact with or sharing of body fluids through needles or razors.
- Use condoms during sexual activity.

Research has shown that effective strategies for the prevention and control of health care–related infections include proper hand hygiene, utilizing barrier techniques when needed such as wearing gowns and gloves, appropriate care of invasive devices, and cautious use of antibiotics (Larson, 2005; Wiseman, 2006).

NURSING PROCESS: Patient Care Plan for Infection

Assessment of Pain

Subjective Data:
Do you hurt?
On a scale of 1 to 10 with 10 being the worst possible pain, how bad is the pain?
Where is the pain located?
How would you describe the pain?
Does anything make the pain better or worse?
What have you tried to relieve the pain and has it worked?
How long have you had the pain?

Objective Data:
Heart and respiratory rate may be increased.
Patient demonstrates a facial grimace or gritting of teeth.
Patient guards painful area.
Diaphoresis and pallor may be present.
Presence of nausea and vomiting.
Patient may be crying or moaning.

Nursing Assessment and Diagnoses	Outcomes and Evaluation Parameters	Planning and Interventions with *Rationales*
Nursing Diagnosis: *Acute Pain* related to tissue inflammation and damage	**Outcomes:** Patient reports pain early. Patient reports no adverse effects from pain or medication. Patient verbalizes pain relief and rates the pain lower on the scale of 1 to 10. Pain decreases, requiring less medication. **Evaluation Parameters:** Patient reports that pain is relieved or improved. Heart rate is <100 beats/min. Respiratory rate is <20 breaths/min. Facial muscles are relaxed. Patient is willing to participate in activities and therapies.	**Interventions and *Rationales:*** Instruct the patient to report and describe pain before it becomes unmanageable. *Pain should be assessed and medication given before pain gets unbearable. Intervention will be more effective if given before the pain is severe.* Describe any adverse effects of unrelieved pain. *Pain may lead to physiological and psychological morbidity factors.* Review patient's chart for frequency of medication administration and overall relief of pain. *Tracking of pain helps the nurse and patient plan ahead and improve pain management.* Support the patient's use of nonpharmacologic measures to control pain such as distraction, imagery, etc. *Some nonpharmacologic strategies can restore the patient's sense of control and help decrease pain.* Plan care activities around periods of greatest comfort. *The presence of pain diminishes the patient's ability to be active.* Assess cultural and religious impact on the patient's responses. *Different cultures and religions respond differently to pain.*

Assessment of Fever

Subjective Data:
Are you feeling unusually warm?
Do you have body aches?
Have you had chills?
Have you taken your temperature and what were the results?

Objective Data:
Temperature >37.2°C (>99°F)
Tachycardia
Respiratory rate of >20 breaths/minute
Decreased alertness
Restlessness
Diaphoresis

Nursing Assessment and Diagnoses	Outcomes and Evaluation Parameters	Planning and Interventions with *Rationales*
Nursing Diagnosis: *Hyperthermia* related to increased metabolic rate from infection	**Outcome:** Normal body temperature **Evaluation Parameters:** Body temperature will be within normal limits. Changes in body temperature will be noted quickly. Patient will remain warm and dry. Patient hydration status will be adequate. Skin will be warm and dry. Alert and oriented without restlessness or malaise. Heart rate <100 beats/min. Respiratory rate <20 beats/min. Resolution of infection.	**Interventions and *Rationales:*** Assess temperature at regular intervals and when the patient complains of chills or myalgia. *Recognize pattern for fever and note when rising or decreasing.* Keep patient comfortable with dry clothing and linens. *Patient in wet clothes and linens will shiver, leading to increased energy needs and possibly increasing fever.* Encourage an intake of eight to ten 8-oz glasses of fluids. *Fluids lost through perspiration need to be replaced.* Administer antipyretics *to decrease temperature.* Administer antibiotics *to treat organism responsible for infection.*

NURSING PROCESS: Patient Care Plan for Infection—*Continued*

Assessment of Fatigue
Subjective Data:
Are you feeling tired?
How much activity makes you tired?
Can you complete activities of daily living?
What makes your fatigue better or worse?

Objective Data:
Inability to stay awake
Unwillingness to participate in activities or therapeutics
Expressionless face.

Nursing Assessment and Diagnoses	Outcomes and Evaluation Parameters	Planning and Interventions with *Rationales*
Nursing Diagnosis: *Fatigue* related to increased energy production	**Outcome:** Increased energy level ***Evaluation Parameters:*** Patient voices an increase in energy. Patient performs only those essential tasks and asks for help with other activities as energy level increases. Patient takes rest periods throughout the day. Patient eats small frequent meals containing high-energy foods if not contraindicated.	**Interventions and *Rationales:*** Assist the patient with activities of daily living as necessary. *Encourage independence and some activity.* Help the patient identify essential from nonessential tasks *to help conserve energy while providing some independence.* Allow the patient to take rest periods without interruption every couple of hours or more often if needed. *Rest will allow energy to be restored.* Teach the patient strategies for conserving energy. *Some activities can be done sitting instead of standing or in ways that require less energy.*

Assessment of Fluid Volume Status
Subjective Data:
Do you feel thirsty?
How often are you urinating?
Do you feel diaphoretic?

Objective Data:
Skin that is moist and warm
Decreased intake of fluids
Decreased urine output
Poor skin turgor
Dry mucous membranes
Increased urine specific gravity
Tachycardia
Tachypnea

Nursing Assessment and Diagnoses	Outcomes and Evaluation Parameters	Planning and Interventions with *Rationales*
Nursing Diagnosis: *Deficient Fluid Volume* related to increased perspiration and inability to drink	**Outcome:** Fluid balance is maintained. ***Evaluation Parameters:*** Urine output is equal to or less than intake. Skin is warm and dry. Skin turgor is normal. Mucous membranes are moist.	**Interventions and *Rationales:*** Monitor trends in output related to intake. Note color and specific gravity of urine. *Provides a picture of the patient's hydration status.* Monitor for decreased skin turgor, thirst, dry mucous membranes, dry skin, sunken eyeballs, weakness, and confusion. *These are signs of fluid deficit.* Provide oral hygiene before each meal and at bedtime. *Oral hygiene decreases unpleasant taste, increasing the patient's desire to eat and drink.* Provide fresh water and oral fluids as requested by the patient evenly distributed over 24 hours. *Helps increase oral intake and counter dehydration. When distributed throughout the day, the intake has a greater chance of being retained.*

Assessment of Anxiety Related to Infection
Subjective Data:
What do you know about your infection and/or disease process?
How does this disease affect your daily life?
Do you have family members or friends to provide support?
Do you feel anxious or afraid?

Objective Data:
Presence of restlessness
Withdrawal from activities
Inability to sleep

(continued)

NURSING PROCESS: Patient Care Plan for Infection—*Continued*

Nursing Assessment and Diagnoses	Outcomes and Evaluation Parameters	Planning and Interventions with *Rationales*
Nursing Diagnosis: *Anxiety* related to threat to health status	**Outcome:** Anxiety level is minimal and coping is effective. ***Evaluation Parameters:*** Acknowledges and verbalizes feelings of anxiety. Verbalizes that anxiety is decreased. Verbalizes that physical manifestations of anxiety are decreased or absent. Participates in activities. Able to sleep without restlessness.	**Interventions and *Rationales:*** Monitor patient's level of anxiety and physical reactions. *Signs of anxiety are very individual. Monitoring those reactions helps in the development of a plan to address the anxiety.* Explore coping skills the patient has used in the past for anxiety. *Methods that have been successful in the past are likely to be successful again.* Encourage the patient to use new techniques to reduce anxiety such as imaging, relaxation techniques, or soothing music. *Many techniques will help patients cope with anxiety.* Encourage the patient to express feelings of anxiety. *Recognizing and expressing feelings sometimes helps to relieve them.* Explain all procedures and allow time for mental preparation. *Increased knowledge decreases anxiety related to the unknown.* Explain the disease process and therapies involved in the treatment. *Increased knowledge decreases anxiety related to the unknown.*

Assessment of Knowledge of Disease Process

Subjective Data:
What do you know about your disease?
What do you know about the treatment involved with your infection?
Do you understand how to prevent infection?
Do you know what symptoms to report immediately?

Objective Data:
Assess knowledge of infection, how it occurred, how to prevent it, and how to treat it.

Nursing Assessment and Diagnoses	Outcomes and Evaluation Parameters	Planning and Interventions with *Rationales*
Nursing Diagnosis: *Deficient Knowledge* related to infection and its prevention	**Outcome:** Verbalizes understanding of condition and treatment plan. ***Evaluation Parameters:*** Patient and family verbalize an understanding of the signs of infection and how to prevent an infection. Patient and family verbalize an understanding of the treatment modalities being used. Patient and family verbalize the signs and symptoms to report to the health care provider.	**Interventions and *Rationales:*** Teach patient and family the signs of infection and what to report to the physician *to allow for early recognition and treatment.* Teach the patient and family causes of infection. *Helps the patient to avoid getting an infection.*

Discharge Priorities

With the movement toward decreasing the length of hospital stays and preference to receive care at home, many patients are being cared for in their homes. Infection control has been a concern of hospitals but consideration should now be given to the home environment as well. The prevention of infection in the home is different than in the hospital. Patients being cared for at home are not exposed to other patients and reservoirs of pathogens that would be present in the hospital setting. Home care patients are usually not as ill as hospitalized patients, so their ability to resist infections may be better. However, other environmental resources in the home, such as plumbing, sanitation, and ventilation, typically are more difficult to control than in an institution.

The basic principles of prevention and control still apply. The focus should not be on getting rid of household germs but on using good hygiene measures such as hand washing to prevent exposure to germs and cross infection. Families must be taught infection control principles so that they can develop their own approaches and make knowledgeable decisions related to reducing the chances of infection. Hand hygiene remains a very important part of preventing infection. Other procedures such as care of catheters and wounds can be adapted to the home. Equipment needs to be cleaned in the dishwasher if possible or with regular household cleaning products. Use of gowns, gloves, and masks is only necessary when family members need to be protected from the patient's infection. The Patient Teaching & Discharge Priorities box (p. 479) outlines the teaching needs of a patient who is discharged with an open wound.

There is a requirement that cases or suspected cases of certain diseases or conditions, called **notifiable diseases,** be reported to

PHARMACOLOGY Summary of Medications to Treat Infectious Disease

Medication Category	Action	Application/Indication	Nursing Responsibility
Antibiotics			
Used to treat infections related to bacterial agents	Act by killing bacteria or by inhibiting their growth.	Each type of antibiotic is effective against a different type of organism.	Assess for history of allergies to the medication. Assess the patient's response to the medication in terms of effectiveness and possible side effects. Patient education should include the importance of completing the entire regimen and the medication and reporting any clinical manifestations related to allergies or side effects.
Specific Types of Antibiotics			
Aminoglycosides • Gentamicin • Streptomycin	Act as bactericidal agents by interrupting the bacteria's protein synthesis.	Used against gram-negative bacilli, some aerobic gram-positive organisms, mycobacteria, and some protozoa. May be used to treat nosocomial infections, urinary tract infections, eye infections, and infections of the central nervous system.	Given intravenously because they are poorly absorbed through the GI tract. Assess kidney and hearing function. Check peak and trough levels so that blood levels are maintained in a narrow margin. Watch for drug interactions.
Penicillins • Penicillin G • Ampicillin • Nafcillin	Bactericidal action is through destruction of the cell wall of the bacteria.	Are broad spectrum and act against gram-positive, gram-negative, and anaerobic organisms. Used for upper respiratory tract infections, syphilis, endocarditis.	Assess for adverse reactions and interactions with other medications. Ensure adequate hydration of the patient. Provide small, frequent meals to minimize stomatitis, and sore mouth. If patient of childbearing age, advise her to use a backup method of birth control.
Cephalosporins • Cefazolin • Cefaclor • Ceftazidime	Inhibit bacterial cell-wall synthesis by binding to protein located on the cell membrane.	Act against gram-positive organisms and gram-negative organisms. Used for patients who are allergic to penicillin. Treat respiratory tract infections, skin infections, otitis media, urinary tract infections, septicemia, endocarditis.	Take on an empty stomach. Refrain from drinking alcohol. Maintain adequate hydration.
Tetracyclines • Doxycycline • Minocycline	Bacteriostatic. Inhibit cell growth by inhibiting protein synthesis leading to prevention of cell division.	Used for infections caused by *Rickettsia* species, *Mycoplasma,* and *Chlamydia.* Treats Lyme disease, *Helicobacter pylori,* acne vulgaris, skin infections.	Must use an additional birth control method while taking. Absorption may be decreased if taken with some over-the-counter medications. Take on an empty stomach. Will cause increased sensitivity to the sun.
Macrolides • Erythromycin • Azithromycin • Clarithromycin	Can prevent the cell from dividing or can kill the bacterial cell. Act by inhibiting RNA-dependent protein synthesis.	More effective against gram-positive organisms than gram-negative organisms. Treats *Staphylococcus, Streptococcus, Chlamydia, Mycoplasma.* Used to treat urethral, endocervical, or rectal infections, bronchitis, pharyngitis, skin infections, respiratory infections, pharyngitis, pneumonia.	Monitor the patient's hearing. Medication should be taken 1 hour before or 2 hours after meals.
Vancomycin	Has bacteriocidal activity that inhibits cell-wall synthesis by altering the cell's permeability.	Used to treat bacterial septicemia, endocarditis, bone and joint infections, and *Clostridium difficile* infections. Effective against streptococci and staphylococci.	Monitor hearing and renal function. Monitor fluid status. Assess peak and trough serum levels.
Carbapenems • Ertapenem • Meropenem	Bactericidal. Work by inhibiting cell-wall synthesis.	Have beta-lactam activity for use against anaerobes. Are broad spectrum and effective against gram-positive and gram-negative organisms. Frequently used for serious or life-threatening infections.	Give with caution in patients with head trauma or brain lesions because they can induce seizures.

(continued)

PHARMACOLOGY **Summary of Medications to Treat Infectious Disease—*Continued***

Medication Category	Action	Application/Indication	Nursing Responsibility
Monobactams • Aztreonam	Inhibits cell-wall synthesis, leading to cell death.	Effective against gram-negative aerobic organisms such as *Pseudomonas aeruginosa*. Also used to treat urinary tract infections, septicemia, skin, and lower respiratory tract infections.	Given IV or IM. Monitor for signs of thrombophlebitis at the insertion site.
Fluoroquinolones • Ciprofloxacin • Levofloxacin • Ofloxacin	Interrupt DNA synthesis during bacterial replication, interfering with replication.	Used to treat urinary tract infections, respiratory tract infections, skin, bone and joint infections, pneumonia, gynecologic infections, sexually transmitted infections.	Antacids will lead to decreased absorption. Avoid sunlight. Tendon rupture is a potential adverse event and should be assessed.
Sulfonamides • Sulfasalazine	Interferes with synthesis of folic acid needed for DNA synthesis. This prevents reproduction of the bacteria.	Treats urinary tract infections, lower respiratory tract infections, diarrhea, skin, bone and joint infections, gynecologic infections.	Antacids will decrease absorption. Monitor folate deficiency. Monitor fluid intake. Photosensitivity can be a problem. Take on an empty stomach with a full glass of water. Monitor hematologic function.
Nitrofurantoin	Is bacteriostatic by inhibiting the energy production of the bacteria.	Is rapidly excreted in the urine and, therefore, is used only for urinary tract infections.	Monitor for peripheral neuropathy and pulmonary reactions.
Antivirals Used to treat viral infections			
Nucleoside analogues • Acyclovir • Famciclovir	Inhibits viral DNA polymerase, leading to disruption of viral growth.	Treat viral syndromes that occur in immunocompromised patients such as herpes simplex.	Monitor for adverse reactions. Monitor for nephrotoxicity. Is expensive so consider referring patient to social services for financial help.
Influenza A and syncytial virus drugs • Amantadine • Zanamivir	Appear to inhibit viral replication by blocking the uncoating of the virus particle and release of viral RNA into the host cell.	Used to treat influenza A infections and respiratory syncytial virus infections.	Should not be used with central nervous system stimulants such as alcohol.

local, county, or state public health departments. This process helps with disease surveillance efforts so that the health of individuals and families can be protected and the diseases controlled or prevented. The National Guidelines box (p. 480) lists diseases that were designated as reportable at the national level as of 2007. Other additional diseases may be reportable to the state as designated by state law and vary from state to state. The list of diseases designated as reportable changes to reflect the needs of the public at any given time. Annual recommendations for what diseases should be on the list are made by the Council of State and Territorial Epidemiologists (CSTE) and the CDC. The reporting of a disease to a public health authority leads to an immediate response that includes case investigation, contact prophylaxis, and outbreak control. Analysis of the information supplied for the notifiable diseases allows for the establishment of public health priorities and the monitoring of trends.

Collaborative Management

The goals of care are to identify the site of the infection and the causative organism so that a cure can be achieved quickly and

without complications. This will require a collaborative approach to care. The multidisciplinary team may consist of nurses, physicians, occupational therapists, physical therapists, nutritionists, psychologists, and pharmacists. A thorough history and physical examination will help identify the system involved. The physician will order diagnostic tests to help narrow the focus and identify the site and causative agent. It is the nurse's responsibility to continually assess the patient as the presenting signs and symptoms become more defined and to ensure that diagnostic tests are completed and specimens collected correctly.

Once the infecting agent has been identified, therapy can be ordered that is narrowly focused on the patient's problem. A pharmacist will help identify the proper medications and educate the patient on the use and side effects of the medications. A viral infection will often resolve with only supportive care. If antibiotics are administered systemically, it is important to watch for any adverse effects caused by the drugs. It also is the nurse's responsibility to protect the patient from obtaining new infections and decrease the potential for spreading the infection to others.

Nutritionists can help provide the patient with a well-balanced diet to help keep the immune system strong. Physical and occupa-

PATIENT TEACHING & DISCHARGE PRIORITIES for Infection

Need	Teaching
Wound care: Patient/family/support system Setting	Perform daily cleansing and dressing changes for open areas.
	Elevate areas where edema formation occurs.
	Avoid scratching the healed areas as this could cause breakdown: • Use liberal amounts of emollient lotions for dryness and flaking. • Use diphenhydramine hydrochloride (Benadryl) for pruritus (itching). • Keep fingernails short and use gloves when sleeping.
	Avoid sunlight because it can cause, among other things, healed wounds to permanently discolor or darken. • Avoid overexposure to sun. • Use sunscreen products when exposed to sunlight. • Use clothing and hats for added protection.
	Avoid exposure to extreme temperatures and harsh chemicals.
	Wear loose-fitting, soft clothing.
	Assess availability, knowledge, and compliance with treatment regimen.
	Assess discharge placement needs for the home, rehabilitation facility, or extended care facility.
	Assess home environment for need for assistive devices.
	Assess for professional home health needs.
	Assess need for follow-up appointments.
Wound infection: Patient/family/support system Setting	Assess for infection of open wounds and healed wound breakdown with each dressing change and report as necessary.
	Signs and symptoms include odor and exudate, fever, increased drainage, swelling, and lack of wound closure.
	Apply antibiotic ointments as prescribed.
	Teach minimization of risk factors for infection.
	Explain signs and symptoms that require medical attention.
	Assess environment for risk factors.
Nutrition: Patient/family/support system Setting	Maintain a high-calorie, high-protein diet.
	Continue taking vitamins and mineral supplements as ordered.
	Observe for appetite and weight loss and food intolerance.
	Taper calorie intake once preinjury or ideal weight has been achieved to prevent excessive weight gain.
	With professional guidance (i.e., physical therapist) institute an exercise program.
	Assess financial resources.
Pain management: Patient/family/support system Setting	Assess pain level and report any increase in pain.
	Assess effectiveness of pharmacologic interventions.
	Wean patient off pain medication when pain lessens.
	Assess environment for safety and promotion of therapeutic needs.
Emotional adjustment: Patient/family/support system Setting	Answer questions honestly.
	Encourage verbalization of frustrations and anger.
	Encourage positive reinforcement from the family.
	Encourage independent functioning as soon as possible.
	Stress that it is not uncommon to feel letdown after discharge.
	Encourage participation in a support group.

tional therapists will be needed to maintain or regain physical functioning. Every member of the health care team along with the patient and the patient's family must be cognizant of the importance of proper hand hygiene and its huge role in the prevention of disease transmission.

Antimicrobials are chosen based on a number of factors. The clinical and diagnostic evaluation is used to decide whether therapy should be instituted as well as what type. If the severity of the infection merits, the physician may decide to begin therapy before the culture results are available. This is known as **empiric therapy.** Data used to decide on the medication of choice in this instance includes the usual susceptibility of the suspected organism, the capability of medication to penetrate the site of infection, and patient factors such as other illnesses, medication allergies, immune status and pregnancy status. Once the culture results are available, the medication is chosen based on what is most effective against the identified organism, with the least risk of toxicity and fewest adverse effects for the patient. The physician, in consultation with the pharmacist, also considers patient compliance, cost, and dosing schedule.

NATIONAL GUIDELINES Diseases Designated as Notifiable at the National Level During 2007

Acquired immunodeficiency syndrome (AIDS)
Anthrax
Arboviral neuroinvasive and nonneuroinvasive diseases
California serogroup virus disease
Eastern equine encephalitis virus disease
Powassan virus disease
St. Louis encephalitis
West Nile virus disease
Western equine encephalitis virus disease

Botulism
Brucellosis
Chancroid
Chlamydia trachomatis, genital infection
Cholera
Coccidioidomycosis
Cryptosporidiosis
Cyclosporiasis
Diphtheria
Ehrlichiosis
Human granulocytic
Human monocytic
Human, other or unspecified agent
Giardiasis
Gonorrhea
Haemophilus influenzae, invasive disease
Hansen disease
Hantavirus pulmonary syndrome
Hemolytic uremic syndrome, postdiarrheal
Hepatitis A, acute
Hepatitis B, acute
Hepatitis B, perinatal infection
Hepatitis C
Hepatitis viral, chronic B and C
Human immunodeficiency virus (HIV) infection
Adult and pediatric HIV
Influenza-associated pediatric mortality
Legionellosis
Listeriosis
Lyme disease

Malaria
Measles
Meningococcal disease
Mumps
Novel influenza A virus infections
Pertussis
Plague
Poliomyelitis, paralytic
Poliovirus infection, nonparalytic
Psittacosis
Q fever
Rabies, animal
Rabies, human
Rocky Mountain spotted fever
Rubella
Rubella, congenital syndrome
Salmonellosis
Severe acute respiratory syndrome– associated coronavirus (SARS-CoV) disease
Shiga toxin-producing *Escherichia coli* (STEC)
Shigellosis
Smallpox
Streptococcal disease, invasive, group A
Streptococcal toxic-shock syndrome
Streptococcus pneumoniae, drug-resistant, invasive disease
Streptococcus pneumoniae, invasive, in children <5 years old
Syphilis
Syphilis, congenital
Tetanus
Toxic-shock syndrome
Trichinosis
Tuberculosis
Tularemia
Typhoid fever
Vancomycin intermediate-resistant *Staphylococcus aureus* (VISA)
Vancomycin-resistant *Staphylococcus aureus* (VRSA)
Varicella
Varicella deaths
Vibriosis
Yellow fever

Source: Centers for Disease Control and Prevention Morbidly and Mortality Weekly Report. Summary of Notifiable Diseases—-United States, 2007. Retrieved June 12, 2008 from http://www.cdc.gov/mmwr/preview/mmwrhtml/mm5553a1.htm.

CRITICAL ALERT *Be sure to assess patient for signs of an allergic reaction or side effects of the medication being given.*

The nurse serves as the patient advocate and liaison between the patient and other members of the health care team. The nurse coordinates and facilitates communication between all members of the health care team and the patient. The educational needs and emotional support needs are the responsibility of the nurse.

 Research

There are many research opportunities in nursing related to infection. The goals of research are to identify more effective means of caring for the patient with infection and to prevent infection from occurring. A list of research topics related to infection is provided in the Research Opportunities and Clinical Impact box.

RESEARCH OPPORTUNITIES AND CLINICAL IMPACT RELATED TO INFECTION

Research Area	Clinical Impact
Immunization	
Effects of nursing role on compliance with immunizations	Increases the numbers of people who are immunized so that the numbers exposed to infectious disease can be decreased.
Effects of laws on compliance with immunization	
Adverse effects of vaccines on the outcomes of pregnancy or the unborn child	
Home Care	
Prevention techniques needed in the home	Little is known about the prevalence of infection in the home and the best techniques to prevent it.
The development of surveillance systems for infection in the home	
Prevention of Nosocomial Infections	
The degree and type of organisms related to environmental surface contamination	More information is needed about where the organisms come from and how to prevent their transmission.
Assessment of prevention strategies at specific sites such as ventilator-associated pneumonia	
Compliance of health care personnel with hand hygiene practices	
What agents are most effective for hand hygiene and what time intervals are needed	
Treatment	
Studies related to improved antibiotic usage and management of antibiotic resistance	Although much progress has been made in the treatment of infection, new problems are developing that need to be addressed.

Effects of Infection and Antibiotic-Resistant Bacteria on Wound Healing

Clinical Problem

Antimicrobial resistance occurs when the antibiotics taken to stop the infection do not kill the bacteria that cause the infection. The bacteria resist the effects of the antibiotic, which allows them to continue to survive and grow causing more harm. After repeated exposure to an antibiotic that does not kill them, microorganisms develop the ability to avoid the inhibitory or lethal activity of an antimicrobial agent through several mechanisms. Research has been done to increase understanding about how bacteria protect themselves. Bacteria can become resistant by neutralizing the antibiotic, pumping the antibiotic out, or changing the antibiotic attack site so the function of the bacteria is not affected. Bacteria that were at one time killed by an antibiotic can become resistant through mutation of their genetic material or by acquiring pieces of DNA that code for the resistance properties from other bacteria. The transfer of one piece of DNA may allow the bacteria to become resistant to many antibiotics.

There are several resistant pathogens on the rise. These include penicillin-resistant *Streptococcus pneumoniae* (DRSP), group A streptococci of enhanced virulence, and vancomycin-resistant enterococci. As long as bacteria are able to mutate, the battle against infection will be a struggle. Infection will become more prominent. One of the areas affected by infection and antibiotic-resistant bacteria is that of wound healing. The presence of bacteria in the wound leads to inflammation, delayed healing, and increased scarring.

Research Findings

Ryan (2007) reviewed research on the effects of infection and antibiotic-resistant bacteria on wound healing. As research continues, new mechanisms have been discovered by which bacteria protect themselves. Research has reported that bacteria use a biofilm cover and that bacteria may mutate their genes and horizontally transfer their genes to other bacteria. The ability of bacteria to make adaptations like these causes concerned about prescribing antibiotics. An understanding of these mechanisms will help to identify other ways of attacking the bacteria.

Bacteria in wounds are initially gram positive, but gram-negative bacteria also play a role in the delay of wound healing. In order for the right antibiotic to be prescribed, it is important to identify the right bacteria. Wounds are often contaminated with other materials or may grow different bacteria in different areas of the wound. A good understanding of how to take samples from the wound for culture is important.

Other factors related to wound healing and preventing contamination of the wound should be considered. The healing of the wound and signs of inflammation can be influenced by factors such as the presence of anemia and malnutrition. Medications that the patient may be taking such as steroids or immunosuppressive agents may delay wound healing and make the patient more susceptible to infection. Good nutrition with adequate amounts of vitamins A and C, iron, and zinc is necessary for wound healing. Accurate diagnosis and assessment is important so that antibiotics will be prescribed correctly and only when needed. The traditional implementation of activities thought to be antibacterial is being questioned. Actions such as preoperative bathing and hair removal have been found in some studies to have no effect on the rate of infection. The one activity that has been shown through research to be effective in preventing infection is proper hand hygiene, especially when alcohol is used.

Implications for Nursing Practice

This study demonstrates the need for nurses to help to prevent infections in wounds so that healing can occur. Nurses need to perform hand hygiene before and after caring for the patient. Gloves should be worn to provide wound care. The patient's overall health should be enhanced through a well-balanced diet, proper hydration, good hygiene, and some exercise, if possible, to increase circulation. The proper use of antibiotics can help reduce the development of antibiotic resistance. Patients should be assessed for their response to antibiotic treatment to help decide if the antibiotic is effective. Patient education about the use of antibiotics is also supported in this research. Patients often want an antibiotic when one may not be indicated. Nurses can help the patient and the patient's family understand when the use of an antibiotic is needed and how to take the antibiotic properly.

Critical Thinking Questions

1. Develop a plan for helping the patient prevent a wound infection preoperatively.

2. Describe the proper assessment of a wound when concerned about the possibility of infection.

3. Identify nursing measures that would decrease the chances for infection in a patient wound.

4. Identify interventions that would help decrease resistance to antibiotics.

Answers to Critical Thinking Questions appear in Appendix D.

Reference

Ryan, T. J. (2007). Infection following soft tissue injury: Its role in wound healing. *Current Opinion in Infectious Disease, 20*(2), 124–128.

Clinical Preparation

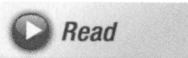 **Read**

- History of Current Illness
- Past Medical History
- Physical Exam
- Admitting Medical Orders
- Laboratory Study Results

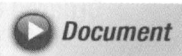 **Document**

- Summary of Hospitalization
- Pathophysiology Form
- Laboratory Values
- Laboratory Results Explanation

 Apply

- List of Potential Nursing Diagnoses
- Concept Map
- Critical Thinking Questions

Log on to MyNursingKit.com to download forms you will need and to complete further steps in the Clinical Preparation assignment.

HISTORY OF PRESENT ILLNESS

Mr. Ralph Newman is a 68-year-old black male admitted with a diagnosis of "infection of right leg wound." Mr. Newman was struck in the right leg with a piece of wood while cutting up firewood. He finished cutting the wood then went in the house and washed off his leg. However, 3 days later the wound began to drain thick greenish, yellow liquid and was painful. He visited his doctor who cleaned the wound and put him on Keflex. However, the wound continued to get worse so he was admitted to the hospital. On the day of admission, Mr. Newman was taken to surgery for a cleaning and debridement of his leg wound.

Medical-Surgical History
Insulin-dependent diabetes mellitus
Myocardial infarction 10 years ago but has been doing well since that time
Allergies: none known
Drug intolerance: none known

Social History
Retired and likes to work outside around his home
Smokes 1 pack of cigarettes per day
Lives with his wife in the country

Physical Exam
Weight: 200 lb; height: 5 ft 8 in.
BP 164/90; P 85; RR 20; T 101°F
HEENT: PERRLA, ears appear normal; pharynx pink with no exudates
Neck: no cervical lymphadenopathy; thyroid nonpalpable
Heart: regular rate and rhythm; no extra heart sounds
Lungs: clear to auscultation
Abdomen: bowel sounds present × 4 quadrants; soft and nondistended; no tenderness or masses; no hepatomegaly
Extremities: left leg 1+ pitting edema; brown discoloration from midcalf down to ankle; toes slightly pink in color
Pedal pulses 1+ left foot
Pulses absent in right foot; toes on right foot pink and cool to touch
Right leg 2+ pitting edema
Open wound on anterior shin approximately 4 inches in diameter. Draining moderate amount of greenish yellow, thick liquid. Necrotic tissue noted in wound bed. Skin around wound red and warm to touch

MS: moves all extremities; full ROM except right ankle due to pain; normal muscle strength
Neuro: sensation slightly diminished in both lower legs. DTRs 2+. CN ii-xii intact

Admitting Medical Orders
Admit to surgical service
Diagnosis: right leg wound infection; status post-incision and drainage of right leg
No known allergies
Vital signs with oxygen saturation q4h
Wet-to-dry dressing with Dakin's solution q4h
Up in chair
Bathroom privileges
ADA diet
Accu-Chek ac and HS
Sequential compression devices (SCD) to lower extremities
Incentive spirometry q hour while awake
IV: saline lock; NS flushes q8h
Intake and output
Call house officer: pulse < 60 & > 110/minute; BP < 90 & > 160 systolic; temperature > 38.5; urine output < 30 mL/hr for 2 hours; respiratory rate > 30/minute: oxygen saturation < 92%; blood sugar < 70 & >130

Scheduled Medications
Insulin 15 units SQ of 70/30 in a.m. and 10 units of 70/30 SQ at HS
Cefoxitin 1 g IV q8h
Aspirin 81 mg po daily
Lipitor 10 mg po daily

PRN Medications

Phenergan 25 mg IV q6h prn nausea
Mylanta 30 mL po q4–6h prn dyspepsia
Triazolam 0.125–0.25 mg po q noc, prn sleep
Ativan 0.5-2 mg IV q6–8h prn anxiety
Milk of Magnesia 30 mL po daily, prn constipation
Tylenol 650 mg po/pr q4h for pain
Vicodin 1-2 tabs po prn q6h for mild to moderate pain
Morphine sulphate 1-8 mg IV q4h prn severe pain

Ordered Laboratory Studies

Wound culture
ESR × 1
Chemistry panel q a.m.
CBC q a.m.

Ordered Diagnostic Studies

Chest x-ray

LABORATORY STUDY RESULTS

Test	Day 1	Day 2	Day 3
Hemoglobin A_1C	9.1%		
Random glucose	160 mg/dL		
Fasting glucose	140 mg/dL	138 mg/dL	142 mg/dL
WBC	12,000/mm³	15,000/mm³	14,000/mm³
Lymphocytes	11%	12%	11%
Monocytes	1%	2%	2%
Bands	12%	18%	17%
Neutrophils	78%	80%	79%
Basophils	10%	10%	9%
RBC	3.08/mm³	3.10/mm³	3.10/mm³
Hemoglobin	9 gl/L	9.5 gl/L	9.7 gl/L
Hematocrit	27%	28%	28%
Wound culture	*Staph. aureus*		
ESR	48 mm/h		
Chest x-ray	Normal		

CRITICAL THINKING QUESTIONS

1. When Mr. Newman is admitted to the unit there are no private rooms available. The choices are as follows: room 110 with Mr. Jonas, diagnosis: leukemia; room 115 with Mr. Smithson who has a GI bleed; or room 122 with Mr. Kendrick who was admitted for deep venous thrombosis. In which room should Mr. Newman be placed?

2. Should Mr. Newman be placed in isolation. If so, why?

3. What factors does Mr. Newman have that make him susceptible to infection?

4. What nursing diagnoses would be appropriate for Mr. Newman?

Answers to Critical Thinking Questions appear in Appendix D.

NCLEX® REVIEW

1. The nurse is caring for a patient with a wound infection. Which of the following would explain an increase in purulent exudate in the wound?
   1. Response of white blood cells to the cellular injury
   2. Temporary vasoconstriction to avoid blood loss after injury
   3. Vasodilatation to increase blood supply to the area
   4. Leakage of fluid and cells out of capillaries into interstitial spaces

2. The nurse is assessing a patient with an infection. Which of the following assessment findings could indicate the cause for the infection?
   1. Inadequate nutrition
   2. Personality disorder
   3. Age 45 and employed
   4. Urban living

3. A patient is admitted with tuberculosis. The nurse realizes that this patient received this infection through which mode of transmission?

1. Contact
2. Airborne
3. Vehicle
4. Vector

4. While providing care to patients, the nurse realizes that preventing the control and spread of infection is a priority. Which of the following should the nurse do when washing the hands between patients?

1. Use water as hot as tolerated.
2. Clean under artificial nails prior to starting the shift.
3. Use a petroleum-based lotion for prevention of dryness.
4. Wash for at least fifteen seconds covering all surfaces.

5. A patient with an indwelling urinary catheter is demonstrating signs of having a urinary tract infection. The nurse realizes this infection is most likely caused by:

1. Group A beta-hemolytic streptococci.
2. *Staphylococcus aureus.*
3. *Neisseria meningitidis.*
4. *Staphylococcus epidermidis.*

6. A patient is experiencing an infectious disease. The nurse realizes that this is an expected result of passive immunity which is characterized by:

1. Providing long-term and possibly lifelong immunity.
2. The introduction of live, killed or attenuated toxin into the body.
3. Injecting already formed antibodies into the body.
4. Being immunized for such diseases as measles and mumps.

7. The nurse is admitting a patient with tuberculosis. Which of the following is a *Healthy People 2010* guideline for this disease process?

1. Eradicate the incidence of tuberculosis in the United States.
2. Increase the proportion of all tuberculosis clients who complete curative therapy within 12 months.
3. Increase the percentage of health care workers who are immunized against tuberculosis.
4. Decrease the communicable spread of tuberculosis among the rural population.

8. The nurse is interviewing a patient for a history of infectious diseases. Which of the following questions would provide the most information about these diseases?

1. How many hours a week do you work out of the home?
2. What types of activities do you participate in for recreation?
3. Have you received chemotherapy for cancer, psoriasis, or rheumatoid arthritis?
4. Explain your exercise routine.

Answers for review questions appear in Appendix D

KEY TERMS

active immunization *p.468*
antigenicity *p.464*
carrier *p.461*
chain of infection *p.461*
community-acquired infection *p.457*
empiric therapy *p.479*
endotoxins *p.465*

exotoxins *p.465*
fever of unknown origin (FUO) *p.471*
infectivity *p.464*
invasiveness *p.464*
mode of transmission *p.461*
nosocomial infection *p.457*
notifiable disease *p.476*

passive immunization *p.468*
pathogenicity *p.461*
portal of entry *p.461*
portal of exit *p.461*
reservoir *p.461*
viability *p.464*
virulence *p.464*

REFERENCES

Centers for Disease Control and Prevention. (2003). *Anthrax: What you need to know.* Retrieved July 14, 2007, from http://www.bt.cdc.gov/agent/anthrax/needtoknow.asp

Centers for Disease Control and Prevention. (2004). *International conference on new and emerging diseases.* Retrieved July 14, 2007, from http:// www.cdc.gov/iceid/2004/index.htm

Centers for Disease Control. (2008). *2008 Child & Adolescent Immunization Schedules.* Retrieved June 12, 2008 from http://www.cdc.gov/vaccines/recs/schedules/child-schedule.htm

Creedon, S. A. (2005). Healthcare workers' hand decontamination practices: Compliance with recommended guidelines. *Journal of Advanced Nursing, 51*(3), 208–216.

Garner, J. S. (1996). *Guidelines for isolation precautions in hospitals: Hospital Infection Control Advisory Committee.* Atlanta, GA: Centers for Disease Control and Prevention.

Kozier, B., Erb, G., Berman, A., & Snyder, S. (2004). *Fundamentals of nursing: Concepts, process, and practice* (7th ed.). Upper Saddle River, NJ: Pearson Prentice Hall.

Larson, E. L. (2005). State-of-the-science 2004: Time for a "no excuses/no tolerance" (NET) strategy. *American Journal of Infection Control, 33*(9),548–557.

Larson, E. L., Girard, R., Pessoa-Silva, C. L., Boyce, J., Donaldson, L., & Pittet, D. (2006). Skin reactions related to hand hygiene and selection of hand hygiene products. *American Journal of Infection Control, 34*(10), 627–635.

Porth, C. M. (2007). *Essentials of pathophysiology: Concepts of altered health status* (2nd ed.). Philadelphia: Lippincott Williams & Wilkins.

Schulster, L., & Chinn, R. Y. W. (2003). Guidelines for environmental infection control in health-care facilities. *MMWR, 52*(RR10), 1–42.

Siegel, J. D., Rhinehart, E., Jackson, M., Chiarello, L., & the Healthcare Infection Control Practices Advisory Committee. (2007, June). *Guideline for isolation precautions: Preventing transmission of infectious agents in healthcare settings 2007.* Retrieved June 6, 2008, from http://www.cdc.gov/ncidod/dhqp/pdf/guidelines/Isolation2007.pdf

Somner, J.E.A., Scott,K. M. & Gibb, A.P. (2007). What is the Optimum Location of Alcohol-Based Hand Cleanser? *Infect Control Hosp Epidemiol 28*:108–109.

Trick, W. E., Vernon, M. O., Hayes, R. A., Nathan, R., Rice, T. W., Perterson, B. J., et al. (2003). Impact of ring wearing on hand contamination and comparison of hand hygiene agents in a hospital. *Clinical Infectious Diseases, 36*(11), 1383–1390.

U.S. Department of Health and Human Services. (2000). *Healthy people 2010: Understanding and improving health.* Retrieved June 5, 2008, from http://www.healthypeople.gov

Widmer, A. F., Conzelmann, M., Tomic, M., Frei, R., & Stranden, A. M. (2007). Introducing alcohol-based hand rub for hand hygiene: The critical need for training. *Infection Control and Hospital Epidemiology, 28*(1), 50–54.

Wiseman, S. (2006). Prevention and control of healthcare-associated infection. *Nursing Standard, 20*(38), 41–45.

Hypertension

Ann Harley

Outcome-Based Learning Objectives

After studying this chapter, the learner will be able to:

1. Compare and contrast the differences between the types of hypertension: prehypertension, stage 1 hypertension, and stage 2 hypertension.
2. Describe the pathophysiology of hypertension.
3. Discuss the risk factors associated with the development of hypertension.
4. Explain the therapeutic agents used to manage hypertension.
5. Compare and contrast how social and cultural influences affect the plan of care for the hypertensive patient.
6. Develop a nursing plan of care with the hypertensive client.
7. Discuss how multidisciplinary therapeutic interventions are associated with patient outcome.

Blood pressure is defined as the pressure created by the circulating blood through the arteries, veins, and the chambers of the heart. Blood pressure readings are classified into four stages: normal tension, prehypertension, stage 1 hypertension, and stage 2 hypertension (National Heart, Lung, and Blood Institute [NHLBI], 2003; Yuan, 2004).

A severe form of hypertension is referred to as malignant hypertension. In the NHLBI's May 2003 publication titled *Seventh Report of the Joint National Committee on Prevention, Detection, Evaluation, and Treatment of High Blood Pressure (JNC 7),* malignant hypertension is referred to as a hypertensive urgency and emergency that reflects the patient's markedly elevated blood pressure and acute target organ damage requiring immediate hospitalization and parental drug therapy.

The various stages of high blood pressure are discussed throughout this chapter. Nurses should monitor patients for hypertension using the assessment points listed in Chart 21–1.

Regulation of Blood Pressure

Due to the pulsating blood flow created by the contraction and relaxation of the heart, there are two readings associated with blood pressure: the systolic and diastolic. The **systolic** blood pressure is the maximum pressure in the aorta and major arteries. It occurs when the left ventricle contracts and ejects blood into the central vascular system. This systolic reading averages 120 mmHg

CHART 21–1	Clinical Awareness and Monitoring

- Anticipate adherence problems for young men.
- Ask about smoking history:
  - Use of "Smoke Ender" or a similar program
  - History of success in quitting smoking.
- Consider nonadherence as cause of:
  - Failure to reach goal blood pressure
  - Resistant hypertension
  - Sudden loss of control.
- Encourage patients to bring all medications from all physicians and other sources, whether prescription, complementary, or over the counter, to each visit to review and cull out iatrogenic causes of high blood pressure.
- Ask what the patient takes for pain.
- Recognize depression and other psychiatric illnesses, including panic attacks, and manage appropriately.
- Be willing to change unsuccessful regimens and search for those more likely to succeed.

in a healthy adult individual. The **diastolic** blood pressure reflects cardiac relaxation, thus it is the minimum pressure in the arteries, which occurs just prior the next cycle of ventricular ejection of blood. This reading is approximately 80 mmHg in healthy individuals. The difference between the systolic and diastolic pressure is about 40 mmHg and is called the **pulse pressure** (Guyton & Hall, 2005). The pulse pressure is the ratio of stroke volume (amount of blood ejected with each heartbeat) to compliance of the arterial system (systemic vascular resistance) (Guyton & Hall, 2005).

Blood pressure is the product of cardiac output (the amount of blood pumped by the heart each minute) and systemic **peripheral vascular resistance** (the resistance to the flow of blood as determined by the vascular musculature and the diameter of the blood vessels and by influences on the ability of the cardiovascular system to adapt). The homeostatic systems that influence blood pressure changes in accordance with body needs are neural regulation, arterial baroreceptors and chemoreceptors, regulation of fluid volume, and humoral regulation (Guyton & Hall, 2005).

Neural Regulation

The pons and medulla of the brain are the neural control centers for the regulation of blood pressure. These areas are where the autonomic nervous system is integrated and modulated and where the vasomotor control center and cardiovascular control center are located. These control centers transmit parasympathetic impulses through the vagus nerve and sympathetic impulses through the spinal cord and peripheral sympathetic nerves to the heart and blood vessels. The parasympathetic impulse slows the heart rate as opposed to the sympathetic impulse dominance, which increases the heart rate and cardiac contractility. Blood vessels also are selectively innervated by the sympathetic nervous system. When this system is stimulated, vasoconstriction occurs, decreasing blood flow to the periphery and shunting blood to critical organs such as the heart and brain.

Arterial Baroreceptors and Arterial Chemoreceptors

Baroreceptors located in the walls of blood vessels are pressure-sensitive receptors that respond to changes in the stretch of the blood vessels by sending impulses to the brain and heart to adjust the heart rate and smooth muscle tone. These stretch receptors are located in various large vessels throughout the body, such as the carotid sinus and the wall of the left ventricle. They respond to changes in arterial pressure (high or low) and signal the central nervous system (CNS). Signals are then transmitted back through baroreceptors to counteract the abnormal changes in the arterial pressure. If the pressure is elevated, the vagus nerve is stimulated, thereby slowing the heart rate and causing vasodilation, which decreases the pressure in the arteries. This system needs to function effectively to prevent hypertension. When failure occurs in regulating the determinants of blood pressure—cardiac output and the total peripheral resistance—the body needs to reset the baroreceptor and chemoreceptor sensitivity to more adequately respond to the changes in the systemic blood pressure.

The chemoreceptors located in the carotid bodies and the aorta respond to changes in oxygen, carbon dioxide, and hydrogen ion content in the arterial blood. Chemoreceptors regulate ventilation and communicate with the brainstem and cardiovascular centers to cause widespread vasoconstriction.

When the sympathetic nervous system detects an inadequate (low) blood pressure, a lack of oxygen, or a buildup of metabolic end products, the baroreceptors and chemoreceptors are activated. Changes in blood pressure are transmitted back to the CNS. A drop in blood pressure causes parasympathetic system inhibition and cardiac sympathetic nerve activation, resulting in an increased heart rate. In a resting position, the heart rate is under the parasympathetic influence and the heart rate is 60 to 80 beats/minute.

Regulation of Fluid Volume

Fluid volume throughout the body is maintained through multiple homeostatic mechanisms. Normal fluid volume is the result of a dynamic equilibrium between oral fluids and other dietary intakes and fluid output, which occurs through perspiration, urination, and respiration. The cardiovascular, renal, and respiratory areas are involved as are the pituitary gland, parathyroid glands, and adrenal glands.

When changes occur in the osmolarity (i.e., the concentration of the solute), the number of particles in fluid is conserved or eliminated in order to maintain a system homeostatic state. Guyton and Hall (2005) state that 80% of the total osmolarity of the interstitial fluid and plasma is due to sodium and chloride ions. The intracellular fluid is composed of potassium ions, which make up 50% of the osmolarity, and the balance is divided among the other intracellular substances (Guyton & Hall, 2005). The difference between plasma and interstitial fluid is due to the osmotic effects of the plasma proteins, which maintain about 20 mmHg greater pressure in the capillaries than the surrounding interstitial spaces (Guyton & Hall, 2005). Fluid balance is essential to maintaining normal blood pressure. When hypovolemia or hypervolemia occurs, it is reflected in the systemic blood pressure. A loss of fluid or hypovolemia results in a decrease in blood pressure due to the loss of circulating blood volume. With an excess of fluid volume, hypervolemia occurs.

Humoral Regulation

A second mechanism that plays a role in blood pressure regulation is the intrinsic hormones of the body. These include the renin-angiotensin-aldosterone mechanism, vasopressin, and epinephrine and norepinephrine. These hormones are essential in maintaining normal blood pressure on an ongoing basis.

Renin-Angiotensin-Aldosterone System

Renin is an enzyme that is produced and stored by the kidney. It is released with:

- Increased sympathetic nervous system stimulation
- Decreased blood pressure
- Increased extracellular fluid volume
- Increased extracellular sodium concentration.

Once in the bloodstream renin acts as an enzyme to the inactive plasma protein substrate angiotensinogen to convert it to angiotensin I. Angiotensin I travels to the lung and is converted to angiotensin II by the angiotensin-converting enzyme present in the blood vessels of the lungs. Angiotensin II is a potent vasoconstrictor hormone, which increases peripheral vascular resistance, thus increasing blood pressure. A second function of angiotensin II is to stimulate the adrenal glands to release aldosterone. Aldosterone, a steroid, increases sodium and water retention by the kidneys, thereby increasing blood pressure (Figure 21–1 ■).

Vasopressin

Vasopressin, also known as antidiuretic hormone (ADH), is a peptide produced by the posterior pituitary gland. Vasopressin is released in response to decreases in blood volume and blood pressure, as well as when an increase in the osmolality occurs. Its major functions are to increase water reabsorption by the kidneys and cause vasoconstriction, thus increasing blood pressure (Guyton & Hall, 2005). Vasopressin also serves as a neurotransmitter to modify the autonomic nervous system response, as discussed later in this chapter.

Epinephrine and Norepinephrine

The catecholamines, epinephrine and norepinephrine, exert their effects on target cells, which impact blood pressure. The

function of the adrenal medulla is to secrete these two catecholamines and depend on the receptor cell designation for their effects. Norepinephrine excites alpha receptors and beta receptors to a lesser degree than does epinephrine. Epinephrine excites both alpha and beta receptors equally. Thus, the effect of norepinephrine and epinephrine differs by the type of receptors in the organs (Guyton & Hall, 2005).

Epinephrine differs from norepinephrine in the following ways: epinephrine stimulates the beta receptors, increasing the effect on cardiac stimulation and weak vasoconstriction (Guyton & Hall, 2005). The heart increases the stroke volume (amount of blood ejected from the ventricle in one systole), the heart rate, and the muscle contractility. Blood vessels are able to constrict and dilate, thus impacting peripheral vascular resistance, which is the resistance to blood flow determined by the tone of the vascular system and the diameter of the blood vessel lumen. Through the action of these catecholamines, blood pressure is maintained. Norepinephrine also increases the heart rate and blood pressure.

■ Epidemiology and Etiology of Hypertension

The National Heart, Lung, and Blood Institute in 2004 reported that 65 million adult Americans—or one-third of the general adult population in the United States—have hypertension (Fields et al., 2004). If high blood pressure remains undiagnosed and untreated, it has a high morbidity and mortality rate.

This universal health dilemma of high blood pressure in the general population is undergoing intense inspection. The health care industry, health insurance groups, pharmaceutical companies, and the federal government are involved in solving this universal problem. The National Guidelines box (p. 490) outlines the *Healthy People 2010* midcourse review objective, target goal, and baseline data for people with hypertension. To make the condition of hypertension more easily understood, the name *hypertension*, a medical term, is gradually being changed to *high blood pressure*. This change is designed to make the term more easily understood in a worldwide multicultural community. The JNC 7 report (NHLBI, 2003b) states that many experts consider high blood pressure a "silent killer." It is a complex syndrome that can occur at any age, involves multiple systems of the body, and requires aggressive treatment.

■ Pathophysiology of Hypertension

Hypertension is diagnosed when the average blood pressure is higher than the accepted norm over a period of time consisting of two or more consecutive office visits. The May 2003 JNC 7 report (NHLBI, 2003b) included revised guidelines for what constitutes hypertension and divided these parameters into three separate classifications for adults over the age of 18 years, as listed in the National Guidelines box (p. 490).

The term **prehypertension,** introduced in the JNC 7 report (NHLBI, 2003b), describes those individuals with a blood pressure finding on two or more office visits of 120–139 mmHg systolic or 80–89 mmHg diastolic. These individuals are at twice the risk of developing hypertension as those with lower values.

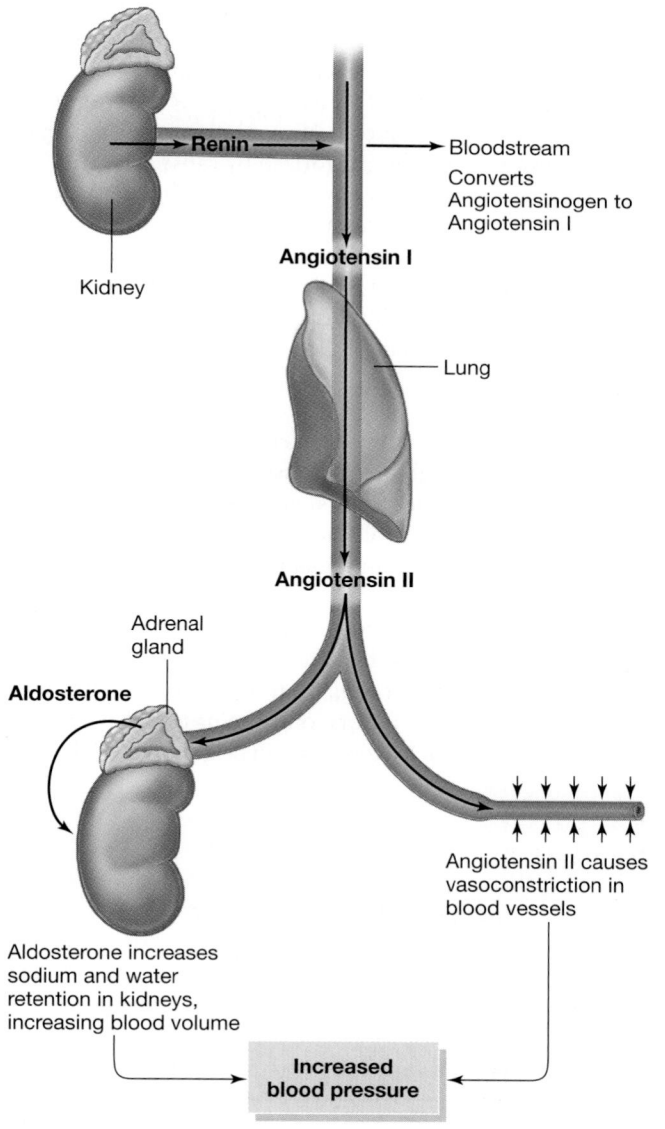

FIGURE 21–1 ■ Renin-angiotensin-aldosterone system.

MyNursingKit Animation: Stages of Hypertension Table

NATIONAL GUIDELINES *Healthy People 2010* **Midcourse Review: Objectives, Target Goals, and Baseline Data**

12.9. Reduce the proportion of adults with high blood pressure.
   Target: 14 percent
   Baseline: 26 percent of adults ages 20 years and older had high blood pressure in 1988–1994 (age adjusted to the year 2000 standard population).

12.10. Increase the proportion of adults with high blood pressure whose blood pressure is under control.
   Target: 68 percent
   Baseline: 25 percent of adults ages 18 years and older with high blood pressure had it under control in 1988–1994 (age adjusted to the year 2000 standard population).

12.11. Increase the proportion of adults with high blood pressure who are taking action (for example, losing weight, increasing physical

activity, or reducing sodium intake) to help control their blood pressure.
   Target: 98 percent
   Baseline: 84 percent of adults ages 18 years and older with high blood pressure were taking action to control it in 1998 (age adjusted to the year 2000 standard population).

12.12. Increase the proportion of adults who have had their blood pressure measured within the preceding 2 years and can state whether their blood pressure was normal or high.
   Target: 95 percent
   Baseline: 90 percent of adults ages 18 years and older had their blood pressure measured in the past 2 years and could state whether it was normal or high in 1998 (age adjusted to the year 2000 standard population).

Source: U.S. Department of Health and Human Services. (2006). *Midcourse review: Healthy People 2010: Heart disease and stroke—12.* Retrieved June 9, 2008, from http://www.healthypeople.gov/data/midcourse/html/focusareas/FA12TOC.htm.

Prehypertension is the early phase when the relationship between the blood pressure measurement and the need for health education is the primary focus of care. The individual demonstrating prehypertension is at risk for development of stage 1 or stage 2 hypertension. The JNC 7 report emphasizes increasing the awareness of the need to reduce blood pressure levels and prevent the development of high blood pressure in the general population through the education of health care professionals.

Stage 1 hypertension and stage 2 hypertension parameters are outlined in the National Guidelines box. **Stage 1 hypertension** is a blood pressure of 140–159 mmHg systolic or 90–99 mmHg diastolic measured during multiple office visits following the guidelines for accurate blood pressure measurement. Lifestyle changes as well as medications would be part of the therapeutic plan.

Stage 2 hypertension is a systolic blood pressure measured on multiple occasions during an office visit of greater than 160 mmHg or a diastolic pressure of greater than 100 mmHg. The measurement of the blood pressure would follow the guidelines for accuracy (Chart 21–2). Both medications and lifestyle changes would be a part of the therapeutic plan.

In addition, **white coat phenomenon** is an elevated blood pressure when the assessment of the blood pressure is done by a physician or another health care professional. If this phenomenon occurs frequently over time, the patient is responding to a

perceived stressful situation and may need early hypertensive treatment. Often the physician will request the patient measure her blood pressure in the home setting and record the findings in order to diagnosis high blood pressure. This process is used to determine if the patient is demonstrating white coat phenomenon.

Hypertension is further categorized by cause. There are two types: essential and secondary hypertension. *Essential hypertension* is defined as a chronic elevation in blood pressure that occurs without the evidence of disease. *Secondary hypertension* is high blood pressure that is a result of some other disorder such as kidney disease. Essential hypertension may be systolic, diastolic, or both systolic and diastolic.

Risk Factors

Certain identifiable contributing elements increase the risk of the development of high blood pressure. These risk factors are classified as modifiable factors and nonmodifiable factors (Chart 21–3). The modifiable factors are those that the patient can control, whereas nonmodifiable factors cannot be controlled by the patient.

A patient evaluation includes determining the risk factors, lifestyle, possible causes of hypertension, and target organs for damage including the heart (e.g., from coronary heart disease). A review of the multiple risk factors contributing to high blood pressure, as listed in the Risk Factors box, can be done while taking the

NATIONAL GUIDELINES JNC 7 Classification of Blood Pressure for Adults

BP Classification	SBP (mmHg)	DBP (mmHg)	Lifestyle Modification Encouraged
Normal	<120	and <90	
Prehypertension	120–139	Or 80–89	Yes
Stage 1 hypertension	140–159	Or 90–99	Yes
Stage 2 hypertension	>160	Or >100	Yes

Note: DBP, diastolic blood pressure; SBP, systolic blood pressure. Treatment determined by highest BP level.
Source: National Heart, Lung, and Blood Institute. (2003, May). *Seventh report of the Joint National Committee on Prevention, Detection, Evaluation, and Treatment of High Blood Pressure (JNC7).* Retrieved June 9, 2008, from http://www.nhlbi.nih.gov/guidelines/hypertension/jnc7full.pdf.

CHART 21–2 Guidelines for Assessing Blood Pressure in Adults

QUESTIONS TO BE ASKED BEFORE A BLOOD PRESSURE ASSESSMENT IS DONE

- Have you drunk any caffeinated beverages within the last hour?
- Have you eaten any chocolate within the last hour?
- Have you smoked within the last 15 minutes?
- Are you using any nasal decongestants? (If yes, assess whether the decongestant contains phenylephrine.)
- Do you use eyedrops for pupillary dilation?
- Does the environment feel cold to you?
- Have you just eaten a meal?
- Do you need to use the restroom?
- Do you exercise? If so, what do you do, for how long and how many times per week?

ENVIRONMENT

- A quiet, warm and comfortable setting.
- Home readings.

EQUIPMENT

- *Cuff size for adult:* The bladder should encircle and cover two-thirds of the length of the arm. If the bladder is too small, a high reading may result.
- *Manometer:* Aneroid gauges should be calibrated every 6 months against a mercury manometer.
- *Infants and children:* Use a Doppler method.

POSTURE

- *Initial assessment:* For patients over age 65 receiving antihypertensive therapy or a diabetic check for postural changes in blood pressure, the first reading is taken after the patient has been supine for 5 minutes and then immediately and 2 minutes after the patient stands.

- *Follow-up:* For a follow-up, a sitting pressure is recommended. The patient should be seated quietly for 5 minutes with the back supported. The arm is then supported at the level of the heart.

TECHNIQUE

- Initially, the blood pressure assessment is taken in both arms. The findings are recorded, identifying the arm and the pressure reading.
- On each occasion, take at least two readings. These are separated by as much time as practical. When readings vary more than 5 mmHg, take additional readings until two readings are close.
- When making the diagnosis of high blood pressure, three sets of readings are obtained at least 1 week apart.
- When the arm pressure is elevated in a patient younger than 30, take the blood pressure in the leg.

PERFORMANCE

- Find the brachial artery.
- Inflate the bladder quickly to a pressure at least 20 mmHg above the systolic pressure. This can be checked by determining that the radial pulse has disappeared.
- Deflate the bladder at about 3 mmHg every second.
- Record the Korotkoff phase V (disappearance) in adults. In children use phase IV (muffling).
- If the Korotkoff sounds are weak, have the patient raise the arm, open and close the hand 5 to 10 times, and then inflate the bladder quickly.
- Recording the findings.
  - Note the pressure obtained.
  - Note which arm was used.
  - Note the patient's position.
  - Note the cuff size.

Example: 140/90, seated, right arm, large adult cuff

Source: This article was published in Cecil essentials of medicine, 6th Ed., Andreoli, T. E., Carpenter, C. C. J., Griggs, R. C. & Loscalzo, J., pp. 38–39 (2004). Cecil essentials of medicine. (6th Ed.) Philadelphia: Saunders, pp. 38–39.

CHART 21–3 Factors Contributing to Hypertension

MODIFIABLE FACTORS

- High sodium dietary intake
- Overweight
- Excessive alcohol consumption
- Low potassium intake
- Smoking

NONMODIFIABLE FACTORS

- Family history
- Age
- Race

Source: National Heart, Lung, and Blood Institute. (2003, May). *Seventh report of the Joint National Committee on Prevention, Detection, Evaluation, and Treatment of High Blood Pressure (JNC7).* Retrieved June 9, 2008, from http://www.nhlbi.nih.gov/guidelines/hypertension/jnc7full.pdf.

RISK FACTORS for Hypertension

Cigarette smoking

Obesity (BMI > 30 kg/m^2)

Physical inactivity

Dyslipidemia

Diabetes mellitus

Microalbuminuria or estimated GFR < 60 mL/min

Age (older than 55 years for men and 65 years for women)

Family history of premature cardiovascular disease (men under age 55 and women under age 65)

Gender

Sodium intake

Excessive alcohol consumption

Atherosclerosis

Source: Adapted from National Heart, Lung, and Blood Institute. (2003, May). *Seventh report of the Joint National Committee on Prevention, Detection, Evaluation, and Treatment of High Blood Pressure (JNC7).* Retrieved June 9, 2008, from http://www.nhlbi.nih.gov/guidelines/hypertension/jnc7full.pdf.

patient and family history. The nurse needs to evaluate the patient's stress level in terms of physical and emotional stresses, the reported amount of sodium intake, the patient's weight, the amount of alcohol consumed, the serum potassium level, and use of tobacco. Chart 21–4 outlines the causes of high blood pressure.

Culture, Environment, Race, Genetics, and History

The assessment of an individual's culture, environment, and race is obtained from the patient and family. It is essential for these factors to be assessed during the interview because diversity is well established in the American lifestyle. It is estimated that half of the population in the United States in the year 2050 will be from a minority group (Donnelly, 2000). For example, the health care provider needs to be cognizant that African American individuals have twice as high a possibility of developing high blood pressure than do Caucasian Americans. If the patient lives in the southeastern portion of the United States as opposed to other parts of the country, the incidence of high blood pressure also is higher. In addition, environmental factors such as obesity, cigarette smoking, sedentary lifestyle, use of illegal drugs, and sodium intake have an impact on blood pressure.

The family may contribute medically historic information and report on any therapies the patient may have used. The interview may be both a teaching and learning opportunity, giving the nurse a further opportunity to gather data concerning the lifestyle of the patient and family. The Genetic Considerations box addresses how genetics might affect a patient's propensity for high blood pressure.

Psychosocial Assessment

When the nurse is obtaining a patient's psychosocial data, care must be used when listening to how the patient describes the meaning of the diagnosis of high blood pressure. Life stresses can make the patient's ability to participate in a partnership of care difficult. Areas of stress may be related to job stresses, economic position, losses and/or gains of any kind, and many other issues of life. The activation of the sympathetic nervous system

GENETIC CONSIDERATIONS Related to Hypertension

Despite the advances in medical science, the causes of prehypertension and stage 1 and stage 2 hypertension are not discernible in most cases (Andreoli, Carpenter, Griggs, & Loscalzo, 2004). The genetic profile may assist by providing information about alterations in the genetic coding of angiotensinogen in the hypertensive population. Hypertension is seen most often with persons who have a family history of hypertension, thus implicating a genetic predisposition. If an individual has two or more family members with hypertension before the age of 55 years, there is a 3.8 times greater risk for the development of hypertension (Porth, 2005). A family history of high blood pressure and heart disease may suggest a genetic predisposition for the development of these disorders.

is a significant response to stress. When a patient experiences severe stress, the amount of catecholamines is increased. This is frequently referred to as the "fight-or-flight" response. This response increases the blood pressure.

The assessment of anger and the patient's coping skills need to be incorporated into any care plan. Good patient participation and ownership of the negotiated therapeutic plan are essential to the success of lifestyle changing strategies.

■ Clinical Manifestations

High blood pressure is asymptomatic in the initial period. The patient may be of any age ranging from early childhood to elderly. It is estimated that high blood pressure may be present in some individuals for many years prior to discovery. During this time, the major organs may be slowly damaged.

Clinical signs and symptoms the patient describes may be nonspecific such as a headache or dizziness, sleepiness, nausea and vomiting, irritability, and visual disturbances. More serious complications may occur when a patient remains undiagnosed for years. Myocardial infarction, heart failure, cerebral vascular accidents, and renal failure may all be the result of untreated high blood pressure and occur without further warning.

Assessment

The assessment of a patient includes a review of history, signs, symptoms, prescribed medications, alternative therapies, and over-the-counter (OTC) medicines. The purpose of this assessment is to determine what risk factors are present, what concomitant therapies may have been used, the patient's lifestyle choices, and family history. The nurse records any signs and symptoms such as weakness, muscle cramps, polyuria (possible diabetes mellitus), headache, palpitations, or hyperhidrosis (possible excess of catecholamines). If end-organ involvement is suspected, the history should include symptoms of coronary artery disease, heart failure, cerebral vascular disease, and uremia.

Blood Pressure Measurement

The blood pressure is properly measured using both arms on two or more different occasions, when the patient has been seated for at least 5 minutes prior to measurement. Chart 21–2 (p. 491) includes the guidelines for assessing blood pressure in the adult.

CHART 21–4	Identifiable Causes of Hypertension

Sleep apnea

Drug-induced or -related causes

Chronic kidney disease

Primary aldosteronism

Renovascular disease

Chronic steroid therapy and Cushing's syndrome

Pheochromocytoma

Coarctation of the aorta

Thyroid or parathyroid disease

Cause may be unknown

Source: Adapted from National Heart, Lung, and Blood Institute. (2003, May). *Seventh report of the Joint National Committee on Prevention, Detection, Evaluation, and Treatment of High Blood Pressure (JNC7)*. Retrieved June 9, 2008, from http://www.nhlbi.nih.gov/guidelines/hypertension/jnc7full.pdf.

Diagnostic Tests

There are no specific diagnostic tests for hypertension, except the tracking of serial blood pressures. When any stage of hypertension is diagnosed, a complete workup needs to be completed to determine target organ damage. This provides a baseline from which to assess future changes. The Diagnostic Tests box (p. 494) outlines tests that can be used during the initial workup of a newly diagnosed hypertensive patient.

Medical Management

The outcome of the therapeutic plan is to effectively lower and maintain the systemic blood pressure at a normal level. The plan needs to be individualized for each patient. The following factors should be considered when tailoring a plan for a given patient:

- Culture
- Age
- Risk factors
- Degree of blood pressure elevation
- Coexisting diseases
- Cost of prescribed pharmacologic agents
- Family/social support
- Amount and type of follow-up care needed.

A comprehensive plan includes addressing all factors that influence the occurrence of hypertension. This includes dietary restrictions, weight reduction where appropriate, medication regimen, exercise program, and finally stress reduction. Additionally, an evaluation needs to be made to determine if the patient is able to follow through with the lifestyle changes, monitoring of his blood pressure, and maintaining contact with the health care team.

Diet

The Dietary Approaches to Stop Hypertension diet, known as the **DASH** diet, is low in sodium, saturated fat, cholesterol, and total fat. The diet focuses on fruits, vegetables, nuts, and low-fat dairy products. This plan is rich in potassium and calcium. Although, lowering total and saturated fats has no direct effect on controlling blood pressure, it will lower cholesterol and have an effect on the development of coronary artery disease. Therefore, it is an important adjunct to the dietary plan.

There are two versions of the DASH plan in relation to sodium restrictions. Plan 1 limits the patient to 2,400 mg of sodium per day, whereas plan 2 limits the patient to 1,500 mg of sodium per day. The health care provider would assess the stage of hypertension in order to determine the degree of sodium restriction that is necessary. Increasing the intake of potassium-rich foods also is encouraged, due to the side effect of some of the antihypertensive medications and because it is known that a low potassium level is linked to increased blood pressure (Welton, 2003). It is thought that one of the major benefits of a potassium-rich diet is increased elimination of sodium (natriuretic effect) and suppression of the renin-angiotensin system. Note that many processed foods tend to be low in potassium and high in sodium. Thus, patients should be encouraged to consume natural foods and avoid processed foods.

The patient with stage 1 or stage 2 high blood pressure should be encouraged to make the following lifestyle changes: Eat a low-sodium diet (DASH meal plan), reduced-calorie diet (weight re-duction diet), or low-cholesterol diet; decrease the intake of saturated fats; limit the use of alcohol; and stop smoking. The DASH diet plan is considered to be equivalent to a single-drug therapy (NHLBI, 2003b). Chapter 14 provides an overall description of healthy sensible eating plans, using the Food Guide Pyramid and a description of the DASH diet.

Exercise

Regular physical activities assist in the promotion of cardiovascular fitness and beneficial changes: They lower blood pressure and raise a person's high-density lipoproteins (the good cholesterol). It is essential to have an organized aerobic exercise program, approved by a health care provider, which is completed on a regular basis for 30 to 45 minutes three to five times per week. This plan is begun slowly and stopped if the patient develops shortness of breath, fainting, or chest pain. Physical conditioning has a positive impact on both lowering and maintaining normal blood pressure, as further discussed in the Complementary and Alternative Therapies box (p. 495). Chapter 40 includes an in-depth discussion of the lipids and the benefit of exercise on the heart.

Light weight training is recommended to lower blood pressure, but heavy lifting is known to raise blood pressure due to the vasovagal response that occurs with intense isometric exercise. Thus, heavy lifting should be avoided in hypertensive individuals.

Weight Control

According to the Centers for Disease Control and Prevention (2008) obesity has risen to epidemic proportions in the past 20 years. A standard measurement for expressing the relationship (or ratio) of weight-to-height is the body mass index (BMI). The BMI is calculated by dividing the body weight in kilograms by the square of height in meters. A person with a BMI of 25 to 29.9 is considered overweight, and individuals with a BMI of 30 or more are considered obese. A BMI of 27 or greater correlates closely with high blood pressure.

A second risk factor for the development of high blood pressure is the presence of excess fat accumulated in the torso that is out of proportion to the rest of the body fat distribution. Men with a waist circumference of 40 inches or more and women with a waist circumference of 35 inches or more are at risk for developing high blood pressure (National Heart, Lung, and Blood Institute, 1998).

For individuals who are 10% or greater above ideal body weight, as little as a 10-pound reduction in weight will lower the blood pressure. Additionally, antihypertensive medication effectiveness is enhanced with weight reduction. During the weight reduction process, the blood pressure needs to be assessed regularly and medications adjusted appropriately.

Stress Reduction

A priority for the nurse is discussion of the issue of stress with both the patient and family. Often individuals are not totally aware of the impact of stress on the development of high blood pressure. Frequently, individuals may feel helpless about how to control their stress levels. It is important for the nurse to explain clearly the impact of stress on the development of high blood pressure. Teaching the patient stress reduction techniques is an essential part of the plan for controlling high blood pressure. Exercise, the use of support systems, and some alternative therapies have all been identified as stress reduction techniques.

DIAGNOSTIC TESTS for Hypertension

Test and Normal Values	Expected Abnormality	Rationale for Abnormality
Aldosterone (blood) *Supine:* 3–20 ng/dL *Upright* (sitting for at least 2 hr): *Males:* 6–22 ng/dL *Females:* 5–30 ng/dL	An increased aldosterone serum level is associated with hypertension and hypokalemia.	Primary aldosteronism may be due to aldosterone-producing adenomas. Aldosterone causes the kidneys to retain salt and excrete potassium, causing the retention of water and, thus, increasing the blood volume and blood pressure (Nicoll, McPhee, & Pignone, 2004, p. 44).
Renin assay, plasma (PRA) (Plasma renin concentration [PRC]) *Adult/Elderly:* *Upright* (sodium-restricted diet): *Age 20–39 years:* 2.9–24 ng/mL/hour *Age >40 years:* 2.9–10.8 ng/mL per hour *Upright* (normal sodium diet): *Age 20–39 years:* 0.1–4.3 ng/mL per hour *Age >40 years:* 0.1–3.0 ng/mL per hour	Increased in some hypertensive states (e.g., renal artery stenosis). Decreased in hyporeninemic hypoaldosteronism, and some hypertensive states: primary aldosteronism, severe preeclampsia.	PRA is helpful in the differential diagnosis of aldosteronism and the evaluation of hypertension. The PRA is increased in dehydration, edematous states due to cirrhosis, nephritic syndrome, heart failure, hypokalemic states, adrenal insufficiency, chronic renal failure, and left ventricular hypertrophy. Test is useful in the evaluation of hypoaldosteronism (low-sodium diet and patient standing) (Nicoll et al., 2004, p. 158).
Glucose (blood) *Adult:* 70–110 mg/dL	The expected finding is an increase in renal damage as a result of hypertension and the acceleration of atherosclerosis, arteriosclerosis, and renal failure.	Prevalence, prematurity, and severity of coronary atherosclerosis are demonstrated among patients with diabetes. When this occurs, the peripheral resistance in the blood vessels increases and the clinical sign is hypertension. Diabetes mellitus may be associated with accelerated arteriosclerosis and primary aldosteronism (Kasper et al., 2005, p. 1469).
Creatinine (blood) *Males:* 0.6–1.2 mg/dL *Females:* 0.5–1.1 mg/dL *Elderly:* decreased values due to decreased muscle mass	Increased in acute renal failure. Decreased when there is a reduced muscle mass.	Nitrogenous end product of protein metabolism. As creatinine and BUN rise, the glomerular filtration rate decreases. With deterioration of renal function occurring, glomerular hypertension occurs within the nephrons.
Sodium (blood) 135–145 mEq/L	Increased sodium levels increases fluid retention, which increases blood pressure.	Link between sodium intake and high blood pressure is described as increased renal vascular resistance, which reduces renal blood flow and GFR mainly in the cortical collecting tubules (Guyton & Hall, 2005, p. 376).
Cholesterol (serum) *Desirable:* <200 mg/dL *Borderline:* 200–239 mg/dL *High risk:* >240 mg/dL	Increased	Associated with hypertension, predisposition to arteriosclerosis.
Calcium *Total calcium, adult:* 9.0–10.5 mg/dL *Ionized calcium, adult:* 4.5–5.6 mg/dL	Decreased calcium intake is associated with increased blood pressure.	Increased calcium excretion occurs in chronic renal insufficiency. There is a potential link between salt sensitive forms of high blood pressure and calcium (Kasper et al., 2005, p. 1464).
Lipoprotein (HDL [alpha lipoproteins]) *Males:* >45 mg/dL *Females:* >55 mg/dL	HDL is a carrier of cholesterol. It is thought to be the protective cardiac characteristic. Low levels are found with heart disease.	Measurement of the lipoproteins is essential in the therapeutic management of a patient with hypertension because an increase in lipoproteins indicates a risk of atherogenic heart disease and peripheral vascular disease, which may further increase high blood pressure.
LDL (beta lipoproteins) and VLDL (pre-beta-lipoproteins) *LDL:* 60–180 mg/dL *VLDL:* 25–50%	Increased LDL is associated with atherosclerotic heart disease and peripheral vascular disease, which increase the peripheral resistance and blood pressure.	LDL is carried to peripheral tissues and is associated with an increased risk of arteriosclerotic hypertension and peripheral vascular disease.
Urinalysis *Color and appearance:* amber yellow and clear *Odor:* aromatic *pH:* 4.6–8.0 *Protein:* 0–8 mg/dL *Glucose:* none with fresh specimen.	Urine is tested for protein blood and glucose to determine if target organ damage is present.	Part of the screening test for hypertension is to gain information about the potential target organ damage and the etiology of the patient's high blood pressure. Concentration of urine is controlled by secretion of ADH and the renin-angiotensin feedback.

Source: Adapted from National Heart, Lung, and Blood Institute. (2003, May). *Seventh report of the Joint National Committee on Prevention, Detection, Evaluation, and Treatment of High Blood Pressure (JNC7).* Retrieved June 9, 2008, from http://www.nhlbi.nih.gov/guidelines/hypertension/jnc7full.pdf.

COMPLEMENTARY & ALTERNATIVE THERAPIES
Exercise

Description:

Exercise need not be complex. A patient can create an effective exercise program that is as simple as setting up a treadmill in the bedroom. Other exercise options that are more structured include working with a personal trainer, joining a class, or walking with a group of neighbors. Many organizations offer participatory classes that can promote program adherence and provide instruction in the proper exercise technique. Such organizations include Jazzercise, YMCA, Curves, as well as local gyms.

Research Support:

When the human body is under threat, it exhibits a set of neuroendocrine responses collectively known as the "fight or flight" response. These responses include an increased secretion of glucocorticoids (GCs) and catecholamines from the adrenal gland and the activation of the sympathetic nervous system. These hormones mobilize endogenous substrate and induce a state of insulin resistance in the liver and skeletal muscles. This stress response was essential to survival in ancient times, where the increased metabolic demand was put to immediate use. However, in modern times, one can no longer fight or flee the most common stressors, which often involve emotional, professional, and social stressors. These types of psychological stressors may be protracted and create long-term metabolic disturbances. These metabolic disturbances can lead to a number of comorbidities including central obesity and hypertension. The stress response is a neuroendocrine mechanism that was intended to provide the energy needed for survival-focused physical action. Therefore, physical activity should be the natural means to prevent the comorbid consequences of stress. Indeed, there is a great deal of evidence that documents the beneficial effects of regular exercise in preventing or ameliorating the stress-induced metabolic and psychological comorbidities. It is believed that exercise reduces the body's sensitivity to stress and also the peripheral actions that influence metabolic functions. Of particular importance are the documented effects of exercise on insulin sensitivity and metabolizing calories for fuel rather than storage. It is concluded that when chronic psychosocial stress accompanies physical inactivity, it contributes to our current epidemic of cardiometabolic and emotional disease. Regular exercise provides a way to prevent and combat this burden (Tsatsoulis & Fountoulakis, 2006).

There is evidence that two conditions in particular, hypertension and stroke, are improved with increased physical activity. The following two paragraphs discuss this evidence.

Rates of hypertension and hypertension-related death in older African Americans are very high versus all other American ethnic groups. A lifestyle factor in this population that contributes to their hypertension-related health problems is that they are also one of the most physically inactive groups. Interventions can assist them to increase their exercise activities and thereby gain better hypertension control. Findings of one study by Cromwell and Adams (2006) supported a strong association between physical activity level and exercise self-efficacy in this population. These findings suggest that interventions that address exercise self-efficacy would be helpful for increasing the level of exercise in older African Americans (Cromwell & Adams, 2006).

Stroke is another condition that may be improved through increased physical activity. In order to prevent a first-time stroke, it is vital to identify at-risk patients and control as many risk factors as possible. Some risk factors, such as lifestyle factors, can be eliminated; others, such as hypertension, can be controlled or treated. Exercise provides one way to control the risk of stroke (Sauerbeck, 2006). In the general as well as elderly populations, aerobic exercise is effective for reducing blood pressure (McDonald, Blackwell, & Meurer, 2006). Researchers have found that, when a patient adheres to either supervised or unsupervised moderate-intensity exercise, it is sufficient to reduce short- and long-term blood pressure (Cox, 2006).

References

Cox, K. L. (2006). Exercise and blood pressure: Applying findings from the laboratory to the community setting. *Clinical and Experimental Pharmacology and Physiology, 33*(9), 868–871.

Cromwell, S. L., & Adams, M. M. (2006). Exercise, self-efficacy, and exercise behavior in hypertensive older African-Americans. *Journal of National Black Nurses Association, 17*(1), 17–21.

McDonald, K. C., Blackwell, J. C., & Meurer, L. N. (2006). Clinical inquiries. What lifestyle changes should we recommend for the patient with newly diagnosed hypertension? *Journal of Family Practice, 55*(11), 991–993.

Sauerbeck, L. R. (2006). Primary stroke prevention. *American Journal of Nursing, 106*(11), 40–41, 43–45, 48–50.

Tsatsoulis, A., & Fountoulakis, S. (2006). The protective role of exercise on stress system dysregulation and comorbidities. *Annals of the New York Academy of Sciences, 1083,* 196–213.

Alcohol Consumption

Research indicates that regular consumption of three or more drinks per day increases the risk of hypertension. The systolic blood pressure is more affected by alcohol than the diastolic. The exact mechanism whereby alcohol exerts it effect on blood pressure is unclear, but elevated blood pressure may improve and return to normal when alcohol consumption ceases. Patients tend to understate the amount of alcohol consumed. The nurse needs to realize the amount may be more and tailor the teaching to the possibility of greater consumption.

Pharmacologic Agents Used to Treat Hypertension

The care of the patient with high blood pressure includes the use of pharmacologic agents. These agents have reduced the morbidity and mortality associated with high blood pressure as well as the incidence of cerebrovascular accident. The Pharmacology Summary (p. 497) outlines the eight classifications of medications

used to treat high blood pressure. The summary also includes the nursing responsibilities for patient and family teaching that are necessary for the safe use of these medications. Chart 21–5 (p. 496) outlines herbal therapies for treatment of hypertension.

Complementary and Alternative Therapies

The use of complementary or alternative therapies may be attractive to the patient because of the ease of availability and the lower cost of medicinal herbs as opposed to pharmacologic agents. Eisenhower (2002) reported the finding from the *Descriptive Study of Client Use of Herbal Substances and Over-the-Counter Medications* that 100% of the study subjects took herbs and OTC drugs. In addition, Eisenhower reported (1) that 95% of the subjects mixed herbal and OTC drugs with prescription medications, (2) that the subjects reported they believed these herbal remedies helped 80% of the time, and (3) that 55% of subjects had not told their health care provider of these practices.

Complementary and/or alternative therapies include autogenic therapy, healing, hypnosis, exercise, relaxation and visualization,

CHART 21–5	Selected Herbal Products for Treating Hypertension		
Name	**Action**	**Application/Indications**	**Nursing Responsibility**
Black cohosh	Unknown. Therapeutic effect produced by glycosides isolated from fresh or dried rhizome with attached roots. May decrease symptoms of menopause, including hot flashes, sweating, sleep disturbances, and anxiety.	May potentiate hypertensive drugs and hypertension. Patients need to be warned not to take this drug as a supplement with other antihypertensive drugs without consulting with the health care provider.	Teach patient to monitor blood pressure when taking antihypertensive drugs. Assess for reports of nausea and vomiting, history of seizures, liver disease, and alcohol intake.
Hawthorne	Active compounds are flavonoids and procyanidins that increase coronary blood flow and have positive inotropic and chronotropic effects due to increased permeability to calcium and inhibition of phosphodiesterase. Cardiac output increases; myocardial workload and oxygen consumption decrease. The pharmacokinetics of hawthorne are unknown.	Hawthorne does not cure heart failure but keeps control of symptoms. Do not take hawthorne unless you have the approval of a health care professional. The substance may cause hypertension.	Assess the patient's lung sounds for signs of heart failure. Teach importance of taking daily weights and of taking the pulse for rate and rhythm. Teach symptoms of "heart attack" and heart failure. Instruct therapy may not take effect for 6–8 weeks. Adverse responses to hawthorne may cause drowsiness, profuse sweating, and dehydration leading to severe hypotension. Teach that during hot weather exercise should always be minimized.

Sources: Deglin, J. H., & Vallerand, A. H. (2005). *Davis's drug guide for nurses* (10th ed.) Philadelphia: F. A. Davis Company; Rankin-Box, D. (2001). *The nurse's handbook of complementary therapies* (2nd ed.) London: Bailliere Tindall.

and therapeutic touch. Other therapies include animal-assisted therapy, aromatherapy, biofeedback, herbs (e.g., garlic and hawthorn), message, meditation, qi gong, vitamin C and calcium supplements (if high blood pressure is pregnancy induced), t'ai chi, and yoga. Lily of the valley, an herb containing cardioactive glycosides, would not be prescribed with digitalis because it increases the action of each product (Rankin-Box, 2001). The Complementary and Alternative Therapies box (p. 499) outlines the most common alternative therapies for high blood pressure.

 *Assessment of the patient's treatment routine must include the determination of use of herbal and complementary therapies. Nurses are responsible for teaching patients about the use of herbal products and their interactions with prescription drugs.*

Nursing Management

A partnership of care with the hypertensive patient involves the process of devising a role for each patient, family member, and the nurse. The nurse is the coordinator of care and provider of information concerning risk reduction, health promotion, disease prevention, and the nursing care plan. The nursing needs of the individual with prehypertension or stage 1 or stage 2 hypertension focus on educating the patient about lifestyle changes and implementing the therapeutic regimen.

The nurse functions with autonomy and creativity in providing the patient with information that the patient/family can use to make informed choices and decisions. Throughout this process, the nurse will use assessment data and technical skills to maintain pri-

vacy, cultural sensitivity, and confidentiality. Jhala (2001) suggested that individuals of a different culture view themselves differently and reflect their own culture in the area of attitudes, beliefs, and values that are embedded in their own world. In addition, language barriers play a large role in the feelings of vulnerability and helplessness (Jhala, 2001). The Cultural Considerations box (p. 499) discusses various cultures' susceptibility to high blood pressure.

As the patient's hypertension moves from one stage to the next, the nursing process provides a framework for assessing, following clinical data, and evaluating the patient outcomes. The nursing care needs of the individual with any classification of high blood pressure are complex and multifaceted. Use of the nursing process will facilitate a comprehensive approach to patient assessment and care. The Nursing Process: Patient Care Plan (p. 500) feature applies the nursing process to the applicable nursing diagnoses and provides a comprehensive care plan for a hypertensive patient.

Health Promotion

Health care providers are beginning to place more responsibility with the individual for healthy lifestyle choices across the life span because, as mentioned earlier, a healthy lifestyle assists in controlling high blood pressure. A healthy lifestyle includes eating three balanced meals per day, eating to maintain a healthy weight, exercise, limited use of alcohol, no smoking, adequate sleeping time (7 to 8 hours per night), and reduction of stress. The individual and family need to be familiar with their current blood pressure measurements. If the findings are higher than 120/80 mmHg, the nondiabetic individual needs to seek medical advice. If an individual has diabetes and her blood pressure is higher than 130/80 mmHg, she too should seek medical advice.

PHARMACOLOGY Summary of Medications to Treat High Blood Pressure

Medication Category	Action	Application/Indication	Nursing Responsibility
Thiazide diuretics: • Chlorothiazide • Hydrochlorothiazide	Prevents sodium and water reabsorption in the distal tubules, thus facilitating excretion of fluid and electrolytes, which decreases the blood volume, thereby decreasing the blood pressure.	Treatment goal is prevention of end-organ damage. Used to lower the blood pressure to the lowest diastolic pressure the patient can tolerate.	Instruct the patient to take this medication at the same time daily. Encourage the intake of foods high in potassium such as bananas and orange juice. Review the frequency of prescription renewal as a measure of compliance. Teach that abrupt withdrawal will cause rebound hypertension.
Potassium-sparing diuretics • Spironolactone • Triamterene	Causes the loss of sodium bicarbonate and calcium while preserving the potassium and hydrogen ions. The fluid follows sodium, facilitating the loss of volume, leading to a decrease in blood pressure while preventing diuretic-induced hypokalemia.	Medication used singly or with another agent to treat hypertension or edema.	Teach to monitor blood pressure daily and report sudden weight gains over a 2-day period to health care provider. Teach regular monitoring of serum electrolytes.
Beta-adrenergic blocking agents • Propranolol • Atenolol • Nadolol	Agents block stimulation of the beta-1 (myocardial) and beta-2 (pulmonary), vascular, and uterine adrenergic receptor sites. This blockage causes vasodilation, decreasing intravascular pressure and blood pressure.	Used in the management of hypertension, heart failure, and angina pectoris. Blocks the stimulation of beta and beta-adrenergic receptor sites.	Teach blood pressure and pulse taking prior to medication. If pulse is below 60, inform the health care provider prior to taking the medication. Medication to be taken at the same time each day. Teach that rapid withdrawal of medication may cause life-threatening dysrhythmias. Instruct patient to report to health care provider any fatigue, difficulty with sexual activity, weakness, or depression. Assess for reported orthostatic hypotension, cough, and shortness of breath.
Calcium channel blockers • Diltiazem hydrochloride • Nifedipine • Verapamil	Agents block the calcium ion from entering the cells of the smooth muscle and myocardium, causing a loss of cell excitation. This results in dilation of the arteries and slowing of the SA node excitation and conduction. These actions decrease both heart rate and blood pressure.	Alone or with other agents for the management of hypertension, angina pectoris, vasospastic angina, supraventricular tachyarrhythmias, and rapid supraventricular rates in atrial flutter and fibrillation.	Instruct that sustained-action capsules or tablets cannot be crushed, broken up, or chewed. Teach monitoring pulse, blood pressure, and weight at regular intervals. Teach that if irregular heartbeats occur, notify the health care provider quickly. Assess the patient's reports of dizziness and use of OTC medications and alcohol unless approved by the health care professional. Teach patient to wear sunscreen to avoid a photosensitive reaction.

(continued)

PHARMACOLOGY Summary of Medications to Treat High Blood Pressure—*Continued*

Medication Category	Action	Application/Indication	Nursing Responsibility
Angiotensin-converting enzyme (ACE) inhibitors • Captopril • Enalapril • Lisinopril	Action blocks the conversion of angiotensin I to vasoconstrictor angiotensin II. Because angiotensin II is a potent vasoconstrictor, the primary vasoactive hormone of the renin-angiotensin-aldosterone system, when it is blocked vasodilation occurs, resulting in a decrease in blood pressure. It also inactivates the vasodilator bradykinin and other vasodilator prostaglandins. ACE inhibitors increase the plasma renin levels and reduce aldosterone levels, causing systemic vasodilation.	Used in the management of hypertension as a single medication or in combination with other agents. It reduces the risk of heart failure following a myocardial infarction.	Encourage the patient to practice good dental hygiene. Instruct patient to contact the health care professional if any of the following occur: irregular heartbeat, chest pain, difficulty breathing, dry cough, sore throat, mouth sores, rash, fever, swelling of the hands and feet and/or face. Teach monitoring of blood pressure daily. Monitoring of renal function tests should be done regularly. Instruct about danger of double medication dosing.
Central alpha agonists • Clonidine	Stimulates the alpha-adrenergic receptors in the CNS, resulting in decreased sympathetic outflow and, hence, inhibition of cardioacceleration and vasoconstriction centers, and also prevents the reuptake of norepinephrine. This results in a drop in blood pressure.	Used in the management of hypertension.	Instruct patient to monitor blood pressure and pulse. Instruct that sudden changes in position may produce dizziness. Instruct that medication is administered at bedtime because of the sedative effect at the beginning of therapy and/or when the dosage is changed. Assess for skin rash when using the transdermal route. Men may have sexual difficulty, which should be reported to the health care professional.
Vasodilators • Hydralazine • Fenoldopam • Nitroprusside	The vasodilator lowers the blood pressure by relaxing the smooth muscle tone of the blood vessel, thus reducing the peripheral resistance.	Short-term hospital management in hypertensive emergencies includes malignant hypertension and end-organ deterioration.	Monitor the blood pressure 2–6 hour after initiating therapy or dosage adjustment. Assess patient for reports of dizziness. Teach that medication should be taken at bedtime to reduce effect of hypotension. If the patient experiences tinnitus, dyspnea, dizziness, headache, and/or blurred vision, these conditions need to be reported to the health care provider.
Angiotensin II receptor blockers • Candesartan • Valsartan	Blocks vasoconstriction and aldosterone-producing effects of angiotensin II at receptor sites, vascular and smooth muscle, and adrenal glands.	Lowers blood pressure and risk of stroke. Decreases hospitalization in patients with heart failure. Used in the management of hypertension.	Teach patient to take medication as directed, not to double dose. Instruct patient to take blood pressure weekly and report any significant changes to the health care provider. Instruct that medication may cause dizziness. Instruct to check with health care provider prior to taking any OTC medications, herbals, cough, cold, or allergy medications. Instruct on the need for follow-up with health care provider. Check for compliance via frequency of refills.

Sources: Deglin, J. H., & Vallerand, A. H. (2007). *Davis's drug guide for nurses* (10th ed.). Philadelphia: F. A. Davis; Rankin-Box, D. (2001). *The nurse's handbook of complementary therapies* (2nd ed.) London: Bailliere Tindall.

COMPLEMENTARY & ALTERNATIVE THERAPIES

Management of High Blood Pressure

Type of Therapy	Purpose	Comments
Healing "is the practice of conscious intentionality to improve health and well-being" (Rankin-Box, 2001, p. 171).	To instill a feeling of relaxation and calm to improve the patient's health and well-being.	*Contraindication:* May cause light-headedness or faintness in some patients. Patient must give informed consent prior to participating in this method of healing when it involves spiritual and/or cultural belief systems.
Relaxation and visualization are "techniques using the imagination to create any desired changes in the individual's life" (Rankin-Box, 2001, p. 276).	Relaxation helps patient feel peaceful and free from anxiety and fear. Visualization creates positive changes in the patient's life.	*Contraindication:* Patient may have difficulty learning the skill, or may be too weak to use the energy to concentrate to elicit a response. A patient with breathing difficulties or cardiac arrhythmias may have increased problems; use should be limited to two to three times per day for 20 minutes because some may experience withdrawal from life, experiencing insomnia or hallucinations. These techniques are to be taught by an individual experienced with these techniques.
Therapeutic touch "is the interaction between energy fields of two or more people with the focus of rebalancing the energy field to enable relaxation and self healing" (Rankin-Box, 2001, p. 276).	To promote relaxation, pain relief, and self-healing through the interaction of people's energy fields, which rebalances or repatterns the energy field.	*Contraindication:* Caution should be used when using the therapy with babies, frail elderly, pregnant women, people with head injuries, emaciated patients, people experiencing psychosis, and patients in shock. The practice of therapeutic touch is taught through course work or home study. Certification as a healing touch practitioner is available through the American Holistic Nurses Association.
Hypnosis is a deliberate use of a trance state to increase the feeling of health and well-being (Rankin-Box, 2001).	To use a trance state to foster a sense of well-being and health.	The therapist must be competent in the technique. Hypnosis gives the patient responsibility for his own healing.
Animal-assisted therapy is the use of selected animals as a treatment modality in health care settings.	To promote human–animal interactions such as bonding, attachment, and to provide cardiovascular and other benefits.	Research supports the value of human–animal interaction in the management of high blood pressure.
Qi gong T'ai chi is a series of postures and exercises developed by the Chinese characterized by relaxed, circular motions.	To foster the generation of energy and conserves their energy to maintain health or to treat illness. As a health discipline, t'ai chi combines physical fitness, meditation, and self-defense. Considered to be the "root of motion."	These are individual personal disciplines. It is best when learning these skills to have an instructor. The teacher is considered to be the only way to advanced skill. Honor and reverence of the teacher is part of the belief system that empowers the disciple.

Sources: Rankin-Box, D. (2001). *The nurse's handbook of complementary therapies* (2nd ed.). London: Bailliere Tindall; Fontaine, K. L. (2004). *Healing practices: Alternative therapies for nursing.* Upper Saddle River, NJ: Pearson Prentice Hall.

CULTURAL CONSIDERATIONS for Hypertension

African Americans have a three to four times higher risk than Caucasians of angioedema and cough attributed to ACE inhibitors. American Indian and Asian populations undergoing Westernization will have significant increases in high blood pressure. Individuals living in the southeastern region (sometimes called the Salt Belt) of the United States have a higher percentage of high blood pressure.

Discharge Priorities

The discharge priorities represent a cooperative effort among the patient, family, and nurse. The focus is to determine if the patient knows the rationale for the prescribed therapy. The pa-

tient should also know how to monitor his blood pressure to maintain it at <120/80 mmHg (or with diabetes mellitus, <130/80 mmHg). In addition, the patient should demonstrate no signs or symptoms of target organ damage. The Patient Teaching & Discharge Priorities box (p. 502) outlines the necessary teaching for discharging a patient with hypertension.

 Collaborative Management

The outcome goal of therapy for high blood pressure is to reduce the cardiovascular, cerebral vascular, and renal morbidity and mortality through achieving a systolic blood pressure of <120 mmHg and a diastolic blood pressure of <80 mmHg. However, if the patient has diabetes mellitus, the systolic blood

NURSING PROCESS: Patient Care Plan for Hypertension

Assessment of Knowledge Related to Hypertension
Subjective Data:
What did the health care provider tell you about the family member's prognosis?
Do you know the meaning of high blood pressure to the patient?

Do you know if family members understand the diagnosis of high blood pressure?

Nursing Assessment and Diagnoses	Outcomes and Evaluation Parameters	Planning and Interventions with *Rationales*
Nursing Diagnosis: *Deficient Knowledge* related to the relationship between lifestyle choices and the management of hypertension	**Outcome:** The patient/family has a clear understanding of the modification of lifestyle choices. **Outcome:** States understanding of the long-term nature of the partnership between the health care team and the patient. ***Evaluation Parameters:*** The patient/family states an understanding of: Disease process. Modifiable elements of lifestyle. Cultural influences. Blood pressure measurement. Monitoring of condition. Therapeutic plan with its rationale. Signs and symptoms of noncompliance and/or complications. Patient states an understanding of the partnership between the health care team and the patient over the long term. Patient states preferences in modifying lifestyle.	**Interventions and *Rationales:*** Teach patient that health beliefs and practices influence lifestyle choices. *Build a trusting and sharing relationship between the patient and health care team.* Monitor blood pressure in the health care office and home. Monitoring is done by the nurse, patient, and/or family member. *Blood pressure findings may vary dependent on the lifestyle choices, time of day, and degree of stress experienced by the patient.* Monitor exercise and weight patterns. *Weight may be in excess of the body's needs and can lead to potential complications of therapy.* Assess the degree of patient anger. *Self-concept changes when the individual is physiologically and psychologically threatened as reflected by ineffective coping and high blood pressure.* Teach the patient to report to the health care provider the use of herbal products and OTC medications prior to taking them because they frequently change the action of the hypertensive drugs. *Herbal substances are not regulated by the federal Food and Drug Administration and may vary in strength. OTC medicines may interact with prescription medications either by increasing or decreasing the therapeutic effect.* Teach the patient to monitor the amount of alcohol consumed per day/week because many hypertensive drugs labels warn about the consumption of alcohol. *Alcohol consumption elevates arterial blood pressure and adds "empty" calories to the patient's diet.* Teach that smoking cessation is important. *Cigarette, cigar, and pipe smoking affects the cardiovascular system through the action of inhaled nicotine.*

Assessment of Fatigue
Subjective Data:
What symptoms of fatigue do you have?
How many hours of sleep do you require?

Objective Data:
Family reports increasing fatigue.
Patient appears tired.

Nursing Assessment and Diagnoses	Outcomes and Evaluation Parameters	Planning and Interventions with *Rationales*
Nursing Diagnosis: *Fatigue* related to biochemical changes due to chronic disease	**Outcome:** Patient's fatigue level is manageable. ***Evaluation Parameters:*** Patient states an understanding of the use of prescribed therapeutic agents. Patient states the possible side effects of the therapeutic agents.	**Interventions and *Rationales:*** Instruct the patient/family about potential side effects of the prescribed therapeutic agents *to identify any areas of misunderstanding or misinformation concerning the therapeutic plan.* Instruct the patient to read medicine bottle labels and to follow the directions for pulse and blood pressure assessment prior to taking the dose of medication *to promote the therapeutic medication dose levels and the safe physiological levels when administering the pharmaceutical treatment.* Instruct the patient to report and have approved by the health care professional prior to taking any OTC medications, herbal substances, alcohol, diet supplements, or stimulants *to identify any untoward reactions like fatigue between the therapeutic regime and other substances.* Plan rest periods to decrease fatigue level.

Assessment of Nutrition

Subjective Data:
What diet are you currently following?
What is your weight pattern during the past 6 months?

Objective Data:
What are the following measurements: weight, height, and abdominal girth?

Nursing Assessment and Diagnoses	Outcomes and Evaluation Parameters	Planning and Interventions with *Rationales*
Nursing Diagnosis: *Imbalanced Nutrition: More than Body Requirements* related to excessive caloric intake	**Outcome:** Demonstrates the ability to select a diet to meet nutritional requirements. **Evaluation Parameters:** The patient states an understanding of modifications needed in lifestyle. The health care team verbalizes the importance of cultural influences, the meaning of food, financial concerns, and the patient's choices.	**Interventions and *Rationales:*** Discuss with the patient realistic goals for weight reduction and an exercise program. This plan is age dependent. *Weight is a modifiable cause of high blood pressure. A relationship between saturated fat and cholesterol to weight is well established.*

Assessment of Perfusion

Subjective Data:
Do you have difficulty walking around home, a grocery store, or a shopping mall/center?
Do you have difficulty breathing after exercising?

Objective Data:
Does the patient cough after exercising? Have a flushed face?
Does the patient have edema of the extremities?

Nursing Assessment and Diagnoses	Outcomes and Evaluation Parameters	Planning and Interventions with *Rationales*
Nursing Diagnosis: *Impaired Tissue Perfusion* related to resistance to blood flow	**Outcome:** The patient has a clear understanding of the adequacy of perfusion and pulmonary gas exchange. **Evaluation Parameters:** Patient verbalizes an understanding of the seriousness of adequate systemic perfusion.	**Interventions and *Rationales:*** Teach combination of medications, diet, and exercise for the protection of the target organs. *Knowledge and ownership of the treatment plan by the patient will increase the patient's motivation to modify lifestyle.*

Assessment of Noncompliance

Subjective Data:
Do you have a support system?
Do you consider the treatment plan to be requiring too many lifestyle changes?

Objective Data:
How many missed appointments have been recorded?
Does the patient refill prescriptions promptly?
Does the patient have transportation to the medical office?
Does the patient have financial problems?

Nursing Assessment and Diagnoses	Outcomes and Evaluation Parameters	Planning and Interventions with *Rationales*
Nursing Diagnosis: *Risk of Noncompliance* related to the medical treatment plan	**Outcome:** Demonstrates the ability to make decisions regarding compliance with the therapeutic plan. **Evaluation Parameters:** Partnership between patient and health care team evolves with the patient verbalizing the meaning of the therapeutic plan.	**Interventions and *Rationales:*** Teaches and demonstrates a partnership with the patient/family so that the treatment regimen is understood. Teaches the goals of therapy and the dangerousness of a relapse in the treatment plan. *Compliance is a positive behavior that patients demonstrate when therapeutic goals are mutually agreed on. Compliance is a continuum of coordinated action.*

Assessment of Ineffective Sexual Patterns

Subjective Data:
Have you experienced any changes in sexual performance?
When did these sexual patterns change?

Objective Data:
Observe interactions between family and/or significant other.

Nursing Assessment and Diagnoses	Outcomes and Evaluation Parameters	Planning and Interventions with *Rationales*
Nursing Diagnosis: *Sexual Dysfunction* related to disease and/or therapy	**Outcome:** Verbalizes effective patterns of sexual relationship. **Evaluation Parameters:** Patient verbalizes satisfaction with the quality of life.	**Interventions and *Rationales:*** When assisting with patient discussion of sexuality, teach that it is part of the plan of care and may be discussed at any health care visit. The patient needs reassurance that the information is confidential. *It is important that the health care provider be educated concerning sexual health and sexuality throughout the life span. The health care provider needs to know his or her feelings and beliefs concerning sexuality within the culture. Patients want to know if their feelings are normal versus abnormal concerning this important information.*

PATIENT TEACHING & DISCHARGE PRIORITIES for Hypertension

Need	Teaching
Prior to discharge the nurse instructs the patient and family on how to measure the blood pressure.	The patient and family will demonstrate to the nurse how to take the blood pressure. The interaction may be in a clinic, health provider's office, patient's home, or hospital.
The nurse teaches the patient and family about the medications prescribed. The patient and family know the name of each medication and: 1. Dosage for each medication 2. Time of medication administration 3. Precautions, such as foods to avoid, medication interactions, and the need to take blood pressure and pulse prior to taking the medication 4. Possible side effects 5. What to do if side effects do occur 6. Cautions about using OTC medications, herbals, stimulants, diet supplements, alcohol, and tobacco.	Patient and family need to be knowledgeable about the medications prescribed. Frequently, the nurse may supplement the teaching plan by giving the patient a written guide outlining the medications with a list of do's and don'ts. If the patient has difficulty reading the information, pictures may be used. In addition, tape recording or video recording the teaching session for the patient and family may be very helpful.
The nurse needs to review all of the medications the patient is taking such as vitamins, herbal products, prescribed medications, "cold medicines," stimulants, and diet supplements because these products may cause elevation in the systemic blood pressure. In addition, herbal substances such as black cohosh and hawthorne may lower blood pressure. The patient and family will demonstrate to the nurse how to take the blood pressure.	The nurse has a responsibility to teach the patient and family about the hazards of mixing OTC products, herbal substances, diet substances, stimulants, alcohol, and tobacco with prescription medications.
The nurse demonstrates how menu planning is carried out using a prescribed diet plan such as the DASH diet. Frequently, a referral needs to be made to a therapeutic dietitian for assistance in initiating and maintaining these lifestyle changes. Suggestions for lifestyle changes include: 1. Weight reduction 2. Exercising 3. Stopping smoking 4. Reducing alcohol consumption 5. Reducing stress. The patient may need referrals to support groups for making these lifestyle changes.	Family and patient meet with the nurse and/or the therapeutic dietitian for instruction in how to structure the diet plan. Personal preferences and cultural sensitivity are important because food is an essential part of lifestyle. Family and patient are given the necessary referrals to approved organized groups within their community. With full permission of the patient, involve caring family members or social support (e.g., faith based or community organizations) in the treatment process. Suggest common interest group activities (e.g., walking group) to enhance natural support and motivation.
Reasons for the patient/family to call the health care provider include: 1. Experiencing a headache 2. Fainting 3. Dizziness 4. Need for a follow-up appointment 5. Medication renewal of prescription.	Family and patient need to be aware that there are specific reasons to call the health care provider. These symptoms are potential signs of an elevated blood pressure.
The patient needs to join a community support group.	Family and patient visit and join support group(s) for continuing encouragement and community.

pressure should not be greater than 130 mmHg and the diastolic blood pressure less than 80 mmHg.

The objective of care for the patient with high blood pressure requires a multidisciplinary approach to begin to facilitate the patient and family in making lifestyle changes. The nurse is the coordinator of care, accessing the health team members to facilitate the ongoing care of the patient and family. Ingle (2001) reported from *Factors Assisting with Management of Hypertension* that male subjects stated they cannot trust their body anymore, living with hypertension is dangerous, and it requires learning to live with hypertension on a daily basis. Multiple resources may be needed to support the patient and family during the

management of this chronic illness. The roles of resource individuals for the patient are as follows:

- **Clinical dietitians**—The patient/family will be making a number of lifestyle changes including the selection of food and the amount to be eaten. The patient needs the clinical expertise of a therapeutic dietitian to assist in the modification of diet, menu planning, and modification of recipes. This is viewed as a major lifestyle change with many cultural consequences.

- **Fitness/exercise leader**—The fitness/exercise leader is one employed by a recognized, organized health care system. The leader is able to assess, follow a physician's prescription, and modify the types and kind of activities for the individual with hypertension.

- The pharmacist provides information about the action of the antihypertensive medications as well as precautions and side effects.

Throughout this process, the patient must take ownership and responsibility for maintaining the regimen over the long term.

Complications of High Blood Pressure

The impact of uncontrolled high blood pressure on organs occurs insidiously over an extended period of time throughout the body. The JNC 7 report (NHLBI, 2003b) referred to certain complications of hypertension as target organ damage, with the heart, kidney, brain, peripheral vasculature, and retina considered to be target organs. Prolonged untreated hypertension causes both large and small blood vessels to become sclerotic, tortuous, and weak. These changes cause narrowing of the artery lumen, decreased blood flow to organs, and increased blood pressure. Additionally, the weakened arteries are more prone to rupture. Large arteries tend to occlude or rupture, causing a loss of the blood supply to organs and tissues. Small arteries that are damaged decrease the blood supply to organs, resulting in structural changes. An increased diastolic blood pressure causes injury to the intimal wall of the arteries, resulting in plaque buildup and local inflammation, which in turn results in plaque rupture, platelet aggregation, and subsequent vessel occlusion. The result is a decreased blood supply to organs, leading to progressive loss of function. The organs that are the most affected by these changes are the heart, brain, kidney, and retina. Chart 21–6 outlines the target organs that are most prone to damage.

CHART 21–6	**Target Organ Damage**

Heart

Left ventricular hypertrophy

Angina or prior myocardial infarction

Prior coronary revascularization

Heart failure

Brain

Stroke or transient ischemic attack

Chronic kidney disease

Renal failure

Peripheral arterial disease

Peripheral ischemia

Retinopathy

Vision changes leading to blindness

Source: Adapted from National Heart, Lung, and Blood Institute. (2003, May). *Seventh report of the Joint National Committee on Prevention, Detection, Evaluation, and Treatment of High Blood Pressure (JNC7)*. Retrieved June 9, 2008, from http://www.nhlbi.nih.gov/guidelines/hypertension/jnc7full.pdf.

Ischemic heart disease is the most common site of target organ damage associated with high blood pressure (NHLBI, 2003b). As a result of prolonged hypertension, the coronary arteries are unable to deliver an adequate blood supply to the myocardium. This loss causes the heart muscle to lose its ability to contract sufficiently, resulting in decreased cardiac output. The shearing force of blood flowing with increased pressure over time causes irregularities in the intima of the lumen of the arteries. This causes an increased buildup of plaque, ultimately narrowing the lumen of the artery and decreasing blood flow to the myocardium, resulting in ischemic heart disease.

Heart failure occurs because of the increased cardiac workload due to pumping against an increased afterload, which is the increased pressure created by the narrowed lumen of diseased blood vessels, as the heart attempts to eject its blood supply. Eventually the left ventricle hypertrophies to compensate for increased pressure. Left ventricular hypertrophy increases with age and is most prevalent in persons with blood pressure of 160/95 mmHg (Porth, 2005). Heart failure is a systolic or diastolic ventricular impairment, which can be caused by both ischemic heart disease and long-standing uncontrolled high blood pressure. Heart failure leads to a backup of blood into the pulmonary circulation, causing pulmonary edema and left-sided heart failure. Serous fluid is forced back through the pulmonary capillaries into the alveoli and quickly enters the bronchioles and bronchi. The patient will experience tachypnea, restlessness, apprehensiveness, air hunger or cyanosis, and frothy, blood-tinged sputum. The peripheral and neck veins are engorged and the blood pressure and heart rate are increased. Edema may be present in the extremities and crackles in the lung; respiratory acidosis and profuse diaphoresis may also be present (Andreoli et al., 2004). Ventricular hypertrophy and an increased workload of the heart contribute to approximately 50% of high blood pressure deaths due to myocardial infarction or myocardial failure.

Hypertension leads to nephrosclerosis, which is a common cause of renal insufficiency. This condition is caused by diseased blood vessels that are no longer able to deliver adequate blood supply to the kidneys, resulting in decreased renal function. Additionally, high blood pressure accelerates other types of kidney diseases, particularly in diabetes. The American Diabetic Association recommends that diabetic's maintain a blood pressure of less than 130/80 mmHg (Porth, 2005).

The patient with diabetes may have high levels of circulating cholesterol and other lipids, which impacts the development of atherosclerosis, arteriosclerosis, and severe coronary heart disease, as well as multiple microcirculatory lesions. Due to the complications of diabetes, atherosclerosis increases the probability of developing hypertension, diabetic retinopathy, cataracts, and chronic renal disease (Guyton & Hall, 2005).

Metabolic syndrome is being diagnosed more frequently within the adult obese population. It is estimated that one-fourth of the U.S. population has this syndrome. The characteristics are insulin resistance, hypertension, dyslipidemia, high triglyceride levels, diabetes mellitus, low HDL cholesterol level, and a tendency for the patient to form blood clots (NHLBI, 2003b). Metabolic syndrome is discussed in detail in Chapter 40 ☞.

Cerebral vascular disease is caused by arteriosclerotic plaques that occur in the feeder arteries to the brain. When these arteries are damaged by prolonged hypertension, plaque forms and it becomes vulnerable to rupture away from the wall of the artery. Ruptured plaque activates the clotting mechanism and platelets aggregate, causing a clot to form and block the artery, thus leading to an acute loss of brain function in the local area (Guyton & Hall, 2005). High blood pressure may cause the vessel to rupture. Hemorrhage follows, compressing the local brain tissue. Subsequent clotting of the blood vessel leads to blood vessel blockage (Guyton & Hall, 2005).

Hypertensive eye disease includes the retinal arterioles, retinal parenchyma, choroids, and optic nerve. High blood pressure can be detected in the eye by the presence of diffuse arteriolar narrowing, bleeding, cotton wool patches, hard exudates, microaneurysms, zones of nonperfusion, and flame-shaped bleeding at or near the retina (NHLBI, 2003b). All of these conditions are visible through an ophthalmoscope. The ability of the patient to have visual acuity is dependent on the degree of pathology.

Aortic artery disorders are commonly associated with hypertension. An aortic aneurysm is a weakened area in the wall of an artery that bulges out over time. This disorder is associated with vessel wall degeneration and high blood pressure. It is estimated that approximately 50% of the population with aortic aneurysms have high blood pressure (Porth, 2005). Controlling blood pressure will help diminish vessel degeneration.

Hypertensive Emergencies

If left untreated on rare occasions high blood pressure can become a life-threatening emergency. Approximately 90% of the cases of untreated hypertension will lead to death from myocardial infarction, stroke, renal failure, or aortic dissection. The most common emergencies are discussed next.

Hypertensive Crisis

Hypertensive crisis is rare and sometimes has a fatal occurrence characterized by the sudden onset of a diastolic blood pressure of between 120 and 130 mmHg, the clinical manifestation of target organ vascular damage, and the presence of retinal exudates and hemorrhage. A diastolic blood pressure of greater than 120 mmHg causes acute vascular damage, and structural organ changes begin to occur. The release of catecholamines and the activation of the renin-angiotensin mechanism occur, raising the blood pressure even further. The symptoms may include unstable angina, pulmonary edema, myocardial infarction, eclampsia, stroke, life-threatening arterial bleeding, aortic dissection, morning headache, blurred vision and dyspnea, and potential signs of uremia.

The causes of a hypertensive crisis include acute and chronic renal failure, exacerbation of chronic hypertension, sudden withdrawal of antihypertensive medications, and vasculitis. The management of a hypertensive crisis includes immediate hospitalization in a special care area such as a coronary care unit. The goal of management is to bring the blood pressure down within 1 hour of the crisis, without sending the blood pressure too low. Decreasing the blood pressure too severely can cause cerebral and/or myocardial infarcts and renal failure. Intravenous **vasodilator** medications and adrenergic inhibitors are used to treat the hypertension (Yuan, 2004). Sodium nitroprusside has

been the drug of choice in these situations because it has an instantaneous onset and a short half-life. If the blood pressure begins to drop too severely, its effect is short acting.

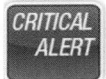 *Hypertensive crisis is a medical emergency. Rapid onset: a systolic blood pressure of greater than 240 mmHg and/or a diastolic blood pressure of greater than 130 mmHg.*

Hypertensive Encephalopathy

Hypertensive encephalopathy is a very dangerous state of multifocal cerebral ischemia due to a severely acute or subacute elevated blood pressure. The pathogenesis of hypertensive encephalopathy is the effect of high blood pressure on the brain's arterioles. "If [the] elevated pressure exceeds the upper limits of normal cerebral autoregulation, a combination of multifocal arteriolar vasodilatation and vasoconstriction occurs, producing diffusely distributed small zones of microhemorrhages and ischemia" (Andreoli et al., 2004). The patient with this diagnosis needs urgent and immediate treatment. The decreasing incidence of this emergency is due in part to the use of effective antihypertensive drugs.

Dissecting Aortic Aneurysm

Dissecting aortic aneurysm is a localized dilation of the aorta that has a longitudinal dissection between the outer and middle layers of the vascular wall. A patient demonstrating signs and symptoms of a dissecting aortic aneurysm needs to be admitted to an intensive care unit for hemodynamic monitoring and the monitoring of urinary output.

High blood pressure generally precedes the dissecting aortic aneurysm. Blood penetrates the tear in the aortic intimal lining, forming a false channel with the aortic media. Blood in this false channel may reenter the true aortic channel via a second intimal tear or rupture through the adventitia into the periaortic tissues. Aortic dissection occurs suddenly with severe chest pain, which radiates to the back. The symptoms will vary depending on the location of the dissection (Andreoli et al., 2004). Kasper and colleagues (2005) stated that a type A aneurysm is an ascending aortic dissection that requires emergency surgical repair with a composition graft. A type B aneurysm is described as the compromising of the aortic branches, leading to impending rupture and pain. Transcatheter techniques may be used with stenting of narrow vessels to preserve blood flow to compromised organs. In both cases, long-term therapy includes careful control of hypertension and decrease of cardiac contractility.

Research

Research into the diagnosis, treatment, and prevention of high blood pressure is a universal high priority. The topic is being approached using a variety of methods and by multiple disciplines (see the Evidence-Based Practice feature). Much information is being revised to reflect the need for prevention of high blood pressure by living a healthy lifestyle from birth to old age. Studies about care models to assist patients and families to maintain motivation for a lifetime of health are beginning to be reported in the literature. The reported research indicates that meaningful and positive relationships assist in gaining and nurturing trust between patient and health care provider. There is recognition that diversity of beliefs, culture, and previous experiences within the environment will influence the meaning the patient attributes to the experience with high blood pressure. The patient's ownership of the treatment plan and lifestyle changes is essential. There is gathering evidence that when patient and health care professionals work collaboratively in communicating, exploring, setting goals, and reinforcing them, the patient's management is more successful.

The numbers of therapeutics available to provide protection of the target organs against vascular damage due to high blood pressure are increasing. Teaching aids that use multimedia techniques and information sources need to be devised and made available to the patient and family in their native languages. The Research Opportunities and Clinical Impact box (p. 506) outlines various topics on hypertension that are either under current investigation or in need of investigation.

Impact of Hypertension

Clinical Problem

In the adult practice setting, patients learning to live with hypertension were asked to tell their story concerning what factors have assisted them in managing their hypertension on a daily basis. What do hypertensive adults describe as useful to them in managing their high blood pressure and finding the meaning in their everyday life? Measurement techniques used in a quantitative approach do not reveal a meaningful whole for understanding the hypertensive patient's lived experience. The essence of the hypertensive patient's experience was unveiled through the description of the experiences by the participant using qualitative techniques.

Research Findings

DeWitt and Ploeg (2006) reported that the interpretative phenomenology method should be used to assist in the expression of rigor in the preservation of integrity and legitimacy of nursing research. In a study by Ingle (2001) participants described the everydayness of hypertension, their realization that they were no longer in control of their life, and their learning that life was dangerous. Participants said that individuals with hypertension can no longer take their health for granted. Health becomes a choice made each day by the patient. The therapeutic plan of medication management and care was not part of the patient's narrative. Each patient was describing how they wanted to live in this world.

In a study reported by Peters (2006), the relationship between the factors of perceived racism, emotion-focused stress, and blood pressure were examined within the African American community. This descriptive-correlational, causal modeling study with a convenience sample of 162 community-dwelling adults reported bias, prejudice, and stereotyping by health care providers in conjunction with other racially discriminatory experiences that lead to health care disparities among minorities. Further study is needed to determine the relationship between racism, emotions, psychological factors, and hypertension.

Implications for Nursing Practice

Findings from qualitative and quantitative research studies reveal the need for an increased awareness of the multiple factors that influence the care of patients with hypertension. Assessing the hypertensive patient using narrative interviewing techniques can provide an understanding of the situation. Patients and family were experiencing anger and denial that a problem exists, and that hypertension is perceived as "no big deal." Physical factors were reported to be less significant and did not emerge as a theme (Ingle, 2001). The acronym NURSE is a useful assessment tool.

Acronym	Request	Example
N	Narrative *Assist the patient to understand and state her feelings about hypertension.*	Tell me your story about having high blood pressure.
U	Understanding *Listen with empathy to the situation.*	It is important for me to know what this diagnosis means to you.
R	Reflect *When a patient tells his story, it is difficult to acknowledge it.*	It is difficult to acknowledge and support the various emotions of the story.
S	Silence *During the conversation, pauses will occur.*	Take your time and process both your and the patient's thoughts.
E	Explain *Take time to clarify any misconceptions or to answer any questions.*	I am here to answer any questions.

Critical Thinking Questions

1. After the narrative interview, the patient asks if you would listen to some insights that have become apparent through the process. How would you answer this individual?

2. How will you use silence with the patient?

Answers to Critical Thinking Questions appear in Appendix D.

References

De Witt, L., & Ploeg, J. (2006). Critical appraisal of rigor in interpretive phenomenological nursing research. *Journal of Advanced Nursing, 55*(2), 215–229.

Ingle, E. A. (2001). *Factors assisting with client management of hypertension.* Unpublished master's thesis, Carson-Newman College, Jefferson City, TN.

Peters, R. M. (2006). The relationship of racism, chronic stress emotions, and blood pressure. *Journal of Nursing Scholarship, 38,* 234–240.

EVIDENCE-BASED PRACTICE

RESEARCH OPPORTUNITIES AND CLINICAL IMPACT RELATED TO HYPERTENSION

Research Area	Clinical Impact
How do hypertensive drug actions vary between men versus women?	Selection of gender-specific pharmaceutical packages may decrease target organ injury.
What is the difference between men and women in the description of their symptoms of high blood pressure?	Men and women describe their symptoms differently.
How do childhood obesity and hypertension affect the rate of development of end-organ damage?	Children's physiological response to obesity and hypertension is different than that of adults and the elderly.
What are the roles of heredity and environment in the prevention of hypertension?	Determine the role of genetics and the environment in prevention and treatment of hypertension.
Describe the relationship between aging and hypertension.	Determine the relationship between the aging process and the progression of hypertension.
How does the meaning of living with a diagnosis of hypertension influence the patient's prognosis?	Knowing the meaning and significance of the diagnosis of hypertension to the patient will enhance teaching and learning opportunities.
How does the family cope with the long-term burden of the chronic illness of hypertension?	Knowing the meaning of a chronic illness to a patient will facilitate the partnership care of this individual and the family.
How do the ethics of hypertension, a long-term illness, determine care?	Potential justification of care for patients with chronic long-term illnesses.
How can assessment tools for the measurement of anger be incorporated into adult health assessments?	Such tools could help determine the effect of anger on the blood pressure.
Do hypertensive patients beginning pharmaceutical interventions make self-modifications to maintain sexual performance?	Impact on lifestyle and potential need for intervention.
How does the community function as a long-term support group?	Long-term impact on target organs, body image, and compliance with the therapeutic plan.
How can cultural sensitivity in the care of the patient with hypertension be improved?	Such knowledge would help promote cultural insight surrounding chronic hypertensive care.

Clinical Preparation

 Read

- History of Current Illness
- Past Medical History
- Physical Exam
- Admitting Medical Orders
- Laboratory Study Results

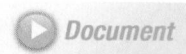 **Document**

- Summary of Hospitalization
- Pathophysiology Form
- Laboratory Values
- Laboratory Results Explanation

 Apply

- List of Potential Nursing Diagnoses
- Concept Map
- Critical Thinking Questions

Log on to MyNursingKit.com to download forms you will need and to complete further steps in the Clinical Preparation assignment.

HISTORY OF PRESENT ILLNESS

Ms. Grace Bell is a 65-year-old Caucasian female with hypertension. She is of German-American heritage. For the past year and a half, she has been experiencing headaches, irritability, anger, and fatigue. She arrived at the nurse practitioner office for an appointment 1 month ago to discuss the recent death of her husband. She also stated "I'm not feeling too great." Her sitting blood pressure in the left arm was 190/92, her height was 5'2" and she weighed 150 pounds. Ms. Bell was asked if she was taking any over-the-counter medications or any alternative or complementary medications. Her response was "No. I'm allergic to everything." At the first appointment she was advised to reduce her intake of cholesterol-rich foods and to reduce her intake of salt by not adding it to food during preparation or at the table. She indicated she had become a "couch potato" and did little exercising. She was given a return appointment for the following week. Ms. Bell's admitting diagnosis to the nurse practitioner's practice was "rule out stage 2 hypertension and white coat hypertension."

Ms. George, FNP, notes that Ms. Bell's voice is loud and her speech fast, she is apparently angry with the office wait, and she reports she has a bad headache. She also wants to know why everyone is so interested in her blood pressure. Ms. Bell states, "It will come down, if you could just let me rest a minute."

Medical–Surgical History

Ms. Bell's medical history includes one vaginal birth of a live female. There is no history of hypertension in the family.

Social History

Ms. Bell reports she has just lost her husband. Her daughter lives nearby and very helpful.

Physical Exam

Weight: 150 lb; height: 5 ft 2 in.
T 98.0; P 120; R 22
Blood pressure: left arm and right arm have a 5-point discrepancy: lying 200/100; sitting 190/95; standing 184/90
Capillary refilling times: 3 seconds in both hands

Laboratory Studies

Total cholesterol
HDL
LDL
Glucose
Creatinine
Urinalysis

Scheduled Medications

Atenolol 50 mg once per day
Quinapril 40 mg once per day

PRN Medications

Tylenol 500mg for headache

LABORATORY STUDY RESULTS

Test	Week 1	Week 2	Week 3
Total cholesterol	300 mg/dL	310 mg/dL	295 mg/dL
HDL	50 mg/dL	45 mg/dL	49 mg/dL
LDL	250 mg/dL	275 mg/dL	255 mg/dL
Glucose (fasting)	175 mg/dL	182 mg/dL	170 mg/dL
BUN	25 mg/dL	25 mg/dL	23 mg/dL
Creatinine	2.0 mg/dL	2.0 mg/dL	1.9 mg/dL
Urinalysis	Protein 2+ Glucose 2+	Protein 2+ Glucose 2+	Protein 2+ Glucose 2+

CRITICAL THINKING QUESTIONS

1. Ms. Bell just entered the office for her third appointment and states "I've just become unemployed, I have no health insurance and no income. What shall I do?" What essential recommendations does Ms. Bell need to maintain control of her hypertension? What would you do if Ms. Bell relapses into noncompliant behavior?

2. What process would you use to help Ms. Bell accept responsibility for her own health care?

3. How are you as Ms. Bell's nurse going to listen to her therapeutically?

4. Using the nursing process, develop a plan of care for Ms. Bell related to the impact of chronic illness and ineffective coping with changes in lifestyle.

Answers to Critical Thinking Questions appear in Appendix D.

NCLEX® REVIEW

1. The nurse recognizes that a patient with two consecutive blood pressure readings, a month apart, of 132/80 and 130/88 is considered to have:
1. Normal blood pressure.
2. Prehypertension.
3. Stage 1 hypertension.
4. Stage 2 hypertension

2. From the list provided, choose the factors having a direct influence on regulation of blood pressure. (Select all that apply.)
1. Cardiac output
2. Peripheral vascular resistance
3. Production of adrenocorticotropic hormone
4. Baroreceptors
5. Chemoreceptors
6. Body fluid volume

3. Which of the following patients represents the highest risk for development of hypertension?
1. 46-year-old female, African American, recently fired from her job
2. 46-year-old female, Caucasian, 50 pounds over ideal body weight
3. 56-year-old male, African American, insulin dependent diabetic
4. 56-year-old male, Caucasian, excessive alcohol consumption

4. The nurse would teach a patient prescribed nifedipine (procardia XL) to:
1. Add foods high in potassium such as bananas and orange juice to the diet.
2. Report the common adverse effect of dry cough to the health care provider.
3. Not crush, break in half, or chew the extended release form of the drug.
4. Assess the pulse prior to taking the medication with each dose.

5. The nurse is aware which of the following cultural components play a role with hypertension? Select all that apply.
1. Asian populations undergoing Westernization will have significant increases in high blood pressure.
2. Individuals living in southeastern region of the United States have a higher percentage of high blood pressure.
3. Caucasians adapt more readily to following the DASH diet and starting a routine exercise program.
4. African Americans tolerate using the ACE inhibitor drug group better than any other ethnicity.

6. A nurse developing a plan of care for an individual with prehypertension would emphasize the need for which of the following? Select all that apply.
1. A sedentary lifestyle will lower the body's oxygen needs and manage hypertension.
2. Set a goal to reduce cigarette smoking from two packs, to a half pack a day.
3. Developing a diet plan that is low in saturated fats and sodium.
4. Avoid any activities or relationships which are stress-producing.
5. Target weight loss at five pounds per week until ideal body mass index is obtained.
6. Eliminating or reducing alcohol consumption to one ounce a day.

7. A priority patient outcome for an individual with long-term Stage 2 hypertension would include:
1. Avoiding use of generic brands of anti-hypertensive medications.
2. Verbalizing the warning signs and symptoms of cerebral vascular accident.
3. Maintaining healthy, supportive relationships among friends and family.
4. Recording blood pressure measurements once a month with home monitoring.

Answers for review questions appear in Appendix D

KEY TERMS

blood pressure *p.487*
DASH diet *p.493*
diastolic *p.487*
dissecting aortic aneurysm *p.504*
hypertensive crisis *p.504*

hypertensive encephalopathy *p.504*
peripheral vascular resistance *p.488*
prehypertension *p.489*
pulse pressure *p.488*
stage 1 hypertension *p.490*

stage 2 hypertension *p.490*
systolic *p.487*
vasodilator *p.504*
white coat phenomenon *p.490*

EXPLORE   **mynursingkit**   PEARSON

MyNursingKit is your one stop for online chapter review materials and resources. Prepare for success with additional NCLEX®-style practice questions, interactive assignments and activities, web links, animations and videos, and more!

Register your access code from the front of your book at
www.mynursingkit.com

REFERENCES

Andreoli, T. E., Carpenter, C. C. J., Griggs, R. C., & Loscalzo, J. (2004). *Cecil essentials of medicine* (6th ed.). Philadelphia: W. B. Saunders.

Centers for Disease Control and Prevention. (2008). *Overweight and Obesity Trends Among Adults.* Retrieved June 13, 2008 from http://www.cdc.gov/nccdphp/dnpa/obesity/trend/

Donnelly, P. (2000). Ethics and cross-cultural nursing. *Journal of Transcultural Nursing, 11,* 119–125.

Eisenhower, J. S. (2002). *Descriptive study of client use of herbal substances and over-the-counter medications.* Unpublished master's thesis, Carson-Newman College, Jefferson City, TN.

Fields, L. E., Burt, V. L., Cutler, J. A., Hughes, J., Roccella, E. J., & Sorlie, P. (2004). The burden of adult hypertension in the United States 1999 to 2000: A rising tide. *Hypertension, 44,* 1–7.

Guyton, A., & Hall, J. E. (2005). *Textbook of medical physiology* (11th ed.). Philadelphia: W. B. Saunders.

Ingle, E. A. (2001). *Factors assisting with client management of hypertension.* Unpublished master's thesis, Carson-Newman College, Jefferson City, TN.

Jhala, S. (2001). *The healthcare needs of Asian Indian females.* Unpublished master's thesis, Carson-Newman College, Jefferson City, TN.

Kasper, D. L., Braunwald, E., Fauci, A. S., Hauser, S. L., Longo, D. L., & Jameson, J. L. (2005). *Harrison's principles of internal medicine* (16th ed.). New York: McGraw-Hill.

National Heart, Lung, and Blood Institute. (1998). *Clinical guidelines on the identification, evaluation, and treatment of overweight and obesity in adults.* Bethesda, MD: Author.

National Heart, Lung, and Blood Institute. (2003, May). *Seventh report of the Joint National Committee on Prevention, Detection, Evaluation, and Treatment of High Blood Pressure (JNC7).* Retrieved June 9,

2008, from http://www.nhlbi.nih.gov/guidelines/hypertension/jnc7full.pdf

Nicoll, D., McPhee, S. J., & Pignone, M. (2004). *Pocket guide to diagnostic tests* (4th ed.). New York: Lange Medical Books/McGraw-Hill.

Porth, C. M. (2005). *Pathophysiology: Concepts of altered health status* (7th ed.). Philadelphia: Lippincott Williams & Wilkins.

Rankin-Box, D. (2001). *The nurse's handbook of complementary therapies* (2nd ed.). Edinburgh: Bailliere Tindall.

Welton, P. K. (2003). Potassium and blood pressure. In J. E. Izzo & H. R. Black (Eds.), *Hypertension primer* (3rd ed., pp. 280–283). Dallas: American Heart Association.

Yuan, S. Y. (2004). *Handbook of diseases* (3rd ed.). Philadelphia: Lippincott Williams & Wilkins.

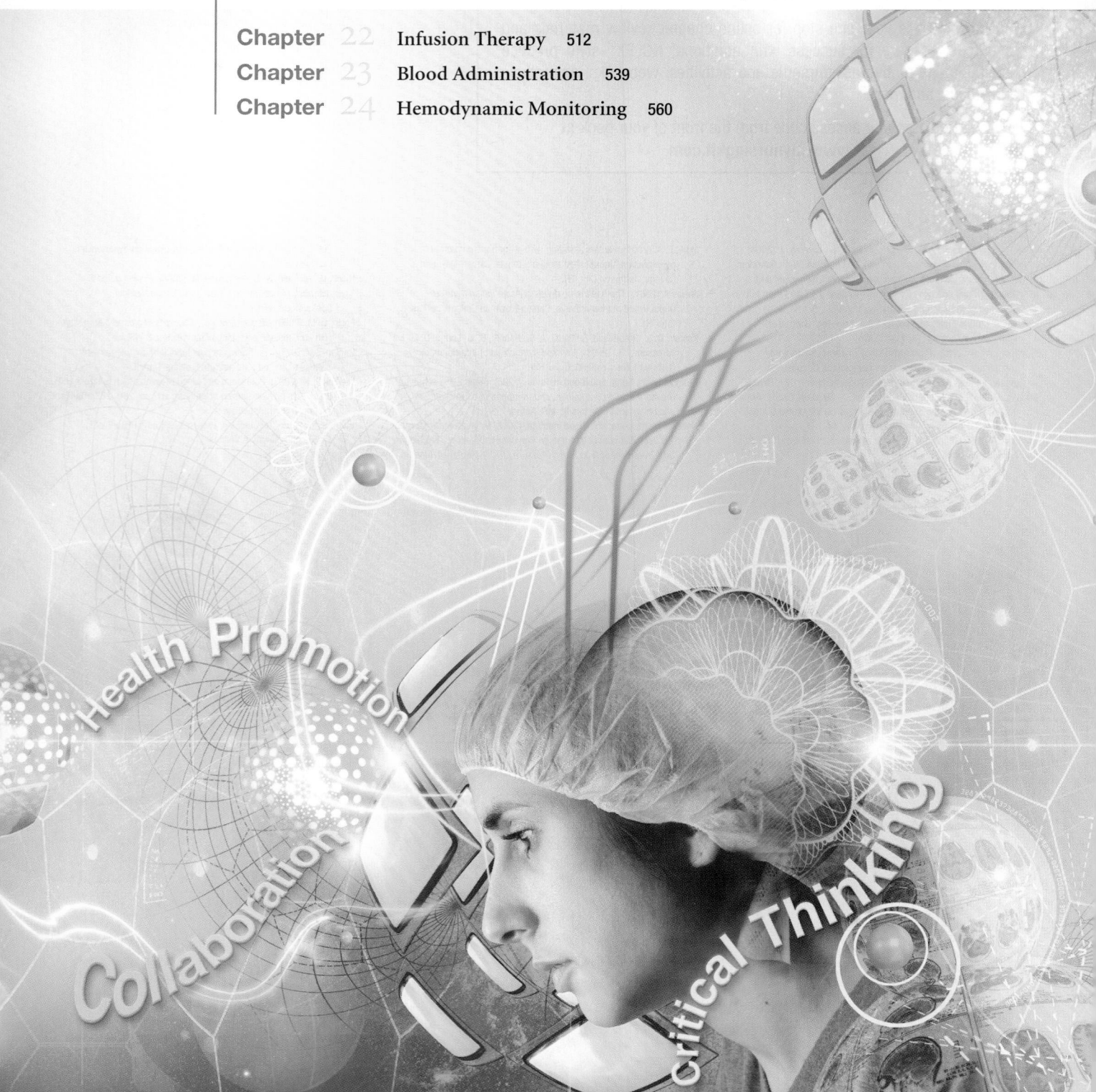

UNIT 4

Complex Skills Related to Nursing Practice

Health Promotion

Collaboration

Critical Thinking

Profiles in Nursing

CINDY My name is Cindy and I am the nurse manager of the Apheresis/Transfusion and Infusion Unit at the Albany Medical Center hospital in Albany, New York. I am also presently comanaging the Surgical Intensive Care Unit (ICU), while a new nurse manager is being recruited and trained. Albany Medical Center is a large 614-bed Level I trauma center with an extremely busy flight program, a medical college involved in educating physicians, and a nationally recognized research program.

I began work at this hospital approximately 28 years ago, in the Burn Unit. This experience provided me with the opportunity to embrace **compassion, commitment,** and **confidence** in my practice as a health care professional. This was when I first began to appreciate the importance of critical thinking skills and clinical reasoning; as a result, I looked for any and all opportunities to float to other critical care areas within the facility to enhance my clinical skills.

I now work full time in the Apheresis Unit as a hands-on manager. I have always lived by the notion that managers should never ask of staff what they themselves are not willing to do. Therefore, I am actively involved in the coordination of care for all of our patients, while ensuring a collaborative team-centered approach to the care. Quality is of the highest priority not only for our patients, but for the staff working in the unit as well. We collaborate on a daily basis with a variety of constituents in order to ensure positive patient outcomes and coordination of care.

Our patient population is as diverse as the age range of the patients that we serve. They have hematologic, immunologic, and oncologic challenges and are in various stages of their disease processes. The goal of the program is to foster an environment that allows patients to spend as much time at home with their families as possible, while addressing their emotional and physical health care needs.

I cherish the memory of a 5-year-old boy whom I had cared for during the last 3 years of his very short life. He had become so riddled with pain that during treatments his mother would lie next to him in bed and rub his tiny spine to make the pain tolerable. During his care one day, the doctors wanted to discuss with the family his next phase of treatment, which meant the parents would have to leave the unit. The child became very distraught at the idea that he would be left and not held. I remember climbing into bed next to him and rubbing his spine as I had watched his mother do. The child immediately calmed; he reached up and started twisting my hair, as he often did with his mother. When his parents arrived back to the unit, the child looked up at me and said "Cinny, I love you." A few days later Michael lost his battle with cancer and when I went to the wake, I was overwhelmed to see that laying there beside him was a picture that his parents had taken of the two of us, lying together in bed. This situation emulates our need to respond not just as health care providers in the clinical sense, but to be able to utilize our compassion in a way that provides for the emotional support that our patient's need.

Most recently we were caring for a patient who had been diagnosed with cancer and required a blood transfusion. To many this process appears quite benign on the surface; I even had an orientee tell me that this "wasn't rocket science." The patient had no indicators that would preclude us from going forward with the plan of care; therefore, the first unit of blood was hung. I remember being only about 10 paces outside of the room when I overheard the patient say "Gee, my lower back hurts." I called for help and immediately stopped the transfusion. Because of the team approach our unit has to nursing, everyone assumed a role: vital signs, oxygen applied, crash cart at bedside, physician called, epinephrine and steroids drawn and ready to administer. Because of their knowledge and expertise, everyone involved recognized that a transfusion reaction was taking place.

You see, what the orientee learned that day was that a mere 2 mL of blood caused this patient to have a true anaphylactic response to blood and that the staff demonstrated how critical thinking, collaboration, and respect could salvage a potentially life-threatening outcome. This patient had an unknown IgA antibody problem and 3 mL of blood would have been enough to cause a lethal situation.

I'd like to conclude by saying that it is the work that we do every day as health care professionals—work that involves thoughtful action, critical thinking, mindfulness, and an ability to understand through reflection and discussion while making sound judgments that lead to justifiable actions—that is true nursing praxis.

> "Quality is of the highest priority not only for our patients, but for the staff working in the unit as well. We collaborate on a daily basis with a variety of constituents in order to ensure positive patient outcomes and coordination of care."

Infusion Therapy

Deborah Benvenuto
Mary Alexander

Outcome-Based Learning Objectives

After studying this chapter, the learner will be able to:

1. Compare and contrast the types and uses of catheters for parenteral administration of solutions and medications.
2. Describe the types and uses of parenteral administration equipment and infusion devices.
3. Evaluate the tenets of infusion nursing practice including competencies, skill validation, and patient assessment.
4. Describe components of infusion-specific documentation.
5. Discuss the recognition and management of infusion-related complications, and strategies to prevent complications for the patient receiving infusion therapy.

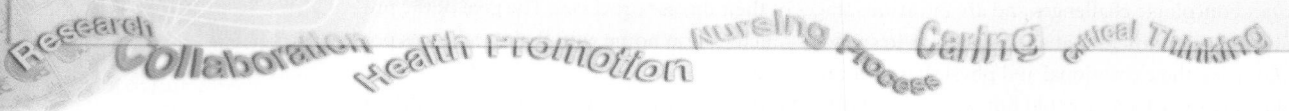

Research   Collaboration   Health Promotion   Nursing Process   Caring   Critical Thinking

INFUSION THERAPY began in the late 1400s when the vascular system was accessed with crude hollow-bore instruments that consisted of feather quills, animal veins, and bladders. Today, research and technology have produced devices that can be easily inserted into vascular and nonvascular spaces and allowed to **dwell** (remain in place) for periods of several days to many months and sometimes years. These devices are used for delivery of prescribed **infusates** (solutions and medications) over a period of time for specific therapeutic indications or diagnostic evaluations. This method of delivery is referred to as the **parenteral** route, which means that the alimentary canal is bypassed and medications and solutions are instead delivered by subcutaneous, vascular, intramuscular, or nonvascular routes. This chapter discusses these infusion therapies and focuses on the administration of infusates via the subcutaneous, vascular, and nonvascular routes.

Because infusion therapy requires that specific sterile compartments within the body be accessed, standard precautions and sterile technique are to be practiced with all infusion-related procedures. More information about standard precautions is given in Chapter 20 ☜. Single-use catheters and infusion-specific products are used to promote safety for the patient and health care provider and to prevent and minimize development of infusion-related complications such as infection.

Pathogens associated with infusion therapy causing the greatest health care risk are the hepatitis B and C viruses (HBV and HCV) and the human immunodeficiency virus (HIV). Hollowbore needles, which are commonly used for obtaining blood samples, administering injections, or accessing vascular and nonvascular structures, are implicated in the transmission of bloodborne diseases because contaminated blood can become lodged within the internal space, or **lumen**, of the device.

■ Vascular Access Devices

A **vascular access device (VAD)** or **catheter** is a device that is introduced through the skin, into the vascular network, for the purpose of infusing parenteral solutions and medications. These devices require the nurse to become proficient in not only insertion techniques for the devices, but patient assessment and monitoring practices, and care and maintenance strategies for these devices.

Peripheral Vascular Access Devices

Vascular access devices that are used primarily for infusion therapies administered via locations found on the upper extremities, or the peripheral vasculature, are addressed in the following sections. These devices are used with parenteral therapies administered in a variety of care settings.

Peripheral-Short Catheters

Peripheral-short catheters are VADs that are less than 7.5 cm (3.0 in.) in length and are placed in the superficial peripheral vasculature of the arms of adult and pediatric patients. In children, VADs also may be inserted in other locations such as the occipital, superficial temporal, posterior auricular, and saphenous veins.

Peripheral short catheters are manufactured with various configurations, lengths, and sizes, and from polyurethane-based and silastic materials. Certain materials such as Teflon (polytetrafluoroethylene) decrease the occurrence of catheter-related phlebitis and thrombogenesis. Another material, Vialon, is considered hemocompatible, and becomes "slick" when moistened. It softens soon after insertion, which minimizes intimal trauma and thrombus formation. Typically, the lengths of peripheral-short catheters vary from 1.5 to 7.5 cm (5/8 to 3.0 in.). Needles range in size, or **gauge**, from a 24-gauge needle, which is the smallest size, to 10- and 12-gauge needles, which are used for large-volume replacement and emergency and trauma care procedures.

During catheter insertion, the stylet is held stationary with the bevel up to prevent vein trauma and facilitate adequate blood flashback. The **bevel** is the slant or angle of the needle that facilitates puncture of the skin and cannulation of the vascular lumen. The **flashback chamber** is a small space in the hub of the stylet that allows for confirmation of the presence of blood and indicates access to the vascular lumen. The nurse must be able to stabilize the stylet assembly during insertion in order to minimize vein trauma and patient discomfort and to prevent accidental exposure to blood or body fluids.

As a result of the Needlestick Safety and Prevention Act of 2000, manufacturers have made great strides in redesigning catheters to afford a measure of safety against accidental blood exposure and possible sharps-related injuries. One type of engineered safety mechanism is identified by the **self-sheathing** stylet, which causes the needle to become encased in a protective chamber upon removal from the inserted catheter. These protective devices require the nurse to purposefully activate the safety mechanism after the needle is withdrawn. Other devices, after withdrawal from the catheter, capture the tip of the exposed stylet with a protective metal casing.

Dwell times for peripheral-short catheters usually range from 72 to 96 hours. Dwell times for winged steel infusion sets (see next section) should be kept under 4 hours and relegated to single-dose therapies due to the increased incidence of complications associated with rigid devices, such as **infiltration** (the inadvertent administration of nonvesicant solutions or medications into surrounding tissues), or for such procedures as phlebotomy procedures.

Removal or discontinuance of the catheter should be accomplished using standard precautions, and aseptic technique must be observed. The dressing materials should be removed from the catheter insertion site followed by gentle retraction of the catheter. Close assessment of the exit site is necessary to detect complications such as phlebitis or drainage, and a dry sterile dressing is applied to the site until hemostasis occurs. The nurse should also inspect the catheter for its condition upon removal. Patients must be educated as to the scope of activities they may engage in and should be instructed to report any drainage or tenderness from the catheter's former site.

The various types of peripheral-short catheters are discussed next. Figure 22–1 ■ shows the most common veins used for intravenous infusions.

Winged Steel Infusion Set

The **winged steel infusion set** is identified by its flexible plastic attachments, or "wings," that extend from either side of the steel needle to facilitate its insertion (Figure 22–2 ■, p. 514). The needle of this device comes in several lengths, from approximately 3/8 to 1.5 inches. Needle gauges vary from 19 to 27. Steel needle gauges are often odd numbered, with the lower number being the larger lumen. Fastened to the winged attachments and needle is plastic tubing generally made of polyvinyl chloride (PVC). This tubing or extension ranges in length from several inches to usually no more than 12 inches. At the distal portion of the extension is an **adapter** to which the administration equipment may be attached. Winged steel infusion sets are now manufactured with safety sheaths that must be activated by the clinician to prevent accidental needlesticks. The winged steel infusion set is biocompatible; therefore, low rates of device-related phlebitis are documented with this infusion product.

Insertion techniques require the nurse to be knowledgeable about vascular anatomy, proficient in desired site selection, and skilled at insertion procedures. Due to the rigidity of the steel

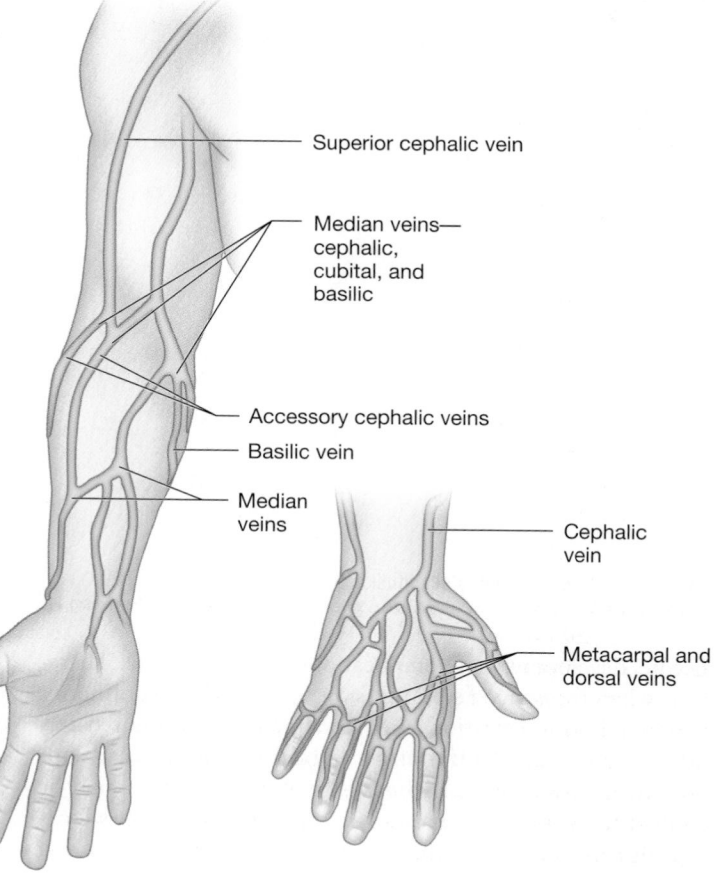

FIGURE 22–1 ■ Common veins used for intravenous therapy.

CRITICAL ALERT *Winged steel infusion sets have demonstrated a tendency to infiltrate easily due to rigidity of the steel needle. Observe the patient closely for sudden development of complications such as bruising and infiltration during venipuncture and infusion procedures.*

retraction on the wings will facilitate device removal. Hemostasis will be achieved with the application of sterile dressing material and gentle pressure applied to the exit wound.

Over-the-Needle Peripheral-Short Catheters

Over-the-needle peripheral-short catheters (Figure 22–3 ■) are commonly used for short-term infusion therapies. They are less than or equal to 7.5 cm (3.0 in.) in length. They are made of radiopaque materials for ease of x-ray visualization. During the manufacturing process, a hollow-bore metal stylet needle is inserted through the lumen of the flexible catheter. This provides stability to the plastic catheter and facilitates penetration of the skin and vascular or nonvascular structures during device insertion. The presence of blood in the flashback chamber, situated on the posterior aspect of the catheter, indicates when the lumen of the vessel has been accessed. The stylet is then withdrawn as the catheter is moved forward into the vein.

Through-the-Needle Peripheral-Short Catheters

A **through-the-needle peripheral-short catheter** allows passage of the catheter through the lumen of the steel introducer needle, which is the rigid device that allows passage into the vessel. The introducer is withdrawn after successful penetration and positioning within the vessel lumen, leaving the flexible catheter in place. Because the introducer needle cannot be separated from the catheter, it is covered with a protective clip or sleeve to prevent inadvertent catheter shearing or patient injury.

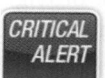 **CRITICAL ALERT** *When inserting a catheter via this method, be extremely careful **not** to withdraw the catheter back through the steel introducer needle in order to prevent accidental shearing of the catheter. After catheter placement is confirmed, withdraw the introducer needle carefully from the venipuncture site, taking care not to accidentally cut the catheter, and secure with a sterile clip to stabilize the device.*

Midline Catheters

Another example of a peripherally inserted VAD is the midline catheter. Made of materials similar to peripheral-short catheters, the **midline (ML) catheter** is approximately 7.5 to 20 cm (3.1 to

FIGURE 22–2 ■ Winged steel infusion set.
Source: (bottom) Winged safety steel infusion set. Courtesy Exel International Inc., St. Petersburg, FL

needle, development of complications is a serious risk. Therefore, when the winged steel infusion set is used for continuous parenteral administration, the site should be monitored frequently for signs of infiltration or bruising. Temporary supportive devices such as arm boards or splinting surfaces may be applied to assist in preservation of the infusion device's location during short-term therapy. Care should be used during device removal to prevent injury to sensitive or fragile anatomic structures. Adherence to standard precautions and observation of aseptic technique are required. Smooth gentle

FIGURE 22–3 ■ Introcan safety over-the-needle peripheral-short catheters.

8.0 in.) in length. Dwell periods of these devices are usually recommended not to exceed 4 weeks. Insertion location of the catheter is the antecubital fossa, with alternate sites considered for pediatric patients such as the saphenous, posterior auricular, and superficial temporal veins. The distal tip dwells in the basilic, cephalic, or brachial veins, and is level with the axilla and distal to the shoulder. Because of the extended dwell time, insertion preparations are more extensive than those of the peripheral-short VADs in an effort to minimize development of complications.

ML catheters are generally inserted using an introducer technique, described above. The vein is selected and prepared for venipuncture with appropriate antiseptic agents. An introducer is inserted into the selected vein. The stylet is withdrawn once a positive blood aspirate is confirmed. The ML catheter is then threaded through the introducer. Once the full length of the ML has been inserted, the introducer is withdrawn. Due to its specialized design, the introducer is next peeled apart or separated, allowing its removal from around the ML without disruption to the catheter's location.

A nurse may remove an ML catheter at completion of therapy provided the nurse is educated and skilled in ML catheter removal. It is recommended that antiseptic ointment and an occlusive sterile dressing be applied to the exit wound after removal. This aids hemostasis by occluding the original catheter pathway, and provides a measure of antimicrobial activity due to the extended dwell time of the ML catheter. Due to the length of the device, the catheter must be measured upon removal and be compared to preinsertion documentation.

Therapies infused through a ML catheter are the same as for peripheral-short catheters since the tip of the ML catheter does not pass beyond the peripheral circulatory system. Peripheral infusion prescriptions restricted to ML catheter use are those with pH ranges of 5 to 9, osmolarities of less than 500 mOsm/L, and solutions not to be administered for greater than 4 weeks of therapy.

Central Vascular Access Devices

The **central vascular access device (CVAD)**, defined as a catheter inserted into a centrally located vein with the tip residing in the vena cava, was once relegated to emergent resuscitative procedures and therapies for critically ill patients. Today, their use has evolved to patients in multiple care settings including those outside of the traditional confines of the acute care setting. After insertion, but prior to initiation of therapy, the catheter tip location must be confirmed by radiologic examination.

Nontunneled and Noncuffed CVADs

CVADs are typically divided into three separate and distinct categories for product identification and access configuration purposes. The **nontunneled and noncuffed device** (Figure 22–4 ■) is one that is inserted **percutaneously** via a direct skin puncture with passage of the catheter directly into the vasculature. A catheter inserted using this method is generally not considered a long-term device because it is not tunneled under the skin. A percutaneous catheter may have a single or multiple lumens and is made of polyurethane- or silastic-based materials. A common misnomer is to identify the catheter product by its vascular point of entry such as "subclavian," "jugular," or "femoral" rather than by product name.

FIGURE 22–4 ■ Triple-lumen noncuffed central catheters.
Source: Reprinted with permission of Arrow International, Inc.

Typically, most CVADs are inserted by physicians or by advanced practice clinicians who are skilled and competent to perform the procedure. Once inserted, the device must be secured, usually with sutures, to prevent inadvertent dislodgment and loss of access. Insertion procedures require sterile technique and maximal barrier precautions.

Removal of nontunneled and noncuffed devices may be done by a nurse skilled and educated in the procedure. Adherence to standard precautions and observation of aseptic technique are required. The patient is placed in a recumbent position and is instructed to perform the Valsalva maneuver, which is to take a deep breath, hold it, and bear down as if to defecate. When the patient bears down, air is prevented from entering the catheter wound and pathway, preventing an **air embolism**, which is caused by the entry of air into the vascular system. While the patient is performing the maneuver, the nurse, having already removed the dressing and released the securement devices, removes the catheter and applies pressure to the catheter exit wound, followed by immediate application of an antiseptic ointment and a sterile occlusive dressing to the site. Then, the nurse instructs the patient to breathe normally and remain inactive and recumbent for approximately 30 minutes, in order to achieve hemostasis and allow monitoring for untoward events related to CVAD removal. The nurse also must inspect the integrity of the device and measure for preinsertion catheter length. This confirms whether the catheter has fractured, leaving a segment in the patient's circulation.

Another type of CVAD that falls into the category of percutaneously inserted nontunneled and noncuffed devices is the **peripherally inserted central catheter (PICC)** (Figure 22–5 ■, p. 516). This is classified as a long-term catheter that is typically inserted at the patient's bedside by nurses educated and skilled in the procedure. Therapies to be infused through a PICC include the following:

- Therapies that require vascular access for several weeks to many months to as long as 1 year
- Therapies with extreme variations in solution pH (>5 and <9) and osmolarity (>600 mOsm/L) and including those solutions with irritant and **vesicant** (causes blistering) properties
- Therapies commonly associated with CVADs such as parenteral nutrition and antineoplastic, anti-infective, and inotropic therapies.

Radiologic confirmation of the catheter tip location prior to therapy initiation is mandatory. Due to the insertion location in

FIGURE 22–5 ■ Peripherally inserted central catheters.
Source: Courtesy of Infusion Nurses Society, PICC Education Module 2003, Norwood, MA.

the antecubital region for most PICCs and ML catheters, the ability of the patient to participate in self-care and self-administration practices makes these popular devices among both patients and health care providers.

The PICC is also less commonly associated with development of complications such as site infection, due to the decreased bacterial ecosystem of the antecubital region, and air embolism, because the device does not externally penetrate the thorax during its dwell time. It does lend itself, however, to other complications associated with VADs such as device fracture, tip malposition, device occlusion, and thrombus formation. When removing a PICC, the educated and skilled nurse instructs the patient in the Valsalva maneuver, places the patient in a recumbent position, and performs the removal procedure following the same procedure indicated for removal of other CVADs. Documentation must include measurement of the PICC and preinsertion length comparisons.

Tunneled and Cuffed CVADs

A second category of CVAD is the **tunneled and cuffed device** (Figure 22–6 ■). The cuff is the manufactured piece of the catheter generally made of synthetic materials such as nylon or Dacron. It is attached to the catheter in such a manner that the device is stabilized during its dwell time, and it reduces the risk of catheter-related infection by inhibiting the migration of microorganisms along the catheter track. Some cuffs are impregnated with antimicrobial agents such as a silver-impregnated collagen matrix. The catheter is usually made of silastic-based

materials for its durability and antithrombogenic characteristics. It is configured with either single or multiple lumens. These CVADs are often identified by the physician(s) who developed such clinical devices: Broviac, Hickman, Raaf, and Groshong.

Tunneled and cuffed catheters are typically inserted in the surgical or radiology suite. Tunneling under the skin is the technique used to access the vasculature. An entrance wound is created at a point generally near a large vein, typically the subclavian or femoral vein. The catheter is inserted into the vena cava and radiologic confirmation of tip placement is mandatory prior to initiation of therapy. After tip insertion, the catheter's remaining length is drawn though an exit wound located lower on the chest wall. This technique minimizes the potential for microorganisms gaining access into the body by establishing mechanical barriers (the skin), as well as enabling the cuff to act as a securement device once the tissues heal from the procedure. These CVADs are intended for long-term infusion therapies, with the patient often participating in self-care in the home setting.

Implanted Ports

Implanted ports comprise the third category of central vascular access devices. Implanted ports are indicated for long-term or chronic therapies such as antineoplastic, inotropic, antimicrobial, and blood replacement therapies. An **implanted port** is a chambered device, containing either single or double reservoirs, with an attached silastic catheter (Figure 22–7 ■). The catheter may be a single- or a double-lumen catheter, depending on the configuration of the port. The catheter's tip is directed to dwell in a designated structure, which could be either vascular or nonvascular, depending on the intended infusion prescription.

Implanted ports are in their own category because of their unique physical structure, implantation procedures, clinical indications, and recommended lengths of dwell time. Typically, these devices are surgically placed either in the operating or radiology suite by physicians or advanced practice clinicians. The device is considered long term because it can remain in place for several years. It is inserted, or implanted, under the skin in a surgically designed pocket of skin, and placement of the port or reservoir portion is usually located over a bony surface to enhance port stability and facilitate access. When the port is not in use, it requires very little maintenance.

The port chamber, or reservoir, will have one or two chambers leading to either a single- or double-lumen catheter with the catheter tip located in the vena cava (Figures 22–8 and 22–9 ■).

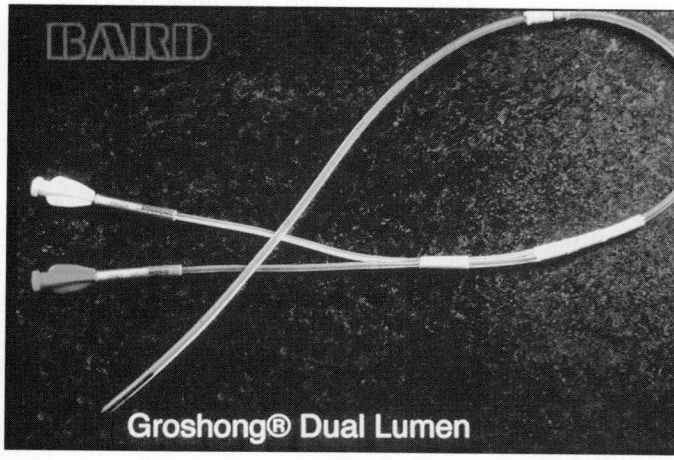

FIGURE 22–6 ■ Tunneled and cuffed CVAD device.
Source: Courtesy of Bard Access Systems, Salt Lake City, UT

FIGURE 22–7 ■ Implanted port.
Source: Courtesy of Infusion Nurses Society, PICC Education Module, 2003.

FIGURE 22–8 ■ Double-lumen implanted ports.
Source: Courtesy of Bard Access Systems, Salt Lake City, UT

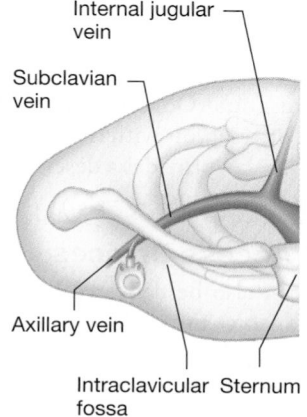

FIGURE 22–9 ■ Single-lumen implanted ports.
Source: Courtesy of Bard Access Systems, Salt Lake City, UT

The port is usually less than 1 inch in height and diameter. There also are low-profile ports that are smaller, less than 1/2 inch in height and width, allowing for placement in children or the inner aspect of the adult's upper arm or ventral surface of the forearm.

The septum is a key factor for optimal functioning of the port. The **septum** is the access point of the port and is usually made of highly compressed silicon. If the septum becomes damaged in any way, then the whole device must be surgically removed and replaced. The septum is designed to accommodate a **noncoring needle** (Figure 22–10 ■). The bevel of the noncoring needle opens on the *side* of the needle, preventing coring of the septum. Damaging the septum would allow leakage of infusate from the septum, placing the patient at potential risk for infiltration and extravasation, air embolism, and infectious processes. It would also cause the patient to face another surgical procedure in order to replace the port.

Removal of tunneled and cuffed catheters and implanted ports and reservoirs is performed by the physician or by advanced practice clinicians who are competent in performing the procedure, and are therefore not included within the scope of practice for most nurses.

In summary, CVADs are indicated for critical care and long-term therapies. These devices are used in all care settings such as hospitals; homes; long-term, rehabilitation, and subacute facilities; ambulatory infusion centers; and physicians' offices. Certain properties of solutions and medications mandate the use of CVADs to avoid damaging the sensitive peripheral vascular structures. Additionally, CVADs are useful for medications, such as inotropics and antineoplastic therapies, that are administered in cycles and over many months. Medications for chronic conditions or illnesses such as immunodeficiency diseases or genetic conditions such as cystic fibrosis are amenable to longer dwell infusion devices.

Specialized Infusion Catheters and Devices

Some VADs are indicated for hemodynamic monitoring in the critical care setting. These types of catheters are used exclusively

FIGURE 22–10 ■ Noncoring needles.
Source: Courtesy of Bard Access Systems, Salt Lake City, UT

for cardiac monitoring and hemodynamic analyses. They have multiple lumens and are used to measure central venous pressure, pulmonary artery pressure and cardiac output, pulmonary wedge pressure, and temporary heart pacing and for parenteral administrations.

The most common is the pulmonary artery catheter, which is inserted into the pulmonary artery via the right atrium and ventricle. This device is indicated for patients in need of critical monitoring, such as those experiencing acute cardiac and respiratory failures. The brand name is **Swan-Ganz catheter**, named after the two physicians, Drs. Harold James Swan and William Ganz, who developed it. Chapter 24 👁 provides a complete description of the many uses and functions of pulmonary artery catheters.

Dialysis and Pheresis Catheters

Dialysis and pheresis catheters are rarely considered for routine infusion administrations. They are instead used for procedures where large volumes of blood need to be treated for specific medical indications. They may be inserted at the bedside or in the radiology or operating suite. The **dialysis catheter** is inserted and used for dialysis until a permanent shunt can be inserted. A **pheresis catheter** may be inserted for plasmapheresis procedures where large volumes of blood are filtered in attempts to remove undesired plasma components. The lumen of the catheter is large enough for blood flow in both directions, thereby facilitating flow through a dialysis or pheresis machine. Dialysis catheters that are inserted for temporary kidney dialysis are reserved for that function only due to the prevalence of high infection rates and problems associated with device occlusion. This also holds true for pheresis catheters. Pheresis and dialysis catheters are known by many brand names, including Quinton, Hohn, Tesio, and Perma-Cath. Pheresis catheters can be used interchangeably for infusions and pheresis procedures, again depending on patient condition, available vascular access, and the infusion prescription.

Both devices are available in silastic and polyurethane materials. The softer silastic devices are reserved for long-term dwell times. These catheters are generally shorter in overall length than typical tunneled and cuffed devices ranging in length from 7.5 to 20 cm (about 3 to 8 in.), and they have larger gauge sizes (12 to 16). The catheter tip resides in the vena cava allowing for high flow rates, which are necessary for fluid and blood volume exchange. Chapter 47 👁 provides a description of dialysis.

Arterial-Venous Shunts

Arterial-venous shunts are Gor-Tex or silicone-based devices that are used to anastomose venous and arterial structures, usually located in the arm, such as the radial artery and the cephalic or brachial veins. These shunts are used for specific infusion and exchange therapies and as VADs. When used for dialysis, the shunt is accessed with a large-bore needle. Occasionally these access devices can be used for other infusion therapies such as parenteral nutrition or fluid rehydration.

Assessment for patency is done by placing a stethoscope over the top of the shunt and listening for a bruit, or by placing the fingers of the hand over the site and palpating for a vibration feeling. If present, the shunt is patent. This is necessary when assessing the patient for additional vascular access device placement because no other VADs should be placed in the extremity with an AV shunt for fear of complication development such as infection, compromise and rupture of the shunt, and thrombo-

sis of the peripheral vasculature. If a shunt is damaged, surgical repair and/or replacement are the only options available.

Arterial Catheters

Arterial catheters are used for two primary indications: blood pressure monitoring and vascular access for obtaining blood samples. The catheter is usually made from stiff material such as polyurethane because it must withstand dwell time–limiting effects such as kinking and softening. Peripherally located arterial catheters are most commonly inserted into the radial artery and attached to pressure transducers and monitors. These catheters provide an ongoing assessment of blood pressure as well as access to arterial blood for laboratory testing. No medications are delivered through these catheters because that would cause severe injury to tissues and areas distal to the catheter insertion site. Chapter 24 👁 provides a complete description of the use and care of arterial catheters.

Hepatic Artery Catheters

The **hepatic artery catheter**, in contrast to the arterial catheters just discussed, is used to deliver specific, or targeted, antineoplastic therapy. Regionalized antineoplastic therapy is best delivered by this route. Other infusions may be attached to an implanted port or reservoir with the catheter tip positioned arterially. Chapter 46 👁 provides a description of the diagnosis and treatment of liver cancer.

Nonvascular Access Devices

Infusion therapy can also be delivered by nonvascular routes such as the subcutaneous, intraosseous, and intraspinal routes. Although many of the prescribed therapies are complicated, the catheter products used in conjunction with these modalities are the same as those used with vascular access.

Subcutaneous Infusion Therapy

Subcutaneous infusion therapy involves the infusion of parenteral solutions and medications via absorption through the subcutaneous tissues. The technique used to infuse a large amount of isotonic solutions in this manner is known as **hypodermoclysis**. Infusing smaller volumes such as medications prescribed for pain control or diabetes mellitus is known as **continuous subcutaneous infusions (CSI)**. The infusion devices are manufactured with extremely small gauge sizes (25 to 27 gauge) and are approximately 1/2 inch in length.

The needle may be positioned at a 90-degree angle and attached to an adhesive disk or may appear as a winged steel infusion set used for vascular access (Figure 22–11 ■). The device is inserted over an area where there is adequate subcutaneous tissue and capillary beds to absorb the infusate. These areas include the abdomen, outer aspects of the thigh and upper arm, and subclavicular and subscapular regions. These areas allow adequate visualization of the infusion site in addition to allowing the patient unfettered mobility.

Even though these are nonvascular insertion procedures, the nurse must prime the administration set and access device with the prescribed parenteral solution prior to initiation of therapy. The intended site is prepared with the appropriate antiseptic agent, allowed to dry, and the device inserted. The device must be aspirated with a syringe to confirm the absence of blood in the area of insertion. If no blood is found, then the device is se-

FIGURE 22–11 ■ Clysis infusion set.
Source: Aqua-C Hydration System. Courtesy of Norfolk Medical Products, Inc. Skokie, IL

cured with sterile dressing material and the infusion started. If blood is obtained, the device is removed and another infusion site selected and prepared. A new device is then readied and inserted, once again aspirating to confirm the absence of blood at the insertion site.

Common complications associated with this type of treatment are localized skin irritation including erythema and itching, infection, and dislodgment of the access device. Systemic complications are associated with the medication or solution being infused. Ineffective dosing may require another infusion site or route to be secured. Site rotation usually occurs every 3 to 5 days, depending on the concentration and rate of the fluid or medication being administered.

Hypodermoclysis has been found to be an effective treatment for older patients who require short-term isotonic fluid resuscitation to treat dehydration. Additional criteria for this treatment modality include fluid needs of less than 3 liters per day, no evidence of existing coagulopathies, and intact skin sites.

Intraosseous Therapy

Intraosseous therapy is the insertion of a hollow-bore needle into the bone, with the device tip accessing the marrow space. The tip of the needle is protected by an obturator, which has screw-like threads, facilitating penetration of the bony structure. The long bones of the leg or iliac crest are usually preferred in the pediatric patient, while the sternum has been used equally effectively in adults. Children less than 6 years of age and patients with thermal injuries, trauma, cardiac arrest, or other life-threatening illnesses can be treated in this manner until traditional vascular access can be obtained. Complications include bone fracture, infiltration, osteomyelitis, and cellulitis, in addition to occlusion of the obturator or needle and needle breakage. Emergent access of the bone core allows rapid infusion of large volumes of parenteral fluids and medications until vascular access can be obtained.

Intraspinal Catheters

Intraspinal catheters are located within the spinal spaces such as the epidural and intrathecal spaces. The intraspinal space has been used with great reliability for many procedures such as delivery of anesthesia, diagnostic testing, and infusions. Catheters

used for the intraspinal route have 22- to 26-gauge lumens and vary from 10 to 30 inches in length. They are made of biocompatible materials such as polyurethane and silastic. For temporary placement the catheter is inserted percutaneously into the desired spinal space and secured externally. For more stable long-term placement and as an infection control measure, the catheter can be tunneled to an isolated exit site.

Implanted infusion ports also can be used for intraspinal access. These are usually reserved for those patients with intractable pain who require lifelong pain control and who have a life expectancy of months to a year, or for those patients diagnosed with terminal cancer who require ongoing pain control. The device consists of a catheter whose tip is located in the epidural space. The catheter is attached to an infusion pump that is often implanted under the skin, in the vicinity of the abdominal region or chest wall. A blood return should never be obtained from these devices because the device tip is located in the epidural space where there should not be any blood. Additionally, epidural catheters should have a negative aspirate for spinal fluids because the epidural compartment does not communicate directly with the subarachnoid space, where the spinal cord resides.

Infusates, drugs, and diluents must be preservative free due to the neurotoxic effects of preserving agents. The epidural space can usually accommodate an infusion rate no greater than 15 mL/min due to limitations imposed by physical structures and restrictions of the epidural space. Medications and solutions given via this route have the ability to cross the dura mater, and have direct effects on the central nervous system (CNS). Complications such as infection and catheter malposition must be avoided through skilled manipulation of these infusion systems and observation of sterile technique. Surfactant-free filters on the administration system and alcohol-free skin antiseptic agents are used to prevent potential neurotoxic agents from entering the CNS.

Intrathecal Therapy

Intrathecal therapy involves the administration of medications directly into the cerebrospinal fluid (CSF) via an implanted reservoir system. The most common device, the **Ommaya reservoir**, allows delivery of medications directly into the CSF without relying on diffusion. Unlike epidural catheter systems where medications and solutions enter the CNS by diffusing across the dura mater, medications are injected directly into the CSF, permitting immediate therapy. The catheter attached to the reservoir terminates in the ventricular space of the cerebrum. Not all medications can pass the blood–brain barrier and target specific areas of the brain for treatment. The Ommaya reservoir is very effective for the following therapies:

- Delivering medications such as preservative-free opioids
- Administering selected antineoplastic agents such as methotrexate and cytarabine
- Measuring CSF pressures
- Draining excess CSF
- Obtaining CSF samples for laboratory assay.

The reservoir is surgically placed via a burr hole in the skull and the skin is secured over the device. Care and maintenance practices are dependent on the intended therapy, and standard precautions and sterile technique must be maintained. Complications are the same as those associated with intraspinal devices.

Infusion Delivery Systems

Vascular access devices are just one piece of the entire infusion delivery system. Fluid containers, administration sets, infusion flow control devices, and add-on devices also are integral components to effective therapy delivery.

Fluid Containers

Fluid containers are made of either glass or plastic. Glass containers allow for easy visualization and accurate recording of contents, but are heavy, bulky to store, and may break. Glass containers require a venting mechanism to be inserted into the container in order to facilitate solution delivery. Venting permits movement of air into the fluid container, facilitating flow of parenteral fluid. One such design is an *open airway*, in which a tube is attached to the inside of the bottle stopper. When the bottle is inverted, environmental air moves up the tube and displaces the fluid in the container. A vented administration set is not necessary. The second type of container, a closed system, does require a venting mechanism on the administration set. Air is allowed to access the bottle through a filter attached to the administration set spike.

Plastic containers are the preferred type of container because of easy portability, storage, and reduced manufacturing costs. Due to the flexibility of plastic containers, however, volume and dose administrations may be inaccurate. Plastic containers collapse as the fluid drains, which eliminates the need for vented administration sets. Plastic containers are highly amenable to fluctuations in temperature, which makes freezing of drugs post-admixture advantageous for availability and storage.

Administration Sets

The **administration set** is the tubing that delivers the parenteral fluid from the infusate container to the catheter that is in the patient's vein. *Primary* and *secondary sets* are terms used to describe the function of the set. The **primary set** is typically the main tubing that extends from the infusate container to the access device. It permits fluid passage by using gravity, an electronic infusion device set, or specialized microbore tubing attached to a syringe pump-delivery system.

Any extra equipment such as filters, stopcocks, extensions, connectors, and injection ports or caps added to the primary set are called **add-on devices** (see later section). The use of multiple add-on devices is not recommended because interruption in the fluid pathway increases the risk of system malfunction, inadvertent separation of component elements, and infusion-related complications such as air embolism and infection. All connections to the catheter adapter and for add-on devices should be Luer-Lok attachments to prevent inadvertent separation of administration equipment. A **Luer-Lok** is an attachment mechanism that is threaded to prevent inadvertent separation of equipment.

The **secondary set** is tubing that attaches to the primary set and permits additional infusion administrations. Typically, secondary sets are used to infuse medications and solutions that are administered on an intermittent basis, for example, every 4 hours. The secondary set is attached to a small bag of intravenous solution and then it is "piggybacked" into the primary set and hung up higher than the primary solution so it infuses instead of the primary solution (Figure 22–12 ■). When the bag is empty, the primary solution simply takes over again. Both the primary infusate and the secondary infusate must be compatible in order to prevent complications such as precipitate formation, which can result in occlusion of the fluid pathway.

The drip factor in either set can be described as macrodrip or microdrip, with the set being vented or nonvented. The **drip factor** is the number of drops that will equal 1 milliliter (mL) of infusate. Drip factor sizes vary from 10 to 60 drops/mL. A macrodrip calculation varies from 10 to 20 drops/mL and a microdrip is 60 drops/mL, depending on the manufacturer. This information is critical when calculating the exact amount of solution to be infused. Several formulas are used for fluid delivery calculations and these are dependent on drip factors, prescribed drug, and infusate solutions, as well as other parameters such as body surface area and weight.

Metered-volume chambered sets consist of an administration set topped with a metered, small-volume container that is attached to a fluid container (Figure 22–13 ■). Markings on the chamber vary from 1- to 5-mL increments. The use of this type of administration set is often seen in special patient populations, such as neonate and pediatric groups, in critical care units, and for those older adults with fluid control issues requiring close observation and monitoring. Metered-volume chambered administration sets also are often used with drugs and solutions that require significant control or intermittent delivery, with titrated medications, and for patients with fluid restrictions. Medications can be added to the chamber and diluted with the infusate, thereby not increasing the amount of fluid the patient is receiving.

Clamping mechanisms are features of administration sets that regulate the prescribed infusion rates (Figure 22–14 ■). *Roller clamps*, generally found on primary infusion sets, allow the nurse to regulate the parenteral fluid by either opening or closing the clamp. *Slide and pinch* clamps are not volume controlling, but instead provide an "on–off" feature to the set. These

FIGURE 22–12 ■ Piggyback system.

FIGURE 22–13 ■ Metered-volume chambered set.

clamps are seen often on add-on equipment and secondary sets. *Screw* clamps may also be found on administration sets and offer "on–off" and flow regulation functions comparable to those of roller clamps.

Flow Control Device

An add-on device that can be used for regulation of fluid administration is the **flow control device**. This device is added to a gravity infusion system at the point closest to the patient, and used to regulate fluid flow instead of using the clamp provided on the set. (A *gravity* infusion is one in which the infusion is regulated by hand and is affected by the container position above the patient and by patient activities.) At issue is the efficacy of calibrations and effective rate adjustments. Accuracy and consistency of infusion rates are affected by patient activity, height of the fluid container above the patient, and fluid composition and temperature.

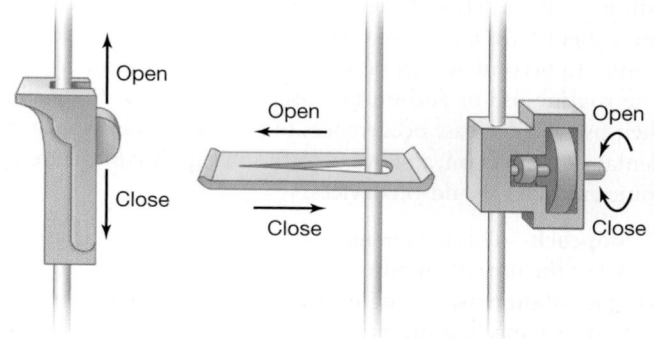

FIGURE 22–14 ■ Administration set clamps.

Once the flow rate is "dialed" or set, it is subject to wide variations in fluid delivery if the patient is ambulatory or the fluid container's height is adjusted. Clamping mechanisms do not negate the effect of close monitoring and fluid regulation by the nurse.

Some infusion products and medications, such as nitroglycerin, lipid emulsions, and blood products, have specific requirements associated with their delivery. Specialized administration sets are manufactured with features that meet these requirements, as discussed here:

- Nitroglycerin is incompatible with standard PVC tubing. Hence, nitroglycerin administration sets are manufactured from non-PVC materials. Also, nitroglycerin is admixed in glass containers for medication delivery to minimize drug loss.
- According to recent controversial reports, lipids are affected by containers and administration sets that contain DEHP (a *plasticizer* in manufacturing of articles made of polyvinyl chloride) (Hankins, Lonsway, Hedrick, & Perdue, 2001). Lipid emulsions are manufactured in glass containers. Due to the limited hang time for the infusion itself, researchers believe the limited contact with plastic tubing does not place the patient at risk (Hankins et al., 2001).
- Blood infusion sets are designed to accommodate the specific properties of blood and its components. Blood administration sets may have Y-shaped tubing and will contain filter systems to remove debris and accumulated by-products that result from blood storage. Other systems require the nurse to attach a separate filter product to a standard administration set. The Y-tubing permits a container of 0.9% sodium chloride to be connected to one access spike of the set and the blood container to be connected to the second access spike. Some sets can be used for gravity infusion while others are compatible with electronic infusion devices. When rapid infusion is indicated, some sets are equipped with an in-line hand pump. These sets should only be used in areas such as emergency departments, surgical suites, and intensive care units. Chapter 23 💿 provides a description of the blood administration procedure.

Add-on-Devices

Add-on devices are pieces of equipment that extend the efficacy of the existing administration set. Devices are added to the administration set either proximally at the spike end, or distally at the patient end. Devices can also be added at side ports along the administration set. Add-on devices are used to add length to the administration set, add filter infusates, and increase access to the patient's VAD. Add-on devices should contain a Luer-Lok feature to prevent accidental separation of the infusion system. The routine use of add-on devices is discouraged. Restricting their use will decrease occurrences of fluid contamination, accidental disconnection, and overall infusion supply costs. Here are some examples of add-on devices:

- **Stopcock**—This is a manually operated device that is used to direct the flow of an infusate. Stopcocks are used when multiple solutions are being infused. They have a three-way or four-way mechanism, permitting infusions to be connected at a common aperture, which is located at the VAD's hub. The

FIGURE 22–15 ■ Three-way stopcock.

stopcock requires the nurse to manually direct the infusion by turning the valve toward a specific infusion in order to initiate fluid flow (Figure 22–15 ■).
- **Extension set**—Device used to add length as well as additional side access ports to the existing administration set.
- **Multiflow adapter** and **Y set**—Devices used for administration of two or more infusates simultaneously. Access to the multiflow adapter is usually via a cap that maintains sterility of the fluid pathway. Each access of the adapter must be primed before attachment to the administration system and prior to attachment to the infusion catheter (Figures 22–16 and 22–17 ■).
- **Injection port or cap**—Device used to gain access to the indwelling catheter. Manufactured with resealable rubber caps, the device permits access with either needles or needleless safety infusion cannulas. Typically, they are lightweight and vary in length from 1/2 to 2 inches (Figure 22–18 ■).
- **Filter**—The purpose of filters is to provide sterility to the infused parenteral medications or solutions. Filters remove particulate matter, eliminate air, and retain or capture microorganisms. Filters are not used when certain medications, such as amphotericin B, are prescribed because the medication may become trapped on the filter bed and not reach the patient. Additionally, filters should not be used in line when administering IV push medications or very small volumes because these medications can also become trapped on the filter bed.

Infusion Delivery Devices

As discussed in the following sections, several methods other than gravity are used to enhance effective delivery of prescribed parenteral solutions. Note, however, that infusion delivery devices should never be used to replace nursing care, but as an adjunct to that care.

Mechanical Infusion Devices

Mechanical infusion devices (MIDs) are devices that do not require the use of an external power source to operate. MIDs are relatively easy to use and monitor, but the nurse should realize that they cannot detect flaws in the administration system such as air in the set, infiltration, or catheter occlusion.

FIGURE 22–16 ■ Three-lumen multiflow adapter.

FIGURE 22–17 ■ (A) Two-lumen multiflow adapter.

FIGURE 22–18 ■ Injection cap.

Mechanical infusion devices include these types:

- **Elastomeric balloons** are made of soft, expandable material contained within a transparent hard plastic casing. The prescribed medication is contained within the balloon-like container. Microbore tubing is attached to its outlet and, depending on its bore size, delivers the fluid at a corresponding rate over 30 minutes or more, depending on the volume

of the fluid. The small size of the tubing impedes the flow, preventing undue pressure on the patient's catheter. These MIDs are usually reserved for home care situations. These devices tend to be costly because they are a one-time-use product.

- The **spring-coil syringe** acts by powering the plunger of a syringe and delivering the medication to the patient. Once the syringe is empty, a new syringe must be fitted into the locking mechanism. This type of delivery system is more bulky than elastomeric balloons, and its function is relegated to a specific syringe size.

- The **spring-coil container** is a combination of the spring coil and a collapsible disk. The mechanism is activated by applying pressure on the top and bottom disk, causing collapse of the container and allowing its contents to infuse with flow being controlled by microbore tubing. Both the spring-coil syringe and container are used for small-volume parenteral administrations and are seen in acute and home care settings.

Electronic Infusion Devices

Electronic infusion devices (EIDs) can be divided into two categories, pumps and controllers. The *pump* is a device that delivers its solutions via positive pressure, whereas the *controller* is a device that relies on gravity to assist its action. A controller is often seen in general patient populations where uncomplicated therapies are used. Controllers usually do not contribute to infusion-related complications such as infiltration and vascular injury so they are safe for special populations such as geriatrics, neonates, pediatrics, and patients with most antineoplastic therapies. Most controllers use a drop sensor that attaches to the drip chamber of the administration set.

Positive Pressure Infusion Pump

Pressure is expressed in pounds per square inch (psi). One psi is equal to 50 mmHg. This pressure is exerted through the system and culminates at the infusion catheter site within the patient. The psi is an important consideration because it affects the integrity of the entire system and is a factor when undue infusion pressures cause a catheter to burst, an unfortunate and sometimes life-threatening complication of infusion therapy. Gravity-initiated pressures usually average around 2 psi if the infusate container is maintained approximately 60 cm (2 feet) above the patient's head. The higher the container, the greater the pressure exerted.

The **positive pressure infusion pump** creates pressure to infuse the fluid and overcome vascular resistance (Figure 22–19 ■). Pumps have psi parameters somewhere in the vicinity of 10 psi. Pumps are used in high acuity care areas such as critical care where the therapies are complex. Depending on hospital policy, pumps may be used in the general medical–surgical

FIGURE 22–19 ■ Positive pressure pump.

areas or when medications are being delivered that require strict monitoring, such as anticoagulation, parenteral nutrition, and inotropic therapies. The pump delivers infusate at an accurate prescribed rate and has an alarm system that detects infusion-related errors of delivery such as free flow, air in the line, and changes in vascular resistance such as occlusion or infiltration.

A **volumetric pump** is one that calculates the infusion volume delivered by the amount displaced in a reservoir. Drop sensors can also be included in this pump category. The sensor may be located internally in the pump where the fluid passes through a chamber, but it is usually found externally attached to the drip chamber. Syringe pumps are infusion specific and are limited to small-volume parenterals such as anti-infectives or pain medications. Syringe pumps are unable to detect "no flow" unless significant back pressure is generated from the distal set or indwelling catheter.

Alarms on infusion delivery devices indicate pending disruptions in fluid delivery. Not all devices have comparable alarms or a full array of similar controls. In effect, these systems serve to protect the patient and alert the nurse to evaluate the patient and the patient's infusion system. The following are some alarm features:

- **Air in the line**—Detects the presence of air in the fluid pathway of the set.
- **Occlusion**—Infusion pumps detect disruption of flow above the catheter and resistance to flow occurring below the device.
- **Infusion complete**—This alarm sounds when a preset volume limit has been reached.
- **Free flow**—This alarm is *essential* for preventing the inadvertent bolus dosing of fluid or medications. The administration set, upon its removal from the EID, must have a self-clamping mechanism that prevents free flow of infusate. The alarm detects rapid infusion of fluid as a result of partial disengagement of the pumping mechanism.
- **Other alarms**—Alarms indicating low battery; nonfunctional; not infusing; door open; pressure capabilities; programming capabilities: rate, volume to be infused, and volume infused; ramping; and timed infusion are but a few of the alarms integral to EIDs.

Several types of infusion pumps are designed for very specific care settings or infusions. Ambulatory infusion pumps are lightweight and small enough to be easily carried. They may be attached to the patient's belt, contained within a backpack, or placed on a table top. The power supply is usually a disposable battery. **Patient-controlled analgesia (PCA) pumps** are available in ambulatory, semiportable, or pole-mounted versions. The PCA pump is capable of delivering medication continuously or on patient or clinician demand. **Multichannel** and **dual-channel pumps** are pole-mounted EIDs that can be operated by manufactured housing or channels within a single device. Each channel can be operated independently of each other. Different medications and solutions can be programmed for delivery at assigned times for predetermined doses via a single infusion pathway to the patient.

In addition to the type of VAD, the infusion prescription(s), and care setting, particular features of infusion delivery devices are highly important when selecting the appropriate device.

Specific controls and alarm systems are integral to the infusion delivery device as safety measures for the patient and they also ensure accurate administration of solutions and medications. Infusion delivery devices are never to be considered a substitute for nursing care, but rather an adjunct. Monitoring and evaluation of response to therapy, in addition to effective care and maintenance strategies for the infusion patient, will provide the foundation for positive outcomes.

Infusion Nursing Practice

Competency and skill validation are required for nurses providing infusion therapy in order to be proficient in its technical aspects, demonstrate competency in clinical judgment, and practice in accordance with their state's nurse practice act. Basic competencies are intended to serve as guidelines and define the knowledge, skill, and abilities necessary to fulfill the expectations of the nurse practicing infusion therapy. Clinical skill validation and competency are vital to health care organizations that participate in annual reviews to ensure that their policies and procedures agree with those of regulatory and nonregulatory agencies (Infusion Nurses Society [INS], 2006b).

Calculations

Infusion therapy is ordered by the health care provider or by a legally authorized prescriber. It is the responsibility of the nurse to be knowledgeable about the drugs' and solutions' properties, intended outcomes, and potential side and adverse effects that may occur. Although many formulations are available for deriving correct dosing volumes and amounts, certain methods are relatively easy to use and are used consistently.

Keep in mind that certain patient conditions and patient populations (i.e., pediatric and geriatric patients and patients receiving antineoplastic or antimicrobial therapies) have specific restrictions and requirements based on body surface area, weight, and age. Medication error reduction and patient safety should remain in the forefront of nursing practice when administering infusion therapies. The nurse should be skilled and knowledgeable about the Joint Commission's approved abbreviations and medication ordering procedures.

Flow rate determination is used to calculate the amount of fluid to be delivered over a specific time period. Flow rates can be ordered as milliliters per hour or minute, total volume over a set period such as multiple hours or a 24-hour period, or number of drops per minute. The nurse must be knowledgeable of the available drop factor of the administration sets on hand and select the most appropriate for the infusion prescription.

One simplified order conversion technique is to divide the milliliter rate per hour by a specific number associated with the drop factor. The formula and an example are given in Chart 22–1. Consistent use and knowledge of the variety of calculations associated with accurate dosing and therapy administration criteria will result in safe nursing practice for the clinician, fewer medication errors, increased patient safety, and positive infusion outcomes.

Infusion Nursing Standards of Practice

Standards of practice enable those outside of a profession to measure a practitioner's performance; thus, standards protect

---

| CHART 22–1 | Infusion Rate Calculation Formula |

Example: The flow rate of therapy is ordered at 120 mL per hour via gravity. The administration set on hand has a drip factor of 15 gtts/mL. To calculate drops per minute:

$$\frac{120 \ (\text{mL/hr}) \times 15 \ (\text{gtt factor})}{60 \ (\text{time in minutes})} = 30 \ \text{drops per minute}$$

Typically the 30 is divided by 4 and the nurse counts the number of drops in 15 seconds.

---

both patients and practitioners. Standards of practice focus on the provider and define the activities and behavior needed to achieve patient outcomes. They are consistent with valid research findings, national norms, legal guidelines, and complement expectations of regulatory agencies. The goal of the *Infusion Nursing Standards of Practice* is to preserve the patient's right to safe, quality care, and protect the nurse who administers infusion therapy (INS, 2006a). The INS standards define the criteria relative to nursing accountability in the delivery of infusion therapies. They provide a framework to use in evaluating patient outcomes and are used as a mechanism for evaluating the quality of patient care and the competency of the nurse delivering infusion therapy. The INS standards are applicable in all practice settings, such as hospitals, homes, long-term care facilities, and physician offices. Therefore, nurses are accountable for adherence to them regardless of the care setting.

National guidelines are also incorporated into infusion practice. An example related to infusion nursing is the *CDC Guidelines for the Prevention of Intravascular Catheter-Related Infections* (Centers for Disease Control and Prevention [CDC], 2002). This publication provides recommendations that, when incorporated in practice, are designed to reduce infectious complications associated with infusion therapy (see the National Guidelines box).

Required Order and Informed Consent

Before initiation of any type of infusion therapy, the nurse must obtain an order from a health care provider. A medication order needs to include the type of medication or solution, dose of the medication, volume to be infused, duration of therapy, frequency, rate, and route of administration. An order must also be obtained to discontinue infusion therapy. For example, in infusion therapy, informed consent would be obtained prior to inserting a PICC.

NATIONAL GUIDELINES Prevention of Intravascular Catheter-Related Infections

The CDC's guidelines for the prevention of intravascular catheter-related infections were developed for practitioners who insert catheters and for persons responsible for surveillance and control of infections in hospital, outpatient, and home health care settings. A complete copy of the guidelines can be found at http://www.cdc.gov/ncidod/dhqp/gl_intravascular.html.

Source: Centers for Disease Control and Prevention. (2002). *CDC Guidelines for the Prevention of Intravascular Catheter-Related Infections.* Retrieved June 12, 2008, from http://www.cdc.gov/ncidod/dhqp/gl_intravascular.html.

The nurse would provide the patient with accurate and complete information, including a description of the procedure, potential benefits of such a device, possible risks associated with the procedure, and available alternatives. The consent must reflect the patient's voluntary agreement and understanding of the procedure.

Patient Assessment

Patient assessment is an ongoing process to determine the appropriateness of the therapy and ensure desired patient outcomes. The results of the initial assessment identify the baseline for the patient's care and treatment. Ongoing assessment chronicles the patient's response to treatment and provides data to measure outcomes. Pertinent information obtained during assessment and monitoring should be communicated to other health care professionals responsible for the patient's care.

Patient assessment should include the patient's past and present medical history, including diagnosis, medical and surgical histories, age, allergies, vascular access history, and patient preferences regarding VAD types and site locations. Prior to initiation, the prescribed therapy should be assessed for appropriate dose, route, and rate of infusion; potential incompatibilities among infusates, oral medications, and food; and appropriateness of the care setting.

Because infusion therapy is directly related to the patient's fluid volume and electrolyte status, reviewing laboratory data is an important component of the assessment process. Necessary components of the process include, but are not limited to, the patient's electrolytes, serum proteins, blood chemistries, and renal function tests. Clinical assessment of the patient may include height and weight, body surface area, nutritional status, pain threshold, skin turgor, vital signs, intake and output, and vascular access integrity.

The type and frequency of patient monitoring will be determined by the prescribed therapy, access device, patient's condition and age, and care setting. In addition, the nurse must monitor the catheter–skin junction site and surrounding area, flow rate, clinical data, patient response, side effects, and the patient's compliance with the prescribed therapy.

Hand Hygiene

Because of the inherent risks associated with the invasive nature of infusion therapy, knowledge of infection control principles is essential for minimizing and preventing complications from infection. Hand hygiene is a fundamental practice that reduces the transmission of pathogenic microorganisms. Hand hygiene should be done before and after performing patient care procedures, and before donning and after removal of gloves. The use of gloves does not preclude the need to perform hand hygiene. Acceptable products for decontaminating hands include antiseptic soap and water as well as waterless alcohol-based gels and foam (Boyce & Pittet, 2002; O'Grady et al., 2002).

Site Selection

Vein selection for cannulation will need to accommodate the gauge and length of the catheter. Site selection is based on the patient's condition, age, and diagnosis; the vein condition, size, and location; the type and duration of prescribed therapy; and the patient's history. Veins that should be considered for peripheral cannulation are those found on the dorsal and ventral surfaces of the upper extremities including the metacarpal, cephalic, and basilic veins (see Figure 22–1 ■, p. 513). Use of veins of the lower extremities of adults should be avoided due to the risk of embolism and thrombophlebitis formation.

Site selection should be routinely initiated in the distal areas of the upper extremities with subsequent cannulations made proximal to previous cannulated sites. Areas of flexion should be avoided, except when placing a ML catheter or PICC. Also, avoid veins in arms with compromised circulation, postmastectomy or postaxillary node dissection, or fistulated extremities as potential venipuncture sites.

Assess vascular access by applying a tourniquet 10 to 20 cm (4 to 8 in.) proximal to the intended venipuncture site. Palpate the extremity to assess the condition of the vein. An appropriate vein for venipuncture will feel soft and bouncy. A hard, cordlike feeling indicates a sclerosed or compromised vein. Valves can be detected by a hard lump or "knot-like" feeling. Resilient veins that are easily depressed are required for successful venipuncture. Palpation also differentiates arteries from veins, because veins do not pulsate.

Site Preparation

While adhering to standard precautions during site preparation, disinfect the skin with an antiseptic solution before catheter insertion. Apply the agent using friction and allow it to dry thoroughly before making the venipuncture. Fanning, blowing, or blotting the prepared area is contraindicated. Agents recommended for skin preparation include 2% chlorhexidine-based solutions, 1% to 2% tincture of iodine, 10% povidone-iodine, or 70% alcohol as single agents or in combination preparations.

Dressings

Dressings are used to protect the catheter from external environmental contamination. Sterile dressings should be aseptically applied at the initiation of vascular access, when the integrity of the dressing is compromised, and at specified time intervals determined by organizational policy and procedure. Dressings should not be reinforced if they become damp, loose, or visibly soiled, but replaced with new dressing materials. Types of dressings include the following:

- Gauze and tape dressings can be used to cover the venipuncture site. To adequately assess the catheter–skin junction and monitor for development of complications, a gauze dressing needs to be changed according to hospital protocol.
- Transparent semipermeable membrane (TSM) dressings facilitate daily catheter–skin junction inspection without disruption of the therapy, and allow direct observation of the insertion site. For peripheral-short catheter sites, a TSM dressing should be changed at the time of catheter site rotation and immediately if the integrity of the dressing is compromised. For other VADs, the TSM dressing should be changed per protocol or if the dressing has lost its integrity. It is not recommended that topical ointments be placed on the insertion site, because their efficacy at reducing infections is not proven (O'Grady et al., 2002).

Research supporting the choice of dressings is limited, and evidence does not support one choice over the other. In a systematic review of controlled trials that compared the effects of gauze and tape with transparent dressings, there was no evidence of differences in the incidence of infectious complications between dressing types. Because the studies were from small samples, however, the authors recommend the need for more research (Gillies et al., 2003).

Antiseptic dressings, such as the chlorhexidine-impregnated foam dressing, are being used more frequently. A small, round disk is placed around the catheter at the exit site, covered with a transparent dressing. In a meta-analysis published by Ho and Litton in 2006, chlorhexidine-impregnated dressings were found to be effective in reducing bacterial colonization at vascular sites, although they were also identified with a trend toward catheter-related bloodstream infections. As more research becomes available, it will be important that nurses evaluate the technology and incorporate that which will make a positive impact in patient care.

Catheter Securement

Catheters are to be stabilized so as not to interfere with assessment and monitoring of the site or impede delivery of the prescribed therapy. Devices used to secure and stabilize catheters include sterile tapes, sterile surgical strips, and sterile manufactured stabilization devices. Minimizing catheter movement helps prevent mechanical irritation to the vein lining and reduces the risk of phlebitis formation. When feasible, using a manufactured stabilization device is preferred, because it prevents the catheter from telescoping within the vein or becoming dislodged (INS, 2006a).

Flushing

Flushing, which is the infusion of a sterile solution, is performed to ensure and maintain patency of the VAD and to prevent mixing of incompatible medications and solutions. Routine flushing should be performed in the following situations:

- Administration of blood and blood components
- Sampling of blood
- Administration of incompatible medications or solutions
- Intermittent therapy
- Converting the VAD from continuous to intermittent therapies.

Patency flushing is performed at established intervals determined by organizational policy and procedure and the patient's condition. Acceptable flush solutions are saline (preservative-free 0.9% sodium chloride, injection) and heparin in the lowest concentration to achieve patency, while not affecting the patient's clotting factors. Many organizations flush intermittent peripheral devices with 0.9% sodium chloride solution only. Most studies that have compared the use of normal saline versus heparin recommend normal saline for use with peripheral VADs (Hankins et al., 2001). The volume of the flush should be equal to two times the volume capacity of the catheter plus any add-on devices that are attached to the system.

The equipment being used will dictate the correct flushing procedure. If positive pressure is to be exerted to prevent reflux of blood in the catheter lumen, then a forward motion is applied to the syringe plunger as it is removed from the injection port, or the clamping mechanism on the device is activated prior to removal of the syringe.

An occluded or partially occluded catheter should never be forcibly flushed to restore patency because of the potential risk of embolizing the contents into the patient's circulation. The size of the syringe must be considered, because the smaller the syringe, the greater the pressure exerted on the catheter. Excessive pressure may cause the catheter or the vessel to rupture.

Compatibility flushing is accomplished by using 0.9% sodium chloride solution before and after medication administration. Flushing the catheter should prevent incompatible medications and solutions from forming precipitates that can occlude the device. When heparin is used to complete the flushing procedure, *SASH* criteria are used, as outlined in Chart 22–2.

Documentation

Accurate documentation in the patient's medical record objectively describes the care rendered and the patient's response. It also allows for tracking patient outcomes and monitoring care. Chart 22–3 (p. 528) lists the pertinent information that should be documented when an infusion therapy-related procedure has been performed

■ Complications Associated with Infusion Therapy

Due to the invasive nature of infusion therapy, there is a risk for the development of complications that range from minor to severe problems. Complications increase hospital stays, length of therapy, cost of treatment, and nursing responsibilities, and can put the patient at risk for other medical problems. Most infusion-related complications are preventable, but knowledge and understanding of the risks involved with infusion therapy and the use of measures to prevent their occurrence can eliminate many of the problems associated with this treatment. If appropriate interventions are not implemented in a timely manner to treat serious complications, death can result.

Complications associated with infusion therapy are classified by their location. Local complications are generally recognized at the site of venipuncture or occur as a result of mechanical failure. Timely recognition and nursing intervention can often prevent escalation into more serious occurrences. Systemic complications are defined as those that occur within the vascular system distant from the venipuncture site. Although these complications are less common than local complications, they are often more difficult to treat. Prevention of complications is a primary responsibility of the nurse caring for the infusion patient.

 CHART 22–2　**Intermittent VAD Flushing: The SASH Criteria**

S: Saline

A: Administer medication/solution

S: Saline

H: Heparin (if necessary)

CHART 22–3 **Documentation for Insertion and Removal of VADs**

- Patient consent and education
- Variations in the procedure such as patient sensitivity or allergy to preparatory agents, latex, or securement adhesives
- Use of anesthetics for preprocedure medications
- Size, length, and type of catheter
- Name of vein used for access and number of insertion attempts (successful and unsuccessful)
- Securement method and dressing
- Administration set, extension equipment, and access caps used
- Flush or infusate initiation
- Patient's response to the procedure
- Name and title of the nurse

Similar documentation should occur when a VAD is removed including:

- Patient consent and education
- Size, length, and type of catheter and condition (e.g., was the catheter intact or fractured upon removal?)
- Condition of the venipuncture site (evidence of erythema, drainage, bleeding, skin tears)
- Dressing materials applied
- Patient's response to the procedure
- Name and title of the nurse

Local Complications

Local complications are usually associated with mechanical failure of the infusion system or traumatic injury to the vasculature. Mechanical difficulties may lead to the inability to deliver or infuse solutions and medications to the patient as prescribed. Trauma to the vasculature may occur with unskilled venipuncture techniques, patient agitation, and noncompliance with infusion therapy. The injured vein will become edematous as a result, which can lead to interruption in the infusion prescription, tissue injury, phlebitis, thrombus formation, and possibly sepsis.

Mechanical Complications

Mechanical complications usually are the result of failure of the infusion administration system to deliver the prescribed therapy, as opposed to the venous access. They are typically the most easy to identify and correct. Areas to be evaluated when determining the causal factors include the patient and the cannulated extremity, the venipuncture site, the catheter, the administration set, and the infusate container and its contents.

The patient's extremity should be checked for constricting clothing, identification bands or bracelets, jewelry, tapes, physical positioning, and restraints. The catheter–skin junction at the venipuncture site and the immediate surrounding area should be assessed for swelling that can impede flow. Verification of catheter placement should be confirmed prior to initiation and periodically throughout the infusion period. A catheter that is inserted so that the tip is against a valve or venous bifurcation may impede the infusion by slowing or stopping the flow. The catheter may become dislodged, bent, or kinked due to patient activity or inadequate device securement.

Placement of a catheter in an area of flexion may adversely affect the infusion rate and the dwell time of the device. If the flow rate slows or increases, the catheter can be stabilized by applying an armboard. The use of restraints and armboards needs to be in accordance with the organization's policies.

Administration sets can easily be pinched, bent, kinked, or crimped. The infusion pathway will be affected and not allow delivery of fluid from the infusion container to the patient. In-line filters or add-on equipment may become clogged due to undissolved medications or precipitate formation from the introduction of incompatible medications into the administration system.

The infusate container and its contents need to be assessed as a contributing factor of mechanical failure. Inadequate height of the fluid container in relation to the patient and catheter insertion site can adversely affect gravity flow, or an empty container can lead to diminished flow or cessation of flow. Rigid containers, such as those made from glass, should be checked for the presence of a venting mechanism. Soft, flexible plastic containers do not need to be vented. The entry port on a container must be completely penetrated in order for the solution to infuse into the patient. Refrigerated solutions need to be brought to room temperature prior to administration. Cold infusates not only cause discomfort for the patient but also may cause venospasm resulting in vasoconstriction and decrease or cessation of flow.

Catheter-Related Complications

Complications related specifically to the vascular access device versus those related to the infusion system and infusate are readily identifiable. Addressing catheter-related complications should begin with the evaluation of the inserter's skill and technique.

Bruising

Bruising (skin discoloration due to infiltration of blood into the subcutaneous tissue) may be attributed to unskilled insertion technique, tourniquet placement (too tight), vigorous device securement and restraining techniques, or preexisting poor skin integrity. For example, patients who are prescribed long-term steroid or anticoagulant therapies are more susceptible to bruising.

Bruising may be particularly notable after multiple attempts at device insertion during a prescribed therapy period. These injuries adversely impact future visualization of intended venipuncture sites. Bruising may predispose the patient to development of cellulitis and other localized infections. The term *ecchymosis* is used to define generalized bleeding into the tissues, whereas *hematoma* describes uncontrolled bleeding at the venipuncture site that usually creates a hard painful lump (Figure 22–20 ■).

Infiltration

Infiltration, as mentioned earlier, is the inadvertent administration of nonvesicant solutions or medications into surrounding tissues. It is manifested by swelling either along the venous pathway or generally located around the venipuncture site (Figure 22–21 ■). The patient may complain of "heaviness" or coldness in the extremity, or may observe generalized swelling. The patient may realize that he cannot remove a ring or other piece of jewelry or cannot close the hand. The extremity will appear enlarged with the skin appearing stretched or shiny. The venipuncture site dressing may appear taut.

The amount of discomfort experienced by the patient is proportional to the type of infusate, rate of infusion, and infusion

FIGURE 22–20 ■ Hematoma.
Source: Johnson & Johnson—Ethicon Inc.

FIGURE 22–21 ■ Intravenous infiltration.
Source: Johnson & Johnson Medical, Inc. 1997. Used by permission of the copyright owner

history. Isotonic solutions generally do not produce much discomfort when an infiltration occurs. Solutions with acidic or alkaline pH or those that are slightly more hypertonic are more irritating and usually cause discomfort (Hankins et al., 2001). If left undetected, infiltration may cause compression of pressure-sensitive tissues such as neurological and arterial structures.

A complete assessment of the patient, the venipuncture site and surrounding area, the involved extremity, and the infusion system may be necessary to determine the presence of an infiltration. The site around the tip of the catheter and the extremity should be inspected for swelling, blanching, stretched skin, firm tissues, and coolness. It may be helpful to compare the site with the same area on the opposite extremity. If both extremities appear edematous, the patient's medical status should be evaluated.

In determining the presence of an infiltration, pressure should be applied to the vein with a finger or tourniquet about 5 cm (2 in.) proximal to the insertion site. If the catheter is in the vein, manual pressure will slow or stop the infusion. If the infusion continues despite venous obstruction, an infiltration has occurred.

If infiltration is noted or suspected, discontinue the infusion immediately and remove the catheter. Elevation of the affected extremity relieves patient discomfort and assists in absorption of excess fluids and improving circulation.

Preventive measures can minimize the severity of the infiltration. When inserting a VAD, areas of flexion should be avoided if possible. The catheter should be secured adequately and the site protected from excessive movement or pressure by use of an armboard or restraint.

 CRITICAL ALERT *Be aware that despite the presence of a positive blood aspirate, an infiltration may have occurred. Remove the VAD immediately and restart it, preferably in the opposite extremity.*

Extravasation

Extravasation is the inadvertent administration of a vesicant solution or medication into the surrounding tissues. The solution produces tissue damage by causing blister-like formations with subsequent tissue sloughing (Figure 22–22 ■). Initially the patient may complain of pain or burning along the vein pathway or at the venipuncture site. Fluid can also seep into adjacent tissues as it passes through a previous proximal venipuncture site.

Tissue sloughing may take several weeks to occur as it progresses from edema and erythema to necrosis. Necrosis may involve not only superficial skin layers but may penetrate into basement supporting tissues, muscles, tendons, and bones. The severity of the injury is related to the type, concentration, and volume of the medication or solution infiltrated. This is an adverse condition that could severely impact the future of the patient, resulting in loss of the extremity, prolonged hospitalization, protracted treatments involving surgery and rehabilitation, and potentially loss of life.

When an extravasation is suspected, discontinue the infusion immediately and remove the catheter. Treatment protocols established in written policies and procedures are initiated and a new site is established, preferably in the opposite extremity or in a site above and away from the extravasated site.

Prevention is the key in minimizing extravasation episodes. Only qualified, skilled nurses who have demonstrated proficiency and knowledge in infusion therapy along with knowledge of medications that have the potential for causing injury should be allowed to administer vesicant medications. The venipuncture site must be observed for signs of pending extravasation prior to, during, and after the infusion treatment. Many organizations require

FIGURE 22–22 ■ Extravasation.
Source: Johnson & Johnson Medical, Inc. 1997. Used by permission of the copyright owner

that a new VAD be placed prior to the administration of vesicants in order to avoid questionable patency issues.

If a vesicant medication is delivered directly into a vein via a syringe, the patency of the catheter should be ascertained intermittently throughout the infusion by gently pulling back on the syringe plunger to confirm the presence of a blood return. The catheter should be appropriately secured so as to prevent movement in the vein, while allowing for frequent visualization of the site and venous pathway throughout the administration procedure. Areas of flexion, bony prominences, and the hands should be avoided as access sites for vesicant therapies. Consideration should be given to the possibility of using a CVAD for vesicant therapies given the chronicity of many antimicrobial, inotropic, or antineoplastic therapies.

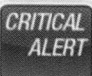 **CRITICAL ALERT** *Continuous observation of the venipuncture site is necessary prior to, during, and after administration of a vesicant. Have knowledge of the protocols needed to treat an extravasation.*

Phlebitis

Phlebitis is defined as an inflammation of the vein's tunica intima (Figure 22–23 ■). It is a common catheter-related complication that is often associated with erythema along the venous pathway, discomfort and tenderness of varying intensities, and inflammation and warmth at the site. Causes of phlebitis include:

- Inappropriate catheter length, gauge, or material
- Inexperience at insertion by the nurse
- Inappropriate site selection
- Prolonged dwell time for the catheter
- Ineffective device securement
- Chemical properties of the infusate(s)
- Patient age, infusion history, compliance, existing disease, or conditions.

Phlebitis can be classified by causative factors: chemical, mechanical, bacterial, and post-infusion phlebitis.

Chemical phlebitis is often associated with infusates with varying ranges of pH values or osmolarities. Improper admixing

or dilution of some medications can result in incompatibilities that may cause irritation. Infusion rates may cause irritation. For example, rapid fluid delivery can cause a higher concentration of medication within a localized area, resulting in poor or inadequate hemodilution leading to inflammation. Particulate matter has been demonstrated to cause irritation of the vein wall.

Mechanical phlebitis is primarily associated with the catheter, its insertion, and the selected site. Using areas of flexion and too large a gauge size for the intended vein and prescribed therapy can result in the development of mechanical phlebitis. Poor device securement allows telescoping of the catheter within the vein. Patient noncompliance insofar as unrestricted physical activity will enhance the development of phlebitis. The skill of the nurse inserting the device may contribute to the development of mechanical phlebitis.

Bacterial phlebitis is associated with infectious processes. It is a very serious condition because it may progress to a systemic infection that is potentially life threatening. Hand hygiene and the observance of aseptic techniques throughout the catheter insertion procedure are mandatory for the prevention of catheter- and infusion-related infections. All infusion-related equipment must be inspected prior to use to confirm product integrity and detect any presence of contaminants. Expiration dates, damaged packaging, particulate matter, and presence of color or cloudiness are signs that may indicate compromised products. Appropriate site selection and preparation reduces the opportunity for catheter-related infections to occur. Shaving the intended venipuncture site is not recommended because of the potential to cause microabrasions that would allow for the entry of microorganisms into the circulation. If hair removal is necessary, clipping should be performed.

Postinfusion phlebitis is commonly seen 2 to 4 days after the catheter has been removed. Occurrence is often attributed to the original insertion technique, patient condition, condition of the vein that was cannulated, the properties of the infusate that was delivered, size and length of the catheter, and the dwell time of the device. It is recommended that the identification of phlebitis be standardized and classified according to the phlebitis scale (Chart 22–4) published in the *Infusion Nursing Standards of Practice* (INS, 2006a).

FIGURE 22–23 ■ Phlebitis.
Source: Johnson & Johnson Medical, Inc. 1997. Used by permission of the copyright owner

CHART 22–4	**Phlebitis Scale**

Grade	Clinical Criteria
0	No symptoms
1	Erythema at access site with or without pain
2	Pain at access site with erythema and/or edema
3	Pain at access site with erythema and/or edema Streak formation Palpable venous cord
4	Pain at access site with erythema and/or edema Streak formation Palpable venous cord >1 in. in length Purulent drainage

Source: From Infusion Nurses Society. Infusion Nursing Standards of Practice. JIN Supplement. 29 (IS) Standard 53: Phlebitis, p. S59

The most effective treatment for phlebitis is prevention. Venipuncture sites should be assessed frequently. At the first signs of phlebitis, remove and relocate the catheter. Gently palpate the venous pathway at the tip of the catheter to ascertain tenderness while observing for warmth, edema, and induration. If an infection is suspected, remove the catheter and obtain a health care provider order to culture the catheter tip. Establish a new venipuncture site, preferably in the opposite extremity. Document the degree of phlebitis in the patient's medical record and monitor the site frequently at specified intervals.

Thrombosis

Thrombosis is the formation of a blood clot within the vein. It is caused by an injury to the cells lining the vein, usually occurring at the junction where the catheter comes into contact with the tunica intima of the vessel. The causes of thrombus formation are similar to those of phlebitis:

- Poor insertion technique
- Multiple attempts at venipuncture
- Inappropriate catheter gauge and length for the patient and/or prescribed therapy
- Poor circulation
- Administration of incompatible medications and solutions, or those with extreme variations in pH and osmolarity
- Catheter material.

Thrombophlebitis is the combination of thrombus formation in association with inflammation of the vein. Figure 22–23 ■ shows an arm with phlebitis from an intravenous infusion complication. The inflammation may be first detected along the venous pathway, followed by edema, pain, and warmth. The vein will become markedly hardened as the thrombosis progresses.

The patient should be assessed for causative factors that may lead to the development of thrombosis and thrombophlebitis. Slowing or cessation of the infusion may be the first sign that complications are developing. Mechanical problems should be eliminated. If the infusion is being administered via an EID, occlusion alarms may offer an important clue. Patient complaints of discomfort and generalized swelling in the involved extremity are important clinical indications of this pending complication.

The degree of circulatory involvement should be monitored because deprivation of blood flow could seriously impact the functional use of the extremity. Thrombus formation has also been a precursor to systemic infections and embolic events. If thrombosis or thrombophlebitis is detected, remove the catheter and establish a new venipuncture site in the opposite extremity, if possible.

To prevent these complications, skilled insertion techniques are necessary. Avoid cannulation of veins in the lower extremities, particularly in adults, because these veins are very small and allow pooling of blood with subsequent damage to the vein intima and clot formation. Appropriate catheter selection, avoidance of insertions over bony prominences and points of flexion, and proper catheter securement are nursing interventions that have proven to be effective preventive measures against thrombus formation.

Infection

Infection is considered a localized event when it occurs at the insertion site. Evidence of phlebitis may not be apparent. Typical signs of infection such as erythema, tenderness, and drainage will be detected at the catheter–skin junction. The cause of this type of infection is usually due to a faulty insertion technique, such as nonadherence to aseptic technique during catheter insertion, site care, or device removal. The use of contaminated equipment, improper hand hygiene, or patient manipulation may also contribute to the development of an infection. There are instances when infection becomes apparent only after catheter removal.

If an infection is suspected, remove the catheter immediately, obtain a health care provider order to culture the site, and establish a new site. Place a sterile dressing over the site, notify the health care provider, and document appropriately. Topical antimicrobial ointments with sterile dressings may be ordered. Antimicrobial infusions may be required, and surgical intervention may be necessary to treat the infection.

Occlusion

Occlusions are caused by thrombus formation, drug precipitates, or lipid deposits. Slowing of the flow or cessation of the flow from the solution container and an inability to flush the device are signs of possible occlusion. Catheters will become occluded if infusion containers are allowed to "run dry" or when incorrect flushing techniques are used. The administration of incompatible infusates may contribute to the development, causing occlusion of the fluid pathway.

When attempting to restore catheter patency, never forcibly flush the catheter because catheter fracture or embolization of the catheter contents can occur. The occluded catheter must be removed and another site located for the continuation of the prescribed therapy. Containers of solution should be replaced when the contents are nearly empty. Frequent monitoring of the entire infusion system should occur at specified intervals. Establish compatibility of prescribed infusates prior to initiation. Follow policies and procedures for flushing intermittent infusion devices.

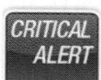 *Never use force when flushing an occluded VAD. Administer the appropriate flushing solution and technique to maintain VAD patency.*

Systemic Complications

Systemic complications are those complications that occur in the circulation and have the potential to affect the entire body. Although these complications can occur in patients receiving peripheral infusion therapy, they are more frequently seen in those receiving therapies through a CVAD.

Air Embolism

The symptoms of an air embolism, which is caused by entry of air into the vascular system, include chest pain, shortness of breath, shoulder or low back pain, anxiety, cyanosis, hypotension, weak rapid pulse, and loss of consciousness. If left untreated, shock or cardiac arrest may result.

If an air embolism is suspected, the patient should be placed on the left side in the Trendelenburg position. Identify the source of air intake and correct the problem immediately. If the air embolism results from an open or leaking administration system, the administration set should be changed immediately and replaced with a new one flushed with solution.

Measures need to be incorporated to prevent the occurrence of an air embolism.

Administration sets should be clamped when they are being changed. Solution containers should be changed before they are completely empty. Luer-Lok connections should be used to prevent the accidental disconnection of infusion systems. Infusion systems need to be purged of air prior to the initiation of an infusion. Infusions using EIDs with "air-in-line" alarm systems should be used.

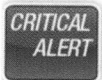 **CRITICAL ALERT** *Accidental disconnection of the administration set can lead to an air embolism. The nurse must be able to recognize symptoms of an air embolism and be prepared to administer resuscitative measures.*

Catheter Embolism

A **catheter embolism** occurs when a piece of catheter is fractured and enters the circulatory system. The catheter may block a major vein, causing loss of circulation, or may travel to the heart, causing cardiac irritability and cardiac arrest. Catheter fracture is commonly associated with poor insertion technique such as retracting a catheter back through an introducer, partially withdrawing a stylet from a catheter, then reinserting and advancing the now-torn catheter, or forcibly flushing an occluded catheter.

Signs that a peripheral catheter has broken are separation of the catheter and hub or a severed catheter on withdrawal from the venipuncture site. A rupture of a CVAD may not be noted until the device is used and the patient is symptomatic. If a catheter embolism is suspected, the nurse should observe the patient for signs of cyanosis, chest pain, hypotension, increased central venous pressure, tachycardia, fainting, and loss of consciousness.

For a peripheral catheter that has embolized, immediate interventions need to be initiated. Secure a tourniquet on the patient's arm proximal to the venipuncture site, and place the patient on bed rest to minimize the movement of the catheter within the vascular system. If a central venous catheter embolism is suspected, place the patient on bed rest, notify the health care provider, and monitor the patient for signs of shock. Radiographic studies will be ordered to detect the location of the catheter fragment. Medical intervention will depend on the catheter location.

Knowledge of measures to employ to prevent a catheter embolus is important. Inspect catheters for defects before use. Never pull through-the-needle catheters back through the needle once it has been inserted into the patient. Also, never withdraw or reinsert over-the-needle catheters once they have been partially or fully threaded in the vein.

Pulmonary Edema

Pulmonary edema is caused by the presence of excess fluid volume in the circulatory system. If the condition persists, the patient can develop heart failure, shock, and cardiac arrest. This condition is frequently caused by too rapid infusion rates or too much volume infused within a given time period. Patients prone to developing pulmonary edema are pediatric and elderly patients, and those patients with cardiac and renal disease.

Signs of pulmonary edema include shortness of breath, cough, increased pulse, dyspnea, hypertension, moist rales, frothy sputum, and periorbital edema. If pulmonary edema is suspected, the infusion should be slowed immediately to a rate that maintains vascular access, and the patient placed in high Fowler's position. The health care provider should be notified and oxygen administered as ordered. Emergency treatment may include the administration of diuretics, vasodilators, and opiates. Chapter 36 includes an in-depth discussion of pulmonary edema.

Before initiating infusion therapy, assess the patient's cardiac and respiratory history, ability to tolerate fluid volume, and any previous problems associated with fluid volume while receiving infusion therapy. Closely monitor patients receiving infusion therapy for tolerance of the amounts of fluids being administered. Maintain infusion rates as ordered and do not increase rates for solutions that are behind schedule. Use volumetric devices and infusion controllers when accurate measurements are required or when the patient's condition warrants management to prevent fluid overload.

Septicemia

Septicemia is caused when pathogenic bacteria enter the bloodstream. Contributing factors placing the patient at risk for septicemia can lead to increasing the patient's susceptibility to infection and allowing microorganisms to enter the infusion system. Risk factors associated with septicemia are outlined in the Risk Factors box.

Early symptoms of septicemia must be evaluated for possible causes. Fever in a patient with a CVAD should be attributed to the device until proven otherwise. Erythema at the insertion site could indicate an infectious process that could lead to sepsis. The health care provider should be notified and cultures of the catheter and the patient's blood may be ordered.

The most effective treatment for septicemia is prevention. Appropriate hand hygiene and strict adherence to aseptic technique should be used when initiating or manipulating an infusion system. All solutions and equipment should be inspected for intact packaging and product integrity. Venipuncture sites should be disinfected with approved antimicrobial agents. Catheter sites are to be rotated, dressings and administration sets changed, and sites

RISK FACTORS for the Development of Septicemia

- Patient susceptibility
- Alteration in host defenses
- Presence of other infectious processes
- Contaminated infusion equipment
- Inexperience of the nurse inserting the VAD
- Inadequate site preparation
- Manipulations of the administration delivery system
- Dwell time of the device
- Lack of or improper hand hygiene

monitored according to the *Infusion Nursing Standards of Practice* (INS, 2006a) and organizational policy and procedure.

Allergic Reactions

An allergic reaction is a response to a medication or solution to which the patient is sensitive. The most common reactions are those seen as a result of administering antimicrobial, biologic, and blood products. The patient may experience chills, fever, urticaria, erythema, itching, shortness of breath, or wheezing. Patients should be assessed for a complete allergy history. Use of identification bracelets and special identifying labels on the patient's medical record serve to inform all health care providers about patient allergies.

 **CRITICAL ALERT** *Be aware of the risk of an allergic reaction occurring when administering antimicrobial, biologic, or blood products. Maintain vascular access and be prepared to treat an anaphylactic event.*

If an allergic reaction is suspected, the infusion should be stopped immediately, the administration set and solution container changed, and vascular access maintained to allow for emergent treatment for possible anaphylactic shock. The health care provider should be notified and the nurse prepared to administer resuscitative measures.

Needlestick Complications

Sharps-related injuries take place at an alarming rate with an estimate of more than 800,000 needlesticks occurring annually among more than 5.6 million health care workers (Perry, Parker, & Jagger, 2003). Unfortunately, it is also estimated that at least one-half of these injuries go unreported. Additionally, of those injured, more than 1,000 reportedly contract a serious infection from the injury (Perry et al., 2003). Data collection for statistical information concentrates on the categories listed in Chart 22–5 for risk of injury with nurses reporting the most percutaneous injuries at 43.6% (Perry et al., 2003). The International Healthcare Worker Safety Center at the University of Virginia Health System provides extensive resources on sharps safety and occupational exposure prevention: tools for conducting exposure surveillance, a list of safety-engineered sharp devices, and statistics.

The Needlestick Safety and Prevention Act was signed into law November 6, 2000, and was incorporated into the revised bloodborne pathogen directive published January 2001 by the Occupational Safety and Health Administration (OSHA). The act changed OSHA's original 1991 *Bloodborne Pathogens Standards* from a directive to law, enforceable in the same manner as any other safety law enforced by OSHA. This legislation, effective on April 18, 2001, with final enforcement and implementation July 17, 2001, clarified OSHA's previous bloodborne standard that required health care workers to use devices that

CHART 22–5 **Data Collection Categories**

- Injection devices
- Blood-drawing and vascular access devices
- Glass containers
- Surgical instruments

eliminate or minimize chances of exposure or injury by needles and other sharps.

The needlestick act was introduced as a response to two issues: increased concern over inadvertent or accidental needlestick injuries in health care settings, and advancements in technology to prevent health care professionals, patients, and caregivers from sharps-related injuries. The importance of using safety-engineered technologies in an effort to deliver safe infusion therapies is not diminished with the implementation of the act, because it also requires employers currently covered by the *Bloodborne Pathogens Standards* to continually evaluate and use devices that reduce the risk of injuries.

Needleless Infusion Systems

Needlestick injuries can occur as a result of unsafe products or improper use of a product. Factors that contribute to exposure to body fluids include equipment without adequate safety features, failure to observe standard precautions, and actively engaging in hazardous activities such as recapping needles. Needled syringes, winged steel infusion sets, vacuum blood collection tubes, and vascular access devices are often associated with high rates of injury. Other devices or equipment such as infusion connectors and Luer slip tips are considered high risk due to the potential for inadvertent separation of the equipment during a procedure. Needles manufactured as permanent components attached to infusion administration sets are difficult to dispose of without causing injury. Equipment such as blood collection systems may cause inadvertent exposure due to disassembly practices.

Improperly disposing of needles or other sharps often places at risk many employees, patients, and visitors within the health care organization. Expended sharps should never be temporarily placed on food service trays or stuck into bed linens prior to disposal because those procedures greatly increase the risk of injury to others. Procedures that require the use of multiple needles such as flushing intermittent infusion devices are often associated with injury. Needles and syringes should be disposed of immediately after use, and not stored in a uniform pocket to be dropped into the sharps box when next at the medication cart or closet.

Drawing blood poses special risks to the health care worker. Vacuum tubes are frequently associated with higher than normally expected injury rates; recapping needles and removing needles from reusable tube holders for disposal hold risk for personal injury.

Other procedures can pose a risk of exposure to blood or injury. Glass-based tubes may crack and break during phlebotomy procedures or during transport. Administration of infusates and medications presents special risks when piggybacking into primary infusion systems or when connecting to intermittent infusion devices. Equipment with longer lengths of extension tubing can become entangled and expose the clinician and other staff members to sharps-related injury. Injuries may occur when equipment is not properly attached and must be forced apart, or when unfamiliar equipment is not used appropriately. Nurses who are not skilled at certain tasks, such as inserting infusion catheters or performing such procedures on specific patient populations such as pediatrics or confused, combative, or elderly patients, are more susceptible to injury.

In response to these issues, manufacturers have devised engineered controls for sharps injury protection. Engineered safety products have demonstrated a reduction in needlestick injuries and subsequent exposure to bloodborne pathogens. Needleless systems are examples of engineering controls. A **needleless system** is a device that does not use needles for the collection of body fluids or withdrawal of such fluids after initial access is established or for the administration of medications or fluids or any other procedure involving the potential for occupational exposure to pathogens due to percutaneous injuries from contaminated sharps.

More than 200 needleless products have been approved by the Food and Drug Administration (FDA). These products are classified by the mode of engineered safety incorporated into the device or equipment:

- Elimination of sharps:
  - ✓ Needleless injection system
  - ✓ Presplit septum and blunted cannula
  - ✓ Threaded Luer-Lok adapter.
- Passive (the engineered safety mechanism is a component within the system):
  - ✓ Recessed needles
  - ✓ Self-advancing sheathing syringe
  - ✓ Self-blunting cannula
  - ✓ Vascular access device.
- Active (the safety mechanism must be activated by the nurse):
  - ✓ User-activated needle cover
  - ✓ Sheathing vascular access device, winged steel infusion set, syringe.
- Disposal (safe disposal via nonpermeable, tamper-proof, puncture-resistant containers):
  - ✓ Mailbox or drop-in style.

Using prefilled syringes and other commercially prepared solutions and medications negates the occurrence of injuries during preparation. Needle-free systems using vial adapters can prevent percutaneous injury. Vacuum tubes for laboratory analysis are now available in glass-free materials. Sharps disposal containers should be at eye level and near the patient's bedside. They should also be emptied according to manufacturer's instructions, specifically when the container is three-quarters full. All sharps are to be accounted for at the completion of any procedure. Needles are not to be recapped.

The use of needleless systems does not negate the fact that sterile technique is *always* observed when accessing and manipulating the infusion delivery system. Infection control practices must be adhered to throughout all infusion therapy administrations.

Nursing Management

Infusion therapy is prescribed to deliver many types of solutions and medications to patients in all care settings via vascular and nonvascular routes. Disruptions and variances in accepted standardized care and maintenance practices will adversely impact the patient by jeopardizing the safety, therapy delivery, and prescription compliance. Additionally, ineffective nursing skill and care competencies will negatively impact intended outcomes. Thus, the nurse must possess a variety of skills and knowledge in order to safely manage patients receiving infusion therapies. These include:

- Knowledge of aseptic technique in order to prevent both local and systemic infections
- Skill in venipuncture
- Knowledge of care and maintenance procedures to preserve vascular access sites and devices
- Knowledge of the impact that solutions and infusion rates have on the body systems, especially in the presence of disease
- Ability to identify and treat catheter-related complications
- Critical thinking skills necessary to troubleshoot equipment problems when they occur
- Knowledge of the impact of medication administration via the intravenous route, including administering more than one medication simultaneously
- Ability to provide emotional support to the patient and family members.

The Nursing Process: Patient Care Plan uses the nursing process to provide a comprehensive plan of care for patients receiving infusion therapy.

Collaborative Management

With emphasis on clinical care and performance competence, collaboration with members of the health care team and the patient and her family will provide the patient with specialized support through education and technical expertise. Members of the health care team, include the primary care physician, the nurse and members of the infusion team, the infection control practitioner, the pharmacist, and the case manager, will collaborate on specific issues such as appropriate VAD selection for the prescribed therapy and home-based infusion services and other indicated support systems as appropriate.

Once the health care provider discusses the purpose of the treatment and orders the patient's therapy, the nurse is responsible for the continued assessment of the patient's infusion needs. The nurse educates the patient about the treatment plan and determines the level of participation the patient can be engaged in. The patient's caregiver is also included in the education process and taught the necessary skills if needed to assist the patient with the infusion care.

Others on the health care team involved with infusion therapy include infection control practitioners and pharmacists. The infection control specialist monitors sharps injuries, infection rates, and disseminated infection control practices. Pharmacists have knowledge of medication and solution concentrations and compatibility issues. The case manager plays an integral role in the care coordination for the patient within the care setting. Knowledge of the intricacies of insurance benefits, availability of health care providers, and logistics coordination activities falls within the purview of the case manager.

NURSING PROCESS: Patient Care Plan for Infusion Therapy

Assessment of Potential for Injury Secondary to Placement and Dwell Time of VAD and Disruption of the Infusion Delivery System

Subjective Data:

Do you know why you are having infusion therapy, and how long do you expect to have it?

Have you ever had an intravenous catheter? If so, did you ever experience any problems with it?

What "handedness" are you?

Have you ever had a stroke (CVA) or surgery on your arm or chest, such as mastectomy, fracture, vascular surgery, AV fistula or shunt?

Are you sensitive to tape or any antiseptic agents?

Do you use any ambulatory aids?

Objective Data:

Does the patient have a preference for VAD location?

Does the patient have observable physical limitations or conditions that will impact site selection, site preparation, and dwell time of the VAD?

Nursing Assessment and Diagnoses	Outcomes and Evaluation Parameters	Planning and Interventions with *Rationales*
Nursing Diagnosis: *Deficient Knowledge* related to therapeutic infusion management and maintenance practices	**Outcomes:** Patient and/or caregiver will successfully demonstrate VAD care and maintenance practices. Patient and/or caregiver will be educated in disease process and progression, signs and symptoms of distress, and indicated infusion-specific treatment regimen(s). *Evaluation Parameter:* Verbalizes understanding of complications associated with infusion therapy.	**Interventions and *Rationales:*** Patient/caregiver will be able to: Explain rationale for VAD placement. Explain rationale for hand hygiene. Describe appropriate condition of VAD location, i.e., intact dressing, clean securement device, intact skin integrity. Describe symptoms of pending complications secondary to VAD dwell, i.e., infiltration, phlebitis, leaking of fluids (bloody drainage, exudates) from catheter–skin junction, pain, and erythema. Describe signs and symptoms of potential infusion-related complications, i.e., air in the line, occlusion, empty infusion container, retrograde blood flow, nonflow of infusate, alarming of infusion assistive device. *Patient and/or caregiver will be able to identify signs and symptoms of possible catheter-related complications through education processes. Patient/caregiver will be able to identify and seek emergency assistance as appropriate.*

Assessment of Knowledge Deficit Related to Infection Control Measures Pertaining to Infusion-Specific Care and Maintenance Practices

Subjective Data:

Have you ever had an infection related to an earlier infusion?

Have you needed an infusion catheter replaced due to an occlusion or infiltration, infection, or catheter malposition?

Have you ever been assessed for a VAD reserved for long-term therapy such as a PICC or implanted port?

Objective Data:

Is the VAD dressing dry and intact?

Is there presence of erythema, swelling, or drainage along the vascular pathway or at the catheter–skin junction?

Is the patient complaining of discomfort or pain along the vascular pathway or at the catheter–skin junction?

Are the EID alarms going off frequently for "occlusion" or "no flow"?

Is there a lack of blood return?

Nursing Assessment and Diagnoses	Outcomes and Evaluation Parameters	Planning and Interventions with *Rationales*
Nursing Diagnoses: Infection, risk for Injury, risk for	**Outcomes:** The VAD will dwell according to established organizational policies and procedures. The VAD will be asymptomatic for the length of dwell time. The patient will achieve intended infusion-related outcomes. *Evaluation Parameters:* The patient will be able to verbalize understanding of care and maintenance practices associated with the prescribed infusion therapy and mode of delivery to prevent catheter-related complications.	**Interventions and *Rationales:*** Patient/caregiver will be able to: Explain rationale for hand hygiene. Explain rationale for use of aseptic technique when changing infusion containers and administration sets. Explain rationale for use of antiseptic agent(s) when preparing injection cap/access port for injection. *Patient and/or caregiver will be able to identify signs and symptoms of possible infusion-related complications through education processes. Patient/caregiver will be able to identify and seek emergency assistance as appropriate. Patient and/or caregiver will be able to identify sources for information and nursing support, and will be able to make informed decisions regarding infusion care.*

(continued)

NURSING PROCESS: Patient Care Plan for Infusion Therapy—*Continued*

Assessment of Knowledge Deficit Related to Information Pertaining to Parenteral Medication Use and Administration at Home

Subjective Data:
Do you wear a hearing aid or glasses?
Do you have trouble using your hands due to disease (arthritis) or injury?
Do you have pets?
Do you have someone who can assist you at home?
Do you have running water, refrigeration, electricity, a telephone?
Can you read?
What is the language spoken in your home?
Do you know how long the doctor has prescribed this therapy?

Objective Data:
Do pediatric patients have arrangements for tutoring or for monitoring the infusion in the school setting?

Nursing Assessment and Diagnoses	Outcomes and Evaluation Parameters	Planning and Interventions with *Rationales*
Nursing Diagnosis: *Effective Therapeutic Regiment Management* related to home environment	**Outcome:** Patient and/or caregiver will successfully demonstrate infusion system care and maintenance practices, and safe infusion administration procedures. **Evaluation Parameter:** Patient demonstrates competency related to prescribed infusion therapy.	**Interventions and *Rationales:*** Patient and /or caregiver will be able to: Describe prescribed infusion treatment regimen including anticipated outcomes. Describe expected care and maintenance procedures for prescribed infusion therapy including, but not limited to: 1. Parenteral solution and/or medication use and action. 2. Storage of parenteral medication(s) and solution(s), and equipment. 3. Elements of effective infection control practices including hand hygiene, standard precautions and aseptic technique, and disposal of expended equipment and supplies. 4. Preparation and administration practices for infusion therapy. 5. Signs and symptoms of untoward medication reactions. 6. Use of infusion-specific equipment. *Patient and/or caregiver will successfully describe parenteral infusion treatment protocols and seek interventions and assistance as appropriate.* *Patient and/or caregiver education processes will be documented in the patient's permanent medical record.*

Research

Research within the specialty nursing field of infusion therapy is essential in order to advance the practice, but also to identify areas requiring specific data, supporting performance improvement indicators, and identifying concerns and considerations that affect anticipated outcomes and patient safety. Although ongoing assessment is critical for the patient receiving infusion prescriptions, post-therapy assessments and achievement and evaluation of indicators will continue to suggest improved methods of infusion care. Advances in technologies affecting infusion care delivery will need to be addressed in all care settings. Examples of promising areas of research are presented in the Research Opportunities and Clinical Impact box.

Summary

Infusion therapy will continue to be practiced in all care settings and administered to patient populations of all ages. Technologic advances affecting insertion, care and maintenance, and research-based practices will continue to shape this nursing specialty. Education and continued competence are necessary to keep nurses abreast of proper techniques and new technology that are essential components of the specialty practice of infusion therapy.

RESEARCH OPPORTUNITIES AND CLINICAL IMPACT RELATED TO INFUSION THERAPY

Research Area	Clinical Impact
Evaluate the process of early patient assessment related to VAD selection.	Timely initiation of therapy
	Appropriate site and VAD selection to preserve sites and minimize the number of venipunctures
	Patient education to promote therapy compliance
Determine the efficacy of saline versus heparin flushes of CVADs in the home care patient.	Prevention of VAD occlusion
	Continuation of therapy without impacting patient's clotting mechanisms
Determine whether a 72- to 96-hour site rotation interval for peripheral-short catheters is appropriate.	Site preservation
	To minimize number of venipunctures
	To decrease risks associated with catheter-related complications

NCLEX® REVIEW

1. A patient, being discharged, will need to receive antibiotic therapy for an additional three weeks. The peripheral vascular access device that would be the best for this patient would be:
   1. A peripheral-short catheter
   2. A winged steel infusion set
   3. A midline catheter
   4. A PICC line

2. A patient receiving parenteral fluids is prescribed an intravenous medication to be infused every 6 hours. Which of the following infusion devices should the nurse use for this medication?
   1. Stop cock
   2. Extension set
   3. Elastomeric balloon
   4. Secondary administration set

3. The staff development department is planning an annual skills review day for the basics of intravenous therapy. If the Infusion Nursing Standards of Practice are being followed, the purpose of this skills day would be to:
   1. Ensure all nurses follow standard precautions.
   2. Preserve the patient's right to safe, quality care and protect the nurse who administers infusion therapy.
   3. Ensure the nurses are in compliance with all regulatory agencies.
   4. Ensure the nurses' skill levels are adequate.

4. A patient is prescribed parenteral fluid therapy. Which of the following should the nurse do first?
   1. Wash hands.
   2. Gather the equipment to insert the peripheral access device.
   3. Prepare the flush to use once the peripheral access device is in place.
   4. Review the procedure with the patient and obtain consent.

5. A patient receiving parenteral fluid therapy complains of the arm "feeling cold" and the dressing "feeling tight." What should the nurse do?
   1. Check for a blood return in the catheter.
   2. Stop the infusion and remove the catheter.
   3. Turn off the infusion, reposition the catheter.
   4. Change the dressing and observe the site.

Answers for review questions appear in Appendix D

KEY TERMS

adapter *p.513*
add-on devices *p.520*
administration set *p.520*
air embolism *p.515*
arterial-venous shunts *p.518*
bacterial phlebitis *p.530*
bevel *p.513*
catheter *p.512*

catheter embolism *p.532*
central vascular access device (CVAD) *p.515*
chemical phlebitis *p.530*
continuous subcutaneous infusion (CSI) *p.518*
dialysis catheter *p.518*
drip factor *p.520*
dual-channel pump *p.524*

dwell *p.512*
elastomeric balloon *p.523*
electronic infusion device (EID) *p.523*
extension set *p.522*
extravasation *p.529*
filter *p.522*
flashback chamber *p.513*
flow control device *p.521*

PEARSON
EXPLORE mynursingkit™

MyNursingKit is your one stop for online chapter review materials and resources. Prepare for success with additional NCLEX®-style practice questions, interactive assignments and activities, web links, animations and videos, and more!

Register your access code from the front of your book at
www.mynursingkit.com

REFERENCES

Boyce, J. M., & Pittet, D. (2002). Guideline for hand hygiene in health-care settings: Recommendations of the Healthcare Infection Control Practices Advisory Committee and the HICPAC/SHEA/APIC/IDSA Hand Hygiene Task Force. *Infection Control and Hospital Epidemiology, 23*(12 Suppl.), S1–S40.

Centers for Disease Control and Prevention. (2002). *CDC Guidelines for the Prevention of Intravascular Catheter-Related Infections.* Retrieved June 12, 2008, from http://www.cdc.gov/ncidod/dhqp/gl_intravascular.html

Gillies, D., O'Riordan, L., Carr, D., Frost, J., Gunning, R., & O'Brien, I. (2003). Gauze and tape and transparent polyurethane dressings for central venous catheters. *Cochrane Database of Systematic Reviews, 4,* CD003827.

Hankins, J., Lonsway, R. A., Hedrick, C., & Perdue, M. (Eds.) (2001). *Infusion therapy in clinical practice.* (2nd ed.). Philadelphia: W. B. Saunders.

Infusion Nurses Society. (2006a). Infusion nursing standards of practice. *Journal of Infusion Nursing, 29*(Suppl.1).

Infusion Nurses Society. (2006b). *Policies and procedures for infusion nursing* (3rd ed.). Norwood, MA: Author.

O'Grady, N. P., Alexander, M., Patchen Dellinger, E., Gerberding, J. L., Heard, S. O., Maki, D. G., et al. (2002, August 9). Guidelines for the prevention of intravascular catheter-related infections. *Morbidity and Mortality Weekly Report, 51*(RR-10), 1–26.

Perry, J., Parker, G., & Jagger, J. (2003). EPINet report: 2001 percutaneous injury rates. *Advances in Exposure Prevention, 6*(3), 32–36.

Blood Administration

Kathleen Osborn

Outcome-Based Learning Objectives

After studying this chapter, the learner will be able to:

1. Describe the rationale for blood donation requirements and restrictions.
2. Describe the advantages of blood component therapy and the therapeutic uses for each component.
3. Compare and contrast the hazards of transfusion therapy and the nursing measures used to assess and prevent them.
4. Using the nursing process, describe the administration procedure for blood administration.
5. Delineate the critical thinking and clinical judgment nursing skills necessary to appropriately treat adverse reactions to blood transfusions.

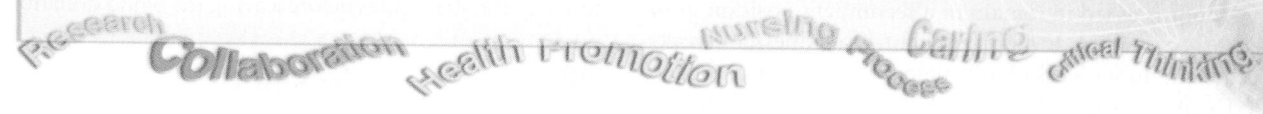

Blood transfusion is defined as the infusion of blood products for the purpose of restoring circulating volume and thereby increasing oxygen carrying capacity. The benefit of a blood transfusion is that it reverses the tissue hypoxia caused by clinically significant anemia and/or blood loss. This reversal can be lifesaving. Blood transfusions are given to approximately 5 million people in the United States annually (Mayo Clinic, 2005). Approximately 14 million units of blood are collected annually in the United States and of these 12 million are transfused (Pearl & Pohlman, 2002). About 60% of the population in the United States is eligible to donate blood; only 5% do (America's Blood Centers, 2006). As the population ages, it is expected that the demand for blood products will increase, perhaps exceeding the supply. The specialty of transfusion medicine is no longer just the practice of storing and administering blood; it now also includes the management of blood resources to ensure the right patients receive transfusions appropriately.

Blood may be administered as either whole blood or blood components. **Whole blood** is obtained from a donor, processed, and infused into a recipient. Whole blood contains red blood cells (RBCs), white blood cells (WBCs), and **platelets**, which are suspended in the **plasma**. Because patients seldom require all of the components of whole blood, in recent years blood component therapy has become the more frequently used method of transfusion. It is more appropriate and economical to separate

blood into its component parts and use only that portion needed by the patient for a specific condition or disease. Two advantages of blood component therapy are (1) conservation of blood resources, because one unit can be used for multiple recipients; and (2) the patient receives only the needed components, thereby decreasing volume overload and reducing side effects and complications.

Blood is fractioned into component parts by either a centrifuge or a cell separator. Each component is then processed and stored appropriately, so as to maximize longevity and cell viability. (See discussion later in the chapter about blood storage.)

Another type of transfusion is **apheresis,** a technique in which blood is withdrawn from a donor, a portion is separated out, and the remainder is returned to the donor. This is useful when a blood donor has been in, say, a malaria-active area of the world. The RBCs from such a donor cannot be used because they may carry the malaria virus, but the plasma portion of the blood can be used.

▊ Donor Considerations

To protect both the donor and the recipient, every potential donor is examined and interviewed. According to the American Red Cross (2005), to be a donor of blood the individual must be healthy, at least 17 years old or 16 years old if allowed by state law, weigh at least 110 pounds, and not have donated blood in the last 8 weeks (56 days). "Healthy" is defined as the ability to perform normal activities. In the presence of a chronic disease such as diabetes or high blood pressure, "healthy" means that the condition is being treated and is under control.

Both the federal Food and Drug Administration (FDA) and the American Association of Blood Banks (AABB) have specific criteria that must be met before a person is accepted for blood donation. The donor must complete a donor history questionnaire. The FDA approved a revised version of a donor history questionnaire developed by the AABB in 2005. A summary of the questions included on the questionnaire are outlined in the National Guidelines box.

Following the history, donors undergo a brief medical examination to evaluate for any obvious signs of illness or conditions that would disqualify them from blood donation. Vital signs are checked and individuals with a fever, high blood pressure, very high or very low pulse rate (with the exception of highly conditioned athletes), and irregular heartbeat are not permitted to donate blood.

Donation Procedure

Blood is obtained from the donor using standard precautions for both donor and phlebotomist. Typically the donor sits in a reclining chair and the antecubital fossa is cleansed with an antiseptic solution. Withdrawal of 450 mL of blood typically takes about 15 minutes. After completion, a firm bandage is applied and the donor is asked to remain in a recumbent position until she feels ready to sit up. If dizziness, light-headedness, or weakness occurs, the donor is asked to remain seated for awhile longer.

Blood banks typically offer donors both food and fluids and ask them to remain for about 15 minutes after standing up. Follow-up donor instructions include (1) leave the dressing in place and avoid heavy lifting for several hours, (2) increase fluid intake for 2 days, (3) avoid alcoholic beverages for 3 hours, (4) avoid smoking for 1 hour, and (4) eat healthy meals for 2 weeks.

Complications of Donation

Many individuals have the misconception that diseases are transmitted during blood donation. Education of potential donors is necessary to ensure understanding that the equipment is sterile, used once, and that it is a closed system from the beginning to the end of the blood collection process.

Excessive bleeding at the donor venipuncture site is a complication of blood donation. Causes include donor bleeding disorder, laceration of the vein during the puncture, excessive tourniquet pressure, and/or failure to apply adequate pressure after the needle is withdrawn. The phlebotomist must ensure that the bleeding has completely stopped before allowing the donor to leave the blood donation center.

Other complications of blood donation include anginal chest pain in unsuspected individuals with coronary artery disease, and on rare occasions, a blood donation can precipitate a seizure in people with epilepsy. Both of these complications require medical evaluation prior to leaving the blood donation center.

The most common complication of blood donation is fainting, typically due to emotional factors, vasovagal reaction, or inadequate fluid or food intake before donation. Hypotension and syncope also may occur due to loss of blood volume when the donor assumes a standing position. These individuals need to lie down or sit with their head between the knees. The donor needs to be symptom free for 30 minutes before leaving the blood donation center.

◼ Blood Supply Safety

The FDA is responsible for ensuring the safety of the blood supply in the United States. Specifically, the Center for Biological Evaluation and Research (CBER) regulates the collection of

---

NATIONAL GUIDELINES for Minimum Requirements for Blood Donation

Oral temperature must be less than 37.5°C (99.6°F).

Regular pulse rate between 50 and 100 beats per minute.

Systolic blood pressure between 90 and 180 mmHg.

Diastolic blood pressure between 50 and 100 mmHg.

Hemoglobin greater than 13.5 g/dL for men and 12.4 g/dL for women.

Body weight must be greater than 50 kg (110 lb) to donate 450 mL. Donors weighing less than 50 kg may donate proportionately less blood.

Age of 17 to 65 years old.

Normal liver function tests.

No blood or plasma donations in the previous 8 weeks.

Medication use (prescription, over the counter, blooding thinners, recent immunization, and illicit).

Exposure to illnesses.

Travel to high-risk areas of the world.

Pregnancy.

Transfusion history.

Surgical history.

Sexual preferences and history (including male-to-male contact even once).

Body piercing and/or tattoos in the last 12 months.

Treatment for syphilis or gonorrhea.

Prison or juvenile hall in the last 12 months.

Residing in the United Kingdom from 1980 to 1996 for greater than 3 months.

Residing in Europe for greater than 5 years.

Lived in Africa or had sex with someone who was born or lived in Africa.

Tested for HIV/AIDS.

History of hepatitis, malaria, Chagas' disease, babesiosis, cancer, leukemia, heart or lung disease, bleeding disorder, Creutzfeldt-Jakob disease.

History of selling illicit drugs.

History of IV drug use.

Source: American Red Cross. (2005). *Blood donation eligibility guidelines.* Retrieved November 7, 2006, from http://www.redcross.org/services/biomed/0,1082,0_557_,00.html#top.

blood and blood components, including manufactured pharmaceuticals derived from blood, such as clotting factors (FDA, 2006a). Additionally, CBER develops and enforces quality standards, inspects blood donation centers, and monitors reports of errors, accidents, and adverse clinical events. This organization also works closely with the federal Public Health Service to identify and respond to potential threats to the blood supply and to develop safety and technical standards to ensure consistent monitoring of the blood supply.

Once blood has been received from the donor it is immediately tested for blood type and infectious diseases. A negative result for the disease testing is required before the blood is used, and each unit is labeled to certify the results.

ABO and Rh Factor Testing

Equally important as disease testing is accurate determination of blood type. Each individual has one of four types of blood: A, B, AB, or O. In a large percentage of the population, two related inherited antigens, A and B, occur on the surface of RBCs and form the basis for the ABO blood typing. Those individuals with A antigen have **type A blood** (41%), those with B antigen have **type B blood** (12%), and those with both A and B have **type AB blood** (3%). If neither A nor B antigens are present, the individual has **type O blood** (44%). Type O blood does not have the genetic information required to make any antigenic formation (Josephson, 2004; Porth, 2005).

Antibodies develop in the serum of people who do not have the corresponding antigen, referred to as anti-A and anti-B. The person with blood type A has B antibodies, someone with type B has A antibodies, someone with type AB has no antibodies, and a person who has type O blood has both antibodies. Therefore, the person with type AB blood can receive any type of blood in an emergency situation and is referred to as the universal recipient. A person with the O blood type is considered a universal donor in an emergency situation. Chart 23–1 outlines each blood type, its antigens and antibodies, and what type of blood a person with each blood type can safely receive. Even though a person is a universal donor or recipient, unless there is an emergency, blood typing should be done to avoid transfusion reactions. ABO incompatibility is an immediate and often fatal cause of transfusion reaction.

 CRITICAL ALERT *In emergency hemorrhage situations, O negative blood can be lifesaving. This is referred to as "uncrossed matched blood," which means that the patient will not react to type O blood because there are no antigens or Rh factor. However, the number of units of O negative blood that can be given is still restricted because of the other antibodies in the blood that can be received. The uncross matched blood places the patient at high risk for transfusion reaction because of these other antibodies.*

The **Rh factor,** also called factor D, is made up of numerous complex antigens. When it is present on the surface of RBCs, the person is Rh positive (Rh$^+$); if not present, the person is Rh negative (Rh$^-$). The designation of Rh positive or negative is influenced by race, with African Americans being approximately 95% Rh$^+$, Native Americans 100% Rh$^+$, and about 85% of Caucasians Rh$^+$ (Guyton & Hall, 2000). An Rh$^-$ person must receive only Rh$^-$ blood to avoid antibody formation from Rh$^+$ blood. An Rh$^+$ person may receive either negative or positive blood. The first time an Rh$^-$ person receives Rh$^+$ blood, there is usually no reaction. But antibodies will form during the next 2 to 4 weeks and if another transfusion of Rh$^+$ blood is given, the antibodies will agglutinate or clump with the Rh antigens of the blood being transfused. Agglutination of cells causes obstruction of the capillaries and blockage of blood flow to the organs. Agglutination and antibody testing are done using the direct Coombs' test (see Chart 23–2, p. 542).

After the blood is taken from the donor, a series of procedures determines both donor and recipient ABO and Rh types. These procedures are referred to as "type and crossmatch" and are listed in Chart 23–2 (p. 542). Typing the blood determines the ABO and Rh factor, whereas crossmatching determines compatibility between donor and recipient blood. To determine blood compatibility, the donor's blood is mixed with the recipient's and observed for agglutination of the cells. If the cells do not agglutinate, and the blood tests negative for diseases, then the blood is compatible and ready to transfuse into the recipient. The blood is stored in a blood bank until needed.

Disease Testing

The blood also is tested for the diseases outlined on Chart 23–3 (p. 542) prior to be being released for patient use. A blood-screening test using nucleic acid technology (NAT) is able to detect minute amounts of the RNA and DNA of specific viruses in blood. Prior to NAT testing, blood could only be tested for antibodies to the virus. There is always a lag time between infection and production of antibodies during which the blood could test negative even though the virus is present. NAT testing markedly reduces this time period, thus making the blood supply safer. NAT testing has been approved by the FDA for hepatitis C, human immunodeficiency virus (HIV), and most recently West Nile virus.

■ Therapeutic Uses of Blood Products

Major therapeutic uses for blood, as stated earlier, are to restore circulating volume and oxygen carrying capacity. This makes blood transfusions useful to replace blood volume during and after surgery. Many surgeries could not be performed without blood transfusions. Additionally, blood replacement is essential in the treatment of trauma when large amounts of blood have been lost.

CHART 23–1	Blood Types, Antigens and Antibodies, and Transfusion Types	
Blood Type with Antigen	**Antibody Produced**	**Type for Transfusion**
Blood type A Antigen A	Antibody B	Can receive A or O blood
Blood type B Antigen B	Antibody A	Can receive B or O blood
Blood type AB Antigen AB	None	Can receive A, B, or O type blood Universal recipient
Blood type O No antigens	Antibodies A and B	Can receive O type blood only Universal donor

CHART 23–2 Blood Type and Crossmatch and Antigen Testing

Name of Test	Purpose of Test	Test Results
Blood type and crossmatch Mandatory test prior to blood transfusion (exception in extreme medical emergency/hemorrhage)	Tests for antigens on the patient's RBCs: ABO antigens on RBCs determine blood type. Rh antigen determines negative or positive Rh factor.	Type A Type B Type AB Type O Rh– Rh+
Indirect Coombs' test Screening prior to blood transfusion	Tests for antibodies present in the patient's serum. Patient's serum is mixed with donor's RBCs. If the patient has antibodies to a specific antigen on the donor RBCs, an antigen–antibody complex is formed and agglutination (clumping) occurs. Blood is tested for more than 40 antibodies.	Normal results: no agglutination; negative for a specific antibody. Abnormal results: agglutination; positive for a specific antibody.
Direct Coombs' test Usually only tested if a transfusion reaction is suspected	Tests for antibodies on the patient's RBCs (not in the serum). Used to detect antibodies from the donor blood that are coating and destroying the patient's RBCs. Patient blood is mixed with Coombs' serum that contains various components of complement and antibodies to IgG to determine antigen–antibody reaction and agglutination.	Normal results: no agglutination; negative for antibodies. Abnormal results: agglutination; positive for antibodies.

Source: Kozier, Barbara J; Erb, Glenora: Berman, Audrey; Snyder, Shirlee. Fundamentals of Nursing: Concepts, Procedures, & Practices, 7th, © 2004. Electronically reproduced by permission of Pearson Education, Inc., Upper Saddle River, New Jersey.

CHART 23–3 Transmission of Bloodborne Diseases

Disease	Test	Safety Margin
Hepatitis B	Core antibodies (anti-HBc) and surface antigen (HbsAG) are tested. Not for the virus itself. Research has just begun on the use of NAT (DNA) testing of blood products that will detect the virus itself.	There is still a window from the time an individual is infected to the time the antibodies are produced. Risk of transmission is 1 in 220,000. There is a 7- to 10-day window.
Hepatitis C	NAT testing for the DNA in the virus. Anti- HCV.	If the blood tests positive, it is sent out for confirmatory testing. If it confirmed positive, it is not used. Risk of transmission is 1 in 1.6 million. There is a 7- to 10-day window.
HIV-1	NAT testing for the DNA in the virus. If the test comes out positive, the blood is sent for confirmatory testing.	This test reduces the period of time from infection to detecting the presence of antibodies from 12 weeks to 11 days. Risk of transmission is 1 in 1.8 million.
Human T-lymphocyte virus-1 (retrovirus present with leukemia)	Screened with EIA for HTLV antibodies. If the test comes out positive, the blood is sent for confirmatory testing.	It is possible to have both false positives and negatives. If the blood tests positive, it is sent out for confirmatory testing. If it is confirmed positive, it is not used.
West Nile virus	NAT testing for the DNA in the virus.	If the blood tests positive, it is not used.
Syphilis	PK 7200 with RPR backup. PK 7200: Tests IgM and IgG antibodies for syphilis (*Treponema pallidum*). Immucor Captive CMV: Also tests for IgM and IgG antibodies. RPR test for reagent antibodies. If the test comes out positive, the blood is sent for confirmatory testing.	It is possible to have both false positives and negatives. If the blood tests positive, it is sent out for confirmatory testing. If it is confirmed positive, it is not used.
Malaria	If a donor has been in a malaria-active area of the world in the last 3 years blood is not accepted.	The only exception is if an individual has taken prophylactic medication. Plasma apheresis (using the plasma portion of the blood only) is still possible because malaria is only carried on the RBCs.
Creutzfeldt-Jakob disease (mad cow disease)	If an individual has spent an extended period of time in Great Britain and Europe from 1980 to 1996, the blood is refused.	If the blood tests positive it is not used. No further testing is done. Diagnosis is usually made by autopsy, biopsy, or process of elimination.
Cytomegalovirus	PK 7200 and Immucor Captive CMV as performed as backup.	Transmission risk greater for premature newborns and immunocompromised recipients who are CMV negative. Leukocyte reduction helps reduce transmission of virus. CMV-negative blood is frequently specifically ordered.

Sources: American Association of Blood Banks. (2003). *Testing of donor blood for infectious disease.* Retrieved November 9, 2006, from http://www.aabb.org/Content/About_Blood/Facts_About_Blood_and_Blood_Banking/fabloodtesting.htm; Josephson, D. (2004). *Intravenous infusion therapy for nurses* (2nd ed.). Clifton Park, NY: Thompson Delmar Learning.

Additional therapeutic uses for blood products are to replace platelets and other clotting factors, which is lifesaving for hemophiliacs. Platelet replacement also is important for cancer patients receiving radiation and chemotherapy. Cancer treatments can cause bone marrow depression and platelet depletion. Blood also can provide protein and other nutrients in severely undernourished patients. Each unit of blood contains approximately 35 grams of protein in the form of plasma proteins, and further sources of protein are found in the cellular elements.

Note that some individuals may refuse blood transfusions for cultural or religious reasons, as discussed in the Cultural Considerations box.

Types of Blood Products

Administering blood products has become more complex with the advent of blood component therapy. It is essential for the nurse to know the correct blood type, the specific rationale for administration, as well as any special considerations of a given blood product and patient. Chart 23–4 (p. 544) outlines the various types of blood products and their volume, storage, and uses. Chart 23–5 (p. 546) lists the necessary information needed by the nurse to safely administer blood. In addition, the nurse must follow strict institutional guidelines and protocols to ensure safe administration with the fewest number of side effects.

CULTURAL CONSIDERATIONS Related to Refusal of Blood Products

It is not unusual for persons to refuse blood transfusions. Many people are frightened of disease transmission and therefore opt to instead replenish their blood supply with blood alternatives, iron supplements, and diet. Although slower, these treatments are effective unless there has been significant blood loss in a short period of time.

Certain religions ban the use of blood products. For example, Jehovah's Witnesses strictly prohibit receiving blood or agents in which blood is an ingredient in any form. This belief is based on scriptural references and precedents in the history of Christianity (Andrews & Boyle, 2003; Lipson, Dibble, & Minarik, 1996). Jehovah's Witnesses do accept blood volume expanders and vigorously pursue blood alternative therapies as long as they do not contain any derivative of blood. Mechanical devices for circulating blood are acceptable as long as they have not been primed with blood.

Other religions' rules vary with regard to blood transfusion. For example, Christian Scientists generally do not believe in any type of medical interventions except those mandated by law such as immunizations. Thus, they do not accept or donate blood products (Andrews & Boyle, 2003). The Jewish religion prohibits the ingestion of blood (blood sausage, raw meats); however, this belief does not apply to receiving blood products. The following religions have no restrictions on the use of blood or blood products (Andrews & Boyle, 2003):

- Amish
- Baha'i
- Catholic
- Hindu
- Mennonite
- Muslim
- Seventh-Day Adventist
- Unitarian.

Each product has its own special consideration beginning with simple administration of whole blood.

Whole blood contains the normal constituents of blood. After being obtained from a donor, anticoagulants and preservatives are added, and the blood is ready for the recipient. Most of the platelets and WBCs are removed or destroyed during the processing of the blood. **Packed RBCs** have had the plasma portion of the blood removed by a centrifuge process. This is the most common blood product given in the hospital. **Washed RBCs** are indicated when previous transfusion reactions have occurred. The washing process increases the removal of immunoglobulins and proteins that cause reactions. **Frozen RBCs** are coated in glycerol prior to freezing and then washed after thawing to remove the glycerol prior to administration.

Leukocyte-poor RBCs have had most of the WBCs removed as soon as the blood has been taken from the donor (prior to storage). The reason the reduction is done prior to storage is because the storage process causes necrosis of the WBCs, creating by-products that can cause serious adverse signs and symptoms for the recipient of the blood. White blood cells do not contribute to the efficacy of blood transfusions and are generally regarded as contaminants that potentially reduce transfusion safety. Until recently, the use of blood with fewer WBCs has been reserved for patients who are considered a high risk for developing problems from the presence of WBCs. That would include immunocompromised individuals who have cancer or acquired immunodeficiency syndrome (AIDS), and transplant patients. Currently the majority of the blood banks in the United States reduce the WBCs from every unit of blood.

Fresh frozen plasma (FFP) is prepared from whole blood by separating it from the cell portion and freezing it within 4 to 6 hours of taking it from the donor. Platelets are prepared from individual units of whole blood by a centrifuge process. Usually 6 to 10 units are given at one time and the units are usually pooled into one bag for easier administration. **Albumin** is derived from the plasma portion of the blood. It is a commercially prepared product that has no risk of disease transmission and does not require ABO compatibility screening. **Cryoprecipitates** are collected by thawing FFP and collecting the white precipitate that remains (May & Kauder, 2006). This precipitate, which is rich in von Willebrand's factor, **factor VIII,** and fibrinogen are given to treat bleeding associated with hemophilia and disorders that cause a depletion of the clotting factors.

 *The platelet count must be assessed within 1 hour following all types of platelet transfusions. This is the best way to accurately assess the therapeutic effect.*

Homologous Transfusion

A **homologous transfusion** is one in which blood is collected from a donor for transfusion into other individuals who are in need of blood. The blood may come from volunteers, designated donors, and/or cadavers. Volunteer donors visit a blood bank periodically and donate a unit of blood to be used by an unspecified person. This blood is labeled "volunteer donor." Designated donors are individuals chosen by the intended recipient to donate blood. Cadaver blood is usually collected with the body still on artificial life support. Regardless of which method is used to

CHART 23–4	Types of Blood Components

Type of Blood Product	Amount	Action	Uses	Storage	Special Considerations
Whole blood	500 mL.	Increases RBCs to carry the oxygen (O_2) to the tissues. Increases plasma to augment intravascular volume and protein and clotting factors.	Shock, hemorrhage, low hemoglobin, hematocrit, and circulating volume.	For up to 35 days at 0–10°C. Warm for 20–30 minutes prior to administration.	Monitor for volume overload. Give slowly. Use fresh blood when possible to avoid increased amounts of potassium, ammonia, and cellular debris that accumulates in stored blood.
Packed RBCs	250–300 mL. 80% of plasma removed. Hematocrit 70%.	Increases RBCs, hematocrit. Increases O_2 carrying capacity.	Anemia associated with cancer, liver, and cardiac disease, renal disease, and for moderate blood loss. Useful when volume overload is a risk.	Same as whole blood.	More viscous than whole blood; slows transfusion. Most common blood product given.
Washed RBCs	250–300 mL. 80% of plasma removed. Hematocrit 70%.	Increases RBCs, hematocrit. Increases O_2 carrying capacity.	Same as packed RBCs, except previous transfusion reactions have occurred. Decreased fibrinogen coating.	Same as whole blood.	RBCs washed with sterile isotonic saline before transfusion. More viscous than whole blood; slows transfusion.
Frozen RBCs	250–300 mL. 80% of plasma removed. Hematocrit 70%.	Increases RBCs, hematocrit. Increases O_2 carrying capacity.	Storage of rare blood type or frequent transfusion reactions. Storage for autologous future use.	Frozen up to 3 years at −87°C (−188.6°F). Must be used within 24 hours of thawing. Storage in liquid state after 24 hr results in loss of clotting factors.	Relatively free of WBCs and microemboli. Expensive.
Leukocyte-poor RBCs	200–325 mL. 80% of plasma removed. Hematocrit 70%.	Increases RBCs, hematocrit. Increases O_2 carrying capacity.	Previous sensitivity to WBC antigens from prior transfusions or pregnancy.	Same as whole blood.	Decreases transfusion reactions.
Fresh frozen plasma	200–250 mL.	Restores plasma volume in shock without increasing RBCs. Increases factors V, VII, VIII, IX, and X.	Bleeding due to liver disease and hemophilia disseminated intravascular coagulation (DIC), hemorrhage, massive transfusion.	Frozen up to 1 year. Must be used within 24 hours after thawing to prevent deterioration of factors V and VIII.	Effective for rapid volume replacement. Give through a filter. No platelets in FFP.
Platelets	50–70 mL.	Increases platelets and maintains normal blood coagulability. Expected increase of 10,000 mm^3	Bleeding due to thrombocytopenia (<10,000 to 20,000 mm^3) and thrombocytopathy. Bone marrow depression and DIC.	Five days at room temperature depending on type of collection and storage bag.	Can be made packed, washed, or leukocyte poor. Bag needs to be agitated periodically. Failure to increase platelets after administration could be due to fever, sepsis, splenomegaly, and DIC.

CHART 23–4	Types of Blood Components—*Continued*

Type of Blood Product	Amount	Action	Uses	Storage	Special Considerations
Albumin (5% or 25% solution)	25-mL, 50-mL, and 100-mL bottles.	Increases plasma colloid osmotic pressure. Increases plasma volume.	Hypovolemic shock and chronic liver failure. Hypoalbuminemia. Burns. Pulmonary and peripheral edema and hypoproteinemia.	Up to 5 years. Check expiration date prior to administration.	No preservatives so each bottle must be used at once. Rapid infusion can cause volume overload. Rate of infusion should not exceed 1 mL/min. Potential capillary leakage in shock due to increased permeability. Often administered with diuretic to prevent fluid overload.
Cryoprecipitate	5–20 mL/unit.	Increases factors VIII and XIII, von Willebrand's factor, and fibrinogen.	Hemophilia, congenital or acquired fibrinogen deficiency, von Willebrand's disease.	Frozen up to 1 year. When thawed must be used within 6 hours.	Multiple units (8–15) typically given depending on reason for administration.
Factor VIII	Number of units is stated on each vial.	Increases factor VIII.	Hemophilia A.	Given either IV push or IV drip.	A factor VIII coagulant level of 30–50% is common end point therapy.
Factor IX	Number of units is stated on each vial.	Increases factor IX.	Hemophilia B or Christmas disease, congenital factor VII or X deficiency.	IV push.	Factor IX levels need to be performed at appropriate intervals to determine response.

Sources: U.S. Department of Health and Human Services, 2000; Josephson, D. (2004). *Intravenous infusion therapy for nurses* (2nd ed.). Clifton Park, NY: Delmar Cengage Learning.

obtain the blood, it must be ABO and Rh typed and tested for all of the diseases outlined earlier in Chart 23–3 (p. 542).

Designated (Directed) Blood

Designated, or directed, blood is collected from a donor designated by the intended recipient. Compatibility testing is required and the blood must meet all of the requirements of homologous blood including being free from transfusion-transmitted diseases. This method of blood donation is controversial due to the risk of a donor whom the recipient knows not disclosing high-risk behaviors.

Autologous Transfusion

Autologous transfusion is the process of collection and reinfusion of the patient's own blood. There are three forms of autologous transfusion; (1) preoperative donation, (2) perioperative blood salvage, and (3) postoperative blood salvage. The advantages to this type of blood replacement are:

- Elimination of infectious disease transmission
- No risk of transfusion reaction
- Provides a source of blood for persons with a rare type or antibodies that make it difficult to find compatible blood.

These blood products require special handling and labeling under strict guidelines by trained personnel before storage and reinfusion; therefore, an autologous transfusion is more expensive than blood obtained from a volunteer donor (Josephson, 2004).

Preoperative Donation

The blood is collected from individuals who are preparing for surgery at a later date. This method is useful for healthy patients who are having elective surgery where the potential need for transfusion is high (e.g., orthopedic surgery). Typically the blood is collected 1 to 6 weeks prior to surgery and stored for reinfusion. The patients are given iron supplements to help build up the RBCs. Occasionally erythropoietin (Procrit, Epogen) is given to stimulate erythropoiesis to maintain the required hematocrit.

CHART 23–5 Blood Administration Procedure

PURPOSE

- To administer blood products safely to patients with altered hematologic function.
- To replace circulating blood volume.
- To restore oxygen carrying capacity.
- To stop and prevent bleeding.

EQUIPMENT

- Y-type blood transfusion tubing (see Figure 23–1 ■, p. 552).
- 250- to 500-mL bag of normal saline (0.9% NaCl).
- Blood product from blood bank.
- Blood administration record for vital sign assessment (Figure 23–2 ■, p. 553).
- Nonsterile gloves.
- Alcohol wipes.
- Tape.
- 18- to 20-gauge IV catheter.
- IV pole.

ASSESSMENT PARAMETERS

- Size of IV catheter (18 to 20 gauge).
- Health care provider's order for type, amount, and rate of blood administration.
- History of blood transfusion reactions.
- Religious or other personal objections to receiving blood products.
- Compatibility of blood product to recipient blood type.
- Circulatory and respiratory status.
- Vital signs before, during, and after transfusion.
- Presence of rash prior to transfusion.

SPECIAL CONSIDERATIONS

- No medications are to be piggybacked into a transfusion.
- The transfusion is never interrupted for medication administration.
- Only 0.9% NaCl is to be infused in the same line as the blood.

PLANNING FOR BLOOD ADMINISTRATION

- Obtain patient transfusion history (previous transfusions, transfusion reactions).
- Ensure the patient understands the need for blood administration and is willing to sign the informed consent. Informed consent is obtained by the health care provider. The blood is not given without the consent.
- Check health care provider's order for type of blood product to be administered.
- Check size and insertion date of the IV catheter:
  - 18- or 20-gauge catheter, depending on the hospital protocol.
  - If the catheter is more than 48 hours old, it should not be used for administration of blood products. (*Note:* Specific agency protocols supersede this procedure.)

NURSING IMPLEMENTATION: ADMINISTRATION PROTOCOL

- Wash hands and assemble appropriate equipment.
- Explain to patient/family the procedure and rationale, length of transfusion, as appropriate. Assess understanding.
- Instruct patient to report *any* unusual symptoms.

- Follow hospital protocol for obtaining blood products from the laboratory.
- Close all three clamps on the Y-type blood tubing with filter and attach the 0.9% NaCl (NS) bag, open the clamp to the NS, and purge the Y-tubing (see Figure 23–1 ■, p. 552).
- Make sure the filter chamber is completely filled with saline.
- Using aseptic technique, connect tubing to IV catheter or to saline lock.
- Check identification of blood product with two (2) *licensed staff nurses* and the patient:
  - Patient name and medical record number (in chart and on the blood product). (*Note:* It is often useful to check the birth date as well.)
  - Blood product type and unit number.
  - Blood ABO group and Rh factor of both donor blood and patient.
  - Expiration date of blood product (may be given up to midnight on expiration day).
  - Both nurse's sign and date blood bank slip that is attached to the blood bag.
- Compare the above patient identification information with the patient's name band.
- Obtain baseline vital signs (TPR, BP) and document on the chart. Follow hospital protocol for frequency of reassessing vital signs.
- Prior to handling any blood products, put on nonsterile gloves and use standard precautions.
  - Connect blood bag to the free arm of the Y-tubing (see Figure 23–1 ■, p. 552) and open the roller clamp on the same arm of the Y.
  - Close the clamp on the NS side of the Y tubing before opening the clamp on the blood side of the Y tubing.
  - Begin infusion of blood product by adjusting the roller clamp closest to the patient's IV site.
  - Take vital signs prior to the infusion of the blood.
  - The nurse must remain with the patient for this 15-minute period and observe the patient for transfusion reactions (Chart 23–6, p. 549). Blood products should be infused very slowly for the first 15 minutes of the transfusion.
  - Vital signs are taken after the first 15 minutes.
  - If there are no indications of a transfusion reaction, increase the infusion rate to the prescribed rate or the standard hospital infusion rate.
- Continue observation for transfusion reactions until the blood product has completely infused.
- Terminating the transfusion:
  - Flush the IV tubing with normal saline by closing the blood product roller clamp and opening the saline roller clamp.
  - Follow hospital protocol for discarding blood product bag and tubing.
  - Flush IV catheter after discontinuing blood tubing.

DOCUMENTATION IN PATIENT RECORD AND BLOOD ADMINISTRATION RECORD (SEE FIGURE 23–2 ■, P. 553)

- Date.
- Time the infusion was started and completed.
- Volume of blood product and normal saline infused (Intake and output record).
- Blood product and number.
- Signature of the two nurses who checked the blood product.
- Baseline and continuing patient assessment.

CHART 23–5	**Blood Administration Procedure—**_Continued_

SPECIAL EQUIPMENT USED FOR TRANSFUSION THERAPY

- Blood warmers are used when blood is infused rapidly.
- Infusion pumps are used when blood needs to be given at a very specific rate to prevent fluid overload.

NURSING EVALUATION

- Vital signs before, during, after the transfusion.
- Lung assessment during and after the transfusion.
- Hemoglobin and hematocrit.
- Transfusion reaction.
- Changes in fatigue levels.
- Increased tissue perfusion.
- Clinical manifestations of anemia.

Source: Kozier, Barbara J; Erb, Glenora; Berman, Audrey; Snyder, Shirlee. Fundamentals of Nursing: Concepts, Procedures, & Practices, 7th, © 2004. Electronically reproduced by permission of Pearson Education, Inc., Upper Saddle River, New Jersey.

One unit of blood is typically collected each week, up to 72 hours prior to surgery. The number of needed units varies depending on the surgical procedure. Individual units of blood components also can be collected and stored for future use. The American Red Cross (ARC) requires that autologous blood be given only to the donor. If the blood is not used, it can be stored up to 10 years for future surgeries. It can never be placed in the general donor supply to be used by someone else.

Criteria for donation include a minimum hemoglobin of 11 g/dL, hematocrit of 33%, and no presence of infection. Individuals with unstable angina, acute cardiovascular and cerebrovascular disease, and hypertension may not donate. Cancer patients may donate provided they meet the minimum criteria for donation, as listed earlier in the National Guidelines box (p. 540). Before the transfusion the patient and blood are typed and crossmatched to confirm the ABO and Rh factors and tested for diseases (see Chart 23–3, p. 542) to protect the people handling the blood. The blood is processed and stored in designated blood banks until reinfusion.

Most patients take iron supplementation (ferrous sulfate 325 mg three times per day or ferrous gluconate 325 mg five times daily) starting 1 week before donation and continuing until surgery.

Perioperative Blood Salvage

Perioperative blood salvage is defined as the collection and reinfusion of blood lost during both the intraoperative and early postoperative periods. This is a common procedure employed for major surgeries such as cardiovascular bypass, orthopedic, and vascular surgeries, splenectomy, organ transplantation, and trauma when major blood loss has occurred (Josephson, 2004). The blood is collected under sterile conditions and may be reinfused back into the patient with a standard blood filter and gravity. Suction is used to salvage the blood but it does not traumatize the RBCs. The viability of recovered RBCs is comparable to that obtained with homologous transfusions. This salvage process has all the advantages of an autologous transfusion as outlined earlier, except that the blood has to be given within 12 hours after collection. The amount of blood recovered is usually about 50% of what is lost, so it often precludes the need for a transfusion.

Perioperative blood salvage, however, has a number of disadvantages, the main one being a considerable loss of coagulation factors and platelets. Due to the risk of spreading infection, blood is not used if there is an infection present or if intestinal contents have contaminated the sterile surgical field. Washing and filtering the blood does not eliminate bacteria from the salvaged blood. If malignancy is present, the blood is not used due to risk of causing the cancer to metastasize to other organs.

Postoperative Blood Salvage

Postoperative blood salvage is used following major surgeries, typically cardiovascular, thoracic, and some orthopedic procedures. Blood is obtained from mediastinal and chest tubes and then reinfused. Even though the blood has been diluted with normal saline, it still has viable RBCs, making it useful for increasing tissue perfusion.

Therapeutic Apheresis

As mentioned earlier, apheresis, a Greek word meaning to "separate," is a process in which blood is removed from the donor and passed through an automated cell separation device that removes specific components. The remaining blood is then returned to the donor. Apheresis platelets are collected from a single donor rather than multiple donors, and each unit contains 200 to 400 mL. This is equivalent to six to eight units of platelets obtained from separate donors. Donors can have platelets apheresed about 24 times per year (Kleinman, 2006b).

White blood cells can be obtained in a similar manner, typically after the donor has received growth factors (G-CSF, GM-CSF) to stimulate WBC formation. Growth factors also release stem cells into the circulation that can be harvested over a period of several days and used for a peripheral blood stem cell transplant (Chapter 60).

Another use for apheresis is to remove specific components of the blood to treat certain diseases. For example, WBCs and platelets can be removed by a centrifuge process and the remaining blood given back to the patient. When platelets and WBCs are removed, the temporary reduction in the number of these cells decreases immunity, thus allowing time for chemotherapy to have a therapeutic effect. Finally, removal of plasma is typically done so that specific abnormal proteins can be transiently lowered until long-term therapy is initiated. This process is performed for many reasons some of which include autoimmune diseases such as Raynaud's phenomenon (Chapter 43), hematologic disorders such as sickle cell anemia (Chapter 65), and some neurological conditions including myasthenia gravis and multiple sclerosis (Chapter 31) (McLeod, 2000).

Risks Associated with Transfusion Therapy

Transfusion therapy is associated with a variety of risk factors that need to be evaluated prior to and monitored during the transfusion to ensure patient safety. Risks of transfusion therapy include disease transmission, bacterial contamination, acute or delayed transfusion reactions, and circulatory overload. When it is necessary to administer massive transfusions (replacement of greater than one blood volume in 24 hours), the risks include hypothermia, hemodilution, and platelet dysfunction (Rose, 2007). Finally, there is also a somewhat rare risk for the development of a pulmonary reaction to blood administration, referred to as *transfusion-related acute lung injury*, which is discussed in a later section. When informing the recipient about the reason for the transfusion, it is important for the nurse to explain the risks, the benefits, and what to expect during and after the transfusion. Patients must understand that the blood supply is not completely risk free. Each of the risks of transfusion therapy is discussed next. Note also that the nurse must be aware of how blood transfusions can affect the elderly, as discussed in the Gerontological Considerations box.

Disease Transmission

The FDA (2006b) states that the blood supply in the United States is not without risk of transmitting infectious disease, although the blood supply is safer than ever before. Currently tests for the nine diseases outlined earlier in Chart 23–3 (p. 542) are conducted on each unit of blood (AABB, 2003). It remains a nursing responsibility to inform the patient that there are still some risks associated with blood transfusion therapy.

Bacterial Contamination

Bacterial contamination of blood products is very rare, but may occur at any point from procurement to processing and during administration. A unit of contaminated blood product may appear normal or it may have an abnormal color. The refrigeration process helps prevent the growth of bacteria in the donated blood because most bacteria cannot survive the cold temperatures. Platelets are stored at room temperature and therefore are more susceptible to bacterial growth. Besides refrigeration, other

measures that help prevent bacterial contamination and growth include meticulous care in the handling of blood products and following time guidelines when administering the blood. For example, whole blood and RBCs need to be infused within 4 hours because room temperature promotes bacterial growth.

The clinical manifestations of bacterial contamination may not occur until the transfusion is complete, or in some instances several hours later depending on the virulence of the infecting organism. Fever, chills, and hypotension are common initial symptoms. Endotoxic shock and even death will occur if the infection is left untreated (Brown & Whalen, 2000). Fluid replacement, antibiotics, and vasopressors (for blood pressure) are needed immediately to prevent irreversible shock and death.

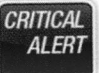 *As soon as abnormal clinical manifestations occur when transfusing blood, the transfusion is stopped, the doctor is notified, and the blood and tubing are sent to the laboratory for testing and culturing. The nurse may not know the exact reason for the clinical manifestations, but when they occur, the focus is on preventing complications and, at times death.*

Transfusion Reactions

With blood administration there is always the risk of having a transfusion reaction occur. It is essential for the nurse to know the signs and symptoms of each type of transfusion reaction and comprehend the importance of immediate treatment in order to prevent potentially fatal complications. During and after the transfusion, it is vital for the nurse to observe the patient for complications of transfusion therapy and know how to carry out the necessary interventions to reverse the reaction, if possible.

Transfusion reactions may be acute or delayed. Acute or immediate reactions can occur as soon as 5 minutes after starting the transfusion, whereas delayed transfusion reactions may occur from 48 hours to 6 months later. There also may be a reaction when a patient receives multiple units of blood products due to preservatives used to store the blood. If possible prior to administering blood, the nurse needs to obtain a health history including allergies and reactions to previous transfusions. Patients with allergies potentially have a higher risk of transfusion reaction and need to be observed closely. Patients who have had previous transfusion reactions or have received multiple transfusions frequently are medicated with antipyretics and/or antihistamines prior to the transfusion due to the presence of antibodies. Chart 23–6 outlines the essential information related to transfusion reactions and the associated nursing care requirements. The Critical Alert discusses the essential nursing actions required during an acute transfusion reaction.

 When a transfusion reaction is occurring and it is necessary to stop the transfusion, it is essential for the nurse to keep the intravenous (IV) line patent. It may be needed to administer emergency medication to treat the presenting signs and symptoms. The line will need to be flushed with normal saline and/or a continuous infusion of fluid initiated by the nurse as soon as the blood transfusion is disconnected from the IV site.

White Blood Cell Reduction

White blood cells do not contribute to the efficacy of blood transfusions. They are generally regarded as contaminants that

---

GERONTOLOGICAL CONSIDERATIONS for Blood Transfusions

The nurse must possess critical thinking and clinical judgment skills in order to assess the patient's tolerance of a transfusion. Unless the patient is acutely hemorrhaging or is significantly hypovolemic, blood is administered slowly to prevent fluid overload. The nurse needs to know the patient's medical history in order to be aware of the risk for this development. This is especially true for elderly patients with a history of heart failure or renal insufficiency/failure who would be more at risk than a young patient with a healthy heart. Frequent monitoring of high-risk patients will typically prevent complications. Often with elderly patients with previous heart failure problems, the health care provider orders furosemide (diuretic) to be given before or after the transfusion. If the patient is to receive more than one unit, furosemide is often ordered to be given between the two units.

| CHART 23–6 | Transfusion Reactions | | |

Class	Cause	Clinical Manifestations	Nursing Care
Allergic reaction	Recipient's sensitivity to foreign plasma proteins. Common in patients with allergies.	Itching, hives, flushing, and chills.	Slow the transfusion. Take vital signs. Notify the health care provider. May be necessary to medicate with antipyretic and/or antihistamine. Then resume the transfusion.
Febrile nonhemolytic reaction	Due to leukocyte or thrombocyte incompatibility (donor's WBCs or platelets react with recipient's antibodies). Usually occurs after multiple transfusions. Accounts for 90% of transfusion reactions. Fever begins about 2 hours after the transfusion. WBC reduced blood helps prevent these reactions.	Increased pulse rate, temperature > 1°C, chills, headache, nausea and vomiting, anxiety, flushing, back pain, muscle aches.	Stop transfusion, but maintain IV site. Give antipyretics as prescribed. Take vital signs. Notify health care provider. Obtain urine and blood sample. Send blood bag, normal saline, and IV tubing to the laboratory. Consider using leukocyte-poor blood.
Delayed hemolytic reaction	May occur up to 14 days after a transfusion when the level of the antibodies has increased to the extent that a reaction occurs.	Fever, anemia, increased bilirubin level, decreased or absent haptoglobin, and jaundice.	Generally not dangerous, but it is important to recognize the reaction because subsequent transfusions may cause a more severe hemolytic reaction. Typically not recognized or treated due to the mild nature of the reaction.
Acute hemolytic reaction	ABO incompatibility of the blood and recipient. May be due to a mistake in labeling by laboratory or blood bank or nursing error. Causes agglutination of cells, which causes obstruction of the capillaries and blockage of blood flow.	Bloody urine and decreased urine output. Petechiae, jaundice, decreased BP, chest tightness, low back pain, nausea, anxiety, and dyspnea. Hypotension, bronchospasm, and vascular collapse may occur. Hemoglobinemia, acute renal failure, shock, cardiac arrest, death. Symptoms typically occur within the first 15 minutes of the transfusion.	Emergent life-threatening situation. Stop transfusion, but maintain IV site and infuse IV colloid solutions to maintain BP. Give diuretics as prescribed to maintain urine flow. Insert urinary catheter to assess output and color. Obtain vital signs. Treat shock. Start CPR if necessary. Give epinephrine. Notify health care provider. Obtain urine and blood sample. Send blood bag, normal saline, and IV tubing to the laboratory.
Hemolytic or anaphylactic reaction	Reaction to donor plasma proteins. Specifically, infusion of IgA proteins to an IgA-deficient recipient who has an IgA antibody.	Wheezing, restlessness, anxiety; progressing to cyanosis, shock, and possibly cardiac arrest.	Stop infusion, but maintain IV site. Give epinephrine per doctor's order. Initiate CPR if necessary. Notify health care provider. Obtain urine and blood sample. Send blood bag, normal saline, and IV tubing to the laboratory.

Sources: Josephson, D. (2004). *Intravenous infusion therapy for nurses* (2nd ed.). Clifton Park, NY: Delmar Cengage Learning; Porth, C. M. (2005). *Pathophysiology: Concepts of altered health status* (7th ed.). Philadelphia: Lippincott Williams & Wilkins.

potentially reduce transfusion safety (ARC, 2006). As mentioned earlier, until recently, reducing WBCs has been reserved for patients who are considered high risk for developing problems from the presence of WBCs, including immunocompromised patients. Recent advances in leukocyte reduction technology have contributed to the ease and effectiveness of removing leukocytes from blood and blood products including whole blood and RBCs (FDA, 2006b). Currently most blood banks reduce WBCs for every recipient. White blood cell reduction reduces the incidence of febrile transfusion reactions (see Chart 23–6) and the transmission of cytomegalovirus (ARC, 2006). The FDA concluded that there are no significant adverse effects with leukocyte reduction. All leukocyte-reduced blood products are specifically labeled "leukocyte reduced."

Noninfectious Serious Hazards of Transfusion Therapy

According to the AABB (2003) there has been a 10,000-fold reduction in transfusion-transmitted infectious diseases in recent decades, but there has been very little progress in reducing the risk of noninfectious serious hazards from transfusions. As a result patients are harmed from noninfectious hazards at a rate of 100-fold to 1,000-fold. The most common noninfectious transfusion-related problems include:

- Mistransfusion and ABO/Rh incompatible transfusion
- Cardiopulmonary toxicity/circulatory overload
- Transfusion-related graft versus host disease
- Transfusion-related acute lung injury
- Metabolic derangements in pediatric and massive transfusion
- Undertransfusion.

Mistransfusion and ABO/Rh Incompatible Transfusion

Transfusion of incompatible blood (see Chart 23–6, p. 549) or mistransfusion is the most common cause of serious morbidity and mortality associated with transfusions (AABB, 2003). Errors may occur at the time of sample collection, within the laboratory, when the blood is issued from the laboratory, or at the bedside. This type of transfusion reaction is typically fatal and the incidence has not significantly decreased. One study by the New York State Department of Health reported that the incidence of these fatal reactions has not decreased significantly in decades in New York State (Linden, Wagner, Voytovich, & Sheehan, 2000).

Circulatory Overload

Circulatory overload can occur with transfusions when the blood is infused too rapidly or in too large a quantity, thus causing hypervolemia. The osmotic makeup of the blood causes fluid to be mobilized from the interstitial space, thereby increasing intravascular volume well beyond that given during the transfusion. High-risk patients include the elderly and those individuals who already have increased circulatory volume or who have a history of heart failure. Clinical manifestations of circulatory overload include dyspnea, tachycardia, distended neck veins, crackles in the lungs, and a rise in blood pressure. If the transfusion is not slowed down or stopped, pulmonary edema will result. A complete description of heart failure and the impact of fluid volume are discussed in Chapter 42 🔗 .

If the blood is administered slowly, typically circulatory overload can be prevented. The only time blood is given rapidly is when a patient is hemorrhaging or is severely volume depleted. Packed RBCs are safer than whole blood for high-risk individuals because the plasma portion of the blood has been removed, which decreases the volume of the unit by approximately one-half. Frequently diuretics are administered between units or after the transfusion to high-risk individuals to decrease the circulating volume. If pulmonary edema is present, oxygen, diuretics, morphine, and in severe cases mechanical ventilation may be necessary.

Transfusion Related Graft Versus Host Disease

Graft versus host disease (GVHD) occurs in severely immunocompromised patients when transfused lymphocytes attack host lymphocytes or body tissues. Clinical manifestations include diarrhea, fever, diffuse red skin rash, nausea, vomiting, and hepatitis. The primary prevention is to administer leukocyte-reduced blood products. There is no effective therapy or cure for GVHD, thus nursing care focuses on managing the signs and symptoms. Mortality resulting from acute GVHD is directly related to severity, with overwhelming sepsis being the primary cause of death in patients with acute GVHD (Kuechle, 2005).

Transfusion-Related Acute Lung Injury

See Evidence-Based Practice box for Transfusion of Blood Products (p. 554). **Transfusion-related acute lung injury (TRALI)** is a serious, life-threatening clinical syndrome that is a complication of blood transfusions (Silliman, Ambruso, & Boshkov, 2005). In fact, TRALI is the most commonly reported cause of transfusion-related deaths in the United States, surpassing those caused by ABO incompatibility and bacterial contamination (Silliman et al., 2005). Due to the difficulty of specifically identifying the disorder, it is difficult to calculate the incidence. One group of investigators calculated that it occurs in approximately 1 in every 1,000 to 2,400 units of blood (Finlay, Cassorla, Feiner, & Toy, 2005). No identifiable risk factors have been found.

The exact cause of this complication is not fully understood. One prevailing theory is that TRALI is thought to be caused by the presence of granulocyte antibodies and biologically active lipids in the donor plasma that the recipient reacts to. If antibodies are present in the donor's plasma, they stimulate the WBCs in the recipient's blood. Aggregates of WBCs form and occlude the microvasculature of the lungs (Halpern, Taichman, & Hansen-Flaschen, 2005). Whatever the cause, the end result is increased pulmonary vascular permeability leading to the clinical manifestations described next. All plasma-containing blood components, including RBCs, platelets, FFP, and cryoprecipitates, can be a cause of TRALI.

Clinical manifestations include sudden onset of respiratory distress during or shortly after a transfusion. Hypoxemia, hypotension, severe pulmonary edema, cyanosis, and fever may also occur. Diffuse crackles and decreased breath sounds in the lungs are typically present. In its most severe form, TRALI is indistinguishable from adult respiratory distress syndrome (Chapter 36 🔗). It can occur during the transfusion and as late as 6 hours after a plasma-containing transfusion, but most frequently occurs 1 to 2 hours after the transfusion. The severity of symptoms can range from mild to severe. The symptoms usually last about 96 hours and then begin to resolve. Treatment is supportive and related to the severity of symptoms. Frequently patients need ventilatory support, and diuretics are indicated if pulmonary edema is present (Halpern et al., 2005). Once TRALI has occurred the recipient should not receive any more transfusions from the same donor. Transfusion from other donors poses no increased risk.

Less Common Noninfectious Transfusion-Related Hazards

Other less common noninfectious hazards of transfusion therapy include iron overload and the side effects of multiple and massive transfusions. Repeated exposure to blood transfusion not only carries an increased risk of the transmission of blood-borne diseases but also can cause iron overload.

Iron Overload

Iron overload, referred to as hemochromatosis, may occur in patients who have chronic transfusion requirements. One unit of RBCs contains 250 mg of iron. Patients who receive repeated transfusions acquire more iron than they need and the excess builds up in the tissues. Over time these deposits can cause organ damage, particularly to the pancreas, liver, heart, and testes. Laboratory tests conducted to diagnose hemochromatosis are the total iron binding capacity (TIBC), serum iron (SI), and serum ferritin (SF) tests. These values will all be elevated in iron overload.

The treatment goal is to induce a mild anemia and maintain it until the stored iron is greatly reduced. The SF test value is a measure of stored iron and this number needs to come down to normal range. This is accomplished by bloodletting, that is, therapeutic phlebotomies. Phlebotomy refers to the removal of a full unit of blood from the patient, approximately 500 mL. This should be done in a medical setting. The schedule of this treatment should be twice a week or a minimum of once a week. Chelation therapy that is promptly initiated can prevent end-organ damage from iron toxicity.

Multiple and Massive Transfusion Reactions

A massive transfusion is defined as the replacement by transfusion of more than 50% of a patient's blood volume in 12 to 24 hours. Patients who have repeated exposure to blood products and the preservatives used to store blood products have an increased risk of developing elevated blood ammonia titers, coagulation imbalances, hypocalcemia, acid–base imbalance, and hyperkalemia (Kleinman, 2006a). The ammonia level increases in stored blood due to decomposition of the blood products. Coagulation imbalance occurs due to dilutional thrombocytopenia and decreased platelets that are destroyed in stored blood. Depending on the age of the blood product, it may have few viable clotting factors; therefore, an inability to clot normally may result from multiple transfusions. The longer the blood is stored, the more ineffective the clotting factors become. Replacement of clotting factors, plasma, and platelets is typically necessary (Kleinman, 2006a). The decrease in calcium is due to its binding with the citrate (the preservative), and hyperkalemia occurs when potassium leaks from the stored RBCs. Finally, hypothermia may occur with massive transfusions if refrigerated blood is rapidly transfused. This can be prevented by the use of a blood warming device. It is essential for the nurse to monitor for all of the potential side effects when a patient is receiving repeated transfusions.

Nursing Responsibilities Before, During, and After Transfusions

Nursing care of the patient receiving a blood transfusion requires the nurse to follow strict protocols set forth by the AABB, state licensing boards, individual employers, the Infusion Nurses Society (INS), and the American Nurses Association nurse practice act. The nurse is responsible for all aspects of blood transfusion therapy and must continually assess the patient's response to the transfusion. Knowledge specific to blood transfusions includes blood types, blood component therapy, administration equipment, specific techniques for administer-ing each component, and hazards of transfusion therapy. Critical thinking and clinical judgments skills are necessary because the clinical manifestations of a transfusion reaction are not always "textbook." Therefore, the nurse is responsible for evaluating each situation and being knowledgeable about and able to respond with the appropriate care when problems occur.

Nursing Management

Blood transfusion therapy occurs most frequently in the acute care setting, although under certain circumstances patients will receive blood in other settings. Patients who need chronic transfusions may use free-standing infusion centers, ambulatory care settings, doctor's offices, and even private homes for their transfusions. Nurses need to have the skill and knowledge to adapt to any of these settings when performing a blood transfusion. Use of the nursing process provides the template that enables the nurse to safely perform transfusion therapy in multiple settings. Outlined next are the necessary steps within the nursing process for safe blood administration.

Patients are required to sign a consent form prior to the transfusion. It is the health care provider's responsibility to explain why the transfusion is needed and what risks are associated with the procedure. The nurse's responsibility includes verifying that the patient understands the health care provider's explanation prior to signing the consent form. It is essential for the patient to understand that once the transfusion begins, any unusual signs or symptoms must be reported to the nurse.

Assessment

Prior to beginning a transfusion, the nurse needs to obtain a transfusion history from the patient. This includes information about previous transfusions, allergies, and any transfusion reaction. Information about the type of transfusion reaction, its manifestations, and treatment also is necessary and must be documented in the patient's record. This will alert the nurse about the risk of transfusion reactions and possibly the need for premedication to prevent an allergic reaction.

The physical assessment includes vital signs prior to beginning the transfusion. This provides a baseline for vital sign assessment during the transfusion. An acute rise in the body temperature may indicate a transfusion reaction, thus it is essential to know the baseline temperature. Fluid overload causes changes in both pulse and blood pressure, therefore obtaining baseline vital signs enables the nurse to monitor and assess significant changes. Additionally, lung sounds need a baseline assessment. The development of rales may also indicate fluid overload. Any concurrent health problems relating to cardiac, respiratory, or renal diseases need to be assessed.

 During a transfusion it is essential for the nurse to assess the patient's vital signs and lungs sounds. The heart rate and respiratory rate increase when fluid overload occurs and rales can be heard in the lungs. Additionally, these patients tend to develop cardiac dysrhythmias. If these changes occur, the nurse needs to slow the transfusion and notify the health care provider.

Nursing Diagnosis

The nursing diagnoses associated with the need for blood administration include:

1. *Fluid Volume Deficit* related to blood loss.
2. *Gas Exchange Impaired* related to low hemoglobin.
3. *Ineffective Tissue Perfusion* related to hypovolemia.
4. *Fatigue* related to low hemoglobin.
5. *Decreased Cardiac Output* related to hypovolemia.
6. *Risk of Injury* related to complications of blood transfusion.

Planning

In addition to reviewing the patient's medical history, the nurse must plan for and prepare the equipment that will be used during blood administration.

Equipment Preparation

A 16- to 20-gauge catheter is required for RBCs to pass through without being damaged. Using a smaller gauge needle also may slow or stop the transfusion. Special Y-type blood tubing with an in-line filter is always used for the administration of blood products (Figure 23–1 ■). Normal saline (0.9% NaCl) is attached to one of the Y sites and the tubing is primed with normal saline prior to blood administration.

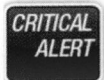 **CRITICAL ALERT** *Only normal saline can be administered with blood. Dextrose solutions cause hemolysis of the cells. Calcium, which is present in lactated Ringer's solutions, can cause coagulation in citrated (preservative) blood. To increase the rate of the transfusion and decrease the viscosity of the blood, normal saline may run simultaneously to help thin the blood product.*

The purpose of an in-line filter is to trap clots and other debris from all blood components older than 5 days. Some institutions require additional in-line filters to be added to the blood tubing. There are basically two purposes for these additional filters. One type of filter augments the in-line filter in trapping clots and debris, and the other filter removes leukocytes for patients with a history of febrile reactions.

Other optional equipment used for transfusions includes electronic infusion pumps, pressure cuffs, and blood warmers. Electronic pumps regulate the rate or speed of the transfusion and are used when blood needs to be given very rapidly or very slowly. Special blood tubing can be inserted into infusion pumps, and the rate of administration is dialed into the pump. External cuffs may be applied to the outside of the blood bag and the cuffed bag is inflated, which pushes the blood in and therefore increases the rate of infusion. These bags are contraindicated unless large-bore catheters are used. The bag pressure should never exceed 300 mmHg. Blood warmers are used when rapid infusion of blood products is necessary and there is an increased risk of hypothermia. Cold blood may precipitate cardiac dysrhythmias and cardiac arrest associated with rapid, massive infusion of cold blood products. Blood warmers have a preset maximum temperature of 38°C (100.4°F) so as not to damage the RBCs. Blood should never be immersed under hot water or placed in a microwave oven for warming.

Outcome and Evaluation Parameters

The outcome of blood administration is dependent on the reason for the transfusion. For example if it is needed for a low red

FIGURE 23–1 ■ Y-type blood tubing.

blood cell count, then the outcome is to normalize the value. If the need for the transfusion is due to low platelets resulting in bleeding, the outcome is to normalize the platelet count and stop or prevent blood loss. Since blood administration is just part of a treatment plan, it is imperative that the reason for the abnormality be identified and corrected, if possible. Evaluation parameters include a normal red blood cell count, hemoglobin, hematocrit, platelet count, and clotting factors. Additionally, part of the evaluation would be relief from the clinical manifestations that resulted from the abnormality. These manifestations are the nursing diagnoses listed above.

Interventions and Rationales

Once the blood has been taken from the blood bank, it must be administered within 30 minutes. It cannot be stored in the refrigerator on the nursing unit because a lack of temperature control may damage the blood. When administering a blood product, it is essential to follow institutional policy. The nurse must ensure positive patient identification, appropriateness of blood component, blood product inspection, verification of donor–recipient compatibility, and verification of product expiration date.

Additionally the nurse must have knowledge of the appropriate rate at which to infuse the blood product. Occasionally the health care provider will order a specific rate; otherwise, the institution will identify safe rates of infusion of various blood products in their blood administration policy and procedure. For example, a common infusion rate for a unit of whole blood is 4 hours. Chart 23–5 (p. 546) earlier in the chapter outlines the blood administration procedure, and Figure 23–2 ■ shows a sample blood administration record.

 CRITICAL ALERT To protect both the patient and the nurse, strict hospital protocols must be followed when checking blood in order to prevent fatal transfusion reactions. It is the nurse's responsibility to know and follow the hospital protocol when checking blood. The protocols vary from institution to institution. Most agencies require that two registered nurses verify the right unit, patient, blood type, and blood product.

Evaluation

During and after the transfusion, the nurse needs to evaluate the patient for response to the transfusion. The nurse must stay with the patient for the first 15 minutes of the transfusion to assess for any clinical manifestations of a transfusion reaction (see Chart 23–5, p. 546). If the patient begins to have clinical manifestations that indicate an abnormal response, the nurse must have knowledge of the appropriate interventions. It is a nursing responsibility to possess the necessary clinical judgment to evaluate a normal versus abnormal response during a blood transfusion. For example, vital signs are monitored at frequencies prescribed by the institution. Both immediate and delayed reactions are manifested by altered vital signs and indicate an abnormal response to the blood. Additionally, the lungs are monitored during and after the transfusion to assess for fluid overload.

The alteration in tissue perfusion that was occurring prior to the transfusion may be assessed by evaluating the hemoglobin and hematocrit. After administration of one unit of packed RBCs in a nonbleeding adult, the hemoglobin increases by 1 g/dL and the hematocrit by 3 percentage points (U.S. Department of Health and Human Services, 2000). The patient should have

UNIVERSITY OF CALIFORNIA DAVIS
MEDICAL CENTER,
SACRAMENTO, CALIFORNIA

Blood Administration Record

PATIENT PROGRESS RECORD

Date	Product Type	Unit#	Blood Type	Time Beg.	Time End	Pre-meds? Y	Pre-meds? N	Pre-Infusion T	Pre-Infusion HR	Pre-Infusion RR	Pre-Infusion BP	15 minutes T	15 minutes HR	15 minutes RR	15 minutes BP	30 minutes T	30 minutes HR	30 minutes RR	30 minutes BP	End of Infusion T	End of Infusion HR	End of Infusion RR	End of Infusion BP	Bld Wmr? Y	Bld Wmr? N	S/S Reaction? Y	S/S Reaction? N	Signature

RECORD REACTION # IN THE "S/S REACTIONS?" COLUMN

Acute Reactions:
1 = fever
2 = temperature of > 1°C during or immediately following transfusion
3 = chills, mild itching or urticaria, sometimes confluent
4 = pain, sudden onset of dyspnea or complaints of inability to breathe
5 = hypotension
6 = sudden drop of systolic blood pressure 40 mmHg
7 = hemoglobinuria
8 = patient complaining of sense of impending doom (particularly for possible acute hemolytic reaction)
9 = abrupt change in urine color to a deep red/brown color or unexpected, sudden decrease in urine output
10 = unexplained bleeding or unexpected oozing from puncture/incision sites, chest pain, shock, pulminary edema

Delayed Reactions:
11 = unexplained onset of jaundice
12 = unexpected decrease in (or failure to increase) hemoglobin level occurring 5–13 days after transfusion
13 = unexpected elevations in liver function tests
14 = sudden and unexplained appearance of rash or diarrhea occuring 6–10 days

Transfusion Reaction Workup:
1. Send ASAP: 7mL clotted blood, and 10mL urine collected after reaction.
2. Six (6) hours post blood sample is required only for acute hemolytic transfusion reaction (HTR) or requested by Medical Director.
3. Send the remainder of the implicated unit(s) or empty blood bags, attached to administration set, all "Y" tubing with Transfusion Reaction investigation form to the Blood Bank.

FIGURE 23–2 ■ Sample blood administration record.
Used with permission from UC Davis Medical Center.

increased endurance and less fatigue after the transfusion due to the increased oxygen carrying capacity.

Blood Alternatives

Due to the risks associated with blood transfusion, alternative treatments for replacement of hemoglobin are sought. Recombinant technology has provided a means to augment the pro-

duction of blood cells within functioning bone marrow. Referred to as *blood modifier medications,* these drugs are being used in place of transfused blood in certain groups of patients. These medications have the same biological activity as endogenous human erythropoietin. They induce erythropoiesis by stimulating the division and differentiation of cells in the bone marrow. Indications for their use are the same as for blood transfusions: anemia associated with blood loss, HIV, cancer, and renal failure. These drugs are being used in place of a blood transfusion

EVIDENCE-BASED PRACTICE

Transfusion of Blood Products

Clinical Problem

Transfusing blood products is beneficial and often lifesaving, especially in the critically ill population. Blood transfusions are not without risk, however. Anemia is common among patients admitted to intensive care units (ICUs), and studies indicate that more than 40% of patients receive RBC transfusions while in the ICU (Corwin et al., 2004; Walsh et al., 2004). Two life-threatening risks include transfusion-related acute lung injury (TRALI) and fluid overload resulting in pulmonary edema. Nurses need to understand and apply evidence-based findings when administering blood in order to mitigate the occurrence of these complications.

Research Findings

Rena and colleagues (2006) conducted a study to assess the incidence of transfusion-related acute lung injury (TRALI) and transfusion-associated circulatory overload (TACO) in critically ill patients. Patients in four different ICUs who were not on ventilatory support at the time of transfusion were followed by a custom electronic surveillance system that tracked the time of transfusion and onset of respiratory failure. For this study respiratory failure was defined as the need for noninvasive or invasive ventilator support within 6 hours of transfusion.

The study evaluated 8,902 units that were transfused in 1,351 patients. From this sample, 94 patients required new respiratory support within 6 hours of transfusion. For analysis the data were separated into categories of (1) suspected TRALI, (2) possible TRALI, and (3) TACO. The incidence of suspected TRALI was 1 in every 1,271 units transfused; possible TRALI, 1 in 534 per unit transfused; and TACO, 1 in 356 per unit transfused. It was noted that suspected and possible TRALI patients received larger amounts of plasma. The authors concluded first that in the ICU, pulmonary edema frequently occurs after blood transfusion, requiring some form of ventilatory support. Secondly, they concluded that there is an association between infusion of plasma and the development of suspected or possible TRALI, which may have important implications with regard to etiology and prevention of this syndrome.

Implications for Nursing Practice

The impact on nursing practice from the findings of this research is multidimensional and requires critical thinking skills. The nurse must be vigilant of the transfusion infusion rate for a given patient. The patient's age, medical history, current diagnosis, and hemodynamic stability all influence the infusion rate. Except in emergent situations where acute blood loss impacts hemodynamic stability, blood is transfused slowly in order to prevent fluid overload. Monitoring the patient's response to the transfusion also is of critical importance. Vital signs, lung sounds, and oxygen saturation are assessed during and after the transfusion in order to evaluate the patient's tolerance. It is essential for the nurse to report to the health care team the

occurrence of abnormal lung sounds and/or a change in the rate and depth of respirations, as well as a decrease in oxygen saturation levels. The nurse needs to understand when ventilatory support is required and facilitate the plan to get it instituted.

The nurse also must be aware of the clinical manifestations of TRALI. Because this complication is often difficult to diagnose and can occur several hours after the transfusion, the nurse must continue ongoing monitoring of the patient subsequent to the transfusion. It is essential for the next shift of nurses to be told that the patient had a transfusion, especially if it was plasma, so that monitoring for side effects will be continued. Typically it is easier to limit the progress of the disorder if it is diagnosed and treated early in its development. Typically it is the nursing staff that picks up the clinical manifestations.

Critical Thinking Questions

1. You are the nurse caring for a patient who received a blood transfusion during the last shift. The nurse reported that the transfusion had occurred without incidence and that the follow-up blood work indicated that there was no need for another transfusion right now. When you assess your patient, you note that the heart respiratory rates are increased and the oxygen saturation has dropped. You suspect that the patient may be experiencing TRALI. Your nursing actions are based on:
   a. Symptoms will last a few minutes and then begin to subside.
   b. The symptoms usually last about 96 hours and then begin to resolve.
   c. Frequently patients need ventilatory support and diuretics.
   d. Since the symptoms are self limiting no medical intervention is needed.
   e. a & d
   f. b & c

2. You are caring for an 86-year-old patient with cardiac problems who is receiving his second unit of packed RBCs. During the transfusion he becomes short of breath and develops wheezes in his lung bases. What are the appropriate nursing actions?

Answers to Critical Thinking Questions appear in Appendix D.

References

Corwin, H. L., Gettinger, A., Pearl, R. G., et al. (2004). The CRIT study: Anemia and blood transfusion in the critically ill—Current clinical practice in the United States. *Critical Care Medicine, 32,* 39.

Rena, R., Fernandez-Perez, E. R., Khan, S. A., Rana, S., Winters, J. L., Lesnick, T. G., et al. (2006). Transfusion-related acute lung injury and pulmonary edema in critically ill patients: A retrospective study. *Transfusion, 46*(9), 1478–1483.

Walsh, T. S., Garrioch, M., Maciver, C., et al. (2004). Red cell requirements for intensive care units adhering to evidenced-based transfusion guidelines. *Transfusion, 44,* 1405.

because they are a safe and effective way to improve oxygen up-take and therefore tissue perfusion (Vernon & Pfeifer, 2003). In cases of massive hemorrhage, blood transfusion is still the treat-ment of choice due to the acute need for circulating volume and hemoglobin. See Chapter 64 🔗 for a complete description of blood modifier therapy.

A second method used to minimize the use of blood products is recombinant factor VIIa. Clotting occurs with the administra-tion of factor VIIa due to the activation of factor X, which causes additional generation of thrombin, resulting in the conversion of fibrinogen to fibrin. It is useful for a variety of clinical situa-tions including (Rose, 2007):

- Massive hemorrhage
- Thrombocytopenia
- Trauma
- Liver failure

- Oral anticoagulant toxicity
- Surgical, intracranial, and obstetrical hemorrhage
- Hemophilia.

Administration of factor VIIa has resulted in cessation of bleeding, reduced blood product use, and an improved coagulation profile (Bliss & Hanley, 2005; Growers & Parr, 2005; Mayo et al., 2004).

Research

Research is essential in order to continue improving the safety and efficacy of blood transfusion therapy. The goal of research is to identify areas where current practice could improve and then evaluate and test methods to improve these areas. The Research Opportunities and Clinical Impact feature provides a list of re-search topics still under investigation. Electronic databases also are a source for finding specific studies related to these topics.

RESEARCH OPPORTUNITIES AND CLINICAL IMPACT RELATED TO BLOOD ADMINISTRATION

Research Area	Clinical Impact
Prevention of disease transmission.	Ensure a safe blood supply.
Development of a synthetic product that can be used to raise hemoglobin and replace volume quickly in emergent situations and for persons who refuse blood transfusions.	Would provide a safe method for volume and cell replacement when blood products are not available due to the type and crossmatch process. Will provide a safe effective blood replacement for persons who refuse blood transfusions.
Development of a method to prevent ABO incompatibility errors.	Prevent the wrong blood being given to a patient.
A storage process that prevents the loss of viable cells and clotting factors.	Increase the therapeutic effectiveness of blood products.
Evaluate the impact of infusion devices (IV pumps) on cell integrity.	Obtain evidence that supports or negates the use of infusion pumps.
The need for additional in-line blood filters to prevent the infusion of clots and other debris.	Obtain a safer blood product.
Stimulating production of RBCs.	Treat anemia and decrease the need for a blood transfusion.
Measures to prevent or reduce blood transfusion reactions.	Increase safety of blood supply.

Clinical Preparation

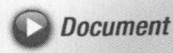 **Read**

- History of Current Illness
- Past Medical History
- Physical Exam
- Admitting Medical Orders
- Laboratory Study Results

 Document

- Summary of Hospitalization
- Pathophysiology Form
- Laboratory Values
- Laboratory Results Explanation

Apply

- List of Potential Nursing Diagnoses
- Concept Map
- Critical Thinking Questions

Log on to MyNursingKit.com to download forms you will need and to complete further steps in the Clinical Preparation assignment.

HISTORY OF PRESENT ILLNESS

Mr. B., an 86-year-old male, is admitted to the medical–surgical floor after being seen and evaluated in the emergency department (ED). His chief complaint is abdominal pain, nausea, and vomiting of moderate to large amounts of dark red liquid. Mr. B. has moderate to severe abdominal pain and nausea. He states he has been vomiting for 2 days and taken in very little food or water in 3 days. ED laboratory work: complete blood count (CBC), complete metabolic panel, UA, PTT, PT, and INR; liver function studies; troponin; type and crossmatch for 4 units packed cells. Vital signs in the ED were BP 90/60, HR 118, RR 28, T 37°C. On admission to the floor, the patient is awake and alert. He states he feels weak and light-headed. Two 500-mL fluid boluses of 0.9% NS were administered in the ED.

You are the nurse caring for Mr. B on his second day of hospitalization. The night nurse reported that there had been no vomiting or bloody stools since his admission. He does continue to complain of abdominal tenderness. After morning report you evaluate the patient's morning laboratory values. All laboratory work except the hemoglobin and hematocrit are normal. When you note that the hemoglobin is 8 g/dL and the hematocrit is 24%, you call the health care provider. Two units of packed RBCs are ordered to be given this a.m. followed by an Hgb & Hct and potassium. An endoscopy is scheduled for today.

Medical–Surgical History

Non-Q wave MI: 1998
Osteoarthritis
No known allergies
Denies a history of syncope
Denies history of gastric ulcers
Denies fever, chills, and night sweats

Home Medications

ASA 81 mg po daily
Lipitor 50 mg po daily
Lopressor 100 po mg bid
Celebrex 200 mg po daily
MVI po daily
Surgeries: appendectomy in 1982

Social History

He lives with his wife; has three grown children who live in the local area

Physical Exam

Elderly male, mild discomfort due to abdominal pain
Oxygen sat 94% on RA
BP: 90/62   HR 118   RR 26
HEENT: normal
Neck: negative JVD, no bruits
Heart: NL S1, S2

Lungs: clear
Abdomen: mildly distended soft, tender, hyperactive bowel sounds
Pulses: present in all extremities; strong throughout; good cap refill
Normal neuro exam
No rash
Poor skin turgor
Osteoarthritis
12-lead EKG showed sinus tachycardia, low voltage, and nonspecific ST wave changes
Chest x-ray is within normal limits

Admitting Medical Orders

Medicine Service
Admit to Telemetry Unit
Admitting diagnosis: GI bleed of unknown etiology
No known allergies
Vital signs and oxygen saturation: q2h
Daily weight
Foley catheter
Strict I&O
NPO
Full code status
Call house officer: BP systolic < 90 > 150 & diastolic > 90; HR > 120 & < 60; RR > 30; < 30 mL of urine per hour × 2 hours; oxygen saturation < 92%

NG: Salem sump lavage until clear and clamp; if vomiting occurs, apply low wall suction
Bed rest: out of bed to bedside commode with assist only
Incentive spirometer q2h
Sequential compression device (SCD) to lower extremities
IV: 0.9 normal saline with 20 mEq of KCl via infusion pump at 125 mL/hr
Keep 2 units of RBCs on hold at all times
GI consult ordered

Scheduled Medications
Protonix 40 mg IV q12h

PRN Medications
Morphine sulfate 2–4 mg IV push q2h prn for pain
Zofran 4 mg IV q8h prn nausea and vomiting

Ordered Laboratory Studies
Amylase and lipase now
Hgb & Hct now and q6h
Chem 7 panel now and in a.m.
Liver function studies now
PT, PTT and INR in a.m.
Potassium after blood

Ordered Diagnostic Studies
Abdominal CT scan

LABORATORY STUDY RESULTS

Test	Pt. Values # 1	Pt. Values #2	Pt. Values #3
Chemistry	Emergency Department	Pre-blood	Post-blood
Sodium	148 mEq/L	143 mEq/L	
Potassium	3.5 mEq/L	3.7 mEq/L	4.2 mEq/L
Chloride	113 mEq/L	110 mEq/L	
Carbon dioxide (CO_2)	25 mEq/L	24 mEq/L	
Blood urea nitrogen (BUN)	40 mg/dL	9 mg/dL	
Creatinine	1.0 mg/dL	1.0 mg/dL	
Blood, glucose	150 mg/dL	136 mg/dL	
Calcium	8.1 mg/dL		
Amylase		60 units/L	
Lipase		82 units/L	
Magnesium	2.2 mEq/L		
Troponin I	0.2 ng/mL		
Albumin	3.9		
Alkaline phosphorus	100 units/L		
GGT (0–65)	56 units/L		
Total bilirubin	1 mg/dL		
CPK total	200 units/L		
CPK MB	2.5%		
LDH	166 units/L		
AST	42 units/L		
ALT	60 units/L		
Hematology			
WBC	8000/mm³	7000/mm³	7000/mm³
Hemoglobin	10.2 g/dL	8 g/dL	10 g/dL
Hematocrit	32%	24%	37.9%
RBC	5/mm³		
Platelets	395/mm³	325/mm³	250/mm³
PTT	24 second		
PT	16.4 second	12 seconds	
INR (<1.19)	1.5	1.19	
Urine analysis	Normal		

CRITICAL THINKING QUESTIONS

1. What might be one cause of the gastric bleeding?

2. What are some possible reasons for the hemoglobin/hematocrit to decrease on the second hospital day?

3. What are critical nursing assessments during blood administrations?

4. What might Mr. B. be at high risk for during blood administration?

5. In the presence of dehydration, why would this patient's heart rate not be more elevated?

6. Compare and contrast the first and second set of labs. What lab data indicate that the patient was dehydrated when he came into the ED?

7. Why is the health care provider ordering an amylase and lipase study?

8. Why is the first PT/INR elevated?

Answers to Critical Thinking Questions appear in Appendix D.

NCLEX® REVIEW

1. A patient is prescribed to receive a transfusion of albumin. The nurse realizes that this transfusion will:
   1. Increase plasma colloidal osmotic pressure and plasma volume.
   2. Increase platelets and increase coagulation.
   3. Increase circulating RBCs.
   4. Increase plasma volume without increasing RBCs.

2. The teenage daughter of a patient asks for information to donate blood for her mother's health care needs. Which of the following should the nurse include in this information?
   1. Family members are discouraged from donating blood for patients.
   2. The youngest age for a blood donor is 17.
   3. A donor's blood pressure has to be greater than 180/90.
   4. A donor's blood count has to be greater than 13.5 mg/dL.

3. The nurse is planning to administer a unit of PRBCs to a patient. Which of the following should be included in this planning?
   1. History of blood transfusion reactions
   2. Circulatory and respiratory status
   3. Assemble appropriate equipment
   4. Patient provides informed consent for the transfusion

4. An elderly patient receiving a blood transfusion begins to cough and has an increase in blood pressure. What should the nurse do to help this patient?
   1. Stop the blood transfusion.
   2. Administer an antipyretic.
   3. Administer epinephrine.
   4. Stop the transfusion, flush the peripheral access device, and resume the transfusion.

5. A patient receiving a unit of PRBCs complains of chest pain within 5 minutes of the start of the transfusion. What should the nurse do?
   1. Slow the transfusion rate.
   2. Stop the transfusion, call for help and begin life-supporting measures.
   3. Administer epinephrine as according to the health care provider's order.
   4. Provide antipyretics.

Answers for review questions appear in Appendix D

KEY TERMS

albumin *p.543*
apheresis *p.539*
autologous transfusion *p.545*
blood transfusion *p.539*
cryoprecipitates *p.543*
factor VIII *p.543*
fresh frozen plasma *p.543*
frozen RBCs *p.543*

homologous transfusion *p.543*
leukocyte-poor RBCs *p.543*
packed RBCs *p.543*
perioperative blood salvage *p.547*
plasma *p.539*
platelets *p.539*
postoperative blood salvage *p.547*
Rh factor *p.541*

transfusion-related acute lung injury (TRALI) *p.550*
type A blood *p.541*
type AB blood *p.541*
type B blood *p.541*
type O blood *p.541*
washed RBCs *p.543*
whole blood *p.539*

PEARSON
EXPLORE mynursingkit™

MyNursingKit is your one stop for online chapter review materials and resources. Prepare for success with additional NCLEX®-style practice questions, interactive assignments and activities, web links, animations and videos, and more!

Register your access code from the front of your book at
www.mynursingkit.com

REFERENCES

American Association of Blood Banks. (2003). *Testing of donor blood for infectious disease.* Retrieved November 9, 2006, from http://www.aabb.org/Content/About_Blood/Facts_About_Blood_and_Blood_Banking/fabloodtesting.htm

American Red Cross. (2005). *Blood donation eligibility guidelines.* Retrieved November 7, 2006, from http://www.redcross.org/services/biomed/0,1082,0_557_,00.html#top

American Red Cross. (2006). *Leukocyte reduction Q&A.* Retrieved November 9, 2006, from http://www.redcross.org/services/biomed/blood/supply/ulr/qanda.html

America's Blood Centers. (2006). *56 facts about blood.* Retrieved November 7, 2006, from http://www.americasblood.org/go.cfm?do=Page.View&pid=12

Andrews, M. M., & Boyle, J. S. (2003). *Transcultural concepts in nursing care.* Philadelphia: Lippincott Williams & Wilkins.

Bliss, T., & Hanley, J. (2005). Recombinant activated factor VII (rFVIIa/NovoSeven) in intractable haemorrhage: Use of a clinical scoring system to predict outcome. *Vox Sang, 90,* 45–52.

Brown, M., & Whalen. P. K. (2000). Red blood cell transfusion in critically ill patients. *Critical Care Nurse* (Suppl.).

Finlay, H. E., Cassorla, L., Feiner, J., & Toy, P. (2005). Designing and testing a computer-based screening system for transfusion-related acute lung injury. *American Journal of Clinical Pathology, 124,* 601.

Food and Drug Administration. (2006a). *About CBER.* Retrieved November 8, 2006, from http://www.fda.gov/cber/blood.htm

Food and Drug Administration. (2006b). *Blood.* Retrieved November 9, 2006, from http://www.fda.gov/cber/blood.htm

Growers, C., & Parr, M. (2005). Recombinant activated factor VIIa use in massive transfusion and coagulopathy unresponsive to conventional therapy. *Anesthesia Intensive Care, 33,* 196–200.

Guyton, A., & Hall, J. (2000). *Textbook of medical physiology* (10th ed.). Philadelphia: W. B. Saunders.

Halpern, S. D., Taichman, D. B., & Hansen-Flaschen, J. (2005). *Transfusion-related acute lung injury (pulmonary leukoagglutinin reactions).* Retrieved November 16, 2006, from http://www.uptdol.com

Josephson, D. (2004). *Intravenous infusion therapy for nurses* (2nd ed.). Clifton Park, NY: Thompson Delmar Learning.

Kleinman, S. (2006a). *Massive blood transfusion.* Retrieved November 16, 2006, from http://www.uptdol.com

Kleinman, S. (2006b). *Patient information: Blood donation and transfusion.* Retrieved November 8, 2006, from http://patients.uptodate.com/topic.asp?file=blood_dis/2419

Kuechle, M. (2005). *Graft versus host disease.* Retrieved November 10, 2006, from http://www.emedicine.com/derm/topic478.htm

Linden, J. V., Wagner, K., Voytovich, A. E., & Sheehan, J. (2000). Transfusion errors in New York State: An analysis of 10 years' experience. *Transfusion, 40,* 1207–1213.

Lipson, J. G., Dibble, S. L., & Minarik, P. A. (1996). *Culture and nursing care: A pocket guide.* San Francisco: UCSF Nursing Press.

May, A. K., & Kauder, D. R. (2006). *Use of blood products in the critically ill.* Retrieved November 18, 2006, from http://www.uptodate.com

Mayo, A., Misgav, M., Kluger, Y., et al. (2004). Recombinant activated factor VII (NovoSeven): Addition to replacement therapy in acute, uncontrolled and life-threatening bleeding. *Vox Sang, 87,* 34–40.

Mayo Clinic. (2005). *Blood donation: A life saving gift.* Retrieved November 7, 2006, from http://www.mayoclinic.com/health/blood-donation/GA00039

McLeod, B. C. (2000). Introduction to the third space issue: Clinical applications of therapeutic apheresis. *Journal of Clinical Apheresis, 15*(1/2), 1–5.

Pearl, R. G., & Pohlman, A. S. (2002). Understanding and managing anemia in critically ill patients. *Critical Care Nurse* (Suppl.), 1–14; quiz 15–16.

Porth, C. M. (2005). *Pathophysiology: Concepts of altered health status* (7th ed.). Philadelphia: Lippincott Williams & Wilkins.

Rose, L. (2007). Recombinant factor VIIa. *AACN Advanced Critical Care, 18*(2), 141–148.

Silliman, C., Ambruso, R., & Boshkov, L. (2005). Transfusion-related acute lung injury. *Blood, 105,* 2266–2273.

U.S. Department of Health and Human Services. (2000). *Healthy people 2010: Understanding and improving health.* Retrieved June 11, 2008, from http://www.healthypeople.gov

Vernon, S., & Pfeifer, G. M. (2003). Blood management strategies for critical care patients. *Critical Care Nurse, 23*(6), 34–41.

Hemodynamic Monitoring

Patricia A. Baker

Outcome-Based Learning Objectives

After studying this chapter, the learner will be able to:

1. Explain the concept of hemodynamic monitoring.
2. Identify components of a hemodynamic monitoring system.
3. Compare and contrast arterial, central venous, and pulmonary artery pressure monitoring.
4. Identify adequate central venous and pulmonary artery pressures.
5. Evaluate nursing management of arterial lines and central venous and pulmonary artery catheters.
6. Discuss how alterations in preload, afterload, and contractility affect cardiac output.
7. Compare and contrast how measurements obtained from a central venous catheter differ from the data obtained from a pulmonary artery catheter.

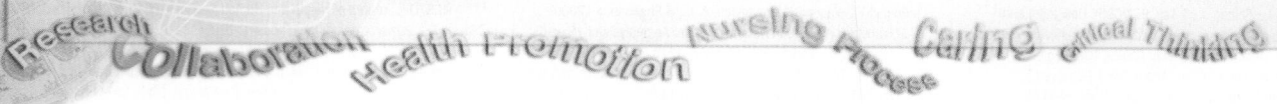

Research   Collaboration   Health Promotion   Nursing Process   Caring   Critical Thinking

Hemodynamic monitoring is the monitoring of blood flow and pressures within the body. Current technology allows for the monitoring of both the cardiac and neurological systems. This chapter describes invasive and noninvasive hemodynamic monitoring techniques used for the cardiovascular system. The purposes of hemodynamic monitoring are to (1) aid in the diagnosis of various disorders, (2) assist in guiding therapies to minimize or correct dysfunction, and (3) evaluate the patient's response to therapy. For safe operation of hemodynamic monitoring devices, nurses must be familiar with the anatomy and physiology of the system being monitored. Moreover, the nurse must be knowledgeable about therapeutic interventions and their rationales in order to achieve optimal, patient-specific stable outcomes. Nurses must be prepared to provide care based on the findings obtained from the hemodynamic monitoring, to institute interventions, and to report changes to the health care provider when they occur.

Hemodynamic monitoring capability is not restricted to the intensive care unit (ICU). Patients who require hemodynamic assessment are treated in emergency departments, postanesthesia care units, and intermediate care units. The level of intervention differs depending on the patient's diagnosis and hemodynamic stability, but may include monitoring arterial blood pressure, central venous pressure, or intracardiac pressures, all of which are discussed throughout this chapter.

Equipment

Both noninvasive and invasive devices are available for hemodynamic monitoring. The required equipment depends on the parameter monitored. Noninvasive monitoring often involves a stethoscope and sphygmomanometer; however, technologies such as ultrasound, and impedance cardiography are also considered noninvasive.

Invasive monitoring necessitates the insertion of a catheter into an artery or vein for direct and ongoing measurement of vascular pressures and volumes. Hemodynamic pressures are transmitted from the intravascular space via this specialized catheter into the monitoring system for the health care team to read and interpret. Invasive monitoring requires informed consent and staff who are knowledgeable about the equipment and techniques for safe use during the procedure. Assembling the equipment and maintaining the system are usually the responsibilities of the bedside nurse.

Informed Consent

Hemodynamic monitoring is not without risk. The physician or licensed provider who will be performing the procedure is responsible for discussing its risks with the patient. The nurse assesses the patient's understanding, reinforces the information as part of ongoing patient and family education, and witnesses a signature on the consent form. Consent in the critical care environment can be implied if a patient experiences an acute, life-threatening event. Chapter 6 discusses informed consent.

CRITICAL ALERT *Analgesics, sedatives, anxiolytics, and hypnotic medications impair judgment and thinking. The elderly are particularly susceptible to adverse reactions (confusion and disorientation) with other classes of medications. Nurses should inform the medical team if there is suspicion of cerebral impairment that would preclude informed consent.*

Components of the Monitoring Equipment

An invasive hemodynamic monitoring system has five basic components: the monitor, flush system, transducer, high-pressure tubing, and catheter (Figure 24–1 ■). The system is referred to as a transducer system and is assembled in an identical fashion whether used for an artery or vein. Chart 24–1 describes the step-by-step process for setting up the hemodynamic monitoring system.

These systems require a constant flow of sterile solution in order to maintain patency and decrease the risk of clot formation. The most common solution used is 0.9% normal saline (NS). Because these catheters are placed into high-pressure systems in the body, a sleeve is placed over the NS bag that is

---

CHART 24–1 Setup of Pressure Transducer System

1. Obtain an intravenous (IV) flush solution of normal saline and a transducer system.
2. Attach the transducer system to the IV flush solution and prime all tubing, ensuring that air bubbles are removed from the system.
3. Replace all vented caps with nonvented (dead-end) sterile caps.
4. Inflate the pressure bag to 300 mmHg.
5. Assist the patient to the supine position with the head of the bed elevated no more than 45 degrees.
6. Accurately measure and mark the patient's phlebostatic axis with an indelible marker.
7. Level the air–fluid interface to the phlebostatic axis.
8. Zero the system.
9. Set alarm limits.

Source: Adapted from American Association of Critical-Care Nurses. (2005). AACN Procedure manual for critical care. (5th Ed). D. J. Lynn-McHale Wiegand & K. K. Carlson. (Eds). Philadelphia: Elsevier, p. 591.

MyNursingKit | Video: Peripheral Vascular: Arterial Pressure Monitoring

FIGURE 24–1 ■ Components of the hemodynamic monitoring system.

inflated to 300 millimeters of mercury (mmHg) to counteract the pressure in the vessel and allow the solution to flow into the patient. High-pressure tubing instead of flexible intravenous (IV) tubing is necessary to withstand the external pressure exerted by the sleeve and to decrease the distortion of the waveform.

After the transducer system has been assembled and attached to the catheter, the infusion rate is held constant by the transducer system and the pressure sleeve. The information on the transducer package insert will indicate the constant infusion rate, but 1 to 3 mL/hour is common (Lynn-McHale Weigand & Carlson, 2005). The transducer converts pressure detected at the catheter tip into an electrical signal. This signal is displayed on a bedside or portable monitor. Both reusable and disposable transducers are available. Reusable transducers must be disinfected between patients in accordance with institutional policy.

Heparin versus No Heparin Flush Bags

The effect of heparinized versus nonheparinized flush solution on the patency of arterial catheters has been studied. Nursing research has demonstrated that heparin does influence the patency of arterial lines (Urden, Stacy, & Lough, 2006). When heparinized flush solutions were used on arterial lines in place for 72 hours, a greater percentage of arterial lines remained patent; however, heparin in the flush solution did not guarantee patency. Caution should be taken when exposing patients to heparin unnecessarily because the risk of heparin-induced thrombocytopenia increases with every exposure. Some institutions utilize only NS flush bags for all hemodynamic pressure lines.

 Heparin-induced thrombocytopenia occurs 4 to 7 days after exposure to heparin. Any exposure to heparin places the patient at risk of an immune response. The heparin stimulates an antibody that reacts with circulating platelets. This causes platelet aggregation and thrombosis. Diagnosis of heparin-induced thrombocytopenia is made when, during or after reexposure to heparin, the platelet count drops to <50% of baseline or the platelet count is <100,000/μL and other potential causes of thrombocytopenia are excluded. All heparin must be discontinued including heparin-coated invasive catheters.

Leveling, Zero Referencing, and Performing the Dynamic Response Test

Leveling the transducer, zero referencing, and performing the dynamic response test are nursing responsibilities when patients have hemodynamic monitoring catheters in place. Variability in technique among clinicians conducting these operator-dependent procedures influences the accuracy of the hemodynamic data (Urden et al., 2006). Each of these variables is discussed next.

Leveling the Transducer

Leveling the transducer means placing the transducer at the same level as the tip of the catheter sitting in the patient. A reference point on the patient, referred to as the **phlebostatic axis**, is identified to use as a baseline for consistent transducer height placement. To locate the phlebostatic axis, a horizontal line is identified that is halfway between the anterior and posterior di-

ameter of the chest. This horizontal line intersects with a vertical line from the fourth intercostal space (Figure 24–2 ■). Marking this reference point with an indelible marker permits ready identification by others.

The transducer is typically mounted on an IV pole beside the bed and a yardstick with a carpenter level aids the nurse in aligning the transducer with the phlebostatic point. Figure 24–3 ■ illustrates adjustment of the reference point for a patient in a lateral position. Research has shown that when the patient is supine, with the head of the bed elevated up to 45 degrees, the accuracy of pressure readings does not change (Giuliano, Scott, Brown, & Olson, 2003).

The importance of using the same reference point cannot be overstated. Incorrect transducer placement results in invalid pressure readings. Positioning the transducer above the reference point will decrease the pressure reading, and lowering the transducer will increase the reading. This discrepancy can expose a patient to unnecessary or erroneous treatment.

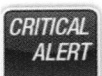 *To ensure accurate pressure readings, it is imperative that when the patient is repositioned, including raising or lowering the head of the bed, the transducer must be zeroed out again at the phlebostatic point. When the transducer is pole mounted and the bed height is raised or lowered, the zeroing out process should be repeated.*

Zero Referencing the Transducer

Once the transducer is level with the reference point, the next step is to zero reference the system. Prior to performing this procedure, ensure the transducer system is intact, the tubing is without air bubbles, and connections are tight. **Zero referencing** the transducer calibrates the equipment to atmospheric pressure. Figure 24–4 ■ illustrates the concept of zero referencing. To zero the transducer, turn the stopcock closest to the patient to

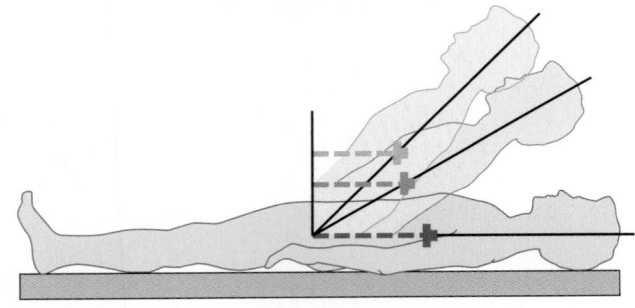

FIGURE 24–2 ■ Phlebostatic axis.

FIGURE 24–3 ■ Identification of phlebostatic axis when patient is in the lateral position.

FIGURE 24–4 ■ Leveling and zero referencing the transducer to the phlebostatic axis.

the off position. This turns the transducer off to the patient. Remove the cap from the transducer to allow for equilibration of the transducer with atmospheric pressure. Initiate the zero function on the monitoring system. Wait for the display to read zero then turn the stopcock knob back to the neutral position. The frequency of zeroing the transducer varies between institutions; however, zeroing should be done once per shift, after turning a patient, and whenever pressure readings are questionable (Darovic, 2004).

Dynamic Response Test/Square Wave Test

To test whether the transducer system is accurately transmitting the pressure detected in the vessel, a **dynamic response test** is performed. Poor dynamic response affects readings, making them either appear lower or higher than the actual reading. Dynamic response testing, also called the square wave test, is initiated by using the built-in flush system (pigtail) in the transducer. The nurse quickly pulls the pigtail and releases it, a process that is referred to as "fast flushing" the catheter. This results in a "square wave" in place of the normal waveform. If the test is normal, one or two oscillations will appear below the baseline (Kaplow & Hardin, 2007). The dynamic response test should be performed every 8 to 12 hours, after the system is opened for blood sampling, or whenever the accuracy of readings is questioned (Lynn-McHale Weigand & Carlson, 2005). The waveforms in Figure 24–5 ■ compare an appropriate dynamic response test with abnormal findings.

■ Hemodynamic Terminology

Invasive and noninvasive hemodynamic monitoring provide for close examination of cardiac function. This section explains the terms referred to in hemodynamic monitoring and provides examples to clarify their use. Chart 24–2 (p. 564) summarizes these terms.

Stroke Volume

Stroke volume (SV) is the amount of blood leaving the left ventricle with each contraction. For a healthy heart, the expected SV is 60 to 100 mL per beat. Stroke volume is sensitive to alterations in preload, afterload, and contractility, which are discussed later.

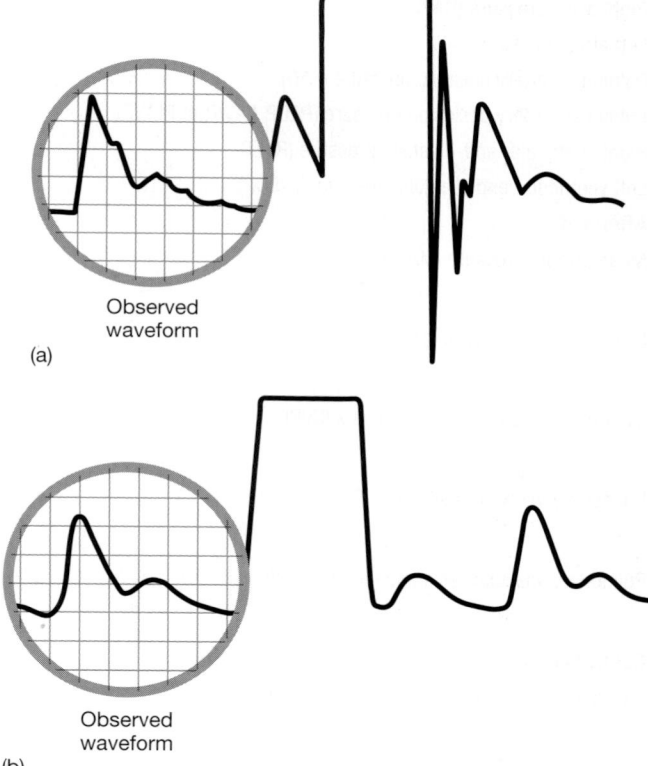

Observed waveform

(a)

Observed waveform

(b)

Square wave test configuration

Observed waveform

FIGURE 24–5 ■ Dynamic response testing: (A) normal response; (B) abnormal response.

CHART 24–2	Hemodynamic Parameters	
Parameters	**Calculation**	**Expected Value**
Cardiac Output (CO)		
Stroke volume (SV)	$\dfrac{CO \times 1000}{HR}$	60–100 mL per beat
Stroke volume index (SVI)	$\dfrac{SV}{BSA}$	35–75 mL/m² per beat
Cardiac index (CI)	$\dfrac{CO}{BSA}$	2.8–4.2 L min m⁻²
Heart rate (HR)		60–100 beats/min
Cardiac output	$HR \times SV$	4–8 liters/min
Preload		
Central venous pressure (CVP)		2–6 mmHg
Right atrial pressure (RAP)		4–6 mmHg
Left atrial pressure (LAP)		4–12 mmHg
Pulmonary artery diastolic pressure (PAD)		5–15 mmHg
Pulmonary artery occlusion pressure (PAOP, PAWP, or PCWP)		4–12 mmHg
Right ventricular end-diastolic pressure (RVEDP)		0–8 mmHg
Left ventricular end-diastolic pressure (LVEDP)		4–10 mmHg
Afterload		
Mean arterial pressure (MAP)	$DBP + \dfrac{(SBP - DBP)}{3}$	
Systemic vascular resistance (SVR)	$\dfrac{MAP - CVP \ (or \ RAP) \times 80}{CO}$	900–1600 dyn sec cm⁻⁵
Systemic vascular resistance index (SVRI)	$\dfrac{MAP - CVP \ (or \ RAP) \times 80}{CI}$	1970–2390 dyn sec cm⁻⁵
Pulmonary vascular resistance (PVR)	$\dfrac{PAM - PAOP \ (or \ PAWP) \times 80}{CO}$	155–255 dyn sec cm⁻⁵
Pulmonary vascular resistance index (PVRI)	$\dfrac{PAM - PAOP \ (or \ PAWP) \times 80}{CI}$	255–285 dyn sec cm⁻⁵
Contractility		
Ejection fraction (EF)	$\dfrac{LVEDV \times 100}{SV}$	60–75%
	$\dfrac{RVEDV \times 100}{SV}$	45–50%

Source: Adapted with permission from Whalen, D. A., & Kelleher, R. M. (1998). Cardiovascular patient assessment. In M. R. Kinney et al. (Eds.), *AACN clinical reference for critical care nursing* (4th ed., p. 279). St. Louis: Mosby.

Cardiac Output

Cardiac output (CO) is defined as the amount of blood leaving the left ventricle per minute. Cardiac output is calculated by multiplying heart rate (HR) by stroke volume (HR × SV). With a healthy ventricle, this amount is between 4 and 8 L/min. Adequate cardiac output is essential for circulation and tissue oxygenation. A drop in CO or when the heart is failing and cannot pump effectively reduces the amount of oxygen and nutrients delivered to the tissues.

Cardiac Index

Cardiac index (CI) is a more accurate measurement of circulation than cardiac output. The calculation for cardiac index incorporates the patient's body surface area (BSA). The cardiac index is the CO per square meter of the body. Body surface area can be calculated using the DuBois scale, software in a personal digital assistant (PDA), or by computing it as follows:

$$BSA = (weight \ in \ kg \times 0.425) \times (height \ in \ cm \times 0.725) \times 0.007184$$

If using the DuBois scale, a line is drawn between the patient's height and weight to obtain a BSA.

Whichever method is used to obtain a BSA, the BSA value is then divided into the cardiac output to obtain the cardiac index. An adequate CI is between 2.8 and 4.2 L/min. Most bedside monitors automatically calculate the BSA during a cardiac output measurement, provided the patient's height and weight have been preprogrammed into the monitor. The nurse is responsible for entering the correct height and weight into the bedside monitoring system. Frequently, the patient's admission weight is used. The CO and CI are hemodynamic parameters obtained with a pulmonary artery catheter, discussed later in this chapter.

Ejection Fraction

With each contraction, the left and right ventricles of the heart do not empty completely. The percentage of the total volume that is ejected with each beat is called the **ejection fraction (EF)**. Ejection fraction is a calculation that compares the end-diastolic volume to the stroke volume. It is expressed as a percentage. A normal EF is 65%, meaning that 65% of the blood in the left ventricle is ejected under normal circumstances with each heartbeat and 35% is left for periods of high demand.

The volume of blood remaining in the ventricle is considered a reserve. During periods of stress or exercise, this cardiac reserve, combined with a healthy ventricular contraction, assists in meeting the increased demand for adequate tissue oxygenation. Myocardium with abnormal contractile fibers is unable to pump as effectively as usual; thus, more blood remains in the ventricle with each beat, thereby decreasing the EF. Ejection fraction is an important parameter because a low EF value indicates ventricular dysfunction. An EF of less than 35% indicates serious ventricular failure. In patients with right or left ventricular failure, the administration of volume to improve stroke volume is poorly tolerated and may actually lead to a further decrease in cardiac performance.

Contractility

Contractility is the force generated by the contracting myocardium. The ability of the ventricles to contract or squeeze against resistance is determined by the contractile force of the ventricle. The force of contraction is related to the ability of the ventricular muscle fiber to lengthen or stretch. According to the **Frank-Starling law**, the muscle fibers in healthy ventricles will stretch to accommodate the venous return received during diastole. Generally, if the ventricle receives excess venous blood return during diastole, the ventricular contraction will be more forceful, resulting in an increased stroke volume. A filling pressure between 10 and 12 mmHg is considered optimal (Porth, 2007). When the pressure exceeds 12 mmHg and the myocardial fibers are overstretched, the force of ventricular contraction will decrease, eventually resulting in heart failure.

Contractility is enhanced by circulating catecholamines, sympathetic nervous system stimulation, and certain positive inotropic medications such as digoxin, dopamine, or dobutamine. Contractility is depressed with acidosis, hypoxemia, and beta-adrenergic blocking medications.

Preload

Preload is the volume of blood in the ventricle at the end of diastole. Although reflective of volume, preload is referred to as an end-diastolic pressure (EDP). Right ventricular preload is dependent on total blood volume returning to the heart, cardiac output, and venous vascular resistance (Porth, 2007). **Central venous pressure (CVP)** and right atrial pressure (RAP) are measurements that reflect venous return to the right side of the heart. A central venous pressure of less than 2 mmHg or a RAP of less than 4 mmHg is indicative of hypovolemia. True hypovolemia results from fluid losses such as excess diuretic therapy or the blood losses associated with hemorrhage. Relative hypovolemia occurs with venodilation. Venodilation results in less blood volume being returned to the heart. In patients with increased capillary permeability, as exhibited with sepsis, there is a generalized movement of fluid out of the vascular space and into the transcellular space referred to as "third spacing" of fluid (Porth, 2007). In these patients the CVP or RAP may be an unreliable indicator of preload, but can be monitored for an increasing or decreasing trend.

Hypervolemia, a CVP or RAP of more than 6 mmHg indicates that an increased volume of blood is being returned to the right atrium. Increased preload may be the result of volume overload, renal failure, or cardiac tamponade. Usually the volume of increased preload is the result of intravascular excess. An increase in preload may be noted after a rapid, large-volume IV infusion; however, a patient in renal failure or in heart failure will also exhibit an elevated CVP due to either an inability to excrete fluid or to the buildup of excess pressure in the heart due to poor ventricular function. An elevation in the CVP or RAP also occurs when fluid accumulates in the pericardial sac and exerts external pressure on the heart chambers, as in cardiac tamponade (Chapter 41 ☞). Further investigation is required to determine the exact cause. When assessment of preload must be more precise, a pulmonary artery catheter with a lumen in the right ventricle provides measurement of right ventricular volume using the previously described transducer system.

Afterload

Afterload is the pressure or resistance the ventricles must overcome to eject blood during systole. Vascular resistance is the major determinant of afterload. The right ventricle pumps blood into the pulmonary system through the pulmonic valve into the pulmonary artery (Kaplow & Hardin, 2007). Afterload of the pulmonary system is termed pulmonary vascular resistance (PVR). The left ventricle pumps blood into systemic circulation through the aortic valve. Systemic afterload is termed systemic vascular resistance (SVR). Elevations in vascular resistance are the result of vasoconstriction, which has many causes such as hypothermia or hypoxemia. Vascular resistance can also be elevated from mechanical barriers such as aortic or pulmonary artery stenosis. Decreases in vascular resistance are noted in hyperthermia or when vasodilators are administered. Unlike the direct measurement of preload, afterload is a calculated value.

■ Normal Hemodynamic Pressures

Human physiology relies on a dynamic balance between blood flow, resistance, and pressure. Hemodynamic monitoring provides

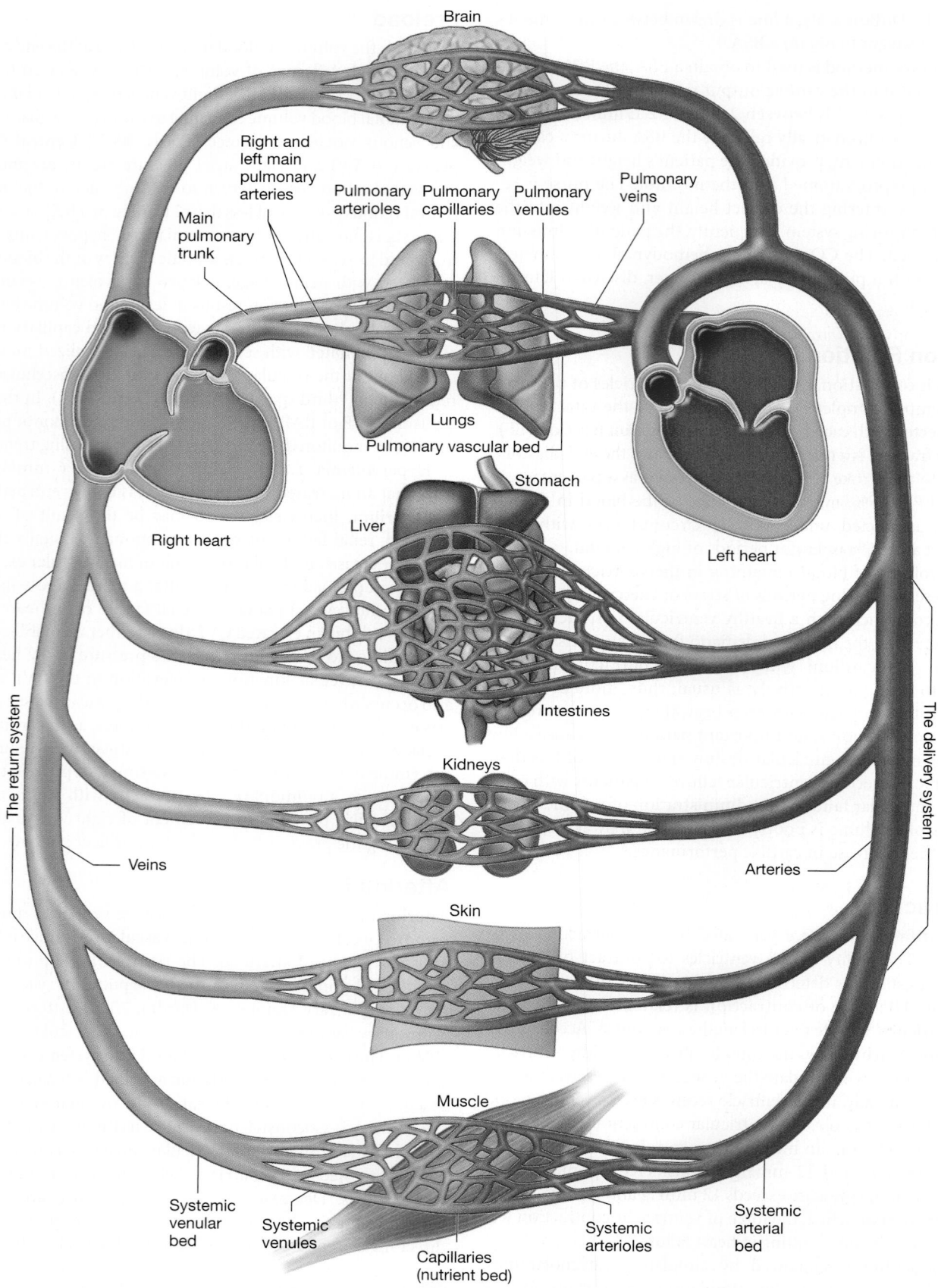

FIGURE 24–6 ■ Vascular circuit.

an overall assessment of this balance with individual components focusing on circulation, perfusion, and tissue oxygenation. This in-depth assessment of these interactions helps health care providers as they diagnose, guide, and evaluate therapies.

The Pump and the Circuit

The closed loop of the cardiovascular system relies on pressure gradients to maintain the normal forward movement of blood flow (Figure 24–6 ■). The low-pressure pulmonary and systemic venous systems deliver blood to their respective atria. Pressure changes in the atria and ventricles are the end result of electrical and mechanical activities. When atrial pressure exceeds ventricular pressure, the tricuspid and mitral valves open and blood passively flows into the ventricle. At the end of this passive flow, when the tricuspid and mitral valves are open, the mean pressure between the atria and the ventricles is equal. When ventricular pressure exceeds pressure in the atria, the tricuspid and mitral valves close. When ventricular pressure exceeds the pressure in the pulmonary artery and aorta, the pulmonic and aortic valves open. Disruption to any segment in the closed loop or cardiac dysfunction can cause an alteration in preload and afterload.

Waveforms and the Cardiac Cycle

When an invasive catheter senses the cardiovascular system's pressures, they are displayed on a monitor as pressure readings. Pressure changes produce positive waves and negative deflections. The waveform correlates with the cardiac cycle, but because the pressures are being transmitted through fluid-filled tubing, there is a slight delay. Simultaneous dual-channel recording of the electrocardiogram (ECG) and pressure waveforms improves the accuracy of the pressure readings, or tracings (Figure 24–7 ■) (Dietz & Smith, 2002). Pressure readings are most accurate at the end of expiration when the effect of intrathoracic pressure is negligible. The location of end expiration on a pressure tracing differs between a spontaneously breathing patient and a patient on positive pressure mechanical ventilation. When a patient is spontaneously breathing, end expiration on a pressure tracing will be higher. With less intrathoracic pressure compressing the great vessels, there is a corresponding increase in preload. Conversely, when a patient is receiving positive pressure ventilation, the intrathoracic pressure is lower during expiration due to the reduction in intrathoracic pressure during exhalation. Figure 24–8 ■ (p. 568) illustrates the differences between the end expiration point in a

spontaneously breathing and a mechanically ventilated patient. Identification of end expiration is important due to its influence on preload, with a falsely elevated preload leading to a falsely elevated cardiac output measurement.

Invasive Pressure Monitoring

Invasive hemodynamic monitoring provides a method of direct measurement of vascular pressures. Medical therapies are based on the interpretation of the parameter being assessed. Systemic, central venous, and pulmonary artery monitoring devices are frequently used for this purpose. Each of these is discussed in this section along with information on complications and nursing management.

Intra-arterial Catheters

An **arterial line** is an indwelling catheter inserted into an artery by a physician or an advanced practice nurse in order to monitor blood pressure. These catheters, which are inserted either percutaneously or by a surgical cutdown technique, are recommended for patients whose blood pressure is unstable and therefore require frequent monitoring. These patients include those who are hypotensive, hypertensive, or receiving vasoactive medications requiring titration and careful monitoring. Arterial lines also provide access for obtaining frequent blood specimens.

CRITICAL ALERT   *An arterial line is never used for infusion of IV solutions or medications. Both IV solutions and medications are irritating to the vessel and may compromise tissue perfusion distal to the catheter.*

Insertion of Arterial Catheters

The radial artery is the most common site for arterial catheter placement. Other sites such as the brachial, axillary, femoral, dorsalis pedis, and posterior tibial are possible alternatives. Although the diameter of the radial artery is smaller than that of the ulnar artery, the radial artery is easily accessible because of its proximity to the skin surface, making it the preferred site. An **Allen's test** is performed prior to insertion of the radial arterial catheter to assess ulnar circulation in the hand (Figure 24–9 ■, p. 568). To perform an Allen's test, raise the patient's hand above his head and ask the patient to make a tight fist. While the fist is tight, apply pressure to occlude the radial and ulnar arteries simultaneously. Lower the patient's hand and ask him to release the tight fist. The nurse then releases the pressure over the ulnar

FIGURE 24–7 ■   Single-lead ECG and arterial pressure waveform.

ECG

PAP

PAP = 72/36

72

36

(a)

ECG

Ventilator   Ventilator   Ventilator

PAWP=20

(b)

FIGURE 24–8 ■ End expiration: (A) spontaneously breathing patient; (B) mechanically ventilated patient.

Radial artery — Ulnar artery

(a)   **(b)**   **(c)**

FIGURE 24–9 ■ Performing the Allen's test.

artery and observes the return of color to the hand. An Allen's test is positive if the color returns to the hand in 7 seconds or less after release of the ulnar artery. If return time is greater than 7 seconds, the test is inconclusive, but if greater than 15 seconds, the test is negative. If color does not return to the hand after re-

leasing the ulnar artery, the health care provider should be notified prior to an arterial puncture. If the test is negative, the radial artery should not be used for an arterial line because the superficial palmar arch is not intact. This may place the patient at risk for vascular thrombosis and arterial occlusion, which may lead to necrosis and in severe cases amputation of the hand. The nurse must always document that the Allen's test was performed, the results, and any action taken if the test is negative. Ongoing assessment of circulation distal to the insertion site is the responsibility of the bedside nurse.

 The Allen's test can be performed on an unconscious patient by holding the patient's arm above her head and clenching her hand into a fist. Apply pressure to both ulnar and radial arteries while the arm is overhead. Lower the arm and release the pressure from the radial artery.

Ensuring the integrity of the monitoring system, preventing infection, and assessing for thrombus formation also are fundamental nursing responsibilities associated with arterial line placement (Urden et al., 2006). Once the catheter is secured, an occlusive dressing is applied. The arterial catheter can be sutured in place prior to the application of the dressing. Also prior to applying the dressing, ensure the arterial catheter is tightly attached to the hub on the pressure tubing. The monitoring system has upper and lower limit alarming capabilities, and it is the responsibility of the nurse to set, adjust, and ensure these alarms are engaged at all times.

 Always set the patient's alarms based on the patient's baseline hemodynamic pressures and the abnormality being monitored. Never turn the alarms off entirely. To allow alert patients periods of uninterrupted rest, the intensity or volume of the alarm can usually be adjusted on bedside monitors without affecting the alarm signal or message from the central station.

Arterial Pressure Waveforms

When the pressure transducer system is attached to the arterial catheter, an identifiable arterial waveform appears on the monitor. This waveform represents systolic and diastolic pressures generated by the mechanical activity of the heart (Figure 24–10 ■). The systolic pressure represents maximum left ventricular systolic pressure. The dicrotic notch represents closure of the aortic valve and distinguishes the end of systole and beginning of diastole. The beginning of diastole is a significant cardiac event. Diastolic pressure indicates the pressure in the ventricle at rest and is directly related to blood vessel elasticity (Darovic, 2004).

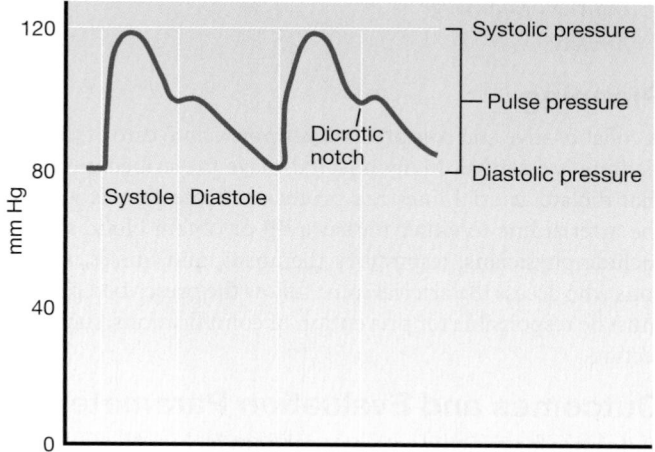

FIGURE 24–10 ■ Analyzing arterial pressure waveform.

Complications of Arterial Blood Pressure Monitoring

Complications of arterial blood pressure monitoring include hemorrhage, emboli, vascular occlusion or spasm, and infection. Occult hemorrhage may occur, particularly after a femoral artery catheter has been inserted. Signs of hypovolemia, lower abdominal firmness, or swelling or bruising at the site should alert the nurse to notify the health care provider immediately. Due to high pressure in arteries, massive blood loss can occur if the catheter dislodges or is disconnected from the patient or if the connections are loosened. Assessment of circulation distal to the insertion site, prior to insertion of the catheter, does not preclude vascular ischemia and necrosis. Arterial clots, fibrin, or air may cause emboli. Risk factors include multiple arterial punctures of the same limb or site, vasoconstriction, low cardiac output, severe peripheral vascular disease, prolonged duration of catheter, and an active infectious process (Darovic, 2004). Vascular occlusion or spasm cannot be predicted and risk factors for spasm are the same as embolic events. Aseptic technique is used for all dressings and sterility is maintained when obtaining blood specimens.

Factors Influencing Arterial Pressure

Alterations in the conduction system of the heart influence arterial pressure. Patients who have irregular cardiac rhythms, such as atrial fibrillation or premature contractions, demonstrate arterial waveforms with varying systolic pressures. These patients experience a decrease in systolic pressure as a result of the decrease in diastolic filling time. Premature contractions prevent complete filling of the ventricle during diastole. With less blood volume filling the heart, there is less volume to eject on the next systole, which results in the lower arterial systolic pressure. Figure 24–11 ■ (p. 570) illustrates this phenomenon. Chapter 38 ☞ provides an in-depth discussion of these dysrhythmias.

As the distance between the heart and the catheter site increases, the shape of the arterial waveform will change: The systolic pressure waveform becomes higher and the diastolic pressure waveform becomes lower. Figure 24–12 ■ (p. 570) illustrates the changes in the shape of an arterial waveform as distance from the heart increases. The mean arterial pressure, however, remains constant irrespective of the arterial catheter site. **Mean arterial pressure (MAP)** is the average pressure in the arteries during one cardiac cycle. When administering vasoactive medications, the MAP is usually specified as the titration parameter. Mean arterial pressure is used in the equation to calculate afterload or SVR.

Pulsus paradoxus refers to a pattern in the arterial waveform in which the systolic pressure decreases by 10 mmHg or more during the inspiratory phase of ventilation. This pattern is the classic sign of cardiac tamponade, but can also be present in any condition that results in compression of the right side of the heart (Urden et al., 2006). In tamponade, fluid or blood has accumulated in the pericardial sac causing compression of the heart. This compression is temporarily relieved during the inspiratory phase of ventilation. During inspiration, a drop in intrathoracic pressure occurs that allows for an increase in venous return. The increased venous return translates into an increase in stroke volume during the next systole. Chapter 41 ☞ describes the causes of pulsus paradoxus and cardiac tamponade.

FIGURE 24–11 ■ Effect of atrial tachycardia on arterial pressure.

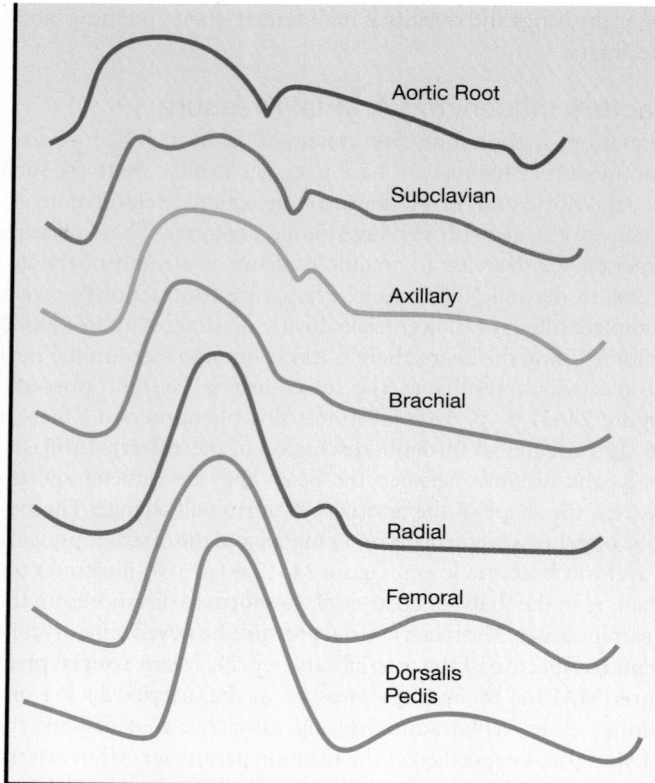

FIGURE 24–12 ■ Changes in arterial pressure waveform.

◼ Nursing Management

Explaining the procedure to the patient and family will assist in decreasing their anxiety and elicit their cooperation. Prior to insertion a modified Allen's test must be performed and documented. The bedside nurse can facilitate radial artery cannulation by hyperflexion of the patient's wrist during insertion. After insertion a padded armboard is sometimes necessary after an arterial line is placed to keep the wrist hyperflexed and to optimize the waveform. The nursing process serves as a guideline for nursing management of patients with arterial lines.

Assessment

An in-depth assessment can identify patients at risk, so that actions can be taken to prevent complications from the arterial line. The nurse needs to assess the arterial line insertion site for redness, pain, and swelling, because this is an indication of infection. Assessment of the circulation also is essential to prevent ischemic changes due to compromised circulation. Note the presence and quality of pulses in the extremity. Regularly observe for changes in skin color and assess for motor and sensory changes in the extremity distal to the insertion site. Assessment of the blood pressure (BP) is done on a continuous basis and documented per health care provider orders or unit guidelines. The nurse must note the waveform, and when changes occur the patient should be reassessed and troubleshooting done on the equipment.

Nursing Diagnosis

Nursing diagnoses related to arterial line placement include:

* *Risk for Infection*
* *Impaired Tissue Integrity*
* *Ineffective Tissue Perfusion*
* *Deficient Knowledge*
* *Anxiety.*

Planning

A collaborative and comprehensive approach to care of the arterial line is essential. Many hospitals have prescribed guidelines that dictate arterial line care protocols. Professionals who use the arterial line to either measure BP or obtain blood samples include physicians, respiratory therapists, and nurses. All persons who access the arterial must follow the prescribed plan and must be responsible for prevention of complications, such as infection.

Outcomes and Evaluation Parameters

Outcomes for patients with arterial lines include the following:

* Stabilization of the BP without vasoactive drugs
* No infection at the catheter site or in the bloodstream

- No bleeding from the arterial line site or catheter
- Having the arterial discontinued due to BP stabilization.

Interventions and Rationales

An arterial line can be inserted for the sole purpose of obtaining blood specimens. More commonly, however, a catheter is placed so that blood pressure can be closely monitored. Nursing interventions include monitoring the blood pressure and, if administered, assessing the effectiveness of vasoactive therapy. When a patient is receiving vasoactive medications, which either increase or decrease BP, the bedside nurse is responsible for medication titration to keep the blood pressure within the parameters ordered by the health provider. Frequent assessment of blood pressure (usually at 5- to 10-minute intervals) and documentation of amount of medication infusing are required. When the goal blood pressure is achieved and maintained, then the institutional policy related to documentation is followed.

Each monitor has the ability to notify the nurse that the blood pressure is too high or too low. After the arterial line is inserted, set the high and low alarm limits. These alarms should never be turned off when the nurse leaves the room. When high or low alarms occur, assess the patient for changes. If changes occur in the arterial waveform, *first* assess the patient and take a manual cuff pressure. If the cuff pressure varies from the arterial pressure, it is necessary to troubleshoot the equipment by systematically inspecting and, if necessary, tightening all connections and tubing from insertion site to pressure bag.

Care of an arterial line site includes changing the dressing per unit protocol or whenever the occlusive dressing becomes loose or when contamination is suspected. If infection is suspected, the health care professional should be notified and preparation for a new line instituted. After the dressing is applied, obtain a strip of the arterial line tracing and document the procedure in the patient's record.

Nurses can remove an arterial catheter according to institutional policy and on order by the health care provider. Explain to the patient that the catheter is being removed and pressure will be applied to the site. Prior to removing a radial artery catheter, don goggles and apply nonsterile gloves. Remove the dressing, then remove the suture, if present, with a suture removal kit. With one hand, gently remove the catheter, and apply direct site pressure as soon as the catheter is removed. Continue to apply pressure until hemostasis is achieved, then apply a sterile dressing. The procedure is the same when removing a femoral arterial catheter; however, with the large femoral artery more time is required to achieve hemostasis by direct pressure. Routinely sending catheter tips for culture after removal is not recommended (Centers for Disease Control and Prevention [CDC], 2002). Observe the catheter site regularly for bleeding and/or hematoma formation after the catheter has been removed.

Evaluation

While the arterial line is in place, the nurse should correlate the cuff blood pressure with the arterial line pressure by simultaneously obtaining a reading from the arterial line and a sphygmomanometer. The pressure reading obtained by the arterial line is higher than the cuff pressure because the arterial catheter is a direct measurement rather than an indirect measurement obtained with a sphygmomanometer or by an automated noninvasive

blood pressure machine. Evaluation of the arterial line site should be done every shift and clinical manifestations of infections need to be reported to the health care professional.

Central Venous Catheters

Single- or multiple-lumen catheters are inserted for monitoring central venous pressure, which is the pressure in the right atrium. The subclavian, internal or external jugular, and femoral veins are potential insertion sites. Depending on the selected site and the length of the catheter, the tip transmits pressure from the right atrium, superior vena cava, or inferior vena cava. Specialized central venous catheters with a fiber-optic sensor allow for measurement of systemic central venous oxygen saturation ($ScvO_2$) (Kaplow & Hardin, 2007). The use of central venous oxygen saturation readings for the treatment of severe sepsis is discussed in Chapter 61 .

Insertion of Central Venous Catheters

After obtaining consent, the patient is placed supine. Positioning the patient during line placement is important. If the subclavian or a jugular vein site is selected and if tolerated by the patient, then the nurse may be asked to place the patient in the Trendelenburg position. This position facilitates venous dilation of the central veins and reduces the risk of an air embolus. Also, a rolled-up towel placed between the shoulder blades and parallel with the spine aids in landmark identification and reduces the risk of a pneumothorax. The patient may be asked to turn her head away from the insertion site to minimize contamination of the site. Patients should be informed of the necessity of maintaining a sterile barrier, which for upper torso sites, involves temporarily covering the patient's face with sterile drapes. The health care provider and anyone assisting with catheter insertion wear a cap, mask, sterile gown, and gloves. The nurse and anyone present in the room during the procedure wear a cap and mask. If, at any point during the procedure, the nurse expects to be in contact with the sterile field, then sterile attire is required for the nurse.

When the catheter is secured, the sterile drapes are removed and a sterile dressing is placed over the insertion site. Despite blood return from the central venous catheter port(s) after insertion, the catheter should not be accessed for intravenous infusions or monitoring until a chest x-ray confirms correct placement and a pneumothorax is ruled out. A chest x-ray is not necessary for femoral lines. Reassess the patient and compare the postinsertion findings with the preinsertion assessment.

CRITICAL ALERT *If in doubt as to whether the catheter is in a vein or artery, remove a sample of blood and send or test it for oxygen saturation. This can be included in the line insertion procedure.*

Central Venous Pressure Monitoring

The central venous pressure reflects the blood pressure of the vena cava and the right atrium. CVP monitoring requires the insertion of a catheter into a central vein that is used for monitoring volume status and venous return to the heart. When a central venous catheter is attached to a transducer system, a CVP or RAP waveform can be obtained. The CVP or RAP waveform should be continually displayed on the bedside monitor. A venous pressure of 2 to 6 mmHg is adequate; however, patients may be hemodynamically stable or unstable with lower or higher pressures. Monitoring the trend in CVP, either increasing or decreasing, is of more importance than one observed value. As with other measurements, correlation of findings with patient assessment is essential.

The CVP may be intermittently monitored. When the central venous catheter is the sole IV access and CVP monitoring is required, a stopcock connector may be used in combination with the transducer system. It is important to understand that when the knob on the stopcock is turned so that the CVP can be checked, any IV infusion at the stopcock is stopped until the stopcock is returned to its original position, allowing for infusion therapy to continue.

Central Venous Pressure Waveform

The normal CVP waveform has three positive waves that correspond to atrial cardiac events. The *a* wave correlates with the P wave or atrial contraction (systole). The next positive wave, the *c* wave, may not be visible on the tracing. The *c* wave reflects retrograde swelling of the tricuspid valve into the right atrium, which occurs during ventricular contraction. The *v* wave represents atrial filling (diastole) and the increased pressure against the closed tricuspid valve in early diastole. Figure 24–13 ■ illustrates these relationships.

Complications of Central Venous Pressure Monitoring

Infection can occur any time the catheter is in place, therefore prevention of infection is an important nursing responsibility. The transmission of organisms is preventable when strict aseptic technique is maintained during catheter insertion and dressing changes (see the National Guidelines box about prevention of catheter-related infections). An air embolus is a complication that may occur during insertion or removal of a central catheter, if the IV disconnects from the catheter hub, or when obtaining blood specimens. Assessment findings that may indicate an air embolus include dyspnea, tachypnea, cyanosis, hypotension, and chest pain. A pneumothorax is another risk associated with thoracic central line placement. It can occur when a needle or introducer penetrates the vessel wall, causing air to enter the pleural space. Assessment findings associated with a pneumothorax include those for an air embolus, plus absence of breath sounds on the side of insertion.

FIGURE 24–13 ■ Correlation of cardiac cycle to CVP and pulmonary artery waveforms.

■ Nursing Management

Nursing management of central venous catheters focuses on preventing complications, starting with catheter insertion and ending with catheter removal. When compared to arterial catheters and pulmonary artery catheters, the rate of catheter-related infections is highest for central venous catheters (CDC, 2002). The National Guidelines box provides a synopsis of key points from the national guidelines released in 2002 by the CDC.

Further recommendations include replacing all central venous catheters if the patient is hemodynamically unstable and catheter-related bloodstream infection is suspected. In this instance, the bedside nurse alerts the health care team to the catheter replacement need and assists with new central line placement.

NATIONAL GUIDELINES Prevention of Intravascular Catheter-Related Infections

1. Sterile barrier precautions are necessary for all personnel assisting with central venous access insertion.
2. A 2% chlorhexidine preparation is the preferred antiseptic before catheter insertion and during dressing changes.
3. The antiseptic should remain on the insertion site and be allowed to air dry before catheter insertion.
4. Inspect catheter sites visually or manually palpate on a regular basis. Remove dressing to examine if site is tender to palpation.
5. Remove any vascular device that is no longer essential to patient care.
6. Replace disposable transducers, tubing, flush devices, and flush solution at 96-hour intervals.
7. Replace administration sets, including secondary sets and add-on devices, no more frequently than at 72-hour intervals.
8. To prevent infection, avoid routine replacement of central venous catheters.
9. Clean injection port with 70% alcohol or iodophor before accessing.
10. Do not routinely culture catheter tips.

Source: Adapted from Centers for Disease Control and Prevention. (2002). Guidelines for the prevention of intravascular catheter-related infections. *Morbidity and Mortality Weekly Report, 51,* 1–26.

Assessment

Nursing management of a central venous catheter, whether new or *in situ*, involves patient education, assessing the site for infection and leakage, dressing changes, and monitoring of pressures. Prior to insertion of a central venous catheter, the nurse is responsible for assessing the patient for contraindications to the procedure. These include assessing the insertion site, assessing potential difficulties in positioning the patient, and obtaining a baseline physical assessment, including vital signs, pulse oximetry, and heart and breath sounds. Preassessment provides a point of reference for comparison when the procedure is complete. Ensure that external monitoring devices such as ECG wires and electrodes, noninvasive blood pressure cuffs, and pulse oximetry cables are clear of the insertion site. Check the ECG electrodes for good skin contact. If necessary due to the choice of insertion site, relocate ECG electrodes prior to the procedure and before the patient is covered with sterile drapes.

Nursing Diagnosis

Nursing diagnoses related to hemodynamic monitoring include:

- *Anxiety*
- *Risk for Imbalanced Fluid Volume*
- *Ineffective Health Maintenance*
- *Risk for Injury*
- *Deficient Knowledge*
- *Risk for Infection*

Planning

Patient education decreases anxiety and increases patient participation in care. Inform the patient that routine dressing changes and close examination of the insertion site will occur. Before the procedure patients should be informed of the risks of the procedure, the expected duration of the procedure, and that repositioning may be required. Planning for interventions for care for the patient with invasive lines is multifaceted. Each institution has specific procedures for maintaining a sterile occlusive dressing over the line insertion site. The nurse must be knowledgeable of these procedures and carry them out within the required time frames.

Outcomes and Evaluation Parameters

Outcomes associated with central venous catheters include:

- Stabilization of the central venous pressure readings to within normal limits
- No infection at the catheter site or in the bloodstream
- No bleeding from the site or catheter
- Having the central venous catheter discontinued due to patient stabilization.

Interventions and Rationales

Once the central venous catheter is in place, the nurse is responsible for site care and dressing changes. Routine site inspection includes assessing the insertion site and surrounding skin for signs of infection or leakage. Institutional policies vary as to the type of dressing applied; however, hand hygiene and nonsterile gloves are always used to remove the old dressing. If using a prepackaged dressing kit, don the sterile gloves and clean the insertion site and catheter using the disinfectant provided. Allow the disinfectant to air dry. Do not fan the area to speed the drying time because this may lead to site contamination. After the new dressing has been applied, document the procedure, including patient education, date and time of procedure, description of the catheter site, and type of dressing. Some institutions require the date and time of dressing change plus the initials of the person changing the dressing to be placed on the dressing. After assisting with placement of a central venous line, do not access the line until a chest x-ray has confirmed correct placement.

Monitoring the CVP, interpreting the information, and correlating the data collected with the patient's condition are nursing responsibilities. Monitoring the CVP is accomplished with the previously described transducer system. By leveling and zero referencing the transducer and performing the dynamic response test, the nurse can help ensure that the CVP values are accurate.

The CVP reflects preload. Conditions causing an increased CVP include venoconstriction, fluid volume overload, cardiac tamponade, pulmonary hypertension, or depressed cardiac function, especially right ventricular function. Corroborate elevations in CVP with physical assessment findings, which include dependent edema; tachypnea, dyspnea, or orthopnea; anxiety; crackles; and jugular vein distention. Central venous pressures below normal are indicative of venodilation or hypovolemia. Low pressures are frequently seen with major burn injuries, hemorrhage, and spinal cord injuries. Physical findings include postural hypotension, tachycardia, and decreased mean arterial pressure. If continuous monitoring of CVP is not routine, then institutional policy and the health care provider's orders dictate the frequency of obtaining readings. A single CVP value that is less than or more than normal is not as alarming as is a trend in values up or down coupled with a change in the physical assessment findings. Contacting the health care provider is indicated when an abnormal CVP measurement correlates with assessment findings.

Removal of a central venous catheter is done in much the same manner as an arterial line catheter. However, when removing a central venous catheter from the subclavian or jugular site, the removal is timed with the inspiratory phase of the respiratory cycle. When the patient takes a deep breath, the intrathoracic pressure is increased. This maneuver decreases the potential for air embolus. At the peak of inspiration, gently remove the catheter and tell the patient to breathe normally. Continue to hold pressure until hemostasis is achieved and then apply a sterile dressing.

Although CVP and RAP assess preload based on volume status and venous return to the heart, these measurements are often insufficient. When medical therapies depend on accurate evaluation of cardiac output, then measurement of preload, afterload, and contractility is required. Invasive and noninvasive methods are available for this purpose.

Evaluation

Due to the risk of infection, the expected outcome for these patients is stabilization with the intent of getting the invasive catheters removed as soon as possible. Fluid balance as determined by heart rate, BP, and urine output is the evaluation parameter. Not every patient will have normal readings, thus, the goal is to achieve readings that are tolerated by the patient.

Measuring Cardiac Output

Variations in heart rate, preload, afterload, or contractility influence cardiac output. Healthy individuals maintain homeostatic balance through intact compensatory pathways. Athletes, for example, are frequently bradycardic (heart rate below 60 beats/min), but their CO is maintained with above-normal stroke volumes. Critically ill patients either lack reserve or have exhausted their compensatory responses. In other words they are unable to significantly increase contractility to increase the stroke volume. The bedside nurse should be knowledgeable about the components that influence cardiac output, because these factor into determining not only initial therapy, but also evaluation of therapy.

Invasive Methods with Pulmonary Artery Catheters

A **pulmonary artery catheter (PAC)** is a flow-directed, balloon-tipped catheter. The brand name for this catheter is Swan-Ganz, so named for the inventors (Urden et al., 2006). Since the development of the PAC, multiple generations have evolved, although the basic technologies of the catheter remain identical. These catheters allow for assessment of cardiac function, calculation of vascular resistance, measurement of cardiac output, and infusion of IV fluids. The readings obtained with the PAC assist the health care team in diagnosing, treating, and estimating the prognoses of patients who are critically ill. When the PAC was

introduced into critical care, little research existed on its therapeutic use and, yet, the catheter became commonplace in the care of critically ill patients (Adams, 2004). Controversy exists over which patient groups benefit from pulmonary artery catheter guided therapy and if insertion of a PAC decreases mortality rates (Urden et al., 2006).

The American Society of Anesthesiologists (ASA) recommends the use of a PAC for patients undergoing surgical procedures associated with an increased risk of complications from hemodynamic changes (ASA, 2003). Observational studies report mixed results concerning the use of PACs. Chittock and associates (2004) reported that the "mortality rate associated with use of the PAC may be greater if used in a lower severity of illness group but of potential benefit when used in an extremely ill population."

Because controversy still exists over whether the benefits of PACs outweigh the risks, major educational efforts are under way to ensure that patients receive appropriate care based on information derived from the pulmonary artery catheter. The Pulmonary Artery Catheter Education Project is a web-based program for critical care clinicians that focuses on interpretation and application of data obtained from a PA catheter.

Ports and Lumens on a Pulmonary Artery Catheter

The pulmonary artery catheter is a multiple-lumen catheter, with each lumen having a specific purpose (Figure 24–14 ■). The external ports of the catheter correspond to internal lumens that lie either in the right side of the heart or pulmonary artery. There are several types of PACs, some of which have more ports and lumens than others, depending on the intended purpose of the catheter and the manufacturer. Newer multifunction PACs

FIGURE 24–14 ■ Ports and lumens of a pulmonary artery catheter.

with additional lumens are used to measure continuous mixed venous oxygen saturation (SvO_2), right ventricular volume, continuous cardiac output, or additional ports for insertion of transvenous pacing electrodes. Specialized pulmonary artery catheters are discussed later in the chapter.

The proximal port of the PAC sits in the right atrium and is used to infuse IV fluids and nonvasoactive medications. If a transducer is attached to this port, right atrial pressures can be obtained. The second port, which also sits in the right atrium, is the proximal injectate port, used for measuring cardiac output, which is discussed later. The distal port located at the end of the catheter is positioned in the pulmonary artery. The distal port is connected to the pressure transducer system with the flush solution and used for continuous monitoring of pulmonary artery pressures. The tip of the PAC also contains a thermometer, referred to as a **thermistor**. The thermistor permits measurement of the blood temperature in the pulmonary artery, termed the core temperature. The external thermistor connector is attached to the cardiac output computer.

The final port is the balloon inflation port, which is used to inflate the balloon at the distal end of the catheter. The balloon is inflated during insertion to assist with "floating" the catheter through the heart. The balloon port is also used to obtain pulmonary capillary pressure or the **pulmonary artery occlusion pressure (PAOP)**. The amount of air used to inflate the balloon differs among manufacturers. Usually this volume of air is up to 1.5 mL; however, the capacity of the balloon is limited by the catheter size. Manufacturers of PACs usually indicate the maximum balloon inflation volume on the catheter hub and provide a volume-limiting syringe to prevent accidental overinflation. Overinflation may cause rupture of the balloon or pulmonary artery. Once insertion of the catheter is complete, the balloon *never* remains inflated but rather lies uninflated in the pulmonary artery until it is necessary to obtain the PAOP.

Insertion of the Pulmonary Artery Catheter

For insertion the patient is prepped and draped in a similar manner as for any central venous access because strict sterile technique is required. An introducer is inserted in either the jugular, subclavian, or femoral vein. A protective sheath should be placed over the PAC prior to insertion through the introducer. The sheath is an infection control barrier and allows for repositioning of the PAC after insertion. The PAC is passed through the introducer and advanced into the selected vessel to the right atrium. Once the catheter is in the right atrium, the balloon is inflated to allow it to flow with the blood through the heart chambers. This facilitates passage of the PAC through the tricuspid valve, right ventricle, pulmonic valve, and into the pulmonary artery. The balloon is then deflated and the introducer is sutured in place. Right atrial and right ventricular pressures are measured during the insertion of the catheter.

Hemodynamic pressures and waveforms are generated by myocardial contraction (systole) and relaxation (diastole). When the PAC is advanced through the heart, each chamber has a characteristic waveform (Figure 24–15 ■). As the catheter enters the right atrium, the waveform appears similar to a CVP waveform. The identification of the *a, c,* and *v* waves of the RAP is the same as with a CVP tracing. The normal mean RAP is 4 to

Interpreting hemodynamic waveforms

Right atrium

Right ventricle

Pulmonary artery

Pulmonary capillary wedge

FIGURE 24–15 ■ Cardiac pressures during PAC insertion.

6 mmHg. Normal systolic pressures in the right ventricle (RV) are between 20 and 30 mmHg, and diastolic pressures are between 0 and 8 mmHg (Lynn-McHale Weigand & Carlson, 2005). As the PAC passes through the RV, the tip of the catheter can irritate the ventricle. Monitor the ECG closely for ectopy. Patients may exhibit premature ventricular contractions (PVCs). This ectopy usually ceases when the catheter is advanced into the pulmonary artery or withdrawn from the right ventricle.

As the catheter enters the pulmonary artery, the waveform resembles an arterial pressure waveform with not only systolic and diastolic pressures but also a dicrotic notch. The dicrotic notch represents closure of the pulmonic valve. The normal pulmonary artery systolic (PAS) pressure is 20 to 30 mmHg and the pulmonary artery diastolic (PAD) pressure is 5 to 15 mmHg. Notice that the normal right ventricular systolic pressure and the pulmonary artery systolic pressure are the same

Nursing Management

Nursing management of patients needing pulmonary artery catheters requires critical thinking and clinical judgment. These patients are typically critically ill and hemodynamically compromised. Insertion of a PAC is an intervention that will provide the nurse with advanced assessment parameters as well as a central intravenous line to administer the necessary medications and fluid.

Assessment

Prior to insertion of a pulmonary artery catheter, the nurse is responsible for assessing the patient in the same manner as for a central venous catheter. Inform the health care provider or person inserting the catheter if the patient is coagulopathic, has an electrolyte imbalance (particularly magnesium, potassium, or calcium), or has an acid–base imbalance. Patients with a coagulopathy are more likely to have bleeding complications, and patients with electrolyte or acid–base imbalances are at increased risk for cardiac irritability that may lead to intractable arrhythmias.

Interventions and Rationales

Prepare the transducer system as previously described. Flush all ports with normal saline to remove air from the lines. The normal saline flush syringe may remain attached to the lumen until after the procedure. Attach the distal end of the PAC to the transducer system and zero balance the system. Test the balloon on the PA catheter by inflating the syringe with the appropriate amount of air.

Assist with setup of the sterile field and opening of sterile kits. Sterile barriers identical to those used for central venous catheters are employed for insertion of PACs. Once the central venous access is obtained and the introducer inserted, the port end of the PAC is given to the bedside nurse. Flush all of the ports with normal saline to remove air from the lines. Test the balloon on the PAC by inflating the syringe with the appropriate amount of air. Attach the distal end of the PAC to the transducer system and zero balance the system.

During catheter insertion, watch the monitor for waveform changes as the PAC passes through the chambers of the heart. When the catheter is in the right atrium, the nurse inflates the balloon. This facilitates passage of the catheter through the tricuspid valve. During this time, watch closely for ventricular ectopy.

Note the distance the catheter is inserted. The PAC has thin and wide black lines on the exterior. The thin line represents 10-cm increments and the wide line signifies 50 cm. Document the number of centimeters. This will serve as a reference to others caring for the patient.

Evaluation

After the catheter is placed, secure the site with an occlusive dressing. Reassess the patient to determine tolerance to procedure. Follow through with the health care provider on orders for

a chest x-ray. Once the x-ray confirms proper placement and rules out a pneumothorax, the bedside nurse connects the IV infusions to the remaining ports of the PAC and obtains pulmonary artery occlusion pressures and cardiac output measurements, as discussed in a later section.

Complications of a Pulmonary Artery Catheter

As with central venous catheters, complications from a pulmonary artery catheter include infection, air embolus, and pneumothorax (Urden et al., 2006). However, with a PAC there are additional risks of pulmonary artery rupture, pulmonary infarction, balloon rupture, catheter coiling or displacement, arrhythmias, and conduction defects. Pulmonary artery rupture is a life-threatening complication and, although rare, the mortality rate is 45% to 65% (Weininger, Ginosar, Sprung, & Weiss, 2002). Rupture of the pulmonary artery may occur when the balloon is overfilled or if the tip of the PAC migrates through the pulmonary artery intima. In most cases, hemoptysis is the presenting symptom (Weininger et al., 2002). If a pulmonary artery rupture is suspected, immediately place the patient with the affected side down to prevent blood from leaking into the unaffected lung and notify the health care provider.

Balloon rupture may cause air or balloon pieces to embolize the pulmonary vasculature. The likelihood of balloon rupture increases with catheter duration, because the balloon loses its elasticity over time. If blood is noted in the air inflation port or if no PAOP tracing appears with balloon inflation, then after placing the patient with the affected lung down, notify the health care provider.

Pulmonary infarction can occur if the balloon accidentally remains inflated or if the PA catheter tip occludes a branch of the artery. Continuous monitoring of the PAC waveform noting the contour of the wave and the corresponding numeric values is an important nursing intervention to detect pulmonary infarcts. It is especially important to note the return of the normal pulmonary artery waveform after obtaining the PAOP or wedging of the catheter, which is discussed later. If the nurse suspects that the PAC is remaining wedged despite balloon deflation, then turning the patient side to side or having the patient cough may unwedge the catheter. If these techniques are unsuccessful, the catheter may need repositioning by the health care provider or advanced practice nurse.

 After obtaining the PAOP, remove the syringe from the balloon inflation port and allow passive deflation of the balloon. Using the syringe to remove the air causes damage to the balloon and may lead to rupture.

The PAC may coil on itself at any time. Usually the coiling occurs within the right atrium or right ventricle. An x-ray is necessary to detect this complication and requires an invasive procedure to correct. Arrhythmias and conduction defects result when the PAC is touching the endocardium and septal wall. Conduction defects, especially right bundle branch blocks, can occur when the PAC is advanced through the right ventricle. In patients with a preexisting left bundle branch block (LBBB), a new right bundle branch block (RBBB) places the patient at risk for developing a complete bundle branch block. For a patient with a preexisting LBBB, having transcutaneous pacing equipment available is advisable. As previously discussed, electrolyte or acid–base imbalances should be corrected prior to PAC insertion in an effort to decrease the likelihood of arrhythmias from these sources.

Pulmonary Artery Occlusion Pressure

The pulmonary artery occlusion pressure (PAOP), also referred to as pulmonary artery wedge pressure (PAWP) and pulmonary capillary wedge pressure (PCWP), is an indirect measurement of left ventricular end-diastolic pressure (LVEDP), or left-sided preload. To obtain this measurement, the balloon of the PAC is inflated, which facilitates forward movement of the catheter until it wedges in the pulmonary capillary (Figure 24–16 ■). The pressure is measured at the tip of the catheter; thus, when the balloon is inflated, blood flow in through the pulmonary artery is temporarily stopped and only pressures in front of the balloon are measurable. Therefore, the PAOP is the most direct bedside measurement of left heart function. A normal PAOP reading is between 4 and 12 mmHg.

Left ventricular (LV) failure and myocardial ischemia, constrictive pericarditis, mitral valve disease, or volume overload are conditions that elevate the PAOP. The diminished contractility and ensuing increase in left ventricular volume seen with LV failure and ischemia are reflected in an increased PAOP. Constrictive pericarditis, like pericardial tamponade, causes an increase in PAOP when the external pressure exerted on the left side of the heart in-

creases. Infectious processes, trauma, and uremia secondary to renal disease are examples of conditions causing constrictive pericarditis. Mitral valve disease increases the PAOP when either the mitral valve does not allow for complete emptying of the left atrium due to stenosis (narrowing of the outlet) or when the valve leaflets cannot close completely (insufficiency), causing a reflux of blood into the left atrium during left ventricular contraction. The volume overload of the left heart is usually secondary to LV failure. PAOPs decrease when patients are hypovolemic, in shock, or when receiving vasodilating medications. Vasodilators decrease SVR, making it easier for left ventricular ejection and improvement in ejection fraction (Urden et al., 2006).

Correlating the PAOP Waveform with the Cardiac Cycle

There is a delay in the transmission of pressure changes in the PAOP waveform. Therefore, the *a* wave occurs 0.20 to 0.24 seconds after the P wave, near the end of the QRS complex as illustrated earlier in Figure 24–13 ■ (p. 572). The *v* wave corresponds with the T-P interval. The *c* wave occurs with closure of the tricuspid valve and is found on the *a* to *x* downslope. Identification of the *c* wave is important because prior to the *c* wave occurring, the pressure equilibrates between the atrium and the ventricle. This is the point where the PAOP left ventricular end diastolic volume (LVEDV) is measured. If the *c* wave is indistinguishable, the PAOP is obtained by averaging the *a* and the *x* wave.

Thermodilution Cardiac Output

With the thermodilution method of obtaining a cardiac output reading, a specified amount of solution, typically 5 to 10 mL, is injected through the proximal injectate port of the PAC (see Figure 24–14 ■, p. 574). This process is commonly referred to as "shooting" a cardiac output. The injectate is at room temperature (about 21°C [70°F]) when it enters the right atrium and mixes with blood (about 37°C [98.6°F]). The CO computer calculates the time required for the solution of a different temperature to reach the thermistor, located at the end of the catheter in the pulmonary artery. The change of temperature occurs over time to

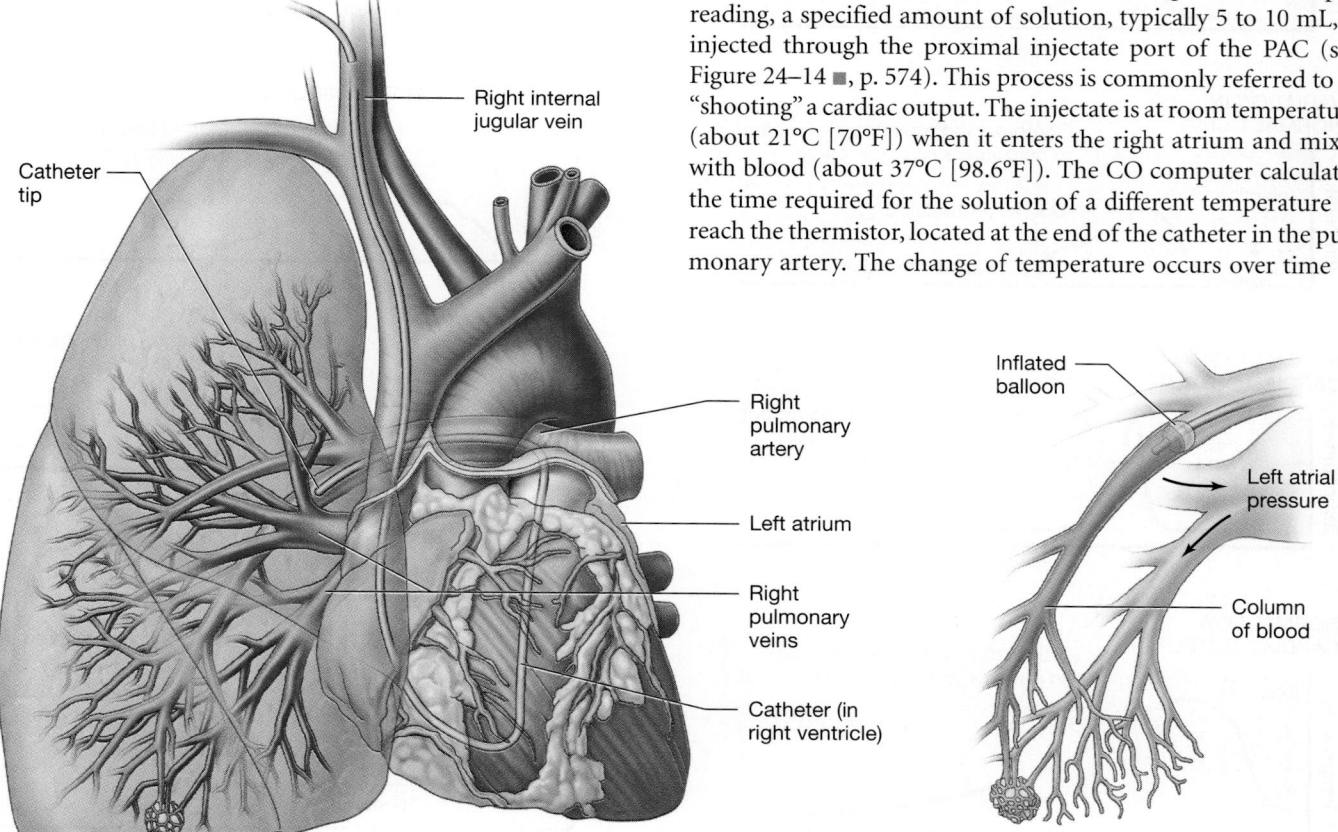

FIGURE 24–16 ■ Position of pulmonary artery catheter during PAOP.

yield a CO curve, as shown in Figure 24–17 ■. The area under the CO curve inversely corresponds to the cardiac output. When the area under the curve is large, the CO is low. Conversely, when the area under the curve is small, the CO is high.

Awareness of what constitutes a normal curve is important. Assessment of the shape of the cardiac output curve is necessary to determine if the CO measurement should be accepted or rejected. A normal CO curve starts at the baseline and has a smooth incline and decline. Hesitation or starting and stopping during a CO injection would yield an invalid curve. The injectate should be injected smoothly and in less than 4 seconds. This prevents prolonged injection times that would yield a lower CO result. Additionally, injecting less than or greater than the recommended amount of injectate invalidates the measurement. Cardiac output measurements are performed 1 to 2 minutes apart with an average of three measurements obtained. Also, the injectate should be timed to the end-expiratory phase of respiration. This will minimize the variation in intrathoracic pressure during respiration. Any CO that is questionable based on the curve or two CO measurements differing by 10% should be discarded (Lynn-McHale Weigand & Carlson, 2005).

Influence of Heart Rate on Cardiac Output

A slow or rapid heart rate affects cardiac output. Heart rates greater than 100 decrease diastolic filling time. For example, a heart rate of 150 beats/min and a reduced stroke volume to 20 mL is detrimental to CO:

$$HR\,(150) \times SV\,(20) \;=\; 3,000 \; mL \; or \; 3.0 \; L/minute$$

Dysrhythmias such as atrial fibrillation and atrial flutter cause not only a decreased diastolic filling time but also a loss of atrial kick, which is responsible for up to 25% of the total cardiac output (Chapter 38 🔗).

Bradycardia allows sufficient time for the ventricles to fill and usually is not detrimental to cardiac output because of compensatory mechanisms. However, when patients have lost their compensatory mechanisms, a bradycardic rhythm may not provide sufficient cardiac output. For example, a heart rate of 35 beats/min and a normal stroke volume of 60 mL/beat yields a CO of 2.1 L/min:

$$HR\,(35) \times SV\,(60) \;=\; 2,100 \; mL \; or \; 2.1 \; L/minute$$

Additionally, consider a patient with frequent premature ventricular contractions. If a patient has a heart rate of 80 but every other beat is a PVC, the heart rate is effectively reduced by one-half, due to little or no cardiac output with PVCs.

Influence of Preload on Cardiac Output

Reduced preload (CVP < 2, RAP < 4, PAOP < 4) signals vasodilation or volume loss. Exploration of cause is essential so that appropriate action is taken. Treatment of hypovolemia is the

FIGURE 24–17 ■ Normal and abnormal cardiac output curves.

administration of crystalloids, volume expanders, and/or blood products. Examples of obvious fluid losses occur after trauma, during surgery, with diuretic therapy, profuse sweating, or excessive upper or lower gastrointestinal losses. Internal, nonvisible blood loss is an example of insidious hypovolemia and may go undetected unless considered as a suspected cause of preload reduction.

Vasodilation and loss of venous tone demonstrated in neurogenic or anaphylactic shock have a profound effect on preload. In neurogenic shock, the loss of vasomotor tone is secondary to the loss of neural output or from spinal cord damage. This can result from general or spinal anesthesia or, in the case of spinal cord injury, from loss of sympathetic tone. In anaphylactic shock, the antigen–antibody response triggers the release of vasoactive chemicals in the body (histamine, bradykinin), which create massive vasodilation. Shock is discussed in Chapter 61 .

Excess preload (CVP/RAP > 6, PAOP > 12) may indicate hypervolemia or ventricular failure. Excessive circulating volume strains the heart and compromises adequate tissue oxygenation. Excess preload increases the workload of the heart and increases myocardial oxygen demands. Diuretics and venodilators are ordered if the cause is hypervolemia. If patients do not respond to diuretic therapy or renal failure is diagnosed, then continuous renal replacement therapy utilizing ultrafiltration or dialysis may be considered. If ventricular failure is determined to be the cause, inotropic medications are prescribed.

Influence of Afterload on Cardiac Output

Reduced afterload (PVR < 155, SVR < 900) suggests vasodilation of the pulmonary and systemic vasculature. Decreased afterload lessens the workload on the heart and reduces myocardial oxygen requirements. With reduced resistance to ventricular ejection, an increase in stroke volume occurs as the ventricles empty. For example, patients with sepsis present with hypotension, fever, and vasodilatation, which reduce the SVR. The cardiac output of a patient with sepsis can elevate to as much as 10 L/min.

Excessive afterload (PVR > 255, SVR > 1,600) imposes great strain on the ventricles, increases the myocardial oxygen requirement, and decreases the stroke volume. Conditions that increase pulmonary resistance include hypoxia, acute respiratory distress syndrome, positive end-expiratory pressure, pulmonary embolism, chronic obstructive pulmonary disease (COPD), increased interstitial lung water, and pulmonary fibrosis (Urden et al., 2006). Left ventricular afterload is the resistance to ejection into the systemic circulation. Conditions that increase resistance include aortic valve stenosis, hypertension, and vasoconstriction of the peripheral vasculature.

Influence of Contractility on Cardiac Output

Contractility, the intrinsic ability of the myocardium to contract, occurs independent of changes in preload and afterload. Myocardial damage during an infarction or the presence of cardiomyopathy decreases contractility. Cardiomyopathy is discussed in detail in Chapter 41 . Positive inotropic medications, such as dobutamine and epinephrine, stimulate the sympathetic nervous system and increase contractility, but these events also increase myocardial oxygen demand. Negative inotropic medications, such as beta-adrenergic blockers, are administered when myocardial work and oxygen consumption are detrimental, such as with a myocardial infarction.

Specialized Pulmonary Artery Catheters

Subsequent to the development of the generic thermodilution catheter, multiple generations evolved. This section explains different PAC models and provides supplemental information. Although presented as separate entities, many of these features are combined on one PAC model. Model variations are usually not available within one institution. The available model is dependent on hospital contracts, health care provider preference, and the patient population needs.

Continuous Cardiac Output PAC

This catheter modifies the thermodilution PAC by adding a thermal filament that slightly warms the blood. This warmed blood is sensed at the thermistor in the catheter tip. The CO result is based on temperature changes at preset intervals, usually every minute (Urden et al., 2006). The updated calculation is then displayed on a CO monitor. The advantages to this system include recognition of CO as a dynamic, fluctuating parameter, the elimination of "shooting" cardiac outputs with the inherent risk of operator variability, plus the elimination of extra fluid a patient receives during that process.

Continuous Mixed Venous Oxygen Saturation

A **mixed venous oxygen saturation** (SvO_2) PAC provides information about the supply of oxygen to the tissues and demand for oxygen by the tissues (Kaplow & Hardin, 2007). This catheter is positioned like a thermodilution catheter with the distal end in the pulmonary artery. These specialized catheters have fiber-optic fibers. One fiber emits a light wave to illuminate red blood cells (RBCs) and the second fiber receives the reflected light signal. The amount of light reflected by the RBCs is determined by their hemoglobin saturation. Because this analysis occurs in the pulmonary artery, it reflects the saturation of all venous blood returned to the right side of the heart. This means that the SvO_2 reflects the consumption of oxygen at the tissue level. The numeric value displayed on the SvO_2 monitor reflects the saturation of mixed venous blood or the amount of deoxygenated blood that returns to the heart. The normal SvO_2 value is 60% to 80%.

Four factors affect mixed venous oxygen saturation: cardiac output, hemoglobin, arterial oxygen saturation, and oxygen consumption. Mixed venous oxygen saturation parallels cardiac output, hemoglobin concentration, and arterial oxygen saturation: A drop in cardiac output, hemoglobin, or oxygen saturation will cause a decrease in SvO_2; an increase in cardiac output, hemoglobin, or oxygen saturation will elevate SvO_2. High tissue extraction of oxygen (low SvO_2) occurs when patients are in pain (high oxygen demand) or when patients are experiencing respiratory failure (low oxygen supply). Low tissue extraction (high SvO_2) occurs when patients are sedate (low oxygen demand) or after blood transfusions (high oxygen supply). Nursing procedures such as patient repositioning and dressing or linen changes are oxygen-consuming activities for the patient and correspondingly lower the SvO_2.

CRITICAL ALERT *Use the information offered by the SvO_2 catheter to prioritize and plan nursing interventions. Patients who are compromised do not tolerate turning, suctioning, and dressing changes in a short time interval.*

Right Ventricular Ejection Fraction Volumetric Catheter

This catheter provides data on right ventricular systolic and diastolic volumes. Two sensors in the catheter, one in the right ventricle (RV) and one in the pulmonary artery, detect ventricular depolarization, heart rate, and temperature change. Using the information on systolic volume and diastolic volume, the ejection fraction is calculated. Accurate measurement of preload using the right ventricular end-diastolic volume instead of estimation of preload by CVP or PAOP is helpful in assessing the fluid requirement after right ventricular infarction and during high levels of positive end-expiratory pressure (PEEP) on mechanically ventilated patients (Weininger et al., 2002). Accurate calculation of RV systolic and diastolic volumes relies on temperature consistency. Large-volume resuscitations with room temperature IV fluid or cool blood components diminish the accuracy of RV end-diastolic volumes and influence the calculation.

Transpulmonary Thermodilution with Pulse Contour Analysis

Using a special thermistor-tipped catheter inserted in the femoral or brachial artery and a regular central venous catheter, intermittent and continuous cardiac outputs can be evaluated. For an intermittent CO, a preset volume of cold injectate is injected into the central venous catheter. After completion of the vascular circuit, the temperature change is detected by the thermistor in the arterial catheter. As with the previously described thermodilution method, the calculation of CO is based on temperature change over time. For continuous cardiac output monitoring, the value obtained by an intermittent CO is used to calibrate the monitoring equipment. An internal algorithm combines this information with continual analysis of the arterial pressure wave contour to determine CO. Rather than measuring preload, afterload, and stroke volume, this device calculates intrathoracic volume and pulmonary volume by analysis of the CO distribution curve. End-diastolic volumes are automatically calculated. The advantage of measuring end-diastolic volume during fluid resuscitation without a PAC is useful. Nursing care requires knowledge of cardiac and pulmonary physiology plus a shift in thinking from hemodynamic pressure monitoring to hemodynamic volume monitoring (Genahr & McLuckie, 2004).

Nursing Management

The bedside nurse is responsible for management of the pulmonary artery catheter from preinsertion until removal. These responsibilities include patient and family education, assisting with insertion, site care, assessment and interpretation of hemodynamic waveforms and parameters, and titration of vasoactive medications. The nurse should provide information about the PAC and how the measurements obtained will direct therapy. Use of the nursing process facilitates an organized approach for management of patients with invasive catheters.

Assessment

Assessment includes monitoring the insertion site for infection, monitoring of PA pressures, measuring PAOP, and cardiac outputs, and monitoring the patient when changes occur.

Nursing Diagnosis

Nursing diagnoses related to hemodynamic monitoring include:

- *Anxiety*
- *Decreased Cardiac Output*
- *Risk for Imbalanced Fluid Volume*
- *Ineffective Health Maintenance*
- *Risk for Injury*
- *Deficient Knowledge*
- *Risk for Infection.*

Planning

Planning for interventions for care for the patient with invasive lines is multifaceted. Each institution has specific procedures for maintaining a sterile occlusive dressing over the line insertion site. The nurse must be knowledgeable of these procedures and carry them out within the required time frames.

Outcomes and Evaluation Parameters

Outcomes and evaluation parameters associated with pulmonary artery catheters include:

- Stabilization of the pulmonary artery readings to within normal limits
- Normal or stable cardiac output
- No infection at the catheter site or in the bloodstream as evidenced by no fever and a negative blood culture
- No bleeding from the site or catheter
- Having the PAC discontinued due to patient stabilization.

Interventions and Rationales

Appropriate interventions include changing the occlusive dressing if loosened and inspecting the site for redness, swelling, and leakage. The nurse must also possess the knowledge required to operate and troubleshoot the catheter. The transducer system must be inspected for kinks and air bubbles from site to pressure bag. After leveling, zero referencing, and checking the dynamic response, the pulmonary artery systolic, diastolic, and mean pressures are usually documented hourly and after changes in therapies. PAOP and CO readings are obtained when changes occur in the patient's clinical status; with initiation, titration, or discontinuation of vasoactive medications; when significant changes occur in heart rate or rhythm; or when greater than 5 cm of PEEP is applied during mechanical ventilation. Increases in PEEP over 5 cm are associated with increased intrathoracic pressure, which may decrease cardiac output. PEEP is discussed in detail Chapter 36 ☞.

Evaluation

The expected outcome for these patients is hemodynamic stabilization with the intent of getting the invasive catheters removed as soon as possible. Not every patient will have normal readings; thus, the goal is for readings that are tolerated by the patient. One gauge of tolerance is the patient's ability to perform activities of daily living.

Health Promotion During Invasive Procedures

Family members should be given the opportunity to stay during invasive procedures, if desired. Based on evaluations conducted in emergency department settings from family presence programs for pediatric patients, family members are grateful and voice their approval (American Heart Association [AHA], 2000). However, there is a lack of evidence related to family presence during adult resuscitations and invasive procedures. Nursing research on family presence is progressing. Initial results indicate that families and patient's favor this practice change (Eichhorn et al., 2001; Meyers et al., 2000). The success of these programs in adult populations is predictable, according to the AHA (2000), when health care workers demonstrate the same level of care and concern seen in pediatric programs.

 **CRITICAL ALERT** *If family members wish to be present during invasive procedures, a staff member should stay with them to answer questions and clarify what is happening.*

■ Alternative Methods of Determining Cardiac Output

Patients who are coagulopathic or immunosuppressed are at high risk of complications from invasive devices. Additionally, patients who may not tolerate positioning for a pulmonary artery catheter or are clinically unstable may be candidates for noninvasive determination of cardiac output. Minimally invasive and noninvasive monitoring devices estimate hemodynamic pressures in patients who are critically ill and are used in ICUs. Some devices are gaining acceptance in intermediate care units, emergency departments, and outpatient clinics to evaluate and treat patients with congestive heart failure and to optimize pacemaker settings. These devices, the supporting hardware, and monitoring systems are incompatible with the transducer systems used in invasive monitoring. Therefore, separate supporting hardware must be available.

Transesophageal Ultrasound

Transesophageal ultrasound is a minimally invasive method for continuous monitoring of cardiac function. An ultrasound probe is inserted into the esophagus similar to the insertion of a nasogastric tube. When the probe is properly positioned, the ultrasound waves detect red blood cells descending through the aorta. Figure 24–18 ■ illustrates probe position in the aorta. The blood flow and velocity are transmitted to a display monitor where an internal algorithm converts blood flow, velocity, heart rate, and diameter of the aorta into estimations of cardiac output and stroke volume (Turner, 2003). Sedation is recommended before passage of the probe. Nurses assisting with this procedure must have knowledge of conscious sedation protocols.

Thoracic Impedance

Thoracic impedance cardiography is an external, noninvasive method of hemodynamic monitoring. Impedance electrodes are applied to the body, one set at the base of the neck and another set to both sides of the thorax (Figure 24–19 ■, p. 582). These electrodes work in tandem: The outer electrodes inject a

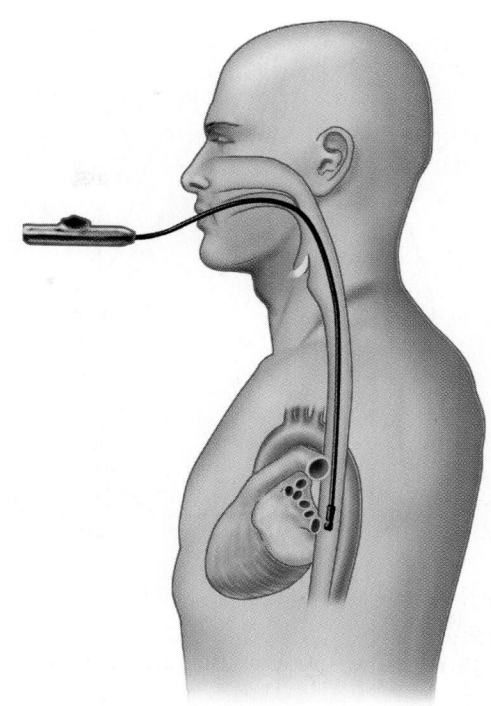

FIGURE 24–18 ■ Transesophageal ultrasound.

low-level electric current (harmless current) and the inner electrodes sense thoracic impedance. Changes in thoracic impedance are associated with changes in aortic blood flow during systole and diastole. Peak blood flow during systole, combined with heart rate analysis from the ECG, is used to compute stroke volume and cardiac output. Unlike invasive monitoring, which hinders patient mobility, when thoracic impedance monitoring is used, patients can be mobilized, including ambulation, by disconnecting the monitoring leads from the system.

The evolution of hemodynamic monitoring does not preclude investigations of current technology. The nursing research discussed in this chapter needs replication, because study replication produces a body of knowledge that enhances nursing science and produces evidence-based practice. All nurses make a contribution in the research process, whether by collecting data or explaining in lay terms the research behind relocating a transducer after turning a patient. Bedside nurses are prime candidates for identification of potential research projects, as outlined in the Research Opportunities and Clinical Impact box (p. 582).

■ Summary

Exposure to patients who are critically ill and experience with invasive technologies enables the nurse to initiate and actively participate in discussions regarding utilization of invasive devices. As health care team members, nurses' responsibilities include patient advocacy. Nurses are not just accountable for safe care, but also for reasonable care. The nurse should always ask, "What information will be obtained if this catheter is inserted?" and "How will having that information enhance this patient's quality of life?" These questions are not easy to answer, nor is the answer always evident.

(a)   **(b)**

FIGURE 24–19 ■ Electrode placement for thoracic impedance cardiography: (A) anterior view; (B) lateral view.

Although hemodynamic monitoring technology has evolved (and will continue to do so), the clinical assessment combined with laboratory data analysis and patient history are equally important in the provision of quality care. Linking a clinical presentation with hemodynamic data requires repeated exposure.

With each experience managing critically ill patients, nursing actions will be become incorporated into daily practice even before an invasive catheter is inserted so that treatment can be initiated quickly.

RESEARCH OPPORTUNITIES AND CLINICAL IMPACT RELATED TO HEMODYNAMIC MONITORING

Research Area	Clinical Impact
Exploration of cultural beliefs about medical decision making	Improves the delivery of care, patient satisfaction, and health care providers' knowledge of other cultures.
Comparison of techniques used to secure arterial catheters	Results in fewer dislodged or accidentally removed arterial catheters, improved patient safety.
Techniques to decrease the infection rates associated with central venous catheters	Prevention of infections will decrease patient morbidity and mortality rates.
Continuous monitoring of left ventricular ejection fraction	Provides immediate information about cardiac function.
Noninvasive methods to accurately measure cardiac output	Decreases exposure to invasive catheters and the associated complications and risks.
Methods of facilitating family presence programs	Recognizes the impact of family systems on patient health and well-being.
The effect of prone positioning on hemodynamic pressures	Provides for accurate hemodynamic assessment during therapeutic proning.

NCLEX® REVIEW

1. A patient is admitted to the ICU in critical condition. The use of hemodynamic monitoring for this patient will be to:
   1. Make measuring the patient's blood pressure more accurate.
   2. Help with diagnosis, treatment, and evaluation of care.
   3. Reduce the amount of nursing time needed to provide care.
   4. Determine when the patient can be transferred to a step-down unit.

2. The nurse is assessing the waveform created after the placement of a hemodynamic monitoring device. The waveform appears distorted. What can the nurse do?
   1. Increase the flow rate through the device.
   2. Reposition the catheter.
   3. Find out if the correct type of tubing was used.
   4. Check the patient and alert the health care provider and begin interventions to improve hemodynamic stability.

3. During the placement of a hemodynamic monitoring device the patient demonstrates premature ventricular contractions upon ECG. Which of the following should be done?

1. Flush the arterial line with normal saline.

2. Reposition the CVP monitor.

3. Zero the transducer.

4. Advance the catheter into the pulmonary artery.

4. A patient's central venous pressure is 10 mmHg. What should the nurse do?

1. Report the measurement to the health care provider and prepare for interventions.

2. Access the algorithm for an elevated CVP and begin the protocol.

3. Adjust the catheter tip.

4. Compare the result with other measurements.

5. While shooting a patient's cardiac output, the nurse obtains readings that are inconsistent. What should the nurse do?

1. Begin again and inject the injectate over 10 seconds.

2. Eliminate any values that differ by 10%.

3. Warm the injectate to body temperature.

4. Use 45 mL of injectate.

6. A patient's central venous pressure reading is 12 mmHg with a right atrial pressure of 14 mmHg. The nurse realizes these pressures reflect:

1. Fluid volume overload or ventricular failure.

2. Hypotension.

3. Vasodilation.

4. Anaphylactic shock.

7. During the placement of a pulmonary artery catheter a tracing begins to resemble an arterial line tracing but with a dicrotic notch. The nurse realizes that this notch indicates:

1. Atrial contraction.

2. Retrograde swelling of the tricuspid valve.

3. Atrial filling.

4. Closure of the pulmonic valve.

Answers for review questions appear in Appendix D

KEY TERMS

afterload *p.565*
Allen's test *p.567*
arterial line *p.567*
cardiac index (CI) *p.564*
cardiac output (CO) *p.564*
central venous pressure (CVP) *p.565*
contractility *p.565*
dynamic response test *p.563*

ejection fraction (EF) *p.565*
Frank-Starling law *p.565*
hemodynamic monitoring *p.560*
leveling *p.562*
mean arterial pressure (MAP) *p.569*
mixed venous oxygen saturation *p.579*
phlebostatic axis *p.562*
preload *p.565*

pulmonary artery catheter (PAC) *p.574*
pulmonary artery occlusion pressure (PAOP) *p.575*
stroke volume (SV) *p.563*
thermistor *p.575*
thoracic impedance *p.581*
transesophageal ultrasound *p.581*
zero referencing *p.562*

EXPLORE PEARSON mynursingkit™

MyNursingKit is your one stop for online chapter review materials and resources. Prepare for success with additional NCLEX®-style practice questions, interactive assignments and activities, web links, animations and videos, and more!

Register your access code from the front of your book at
www.mynursingkit.com

REFERENCES

Adams, K. L. (2004). Hemodynamic assessment: The physiologic basis for turning data into clinical information. *AACN Clinical Issues, 15,* 534–546.

American Heart Association. (2000). Guidelines 2000 for cardiopulmonary resuscitation and emergency cardiovascular care. *Circulation, 102*(8), I-136–I-139.

American Society of Anesthesiologists. (2003). Practice guidelines for pulmonary artery catheterization: An updated report by the American Society of Anesthesiologists Task Force on Pulmonary Artery Catheterization. *Anesthesiology, 99,* 988–1014.

Centers for Disease Control and Prevention. (2002). Guidelines for the prevention of intravascular catheter-related infections. *Morbidity and Mortality Weekly Report, 51.*

Chittock, D. R., Dhingra, V. K., Ronco, J. J., Russell, J. A. Forrest, D. M., Tweeddale, M., et al. (2004). Severity of illness and risk of death associated with pulmonary artery catheter use. *Critical Care Medicine, 32,* 911–915.

Darovic, G. O. (2004). *Handbook of hemodynamic monitoring.* St. Louis, MO: W. B. Saunders.

Dietz, B., & Smith, T. T. (2002). Enhancing the accuracy of hemodynamic monitoring. *Journal of Nursing Care Quality, 17,* 27–34.

Eichhorn, D. J., Meyers, T. A., Guzzetta, C. E., Clark, A. P., Klein, J. D., Taliaferro, E., et al. (2001). Family presence during invasive procedures and resuscitation: Hearing the voice of the patient. *American Journal of Nursing, 101,* 48–55.

Genahr, A., & McLuckie, A. (2004, Spring). Transpulmonary thermodilution in the critically ill. *British Journal of Intensive Care,* 6–10.

Giuliano, K. K., Scott, S. S., Brown, V., & Olson, M. (2003). Backrest angle and cardiac output measurement in critically ill patients. *Nursing Research, 52,* 242–248.

Kaplow, R., & Hardin, S. R. (2007). *Critical care nursing: Synergy for optimal outcomes.* Sudbury, MA: Jones and Bartlett.

Lynn-McHale Weigand, D. J., & Carlson, K. K. (Eds.). (2005). *AACN procedure manual for critical care* (5th ed.). Philadelphia: Elsevier.

Meyers, T. A., Eichhorn, D. J., Guzzetta, C. E., Clark, A. P., Klein, J. D., Taliaferro, E., et al. (2000). Family presence during invasive procedures and resuscitation: The experience of family members, nurses, and physicians. *American Journal of Nursing, 100,* 32–43.

Porth, C. M. (2007). *Essentials of pathophysiology: Concepts of altered health states* (2nd ed., p. 36). Philadelphia: Lippincott Williams & Wilkins.

Turner, M. A. (2003). Doppler-based hemodynamic monitoring. *AACN Clinical Issues, 14,* 220–231.

Urden, L. D., Stacy, K. M., & Lough, M. E. (2006). *Thelan's critical care nursing: Diagnosis and management* (4th ed., pp. 355–359). St. Louis: Mosby.

Weininger, C. F., Ginosar, Y., Sprung, C. L., & Weiss, Y. (2002). Arterial and pulmonary artery catheters. In J. E. Parillo & R. P. Dellinger (Eds.), *Critical care medicine* (2nd ed., pp. 36–63). St. Louis: Mosby.

Research

Nursing Process

Caring

Profiles in Nursing

BETTY   My name is Betty and I am a staff nurse in the Ambulatory Surgery Center at Stanford Hospital and Clinics in Stanford, California. Stanford has 600 beds and is the primary teaching hospital for the Stanford University School of Medicine. The Ambulatory Surgery Center has 12 operating rooms, two procedure rooms, and three interventional radiology suites. We care for patients ranging from 1 year old to more than 100 years old. The majority of our patients are admitted for surgery and discharged the same day, but because we are part of Stanford Hospital, our surgery schedule also includes patients who are scheduled to be admitted to the hospital. In a typical day we may have 50 surgeries and procedures scheduled.

At Stanford, I am encouraged to advance in my nursing career. The hospital supports nurses in obtaining advanced degrees or certification in a nursing specialty, or promotion to a management position. I knew I always wanted to remain a "bedside" nurse, but was looking for that next challenge. As the clinical nurse educator for preoperative care and PACU in the Ambulatory Surgery Center, I found a good balance. I coordinate the orientation needs of new staff and provide ongoing education to staff for new procedures in our department. I am also a member of our Nursing Practice Council, led by staff nurses to establish and implement standards of practice for our department. We collaborate with other departments to ensure we give the best care possible. For example, the PACU nurses are currently working on a project with the anesthesiologists to redefine our extubation policy.

I enjoy being a perianesthesia nurse and I appreciate the opportunities it affords me to practice all components of caring. The competence of the preoperative nurse in assessing the patient ensures that the patient meets all of the criteria necessary for a safe and successful surgery. The **commitment** to teaching is evident throughout the perioperative experience. It begins with the preoperative call the night before surgery, then continues in the preoperative area. Questions are answered and learning needs are assessed. Every patient is assessed to make sure he or she has the knowledge and support to ensure successful care once he or she returns home. Each patient and caregiver is given detailed instructions regarding postoperative care before the patient is discharged from our facility.

When a patient first arrives from surgery, many things are done simultaneously. The first priority is to ensure that the airway is unobstructed and the patient is breathing adequately. Monitors are applied and the patient is assessed and appropriate interventions are initiated.

Many patients are confused or frightened when they emerge from anesthesia. One of the most important aspects of our care is to assure patients that their surgery is completed and they are doing well. Patients always remember the **compassion** and comfort care you give—I recall taking care of a patient who had a very unstable course in the PACU, requiring extensive monitoring and critical care. On a subsequent visit to our unit, he did not remember how sick he had been, but he thanked me for giving him the warm blanket after surgery.

Taking care of patients after they have undergone a general anesthetic requires critical thinking skills and clinical reasoning. A patient who is difficult to arouse after anesthesia might be hypercarbic or simply sleeping deeply because he worked the night shift. Pain management can be quite challenging, especially in patients on chronic opiates. It is easy to just give more narcotics, but looking for other reasons and solutions can sometimes be more beneficial. PACU nurses often consult with anesthesiologists about these issues.

Most of the pediatric patients we care for in our PACU are healthy children undergoing tonsillectomies, placement of myringotomy tubes, or hand surgery. It is a frightening experience for the child and the parents. Children often wake up quite agitated, but by **confidently** handling the child and reassuring the parents that this is normal, I can make their surgical experience a positive one.

My **comportment** while charge nurse in the PACU sets the tone for the other members of the PACU team. When critical situations arise, the team pulls together to handle the situation. New staff members are given autonomy in caring for their patients, but always have the backup of a more experienced PACU nurse.

"The competence of the preoperative nurse in assessing the patient ensures that the patient meets all of the criteria necessary for a safe and successful surgery. The **commitment** to teaching is evident throughout the perioperative experience."

Preoperative Nursing

Jane Ashley

Outcome-Based Learning Objectives

After studying this chapter, the learner will be able to:

1. Describe the components and significance of preoperative assessments.
2. Identify critical preoperative assessment findings that require further intervention.
3. Discuss the elements of preoperative preparation.
4. Prioritize nursing interventions for the preoperative patient.
5. Develop a teaching plan for the preoperative patient.
6. Identify and discuss areas of future research relevant to the preoperative patient.

Research   Collaboration   Health Promotion   Nursing Process   Caring   Critical Thinking

ACCORDING TO data from the National Center for Health Statistics, approximately 71 million surgeries were performed in the United States in the year 2004. Of these, 40 million were inpatient procedures and 31 million were outpatient procedures. Surgeries performed on the digestive tract, including endoscopy, colonoscopy, colectomy, appendectomy, and cholecystectomy, are the most common followed by surgeries on the musculoskeletal system, cardiovascular system, and eye. Surgeries are performed in hospital-based inpatient or outpatient settings or in free-standing surgical centers. **Same-day admission,** in which the patient reports from home directly to the reception area of the operating room is becoming standard procedure for many surgeries including complex cardiac procedures.

Categories of Surgery

Surgical procedures are categorized in a variety of ways, and any given procedure will fall into several of the categories. Each of the categorizations provides a small piece of information about the patient who is having surgery. For example, knowing the specific procedure to be performed allows the nurse to begin formulating plans for preoperative teaching. Knowing that a procedure needs to be done emergently gives information about patient acuity. Commonly, procedures are categorized according to the:

- General anatomic location of the surgery (e.g., abdominal, gynecological)
- Specific procedure to be performed (e.g., colectomy, total hip replacement)
- Purpose of the surgery (e.g., diagnostic, cosmetic)
- Urgency of the surgery (e.g., elective, urgent, emergent)
- Degree of risk associated with the surgery (low, moderate, high).

Surgery may also be performed for diagnostic, curative, reconstructive, palliative, or cosmetic purposes. **Diagnostic procedures** are those that are performed for the purpose of making or confirming a medical diagnosis. These procedures frequently require the removal of tissue or cells for analysis. Examples of diagnostic surgeries include procedures such as breast biopsy, arthroscopy, and laparotomy. In some cases, diagnostic surgery is referred to as **exploratory surgery** because the surgeon examines or explores the tissues and structures in order to decide what further procedures or treatments needs to be done.

Curative procedures are those that are done for the purpose of affecting a cure, for example, the successful treatment of a disease or condition. Many surgeries are done for this purpose including cholecystectomy, hernia repair, open reduction of a fracture, and mammoplasty.

Reconstructive surgery is done for the purpose of rebuilding tissues or body structures to achieve a more normal function and appearance. Examples include skin grafting and breast reconstruction following mastectomy.

Palliative procedures are those that are done for the purpose of alleviating symptoms caused by disease or a condition. Palliative surgery does not affect a cure, but it frequently improves quality of life. Examples include tumor debulking, performing a laminectomy to reduce spinal cord compression in a patient with metastatic cancer, and creation of a colostomy in a patient with severe inflammatory bowel disease.

Cosmetic surgery is performed for the primary purpose of improving physical appearance. Examples include liposuction, rhinoplasty, and breast augmentation.

Surgeries are also classified according to the urgency with which the procedure needs to be performed. **Elective procedures** are those that are scheduled in advance for a nonacute condition. Performing a procedure electively is always preferred because the patient will be in better health than he would be during an acute illness, and it allows optimum physiological and psychological preparation of the patient. There also is a technical advantage to elective procedures because the tissues are not distorted by inflammation or infection.

Urgent procedures are those that require prompt attention, within the next 24 to 48 hours, but they describe situations where the patient's condition is not currently life threatening. An appendectomy performed for a ruptured appendix is an example of an urgent procedure. An **emergent** (or emergency) **surgery** is a procedure that must be performed immediately to prevent serious consequences. Failure to perform emergency surgery in a timely manner can result in a patient's death or disability. A fas-

ciotomy performed to treat compartment syndrome in a fractured leg is an example of an emergent procedure.

Surgical procedures are accompanied by varying levels of risk. This risk is sometimes characterized using the terms *minor* or *major surgery*. Minor surgery refers to procedures associated with minimal risks. These procedures are often done under local anesthetic and do not require hospitalization. Major surgery describes procedures accompanied by more significant risks. The surgical risk associated with particular procedures can also be described as low, moderate, or high. Low-risk surgeries refer to those that have few complications, and when complications do occur, they are not serious. High-risk surgery describes procedures that are associated with a larger number of and more serious complications. One practice guideline developed by the American College of Cardiology (ACC) and the American Heart Association (AHA), classifies surgical procedures as high, intermediate, or low risk according to how much hemodynamic stress the procedure places on the heart (Eagle et al., 2002). In the guidelines, risk refers specifically to the perioperative development of a myocardial infarction, heart failure, or sudden death. In high-risk surgeries, cardiac events occur more than 5% of the time; in intermediate-risk surgeries, they occur between 1% and 4% of the time; and in low-risk surgeries, they occur less than 1% of the time. The National Guidelines box shows the ACC/AHA surgery-specific classification (Eagle et al., 2002).

Common Surgical Suffixes

There is no standardization for the naming of surgical procedures. Consequently, any given surgical procedure may have several names that are used interchangeably. Knowing the meaning

---

NATIONAL GUIDELINES ACC/AHA Surgery-Specific Classification

High-Risk Surgical Procedures	Emergent operations, particularly in elderly
	Aortic and other major vascular surgery
	Peripheral vascular surgery
	Prolonged surgical procedures, usually longer than 2 hours, associated with large fluid shifts and/or blood loss (e.g., major spinal surgery, pancreas resection)
	Cardiac procedures
Intermediate-Risk Surgical Procedures	Carotid endarterectomy
	Head and neck surgery
	Intraperitoneal and intrathoracic surgery
	Orthopedic surgery
	Prostate surgery
Low-Risk Surgical Procedures	Endoscopic procedures
	Superficial procedures
	Cataract surgery
	Breast surgery
	Cosmetic surgery

Source: Reprinted from ACC/AHA Guideline update for perioperative cardiovascular evaluation for non-cardiac surgery: A report of the American College of Cardiology/American Heart Association Task Force on Practice Guidelines (Committee to Update the 1996 Guidelines on perioperative cardiovascular evaluation for non-cardiac surgery). Eagle, K., Berger, P., Calkins, H., Chaitman, B., Ewy, G., Fleischmann, K., Fleisher, L., Froehlich, J., Gusberg, R., Leppo, J., Ryan, T., Schlant, R., & Winters, W. (2002). Reprinted with permission from Elsevier. American College of Cardiology Web site. Available at http://www.acc.org/clinical/guidelines/perio/dirlndex.htm

of common surgical suffixes, however, provides some help in understanding what type of surgery is to be performed:

- **ectomy**—removal of, surgical excision to remove (e.g., colectomy)
- **ostomy**—surgical creation of permanent opening (e.g., colostomy)
- **otomy**—surgical incision of or cutting into (e.g., thoracotomy)
- **plasty**—surgical repair or reconstruction of (e.g., rhinoplasty)
- **orraphy**—surgical repair or suture of (e.g., herniorrhaphy)
- **scopy**—use of a scope to view an area, looking into (e.g., laparoscopy).

Perioperative Nursing and Perioperative Nursing Practice Standards

The term **perioperative** encompasses the entire surgical experience: preoperative, intraoperative, and postoperative. The nurse's role in a perioperative setting includes preparing the patient for surgery, assisting and observing the patient during the operation, preventing and treating postoperative complications, and preparing the patient for discharge. Practice standards and practice guidelines are the basis for providing consistent, high-level care for the patient who is undergoing surgery. Practice standards developed by professional organizations set the expectations and responsibilities of professional nursing performance.

Standards are subject to ongoing evaluation and refinement so that they reflect current and best practices. The American Nurses Association's (ANA's) *Standards of Clinical Nursing Practice* and the *Code of Ethics for Nurses with Interpretive Statements* describe the roles and responsibilities of nurses regardless of practice setting. These standards are presented in Chapter 1 🔗. Specialty organizations in nursing use the ANA's conceptual framework for developing practice guidelines specific to the specialty. An example of this is the *Standards, Recommended Practices and Guidelines* developed by the Association of periOperative Registered Nurses (AORN, 2005). One part of the AORN standards, the *Standards of Perioperative Clinical Practice,* uses the nursing process (assessment, nursing diagnosis, outcome, planning, implementation, and evaluation) to describe how the perioperative nurse provides care to the surgical patient. Another part of the AORN standards, the *Standards of Perioperative Professional Performance,* focuses on professional role activities.

Several critical beliefs underlie AORN's standards. Among these is the belief that quality nursing care:

- Is a partnership between the nurse and the patient
- Is individualized
- Respects the patient's personal, cultural, and religious beliefs
- Respects the patient's autonomy
- Incorporates the patient's goals and preferences
- Focuses on collaboration, education, and advocacy.

Another organization important to perioperative nurses is the American Society of PeriAnesthesia Nurses (ASPAN). This organization develops and publishes standards of practice for care of the patient during recovery from surgery (ASPAN, 2006b).

Perioperative nurses need to be familiar with standards developed by groups interested in promoting quality care. Such groups include the National Council of State Boards of Nursing (NCSBN), the Joint Commission, the Institute for Healthcare Improvement (IHI), and the Medicare Quality Improvement Community. Hospitals also develop policies and procedures for the purpose of defining quality care. Hospital policies need to be rational, reasoned, current, and consistent with state and nationwide clinical and evidence-based practice (Meeker & Rothrock, 1999). Practice guidelines and clinical pathways are used to promote quality care. Clinical pathways are evidence-based and reflect critical activities, interventions, time frames, and desired outcomes for specific surgeries or diseases. It is the responsibility of perioperative nurses to use standards, guidelines, pathways, and policies in conjunction with their expertise and judgment when delivering high-level nursing care.

Collaborative Management

A successful surgical experience includes all members of the health care team. The surgeon and anesthesia care providers assess the patient prior to surgery. Consults from specialty areas such as cardiology, endocrinology, or neurology may be required depending on the patient's past or current medical condition. Some surgeries, such as organ transplantation or the creation of an ostomy, will require the patient to learn a whole new set of health maintenance skills. In these situations, the health care team may include a nurse who works directly with the surgeon and specializes in health care teaching for those surgeries.

A **preoperative health evaluation** is done within 30 days of a planned operation and must be documented in the patient's chart per the Joint Commission requirements (American Society of Anesthesiologists [ASA], 2006a; Institute for Clinical Symptoms Improvement [ICSI], 2006). An internist, surgeon, or anesthesia provider performs the evaluation, and it frequently is done as an outpatient examination. This evaluation is performed specifically to clear the patient for the planned surgical procedure. It provides data for confirming the overall appropriateness of performing the planned surgery (by answering questions such as "Is the patient healthy enough to have surgery?"), and confirms the plan to perform the surgery either as an outpatient, as a same-day admission, or as an inpatient. If abnormal findings are identified during this evaluation, further tests may be required prior to having the surgery. The preoperative evaluation includes a medical history; a focused review of issues pertinent to the planned anesthesia and surgical procedure; an abbreviated physical exam including height, weight, vital signs, cardiac and pulmonary systems; and an assessment of the patient's overall functional ability (ICSI, 2006). The preoperative health evaluation and any recommendations from the evaluation must be sent to the site where the surgery will be conducted.

The anesthesia provider also conducts a preoperative history and physical exam. This preprocedure assessment includes a review of systems with a focus on issues that affect the choice and administration of anesthesia. The patient is asked about any family history of anesthetic problems and any history of motion sickness or anesthesia-related nausea and vomiting. The latter two are risk factors for postoperative nausea and vomiting. The anesthesia assessment includes an examination of the patient's airway, neck (for range of motion), and teeth. Permanent dental prostheses may be documented during the exam. Chart 25–1 lists the ASA guidelines for classifying a patient's physical status and operative risk. Patients are classified in one of six categories, with lower classifications (e.g., I and II) representing those who are healthy or with mild systemic disease and good operative risks, and higher classifications (V and VI) representing patients who have severe disease and who are unlikely to survive surgery (ASA, 2006a).

A newer approach to surgery, accelerated recovery programs, relies on a multidisciplinary team approach with emphasis on collaboration. At the center of accelerated recovery programs, also referred to as fast-track surgery, is the view that patient outcomes are improved by expediting postoperative recovery. Key elements of accelerated programs include the following (Pasero & Belden, 2006):

- Preoperative education to prepare patients to take an active part in their recovery
- Use of anesthetics, analgesics, and surgical techniques that minimize surgical trauma and physiological stress, thereby allowing faster recovery
- Aggressive postoperative rehabilitation including early feeding and intensive ambulation
- Selective and evidence-based use of traditional postoperative practices such as the use of drains, tubes, and monitoring.

In accelerated recovery programs, patient assessment and education are important collaborative roles for nurses working in preoperative care.

Nursing Management

Nursing management in the preoperative setting is a cluster of activities (e.g., assessing, planning, teaching, and evaluating) performed by the nurse in anticipation of surgery. The purpose of preoperative care is to evaluate the patient's readiness for surgery,

to identify potential risks and hazards of the surgery, to advise the patient about the surgical procedure, to prepare the patient for the postoperative experience, to plan for home care, and to provide emotional support.

Nursing Assessment of the Preoperative Patient

Assessment of the preoperative patient is a nursing responsibility identified in practice standards (AORN, 2005). A complete and thorough preoperative assessment serves several purposes. The assessment identifies risk factors for intraoperative and postoperative problems. The risk of surgery is influenced by several factors including the patient's age, health history, current cardiac and pulmonary status, functional ability, and the type of surgery planned (Eagle et al., 2002). Once risk factors have been identified, the nurse takes steps to correct, minimize, or prevent potential problems. The assessment also provides the data necessary for developing preoperative and postoperative teaching plans. Importantly, the preoperative assessment provides a baseline of physical and functional ability. Nurses caring for the patient postoperatively will use preoperative assessments in deciding if a sign or symptom is a new finding, if the patient is progressing as expected, or if the patient needs specialized care, rehabilitation, or follow-up home services.

The preoperative assessment may be done in a separate appointment before the surgery or on the morning of the surgery. Many hospitals use their own forms for preoperative assessment to ensure completeness and simplicity. Most of these forms will represent an abbreviated version (using checklists for example) of the assessment described next. Figure 25–1 ■ (p. 590) is an example of a nursing assessment form. Preoperative assessment includes a patient history with physical examination and functional assessment. Patient history includes:

- Age
- Allergies
- Current health problem
- Type of surgery planned
- Plans for autologous blood donation
- Family history
- Past medical history
- Past surgical history and experiences with anesthesia
- Current medications
- Current herbal medications and nutritional supplements
- Alcohol, cigarette, social drug use.

Each of the areas listed is discussed in more detail in the following subsections.

Age

Approximately one-third of all surgeries are performed on elderly people. Age alone is not a contraindication for surgery; however, the risks of surgery increase with advancing age. (For more information refer to the Gerontological Considerations section later in this chapter, p. 599.)

CHART 25–1	ASA Physical Status Classification
ASA I	A normal healthy patient
ASA II	A patient with mild systemic disease
ASA III	A patient with severe systemic disease that limits disease but is not incapacitating
ASA IV	A patient with severe systemic disease that is a constant threat to life
ASA V	A moribund patient who is not expected to survive 24 hours without the operation
ASA VI	A patient declared brain dead and whose organs are being removed for transplantation

Source: Adapted from American Society of Anesthesiologists Classification of Physical Status. ASA Relative Value Guide, 2008. http://www.asahq.org/clinical/physicalstatus.htm

PRE PROCEDURE ASSESSMENT

Date:	PROCEDURE:

Confirmation of Procedure Including Site and Side if Applicable

☐ Patient procedure confirmed

☐ Patient identified using two identifiers

☐ ID Bracelet on   ☐ N/A

Patient states: _____

Patient points to: _____

Consent form states: _____

☐ Outpatient
☐ Inpatient

☐ Waive

☐ Telephonic Interview

☐ Consent not available

Height:_____ Weight:_____

PAT ONLY

Arrival Time _____

Start Time _____

End Time _____

☐ **Discrepancy noted, surgeon notified   Date __/__/__   Time_____   RN Initials_____**   Visit Level _____

ALLERGIES:

Latex Allergy ☐ No

☐ Yes ☐ O.R. aware   Precautions: _____

Review of Systems	☐ Refer to Nursing Assessment in patient's medical record dated: _____ (if within 30 days of procedure)
Cardiovascular & Respiratory	☐ Heart/valve ☐ Hypertension ☐ Angina ☐ Dyspnea ☐ Asthma
GI/Endo/Renal	☐ Diabetes ☐ Digestive/Reflux ☐ Kidney ☐ Liver
Neuromuscular	☐ CVA ☐ Seizures
Other	☐ Anemia ☐ Bleeding/Clotting ☐ Cancer
Habits	Tobacco Use ☐ No ☐ Yes Amount: _____ ETOH ☐ No ☐ Yes Amount: _____ Recreational Drug Use ☐ No ☐ Yes Amount: _____
Surgical History	
Anesthesia History	TMJ/Neck Problems? ☐ No ☐ Yes _____ Past Anesthesia? ☐ No ☐ Yes _____ Problems? ☐ No ☐ Yes _____

MEDICATIONS (Include herbal supplements)

Medication	Dose	Frequency	Medication	Dose	Frequency

Psycho/Social

Lives: ☐ Alone   ☐ w/Family ☐ w/Spouse   ☐ Other

Occupation: _____

Cultural/Religious Preference: _____

Do you feel safe in your relationships?   ☐ Yes   ☐ No

If patient answers no, contact   ☐ Safe Transitions (#31389) and/or
☐ Social Work for assistance

Pain

Baseline Pain score (0-10): _____ Location:_____

Quality: _____

Daily Narcotic use: ☐ No   ☐ Yes

Type and daily dosage: _____

Cognitive/Perceptual

Visual/Hearing Deficit: ☐ No   ☐ Yes _____

Primary language other than English: _____

Interpreter: ☐ No   ☐ Yes   ☐ Requested

Nutrition/Elimination

Difficulty Swallowing	☐ No	☐ Yes ____
Bladder/Bowel Problems	☐ No	☐ Yes ____
Unintentional Weight Loss > 10lbs:	☐ No	☐ Yes ____

Activity/Mobility

Self ADL   ☐ Yes   ☐ No _____

Balance   ☐ Steady   ☐ Unsteady

Hx Slips & Falls ☐ No   ☐ Yes

Judgement   ☐ Intact   ☐ Impared

Patient has Health Care Proxy   ☐ Yes   ☐ No

If no, Proxy Explained & Patient Advised how to Obtain

☐ No   ☐ Yes   Name of Proxy:_____

Phone Number: _____

Advanced Directives   ☐ Yes   ☐ No

If no, directives explained & patient advised how to obtain

Preoperative teaching completed, patient verbalizes understanding ☐ Yes ☐ PAT Communication Form No ___ Completed and Sent ☐ N/A

Nursing Diagnoses 1-2 Outcomes Met   ☐ Yes   ☐ No

Notes: _____

Signature: _____ RN   Printed name: _____ RN   Date: ____ / ____ / ____

FIGURE 25–1 ■ Preoperative nursing assessment form.

Source: Courtesy of Beth Israel Deaconess Nursing Department

PREOPERATIVE ASSESSMENT

Allergies: _____

Precautions: _____

ID verified: ☐ Patient identified using two identifiers   ☐ Bracelet on   NPO since: Date _____   Time _____

Last void: Time _____   ☐ Foley cath.   ☐ Other _____

Meds. taken today: _____

_____

V.S.   T _____   P _____   R _____   SpO2 _____   O2 Source _____   B/P in _____ arm: _____

Test results drawn in Holding Area: Hgb. _____   Glucose _____   K _____   T&S _____
Other _____

Consents: ☐ H&P   ☐ Surgical   ☐ General Agreement   ☐ Anesthesia [☐ N/A]

☐ Patient Procedure Confirmed   ☐ No Laterality
☐ No discrepancy, preadmission testing documentation reviewed
OR schedule says _____
Consent form says _____
Patient states & points to _____
Side/site marked is _____

☐ **Discrepancy noted, Surgeon notified**   date ___ / ___ / ___   time ___ : ___
Surgeon's final side/site directive with surgeon's signature _____   RN Initials _____

Implants: _____

Level of Consciousness: ☐ alert   ☐ unresponsive   ☐ oriented   ☐ disoriented   ☐ somnolent but arousable

Emotional status: ☐ calm   ☐ anxious   ☐ agitated

Pain: ☐ Reviewed baseline pain from pre-procedure assessment.   Current baseline pain score (0-10): _____
Location/Quality & pain relief methods in use today: _____

Interpreter: Name _____

Escort/Contact: Name _____   ☐ N/A
Phone number: _____   Location: _____

Nursing Diagnoses 1-4 Outcomes Met: ☐ Yes   ☐ No   Notes: _____

_____

_____   _____ RN Initials

Medication: dose/route/time/by
1. _____
2. _____

Medication: dose/route/time/by
3. _____
4. _____

PATIENT BELONGINGS	Transport	To PACU	w/Patient	w/Escort	PACU Safe	BIDMC Safe	N/A	Locker
Dentures: ☐ upper ☐ lower								
Glasses								
Contact lenses								
Hearing Aid: ☐ right ☐ left								
Prosthesis								
Jewelry:								
Clothing								
Cash ($)								
Credit Cards								
Other:								
Medications brought from home:								

☐ Patient aware of policy, but declines to place valuables in safekeeping.

Signature of Patient/Family   **RN Initials**   **Signature of Recipient**   **RN Initials**

1. _____   RN _____   RN _____   ___ / ___ / ___
   Signature   **Printed name**   **Initials**   **Date**

2. _____   RN _____   RN _____   ___ / ___ / ___
   Signature   **Printed name**   **Initials**   **Date**

Patient's name   Med. Rec. #   DOB

Allergies

Allergies and allergic reactions to medications, chemicals, and foods must always be identified and prominently displayed on the patient's wristband, in the chart, and in the medication record. Patients with histories of allergic reactions have a greater risk of hypersensitivity to anesthesia, so the type of allergic reaction is very important. They also are much more likely to develop latex allergies. A special operating room setup is required for patients with latex allergy. Latex skin allergy is discussed in detail in Chapter 60 ☺. Patients who are allergic to shellfish or iodine may also be allergic to the solution for surgical preparation, povidone-iodine.

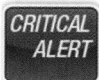 *Allergic responses to latex range from mild dermatitis to anaphylaxis. If latex allergy is suspected, a blood or skin test can be performed to confirm the allergy. A latex-reduced environment must be created for individuals who are allergic to latex.*

Current Health Problem

The patient's current health problem may influence various aspects of perioperative care. It may affect the type of anesthesia used, the type and amount of fluid replacement given, and the type of intraoperative monitoring performed. It may also determine priorities of postoperative care.

For women, anesthesia should be avoided during the first trimester of pregnancy. It is important to know the date of the last menstrual period. A pregnancy test is done if there is uncertainty about whether or not the patient is pregnant.

Type of Surgery Planned

The surgical procedure planned influences every aspect of perioperative care including the preoperative assessment, preoperative teaching and preparation, the setup of the operating room, the type of anesthesia used, and priorities of postoperative care. The preoperative assessment is a good time for the nurse to review the operative permit (e.g., consent), to evaluate the patient's understanding of the surgical procedure to be performed, and to clarify questions for the patient.

Plans for Autologous Blood Donation

Patients scheduled for elective surgery may make arrangements to donate their own blood in advance of the surgery. To be eligible for preoperative autologous donation, the patient must be in good health, be afebrile, have a hemoglobin of 11 g/dL or higher, and have the approval of her physician or surgeon. Chapter 23 ☺ includes a complete description of autologous blood donation and its administration procedures and nursing interventions.

Family History

Family history is important to determine the presence of possible genetic predispositions. It is particularly important to ask about family history of diabetes, heart disease, sudden cardiac death, and malignant hyperthermia (MH). Malignant hyperthermia is a life-threatening condition of sustained muscle contraction precipitated by common agents of anesthesia such as inhalation agents and the muscle relaxant succinylcholine. Malignant hyperthermia is an autosomal dominant trait so that each child of an MH parent has a 50% chance of inheriting the susceptibility. MH is discussed in detail in Chapter 26 ☺.

Past Medical History

Past medical history (PMH) can increase the risk associated with surgery as well as the possibility of postoperative complications. Patients are asked about all previous diseases and conditions. Preexisting disease influences many perioperative decisions including whether or not to proceed with the operation, the type of anesthesia used, the need for additional testing or procedures prior to surgery, and the need for intraoperative and postoperative monitoring. The implications of specific conditions are discussed next.

Neurological conditions assessment includes asking about any history of stroke or transient ischemic attacks (TIAs). If a patient has a history of a stroke, it is important to determine what, if any, deficits remain and whether or not the patient is receiving anticoagulation therapy. Deficits in cognitive functioning may affect the patient's ability to understand preoperative and postoperative instructions. Mobility deficits may place the patient at increased risk for postoperative atelectasis, pneumonia, abdominal distention, constipation, skin breakdown, and deep venous thrombosis (DVT). DVT is discussed in Chapter 43 ☺. Patients who have neuromuscular disorders (myasthenia gravis, multiple sclerosis) or spinal cord injury also may be at a higher risk for postoperative complications associated with limited mobility. Patients who are experiencing transient ischemic attacks (TIA) may need to have a procedure to improve blood flow to the brain (carotid endarterectomy) prior to having any other surgical procedure in order to decrease the risk of a perioperative stroke. Seizure disorder also is a significant surgical factor because some anesthetic agents are known to lower the threshold for seizures.

The *cardiovascular disorders* assessment is important because surgery is a major stress to the heart as a result of the hemodynamic changes that occur with tissue injury and fluid loss. All anesthetic drugs have known cardiovascular affects. Disorders of the cardiovascular system are particularly important in establishing surgical risk for the patient. The highest risk is associated with acute myocardial infarction (AMI) (within 7 days preceding the operation), recent MI (occurred in the month prior to the operation), unstable angina, heart failure, significant arrhythmia, and severe valvular disease (Eagle et al., 2002). It is recommended that patients wait a minimum of 4 to 6 weeks after an MI to have elective surgery to prevent the likelihood of reinfarction. Patients with unstable angina may require stabilization either with medications or coronary revascularization prior to having any other surgical procedures. Patients with heart failure are at increased risk of postoperative pulmonary complications and fluid and electrolyte imbalances (Qaseem et al., 2006). These patients will need to have their fluid status monitored closely during the intraoperative and postoperative periods. Brain natriuretic peptide (BNP) is a chemical that is released when the heart ventricle is stretched. Serum BNP is used preoperatively to screen or monitor heart failure. Postoperatively, it is used to decide whether dyspnea is caused by heart failure or some other condition (Pagana, 2007). Patients with valvular disorders may require antibiotic prophylaxis to reduce the risk of bacterial endocarditis (Chapter 41 ☺). Also, these patients must be monitored postoperatively for the development of worsening heart failure.

Patients with a history of dysrhythmias will require postoperative cardiac telemetry. Patients with pacemakers or implantable cardioverter defibrillators (ICDs) present specific concerns during surgery. The presence of a pacemaker affects placement of the electrocautery grounding pad and choice of anesthetic agents. Electrocautery, used in the operating room, can create an electromagnetic interference that may cause pacemaker dysfunction or damage (Rooke, 2007). The use of succinylcholine, a depolarizing muscle relaxant sometimes used during anesthesia, causes muscle fasciculations and postoperative shivering that can suppress pacemaker function (Rooke, 2007). Preoperative information required for patients with pacemakers includes identification of the underlying cardiac rhythm that necessitates pacemaker, and information about the pacemaker itself (e.g., type, device, lead system, availability of technical support). All patients with pacemakers need to have the unit interrogated (i.e., tested to check battery status, and thresholds for sensing and pacing leads) within 3 months of scheduled surgery. Pacemaker interrogation after surgery is also recommended. Patients with ICDs also need to supply information about the device as well as evidence of unit interrogation prior to surgery. It is recommended that the tachyarrhythmia detection of the ICD unit be turned off prior to surgery (Rooke, 2007). Electromagnetic noise from electrocautery can mimic the signal for ventricular tachycardia or ventricular fibrillation, causing the ICD to deliver an unnecessary shock during surgery. A magnet is used to turn off the tachycardia detection feature on the morning of surgery. Postoperatively, the unit must be turned back on.

Patients undergoing cardiac surgery may have a beta-adrenergic blocking medication prescribed preoperatively to reduce the risk of developing atrial fibrillation postoperatively (Bradley et al., 2005) and statin drugs to improve surgical outcomes (Pan et al., 2004). Generally, patients with hypertension will continue to receive antihypertensive medications throughout the perioperative period especially in patients with hard to control hypertension.

Patients with *chronic respiratory conditions* such as chronic obstructive pulmonary disease (COPD) and severe asthma, as well as the elderly and people who smoke cigarettes, have an increased risk of postoperative atelectasis and pneumonia (Qaseem et al., 2006). Preoperative pulmonary function tests may need to be performed on patients with COPD. Patients with an upper respiratory infection may have surgery postponed. Obstructive sleep apnea (OSA) is a serious condition that is evaluated in the preoperative assessment. OSA is associated with airway collapse, hypoventilation, and sensitivity to the respiratory depressant effects of medications such as anesthetics, narcotics, and sedatives (ASA, 2006b).

 Notify the anesthesia care provider of patients with suspected or documented OSA. It may be difficult to intubate this patient and he will require continuous monitoring for hypoventilation and hypoxemia during surgery and postoperatively until he is stable.

Patients with *chronic renal failure* (CRF) will require close monitoring of fluid and electrolyte balance and medication administration. The effectiveness of drugs may be altered because the kidney excretes most drugs. Patients with CRF are at a higher than expected risk of an intraoperative cardiac event (Eagle et al., 2002). Patients with benign prostatic hypertrophy (BPH) should be monitored postoperatively for problems with urinary retention.

Musculoskeletal conditions such as arthritis can have a major impact on the ability to properly position a patient intraoperatively and postoperatively. Care must be taken not to injure arthritic joints. Temporomandibular joint (TMJ) syndrome and limitations of neck mobility can interfere with intubation for general anesthesia. Myotonic dystrophy, a rare form of muscular dystrophy, increases the patient's sensitivity to anesthesia and narcotics.

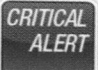 *Patients with a history of certain neuromuscular disorders, such as myotonic dystrophy, may be highly sensitive to anesthesia and require special precautions when planning surgery. The patient should wear a medical alert bracelet and all health care providers need to be aware of this condition. Monitor the use of narcotics carefully.*

Several issues must be considered in caring for the surgical patient with an *endocrine disorder* such as diabetes. Type I diabetes is associated with an increased risk of perioperative cardiac morbidity (Eagle et al., 2002). Poor glucose control is associated with higher rates of surgical site infections (IHI, 2006; Schweon, 2006). Patients with diabetes also experience slower wound healing. The physiological stress of surgery changes the insulin requirement. Careful monitoring of blood sugar is needed to prevent hypoglycemia and ketosis.

Patients who are immunocompromised present a special surgical challenge. Examples of patients at high risk for immune system dysfunction include those with human immunodeficiency virus (HIV) or cancer, those who have undergone chemotherapy, splenectomy, or organ transplantation, those taking immunosuppressive drugs such as prednisone, and those who are malnourished, experience chronic pain, or abuse alcohol (Neil, 2007). Surgery depresses the normal immune system for up to a week, and this effect is heightened in patients already immunocompromised. Immunosuppression increases the surgical risks for hypothermia, infection, and hypoadrenal function. Preoperative assessment for immunosuppressed patients includes weight, blood pressure, a complete blood count, liver and renal function tests, and chest x-ray (Neil, 2007).

Other disorders that may impact surgery include anemia, bleeding or clotting disorders, cancer, and morbid obesity. Skin and tissues that have been irradiated, as a treatment for cancer, are more easily damaged and heal more slowly than other tissues. The effects of chemotherapy depend on the drugs given. Morbid obesity, a body mass index of 40 or greater, is associated with significant comorbidities including diabetes mellitus, hypertension, gastroesophageal reflux disease, and OSA (Owens, 2006). Surgical procedures may also take longer, requiring a longer period of anesthesia (Rogers et al., 2006).

Past Surgical History and Experience with Anesthesia

A patient's previous experience with surgery and anesthesia will influence decisions about the current surgery. A complete surgical history should be obtained, focusing specifically on previous surgeries, dates they were performed, problems with anesthesia, and postoperative complications. Some problems are likely to repeat themselves. If it was difficult to intubate the patient with a previous surgery, it will likely be difficult with the current surgery. Difficulty with intubation needs to be prominently noted in the medical record, and the patient should wear a colored wristband identifying the problem. Other problems with prior surgery may not reoccur because of changes in surgical techniques, improved technologies, better anesthetic agents, or new medications.

 CRITICAL ALERT *Alert the anesthesia care provider if the patient reports a history of difficult intubation with a prior surgery. This patient needs an airway examination and specialized airway equipment must be available.*

A preoperative risk assessment for postoperative nausea and vomiting (PONV) needs to be completed. Risk factors for PONV are outlined in the Risk Factors box. The preoperative risk assessment is used to plan for surgery and prophylaxis for postoperative nausea and vomiting. Patients with multiple risk factors may be given different anesthetics (e.g., total intravenous anesthesia or regional blocks) and preoperative medications (ASPAN, 2006a). Patients with moderate to high risk of PONV need a multimodal approach to prevention. Some medications are given to the patient in the presurgical area, whereas others such as a transdermal scopolamine patch are applied by the patient the night before surgery.

Current Medications

Patients are asked to provide a specific and detailed list of regularly taken medications, including over-the-counter (OTC) medications and herbal preparations. The list includes the name of the medication, as well as the amount and how often it is taken. Information on medications is used in numerous ways. Many medications have the potential to either increase or decrease the effect of anesthetic agents. Certain medications may necessitate specific preoperative tests. For example, patients taking digoxin or a diuretic (furosemide, hydrochlorothiazide) may need to have potassium levels tested prior to surgery.

Some medications require dose adjustments prior to surgery. Examples of drugs that may be adjusted prior to surgery include insulin, oral hypoglycemic agents, corticosteroids, and antihypertensive agents. Medications that slow coagulation are frequently discontinued prior to surgery. Examples of these are aspirin, enoxaparin, heparin, vitamin E, and warfarin. Chart 25–2 (p. 595) shows selected medications and the implications for surgery.

RISK FACTORS for Postoperative Nausea and Vomiting

Gender (women more than men)

History of nausea and vomiting with a previous surgery

History of motion sickness

Nonsmoker

Use of certain inhalation anesthetics (volatile anesthetic gases and nitrous oxide)

Use of opioid analgesics

Type of surgery (gynecologic, abdominal, and those on the ear or eye)

Longer surgeries.

Sources: American Society of PeriAnesthesia Nurses. (2006). ASPAN's evidence-based clinical practice guideline for the prevention and/or management of PONV/PDNV. *Journal of PeriAnesthesia Nursing, 21*(4), 230–250; Murphy, M., Hooper, V., Sullivan, E., Clifford, T., & Apfel, C. (2006). Identification of risk factors for postoperative nausea and vomiting in the perianesthesia adult patient. *Journal of PeriAnesthesia Nursing, 21*(6), 377–384.

Current Herbal Medications and Nutritional Supplements

The use of herbal remedies and nutritional supplements is becoming increasingly common in the United States. Studies show that between 40% and 70% of patients do not tell their health care providers or pharmacists about the use of herbal remedies (Bennett & Brown, 2000; Pribitkin & Boger, 2000; Roberts et al., 2005; Vallerand, Fouladbakhsh, & Templin, 2005; Yoon, Horne, & Adams, 2004). Often, patients combine herbs, prescription medications, and OTC products in treating health problems (Roberts et al., 2005; Yoon et al., 2004).

Patients need to be asked specifically about the use of herbs and nutritional supplements in a preoperative assessment. Although herbs are considered relatively safe, they do have pharmacologically active properties that can produce drug interactions or adverse effects. For example, several herbs are known to inhibit platelet function and delay clotting time (Hatcher, 2001). In the United States, herbs are classified as diet supplements; they are not subject to federal regulation and there is no standardization in herb potency. Consequently, it is difficult to know how much of a pharmacologic effect is exerted by any given herbal product. The ASA (1999a) recommends discontinuing all herbal products 2 to 3 weeks prior to surgery.

The use of nutritional supplements can also affect surgery. Fish oil, a popular supplement thought to reduce the effects of atherosclerosis and prevent myocardial infarction and angina, may slow blood clotting. Patients should stop taking fish oil 2 to 3 weeks before surgery. Chart 25–3 (p. 596) lists some common herbs, their uses, and the implications for surgery.

Alcohol, Cigarette, and Drug Use

A careful history of alcohol and illicit drug use is important because excessive and chronic use of these substances can interfere with anesthesia, increase the patient's tolerance to anesthesia, reduce the effectiveness of postoperative pain medication, and cause serious physiological issues such as drug or alcohol withdrawal syndromes. If surgery must be performed on patients who are addicted to alcohol or narcotics, then the careful titration of benzodiazepines (for alcohol) and methadone (for narcotics) may be used to prevent withdrawal symptoms.

 CRITICAL ALERT *When the possibility of alcohol withdrawal exists, the nurse and surgical team need to monitor the patient closely. A standardized alcohol withdrawal rating scale, such as the Clinical Institute Withdrawal Assessment (CIWA) scale, helps in identifying serious withdrawal symptoms and in monitoring treatment for alcohol withdrawal syndrome.*

A lifetime history of cigarette smoking is described in pack-years, the number of packs smoked per day multiplied by the number of years smoked. Cigarette smoking increases surgical risk for several reasons. Smoking damages the mucociliary clearance system, resulting in increased secretions and a higher risk of postoperative atelectasis and pneumonia (Barrera et al., 2005). Smoking increases circulating carboxyhemoglobin, which reduces circulating oxygen resulting in less oxygen delivery to body tissues. Smoking causes vasoconstriction, a serious concern for patients undergoing cardiac or vascular surgery. Smoking cessation is thought to reduce sputum production, increase ciliary action and clearance of secretions, and improve small airway function. Patients are asked to stop smoking 6 to 8

CHART 25–2 Medications and Their Implications for Surgery

Drug Classification and Sample Medications	Implications for Surgery
ACE inhibitors Enalapril Lisinopril (Zestril) Quinapril (Accupril)	Inhibit angiotensin-aldosterone system, resulting in decreased peripheral resistance. Can cause hypotension. Monitor blood pressure closely. Surgeon may recommend holding drug on the morning of surgery unless prescribed for heart failure.
Antiarrhythmics Amiodarone Procainamide (Pronestyl) Quinidine	Depress myocardial excitability and contractility and slows heart rate. Some agents can cause hypotension. Can increase the cardiac effects of anesthetic agents.
Anticoagulants Enoxaparin sodium Heparin sodium Warfarin sodium (Coumadin)	Increase the risk of bleeding intraoperatively and postoperatively. Coagulants may be discontinued 24 to 48 hours before surgery. Monitor coagulation studies (PT, INR, aPTT). Watch for signs of bleeding.
Antidepressants Citalopram (Celexa) Paroxetine (Paxil) Sertraline (Zoloft)	Restart the medication as soon as possible once the patient is able to tolerate oral intake.
Antidiabetic agents Glyburide (Glibenclamide) Glipizide (Glucotrol XL) Insulin Metformin (Glucophage)	The physiological stress of surgery increases serum glucose levels and insulin requirements. Hospitals have standard protocols to guide insulin and glucose administration in the perioperative period. Monitor serum glucose levels closely during postoperative period. Expect patients with diabetes to be on regular insulin sliding scale coverage during periods of acute stress and infection. Surgeon may recommend that patient hold the medication at least 8 hours prior to surgery.
Antihypertensives Amlodipine (Norvasc) Atenolol Metoprolol (Lopressor)	Side effects include hypotension and bradycardia. Monitor blood pressure and heart rate. Frequently taken on the morning of surgery especially when hypertension is difficult to manage.
Antiplatelet drugs Clopidogrel (Plavix)	Inhibit platelet aggregation, increasing the risk of bleeding postoperatively. Monitor platelet count. Surgeon may want the drug stopped 2 weeks before surgery.
Antiseizure medications Gabapentin (Neurontin)	Dose may need to be adjusted for surgery. Some anesthetic agents can lower the potential for seizures.
Corticosteroids Dexamethasone (Decadron) Hydrocortisone (Solu-Cortef) Prednisone	Steroids decrease inflammation, delay wound healing, and mask signs of infection. Steroids increase serum glucose levels and insulin requirements. Steroids increase risk of postoperative bleeding. Surgery increases the need for steroids and patients may need to have their steroid dose adjusted.
Diuretics Furosemide (Lasix) Hydrochlorothiazide	Diuretics cause urinary excretion of sodium, chloride, potassium, bicarbonate, magnesium, and calcium. Serum electrolytes should be checked regularly. Monitor intake and output. Surgeon may recommend holding medication on the morning of surgery unless the patient is taking for heart failure.
Gastric acid inhibitors Lansoprazole (Prevacid) Omeprazole (Prilosec)	Proton pump inhibitors also inhibit a liver enzyme needed for the metabolism of other drugs. They can prolong the half-life of some drugs including benzodiazepines. Usually taken on the morning of surgery.
Hormones Levothyroxine (Synthroid)	Should be given intravenously while the patient is NPO.
NSAIDs Aspirin Celecoxib (Celebrex) Ibuprofen	Increase the risk of intraoperative and postoperative bleeding. Aspirin inhibits platelet aggregation and the effect lasts the duration of the thrombocyte life span (7 to 10 days). NSAIDs are stopped 2 weeks before surgery.

weeks prior to surgery. For patients who are unable to quit before surgery, a nicotine patch can be applied postoperatively to prevent nicotine craving and withdrawal.

Physical and Functional Assessment

An important part of the preoperative assessment is the physical examination and functional assessment. During this assessment the nurse documents the patient's baseline physical findings such as vital signs and mental status as well as his baseline functional ability. The components of the assessment remain the same regardless of the type of surgery being performed, but the level of detail provided in certain categories may change by type of surgery. Patients admitted for neurosurgery will have a more thorough reporting of their neurological exam, whereas patients admitted for gastrointestinal surgery will need a more detailed abdominal and nutritional assessment. The patient's past medical

CHART 25–3	Herbs, Their Common Uses, and Implications for Surgery	

Herb	Common Use	Implications for Surgery
Black cohosh	Hot flashes, dysmenorrhea	Unknown
Cayenne	Neuropathy, cluster headaches	Unknown
Echinacea	Cold, sore throat	Unknown
Ephedra	Weight loss	Cardiac stimulation with tachycardia and elevated blood pressure.
Feverfew	To control migraine headache	Impairs platelet function.
Garlic	Cold, flu, hypertension	Interferes with platelet aggregation and prolongs clotting time with risk of bleeding. May decrease blood glucose levels.
Ginger	Nausea, motion sickness	Prolongs clotting time with risk of bleeding.
Ginkgo biloba	Vertigo, tinnitus, intermittent claudication, Alzheimer's disease	Interferes with platelet aggregation. May increase seizure potential.
Ginseng (American)	To strengthen the immune system	May lower serum glucose levels in patients with diabetes.
Ginseng (Asian)	To improve stamina and vitality	Inhibits platelet function.
Guargum	To lower cholesterol	May interfere with gastrointestinal absorption of some antibiotics.
Milk thistle	Liver disease	Unknown
Saw palmetto	Benign prostatic hypertrophy	Increases risk of bleeding.
St. John's wort	Depression, anxiety	Unknown
Valerian	Sedative, anxiety	May potentiate sedative effects of anesthetic agents.

Sources: Flanagan, K. (2001). Preoperative assessment: Safety considerations for patients taking herbal products. *Journal of PeriAnesthesia Nursing, 16*(1), 19–26; Hatcher, T. (2001). The proverbial herb. *American Journal of Nursing, 101*(2), 36–43; Miller, L. (1998). Herbal medicinals: Selected clinical considerations focusing on known or potential drug–herb interactions. *Archives of Internal Medicine, 158*(20), 2200–2211; Pribitkin, E., & Boger, G. (2000). Surgery and herbal therapy: Essential guidelines on bleeding, skin reactions, and wound healing. *Complementary Health Practice Review, 6*(1), 29–40.

history will also direct the nurse's attention toward specific categories of assessment.

Neurological Assessment

The neurological examination includes a baseline mental status examination as well as an assessment of motor and sensory function. An evaluation of mental status includes level of consciousness, judgment, ability to follow commands, appropriateness of behavior, speech, and the ability to express oneself and to understand what is being said. These data are especially helpful in designing pre- and postoperative teaching plans. It is particularly important to document baseline performance for older patients because they are at a higher risk than other adults of experiencing a surgery-related change in mental status. Evaluation of motor function includes strength, movement, balance, and gait. Any physical limitations or impairments such as difficulty with hearing, vision, speech, swallowing, or walking should be noted as well as any history of falls. The risk of falls is associated with many factors, but two factors consistently identified across studies are altered mental status and impaired mobility (Chang et al., 2004; Evans, Hodgkinson, Lambert, & Wood, 2001). During the evaluation, the nurse makes a determination about the patient's fall risk and begins developing a safety plan. A patient's neurological status may affect a patient's ability to carry out activities of daily living (ADLs) independently such as bathing, dressing, toileting, feeding, walking, and transferring.

 CRITICAL ALERT *The reduction of patient falls is a Joint Commission National Patient Safety Goal. A multifactorial falls assessment combined with a fall reduction program is an effective means of reducing falls in the hospital setting.*

The patient is asked about issues of pain and pain tolerance. The location, description, and rating of preoperative pain are noted, and the patient is asked about successful strategies for dealing with pain. This is a good time to discuss postoperative pain, to teach about using a numeric rating scale, and to reassure the patient that pain control is a key concern for health care providers. Patients who are taught preoperatively how to use a pain rating scale are better able to describe their pain postoperatively (Bond et al., 2005). Pain assessment and management is discussed in detail in Chapter 15 😊 .

Cardiovascular Assessment

Baseline vital signs are established for the preoperative patient. It is helpful to know baseline pulse and blood pressure because postoperative problems such as anxiety, pain, hypoxia, and dehydration can manifest via a change in vital signs. The nurse assesses heart rate and rhythm, blood pressure, and peripheral pulses in addition to observing the extremities for color, sensation, capillary refill, and the presence of edema. The physician is made aware of any cardiac-specific abnormalities present on exam such as hypertension, chest pain, dyspnea, pedal edema, or heart rhythm irregularities.

Cardiac abnormalities may need further evaluation prior to surgery to prevent an intraoperative cardiac event (Eagle et al., 2002). Additional evaluation may include an electrocardiogram, echocardiogram, cardiac stress test, and pacemaker or ICD interrogation. In patients with a history of cardiovascular disease, the effect of the disease on the patient's ability to walk, exercise, and participate in ADLs is investigated. It is important to document baseline activity levels for all patients. Research suggests that those who participate in exercise and muscle strengthening activities preoperatively walk greater distances postoperatively and are discharged earlier than those with more sedate lifestyles (Whitney & Parkman, 2002).

Respiratory Assessment

Baseline findings of respiratory rate and depth, quality of respiratory effort, lung sounds, and oxygen saturation level with room air and with oxygen, if the patient requires oxygen, are established. The nurse also asks the patient about any problems breathing, whether or not shortness of breath interferes with ADLs, and about the use of inhalers, oxygen, or continuous positive airway pressure (CPAP) devices at home. Baseline information is important because postoperative atelectasis is a common problem and because the nurse is usually responsible for weaning patients off oxygen in the postoperative period.

Gastrointestinal Assessment

Physical exam includes palpation of the abdomen and auscultation of bowel sounds. Patients are asked about the usual pattern and consistency of bowel movements, the date of the last bowel movement, and what, if any, medications they take for their bowels. Abdominal distention and constipation can occur postoperatively as a result of factors such as anesthesia, limited physical mobility, and the use of narcotics for pain. A patient who has an ostomy is asked about any ostomy-specific issues such as skin care and regularity and about the required supplies during the hospitalization.

Genitourinary Assessment

Patients are asked about their usual pattern of urinary elimination as well as urinary issues such as any difficulty starting a stream, controlling continence of urine, completely emptying the bladder, and dysuria. Patients with chronic renal failure are asked if they are anuric (no urine production) and their usual schedule for dialysis. If a patient is on dialysis, then the arteriovenous (AV) fistula or graft, if present, is documented and checked for patency. The AV fistula or graft is palpated for the presence of a thrill and auscultated for a bruit. Baseline data are important for interpreting postoperative findings and anticipating potential problems. Postoperatively, fluid balance is monitored using urinary output. Urinary retention is a postoperative problem that is associated with certain surgeries, such as gynecologic and genitourinary procedures.

Musculoskeletal Assessment

Musculoskeletal assessment is concerned with patients' ability to move themselves and their extremities. The nurse notes any problems with range of motion, arthritic joints, or mobility restrictions. These data are important to the proper positioning of the patient intraoperatively as well as postoperatively. If a patient uses a prosthetic device, electrocautery grounding pads, which are used in surgery, should be placed away from the site of prosthesis to prevent potential injury to the tissue. Assistive devices (e.g., prostheses, crutches, a walker, a wheelchair) that the patient requires for mobilization need to be available to the patient postoperatively to facilitate early mobilization.

Endocrine Assessment

Patients with diabetes are asked about the frequency of glucose testing and use of oral hypoglycemic agents and insulin. Surgery and anesthesia can affect the regulation of glucose. The physiological and psychological stress of surgery and illness tend to elevate serum glucose levels, whereas factors such as preoperative restriction of food and fluids tend to lower glucose levels. The patient with diabetes should be scheduled for surgery early in the day to limit prolonged fasting. The patient will need frequent monitoring of serum glucose with insulin coverage using a sliding scale. Patients who ordinarily take oral hypoglycemic agents may need the temporary coverage of insulin during periods of stress and illness.

Nutritional Assessment

The nutritional assessment includes a baseline height and weight. The nurse asks specific questions about the patient's appetite, usual diet, food preferences, recent weight loss or gain, and any problems with chewing or swallowing. The nurse notes signs of poor nutrition including brittle nails and dry, flaky, skin. The patient's nutritional status has a profound effect on surgical outcomes. Surgery increases basal metabolic rate and the need for proteins, vitamins, and calories. Patient's who are malnourished with a negative nitrogen balance and deficits of vitamins A, C, and B complex are at risk for experiencing problems with their wound including infection, delayed healing, and dehiscence. A low serum albumin (less than 3.5 mg/dL) or a low or declining prealbumin are markers of poor nutrition and are associated with a higher risk of postoperative pulmonary complications (Qaseem et al., 2006). Prealbumin or a transthyretin test is considered a more sensitive marker of nutrition than albumin and correlates with patient outcomes (Beck & Rosenthal, 2002). Postoperatively, a dropping prealbumin alerts the caregiver to a declining nutritional status.

Patients who are morbidly obese face a number of potential postoperative problems. Access to the operative site is difficult and may prolong the operation and length of time anesthesia is used. Anesthetic agents are absorbed by adipose tissue, prolonging the effects of anesthesia on all body systems. Research shows obesity to be a significant risk factor in the development of postoperative complications (Brooks-Brunn, 2000; Owens, 2006). Wound approximation during surgical closure is difficult and decreased tissue vascularity contributes to slower healing. These factors and others such as insulin resistance increase the potential for wound infection, dehiscence, and evisceration in the obese patient.

Integumentary Assessment

The nurse asks about skin sensitivities and problems, and observes the condition of the skin for moisture, turgor, and color. Any area of injury or breakdown is noted. Many hospitals adopt the use of a tool or scale to measure the risk or likelihood of pressure ulcer development. Chapter 67 ⊙ has an example of the Braden Scale as well as other skin breakdown assessment data.

Maintaining skin integrity is a priority of care in the operating room. Surgical cleansing materials, surgical tape, electrodes, and other materials have the potential to cause allergic skin reactions. The grounding pad used with electrocautery can cause a burn if improperly placed. Pressure ulcers can develop within 2 to 3 hours of unrelieved pressure (Heizenroth, 1999). Preoperative risk factors for development of skin breakdown include older age; the presence of comorbidities such as diabetes, hypertension, and vascular disorders; poor nutritional status; and low hemoglobin and hematocrit levels (Price, Whitney, & King, 2005).

Psychosocial Assessment

Surgery is a stressful life event for patients and their significant others. Among the reported sources of anxiety are fears—of the unknown, of death, of mutilation, of disability and loss of independence, of loss of sexuality, of waking up during the surgery, of pain, of separation from family, and of the financial impact. The nurse asks open-ended questions to illicit the patient's concerns about surgery and anesthesia. The nurse also assesses for physiological indicators of stress and anxiety including crying, restlessness, tachycardia, tachypnea, diaphoresis, complaints of inability to sleep, stomach upset, nausea, and diarrhea. Numeric rating scales of anxiety, similar to those used to rate pain, are an effective, easy, and valid way to measure anxiety (Elkins, Staniunas, Rajab, Marcus, & Snyder, 2004). Patients' level of stress will influence their ability to listen and absorb perioperative instruction. It can also affect their response to anesthesia and pain medication and their ability to comply with postoperative care. Patients who are highly anxious about surgery may benefit from receiving premedication with an antianxiety agent. A meta-analysis of 16 studies in which medication for anxiety was used preoperatively showed that using an antianxiety agent did not slow down the time frame for postoperative ambulation or discharge from the postanesthesia care unit (Walker, Smithy, & Pittaway, 2003).

The nurse asks about patients' support systems including family (traditional and nontraditional), friends, and other sources of support such as neighbors and religious affiliations. Patients are also asked if there are spiritual or cultural rituals or traditions that they would like to maintain during their hospitalization. The nurse is sensitive to the view that the hospital culture and its routines and food may be alien to some patients. All cultures hold beliefs about health, illness, and healing. Culturally competent nurses support and build positive cultural health care practices (Spector, 2004). The Cultural Considerations box identifies cultural and ethnic concerns for the perioperative nurse.

Diagnostic Tests

Laboratory tests are not required for routine, non–high-risk surgical procedures unless there is a specific reason for performing the test (ICSI, 2006). Nevertheless, many patients have preoperative laboratory testing as part of a routine examination. Some hospitals require a complete blood count on all patients over a certain age, usually 55 years old. Generally, a hematocrit and hemoglobin as well as a urine pregnancy test are performed on all menstruating females. It is recommended that all patients with diabetes have a hemoglobin A1C level drawn as part of preoperation testing and a fasting blood sugar drawn immediately before the surgical procedure (IHI, 2006). A patient may have a specific indication for performing a laboratory test. A patient taking digoxin (Lanoxin) or a diuretic may need to have a potassium level checked. When laboratory tests are indicated, they should be performed within 30 days of the planned procedure, although many surgeons prefer laboratory tests to be performed within the 1 to 2 weeks prior to surgery. If the need for a blood transfusion is anticipated, the patient will require a blood type and cross-match test to be processed at the facility performing the surgery.

Diagnostic studies performed preoperatively depend on the patient and the surgery to be performed. These studies are de-

CULTURAL CONSIDERATIONS for Perioperative Nurses

Use an interpreter for preoperative teaching. If a patient does not speak English and the nurse does not speak the patient's primary language, schedule an interpreter to assist with the assessment and teaching rather than relying on the patient's family member or significant other. The interpreter should be the same gender as the patient and the nurse should speak directly to the patient regardless of the presence of an interpreter.

Ask the patient about any special needs concerning the scheduling of surgery. In some cultures, the patient may need to consult a religious leader or healer, a special reader, or the zodiac in order to schedule surgery at the most opportune time. In some religions (e.g., Orthodox Jewish, Seventh-Day Adventist, Muslim) Friday evening and Saturday are times of observance and are avoided when scheduling elective surgery.

Consider the patient's view of "time" when scheduling surgery and preoperative appointments. Not all cultures view the concept of time as "clock" time. In some cultures, time is seen in relation to an activity that needs to be completed. The nurse needs to understand that cultures may view time differently and provide an explanation that an appointment time in this culture is an actual time period that is set aside for the patient.

Respect the family structure in getting surgical consent. In some cultures, there is a strict family hierarchy that is based on gender (e.g., the male is head of household) or age (e.g., the oldest member of the family is head of household). Be respectful of family hierarchies when getting consent for surgery and in teaching the patient.

Respect the patient's beliefs. Certain culturally held beliefs will affect preparations for surgery. An amulet may be worn, in some cultures, to ward off evil or bad spirits. When possible, patients should be allowed to wear the amulet into the operating room. If the amulet needs to be removed, remove it after induction of anesthesia and replace it as soon as the surgery is complete. In some cultures or religions (e.g., East Indian, Sikh) there are prohibitions against shaving body hair.

Find out the patient's view of the surgery. Surgery and anesthesia may be viewed as harbingers of death in some cultures (e.g., Roma). Allow family members to stay with the patient as long as possible in the preoperative area, and teach the patient and family about the surgical procedure to reduce anxiety.

Individualize your preoperative teaching. In some cultures, preoperative teaching is not a routine part of preoperative care, therefore, teaching can actually increase the patient's anxiety level. Find out what kind of information and how much information the patient wants and tailor the teaching to meet the patient's needs.

Source: Deyirmenjian, M., Karam, N., & Salameh, P. (2006). Preoperative patient education for open-heart patients: A source of anxiety? *Patient Education and Counseling,* 62(1), 111–117; Galanti, G. A. (2006). Applying cultural competence to perianesthesia nursing. *Journal of PeriAnesthesia Nursing,* 21(2), 97–102; Quinn, D. (2006). How religion, language and ethnicity impact perioperative nursing care. *Nursing Clinics of North America,* 41, 231–248; Spector, R. (2004). *Cultural diversity in health and illness.* Upper Saddle River, NJ: Pearson Prentice Hall.

termined by factors such as the reason the surgery is being done, the patient's overall health, surgeon's preference, and significant past medical history. In addition to any studies performed as part of the work-up of the patient's health problem, a chest x-ray, an electrocardiogram, and pulmonary function tests may be part of the preoperative tests for certain patients. A preoperative chest x-ray is not required for routine, low- to moderate-risk surgery but may be performed on patients who are older or who have a history of respiratory or cardiac disease. Similarly, pulmonary function tests are only done preoperatively if there is a specific indication such as in a patient with severe asthma or chronic obstructive pulmonary disease or a patient scheduled for removal of lung tissue (e.g., lobectomy, pneumonectomy). Electrocardiograms are recommended for all preoperative patients who are 55 years or older or in younger patients with a specific indication (ICSI, 2006). Common preoperative laboratory and diagnostic tests and rationales are presented in the Diagnostic Tests box (p. 600).

◼ Gerontological Considerations

Age is a major consideration in the nursing management of patients scheduled for surgery. Age-related changes to the body make it less able to respond and adapt to the physiological demands of surgery. Older people have less reserve capacity and less of a safety margin during times of higher demand (Muravchick, 2004). Also, older persons are more likely than others to have coexisting illnesses that increase surgical risk. A 2005 profile of older Americans by the Administration on Aging (AOA) notes that most people age 65 or older have one chronic illness and many have more than one. The most common conditions reported are arthritis, hypertension, hearing impairment, heart disease, cataracts, orthopedic impairments, sinusitis, and diabetes (AOA, 2005). Heart disease (i.e., angina, hypertension, heart failure, valve disease, and arrhythmias) is a particular concern because it is a significant predictor of surgical risk (Eagle et al., 2002).

Coexisting disease also is likely to place the older patient in a higher category of the ASA's Physical Status Classification (see Chart 25–1, p. 589) (ASA, 2006a). Patients in higher physical status categories experience greater surgical morbidity and mortality than those in lower categories. Some older adults experience memory impairment and depressive symptoms that can interfere with their ability to learn and comply with perioperative instruction. Other factors that increase the risk of surgery for older persons include preoperative anemia, malnutrition, and dehydration, as well as limitations of mobility. Chart 25–4 (p. 601) presents some of the normal changes associated with aging and the associated potential perioperative problems. Chart 25–5 (p. 602) lists the most common surgeries performed on patients age 65 or older as reported by the CDC, 2008).

◼ Health Promotion: Nursing Diagnoses and Outcomes

Nursing diagnoses will emerge from the preoperative assessment. Common diagnoses in the preoperative patient include:

- *Deficient Knowledge* (*Outcome:* The patient will demonstrate knowledge of the surgery, preoperative preparation, and postoperative exercises.)
- *Anxiety* (Outcome: The patient will verbalize decreased or tolerable levels of anxiety.)

- *Pain Acute* (*Outcome:* The patient will report an acceptable level of pain.)
- *Risk for Perioperative Positioning Injury* (*Outcome:* The patient will remain safe from perioperative injury.)
- *Ineffective Thermoregulation* (*Outcome:* The patient will maintain a normal body temperature throughout surgery.)
- *Impaired Home Maintenance* (*Outcome:* The patient will demonstrate an understanding of discharge instructions.)

Preoperative Instructions

Preoperative teaching is an important role of the perioperative nurse. The overall goal of preoperative teaching is to best prepare the patient for surgery, postoperative care, and discharge, and to protect the patient's safety. Depending on where and how teaching is conducted, teaching serves the purposes of clarifying a patient's preoperative concerns, reducing the patient's anxiety about the perioperative experience, increasing the patient's compliance with perioperative care, decreasing patient-controlled risk factors of postoperative complications, and increasing the patient's satisfaction with nursing and with the surgical experience.

Preoperative education is shown to decrease preoperative anxiety (Guruge & Sidani, 2002; Johansson et al., 2004; Lin & Wang, 2005; and McDonald, Hetrick, & Green, 2006), but it may also create worries perhaps more so in individuals who feel healthy but are scheduled for major elective procedures (Letterstal, Sandstrom, Olofsson, & Forsberg, 2004). This highlights the need to individualize teaching. Preoperative education can improve patient outcomes (Asilioglu & Celik, 2004; Deyirmenjian, Karam, & Salameh, 2006; Hering, Harvan, Dangelo, & Jasinski, 2005; Hulzebos et al., 2006; Yung et al., 2005) although more studies, particularly with experimental designs and those using subjects from various cultural groups, are needed to document which outcomes are most amenable to educational programs (Johansson et al., 2004).

Preoperative teaching and support can be categorized into five dimensions (Bernier, Sanares, Owen, & Newhouse, 2003):

- Situational and procedural information refers to teaching about the surgery and anesthesia.
- Sensation and discomfort information refers to teaching about what the patient can expect to see, hear, or feel.
- Patient role information refers to teaching patients how to participate in their own care.
- Skills training information refers to teaching about specific skills to be used postoperatively such as how to get out of bed with less pain or how to use the incentive spirometer.
- Psychosocial support refers to interactions aimed at alleviating fears and anxieties.

Patient teaching is accomplished in several ways. Many hospitals schedule a preoperative appointment days or weeks prior to the surgery for the purpose of conducting preoperative assessment and patient education. It is increasingly common for patients to receive written instructions either at the time of the appointment or mailed to their home that reinforce important aspects of care. Some hospitals and surgical centers use videotapes that explain the surgical procedure as well as preoperative

DIAGNOSTIC TESTS Commonly Performed Preoperatively

Laboratory Test	Abnormalities Preventing Surgery	Rationale for Performing the Test
COMPLETE BLOOD COUNT		
Red blood cell, hemoglobin, hematocrit	Significantly low hematocrit and hemoglobin.	Check for preoperative anemia; patient may need transfusion before surgery.
White blood cell (WBC)	Significantly elevated WBC. Presence of infection may delay or cancel the procedure. Neutropenia may delay surgery due to an increased risk of infection.	Provides information on the patient's immune status. Check for preoperative infection or inflammation. Preexisting infections, even those distant to the site of the operation, increase the risk of surgical site infection.
ELECTROLYTES AND OTHER TESTS		
Sodium, potassium, chloride, bicarbonate, glucose	Electrolyte imbalances, especially potassium, are corrected prior to surgery.	Check for electrolyte imbalances, metabolic status, and glucose regulation.
Blood urea nitrogen (BUN) and creatinine	Elevated creatinine and BUN are noted prior to surgery because renal function affects selection and dosage of medications. Renal failure patients may need to be dialyzed prior to surgery.	Gives information about renal function. Many drugs are excreted by the kidneys.
Brain natriuretic peptide (BNP)	Elevated levels indicate heart failure.	Rapid, bedside test to identify heart failure. Used in the differential diagnosis of shortness of breath.
Albumin	Marker of nutritional status.	Low serum albumin is associated with higher postoperative pulmonary complications.
Prealbumin or transthyretin test	Marker of nutritional status.	Low prealbumin levels are associated with higher postoperative complications and risk of pressure ulcers.
Hemoglobin A1C	A more stable measure of glucose. Indicates the level of diabetic control over the previous 6 weeks.	Poor glucose control is associated with an increased risk of surgical-site infection.
COAGULATION STUDIES		
International normalized ratio (INR), prothrombin time (PT), partial thromboplastin time (PTT)	Elevated levels may delay or cancel surgery.	Provides information about bleeding tendencies and ability to clot.
Arterial blood gas	May be performed preoperatively in patients with severe lung disease.	Provides information on oxygenation and acid–base status.
Type and crossmatch (T&C) for blood replacement	Performed preoperatively in patients who are bleeding or for surgeries that are expected to have large amounts of blood loss.	Patient's blood type is identified and matched with specific blood units for transfusion. For a T&C to be active, it must be recent (within 48 hours).
Pregnancy test	Surgery is avoided, if possible, during the first trimester of pregnancy.	Performed when there is uncertainty about whether or not the patient is pregnant. May be performed on all menstruating females.
Urinalysis	Abnormal results may require additional follow-up prior to surgery.	Provides screening information about the presence of protein, glucose, blood, and bacteria in the urine. Provides an indication of renal function and urinary tract infection.
Chest x-ray	Surgery may be postponed in patients with pneumonia or who have significant heart failure.	Provides baseline data on pulmonary and cardiac function. Can detect cardiac enlargement, heart failure, infiltrates, pneumonia, pleural effusions.
Electrocardiogram	Indications of cardiac injury (elevated ST segment), ischemia (T wave inversion), or myocardial infarction may delay surgery. Abnormal heart rate and rhythm are corrected preoperatively if possible.	Provides baseline data on cardiac rhythm and cardiac disease. Recommended for all preoperative patients 55 years or older.
Pulmonary function tests	Chronic lung conditions increase the risk of surgery.	Provides preoperative information on lung volumes and condition of airways.

Normal Changes of Aging, Perioperative Risk, and Nursing Implications

Normal Changes of Aging	Impact on Perioperative Risk	Implications for Nursing Care
Overall		
Decreased reserve capacity of all body organs, which causes various systems to be overwhelmed during periods of physiological stress	Places the patient at a higher risk for many postoperative problems and complications	Minimize physiological stress as much as possible. Provide adequate oxygen, rest, nutrition, hydration, emotional support, and monitor and correct electrolyte imbalance.
Neurological		
Decreased reserve and increased sensitivity to physiological stressors such as fever and hypoxia Lowered ability to adjust to environmental changes and stimuli Slower reaction times Slower cognitive processes	Potential for acute confusion postoperatively that can take months to resolve Potential for sleep–wake disturbances while in the hospital Potential for knowledge deficit	Assess mental status every shift. Avoid using medications known to cause changes in mental status in the elderly (CNS depressants, H2–receptor antagonists, lidocaine, Dilantin, anticholinergics). Provide for uninterrupted sleep. Avoid unnecessary room or unit changes. Encourage ambulation and participation in activities of daily living (ADLs). If acute confusion develops, look for and treat physiological stressors such as fever, hypoxemia, anemia, pain, and dehydration.
Cardiovascular		
Increased workload of the heart Increased arterial resistance Decreased cardiac output Reduction in the maximum attainable heart rate and cardiac output Decreased peripheral circulation Lowered ability to respond to demands for increased blood, oxygen, and nutrients	Potential for decreased cardiac output Potential for intraoperative cardiac complications Potential for activity intolerance postoperatively	Prevent or treat factors such as anemia that increase cardiac workload. Keep warm to prevent shivering. Apply oxygen to keep oxygen saturation above 93%. Monitor fluid balance to prevent dehydration or fluid overload. Monitor BP, heart rate, oxygen saturation, fatigue, and dyspnea with activity.
Respiratory		
Decreased elasticity of lungs Loss of muscle mass, which weakens muscles of respiration Stiff chest wall, which reduces the ability to expand the lungs Less effective protective mechanisms such as coughing and mucociliary transport	Potential for postoperative pulmonary complications Potential for impaired gas exchange Potential for ineffective airway clearance	Encourage deep breathing postoperatively. Monitor for dyspnea as a sign of ventilatory dysfunction. Control pain but avoid overmedication with narcotics.
Gastrointestinal		
Decreased saliva Loss of teeth and changes in dentition More difficulty with swallowing Decreased peristalsis Decreased blood flow to internal organs	Risk of aspiration Potential for poor nutrition Potential for constipation	Follow aspiration precautions. Make sure dentures are in place when patient is allowed to eat. Encourage mobility postoperatively to prevent abdominal distention and constipation.
Genitourinary		
Decreased renal blood flow Decreased renal function Decreased elasticity of bladder Decreased bladder capacity Enlarged prostate	Risk for impaired renal function postoperatively Risk of fluid and electrolyte imbalances	Monitor intake & output, BUN, and creatinine postoperatively. Ensure adequate hydration. Effects of drugs may be prolonged; choose drugs with short half-lives.
Musculoskeletal		
Loss of bone mass and height Changes in balance and gait Decreased range of motion in joints	Potential for falls	Perform a risk assessment for falls. Assist with ambulation. Use assistive devices as necessary. Physical therapy consult after surgery. Home safety evaluation at discharge.

(continued)

CHART 25–4 **Normal Changes of Aging, Perioperative Risk, and Nursing Implications—*Continued***

Normal Changes of Aging	Impact on Perioperative Risk	Implications for Nursing Care
Sensory		
Decreased visual acuity and accommodation	Potential for falls	Make sure that glasses, hearing aids, and dentures are
Decreased ability to adapt to changes in light	Potential for acute confusion	available postoperatively.
Hearing loss and change in taste	Potential for alterations in	Assess pain frequently.
Atypical pain response	communication	
Skin		
Slow replacement of epithelial cells	Potential for tissue injury and	Document preoperative condition of the skin.
Decreased elasticity of skin	pressure ulcers	Keep warm postoperatively.
Loss of subcutaneous tissue	Potential for hypothermia	Encourage adequate nutrition.
Decreased circulation	Delayed wound healing and	Offer nutritional supplements as necessary.
	risk of infection	

CHART 25–5 **Common Surgical Procedures in Older Patients**

Gender	Common Procedures in Older Patients
Men	Prostatectomy
	Cardiac catheterization
	Coronary bypass
	Pacemaker insertion
	Repair of inguinal hernia
	Digestive system biopsies
	Cataract extraction
Women	Cardiac catheterization
	Reduction of fracture
	Pacemaker insertion
	Digestive system biopsies
	Cholecystectomy
	Cataract extraction

and postoperative care. Telephone interviews also are used for preoperative assessment, teaching, and follow-up after discharge. Depending on circumstances surrounding the surgery, preoperative teaching may be done at the patient's bedside the night before surgery if the patient is an inpatient, or on the morning of the surgery if the patient is an outpatient.

Preoperative teaching is best accomplished in a calm, quiet, and private environment that facilitates discussion and questions, and reduces the patient's anxiety or embarrassment. The nurse needs to be sensitive to the patient's level of anxiety, her ability to understand instructions and express herself, and to cultural issues.

Written instructions are important in reinforcing teaching and serving as a reference. When written instructions are given to patients, they should not use medical jargon, be written at a level that is easy to understand, and be available in various languages. The nurse assesses whether or not a patient is literate in English or in another language before giving written instructions.

General Preoperative Teaching

A preoperative patient needs information about the surgery and surgical routines, home preparation for the surgery, what to ex-

pect postoperatively, and preoperative exercises to prevent postoperative complications. Many operations are scheduled as a same-day procedure, so an easy way to start the teaching is to discuss some of the logistics that surround surgery. Provide the patient with information about transportation to the hospital, where to park a car, the cost of parking, what to wear, when to arrive at the hospital, where to report, where significant others may wait during the procedure, and how hospital personnel will communicate with significant others during and after the surgery. Many hospitals are incorporating surgical liaison programs to facilitate better ongoing communication and support for family members and significant others who are waiting for the patient during the surgical procedure. It has been shown that providing the family with updates on the progress of the patient during surgery and early in the recovery period results in better coping and problem-solving skills and reduced anxiety in family members (Cunningham, Hanson-Heath, & Agre, 2003; Leske, 2000).

Similarly, there is a trend to allow and even encourage family members and significant others to visit the patient in the postanesthesia care unit (PACU), recognizing that this can reduce anxiety for the family and provide comfort and support to the patient. Studies report that the presence of others during the perioperative period provides patients with a sense of comfort, safety, and control (Costa, 2001; Susleck et al., 2007). Hospitals that have adopted PACU visitation often have an information sheet that instructs family and significant others about the experience (e.g., keep the visit short, no cell phones, respect the privacy of other patients, comply with requests to leave) (Smykowski & Rodriguez, 2003).

Patients who will be discharged home rather than admitted to the hospital are not allowed to drive after the procedure and must be transported home by a responsible adult.

Teaching About the Surgery

Patients need to be prepared for how they will feel and how things will progress postoperatively. The patient should receive information about the surgery including what is done during the surgery, what the surgery will accomplish, where the incision(s) will be located, the anticipated length of the procedure, and the expected recovery trajectory. It is important that nurses give patients an honest, realistic view of the surgery without creating heightened anxiety. In one study, 89 subjects who had cardiac surgery were interviewed 6 weeks after discharge from the hospital. Researchers found that these subjects were surprised about the intensity of the surgery and wished that they had received more detailed information about such things as the location of incisions, breathing exercises, and what recovery would be like (Doering, McGuire, & Rourke, 2002). Patients need to know that their initial recovery from anesthesia occurs in a PACU where they will be monitored frequently until they are stable enough to be transferred to a surgical unit, or home in the case of outpatient procedures. If a patient is expected to go to an intensive care unit following the surgical procedure, the patient needs to know the routines of intensive care and the length of the anticipated stay.

It is important to prepare the patient and family for any tubes, drains, devices, or attachments that may be present postoperatively. Some of these devices have alarms that can frighten patients unless they are expecting them. In the PACU, the patient will have an intravenous catheter and intravenous fluid and will be attached to a cardiac monitor, blood pressure cuff, and pulse oximeter. Many patients will also have a Foley catheter to accurately measure postoperative urinary output, and pneumatic compression boots or an alternative device to reduce the

risk of deep venous thrombosis. Depending on the type of surgery performed, the patient may have a nasogastric tube for abdominal decompression, wound drains (e.g., Jackson-Pratt, Anderson sump, Hemovac), other drainage devices (e.g., chest tube, biliary tube, gastrostomy tube), or devices for pain control (e.g., PCA pump or epidural catheter).

If the patient is having orthopedic surgery, he may have equipment such as traction, continuous motion devices, or joint immobilizers. Patients should be prepared for postoperative routines so that they do not become excessively anxious with frequent assessments, measures of vitals signs, and observation and manipulation of the accompanying equipment and devices. Teaching is an important piece of health promotion and must be individualized for the patient and the surgery being performed. Chart 25–6 (p. 604) provides an overview of health promotion teaching content for patients experiencing common surgical procedures. The Evidence-Based Practice box provides information about the benefit of preoperative patient teaching for pain management.

Preoperative Fasting Requirements
Patients are instructed to abstain from food and fluids prior to the operation for the primary purpose of reducing the risk of

---

The Benefit of Preoperative Patient Teaching for Pain

Clinical Problem

Although health care professionals agree that preoperative teaching is important, research studies do not consistently demonstrate a specific benefit (Johansson et al., 2004; McDonald, Hetrick, & Green, 2006). Preoperative education studies often focus on increasing patient knowledge and/or on reducing patient anxiety, with fewer studies looking at the effects of preoperative education on functional outcomes such as pain, nausea, or fatigue (Johansson et al., 2004). Can a preoperative education program improve postoperative outcomes?

Research Findings

A small study conducted by Lin and Wang (2005) set out to determine whether or not a preoperative nursing intervention for pain reduces postoperative pain. This study randomly assigned adult patients scheduled for abdominal surgery to a control group who received routine care comprised of physical preparation and education on postoperative coughing and deep breathing and an experimental group who received routine care as well as a nursing intervention. The nursing intervention was a 20- to 30-minute individual educational session where postoperative pain and pain management were discussed. The session encouraged patients to set a postoperative pain goal and to select a favorite nonpharmacologic method of pain control that could be used in addition to pain medication. The researchers found that the two groups used similar amounts of medication postoperatively, but the experimental group reported significantly lower pain scores after surgery, and reported significantly less pain with activities such as repositioning, coughing, and deep breathing than did the control group. The group that received the nursing intervention got out of bed sooner than the other group. There was no difference between the groups in length of hospital stay.

Implications for Nursing Practice

These findings suggest that a preoperative nursing intervention for pain can decrease postoperative pain and the pain associated with

certain postoperative activities. The intervention can serve as a model for other individualized preoperative teaching strategies. The research findings add to the small, but growing, body of knowledge regarding the functional effects of preoperative teaching. Further, an intervention that speeds up postoperative ambulation and reduces pain associated with deep breathing and coughing could, ultimately, help reduce the incidence of postoperative pulmonary complications.

Critical Thinking Questions

1. This study was conducted in Taiwan, a country that provides national health insurance. What are the implications of this information? What further information would you need to fully answer the first question?

2. In this study, pain was measured using a questionnaire and visual analog scales, measures that are appropriate because pain is a subjective experience. Give examples of objective measures the researchers could include in their study to bolster the findings that the intervention reduced pain or the effects of pain. Provide a rationale for your answers.

Answers to Critical Thinking Questions appear in Appendix D.

References
Johansson, K., Salantera, S., Heikkinen, K., Kuusisto, A., Virtanen, H., & Leino-Kilpi, H. (2004). Surgical patient education: Assessing the interventions and exploring the outcomes from experimental and quasiexperimental studies from 1990 to 2003. *Clinical Effectiveness in Nursing, 8*(2), 81–92.

Lin, L. Y., & Wang, R. (2005). Abdominal surgery, pain and anxiety: Preoperative nursing intervention. *Journal of Advanced Nursing, 51*(3), 252–260.

McDonald, S., Hetrick, S., & Green, S. (2006). Pre-operative education for hip or knee replacement. *The Cochrane Library, 4* (CD003526).

EVIDENCE-BASED PRACTICE

| CHART 25–6 | **Health Promotion Teaching for Common Surgical Procedures** |

Surgery	Incision Site	Drains	Pain Control	Activity	Diet After Surgery	Special Concerns or Instructions	Length of Stay
Abdominal hysterectomy	Pfannenstiel	Foley is removed first day	Patient-controlled analgesia (PCA)/Intra-muscular (IM)/per oral (po)	Ambulate the evening of surgery	Clear liquids with advance diet as tolerated (ADAT)	Urinary retention sometimes occurs. Risk of DVT.	2–3 days
Appendectomy, open	Lower right quadrant of abdomen	Wound drain if abscess or perforation present	PCA/IM	Ambulate the evening of surgery	Clear liquids first day if no perforation	Wound infection is more likely with perforation of appendix. Hospital stay longer (4 to 7 days) with perforation.	1–2 days if no perforation
Carotid endarterectomy	Right or left neck	None but may have wound drain	PCA/IM/po	Ambulate evening of surgery or first day postop	Clear liquids with ADAT	May overnight in ICU or PACU. Neurological assessment is critical. Check incision for edema or hematoma. Monitor BP.	2–3 days
Cholecystectomy, open	Right upper quadrant of abdomen	T-tube if common bile duct explored, Foley, wound drain, and sometimes a nasogastric tube (NGT)	PCA	Ambulate evening of surgery or first day postop	Nothing per oral (NPO) for 2–3 days.	Risk of atelectasis is increased because of subcostal incision. Encourage deep breathing, ambulation, and pain control.	3–5 days
Colon resection	Abdomen, lower midline, or transverse	Foley, may have NGT, may have temporary colostomy	PCA/PCEA	Ambulate first day postop	NPO for several days	Encourage deep breathing; may have temporary colostomy if bowel perforation present.	5–7 days
Inguinal hernia	Right or left lower quadrant of abdomen	None	po	Ambulate day of surgery	Clear liquids with ADAT	Men may experience swelling of scrotum. Ice applications to decrease swelling.	Outpatient
Lumbar laminectomy	Back, 5–13 cm (2–5 in.) long	Foley, may require wound drain	PCA/PCEA	Ambulate evening of surgery	Clear liquids with ADAT	Back brace may be required when out of bed. Expect involvement of physical therapy. No bending or twisting of the back.	1–4 days
Mastectomy	Right or left chest	1 to 2 Jackson-Pratt drains	PCA/Patient Controlled Epidural Analgesia (PCEA) first day	Ambulate evening of surgery or first day postop	Clear liquids with ADAT	May be discharged with wound drains. Check with MD about arm and shoulder exercises on the affected side. Body image may be concern.	1–2 days
Transurethral resection of the prostate	None	Three-way Foley with continuous bladder irrigation	IV/IM/po	Ambulate evening of surgery	Clear liquids with ADAT	Run bladder irrigant to keep urine clear. Catheter removed day 1 or 2. Bladder spasms common.	1–2 days

pulmonary aspiration of stomach contents associated with anesthesia. Traditionally, patients were told to take nothing by mouth (NPO) after midnight on the night preceding surgery, but 1999 ASA guidelines loosened these requirements because the evidence showed that pulmonary aspiration rarely occurs with modern anesthesia (ASA, 1999b). Current guidelines recommend that patients fast from the intake of solid food (i.e., a light meal) for 6 or more hours before procedures and from clear liquids for 2 or more hours. Fasting is implemented for patients who will have general anesthesia, regional anesthesia, or conscious sedation. Clear liquids (nonparticulate fluids without fat) include water, fruit juices, carbonated drinks, broth, coffee, and tea. Studies show that despite the change in standards, many patients are instructed to fast longer than is necessary, creating feelings of thirst and hunger and sometimes resulting in dehydration, hypovolemia, and hypoglycemia (Crenshaw & Winslow, 2002; Madsen, Brosnan, & Nagy, 1998; Murphy, Ault, Wong, & Szokol, 2000). The new standards allow individualization of fasting instructions so that a patient scheduled for an afternoon procedure is not fasting excessively before the procedure. Patients with known delay in gastric emptying should be assessed on an individual basis and may require longer fasting periods (Soreide & Ljungqvist, 2006). On the day of surgery, patients are asked about the last time that they ate or drank and surgery may need to be delayed or canceled if a patient has not complied with fasting requirements.

 *Notify the anesthesia care provider immediately if the patient has not followed the preoperative food or fluid restrictions. This patient will be at a higher risk for aspiration and the surgery may need to be postponed. In some states, patients must sign a document to confirm that they have followed food and fluid restrictions.*

Other Home Instructions

Patients may be given other instructions to follow at home prior to the surgery. Patients who smoke cigarettes are instructed to stop smoking. Eight weeks prior to surgery is suggested as the optimal time frame, although research has not established if there is any benefit to a patient who quits smoking days or even a few weeks before surgery (Barrera et al., 2005; Brooks-Brunn, 2000). It is recommended that patients stop taking any herbal remedies 2 to 3 weeks before surgery because of the uncertain effect of herbs on anesthesia and in some cases on blood clotting. Medications that interfere with blood clotting, such as heparin, enoxaparin, warfarin, clopidogrel, aspirin, and vitamin E are usually stopped before surgery although the time frame for stopping will vary according to the drug taken, the reason it is being taken and laboratory tests.

Some experts recommend stopping warfarin 5 to 6 days before surgery depending on the patient's INR, stopping enoxaparin 12 to 18 hours before procedures, and stopping heparin 6 to 8 hours before an operation (Merli, 2000). Time frames for stopping anticoagulation are under investigation. A recent study of 80 patients taking enoxaparin found markedly elevated levels of anti-Xa heparin (a marker of anticoagulation activity) 14 hours after the last dose (O'Donnell et al., 2007). The finding suggests that stopping enoxaparin the evening before surgery may not be long enough to minimize the risk of surgical bleeding. Some patients may need to be admitted to the hospital 2 to

3 days in advance to make a safe transition from warfarin to heparin in the preoperative period.

Usually, it is acceptable for patients to take their regular oral medications with a small amount of water, not more than 150 mL, on the morning of surgery, but patients should check with the surgeon and the anesthesiologist. Patients who take insulin need to check with their doctor about proper preoperative dosage. The ASA established diabetic protocols to guide the administration of insulin and glucose during the perioperative period (Maurer, Borkowski, & Parker, 2004). Usually one-half the usual morning dose is administered on the morning of surgery. Frequent monitoring of blood glucose levels will determine the need for additional sliding scale insulin coverage. Some research suggests that tight glucose control (e.g., maintaining blood glucose levels at 80 to 110 mg/dL) using continuous intravenous insulin during certain surgeries is beneficial to patients (Van den Berghe et al., 2001), but other studies not only challenge these results but also found a deleterious effect with the practice of continuous intravenous insulin (Gandhi et al., 2005, 2007). Clearly more research is needed to determine how best to manage intraoperative glucose levels. Other medications may also need adjustment with surgery. For example, the dose of a corticosteroid might need to be increased depending on the reason it is taken.

 *All diabetic medications taken in the 24 hours prior to surgery need to be carefully documented in the patient's record.*

Patients will receive surgery-specific instructions to follow at home. For example, patients who are scheduled for colorectal surgery may be asked to follow a special diet, take a laxative, and administer an enema on the night before and morning of surgery to empty the bowel of stool and reduce microorganisms (Nichols, 2001). Some studies question the effectiveness of mechanical bowel preparation (Guenaga, 2002), and in some elective colon resections, patients are allowed a normal diet and require no routine bowel preparation ahead of time (Soreide & Ljungqvist, 2006). The Centers for Disease Control and Prevention (CDC) guidelines recommend that patients take a shower the night before a surgical procedure with an antimicrobial body wash containing 2% chlorhexidine gluconate, although this practice has not yet been shown to reduce surgical-site infections (Schweon, 2006; Seltzer, Horsman, & Korniewicz, 2002).

Preoperative Teaching to Prevent Postoperative Complications

Patients who are scheduled for major surgery that reduces mobility and requires inpatient recovery should be taught breathing exercises, how to splint the incision, coughing (to help clear airways), leg exercises, and the importance of postoperative ambulation. The patient may also benefit from the use of an alternative therapy, such as the mind/body practice of eliciting the relaxation response, as discussed in the Complementary and Alternative Therapies box (p. 606).

Breathing Exercises

Deep breathing is taught as an intervention to decrease the risk of the postoperative pulmonary complications of hypoxemia, atelectasis, and pneumonia. In one small study of patients scheduled for coronary artery bypass graft surgery, patients who received inspiratory muscle training preoperatively were much less likely to develop postoperative pulmonary complications than a comparison group (Hulzebos et al., 2006). To perform deep breathing, the patient breathes out normally then takes a deep breath through the nose or mouth, holds inspiration to the count of three or longer, and slowly releases the breath. Postoperatively, the patient is asked to take 5 to 10 deep breaths every hour.

Research suggests that the effects of deep breathing are not sustained over time and must be performed regularly to achieve physiological outcomes (Orfanos, Ellis, & Johnston, 1999). Deep breathing slows the respiratory rate and produces a sustained maximal inspiration. It is thought that deep breathing increases lung volumes by increasing tidal volume and minute ventilation. It also generates higher flow rates, and stimulates surfactant to help keep alveoli open (Brooks et al., 2001; Orfanos et al., 1999).

Deep breathing can also be used as a technique to reduce pain when moving. Encouraging the patient to focus on taking continuous deep breaths while moving or changing positions may help to prevent the patient from tensing muscles, which tends to worsen postoperative pain. One study found that patients who had received videotape instruction on how to use breathing and

COMPLEMENTARY & ALTERNATIVE THERAPIES

Relaxation Response

Description:

More than 30% of American adults use mind–body practices that elicit the relaxation response (RR). Although the mechanisms that mediate the RR remain unknown, eliciting the RR reduces volumetric oxygen consumption from rest and counteracts the effects of stress (Dusek et al., 2006). RR is an integrated psychophysiological response that originates in the hypothalamus and is the direct operate of the stress response. It leads to a generalized decrease in central nervous system arousal. The RR is a hypometabolic state that can be useful in many situations. The patient who activates the RR can use the body's own innate mechanisms to calm and slow down. The RR can occur through the repetition of a word or short phrase. The patient can return to this gentle repetition whenever distracting thoughts occur. This technique triggers a series of physiological changes (slower breathing, heart rate, blood pressure, etc.) that reduce stress.

The pre- and perioperative areas are excellent settings in which to instruct the patient in various RR techniques, such as how to slow down, focus on breathing techniques, and repeat a simple relaxing phrase. The nurse can utilize this technique at the bedside or in the perioperative area prior to anesthesia. A good place for the nurse to begin is to instruct the patient to breathe in through the nose, out through the mouth, and "focus on my voice." The nurse should practice this technique often to help in its delivery. This technique is also used as a preliminary step in many other CAM therapies.

Research Support:

One study investigated whether brief psychologic interventions to reduce perioperative stress in patients undergoing abdominal surgery would improve the patients' postoperative recovery. Participants involved 60 elderly cancer patients undergoing conventional resection of colorectal carcinoma. Researchers used a randomized, controlled, partially blinded trial to evaluate the differential effectiveness of guided imagery and progressive muscle relaxation on analgesic requirement, pain perception, pulmonary function, duration of postoperative ileus, and fatigue after surgery. Of the 60 patients, 20 used guided imagery, 22 used relaxation, 18 were the control. The effects on analgesic consumption and subjective pain intensity at rest and while coughing did not differ between groups. Pulmonary function recovery, postoperative ileus duration, and subjective postoperative fatigue were also not influenced. Results did not show a clinically relevant influence on the postoperative physiologic course. However, the results showed that imagery and relaxation yielded a very positive patient response. Ninety percent of the patients indicated that they would recommend the techniques to other patients (Haase, Schwenk, Hermann, & Muller, 2005).

Another study investigated whether nitric oxide (NO) mediates RR elicitation. Researchers measured percentage changes in fractional exhaled nitric oxide to evaluate whether depth of RR elicitation was correlated with changes in NO. In this randomized, controlled trial, 46 participants were randomized to either 8 weeks of RR training using audiotapes (n = 34) or 8 weeks of exposure to a control condition in which participants received health education by audiotapes (n = 12). Prior to randomization, participants' volumetric oxygen consumption and fractional exhaled nitric oxide levels were measured while the participants listened to a control audiotape. Eight weeks later, researchers measured participants' volumetric oxygen consumption and fractional exhaled nitric oxide levels while the RR group listened to a RR-eliciting audiotape and the control group listened to a control audiotape. There was no association between volumetric oxygen consumption slope and fractional exhaled nitric oxide prior to the training. However, after training, the results showed an inverse correlation between volumetric oxygen consumption slope and fractional exhaled nitric oxide in the RR group, but not in the control group. Based on these results, the researchers concluded that the depth of RR elicitation was associated with increased concentrations of fractional exhaled nitric oxide after RR training. Their further conclusion was that the RR may be mediated by NO, which helps to explain its clinical effects in stress-related disorders (Dusek et al., 2006).

Another group of investigators conducted a single-blind, 3-arm, randomized controlled trial by evaluating the efficacy of an RR intervention program on the quality of life (QOL) and exercise capacity of CHF patients. Study intervention group patients (n = 95) attended a weekly RR group for 15 weeks and were requested to practice the techniques at home twice a day. An alternative intervention was a 15-week cardiac education (EDU) program. The control group was involved usual care (UC). Researchers administered the QOL questionnaires and a bicycle test at baseline and after intervention (or 15 to 19 weeks). Results were adjusted for baseline scores, time between assessments, age, education, diet, and medication. After these adjustments, results showed that the RR group had significantly better QOL change scores in peace–spiritual scales than did the UC group. However, no significant difference was observed between the EDU and UC groups. Researchers observed a similar trend in emotional QOL. The researchers found no statistically significant intervention effect on physical QOL or exercise capacity (Chang et al., 2005).

References

Chang, B.H., Hendricks, A., Zhao, Y., Rothendler, J. A., LoCastro, J. S., & Slawsky, M. T. (2005). A relaxation response randomized trial on patients with chronic heart failure. *Journal of Cardiopulmonary Rehabilitation, 25*(3), 149–157.

Dusek, J. A., Chang, B. H., Zaki, J., Lazar, S., Deykin, A., Stefano, G. B., et al. (2006). Association between oxygen consumption and nitric oxide production during the relaxation response. *Medical Science Monitor, 12*(1), CR1–10.

Haase, O., Schwenk, W., Hermann, C., & Muller, J. M. (2005). Guided imagery and relaxation in conventional colorectal resections: A randomized, controlled, partially blinded trial. *Diseases of the Colon and Rectum, 48*(10), 1955–1963.

imagery while performing postoperative activities reported significantly less pain, more mobility, and more independent mobility than patients who had not received the instruction (Heye, Foster, Bartlett, & Adkins, 2002).

Incentive Spirometry

The use of incentive spirometry (IS) as a mechanism to encourage deep breathing is widespread. An incentive spirometer is a device that is activated by the inspiratory effort of the patient. Incentive spirometers come in many different models but there are two basic types, flow oriented and volume oriented. To operate the IS, the patient takes a deep breath, which causes a plate or a ball to rise up a calibrated cylinder. The cylinder displays either the inspired volume (a volume-oriented incentive spirometer) or the generated flow (a flow-oriented incentive spirometer) (Weindler & Kiefer, 2001). An incentive spirometer can be helpful postoperatively because it provides a numeric reading of how effectively patients are taking deep breaths, and the use of IS encourages patients to take responsibility for their care, but it is probably not any better than deep breathing in preventing postoperative complications (Overend et al., 2001).

Splinting the Incision

Patients with thoracic or abdominal incisions can be taught preoperatively how to splint the incision to prevent painful stress on the area. The patient can use a small, flat pillow or a small, folded blanket, sometimes referred to as a "cough pillow," to apply gentle, firm pressure over the incision when performing activities that tend to pull the incision such as when getting out of bed, getting up from a chair, or coughing. Splinting the incision is helpful in reducing pain.

Coughing

Postoperative patients have an increase in mucous production and a decreased ability to clear mucus from the airways as a result of anesthesia (Smith & Ellis, 2000). Retained mucus places patients at risk for the development of atelectasis and pneumonia. Coughing can help to clear mucus from the airways and facilitate full expansion of the lungs because it requires an increase in intrathoracic pressure and a rapid expiratory flow (Smith & Ellis, 2000). Coughing can be quite painful for some patients because of the stress it places on the suture line. Splinting the incision will help protect it and reduce some of the pain that occurs with movement of the incisional area. Coughing may be contraindicated after some surgeries because of the stress it puts on the incision (e.g., hernia) or because it increases intracranial pressure (e.g., craniotomy). Generally a health care provider's order will be written to avoid coughing for surgical procedures where it is contraindicated.

Leg Exercises

Guidelines on prevention of venous thromboembolism recommend that a risk assessment be performed on all surgical patients (Blondin, 2006). Most patients receive some form of prophylaxis against the development of DVT (i.e., venous blood clot in the leg) postoperatively. Leg exercises are a simple way of stimulating venous return in the patient with limited mobility. They are used in addition to other devices to prevent venous stasis.

Several types of leg exercises can be performed. The exercises should be done on each leg and should be repeated several times before moving to the next exercise. Descriptions of various leg exercises follow:

- Alternate between flexing the foot and dorsiflexing the foot.
- Lift the foot off the bed and make circles with the ankle several times.
- Bend the knee and lift the leg off of the bed holding the position for a few seconds.
- With knees bent, push the ball of the foot into the bed or floor, contracting the calf and thigh muscles.

Ambulation and Mobility

Early ambulation is beneficial to the postoperative patient for a number of reasons. Ambulation increases heart rate and cardiac output and stimulates circulation to all body systems. The increase in circulation helps to rid the body of the effects of anesthesia. Ambulation increases respiratory rate and minute ventilation, and it helps to mobilize respiratory secretions. Increased circulation to the intestinal tract helps to stimulate peristalsis, and increased blood flow through the kidneys stimulates the production of urine. Blood flow to skin and muscles brings nutrients needed for wound healing. Ambulation stimulates calf muscles and increases venous return. Frequent ambulation, a minimum of three times per day, may help prevent some of the complications associated with immobility. Patients need to understand the importance and emphasis that is placed on walking after an operation and be shown effective ways of getting out of bed postoperatively. In one intervention study, women who were scheduled for abdominal hysterectomy were taught a specific technique for getting out of bed, practiced the technique preoperatively, and were encouraged to use the skill after surgery. The authors reported that the women who received coaching and skill training ambulated for longer periods of time postoperatively than the women who did not receive the training (Oetker-Black et al., 2003). Most patients will be allowed to walk with assistance on the evening of surgery or the first postoperative day. For some surgeries, ambulation is initially restricted. These patients need to turn and reposition every 1 to 2 hours to prevent complications of immobility until they are allowed to ambulate. Older patients have the same informational needs as other adults, but the teaching process may require a different approach, as discussed in the Gerontological Considerations box.

GERONTOLOGICAL CONSIDERATIONS
for Preoperative Teaching

Teaching techniques for older adults who are scheduled for surgery include going over the material more slowly, repeating the material, asking the patient to confirm their understanding of the instruction, and reinforcing verbal instructions with written materials and instructions. Including someone from the elder's social support system in the preoperative teaching session can be helpful as well. Older patients may have more worries about surgery than others because the surgery presents very real threats to their physical function and a potential loss of independence. Older patients having surgery may also worry about the care of an elderly spouse, partner, or sibling during their absence. The nurse must be sensitive to these issues and encourage patients to discuss concerns they may have. A social worker may need to be consulted for assistance in problem solving.

Legal Preparation and Ethical Considerations

The nurse must consider both legal and ethical considerations when preparing a patient for surgery. Patients have a right to be informed about the risks of surgery and anesthesia and to make treatment decisions. They also have the right to decide what course of treatment to follow in the event that they experience a serious postoperative complication.

Informed Consent

The patient must sign an informed consent form prior to surgery. The informed consent protects all parties involved: the patient, the surgeon, and the hospital. In order for the consent to be valid, there must be full disclosure of the treatment to be performed, the patient must sufficiently understand the information provided (i.e., must be competent), and the patient must voluntarily consent to the treatment. Full disclosure includes a description of the condition requiring surgery, the surgical procedure, the possible risks and benefits, alternative treatments, and prognosis. The surgeon is responsible for discussing the procedure with the patient and securing an informed consent. If a patient is unable to sign, an "X" is an acceptable substitute provided there are two witnesses. Consent is voluntary and can be withdrawn at any time. The surgical consent form may include additional consents such as consent for a blood transfusion and for the disposal of body tissues. The nurse's role in the process is to clarify information for the patient and advocate for the patient as needed.

In cases where the patient is unable to participate in informed consent (e.g., an unconscious or incompetent patient), the consent is obtained from the legally responsible person. This person might be the health care proxy, the next of kin, or a court-appointed legal guardian. In emergencies, telephone consent is acceptable. In cases of extreme emergency where the legally responsible person is not available and delaying the operation might result in death or serious impairment, the medical emergency overrides the need for consent and the surgery proceeds without consent. In such circumstances, hospitals have set protocols for documenting in the patient's chart the gravity of the situation and the nature of the emergency.

Frequently, the consent for anesthesia is a separate process performed by the anesthesia care provider. The patient receives information about the type of anesthesia planned and the possible risks associated with it. Figure 25–2 ■ is an example of an informed consent form for surgical treatment. Chapter 4 ⊕ provides a complete description of informed consent.

Resuscitation Orders

It is not unusual for a patient with a do-not-resuscitate (DNR) order to require surgery. Surgery might be done for palliative reasons (e.g., to decrease pain associated with tumor growth) or to facilitate care (e.g., the insertion of a feeding tube) or to improve quality of life. Some older patients who are in reasonably good health request a DNR order in case of an untoward event even though the surgery to be performed is elective. In the past, DNR orders were suspended for the length of the surgery and early postoperative period.

Professional organizations of surgeons, anesthesiologists, and perioperative nurses have challenged the routine suspension of DNR orders (AORN, 1999; ASA, 2001). The position of the AORN is that a patient's autonomy should be respected in the operating room and therefore DNR orders should not be routinely suspended for surgery. Instead, AORN recommends that there be a required reconsideration of the DNR order with the scheduling of surgery. The patient is given the opportunity to consider the consequences of withholding resuscitation efforts during surgery and what, if any, resuscitation efforts she might want performed. The ultimate DNR decision falls with the patient and must be clearly documented in the record. If the patient decides to suspend DNR orders intraoperatively, then the point at which the DNR is to be reinstituted needs to be clearly stated.

Common Routines and Medications

Preoperative care and routines are designed to protect the safety of patients and to minimize the likelihood of postoperative complications. Surgical preparation may include bowel preparation, skin preparation, and hair removal. Bowel preparation is usually ordered for major abdominal surgery of the colon or rectum. The goal of preoperative bowel cleansing is to clear the intestine of feces and to decrease intestinal bacteria. It is thought that this preparation reduces the risk of contamination of the operative site with stool, however, some studies question the necessity and effectiveness of mechanical bowel preparation (Guenaga, 2002). Most surgeons continue to use mechanical bowel preparation prior to colorectal surgery. There are several methods to clear the colon of fecal material. Conventional bowel preparation requires a low-residue diet for several days prior to surgery, administration of laxatives 1 to 2 days before surgery, and the administration of enemas on the evening before surgery (Guenaga, 2002). Bowel preparation also may include the administration of oral antibiotics (e.g., neomycin and erythromycin, or metronidazole). Bowel preparation is a time-consuming and exhausting process, and it can contribute to preoperative dehydration in older patients.

Skin preparation may require the patient to shower the night before surgery or the morning of surgery with an antiseptic solution (i.e., 2% chlorhexidine gluconate). Hair removal prior to surgery is a controversial practice. If hair is to be removed for an operation, the CDC recommends using sterile supplies, clipping rather than shaving, in the direction of hair growth, and performing the procedure as close to the time of operation as possible (Mangram, Horan, Pearson, Silver, & Jarvis, 1999; Niel-Weise, Willie, & van den Broek, 2005; Schweon, 2006). Figure 25–3 ■ (p. 610) shows the areas of skin preparation for common surgical sites.

Preoperative Medications

Preoperative medications refer to those that are given specifically in preparation for surgery. It is increasingly common for preoperative medications to be given in the **holding area** of the surgical suite immediately prior to the operation. The Pharmacology Summary box (p. 611) lists common preoperative medications and the rationale for their administration.

County General
Hospital

Patient's name _____

Med. Rec. # _____

DOB _____

Consent for Medical/Surgical Procedure

_____ has explained that I have a condition called _____ and
(Name of Healthcare Provider)

has recommended a medical or surgical treatment called _____
_____ .

Benefits and Alternatives to Treatment: My doctor has spoken with me about the benefits I may expect from this treatment,
such as _____ but has made no guarantees or promises. My doctor has also spoken about what
could happen if I do not get this treatment, and explained other options for my care including _____
_____ .

Risks:

My doctor has explained that there are some risks to this treatment. The risks include, but are not limited to, allergic reactions, drug reactions, bleeding, blood clots, nerve injury, brain damage, infection, loss of bodily function or life, or the need for more procedures or treatments. My doctor has also explained that there may be other risks or complications. Particular risks include, but are not limited to _____
_____ .

☐ **N/A   Blood Transfusion:**

I may also need a blood transfusion. There are risks to this, even when all safety measures are taken. The risks of getting blood transfusion include (but are not limited to) fever; chills; allergic reactions (rashes including hives); heart failure; hemolysis (destruction of the transfused red blood cells) with fever; shock; chest pain; red urine; transmission of infectious agents such as bacteria, hepatitis virus, or HIV (human immunodeficiency virus).

☐ **N/A   Disposal of Tissues:**

I give permission to County General Hospital to dispose of any tissue, fluid, or bone that may be removed during my treatment. I understand that this tissue, fluids, or bone may be used, saved, or transferred to others for scientific or teaching purposes.

☐ **N/A   Non-Anesthesiologist Delivered Moderate Sedation:**

I understand that I will receive sedation through my intravenous line (IV) in order to help me feel more comfortable during my procedure. This sedation is not general anesthesia and is not administered by an anesthesiologist. With this sedation I may still be aware of what is happening. There are risks to sedation, including (but are not limited to) allergic reactions, drug reactions, bleeding, blood clots, breathing problems that require a breathing tube, nerve injury, brain damage, infection, or loss of bodily function or life.

☐ **N/A   Industry Representative:**

I understand that an industry representative(s) will be present during my procedure. My doctor has explained the reasons why the industry representative(s) will be present.

☐ **I do not** consent to the presence of an Industry Representative(s).

☐ **N/A   Tracking Medical Devices:**

Some surgical treatments include putting in (implanting), or taking out (removing) a medical device. The hospital is asked, by law, to track this device. This means that the hospital is asked to give my name, address, and social security number to the medical device manufacturer, and/or the Food and Drug Administration (FDA). It is my decision whether the hospital can give out this information.

☐ **I refuse** to let the hospital give information to the manufacturer and/or FDA.

Trainees & Observers:

County General Hospital is a teaching facility. This means that health care trainees such as resident physicians and students may be involved in or observe my care. All trainees are supervised by professional staff.

Patient Consent:

My questions have been answered. I have read and understood the content of this form. I consent to treatment and medical care.

X_____ or X_____   X __ / __ / __
Patient   Person authorized to sign for patient and relationship to patient   Date

I have explained the above statements, and answered all the patient's questions.

X_____ or X_____   X __ / __ / __
Physician/Surgeon/Other Healthcare Provider   Print Name   Date

FIGURE 25–2 ■ Consent for medical–surgical treatment.
Source: Courtesy of Beth Israel Deaconess Nursing Department

Head surgery

Unilateral chest surgery

Thoracoabdominal surgery

Abdominal surgery

Forearm, elbow, or hand surgery

Gynecologic surgery

Genitourinary surgery

Hip surgery

Thigh and leg surgery

Foot/lower leg surgery

Ankle, foot, or toe surgery

FIGURE 25–3 ■ Skin preparation for common surgical sites.

Antianxiety agents are often given to relax the patient. Prophylactic antibiotics are given in many, but not all, surgical cases. Antibiotics are frequently given intravenously in the surgical holding area or at induction of anesthesia. Research supports the view that the antibiotic must be in the target tissues before bacterial contamination if it is to prevent subsequent infection (Nichols, 2001). Ideally, antibiotics should be given 30 to 60 minutes before an incision is made (Golembiewski, 2004). Cefazolin, a first-generation cephalosporin, is often the drug of choice for surgical prophylaxis, although cefoxitin may be used in colon surgeries. If vancomycin is to be given, it should be started 2 hours before the incision because it takes 60 minutes to administer. In uncomplicated, short, clean surgical cases, one dose of parenteral antibiotic may be sufficient to prevent infection. Additional doses of antibiotics may be given during surgical procedures that last more than 2 to 3 hours or where contamination is suspected (Golembiewski, 2004; Nichols, 2001). Postoperative antibiotic prophylaxis is not recommended beyond 24 hours because studies do not show any benefit and it may contribute to the development of drug resistance (Bratzler & Houck, 2004).

Other preoperative medications that may be given include gastrointestinal stimulants, gastric acid blockers for gastric ulcer prophylaxis, or antiemetics to decrease nausea and vomiting. These medications are not recommended for the purpose of decreasing risk of pulmonary aspiration (ASA, 1999b). Beta-adrenergic blockers are given to patients prior to cardiac surgery to reduce the incidence of postoperative atrial fibrillation. Beta-adrenergic blocker therapy may also be given to high-risk cardiac patients or to those undergoing vascular procedures to reduce the risk of perioperative cardiovascular complications (Fleisher et al., 2006). Currently, it is recommended that beta-adrenergic blocker therapy be started days to weeks before elective surgery although the ideal dose, drug, and timing has not been established.

Preoperative Checklist

Most hospitals use preoperative checklists, like that shown in Figure 25–4 ■ (p. 612), to ensure and document the readiness of the patient for surgery. The admitting nurse completes the preoperative checklist for a patient who is having same-day admission surgery. If the patient is an inpatient, the clinical nurse

PHARMACOLOGY Summary of Common Preoperative Medications

Medication Category	Rationale for Administering Medication to Preoperative Patient
Antibiotics	
• Cefazolin: recommended for many different types of surgery (e.g., neurosurgical, cardiothoracic, vascular, gastric, biliary tract, urologic, gynecologic, orthopedic procedures) • Erythromycin: may be given orally for surgery on colon and rectum • Neomycin: may be given orally for surgery on colon and rectum • Trimethoprim 160 mg and sulfamethoxazole 800 mg (Bactrim DS) may be given orally to patients having urologic surgery	Antibiotics are given for prophylaxis against infection. Recommendations for the selection of an antibiotic and how it is administered vary according to the surgery and the patient. Prophylactic antibiotics may be given to patients with heart valve abnormalities to prevent bacterial endocarditis. Prophylactic antibiotics are frequently given to patients receiving prostheses (e.g., vascular graft, joint replacement) or transplants (e.g., heart, kidney, pancreas, liver).
Anticholinergics	
• Atropine • Glycopyrrolate • Scopolamine eyedrops	Given to suppress oral, respiratory, and gastric secretions during surgery. Atropine and glycopyrrolate increase heart rate (prevent bradycardia). Atropine and scopolamine eyedrops may be used in ophthalmic procedures to dilate pupils.
Antiemetics	
• Droperidol (Inapsine) • Ondansetron (Zofran) • Metoclopramide (Reglan)	Given to reduce nausea and vomiting. Metoclopramide speeds gastric emptying.
Anticoagulants, Low-Dose	
• Low-dose heparin • Low-molecular-weight heparin (e.g., enoxaparin, dalteparin, ardeparin)	Given to prevent the development of thrombus formation and pulmonary emboli in surgeries or patients who are high risk (e.g., orthopedic procedures). Usually not recommended for patients having neurosurgery, spinal needles, or epidural catheters.
Benzodiazepines	
• Midazolam (Versed) • Lorazepam (Ativan) • Diazepam (Valium)	Given to reduce anxiety, increase sedation, and smooth induction of anesthesia.
Beta-adrenergic Blocker Therapy	
• Atenolol • Metoprolol • Propranolol	Given in cardiac surgery to reduce the risk of atrial fibrillation. Given in noncardiac surgery to select patients to reduce the risk of cardiovascular complications.
Gastric Acid Blockers	
• Proton-pump inhibitor (e.g., Protonix) • H2-receptor antagonist (e.g., famotidine, ranitidine, cimetidine)	Given to decrease gastric acid production as prophylaxis against development of gastric/duodenal ulcer from physiological stress. May be given to raise gastric pH in specific situations where the patient is high risk for pulmonary aspiration. If aspiration occurs the higher pH of gastric secretions does less damage than those that are very acidic.
Narcotics	
• Fentanyl • Morphine sulfate • Meperidine	Given to reduce pain and discomfort associated with preoperative procedures, and to reduce anesthesia requirements.

Sources: American Society of Anesthesiologists. (1999). Practice guidelines for preoperative fasting and the use of pharmacologic agents to reduce the risk of pulmonary aspiration: Application to healthy patients undergoing elective procedures. A report by the American Society of Anesthesiologists Task Force on Preoperative Fasting. *Anesthesiology, 90*(3), 896–905; American Society of Health System Pharmacists. (1999). ASHP therapeutic guidelines on antimicrobial prophylaxis in surgery. *American Journal of Health System Pharmacists, 56*(18), 1839–1888; Adams, M., Josephson, D., & Holland, L. (2005). *Pharmacology for nurses: A pathophysiological approach.* Upper Saddle River, NJ: Pearson Prentice Hall; Fleisher, L., Beckman, J., Brown, K., Calkins, H., Chaikof, E., Fleischmann, K., Freeman, W., Froehlich, J., Kasper, E., Kersten, J., Riegel, B., & Robb, J. et al. (2006). ACC/AHA 2006 guideline update on perioperative cardiovascular evaluation for noncardiac surgery: Focused update on perioperative beta-blocker therapy. *Journal of the American College of Cardiology, 47*(11).

County General Hospital

PRE-PROCEDURE REPORT

Patient Identification Area

SECTION 1

PROCEDURE: ☐ Surgical ☐ Cardiac Cath ☐ Angiography ☐ Arteriogram ☐ Tips ☐ Other _____

CHART PREPARATION	Completed			PHYSICAL PREPARATION	Completed		
	Yes	No	N/A		Yes	No	N/A
Health care Proxy				ID band on			
Surgical/Procedure Consent				Nail polish/hairpins/makeup removed			
Anesthesia Consent				Hospital gown ONLY			
Hemoglobin/Hematocrit				Valuables, jewelry removed			
Interpreted EKG				Prosthesis removed			
Interpreted CXR				Dentures removed			
Addressograph plate				Contact lenses removed			
Medication Adminstration Record				Eyeglasses removed			
Old record				Hearing aide in place L / R			
Insulin record				Preop scrub/prep done			

SECTION 2: PRE-PROCEDURE ASSESSMENT   To be completed on the day of surgery/procedure.

VITAL SIGNS:

T_____ BP _____ HR _____ RR _____

O2 SAT_____ ☐ ROOM AIR _____ ☐ NP @ _____ L/M

WEIGHT:_____ HEIGHT:_____

ALLERGIES:

_____

_____

PRECAUTION STATUS:

_____

PRIMARY LANGUAGE:

_____

NEURO:

LOC
  ☐ ORIENTED X 3   ☐ CONFUSED
  ☐ SEDATED   ☐ OTHER _____

PAIN
  LOCATION_____
  MEDICATION _____

IMPAIRMENTS: ☐ VISUAL   ☐ HEARING   ☐ COGNITIVE

MEDICATIONS TAKEN THIS MORNING (ROUTINE):

_____

_____

_____

PREOP MEDS:

_____

_____

ENDOCRINE:

  ☐ IDDM   ☐ NIDDM   ☐ AM BS _____
  PRE OP INSULIN (Date, Time)_____

LOCATION OF FAMILY:

  CONTACT TO BE CALLED:_____
  PHONE #:_____

LOCATION OF BELONGINGS:

_____

GI:
  NPO SINCE _____

GU:
  LAST VOIDED _____ FOLEY _____
  ☐ CRF/LAST DIALYSIS _____
  ACCESS SITE: _____

TRANSFER NURSE:

_____ RN

DATE: _____ TIME: _____

COMMENTS: _____
_____
_____
_____

FIGURE 25–4 ■ Preprocedure report form.
Source: Courtesy of Beth Israel Deaconess Nursing Department

caring for the patient completes the checklist. The patient scheduled for surgery is identified using two indicators (e.g., asking the patient his name and date of birth and checking the wristband). The patient must have a hospital identification wristband in place and allergy band if applicable. Prior to sending the patient to the operating room, the nurse checks to see that signed surgical and anesthesia consents are on file. If consent for surgery or anesthesia is missing, the appropriate physician is contacted. The nurse also checks that the medical record is complete including recent laboratory tests, diagnostic tests, medication records, intake and output sheets, and vital sign graphic records. The nurse records the patient's current level of consciousness and a recent set of vital signs. The nurse notes the medications, routine and preoperative, taken before surgery. Patients should void before going to the operating room.

Commonly cosmetics, including nail polish, are removed preoperatively in order to observe skin color and capillary filling. All jewelry is removed from the patient and locked up with other valuables per hospital policy. It is particularly important to note on the preoperative checklist where valuables are located to prevent loss. Most facilities allow the patient to wear a wedding band that has been taped to the finger to the operating room, but the patient may want to remove the ring if postoperative swelling is expected (e.g., mastectomy with lymph node dissection). Pierced earrings and other body piercings must be removed to prevent accidental burns from electrocautery (Bray, 2006).

All prosthetic devices including dentures, removable bridges, and contact lens are removed prior to surgery. On occasion, the anesthesia care provider may prefer that the patient leave dentures in place to assist in airway maintenance. The presence of dentures in the mouth can assist in creating a tighter seal between the mouth and the oxygen mask (Bray, 2006). When dentures are removed, they must be labeled and stored safely to prevent loss. Patients may want to wear glasses or hearing aids to the holding area, this is acceptable although they will be removed before the surgery. Patients are transported with their medical record, including the medication administration record, to the operating room holding area via gurney.

Additional guidelines for the preoperative phase that deal with pain and comfort are listed in the National Guidelines box (p. 614).

◼ Research

Research is important to improving the care of surgical patients. Advances in technology and changes in surgical technique create the need to research the effects of the change. For example, patients today are sent home earlier after surgery because surgical procedures have become less invasive. What effect does this have on the patient, his or her family, and the home health agency that provides the care that was once provided in the hospital? Research is critical to nurses who want to know that the interventions they perform are based on scientific evidence. The Research Opportunities and Clinical Impact box (p. 615) lists some of the research problems that are important to the care of the preoperative patient. An example of a research study that could have a positive effect on perioperative nursing practice is described in the Evidence-Based Practice feature (p. 603).

NATIONAL GUIDELINES American Society of PeriAnesthesia Nurses Pain and Comfort Clinical Guidelines

Preoperative Phase

Assessment

1. Vital signs including pain and comfort goals (e.g., 0 to 10 scale).

2. Medical history (e.g., neurological status, cardiac and respiratory, instability, allergy to medication, food and objects, use of herbs, motion sickness, sickle cell, fibromyalgia, use of caffeine/substance abuse, fear, and anxiety).

3. Pain history (e.g., preexisting pain, acute, chronic, pain level, pattern, quality, type of source, intensity, location, duration/time, course, pain effect, and effects on personal life).

4. Pain behaviors/expressions or history (e.g., grimacing, frowning, crying, restlessness, tension, and discomfort behaviors, such as shivering, nausea, and vomiting. Note that physical appearance may not necessarily indicate pain/discomfort or its absence.)

5. Analgesic history: type (i.e., opioid, nonopioid, and adjuvant analgesics), dose, frequency, effectiveness, adverse effects, other medications that may influence choice of analgesics (e.g., anticoagulant, antihypertensive, muscle relaxants).

6. Patient's preferences (e.g., for pain relief/comfort measures, expectations, concerns, aggravating and alleviating factors, and clarification of misconceptions).

7. Pain/comfort acceptable levels (e.g., patient and family, as indicated, agree to plan of treatment/interventions postoperatively).

8. Comfort history (i.e., physiological, sociocultural, psychospiritual, and environment, such as spiritual beliefs/symbols, warming measures, music, comfort objects, privacy, positioning, factors related to nausea/vomiting).

9. Educational needs (i.e., consider age or level of education, cognitive and language appropriateness, and barriers to learning).

10. Cultural language preference, identification of personal beliefs, and resulting restrictions.

11. Pertinent laboratory results (e.g., prolonged prothrombin time, partial thromboplastin time, and abnormal international normalized ratio and platelet count to determine risk for epidural hematoma in patients with epidural catheter).

Interventions

1. Identify patient, validate surgeon's order and procedure (i.e., correct name of drug, dose, amount, route, and time), and validate type of surgery and correct surgical site as applicable.

2. Discuss pain and comfort assessment (i.e., presence, location, quality, intensity, age, language, condition, and cognitively appropriate pain rating scale [e.g., a 0 to 10 numerical scale or FACES scale] and comfort scale). Assessment method must be the same for consistency.

3. Discuss with patient and family, as indicated, information about reporting pain intensity using a numerical or FACES rating scales and available pain relief and comfort measures. Include discussion of patient's preference for pain and comfort measures; implement comfort measures (i.e., physiological, sociocultural, spiritual, environmental support as indicated by patient).

4. Discuss and dispel misconceptions about pain and pain management.

5. Encourage patient to take a preventive approach to pain and discomfort by asking for relief measures before pain and discomfort are severe or out of control.

6. Educate purpose of intravenous or epidural patient-controlled analgesia (PCA) as indicated; educate about use of nonpharmacologic methods (e.g., cold therapy, relaxation breathing, music).

7. Discuss potential outcomes of pain and discomfort treatment approaches.

8. Establish pain relief/comfort goals with the patient (e.g., a pain rating of less than 4 on a scale of 0 to 10 to make it easy to cough, deep breathe, and turn). Premedicate patients for sedation, pain relief, and comfort (e.g., nonopioid, opioid, antiemetics as ordered; consider needs of chronic pain patients).

9. Arrange interpreter throughout the continuum of care as indicated.

10. Utilize interventions for patients with sensory impairments (e.g., device to amplify sound, sign language, and interpreters).

11. Report abnormal findings including laboratory values (prolonged PT/PTT and abnormal INR and platelet count among epidural patients).

12. Arrange for parents to be present for children.

Expected Outcomes

1. Patient states understanding of care plan and priority of individualized needs.

2. Patient states understanding of pain intensity scale, comfort scale, and pain relief/comfort goals.

3. Patient establishes realistic and achievable pain relief/comfort goals (e.g., a pain rating of less than 4 on a scale of 0 to 10 to make it easier to cough, deep breathe, and turn upon discharge).

4. Patient states understanding or demonstrates correct use of PCA equipment as indicated.

5. Patient verbalizes understanding of importance of using other nonpharmacologic methods of alleviating pain and discomfort (e.g., cold therapy, relaxation breathing, music).

Source: Reprinted from American Society of PeriAnesthesia Nurses. ASPAN pain and comfort guideline. Journal of PeriAnesthesia Nursing, *18*(4), 232–236, 2003, with permission from Elsevier.

RESEARCH OPPORTUNITIES AND CLINICAL IMPACT RELATED TO CARE OF THE PREOPERATIVE PATIENT

Research Area	Clinical Impact
General Preoperative Teaching	
What is the effect of preoperative education on patients' self-care behaviors postoperatively?	A goal of preoperative education is to increase patients' self-care behaviors and participation in desired postoperative activities.
Is there a difference in knowledge outcomes of preoperative education presented in written versus oral versus video formats?	Provides data for selecting an appropriate format(s) for the presentation of preoperative information.
How does the availability of Internet information on surgical procedures change preoperative education provided by the nurse?	Increased use of the Internet by patients and family members may change the focus of preoperative teaching. It may also affect the type and amount of information desired.
Is there an optimal time for preoperative education?	Provides rationale for scheduling preoperative appointments and for providing written materials to the patient.
What factors (nurse, environment, patient) increase the effectiveness of preoperative education?	Provides background information necessary for understanding the educational process and for creating an effective teaching environment.
Does preoperative education improve patient outcomes postoperatively?	A critical desired outcome of preoperative education programs.
Psychosocial Aspects of Preoperative Care	
How does the timing of preoperative teaching affect patient and family anxiety levels and coping strategies?	Provides information about an optimal time of psychological readiness for preoperative information.
Does family presence in the surgical holding area enhance the well-being of patients and family members?	Provides a rationale for designing a patient/family-friendly environment for surgery.
How do the communication skills of novice nurses in the preoperative area compare to those of experienced nurses?	Provides a basis for understanding the development of therapeutic communication in nurses.
How does a nurse's skill in communication affect preoperative teaching?	Provides a basis for understanding how specific skills affect the teaching–learning process.
What is the effect of an emergency surgery on the informational needs of patients, families, and significant others?	Provides background information for prioritizing information in specific situations.
Culture	
What interventions can be done to support culturally appropriate care preoperatively?	Provides a rationale for developing a range of culture-specific interventions.
What are the differences across cultures regarding the type and amount of preoperative education desired by patients?	Provides information needed for designing culturally sensitive preoperative teaching plans.
Specific Preoperative Instructions	
What is the optimal time frame to quit smoking prior to surgery?	Provides important information about the time frame necessary to achieve positive outcomes.
Does a preoperative shower using antimicrobial soap decrease the risk of surgical-site infection?	Provides rationale for a common preoperative instruction.
What are the physiological effects of a "good nights sleep" before surgery on the preoperative patient?	Provides important psychological and physiological information about the patient going into surgery.
Should gender, ethnicity, and body weight make a difference in the instructions for mechanical bowel preparation for surgery?	Provides information about differences in physiological responses that might support individualizing preoperative preparation.
Does the use of a preoperative risk assessment for venous thromboembolism correlate with reduced incidence of deep vein thrombosis (DVT) postoperatively?	Provides the evidence for a current nursing practice recommendation.
Does specific information about deep vein thrombosis (DVT) prophylaxis increase patients' compliance with leg exercises, ambulation, and use of intermittent pneumatic compression devices postoperatively?	Provides a rationale for preoperative teaching.

NCLEX® REVIEW

1. The nurse asks a preoperative patient about the presence of allergies. The purpose of this information is to:
   1. Reduce allergic reactions to medications or to latex.
   2. Determine the type of anesthesia to be used.
   3. Determine the care area to transfer the patient after the surgical procedure.
   4. Ensure blood products are available for the patient.

2. The nurse is assessing the cardiovascular status of a preoperative patient and learns of the patient's history of valve disease. Which of the following might be indicated for this patient?
   1. Monitor fluid status
   2. Monitor electrolyte status
   3. Antibiotic prophylaxis
   4. BNP level

3. A 40-year-old patient is scheduled for a total knee replacement. Which of the following would be indicated for this patient?
   1. Preoperative arterial blood gas
   2. Stop all NSAIDs two weeks before the scheduled surgery
   3. Recent hemoglobin A1c level
   4. Recent electrocardiogram

4. The nurse is planning preoperative care for an elderly patient. Which of the following should be included to reduce the risk of pulmonary complications?
   1. Encourage deep breathing and coughing
   2. Monitor oxygen saturation
   3. Monitor intake and output
   4. Follow aspiration precautions

5. While providing preoperative instructions in the waiting room, the patient says to the nurse "I don't want to be cauterized." Which of the following should the nurse respond to this patient?
   1. Everyone is cauterized.
   2. Can you explain to me what you mean by cauterized?
   3. The surgeon will cauterize in the operating room if it's necessary.
   4. Who said anything about being cauterized?

6. A preoperative patient tells the nurse that he researched the surgical procedure on the Internet and has no questions at this time. Which of the following should the nurse do?
   1. Document that the patient studied the surgical procedure on the Internet.
   2. Assess the patient's understanding of the procedure to supplement any areas not reviewed through the Internet.
   3. End the preoperative teaching session.
   4. Encourage the patient to use the call light in the event he decides he wants to discuss the procedure.

Answers for review questions appear in Appendix D

KEY TERMS

cosmetic surgery *p.587*
curative procedures *p.586*
diagnostic procedures *p.586*
elective procedures *p.587*
emergent (emergency) surgery *p.587*

exploratory surgery *p.586*
holding area *p.608*
palliative procedures *p.587*
perioperative *p.588*

preoperative health evaluation *p.588*
reconstructive surgery *p.586*
same-day admission *p.586*
urgent procedures *p.587*

EXPLORE   PEARSON **mynursingkit**™

MyNursingKit is your one stop for online chapter review materials and resources. Prepare for success with additional NCLEX®-style practice questions, interactive assignments and activities, web links, animations and videos, and more!

Register your access code from the front of your book at
www.mynursingkit.com

REFERENCES

Administration on Aging. (2005). *A profile of older Americans: 2005.* Retrieved on October 21, 2008 from http://www.aoa.gov/prof/Statistics/profile/2005/2005profile.pdf

American Society of Anesthesiologists. (1999a). *Anesthesiologists warn: If you're taking herbal products, tell your doctor before surgery.*

Retrieved on October 21, 2008 from http://www.asahq.org/publiceducation/herbal.html

American Society of Anesthesiologists. (1999b). Practice guidelines for preoperative fasting and the use of pharmacologic agents to reduce the risk of pulmonary aspiration: Application to healthy patients undergoing elective procedures. A report by the American Society

of Anesthesiologists Task Force on Preoperative Fasting. *Anesthesiology, 90*(3), 896–905.

American Society of Anesthesiologists. (2001). Ethical guidelines for the anesthesia care of patients with do-not-resuscitate orders or other directives that limit treatment. In *ASA standards, guidelines, and statements* (pp.10–11). Park Ridge, IL: Author.

American Society of Anesthesiologists. (2006a). *ASA standards, guidelines, and statements.* Park Ridge, IL: Author.

American Society of Anesthesiologists. (2006b). Practice guidelines for the perioperative management of patients with obstructive sleep apnea: A report by the American Society of Anesthesiologists Task Force on Perioperative Management of Patients with Obstructive Sleep Apnea. *Anesthesiology, 104*(5), 1081–1093.

American Society of PeriAnesthesia Nurses. (2006a). ASPAN's evidence-based clinical practice guideline for the prevention and/or management of PONV/PDNV. *Journal of PeriAnesthesia Nursing, 21*(4), 230–250.

American Society of PeriAnesthesia Nurses. (2006b). *Standards of perianesthesia nursing practice.* New Jersey: Author.

Asilioglu, K., & Celik, S. (2004). The effect of preoperative education on anxiety of open cardiac surgery patients. *Patient Education and Counseling, 1*, 65–70.

Association of periOperative Registered Nurses. (1999). *Perioperative care of patients with do-not-resuscitate (DNR) orders.* Adopted 1995; reaffirmed October 1999. Retrieved from http:// www.aorn.org/about/positions/dnr.htm

Association of periOperative Registered Nurses. (2005). *AORN standards, recommended practices, and guidelines.* Denver: Author.

Barrera, R., Shi, W., Amar, D., Thaler, H., Gabovich, N., Bains, M., et al. (2005). Smoking and timing of cessation: Impact on pulmonary complications after thoracotomy. *Chest, 127*, 1977–1991.

Beck, F., & Rosenthal, T. (2002). Prealbumin: A marker for nutritional evaluation. *American Family Physician, 65*, 1575–1578.

Bennett, J., & Brown, C. (2000). Use of herbal remedies by patients in a health maintenance organization. *Journal of the American Pharmacology Association, 40*(3), 353–358.

Bernier, M., Sanares, D., Owen, S., & Newhouse, P. (2003). Preoperative teaching received and valued in a day surgery setting. *AORN Journal, 77*, 563–582.

Blondin, M. (2006). *Prevention of deep vein thrombosis.* Iowa City, IA: University of Iowa Gerontological Nursing Research Center, Research Dissemination Core.

Bond, L., Flickinger, D., Aytes, L., Bateman, B., Chalk, M. B., & Aysse, P. (2005). Effects of preoperative teaching of the use of a pain scale with patients in the PACU. *Journal of PeriAnesthesia Nursing, 20*(5), 333–340.

Bradley, D., Creswell, L., Hogue, C., Epstein, A., Prystowsky, E., & Daoud, E. (2005). Pharmacologic prophylaxis: American College of Chest Physicians guidelines for the prevention and management of postoperative atrial fibrillation after cardiac surgery. *Chest, 128*, 39S–48S.

Bratzler, D., & Houck, P. (2004). Antimicrobial prophylaxis for surgery: An advisory statement from the National Surgical Infection Prevention Project. *Clinical Infectious Disease, 28*(12), 1706.

Bray, A. (2006). Preoperative nursing assessment of the surgical patient. *Nursing Clinics of North America, 41*, 135–150.

Brooks, D., Crowe, J., Kelsey, C., Lacy, J., Parsons, J., & Solway, S. (2001). A clinical practice guideline on peri-operative cardiorespiratory physical therapy. *Physiotherapy Canada, 53*(1), 9–25.

Brooks-Brunn, J. (2000). Risk factors associated with postoperative pulmonary complications following total abdominal hysterectomy. *Clinical Nursing Research, 9*(1), 25–46.

Centers for Disease Control and Prevention. (2008). *National Center for Health Statistics: Monitoring this nations health.* Retrieved on June 24, 2008 from http://www.cdc.gov/nchs

Chang, J., Morton, S., Rubenstein, L., Mojica, W., Maglione, M., Suttorp, M., et al. (2004). Interventions for the prevention of falls in older adults: Systematic review and meta-analysis of randomized clinical trials. *BMJ, 328*(7441), 653–657.

Costa, M. (2001). The lived perioperative experience of ambulatory surgery patients. *AORN Journal, 74*, 874–881.

Crenshaw, J., & Winslow, E. (2002). Preoperative fasting: Old habits die hard. *American Journal of Nursing, 102*(5), 36–44.

Cunningham, M. F., Hanson-Heath, C., & Agre, P. (2003). A perioperative nurse liaison program: CNS interventions for cancer patients and their families. *Journal of Nursing Care Quality, 18*(1), 16–21.

Deyirmenjian, M., Karam, N., & Salameh, P. (2006). Preoperative patient education for open-heart patients: A source of anxiety? *Patient Education and Counseling, 62*(1), 111–117.

Doering, L., McGuire, A., & Rourke, D. (2002). Recovering from cardiac surgery: What patients want you to know. *American Journal of Critical Care, 11*(4), 333–343.

Eagle, K., Berger, P., Calkins, H., Chaitman, B., Ewy, G., Fleischmann, K., et al. (2002). *ACC/AHA guideline update for perioperative cardiovascular evaluation for non-cardiac surgery: A report of the American College of Cardiology/American Heart Association Task Force on Practice Guidelines (Committee to Update the 1996 Guidelines on perioperative cardiovascular evaluation for non-cardiac surgery).* Retrieved from American College of Cardiology website: http://www.acc.org/clinical/guidelines/perio/dirIndex.htm

Evans, D., Hodgkinson, B., Lambert, L., & Wood, J. (2001). Fall risk factors in the hospital setting: A systematic review. *International Journal of Nursing Practice, 7*, 38–45.

Elkins, G., Staniunas, R., Rajab, H., Marcus, J., & Snyder, T. (2004). Use of a numeric visual analog anxiety scale among patients undergoing colorectal surgery. *Clinical Nursing Research, 13*(3), 237–245.

Fleisher, L., Beckman, J., Brown, K., Calkins, H., Chaikof, E., Fleischmann, K., et al. (2006). ACC/AHA 2006 guideline update on perioperative cardiovascular evaluation for noncardiac surgery: Focused update on perioperative beta-blocker therapy. *Journal of the American College of Cardiology, 47*(11).

Gandhi, G., Nuttall, G., Abel, M., Mullany, C., Schaff, H., O'Brien, P., et al. (2007). Intensive intraoperative insulin therapy versus conventional glucose management during cardiac surgery: A randomized trial. *Annals of Internal Medicine, 146*(4), 233–243, I29–I32.

Gandhi, G., Nuttall, G., Abel, M., Mullany, C., Schaff, H., Williams, A., et al. (2005). Intraoperative hyperglycemia and perioperative outcomes in cardiac surgery patients. *Mayo Clinic Proceedings, 80*, 862–868.

Golembiewski, J. (2004). Antibiotic prophylaxis for preventing surgical site infection. *Journal of PeriAnesthesia Nursing, 19*(2), 111–113.

Guenaga, K. (2002). Preoperative bowel cleansing. *Seminars in Colon & Rectal Surgery, 13*(1), 53–61.

Guruge, S., & Sidani, S. (2002). Effects of demographic characteristics on preoperative teaching outcomes: A meta analysis. *Canadian Journal of Nursing Research, 34*(4), 25–33.

Hatcher, J. (2001). The proverbial herb. *American Journal of Nursing, 101*(2), 36–43.

Heizenroth, P. A. (1999). Positioning the patient for surgery. In M. Meeker & J. Rothrock (Eds.), *Care of the patient in surgery* (pp. 153–172). Philadelphia: Mosby.

Hering, K., Harvan, J., Dangelo, M., & Jasinski, D. (2005). The use of a computer website prior to scheduled surgery: Impact on patient information, acquisition, anxiety level, and overall satisfaction with anesthesia care. *AANA Journal, 73*(1), 29–33.

Heye, M., Foster, L., Bartlett, M. K., & Adkins, S. (2002). A preoperative intervention for pain reduction, improved mobility, and self-efficacy. *Applied Nursing Research, 16*(2), 174–183.

Hulzebos, E., DeBie, R., Favie, N., Helders, J., De La Riviere, A., & Van Meeteren, U. (2006). Preoperative intensive inspiratory muscle training to prevent postoperative pulmonary complications in high-risk patients undergoing CABG surgery: A randomized clinical trial. *JAMA, 296* (15), 1851–1858.

Institute for Clinical Symptoms Improvement. (2006). *Preoperative evaluation.* Retrieved on October 21, 2008 from http://www.icsi.org/preoperative_evaluation/preoperative_evaluation_2328.html. Bloomington, MN: Author.

Institute for Healthcare Improvement. (2006). *Reducing surgical complications.* Retrieved on October 21, 2008 from http://www.ihi.org/IHI/Programs

Johansson, K., Salantera, S., Heikkinen, K., Kuusisto, A., Virtanen, H., & Leino-Kilpi, H. (2004). Surgical patient education: Assessing the interventions and exploring the outcomes from experimental and quasiexperimental studies from 1990 to 2003. *Clinical Effectiveness in Nursing, 8*(2), 81–92.

Leske, J. S. (2000). Family stresses, strengths and outcomes after critical injury. *Critical Care Nursing Clinics of North America, 12*(2), 237–244.

Letterstal, A., Sandstrom, V., Olofsson, P., & Forsberg, C. (2004). Postoperative mobilization of patients with abdominal aortic aneurysm. *Journal of Advanced Nursing, 48*(6), 560–568.

Lin, L. Y., & Wang, R. (2005). Abdominal surgery, pain and anxiety: Preoperative nursing intervention. *Journal of Advanced Nursing, 51*(3), 252–260.

Madsen, M., Brosnan, J., & Nagy, V. (1998). Perioperative thirst: A patient perspective. *Journal of PeriAnesthesia Nursing, 13*(4), 225–228.

Mangram, A., Horan, T., Pearson, M., Silver, L., & Jarvis, W. (1999). Guideline for prevention of surgical site infection. Centers for Disease Control and Prevention, Hospital Infection Control Practices Advisory Committee. *Infection Control and Hospital Epidemiology, 20*(4), 247–280.

Maurer, W., Borkowski, R., & Parker, B. (2004). Quality and resource utilization in managing preoperative evaluation. *Anesthesiology Clinics of North America, 22*, 155–175.

McDonald, S., Hetrick, S., & Green, S. (2006). Pre-operative education for hip or knee replacement. *The Cochrane Library, 4* (CD003526).

Meeker, M., & Rothrock, J. (1999). *Care of the patient in surgery.* Philadelphia: Mosby.

Merli, G. (2000). Prophylaxis for deep venous thrombosis and pulmonary embolism in the surgical patient. *Clinical Cornerstone, 2*(4), 15–25.

Muravchick, S. (2004). *Geriatric anesthesia—Are you ready?* Retrieved April 26, 2004, from ASA Syllabus on Geriatric Anesthesiology, http://www.asahq.org/clinical/geriatrics/geron.htm

Neil, J. (2007). Perioperative care of the immunocompromised patient. *AORN Journal, 85*(3), 544–565.

Nichols, R. L. (2001). Preventing surgical site infections: A surgeon's perspective. *Emerging Infectious Diseases, 7*(2), 220–224.

Niel-Weise, B., Willie, J., & van den Broek, P. (2005). Hair removal policies in clean surgery: Systematic review of randomized, controlled trials. *Infection Control and Hospital Epidemiology, 26*(12), 923–928.

O'Donnell, M., Kearon, C., Johnson, J., Robinson, R., Zondag, M., Turpie, I., et al. (2007). Preoperative anticoagulant activity after bridging low-molecular-weight heparin for temporary interruption of warfarin. *Annals of Internal Medicine, 146*(3), 184–187.

Oetker-Black, S., Jones, S., Estok, P., Ryan, M., Gale, N., & Parker, C. (2003). Preoperative teaching and hysterectomy outcomes. *AORN Journal, 77*(6), 1215–1227.

Orfanos, P., Ellis, E., & Johnston, C. (1999). Effects of deep breathing exercises and ambulation on pattern of ventilation in post-operative patients. *Australian Journal of Physiotherapy, 45*(3), 173–182.

Overend, T., Anderson, C., Lucy, S. D., Bhatia, C., Jonsson, B., & Timmermans, C. (2001). The effect of incentive spirometry on postoperative pulmonary complications. *Chest, 120*(3), 971–978.

Owens, T. (2006). Bariatric surgery risks, benefits, and care of the morbidly obese. *Nursing Clinics of North America, 41*, 249–263.

Pagana, K. (2007). Laboratory and diagnostic testing: A perioperative update. *AORN Journal, 85*(4), 754–762.

Pan, W., Pintar, T., Anton, J., Lee, V., Vaughn, W., & Collard, C. (2004). Statins are associated with a reduced incidence of perioperative mortality after coronary artery bypass graft surgery. *Circulation, 110*(11), S45–S49.

Pasero, C., & Belden, J. (2006). Evidence-based perianesthesia care: Accelerated postoperative recovery programs. *Journal of PeriAnesthesia Nursing, 21*(3), 168–176.

Pribitkin, E., & Boger, G. (2000). Surgery and herbal therapy: Essential guidelines on bleeding, skin reactions, and wound healing. *Complementary Health Practice Review, 6*(1), 29–40.

Price, M., Whitney, J., & King, C. (2005). Development of a risk assessment tool for intraoperative pressure ulcers. *The Journal of Wound, Ostomy and Continence Nursing, 32*(1), 19–30.

Qaseem, A., Snow, V., Fitterman, N., Hornbake, R., Lawrence, V., Smetana, G., et al. (2006). Risk assessment and strategies to reduce perioperative pulmonary complications for patients undergoing noncardiothoracic surgery: A guideline from the American College of Physicians. *Annals of Internal Medicine, 144*(8), 575–580.

Roberts, C., Baker, F., Hann, D., Runfola, J., Witt, C., McDonald, J., et al. (2005). Patient–physician communication regarding use of complementary therapies during cancer treatment. *Journal of Psychosocial Oncology, 23*(4), 35–60.

Rogers, R., Lebkuchner, U., Kammerer-Doak, D., Thompson, P., Walters, M., & Nygaard, E. (2006). Obesity and retropubic surgery for stress incontinence: Is there really an increased risk of intraoperative complications? *American Journal of Obstetrics and Gynecology, 195*(6), 1794–1798.

Rooke, G. A. (2007). *Pacemakers.* Retrieved August 8, 2007, from Association of Veterans Affairs Anesthesiologists, http://www.vaanes.org/FORUMS/pacer.html

Schweon, S. (2006). Stamping out surgical site infection. *RN, 69*(8), 37–40.

Seltzer, J., Horsman, A., & Korniewicz, D. (2002). Awareness of surgical site infections for advanced practice nurses. *AACN Clinical Issues, 13*(3), 398–409.

Smith, M., & Ellis, E. (2000). Is retained mucus a risk factor for the development of postoperative atelectasis and pneumonia? Implications for the physiotherapist. *Physiotherapy Theory and Practice, 16*(2), 69–80.

Smykowski, L., & Rodriguez, W. (2003). The post anesthesia care unit experience: A family centered approach. *Journal of Nursing Care Quality, 18*(1), 5–15.

Soreide, E., & Ljungqvist, O. (2006). Modern preoperative fasting guidelines: A summary of the present recommendations and remaining questions. *Best Practice & Research Clinical Anaesthesiology, 20*(3), 483–491.

Spector, R. (2004). *Cultural diversity in health and illness.* Upper Saddle River, NJ: Pearson Prentice Hall.

Susleck, D., Willocks, A., Secrest, J., Norwood, B., Holweger, J., Davis, M., et al. (2007). The perianesthesia experience from the patient's perspective. *Journal of PeriAnesthesia Nursing, 22*(1), 10–20.

Vallerand, A., Fouladbakhsh, J., & Templin, T. (2005). Patients' choices for the self-treatment of pain. *Applied Nursing Research, 18*(2), 90–96.

Van den Berghe, G., Wouters, P., Weekers, F., Verwaest, C., Bruyninckx, F., Schetz, M., et al. (2001). Intensive insulin therapy in critically ill patients. *New England Journal of Medicine, 345*, 1359–1367.

Walker, K., Smithy, A., & Pittaway, A. (2003). Premedication for anxiety in adult day surgery. *Cochrane Database of Systematic Reviews, 1* (CD002192).

Weindler, J., & Kiefer, R. (2001). The efficacy of postoperative incentive spirometry is influenced by the device-specific imposed work of breathing. *Chest, 119*(6), 1858–1864.

Whitney, J. A., & Parkman, S. (2002). Preoperative physical activity, anesthesia, and analgesia: Effects on early postoperative walking after total hip replacement. *Applied Nursing Research, 15*(1), 19–27.

Yoon, S., Horne, C., & Adams, C. (2004). Herbal product use by African American older women. *Clinical Nursing Research, 13*(4), 271–289.

Yung, W., Mok, Y., Ling, S., Poon, Y., Wong, K., & Yim, C. (2005). Does preoperative intervention program improve postoperative outcome in high-risk patients undergoing thoracic surgery? *Chest, 128*, 337S–339S.

Intraoperative Nursing

Krista Brecht
Krisna Ogerio
Donna Stanbridge
Danielle Vigeant
Suzanne Watt

With contributions by:
Jane Ashley
Kathleen Osborn

Outcome-Based Learning Objectives

After studying this chapter, the learner will be able to:

1. Discuss the sequence of events for the patient from the beginning of surgery to arrival in the postanesthesia care unit.
2. Differentiate the roles of the surgical team.
3. Describe the interplay between each team member in the success of the surgical intervention.
4. Prioritize nursing interventions to maximize patient safety in the operating room.
5. Evaluate effective nursing measures for patient advocacy in the operating room.
6. Prioritize the nursing care of patients experiencing selected intraoperative complications.
7. Differentiate the role of the certified nurse and the anesthesiologist for the anesthetized patient.

Research   Collaboration   Health Promotion   Nursing Process   Caring   Critical Thinking

THE GOAL of perioperative or intraoperative nursing practice is to assist patients and their families to achieve a level of wellness equal to or greater than that which they had prior to the procedure (Association of periOperative Registered Nurses [AORN], Perioperative Nursing Data Set (PNDS-2007). The most important role of the perioperative nurse is to be a patient advocate. The essence of the advocacy in the perioperative role is defined as protection, communication (giving a voice), doing, comfort, and caring.

Advocacy is described as an act of informing and supporting the individuals so that they may make the best decisions possible for themselves. It is also speaking up for someone who is unable to speak for himself. Advocacy is a critical issue for surgical patients who are unconscious or sedated and unable to make decisions related to their care. Protecting patients from harm is the essence of the advocacy role of nurses, and it is a critical component for patients whose family members are not readily accessible and whose only possible advocate is the nurse. This is often the case for the patient having surgery. Many perioperative issues involve advocacy. These may include helping patients who are uninformed or have not given adequate consent for surgical procedures, confronting an incompetent colleague, pressing for more analgesia for

a patient in pain, or supporting the patient's view toward prolonging life with extraordinary treatment or technology.

 CRITICAL ALERT *Surgical patients can be compromised by stress, disease process, and sedation or general anesthesia, and they trust that a perioperative nurse will advocate in their best interest to ensure their privacy, dignity, rights, and safety.*

The nurse must accept accountability for nursing actions that safeguard the rights of the surgical patients. Perioperative nurses act as patient advocates by protecting, and they must be able to quickly and accurately identify advocacy issues and be ready to intervene on behalf of their patients. In recent years, the acceptance of a conceptual model for patient care, published by AORN, has helped to distinguish the relationship of various components of nursing practice and the effect on patient outcomes (Beyea, 2000) (Figure 26–1 ■).

Guidance for Professional Practice

The practice of perioperative nursing is guided by its own professional organization, the Association of periOperative Registered Nurses, as well as the Centers for Disease Control and

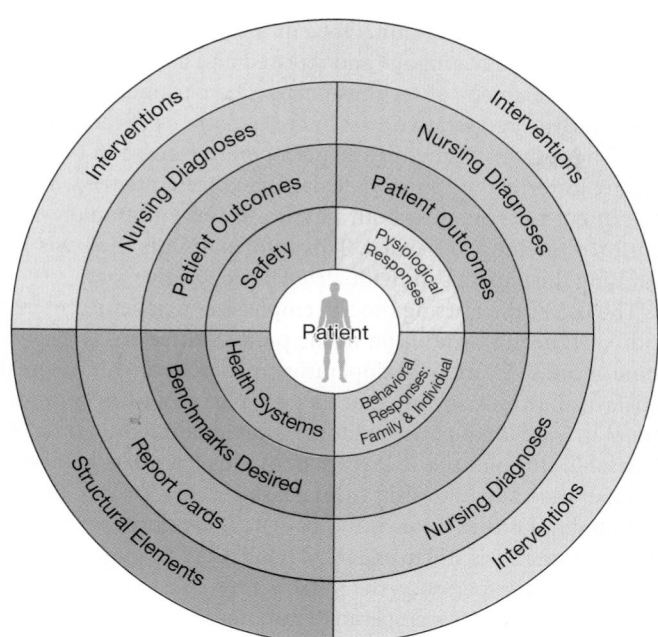

FIGURE 26–1 ■ Perioperative patient-focused model.

Source: Reprinted with permission from "The PNDS model," http://www.aorn.org/PracticeResources/
PNDSAndStandardizedPerioperativeRecord/PNDSModel. Copyright © 2002 AORN, Inc., 2170 South
Parker Road, Suite 300, Denver, CO 80231. All rights reserved.

Prevention (CDC) and the Joint Commission. AORN defines its
mission as follows: "to promote safety and optimal outcomes for
patients undergoing operative and other invasive procedures by
providing practice support and professional development opportunities to perioperative nurses." AORN is composed of approximately 41,000 perioperative registered nurses in the United States
and abroad who manage, teach, and practice perioperative nursing; who are enrolled in nursing education; and who are engaged
in perioperative research (AORN, 2007a). This professional organization has developed a conceptual framework and vocabulary
called the Perioperative Nursing Data Set (PNDS). The data set
addresses the domains of safety, physiological responses, behavioral responses of the patient and family, and the environment of
the perioperative setting within the health system.

The CDC's mission is to promote health and quality of life by
preventing and controlling disease, injury, and disability. It also
influences perioperative practice. In 1999, the CDC issued
guidelines for the prevention of surgical infection. Additionally,
it reflected the mission statement of the Joint Commission to
continuously improve the safety and quality of care provided to
the public through the provision of health care accreditation
and related services that support performance improvement in
health care organizations (Joint Commission, 2007). The Joint
Commission is an independent, not-for-profit organization that
is the United States' predominant accrediting body charged with
maintaining and improving health care delivery. The Joint
Commission's comprehensive accreditation process evaluates
an organization's compliance with its standards and other accreditation requirements. Joint Commission accreditation is
recognized nationwide as a symbol of quality that reflects an organization's commitment to meeting certain performance standards. To earn and maintain the Joint Commission's Gold Seal
of Approval, an organization must undergo an on-site survey by

a Joint Commission survey team at least every 3 years. A complete discussion of the Joint Commission is presented in
Chapter 3 ⊕.

■ Surgical Team

Successful surgery relies on the interplay of many individuals
working as a team, complementing each other's skills and responsibilities. This multidisciplinary team includes the surgeon and
assistants, anesthesiologist and assistants, the nursing team, and
support staff. Each of these professionals is responsible for specific
functions and plays a role in supporting the other groups. This
overlap of responsibilities ensures the safety of patients while they
are in a most vulnerable situation of not being able to give any
personal input. The roles of each member are described next.

Surgeon

The surgeon heads the surgical team and is responsible for making decisions related to the surgical procedure. Depending on the
procedure, an assistant might be required. This assistant could be
another surgeon, physician, resident in a university teaching hospital, or the registered nurse first assistant. The surgeon is responsible for performing the procedure and for coordinating the team.

An expanded role for perioperative nurses is that of registered
nurse first assistant (RNFA). The RNFA collaborates with the
surgeon and performs the role of first assistant during the operation. This role includes handling tissue, providing exposure, using instruments, suturing the wound, and providing hemostasis.
The role of an RNFA is highly specialized and demanding. In
2008, AORN approved a policy statement that defines the RNFA
role, scope of practice, and qualifications.

Anesthesia Care Provider

The anesthesiologist is a health care provider who specializes in
the administration of anesthetic agents and provides care to alleviate pain and promote relaxation. This professional is responsible for maintaining the airway; monitoring and ensuring gas
exchanges, respiration, and circulation; estimating and replacing
blood and fluid losses; administering medications to maintain hemodynamic stability; managing care in the event of a physiological crisis; and constantly communicating with the surgical and
nursing team. The anesthesiologist heads the anesthesia team and
might be assisted by a respiratory therapist, anesthesia resident or
fellow in a university teaching hospital, or a certified registered
nurse anesthetist (CRNA). As Chapter 1 ⊕ discussed, the CRNA
is an advance practice nurse, educated with a master's degree from
an accredited nurse anesthesia educational program. CRNAs administer anesthesia and anesthesia-related care in four general categories: (1) preanesthetic preparation and evaluation;
(2) anesthesia induction, maintenance, and emergence; (3) postanesthesia care; and (4) perianesthetic and clinical support functions. The CRNA works under the supervision of the
anesthesiologist. In a large study examining morbidity associated
with anesthesia, researchers found several factors that significantly reduce the risk of anesthesia. Among these are the direct
availability of an anesthesiologist during surgery, the presence of
a consistent anesthesia care provider throughout the case, and the
presence of an anesthetic nurse (Arbous et al., 2005).

Nurses

The perioperative nurse's primary role in the operating room (OR) is that of the circulating nurse. Most states have taken legislative measures in order to ensure the presence of a registered nurse in the circulator role in the OR for every surgical procedure. The circulating nurse's duties are performed outside the sterile field and encompass responsibilities of nursing care management within the OR. The **circulating nurse** observes the surgical team from a broad perspective and assists the team to create and maintain a safe, comfortable environment for surgery. The circulating nurse communicates patient care needs to each member of the surgical team, facilitating a united effort while being the patient advocate whose actions are dedicated to ensuring that the patient's rights and wishes are respected and carried out.

The **scrub nurse** works directly with the surgeon within the sterile field passing instruments, sponges, and other items needed during the surgical procedure. The sterile field is the area closely surrounding the OR table. Surgical team members who work within the sterile field perform a surgical scrub of their hands and arms with special disinfecting solution and, in addition to the regular surgical attire, don a sterile gown and gloves. This role can also be performed by other personnel than an RN, in which case the person is then called a scrub technician. Other roles for RNs are team leader, assistant head nurse, head nurse or nurse manager, nurse educator, and clinical nurse specialist.

As with any specialty, the perioperative nursing assessment is the first step in providing individualized care for perioperative patients. The nursing process serves as a guide to make perioperative nursing assessments comprehensive and holistic in nature. The focus is aimed at promoting and maintaining wellness as well as identifying and preventing illness (Hurley & McAleavy, 2006). These assessments provide valuable information to the entire perioperative team. The nursing care plans that are developed based on the assessment data are utilized to ensure continuity of care during each phase of the individual's perioperative experience. The assessment provides a baseline against which information about the individual's stability can be measured and monitored at any stage of her perioperative experience.

Perioperative Nursing Education

Given that most nursing programs offer limited or no operating room experience in their curricula, nurses initiating a career in the OR get their perioperative education either at the hiring institution or by enrolling in a postgraduate or fellowship perioperative program. It is estimated that a minimum of 3 to 6 months of instruction is required to adequately educate nurses with no previous OR experience depending on the OR's activities (AORN, 2007a). Programs may include the surgical environment, aseptic technique, perioperative assessment, anesthesia, positioning the surgical patient, sterilization and disinfection, surgical instruments, safety considerations, patient teaching, teamwork, scrubbing and circulating, and wound healing and hemostasis (AORN, 2007a). In addition to didactic modules, nurses are often instructed through a cognitive apprenticeship model in the OR in which they take on increasingly complex responsibilities over time.

Health Promotion

Patient teaching for the **intraoperative** patient is usually done in a preadmission testing clinic or the day before the surgery in a patient general surgical unit. Once in the preoperative area, the patient is normally anxious and stressed and assumes a passive role as the recipient of technical care. The perioperative nurse performs the preoperative assessment of patients in the holding area. The responsibilities of the perioperative nurse in this setting are to verify the appropriate data have been obtained, assess the patient for readiness both physically and emotionally, and reinforce teaching as needed. This information is the basis for planning the patient's individualized perioperative care.

The use of the nursing process emphasizes a patient-centered approach; health promotion in the perioperative arena has become more evident as perioperative nurses have gained great satisfaction from knowing that they are part of a team committed to an individual patient with an individualized outcome. As illustrated through the PNDS (p. 624), this framework enables perioperative nurses to shift from a task-oriented role to that of providing a holistic view of the patient. Therefore, even if the nurse's main role is still to ensure patient safety throughout a patient's surgical experience, the nurse is now able to demonstrate the caring aspect of perioperative nursing by participating in a preoperative assessment of the patient.

Surgical Areas

Patients needing surgery go to the operating room for a surgical procedure after having been admitted to the hospital on the same day as surgery, unless an extensive work-up or in-hospital treatments or tests are required prior to surgery. Patients also access the operating room emergently through the emergency department. The practice of same-day admission has become popular for both financial reasons and because evidence suggests that surgical-site infection rates are reduced when the preoperative stay is reduced (Nichols, 2001).

Prior to being admitted to the surgical setting, the patient dons a gown and cap. Surgical-site skin preparation includes a baseline assessment, cleaning of the surgical site and surrounding area, hair removal, and application of an antiseptic agent when required. Traditionally hair removal was extensive and often performed the day prior to surgery. Research studies have revealed that hair removal does not reduce the incidence of surgical-site infections (SSIs). In fact, today, hair removal is instead performed to improve access to surgical site, improve the field of view, or per the institution's policy or surgeon's preference (Evidence-based practice information sheets, 2003; Niel-Weise, Willie, & van den Broek, 2005). Should hair removal be indicated, care needs to be taken to maintain skin integrity and minimize injury. The removal is ideally done outside of the surgical suite as close to the surgery time as possible (AORN, 2007b). There is some evidence that use of hair clippers is superior to use of a razor, but more research is needed (Niel-Weise et al., 2005).

Presurgical or Preoperative Holding Area

The surgical area typically has a presurgical or preoperative holding area next to the operating rooms. The preoperative holding area is a *semirestricted* area usually just inside of the surgical area. This area provides a quiet, calm transition area for the patient to wait immediately before surgery. It provides a shield from the sights and sounds of the busy surgical suite and allows personnel to interview the patient and verify the documentation. Equipment should be readily available in the preoperative holding area for patient care and monitoring. This includes oxygen, suction, electrocardiogram machine, pulse oximetry, and a blood pressure cuff; an emergency medical cart and defibrillator should be nearby (Bailey, McVey, & Pevreal, 2005; Sullivan, 2000).

In the holding area, the nurse must verify that all the relevant documents and studies (films, scans, etc.) are available prior to the start of the procedure, that they have been reviewed and are consistent with each other, and with the patient involved. Team consensus about the intended patient, procedure, and site and as applicable implant is also needed. This verification should occur before the patient leaves the preoperative area and enters the procedure/surgical room.

When the operating room suite is ready to receive the patient, the patient is asked to empty the bladder to prevent incontinence or overdistention because an overly full bladder can hinder access to the surgical site and predispose the patient to inadvertent surgical bladder injury. Urinary catheterization is performed in the OR as necessary (Iorio et al., 2005). The nurse accompanies the patient to the operating room where the patient will be placed on the operating table and prepared for surgery.

Preoperative Operating Room Checklist

The preoperative checklist is a tool for continuing the patient assessment. On it, allergies are documented as per facility policy. Accurate documentation of height and weight is important for proper dosage calculation of the anesthetic agents. The perioperative nurse ensures that the results of all laboratory, radiographic, and diagnostic tests are on the patient's chart.

Any abnormal results are documented and reported to the surgical team as well as any special needs, concerns, or instructions especially with regard to cultural or spiritual beliefs, physical impairments or limitations, and psychosocial conditions. For example, advise the surgical team whether the patient is a member of Jehovah's Witnesses and does not accept blood products or whether the patient is hard of hearing and does not have his hearing aid (Hurley & McAleavy, 2006). Showing respect for patients' spiritual beliefs, psychosocial conditions, and physical limitations facilitates rapport and trust that enable nurses to understand the important role these factors play in how people cope with fear and anxiety related to their perceived perioperative experience.

The perioperative nurse also notes the medical diagnosis, previous surgical experience, patient's physical appearance, visual skin assessment, medical devices accompanying the patient or indwelling medical devices, and any prostheses, jewelry, dentures, and/or capped teeth. The nurse also ensures that prescribed preoperative medications have been taken by the patient and any medications that have been ordered to be given just prior to surgery such as antibiotics are documented on the chart accompanying the patient. The NPO status of the patient is also confirmed by the nurse to assess any potential risk of aspiration. All relevant information is communicated to the surgical team.

Operating Room

Surgery may involve the removal, repair, drainage, replacement, or exploration of body tissue or organs. The operating room or suite is where the surgery will be performed. This room is a *restricted* area where the team of health care professionals wears attire that was donned in the surgery dressing room. This attire, commonly referred to as "scrubs," includes a shirt, trousers, cap, shoe covers, and mask. Those directly involved in the surgical procedure will have scrubbed and will be wearing sterile gowns.

Surgical hand preparation, previously known as a "surgical scrub," is performed prior to participating in a surgical procedure in order to reduce the potential risk of SSI by reducing the number of microorganisms on intact skin of the hands and forearms. Hand preparation considerations include use of a broad-spectrum, fast-acting, nonirritating, FDA-approved antiseptic agent. Traditional scrub techniques with prolonged use of detergent, water, and brushes have contributed to the deterioration of skin, sometimes leading to undesirable changes of hand skin flora and colonization. Additionally, surgical facilities are examining ways to improve the use of physical resources and health care professionals' time. Compared to the traditional surgical scrub, waterless hand preparation boasts a reduction in microbial counts of hands, improved skin health, and reduced use of time and resources (Larson et al., 2001). Below is a list of recommended surgical hand preparation practices (AORN, 2007b), and Chart 26–1 (p. 622) highlights the differences between a surgical scrub and hand rub preparation method:

- Do not wear artificial nails.
- Keep skin free from open lesions and breaks.
- Remove all jewelry from hands and forearms before performing hand hygiene.
- Use only lotions that are approved by infection control staff; lotions must be compatible with the hand antiseptic and gloves, and be stored in disposable, hands-free dispensers.
- Use a standardized hand scrub procedure that follows manufacturer's written guidelines and is approved by the health care facility.

Due to the rapid growth of surgical technologies and innovation during the past decade, many operating rooms have been renovated or reconstructed. This has been done in part to address the abundance of equipment needed in today's operating rooms as well as ergonomic issues. Recent trends in surgery include the move toward less invasive techniques with shorter hospital stays and faster recovery periods. One of the newest trends promising to transform surgery is the *intelligent OR*. The intelligent OR incorporates advanced robotic surgical systems. A speech recognition robot allows the surgeon to control the operating bed, lighting, video displays, and other devices with simple voice commands. A robotic endoscopic camera facilitates optimal views of the surgical field, and the robotic surgical assistant enables the surgeon to control precise technical movements of a robotic arm from a console station. Robotic systems are currently in use for certain cardiac procedures with plans for expansion on the horizon. Surgical robots make it likely that future surgeries could be performed at one facility with the surgeon operating the console from a distant facility. One of the nurse's roles in robotic surgery is to assist the surgeon at the patient's side during the operation.

In addition digital information is becoming the standard format for accessing patient information and images, for communicating with other areas of the hospital or consultants, and for conferring with other health care providers. The operating

| CHART 26–1 | Traditional and Waterless Surgical Hand Preparation |

Traditional Surgical Hand Preparation

1. Wash hands with soap and water.
2. Use a disposable nail cleaner to clean nail beds under running water. Discard nail cleaner after use.
3. Rinse. Wash hands, then forearms, using antimicrobial-impregnated sponge. Use the counted stroke technique or the recommended amount of time according to the manufacturer's instructions.
4. Rinse.
5. Proceed to operating room.

Note: Step 2 is performed for the first scrub of the day or as required.

Scrub time for step 3 may vary according to product instructions from 3 to 5 minutes.

Waterless Surgical Hand Preparation

1. Wash hands with soap and water.
2. Use a disposable nail cleaner to clean nail beds under running water. Discard nail cleaner after use.
3. Rinse and thoroughly dry hands and arms. Apply alcohol-based surgical hand scrub product according to manufacturer's instructions.
4. Proceed to operating room.

Note: Step 2 is performed for the first scrub of the day or as required. Hand preparation time for step 3 generally requires 2 minutes.

room requires convenient real-time access to these digital data and a way to manage the digital information acquired within the operating room. OR design may be categorized into three major areas: physical, information and communication systems, and management.

To accommodate an optimal workflow and facilitate observation of aseptic technique, certain physical considerations need to be taken into account, including the dimensions of the OR suite, positions of exits and entrances, and location of support services. In addition, integration systems are available that permit the control of medical devices, lighting, and the OR bed; access to images; and the routing of all this digital information to any particular monitor for display or to one or more recording devices for archiving, or to pathologists or radiologists via teleconferencing links. Control can be maintained from the surgical field by touch-screen or voice control interfaces, or from a nursing station (Figure 26–2 ■).

Intentional OR design considers the logistics of flow, maintains versatility, optimizes the use of resources, promotes communication, synchronizes services, and adopts technological advances while including all stakeholders in order to promote

successful adoption. The ultimate goal of surgical technology adoption is to enhance patient care and improve patient outcomes.

Surgical table setup is specific to the procedure, facility, and surgeon preference. Scrub tables are often standardized in order to facilitate efficiency and changeover of staff. Instruments vary according to specialty and type of procedure. Figure 26–3 ■ displays the contrast between traditional open surgery and endoscopic instrumentation.

Other perioperative nursing responsibilities include ensuring proper instrument functionality intraoperatively through cleaning and inspection. Inadvertent patient injury may occur due to an instrument malfunction, resulting in an undesirable effect such as tearing tissue, loss of small parts inside the patient, or improper reprocessing leaving a residue of bioburden that can result in postoperative complications. The use of protocols, checklists, and detailed documentation of OR equipment is associated with a significant decrease in perioperative patient injury (Arbous et al., 2005). The majority of surgical instruments are composed of high-grade stainless steel, although advances in surgery such as robotics and minimally invasive surgery (MIS) have resulted in in-

FIGURE 26–2 ■ Layout of a typical surgical unit. (Note: SDA=Same day surgery, DS=day surgery)

FIGURE 26–3 ■ Surgical instruments : (A) traditional versus (B) endoscopic.
Source: © J. Barabe/Custom Medical Stock Photo

novative discoveries of surgical materials and instruments. Surgical instruments are costly and require proper maintenance and care in order to preserve their longevity.

Patient Preparation

Once they enter the surgical suite, patients are cared for by the anesthetist, surgeons, and nurses. Members of the team ask the patient questions, apply electrocardiogram (ECG) leads, remove arms from gown, and so forth. Every effort should be made to limit activity with the patient until she has received a general anesthetic or been given a relaxant if warranted. For example, a patient should have the bladder catheterized following the general anesthetic whenever possible. Also, patients should be kept informed on an ongoing basis. This will prevent and limit anxieties created by the already stressful surgical experience. If regional anesthesia is being used, the patient will remain awake; therefore, a screen is placed in front of the patient's face. Sedatives, hypnotics, or tranquilizers are administered in order to decrease feelings of anxiety and provide sedation.

The perioperative nurse greets the patient on arrival by first asking the patient his name and checks this with the patient's identification bracelet, chart, and hospital card using at least two identifiers, for example, name and date of birth. The nurse reviews the patient's chart, the medical record, and preoperative checklist, and ensures that the consent is signed and that all documentation, preoperative procedures, and orders have been completed. The nurse conducts the preanesthetic assessment by looking at the patient from a holistic viewpoint. This means recognizing the individual person as a dynamic entity made up of components that are continuously interacting with one another. The perioperative nursing assessment is the first step in providing individualized care to the perioperative patient. To harmonize care in all perioperative settings, the Perioperative Nursing Data Set vocabulary can be used as part of the data collection tool (Chart 26–2, p. 624). The PNDS describes the practice of perioperative nursing practice in four domains: safety, physiological responses, behavioral responses, and health care systems. The first three domains reflect phenomena of concern to perioperative nurses and are composed of nursing diagnoses, interventions, and outcomes that surgical patients and their families experience. The fourth domain, the health care system, comprises structural data elements and focuses on clinical processes and outcomes. The model is used to depict the relationship of nursing process components to the achievement of optimal patient outcomes (AORN, 2002).

Comprehensively written nursing care plans have been specifically adapted to the perioperative environment as clinical pathways. Because of the fast-paced environment of the OR, patients' short lengths of stay, and the many routines, some procedures and protocols can be documented on a flow sheet.

Surgical Approaches

Minimally invasive surgery became widespread when the laparoscopic cholecystectomy became a standard of surgical care in the early 1990s. Initial reservations included the limitations of equipment, introduction of new instruments, and the ability of surgeons to adapt and acquire these new surgical skills. Other concerns included performing surgery on larger patients and the spreading of cancer cells intraoperatively. The latter concerns have been overcome through advances in equipment and instrumentation and adaptive surgical techniques that have enabled the use of laparoscopic gastric bypass surgery for bariatric patients. Study reports confirm MIS to be oncologically safe (Bonjer et al., 2007). The laparoscopic cholecystectomy will be used to illustrate the differences between MIS and open surgery. Open surgery involves an incision under the rib cage on the right side of approximately 15 to 38 cm (6 to 15 in.) in order to allow surgeons access with their hands to perform surgery.

Laparoscopic removal of the gallbladder involves several small incisions, usually four, that are one-quarter to one-half inch in size. Trocars or ports (tubes with valves) are then inserted through these small incisions in order to provide imaging through a telescope attached to a camera for viewing on a monitor while other ports are accessed for instruments used to perform the surgery. To provide space to view and perform surgery, the abdomen is inflated with gas (usually carbon dioxide). Carbon dioxide is used because it is readily accessible, inexpensive, does not support combustion when using surgical energy sources, and is easily absorbed and excreted by the body through the circulatory and respiratory system. In addition, the smaller incisions available with MIS require the use of finer instruments as shown in Figure 26–3b ■ (p. 622) resulting in less surgical trauma and immunosuppression than open surgery (Boo et al., 2007).

Advantages of a laparoscopic surgery over open surgery include less scarring, quicker recovery, shorter hospitalization, faster return to normal activities (work), fewer problems with incisions, less pain, and less use of opioids, which reduces the negative secondary effects associated with opioid use. Often patients undergoing laparoscopic surgery will be discharged the same day as surgery, whereas open surgery procedures can require 3 to 5 days of hospitalization. The intraoperative cost of MIS surgery is often more, but is offset by the reduced hospital stay and quicker recovery (Noblett & Horgan, 2007).

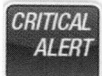 *Many patients complain of discomfort similar to muscle ache in the shoulder area following laparoscopic surgery. This is a referred pain and is due to the distention of the diaphragm, which results from the insufflation of the abdomen with gas that is required for laparoscopic procedures. The discomfort usually subsides within 24 to 48 hours postoperatively.*

The Future of Surgery: Natural Orifice Transluminal Endoscopic Surgery

Natural Orifice Transluminal Endoscopic Surgery (NOTES) is the exploration of methods to perform surgery through any of the body's natural orifices (e.g., oral, rectal, urethral, vaginal). NOTES attempts to further minimize the effects of surgery through a totally noninvasive technique.

Anesthesia

Advances in anesthesia, such as improvements in airway devices, use of quickly reversible inhalation agents, and selection of short-acting anesthetic agents, have improved patient outcomes (Arbous et al., 2005; Tarrac, 2006). Anesthesia needs to accomplish several things. It must produce sleep (hypnosis), lack of

CHART 26–2	**Perioperative Nursing Data Set**			
Code	**Diagnosis/Intervention/Outcome**	**Yes**	**No**	**Comments**
X29	Diagnosis: *Risk of Injury* related to transfer and transport			
I26	Intervention: Confirms identity before the operative or invasive procedure.			
I126	Intervention: Verifies operative procedure.			
I60	Intervention: Identifies baseline tissue perfusion.			
I65	Intervention: Identifies physiological barriers to communication.			
I66	Intervention: Identifies physiological status.			
I59	Intervention: Identifies baseline cardiac function.			
I64	Intervention: Identifies physical alterations that may affect procedure-specific positioning.			
	AORN Outcome: Patient is free from signs and symptoms of injury related to transfer/transport.			
X4	Diagnosis: *Risk for Anxiety* related to knowledge deficit and stress of surgery			
I13	Intervention: Assesses coping mechanisms based on psychological status.			
I27	Intervention: Provides continuity of care.			
I30	Intervention: Develops individualized plan of care.			
I57	Intervention: Identifies and reports philosophical, cultural, and spiritual beliefs and values.			
I85	Intervention: Minimizes the length of invasive procedure by planning care.			
I101	Intervention: Provides care to each individual in a manner that preserves and protects the patient's autonomy, dignity, and human rights.			
I106	Intervention: Provides instruction based on age and identified need.			
I56	Intervention: Explains expected sequence of events.			
I50	Intervention: Evaluates response to instructions.			
	AORN Outcome: Patient participates in decision making affecting the perioperative plan of care.			
X38	Diagnosis: *Risk for Acute/Chronic Pain*			
I24	Intervention: Collaborates in initiating patient-controlled analgesia.			
I51	Intervention: Evaluates response to medication.			
I61	Intervention: Identifies cultural and value components related to pain.			
I69	Intervention: Implements alternative methods of pain control.			
I71	Intervention: Implements pain guidelines.			
I108	Intervention: Provides pain management instructions.			
I16	Intervention: Assesses pain control.			
I54	Intervention: Evaluates response to pain management interventions.			
	AORN Outcome: Patient demonstrates and/or reports adequate pain control throughout the perioperative period.			
X28	Diagnosis: *Risk for Infection*			
I3	Intervention: Administers care to invasive device sites.			
I21	Intervention: Assesses susceptibility for infections.			
I22	Intervention: Classifies surgical wound.			
I94	Intervention: Performs skin preparation.			
I31	Intervention: Dresses wound at completion of procedure.			
	AORN Outcome: Patient is free from signs and symptoms of infection.			
X29	Diagnosis: *Risk for Injury*			
I11	Intervention: Applies safety devices.			
I39	Intervention: Evaluates for signs and symptoms of injury to skin and tissue.			
I72	Intervention: Implements protective measures to prevent injury due to electrical sources.			
I73	Intervention: Implements protective measures to prevent injury due to laser sources.			
I77	Intervention: Implements protective measures to prevent skin/tissue injury due to mechanical sources.			
I93	Intervention: Performs required counts.			
I84	Intervention: Manages specimen handling and disposition.			
I112	Intervention: Records devices implanted during the operative or invasive procedure.			
	AORN Outcome: Patient is free from signs and symptoms of physical injury.			
X40	Diagnosis: *Risk for Injury: Positioning*			
I38	Intervention: Applies safety devices.			
I39	Intervention: Evaluates for signs and symptoms of injury to skin and tissue.			
I77	Intervention: Implements protective measures to prevent skin/tissue injury due to mechanical devices.			
	AORN Outcome: Patient is free from signs and symptoms of injury related to positioning.			

CHART 26–2 Perioperative Nursing Data Set—*Continued*

Code	Diagnosis/Intervention/Outcome	Yes	No	Comments
X30	Diagnosis: *Deficient Knowledge*			
I19	Intervention: Assesses readiness to learn based on physiological status.			
I20	Intervention: Assesses readiness to learn based on psychological status.			
I79	Intervention: Includes family and support persons in the preoperative teaching.			
I103	Intervention: Provides information and explains Patient Self-Determination Act.			
I67	Intervention: Identifies psychological barriers to communication.			
I63	Intervention: Identifies individual values and wishes concerning care.			
I30	Intervention: Develops individualized plan of care.			
I104	Intervention: Provides instruction about prescribed medications.			
I105	Intervention: Provides instruction about wound healing and wound care.			
	AORN Outcome: Patient demonstrates knowledge of the expected responses to the operative or other invasive procedure.			

Source: Reprinted with permission from "PNDS unique coding document, in *Perioperative Nursing Data Set*; http://www.aorn.org/PracticeResources/PNDSAndStandardizedPerioperativeRecord/PNDSResources. Copyright © 2007 AORN, Inc., 2170 South Parker Road, Suite 300, Denver, CO 80231. All rights reserved. Note that the PNDS codes are being extensively restructured and revised; this example is for illustration purposes only.

awareness and recall (amnesia), freedom from pain (analgesia), and muscle relaxation. A variety of anesthetic agents can produce these effects. The anesthesia care provider considers the patient and selects the agent or a combination of agents that will produce the best anesthesia with the fewest negative effects for the patient.

Inhalation Agents

Inhalation agents are frequently used for anesthesia because they are fast acting and easily controlled. Anesthetic agents pass through a vaporizer and are mixed with oxygen. The patient inhales the vapors into the lungs. The gas crosses the alveolar membrane, dissolves in the blood, and is carried to body tissues via circulation where it attaches to receptor sites on the cells to produce its effects, primarily depression of the central nervous system (CNS). Frequently, a mixture of gases is used to maintain anesthesia.

A number of theories have been proposed to explain how inhaled anesthetic agents work, but no single theory explains the various effects seen with these agents (Hoffer, 1999). The effects of anesthesia diminish as the gas is washed out of the lungs with 100% oxygen and the remainder is metabolized by the liver. The Pharmacology Summary box (p. 626) lists the advantages, the side effects, and implications of commonly used anesthetic gases.

Intravenous Agents

A variety of intravenous (IV) agents are used to induce and maintain anesthesia. The Pharmacology Summary box (p. 627) lists common intravenous medications used for anesthesia or as adjuncts to anesthesia. Induction of anesthesia may be accomplished with the administration of a sedative hypnotic or anxiolytic drug. Common drugs include barbiturates such as thiopental sodium (Pentothal) and sodium methohexital (Brevital). These drugs cause rapid, short-acting depression of the CNS (sedative hypnotic), but they have limited analgesic effects. A smaller test dose is initially given to make sure the patient tolerates the mediation without reaction. These drugs quickly (within seconds) produce sedation and unconsciousness. Both drugs can cause respiratory and cardiovascular depression.

Nonbarbiturate drugs that depress the CNS may also be used to induce anesthesia. Etomidate (Amidate) produces rapid hypnosis but with less effect on the respiratory and cardiovascular systems than the barbiturate drugs. This makes it an attractive alternative for use with high-risk patients. Etomidate suppresses cortisol secretion causing hypotension. These effects are not significant in short procedures but can be an issue in longer surgeries. Etomidate is used primarily in short procedures. Ketamine hydrochloride (Ketalar) is a fast-acting CNS depressant that causes profound anesthesia but little skeletal muscle relaxation. It is associated with a difficult emergence phase that is characterized by hallucinations and disassociative feelings (feeling separate from the environment). The patient who is recovering from ketamine will do better in a quiet, supportive environment. Propofol (Diprivan) is a rapid-acting hypnotic that causes minimal excitation effects during induction. Risk of the patient's vomiting or thrashing during induction is reduced. A test dose is initially given to test for allergy. Propofol is metabolized rapidly so it does not accumulate in the blood when used to maintain anesthesia. Patients emerge from propofol quite quickly during the recovery period.

Other IV medications used in anesthesia include benzodiazepines and opioid analgesics. Examples of benzodiazepines include midazolam (Versed), lorazepam (Ativan), and diazepam (Valium). The benzodiazepines are antianxiety agents that also have hypnotic, sedative, and muscle relaxant effects. Midazolam is sometimes used to induce anesthesia but these drugs are more commonly used as premedication to reduce the patient's anxiety because they have an amnesic effect. Benzodiazepines are used in combination with other drugs to produce **conscious sedation** or as adjuncts to regional anesthesia to produce sedation and muscle relaxation. Opioids are used in anesthesia for their analgesic effect. Common medications include morphine sulfate, fentanyl citrate (Sublimaze), sufentanil, and alfentanil. Fentanyl is more potent than morphine and is the most commonly used analgesic in anesthesia. The opioid analgesics have good cardiovascular stability but cause respiratory depression.

PHARMACOLOGY Summary of Anesthetic Gases Used During Surgery

Agent	Action and Advantages	Disadvantages and Side Effects	Nursing Responsibility
Desflurane (Suprane)	Maintenance of anesthesia. Very rapid emergence. Good degree of muscle relaxation.	Must be heated to vaporize. Causes increase in heart rate and decrease in blood pressure. Has a strong odor precluding its use for induction of anesthesia. May cause coughing if used for induction.	Monitor for hypotension.
Enflurane (Ethrane)	Maintenance of anesthesia. Good degree of muscle relaxation.	May lower the threshold for seizures. Increases heart rate and decreases blood pressure.	Monitor for hypotension. Contraindicated in patients with seizure disorders.
Halothane (Fluothane)	Maintenance of anesthesia. Rapid induction and emergence but less than that of isoflurane. Low incidence of postoperative nausea and vomiting.	Fair degree of muscle relaxation. Increases heart rate and triggers arrhythmias. Requires a higher degree of liver metabolization than other agents. Causes postoperative shivering.	Can cause hypotension. Monitor for premature ventricular contractions, ventricular tachycardia, and ventricular fibrillation with use of epinephrine. Provide warm blankets during recovery period.
Isoflurane (Forane)	Induction and maintenance of anesthesia. Faster induction and recovery than enflurane or halothane. Minimal metabolization by the liver.	Causes increase in heart rate and hypotension. Hypotension can be unpredictable and severe if concomitant use of antihypertensive agents. Weak stimulation of secretions.	Monitor for hypotension.
Nitrous oxide	Rapid induction and recovery of anesthesia. When used with other inhalants, it reduces the concentration of other agent.	Does not produce muscle relaxation.	
Sevoflurane (Ultane)	Induction and maintenance of anesthesia. Very rapid induction and recovery (3–4 minutes faster than Isoflurane). Minimal metabolization by the liver.		

Sources: Adams, M., Josephson, D., & Holland, L. (2008). *Pharmacology for nurses: A pathophysiological approach.* Upper Saddle River, NJ: Pearson Prentice Hall; Ebert, T. J. (2004). *Physiology of the cardiovascular effects of general anesthesia in the elderly.* Retrieved April 26, 2004, from the ASA Syllabus on Geriatric Anesthesiology website: http://www.asahq.org/clinical/geriatrics/phy. htm; Hoffer, J. L. (1999). Anesthesia. In M. Meeker & J. Rothrock (Eds.), *Care of the patient in surgery* (pp. 203–238). Philadelphia: Mosby; Thompson, A. M. (2002). Anaesthesia. In L. Shields & H. Werder (Eds.), *Perioperative nursing* (pp. 79–105). San Francisco: Greenwich Medical Media.

Muscle Relaxants

Muscle relaxants (neuromuscular blocking agents) primarily affect skeletal muscle and they are used in surgery to facilitate endotracheal intubation and to provide optimal operating conditions. A rapid-acting neuromuscular blocking agent is administered before intubation to paralyze the muscles of the jaw and vocal cords making placement of the endotracheal tube easier. Muscle relaxation is used throughout the surgery to facilitate dissection of tissue. During surgery, the anesthesia care provider monitors the effects of muscle relaxant drugs with a peripheral nerve stimulator. Recovery from neuromuscular blocking agents after surgery is evidenced by the patient's ability to breathe on her own and hold her head upright as well as the presence of a strong hand grasp. There are two types of neuromuscular blocking agents, depolarizing and nondepolarizing.

Succinylcholine is a depolarizing agent and the only one in clinical use. The drug has a strong affinity for acetylcholine receptor sites and once it attaches to the site causes continuous depolarization of the motor end plate. Continuous muscle contractions and fasciculations are followed by flaccid paralysis of the muscles. The onset of paralysis is quick with intravenous administration, 30 to 60 seconds, and the effects last up to 10 minutes. Often succinylcholine is used for intubation because it works very quickly and wears off quickly, but there are disadvantages to the drug. The depolarization of muscle cells causes a transient increase in serum potassium that can produce cardiac dysrhythmia. Muscle fasciculation (twitching) leads the patient to complain of muscle soreness postoperatively. Succinylcholine is known to trigger malignant hyperthermia in susceptible individuals. The drug is broken down by the plasma enzyme cholinesterase. Prolonged paralysis occurs in individuals with insufficient amounts of cholinesterase although this condition is rare.

Nondepolarizing agents work by blocking the depolarizing action of acetylcholine at the motor end plate of the neuromuscular junction, thereby producing muscle paralysis. Muscle fasciculations do not occur with these drugs, eliminating postoperative myalgia. Another advantage is that these agents can be antagonized or reversed with the administration of neostigmine, edrophonium, or pyridostigmine. Use of reversal agents reduces the risk of morbidity associated with anesthesia

PHARMACOLOGY Summary of Intravenous Anesthetic Agents and Other Adjuncts to Anesthesia Used During Surgery

Agent	Action and Advantages	Disadvantages and Side Effects	Nursing Responsibility
Intravenous Anesthetic			
Etomidate (Amidate)	CNS depressant used for induction and maintenance of anesthesia for short procedures. Hypnotic effect but no analgesia. Fewer respiratory and cardiovascular effects than other agents. Onset is 60 seconds with duration of 3–5 minutes.	Suppresses cortisol secretion. Postoperative nausea and vomiting. May cause transient skeletal muscle movements. Metabolized in the liver.	Good anesthetic for patients with asthma or cardiovascular disease. Used in neurosurgery because it causes a slight decrease in intracranial pressure. Monitor cortisol levels and blood pressure.
Diazepam (Valium)	Benzodiazepine with hypnotic and amnesiac properties. Used as adjunct drug in induction of anesthesia and as a preoperative medication to reduce anxiety.	May cause hypotension and tachycardia. Prolonged effect.	Monitor sedation postoperatively.
Ketamine (Ketalar)	CNS depressant used for induction of anesthesia. May supplement nitrous oxide anesthesia. Fewer postoperative nausea and vomiting than other agents.	Increases salivary secretions. Does not produce muscle relaxation. May increase heart rate and blood pressure. Depresses respirations and increases intracranial pressure. Associated with emergence reactions including hallucinations, dissociative feelings, and irrational behavior. Recovery can be prolonged.	Premedicate with anticholinergic agent to reduce secretions. Provide a quiet, calm, reassuring environment for recovery. Monitor heart rate and blood pressure. Monitor airway to prevent aspiration.
Midazolam (Versed)	Benzodiazepine with hypnotic, amnesiac, anxiolytic, and muscle relaxant properties. Used for induction of general anesthesia and for conscious sedation.	Slower induction than with barbiturates. May cause hypotension and tachycardia.	Prepare patient for amnesia. Monitor for respiratory depression.
Propofol (Diprivan)	CSN depressant used for induction and maintenance of anesthesia. Rapid onset with minimal excitation during induction.	Abnormal muscle movement. May cause hypotension.	Monitor blood pressure. Cautious use in patients with allergies to eggs.
Sodium methohexital (Brevital)	Barbiturate used for induction and maintenance of anesthesia. More potent and with a shorter onset and quicker recovery than thiopental.	May cause abnormal muscle movements, coughing, and laryngospasm. Hypotension occurs in some patients. Hiccups may persist postoperatively.	Patient should be recumbent during administration. Monitor blood pressure.
Thiopental sodium (Pentothal)	Barbiturate used for induction and maintenance of anesthesia. Depresses CNS causing sedation and hypnosis. Ultrashort acting with onset in 10–20 seconds and duration of 20–30 minutes.	Depresses respiratory and circulatory function. Can cause anaphylaxis and laryngospasm. Metabolized by the liver.	Test dose given first.
Opioid Analgesics			
Alfentanil (Alfenta)	Narcotic used for induction, analgesia, and balanced anesthesia. Rapid onset and short duration make it a good choice for short surgical procedures.	Causes respiratory depression. Can cause bradycardia and hypotension. Bradycardia is more likely in patients who are taking a beta-blocking drug. Nausea and vomiting common.	Monitor vital signs. Report bradycardia.

(continued)

PHARMACOLOGY **Summary of Intravenous Anesthetic Agents and Other Adjuncts to Anesthesia Used During Surgery—*Continued***

Agent	Action and Advantages	Disadvantages and Side Effects	Nursing Responsibility
Fentanyl (Sublimaze)	Narcotic used as adjunct for induction to anesthesia and for analgesia supplement. The drug of choice for epidural analgesia. Short acting. Causes less nausea and vomiting than morphine.	Causes sedation and respiratory depression. May also cause bradycardia and hypotension.	Monitor vital signs. Watch for signs of respiratory depression.
Morphine sulfate	Narcotic used as premedication and for postoperative analgesia. Long-lasting effect.	Causes respiratory depression. Histamine release causes peripheral vasodilation and hypotension. Nausea and vomiting common.	Monitor vital signs.
Sufentanil (Sufenta)	Narcotic used for analgesic supplement in balanced anesthesia. More potent than fentanyl. Has a quicker onset and shorter recovery than fentanyl. Not associated with histamine release so there is less hypotensive effect.	Prolonged respiratory depression.	Monitor vital signs. Watch for signs of respiratory depression.
Depolarizing Muscle Relaxants			
Succinylcholine	Depolarizing neuroblocking agent with high affinity for acetylcholine receptor sites. Produces muscle relaxation and paralysis. Used to facilitate endotracheal intubation and to produce skeletal muscle relaxation for short surgical procedures. Short-acting agent with onset in 30–60 seconds and duration of several minutes.	Causes muscle fasciculations, bradycardia, and respiratory depression. May precipitate malignant hyperthermia in susceptible individuals.	Monitor vital signs. Maintain airway and clear secretions. Patient may complain of muscle soreness postoperatively.
Nondepolarizing Muscle Relaxants—Intermediate			
Mivacurium (Mivacron)	Intermediate, nondepolarizing muscle relaxant used for endotracheal intubation and to produce relaxation of skeletal muscles for surgery. Effect lasts 15–20 minutes.	Transient hypotension and bradycardia. Metabolized by plasma cholinesterase.	Monitor vital signs.
Vecuronium (Norcuron)	Intermediate, nondepolarizing muscle relaxant used for endotracheal intubation and to produce relaxation of skeletal muscles for surgery. Effect lasts 20–40 minutes.	Metabolized by the liver. Causes respiratory depression. Minimal cardiovascular effects.	Monitor for delay of recovery postoperatively.
Nondepolarizing Muscle Relaxants—Long Acting			
Tubocurarine	Long-acting, nondepolarizing muscle relaxant used for maintenance of relaxation during surgery. Muscle relaxant effects last 30–40 minutes.	Causes histamine release with hypotension. Increases bronchial and salivary secretions.	Monitor blood pressure and airway until full recovery from drug. Observe for residual muscle weakness.
Metocurine (Metubine)	Long-acting, nondepolarizing muscle relaxant used for maintenance of relaxation during surgery. Muscle relaxant effects last 30–90 minutes.	Hypotension, increased salivary secretions, and respiratory depression.	Monitor blood pressure and airway until full recovery. May take several hours for complete neuromuscular recovery.

PHARMACOLOGY Summary of Intravenous Anesthetic Agents and Other Adjuncts to Anesthesia Used During Surgery—*Continued*

Agent	Action and Advantages	Disadvantages and Side Effects	Nursing Responsibility
Pancuronium (Pavulon)	Long-acting, nondepolarizing muscle relaxant used for maintenance of relaxation during surgery. Muscle relaxant effects last 30–60 minutes.	Tachycardia, hypertension, and premature ventricular contractions.	Monitor vital signs.
Anticholinergics			
Atropine	Anticholinergic agent used to decrease salivary and respiratory secretions, to treat bradycardia and/or hypotension, and to reverse muscle relaxants.	Tachycardia, hypertension, urinary retention, and dry mouth. May cause cardiac arrhythmias.	Monitor heart rate and blood pressure. Heart rate is best indicator of response to the drug.
Glycopyrrolate (Robinul)	Anticholinergic agent used to decrease salivary and respiratory secretions and to reverse neuromuscular block.	Tachycardia, urinary retention, and dry mouth. Fewer problems with cardiac arrhythmias than atropine.	Monitor heart rate.

Sources: Adams, M., Josephson, D., & Holland, L. (2005). *Pharmacology for nurses: A pathophysiological approach.* Upper Saddle River, NJ: Pearson Prentice Hall; Ebert, T. J. (2004). *Physiology of the cardiovascular effects of general anesthesia in the elderly.* Retrieved April 26, 2004, from the ASA Syllabus on Geriatric Anesthesiology website: http://www.asahq.org/clinical/geriatrics/phy. htm; Hoffer, J. L. (1999). Anesthesia. In M. Meeker & J. Rothrock (Eds.), *Care of the patient in surgery* (pp. 203–238). Philadelphia: Mosby; Thompson, A. M. (2002). Anaesthesia. In L. Shields & H. Werder (Eds.), *Perioperative nursing* (pp. 79–105). San Francisco: Greenwich Medical Media.

(Arbous et al., 2005). Reversal drugs cause bradycardia, which is treated with atropine or glycopyrrolate. Nondepolarizing agents are divided into intermediate acting and long acting. Intermediate-acting agents have a quick onset, 60 seconds or less, and last 25 to 40 minutes. Examples of intermediate-acting nondepolarizing agents are vecuronium, atracurium, and mivacurium. Longer acting nondepolarizing muscle relaxants also have a rapid onset but last 45 to 60 minutes. Examples include pancuronium, metocurine, and tubocurarine.

Complications of General Anesthesia

The majority of patients experience **general anesthesia** without problems except for the complaint of a sore throat from the endotracheal tube. Other problems that may occur with intubation are damage to teeth or dental work and trauma to the vocal cords. Complications that arise from general anesthesia include hypoxia, hypotension, hypertension, cardiac dysrhythmia, residual muscle paralysis, hypothermia, and malignant hyperthermia.

A drop in body temperature is common during surgery. Anesthesia interferes with the physiological mechanisms of thermoregulation. This effect combined with environmental factors such as the ambient temperature in the OR, the exposure of body cavities, and the administration of cold solutions (e.g., blood products, IV fluids) or irrigants leads to a reduction in core body temperature. Studies show the most significant drop in body temperature occurs during the first hour of anesthesia (Hasankhani, Mohammadi, Moazzami, Mokhtari, & Naghgizadh, 2007; Sessler & Todd, 2000; Wagner, 2006). Monitoring body temperature and using warming devices during surgery (e.g., blankets, thermal drapes, fluid warmers) is imperative (Hasankhani et al., 2007; Wagner, 2006). Research supports the use of forced-air warming blankets as the most effective method of preventing or treating hypothermia (American Society of

PeriAnesthesia Nurses, 2001). Some suggest that using a forced-air warming blanket for 30 minutes prior to surgery helps prevent intraoperative hypothermia and improve patient outcomes (Bitner, Hilde, Hall, & Duvendack, 2007).

Malignant Hyperthermia

Malignant hyperthermia (MH) is a rare but life-threatening complication of anesthesia. The predisposition for MH is genetically transmitted by an autosomal dominant trait. It is thought that MH is triggered by the medications or agents used in general anesthesia with the most common being succinylcholine or one of the inhalant anesthetics. Other factors such as stress, trauma, fatigue, or muscle injury may play a role in increasing susceptibility to the condition or in modifying the patient's response to the condition. Malignant hyperthermia occurs most commonly during induction of anesthesia although it may present anytime during the surgery or early postoperative period.

Malignant hyperthermia is not well understood. With MH, calcium levels within skeletal muscle cells increase, although the reasons for this are not known. The elevation in intracellular calcium activates muscle rigidity and spasm and a hypermetabolic state. The increase in cellular metabolism leads to an increase in carbon dioxide production (hypercarbia) and a metabolic acidosis. As the process continues, the patient becomes hypoxic, hyperthermic, and develops dysrhythmias and hypotension. Muscle breakdown with the release of myoglobins leads to myoglobinuria and an increased risk of renal failure. Damaged muscle cells release intracellular potassium and creatinine phosphokinase (CPK) into the circulation.

The presentation of MH is variable. Early signs are masseter spasm (contracture of jaw), sinus tachycardia, and an increase in expiratory carbon dioxide levels. The anesthesia provider first suspects MH by the rise in the patient's expired CO_2, which is monitored throughout the surgery. An end-tidal carbon dioxide level that is two to three times normal is the earliest and most definitive sign of MH (Redmond, 2001). Other signs are rigor of muscles, hypoxemia evidenced by a drop in oxygen saturation, and tea-colored urine, indicating the presence of myoglobins. Laboratory blood tests results show metabolic acidosis and increases in serum calcium, potassium, and creatinine phosphokinase. Hyperthermia is a late sign and temperature elevations can be extreme with increases of 1 to 2 degrees every few minutes. Other late signs are cardiac dysrhythmia and hypotension.

Malignant hyperthermia can be fatal. The key to treatment is early recognition of the syndrome, immediate discontinuation of the triggering agent, administration of dantrolene sodium to produce muscle relaxation, and providing supportive care. Following emergency treatment, the patient is monitored in the intensive care unit for 24 hours or longer because a small percentage of patients experience a reoccurrence of MH (Redmond, 2001). Chart 26–3 summarizes the management of the patient with malignant hyperthermia.

Other Complications

Other adverse events or complications may occur in the operating room as a result of the surgical procedure. Examples include such things as bleeding with excessive blood loss or inadvertent injury to surrounding organs or tissues. Intraoperative complication rates depend on the surgery, the type of anesthesia, and the patient's physical status. In studies of complications associated with various procedures (e.g., abdominal, spinal, orthopedic, and urologic), 3% to 4% of patients experience intraoperative complications (Rampersaud et al., 2006; Tarrac, 2006).

CHART 26–3	**Management of the Patient with Malignant Hyperthermia**

- Immediately discontinue triggering agent.
- Stop surgery if possible. Otherwise, deepen anesthesia with opioids, sedatives, nondepolarizing muscle relaxants.
- Hyperventilate with 100% oxygen.
- Administer a bolus of dantrolene sodium (Dantrium) 2 to 3 mg/kg intravenously with additional bolus doses up to 10 mg/kg until decreased signs of hypercarbia.
- Administer cooling devices: Apply cooling blanket, use iced normal saline intravenously, lavage open body cavities with iced saline.
- Hydrate with intravenous normal saline.
- Maintain a urine output greater than 2 mL/kg per hour. Administer furosemide and/or mannitol if urine output is less than goal.
- Treat metabolic acidosis with intravenous sodium bicarbonate if it does not self-correct with treatment.
- Treat hyperkalemia with intravenous sodium bicarbonate, 10 units of regular insulin with dextrose intravenously.
- Treat cardiac arrhythmia if it does not self-correct with treatment. Do not use calcium channel blockers.
- Continue to monitor vital signs, oxygen saturation, electrocardiogram, urine output, arterial blood gases, and blood chemistry.
- Transfer to Intensive Care Unit for postoperative care.

Source: Reprinted from Perianesthesia recognition, treatment and care. Redmond, M.C. Copyright 2007, with permission from Elsevier. Retrieved on July 2, 2008 from http://aspan. org/EdCeMalHyper.htm#head 11

Regional Anesthesia

Regional anesthesia is a general classification of anesthesia that includes spinal and epidural anesthesia, peripheral nerve blocks, Bier blocks, and local anesthesia. The common feature of all types of regional anesthesia is the local injection of a medication to block the transmission of sensory impulses from that area to the brain, thus, effectively blocking the sensation of pain. Regional anesthesia has some advantages over general anesthesia. Usually, regional anesthesia does not depress respirations so the patient is at lower risk of postoperative respiratory complications. This makes regional anesthesia a good choice for patients with severe cardiopulmonary disease. Patients who receive a regional anesthetic usually experience less postoperative nausea and vomiting.

Regional anesthesia can be used for any number of surgeries. It is commonly used for repair of inguinal hernia, transurethral resection of the prostate, gynecologic procedures, and arthroscopies and other orthopedic surgeries including repair of hip fractures in the elderly. Typically, patients scheduled for regional anesthesia are premedicated in the holding area with an antianxiety agent to produce mild to moderate sedation. Opioid analgesics may be administered to reduce the pain associated with the insertion of needles and the administration of numbing agents.

Spinal Anesthesia

Spinal anesthesia, also called **intrathecal anesthesia**, is the injection of a local anesthetic into the subarachnoid space and directly into the cerebrospinal fluid (CSF). The anesthetic blocks nerve fibers (i.e., sensory, motor, and sympathetic) at the level of the spinal cord. Spinal anesthesia effectively blocks motor and sensory nerves so that the patient cannot move the affected area (temporary paralysis) or feel pain, touch, temperature, or pressure. The spinal needle is inserted between the 2nd and 3rd lumbar vertebrae (L^2–L^3) or the 3rd and 4th vertebrae (L^3–L^4). For insertion, the patient is placed in a sitting position or in a side-lying position with their head and knees flexed (i.e., fetal position). A spinal needle is inserted in the intervertebral space through the dura mater and into the subarachnoid space. Special spinal needles called *pencil point needles* enter the dura mater by separating the fibers rather than cutting them, reducing the risk of a CSF leak after the needle is removed.

Commonly, spinal anesthesia includes the administration of local anesthetics such as lidocaine, bupivacaine (Marcaine), or chloroprocaine combined with an opioid analgesic such as fentanyl or preservative-free morphine. The medication may be mixed with a dextrose solution to create a hyperbaric solution (i.e., a solution that is heavier than CSF). Once a hyperbaric solution is injected into the CSF, it travels by gravity. The anesthesiologist may have the patient sit for a few minutes to create a block in the lower extremities or place the patient supine with the head tilted slightly downward to create a higher block. After 10 to 15 minutes, the block sets and does not extend further.

Epidural Anesthesia

Epidural anesthesia is the injection of a local anesthetic into the epidural space. The epidural space is located adjacent to the dura mater and contains fat, tissue, and blood vessels. Anesthetic injected into the epidural space affects nerve roots as they leave the spinal cord and some medication diffuses across the dura mater into the subarachnoid space and the CSF. The anesthetic spreads in both directions (i.e., cephalad and caudad) from the site of the injection, and positioning has less effect on movement of the medication than it does with spinal anesthesia.

The same medications used in spinal anesthesia are used in epidural anesthesia, but the concentration of the drugs is greater because they must diffuse across several layers of tissue. The onset of epidural anesthesia is slower than that of spinal anesthesia. A test dose of lidocaine with epinephrine is injected to make sure that the needle is correctly placed in the epidural space and not in the subarachnoid space or in a vein. If the needle is mistakenly in a vein, the test dose produces transient tachycardia; if it is in the subarachnoid space, it produces mild numbness. Frequently, an epidural catheter remains in place after the operation to provide postoperative pain control. Caudal anesthesia is the administration of a local anesthetic into the epidural space, but the approach is through the caudal canal in the sacrum rather than through the lumbar vertebrae.

Complications of Spinal or Epidural Anesthesia
Spinal anesthesia may be complicated by the development of headache, hypotension, and meningitis. Spinal headache or post–dural puncture headache (PDPH) is a common postoperative complaint. PDPH is caused by the leaking of CSF through the hole in the dura (e.g., the puncture site). The loss of CSF causes irritation of meningeal nerves and vessels (Hyderally, 2002). Because PDPH develops or worsens when the patient moves to an upright position, patients may be restricted to bed rest for the first 8 to 24 hours postoperatively to reduce the incidence of spinal headache. When headache develops, it is located in the occipital area and resolves in 1 to 3 days. Patients who develop a headache are treated with hydration and analgesics. The patient is placed on bed rest with the head of the bed maintained at less than 30 degrees to reduce CSF leak. PDPH that does not resolve quickly or that produces an intolerable headache may be treated with a "blood patch." The anesthesiologist injects 5 to 10 mL of autologous blood into the epidural space at the site of puncture to seal the leak.

Whereas PDPH occurs postoperatively, hypotension is more likely to occur while anesthesia is still being administered. Hypotension is caused by vasodilation associated with the blocking of sympathetic nerves. When sympathetic nerves are blocked by anesthesia, arteries and veins lose muscle tone and the ability to constrict. This decreases venous return from the extremities and reduces cardiac output. Hypotension can occur with both spinal and epidural anesthesia. Hypotension is avoided with the administration of fluid volume usually normal saline. Medications with strong alpha-adrenergic stimulation effects, such as ephedrine or phenylephrine, are used to prevent or treat hypotension.

Spinal anesthesia is associated with a low risk of aseptic meningitis. When it does occur, signs develop within the first 24 hours after surgery (Hyderally, 2002). The patient presents with the typical signs of meningitis, fever, headache, nuchal rigidity, and photophobia.

Peripheral Nerve Blocks
A **peripheral nerve block** is the injection of a local anesthetic into or around a nerve plexus to produce anesthesia of a selected area. The major advantage of a nerve block is that anesthesia is confined to the area of the surgery and does not have a systemic effect. Long-acting local anesthetics used in the nerve block provide extended control of pain postoperatively. The local anes-

thetic blocks motor, sensory, and sympathetic nerves. Frequently, epinephrine is administered with the local anesthetic. Epinephrine causes vasoconstriction of the area and decreases vascular uptake of the medication, thus prolonging the effect of the local anesthetic. The duration of the block depends on the choice of anesthetic, the volume and concentration of the drug, and the site being injected. Frequently, nerve blocks are administered by anesthesia in the holding area because they may take anywhere from 5 to 30 minutes to take effect.

A nerve block can be performed in a number of different sites. For example, an interscalene or axillary block of the brachial plexus is done for surgeries on the shoulder, forearm, or elbow. Surgery on the lower leg may be accomplished using a femoral or sciatic block. Peripheral nerve blocks are used alone or in combination with general anesthesia. When used with general anesthesia, the amount of general anesthesia can be reduced. Complications that can occur with nerve blocks include hematoma at the site of the block, nerve damage, and toxicity from systemic absorption of local anesthetic. Other, specific complications depend on the site where the block is administered.

Peripheral nerve blocks may be performed as outpatient surgeries. Patients are taught that recovery of motor function occurs first followed by recovery of sensation. Note that while the area is numb, the patient is at risk for inadvertently injuring the area.

A **Bier block** is a specific type of peripheral nerve block that is administered intravenously, but certain techniques are used to trap the anesthetic in the local area. Bier blocks may be used for surgeries on an extremity, usually the arm. An IV catheter is inserted in the extremity at the most distal site possible. A pneumatic tourniquet is applied proximal to the surgical site and inflated higher than the patient's systolic blood pressure. When the local anesthetic (lidocaine) is injected intravenously, the obstruction of blood by the tourniquet prevents it from leaving the surgical area. At the completion of the surgery, the tourniquet is intermittently deflated so that the lidocaine enters the patient's general circulation slowly, preventing a toxic reaction to the anesthetic.

■ Nursing Management

The verification process consists of information gathering and verification, which begins with the determination to do the procedure and continues through all settings and interventions involved in the preoperative preparation of the patient, up to and including the time-out (discussed later) just before the start of the procedure.

Assessment

The nurse asks the patient to confirm the procedure to be completed, the surgical site, and the surgeon. The nurse verifies this information with the surgical consent form, a site verification form per organization policy, and the operating room schedule. In some cases, especially when there is a left or right side involved in the procedure, the correct area for surgery is marked on the patient. Per the AORN (2008) correct site surgery position statement, a comprehensive approach is needed in each health care delivery system to prevent wrong site surgery. In 2003 AORN and the American College of Surgeons developed national guidelines that are to be used with every patient having surgery to eliminate inadvertently operating on the wrong surgical site (see the National Guidelines box, p. 632).

NATIONAL GUIDELINES AORN Guidelines for Eliminating Wrong Site Surgery

The following guidelines are supported by both AORN and the American College of Surgeons.

1. Verify that the correct patient is being taken to the operating room. This verification can be made with the patient or the patient's designated representative if the patient is underage or unable to answer for him/herself.

2. Verify that the correct procedure is on the operating room schedule.

3. Verify with the patient or the patient's designated representative the procedure that is expected to be performed, as well as the location of the operation.

4. Confirm the consent form with the patient or the patient's designated representative.

5. In the case of a bilateral organ, limb, or anatomic site (for example, hernia), the surgeon and patient should agree and the operating surgeon should mark the site prior to giving the patient narcotics, sedation, or anesthesia.

6. If the patient is scheduled for multiple procedures that will be performed by multiple surgeons, all the items on the checklist must be verified for each procedure that is planned to be performed.

7. Conduct a final verification process with members of the surgical team to confirm the correct patient, procedure, and surgical site.

8. Ensure that all relevant records and imaging studies are in the operating room.

9. If any verification process fails to identify the correct site, all activities should be halted until verification is accurate.

10. In the event of a life- or limb-threatening situation, not all of these steps may be followed.

Source: Reprinted from Evolution of Wrong Site Surgery Prevention Strategies. AORN, Carney, B., Volume 83, Issue 5, pp. 1115–1122. Copyright 2006 with permission from Elsevier.

Nursing Diagnoses

The actual and potential nursing diagnoses related to surgery include:

1. *Stress, Overload*
2. *Surgical Recovery Delayed*
3. *Fear*
4. *Infection, Risk for*
5. *Pain, Acute.*

Planning

To provide the safest and least stressful experience for the patient, planning is essential. Planning for the surgical experience typically begins with the admission to the hospital. A comprehensive plan that organizes the care of the patient and family will facilitate the surgical process. The plan includes preoperative, intraoperative, and postoperative management and teaching. Communication is as essential part of executing the plan. Each hospital has specific forms that are used to guide the nurse through the process. Chapter 25 ☞ includes an example of a preoperative checklist.

Outcomes and Evaluation Parameters

The desired outcome for patients having surgery is that the patient safely transitions through the entire process. Evaluation parameters include: airway is maintained, oxygen levels are within normal limits, pain is managed and any postoperative complications are effectively mitigated or controlled as much as possible.

Interventions and Rationales

The nurse must communicate pertinent information to the anesthesia team. Information may include allergies, lab/test results, skin condition, NPO status, sensory/mobility impairments, physical particularities, restrictions to jaw and neck range of motion, history of drug use including herbal medication, anticoagulants held for number of days, implanted electronic devices (IEDs),

other implants, previous anesthesia/surgery history, artificial or loose teeth, previous surgery, comorbidities, particular patient requests, or any other information deemed crucial to intraoperative patient care. Although this verification takes place in the same-day admission unit or the surgical unit, many ORs have developed a presurgical checklist to ensure that all pertinent information is reviewed and communicated.

Preventing Wrong Site Surgery

When a procedure involves a left/right distinction, multiple structures (such as finger and toes), or multiple levels (such as spinal procedures), the intended site must be marked so that the mark will be visible after the patient has been prepped and draped. The purpose is to identify unambiguously the intended site of incision or insertion. The mark must be made using a marker that is sufficiently permanent to remain visible after the skin preparation. The Joint Commission (2004) recommends that the method and the type of marking should be consistent throughout the organization and that the person doing the marking should be the one doing the procedure. Marking must take place with the patient involved and aware.

 Exemptions to the marking procedure may include single-organ cases, interventional cases where the point of insertion is not predetermined (such as cardiac catheterization), teeth extractions (although the involved tooth should be documented), and premature infants, for whom the mark may cause a permanent tattoo.

As the patient's advocate, the perioperative nurse should communicate with all members of the surgical team to verify the correct surgical site. Individual facility policy should clearly delineate the role and responsibility of the health care provider and other team members in marking and verifying the correct surgical site. The 2006 statistics on sentinel events from the Joint Commission identify wrong site surgery as the second most reported sentinel event, accounting for 13% of reported sentinel events (Beyea,

2000). Although it is the surgeon's role to diagnose a patient's need for surgery and to delineate the surgical site, verifying the surgical site at the time of surgery is the responsibility of perioperative nurses and every member of the health care team (AORN, 2008). To this effect, the Joint Commission has issued regulations and is endorsing the Universal Protocol as part of the 2007 National Patient Safety Goals (Joint Commission, 2007).

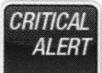 **CRITICAL ALERT** *The goal of the universal protocol is to prevent wrong site, wrong procedure, and wrong person surgery. The Joint Commission's national guidelines to prevent wrong site surgery are based on the consensus of experts from the relevant clinical specialties and professional disciplines and is endorsed by more than 40 professional medical associations and organizations. The active involvement of the team and the patient or patient's representative and effective communication among all members of the operating room team are important for success.*

Surgical Time-Out

Safety initiatives that address communication issues such as the time-out are designed to promote correct site surgery. The time-out checklist has been adopted from the aviation industry model and requires surgical team members to cease all other activities in order to actively, verbally, and mutually verify information such as the correct patient, correct surgery, correct site/side, correct patient position, and possibly additional information such as prophylactic medications being administered at the appropriate time prior to surgery. Figure 26–4 ■ shows a sample of a time-out checklist.

Wrong site surgery may be the result of operating on the wrong patient or performing the wrong procedure, but most commonly it is the result of operating on the wrong site/side; for example, the left hand is operated on instead of the right (Joint Commission, 2007). Although rare, the consequences of wrong site surgery can

---

AORN

Guidelines for Implementing *JCAHO Universal Protocol* To Promote Correct Site Surgery

PREOPERATIVE VERIFICATION

2 Patient Identifiers Must be Used (for example)*
- Ask patient to state their full name.
- Ask patient to state their date of birth.
- Ask patient to state their planned procedure and document it in the patient's own words.
- The patient's room number is <u>not</u> an acceptable patient identifier:

Confirm and Verify
- Patient's name on their ID band, date of birth, and other documents that correspond with the patient's responses.
- Medical record number.
- Consents.
- Availability of implant if required.
- Availability of blood if ordered.
- Radiologic exams (x-ray, CT scan, MRI, etc.).

> PATIENT RESPONSES MUST MATCH:
> MARKED SITE * ID BAND * CONSENTS * RADIOLOGIC EXAMS * SCHEDULED PROCEDURE

> In the case of pediatric patients and patients unable to verify information for themselves, the RN identifies the patient's legal guardian and verifies with them the following protocol.

SITE MARK:
- Use a permanent marker that is visible after skin is prepped and draped
- Have operating physician/surgeon mark the site with his or her **initials, prior to** patient entering the OR suite. ***
- Mark site(s) with patient participation (e.g., verbal confirmation or visual pointing).
- Use an additional mechanism for identifying site(s) exempt from marking according to facility policy and JCAHO guidelines (For example, an ID band with the procedure written on it is an alternative for site marking. When possible the ID band should be verified during the time out phase similar to the site mark).

When marking the site DO NOT USE:
The letter X or the word NO
Do NOT mark the Non-Operative Site

According to AORN standards, the patient is identified by the circulating RN when the patient enters the OR suite. The procedure and surgical site are validated at this time as well.

"TIME OUT"
Takes place in the procedure/OR room, after the patient is prepped and draped and it involves the ENTIRE TEAM.

All team members must verbally verify their agreement on:
- The name of the patient.
- The procedure to be performed.
- The site of the procedure, including laterality, implant to be used and radiologic exams, if applicable.

Validate site mark after draping or confirm ID band with the procedure written on it if used in cases of exemption.

> **DISCREPANCIES/ISSUES**
> ✓ Procedure does not start until patient verification & missing information is completed and agreed upon by all team members.
> ✓ If a disagreement is not resolved, follow your facility policy and notify your manager or administrator.
> ✓ All issues resolved are documented in the medical record.

DOCUMENTATION of "TIME OUT"
Should indicate the following was verified:
- Correct patient.
- Correct site and side.
- Agreement to procedure.
- Correct patient position.
- Implants and/or special equipment or special requirements available.

 * Facility determined identifiers should be used.
 ** Remove the mark at the end of procedure, especially for patients returning for subsequent procedures (e.g., trauma).
 *** If operating physician does not mark site, an individual identified by facility policy with knowledge of the patient and planned procedure to be performed may mark the site.

FIGURE 26–4 ■ AORN guidelines for verifying the correct surgical site.

AORN SAMPLE Patient Record
(Facility Name and Address)

This record is a sample only. Clinical records should be customized to incorporate data fields that represent the setting, facility, procedure, and patient. Reproductions and variations are encouraged, provided credit is given to AORN.

Addressograph

(Patient Information: name, age, gender, medical record number, date)

Structural Data:

Operating Room Progress Notes

Room #:	ASA:	Pt. in room:	Anes. start:
Procedure start:	Procedure finish:	Pt. out of room:	Anes. finish:

Anesthesia type:

☐ General   ☐ MAC   ☐ Spinal   ☐ Epidural

☐ Local block, Type: _____   ☐ Other:

Op Dx: _____

Procedure(s): _____

Op Dx: _____

Surgeon 1:	Circulating nurse 1:
Surgeon 2:	Circulating nurse 2:
Assistant 1:	Circ. 1 relief: Time in: ___ Time out: ___
Assistant 2:	Circ. 2 relief: Time in: ___ Time out: ___
Anesthesia care provider 1:	Scrub 1:
Anesthesia care provider 2:	Scrub 2:
Laser operator:	Scrub 1 relief: Time in: ___ Time out: ___
Other authorized personnel:	Scrub 2 relief: Time in: ___ Time out: ___

Nursing Data Elements - Preoperative:

Preoperative checklist reviewed/evaluated

Risk for injury related to transfer and transport (X29):

☐ ID confirmed   ☐ Consent verified   ☐ Site verified
Allergies verified   ☐ Procedure verified
Latex allergy: ☐ Yes   ☐ No   ☐ NPO verified
Time: _____

☐ Alert/oriented   ☐ Drowsy   ☐ Sedated
☐ Asleep   ☐ Unresponsive   ☐ Disoriented
☐ Other: _____

☐ Cool   ☐ Warm   ☐ Intact
☐ Dry   ☐ Moist   ☐ Body jewelry removed
☐ Tattoos: _____

Sensory impairment: ☐ No limitations   ☐ Hearing
☐ Language barrier   ☐ Sight

Musculoskeletal status: ☐ No limitations   ☐ Paralysis   ☐ Traction

Prosthetics/Assistive devices: ☐ Hearing aid   ☐ Glasses
☐ AICD
☐ Prosthetics: _____

Cardiopulmonary status:
Peripheral edema: ☐ Yes Location: _____
☐ No

DVT/PE risk: ☐ High   ☐ Med.   ☐ Low
Respiratory: ☐ Tracheotomy   ☐ Intubated   ☐ Chest tube
☐ Regular   ☐ Labored   ☐ Other findings

Risk for anxiety related to knowledge deficit and stress of surgery (X4):

Psychosocial status:
☐ Calm/relaxed   ☐ Anxious   ☐ Talkative
☐ Crying   ☐ Restless
☐ Other: _____

☐ Provided instruction based on age and identified needs (I106).
☐ Communicated patient concerns to appropriate members of health care team (I128).
☐ Explained sequence of events and preoperative routine (I56).
☐ Evaluated response to instructions (I50).

Risk for acute/chronic pain (X38, X74):

☐ Instructed on use of pain scale
☐ Pain assessment (0-10): _____
Location: _____

Outcomes:

☐ Verbalizes/indicates decreased anxiety, ability to cope, understanding of procedure and sequence of events. Questions answered.
☐ Demonstrates adequate pain management.
☐ Verbalizes comfort related to transfer/transport.

Transfer to suite via:

☐ Stretcher   ☐ W/C   ☐ Bed
☐ Isolette   ☐ Crib

FIGURE 26–5 ■ Sample of intraoperative nursing documentation.

Intraoperative Structural Data:

☐ EKG ☐ Oximeter ☐ NIAPB ☐ Temp monitor

Implants/Prosthesis: ☐ Yes ☐ No Exp. Date:_____

Manufacturer:_____

Type:_____

Size:_____

Lot/Serial #:_____

OR medications: (other than those given by anesthesia care provider)

Time	Medication	Dosage	Route	Initials

Blood products: ☐ Yes ☐ No Blood band #: _____

Unit #:_____ Start time:_____ Finish time:_____
Unit #:_____ Start time:_____ Finish time:_____
Unit #:_____ Start time:_____ Finish time:_____

Blood recovery: ☐ Yes ☐ No Unit #:_____
CCs reinfused: _____

Irrigation:

Type: _____

Amount: _____

X-rays: ☐ Yes ☐ No
Site:_____
Type:_____
Protective devices:
☐ Gonadal ☐ Thyroid
Other:_____

Grafts: ☐ Yes ☐ No
Type:_____
Donor site: _____
Recipient site:_____

Pathology specimens:

Routine: ☐ Yes ☐ No
#:_____

Frozen section: ☐ Yes ☐ No
#:_____

Cultures: ☐ Yes ☐ No
#:_____

Comments:_____
_____
_____
_____
_____

Intraoperative Nursing Data:

Risk for infection (X28):

☐ Skin Pre-op intact ☐ Other:_____
☐ Surgical clippers:_____
  Area:_____
☐ Skin prep By:_____
  ☐ Povidone-iodine ☐ Chlorhexidine
  ☐ Other:_____

Wound classification:
☐ 1-Clean   ☐ 3-Contaminated
☐ 2-Clean/contaminated   ☐ 4-Dirty
☐ Urinary catheter:
  (size/type/site):_____
  OR output:_____ Inserted by:_____
☐ Drains/tubes (size/type/site):_____
  OR drainage amount:_____
☐ Packing (size/type/site):_____
☐ Cast (type/site):_____
☐ Dressing (type/site):_____

Risk for hypothermia (X26):

☐ Apply warming blanket #:_____
  Temp setting:_____
  Applied by:_____
☐ Warm IV fluid
☐ Warm irrigation
☐ Other:_____

Risk for impaired skin integrity (X50):

Position for surgery: ☐ Supine ☐ Prone ☐ Mod. lithotomy ☐ Jackknife
  ☐ Lt. lateral ☐ Rt. lateral ☐ Other:_____

Positioning devices: ☐ Chest roll ☐ Shoulder roll ☐ Axillary roll
  ☐ Pillow/wedge ☐ Stirrups ☐ Leg holder

Pad bony prominences: ☐ Elbows ☐ Heels ☐ Arms tucked/padded
  ☐ Other:_____

Positioned by: _____

Risk for injury (X29):

☐ Apply safety strap to: _____
☐ Apply grounding pad Site: _____
☐ Electrosurgical unit #: _____ ☐ Bipolar #:_____
  Setting: Coag:_____ Cut:_____
☐ Laser Type: _____ Unit #:_____ Settings:_____ Time:_____
  ☐ Safety measures implemented Operator:_____
☐ Tourniquet checked & applied #: _____ Site:_____ Applied by:_____
  ☐ Inflated:_____ ☐ Deflated:_____ Pressure:_____
Sequential stockings: ☐ Yes ☐ No Other:_____ Unit #:_____

Counts:	Sponge	Needles	Instruments
1st count:	☐ Correct	☐ Correct	☐ Correct
2nd count:	☐ Correct	☐ Correct	☐ Correct
3rd count:	☐ Correct	☐ Correct	☐ Correct
	☐ Unresolved	☐ Unresolved	☐ Unresolved
	☐ N/A	☐ N/A	☐ N/A

☐ Surgeon notified of counts If counts unresolved, X-ray taken: ☐ Yes ☐ No
Signature: _____ If no, explain: _____

Postprocedure Assessment/Evaluation:

Outcomes: ☐ Patient's surgery performed using aseptic technique and in a manner to prevent cross-contamination (O10).
☐ Skin remains smooth, intact, non-reddened, non-irritated, free of bruising (O5, O2, O8).
☐ Core body temperature remains in expected range (O12).

be devastating and warrant improved systems that promote effective communication such as the time-out initiative.

Intraoperative Patient Record

Most facilities have an intraoperative patient record, like that shown in Figure 26–5 ■, that is used to record intraoperative information. In addition, perioperative nurses may chart information in the nurse's notes when warranted. For example, information may include personnel involved, length of surgery, position and accessories implemented, wound classification, anesthesia classification, and monitoring devices to name a few.

Protecting the Patient from Infection

Surgical-site infections are the third most frequently reported type of iatrogenic (hospital-acquired) infection (Engemann et al., 2003). Preventing and minimizing associated risks of SSI are fundamental perioperative nursing diagnoses of the surgical patient. According to Nichols (2001), the most critical factor in postoperative infection is the sound judgment and proper practice of the surgical team in addition to the general health and disease state of the patient. It is for this reason that perioperative nurses have become quite expert in the areas of aseptic technique and sterile conscience. Surgical aseptic practice is based on the premise that most infections are caused by exogenous organisms or organisms that are external from the body.

Asepsis is the absence of infectious organisms. In the OR aseptic techniques are practices that minimize contamination due to microorganisms. Frequently aseptic techniques and practices are criticized for being ritualistic in nature and lacking in scientific rigor, but until empiric evidence demonstrates a technique is otherwise unnecessary or ineffective, basic aseptic principles should be observed.

There are no sterilization processes that completely eliminate all microorganisms. The best technologies to date can only limit and reduce the presence of microbial life such as bacteria, viruses, fungi, and spores to an acceptable sterility assurance level. It is for this reason that nurses and surgical team members in the OR need to continually monitor the surgical field and develop strategies to minimize patient risk. An example may include inspecting sterile packaging, delivering items using proper aseptic technique, and ensuring items have been appropriately sterilized.

SSIs may also be predicted based on the surgical wound classification. The CDC publishes norms for SSI rates based on certain indicators, including wound classification (see the National Guidelines box). The CDC data provide benchmarks for health care professionals to evaluate their SSI rates so they can further investigate the problem and implement initiatives should the rates be unusually high.

 CRITICAL ALERT *The purpose of surgical wound classification is to track and learn the cause of infections in order to prevent future incidence. This information is generally recorded on the patient's intraoperative record.*

Over time, surgical team members will in fact develop a surgical conscience. Surgical conscience is defined as "An inner commitment to strictly adhere to aseptic practice, to report any break

in aseptic technique, and to correct any violation whether or not anyone else is present or observes the violation. A surgical conscience mandates a commitment to aseptic practice at all times" (Spry, 2005). This allows personnel to function in a more efficient and safe manner.

One of the strategies employed is the creation of the sterile field. The sterile field begins at the surgical site (incision), and extends to the rest of the patient, OR table, surgical team, scrub table, and to a 1-foot parameter around the draped areas (Figure 26–6 ■). This principle is applied to application of prepping solutions, patient draping, room setup, and so forth. It is commonly referred to as the *clean to dirty principle*.

Surgical attire, scrubbing, gowning, and gloving are all functions of OR aseptic technique. Figure 26–7 ■ shows a nurse in

FIGURE 26–6 ■ OR table.
Source: Custom Medical Stock Photo, Inc.

NATIONAL GUIDELINES for Surgical Wound Classification

Clean wounds	An uninfected operative wound in which no inflammation is encountered and the respiratory, alimentary, genital, or uninfected urinary tracts are not entered. In addition, clean wounds are primarily closed and, if necessary, drained with closed drainage. Operative incisional wounds that follow nonpenetrating (blunt) trauma should be included in this category if they meet the criteria.
Clean-contaminated wounds	Operative wounds in which the respiratory, alimentary, genital, or urinary tracts are entered under controlled conditions and without unusual contamination. Specifically, operations involving the biliary tract, appendix, vagina, and oropharynx are included in this category provided no evidence of infection or major break in technique is encountered.
Contaminated wounds	Includes open, fresh, accidental wounds. In addition, operations with major breaks in sterile technique (e.g., open cardiac massage) or gross spillage from the gastrointestinal tract, and incisions in which acute, nonpurulent inflammation is encountered are included in this category.
Dirty or infected wounds	Includes old traumatic wounds with retained or devitalized tissue and those that involve existing clinical infection or perforated viscera. This definition suggests that the organisms causing postoperative infection were present in the operative field before the operation.

Source: Devaney, L., & Rowell K. S. (2004). *Improving surgical wound classification—why it matters.* AORN Journal. Retrieved on July 2, 2008 from http://findarticles.com/p/articles/mi_m0FSL/is_2_80/ai_n6159709.

FIGURE 26–7 ■ Correct surgical attire.
Source: Custom Medical Stock Photo, Inc.

proper OR attire and a surgical team member in scrub apparel, highlighting important standards and principles.

Positioning the Patient to Prevent Injury

Patient positioning in the OR is chosen to accommodate surgical access, staff ergonomics, and surgical view while maintaining the patient's skin integrity. It is for this reason that OR tables are narrow (ergonomic for surgeon) and firm (limits movement and allows for CPR). OR tables and accessories are designed to accommodate a wide range of positions in order to allow for the use of gravity to displace organs in order to provide additional working space, surgical access, enhanced ergonomics for professionals, and prevent patient complications.

Complications secondary to positioning include compromised respiratory or circulatory responses, injury to nerves and muscles, and the development of pressure ulcers. Chart 26–4 lists common intraoperative positioning complications and potential causes. Nurses may review patient's intraoperative position via the OR record and assess any relevant patient outcomes. Of these, pressure ulcers have received much attention as a preventable intraoperative complication. The incidence of pressure ulcers in

surgical patients ranges from 4% to a high of 45% depending on the study (Feuchtinger, Halfens, & Dassen, 2005; Price, Whitney, & King, 2005). Researchers report conflicting data on risk factors for the development of pressure ulcers. However, preoperative risk factors commonly cited across studies include age (e.g., older patients); presence of comorbidities particularly diabetes, hypertension, and vascular disorders; and poor nutritional status as measured by low serum albumin and anemia (Feuchtinger et al., 2005; Price et al., 2005). Further research is needed to clarify intraoperative risk factors but those that are suggested include type of surgery (e.g., higher risk with vascular, cardiac, thoracic, and spinal surgery), length of operation (e.g., longer surgeries), care taken during perioperative skin preparation to reduce unnecessary moisture collection under the skin, hypotensive episodes during surgery reducing the blood available to tissues, and the type of anesthetic used. Perioperative nurses need adequate knowledge of anatomy and an understanding of the physiological effects of specific surgical positions. Appropriate positioning accessories and excellent communication between the anesthesia team monitoring physiological responses and the surgical team often requesting position changes is essential in order to prevent patient injury.

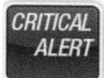 *The primary objective of patient positioning for surgery is to provide maximize exposure while ensuring patient safety. For example, proper positioning can help maintain proper body alignment and access to intravenous and anesthesia support devices.*

Preventing the Retention of Foreign Objects

Surgical counts are the responsibility of perioperative nurses and are performed in order to prevent patient injury due to the high risk of retained foreign body, which can include gauzes, needles, or instruments. Retained foreign objects in patients have resulted in major injuries such as sepsis, bowel perforation, and death. Most facilities follow a legal counting procedure based on the AORN (2007b) recommended standards and practices. The desired patient outcome is a patient free from injury related to extraneous objects. It seems to be a much greater issue than reported, leading to an initiative by health care professional organizations, such as AORN, American College of Surgeons (ACS),

CHART 26–4	**Intraoperative Positioning Complications**
Potential Complications Secondary to Intraoperative Positioning	**Potential Intervention**
Decreased lung expansion due to supine position resulting in compromised respiratory effects	Position bolsters correctly to minimize compression of thorax, facilitating full lung expansion.
Brachial plexus nerve injury	Position arm correctly to ensure proper arm alignment of less than 90 degrees, supinated, and adequately padded and protected.
Circulatory obstruction due to position resulting in increased risk of postoperative deep vein thrombosis	Apply antiembolic stockings and sequential compression leggings. Use appropriate prophylactic anticoagulant medication administration.
Integumentary injury resulting in pressure ulcers, abrasion, and blistering	Use OR table equipment that will minimize pressure and maximize capillary refill. Appropriate equipment includes gel mattresses. Ensure proper lifting and securing of patient to prevent friction-related injuries.
Dislocation of acetabulum	Ensure proper placement of stirrups and ensure that two health care professionals simultaneously lift, support, and place legs onto stirrups observing correct alignment.

and the Joint Commission, to develop improved methods of accounting for surgical items. One technology that is currently being tested is radio-frequency identification (RFID). This involves RF tags being implanted in surgical sponges (Figure 26–8 ■). This permits the surgical team to pass a wand over the patient following a procedure to verify that no sponges have been left in the patient (Medline, 2006).

The presence of foreign materials in the body can lead to infection, abscess, and other serious problems. Multiple procedures are in place to prevent leaving an instrument or a sponge or other material in the patient when the wound is closed. Sponges, swabs, instruments, and sharps are counted many times during the surgical procedure. Hospitals have written policies describing what is counted, when it is counted, who does the counting, where the counting is documented, and how to resolve a discrepancy in the count. To prevent a foreign object from being left behind:

- All items brought to the operating room are documented.
- No items are removed from the operating room until the final count is complete and verified.
- Sponges, swabs, and other items are counted before surgery, before wound closure begins, and before skin closure begins.
- The circulating nurse and scrub nurse count items in unison.
- The circulating nurse and scrub nurse document the count in the record.

If there is a discrepancy in the count, all personnel try to locate the missing item. If it cannot be found, the patient may be x-rayed. Surgical instruments can be seen by x-ray and soft materials, such as surgical sponges, have a radio-opaque stripe for x-ray identification.

Estimating Blood Loss

The patient is monitored throughout the operation for blood loss. The calculation of blood loss is referred to as the estimation of blood loss (EBL). Blood in suction containers, wound drains, chest tubes, and nasogastric tubes is measured directly at frequent intervals during the surgery. If irrigating fluid is used, it is subtracted from the total amount of drainage to determine the amount of actual blood loss. Blood in sponges can be approxi-

mated from their weight with 1 gram of weight being equal to 1 mL of blood. Blood-soaked sponges are collected in a plastic bag and weighed. The weight of the dry sponge(s) and plastic container is subtracted from the total weight to determine blood loss.

Whether or not the patient needs a transfusion during surgery depends on blood loss as well as on other factors such as age, general level of health prior to surgery, history of cardiovascular disease, how well the patient tolerates the blood loss, and the availability of autologous blood. Some religions, such as Christian Science and Jehovah's Witnesses, restrict the administration of blood products.

Adult patients who are generally healthy can tolerate surgical blood loss of up to 500 mL without the need for a transfusion. Blood loss is treated with the administration of packed red blood cells. Chapter 23 ∞ provides a complete description of blood administration indications and procedures.

Latex Allergy

There has been a significant increase in the number of latex allergies seen in the hospital, including the operating room. Some suggest the increase correlates with the adoption of universal precautions and the increased use of latex gloves. Patients are asked preoperatively about the possibility of latex allergy. A latex sensitivity questionnaire can be used to identify those who have a latex allergy or who are likely to develop the allergy. A high incidence of latex allergy is found in people with spina bifida, patients who have had multiple surgeries, those who work with latex products (health care workers, dental industry workers, rubber workers), and those with a genetic predisposition to allergies (atopy). Patients who report allergies to kiwis, bananas, and avocados are also at an increased risk of latex allergies due to the cross reactivity of the proteins present in these fruits and latex. Blood or skin tests can detect latex-specific IgE antibodies and are performed preoperatively when latex allergy is suspected. Latex allergy is discussed in detail in Chapter 60 ∞ .

It is virtually impossible to create a latex-free environment in the operating room—although it may be possible in the future as more products are being manufactured without latex. For patients with known allergy, a latex-reduced environment is created. Elements of a latex-reduced environment in the operating room include (1) scheduling elective cases as the first cases of the

(a)

(b)

(c)

FIGURE 26–8 ■ RFID technology: (A) RF tag implanted in surgical gauze; (B) wand to detect the RF tag in surgical gauze; (C) surgical RFID detection console.
Source: RF Surgical Systems, Inc. @http://www.rfsurg.com/features.htm

day to minimize contact with aerosolized allergen from latex gloves, (2) using vinyl gloves rather than latex gloves, (3) using powder-free gloves to limit the aerosolization of latex antigens, (4) avoiding latex on the sterile field, (5) using a plastic anesthesia mask, (6) using a stopcock rather than the rubber port for injection of intravenous drugs, (7) removing the rubber cap on medication vials rather than drawing a medication through the cap, (8) using nonlatex equipment such as blood pressure cuff, stethoscope, and electrocardiogram leads, and (9) using nonlatex tape. Premedication of allergic patients with steroids or antihistamines is not recommended.

Allergic responses to latex can range from mild cases of contact dermatitis evidenced by a rash and urticaria to serious cases of anaphylaxis. When a latex allergy is suspected in the operating room, the source of latex in direct contact with the patient is immediately removed. Follow-up treatment includes the administration of 100% oxygen, intravenous fluids to support the blood pressure, and the administration of intravenous epinephrine. Diphenhydramine and steroids may also be given intravenously to attenuate the allergic response.

■ Postanesthesia Care Unit

Once the surgery is completed, the anesthetist and the nurse will accompany the patient to the postanesthesia care unit (PACU) for further monitoring. Concerns along this route will focus on safety, infection control, medication, communication, positioning, and equipment. The PACU is where the patient will recover from the anaesthetic he has received. This is an unrestricted area where the patient will no longer need to wear a head cover and the nurses will wear regular uniforms. Visitors may be allowed in certain parts of the PACU under certain circumstances.

Poor communication is one of the top contributing factors to medical errors. Therefore, nurses must strive to provide effective and consistent information during patient handoff to a transition unit such as the PACU or Intensive Care Unit (ICU). It is important to give any pertinent information to the unit members where the transfer of responsibility for the surgical patient is occurring and provide an interactive communication that is free of interruptions and includes a systematic process of verification. Figure 26–9 ■ (p. 640) shows a mnemonic that highlights the handoff principles and verification process. PACU is dicussed in detail in Chapter 27 ☺.

■ Gerontological Considerations

Persons 65 years of age and older, require surgical interventions more often than younger persons because of age-related system changes and comorbid conditions. Degeneration of multiple systems such as the musculoskeletal, nervous, cardiovascular, respiratory, genitourinary, endocrine, and hematopoietic systems and hearing and vision can influence intraoperative and postoperative outcomes. Changes in pharmacokinetics result in changes in drug absorption, distribution, metabolism, and excretion by the body. At this stage of life, both physical and cognitive abilities may vary greatly. Appropriate age-specific interventions should be considered for the geriatric population taking into consideration both physical, cognitive, sensorimotor, and psychosocial factors. The Gerontological Considerations box highlights the special considerations for the gerontological population.

Assess the geriatric patient's history and general health status, in particular medications, previous surgeries, and comorbidities. Promote patient warmth through warming devices and assess range of motion prior to patient being anesthetized in order to ensure correct positioning accessories are available. Additional padding may be necessary due to decreased adipose tissue and circulation, predisposing the patient to the development of pressure ulcers. Efforts should be made to diminish the use of tapes that may lead to denuding of geriatric fragile thinner skin. Ensure adequate time is available to communicate clearly and slowly, keeping in mind possible hearing impairment and need for additional processing and response time.

Hyperglycemia is known to be associated with increased sepsis, suggesting that careful monitoring of glucose levels may be a way to reduce serious postoperative infections. Infections are a major concern for all hospitalized patients, but are especially dangerous for elderly persons. General risk factors for infection in elderly patients are known to include frailty, chronic undernutrition, reduced muscle mass, and poor dentition. Other more general factors common to all age groups are diabetes, aspiration, and the presence of an indwelling urinary catheter.

Patients with postoperative cognitive dysfunction (POCD) experience deterioration in cognitive function that persists for years after the operation. POCD may be related to brain oxygenation during anesthesia, anesthetic agents, and hospital environment (Prough, 2005).

GERONTOLOGICAL CONSIDERATIONS for Elderly Patients Having Surgery

Physical Factors	Cognitive Factors	Sensorimotor Factors	Psychosocial Factors
• Decreased tolerance to heat and cold • Loss of skin tone • Declining cardiac/renal function • Atrophy of reproductive organs • Increased incidence of preexisting health conditions	• Decline dependent on pregeriatric state and general health and social involvement • Decreased memory, inductive reasoning, and figural relations may occur • Cognitive tasks may require more time to complete	• Decreased visual acuity • Diminished hearing • Altered tactile sensation • Changes in taste and smell • Diminished response to stress and sensory stimuli • Decreased mobility	• Ego integrity important • Stressors: end of life, changes in environment, increased cognitive demands • Death of loved ones • Concerns for general health increase

Handoff Communications

"I PASS THE BATON"

	Handoffs and Healthcare Transitions with opportunities to ask QUESTIONS, CLARIFY AND CONFIRM

I	**Introduction**	Introduce yourself and your role/job (include patient)
P	**Patient**	Name, identifiers, age, sex, location
A	**Assessment**	Presenting chief complaint, vital signs and symptoms and diagnosis
S	**Situation**	Current status, medications, circumstances, including code status, level of (un)certainty, recent changes, response to treatment
S	**SAFETY Concerns**	Critical lab values/reports, socio-economic factors, alllergies, alerts (falls, isolation, etc.)
THE		
B	**Background**	Co-morbidities, previous episodes, past/home medications, family history
A	**Actions**	What actions were taken or are required AND provide brief rationale
T	**Timing**	Level of urgency and explicit timing, prioritization of actions
O	**Ownership**	Who is responsible (nurse/doctor/team) including patient/family responsibilities
N	**Next**	What will happen next? Anticipated changes? What is the PLAN? Contingency plans?

FIGURE 26–9 ■ Handoff protocol to improve communication when transferring a patient from the OR to another unit.

Source: Joint Commission (2008). National Patient and Safety Goals. Retrieved July 3, 2008 from http://www.jointcommission.org/NR/rdonlyres/ACA4DBF6-90FD-4400-BE7E-4C6F881E5DCD/0/08_OBS_NPSG_Master.pdf. From the Department of Defense Safety Program.

Prevention of Infection

Clinical Problem

Mild perioperative hypothermia, which is common during major surgery, may promote surgical-wound infection by triggering thermoregulatory vasoconstriction, which decreases subcutaneous oxygen tension. Reduced levels of oxygen in tissue impair oxidative killing by neutrophils and decrease the strength of the healing wound by reducing the deposition of collagen. Hypothermia also directly impairs immune function.

Research Findings

Research was done testing the hypothesis that hypothermia both increases susceptibility to surgical-wound infection and lengthens hospitalization. Good et al. (2006) report that hypothermia itself may delay healing and predispose patients to wound infections. Maintaining normothermia intraoperatively is likely to decrease the incidence of infectious complications in patients undergoing colorectal resection and to shorten their hospitalizations.

Other research was done on prewarming of patients' skin and its influence on core hypothermia (Cooper, 2006; Vanni et al., 2003). Camus et al. (1995) found that a single hour of preoperative skin surface warming reduced the rate at which core hypothermia developed during the first hour of anesthesia.

Antibiotic Administration

Another measure to reduce infection in the operating room is proper timing for antibiotic administration. Antibiotic prophylaxis is being used in a variety of surgical procedures to reduce the incidence of surgical-site infections. Antibiotics should be chosen on the basis of their effectiveness against the pathogens most likely to be encountered. Skin floras (e.g., *Staphylococcus* organisms) are the usual target, so first-generation cephalosporins are most often chosen. Preoperative prophylactic antibiotics should be administered within 60 minutes before the initial incision is made to ensure that antimicrobial levels in the tissue are adequate and maintained for the duration of the procedure (Gordon, 2006; White & Schneider, 2007). To comply with the recommendations of administration within 60 minutes of incision, the holding area was identified as the preferred location (Olin, 2006).

Implications for Nursing Practice

The latest research results have and will influence a change of practice in the perioperative setting based on evidence. In the preoperative setting nurses can use blankets and warming to maintain normothermia. For maintaining normothermia in the OR policies and procedures could be implemented such as use of warming devices under the patient as well as the use of warm solutions. In addition the temperature of the OR suite could be increased.

Nurses also can coordinate the timing of preoperative antibiotic administration. This will necessitate cooperation with both the surgeon and the OR staff to determine the optimal timing of antibiotic administration.

Critical Thinking Questions

1. What nursing interventions will decrease the risk of infection?

Answers to Critical Thinking Questions appear in Appendix D.

References

Camus, Y., Delva, E., Sessler, D., & Lienhart, A. (1995). Pre-induction skin surface warming minimizes intraoperative core hypothermia. *Journal of Clinical Anesthesia, 7,* 384–388.

Cooper, S. (2006). The effect of preoperative warming on patient's postoperative temperatures. *AORN Journal, 83*(5) 1074–1076, 1079–1084.

Good, K. K., Verble, J. A., & Norwood, B. R. (2006). Postoperative hypothermia—The chilling consequences. *AORN Journal, 83*(5), 1055–1066.

Gordon, S. M. (2006). Antibiotic prophylaxis against postoperative wound infections. *Cleveland Clinic Journal of Medicine, 73,* S42–S45.

Olin, J. (2006). Multidisciplinary approach to optimizing antibiotic prophylaxis of surgical site infections. *American Journal of Health-System Pharmacy, 63,* 2312–2314.

Vanni, S. M., Braz, J. R., Modolo, N. S., Amorim, R. B., & Rodrigues, G. R. (2003). Preoperative combined with intraoperative skin surface warming avoids hypothermia caused by general anesthesia and surgery. *Journal of Clinical Anesthesia, 15*(2), 119–125.

White, A., & Schneider, T. (2007). Improving compliance with prophylactic antibiotic administration guidelines. *AORN Journal, 85*(1), 173–180.

EVIDENCE-BASED PRACTICE

NCLEX® REVIEW

1. A preoperative patient is taken into the holding area. The nurse will utilize this time with the patient to do which of the following?
   1. Ensure surgical instruments are operational.
   2. Clean and inspect surgical instruments.
   3. Conduct an interview.
   4. Insert an indwelling urinary catheter if necessary.

2. A registered nurse first assistant is scheduled to assist a surgeon with a surgical procedure. This nurse will be responsible for:
   1. Administering anesthetic agents.
   2. Serving as the patient advocate.
   3. Providing the surgeon with instruments.
   4. Collaborating with the surgeon and suturing the wound closed.

3. During the course of a surgical procedure, the patient's heart rate increases and the blood pressure drops. The care provider who would address these physiological changes to the patient would be the:
   1. Surgeon.
   2. Anesthesiologist.
   3. RNFA.
   4. Scrub nurse.

4. While conducting a surgical time-out, the nurse says that the site of surgery is the right knee whereas the left knee was marked as the site of the surgery. Which of the following should be done?
   1. Operate on the right knee.
   2. Operate on the left knee.
   3. Ask a family member which knee is the site of surgery.
   4. Stop all preparations until it can be verified which knee is the site of surgery.

5. While an anesthetized patient is being moved to the operating room table, the patient's lower left leg drops and hits the side of the table. Which of the following should the nurse do?
   1. Move the leg and place it on the table.
   2. Examine the leg for possible or extent of injury and document the event.
   3. Nothing because this is considered an acceptable hazard of surgery.
   4. Elevate the leg on a pillow.

6. During a surgical procedure the patient begins to demonstrate signs of malignant hyperthermia. Which of the following should be done to support this patient?
   1. Administer calcium channel blockers.
   2. Stop the surgery or deep the anesthesia.
   3. Transfer to the PACU for postsurgical care.
   4. Provide 21% oxygen.

7. During a surgical procedure the anesthesiologist directs another care provider to change the oxygen mix being provided to the patient. The care provider most likely to make this oxygen change would be the:
   1. RN First Assistant.
   2. Scrub nurse.
   3. CRNA.
   4. Respiratory therapist.

Answers for review questions appear in Appendix D

KEY TERMS

Bier block *p.631*
circulating nurse *p.620*
conscious sedation *p.625*
epidural anesthesia *p.630*

general anesthesia *p.629*
intraoperative *p.620*
intrathecal anesthesia *p.630*
malignant hyperthermia (MH) *p.629*

peripheral nerve block *p.631*
regional anesthesia *p.630*
scrub nurse *p.620*
spinal anesthesia *p.630*

PEARSON
EXPLORE mynursingkit™

MyNursingKit is your one stop for online chapter review materials and resources. Prepare for success with additional NCLEX®-style practice questions, interactive assignments and activities, web links, animations and videos, and more!

Register your access code from the front of your book at
www.mynursingkit.com

REFERENCES

American Society of PeriAnesthesia Nurses. (2001). Clinical guideline for the prevention of unplanned perioperative hypothermia. *Journal of PeriAnesthesia Nursing, 16*, 305–314.

Arbous, M., Meursing, A., van-Kleef, J., de-Lange, J., Spoormans, H., Touw, P., et al. (2005). Impact of anesthesia management characteristics on severe morbidity and mortality. *Anesthesiology, 102*(2), 257–268.

Association of periOperative Registered Nurses. (2002). *PNDS Resources*. AORN. Retrieved June 29, 2008 from http://www.aorn.org/

PracticeResources/PNDSAndStandardizedPerioperativeRecord/PNDSResources/

Association of periOperative Registered Nurses. (2007a). *About AORN*. Retrieved February 16, 2007, from http://www.aorn.org/AboutAORN

Association of periOperative Registered Nurses. (2007b). *Standards, recommended practices and guidelines. Orientation of the registered professional nurse to the perioperative setting*. Denver, CO: Author.

Association of periOperative Registered Nurses. (2008). *RN First Assistant*. AORN. Retrieved on June 29, 2008 from http://www.aorn.org/CareerCenter/CareerDevelopment/RNFirstAssistant/

Bailey, J., McVey, L., & Pevreal, A. (2005). Surveying patients as a start to quality improvement in the surgical suites holding area. *Journal of Nursing Care Quality, 20*(4), 319–326.

Beyea, S. (2000). Preventing surgical site infections—Guiding practice with evidence *AORN Journal*. Retrieved on June 29, 2008 from http://findarticles.com/p/articles/mi_m0FSL/is_2_72/ai_64424354/pg_3

Bitner, J., Hilde, L., Hall, K., & Duvendack, T. (2007). A team approach to the prevention of unplanned postoperative hypothermia: Clinical report. *AORN Journal, 85*(5), 921–928.

Bonjer, H. J., Hop, W. C., Nelson, H., Sargent, D. J., Lacy, A. M., et al. (2007). Laparoscopically assisted vs open colectomy for colon cancer: A meta-analysis. *Archives of Surgery, 142*(3), 298–303.

Boo, Y. J., Kim, W. B., Kim, J., Song, T. J., Choi, S. Y., et al. (2007). Systemic immune response after open versus laparoscopic cholecystectomy in acute cholecystitis: A prospective randomized study. *Scandinavian Journal of Clinical & Laboratory Investigation, 67*(2), 207–214.

Engemann, J. J., Carmeli, Y., Cosgrove, S. E., Fowler, V. G., Bronstein, M. Z., et al. (2003). Adverse clinical and economic outcomes attributable to methicillin resistance among patients with *Staphylococcus aureus* surgical site infection. *Clinical Infectious Disease, 36,* 592–598.

Evidence based practice information sheets for health professionals. The impact of preoperative hair removal on surgical site infection. (2003). *Best Practice, 7*(2), 1–6.

Feuchtinger, J., Halfens, R., & Dassen, T. (2005). Pressure ulcer risk factors in cardiac surgery: A review of the research literature. *Heart & Lung: The Journal of Acute and Critical Care, 34*(6), 375–385.

Hasankhani, H., Mohammadi, E., Moazzami, F., Mokhtari, M., & Naghgizadh, M. (2007). The effects of intravenous fluid temperature on perioperative hemodynamic situation, post-operative shivering, and recovery in orthopaedic surgery. *Canadian Operating Room Nursing Journal, 25*(1), 20–24, 26–27.

Hoffer, J. L. (1999). Anesthesia. In M. Meeker & J. Rothrock (Eds.), *Care of the patient in surgery* (pp. 203–238). Philadelphia: Mosby.

Hurley, C., & McAleavy, J. (2006) Preoperative assessment and intraoperative care planning. *British Journal of Perioperative Nursing, 16*(1), 187–194.

Hyderally, H. (2002). *Complications of spinal anesthesia.* The Mount Sinai Journal of Medicine. Retrieved June 29, 2008 from http://www.mssm.edu/msjournal/69/v69_1&2_055_056.pdf

Iorio, R., Whang, W., Healy, W. L., Patch, D. A., Najibi, S., & Appleby, D. (2005). The utility of bladder catheterisation in total hip arthroplasty. *Clinical Orthopedics and Related Research, 432,* 148–152.

Joint Commission. (2007). *Facts about the Joint Commission.* Retrieved February 16, 2007, from http://www.jointcommission.org/AboutUs/Fact_Sheets/joint_commission_facts.htm

Larson, E. L., Aiello, A. E., Heilman, J. M., Lyle, C., Cronquist, A., Stahl, A., et al. (2001). Comparison of different regimens for surgical hand preparation. *AORN Journal, 73*(2), 412–432.

Medline. (2006). *RF Surgical Systems, Inc. and Medline Announce Regulatory Clearance to Market RF-Detect, a Breakthrough Surgical Detection System.* Retrieved July 2, 2008 from http://www.medline.com/News/press.asp?ID=39

Nichols, R. L. (2001). Preventing surgical site infections: A surgeon's perspective. *Emerging Infectious Diseases, 7*(2), 220–224.

Niel-Weise, B., Willie, J., & van den Broek, P. (2005). Hair removal policies in clean surgery: Systematic review of randomized, controlled trials. *Infection Control and Hospital Epidemiology, 26*(12), 923–928.

Noblett, S. E., & Horgan, A. F. (2007). A prospective case-matched comparison of clinical and financial outcomes of open versus laparoscopic colorectal resection. *Surgical Endoscopy, 21*(3), 404–408.

Price, M., Whitney, J., & King, C. (2005). Development of a risk assessment tool for intraoperative pressure ulcers. *Journal of Wound, Ostomy and Continence Nursing, 32*(1), 19–30.

Prough, D. S. (2005). Anesthetic pitfalls in the elderly patient. *Journal American College of Surgeons, 200*(5), 784–794.

Rampersaud, Y., Moro, E., Neary, M., White, K., Lewis, S., Massicotte, E., et al. (2006). Intraoperative adverse events and related postoperative complications in spine surgery: Implications for enhancing patient safety founded on evidence-based protocols. *Spine, 31*(13), 1503–1510.

Redmond M. (2001). Malignant hyperthermia: perianesthesia recognition, treatment, and care. *Journal of Perianesthesia Nursing. 16,* 259–270.

Sessler, D., & Todd, M. (2000). Perioperative heat balance. *Anesthesiology, 92*(2), 578–596.

Spry, C. (2005). *Essentials of perioperative nursing* (3rd ed.). Sudbury, MA: Jones & Bartlett.

Sullivan, E. E. (2000). Preoperative holding area, *Journal of PeriAnesthesia Nursing, 15*(5), 353–354.

Tarrac, S. (2006). A description of intraoperative and postanesthesia complication rates. *Journal of PeriAnesthesia Nursing, 21*(2), 88–96.

The Joint Commission (2004). *Procedures Requiring Surgical Site Marking.* Retrieved on July 2, 2008 from http://www.jointcommission.org/AccreditationPrograms/Hospitals/Standards/FAQs/Provsion[plus]of[plus]Care/Operative_HRP_Sed_Anesth/Surgical_Site_Marking.htm

Wagner, D. (2006). Unplanned perioperative hypothermia. *AORN Journal, 83*(2), 470–476.

Postoperative Nursing

Jane Ashley

Outcome-Based Learning Objectives

After studying this chapter, the learner will be able to:

1. Prioritize nursing diagnoses and interventions for the patient in the postanesthesia care unit.
2. Discuss criteria for moving patients through the phases of recovery.
3. Discuss the assessment, prevention, and nursing management of common postoperative problems.
4. Develop a teaching plan for the discharge of a patient after surgery.
5. Identify and discuss areas of future research relevant to the care of the postoperative patient.

Research Collaboration Health Promotion Nursing Process Caring Critical Thinking

THE POSTOPERATIVE period begins with the completion of surgery and the transfer of the patient to the **postanesthesia care unit (PACU)**, where the patient recovers from the effects of anesthesia. The PACU, located close to the operating room, is designed to care for patients as they stabilize and recover from surgery and anesthesia. Following surgery, the patient is moved to the PACU accompanied by the circulating nurse and a member of the anesthesia care team. In some circumstances, a surgical patient may be transferred directly to an intensive care unit (ICU) for recovery rather than to the PACU, but most surgical patients stabilize in the PACU before discharge home or transfer to a clinical unit. After discharge from the PACU, postoperative care continues in the home for ambulatory surgical patients, or in the hospital for patients requiring a more monitored recovery.

Nursing Management

Nursing assessment and intervention immediately following surgery focus on patient safety, hemodynamic stability, and the recognition and prevention of postoperative complications. Care in the PACU is organized around postanesthesia phases I and II. Phase I begins with the arrival of the patient and focuses on the recovery of physiological homeostasis and protective mechanisms. During this phase, the patient requires intensive nursing observation and care.

Phase II begins when the patient becomes more alert and functional. The patient requires less intensive nursing and the focus of interventions is on preparing the patient and significant others for the patient's discharge home. As such, phase II refers most specifically to ambulatory surgery. The term **fast-tracking** describes a situation in which the patient is transferred from the operating room to PACU phase II bypassing PACU phase I. Fast-tracking is possible when surgical techniques are minimally invasive and anesthesia is of a short duration. More research is needed to identify which patients are appropriate for fast-tracking, to standardize guidelines and develop protocols used in fast-tracking, and to follow patient outcomes (Ead, 2006).

Nurses should also be aware of certain specifics related to caring for postoperative patients from various cultures, as discussed in the Cultural Considerations box.

Collaborative Management

The PACU nurse works in close collaboration with the anesthesia provider and surgeon. Nurse–physician collaboration in ICUs is linked to better patient outcomes including a reduction in mortality rates (Wheelan, Burchill, & Tilin, 2003). Generally, the anesthesia provider assumes responsibility for coordinating the medical and surgical care of the patient in the PACU. The patient's

CULTURAL CONSIDERATIONS for the Postoperative Patient

- Modesty is extremely important in some cultures and in some religions (e.g., Hispanic, Arab, Muslim). Keep women modestly covered and expose only the body area necessary for examination or treatment. Provide a cover for the head to female patients who desire it. Provide same-gender caretakers when possible.

- Pain assessment may need to be modified for some patients. Numeric rating scales may not be appropriate for all cultures. In some situations, the FACES pain rating scale that uses facial expressions to assess pain may be more useful than numeric rating scales. Some patients may be reluctant to talk about their pain or to take pain medication.

- Pain expression is culturally influenced. In some cultures pain may be openly expressed in words, sounds (e.g., moaning), and physical movement, whereas in other cultures, patients are expected to be stoic about the presence of pain. Nurses need to be aware of and sensitive to cultural expressions of pain.

- Consider cultural beliefs in the selection and use of pain medications. In some cultures, patients may be reluctant to talk about pain and to take pain medication for fear of addition, dependence, or sedation. Explain to patients the importance of treating pain and be sensitive to alternative pain therapies.

- Be aware of and sensitive to treatment restrictions. Some cultures or religions restrict or discourage the use of certain medical treatments such as blood transfusions or organ transplantation.

- Recognize and support the dietary practices in cultures and religions. Many religions (Orthodox Jewish, Muslim, Seventh-Day Adventist, Catholic) have dietary requirements such as vegetarianism or Kosher food preparation, or dietary restrictions such as avoidance of pork, shellfish, or caffeinated products. Hospital kitchens and health care providers need to accommodate these practices. Encourage family members who wish to bring in specially prepared foods to do so. Ask your patient about and be sensitive to special dietary needs.

- Ask about and support the use of alternative healing treatments when possible. Some alternative therapies such as the use of prayer, anointment, healing touch, or communion can be accommodated with little problem. Other therapies such as the use of herbal products to promote healing may need to be evaluated for their effects on wound healing or medications. Talk with patients about what, if any, alternative treatments they believe are important to their recovery.

- Visitors should be encouraged. In some cultures, it is important for family members and extended family members to be present in the hospital with the patient. Consider ways to include family members in the care of the patient.

Sources: Galanti, G. A. (2006). Applying cultural competence to perianesthesia nursing. *Journal of PeriAnesthesia Nursing, 21*(2), 97–102; Lovering, S. (2006). Cultural beliefs about pain. *Journal of Transcultural Nursing, 17*(4), 389–395; McDonald, D. D., McNulty, J., Erickson, K., & Weiskopf, C. (2000). Communicating pain and pain management needs after surgery. *Applied Nursing Research, 13*(2), 70–75; Quinn, D. (2006). How religion, language and ethnicity impact perioperative nursing care. *Nursing Clinics of North America, 41*, 231–248; Spector, R. (2009). *Cultural diversity in health and illness.* Upper Saddle River, NJ: Pearson Prentice Hall.

trajectory in the PACU moves from instability to stability over the course of an hour to several hours (Prowse & Lyne, 2000). Chart 27–1 shows the typical trajectory of a postoperative patient.

Assessment

The PACU nurse ensures patient safety during the transition from the operating room to home or to the clinical unit. The PACU nurse is an intensive care nurse who is prepared to identify and prevent the acute problems and complications associ-

ated with surgery and anesthesia. The nurse is skilled in the management of situations where the patient's physiological condition is rapidly changing and the nurse is especially attentive to **surveillance** (the systematic and continuous assessment of the patient) and to the recognition and management of potentially catastrophic events (Clarke & Aiken, 2003). The nurse also is prepared to respond to patients' psychological responses to surgery and anesthesia providing reassurance and comfort. Care in the PACU is guided by the *Standards of Perianesthesia Nursing Practice* developed by the American Society of PeriAnesthesia Nurses (ASPAN), the professional organization for PACU nurses (ASPAN, 2006b), the *Standards for Post Anesthesia Care* (ASA, 2004), hospital policies, and clinical guidelines.

The PACU nurse receives a report about the patient's condition from the anesthesia provider. The report provides a description of pertinent medical and surgical history, the condition requiring surgery, the surgical procedure and any complications, the anesthesia, medications given during surgery, any difficulties with intubation, the estimated blood loss from surgery, fluid status of the patient, transfusions, and vital signs. Other pertinent information communicated to the nurse includes the type and location of incisions and drains, intravenous fluids, current medications and medications held prior to surgery, impairments in skin integrity, swallowing, mobility, or communication. The PACU nurse is apprised of concerns the patient expressed preoperatively, any special requirements, and the presence of significant others waiting for the patient.

A complete system assessment of the patient is conducted immediately on arrival to the PACU. The nurse uses the ABCs

CHART 27–1 Postanesthesia Patient Trajectory

Level of Consciousness
Unconscious → Semiconscious → Conscious

Airway
Unable to maintain airway → Rejects airway support → Supports own airway

Cardiovascular
Cardiovascular instability → Cardiovascular lability → Cardiovascular stable

Pain
No pain perception → Awareness of pain → Adequate pain control

Body Temperature
Hypothermia → Normothermia

Source: Adapted from Prowse, M., & Lyne, P. (2000). Clinical effectiveness in the post-anesthesia care unit: How nursing knowledge contributes to achieving intended patient outcomes. *Journal of Advanced Nursing, 31*(5), 1115–1124.

(i.e., airway–breathing–circulation) to prioritize the initial assessment of the surgical patient starting with observation of the airway for patency. Unless contraindicated, recovering patients are placed in a lateral position to reduce the risk of aspiration. An artificial airway (oral or nasal) prevents the tongue from falling backward and occluding the airway. It may be used until the patient is able to support her airway unassisted. Humidified oxygen is placed via face mask and titrated to keep oxygenation saturation levels above 93% or at a level determined by the health care provider. For the first 2 hours after surgery, the patient may be placed on high levels of oxygen (e.g., FIO_2 greater than 80%) because evidence suggests that this will destroy pathogens and reduce the risk of surgical-site infections (Greif, Akca, Horn, Kurz, & Sessler, 2000; Hopf et al., 2004; Schweon, 2006). The nurse assesses the patient's respiratory rate and depth, breath sounds, and oxygen saturation via a continuous pulse oximeter.

Some patients will remain intubated and on mechanical ventilation following the surgery. In such cases, the nurse performs the respiratory assessments described above and, in addition, checks the endotracheal tube and ventilator settings. A cardiac monitor is attached to the patient as well as a blood pressure cuff. Apical pulse and blood pressure are taken and the patient's heart rhythm is noted. If the patient has a pulmonary artery catheter in place, pulmonary artery pressures and cardiac output are measured and recorded. The nurse assesses peripheral pulses and the patient's color as indices of the adequacy of circulation.

The patient's core body temperature is measured using the monitoring device considered best according to agency policy and the nurse's judgment. Temperature can fluctuate rapidly during recovery. Core body temperature can be measured in the tympanic membrane using a tympanic thermometer. Oral and axillary temperatures provide only an estimate of the core body temperature, and a rectal temperature is considered unreliable in hyperthermic crisis (ASPAN, 2002). A temporal scanner, a device that relies on an infrared scanner to detect the highest temperature of forehead skin, provides a rapid measurement of body temperature, but may not be accurate in recording core body temperatures under some circumstances (Low et al., 2007).

The PACU nurse performs a systematic, head-to-toe assessment of the patient. Figure 27–1 ■ is an example of a PACU assessment form. The following areas are assessed during the head-to-toe examination.

- **Level of consciousness (LOC)**—Is the patient unconscious, arousable, fully awake? LOC is documented every 15 minutes for the first hour, then hourly thereafter. Describe pupil size and response. If awake, is the patient oriented to person, place, and time? Is the patient's speech clear? Intracranial pressure will be measured following selected cranial surgeries.
- **Cardiovascular**—Record the patient's vital signs and cardiac rhythm. If applicable, measure and record cardiac output, pulmonary artery pressures, and central venous pressure. Examine the extremities for color, sensation, motion, and pulses. An ankle-brachial index may be measured in vascular procedures (Chapter 43 ⊘).
- **Respiratory**—Describe patient's airway and need for artificial airway, respiratory rate, depth, breath sounds, oxygen

saturation, cough, secretions, arterial blood gases, chest tubes, and need for suctioning, if applicable.
- **Pain management**—Describe the location, quality, and rating of pain. If a spinal or epidural was used, describe the sensory level of numbness and the motor ability of the extremities.
- **Gastrointestinal**—Describe abdominal assessment (Is the abdomen flat and soft or firm and distended? Are bowel sounds present?). If the patient is nauseated, describe whether the nausea is mild, moderate, or severe. Is the patient vomiting?
- **Genitourinary**—Does the patient have a urinary catheter? Describe the amount and color of urine output. If no catheter, is the bladder distended? Has the patient voided? Note when the patient is due to void. If a gynecologic procedure was performed, describe vaginal bleeding.
- **Skin integrity**—Describe skin color, temperature, areas of bruising, redness, or ulceration.
- **Temperature**—Record core body temperature.
- **Incision**—Describe location and condition of incision. Describe any bleeding, wound drainage, or the presence of a hematoma. If the suture line is not visible, describe the condition of the dressing. Describe the type and drainage from any wound drains.
- **Activity/movement**—Is the patient able to hold his head up? Is the patient able to move all extremities? Are movements voluntary or on command? Describe strength of extremities; is it equal on both sides? Does the patient have compression stockings, pneumatic compression boots, or another type of deep venous thrombosis (DVT) prophylaxis device in place?
- **Psychosocial**—If the patient is awake, describe the level of psychosocial comfort. Is the patient calm, relaxed, and sleeping or anxious and distressed?
- **Intravenous fluids**—Describe the location of intravenous catheters, the type of catheter, and the type and rate of intravenous fluid.
- **Drains and other tubes**—Describe the type, location, and drainage of any tubes.
- **Other medical devices**—Describe any other devices the patient may have such as an arterial line, pulmonary artery catheter, or traction.

The American Society of Anesthesiologists (ASA, 2004) recommends using a scoring system as part of the continuous evaluation of PACU patients. Numerical rating systems are endorsed by the Joint Commission and they have several advantages. Scoring systems are easy to use, reliable, and they provide objective data for monitoring how well the patient is progressing. Additionally, data from scoring systems can be used in research studies to compare the postoperative progression associated with particular patient characteristics or specific types of surgeries.

Various numerical rating systems are available but the most commonly used system is the Aldrete Post Anesthesia Recovery Score (PARS) (Figure 27–2 ■, p. 655). In this scoring system, the patient receives a score of 0 to 2 for respirations, oxygen saturation, consciousness, circulation, and activity. Total scores range from 0 to 10 with higher scores indicating a higher level of func-

Patient's name _____
Med. Rec. # _____
DOB _____

POSTOPERATIVE ASSESSMENT

TIME																	

POST ANESTHETIC SCORE

POST ANESTHESIA RECOVERY SCORE

ACTIVITY		
Able to move 4 extremities voluntarily or on command	2	
Able to move 2 extremities voluntarily or on command	1	
Unable to move extremities voluntarily or on command	0	
RESPIRATION		
Able to breathe deeply and cough freely	2	
Dyspnea, limited breathing, or tachypnea	1	
Apneic or on mechanical ventilator	0	
CIRCULATION		
BP plus or minus 20% of preoperative baseline	2	
BP plus or minus 20%–40% of preanesthetic level	1	
BP plus or minus 40% of preanesthetic level	0	
CONSCIOUSNESS		
Fully awake	2	
Arousable on calling	1	
Not responding	0	
O2 Saturation		
Able to maintain O2 saturation > 92% on room air	2	
Needs O2 inhalation to maintain O2 saturation > 90%	1	
O2 saturation <50% even with O2 supplement	0	

TOTAL PAR SCORE

POST ANESTHESIA DISCHARGE SCORE

VITAL SIGNS		
BP and pulse within 20% of preoperative baseline	2	
BP and pulse 20%–40% of preoperative baseline	1	
BP and pulse <40% of preoperative baseline	0	
ACTIVITY LEVEL		
Steady gait, no clumsiness, or meets preoperative level	2	
Requires assistance	1	
Unable to ambulate	0	
NAUSEA & VOMITING		
Minimal to none	2	
Moderate	1	
Severe	0	
PAIN		
Minimal to pain free	2	
Moderate pain handeled by oral medication	1	
Severe pain requiring parenteral medication	0	
SURGICAL BLEEDING		
Minimal to none	2	
Moderate	1	
Severe	0	

TOTAL PAD SCORE

LABORATORY RESULTS

Hematology				Coagulation			Chemistry									Miscellaneous TEST RESULTS
Time	Hct	WBC	Plts	PT	PTT	INR	BS	BUN	Cr	Na	K	Cl	CO2	Mg	iCa	

FIGURE 27–1 ■ Sample PACU assessment form.

tioning. A patient receives a score on admission and every 30 minutes until a score of 8 or higher is achieved. The PARS score is the criterion by which patients progress from phase I PACU recovery to phase II PACU recovery (Ead, 2006).

The frequency of patient assessment in the PACU depends on the stability of the patient. A patient's physiological status can change rapidly during recovery. In acute crisis, patients are con-tinuously monitored (every 1 to 5 minutes) until the situation no longer warrants such close observation. For the person who is stable, vital signs and patient assessment are performed on admission and every 15 minutes for the first hour (i.e., four assessments). This is followed by every 30 minutes for the next 2 hours (i.e., four assessments), then every hour until discharge from the unit. Chart 27–2 (p. 655) lists abnormal findings on assessment

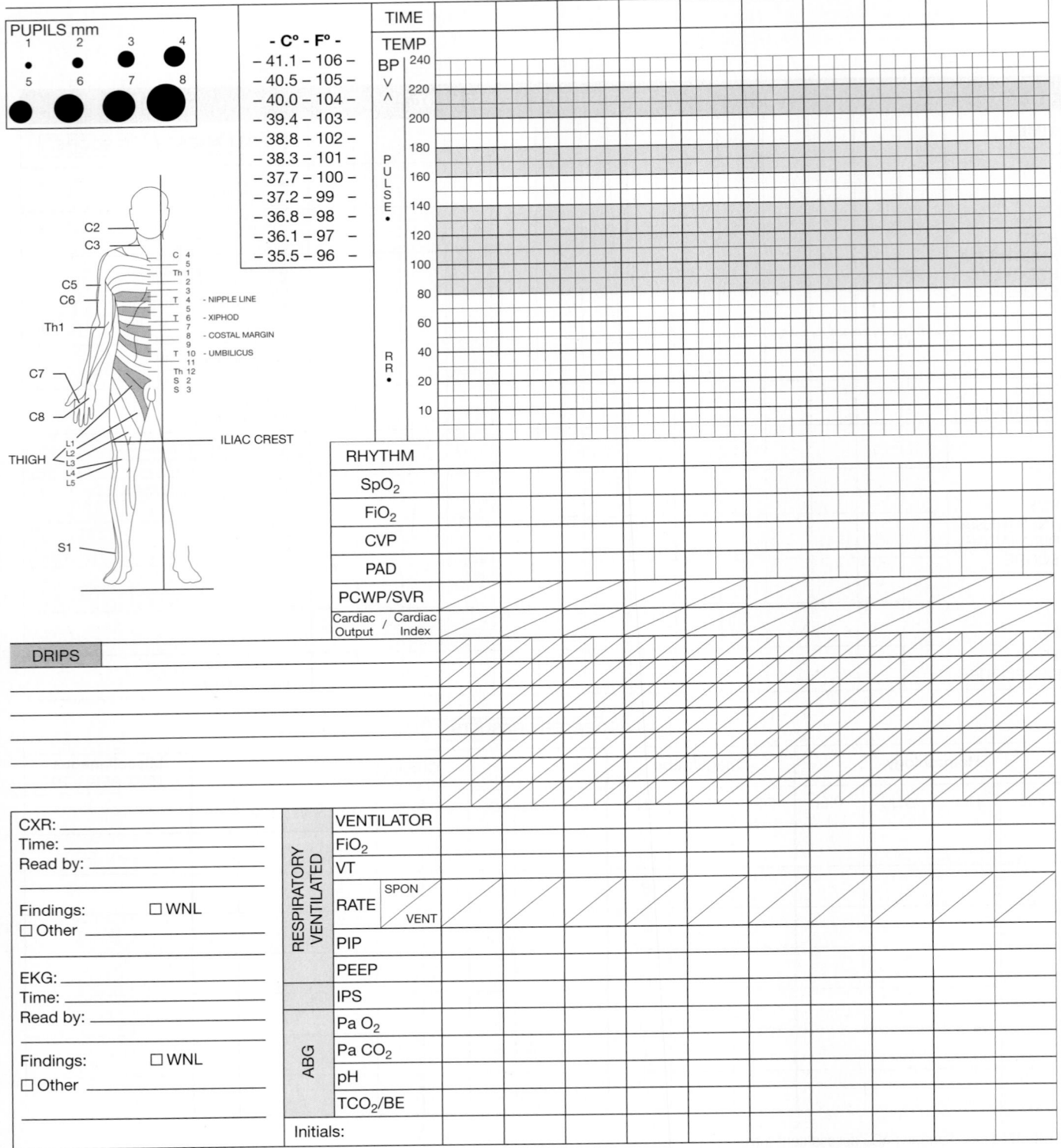

FIGURE 27–1 ■ *Continued*

that suggest the need for closer observation and consultation with the anesthesiologist.

Initially, patients are placed in a lateral position. As they become more awake, they are placed with the head of the bed elevated if not contraindicated by the surgery. Patients are repositioned every 1 to 2 hours or as needed. A patient who is experiencing nausea and vomiting may remain in a lateral position to prevent aspiration.

Nursing Diagnoses and Expected Outcomes

The patient recovering from anesthesia and surgery is at risk for a number of problems. Some of these problems occur early in the course of recovery and are much more likely to be seen in the PACU than elsewhere. Others may occur both in the PACU and on the clinical unit. Some problems occur later in recovery and

Patient's name _____

Med. Rec. # _____

DOB _____

TIME											
TEMP											

BP V ∧ PULSE • RR • (graph 10–240)

RHYTHM											
SpO$_2$											
FiO$_2$											
CVP											
PAD											
PCWP/SVR											
Cardiac Output / Cardiac Index											

DRIPS												

CXR: _____

Time: _____

Read by: _____

Findings: ☐ WNL

☐ Other _____

EKG: _____

Time: _____

Read by: _____

Findings: ☐ WNL

☐ Other _____

RESPIRATORY VENTILATED	VENTILATOR										
	FiO$_2$										
	VT										
	RATE SPON / VENT										
	PIP										
	PEEP										
	IPS										
ABG	Pa O$_2$										
	Pa CO$_2$										
	pH										
	TCO$_2$/BE										
Initials:											

FIGURE 27–1 ■ *Continued*

are more likely to be seen on the clinical unit or at home after discharge. Common nursing diagnoses with expected outcomes in the PACU are as follows:

- *Risk for Impaired Gas Exchange* (airway obstruction, laryngospasm, hypoxia).

  Outcomes: The patient will have an open airway. The patient will have breathing patterns consistent with or improved from baseline. The patient will demonstrate adequate oxygen saturation levels.

- **Risk for Imbalanced Fluid Volume** (bleeding, hypovolemia, fluid overload)

  Outcomes: The patient will achieve adequate hemostasis. The patient will demonstrate normal fluid and electrolyte balance.

FIGURE 27–1 ■ *Continued*

- *Risk for Decreased Cardiac Output:* (dysrhythmia, hypotension, hypertension).

  Outcomes: The patient will have normal cardiac rhythm. The patient will achieve adequate cardiac output. The patient's blood pressure and heart rate will return to normal or be consistent with baseline values.

- *Risk for Imbalanced Body Temperature:* *Hypothermia*

  Outcome: The patient will demonstrate a normal core body temperature.

- *Readiness for Enhanced Comfort:* *Nausea and Vomiting*

  Outcome: The patient will report adequate relief from nausea and vomiting.

- *Readiness for Enhanced Comfort:* *Pain*

  Outcome: The patient will report an acceptable level of pain control.

- **Anxiety**

  Outcomes: The patient will report diminished anxiety levels. The patient will report an acceptable level of anxiety.

Interventions, Rationales, and Evaluation

The interventions and rationales for the nursing diagnoses often seen with patients in the PACU are discussed next, and additional guidelines for patients in postoperative phase I that deal with pain and comfort are listed in the National Guidelines box (p. 656).

TIME (?) Yes (-) No (*) See Notes (N/A) Not applicable																				
☐Patient identified using two indicators																				
LEVEL OF CONSCIOUSNESS																				
Fully awake																				
Arousable upon calling																				
Not responding																				
PUPIL SIZE (mm) REACTION R																				
SL = sluggish R = reactive NR = nonreactive L																				
PAIN: Location & Level (0-10) (Quality*)																				
SPEECH CLEAR & APPROPRIATE																				
BREATH SOUNDS																				
SYMMETRICAL																				
COUGH/DEEP BREATHE																				
AIRWAY																				
Patent																				
___ oral ___ nasal D/C___																				
CPT/IS																				
SUCTIONING																				
EXTREMITIES WARM & WNL																				
PERIPHERAL PULSES R																				
L																				
SEQUENTIAL COMPRESSION DEVICE 45 mmHg																				
POSITION																				
SPINAL/EPIDURAL SENSORY LEVEL R																				
L																				
MOTOR RESPONSE R Arm																				
3 = Lifts & holds L Arm																				
2 = Lifts & falls back R Leg																				
1 = Moves on bed L Leg																				
0 = No movement																				
DRESSING D&I: Site(s)																				
DRAINS PATENT/DRAINAGE																				
1. Type drain/site:																				
1. Type drainage:																				
2. Type drain/site:																				
2. Type drainage:																				
SKIN INTEGRITY:																				
ARTERIAL LINE Dressing D&I																				
CENTRAL LINE Dressing D&I																				
PERIPHERAL IVs:																				
REWARMING DEVICE:																				
VAGINAL FLOW																				
NAUSEA OR VOMITING																				
NGT -> CONTINUOUS SUCTION																				
-> Type drainage																				
ABDOMEN SOFT																				
FOLEY CATHETER PATENT																				
Type drainage																				
BLADDER NOT PALPABLE																				
Voided QS																				
No void. Discharge voiding instructions reviewed.																				
DTV@																				
INITIALS																				

(Left vertical label: NURSING OBSERVATIONS AND INTERVENTIONS)

FIGURE 27–1 ■ *Continued*

TIME (?) Yes (-) No (*) See Notes (N/A) Not applicable	/	/	/	/	/	/		TIME	NOTES
☐ Patient identified using two indicators									
LEVEL OF CONSCIOUSNESS									
Fully awake									
Arousable upon calling									
Not responding									
PUPIL SIZE (mm) /REACTION R	/	/	/	/	/	/			
SL = sluggish R = reactive NR = nonreactive L	/	/	/	/	/	/			
PAIN: Location & Level (0-10) (Quality*)									
SPEECH CLEAR & APPROPRIATE									
BREATH SOUNDS									
SYMMETRICAL									
COUGH/DEEP BREATHE									
AIRWAY									
Patent									
____ oral ____ nasal D/C ____									
CPT/IS									
SUCTIONING									
EXTREMITIES WARM & WNL									
PERIPHERAL PULSES R									
L									
SEQUENTIAL COMPRESSION DEVICE 45 mmHg									
POSITION									
SPINAL/EPIDURAL SENSORY LEVEL R									
L									
MOTOR RESPONSE R Arm									
3 = Lifts & holds L Arm									
2 = Lifts & falls back R Leg									
1 = Moves on bed									
0 = No movement L Leg									
DRESSING D&I: Site(s)									
DRAINS PATENT/DRAINAGE									
1. Type drain/site:									
1. Type drainage:									
2. Type drain/site:									
2. Type drainage:									
SKIN INTEGRITY:									
ARTERIAL LINE Dressing D&I									
CENTRAL LINE Dressing D&I									
PERIPHERAL IVs:									
REWARMING DEVICE:									
VAGINAL FLOW									
NAUSEA OR VOMITING									
NGT -> CONTINUOUS SUCTION									
-> Type drainage									
ABDOMEN SOFT									
FOLEY CATHETER PATENT									
Type drainage									
BLADDER NOT PALPABLE									
Voided QS									
No void. Discharge voiding instructions reviewed.									
DTV@									
INITIALS									

(Left margin vertical label:) NURSING OBSERVATIONS AND INTERVENTIONS

FIGURE 27–1 ■ *Continued*

MEDICATIONS							
MEDICATION	DOSE	ROUTE	TIME				

Patient's name _____

Med. Rec. # _____

DOB _____

MEDICATION	DOSE	ROUTE	TIME				

TIME	NOTES	TIME	NOTES

_____ RN   _____ RN   _____ ___/___/___
Signature   Printed name   Initials   Date

_____ RN   _____ RN   _____ ___/___/___
Signature   Printed name   Initials   Date

_____ RN   _____ RN   _____ ___/___/___
Signature   Printed name   Initials   Date

_____ RN   _____ RN   _____ ___/___/___
Signature   Printed name   Initials   Date

FIGURE 27–1 ■ *Continued*

INTAKE & OUTPUT														
ENTERAL		CRYSTALLOID				COLLOID			OUTPUT					
TIME	AMT	TIME	AMT		ABS	TIME		ABS	TIME	IRRIGATION		HOURLY URINE		
										UP	IN		TOTAL	NG/EMESIS	CHEST	HEMOVAC/ JP

(Note: the OUTPUT section has sub-columns: TIME, IRRIGATION (UP, IN), HOURLY URINE (TOTAL), NG/EMESIS, CHEST, HEMOVAC/JP)

ENTERAL TIME	AMT	CRYSTALLOID TIME	AMT		ABS	COLLOID TIME		ABS	TIME	UP	IN	HOURLY URINE	TOTAL	NG/EMESIS	CHEST	HEMOVAC/JP
O.R. →						EBL=										

DISCHARGE SUMMARY

NURSING DIAGNOSES 1-14 OUTCOMES MET: ☐ Yes ☐ No _____

SURGICAL CRITERIA MET: ☐ Yes ☐ No _____

Time Ready for Discharge:_____ Discharged: _____

☐ Room #: _____ ☐ Transfer Communication Completed

Discharge ☐ Home Time:_____ ☐ Valuables Returned to Patient

_____ _____
Signature of Recipient   RN Initials

Discharge teaching completed. Patient verbalizes understanding.
☐ Yes ☐ No (See note)
Prescriptions: _____
_____
Copy of instructions given to patient: ☐ Yes ☐ No

OUTPATIENT POST-OP PHONE CALL

Phone #: _____
Date: _____ Time: _____
Pain: Score (0-10) _____ : Location/Quality _____
Nausea/Vomiting: ☐ No ☐ Yes _____
Voiding: ☐ Yes ☐ No _____
Any problem with procedure site? ☐ No ☐ Yes _____
Any concerns? ☐ No ☐ Yes _____
Did you need to call MD? ☐ No ☐ Yes _____
☐ Voice mail left. Patient to call with questions.
Comments: _____
_____

Signature RN _____ Print Name _____

FIGURE 27–1 ■ *Continued*

Source: Courtesy of Beth Israel Deaconess Nursing Department

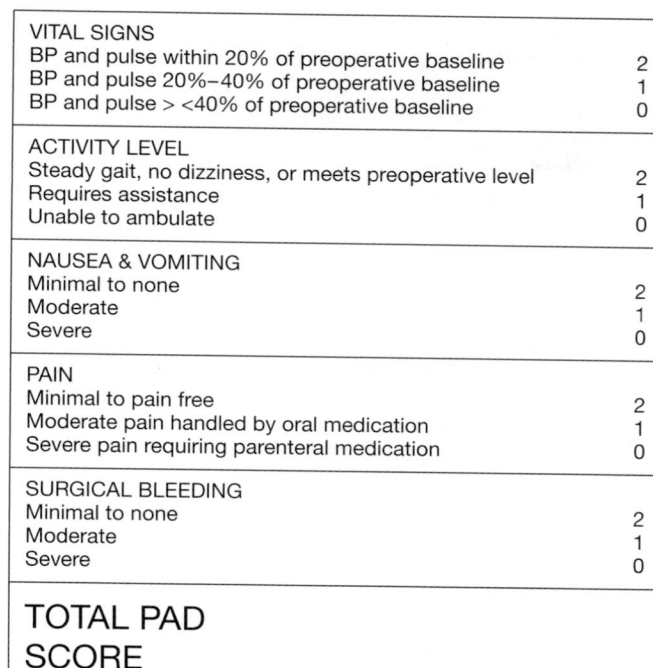

VITAL SIGNS	
BP and pulse within 20% of preoperative baseline	2
BP and pulse 20%–40% of preoperative baseline	1
BP and pulse > <40% of preoperative baseline	0
ACTIVITY LEVEL	
Steady gait, no dizziness, or meets preoperative level	2
Requires assistance	1
Unable to ambulate	0
NAUSEA & VOMITING	
Minimal to none	2
Moderate	1
Severe	0
PAIN	
Minimal to pain free	2
Moderate pain handled by oral medication	1
Severe pain requiring parenteral medication	0
SURGICAL BLEEDING	
Minimal to none	2
Moderate	1
Severe	0
TOTAL PAD SCORE	

FIGURE 27–2 ■ Aldrete Post Anesthesia Recovery Score.
Source: Courtesy of Beth Israel Deaconess Nursing Department

Impaired Gas Exchange

Most patients will arrive in the PACU with supplemental oxygen to prevent **hypoxemia**, insufficient oxygen content in the blood. Common causes of hypoxemia in the early postoperative period include airway obstruction, hypoventilation, and laryngospasm. Respiratory complications, especially the need for upper airway support, are the most frequent postoperative problem in the PACU (McAlister, Bertsch, Man, Bradley, & Jacka, 2005; Tarrac, 2006).

Airway obstruction occurs most often because medications used in anesthesia cause the muscles to relax. When the tongue relaxes, it can fall backward blocking the airway. Signs of an obstructed airway include snoring, stridor, retraction of intercostal muscles, and a fall in oxygen saturation levels. To prevent airway obstruction, patients are positioned on their side and an artificial airway is inserted. An oral airway is effective with the patient who is minimally responsive, but a patient who is more arousable may gag, choke, or spit out the airway. For these patients, a nasal airway may be more effective and comfortable. A patient who is experiencing an acute airway obstruction needs to be stimulated. If a patient is arousable, the problem can often be resolved by speaking to the patient, encouraging her to take deep breaths, and turning up the oxygen level if necessary. Patients who are not arousable may need to have their airway opened. The nurse can perform the chin-tilt/jaw-thrust maneuver used in cardiopulmonary resuscitation to open the airway. An oral airway is inserted to maintain patency. Airway occlusion becomes less of a threat once the patient is more responsive and regains protective mechanisms.

In some patients, a delay in the excretion of neuromuscular blocking agents used in anesthesia can result in weakened respiratory muscles causing *hypoventilation*, insufficient inspiratory

CHART 27–2 Abnormal PACU Assessments That Are Reported to the Anesthesiologist

NEUROLOGICAL FINDINGS

- Prolonged unresponsiveness
- Change in level of consciousness
- Abnormal responses such as slurred speech, asymmetrical smile, weak hand grasps, inability to move all extremities

CARDIOVASCULAR FINDINGS

- Heart rate >120 beats/min
- Hypotension (e.g., systolic blood pressure of less than 90 mmHg)
- New cardiac dysrhythmia
- Hypertension (e.g., systolic blood pressure 20% to 30% higher than baseline)
- Absence of peripheral pulses

RESPIRATORY FINDINGS

- Oxygen saturation < 93%
- Respiratory rate <10 breaths/min
- Indications of respiratory distress and/or hypoventilation such as stridor, retraction of intercostal muscles, minimal respiratory effort

OTHER FINDINGS

- Urine output < 30 mL hour or < 5 mL/kg per hour
- More than the expected amount of bleeding at the incision site
- Enlarging hematoma
- Loss of pulse(s) in a graft site
- Unexpected presence of blood in drainage tubes
- More than the expected amount of drainage from chest tubes or wound drains
- Vomiting associated with possible aspiration

and expiratory effort. This should be suspected in patients who are unable to sustain a head lift or have weak hand grasps although this may be hard to evaluate in a patient who is obtunded. The prolonged effects of anesthetic agents also can produce a slow respiratory rate (i.e., less than 10 per minute) and shallow breathing. The continuous assessment of oxygen saturation helps to identify the patient who is becoming hypoxemic as a result of poor ventilatory effort. The nurse reports to the anesthesiologist a respiratory rate of less than 10 or oxygen saturation rate of less than 93% or less than a health care provider–prescribed value. Some patients experiencing hypoxemia may benefit from the application of continuous positive airway pressure (CPAP) to keep airways open (Squadrone et al., 2005).

Laryngospasm occurs when the muscles of the larynx contract forcefully, causing a closure or partial closure of the airway. It can be caused by irritation from secretions, inhalants, or medications and is an emergency situation because the patient can quickly become hypoxic. Treatment may include opening the airway, suctioning secretions, administering oxygen, administering an aerosolized epinephrine solution, and in severe cases reintubation.

NATIONAL GUIDELINES American Society of PeriAnesthesia Nurses Pain and Comfort Clinical Guidelines

Postanesthesia Phase I

Assessment

1. Refer to preoperative phase assessment, interventions, and outcomes data.

2. Type of surgery and anesthesia technique, anesthetic agents, reversal agents.

3. Analgesics (i.e., nonopioid, opioid, adjuvants given before and during surgery, time and amount at last dose, and regional [e.g., spinal/epidural]).

4. Pain and comfort levels on admission and until transfer to receiving unit or discharge to home. Reassess frequently until pain or discomfort is controlled. During sedation procedure, assess continuously.

5. Assessment parameters:
   A. Functional level and ability to relax.
   B. Pain: type, location, intensity (i.e., using self-report pain rating scale whenever possible [age, language, condition, and cognitive appropriate tools], quality, frequency [continuous or intermittent], and sedation level; patient's method of assessment and reporting need to be the same during the postoperative continuum of care for consistency). Note pain level at rest and during activity.
   C. Self-report of comfort level using numerical scale (0 to 10 scale) or other institutionally approved instruments.
   D. Physical appearance (e.g., pain/discomfort behaviors. [*Note:* Pain behaviors are highly individual and the absence of any specific behavior, e.g., facial expression or body movement, does not mean the absence of pain.].)
   E. Other sources of discomfort (e.g., position, nausea and vomiting, shivering, environment such as noise, noxious smell, anxiety).
   F. Achievement of pain relief/comfort treatment goals.

6. Age, cognitive ability, and cognitive learning methods.

7. Status/vital signs:
   A. Airway patency, respiratory status, breath sounds, level of consciousness, and pupil size as indicated and other symptoms related to the effects of medications.
   B. Blood pressure.
   C. Pulse/cardiac monitor rhythm.
   D. Oxygen saturation.
   E. Motor and sensory functions postregional anesthesia technique.

Interventions

1. Identify patient correctly; validate health care provider's order; implement correct drug, dose, amount, route, and time; include type of surgery and surgical site as applicable.

2. Pharmacologic (medicate as ordered).
   A. *Mild to moderate pain:* Use nonopioids and may consider opioid (e.g., acetaminophen, NSAIDs, cyclooxygenase 2 [Cox-2] inhibitors). All of the patient's regular nonopioid prescription medications should be made available unless contraindicated and per institutional approval.
   B. *Moderate to severe pain:* Use multimodal therapy (e.g., combine nonopioid and opioid).
   C. Utilize the three analgesic groups appropriately (consider multimodal therapy):
      i. Nonopioids (e.g., acetaminophen, NSAIDs, Cox-2 inhibitors); adjuvants nonopioids (acetaminophen and NSAIDs, such as aspirin, ketorolac, ibuprofen, Cox-2 inhibitors).
      ii. Beta-agonist opioids (e.g., morphine, hydromorphone, fentanyl).
      iii. Adjuvants:
         a. Multipurpose for chronic pain (e.g., anticonvulsants, tricyclic antidepressants, corticosteroids, antianxiety medication).
         b. Multipurpose for moderate to severe acute pain (e.g., local anesthetics, ketamine).
         c. Neuropathic continuous pain (antidepressants, tricyclic antidepressants, oral or local anesthetic).
         d. Neuropathic lancinating pain, e.g., stabbing, knifelike pain (anticonvulsant, baclofen).
         e. Malignant bone pain (corticosteroids, calcitonin).
         f. Post–orthopedic surgery: Consider muscle relaxants if patient experiences muscle spasm.

3. Initiate and adjust IV and regional infusions, i.e., patient controlled analgesia (PCA) as indicated and ordered, and based on hemodynamics status. (Refer to institutional permissive procedure.)

4. Nonpharmacologic intervention use to complement, not replace, pharmacologic interventions.

5. Administer comfort measures as needed:
   A. Physiological (e.g., positioning, pillow, heat and cold therapies, sensory aids [e.g., dentures, eye glasses, hearing aids]; use meperidine [Demerol] for shivering, antiemetics [e.g., Reglan, Zofran] as ordered).
   B. Sociocultural (e.g., family/caregiver, interpreter visit).
   C. Psychospiritual (e.g., chaplain or cleric of choice, religious objects/symbols).
   D. Environmental (e.g., confidentiality, privacy, reasonably quiet room).

6. Cognitive behavioral (e.g., education/instruction, relaxation, imagery, music, distraction, biofeedback).

Expected Outcomes

1. Patient will maintain hemodynamic stability including respiratory/cardiac status and level of consciousness.

2. Patient will state achievement of pain relief/comfort treatments goals (e.g., acceptable pain relief with mobility at time of transfer or discharge).

3. Patient will state he/she feels safe and secure with the instructions (e.g., use of PCA machine).

4. Patient will show effective use of at least one nonpharmacologic method (i.e., breathing relaxation techniques).

5. Patient will show effective use of PCA as indicated and discuss expected results of regional techniques.

6. Patient will verbalize evidence of receding pain level and increased comfort with pharmacologic and nonpharmacologic interventions.

NATIONAL GUIDELINES American Society of PeriAnesthesia Nurses Pain and Comfort Clinical Guidelines—*Continued*

Postanesthesia Phase II/III
Assessment

1. Refer to preoperative phase and phase I assessments, interventions, and outcomes data.

2. Achievement of pain/comfort treatment goals and level of satisfaction with pain relief and comfort management.

3. Pain relief/comfort management plan for discharge and patient agreement.

4. Educational and resource needs, considering age, language, condition, and cognitive appropriateness.

Interventions

1. Identify patient correctly; validate health care provider's order; implement correct drug, dose, amount, route, and time.

2. Pharmacologic interventions (medicate as ordered): nonopioid (e.g., acetaminophen, NSAIDs, Cox-2 inhibitors), beta-agonist opioids (e.g., morphine, hydromorphone, fentanyl), and adjuvant analgesics (e.g., local anesthetics).

3. Continue and/or initiate nonpharmacologic measures from phase I.

4. Educate patient and family/caregiver:
   A. Pain and comfort measures.
   B. Untoward symptoms to observe.
   C. Regional or local anesthetic effects dissipating after discharge (e.g., numbness, motor weakness, or inadequate relief) and potential adjustments as applicable.
   D. Availability of resources as needed.

5. Discuss misconceptions and expectations and implement plan of action satisfactory to patients.

6. Address nausea with pharmacologic interventions or other techniques and discuss expectations.

Expected Outcomes

1. Patient will state acceptable level of pain relief and comfort with movement or activity at time of transfer or discharge to home.

2. Patient will verbalize understanding of discharge instruction plans:
   A. Specific drug to be taken.
   B. Frequency of drug administration.
   C. Potential side effects of medication.
   D. Potential drug interactions.
   E. Specific precaution to follow when taking medication (e.g., physical limitation, dietary restrictions).
   F. Name and telephone number of the health care provider/resource to notify about pain, problems, and other concerns.

3. Patient will state understanding or show effective use of nonpharmacologic methods (e.g., cold/heat therapy, relaxation breathing, imagery, music).

4. Patient will state achievement of pain/comfort treatment goals and level of satisfaction with pain relief and comfort management in the perianesthesia setting.

Source: Reprinted from American Society of PeriAnesthesia Nurses. ASPAN pain and comfort guideline. *Journal of PeriAnesthesia Nursing, 18*(4), 232–236, 2003, with permission from Elsevier.

Risk for Imbalanced Fluid Volume

The patient is monitored postoperatively for evidence of bleeding, hypovolemia, and fluid overload. Bleeding is identified in several ways depending on the specific surgery performed. Bleeding can be seen on surgical wound dressings and in drainage tubes such as a nasogastric tube, a chest tube, a urinary catheter, or a wound drainage tube. The nurse examines the wound and dressing for signs of bleeding every hour or more frequently as needed.

Often, the surgical wound is expected to ooze small to moderate amounts of blood or sanguineous drainage. The nurse does *not* take off the surgical dressing, because it aids in hemostasis. Instead, an area of drainage is marked (e.g., circled in pen) on the dressing, monitored for enlargement, and reported to the surgeon. The sheets under the patient are examined for evidence of bleeding because gravity may cause blood to leak from the dressing and pool underneath the patient. If blood soaks through a dressing, the dressing should be reinforced and the event reported to the surgeon. Drains are monitored with dressing checks. The nurse reports the presence of blood or sudden increased amounts of drainage in a drain as a new finding to the surgeon. Certain tubes, such as chest tubes following a lung resection, a nasogastric tube following a gastrectomy, or wound drainage tubes, might be expected to drain blood initially with the drainage gradually changing from sanguineous to serosanguineous drainage during the next several hours or days. The

nurse needs to have a sense of the expected amount and type of drainage from a drainage tube in order to respond promptly to any increases in drainage. The surgeon must be notified of any changes.

Internal bleeding is sometimes seen as distention of tissues or the formation of a bruise or hematoma. A hematoma forms in an area where blood is collecting, and often causes increased pain. Generally this will be in the area surrounding the wound but in some cases, a hematoma may form in what appears to be a distant site. Other signs of internal bleeding are seen when blood loss is large enough to produce a drop in blood pressure, an increase in heart rate, or a decrease in cardiac output (Clancy, McVicar, & Baird, 2002). Initially the heart rate increases in an attempt to maintain a normal cardiac output and blood pressure; thus, it is an early sign of bleeding. Other indications of bleeding include a change in the patient's level of consciousness (anxiety, agitation, and confusion), a decrease in blood pressure (hypotension) with an increase in heart rate (tachycardia) and respiratory rate (tachypnea), and a drop in oxygen saturation. The patient may appear pale, cold and clammy, or cyanotic. Urine output may decrease as a result of poor renal perfusion.

Significant postoperative bleeding is an emergency and is always reported immediately. It may require an operation to explore the surgical site. The patient is monitored continuously until arrangements for the operating room are complete. If needed and not contraindicated, the patient is positioned with the head flat and the legs elevated or in Trendelenburg position (head lowered and feet elevated) to increase venous return and raise the blood pressure. The patient is supported with supplemental oxygen to prevent hypoxemia and the administration of intravenous fluids, blood transfusions, and/or plasma expanders to replace blood volume. Chapter 61 ⊕ provides a complete description of nursing care for the patient experiencing shock.

Surgery has a significant effect on a patient's fluid balance and it is unlikely that the patient will have a normal urinary output in the first 24 to 48 hours postoperatively (Clancy et al., 2002). The surgical patient is affected by factors that can lead to dehydration or fluid overload. Factors that contribute to fluid loss and dehydration in the surgical patient include preoperative fasting from foods and fluids, preoperative bowel preparation, hyperventilation from anxiety, blood loss intraoperatively, wound drains, nasogastric drainage, vomiting, evaporative water loss from exposed tissues during the operation, and decisions about intravenous (IV) fluid replacement. Some surgeons prefer a conservative approach to the administration of IV fluids in the operating room because research shows that these patients progress better postoperatively than patients who receive more liberal amounts of IV fluid (Nisanevich et al., 2005). Another factor in fluid balance is that tissue injury can cause a third spacing of fluids that contributes to dehydration initially because the fluid is not in the intravascular space. Postoperatively, fever, hypermetabolism, and sweating can significantly increase insensible water losses from an average of 600 to 800 mL/day to as high as 1,500 mL/day (Arieff, 1999).

Alternatively, certain factors contribute to overhydration and *fluid overload*. The primary factor is the secretion of hormones that occurs with physiological stress. Stress, pain, and anxiety stimulate the release of epinephrine, aldosterone, and antidiuretic hormone (ADH). These hormones affect fluid balance by causing the retention of sodium and water. Fluid overload may also occur as a result of the administration of intravenous fluid. The replacement of fluids during surgery is a clinical approximation of fluid loss, and monitoring is needed to prevent fluid overload.

Although dehydration is more common than fluid overload postoperatively, patients are monitored for signs of overhydration. The risk of overload is highest during the first 24 to 48 hours postoperatively when hormonal influences are at their peak. Most healthy patients can tolerate an overexpansion of fluid volume but the problem can be serious in those with altered physiological reserves. For those patients, the increased cardiac workload associated with fluid overload can precipitate heart failure or pulmonary edema. Patients who are at an increased risk of fluid overload are the elderly and those with preexisting cardiac, pulmonary, or renal disease. Early indicators of fluid retention are heavy, swollen eyelids, edema in the hands and feet, weight gain, and an intake that is greater than output. The patient may complain of headache, apprehension, or dyspnea. Other signs are agitation, distended neck veins, crackles in the lungs, and a drop in urinary output. Vital sign changes include an increase in heart rate, blood pressure, and respiratory rate. Treatment of fluid overload depends on the severity. Continuous close monitoring of weight, intake and output, and lung sounds is paramount, and the administration of IV fluids may be slowed or discontinued. In some cases, the patient may be given a diuretic, such as furosemide, intravenously to facilitate fluid excretion.

It is more common, however, for a patient to be dehydrated after surgery rather than overhydrated (Clancy et al., 2002). Intake may exceed output for approximately 24 to 48 hours. Fluid balance begins to correct approximately 48 to 72 hours after surgery. At this time, fluid in the interstitial space begins to shift back into the vascular space and the effect of stress hormones decreases, producing a urinary diuresis.

Careful assessment of fluid balance is the key to maintaining adequate hydration and preventing fluid overload. Intravenous fluid is monitored closely. A number of formulas are available for calculating postoperative fluid replacement. As an example, approximately 2,500 mL/day (or 30 to 35 mL/kg body weight per day) is needed for routine fluid replacement with additional amounts, from 500 to 3,000 mL/day, for replacement of losses from third spaced fluid, drains, or other sources (Arieff, 1999). Isotonic solutions (normal saline, Ringer's lactate) are frequently used for routine IV fluid replacement.

In the PACU, urine output is measured hourly. A urine output that is less than 30 mL/hr or 0.5 mL/kg per hour is reported to the health care provider as a significant finding. Frequently, a low urine output in the postoperative patient is the result of depressed renal function from dehydration. Other indications of dehydration include dry mouth, dry tissues, poor skin turgor, and complaints of headache. Tachycardia occurs as a compensatory mechanism for dehydration and the blood pressure tends to decrease as a result of too little blood volume.

A patient with low urine output or other signs of hypovolemia may be given a fluid bolus to expand blood volume and increase renal blood flow. A typical fluid bolus is 250 to 1,000 mL of 9.9% sodium chloride administered over 30 to 60 minutes. The nurse monitors urine output to determine the effectiveness of the fluid bolus. If effective, urine output increases. Vital signs may return to normal although issues other than dehydration (e.g., anxiety, pain) affect vital signs. In some patients, particularly the elderly, a fluid bolus can overwhelm the pumping ability of the heart, resulting in heart failure and pulmonary edema. Older patients need to be monitored during a fluid bolus to ensure that they are able to tolerate the rapid administration of fluid. Crackles (i.e., rales) in the lungs, dyspnea, or a drop in oxygen saturation indicate that the patient is unable to tolerate the fluid.

Risk for Decreased Cardiac Output

Following surgery, patients may have problems with cardiac irregularities, hypotension, or hypertension. Abnormal cardiac rhythms are a frequent finding after surgery. Most abnormal rhythms are a result of expected postoperative issues such as pain or fluid and electrolyte imbalances but an abnormal rhythm can also indicate a more serious problem such as cardiac ischemia. Cardiac telemetry is used to monitor heart rhythms and abnormal beats in the PACU. Telemetry is discontinued when the patient is transferred to a clinical unit, but it will be continued for patients who have signs of myocardial ischemia or abnormal cardiac rhythms or for those who need monitoring for heart or blood pressure medications.

The apical pulse is a more reliable measure than a peripheral pulse of heart rate and rhythm in the postoperative patient. The health care provider usually writes parameters that specify vital signs to report. The nurse relies on these parameters as well as on clinical judgment in reporting changes in the patient's condition. In addition to changes in heart rate, the nurse reports and investigates evidence of new irregularity in the heart rhythm. Irregularity in the heart rhythm may indicate premature ventricular contractions or new-onset atrial fibrillation.

Sinus tachycardia (i.e., a heart rate greater than 100 beats/min) is the most common dysrhythmia and it is caused by fever, anxiety, pain, hypovolemia, anemia, and hypoxia among other reasons. As a rule of thumb, a heart rate greater than 100 beats/min in a postoperative patient is investigated initially to determine the likely cause. If the patient is persistently tachycardic, the nurse must assess for other signs and symptoms (e.g., vertigo, syncope, hypotension, hypoxemia, chest pain) and report heart rates greater than 120 beats/min. The goal is to treat the underlying cause (e.g., give pain medication, fluids, oxygen, or blood transfusion). Although many patients experience tachycardia in the postoperative period, it is important to remember that an increase in heart rate increases the workload of the heart, so in compromised patients decompensation can occur rapidly.

Sinus bradycardia (i.e., a heart rate less than 60 beats/min) occurs postoperatively as a result of anesthetic medications or vagal stimulation. Patients with bradycardia are observed for its effect on cardiac output. If the patient is asymptomatic, further treatment is not usually necessary. Bradycardia that produces hypotension, syncope, or other symptoms may need to be treated with medications such as atropine or with a pacemaker.

Premature ventricular contractions (PVCs) are not unusual after surgery. PVCs may be caused by anxiety, pain, hypoxia, hypovolemia, and electrolyte imbalances particularly hypokalemia or hypomagnesia. Occasional PVCs are often benign and do not require treatment. The nurse reports an increase in the frequency of PVCs, the clustering of PVCs (i.e., couplets, triplets), and episodes of ventricular tachycardia (i.e., four or more PVCs in a row). Treatment is directed toward the underlying cause of the abnormal beats, but an antiarrhythmic drug such as amiodarone may be used to suppress episodes of ventricular tachycardia. It is important to remember that an antiarrhythmic drug given intravenously is also proarrhythmic (i.e., it has the potential to trigger an abnormal rhythm), therefore, these drugs are used cautiously. Chapter 38 includes a complete discussion of cardiac dysrhythmias.

Hypotension is a systolic blood pressure of less than 90 mmHg or a drop in the patient's systolic blood pressure of more than 20% from baseline. Hypotension can occur for a variety of reasons including bleeding, hypovolemia, depressed myocardial function, abnormal heart rhythm (e.g., atrial fibrillation), pulmonary emboli, and medications. Hypovolemia is the most likely cause of postoperative hypotension. The nurse reports hypotension and monitors the patient for other signs of decreased tissue perfusion. Interventions to treat hypotension depend on the underlying cause, but include placing the patient in Trendelenburg position and administering IV fluids rapidly to increase blood volume.

Hypertension is a systolic blood pressure equal to or greater than 140 mmHg, a diastolic blood pressure equal to or greater than 90 mmHg, or an increase greater than 20% from baseline in the patient's blood pressure. There are many reasons for a postoperative patient to be hypertensive including pain, anxiety, hypothermia, fluid overload, and distention of the bladder. Interventions are focused on treating the cause. If the patient was on antihypertensive medications at home, these are restarted as soon as possible. Patients who are NPO are sometimes allowed to take medications with small sips of water or they may be temporarily switched to an antihypertensive medication that can be given intravenously.

Risk for Imbalanced Body Temperature: Hypothermia

Hypothermia is defined as a core body temperature of less than 36°C (96.8°F) or a condition, regardless of body temperature, in which a person experiences shivering, peripheral vasoconstriction, piloerection, and feeling cold. Hypothermia is a common problem in the PACU, and it can have significant consequences for patients. Hypothermia is linked to patient discomfort, sympathetic stimulation, altered drug metabolism, increased intraoperative blood loss and the need for postoperative transfusions, impaired platelet function and clotting ability, slowed wound healing, increased susceptibility to infection, and untoward cardiac events such as angina (ASPAN, 2002; Scott & Buckland, 2006). Slow drug metabolism means that the hypothermic patient remains anesthetized longer than necessary.

Patients at risk for hypothermia include those with history of vascular and endocrine diseases, those who are immunocompromised, those with open wounds, older patients, and persons who are malnourished with low reserves of body fat. Also, longer surgeries (those lasting more than 1 hour) and the use of cold irrigation solution intraoperatively contribute to the development of postoperative hypothermia. On admission to the PACU, the patient is assessed for evidence of hypothermia and the core body temperature is taken. Clinical guidelines for the prevention of hypothermia recommend maintaining ambient room temperature between 20° and 24°C (68° and 75°F) and using passive insulation such as warm cotton blankets, socks, head coverings, limiting skin exposure, and a circulating water mattress for all patients (ASPAN, 2002; Good, Verble, Secrest, & Norwood, 2006; Wadlund, 2006; Wagner, 2006). Hypothermic patients must be actively rewarmed using a forced-air warming system. These systems help to raise body temperature because they blow warm air through a blanket that covers the patient. Other warming techniques include warming IV fluids and applying warm, humidified oxygen (Hasankhani, Mohammadi, Moazzami, Mokhtari, & Naghgizadh, 2007).

Patients who are hypothermic require more oxygen than they would if they had a normal temperature because shivering increases oxygen demand of the tissues and workload of the heart. Meperidine (Demerol) 12.5 to 25 mg IV is given to treat postoperative shivering, thus reducing oxygen demand. Achieving **normothermia** (i.e., a normal body temperature) reverses the immediate effects of hypothermia (e.g., shivering), but patients who experience perioperative hypothermia develop more cardiac events and wound infections postoperatively than patients who do not experience hypothermia (Scott & Buckland, 2006). Assessment of the patient's comfort and temperature are made every 30 minutes until discharge. The patient must achieve a minimum core body temperature of 36°C (96.8°F) prior to PACU discharge.

Readiness for Enhanced Comfort:
Nausea and Vomiting

Postoperative nausea and vomiting (PONV) is a significant problem that can be more debilitating than the surgical procedure. Despite advances in anesthesia, a large number of patients are affected by nausea and vomiting. Incidence of postoperative nausea and vomiting ranges from 40% to 84% depending on the surgery (Goldman & Ausiello, 2004; Schultz, Andrews, Goran, Mathew, & Sturdevant, 2003). Nausea and vomiting contribute to the development of fluid and electrolyte imbalances, poor nutritional intake, and patient discomfort. Often, patients who experience nausea and vomiting are reluctant or unable to ambulate, increasing the likelihood of other postoperative complications. Predisposing factors for postoperative nausea and vomiting include gender (women more than men), the surgery (there is a higher risk with gynecologic, abdominal, eye, and ear surgeries), longer surgeries (increased risk with surgeries longer than 2 hours), use of opioid analgesics, use of inhalation agents during anesthesia, a history of motion sickness, a history of nausea and vomiting with previous surgery, and a nonsmoking status (ASPAN, 2006a; Gunta, Lewis, & Nuccio, 2000; Murphy, Hooper, Sullivan, Clifford, & Apfel, 2006).

There are three types of PONV. Early postoperative nausea and vomiting occurs quickly, within 2 to 6 hours after the surgery. Late PONV develops 6 to 24 hours after the surgery, and delayed PONV extends beyond the first 24 hours after surgery. The causes of nausea and vomiting are complex and it may be that different types of PONV are caused by different factors and stimuli. PONV occurs as a result of stimulation of the vomiting center in the brain (Goldman & Ausiello, 2004). The vomiting center is activated by pathways from (1) the chemoreceptor trigger zone (CTZ) in the brain, (2) the gastrointestinal (GI) tract and other viscera via the vagus nerve, (3) the vestibular apparatus in the ear, and (4) the cerebral cortex. The CTZ contains serotonin and dopamine receptors that, when stimulated by certain toxins, substances, and drugs, activate nausea and vomiting in the vomiting center. The gastrointestinal (GI) tract also contains receptors—serotonin (5-HT3), dopamine (D2), and histamine (H1)—that when stimulated send messages to the brain via the vagus nerve to trigger nausea and vomiting. Factors such as GI irritation, gastric distention, inflammation, or ischemia can cause nausea and vomiting. For the postoperative patient, anesthesia and medications, especially narcotics, are important triggers of nausea.

Most postoperative nausea and vomiting occur early in the course of recovery and improve over time. One study of 300 postoperative patients found the highest incidence of nausea and vomiting occurred within 2 hours following surgery (Gunta et al., 2000). Interventions to reduce nausea and vomiting begin in the preoperative or intraoperative period with the administration of antiemetic medication. It is thought that early administration of antiemetic drugs (i.e., the drug is administered before emesis is triggered) is more effective than waiting until the patient experiences nausea and vomiting (Clancy et al., 2002). When preventative therapy fails, experts recommend rescue therapy using an agent from a different antiemetic class (ASPAN, 2006a). All patients with PONV need to be well hydrated with IV fluid.

The various antiemetic drugs that are available have different modes of action, and the ideal drug or drug combination has yet to be found. In some cases, a combination of drugs may work more effectively than a single drug (Wallenborn et al., 2006). One large study compared the effectiveness of six different two-drug combinations (e.g., dexamethasone, droperidol, ondansetron) in reducing PONV. The researchers reported that all of the drug combinations reduced PONV by 25% to 30%, but none of the combinations proved superior (Apfel et al., 2004). Not all antiemetics are effective for the nausea and vomiting associated with anesthesia, and all of the drugs have limitations. Some researchers are investigating the antiemetic effects of drugs not generally used for this purpose. In a small trial of patients having laparoscopic surgery, the prophylactic use of gabapentin, an antiseizure drug, decreased PONV (Pandey et al., 2006). The Pharmacology Summary describes common antiemetics used for postoperative nausea and vomiting.

Unfortunately, antiemetic medication does not work for everyone and there are few effective alternatives to the use of drugs. One study found that ginger (1 gram) was better than placebo in decreasing PONV (Chaiyakunapruk, Kitikannakorn, Nathisuwan, Leeprakobboon, & Leelasettagool, 2006), although other studies do not support the finding (Pittler & Eberhart, 2003). Acupuncture, P6 acupoint stimulation bands, aromatherapy, music, and self-hypnosis have limited success in reducing nausea and vomiting (Ezzone, Baker, & Terrepka, 1998; King, 1997; Lee & Done, 2004; Odom-Forren, Fetzer, & Moser, 2006; Phillips & Gill, 1994; Schultz et al., 2003). The nurse provides comfort by allowing the patient periods of uninterrupted rest, offering empathy and support, and encouraging deep breathing. The nurse also offers applications of a cool washcloth, frequent mouth care, and ice chips. Patients frequently report increased nausea with head elevation and movement. Slow position changes may help to prevent this trigger.

Pain

Achieving adequate pain control and comfort are major goals of postoperative care. The physiological effects of pain are well known and include an increase in sympathetic stimulation with an increase in blood pressure, heart rate, respiratory rate, and cardiac workload. The body enters a catabolic state that uses up physiological reserves. From a psychological standpoint, pain contributes to loss of sleep, lack of appetite, depression, anxiety, anger, helplessness, and hopelessness. Postoperative pain is associated with delayed ambulation and diminished functional performance (Horvath, 2003; Morrison, Magaziner, & McLaughlin, 2003). Pain control is necessary in promoting mobility and preventing complications such as atelectasis, ileus, DVT, and poor wound healing. The goal in postoperative pain control is to achieve a level of comfort without producing too much sedation or other side effects. Patients who are sedated will not be able to participate in postoperative breathing exercises or ambulation.

Incisional pain is expected to be highest in the first 24 to 48 hours postoperatively followed by a gradual reduction in pain, but the course of pain varies with the surgery and the individual. In one study, subjects with abdominal surgery reported more pain than those with cardiac surgery, and neither group experienced a reduction in pain 3 days postoperatively as might be expected (Puntillo & Weiss, 2003). Activities and procedures can also alter the course of pain. In a large study of more than

PHARMACOLOGY Summary of Common Drugs Used to Control Postoperative Nausea and Vomiting

Drug	Class and Action	Major Side Effect	Nursing Responsibility
Aprepitant	Neurokinin-1 (NK-1) receptor antagonist. Blocks NK-1 receptors in the central pathway of the vomiting center.	Headache, hypotension, bradycardia, pruritus, constipation.	Used only for prophylaxis. Give as a single dose 3 hours before surgery.
Dexamethasone	Corticosteroid. Augments the antiemetic effect of 5HT3 blockers. May also antagonize prostaglandins or release endorphins that increase mood and well-being.	Headache, gastrointestinal irritation, glucose elevation, retention of sodium and water.	Used in combination with other antiemetics. Watch for GI bleeding.
Diphenhydramine (Benadryl)	Blocks effects of histamine at H1 receptor sites.	Sedation, vertigo, hypotension.	Used more often for nausea associated with motion sickness or chemotherapy. Elderly may be very sensitive to the sedative effects of the drug.
Droperidol (Inapsine)	Blocks dopamine type 2 receptors in the chemoreceptor trigger zone in brain to reduce nausea and vomiting.	Sedation, hypotension, tachycardia, extrapyramidal symptoms (restless, tremor).	Low doses are used for postoperative nausea and vomiting. Watch for sedation and respiratory depression in patients receiving other CNS depressants. Monitor heart rate and blood pressure.
Metoclopramide (Reglan)	Increases gastric emptying and raises threshold for triggering the chemoreceptor trigger zone.	Mild sedation, extrapyramidal symptoms, (dystonia, restless, tremor).	Drug should be discontinued if extrapyramidal symptoms occur. Has not been shown to be effective in prophylactic management of PONV.
Ondansetron (Zofran) Dolasetron Granisetron	Serotonin receptor antagonist. Blocks 5HT3 receptor sites in the CTZ and peripherally to reduce nausea and vomiting.	Headache, diarrhea, or (more commonly) constipation.	Headache may be treated with Tylenol. Give stool softener or laxatives to prevent constipation.
Prochlorperazine (Compazine)	Phenothiazine that depresses CTZ in the brain.	Extrapyramidal symptoms, suppresses cough.	Be alert for development of extrapyramidal symptoms such as motor restlessness and parkinsonism.
Promethazine (Phenergan)	Long-acting phenothiazine derivative that depresses the chemoreceptor trigger zone.	Sedation, dizziness, dry mouth.	Monitor for increased sedation when administered with other CNS depressants. Monitor patient safety.
Scopolamine	Antagonizes muscarinic type 1 receptors in hypothalamus and vomiting center.	Visual disturbances, dry mouth, mydriasis.	Used for prophylaxis of PONV, limited use in rescue because of delayed action.

6,000 subjects, an increase in pain was reported with activities such as turning, drain removal, wound care, and suctioning (Puntillo et al., 2002). Cardiac surgical subjects reported coughing as the most painful activity followed by moving or turning in bed, getting out of bed, and using the incentive spirometer (Milgrom et al., 2004).

Pain may come from sources other than the incision. Residual carbon dioxide, used to inflate the surgical area in laparoscopic procedures, can produce shoulder or back pain. The position used during surgery may cause specific muscle aches. In one research study, 52% of patients placed in the lithotomy position for surgery reported back pain postoperatively (Pietrocola, Riley, Beanland, Kelly, & Radnell, 2004). Studies continue to report the undermedication of pain in postoperative patients (Cheever, 1999; Puntillo & Weiss, 2003; Puntillo et al., 1997, 2002; Sjostrom, Dahlgren, & Haljamae, 2000).

The PACU nurse continuously assesses the patient's level of comfort. The Agency for Health Care Policy and Research (AHCPR; now known as the Agency for Healthcare Research and Quality, AHRQ) developed guidelines for the management of acute pain in 1992. These guidelines recommend the use of a rating scale to measure the patient's self-report of pain. Most hospitals use a numeric rating system where patients report their level of pain on a scale of 0 (no pain) to 10 (the worst pain imaginable) (ASPAN, 2003). Postoperative patients rate their pain at rest and with movement.

Self-report is the best indicator of pain (AHCPR, 1992). Studies suggest that nurses and health care providers consistently underestimate patients' pain (Puntillo et al., 1997; Sjostrom et al., 2000) or have difficulty separating pain from anxiety (Stannard et al., 1996) except in situations where they use a pain scale and listen to the patient's response (Sjostrom et al., 2000). Pain assessment in patients who cannot self-report is more complicated and relies on clinical judgment. The nurse needs to consider the usual pain associated with a particular procedure or surgery and assess the patient for behavioral indicators of pain. Based on these factors, an analgesic trial is used and evaluated for effectiveness (Pasero & McCaffery, 2005).

The American Society of PeriAnesthesia Nurses published pain and comfort guidelines for postoperative patients (ASPAN, 2003). The nurse documents the location and character of the pain. The patient is expected to feel pain at the area of the surgical incision, but pain located in other areas requires further investigation. Pain in other sites may be caused by any number of factors and can be benign. Examples include pain referred from the incision, pain as a result of positioning during the operation, or pain caused by the accumulation of carbon dioxide gas from a laparoscopic procedure. Chest pain not related to an incision can be serious indicating cardiac ischemia and it requires further evaluation.

Postoperative pain should be well controlled with medications and other strategies. Early postoperative pain control is important for patient comfort, but it may also play a role in reducing persistent postsurgical pain, a phenomenon in which pain continues long after the incision heals (Kehlet, Troels, Woolf, & Woolf, 2006). The nurse consults with the health care provider when the patient is not getting acceptable pain relief. Another situation requiring consultation is the report of increased pain when the pain was previously well controlled. This finding suggests the possibility of surgical complications, such as infection or hematoma formation, and requires prompt evaluation.

Uncontrolled postoperative pain or a sudden increase in postoperative pain warrants an immediate investigation. These signs can signal a postoperative complication such as bleeding or leaking of the surgical anastomosis. Report findings to the surgeon immediately.

Initially, most patients in the PACU receive small doses of intravenous narcotic analgesics for pain control. Common medications include morphine sulfate, hydromorphone, and fentanyl. A typical standing order may be written for morphine sulfate 1 to 5 mg IV every 5 minutes as needed to a maximum total dose of 0.3 mg/kg body weight. Fentanyl also is used in the PACU because it provides comparable analgesia to morphine, but it has a more rapid onset and excretion (Golembiewski, Torrecer, & Katke, 2005). A typical standing order might read: fentanyl 25 mcg IV as needed to a maximum of 100 mcg. The nurse assesses patients' responses to interventions every 15 to 30 minutes or more frequently if appropriate. Patients are monitored for respiratory depression and narcotics are withheld or even reversed if the respiratory rate falls to 10 per minute or less.

Patients who require close neurological monitoring need an individualized regimen for pain control. Check with the anesthesiologist for special orders if the patient has major head trauma, increased intracranial pressure, a recent cerebrovascular accident, or recent seizures.

Patient-controlled analgesia (PCA) or patient-controlled epidural analgesia (PCEA) is commonly used to control postoperative pain. With PCA, a narcotic analgesic can be administered continuously at a basal rate although continuous infusion is not standard because it increases the risk of adverse effects and opioid overdose (Golembiewski et al., 2005). More common is PCA using small boluses when the patient pushes the control button. The PCA delivers a set amount of medication at specified intervals until a maximum amount of medication is reached. The computerized pump keeps a record of how often the patient attempts to access the medication and how many injections the patient receives. The nurse uses this information to determine whether the patient is using the pump effectively. A typical PCA order for a postoperative patient might read: PCA morphine sulfate 1 mg every 6 minutes with a lockout maximum of 10 mg/hour.

Patients receiving PCA are monitored for pain relief and for the untoward effects of the narcotic, including a depressed respiratory rate, sedation, nausea, pruritus, and slowed gastrointestinal function. In a review of studies comparing PCA with nurse-administered analgesics, researchers found consistent evidence that PCA provides better pain control and increased patient satisfaction with very few adverse effects (Hudcova, McNicol, Quah, Lau, & Carr, 2006).

Patient-controlled epidural analgesia delivers medication via a catheter to the epidural space. PCEA, like PCA, can be set to deliver medication continuously, as a bolus, or both. PCEA is used to deliver a local anesthetic such as bupivacaine (0.0625% to 0.125%) or ropivacaine (0.1% to 0.2%) alone or in combination with a narcotic. Fentanyl is used frequently as the narcotic of choice because it is lipid soluble and easily dissolves in epidural fat, but preservative-free morphine also can be given as an epidural medication. It is thought that local anesthetics and opioids work synergistically to provide better pain relief in smaller doses.

The nurse checks the site of the epidural catheter for signs of infection and patency. Infection is uncommon, but the catheter is taped not sutured and displacement can occur. Catheter displacement is suspected by new complaints of pain in a patient who previously had good pain control with the epidural. The nurse monitors the patient for overall pain control and also notes the sensory level of the epidural (i.e., the area of the body where the patient reports diminished sensation). In the PACU, these assessments are made hourly; on the clinical unit, they are made every 4 hours unless the situation warrants more frequent assessments. It is also important to note any areas of motor deficit. The goal of epidural analgesia in the postoperative patient is to reduce sensation and pain without affecting motor ability. If the epidural is affecting motor ability, it will need to be adjusted downward so that the patient will be able to ambulate safely. Other possible side effects include nausea, pruritus, hypotension, and urinary retention. Some health care providers elect to leave a urinary catheter in place while a patient is receiving epidural medication to avoid urinary retention although others believe this practice to be unnecessary.

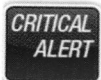 *If a patient with patient-controlled epidural analgesia is unable to lift his legs off of the bed or describes heaviness in their lower extremities, the health care provider should be consulted. These assessments suggest that the dose of medication is too high, causing motor blockade.*

The use of PCA and PCEA is an important advance in control of postoperative pain. Many studies show that PCEA provides better pain control with fewer side effects and better functional outcomes than PCA (Carli et al., 2002; Mann et al., 2000; Mann, Pouzeratte, & Eledjam, 2003; Nishimori, Ballantyne, & Low, 2006; Pasero, 2003a, 2003b, 2005; Schumann et al., 2003). Continuous epidural analgesia with local anesthetics for 24 to 72 hours postoperatively is associated with faster return of GI function, improved respiratory function, and a reduced stress response (Brown, Christo, & Wu, 2004; Holte & Kehlet, 2002). As soon as appropriate, the patient is transitioned away from intravenous or parenteral medications to oral medications.

Experts recommend a multimodal approach (e.g., using multiple agents with different modes of action) for postoperative pain management. When multiple medications are used, pain control can be achieved with smaller doses of narcotics and with fewer adverse effects (Pasero & McCaffery, 2007; Richman, Liu, & Courpas, 2006). For example, infusions of local anesthetics may be used along with intravenous or oral opioids. A continuous wound infusion is the administration of a local anesthetic through a catheter implanted directly into the surgical site. An alternative is the use of continuous perineural infusion. In this type of infusion, a catheter is inserted near the peripheral nerves affected by surgery. An infusion of a short-acting local anesthetic in this area effectively blocks the pain from these nerves (Pasero & McCaffery, 2007).

Nonsteroidal anti-inflammatory drugs (NSAIDs) are used in conjunction with opioids for pain control except where contraindicated. Acetaminophen does not affect postoperative bleeding, so it can be added to most pain control regimens (Kuchta & Golembiewski, 2004). Ketorolac (Toradol) is a particularly effective anti-inflammatory agent but its use is often limited to 72 hours because of its deleterious effect on kidney function. The anticonvulsant agents, pregabalin and gabapentin, may be used postoperatively when there is a neuropathic component to pain as is frequently the case with orthopedic conditions (Pasero & McCaffery, 2007).

Other pain control techniques include the application of heat or cold, primarily cold for the postoperative patient, and elevation. Application of ice or a cold pack helps reduce tissue swelling, one factor that contributes to postoperative pain. Ice packs are applied for 20 minutes then removed for 20 minutes and repeated as necessary. The application of cold is seen with various orthopedic procedures as well as some plastic surgeries. Elevation of an affected area above the level of the heart reduces edema and assists with pain control. Elevation is used most often with open reduction of an extremity fracture. Chapter 15 🌐 provides a complete description of pain management techniques.

Nurses use nonpharmacologic interventions to reduce pain, but these interventions should complement medications not replace them. The evidence of the effectiveness of selected nonpharmacologic approaches to pain is inconsistent. In two studies, for example, patients reported that the use of positioning, massage, distraction, and relaxation techniques combined with pain medication is more effective than pain medication alone in providing pain relief and comfort (Smith, Kemp, Hemphill, & Vojir, 2002; VanKooten, 1999). In a systematic review of relaxation interventions, researchers found support for the effectiveness of these techniques in reducing pain in approximately half of the 15 studies they examined (Kwekkeboom & Gretarsdottir, 2006). Similarly, research on the effects of healing touch on postoperative pain control show mixed results (Wardell & Weymouth, 2004). Clearly more studies are needed to establish the efficacy of nonpharmacologic approaches in the management of postoperative pain.

Anxiety

Anxiety is an unpleasant emotional response. Anxiety is associated with increased morbidity and mortality and longer, more complicated hospitalizations in the postoperative patient. Anxiety causes stimulation of the sympathetic nervous system, which can increase blood pressure by 30% to 40% and heart rate by 20% (Frazier et al., 2003). Anxiety depresses the immune system, delays wound healing, and alters blood coagulation. Other reported physiological responses to anxiety include increases in myocardial ischemia, cardiac dysrhythmias, and postoperative pain. The nurse assesses the patient for signs of anxiety, similar to pain assessment. The best indicator of anxiety is patient reports of how anxious they feel. Patients are encouraged to verbalize fears and concerns.

Nurses play a critical role in reducing the anxiety of postoperative patients. The PACU nurse provides frequent reassurance to patients about their condition and how well they are progressing. Reassurance and caring are major factors in reducing anxiety. In one study of critically ill medical and surgical patients, subjects reported an overwhelming need to "feel safe" in their environment, and they identified nurses as the key to either feeling safe or not feeling safe (Hupcey, 2000). The researcher found that nurses who came right away when called, who listened, who expressed genuine interest, and who explained what was happening to the patient were deemed trustworthy and fostered patients' beliefs that they were being "watched over" and therefore safe. Other studies supporting these findings show that nurses' caring behaviors are associated with patients' sense of emotional comfort, well-being, and security, and lead to better functional outcomes (Doering, McGuire, & Rourke, 2002; Meade, Bursell, & Ketelsen, 2006; Swan, 1998; Werner et al., 2002; Williams & Irurita, 2005). Whenever possible, patients should be given choices regarding their care. Regaining a sense of control helps the patient to feel a sense of security (Susleck et al., 2007; Williams & Irurita, 2005).

The nurse individualizes nursing interactions with patients and provides information consistent with the individual's preference for information and personal coping style. Some patients will want and need detailed information about their status, whereas others may become more anxious if the nurse provides too much information or explanations that are too explicit. Nurses should speak slowly and calmly, and maintain a quiet and restful environment. The trend toward allowing significant others to visit with the patient in the PACU is likely to be beneficial in reducing the anxiety of the patient and the significant other. Family and friends are an important source of support and comfort

(Cunningham, Hanson-Heath, & Agre, 2003; Hupcey, 2000; Leske, 2003; Smykowski & Rodriguez, 2003; Susleck et al., 2007).

Other techniques that are helpful in reducing anxiety are sitting with the patient, touch, massage, distraction, meditation, guided imagery, relaxation exercises, and music. It may be very useful to incorporate music into a plan of care. Music therapy is presented in the Complementary and Alternative Therapies box in Chapter 41 ☺. One study found that 20 minutes of music significantly reduced anxiety, heart rate, respiratory rate, and cardiac workload in patients admitted to a coronary care unit (White, 1999).

Despite nonpharmacologic interventions, some patients may require antianxiety agents. A number of antianxiety agents are available. Lorazepam (Ativan) works quickly (1 to 5 minutes) when given intravenously, but can also be administered as an intramuscular (IM) injection or given orally. The dose is titrated to produce desired effects so that oversedation of the patient is avoided. It is important for the nurse to follow up on the effectiveness of interventions to reduce anxiety. In a study of 843 postoperative patients and their nurses, the nurses tended to overrate the amount of anxiety relief that the patient received from interventions (Leinonen, Leino-Kilpi, Stahlberg, & Lertola, 2003).

Discharge from the Postanesthesia Care Unit

Patients are discharged from the PACU to home or to an inpatient unit. PACUs use written criteria and a numeric rating scale to determine the patient's readiness for discharge home or to an inpatient unit. The Aldrete Post Anesthesia Discharge Score (PADS) (Figure 27–3 ■) is one measure of a patient's readiness

POST ANESTHETIC SCORE	
ACTIVITY	
Able to move 4 extremities voluntarily or on command	2
Able to move 2 extremities voluntarily or on command	1
Unable to move extremities voluntarily or on command	0
RESPIRATION	
Able to breathe deeply and cough freely	2
Dyspnea, limited breathing or tachypnea	1
Apneic or on mechanical ventilator	0
CIRCULATION	
BP plus or minus 20% of preoperative baseline	2
BP plus or minus 20%–40% of preanesthetic level	1
BP plus or minus 40% of preanesthetic level	0
CONSCIOUSNESS	
Fully awake	2
Arousable on calling	1
Not responding	0
O2 Saturation	
Able to maintain O2 saturation > 92% on room air	2
Needs O2 inhalation to maintain O2 saturation > 90%	1
O2 saturation <90% even with O2 supplement	0
TOTAL PAR SCORE	

FIGURE 27–3 ■ Aldrete Post Anesthesia Discharge Score.
Source: Courtesy of Beth Israel Deaconess Nursing Department

for discharge. The PADS assigns a numerical rating of 0 to 2 for each of the following: vital signs, activity level, nausea and vomiting, pain, and surgical bleeding. Patients can be transferred to an inpatient unit with a PADS of between 8 and 10, but a score of 9 or better is required if the patient is being discharged home. If patients have a baseline PADS of less than 8 due to a preexisting condition, the anesthesia provider makes the decision to discharge on an individual basis.

Ambulatory Surgery Discharge

Ambulatory settings require a PADS of 9 or higher for discharge, but other criteria may need to be met before the patient is allowed to go home. Discharge criteria vary depending on the surgery, the patient, and health care provider preference. Additional discharge criteria may include the following:

- Stable vital signs for 1 hour
- Baseline level of consciousness
- Wound is stable with minimal bleeding
- Able to take fluids orally (applicable to selected patients)
- Able to void (applicable to certain surgeries or selected patients)
- Pain is at an acceptable level
- Able to dress and ambulate with assistance
- Adult caretaker available to accompany the patient home.

Patients are no longer required to void or to take oral fluids prior to discharge. Evidence from research studies found that many patients can be safely discharged home without voiding or drinking fluids (Ead, 2006; Mulroy, Salinas, Larkin, & Polissar, 2002). Patients who are considered at low risk for urinary retention may be discharged home without voiding as long as their bladder is not distended. Patients are given explicit instructions to seek medical attention in the emergency room if they have not voided after 8 hours at home. Patients who do not void and who have bladder distention need an ultrasonic bladder scan and may require an intermittent catheterization before discharge. Patients at high risk of postoperative urinary retention are still required to void before discharge. Many patients will be able to drink fluids before discharge, but in most cases, it is not necessary to delay discharge for those who do not tolerate oral fluids. Certain patients, such as those with diabetes, the elderly and the frail, remain under observation until they are able to drink fluids postoperatively.

Patients discharged home need to have complete and concise information about performing self-care. The information is presented verbally as well as in writing using simple language. When home care involves performing a procedure, the nurse demonstrates the technique then asks the patient to return the demonstration (Ross, 2007). The nurse reviews any new medications including the purpose of the drug, the dose, the frequency of administration, and any significant side effects. Pain management is discussed as well as wound care. The nurse reviews any restrictions on bathing, activity, and diet. Patients should be clear about how they are expected to feel after surgery and what symptoms require follow-up with their surgeon. Patients are given instructions about how to contact their health care provider should a problem develop. Information about follow-up appointments is also given to patients. The Patient Teaching & Discharge Priorities box pro-

PATIENT TEACHING & DISCHARGE PRIORITIES Following a Breast Biopsy

Need	Teaching
Care of Incision	Your incision is covered with Steri-Strips and a bandage. Leave the bandage in place tonight. Tomorrow, you may remove the bandage (but not the Steri-Strips) and shower. Gently wash the area and pat it dry. Leave the Steri-Strips in place until they fall off by themselves. If you have sutures, they will be removed during your follow-up appointment. It is not unusual to have mild bruising around the area of the incision.
Pain control	You should have very little pain after your biopsy. Your health care provider has given you a prescription for pain medication if you need it. Do not drive while taking the prescription medication. If your pain is mild, you may take acetaminophen (Tylenol) regular or extra strength every 4 to 6 hours as needed instead of the prescription medication. Do *not* take aspirin or ibuprofen because these medications may cause you to bleed.
	Ice will help to reduce swelling and discomfort. An ice pack can be inserted in the bra. Leave the ice pack in place until it gets warm, then remove and replace. Apply ice packs off and on for the remainder of today.
	You should wear a bra for the next 24 to 36 hours to support your breast. This means that you should sleep in the bra tonight. A soft, front-closing bra may be more comfortable for you than other types.
Activity level	Do not drive on the day of your surgery. You should rest and take it easy for the remainder of the day. You received medications during surgery that may make you feel tired. You may return to work when you feel able. For most people, this will be in 1 or 2 days after the procedure. You can begin performing normal activities tomorrow but avoid strenuous exercise until the follow-up appointment with your health care provider.
Possible problems that require attention	You should watch for signs of infection. If your incision becomes red, painful, or develops drainage you should call your health care provider. You should also call if you develop a fever (>38°C [100.4°F]) or if you have pain that is not relieved by pain medication.
Follow-up with the health care provider	The results of your biopsy will be available in 2 or 3 days. Your health care provider will call you at home with the results. If you have sutures, you should make a follow-up appointment for 7 to 10 days after the procedure. If you do not have sutures, you should make a follow-up appointment for 1 month after the procedure.

vides examples of discharge priorities following ambulatory surgery for a breast biopsy.

Many ambulatory surgery centers contact the patient by telephone the day after surgery. The nurse performs the telephone follow-up and inquires about the patient's recovery. The nurse asks questions about pain, nausea and vomiting, voiding, and the surgical site, and gives the patient the opportunity to ask questions. Often, the surgeon or surgical assistant will also contact the patient at home to monitor recovery. Follow-up phone calls help to ensure patient safety. Also, they may be helpful in reducing emotional stress and improving self-care abilities after surgery although more research is needed in this area (Allard, 2007).

Transfer to an Inpatient Unit

The surgeon and anesthesiologist discharge patients from the PACU to an inpatient unit when the patient meets specific discharge criteria including an acceptable PADS. Other criteria for PACU discharge may require the patient to be normothermic, with pain and bleeding controlled, and all tubes, drains, catheters, and IV lines patent and functioning.

Postoperative orders are written before transfer to the nursing unit. The PACU nurse reports to the receiving nurse all pertinent information about the patient. The report includes relevant past history, a description of the surgery and type of anesthesia, any significant postoperative events, estimated blood loss from surgery, recent laboratory data, a summary of OR and PACU fluid status, recent vital signs, a description of the dressing, drains, pain medication, and antiemetics given, and any equipment required postoperatively. Figure 27–4 ■ (p. 666) is an example of a PACU report. The PACU report may be given verbally or in written form.

■ Nursing Management

The nurse on the clinical unit admits the PACU patient and performs a head-to-toe assessment beginning with vital signs and an admitting weight. The elements of the assessment are similar to the PACU admission assessment described earlier. The nurse makes sure that all equipment is set up correctly and functioning well. The safety of the patient is assessed using a fall risk assessment tool. Patients at risk for falls need an individual plan to prevent a fall. Such plans often include simple strategies such as putting the call light within reach, placing the bed in the low position, monitoring the patient frequently, educating the patient and family about falls, and activating the bed alarm if needed (Lyons, 2004; Resnick, 2003).

Postoperative patients are assessed often because their condition can change rapidly. The usual routine on a surgical unit includes a full head-to-toe assessment at the beginning of a shift followed by frequent follow-up assessments as the day progresses. Vital signs with oxygen saturation are taken every 4 hours, although the timing of postoperative observations is

PACU FAX REPORT   RM# _____

OR PROCEDURE: _____
_____
_____

ANESTHESIA:

☐ General   ☐ Spinal   ☐ Epidural   ☐ MAC   ☐ Other

(ADDRESSOGRAPH)

SIGNIFICANT POST OP EVENTS:

ALLERGIES: _____
_____
_____

HISTORY

| I & O | OR/PACU TOTAL | | | | CV | ☐ WNL | ☐ CABG ☐ VASCULAR BYPASS ☐ MI ☐ ANGINA ☐ HYPERTENSION ☐ OTHER |

CRYST   COLLOID   EBL   UOP

PULM   ☐ WNL   ☐ THORACOTOMY
☐ SMOKING
☐ OTHER
☐ PRE-OP O2 SAT

VITAL SIGNS:

T _____ BP _____ HR _____ RHYTHM _____ RR _____
O2 SAT _____   ☐ ROOM AIR   ☐ NP @ _____ L/M

RENAL   ☐ WNL   ☐ TRANSPLANT
☐ CRF/DIALYSIS
☐ OTHER

IV: _____ mL/hr   AMT. REMAINING _____
☐ D5 1/2 S   ☐ D5 1/2 + 20Kcl   ☐ LR

NEURO   ☐ WNL   ☐ CVA
  ☐ RESIDUAL
  ☐ NO RESIDUAL
☐ OTHER

OTHER: _____

DRESSING:

☐ D & I   ☐ SM TO MOD SEROSANG
☐ REINFORCED   ☐ CHANGED IN PACU

GI   ☐ WNL   ☐ GERD
☐ OTHER

DRAINS:

☐ NG   ☐ FOLEY   ☐ CT X _____   ☐ JP x _____
☐ HEMOVAC   ☐ DAVOL X _____   ☐ OTHER

SUCTION   ☐ WALL   ☐ SELF

ENDOCRINE   ☐ WNL   ☐ IDDM
☐ NIDDM
☐ OTHER

PAIN MEDICATIONS:	ANTI-EMETICS:
MSO$_4$ _____	DROPERIDOL _____
DEMEROL _____	ZOFRAN _____
KETOROLAC _____	REGLAN _____
OTHER _____	OTHER _____
☐ PCA	
☐ EPIDURAL	
APS ☐ YES ☐ NO	

OTHER

EQUIPMENT

☐ IV POLE   ☐ SUCTION
☐ OXYGEN   ☐ BOOT MACHINE
☐ IMED/IVAC
☐ OTHER _____

☐ PLEASE REMOVE BED FROM ROOM
  THANK YOU!

LABS: HCT _____   K+ _____   BS _____
OTHER _____

PRIMARY NURSE

_____ RN

INSULIN: PRE-OP _____   POST-OP _____

FAX TIME _____   ETA TO FLOOR _____

FIGURE 27–4 ■ Sample PACU report.

PACU Report Sheet   Name:

Hx: _____
_____
_____
_____

Anes: GA   ETT   Pre-med: _____
                                                  _____
        LMA

        Mac   Epidural _____
                                                  _____
        Spinal

Intra-op Events of note: _____
_____
_____
_____

Intra-op meds: _____   Antiemetics _____
               _____   _____
               _____   _____

Fluids: Cryst: _____   Colloid: _____

FIGURE 27–4 ■ *Continued*
Source: Courtesy of Beth Israel Deaconess Nursing Department

based on tradition rather than on empirical evidence (Dip, Dip, & McCutcheon, 2006; Zeitz & McCutcheon, 2006). Hospital policy or a health care provider's order may specify parameters for reporting changes in vital signs. Policies do not cover the range of events that can occur in the postoperative period.

The nurse uses clinical judgment in deciding which data require health care provider notification. Chart 27–3 (p. 668) describes findings that are usually reported to the health care provider. Initially, postoperative patients may run a low-grade fever as a result of tissue injury, inflammation, and mild dehydration so mild temperature elevations are not cause for alarm (Vermeulen, Storm-Versloot, Goossens, Speelman, & Legemate, 2005). The nurse reports a fever of 38°C (100.4°F) or higher unless otherwise directed by the health care provider. Atelectasis is often associated with the development of a fever in the first 24 to 48 hours after surgery, so the nurse assesses breath sounds and encourages deep breathing if fever is present. Oxygen saturation is also an important postoperative measurement. Many patients arrive from the PACU with oxygen in place and orders to maintain oxygen saturation above 93%. If the patient's oxygen saturation is acceptable, the nurse begins the process of titrating the oxygen downward.

While performing the head-to-toe assessment, the nurse asks specific questions to assess the patient's level of consciousness, orientation, and cognition. The nurse also asks about the patient's ability to sleep in the hospital. There is a high rate of sleep disturbance in the hospital and sleep is thought to have restorative functions (Redeker, 2000). The nurse asks the patient to rate his pain and assesses the adequacy of pain control measures. If the patient is using PCA for pain control, the nurse checks the

accuracy of the settings on the pump and reviews the history to see how frequently the patient is using the PCA. If the patient has an epidural catheter, the nurse assesses the insertion site on the patient's back for redness, swelling, leaking, or kinking of the tubing. The nurse also reviews the pump settings, and evaluates the level of sensation and the patient's ability to move and use his extremities. The nurse listens to lung sounds, asks about sputum production, and evaluates the patient's ability to perform deep breathing exercises.

The nurse listens to bowel sounds, palpates the abdomen, and asks the patient about nausea, vomiting, passing flatus, and moving of his bowels. General anesthesia and narcotics slow peristalsis but bowel function is expected to return within several hours after surgery unless the patient has had pelvic or abdominal surgery. In these surgeries, peristalsis may be delayed for 24 to 48 hours or longer. Patients are expected to void 6 to 8 hours after surgery and urine output is measured and recorded with each void. If the patient has a urinary catheter in place, urine output is measured frequently and a urine output of less than 30 mL/hr or less than 0.5 mL/kg per hour is reported to the health care provider.

The nurse examines the patient's wound dressing and notes the color and amount of any drainage. The nurse checks the color, sensation, and motion of the extremities and the presence of pedal pulses. The nurse teaches the patient how to perform leg exercises and makes sure that any devices ordered to prevent DVT are in place and functioning properly.

At the conclusion of the assessment, the nurse works with the patient to establish goals for the day and a specific plan to accomplish the goals. One of the most important tasks for the nurse to

CHART 27–3 Abnormal Postoperative Assessments That Need to Be Reported to the Surgeon

METABOLIC
- Temperature >38°C (100.4°F)

NEUROLOGICAL FINDINGS
- Change in level of consciousness

CARDIOVASCULAR FINDINGS
- Heart rate < 60 or >120 beats/min
- Hypotension (e.g., systolic blood pressure of less than 90 mmHg)
- New cardiac arrhythmia
- Hypertension (e.g., systolic blood pressure 20% to 30% higher than baseline)
- Chest pain
- Loss of pulses

RESPIRATORY FINDINGS
- Oxygen saturation < 93%
- Respiratory rate < 10 breaths/minute or >24 breaths/minute
- Indications of respiratory distress such as dyspnea, crackles, wheezing

GASTROINTESTINAL
- Abdominal distention
- Vomiting uncontrolled by antiemetics

FLUID BALANCE
- Urine output < 30 mL/hr or < 0.5 mL/kg per hour
- Unable to void in 6 to 8 hours

WOUND
- More than the expected amount of bleeding at the incision site
- More than the expected amount of drainage from chest tubes or wound drains
- Incision with redness, purulent drainage, or opened areas

PAIN
- Pain not adequately controlled

EXTREMITIES
- Absence of peripheral pulses
- Swelling, redness, pain in calf

OTHER
- Unexpected presence of blood in tubes

accomplish is to assist the patient with rest and ambulation. It can be difficult to plan uninterrupted periods of rest, given frequent nursing assessments, health care provider visits, blood draws, and consultations by physical therapists, nutritionists, case managers, and social workers among others, visits with family and friends, and the noise level of the clinical unit. Despite these problems, the nurse creates periods where the patient is able to rest because rest is thought to be important in immune function, wound healing, and mental outlook (Redeker, 2000).

Early ambulation is one of the most important interventions that can assist in recovery from anesthesia and surgery. Unless contraindicated, ambulation begins on the evening of surgery or on the first postoperative day. The nurse is present to assist patients with their first attempt at ambulation. Patients may feel dizzy or nauseated when they first move to a sitting or standing position. Splinting the incision, deep breathing, moving slowly, and moving at the patient's pace may help to minimize pain, nausea, and vertigo. Allow patients to sit on the side of the bed for a few minutes before moving to a standing position. Some patients may be inclined to hunch over in a move designed to protect their incisions, but this posture creates muscle tension and distorts balance, so patients are encouraged to relax and assume the correct posture. Patients may be able to ambulate only a short distance initially, but the nurse provides reassurance that the distance will gradually lengthen. Postoperative patients need to ambulate at least three times daily. Early ambulation and physical therapy correlates with faster functional recovery after some surgeries (Kondo et al., 2005; Oldmeadow, McBurney, Robertson, Kimmel, & Elliott, 2004), particularly orthopedic procedures, and early and aggressive ambulation is an important element of accelerated recovery programs (Pasero & Belden, 2006).

Evidence-based demonstration projects are being used to develop models of nursing care delivery (Smith et al., 2002). The Evidence-Based Practice feature describes a model of nursing care delivery that was successful in creating a healing environment for its patients.

Collaborative Management

It is important for the nurse to work closely with the surgeon and other members of the health care team in order to facilitate the patient's rapid recovery from surgery and to prevent complications. Some hospitals are using a collaborative, comanagement approach that teams the surgeon and nurse with a hospitalist in managing postoperative patients. One study of more than 500 patients showed a decrease in minor postoperative complications for patients managed in this type of system (Huddleston et al., 2004).

Other members of the health care team are also closely involved in the patient's care. Clinical nurse specialists provide assistance regarding selected aspects of a patient's recovery such as wound care for more complicated wounds or teaching for a new ostomy or organ transplantation. Physical therapy and occupational therapy provide valuable information about postoperative exercises, ambulation, transfer, and use of assistive devices. A nutritionist may be consulted to make specific recommendations about diet or diet supplementation. Social workers are consulted to provide support and counseling for patients and their families. Case managers help provide a seamless transition from hospital to rehabilitation facility or to home with services. Many patients will be discharged home after surgery without the need for home services. Some postoperative patients, however, will require services at

Impact of Scheduled Nursing Rounds on Use of Call Light

Clinical Problem

Hospital environments, with their noise, restrictions, and loss of personal control, are not generally conducive to patient recovery. Patients report feeling a loss of personal control in the hospital and that this feeling leads to a sense of vulnerability and a poor outlook on their health status. Factors that contribute to the loss of personal control include such things as having to wait for assistance in going to the bathroom or in performing personal care, an inability to reach needed objects, such as a call light, and having to wait to receive a response to requests made (Williams & Irurita, 2005). Can a routine nursing intervention create a more therapeutic environment for patients?

Research Findings

A multisite, quasi-experimental study set out to determine the effect of making "nursing rounds" on patients' use of call lights and on patient satisfaction (Meade, Bursell, & Ketelsen, 2006). In this study, 27 nursing units at 14 hospitals implemented regular nursing rounds for a period of 4 weeks. The nursing units could opt to conduct the rounds every hour from 6 a.m. to 10 p.m. or every 2 hours from 10 p.m. to 6 a.m. A protocol for the rounds was established that included a pain assessment, offers to toilet and reposition patients, placing needed items such as the call light, telephone, and water within patient reach, and concluding the round by asking whether the patient needed anything else and indicating the time of the next scheduled round.

The researchers found that regularly scheduled rounds significantly decreased patients' use of call lights while increasing patient satisfaction. The nursing units that conducted hourly rounds also reported significant reductions in patient falls. Interestingly, even nurses who were initially reluctant to add "nursing rounds" to an already busy day were satisfied with the protocol because it increased their contact with patients in more productive ways. Perhaps most impressive is the finding that 1 year after the study was completed,

85.7% of the nursing units involved in the study continued to use nursing rounds.

Implications for Nursing Practice

This study is important because it takes a cluster of common nursing activities and demonstrates that the performance of these activities in a consistent, caring way has positive patient outcomes. The findings of the study suggest that simple changes in the delivery of nursing care can make a difference to patients—and perhaps to nurses. Understanding how and why this simple intervention worked and testing the intervention with different outcome measures is the next step in the process.

Critical Thinking Questions

1. Explain, using a theory of nursing or of growth and development, why conducting nursing rounds was an effective intervention.

2. An outcome of this study was the reduction of falls on the units that used an hourly nursing rounds protocol. If the study were replicated, what other patient outcomes might be influenced by a nursing rounds protocol?

3. Suggest specific changes in the sample or intervention that might be helpful if the study were replicated.

Answers to Critical Thinking Questions appear in Appendix D.

References

Meade, C., Bursell, A., & Ketelsen, L. (2006). Effects of nursing rounds on patients' call light use, satisfaction, and safety. *American Journal of Nursing, 106*(9), 58–70.

Williams, A., & Irurita, V. (2005). Enhancing the therapeutic potential of hospital environments by increasing the personal control and emotional comfort of hospitalized patients. *Applied Nursing Research, 18*(1), 22–28.

EVIDENCE-BASED PRACTICE

---

home such as physical therapy, speech therapy, intravenous antibiotics, wound and drain checks, or teaching. The surgical nurse collaborates with home health agencies to make sure that the patient's discharge to home is a successful one.

Preventing Postoperative Complications

A significant role of the nurse on a surgical unit is to prevent postoperative complications when possible. Chart 27–4 (p. 670) lists postoperative problems that are common to many surgeries. Common problems that occur after surgery include atelectasis, pneumonia, abdominal distention, constipation, urinary retention, wound infection and venous stasis among others. The Nursing Process: Patient Care Plan (p. 671) feature is for a patient following general surgery. Examples of appropriate nursing diagnoses in the postoperative period are described in the care plan.

Atelectasis and Pneumonia

Atelectasis refers to the collapse of alveoli and the surrounding airways. When alveoli collapse, lung volume is reduced, and mucus accumulates, causing localized airway obstructions from mucous plugs. If atelectasis remains untreated, it leads to fever and hypoxia. Although it is not entirely clear, some theorize that the re-

tention of secretions associated with atelectasis increases the risk of developing pneumonia (Smith & Ellis, 2000). Pneumonia is the inflammation of lung parenchyma caused by a virus, bacteria, or other organism. The invasion of lung tissue by an organism causes an inflammatory response and the alveoli fill with inflammatory exudates. These changes are seen on chest x-ray as new infiltrates. Signs of pneumonia include fever, dyspnea, crackles in the lung fields, purulent sputum, congested cough, hypoxia, and an elevation in the white blood cell count. The incidence of postoperative atelectasis varies according to the surgery performed, but it is estimated to be as high as 84% (Smith & Ellis, 2000). The incidence of postoperative pneumonia is much lower, around 15%, although certain surgeries such as abdominal or thoracic procedures have much higher rates (as high as 40%) (Brooks, 2001).

Atelectasis and pneumonia are referred to collectively as postoperative pulmonary complications. Some researchers also include hypoxia in that description. It can be difficult to distinguish atelectasis from pneumonia initially, and the factors that predispose patients to atelectasis also predispose them to postoperative pneumonia. Older age, preexisting respiratory conditions, heart failure, decreased level of consciousness, poor functional ability, a history of cigarette smoking, and malnutrition predispose the patient to postoperative pulmonary complications (Qaseem et al., 2006).

| CHART 27–4 | **Common Postoperative Problems** | | | |

Problem	Cause/High Risk	Goal	Assessment	Interventions
Pain	Cell injury, muscle spasm, drains, anxiety.	Pain free, rate pain a 3 or less.	Pain rating scale 0–10 Increased HR, BP, RR Guarding, grimacing	Narcotics: PCA or epidural NSAIDS: Tylenol, Toradol Comfort measures
Fluid retention (overload)	Stress response, excess IV fluid, medical diagnosis such as heart failure.	Ensure adequate perfusion without causing overload. (Diuresis is expected by day 3 postop.)	Swelling in hands, feet, eyelids. Weight gain. Decreased urine output of <30 mL/hour or < 0.5 mL/kg per hour. Crackles or rales.	Monitor urine output every 1–4 hours. Check breath sounds. Monitor IV fluid.
Fluid deficit (dehydration)	Excess fluid losses during surgery, from wound, drains; vomiting, fever.	Ensure adequate tissue perfusion.	Dry skin, mucous membranes. Decreased urine output of <30 mL/hour or < 0.5 mL/kg per hour. HR >100, SBP < 90 mmHg, narrow pulse pressure.	Fluid bolus: normal saline (NS) 250–500 mL over 1 hour. Monitor urine output, heart rate, and BP.
Bleeding	High risk for surgery on vascular tissue or on patient with history of clotting disorder, use of anticoagulants, malnourished.	Hemodynamic stability.	Cool, clammy skin. HR >100, SBP < 90 mmHg, narrow pulse pressure. Decreased Hct/Hgb. Decreased urine output of <30 mL/hr or < 0.5 mL/kg per hour. Swelling or distention, oozing from wounds, hematoma, bloody drainage.	Fluid replacement: NS bolus. Transfusion packed red blood cells if active bleeding. Transfusion with fresh frozen plasma (if clotting factors need replacing).
Atelectasis (risk of pneumonia)	Most common problem in first 48–72 hours postop. Primary cause is anesthesia. Risk increases with surgery on chest or abdomen, with uncontrolled pain, decreased mobility, obesity, smoker, chronic obstructive pulmonary disease, asthma.	Patient will demonstrate adequate oxygenation and will not develop postop pneumonia.	Fever is most common sign. Breath sounds diminished or crackles. Increased RR Oxygen (O_2) saturation< 93%. Sputum: increased production and consistency.	Incentive spirometer or turn–cough–deep breathe 10 times per hour. Turn every 1–2 hours. Adequate pain relief. Splint incision during movement. Increase head of bed 30 degrees or higher. Ambulate 3 times per day (tid). Titrate oxygen to maintain O_2 saturation >93%.
Nausea and vomiting (N&V)	Most N&V peaks in 24–36 hours postop. Anesthesia, narcotics, antibiotics, retained gastric secretions.	Will not experience N&V or N&V will be relieved.	Nausea and vomiting. Nausea increases with movement. Abdominal distention.	IV fluid to maintain hydration. Medicate with antiemetic: droperidol, ondansetron, promethazine, metoclopramide. Maintain function of nasogastric tube if needed for comfort. Minimize use of opioids and increase use of nonopioids for pain. Advance diet slowly (ice chips—clear liquids—full liquids—regular diet).
Abdominal distention (postoperative ileus)	Following surgery on the bowel, it will take 3–5 days for return of GI function. Factors that decrease bowel function: anesthesia, surgical trauma, narcotics, decreased mobility.	Return of bowel peristalsis.	Abdomen is distended. No stool or flatus. Nausea and vomiting. No bowel sounds or hypoactive bowel sounds.	NPO until flatus; may be 3–5 days post-gastrointestinal (GI) surgery. NGT to suction for comfort if vomiting. Ambulate tid. Advance diet slowly.

CHART 27–4   Common Postoperative Problems—*Continued*

Problem	Cause/High Risk	Goal	Assessment	Interventions
Syncope (orthostatic hypotension)	Anesthesia, immobility, dehydration, some medications.	Patient will not experience orthostatic hypotension.	Complaints of dizzy, light-headedness, diaphoresis. Increased symptoms with standing or sitting. Orthostatic (postural) vital sign changes: HR increases at least 10 beats/minute (from lying to standing); BP decreases by at least 10 mmHg (from lying to standing).	Get out of bed slowly; dangle legs before standing. If symptomatic, take orthostatic vital signs. If syncope is from dehydration, give patient a fluid bolus.
Urinary retention	Anesthesia, narcotics, anticholinergics, spasm of abdominal or pelvic muscles.	Patient will void (minimum 200 mL) after surgery or 6–8 hours after removal of Foley catheter.	No voiding or small, frequent voids. Fullness above symphysis pubis.	Ambulate. Avoid use of bedpan. Check intake and output and offer fluids. Bladder scan. Catheterize (per order) if not void in 8–12 hours.
Wound healing: risk of infection Dehiscence Evisceration	Infection usually not evident until 3–7 days after surgery. High risk with obesity, poor circulation, diabetes, malnourishment.	Wound well approximated and without drainage. Wound heals.	Local: redness, swelling, increased pain, edges not approximated, increased drainage from incision. Systemic: fever, elevated white blood cells count.	Adequate nutrition. Limit stress on wound. Prophylactic antibiotic for 24 hours only. Use sterile technique.
Deep venous thrombosis (DVT)	Occurs 5–7 days after surgery and is caused by venous stasis and pressure. DVT can dislodge and become a pulmonary embolus.	Adequate circulation without evidence of venous stasis.	Calf: red, painful, swollen. Positive Homans' sign.	Ambulate tid. Leg exercises. Antiembolism stockings or pneumatic compression boots. Antithrombotic medication. Avoid pressure under the knees.

NURSING PROCESS: Patient Care Plan for the Postoperative Patient Following General Surgery

Assessment of Discomfort

Subjective Data:
Ask the patient to describe the pain, its location and intensity.
Ask patient to rate pain from 0–10 on the pain scale.

Objective Data:
Watch for physical signs of pain including guarding, grimacing, crying, increased blood pressure (BP), heart rate (HR), and respiratory rate (RR).

Nursing Assessment and Diagnoses	Outcomes and Evaluation Parameters	Interventions with *Rationales*
Nursing Diagnosis: *Readiness for Enhanced Comfort* related to surgical incision, muscle spasm, positioning in the operating room, the presence of drains, and anxiety	**Outcome:** The patient will be comfortable and rate the pain at a 3 or less. ***Evaluation Parameters:*** Patient is comfortable. Patient participates in postoperative activities and exercises without discomfort.	**Interventions and *Rationales:*** Use pain scale (0–10) to assess pain every 2–4 hours. *Increases consistency in quantifying pain.* Watch for physical signs of pain including guarding, grimacing, crying, increased BP, HR, and RR. *Some patients are reluctant to ask for pain medication. Different cultures respond to and express pain differently.* Administer pain medication, narcotics and anti-inflammatory agents as prescribed. *Postoperative pain is highest in the first 48 hours after surgery.* Provide teaching about patient controlled analgesia (PCA) or patient controlled epidural analgesia (PCEA) if prescribed. Elevate affected area if appropriate *to decrease tissue swelling.* Apply ice to affected area if appropriate *to decrease tissue swelling.* Teach to splint the incision. *Provides stability to injured area.* Use nonpharmacologic interventions such as massage, distraction, relaxation techniques. *These measures augment other pain control measures.*

(continued)

NURSING PROCESS: Patient Care Plan for the Postoperative Patient Following General Surgery—*Continued*

Assessment of Nausea and Vomiting

Subjective Data:
Ask patient about feeling nauseated.

Objective Data:
Patient vomits.
Abdomen is firm, distended with hypoactive bowel sounds.

Nursing Assessment and Diagnoses	Outcomes and Evaluation Parameters	Interventions with *Rationales*
Nursing Diagnosis: *Alteration in Nausea* related to anesthesia, narcotics, antibiotics, slowed peristalsis	**Outcomes:** Patient will get relief from nausea and vomiting. Patient will have a soft abdomen and pass flatus. Patient will have adequate intake of fluids. ***Evaluation Parameters:*** Abdomen soft. Appetite is present. Oral fluid intake is 1,500– 2,500 mL in 24 hours. Passing flatus and stool.	**Interventions and *Rationales:*** Assess for nausea, vomiting, abdominal distention, and flatus. *Most nausea and vomiting peaks in 24 to 36 hours after surgery.* Maintain nasogastric tube (NGT) as prescribed for comfort. *An NGT decompresses the stomach and prevents vomiting.* Maintain NPO status until nausea recedes and bowel function returns. *Flatus and passing stool are the best indicators that bowel function has returned.* Advance diet slowly from ice chips to clear liquids to full liquids and regular diet. *Vomiting can occur when the diet is advanced too rapidly.* Medicate with antinausea medication as prescribed. *Early administration of medication is more effective than waiting until the patient experiences nausea and vomiting.* Encourage patient to change positions slowly. *Movement is a trigger for nausea and vomiting.* Provide comfort measures such as rest, a cool washcloth, mouth care, and deep breathing.

Assessment of Fluid Volume

Subjective Data:
Patient reports vertigo.
Are you thirsty?

Objective Data:
Watch for signs of active bleeding including blood on dressing, hematoma, presence of blood in drainage tubes, and decreased hematocrit and hemoglobin.
Watch for signs of dehydration including heart rate (HR) >100, systolic blood pressure (BP) <90, narrow pulse pressure, decreased urine output of <30 mL/hour or <0.5 mL/kg per hour.

Nursing Assessment and Diagnoses	Outcomes and Evaluation Parameters	Interventions with *Rationales*
Nursing Diagnosis: *Deficient Fluid Volume* related to hemorrhage, blood loss with surgery, fluid loss, wound drains, vomiting, or fever	**Outcome:** Patient will have adequate hemostasis and normal intravascular volume. ***Evaluation Parameters:*** Normal vital signs. Urine output >0.5 mL/kg per hour. No evidence of active bleeding.	**Interventions and *Rationales:*** Assess for indications of bleeding and dehydration every 1–4 hours. *There is a higher risk of bleeding if surgery is performed on tissue that is vascular. The patient is most at risk for dehydration in the first 24–48 hours postop.* Report HR >120, systolic blood pressure (SBP) <90, urine output <30 mL/hour or <0.5 mL/kg per hour, or more drainage than expected on dressing or in tubes. *Indicators or risk of imbalanced fluid volume and possible postoperative bleeding.* Check dressing and circle any new drainage with pen *to monitor for bleeding.* Reinforce dressing as needed. *The surgeon changes the primary dressing.* Administer IV fluids as ordered *to replace fluids lost during surgery.* Administer normal saline fluid bolus if required. *Used to expand blood volume and increase urine output.*

NURSING PROCESS: Patient Care Plan for the Postoperative Patient Following General Surgery—*Continued*

Assessment of Fluid Volume
Subjective Data:
Patient reports dyspnea.

Objective Data:
Swelling in hands, feet, and eyelids, weight gain, urine output < 30 mL/hr or <0.5 mL/kg per hour crackles in the lungs.

Nursing Assessment and Diagnoses	Outcomes and Evaluation Parameters	Interventions with *Rationales*
Nursing Diagnosis: *Risk for Imbalanced Fluid Volume* related to response to stress hormones, excess intravenous fluids, or preexisting medical condition such as congestive heart failure	**Outcome:** Patient will have adequate fluid volume without evidence of overload. *Evaluation Parameters:* Urine output is >30 mL/hr or >0.5 mL/kg per hour. Intake and output (I&O) is balanced. Clear breath sounds. Normal vital signs without tachycardia or tachypnea.	**Interventions and *Rationales:*** Assess for swelling, weight gain, urine output <30 mL/hr or <0.5 mL/kg per hour, crackles in lungs, and dyspnea every 1–4 hours. *The effect of stress hormones is greatest in the first 24–48 hours.* Monitor IV fluid administration carefully. *Fluid given too rapidly can exacerbate fluid overload.*

Assessment of Respiratory Status
Subjective Data:
Patient states it is painful to take deep breaths.

Objective Data:
Watch for fever, diminished breath sounds, crackles in the lungs, sputum production, increased respiratory rate, and decreased oxygen saturation.

Nursing Assessment and Diagnoses	Outcomes and Evaluation Parameters	Interventions with *Rationales*
Nursing Diagnosis: *Ineffective Breathing Pattern* related to anesthesia, surgical pain, location of the surgery, limited mobility, a history of smoking, or preexisting medical condition	**Outcome:** Respiratory status will be stable and within normal limits. *Evaluation Parameters:* Afebrile. Clear lung sounds. Oxygen saturation >93%. Normal respiratory rate. Denies shortness of breath and air hunger.	**Interventions and *Rationales:*** Monitor respiratory rate, depth, breath sounds, and oxygen saturation every 4 hours *to assess for atelectasis.* Encourage deep breathing or use of incentive spirometry 10 times every hour *to increase maximal inspiration and stimulate surfactant.* Encourage patient to cough every hour. Splint incision if appropriate. *Coughing clears mucous secretions.* Elevate head of the bed 30 degrees or higher *to lower the diaphragm and facilitate lung expansion.* Provide adequate pain relief. *Patients consistently give high pain ratings to coughing and deep breathing.* Ambulate three times daily. *Increases RR, minute ventilation, and tidal volume.* Titrate oxygen (O_2) to maintain the O_2 saturation at or >93%. *Oxygen dries the airways and reduces mucociliary clearance.*

Assessment of Urine Output
Subjective Data:
Patient states he cannot void or is only able to void small amounts.

Objective Data:
Patient does not void or voids only small amounts. Palpable fullness above symphysis pubis or a bladder scan showing a full bladder.

Nursing Assessment and Diagnoses	Outcomes and Evaluation Parameters	Interventions with *Rationales*
Nursing Diagnosis: *Urinary Retention* related to anesthesia, narcotics, anticholinergic medications, or spasm of abdominal or pelvic muscles	**Outcome:** Patient voids >100–150 mL within 6–8 hours after surgery or after removal of Foley catheter. *Evaluation Parameters:* I&O is balanced. Voids adequate amounts without difficulty.	**Interventions and *Rationales:*** Monitor I&O *to determine adequacy of urine output.* Encourage oral fluids if appropriate. *Inability to void may be due to dehydration.* Ambulate frequently *to stimulate circulation and production of urine.* Perform measures to stimulate voiding reflex (i.e., use commode rather than bedpan; have male patients stand to use urinal; run water; run warm water over perineum; use spirits of peppermints). If patient is unable to void 8 hours after surgery or after Foley catheter is removed, perform a bladder scan and call the surgeon for an order to perform catheterization. *The patient should feel the urge to void when the bladder has 300 mL of urine.*

(continued)

NURSING PROCESS: Patient Care Plan for the Postoperative Patient Following General Surgery—*Continued*

Assessment of Activity Level

Subjective Data:
Patient states he has vertigo, fatigue, or dyspnea with activity.

Objective Data:
Positive orthostatic vital signs with activity or an increased heart rate of >10 beats/minute, increased respiratory rate of >10 beats/minute, decreased oxygen saturation, or labored breathing with activity.

Nursing Assessment and Diagnoses	Outcomes and Evaluation Parameters	Interventions with *Rationales*
Nursing Diagnosis: *Activity Intolerance* related to anesthesia, narcotics, surgery, and limited mobility	**Outcome:** Patient will carry out postoperative activities and activities of daily living without signs of activity intolerance. **Evaluation Parameters:** Ambulates without experiencing symptoms. Completes activities of daily living without experiencing symptoms. Postactivity vital signs and oxygen saturation are within normal limits.	**Interventions and *Rationales:*** Encourage muscle strengthening activities every shift *to increase circulation.* Encourage use of slow changes in position. Dangle legs at bedside before attempting to ambulate. Assist with two people during first attempt at ambulation *to provide for patient safety.* If symptomatic, take orthostatic vital signs and notify surgeon. Anticipate administering a fluid bolus. *Positive orthostatic vital signs are an indication of dehydration.* Ambulate a minimum of three times daily.

Assessment of Wound

Subjective Data:
Patient states that incision feels painful and swollen.

Objective Data:
Incision is red, painful, or swollen. Wound edges are not approximated and the wound has increased drainage.
Elevated white blood cells count (WBC) and fever.

Nursing Assessment and Diagnoses	Outcomes and Evaluation Parameters	Interventions with *Rationales*
Nursing Diagnosis: *Risk for Infection* related to altered skin integrity, and high-risk factors (e.g., diabetes, obesity, diminished arterial circulation, malnutrition)	**Outcomes:** The patient will be free from infection. The wound will heal within appropriately 7–10 days. **Evaluation Parameters:** The patient is afebrile. The wound edges are well approximated without drainage, redness, or swelling.	**Interventions and *Rationales:*** Monitor temperature, WBC count, and serum glucose. *Infection causes a fever and increased WBC and glucose.* Change dressing every shift using sterile technique and monitor for signs of infection. *The inflammatory response in an infected wound will cause redness, pain, swelling, and drainage.* Encourage adequate nutrition that is high in protein and vitamins. *Protein, calories, calcium, iron, zinc, and vitamins A, B_6, B_{12}, and C are needed for wound healing.*

Assessment of Blood Flow to the Extremities

Subjective Data:
Patient complains of pain in calf.

Objective Data:
Calf is red, painful, and swollen. Patient reports a positive Homans' sign.

Nursing Assessment and Diagnoses	Outcomes and Evaluation Parameters	Interventions with *Rationales*
Nursing Diagnosis: *Ineffective Tissue Perfusion, Venous Stasis* related to immobility, surgical procedure, and high-risk factors (e.g., age, use of estrogen, cancer, history of previous deep vein thrombosis [DVT])	**Outcome:** The patient will have adequate peripheral circulation and no evidence of DVT. **Evaluation Parameters:** Palpable dorsal pedis and posterior tibialis pulses. Calf is pain free without evidence of redness or swelling.	**Interventions and *Rationales:*** Assess for signs of DVT. A red, warm, swollen, or painful calf alerts the nurse to the possibility of a venous clot. *Venous thrombosis is most likely to occur 5 to 7 days after surgery.* Administer anticoagulant medication as prescribed *to prevent clot formation.* Measure the circumference of the calf and thigh of each leg and compare them prn. *The leg will increase in size with DVT formation.* Any indication of a clot is reported immediately to the health care provider. *Early treatment will decrease the risk of further clot formation.* The patient is placed on bed rest until the possibility of a clot is evaluated. *There is an increased chance of clot migration with activity.* Encourage ambulation and leg exercises three times daily *to stimulate circulation.* Apply pneumatic compression boots, antiembolism stockings or other antithrombotic devices as ordered *to increase venous return and prevent venous stasis.* Avoid pressure under the knees. *Venous compression contributes to the development of DVT.*

NURSING PROCESS: Patient Care Plan for the Postoperative Patient Following General Surgery—*Continued*

Assessment of Knowledge Regarding Surgery and Postoperative Care

Subjective Data:
Patient states that she needs information on how to care for herself at home.

Objective Data:
Patient is being discharged home following a recent surgery.

Nursing Assessment and Diagnoses	Outcomes and Evaluation Parameters	Interventions with *Rationales*
Nursing Diagnosis: *Deficient Knowledge* related to postoperative care	**Outcomes:** The patient will recover from surgery without complications. The patient is knowledgeable about how to care for herself at home. *Evaluation Parameters:* Demonstrates appropriate care of her wound and drains (if applicable). Verbalizes an understanding of pain management. Verbalizes an understanding of activity restrictions and other discharge instructions. Verbalizes an understanding of danger signs and what to do about them.	**Interventions and** *Rationales: The specific information taught depends on the surgery (refer to the appropriate disorder chapter in this text for specific information) and the preferences of the surgeon. General areas for teaching are listed below.* Teaching is done in the patient's native language, through an interpreter, if necessary. • General information about recovery • Wound care • Activity • Specific exercises to aid recovery • Diet • Medication • Symptom management: pain, constipation, fatigue • Recognition and prevention of complications • Follow-up appointments • Who to call with questions

There is a higher risk of postoperative atelectasis and pneumonia with surgeries of the chest and abdomen because the incision is located close to the diaphragm, making it painful to take deep breaths, turn, and ambulate. Studies show that vital capacity can decrease by as much as 60% in the first 24 hours following abdominal surgery (Brooks-Brunn, 1998; Shea, Brooks, Dayhoff, & Keck, 2002). Immobility increases risk because the movement of the diaphragm and chest wall are restricted, resulting in diminished lung volumes (Brooks, 2001). Longer surgeries, those that take more than 4 hours, also increase risk as a result of prolonged anesthesia (Smith & Ellis, 2000). Other procedures associated with increased risk of postoperative pulmonary complications are neurosurgery, head and neck surgery, vascular surgery, and emergency surgery (Qaseem et al., 2006).

The nurse assesses the patient's respiratory rate, depth, lung sounds, and oxygen saturation at frequent intervals. Postoperative atelectasis most often occurs in the lower lobes of the lungs. Lung sounds may be diminished as a result of shallow respirations or crackles, which are most noticeable on inspiration and may be heard as collapsed alveoli are forced open. Crackles also occur with pneumonia as air is forced through mucus and fluid in the alveoli. The crackles with pneumonia may be present throughout the respiratory cycle. Atelectasis can clear with repeated deep breathing, so the nurse assesses lung sounds before and after use of incentive spirometry or deep breathing. Fever can be present with either atelectasis or pneumonia and is caused by inflammatory mediators.

A number of interventions are designed to decrease postoperative pulmonary complications. Unless contraindicated, the patient is placed in semi-Fowler's, Fowler's, or high-Fowler's position. Elevating the head of the bed 30 to 90 degrees lowers the diaphragm, thus facilitating chest expansion.

The patient is encouraged to use lung expansion therapies, deep breathing, or incentive spirometry. Deep breathing reverses alveolar collapse by forcing and holding maximal inspiration. Techniques for deep breathing and incentive spirometry are discussed in Chapter 26 ⊚. Deep breathing is most effective when maximal inspiration is held for 3 seconds or longer and when the exercises are performed frequently. Patients are encouraged to take 5 to 10 deep breaths every hour, but more is better. Nasal continuous positive airway pressure, a specially designed face mask and pump that forces air into the nasal passages at pressures high enough to keep the airway open, may be helpful to patients who are unable to perform deep breathing (Qaseem et al., 2006).

Forced coughing is used postoperatively to clear secretions. To have an effective cough, the patient must take a deep breath, increase intrathoracic pressure, and produce a high expiratory flow rate. Both volume and force of airflow are required to remove secretions. Coughing can be painful and the incision should be splinted with a pillow or small rolled blanket held firmly across the incision to prevent undue stress. Coughing is usually performed with deep breathing exercises, but the practice is contraindicated in some situations (e.g., cranial surgery, eye surgery) because it can increase intracranial and intraocular pressures and in other circumstances because it places too much stress on the incision (e.g., hernia surgery). Interventions to loosen and remove secretions such as percussion and postural drainage are recommended in specific situations but they are not employed universally after surgery (Brooks et al., 2001).

Ambulation is an important intervention to prevent postoperative pulmonary complications. Ambulation increases respiratory rate, minute ventilation, tidal volume, and inspiratory flow rates (Orfanos, Ellis, & Johnston, 1999). Patients who walk more and who walk longer distances tend to recover quicker and are discharged sooner than patients who are less mobile (Whitney & Parkman, 2002). There are no practice guidelines describing optimal postoperative ambulation. As soon as allowed by the surgeon, patients are encouraged to walk a minimum of three times daily. Patients are encouraged to walk with good posture and to take deep breaths with ambulation. More ambulation is likely to be better, provided that the patient does not overexert. Patients are monitored during ambulation for signs of activity intolerance. Signs include shortness of breath, tachypnea, hypoxia, tachycardia, chest pain, and fatigue. It is also beneficial for patients to get out of bed to a chair several times each day (Markey & Brown, 2002). Sitting facilitates excursion of the diaphragm, and it is associated with improved respirations and lung volumes (Brooks, 2001; Smith & Ellis, 2000).

Pain control is absolutely essential to getting patients to participate in pulmonary exercises and ambulation. Postoperative patients consistently give high pain ratings to turning, movement, coughing, and deep breathing (Puntillo, 2003; Puntillo et al., 2002; Stanik-Hutt, Soeken, Belcher, Fontaine, & Gift, 2001). Higher pain scores are associated with reluctance to walk and to take deep breaths and with higher rates of atelectasis and pneumonia (Edelen & Perlow, 2002; Puntillo & Weiss, 2003; Shea et al., 2002). Patients are medicated prior to periods of mobility and, when possible, the nurse plans to ambulate patients when pain medication is at its peak. Encouraging the use of nonpharmacologic interventions for pain control is also useful. In one study, the use of relaxation techniques 15 minutes before deep breathing exercises was associated with higher inspiratory volumes (Edelen & Perlow, 2002).

The use of nasogastric tubes for patients with nausea and vomiting or symptomatic abdominal distention is shown to reduce the incidence of postoperative atelectasis and pneumonia (Lawrence et al., 2003; Qaseem et al., 2006). Conversely, quick removal of the nasogastric tube when it is no longer necessary may reduce microaspiration and bacterial colonization of the oropharyngeal area, both of which are risk factors for postoperative pneumonia (Brooks, 2001; Smith & Ellis, 2000).

Other interventions may be helpful in reducing atelectasis and pneumonia although the benefit is not established through research. Titrating the patient off of oxygen may be helpful because supplemental oxygen can dry airways and reduce mucociliary clearance (Smith & Ellis, 2000). The Centers for Disease Control and Prevention (CDC, 1997) recommends using sterile water to fill oxygen humidifiers and to rinse medication nebulizers to reduce the introduction of microorganisms to the respiratory tract. Poor nutrition correlates with postoperative pulmonary complications but the routine use of enteral feedings using a gastrostomy, jejunostomy tube, or total parenteral nutrition is not recommended. Enteral feedings pose a risk of aspiration and are discontinued as soon as possible. While feeding tubes are needed, interventions are used to reduce the risk of aspiration including elevating the head of the bed a minimum of 30 degrees and checking tube placement regularly (CDC, 1997). Dental plaque and poor oral care provide a site for bacterial growth and are thought to predispose patients to pneumonia. Good oral hygiene may stimulate salivary flow, reducing the growth of microorganisms in the mouth. Adequate hydration aids in mucous clearance.

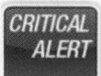 *A fever in the first 48 hours after surgery is commonly related to atelectasis. Encourage the patient to cough, deep breathe, and ambulate, if appropriate. If the fever is accompanied by crackles in the lungs, respiratory congestion, respiratory distress or low oxygen saturations, contact the health care provider because these signs are consistent with pneumonia.*

Abdominal Distention, Ileus, and Risk for Constipation

As part of a routine gastrointestinal assessment, the nurse palpates the abdomen for firmness and tenderness and asks about the presence of nausea and vomiting, passing of flatus, and recent bowel movement. Multiple factors place postoperative patients at risk for abdominal distention, a bloated abdomen, and **ileus**, a hypoactive bowel with delay in peristalsis. Surgical trauma, physiological stress, and the inflammatory process stimulate the release of catecholamines, neurotransmitters, and hormones that slow gastrointestinal motility. The inhibitory effects of anesthesia and opioids further reduce peristalsis. Despite these factors, most patients regain bowel function several hours after surgery except in abdominal procedures where the return of bowel function is delayed for several days.

A postoperative ileus (POI) occurs when peristalsis does not return as expected after surgery. An ileus is more likely to occur in patients who have had major abdominal surgery, particularly if inflammation or leakage of an abdominal organ was involved (e.g., leaking appendix or ruptured gallbladder). Other factors such as postoperative fluid and electrolyte imbalance can cause POI. Minimally invasive surgical approaches (laparoscopy), epidural analgesia, and lower doses of opioids are associated with lower rates of POI (Ead, 2006; Saclarides, 2006; Zutshi, Delaney, Senagore, & Fazio, 2004). Indications of an ileus include a hard, firm abdomen, hypoactive or absent bowel sounds, and no passing of flatus or stool. Patients with severe abdominal distention may also experience nausea, vomiting, pain, and hiccups caused by irritation of the diaphragm. Research efforts are focused on preventing postoperative ileus and on speeding resolution of ileus after abdominal surgery. Chart 27–5 lists some of the strategies used to prevent or correct postoperative ileus.

 The nurse gives priority to performing an abdominal assessment early in the shift on patients who are recovering from abdominal surgery. A hard, distended, painful abdomen can indicate internal bleeding and the surgeon should be notified.

There are many approaches to treatment of postoperative ileus although not all treatments are evidence based. POI may resolve with time alone or with the correction of dehydration or electrolyte imbalance. In some cases, a nasogastric tube (NGT) or a longer intestinal tube is used to decompress the stomach and/or intestine. Studies show that nasogastric intubation does not improve postoperative ileus (Person & Wexner, 2006; Saclarides, 2006), but it may provide comfort by reducing abdominal bloating and nausea and vomiting. The NGT is attached to suction and the nurse checks that the suction is functioning correctly. NGT drainage is measured every shift. If a disposable

CHART 27–5 Strategies Used to Reduce Postoperative Ileus

Good Evidence that Strategies Are Effective in Reducing POI	Some Evidence that Strategies Might Be Effective in Reducing POI, But Further Research Is Needed
Use of minimally invasive surgical techniques	Use of laxatives postoperatively
Use of epidural analgesia	Chewing gum
NSAIDS for pain control	Early feeding of patient postoperatively
Opioid antagonists for pain control	Sham feeding: allowing patients to chew food without swallowing it
	Alternative therapies: guided imagery, mechanical massage, acupuncture

system is being used, the entire setup is replaced, rather than emptied, once a day or as often as needed. The NGT is taped firmly to the patient's nose to prevent dislodgement. Usually, an NGT can be flushed with 30 mL of normal saline to maintain patency except when contraindicated by the presence of internal sutures. The nurse does not flush an NGT if the patient has had esophageal or gastric surgery except by order of the health care provider because a strong flush could disrupt sutures and stimulate bleeding. Ambulation helps to stimulate peristalsis and return the bowel to normal function. Usually, it is acceptable to clamp an NGT temporarily for the purpose of ambulation or transfer to a chair.

The passing of flatus and stool marks the return of bowel motility and function. The presence of bowel sounds is not a good marker of the return of bowel function in the postoperative patient and is probably an unnecessary assessment (Madsen et al., 2005). The trend in postoperative care is toward early feeding. Most patients (except those with abdominal surgery) will be started on clear fluids the evening of surgery. Traditionally, patients begin on clear liquids and the diet is advanced if the patient tolerates clear liquids without nausea and vomiting, but this practice may be unnecessary. Studies show that many postoperative patients, perhaps 80% to 90%, tolerate oral feedings without problems (Basse, Billesbolle, & Kehlet, 2002; Person & Wexner, 2006; Rimmele et al., 2005; Saclarides, 2006). In a review of 15 research studies, 86% of patients progressed well with early feeding without problems of aspiration, bowel obstruction, anastomotic leak, or pneumonia (Ng & Neill, 2006). Further, early feeding may stimulate gastric emptying, help with tissue repair, and improve patient comfort (Ead, 2006; Saclarides, 2006), but further research is needed to substantiate these benefits.

Many postoperative patients experience constipation. Most patients receive a stool softener such as docusate sodium (Colace). Fluids, ambulation, and bulk laxatives such as Metamucil or MiraLax are also helpful with postoperative bowel regularity. If a patient is unable to move her bowels, she may require a laxative such as milk of magnesia or bisacodyl or an enema, but health care provider approval is necessary.

Urinary Retention

Many patients will have a urinary catheter for the first 12 to 24 hours after surgery. Urine output is observed frequently in patients with a Foley catheter. If urine output falls below 30 mL or .5 mL/kg per hour, the health care provider is notified. The catheter will be removed as soon as possible to avoid the possibility of a urinary tract infection (UTI). Once the catheter is removed, the patient is at risk for development of urinary retention. Urinary retention is common and occurs as a result of general anesthesia from relaxation of the detrusor muscle, spinal anesthesia from blocking parasympathetic fibers in the sacral region of the spine controlling micturition, certain preoperative medications, and narcotics. Urinary retention is also more likely to occur in surgeries of the lower abdomen, pelvis, and genitourinary tract where manipulation of tissues may cause swelling of or around the urethra.

Once the urinary catheter is discontinued, the patient must void within the next 6 to 8 hours. The time when the patient is due to void (DTV) is noted on the intake and output (I&O) record and in the nursing note. The void must be substantial, a minimum of 100 to 150 mL, to be considered adequate. A patient who only voids small amounts may have urinary retention with overflow or a UTI.

When a patient is unable to void, the nurse palpates the bladder. A bladder scan can be used to estimate the amount of urine in the bladder and to determine the need for catheterization. The I&O record is also reviewed because dehydration may be partially to blame. Techniques to help patients void include running warm water over the perineum, allowing the patient to stand or use the bathroom rather than a bedpan, running water in the bathroom, and allowing the patient to smell spirits of peppermint. These techniques may help, however, their efficacy has not been demonstrated through research.

Patients who do not void within the specified time frame are usually straight catheterized to empty the bladder. The nurse needs a health care provider's order to perform urinary catheterization. Sometimes the catheter is left in place if more than 1,000 mL is drained during the catheterization. The patient is reassured and encouraged to continue to drink fluids. Urinary retention resolves over time, but it may take one or two straight catheterizations before the patient is able to void on his own.

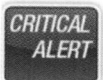 **CRITICAL ALERT** *Urinary retention can place pressure on internal sutures in a patient recovering from some types of urological surgery. Contact the surgeon immediately if a patient is unable to void within the prescribed time period.*

Wound Infection

Wound healing begins immediately after tissue injury. In the first stage (days 1 to 4), the inflammatory process is triggered bringing blood, lymph, and fibrin to the area. Fibrin strands form along the area of injury, creating a blood clot that holds the wound edges together. Increased blood flow to the site brings white blood cells (WBCs) that remove damaged tissue and fight off microorganisms. In the second stage (days 5 to 14 or longer), epithelial cells migrate to the area and proliferate, forming a protective barrier at the wound site. While the process of epithelialization is occurring, collagen synthesis is taking place, filling in tissue gaps and giving the wound added strength. Collagen synthesis helps contract the wound, making it smaller than its original size. The last stage of healing begins 2 to 3 weeks after injury and lasts a year or longer as the wound is reshaped. As collagen breaks down and is replaced, the new fibers become more closely packed shrinking the scar and making it less bulky. Until the wound is completely healed, infection is a concern.

Surgical-site infections (SSIs) continue to be a serious postoperative problem. To qualify as a SSI, the infection occurs within 30 days of the operation. In 1992, the CDC classified surgical site infections into those that are incisional (superficial or deep) and those that are in an organ or organ space (Horan, Gaynes, Martone, Jarvis, & Emori, 1992). The CDC has established definitions for each of the classifications, as shown in the National Guidelines box.

The risk of developing a SSI is affected by characteristics of the patient, the operative procedure, and the type of surgery performed. Older patients, smokers, those who are obese, and those who are malnourished are at a higher risk of developing a wound infection. Patients with diabetes or peripheral vascular disease heal more slowly and are at increased risk. Patients who are immunocompromised have insufficient defenses to fight infection and to repair tissues (Neil, 2007). Factors associated with operative procedures that increase the risk of infection include ineffective preoperative skin preparation, breaks in sterile technique, inadequate sterilization of instruments, hypothermia during surgery, failure to administer appropriate antibiotic coverage, and procedures that last significantly longer than expected according to a preestablished standard (Seltzer, Horsman, & Korniewicz, 2002). The type of surgery also affects the risk of SSI. The National Guidelines for Surgical Wound Classification box in Chapter 26 🔗 lists the CDC's classifications for surgical wounds. The classification is standardized and documented in the surgical record. The CDC's National Nosocomial Infections Surveillance (NNIS) program uses three criteria to assess risk of SSI: wound classification, duration of the surgical procedure, and the ASA physical status classification (described earlier).

Best practices for preventing SSIs come from the CDC and the American College of Surgeons. The CDC clinical guidelines recommend protecting the surgical wound with a sterile dressing for 24 to 48 hours postoperatively. They also recommend using sterile technique for dressing changes. The question of whether clean technique is as effective as sterile technique in the incidence of wound infection is being researched. At present, there is not enough evidence to recommend clean technique over sterile technique (Horan et al., 1992; St. Clair & Larrabee, 2002). Dressings are used postoperatively for a number of reasons. Dressings act to reduce contamination of the incision by microorganisms (i.e., dry sterile dressing), to reduce bleeding or swelling (i.e., pressure dressing), to cushion the wound and absorb drainage, and in some cases to debride the wound (i.e., wet to dry dressing).

Traditionally, the surgeon performs the first dressing change. Until then, the nurse monitors the surgical site for evidence of bleeding or drainage. Some amount of drainage is normal after surgery. Small to moderate amounts of drainage are circled with a pen directly on the dressing. This allows the nurse to watch for an increase in the amount of drainage. The dressing can also be reinforced. Excessive amounts of bleeding or drainage are reported to the surgeon. After the first dressing change, the wound may be left open to air or covered with a dry sterile dressing according to health care provider preference. Dressing changes are usually performed once or twice a shift using sterile technique. During the dressing change, the nurse notes the condition of the incision. It should be well approximated, slightly pink, and free of purulent drainage. Crusting along the incision is a normal finding. The nurse reports signs of wound infection including pain and tenderness at the site, swelling, redness, purulent drainage, odor, or evidence of dehiscence to the surgeon. Systemic indicators of infection include fever (38°C [100.4°F] or higher), elevated WBC count, and elevated serum glucose. Studies confirm that fever is a nonspecific and insensitive measure of infection. In one study of 284 general surgical patients, 63% of infected patients did not have a fever (Vermeulen et al., 2005).

NATIONAL GUIDELINES CDC Criteria for Defining Surgical Site Infection

Infection Site	Time Frame for Developing Symptoms	Patient Symptoms (Patient Must Have at Least One of These)
Superficial incisional (involves only the skin and subcutaneous tissue)	Infection occurs within 30 days of the surgery.	Purulent drainage from the site. Organisms isolated from a culture of fluid or tissue from the site. One sign and symptom of infection: pain, tenderness, redness, localized swelling and heat.
Deep incisional (involves deep soft tissue such as fascia and muscle layers of incision)	Infection occurs within 30 days of surgery or if an implant is placed within 1 year and the infection appears to be related to operative procedures.	Purulent drainage from the deep incision but not from an organ or body cavity. A deep incision dehisces, or is deliberately opened by the surgeon when the patient presents with at least one of the symptoms of infection: fever, localized pain, or tenderness. Abscess or other evidence of infection involving the deep incision.

Source: Adapted with permission from Mangram, A., Horan, T., Pearson, M., Silver, L., & Jarvis, W. (1999). Guideline for prevention of surgical site infection. Centers for Disease Control and Prevention (CDC), Hospital Infection Control Practices Advisory Committee. *Infection Control and Hospital Epidemiology, 20*(4), 247–280.

Fever that starts or persists after the fifth postoperative day is more likely to be clinically significant for wound infection than is a fever earlier in the postoperative course (Dellinger, 2005).

Parenteral antibiotic prophylaxis may continue for 24 hours after surgery but should not extend beyond this period because it is thought to be unnecessary and may lead to the development of drug resistance (Golembiewski, 2004). Prophylactic antibiotics may be necessary in situations where an organ ruptured or leaked prior to surgery because these wounds are more likely to become infected. Other factors that may aid in wound healing include improving the patient's nutritional status. Protein, calories, calcium, iron, zinc, and vitamins A, B_6, B_{12}, and C are needed for wound healing. Chapter 14 🔗 provides a complete description of adequate nutrition. Chapter 67 🔗 discusses normal and abnormal wound healing.

Wound Dehiscence and Evisceration

Two potential problems of the wound site are wound dehiscence and wound evisceration (Figure 27–5 ■). Wound dehiscence is a partial or complete separation of the wound layers with an opening of the wound. Evisceration is a complete separation of the wound layers and the protrusion of internal organs or viscera. Any wound can dehisce, but it occurs most frequently with abdominal incisions and it occurs most often 5 to 10 days postoperatively. Wound disruption can occur because of poor surgical closure, poor wound healing, or increased stress on the surgical incision.

Risk factors for dehiscence and evisceration are the same (see Rick Factors box). Patients may report "feeling like something popped" and dehiscence is sometimes preceded by a gush of serosanguineous drainage. Wound dehiscence and wound evisceration are emergencies. The nurse calls for help and assists the patient back to bed. The patient is positioned supine with knees bent, and the nurse covers the wound and internal organs with sterile towels or gauze soaked in normal saline. The nurse keeps

RISK FACTORS for Wound Dehiscence and Evisceration
Age (elderly patients)
Diabetes
Obesity
Current wound infection
Preoperative malnutrition
Low serum albumin
Coughing
Vomiting
Straining
Moving

the wound moist and does *not* attempt to replace the organs. The surgeon is called and the patient's vital signs are taken every 5 minutes. Wound dehiscence may be treated medically with dressings or surgically with wound closure. Evisceration is treated with surgical closure.

Wound Drains

Drains are used for a variety of reasons. Wound drains are inserted through an intentional stab wound into an area close to the incision and site of the operation. The purpose of the drain is to remove inflammatory fluid (serum, blood, lymph) that might otherwise accumulate at the operative site causing infection or abscess. The surgeon inserts a closed, suction-type drain such as a Jackson-Pratt or a Hemovac. Applying negative pressure in the drain reservoir creates suction in the drain and speeds the removal of fluid. The nurse empties the drain and records the color and amount of drainage every 8 hours or as often as necessary. The drainage may be sanguineous initially but progresses to serosanguineous and sometimes serous. The nurse reports an increase in the amount of drainage and any unexpected change in the type of drainage. Wound drains are removed when there is minimal drainage (e.g., less than 30 mL in 24 hours). Patients report that the removal of wound drains is quick but very painful (Mimnaugh, Winegar, Mabrey, & Davis, 1999; Puntillo et al., 2002). Patients should be medicated prior to the discontinuation of a drain. Many patients are now discharged to home with wound drains in place. The nurse teaches patients how to empty and measure the drainage so they will be able to continue the care at home.

Other drains and tubes may be inserted during surgery. Chest tubes are used to drain fluid and air from the pleural space and to reestablish a negative intrapleural pressure after thoracotomy. A biliary tube (or T-tube) may be inserted in the common bile duct to prevent biliary obstruction after surgery on the common bile duct. A jejunostomy tube may be inserted during surgery on the pancreas to provide an alternative method of feeding the patient. Chart 27–6 (p. 680) lists common tubes with their purpose and expected drainage. Chapter 67 🔗 further discusses drains and provides pictures.

Venous Thromboembolism

Deep venous thrombosis is the formation of a venous blood clot in a deep vein, usually in the lower leg or pelvis, and it is a serious

Dehiscence

Evisceration

FIGURE 27–5 ■ (A) Wound dehiscence; (B) wound evisceration.

| CHART 27–6 | **Common Tubes and Expected Drainage** |

Tube	Purpose	Drainage Amount	Drainage Color	Other
Foley (bladder)	Drains urine and decompresses the bladder.	1,500–2,500 mL in 24 hours or a minimum of 30 mL/hour	Clear, yellow	Report hematuria, or cloudy urine. Report low urine output.
Three-way Foley (bladder) May have a 30-mL balloon rather than a 5- to 10-mL balloon.	Drains urine and is used for continuous bladder irrigation (CBI).	1,500–2,500 mL/24 hour and any irrigating fluid that is instilled	If used for CBI then expect urine to be pink.	Normal saline is used to irrigate. Regulate the CBI to keep the urine clear. Watch for bladder spasms and clots. Careful intake & output (I&O).
Suprapubic tube (bladder)	Drains urine.	1,500–2,500 mL/24 hour or 30 mL/hour	Clear, yellow	Report no urine output. Report dislodgement.
Nephrostomy tube (kidney pelvis)	Drains urine from the kidney.	Amount depends on function of the kidney.	Clear, yellow	Can be gently flushed with 5 to 10 mL of normal saline.
Nasogastric tube (NGT) Salem sump (stomach) Levine tube (stomach)	Decompress the stomach Low, continuous, or intermittent suction is used; intermittent use if the tube does not have an air vent.	Depends on the situation; up to 1,500 mL/24 hour	Usually pale, yellow-green	Expect some blood in the drainage for 8 hours after gastrectomy. NGT can be flushed with 30 mL or more of saline except after gastric or esophageal surgeries.
Gastrostomy tube	Drainage or feeding.	Varies	Green to dark brown, bloody	Flush with normal saline to keep patent.
Jejunostomy tube	Drainage or feeding.	Varies	Green to dark brown, bloody	Flush with normal saline to keep patent.
Blakemore-Sengstaken tube (triple lumen Esophageal balloon, gastric balloon, drainage	Drains stomach and compresses esophageal or stomach varices.	Varies	Green to dark brown, bloody	Measure pressure in esophageal balloon. Balloon is only inflated for a 48-hour period. Periodic release of balloon pressure.
Wound drains, such as Jackson-Pratt, Hemovac	Drains inflammatory fluid from area surrounding incision.	Varies, but the need to empty the drain frequently (e.g., more than every 4 hours) should be cause for concern.	Sanguineous to serosanguineous. Drainage should become more serous over time.	Drains usually removed when drainage is < 30 mL in 24 hours.
Chest tube (pleural space)	Drains fluid or air from pleural space, restores negative intrapleural pressure. Reexpands the lung.	Not more than 100 mL/hour	Drainage varies from sanguineous to serosanguineous to serous.	Must have a water seal. Record drainage at least every 8 hours. Clamp the chest tube *only* prior to changing the drainage system.
T-tube (common bile duct)	Drains bile if the common bile duct (CBD) is obstructed. Maintains patency of CBD after surgery on the bile duct.	Varies from 0 to 500 mL in 24 hours.	Green, yellow, or brown	Normal bile production is 500–800 mL in 24 hours.

postoperative problem. Once the clot forms, there is a danger of detachment and the possibility of a pulmonary embolus (PE), a serious condition in which the clot obstructs an artery in the lungs. Venous thromboembolism (VTE) is the collective term for DVT and PE. It describes the process of blood clot formation and travel through the veins. The overall incidence of DVT is around 9% to 10% but the rate in some surgeries is much higher. The in-

cidence of DVT following general surgery has been reported at 20% to 30%, and the incidence of DVT following hip fracture may be as high as 50% (Clagett et al., 1998).

DVT occurs as a result of vascular stasis (injury to the intimal layer of the vein) and hypercoagulability. The postoperative patient is at risk for DVT because anesthesia vasodilates vessels, leading to stasis and decreased venous return. Longer surgeries cause prolonged immobilization of the patient during the procedure and are associated with a higher risk of blood clot formation. Reduced mobility after surgery contributes to vascular stasis and DVT. Major orthopedic surgery, multiple trauma, and pelvic surgeries are associated with a higher risk of DVT than other procedures (Geerts et al., 2004; Merli, 2000). Other risk factors include age (over age 60), obesity, prolonged immobilization, use of estrogen, cancer, and history of previous DVT.

Prevention of venous thromboembolism is a goal for all postoperative patients and the nurse should discuss prophylaxis with the health care provider if a postoperative patient arrives on the clinical unit without such orders (Blondin, 2006). The American College of Chest Physicians (ACCP) established guidelines for the prevention of DVT and PE at a consensus conference (Geerts et al., 2004). Several methods of DVT prophylaxis are recommended. Chart 27–7 summarizes some of the recommendations for surgical patients.

Antithrombotic drug therapy is frequently used to prevent DVT. Low-dose unfractionated heparin (LDUH) or low-molecular-weight heparin (LMWH) is given subcutaneously in large enough doses to prevent clot formation but the dose is not large enough to produce systemic anticoagulation. LDUH, as a fixed dose, is given as 5,000 units subcutaneously every 8 hours for high-risk patients, or every 12 hours for moderate-risk patients. LMWHs are better absorbed, have longer action, are more effective in producing anticoagulation, and cause bleeding less often than unfractionated heparin, but they are substantially more expensive (Merli, 2000). There are at least six types of LMWH but the most common are enoxaparin, dalteparin, and ardeparin. Enoxaparin is given 30 to 40 mg subcutaneously daily or twice a day. An alternative to LMWH is fondaparinux. This drug inhibits Factor X and has a longer half-life, a more predictable response, and fewer adverse effects than does LMWH (Finnish Medical Society, 2006).

Oral medication, such as warfarin (Coumadin), can also be used for DVT prophylaxis in some situations but the dose must be titrated to achieve a target INR of 2.5 (Geerts et al., 2004). Patients in higher risk categories for venous thromboembolism may need to continue antithrombotic drug therapy for 2 to 4 weeks after hospital discharge. Examples of surgeries that are higher risk for VTE and therefore require extended DVT prophylaxis include hip fracture repair, total hip or knee replacement surgeries, and major gynecologic surgeries.

Some patients should not receive either LDUH or LMWH even in low doses because if bleeding does occur, it could be catastrophic. Patients having cranial surgery (risk of intracranial bleed) or spinal surgery (risk of spinal cord compression from hematoma) might be better served with another form of prophylaxis.

Other ways to decrease the risk of DVT include intermittent pneumatic compression devices (IPCs) or graduated compression stockings (GCSs). There are several manufacturers of **intermittent pneumatic compression devices** and all of them work on the basis of applying intermittent compression of the calf muscle, thereby increasing venous return. The pump is set to apply 45 mmHg of pressure with inflation. Pneumatic compression devices may be applied in the operating room and worn almost continuously (except when ambulating or bathing) for the next several days. Patients sometimes complain that the plastic leg sleeves are hot, cause sweating, or interrupt sleep. Some machines have a switch that cools the airflow through the sleeves. Experts suggest that pneumatic compression devices not be used on patients who are immobilized for 72 hours without prophylaxis. If a clot has formed, the device could dislodge it (Merli, 2000).

Graduated compression stockings are elastic stockings that apply varying degrees of pressure on the lower leg with the greatest exertion of pressure at the ankle and the lowest pressure at the thigh (or knee in shorter stockings). GCSs increase venous return and velocity, thereby reducing venous wall distention and venous stasis (Evans et al., 2001). GCSs have been shown through research to be effective in reducing the incidence of DVT (Amaragiri & Lees, 2006). Pneumatic compression devices and gradient stockings may be used in conjunction with antithrombotic drug therapy or as an alternative to it in patients who should not receive any type of anticoagulation.

CHART 27–7 **Summary of Recommendations for DVT Prophylaxis in the Surgical Patient**

Level of Risk for Venous Thromboembolism	Recommendation
Low risk: minor procedure, age < 40 years, no other risks OR Gynecologic procedures lasting < 30 minutes OR Low-risk urological procedures (TURP)	Early and persistent ambulation
Moderate risk: non–major general surgery, age 40 to 60 years Gynecologic surgery (benign disease)	LDUH 5,000 units bid OR LMWH <3,400 units daily
Higher risk: non–major surgical procedure and age >60 years Extensive gynecologic surgery	LDUH 5,000 units tid OR LMWH >3,400 units daily
Very high risk: major surgery with multiple risk factors	LDUH tid OR LMWH (higher doses) daily AND Graduated compression stockings OR Intermittent pneumatic compression boots
High risk for bleeding	Intermittent pneumatic compression boots OR Graduated compression stockings

Source: Adapted from Geerts, W., Pineo, G., Hit, J., Bergqvist, D., Lassen, M., Colwell, C., et al. (2004). Prevention of venous thromboembolism: The Seventh AACP Conference on Antithrombotic and Thrombolytic Therapy. *Chest, 126*(3 Suppl), 338S–400S.

Early ambulation is important in preventing deep venous thrombosis. Patients are encouraged to ambulate several times a day and to change positions in bed every 1 to 2 hours. Leg exercises can be done while the patient is in a chair or in bed. Chapter 43 ☺ contains a complete description of DVT cause and treatment.

■ Gerontological Considerations

Care of the older adult after surgery is similar to care of younger adult patients with a few exceptions. Older adults have decreased physiological reserves, making them less able or slower to respond to the specific demands of surgery (Mamaril, 2006). It may take older patients 48 hours or longer to fully recover from the effects of anesthesia (Asher, 2004). Also, older adults tend to experience more postoperative complications than younger people because of preexisting illness, nutritional deficits, and altered drug metabolism and, when complications occur, the elderly experience higher death rates (Hamel, Henderson, Khuri, & Daley, 2005). The risk of postoperative complications varies depending on the surgery; however, in a large study (>500,000), 20% of seniors over the age of 80 years developed postoperative complications (Hamel et al., 2005).

The assessment of older patients may show slight variations from those of younger adult patients. For example, older adults tend to run slightly lower body temperatures or oxygen saturation levels (i.e., 93% to 95%) than younger patients, but the nurse needs to use the same parameters of concern for older adults that would be used for others. The nurse also uses the same priorities of postoperative care. The older adult does have special needs (e.g., replace hearing aids, dentures, and glasses as soon as possible) and problems. Major issues to address include pain management, postoperative delirium, medication management, restoring functional ability, and discharge planning. Older patients also have an increased risk for falls, as discussed in the Gerontological Considerations box.

Pain management is a challenge in older adults, and some studies report that postoperative pain is undertreated (Sauaia et al., 2005) or inappropriately treated (Titler et al., 2003). Teaching older patients about communicating their pain may im-

prove pain treatment (McDonald, Thomas, Livingston, & Severson, 2005), and studies show that even elders with mild or moderate cognitive impairments can accurately report pain using a verbal or numeric rating scale (Kaasalainen & Crook, 2004).

The rule of thumb in treating pain in older patients is to start low and go slow (i.e., use the lowest doses first and slowly titrate medications upward) (Mamaril, 2006). Opioids are used to control postoperative pain, but the concurrent use of NSAIDS can decrease the amount of narcotics required. All older patients receiving narcotics should also receive a stool softener to offset the constipating effect of the narcotic (Asher, 2004). Certain narcotics, such as meperidine (Demerol), are avoided in older adults because they produce toxic metabolites that can cause seizures or confusion. Nurses and health care providers need more training in pain management for older adults. In one study of more than 700 patients being treated for hip fracture, pain management was a serious problem. The study reported that acetaminophen, the drug of choice for pain treatment, was administered in subtherapeutic doses; that half of the patients received at least one dose of meperidine, although the drug is not recommended for the elderly; and that only 27% of patients received pain medication around the clock even though this is a suggested practice for postoperative pain control (Titler et al., 2003).

Postoperative delirium, an acute change in cognitive function with decreased ability to focus or sustain attention and altered perceptions, is a serious problem for older adults. Postoperative delirium increases morbidity and mortality for those affected. The incidence of postoperative delirium ranges from 3.8% in low-risk patients (Kalisvaart et al., 2006) to as high as 60% in higher risk patients (Milisen, Lemiengre, Braes, & Foreman, 2005). Postoperative delirium can occur at any time during hospitalization but it is more likely to occur shortly after surgery. In one small study of orthopedic patients, the highest incidence of postoperative confusion occurred on postoperative days 1 and 2 (35% and 37%, respectively) compared with a 12% incidence on postoperative day 4 (Wong, Wong, & Brooks, 2002).

The development of postoperative delirium is multifactorial with the most vulnerable and frail elders being at highest risk. Risk factors include prior cognitive impairment, severity of illness on admission, depression, increased age, sensory deficits, impaired functional ability, and use of certain medications (Kalisvaart et al., 2006; Leung, Sands, Mullen, Wang, & Vaurio, 2005; Milisen et al., 2005; Wong et al., 2002). Patients needing emergency surgery may be more likely to develop acute confusion than those admitted for elective procedures (Kalisvaart et al., 2006).

Programs designed to prevent postoperative delirium have had some success in preventing delirium, reducing the severity of it, or shortening the course (Marcantonio, Flacker, Wright, & Resnick, 2001; Milisen et al., 2001, 2005). Such programs generally include identification of high-risk patients preoperatively, daily consultation with a geriatrician or advanced practice nurse specializing in geriatrics, reducing the use of unnecessary medications, training of bedside nurses in the early recognition of acute confusion, and aggressive correction of factors that may be contributing to confusion (e.g., hypoxia, fluid and electrolyte imbalance, pain). Some have tried to prevent postoperative delirium by administering low doses of haloperidol prophylactically; however, haloperidol does not seem to prevent delirium

---

GERONTOLOGICAL CONSIDERATIONS Related to Falls

The Joint Commission's 2007 National Patient Safety Goals require hospitals to implement a fall reduction program. Older surgical patients are more likely to fall than younger patients. Risk factors for falls include a prior history of falls, fear of falling, cognitive impairment, bowel and bladder incontinence, and functional impairment (Lyons, 2004; Resnick, 2003). The older postoperative patient will likely have additional risk factors associated with surgery or anesthesia including the use of narcotics for pain control, the attachment of medical equipment (e.g., intravenous lines, urinary catheters) that can limit ambulation, and a temporary functional impairment from the presence of incisions. All postoperative patients are assessed for their risk for falls after surgery and at other times as their condition warrants. The hospital-based fall reduction program must be implemented for all patients who are identified as being at risk.

but it may decrease the severity and duration of it (Kalisvaart et al., 2005).

Older patients experience more adverse effects with medications than do younger adults. Aging causes changes in the absorption, distribution, protein binding, metabolism, and elimination of drugs (Kuchta & Golembiewski, 2004). These changes tend to increase the plasma concentration of some drugs and narrow the therapeutic range. In general, giving smaller doses of drugs or increasing the dosing interval may help reduce adverse effects. Certain drugs should be used sparingly or avoided altogether because of their propensity for causing sedation or confusion in older patients. Examples of these medications include meperidine, cimetidine, long-acting benzodiazepines (e.g., diazepam), and diphenhydramine (Kuchta & Golembiewski, 2004).

It is important to restore functional ability to the older surgical patient as soon as possible. A collaborative effort among health care providers, nurses, physical therapists, and others is required to optimize the elder's recovery. Postoperative imbalances such as dehydration, electrolyte disturbances, or anemia should be corrected. Older patients are not routinely transfused with red blood cells postoperatively, but anemia will impair functional ability. A large study (n = >5,700) of older patients recovering from hip fracture surgery showed that those with higher hemoglobin levels were able to walk further distances postoperatively than those with lower levels (Lawrence et al., 2003).

Early mobilization and muscle strengthening can have positive effects. In one small study, elders who received muscle resistance training after hip surgery showed increased muscle mass, muscle strength, and functional ability over those who did not receive the training (Suetta et al., 2004). Other studies support these findings. A study of 224 patients suffering hip fracture showed that those who began weight bearing and ambulation training early in the postoperative course were more likely to be able to walk independently within a month of hospital discharge (Kondo et al., 2005). Some older patients may be able to be discharged home rather than to rehabilitation when an increased emphasis is placed on muscle strengthening and physical therapy (Oldmeadow et al., 2004).

There are special concerns when discharging an older person home. The nurse needs to ask the patient about the availability of social support, the specifics of the home environment, and any surgery-related needs (Burden, 2004). Specific concerns include the following:

- Is the elder able to perform self-care?
- Who is available to assist the elder in meeting her needs?
- Is the elder a primary caretaker for someone else?
- What is the condition of the home environment (e.g., stairs, location of bedrooms and bathrooms, availability of telephone, presence of a lifeline)?
- Does the home environment need a safety evaluation?
- What supplies, medications, or other equipment (wheelchair, hold bars, raised toilet seat, etc.) does the elder need at home?
- How will the elder get to follow-up appointments?

Another concern for the nurse is the patient's psychological readiness for discharge. Patients need to feel that they will be safe at home. The sense of safety is related to patients; confidence in their ability to care for themselves and in the support they will have from others (Heine, Koch, & Goldie, 2004; Nilsson, Unosson, & Kihlgren, 2006). Nurses need to work closely with patients so that the patient develops the confidence needed to feel safe and ready for discharge.

Health Promotion

Discharge teaching is critical now that the length of hospitalization is shorter. Surgeries that once required a 10-day hospital stay now require a 3- to 4-day stay. Minimally invasive surgical techniques allow some patients to go home on the same day as surgery. It is not unusual to discharge patients home with dressings, drains, and even IV antibiotics or parenteral nutrition. Understandably, patients are concerned about how to care for themselves after discharge. Patients want information about wound care, medications, activities, diet, symptom management, and other aspects of self-care.

Teaching is provided to the patient as well as to others who will be involved in providing care for the patient. It is important to use language the patient understands and to check the patient's understanding of the information. In one study that compared nurses' perceptions of discharge teaching with patients' perceptions, there were significant differences in the understanding of discharge information, with nurses overestimating patients' understanding of the material (Reilly et al., 1996). It is critical to provide written instructions. Research suggests that written information fosters the patient's understanding and compliance with discharge instructions (Holmes & Lenz, 1997; Jacobs, 2000). Also, being able to call the nurse with questions may be especially important to patients in their adjustment after surgery (Burt, Caelli, Moore, & Anderson, 2005; Oermann, Harris, & Dammeyer, 2001; Ross, 2007). The teaching needs of the patient vary according to the surgery and other factors, but general areas to be covered in discharge teaching are discussed next.

Patients need to be advised about the trajectory of recovery. It is theorized that postoperative recovery includes four dimensions: physiological recovery, marked by a return of bodily functions; psychological recovery, a return of well-being; social recovery, a return to social activities and independence; and habitual recovery, a point at which the person returns to a full range of normal activities (Allvin, Berg, Idvall, & Nilsson, 2007). Patients need to know that recovery takes time. One study of patients following cardiac surgery found that patients were surprised to find that recovery took much longer than expected and they felt unprepared for prolonged symptoms such as fatigue (Doering et al., 2002). Uncomplicated surgery often takes 4 to 6 weeks or even longer for recovery. The effects from general anesthesia can linger, wound healing requires energy, it takes weeks to make sufficient red blood cells to replace those lost in surgery, and patients may experience pain or soreness until healing is well on its way. Patients may lack their usual level of energy during recovery. Pain, fatigue, and depression are common symptoms during recovery from major surgery (Hodgson & Given, 2004; Horvath, 2003; Lupien, Schoneboom, & Wren, 2000; Nilsson et al., 2006; Zalon, 2004), but these symptoms will gradually resolve. Social support is important to the psychological well-being of patients as they recover from surgery (Nilsson et al., 2006).

Information on how to care for the wound following discharge is a common need for postsurgical patients. The nurse checks with the surgeon about any special requirements of wound care. Some patients will have a dressing in place that is kept clean and dry until the follow-up appointment with the surgeon. In other situations, incisions are kept covered for the first 24 to 48 hours and then the dressing is removed and the wound left open to the air. These wounds are gently cleaned each day and the dressing replaced if there is risk of contamination. Staples and sutures are often removed 7 to 10 days after the surgery in a follow-up appointment with the nurse or health care provider. If Steri-Strips cover the wound, they are left in place until they fall off naturally. Wound drains are emptied as often as needed and the amount and type of drainage recorded. Any sudden increase in the amount of drainage or a change in the character or color of the drainage needs to be reported to the surgeon.

Information about those activities that are allowed and those that are not allowed after surgery is especially important to provide. Research consistently finds that patients are unclear about what activities are allowed at home and they want specific information on this topic (Doering et al., 2002; Hughes, Hodgson, Muller, Robinson, & McCorkle, 2000; Jacobs, 2000; Reilly et al., 1996). This information also is important because patients may judge their postoperative progress on the activities they are able to perform. Examples of the type of questions that patients' have are as follows:

- When can I bathe or shower?
- When can I exercise? Are there any restrictions on exercising?
- Can I do housework?
- When can I start driving?
- When can I resume sexual activity?
- How much rest should I get?
- When can I return to work?

Usually, patients are encouraged to bathe or shower daily. If a dressing is in place, it is kept clean and dry. For most surgeries, the patient is discouraged from lifting anything heavier than 10 to 15 pounds until the incision has healed in 4 to 6 weeks. Walking at a reasonable pace is encouraged and limited only by pain and fatigue, but heavier aerobic-type workouts are restricted until approved by the surgeon. Similarly, light housework is generally acceptable when the patient feels able but heavier housework may be restricted. Most restrictions on driving are based on the need for road safety rather than potential injury to the wound. Often patients are allowed to drive when their ability to move is no longer restricted by pain or soreness. For some surgeries driving is restricted for several days and for others, it may be several weeks. Once patients are able to drive, they are cautioned not to drive while taking narcotic analgesics. Except with certain gynecologic or genitourinary surgeries, sexual activity after surgery is restricted as a result of pain. Most people will be able to resume sexual activity in 2 to 3 weeks. The time frame for returning to work will depend on the surgery and the type of work performed. For less invasive procedures such as arthroscopy, patients can return to work in 2 to 4 days. Most patients will be out of work for 3 to 6 weeks following major surgery and up to 10 weeks for major abdominal or thoracic resections.

The postoperative diet for most patients emphasizes good nutrition for wound healing. Patients are encouraged to get adequate calories, proteins, and vitamins. Diet restrictions or recommended modifications are made for some surgeries. Examples of these include Nissen's fundoplication, gastrojejunostomy (Bilroth II), pancreatic resection (Whipple), radical neck dissection, and ileostomy.

Research suggests that patients may not feel adequately prepared to manage their medication regimens at home (Cutilli, 2007; Jacobs, 2000; Reilly et al., 1996). Discharge teaching includes a discussion of medications including purpose, how to take the medication, and key side effects. Most postoperative patients will be discharged with an oral narcotic for pain control and some will have antibiotics prescribed. They need to know when to take pain medication, how much medication to take, alternative strategies for pain control such as elevation and ice applications, and how to prevent constipation, a common side effect of narcotics.

Early discharge puts the burden of recognizing and responding to potential complications on the patient. Often, signs of wound infection take several days to develop and may not show up until after the patient is discharged home. Research studies show that patients feel unprepared to identify possible postoperative complications (Hughes et al., 2000; Jacobs, 2000) or to manage expected postoperative problems (Burt et al., 2005). Chart 27–8 lists some of the danger signs that patients should report to their surgeons. Discharge information includes contact phone numbers for emergencies. Most patients will have a follow-up appointment in 7 to 10 days after discharge.

The information needs of surgical patients are complex and it is unrealistic to think that the needs of every patient can be met on discharge from the hospital. Patients need to be carefully evaluated on their ability to provide care for themselves at home, and nurses must make referrals to community services (e.g., visiting nurses association [VNA], physical therapy, hospice) when home assistance is required. Appropriate referrals not only improve patient care but can prevent hospital readmission. Nurses need to develop skills in evaluating patients for discharge.

One study found that nurses and health care providers did not always recognize the needs of their patients on discharge. The study concluded that health care professionals need increased knowledge of the discharge process, of the community services available, training in identifying patients' needs and improved collaboration among themselves with regard to patient discharge (Bowles, Foust, Naylor, & Ware, 2003). Surgical patients may need the services of a VNA or other home health agency to assist

CHART 27–8 Danger Signs That Patients Should Report to Their Health Care Provider

- Temperature greater than 38°C (100.4°F)
- Fever with chills
- Pain that is increasing or that is not adequately controlled by medication
- Incision that is red, painful, or has drainage
- Difficulty voiding or unable to void
- Painful urination

with their recovery. Services that may be appropriate, particularly for the elderly, include home nursing care for dressing changes, wound checks, antibiotic administration, home safety evaluation, and the coordination of other services such as a home health aide to assist with meeting personal care needs, home physical therapy to assist with rehabilitation, homemaker services for housekeeping, and meal preparation.

Patients are discharged home when the health care provider and health care team determines they no longer need the care and close attention of an acute care hospital and they are safe to care for themselves at home. The nurse has an obligation to speak with the health care provider and advocate for patient safety in situations where the nurse questions the readiness of the patient for discharge. There are no set criteria for determining readiness for discharge; it is a clinical judgment, but the nurse can use indicators to assist in making this judgment. Indicators of stability and readiness for discharge are:

- Stable vital signs; vital signs at patient's baseline
- Baseline level of consciousness
- Wound is stable without bleeding
- Able to take food and fluids orally without nausea and vomiting
- Able to void and move bowels

- Pain is at an acceptable level
- Able to ambulate without assistance
- Able to perform ADLs independently or at baseline
- Home services are adequate to meet the needs of the patient.

Discharge teaching for both the patient and the family/support system is outlined in Patient Teaching & Discharge Priorities box.

Research

Research is changing the way nurses care for postoperative patients. Nurses are looking for evidence to support their practice. It is important to know whether or not nursing interventions are having the desired outcome. A culture of answering practice questions by using the best available research evidence or by designing a research study is evolving. The Research Opportunities and Clinical Impact box (p. 686) lists research problems that are important to the care of the postsurgical patient.

Research is also being used to design structures and nursing care delivery models to create healing environments. Single rooms in hospitals create space for privacy and personal control and provide a place for family to stay overnight. Researchers are examining the effects of single rooms on outcomes such as infection control, pain management, and rest and recovery (Chaudhury, Mahmood, & Valente, 2006).

PATIENT TEACHING & DISCHARGE PRIORITIES for Postoperative Nursing

Need	Teaching
Incision and drain care	Inspect wound daily.
	Assess for redness, warmth, swelling, increased pain, or drainage. Mild bruising around the wound is often normal.
	Keep wound dry for first 48 hours or as directed by the surgeon.
	After 48 hours, wash gently around the incision site(s) and pat dry.
	If Steri-Strips are in place, allow them to fall off by themselves.
	Sutures are usually removed in 7 to 10 days.
	If drains are in place, empty daily or as often as indicated. Note color and amount of drainage.
	Assess availability, knowledge, and comfort with treatment regimen.
	Report a fever >38°C (>100.4°F) or an incision that becomes red, painful, swollen, or has increased drainage.
	Assess respite needs and resources.
	Assess need for follow-up appointments.
	Assess need for wound checks by health professional.
Pain control	Take pain medication as prescribed.
	Do not drive while taking prescription pain medication.
	Increase fluids and take a stool softener to prevent constipation from prescription pain medication.
	Take acetaminophen (Tylenol) regular or extra strength for mild pain.
	Do *not* take aspirin or ibuprofen unless approved by your surgeon.
	Assess pain level and report any increase in pain.
	Assess environment for safety.
Activity	Expect that the effects of surgery, anesthesia, wound healing, and pain medication will make you feel more tired than usual.
	Fatigue may last several weeks. Plan rest periods and pace your activities.
	Avoid strenuous exercise until the follow-up appointment with the surgeon.
	You will need to check with the health care provider about a time frame for returning to work and normal activities.
	Assess support systems for meal preparation, household chores, child care, or spousal care.
	Assess need for home care services.

RESEARCH OPPORTUNITIES AND CLINICAL IMPACT RELATED TO CARE OF THE SURGICAL PATIENT

Research Area	Clinical Impact
Comparison of deep breathing exercises and incentive spirometry in reducing postoperative pulmonary complications.	Important for evidenced-based practice.
Effectiveness of alternative interventions (e.g., relaxation techniques) in reducing postoperative pulmonary complications.	Provides rationale for common nursing interventions performed after surgery.
Effectiveness of ambulation (distance and frequency) in reducing the incidence of postoperative complications (e.g., pneumonia, abdominal distention, urinary retention).	Provides data to support or refute the use of innovative approaches to common postoperative problems.
Effectiveness of various interventions in treating postoperative urinary retention.	
The effect of early feeding after surgery in stimulating the return of bowel function.	
Factors that increase wound healing postoperatively.	
Comparison of wound dressing technique, clean technique versus sterile technique, in the incidence of postoperative wound infection.	
The effectiveness of interventions in the treatment of postoperative nausea and vomiting.	
Effectiveness of interventions to prevent postoperative confusion in older patients.	
Critical Thinking	
Factors influencing nurses' decisions in weaning patients off of oxygen postoperatively.	Provides a basis for understanding how nurses develop clinical judgment.
Factors influencing nurses' decisions in postoperative pain management.	
Comparison of nursing management to prevent postoperative complications by experienced and novice nurses.	
Comparison of decisions to report abnormal findings to surgeons by experienced and novice nurses.	
Factors influencing the use of "alternative" nursing interventions in the prevention of postoperative complications.	
Strategies used to increase patient compliance with postoperative interventions (e.g., ambulation, coughing, and deep breathing).	
Pain Management	
Effectiveness of nonpharmacologic interventions (e.g., splinting, elevation, application of ice, relaxation techniques) in reducing postoperative pain.	Increased patient comfort.
Evaluation of pain and discomfort associated with common postoperative interventions.	Improve interventions to decrease pain associated with the surgical experience.
Strategies to reduce pain associated with procedures.	
Factors that influence the effectiveness of patient-controlled analgesia in the postoperative patient.	
Factors that reduce persistent postoperative pain.	
Psychosocial Responses	
Predictors of anxiety in surgical patients.	Improve the psychological well-being of postoperative patients.
Factors that influence anxiety levels in the older surgical patient.	
Strategies to reduce anxiety in postoperative patients.	Understand the impact of sleep and rest on postoperative recovery.
Effect of family visits on postoperative anxiety.	
Description of the sleep and rest patterns in postoperative patients.	
Influence of sleep on postoperative recovery.	
Factors important to patients and families in selecting a rehabilitation facility.	
Discharge	
Common problems experienced by the patient following discharge home.	Improve health care professionals' understanding of the issues that patients face following discharge.
Interventions used by patients to manage problems at home (e.g., fatigue, depression, constipation, pain, wound healing).	
Strategies to increase the patient's ability to manage symptoms at home.	Increase patient's competence in managing their own recovery.
Adjustment of discharge teaching to accommodate cultural differences.	

Clinical Preparation

 Read

- History of Current Illness
- Past Medical History
- Physical Exam
- Admitting Medical Orders
- Laboratory Study Results

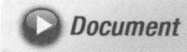 **Document**

- Summary of Hospitalization
- Pathophysiology Form
- Laboratory Values
- Laboratory Results Explanation

 Apply

- List of Potential Nursing Diagnoses
- Concept Map
- Critical Thinking Questions

*Log on to MyNursingKit.com to download forms you will need and to complete further steps in the Clinical Preparation assignment.

HISTORY OF PRESENT ILLNESS

Ryan Landry is a 67-year-old man who is admitted to the surgical unit following a left hemicolectomy. Mr. Landry was in reasonably good health until 2 months ago when he began to experience cramping abdominal pain that he attributed to constipation and gas. When the abdominal cramping continued and he noticed that his stools were narrower than usual, he made an appointment with his primary health care provider. A routine exam uncovered occult blood in the stool, and Mr. Landry was referred for a colonoscopy.

Several polyps were removed during the colonoscopy and biopsy results revealed adenocarcinoma of the colon. A left hemicolectomy without colostomy was performed. Once the results of lymph node biopsies taken during surgery are available, Mr. Landry will be referred to an oncologist for discussion of follow-up treatment, including possible chemotherapy. Currently Mr. Landry is second day postoperative from the hemicolectomy.

Medical–Surgical History
Patient has hypertension and elevated cholesterol. He smokes 1 pack per day and has done so for the past 40 years. His father died of colon cancer at the age of 70. His hypertension is treated with metoprolol 50 mg daily and the elevated cholesterol levels are treated with atorvastatin 80 mg daily. He has failed many times to quit smoking.

Social History
He lives with his wife and a grown son.

Physical Exam
Vital signs: T 101.4, HR 108, RR 20, BP 142/84

Alert and oriented; reports feeling very anxious; asks frequent questions often repeating them; looks worried and seems overly vigilant any time a health care worker comes into the room

Reports a significant amount of pain, rating it as a 7 at rest and a 10 with movement

Cardiac telemetry: sinus tachycardia with occasional premature ventricular contractions

Taking shallow breaths; crackles in the lung bases bilaterally

Oxygen saturation: 93% on 4 liters of oxygen via nasal cannula; using the incentive spirometer sporadically; weak cough

Abdomen: slightly firm; distended with hypoactive bowel sounds and negative flatus

Nasogastric tube attached to low intermittent suction; draining small amount of green fluid

Complains of being thirsty and having a sore throat; slightly nauseated especially with movement

Foley catheter in place; draining concentrated urine

Urine output in the last 2 hours: 42 mL

Skin: warm and dry

Abdominal incision covered by a primary dressing that is dry and intact

2+ pedal pulses bilaterally and no peripheral edema

Patient requires assistance with ambulation. He complains of severe pain and vertigo when standing. He ambulates a very short distance before requesting to go back to bed. Following activity his respiratory rate was 32 and his heart rate was 118.

Admitting Medical Orders
Surgical service

Admit to Telemetry Unit

No known allergies

Vital signs every 4 hours

Call house officer: pulse < 60 and > 110/minute; BP < 90 and > 160 systolic; temperature > 38.5; urine output < 30 mL/hr for 2 hours; respiratory rate > 30/minute; oxygen saturation > 92%

NPO

Maintain nasogastric tube to low continuous suction

Incentive spirometry 10 times every hour

Foley to gravity drainage

Monitor intake and output

Sequential compression device (SCD) to lower extremities while in bed

Ambulate three times daily

Cardiac telemetry while receiving IV metoprolol

IV: D5½NS with 20 mEq KCl at 125 mL/hr

Scheduled Medications

Heparin 5,000 units subcutaneous twice a day
Nicotine transdermal patch 15 mg daily
PCA morphine sulfate 1 mg/mL incremental dose 1 mg and lock out 6 minutes
Metoprolol 5 mg IV every 6 hours while NPO

PRN Medications

Phenergan 25 mg IV q6h prn nausea
Mylanta 30 mL po/NG q4–6h prn dyspepsia

Lorazepam 0.5 to 2 mg IV q6–8h prn anxiety
Tylenol 650 mg po/pr q4h prn pain/fever
Milk of magnesia 30 mL po/NG q4h prn constipation

Ordered Laboratory Studies

Chemistry 20 and CEA on admission
Chemistry 7 with magnesium, phosphorus, and calcium every 48 hours postoperatively
CBC daily

LABORATORY STUDY RESULTS

Test	Day 1 (Preop)	Day 2 (Postop Day 1)	Day 3 (Postop Day 2)
Sodium	136 mEq/L		142 mEq/L
Potassium	4.1 mEq/L		3.9 mEq/L
Chloride	102 mEq/L		106 mEq/L
Bicarbonate	26 mEq/L		21 mEq/L
Blood urea nitrogen (BUN)	24 mg/dL		33 mg/dL
Creatinine	0.8 mg/dL		1.1 mg/dL
Glucose	113 mg/dL		153 mg/dL
Magnesium	2.2 mEq/L		2.4 mEq/L
Phosphorus	3.2 mg/dL		2.5 mg/dL
Calcium	9.3 mg/dL		10.1 mg/dL
White blood cell (WBC)	7,000/mm^3	11,000/mm^3	13,000/mm^3
Hematocrit	37%	32%	27%
Hemoglobin	13 g/dL	10.6 g/dL	9.2 g/dL
Carcinoembryonic antigen (CEA)	6.0 ng/mL		

CRITICAL THINKING QUESTIONS

1. What five nursing diagnoses are of the highest priority for Mr. Landry today? Why?

2. Review Mr. Landry's current physical examination. What postoperative problems, if any, is Mr. Landry currently experiencing?

3. The following activities need to be performed with or for Mr. Landry: Change the syringe in the PCA pump, empty and record urine output, perform a.m. care, teach use of the incentive spirometer, and call the surgeon for an additional antiemetic order. In which order should the nurse perform these activities? Why?

4. Later in the day, Mr. Landry says to the nurse, "The surgeon told me he's pretty sure he got all of the cancer. I guess I won't need that appointment with the oncologist." What is the nurse's best response to this situation?

Answers to Critical Thinking Questions appear in Appendix D.

NCLEX® REVIEW

1. A postoperative patient in the PACU begins to demonstrate an increased heart rate. The nurse realizes this increase is most likely because of:
   1. Bleeding.
   2. Anxiety.
   3. Nausea.
   4. Pain.

2. The nurse is assessing a postoperative patient in the PACU. Which of the following would indicate the patient is stable enough for transfer to another inpatient care area?
   1. Breathing with an oral airway
   2. Easily arousable and moving all four extremities
   3. Lower extremities without sensation post spinal anesthesia
   4. Moderate amount of vomiting

3. A postoperative patient is demonstrating a distended abdomen with no bowel sounds. Which of the following should the nurse do to help this patient?
   1. Advance to full diet.
   2. Restrict fluids.
   3. Ambulate three times a day.
   4. Administer antiemetic medication.

4. The nurse is instructing a postoperative patient about care needed when at home. Which of the following should the nurse include in these instructions?
   1. Habitual recovery will occur in a short period of time.
   2. Keep the wound open to air and permit the Steri-Strips to fall off on their own.
   3. Return to the doctor's office to have the staples removed in 3 weeks.
   4. Full recovery from surgery will be unexpectedly short.

5. The nurse would like to study how a nurse's critical thinking skills can be improved when working with a postoperative patient. Which of the following research topics would provide information on nurses' critical thinking skills?
   1. Factors that influence anxiety levels in the older surgical patient
   2. Strategies to increase the patient's ability to manage symptoms at home
   3. Nurse's ability to manage post operative pain
   4. Adjustment of discharge teaching to accommodate cultural differences

Answers for review questions appear in Appendix D

KEY TERMS

airway obstruction *p.655*
fast-tracking *p.644*
graduated compression stockings *p.681*
hypothermia *p.659*

hypoxemia *p.655*
ileus *p.676*
intermittent pneumatic compression devices *p.681*

laryngospasm *p.655*
normothermia *p.659*
postanesthesia care unit (PACU) *p.644*
surveillance *p.645*

PEARSON

EXPLORE **mynursingkit**™

MyNursingKit is your one stop for online chapter review materials and resources. Prepare for success with additional NCLEX®-style practice questions, interactive assignments and activities, web links, animations and videos, and more!

Register your access code from the front of your book at
www.mynursingkit.com

REFERENCES

Allard, N. (2007). Day surgery for breast cancer: Effects of a psychoeducational telephone intervention on functional status and emotional distress. *Oncology Nursing Forum, 34*(1), 133–141.

Allvin, R., Berg, K., Idvall, E., & Nilsson, U. (2007). Postoperative recovery: A concept analysis. *Journal of Advanced Nursing, 57*(5), 552–558.

Amaragiri, S., & Lees, T. (2006). Elastic compression stockings for prevention of deep vein thrombosis. *Cochrane Library, 4* (CD001484).

American Society of Anesthesiologists. (2004). *Standard for post anesthesia care.* Park Ridge, IL: Author.

American Society of PeriAnesthesia Nurses. (2002). *Clinical guideline for the prevention of unplanned perioperative hypothermia.* Cherry Hill, NJ: Author.

American Society of PeriAnesthesia Nurses. (2003). ASPAN pain and comfort clinical guideline. *Journal of PeriAnesthesia Nursing, 18*(4), 232–236.

American Society of PeriAnesthesia Nurses. (2006a). ASPAN's evidence-based clinical practice guideline for the prevention and/or management of PONV/PDNV. *Journal of PeriAnesthesia Nursing, 21*(4), 230–250.

American Society of PeriAnesthesia Nurses. (2006b). *Standards of perianesthesia nursing practice.* Cherry Hill, NJ: Author.

Apfel, C., Korttila, K., Abdalla, M., Kerger, H., Turan, A., Vedder, I., Zernak, C., Danner, K., Jokela, R., Pocock, S., Trenkler, S., Kredel, M., Biedler, A., Sessler, D., & Roewer, N., et al. (2004). A factorial trial of six interventions for the prevention of postoperative nausea and vomiting. *New England Journal of Medicine, 350*(24), 2441–2451.

Arieff, A. (1999). Fatal postoperative pulmonary edema. *Chest, 115*(5), 1371–1377.

Asher, M. (2004). Surgical considerations in the elderly. *Journal of PeriAnesthesia Nursing, 19*(6), 406–414.

Basse, L., Billesbolle, P., & Kehlet, H. (2002). Early recovery after abdominal rectopexy with multimodal rehabilitation. *Diseases of the Colon and Rectum, 45*(2), 195–199.

Blondin, M. (2006). *Prevention of deep vein thrombosis.* Iowa City: University of Iowa Gerontological Nursing Research Center, Research Dissemination Core.

Bowles, K., Foust, J., Naylor, M., & Ware, M. (2003). Hospital discharge referral decision making: A multidisciplinary perspective. *Applied Nursing Research, 16*(3), 134–143.

Brooks, D., Crowe, J., Kelsey, C., Lacy, J., Parsons, J., & Solway, Sherra. (2001). A clinical practice guideline on peri-operative cardiorespiratory physical therapy. *Physiotherapy Canada, 53*(1), 9–25.

Brooks, J. (2001). Postoperative nosocomial pneumonia: Nurse-sensitive interventions. *AACN Clinical Issues, 12*(2), 305–323.

Brooks-Brunn, I. (1998). Validation of a predictive model for postoperative pulmonary complications. *Heart & Lung, 27,* 151–158.

Brown, A., Christo, P., & Wu, C. (2004). Strategies for postoperative pain management. *Best Practices & Research. Clinical Anesthesiology, 18,* 703–717.

Burden, N. (2004). Discharge planning for the elderly ambulatory surgical patient. *Journal of PeriAnesthesia Nursing, 19*(6), 401–405.

Burt, J., Caelli, K., Moore, K., & Anderson, M. (2005). Radical prostatectomy: Men's experiences and postoperative needs. *Journal of Clinical Nursing, 14*(7), 883–890.

Carli, F., Mayo, N., Klubien, K., Schricker, T., Trudel, J., & Belliveau, P. (2002). Epidural analgesia enhances functional exercise capacity and health-related quality of life after colonic surgery: Results of a randomized trial. *Anesthesiology, 97*(3), 540–549.

Centers for Disease Control and Prevention. (1997). Guidelines for the prevention of nosocomial pneumonia. *Morbidity and Mortality Weekly Report, 46* (RR-1), 1–79.

Chaiyakunapruk, N., Kitikannakorn, N., Nathisuwan, S., Leeprakobboon, K., & Leelasettagool, C. (2006). The efficacy of ginger for the prevention of postoperative nausea and vomiting: A meta-analysis. *American Journal of Obstetrics and Gynecology, 194*(1), 95–100.

Chaudhury, H., Mahmood, A., & Valente, M. (2006). Nurses' perception of single-occupancy versus multioccupancy rooms in acute care environments: An exploratory comparative assessment. *Applied Nursing Research, 19,* 118–125.

Clagett, G. P., Anderson, F., Geerts, W., Heit, J. A., Knudson, M., Lieberman, J. R., Merli, G. J., & Wheeler, H. B., et al. (1998). Prevention of venous thromboembolism. *Chest, 114*(5, Suppl.), 531S–560S.

Clancy, J., McVicar, A., & Baird, N. (2002). *Perioperative practice: Fundamentals of homeostasis.* New York: Routledge.

Clarke, S., & Aiken, L. (2003). Failure to rescue. *American Journal of Nursing, 103*(1), 42–47.

Cheever, K. (1999). Pain, analgesic use, and morbidity in appendectomy patients. *Clinical Nursing Research 8*(3), 267–282.

Cunningham, M. F., Hanson-Heath, C., & Agre, P. (2003). A perioperative nurse liaison program: CNS interventions for cancer patients and their families. *Journal of Nursing Care Quality, 18*(1), 16–21.

Cutilli, C. (2007). Health literacy in geriatric patients: An integrative review of the literature. *Orthopedic Nursing, 26,* 43–48.

Dellinger, E. (2005). Should we measure body temperature for patients who have recently undergone surgery? *Clinical Infectious Diseases, 40*(10), 1411–1413.

Dip, K., Dip, G., & McCutcheon, H. (2006). Observations and vital signs: Ritual or vital for the postoperative monitoring of postoperative patients? *Applied Nursing Research, 19*(4), 204–211.

Doering, L., McGuire, A., & Rourke, D. (2002). Recovering from cardiac surgery: What patients want you to know. *American Journal of Critical Care, 11*(4), 333–343.

Ead, H. (2006). From Aldrete to PADSS: Reviewing discharge criteria after ambulatory surgery. *Journal of PeriAnesthesia Nursing, 21*(4), 259–267.

Edelen, C., & Perlow, M. (2002). A comparison of the effectiveness of an opioid analgesic and a nonpharmacologic intervention to improve incentive spirometry volumes. *Pain Management Nursing, 3*(1), 36–42.

Evans, D., Read, K., Charles-Barks, C., Edwards, S., Gill, S., Leith, S., Morrison, H., Nelson, J., Sandison, S., & Wilkie, A., et al. (2001). Graduated compression stockings for the prevention of postoperative venous thromboembolism. *Best Practice, 5*(2), 1–5.

Ezzone, S., Baker, R., & Terrepka, E. (1998). Music as an adjunct to antiemetic therapy. *Oncology Nursing Forum, 25,* 1551–1556.

Finnish Medical Society Duodecim. (2006). Prevention of venous thrombosis. In *EMB guidelines: Evidenced-based practice.* Helsinki: Duodecim Medical Publications.

Frazier, S., Moser, D., Daley, L., McKinley, S., Riegel, B., Garvin, B., & An, K., et al. (2003). Critical care nurses' beliefs about and reported management of anxiety. *American Journal of Critical Care, 12*(1), 19–27.

Geerts, W., Pineo, G., Hit, J., Bergqvist, D., Lassen, M., Colwell, C., & Ray, J., et al. (2004). Prevention of venous thromboembolism: The Seventh AACP Conference on Antithrombotic and Thrombolytic Therapy. *Chest, 126*(3 Suppl.), 338S–400S.

Goldman, L., & Ausiello, D. (Eds.). (2004). *Cecil textbook of medicine.* Philadelphia: W. B. Saunders.

Golembiewski, J. (2004). Antibiotic prophylaxis for preventing surgical site infection. *Journal of PeriAnesthesia Nursing, 19*(2), 111–113.

Golembiewski, J., Torrecer, S., & Katke, J. (2005). The use of opioids in the postoperative setting: Focus on morphine, hydromorphone, and fentanyl. *Journal of PeriAnesthesia Nursing, 20*(2), 141–143.

Good, K., Verble, J., Secrest, J., & Norwood, B. (2006). Postoperative hypothermia—The chilling consequences. *AORN Journal, 83*(5), 1054–1069.

Greif, R., Akca, O., Horn, E., Kurz, A., & Sessler, D. (2000). Supplemental perioperative oxygen to reduce the incidence of surgical-wound infection. *New England Journal of Medicine, 342*(3), 161–168.

Gunta, K., Lewis, C., & Nuccio, S. (2000). Prevention and management of postoperative nausea and vomiting. *Orthopaedic Nursing, 19*(2), 39–48.

Hamel, M., Henderson, W., Khuri, S., & Daley, J. (2005). Surgical outcomes for patients aged 80 and older: Morbidity and mortality from major noncardiac surgery. *Journal of the American Geriatrics Society, 53*(3), 424–429.

Hasankhani, H., Mohammadi, E., Moazzami, F., Mokhtari, M., & Naghgizadh, M. (2007). The effects of intravenous fluids temperature on perioperative hemodynamic situation, post-operative shivering, and recovery in orthopaedic surgery. *Canadian Operating Room Nursing Journal, 25*(1), 20–24, 26–27.

Heine, J., Koch, S., & Goldie, P. (2004). Patients' experiences of readiness for discharge following a total hip replacement. *Australian Journal of Physiotherapy, 50*(4), 227–233.

Hodgson, N., & Given, C. (2004). Determinants of functional recovery in older adults surgically treated for cancer. *Cancer Nursing, 27*(1), 10–16.

Holmes, K., & Lenz, E. (1997). Perceived self-care information needs and information-seeking behaviors before and after elective spinal procedures. *Journal of Neuroscience Nursing, 29,* 79–85.

Holte, K., & Kehlet, H. (2002). Epidural anaesthesia and analgesia on perioperative outcome: Effects on surgical stress responses and implications for postoperative nutrition. *Clinical Nutrition, 21,*199–206.

Hopf, H., Hunt, T., Rosen, N., Akca, O., Sessler, D., Greif, R., Sessler, D.I., Harten, J., Anderson, K., Kinsella, J., Lee, J., O'Neill, M., Pryor, K., Fahey, T., Lien, C., & Goldstein, P., et al. (2004). Surgical site infection and the routine use of perioperative hyperoxia in a general surgical population: A randomized controlled trial. *Journal of the American Medical Association, 291*(16), 1956–1965.

Horan, T., Gaynes, R., Martone, W., Jarvis, W., & Emori, T. (1992). CDC definitions of nosocomial surgical site infections. *Infection Control Hospital Epidemiology, 13,* 606–608.

Horvath, K. (2003). Postoperative recovery at home after ambulatory gynecologic laparoscopic surgery. *Journal of PeriAnesthesia Nursing, 18*(5), 324–334.

Hudcova, J., McNicol, E., Quah, C., Lau, J., & Carr, D. (2006). Patient controlled opioid analgesia versus conventional opioid analgesia for postoperative pain. *Cochrane Library, (4)* (CD003348).

Huddleston, J., Long, K., Naessens, J., Vanness, D., Larson, D., Trousdale, R., Plevak, M., Cabanela, M., Ilstrup, D., & Wachter, R., et al. (2004). Improving patient care. Medical and surgical comanagement after elective hip and knee arthroplasty: A randomized, controlled trial. *Annals of Internal Medicine, 141*(1), 28–38.

Hughes, L., Hodgson, N., Muller, P., Robinson, L., & McCorkle, R. (2000). Information needs of elderly postsurgical cancer patients during the transition from hospital to home. *Journal of Nursing Scholarship, 32*(1), 25–30.

Hupcey, J. (2000). Feeling safe: Psychosocial needs of ICU patients. *Journal of Nursing Scholarship, 32*(4), 361–367.

Jacobs, V. (2000). Informational needs of surgical patients following discharge. *Applied Nursing Research, 13*(1), 12–18.

Kaasalainen, S., & Crook, J. (2004). An exploration of seniors' ability to report pain. *Clinical Nursing Research, 13*(3), 199–216.

Kalisvaart, K., de Jonghe, J., Bogaards, M., Vreeswijk, R., Egberts, T., Burger, B., Eikelenboom, P., & van-Gool, W. et al. (2005). Haloperidol prophylaxis for elderly hip-surgery patients at risk for delirium: A randomized placebo-controlled study. *Journal of the American Geriatrics Society, 53*(10), 1658–1666.

Kalisvaart, K., Vreeswijk, R., de Jonghe, J., van der Ploeg, T., van Gool, W., & Eikelenboom, P. (2006). Risk factors and prediction of postoperative delirium in elderly hip-surgery patients: Implementation and validation of a medical risk factor model. *Journal of the American Geriatrics Society, 54*(5), 817–822.

Kehlet, H., Troels, S., Woolf, J., & Woolf, C. (2006). Persistent postsurgical pain: Risk factors and prevention. *Lancet, 367,* 1618–1626.

King, C. (1997). Nonpharmacologic management of chemotherapy-induced nausea and vomiting. *Oncology Nursing Forum, 24*(Suppl.7), 41–47.

Kondo, A., Kanda, K., Isokawa, Y., Nishibayasi, K., Nanpo, S., Kadowaki, R., Anai, K., & Mibu, Y., et al. (2005). The relationship in hip fracture patients of post-operative days to initial rehabilitation activities and their ambulatory ability on postoperative day 20. *Journal of Orthopaedic Nursing, 9*(3), 146–156.

Kuchta, A., & Golembiewski, J. (2004). Medication use in the elderly patient: Focus on the perioperative/perianesthesia setting. *Journal of PeriAnesthesia Nursing, 19*(6), 415–427.

Kwekkeboom, K., & Gretarsdottir, E. (2006). Systematic review of relaxation interventions for pain. *Journal of Nursing Scholarship, 38*(3), 269–277.

Lawrence, V., Silverstein, J., Cornell, J., Pederson, T., Noveck, H., & Carson, J. (2003). Higher Hb level is associated with better early functional recovery after hip repair. *Transfusion, 43*(12), 1717–1722.

Lee, A., & Done, M. (2004). Stimulation of the wrist acupuncture point P6 for preventing postoperative nausea and vomiting. *Cochrane Database of Systematic Reviews, 3* (CD003281).

Leinonen, T., Leino-Kilpi, H., Stahlberg, M., & Lertola, K. (2003). Comparing patient and nurse perceptions of perioperative care quality. *Applied Nursing Research, 16*(1), 29–37.

Leske, J. S. (2003). Comparison of family stresses, strengths, and outcomes after trauma and surgery. *AACN Clinical Issues, 14*(1), 33–41.

Leung, J., Sands, L., Mullen, E., Wang, Y., & Vaurio, L. (2005). Are preoperative depressive symptoms associated with postoperative delirium in geriatric surgical patients? *Journals of Gerontology Series A: Biological Sciences and Medical Sciences, 60A*(12), 1563–1571.

Low, D., Vu, A., Brown, M., Davis, S., Keller, D., Levine, B., & Crandall, C., et al. (2007). Temporal thermometry fails to track body core temperature during heat stress. *Medicine & Science in Sports and Exercise, 39*(7), 1029–1035.

Lupien, A., Schoneboom, B., & Wren, K. (2000). Limitations to self-care in the ambulatory surgical patient. *Journal of PeriAnesthesia Nursing, 15*(2), 102–107.

Lyons, S. (2004). *Fall prevention for older adults.* Iowa City: University of Iowa Gerontological Nursing Interventions Research Center, Research Dissemination Core.

Madsen, D., Tamara, S., Cullen, L., Folkedahl, B., Mueller, T., Richardson, C., & Titler, M., et al. (2005). Listening to bowel sounds: An evidence-based practice project. *American Journal of Nursing, 105*(12), 40–49.

Mamaril, M. (2006). Nursing considerations in the geriatric surgical patient: The perioperative continuum of care. *Nursing Clinics of North America, 41,* 313–328.

Mann, C., Pouzeratte, Y., Boccara, G., Peccoux, C., Vergue, C., Brunat, G., Domergue, J., Millat, B., & Colson, P., et al. (2000). Comparison of intravenous or epidural patient-controlled analgesia in the elderly after major abdominal surgery. *Anesthesiology, 92*(2), 433–441.

Mann, C., Pouzeratte, Y., & Eledjam, J. (2003). Postoperative patient-controlled analgesia in the elderly: Risks and benefits of epidural versus intravenous administration. *Drugs and Aging, 20*(5), 337–345.

Marcantonio, E., Flacker, J., Wright, R., & Resnick, N. (2001). Reducing delirium after hip fracture: A randomized trial. *Journal of the American Geriatrics Society, 49,* 516–522.

Markey, D. W., & Brown, R. J. (2002). An interdisciplinary approach to addressing patient activity and mobility in the medical-surgical patient. *Journal of Nursing Care Quality, 16*(4), 1–12.

McAlister, F., Bertsch, K., Man, J., Bradley, J., & Jacka, M. (2005). Pulmonary complications after noncardiac surgery. *American Journal of Respiratory and Critical Care Medicine, 171*(5), 514–517.

McDonald, D., Thomas, G., Livingston, K., & Severson, J. (2005). Assisting older adults to communicate their postoperative pain. *Clinical Nursing Research, 14*(2), 109–127.

Meade, C., Bursell, A., & Ketelsen, L. (2006). Effects of nursing rounds on patients' call light use, satisfaction, and safety. *American Journal of Nursing, 106*(9), 58–70.

Merli, G. (2000). Prophylaxis for deep venous thrombosis and pulmonary embolism in the surgical patient. *Clinical Cornerstone, 2*(4), 15–25.

Milgrom, L. B., Brooks, J. A., Qi, R., Bunnell, K., Wuestefeld, S., & Beckman, D. (2004). Pain levels experienced with activities after cardiac surgery. *American Journal of Critical Care, 13*(2), 116–125.

Milisen, K., Foreman, M., Abraham, I., deGeest, S., Godderis, J., Vandermeulen, E., Fischler, B., Delooz, H., Spiessens, B., & Broos, P., et al. (2001). A nurse-led interdisciplinary intervention program for delirium in elderly hip-fracture patients. *Journal of the American Geriatrics Society, 49,* 523–532.

Milisen, K., Lemiengre, J., Braes, T., & Foreman, M. (2005). Multicomponent intervention strategies for managing delirium in hospitalized older people: Systematic review. *Journal of Advanced Nursing, 52*(1), 79–90.

Mimnaugh, L., Winegar, M., Mabrey, Y., & Davis, J. (1999). Sensations experienced during removal of tubes in acute postoperative patients. *Applied Nursing Research, 12,* 78–85.

Morrison, R., Magaziner, J., & McLaughlin, M. (2003). The impact of post-operative pain on outcomes following hip fracture. *Pain, 103,* 303–311.

Mulroy, M., Salinas, F., Larkin, K., & Polissar, N. (2002). Ambulatory surgery patients may be discharged before voiding after short-acting spinal and epidural anesthesia. *Anesthesiology, 97*(2), 315–319.

Murphy, M., Hooper, V., Sullivan, E., Clifford, T., & Apfel, C. (2006). Identification of risk factors for postoperative nausea and vomiting in the perianesthesia adult patient. *Journal of PeriAnesthesia Nursing, 21*(6), 377–384.

Neil, J. (2007). Perioperative care of the immunocompromised patient. *AORN Journal, 85*(3), 544–565.

Ng, W., & Neill, J. (2006). Evidence for early oral feeding of patients after elective open colorectal surgery: A literature review. *Journal of Clinical Nursing, 15*(5), 696–709.

Nilsson, U., Unosson, M., & Kihlgren, M. (2006). Experience of postoperative recovery before discharge: Patients' views. *Journal of Advanced Perioperative Care, 2,* 97–106.

Nisanevich, V., Felsenstein, I., Almogy, G., Weissman, C., Einav, S., & Matot, I. (2005). Effect of intraoperative fluid management on outcome after intraabdominal surgery. *Anesthesiology, 103*(1), 25–32.

Nishimori, M., Ballantyne, J., & Low, J. (2006). Epidural pain relief versus systemic opioid-based pain relief for abdominal aortic surgery. *Cochrane Library, (4)* (CD005059).

Odom-Forren, J., Fetzer, S., & Moser, D. (2006). Evidence-based interventions for post discharge nausea and vomiting: A review of the literature. *Journal of PeriAnesthesia Nursing, 21*(6), 411–430.

Oermann, M. H., Harris, C. H., & Dammeyer, J. A. (2001). Teaching by the nurse: How important is it to patients? *Applied Nursing Research, 14*(1), 11–17.

Oldmeadow, L., McBurney, H., Robertson, V., Kimmel, L., & Elliott, B. (2004). Targeted postoperative care improves discharge outcome after hip or knee arthroplasty. *Archives of Physical Medicine and Rehabilitation, 85,* 1424–1427.

Olsson, U., Bergbom, I., & Bosaeus, I. (2002). Patients' experiences of the recovery period 3 months after gastrointestinal cancer surgery. *European Journal of Cancer Care, 11,* 51–60.

Orfanos, P., Ellis, E., & Johnston, C. (1999). Effects of deep breathing exercises and ambulation on pattern of ventilation in post-operative patients. *Australian Journal of Physiotherapy, 45*(3), 173–182.

Overend, T., Anderson, C., Lucy, S. D., Bhatia, C., Jonsson, B., & Timmermans, C. (2001). The effect of incentive spirometry on postoperative pulmonary complications. *Chest, 120*(3), 971–978.

Pandey, C., Priye, S., Ambesh, S., Singh, S., Singh, U., & Singh, P. (2006). Prophylactic gabapentin for prevention of postoperative nausea and vomiting in patients undergoing laparoscopic cholecystectomy: A randomized, double-blind, placebo-controlled study. *Journal of Postgraduate Medicine, 52,* 95–99.

Pasero, C. (2003a). Epidural analgesia for postoperative pain, Part 1. *American Journal of Nursing, 103*(10), 62–64.

Pasero, C. (2003b). Epidural analgesia for postoperative pain, Part 2. *American Journal of Nursing, 103*(11), 43–45.

Pasero, C. (2005). Improving postoperative outcomes with epidural analgesia. *Journal of PeriAnesthesia Nursing, 20*(1), 51–55.

Pasero, C., & Belden, J. (2006). Evidence-based perianesthesia care: Accelerated postoperative recovery programs. *Journal of PeriAnesthesia Nursing, 21*(3), 168–176.

Pasero, C., & McCaffery, M. (2005). No self-report means no pain-intensity rating: Assessing pain in patients who cannot provide a report. *American Journal of Nursing, 105*(10), 50–53.

Pasero, C., & McCaffery, M. (2007). Orthopaedic postoperative pain management. *Journal of PeriAnesthesia Nursing, 22*(3), 160–174.

Person, B., & Wexner, S. (2006). The management of postoperative ileus. *Current Problems in Surgery, 43*(1), 12–65.

Phillips, K., & Gill, L. (1994). The use of simple acupressure bands reduces postoperative nausea. *Complementary Therapies in Medicine, 2,* 158–160.

Pietrocola, P., Riley, R., Beanland, C., Kelly, C., & Radnell, J. (2004). A randomized controlled trial to measure the effectiveness of a sacral wedge in preventing postoperative back pain following trans-urethral resection of the prostate in lithotomy position. *Journal of Clinical Nursing, 13*(8), 977–985.

Pittler, M., & Eberhart, L. (2003). No effect of *Zingiber officinale* (ginger) on postoperative nausea and vomiting. *Focus on Alternative and Complementary Therapies, 8*(4), 416–418.

Prowse, M., & Lyne, P. (2000). Clinical effectiveness in the post-anaesthesia care unit: How nursing knowledge contributes to achieving indented patient outcomes. *Journal of Advanced Nursing, 31*(5), 1115–1124.

Puntillo, K. (2003). Pain assessment and management in the critically ill: Wizardry or science? *American Journal of Critical Care, 12*(4), 310–316.

Puntillo, K., Miaskowski, C., Kehrle, K., Stannard, D., Gleeson, S., & Nye, P. (1997). The relationship between behavioral and physiological indicators of pain, critical care patients' self reports of pain and opioid administration. *Critical Care Medicine, 5,* 1159–1166.

Puntillo, K., & Weiss, S. J. (2003). Pain: Its mediators and associated morbidity in critically ill cardiovascular surgical patients. *Nursing Research, 43,* 31–36.

Puntillo, K., Wild, L., Morris, A., Stanik-Hutt, J., Thompson, C., & White, C. (2002). Practices and predictors of analgesic interventions for adults undergoing painful procedures. *American Journal of Critical Care, 11*(5), 415–429.

Qaseem, A., Snow, V., Fitterman, N., Hornbake, R., Lawrence, V., Smetana, G., Weiss, K., Owens, D., Aronson, M., Barry, P., Casey, D., Cross, J., Fitterman, N., & Sherif, K., et al. (2006). Risk assessment for and strategies to reduce perioperative pulmonary complications for patients undergoing noncardiothoracic surgery: A guideline from the American College of Physicians. *Annals of Internal Medicine, 144*(8), 575–580.

Redeker, N. (2000). Sleep in acute care settings: An integrative review. *Journal of Nursing Scholarship, 32*(1), 31–38.

Reilly, P., Iezzoni, L., Phillips, R., Davis, R., Tuchin, L., & Calkins, D. (1996). Discharge planning: Comparison of patients' and nurses' perceptions of patients following hospital discharge. *Journal of Nursing Scholarship, 28*(2), 143–147.

Resnick, B. (2003). Preventing falls in acute care. In M. Mezey, T. Fulmer, & A. Zwicker (Eds.), *Geriatric nursing protocols for best practice* (pp. 141–164). New York: Springer.

Richman, J., Liu, S., Courpas, G., et al. (2006). Does continuous peripheral nerve block provide superior pain control to opioids? A meta-analysis. *Anesthesia and Analgesia, 102,* 248–257.

Rimmele, T., Combourieu, E., Wey, P., Boselli, E., Allaouchiche, B., Chassard, D., & Escarment, J., et al. (2005). Immediate postoperative refeeding in orthopedic surgery is safe. *Journal of Anesthesia, 19*(4), 323–325.

Ross, J. (2007). Health literacy and its influence on patient safety. *Journal of PeriAnesthesia Nursing, 22*(3), 220–223.

Saclarides, T. (2006). Current choices—good or bad—for the proactive management of postoperative ileus: A surgeon's view. *Journal of PeriAnesthesia Nursing, 21*(2, Suppl. 1), S7–S15.

Sauaia, A., Min, S., Leber, C., Erbacher, K., Abrams, F., & Fink, R. (2005). Postoperative pain management in elderly patients: Correlation between adherence to treatment guidelines and patient satisfaction. *Journal of the American Geriatrics Society, 53*(2), 272–282.

Schultz, A. A., Andrews, A. L., Goran, S. F., Mathew, T., & Sturdevant, N. (2003). Comparison of acupressure bands and droperidol for reducing post-operative nausea and vomiting in gynecologic surgery patients. *Applied Nursing Research, 16*(4), 256–265.

Schumann, R., Shikora, S., Weiss, J. M., Wurm, H., Strassels, S., & Carr, D. B. (2003). A comparison of multimodal perioperative analgesia to epidural pain management after gastric bypass surgery. *Anesthesia & Analgesia, 96*(2), 469–474.

Schweon, S. (2006). Stamping out surgical site infection. *RN, 69*(8), 37–40.

Scott, E., & Buckland, R. (2006). A systematic review of intraoperative warming to prevent postoperative complications. *AORN Journal, 83*(5), 1090–1112.

Seltzer, J., Horsman, A., & Korniewicz, D. (2002). Awareness of surgical site infections for advanced practice nurses. *AACN Clinical Issues, 13*(3), 398–409.

Shea, R., Brooks, J. A., Dayhoff, N., & Keck, J. (2002). Pain intensity and postoperative pulmonary complications among the elderly after abdominal surgery. *Heart & Lung, 31*(6), 440–449.

Sjostrom, B., Dahlgren, L., & Haljamae, H. (2000). Strategies used in post-operative pain assessment and their clinical accuracy. *Journal of Clinical Nursing, 9,* 111–118.

Smith, M., & Ellis, E. (2000). Is retained mucus a risk factor for the development of postoperative atelectasis and pneumonia? Implications for the physiotherapist. *Physiotherapy Theory and Practice, 16*(2), 69–80.

Smith, M., Kemp, J., Hemphill, L., & Vojir, C. (2002). Outcomes of therapeutic massage for hospitalized cancer patients. *Journal of Nursing Scholarship, 34*(3), 257–262.

Smith, T., White, M., O'Connor, C., Salinas, T., Lucas, J., Bowar-Ferres, S., & Fitzpatrick, J., et al. (2002). Nursing care quality initiative (NCQI) for hospitalized elders and their families: A demonstration and quality improvement model of nursing care. *Applied Nursing Research, 15*(1), 48–51.

Smykowski, L., & Rodriguez, W. (2003). The post anesthesia care unit experience: A family centered approach. *Journal of Nursing Care Quality, 18*(1), 5–15.

Squadrone, V., Coha, M., Cerutti, E., Schellino, M., Biolino, P., Occella, P., Belloni, G., Vilianis, G., Fiore, G., Cavallo, R., & Ranieri, V., et al. (2005). Caring for the critically ill patient. Continuous positive airway pressure for treatment of postoperative hypoxemia: A randomized controlled trial. *Journal of the American Medical Association, 293*(5), 589–595.

Stanik-Hutt, J., Soeken, K., Belcher, A., Fontaine, D., & Gift, A. (2001). Pain experiences of traumatically injured individuals in a critical care setting. *American Journal of Critical Care, 10,* 252–259.

St. Clair, K., & Larrabee, J. (2002). Clean versus sterile gloves: Which to use for postoperative dressing changes? *Outcomes Management, 6*(1), 17–21.

Suetta, C., Magnusson, S., Rosted, A., Aagaard, P., Jakobsen, A., Larsen, L., Duus, B., & Kjaer, M., et al. (2004). Resistance training in the early postoperative phase reduces hospitalization and leads to muscle hypertrophy in elderly hip surgery patients: A controlled, randomized study. *Journal of the American Geriatrics Society, 52*(12), 2016–2022.

Susleck, D., Willocks, A., Secrest, J., Norwood, B., Holweger, J., Davis, M., Myhan, G., & Trimpey, M. et al. (2007). The perianesthesia experience from the patient's perspective. *Journal of PeriAnesthesia Nursing, 22*(1), 10–20.

Swan, B. (1998). Research utilization: Postoperative nursing care contributions to symptom distress and functional status after ambulatory surgery. *Medsurg Nursing, 7,* 148–151, 154–158.

Tarrac, S. (2006). A description of intraoperative and postanesthesia complication rates. *Journal of PeriAnesthesia Nursing, 21*(2), 88–96.

Titler, M., Herr, K., Schilling, M., Marsh, J. L., Xie, X.-J., Ardery, G., Clarke, W., & Everett, L., et al. (2003). Acute pain treatment for older adults hospitalized with hip fracture: Current nursing practices and perceived barriers. *Applied Nursing Research, 16*(4), 211–227.

VanKooten, M. (1999). Non-pharmacologic pain management for postoperative coronary artery bypass graft surgery patients. *Journal of Nursing Scholarship, 31*(2), 157.

Vermeulen, H., Storm-Versloot, M., Goossens, A., Speelman, P., & Legemate, D. (2005). Diagnostic accuracy of routine postoperative body temperature measurements. *Clinical Infectious Disease, 40,* 1404–1414.

Wadlund, D. (2006). Prevention, recognition, and management of nursing complications in the intraoperative and postoperative surgical patients. *Nursing Clinics of North America, 41,* 151–171.

Wagner, D. (2006). Unplanned perioperative hypothermia. *AORN Journal, 83*(2), 470–476.

Wallenborn, J., Gelbrich, G., Bulst, D., Behrends, K., Wallenborn, H., Rohrbach, A., Krause, U., Kuhnast, T., Wiegel, M., & Olthoff, D., et al. (2006). Prevention of postoperative nausea and vomiting by metoclopramide combined with dexamethasone: Randomized double blind multicentre trial. *British Medical Journal, 333,* 324–328.

Wardell, D., & Weymouth, K. (2004). Review of studies of healing touch. *Journal of Nursing Scholarship, 36*(2), 147–160.

Werner, J., Wendler, M., McCormick, J., Paulus-Smith, S., Jackson, C., & Nie, J. (2002). Human response outcomes influenced by nurse caring. *International Journal for Human Caring, 6*(3), 15–23.

Wheelan, S., Burchill, C., & Tilin, F. (2003). The link between teamwork and patients' outcomes in intensive care units. *American Journal of Critical Care, 12*(6), 527–534.

White, J. (1999). Effects of relaxing music on cardiac autonomic balance and anxiety after acute myocardial infarction. *American Journal of Critical Care, 8,* 220–230.

Whitney, J. A., & Parkman, S. (2002). Preoperative physical activity, anesthesia, and analgesia: Effects on early postoperative walking after total hip replacement. *Applied Nursing Research, 15*(1), 19–27.

Williams, A., & Irurita, V. (2005). Enhancing the therapeutic potential of hospital environments by increasing the personal control and emotional comfort of hospitalized patients. *Applied Nursing Research, 18*(1), 22–28.

Wong, J., Wong, S., & Brooks, E. (2002). A study of hospitalized recovery pattern of acutely confused older patients after hip surgery. *Journal of Orthopaedic Nursing, 6*(2), 68–78.

Zalon, M. (2004). Correlates of recovery among older adults after major abdominal surgery. *Nursing Research, 53*(2), 99–106.

Zeitz, K., & McCutcheon, H. (2006). Observations and vital signs: Ritual or vital for the monitoring of postoperative patients? *Applied Nursing Research, 19*(4), 204–211.

Zutshi, M., Delaney, C., Senagore, A., & Fazio, V. (2004). Shorter hospital stay associated with fastrack postoperative care pathways and laparoscopic intestinal resection are not associated with increased physical activity. *Colorectal Disease, 6,* 477–480.

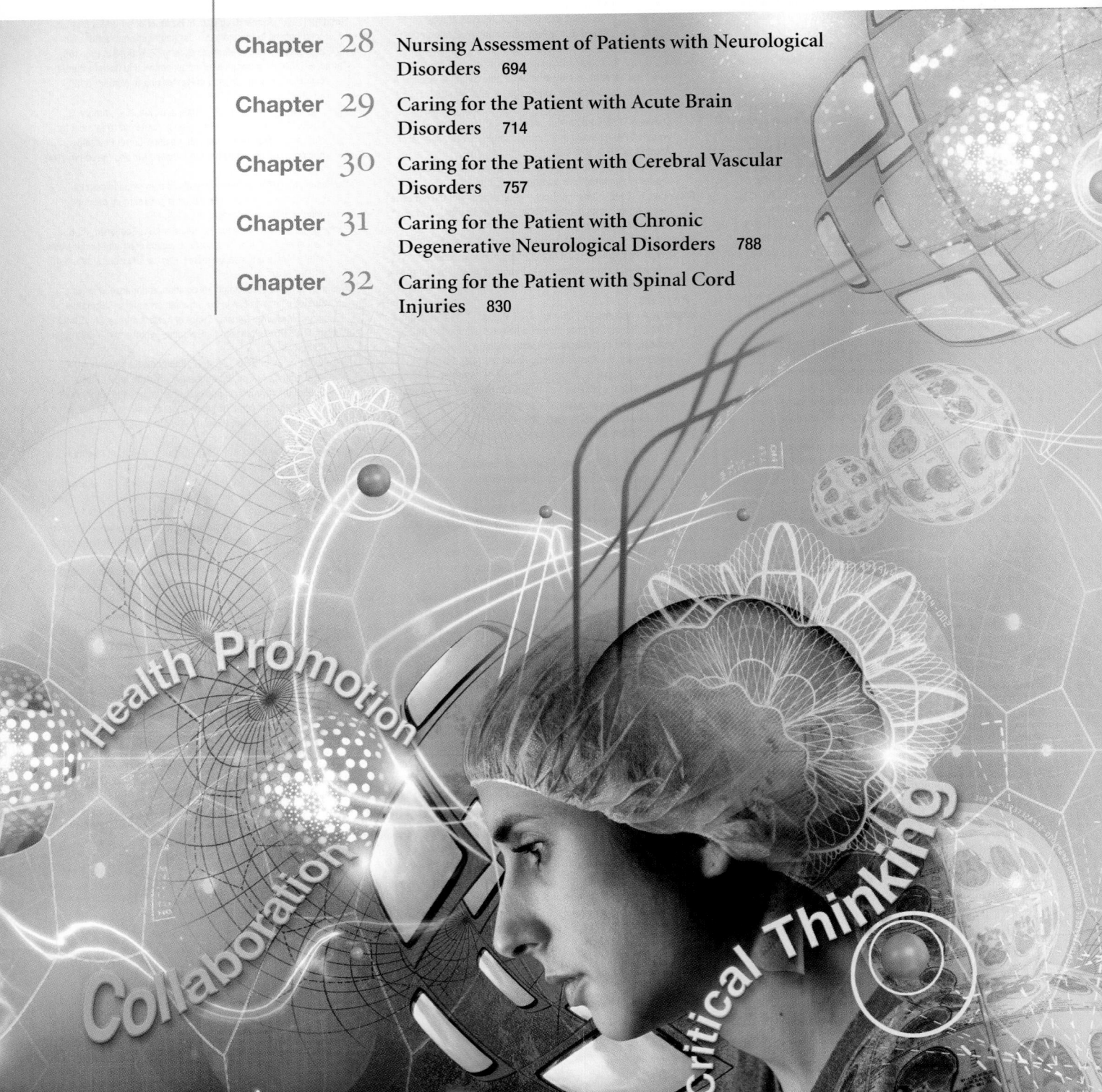

Nursing Management of Patients with Neurological Disorders

Health Promotion

Collaboration

Critical Thinking

MARY KAY BADER, MSN, CCNS, CNRN, CCRN, FAHA, Neurosurgical Clinical Nurse Specialist, Mission Hospital, I have worked as the neuroscience/critical care clinical nurse specialist (CNS) for 10 years. As the CNS, my position incorporates the multiple roles of clinical expert, educator, leader, change agent, researcher, mentor, and team builder. To be a CNS, I must be master's prepared and clinically competent in the specialty area in which I work.

On a typical day, I conduct clinical rounds in the 12 bed Surgical-Trauma ICU. The purpose of the morning rounds is to assess each patient's clinical status, discuss any issues with the patient's nurse, and talk with family members present about the previous 24 hours. The team in the ICU uses a series of algorithms/clinical guidelines to direct the care of the severe traumatic brain injury (TBI). As the primary developer of these hospital-based guidelines, my role involves educating and collaborating with the nurses, respiratory therapists, and pharmacists on the application of the complex interventions.

I also work with a multidisciplinary vascular team made up of vascular surgeons, interventional radiologists, cardiologists, interventional technologists, and nurses. My role as CNS involves assisting with the development of the IRB research proposal, conducting preprocedure neurological examinations, assisting with the pre- and postprocedure patient/family education, monitoring the neurological status during the procedure, briefing the ICU nursing team on the patient status, following the patient in the hospital, collecting data for the study, and tracking patient visits postprocedure for the year following carotid stent placement.

I have the privilege of following the neurosurgical patients throughout their hospitalization. This helps me build a strong rapport with the patient and family. As I check on patients, I collaborate with the floor nurse and discuss each patient's progress. We advance patients activities and evaluate their responses to therapies.

In the role of CNS, I respond to a "Code Trauma" on all neurological cases, and whenever the team needs an extra hand. I help the trauma nurse with patient care, accompany them to the CT scanner, and await the results. Upon completion of the CT scan I collaborate with the team to develop a plan of care.

The CNS role participates in hospital committees. I attend the Collaborative Practice Council (CPC) meeting. I have been working closely with the CPC as a consultant on the revision of the clinical practice manuals containing procedures, standards of care, patient education plans, and protocols.

In the afternoon I round with the neurosurgeons. I value this time each day as it is an opportunity to engage the team in conversation about the patients. I also participate in the afternoon rehabilitation rounds which is a multidisciplinary team meeting held in the ICU each Wednesday involving nursing members from the various units, therapists, psychiatrist, social worker, and discharge planner. Reviewing the in-house trauma and neurosurgical patients allows the team to anticipate progression of the patients and coordinate timing of referrals.

As an advanced practice nurse, I have the privilege of working with great physicians, nurses, therapists, and other health care providers. I am part of a team in which the whole is greater than the sum of its parts. I consider it an honor to be part of this collaborative team who welcomes the knowledge and skills I can share with them. I would never be able to impact patient care outcomes alone. It takes a synergistic team to save a life when the odds are against them, heal the sick, comfort the dying, and empower families to make tough end-of-life decisions. I am honored and humbled to be part of the nursing profession.

> "As the primary developer of these hospital-based guidelines, my role involves educating and collaborating with the nurses, respiratory therapists, and pharmacists on the application of the complex interventions."

28 Nursing Assessment of Patients with Neurological Disorders

Michele Grigaitis

Outcome-Based Learning Objectives

After studying this chapter, the learner will be able to:

1. Correlate the anatomic and physiological aspects of the nervous system with the neurological examination.
2. Explain the importance of history taking in the neurological assessment.
3. Categorize the cranial nerves with common functional deficits seen in neurological disease.
4. Describe the components of the mental status exam and methods to complete the assessment.
5. Explain the rationale for and methods of measuring and documenting muscle stretch reflexes.
6. Explain the methods of assessing the presence of pathologic reflexes and the method of documentation.
7. Explain the normal age-related differences in the neurological examination of the elderly patient.

IN THE CARE OF THE PERSON with a known or suspected neurological disorder, the initial neurological assessment becomes the baseline against which all further examination is compared. The need for a thorough and accurate assessment cannot be overemphasized. Patient management is guided by the use of evidence-based medicine, standardized clinical pathways, policies and procedures, or predetermined protocols. The initiation of the management strategy is based on the initial assessment completed by the nurse.

The nursing process is the framework within which the nurse is able to generate a database from the patient's history; construct a list of problems using nursing diagnoses with expected outcomes; design a plan of care; initiate interventions; and evaluate desired patient outcomes. This chapter presents guidelines for the assessment of the adult patient in a variety of clinical settings. The American Nurses Association *Scope and Standards of Neuroscience Nursing Practice* (2002) were used as a framework in determining neurological assessment guidelines.

■ Anatomy and Physiology of the Nervous System

It is necessary for the nurse to correlate knowledge of normal neuroanatomy and physiology with clinical findings to identify clinically significant abnormalities of the nervous system. The

nervous system is, to many, the most complex of the body systems. Separated into three areas, the nervous system consists of the central nervous system (CNS), the peripheral nervous system (PNS), and the autonomic nervous system (ANS). Although complex, a basic understanding of the structure and function of the nervous system is critical to the nurse in order to competently assess a patient.

The basic unit of the nervous system is the **neuron.** The primary function of the neuron is to receive information and subsequently transmit this information to other neurons. This information transmission takes place in the **synapse**, the channel between neurons, as shown in Figure 28–1 ■. The size and shape of neurons are different based on the location in the nervous system, but conceptually they are the same. Each neuron is a single cell body. From this body, several branches, or dendrites, extend. These branches communicate through the synapse to other dendrites.

A nerve fiber originating in the body is the axon. The axon can divide into several branches, through which impulses can be distributed to a number of destinations simultaneously. Information transmitted neuronally is dependent on cellular changes in electrical activity. When a neuron is stimulated, the electrical stimulus proceeds down the axon, stimulating vesicles containing chemicals called neurotransmitters. Neurotransmitters act in the synapse, causing the stimulation of the next neuron.

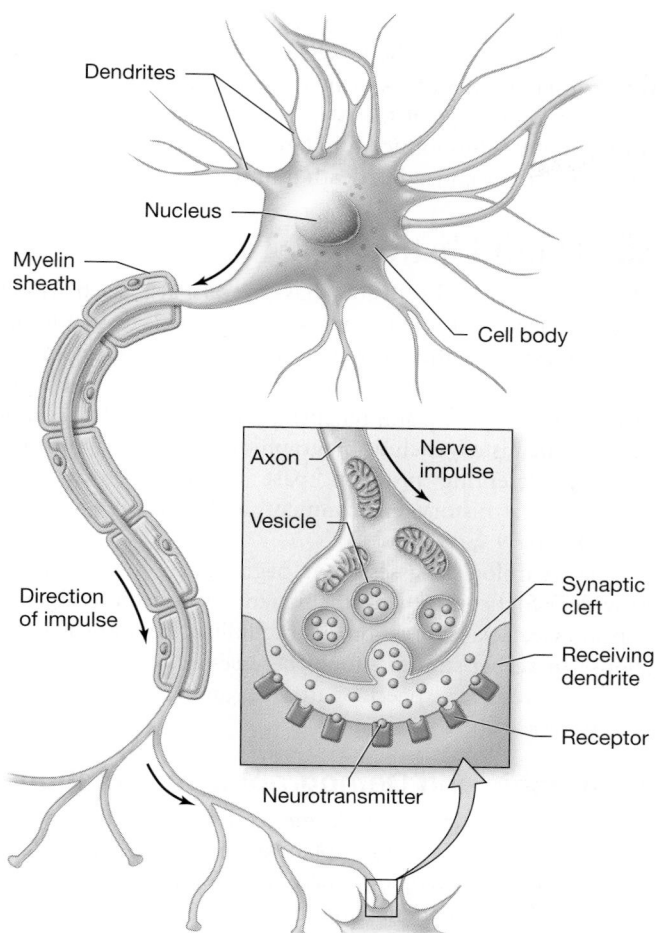

FIGURE 28–1 ■ Two neurons with a synapse between.

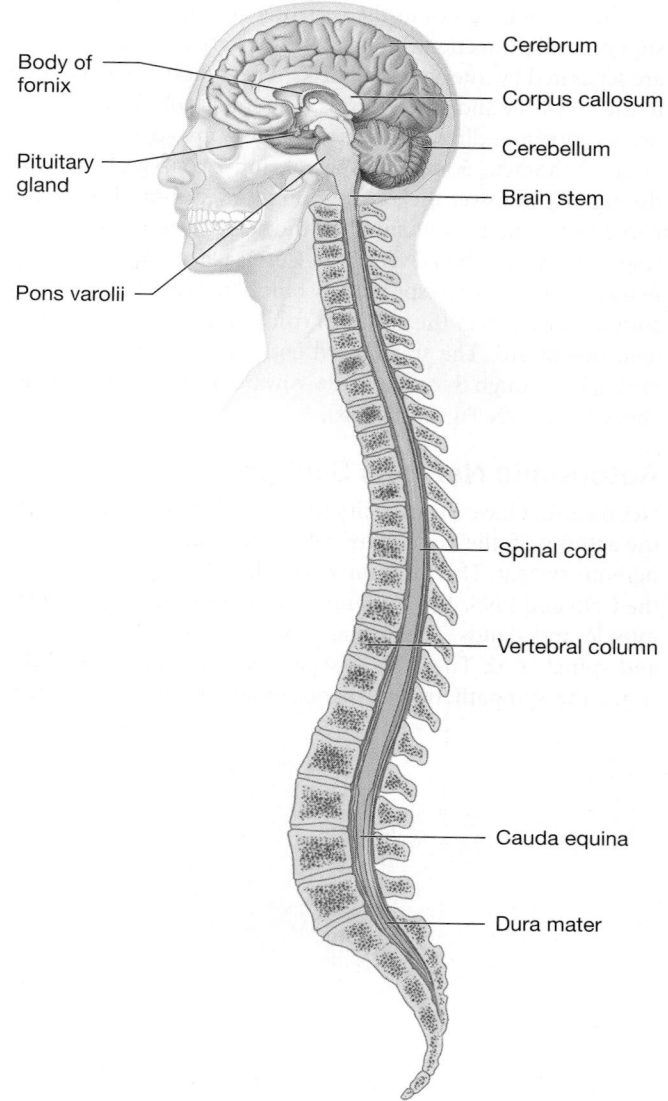

FIGURE 28–2 ■ Brain and spinal cord.

Neuroglia comprise the other major cellular component of the nervous system. Unlike neurons, neuroglia do not directly transmit information. There are three main types of neuroglia: oligodendrocytes, astrocytes, and microglia. Oligodendrocytes form the myelin sheath that covers many neuronal axons. Astrocytes are a key component of the blood–brain barrier, and microglia have a role in removing cellular debris in nervous system damage. Knowledge of the cellular components of the nervous system assists the nurse in understanding the etiology of disease states, such as multiple sclerosis or a primary neoplastic condition. Neurological disorders are discussed in Chapters 29 through 32 👁.

Central Nervous System

The central nervous system consists of the brain and spinal cord, as shown in Figure 28–2 ■. It contains the majority of axons and synapses. The CNS is consistent in its apportionment of neurons. Areas with a high density of cell bodies are called gray matter; those primarily containing axons are referred to as white matter. Axons are generally myelinated, which results in a pale color, hence the term *white matter*.

In general, CNS pathways conveying sensory information to the cerebral hemisphere cross over, or decussate, from one side of the CNS to the other. This holds true of descending pathways

also. Therefore, each cerebral hemisphere generally perceives sensation from and controls the movement of the contralateral side of the body.

Three protective membranes called the meninges cover the brain and spinal cord. Specifically these membranes are the dura mater, arachnoid mater, and the pia mater. The space between the arachnoid and pia is known as the subarachnoid space. This is the space through which cerebrospinal fluid (CSF) flows. Blood is supplied to the brain through the internal carotid and vertebral arteries.

Peripheral Nervous System

The peripheral nervous system is the link between the CNS and structures of the body from which it receives information and to which it sends information. The PNS consists of nerves joined to the brain and spinal cord, for example, the cranial nerves and spinal nerves. The spinal nerves are shown in Figure 28–3 ■ (p. 696). The spinal nerves branch and combine in areas called plexuses and in groups of cell bodies in structures called ganglia.

The spinal cord lies in the vertebral column, which provides support and protection (Figure 28–3 ■). Vertebrae are bones that are separated by intervertebral disks. These disks act as a cushion to the vertebrae and absorb stress. The spinal cord has 31 pairs of nerves corresponding to the vertebrae they are adjacent to: 8 cervical, 12 thoracic, 5 lumbar, 5 sacral, and 1 coccygeal. Nerves C_1 through C_7 exit over their corresponding vertebrae, but thoracic nerve 1 (T_1) and the remainder of the nerves exit below their correspondingly numbered vertebrae. Cervical nerve 8 (C_8) is unique in that there is no correspondingly numbered vertebra. The spinal cord is shorter than the vertebral column so the spinal roots extend downward. The spinal cord ends at vertebral level L_2, but nerves L_2 through S_5 continue downward as the *cauda equina* or "horse's tail" (see Figure 28–3 ■).

Autonomic Nervous System

Neurons that have the capacity to detect changes in, and control the activity of, the viscera are collectively called the autonomic nervous system. The components of the ANS are found in both the CNS and PNS. The ANS innervates smooth muscle, cardiac muscle, and glands. The primary control of the ANS is the brain and spinal cord. The ANS is separated into two distinct divisions, the sympathetic and parasympathetic nervous systems.

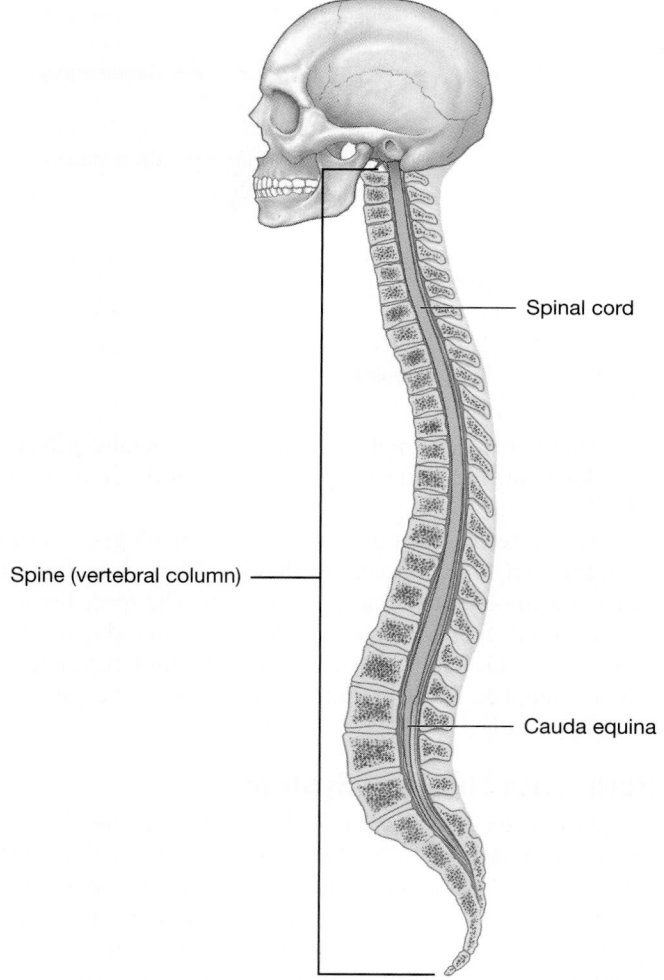

Spinal cord

Spine (vertebral column)

Cauda equina

FIGURE 28–3 ■ Spinal nerves with corresponding vertebrae, to include the cauda equina.

The sympathetic nervous system is the system used to mediate stress. The parasympathetic system, conversely, is associated with conservation and restoring energy. The nurse must have a thorough knowledge of the ANS when dealing with the spinal cord patient. Autonomic dysreflexia (AD) is a hypertensive emergency that can lead to death if untreated.

■ Health History

The traditional health history has several parts, each with its specific purpose. In the patient with neurological symptoms it has been said that the most critical aspect of the assessment is the history (Fuller, 2004). Special care, then, must be taken to ensure the history is comprehensive and accurate. The components of the history include biographic and demographic information, presenting problem, past medical history, family history, social history, environment, and cultural assessment. (See Chapter 9 ☞ .)

The neurological assessment begins with the health care provider's first contact with the patient. Observation of general appearance, facial expression, distractibility, eye contact, and response to verbal stimuli should be assessed. Cognition, emotional expression, speech patterns, and ability to follow directions are noted.

Biographic and Demographic Information

Biographic and demographic data refer to identifying facts. These include age, sex, race, place of birth, current residence, marital status, and religion. These data points serve not only to establish who the patient is but also to give the nurse tentative suggestions as to what areas to further explore. Many neurological conditions occur in specific populations, for example, Alzheimer's disease in the elderly or multiple sclerosis in the young adult. Ethnicity plays a role in cerebral vascular accidents, as epidemiological studies indicate minority populations are at higher risk (Centers for Disease Control and Prevention [CDC], 2007). Current residence is an important piece of information when looking at region-specific diseases such as West Nile virus or cystosarcosis (CDC, 2007).

Presenting Problem

The presenting problem is the reason the individual is seeking care. This reason is best documented in the patient's own words, in quotations. Often, patients with neurological problems have a spouse, family member, or friend present at the time of initial assessment. This should be allowed if possible, because this may provide both support and reassurance to the patient as well as offer validation of the history. In the acute setting, the patient may not be capable of conveying information if the patient is elderly or cognitively impaired or has experienced a traumatic injury; validation of information may be necessary.

History of Presenting Problem

The presenting problem is followed by the history of the presenting problem. The nurse should begin with the initial presentation of the symptom and proceed to the present. If the patient has a single complaint, it is necessary to ascertain when the symptom began and how it evolved over time. If the patient has multiple complaints, a common occurrence in the neurological population, the nurse should explore each symptom individually. One should obtain as full a description as possible. Use of the mnemonic OLD CARTS can be helpful in ensuring all necessary information is obtained. The system of OLD CARTS is designed to assist the health care provider in remembering an assessment order by the use of sequential initials and what they stand for. This tool is shown in Chart 28–1.

When gathering historical information, it is necessary to be very specific. For example, the term *dizziness* can be used to describe vertigo (a sensation of the environment spinning around the patient or spinning of the patient in an immobile environment), light-headedness (a feeling of faintness), momentary visual loss, or overall weakness. The term *weakness* can be used to describe loss of muscle strength, but also imbalance, lack of coordination, or a sensory disturbance. Using the symptom of *headaches* as an example, the questions the nurse would ask include these:

- When did it start?
- What is the location of your headache (frontal, temporal, occipital, global)?
- How long does your headache last?
- How often do the headaches occur (if monthly, related to menses? daily?)? Is the pain throbbing (as with vascular or migraine headaches) or dull (as with chronic daily headaches or rebound headaches)?
- Is a visual disturbance associated with the headache?
- Do the symptoms change with position, for example, are they worse when sitting or standing, and improve with lying flat? (This can indicate increased intracranial pressure caused by, e.g., a tumor, or low-pressure headaches, commonly seen with cerebral spinal fluid leakage.)
- What makes the headache better?
- Has the patient taken any medication, herbal remedy, or supplement to help the headache in the past?
- Rate the pain on a scale of 1 to 10.

 **CRITICAL ALERT** *When evaluating a patient presenting with headache in the ambulatory setting, difficulty with vision, large palpable temporal arteries, and temporal tenderness are the hallmark of temporal arteritis. This is a neurological emergency and will result in blindness if not treated.*

 CRITICAL ALERT *A patient with the "worst headache of my life" with or without photophobia and meningeal signs could have a subarachnoid hemorrhage. This is a neurological emergency and can result in death if not treated immediately.*

Past Medical History

The past medical history includes major illnesses, which encompass all hospitalizations, surgeries, ambulatory procedures, and illnesses, both acute and chronic. In addition, childhood diseases, immunizations, medications, and allergies are explored.

Childhood Diseases and Immunizations

Many diseases associated with neurological sequelae commonly occur in childhood. Rubella, rubeola, cytomegalovirus, herpes, influenza, and meningitis are examples. It is important to determine vaccination status. Has the patient received adequate vaccination? Vaccines have proven effective against development of certain types of bacterial meningitis. For patients older than 65 years of age, the pneumococcal vaccine should be considered due to the risk of pneumococcal meningitis. Is the patient an immigrant? Many diseases eradicated in the United States occur in other countries. Poliomyelitis, for example, occurs in Africa and South Asia (World Health Organization, 2007).

Major Illness

Several medical conditions are associated with neurological dysfunction. Diabetes mellitus can result in peripheral neuropathy (see Chapter 53 🔗). Hypertension is a risk factor for cerebrovascular disease (see Chapter 30 🔗). Infections and neoplastic conditions can result in a myriad of neurological symptoms. Metabolic conditions, such as vitamin deficiency or electrolyte imbalance, can cause neurological symptoms and also exacerbate existing disorders.

A history of trauma is important, as are seizures, stroke, and cranial nerve problems. Important also is the history of surgical procedures. Cognitive impairment has been noted in up to three-quarters of all cardiac surgery patients (Newman, 2007).

Medications

The medication history should include all medications the patient currently is taking or historically has taken. Herbal, over-the-counter, home remedies, and supplements need to be listed as well as prescribed medications. The nurse will need to specifically ask

---

CHART 28–1 **OLD CARTS Mnemonic for Assessment of Presenting Problem**

Onset of symptom:	When did the symptoms begin?
Location of symptom:	Note the location of the manifestation.
Duration of symptom:	How long has the manifestation been affecting you?
Characteristics:	Describe the characteristics of the manifestation in common language.
Aggravating/**A**ssociated factors:	What factors make the situation worse? What symptoms occur that are associated with the main symptom or manifestation?
Relieving factors:	What factors alleviate the symptoms or make you feel better?
Temporal factors:	Is the onset of the manifestation gradual or sudden? When does it occur? How frequently does it occur? Does it occur in specific settings or environments, e.g., usually after breakfast?
Severity of symptoms:	How severe is the problem? Rate on a scale of 1 to 10 with 10 being the most severe.

if any of these preparations are taken, because many people do not associate them with the term *medication*. This is especially important in the minority and elderly populations. Many ethnic groups commonly use herbs, poultices, tisanes, and teas for medicinal use, both orally and as inhalants. The elderly frequently take "memory-enhancing" supplements. This can be critical information because many of these compounds contain antioxidants, some of which can interfere with prescriptive drugs such as warfarin. When obtaining the medication history, the dose, route, reason for taking, length of time taken, and last dose taken are necessary pieces of information.

Allergies

Many patients believe they have "allergies" to medication, when in fact they are experiencing an adverse drug reaction. Explore the response the patient experienced and list the medication involved. The health care provider should specifically ask about iodine allergies, because many neurological conditions are best ruled in or out with a contrasted imaging study, which uses iodine. All patients should be questioned regarding an allergy to latex.

Family History

A thorough family history includes age, if living, and cause of death if deceased, of all immediate biological family members: parents, grandparents, siblings, and children. Many neurological disorders are inherited. In others, a positive family history represents a risk factor. Examples of inherited disorders are those with autosomal dominant inheritance, such as Huntington disease, or autosomal recessive inheritance, such as Friedreich's ataxia (Victor & Ropper, 2001). An example of a neurological disorder that includes a positive family history as a risk factor is Alzheimer's disease of the late-onset sporadic type (Reyes, Nowak, & Rice, 2006). CADASIL (cerebral autosomal dominant arteriopathy with subcortical infarcts and leukoencephalopathy) is the most common form of hereditary stroke disorder (Joute, Corpechot, & Ducros, 1996). Oftentimes these patients have family members with diagnoses of multiple sclerosis, strokes, and/or dementia. A thorough family history can lead the treating health care provider to these disorders.

Social History

It is important that the social history be obtained in a nonjudgmental fashion. The social history begins with determining the highest level of education the patient has attained, as well as performance in school. The history of current and past employment indicates possible occupational toxin exposure. Marital status and sexual orientation are necessary data points. Drug and alcohol use is critical in the assessment of patients with cognitive impairments. For example, it is necessary to know the answers to these questions: What is the drug/drink of choice? When was it last used? How often is it used? This information will be essential in mediating withdrawal symptoms in the acutely ill hospitalized patient. Tobacco use should be explored as well.

Given the disabling consequences of trauma to the CNS with head and spinal cord injury, the nurse should establish if high-risk factors are present such as drinking and driving, or using recreational drugs and driving. It also is necessary to determine if the patient undertakes high-risk endeavors without appropriate safety equipment, such as not wearing a helmet when riding a motorcycle.

Environment

The home and workplace environment should be assessed for possible exposure to industrial toxins (lead, arsenic, asbestos, benzene, polyvinylchloride, and other carcinogens), as well as the use of any protective safety devices. Potential for falls should be evaluated. Travel or exposure to contagious diseases also should be explored.

Cultural Considerations

Cultural components are present in all patients. Differences, both subtle and obvious, exist. The nurse must take care not to assume that any patient has a prescribed cultural behavior pattern, because this would constitute stereotyping. It is important to explore communication styles, nutrition, family relationships, health beliefs, and religion. This exploration can occur concurrently with the history portion of the assessment. The nurse should ascertain the patient's beliefs regarding the presenting problem. What does the patient believe the cause of the problem is? Being culturally aware is important to the nursing process, as discussed in the Cultural Considerations box.

■ Physical Examination

The physical examination of the patient with neurological symptoms is conceptually the same as any other system physical examination. The findings of the physical exam are interpreted with the focus on the nervous system.

General Appearance

The physical examination begins when the nurse first encounters the patient. What is the patient's expression? Are there signs of distress, anger, depression, or apathy? Does the patient appear the stated age? The patient's body habitus and nutrition, skin color, amount and distribution of hair, and grooming of hair and nails should be observed. Many chronic illnesses are associated with pallor and weight loss, leading to emaciation.

Vital Signs

Vital signs should be taken by measuring height and weight, and obtaining a temperature. Blood pressure, pulse rate, and respiratory rate also should be obtained. Many cardiovascular anomalies can result in neurological symptoms (see Chapters 40, 42, and 43).

CULTURAL CONSIDERATIONS Related to the Health History

Maintaining cultural awareness indicates a nurse's recognition that patients' attitudes and reactions to illness are reflective of their beliefs as well as practices. Being aware of cultural beliefs and practices enables the nurse to more effectively evaluate and plan appropriate nursing interventions. Medication administration may need to be modified for various cultural groups in order to enhance communication and decrease misconceptions. When patients are evaluated within the context of their cultural orientation and current health care beliefs, improved assessment and planning for interventions are more likely to occur. Chapter 1 ☺ contains a full discussion of cultural considerations and cultural competence.

Skin

It is necessary to examine the skin of the face, extremities, trunk, and legs, and note the color, temperature, moisture, and dryness in order to detect any signs indicative of a neurological problem. In Parkinson's disease, for example, the face is often oily, a condition called seborrhea (Victor & Ropper, 2001). Sebaceous adenomas following a butterfly area distribution over the bridge of the nose may suggest tuberous sclerosis (Victor & Ropper, 2001).

The nurse also should check for café au lait spots, which can be indicative of neurofibromatosis. Café au lait spots are more or less oval, with the long axis situated along a cutaneous (skin) nerve tract. They are light to medium brown, as reflected by the name, which means "coffee with milk" in French. They usually are present at birth, but may arise later in the first few years of life. They are much more common in black infants. To have a few such spots is totally normal. However, more than six such spots of greater than 1.5 mm in diameter in prepubertal or greater than 5 mm in diameter in postpubertal children will get the doctor's attention, because they are then essentially diagnostic of neurofibromatosis (although other features are required to make the diagnosis and some individuals may have multiple spots without having the disease—a trait that is itself inherited).

The nurse should also pay special attention to the lower lumbar area at the base of the spine. A dimple, with or without a tuft of hair, in that area can signify spina bifida or meningocele (Fuller, 2004).

Head, Neck, and Extremities

The health care provider should observe the responsiveness of the patient's facial expression and look for asymmetry. Parkinson's disease results in a poverty of facial expression, called **masked facies**, and facial asymmetry can be a subtle indication of facial weakness. Other assessment factors include the following:

- Listen to the patient speak to determine whether the speech is clear and fluent or hesitant. Is the patient able to find the correct words to express himself?
- Examine the head to determine whether the skull is abnormally large (**macrocephalic**) or small (**microcephalic**).
- Inspect the scalp for old incisions and palpate the skull to detect deformities that may suggest previous surgery or fractures.
- Palpate the temporal arteries, noting if the patient experiences tenderness.
- Inspect and palpate the neck, looking for thyroid enlargement or cervical lymphadenopathy (disease of the lymph nodes, synonymous with swollen or enlarged lymph nodes).
- Passively flex the neck to detect pain or limitation of movement, which suggests meningeal irritation.

 CRITICAL ALERT *When examining the neck of the patient, note if the patient has pain on flexion or extension. Brudzinski sign is flexion of the hips when the neck is flexed from a supine position. This is consistent with meningitis, and must be evaluated further.*

- Inspect for **Battle's sign** bruising immediately behind the ears, which refers to ecchymosis on the mastoid bone. **Raccoon sign** (or **eyes**), a darkening around the periorbital area that generates the appearance of a raccoon, refers to periorbital ecchymosis. These signs raise suspicion of basal skull fracture.

- Inspect the hands and fingers to detect deformity. Multiple ungula fibromas are a primary feature of tuberous sclerosis (Victor & Ropper, 2001).
- Inspect the legs to detect abnormally high arches or hammer toe deformity. Friedreich's ataxia, an inherited disease that causes progressive damage to the nervous system resulting in symptoms ranging from gait disturbance and speech problems to heart disease, and some of the hereditary sensor motor neuropathies are associated with high arches and hammer toes (Victor & Ropper, 2001).
- Observe hair distribution over the lower portion of the legs. Loss of hair from these regions occurs with autonomic neuropathies, frequently diabetic neuropathy.
- Use an otoscope to observe the canals and tympanic membrane. Cholesteatoma, or "pearly tumor," though rare, can be seen in the middle ear (Victor & Ropper, 2001). These tumors involve cranial nerve XII (discussed later in the chapter), and are associated with a history of chronic middle ear infections.
- Inspect the lips for cyanosis or pallor, and then look at the gingivae and teeth to detect **gingival hyperplasia**, proliferation of cells causing enlargement, pyorrhea, redness, or erosion. Examine the gums for hyperplasia, which can occur with phenytoin ingestion and ascorbic acid deficiency. Discoloration of the gums can result from heavy metals, notably copper and arsenic, and adrenocorticotrophic hormone.
- Note the color of the tongue and determine whether it is abnormally red, smooth, or fissured. Several vitamin deficiencies, such as niacin, riboflavin and cyanocobalamin are associated with a red, smooth tongue.

Lungs, Cardiac, and Abdomen

The nurse should assess for dyspnea, orthopnea, or shortness of breath. Heart sounds should be auscultated, noting the rate, rhythm, and tone and listening for murmurs. The carotid and subclavian arteries should be auscultated, listening for bruits.

The abdomen should be inspected and palpated to detect tenderness, masses, and abnormal pulsations. The nurse also should listen for bowel sounds. In the hospitalized patient with neurological disorders, bowel function is important to monitor. Ileus, or sluggishness of the bowel, can be common postoperatively.

◼ Neurological Examination

The neurological examination can be divided into five areas: the evaluation of mental status, cranial nerves, motor system, sensation, reflexes, and cerebellar function. In taking the history from the patient, the nurse has developed an impression of the mental status of the patient. However, formal mental status testing must be completed.

Mental Status Examination

Mental status is defined as "the functional state of the mind as judged by the individual's behavior, appearance, responsiveness to stimuli of all kinds, speech, memory, and judgment" (Thomas, 1997). The mental status examination assesses the higher cortical functions of thinking and reasoning as well as level of consciousness, orientation, attention, memory, affect and insight, speech and language, fund of knowledge, and abstraction.

Level of Consciousness

Level of consciousness (LOC) is a critical component of the neurological assessment. Consciousness is a state of awareness and can be a sensitive indicator of cortical function. Consciousness is disrupted easily by neurological damage or disease. Coma is the opposite state to consciousness, and between the two are a variety of altered states of awareness. Arousal is a state of responsiveness to sensory stimulation. Arousal requires both hemispheres and the upper brainstem to be intact (Stewart-Amidei & Bader, 2004). The health care provider should observe the patient's ability to respond to noxious stimuli in an appropriate manner. Awareness is the orientation to person, place, and time, and implies interaction with, and reaction to, environmental stimuli. In documenting the patient's LOC, the health care provider should include both the response and the stimulus that was required to produce the response. Evaluation of the LOC is most accurate when the patient is stimulated to a maximal state of arousal.

The Glasgow Coma Scale (GCS) is the most widely recognized LOC assessment tool (Chart 28–2). It is commonly used in emergency departments, trauma units, and intensive care areas (Teasdale & Jennett, 1974). This tool evaluates three areas: eye opening, verbal response, and best motor response. The highest score that can be attained is 15, and the lowest is 3. In general, a GCS of 8 or lower indicates a coma. When using the GCS for serial assessment, the clinician should note that it is not a sensitive tool for evaluation of altered sensorium. It does not account for aphasia and is not an indicator of lateralization of neurological deterioration. When completing the GCS it is important to score the best response for each category. For the motor response, the upper extremities are scored.

Another validated tool that has been developed more recently than the GCS is the FOUR Score Consciousness Scale (Wijdicks, Bamlet, Maramattom, Manno, & McClelland, 2005). This scale evaluates four components: eye, motor, brainstem, and respiration). Each component has a maximal score of 4. This scale provides greater neurological detail than the GCS. In contrast to the GCS, verbal response is not a component of the FOUR Score Consciousness Scale, making it fully applicable in intubated patients. See Chart 28–3 for a description of the scale.

Orientation

The patient is assessed for orientation to time, place, and person. Time orientation is assessed by evaluating awareness of the year, season, month, day of the week, and date. Place orientation is assessed via awareness of the state the patient is in, followed by city, county, name of the current location (hospital or medical office), and the floor the patient is currently on (or office number).

CHART 28–2	**Scoring for Glasgow Coma Scale**

Eye Opening (E)	Verbal Response (V)	Motor Response (M)
4 = Spontaneous	5 = Normal conversation	6 = Normal
3 = To voice	4 = Disoriented conversation	5 = Localizes to pain
2 = To pain	3 = Words, but not coherent	4 = Withdraws to pain
1 = None	2 = No words; only sounds	3 = Decorticate posture
	1 = None	2 = Decerebrate
		1 = None

Total = E + V + M

With the Glasgow Coma Scale, one determines the best eye opening response, the best verbal response, and the best motor response. The score represents the sum of the numeric scores of each of the categories. There are limitations to its use. If the patient has an endotracheal tube in place, she cannot talk. For this reason, many prefer to document the score by its individual components; so a patient with a Glasgow Coma Scale score of 15 would be documented as follows: E4 V5 M6. An intubated patient would be scored as E4 V intubated M6. Of these individual factors, the best motor response is probably the most significant.

Source: American College of Surgeons Committee on Trauma (2004). Advanced Trauma Life Support for Doctors (7th ed). Chicago: American College of Surgeons.

Time orientation often is impaired early, and many times may be the first sign of neurological change. In the hospitalized patient this may be the result of a sleep disturbance and/or sensory overload. Impaired orientation to place may occur with moderate cerebral dysfunction (Stewart-Amidei & Bader, 2004). Impaired orientation to person is generally the last parameter lost and occurs with severe dysfunction such as delirium or dementia.

Confusion is defined as not being aware of or oriented to, time, place, or self (*Dictionary of Cell and Molecular Biology*, 2008; Thomas, 1997). Confusion may be acute or chronic, and etiologies include metabolic disorders, infections, changes in underlying neurological disorder, and drug or alcohol intoxification. A list of validated tools to assess cognition is shown in Chart 28–4.

Attention and Concentration

Attention refers to the ability to focus on a particular stimulus, task, or situation. Concentration refers to the ability to sustain attention. Alteration in attention and concentration can be early indicators of delirium. To evaluate attention and concentration, the nurse asks the patient to count backwards from 100 by 7 (93, 86, 79, 72, 65). In the patient who is lacking in formal education, the nurse can ask for the days of the week or the months of the year backwards.

CHART 28–3	**FOUR Score Consciousness Scale**

Eye Response	Motor Response	Brainstem Reflexes	Respiration
4 = Eyelids open, tracking or blinking on command	4 = Thumbs up or fist to command	4 = Pupil and corneal reflex present	4 = Not intubated, regular breathing
3 = Eyelids open, not tracking	3 = Localizing to pain	3 = One pupil wide and fixed	3 = Not intubated, Cheyne-Stokes pattern
2 = Eyelids closed, but open to loud noise	2 = Flexion to pain	2 = Pupil **or** corneal reflex absent	2 = Not intubated, irregular pattern
1 = Eyelids closed, but open to pain	1 = Extensor posturing	1 = Pupil **and** corneal reflex absent	1 = Breathes above ventilator rate
0 = Eyelids closed with pain	0 = No response to pain or myoclonus status epilepticus	0 = Absent pupil, corneal, and cough reflex	0 = Breathes at ventilator rate or apnea

CHART 28–4 **Cognitive Assessment Tools**

Test Name	Evaluation	Scoring
Mini-Mental Status Examination (MMSE)	Evaluates orientation, language, memory, writing, ability to follow commands, calculations, constructional abilities.	30-item examination scored by correct responses: Maximum score = 30 Average score = 27.6 Cognitive impairment = 25 or less.
Short Portable Mental Status Questionnaire (SPMSQ)	Evaluates orientation, language, personal history, awareness and remote memory, and calculational ability.	Ten-item instrument scored by errors. Score of 3 or greater indicates impairment. Able to adjust for educational level. Add one error if person has completed 12th grade. Delete one error if person has not completed 12th grade.
Cognitive Capacity Screening Examination (CCSE)	Evaluates orientation, memory, attention, calculation, and extracting abilities. Most reliable for distinguishing between delirium and dementia.	30-item instrument scored by correct responses. Most reliable for distinguishing between acute and chronic disorders. Maximum score = 30. Score of 20 or below indicates cognitive impairment.

Memory

Memory, the ability to recover information about past events or knowledge, can be subdivided into remote, intermediate, and recent. Most questions related to memory can be asked in the context of obtaining the history.

Remote Memory

Some of the following questions can be asked to evaluate remote memory. The information from the patient can be validated by family or friends.

• Where and when were you born?
• How old are you?
• When did you graduate from high school?
• When were you married?
• What are the names, ages, and birth dates of your children?

Intermediate Memory

Intermediate memory can be evaluated by referring to personal and general events of the previous 5 years; for example, the patient could be asked to give a chronological account of the presenting illness including dates. The nurse could also inquire about common events of the previous 5 years, such as presidential elections.

Recent Memory

Recent memory can be tested in a variety of ways. The nurse could name three objects (i.e., apple, penny, table) and ask the patient to repeat them. Inform the patient you will be asking later for the patient to repeat the names of these objects. Wait 5 minutes, completing other aspects of the assessment, and then ask the patient to recall the three objects named previously. A person without cognitive deficit should be able to correctly recall the three objects. Another method is to ask the patient how she arrived at the place of assessment and with whom, or to name what she had for breakfast that day.

Affect and Insight

Assessment of affect, or display of emotions, begins with observation. **Euthymia** refers to a normal state; that is the patient is calm and appropriate. **Euphoria** is excessively cheerful or inappropriately cheerful. **Apathetic** is used to describe the patient who is flat or dull in appearance. **Dysphoria** is noted as being depressed, despondent, or sad. Validated tools to assess mood or affect are listed in Chart 28–5.

Insight refers to the ability to assess and monitor one's own cognitive, motor, or sensory function. Insight and reality orientation are frequently impaired in neurological diseases. The nurse

CHART 28–5 **Affective Assessment Tools**

Test Name	Evaluation	Scoring
Beck Depression Inventory (BDI)	Measures manifestations of depression. The BDI takes approximately 10 minutes to complete, although patients require a fifth to sixth grade reading age to adequately understand the questions. Is considered the gold standard for self-rating depression.	21-item self-report scale.
Hamilton Depression Rating Scale	Assesses the severity of depression for clinical purposes in adults of any age.	17-item scale that is rated by semistructured interview with trained interviewer.
Duke Anxiety-Depression Scale (DUKE-AD)	Brief screen for clinical anxiety and depression.	Seven items measured with a score of 5 or above indicates high risk for anxiety or depression.

can assess insight by asking the patient "Why are you being seen today?" or "Why are you in the hospital?"

Speech and Language

Fluency refers to the spontaneity, articulation, hesitancy, and duration of the patient's response. The nurse has evaluated the fluency of speech throughout the assessment. **Aphasia** is a disorder of speech and language due to cerebral dysfunction. The three primary aphasic deficits are in comprehension of spoken language, expressive language, and naming. Aphasic deficits can be localized to the area of dysfunction. Approximately 90% of the U.S. population is right-handed and left hemisphere dominant for language. Among people that are left-handed, two-thirds are thought to have left hemisphere language dominance, while the remainder has varying degrees of mixed or right hemisphere dominance (Fuller, 2004).

Most patients with neurological disorders have some communication function left intact. Carefully evaluating the patient's ability to communicate can aid in localizing a lesion to a specific area of the brain. The various aphasias can be subdivided into categories, and are listed in Chart 28–6 along with the respective areas of involvement.

To assess comprehension, or the ability to understand the spoken word, the patient is first asked to follow a simple instruction, such as "Close your eyes." If the patient is able to do so, increasing complex commands are given, "Touch your right ear with your left index finger." If the patient is able to carry out complex commands, this portion of the communication system appears intact.

- To evaluate the ability to understand the written word, commands of increasing difficulty are written on cards that are shown to the patient, who is asked to follow the instructions. Examples include "Open your mouth," "Stick out your tongue," and "Point to your right ear."
- To assess the ability to express ideas verbally, the patient is asked to identify common objects, such as a pencil or watch. The nurse then proceeds to ask open-ended questions, such as "Tell me about the kind of work you do" or "What types of activities do you enjoy in your free time?" or "Tell me about your illness."
- To test for naming, also called word finding difficulty, the patient is shown common objects such as a pen and watch, and asked to name the object.

CHART 28–6	Aphasias by Location
Aphasia	**Location**
Auditory receptive aphasia	Lesion at Wernicke's area of the temporal lobe
Visual receptive aphasia	Lesion at parietal-occipital area
Expressive speaking aphasia	Lesion at Broca's area of frontal lobe
Expressive writing aphasia	Lesion at posterior frontal area
Global aphasia (a form of aphasia that involves both expressive and receptive aphasias)	Lesions (extensive) of Broca's area, Wernicke's area, parietal-occipital area, and posterior frontal area

- If there is a question about the inability to express oneself in writing, the patient is given paper and pencil and asked to write his name and address. As with other aphasia evaluations, complexity is increased. The patient could be asked to write an account of a current news event or to describe the weather.

Fund of Knowledge and Abstraction

General fund of knowledge refers to the patient's knowledge base—an understanding of one's natural and social environment. This may be tested by asking questions such as, "How many nickels are in $1.15?" or asking the patient to list the last five presidents of the United States, or to list five major U.S. cities. The higher the number of correct answers, the better the understanding and knowledge base, taking into consideration the individual's educational background and other training.

Abstraction is measured by assessing the patient's ability to determine similarities. For example, one may ask the patient how two items are alike, an apple and an orange or a car and an airplane. The first answer would be good if the patient said "fruit"; it would be poor if the patient said "round." The second answer would be good if the patient said, "modes of transportation." The patient also may be asked the interpretation of proverbial phrases, e.g., what is the meaning of "do not cry over spilt milk?" A good response would be "do not get upset over the little things"; whereas a poor response might be "spilling milk is bad."

Cranial Nerve Examination

The cranial nerves (CNs) are referred to by specific name, as well as an assigned Roman numeral. For documentation purposes, they are referred to by the Roman numeral. They are called cranial nerves because they emerge from the cranium and can have sensory function, motor function, or both ability to recover information about past events or knowledge (Wilson-Pauwels, Akesson, Stewart, & Spacey, 2002). Cranial nerves numbered II through XII arise from the brainstem, as shown in Figure 28–4 ■.

Olfactory Nerve (CN I)

CN I has sensory function only. The sense of smell is tested by occluding one nostril while testing the other. A common odoriferous substance is placed under the unobstructed nostril. Coffee, lemon oil, and peppermint are common substances used. **Anosmia** is the inability to smell. Common neurological causes of anosmia include tumors of the frontal lobe, fractures of the anterior fossa, meningitis, hydrocephalus, and traumatic brain injury. Common nonneurological causes of anosmia include the common cold and inflammation of the nasal cavity. Recently, olfactory deficits have been described early in both Alzheimer's disease and Parkinson's disease (Luzzi, Snowden, Neary, Coccia, Provinciali, & Lambon, 2007). (See Chapters 33, 34, and 69 ☉.)

Optic Nerve (CN II)

CN II has sensory function only. Assessing the optic nerve involves inspecting the globe for cataracts, foreign bodies, or other obvious abnormalities; testing visual acuity; testing visual fields; and completing a funduscopic examination (see Chapter 71 ☉). To assess CN II, each eye is evaluated separately. Visual acuity can be assessed by asking the patient to read from a newspaper, or in the ambulatory setting a Snellen chart is frequently used. A Snellen chart is an eye chart used by eye care professionals and

FIGURE 28–4 ■ Dorsal aspect of brain with cranial nerves noted.

others to measure visual acuity. Normal vision is 20/20, which means the patient can read the Snellen chart from a distance of 20 feet. A reading of 20/30 means the patient can read at 30 feet what the normal eye can read at 20 feet.

A visual field extends 60 degrees to the nasal side, 110 degrees to the temporal side, and 130 degrees vertically (Digre & Corbett, 2003). Visual fields are assessed using the confrontation test, whereby the patient and nurse face each other 2 feet apart. The patient is directed to cover one eye and look directly at the nurse. The nurse brings an object, such as a pencil, into each cardinal gaze and the patient indicates when she first sees the object. This test reveals only gross defects. Further testing would be indicated.

The funduscopic examination requires the use of an ophthalmoscope. The ophthalmoscope has a special lens that is used to visualize the inside of the eye by shining light directly into the eye. The room should be dimmed while performing this exam for best results. The nurse examines the patient's right eye by holding the ophthalmoscope in the right hand and using his right eye. The opposite is the case with the left eye. Figure 28–5 ■ illustrates obtaining a pupil response.

The fundus includes the optic disc, macula, and blood vessels on the back wall of the eye. The funduscopic examination is perceived as a difficult task, and is avoided by many nurses. It is essential, however, for the assessment of papilledema, or optic disc swelling, which is a hallmark of increased intracranial pressure.

FIGURE 28–5 ■ Obtaining a pupil response.
Source: © Timothy Tadder/CORBIS All Rights Reserved

As with all things, practice increases comfort level, so the nurse is encouraged to practice funduscopic exams when possible. (See Chapter 71 .)

Oculomotor (CN III), Trochlear (CN IV), and Abducens (CN VI) Nerves

Cranial nerves III, IV, and VI are usually tested together because they supply the various muscles that move the eye, and have motor function only. These three nerves supply the extraocular muscles, pupils, and eyelids. The first step in assessing these nerve functions is to observe the eyes. Note the position of the eyeball within the head. Are the eyes symmetrical? The abnormal protrusion of one or both eyeballs is called **proptosis** or **exophthalmos**. This is commonly seen in hyperthyroidism. Next, note the position of the upper eyelid in relation to the pupil and iris in each eye and compare. **Ptosis** is the term for a drooping upper eyelid, and can be seen in Horner's syndrome and myasthenia gravis.

Extraocular movements are evaluated by asking the patient to follow a finger or pencil through the six cardinal fields of gaze. In the patient without deficits, both eyes move at the same time in the same direction. This is referred to as **conjugate gaze**. If the eye movements are not the same, this is called **dysconjugate gaze**. Double vision may be present if the patient cannot move the eye in a particular direction. The loss of function of the muscles necessary for these movements may be caused by direct damage to the muscle or by injury of the cranial nerve. **Nystagmus** is an involuntary movement of the eyes that may be horizontal, vertical, or mixed in direction. There are multiple types of nystagmus; however, all involve a "jerky" movement of the eyes. Nystagmus is not uncommon in patients taking phenytoin for seizures.

In assessing the unconscious patient, the oculocephalic reflex (doll's eye response) and the oculovestibular reflex (cold calorics) are evaluated for reflex movement of the eye. The **oculocephalic reflex**, or **doll's eyes reflex**, is one in which the eyes move opposite the direction the head is turned, thus maintaining a more or less steady gaze. It is produced by moving the patient's head left to right or up and down. When the reflex is present, the eyes of the patient remain stationary while the head is moved, thus moving in relation to the head. In a normal, alert person, this brainstem reflex is inhibited by gaze control mechanisms. The eyes go wherever the cortex wants them to go. In the comatose patient, this inhibition is lost, and the oculocephalic reflex becomes disinhibited, and clinically demonstrable. Therefore, the eyes deviate in the direction opposite the head turning. This is a positive doll's eyes response. Eyes stay focused on whatever they were looking at before head turning.

The **oculovestibular reflex**, or cold calorics, is a reflex movement that stabilizes images on the retina during head movement by producing an eye movement in the direction opposite to head movement. This can be produced by placing the patient's upper body and head at 30 degrees off horizontal, and injecting 50 to 100 mL of cold water into an ear. The water has the same effect on the semicircular canal as if the patient's head was turned to the opposite side of the injection. Therefore, the patient's eyes will look toward the ear of injection. The eye deviation lasts for a sustained period of time. This is an excellent maneuver to assess extraocular muscles in the comatose patient with possible cervical spine injury. If the oculovestibular reflex is absent, a lesion of the pons, medulla, or less commonly the III, IV, IV, or VIII nerves is present. Unlike the oculocephalic reflex, the oculovestibular reflex is present in patients who are awake. In alert patients, this reflex not only induces eye deviation, it also produces nystagmus in the direction of the noninjected ear. The slow phase is toward the injected ear and the fast

phase is away. The presence of these reflexes indicates the brainstem is intact.

To assess the pupils, the patient is directed to look at an object in the room, preferably straight ahead. In the unconscious patient, the pupils are examined as found. Pupils are examined for size, shape, and equality. The normal size of the pupil ranges from 2 to 6 mm. When the pupils are compared to each other, they should be equal; however, approximately 17% of the population has unequal pupil size without the presence of pathology (Wilson-Pauwels et al., 2002). This is called **anisocoria**. The normal pupil is round. Patients who have had cataracts removed will have a "keyhole"-shaped pupil of the affected eye.

 An ovoid pupil indicates papillary dysfunction, and is seen in early herniation. This is a neurological emergency and must be addressed immediately.

The pupils are next tested for reaction to light. This is called the direct light reflex. A light is directed into each pupil and then withdrawn. When the light is shone in the eye, the pupil should constrict; conversely, when the light is withdrawn, it should dilate. Additionally, when the light is directed to the eye, the opposite eye should constrict slightly. This is called the consensual light reflex.

 A unilateral papillary dilation may represent excessive pressure and ultimately herniation of the medial temporal lobe. The nurse must communicate the assessment and observe the patient closely with serial assessments.

The accommodation reflex is evaluated next. The patient is asked to focus on an object, such as the nurse's finger, that is positioned 2 or 3 feet directly in front of her and asked to follow it with her eyes. The finger is rapidly moved toward the patient's nose. The pupils should constrict when looking at the finger near her face.

In the unconscious patient, the maneuver to assess these nerves is called the doll's eyes maneuver, as previously discussed. To complete, the nurse must first ensure that cervical injury has been ruled out. The nurse then holds the eyelids open and briskly turns the head from side to side. If the eyes lag to the opposite side to which the head is turned, that is considered a positive response. Positive in this instance means the brainstem is intact. If the eyes are fixed, and move with the direction of the head, that is considered a negative response. Negative in this instance means there is a brainstem lesion.

Trigeminal Nerve (CN V)

The trigeminal nerve has both a sensory and motor component. The sensory component is tested with the patient's eyes closed as follows:

- The nurse places warm and cold objects on each side of the face randomly and asks the patient to identify the temperature.
- Touch is evaluated by using a piece of cotton or gauze and lightly touching each side of the face randomly, again asking the patient to identify the sensation.
- Pain is tested by using a sharp object to lightly touch each side of the face.
- The corneal reflex is tested by lightly touching the cornea with cotton, resulting in the patient blinking the stimulated eye.

The motor aspect of the fifth nerve innervates the muscles used for chewing. The patient is asked to tightly clamp the jaw and close the mouth. Palpate the muscles of the jaw, looking for symmetry.

Facial Nerve (VII)

The facial nerve has a sensory and motor function. The seventh nerve innervates the sense of taste in the anterior two-thirds of the tongue. Each side of the tongue is tested separately. The patient is asked to stick out his tongue and identify the taste of sugar. Water is then given and then repeated with a salty or sour substance.

The motor component is tested by observing the face at rest and while completing deliberate movements such as smiling, blowing air into the cheeks, wrinkling the forehead, and raising the eyebrows. If weakness or asymmetry is noted, it is essential to determine if the lesion involved is central or peripheral. Central facial weakness, indicated by weakness below the eyes indicates the cause is in the central nervous system, and can be related to a lesion in the contralateral frontal lobe, such as a patient with a stroke. The patient with central facial weakness is unable to lift the corner of the mouth to smile, but can wrinkle the forehead. If the entire side of the face is involved, the patient has a peripheral facial weakness, involving CN VII, such as Bell's palsy. In this case, the patient may have lost the ability to close the eyelids. The nurse must be aware of this and ensure that the eye is kept moist and protected. During sleep, the use of an "eye bubble" is appropriate. These are clear plastic devices that allow moisture to remain, yet protect the eye from trauma. Use of an eye patch or taping the lid closed while sleeping is appropriate as well.

Vestibulocochlear or Acoustic Nerve (CN VIII)

The acoustic nerve is a pure sensory nerve that is divided into two branches. The cochlear branch deals with hearing, and the vestibular branch is involved with balance. The vestibular branch is not routinely assessed. If the patient identifies symptoms of vertigo, tinnitus, or disturbed balance, more specific testing can be done, generally by the neurologists. These symptoms are common in Ménière's disease and acoustic neuromas (see Chapter 70 ☺).

The cochlear branch is tested by the nurse whispering numbers and the patient repeating them, or by asking the patient to close her eyes while the nurse rubs the thumb and first two fingers together testing each ear separately, and asking the patient to identify on which side they hear the noise. Bone and air conduction tests, using a tuning fork, though not routine, can be done as well. Damage to this nerve can result in impaired hearing, tinnitus, vertigo, nystagmus, and unilateral or bilateral deafness.

Glossopharyngeal (CN IX) and Vagus (CN X) Nerves

The glossopharyngeal and vagus nerves are generally tested together because their innervation overlaps in the pharynx. They have both sensory and motor functions. The glossopharyngeal nerve supplies sensory function to the pharynx, tonsils, and posterior third of the tongue. The motor component elevates the pharynx. To test, the patient is directed to open the mouth and say "aaah." The palate and uvula should move upward. The pharyngeal (gag) reflex is innervated by both the 9th and 10th nerves. To evaluate, the posterior pharynx is stimulated with a tongue blade. The pharynx should elevate and constrict and the tongue should

retract, or "gag." In the unconscious patient, the suction catheter can be used.

The vagus nerve controls swallowing and speaking by innervating the larynx and pharynx. When the patient has the mouth open and is saying "aaah," the uvula should be midline. The quality of the voice is assessed for hoarseness. The patient can be asked to repeat "No ifs, ands, or buts." Damage to this nerve can result in impaired sensation, dysphasia, dysarthria, dysphonia, excessive drooling, and stridor (see Chapter 34 ☺).

Spinal Accessory Nerve (CN XI)

The spinal accessory nerve has motor function only. This nerve innervates the sternocleidomastoid and trapezius muscles. To assess function, the patient is first asked to shrug the shoulders while the nurse uses resistance. The patient is then asked to turn the head to one side and push the chin against the nurse's hand. Damage to this nerve can result in impaired strength in lifting the shoulders or difficulty in turning the head to either side.

Hypoglossal Nerve (CN XII)

The patient is asked to open the mouth and stick out the tongue. The tongue is observed for deviation, atrophy, and **fasciculation,** a small, local involuntary muscle contracting or twitching visible under the skin. Next, the patient is asked to push the tongue against a tongue blade, to each side, to assess strength.

Motor Examination

The motor examination consists of assessing gait, muscle bulk, tone, and strength. The first aspect of the motor examination is the evaluation of the patient's gait. The patient is asked to walk naturally in the examination room. It is necessary to note posture, movement of body parts, and the type of steps taken. See Chart 28–7 for a description of gaits.

Each of the muscles to be evaluated is inspected. Each side of the body is compared against the other. Palpating the muscles can assist with detecting atrophy. Observe for fine or gross involuntary movements such as fasciculations, tremors, or myoclonic jerks. If muscles in an extremity appear asymmetric, each limb should be measured. A difference of 1 cm or less is not significant. As a general rule, loss of muscle bulk may be due to a peripheral nerve dysfunction such as brachial plexus or Guillain-Barré

CHART 28–7	Types of Gait

Gait	Description
Steppage	Associated with flaccidity of the leg and foot drop. The patient lifts the thigh and leg high, and the foot slaps against the floor. The patient looks as if he is walking up stairs.
Ataxic	Wide-based, staggering, and uncoordinated. Cannot stand with feet together.
Spastic	Leg extension, and shuffles with the legs stiff without lifting the feet.
Parkinsonian	In this gait, the hallmark is the loss of arm swing while walking. The head and body can be flexed forward and the legs are rigid. The feet shuffle, and the gait is slow.

syndrome. Guillain-Barré syndrome is a disorder in which the body's immune system attacks part of the peripheral nervous system. The first symptoms of this disorder include varying degrees of weakness or tingling sensations in the legs. In many instances the weakness and abnormal sensations spread to the arms and upper body. These symptoms can increase in intensity until certain muscles cannot be used at all and, when severe, the patient is almost totally paralyzed. In these cases the disorder is life threatening—potentially interfering with breathing and, at times, with blood pressure or heart rate—and is considered a medical emergency.

Muscle tone represents muscle resistance to passive movements. Tone is assessed by passive range of motion. Slight resistance on movement is indicative of normal muscle tone. Each extremity should be assessed, and should demonstrate smooth movement without change. Rigidity is a state of resistance that can be intermittent, such as cogwheel rigidity, when small regular jerks are felt. Flaccidity describes decreased muscle tone, or hypotonia. The muscle is weak and flabby.

In the unconscious patient, stimuli may elicit an abnormal motor response. Passive range of motion is done to assess muscle tone in these patients. Additionally response to pain is evaluated. Pain is elicited by means of a sternal rub, squeezing of a nail bed, or pinching of the sternocleidomastoid muscle. When painful stimuli are applied, if the patient demonstrates flexion of the arm, wrist, and fingers while adducting the upper extremity, this is known as **decorticate posturing**, or abnormal flexion. The lower extremities are extended, internally rotated, and plantar flexed. **Decerebrate posturing**, an abnormal body posture that involves rigid extension of the arms and legs, downward pointing of the toes, and backward arching of the head, is seen in the presence of noxious or painful stimuli. The patient clenches his teeth with arm extension in an adducted and hyperpronated fashion. Lower extremities are extended with plantar flexion. Because the lower extremities have similar positions in both motor responses, the upper extremities are used to identify the posturing. It is possible to demonstrate both abnormal responses simultaneously, or each intermittently. Abnormal extension is believed to be the more grave of the two responses (Wilson-Pauwels et al., 2002). It is imperative that the nurse caring for the unconscious patient notify the responsible health care provider treating the patient for immediate intervention.

 CRITICAL ALERT *When caring for the unconscious patient, it is imperative for the nurse to contact the treating clinician when a patient begins to demonstrate abnormal flexion or extension, or if the patient alternates between one and the other.*

Muscle strength is evaluated in both the upper and lower extremities. Each muscle group is assessed by using passive range of motion against gravity followed by active resistance positioned by the nurse and graded based on the ability to move against resistance. Chart 28–8 shows gradations of muscle strength.

To evaluate the upper extremities begin by observing for mild hemiparesis. Direct the patient to close his eyes and place the arms straight out in front of him with the palms up. Observe for 20 to 30 seconds. If one arm lowers slowly, this is referred to as drift. If the hand pronates, this is noted as pronator drift. These are subtle signs of hemiparesis (muscle weakness on one side of the body). Ask the patient to place the arms at the side

CHART 28–8 Muscle Strength

Muscle Function Level	Grade	Percentage of Normal
No evidence of contractility	0	0
Slight contractility, no movement	1	10
Muscle able to move with support against gravity	2	25
Muscle able to move without support against gravity	3	50
Muscle able to move without support against gravity with weakness to applied resistance	4	75
Muscle able to move through full range of motion with no weakness to applied resistance	5	100

with elbows flexed and abducted to 90 degrees. Resistance is applied. This assesses the deltoid muscle. The biceps is tested by flexing the elbow and, with the forearm supinated, the patient is directed to pull in against resistance. The patient is then directed to push the arm away against resistance, testing the triceps.

To evaluate the lower extremities, the patient is asked to sit on the examination table, or on the edge of the hospital bed, with the legs dangling freely. The patient is asked to lift the knee up as if walking up a stair. Resistance is then applied, allowing the nurse to assess the iliopsoas muscle. The patient is then asked to pull the lower leg back toward the table, which tests the hamstring group. This is followed by directing the patient to push the lower leg out toward the nurse applying resistance, thereby testing the quadriceps.

Next the feet are examined. The patient is directed to pull the toes up; this dorsiflexion tests the tibialis anterior; the patient then follows up with plantar flexion, which tests the gastrocnemius. These are important in assessing for foot drop. Chart 28–9 indicates major spinal cord segments with the corresponding functional ability and specific muscles to be tested.

Muscle strength assessment is a key factor in determining a diagnosis. Weakness or asymmetry can be seen in neuromuscular disorders such as myasthenia gravis, cerebral vascular accidents, cranial space–occupying lesions, spinal cord lesions or compression, and many others.

Sensory Examination

In the evaluation of sensory function, the patient is tested with the eyes closed. As with muscle testing, each side of the body is

CHART 28–9 Muscle Innervation

Reflex	Spinal Level
Biceps	C_5–C_6
Triceps	C_6–C_7
Patellar	L_4
Achilles	S_1

compared to the opposite. The examination is completed in a distal to proximal fashion. Areas for evaluation include hands, forearms, upper arms, trunk, thighs, legs, feet, and perineal and perirectal regions. Primary sensory modalities include light touch, superficial pain, temperature, position sense, and vibratory sense. A dermatome chart is helpful to use as a reference when assessing sensation and the patient's response to testing (Figure 28–6 ■).

Light touch is tested by using a wisp of cotton as the stimulus. The patient is asked to identify when he feels something. The nurse lightly touches the skin with the cotton beginning at the head and moving downward. Light touch can be preserved while other modalities are compromised in lesions of the spinal cord (see Chapter 32 ⊖). Superficial pain is assessed in the same manner as light touch; however, the nurse uses a pin or other disposable sharp instrument for the stimulus. Temperature sensation is assessed in the same fashion as pain and touch. Test tubes filled with warm and cold water can be used. Others prefer to run warm and cold water over tuning forks. The disparate temperature objects are used as the stimuli.

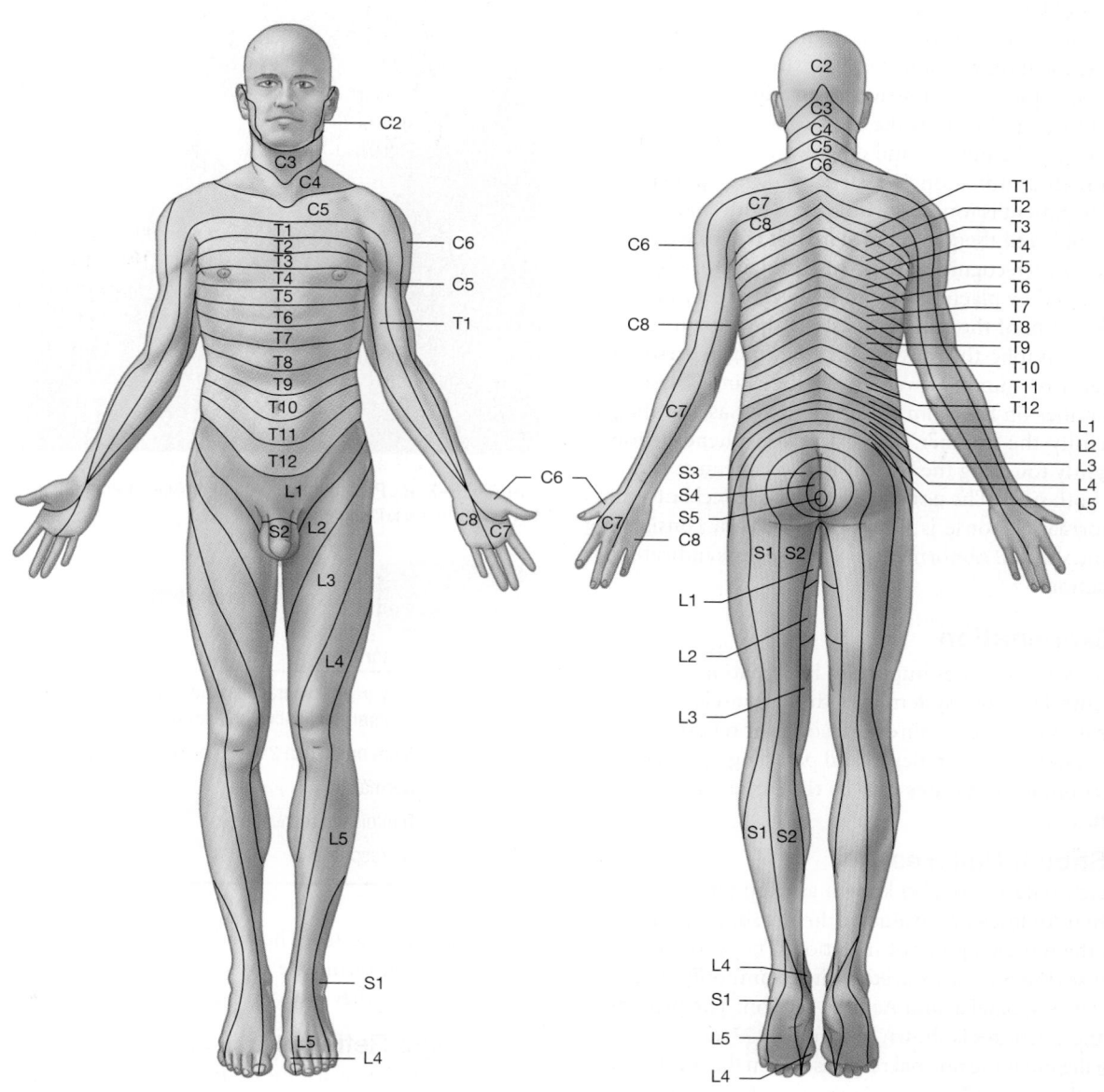

Levels of principal dermatomes

C5	Clavicles	**T10**	Level of umbilicus
C5, 6, 7	Lateral parts of upper limbs	**T12**	Inguinal or groin regions
C8, T1	Medial sides of upper limbs	**L1, 2, 3, 4**	Anterior and inner surfaces of lower limbs
C6	Thumb	**L4, 5, S1**	Foot
C6, 7, 8	Hand	**L4**	Medial side of great toe
C8	Ring and little fingers	**S1, 2, L5**	Posterior and outer surfaces of lower limbs
T4	Level of nipples	**S1**	Lateral margin of foot and little toe
		S2, 3, 4	Perineum

FIGURE 28–6 ■ Dermatome man.

Vibratory sense is tested using a tuning fork. The bony prominences are used, such as the great toe, malleolus, patella, elbow, and wrist. The vibrating tuning fork is placed on these areas and the patient is asked to describe the feeling. Many will use the word "buzzing" to describe the sensation. The patient is then asked to tell the nurse when the feeling stops. Diminished distal vibratory sense is commonly seen in diabetic neuropathy and involves the dorsal columns of the spinal cord (Ziegler, Siekeirka-Kleiser, & Schweers, 2005). (See Chapters 31 and 32 🌐.)

To assess **proprioception**, the ability to determine spatial body position, the patient again is instructed to close the eyes. The nurse should grasp the great toe by the side of the joint and move the toe in a forward-to-backward manner. This also may be done using the thumb as well. Once the thumb or great toe is pointing in an upward or downward position, the patient is asked to state which direction the digit is pointing. This is repeated using both the upward and downward positions.

Two-point discrimination is tested by using calipers or a compass. The patient is touched with one or both sharp objects at the same time and then asked to state if it was one object or two. Stereognosis (recognition of form and shape of objects by touch) is assessed by placing common objects, such as a pencil or key, in the palm of the hand and asking the patient to identify the object. Graphesthesia (the sense by which a person recognizes figures or numbers written on the skin) is tested by tracing a number on the palm of the hand and asking the patient to identify the number. The extinction phenomenon is tested by lightly touching the patient in the same area simultaneously on both sides. The normal response is to feel both stimuli; an abnormal response is noted if the patient consistently feels only one stimuli. Abnormalities in these tests indicate cortical dysfunction.

Reflex Examination

Evaluating reflexes provides important information on the status of the central nervous system in both the conscious and unconscious patient. There are three categories of reflexes: muscle stretch reflexes, superficial reflexes, and pathologic reflexes. Abnormalities in reflex responses may be the earliest sign of CNS dysfunction.

Muscle Stretch Reflexes

Muscle stretch reflexes are also known as deep tendon reflexes (DTRs). These reflexes are evaluated first, using a percussion hammer at the muscle's point of insertion. The stimulus of the hammer causes the muscle to stretch. Sites commonly tested are the biceps, triceps, patella, and Achilles tendon. The procedure for testing these reflexes is shown in Figure 28–7 ■.

Forearm flexion is the normal response when the brachial tendon is tapped with the hammer. Forearm extension is the response to the triceps stimuli. Stimuli to the area just below the patella results in leg extension, and plantar flexion of the foot is seen when the Achilles is tapped. Muscle stretch reflexes are graded based on the briskness of the response. The grade ranges from zero (no response) to four (hyperactive). Chart 28–10 illustrates muscle stretch reflexes.

Superficial Reflexes

Superficial reflexes are elicited by lightly stroking the skin or mucous membrane of the area tested. Chart 28–11 lists the most

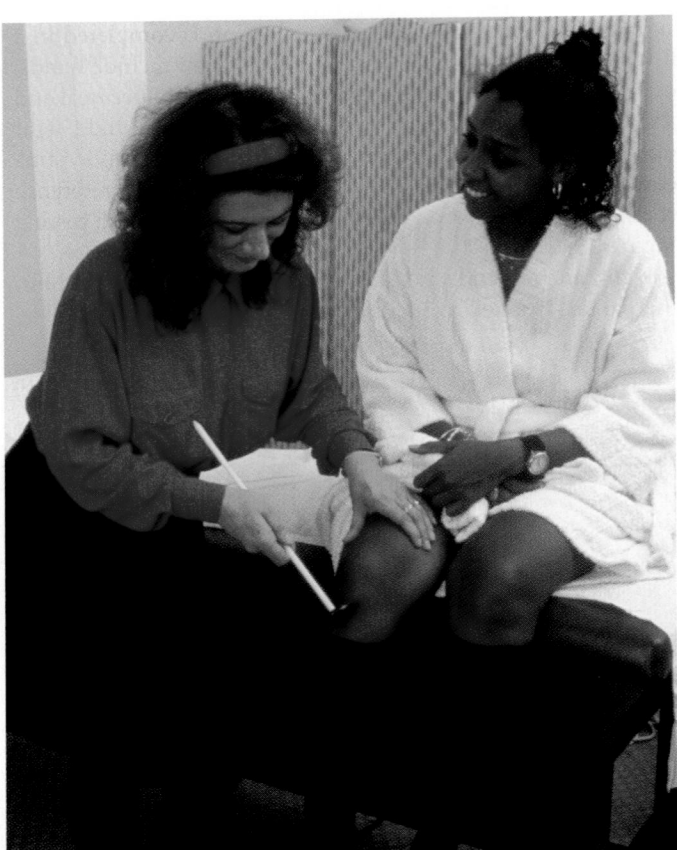

FIGURE 28–7 ■ Procedure for testing muscle stretch reflexes.
Source: © Hattie Young/Photo Researchers, Inc.

CHART 28–10	Muscle Stretch Reflexes and Scoring

Grade	Description
4+	Very brisk, hyperactive; muscle contracts multiple times, generally indicative of disease
3+	More brisk than 2+, can be normal for the individual
2+	Normal
1+	Diminished response
0	No response

common reflexes tested. The grading of superficial reflexes is different from that of muscle stretch reflexes. When evaluating superficial reflexes, they are scored as present (+) or absent (−).

Pathologic Reflexes

Pathologic reflexes, as the name implies, are abnormal responses. The extensor plantar response is also known as the Babinski reflex. It is tested by using a moderately sharp object, such as the handle of the percussion hammer, and stroking the lateral aspect of the sole of the foot from the heel to the ball of the foot, curving medially across the ball. Observe the movement of the toes, normally in flexion. Dorsiflexion of the great toe, with fanning of the other toes is seen. Figure 28–8 ■ shows pathologic reflexes.

Additional pathologic reflexes include the grasp reflex, snout reflex, and sucking reflex. These reflexes also are known as prim-

CHART 28–11   Superficial Reflexes

Reflex	Corresponding Spinal Nerve	Description
Abdominal	$T_8, T_9, T_{10}, T_{11}, T_{12}$	Each side of the abdomen is stroked lightly. Each quadrant is tested separately. The umbilicus should move in the direction of the skin stimulated.
Anal	S_3, S_4, S_5	The skin at the side of the anus is scratched with a blunt instrument or pin. There should be puckering of the anus.
Bulbocavernous	S_3, S_4	Direct pressure is applied to the muscle behind the scrotum and pinching the glans penis. The muscle should contract.
Cremasteric	L_1, L_2	The inner aspect of the thigh or lower abdomen is stroked lightly. There should be elevation of the opposite testicle, or both testicles.

FIGURE 28–8 ■ Procedure for testing pathologic reflexes.

itive reflexes because they are normally seen in early stages of development and disappear. The grasp reflex is elicited by placing two fingers in the palm of the patient's hand. The hand grasps the fingers involuntarily. The snout reflex is seen when the oral region is gently percussed. The response is the puckering of the lips. The sucking reflex is seen when the oral region is stimulated. This may be seen when the patient's mouth is suctioned, or when oral care is done. Pathologic reflexes are graded in the same fashion as the superficial reflexes, in that the reflex is either present or absent. The difference is that in pathologic reflexes, present (+) is abnormal and absent (−) is normal.

Cerebellar Examination

The cerebellar system is important in the coordination of movement. The cerebellum can be separated into two clinically useful divisions: the midline and lateral. The midline aspect of the cerebellum is concerned mainly with head position, maintenance of posture, and oculomotor function. The lateral aspect is involved with limb use and execution of fine coordinated movements. Patients with cerebellar pathology can exhibit dysfunction of both divisions.

Various methods are used to assess balance and coordination. The following are some of the more commonly used methods:

1. Starting with the arms outstretched, the patient is asked to touch her nose. Then the patient is asked to repeat the maneuver with her eyes closed.

2. The nurse, using his index finger, asks the patient to touch the nurse's index finger with the patient's own index finger while the nurse is moving the finger, essentially asking the patient to touch a moving target.

3. In the Romberg test the patient is asked to stand with the feet together, first with the eyes open, and then closed. If the patient can stand with the eyes open, but sways or loses balance with them closed, she is said to have a positive Romberg's test.

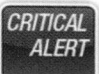 When performing the Romberg test, it is important for the nurse to stand close to the patient to prevent the patient from falling.

4. In the patient who is supine, the patient is directed to run the heel of the foot down the shin of the opposite leg. The procedure is repeated on the opposite leg.

A composite list of neurological assessment guidelines is shown in Chart 28–12 (p. 710).

■ Gerontological Considerations

Neurological disorders are the primary cause of disability in older adults. These disorders account for 50% of disability in those over 65 years of age and greater than 90% of serious dependency (Drachman, Long, & Swearer, 1994; Partners in Research, 2008). The impact of neurological diseases and disorders in the older adult is significant. Whether the older adult is experiencing an acute neurological event or a chronic disabling condition, nurses are pivotal in assessment, treatment, and continuing care. The assessment guidelines are derived from the American Association of Neuroscience Nurses' *Neurological Assessment of the Older Adult: A Guide for Nurses* (2007), a publication in its Clinical Practice Guidelines Series.

History

When obtaining a history from patients over 65 years of age, it is important to use a calm, ordered approach. Due to decreased processing speed, it is helpful to allow adequate time for the patient to respond and for giving verbal instructions (Whitney, Pugh, & Mortimer, 2004). If the patient uses adaptive devices, such as hearing aids, glasses, or walkers, one should attempt to have them in place during the assessment (Pepper, 2006).

CHART 28–12 **Neurological Assessment Guidelines**

Function	Neuroanatomic Correlate	Assessment Strategy	Common Disorders

Mental Status
1. Consciousness
2. Cognition
3. Affect
4. Speech and language
  4a. Dysarthria
  4b. Aphasia
	1. CNS: bilateral hemispheres, reticular activating system
	2. CNS: Bilateral hemispheres, primarily cortical areas
	3. CNS: limbic system, specific cortical areas
	  4a. CNS and PNS: subcortical lesions— brainstem, cerebellar, CN V, VII, IX, X, XII
	  4b. CNS: specific areas of the left frontal, temporal, parietal, and occipital lobes
		Observation: Is the patient alert? Responding to environment? Requiring painful stimuli to respond?
		Assessment: Does the patient know the date? Time? Month? Can he recall how he arrived at the point of care? Is the mood congruent with affect? Does he see things others do not see (hallucinations)? Can he repeat this sentence: "Around a rugged rock the ragged rascal ran"? Is speech free flowing? Can he identify objects correctly?
			Delirium, dementia, coma, accidents, trauma, infection, cerebral vascular accidents, tumors, neurodegenerative disorders

Cranial Nerves 1. Motor 2. Sensory 3. Motor and sensory	PNS 1. CN III, IV, VI supply the extraocular muscles, pupils, and eyelids. CN XI innervates the sternocleidomastoid and trapezius muscles. CN XII innervates the tongue. 2. CN I, II supply the sense of smell, visual acuity, and visual fields. CN VIII supplies hearing and balance. 3. CN V is responsible for facial temperature, touch, pain, and corneal reflex. Jaw muscles are innervated. CN VII innervates taste in the anterior 2/3 of tongue, and facial movements. CN IX , X supply the pharynx including gag reflex. Voice quality, including hoarseness, is involved.	*Examination:* Necessary equipment includes odiferous substance, ophthalmoscope, pen light, Snellen chart (or other acuity method), tongue blade, cotton ball, tuning fork.	Brainstem lesions, pituitary lesions, cerebral vascular accidents, neoplasm, neurodegenerative disorders, Bell's palsy, Ménière's syndrome, acoustic neuromas, schwannoma, local trauma
Motor 1. Gait 2. Bulk 3. Tone 4. Strength	CNS, PNS: Involves the cortical motor strip, pyramidal tracts, cerebellum and spinal cord as well as the innervation of peripheral muscles.	*Observation:* Is there a normal gait? Does she walk straight? Does she need an assistive device? Is her stance wide based? Do her feet leave the floor? Are involuntary movements present? Is muscle tone normal?	Cerebral vascular accidents, spinal cord injury, demyelinating disorders such as multiple sclerosis, transverse myelitis, neurodegenerative-normal pressure hydrocephalus, multisystem atrophy, Parkinson's disease, familial ataxic disorders, neuromuscular disorders such as amyotrophic lateral sclerosis
Sensory/Reflex 1. Light touch 2. Superficial pain 3. Temperature 4. Proprioception 5. Vibratory sense 6. Muscle stretch reflex Superficial reflex Pathologic reflex	CNS, PNS: Involves spinothalamic tracts, postcentral gyrus, parietal lobe, dermatomes.	*Examination:* Necessary equipment includes cotton ball, lancet (or other disposable sharp object), test tubes with disparate temperature liquid, and tuning fork, reflex hammer.	Spinal cord injury, polyneuropathy (B_{12} deficiency, anemias, diabetes), neurodegenerative disorders, cerebral vascular accidents, coma
Elimination 1. Bowel 2. Bladder	CNS, ANS 1. ANS: spinal nerves S_3–S_5, cortical areas 2. ANS: spinal nerves T_9–L_2, S_4, cortical areas	*Examination:* Check for incontinence or impaction, assess muscle tone and sensation, bladder scan for postvoid residual.	Spinal cord injury, cerebral vascular accident

In the geriatric population, the use of anticoagulant mediation is common. The use of an anticoagulant, in the presence of fall risk, can lead to a subdural hematoma if the patient were to fall and strike his head. The nurse must evaluate the fall potential of all older patients who are on anticoagulant medication.

Mental Status Examination

Older patients generally have normal levels of consciousness and are alert. It is an abnormal finding if the patient is not oriented to situation, time, and place (Sirven & Mancall, 2002). Similarly, it is an abnormal finding if the patient has difficulty with calculations or impaired judgment. Remote and recent memory are normal; however, the processing speed and information retrieval capability are slowed (Sirven & Mancall, 2002; Whitney et al., 2004). Therefore, if problems are noted with speech and language, underlying pathology must be considered. Mood and affect should be evaluated. Two questions to ask are "During the past month have you been bothered by feeling sad, depressed, or hopeless?" and "During the past month have you often been bothered by decreased interest or pleasure in doing things?" These questions have 96% sensitivity for detecting major depression, signifying the need for further follow-up (Johnston, Covinsky, & Landefeld, 2005).

Cranial Nerve Assessment of the Elderly

Cranial assessment of the elderly provides a basis for a functional assessment, which provides data regarding possible and potential impairments as well as ability to care for self.

Cranial Nerve	Comment
CN I	Deficits are common with aging (Larner, 2006).
CN II	Presbyopia. Depth, motion perception, and contrast sensitivity decreased (Larner, 2006).
CNs III, IV, VI	Pupils are generally smaller, known as *senile myosis*, and reflexes to light and accommodation become slower. This is due to aging changes in the muscles of the sphincter pupillae and lens, not neurological changes. Restricted upward motion may also result in convergence difficulties (Benassi, D'Alessandro, Gallassi, Morreale, & Lugaresi, 1990; Larner, 2006).
CN V	Decreased lacrimal secretions (Hobdell et al., 2004).
CN VII	Presbycusis (a progressive bilaterally perceptive hearing loss) (Larner, 2006).
CNs VII, IX, X	Decreased taste bud number, but increased perception of salty, sweet, sour, and bitter (Hobdell et al., 2004).
CN XI	Delay in swallowing (Hobdell et al., 2004).

Motor Examination

Muscle tone can alter with age, with increased tone being the most common. Strength is preserved except for a mild reduction in power proximally with advancing age (Sirven & Mancall, 2002). Action tremors often occur; however, they are not a normal aspect of aging. Motor reaction time is decreased with older age (Sirven & Mancall, 2002).

Sensory Examination

The most common expression of aging seen on the neurological examination is in the sensory evaluation. Impairment of loss of vibratory sense in the distal aspect of the lower extremities is a well-known finding. Conversely, proprioception is preserved. Decreases in two-point discrimination and stereognosis have been reported, but are not well characterized (Sirven & Mancall, 2002).

Reflex Examination

Muscle stretch reflexes are generally preserved in the elderly, and absence or asymmetry generally indicates disease. Decreased or absence of ankle jerks are common but thought to be due to Achilles tendon inelasticity versus true neurological change (Sirven & Mancall, 2002). Superficial reflexes may be diminished or absent, likely due to other causes such as pregnancies, history of abdominal surgery, and the like. The snout reflex may return, and is not considered pathologic. However, the suck and grasp reflex are indicative of frontal lobe disease.

Summary

The neurological assessment of a patient begins in the same fashion as any other type of system assessment, and that is with the history. The examination consists of the evaluation of cognition, cranial nerves, motor function, sensation, and reflexes. The techniques described in this chapter will assist the nurse in the incorporation of the nursing process and the development of a problem list and a plan of care.

NCLEX® REVIEW

1. The nurse, providing care to a patient with multiple sclerosis, realizes the patient has a disorder within which of the following areas of the neurological system?
   1. Central nervous system
   2. Peripheral nervous system
   3. Sympathetic nervous system
   4. Autonomic nervous system

2. The nurse is assessing a patient who is demonstrating a neurological disorder. In which area of the health history would the nurse document current medications?
   1. Presenting problem
   2. History of presenting problem
   3. Medication history
   4. Past medical history

3. While assessing a patient's neurological status, the nurse notes the patient is unable to move his head from left to right. This finding could indicate a disorder with which of the following cranial nerves?
   1. Vagus
   2. Hypoglossal
   3. Spinal accessory
   4. Facial

4. While assessing a patient's neurological status, the nurse uses the Glasgow Coma Scale. For which part of the mental status examination is this tool most likely used?
   1. Level of consciousness
   2. Language
   3. Memory
   4. Attention

5. After assessing a patient's patellar reflex, the nurse documents +2 on the patient's medical record. This document indicates the patient's reflex is:
   1. Indicative of disease.
   2. More brisk.
   3. Normal.
   4. Diminished.

6. The nurse is going to assess for the presence of a Babinski reflex. Which of the following will the nurse use to assess this reflex?
   1. Rubber triangle end of the reflex hammer
   2. Handle of the reflex hammer
   3. Safety pin
   4. Cotton swab

7. While assessing an elderly patient's cranial nerves, the nurse notes a sluggish pupilary response to light and accommodation. This finding could be indicative of:
   1. Cranial frontal lobe disease.
   2. Cerebellar disease.
   3. A pending stroke.
   4. Nothing; this can be a normal finding.

Answers for review questions appear in Appendix D

KEY TERMS

anisocoria *p.704*
anosmia *p.702*
apathetic *p.701*
aphasia *p.702*
Battle's sign *p.699*
conjugate gaze *p.704*
decerebrate posturing *p.706*
decorticate posturing *p.706*
doll's eye reflex *p.704*
dysconjugate gaze *p.704*

dysphoria *p.701*
euphoria *p.701*
euthymia *p.701*
exophthalmos *p.704*
fasciculation *p.705*
gingival hyperplasia *p.699*
macrocephalic *p.699*
masked facies *p.699*
microcephalic *p.699*

neuron *p.694*
nystagmus *p.704*
oculocephalic reflex *p.704*
oculovestibular reflex *p.704*
proprioception *p.708*
proptosis *p.704*
ptosis *p.704*
raccoon sign (eyes) *p.699*
synapse *p.694*

REFERENCES

American Association of Neuroscience Nurses. (2007). *Neurological assessment of the older adult: A guide for nurses.* Glenview, IL: Author.

American Nurses' Association. (2002). *Scope and standards of neuroscience nursing practice.* Silver Spring, MD: Author.

Centers for Disease Control and Prevention. (2007). Prevalence of stroke—United States, 2005. *Morbidity and Mortality Weekly Report.* Retrieved April 15, 2008, from http://www.cdc.gov/MMWR/previdw/mmwrhtml/mm5619a2.htm

Dictionary of Cell and Molecular Biology. (2008). Confusion. Retrieved June 24, 2008, from the Centre for Cancer Education, University of Newcastle, website: http://cancerweb.ncl.ac.uk/cgi-bin/omd?confusion

Digre, K. B., & Corbett, J. B. (2003). *Practical viewing of the optic disc.* New York: Butterworth-Heinemann.

Fuller, G. (2004). *Neurological examination made easy* (3rd ed.). Philadelphia, PA: Churchill Livingstone.

Johnston, C. B., Covinsky, K. E., & Landefeld, S. (2005). Geriatric medicine. In L. M. Tierney, Jr., S. J. McPhee, & M. A. Papadakis (Eds.), *Current medical diagnosis and treatment.* New York: Lange.

Joute, A., Corpechot, C., & Ducros, A. (1996). Notch 3 mutations in CADASIL, a hereditary adult-onset condition causing stroke and dementia. *Nature, 383,* 707–710.

Luzzi, S., Snowden, J. S., Neary, D., Coccia, M., Provinciali, L., & Lambon, R. (2007). Distinct patterns of olfactory impairment in Alzheimer's disease, semantic dementia, frontotemporal dementia, and corticobasal degeneration. *Neuropsychologia, 45*(8), 1826–1831.

Newman, M. F. (2007). Open heart surgery and cognitive decline. *Cleveland Clinic Journal of Medicine, 74*(1) 52–55.

Pepper, G. A. (2006). Critical care patient with special needs: Geriatric patients. In J. G. Alspach (Ed.), *Core curriculum for critical care nurses* (6th ed.). Philadelphia: W. B. Saunders.

Reyes, P. F., Nowak, L. A., & Rice, S. G. (2006). Alzheimer's disease: Clinical diagnosis and treatment. *Barrow Quarterly, 22*(1), 9–15.

Sirven, J. I., & Mancall, E. (2002). Neurological examination of the older adult. In J. I. Sirven & B. L. Malamut (Eds.), *Clinical neurology of the older adult.* Philadelphia: Lippincott.

Stewart-Amidei, C. (2006). Why bother with practice guidelines? *Journal of Neuroscience Nursing. 38:*3.

Teasdale, G., & Jennett, B. (1974). Assessment of coma and impaired consciousness: A practical scale. *Lancet, 2,* 81.

Thomas, C. L. (Ed.), (1997). *Taber's cyclopedic medical dictionary.* Philadelphia: F. A. Davis.

Victor, M., & Ropper, A. (2001). *Adams and Victor's principles of neurology* (7th ed.). New York: McGraw-Hill.

Whitney, F., Pugh, D., & Mortimer, D. (2004). Geriatric issues. In M. K. Bader & L. R. Littlejohn (Eds.), *AANN core curriculum for neuroscience nursing* (4th ed.). St. Louis, MO: W. B. Saunders.

Wijdicks, E. F., Bamlet, W. R., Maramattom, B. V., Manno, E. M., & McClelland, R. L. (2005). Validation of a new coma scale: The FOUR Score. *Annals of Neurology, 58*(4), 585–593.

Wilson-Pauwels, L., Akesson, E. J., Stewart, P. A., & Spacey, S. D. (2002). *Cranial nerves in health and disease* (2nd ed.). Hamilton, Ontario: BC Decker.

World Health Organization. (2007). *Weekly epidemiological record.* No. 12, *82,* 93–194.

Ziegler, D., Siekeirka-Kleiser, E., & Schweers, M., (2005). Validation of a novel screening device (NeuroQuick) for quantitative assessment of small nerve fiber dysfunction as an early feature of diabetic polyneuropathy. *Diabetes Care, 28*(5), 1169–1174.

29

Caring for the Patient with Acute Brain Disorders

Denita Ryan

Outcome-Based Learning Objectives

After studying this chapter, the learner will be able to:

1. Describe basic pathophysiology of increased intracranial pressure as presented in this chapter.
2. List possible signs or symptoms of increased intracranial pressure.
3. Explain rationale of nursing interventions in caring for patients with increased intracranial pressure.
4. Identify various types and causes of head trauma according to level of injury.
5. Compare and contrast differences between bacterial meningitis and viral meningitis, including causes, signs and symptoms, diagnostic evaluation, and treatment.
6. Identify and distinguish between the major types of brain tumors: intra-axial, extra-axial, and metastatic.
7. Explain treatment options for brain tumors.
8. Explain the role of the nurse in family teaching of patients with acute brain disorders.

Research Collaboration Health Promotion Nursing Process Caring Critical Thinking

ACUTE BRAIN disorders include a wide range of conditions, such as traumatic injuries, brain tumors, and infectious diseases of the brain. Each of these disorders may affect not just the central nervous system, but every other system of the body as well. The symptoms of the disorders have a tremendous effect on not only the patient, but also on family, friends, and their community.

Intracranial Pressure

An important and underlying physiological concept in the care of any patient with an acute neurological disorder is that of **intracranial pressure (ICP)** or pressure in the head and the mechanisms of its alteration. Any disorder of the brain can cause an increase in intracranial pressure, which may have wide-reaching effects on the patient's neurological status and overall health.

Healers throughout history have known, or at least suspected, that pressure in the head causes harmful outcomes. Trepanations, or the creation of holes in the skull, were apparently performed for thousands of years to relieve pressure in the brain. A historic archeological find in France discovered 120 skulls, 40 of which had been trepanned. The trepanation tools found in Europe were thought to be 4,000 to 5,000 years old. Trepanations have also been attributed to the Incas and a large number of other ancient civilizations throughout the world (Walker, 1967). Hippocrates acknowledged in his early writings on ancient medicine

that relieving pressure in the head must be done to relieve "dropsy of the brain" (Key, Rothrock, & Falk, 1997).

Monro-Kellie Doctrine

Monro wrote in 1783 "brine enclosed in a case of bone ... the substance of the brain ... is nearly incompressible, the quantity of blood in the head must be the same ... those cases only excepted in which water or other matter is effused or secreted from the blood vessels, for in these, a quantity of blood, equal in bulk to the effused matter will be pressed out of the cranium" (cited in Maramou & Beaumont, 2004). This statement became the precursor to the **Monro-Kellie doctrine**, which is the foundation for understanding increased ICP. The Monro-Kellie doctrine has two basic tenets. The first tenet is the relative incompressibility of the intracranial contents, such as the brain tissue, blood, and cerebrospinal fluid (CSF). The second basic tenet is that changes in the volume of one component must cause a reciprocal change in the other components (Maramou, 1996). Once the sutures in the developing cranium become closed, the brain is sealed within a nonexpandable vault.

In some instances brain volume actually decreases. This can occur, for instance, as part of the normal aging process, and it is detected on imaging studies of the brain as cerebral atrophy. The Monro-Kellie doctrine, however, holds true in this condition as well, with the amount of CSF usually increasing to offset the decreasing brain volume.

Pathophysiology

The fixed nature of the skull is the reason that the volume of its contents, brain tissue, blood, and CSF must remain constant. If the volume of any one of the three components of the brain changes, the volume of the other components also may change (be displaced), but the total volume will not change. ICP is the pressure exerted within the skull, in association with the volume of its three components: brain tissue, blood, and CSF. A normal ICP ranges from 0 to 15 mmHg. Brain tissue itself, known as the parenchyma, is a relatively fixed mass. Thus, the presence of a space-occupying lesion, such as a hematoma, tumor, hydrocephalus, or edema, will ultimately cause compression and/or displacement of the two other components, the vasculature and CSF. The body has several compensatory mechanisms that it can access to adapt to changes.

Compensatory Mechanisms

In order for the brain to maintain a normal ICP, attempts are made to compensate for changes in any of the three components within the brain. Initial mechanisms may include changing the volume of CSF by decreasing production or altering absorption. A decrease in brain tissue may be exhibited by the compression of tissue. Alterations in blood volume may occur as a result of local changes in cerebral vasculature, cerebral perfusion pressure, and cerebral blood flow.

Cerebral Blood Flow

Cerebral blood flow (CBF) is the amount of blood that passes through 100 grams of brain tissue in 1 minute. Normal CBF is approximately 50 mL per minute per 100 grams of brain tissue. Because the brain has a high requirement for the oxygen and glucose found in blood, the maintenance of an adequate level is extremely important. The brain utilizes 20% of the body's oxygen, and 25% of its glucose supply. The brain has the ability to alter its blood flow in response to its needs for oxygen and glucose. The process by which this is done is referred to as **autoregulation**. Autoregulation is defined as the process by which the brain is able to alter its vasculature to accommodate changes in ICP.

Cerebral Perfusion Pressure

Cerebral perfusion pressure (CPP) is defined as the pressure gradient that drives cerebral blood flow. It is the amount of pressure needed to provide adequate blood flow to the brain. The purpose of autoregulation is to provide consistent CBF to ensure adequate CPP to meet the metabolic needs of the brain. When the systemic arterial blood pressure is normal, and ICP is normal, there is very little difference between the mean arterial blood pressure (MAP) and the CPP. In the damaged brain however, the compensatory mechanisms that usually preserve CPP are compromised (Feldman & Robertson, 1997). The initial mechanisms used by the various components within the brain to maintain normal ICP begin to fail. Chart 29–1 shows the calculations used to determine CPP.

When the CPP decreases, CBF also decreases due to failure of autoregulation. Normal CPP is 70 to 100. As the CBF and CPP

CHART 29–1   Calculation of Cerebral Perfusion Pressure

CPP = MAP − ICP

MAP = DBP + 1/3 (SBP − DP)

  where
    CPP = cerebral perfusion pressure
    MAP = mean arterial blood pressure
    ICP = intracranial pressure
    DBP = diastolic blood pressure
    SBP = systolic blood pressure.

Normal CPP = 70–100 mmHg

Normal ICP = 0–15 mmHg

fall, neuronal ischemia, or lack of oxygen to nerve cells, and death occur. CPP of 50 to 60 mmHg is necessary to adequately perfuse brain tissue. CPP of less than 30 is considered incompatible with neuronal life.

In a normal brain, autoregulation maintains adequate tissue perfusion by adjusting metabolic needs and by altering cerebral vasculature, either by vasoconstriction or vasodilation. These adjustments are made to maintain normal ICPs. When ICP is elevated, it is of utmost importance to maintain an adequate MAP. Though CPP strives to maintain adequate tissue perfusion, this may not be the case in all areas of the brain. The damaged brain may have areas of increased edema, causing a localized area of limited tissue perfusion, resulting in ischemia and further neurological compromise.

Increased Intracranial Pressure

Increased ICP is caused by an increase in the volume of any of the intracranial compartments. Many conditions can cause an increase in ICP (Chart 29–2). Examples of these are craniocerebral trauma (blood), vascular abnormalities, tumors, or edema. ICPs are considered elevated when sustained at greater than 20 mmHg.

At approximately 25 mmHg, increased ICPs become evident by decreased CBF, decreased CPP, and distortion of brain tissue (Geraci & Geraci, 1996). Increased ICPs are associated with increased mortality and morbidity. In the presence of increased ICP, many events take place to perpetuate the process. The **vasodilatory cascade** is a series of events triggered by hypoxia, with the result being increased ICP. Common causes of hypoxia are decreased blood volume and decreased respiratory effort. Hypoxia, from any cause, is a potent vasodilator. Vasodilation

CHART 29–2   Conditions Associated with Increased ICP

Intracranial tumors

Hematomas

Stroke

Subarachnoid hemorrhage

Hydrocephalus

Abscess

TBI

stimulates increased CBF and increased ICP. In acute brain injury, the common pathway toward the progression of increased ICP is the failure of the oxygen delivery system, or ischemia (Andrews, 2005) (Figure 29–1 ■).

Cerebral Edema

Several pathological conditions affect the brain tissue, or parenchyma. It is rare, however, that these conditions occur in the absence of effect on the other components, that is, the CSF and the vasculature. The most typical process capable of increasing brain tissue volume is cerebral edema. **Cerebral edema** is defined as an increase in the water content of the brain. There are two separate forms of cerebral edema: cytotoxic and vasogenic.

Cytotoxic edema is the accumulation of intracellular water. This type of edema occurs as a result of a hypoxic, or possibly toxic event, which damages the cells' ability to pump water out of the intracellular space. Examples include anoxic events such as cardiac arrest or asphyxiation. It is also seen in severe water intoxication due to hyponatremia. This process may or may not be reversible (Farrell & Bower, 2003; Quinn, 2008; Smith & McIntosh, 1996). **Vasogenic edema** represents an alteration in vascular permeability, with disruption of the blood–brain barrier. This results in increased extracellular space. Vasogenic edema frequently is seen in neoplastic diseases, and may be treated with corticosteroids, such as dexamethasone. It also may be treated with osmotic agents such as mannitol.

Cytotoxic edema and vasogenic edema may be seen together. An example of this is a malignant brain tumor in which vasogenic edema exists, causing increased ICP. This in turn decreases tissue perfusion, causing hypoxia to the brain, resulting in cytotoxic edema. Regardless of the process, an increase in brain mass mandates the displacement of other components, which results in increasing ICPs.

Herniation Syndromes

When cerebral edema occurs as a result of a space-occupying lesion, such as a tumor or a hematoma, the pressure exerted on surrounding tissue may not be evenly distributed. The result is a movement of brain mass from an area of high pressure to an area of lower pressure. This movement of brain tissue is referred to as mass effect. The term **herniation** refers to the protrusion of brain structures under pressure into areas causing compression and damage of the brain tissue, with possible catastrophic results. The three most common forms of herniation are cingulate, transtentorial, and uncal and are described by Plum and Posner in their early works and most recent editions (Plum and Posner, 1980; Posner, Saper, Schiff, & Plum, 2007). Herniation syndromes are shown in Figure 29–2 ■.

Cingulate Herniation
Cingulate herniation, also referred to as falcine herniation, is caused by an expanding lesion located in one hemisphere that shifts toward the opposite hemisphere, forcing the cingulate gyrus under the falx cerebri and displacing it to the opposite side. This shift causes displacement of the local blood supply, resulting in compression of the local blood supply, often that of the anterior cerebral artery. Cerebral edema, local cerebral tissue ischemia, and increased ICP follow. Cingulated herniation is common in head trauma and brain tumors; the signs and symptoms are dependent on the specific location affected.

Transtentorial Herniation
Transtentorial herniation, also referred to as central herniation, is caused by lesions that precipitate downward displacement of the cerebral hemispheres, the basal ganglia, the diencephalons, and the brainstem through the tentorial notch (Posner et al., 2007). Cerebral edema, ischemia, and possibly hemorrhage may occur. Signs and symptoms of transtentorial herniation may include decreasing levels of consciousness, altered respiratory patterns, and contralateral motor weakness.

Uncal Herniation
The most common herniation syndrome is uncal herniation. Uncal herniation is caused by an expanding lesion, often located in the temporal lobe. Pressure is exerted across the midline, pushing the medial edge of the uncus into the edge of the tentorium. Brainstem compression may occur. The third cranial nerve (oculomotor nerve) may become compressed, causing ipsilateral pupillary abnormalities, such as a dilated pupil, a common early sign in uncal herniation (Posner et al., 2007).

Often, the first sign of impending uncal herniation is a sluggishly reactive pupil on the ipsilateral side of the lesion (Chart 29–3). This is an early sign, and may be present before any other clinical symptom. Later signs and symptoms of uncal herniation are contralateral hemiparesis, altered levels of consciousness, beginning with restlessness, and progressing through sleepiness, obtundation, and coma. Late signs are altered respiratory patterns, such as Cheyne-Stokes, or pathological positioning, such as decorticate or decerebrate positioning. Very late signs are dilated, fixed pupils.

FIGURE 29–1 ■ Progression of increased ICP.
Source: ISM/Phototake NYC

Normal

1. Herniation of cingulate gyrus under the falx

3. Downward displacement of the brain stem through notch

2. Herniation of the temporal lobe into the tentorial notch

Herniation syndromes

FIGURE 29–2 ■ Herniation syndromes.

CHART 29–3	**Pupillary Changes Associated with Herniation**
Location of Herniation	**Pupillary Change**
Compression on CN III	Unilateral dilating pupil Sluggishly reactive Usually ipsilateral to lesion
Compression on midbrain to upper pons	Midposition Fixed
Compression on lower pons to upper medullary	Midposition Fixed
Compression on medulla	Dilated Fixed

Urgent surgical intervention to decompress the brain is often the treatment of choice. This may include surgical resection of a mass lesion with or without craniectomy (removal of the bone flap) to allow the brain to swell. Often an intermediate intervention is the placement of a ventriculostomy (catheter placed within the ventricles to drain the CSF) to relieve pressure by allowing CSF to travel another path of less resistance. It also is a valuable tool to measure the ICP. Prior to surgical treatment, hyperosmolar drugs, such as mannitol, can be used to decrease extracellular volume as a temporizing measure.

Herniation syndromes are life-threatening neurological emergencies that, left untreated, can progress rapidly to death. Nursing intervention is aimed at prevention by careful monitoring of neurological status and early recognition of impending problems.

New onset of restlessness, agitation, or confusion may be early signs of increased ICP and possible impending herniation. Monitor neurological assessment hourly, and notify MD of any changes in neurological status.

Clinical Manifestations

The effect of increased ICP on the brain and the corresponding neurological exam is dependent on several common factors: the rate of the pressure increase and the location within the brain that is exerting the pressure. Different parts of the brain, such as the brainstem, are less tolerant of pressure increases than others. The rate and location of pressure increase are reflected in the patient's neurological examination, as well as other body systems.

A complete neurological assessment as described in Chapter 28 🖙 is essential to detecting increasing ICP. Alterations in the patient's level of consciousness (LOC) are usually the first sign of impending changes. These changes may be subtle, such as restlessness or slight confusion. They also may be catastrophic, presenting as coma or even death. The earlier the change is detected and treated, the better the prognosis.

Changes in the cranial nerve exam also may be an early sign of increased ICP. Pressure on the oculomotor nerve (CN III) may result in the impaired ability of the pupil on the affected side to constrict, resulting in a dilated, unreactive (or slow-reacting) pupil. Decrease in motor function with presenting weakness in the extremities also may result, depending on the location of the pressure.

Unrelieved increased ICPs may result in pathologic posturing of the body. These may be seen when a patient no longer is able to follow commands or display purposeful movements. Decorticate (flexor) positioning is described as flexion of the arms and wrists in an adduction posture when the patient is exposed to noxious stimuli, such as pain. A more ominous sign is seen with decerebrate (extensor) posturing. This is seen when all four extremities are in rigid extension, with outward pronation of the forearms, and plantar flexion of the feet, when exposed to noxious stimuli. Both of these postures are indicators of brainstem damage and may indicate more serious conditions, such as herniation.

Other signs, such as headache and vomiting, are less specific. Headaches are generally not a specific indication of ICP problems. Headaches that are "different," such as more severe, unrelenting, and not responsive to modalities that are usually effective, may warrant notification of the health care provider. An example of a "different" headache is one that is "worse in the morning," which may be present with tumors in the posterior fossa. Vomiting, without prior nausea, may be an indication of increased ICP. Vomiting may be without warning, and projectile.

Changes in vital signs may be caused by pressure on the brainstem and/or the hypothalamus. They may be seen as increasing systolic pressure (widening pulse pressure), bradycardia, and/or irregular respiratory patterns. These are known as **Cushing's triad** and are a late indicator of increased ICP. Alterations in respiratory patterns may be a sign of impending neurological decline, especially when associated with a decrease in LOC.

Medical Management

The major goal of medical management of ICP is the prevention of secondary injury due to cerebral edema and increased ICP. This is accomplished by close monitoring of the ICP. The management of increased ICP requires an understanding of the various compensatory systems involved in the regulation of ICP. The goal is the monitoring of ICP dynamics, identifying normal and abnormal values, and the correction of abnormal values. Systemic blood pressure, ICP, volume status, and oxygenation must all be known to provide adequate management. Treatment may be medical or surgical.

Various modalities are available to determine, monitor, and treat ICP. These vary by institution and by health care provider preference. Examples of these are external ventricular drains (EVDs) and parenchymal wires or bolts. An EVD is a catheter placed into the ventricle and connected to a continuous monitoring device. The EVD allows the practitioner to monitor ICP at any given time, including trends. It also allows drainage of excess CSF if necessary to lower the ICP. Another purpose of the EVD is to allow the practitioner to collect CSF for the purpose of sending it to a laboratory for evaluation. The desired range of ICP is 0 to 15 mmHg.

Other monitoring devices also can be used to monitor ICP. In most institutions, the EVD described above is the most commonly used intervention, but it also is possible to place a monitoring device into the brain tissue, or parenchyma, to monitor ICP. Although it is easier to place than an EVD, it is less accurate and allows only monitoring of pressure, without the possibility of CSF drainage that is possible with an EVD (Bader, 2006a). Placement of monitoring devices, such as a catheter or bolt into the ventricle, or the brain parenchyma, usually is done in an intensive care setting, emergency room, or operating room. It usually is reserved for patients with decreased LOC or ones in which elevated ICPs are suspected. Although there are many advantages to the placement of these monitoring devices, they are both invasive and require an intensive level of nursing care.

One type of noninvasive monitoring device is the pupillometer. This is a small, handheld device that measures the dynamics of pupil reactivity. The idea is that patients with ICPs higher than 20 mmHg are thought to have lower constriction velocities than those with normal ICPs. This device is used in limited markets at this time, and data are being collected regarding its use. At this time, the pupillometer is being used in some institutions as a supplemental monitoring device (Bader, 2006b).

Another type of monitoring device is the brain tissue oxygen monitor, which may be used in conjunction with other methods of monitoring. The purpose is to recognize and treat ischemic injuries to the brain. Following an insult to the brain, compensatory mechanisms attempt to maintain autoregulation. The two most frequent causes of secondary injury are hypotension and hypoxia. Therefore, the measurement of oxygenation in brain tissue ($PbtO_2$) leads to valuable information regarding the supply and demand of oxygen within the brain. Measurement of $PbtO_2$ is accomplished by the placement of an oxygen-sensitive probe into the brain tissue. This probe is able to monitor both the level of oxygen and the temperature of the brain tissue. The probe must be placed in healthy tissue, not in area of damage or injury. The measurements are displayed in millimeters of mercury. The type of system used to measure $PbtO_2$ impacts the range of normal levels. However, lower levels of $PbtO_2$ correspond with lower levels of tissue oxygenation, translating to poor neurological outcome.

Jugular bulb venous oxygenation saturation is another method of monitoring cerebral oxygenation. This method consists of a catheter inserted into the jugular bulb of the internal jugular vein. The purpose is to obtain a continuous measurement of jugular venous oxygen saturation (SjO_2). This method provides a measurement of the oxygen saturation of venous blood leaving the brain. The goal of the measurement of SjO_2 is early identification of cerebral hypoxia. A low SjO_2 saturation (less than 54%) is indicative of ischemia (Bader, 2006a). However, measurements are not indicative of specific areas of cerebral tissue oxygenation, but are global readings.

The cerebral microdialysis system is being researched for its effectiveness as a method for measuring extracellular levels of cerebral metabolites. Energy metabolites, such as glucose, pyruvate, lactate, and glycerol, and amino acids, such as aspartate and glutamate, are produced when the brain experiences ischemia (Sarrafzadeh et al., 2002). A tiny microcatheter is inserted into the brain parenchyma, and a dialysate fluid is pumped into the brain. The dialysate fluid is recovered at set intervals and analyzed for levels of chemical metabolites. Changes in the cerebral metabolites indicate the presence of cerebral ischemia, with or without tissue damage. Microdialysis is an emerging technology, but at this point, not widely used. It is an area in which more research is needed (Bader, 2006a).

Various pharmacologic agents may also be used in the management of ICP. Hyperosmotic fluids, such as mannitol or hypertonic saline solutions, can be used to decrease ICP. These are effective in that they move water from cerebral tissue into the circulation. Hemodilution of red blood cells (RBCs) occurs, reducing viscosity and allowing more blood flow to occur within smaller vessels. Vasoconstriction follows, which decreases ICP. It is important to closely monitor the patient's fluid status, including electrolytes and serum osmolality, to avoid negative fluid balance.

Maintenance of adequate vascular volume is of utmost importance in the maintenance of adequate CPP. Central venous catheters and pulmonary artery catheters also may be used to adequately monitor volume status. Also important in the management of CPP is close monitoring of arterial blood pressure with the use of an arterial line. Vasopressors such as phenylephrine and dopamine may be necessary to elevate the systemic arterial blood pressure to support adequate CPP. The goal of treatment is based on the relationship of ICP and CPP.

Patients at risk for neurological deterioration due to ICPs refractory to other methods of treatment may be placed in a barbiturate coma. Patients are given a barbiturate such as pentobarbital, via a loading dose, then a maintenance dose. This method is used in order to decrease LOC, thus decreasing cerebral metabolic needs. The negative aspect of barbiturate coma is that the neurological assessment, including the most basic reflexes, such as gag, swallow, and cough, are lost. The patient in pentobarbital coma must be mechanically ventilated, with intensive nursing care. It also is necessary to monitor patients in pentobarbital coma with continuous electroencephalography (EEG) monitoring. This is done to ensure proper barbiturate dosage. The EEG pattern that is used to regulate appropriate dosing is called burst suppression (BS). The BS pattern is a characteristic signal in the EEG. It is recognized by a period pattern of low voltage of less than 10 μv and a relatively shorter pattern

of higher amplitude complexes. The BS pattern is classified as an EEG abnormality because of its relation to severe encephalopathy. It can be generalized or lateralized. Depending on the initial cause, the state is reversible in some instances (Burst Suppression Tutorial, 2003). The BS pattern may indicate that the barbiturate dose is adequate to suppress brain activity. Continuous monitoring of ICP and hemodynamic and respiratory functions also is vital.

Other, less aggressive means of sedation, such as use of propofol, can be used to keep patients' pain and/or anxiety under control. The goal of sedation is to decrease ICP, CBF, and oxygen demand. Propofol has a short half-life, allowing practitioners to suspend infusion temporarily to accurately assess neurological status.

In some circumstances the best method of treating increased ICP is surgical intervention. In cases of extreme cerebral edema, a hemicraniectomy may be performed. This is a surgical procedure in which a portion of the skull (bone flap) is removed. This method allows room for the swollen brain, lessening the risk for brain tissue damage. The bone flap often is replaced 2 to 4 months later when the patient's condition has stabilized.

■ Nursing Management

The nursing management of patients with elevated ICP is complex and requires constant vigilance in terms of the neurological exam and trending of monitoring data. An increased ICP affects the brain's overall function and leads to dysfunction in many body systems, including the respiratory, cardiovascular, metabolic, and neurological systems. Therefore, nursing assessment of ICP management must encompass all of these systems.

Assessment

Any patient with neurological compromise must be assessed for adequate respiratory function. Patients with a decreased LOC may have a decreased level of respiratory function. Adequate oxygenation is essential to neurological function. Patients with a Glasgow Coma Scale (GCS) score of 8 or less should be considered for intubation, with possible mechanical ventilation. The GCS is a scale that measures the level of consciousness and is explained in detail in Chapter 28 ⬀. Pulse oximetry should be used with supplemental oxygen to maintain oxygen saturations of 95% or greater.

Normocapnia, the normal level of carbon dioxide in the blood, is an important nursing implication. In the past, hypocapnia was the standard of care after head injury. However, recent studies have shown that aggressive hyperventilation and hypocapnia ($PaCO_2 < 30$ mmHg) may actually aggravate secondary brain injury. This occurs through a process where the brain compensates for decreased levels of carbon dioxide, altering the pH of the CSF and initiating autoregulatory responses (Wong, 2000). Ultimately, this leads to increased CBF, increased ICP, decreased CPP, and decreased oxygen to the already ischemic brain tissue (see Figure 29–1 ■, p. 716).

The role of hyperventilation in the management of early brain injury is limited. Prophylactic use of hyperventilation should be avoided. Normocapnia (i.e., PCO_2 values between 35 and 40 mmHg) is recommended to avoid further brain injury. Another important nursing implication is that of monitoring and maintaining the patient in a euglycemic state. Brain trauma induces the increased release of glutamate, which increases cerebral metabolism. This, in turn, increases the metabolic breakdown of glucose, the major energy source for the brain. Decreased CBF results in inadequate oxygen delivery for the increased cerebral demands. This process leads to tissue acidosis, ischemia, and a worsened neurological outcome due to secondary injury.

Hyperglycemia in the setting of an ischemic brain has been shown to be an independent predictor of poor outcome. The goal of nursing is to maintain a normal blood glucose level. Blood levels should be monitored closely, approximately every 4 hours or less. Insulin should be administered to keep the blood levels within parameters associated with normal blood glucose levels, usually between 80 and 120 mg/dL.

Normothermia, the normal body temperature, is another important implication for nursing. Fever is a relatively common finding in neurological patients. It is estimated that between 70% and 100% of patients with traumatic brain injury experience fever during their hospitalization (McIlvoy, 2005). Increases in body temperature may increase metabolic demands, causing an increase in CBF, cerebral blood volume, and ICP. Hyperthermia may lead to ischemia and further brain injury. It is understood that fever in patients with neurological injury is associated with poor outcomes (Thompson, Kirkness, Mitchell, & Webb, 2007). Nursing interventions in maintenance of normal temperature include close monitoring of the patient's temperature. Measuring accurate core temperature is essential, and may require taking rectal temperatures, unless more accurate methods are available. Treatment should be considered as early as a temperature of 37.5°C (99.5°F). Cooling mechanisms may be implemented, if necessary. These include ice packs, cooling blankets, or bathing with tepid water. Care should be taken to prevent the patient from shivering, because this raises temperatures and metabolic demands. Skin integrity also should be monitored closely. Use of acetaminophen is appropriate to lower temperature, if not contraindicated.

The maintenance of normal blood pressure also is an important nursing intervention. To prevent cerebral ischemia, adequate CBF is mandatory. Hypotension in the presence of brain trauma has a strong negative effect on outcome. Patients with hypotension (systolic blood pressure <90 mmHg) in the early phase of brain trauma demonstrate a mortality rate twice as high as those who remain normotensive (Carroll, 1994; Manley et al., 2001; Olson, 2006). Therefore, maintenance of adequate CPP (>60 mmHg) is imperative to prevent further brain injury. Invasive lines, such as arterial lines and Swan-Ganz catheters, may be warranted to adequately monitor blood pressure and hemodynamic status. If necessary, vasopressive or inotropic agents may be necessary to maintain adequate blood pressure. The nursing implications for the management of ICP are summarized in Chart 29–4.

Interventions and Rationales

Many studies have been done to explain the relationship of various nursing activities such as turning, suctioning, and bathing to ICP. Most activities demonstrate only transient increases in ICP; however, this suggests that nurses be aware of such tendencies for increasing ICP and to administer these activities cautiously. Fan (2004) suggests that head positioning in the brain-damaged patient has both positive and negative effects on ICP. The suggestion is that head positioning, both in terms of elevation and rotation, has a definite effect on ICP. Winkleman (2000) studied bed positioning in patients with head injuries and found that elevation of the head of the bed provided optimal CPP and ICP in adults with brain injuries not vascular in

---

CHART 29–4 **Nursing Implications and Interventions for Management of ICP**

Actual and Potential Problems	Nursing Action	Rationale for Action
Monitoring of ICP	Monitor ICP via EVD or other intracranial pressure device.	Maintenance of normal ICP is essential to prevent further brain injury.
Patient positioning	Keep head of bed at 30°. Maintain head and neck in neutral position.	Decreases resistance to venous return. Prevents pulmonary complications.
Euglycemia	Monitor blood glucose levels. Administer insulin when appropriate.	Prevents increased cerebral metabolic needs and resulting ischemia.
Normocapnia	Maintain PCO_2 between 35 and 40 mmHg.	Avoids hyperventilation and potential for rebound increase in ICP.
Normothermia	Monitor body temperature. Use cooling devices if necessary. Administer appropriate antipyretics, if warranted.	Normothermia protects cerebral metabolic needs.
Normotension	Monitor blood pressure, using arterial line, if necessary. Administer vasopressors or inotrope if indicated.	Hypotension increases mortality. Adequate blood pressure is necessary to maintain adequate CPP.
Adequate oxygenation	Monitor oxygen saturations. Maintain adequate oxygenation via pulmonary toilet. Prevent deep vein thrombosis (DVT) through use of sequential compression devices and ambulation as appropriate.	Increased oxygen demands of the brain require adequate oxygenation to prevent further cerebral hypoxia.
Regulate nursing activities	Decrease external stimulation. Coordinate activities, to limit stimulation.	Helps prevent increased ICP.

origin. However, it is recommended that head position be established on an individual basis, with the help of monitoring devices to avoid the possible elevation of ICP.

Traumatic Brain Injury

A damaged skull from the species *Australopithecus africanus*, found in South Africa, provides the first evidence of brain injury, in a murder committed more than 1 million years ago. In this case, the cause of death was probably skull fracture, caused by clubbing (Evans, 1996).

Injuries to the brain have long been considered fatal. In 1682, Younge published a literature review of all recorded medical literature dating from approximately 500 A.D., and found reports of only 100 patients who had survived a brain wound (Evans, 1996). As recently as the 1970s, approximately 90% of all patients with brain injuries died (Senelick & Dougherty, 2001).

Epidemiology and Etiology

Traumatic brain injury (TBI) is and has always been a major health problem globally. In the United States, the Centers for Disease Control and Prevention (CDC) estimate the incidence of patients with closed-head injuries admitted to hospitals is conservatively 1.5 million each year. Approximately 235,000 cases of TBI are admitted to hospitals every year, with approximately 50,000 deaths (CDC, 2007). Although the causes of TBI differ by region, gender, and age group, the largest number of TBI appears to be secondary to motor vehicle crashes, falls, and acts of violence, such as gunshot wounds and assault. Studies have shown that African American men have higher rates of brain injury than other groups. Penetrating head injuries in the United States, such as gunshot wounds and skull fractures, are estimated to be 12 per 100,000, the highest of any developed country in the world (Langlois, Rutland-Brown, & Thomas, 2006). Motor vehicle crashes account for the largest percentage, followed by acts of violence and auto–pedestrian collisions (Burnett et al., 2003). Military personnel in combat zones are most likely to sustain a TBI from a blast (Defense and Veterans Brain Injury Center, 2005). Males are 1.5 times as likely as females to sustain a TBI (Langlois, Rutland-Brown, & Walk, 2006). For some ethnic and socioeconomic groups, risk exposure for TBI is elevated in various ways:

- Increased exposure to physically demanding employment settings (such as construction and manual labor)
- Increased exposure to personal violence
- Increased exposure to older homes and vehicles
- Greater reliance on substandard housing (Evans, 1996; Mayo Clinic Staff, 2008).

The Risk Factors box summarizes the risks for TBI.

The direct and indirect costs of treatment and rehabilitation for TBI patients were estimated at about $60 billion in the United States in 2000 (Finkelstein, Corso, & Miller, 2006). The effect on the lives of the patient, the family, and the entire community is beyond comprehension and is impossible to calculate or predict.

RISK FACTORS for Traumatic Brain Injury

Age 18–25 or over age 70

Alcohol intake

Males (1.5:1)

Military

Participation in certain sports activities

Classification of Acute Head Trauma

Acute head trauma occurs in varying degrees of severity and complexity. It can range from minor scalp lacerations requiring little to no treatment, to severe TBIs resulting in prolonged hospitalization, permanent disabilities, or death.

Superficial Injuries

Injuries to the scalp are relatively common. Although usually minor, they must be carefully assessed and treated diligently. The degree of subsequent treatment is dependent on the extent and depth of the injury. The scalp consists of five layers that cover the skull (Figure 29–3 ■, p. 722). The skin, or dermal, layer contains hair and protects the scalp. The subcutaneous fascia is a fatty, vascular layer, and contains blood vessels that may bleed profusely. The galea aponeurotica is a thick, flexible, and fibrous tissue. The subgaleal space is below the galea, and is a potential space for blood to collect and form cephalohematomas, or "goose eggs." Below the subgaleal space is the periosteum, a thin layer of tissue, covering the skull.

The most common and least severe scalp injury is a simple abrasion. An abrasion is a simple scraping of the skin. It may bleed slightly. A contusion is a bruise of the skin. Treatments for both abrasions and contusions include a thorough cleansing of the wound with possible application of an antibiotic ointment.

Scalp lacerations account for a large number of emergency department visits. The scalp is extremely vascular, and exsanguination has been known to occur in extreme cases. This vascularity is what allows the scalp to heal well in most cases. With any scalp laceration, the possibility of an underlying skull fracture must be addressed. An accurate history of the event surrounding the injury is very important. Based on the mechanism of injury, if there is any reason to suspect a skull fracture, a computerized tomography (CT) scan or, at the very least, a plain x-ray of the skull should be obtained. Once the degree and extent of the scalp injury have been determined, the wound should be carefully cleaned with a standard skin-sterilizing solution, such as a povidone-iodine compound. The wound may require suturing and antibiotic ointment. In addition to a careful history of the event, the immunization history of the patient should be obtained, and a tetanus toxoid should be administered, if appropriate.

Skull Fractures

The skull, or calvarium, is the bony structure that houses the brain. It is composed of the frontal, parietal, temporal, and occipital bones. It also includes the multiple facial bones that make up the facial structure. Of these facial bones, only the mandible is movable. The skull itself is asymmetrical and varies in thickness. The temporal bone is the thinnest; the occipital bone is the thickest. The floor of the skull, known as the

FIGURE 29–3 ■ Cross section of skull.

currence of CSF leak, while not unexpected, must be reported to the health care provider because the patient is at high risk for meningitis.

> **CRITICAL ALERT** *The presence of CSF leaking from the nose (rhinorrhea) or ears (otorrhea) is a serious complication. The patient with CSF leak is at risk or meningitis. Place head of bed at 30 to 45 degrees (unless contraindicated) and call MD.*

Other characteristic signs and symptoms of basal skull fractures are Battle sign, which is ecchymosis, or bruising, over the mastoid bone (Figure 29–4 ■); bulging tympanic membranes; and the presence of raccoon eyes, or periorbital ecchymosis (Figure 29–5 ■). Cranial nerve deficits, due to damage to various cranial nerves, also may occur. Damage to the olfactory nerve (CN I) may result in decreased sense of smell. Visual deficits, due to damage to the optic nerve (CN II), facial weakness, due to damage to the facial nerve (CN VII), and decreased hearing, due to damage to the acoustic nerve (CN VIII), also may be seen.

• **Depressed skull fractures** are the displacement of a comminuted skull fracture (Figure 29–6 ■). They frequently are seen with other injuries to the brain, such as contusions and/or lacerations of the brain. The degree of neurological symptoms depends on the degree and location of brain involvement. Hair, dirt, and other debris may be found within the wound and present risk for infection.

Clinical Manifestations

Skull fractures alone do not cause neurological symptoms, but frequently they are seen in conjunction with other, more serious

skull base, is rough and uneven, attributing to an important role in brain injury. Skull fractures are categorized according to type of break and severity of the fracture as listed here:

• **Linear skull fractures** are the most common type of skull fracture. They are simple breaks in the continuity of bone, with no displacement, and most commonly are seen in low-velocity impact situations. Linear fractures of the temporal bone may result in a tear of the middle meningeal artery, resulting in more serious brain injury, such as an epidural hematoma.

• **Comminuted skull fractures** are fragmented interruptions of the skull resulting from multiple linear fractures. An area of bone depression at the point of impact is characteristic of a comminuted fracture.

• **Basal skull fractures** usually are an extension of a linear fracture into the skull base. The mechanism of injury generally is the same as linear skull fractures with a more serious result. The inner aspect of the skull is closely associated with the dura, the thin membrane that covers the brain. The skull base is rough and uneven, and its texture may cause tears to the delicate dura. Consequently, CSF may leak through the tear in the dura. This may result in CSF leaking from the nose or the ear. CSF leaking from the nose is called rhinorrhea. CSF leaking from the ear is called otorrhea. Drainage of CSF may be visualized directly, or may be seen on dressings or bed linens. It is distinguishable by its characteristic halo sign, which appears as blood with a yellow ring around it. The oc-

FIGURE 29–4 ■ Battle sign.

FIGURE 29–5 ■ Raccoon eyes.

FIGURE 29–6 ■ Depressed skull fracture.

brain injuries, such as hematomas or contusions. Clinical manifestations then are representative of the other brain injuries that may be present.

Laboratory and Diagnostic Procedures

Diagnosis of skull fractures can be made with plain skull x-rays. However, if a skull fracture is suspected based on the physical assessment and knowledge of the mechanism of injury, a CT scan of the head should be obtained, because the question of underlying brain trauma must be addressed. Fractures of the facial bones and basal skull fractures may be seen best with a thin-cut

CT scan. The Diagnostic Tests box provides more details about appropriate tests for skull fractures.

Medical Management

Treatment depends on the type of fracture. Linear fractures usually do not require treatment, other than close observation of the patient for neurological deterioration. Open or comminuted

DIAGNOSTIC TESTS for Acute Brain Disorders

Test	Expected Abnormality	Rationale for Abnormality
Plain skull films	Fracture lines, linear, basal, depressed, or comminuted	Skull fractures are best seen in plain films.
CT of head	Hematomas (SDH, EDH), contusions, hydrocephalus. Test is time sensitive, as the presence of blood (in SDH) changes characteristics with time	CT scans are best suited to examining presence of blood, edema, CSF.
MRI	DAI (late) tumors	MRI will demonstrate small lesions not seen on CT scan. Best suited to demonstrate heterogeneity of tumors.
Lumbar puncture	Blood in CSF (subarachnoid blood) Abnormalities in fluid chemistry	**Contraindicated** until space-occupying lesions are ruled out—possibility of induced brain herniation. Bacterial or viral pathogens affect glucose, protein, cell counts, RBCs, and WBCs.
Electroencephalogram (EEG)	Seizure activity	Common in head trauma, brain tumors, and infectious process due to altered electrical activity in brain.
Serum electrolytes	Hyponatremia (serum Na+ less than 134 mEq/L) or hypernatremia (Na greater than 145)	Risk factor for increased cerebral edema.
Blood glucose	May be elevated	Indicative of steroid use (dexamethasone).
Complete blood count (CBC)	Elevated WBC count Alteration in hemoglobin/hematocrit	Indicates infection. Also may be present with steroid use. Important for accurate hemodynamic monitoring, especially in patients at risk for vasospasm.
Culture of CSF	Presence of pathogens	Indicated for suspicion of infectious CNS process.
Tissue pathology	Presence of malignancy, pathogen	Indicated for suspicion of tumor or abscess.
Arterial blood gases	Hypoxia, hypercapnia	Depressed neurological state may also indicate depressed respiratory drive. Decreased levels of oxygen and increased levels of CO_2 are a concern for increasing ICPs.

fractures should be considered contaminated, and careful wound debridement with surgical closure often is required. Depressed skull fractures may require elevation of the depressed bone as well as debridement of the wound. The possibility of infection must be considered, and antibiotics are started if considered appropriate.

Hematomas

Hematomas are collections of blood. Intracranial hematomas are defined by their location, either epidural or subdural. Chart 29–5 summarizes the types of hematomas, which are discussed in more detail in the following subsections.

Epidural Hematoma

An **epidural hematoma (EDH)** refers to bleeding into the space between the skull and the dura, caused by the laceration of an artery or a vein (Figure 29–7 ■). Approximately 85% of EDHs are caused by arterial lacerations (Greenberg, 2001), most commonly the middle meningeal artery, with or without fracture of the temporal bone. As bleeding occurs, an enlarging hematoma develops as the dura is stripped away from the inner table of the skull. Pressure is exerted on the brain tissue by the expanding lesion, with resulting neurological compromise.

CHART 29–5	Types of Hematomas	
Hematoma	**Onset of Symptoms**	**Characteristic on CT Scan**
Epidural	Immediate loss of consciousness, followed by lucid interval (considered "textbook presentation")	Hyperdense, elliptical
Subdural, acute	Up to 48 hours after injury	Hyperdense
Subdural, subacute	48 hours to 3 weeks	Isodense
Subdural, chronic	3 weeks to several months	Hypodense

EDHs most frequently occur in children and young adults and account for approximately 2% to 6% of intracerebral trauma (Hickey, 2003). It is seen rarely in children younger than 2 years old, or the elderly, possibly because the dura is more adherent to the skull at those ages. The male-to-female ratio of EDH is approximately 4 to 1 (Greenberg, 2001).

Clinical Manifestations of EDH   Classic clinical presentation of EDH is characterized by an immediate post-traumatic period of unconsciousness, followed by a lucid interval, which can last from minutes to hours. The "lucid interval" is considered a textbook presentation of EDH, seen in approximately 85% of patients with EDH. A rapid deterioration in LOC may follow, characterized by sleepiness, confusion, obtundation, coma, and possibly death. Neurological decline is caused by the rapidly increasing pressure, or mass effect, caused by the enlarging hematoma. Other possible signs and symptoms are an enlarging pupil on the same side of the injury (ipsilateral), increasing headache, seizures, motor weakness, and/or pathological positioning (refer to Chapter 28 ☺ on assessment).

Subdural Hematoma

Subdural hematoma (SDH) is defined as bleeding between the dura and the arachnoid layers of the meninges (Figure 29–8 ■). Approximately 30% of intracranial traumatic lesions are SDHs (Hickey, 2003). They usually are caused by the tearing of bridging veins located over the surface of the brain. SDHs are divided into three categories based on the amount of time between the initial injury and the presentation of signs and symptoms.

Acute Subdural Hematoma   Acute SDH is characterized by the presentation of neurological signs and symptoms up to 48 hours after injury. On CT of the head, the acute SDH appears as a hyperdense lesion. The most common signs are severe headache with possible gradual deterioration of LOC, starting with drowsiness and progressing through confusion, obtundation, and coma. Pupillary signs also may be present, most commonly an ipsilateral dilation, and sluggish reactivity. Hemiparesis of the contralateral arm and leg also may be present.

FIGURE 29–7 ■ Epidural hematoma.

FIGURE 29–8 ■ Subdural hematoma.

Subacute Subdural Hematoma With subacute subdural hematoma neurological signs and symptoms develop from 48 hours postinjury up to about 3 weeks. They are associated with less serious lesions, perhaps due to bleeding at a much slower rate. The blood in a subacute SDH appears isodense with hyperdense areas and a clear blood–fluid level on a CT scan.

Chronic Subdural Hematoma With chronic subdural hematoma neurological signs and symptoms develop over 3 weeks to several months. These are associated with minor head injuries, possibly occurring weeks to months prior to the presentation of neurological signs. The SDH increases slowly in size, possibly from repeated small venous bleeds, until a significant mass effect develops and symptoms occur.

Chronic subdural hematomas also are associated with the elderly, who may have atrophic brains that provide more free space to bleed into. Also of significance in the aging brain, bridging veins are stretched as the brain atrophies, which also may cause bleeding into the subdural space. Because there is more room for the clot to expand, the SDH may become quite large before symptoms occur. On CT scan, the chronic SDH appears isodense. However, because chronic SDH may occur from repeated small episodes of subdural bleeding, it is not uncommon to have acute or chronic SDH, as evidenced by areas of varying density demonstrated on CT scan. Chronic SDHs usually do not present with the rapid and dramatic deterioration of neurological function as do acute SDHs. The most common symptom is increasing headache, slowing mentation, confusion, and drowsiness. Seizures are a common presenting symptom.

 Patients with a diagnosis of SDH are at risk for expanding hematoma. Therefore, frequent neurological assessments are required (i.e., hourly until stable, then q2h). A decrease in neurological function, such as increasing confusion or lethargy, increasing motor weakness, or an enlarging pupil is a medical emergency. The doctor should be notified immediately.

Laboratory and Diagnostic Procedures

CT scan of the head remains the most accurate diagnostic tool, along with a thorough and accurate history of the event. EDH is characterized by a high-density elliptical-shaped mass adjacent to the skull. Mass effect also is seen with a shift of the brain from the side with the EDH to the opposite side. CT scan is highly diagnostic for SDH, as well as for the determination of the acute, subacute, or chronic type of hematoma.

Medical Management

The treatment for EDH is almost always surgical. The exception to surgical management is a small lesion that is causing little to no neurological impairment. The patient is hospitalized, possibly in the intensive care unit (ICU), with frequent neurological assessment, and serial CT scans are taken to monitor the size of the hematoma. A decline in the neurological assessment of the patient, with or without radiographic evidence of increased size, warrants emergent surgical evacuation of the hematoma. Mortality rates are dependent on the availability of neurosurgical treatment.

The treatment for SDH is dependent on several factors. Observation with medical management may be appropriate for a small SDH with little to no neurological deterioration, because

a small SDH may reabsorb with time. However, a large SDH, with significant neurological compromise requires immediate surgical evacuation. SDH is commonly associated with therapeutic anticoagulation, and correction of coagulopathy is a critical step in preparing the patient for operative care. It is possible to drain a small liquefied hematoma with twist drill burr holes. Burr holes are small holes made with a twist drill into the skull, over the area of hematoma. Commonly, a drain is left in to drain the hematoma over time. Larger acute, subacute, and chronic SDH may require an open craniotomy for evacuation of the hematoma. Twist drill drainage of chronic SDH may not be possible, because the clotted blood is the consistency of motor oil and may be too gelatinous to be successfully evacuated with burr holes.

Postoperatively, the patient should remain in the ICU, with close monitoring of neurological status. Use of intracranial monitoring is done with caution, because an EVD may cause the SDH to worsen. The patient may require hemodynamic monitoring and/or ventilatory assistance, depending on the size and location of the lesion, as well as the presence of any accompanying injuries.

Because seizures are a common occurrence in SDH, the use of antiepileptic drugs (AEDs) may be warranted. The prophylactic use of AEDs is controversial, because they have many side effects and contraindications. If a patient has a seizure due to a lesion, the patient should be started on an AED such as phenytoin (Dilantin). Seizures and their management are addressed later in the chapter.

Cerebral Contusions

Contusions of the brain are defined as bruising of the brain tissue, often associated with other neurological injuries, such as skull fractures or hematomas. They may occur from blunt trauma, penetrating wounds, or acceleration/deceleration injuries. Causes may include motor vehicle crashes, falls, and assault. The injuries are referred to as coup, in which bruising occurs directly below the point of impact on the skull, or contrecoup, which occurs directly on the opposite point of impact. Contrecoup contusions usually have a coup component, in which case they are referred to as coup-contrecoup contusions. Contrecoup contusions occur as a result of the brain moving with the skull, and bruising itself during acceleration/deceleration movement.

Clinical Manifestations

The clinical presentation of cerebral contusion is highly dependent on the location, size, and the amount of cerebral edema associated with the lesion. For example, a patient with temporal contusions, especially bilateral contusions, may have a significant decrease in LOC with motor and speech deficits. This patient is at high risk for cerebral edema and herniation. A patient with a frontal contusion may be alert, possibly confused, and may be monitored in the hospital for a short period of time with no obvious consequences. However, the patient may experience more obvious neuropsychological deficits such as disinhibition in social situations; therefore, careful observation of the patient's cognitive status is warranted. Patients with neurocognitive deficits often require 24-hour care following discharge for this reason.

Laboratory and Diagnostic Procedures

As with all cerebral traumas, a thorough and accurate history is important. Diagnosis is made by radiographic detection on imaging studies to evaluate for the presence of contusion and possibly edema.

Medical Management

Once the diagnosis of cerebral contusion(s) is made, along with determination of the location and size of the contusion, treatment is dependent on the neurological condition of the patient. Close monitoring of the patient's neurological assessment is important. Monitoring of ICP may be necessary since cerebral edema may be present. Serial CT scans over several days may be warranted to assess the size of the contusion as the brain heals. "Blossoming" or expansion of the contusion may occur at approximately 3 days.

Seizures may be a presenting sign; therefore, use of AEDs may be necessary. Prophylactic use of AEDs is controversial, though some health care providers believe their use is warranted for a limited time (usually 7 days) due to the potential risk of seizures.

Hyponatremia is another common sequelae to TBI, often requiring both salt supplementation and fluid restriction for management.

Concussion

Concussion refers to a recognized collection of symptoms as a result of mild head injury. It is described as a temporary, neurological dysfunction caused by an external force to the head. It is also described as a "shaking of the brain."

Clinical Manifestations

Concussion is associated with a myriad of symptoms, including confusion, possible brief loss of consciousness, headache, intellectual impairment, and memory loss. Concussion is characterized by a nonfocal neurological exam. The American Academy of Neurology Practice has issued a grading scale to define levels of concussion and make recommendations for treatment, as described in the National Guidelines box.

Laboratory and Diagnostic Procedures

An accurate history of the event is essential, including questions such as length of period of loss of consciousness, if any; presence of confusion; and length of time until symptoms subside. No radiographic findings are associated with concussions. However, if the patient has a focal neurological exam, or an extended period of unconsciousness, the patient should be admitted to the hospital, and a CT of the head should be obtained to rule out other, more serious brain trauma.

Medical Management

The management of the concussion is dependent on the grade determined. However, the treatment recommendations are guidelines, and each patient should be assessed individually.

Second-Impact Syndrome

Second-impact syndrome is characterized by a second concussion, in an indeterminate time frame, that occurs before the brain can completely recover from the first concussion. It is caused by a loss of disordered autoregulation of the brain's blood supply as a result of the first injury (Bowen, 2003; Terrell, 2004). Because of poor brain compliance, persistent vascular congestion and increased ICP persist. This condition may persist for an indeterminate length of time. Because second-impact syndrome is the result of a second injury before the brain has recovered from the first injury, the result can be massive cerebral edema and possibly death. The mortality rate is 50% and the morbidity rate is 100% (Proctor & Cantu, 2000). It is for this reason that consideration must be made of the advisability of continuing risk-taking activities after receiving an initial concussion. An example of this is the athlete who continues playing football after receiving one or more concussions and then collapses and dies on the sidelines after an apparent mild injury. For these reasons, well-recognized return-to-play guidelines are now used that progress in a stepwise fashion. The athlete has a period of rest and when symptom free may return to limited noncontact activity and progress each week to full play if no symptoms such as headache or recurrent cognitive problems are experienced. The player must return to repeat the previous step if symptoms recur (Aubry et al., 2001; Terrell, 2004).

Postconcussion Syndrome

Postconcussion syndrome is a condition that follows mild head injury and is characterized by one or more of the following symptoms: headaches, dizziness, vertigo, tinnitus, hearing loss, blurred vision, light and/or noise sensitivity, alteration in smell, anxiety, depression, personality change, sleep disorders, decreased libido, decreased appetite, memory loss, alteration in cognitive function, personality changes, and physical or cognitive decline (Rees & Bellon, 2007). It was once thought that these symptoms were psychological, and the patient perhaps malingering. However, current literature supports a physiological basis for this condition. Symptoms usually subside with time; however, it can take months for total resolution (Mittenberg & Strauman, 2000).

The only treatment for postconcussive syndrome is education and support for the patient and family members. Counseling may be helpful to cope with personal and work-related problems.

Diffuse Axonal Injury

Diffuse axonal injury (DAI) is defined as a primary injury of diffuse white matter that results in tearing or shearing of axons and small blood vessels. Presentation of the patient with DAI is

---

NATIONAL GUIDELINES American Academy of Neurology Practice Parameter Grading System for Concussion

Grade	Type of Concussion
Grade 1	Transient confusion, no loss of consciousness, symptoms of mental status abnormalities on examination resolve in less than 15 minutes.
Grade 2	Transient confusion, no loss of consciousness, symptoms of mental status abnormalities on examination last more than 15 minutes.
Grade 3	Any loss of consciousness, either brief or prolonged.

Source: Kelly, P., & Rosenburg, J. H. (1997). Diagnosis and management of concussion in sports. *Neurology, 483,* 575–580.

frequently seen as neurological compromise, possibly coma, with decerebrate or decorticate posturing as described in Chapter 28 . DAI lesions may be microscopic, and not initially detected by CT scan. Magnetic resonance imaging (MRI) is more appropriate for the detection of small DAI lesions. Surgery is not indicated because the injury is diffuse. Treatment is determined by the neurological presentation of the patient and is usually supportive. Support of respiratory and hemodynamic functions may be warranted. DAI is classified as mild, moderate, and severe. Patients with mild DAI may have only mild long-term cognitive disabilities, whereas severe DAIs are associated with significant mortality and long-term disabilities.

Primary/Secondary Injuries

Head injuries can be divided into primary and secondary injuries. **Primary injury** refers to the mechanical injury to the brain. The injury is a direct result of the initial insult to the brain and may be localized, such as occurs with a laceration or contusion, or diffuse, such as with a concussion or DAI.

Secondary injury is a result of the body's response to the primary insult to the brain. It is caused by a flow–metabolism mismatch, which results in **cerebral ischemia**, which then triggers the **ischemia cascade**, which is a series of events that results in changes on the cellular level, which then results in **cerebral infarction** (Goldman & Ausiello, 2004; Porth, 2007). It can be the result of a single event or a series of events. Deficits in cellular metabolism in the brain can cause cell death, leading to death of brain tissue, compromised neurological function, and poor patient outcomes. Causes of secondary injury are many, and include respiratory insufficiency, hypoxia, sepsis, hypotension, metabolic dysfunction, cerebral edema, and increased ICP. It has been estimated that 50% of patients with head trauma succumb to effects of secondary injury (Hilton, 2000; Porth, 2007).

Nursing Management

Nursing care of TBI patients has several goals. The first is protection of the patient's neurological function. This is accomplished by a thorough neurological assessment aimed at determining the patient's level of consciousness and possible focal neurological deficits.

Assessment

A good neurological assessment is essential for communication between medical personnel, as well as for a baseline to detect changes. A tool, such as the Glasgow Coma Scale, is helpful to provide standardized information to other medical personnel. The GCS is a widely used scoring system used in quantifying level of consciousness following traumatic brain injury. The scale and its scoring mechanism is discussed in detail in Chapter 28 . Any unfavorable change in a neurological exam, even the most subtle, may indicate deterioration in the patient's condition and is reportable. The National Guidelines box lists the questions used by the CDC to screen for detection of mild TBI.

TBI may be a mild head injury, such as a concussion, or cerebral contusion. TBI also may be a severe, life-threatening situation. It is not uncommon for other serious conditions also to be present,

NATIONAL GUIDELINES CDC Screening Instrument for Detection of Mild TBI

Questions

1. At the time of your trauma, did you experience any period of transient confusion, disorientation, or impaired consciousness?
2. At the time of your trauma, did you experience any dysfunction of memory?
3. Did you experience any of the following in relation to your trauma: seizures, headache, dizziness, irritability, fatigue, or poor concentration?
4. At the time of your trauma, did you experience any loss of consciousness lasting 30 minutes or less?

An answer of "yes" on any of these questions indicates mild TBI.

Source: Bay, E., & McLean, S. A. (2007). Mild traumatic brain injury: an update for advanced practice nurses. *American Association of Neuroscience Nurses, 39*(1), 43–51; Centers for Disease Control and Prevention. (2005). *CDCt toolkits.* Retrieved September 25, 2006 from http://www.cdc.govncipe/pub-res/tbi_toolkit/toolkit.htm/.

which also may be life threatening. Patients with severe injury or potentially severe conditions are usually admitted to the ICU and monitored carefully. It is imperative to remember the ABCs of patient management with any trauma patient. Assessing and securing an adequate airway are always of primary consideration. Trauma victims frequently have respiratory compromise due to a number of factors, including other injuries. Whether a patient is severely injured and intubated, or awake and talking, maintenance of an adequate airway is essential. Rate and quality of respirations should be assessed initially, and ongoing. A pulse oximeter may be of assistance in early determination of respiratory decline. This is especially important if the patient has an altered LOC. Any patient with a GCS of 8 or less, with 15 being considered normal, should be considered for intubation. Maintenance of adequate oxygenation is an important tenet of ICP management.

 CRITICAL ALERT *Patients with a decreased level of consciousness are at risk for aspiration and respiratory compromise. Monitor respiratory status carefully, suction as needed, and ensure airway protection.*

Assessment of adequate circulation is the last part of the ABCs of life support. Patients with TBI may exhibit alterations in circulatory function, such as bradycardia, hypotension, or hypertension. They may also be hemodynamically unstable due to blood loss secondary to trauma. Therefore, the initial nursing assessment must include a complete set of vital signs and a thorough assessment of the circulatory status of the TBI patient. After the initial ABCs of patient management, the most common concern for nurses caring for patients with TBI is that of ICP. Many patients with TBI require placement of a device to monitor ICP. The nursing management of patients with increased ICP was addressed earlier in this chapter.

Interventions and Rationales

Nursing is in a good position to recognize signs and symptoms, or the potential, of cognitive impairment due to TBI. It is often in the

EVIDENCE-BASED PRACTICE

Traumatic Brain Injury

Clinical Problem

Traumatic brain injury is a major health problem globally. It occurs with varying degrees of severity and disability. It can affect all ages, but the National Institutes of Health (NIH) states that the majority of those with TBI are between the ages of 18 and 25 (NIH Consensus Panel, 1999).

Although the causes of TBI differ by region, gender, and age group, the largest number of TBIs appears to be secondary to motor vehicle crashes, falls, and acts of violence, such as gunshot wounds and assault. In the United States, the incidence of people with closed head injuries admitted to hospitals is conservatively estimated to be 1.5 million each year. Approximately 235,000 cases of TBI are admitted to hospitals every year, with approximately 50,000 deaths (Langlois, Rutland-Brown, & Thomas, 2006).

Mild TBI accounts for approximately 75% of all diagnosed TBI (Bazarian et al., 2005). Persons experiencing mild TBI may enter the health care system through emergency departments; others may present through their primary care health care providers. The signs and symptoms may be mild or even unnoticed. It has been estimated that approximately 25% of those with mild TBI do not seek medical treatment at all (Dawodu, 2007).

The symptoms of mild TBI are frequently cognitive and may consist of memory problems, difficulty with concentration, personality changes, or other alterations in thought processes. These deficits may lead to problems with relationships, education, and/or occupation. For these patients, it is essential that signs and symptoms of mild TBI are recognized early to provide appropriate management. Diagnosis of mild TBI may be obtained through screening procedures, cognitive assessment, and accurate and thorough interviewing and history-taking. A management plan for the patient with mild TBI is based on evidence-based practices.

Research Findings

Management of the patient with mild TBI is based on symptom management. This includes environmental modifications, compensatory strategies, and support and education of the patient and family while gradually returning to work and home responsibilities (Bay & McLean, 2007).

Many of these compensatory strategies are the focus of speech and occupational therapists, either in an acute or outpatient setting. An evidence-based review article published by Cicerone et al. (2005) found evidence to support the use of aids, such as voice organizers and memory journals, to help patients with memory impairment after TBI.

A study by Mittenberg and colleagues (1996) described a printed manual and a 1-hour treatment session regarding symptom management to a small group of patients with mild TBI. They compared this group to a usual treatment group. They compared the two groups 6 months later and found that the first group reported fewer and less severe symptoms. They suggest that even brief educational interventions are beneficial to reducing prolonged symptoms post-TBI.

A review of the literature regarding screening and symptom management of patients with mild TBI suggests that awareness of actual and potential cognitive deficits and subsequent education regarding symptom management are beneficial to reducing prolonged symptoms. There is great need for continued research in the management of mild TBI patients.

Implications for Nursing Practice

Patients with mild TBI may exhibit a vast array of symptoms, including headache, dizziness, and/or subtle symptoms of cognitive impairment. Some of these symptoms include difficulty with concentration, memory, or attention. Personality changes may also be seen. Nurses are in an excellent position to identify signs and symptoms of mild TBI. Screening tools can assist in determining the severity of TBI (see the National Guidelines box titled CDC Screening Instrument for Detection of Mild TBI, p. 727). Nursing staff should also assist patients in obtaining the appropriate therapies, including support and education of patients and their families.

Critical Thinking Questions

1. What patient complaints might be suspicious for signs and symptoms of mild TBI?

2. What part of a patient's history would lead to concern about a possible mild TBI?

3. What would be appropriate management strategies for patients with mild TBI?

Answers to Critical Thinking Questions appear in Appendix D

References

Bazarian, J., McClung, J., Shah, M., Cheng, Y., Flesher, W., & Kraus, J. (2005). Mild traumatic brain injury in the United States, 1998–2000. *Brain Injury, 19*(2), 85–91.

Cicerone, K. D., Dahlberg, C., Malec, J., Langenbahn, D., Felicetti, T., Kneipp, S., et al. (2005). Evidence-based cognitive rehabilitation: Updated review of the literature from 1998 through 2002. *Archives in Physical Medicine Rehabilitation, 86,* 1681–1692.

Dawodu, S.T. (2007). Traumatic brain injury: definition, epidemiology, pathophysiology. *EMedicine.* Retrieved July 14, 2008 from http://www.emedicine.com/pmr/TOPIC212.HTM.

Langlois, J. A., Rutland-Brown, W., & Thomas, K. E. (2006). *Traumatic brain injury in the United States: Emergency department visits, hospitalizations, and deaths.* Atlanta, GA: Centers for Disease Control and Prevention, National Center for Injury Prevention and Control.

Mittenberg, W., Tremont, G., Zielinski, R., Fichera, S., & Rayls, K. (1996). Cognitive-behavioral prevention of post-concussion syndrome. *Archives of Clinical Neuropsychology, 11*(2), 139–145.

National Institutes of Health Consensus Panel. (1999). NIH consensus statement: Rehabilitation of persons with traumatic brain injury. *Journal of the American Medical Association, 282,* 974–983.

Source: From "Mild Traumatic Brain Injury: An Update for Advanced Practice Nurses," E. Bay and S. McLean (2007). *Journal of Neuroscience Nursing, 39*(1), 43–51.

---

patient's best interest to obtain therapy consults in order to recognize and define possible cognitive problems. Evidence-based practice asserts that early recognition and education regarding possible cognitive deficits may aid in the patient's rehabilitation and recovery (see the Evidence-Based Practice box).

A second goal for the neuroscience nurse is the prevention of complications, many of which are common and known to be complications common to patients with TBI. Examples of these are respiratory failure, development of deep venous thrombosis, and other systemic complications. These complications can be extremely serious and may even be life threatening. Many of these systemic complications are addressed later in this chapter.

TBI is almost always unexpected and usually comes at a time that finds both patients and their families unprepared. The early period of hospitalization requires critical thinking and astute assessment skills. It always requires understanding, empathy, and strong emotional support. Nurses may be equipped with the skills needed to care for TBI patients efficiently, but skills to appropriately care for families of patients with devastating, perhaps potentially fatal injuries also is extremely important. Families of severely injured patients are frequently overwhelmed, often angry, and not uncommonly in denial. The nurse caring for the patient's family members may be their only link for communication, support, and encouragement. It is important to keep them as involved as they want to be in the care of their family member, as informed as possible, and given as much control as is possible. Experienced nurses often relate that the most frequent complaint heard from families is that they "don't know what is going on." It also is important to answer questions honestly, educating the family about the treatment plan and the expected rehabilitation process. It is important to encourage, educate, and offer hope, without misleading. Determining brain death in patients and working with patients' family members are discussed in the Ethical Issues box.

Collaborative Management

The patient with TBI is one with multifaceted challenges. TBI patients require the collaboration of many specialists and ancillary services. Medically, it is not uncommon for a TBI patient to be under the care of several health care providers, such as a pulmonologist to manage respiratory problems, a neurologist to manage seizures, an orthopedic surgeon and/or a trauma surgeon to manage coexisting injuries, and possibly a critical care specialist.

It also is important to have a dietitian involved in the TBI patient's care. Metabolic needs should be determined in order to ensure that caloric needs are met. TBI patients often require enteral feedings, and the type and amount are important to ensure the patient receives the appropriate nutrition for his needs. Nutrition should be started as soon as it is medically possible (see Chapter 14).

Most TBI patients will, at some point in their hospital stay, require therapists. In many hospitals this may consist of physical therapists, occupational therapists, and possibly recreation therapists. Speech pathologists also may be called on to assess swallow function as well as cognitive function. Sometimes a neuropsychologist will be consulted to assess higher cognitive function and to help determine the safety and feasibility of returning home or to a previous occupation. In some hospitals, a psychiatrist, specializing in rehabilitation, may be consulted to facilitate post-hospital therapies. Many TBI patients benefit from a post-hospital stay in a rehabilitation facility to prepare them for return to home and their previous lives.

Social services may be called on to assist in attaining resources the patient and her family may need. Many patients and their families find TBI support groups to be helpful. This is especially important for the families of patients experiencing long-term rehabilitation or those experiencing significant changes in their jobs and/or lifestyles. Nursing support is important in providing and encouraging care for the caregiver.

ETHICAL ISSUES Related to Brain Death

Brain death can be defined as damage to the brain that is irreversible and extensive to the point that there is no potential for recovery. Brain damage can result from numerous causes, including trauma, stroke, or tumor.

Brain death determination is done by a physician and includes the following criteria:

- Absence of brainstem reflexes: fixed pupils, absent corneal reflexes, absent oculovestibular reflexes, absent gag reflex, no spontaneous respirations with apnea challenge
- No response to deep central pain
- Core temperature less than 32.2°C (89.9°F)
- SBP > 90 mmHg.

Determination of brain death is not appropriate in patients with possibility of intoxication, either alcohol or drug.

Consider organ donation for patients in which brain death is a possibility.

Persistent Vegetative State

The term *persistent vegetative state* (PVS) was proposed by Jennett and Plum (1972) to describe the state following coma in some patients who have experienced severe brain injury. This is a state following coma characterized by an awakened state, without cognitive awareness. Patients in a PVS have sleep–wake cycles, with eyes open spontaneously. Normal vital signs, including respiratory function, are maintained. There is no attempt to follow commands, or to communicate. There is no evidence of cognition.

Patients in a PVS may survive many years following a brain injury. This often presents a very difficult situation for family. It is helpful if a living will is available and the patient and family have had discussions regarding the prolongation of life in a situation where quality of life appears minimal at best.

Family conferences with physicians, nursing, therapists, social work, and clergy are frequently helpful in determining prognosis, including quality of life. Discussions involving discontinuance of medical treatment, including nutrition, are difficult at best, and should be done with the patient's living will and/or advance directive. Assuring the family that such decisions are reflections of the patient's own wishes may be comforting and may assuage feelings of guilt or responsibility.

Health Promotion

The most important principle of TBI management is prevention. A vast number of programs in hospitals and communities nationwide are aimed at the prevention of TBI. Community education and public awareness programs are essential in the prevention of TBI. Such programs include the promotion of helmets for bicycle and motorcycle riders and seat-belt laws, which are known to have an effect on the severity of TBI due to motor vehicle collisions.

Infectious Diseases of the Central Nervous System

Many infectious diseases may affect the nervous system. Meningitis, encephalitis, and cerebral abscesses are examples of infections of the central nervous system (CNS) that can be caused by a number of pathogens including common bacteria, fungi, and viruses. Infectious diseases may be acquired or nosocomial. Nosocomial infections are those that are acquired due to hospitalization; they were not present or in the incubation period prior to admission. The nationwide rate of nosocomial infections is about 7% to 10%. It is estimated that approximately 20% of all hospital-acquired infections occur in critical care areas (Smith et al., 2005).

Meningitis

Meningitis is defined as an inflammation of the meninges. **Bacterial meningitis** is an inflammation of the meninges caused by a bacterial pathogen. **Viral meningitis** is an inflammation of the meninges caused by viral pathogens, such as herpes simplex virus, mumps, measles, or any other virus.

Epidemiology

Before the introduction of antibiotics in the 1930s and 1940s, acute bacterial meningitis was fatal in most cases (Koedel, Scheld, & Pfister, 2002). Nowadays, most cases of meningitis are curable, with variable morbidity related to variable pathogens. Bacterial meningitis occurs most often in three patient populations, the very young and the very old, and those with head trauma or surgery. According to the American Association of Neuroscience Nurses (AANN), 70% of all cases of bacterial meningitis occur in children under the age of 5 years old. In adults over age 40, the incidence is 5 to 10 per 100,000. It also has been noted that patients with diabetes mellitus appear to have a higher than average incidence of acquired bacterial meningitis (Huang et al., 2002). Prognosis is good if treated early; however, if left untreated, it has a mortality rate of greater than 70% (Bader & Littlejohns, 2004). Viral meningitis also affects all age groups, including children. Incidence and type of pathogen are highly dependent on geographic locale. An example of a region-specific virus is that which is arthropod-borne, such as the West Nile virus. This virus is more prevalent around water and in humid locales. Viral meningitis may occur as an epidemic or as an isolated occurrence.

Etiology and Pathophysiology

Meningitis involves the layers of the meninges, and the subarachnoid space. Through a complex physiological process, the response of the meningeal tissue causes an alteration in the blood–brain barrier. This process may result in vasogenic edema with an increase in ICP.

Bacteria can enter the meninges by various methods and structures. Bloodborne pathogens are the most common, entering via the bloodstream. Other bacteria enter the body via other structures, such as the sinuses or the inner ear, by dental procedures, or endocarditis. Cerebrospinal fluid is a common route for infection. A dural tear caused by trauma or surgery can create a route for the introduction of pathogens. Patients with skull fractures, for example, may experience rhinorrhea or otorrhea. If a route is available for CSF to leave the body, organisms have a route to enter the body. Unsterile technique during surgical procedures, including lumbar puncture, placement of an EVD, or collection of CSF from an EVD, is a method of introducing organisms into the CSF.

The most common causative agents differ in children and adults. The age of the patient directs suspicion toward the identity of the pathogen. Adults contract bacterial meningitis most frequently from trauma and/or brain surgery. *Staphylococcus aureus*, *Staphylococcus epidermidis*, and gram-negative bacilli are common causative agents as introduced by neurological procedures, such as surgery or lumbar puncture.

Clinical Manifestations

A common and early sign of bacterial and viral meningitis is that of meningeal irritation, or **meningismus**. Symptoms of meningismus include photophobia, nuchal rigidity, or stiff neck, Kernig's sign, and Brudzinski sign. Kernig's sign is elicited by flexing the patient's hip to approximately 90 degrees, then straightening the leg at the knee. Pain in the hamstring area prevents the straightening of the leg. This is referred to as a positive Kernig's sign, and must be present bilaterally to be considered positive. Brudzinski sign is positive when flexion of the patient's neck elicits flexion of the hips and knees. The discomfort associated with meningismus is caused by inflammation of the meninges.

Headache is another common and early symptom of meningitis. These headaches are usually described as severe and difficult to control. Fever also is common, and is usually high. Altered levels of consciousness, such as lethargy, irritability, and confusion, may occur as the disease progresses. Seizures may be seen at the onset.

Laboratory and Diagnostic Procedures

A thorough and accurate history is very important, focusing on recent illnesses, such as any "flu-like" illness. The presence of systemic viral infections is significant. A history of recent dental procedures, head trauma, and/or brain surgery also is pertinent.

Once meningitis is suspected, lumbar puncture must be done to determine the presence and identity of organisms as well as other diagnostic criteria of CSF. Before a lumbar puncture can be done, however, a CT scan of the head should be done to ascertain that no space-occupying lesion is present to cause mass effect. A lumbar puncture done in the presence of a space-occupying lesion could cause downward shifting of the brain and herniation through the foramen magnum, with neurologically devastating results as described earlier in the chapter (herniation syndromes).

Lumbar puncture can prove with certainty if pathogens are present in the CSF. Also of benefit is examination of the fluid for other diagnostic factors. The CSF may be turbid or cloudy in the presence of bacteria. Other chemical constituents are diagnostic for bacterial meningitis, that is, protein and glucose. The amount of protein in the CSF is usually high, whereas the glucose level is low. Viral meningitis differs in that the glucose count is usually normal, whereas the protein count remains elevated. The CSF appears clear. Intracranial pressure also may be measured via lumbar puncture. Chart 29–6 lists CSF findings under various conditions.

Medical Management

The treatment for bacterial meningitis is antibiotics. They are usually given intravenously, but may be given intrathecally in certain circumstances. The type and route of antibiotics used are determined by the identity of the pathogen. For appropriate antibiotic determination, a CSF Gram stain and culture is very important. It also is important to obtain blood cultures to assist with therapy determination. For an antibiotic to be effective in

CHART 29–6   **CSF Findings in Various Pathologic Conditions**

Condition	Opening Pressure (cm H$_2$O)	Appearance	Cells (per mm^3)	Protein (mg %)	Glucose (% serum)	Cultures
Normal	7–18	Clear, colorless	0	15–45	50	No organisms
Bacterial meningitis	Frequently increased	Turbid, cloudy	20–50+	100–1,000	Less than 40	Bacterial organisms
Viral meningitis/encephalitis	Normal	Normal, may be cloudy	Few–350	40–100	Normal	No bacterial organisms; viral organisms present on viral cultures only
Subarachnoid hemorrhage	Increased	Bloody	Increased RBCs	50–400	Normal	No organisms

treating meningitis, it must have a bactericidal effect against the causative organism, and it must be able to penetrate the blood–brain barrier. The antibiotic most sensitive to the causative agent is the drug of choice. Because recovery depends on the timeliness of treatment, it usually is important to start treatment as soon as possible, even before the causative agent is identified.

It is important to note that some antibiotics interfere with the metabolism of other drugs, including phenytoin. This is significant because it generally decreases the blood levels of phenytoin, leaving the patient more susceptible to seizure activity.

 Seizure precautions must be taken with any patient having seizures or the potential for seizures. While the patient is in bed, the rails should be padded and in the upright position. All patients should be on AEDs, unless contraindicated. Drug levels should be monitored to maintain therapeutic range.

Because meningitis may cause vasogenic edema, the use of dexamethasone is strongly recommended. Studies also have shown that dexamethasone has been found to decrease mortality when given early (van de Beek et al., 2002). Prognosis also appears to correlate with the causative agent, age, degree of neurological impairment, the presence of underlying disease, such as diabetes, and the general health condition. Mortality and morbidity rates range from 10% to 30%, but if left untreated, the morbidity is greater than 70% (Bader & Littlejohns, 2004). Prognosis depends on many factors: the causative agent, the severity of the infection, the age and general health condition of the patient, and the timeliness of effective treatment.

Treatment of viral meningitis consists mainly of supportive measures. These measures may consist of relief of symptoms, such as fever or pain. A more seriously ill patient may require respiratory and/or circulatory support. AEDs may also be necessary. Frequent monitoring of the patient's neurological status is important, with any decline in the neurological exam reported. Prognosis is dependent on variable factors, similar to those with the bacterial form of meningitis. Occasional neurological impairment has been reported, but full recovery is frequent.

Isolating the patient with a CNS infection usually is not necessary. In the acute phase of meningococcal meningitis, it is possible to spread the infection to others by respiratory droplets. In such a situation, respiratory isolation of these patients may be needed to protect other patients and the nursing staff for a short period of time. Universal precautions are usually adequate protection from the spread of CNS infections.

Encephalitis

Encephalitis refers to an inflammation of the brain tissue. The cause may be bacterial, viral, fungal, or parasitic. There are many causes of encephalitis worldwide. Like meningitis, the specific pathogen is highly influenced by geographic location. The most common form of encephalitis in the United States is viral. The most common of these viruses is herpes simplex virus (HSV). Other types of viruses include arthropod-borne, such as those carried by mosquitoes. Another cause of viral encephalitis is postviral disease, from measles, mumps, or chickenpox.

HSV exists as type 1 and type 2. HSV-1 is the virus that causes cold sores, and exists in the dormant form in most adults. HSV-1 is the virus that causes HSV encephalitis. It is unknown how or why the virus changes from the dormant phase to the active phase. HSV-2 is the virus that causes genital herpes through sexual transmission.

Pathophysiology

The mechanism by which a virus infects the brain varies with the type of virus. Effects include degenerative changes within the nerve cell. Also seen are localized edema, hemorrhages, and areas of necrosis. HSV has a special affinity for the frontal and temporal lobes. Increased ICP may be present.

Clinical Manifestations

Symptoms are usually more pronounced than those with meningitis. They also are dependent on the type of virus infecting the brain. Symptoms include severe headache, fever, nausea and vomiting, confusion, alterations in LOC, such as lethargy, and focal deficits, such as motor weakness. It is not unusual for patients to have seizures and bizarre behavior. If the virus is causing cerebral edema, the patient will have signs and symptoms of increased ICP, as discussed earlier in this chapter. Death or severe neurological deficits can occur if the condition is left untreated.

Laboratory and Diagnostic Procedures

Diagnosis is made primarily by examination of CSF. Glucose levels are low, protein levels are high, and white blood cells (WBCs) are elevated. Opening pressure is elevated during lumbar puncture. It is important to make a diagnosis as quickly as possible to initiate treatment. A thorough history is important to rule out other causes of the current illness. MRI scan may show early evidence of small localized hemorrhagic lesions. Definitive diagnosis of HSV is accomplished only by brain biopsy.

Medical Management

Treatment is supportive management of symptoms, such as support of respiratory system, and management of increased ICP, nutritional support, and close evaluation of intake and output. Laboratory values, such as a complete blood count (CBC), also should be monitored to assess systemic response to the disease.

Antiviral agents, such as acyclovir or famciclovir, are the standard for treatment of HSV. They are given intravenously and must be started early in the disease process to be effective. Other important medications include dexamethasone to reduce cerebral edema, phenytoin for seizure management, and medication for pain and fever control. Medications used in treatment of seizures are shown in the Pharmacology Summary box. Prognosis is dependent on early diagnosis and treatment. Neurological deficits such as cognitive impairment, motor weakness, seizure disorder, swallowing difficulties, and personality changes are common.

Brain Abscess

A **brain abscess** is a localized infection carried from other sites of the body extending into the cerebral tissue. There are several mechanisms by which an abscess can be introduced into the brain, such as infection, congenital abnormalities, or by penetrating wounds. An abscess may be caused by various agents, including bacteria, fungus, virus, and parasites.

Epidemiology and Etiology

Brain abscesses occur most often in the cerebellum, but can occur in the frontal, parietal, or occipital lobes. They can occur at any age. There is a 2:1 male-to-female ratio in the occurrence of brain abscesses (Greenberg, 2001). Forty percent of all brain abscesses result from the mastoid, or inner ear; 10% come from the sinuses. Penetrating head wounds, such as trauma, or intracranial surgery account for a small number. Almost half of all abscesses are carried through the blood from other infected sources, as with pneumonia or endocarditis (Hickey, 2003). It is believed that in approximately 25% of all brain abscesses, no primary focus is identified (Bader & Littlejohns, 2004). Note, however, that brain abscess in intravenous (IV) drug users carries especially high morbidity and mortality rates (Tunkel & Pradhan, 2002).

Pathophysiology

Brain abscesses begin as an infectious organism that invades the brain from a nearby location, such as the sinuses, mastoid, or inner ear. The initial focus for infection also may be head or facial trauma or a neurosurgical procedure. Bacteremia in IV drug users may seed in the brain tissue or the epidural space. The invading bacteria cause inflammation, cerebral edema, increased ICP, and necrosis. With time, the necrosis liquefies and capsulates. If untreated, it is possible the abscess could rupture, causing more widespread disease.

Clinical Manifestations

Initial symptoms are directly related to the location of the forming abscess. Headache is common, as well as generalized malaise, fever, nausea and vomiting, and chills. Neurological deficits correspond to the location of the lesion, and may include motor weakness, sensory deficits, cranial nerve weakness, speech disturbances, and alterations in LOC, such as confusion and lethargy. The patient may experience seizures.

As the abscess develops, secondary symptoms may occur due to the expansion of the space-occupying lesion. Symptoms are dependent on the location of the lesion. Cerebellar lesions may result in ataxia, nystagmus, or postoccipital headache. Frontal lesions may result in contralateral hemiplegia, aphasia, or personality changes. Headaches may become more severe, and signs of increased ICP may occur. Herniation syndromes may occur if the abscess is left untreated.

Laboratory and Diagnostic Procedures

Diagnosis is made by history and by imaging studies such as CT scan or MRI. Imaging studies show the encapsulated abscesses. CT scan also is helpful in identifying hydrocephalus, mass effect, and cerebral edema. Occasionally abscesses in the brain may appear to be cystic brain tumors. Diffusion-weighted MRI can be used to identify infectious brain lesions and to differentiate between cystic lesions and abscesses (Guzman et al., 2002). Lumbar puncture usually is not performed because abscesses are space-occupying lesions, capable of causing herniation in certain circumstances. If examination of the CSF is possible, the glucose usually would be normal, with an increased protein and WBC count.

Medical Management

Treatment is surgical drainage of the abscess if possible. Medical management consists of administering the appropriate antibiotics, along with steroids. Support of symptoms, such as ICP management, and respiratory and cardiovascular systems is important. Management of fever and pain issues is warranted. Prognosis is excellent if treated early and aggressively. Also significant in determining prognosis is the number of abscesses noted. Patients with single lesions do considerably better than those with multiple lesions. Patients who survive brain abscess have an approximately 30% chance of neurological deficits, seizures being the most common (Hickey, 2003).

■ Nursing Management

The single most important intervention on the part of nursing and every hospital employee is prevention. The advent of universal precautions has been successful to educate employees in ways to prevent, or at least reduce, the occurrence of infections. The population of patients with neurological disorders appears to have an affinity for infections. One reason for this is the drugs common to patients in this environment. Many patients are given steroids such as dexamethasone, which is an immunosuppressant. Radiation and chemotherapy also act as immunosuppressants. Many patients with neurological disorders have respiratory compromise, requiring intubation and possibly mechanical ventilation. These patients are at high risk for developing nosocomial infections.

Nutritional deficits also are predisposing factors for infection. Many patients enter the hospital in debilitated conditions, in advanced stages of brain tumor, vegetative conditions, or stroke. The widespread use of antibiotics for hospitalized patients plays a role in diminishing the normal flora of a person's

PHARMACOLOGY Summary of Medications to Treat Acute Brain Disorders

Drug	Category	Application/Indication	Nursing Concerns
Dexamethasone	Corticosteroid	Reduce vasogenic edema.	Can cause psychosis, alteration in sleep, GI upset, leukocytosis, hyperglycemia
Mannitol	Osmotic solution	Reduce vasogenic edema.	Monitored unit; monitor serum sodium, osmolality levels
Famotidine (Pepcid) Ranitidine (Zantac) Omeprazole (Prilosec)	H2-blocker	Reduce acid in the stomach.	Thrombocytopenia
Phenytoin (Dilantin) Carbamazepine (Tegretol) Divalproex (Depakote) Gabapentin (Neurontin) Lamotrigine (Lamictal) Phenobarbital Clonazepam (Klonopin) Ethosuximide (Zarontin)	Antiepileptic drug	Prevent seizures.	Thrombocytopenia, gingivitis; allergic reactions can be severe
Diazepam (Valium) Lorazepam (Ativan)	Benzodiazepines	Treatment for seizure cessation, status epilepticus.	Oversedation, respiratory depression
Oxycodone (Percocet, Oxy-IR, OxyContin) Hydromorphone (Dilaudid) Hydrocodone (Vicodin, Lortab) Morphine Fentanyl (Sublimaze, Duragesic)	Opioids	Provide pain control for moderate to severe pain.	Respiratory depression, oversedation, constipation, difficulty with urination
Codeine Tramadol (Ultram)	Opioids	Provide pain control for mild to moderate pain.	Respiratory depression, oversedation
Ketorolac (Toradol) Indomethacin (Indocin) Ibuprofen (Motrin, Advil) Naproxen (Naprosyn)	Nonsteroidal anti-inflammatory drug (NSAID)	Provide pain control and fever reduction.	GI upset
Acetaminophen	Analgesic and anti-inflammatory	Provide pain control and fever reduction.	Liver toxicity
Naloxone (Narcan) Flumazenil (Romazicon)	Opioid antagonist; benzodiazepine antagonist	Reverse opiate effects and benzodiazepine effects.	
Propofol (Diprivan)	Sedative hypnotic	Provide sedation.	Short-acting, reverses quickly, oversedation
Ondansetron (Zofran) Metoclopramide (Reglan) Trimethobenzamide (Tigan) Prochlorperazine (Compazine) Promethazine (Phenergan)	Antiemetics (nonphenothiazines, phenothiazines)	Reduce/prevent nausea.	Psychosis, extrapyramidal symptoms
Carisoprodol (Soma) Cyclobenzaprine (Flexeril) Diazepam (Valium)	Antispasmodics	Muscle relaxants	Oversedation, respiratory depression
Temozolomide (Temodar) Procarbazine Cisplatin/carboplatin Vincristine Methotrexate	Chemotherapy	Treat malignant primary brain tumors.	Thrombocytopenia, neutropenia, anemia, nausea and vomiting

immune system, leaving the patient vulnerable to hospital-acquired infection. Nursing plays a vital role in the prevention of nosocomial infections. The most obvious actions might be the observation of universal precautions, the practice of meticulous hand hygiene, and the monitoring of signs and symptoms of impending infection.

Assessment

Patients with infectious diseases of the brain such as meningitis, encephalitis, or brain abscess initially may appear to be neurologically intact, but systemically ill. They and their families are usually frightened by the intensity of their illness. Often, it is the nurse who identifies that the patient is becoming ill with symptoms such as fever or signs of nuchal (back of neck) rigidity and brings it to the attention of the physician so that diagnostic testing can be done (see the Diagnostic Tests box, p. 723). Meningeal signs, such as nuchal rigidity (neck stiffness that prevents flexion), often are the first symptom. Patients not only experience headache and neck discomfort, they usually are photophobic, complaining of light sensitivity. A careful neurological exam, including testing for nuchal rigidity, Kernig's sign (severe stiffness of the hamstrings), and Brudzinski sign, yields important information.

Interventions and Rationales

The patient with suspected meningitis will need a lumbar puncture for diagnostic purposes. A nurse assisting with this procedure can help alleviate some of the fears of the patients, informing them of the procedure, the purpose of the procedure, and what is expected of them. It also is important for the patient to stay flat for approximately 4 hours after the lumbar puncture to avoid low-pressure spinal headaches. Once the lumbar puncture has been done, the CSF is sent to the laboratory for chemistry tests such as glucose, protein, cell count, and microbiology cultures.

It is important to monitor vital signs closely to watch for fever. The patient should be treated with antipyretics for fever reduction and kept cool and comfortable. Pain management also is important, because headaches may be severe. Use of narcotics to relieve pain must be balanced with the need to preserve the patient's clinical examination. Excessive use of narcotics will result in sedation and an inability to distinguish deterioration from medication effect.

Nursing management of patients with infectious processes of the CNS includes consideration of family members by keeping them involved and informed of their family member's condition. There is a great deal of fear involving diseases such as meningitis, encephalitis, and brain abscesses. There is concern about these conditions being contagious. Sometimes meningitis is contagious, such as in meningococcal meningitis caused by *Neisseria meningitidis*. When cultures are negative for unusual strains passed by contact, family and friends can be reassured that they cannot "catch" these diseases from the patient.

Medications for these disease processes include dexamethasone to decrease cerebral edema, an AED such as phenytoin, for seizure treatment or prophylaxis, antipyretics, and medications for pain control. The use of these medications is described in the Pharmacology Summary box (p. 733). It also is extremely important to start the patient on the appropriate antibiotic as soon as possible to combat the suspected pathogen.

These antibiotics should be started as soon as the CSF has been obtained.

Patients with brain abscess may present with symptoms such as those with any space-occupying lesion in their brain. They may have neurological compromise dependent on the size and location of the lesion. The abscess may cause mass effect and possible cerebral edema. Accurate and thorough neurological assessments are essential to identifying even a slight change in the patient's neurological status. These changes may be caused by an increase in the mass effect caused by an abscess or increased edema.

Evaluation

Brain abscess, once diagnosed, may require removal, with identification of the causative pathogen. Once identified, an aggressive regiment of IV antibiotic therapy is required under the guidance of an infectious disease specialist, if available. Postoperatively, patients will be admitted to the ICU. Though not usually the case, they may require monitoring of ICP and/or hemodynamic monitoring. They certainly will require close monitoring of their neurological status, with frequent, perhaps hourly, neurological assessment, as well as monitoring of their heart rate, blood pressure, respiratory rate, and oxygen saturation. A postoperative MRI is usually done to assess the degree of resection and to look for postoperative changes, such as hemorrhage or edema.

Collaborative Management

Consultation with an infectious disease specialist may be indicated, if available. Commonly, antibiotic courses are 4 to 6 weeks in the duration of the cerebral abscess. Infectious disease health care providers specialize in the management of infections, including method of transmission, appropriate antibiotics, and drug interactions. They also monitor disease trends and outbreaks.

Future Directions

It is important to continue to monitor the epidemiological trends of CNS infections to understand infection dynamics and to develop appropriate medical interventions. Although the mortality rate for meningitis and encephalitis is still significant, it appears that the rate is decreasing. One important trend is that of vaccines for meningococcal infections (Moura, Pablos-Mendez, Layton, & Weiss, 2003).

Another important consideration is that of antimicrobial resistance. The large volume of antibiotics prescribed has contributed to the emergence of highly resistant pathogens, among them vancomycin-resistant enterococci and methicillin-resistant *Staphylococcus aureus*. Some clinicians are very concerned that unless preventive measures are taken and new drugs are developed, at some point in the future, pathogens will appear that are not responsive to antibiotics (Yoshikawa, 2002). It is easy to imagine the high mortality rates we would face if bacterial meningitis could not be treated.

Other studies have demonstrated an inflammatory cascade evident in the tissue destruction in bacterial meningitis. Genetic targeting or pharmacologic blockage of these pathways may be beneficial in developing treatment or vaccines for bacterial pathogens (Koedel et al., 2002).

Brain Tumors

The diagnosis of a brain tumor often brings feelings of fear and uncertainty to the patient and his family. Most patients have little understanding of the concept of brain tumors, and many harbor misconceptions about the cause, treatment, and prognosis of their disease.

Epidemiology

According to the American Cancer Society (ACS), it was estimated that more than 20,000 people in the United States would be diagnosed with a malignant CNS tumor in the year 2007. In the same period approximately 13,000 people will die from brain, spinal cord, or other CNS malignancies (ACS, 2006). Although possible at any age, brain tumors are most commonly seen in children under the age of 10 and in adults from 30 to 50 years old. The average age at onset of all primary brain tumors is 53 years. Age prevalence differs with tumor type (Central Brain Tumor Registry of the United States, 2000). Incidence of gliomas is 40% higher among males; incidence of meningiomas is 80% greater in females (Surawicz, McCarthy, & Kupelian, 1999). Malignant brain tumors account for approximately 1% of all cancers, and 2% of all cancer-related deaths (ACS, 2006).

Etiology

The cause of CNS tumors is not well understood. It is known that brain tumors, like other tumors, are caused by abnormal changes in the genes. DNA, found in all genes, is considered the "building block of life." Genes are inherited from parents, and they literally make people what they are. Abnormal genes are called **gene mutations**, and also are inherited. Mutations can develop into diseases, including tumors. Cancer is believed to develop through an accumulation of genetic mutations or alterations, which allow the cells to grow out of control of normal regulatory mechanisms or to escape destruction by the immune system (see Chapter 64 🔗) (Minn, Wrensch, & Bondy, 2002).

Some inherited diseases, such as neurofibromatosis, are associated with increased risk of developing CNS tumors. It also is known that some gene mutations are not inherited. Research into these mutations has led to experimental laboratory treatments for brain tumors, with further refinement expected in the future (ACS, 2006).

It is not known why some people have gene mutations that cause brain tumors. Much research has been done looking for causes for brain tumors, such as cell phone use or environmental factors. There has been no link confirmed for the development of brain tumors with the use of cellular phones (Inskip, Tarone, & Hatch, 2001). However, children living in the vicinity of electromagnetic fields and having high exposure to them have shown increased risk for brain tumors, as have exposed workers (Meinert & Michaelis, 1996). Environmental factors, such as cigarette smoke, are known to cause lung cancer, which can metastasize to the brain to form metastatic lesions; however, no link has been found for primary disease (Wrensch, Minn, & Bondy, 2000).

Classification of Brain Tumors

The term *benign* can be misleading. Benign refers to microscopic cells that are well differentiated and resemble normal cells, but do not carry out the functions of normal cells. Instead they form slow-growing, space-occupying tumors. Histologically, although a tumor may be benign, if it is in a deep, eloquent area of the brain that is not accessible surgically, the tumor is not resectable. A tumor that is not resectable can continue to grow, producing neurological symptoms and possibly death. Some benign tumors also may progress into more malignant tumors if left untreated. A patient whose benign tumors are surgically resected can be considered cured.

Malignant tumors are those with poorly differentiated cells. Malignant tumors tend to be both aggressive and invasive. Although surgical resection may reduce the tumor, it is not curative. The prognosis for malignant tumors usually is poor.

Brain tumors may be primary or metastatic. **Primary tumors** are those that originate in the brain. These tumors rarely, if ever, travel to other areas of the body, remaining only in the brain. **Metastatic tumors** are those that originate in other areas of the body and travel to the brain. Examples of these are tumors that originate in the lung or breast tissue and metastasize to the brain. Tumors within the brain are classified as intra-axial, extra-axial, or metastatic.

Intra-Axial Tumors

Intra-axial tumors, located in the cerebrum, the brainstem, and the cerebellum, arise from glial cells, astrocytes, primitive brain structures, and ependymal structures. Glial cells are the supportive or nourishing cells of the brain. Any tumor arising from glial cells is referred to as a glioma. There are several types of gliomas: astrocytomas, oligodendrogliomas, and ependymomas. They are named for the type of cells they originate from and are graded for their degree of malignancy. Some tumors exist in a homogeneous form; others exhibit heterogeneous, or mixed, cell types.

Astrocytomas

Astrocytomas arise from the astrocyte cell. They have varying degrees of differentiation and are graded dependent on their degree of malignancy. Astrocytomas range from low grade (grades I and II), to anaplastic astrocytoma (grade III), to the most aggressive form of astrocytoma (grade IV), also known as glioblastoma multiforme. Low-grade astrocytomas, grade I or II, have well-differentiated cells. As the tissues become more malignant, cellularity increases, cell atypia increases, and mitotic activity increases. An astrocytoma with these cellular characteristics is termed anaplastic astrocytoma and is considered to be more malignant.

Astrocytomas account for approximately 50% of all primary brain tumors (Adesina, Leech, & Brumback, 2002). They are seen most commonly in the 30- to 50-year-old population, though they do occur in all age groups. Though astrocytomas may spread into surrounding normal brain tissue, it is rare for them to spread outside the brain and CSF system. Some astrocytomas spread throughout the CNS via CSF pathways.

Survival rates are dependent on many factors. These include grade, age of patient, extent of surgical resection, and response to treatment. The strongest predictor of survival with low-grade gliomas is age. One study reported a mean survival time of 8.5 years for adults less than 40 years of age. This contrasts with 4.9 years for adults 40 years of age and older (Piepmeier, 1987). Though this study is approximately 20 years old, the age factor has remained a strong prognostic factor.

MyNursingKit | Central Brain Tumor Registry

Anaplastic astrocytomas (grade III) are noted to be more aggressive than lower grade astrocytomas. They have a median survival rate of approximately 3 to 5 years (Burton & Prados, 2002). Clinical manifestations are dependent on many factors including location and size of the lesion. They may include a single seizure, behavior changes, headaches, or sensorimotor alterations.

Glioblastoma Multiforme   A grade IV astrocytoma also is referred to as a glioblastoma multiforme (GBM). These are the most malignant of the astrocytic tumors. Though they too arise from astrocytes, as do all astrocytomas, they are characterized by much more aggressive and invasive cellularity. They are rapidly growing, sometimes doubling in size in as little as 10 days. The GBM is composed of heterogeneous cells, which demonstrate the transformation of cells within this tumor from a low-grade to a high-grade or more malignant tumor. They are characterized by the presence of necrosis and hemorrhage within the tumor.

GBMs account for approximately 50% of all gliomas, and approximately 35% to 45% of all adult brain tumors. They are found most commonly in adults in their fourth to seventh decade, although they can be seen in young adults. The average age of patients with a GBM is 62 years, and they occur more often in men than women (Cox & Ang, 2003). The clinical history of GBM is relatively short. It frequently is less than 3 months before the patient presents with symptoms. The most common presenting symptoms are seizure, focal symptoms, such as motor weakness or aphasia, or nonfocal symptoms, such as headache or personality changes. The most dangerous aspect of symptomatology is the potential for rapidly increasing ICP caused by the rapid growth potential of this tumor (Kleihues, Davis, Coons, & Burger, 2000).

GBMs are the most malignant of all brain tumors. Despite improvements in surgical techniques, and the advancement of adjunctive therapies such as radiation therapy, chemotherapy, and radiosurgery, the prognosis is grim. The median survival rate is approximately 12 months (Burton & Prados, 2002). Although the prognosis is bleak, there is reason for hope in the treatment of high-grade gliomas. Research is ongoing, and new treatment protocols are being developed to treat this difficult and devastating disease.

Treatment is aimed at prolonging quality of life and may include the following strategies: surgical resection, radiation therapy, stereotactic radiosurgery, and chemotherapy. Despite what appears to be complete gross total resection, it is felt that this group of tumors is highly invasive at a microscopic level. This accounts for tumor recurrence despite resection in most cases. Radiation therapy (RT) is considered adjunctive. The most common form of radiation is focal external beam RT or conformal RT. Gamma knife radiosurgery has been shown to increase survival time in some cases. It can be used as a boost, or at tumor recurrence.

In some institutions, the implantation of radioactive materials, or a localized chemotherapeutic agent is used. This has met with mixed results, extending life by 4 to 10 weeks, but may be associated with seizures and craniotomy wound breakdown requiring additional hospital care. Chemotherapy also is an option for treatment of GBMs. Most treatment decisions are made based on the life expectancy and personal goals of the patient.

Some patients choose biopsy only and decide to spend their remaining time in their home with their family, whereas others prefer to exhaust all treatment measures. Nursing support for the family during their difficult decision process is essential.

Oligodendrogliomas

Tumors originating in brain cells are called oligodendrocytes. They grow and spread in much the same manner as astrocytomas. Specific to oligodendrogliomas is the frequent presence of calcification noted in diagnosed lesions (Adesina et al., 2002). They are slow growing, and can also spread to the CSF pathways, but rarely outside of the brain or spinal cord. Presenting signs and symptoms of oligodendrogliomas are dependent on the size and location of the tumor. Frequently, the initial presenting symptom is seizures. Oligodendrogliomas occur mostly in middle-age adults, but are occasionally seen in children. Treatment is surgical resection and radiation therapy. Prognosis for survival is thought to be approximately 7 years (Shaw, 2002).

Ependymomas

Ependymomas are tumors that originate in the ependymal cells lining the ventricles. They can be found in the brain or spinal cord. They do not spread into normal brain tissue, but they may spread along the CSF pathways. Therefore, there is a much better chance for complete surgical resection of ependymomas, especially from the spinal cord. Because these tumors are found in and around the ventricles and the CSF pathways, they occasionally cause obstruction of CSF flow, and hydrocephalus may occur.

Signs and symptoms are related to the location of the lesion. Seizures, motor weakness, cranial nerve deficits, or alterations in LOC may be present. If hydrocephalus is present, symptoms of increased ICP also may be present. Treatment consists of surgical resection and placement of a shunt if hydrocephalus is present. Radiation may be beneficial. Prognosis is excellent with surgical resection.

Extra-Axial Tumors

Extra-axial tumors are those that originate outside of the brain. The most common extra-axial tumors are meningiomas, schwannomas, and pituitary tumors.

Meningiomas

Meningiomas are the most common type of brain tumor, accounting for approximately 15% of all primary adult brain tumors (Cox & Ang, 2003). They arise from the meninges, the layer of tissue covering the brain and spinal cord. They are firm, encapsulated tumors that are extremely slow growing. Because they grow so slowly, they can grow to become quite large before they start causing symptoms. Meningiomas are most common in the middle-aged and the elderly. The peak occurrence is in the sixth and seventh decade of life. In middle-aged patients, there is a 3:2 female-to-male prevalence (Louis, Scheithauer, Budka, von Deimling, & Kepes, 2000). Presenting signs and symptoms depend on the location and size of the lesion.

Treatment is surgical resection in most cases. Occasionally, a complete resection is not possible because of the size of the lesion and its proximity to vital structures within the brain. In this case, radiation and/or gamma knife radiosurgery may be necessary. It also is necessary to follow these patients closely with yearly MRI scans to monitor the possible growth of the tumor. Tumor recurrence occurs in approximately 50% of patients with subtotal resection (Cox & Ang, 2003). In some cases, a lesion may be considered too small to warrant a surgical procedure. In these cases, monitoring of the lesion may be sufficient. Though considered benign, there is an atypical form and a malignant form of this disease, which may cause recurrence. It also is possible to have multiple meningiomas, which carries a high morbidity. Although the prognosis is extremely favorable with complete resection, it also is highly dependent on the degree of cell differentiation.

Schwannomas

Schwann cells are those that surround cranial nerves and other nerves. **Schwannomas** usually are benign tumors. The most common are schwannomas of the acoustic nerve (CN VIII), also referred to as **acoustic neuromas**. Acoustic neuromas usually are diagnosed when the patient experiences gradual hearing loss. Tinnitus and/or dizziness may also be noted. If left untreated, these lesions can become quite large, causing compression of the facial nerve (CN VII) or the trigeminal nerve (CN V).

For symptomatic lesions, gamma knife radiosurgery is the preferred treatment due to the ease of treatment, the excellent control of tumor growth, and reduction in unfavorable cranial nerve defects. Gamma knife treatment can also be planned to preserve hearing in those patients who still have functional hearing.

Open surgery is more appropriate for lesions that exceed 3 cm (about 1 in.). Surgical resection of acoustic neuromas can cause damage to cranial nerves in proximity to the tumor. In some instances, hearing may be sacrificed in the attempt to remove the tumor. The proximity of the brainstem and cranial nerves may result in damage to these nerves. Acoustic neuromas are located in the cerebropontine angle (CPA) with cranial nerves in proximity. Damage to the facial nerve (CN VII) may be present before surgery or as a result of surgery. Other cranial nerves also may be affected, specifically those involved with swallowing (CN IX, X, and XII). Therefore, a thorough cranial nerve assessment is important, both preoperatively and postoperatively.

If the facial nerve is damaged, it is important to note the degree of facial weakness exhibited. A facial weakness scale, known as the House/Brackmann scale, is used to note the degree of weakness (House & Brackmann, 1985). If significant facial weakness is observed, special care should be taken to protect the eye that does not close adequately. It is important to protect the eye from dryness and even abrasions by keeping it well lubricated with eyedrops. Occasionally, complete resection is not possible due to the size and location of the tumor. Residual tumor may be radiated and/or monitored with serial MRIs. Gamma knife radiosurgery may be a beneficial adjunctive treatment.

Pituitary Adenomas

Tumors of the pituitary gland occur most frequently in the anterior lobe, but both lobes may show symptoms. Tumors are classified by the type of hormone secreted (Chart 29–7, p. 738). Examples of these are prolactin, growth hormone, or ACTH secreting tumors. Pituitary tumors also are classified as functioning, hormone secreting, or nonfunctioning. Functioning pituitary adenomas produce endocrine symptoms, such as acromegaly, hyperprolactinemia, or Cushing's syndrome. Nonfunctioning pituitary adenomas produce symptoms caused by pressure of the tumor on surrounding structures, such as the optic nerve. Frequently, visual loss is the presenting symptom. It may be in the form of decreased acuity, hemianopsia, or scotomas. Headaches frequently accompany visual symptoms. Treatment may be medical and/or surgical. With treatment, prognosis is excellent.

Metastatic Tumors

Metastatic brain tumors originate in another part of the body from another type of cancer and travel to the brain. They are not considered to be cancer of the brain, but rather cancer from another source that has migrated to the brain.

Epidemiology and Etiology

Metastases to the brain come from many sources. The most common sites of primary disease are lung, breast, and skin. Metastatic lesions are probably more common than primary lesions. Males and females are represented equally, most commonly seen between the fifth and seventh decade of life (Sneed, 2002). The method of spread of metastatic lesions varies by the type of primary disease. Lesions most commonly spread from their primary site via the arterial route. They also may spread via the meninges. Occasionally, direct extension of melanoma lesions of the head or neck may lead to melanoma in the brain.

Other characteristics of metastatic lesions vary by primary disease. The number and location of lesions also vary by primary disease. Single lesions are more common, but multiple lesions occur frequently in some types of primary disease, such as lung cancer. The cerebral cortex is the most common site of metastatic disease, with the cerebellum less so.

Clinical Manifestations

Presenting symptoms of metastatic tumors are dependent on the location of the tumors. Most common symptoms are similar to those of primary tumors, and include headache, motor weakness, alteration of mentation, and/or behavioral changes. Seizures are the presenting symptom in many cases.

Laboratory and Diagnostic Procedures

Diagnosis of brain tumors always begins with an accurate and thorough history and physical. Symptom analysis, including duration and frequency of symptoms, is a valuable tool for determining presence and onset of symptoms. It also is important to have an accurate accounting of seizure events, including type, and frequency.

The actual diagnosis of a brain tumor is made by MRI of the suspected region, with and without gadolinium. It is possible with this test to determine the location, size, and characteristics of the lesion, including heterogeneity and presence of necrosis or hemorrhage. MRI also will determine the presence of calcification, cystic qualities, or enhancement. Ventricle size also is seen, as hydrocephalus is a potentially dangerous side effect of the presence of tumor, and the presence of edema and/or mass effect also can be determined. Although it is possible to diagnose a brain tumor with the aid of MRI, it only is possible to assume the type of tumor, not to diagnose the type of tumor. The only positive diagnosis of tumor type is by obtaining tissue for pathology diagnosis.

Medical Management

Once the diagnosis of brain tumor is made, treatment options must be explored. As just stated, the only means for positive

| CHART 29–7 | **Classification of Brain Tumors** | | | |

Type	Average Age at Onset	Symptoms	Treatment	Prognosis
Meningioma	Age 40–60s	Dependent on location and size Seizures Headaches	Surgery Radiation for residual or recurrence (gamma knife, cyberknife)	Excellent with resection
Astrocytoma	Variable	Dependent on location and size	Surgery Radiation for residual recurrence	3–7 years with treatment, dependent on grade and extent of resection
Glioblastoma multiforme (GBM)	Age 50–60s	Dependent on location and size	Surgery Radiation Chemotherapy	12–18 months with treatment
Oligodendroglioma	Age 40–50s	Dependent on location Seizures	Surgery Radiation Chemotherapy	5–10+ years with treatment
Ependymoma	All ages (60% are children)	Signs and symptoms Increased ICP Hydrocephalus	Surgery Radiation Chemotherapy for recurrence May need shunt	7–8+ years with surgery, less with recurrence
Pituitary adenomas	Variable	Hormone abnormalities dependent on area of pituitary affected Visual disturbances Headaches	Medical Surgical possible Radiation possible	Excellent
Acoustic neuromas	Age 40–50s	Hearing loss	Surgery Radiation for residual (gamma knife)	Excellent
Metastatic tumors	Variable	Dependent on location, size, single or multiple	Surgery if single metastasis or symptomatic Radiation (gamma knife) Chemotherapy	Usually poor, dependent on single or multiple and identification of primary disease

diagnosis is pathologic examination of the tissue. Neurosurgical consultation is imperative if a brain tumor is suspected. In addition to surgical intervention, options of radiation therapy, chemotherapy, and/or radio surgery may be available.

Surgical Excision

The role of surgical excision has several goals. The first is to establish a pathology diagnosis. As previously stated, the only way to obtain a positive diagnosis is to have a pathologist specializing in neuropathology make a positive identification of tumor type. Tumor type and grade, if appropriate, are necessary to establish an appropriate treatment plan. The second goal of surgery is to obtain the maximum tumor debulking possible while maintaining function. In many cases, the success of the treatment—and the prognosis—is based on the amount of tumor resection.

Surgical excision of a brain tumor requires monitoring in an ICU setting initially. Some patients may require ICP monitoring postoperatively. A postoperative MRI usually is done to assess the extent of resection and to assess the presence of hemorrhage, edema, and the status of the ventricles. The National Guidelines box provides the AANN national guidelines for the care of craniotomy patients.

Radiation Therapy

Once a pathologic diagnosis is made, some patients will require a consultation for a radiation oncologist. Brain tumors that cannot be cured by surgery alone may be treated with radiation. Recurrent, intermediate, or high-grade astrocytomas, metastatic tumors, incomplete or subtotal resections, or any other tumor deemed appropriate by the neurosurgeon or the neuro-oncologist may benefit from recommendations from a radiation oncologist. There are many types of radiation, and radiological treatment varies by pathologic diagnosis.

Radiation from an external source focused directly on the tumor is called external beam radiation. These treatments are given over a period of several weeks. Three-dimensional treatments are referred to as conformal radiation. Whole-brain radiation is given over a period of weeks. It generally is reserved for patients with several metastatic lesions for whom other methods of radiation would not be appropriate. Radiation therapy using any of these methods is used after surgical resection. The purpose is to slow growth, or to stabilize the residual tumor. It also may be used to prevent recurrence. The addition of RT to the treatment regimen of brain tumor patients adds to the comfort and quality of life and also increases survival time.

NATIONAL GUIDELINES AANN Guidelines for the Care of Craniotomy Patients for Brain Tumor

Neurological

- Most complications occur within the first 6 hours postoperative
- ICU admission postoperative
- Frequent neurological assessments
  - Ask the neurosurgeon what complications or deficits are expected
- Incision care
  - Monitor incision for drainage
  - Keep incision dry
- Drains
  - Make sure the location of each drain is known; label clearly

Cardiovascular

- Cardiac arrhythmias
- Hypovolemic shock
- Monitor rate and rhythm
- Monitor blood pressure and maintain ordered parameters

Respiratory

- Related to decreased level of consciousness/inability to protect airway
- Especially relevant to surgery near brainstem
- Prevent atelectasis and pneumonia
- Maintain $SaO_2 > 94\%$
- Incentive spirometry unless contraindicated (transsphenoidal surgery)

Gastrointestinal

- Prevention of gastric ulceration (antacids, proton pump inhibitor, H2-blockers)
- Some drugs used in neurological treatment can contribute to gastric irritation (dexamethasone, phenytoin, some antibiotics)

Nutrition

- May require swallow evaluation
- May require enteral feedings

Serum Glucose

- Hyperglycemia may increase cerebral edema
- Hyperglycemia may result from steroid therapy
- Monitor blood glucose as ordered
- Maintain euglycemia

Serum Sodium

- Diabetes insipidus
  - Especially relevant to surgery involving or near the pituitary gland
  - Monitor intake/output and specific gravity
  - Notify health care provider for urine output > 200 mL/hr × 2 consecutive hours
- Syndrome of inappropriate antidiuretic hormone
  - Monitor sodium levels; treat as ordered

Activity

- Population at risk for deep vein thrombosis (DVT)
  - Early ambulation
  - DVT prophylaxis, such as low-molecular-weight heparin, when ordered
  - Therapy consults
- Pain control
  - Assess per hospital protocol
  - Administer pain medication as ordered
  - Offer other techniques for pain management, such as deep breathing or music

Source: Adapted from American Association of Neuroscience Nurses, AANN Reference Series for Clinical Practice. (2006). *Guide to the Care of the Patient with Craniotomy Post-Brain Tumor Resection.* Glenview, IL: American Association of Neuroscience Nurses.

Stereotactic Radiosurgery

Stereotactic radiosurgery is another treatment option. It is a form of radiation therapy that delivers a single, high dose of radiation directly at the tumor or tumor bed. Despite the terminology, it is not a surgical procedure; however, it is meant to provide a highly conformed dose of radiation to the lesion. It may be used as the first preferred treatment or it may be used as a follow-up to other forms of treatment. The goal of radiosurgery is to treat all tumor cells in its path. Two types of radiosurgery most commonly used for treatment of brain tumors are gamma knife and cyber knife radiosurgery.

Gamma knife radiosurgery is a system that uses focused radiation in a single dose. It is used to irradiate very specific areas of tumor, such as the tumor bed of a metastatic lesion. This is a system developed by Lars Leksell that delivers multiple source beams (more than 200) to a specific, small target (Hickey, 2003). The name, however, is misleading because it is not really surgery and it is not really a knife. It may be used as the "first line" of treatment, or it may be used as adjunctive therapy. It may be used to "shrink" the residual tumor when complete resection is not possible. Gamma knife radiosurgery also may be beneficial

in treating tumors that are considered inoperable or small enough that a surgical procedure is not necessary.

Cyber knife radiosurgery is a relatively new addition to the radiation arsenal. It is a radiosurgical system that consists of a linear accelerator and a robotic arm. This system can locate tumors using image guidance, and then deliver multiple beams of radiation directly to the tumor site. This system has some important advantages. It minimizes radiation exposure to surrounding tissue and has the capacity to treat tumors up to 6 cm (2.4 in.) in size (Quinn, 2002). It has proven beneficial in treating metastatic brain tumors (Shimamoto et al., 2002).

Brachytherapy is referred to as an internal form of radiation therapy. It is the surgical implantation of radioactive capsules, or "seeds," directly into the tumor bed. These may be temporary or permanent. This procedure is generally reserved for high-grade gliomas.

Radiation is more damaging to cancer cells than to normal tissue, but it can cause damage to normal tissue. Sometimes an area of dead tissue forms at the site of an irradiated tumor. This is referred to as tissue necrosis and can appear as a mass on MRI, making it difficult to differentiate between dead tissue and tumor.

Positron emission tomography (PET) imaging may be used to aide in differentiating tissue necrosis, which has no metabolic activity, from new tumor growth, which has a high metabolic activity. Surgical resection may be necessary to debulk the mass and to differentiate between tumor regrowth and treatment effect. Radiation therapy is not without risk for adverse symptoms. However, the benefits of tumor suppression may outweigh the risks of radiation.

Chemotherapy

The purpose of chemotherapy is to destroy tumor cells, either by destroying the cells themselves or by destroying their capacity to reproduce themselves. Chemotherapy uses anticancer drugs, which are given intravenously or orally. They also may be given intrathecally, usually into an implanted reservoir. The implantation of a wafer soaked in a chemotherapeutic agent is occasionally used in the treatment of GBMs. The types of drugs used, dosage, and route are determined by the tumor type. Special concerns when treating malignant brain tumors with chemotherapeutic agents include the following:

- The location of the tumor in the brain affects choice of treatment.
- Cerebral edema affects drug entry into the brain.
- Brain tissue has a low capacity to remove dead tissue, cell debris, fluid, and drugs because there is no lymphatic drainage in the brain.
- Tumor cell resistance can occur (when tumor cells are no longer susceptible to damage by a particular drug).
- Malignant tumors (GBM) are composed of diverse (heterogeneous) cells, resulting in differences in the chemosensitivity of cells within the tumor.
- Many drugs cannot cross the blood–brain barrier (Shapiro & Shapiro, 1986).

Chemotherapy drugs kill cancer cells, but also can damage normal cells. Some normal tissue, such as bone marrow, the lining of the mouth and intestines, and hair follicles, grow rapidly to replace cells that wear out naturally. These cells are the ones most affected by chemotherapy drugs. Although care is taken to avoid or reduce the side effects of chemotherapy, these patients may experience hair loss, decreased white cell counts, fatigue, mouth sores, decreased appetite, and nausea and vomiting. These side effects are temporary and generally cease once treatment is over.

The survival of patients with brain tumors has improved somewhat with the addition of chemotherapy. However, the most effective drugs or combination of drugs is not yet known. At this point in time, the most common chemotherapeutic drugs are the alkylating agents such as carmustine (BCNU), lomustine (CCNU), procarbazine, vincristine, and temozolomide. They are typically used in combination with other therapies, such as RT. The use of chemotherapy in the treatment of cancer also is discussed in Chapter 64 ☻.

▮ Nursing Management

Nursing management of the patient with a brain tumor includes the opportunity to support patients and their families through one of the most difficult experiences they will experience. The patient and her family are presented with a life-altering diagnosis, which will affect every facet of the patient's life and every member of the patient's family. Innumerable factors can affect the patient's needs, both emotional and physical. The response to the diagnosis by the family and the patient is dependent on many factors, including the type of tumor, the location of the tumor, treatment plan, degree of neurological deficits, age of the patient, numerous family dynamics, educational status of the patient and family, and many other factors that change as the course of the disease changes.

Assessment

When the patient is initially diagnosed with a brain tumor, it may be because of an initial event that brought the patient into the emergency room, such as a seizure. Respiratory status must be monitored carefully, especially if the patient is admitted with a decreased level of consciousness. The ABCs of any emergency assessment (airway–breathing–circulation) are equally as important in patients with neurological deterioration. Monitoring of respiratory rate, rhythm, and effort are paramount, with preparations made for emergency intubation should the patient's respiratory status decline.

Usually, however, the patient is not in medical distress or even particularly ill. The patient's first exposure to a hospital setting may be on admission for surgery to remove the brain tumor. It may be unknown as to the patient's level of knowledge regarding his diagnosis or plan. An important nursing intervention is education, both of the surgical experience and what to expect postoperatively. The surgeon will review the planned surgery, surgical approach, projected length of hospital stay, and possible side effects with the patient and family. However, most patients and their families have many other questions that they do not ask their surgeon. Examples of these are: Will I have my head shaved? When will I be able to eat, or get out of bed, or go to the bathroom by myself? Will I be in pain? When can I go back to work? What's going to happen to me when I go home? It is not uncommon for the patient and family to depend on the nurse to provide them with the information that will affect their everyday lives.

Interventions and Rationales

As with other types of acute brain disorders, it is of utmost importance to adhere to the nursing care regimen associated with increased ICP, discussed earlier in this chapter. Certain tumor types are more prone to cause vasogenic edema. This may lead to cerebral edema, and increased ICP causing a variety of neurological deficits (refer to Chart 29–4, p. 720, on the nursing implications and interventions for management of ICP earlier in the chapter). These deficits include personality changes, decreased level of consciousness, aphasia, motor deficits, sensory deficits, visual deficits, and/or cranial nerve deficits. These deficits are dependent on the location and size of the lesion. Cerebral edema can be seen with almost any tumor type, but is most common with GBM, metastatic lesions, and even some "benign" tumors, such as meningiomas. The medical treatment of choice is dexamethasone. It is important that this drug be given exactly as ordered, because an abrupt halt—or even a decrease in dose—can cause an increase in edema and associated neurological symptoms. A patient care plan for patients with acute brain disorders applies to this clinical discussion, as it does with other types of acute brain disorders, and is discussed in the Nursing Process: Patient Care Plan for Acute Brain Disorders.

NURSING PROCESS: Patient Care Plan for Acute Brain Disorders

Assessment of Altered Levels of Consciousness

Subjective Data:

Does the patient have any history of health problems, such as hypertension, heart disease, bleeding disorders, renal disease, or cancer?

What were the patient's presenting symptoms/complaints?

How long ago did the first symptoms present?

Objective Data:

Neurological assessment, including mentation, cranial nerve examination, motor and sensory examination.

Imaging studies, including magnetic resonance imaging (MRI), computed tomography scan (CT), and/or lumbar puncture.

Laboratory data, including complete blood count (CBC), cerebral perfusion pressure (CPP), and drug levels.

Nursing Assessment and Diagnoses	Outcomes and Evaluation Parameters	Planning and Interventions with *Rationales*
Nursing Diagnoses: *Actual and Potential Alteration in Level of Consciousness* related to traumatic brain injury (TBI), intracranial tumor, or infectious process	**Outcome:** Improvement to optimum level of function. *Evaluation Parameters:* Stable neurological examination. Glasgow Coma Scale. Laboratory tests, including serum sodium and cultures of blood and cerebrospinal fluid (CSF) if suspicious for infection.	**Interventions and *Rationales:*** Monitor neurological examination hourly, or as directed. *Allows early recognition of pending neurological deterioration.* Monitor lab values, including serum sodium levels and cultures. *Early recognition and treatment of hyponatremia or infection.*
Impaired Physical Mobility related to altered level of consciousness	**Outcome:** Improvement to optimum level of motor function. *Evaluation Parameters:* Neurological motor and sensory examination. Level of participation in therapies and ADLs.	**Interventions and *Rationales:*** Monitor motor strengths and limitations. *Allows early recognition of neurological changes.* Initiate therapies, such as physical and occupational unless contraindicated. *Early initiation of therapies helps to identify deficits and needed areas for improvement.* Initiate activity as tolerated, unless contraindicated. *Physical activity will increase strength and endurance, as well as decrease complications, such as pneumonia or blood clots.*
Ineffective Tissue Perfusion related to immobility	**Outcome:** Adequate tissue perfusion. *Evaluation Parameter:* Absence of deep vein thrombosis (DVTs) or pulmonary embolus.	**Interventions and *Rationales:*** Encourage activity as tolerated, unless contraindicated. *Physical activity will prevent immobility and the formation of blood clots.* Apply thigh-high elastic stockings and sequential compression stockings *to increase venous circulation.* Administer subcutaneous injections of low-molecular-weight heparin, if indicated *to discourage the formation of blood clots.* Monitor lower extremities frequently for signs/symptoms of DVT. *Early recognition and treatment of a DVT may prevent extension of the clot or pulmonary embolus.*
Impaired Verbal Communication related to anatomical defect.	**Outcome:** Maximum level of communication. *Evaluation Parameter:* Ability to adequately communicate with others.	**Interventions and *Rationales:*** Assess type and degree of communication deficit *to determine patient needs and establish a baseline.* Arrange a speech therapy consult. *Early intervention and therapy optimizes results.*
Actual or Potential Alteration in Visual Perception related to TBI or brain tumor	**Outcome:** Maximum level of vision/visual acuity. *Evaluation Parameter:* Formal and informal vision screening including visual fields.	**Interventions and *Rationales:*** Assess vision by informal testing (i.e., counting fingers, reading the clock) *to assess type and degree of visual deficit present.* Institute safety measures, such as placing call light within reach, orienting patient to surroundings, *to prevent accidents/falls.* Obtain occupational therapy evaluation if warranted. *Evaluation of visual deficits and education regarding coping mechanisms.*
Ineffective Cerebral Tissue Perfusion related to electrolyte imbalances in TBI, brain tumors, or infectious process	**Outcome:** Optimum neurological function. *Evaluation Parameters:* Stable neurological examination. Electrolyte levels, specifically sodium.	**Interventions and *Rationales:*** Monitor serum sodium as indicated, at least daily *to assess for hyponatremia.* Conduct neurological assessments frequently *to assess for decreased level of consciousness.* Administer fluids as directed *to maintain adequate fluid balance.* Notify health care providers immediately of abnormal lab values or change in neurological examination. *Such changes may indicate hyponatremia.*

(continued)

NURSING PROCESS: Patient Care Plan for Acute Brain Disorders—*Continued*

Assessment of Airway and Gas Exchange

Subjective Data:
Does the patient have any preexisting medical problems such as emphysema or asthma, or any cardiac diseases?

Objective Data:
Respiratory rate
Oxygen saturation
Arterial blood gases

Vital signs
Lung sounds
Skin/nail bed/lip color

Nursing Assessment and Diagnoses	Outcomes and Evaluation Parameters	Planning and Interventions with *Rationales*
Nursing Diagnoses: *Ineffective Airway Clearance* related to altered level of consciousness	**Outcome:** Adequate respiration status. ***Evaluation Parameters:*** Adequate arterial blood gases. Respiratory rate within normal limits. Normal oxygen saturation levels. Clear lung sounds. Mental status, such as confusion or agitation.	**Interventions and *Rationales:*** Monitor respiratory status (i.e., rate, rhythm, and quality). *Changes in respiratory rates or patterns may indicate pending respiratory failure. It may also indicate neurological change.* Monitor mental status. *Restlessness, agitation, or confusion may indicate hypoxia.* Monitor oxygen saturation *to assess adequacy of gas exchange.* Encourage deep breathing or use of an incentive spirometer *to promote adequate gas exchange.* Position with head in neutral position, head of bed elevated at 30 degrees, unless contraindicated *to promote adequate gas exchange.* Suction as necessary. *Patients with decreased neurological status may be unable to protect their airways.* Report changes in respiratory patterns to MD. *Such changes indicate possible risk for respiratory failure.* If patient not intubated, have necessary intubation equipment available. *Protecting the airway is the priority. Intubation may be necessary to protect airway.*
Risk for Aspiration related to altered level of consciousness	**Outcome:** No aspiration. ***Evaluation Parameters:*** Adequate oxygen saturation. Safe swallowing techniques.	**Interventions and *Rationales:*** Keep NPO until alert and/or swallow reflex is assessed and deemed safe. *Altered level of consciousness may depress the cough and/or swallow reflex.*

Assessment of Hemodynamic Status

Subjective Data:
Does the patient have any preexisting cardiac or respiratory problems?

Objective Data:
Vital signs, including heart rate, blood pressure, respiratory rate, and central venous pressure, if available
Oxygen saturation
Skin, lips, and nail bed color
Lung sounds
Cardiac rhythm strips or ECG

Nursing Assessment and Diagnoses	Outcomes and Evaluation Parameters	Planning and Interventions with *Rationales*
Nursing Diagnoses: *Decreased intracranial adaptive capacity* related to increased intracranial pressure	**Outcome:** Hemodynamic stability. ***Evaluation Parameters:*** Adequate blood pressure to maintain central perfusion pressure (CPP). Stable vital signs, including central venous pressure (CVP), Pulmonary Arterial Pressure (PAP), and intracranial pressure (ICP).	**Interventions and *Rationales:*** Monitor vital signs as directed *to establish a baseline and note changes in vital signs.* Administer fluids and medications as directed *to assist in maintaining blood pressure as ordered to maintain adequate CPP.* Monitor ECG rhythm *to assess for alterations in rhythm or rate.* Monitor intake and output *to assess fluid balance to maintain hemodynamic parameters.* Notify health care provider of hemodynamic changes. *Medical intervention may be necessary to prevent hemodynamic instability leading to neurological decline.* Monitor neurological assessments closely. *Hemodynamic stability is closely related to CPP and ICP changes in neurologically compromised patients.*

Assessment of Pain

Subjective Data:
Does the patient complain of pain?
Facial expressions (i.e., grimacing).

Objective Data:
Increased heart rate, blood pressure, or respiratory rate?

Nursing Assessment and Diagnoses	Outcomes and Evaluation Parameters	Planning and Interventions with *Rationales*
Nursing Diagnosis: Readiness for enhanced comfort related to brain tumor, head injury, meningitis, or surgical procedure	**Outcome:** Adequate pain control. **Evaluation Parameters:** Vital signs within normal limits. Patient verbalizes pain control.	**Interventions and *Rationales:*** Assess presence of pain or efficacy of pain control frequently *to ensure patient comfort.* Administer pain medications as ordered *to ensure patient comfort.*

Assessment of Coping

Subjective Data:
What are patient's complaints?
What is the patient's understanding of present condition or disease?
What are patient's concerns for the future?

Objective Data:
What is the patient's level of education?
What is the patient's occupation?
What is the patient's family support system?
Does the patient have a religious affiliation?

Nursing Assessment and Diagnoses	Outcomes and Evaluation Parameters	Planning and Interventions with *Rationales*
Nursing Diagnoses: *Ineffective Coping* related to knowledge deficit	**Outcome:** Patient and family will have information needed. **Evaluation Parameter:** Discussions with patient, with verbalization of condition and treatment.	**Interventions and *Rationales:*** Provide information as needed and answer questions honestly and completely. *Information and education are important to the patient.* Involve family as appropriate. *Family support is important for recovery.*
Readiness for Enhanced Family Coping related to neurological deficits	**Outcome:** Family will have improved coping with neurological disability. **Evaluation Parameters:** Discussions with patient and family with verbalization of concerns. Observation of family/patient interactions.	**Interventions and *Rationales:*** Reassure patient and family with honesty and compassion *to provide encouragement and information needed for coping.* Encourage family members to voice concerns *to help with assessment of family needs.* Provide family with support as needed, such as spiritual, therapies, or psychological. *Neurological disability affects the whole family and community.*

These patients usually are started on corticosteroids, such as dexamethasone (Decadron). The most common dose is 4 mg every 6 hours, but it may be necessary to give 10 mg every 6 hours in the presence of cerebral edema. Use of steroids such as dexamethasone usually increases blood glucose levels, possibly requiring treatment. It also raises white blood counts, which may mask underlying infectious processes. Steroids can cause significant alterations in behavior and produce insomnia, elation, and even psychosis. Nursing care should include careful monitoring to detect behavioral changes. Refer to the Pharmacology Summary (p. 733) for more explanation of these medications.

Patients undergoing chemotherapy may experience many side effects. Common side effects of the various chemotherapeutic drugs include fatigue, nausea and vomiting, loss of appetite, rash, neuropathies, myelosuppression, constipation, and immunosuppression. Side effects differ with the agent, and may range from mild to severe. Occasionally treatment cannot be continued due to the severity of the reaction. It is important for nurses to be aware of side effects specific to the treatment of each patient. All side effects should be reported to the health care provider.

Also associated with some brain tumors are seizures. Although seizures may be seen with other acute brain disorders, they are closely associated with certain types of brain tumors. Seizures are the most common presenting symptom of patients with oligodendrogliomas. They also are seen frequently with other tumor types, especially those located in the temporal region, due to the high intensity of seizure focus in that area. These seizures are treated with antiepileptic drugs such as phenytoin. The nursing implications of seizure treatment are discussed later in this chapter.

Patients with newly diagnosed brain tumors may present with overwhelming emotional needs. Nursing intervention comes in the form of education and support. An important discharge intervention may be acquainting patients and their families with available brain tumor support groups. Many patients and families feel that the diagnosis of brain tumor is one without hope. Providing the patient and their family with education and support may be helpful in relieving the fear of the unknown.

■ Collaborative Management

The diagnosis, treatment, and management of patients with brain tumors require the expertise of multiple disciplines. These include, but are not limited to, nursing, neurosurgery, neuro-oncology, radiation oncology, physical therapy, speech and cognitive therapy, occupational therapy, pathology, rehabilitation specialists, neuropsychologists, research scientists and nurses, dietitians, and support groups. Once the diagnosis of brain tumor is made, the patient should be referred to a neurosurgeon. Postoperatively, the patient may require the services of various therapists, such as physical, occupational, and/or speech therapists. Therapies are important for evaluation, and treatment if necessary. It is also important for discharge recommendations. Dependent on the pathology of the tumor, consultations with neuro-oncology, medical-oncology, and/or radiation oncology may be warranted. These consultations may be for the purpose of recommendations, with or without treatment.

Upon discharge from the hospital, the patient may need further therapy. This may be in the form of outpatient therapies, home health therapy, or an acute inpatient rehabilitation stay. Determination of the patient's need for further therapy is usually made by specialists in rehabilitation medicine. (For more on patient education regarding discharge, see the Patient Teaching & Discharge Priorities box.)

At the center of the brain tumor patient's plan of care is nursing. As stated previously, newly diagnosed brain tumor patients are frequently in a state of confusion and emotional upheaval. Their lives are full of changes: physical, emotional, practical, and possibly financial. They may be facing the loss of a job and fi-

PATIENT TEACHING & DISCHARGE PRIORITIES for Acute Brain Disorders

Need	Teaching

Wound infection:
Patient
Family support system
Setting
	Assess surgical wound for signs/symptoms of infection.
	Signs and symptoms of infection include:
	  Redness
	  Tenderness
	  Exudate and/or odor
	  Swelling
	  Poor healing.
	The presence of fever or any of the above symptoms should be reported.
	Assess family support for needed assistance.

Mobility assistance: Patient Family support system Setting	Assess motor strengths and ability for ambulation. Obtain consults for physical and occupational therapy. Assess need for assistive devices, such as wheelchair, walker, or splints. Assess availability of family for support with mobility and ADLs. Conduct family teaching. Assess environment for risk factors.
Pain control: Patient Family support system Setting	Assess need for pain control. Is present medication regimen adequate? Is pain controlled sufficiently to allow patient to participate in ADLs? Assess need for family intervention in dispensing pain medication. Assess patient/family understanding of medication instructions.

Safety:
Patient
Family support system
Setting
	Assess patient cognitive status:
	  Is patient a fall risk?
	  Assess safety awareness.
	Assess patient understanding of medication schedule and needs.
	Assess patient need for supervision.
	Obtain consults for speech/cognitive evaluation.
	Obtain social service consult.
	Obtain home health consult.
	Assess family involvement in patient's recuperative period.
	Conduct family teaching regarding possible cognitive impairments.
	Conduct family teaching regarding need for supervision.
	Assess environment for safety. May require home health or social service involvement.

Follow-up needs:
Patient
Family support system
Setting
	Assess need for follow-up appointments for needed therapies or interventions:
	  Radiation therapy
	  Outpatient therapies: physical, occupational, speech
	  Physician appointments
	  Laboratory visits for evaluation of drug levels or electrolytes
	  Follow-up x-rays.
	Assess family understanding and need for further explanation.
	Assess availability of resources for follow-up.

nancial security and changes within their family structure (e.g., spouses becoming caregivers). It is important to supply these patients with as much education and support as they require. If support groups are available, it is usually helpful to give this information to the patients and their families.

Health Promotion

Much research has been done to look for causes of brain tumors. These research inquiries include genetic research, environmental factors, dietary factors, and hereditary factors. As mentioned earlier, attention has been given to the use of cellular phones and a possible connection with the development of brain tumors. Use of cellular phones has not been shown to be harmful (Inskip et al., 2003). Studies have been completed to answer the concern about the possibility that exposure to the polio vaccine in the 1950s may have exposed millions to a precursor to the development of brain tumors. No evidence was found to link polio vaccine with the development of brain tumors (Brenner et al., 2002).

Some of the stronger leads concerning potential causes of brain tumors have come from studies of occupation. Suspected occupations of high risk include employment in the petroleum industry, electricity-related jobs, farming, and work involving pesticides, and electric and magnetic fields (DeRoos et al., 2003). Because there are inconsistencies among study results, there is a defined need for further study in certain fields, such as environmental and occupational hazards.

Despite much attention to the potential risk factors of brain tumors, the etiology of brain tumors remains largely unknown. There are some familial genetic cancer syndromes, such as neurofibromatosis and tuberous sclerosis, but these account for a very small number. The only environmental risk factor that is well established is that of ionizing radiation. It is therefore important to continue research to look for factors that may cause brain tumors, and factors that may protect us from brain tumors (Brenner et al., 2002).

Future Directions

A diagnosis of brain tumor is life altering, at best. Even with more than 20 years of clinical trials and new technologies to combat this disease, few improvements in prognosis have been seen, especially in the treatment of high-grade tumors. However, the team of professionals aligned to fight this disease and find a cure, or at very least improved treatment, also is formidable. Neuro-oncologists are facing great challenges in the management of brain tumors. They are joined by radiation oncologists, geneticists, cellular biologists, neurologists, and neurosurgeons.

Pueschel, Ashby, and Shapiro (2003) described the results of clinical trials in the treatment of adult and pediatric CNS tumors published in a single year (2001). These studies described various chemotherapy regimens, delivered with and without adjunctive RT. There is no doubt that these trials will continue examining new and different drug and treatment combinations until one is found that will successfully treat, and, it is hoped, cure brain tumors.

The Radiation Therapy Oncology Group (RTOG) (2008) protocols also are important in identifying optimal RT programs for various tumor types. Radiosurgery has become and will continue to be important in the treatment of various tumor types. Information is being obtained and processed continually to determine the efficacy of various treatment plans.

Research into the genetics of brain tumors is dynamic. Genetic aberrations are being defined for the various glial tumors previously described. It is known that tumors can evolve by different pathways. Genetic aberrations differ from grade of malignancy and the type of tumor. Additional research is needed to continue in this field of brain tumor research to identify causes and look for treatment (Shapiro, 2001). Immunotherapy and gene therapy offer exciting challenges for future investigation of treatment for brain tumors (Pueschel et al., 2003).

Hydrocephalus

Cerebrospinal fluid is a clear, colorless fluid produced within the ventricles, in the choroid plexus. Its purpose is to circulate within the subarachnoid space and bathe the brain and spinal cord in fluid to cushion it. A normal adult has approximately 125 to 150 mL of CSF at any one time. It is normally produced at approximately 25 mL an hour. The most common pathologic condition concerning CSF is hydrocephalus. Hydrocephalus is an excessive accumulation of CSF in the intracerebral ventricles. It may be caused by overproduction or inadequate drainage or absorption. Two types of hydrocephalus are communicating and noncommunicating.

Communicating hydrocephalus refers to large ventricles in a system with communication between all of the ventricles and the pathway for CSF. The size of the ventricles is relatively proportional. The cause of communicating hydrocephalus usually is due to blockage or malabsorption of CSF by the arachnoid granulations. Common causes include subarachnoid hemorrhage (SAH) or the presence of infection, such as coccidiomycosis.

Noncommunicating (also referred to as obstructive) hydrocephalus refers to a blockage somewhere within the CSF pathway. One or more of the ventricles may be larger than the other ventricles, depending on the level of the obstruction. The most common cause of noncommunicating hydrocephalus is space-occupying lesions, such as tumors.

The most important concept to understanding hydrocephalus is that of resistance to the absorption of CSF, which can cause hydrocephalus and the increase of ICP. The most common cause of malabsorption of CSF is subarachnoid hemorrhage, in which protein from blood product breakdown clogs the arachnoid granulations, hindering absorption of CSF. In the absence of a lymphatic drainage system in the CNS, open communication between the CSF and the interstitial fluid is necessary for maintenance of homeostasis (Sato, Takei, & Yamada, 1994).

In the presence of cerebral edema, there may be no increase in ventricular size, due to the pressure of the brain tissue (parenchyma) against the ventricular system. Ventricular size is a balance between brain tissue forces attempting to compress the ventricles and intraventricular pressure, attempting to enlarge the ventricles This concept of intracranial pressure was discussed earlier in the chapter. Hydrocephalus is a common occurrence in brain trauma, some brain tumors, subarachnoid hemorrhage, and some encephalopathic conditions, including meningitis, encephalitis, and brain abscess.

Clinical Manifestations

The presentation of increasing ventricular size in adults is dependent on the type of hydrocephalus. Examples of symptoms are similar to those of increased ICP and include papilledema, headache, nausea and vomiting, incontinence, gait changes, difficulty with extraocular movements particularly upgaze, and alterations in LOC.

Laboratory and Diagnostic Procedures

A CT scan of the head, without contrast, is the quickest and most definitive means of diagnosing hydrocephalus. MRI is also an effective diagnostic study, and may be a better choice for imaging when pathology, such as a brain tumor, is suspected. As always, close clinical correlation of the patient's history and presenting symptoms is recommended.

Medical Management

Hydrocephalus is a surgically treated condition. In emergency situations, removal of spinal fluid by means of an external ventricular drain is a temporary solution. However, placement of a shunting device to remove extra spinal fluid is the gold standard for treatment of hydrocephalus. There are several types of shunts; the most common are the ventriculo-peritoneal shunt and the lumbo-peritoneal shunt. Other less commonly used shunts include the ventriculo-atrial shunt, the ventriculo-gallbladder shunt, and the ventriculo-cyst shunt. These are used most commonly when the more common types of shunts are not successful or their use is not possible for some reason.

Disadvantages of shunts are obstruction of the proximal or distal end, infection, or failure due to disconnection. There also is the possibility of overshunting, that is, the drainage of too much CSF, resulting in slit ventricles and headaches for the patient. In extreme cases, subdural hematoma (SDH), caused by tearing of bridging veins, may occur. Undershunting, or too little fluid removal, results in the ventricles remaining large. A CT scan after the placement of a shunt is recommended to document appropriate placement of the shunt and to assess the efficiency of the shunt by checking for decrease in ventricle size.

◼ Nursing Management

Nursing management of patients with hydrocephalus consists primarily of accurate neurological assessment. Hydrocephalus can occur with virtually any neurological condition. Decrease in mental status can occur slowly, over days, or rapidly. Any change in neurological status is significant and should be reported. These changes include a decrease in LOC, decrease in ability to speak, decrease in ability to ambulate, and/or incontinence of bowel or bladder. Please refer to the Nursing Process: Patient Care Plan for Acute Brain Disorders (p. 741) for the details of how to care for a patient with hydrocephalus.

◼ Seizures

Seizures are described as a single, temporary event that consists of uncontrolled, electrical neuronal discharge of the brain that interrupts normal brain function. Seizures may occur as a result of most acute brain disorders: a brain tumor, brain trauma such as a hematoma or concussion, or in conjunction with an infectious process such as meningitis, encephalitis, and abscesses. They also may be seen with other, nonneurological disorders, such as metabolic disorders including severe dehydration, electrolyte imbalances, or withdrawal from alcohol or drugs. Idiopathic seizures also may occur in the absence of underlying abnormalities. Epilepsy is a condition in which seizures occur spontaneously, and they can recur due to an underlying condition or without a known cause.

Epidemiology and Etiology

There are many causes of seizures. These causes are different with age of the patient at onset. In newborns, birth trauma is the most common cause for seizures. In children, fever, trauma, and CNS infections are the most common. Structural abnormalities, such as tumors, strokes, and trauma, are the most common cause in adults. Genetic causes account for approximately 30% of epilepsy in adults and approximately 60% of epilepsy in children (Hirose, Okada, Kaneko, & Mitsudome, 2000).

Clinical Manifestations

The clinical manifestations of seizures are dependent on the location of the seizure focus, or electrical aberrancy. Seizures are divided into two main divisions: generalized and partial (Chart 29–8). Generalized seizures affect the whole brain (Shapiro & Shapiro, 1986). They may be characterized by alterations in mentation, behavior, sensation, or motor tonic–clonic, or grand-mal, seizures. They are characterized by bilateral, symmetric electrical discharges, and are described as a stiffening of the body, with jerking of all extremities (Shapiro & Shapiro, 1986). The patient may become cyanotic, have excessive drooling, and bite the inside of the mouth and/or tongue. Urinary incontinence is common with this type of seizure. The patient loses consciousness and is not communicative or interactive during the event. There may be pupillary changes, with a gaze deviation (away from the side of a structural abnormality, if present). After the seizure, the patient enters the postictal stage, which usually is characterized by extreme lethargy, allowing the patient to sleep. The patient has no memory of the seizure event.

Partial seizures are further divided into simple or complex, with the differentiating factor being consciousness. Simple partial seizures are described as those with specific motor or sensory abnormalities. These would include focal motor seizures or those with somatosensory components, such as the visualization of flashing lights or hearing of noises that are not real. There is no loss of consciousness. Complex partial seizures may begin as a simple partial seizure. They may share many of the same features as simple partial seizures, but consciousness is impaired. They also may progress to a generalized seizure.

Status Epilepticus

Status epilepticus has been described as "either continuous seizures lasting at least five minutes or two or more discrete

CHART 29–8	Types of Seizures			
Type of Seizure	**Characteristics**	**Consciousness**	**Medications**	**Age Groups**
Tonic–clonic Generalized Grand mal Absence	Bilateral Symmetric No warning Stiffening of the body Jerking Cyanosis Tongue-biting Incontinence Abnormal behavior Staring spells	Loss of consciousness for seconds to minutes	Phenytoin (Dilantin) Carbamazepine (Tegretol) Levetiracetam (Keppra) Lamotrigine (Lamictal) Phenobarbital Topiramate (Topamax) Divalproex (Depakote) Klonopin Divalproex (Depakote)	All children
Partial, simple	Focal Motor and/or sensory May progress	No loss of consciousness	Same as above Pregabalin (Lyrica) Gabapentin (Neurontin) Oxcarbazepine (Trileptal)	All
Partial, complex	Focal Motor and/or sensory Automatisms	Altered state of consciousness Clouding or confusion Déjà vu	Same as above	All

seizures between which there is incomplete recovery of consciousness" (Sirven, & Waterhouse, 2003). Status epilepticus is a medical emergency, because continued seizure activity could result in severe neurological injury due to cerebral hypoxia. It also may result in respiratory and/or cardiovascular failure.

Laboratory and Diagnostic Procedures

The diagnosis of seizures is dependent on many factors. First, a detailed account of the event must be available. This includes clinical presentation, medications, and past medical history. A physical examination, with a focus on neurological assessment is essential.

Diagnostic tests include, but are not limited to, imaging studies, such as MRI or CT scan, to rule out structural abnormality as a cause (see the Diagnostic Tests box, p. 723). This does not address whether or not a seizure has occurred, but rather is used to determine if there is an underlying cause present that could potentiate a seizure. EEGs record the electrical potential of the brain. This is done by placing electrodes on the patient's scalp and recording tracings of the electrical activity of the brain. Patients with epilepsy have abnormal electrical tracings. EEGs should be used in conjunction with other diagnostic tests, such as MRI, PET scans, or other tests that determine potential organic causes for seizures, such as a tumor. EEGs are very helpful in recording abnormal electrical activity if a seizure occurs during the tracing. However, these tracings can be normal in the interictal period, between seizure events. Other tests may be used to help determine the exact location of a seizure focus and the area and function of the brain affected. Wada tests, officially known as the intracarotid sodium amobarbital procedure (ISAP), are used to determine which side of the brain controls language function and also how important each side of the brain is with regard to memory function. Functional MRIs also are very helpful to determine where specific functions lie in the brain.

Medical Management

Treatment of seizures begins with treatment of an underlying condition, if present. Medical treatment of seizures should begin immediately, and it depends on the type of seizure. Antiepileptic drugs should be started immediately to prevent further seizures. Many antiepileptic drugs are available, and research is being done to best determine the most efficacious according to seizure types. Antiepileptic drugs are described in the Pharmacology Summary box (p. 733) earlier in the chapter.

In some circumstances, surgical resection of an identifiable seizure focus is warranted. To determine suitability for resection, these patients may be evaluated extensively in a specialized monitoring unit (e.g., the Epilepsy Monitoring Unit) equipped with 24-hour EEG and surveillance monitors to identify the seizure focus. Invasive EEG electrodes may be placed surgically. These data are reviewed along with continuous video surveillance of the patient and all possible seizure activity. This information, along with diagnostic imaging studies, gives useful information to specialists in seizures, called epileptologists. These specialized neurologists work closely with neurosurgeons to determine if surgical resection of a seizure focus would be warranted. This surgery is referred to as a selective amygdalohippocampectomy (SAHC).

Management of status epilepticus consists of two important points. Termination of the seizure is of primary importance. This usually is accomplished with medications, such as short-acting benzodiazepines. Secondly are the ABCs of life support, such as assessment of the patient's respiratory status, with administration of oxygen by mask or nasal cannula and ventilatory support if necessary.

■ Nursing Management

One of the most important factors in the management of seizures is the reporting of the seizure event. Often, nursing staff are the ones who witness a seizure.

Assessment

Accurate and thorough assessment and reporting of the characteristics of the event is important to the classification of the seizure type and its management. See Chart 29-9 for assessment guidelines.

Interventions and Rationales

Certain tumor types, such as high-grade gliomas and metastatic melanoma to the brain, cause the patient to be at high risk for seizures. All TBI patients are at risk for seizures, as are patients with any type of infectious process in the brain. If the patient is admitted to the hospital after having his first seizure, an important nursing intervention is to prevent further harm to the patient having a seizure. Padding the rails of the bed is one simple nursing action. Administering the necessary antiepileptic drug is another.

 It is important to be aware of precautions and adverse risks concerning the administration of phenytoin. Phenytoin must be administered at a rate of no more than 50 mg/min when given intravenously to avoid pain at the administration site, or hemodynamic compromise, such as bradycardia or hypotension.

Phenytoin may cause drowsiness. When given as routine dosing, it may be necessary to give full daily dose at night to avoid drowsiness during day.

Phenytoin is thought to work by maintaining adequate blood levels of the drug. It is important to monitor drug levels periodically. Most seizures are controlled with a serum level between 10 and 20. Certain drugs interfere with the metabolism of phenytoin, altering the blood levels. It is important to be aware of drugs that interact with phenytoin.

Unexplained rash and/or fever may be attributed to allergy to phenytoin. Report to MD if patient develops rash or fever while on phenytoin.

A common first line AED is phenytoin (Dilantin). Phenytoin is given as a loading dose of 1 gram, or 17 mg/kg intravenously over a period of 30 minutes to 1 hour. The patient is then started on a maintenance dose of 100 mg three times a day. The efficacy of phenytoin is determined by seizure control. Blood testing also is done to measure the serum level of phenytoin. Seizure control is often achieved with a level between 10 and 20, but phenytoin levels are managed based on seizure control and the occurrence of

side effects. Occasionally a patient will be started on phenytoin without having had a seizure when health care providers feel that the patient is at risk for seizures. If the patient has a seizure while on phenytoin and while blood levels appear to be in the therapeutic range, a second AED may be necessary.

Phenytoin is not without side effects. It has been known to cause fatigue, which can be alleviated by giving the patient his entire dose at nighttime. Therapeutic drug levels may be achieved with a once daily dose if it is easier for the patient and causes him fewer side effects. Other side effects include nausea, dizziness, gait and balance problems, gingival hyperplasia, and drug-induced fever. Occasionally phenytoin has been associated with severe allergic reactions, ranging from a mild rash to a severe hypersensitivity condition known as Steven-Johnson syndrome (Greenberg, 2001). This condition can be severe and can lead to multisystem failure.

 Confusion, lethargy, and/or seizure may be a sign of hyponatremia. Check recent serum Na+ level, check intake and output, and determine which intravenous fluids are running, if any. Notify health care provider of suspicions of Na+ level less than 135 mEq/L.

Patients with hyponatremia are at risk for seizures. Institute seizure precautions.

Many other AEDs are available. Research is ongoing to determine the most appropriate and efficacious AED for each seizure type. Many patients do not tolerate the first AED prescribed and must switch to another. Some patients require more than one drug to effectively treat their seizures. It should also be recognized that many drugs interact with AEDs. These drugs can increase or decrease the action of AEDs, particularly phenytoin. They include many antibiotics, warfarin, hormones such as estrogen, antihistamines, and various cardiac drugs. It is important that a thorough record be made of all medications taken by any patient taking AEDs.

Protecting the patient from secondary injury is an important concern regarding patients with seizures. It is imperative that the patient not be left alone while having a seizure. It is also important never to force anything into the patient's mouth, such as a "bite stick." Occasionally, a patient may stop breathing after a seizure, especially if the patient is in status epilepticus. This is a medical emergency, and CPR should be started immediately. Oxygen should be administered by nasal cannula or face mask. The ABCs of life support may be instituted. The health care provider should always be notified in the case of seizure. (See also the Nursing Process: Patient Care Plan for Acute Brain Disorders, p. 741.)

Collaborative Management

Seizure management, specifically AED management, is a specialty area in some institutions. If epileptologists or neurologists specializing in seizure management are available, consulting this service may be helpful, especially if seizure management proves to be difficult. Phenytoin dosing services are available in some institutions, and are a welcome addition to management of this drug, dosing in accordance to laboratory drug levels.

Pharmacists also may be of assistance with the many drug interactions associated with AEDs. Many common drugs, as well

---

CHART 29-9 Nursing Assessment of Seizure Event

- Was the seizure witnessed? If so, by whom?
- Were there precipitating events?
- Where did the seizure start and did it progress to other areas?
- What type of movement of the extremities?
- Were there pupillary changes?
- Was there gaze deviation? If so, which direction?
- Was there incontinence of bowel or bladder?
- What was the patient's mental status (unconscious or awake and talking)?
- How long did the event last?
- After the seizure, what was the patient's mental status?
- Was there any motor weakness after the seizure?
- Did the patient experience an injury from the event?

as foods, can interact with and potentiate or diminish the effects of AEDs. It is important for the patient and family to be aware of these common foods and drugs and the effect they may have on seizure management.

Systemic Response to Acute Brain Disorders

Although the primary nursing focus for patients with acute brain disorders is the neurological status, other systems also must be considered to ensure the best possible outcome for the patient. Insults to the brain affect many other major organ systems and must be carefully evaluated and monitored.

Respiratory Effect

Patients with decreased neurological status frequently have compromised respiratory status. Protecting the patient's airway must be of paramount importance. The patient with decreased level of consciousness is at risk for aspiration, ineffective airway clearance, and respiratory failure. Injuries to the brainstem can cause altered respiratory patterns, which can increase the risk of cerebral hypoxia, extending the neurological damage. The nurse must carefully assess respiratory status by monitoring respiratory patterns, effectiveness of respiration, O_2 saturation, respiratory rates, and arterial blood gases. The possibility of intubation and mechanical ventilation must be considered, especially for patients with GCS $\leq$ 8.

Neurogenic pulmonary edema is a phenomenon associated with head injury. This is due to a systemic response of the body to shunt blood away from the brain and to the lungs as a result of brain trauma. Treatment is supportive, with possible mechanical ventilation, management of increased ICP, and the use of pharmacologic agents such as dobutamine (Pyeron, 2001).

Pneumonia is a frequent complication of brain injury. The patient is at risk for more than one type of pneumonia, whether it is from bacteria introduced to an already compromised patient, nosocomial from the hospital environment, or aspiration, from a compromised swallow reflex. Ventilator-acquired pneumonia (VAP) is a specific risk for patients in this population. For this reason it is imperative that nursing staff take specific precautions when treating neurologically compromised patients requiring mechanical ventilation.

Of utmost importance is the monitoring of respiratory parameters, such as rate, rhythm, and breath sounds. Accurate monitoring of arterial blood gases is important to recognize patterns of abnormal ventilation. One of the most important nursing functions in supporting respiratory status is turning the patient frequently, if not contraindicated (such as a patient with a potential neck injury). Encouraging the patient to move as much as her condition warrants is helpful to avoid pneumonia.

Mechanically ventilated patients are especially at risk for developing VAP. Intubated patients may require suctioning of their endotracheal or tracheal tubes to clear out excess secretions. Also of importance in reducing VAP is aggressive oral care. Patients with a decreased LOC are at an increased risk for aspiration. This may be due to impairment of the swallow reflex or because of extreme lethargy. The potential for aspiration and/or pneumonia due to an unprotected airway mandates close observation of respiratory status and immediate reporting to the health care provider of any changes. A nurse caring for a patient with an acute brain disorder should be prepared for sudden changes, and the possibility of intubation to protect the airway. (See also the Nursing Process: Patient Care Plan for Acute Brain Disorders, p. 741.)

Cardiovascular Effect

It is common for patients with TBI to experience alterations in cardiovascular function. Arrhythmias are seen, some potentially lethal, such as premature ventricular beats. Bradycardia and tachycardia also are seen. Most common, however, is hypertension. This may indicate increasing intracranial pressure. Hypotension is not frequently associated with head injury, but may be seen in conjunction with an associated injury, such as bleeding. As discussed in the section on ICP management, prevention of hypotension is essential to maintenance of adequate CPP.

Nurses caring for TBI patients, especially in the acute phase, must carefully monitor vital signs, including heart rate and rhythm and blood pressure. Close monitoring of electrocardiograph (ECG) patterns also are essential, including changes in pattern. Acute changes in vital signs may be signs of increasing ICP or changes in nonneurological systems. This is especially important in trauma patients and should be reported without delay.

Monitoring of hemodynamic functions frequently is warranted. To adequately assess cardiovascular function, the placement of invasive lines is common. Arterial lines may be inserted to continually monitor blood pressure. Central venous pressure (CVP) and Swan-Ganz catheters allow practitioners to closely monitor cardiovascular parameters, such as volume, which is essential to the maintenance of adequate CPP. Alterations in blood pressure pose a frequent problem for nurses caring for this population. It is important to know the patient's previous medical history including medications. A trauma patient may experience hypotension due to blood loss from injuries. As observed in the section on ICP management earlier in the chapter, hypotension has a strongly negative effect on CPP and ICP. The use of vasopressors, blood transfusions, and/or fluid challenges may be warranted. Hypertension also may be seen and treated as appropriate. Laboratory values such as serial hemoglobin and hematocrit levels should be monitored closely. (See also the Nursing Process: Patient Care Plan for Acute Brain Disorders, p. 741.)

Gastrointestinal Effect

The most common gastrointestinal (GI) problem is stomach ulcers (Cushing's ulcer). In the initial stage of head injury, GI bleeding may be common due to an increase in gastric acid production. Use of H2-blockers that work to reduce acid in the stomach, such as famotidine, is recommended early in the hospital course to avoid this unnecessary complication. Another potential complication involving the GI system is that of constipation. Patients may be receiving an alternate form of nutrition, such as enteral feedings. Coupled with medications, such as narcotics, and relative immobility, constipation is a constant possibility.

If not closely monitored, constipation may progress to bowel obstruction, a serious (and preventable) complication. Nursing should be aware of elimination patterns and in the event of constipation, stool softeners and laxatives should be given as ordered.

Support of nutritional needs also is of paramount importance to the patient with neurological disease or trauma. It is especially important for the neurologically compromised patient.

A complete nutritional assessment should be done and nutrition should be started as early as possible. Often this means the placement of a feeding tube to provide enteral nutrition. If available, a dietitian can assist in determining caloric needs and optimal nutritional options. If the patient is able to take oral nutrition, it may be necessary to do a calorie count to ensure the patient's caloric support. For more on nutrition, see Chapter 14 . (See also the Nursing Process: Patient Care Plan for Acute Brain Disorders, p. 741.)

Metabolic Effect

The occurrence of brain injury may cause alterations to electrolyte balance. Of primary concern is the maintenance of appropriate sodium levels. Hyponatremia, low serum sodium, is relatively common in head injury. Syndrome of inappropriate antidiuretic hormone (SIADH), an electrolyte imbalance caused by excessive ADH release from the pituitary, must be considered and sodium levels monitored. Hyponatremia is associated with cerebral edema, manifesting symptoms such as lethargy, confusion, seizures, and neurological decline. Diabetes insipidus also must be considered, although it is much less common. Diabetes insipidus is characterized by hypernatremia and low urine specific gravities and is seen with pituitary tumors (see Chapter 18).

Normal levels of serum sodium are between 135 and 145 mEq/L in most institutions. Close monitoring of serum sodium levels and serum osmolality is important because low levels of serum sodium, especially less than 130 mEq/L, can facilitate cerebral edema, causing decreased levels of consciousness, confusion, seizures, and even death.

Fluid restriction, especially of free water, is the treatment of choice of SIADH, while administration of salt tablets, and hyperosmolar saline is the preferred treatment for cerebral salt wasting. Sodium levels should be checked every 6 hours if there is concern for SIADH, or if the patient is receiving treatment for SIADH to prevent overcorrecting. Accurate intake and output is an important nursing function. (See also the Nursing Process: Patient Care Plan for Acute Brain Disorders, p. 741.)

Hematologic Effect

Occasionally patients with an acute brain disorder may develop clotting abnormalities. The most devastating of these is disseminated intravascular coagulopathy (DIC). This is caused by the release of large amounts of thromboplastin by the injured brain. Treatment is the normalization of clotting factors and the maintenance of adequate blood volume.

The development of deep venous thrombosis (DVT) is another potentially dangerous hematologic complication. The cause of DVT usually is immobility; it is, therefore, usually preventable. DVT can lead to the potentially fatal development of a pulmonary embolus. Some brain tumors, especially high-grade gliomas, seem to be a risk factor for the development of DVT and/or pulmonary embolus. Diagnosis is made by ultrasound of the lower extremities.

CRITICAL ALERT *Patients with acute brain disorders, especially those with lower extremity weakness, are prone to formation of DVT. Activity is extremely important. Patients should get out of bed and into a chair or ambulate with assistance, unless contraindicated.*

All patients who are not ambulating independently should wear antiembolism stockings and compression stockings. Subcutaneous injection of low-molecular-weight heparin or enoxaparin should be considered. Notify health care provider for any signs of DVT (i.e., calf pain).

If the patient is experiencing motor weakness postoperatively, great care must be taken to avoid DVT due to immobility. Prevention is the ideal treatment.

The use of antiembolism hose or pneumonic stockings is highly recommended and should be applied as soon as possible, even before the patient goes to surgery. Frequent turning of the patient and early mobilization, with health care provider approval, is of utmost importance. Prophylactic use of subcutaneous enoxaparin also is recommended in instances of motor deficits that cause immobility of the limb and when it is not otherwise contraindicated. Early mobilization is a key preventive strategy in avoiding DVT; however, patients must be able to ambulate a minimum of 150 feet per day to discontinue adjunctive prevention treatment.

Any patient with an acute brain disorder, especially one associated with immobility, should be assessed frequently for DVT. Pain in the lower extremity, especially the calf, is a frequent complaint in the presence of DVT. However, many patients in this population may be unaware of, or unable to complain of, this discomfort. Therefore, it is important for nursing to include an examination of the patient's lower extremities in the routine assessment of patients with any neurological disorder. This includes observation for the presence of edema, redness, warmth of calf, and/or pain in the lower extremity. Any abnormality, including patient complaint, should be reported. (See also the Nursing Process: Patient Care Plan for Acute Brain Disorders, p. 741.)

◼ Gerontological Considerations for Acute Brain Disorders

Acute brain disorders, such as traumatic brain injury, brain tumors, or infectious diseases, can cause substantial injury to patients across the age continuum. TBI in the elderly, however, has some specific considerations. The incidence of TBI in the elderly may be influenced by age-related changes, such as decreased vision, decreased mobility, decreased muscle and bone mass, and decreased physical agility. Adding to the increased fall risk of the elderly is the fact that many elderly patients live alone.

TBI in the elderly carries a higher percentage of mortality and morbidity than other age groups. Ritchie and colleagues (2000) found that overall mortality of TBI in the elderly is approximately 33.5%, with overall poor functional outcomes. Less favorable outcomes may be due to several factors including chronic, preexisting comorbidities, such as pulmonary or cardiovascular problems. Preexisting cognitive impairment is another factor influencing outcome. Medication, specifically anticoagulation, also plays a significant role in outcome.

According to the U.S. Census Bureau (2000), the number of people age 65 or older approximated 13% of the total population. Those over the age of 85 are projected to be the fastest growing age group in America, with a projected population of more than 8.5 million by the year 2030. Mild or moderate TBI is associated with 2.3% and 4.5%, respectively, increased risk over Alzheimer's disease in the elderly (Langlois, Rutland-Brown, & Walk, 2006). These numbers support the importance of recognizing the specific considerations of TBI in the gerontological population.

Other acute brain disorders, such as brain tumors also may have age-specific characteristics. As noted, brain tumors affect all ages, but certain tumor types are more common in the elderly. Meningiomas are found most commonly in the sixth or seventh decade.

■ Rehabilitation

During the patient's hospitalization, the patient's nurse may be the one he sees the most often, and the one who is looked to for support and encouragement. Often, the realization that life may be changed, perhaps drastically, is overwhelming. Patients need to know that there is support and resources available to help them and their family through whatever the future holds.

At the time of discharge, it may be necessary to transfer the patient to another facility for rehabilitation, or perhaps to arrange for rehabilitation as an outpatient. For patients with brain tumors, this may be coordinated with radiation therapy and possibly chemotherapy. It is helpful to be able to provide the patient and family with information about the benefits of rehabilitation, and what is available to that patient. In many cases, rehabilitation is very important to allow the patient to return home with optimum independence. According to a study done by Mukand and colleagues (2001), impaired cognition, motor weakness, and visual-perceptual deficits were the most common problems in the population studies. Their study supports the benefits of a comprehensive and interdisciplinary rehabilitation program for patients with primary or metastatic brain tumors.

For patients with altered level of consciousness or deficits, rehabilitation also is necessary to provide the patient with the opportunity to maximize functional abilities. The goal for all rehabilitation is to return patients to their optimum level of independence. According to Jennett and Teasdale (1981) in their classic work on level of consciousness, the six aspects of living must be addressed for rehabilitation purposes: activities of daily living (ADLs), mobility and life organization, social relationships, work or leisure activities, present satisfaction, and future prospects. These factors cannot be measured quantitatively, although several outcome measurement scales are available that can be used to address outcomes. The Glasgow Outcome Scale (Jennett & Bond, 1975) and the Karnofsky Performance Status Scale (Karnofsky & Burchenal, 1949) are two such examples.

RESEARCH OPPORTUNITIES AND CLINICAL IMPACT RELATED TO ACUTE BRAIN DISORDERS

Research Area	Clinical Impact
Examine the advantage of various modalities to prevent venous stasis in patients with TBI and brain tumors, such as antiembolism stockings, early ambulation, and the use of low-molecular-weight heparin.	DVTs and pulmonary embolisms are a worrisome complication of head injury and are fairly common in patients with brain tumors. Identifying and implementing DVT prophylaxis may reduce the rate of thromboembolic events, such as DVTs and pulmonary embolisms.
Examine various treatment modalities for hyponatremia (i.e., hypertonic saline, salt tablets, fluid restriction, or other medications) and their impact on the treatment of hyponatremia in the presence of brain tumors.	Hyponatremia is relatively common in the presence of brain tumors and head injury, and it also is associated with cerebral edema. The appropriate treatment of hyponatremia may be significant to a positive patient outcome.
Examine the outcome of patients with TBI or brain tumor who are provided with rehabilitation services versus patients who receive no rehabilitation after discharge (retrospective study).	Define the benefits of therapies and rehabilitation to patients with brain injury due to TBI or tumor.
Examine different monitoring devices for the maintenance of adequate brain oxygenation.	Maintenance of adequate brain oxygenation, with the reduction of neurological injury.
Examine various administration routes (oral, enteral, IV) for the administration of phenytoin and any possible differences in maintenance of adequate blood levels of the drug.	Maintenance of adequate blood levels of phenytoin, possibly reducing the risk of seizures.

Clinical Preparation

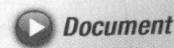 **Read**

- History of Current Illness
- Past Medical History
- Physical Exam
- Admitting Medical Orders
- Laboratory Study Results

 Document

- Summary of Hospitalization
- Pathophysiology Form
- Laboratory Values
- Laboratory Results Explanation

Apply

- List of Potential Nursing Diagnoses
- Concept Map
- Critical Thinking Questions

Log on to MyNursingKit.com to download forms you will need and to complete further steps in the Clinical Preparation assignment.

HISTORY OF PRESENT ILLNESS

As a nurse in the neuroscience ICU of a large metropolitan teaching hospital, you receive a phone call from the charge nurse of the emergency department (ED). The nurse is calling to give a report on a new patient being admitted to your unit. The patient is a 32-year-old Hispanic male brought to the ED by his brother, who found him wandering outside their home, confused and disoriented. He also noted that his brother had trouble opening the car door with his right hand. He stated that his brother had come home from his job stocking supplies in a grocery warehouse complaining of a headache. Coworkers told his brother that they had seen several boxes that had fallen, but were unaware that any had actually struck the patient.

On admission to the ED, a CT scan was done and a moderate-sized subdural hematoma was noted in the left temporal area. A skull fracture was ruled out. The patient is now being admitted to the neuroscience ICU for close monitoring of his neurological status. A craniotomy for evacuation of the left temporal subdural hematoma is planned for early the following morning. The ED nurse tells you that the patient is on his way, and his family is accompanying him. His family consists of several siblings, his wife, his parents, and two small children. They are very concerned and do not speak English.

Medical–Surgical History

This history was obtained from multiple family members: On examination of the patient's records, you note that the patient, whose name is Jose R., has no past medical history and has, in fact, never been in the hospital for any reason. He has no allergies and takes no medication. Illnesses: none, with the exception of "usual" childhood illnesses, per parents

Social History

His social history, according to his family, includes a wife, two small children, and multiple family members. His wife denies any drug or alcohol use; however, his brother relates moderate alcohol consumption "on the weekends." He works in a warehouse stocking groceries and supplies. He has completed high school. He has lived in this country for many years and is a citizen of this country. He has not traveled outside of the country since he was a young child.

Physical Exam

His emergency department assessment and orders are as follows:
Young Hispanic male, resting quietly, appears in no distress
Vital signs: afebrile; HR 62 regular, RR 16, BP 134/74
HEENT: normocephalic, with small tender, bruised area near L temple
Heart: rhythm and rate regular, S_1S_2 heard, no abnormal murmurs, good capillary refill, pulses 2+ all extremities, no pitting edema
Lungs: clear to auscultation bilaterally

O_2 sat at 97% on room air
Abdomen: soft, nontender, bowel sounds heard all quadrants

Neurological Exam

GCS = E4 M6 V4 = 14; oriented to name only, confused to date and surroundings
Pleasant, cooperative, and attentive
Speech clear and fluent
Cranial nerves: CN II–XII intact bilaterally
Motor:
Right upper extremity 5/5
Right lower extremity 5/5
RUE pronator drift
Left upper extremity 5/5
Left lower extremity 5/5
Sensory: grossly intact to light touch bilaterally

Imaging Studies

Head CT scan done in the ED reveals an acute left-sided subdural hematoma
Chest x-ray: negative for abnormal pathology

Admitting Medical Orders

Admit to Neuroscience ICU
Diagnosis: acute left subdural hematoma
Condition: guarded
Allergies: none known
Vital signs and neuro assessment: q1h

Bed rest

Diet: NPO

Notify resident on call: any change in neurological status; increase in severity of headache or nausea, temperature > 38ºC, HR < 60 or > 120, systolic BP < 100 or > 160, RR < 10 or > 30, O_2 sat less 92%, urine output < 30 mL/hr × 2

Sequential compression devices (SCDs) to lower extremities prior to surgery

IV: D5/0.45NS @ 75 mL/hr

Continuous ECG, pulse oximetry

Foley catheter

Intake and output q2h

Consent for craniotomy for evacuation of left subdural hematoma by Dr. XYZ

Scheduled Medications

Pepcid 20 mg IV q12h

PRN Medications

Acetaminophen 650 mg po/PR q4h for pain or fever

Morphine sulfate 2–4 mg IV q2h for pain

Promethazine 25–50 mg po/IV/PR q4h for nausea

Ordered Laboratory Studies

ABG × 1 now

Serum and urine osmolality × 1 now

CBC now and q a.m.

PTT, INR. Chem 7 panel, magnesium, phosphorous, and ionized CA now and q12h

Urinalysis now

Ordered Diagnostic Studies

Preoperative ECG

After Jose is settled in your unit, you examine the patient. His vital signs and neurological assessment are unchanged from the admitting assessment. (Refer to Chapter 28 🔗 for a review of neurological assessment.)

Jose is resting comfortably, talking with the nursing staff, and is quite pleasant and cooperative. He is complaining of a headache and is medicated with intravenous morphine. He has an IV line running. He is denying nausea at this time, but is not hungry. He is in the ICU for close monitoring. He is considered to be stable, and safe to wait the few hours until morning to evacuate his hematoma.

About 2 hours after Jose is admitted, he requests more pain medication, because his headache is worse. Before you can bring his medication, he attempts to crawl over the side rails of his bed. He is clearly agitated, worried about his family, and wants to go home. You convince him to return to bed. Within minutes, he has projectile emesis, and now is clearly confused. He is unable to tell you his name or where he is. His vital signs are essentially unchanged, although his heart and respiratory rate are slightly elevated. His neurological examination is as follows: He is alert, restless, and agitated. He is clearly confused, unable to state name or where he is. His pupils are equal, but his left pupil is slow to react. His right pronator drift is still present, but does not appear to be any worse. The neurosurgical resident you call wants another CT scan, but states that he may go straight to surgery after his scan. As you are preparing to take the patient to radiology, you look up his labs, and check his paperwork to make sure the surgical consent is in the chart. As the patient is receiving his scan, you go to the waiting room to speak to the family and keep them aware of events.

LABORATORY STUDY RESULTS

Test	On Admission
pH	7.36
$PaCO_2$	40 mmHg
PaO_2	80 mmHg
SO2	96%
HCO_3	24 mEq/L
Sodium	140 mEq/L
Potassium	3.6 mEq/L
Chloride	92 mEq/L
Carbon dioxide	23 mEq/L
Blood urea nitrogen (BUN)	26 mg/dL
Creatinine	1.4 mg/dL
Blood glucose	93 mg/dL
Blood alcohol	NA, 00.0%
White blood cells	9200 /µL
Hemoglobin	14.2 g/dL
Hematocrit	39.8%
Platelets	312,000 µL
Protime (PT)	11.8 seconds
International normalized ratio (INR)	0.9 INR
Partial thromboplastin time (PTT)	34 seconds
Serum osmolality	280 mOsm/kg
Urine osmolality	600 mOsm/kg H_2O

CRITICAL THINKING QUESTIONS

1. What neurological findings might you expect in a patient with an injury to the left temporal area?

2. At what point did Jose's neurological status change?

3. What is the significance of Jose's change in mental status?

4. Based on the change in Jose's condition, what might the nurse expect Jose's CT scan to show?

5. What other clinical findings might support the nurse's concern about rising ICPs?

Answers to Critical Thinking Questions appear in Appendix D.

NCLEX® REVIEW

1. The encased structure of the adult brain is the reason that the relationship between brain mass, cerebrospinal fluid (CSF), and blood must remain constant. Initial mechanisms to compensate for pressure changes in any of these components include which of the following?

   1. Increasing production of CSF
   2. Expansion of brain tissue
   3. Blocking the auto-regulation of cerebral blood flow
   4. Increasing absorption of CSF

2. A patient is admitted with a gradual increase in intracranial pressure due to an enlarging tumor. Early signs of increased intracranial pressure may include which of the following?

   1. Changes in the optic nerve (CN VIII) may result in ringing in the ears
   2. Decorticate movement observable in the arms
   3. Complaints of a 'different' headache and projectile vomiting
   4. Cushing's triad

3. The nursing management for the patient with increased intracranial pressure involves assessment of respiratory, cardiovascular, metabolic, and neurological processes. Desired parameters to avoid complications include which of the following? Select all that apply.

   1. Pulse oximetry should be used with supplemental oxygen to maintain saturations of 90% or greater
   2. Normocapnia levels ($PaCO_2$ levels of 35–40mm Hg)
   3. Euglycemic levels of 80–120 mg/dL
   4. Normothermia and interventions for body temperatures >99.5°F rectally

4. A 50-year-old patient is admitted to the ED with a scalp laceration that was bleeding profusely and was bandaged at the scene by emergency personnel. The patient is currently stable. The nurse is aware that before wound closure is initiated, which of the following activities is a priority?

   1. A complete neurological assessment to rule out cerebral contusion
   2. A CAT scan of the head to rule out skull fracture
   3. A cerebral arteriogram to identify which vessel has been ruptured
   4. A skull series to determine the presence of hematomas

5. The presenting signs and symptoms for bacterial and viral meningitis are the same. It is important, therefore, for the nurse to utilize laboratory data to differentiate between these acute processes. Which of the following is true concerning bacterial meningitis?

   1. In the spinal fluid, protein levels will be high and glucose levels will be low.
   2. In the spinal fluid, the color will be clear.
   3. In the spinal fluid, the protein and glucose levels will be low.
   4. The spinal fluid will be bloody.

6. Brain tumors are a threat to life whether they are benign or malignant. Which of the following statements reflects the characteristics of benign tumors of the brain?

   1. These tumors are nonmalignant and are easily removed by surgery.
   2. The tumors are self-limiting and do not influence the function of surrounding tissues.
   3. Benign tumors may be surgically difficult to remove and may compress vital structures.
   4. These tumors do not progress into malignant tumors.

7. Chemotherapy in the treatment of brain tumors may be administered intrathecally, intravenously, or orally. Special concerns with the use of chemotherapy for brain tumors include:

   1. Brain tissue, due to increase lymph flow, has an improved mechanism to remove cellular debris.
   2. Chemotherapy is the treatment of choice because all of these drugs readily cross the blood–brain barrier.
   3. Malignant cells are homogenous and are consistent in their sensitivity to chemotherapeutic agents.
   4. A flexible approach due to the changing resistance patterns to specific drugs.

8. The role of the nurse in family teaching of patients with acute brain disorders is:

   1. Limited to teaching the early detection of cognitive impairment.
   2. Different than other long term-care patients because of the early implementation of rehabilitative therapies.
   3. Provide answers to questions honestly as they arise, educate them about the treatment plan, and involve them in discussions of the rehabilitation process.
   4. Geared to offering the family a realistic perspective of the limited abilities of the patient.

Answers for review questions appear in Appendix D

KEY TERMS

acoustic neuromas *p.737*
autoregulation *p.715*
bacterial meningitis *p.730*
basal skull fracture *p.722*
brain abscess *p.732*
cerebral blood flow (CBF) *p.715*
cerebral edema *p.716*
cerebral infarction *p.727*
cerebral ischemia *p.727*
cerebral perfusion pressure (CPP) *p.715*
comminuted skull fracture *p.722*
concussion *p.726*
contusions *p.725*
Cushing's triad *p.718*

cytotoxic edema *p.716*
depressed skull fracture *p.722*
diffuse axonal injury (DAI) *p.726*
encephalitis *p.731*
ependymomas *p.736*
epidural hematoma (EDH) *p.724*
extra-axial tumors *p.736*
gene mutations *p.735*
herniation *p.716*
intra-axial tumors *p.735*
intracranial pressure (ICP) *p.714*
ischemia cascade *p.727*
linear skull fracture *p.722*
meningiomas *p.736*

meningismus *p.730*
metastatic tumors *p.735*
Monro-Kellie doctrine *p.714*
postconcussion syndrome *p.726*
primary injury *p.727*
primary tumors *p.735*
schwannomas *p.737*
second-impact syndrome *p.726*
secondary injury *p.727*
subdural hematoma (SDH) *p.724*
traumatic brain injury (TBI) *p.721*
vasodilatory cascade *p.715*
vasogenic edema *p.716*
viral meningitis *p.730*

EXPLORE PEARSON mynursingkit™

MyNursingKit is your one stop for online chapter review materials and resources. Prepare for success with additional NCLEX®-style practice questions, interactive assignments and activities, web links, animations and videos, and more!

Register your access code from the front of your book at
www.mynursingkit.com

REFERENCES

Adesina, A. M., Leech, R. W., & Brumback, R. A. (2002). Histopathology of primary tumors of the central nervous system. In M. Prados (Ed.), *Brain cancer* (pp. 16–45). London: B. C. Decker.

American Cancer Society. (2006). Detailed guide: brain/cnss tumors in adults. What are the key statistics for brain and spinal cord tumors in adults. *Cancer Reference Information*. Retrieved July 13, 2008 from http://www.cancer.org/docroot/CRI/content/CRI_2_4_1X_What_are_the_key_statistics_fo…

Andrews, P.J.D. (2005). Cerebral perfusion pressure and brain ischemia: Can one size fit all? *Critical Care, 9*, 638–639.

Aubry, M., Cantu, R. C., Dvorak, J., Graf-Baumann, T., Johnston, K., & Kelly, J. (2001). *Concussion in sport group: Summary and agreement statement of the First International Concussion in Sport.* Vienna, Austria.

Bader, M. K. (2006a). Gizmos and gadgets for the neuroscience intensive care unit. *Journal of Neuroscience Nursing, 38*(4), 248–260.

Bader, M. K. (2006b). Recognizing and treating ischemic insults to the brain: The role of brain tissue oxygen monitoring. *Critical Care Nursing Clinics of North America, 18*, 243–256.

Bader, M. K., & Littlejohns, L. (Eds.). (2004). *Core curriculum for neuroscience nursing* (4th ed.). Chicago: American Association of Neuroscience Nurses.

Bay, E., & McLean, S. A. (2007). Mild traumatic brain injury: An update for advanced practice nurses. *Journal of Neuroscience Nursing, 39*(1), 43–51.

Bowen, A. P. (2003). Secondary impact syndrome. *Journal of Emergency Nursing, 29*(3), 287–289.

Brenner, A. V., Linet, M. S., Fine, H. A., Shapiro, W. R., Selker, R. G., Black, P. M., et al. (2002). History of allergies and autoimmune diseases and risk of brain tumors in adults. *International Journal of Cancer, 99*, 252–259.

Burnett, D. M., Kolawkowky-Hayner, S. A., Slater, D., Stringer, A., Bushnik, T., Zafonte, R., et al. (2003). Ethnographic analysis of traumatic brain injury patients in the National Model Systems Database. *Archives of Physical Medicine and Rehabilitation, 84*(2), 263–267.

Burst suppression tutorial. (2003, December). Reykjavik, Iceland: Taugagreininghf.

Burton, E., & Prados, M. (2002). Management of primary malignant brain tumors in adults. In Prado, M. (Ed.), *Brain cancer* (pp. 262–277). London: B. C. Decker.

Carroll, S. (1994). Secondary brain injury and the role of neuroprotective agents. *Journal of Neuroscience Nursing, 26*, 251–254.

Centers for Disease Control and Prevention. (2007). *Brain injuries and mass casualty events.* Retrieved June 25, 2007, from http://www.bt.cdc.gov/masscasualties/braininjuriespro.asp

Central Brain Tumor Registry of the United States. (2000). *Statistical report: Primary brain tumors in the United States, 1992–1997.* Chicago: Author.

Cox, J. D., & Ang, K. K. (2003). *Radiation oncology* (pp. 801–806). St. Louis: Mosby.

Defense and Veterans Brain Injury Center. (2005). *Living with Brain Injury*, Brain Injury Association of America, Washington, DC: Walter Reed Army Medical Center.

DeRoos, A. J., Stewart, P. A., Linet, M. S., Heineman, E. F., Dosemeci, M., Wilcosky, T., et al. (2003). Occupation and the risk of adult glioma in the United States. *Cancer Causes and Control, 14*, 139–150.

Evans, R. W. (1996). *Neurology and trauma.* Philadelphia: W. B. Saunders.

Fan, J. (2004). Effect of backrest position on intracranial pressure and cerebral perfusion pressure in individuals with brain injury: A systematic review. *Journal of Neuroscience Nursing, 36*(5), 278–288.

Farrell, D. J., & Bower, L. (2003). Fatal water intoxication. *Journal of Clinical Pathology, 56*(10), 803–804.

Feldman, Z., & Robertson, C. S. (1997). Monitoring of cerebral hemodynamics with jugular bulb catheters. *Critical Care Clinics, 13*(1): 55–77.

Finkelstein, E., Corso, P., & Miller, T. (2006). *The incidence and economic burden of injuries in the United States.* Oxford University Press: New York.

Geraci, E. B., & Geraci, T. A. (1996). A look at recent hyperventilation studies: Outcomes and recommendations for early use in the head injured patient. *Journal of Neuroscience Nursing, 28*(4), 222–233.

Goldman, L., & Ausiello, D. (2004). *Cecil textbook of medicine* (22nd ed.). Philadelphia, PA: W. B. Saunders.

Greenberg, M. S. (2001). *Handbook of neurosurgery* (5th ed.). New York: Thieme.

Guzman, R., Barth, A., Lovblad, K. O., El-Koussy, M., Weis, J., Schroth, G., et al. (2002). Use of diffusion-weighted magnetic resonance imaging in differentiating purulent brain processes from cystic brain tumors. *Journal of Neurosurgery, 97*(5), 1101–1107.

Hickey, J. (2003). *The clinical practice of neurological and neurosurgical nursing* (5th ed.). Philadelphia: Lippincott.

Hilton, G. (2000). Cerebral oxygenation in the traumatically brain-injured pateint: Are ICP and CPP enough? *Journal of Neuroscience Nursing, 32*(5): 278–281.

Hirose, S., Okada, O., Kaneko, S., & Mitsudome, A. (2000). Are some idiopathic epilepsies disorders of ion channels? A working hypothesis. *Epilepsy Research, 41*, 191–204.

House, J. W., & Brackmann, D. E. (1985). Facial nerve grading scale. *Otolaryngology, 93*(2), 146–147.

Huang, C. R., Lu, C. H., Chang, H. W., Lee, P. Y., Lin, M. W., & Chang, W. N. (2002). Community-acquired spontaneous bacterial meningitis in adult diabetic patients: An analysis of clinical characteristics and prognostic factors. *Infection, 30*(6), 346–350.

Inskip, P. D., Tarone, R. E., & Hatch, E. E. (2001). Cellular-telephone use and brain tumors. *New England Journal of Medicine, 344*, 79–86.

Inskip, P. D., Tarone, R. E., Hatch, E. E., Wilcosky, T. C., Selker, R. G., Fine, H. A., et al. (2003). Laterality of brain tumors. *Neuroepidemiology, 22*(3): 130–138.

Jennett, B., & Teasdale, G. (1981). *Management of head injuries.* Philadelphia: F. A. Davis.

Jennett, W. B., & Bond, M. (1975). Assessment of outcome after severe brain damage: A practical scale. *Lancet*, 480–484.

Jennett, W. B., & Plum, F. (1972). The persistent vegetative state: A syndrome in search of a name. *Lancet, 1*, 734–737.

Karnofsky, D. A., & Burchenal, J. H. (1949). In C. M. Macleod (Ed.), *Evaluation of chemotherapeutic agents* (pp. 191–205). New York: Columbia University Press.

Key, C. B., Rothrock, S. G., & Falk, J. L. (1997). Cerebrospinal fluid shunt complications: An emergency medicine prospective. *Pediatric Emergency Care, 11*(5), 265–272.

Kleihues, P., Davis, R. L., Coons, S. W., & Burger, P. C. (2000). Anaplastic astrocytoma. In P. Kleihues & W. K. Cavenee (Eds.), *Pathology & genetics of tumours of the nervous system* (pp. 27–28). Lyon, France: IARC Press.

Koedel, U., Scheld, W. M., & Pfister, H. W. (2002). Pathogenesis and pathophysiology of pneumococcal meningitis. *Lancet Infectious Disease, 2*(12), 721–736.

Langlois, J. A., Rutland-Brown, W., & Thomas, K. E. (2006). *Traumatic brain injury in the United States: Emergency department visits, hospitalizations, and deaths.* Atlanta, GA: Centers for Disease Control and Prevention, National Center for Injury Prevention and Control.

Langlois, J., Rutland-Brown, W., & Walk, M. (2006). The epidemiology and impact of traumatic brain injury: A brief overview. *Journal of Head Trauma Rehabilitation, 21*(5), 375–378.

Louis, D. N., Scheithauer, B. W., Budka, H., von Deimling, A., & Kepes, J. J. (2000). Meningiomas. In P. Kleihues & W. K. Cavenee (Eds.), *Pathology & genetics of tumours of the nervous system* (pp. 176–184). Lyon, France: IARC Press.

Manley, G., Knudson, M. M., Morabito, D., Damron, S., Erickson, V., & Pitts, L. (2001). Hypotension, hypoxia, and head injury. *Archives of Surgery, 136*(10): 1118–1123.

Maramou, A. (1996). Physiology of intracranial pressure. In R. K. Narayan, J. E. Wilberger, & J. T. Povlishock (Eds.), *Neurotrauma.* New York: McGraw-Hill.

Maramou, A., & Beaumont, A. (2004). Physiology of the cerebrospinal fluid and intracranial pressure. In M. Kliot (Ed.), *Youman's neurological surgery* (5th ed., pp. 175-194). Philadelphia: W. B. Saunders.

Mayo Clinic Staff. (2008). *Traumatic Brain Injury.* Retrieved July 13, 2008 from http://www.mayoclinic.com/health/traumatic-brain-injury/DS00552/DSECTION=risk-fact...

McIlvoy, L. (2005). The effect of hypothermia and hyperthermia on acute brain injury. *AACN Clinical Issues, 16,* 488–500.

Meinert, R., & Michaelis, J. (1996). Meta-analyses of studies on the association between electromagnetic fields and childhood cancer. *Radiation & Environmental Biophysics, 35,* 11–18.

Minn, Y., Wrensch, M., & Bondy, M. L. (2002). Epidemiology of primary brain tumors. In M. Prados (Ed.), *Brain cancer.* London: B. C. Decker.

Mittenberg, W., & Strauman, S. (2000). Diagnosis of mild head injury and the postconcussion syndrome. *Head Trauma Rehabilitation, 15*(2), 783–791.

Moura, A. S., Pablos-Mendez, A., Layton, M., & Weiss, D. (2003). Epidemiology of meningococcal disease, New York City, 1989–2002. *Emerging Infectious Disease, 9*(3), 355–361.

Mukand, J. A., Blackinton, D. D., Crincoli, M. G., Lee, J. J., & Santos, B. B. (2001). Incidence of neurologic deficits and rehabilitation of patients with brain tumors. *American Journal of Physical Medicine and Rehabilitation 80*(5), 346–350.

Olson, D. A. (2006). Head injury. *EMedicine.* Retrieved July 13, 2008 from http://www.emedicine.com/neuro/TOPIC143.HTM

Piepmeier, J. M. (1987). Observations on the current treatment of low-grade astrocytic tumors of the cerebral hemispheres. *Journal of Neurosurgery, 67,* 177–181.

Plum, F., & Posner, J. (1980). *Diagnosis of stupor and coma* (3rd ed., Contemporary Neurology Series). Philadelphia: F. A. Davis.

Porth, C. M. (2007). *Essentials of pathophysiology: Concepts of altered health states.* (2nd Ed.). Philadelphia: Lippincott Williams & Wilkins..

Posner, J. B., Saper, C. B., Schiff, N., & Plum, F. (2007). *Plum and Posner's diagnosis of stupor and coma* (4th ed.). New York: Oxford University Press.

Proctor, M. R., & Cantu, R. C. (2000). Head and neck injuries in young athletes. *Clinics of Sports Medicine, 19*(4).

Pueschel, J. K., Ashby, L. S., & Shapiro, W. R. (2003). Brain tumors. In G. Giaccone, R. Schilsky, & P. Sondel (Eds.), *Cancer chemotherapy and biological response modifiers* (Annual 21). New York: Elsevier Science.

Pyeron, A. M. (2001). Respiratory failure in the neurological patient: The diagnosis of neurogenic pulmonary edema. *Journal of Neuroscience Nursing, 33*(4), 203–207.

Quinn, A. M. (2002). CyberKnife: A robotic radiosurgery system. *Clinical Journal of Oncology Nursing, 6*(3), 149–156.

Quinn, E. (2008). Water intoxication—hyponatremia. *Sports Medicine.* Retrieved March 30, 2008, from http://sportsmedicine.about.com/od/hydrationandfluid/a/Hyponatremia.htm

Radiation Therapy Oncology Group (RTOG). (2008). *Brain tumor protocols.* Retrieved July 14, 2008 from http://www.rrtog.org/summaries/brain.html

Rees, R. J., & Bellon, M. L. (2007). Post concussion syndrome ebb and flow: Longitudinal effects and management. *NeuroRehabilitation, 22*(3), 229–242.

Ritchie, P. D., Cameron, P. A., Ugoni, A. M., & Kaye, A. H. (2000). A study of the functional outcome and mortality in elderly patients with head injuries. *Journal of Clinical Neuroscience, 7*(4), 301–304.

Sarrafzadeh, A. S., Sakowitz, O. W., Kiening, K. I., Benndorf, G., Lanksch, W. R., & Unterberg, A. W. (2002). Bedside microdialysis: A tool to monitor cerebral metabolism in subarachnoid hemmorrhage patients? *Critical Care Medicine, 30,* 1062–1070.

Sato, O., Takei, F., & Yamada, S. (1994). Hydrocephalus: Is impaired cerebrospinal fluid circulation only one problem involved? *Child's Nervous System, 10*(3), 151–154.

Senelick, R., & Dougherty, K. (2001). *Living with brain injury: A guide for families* (2nd ed., p. 3). Birmingham, AL: Healthsouth Press.

Shapiro, J. R. (2001). Genetics of nervous system tumors. *Hematology/Oncology Clinics of North America, 15*(6), 961–977.

Shapiro, W. R., & Shapiro, J. R. (1986). Principles of brain tumor therapy. *Seminars in Oncology, 13*(1), 56–69.

Shaw, E. G. (2002). Management of low-grade gliomas in adults. In M. Prados (Ed.), *Brain cancer.* London: B. C. Decker.

Shimamoto, S., Inoue, T., Shiomi, H., Sumida, I., Yamada, Y., & Tanaka, E. (2002). CyberKnife stereotactic irradiation for metastatic brain tumors. *Radiation Medicine, 20*(6), 299–304.

Sirven, J. I., & Waterhouse, E. (2003). Management of status epilepticus. *American Family Physician, 68*(3), 469–476.

Smith, D. H., & McIntosh, T. K. (1996). Traumatic brain injury and excitatory amino acids. In R. K. Naryan, J. E. Wilberger, & J. T. Povlishock (Eds.), *Neurotrauma.* New York: McGraw-Hill.

Smith, D. L., Levin, S. A., & Laxminarayan, R. (2005). Strategic interactions in multi-institutional epidemics of antibiotic resistance. *Proceedings. National Academy of Sciences. USA 102,* 3153–3158.

Sneed, P. K. (2002). Metastatic brain tumors. In M. Prados (Ed.), *Brain cancer.* London: B. C. Decker.

Surawicz, T. S., McCarthy, B. J., & Kupelian, V. (1999). Descriptive epidemiology of primary brain and CNS tumors: Results from the Central Brain Tumor Registry of the United States, 1990–1994. *Neurooncology 1999, 1,* 14–25.

Terrell, T. R. (2004). Concussion in athletes. *Southern Medical Journal, 97*(9), 837–842.

Thompson, H. J., Kirkness, C. J., Mitchell, P. H., & Webb, D. J. (2007). Fever management practices of neuroscience nurses: National and regional perspectives. *Journal of Neuroscience Nursing, 39*(3), 151–161.

Tunkel, A. R., & Pradhan, S. K. (2002). Central nervous system infections in injection drug users. *Infectious Disease Clinics of North America 16*(3): 589–605.

U.S. Bureau of the Census. (2000). *United States census 2000: Your gateway to census 2000.* Retrieved October 20, 2008. http://www.census.gov/main/www/cen2000.html

van de Beek, D., Schmand, B., de Gans, J., Weisfelt, M., Vaessen, H., & Vermeulen, M. (2002). Cognitive impairment in adults with good recovery after bacterial meningitis. *Journal of Infectious Disease, 186*(7), 1047–1052.

Walker, J. T. (1967). *History of neurological surgery.* New York: McGraw-Hill.

Winkleman, C. (2000). Effect of backrest position on intracranial and cerebral perfusion pressures in traumatically brain-injured adults. *American Journal of Critical Care, 9*(6), 373–380.

Wong, F. W. H. (2000). Prevention of secondary brain injury. *Critical Care Nurse, 20*(5), 18–27.

Wrensch, M., Minn, Y., & Bondy, M. L. (2000). Epidemiology. In M. Bernstein & M. Berger (Eds.), *Essential neuro-oncology* (pp. 1–17). New York: Thieme.

Yoshikawa, T. T. (2002). Antimicrobial resistance and aging: Beginning of the end of the antibiotic era? *Journal of American Geriatric Society, 50*(7), 226–229.

Caring for the Patient with Cerebral Vascular Disorders

Denita Ryan

Outcome-Based Learning Objectives

After studying this chapter, the learner will be able to:

1. Identify and distinguish between the different types of stroke and their reported impact on rehabilitation and recovery to a functional status.
2. Describe the basic pathophysiology of each type of identified stroke.
3. Explain the events of the ischemic cascade as it relates to the pathophysiology of stroke.
4. Compare and contrast the different medical management options for the treatment of ruptured aneurysms.
5. Explain nursing interventions associated with management of vasospasm.

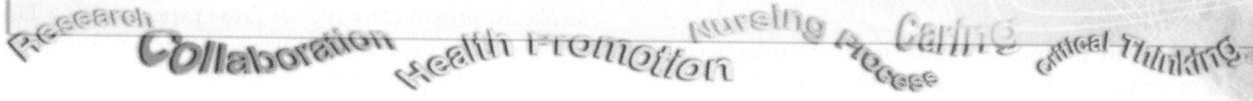

THE CEREBRAL VASCULAR disorders discussed in this chapter consist of stroke and arterial venous malformations. Both represent major disorders that cause an assault on the brain, and in many ways they manifest symptoms similar to the disorders discussed in Chapter 29 ⊛ on acute brain disorders. The prevalence, current modes of diagnosis and treatment, and nursing management of these disorders are discussed, as are the societal implications.

◼ Stroke

Stroke is brain attack. This strong statement is indicative of the new definition for stroke. "Time is brain" is another strong statement exclaiming the importance of timely treatment before neurological deterioration. Hickey (2003) defines stroke as "a heterogeneous, neurological syndrome characterized by the gradual, or rapid, nonconvulsive onset of neurological deficits that fit a known vascular territory and that last for 24 hours or more."

A stroke, or brain attack, occurs in one of two ways. A blood vessel or artery is clogged or obstructed, which interrupts blood flow to a certain area of the brain. The second method of stroke is when the vessel or artery hemorrhages, with the blood itself interrupting blood flow to a certain area of the brain. Both methods cause ischemia, or a lack of oxygen to the brain cells. Cells that are deprived of oxygen for an undetermined amount of time begin to die; this area of dead tissue is called an **infarction**.

As certain areas of the brain become damaged or infarcted, the control of various bodily functions may become affected. These functions include motor function, sensory function, speech, memory, and other cognitive mechanisms. The type and extent of neurological disabilities are dependent on the location of the stroke. Strokes are divided into two categories: ischemic stroke and hemorrhagic stroke. Ischemic strokes are further divided by mechanism, embolic, arteriosclerotic cerebrovascular disease, or lacunar infarct. A lacunar infarct is a thrombosis of a small penetrating artery that results in tissue death. The outcome is a small cavity in the deep white matter of the brain, referred to as a *lacuna*.

 The onset of neurological symptoms indicating stroke is a medical emergency. Notify health care provider immediately for any new symptoms indicating possibility of a stroke. Stroke protocols must be initiated immediately.

Public awareness has changed the outlook for stroke. No longer is stroke viewed as fatal or devastating. Education has broadened public knowledge about stroke and clarified some misconceptions. The term *cerebrovascular accident*, or *CVA*, implies that stroke is an isolated event, somehow unexpected and random. Stroke actually is a vascular event that results from an actual disease of the blood vessels (Adams, del Zoppo, & von Kummer, 2006). Education has taught the public that they have some control over their own health. Research has brought public new sets of guidelines and recommendations for the prevention and management of brain attack.

Epidemiology

Stroke is a leading cause of death and disability in many developed nations. In the United States, it is the third leading cause of death, after heart disease and cancer (American Heart Association [AHA], 2005a). There are approximately 750,000 cases of stroke each year (American Heart Association [AHA], 2004), of which 160,000 are fatal (AHA, 2008a).

Approximately 4 million people in the United States have survived a brain attack and are living with the aftereffects. Although stroke is considered a condition of the elderly, stroke can happen to anyone—28% of its victims are under the age of 65 (AHA, 2008a). The annual cost of ischemic stroke is approximately $71.8 billion (Matchar & Samsa, 2000; Rosamond et al., 2007). The prevalence for stroke is almost twice as high for African Americans than Caucasians, and more men than women experience stroke. However, women account for approximately 60% of all stroke deaths (AHA, 2005b). Stroke kills almost twice as many women as breast cancer (Adams et al., 2006).

Etiology and Classification

As mentioned earlier, strokes generally are classified according to two main categories, ischemic and hemorrhagic, contingent on the pathology of the lesion or infarct that develops. Each category of stroke is further broken down into specific types.

Ischemic Stroke

Ischemic strokes are the most common form of stroke, accounting for approximately 400,000 cases or 80% (Rosamond et al., 2007). Ischemic strokes are further divided into several subtypes, including atherosclerotic thrombotic strokes, cardioembolic strokes, and lacunar strokes. A small percentage of ischemic strokes are caused by other vascular conditions.

Thrombotic Strokes

Thrombotic strokes occur most commonly in older individuals with underlying atherosclerosis (Alberts, 1999; Rosamond et al., 2007). Atherosclerosis is a condition in which the large arteries, both extracranial and intracranial, are subject to a buildup of "plaque," which narrows the lumen of the artery. Narrowing of the arteries is referred to as stenosis. Blood clots may form on an atherosclerotic vessel, further narrowing the lumen of the artery and causing severe stenosis. Large arteries, such as the internal carotid artery or the vertebral artery, can become stenotic, as can small, deep intracerebral vessels. Hypercoagulable states, conditions which promote platelet aggregation and clotting, also contribute to stenotic arteries.

Embolic Strokes

Embolism results when a clot breaks off and travels to an area of decreased circulation, blocking off blood flow. The tissue may then become hypoxic and finally infarcted, or dead. This embolism could be made of plaque from within the arterial lumen, or a blood clot from a faulty heart valve. Embolisms from cardiac sources are referred to as **cardiogenic embolisms**. The most common cause is atrial fibrillation, which accounts for almost 20% of all ischemic strokes (Hickey, 2003). Any condition that can cause a reduction in systemic blood flow can cause an ischemic event.

Examples of this are shock, hypotension, or cardiac arrest. Extremely low rates of blood flow may be responsible for the lack of cerebral oxygenation, resulting in ischemia and infarction.

Lacunar Strokes

Lacunar strokes also are known as small artery occlusive disease, or penetrating artery strokes. As mentioned earlier, the term *lacuna* refers to a small cavity that remains in brain tissue after dead tissue that results from an infarct has sloughed away. Lacunar strokes occur primarily in the deep areas of the brain, such as the basal ganglia or the thalamus. Although lacunar strokes usually are small, they are usually in eloquent, or highly functional, areas of the brain and can cause significant deficits. Hypertension is the predominant risk factor.

Transient Ischemic Attacks

Transient ischemic attacks (TIAs) are episodes of neurological deficit resulting from ischemia that is temporary and resolves in minutes to hours. This ischemia is a result of vascular disease and is specific to a defined vascular territory. Neurological deficits are a result of ischemia in a specific vascular territory. Examples of focal neurological deficits are weakness or sensory loss to one side of the body, unilateral visual deficits, loss of speech, and/or facial droop. Global deficits, such as confusion or lethargy, are not indicative of TIAs.

Onset is usually rapid. Resolution of accompanying neurological deficits occurs in less than 24 hours, often in less than 1 hour. Waxing and waning symptoms are not common with TIAs. Many patients have TIAs before having a large-vessel stroke. Approximately 10% of those experiencing a TIA will experience a major stroke within a year. The risk for stroke is greatest within the first 48 hours after a TIA (Howard et al., 2006; Johnson, Gress, Browner, & Sidney, 2000). TIAs are an important warning sign of impending stroke.

Hemorrhagic Strokes

Hemorrhagic strokes also are referred to as intracerebral or intraparenchymal hemorrhages. Approximately 20% of all strokes are hemorrhagic. The most common causes of intracerebral hemorrhage are hypertension or amyloid angiopathy. Intracerebral hemorrhage is seen most often in the elderly, although it is seen in the younger population with certain high-risk factors. Trauma, such as motor vehicle crashes, assaults, and falls, also accounts for intracerebral hemorrhage. When intracerebral hemorrhage is seen in a young adult, and trauma is ruled out as the cause, drug use should be suspected, specifically cocaine or amphetamines.

Another type of hemorrhagic stroke is subarachnoid hemorrhage (SAH). Rupture of an intracerebral aneurysm, with hemorrhage into the subarachnoid space, is the most common case of SAH. SAH and cerebral aneurysms are discussed later in the chapter.

Pathophysiology

The pathophysiology of stroke varies contingent on the different types of strokes. Factors that need to be considered include predisposing factors, including risk factors, comorbidities, duration of symptoms, and age (Stanford School of Medicine, 2008).

Ischemic Strokes

Atherosclerosis is the strongest contributing factor to ischemic stroke. The term **atherogenesis** refers to the development of the condition of atherosclerosis. The most fundamental lesion of atherosclerosis is a fatty streak, located in the intimal layer of large arteries. Fatty streaks may be in existence for many years, possibly starting in the early adult years. As years pass, the fatty streak becomes a fatty plaque. The growth and enlargement of the plaque occurs over years and decades. The patient is unaware of the presence of plaque until the plaque starts to invade the diameter of the artery and interfere with blood flow. The plaque disrupts the integrity of the arterial lining, causing blood to enter the plaque, which in turn causes thrombus (Hickey, 2003).

Smaller arteries are probably affected by a different process. It is thought that the smaller vessels become coated with a lipid compound in a process called lipohyalinosis. **Lipohyalinosis** is indicative of a vascular abnormality due to hypertension (Greenberg, 2001). This lipid coating causes the vessel walls to gradually become thicker, until the lumen becomes extremely narrow and blood flow is obstructed. Lipohyalinosis is believed to be the mechanism behind lacunar strokes.

Regardless of the mechanism involved—plaque, embolus, or thrombus—the result is the same. As the vessel becomes obstructed, blood flow becomes inadequate to perfuse brain tissue, and ischemia results. If this ischemia is left untreated, the tissue dies, which is referred to as cerebral infarction. Dead tissue is referred to as necrotic.

Ischemia causes injury at the cellular level because of lack of blood flow. The brain is extremely sensitive to lack of blood flow, and ischemic injury can occur within minutes. Further (secondary) injuries are due to the effects of the molecular changes due to ischemia. In cerebral infarction, an area of dead, necrotic tissue exists at the core of the damage. Around the necrotic core, there exists an area referred to as the penumbra. The cells within the penumbra are damaged, but not destroyed, and may be salvaged if blood flow is restored. The ischemic penumbra was described for the first time in 1970 as the hypoperfused zone surrounding an area of infarction. It is referred to as functionally silent tissue that is able to regain its function if promptly reperfused (Pestalozza, DiLegge, Calabresi, & Lenzi, 2002).

The ischemic penumbra that surrounds the necrotic core is comprised of edematous, oxygen-starved brain cells. A process known as the ischemic cascade refers to a series of events that occur in response to cellular hypoxia. This process induces intracellular swelling, further propagating cerebral edema, cerebral ischemia, and, finally, cerebral infarction and cell death. This further extends the area of infarction, or the necrotic core. Chart 30–1 depicts the ischemic cascade. The concept that cells within the ischemic penumbra are viable and can be saved if blood flow is returned quickly cannot be overstated. Time *is* indeed brain.

Reperfusion injury refers to injury to cells due to released oxygen free radicals that occurs after the blood supply has been reestablished to the ischemic area. Reperfusion injury results in further injury to already damaged tissue that is compromised, but viable (Ayata & Ropper, 2002; Clark, 2007). Reperfusion injury is seen most often with thrombolytic therapy.

Hemorrhagic Stroke

The pathology of hemorrhagic stroke is associated with increased intracranial pressure (ICP). This event triggers a series of conditions, such as increased mass effect, decreased cerebral blood flow, and cerebral edema. It may further increase ICP and possibly lead

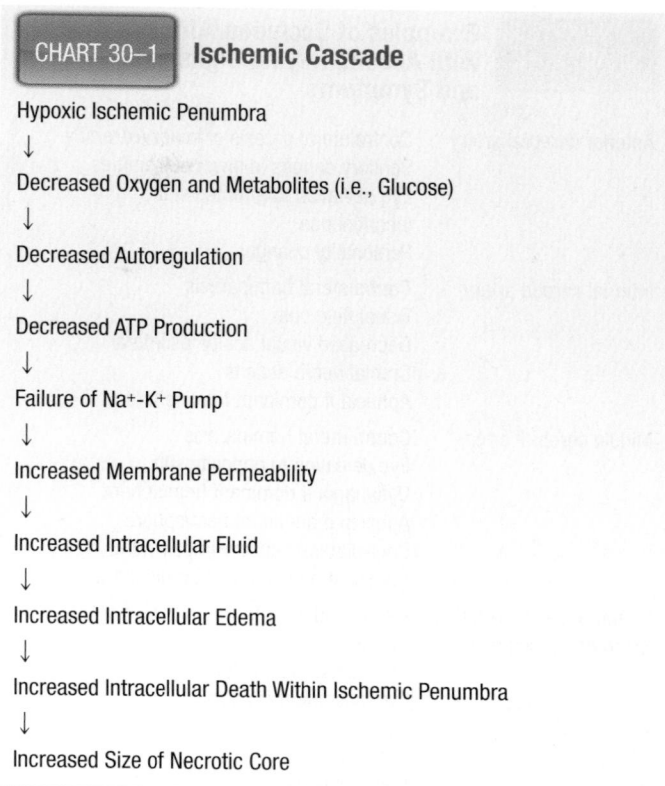

CHART 30–1   **Ischemic Cascade**

Hypoxic Ischemic Penumbra
↓
Decreased Oxygen and Metabolites (i.e., Glucose)
↓
Decreased Autoregulation
↓
Decreased ATP Production
↓
Failure of Na⁺-K⁺ Pump
↓
Increased Membrane Permeability
↓
Increased Intracellular Fluid
↓
Increased Intracellular Edema
↓
Increased Intracellular Death Within Ischemic Penumbra
↓
Increased Size of Necrotic Core

to herniation. The events associated with hemorrhagic stroke are closely related to the pathophysiology of increased ICP and herniation syndromes (see Chapter 29 for a review of herniation syndromes).

Clinical Manifestations

The signs and symptoms of ischemic stroke vary widely, and are dependent on the location of the vessel involved and the extent of the occlusion. Examples of occluded arteries and their associated signs and symptoms are found in Chart 30–2 (p. 760).

In hemorrhagic strokes, intracerebral bleeds happen quickly. Therefore, the presenting signs and symptoms occur rapidly. There may be little to no warning. Severe headache is a common sign. The other signs and symptoms are dependent on the region of the brain affected and the size of the hemorrhage. The most common areas for hemorrhagic stroke are the putamen and the surrounding internal capsule. These are the very deep structures, and account for approximately 50% of all hemorrhagic strokes due to hypertension (Hickey, 2003). Other areas in which hemorrhages frequently are found are the thalamus, the cerebellum, the brainstem, and the white matter of the frontal, temporal, and the parietal lobes.

As stated, hemorrhagic strokes occur rapidly. Often, there is no warning sign, and the patient presents with loss of consciousness and severe neurological impairment, possibly death. The area of hemorrhage may represent a large volume, which gathers quickly, causing rapid displacement of brain tissue. The presenting signs and symptoms of hemorrhagic stroke may be focal signs associated with the specific location of the hemorrhage, but also may be those of increased ICP and herniation syndromes.

CHART 30–2	Examples of Occluded/Affected Arteries with Accompanying Signs and Symptoms
Anterior cerebral artery	Contralateral paresis of lower extremity Sensory deficits in lower extremities Eye deviation to affected side Incontinence Personality changes
Internal carotid artery	Contralateral hemiparesis Visual field cuts Decreased visual acuity ipsilateral Cranial nerve deficits Aphasia if dominant hemisphere
Middle cerebral artery	Contralateral hemiparesis Eye deviation to opposite site Dysphagia if dominant hemisphere Aphasia if dominant hemisphere Contralateral sensory impairment Apraxia if nondominant hemisphere
Vertebral/basilar arteries (posterior circulation)	Visual field deficits Ataxia Cranial nerve deficits: Eye movement disorders Dysphagia Dysarthria Quadriparesis Vertigo Sensory deficits Mutism

RISK FACTORS for Stroke

Hypertension
Family history
Atrial fibrillation
Hyperlipidemia
Diabetes mellitus
Stress
Excessive alcohol use
Sedentary lifestyle
Obesity
Smoking
Valvular disease
Coronary artery disease

Laboratory and Diagnostic Procedures

Diagnosis of stroke is made by a careful and accurate history of events, and presentation of symptoms. It also is important to determine a patient's risk factors for stroke (see the Risk Factors for Stroke box). A noncontrast computerized tomography (CT) scan of the head should be obtained as soon as possible to rule out hemorrhagic stroke. This is especially important if any condition exists that may predispose the patient to hemorrhage. Examples of these conditions are anticoagulation, known presence of lesions such as brain tumors, or a rapid deterioration of neurological status. It is important to rule out hemorrhage in order to provide the patient with the optimum treatment plan.

Once hemorrhage has been ruled out, diagnosis of ischemic stroke is made by cerebral angiography. Angiography provides details of the vasculature, which artery is occluded, and the extent of occlusion. Note that a CT scan does not immediately show infarcted tissue, and the patient may have a normal CT scan, yet have an occluded artery.

Another important imaging tool for the diagnosis of carotid stenosis is duplex sonography with Doppler imaging. Koga and colleagues (2001) studied diagnostic tools for imaging of carotid arteries and asserted that carotid ultrasound was an effective tool for the diagnosis of carotid stenosis.

Medical Management of Ischemic Stroke

Both medical and surgical approaches are used to treat ischemic stroke. The medical treatment for ischemic stroke is antiplatelet and antithrombotic therapy. **Antiplatelet therapy** inhibits platelet adhesion and aggregation and is the cornerstone of therapy for occlusive artery disease. For more than 100 years, the only antiplatelet drug available was aspirin (Lubbe & Berger, 2002). Recently, the addition of a second-line drug, clopidogrel (Plavix), a thienopyridine, has added benefits to the patient at risk for progression of a stroke or the possibility of another stroke. Dual antiplatelet drug therapy, with the addition of clopidogrel (Plavix), has significantly improved clinical outcomes in reducing ischemic events. One limitation of dual antiplatelet therapy is an increased risk of bleeding (Lubbe & Berger, 2002).

Another class of drug that has gained much attention is the glycoprotein receptor antagonist, abciximab (ReoPro). Abciximab inhibits platelet aggregation and leukocyte adhesion. When used with aspirin and heparin, it has been shown to reduce the risk of ischemic complications for patients undergoing endovascular intervention. Abciximab appears to be particularly beneficial to high-risk patients, including those with diabetes mellitus (Ibbotson, McGavin, & Goa, 2003). In clinical trials, abciximab has been shown to dissolve intravascular thrombi and to improve neurological outcomes after stroke and endovascular intervention (Winkley & Adams, 2000). It appears that the use of antiplatelet drugs, such as aspirin, clopidogrel, and glycoprotein inhibitors, provides strategies that block multiple platelet activation pathways, providing increased safety for patients with vascular disease (Brinkman, Terramani, Najibi, & Chaikof, 2002).

Recent studies of angiotensin-converting enzyme (ACE) inhibitors have identified an important role for the secondary prevention of stroke, even in patients who are not hypertensive (MacWalter & Shirley, 2002). Lipid-lowering drugs, such as the statins, also have an important role in the prevention of stroke. These drugs also have a role in the reduction of risk factors of those patients who are at risk for stroke or who have already had a stroke.

The term **neuroprotection** refers to therapies, both pharmacologic and nonpharmacologic, that are used to arrest the sequence of events that occur during the ischemic cascade (Hinkle & Bowman, 2003). During an ischemic stroke, the cerebral blood flow (CBF) decreases, causing ischemic tissue to become infarcted, with an ischemic penumbra around it. At this point, it is important to restore blood flow to the ischemic tissue that still has potential for revitalization. Currently, the only available treatment is tissue plasminogen activator (t-PA), which lyses the clot and restores blood flow to the ischemic penumbra (Alberts, 1999). See the Evidenced-Based Practice box which presents the latest research on treating ICH (p. 782).

Administration of t-PA is approved by the U.S. Food and Drug Administration (FDA) and must be administered within 3 hours of onset of symptoms. Note that the administration of t-PA does not affect the infarcted, necrotic core, but may revitalize the penumbra and limit the extent of damage caused by ischemic stroke (National Institute of Neurological Disorders and Stroke t-PA Study Group, 1995). t-PA is given intravenously, although it also may be given via an intra-arterial route. The advantage of the intra-arterial route is that the agent can be given directly into the clot. It also may be given within a longer time frame, 6 hours, rather than 3 hours for the intravenous (IV) route. The disadvantages to both administration routes are the risk of intracerebral hemorrhage (Saver, 2001).

Anticoagulation with IV infusion of heparin for several days during the acute care management of a patient with ischemic stroke is common. Some institutions are using low-molecular-weight heparin (LMWH) subcutaneously instead of intravenous heparin. It also may be administered at the onset of warfarin therapy until prothrombin time and International Normalized Ratio (INR) levels are therapeutic. The advantage of this method is a shorter length of hospitalization. Warfarin therapy is commonly used for patients with cardioembolic strokes due to atrial fibrillation.

 Anticoagulation is one type of treatment for ischemic stroke due to an embolus. Patients receiving heparin therapy must have partial prothromboplastin times done every 6 hours, with the rate of heparin adjusted appropriately in order to reach the target goal. Patients on warfarin or enoxaparin must have daily prothrombin times taken to ensure therapeutic levels.

Neuroprotective agents are defined as those that protect the brain from further injury. Thrombolytic drugs (that cause the break-up of a blood clot), such as t-PA, are considered neuroprotective. Much research has been done to look for other drugs that can protect the brain from further stroke. Very few have been shown to improve outcome. Glutamate antagonists, calcium channel blockers, gamma-aminobutyric acid (GABA) agonists, and free-radical scavengers are neuroprotective drugs that currently are under investigation for the treatment of ischemic stroke. These drugs interact during the ischemic cascade, and have shown promise in animal studies (Hinkle & Bowman, 2003).

Another neuroprotective strategy is mild hypothermia. Studies have shown that mild hypothermia, even when delayed by as much as 2 hours, decreased inflammatory responses in stroke (Deng, Han, Cheng, Sun, & Yenari, 2003). It is thought that hypothermia may limit the extent of ischemic injury.

Other drugs used in the treatment of strokes and other cerebrovascular disorders are listed in the Pharmacology Summary box (p. 762).

Surgical Management of Ischemic Strokes

Patients with atherosclerotic disease in selected vessels may be candidates for surgical intervention. The diseased vessels can be either intracranial or extracranial. The goal of treatment is to prevent further strokes or TIAs. Surgical intervention may consist of a carotid endarterectomy, percutaneous angioplasty with or without intervascular stenting, or possibly an extracranial to intracranial bypass procedure. A **carotid endarterectomy (CEA)** is a surgical procedure to correct carotid stenosis. Surgical options are dependent on several variables: the location of the stenotic or occluded vessel, the extent of occlusion, and the accessibility of the appropriate facilities and surgical expertise available.

Neurovascular procedures such as CEA, stenting, and bypass procedures are highly specialized. The risks of all three procedures are significant and potentially devastating to the patient. The major risks of CEA are wound hematoma, stroke, or hemorrhage. The risks of percutaneous angioplasty with or without stenting are hemorrhage of the vessel, extravasation of contrast material, or stroke. Bypass procedures carry significant risk to the patient, such as hemorrhage of the vessel, stroke due to clot in the graft, blood pressure instability, or stroke due to a variety of other factors. All surgical procedures carry risks of infection and alteration in wound healing.

Carotid Endarterectomy

Carotid endarterectomy has been proven to be superior to medical treatment alone for the prevention of stroke by the North American Symptomatic Carotid Endarterectomy Trial (NASCET, 1991). The practice of CEA has not always met with favor. In the 1980s, the practice of CEA was controversial. It was not apparent that CEA was performed for appropriate conditions. Since then, several clinical trials have supported the classic study conducted by the NASCET by demonstrating that under appropriate conditions, CEA is the most beneficial treatment for carotid stenosis (Barnett, Taylor, & Eliasziw, 1998). In 1999, more than 130,000 CEAs were performed in the United States alone (Gross, Steiner, Bass, & Powe, 2000). Patients with a greater than 70% stenosis of the internal carotid artery have a greater than 60% risk reduction with CEA, assuming they have no major surgical risk factors. CEA is not recommended for patients with a less than 50% stenosis of the internal carotid artery. These patients are usually placed on antiplatelet therapy (NASCET, 1991).

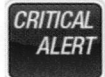 *Patients who have had a carotid endarterectomy are at risk for hematoma at the incision. Monitor the incision at least every 2 hours for the first 24 hours. If hematoma occurs, measure the neck circumference, noting the presence of tracheal deviation, or respiratory distress. Notify health care provider immediately.*

Endovascular Procedures

Endovascular procedures have been a tremendous asset to the treatment of stenotic disease and the prevention of stroke. Endovascular procedures include intravascular stenting and **percutaneous angioplasty**. These are interventional radiological procedures done by endovascular neurosurgeons or interventional radiologists. Angioplasty and stenting may be appropriate alternatives for patients who are at high risk for CEA. Percutaneous angioplasty is a form of catheterization with microcatheters. These catheters are floated into a large vessel, such as the carotids, middle cerebrals, vertebrals, or the basilar

PHARMACOLOGY Summary of Medications to Treat Cerebrovascular Disorders

Drug	Category	Application/Indication	Nursing Concerns
Dopamine Dobutamine (Dobutrex) Phenylephrine (Neo-Synephrine) Norepinephrine (Levophed) Epinephrine	Vasopressors	Increase blood pressure.	Monitored unit Hypertension
Labetalol hydralazine Nitroglycerine (NTG) Nitroprusside (Nipride) Enalapril Metoprolol	Vasodilators	Reduce blood pressure.	May raise ICP Monitored unit for IV use Possible hypotension
Nimodipine (Nimotop) Nicardipine (Cardene)	Calcium channel blockers Triple-H therapy	Reduce blood pressure. Reduce vasospasm.	Hypotension
Clopidogrel (Plavix) Aspirin Warfarin (Coumadin) Heparin	Antithrombotic agents	Reduce platelet aggregation. Provide anticoagulation.	Monitor for bleeding Monitor protime/INR Monitor PTT Family teaching for home care
t-PA Streptokinase	Antithrombotic agents	Recanalize occluded arteries. Restore oxygenation and cerebral blood flow.	Must meet eligibility criteria Increased risk for bleeding or reperfusion injury Monitored unit
Mannitol	Osmotic solution	Reduce vasogenic edema.	Monitored unit Monitor serum sodium, osmolality levels
Famotidine (Pepcid) Ranitidine (Zantac) Omeprazole (Prilosec)	H2-blockers	Reduce acid in the stomach.	Thrombocytopenia
Phenytoin (Dilantin) Carbamazepine (Tegretol) Divalproex (Depakote) Gabapentin (Neurontin) Lamotrigine (Lamictal) Phenobarbital Clonazepam (Klonopin) Ethosuximide (Zarontin)	Antiepileptic drugs	Prevent seizures.	Thrombocytopenia Allergic reactions can be severe Gingivitis Monitor blood levels when appropriate Possible drug interactions
Diazepam (Valium) Lorazepam (Ativan)	Benzodiazepines	Used as treatment for seizure cessation, status epilepticus.	Oversedation Respiratory depression
Oxycodone (Percocet, Oxy-IR, Roxicet, OxyContin) Hydromorphone (Dilaudid) Hydrocodone (Vicodin, Lortab) Morphine Fentanyl (Sublimaze, Duragesic)	Opioids	Control moderate to severe pain.	Respiratory depression Oversedation Constipation Difficulty with urination
Codeine Tramadol (Ultram)	Opioids	Control mild to moderate pain.	Respiratory depression Oversedation
Ketorolac (Toradol) Indomethacin (Indocin) Ibuprofen (Motrin, Advil) Naproxen (Naprosyn)	Nonsteroidal anti-inflammatory drugs	Control pain. Reduce fever.	GI upset, GI bleed
Acetaminophen	Analgesic and anti-inflammatory	Control pain. Reduce fever.	Liver toxicity
Naloxone (Narcan) Flumazenil (Romazicon)	Opioid antagonists Benzodiazepine antagonists	Reverse opiate action. Reverse benzodiazepine action.	
Ondansetron (Zofran) Metoclopramide (Reglan) Trimethobenzamide (Tigan) Prochlorperazine (Compazine) Promethazine (Phenergan)	Antiemetics, nonphenothiazines Antiemetics, phenothiazines	Reduce/prevent nausea.	Psychosis Extrapyramidal symptoms

artery. The catheter then enters the stenosed, or narrowed, vessel, and the atherosclerotic plaque is broken apart by inflation of a balloon within the catheter. The patency of the vessel may be preserved by the use of a **stent**, which is an open-ended tube. The stent supports the vessel wall and widens the lumen of the vessel.

Revascularization

Bypass procedures are highly controversial. These procedures are extracranial to intracranial (EC-IC) anastomosis and, frequently, the superficial temporal artery to the middle cerebral artery (STA-MCA). This is a microsurgical procedure done to improve circulation to the area of the brain served by a specific artery, often the MCA. This procedure was initially looked on as unfavorable because of the negative results reported in the EC-IC Bypass Trial (Barnett et al., 1987). This study was unable to prove that this procedure reduced the risk of stroke (Martin, Kureshi, & Coiteiro, 2004). However, this procedure offers favorable results when done by surgeons who are highly specialized in neurovascular techniques. It is used most often as a refined revascularization technique in the treatment of aneurysms.

Medical Management of Hemorrhagic Stroke

Treatment of hemorrhagic stroke is dependent on the location of the hemorrhage, the extent of the hemorrhage, and the neurological condition of the patient. Management is frequently both medical and surgical. After an initial neurological examination, the patient must be monitored closely in the intensive care unit (ICU), with frequent neurological assessment. The patient's symptoms are usually as a result of increased ICP and mass effect due to a hematoma. Placement of an external ventricular drain (EVD) may be necessary to monitor ICP and to treat elevation of ICP by drainage of cerebrospinal fluid (CSF). Medical support of blood pressure and respiratory effort also may be necessary. If the hemorrhage is large enough to cause a shift due to mass effect, a craniotomy may be done to evacuate the hematoma to relieve mass effect.

■ Cerebrovascular Malformations

Cerebrovascular malformations are congenital lesions composed of a complex tangle of arteries and veins connected by one or more fistulae. They represent several types of complex disorders whose exact etiology is not known, but which typically produce neurological deficits (Schumacher & Marshall, 2006).

Cerebral Aneurysms

The word *aneurysm* comes from the Greek word *aneurysma*, which means "widening" (Khurana & Spetzler, 2006). A **cerebral aneurysm** is defined as a "saccular outpouching of a cerebral artery" (Hickey, 2003). Though aneurysms may consist of varied shapes, the saccular, or **berry aneurysm**, is by far the most common, accounting for approximately 85% to 95% of all intracerebral aneurysms. These aneurysms are generally located on a major artery at the site of maximum hemodynamic stress, and they have a neck (Figure 30–1 ■). Common locations are the middle cerebral artery, the anterior communicating artery, the anterior cerebral artery, and the internal carotid artery. Saccular aneurysms also are located in the posterior circulation, on the vertebral or basilar arteries, although this placement is not as common. Fre-

FIGURE 30–1 ■ Intracerebral saccular aneurysm.

quently seen in the posterior circulation are **fusiform aneurysms**, which are elliptical in shape. Intracerebral aneurysms may occur singularly or in multiples. **Familial intracranial aneurysms** are defined as two or more family members with documented cerebral aneurysms.

Rupture of an intracerebral aneurysm results in **subarachnoid hemorrhage (SAH)**. SAH is defined simply as bleeding into the subarachnoid space. Though SAH can occur from other causes, such as trauma, or be idiopathic, SAH most often occurs from aneurysm rupture. This is referred to as aneurysmal SAH.

Epidemiology

Each year in the United States there are approximately 30,000 new cases of aneurysmal SAH (Schumacher & Marshall, 2006). Autopsy studies demonstrate an incidence of approximately 5% of the population (Khurana & Spetzler, 2006). The morbidity and mortality of SAH is relatively high. Despite vast improvements in medical technology and surgical techniques, outcome of SAH is still poor, with a fatality rate of approximately 40% to 50% (Juvela, 2003). Survivors of SAH may have significant neurological, physical, and/or cognitive deficits (Ballard et al., 2003). The incidence of SAH increases with age, the mean age being approximately 50 years, and is higher in women than in men (Kaminogo, Yonekura, & Shibata, 2003). Literature indicates that African Americans are at higher risk than Caucasians (Sacco et al., 1998). In one study, the author found that heterogeneity, based on ethnicity, was a risk factor for SAH (Kim, 2007). Kim concluded that the ethnic groups involved in the study had a higher propensity for smoking versus the nonethnic participants, and that the harmful health effects of smoking may be one cause for the higher incidence of SAH. The Stanford Stroke Center also identified race as a risk factor; however, they did not elaborate on or describe an interpretation of this factor (Stanford School of Medicine, 2008).

Familial Aneurysms

Familial intracranial aneurysms are defined as the presence of two or more family members among first- and second-degree relatives with proven aneurysms, either ruptured or incidental (Hickey, 2003). Multiple studies have been done regarding familial aneurysms, and they have determined that the incidence is between 7% and 20% (Schievink, 2004). Because family members may have different risk factors and show no signs of other disorders that may predispose them to intracranial aneurysms, it is believed that there is a genetic component to familial intracranial aneurysms (Wills et al., 2003). Multiple aneurysms occur in approximately 10% to 20% of all patients with SAH (Brown & Piepgras, 2004).

Etiology

The etiology of cerebral aneurysms is not clear. Genetic predisposition is one possibility. It is probable that genetic factors, combined with various intrinsic and extrinsic factors, may be an explanation. There are also many intrinsic and extrinsic factors that affect the integrity of the vascular system. Examples of these factors are hypertension and smoking. A genetic predisposition for weakened vasculature, coupled with hypertension and/or smoking that may exacerbate the weakened vessel, could cause rupture (see Risk Factors for Aneurysms).

As stated earlier, the saccular aneurysm, also known as the berry aneurysm, is the most common type of aneurysm. It is formed by a ballooning of the vessel at the weakened portion of the artery. In contrast, fusiform aneurysms are elliptically shaped. They do not have a neck. They look like "swollen" areas of the artery, and are associated with fatty plaque buildup in the artery. Although they do not usually rupture, they may cause neurological compromise due to pressure exerted on surrounding brain. Most fusiform aneurysms are located in the posterior circulation.

The etiology of cerebral aneurysms remains an area where research is warranted; however, the cause for some aneurysms is well understood. Some aneurysms are caused by bacterial or fungal infections, resulting in mycotic aneurysms. These aneurysms do not result in SAH.

Location and Classification of Aneurysms

The location of cerebral aneurysms, their size, and whether or not they have ruptured are the most important factors in determining signs and symptoms of the patient. Four main arteries enter the brain. The two internal carotid arteries enter in the front of the brain. Two vertebral arteries enter from the back. These four arteries form a ring that circles the underside of the brain. This ring is referred to as the circle of Willis. Many smaller arteries branch off from the larger arteries (Figure 30–2 ■). The arteries at the top of the ring are in the **anterior circulation**; the arteries at the lower portion of the ring are in the **posterior circulation**.

RISK FACTORS for Aneurysms

Smoking

Hypertension

Previous aneurysms

Family history of aneurysms

Connective tissue disorder

Age greater than 40 years

Female

Blood vessel injury or dissection

Aneurysms also are classified by their size, with small aneurysms being the most common (Chart 30–3). Small and large aneurysms are more prone to rupture. Although giant aneurysms occasionally rupture, most often giant aneurysms cause patients to be symptomatic due to compression on surrounding brain tissue (Khurana & Spetzler, 2006).

Pathophysiology

The occurrence, natural history, and eventual rupture of intracerebral aneurysms appear to occur as a result of several factors. The formation of an aneurysm seems be precipitated by the integrity of the vasculature. Weakening of the vascular wall may occur due to structural limitations of the vessel. Hemodynamic stressors further influence the formation and growth of aneurysms. Intrinsic and extrinsic factors, such as hypertension, smoking, and various autoimmune diseases, further affect the history of aneurysms.

Once an aneurysm ruptures, the arterial pressure forces blood into the subarachnoid space, creating an SAH. Pressure in the brain tissue stops the bleeding. The blood irritates brain tissue, causing an inflammatory response, which may further cause cerebral edema. The circulating blood in the CSF is an irritant that may inhibit CSF absorption, causing hydrocephalus. The presence of SAH causes hemodynamic changes, with a resultant increase in ICP. The pathophysiology of increased ICP is discussed in Chapter 29 ⊙ .

Clinical Manifestations

Patients with aneurysms of the anterior circulation have different symptoms than those with aneurysms of the posterior circulation. Those patients who experience SAH also have more severe neurological compromise than those without SAH. Clinical manifestations are dependent on the location and size of the hemorrhage. See Chart 30–2 (p. 760) for specific arteries that are occluded or somehow compromised due to stroke and the accompanying symptoms that may be present.

Ruptured Aneurysms

In patients with SAH, the most frequent presenting sign is headache, then progressively deteriorating neurological status. The headaches are described as the "worst headache of my life," almost without exception. Neurological deterioration usually follows, with focal signs dependent on location and the size of the hemorrhage. Seizures are not uncommon. Not infrequently, the presenting sign is death.

SAH in the posterior circulation also produces severe headaches. If the patient is conscious, extreme vertigo and nausea and vomiting usually are present. Neurological deterioration may also be present in posterior circulation aneurysms.

Unruptured Aneurysms

Although most patients are completely asymptomatic until rupture occurs, some aneurysms produce warning signs. They are frequently attributed to other causes and ignored. Occasionally, an aneurysm is found incidentally, when the patient has imaging studies for another purpose. When an aneurysm becomes large enough to cause symptoms, the most frequent symptom appears to be localized headache and/or cranial nerve signs. The most common cranial nerve deficits are dilated pupil, decreased mobility of the eye, or ptosis (drooping of the eyelid), all due to pressure on cranial nerve (CN) III (oculomotor nerve). The aneurysm be-

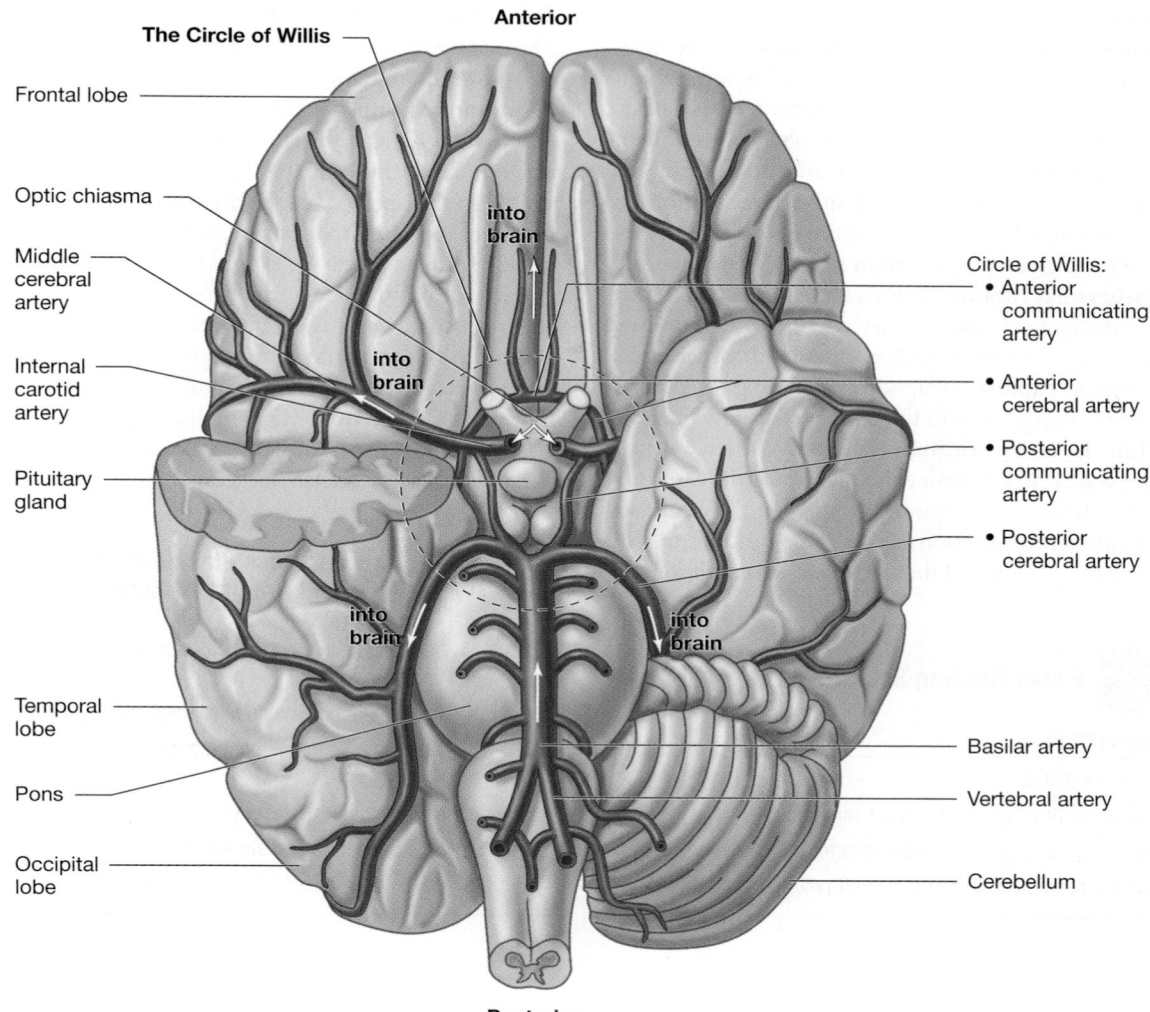

FIGURE 30–2 ■ Circle of Willis.

CHART 30–3	**Classification of Aneurysm Size**

Classification	Size
Small	Up to 10 mm
Medium	10–15 mm
Large	15–25 mm
Giant	>25 mm

comes a space-occupying lesion, causing symptoms dependent on the location and size of the aneurysm. Clinical manifestations of unruptured aneurysms of the posterior circulation are those of dizziness and balance difficulties. The symptoms are caused by the size of the aneurysms exhibiting mass effect.

Risk Factors for Subarachnoid Hemorrhage (SAH)

Risk factors for SAH have been shown to be age, gender, and race, as described earlier. As with other types of stroke, smoking is a strong risk factor for SAH, especially in women (Anderson et al., 2004). In the past, the use of oral contraceptives was felt to be

a strong risk factor, but with the change in the estrogen composition of these drugs, the risk appears significant for thrombotic stroke, but not SAH (Chan et al., 2004). Drug abuse has been associated with SAH, especially use of stimulants, such as cocaine and amphetamines. It appears that while the use of cocaine or amphetamines may not actually cause a hemorrhage, the vasoactive properties of the drugs appear to worsen an already weakened vasculature. There is evidence that the patients who indulged in cocaine use prior to SAH have a greater incidence of vasospasm (Conway & Tamargo, 2001). Smoking, drug use, and hypertension are all modifiable risk factors.

Once an aneurysm ruptures, risk factors differ slightly. Once SAH has occurred, factors such as the patient's initial clinical condition, the amount of subarachnoid blood, and the continued presence of hypertension are strong negative prognostic factors. Cigarette smoking also appears to be a strong risk factor for poor outcome (Juvela, 2003). It is believed that approximately 60% to 70% of all SAH patients are smokers (Juvela, 2000).

Laboratory and Diagnostic Procedures

The patient who comes into the emergency department in a neurologically compromised condition should always receive a CT scan of the head immediately. The CT scan will demonstrate blood in the ventricles and subarachnoid space. The patient is assigned a grade based on the **Fisher grading scale** (Chart 30–4). This scale is used to determine the amount of blood demonstrated on CT scan. It also is used as a predictor for vasospasm. Once SAH is diagnosed, the patient should have a cerebral angiogram to ascertain the location of the ruptured aneurysm. Lumbar puncture no longer is the definitive examination because, even though it will show blood in the CSF, it will not determine the location of the aneurysm or even whether it is caused by aneurysmal rupture. The Diagnostic Tests box provides more information about tests used for determining whether an aneurysm or other cerebral vascular disorder exists.

Once aneurysmal rupture is diagnosed, a grading scale is used to assign an SAH classification to the patient. This SAH grading scale is the **Hunt-Hess classification** (Chart 30–5). The purpose of this grading scale is to determine the severity of the SAH, and possibly assist with treatment options. It also is a common language that health care professionals use to communicate with when discussing the patient and the severity of his condition.

Medical Management

The treatment of aneurysms is highly dependent on many factors, the most important of which is whether the aneurysm is ruptured or unruptured. Other factors include the generalized medical condition of the patient, the Hunt-Hess grade, and the facilities available to the patient. Patients with SAH due to ruptured aneurysm should be transported to facilities with the capabilities and training to appropriately treat patients with ruptured aneurysms. A national study looked at surgery of unruptured aneurysm nationwide, and found that for patients with unruptured aneurysms treated in the United States between 1996 and 2000, surgery at high-volume institutions performed by high-volume surgeons was associated with significantly lower morbidity and mortality (Carter, Amin-Hanjani, Butler, Ogilvy, & Barker, 2003).

Historically, the treatment of choice has been surgical. For years, the neurovascular surgeon treated the aneurysm, both

---

CHART 30–4 **Fisher Grading Scale**

Group	Blood on CT Scan
1	No blood detected
2	Diffuse or vertical layers less than 1 mm thick
3	Localized clot and/or vertical layer greater than 1 mm thick
4	Intracerebral or intraventricular clot with diffuse or no SAH

CHART 30–5 **Hunt-Hess Classification of Subarachnoid Hemorrhages**

Grade	Description
0	Unruptured
I	Asymptomatic, or mild headache and slight nuchal rigidity
II	Cranial nerve palsy, moderate to severe headache, nuchal rigidity
III	Mild focal deficit, lethargy, or confusion
IV	Stupor, moderate to severe hemiparesis, decerebrate rigidity
V	Deep coma, decerebrate rigidity, moribund

DIAGNOSTIC TESTS for Cerebrovascular Disorders

Test	Expected Abnormality	Rationale for Abnormality
CT of head	Hematomas, SAH, hydrocephalus	CT scans are best suited to examine presence of blood, edema, CSF.
Cerebral angiogram	Vascular abnormalities, i.e., cerebral aneurysms, arteriovenous malformations.	Angiogram is gold standard for visualization of the arterial system.
Magnetic resonance angiography (MRA)	Vascular abnormalities	Demonstrates the vascular system, best when large aneurysms are present (>0.5 cm).
MRI, including diffusion-weighted images (DWI)	Ischemic abnormalities, cavernous malformations	MRI will demonstrate small lesions not seen on CT scan. Best suited to demonstrate ischemic areas of stroke.
Lumbar puncture	Blood in CSF (subarachnoid blood) Time-sensitive blood in CSF presents as yellow with passage of time	Contraindicated until space-occupying lesions are ruled out; possibility of induced brain herniation.
Electroencephalogram (EEG)	Seizure activity	Common in head trauma, SAH, vascular malformations due to altered electrical activity in brain.
Serum electrolytes	Hyponatremia (serum Na^+ less than 134 mEq/L)	Risk factor for increased cerebral edema. Significant in the presence of SAH and vasospasm.
Blood glucose	May be elevated	Indicative of steroid use (dexamethasone). Hyperglycemia a significant risk for ischemic brain.
Complete blood count (CBC)	Elevated white blood cell count	Indicates infection. Also may be present with steroid use.
Arterial blood gases	Hypoxia, hypercapnia	Depressed neurological state may also indicate depressed respiratory drive. Decreased levels of oxygen and increased levels of CO_2 raise concerns about increasing ICP.

ruptured and unruptured, by placing a surgical clip across the neck of the aneurysm to completely obliterate it (Figure 30–3 ■). Improvement in outcomes came with the improvement of the clips themselves and with the development of more efficient methods of approaching the aneurysm. Again, the institutions doing a high volume of aneurysm clippings by surgeons doing the highest volume of surgeries were associated with more favorable outcomes than lower volume institutions.

Regardless of the expertise of the surgeons, or the volume of surgery done at various institutions, some aneurysms still were felt to be inoperable. This challenge has led to the innovative use of techniques devised by cardiac surgeons to perform cardiac bypass surgeries. In a limited number of institutions, certain aneurysms are being clipped under cardiac standstill, cooling the body of the patient and stopping blood circulation. Large basilar artery aneurysms that previously were not amenable to being surgically clipped can now at least be considered for treatment in the hands of surgeons skilled in this highly technical procedure. Although the number of institutions that have the capability to perform this intervention is relatively small, it is exciting to realize the possibilities that exist and are constantly being revised.

The advent of endovascular procedures has presented nonsurgical options, such as coiling or stenting. The goal of any treatment is to prevent rebleeding by obliterating the aneurysm with either a surgical clip or a coil.

Unruptured Aneurysms

In 1998, a group of researchers nationwide collaborated to study unruptured aneurysms to determine the most advantageous treatment plan. The International Study of Unruptured Intracranial Aneurysms (ISUIA) studied 1,449 patients with 1,937 unruptured aneurysms from 53 participating centers. In studies published on clipping of unruptured aneurysms, the mortality rate was reported at 2.6%, and the morbidity at 10.9%. The mortality rate for SAH was 66%. The high mortality associated with rupture of aneurysms suggests that preventive surgery for the obliteration of unruptured aneurysms is a good therapeutic option (Raaymakers, Rinkel, Limburg, & Algra, 1998).

FIGURE 30–3 ■ Aneurysm with clip applied.

Ruptured Aneurysms

Patients with ruptured intracranial aneurysms should be treated as soon as possible after the hemorrhage. The purpose of treatment is to prevent rebleeding. It also is important to aggressively manage medical complications associated with SAH, such as **vasospasm**. The choice of treatment—endovascular or surgical—is a source of ongoing debate. The choice of treatment should be based on the angiographic demonstration of the aneurysm. According to the International Subarachnoid Aneurysm Trial [ISAT] Collaborative Group (2002), if the aneurysm is suitable for coiling, that is the preferred method (van den Berg, Rinkel, & Vandertop, 2003). Preferably, treatment would occur at a hospital with neurosurgeons specially trained in the clipping of aneurysms, and interventional neuroradiologists.

The ISAT Collaborative Group (2002) found that in patients with ruptured intracranial aneurysm, for which endovascular coiling and neurosurgical clipping are both options, the outcome for survival free of disability at 1 year is significantly higher with endovascular coiling (Molyneux et al., 2002). Although not a factor in the decision-making process of clip versus coil, both treatment options have financial implications. Bairstow and colleagues (2002) reported that the expense of endovascular coiling was actually higher than that of surgical clipping, but the expense was more than compensated for by the decreased hospital length of stay and the patient's earlier return to work and normal activities of daily living (ADLs).

Complications of Subarachnoid Hemorrhage

The complications of aneurysmal SAH are varied and potentially life threatening. The major risks are rebleeding, vasospasm, hyponatremia, seizures, and hydrocephalus.

Rebleeding

The risk of rebleeding is highest in the first 2 weeks after the initial bleed. Aneurysms rebleed because the area of weakened vasculature is even weaker after it bleeds. Rebleeding is also possible if the risks, such as hypertension, remain. The hemodynamic forces that aided the rupture of an aneurysm will continue to weaken the vessel, causing it to bleed again. The highest incidence of rebleeding is in the first 24 to 48 hours. Seventy percent of patients whose aneurysms rebleed will die (LeRoux & Winn, 2004). Historically, the preferred treatment option is to treat as early as possible to prevent rebleeding.

Cerebral Vasospasm

Cerebral vasospasm is defined as narrowing of the arterial lumen due to overcontraction of the vessel wall (Khurana & Spetzler, 2006). Vasospasm occurs in approximately 30% of all patients with SAH. Vasospasm decreases CBF to the area supplied by the vessel in question, causing signs and symptoms of cerebral ischemia, and infarction if left untreated. In patients already compromised by the SAH itself, vasospasm may introduce additional signs of neurological deterioration (Chart 30–6, p. 768). The peak incidence of vasospasm is from 3 to 14 days from the incidence of SAH, although it may occur up to 21 days after the bleed occurs.

 Patients with SAH are at significant risk for vasospasm. Monitor fluid intake and output carefully. DO NOT discontinue IV fluids even if patient has adequate oral intake. Check with health care provider before discontinuing IV fluids. Monitor blood pressure at least hourly. Do not administer antihypertensive medications without parameters for administration.

CHART 30–6

Clinical Presentation of Cerebral Vasospasm

- Confusion
- Impaired level of consciousness
- Focal neurological impairment, such as hemiplegia, aphasia
- Fever
- Neck stiffness

Diagnosis of vasospasm is made in several ways. The easiest way is through transcranial Doppler studies (TCDs). TCDs monitor the CBF through the cerebral arteries in question and can clearly demonstrate impaired flow. Cerebral angiography shows the artery in vasospasm as a narrowed vessel. Obviously cerebral angiograms are more invasive and take more time than TCDs, but are more definitive about the vessel itself. TCDs can be performed at the bedside and may be ordered routinely on patients with SAH.

It is not uncommon for patients to demonstrate vasospasm by angiogram or TCDs, while being completely asymptomatic. It is estimated that up to 50% of patients with vasospasm are asymptomatic. Usually, however, vasospasm is characterized by a neurological decline distinguished by the specific territory supplied by the vessel in spasm. Patients may experience a decrease in the level of consciousness (LOC), but may also exhibit a focal neurological impairment. Examples of these are motor weakness, aphasia, confusion, and/or cranial nerve deficits.

Treatment of vasospasm is a medical triad of therapies referred to as **triple-H therapy**. Triple-H therapy consists of hypertension, hemodilution, and hypervolemia. The goal of triple-H therapy is to increase cerebral perfusion pressure and CBF, therefore, reducing the risk for further neurological deficits.

Hypertension is one form of therapy to treat vasospasm in the presence of a clipped or coiled aneurysm. Systolic blood pressure should be kept at no less than 160 mmHg, and may be kept as high as 180 to 200 mmHg in patients with vasospasm that does not respond to standard treatment. If necessary, hypertension may be induced with vasopressors, such as dopamine, phenylephrine, or dobutamine. It is also common to use hypervolemia as a method of maintaining blood pressure. Patients must be in a monitored ICU, with a central venous catheter, and a pulmonary artery catheter for hemodynamic monitoring.

Hemodilution increases CBF. The balance of viscosity and oxygen-carrying capability is maintained at a hematocrit of 32% to 35% (Hickey, 2003). To maintain the hematocrit at this range, the infusion of volume expanders, such as albumin, may be used.

Calcium channel blockers, such as nimodipine, have been shown to reduce ischemic neurological deficits after aneurysmal SAH (Rinkel, Feigin, Algra, Vermeulen, & van Gijn, 2002). It also has been shown to increase CBF. In many institutions, nimodipine is given routinely to patients with SAH. Nimodipine has antihypertensive properties, however, that might limit its effectiveness for some patients.

Another neuroprotective strategy for the treatment of vasospasm is hypothermia. The use of mild hypothermia is controversial; however, there is some support for its use for treatment of cerebral ischemia due to vasospasm (Nagao et al., 2003).

Vasospasm is a dangerous complication of SAH, often causing secondary neurological declines. Thirteen percent of patients with SAH die or have serious neurological impairments due to vasospasms (Oyama & Criddle, 2004). However, the treatment for vasospasm is not without risk. Patients with underlying pulmonary or heart disease are at risk for complications from triple-H therapy. Nurses play a critical role in assessment and treatment of vasospasms. Nurses must be aware of pulmonary compromise and congestive heart failure caused by hypervolemic therapy in patients with preexisting pulmonary or heart conditions or those who are at risk due to age or other predisposing factors (Friedman et al., 2003).

Hyponatremia

Hyponatremia is another common complication of SAH. Hyponatremia occurs in approximately one-third of all SAH cases (MacDonald & Weir, 2004). Hyponatremia in SAH is caused by either syndrome of inappropriate antidiuretic hormone (SIADH) or **cerebral salt wasting**. It is very important for the cause of hyponatremia to be determined, because the treatment strategies for SIADH and cerebral salt wasting are very different. The treatment for SIADH is fluid restriction, and the treatment for cerebral salt wasting is the addition of salt. This is an important clinical differentiation, because two of the risk factors for SAH are low volume and hyponatremia. Fluid restriction for patients with SAH can be catastrophic, attributing to increased vasospasm. Generally, the treatment for hyponatremia in SAH is hypertonic saline, with oral salt supplements, if possible. This is in addition to IV fluids, usually normal saline, administered at 100 to 150 mL/hr for the prevention of vasospasm. It is very important for the patient's serum sodium levels to be monitored frequently, every 6 hours if the patient is receiving hypertonic saline. It also is important for the patient's fluid intake and output to be carefully monitored. As stated earlier, hemodynamic monitoring also may be warranted. An important feature of hyponatremia in the presence of SAH is that it frequently accompanies vasospasm, so very careful nursing monitoring of this patient is extremely important.

CRITICAL ALERT *Patients with SAH are at significant risk for hyponatremia. Monitor serum Na^+ levels at least daily. Levels at or below normal should be treated. Standard treatment is the administration of salt, both as oral tablets and as IV hypertonic saline. Fluid restriction in this setting is absolutely CONTRAINDICATED.*

The clinical picture of patients with hyponatremia usually is that of decreased LOC. This patient may become suddenly confused, restless, or lethargic. It is not uncommon for hyponatremia to become evident when the patient has a seizure. Patients with SAH should have sodium levels done at least daily, even if their levels are normal. Those with levels at baseline or slightly below should be treated to avoid worsening hyponatremia because these patients are very sensitive to vasospasm. The normal levels of serum sodium vary from hospital laboratories, and it is important to note the normal levels for any particular institution.

Seizures

Seizures also are not uncommon for patients with SAH. They can occur immediately after the bleed or may be delayed. The seizures may be generalized or focal, depending on the area involved. Treatment for seizures usually consists of phenytoin initially; however, other drugs may be added as needed. Prophylactic use of antiepileptic drugs is controversial.

Hydrocephalus

Hydrocephalus is a common complication of SAH. As the blood products in the CSF break down, the high protein levels actually "clog" the absorption of CSF, causing communicating hydrocephalus (refer to Chapter 29). Symptoms of hydrocephalus include lethargy, confusion, or other focal neurological deficits. Hydrocephalus is diagnosed by a CT scan. Many patients have serial CT scans while hospitalized to monitor ventricle size. The treatment for hydrocephalus is placement of a shunt, usually a ventriculo-peritoneal shunt. Hydrocephalus in SAH patients frequently occurs while the patient is still hospitalized, but it is not uncommon for delayed hydrocephalus to occur weeks after the initial bleed.

Arteriovenous Malformations

Malformations of the cerebrovascular system are believed to be developmental anomalies that result from failure of the embryonic vasculature to develop properly (National Institute of Neurological Disorders and Stroke, 2007a; Tatter & Ogilvy, 1995). The two most common types of cerebrovascular malformations are arteriovenous malformations and **cavernous malformations**.

Arteriovenous malformations (AVMs) are a mass of abnormal blood vessels in which arterial blood flows directly into the venous system. AVMs contain blood vessels that are thin walled and do not have normal characteristics of blood vessels. AVMs appear as a tangled mass of vessels (Figure 30–4 ■). There is no normal brain tissue within the AVM. Because arterial blood is flowing into the venous system, this is a medium- to high-flow system. Therefore, bleeding is often the first symptom.

Epidemiology and Etiology

AVMs account for approximately 8.6% of all SAH. The incidence is approximately 1 per 100,000 person/year. There is a slight male prevalence, with the most common age at diagnosis being between 20 and 40 years old (Soderman, Andersson, Karlsson, Wallace, & Edner, 2003). About half of AVMs are diagnosed with hemorrhage being the presenting symptom. AVMs are congenital, which implies a lifelong risk of hemorrhage (Greenberg, 2001).

FIGURE 30–4 ■ Arteriovenous malformation.

Pathophysiology

There are several important points to consider regarding AVMs. One is that an AVM is actually a mass, which displaces normal tissue as it grows in size. Therefore, the presence of mass effect is possible, even in cases where hemorrhage has not occurred. The result may be increased ICP, as discussed in Chapter 29 . AVMs are considered to be errors in the developing vasculature of the brain that are associated with abnormal connectivity between the venous and the arterial system. The largest concentration of abnormal vessels is located in the center of the AVM, referred to as the **nidus**. The nidus is composed of these abnormal vessels that are a cross between veins and arteries. These AVMs are supplied by one or more arteries and drained by one or more draining veins.

Normal effects of blood flow lead to an atypical shunting of arterial blood into the venous system (Soderman et al., 2003). This results in an elevated intravascular pressure and possible rupture and hemorrhage of vessels. It also is possible for aneurysms to form on the artery that supplies the AVM. These aneurysms are prone to rupture due to high intravascular pressure. Approximately 6% to 7% of patients with AVMs have associated aneurysms (Khurana & Spetzler, 2006). Neurological deterioration may be rapid in the presence of hemorrhage. Diversion of arterial blood to the AVM may increase intravascular pressure, thus decreasing cerebral perfusion pressure. The brain tissue surrounding the AVM may become ischemic. Neurological deficits may progress slowly without the presence of hemorrhage.

Classification of AVMs

AVMs have three distinguishing characteristics: the size of the nidus, the eloquence of the surrounding tissue, and the presence/pattern of draining veins. The presence of aneurysms also is an important diagnostic factor. Nidus refers to the size of the focus of the AVM. Eloquence refers to the location and to the "value" of identifiable neurological function. Eloquent areas are those in which speech, sensory and motor, and vision functions are located. The pattern of venous drainage refers to the characteristics of draining veins, whether they are superficial or located in deep subcortical tissue.

To assist in decision making regarding treatment of a lesion, and to aid in consistency in referring to these lesions, a grading scale has been determined, and each AVM is given a grade based on a standardized scale. Spetzler and Martin (1986) devised a scale based on the degree of surgical difficulty in resecting these lesions. The **Spetzler-Martin AVM grading scale** rates AVMs by assigning points for size, eloquence, and the presence of draining veins (Chart 30–7, p. 770). Lower grade AVMs have a low morbidity and mortality with treatment; higher grade AVMs have a high morbidity and mortality, and treatment is usually restricted to medical management and observation.

Clinical Manifestations

Signs and symptoms of AVMs are dependent on several variables. The most important are size, the location, and the presence of hemorrhage. As previously stated, the AVM is itself a mass lesion. The symptoms exhibited by a patient with an unruptured AVM might be related to the location of the lesion and to the function of the brain it is displacing. This lesion is generally slow growing, and neurological symptoms may be slow in progressing.

CHART 30–7	Spetzler-Martin Grading Scale for Arteriovenous Malformations				
Size of AVM*		**Eloquence of Adjacent Brain†**		**Pattern of Venous Drainage‡**	
Small (<3 cm)	I	Noneloquent	0	Superficial only	0
Medium (3–6 cm)	II	Eloquent	I	Deep component	I
Large (>6 cm)	III		...		...

*Measure the largest diameter of the nidus of the lesion on angiography.
† Eloquent areas include sensorimotor, language, visual, thalamus, hypothalamus, internal capsule, brainstem, cerebellar peduncles, and deep cerebellar nuclei.
‡ The lesion is considered superficial only if all drainage is via the cortical drainage system.

If the AVM has hemorrhaged, the symptoms may be considerably more drastic. For many patients with AVM rupture, severe neurological compromise, even coma or death, are the presenting symptoms. The severity of the neurological deficits depends on the size of hemorrhage and the eloquence of the brain affected. Seizures are not uncommon with AVM hemorrhage.

Laboratory and Diagnostic Procedures

Diagnosis of the presence of an AVM, with or without hemorrhage, is usually by CT scan or MRI. Once the diagnosis of AVM has been made, cerebral angiography is warranted for determination of involvement of cerebral vasculature, including the presence of associated aneurysms.

Medical Management

The treatment options for AVMs are surgical resection, endovascular embolization, radiosurgery, or conservative treatment, such as management of symptoms and observation. The determination of a treatment plan for patients with cerebral AVMs is dependent on the Spetzler-Martin grade given to the AVM. Grades I and II have favorable results with surgical resection in a setting where a large number of neurovascular procedures are routinely done. Grade III may warrant resection, depending on the individual analysis of the case. Grades IV and V, which are not shown on the chart, usually call for alternate treatment, because surgical resection has high morbidity and mortality even in the hands of the most experienced neurovascular surgeon.

Higher grade AVMs may benefit from endovascular treatment, such as **coiling** or **embolization**. Both coiling and embolization are a highly developed specialty of neurosurgery or interventional neuroradiology. The use of flow-directed microcatheters has made the navigation of the arterial system much safer, and a viable option to conventional surgery. In embolization, selected arteries, including aneurysms, may be obliterated with material such as glue.

The coiling of intra-AVM aneurysms with a Guglielmi detachable coil (GDC), such as those used in coiling of other intracerebral aneurysms, also has allowed some AVMs to be surgically resected that may otherwise not be amenable to surgical resection. The goal of embolization or coiling is to occlude aneurysms and other high-flow areas within the AVM. It may be used exclusively or as adjunctive therapy before surgical resection.

Gamma knife radiosurgery is another option. This treatment modality is used to treat surgically inaccessible lesions. It also is used to treat larger lesions in conjunction with other forms of treatment, usually surgical.

Conservative treatment is usually reserved for those AVMs that are a higher grade (grades III through V) and are felt to be unsafe to treat. Patients with these types of AVMs should be watched with serial magnetic resonance images (MRIs) and/or cerebral angiograms (see the Diagnostic Tests box, p. 766). Managing symptoms, such as headaches or seizures, is appropriate.

Cavernous Malformations

Another type of vascular malformation is the cavernous malformation. Historically, cavernous malformations have been called cavernous angiomas, cavernous hemangiomas, capillary hemangiomas, and cavernomas (National Institute of Neurological Disorders and Stroke, 2007a; Zabramski, Henn, & Coons, 1999). Cavernous malformations are composed of clusters of enlarged capillary channels, separated by dense fibrous tissue, with little to no intervening normal brain tissue. These lesions have a characteristic "grape-cluster" type of appearance (Figure 30–5 ■). Unfortunately, cavernous malformations usually are not diagnosed until they bleed, causing neurological deficits specific to the location of lesion. There are two types of cavernous malformations: sporadic and hereditary (or familial).

Epidemiology and Etiology

Cavernous malformations are believed to affect approximately 0.4% of the population (Passacantilli, Zabramski, Lanzino, & Spetzler, 2002). They comprise approximately 5% to 10% of all cerebral vascular malformations (Zabramski & Han, 2004). There is no gender bias and they may be found in all age groups.

Hemosiderin staining

FIGURE 30–5 ■ Cavernous malformation.

Familial Form of Cavernous Malformations

Genetics appears to play a part in the familial form of cavernous malformations. It is an autosomal dominant inheritance and is characterized by the presence of multiple lesions, often presenting with seizures (Passacantilli et al., 2002). It appears to be more prevalent in Mexican American families (Zabramski et al., 1994). Approximately 50% of documented cavernous malformations are felt to be familial (Johnson, Marchuk, & Zabramski, 2004). A gene contributing to cavernous malformations, both sporadic and hereditary, has been identified (Laurans et al., 2003). (See Chapter 11 🔗 for more information on genetics.)

Pathophysiology

Cavernous malformations are clusters of enlarged capillary channels separated by dense fibrous tissue with little to no intervening brain tissue. These malformations grow and increase in size as a result of recurrent bleeding and thrombosis. Gradual buildup of iron and other blood breakdown products occurs as a result of recurrent hemorrhages. There is an abundant amount of hemosiderin, a blood breakdown product, in virtually every cavernous malformation.

Clinical Manifestations

Clinical manifestations of cavernous malformations are dependent on several factors, including location, size of the lesion, and whether the lesion has bled. A cavernous malformation may produce neurological symptoms because it is a space-occupying lesion. It is not uncommon for the patient to be unaware of the cavernous malformation until it bleeds, causing deficits based on its location. The most common presenting symptom of cavernous malformation is seizures. Other symptoms include headaches and/or focal neurological deficits, such as motor and/or sensory deficits or cranial nerve deficits. Repeated hemorrhages usually worsen the neurological deficits, especially if the lesion is in the brainstem (Wang, Liu, Zhang, Sun, & Zhao, 2003). It is not uncommon for the patient to recover from neurological deficits, but rarely does he completely return to baseline.

Laboratory and Diagnostic Procedures

Because cavernous malformations are low-flow lesions, angiography is not diagnostic. Diagnosis is made via an MRI scan. A CT scan may be helpful to determine the presence of a lesion, but is not specific to the type of lesion. CT scans may be falsely negative in 30% to 50% of studies. (See the Diagnostic Tests box, p. 766.)

Medical Management

Treatment almost always is surgical resection if the lesions are in accessible areas. In the hands of an experienced neurovascular surgeon, these lesions are curable if a complete resection is possible (Nakaji, 2004). Indications for surgery include refractory or worsening seizures, or neurological deterioration due to repeated hemorrhages and/or mass effect. Surgery may not be warranted if the lesion(s) are felt to be small and/or not threatening. These lesions are watched with serial MRIs. Gamma knife radiosurgery is not indicated, because these vascular lesions are not radiosensitive.

As seizures are commonly seen with cavernous malformations, the use of antiepileptic drugs may be appropriate. Steroids are not a common treatment for cavernous malformations. (See the Pharmacology Summary box, p. 762.)

Nursing Management

Nursing management of patients with acute brain disorders was discussed in Chapter 29 🔗. Many of the management implications of patients with brain insults, such as tumors, or trauma are identical to those with stroke. All are caused by insults to the brain, whether the mechanism is trauma or stroke. All insults to the brain can cause neurological deterioration due to cerebral edema and increased ICP. Nursing management of ICP is discussed in Chapter 29 🔗. Nursing management that is specific to stroke and cerebrovascular malformations, such as aneurysms, AVMs, and cavernous malformations, is discussed in this chapter.

Nursing management of patients who have had a stroke, either ischemic or hemorrhagic, is a multifaceted endeavor. Strokes may also be seen in the form of an SAH from a ruptured intracerebral aneurysm or AVM. Nursing management requires comprehensive knowledge of the neurological assessment as well as virtually every system of the body (Chart 30–8).

Assessment

Neurological evaluation is important throughout the patient's course. Ischemic stroke may be an ongoing process, with stepwise changes in a patient's neurological condition. Hemorrhagic stroke may be sudden, with subtle or catastrophic results, such as those seen in SAH. In either case, the neurological consequences may be subtle and/or transient, or extreme and life changing. The nurse taking care of patients with cerebrovascular disease must be able to recognize subtle changes in the neurological exam and act appropriately. The patient's course may begin with emergent measures to stabilize both the neurological system, as well as systemic measures. It continues throughout the patient's hospital stay, through the rehabilitation process and beyond.

At the onset of stroke symptoms, the patient should be admitted to the hospital, usually through the emergency department, and ultimately to the ICU. Initially, patients present to the emergency department with symptoms of stroke, the type of which is unknown. It is imperative that nurses do complete and frequent neurological assessments. Any change, regardless of how insignificant it may appear, should be reported. At the very onset, the patient must be assessed for the basic ABCs: airway, breathing, and circulation.

Patients with cavernous malformations require careful neurological assessment in order to determine the full extent of their deficits. It is helpful for the nurse to be aware of the location of the cavernous malformation and what deficits would be expected in that location. It is imperative to know the patient's

---

CHART 30–8	**Nursing Implications in Treatment of Stroke**

- Blood pressure
- Fever
- Blood glucose
- Immobility
- Respiratory compromise
- Cardiac arrhythmias
- Seizures
- ICP management
- Identification and modification of risk factors

history, including the number of hemorrhages the patient may have had, and surgical history, if any. It would also be helpful to know if the patient has family members who have also experienced a hemorrhage from a cavernous malformation.

Planning

Once neurological deficits have been determined, it is important to ensure that the patient is receiving any and all therapy evaluations that might be helpful. For example, a patient with a brainstem cavernous malformation is at risk for swallowing difficulties. These may not be readily apparent, allowing the patient to experience "silent aspiration" with potentially serious consequences. A swallow evaluation by a speech therapist trained in dysphagia is helpful to determine if a patient is able to swallow safely or if alternate forms of nutrition are required.

As stated, patients admitted with stroke should be assessed for airway and breathing. Nursing management of patients with respiratory compromise due to increased ICP or head trauma was discussed in Chapter 29 ⊙ . As with other types of brain insult, patients with hemorrhagic stroke, including SAH, may present with severely compromised LOC. These patients may require intubation and mechanical ventilation. They also may require frequent suctioning to keep their airway clear. Patients with stroke in the brainstem, either hemorrhagic or ischemic, may experience nausea and vomiting, possibly requiring airway protection.

Interventions and Rationales

Management of blood pressure is a very important nursing consideration in patients with stroke. It may be managed differently depending on the type of stroke. Patients with aneurysms also are treated differently, dependent on whether the aneurysm is ruptured or unruptured, or clipped or unclipped. Occasionally, patients with ischemic stroke may have elevated blood pressure. Many clinicians will not only allow the patient to have an elevated blood pressure, but may actually give the patient vasopressors to raise it. It is sometimes felt that the patient's blood pressure needs to be elevated in order to perfuse the ischemic brain. Measures to lower blood pressure could worsen the neurological condition, perhaps increasing the area of stroke.

Hemorrhagic stroke may be treated differently. As stated, the most common cause of hemorrhagic stroke is hypertension. It is important to know any medications the patient was prescribed prior to admission. It also is important to determine if the patient was compliant and took the medication as prescribed. Any other medications, including herbals, may be significant and should be noted, as should any retrievable information regarding the use of any illegal drugs, such as cocaine or methamphetamines, which are known to raise blood pressure.

Management of blood pressure may be treated differently in the presence of an aneurysm. A patient with a ruptured aneurysm may require an elevated blood pressure to ensure adequate cerebral perfusion after the aneurysm has been clipped. It is possible that hypertension may be induced via fluids and/or vasopressors. In the presence of an unruptured aneurysm, or a ruptured, but unclipped aneurysm, blood pressure is usually well controlled.

Cardiac arrhythmias may be present with stroke, especially cardioembolic stroke. It is possible that a cardiac arrhythmia such as atrial fibrillation may not be diagnosed until the patient experiences an embolic stroke due to small clots sent off to the brain as a result of atrial fibrillation. These patients require diligent cardiac monitoring, with cardiac drugs designed to treat and stabilize atrial arrhythmias. Cardiac arrhythmias are not uncommon in the presence of SAH.

The presence of fever is uncommon at the initial onset of stroke. However, it is associated with decreased levels of neurological function over time. Patients with decreased levels of consciousness are prone to aspiration pneumonia due to their inability to protect the airway. Pneumonia due to immobility is a possibility and is another reason to promote early activity.

Central fever also is a possibility for patients with hemorrhage in thermoregulatory centers of the brain. In some cases, fever may be attributed to certain drugs, such as phenytoin. However, it is important to look for the source of fever for appropriate treatment. Efforts to treat fever should be aggressive. The use of antipyretics, such as acetaminophen, and cooling devices is encouraged. Several studies support the idea that the presence of fever promotes undesirable outcomes (Jorgensen et al., 1999). The presence of fever is known to increase the metabolic demands of the brain; thus, every effort should be made to determine the cause of fever.

Other nursing considerations include close monitoring and control of blood glucose levels, and observation of other laboratory values, such as sodium. These implications are addressed in Chapter 29 ⊙ .

Immobility is a strong nursing implication, as previously discussed. The initiation of early activity and therapy evaluations is extremely important to the prevention of deep venous thrombosis (DVT) and pulmonary embolus. These complications are frequently preventable and require appropriate nursing interventions to prevent this potentially serious, even fatal, complication.

If the patient has a new diagnosis of seizure, education regarding antiepileptic drugs is important. Nurses should educate patients and/or their families regarding the administration, side effects, and drug interactions of their medications. They also should be instructed if blood testing is required for evaluation of efficacy. (Refer to the section on the nursing management of seizures in Chapter 29 ⊙ .)

Another important aspect of nursing management is the identification and modification of risk factors. Smoking cessation is an obvious area in which nursing can assist the patient in identifying strategies to quit. Other modifiable risk factors include diet and exercise. Education of the patient and family is an invaluable service to help avoid future stroke.

As part of every discharge plan, the nurse should evaluate the type and extent of family and patient teaching required. Some patients with cavernous malformations, particularly in the brainstem, may have significant neurological deficits. Some deficits may require the patient and/or family member to learn adaptive measures, such as administering enteral feedings. Nursing plays an integral role in teaching and also assessing the need for further education and support.

The nursing care of patients with cerebrovascular disorders is exciting and challenging. This patient has needs that often are complex and multisystemic. Nursing care should address multiple body systems, with many actual and potential problems. Nursing diagnoses are included in the Nursing Process: Patient Care Plan feature. This plan addresses many of the nursing diagnoses, with an appropriate care plan for the patient with a

Assessment for Level of Consciousness

Subjective Data:

Do you have any history of hypertension, heart disease, bleeding disorders, renal disease, or cancer?

What day is it and where are you?

Squeeze my hands.

Push your feet against my hands.

Have you noticed any facial droop?

Do you have any memory loss that you are aware of?

How long ago did the first symptoms present?

Objective Data:

Glasgow Coma Scale number.

Neurological assessment, including mentation, cranial nerve examination, motor and sensory function.

Imaging studies, including MRI, CT, and/or lumbar puncture.

Laboratory data, including CBC, Complete Metabolic Panel CMP, and drug levels.

Nursing Assessment and Diagnoses	Outcomes and Evaluation Parameters	Planning and Interventions with *Rationales*
Nursing Diagnosis: *Decreased Intracranial Adaptive Capacity* related to SAH, stroke, or intracerebral hemorrhage	**Outcome:** Improvement to optimum level of neurological function ***Evaluation Parameters:*** Improved level of consciousness. Intracranial pressure readings within normal limits. Normal or stable Glasgow coma scale score. Oriented to time, place, person, and circumstances. Pupils equal and reactive to light. Normal ICP < 10 mmHg. Normal P_2 ICP wave form. Normal serum sodium level. Vital signs, especially the blood pressure and temperature remain within normal limits.	**Interventions and *Rationales:*** Monitor neurological assessment using the Glasgow Coma Scale hourly, or as ordered by the health care provider. Assess pupil size and reactivity. *To assess changes in motor and sensory function, and orientation to time, place, person, and circumstances. To assess changes in pupil function that reflect an increase in intracranial pressure.* Monitor ICP reading. *To assess changes in intracranial pressure that may be life threatening. To ascertain when medical intervention is necessary to decrease the pressure. To identify which interventions raise or lower the pressure.* Monitor lab values (serum Na+). *To maintain a normal range to prevent fluid retention that would raise intracranial pressure.* Monitor vital signs as ordered by the health care provider and report changes when abnormalities occur. *To prevent a rise in the blood pressure that would increase intracranial pressure. To report any increase in temperature that may indicate an infection.*

Assessment of Airway and Gas Exchange

Subjective Data:

Do you have a history of emphysema or asthma, or any cardiac diseases?

Do you become short of breath with exertion?

How far are you able to walk before having to rest?

How active are you on a daily basis?

Have you ever experienced chest pain or fainting?

Objective Data:

Respiratory rate.

Oxygen saturation.

Arterial blood gases.

Vital signs.

Lung sounds.

Skin, lips, and nail bed color.

Cough reflex and ability to clear secretions.

Nursing Assessment and Diagnoses	Outcomes and Evaluation Parameters	Planning and Interventions with *Rationales*
Nursing Diagnoses: *Ineffective Airway Clearance and Gas Exchange Impaired* related to SAH, stroke, intracerebral hemorrhage, or increased intracranial pressure *Actual or Risk for Aspiration* related to altered neurological status *Actual or Risk for Ineffective Airway Clearance* related to immobility and ineffective cough reflex	**Outcomes:** Respiratory function within normal limits and stable. Gas exchange within normal limits. ***Evaluation Parameters:*** Respiratory rate within normal limits. Airway clear of secretions. Patient will be able to manage secretions. Stable or improved ABGs. No shortness of breath. Patient able to eat without aspiration occurring.	**Nursing Intervention and *Rationales:*** Monitor respiratory status, i.e., rate, rhythm, quality. *To determine changes due to altered cerebral function.* Suction as necessary. *To maintain a clear airway.* Monitor oxygen saturation as ordered and when clinical manifestations such as increased respiratory rate occur. *To determine need for interventions such as oxygen or endotracheal intubation.* Provide respiratory therapy treatments as ordered. Position patient with neck in neutral position. Elevate head to 30 degrees unless contraindicated. If patient is not intubated, have supplies ready for possible intubation. If patient is intubated, suction as necessary, but limit to 10 seconds to avoid increased ICP. Administer oxygen as needed. Monitor ABG results. Notify health care provider if change in respiratory status occurs. *To improve and stabilize oxygen exchange and promote patient comfort.* Keep patient NPO until alert and/or swallow function is assessed and deemed safe. Conduct swallows evaluation *to assess safety.* Initiate aspiration precautions. *To prevent aspiration and allow normal oral intake.*

(continued)

NURSING PROCESS: Patient Care Plan for Cerebral Vascular Disorders—*Continued*

Assessment of Hemodynamic Status

Subjective Data:
Do you have any preexisting cardiac or respiratory problems?
Do you ever experience chest pain?
Do you have high blood pressure?
Are you taking any cardiac or blood pressure medications—if so, what are they?

Objective Data:
Vital signs, including heart rate,
blood pressure, respiratory rate, and central venous pressure, if available.
Oxygen saturation.
Skin, lips, and nail bed color.
Lung sounds.
Cardiac rhythm strips or ECG.

Nursing Assessment and Diagnoses	Outcomes and Evaluation Parameters	Planning and Interventions with *Rationales*
Nursing Diagnoses: *Cardiac Output, Decreased* related to arrhythmias, hemodynamic instability, and hypotension/hypertension *Actual or risk for Ineffective Tissue Perfusion* related to decreased cardiac output	**Outcomes:** Cardiac output within normal limits. Adequate tissue perfusion maintained. *Evaluation Parameters:* Stable rate and rhythm Blood pressure maintenance within established parameters Patient able to perform activities of daily living comfortably and independently.	**Nursing Intervention and *Rationales:*** Monitor ECG continuously. Notify health care provider of changes in rate or rhythm. Administer cardiac and hypertension medications as ordered and monitor for effectiveness. *To assess and treat cardiac dysrhythmia that affect cardiac output.* Monitor vital signs. Measure cardiac output with Swan-Ganz catheter, if in place. Notify health care provider of changes in blood pressure. *To determine cardiac output and tissue perfusion and treat if necessary. To assess for heart failure.*

Assessment of Motor and Sensory Status

Subjective Data:
Can you move your arms and legs?
Where am I touching you?

Objective Data:
Bilateral motor and sensory function.
Orientation and ability to follow directions.
Family member who can assist the patient with mobility and adherence to directions for safe care, verbally and graphically.

Nursing Assessment and Diagnoses	Outcomes and Evaluation Parameters	Planning and Interventions with *Rationales*
Nursing Diagnoses: *Self Care Deficit* related to altered motor and sensory function from neuro deficit. *Actual or Risk for Impaired Physical Mobility* related to decreased strength and endurance *Risk for Injury* related to fall risk. Risk for Tissue Injury related to immobility	**Outcomes:** Patient will attain maximum motor function. Patient will be free from injury. Family/significant other who is able to assist with care. Adequate tissue perfusion. *Evaluation Parameters:* Patient will be safe. Able to progress with ambulation and complete self-care. No deep vein thrombosis (DVT) or pulmonary embolism.	**Nursing Intervention and *Rationales:*** Monitor strengths and limitations. Initiate physical therapy consultation. Initiate activity as tolerated, unless contraindicated. Obtain occupational therapy consult to assist with activities of daily living. *To regain and increase strength on affected side and promote independence.* Encourage family involvement in patient care and mobility. Educate patient and family regarding safety measures. *To promote family involvement and prepare for discharge.* Institute safety measures, i.e., place call light within reach, ask patient to call nurse before getting out of bed. Apply restraints as ordered. Keep bed rails in high position at all times. *To promote safety and prevent falling.* Apply thigh-high elastic stockings. Apply sequential compression stockings. Administer subcutaneous injections of LMWH if indicated. Monitor lower extremities frequently for signs/symptoms of DVT. Notify health care provider for signs/symptoms of DVT. *To prevent, assess for, and treat deep vein thrombosis.*

Skin Assessment

Subjective Data:
Are you having pain on your skin in any area of your body?
Are you able to turn yourself in bed?
Are you able to get out of bed?

Objective Data:
Skin breakdown.
Patient's ability to move.
Patient's activity level.

NURSING PROCESS: Patient Care Plan for Cerebral Vascular Disorders—*Continued*

Nursing Assessment and Diagnoses	Outcomes and Evaluation Parameters	Planning and Interventions with *Rationales*
Nursing Diagnosis: Risk for Impaired Skin Integrity *related to immobility*	**Outcome:** Skin intact and healthy, without evidence of breakdown. ***Evaluation Parameters:*** Patient will maintain skin integrity. Understands importance of changing positions and is able to do it.	**Nursing Intervention and *Rationales:*** Turn and reposition every 2 hours, unless contraindicated. *To take the pressure off bony prominences and promote tissue perfusion.* Provide skin care frequently, keeping skin clean and dry. *To prevent breakdown.* Monitor skin for redness and possible skin breakdown. Do not position patient on areas of redness. *To detect areas that may be beginning to break down and treat them to prevent further deterioration.* Assess need for air mattress or other pressure relief bed. *To prevent break down.* Assess need for nutrition consult. *To provide the necessary nutrients to promote healing.* Monitor vital signs. *To assess for the presence of infection.*

Nutrition Assessment

Subjective Data:

How is your appetite?

Do you have sores in your mouth?

What kinds of foods are you eating?

What kinds of foods do you like or dislike?

Are there any cultural practices that would influence your diet?

Does any type of food make you choke?

Have you noticed a change in your ability to swallow?

Objective Data:

Assess nutritional status.

Assess 24-hour food intake.

Assess for ability to swallow.

Nursing Assessment and Diagnoses	Outcomes and Evaluation Parameters	Planning and Interventions with *Rationales*
Nursing Diagnosis: *Actual or Risk for Imbalanced Nutrition:* Less than Body Requirements related to neuro deficit	**Outcomes:** Stable weight. Adequate nutritional intake. No aspiration. ***Evaluation Parameters:*** Patient will maintain current body weight. Patient will maintain or improve albumin levels. Patient will tolerate diet or tube feedings.	**Nursing Intervention and *Rationales:*** Monitor food intake. *Food intake needs to be adequate for healing.* Serve small amounts of high calorie, high protein food every 2 hours. *Patient is more likely to eat small amounts more frequently than large amounts less often.* Provide a well-balanced diet with foods the patient likes. *Patient will be more likely to eat.* Consult with a dietician. Assess the need for parenteral or enteral feedings. *If the patient is unable to eat enough food orally to keep up with the body's demands, other avenues may need to be explored and utilized.* Keep calorie count. *To assess adequacy of intake.* Assess ability to swallow. Assess which foods make the patient choke—if any. *To prevent aspiration.*

Assessment of Pain

Subjective Data:

Are you in pain, if so where?

What makes the pain better or worse?

Does it radiate anywhere on your body?

Objective Data:

Increased heart rate, blood pressure, or respiratory rate.

Facial expressions, i.e., grimacing.

Use pain scale (0–10) to quantify pain level.

Assess cultural or religious impact on the patient's response. Assess location, duration, and onset of pain.

(continued)

NURSING PROCESS: Patient Care Plan for Cerebral Vascular Disorders—*Continued*

Nursing Assessment and Diagnoses	Outcomes and Evaluation Parameters	Planning and Interventions with *Rationales*
Nursing Diagnoses: *Pain, Acute* related to Impaired Physical Mobility and motor deficits	**Outcome:** Able to ambulate safely with little to no pain. *Evaluation Parameters:* Patient expresses pain control. Attains maximum motor function.	**Nursing Intervention and *Rationales:*** Administer pain medications as ordered. Use pain scale (0–10) to quantify pain level. *Quantifying pain increases consistency.* Instruct patient to inform nurse if pain is not relieved. *Indicates need to change pain management plan.* Assess cultural and religious impact on patient's responses. *Different cultures and religions respond differently to pain.* Correct misconceptions about risk of addiction and overdose. *To decrease anxiety related to medication addiction.* Explain, prepare, and medicate patient for painful procedures (physical therapy) and anticipated discomforts. *To control increased pain level related to procedure.* Provide a supportive environment where patient is able to express pain level. *Opens communication and facilitates pain management.* Use pain control measures before it becomes severe. *This increases comfort and decreases need for medication.* Teach nonpharmacologic method of control, i.e., guided imagery and massage, and breathing exercises. *These measures augment pain relief.* Plan diversional activities. *To augment pain relief measures.*

Assessment of Communication Ability

Subjective Data:
Are you able to speak?
Has it become more difficult?

Objective Data:
Speech clarity.
Is there any slurring?
Does the mouth droop?

Nursing Assessment and Diagnoses	Outcomes and Evaluation Parameters	Planning and Interventions with *Rationales*
Nursing Diagnosis: *Actual or Risk for Impaired Verbal Communication*	**Outcome:** Patient is able to communicate needs and preferences verbally. *Evaluation Parameters:* Patient attains maximum communication. Speech skills begin to return.	**Nursing Intervention and *Rationales:*** Assess type and degree of communication deficit. *To identify the appropriate therapy.* Initiate speech therapy consultation. *To begin speech rehabilitation.* Provide communication board for intubated patient. *To facilitate communication.*

Assessment of Coping

Subjective Data:
What are your complaints?
What is your understanding of present condition or disease?
What are patient's concerns for the future?

Objective Data:
What is the patient's level of education?
What is the patient's occupation?
What is the patient's family support system?
Does the patient have a religious affiliation?
Facial expressions.
Mood.
Verbalization of fear regarding illness, impact on family, and future.

Nursing Assessment and Diagnoses	Outcomes and Evaluation Parameters	Planning and Interventions with *Rationales*
Nursing Diagnoses: *Ineffective Coping* related to sudden change in physiological status *Anxiety related to apprehension regarding potential outcome*	**Outcomes:** Patient/family is coping with illness in a positive manner. Patient displays reduced anxiety.	**Nursing Intervention and *Rationales:*** Provide factual information concerning diagnosis, treatment, disfigurement, disabilities, and prognosis. *Truthful explanations increase trust and potentially decrease anxiety and may increase coping.* Encourage family involvement. *To assist all members to learn to cope by decreasing fear.* Provide spiritual support as needed, if desired.

NURSING PROCESS: Patient Care Plan for Cerebral Vascular Disorders—*Continued*

Nursing Assessment and Diagnoses	Outcomes and Evaluation Parameters	Planning and Interventions with *Rationales*
	Evaluation Parameters: Manifests coping mechanisms with what is happening, verbally if possible, and by facial expression. Appears calm; discusses possible outcomes. Maintains self-composure when discussing the future. Verbalizes what relieves anxiety. Verbalizes absence of sensory perceptual disorders. Verbalizes absence of physical manifestations of anxiety.	Assess and document level of anxiety. *To track trends in anxiety levels.* Explore with the patient/family techniques to reduce anxiety. *This gives the patient a sense of control and opens communication about the subject.* Explain all procedures and allow time for mental preparation. *This decreases fear and anxiety of the unknown.* Explore with patient effective ways to minimize anxiety. *This gives the patient a sense of control.* Instruct patient on use of relaxation techniques. *To relieve anxiety.* Assess need for and administer antianxiety and pain medication. *If alternative measures are not effective, may need antianxiety agents.* Assist patient/family in setting realistic long-term goals for progress. *Indicates effectiveness of emotional adjustment.* Consider psychiatric counseling for patients/families who exhibit inability to accept situation. *Provide an ongoing plan and interventions to promote long-term relief of anxiety.*

Assessment of Knowledge of Disease Condition
Subjective Data:
What do you understand about your illness?
Do you have questions about the treatment program?
What would you like me to tell you about your illness?

Objective Data:
Patient/family verbalizes questions about the seriousness of illness and prognosis.

Nursing Assessment and Diagnoses	Outcomes and Evaluation Parameters	Planning and Interventions with *Rationales*
Nursing Diagnosis: *Deficient Knowledge* related to **diagnosis**.	**Outcome:** Patient and family knowledgeable about condition and long-term ramifications. *Evaluation Parameter:* Patient and family or significant others verbalize understanding of condition and rehabilitative education provided.	**Nursing Intervention and *Rationales:*** Provide patient with information as needed. Provide patient and family education. Provide patient with resources as needed. *To increase their knowledge about all phases of illness and the necessary treatments.*

cerebrovascular disorder, such as stroke, subarachnoid hemorrhage due to aneurysm rupture, arteriovenous malformation, or cavernous malformation.

Collaborative Management

Patients who experience cerebrovascular insults—whether an ischemic stroke or an intracerebral hemorrhage due to a ruptured aneurysm, arteriovenous malformation, or a cavernous malformation—present a complex, multifaceted situation. There is virtually no system within the body that is unaffected. In addition, every aspect of patients' lives is affected, as well as that of their families and the community.

Because the treatment goal of each patient is to maintain an optimum level of function, a team of practitioners typically is required to aid the patient in this endeavor. In addition to nurses, multiple health care providers of various specialties are part of the team: specialists in neurosurgery, neurology, internal medicine or critical care medicine, endovascular surgeons, and rehabilitation specialists, among others. Also playing an integral part of this multidisciplinary team are the therapists (i.e., physical

therapy, occupational therapy, and speech therapy). Other specialists, such as dietitians, radiologists, and pharmacists, may be involved. Once a patient is admitted to the hospital with a diagnosis of a cerebral vascular disorder, the decision regarding treatment is made with the help of the appropriate specialists, usually neurosurgery and/or endovascular surgeons.

During the patient's hospitalization, it is common to use the help of internal medicine or critical care physicians to manage possible medical complications, such as respiratory failure, pneumonia, hypertension, electrolyte imbalances, and other preexisting conditions. After the initial treatment, the patient will require the entire team of nurses, specialists, and therapists to evaluate and assess for possible therapy needs. It is not unusual for patients with cerebral vascular disorders to need physical therapy and occupational therapy to evaluate and treat motor and functional deficits. It also is frequently beneficial for speech therapy to assess for cognitive deficits, some of which may not be readily apparent. Speech therapy also is of great benefit to assess and treat functional speech abnormalities, as well as swallow evaluations. Once the patient is medically stable, the need for further rehabilitation, frequently in an inpatient facility, may be addressed. See the Complementary and Alternative Therapies box for other options for patient treatments.

The patient with cerebrovascular disorder usually experiences a complicated, multisystem disorder. These patients require the expertise of many modalities. Nursing is the center and coordinator of each patient's care. Collaborative care, involving many of the other disciplines mentioned above, may be required to help each patient return to their optimum level of function.

Rehabilitation

Once a diagnosis has been made, and treatment options have been explored and implemented, the promotion of optimum health is centered on rehabilitation. Rehabilitation for patients with brain injury, whether it be a result of stroke, tumor, or trauma, is discussed in Chapter 29 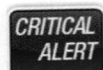. The patient who has had a stroke as a result of a ruptured aneurysm, an intracerebral hemorrhage, or an ischemic infarction may have residual neurological deficits.

CRITICAL ALERT *Patients with cerebral vascular disorders may have residual neurological deficits. These deficits may be subtle cognitive deficits that may hinder the patient's return to school or work. Obtain consults as soon as possible for therapies: physical, occupational, speech, and possibly neuropsychology. Consults for rehabilitation, either in an acute or outpatient setting, may be warranted.*

These deficits may be motor, sensory, learning, or cognitive. It is important that physical, occupational, or speech therapists be consulted and their recommendations initiated early in the patient's hospitalization. It also is important for nursing staff to be diligent in assessing the needs of stroke patients. The nurse is the first line in identifying and assessing deficits and in the education of the patient and family. Several outcome measurement scales that are helpful in determining the type and degree of deficits are available. One such scale from the National Institutes of Health is shown in the National Guidelines box, and another is shown in Chart 30–9.

It is in the patient's best interest to obtain a rehabilitation consult for either inpatient or outpatient therapy. It also is important to obtain information about the patient's home environment

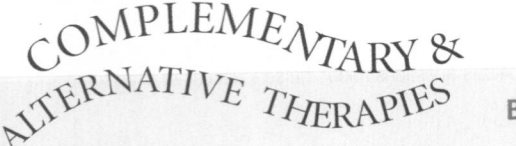

COMPLEMENTARY & ALTERNATIVE THERAPIES   Biofeedback

Description:

Biofeedback employs a way of monitoring changes in one's own body with the aid of sensitive machines. The patient consciously visualizes, relaxes, or imagines while feedback is provided through light, sound, or specialized feedback. This feedback allows the patient to learn to make subtle adjustments to move toward a more balanced internal state. Through repeated practice, a patient can use biofeedback as a self-training therapy to control physical conditions and psychological states. Tension-causing conditions such as hypertension, insomnia, and headaches are also improved by biofeedback.

Research Support:

Many hypertensive patients try CAM therapies, including biofeedback, for blood pressure control (Ernst, 2005). More than 100 randomized controlled trials indicate that behavioral treatments can modestly reduce blood pressure (BP). This reduction in BP is greater than that produced by wait-list or other inactive controls. Greater BP reductions are experienced with multicomponent, individualized psychological treatments than with single-component treatments. There are many types of biofeedback treatments, and two of them—thermal feedback and electrodermal activity feedback—perform better than EMG or direct BP feedback, which tend to produce no effect (Linden & Moseley, 2006).

In one study by Yucha and colleagues (2005), 54 adults with stage 1 or 2 hypertension (78% of which were taking BP medications), researchers administered 8 weeks of relaxation training in addition to thermal, electromyographic, and respiratory sinus arrhythmia biofeedback. Researchers measured blood pressure in the clinic and over 24 hours using an ambulatory BP monitor pretraining and post-training. Results showed that systolic BP dropped from 135.0 +/− 9.8 mmHg pretraining to 132.2 +/− 10.5 mmHg post-training. In addition, diastolic BP dropped from 80.4 +/− 8.1 mmHg pretraining to 78.5 +/− 10.0 mmHg post-training. Researchers developed a prediction model using data from 37 participants with baseline BP of 130/85 mmHg or greater. In this model, regression showed that those who were able to lower their systolic BP 5 mmHg or more:

1. Were not taking antihypertensive medication;
2. Had the lowest starting finger temperature;
3. Had the smallest standard deviation in daytime mean arterial pressure; and
4. Had the lowest score on the Multidimensional Health Locus of Control-internal scale. Researchers concluded that, since these types of persons are most likely to benefit from biofeedback-assisted relaxation (BFAR), they should be offered BFAR prior to starting hypertensive medications (Yucha, Tsai. Calderon, & Tian, 2005).

Another set of researchers, Nakao and colleagues (2003), classified biofeedback interventions into two types: simple biofeedback and relaxation-assisted biofeedback. They found that only the relaxation-assisted biofeedback significantly decreased both systolic and diastolic blood pressures compared with those in sham or nonspecific behavioral intervention controls. These results suggest that biofeedback is more effective in reducing blood pressure in patients with essential hypertension than no intervention. It is important to note, however, that the treatment was only found to be superior to sham or nonspecific behavioral intervention when combined with other relaxation techniques (Nakao, Yano, Nomura, & Kuboki, 2003). Another study concluded that, according to research conducted to date, biofeedback can be a useful alternative or adjunct to conventional forms of treatment (Kranitz & Lehrer, 2004).

References

Ernst, E. (2005). Complementary/alternative medicine for hypertension: A mini-review. *Wiener Medizinische Wochenschrift, 155*(17–18), 386–91.

Kranitz, L., & Lehrer, P. (2004). Biofeedback applications in the treatment of cardiovascular diseases. *Cardiology Review, 12*(3), 177–181.

Linden, W., & Moseley, J. V. (2006). The efficacy of behavioral treatments for hypertension. *Applied Psychophysiology and Biofeedback, 31*(1), 51–63.

Nakao, M., Yano, E., Nomura, S., & Kuboki, T. (2003). Blood pressure-lowering effects of biofeedback treatment in hypertension: A meta-analysis of randomized controlled trials. *Hypertension Research, 26*(1), 37–46.

Yucha, C. B., Tsai, P. S., Calderon, K. S., & Tian, L. (2005). Biofeedback-assisted relaxation training for essential hypertension: Who is most likely to benefit? *Journal of Cardiovascular Nursing, 20*(3), 198–205.

NATIONAL GUIDELINES Outcome Grading Scales: The Modified National Institutes of Health Stroke Scale

Item	Name	Response
1A	Level of consciousness	0 = Alert 1 = Not alert, but arouses easily 2 = Not alert, obtunded 3 = Unresponsive
1B	Questions	0 = Answers both questions correctly 1 = Answers one correctly 2 = Answers neither correctly
1C	Commands	0 = Performs both tasks correctly 1 = Performs one task correctly 2 = Performs neither task correctly
2	Gaze	0 = Normal 1 = Partial gaze palsy 2 = Total gaze palsy
3	Visual fields	0 = No visual loss 1 = Partial hemianopsia 2 = Complete hemianopsia 3 = Bilateral hemianopsia
4	Facial palsy	0 = Normal 1 = Minor paralysis 2 = Partial paralysis 3 = Complete paralysis
5	Motor arm a. left b. right	0 = No drift 1 = Drift before 10 seconds 2 = Falls before 10 seconds 3 = No effort against gravity 4 = No movement
6	Motor leg a. left b. right	0 = No drift 1 = Drift before 5 seconds 2 = Falls before 5 seconds 3 = No effort against gravity 4 = No movement
7	Ataxia	0 = Absent 1 = One limb 2 = Two limbs
8	Sensory	0 = Normal 1 = Mild loss 2 = Severe loss
9	Language	0 = Normal 1 = Mild aphasia 2 = Severe aphasia 3 = Mute or global aphasia
10	Dysarthria	0 = Normal 1 = Mild 2 = Severe
11	Extinction	0 = Normal 1 = Mild 2 = Severe

CHART 30–9 The Barthel Index

1. **Feeding** 10 = Independent; able to apply any necessary device; feeds in reasonable time; 5 = Needs help (i.e., for cutting food); 0 = Inferior performance
2. **Bathing** 5 = Performs without assistance; 0 = Inferior performance
3. **Personal grooming** 5 = Washes face, combs hair, brushes teeth; 0 = Inferior performance
4. **Dressing** 10 = Independent; ties shoes, fastens fasteners, applies braces; 5 = Needs help but does at least half of tasks within reasonable time; 0 = Inferior performance
5. **Bowel control** 10 = No accidents; 5 = Occasional accidents; 0 = Inferior performance
6. **Bladder control** 10 = No accidents; 5 = Occasional accidents; 0 = Inferior performance
7. **Toilet transfers** 10 = Independent with toilet or bedpan; 5 = Needs help for balance, handling clothes or toilet paper; 0 = Inferior performance
8. **Chair/bed transfers** 15 = Independent; 10 = Minimum assistance; 5 = Able to sit, but needs maximum assistance to transfer; 0 = Inferior performance
9. **Ambulation** 15 = Independent for 50 yards; may use assistive devices except for rolling walker; 10 = With help for 50 yards; 5 = Independent with wheelchair for 50 yards; 0 = Inferior performance
10. **Stair climbing** 10 = Independent; 5 = Needs help or supervision; 0 = Inferior performance

and the resources available at home. Whether or not the patient has someone available to provide 24-hour supervision may make the difference between discharge to the home with family supervision and admission to a skilled nursing facility for therapies. Knowledge of a patient's occupation and level of responsibility on discharge also is important. It may be necessary for a patient to have neuropsychological testing prior to returning to the work environment.

It is important to teach the patient and family what to expect on discharge. Patients need to be encouraged with the understanding that there will be disappointments and setbacks, as well as improvement. Encourage questions and give honest answers. It usually is helpful to provide home health visits on discharge to support the family and patient and answer any further questions or concerns they may have. It also is helpful to provide lists of resources for further support. The Patient Teaching & Discharge Priorities box (p. 780) lists some teaching suggestions for patients who have had strokes.

PATIENT TEACHING & DISCHARGE PRIORITIES for Stroke

Need	Teaching
Risk factors: Patient Family Setting	Assess presence of risk factors for patients with atherosclerotic cerebral vascular disease, i.e., smoking, hypertension. Educate patient and family regarding risk factors, and the appropriate interventions. Assess family support and resources.
Wound infection: Patient/family support system Setting	Assess surgical wound for signs/symptoms of infection. Signs and symptoms of infection include: Redness Tenderness Exudate and/or odor Swelling Poor healing. The presence of fever or any of above symptoms should be reported. Assess family support for needed assistance.
Pain control: Patient Family Setting	Assess need for pain control. Is present medication regimen adequate? Is pain controlled sufficiently to allow patient to participate in ADLs. Assess need for family intervention in dispensing pain medication. Assess patient/family understanding of medication instructions.
Safety: Patient Family Setting	Assess patient cognitive status: Is patient a fall risk? Assess safety awareness. Assess patient understanding of medication schedule and needs. Assess patient need for supervision. Obtain consults for speech/cognitive evaluation. Obtain social service consult. Obtain home health consult. Assess family involvement in patient's recuperative period. Provide family teaching regarding possible cognitive impairments. Provide family teaching regarding need for supervision. Assess environment for safety. May require home health or social service involvement.
Anticoagulation: Patient/family support system Setting	If patient requires anticoagulation following an embolic stroke: Assess follow-up plans. How will blood draws be obtained? Which health care provider will be monitoring the lab tests and managing the medication? Assess patient/family understanding of the medication ordered and the reason for the anticoagulation. Assess risk factors concerning anticoagulation: Is patient a fall risk? Will patient be compliant with medication and blood draws? Assess family support. Assess resources. Assess patient ability to follow instructions.
Follow-up needs Patient Family Setting	Assess need for follow-up appointments for needed therapies or interventions: Radiation therapy Outpatient therapies: physical, occupational, speech Health care provider appointments Laboratory visits for evaluation of drug levels, or electrolytes Follow-up x-rays Assess family understanding and need for further explanation. Assess availability of resources for follow-up.

Health Promotion

Stroke is the third leading cause of death in the United States (AHA, 2008b). Many of the risk factors for stroke are preventable. One of the most important defenses against stroke is education. Public awareness of stroke and its risk factors is increasing because of a massive education of not only the public, but health professionals, who are learning that "time is brain." Stroke protocols are being set up in hospitals and in prehospital settings, saving precious time in the treatment of stroke.

Many of the risk factors are genetic and, therefore, unalterable. However, many risk factors are manageable, even preventable. The National Stroke Association's Prevention Advisory Board released its Stroke Prevention Guidelines, a set of recommendations on what the public can do to prevent stroke (NSA, 2008). The guidelines are presented in the accompanying National Guidelines box.

For the majority of patients with diagnosis of vascular malformations and abnormalities, such as aneurysms, arteriovenous malformations, and cavernous malformations, there is no prevention and no warning signs. Patients are unaware of the presence of these lesions until they become symptomatic.

■ Future Directions

With rapidly growing public awareness regarding stroke, the future direction of stroke treatment is education and prevention. As stated earlier in this chapter, many of the risk factors for stroke are preventable. There is hope that with education about the risk factors of stroke, the number of strokes will decrease. Education about the signs and symptoms of stroke will facilitate quicker treatment. Stroke centers are being developed in communities throughout the United States, with protocols for speedy treatment

---

NATIONAL GUIDELINES National Stroke Association Prevention Advisory Board's 1997 Stroke Prevention Guidelines

Guidelines	What You Can Do
1. Know your blood pressure.	Have your blood pressure checked annually.
	If your doctor recommends antihypertensive medication, compliance is critical.
	A diet of low salt and low fat will help lower your blood pressure.
	Start and maintain an exercise program.
	Hypertension is the leading cause of stroke. Fifty million Americans have elevated blood pressure, or are taking antihypertensive medications, yet most do not have their blood pressure adequately controlled. The Systolic Hypertension in the Elderly Program demonstrated that the treatment of systolic hypertension decreased stroke by 36%. A prospective meta-analysis of observational studies showed that a decrease of 10 mmHg in diastolic blood pressure reduced strokes by 50% (NSA, 2008). Compliance with antihypertensive therapy is critical.
2. Find out if you have atrial fibrillation.	Atrial fibrillation is an irregular heartbeat that alters heart function and allows blood to collect in the lower chambers of the heart. Blood clots may form and be pumped into the bloodstream, and into the arterial system, causing embolic stroke. If atrial fibrillation is diagnosed, warfarin or aspirin may be prescribed to thin the blood, making blood less likely to clot and cause stroke. Atrial fibrillation can be diagnosed with a simple electrocardiogram (ECG).
3. If you smoke, STOP.	Smoking doubles the risk for stroke. Cessation of smoking immediately decreases the chance for stroke. Smoking is a completely preventable risk factor for stroke.
4. If you drink, do so in moderation.	If you drink, drink no more than two drinks daily.
	Studies show that drinking one or two alcoholic beverages daily may actually reduce the chance for stroke. However, more than two drinks a day increases the risk for stroke by two to three times. Alcohol also interacts with the actions of many medications, including warfarin.
	If you don't drink, don't start.
5. Know your cholesterol level.	High cholesterol levels, especially of low-density lipoproteins, increase your risk for stroke. High cholesterol can be controlled with diet in most cases. Some people may require cholesterol-lowering medication.
6. If you have diabetes, control it.	Diabetes puts people at increased risk for stroke. By controlling diabetes, via medication or lifestyle modification, patients with diabetes can lower their risk for stroke.
	Maintain an exercise program.
7. Exercise.	Sedentary lifestyle is another preventable risk factor.
8. Reduce salt and fat in the diet.	Increased sodium is associated with hypertension. The role of fat as a stroke risk factor is uncertain, but it may increase the risk of stroke.
9. Develop awareness of circulation problems.	See your doctor if you experience circulatory symptoms, or if you have a history of anemia or sickle cell anemia.
10. Know the symptoms.	Know the signs and symptoms of stroke.
	Call 911 immediately.

MyNursingKit | National Stroke Association

that will minimize neurological deficits. These protocols incorporate not only hospitals, but prehospital personnel and the public.

The area of neurovascular surgery also is growing rapidly. Studies such as the International Subarachnoid Aneurysm Trial, the North American Symptomatic Carotid Endarterectomy Trial Group, the International Study of Unruptured Intracranial Aneurysm, and the Carotid Revascularization Endarterectomy versus Stenting Trial have examined the alternative methods of treatments for aneurysms, and are being reviewed constantly to offer patients the best treatment option. Other trials are in progress to study the differences between coiling and clipping of intracerebral aneurysms and make recommendations for the best possible treatment.

Endovascular neurosurgery is a relatively new field of neurosurgery that is committed to developing new treatment strategies for the treatment of endovascular disease. Intravascular stenting and percutaneous angioplasty are just beginning to be explored as treatment methods for cerebrovascular disease.

Revascularization techniques also are an area in which much research is being committed. The extracranial–intracranial arterial bypass is a procedure that has given patients hope for optimum neurological function that would otherwise have little chance for a functional future. These are procedures that are done by a select group of neurovascular surgeons who are committed to teaching these procedures to surgeons who will continue to expand the capabilities of research and surgery.

EVIDENCE-BASED PRACTICE

Intracerebral Hemorrhage

Clinical Problem

Intracerebral hemorrhage (ICH) is defined as bleeding into brain tissue. Also referred to as hemorrhagic stroke, it accounts for approximately 15% of all strokes. It is a potentially devastating type of stroke, associated with significant mortality and morbidity. The mortality rate in the first 30 days is approximately 35% to 50% (Hickey, 2003). In the United States, an estimated 37,000 to 52,000 people will be affected annually by ICH (Qureshi et al., 2001). Though seen mostly in the elderly, it can also affect people who are middle aged. African Americans and Asians (particularly Japanese) are most often affected (Broderick et al., 1999). It is most commonly associated with uncontrolled hypertension. It is also associated with the use of anticoagulation agents, such as Coumadin.

Clinical manifestations of ICH are usually of sudden onset. Signs and symptoms are dependent on location and size of the hemorrhage. Most common symptoms include severe headache, weakness or numbness on either side of the body, difficulty with speech or understanding speech, or visual disturbances. It is suggested that the size of the hematoma is one of the most important factors in determining outcome for patients with ICH. The use of recombinant-activated Factor VII is a therapy used as medical management of patients with ICH. Nurses caring for patients with ICH must be familiar with this treatment.

Research Findings

It has been suggested that arresting expansion of the hematoma may improve outcome for patients with ICH. The administration of Factor VII to patients with acute ICH may promote coagulation at the site of the hemorrhage and prevent expansion of the clot.

In a Phase IIb randomized, double-blind, placebo controlled trial of 400 patients, Factor VII was administered according to a patient's weight. Single intravenous injections were given within 4 hours of hemorrhage. Treatment with Factor VII was found to decrease the size of the hematoma. A confirmatory, Phase III trial will follow (Mayer et al., 2005).

Implications for Nursing Practice

Nursing responsibilities while caring for the patient with ICH are multiple and varied. As with any medical emergency, the ABCs (airway–breathing–circulation) are of primary concern. Close monitoring of neurological status is critical. Any decline in the patient's neurological status could suggest a worsening condition. This possible decrease in neurological status warrants an emergent CT scan to assess for an increase in the size of the hematoma. Early recognition of neurological decline is necessary to obtain imaging studies, such as CT scans, to alert the medical team of an expanding hematoma. This would allow the patient to be treated with Factor VIIa, if eligible, and hopefully avoiding further neurological deficits.

Other important nursing responsibilities include careful monitoring of blood pressure parameters, optimizing treatment. This would include titration of vasoactive medications. Other neuroprotective mechanisms must be undertaken, if warranted. These include cooling mechanisms, closely controlling blood glucose and other electrolytes, fever management, seizure management, and any other monitoring of physiological processes.

Nurses are in a position to recognize and communicate changes in neurological assessment, sometimes gradual and/or subtle. Nurses skilled in neurological assessment play an important role in the care of patients with ICH, and may prevent further decline due to expanding hematoma.

Critical Thinking Questions

1. What types of patients are at risk for intracerebral hemorrhage?

2. What patient complaints or admitting signs and symptoms are worrisome for ICH?

3. What are appropriate nursing responsibilities for a patient with ICH?

Answers to Critical Thinking Questions are in Appendix D.

References

Broderick, J. P., Harold, A. P., Barsan, W., Feinberg, W., Feldmann, E., & Grotta, J. (1999). Guidelines for the management of spontaneous intracerebral hemorrhage: A statement for healthcare professionals from a special writing group of the Stroke Council, American Heart Association. *Stroke, 30,* 905–915.

Hickey, J. (2003). *The clinical practice of neurological and neurosurgical nursing.* (5th ed.). Philadelphia: Lippincott: Philadelphia.

Mayer, S. A., Brun, N. C., Broderick, J., Davis, S., Diringer, M. N., & Skolnick, B. E. (2005). Safety and feasibility of recombinant Factor VIIa for acute intracerebral hemorrhage. *Stroke, 36,* 74–79.

Presciutti, M. (2006). Nursing priorities in caring for patients with intracerebral hemorrhage. *Journal of Neuroscience Nursing, 38*(4), 296–299.

Qureshi, A. I., Tuhrim, S., Broderick, J. P., Batjer, H. H., Hondo, H., & Hanley, D. (2001). Spontaneous intracerebral hemorrhage. *New England Journal of Medicine, 344,* 1450–1460.

Source: From "Nursing priorities in caring for patients with intracerebral hemorrhage," M. Presciutti (2006). *Journal of Neuroscience Nursing, 38*(4), 296–299.

The role of nursing in the care of patients with cerebral vascular disorders is one of exciting challenges for the future. Nursing has the responsibility and the challenge to explore opportunities to improve the care and possibly the outcome of patients experiencing cerebral vascular insult. There are many opportunities for nursing research, including the treatment of vasospasm, postoperative pain control, and the effect of nursing interventions on ICP (see the Research Opportunities box). Patients who have experienced stroke offer the nurse many opportunities to explore and research treatment modalities to improve patients' quality of life.

RESEARCH OPPORTUNITIES AND CLINICAL IMPACT RELATED TO CEREBRAL VASCULAR DISORDERS

Research Area	Clinical Impact
Examine the various treatment modalities for hyponatremia, such as hypertonic saline, oral salt supplements, diet, or other medicines, and their impact on treating hyponatremia in the presence of subarachnoid hemorrhage.	Hyponatremia in the presence of subarachnoid hemorrhage is common. It is also associated with vasospasm, which is extremely significant to patient outcomes. Evaluation of hyponatremia treatments may be significant to successfully treating vasospasm and having a positive patient outcome.
Examine the differences in postoperative pain in patients who have had a craniotomy for clipping of an aneurysm versus patients who have had aneurysms coiled endovascularly.	Decreased postoperative pain.
Examine the advantages of early ambulation and therapies in patients with stroke.	Earliest possible return to previous level of function.
Examine the impact of ruptured aneurysms in specific arterial locations and the potential for return to previous cognitive function. For example, study the rupture of anterior communicating aneurysms and the long-term cognitive impact.	Identifying cognitive risk factors associated with specific aneurysm locations may lead to early testing and intervention, resulting in improved cognitive function and quality of life.

Clinical Preparation

 Read

- History of Current Illness
- Past Medical History
- Physical Exam
- Admitting Medical Orders
- Laboratory Study Results

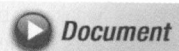 Document

- Summary of Hospitalization
- Pathophysiology Form
- Laboratory Values
- Laboratory Results Explanation

 Apply

- List of Potential Nursing Diagnoses
- Concept Map
- Critical Thinking Questions

*Log on to MyNursingKit.com to download forms you will need and to complete further steps in the Clinical Preparation assignment.

HISTORY OF PRESENT ILLNESS

Mrs. J.M. is a 42-year-old woman admitted to the ICU in a major metropolitan hospital. She was brought into the emergency department (ED) by paramedics who responded to a frantic call from her husband. He reports that she has always been in perfect health until about 3 hours prior to admission. They were about to sit down to dinner with friends when she gasped, grabbed her forehead, and complained of the "worst headache of her life." She then lost consciousness and slid to the floor.

When paramedics arrived, they found Mrs. J.M. moaning and localizing to pain with her left side. She had no obvious movement on her right side. Her respirations were labored, blood pressure 192/110. She was immediately transported to the hospital.

On arrival at the ED, her respirations became labored, and she required intubation to protect her airway. She was placed on a ventilator, and a neurosurgical consult was requested.

She was immediately sent for a CT scan of her head that revealed a subarachnoid hemorrhage (SAH). The neurosurgical resident immediately sent her for cerebral angiography, which revealed a ruptured aneurysm of the left middle cerebral artery. The surgeon discussed the findings with the patient's husband and obtained permission for the patient to go to surgery for a clipping of the left middle cerebral artery aneurysm. While the surgical team assembles, the patient is admitted to the ICU, where you assume care of her.

Medical–Surgical History

Obtained from husband

No known allergies

Medications: regular insulin, per sliding scale; occasional over-the-counter medications, such as acetaminophen

No past surgical history

Social History

No tobacco use; rare social alcohol use

Married, with two daughters, ages 8 and 10

Works as a hotel manager

Physical Exam

Young woman, appearing stated age, sedated, appears in no distress

Vital signs: temp 37.0°C degrees rectally, heart rate 62, respiratory rate 12 (assisted), blood pressure 174/80

HEENT: rhythm and rate regular, S_1S_2 heard, no abnormal murmurs, good capillary refill, pulses 2+ all extremities, no pitting edema

Lungs: clear to auscultation bilaterally

Abdomen: soft, nontender; bowel sounds heard in all quadrants

Neurological Exam

GCS = E3 M4 VT1 = 8T (eyes open to speech only, withdraws her left side to pain, no verbal response, intubated)

Cranial nerves: CN II–XII intact bilaterally

Motor:

   Left upper extremity: withdraws to pain

   Left lower extremity: withdraws to pain

   Right upper extremity: no response to pain

   Right lower extremity: no response to pain

Sensory: Unable to examine

Cerebellar: Unable to examine

Imaging Studies

CT scan done in the ED reveals subarachnoid blood

Cerebral angiogram reveals the presence of a left middle cerebral aneurysm

Chest x-ray: no abnormal pathology

ECG: normal

Admitting Medical Orders

Admit to Neuroscience ICU

Diagnosis: subarachnoid hemorrhage; status postinsertion EVD

Condition: critical

Allergies: none known

Vital signs and neuro assessment q1h

Bed rest

NPO

NG tube to low intermittent suction

Foley catheter

Intake and output: q1h

Continuous ECG, arterial pressure, ICP monitoring

Keep EVD (external ventricular drain) at the level of the EAC (external auditory canal) open to drain for ICP > 20 until ICP is less than 20; then resume monitoring

Call resident on call: any change in neurological status; any change in vital signs: HR < 60 or > 120; systolic blood pressure < 100 or > 140; RR < 12 or > 30; temperature > 38°C; O_2 saturation < 92%; ICP > 20; CPP < 80 or > 100; glucose < 70 or > 120 mg/dL

IV: NS with 20 mEq KCl @ 75 mL/hr

Ventilatory settings: O_2: 40%, TV: 600, IMV: 12

Consent for: craniotomy for clipping of left middle cerebral artery aneurysm by Dr. XYZ

Sequential compression stockings (SCDs) to lower extremities prior to surgery

Internal medicine consult for management of diabetes

Scheduled Medications

Sliding scale regular Insulin, dosage to be determined by internist

Pepcid 20 mg IV bid

PRN Medications

Acetaminophen 650 mg rectal q4h prn fever

Morphine sulfate 2–6 mg IV q1h prn pain

Ativan 0.5–2 mg IV q2h prn agitation

Zofran 4 mg IV q8 prn nausea

Ordered Laboratory Studies

CBC, Chem 7 panel, PTT, PT, INR on admission and q a.m.

Accu-Chek q6h

Ordered Diagnostic Studies

Head CT scan in the morning postoperatively

Head CT scan stat prn if neuro signs change and notify physician

Trans cranial Doppler study every other day

An external ventricular drain (EVD) is placed to monitor and assist with controlling her ICP. Her opening pressure is 26 and her cerebrospinal fluid (CSF) is grossly bloody. A central line is placed to assist with hemodynamic monitoring. An arterial line is also being placed to assist with blood pressure monitoring. Laboratory tests, including coagulation studies done in the ED, are reviewed and are unremarkable. Mrs. J.M. is sent to surgery.

Postoperatively, when Mrs. J.M. returns to the ICU, she is still sedated, but waking up. She opens her eyes and moves her left side purposefully. She does not move the right arm or leg. She remains intubated and ventilated with her EVD in place.

Mrs. J.M. is extubated on postop day 3. She is no longer sedated. Her neurological exam is as follows: GCS = E4 M6 V3. Her pupils are equal and reactive, and her gaze is conjugate. Her face shows some weakness on the right side. She follows commands by showing two fingers on the left side. She is unable to move the right arm or leg. Her speech consists of barely intelligible words. Her EVD is closed to drainage and a follow-up CT scan the following morning shows no increase in ventricular size with the EVD closed, so it is removed.

Transcranial Doppler studies are being performed every other day to monitor blood flow in the affected arteries, and to assess for vasospasm. Her laboratory values are stable, her sodium level is 136 mEq/L. Medications include nimodipine 30 mg sublingual every 2 hours; Pepcid 20 mg orally bid; salt supplements, 2 grams three times a day with food; sliding scale insulin; and prn medications for pain, nausea, and fever. Her vital signs have been stable: afebrile, heart rate in the 70s, blood pressure 140/82–150/90, respirations stable at 16. She does not require supplemental oxygen. She is eating a pureed diet (due to impaired swallow reflex), and nursing is getting her out of bed to sit in a chair. Her IV is running at 100 mL/hr with a solution of NS.

She is transferred to general floor care on postop day 4. She has orders to increase her activity as tolerated and to attempt to eat solid foods. Her IV has been discontinued. Physical therapy and occupational therapy are ordered to assist with mobility and ambulation. Speech therapy is consulted to assist with the evaluation of her swallowing and to assist with her severe aphasia.

On postop day 5, the nurse notes that she is slightly agitated. On questioning her, it is noted that her speech has deteriorated to moans only. Her vital signs are unchanged with the exception of a blood pressure of 100/62. The rest of her exam is unchanged. Laboratory values reveal a sodium level of 130 mg/L. The MD is called, and the patient is sent for a stat angiogram. The angiogram results prove that Mrs. J.M. has vasospasm of her left middle cerebral artery. She is placed on hy-

pertonic saline for her hyponatremia. She is transferred back to the ICU and her triple-H therapy (for hypervolemia, hypertension, and hemodilution) is resumed.

LABORATORY STUDY RESULTS

Test	Day 1	Day 2	Day 3
Sodium	142 mEq/L	138 mEq/L	135mEq/L
Potassium	3.8 mEq/L	3.5 mEq/L	3.6 mEq/L
Chloride	98 mEq/L	97 mEq/L	98 mEq/L
Carbon dioxide	22 mEq/L	22 mEq/L	23 mEq/L
Blood urea nitrogen (BUN)	22 mg/dL	21 mg/dL	22 mg/dL
Creatinine	1.2 mg/dL	1.2 mg/dL	1.2 mg/dL
Blood glucose	290 mg/dL	240 mg/dL	180 mg/dL
White blood cells	8200 µL	8100 µL	8200 µL
Hemoglobin	12.3 g/dL	12.2 g/dL	12.4 g/dL
Hematocrit	35.4%	33%	34%
Platelets	210,000 µL	200,000 µL	205,000 µL
Protime (PT)	10.6 seconds	10.5 seconds	10.5 seconds
International Normalized Ration (INR)	0.8 INR	0.8 INR	0.75 INR
Partial thromboplastin time (PTT)	33 seconds	34 seconds	32 seconds

CRITICAL THINKING QUESTIONS

1. What is the significance of Mrs. J.M. complaining of "the worst headache of her life"?

2. What symptoms did Mrs. J.M. experience that specified the location of the affected artery?

3. What symptoms of vasospasm did Mrs. J.M. exhibit?

4. What interventions could be expected to treat vasospasm?

Answers to Critical Thinking Questions appear in Appendix D.

NCLEX® REVIEW

1. Of the 500,000 strokes that occur annually, 80% of them are ischemic strokes. Which of the following accurately reflects this type of stroke?

   1. The strokes are hemorrhagic in nature.
   2. The signs and symptoms, though acute, resolve without permanent disability.
   3. The strokes are commonly caused by artherosclerosis.
   4. Patients experiencing this type of stroke are usually younger.

2. The pathophysiology of a stroke differs according to its underlying process. In the following selections, identify those processes that can cause a brain attack. Select all that apply.

   1. Plaque formation that alters the internal diameter of a cerebral artery
   2. Embolus that separated from a deep venous thrombosis in the left leg
   3. Thrombus formation as a result of plaque formation
   4. Lipohyalinosis, a vascular abnormality, caused by hypertension

3. The ischemic cascade is a response to cellular hypoxia and may result in additional cell damage. In describing this process, the nurse understands that:

    1. Tissues that surround the necrotic area have themselves undergone anoxia.

    2. Ischemic cascade further extends the area of infarction.

    3. This tissue may be reperfused, but its ability to function has been permanently impaired.

    4. The penumbra of a stroke is the necrotic core.

4. Nurses play a crucial role in the management of patient with vasospasm associated with subarachnoid hemorrhage treated with Triple–H therapy. The nurse must continuously assess for the complications. Assessment parameters include:

    1. Assessing renal output to detect the onset of cerebral salt wasting.

    2. Assessing lung and heart sounds to detect fluid overload.

    3. Detection of the nidus which can warn of impending seizure onset.

    4. Monitoring for focal seizure onset as these warn of a dire complication.

5. There are two major medical management options for the treatment of ruptured aneurysm. When diagnostic testing has found that both endovascular coiling and neurosurgical clipping are treatment options, the choice is based upon which of the following factors?

    1. Endovascular coiling is associated with a longer length of hospital stay.

    2. Neurosurgical clipping is associated with a higher survival and lower morbidity rates one year after procedure.

    3. Endovascular coiling is associated with the patients being able to return to their activities of normal living and work earlier than patients who had undergone neurosurgical clipping.

    4. There is little difference in either treatment option other than the availability of an interventional neuroradiologist.

Answers for review questions appear in Appendix D

KEY TERMS

anterior circulation *p.764*
antiplatelet therapy *p.760*
arteriovenous malformation (AVM) *p.769*
atherogenesis *p.758*
berry aneurysm *p.763*
cardiogenic embolism *p.758*
carotid endarterectomy (CEA) *p.761*
cavernous malformation *p.769*
cerebral aneurysm *p.763*
cerebral salt wasting *p.768*
coiling *p.770*

embolization *p.770*
familial intracranial aneurysms *p.763*
Fisher grading scale *p.766*
fusiform aneurysms *p.763*
Hunt-Hess classification *p.766*
infarction *p.757*
lacunar stroke *p.758*
lipohyalinosis *p.759*
neuroprotection *p.760*
nidus *p.769*

percutaneous angioplasty *p.761*
posterior circulation *p.764*
reperfusion injury *p.759*
Spetzler-Martin AVM grading scale *p.769*
stent *p.763*
stroke *p.757*
subarachnoid hemorrhage (SAH) *p.763*
transient ischemic attack (TIA) *p.758*
triple-H therapy *p.768*
vasospasm *p.767*

EXPLORE PEARSON mynursingkit™

MyNursingKit is your one stop for online chapter review materials and resources. Prepare for success with additional NCLEX®-style practice questions, interactive assignments and activities, web links, animations and videos, and more!

Register your access code from the front of your book at
www.mynursingkit.com

REFERENCES

Adams, H. P., del Zoppo, G. J., & von Kummer, R. (2006). *Management of stroke: A practical guide for the prevention, evaluation, and treatment of acute stroke* (3rd ed.). West Islip, NY: Professional Communications.

Alberts, M. J. (1999). Diagnosis and treatment of ischemic stroke. *American Journal of Medicine, 106*, 211–221.

American Heart Association. (2004). *Heart disease and stroke statistics—2004 update.* Dallas, TX: Author.

American Heart Association. (2005a). *Heart disease and stroke statistics.*—2005 update. Dallas: Author.

American Heart Association. (2005b). American Heart Association and American Stroke Association national survey of stroke risk awareness among women. *Circulation, 111*, 1321–1326.

American Heart Association. (2008a). *Heart disease and stroke statistics: 2008 update at-a-glance.* Dallas, Texas: American Heart Association.

American Heart Association. (2008b). Heart disease and stroke statistics—2008 update. *Circulation, 117*, e25–e146.

Anderson, C. S., Feigin, V., Bennett, D., Lin, R. B., Hankey, G., & Jamrozik, K., et al. (2004). Active and passive smoking and the risk of subarachnoid hemorrhage: An international population-based case-controlled study. *Stroke, 35*(3), 633–637.

Ayata, C., & Ropper, A. H. (2002). Ischaemic brain oedema. *Journal of Clinical Neuroscience, 9*(2), 113–124.

Bairstow, P., Dodgson, A., Linto, J., & Khangure, M. (2002). Comparison of cost and outcome of endovascular and neurosurgical procedures in the treatment of ruptured intracranial aneurysms. *Australian Radiology, 46*(3), 249–251.

Ballard, J., Kreiter, K. T., Claassen, J., Kowalski, R. G., Connolly, E. S., & Mayer, S. A. (2003). Risk factors for continued cigarette use after subarachnoid hemmorrage. *Stroke, 34*, 1859–1863.

Barnett, H. J. M., Sackett, D., Taylor, D. W., Haynes, B., Peerless, S. J., Meissner, I., et al. (1987). Are the results of the extracranial–intracranial bypass trial generalizable? *New England Journal of Medicine, 316*(13), 800–824.

Barnett, H. J., Taylor, D. W., & Eliasziw, M. (1998). Benefit of carotid endarterectomy in patients with symptomatic moderate or severe stenosis: North American Symptomatic Carotid Endarterectomy Trial Collaborators. *New England Journal of Medicine, 339*, 1415–1425.

Brinkman, W. T., Terramani, T. T., Najibi, S., & Chaikof, E. L. (2002). Platelets: Is aspirin sufficient or must we know how to pronounce abciximab? *Seminars in Vascular Surgery, 15*(4), 245–255.

Brown, R. D., & Piepgras, D. G. (2004). Screening for intracranial aneurysms after subarachnoid hemorrhage: do our patients benefit? *Neurology, 62*, 354–356.

Carter, B. S., Amin-Hanjani, S., Butler, W. E., Ogilvy, C. S., & Barker, F. G. (2003, February). *In-hospital mortality and morbidity after surgical treatment of unruptured intracranial aneurysms in the United States from 1996 to 2000: The effect of hospital and surgeon volume.* Oral abstract presentation at the Sixth Joint Meeting of the AANS/CNS Section on Cerebrovascular Surgery and the American Society of Interventional & Therapeutic Neuroradiology, Phoenix, AZ.

Chan, W. S., Ray, J., Wai, E. K., Ginsburg, S., Hannah, M. E., Corey, P. N., et al. (2004). Risk of stroke in women exposed to low-dose oral contraceptives: A critical evaluation of the evidence. *Archives of Internal Medicine, 164*(7), 741–747.

Clark, W. M. (2007). Reperfusion injury in stroke. *eMedicine.* Retrieved April 2, 2008, from http://www.emedicine.com/neuro/topic602.htm

Conway, J. E., & Tamargo R. J. (2001). Cocaine use is an independent risk factor for cerebral vasospasm in aneurysmal subarachnoid hemorrhage. *Stroke, 32*(10), 2338–2343.

Deng, H., Han, H. S., Cheng, D., Sun, G. H., & Yenari, M. A. (2003). Mild hypothermia inhibits inflammation after experimental stroke and brain inflammation. *Stroke 34*, 2495–2501.

Friedman, J. A., Pichelmann, M. A., Piepgras, D. G., McIver, J. I., Toussaint, L. G., McClelland, R. L., et al. (2003). Pulmonary complications of aneurysmal subarachnoid hemorrhage. *Neurosurgery, 52*(5), 1025–1031.

Greenberg, M. S. (2001). *Handbook of neurosurgery* (5th ed.). New York: Thieme.

Gross, C. P., Steiner, C. A., Bass, E. B., & Powe, N. R. (2000). Relation between prepublication release of clinical trial results and the practice of carotid endarterectomy. *Journal of the American Medical Association, 284*, 2886–2893.

Hickey, J. (2003). *The clinical practice of neurological and neurosurgical nursing* (5th ed.). Philadelphia: Lippincott.

Hinkle, J. L., & Bowman, L. (2003). Neuroprotection for ischemic stroke. *Journal of Neuroscience Nursing, 35*(2), 114–118.

Howard, V. J., McClure, L. A., Meschia, J. F., Pulley, L., Orr, S. C., & Friday, G. H. (2006). High prevalence of stroke symptoms among persons without a diagnosis of stroke or transient ischemic attack in a general population: The Reasons for Geographic And Racial Differences in Stroke (REGARDS) study. *Archives of Internal Medicine, 166*(18), 1952–1958.

Ibbotson, T., McGavin, J. K., & Goa, K. L. (2003). Abciximab: An updated review of its therapeutic use in patients with ischaemic heart disease undergoing percutaneous coronary revascularization. *Drugs, 63*(11), 1121–1163.

International Subarachnoid Aneurysm Trial Collaborative Group. (2002). International Subarachnoid Aneurysm Trial (ISAT) of neurosurgical clipping versus endovascular coiling in 2143 patients with ruptured intracranial aneurysms: A randomized trial. *Lancet, 360*, 1267–1274.

Johnson, E. W., Marchuk, D. A., & Zabramski, J. M. (2004). The genetics of cerebral cavernous malformations. In R. F. Spetzler & F. B. Meyer (Eds.), *Youman's neurological surgery* (5th ed., pp. 2299–2303). Philadelphia: W. B. Saunders.

Johnson, S. C., Gress, D. R., Browner, W. S., & Sidney, S. (2000). Short-term prognosis after emergency department diagnosis of TIA. *Journal of American Medical Association, 284*, 2901–2906.

Jorgensen, H. S., Reith, J., Nakayama, H., Kammersgard, L. P., Raaschous, H. O., & Olsen, T. S. (1999). What determines good recovery in patients with the most severe strokes? The Copenhagen Stroke Study. *Stroke, 30*, 2009–2012.

Juvela, S. (2000). Risk factors for multiple intracranial aneurysms. *Stroke, 31*, 392–397.

Juvela, S. (2003). Prehemorrhage risk factors for fatal intracranial aneurysm rupture. *Stroke, 34*, 1852–1858.

Kaminogo, M., Yonekura, M., & Shibata, S. (2003). Incidence and outcome of multiple intracranial aneurysms in a defined population. *Stroke, 34*(1), 16–21.

Khurana, V. G., & Spetzler, R. F. (2006). *The brain aneurysm: A comprehensive resource for brain aneurysm patients, their families, and physicians.* Bloomington, IN: AuthorHouse.

Kim, K. V. (2007). Ethnic differences in risk factors for subarachnoid hemorrhage. *Neurosurgery, 107*(3), 522–529.

Koga, M., Kimura, K., Minematsu, K., & Yamaguchi, T. (2001). Diagnosis of internal carotid artery stenosis greater than 70% with power Doppler duplex sonography. *American Journal of Neuroradiology, 22*(2), 413–417.

Laurans, M. S., DiLuna, M. L., Shin, D., Niazi, F., Voorhees, J. R., Nelson-Williams, M., et al. (2003). Mutational analysis of 206 families with cavernous malformations. *Journal of Neurosurgery, 99*(1), 38–43.

LeRoux, P. D., & Winn, H. R. (2004). Surgical decision making for the treatment of cerebral aneurysms. In R. F. Spetzler & F. B. Meyer (Eds.), *Youman's neurological surgery* (5th ed., pp. 1793–1809). Philadelphia: W. B. Saunders.

Lubbe, D. F., & Berger, P. B. (2002). The thienopyridines. *Journal of Interventional Cardiology., 15*(1), 85–93.

MacDonald, R. L., & Weir, B. (2004). Perioperative management of subarachnoid hemorrhage. In R. F. Spetzler & F. B. Meyer (Eds.), *Youman's neurological surgery* (5th ed., pp. 1813–1835). Philadelphia: W. B. Saunders.

MacWalter, R. S., & Shirley, C. P. (2002). A benefit-risk assessment of agents used in the secondary prevention of stroke. *Drug Safety, 25*(13), 943–963.

Martin, N. A., Kureshi, I., & Coiteiro, D. (2004). Revascularization techniques for complex aneurysms and skull base tumors. In R. F. Spetzler & F. B. Meyer (Eds.), *Youman's neurological surgery* (5th ed., pp. 2107–2119). Philadelphia: W. B. Saunders.

Matchar, D. B., & Samsa, G. P. (2000). *Secondary and tertiary prevention of stroke: Patient Outcomes Research Team (PORT) final report phase 1.* (AHRQ Pub. No. 00-N001). Rockville, MD: Agency for Healthcare Research and Quality.

Molyneux, A., Kerr, R., Stratton, I., Sandercock, P., Clarke, M., Shrimpton, J., et al. (2002). International Subarachnoid Aneurysm Trial (ISAT) of neurosurgical clipping versus endovascular coiling in 2143 patients with ruptured intracranial aneurysms: A randomised trial. *Lancet, 360*(9342), 1267–1274.

Nagao, S., Irie, K., Kawai, N., Nakamura, T., Kunishio, K., & Matsumoto, Y. (2003). The use of mild hypothermia for patients with severe vasospasm: A preliminary report. *Journal of Clinical Neuroscience, 10*(2), 208–212.

Nakaji, P. (2004). Management of brainstem cavernous malformations. For the Proceedings of the 29th Stroke Conference of the Japan Stroke Society. Submitted for publishing.

National Institute of Neurological Disorders and Stroke. (2007a). *NINDS arteriovenous malformation information page.* Retrieved April 3, 2008, from http://www.ninds.nih.gov/disorders/avms/avms.htm

National Institute of Neurological Disorders and Stroke t-PA Study Group. (1995). Tissue plasminogen activator for acute ischemic stroke. *New England Journal of Medicine, 333*, 1581–1587.

National Stroke Association. (2008). *Stroke risk factors.* Retrieved April 5, 2008, from http://www.stroke.org/site.PageServacer?pagename=RISKN

North American Symptomatic Carotid Endarterectomy Trial Collaborators. (1991). Beneficial effect of carotid endarterectomy in symptomatic patients with high-grade stenosis. *New England Journal of Medicine, 325*(7), 445–453.

Oyama, K., & Criddle, L. (2004). Vasospasm after aneurysmal subarachnoid hemorrhage. *Critical Care Nurse, 24*(5), 58–60.

Passacantilli, E., Zabramski, J., Lanzino, G., & Spetzler, R. F. (2002). Cavernous malformations: Genetic, molecular biology, and familial forms. *Operative Techniques in Neurosurgery, 5*(3), 145–149.

Pestalozza, I. F., DiLegge, S., Calabresi, M., & Lenzi, G. L. (2002). Ischaemic penumbra: Highlights. *Clinical Experience with Hypertension, 24*(7–8), 517–529.

Raaymakers, T. W. M., Rinkel, G. J. E., Limburg, M., & Algra, A. (1998). Mortality and morbidity of surgery for unruptured intracranial aneurysms: A meta-analysis. *Stroke, 29*, 1531–1538.

Rinkel, G. J., Feigin, V. L., Algra, A., Vermeulen, M., & van Gijn, J. (2002). Calcium antagonists for aneurysmal subarachnoid hemorrhage. *Cochran Database System.*

Rosamond, W., Flegal, K., Friday, G., Furie, K., et al. (2007). Heart disease and stroke statistics—2007 update: A report from the American Heart Association Statistics Committee and Stroke Statistics Subcommittee. *Circulation, 115*(5), e69–e171.

Sacco, R. L., Boden-Albala, B., Gan, R., Chen, X., Kargman, D. E., Shea, S., et al. (1998). Stroke incidence among white, black, and Hispanic residents of urban community: The Northern Manhattan Stroke Study. *American Journal of Epidemiology, 147*(3), 259–268.

Saver, J. (2001). Intra-arterial thrombolysis. *Neurology, 57*, 58–60.

Schievink, W. I. (2004). Genetics of intracranial aneurysms. In R. F. Spetzler & F. B. Meyer (Eds.), *Youman's neurological surgery* (5th ed., pp. 1769–1777). Philadelphia: W. B. Saunders.

Schumacher, H. C., & Marshall, R. S. (2006). Arteriovenous malformations. *eMedicine.* Retrieved April 2, 2008, from http://www.emedicine.com/NEURO/topic21.htm

Soderman, M., Andersson, T., Karlsson, B., Wallace, M. C., & Edner, G. (2003). Management of patients with brain arteriovenous malformation. *European Journal of Radiology, 46*(3), 195–205.

Spetzler, R. F., & Martin, N. A. (1986). A grading system for arteriovenous malformations. *Journal of Neurosurgery, 65*, 476–483.

Stanford School of Medicine. (2008). Stroke prevention. Retrieved April 2, 2008, from Stanford Stroke Center website: http://strokecenter.stanford.edu/guide/prevention.html

Tatter, S. B., & Ogilvy, C. S. (1995). Vascular malformations: General considerations. In C. W. Mitchell (Ed.), *Surgical management of neurovascular disease.* Baltimore: Williams & Wilkins.

Van den Berg, R., Rinkel, G. J., & Vandertop, W. P. (2003). Treatment of ruptured intracranial aneurysms: Implications of the ISAT on clipping versus coiling. *European Journal of Radiology, 46*(3), 172–177.

Wang, C. C., Liu, A., Zhang, J. T., Sun, B., & Zhao, Y. L. (2003). Surgical management of brain-stem cavernous malformations: Report of 137 cases. *Surgical Neurology, 59*(6), 444–454.

Wills, S., Ronkainen, A., van der Voet, M., Kuivaniemi, H., Helin, K., Leinonen, E., et al. (2003). Familial intracranial aneurysms: An analysis of 346 multiplex Finnish families. *Stroke, 34*, 1370–1374.

Winkley, J. M., & Adams, H. P. (2000). Potential role of abciximab in ischemic cerebrovascular disease. *American Journal of Cardiology, 85*, 47C–51C.

Zabramski, J. M., & Han, P. P. (2004). Epidemiology and natural history of cavernous malformations. In R. F. Spetzler & F. B. Meyer (Eds.), *Youman's neurological surgery* (5th ed., pp. 2292–2298). Philadelphia: W. B. Saunders.

Zabramski, J. M., Henn, J. S., & Coons, S. (1999). Pathology of cerebral vascular malformations. *Neurosurgery Clinics of North America, 10*, 395–410.

Zabramski, J. M., Spetzler, R. F., Johnson, B., Golfinos, J., Drayer, B. P., Brown, B., et al. (1994). The natural history of familial cavernous malformations: Results of an ongoing study. *Journal of Neurosurgery, 80*, 422–432.

Caring for the Patient with Chronic Neurological Disorders

Gale Kittle

Outcome-Based Learning Objectives

After studying this chapter, the learner will be able to:

1. Distinguish among the neurodegenerative disorders of Alzheimer's disease, Parkinson's disease, multiple sclerosis, amyotrophic lateral sclerosis, and myasthenia gravis by describing the etiology and pathophysiology of each disorder.
2. Compare and contrast the presenting signs and symptoms of each of the neurodegenerative disorders discussed in the chapter.
3. Develop a generalized plan of care for each of the neurodegenerative disorders discussed.
4. Develop a comprehensive discharge teaching plan for each of the neurodegenerative disorders discussed.
5. Describe generalized health promotion needs for each neurodegenerative disorder discussed.
6. Explain gerontological implications for each neurodegenerative disorder discussed.
7. Evaluate research implications for nursing practice when caring for persons with a neurodegenerative disorder.

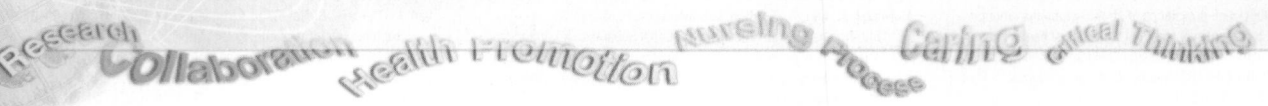

Research Collaboration Health Promotion Nursing Process Caring Critical Thinking

CARING for patients with the neurodegenerative disorders of Alzheimer's disease, Parkinson's disease, multiple sclerosis, amyotrophic lateral sclerosis, and myasthenia gravis challenges the nurse's ability to manage diverse conditions. Characterized by neuronal loss in specific areas of the central nervous system (CNS), neurodegenerative disorders are chronic, progressive, and without cure. Although these disorders manifest with differing signs and distinctive symptoms, they share many common aspects that contribute to the complexity of diagnosing and treating them.

In many cases, a diagnosis cannot be confirmed without autopsy. Clinically, neurodegenerative diseases often have a variable course. Families face a future of uncertain prognosis—other than the knowledge that symptoms will worsen. Complicated treatment strategies only compound the difficulty of these cases. As patients' mental and/or physical symptoms progress and as they lose more and more of their ability to care for themselves, these patients begin to rely on a spouse, a close family member, or another lay caregiver. The ongoing and long-term care of a person with a degenerative disorder is labor intensive and can carry over to threaten the physical and mental well-being of the patient's family.

Nurses caring for patients with neurodegenerative disorders find themselves in a dual role of caring for both the patient and the caregiver, often becoming a vital link among the patient, caregiver, and health care system in a variety of environments.

Because of the prolonged, chronic nature of these diseases, the common settings in which one finds these patients are the home, outpatient clinic, or long-term care facility. Patients may be hospitalized during the initial diagnostic phase or for complications associated with their condition. The wide range of care for those with neurodegenerative disorders creates a unique opportunity for a nurse to have a profound impact on the patient and family response to a seemingly hopeless condition.

Alzheimer's Disease and Related Dementias

Dementia is a general term for brain dysfunction characterized by deterioration of memory and cognition (Desai & Grossberg, 2005). Although other forms of dementia are addressed, this chapter focuses primarily on the most common form of dementia, Alzheimer's disease. **Alzheimer's disease (AD)** is a chronic, progressive, irreversible brain disorder. Long-term care of AD patients is as likely to take place in the home as it is in a nursing facility. Obviously, nurses who specialize in treatment of neurological disorders most often are the providers of ongoing, clinical care in these settings; however, hospital nurses working in other specialties may see AD patients with concurrent health issues.

Epidemiology and Etiology

Alzheimer's disease is found most frequently in adults ages 65 and older (Desai & Grossberg, 2005). The onset of AD begins with subtle lapses of memory, which gradually and progressively develop into a chronic loss of personality, recognition, reasoning, and independence. Neurologists estimate that approximately 4 million Americans have this disease. As the general population grows, the projected number is expected to double by the year 2030 and nearly quadruple by 2050. AD is now emerging as a major public health crisis based on the projected number of people expected to be affected (Leifer, 2003). The causes of dementia are numerous and are listed in Chart 31–1.

Pathophysiology

The pathology of AD is marked by the profusion of amyloid plaques and neurofibrillary tangles, which form in the hippocampus and other parts of the brain critical to memory (Figure 31–1 ■). While normal aging of the brain can cause plaques and tangles, they develop at a much greater rate and mass in those affected with AD (National Institute on Aging [NIA], 2007).

Neurofibrillary tangles were one of the initial discoveries that first described hallmark pathology in AD. The findings revealed a specialized protein known as **tau**. A key component of tangles, tau normally helps maintain the health of neurons. In AD, mutations in tau cause it to distort and twist, creating tangled threads of the protein within neurons (NIA, 2007; Porth, 2007). These neurofibrillary tangles eventually lead to cell death, neuronal degeneration, and the symptoms associated with AD (DeKosky, 2003). Figure 31–2 ■ (p. 790) depicts this process.

FIGURE 31–1 ■ An AD neurofibrillary tangle.
Source: Photo from Alzheimer's Disease: Unraveling the Mystery, U.S. National Institute on Aging, 2002

MyNursingKit | Video: Neurological: Alzheimer's—Etiology and Pathophysiology

Most recently, researchers have focused on the impact amyloid plaques have on determining other pathologic characteristics of AD. Composed of the protein beta-amyloid and clipped from the larger amyloid precursor protein, these thick, insoluble plaques form around neurons, causing oxidative stress and inflammatory changes. Cholesterol also may play a part in the formation of amyloid plaques, and it has become suspect in the development of AD (DeKosky, 2003). It is not known whether amyloid plaques cause AD or if they are a product of the disease process. Research continues to focus on oxidative stress, inflammation, and cholesterol and their relationship to the formation and presence of amyloid plaques in AD (NIA, 2007). The accompanying Risk Factors and Genetic Considerations boxes (p. 790) provide more information about Alzheimer's disease.

Clinical Manifestations

Slow and insidious in onset and ranging over a course of 3 to 20 years, AD progressively degrades cognitive function (Feldman & Woodward, 2005). While the span of the disease varies in length and severity from patient to patient, its symptoms develop in stages corresponding to the area of the brain where degeneration is present (NIA, 2007). Typically, neuronal degeneration starts in the hippocampus, an area of the brain critical to short- and long-term memory. From there, it spreads to other regions that control cognition, judgment, behavior, and physical movement. General descriptions of each of the four basic stages of AD are given below (NIA, 2002).

Preclinical AD

Researchers suspect that the damaging effects of AD on the brain start 10 to 20 years before signs of the disease begin to show. Initially, the degeneration originates in the entorhinal cortex, an area adjacent to the hippocampus (Figure 31–3 ■, p. 791). The first symptom is likely to be an elusive, difficult-to-distinguish

---

CHART 31–1	**Causes of Dementia**

Alzheimer's disease

Vascular dementia

Diffuse Lewy body dementia

Frontotemporal atrophy/Pick's disease

Parkinson's disease

Huntington's disease

Postcortical or post-thalamic stroke

Postanoxic encephalopathy

Hydrocephalus

Brain tumors

Infectious disorders: meningitis, Creutzfeldt–Jakob disease, HIV, neurosyphilis

Toxins: drugs, alcohol, heavy metals

Delirium

Depression

Vitamin B_{12} deficiency

Polypharmacy

Sources: Desai, A. K., & Grossberg, G. T. (2005). Diagnosis and treatment of Alzheimer's disease. *Neurology, 64*(Suppl. 3), S34–S39; Leifer, B. P. (2003). Early diagnosis of Alzheimer's disease: Clinical and economic benefits. *Journal of the American Geriatrics Society, 51,* S281–S288.

Cell membrane

APP molecule

Cell interior

Beta-amyloid

Enzymes

Beta-amyloid plaque

FIGURE 31–2 ■ From amyloid precursor protein (APP) to beta-amyloid and formation of amyloid plaque.

RISK FACTORS for Alzheimer's Disease

- Growing old is the most significant risk factor for developing AD. Late-onset AD occurs in those over the age of 65. Statistics show that, after 65, the prevalence of AD cases doubles every 5 years.
- Other risk factors that have been linked to AD include:

  Genetics/family history

  Atherosclerosis

  High cholesterol

  Elevated plasma homocysteine

  Diabetes

  Down syndrome

  Mild cognitive impairment (MCI)

Sources: National Institute on Aging, U.S. Nation Institutes of Health. (2007). Frontotemporal dementia connections reprint. Retrieved July 18, 2008 from http://www.nia.nih.gov/Alzheimers/Publications/FTDreprint.htm; National Institute of Neurological Disorders and Stroke. (2004). *The dementias: Hope through research.* Bethesda, MD: National Institutes of Health.

GENETIC CONSIDERATIONS Related to Alzheimer's Disease

A genetic predisposition to AD also can add to susceptibility of developing the disease. In familial cases of early-onset AD, genetic mutations are known to produce abnormal amyloid precursor protein, the parent protein of beta-amyloid, and other abnormal proteins called presenilin-1 and presenilin-2. These mutations appear to increase the production of beta-amyloid, the protein found in amyloid plaques. While these findings help delineate a genetic link to AD, familial early-onset cases are rare and do not account for the more common occurrence of late-onset AD.

Also associated with genetic risk of AD is the protein apolipoprotein E (ApoE), which may play a role in determining the age of onset. The gene that produces ApoE has three alleles, e2, e3, and e4. The ApoE e4 allele has been linked to an increased risk of developing AD. This allele occurs in approximately 40% of late-onset cases regardless of whether or not there is a family history. A caveat to this discovery is that the presence of one or two ApoE e4 alleles does not predetermine the development of AD. Conversely, some people who develop AD show no ApoE e4 alleles. Therefore, the ApoE e4 genotype represents an increased vulnerability for developing AD, rather than a causative factor for AD.

Sources: National Institute on Aging, U.S. Nation Institutes of Health. (2007). Frontotemporal dementia connections reprint. Retrieved July 18, 2008 from http://www.nia.nih.gov/Alzheimers/Publications/FTDreprint.htm; Nussbaum, R. L., & Ellis, C. E. (2003). Alzheimer's disease and Parkinson's disease. *New England Journal of Medicine, 348*(14), 1356–1364.

loss of memory. If the patient's memory loss appears to be greater than might be expected for his or her age, while other functions of cognition remain intact, then a diagnosis of **mild cognitive impairment (MCI)** may be rendered. In cases of MCI, the patient's experience of cognitive impairment may be uncorroborated by friends or family who do not notice the subtle behavior changes and memory anomalies of which the patient complains. The relationship between MCI and AD is not fully understood; however, MCI is sometimes considered a precursor to AD.

Mild AD

Once the degeneration of neurons spreads to the cerebral cortex (Figure 31–4 ■), the escalating problems with memory and cognitive function become obvious. Friends and family who do recognize the patient's transitory condition corroborate these difficulties. Clinical testing will reveal the following signs of mild AD:

- Confusion about the location of familiar places
- Slow to accomplish simple tasks
- Difficulty handling money matters
- Loss of spontaneity and sense of initiative
- Mood swings and personality changes.

FIGURE 31–3 ■ Preclinical AD.

Moderate AD

At this stage of the disease, neuronal degeneration expands to areas that control language and reasoning. The symptoms worsen as atrophy continues to spread. The patient may have a bout of wandering and can be easily agitated by the routines of daily living. The following symptoms are indicators of moderate AD:

- Progressive memory loss and confusion
- Unable to recognize friends and family
- Language difficulties

- Difficulties with reading, writing, and simple math
- Problems learning new material, aligning thoughts, and thinking logically
- Hallucinations, delusions, paranoia.

Severe AD

In the most advanced phase of AD, plaques and tangles have spread throughout the brain, causing generalized atrophy (Figure 31–5 ■, p. 792). The patient becomes completely dependent and

FIGURE 31–4 ■ Mild AD.

Extreme shrinkage
of cerebral cortex

Severely
enlarged
ventricles

Extreme shrinkage
of hippocampus

FIGURE 31–5 ■ Severe AD.

is not able to recognize loved ones. Other characteristics of advanced AD include:

- Inability to communicate
- Weight loss secondary to difficulty eating and swallowing
- Bowel and bladder incontinence
- Increased sleeping.

Death usually occurs as a result of aspiration pneumonia or from other concurrent health conditions.

Laboratory and Diagnostic Procedures

A definitive diagnosis of AD can be made only following a brain autopsy, which can determine the presence of the hallmark plaques and tangles. However, diagnostic tools are available that can assist in a preliminary diagnosis of AD (Leifer, 2003). The *Diagnostic and Statistical Manual of Mental Disorders, Fourth Edition*, Text Revision (*DSM-IV-TR*; American Psychiatric Society, 2000) outlines the criteria used to diagnose Alzheimer's dementia (see the National Guidelines box).

Routine laboratory and radiological tests are used to rule out other causes of dementia. These other causes can include metabolic imbalances, vitamin B_{12} deficiency, stroke, and brain tumor. Magnetic resonance imagining (MRI) of the brain is performed primarily to rule out other conditions such as normal pressure hydrocephalus or subdural hematoma, which also can cause dementia symptoms (Leifer, 2003). In early stages, an MRI may show atrophy in the hippocampal

---

NATIONAL GUIDELINES DSM-IV-TR Criteria for Dementia of the Alzheimer's Type

A. Multiple cognitive deficits manifested by both:
  1. Memory impairment (impaired ability to learn new information or to recall previously learned information)
  2. One or more of the following cognitive disturbances:
    a. Aphasia (language disturbance)
    b. Apraxia (impaired ability to carry out motor activities despite intact motor function)
    c. Agnosia (failure to recognize or identify objects despite intact sensory function)
    d. Disturbance in executive functioning (i.e., planning, organizing, sequencing, abstracting).

B. The cognitive deficits cause significant impairment in social or occupational functioning and represent a significant decline from a previous level of functioning.

C. The course is characterized by general onset and continuing cognitive decline.

D. Cognitive deficits are not due to:
  1. Other CNS conditions that cause progressive memory and cognition deficits (i.e., cerebrovascular disease, Parkinson's disease, Huntington's disease, subdural hematoma, normal pressure hydrocephalus, brain tumor).
  2. Systemic conditions that are known to cause dementia (e.g., hypothyroidism, vitamin B_{12} deficiency, neurosyphilis, HIV infection).

Source: Adapted from American Psychiatric Association. (2000). *Diagnostic and statistical manual of mental disorders* (4th ed.). Washington, DC: Author.

area, while later stages will show generalized atrophy (Desai & Grossberg, 2005). Positron emission tomography (PET) has been shown to detect significant alterations in brain metabolism produced by AD and is increasingly being used as a diagnostic tool, especially in cases where a diagnosis of dementia remains uncertain despite a thorough evaluation (Desai & Grossberg, 2005; Silverman, et al., 2001). Functional MRI (fMRI) is used primarily for research purposes to measure changes in brain function and structure, although it has future potential as a diagnostic and monitoring tool (NIA, 2007). In addition to the test results and patient assessment, interviewing a close relative or associate is considered to be another important diagnostic tool. Other tests are listed in the Diagnostic Tests box.

The diagnostic process includes a detailed medical history, physical examination, and neurological assessment, paying particular attention to the duration and progression of the patient's memory loss. Complete and accurate charting of former and current medical conditions, medications, and behavioral symptoms are necessary considerations when prescribing treatments.

Whenever the patient has cognitive and memory difficulties, interviewing the primary caregiver and/or other family members can help to supplement the history. Cognitive status is often evaluated using the Folstein Mini-Mental Status Exam (MMSE). The MMSE is an 11-question measure that tests five areas of cognitive function: orientation, registration, attention and calculation, recall, and language. The maximum score is 30. A score of 23 or lower is indicative of cognitive impairment. The MMSE takes only 5 to 10 minutes to administer and is, therefore, practical to use repeatedly and routinely. The MMSE is considered to be a national standard as a screening device to identify patients with cognitive impairment from those without it in both clinical practice and research (Kurlowicz & Wallace, 1999).

For a detailed evaluation of cognitive functioning, a neuropsychological evaluation of language, memory, problem-solving skills, and visuospatial skills provides a cognitive baseline and measures performance in comparison with an age-matched cohort. The diagnostic work-up concludes with an evaluation of the patient's ability to perform self-care and function normally in daily living (Cummings, Frank, Cherry, Kohatsu, & Kemp, 2002a, 2002b).

After the initial diagnosis, biannual follow-up assessments are recommended. These ongoing examinations are necessary to evaluate response to medications, concurrent medical conditions, and progression of memory impairment (Cummings et al., 2002a, 2002b). When monitoring MMSE results in cases of AD, scores drop at an average rate of 4 points per year (Leifer, 2003).

The presence of depression can complicate the diagnosis of dementia or AD. Depression is the most common form of psychiatric illness in the elderly. Symptoms common to both AD and depression include behavioral slowing, complaints of cognitive difficulties, fatigue, and changes in sleep and appetite. Depression also can occur concurrently with AD, making it critical to separate the diagnosis of AD and depression before appropriate treatments can be implemented (Cummings et al., 2002a, 2002b).

Delirium also could manifest symptoms similar to dementia. Delirium is a transient and potentially reversible condition with fluctuating levels of awareness, hallucinations, and cognitive impairment (Gleason, 2003). Delirium also is discussed in Chapter 10 🔗 as relevant to the aging patient.

The critical difference between dementia and delirium is that delirium is transient and caused by an underlying medical condition, whereas dementia is progressive and irreversible. Common causes of delirium include renal or liver failure, vitamin B_{12} deficiencies, trauma such as hip fractures and head injuries, and medications.

Other Forms of Dementia

Besides AD, other primary dementias include vascular dementia, Lewy body dementia, and frontotemporal dementia. While

DIAGNOSTIC TESTS for Alzheimer's Disease

Test	Expected Result	Rationale
Complete blood count (CBC), electrolytes, blood urea nitrogen (BUN), creatinine, random blood glucose, calcium	Within normal limits (WNL)	Rule out metabolic abnormalities.
TSH	WNL	Rule out hypothyroidism.
Vitamin B_{12}	WNL	Rule out vitamin B_{12} deficiency.
Syphilis serology*	Negative	Rule out syphilis.
HIV*	Negative	Rule out HIV.
Heavy metals*	Negative	
MRI or CT scan	WNL for age; in early stages, mild atrophy may be present in hippocampal regions; in moderate to severe stages, atrophy may be more generalized	Rule out stroke, brain tumor, hydrocephalus, or other structural abnormalities.

*If history indicates.

Sources: Adapted from Alzheimer's Association. (2003). *Provider checklist for treating a confused elder.* Retrieved April 30, 2008, from http://alzla.org/medical/Checklisthtml.html; Farlow, M. R. (2005). The search for disease modification in moderate to severe Alzheimer's disease. *Neurology, 65*(Suppl. 3), S25–S30; Knopman, D. S., DeKosky, S. T., Cummings, J. L., Chui, H., Corey-Bloom, J., Relkin, N., et al. (2001). Practice parameter: Diagnosis of dementia (an evidence-based review). *Neurology, 56,* 1143–1153; Leifer, B. P. (2003). Early diagnosis of Alzheimer's disease: Clinical and economic benefits. *Journal of the American Geriatrics Society, 51,* S281–S288.

MyNursingKit | Alzheimer's Association

CHART 31–2	**Overview of Other Common Types of Dementia**	
Type	**Characteristics**	**Pathology**
Vascular dementia	Most common form of dementia after AD Abrupt onset with stepwise deterioration Focal neurological symptoms; signs or history of stroke	Multiple infarcts on MRI
Lewy body dementia (LBD)	Gradual onset Fluctuating cognitive deficits Parkinsonian symptoms (rigidity, bradykinesia) not responsive to levodopa Visual hallucinations	Lewy bodies (identified on brain autopsy) present in cytoplasm of cortical neurons
Frontotemporal dementia (FTD)	Insidious onset Slowly progressive Psychiatric symptoms include disinhibition, delusions, and social inappropriateness Neglect of hygiene/grooming Incontinence	Atrophy of frontal lobes and anterior temporal lobes Neuronal loss Tau tangles Gliosis

Sources: Leifer, B. P. (2003). Early diagnosis of Alzheimer's disease: Clinical and economic benefits. *Journal of the American Geriatrics Society, 51,* S281–S288; National Institute on Aging, U.S. Nation Institutes of Health. (2007). Frontotemporal dementia connections reprint. Retrieved July 18, 2008 from http://www.nia.nih.gov/Alzheimers/Publications/FTDreprint.htm.

the diagnostic work-up for any form of dementia is the same, treatments for some types will make symptoms worse in other types, thereby making it important to distinguish the type of dementia afflicting the patient. The unique clinical and pathologic characteristics of various forms are summarized in Chart 31–2.

Medical Management

A handful of medications are available to treat AD. At best, these drugs only temporarily slow cognitive and functional loss. As AD continues to progress, treatment increasingly focuses on non-pharmacologic approaches to managing behavioral symptoms.

Drug Therapy

The goals of pharmacologic treatment for AD are to preserve cognitive and functional abilities, minimize behavioral disturbances, and slow the progression of the disease (Geldmacher, 2003). With AD, levels of **acetylcholine**, a neurotransmitter critical in the process of memory formation and especially important to neurons in the hippocampus and cerebral cortex, are lowered as neuronal degeneration occurs. The resulting decreases of acetylcholine and cholinergic activity in general are associated with memory impairment. Increasing available acetylcholine can potentially improve memory symptoms. The only medications approved by the Food and Drug Administration (FDA) for the treatment of mild to moderate AD are acetyl-cholinesterase inhibitors (AChEIs), which increase cholinergic activity and can improve cognitive symptoms of AD (DeKosky, 2003). Although these medications do not reverse or prevent cell death (Geldmacher, 2003), there is evidence that they may improve cognitive functioning and decrease behavioral symptoms, at least in the mild to moderate stages (Cummings et al., 2002a, 2002b). Three FDA-approved AChEIs, donepezil (Aricept), rivastigmine (Exelon), and galantamine (Reminyl), are currently used in the treatment of AD. See the Pharmacology Summary for a description of these medications, including common dosages and side effects.

Late in 2003, the FDA approved the first *N*-methyl-D-aspartate (NMDA) receptor antagonist, memantine (Namenda), for the treatment of moderate to severe AD. Memantine is thought to block the action of **glutamate**, an excitatory neurotransmitter. Glutamate activates NMDA receptors, which modulate the chemical environment necessary for memory. An excess of glutamate overstimulates NMDA receptors, which can lead to cell death. Memantine may protect cells from excess glutamate by partially blocking NMDA receptors (Alzheimer's Association, 2004). While memantine and AChEIs may help symptoms of AD, it does not prevent or slow the neurological degeneration associated with it (FDA, 2003).

Treating Behavioral Symptoms

Behavioral symptoms that present with the disease often are the most difficult for caregivers to manage (Cummings et al., 2002a, 2002b). Restlessness, agitation, anger, anxiety, wandering, or psychotic symptoms may require treatment with psychotropic medications (Geldmacher, 2003). Nonpharmacologic approaches to managing behavioral symptoms center on reducing environmental stimuli, establishing predictable routines, simplifying tasks, and using distraction and redirection (Cummings et al., 2002a, 2002b). See the Pharmacology Summary for a list of drugs used to treat behavioral symptoms of AD.

Before implementing psychotropic medications, other conditions that may contribute to behavioral symptoms should be disqualified. These include, but are not limited to, delirium, pain, infection, or other acute medical conditions (Cummings et al., 2002a, 2002b).

Potential Treatments Undergoing Research

Several agents are undergoing research as potential treatments or preventive therapies for AD. Cholesterol has been associated with ApoE, beta-amyloid, and vascular damage. Studies have shown a decreased AD prevalence and risk reduction in those patients taking statin drugs. Prospective research trials are in process to further delineate the potential role of cholesterol in the prevention of AD (DeKosky, 2003). Because inflammatory changes are associated with the disease process, anti-inflammatory medications may have a role in preventing AD. Large-scale studies examining

PHARMACOLOGY Summary of Medications to Treat Alzheimer's Disease

Medication Category	Action	Application/Indication	Nursing Responsibility
Acetylcholinesterase Inhibitors • Galantamine (Reminyl) • Rivastigmine (Exelon) • Donepezil (Aricept)	Increase acetylcholine levels in the brain.	Treatment of mild to moderate disease	Monitor for nausea, vomiting, diarrhea, weight loss.
NMDA Receptor Antagonist • Memantine (Namenda)	Blocks action of glutamate, decreasing activation of NMDA receptors.	Treatment of moderate to severe disease	Monitor for headache, constipation, confusion, dizziness.
Behavioral Symptoms of Alzheimer's Disease **Atypical Antipsychotics** • Olanzapine (Zyprexa) • Quetiapine (Seroquel)	Act as antagonists of dopamine and serotonin.	Delusions, hallucinations, agitation, combativeness	Monitor mental status and response to drug therapy. Monitor for orthostatic hypotension, somnolence.
Selective Serotonin-Reuptake Inhibitors • Sertraline (Zoloft) • Citalopram (Celexa)	Inhibit uptake of the neurotransmitter serotonin in CNS, potentiating the effects of serotonin. Has little or no effect on other neurotransmitters.	Depression, irritability	Monitor for mood changes, somnolence, and insomnia.

anti-inflammatory drugs and their potential use as a treatment are being conducted now (DeKosky, 2003).

Researchers also are looking at folate. Deficiencies of folate have been associated with increased levels of homocysteine, which is another possible risk factor for developing AD (DeKosky, 2003). Estrogen also could be a possible preventive therapy. Studies suggest that it may protect against AD. More research is needed and in process (DeKosky, 2003). Antioxidants vitamins C and E are believed to be neurologically protective against oxidative damage, again present in AD. Clinical trials to evaluate the role of vitamin E in slowing disease progression are under way. The herbal supplement gingko biloba also has been considered as a treatment, as discussed in the Complementary and Alternative Therapies box.

COMPLEMENTARY & ALTERNATIVE THERAPIES Ginkgo Biloba

Ginkgo biloba has undergone research as a potential treatment for AD. It is thought to have antioxidant and possibly anti-inflammatory and antiplatelet activity (DeKosky, 2003). It is commonly used in Germany to treat AD; however, insufficient studies preclude recommended use in the United States. Results are pending from the Ginkgo Evaluation of Memory Study, sponsored by the National Center for Complementary Medicine, the National Institute on Aging, and the National Heart, Lung, and Blood Institute. This interventional study will help determine the effect of ginkgo biloba in decreasing the incidence of AD and slowing cognitive decline and functional disability (Alzheimer's Disease Education and Referral Center, 2003). Ginkgo biloba should only be taken under the direction of a health care provider, as the risk of spontaneous bleeding increased when it is taken with non-steroidal anti-inflammatory drugs (NSAIDS) and anticoagulants such as heparin or warfarin (De Smet, 2002).

References
Alzheimer's Disease Education and Referral Center. (2003). *Gingko biloba fact sheet*. Retrieved April 14, 2008, from http://www.alzheimers.org.

De Smet, P. (2002). Herbal remedies. *New England Journal of Medicine, 347*(25), 2046–2076.

DeKosky, S. T. (2003). Pathology and pathways of Alzheimer's disease with an update in new developments in treatment. *Journal of the American Geriatrics Society, 51,* S314–S320.

Gerontological Considerations

Because dementia affects primarily the elderly, its signs are often characterized as naturally occurring senility common to old age. This misunderstanding could confuse the signs of dementia and AD with normal aging. This not only perpetuates fallacies of aging, it runs the risk of delaying early, accurate diagnosis and prompt treatment.

With the highest prevalence rates in the oldest segment of the population, nurses will need to recognize the factors that influence an elderly person's response to drugs prescribed for AD. Inevitably, the aging patient likely may have concurrent medical conditions that require multiple medications, presenting the potential for drug interactions and adverse effects. Slowed renal clearance and hepatic metabolism may influence medication tolerance. Drugs that cause sedation have an adverse effect on cognition.

The crippling effect AD has on those who develop it also comes with significant psychosocial ramifications. Often it will impact an elderly spouse or adult children who are called on to provide care and support. Research has demonstrated that the implications of the elderly caring for the elderly in terms of stress and burden on an older caregiver's physical, mental, and financial well-being are substantive.

Special nursing interventions for this population include a complete medical history with special attention to concurrent medical problems and to polypharmacy. Caregiver burden and stress should be periodically assessed, with assistance to develop coping mechanisms. Referrals should be made to appropriate community resources for example, the local area agency on aging.

Nursing Management

Use of the nursing process will facilitate a comprehensive approach to patient and caregiver support throughout the course of the disease (see the Nursing Process: Patient Care Plan for Alzheimer's Disease feature). Protecting the patient from injury, managing dysfunctional behaviors, and supporting the patient and caregiver in activities of daily living (ADLs) are the primary focus of nursing care. Nurses must be prepared to assist family caregivers in dealing with denial, anger, guilt, grief, or clinical depression as the patient progresses, with the goal of helping the caregiver adjust and adapt to the changes associated with the progressive stages (Volcifer & McKee, 2001). See the Cultural Considerations box for a discussion related to the care of the patient and family with AD.

Collaborative Management

Throughout the disease process, a multidisciplinary approach facilitates optimal disease management. In the early and mid-stages of the disease, periodic outpatient visits to the neurologist will be required for medication management. Neuropsychologists play critical roles in the periodic evaluation of cognitive function. Geriatric psychiatrists may become involved either at the time of diagnosis or as the behavioral symptoms increase.

CULTURAL CONSIDERATIONS Related to Alzheimer's Disease

Throughout the nursing process, cultural sensitivity is imperative. The meaning of dementia, how families care for elders, and help-seeking methods can all vary depending on ethnicity. Recent studies suggest that ethnically diverse older people frequently subscribe to folk beliefs to explain dementia, rather than the biomedical explanation of a physical disease or condition. Such folk explanations might include that AD is caused by psychosocial stress or that it is a normal part of aging (Hinton, Franz, Yeo, & Levkoff, 2005). Nurses need to consider the patient's and family's perspective of dementia, and approach the provision of care in a way that considers those views and values.

Sources: Ackley, B. J., & Ludwig, G. B. (Eds.). (2003). *Nursing diagnosis handbook: A guide to planning care* (6th ed.). St. Louis: Mosby; Doenges, M. E., & Moorhouse, M. F. (2003). *Application of nursing process and diagnosis: An interactive text for diagnostic reasoning* (4th ed.). Philadelphia: F. A. Davis.

Physical therapy may be needed as mobility becomes affected and to counteract contractures in the end stages. Occupational therapy will help the patient and caregiver accomplish ADLs. A psychologist, social worker, or mental health professional is needed to help the family work through altered dynamics and to plan for long-term care.

Discharge Priorities

Discharge plans for the patient with AD, as discussed in the Patient Teaching & Discharge Priorities box (p. 799), are extremely important to maintaining functional goals.

Health Promotion

The physical and mental health of the primary family caregiver is critical to the care of the Alzheimer's patient. Caregivers suffer from higher rates of depression and physical illness than persons not functioning in a caregiver role (Schultz, O'Brien, Bookwala, & Fleissner, 1995). Nurses can optimize both patient and caregiver health by (Cummings et al., 2002a, 2002b):

- Providing pertinent information, both written and verbal, about AD
- Referring to organizations for assistance with finding community resources, support groups, financial and legal advice, respite, and long-term care options
- Encouraging discussion about advance directives for management of advanced stages of AD
- Assisting the primary caregiver in managing stress and developing coping mechanisms through psychoeducational interventions and individual and/or group therapy.

In its attempt to produce excellence in the care of Alzheimer's patients, the Alzheimer's Foundation of America (AFA) has developed a nationwide standard of excellence for settings that provide care to individuals with Alzheimer's disease or related dementias. This new initiative, called Excellence in Care, involves on-site evaluations of dementia care settings and assistance in meeting the comprehensive set of standards. The standards reflect what AFA believes to be essential components of any quality dementia care program. Areas of evaluation include the physical environment, safety procedures, program activities, staff–client interaction, and training of staff and families (AFA, 2006).

Parkinson's Disease

Parkinson's disease (PD) is second to Alzheimer's disease as the most common of the neurological degenerative disorders (Nussbaum & Ellis, 2003). It is recognized as the most common movement disorder (Dawson & Dawson, 2003).

Epidemiology and Etiology

With the cardinal symptoms of tremor, rigidity, bradykinesia, and postural instability, PD is estimated to afflict about 1,000,000 Americans (Nutt & Wooten, 2005), with a lifetime risk of 1 in 40 to 50 (Schapira, 2006). Incidence increases with age, rising sharply after age 60; about 4% of the cases occur before age 50 (Van Den Eeden et al., 2003).

Although the cause of idiopathic PD is not known, both genetic and environmental factors have been implicated (Schapira,

NURSING PROCESS: Patient Care Plan for Alzheimer's Disease

Assessment of Safety and Self-Care Ability

Subjective Data:
(Involve family members.)
Does the patient fall frequently?
Has the patient been hurt as a result of falling?
Does the patient wander?
Does the patient wear glasses or a hearing aid?
Does the patient use a walker?

Objective Data:
Neurological status, including orientation, memory, sensory, gait judgment, insight
Wandering behavior

Nursing Assessment and Diagnoses	Outcomes and Evaluation Parameters	Planning and Interventions with *Rationales*
Nursing Diagnosis: *High Risk for Injury* related to poor memory, insight, judgment, and self-control; unstable gait	**Outcome:** Patient remains injury free. *Evaluation Parameters:* Patient uses sensory aids and assistive devices. Family identifies potential environmental hazards. Patient does not fall. Patient does not wander.	**Interventions and *Rationales*:** Encourage use of eyeglasses, hearing aids, and assistive devices such as a walker. *Optimal eyesight and hearing will help patient with environmental awareness; assistive devices will stabilize gait.* Remove potential hazards from environment such as sharp objects and medications *to prevent patient from harming self.* Ensure that patient has identification bracelet. Encourage family to register patient with Safe Return program of the Alzheimer's Association. *Patient may wander and cause harm to self or others.*

Assessment of Cognition and Thought Processes

Subjective Data:
(Involve family members.)
Does the patient hear voices or see things that are not there?
Is the patient easily agitated?
Does the patient act impulsively?

Objective Data:
Neurological status, including orientation, memory, sensory, gait judgment, insight
Ability to follow instructions
Agitation/restlessness
Paranoia

Nursing Assessment and Diagnoses	Outcomes and Evaluation Parameters	Planning and Interventions with *Rationales*
Nursing Diagnosis: *Disturbed Thought Processes* (inappropriate reactions, dysfunctional behavior, delusions and paranoia) related to cognitive decline	**Outcome:** Remains oriented to extent possible given stage of disease. *Evaluation Parameter:* Demonstrates fewer episodes of agitation, delusions, paranoia, or other dysfunctional behavior.	**Interventions and *Rationales*:** When communicating with patient: Approach patient in a gentle, calm manner *to prevent patient from being startled or frightened.* Communicate using short, simple sentences, yes/no questions. *Negative feedback leads to increased confusion and agitation.* Break directions down into short, simple steps. *Unable to follow complex directions; decreases frustration.* Redirect conversation without contradicting or criticizing the patient's statements *to decrease anxiety, frustration.* Maintain consistent daily schedule *to decrease anxiety; situational anxiety due to change can lead to agitation.* Monitor for nonverbal behaviors such as grimacing or increased restlessness. *May indicate pain or discomfort, which may increase agitation.* Create calming environment. Eliminate noise and clutter. *Sensory overload can contribute to disruptive behavior and agitation.* Provide cues to orientation including verbal cues, clocks, and calendars. *Reorients patient to reality as much as possible.* Display pictures, mementos, and encourage reminiscence. *Can comfort patient and trigger memories.*

(continued)

NURSING PROCESS: Patient Care Plan for Alzheimer's Disease—*Continued*

Assessment of
Subjective Data:
(Involve family members.)
Does the patient bathe, groom, and dress independently?
Are these activities accomplished appropriately?
Does the patient become agitated during these activities?
Does the patient require assistance with self-care activities?
Do you have an established schedule for these activities?

Objective Data:
Neurological status, including orientation, memory, sensory, gait judgment, insight, apraxia, agnosia
Appearance
Ability to draw bath or start shower, brush teeth, select and put on clothing
Ability to follow instructions

Nursing Assessment and Diagnoses	Outcomes and Evaluation Parameters	Planning and Interventions with *Rationales*
Nursing Diagnosis: *Self-Care Deficits* (bathing, hygiene, dressing, grooming) related to cognitive losses, impaired judgment	**Outcome:** Self-care needs are met. **Evaluation Parameters:** Performs self-care independently to the extent possible given disease progression. Daily routine of bathing, hygiene, dressing, and grooming is established with patient and family. Staff and family assist with self-care needs.	**Interventions and *Rationales*:** Assist patient to perform self-care such as bathing, dressing, and toileting *to obtain a baseline assessment of ability.* Keep instructions short, simple, and repeat frequently *to allow patient to perform activities; complicated directions can lead to frustration and agitation.* Avoid distractions during bathing, toileting, and dressing. *Sensory overload contributes to agitation and confusion.* Allow sufficient time to perform activities. *Rushing the patient may lead to agitation.* Provide privacy during self-care activities *to demonstrate respect for patient.* Maintain consistent schedule for bathing, dressing, and toileting. *Establishing routine may help decrease agitation during self-care tasks.* Provide care that patient is not able to do *to ensure that all care tasks are completed.*

Sources: Jankovic, J. (2006). Therapeutic strategies in Parkinson's disease. *Geriatrics, 61,* 3–7; Schapira, A. H. V. (2006). Etiology of Parkinson's disease. *Neurology, 66* (Suppl. 4).

2006). It is thought that the resulting disease process results from a complex interaction between genetic and environmental factors that differ from one individual to another (Jankovic, 2006) (see the Genetic Considerations and Risk Factors boxes, p. 800).

Pathophysiology

PD is a disease of the basal ganglia, a structure deep in the brain that includes the corpus striatum and globus pallidus (Figures 31–6 and 31–7 ■, p. 800). These structures are critical to the system of connections that joins the cerebral cortex and the thalamus and allows for ease of movement. The origin of PD pathology lies in the **substantia nigra**, a structure located in the midbrain, beneath the basal ganglia. Neurons in the substantia nigra produce **dopamine**, a neurotransmitter that is necessary for smooth, voluntary movement. Through the connections of the nigral striatal pathway, dopamine is transmitted from the substantia nigra to the striatum. This cycle allows for the smoothness and ease of normal, voluntary movement. In PD, the neurons of the substantia nigra inexplicably begin to degenerate and die. The resulting lack of dopamine production leads to difficulty with movement, tremor, rigidity, and difficulty maintaining posture.

When approximately 70% of the neurons in the substantia nigra have degenerated and/or died, the symptoms of PD begin to appear. Acetylcholine, another neurotransmitter, also is believed to be involved in the pathology. The lack of dopamine upsets the delicate balance between these two neurotransmitters. The defining pathologic feature of PD is the presence of Lewy bodies and neuronal loss in the substantia nigra (Schapira, 2006). Lewy bodies are detected only at brain autopsy, which is required for a definitive diagnosis of PD.

Several medications can cause parkinsonian symptoms, although they do not cause the idiopathic form of PD. These symptoms are often called drug-induced parkinsonism, or pseudo-parkinsonism. Drugs that can cause symptoms of PD include neuroleptics, such as haloperidol and risperidone, and antiemetics, such as Compazine and metoclopramide. Withdrawal from the offending agents will reverse the parkinsonian symptoms, although it may take weeks and possibly months. These medications should be avoided in patients with PD (Nutt & Wooten, 2005).

 Common drugs contraindicated in Parkinson's disease include:

Antiemetics
Prochlorperazine (Compazine)
Metoclopramide (Reglan)
Neuroleptics
Chlorpromazine (Thorazine)
Haloperidol (Haldol)
Nutt & Wooten (2005)

PATIENT TEACHING & DISCHARGE PRIORITIES for Alzheimer's Disease

Need	Teaching
Medication management: Patient/family	Adhere to medication schedule. Monitor response to medication. Monitor and report side effects.
Disease process: Patient/family	Describe diagnostic tests and need for brain autopsy for confirmation. Describe pathophysiology; cause not known. State signs, symptoms, and stages of disease progression. Describe possible treatments.
Activities of daily living: Family Setting	Use wall calendar to mark events and activities to aid orientation and mark passage of time. Place clocks prominently around house. Keep belongings consistently in one place. Use automatic dialing phone. Keep bathing and dressing routines consistent.
Safety: Family Setting	Remove potential hazards: • Cover electrical outlets to prevent shock. • Put locks on cabinets that contain potentially hazardous materials such as medications, cleaning agents, kitchen appliances, knives, or razor blades. • Store firearms in locked area. • Lower water heater temperature to avoid burns. • Remove furniture with sharp corners or pad the corners. • Serve food on plastic plates to prevent breakage. • Use professionally installed safety rails in bathroom and stairway. Hide car keys if necessary. Use signaling device if wandering is a problem. Enroll in Alzheimer Association's Safe Return program.
Managing wandering, aggression, agitation: Family	Reduce stressful situations. Establish daily routines. Simplify surroundings. Look for signs of pain or illness. Encourage light exercise, walking if possible.
Communication: Family	Listen and communicate patiently and in calm, relaxed manner. Replace contradicting with listening and questioning in caring manner. Use words or pictures to cue memories.
Community resources: Family	Contact the Alzheimer's Association (1-800-272-3900) and its local chapter for information about disease process, managing symptoms, and local support groups. Enroll in Alzheimer Association's Safe Return if wandering is a problem. Contact local area agency on aging for home care, respite, or adult day care referrals.
End-of-life issues: Patient/family	Establish advance directive, living will. Explore option of using hospice services.
Caregiver issues: Family	State signs/symptoms of increasing stress and burnout. Get adequate rest. Eat balanced meals and nutritious foods. Exercise. Use relaxation techniques such as deep breathing or meditation. Use community resources for assistance and respite. Attend caregiver support groups.

Sources: Fischer Center for Alzheimer's Research Foundation. Alzheimer's Research Foundation. (2002–2008). Alzheimer's Disease Cause, Care, & Cure. Retrieved July 18, 2008 from http://www.alzinfo.org.

FIGURE 31–7 ■ Main connections of the basal ganglia.

FIGURE 31–6 ■ Cerebral hemispheres and brainstem.

Clinical Manifestations

PD is characterized by four primary symptoms: resting tremor, rigidity, bradykinesia, and postural instability. Secondary and autonomic symptoms also may be present. Secondary symptoms often result from combinations of the primary symptoms.

Primary Symptoms

A parkinsonian tremor characteristically occurs at rest and manifests as involuntary shaking in the hand and wrist or feet while the muscles are relaxed. The tremor may decrease with activity. Although a resting tremor is commonly the first symptom, about 20% of patients do not exhibit this symptom (Nutt & Wooten, 2005). The tremor usually is present only on one side of the body in the early stages of PD, but may spread to the other side as the disease progresses. A "pill-rolling" tremor is particu-larly characteristic and appears as though a person is rolling a pill between his thumb and forefinger (National Institute of Neurological Disorders and Stroke [NINDS], 2006).

Rigidity, or muscle stiffness, may be felt throughout any given range of movement. Typically, Parkinsonian rigidity is characterized as hypertonicity of muscles resulting in stiffness of motion and is often associated with aching and discomfort (Nutt & Wooten, 2005).

Bradykinesia, one of the more disabling symptoms of PD, refers to slowness of movement. Bradykinesia is often the most prominent and disabling symptom, causing difficulty with walking, changing positions, and speaking and swallowing (NINDS, 2006).

Postural instability refers to the balancing difficulties that result from the diminishing of the reflexes that allow a person to maintain her balance (NINDS, 2006). The patient will have difficulty staying balanced and may even fall when changing positions.

Secondary Symptoms

Secondary symptoms usually are the result of the overarching, primary symptoms. Rigid facial muscles combined with bradykinesia lead to **hypomimia**, or decreased facial expression, resulting in the characteristic "masked" face of a PD patient. The decrease in facial expression often conveys lack of emotion, or a depressed affect, which may or may not actually be present. Muscle rigidity, bradykinesia, and postural instability may combine to produce gait abnormalities, like a shuffled walk, difficulty turning while walking, and stooped posture. Face and neck muscles used for talking may be affected as well. Voice changes associated with PD are known as **hypokinetic dysarthria**. They include **hypophonia**, or a soft, muffled speech. Similarly, the muscles used for swallowing become rigid, leading to dysphagia, or difficulty swallowing. **Micrographia**, or small, cramped handwriting, results from rigidity and bradykinesia in the hands (Jankovic, 2006).

Autonomic Symptoms

PD affects the autonomic nervous system, which can lead to symptoms not related to movement. Constipation is common and PD medications may exacerbate it. Orthostatic hypotension, sexual dysfunction, excessive sweating, and urinary incontinence are other common symptoms (Jankovic, 2006).

Neuropsychiatric Symptoms

Neuropsychiatric changes and cognitive impairments including dementia are estimated to occur in 30% of patients. Up to 60% of people with PD may suffer from depression. Depression in this population may be difficult to detect, since many of the symptoms are similar to PD, such as loss of facial expression, motor and mental slowing, and cognitive difficulties (Calne, 2003).

Disease Progression

As PD progresses, motor complications develop. **Dyskinesias**—involuntary, writhing motions that may involve the limbs, trunk, face, and neck—are a side effect of dopaminergic medications and result from overstimulation of dopamine receptors. Drug therapy regimes can create fluctuations in movement ability, known as **on–off phenomena**. When "on," the patient is experiencing a positive response to medication, but the effects may suddenly wear off, rendering the patient barely able to move, or "off." These reactions are related to building a tolerance to or having an unpredictable response to levodopa (Pahwa et al., 2006). Dyskinesia and the associated motor fluctuations can cause a great diversity and range of physical capacity and disability during the course of an average day. The unpredictable nature of these fluctuations interferes greatly with the patient's ability to plan for and perform routine activities.

As motor function worsens, so can other PD symptoms. Dysphagia often worsens over time and a feeding tube may be required to prevent the aspiration of food. Worsening orthostatic hypotension and postural instability increase the risk of injuries resulting from a fall (Bunting-Perry, 2006). Although PD is not considered a fatal disease, the degrading effect it has on the patient's ability to carry out basic daily functions can cause susceptibility to more threatening conditions such as pneumonia or traumatic injury.

Laboratory and Diagnostic Procedures

There is no definitive laboratory or radiological test to diagnose PD. Diagnosis is based on a neurological exam and clinical history. Laboratory tests and MRI are used to rule out other possible causes of the presenting symptoms. The positive response to dopaminergic medications reassures the PD diagnosis. Diagnostic criteria include the following (Pahwa, Lyons, & Wilkinson, 2003):

- Bradykinesia and either resting tremor or rigidity
- Positive response to levodopa
- Other causes ruled out, such as drugs, stroke, or metabolic abnormalities
- Definite diagnosis only by autopsy.

PD is commonly staged using the Hoehn and Yahr scale (1967):

- **Stage I**—Unilateral disease
- **Stage II**—Bilateral disease with preservation of postural reflexes
- **Stage III**—Bilateral disease with impaired postural reflexes; able to ambulate
- **Stage IV**—Severe disease requiring assistance
- **Stage V**—End-stage disease, confined to bed or chair.

Medical Management

An effective treatment for protecting against the loss of dopamine-producing neurons remains to be discovered. Because PD involves the loss of dopamine-producing neurons and the subsequent diminished supply of dopamine in the striatum, dopaminergic drugs that can increase dopamine levels are the first line of treatment. Novel new surgical procedures also can provide relief in advanced cases. Treatment of the secondary symptoms such as hypotension and constipation also is included in a broad approach to increase mobility, decrease symptoms, and improve quality of life, as the underlying disease progresses despite all treatments.

Also noted are the new guidelines published by the American Academy of Neurology regarding the treatment of Parkinson's disease. The guidelines tend to be more proscriptive than prescriptive (Susman, 2006). The guidelines inform the health care provider, as well as patients, that there is no neuroprotective therapy that has shown any proven value. The guidelines demonstrate that nutritional supplementation, for example, does not work. They do note 20 specific recommendations that are categorized under four broad areas:

- Diagnosis and prognosis of new-onset disease
- Neuroprotective treatments and alternative therapies
- Management of Parkinson's disease with motor fluctuations and dyskinesias
- Depression, psychosis, and dementia that are associated with Parkinson's disease (American Academy of Neurology, 2006; Susman, 2006).

Dopaminergic Drugs

Often referred to as dopaminergic drugs, these medications enhance the levels of dopamine naturally produced in the brain. Levodopa was the first breakthrough in treatment for PD in the 1960s, and it is still considered the most effective drug for PD (Jankovic, 2006; Nutt & Wooten, 2005). Dopamine itself cannot cross the blood–brain barrier (Ahlskog, 2001). **Levodopa** is the amino acid precursor of dopamine, and it can cross the blood–brain barrier. Once in the brain, levodopa is converted to dopamine (Ahlskog, 2001). However, a portion of levodopa is converted into dopamine by dopa-decarboxylase prior to entering the brain, leaving dopamine in the circulating system and causing severe nausea and vomiting.

Levodopa is given with carbidopa, a dopa-decarboxylase inhibitor, which blocks premature conversion of dopa into dopamine and minimizes nausea and vomiting (Jankovic, 2006; Nutt & Wooten, 2005). A combination of carbidopa/levodopa is available in tablet form and it varies in dosage combinations. For example, carbidopa/levodopa 25/100 tablets contain 25 mg of carbidopa and 100 mg of levodopa. The first number indicates milligrams of carbidopa, and the second indicates milligrams of levodopa.

Levodopa therapy effectively manages motor PD symptoms in most patients for 4 to 6 years; after that time, nearly half of the patients will develop motor fluctuations and/or dyskinesia (Ahlskog, 2001). Common side effects that may manifest at initiation of therapy include nausea, vomiting, loss of appetite, hypotension, confusion, and hallucinations (Nutt & Wooten, 2005). The motor complications resulting from levodopa therapy have a lower likelihood of occurring with dopamine agonist therapy (Ahlskog, 2001).

Although slightly less effective than levodopa, dopamine agonists are an alternative to levodopa for initial treatment of PD (Nutt & Wooten, 2005). Dopamine agonists approved for the treatment of PD include bromocriptine (Parlodel), pergolide (Permax), pramipexole (Mirapex), ropinirole (Requip), and apomorphine hydrochloride (Apokyn). While levodopa is converted into dopamine within the brain, dopamine agonists act on dopamine receptors within the brain and essentially mimic the effect of dopamine. The side effects of dopamine agonists are similar to those of levodopa. Dopamine agonists are prescribed initially in very low doses and slowly titrated upward to therapeutic amounts (Nutt & Wooten, 2005).

The older dopamine agonists pergolide and bromocriptine are seldom used nowadays because of adverse effects on the heart and lung (Jankovic, 2006), including pleural fibrosis and thickening of cardiac valves (Nutt & Wooten, 2005). Apomorphine hydrochloride differs from the other dopamine agonists in that it is injectable, and it is used as a rapid "rescue" for the PD patient who is undermedicated or "frozen." Symptoms abate 4 to 8 minutes after injection, although the benefit only lasts for 45 to 60 minutes. This drug can cause hypotension and severe nausea and, hence, must be taken with specific antiemetics (Mylan Bertek Pharmaceuticals, 2004).

 Patients receiving apomorphine injectable should be monitored closely for the following side effects (Bowron, 2004; Mylan Bertek Pharmaceuticals, 2004):

Severe nausea: *This side effect may decrease with continued use. Assess patient for previous use of apomorphine with concomitant nausea and vomiting. If antiemetic is needed, it should be administered prior to injection. Trimethobenzamide is the recommended antiemetic. Phenothiazines such as prochlorperazine and 5HT3 antagonists such as odansetron should NOT be given for nausea.*

Orthostatic hypotension: *Blood pressure should be monitored in supine and standing position. Health care provider notified of drop in systolic BP of > 20 mmHg.*

Dyskinesia: *Notify health care provider of onset of involuntary writhing movements of limbs, face, or trunk.*

Anticholinergic Drugs

Anticholinergics are the oldest class of medications used to treat PD. They were commonly used before the discovery of levodopa. These medications are used primarily to treat tremor (Pahwa et al., 2003). Side effects such as dry mouth, blurred vision, constipation, oversedation, urinary retention, and confusion deter their long-term use. The most commonly prescribed medications in this category are trihexyphenidyl (Artane) and benztropine (Cogentin) (Nutt & Wooten, 2005).

PHARMACOLOGY Summary of Medications to Treat Parkinson's Disease

Medication Category	Action	Application/Indication	Nursing Responsibility
Carbidopa/Levodopa • Immediate release • Controlled release • Carbidopa/levodopa/entacapone (Stalevo)	Levodopa is converted to dopamine in the basal ganglia, increasing dopamine concentration within the brain. Carbidopa blocks the peripheral decarboxylation of levodopa, making more levodopa available to the brain.	Symptomatic treatment of idiopathic Parkinson's disease; may be given alone or in combination with other anti-Parkinsonian drugs	Monitor for nausea, hypotension, confusion, hallucinations, motor fluctuations, dyskinesia.
Dopamine Agonists • Bromocriptine (Parlodel) • Pergolide (Permax) • Pramipexole (Mirapex) • Ropinirole (Requip) • Apomorphine hydrochloride (Apokyn) • Rotigotine	Stimulate dopamine receptors in the brain.	May be given as initial treatment or adjunctively with levodopa in advanced cases	Monitor for postural hypotension, nausea, confusion, hallucinations.
Anticholinergics • Benztropine (Cogentin) • Trihexyphenidyl (Artane)	Block cholinergic activity in CNS.	Tremor	Monitor for dry mouth, constipation, urinary retention, blurred vision, hallucinations, confusion.
Antiviral • Amantadine (Symmetrel)	Exact action not clear; likely potentiates dopaminergic transmission in CNS.	Motor fluctuations, dyskinesia	Monitor for lower extremity edema, livedo reticularis, urinary retention, hallucinations.

PHARMACOLOGY Summary of Medications to Treat Parkinson's Disease—*Continued*

Medication Category	Action	Application/Indication	Nursing Responsibility
MAO-B Inhibitors • Selegiline (Eldepryl) • Rasagiline	Exact action not clear; believed to enhance dopaminergic activity in substantia nigra by blocking the enzyme MAO-B.	Sometimes given as monotherapy for initial treatment for PD; usually given adjunctively	Monitor for agitation, insomnia, vivid dreams, hallucinations, orthostatic hypotension.
COMT Inhibitors • Entacapone • Tolcapone	Blocks COMT, an enzyme that metabolizes levodopa; enhances available dopamine.	Given adjunctively with levodopa/carbidopa	Same as for levodopa.
Management of Selected Nonmotor Symptoms of Parkinson's Disease			
Tricyclic Antidepressants • Amitriptyline (Elavil) **Selective Serotonin Reuptake Inhibitors (SSRIs)** • Fluoxetine (Prozac) • Sertraline (Zoloft) • Paroxetine (Paxil) • Citalopram (Celexa)	Potentiates serotonin and norepinephrine in CNS. Inhibits uptake of neurotransmitter serotonin in CNS, potentiating the effects of serotonin. Has little or no effect on other neurotransmitters.	Depression	*Tricyclics:* Monitor for cognitive changes. May improve insomnia, drooling. Monitor for constipation. *SSRIs:* Monitor for restlessness or agitation. *All:* May take several weeks to reach therapeutic dose. Should not be discontinued suddenly. Assess suicide risk. Encourage concomitant counseling.
Atypical Antipsychotics • Clozapine (Clozaril) • Quetiapine (Seroquel)	Likely act as antagonists of dopamine and serotonin.	Hallucinations	Assess anti-Parkinsonian medication schedule for timing and dosage changes. Assess all current medications for possible cause of hallucinations. Assess for infection. Assess for dehydration or constipation. *Clozapine:* Monitor for agranulocytosis.
Glucocorticoid • Fludrocortisone (Florinef)	Acts on distal renal tubule to promote sodium reabsorption and water retention.	Severe, chronic postural hypotension	Assess medication regime for antihypertensives. Monitor blood pressure sitting and standing. Monitor fluid balance and salt intake. Monitor for signs of fluid retention.
Vasopressor • Midodrine (ProAmatine)	Stimulates alpha$_1$-adrenergic receptors, increasing total peripheral resistance, resulting in increased systolic and diastolic blood pressure.	Severe, chronic postural hypotension	Assess medication regime for antihypertensives. Monitor blood pressure sitting and standing. Monitor fluid balance and salt intake.
Genitourinary Antispasmodic • Oxybutynin (Ditropan) • Tolterodine tartrate (Detrol)	Exert a direct spasmolytic action and an antimuscarinic action on smooth muscle, relaxing bladder smooth muscle.	Urinary symptoms of overactive bladder	Monitor for urinary frequency and urgency. Monitor fluid balance. Monitor for signs of urinary tract infection.

Sources: Alzheimer's Association. (2003). *Provider checklist for treating a confused elder.* Retrieved April 30, 2008, from http://alzla.org/medical/Checklisthtml.html; American Society of Health-System Pharmacists. (2006). *AHFS drug information.* Bethesda, MD: Author; Calne, S. M. (2003). The psychosocial impact of late-stage Parkinson's disease. *Journal of Neuroscience Nursing, 35*(6), 306–313; Calne, S. M., & Kumar, A. (2003). Nursing care of patients with late-stage Parkinson's disease. *Journal of Neuroscience Nursing, 35,* 5, 242–251; Jankovic, J. (2006). Therapeutic strategies in Parkinson's disease. Pahwa, R., Lyons, K., & Wilkinson, B. (2003). *Deep brain stimulation for Parkinson's disease: An update.* Retrieved January 23, 2004, from http://www.medscape.com/viewprogram/2274_pnt.

COMT Inhibitors

Catechol-*O*-methyltransferase (COMT) is an enzyme that metabolizes levodopa and dopamine. Inhibiting COMT decreases levodopa metabolism so that more is available to cross the blood–brain barrier (Pahwa et al., 2003). Because they increase the effective duration of the levodopa dosage, COMT inhibitors are effective only when taken in conjunction with levodopa. They are used most often to counteract wearing-off responses (Jankovic, 2006). Approved COMT inhibitors are tolcapone (Tasmar) and entacapone (Comtan). Tolcapone is used less often because of the risk of liver toxicity. Stalevo combines both levodopa/carbidopa and entacapone into one tablet.

Other Medications

Amantadine, an antiviral drug, has proven to provide modest improvement for PD symptoms. It is particularly useful for treating dyskinesias. Side effects include fatigue, agitation, the red or purple skin blotches of livedo reticularis, and edema of the lower extremities (Nutt & Wooten, 2005).

Inhibition of the enzyme monoamine oxidase type B (MAO-B) interferes with the metabolism of dopamine. Although the MAO-B inhibitor selegiline was thought to prevent degeneration of dopamine-producing neurons and delay the progression of PD, studies have not successfully confirmed this. Nonetheless, selegiline reduces the metabolism of dopamine, does improve PD symptoms, and can reduce total levodopa dosage by 10% to 25% in some patients. Unlike other MAO-B inhibitors, selegiline has no dietary restrictions at the recommended dose of 10 mg/day. Because of its stimulating effects, it should be taken in the morning and not later than noon to avoid disruption of sleep. There is potential for serious and possibly fatal drug interactions when taken concurrently with meperidine (Demerol), and therefore should be discontinued at least 2 weeks before surgery (Jankovic, 2006; Nutt & Wooten, 2005). Other medications can be used to treat secondary symptoms of PD including depression, cognitive changes, sleep problems, and genitourinary issues. The Pharmacology Summary box (p. 802) provides more information about medications for Parkinson's disease.

 CRITICAL ALERT *Meperidine should not be given to patients taking selegiline due to risk of fatal drug interaction (Nutt & Wooten, 2005).*

Surgical Approaches

Neurosurgical intervention is an option reserved for certain carefully selected patients with advanced PD. Surgical treatments include ablative procedures, deep brain stimulation (DBS; Figure 31–8 ■), and cell transplantation. Ablative procedures include thalamotomy and pallidotomy, which is the surgical placement of a permanent lesion in the thalamus or the globus pallidus, respectively. Ablative procedures are older procedures and rarely used today.

Recently, DBS became another viable option. DBS involves surgically placing electrodes in targeted areas of the brain. As with ablative procedures, the most common targets are specific areas within the subthalamic nucleus or globus pallidus. The electrodes are attached to an external pacemaker-like device that is implanted underneath the collarbone. High-frequency stimulation provides effects similar to ablative surgery (Pahwa et al., 2003). Like PD drug treatments, surgical interventions do not cure the disease.

FIGURE 31–8 ■ Parkinson's control therapy: deep brain stimulation.

Transplantation therapy involves transplanting stem cells, in an effort to replace lost substantia nigra cells. Currently, these controversial procedures are experimental and the ongoing focus of research (Pahwa et al., 2003).

Complementary and alternative therapies also may be used to treat PD. One such alternative, t'ai chi, is discussed in the Complementary and Alternative Therapies box.

Gerontological Considerations

People with PD ages 65 and older account for 17% of neurology outpatient visits. After Alzheimer's disease, it is the second most common neurological condition requiring home health care (Pahwa et al., 2003). PD imposes socioeconomic burdens as well. Research studies indicate that the individual costs of PD are estimated as to be as high as $24,000 per year, with the cost of medications alone over $2,000 (Pahwa et al., 2003). Medication expense for patients beyond their productive years can be particularly burdensome.

People can live with PD for many years. The chronic and progressive nature of PD can significantly impact older, spousal caregivers, who may not have the physical strength to handle the weight of a patient with limited mobility. Caregiver stress and burden have been shown to increase as the disease progresses (Carter et al., 1998).

■ Nursing Management

Application of the nursing process will facilitate a comprehensive approach to patient care throughout the disease process. Relevant nursing diagnoses, assessment, outcomes, and interventions are

COMPLEMENTARY & ALTERNATIVE THERAPIES   T'ai Chi

Description:

T'AI CHI is an Asian exercise technique that consists of a series of flowing, graceful movements conducted in a specific pattern. Unlike many other forms of exercise, breathing and balance are central to t'ai chi. There are many different t'ai chi styles throughout the world and it is becoming increasingly used as a part of many preventative and restorative health regimens.

Research Support:

One of the diseases that research has shown t'ai chi to improve is Parkinson's disease. The primary effects associated with Parkinson's disease occur in tandem with the secondary, often preventable, effects of immobility (Kluding & McGinnis, 2006). The majority of studies on t'ai chi show that the method may lead to improved balance, reduced fear of falling, increased strength, increased functional mobility, greater flexibility, and increased psychological well-being for patients with Parkinson's disease (Kuramoto, 2006).

One small study examined the effects of 3 months of various physical activities on two 66-year-old males in early or middle stages of Parkinson's disease. The men participated in balance classes twice weekly during the first month, joined a fitness center and self-directed their exercise program during the second month, and participated in group t'ai chi classes twice weekly during the third month. The results of the 3-month program showed improvements in functional reach for both participants, and both demonstrated improvement in their balance test performance over a 3-month period (Kluding & McGinnis, 2006). Once the program ended, participants were given suggestions for continued physical fitness activities, and both participants continued to exercise regularly for at least 8 months following the program.

Another small study described the effects of an 8-week t'ai chi class on two participants: one with Parkinson's disease, the other with multiple sys-tem atrophy. The results showed that both participants demonstrated improved scores on the Activities-specific Balance Confidence Scale and the Functional Reach Test. Both participants also reported subjective improvements in balance and balance awareness. Based on these results, researchers concluded that t'ai chi may be a viable option for improving balance in patients with mild Parkinsonism (Venglar, 2005).

Another larger study involved 15 participants who received 12 weeks of weekly t'ai chi instruction in 45-minute sessions at a community facility. After the participants completed the program, researchers evaluated their results by administering a survey questionnaire, analyzing themes of a focus group discussion, assessing instructor reflections, and reviewing attendance records. Participants perceived benefits in physical, psychological, and social domains. The results showed that improved balance was reported most frequently. In addition, instructor observations and participant testimony suggest that performing t'ai chi may improve movement capability for individuals with Parkinson's (Klein & Rivers, 2006).

References

Klein, P. J., & Rivers, L. (2006). T'ai chi for individuals with Parkinson disease and their support partners: A program evaluation. *Journal of Neurologic Physical Therapy, 30*(1), 22–27.

Kluding, P., & McGinnis, P. Q. (2006). Multidimensional exercise for people with Parkinson's disease: A case report. *Physiotherapy Theory and Practice, 22*(3), 153–162.

Kuramoto, A. M. (2006). Therapeutic benefits of T'ai Chi exercise: Research review. *Wisconsin Medical Journal, 105*(7), 42–46.

Venglar, M. (2005). Case report: T'ai Chi and parkinsonism. *Physiotherapy Research International, 10*(2), 116–121.

---

all part of the nursing process, as outlined in the Nursing Process: Patient Care Plan for Parkinson's Disease feature (p. 806).

Collaborative Management

With the goal of maintaining independence and quality of life, a multidisciplinary plan will help to effectively manage the symptoms and complications of PD. Physical, speech, and occupational therapy can counteract effects of progressive movement and speech complications. Dietary consultation can address nutritional concerns. In the later stages of PD, a multidisciplinary approach will best address the goals of symptom relief, prevention of complications, maintaining patient dignity, and supporting the family caregivers (Thomas & MacMahon, 2004).

Discharge Priorities

Discharge priorities for the patient with PD involve both the patient and the patient's family, or caretakers (see the Patient Teaching & Discharge Priorities box, p. 807).

Health Promotion

In addition to medicines and treatment specifically designed to alleviate symptoms, a complete care plan for the PD patient will include diet, exercise, and mental health needs of the patient and caregiver. People with PD are at risk for dehydration, weight loss, and constipation. A dietitian or nutritionist who is familiar with dysphagia can assess nutritional needs (see Chapter 14 🌐) and recommend adequate amounts of fluids and proper foods for such conditions (Holden, 2003).

Cardiovascular exercise, strength training, and muscle stretching routines can help combat losses of balance, dexterity, and normal movement. Exercise also will improve the strength, endurance, and compensatory qualities of the unaffected parts of the body. Patients should know that physical exercise may help them improve function (Suchowersky, Gronseth, Perlmutter, Reich, & Zesiewicz, 2006).

Parkinson's support organizations offer understanding and hope for both the patients and their families. Local and national support groups provide information, educational programs, and social activities tailored especially for people with PD. Some PD patients choose to participate in clinical research studies as a way of advancing science while keenly managing their condition with the latest, most promising treatments.

Multiple Sclerosis

A chronic and progressive neuroimmunologic disease, **multiple sclerosis (MS)** is characterized by multiple areas of demyelination in the white matter of the brain and spinal cord. The demyelination leaves sclerotic areas, also known as plaques, and subsequent scarring leading to a variety of neurological symptoms including weakness, spasticity, visual difficulties, and **paresthesias**.

Epidemiology and Etiology

In the United States, an estimated 350,000 cases affect almost twice as many women as men. Typically, symptoms first appear

NURSING PROCESS: Patient Care Plan for Parkinson's Disease

Assessment for Independent Activity

Subjective Data:
Do you have stiffness and slowness of movement?
Do these symptoms interfere with your daily activities?
Do you have trouble with balance?
Have you ever fallen?
Do you need assistance when you walk?
Do you use a cane or walker?
Does your medication regimen help your symptoms?
Do you have times during the day when you function better than at other times?

Objective Data:
Neurological status, including motor status (coordination, gait, balance, tremor, rigidity, bradykinesia)

Nursing Assessment and Diagnoses	Outcomes and Evaluation Parameters	Planning and Interventions with *Rationales*
Nursing Diagnosis: *Impaired Physical Mobility* related to rigidity, bradykinesia, postural instability, altered gait	**Outcomes:** Patient demonstrates maximum independent physical function. Patient is free of immobility complications. ***Evaluation Parameters:*** Patient maintains as much independent mobility as possible given degree of disease progression. Patient uses assistive devices to maximize mobility. ADLs and therapy schedule coincide with medication peak effectiveness.	**Interventions and *Rationales:*** Assist patient to ambulate and perform ADLs *to provide assessment of abilities.* Consult with patient regarding medication schedule. *Medication schedule may be complex and may not fit traditional medication timelines.* Schedule therapies and ADLs to coincide with optimum medication benefit. *Movement will be easier when medications are working at peak effectiveness.* Instruct patient to stand as straight as possible and walk with a wide-based gait while swinging arms *to help maintain balance and momentum.* Perform range of motion to all joints *to counteract the effects of rigidity.* Encourage use of walker or other assistive device *to increase mobility by stabilizing gait.* Use side rails or overhead trapeze on bed. *Both act as grab bars and assist with turning over in bed.* Instruct patient to use straight-back chairs with firm seats and arm rests when possible. *It is difficult for patients to get up from low, soft surfaces such as easy chairs or sofas.* Consult with physical therapist. *Can prescribe and tailor appropriate gait assistive devices and also exercises to counteract stiffness and rigidity.* Consult with occupational therapist. *Can assess need for adaptive aids for ADLs such as specialized eating utensils or button hook for dressing.*

Assessment for Ability to Communicate

Subjective Data:
Do people ask you to repeat things?
Do you frequently feel misunderstood?
Do you get frustrated when trying to converse?

Objective Data:
Difficulty understanding patient
Lack of facial expression

Nursing Assessment and Diagnoses	Outcomes and Evaluation Parameters	Planning and Interventions with *Rationales*
Nursing Diagnosis: *Impaired Verbal Communication* related to voice and speech changes and decreased facial expression	**Outcome:** Patient is able to converse and communicate needs. ***Evaluation Parameters:*** Staff and family members are able to understand verbalizations. Patient and family members verbalize disease process and effect on speech and expression.	**Nursing Interventions and *Rationales:*** Assess and monitor for decreased voice volume, slurred or mumbled speech, difficulties initiating speech. *Common symptoms of PD.* Observe ability of patient to communicate needs and converse with family members. *Provides information about impact of speech changes on family dynamics and assesses need for education.* Consult with speech-language pathologist. *Can evaluate speech difficulties and develop treatment program, including assistive devices.* Eliminate background noise (TV, radio) while patient is speaking. *Decreases environmental interference when listening to patient.* Allow ample time for patient to speak and communicate. *Communicating takes longer for patient; allowing ample time decreases stress and anxiety, which may improve speech.*

NURSING PROCESS: Patient Care Plan for Parkinson's Disease—*Continued*

Assessment for Orientation to Time, Place, and Person

Subjective Data:
States name when asked.

Objective Data:
Neurological status including level of consciousness, orientation, MMSE
Agitation
Visual hallucinations
Medication regimen
Signs of infection: fever
Hydration status, including intake and output
Laboratory studies including blood chemistry and CBCs

Nursing Assessment and Diagnoses	Outcomes and Evaluation Parameters	Planning and Interventions with *Rationales*
Nursing Diagnosis: *Disturbed Thought Processes* (confusion, hallucinations and delusions) related to cognitive changes, medication regimen, and/or infection	**Outcome:** Patient remains oriented. **Evaluation Parameters:** Patient does not exhibit evidence of having delusions or hallucinations. Patient is oriented. Family remains calm in event of visual hallucinations.	**Interventions and *Rationales*:** Assess and monitor patient's level of cognitive functioning using rating scale such as MMSE. *Provides a basis of planning care.* Assess changes in medication dosage and/or schedule and monitor for increased or decreased confusion or hallucinations and physical mobility. *Dopaminergic drugs can stimulate hallucinations or cause confusion and may need to be adjusted; these side effects may preclude a dosage high enough to improve mobility.* Assess for treatable causes of confusion such as infection, recent general anesthesia, dehydration. *Can be sources of delirium or increased confusion.* Assess and monitor response to antipsychotic drugs. *May be prescribed to counteract hallucination and delusions.* Reassure patient and family during hallucinations. *Patient may or may not become frightened during hallucinations; hallucinations can be distressing to family.* Minimize environmental hazards *to decrease risk of injury due to confusion.*

Sources: Ackley, B. J., & Ludwig, G. B. (Eds.). (2003). *Nursing diagnosis handbook: A guide to planning care* (6th ed.). St. Louis: Mosby; Calne, S. M. (2003). The psychosocial impact of late-stage Parkinson's disease. *Journal of Neuroscience Nursing, 35*(6), 306–313; Calne, S. M., & Kumar, A. (2003). Nursing care of patients with late-stage Parkinson's disease. *Journal of Neuroscience Nursing, 35,* 5, 242–251; Doenges, M. E., & Moorhouse, M. F. (2003). *Application of nursing process and diagnosis: An interactive text for diagnostic reasoning* (4th ed.). Philadelphia: F. A. Davis; Holloway, N. (2003). *Medical-surgical care planning* (4th ed.). Philadelphia: Lippincott Wilkins & Williams.

PATIENT TEACHING & DISCHARGE PRIORITIES for Parkinson's Disease

Need	Teaching
Disease process: Patient/family	Assess knowledge of disease process: • PD is chronic and slowly progressive. • No clear cause or cure is known. • General progression through stages but progression varies from person to person. • Treatment approaches.
Educational resources: Patient/family	National Parkinson Foundation (1-800-327-4545) Parkinson Disease Foundation (1-800-457-6676) American Parkinson's Disease Association (1-800-223-2732) Local PD clinical and research centers Local support groups Internet resources

(continued)

MyNursingKit | Parkinson Disease Foundation

MyNursingKit | American Parkinson's Disease Association

MyNursingKit | National Parkinson Foundation

PATIENT TEACHING & DISCHARGE PRIORITIES for Parkinson's Disease—*Continued*

Need	Teaching
Dopaminergic medications: Patient/family	Side effects of dopaminergic medications: • Nausea/vomiting • Light-headedness • Drowsiness • Confusion • Hallucinations. Take as directed, usually starting with low dose and titrating upward. Allow time to reach dosage required for symptom improvement. Take carbidopa/levodopa 30 to 60 minutes before a meal or 1 to 2 hours after a meal for optimal absorption. Do not abruptly stop medications unless directed by health care provider. Use medication diary to track schedule, dosage, and side-effects. Need to work closely with health care provider to arrive at optimal, individualized dosage.
Fall prevention: Family Setting	Remove throw rugs. Move electrical cords out of walkways. Create clear, uncluttered walking paths. Rearrange furniture so that it is easy to get around. Install railings along hallways and on stairways. Minimize sharp edges or corners on furniture, wet floors, and hot surfaces. Install grab bars in shower and next to commode. Do not use towel racks as grab bars.
Nutrition: Patient/family	Hydration is important to counteract low blood pressure, constipation, and for general health. Fiber helps to counteract constipation. Calcium is important for maintaining bone density and decreasing the risk of fracture from falls. Protein may interfere with levodopa absorption in a small percentage of patients. Take levodopa at least 30 minutes before eating or 1 hour after eating. Consult with dietitian for weight loss.
Exercise: Patient/family Setting (home/clinic)	Stress importance of the following in accordance with patient's physical ability: • Resistance training to strengthen muscles and bones • Mild aerobic conditioning for cardiovascular health • Stretching to counteract stiffness and rigidity.
Constipation: Patient/family Setting (home/clinic/hospital)	Part of disease process and worsened by medications. Avoid use of laxatives. May use stool softeners and bulking agents such as psyllium on daily basis. Increase dietary fluid and fiber.
Urinary problems: Patient/family Setting (home/clinic/hospital)	Urinary frequency and/or urgency is common. Signs/symptoms of urinary tract infection (UTI): • Foul-smelling urine • Painful urination. Call health care provider if signs/symptoms of UTI develop. Consult with health care provider regarding urinary problems.
Orthostatic hypotension: Patient/family Setting (home/clinic/hospital)	Signs of low blood pressure include light-headedness, dizziness, fainting. Part of disease process, medications also contribute. Change position slowly when rising from a lying or seated position. Increase fluids and salt if not contraindicated by other conditions. Use support stockings and elevate legs throughout the day. Remain seated for 20 to 30 minutes after a large meal or dose of medication. Sit down to towel after hot bath or shower.

Sources: Calne, S. M., & Kumar, A. (2003). Nursing care of patients with late-stage Parkinson's disease. *Journal of Neuroscience Nursing, 35,* 5, 242–251; Cianci, H. (2004). *Fitness counts* (2nd ed.). Brochure. Miami, FL: National Parkinson Foundation; Holden, K. (2003). *Parkinson's disease: Guidelines for medical nutritional therapy for use by nutrition professionals.* Miami, FL: Five Star Living; Marjama-Lyons, J. & Shomon, M. J. (2003). *What your doctor may not tell you about Parkinson's disease: a holistic program for optimal wellness.* New York, NY: Warner Books, Inc.

RISK FACTORS for Multiple Sclerosis

Research has shown that people who spend their first 15 years of life in temperate climates, at a distance from the equator, are more at risk than those who spend the same time in tropical regions closer to the equator (Schapiro, 2003).

There is evidence that a genetic link may influence susceptibility to MS. Generally, a person's chance of developing MS is about one-tenth of 1%; however, if there is a first-degree relative with MS, the risk jumps up to 3%. In identical twins, the chance that the second twin will develop MS if the first twin does is 30%; in fraternal twins, the risk is decreased to 4%. Many researchers hypothesize that MS is not caused by a single gene, virus, or environmental factor, but is the result of a combination of factors (NINDS, 2002).

between 20 and 40 years of age. Onset of the disease may have a geographical component (Schapiro, 2003). Risk for MS increases geographically from southern to northern latitudes. The highest frequency areas of North America include the northern United States and southern Canada. There is also evidence that migration to and from higher frequency areas in early life influences the risk of developing MS (Franklin & Nelson, 2003).

Pathophysiology

MS is a neuroimmunologic disease that attacks **myelin**, the protective sheath surrounding nerve fibers. Demyelinating lesions or plaques form along nerve fibers in the brain and spinal cord, producing symptoms related to the location of damage. The breakdown of myelin interferes with normal nerve conduction in the affected areas (Schapiro, 2003). Demyelination results from an inflammatory process and also leads to irreversible axonal injury and permanent loss of nerve function (Holland, 2003; O'Connor & Canadian Multiple Sclerosis Working Group, 2002). This process may be triggered by a virus or other environmental stimulus that activates T cells specific for the production of myelin basic protein (MBP). The T cells cross the blood–brain barrier into the CNS, where they release cytokines, initiating an immune response that ultimately damages the myelin sheath and axons (O'Connor et al., 2002). Although viruses and environmental factors are suspect for their role in MS, the cause is still unknown (see the Risk Factors box).

Clinical Manifestations

Because MS can damage different parts of the CNS, symptoms vary, not only from patient to patient, but within the same patient over time. The most common initial signs include fatigue, nystagmus, vertigo, gait disturbances, sensory loss, lower extremity weakness, spasticity, bladder disturbance, and optic neuritis. Other symptoms that may present at any time during the course of the disease include cognitive changes such as euphoria or depression, and physical conditions such as muscle cramping and sexual dysfunction (Holland, 2003).

The symptoms of MS are listed in four categories: sensory, motor, cerebellar, and miscellaneous. The symptoms correspond specifically with the area in the brain or spinal cord that is damaged. Sensory symptoms include numbness, paresthesias, loss of proprioception, and **L'Hermite's sign**, or a shocklike pain that results from flexion of the neck. Motor symptoms include weak-

ness, particularly in the lower extremities, and spasticity. Cerebellar symptoms include **ataxia**, or loss of balance and coordination, as well as speech difficulties including dysarthria or slurred and scanning speech. Other symptoms such as fatigue and loss of vision associated with a central scotoma often are an early sign of the disease. Vertigo, sometimes accompanied by vomiting and nystagmus, affects some patients while bowel and bladder problems beset others. Emotional disturbances and cognitive impairment may be present as well.

As with the wide range of symptoms, the course any particular case might take is varied. The four main types of MS are listed here (O'Connor et al., 2002):

- *Relapsing-remitting MS* is the most common type. It is known for its acute attacks followed by complete or partial remission. It makes up about 85% of initial diagnoses.
- *Primary-progressive MS* progresses without remission, although plateaus or minor improvements can happen. Approximately 10% to 15% of the diagnoses are for this form of the disease.
- *Secondary progressive MS* begins as relapsing-remitting, but then it develops into the primary-progressive course.
- *Progressive-relapsing MS* intersperses the progression of the disease with acute attacks.

Both age and duration of the disease have the greatest influence on the rate of relapse.

Laboratory and Diagnostic Procedures

In addition to a comprehensive medical history and neurological exam, diagnostics for MS include MRI, cerebrospinal fluid (CSF) tests, and visual evoked potentials (VEP) (Chaudhuri & Behan, 2004; Holland, 2003). Lesions that represent inflammation or demyelination often are referred to as plaques and are easily detected with T_2-weighted and flair MRI tests. Enhancing lesions, or those enhanced by the contrast agent gadolinium, are considered new. They may appear and then disappear. Nonenhancing lesions can be seen without gadolinium, and reflect older, permanent damage. CSF studies look for inflammatory proteins and oligoclonal bands. The VEP test is done to measure transmission of impulses across nerve fibers, which are slowed in areas of demyelination (Holland, 2003). Other diagnostics are listed in the Diagnostic Tests box (p. 810).

Medical Management

Treating MS relies on drug therapy, relapse management, and symptom management. The nurse plays a critical role in education and health management in all of these areas (Costello, Halper, Harris, & Kennedy, 2003).

Disease-Modifying Drugs

Disease-modifying drugs reduce the frequency of relapses and potentially delay progression. Interferon beta-1b (Betaseron) is used to treat ambulatory patients with relapsing-remitting MS and secondary-progressive MS. Interferon beta-1a (Avonex) helps relapsing forms of MS as well as the initial MS attack. Another interferon beta-1a (Rebif) treats relapsing forms of MS.

These medications are injected either subcutaneously or intramuscularly. Side effects resulting from these treatments range from flu-like symptoms that subside over time and injection-site

DIAGNOSTIC TESTS for Multiple Sclerosis

Test	Expected Result	Rationale
MRI	White matter lesion(s) identified	Rule out other conditions; look for white matter lesions (plaques).
CSF studies	Elevated IgG index or synthesis rate Presence of oligoclonal bands	Uncovers signs of inflammation and myelin breakdown.
VEP	Slowed conduction	Identifies lesions in sensory pathway; may help identify lesion not easily visualized by MRI; for example, optic nerve.

Sources: Chaudhuri, A., & Behan, P.O. (2004). Multiple sclerosis is not an autoimmune disease. *Archives of Neurology, 61,* 1610–1612; NMSS (2008); Holland, N. (2003). *Urinary dysfunction in multiple sclerosis.* Retrieved May 2, 2008, from http://www.nationalmssociety.org;pdf/forpros/Bladder.pdf.

reactions such as erythema to pain, menstrual irregularities, and nausea (Costello et al., 2003). Depression also is a possible side effect. Flu-like symptoms can be minimized by slowly increasing the dose and use of antipyretics. Teaching correct technique and applying ice to the site can manage injection-site reactions. Blood chemistry and hematology should be checked regularly because, even though abnormalities are rare, they do occur. Particular attention should be given to monitoring liver function tests (Costello et al., 2003).

Glatiramer acetate (Copaxone) is not an interferon; nevertheless, it is a disease-modifying drug used to treat relapsing-remitting MS. Like interferons, glatiramer acetate is injected. Localized site reactions are common and can be minimized in the same way as interferon site reactions. Systemic reactions occur rarely. Although not dangerous, they may invoke tachycardia, sweating, anxiety, dyspnea, faintness, flushing, and nausea. Educating patients about the possibility of a postinjection reaction will help to minimize anxiety (Costello et al., 2003).

Traditionally used as a treatment for cancer, mitoxantrone (Novantrone), an antineoplastic drug, suppresses the activity of T cells, B cells, and macrophages. It is used to treat the secondary progressive, progressive-relapsing, and worsening relapsing-remitting forms of MS (National Multiple Sclerosis Society [NMSS], 2008). The therapy calls for its intravenous administration every 3 months. The blue-colored fluid may cause a bluish tinge in urine and bluing in the whites of the eyes. Use of mitoxantrone for more than 2.5 years increases the risk of cardiac toxicity (Schapiro, 2003).

 **CRITICAL ALERT** *Cardiac output should be recorded prior to starting mitoxantrone drug therapy and periodically thereafter (NMSS, 2008).*

In 2006, the FDA approved natalizumab (Tysabri) for the treatment of relapsing MS. A laboratory-produced monoclonal antibody, this drug inhibits the movement of damaging immune cells across the blood–brain barrier and into the brain and spinal cord. Due to the increased risk of progressive multifocal leukoencephalopathy, an opportunistic viral brain infection, it is available only through a restricted distribution program (FDA, 2006). The Pharmacology Summary box provides more information about drugs used for the treatment of multiple sclerosis.

Relapse Management

A relapse is a new sign or a worsening of neurological symptoms with a duration that is greater than 24 hours. Recovery from relapse is variable. After onset of neurological deterioration,

symptoms plateau and patients recover over weeks or months. Symptoms gradually resolve and patients fully or partially recover. Several conditions are known to precipitate symptoms or relapses. These include, but are not limited to, excessive exertion, extreme temperatures, infections, hot baths, fever, emotional stress, and pregnancy (Costello et al., 2003).

Relapses often are treated with an orally or intravenously administered glucocorticoid, such as methylprednisolone. Common side effects from the use of these types of drugs include weight gain, a metallic taste in the mouth, insomnia, hyperglycemia, and gastrointestinal ulceration and upset. Less common side effects include psychosis and blurred vision (Costello et al., 2003).

Detailing the history of relapse and the consequential symptoms becomes the basis of care and treatment of the MS patient. The record should show when the relapse began, the severity of symptoms, and the impact on the patient's daily activities. The patient care plan should address the patient's understanding of factors that can contribute to the worsening of symptoms, common diagnostic evaluations, and a review of common medical therapy.

Symptom Management

Fatigue is a common symptom in patients diagnosed with MS, and it is the most disabling symptom (Schapiro, 2003). MS fatigue may have sudden onset and interfere with normal function. When managing fatigue, the patient's sleep habits, current and former medications, experiences of depression, and applied coping strategies all need to be collectively, as well as individually, taken into consideration. Patients should understand that a hot ambient temperature can trigger the onset of fatigue and symptoms. Countermeasures such as air conditioning, cool drinks, and ice packs can help to restore a patient's strength. Occupational therapists can teach energy conservation strategies that can help the patient accomplish ADLs. The practices of light exercise, scheduling rest times between activities, and using labor-saving tools and appliances often become part of the therapy. Medications prescribed to combat fatigue include amantadine, pemoline, modafinil, and low-dose antidepressants (Lisak, 2001; Schapiro, 2003).

Muscle spasticity also is common. Infection, disease relapse, incorrect body positioning, and a full bowel and/or bladder all can contribute to spasticity. The nurse should obtain a detailed history of the time, place, and circumstances associated with spasticity. Stretching and breathing exercises, cool-water therapy, and relaxation techniques may be incorporated into strategies

PHARMACOLOGY Summary of Medications to Treat Multiple Sclerosis

Medication Category	Action	Application/Indication	Nursing Responsibility
Immunomodulator/Interferons			
• Interferon beta-1a (Avonex) • Interferon beta-1b (Betaseron) • Interferon beta-1a (Rebif)	Although action is not clear, thought to inhibit proliferation of leukocytes and antigens; modulate production of anti-inflammatory cytokines; inhibit T-cell migration across blood–brain barrier.	Relapsing forms of MS	Assess frequency of exacerbations. Monitor hemoglobin, WBC, platelets, blood chemistries. Instruct patient on correct injection technique.
Immunomodulator			
• Glatiramer acetate (Copaxone)	Although action is not clear, thought to modulate T cells to promote production of anti-inflammatory cytokines.	Relapsing-remitting forms	Assess frequency of exacerbations. After injection, assess for flushing, chest pain, palpitations, and dyspnea. Instruct patient on correct injection technique.
Antineoplastic/Immunosuppressive			
• Mitoxantrone (Novantrone)	Inhibits DNA synthesis.	Rapidly worsening relapsing-remitting, progressive-relapsing, secondary-progressive	Assess frequency of exacerbations. Monitor for cardiotoxicity, fatigue, nausea, immunosuppression.
Monoclonal Antibody			
• Natalizumab (Tysabri)	May hamper the movement of immune cells across the blood–brain barrier.	Relapsing forms in patients who have inadequate response or who cannot tolerate other disease-modifying treatment	Due to risk of progressive multifocal leukoencephalopathy, a serious viral infection of the brain, this drug is only available at select authorized infusion sites requiring mandatory patient registration and follow-up.
Management of Selected Symptoms of Multiple Sclerosis			
CNS Stimulants			
• Pemoline • Modafinil	Produce CNS stimulation.	Fatigue	Monitor for restlessness or sleep disturbances. Counsel patient regarding dosing schedule and titration.
Genitourinary Antispasmodics			
• Oxybutynin (Ditropan) • Tolterodine tartrate (Detrol)	Exert a direct spasmolytic action and an antimuscarinic action on smooth muscle, relaxing bladder smooth muscle.	Bladder dysfunction	Assess for urinary tract infection. Monitor for urinary retention. Monitor intake and output. Monitor overall elimination pattern.
Skeletal Muscle Relaxant			
• Oral or intrathecal baclofen	Acts at spinal cord level to decrease frequency and amplitude of muscle spasms.	Spasticity	Time doses to maintain therapeutic blood levels. Titrate doses up. Monitor for sedation or cognitive symptoms. Intrathecal baclofen requires surgical insertion of programmable pump; monitor closely during titration.
Benzodiazepines			
• Diazepam • Clonazepam	Inhibit polysynaptic afferent pathways.	Spasticity	Assess spasticity. Monitor vital signs during therapy. Assess risk of falls and implement fall prevention strategies. Monitor for psychological/physical dependence during long-term therapy.

Sources: Costello, K., Halper, J., Harris, C., & Kennedy, P. (2003). Multiple sclerosis treatment and the importance of early intervention [online]. *International Journal of MS Care.* Retrieved from http://www.mscare.org/cmsc/Journal-of-MS-Care.html; Food and Drug Administration. (2006). *Natalizumab (marketed as Tysabri) information.* Retrieved April 30, 2008, from http://www.fda.gov/cder/drug/infopage/natalizumab; Forest Pharmaceuticals. (2003). *Namenda (memanatine HCL)* [Package insert]. St. Louis: Author; Rizvi, S. A., & Agius, M. A. (2004). Current approved options for treating patients with multiple sclerosis. *Neurology, 63*(Suppl. 6), S8–S14.

designed to minimize these symptoms. In some cases, orthotic devices are used to prevent contractures and maintain proper body posture and alignment. Medications used to treat spasticity include baclofen, tizanidine, clonazepam, gabapentin, and diazepam (Lisak, 2001; Schapiro, 2003). In some cases, injections of botulinum toxin or implantation of an intrathecal baclofen pump may be necessary (Costello et al., 2003).

Bowel and bladder problems are common in MS. Bladder dysfunction can be classified as failure to store, failure to empty, or a combination of both conditions. Urinary tract infections, urinary urgency, incontinence, and dribbling are typical symptoms (Lisak, 2001; Schapiro, 2003). Medication management includes oxybutynin HCL (Ditropan), propantheline (Pro-Banthine), tolterodine (Detrol), and terazosin (Hytrin). Patients should be encouraged to avoid caffeine, alcohol, and other diuretics. Teaching the Kegel technique of contracting and holding the pubococcygeal muscle and the Credé technique of applying pressure to the lower abdomen to express urine may help patients adjust to retention and elimination anomalies. In cases of urinary retention, intermittent catheterization may be necessary. Patients should be instructed on correct straight catheterization technique and care. In some cases, a Foley or suprapubic catheter may be required (Lisak, 2001; Schapiro, 2003). The management of constipation and bowel incontinence is best served with the help of a dietitian familiar with the needs of the MS patient. Stressing a diet and hydration appropriate for the condition (see Chapter 14) along with moderate exercise is helpful (Lisak, 2001).

About half of the people with MS suffer from some form of cognitive impairment as a result of the disease. Although the symptoms vary, they are most likely to manifest as short-term memory deficits and attention difficulties. At times, the person's mental condition may worsen when tired, stressed, or exposed to hot weather. Many patients turn to list making, calendar keeping, and tape recording to aid them with memory lapses (Schapiro, 2003). As discussed in the Complementary and Alternative Therapies box, some therapies related to temperature control may be useful in relieving some of the symptoms of MS.

Gerontological Considerations

MS most often strikes young adults. There are comparatively few occurrences in older people. Those who have MS can expect to live an average life span (Schapiro, 2003).

Nursing Management

Nursing care needs of the patient with MS are multifaceted and complex, encompassing both inpatient and outpatient care. Symptom management is a major area of focus, with nursing care concentrating on nonpharmacologic management, patient education, and support. The nursing process can effectively help develop a plan of care, as outlined in the Nursing Process: Patient Care Plan for Multiple Sclerosis. Relevant nursing assessments, diagnoses, outcomes, and interventions in the care of the MS patient must be addressed.

Collaborative Management

The MS patient presents with a range of needs that are best addressed by a multidisciplinary team approach. Complicated medication regimens to prevent or treat relapses are managed by the neurology team including a neurologist, neuroscience nurses, and rehabilitation services. Physical therapists often participate in the rehabilitation efforts following relapse. They play a critical role in determining the need for mobility aids and design exercise regimes to combat fatigue and spasticity. Occupational therapy is important for developing energy conservation plans. Neuropsychologists may be called on to evaluate cognitive changes. Urologists may be consulted to manage bladder dysfunction common to MS. Issues related to self-esteem, body image, and interpersonal communication may be referred to a psychologist. Gynecologists or sexual therapists may be needed to address sexual dysfunction.

Discharge Priorities

Discharge priorities for patients with MS focus on adaptive strategies for them and their caretakers in the outpatient or home environment, as addressed in the Patient Teaching & Discharge Priorities box (p. 815).

Health Promotion

Like other chronic, degenerative, neurological conditions, physical and emotional stress can exacerbate the symptoms of MS. Patients should be instructed to avoid extreme temperatures and exposure to infections. Techniques to manage emotional stress should be emphasized.

Patients should be encouraged to engage in a regular exercise program and practice healthy eating habits. Exercise may help manage fatigue, spasticity, and bowel and bladder problems. Good nutrition can aid in resistance to infection. Increasing fluids and fiber is particularly useful for bladder problems and constipation (Lisak, 2001). A low-fat, high-fiber diet (see Chapter 14) should be recommended (NMSS, 2008).

The majority of MS cases occur in women of childbearing age, and the disease does not affect a women's ability to conceive or bear children (Giesser, 2003). However, symptoms such as

COMPLEMENTARY & ALTERNATIVE THERAPIES for Multiple Sclerosis

Heat is known to exacerbate symptoms of MS. A recent study showed that cooling suits may help improve fatigue, strength, and cognition when worn on a daily basis over a month (NASA/MS Study Group, 2003). Cooling suits, which cover the trunk and extremities, work by circulating a cooling liquid throughout the garment, which lowers body temperature and may improve conduction of nerve impulses in people with MS. Studies have not addressed the potential benefits of using passive cooling systems, such as ice packs (Rocky Mountain MS Center, 2003).

NURSING PROCESS: Patient Care Plan for Multiple Sclerosis

Assessment for Self-Care and Safety

Subjective Data:
Have you ever fallen?
Do you have double vision?
Do you have trouble sensing the temperature of water?

Objective Data:
Neurological status including muscle tone, gait, balance, vision, sensory perception

Nursing Assessment and Diagnoses	Outcomes and Evaluation Parameters	Planning and Interventions with *Rationales*
Nursing Diagnosis: *Risk of Injury* related to muscle weakness, ataxia, decreased sensory perception	**Outcome:** Patient remains free of injury. *Evaluation Parameters:* Demonstrates correct use of mobility aids. Practices safety measures to compensate for sensory losses.	**Interventions and *Rationales:*** Ambulate patient *to evaluate gait, ataxia, potential for falling.* Consult with physical therapist. *Can evaluate need for mobility assistive equipment.* Instruct on use of mobility aids such as cane, walker, or wheelchair *to help prevent injury, provide security, and increase independent movement.* Consult with occupational therapist. *Can provide instruction to compensate for sensory deficits while accomplishing ADLs.* Teach patient and caregivers safety measures to compensate for sensory loss, such as the use of a thermometer to test water temperature or the wearing of an eye patch to alleviate visual disturbance such as double vision. *Impaired sensory perception increases risk of injury.*

Assessment for Energy and Ability to Perform Own ADLs

Subjective Data:
How many hours per night do you sleep? Do you nap and if so, how often?
How many times do you get up during the night?
Are you or have you been feeling depressed?
Are you able to accomplish your usual activities during the course of a day?
Do you exercise?
Do you notice that you become very tired in hot temperatures?

Objective Data:
Neurological status including gait, coordination, and spasticity
Nutritional status including appetite and weight
Activity level including exercise/therapy
Medications

Nursing Assessment and Diagnoses	Outcomes and Evaluation Parameters	Planning and Interventions with *Rationales*
Nursing Diagnosis: *Fatigue* related to disease process	**Expected Outcomes:** Patient verbalizes increased energy. Patient is able to accomplish daily routines. *Evaluation Parameters:* Patient verbalizes understanding that fatigue is part of disease process. Patient practices prescribed energy conservation strategies. Patient uses prescribed assistive devices to accomplish ADLs. Patient verbalizes understanding that hot ambient temperatures worsen fatigue.	**Interventions and *Rationales:*** Discuss relationship of fatigue and disease process with patient and family; allow both to verbalize coping mechanisms. *Educates patient and family and assesses needs and coping strategies.* Provide rest periods between physical activity and activities of daily living *to minimize fatigue and conserve energy.* Teach patient and caregivers to avoid prolonged exposure to hot ambient temperatures, hot baths or showers. *Can trigger onset of fatigue.* Consult occupational therapist. *Can develop energy conservation plan, and assess need for and prescribe adaptive equipment to assist with ADLs, which helps to minimize fatigue.* Consult physical therapist. *Can develop light exercise regime, which may increase endurance and minimize fatigue.*

Assessment for Ability to Void Normally

Subjective Data:
How many times per day do you void?
Do you feel like your bladder empties completely?
Are there times when you cannot make it to the bathroom in time?
Do you have sudden urges to void?
Do you dribble in between voiding?
Is it hard to get started when voiding?
Do you have burning when you void?

Objective Data:
Intake and output
Voiding pattern
Bladder distention
Postvoid residual
Urine appearance/odor
Urinalysis, culture, sensitivity

(continued)

NURSING PROCESS: Patient Care Plan for Multiple Sclerosis—*Continued*

Nursing Assessment and Diagnoses	Outcomes and Evaluation Parameters	Planning and Interventions with *Rationales*
Nursing Diagnosis: *Impaired Urinary Elimination* related to spastic or flaccid bladder	**Outcomes:** Patient empties bladder completely by voiding and/or catheterizing. Patient remains free of urinary tract infection. *Evaluation Parameters:* Patient demonstrates correct techniques for bladder emptying. Patient is able to verbalize signs and symptoms of UTI.	**Nursing Interventions and *Rationales*:** Discuss voiding patterns with patient. Encourage patient to verbalize concerns. *Provides opportunity for patient to verbalize coping strategies and assesses voiding patterns.* Monitor voiding patterns *to establish baseline voiding patterns.* Assist patient to use the bathroom *to assess patient mobility status and ability to get to and from bathroom.* Assess for signs of urine retention including bladder distention, and urine overflow and intake greater than output. *Signs of retention.* Assess for signs of urinary tract infection. *Urinary retention and catheterization increase risk of infection.* Teach patient Credé maneuver. *Fully expresses urine from bladder for failure-to-empty difficulties, which decreases risk of infection.* Teach patient Kegel exercises. *Contracting and holding pubococcygeal muscle strengthens it, which helps improve failure-to-store problems.* Teach correct technique for prescribed bladder elimination: intermittent catheterization, suprapubic or indwelling catheter care. *Decreases risk of infection and ensures emptying of bladder.* Monitor medications for therapeutic and side effects *to aid in early detection of side effects or adverse reactions.*

Sources: Holloway, N. (2003). *Medical-surgical care planning* (4th ed.). Philadelphia: Lippincott Wilkins & Williams; Schapiro, R. (2003). *Managing the symptoms of multiple sclerosis* (4th ed.). New York: Demos.

urinary urgency and fatigue may flare during pregnancy and may require special management. The use of disease-modifying agents before and during pregnancy is an issue (Giesser, 2003), and patients will need education and counseling regarding treatment choices and recommendations during this time.

Amyotrophic Lateral Sclerosis

Amyotrophic lateral sclerosis (ALS) is a degenerative disease involving upper and lower motor neurons. Degeneration of motor neurons in the spinal cord, brainstem, and cerebral cortex leads to the characteristic symptoms of weakness, muscular atrophy, and spasticity. ALS, also known as Lou Gehrig's disease, is progressive, incurable, and fatal (Charles & Swash, 2001).

Epidemiology and Etiology

Approximately 20,000 Americans have ALS. Another 5,000 diagnoses are made each year (NINDS, 2008a). In the 1930s Lou Gehrig, a baseball player for the New York Yankees, was diagnosed with ALS, thus explaining why the disease is identified by his name in the United States. His celebrity has brought recognition to this disease in the way of public awareness and research funding. Estimates of prevalence rates range from 3 to 7 cases per 100,000 worldwide, making it one of the most common neuromuscular disorders (Borasio, Voltz, & Miller, 2001; Charles & Swash, 2001). The onset of ALS typically occurs between 40 and 60 years of age; however, it can affect younger and older people. It strikes men more often than women (NINDS, 2003a).

The cause of ALS is unknown. The excitatory neurotransmitter glutamate is believed to have a part in motor neuron degeneration (Charles & Swash, 2001). Other investigations have focused on autoimmune responses, environmental toxins, and infectious agents. Still, there is insufficient evidence to implicate any of these factors as causes of ALS (NINDS, 2003a). A genetic link to ALS is possible, as discussed in the Genetic Considerations box.

Pathophysiology

In ALS, degenerative changes occur in the anterior horn cells of the spinal cord, the motor nuclei of the brainstem, and the corticospinal tracts. Upper motor neuron degeneration leads to spasticity and reduced muscle strength, while lower motor neuron degeneration causes flaccid muscles, paralysis, and atrophy. Cognition, sensory function, vision, and hearing are spared. The bowel and bladder functions are not affected until the later stages of the disease (Borasio et al., 2001).

Clinical Manifestations

Subtle at the onset and slow in progression, the symptoms of ALS include painless muscle weakness and wasting, spasticity, cramping, fatigue, **fasciculation** (involuntary twitching) of the limb and tongue muscles, dysarthria, dysphagia, and dyspnea (Charles & Swash, 2001). Symptoms in an arm first present in roughly half of the cases, with about 20% of the occurrences affecting a leg. Initial complaints range from difficulty walking and problems with tripping and stumbling to trouble performing fine tasks

PATIENT TEACHING & DISCHARGE PRIORITIES for Multiple Sclerosis

Need	Teaching
Disease information: Patient/family	Contact the National Multiple Sclerosis Society (1-800-FIGHTMS). Disease progression is variable; some patients never become incapacitated. MS is rarely direct cause of death; expect fairly normal life span.
Medication information: Patient/family	Purpose, dosage, administration schedule. Correct technique for administering injectable medications. Administer on schedule. Expected side effects.
Exacerbating factors: Patient/family Setting	Mild fever worsens symptoms; take acetaminophen promptly for any fever-associated illness. Prevent infections; use hand hygiene, avoid exposure to infection; get flu shot. Avoid emotional stress, undue fatigue, and exertion. Avoid exposure to heat, include home temperature, hot baths, or showers. Use air conditioning in warm months.
Bladder management: Patient/family	Correct technique for: • Catheterization, if warranted • Credé maneuver • Kegel exercises. Call health care provider if signs/symptoms of UTI arise.
Relapse management: Patient/family	Report new or worsening symptoms to health care provider.
Safety: Patient/family	Use thermometer to track water temperature for bathing.
Health promotion: Patient/family	Mild exercise is beneficial, but do not exercise to point of fatigue. Consume high-fiber, low-fat diet. Adequate hydration.
Mobility: Patient/family Setting	Correct use of mobility aids. Ambulation and transfer techniques. Home evaluation for adaptive equipment needs.

Sources: Chaudhuri, A., & Behan, P.O. (2004). Multiple sclerosis is not an autoimmune disease. *Archives of Neurology, 61,* 1610–1612; Holloway, N. (2003). *Medical-surgical care planning* (4th ed.). Philadelphia: Lippincott Wilkins & Williams.

GENETIC CONSIDERATIONS Related to Amyotrophic Lateral Sclerosis

Genetic research has discovered a defect occurring on the gene responsible for the production of the enzyme superoxide dismutase 1 (SODI1) that may be linked to ALS. SODI1 is a powerful antioxidant that protects against free radicals, which are thought to play a role in cell degeneration. The role of the SODI1 gene mutation in motor neuron degeneration is unclear. The theory is that the malfunctioning gene allows for an excessive accumulation of free radicals.

Ninety to 95% of ALS cases are sporadic, while 5% to 10% are classified as familial. The SODI1 gene mutation accounts for approximately 20% of familial cases. Other familial forms involve mutations on the ALS2 gene, which also is implicated in the death of motor neurons.

Sources: Mitchell, J. D., & Borasio, G. D. (2007). Amyotrophic lateral sclerosis. *Lancet, 369,* 2031–2040; National Institutes of Health. (2003). *Genetics home reference: Amyotrophic lateral sclerosis.* Retrieved April 30, 2008, from http://ghr.nlm.nih.gov/condition=amyotrophiclateralsclerosis; National Institute of Neurological Disorders and Stroke. (2003a). *Amyotrophic lateral sclerosis fact sheet.* Retrieved April 2, 2008, from http://www.ninds.nih.gov/disorders/amyotrophiclateralsclerosis/detail_amyotrophiclateralsclerosis.htm.

such as buttoning clothing and writing (Charles & Swash, 2001; NINDS, 2003a).

As the disease progresses, weakness and atrophy extend throughout the muscles. The arms and legs become severely impaired. Muscles involved with speech and swallowing progressively deteriorate to the point of severe dysarthria and dysphagia (Borasio et al., 2001; Charles & Swash, 2001). Swallowing becomes difficult and increases the risk of aspirating food or saliva into the airway. Difficulties eating lead to weight loss. Because cognitive functions remain intact, patients are highly aware of the disease and its progression. Anxiety or depression is likely to complicate the condition (NINDS, 2003a). In the final stage, speaking is nearly impossible if at all. Acute dyspnea sets in and, eventually, a ventilator is required for breathing. Aspiration, infection, and respiratory failure are usually the ultimate causes of death. Average disease duration is 3 to 4 years (Borasio et al., 2001).

Laboratory and Diagnostic Procedures

Like other neurodegenerative diseases, there is no definitive test that will confirm the presence of ALS. Diagnosis is based on medical history, neurological examination, symptoms, and laboratory tests that rule out other metabolic conditions (NINDS, 2003a). Electromyography (EMG) may distinguish characteristic fibrillations that result from denervation, muscle wasting, and atrophy (Borasio et al., 2001). Brain and spinal MRI can detect structural lesions, herniated disks, or cervical spondylosis in the process of eliminating other conditions that mimic ALS symptoms. In the same manner, nerve conduction velocity (NCV) tests can discount peripheral neuropathy and myopathy (NINDS, 2003a). Several different tests are commonly used to aid in the diagnosis of ALS, as presented in the Diagnostic Tests box.

Medical Management

Like other neurodegenerative diseases, there is no cure for ALS. Medical treatment focuses on slowing the progression and on symptom management. Riluzole (Rilutek), a benzothiazole, is the only drug known to slow the progression of ALS (Mitchell & Borasio, 2007). The drug is thought to protect motor neurons by inhibiting glutamate production. Patients who respond well to riluzole delay the need for ventilatory support and lengthen their life expectancies by an average of 3 months (Mitchell & Borasio, 2007). While generally well tolerated, riluzole should be administered with strict monitoring of liver function. Dizziness, vertigo, and somnolence may result from taking the drug. Medications for symptom management may include diazepam or dantrolene for spasticity and quinine sulfate or baclofen for muscle cramping, as discussed in the Pharmacology Summary box for ALS, p. 817.

 CRITICAL ALERT *Patients taking riluzole should have periodic liver function tests to monitor for elevation of liver enzymes (American Society of Health-System Pharmacists, 2006).*

◼ Nursing Management

A home health care plan is critical for patients and families who will be in particular need of ongoing support and assistance in coping with a progressive and fatal illness. They will be faced with making difficult decisions regarding artificial feeding and ventilation. It is important that the choices be made prior to a crisis so that the individual's wishes regarding end of life are honored. Throughout this process, it is critical to respect cultural differences in the meaning of death and dying. Pertinent nursing assessments, diagnoses, assessment, outcomes, and interventions are all part of the nursing process, as outlined in the Nursing Process: Patient Care Plan for Amyotrophic Lateral Sclerosis (p. 818).

◼ Collaborative Management

Management of ALS requires a multidisciplinary approach to meet the needs of both the patient and family (Charles & Swash, 2001; Van den Berg, Kalmijn, Lindeman, Veldink, & de Visser, 2005). Treatment goals should focus on providing symptom relief and on preserving comfort and dignity, because disease progression renders the patient to a completely dependent state. In addition to the previously mentioned drug therapy, supportive care depends on a multidisciplinary approach as depicted below (Borasio et al., 2001; Charles & Swash, 2001):

- Physical therapists can conduct range-of-motion exercises that are used to combat spasticity. They also can recommend the use of orthopedic equipment such as walkers, wheelchairs, splints, and braces.

- Occupational therapists can suggest devices for performing the routine activities of eating, dressing, and bathing. Specialized eating utensils, shower chairs, and case-specific tools assist the patient in prolonging self-sufficiency. These therapists also teach energy conservation, which helps manage fatigue.

- Speech therapists can teach adaptive strategies and techniques to cope with the effects of dysarthria. They may adapt a computer-based communication system to compensate for loss of speech. In addition, these therapists can evaluate and, more importantly, monitor the patient's ability to swallow.

- Dietitians and nutritionists can assess dietary needs and modify the patient's meals to maintain nutrition and prevent aspiration. Inevitably, as the patient's condition deteriorates, the use of a gastrostomy tube will become an issue for both the patient and family.

- Respiratory therapists manage assistive ventilation based on periodic assessment of the patient's respiratory function. Respiratory therapy can be applied as intermittent positive pressure ventilation (IPPV) or bilevel positive airway pressure (BiPAP). The option of whether or not to apply mechanical ventilation will be a growing concern of both the patient and family.

- Social workers can assist with the social, emotional, and financial ramifications of ALS. Support groups, powers of attorney, living wills, financial assistance, and hospice services are areas where expertise in social services can help patients adjust to extremely difficult concerns.

- Spiritual counselors consistent with patient and family beliefs can help the patient and family accept and cope with inevitable death.

Discharge Priorities

The Patient Teaching & Discharge Priorities box (p. 819) covers a wide range of topics that apply to the patient with ALS.

DIAGNOSTIC TESTS for Amyotrophic Lateral Sclerosis

Test	Expected Result	Rationale
Electromyogram (EMG)	Fibrillations	May show signs of denervation, muscle wasting, and atrophy.
CPK level	May be elevated	Indicates breakdown of muscle tissue.
MRI brain and spine	Normal	Rule out conditions that could mimic symptoms of ALS.

Sources: Borasio, G. D., & Miller, R. G. (2001). Clinical characteristics and management of ALS. *Seminars in Neurology, 21,* 155–166; Muscular Dystrophy Association. (2003). *Facts about ALS.* Retrieved April 30, 2008, from http://www.als-mda.org/publications/fa-als.html; National Institute of Neurological Disorders and Stroke. (2003). *Multiple sclerosis: Hope through research.* Retrieved April 30, 2008, from http://www.ninds.nih.gov.

PHARMACOLOGY Summary of Medications to Treat ALS

Medication Category	Action	Application/ Indication	Nursing Responsibilities
Anti-ALS			
riluzole (Rilutek)	Slows progression of ALS by protecting motor neurons through inhibition of glutamate production.	Treatment of ALS	• Monitor for adverse effects: muscular weakness, dizziness, somnolence, nausea, diarrhea, decreased lung function. • Monitor liver function and blood count. • Be aware of multiple drug interactions; (theophylline, barbiturates, aminoglycosides and others). Monitor riluzole plasma levels and observe for hepatotoxicity. • Warn patient caffeine, cigarette smoking, high fat diet, and charcoal-broiled food affect riluzole level. • Give on an empty stomach.
Skeletal Muscle Relaxants			
centrally acting diazepam (Valium) baclofen (Kemstro, Lioresal)*	Relaxes skeletal muscle most likely by depressing afferent reflex activity at the level of the spinal cord.	Spasticity, muscle spasms	• Monitor for adverse effects: drowsiness, dizziness, weakness, confusion, hypotension, nausea, constipation. • Monitor for psychiatric disturbances, especially in elderly. • Monitor liver and kidney function, especially in elderly or if renal or hepatic disease present. • Warn patient to avoid alcohol and other CNS depressants. • Be aware abruptly stopping drug may result in adverse reactions. • Monitor diabetics for hyperglycemia.*
Peripherally Acting dantrolene (Dantrium)	Relaxes skeletal muscle by interfering with calcium ion release within muscle.	Spasticity	• Monitor for adverse effects: muscle weakness, slurred speech, fatigue, diarrhea, constipation. • Monitor blood count, liver and renal function. • Monitor for signs of pleural effusion and pericarditis in patients with cardiac disease, respiratory depression in patients with pulmonary dysfunction. • Warn patient not to use alcohol, check with health care provider before using OTC medications. • Warn patient about possible photosensitivity and need for sun block. • Teach patient symptoms of hepatitis. Notify health care provider if present.
Antimalarial quinine sulfate (Quinamm, Quiphile)	Reduces muscle cramping by direct action at the neuromuscular junction.	Muscle cramping	• Monitor for adverse effects: headache, sweating, tinnitus, vertigo, visual disturbances, vomiting, diarrhea, abdominal pain, cardiac arrhythmias. • Be aware of multiple drug interactions; monitor for toxicity or decreased drug efficacy (digoxin, antacids, warfarin, anticonvulsants, and others). • Give with food or milk.

Sources: Geriatrics, 61, 3–7; Mylan Bertek Pharmaceuticals. (2004). Apokyn [Package insert]; National Institutes of Health. (2003). *Genetics home reference: Amyotrophic lateral sclerosis.* Retrieved April 30, 2008, from http://ghr.nlm.nih.gov/condition=amyotrophiclateralsclerosis.

NURSING PROCESS: Patient Care Plan for Amyotrophic Lateral Sclerosis

Assessment for Comfort in Breathing

Subjective Data:
Do you feel comfortable?
Do you have a headache?
Do you feel tired?

Objective Data:
Neurological status including level of consciousness, cognition
Vital signs
Respiratory status, including respiration rate, pattern, lung sounds, accessory muscles, pulmonary function studies
Skin and nail bed color
Restlessness

Nursing Assessment and Diagnoses	Outcomes and Evaluation Parameters	Planning and Interventions with *Rationales*
Nursing Diagnosis: *Ineffective Breathing Pattern* related to neuromuscular dysfunction	**Outcome:** Patient receives ventilatory assistance to extent desired. ***Evaluation Parameter:*** Patient reports minimal respiratory discomfort.	**Interventions and *Rationales:*** Discuss wishes with patient and family. Consult with spiritual care. Record advance directives/patient wishes for ventilatory assistance in medical record. *Ensures that patient's wishes are met.* Assess respiratory rate and lung sounds q4h *to assess for respiratory distress.* Monitor pulmonary function studies and arterial blood gases as ordered *to assess adequacy of gas exchange.* Assess for morning headaches, restlessness, nightmares, or poor quality of sleep. *Indicates poor gas exchange with resultant brain hypoxia.* Assess skin and nail bed color. *Indicator of poor gas exchange with resultant tissue hypoxia.* Consult with respiratory therapist for noninvasive ventilatory device. *May be recommended if vital capacity is < 70%.*

Assessment for Ability to Swallow Foods and Liquids

Subjective Data:
Do you feel like you have trouble swallowing food or liquids?
Are you afraid of choking?

Objective Data:
Neurological assessment including swallowing and gag reflex
Vital signs
Respiratory status including rate and lung sounds
Choking on food or liquids
Tube feedings
Swallowing studies

Nursing Assessment and Diagnoses	Outcomes and Evaluation Parameters	Planning and Interventions with *Rationales*
Nursing Diagnosis: *High Risk for Aspiration* related to impaired swallowing muscles	**Outcome:** Patient does not show signs of aspiration. ***Evaluation Parameters:*** Patient is able to swallow food without choking or aspirating. Patient does not aspirate oral secretions. Lung sounds clear. No signs of infection.	**Interventions and *Rationales:*** Monitor for persistent coughing after swallowing liquids. *May indicate aspiration.* Consult with speech-language pathologist. *Can evaluate swallowing ability.* Consult with dietitian. *Can develop diet consistent with patient's swallowing abilities.* Administer and evaluate response to medications. *Medications may be given to dry oral secretions.* Discuss wishes regarding tube feedings with patient and family. Consult with spiritual care if needed. Record advance. directives/patient wishes for nutritional support in medical record *to ensure that patient's wishes are met.*

Assessment for Psychological and Spiritual Comfort

Subjective Data:
Do you have a spiritual counselor?
Has your family ever experienced loss and/or death?

Objective Data:
Patient/family interactions
Patient/family cultural background and religious preferences
Use of spiritual resources

NURSING PROCESS: Patient Care Plan for Amyotrophic Lateral Sclerosis—*Continued*

Nursing Assessment and Diagnoses	Outcomes and Evaluation Parameters	Planning and Interventions with *Rationales*
Nursing Diagnosis: *Anticipatory Grieving*, patient and family, related to fatal illness	**Outcome:** Patient and family move through the grieving process and come to terms with fatal illness. ***Evaluation Parameters:*** Patient and family use culturally appropriate coping mechanisms to deal with loss. Patient and family utilize spiritual resources to cope with pending death. Patient and family verbalize the grieving process and how it relates to their situation. Patient and family express feelings related to fatal illness. Patient and family attend support group. Patient and family formulate advance directives.	**Interventions and *Rationales:*** Discuss cultural beliefs with patient and family. *Provides knowledge of cultural beliefs that may influence the grieving process.* Provide patient and family opportunity to verbalize feelings related to prognosis *to help facilitate acceptance.* Encourage patient/family to consult with spiritual counselor consistent with culture and beliefs. *Can help facilitate acceptance and coping.* Encourage patient and family to attend appropriate support groups. *Such groups provide safe environment to express feelings.* Help patient and family become familiar with the grieving process *to help facilitate acceptance and coping.* Encourage patient and family to formulate advance directives. *Provides a sense of control and ensures that patient's wishes are met.*

Sources: Borasio, G. D., Voltz, R., & Miller, R. G. (2001). Palliative care in amyotrophic lateral sclerosis. *Neurologic Clinics, 19*(4), 829–845; Carter, G., & Miller, R. (1998). Comprehensive management of amyotrophic lateral sclerosis. *Physical Medicine and Rehabilitation Clinics of North America, 9*(1), 271–283; Charles, T., & Swash, M. (2001). Amyotrophic lateral sclerosis: Current understanding. *Journal of Neuroscience Nursing, 33,* 245–253.

PATIENT TEACHING & DISCHARGE PRIORITIES for Amyotrophic Lateral Sclerosis

Need	Teaching
Disease process: Patient/family	Disease symptoms and progression; fatal illness. Notify health care professional of increasing weakness, difficulty swallowing. Cognition is generally not affected by disease process. Contact the Muscular Dystrophy Association (1-800-572-1717; http://www.mdausa.org) or the ALS Association (1-800-782-4747; http://www.alsa.org) for educational materials.
Psychosocial: Patient/family	Encourage consultation with mental health professional. Encourage participation in support group.
Respiratory care: Patient/family	Correct use of respiratory equipment such as oxygen therapy, noninvasive ventilatory devices, and suction equipment. Guidelines for breathing: • Don't lie down after eating. • Avoid eating large meals. • Sleep with head elevated 15 to 30 degrees.
Communication: Patient/family	Develop alternative methods to communicate, such as blinking, if not able to speak.
Diet and oral care: Patient/family	Clean corners of mouth after eating. Soft diet as tolerated. Pureed foods should be placed on posterior tongue. Solid foods should be eaten slowly, in small pieces, and swallowed after every bite. Correct care of feeding tube if utilized.
Activity: Patient/family	Balance activity with rest periods. Mild low-impact aerobic exercise OK if able; do not exercise to exhaustion; stop if experiencing muscle cramping, heaviness in extremities, prolonged shortness of breath. Correct use of braces, splints, or other orthotic devices. Correct positioning and transfer techniques.
End-of-life issues: Patient/family	Need to make proactive decisions regarding mechanical ventilation, artificial hydration, and nutrition. Hospice services can help ensure comfortable death at home in accordance with patient and family wishes. Encourage spiritual guidance in accordance with patient, family, and cultural beliefs.

Sources: Borasio, G. D., Voltz, R., & Miller, R. G. (2001). Palliative care in amyotrophic lateral sclerosis. *Neurologic Clinics, 19*(4), 829–845; Carter, G., & Miller, R. (1998). Comprehensive management of amyotrophic lateral sclerosis. *Physical Medicine and Rehabilitation Clinics of North America, 9*(1), 271–283; Charles, T., & Swash, M. (2001). Amyotrophic lateral sclerosis: Current understanding. *Journal of Neuroscience Nursing, 33,* 245–253.

Health Promotion

People with ALS do maintain careers and interests. They are encouraged to remain active for as long as possible. Referral for psychological and/or spiritual counseling may help the patient and family come to terms with the disease and its prognosis. Many find support groups their most valuable asset in the struggle against the condition. Internet organizations also connect individuals who wish to communicate about the disease.

■ Myasthenia Gravis

Myasthenia gravis (MG) is a chronic, autoimmune neuromuscular disorder in which acetylcholine receptors at the neuromuscular junction are destroyed. The two major clinical forms of MG are ocular and generalized (Awwad & Maluf, 2007). The hallmark feature is fluctuating weakness and fatigability of voluntary muscles.

Epidemiology and Etiology

MG is a relatively uncommon disorder, with an annual incidence of 2 new cases per million people in the United States (Awwad & Maluf, 2007). It occurs at any age, although the age of onset is commonly either at 20 to 40 years of age for women or 60 to 80 years of age for men. Overall, the disorder is more common in women than in men, with a female-to-male ratio of 3:2 (Phillips, 2004).

Although the primary etiology remains speculative, there is increasing evidence that the thymus might play an important role. Histological studies have shown prominent germinal centers (Awwad & Maluf, 2007). Epithelial myoid cells normally present in the thymus do resemble skeletal muscle cells and possess acetylcholine receptor (AChR) on their surface membrane; therefore, it is hypothesized that they may become antigenic and set free an autoimmune attack of the muscular end plate AChR by molecular mimicry. Note also that the majority of people affected by MG also have thymus gland abnormalities. It remains unclear why the disease afflicts first and predominantly the extraocular muscles.

Pathophysiology

Muscle weakness in MG is the result of dysfunction at the neuromuscular junction. Acetylcholine (ACh) is a neurotransmitter vital for the transmission of nerve impulses to skeletal muscles, and it is produced in motor nerve endings. In MG, antibodies generated by an autoimmune response bind to AChRs, blocking the transmission of nerve impulses. This inefficient neuromuscular transmission together with the normally present presynaptic rundown phenomenon results in a decremental amount of nerve fibers being activated by successive nerve fiber impulses. This, then, accounts for the fatigability and characteristic muscular weakness of those with the disease (Augustus, 2000; Awwad & Maluf, 2007).

Clinical Manifestations

Usually the initial complaint is a specific muscle weakness rather than generalized muscle weakness. The severity of the weakness typically fluctuates over hours being least severe in the morning and worsening as the day progresses. It also varies over the course of weeks or months, with exacerbations and remissions. Exposure to sunlight, viral illness, surgery, immunization, emotional stress, menstruation, and physical factors might trigger or worsen exacerbations (Awwad & Maluf, 2007). As MG progresses, symptom-free periods decrease, and muscle weakness fluctuates from mild to severe (Keesey, 2004).

Symptoms are classified by some as ophthalmic and nonophthalmic. A majority of the patients initially complain of ocular disturbance, mainly ptosis and diplopia. Ptosis may be unilateral or bilateral and it may shift from eye to eye. Eventually 90% of patients with MG develop ocular symptoms. About 50% of patients present solely with ocular symptoms, and about 50% to 60% progress to develop generalized disease. Of the nonophthalmic symptoms, oropharyngeal muscle disturbances come second in presentation, with approximately 15% of patients first experiencing difficulty in swallowing, talking, and chewing (Awwad & Maluf, 2007).

MG can affect any skeletal muscle group, with 10% of patients initially complaining of limb and trunk weakness. Weakness in the bulbar muscles produces dysarthria and dysphagia, and a nasal quality to the voice. If facial muscles are involved, the patient may appear expressionless or impart a snarling expression when attempting to smile. Involvement of respiratory muscles may lead to symptoms of respiratory insufficiency, and even respiratory failure, an emergency known as **myasthenic crisis**. Patients also demonstrate incremental weakness upon repeating the motor power test over and over.

Patients with MG are at risk for two life-threatening situations with a similar clinical picture: myasthenic crisis and cholinergic crisis. The patient will present with extreme weakness and respiratory insufficiency. Myasthenic crisis is caused by undermedication (lack of acetylcholine) or stressors such as infection, surgery, or incompatible medications. The less common **cholinergic crisis** results from overmedication (excess acetylcholine). Both conditions are medical emergencies because they require mechanical ventilation (Augustus, 2000).

Laboratory and Diagnostic Procedures

MG is initially diagnosed through a detailed history and physical assessment, including a neurological examination. The Tensilon test may be administered, in which 2 mg of edrophonium chloride (Tensilon), a cholinesterase inhibitor with rapid onset and short duration of action, is administered intravenously at 30- to 60-second intervals up to a total of 10 mg. Patients with MG will demonstrate a distinct increase in muscle strength within 30 to 60 seconds. Administration of cholinergic drugs, however, may precipitate a cholinergic crisis, which is a life-threatening situation. Symptoms of cholinergic crisis include muscle weakness, cramps, difficulty talking, difficulty swallowing, bradycardia, bronchospasm, excessive salivation, vomiting, diarrhea and excessive sweating. A Tensilon test should not be administered without the ready availability of intravenous atropine, an antidote for edrophonium (Augustus, 2000; Hood, 1999).

Though not definitive, EMG may contribute to a diagnosis of MG. Repetitive nerve stimulation may be used to evaluate the decremental response in compound action potentials on EMG. A computerized tomography (CT) or MRI scan may be performed to evaluate the thymus gland and to rule out mass lesions compressing cranial nerves. Laboratory studies will include immunologic assays to detect AChR antibodies (Augustus, 2000). Thyroid function tests are indicated to rule out associated Graves' disease or hyperthyroidism. This is particularly essential in patients with ocular MG where the concomitant hyperthyroidism is most frequent.

Recently, the ice pack test (i.e., placing ice over the eyelid) has gained interest among ophthalmologists to assess improvement in ptosis and diplopia in ocular MG, the rationale being that cooling might improve neuromuscular transmission. This remains questionable by some (Awwad & Maluf, 2007; Larner, 2004), as they have demonstrated that patients with ocular MG actually improve on the ice, heat, and modified sleep tests. Hence, rest might be the cause of the improvement in ocular signs. Benatar & Kaminski, (2007) has countered that both the ice test and the rest test are sensitive and specific in ocular MG.

Medical Management

A wide range of treatments may be used for patients with MG. There is not, however, a consensus about which to start first or which to combine. According to Awwad and Maluf (2007), there is general agreement that medical treatment is administered best by a neurologist, and an ophthalmologist should follow up on the ophthalmic symptoms, such as diplopia and ptosis. Ptosis, when it becomes bothersome, is treated best by lid crutches; surgery is contraindicated because of the fluctuation of the disease. Diplopia is treated with the use of Fresnel prisms unless the deviation is large and variable, in which case an opaque lens over the affected eye is preferred.

Surgical treatment includes thymectomy, strabismus surgery, and blepharoptosis. Thymectomy may be performed in the absence of a thymoma. Approximately 85% of patients experience improvement, and 35% of these patients achieve drug-free remission. Patients often experience some transient worsening of symptoms early in the postoperative period, and improvement usually is delayed for months or years. Strabismus surgery may be used for selected patients with a stable course of MG. If a patient has stable ptosis, which has failed to respond to medical therapy, blepharoptosis may be performed.

Drug Therapy

The neurologist tends to coordinate the pharmacologic treatment. Cholinesterase inhibitors (neostigmine, pyridostigmine, or ambenonium) are used to treat the symptoms of MG by preventing the breakdown of acetylcholine at the neuromuscular junction. Pyridostigmine is the most commonly prescribed cholinesterase inhibitor, because it tends to have the least severe muscarinic side effects, including abdominal cramping, diarrhea, increased peristalsis, increased salivation, bradycardia, and blurred vision. Dosage is adjusted to manage the patient's symptoms (Augustus, 2000).

Patients with MG who remain symptomatic on cholinesterase inhibitors may require immunotherapy. Commonly prescribed immunotherapeutic drugs include corticosteroids, azathioprine, and cyclosporine (Saperstein & Barohn, 2004). Although administration of corticosteroids leads to marked improvement in the majority of patients, there may be an initial worsening of symptoms. For this reason, initiation of corticosteroids is reserved for hospitalized patients (Augustus, 2000).

The Pharmacology Summary discusses other drug therapies for myasthenia gravis (p. 822).

Plasmapheresis

Plasmapheresis may be used when a patient is in crisis or not adequately responding to other therapy. Circulating AChR antibodies are removed from the patient's circulation by removing whole blood, extracting the plasma from it, and returning the blood along with fresh or frozen plasma to the patient. The outpatient procedure is repeated three to four times over a period of 8 to 10 days (Augustus, 2000).

Intravenous Immunoglobulin Therapy

Intravenous immunoglobulin (IVIG) therapy is an alternative to plasmapheresis for treating the patient with MG who is experiencing increasing weakness. It may be used as preoperative treatment before thymectomy. Monthly courses of IVIG therapy may be administered until the slower immunotherapy approaches, such as corticosteroids, take effect. The mechanism of action for IVIG therapy is not certain (Saperstein & Barohn, 2004).

■ Nursing Management

Application of the nursing process will facilitate a comprehensive approach to patient care throughout the disease process. Relevant nursing diagnoses, assessment, outcomes, and interventions are all part of the nursing process.

Assessment

Nursing diagnoses for the patient with MG will depend on the muscles affected for each individual. A thorough history of disease onset and progression should be reviewed. Baseline data for respiratory function, bulbar function, and fatigue should be established, including (Augustus, 2000):

- Vital signs, with special attention to respiratory rate
- Breath sounds and breathing pattern
- Lung vital capacity
- Integrity of gag/swallow reflex
- Ability to chew and swallow
- Ability to see correctly without diplopia, ocular motility disturbance, or ptosis
- Ability to perform self-care activities.

Nursing Diagnoses

Possible diagnoses include (Augustus, 2000):

- *Ineffective Breathing Pattern* related to neuromuscular weakness
- *Alteration in Vision Acuity* related to ocular muscle involvement and ptosis
- *Imbalanced Nutrition: Less Than Body Requirements* related to dysphagia, bulbar weakness
- *Self-Care Deficit* related to weakness
- *Deficient Knowledge* related to disease process, medications, and/or energy conservation.

PHARMACOLOGY Summary of Medications to Treat Myasthenia Gravis

Medication Category	Action	Application/Indication	Nursing Responsibility
Cholinesterase Inhibitors neostigmine (Prostigmin) pyridostigmine (Mestinon) ambenonium (Mytelase) edrophonium chloride (Tensilon)	Increases strength of muscle contraction by preventing the breakdown of acetylcholine at the neuromuscular junction.	Symptomatic treatment of myasthenia gravis diagnosis of myasthenia gravis, differentiation between cholinergic and myasthenic crises (not recommended for maintenance therapy due to short duration of action)	• Monitor for adverse effects: abdominal cramping, nausea, vomiting, diarrhea, diaphoresis, blurred vision, bradycardia, hypotension, bronchospasm. • Monitor for cholinergic crisis. Assess vital signs, respiratory and neuromuscular function. Have atropine and resuscitation equipment immediately available for treatment. • Be aware of drug interactions (corticosteroids, aminoglycoside, antibiotics, and others).
Immunosuppressants azathioprine (Imuran) cyclosporine (Sandimmune, Neoral)	Suppresses immune response by inhibiting lymphocyte replication or disrupting helper T cells.	Treatment of myasthenia gravis	• Monitor for adverse effects: hirsutism, hypertension, nausea, vomiting, infection. • Observe for signs of toxicity: tremors, seizures, altered mental status, visual disturbances. • Monitor CBC, liver and renal function tests, *magnesium, *potassium, *blood sugar. • Be aware of multiple drug interactions (digoxin, NSAIDS, erythromycin, verapamil, cimetidine, and others with cyclosporine; allopurinal, ace inhibitors, warfarin, and others with azathioprine). Monitor for altered drug levels, nephrotoxicity, or leukopenia.
Corticosteroid prednisone	Reduces acetylcholine receptor antibody levels, may enhance neuromuscular transmission.	Myasthenia gravis immunosuppression	• Monitor for adverse effects: mood swings, anxiety, insomnia, nausea, vomiting, weight gain, acne, delayed wound healing. • Monitor clinical response to guide incremental dosing. • Observe for transient steroid induced exacerbation of MG with initiation of drug. • Monitor blood count, glucose, and electrolytes. • Be aware of drug interactions (theophylline, warfarin, and others). Monitor for toxicity or decreased efficacy. • Warn patient of potential need for dose adjustment if ill or stress increases and to not abruptly stop drug.

Planning

The overall goals of nursing care for the patient with MG are to minimize symptoms and to detect early signs of myasthenic or cholinergic crisis.

Outcomes and Evaluation Parameters

The outcomes and evaluation parameters are as follows (Augustus, 2000):

- Respiratory rate of 16 to 20 breaths per minute
- Vital capacity 4,600 mL
- Total lung capacity 5,800 mL
- Intact gag/cough reflex
- Able to read and establish visual field
- Heart rate of 60 to 100 beats per minute
- Weight maintained at baseline
- Patient/family verbalizes understanding of disease process, treatments, and signs of myasthenic or cholinergic crises.

In terms of evaluation parameters, the patient with MG will not show evidence of respiratory insufficiency. Weight will be at baseline. The patient will be able to independently complete ADLs and will verbalize an understanding of the disease process, treatment, and signs of myasthenic or cholinergic crisis.

Interventions and Rationales

Because respiratory muscles are often affected, the patient with MG should be monitored closely for signs of respiratory insufficiency that could indicate impending myasthenic crisis. MG often affects the bulbar muscles involved with chewing and swallowing, so ability to chew and swallow should be monitored closely. Other nutritional parameters such as weight, intake and output, electrolytes, and serum albumin should be monitored. The patient should be educated on energy conservation techniques, such as taking frequent rests when completing ADLs. Assistance with bathing and dressing may be needed.

Discharge Priorities

The importance of taking medications on time and as ordered should be emphasized. If bulbar muscles are affected, the patient should be instructed to eat and chew slowly and to match food consistency to the ability to swallow. Nutritional counseling may be necessary if optimal weight cannot be maintained. Caregivers should be instructed on the Heimlich maneuver technique. Patients should be taught measures to prevent respiratory infection, and to contact their health care provider immediately if signs or symptoms occur. Energy conservation strategies such as undertaking physical activities early in the day, and alternating activity with frequent rest periods should be emphasized. It is critical for the patient to know the signs and symptoms of crisis and to seek immediate help should they occur. The patient should also wear a medic alert bracelet and carry a card stating diagnosis, medication dose, and medication schedule (Augustus, 2000).

Research

Neurodegenerative conditions offer a plethora of opportunities for nursing research. These are summarized in the Research Opportunities feature.

EVIDENCE-BASED PRACTICE

Family Caregiver Assistance

Clinical Problem

It is estimated that there are more than 44 million family caregivers in the United States who provide 80% of home care to chronically ill older adults (Habermann & Davis, 2005; National Alliance for Caregiving, 2005). Family caregivers may provide a multitude of tasks in the daily care of their loved ones, from assisting with ADLs, to tasks requiring problem-solving skills and clinical judgment, such as managing symptoms and carrying out treatments as in medication regimes. In addition, family caregivers are often responsible for coordinating health care and social services (Schumacher, Beck, & Marren, 2006). Decades of research has confirmed that providing care to an older, chronically ill family member is stressful and can negatively affect family caregivers' physical and mental health (Schumacher et al., 2006).

While much of the current knowledge of family caregiving has been learned from studies of caregivers to individuals with AD (Habermann & Davis, 2005), further studies suggest that caregivers of individuals with other illnesses have similar negative physical and mental health outcomes. Nurses, particularly those who care for patients with neurodegenerative diseases, will encounter family caregivers in a variety of health care settings, and are often the primary source for family caregivers to learn how to provide care (Schumacher et al., 2006; Shyu, 2000).

Research Findings

Habermann and Davis (2005) conducted a study to compare the assistance needs of family caregivers for individuals with Alzheimer's disease and Parkinson's disease, with the overarching goal of exploring whether there is a core set of caregiver needs across illness groups. The authors opted to study the needs of caregivers of family members with the neurodegenerative diseases AD and PD. These conditions were selected because, although they have a similar downhill disease trajectory, each condition presents unique challenges for the family caregiver. Forty caregivers took part in the study; twenty of whom cared for a family member with AD, and twenty who cared for a family member with PD. The study participants participated in a semistructured, interview which included a self-scored caregiver needs assessment tool as well as open-ended questions addressing the challenges and satisfaction of caregiving. The caregiver needs assessment tool addressed needs in the following areas: (1) caregiving knowledge and skills, (2) finding and using community resources, and (3) accessing personal assistance. This sample of two groups of family caregivers agreed on 75% of these assistance needs. There was additional agreement between the two groups on the challenges of caregiving.

Implications for Nursing Practice

Although further research needs to be conducted regarding specific interventions to increase knowledge, skills, and self-care for caregivers, nurses should be cognizant that there may be common family caregiver needs and challenges across the span of neurodegenerative disorders. Specifically, family caregivers for individuals with AD and PD identified high needs for information about the illness as well as the need for practical training on how to provide care. When providing education and support to individuals with these conditions, nurses need to identify and include the family caregiver. Furthermore, caregivers need information about self-care for their own health promotion, and encouragement to pursue activities to support their own health and well-being.

Critical Thinking Questions

1. What are the important points that would be included in an education plan for patients and families with a neurodegenerative disorder such as AD or PD?

2. How might a nurse determine that a family caregiver understands education and information that has been provided in the plan of care?

3. What measures could nurses recommend to family caregivers to encourage self-care?

Answers to Critical Thinking Questions appear in Appendix D

References

Habermann, B., & Davis, L. L. (2005). Caring for family with Alzheimer's and Parkinson's disease: Needs, challenges and satisfactions. *Journal of Gerontological Nursing, 31,* 49–54.

National Alliance for Caregiving. (2005). *Caregiving in the U.S.* Bethesda, MD: Author.

Schumacher, K., Beck, C. A., & Marren, J. M. (2006). Family caregivers: Caring for older adults, working with their families. *American Journal of Nursing, 106,* 40–49.

Shyu, Y. L. (2000). Role tuning between caregiver and care receiver during discharge transition: an illustration of role function mode in Roy's adaptation theory. *Nursing Research Quarterly, 13*(4), 323–331.

RESEARCH OPPORTUNITIES AND CLINICAL IMPACT RELATED TO NEURODEGENERATIVE DISEASES

Research Area	Clinical Impact
Quality-of-Life (QOL) Research • Assessing domains of QOL. • Impact of disease progression on QOL. • Factors that mediate QOL. • Interventions that improve QOL. • Cultural implications for QOL.	Established domains of QOL. Improve interventions that enhance QOL in face of degenerative disease.
Patient/Family Education Research • Assessing the changing learning needs of patient/family throughout disease trajectory. • Efficacy of interventions to educate patient/family throughout disease trajectory. • Literacy levels of educational materials versus literacy levels of patient/family. • Use of multimedia educational interventions. • Use of Internet as patient/family education tool. • Factors influencing patient/family learning. • Cultural implications for patient/family education.	Proven interventions for effective patient/family education.
Caregiver Research • Changing education and support needs throughout disease trajectory. • Skill-building educational interventions. • Anticipatory grief. • Factors influencing positive and negative caregiver experience. • Barriers to accessing community resources. • Cultural implications of family caregiving.	Maintain family caregiver health.
Emotional and Psychological Research • Ambiguous loss. • Impact of role change. • Sexuality and intimacy issues. • Successful coping. • Factors that influence patients/families to seek mental health services.	Adaptation to progressing disability.
Complementary/Alternative Approach • Impact of meditation and prayer on disease management and experience. • Factors influencing patients and family members to seek alternative treatments.	Impact of complementary approaches on disease management and experience.

Clinical Preparation

Read
- History of Current Illness
- Past Medical History
- Physical Exam
- Admitting Medical Orders
- Laboratory Study Results

Document
- Summary of Hospitalization
- Pathophysiology Form
- Laboratory Values
- Laboratory Results Explanation

Apply
- List of Potential Nursing Diagnoses
- Concept Map
- Critical Thinking Questions

Log on to MyNursingKit.com to download forms you will need and to complete further steps in the Clinical Preparation assignment.

HISTORY OF PRESENT ILLNESS

You are the on-coming nurse receiving report on Mr. X, a 65-year-old male admitted with a diagnosis of Parkinson's disease (PD). Today he underwent surgery for unilateral deep brain stimulation (DBS) therapy. His surgery lasted approximately 5 hours. Mr. X was awake for the surgery that involved placement of the DBS lead, so he did not have general anesthesia. There were no complications during surgery. The implantable pulse generator (also called the battery or pacemaker) will be placed in 1 week in outpatient surgery. Thus, the leads are not yet generating electrical stimulation.

Medical–Surgical History

Mr. X has been diagnosed with PD for 10 years. His case of PD is staged as Hoehn and Yahr Stage III. He has had peak-dose dyskinesia for the past 3 years, as well as unpredictable on–off fluctuations. His medical and surgical history is negative otherwise. His medications include ropinirole, carbidopa/levodopa LA 50/200, amantadine, citalopram, and apomorphine injections prn. His medical history is significant for an appendectomy at 21 years of age.

Social History

Mr. X is a retired bank manager. He is married and has two adult children.

Physical Exam

Mr. X is sleepy but easily aroused and oriented to person, place, and time. His pupils are equal, round, and reactive to light at 4 mm. His speech is low and muffled, and slightly slurred. He is able to move all four extremities equally although movement is slow and stiff. He denies numbness and tingling in his extremities. He has pronounced tremor in his upper extremities. He denies nausea, and has been sipping on clear liquids with assistance. His abdomen is soft, with bowel sounds present in four quadrants. His lungs are clear. He has voided in a urinal standing at the bedside. He has not had a bowel movement. He has a heparin lock in his right forearm. Mr. X has a 1-cm wound at the top of the cranium. He took his anti-PD medications last evening, but has not had any today. Mr. X needs assistance to sit at the bedside, and is able to turn himself over in bed.

Admitting Medical Orders

Admit to Neurosurgical Floor, Neurosurgery Service
Diagnosis: Parkinson's disease, scheduled DBS surgery
Allergies: none noted
VS q4h
Neuro checks q1h × 4, then q2h × 2, then q4h
Ambulate with assistance
Bathroom privileges
I/O q shift
Diet: advance diet as tolerated
Call house officer: HR < 50 or > 120, systolic BP < 90 or > 160, temperature >38.5°C, RR < 10 or > 30, change in neuro status, urinary output < 240 mL in 8 hours, O_2 saturation < 92%
Saline lock with NS flushes q8h
Wound care: dry sterile dressing to scalp wound daily and prn; if drainage present, notify health care provider

Scheduled Medications

Ropinirole 4 mg po tid
Carbidopa/levodopa CR 50/200 po tid
Amantadine 100 mg po bid
Citalopram 40 mg po daily

PRN Medications

Apomorphine 0.2–0.4 ml sq q4h prn for muscle stiffness or lack of muscle control
Darvocet N-100 i-ii po q6h prn for pain, maximum 8 tabs/day

Ordered Laboratory Studies

CBC, Chem 7 panel, PT, PTT, and INR daily

Laboratory Findings

On admission, all lab values were WNL, including CBC, chemistry panel, and bleeding times.

LABORATORY STUDY RESULTS

Test	On Admission	Postop Day 1	Postop Day 2
Sodium	135 mEq/L	137 mEq/L	140 mEq/L
Potassium	3.5 mEq/L	3.7 mEq/L	3.7 mEq/L
Chloride	97 mEq/L	100 mEq/L	101 mEq/L
Carbon dioxide	22 mEq/L	23 mEq/L	24 mEq/L
Blood urea nitrogen (BUN)	22 mg/dL	23 mg/dL	25 mg/dL
Creatinine	1.3 mg/dL	1.3 mg/dL	1.2 mg/dL
Blood glucose	90 mg/dL	94 mg/dL	100 mg/dL
White blood cells	8000 µL	8200 µL	8200 µL
Hemoglobin	140 g/dL	13.5 g/dL	13.6 g/dL
Hematocrit	50%	53%	50%
Platelets	200,000 µL	210,000 µL	220,000 µL
Protime (PT)	12 seconds	12 seconds	13 seconds
Partial thromboplastin time (PTT)	60 seconds	62 seconds	65 seconds
International Normalized Ratio (INR)	2.0 INR	2.0 INR	2.5 INR

CRITICAL THINKING QUESTIONS

1. What are potential postop complications for which you would want to carefully assess?

2. As Mr. X restarts his oral anti-PD meds postop, what aspects of his neuro check would you carefully assess?

3. What are some of the psychosocial issues that you would assess Mr. X for?

4. If Mr. X requests an injection of Apomorphine, what would you assess before the injection?

Answers to Critical Thinking Questions appear in Appendix D.

NCLEX® REVIEW

1. A patient is demonstrating agnosia. The nurse realizes this impairment is characteristic of which of the following disorders?

1. Multiple sclerosis
2. Alzheimer's disease
3. Parkinson's disease
4. Myasthenia gravis

2. A patient is experiencing a disorder that is caused by demyelinating nerve fibers and plaque formation. The nurse realizes this patient is experiencing:

1. Alzheimer's disease.
2. Myasthenia gravis.
3. Multiple sclerosis.
4. Parkinson's disease.

3. The nurse is devising a plan of care for a patient with multiple sclerosis. Which of the following interventions should the nurse include to help reduce the incidence and frequency of fatigue?

1. Discuss voiding patterns.
2. Plan for a daily hot shower.
3. Minimize the use of assistive devices.
4. Instruct to avoid prolonged exposure to hot temperatures including showers, baths, and environmental temperatures.

4. The nurse is preparing a discharge plan of care for a patient with Parkinson's disease. Which of the following should be included to help the patient with constipation?

1. Restrict fluids.
2. Increase dietary fiber.
3. Take a laxative every evening.
4. Limit protein intake.

5. A patient with Alzheimer's disease is being cared for at home by her adult daughter. Which of the following should the nurse instruct the daughter to support health promotion needs?

1. Discuss advance directives for management of advanced stages of the disease.
2. Encourage getting involved in clinical research studies.
3. Instruct to avoid extreme temperatures and exposure to infections.
4. Refer for psychological and spiritual counseling.

6. A patient with Parkinson's disease tells the nurse that she's worried about her 80-year-old husband's ability to care for her as she gets older. Which of the following would be an appropriate response for the nurse to make to this patient?

   1. That's not something that you should be worried about.
   2. You are so healthy now that I'm sure you won't be a burden to your husband.
   3. Would you like to talk about things that can help you and your husband?
   4. I'll get the doctor for you so you can talk with him about your concerns.

7. The nurse is interested in research that focuses on complementary approaches to neurodegenerative diseases. Which of the following topics would the nurse find the most interesting?

   1. Interventions that improve quality of life
   2. Literacy levels of educational materials versus literacy levels of patient/family
   3. Anticipatory grief
   4. Impact of meditation and prayer on disease management and experience

Answers for review questions appear in Appendix D

KEY TERMS

acetylcholine *p.794*
Alzheimer's disease (AD) *p.788*
amyotrophic lateral sclerosis (ALS) *p.814*
ataxia *p.809*
bradykinesia *p.800*
cholinergic crisis *p.820*
dementia *p.788*
dopamine *p.798*
dyskinesia *p.801*
fasciculation *p.814*

glutamate *p.794*
hypokinetic dysarthria *p.800*
hypomimia *p.800*
hypophonia *p.800*
levodopa *p.801*
L'Hermite's sign *p.809*
micrographia *p.800*
mild cognitive impairment (MCI) *p.790*
multiple sclerosis (MS) *p.805*
myasthenia gravis *p.820*

myasthenic crisis *p.820*
myelin *p.809*
on–off phenomena *p.801*
paresthesias *p.805*
Parkinson's disease (PD) *p.796*
postural instability *p.800*
rigidity *p.800*
substantia nigra *p.798*
tau *p.788*

EXPLORE PEARSON mynursingkit™

MyNursingKit is your one stop for online chapter review materials and resources. Prepare for success with additional NCLEX®-style practice questions, interactive assignments and activities, web links, animations and videos, and more!

Register your access code from the front of your book at
www.mynursingkit.com

REFERENCES

Ahlskog, J. E. (2001). Parkinson's disease: Medical and surgical treatment. *Neurologic Clinics, 19*(3), 579–604.

Alzheimer's Association. (2004). *Fact sheet: Memantine (Namenda).* Chicago: Author.

Alzheimer's Foundation of America. (2006, November 17). Alzheimer's Foundation of America sets standard of excellence for dementia settings. *Medical News Today.* Retrieved April 14, 2008, from http://www.medicalnewstoday.com/articles/56912.php

American Academy of Neurology. (2006). Practice parameters: Parkinson disease diagnosis and treatment. *Journal Watch, 66,* 968–975.

American Psychiatric Association. (1994). *Diagnostic and statistical manual of mental disorders.* (4th Ed.). Washington, DC: Author.

American Society of Health-System Pharmacists (2006). *AHFS drug information.* Bethesda, MD: Author.

Augustus, L. (2000). Crisis: Myasthenia gravis. *American Journal of Nursing, 100,* 24AA–24HH.

Awwad, S., & Maluf, R. (2007). *Myasthenia gravis.* Retrieved April 11, 2008, from Emedicine website: http://www.emedicine.com/oph/topic263.htm

Benatar M., & Kaminski H. J. (2007). Evidence report: the medical treatment of ocular myasthenia (an evidence-based review): report of the Quality Standards Subcommittee of the American Academy of Neurology. *Neurology. 68*(24):2144–2149.

Borasio, G. D., Voltz, R., & Miller, R. G. (2001). Palliative care in amyotrophic lateral sclerosis. *Neurologic Clinics, 19*(4), 829–845.

Bowron, A. (2004). Practical considerations in the use of apomorphine injectable. *Neurology, 62*(Suppl. 4), S32–S36.

Bunting-Perry, L. (2006). Palliative care in Parkinson's disease: Implications for neuroscience nursing. *Journal of Neuroscience Nursing, 38,* 106–114.

Calne, S. M. (2003). The psychosocial impact of late-stage Parkinson's disease. *Journal of Neuroscience Nursing, 35*(6), 306–313.

Carter, J. H., Stewart, B. J., Archbold, P. G., Inoue, I., Jaglin, J., Lannon, M., et al. (1998). Living with a person who has Parkinson's disease: The spouse's perspective by stage of disease. *Movement Disorders, 13*(1), 20–28.

Charles, T., & Swash, M. (2001). Amyotrophic lateral sclerosis: Current understanding. *Journal of Neuroscience Nursing, 33,* 245–253.

Chaudhuri, A., & Behan, P. O. (2004). Multiple sclerosis is not an autoimmune disease. *Archives of Neurology, 61,* 1610–1612.

Costello, K., Halper, J., Harris, C., & Kennedy, P. (2003). Multiple sclerosis treatment and the importance of early intervention [online]. *International Journal of MS Care.* Retrieved from http://www.mscare.org/cmsc/Journal-of-MS-Care.html

Cummings, J. L., Frank, J. C., Cherry, D., Kohatsu, N. D., & Kemp, B. (2002a). Guidelines for managing Alzheimer's disease. Part I: Assessment. *American Family Physician, 65*(11), 2263–2272.

Cummings, J. L, Frank, J. C., Cherry, D., Kohatsu, N. D., & Kemp, B. (2002b). Guidelines for managing Alzheimer's disease. Part II: Treatment. *American Family Physician, 65*(11), 2263–2272.

Dawson, T. M., & Dawson, V. L. (2003). Molecular pathways of neurodegeneration in Parkinson's disease. *Science, 302,* 819–821.

DeKosky, S. T. (2003). Pathology and pathways of Alzheimer's disease with an update in new developments in treatment. *Journal of the American Geriatrics Society, 51,* S314–S320.

Desai, A. K., & Grossberg, G. T. (2005). Diagnosis and treatment of Alzheimer's disease. *Neurology, 64*(Suppl. 3), S34–S39.

Feldman, H. H., & Woodward, M. (2005). The staging and assessment of moderate to severe Alzheimer's disease. *Neurology, 65*(Suppl. 3), S10–S17.

Food and Drug Administration. (2003). *FDA approves memantine (Namenda) for Alzheimer's disease.* Retrieved April 30, 2008, from http://www.fda.gov/bbs/topics/NEWS/2003/NEW00961.html

Food and Drug Administration. (2006). *Natalizumab (marketed as Tysabri) information.* Retrieved April 30, 2008, from http://www.fda.gov/cder/drug/infopage/natalizumab/

Franklin, G. M., & Nelson, L. (2003). Environmental risk factors in multiple sclerosis: Causes, triggers and patient autonomy. *Neurology, 61,* 1032–1034.

Geldmacher, D. S. (2003). Alzheimer's disease: Current pharmacotherapy in the context of patient and family needs. *Journal of the American Geriatrics Society, 51,* S289–S295.

Giesser, B. (2003). *Reproductive issues in persons with multiple sclerosis.* Retrieved from http://www.nationalmssociety.org/download.aspx?id=168

Gleason, O. C. (2003). Delirium. *American Family Physician, 67,5,* 1027–34.

Hinton, L., Franz, C. E., Yeo, G., & Levkoff, S. E. (2005). Conceptions of dementia in a multiethnic sample of family caregivers. *Journal of the American Geriatrics Society, 53,* 1405–1409.

Holden, K. (2003). *Parkinson's disease: Guidelines for medical nutritional therapy for use by nutrition professionals.* Miami, FL: Five Star Living.

Holland, N. (2003). *Urinary dysfunction in multiple sclerosis.* Retrieved May 2, 2008, from http://www.nationalmssociety.org;pdf/forpros/Bladder.pdf

Hood, L. (1999). The Tensilon test. *American Journal of Nursing, 99*(5), 24HH, 24JJ– 24KK.

Jankovic, J. (2006). Therapeutic strategies in Parkinson's disease. *Geriatrics, 61,* 3–7.

Keesey, J. C. (2004). Clinical evaluation and management of myasthenia gravis. *Muscle Nerve, 29,* 2004.

Kurlowicz, L., & Wallace, M. (1999). The mini mental state examination (MMSE). *Best Practices in Nursing Care to Older Adults, 3.*

Larner, A. J. (2004). Case report: The place of the ice pack test in the diagnosis of myasthenia gravis. *International Journal of Clinical Practice, 58*(9), 887–888.

Leifer, B. P. (2003). Early diagnosis of Alzheimer's disease: Clinical and economic benefits. *Journal of the American Geriatrics Society, 51,* S281–S288.

Lisak, D. (2001). Overview of symptomatic management of multiple sclerosis. *Journal of Neuroscience Nursing, 33*(5), 224–230.

Mitchell, J. D., & Borasio, G. D. (2007). Amyotrophic lateral sclerosis. *Lancet, 369,* 2031–2040.

Mylan Bertek Pharmaceuticals. (2004). *Apokyn.* Package insert.

NASA/MS Cooling Study Group. (2003). A randomized, controlled study of acute and chronic effects of cooling therapy for MS. *Neurology, 60,* 12: 1955–1960.

National Institute on Aging, U.S. Nation Institutes of Health. (2007). Frontotemporal dementia connections reprint. Retrieved July 18, 2008 from http://www.nia.nih.gov/Alzheimers/Publications/FTDreprint.htm

National Institute of Neurological Disorders and Stroke. (2003). *Amyotrophic lateral sclerosis fact sheet.* Retrieved April 2, 2008, from http://www.ninds.nih.gov/disorders/amyotrophiclateralsclerosis/detail_amyotrophiclateralsclerosis.htm

National Institute of Neurological Disorders and Stroke. (2004). *The dementias: Hope through research.* Bethesda, MD: National Instititutes of Health.

National Institute of Neurological Disorders and Stroke. (2006). *Parkinson's disease: Hope through research.* Bethesda, MD: National Institutes of Health.

National Institute of Neurological Disorders and Stroke. (2008). *NINDS amyotrophic lateral sclerosis information page.* Retrieved May 7, 2008, from http://www.ninds.nih.gov/disorders/amyotrophiclateralsclerosis/amyotrophiclateralsclerosis.htm

National Institute of Neurological Disorders and Stroke. (2008). *Multiple sclerosis: hope through research.* Retrieved July 18, 2008 from http://www.ninds.nih.gov/disorders/mikltiple_scleerosis/detail_multiple_sclerosis.htm?css=...

National Multiple Sclerosis Society. (2008). *Just the facts 2006–2007.* Washington, DC: Author.

Nussbaum, R. L., & Ellis, C. E. (2003). Alzheimer's disease and Parkinson's disease. *New England Journal of Medicine, 348*(14), 1356–1364.

Nutt, J. G., & Wooten, G. F. (2005). Diagnosis and initial management of Parkinson's disease. *New England Journal of Medicine, 353,* 1021–1027.

O'Connor, P., & Canadian Multiple Sclerosis Working Group. (2002). Key issues in the diagnosis and treatment of multiple sclerosis: An overview. *Neurology, 59*(6), S1–S33.

Pahwa, R., Lyons, K., & Wilkinson, B. (2003). *Deep brain stimulation for Parkinson's disease: An update.* Retrieved January 23, 2004, from http://www.medscape.com/viewprogram/2274_pnt

Pahwa, R. A., Factor, S. E., Lyons, K. E., et al. (2006). Practice parameter: Treatment of Parkinson disease with motor fluctuations and dyskinesia (an evidence-based review). *Neurology, 66,* 983–1005.

Phillips, L. H. (2004). The epidemiology of myasthenia gravis. *Seminars in Neurology, 24,* 17.

Porth, C. M. P. (2007). *Essentials of pathophysiology: concepts of altered health status.* Philadelphia: Lippincott Williams & Wilkins.

Rocky Mountain MS Center (2003). *Cooling.* Retrieved April 30, 2008, from http://www.ms-cam.org

Saperstein, D. S., & Barohn, R. J. (2004). Management of myasthenia gravis. *Seminars in Neurology, 24*(1), 41–48.

Schapira, A. H. V. (2006). Etiology of Parkinson's disease. *Neurology, 66*(Suppl. 4).

Schapiro, R. (2003). *Managing the symptoms of multiple sclerosis* (4th ed.). New York: Demos.

Schultz, R., O'Brien, A. T., Bookwala, J., & Fleissner, K. (1995). Psychiatric and physical morbidity effects of dementia caregiving: Prevalence, correlates, and causes. *Gerontologist, 35,* 771–791.

Silverman, D. H., Small, G. W., Chang, C. Y., Lu, C. S., Kung de Aburto, M. A., et al. (2001). Positron emission tomography in evaluation of dementia: Regional brain metabolism and long-term outcome. *Journal of the American Medical Association, 286*(17), 2110–2127.

Suchowersky, O., Gronseth, G., Perlmutter, J., Reich, S., & Zesiewicz, T. (2006). Practice parameter: Neuroprotective strategies and alternative therapies for Parkinson disease (an evidence-based review). *Neurology, 66,* 976–982.

Susman, E. (2006). *AAN: New Parkinson's disease treatment guidelines issued.* Retrieved April 14, 2008, from http://www.medpagetoday.com/Neurology/ParkinsonsDisease/tb/3025

Tanner, C. M., Ottman, R., Goldman, S. M., Ellenberg, J., Chan, P., Mayeux, R., et al. (1999). Parkinson's disease in twins: An etiologic study. *Journal of the American Medical Association, 281*(4), 341–346.

Thomas, S., & MacMahon, D. (2004). Parkinson's disease, palliative care and older people: Part 1. *Nursing Older People, 16*(1), 22–27.

Van den Berg, J. P., Kalmijn, S., Lindeman, E., Veldink, J. H., & de Visser, M. (2005). Multidisciplinary ALS care improves quality of life in patients with ALS. *Neurology, 65,* 1264–1267.

Van Den Eeden, S. K., Tanner, C. M., Bernstein, A. L., Fross, R. D., Leimpeter, A., Bloch, D. A., et al. (2003). Incidence of Parkinson's disease: Variation by age, gender, and race/ethnicity. *American Journal of Epidemiology, 157*(11), 1015–1022.

Volcifer, L., & McKee, A. (2001). Dementia. *Neurologic Clinics, 19*(4), 867–883.

Caring for the Patient with Spinal Cord Injuries

Laurie Baker

Outcome-Based Learning Objectives

After studying this chapter, the learner will be able to:

1. Compare and contrast the most common causes of acute spinal cord injury in persons under the age of 65 as opposed to persons over the age of 65.

2. Differentiate between a complete and an incomplete spinal cord injury.

3. Explain three complications of spinal cord injury and strategies to prevent these complications.

4. Discuss the psychosocial impact of spinal cord injury on the patient and family.

5. Identify rehabilitative needs and goals for discharge for the patient who has experienced a spinal cord injury.

6. Select three nursing diagnoses and apply the nursing process in the care of the patient who has experienced a spinal cord injury.

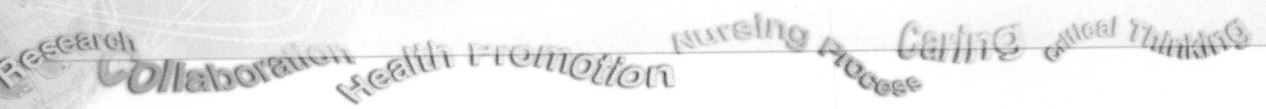

Research   Collaboration   Health Promotion   Nursing Process   Caring   Critical Thinking

SPINAL CORD injury may be caused by trauma, neoplasm, hemorrhage, infection, and even degenerative changes of the spine. Regardless of its etiology, spinal cord injury is a cause of major morbidity and disability. Treatment of this injury and its associated complications is very costly and is estimated to be in the billions of dollars in the United States (National Center for Injury Prevention and Control [NCIPC], 2006). People who have had a spinal cord injury not only experience the physical effects of this injury, but also face significant psychosocial impacts. Patients with spinal cord injury often are faced with major life changes including loss of lifestyle, independence, economic security, and body image.

Patients who have experienced a spinal cord injury can pose a significant challenge to nurses. There may be a profound physiological response as a result of this injury, which can affect all major body systems. The recovery from this injury is variable and can range from no discernible deficit to permanent, severe disability. Nurses caring for this population must have an understanding of the mechanisms of injury and subsequent sequelae, be able to perform an accurate neurological assessment, and institute appropriate interventions to optimize neurological function and avoid potential complications.

Spinal cord injury (SCI) occurs when a mechanical force is applied to the spinal cord, causing either a temporary or permanent loss of sensory, motor, or autonomic function below the level

of injury. The majority of SCIs occur because of trauma to the spinal column. Other traumatic injuries also may be present and can influence outcomes after this injury. Morbidity and mortality after SCI is generally affected by age at the time of injury as well as the level and severity of the injury. Persons of advanced age and those with severe injuries high in the spinal cord generally have higher mortality rates (McIlvoy, Meyer, & McQuillan, 2004).

Epidemiology

It is estimated that more than 200,000 persons are currently living with a SCI in the United States, and approximately 11,000 new cases of SCI occur each year. Young adults are primarily affected, with the majority of SCIs (approximately 78%) occurring among males. The average age at injury currently is 38 years and has been gradually increasing since the 1970s. The percentage of people over the age of 60 who have experienced a SCI has also increased from approximately 5% of the total number of cases in 1980 to 12% in 2000 (National Spinal Cord Injury Statistical Center [NSCISC], 2006). More than 50% of all SCIs occur in the cervical spine. The thoracolumbar juncture is the second most common site for injury because of the relative mobility of the spine at this level (Sekhon & Fehlings, 2001).

The average length of stay for those who are hospitalized in an acute care system that has expertise in treating SCIs is less than 3 weeks. The majority of these patients also will spend an average of 39 days in a rehabilitation facility. Persons with the most severe injuries will have longer lengths of stay. Most people will be discharged eventually to a home environment. The life expectancy for persons who survive at least 1 year after injury is dependent on age and severity of injury, but is steadily increasing. Younger patients with less severe injuries have the best survival rate, whereas older patients, those with severe injuries located high in the spinal cord, and those who are ventilator dependent have the least favorable survival rates (NSCISC, 2006).

Etiology

The vast majority of SCIs are the result of a traumatic event. The most common cause of SCIs in persons under the age of 65 is motor vehicle crashes. Falls rank as the most common cause of SCI in people over the age of 65. Sports and recreation-related SCIs are more likely to occur in people under the age of 30. Spinal cord injuries due to nontraumatic causes are more likely to occur in persons older than 40 years of age (NCIPC, 2006; Spinal Cord Injury Information Network [SCIIN], 2006).

Spinal Tumors

Less than 10% of SCIs are due to medical reasons such as neoplasm or hemorrhage from a vascular abnormality (NCIPC, 2006; SCIIN, 2006). Spinal tumors are broadly classified according to their location within the spine. More specific tumor classifications are based on histology. Intramedullary lesions describe neoplasms that arise from within the spinal cord itself. These types of tumors can cause dilation and distortion of the central portion of the spinal cord or they can infiltrate normal spinal cord tissue. The most common forms of intramedullary spinal cord tumors include ependymoma in adults and astrocytoma in children. Ependymomas are most commonly seen in the conus medullaris and cauda equina. Astrocytomas are most frequently seen in the cervical and thoracic regions of the spinal cord (Bloomer, Ackerman, & Bhatia, 2006; Henson, 2001).

Intradural/extramedullary lesions describe neoplasms that arise between the dura and the spinal cord. These lesions tend to cause compression but do not invade the neural tissue. Schwannoma and meningioma are the most common intradural/extramedullary spinal tumors. Schwannomas can be found anywhere in the spine, but there is a slightly higher incidence in the thoracic spine. Meningiomas are seen most frequently in females after the age of 40 and have a higher incidence of occurring in the thoracic spine (Bloomer et al., 2006).

Extradural lesions, or neoplasms that occur outside of the dural covering of the spinal cord, are the most common form of spinal tumors. The majority of these tumors involve the bony structures of the spine, such as the vertebral bodies, and are metastatic in nature. These tumors cause destruction and weakening of the bone, resulting in spinal instability and collapse. Mass effect from the tumor also may cause compression of the spinal cord. Lung cancer is the most common spinal metastatic lesion followed by breast cancer. Other cancers that commonly metastasize to the spine include myeloma, prostate, and lymphoma (Bloomer et al., 2006).

Pathophysiology

To fully understand the pathophysiology associated with spinal cord injury, it is critical to understand the anatomy and physiology related to the spinal cord. The spinal cord extends from the first cervical vertebra to approximately the first lumbar vertebra in the adult. The spinal nerves exit the spinal cord in pairs. Each nerve has two roots, an anterior or ventral root and a posterior or dorsal root. The anterior root connects to the anterior portion of the spinal cord and contains **efferent** motor fibers, which carry motor information from the brain to the body. The posterior nerve root attaches to the posterior spinal cord and contains **afferent** sensory fibers, which carry sensory information from the body to the spinal cord (Figure 32–1 ■). The spinal cord then transmits this information to the brain (Hickey, 2003a; Mulnard, 2001).

The spinal cord is divided into segments according to region and groups of nerves (Figure 32–2 ■, p. 832). The segments are numbered according to the level of the vertebral column. For example, C_3 denotes the third cervical pair of nerves and the third cervical segment of the spinal column. The spinal cord tapers as it passes through the thoracic region and ends at the conus medullaris at approximately the first lumbar vertebra. Below this is the cauda equina. The cauda equina is comprised of the lumbar and sacral nerve roots as they arise from the conus medullaris (Mulnard, 2001).

A cross section of the spinal cord reveals the gray matter, shaped like an "H" or butterfly, in the center of the cord surrounded by white matter (Figure 32–3 ■, p. 832). The gray matter of the spinal cord contains unmyelinated cells such as the axons and dendrites. It is divided into the anterior (ventral), the posterior (dorsal), and the lateral columns or horns. The lateral columns of the gray matter extend only from T_1 to L_2 or L_3. The motor fibers of the anterior nerve roots originate in the ventral and lateral columns of the gray matter. The posterior columns of the gray matter receive sensory input from the dorsal nerve roots (Hickey, 2003a; Mulnard, 2001).

The white matter serves to link the separate segments of the spinal cord and to link the spinal cord to the brain. It is comprised of ascending and descending tracts that contain mostly myelinated nerve fibers. These tracts are organized into anterior, posterior, and lateral columns. The ascending tracts contain primarily sensory fibers, whereas the descending tracts contain

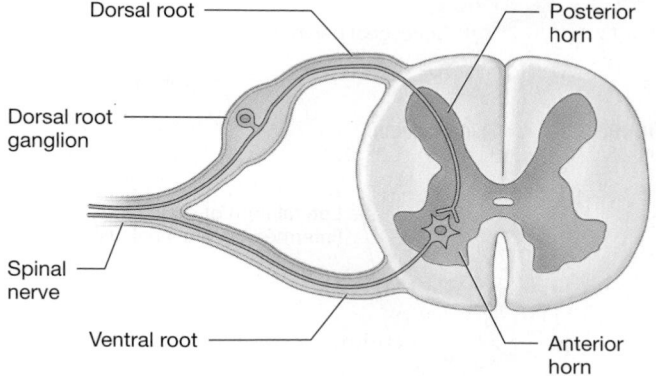

FIGURE 32–1 ■ Ventral and dorsal nerve roots.
Source: Lindsay, K. W. & Bone, I. (2004). Localised neurological disease and its management: peripheral nerves and muscles. In *Neurology and Neurosurgery Illustrated,* 4th Edition

Base of skull

Cervical enlargement

Lumbar enlargement

Internal terminal filum (pial part)

External terminal filum (dural part)

C₁ spinal nerve exits above C₁ vertebra

C₈ spinal nerve exits below C₇ vertebra (there are 8 cervical nerves but only 7 cervical vertebrae)

Conus medullaris (termination of spinal cord)

Cauda equina

Sacrum

Termination of dural sac

Coccygeal nerve

Coccyx

FIGURE 32–2 ■ Spinal column.

Lateral horn of gray matter (intermediolateral nucleus)

T2

FIGURE 32–3 ■ Cross section of the thoracic spinal cord.

primarily motor fibers. The ascending tracts in the anterolateral columns of the white matter are responsible for the conveyance of pain and temperature sensations to the brain. Afferent impulses enter the spinal cord from the dorsal nerve roots. These impulses then cross the midline of the spinal cord to the contralateral side. From here, the impulses travel up the spinal cord to the thalamus. Injury involving the anterolateral columns will result in loss of pain and temperature sensation on the opposite side of the body below the level of the injury. Proprioception includes the sense of position and movement. The ascending tracts responsible for the conveyance of proprioception lie in the dorsal columns of the white matter. These tracts do not cross the spinal cord, but ascend on the same or ipsilateral side to the medulla. Injury involving the ascending tracts in the dorsal column will result in loss of proprioception below the level of injury on the same side. The descending tracts are responsible for motor function and are located in the anterior columns of the white matter. These tracts do not cross in the spinal cord (Connelly, 2001).

The main vessels that provide the blood supply to the spinal cord include the anterior and posterior spinal arteries. These arteries run along the length of the spinal cord and have several vascular feeders. The anterior spinal artery arises from the vertebral arteries and lies along the midline of the anterior surface of the spinal cord. This vessel perfuses the anterior two-thirds of the spinal cord including the anterior and part of the posterior portions of the gray matter. It has a relatively poor collateral blood supply and is therefore susceptible to vascular disease or injury. The posterior spinal arteries are paired arteries that are located laterally on each side of the posterior aspect of the spinal cord. These arteries form a plexus on the posterior aspect of the spinal cord and have a rich collateral blood supply. As a result, the posterior aspect of the spinal cord is less susceptible to vascular disease or injury. The upper cervical spinal cord also is perfused by a plexus of vessels formed by the vertebral and subclavian vessels. The blood supply of the midthoracic region of the spinal cord is augmented by branches of the intercostal artery. The lower portion of the thoracic spinal cord and the conus medullaris receive additional perfusion from the artery of Adamkiewicz. The sacral arteries supply perfusion to the sacrum and cauda equina (Lindsay & Bone, 2004).

Classification

Spinal cord injuries are classified according to the degree of loss of motor and sensory function below the level of injury. Rehabilitation goals and degree of independence after recovery are dependent on the type of SCI.

Complete Spinal Cord Injury

A **complete spinal cord injury** indicates complete loss of voluntary motor and sensory functions below the level of injury. Injuries involving the cervical spinal cord will result in **tetraplegia** (a Greek term; **quadriplegia** is the Latin term) or loss of motor and sensory function involving both upper extremities, both lower extremities, bowel, and bladder. Injuries involving the thoracic or lumbar spinal cord will result in **paraplegia** or loss of motor and sensory function in both of the lower extremities, bowel, and bladder (Chart 32–1). The damage to the spinal cord in this type of injury is irreversible.

| CHART 32–1 | Functional Loss After Complete Spinal Cord Injury | | | |

Level of Injury	Motor Function	Deep Tendon Reflexes	Sensory Function	Bowel and Bladder Function
C_1–C_4	Tetraplegia (quadriplegia) *Lost:* All motor function below the neck	All reflexes lost	*Lost:* All sensation from the neck down	Lost
C_5	Tetraplegia (quadriplegia) *Lost:* All function below the shoulders *Intact:* Sternocleidomastoid Cervical paraspinal muscles Trapezius	C_5, C_6 Biceps	*Lost:* Sensation below the clavicles Most of the arms Hands Chest Abdomen Lower extremities *Intact:* Sensation to head Shoulders Deltoid Clavicle Lateral aspect of the forearm	Lost
C_6	Tetraplegia (quadriplegia) *Lost:* All function below the shoulders and upper arms *Intact:* Deltoid Biceps Rotator muscles of the shoulder	C_5, C_6 Brachioradialis	*Lost:* Sensation below the clavicles Chest Abdomen Lower extremities *Intact:* Sensation to the head Shoulders Arms Palms of hands Thumbs	Lost
C_7	Tetraplegia (quadriplegia) *Lost:* Function in portions of the hands and arms *Intact:* Shoulder depressors Shoulder abductors Shoulder internal rotators Radial wrist extensors	C_7, C_8 Triceps	*Lost:* Sensation below the clavicles Chest Abdomen Lower extremities *Intact:* Sensation to the head Shoulders Most of the arms and hands	Lost
C_8	Tetraplegia (quadriplegia) *Lost:* Function in portions of the hands and arms *Intact:* Elbow extensors Wrist Finger extensors and flexors		*Lost:* Sensation below the chest Portions of the hands *Intact:* Sensation to the head Shoulders Part of the upper chest	Lost
T_1–T_6	Paraplegia *Lost:* Function below the midchest including the muscles of the trunk *Intact:* Shoulders Upper chest Arms Hands		*Lost:* Sensation below the midchest *Intact:* Everything above the midchest T_1, T_2 provide sensation to the inner arm T_4 provides sensation to the nipple area	Lost

(continued)

CHART 32–1	Functional Loss After Complete Spinal Cord Injury—*Continued*			
Level of Injury	**Motor Function**	**Deep Tendon Reflexes**	**Sensory Function**	**Bowel and Bladder Function**
T₆–T₁₂	Paraplegia *Lost:* Function below the waist *Intact:* Shoulders Arms Hands Long trunk muscles		*Lost:* Sensation below the waist *Intact:* Shoulders Arms Hands T₁₀ provides sensation to the umbilicus T₁₂ provides sensation to the groin	Lost
L₁–L₃	Paraplegia *Lost:* Most control of the legs and pelvis *Intact:* Shoulders Arms Hands Torso Hip rotation	L₂–L₄ Knee jerk	*Lost:* Lower abdomen Legs *Intact:* Some sensation to the inner and anterior thigh L₃ supplies the knee	Lost
L₃–L₄	Paraplegia *Lost:* Portions of the lower legs Ankles Feet *Intact:* Increased knee extension		*Lost:* Sensation to portions of the lower legs Ankles Feet *Intact:* Sensation to the upper legs	Lost
L₄–S₅	Incomplete paraplegia *L₄–S₁:* Abduction and internal rotation of the hip Ankle dorsiflexion Foot inversion *L5–S₁:* Foot inversion *L₄–S₂:* Foot eversion *S₁–S₂:* Plantar flexion *S₂–S₅:* Bowel and bladder control	S₁–S₂ Ankle jerk	*L₅:* Medial aspect of the foot *S₁:* Lateral aspect of the foot *S₂:* Posterior aspect of the thigh/calf *Lower sacral nerves:* Perineum	Possibly spared *S₂–S₄:* Urinary control *S₃–S₅:* Bowel control

Source: Adapted from Hickey, J. V. (Ed.). (2003). *The clinical practice of neurological and neurosurgical nursing* (5th ed., pp. 424–425). Philadelphia: Lippincott Williams & Wilkins.

Incomplete Spinal Cord Injury

Patients who have experienced an **incomplete spinal cord injury** will have some preservation of sensory and/or motor function below the level of injury. In these patients, there is sparing of some of the spinal cord tracts, which allows neurotransmission to occur. Five main syndromes are associated with incomplete SCI, each classified according to the portion of the spinal cord damaged and the preservation of function below the level of injury (Figure 32–4 ■) (McIlvoy et al., 2004).

Central Cord Syndrome

Central cord syndrome is the most common incomplete SCI. This injury can occur at any age, but is seen most frequently in older patients who have degenerative bony changes in the cervical spine resulting in narrowing of the overall diameter of the spinal canal (Kirschblum & O'Connor, 2000). It most often is

(a) **(b)** **(c)**

FIGURE 32–4 ■ Incomplete spinal cord injury. a) Central cord syndrome b) Anterior cord syndrome c) Brown & Sequard syndrome.
Source: Hickey, J. (2003). Vertebral and spinal cord injuries. In J. Hickey, *The Clinical Practice of Neurological and Neurosurgical Nursing*, 5th edition, p. 419. Philadelphia, PA: Lippincott/Williams and Wilkins. p. 427. Philadelphia, Pa: Elsevier

caused by a hyperextension injury resulting in damage to the center of the spinal cord. The spinal tracts in the cervical spinal cord are arranged so that the fibers leading to the upper extremities are more centrally located, whereas the fibers leading to the lower extremities are located more laterally. Therefore, there is greater loss of motor and sensory function in the upper extremities than in the lower extremities. Bladder dysfunction is variable (Hickey, 2003b). The overall prognosis for recovery from this injury is generally favorable; however, patients older than 50 years of age have the least favorable prognosis (McIlvoy et al., 2004). The typical pattern of recovery is return of lower extremity function first followed by return of bladder function. Recovery of hand intrinsic function is variable and often the last to return (Kirschblum & O'Connor, 2000).

Anterior Cord Syndrome

Anterior cord syndrome is caused by direct injury to the anterior portion of the spinal cord or disruption of the anterior spinal artery resulting in ischemia and infarction of the anterior two-thirds of the spinal cord (McIlvoy et al., 2004). This is often due to compression from either an acute disk herniation or from a hyperextension injury resulting in fracture-dislocation of the vertebra. Paralysis and loss of pain and temperature sensation are evident below the level of injury. Light touch, vibration, and proprioception are preserved because these tracts are located in the dorsal columns of the spinal cord, which are perfused by the posterior spinal arteries. The prognosis for recovery from this injury is variable, although generally not favorable (Hickey, 2003a; Kirschblum & O'Connor, 2000).

Brown-Séquard Syndrome

Brown-Séquard syndrome occurs usually as a result of a penetrating injury causing transverse hemisection of the spinal cord. This injury accounts for less than 4% of all spinal cord injuries and is rarely seen in its pure form (McIlvoy et al., 2004). Paralysis and loss of proprioception are seen on the ipsilateral side of the injury, and pain and temperature sensation are lost on the contralateral side. The spinal tracts responsible for motor and proprioception do not cross the spinal cord as they travel to the brain; however, the spinal tracts responsible for the conveyance of pain and temperature do cross to the opposite side of the cord (Hickey, 2003a). Functional recovery from this type of injury is variable, although it can be quite favorable (Kirschblum & O'Connor, 2000).

Cauda Equina Syndrome

Compression of the lumbar nerve roots below the level of L_1 can result in **cauda equina syndrome**. This is most commonly seen with large disk herniations at the L_4/L_5 level that cause mass effect on the nerve roots as they descend through the spinal canal. The deficits related to this syndrome are variable depending on specific nerve root involvement, but can involve motor and sensory functions of the pelvic organs and lower extremities. Weakness, sensory deficits, loss of the Achilles reflex, and bowel and bladder dysfunction including bowel incontinence, urinary retention, and overflow urinary incontinence can be seen. Recovery is variable (Hickey, 2003b; McIlvoy et al., 2004).

Spinal Cord Injury Without Radiographic Abnormality

Spinal cord injury without radiographic abnormality (SCIWORA) is defined as spinal cord injury following a traumatic event without signs of fracture, dislocation, or ligamentous injury on plain radiographs, computed tomography (CT), or myelography. This phenomenon was first described in older patients with spondylitic changes of the cervical spine who developed central cord injury or acute **myelopathy** resulting in changes in sensory, motor, and reflex functions after experiencing a hyperextension injury. These patients had no evidence of spinal fracture or dislocation on radiographic evaluation, but were noted to have significantly narrowed spinal canals due to the degenerative changes of the spinal column common in **spondylitic disease** (Kothari, Freeman, Grevitt, & Kerslak, 2000).

This injury pattern also has been described in patients under the age of 16 years. Anatomic and biomechanical characteristics of the immature pediatric spinal column allow it to be hypermobile, increasing the stress on the spinal cord, predisposing it to injury particularly in flexion-extension type mechanisms (Pang & Wilberger, 1982). Magnetic resonance imaging (MRI) provides good imaging of the soft tissue structures of the spinal column including the intervertebral disks, ligaments, and spinal cord itself. Patients who have experienced a SCIWORA type injury often will demonstrate abnormality of the soft tissue structures or spinal cord on MRI that is not evident on standard radiography (Hendy, Wolfson, Mower, & Hoffman, 2002).

Primary Mechanisms of Injury

Regardless of the etiology of SCI, there are five common primary mechanisms of injury including hyperflexion, hyperextension, rotation, compression, and penetrating injury. Each of these mechanisms of injury is related to the type of mechanical force that is applied to the spinal column.

- **Hyperflexion injuries** occur when there is a sudden deceleration in motion such as can occur in a head-on motor vehicle collision or diving accident. As a result, the head and neck are flexed forward in an exaggerated motion. This can result in fracture of the anterior portion of the vertebral body as well as fracture and dislocation of the facets in the posterior aspect of the spinal column. The posterior spinal ligament and the intervertebral disk also may be disrupted (Figure 32–5 ■). The facet joints and the ligaments are important structures in maintaining the stability of the spine. If

Fracture of the vertebral body and disruption of the posterior ligamentous structures.

FIGURE 32–5 ■ Flexion injury.

these structures are compromised, the spine will be unstable and surgical stabilization of the spine may be required. The presence of fracture and dislocation of the facet joints increases the probability of injury to the spinal cord.

- Hyperextension injuries occur when the spine is extended backward as can occur in rear-impact collisions when the head and neck are forcefully extended back, or in forward falls in which the chin or forehead is struck. The spinal cord can be stretched and degenerative changes of the spinal column including the presence of bone spurs and hypertrophy of the ligaments can cause excessive compression of the spinal cord resulting in a SCI. Injury to the ligaments may not be evident and dislocations are relatively uncommon. Fractures involving the posterior elements of the spinal column including the spinous processes may be present (Figure 32–6 ■).

- **Rotational injuries** occur when there is extreme lateral flexion or rotation and flexion of the spine (Figure 32–7 ■). This injury occurs most commonly in the neck because of the relative mobility of the spine in this region. The posterior ligaments may rupture and fracture and dislocation of the facets may occur, resulting in spinal instability. If the facets on both sides of the spine are affected, the incidence of SCI is in-

creased. The fracture and dislocation may need to be reduced with application of traction, and the spine will need to be surgically stabilized.

- **Compression injuries** occur because of axial pressure or loading of the spine. A vertical force is applied to the spine causing fracture of the vertebral body (Figure 32–8 ■). These injuries typically occur as a result of landing on the feet or buttocks after a fall from a significant height or from extreme flexion of the spine (Figure 32–9 ■). A compression fracture also can occur because of weakening of the vertebral body due to infection, malignancy, or osteoporosis. Bone fragments from the fracture can cause compression or mass effect on the spinal cord. These injuries may require decompression of the spinal canal and stabilization of the spine.

- Penetrating injuries occur as a result of a projectile such as a bullet or sharp object entering the spinal column. The spinal

Compression fracture of vertebral body by axial loading forces.

FIGURE 32–8 ■ Compression fracture.

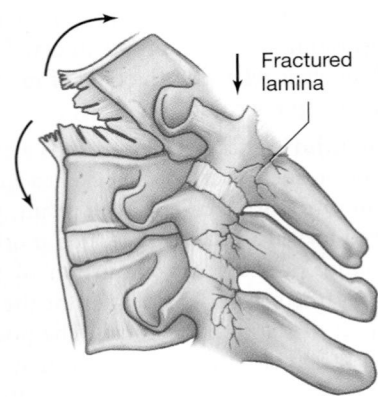

Intervertebral disc and fracturing of the lamina caused by distraction/compression forces.

FIGURE 32–6 ■ Hyperextension injury.

Comminuted fracture of the vertebral body.

FIGURE 32–7 ■ Rotational injury.

FIGURE 32–9 ■ CT scan of thoracic spine compression fracture.
Source: Laurie Baker

cord can suffer a **contusion** (bruising) or even a partial or complete **transection** (severing of the cord). Damage to the bony structures of the spine can also occur resulting in bone fragments in the spinal canal, which can cause additional compression of the spinal cord. The degree of injury to the spinal cord is related to the velocity of the object as it enters the spinal canal.

Types of Injury

The spinal cord may sustain one or a combination of several types of injuries as a result of the above mechanisms of injury:

- **Concussion**—Usually occurs as a result of a blow to the spinal column. The spinal cord is jarred or shaken. A temporary loss of function can be seen for a period of hours or days.

- **Contusion**—Often caused by fracture, dislocation, or direct trauma to the spinal cord. The spinal cord is bruised, resulting in hemorrhage and edema into the cord. Necrosis of spinal cord tissue may occur because of compression from bleeding or edema or because of direct damage of neural tissue. The degree of neurological dysfunction is dependent on the severity of the contusion.

- **Compression**—Occurs as a result of squeezing or pressure on the spinal cord. The pressure can last momentarily as in a hyperextension injury or can be prolonged because of mass effect from bone fragments, neoplasm, hemorrhage, or disk herniation (Figure 32–10 ■). The spinal cord may also suffer contusion, concussion, laceration, or transection as a result.

- **Laceration**—A tear or cut in the spinal cord. Neurological deficits resulting from this type of injury are permanent.

- **Transection**—Severing of the spinal cord.

- **Hemorrhage**—Bleeding that can occur either within the spinal cord or the surrounding tissues. This can result in compression on the spinal cord or irritation to the neural tissues.

FIGURE 32–10 ■ CT axial view of thoracic spine fracture with bone fragments in the canal.
Source: Laurie Baker

- **Infarction**—Ischemia of the spinal cord as a result of interruption of blood flow. This type of injury can occur because of compression or injury to the vessels that perfuse the cord.

Primary Injury

The initial insult to the spinal cord at the time of trauma is known as the primary injury. The spinal cord suffers physical damage as a result of this insult. The degree of damage to the spinal cord is dependent on the amount of force applied to the cord at the time of the initial injury and may range from mild cord concussion resulting in a transient loss of function to severe injury resulting in complete and permanent loss of function. As a result of the initial trauma, the neural elements of the spinal cord, including nerve cells and the ascending and descending spinal tracks, will be disrupted at the level of the injury. The vasculature of the spinal cord also can be affected, resulting in hemorrhage and ischemia of the spinal cord (Kwon, Tetzlaff, Grauer, Beiner, & Vaccaro, 2004; McIlvoy et al., 2004).

Spinal shock is a state of **areflexia** in which there is a loss of all motor, sensory, and reflex activity at the level of the injury and below. Spinal shock occurs as a result of the primary injury. The duration of spinal shock is quite variable, lasting as little as a few hours or as long as several weeks after injury. During this state, it is impossible to determine the extent of the SCI. As spinal shock abates, signs of muscle spasticity and **hyperreflexia** (exaggeration of the deep tendon reflexes) become evident. The return of the perianal reflexes indicates the resolution of spinal shock (Hickey, 2003a; McIlvoy et al., 2004).

Secondary Injury

The initial or primary SCI sets forth a cascade of complex events that can worsen the extent of the injury by causing damage to the adjoining neural tissues. The exact mechanism of this injury is not entirely understood, but many of the current treatment strategies for SCI are directed at reducing the damage caused by this secondary process. The secondary process begins almost immediately after the initial trauma to the spinal cord. Ischemia within the spinal cord at the time of the primary injury leads to additional vascular changes, which worsen the disruption of the normal perfusion of the spinal cord (Kwon et al., 2004). As a result of these vascular changes, cell membrane permeability is affected due to dysfunction of the cellular sodium-potassium pump (see Chapter 18 ☺). Intracellular potassium is depleted and sodium and calcium ions enter into the cell, resulting in cellular edema and subsequent cell death. The increased intracellular calcium triggers the release of enzymes and free radicals, which worsens cellular necrosis and leads to additional tissue damage. An inflammatory response is triggered, resulting in increased vascular permeability, edema, and macrophage activity leading to additional tissue damage and glial scarring (Hickey, 2003a; McIlvoy et al., 2004).

Disruption of autonomic regulation occurs as a result of SCI and can lead to **neurogenic shock**. This is a phenomenon most commonly seen in patients who have had a SCI at T_6 or above and should be differentiated from spinal shock. Spinal shock results in the loss of sensorimotor control and loss of the muscle stretch and cutaneous reflexes below the level of the injury. Neurogenic shock results in the disruption of the sympathetic nervous system. The sympathetic nervous system originates in the thoracolumbar region of the spinal cord and is responsible for elevations in heart rate and blood pressure and for vasoconstriction of the peripheral vascular system during stress situations. Neurogenic shock occurs when the normal impulses from the brainstem, which contribute to the reflexive control of heart rate and blood pressure, are disrupted, resulting in interruption of normal sympathetic outflow. Vagal tone is, therefore, left unopposed (Hickey, 2003a). As a result, bradycardia, peripheral vasodilation below the level of injury resulting in decreased systemic vascular resistance, hypotension, and decreased cardiac output are evident. The resulting hypotension and diminished cardiac output are thought to contribute to ischemia of the spinal cord at the site of injury.

The trauma patient who also is suspected of having a SCI may also experience hypovolemic shock. It is important to distinguish between neurogenic shock and hypovolemic shock in order to ensure that appropriate treatment strategies are implemented. Hypotension is a hallmark sign for both neurogenic shock and hypovolemic shock. The patient experiencing neurogenic shock will exhibit bradycardia with a heart rate of 50 to 70 beats per minute and will often require vasopressor support for treatment. The patient's skin also will be warm and hyperemic. The patient who has hypovolemia will exhibit tachycardia and will usually respond to volume replacement (McIlvoy et al., 2004).

Autonomic Hyperreflexia

Autonomic hyperreflexia occurs as a result of a noxious stimulus below the level of the SCI. Common causes include urinary tract abnormalities such as a distended bladder, abnormalities of the lower intestinal tract such as constipation or fecal impaction, and pressure ulcers. As a result of the noxious stimulus, a sympathetic response is triggered, resulting in vasoconstriction below the level of the SCI. Blood volume is shifted from the vasculature below the SCI to the vasculature above the injury, causing elevation of blood pressure. The baroreceptors in the carotid body and the aortic arch stimulate the vasomotor center of the medulla, which in turn triggers slowing of the heart and vasodilation. The vasculature above the level of injury responds, resulting in flushing of the skin, piloerection, and nasal congestion; however, these impulses are blocked at the level of the SCI and vasoconstriction continues unchecked below the level of injury. This response will continue until the noxious stimulus is removed (Hickey, 2003a; Krassioukov, 2004; McIlvoy et al., 2004; National Guideline Clearinghouse, 2001).

CRITICAL ALERT *It is easy to confuse neurogenic shock and hypovolemic shock in the trauma patient with SCI. Both conditions may be present concomitantly and will manifest with hypotension, but an important distinction is bradycardia. Patients experiencing neurogenic shock will exhibit bradycardia, whereas tachycardia is most often associated with hypovolemia. Patients with neurogenic shock will also exhibit warm, hyperemic skin due to vasodilation. Atropine to increase the heart rate and vasopressor support will be necessary to treat the patient in neurogenic shock.*

■ Clinical Manifestations

The clinical manifestations of spinal cord injury assume a systemic effect. The injury can affect the function of multiple organ systems depending on the level and severity of the injury. It is vi-

tal that nurses caring for this population understand the systemic effects of SCI so that appropriate assessment and interventions can be undertaken to avoid potential medical complications.

Cardiovascular

Neurogenic shock resulting in cardiovascular compromise is most evident in the patient who has sustained a SCI at T_6 or above. Sympathetic innervation is lost leaving vagal tone unopposed. Bradycardia, peripheral vasodilation below the level of injury, decreased systemic vascular resistance, and hypotension are seen. Cardiac preload and afterload subsequently are decreased resulting in decreased cardiac output (see Chapters 37 and 42 ☉). The use of atropine to increase the heart rate and vasopressors such as dopamine or dobutamine may be required to increase the heart rate, promote vasoconstriction, and increase cardiac output (Hickey, 2003a; McIlvoy et al., 2004).

Orthostatic hypotension also may be problematic for this patient population. The loss of sympathetic vascular tone results in blood pooling in the abdomen and lower extremities and a loss of arteriole vasomotor control. Prolonged immobility and decreased intravascular volume also are contributing factors. The patient experiences a drop in blood pressure when placed in an upright position and may complain of dizziness, light-headedness, visual disturbance, or syncope because of diminished blood supply to the brain, a phenomenon referred to as orthostatic hypotension. If this phenomenon if left unchecked, cerebral ischemia is possible (Hickey, 2003a; McIlvoy et al., 2004).

Pooling of blood in the peripheral vascular system, flaccidity of the extremities, and immobility predispose the patient with SCI to the development of venous thrombosis. This condition, if left untreated, could lead to the more serious complication of pulmonary embolus. The risk of development of deep venous thrombosis (DVT) seems to be highest in the first 2 to 3 months after injury (Apuzzo, 2002b). Patients may initially be asymptomatic unless they have some preservation of sensation. Signs of DVT include the presence of low-grade fever, edema in the affected limb, or change in temperature of the affected limb. If patients have sensory sparing, they may complain of pain and tenderness of the site (Hickey, 2003b; McIlvoy et al., 2004).

If signs of DVT are identified, additional testing is required. Venography is the "gold standard" for diagnosing DVT, but it is an invasive procedure and has associated risks, therefore it is rarely used. Duplex Doppler ultrasound screening is most frequently used to evaluate for DVT. This test has a high sensitivity for detecting DVT and carries a low risk to the patient. If a DVT is diagnosed, treatment with anticoagulant therapy should be instituted. Placement of an intravascular filter to prevent migration of the blood clot to the lungs also may be warranted. National guidelines for prevention of thromboembolism after spinal cord injury have been established (see the National Guidelines box).

Pulmonary embolus (PE) is a potentially life-threatening condition. A decline in oxygen saturation may be the only sign of PE; however, other symptoms may include chest pain or dyspnea. If any of these signs are evident and a PE is suspected, additional evaluation such as helical CT scan of the chest should be obtained immediately. Once diagnosed, treatment of PE is supportive with the administration of oxygen therapy and anticoagulation (Apuzzo, 2002c; National Guideline Clearinghouse, 2005b).

NATIONAL GUIDELINES for Prevention of Thromboembolism After Spinal Cord Injury

Risk Factor	Guideline
DVT	Assessment:

Obtain history that could add to the increased risk of DVT after spinal cord injury:

- Age over 40
- Obesity
- Estrogen therapy
- Malignancy
- Congestive heart failure
- History of tobacco use
- Concomitant injuries, specifically fractures of the lower limb
- Previous history of DVT.

Perform physical assessment twice daily and inspect all extremities for signs of DVT:

- Increased circumference of calf or thigh
- Pain, tenderness of the affected extremity
- Low-grade fever of unknown origin
- Erythema of the extremity.

Prophylaxis:

Prophylactic measures should be instituted within 72 hours of injury unless there is a medical contraindication. If application of mechanical prophylactic devices is delayed for >72 hours, the presence of lower extremity DVT should be ruled out prior to employing the following devices:

- Compression stockings
- External pneumatic compression devices
- Anticoagulation with either low-molecular-weight heparin or unfractionated heparin
- Initiation of early mobilization or passive range-of-motion exercises once the patient is medically and surgically stable.

If DVT Is Suspected:

Duplex ultrasound should be obtained of the affected extremity.

Placement of vena cava filter to decrease the risk of development of PE.

Source: National Guideline Clearinghouse. (2005). *Prevention of thromboembolism in spinal cord injury.* Washington, DC: Consortium for Spinal Cord Medicine, Paralyzed Veterans of America. Retrieved April 29, 2008, from http://www.guideline.gov/summary/summary.aspx?doc_id=2965&nbr=002191&string=spinal+AND+cord+AND+injury.

 Pulmonary embolus is a life-threatening disorder that can result in death if not recognized and treated promptly. Common signs and symptoms include decrease in oxygen saturation, shortness of breath, and chest pain. If the patient exhibits any of these symptoms, the managing medical team should be notified immediately.

Pulmonary

Patients who have sustained a SCI above T_{12} have potential for impairment of respiratory function. The degree of this impairment is dependent on the level of injury. Generally, higher level injuries have more significant impairment (McIlvoy et al., 2004). Atelectasis and pneumonia are common complications after SCI regardless of the involved spinal level and also can contribute to decompensation in respiratory function.

The diaphragm receives innervation from the phrenic nerve, which arises above C_5. The diaphragm is responsible for inspiration and deep breathing as well as the initiation of an effective cough. Injuries at C_4 or higher will cause paralysis of the diaphragm, necessitating intubation and ventilation (Hickey, 2003b). Patients who have experienced injuries involving the lower cervical spine, thoracic spine, or lumbar spine usually will not require immediate intubation, but warrant close monitoring for signs of respiratory decompensation because of loss of use of the respiratory accessory muscles. The intercostal and abdominal muscles that aid inspiration, forced expiration, and cough are innervated by the T_1–T_{12} nerves. Loss of use of these accessory muscles will result in a decrease of about 70% of forced vital capacity and maximal inspiratory force in the acute period following SCI (Ball, 2001; McIlvoy et al., 2004).

Gastrointestinal

Gastrointestinal effects of spinal shock include gastroparesis, loss of intestinal peristalsis, and ileus. The resulting abdominal distention places the patient at risk for vomiting and aspiration and also may interfere with respiratory function. Placement of a nasogastric or oral gastric tube will be necessary in the acute phase of SCI for decompression of the stomach and minimization of these risks (Prendergast & Sullivan, 2000).

Patients with SCI also are at risk for gastric stress ulceration. Loss of sensation to the visceral organs, especially in patients with high-level injuries, may interfere with the ability of these patients to feel gastric pain. This may delay early identification of gastric ulceration, which, in turn, will delay appropriate treatment and increase the risk of gastric hemorrhage. A prophylactic medication regimen should be instituted in all SCI patients (Prendergast & Sullivan, 2000).

Patients with SCI will experience abnormalities in both sensory and motor function of the bowel due to disruption of the spinal tracts responsible for bowel control. Generally, patients with injury above T_{12} will experience decreased intestinal peristalsis, absent rectal sensation, and an increase in anal sphincter tone. Anal reflex activity may be preserved. These patients are prone to chronic constipation. Patients with injury at or below L_1 will experience loss of tone throughout the colon and rectal sphincters. These patients are more likely to experience bowel incontinence (Enck, Greving, Klosterhalfen, & Wietek, 2006; Hickey, 2003a).

Genitourinary

The spinal tracts responsible for bladder control also are disrupted in SCI, resulting in loss of the normal bladder reflexes and control of urination. As a result, the bladder becomes atonic and the patient experiences urinary retention and bladder distention. Urinary incontinence may occur as the result of overflow of urine from a distended bladder into the urethra. Overdistension of the bladder can cause impairment of the blood supply to the bladder and reflux of urine into the ureters and kidney because of the increased bladder pressures. These patients are at risk for complications such as urinary tract infection (UTI), hydronephrosis, decline in renal function, and the development of renal calculi. In some cases of incomplete SCI, bladder function may return after recovery of spinal shock. It is important to assess postvoid residuals in these patients to ensure adequate bladder emptying (Hickey, 2003a; Pataki, Woodhouse, Hamid, Shah, & Craggs, 2006).

Integumentary

Patients with SCI are at high risk for development of pressure ulcers because of impairment in sensory and motor functions as well as impairment of tissue perfusion due to hypotension and pooling of blood in the lower extremities. Once these wounds develop, they can be very difficult to heal and can increase the risk of infection. Factors that contribute to the development of pressure ulcers in this population also include fever, infection, poor nutrition, and prolonged immobilization on the firm spinal board used to maintain optimal spinal alignment during transport to the hospital. Prevention is the best strategy to deal with pressure ulcers.

 Autonomic hyperreflexia is a medical emergency that could lead to serious complications if left untreated. When the patient exhibits symptoms of autonomic hyperreflexia, it is important to institute measures to treat the blood pressure and to identify and correct the cause.

■ General Evaluation and Management

Evaluation and management of SCI begins at the scene of the trauma and is carried throughout the acute care hospitalization and rehabilitation phases. Early assessment and management are vital for determining the extent of injury and minimization of secondary injury to the spinal cord. Acute care assessment

and management are directed toward optimizing neurological function and avoidance of early complications. Rehabilitative management and evaluation focus on adaptation and avoidance of long-term complications.

Prehospital

Expert evaluation and management of the trauma victim at the scene can make a difference in the victim's ultimate neurological outcome. Improper mobilization of the trauma victim with an unrecognized, unstable spinal fracture can worsen or even cause injury to the spinal cord. Impairment of respiratory and circulatory function also can worsen SCI. First responders follow the general principles of trauma management including rapid assessment of the victim, evaluation and management of the ABCs (airway–breathing–circulation), stabilization and control of life-threatening injuries, and rapid transport to an appropriate facility for continuation of care.

Spinal precautions are methods of immobilizing the spine and moving patients to prevent or avoid additional spinal injury. Spinal precautions are initiated at the scene of the trauma and are carried out until spinal injury has been ruled out or appropriate treatment strategies have been implemented. Immobilization of the entire spine is necessary because 20% of patients with a spinal injury have injuries at more than one spinal level (Apuzzo, 2002a). Spinal precautions usually are implemented in any trauma patient; however, determination of the mechanism of injury at the scene can prove invaluable in helping to identify potential injuries. Victims of a traumatic event with a significant mechanism of injury have a greater risk for multiple organ injuries and neurological injuries. First responders should have a high suspicion of spinal injury in any victim with multiple injuries, complaint of spinal pain, spinal deformity, or abnormality on sensory and/or motor examination. Also, those victims who have sustained head injury, experienced loss of consciousness, have an altered mental status, have complaint of motor or sensory disturbance at the scene, or are under the influence of drugs or alcohol warrant careful handling until a spinal injury can be definitively ruled out (Apuzzo, 2002a; Hickey, 2003a).

Spinal precautions can be initiated with the patient in an upright position if necessary until extrication and movement to a long back board is possible. A rigid cervical collar is applied and the patient is log rolled onto a back board in the supine position with the spine in a neutral position. Sandbags or blocks are placed on both sides of the head to prevent lateral rotation of the neck. The head is then secured to the back board utilizing tape or straps across the forehead to limit neck flexion. The patient also will be secured to the board utilizing appropriately placed straps.

Pediatric patients pose a special challenge in positioning because of their relatively large sized head. These patients require padding under the torso in order to prevent flexion of the neck. Elderly patients also may also warrant special consideration with positioning due to arthritic changes of the spine affecting spinal alignment. All patients require vigilant monitoring of airway and respiratory function. Immobilization on a back board can contribute to respiratory impairment because forced vital capacity is decreased by 20%. If respiratory function deteriorates and the patient requires ventilatory support, care must be taken to ensure spinal alignment is maintained (Apuzzo, 2002c; Bernbeck & Delamarter, 2000).

Emergency Department

Once the patient arrives in the emergency department, a complete survey of injuries and continued stabilization of the patient will continue while spinal precautions are maintained. A baseline assessment of the patient's physical and neurological status as well as information pertaining to the trauma and the patient's past medical history will be obtained. Efforts should be made to expedite diagnostic testing to facilitate early identification of spinal cord compression or spinal instability so that appropriate surgical measures can be taken if needed or restrictive protective equipment can be removed if not required. After the initial assessment and diagnostic evaluation is complete and the treatment plan established, the patient should be removed from the back board to avoid additional complications related to prolonged immobilization.

Initial Assessment

Evaluation of pulmonary and circulatory function will take precedence in the trauma patient. The patient should be assessed and monitored for adequacy of respiratory efforts and ventilatory function. All patients should receive supplemental oxygen and have oxygenation monitored continuously with pulse oximetry. A baseline arterial blood gas (ABG) should be obtained. Lung sounds should be assessed on admission and repeated periodically. The patient with SCI may initially present with adequate respiratory function but can quickly deteriorate. Apnea, stridorous respirations, use of accessory muscles, rapid, shallow respirations, and decline of oxygen saturation are indicative of inadequate respiratory efforts. Ventilatory support should be considered if the patient exhibits signs of inadequate respiratory function. If intubation is necessary, care should be taken to ensure the spine remains in alignment and extension or flexion of the neck is avoided (Ball, 2001; Hickey, 2003a; Prendergast & Sullivan, 2000).

Circulatory function including heart rate, rhythm, and blood pressure also should be closely monitored. The patient with SCI may be bradycardic and hypotensive on presentation to the emergency department due to disruption in vagal tone because of neurogenic shock. Blood pressure may be further compromised by hypovolemia. Central venous pressure monitoring can be helpful in determining volume status and distinguishing between neurogenic and hypovolemic shock (Hadley, 2002).

Patients with SCI due to trauma also are at risk for other organ injuries. These patients may not be able to experience visceral pain because of the SCI. Therefore, it is vital that emergency department providers be vigilant in assessing for signs of other organ injury during their initial assessment.

A careful baseline neurological examination is crucial in the initial assessment of the patient suspected of having a spinal injury. This assessment will be the basis for management of the patient as well as for determination of change in neurological status. This assessment should take place before the patient receives pain medication, sedatives, or paralytics if possible. These medications can interfere with the ability to obtain an accurate neurological assessment.

The overall level of consciousness should be assessed in all trauma patients utilizing a Glasgow Coma Scale (GCS) score because there is a possibility of concomitant brain injury (Chart 32–2). The GCS score is the sum of scores for the patient's best eye opening, verbal, and motor responses. This score provides a

---

CHART 32–2 Glasgow Coma Scale

Eye Opening (E)	Verbal Response (V)	Motor Response (M)
4 = Spontaneous	5 = Normal conversation	6 = Normal
3 = To voice	4 = Disoriented conversation	5 = Localizes to pain
2 = To pain	3 = Words, but not coherent	4 = Withdraws to pain
1 = None	2 = No words; only sounds	3 = Decorticate posture
	1 = None	2 = Decerebrate
		1 = None

Total = E + V + M

With the Glasgow Coma Scale, one determines the best eye opening response, the best verbal response, and the best motor response. The score represents the sum of the numeric scores of each of the categories. There are limitations to its use. If the patient has an endotracheal tube in place, she cannot talk. For this reason, many prefer to document the score by its individual components; so a patient with a Glasgow Coma Scale score of 15 would be documented as follows: E4 V5 M6. An intubated patient would be scored as E4 V intubated M6. Of these individual factors, the best motor response is probably the most significant.

Source: American College of Surgeons Committee on Trauma (2004). Advanced Trauma Life Support for Doctors (7th ed). Chicago: American College of Surgeons

---

means for monitoring changes in the patient's mental status and predicting a prognosis from the time of injury in patients who have sustained a traumatic brain injury. A score of 15 is the maximum score and indicates a normal level of consciousness; a score of 3 is the lowest score and is indicative of a poor prognosis.

A detailed assessment of motor function of all major muscle groups in both the upper and lower extremities will be obtained as part of the initial assessment and repeated hourly as part of the routine monitoring of vital signs for the first 48 to 72 hours. The strength of each major muscle group is tested individually and compared with the corresponding muscle group on the contralateral side. The muscle strength is graded on a scale of 0 to 5 with 0 indicating no motor function and 5 indicating normal strength (Chart 32–3). Each muscle group is innervated by a corresponding spinal nerve (Chart 32–4, p. 842). Abnormalities in motor function can help with approximating the level of the SCI.

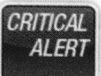 **CRITICAL ALERT** *Frequent monitoring of vital signs and neurological function is necessary for the first 48 to 72 hours after SCI to assess for any change in status. The managing medical team should be notified immediately if any decline in status is noted so that prompt intervention can be initiated to preserve existing function.*

CHART 32–3 Grading of Muscle Strength

Grade	Strength
0	No contraction
1	Trace or flicker contraction
2	Movement with gravity eliminated
3	Movement against gravity
4	Movement against resistance
5	Normal strength

Major Muscle Group Innervation and Function

Spinal Nerve	Muscle	Function
C_5	Deltoid	Abduct arm
C_6	Biceps	Bend elbow
C_6, C_7	Extensor carpi radialis	Extend wrist
C_7	Triceps	Straighten elbow
C_8, T_1	Hand intrinsics	Spread fingers
L_1, L_2	Iliopsoas	Raise knee to chest
L_3, L_4	Quadriceps	Extend knee
L_5	Tibialis anterior	Dorsiflex the foot
S_1	Extensor hallucis longus	Extend the great toe
	Hamstring	Flex knee
	Gastrocnemius	Plantar flex the foot

A sensory examination also is performed assessing the patient's response to pinprick in all dermatomes using a sequential side-to-side manner. Abnormalities in sensation are documented according to the corresponding dermatome. An anatomical dermatome chart is a helpful resource in determining the specific level of sensory abnormality (see Figure 28–6 ■, p. 707 in Chapter 28 ⊜).

Evaluation of the deep tendon reflexes (DTRs) and rectal sphincter tone also will take place as part of the initial assessment. Each reflex is innervated by a corresponding spinal nerve (Chart 32–5). Reflex activity is lost below the level of injury when spinal shock is present. As spinal shock abates, reflexes will generally return. The DTRs usually are not tested on a routine basis after the initial assessment; however, sphincter tone and sensation can be monitored during the routine bowel regimen (McIlvoy et al., 2004).

In addition to the neurological assessment, the entire spine should be palpated as part of the initial evaluation. Bony deformity, alteration in alignment, pain, and focal tenderness should be noted because these signs may be indicative of spinal fracture or dislocation.

Acute Care Hospital

Once the extent of injury has been determined, the patient has been stabilized, and the treatment plan established, the patient will be admitted to the intensive care unit (ICU) where close monitoring and support of neurological, respiratory, and circulatory functions will take place. The patient will be transferred to the general care floor once those functions have stabilized. The treatment plan will then be expanded from physiological

Spinal Reflexes

Spinal Level	Reflex
C_5–C_6	Biceps
C_7	Triceps
L_4	Patellar
S_1	Achilles

support and minimization of secondary injury to prevention of complications, education of the patient and family, and optimization of existing function.

Laboratory and Diagnostic Procedures

All patients who are suspected of having a spinal injury will undergo radiographic evaluation of the spine. Initially, plain x-rays will be obtained of the entire spinal axis to assess spinal alignment and the integrity of the spinal elements. Anterior-posterior (AP) and lateral views will be obtained. The **odontoid process**, the tooth-like projection of C_2 that sits behind the anterior portion of C_1, is difficult to visualize on standard x-ray views; therefore, an x-ray through the patient's open mouth will be necessary for visualization of the odontoid process and the C_1–C_2 junction.

The cervicothoracic junction can also be difficult to visualize with plain radiographs because of interference of the shoulder joint. Visualization of this area of the spine often requires pulling downward on the patient's shoulders or obtaining a lateral swimmer's view with the patient's arm fully abducted. This type of positioning may not be possible if the victim has sustained trauma to the upper extremities.

A CT scan provides detailed imaging of the bony structures of the spine and is very helpful in identifying fractures that may be missed on plain radiographs (Figure 32–11 ■). An MRI may be obtained to provide imaging of the soft tissue structures including the spinal cord, intervertebral disks, and ligaments; however, an MRI is not indicated for all patients (Figure 32–12 ■). Patients who are morbidly obese or have ex-

FIGURE 32–11 ■ CT of C_5–C_6 fracture and subluxation.
Source: Laurie Baker

FIGURE 32–12 ■ MRI of the cervical spine.
Source: Laurie Baker

treme claustrophobia will not be able to undergo an MRI scan. Also, patients with implanted medical devices such as pacemakers or those with retained metal from shrapnel injuries will not be candidates for this test. Another disadvantage of an MRI scan is the length of time it takes to perform this test. A spinal axis MRI can take up to 60 to 90 minutes to

complete. Patients who are medically unstable may be unsuitable for this type of imaging (Apuzzo, 2002e; France, Bono, & Vaccaro, 2005; Hickey, 2003a; National Guideline Clearinghouse, 2005c). See the Diagnostic Tests box for a listing of tests for acute SCI.

■ Medical Management

Decisions regarding treatment strategies for the patient with SCI are guided by the patient's presentation and results of the imaging studies. The ultimate goals of treatment are to stabilize the spine at the level of injury, optimize neurological outcome, and prevent neurological deterioration. Early medical management of the patient with SCI is geared toward stabilization of the spine and lessening of the secondary injury processes.

If stability of the vertebral column or ligaments is in question, immobilization of the spine utilizing an orthotic device will be necessary. Most of these devices are noninvasive and each device is designed to maintain alignment and stability of a particular spinal region. Rigid cervical collars are commonly used to provide stability to the cervical spine (Figure 32–13 ■, p. 844). A halo brace also may be used to stabilize cervical fractures, especially if a collar does not provide adequate stability (Figure 32–14 ■, p. 844). The application of cervical traction with such devices as Gardner-Wells tongs may be necessary to reestablish alignment of the cervical spine or to reduce cervical fractures before surgical stabilization (Figure 32–15 ■, p. 844).

Injuries in the cervicothoracic juncture or high thoracic spine require the use of a device that provides stabilization to both the lower cervical and upper thoracic regions such as a

DIAGNOSTIC TESTS for Acute Spinal Cord Injury

Test and *Normal Values*	Expected Abnormality	Rationale for Abnormality
Spinal x-rays: AP & Lat views Cervical spine x-rays should also include open mouth views and swimmer's view *Normal spinal alignment* *Bony elements of the spine are intact without evidence of fracture*	Subluxation of the vertebral bodies Compression or abnormal shape of the vertebral body Crush deformity of the vertebral body Widening or collapse of the intervertebral space	Injuries to the spinal ligaments or fracture of the stabilizing structures of the spine allow the vertebral body to slip out of alignment. Compression fracture of the vertebra will result in crushing of the vertebral body, altering its normal shape. Disruption of the intervertebral disk will cause changes in the space between the vertebral bodies.
CT scan of the spine *Normal spinal alignment* *Normal configuration of the bony elements of the spine* *No evidence of fracture* *No bone fragments within the canal*	Abnormal alignment of the spine Fracture of the bony elements of the spinal column Bone fragments within the spinal canal	Fracture or ligamentous injuries allow the spine to become unstable and the vertebral bodies to move out of place. Bone fragments from spinal fractures can be propelled or migrate into the canal, causing compression of the spinal cord or nerves.
MRI of the spine *Spinal alignment maintained* *Intervertebral disks intact* *Spinal cord is surrounded by cerebrospinal fluid without evidence of compression or abnormality in signal intensity* *Normal signal intensity of the surrounding ligaments and tissue*	Abnormal alignment of the spine Protrusion of the intervertebral disk into the canal, causing compression of the spinal cord Narrowing of the spinal canal with compression of the spinal cord Hyperintensity within the spinal cord Hyperintensity of the surrounding ligaments and tissues	Brightness or hyperintense signal within the spinal cord or surrounding tissue indicates the presence of swelling or edema due to the inflammatory response of injury. If present only in the surrounding tissue and not the spinal cord, this could be indicative of ligamentous injury, which increases the risk of spinal instability.

FIGURE 32–13 ■ Philly collar.
Source: Courtesy of Ossur

FIGURE 32–15 ■ J tongs.
Source: Courtesy of Ossur

FIGURE 32–14 ■ ReSolve Halo.
Source: Courtesy of Ossur

FIGURE 32–16 ■ SOMI brace.
Source: Courtesy of Trulife

SOMI brace (Figure 32–16 ■). A thoracolumbosacral orthosis will be required to stabilize the thoracic and lumbar regions. This orthotic consists of a fiberglass or rigid plastic vest fitted specifically to the patient.

Methylprednisolone administration in acute SCI has become a standard of care in many treatment centers; however, there is much controversy in the literature regarding the effectiveness of this treatment strategy. Methylprednisolone is thought to provide protection to the neural tissues and lessen the effects of the secondary processes that contribute to the decline in neurological function in the early postinjury period (Hurlbert, 2006). Early studies indicated improvement of both motor and sensory function after administration of high-dose methylprednisolone; however, these results have not been duplicated in subsequent trials. Also, administration of high-dose steroids have associated risks including sepsis, pneumonia, blood sugar elevation, and delayed wound healing (Sayer, Kronvall, & Nilsson, 2006; Walker & Criddle, 2001). Despite the criticism in the literature, it remains a treatment option. The current standardized regimen for the treatment of acute SCI is methylprednisolone 30 mg/kg intravenously (IV) over 15 minutes followed by a continuous infusion of methylprednisolone 5.4 mg · kg^{-1} · hr^{-1} for 23 hours if the patient is seen within 3 hours following injury. For patients who are seen between 3 and 8 hours following injury, the recommendation is to administer 30 mg/kg IV over 15 minutes, then 5.4 mg · kg^{-1} · hr^{-1} for 48 hours (Apuzzo, 2002d, Hickey, 2003b; McIlvoy et al., 2004; Prendergast & Sullivan, 2000). The Pharmacology Summary box lists medication used for treatment of spinal cord injuries.

PHARMACOLOGY Summary of Medications Used in Early Spinal Cord Injury

Medication Category	Action	Application/Indication	Nursing Responsibility
Steroid: • Methylprednisolone	Stabilizes cell membrane permeability. Decreases immune response.	Decreases secondary injury due to inflammatory response.	Assess for side effects including mental status and mood changes. Monitor blood glucose levels. Monitor for symptoms of infection.
Cardiac: • Atropine • Dopamine/dobutamine	Alter autonomic activity of the heart. Act to increase the heart rate. Sympathomimetic. Increases blood pressure and cardiac output.	Bradycardia. Hypotension due to neurogenic shock.	Monitor heart rate and rhythm. Monitor blood pressure. Titrate dosage to keep systolic BP > 90 mmHg and MAP > 85 mmHg.
Anticoagulant: • Low-molecular-weight heparin • Warfarin sodium	Inhibit blood clot formation.	Prevention or treatment of DVT.	Monitor patient for signs and symptoms of DVT formation. Monitor coagulation factors PT, PTT, INR. Assess patient for signs of too much anticoagulation, such as excessive bleeding, bruising, or signs of GI bleed.
Gastrointestinal: *Proton pump inhibitors:* • Lansoprazole • Omeprazole • Pantoprazole *Stool softeners:* • Colace • Peri-Colace • Senokot *Bowel stimulants:* • Dulcolax suppository • Therevac *Osmotic laxative:* • MiraLax *Psychological:* Anxiolytics: • Diazepam • Alprazolam • Lorazepam Antidepressants: • Venlafaxine • Fluoxetine • Duloxetine • Sertraline • Paroxetine	Inhibit gastric acid secretion. Maintain water content of feces. Stimulate bowel activity. Promote water retention in the stool producing a laxative effect. Depress the central nervous system. Inhibit the reuptake of serotonin.	Prevent gastric stress ulceration. Prevent constipation. Encourage regular emptying of the colon. Prevent constipation. Reduces anxiety related to hospitalization, injury, and loss of control over patient's own environment. Mood stabilizers help the patient cope with the injury and focus on rehabilitative goals.	Monitor patient for development of stress ulcer: c/o abdominal pain, signs of GI bleeding. Monitor frequency and quality of bowel movements. Institute bowel program as soon as patient's medical condition warrants. Assess the patient's response to the medication. Monitor patient for alteration in mood.

Current treatment strategies for medical management of acute SCI stress the importance of maintaining adequate oxygenation and blood pressure to ensure perfusion of the spinal cord. Hypotension is thought to be a contributor to worsening spinal cord injury by worsening spinal cord ischemia. Systolic blood pressure should be maintained above 90 mmHg with mean arterial blood pressure targeted above 85 mmHg to ensure adequate spinal cord perfusion (Apuzzo, 2002c; Hadley, 2002; Hickey, 2003a; Hurlbert, 2006; McIlvoy et al., 2004; Prendergast & Sullivan, 2000).

Surgical Management

Surgical management of spinal cord injuries will be considered in patients who have fractures of the spinal column that are unstable and in those patients who have compression of the spinal cord as a result of bone fragments, disk herniation, tumor, or hematoma. There is some controversy among surgeons surrounding the optimal timing for surgical intervention. Advocates for early surgical treatment point to the benefits of early decompression of the spinal cord. These benefits include improvement of spinal cord perfusion, resulting in preservation or possibly even improvement of spinal cord function by decreasing spinal cord ischemia particularly in patients with incomplete injuries. Early stabilization of an unstable spinal column also will allow for earlier mobilization of the patient, resulting in improved pulmonary function and decreased risk of development of DVT and pressure ulcers (Apuzzo, 2002a; Hickey, 2003a).

Surgery often will consist of decompression of the spinal canal and/or fusion to provide structural stability for spine fractures or dislocations. A laminectomy is the surgical procedure of choice for decompression of the spinal canal. This procedure is performed through a posterior approach and consists of removing the ligament and lamina from the back of the spinal column. Bone fragments, disc fragments, tumor, or hematoma resulting in compression of the spinal cord also will be removed when indicated. If the spine is unstable due to fracture, dislocation, or ligamentous injury, spinal instrumentation with fusion will be performed to restore spinal alignment and stability. Spinal fusion with instrumentation consists of placement of a combination of titanium screws, plates, wires, rods, or intervertebral cages and bone from either the bone bank or the patient's iliac crest to bridge fractured, unstable spinal segments with healthy, well-aligned bone. Fusion can be performed through either an anterior, posterior, or lateral approach to the spinal column (Figures 32–17 ■ and 32–18 ■).

Nursing Management

The focus of nursing care for the patient with an SCI is accurate, ongoing assessment of the patient and prevention of complications. Evaluation of the physiological response to the injury and corresponding treatment as well as the patient's emotional response to the injury are important aspects of the nursing assessment. The nursing assessment also is vital in determining the effectiveness of the treatment plan as well as prevention of potential complications and deterioration of the patient's status by allowing for early identification of problems and prompt intervention. The nursing plan of care will reflect the needs of the pa-

FIGURE 32–17 ■ Lateral cervical spine x-ray of C_4–C_6 fusion.
Source: Laurie Baker

tient and family and employ strategies to prevent complications and optimize the patient's function (see the Nursing Process: Patient Care Plan feature, p. 848).

Assessment
Physical Assessment and Interventions

Nursing assessment of the patient with an SCI includes routine assessment of all major organ systems. Neurological assessment includes evaluation of the patient's mental status and motor and sensory functions. Any decline in status warrants additional investigation and should be reported immediately. Range-of-motion exercises and devices such as specialized splints to prevent contracture formation from disuse should be instituted for the affected joints as soon as the patient is stable enough to tolerate these activities.

Routine cardiovascular assessment will include monitoring of blood pressure, heart rate and rhythm, and peripheral circulation including assessment of peripheral pulses and temperature of the extremities. Patients in the ICU may have a pulmonary artery catheter in place to allow for monitoring of the central pressures and cardiac output. The use of vasopressors, cardiotropic medications, and volume replacement should be instituted as ordered to maintain adequate cardiac output and mean arterial blood pressure (MAP). Intake and output should be monitored to evaluate fluid status. Once patients have clearance for mobilization, they should be monitored closely for signs of orthostatic hypotension when upright. If orthostatic hypotension is problematic, measures to prevent blood pooling in the peripheral vascular system and increase venous return to the heart should be instituted. These measures include the use of compression stockings and an abdominal binder. Expansion of intravascular volume also may be helpful. The use of devices such as a tilt table or a reclining

FIGURE 32–18 ■ AP and lateral x-ray of posterior spinal fusion.
Source: Laurie Baker

wheelchair may be necessary to gradually progress the patient into an upright position.

Prophylactic measures to prevent DVT formation, including the use of antiembolic hose and sequential compression boots, should be instituted once the patient is admitted to the hospital. Anticoagulant therapy and mobilization may be initiated after clearance from the surgical team. It is imperative that the nurse be vigilant in assessing for objective signs of DVT including the presence of low-grade fever, change in temperature in an extremity, swelling of an extremity, or loss of a peripheral pulse. All four extremities should be assessed because a DVT can occur in an upper extremity as well as in a lower extremity. If a DVT is suspected, the medical team should be notified immediately so that the appropriate diagnostic study can be performed and treatment initiated.

All patients with SCI should be monitored closely for signs of respiratory impairment. These signs include fever, tachypnea, tachycardia, shortness of breath, use of accessory muscles, increased volume and change in characteristic of secretions, and mental status change including increased anxiety or decrease in mental alertness. Assessment of lung sounds noting the presence of adventitious sounds indicative of pneumonia or atelectasis should be performed routinely and if any change in respiratory function is detected. Respiratory rate and use of accessory muscles in respiration also is to be noted. Pulse oximetry should be monitored on a routine basis and ABGs should be obtained to monitor for the development of hypoxemia in the patient who is at high risk for respiratory decompensation and if a decline in respiratory function or change in mental status not explained by

other means is noted. Assessment of respiratory parameters including tidal volume, vital capacity, and negative inspiratory force can be helpful in determining the need for ventilatory assistance. A chest x-ray should be obtained if alteration in respiratory function is noted (see Chapter 33 ☞).

The patient should be instructed on pulmonary hygiene measures including coughing and deep breathing exercises and the use of an incentive spirometer. Suctioning may be necessary if the patient is unable to clear her own secretions. Assisted coughing techniques may be beneficial as well as chest physiotherapy especially in patients with high-level injuries. The use of continuous positive airway pressure (CPAP) or bilevel positive airway pressure (BiPAP) may also be instituted to assist with reexpansion of lung tissue (Hickey, 2003a; McIlvoy et al., 2004; National Guideline Clearinghouse, 2005c). The National Guidelines box (p. 851) lists guidelines that have been established for respiratory management after spinal cord injury.

Bowel activity should be monitored with routine assessment of bowel sounds and inspection of the abdomen for distention and tenderness. The patient should be monitored for complaints of nausea and/or vomiting. If abdominal distention is present and bowel sounds are absent, an abdominal x-ray may be warranted to evaluate for an ileus. It may be necessary to insert a nasogastric tube for decompression of the stomach if ileus is present. If a drop in hematocrit occurs that is not explained by other means, evaluation for gastrointestinal hemorrhage should be performed by testing for occult blood in the stool. The nurse will need to ensure that a stress ulcer prophylactic regimen has

NURSING PROCESS: Patient Care Plan for Spinal Cord Injury

Assessment of Neurological Status

Subjective Data:
Are you able to move your arms, hand, legs, feet?
Do you have numbness or tingling anywhere?

Objective Data:
Motor strength   Deep tendon reflexes
Sensory level   Sphincter tone

Nursing Assessment and Diagnoses	Outcomes and Evaluation Parameters	Planning and Interventions with *Rationales*
Nursing Diagnoses: *Risk for Constipation* related to spinal cord injury *Disturbed Sensory Perception* related to spinal cord injury *Risk for Injury* due to spinal instability	**Outcomes:** Stabilization or improvement of neurological function. Maintenance of spinal alignment. ***Evaluation Parameters:*** Existing neurological function is preserved. Spine is immobilized with the appropriate orthotic device and mobility restrictions.	**Interventions and *Rationales:*** Spinal precautions maintained as ordered by the treating health care provider. *Measures to limit additional mechanical injury to the spinal cord.* Administer methylprednisolone per hospital protocol. *May limit inflammatory response and secondary injury to the spinal cord.* Maintain adequate oxygenation and mean arterial pressure (MAP) above 85 mmHg and systolic BP above 90 mmHg *to prevent secondary injury due to hypoxia and hypotension.* Monitor motor and sensory function *to assess for change in neurological function allowing for prompt medical attention if needed.*

Assessment of Pulmonary Function

Subjective Data:
Do you feel short of breath?
Do you feel like you are unable to clear your secretions?

Objective Data:
Lung sounds   Adequacy of cough
Monitor respiratory rate   Monitor pulse oximetry
Use of accessory muscles for   Monitor arterial blood gases
breathing   Change in mental status (i.e., anxiety,
Amount and character of secretions   confusion, increased lethargy)

Nursing Assessment and Diagnoses	Outcomes and Evaluation Parameters	Planning and Interventions with *Rationales*
Nursing Diagnoses: *Ineffective Breathing Pattern* related to pulmonary complications of spinal cord injury *Ineffective Airway Clearance* related to the loss of spinal innervation of the respiratory muscles	**Outcome:** Adequate gas exchange. ***Evaluation Parameters:*** Adequate oxygenation is achieved as evidenced by normal blood gases and pulse oximetry. Patient is able to clear airway secretions. Patient is without complaint of dyspnea. Lung sounds remain clear. Patient remains alert and oriented without anxiety or restlessness.	**Interventions and *Rationales:*** Monitor respiratory status. *Evaluate for change indicative of declining respiratory function including increased use of accessory muscles, inability to clear secretions, drop in oxygen saturation, change in mental status, change in respiratory parameters (tidal volume, vital capacity, negative inspiratory force).* Institute pulmonary hygiene, including cough and deep breathing exercises, chest physiotherapy, assisted cough techniques, suctioning *to promote gas exchange and airway clearance.* Administer humidified oxygen as ordered *to increase oxygenation.* Report decline in respiratory function to the medical team. *Medical management including mechanical ventilatory support may be necessary.*

Assessment of Cardiovascular Status

Subjective Data:
Are you dizzy or light-headed?

Objective Data:
Heart rate and rhythm   Blood pressure   Urine output

Nursing Assessment and Diagnoses	Outcomes and Evaluation Parameters	Planning and Interventions with *Rationales*
Nursing Diagnosis: *Risk for Ineffective Tissue Perfusion* related to cardiovascular effects of neurogenic shock	**Outcomes:** Patient maintains hemodynamic stability. Patient is able to tolerate being in an upright position. ***Evaluation Parameters:*** MAP > 85 mmHg SBP > 90 mmHg HR > 50–60 Patient does not complain of dizziness or light-headedness.	**Interventions and *Rationales:*** Monitor hemodynamic status *to assess for change to allow for prompt medical intervention.* Administer vasoactive agents and atropine as ordered *to ensure adequate blood pressure, heart rate, and cardiac output.* Monitor intake and output and replace intravascular volume *to ensure adequate fluid status. Hypovolemia can contribute to hemodynamic instability.* Utilize abdominal binder and thigh-high compression stockings *to increase venous return to the heart and limit blood pooling in abdomen and lower extremities due to vasodilation.* Transition patient slowly into an upright position *to avoid orthostatic hypotension.*

NURSING PROCESS: Patient Care Plan for Spinal Cord Injury—*Continued*

Assessment of Peripheral Tissue Perfusion

Subjective Data:
Do you have any pain or pressure in your extremities?
Have you noticed any abnormal swelling or redness in your extremities?
Have you noticed change in temperature in one or more extremity?

Objective Data:
Peripheral pulses
Temperature and color of the extremities
Unilateral swelling in the extremities

Nursing Assessment and Diagnoses	Outcomes and Evaluation Parameters	Planning and Interventions with *Rationales*
Nursing Diagnosis: *Risk of Ineffective Peripheral Tissue Perfusion* related to deep venous thrombosis (DVT)	**Outcome:** Patient does not develop DVT. **Evaluation Parameters:** The patient does not exhibit signs of DVT: redness, edema, change in temperature of extremity. Patient does not complain of pain or tenderness. Peripheral pulses remain intact.	**Interventions and *Rationales:*** Utilize antiembolic hose and sequential compression boots *to limit blood pooling in the lower extremities.* Administer prophylactic dose of anticoagulant as ordered once cleared by the surgical team *to prevent formation of peripheral DVT.* Begin mobilization of patient including range-of-motion exercises as soon as cleared by the surgical team *to limit the effects of prolonged immobility.* Assess color, temperature, and size of extremities and check peripheral pulses. Report abnormalities to the medical team *to enable early detection and prompt treatment.*

Assessment of Gastrointestinal Function

Subjective Data:
Are you nauseous?
Do you have any abdominal pain?
When was your last bowel movement?

Objective Data:
Abdominal pain
Abdominal distention
Bowel sounds
Frequency of bowel movements
Guaiac stools
Hematocrit
Dietary intake

Nursing Assessment and Diagnoses	Outcomes and Evaluation Parameters	Planning and Interventions with *Rationales*
Nursing Diagnoses: *Risk for constipation* related to impaired gastric motility due to spinal cord injury *Potential for Gastric Ulceration* related to stress of critical injury *Readiness for Enhanced Nutrition* related to increased metabolic need and inadequate caloric intake	**Outcomes:** Gastrointestinal function will be maintained. Patient will be without evidence of gastric stress ulceration. A regular pattern of bowel movements will be established. Patient will receive adequate nutrition to meet caloric requirements. **Evaluation Parameters:** Abdomen will remain soft, nontender, and nondistended. Patient will be without complaints of nausea, vomiting, constipation, or epigastric pain. Hematocrit will remain stable. Nutrition will be implemented.	**Interventions and *Rationales:*** Assess abdomen for tenderness and distention. Auscultate bowel sounds. *Evaluation of gastrointestinal function.* Monitor hematocrit and check stool for occult blood if drop in hematocrit noted without other explanation (i.e., surgery) *to assess for GI bleed due to gastric stress ulceration.* Use nasogastric tube if ileus is present *to provide for decompression of the stomach.* Administer stress ulcer prophylactic regimen as ordered by the medical team. Institute bowel regimen of stool softener, chemical stimulation such as a suppository, and mechanical (digital) stimulation *to establish a regular bowel elimination pattern.* Institute parenteral nutrition until patient is able to tolerate enteral feedings. Call for dietary consult *to determine patient's caloric needs.*

Assessment of Urinary Elimination

Subjective Data:
Are you able to urinate?
Do you feel like your bladder is full?
Have you had any incontinence of urine?

Objective Data:
Urinary output
Bladder scan to assess for urinary retention

(continued)

NURSING PROCESS: Patient Care Plan for Spinal Cord Injury—*Continued*

Nursing Assessment and Diagnoses	Outcomes and Evaluation Parameters	Planning and Interventions with *Rationales*
Nursing Diagnoses: Impaired Urinary Elimination due to neurogenic bladder *Risk for Autonomic Dysreflexia* related to autonomic dysfunction as a result of spinal cord injury	**Outcomes:** The patient will establish a normal pattern of urinary elimination. The patient will be able to recognize the signs of autonomic hyperreflexia, identify potential causes, and describe treatment of hyperreflexia. **Evaluation Parameters:** The patient or caregiver is able to perform clean intermittent catherization (CIC). The patient and caregiver can verbalize common causes of hyperreflexia, common symptoms of hyperreflexia, and actions to take should hyperreflexia occur.	**Interventions and *Rationales:*** Use indwelling catheter during the acute period *to allow for complete bladder emptying and accurate measurement of urinary output*. Check postvoid residuals by either intermittent catheterization or bladder scan *to assess for urinary retention*. Teach CIC to patient and caregiver *to encourage a consistent manner of bladder emptying.* Instruct patient and caregiver on common causes and signs of autonomic hyperreflexia and interventions to institute when these signs occur.

Assessment of Pain

Subjective Data:	Objective Data:	
Are you having pain? Where do you hurt?	Facial grimacing Crying Increased spasticity	Elevated blood pressure Elevated heart rate

Nursing Assessment and Diagnoses	Outcomes and Evaluation Parameters	Planning and Interventions with *Rationales*
Nursing Diagnosis: Readiness for enhanced comfort due to injury and/or surgical procedure	**Outcome:** Effective control of pain. **Evaluation Parameters:** The patient will report improvement of pain. The patient is able to participate in therapies.	**Interventions and *Rationales:*** Assess pain utilizing a pain scale *to provide a method of measuring degree of pain and response to pain control measures.* Administer analgesics as ordered *to provide pharmacologic treatment of pain.* Utilize distraction and repositioning techniques *to augment pharmacologic treatment of pain.*

Assessment of Psychosocial State

Subjective Data:	Objective Data:	
Are you feeling sad, depressed? How have you dealt with stress in the past? Who is your support person?	Refusal to communicate Refusal to participate in activities Avoidance of eye contact	Anger Crying Expressing feelings of hopelessness

Nursing Assessment and Diagnoses	Outcomes and Evaluation Parameters	Planning and Interventions with *Rationales*
Nursing Diagnoses: *Ineffective Coping* related to loss of control over environment and uncertainty of the future	**Outcomes:** Patient will exhibit appropriate coping strategies. Patient will exhibit less anxiety. **Evaluation Parameters:** Patient reports improved mood. Patient participates in care. Patient is able to express feelings.	**Interventions and *Rationales:*** Encourage the patient to express her feelings *to provide for self-expression and identification of feelings.* Allow patient to participate in decisions *so the patient regains some control over self and the environment.* Request psychiatric consultation. *Assist with crisis counseling and to help the patient to identify appropriate coping strategies.* Administer antianxiolytics and antidepressants as prescribed.

Assessment of Adaptation

Subjective Data:	Objective Data:
What are you able to do for yourself? What adaptive equipment do you have available and what will be needed?	Functional assessment based on preserved motor function Patient/caregiver knowledge of use of equipment Patient/caregiver knowledge of available resources

Nursing Assessment and Diagnoses	Outcomes and Evaluation Parameters	Planning and Interventions with *Rationales*
Nursing Diagnoses: *Self-Care Deficit* related to spinal cord injury *Deficient Knowledge* regarding adaptation strategies and resources	**Outcome:** Patient will implement self-care strategies utilizing the appropriate adaptive devices within the limitations of his injury. **Evaluation Parameters:** The patient participates in his own care. The patient will be able to identify available resources to help him to be independent within the limitations of his injury.	**Interventions and *Rationales:*** Schedule nursing care around PT/OT sessions *to ensure patient is able to participate in rehabilitative activities.* Have adaptive equipment readily available and encourage patient to use the equipment in self-care activities. *Encourages self-care strategies and reinforces education on the use of the equipment.* Assist the patient in identifying available community resources *to assist in independent living.*

NATIONAL GUIDELINES for Respiratory Management Following Spinal Cord Injury

Risk Factor	Guideline
Respiratory failure	**Assessment:** **History:** • Relevant past medical history • Prior history of pulmonary disease • Medications • History of substance abuse • Neurological impairment • Coexisting injuries **Examination:** • Physical exam of the respiratory system including lung sounds, respiratory rate, use of accessory muscles • Respiratory complaints • Oxygen saturation with continuous pulse oximetry • Chest x-ray • Measurement of vital capacity, maximal negative inspiratory pressure, forced expiratory volume in 1 second • Neurological level and extent of impairment • Assess risk for aspiration **Initial laboratory and radiographic evaluation:** • Arterial blood gases • CBC, chemistry panel, coagulation profile, cardiac enzymes, urinalysis, toxicology • Chest x-ray • EKG **Intubation Parameters:** • Intractable respiratory failure • High risk for aspiration plus respiratory compromise
Atelectasis and pneumonia	**Assessment:** Monitor indicators for the development of pneumonia or atelectasis: • Rising temperature • Change in respiratory rate • Increasing heart rate • Increasing anxiety • Increased volume and change in character of secretions • Decline in vital capacity • Decline in peak expiratory flow Obtain chest x-ray. If atelectasis or pneumonia present on x-ray, monitor serial x-rays. **Prevention and Treatment:** Incentive spirometry and coughing and deep breathing exercises Chest physiotherapy Assisted coughing techniques Intermittent positive pressure breathing CPAP or BiPAP Turning and alternative positioning when patient is medically and surgically stable Mobilization once patient is medically and surgically stable Prevent aspiration Antibiotic therapy as indicated by sputum culture

Source: National Guideline Clearinghouse. (2005). *Respiratory management following spinal cord injury: A clinical practice guideline for health-care professionals.* Washington, DC: Consortium for Spinal Cord Medicine, Paralyzed Veterans of America. Retrieved April 29, 2008, from http://www.guideline.gov/summary/summary.aspx?doc_id=7198&nbr=004301&string=spinal+AND+cord+AND+injury.

been implemented as part of the medical treatment plan. Nutritional intake should be initiated as soon as possible. A dietary consult may be necessary to ensure adequate caloric intake to meet the patient's metabolic needs.

Regardless of the level of injury, all patients with SCI should have a regular bowel management regimen instituted as part of their ongoing care once the patient's condition allows. This program should be based on the patient's preinjury elimination patterns and provide for a consistent schedule of elimination to avoid such problems as bowel impaction or incontinence. This regimen should include the use of stool softeners, chemical stimulants such as suppositories, and mechanical stimulants such as digital stimulation of the bowel. The patient's bowel elimination pattern should be monitored closely to ensure adequate bowel evacuation. Dietary recommendations to aid in bowel evacuation include ensuring a minimum of 15 grams of dietary fiber per day as well as adequate fluid intake (Enck et al., 2006; Hickey, 2003b; National Guideline Clearinghouse, 2005a).

All patients who have had a SCI will require the use of an indwelling urinary catheter in the acute phase following injury. The catheter allows for bladder decompression and adequate monitoring of intake and output. A catheter can increase the risk of UTI. Urine that is cloudy or has a foul odor may indicate the presence of a UTI and urinalysis and culture should be obtained.

As the patient progresses through the recovery period, the indwelling catheter should be removed. The patient will need to be monitored for signs of urinary retention. Postvoid residuals should be checked either with intermittent catheterization or bladder scan. Urinary incontinence may be due to overflow of urine from a distended bladder. If the patient is unable to void or has high postvoid residual volumes, an alternative method of urinary elimination to allow for complete emptying of the bladder should be implemented. The most common means of urinary management after SCI is the use of clean intermittent catheterization (CIC). Intermittent catheterization should be taught to the patient if there is adequate preservation of hand function or to the patient's primary caregiver if the patient is unable to perform this task.

It is vital that the nurse maintain excellent skin care for the patient with a SCI in order to maintain skin integrity. Patients should be removed from the firm spinal board as soon as the initial trauma assessment is complete and it is deemed safe to move the patient. Routine assessment of the skin particularly in areas over bony prominences and under orthotic devices should be performed a minimum of twice daily. Redness and/or blanching of the skin are early signs of pressure ulcer formation. Areas most vulnerable to pressure ulcer formation include the trochanters, ischial tuberosities, sacrum, coccyx, heels, and occiput. Pressure ulcers can also occur on the elbows and scapula. The patient should be turned every 2 hours with careful attention paid to positioning the patient to avoid pressure over bony prominences and avoidance of shearing forces when moving the patient. The skin, clothing, and sheets should be kept dry and wrinkle free. Devices such as air flotation mattresses, pillows, and wheelchair cushions designed to unload pressure sites should be instituted. Patients also should be instructed in repositioning techniques to unload pressure sites while sitting in the wheelchair.

If the patient requires the use of an orthotic brace for immobilization, the skin under the brace should be routinely inspected. Rigid braces such as cervical collars and thoracic lumbar braces can be removed and the skin underneath can be inspected while the patient is supine in bed. Patients who are immobilized with a halo brace or other traction devices should have the cranial pin sites cleaned with normal saline and inspected for signs of infection twice daily. The vest plates of the halo vest can be removed by an experienced orthotist while the patient is supine, and skin care to the thoracic area can be performed at that time. Incisions and abrasions should be inspected regularly for signs of infection. Nutritional measures should be instituted as soon as possible to ensure the patient receives adequate calories, protein, and micronutrients (Hickey, 2003b; Paralyzed Veterans of America, 2001).

If the patient experiences symptoms of autonomic hyperreflexia, he should be placed in an upright position with the lower extremities dependent to lower the blood pressure. The causative factor should be identified and removed. If hypertension persists, administration of a quick-acting antihypertensive agent may be necessary. The best strategy for managing autonomic hyperreflexia is avoidance of the precipitating stimulus. The patient and family will need to be educated on the signs and symptoms of autonomic hyperreflexia, strategies to avoid this condition, and actions to take should this condition occur (Hickey, 2003b; Krassioukov, 2004; McIlvoy et al., 2004; National Guideline Clearinghouse, 2001). National guidelines for acute management of autonomic hyperreflexia have been established.

Psychosocial Assessment and Intervention

Patients who have experienced a SCI are not only faced with the physical challenges associated with this injury, but also with a significant psychosocial impact. These patients are faced with changes related to loss of body image, loss of independence, loss of control over their immediate environment, loss of economic security, and lifestyle changes. This injury also can place a significant stress and strain on existing relationships. The patient may exhibit a wide range of emotions including denial, grief, anger, hopelessness, and depression.

The nurse should monitor the patient for signs of inadequate coping including withdrawal from social interactions, avoidance of eye contact, and refusal to participate in activities. The patient should be encouraged to discuss her feelings and be allowed to participate in decision making whenever possible. The patient's family members also will need support and ongoing education to help them deal with the stress of having a critically ill loved one and the role changes associated with becoming a primary caregiver. In some cases, consultation with a chaplain, social worker, or psychiatrist may be necessary. Healing touch may also be helpful to patients with SCI, as discussed in the Complementary and Alternative Therapies box (p. 854).

Rehabilitation

Rehabilitation for patients with SCI will consist of a comprehensive, interdisciplinary program designed to help patients adapt to the limitations of their injury, reach the highest level of independence possible, and reintegrate into the home environment and community. During the rehabilitation period, the patient will undergo extensive inpatient physical and occupational

NATIONAL GUIDELINES for Acute Management of Autonomic Hyperreflexia

Risk Factor	Guideline
Autonomic hyperreflexia	Patient's with SCI at or above T_6 are at risk for autonomic hyperreflexia.

Recognize the signs and symptoms of autonomic hyperreflexia:

- Elevated blood pressure: a sudden, significant increase (20–40 mmHg) in both diastolic and systolic blood pressures above the patient's usual level
- Pounding headache
- Bradycardia: may be within normal range but relative slowing compared to the patient's normal heat rate
- Profuse sweating above the level of the lesion, especially the face, neck, and shoulders
- Piloerection above and possibly below the level of injury
- Cardiac dysrhythmias including atrial fibrillation, premature ventricular contractions, and atrioventricular conduction abnormalities
- Flushing of the skin above the level of injury, especially the face, neck, and shoulders
- Patient complaint of visual disturbance such as blurred vision or spots in the visual field
- Nasal congestion
- Feelings of apprehension or anxiety
- Symptoms may be absent or minimal despite significantly elevated blood pressure (silent autonomic hyperreflexia)

Treatment:

- If the person is supine, immediately sit the patient up and lower the legs if possible. This allows the blood to pool in the lower extremities and may lower the blood pressure.
- Loosen any clothing or constricting devices.
- Monitor the blood pressure and pulse frequently. Blood pressure can fluctuate rapidly due to impaired autonomic regulation.
- Quickly assess the patient for the instigating cause and remove it as quickly as possible.
  - The most common cause of autonomic hyperreflexia is bladder distention:
    - Check indwelling catheter for patency and proper placement.
    - If the catheter is blocked, gently irrigate with 10 to 15 mL normal saline at body temperature.
    - Avoid compressing or tapping on the bladder.
    - If the catheter does not drain, remove and replace the catheter.
  - If no catheter is in place, catheterize the patient:
    - Instill 2% lidocaine jelly into urethra and wait 2 minutes if time allows before inserting the catheter to decrease sensory input and relax the urinary sphincter.
  - The second most common cause of autonomic hyperreflexia is fecal impaction:
    - If systolic blood pressure is >150 mmHg, consider pharmacologic treatment to reduce blood pressure without causing hypotension prior to checking for fecal impaction.
    - If systolic blood pressure is <150 mmHg, check for fecal impaction:
      - Instill 2% lidocaine jelly into the rectum.
      - Wait 2 minutes.
      - Insert gloved, lubricated finger into the rectum and check for the presence of stool.
      - If stool is present, gently remove.
      - If autonomic hyperreflexia worsens, stop the manual evacuation, instill additional topical anesthetic, and recheck the rectum after approximately 20 minutes.
  - If urinary and fecal causes of autonomic hyperreflexia have been eliminated and symptoms persist, assess for other instigating causes and treat accordingly:
    - Pressure ulcerations
    - Abdominal pathology
    - Ingrown toenails
    - Long bone fractures
    - Infection

Education:

- Educate the patient and family about common causes of autonomic hyperreflexia and appropriate treatment strategies.

Source: National Guideline Clearinghouse. (2001). *Acute management of autonomic dysreflexia: Individuals with spinal cord injury presenting to a health-care facility.* Washington, DC: Consortium for Spinal Cord Medicine, Paralyzed Veterans of America. Retrieved November 14, 2006, from http://www.guideline.gov/summary/summary.aspx?doc_id=2964&nbr=002190&string=Autonomic+AND+dysreflexia.

therapy to strengthen functioning muscles and optimize functionality. The patient and family will receive instruction regarding strategies for self-care and performance of activities of daily living (ADLs) including proper transfer and mobility techniques. Patients and families also will receive advice regarding appropriate modifications to the home to accommodate the patient's disability and adaptive equipment.

A social worker and psychologist will work with patients and their families to assist with psychosocial issues related to lifestyle including sexuality and recreation. Patients will receive advice on maintaining an active lifestyle within the limitations of their injury. They also will receive instruction specific to sexual activity early in the acute rehabilitative period and this information will be frequently reinforced. It is important that these patients

COMPLEMENTARY & ALTERNATIVE THERAPIES — Healing Touch and Spirituality

Description:

Healing touch is a form of energy-based therapy in which the practitioner's hands move to realign energy that resides just outside the physical body. While it is still a new and somewhat controversial technique, many nurses practice healing touch, and many advocate its use. There are also many anecdotal reports that confirm its beneficial effects. This feature will discuss healing touch as it specifically applies to spinal cord injuries. Many patients with spinal cord injuries experience spiritual crisis during their journey to recovery and a new way of living. Therefore, anything that shows a benefit should be tried to help those suffering this trauma.

Research Support:

A pilot study assessed how healing touch (HT) modulates chronic neuropathic pain and the associated psychological distress from post–spinal cord injury. During six weekly home visits, 12 veterans were assigned to either HT or guided progressive relaxation. Researchers then measured the participants' progress using several instruments: the Brief Pain Inventory, the Profile of Moods, and the Diener Satisfaction with Life Scale. Although there was a large variation among the groups, the instruments did show sensitivity. The composite of interference on the Brief Pain Inventory showed a significant difference. In the fatigue subscale of the Profile of Moods, the mean score decreased (ns) in the HT group, and in the subscale of confusion the mean score remained stable in the control group. The Diener Satisfaction with Life Scale showed increased well-being in the HT group and no change in the control group. Researchers concluded that HT sessions may have benefit in the complex response to chronic pain (Wardell, Rintala, Duan, & Tan, 2006).

A national U.S. sample of insured adults with physical disabilities were examined to estimate the prevalence of CAM practitioner use, assess the reasons for use, and determine the symptoms for which CAM practitioners were consulted. Data for this study were obtained from a longitudinal survey conducted in 2000 and 2001 on a national sample of 830 adults with health insurance. These adults had one of four disabling conditions: multiple sclerosis, cerebral palsy, spinal cord injury, and arthritis. A cross-sectional analysis of the 2001 survey data was used to estimate annual prevalence and reasons and symptoms for which CAM practitioners were consulted. The 2000 survey was used to assess prior use of CAM. Nineteen percent of the sample population consulted CAM practitioners, which is a rate similar to, or higher than, the general population. Results showed that CAM use was more prevalent among women than men (24% versus 10%); in the Western United States (30%) compared to the Midwest (20%), Northeast (14%), and South (10%); and among prior users (62%) compared to nonusers (8%). Results showed no significant differences in CAM use by condition, although individuals with spinal cord injury reported the lowest CAM use (14%). Common symptoms treated included pain (80%), decreased functioning (43%), and lack of energy (24%). Common reasons for using CAM practitioners included lifestyle choice (67%) and because they are perceived to be more effective than conventional medicine (44%). This evidence suggests that a significant proportion of people with physical disabilities consult CAM prac-

titioners. Researchers noted that many of those who use CAM do so because it fits their lifestyle and because they perceive it to be more effective than conventional medicine for treating common symptoms including pain and decreased functioning (Carlson & Krahn, 2006).

An essential component in providing holistic care to patients is spiritual care. Although nursing education often lacks practical guidelines on how to provide culturally competent spiritual care, all nurses are required to provide spiritual care. Rehabilitation patients often face a lengthy recovery time and have special needs; therefore, rehabilitation nurses, in particular, are challenged to be competent in this area (Rieg, Mason, & Preston, 2006).

Nurses must be competent to provide care on a physical, mental, social, and spiritual level in order to deliver spiritual care. In one study, three main nursing competencies associated with the role of the nurse as a professional and as an individual person were identified: delivery of spiritual care by the nursing process; nurses' communication with patients, interdisciplinary team, and clinical/educational organizations; and safeguarding ethical issues in care. Spiritual care is complex, and the Nursing Code of Ethics recommends that nurses increase their awareness of each patient's individual uniqueness and the connection between mind, body, and spirit, and to assess the spiritual status of patients during illness and the implementation of holistic care (Baldacchino, 2006).

Another study investigated the relationship of spirituality and life satisfaction among persons with spinal cord injury. The study involved a nationwide sample of 230 persons with long-term spinal cord injury. These participants completed the Satisfaction with Life Scale (SWLS), the Quality of Life Index (QLI), and a demographic data form. Results indicated a significant positive correlation between life satisfaction and psychological/spiritual factors of the QLI instrument.

The International Council of Nurses, the Joint Commission on Accreditation of Healthcare Organizations, and the Patient's Bill of Rights mandate nurses to provide spiritual care for clients. Rehabilitation nurses, in particular, have the opportunity to support spirituality and life satisfaction when assisting clients with disabilities to redefine their lives and explore new life opportunities (Brillhart, 2005).

References

Baldacchino, D. R. (2006). Nursing competencies for spiritual care. *Journal of Clinical Nursing, 15*(7), 885–96.

Brillhart, B. (2005). A study of spirituality and life satisfaction among persons with spinal cord injury. *Rehabilitation Nursing, 30*(1), 31–4.

Carlson, M. J., & Krahn, G. (2006). Use of complementary and alternative medicine practitioners by people with physical disabilities: Estimates from a national U.S. survey. *Disability and Rehabilitation, 28*(8), 505–13.

Rieg, L. S., Mason, C. H., & Preston, K. (2006). Spiritual care: Practical guidelines for rehabilitation nurses. *Rehabilitation Nursing, 31*(6), 249–56.

Wardell, D. W., Rintala, D. H., Duan, Z., & Tan, G. (2006). A pilot study of healing touch and progressive relaxation for chronic neuropathic pain in persons with spinal cord injury. *Journal of Holistic Nursing, 24*(4), 231–240.

understand they can continue to be active both sexually and recreationally despite their injury. It is even possible for them to have children in the future if they so desire. The ongoing support of a urologist or gynecologist after discharge from the rehabilitation facility will be important in maintaining sexual health.

Once the patient is ready for discharge, identification of community resources for continued support to the patient and family and to assist with reintegration into the home environment and community is beneficial. Other patient teaching priorities are listed in the Patient Teaching & Discharge Priorities box.

◼ Collaborative Management

The patient with a SCI will require a multidisciplinary team approach to treatment throughout the continuum of care. The medical team will often consist of members of the trauma team and surgical team until stabilization of injuries is accomplished. Health care providers specializing in critical care medicine are helpful in management of cardiopulmonary issues in the acute phase after injury. A respiratory therapist will assist with pulmonary management including suctioning and cough and deep breathing strategies. Dietary consultation is helpful to ensure the patient's nutritional requirements are met.

Once the patient has been stabilized, physical and occupational therapy evaluation and treatment are necessary to assist with optimization of function through range-of-motion exercises, strengthening exercises, and instruction regarding mobility and use of adaptive equipment. Involvement of a social worker with expertise in SCI is vital to assist with issues related to lifestyle changes and loss of income as well as identification of resources to assist with transition into the community. The assistance of a

mental health expert, such as a psychologist, will be helpful to assist with issues of depression and adjustment to lifestyle changes related to the injury. Once the acute care issues of hemodynamic and spinal stability have been addressed, involvement of a physiatrist to direct rehabilitation efforts will be necessary.

Nurses are an integral part of the multidisciplinary team, providing a common link for all team members as well as providing education and support to the patient and family through all phases of treatment.

Gerontological Considerations

The number of patients over the age of 60 who have sustained an SCI has gradually increased during the last decade. Falls account for the leading cause of injury in this population. The elderly are at increased risk of injury to the spinal cord because of degenerative changes in the spinal column including ossification and hypertrophy of the spinal ligaments and development of bone spurs within the spinal column leading to narrowing of the spinal canal. Weakening of the bone due to osteoporosis also increases the risk of spinal fracture in these patients. This patient population presents an added challenge to the management of acute SCI because of preexisting medical problems such as diabetes and heart disease, as well as the normal physiological effects of aging (Chart 32–6, p. 856). These factors may affect overall outcomes in this age group (NSCISC, 2006; Villanueva, 2000).

Health Promotion

The majority of SCIs occur as a result of trauma and many of these injuries are preventable. The key to reducing the incidence of these injuries is to decrease high-risk behaviors such as driving while under the influence of drugs or alcohol, lack of seat belt use, and diving into shallow water. Several educational programs geared to both adults and children have been designed to increase

PATIENT TEACHING & DISCHARGE PRIORITIES for Spinal Cord Injury

Need	Teaching
Understanding of bowel/bladder regimen	The patient and family are taught how to perform CIC and how to perform bowel care including insertion of a suppository, digital stimulation of the bowel, and disimpaction of stool.
Prevention of complications	The patient and family are taught strategies such as frequent position changes and skin care to avoid the formation of pressure ulcers.
	The patient and family will understand the importance of maintaining a regular bowel and bladder regimen to avoid complications of UTI and bowel impaction.
Safety	Proper instruction on the use of adaptive equipment and transfer strategies will be given to the patient and family.
	The patient and family will be instructed on the signs and symptoms of autonomic hyperreflexia, common causes of hyperreflexia, and strategies to implement if autonomic hyperreflexia occurs.
Emotional adjustment of patient and family to psychosocial impact of SCI	The patient and family are encouraged to discuss their feelings openly.
	The patient and family will be able to identify supportive resources to help them cope with both the physical and psychosocial changes due to SCI.
Adaptation of environment	The patient and family will be provided instruction on necessary adaptation to the home environment and resources to assist with completion of environmental changes necessary to accommodate the patient's deficits and adaptive equipment.
	If the patient is unable to be discharged to a home environment, arrangements for an assisted living environment will be made.

CHART 32–6 Changes Associated with Aging

System	Associated Changes
Cardiovascular	↓ Contractile strength of the myocardium ↓ Cardiac output and stroke volume ↓ Vessel elasticity
Pulmonary	↓ Vital capacity ↓ Functional residual capacity ↑ Residual volume
Gastrointestinal	↓ Peristalsis ↓ Gastric acid secretion
Integument	↓ Subcutaneous tissue ↑ Thinning of epidermal layer
Musculoskeletal	↑ Osteoarthritic, degenerative joint changes ↓ Muscle mass, tone, and strength

Source: Adapted from Villanueva, N. E. (2000). Spinal cord injury in the elderly. *Critical Care Nurse Clinics of North America, 12,* 509–519.

awareness of those high-risk behaviors as well as to educate the public on simple strategies to decrease the risk of sustaining a SCI. These programs have been implemented in schools, workplaces, and communities, and often are comprised of a team of volunteers including a person who has sustained a permanent SCI and a health care provider who has experience in treating SCIs.

Prevention of complications is important to the maintenance of optimal health for the person with an SCI. Early detection and prompt treatment of problems such as alteration in skin integrity and UTIs are keys in preventing more serious complications such as sepsis and osteomyelitis. The person with an SCI should also be encouraged to obtain regular health maintenance evaluations for screening and treatment of chronic health problems including diabetes and heart disease. Counseling regarding smoking cessation and drug and alcohol use should not be overlooked in this patient population. Many people who have had an SCI are eventually able to return to active productive lives with the appropriate adaptive strategies and optimal health maintenance.

■ Research

Current spinal cord injury research continues to focus on ways to improve outcomes for patients with SCI as well as improving functional ability (see the Research Opportunities and Clinical Impact box). Much of this research is focused on limiting the secondary effects of spinal cord injury as well as restoration of function.

RESEARCH OPPORTUNITIES AND CLINICAL IMPACT RELATED TO SPINAL CORD INJURIES

Research Area	Clinical Impact
Administration of methylprednisolone or GM-1 ganglioside	Reduce secondary effects of spinal cord injury
Early versus delayed surgical decompression	
Cell transplantation into the spinal cord	Repair of spinal cord damage
Restorative therapy techniques	Improvement and restoration of function
Electrical stimulation of muscles below the level of injury	

Respiratory Complications Related to Spinal Cord Injury

Clinical Problem

Respiratory complications account for the most common cause of death in patients who have sustained a spinal cord injury. Patients with injury in the cervical spine are at the highest risk for morbidity and mortality related to respiratory issues due in large part to disruption of innervation to the diaphragm and respiratory accessory muscles; however, aspiration also contributes to pulmonary-related complications (Neville et al., 2005). Patients who have sustained a cervical spinal cord injury are at increased risk for aspiration not only because they are not able to adequately protect their airways due to ineffective protective measures such as cough, but also because these patients experience abnormality in swallowing.

Research Findings

Neville and colleagues (2005) conducted an evaluation of esophageal function in patients who had sustained traumatic cervical spinal cord injury. These authors hypothesized that patients with cervical spinal cord injury had abnormality of esophageal function that put them at risk for aspiration. The study sample consisted of 18 patients who had sustained traumatic cervical spinal cord injury. A control group for comparison was comprised of five patients who had sustained spinal cord injury at T_1 or below. Patients were excluded if they had associated head injury, known history of gastroesophageal reflux disease, previous gastric surgery, or previous antireflux surgery. All patients were subjected to measurement of esophageal pressures utilizing a manometric catheter inserted transnasally into the esophagus. Pressures were obtained at both the upper esophageal sphincter and lower esophageal sphincter. Measurement of peristaltic activity along the length of the esophagus during swallow was also obtained.

All patients in the study group had abnormally elevated pressures of the upper esophageal sphincter on swallow. This was not reflected in the control group. No abnormality of lower esophageal pressures or esophageal peristaltic activity was present for either the study or control group. The authors concluded that patients with cervical spinal cord injury have abnormal pressures of the upper esophageal sphincter necessitating increased force to move secretions or food from the oral pharynx into the esophagus during swallow and increasing the patient's risk for aspiration.

The effect of cervical bracing on swallow also has been evaluated. Stambolis et al. (2003) performed radiographic observation of swallow in 17 normal adults utilizing both solids and liquids without a cervical orthosis and in a rigid cervical collar, a SOMI brace, and in a halo brace. None of the subjects had previous history of swallowing abnormalities. Swallowing abnormalities were apparent in all bracing conditions and were most evident with liquid boluses. The investigators observed changes in the point of initiation of swallow, increased laryngeal penetration, increased residue in the pharynx, and reduced hyoid bone movement. They determined that cervical bracing placed the subjects in an unnatural eating position and limited the use of compensatory swallowing mechanisms. Many people slightly flex their necks when swallowing. This action was limited by the orthoses.

Also, most orthoses placed the subjects in a 90° head position, which caused narrowing of the oropharynx in some of subjects.

Morishima, Ohota, and Miura (2005) also evaluated the effect of halo brace fixation on swallow. Their study sample was comprised of six neurologically intact, healthy volunteers. Radiographic evaluation of swallow with thin liquids was obtained with the subjects in a neutral position without the brace and with the subjects in the halo brace with the head in a neutral position and in a hyperextended position. Activity of the muscles associated with swallow also was observed with electromyography. The investigators demonstrated changes in the activation of the muscles associated with swallow as well as prolonged transit of the liquids in the pharyngeal phase of swallow with the subjects in the halo brace with the head hyperextended. Penetration of liquid into the larynx and aspiration during swallow was also evident.

Implications for Nursing Practice

Based on these studies, the risk of aspiration due to swallowing abnormalities in the patient with cervical spinal cord injury is clearly present. These patients not only have abnormalities in the mechanics of swallow, but treatment modalities such as cervical bracing also contribute to swallowing dysfunction. It is important for nurses caring for this population to be aware of this risk so that appropriate assessment and prevention strategies can be instituted as part of the nursing plan of care. The patient and family also will need to be educated on the risk for aspiration as well as precautions to take to prevent it. If the patient exhibits signs of aspiration such as a wet quality to the voice, coughing with oral intake, or difficulty managing oral secretions, a referral for formal swallow evaluation is warranted. Prevention of aspiration is one of the key strategies in decreasing the risk of pulmonary complications.

Critical Thinking Questions

1. What are the risks for aspiration in the patient with cervical spinal cord injury?

2. What signs may indicate aspiration?

3. What precautions should be taken to avoid aspiration?

Answers to Critical Thinking Questions appear in Appendix D.

References

Morishima, N., Ohota, K., & Miura, Y. (2005). The influences of halo-vest fixation and cervical hyperextension on swallowing in healthy volunteers. *Spine, 30,* E179–E182.

Neville, A., Crookes, P., Velmahos, G., Vlahos, A., Theodorou, D., & Lucas, C. (2005). Esophageal dysfunction in cervical spinal cord injury: A potentially important mechanism of aspiration. *Journal of Trauma, 59,* 905–911.

Stambolis, V., Brady, S., Klos, D., Wesling, M., Fatianov, T., & Hildner, C. (2003). The effects of cervical bracing upon swallowing in young, normal, healthy volunteers. *Dysphagia, 18,* 39–45.

EVIDENCE-BASED PRACTICE

Clinical Preparation

CRITICAL THINKING

 Read

- History of Current Illness
- Past Medical History
- Physical Exam
- Admitting Medical Orders
- Laboratory Study Results

 Document

- Summary of Hospitalization
- Pathophysiology Form
- Laboratory Values
- Laboratory Results Explanation

Apply

- List of Potential Nursing Diagnoses
- Concept Map
- Critical Thinking Questions

Log on to MyNursingKit.com to download forms you will need and to complete further steps in the Clinical Preparation assignment.

HISTORY OF PRESENT ILLNESS

You are the nurse assigned to Mr. H., a 24-year-old male who sustained a spinal cord injury (SCI) 3 days ago. He dove into a pool from the roof of a house while attending a party. When his friends noted he did not surface, they jumped into the pool and brought him out of the water. They estimated he was submerged for 1 to 2 minutes. Once out of the water, Mr. H. was noted to only shrug his shoulders. He was unable to move his arms or legs and complained of feeling "numb" and short of breath. His friends called 911 and Mr. H. was transported to the hospital where he was diagnosed with a compression fracture of C_6, spinal cord contusion at C_6, and a complete SCI. There was no evidence of continued spinal cord compression from bone fragments within the canal, therefore, Mr. H. was placed in a halo brace.

Medical–Surgical History

Mr. H. denies significant past medical or surgical history.

Social History

Mr. H. is single. He lives alone and his parents are out of state. He smokes approximately 1.5 packs of cigarettes per day and drinks 24 to 48 cans of beer on the weekends. He denies recreational drug use.

Physical Exam

Mr. H. has a halo brace in place and the pin sites are clean. He has a triple-lumen, subclavian central line with normal saline infusing at 75 mL/hr in one port, and dopamine infusing at

15 mcg kg^{-1} min^{-1} into a second port to maintain a systolic blood pressure greater than 90 mmHg and O_2 saturation at 90%. He is receiving 50% oxygen via face mask. A nasogastric tube is in place and connected to low intermittent wall suction. An indwelling urinary catheter is draining yellow urine.

Mr. H. is awake, but does not open his eyes to answer questions or acknowledge staff. He is oriented to person, place, time, and current events. He denies complaint of pain, but does report feeling short of breath. Cranial nerve testing is normal. Motor exam reveals 5/5 strength with shoulder shrug and deltoid function bilaterally. Bicep strength is graded as 4/5 bilaterally. He has 0/5 motor function in the triceps, wrist extension, and hand intrinsics bilaterally. His lower extremities are flaccid.

He denies sensation to pinprick below the clavicle including the chest, abdomen, and lower extremities. He has intact sensation in the neck, shoulders, and palmar aspect of the hands. Deep tendon reflexes are 1+ in the biceps, but otherwise absent. Rectal tone is absent. Lung sounds are diminished in the bases. The patient is tachypneic and respirations are shallow. His abdomen is soft, non-tender, with hypoactive bowel sounds. He has not had a bowel movement since admission. His extremities are warm without erythema or edema. Peripheral pulses are intact.

Vital signs reveal a temperature of 37°C (98.6°F). Blood pressure is 90/46. Heart rate is 50 beats per minute, sinus bradycardia. Respiratory rate is 38 and shallow.

Admitting Medical Orders

Service: Neurosurgical

Admit to Neurosurgical ICU

Diagnosis: compression fracture of C_6, spinal cord contusion at C_6, and complete SCI

Allergies: none reported

Vital signs: q1h

Bed rest

Diet: NPO

Nasogastric tube to low intermittent suction

Call house officer: HR < 50 or <120, systolic blood pressure < 90 or > 160, RR < 12 or > 30, temperature < 38.5°C, urinary output less than 30 mL/hr × 2, O_2 saturation < 92%

Respiratory care: incentive spirometer q1h when awake, IPPB respiratory treatment q4h

CVP monitoring q4hours, notify health care provider if < 8 or > 20

Foley catheter

Maintain I&O

Pin site care with 0.5% H_2O_2 and normal saline bid

IVs: Normal saline at 75 mL/hr

Scheduled Medications

Famotidine 20 mg per NG bid

Senokot liquid 15 mL per NG bid

Dopamine titrated to keep the systolic BP above 90 mmHg

PRN Medications

Atropine 0.5–1 mg IV every 3–5 minutes prn heart rate less than 45 beats per minute, and call physician

Ordered Laboratory Studies

Daily ABGs, Chem 7, CBC, and albumin weekly

LABORATORY STUDY RESULTS

Test	Day 1	Day 2	Day 3
ABGs			
PO_2	90 mmHg	88 mmHg	72 mmHg
PCO_2	36 mmHg	38 mmHg	48 mmHg
pH	7.35	7.34	7.31
Chemistry			
Sodium	141 mEq/L	145 mEq/L	142 mEq/L
Potassium	3.8 mEq/L	4.0 mEq/L	4.0 mEq/L
Chloride	95 mEq/L	102 mEq/L	103 mEq/L
CO_2	23 mEq/L	21 mEq/L	21 mEq/L
Glucose	134 mg/dL	121 mg/dL	118 mg/dL
Blood urea nitrogen (BUN)	8 mg/dL	12 mg/dL	16 mg/dL
Creatinine	0.8 mg/dL	1.1 mg/dL	1.0 mg/dL
CBC			
WBC	10.5 µ/L	11.3 µ/L	15.1 µ/L
Hgb	14.7 g/dL	13.8 g/dL	13.0 g/dL
Hct	40.6 ml/dL	39.6 ml/dL	39.8 ml/dL
Platelets	300,000 µL	350,000 µL	300,000 µL
Albumin	2.6 g/dL		

CRITICAL THINKING QUESTIONS

1. What are the indicators in the assessment that should alert the nurse about potential for and/or actual decline in pulmonary status?

2. What measures should be instituted for DVT prophylaxis?

3. What are the possible GI complications for this patient?

4. What are the indicators Mr. H. may be experiencing depression?

5. What are common signs for autonomic hyperreflexia and what are measures to take should this occur?

Answers to Critical Thinking Questions appear in Appendix D.

NCLEX® REVIEW

1. The nurse is teaching a group of nursing students about the causes of spinal cord injury. Which of the following statements made by one of the students indicates a clear understanding of the topic?

   1. "Forward falls in which the chin or forehead strikes the ground might produce compression spinal cord injuries."

   2. "When axial pressure is loaded on the spine, the resultant rotational injuries might include fracture of the vertebral body."

   3. "Hyperextension injuries can cause anterior vertebral body fractures and posterior spinal column facet fracture and dislocation."

   4. "A sudden deceleration injury, such as a head-on motor vehicle collision, is frequently the cause of hyperflexion injuries."

2. The patient was involved in a motor vehicle collision with rear impact and is now experiencing severe neck pain and decreased upper extremity motor function, but there is normal motor function in the lower extremities. The patient complains of parasthesias in both the upper and lower extremities but greater in the arms. Based on these findings you suspect the patient may have which of the following types of injuries?

   1. Anterior cord syndrome

   2. Central cord syndrome

   3. Cauda equina syndrome

   4. Brown-Séquard syndrome

3. Which of the following statements best describes appropriate prophylaxis for some of the most common complications following spinal cord injury?

   1. Use of an abdominal binder and compression stockings to decrease the peripheral venous pooling that can cause neurogenic shock
   2. Use of a Duplex Doppler ultrasound to dissolve deep vein thromboembolisms and reduce the likelihood of pulmonary embolus
   3. Use of a reclining wheelchair to gradually progress the patient into an upright position so as not to cause orthostatic hypotension
   4. Use of sound nutritional measures such as an increased caloric, protein, and micronutrient intake to promote bowel evacuation

4. When planning educational opportunities related to the psychosocial impact of spinal cord injury, the nurse understands that:

   1. The patient's family will need ongoing education to help deal with the stress of any role changes associated with the injury.
   2. The patient may exhibit any number of negative emotions about physical challenges, including elation and jubilation.
   3. The patient should be encouraged to discuss his feelings openly and to support the decisions made for him by the health care provider.
   4. The patient is usually so preoccupied with the physical challenges faced after a spinal cord injury that psychosocial problems rarely occur.

5. The nurse understands that the needs of the patient with a spinal cord injury (SCI) are unique. When planning the discharge of the patient with SCI, the nurse should include which of the following?

   1. Information regarding support systems that can help the patient and his family adjust to the changes in lifestyle and roles
   2. Referral to a rehabilitation program that uses a single, specialized discipline to help the patient adapt to his injury limitations
   3. Strategies such as infrequent position changes that avoid shearing and will help in the prevention of pressure ulcer formation
   4. Instruction on the importance of avoiding use of suppository medication or other bowel stimulation so as to prevent hyperreflexia

6. When planning care for the patient with spinal cord injury, which nursing diagnosis has the highest priority?

   1. Risk for imbalanced nutrition less than body requirements related to increased metabolic need and inadequate caloric intake
   2. Anxiety related to loss of independence, loss of control over environment and uncertainty of the future
   3. Risk for ineffective peripheral tissue perfusion related to the formation of deep venous thrombosis
   4. Ineffective airway clearance related to the loss of spinal innervation of the respiratory and accessory muscles

Answers for review questions appear in Appendix D

KEY TERMS

afferent *p.831*
areflexia *p.837*
autonomic hyperreflexia *p.838*
cauda equina syndrome *p.835*
complete spinal cord injury *p.832*
compression injuries *p.836*
contusion *p.837*
efferent *p.831*

hyperflexion injuries *p.835*
hyperreflexia *p.837*
incomplete spinal cord injury *p.834*
myelopathy *p.835*
neurogenic shock *p.837*
odontoid process *p.842*
paraplegia *p.832*
quadriplegia (*Latin*) *p.832*

rotational injuries *p.836*
spinal cord injury (SCI) *p.830*
spinal precautions *p.840*
spinal shock *p.837*
spondylitic disease *p.835*
tetraplegia (*Greek*) *p.832*
transection *p.837*

REFERENCES

Apuzzo, M. L. (Ed.) (2002a). Cervical spine immobilization before admission to the hospital. Guidelines for the management of acute spine and spinal cord injuries. *Neurosurgery, 50*(Suppl.), S7–S17.

Apuzzo, M. L. (Ed.) (2002b). Deep venous thrombosis and thromboembolism in patients with cervical spinal cord injuries. Guidelines for the management of acute spine and spinal cord injuries. *Neurosurgery, 50*(Suppl.), S73–S80.

Apuzzo, M. L. (Ed.) (2002c). Management of acute central cervical spinal cord injuries. Guidelines for the management of acute spine and spinal cord injuries. *Neurosurgery, 50*(Suppl.), S166–S171.

Apuzzo, M. L. (Ed.) (2002d). Pharmacologic therapy after acute cervical spinal cord injury. Guidelines for the management of acute spine and spinal cord injuries. *Neurosurgery, 50*(Suppl.), S63–S72.

Apuzzo, M. L. (Ed.) (2002e). Radiographic assessment of the cervical spine in symptomatic trauma patients. Guidelines for the management of acute spine and spinal cord injuries. *Neurosurgery, 50*(Suppl.), S36–S43.

Ball, P. A. (2001). Critical care of spinal cord injury. *Spine, 15*(Suppl.), S27–S30.

Bernbeck, J., & Delamarter, R. B. (2000). Pathophysiology and initial treatment of acute spinal cord injuries. In J. M. Cotler, J. M. Simpson, H. S. An, & C. P. Silveri (Eds.), *Surgery of spinal trauma* (pp. 45–60). Philadelphia: Lippincott Williams & Wilkins.

Bloomer, C., Ackerman, A., & Bhatia, R. (2006). Imaging for spine tumors and new applications. *Topics in Magnetic Resonance Imaging, 17,* 69–87.

Connelly, C. (2001). Alterations in affiliative relationships. In C. Stewart-Amidei & J. A. Kunkel (Eds.), *AANN's neuroscience nursing: Human responses to neurologic dysfunction* (2nd ed., pp. 391–405). Philadelphia: W. B. Saunders.

Enck, P., Greving, I., Klosterhalfen, S., & Wietek, B. (2006). Upper and lower gastrointestinal motor and sensory dysfunction after spinal cord injury. *Progress in Brain Research, 152,* 373–384.

France, J. C., Bono, C. M., & Vaccaro, A. R. (2005). Initial evaluation of the spine after trauma: When, what, where, and how to image the acutely traumatized spine. *Journal of Orthopaedic Trauma, 19,* 640–649.

Hadley, M. (2002). Blood pressure management after acute spinal cord injury. *Neurosurgery, 50*(Suppl.), S58–S62.

Hendy, G. W., Wolfson, A. B., Mower, W. R., & Hoffman, J. R. (2002). Spinal cord injury without radiographic abnormality: Results of the national emergency x-radiography utilization study in blunt cervical trauma. *Journal of Trauma, Injury, Infection and Critical Care, 53,* 1–4

Henson, J. W. (2001). Spinal cord gliomas. *Current Opinion in Neurology, 14,* 679–682.

Hickey, J. V. (2003a). Overview of neuroanatomy and neurophysiology. In J. V. Hickey (Ed.), *The clinical practice of neurological and neurosurgical nursing* (5th ed., pp. 45–92). Philadelphia: Lippincott Williams & Wilkins

Hickey, J. V. (2003b). Vertebral and spinal cord injuries. In J. V. Hickey (Ed.), *The clinical practice of neurological and neurosurgical nursing* (5th ed., pp. 407–450). Philadelphia: Lippincott Williams & Wilkins.

Hurlbert, J. R. (2006). Strategies of medical intervention in the management of acute spinal cord injury. *Spine, 31*(Suppl.), S16–S21.

Kirschblum, S. C., & O'Connor, K. C. (2000). Levels of spinal cord injury and predictors of neurologic recovery. *Physical Medicine and Rehabilitation Clinics of North America, 11,* 1–27.

Kothari, P., Freeman, B., Grevitt, M., & Kerslak, R. (2000). Injury to the spinal cord without radiologic abnormality (SCIWORA) in adults. *Journal of Bone and Joint Surgery, 82-B,* 1034–1037.

Krassioukov, A. (2004). Autonomic dysreflexia in acute spinal cord injury: Injury, mechanisms, and management. *SCI Nursing, 21,* 215–216.

Kwon, B. K., Tetzlaff, W., Grauer, J. N., Beiner, J., & Vaccaro, A. R. (2004). Pathophysiology and pharmacologic treatment of acute spinal cord injury. *Spine Journal, 4,* 451–464.

Lindsay, K. W., & Bone, I. (Eds.) (2004). Localized neurologic disease and its management: B. Spinal cord and roots. In *Neurology and neurosurgery illustrated* (4th ed., pp. 385–423). London: Churchill Livingston.

McIlvoy, L., Meyer, K., & McQuillan, K. A. (2004). Traumatic spine injuries. In M. K. Bader & L. R. Littlejohns (Eds.), *AANN core curriculum for neuroscience nursing* (4th ed., pp. 335–402). St. Louis: W. B. Saunders.

Mulnard, R. A. (2001). Sensation: An overview. In C. Stewart-Amidei & J. A. Kunkel (Eds.), *AANN's neuroscience nursing: Human responses to neurologic dysfunction* (2nd ed., pp. 533–556). Philadelphia: W. B. Saunders.

National Center for Injury Prevention and Control (2006). *Spinal cord injury (SCI): Fact sheet.* Retrieved April 28, 2008, from http://www.cdc.gov/ncipc/factsheets/scifacts.htm

National Guideline Clearinghouse. (2001). *Acute management of autonomic dysreflexia: Individuals with spinal cord injury presenting to a health-care facility.* Washington, DC: Consortium for Spinal Cord Medicine, Paralyzed Veterans of America. Retrieved November 14, 2006, from http://www.guideline.gov/summary/summary.aspx?doc_id=2964&nbr=002190&string=Autonomic+AND+dysreflexia

National Guideline Clearinghouse. (2005a). *Neurogenic bowel management in adults with spinal cord injury.* Washington, DC: Consortium for Spinal Cord Medicine, Paralyzed Veterans of America. Retrieved November 14, 2006, from http://www.guideline.gov/summary/summary.aspx?doc_id=850&nbr=000394&string=spinal+AND+cord+AND+injury

National Guideline Clearinghouse. (2005b). *Prevention of thromboembolism in spinal cord injury.* Washington, DC: Consortium for Spinal Cord Medicine, Paralyzed Veterans of America. Retrieved April 29, 2008, from http://www.guideline.gov/summary/summary.aspx?doc_id=2965&nbr=002191&string=spinal+AND+cord+AND+Injury.

National Guideline Clearinghouse. (2005c). *Respiratory management following spinal cord injury: A clinical practice guideline for health-care professionals.* Washington, DC: Consortium for Spinal Cord Medicine, Paralyzed Veterans of America. Retrieved April 29, 2008, from http://www.guideline.gov/summary/summary.aspx?doc_id=7198&nbr=004301&string=spinal+AND+cord+AND+injury

National Spinal Cord Injury Statistical Center. (2006). *Spinal cord injury: Facts and figures at a glance—June 2006.* Retrieved November 14, 2006, from http://www.spinalcord.uab.edu

Pang, D., & Wilberger, J. E. (1982). Spinal cord injuries without radiographic abnormalities in children. *Journal of Neurosurgery, 57,* 114–129.

Paralyzed Veterans of America. (2001). Pressure ulcer prevention and treatment following spinal cord injury: A clinical practice guideline for health-care professionals. *Journal of Spinal Cord Medicine, 24*(Suppl. 1), S40–S101.

Pataki, P., Woodhouse, J., Hamid, R., Shah, J., & Craggs, M. (2006). Lower urinary tract dysfunction in ambulatory patients with incomplete spinal cord injury. *Journal of Urology, 175,* 1784–1787.

Prendergast, V., & Sullivan, C. (2000). Acute spinal cord injury: Nursing considerations for the first 72 hours. *Critical Care Nursing Clinics of North America, 12,* 499–508.

Sayer, F. T., Kronvall, E., & Nilsson, O. G. (2006). Methylprednisolone treatment in acute spinal cord injury: The myth challenged through a structures analysis of the published literature. *Spine Journal, 6,* 335–343.

Sekhon, L., & Fehlings, M. (2001). Epidemiology, demographics, and pathophysiology of acute spinal cord injury. *Spine, 26*(24 Suppl.), S2–S12.

Spinal Cord Injury Information Network. (2006). *Etiology of SCI since 1990.* Retrieved November 22, 2006, from http://www.spinalcord.uab.edu/show.asp?durki=25426.

Villanueva, N. E. (2000). Spinal cord injury in the elderly. *Critical Care Nurse Clinics of North America, 12,* 509–519.

Walker, J., & Criddle, L. M. (2001). Methylprednisolone in acute spinal cord injury: Fact or fantasy? *Journal of Emergency Nursing, 27,* 401–403.

UNIT

7 | Nursing Management of Patients with Respiratory Disorders

Research

Nursing Process

Caring

LINDA   My name is Linda and I am a clinical resource nurse (CN III) in the Trauma/Surgical ICU (SICU-I) at a 540-bed teaching hospital in Northern California. The hospital is a Level I trauma center associated with the University of California Davis, School of Medicine. In my unit we care for the sickest of the adult trauma patients. Although I mainly care for trauma victims, anyone needing intensive monitoring and critical care is a potential patient. In addition to patient care, I also precept new nurses and I am one of a six-member clinical resource team responsible for contributing to the continuing education of all nursing staff in our 12-bed unit.

In the course of performing as a patient-care advocate, six important characteristics of caring have become evident. These characteristics are an integral part of my role as a professional nurse and are incorporated into the daily care of my patients. For example, I cared for a female patient who had been injured in a car crash months ago but whose poor health, chronic back pain, and anxiety were prolonging weaning from the ventilator. She had a tracheostomy and required numerous doses of prn analgesics and frequent repositioning throughout the day to treat her pain. **Compassion** for what I thought was inadequate pain and anxiety control prompted me to obtain an order for a Pharmacy Pain Service consultation. My **conscience** would not allow me to simply give more doses of sedatives without attempting to find a better solution. The pharmacist evaluated her history, spoke with the patient, and developed a plan that added three new medications and cancelled one. The results were impressive. Her need for prn medication in a 24-hour period went from 17 doses of two narcotics down to 6 doses of one narcotic. She appeared much more comfortable and started smiling more. I cannot express how pleased I was to be a part of easing her discomfort after witnessing her previous misery.

Another patient I vividly remember was an elderly Korean pedestrian who had been hit by a car. Her injuries included multiple fractures and a small liver laceration. She had been recently extubated following surgery but still required oxygen at 4 L/min, and her arterial blood gas (ABG) results were of concern because she had documented pneumonia. She had nearly absent breath sounds on the right side. She spoke Korean and was confused and therefore unable to cooperate with incentive spirometry or deep breathing and coughing exercises. There were new physician orders to feed her. After performing an initial morning assessment, I was reluctant to feed her due to concern about her respiratory status and possible compromised swallowing ability. My concern was that if she aspirated her food that she would further compromise her already tenuous respiratory status. I expressed my concerns to the resident who had written the orders to feed her, and he disagreed and wanted her fed.

The patient's daughter was in the room and asking questions about her mother. In answering her, I gave her physiological reasons for my concerns but also let her know about my many years of experience and that of the physicians, to ease her mind. In situations like this, my **comportment** can make a difference in how family members respond to what is happening to their loved ones.

I subsequently verbalized my concerns to the attending physician who put eating on hold until he could view the morning chest x-ray results. **Confidence** in my experience and abilities allows me to pursue patient-care issues like this despite the disagreement with the resident. As it turned out, the x-ray showed a large right pleural effusion. The patient then needed a CT scan of the chest. Taking any critically ill patient to the radiology department involves planning for the worst and hoping for the best. Preparing for any emergency is part of my responsibility as a **competent** critical care nurse. In this case, I took all the emergency equipment and drugs to the radiology department, but fortunately none of it was needed. Although, based on the CT scan a chest tube was placed, which drained a liter of blood. Needless to say, she didn't eat that day.

Being an ICU nurse isn't only about the drama of car crashes, gunshot wounds, and saving lives. It is also about my role as patient advocate and protector. There is no doubt this can be challenging and frustrating, but the rewards include pride in my contribution to helping others and tremendous satisfaction that what I do has value to individuals and to society in general. I also must confess to appreciating the intermittent adrenaline rush and sense of camaraderie that results from working together to save a life. I feel fortunate to have a career for which I continue to have passion.

The internal **commitment** I have made as a nurse is to do as much as I can for my patients on each shift, which includes anything from washing the bloody, glass-riddled hair of an accident victim to doing CPR on a cardiac patient.

Nursing Assessment
of Patients
with Respiratory Disorders

Karen Cooper

Outcome-Based Learning Objectives

After studying this chapter, the learner will be able to:

1. Compare and contrast normal and adventitious breath sounds.
2. Defend the importance of obtaining information on recent travel as a component of the patient history.
3. Describe the relationship of data obtained from the review of a patient's social and occupational history with risk for pulmonary disease.
4. Describe the essential components of a physical assessment of the pulmonary system.
5. Compare and contrast adjuncts used during physical assessment of the pulmonary system.

NURSES IN ALL health care settings require an in-depth knowledge of the pulmonary system and pulmonary skills to be able to rapidly assess the respiratory status of their patients. Breathing and oxygenation are essential to life. The nursing history and physical examination can uncover valuable clues to the origin of actual or potential problems limiting the patient's ability to breathe effectively. Many pathologic conditions can interfere with the body's ability to exchange oxygen and carbon dioxide both within the pulmonary system as well as on a cellular level in all body structures. Nursing assessment of a patient's respiratory status encompasses all of the senses and accurate and appropriate use of a stethoscope as well as information obtained from review of laboratory tests, pulmonary function tests, chest x-rays, and pulse oximetry. Nurses need to be able to recognize normal assessment findings and identify subtle deviations from normal that signal worsening of the patient's condition. Rapid intervention based on assessment findings is crucial to prevent adverse outcomes.

Ventilation is the movement of air into and out of the lungs. As the lung tissue expands, it increases the surfaces available for exchange of oxygen and carbon dioxide. The levels of oxygen in the pulmonary tree set up a gradient forcing the exchange of oxygen on the pulmonary side with carbon dioxide from the vascular side. The act of breathing is regulated by the respiratory centers in the brainstem, voluntary muscle activity, and stimula-

tion of chemoreceptors by changes in pH and oxygen levels in the blood. The respiratory rate and depth are also influenced by these mechanisms. Disease states as well as emotions can also influence these mechanisms. The nurse must utilize knowledge of the patient's history and perform a comprehensive physical assessment to assist in determining the causes of changes in respiratory patterns and findings.

Anatomy and Physiology of the Pulmonary System

Ventilation consists of the movement of air from the environment into the pulmonary system. Respiration consists of the diffusion of oxygen across the alveolar–capillary membrane into the pulmonary circulation, which includes oxygen molecule attachment to hemoglobin molecules and the release of carbon dioxide molecules from hemoglobin across the alveolar–capillary membranes and through the airways out to the environment.

Conducting airways such as the trachea and bronchi do not participate in oxygen–carbon dioxide exchange, but allow passage of these molecules and gases from the bloodstream in and out of the environment. If the conducting airways are blocked by secretions or other conditions causing obstruction, they are unable to permit adequate movement of air and oxygen to the alveoli for gas exchange.

Ventilation is dependent on neurological and musculoskeletal integrity. The central nervous system (CNS) responds to changes in the carbon dioxide and oxygen levels in the blood to influence increases or decreases in the rate and depth of respiration. The medulla and pons respond to changes in respiratory rate and depth as well as changes in the oxygen and carbon dioxide levels in the blood to increase or decrease the rate and depth of respiration. Musculoskeletal structures influencing respiration include the intercostal muscles, diaphragm, abdominal muscles, and thoracic muscles such as the scalene, sternomastoid, and trapezius.

Inspiration and expiration are also influenced by intrapleural pressures. When the pressure of air in the lungs during inspiration reaches capacity, expiration occurs. Inspiration is an active procedure related to neuromuscular activities, but expiration is essentially passive, related to reaching the maximum elastic stretch of the respiratory muscles and the recoil of these muscles. The movement of air in one breath is the tidal volume. The movement of air over 1 minute is the minute ventilation. Tidal volume is usually about 500 mL during normal ventilation, but can increase if more is demanded by the body, as can occur during exercise or times of stress.

The alveoli are the structures where exchange of oxygen and carbon dioxide occurs. For adequate exchange of these gases, the alveoli must be adequately expanded by air and have adequate contact with hemoglobin molecules in the capillaries. If the alveoli are fully expanded but unable to exchange oxygen with the capillaries due to edema or secretions lining the alveoli, a ventilation/perfusion mismatch occurs and the patient will exhibit signs and symptoms of hypoxia. If the alveoli are not able to distend adequately, despite adequate blood flow (perfusion), ventilation/perfusion mismatch will again occur and the patient will exhibit signs and symptoms of hypoxia.

Perfusion, the movement of oxygen across the alveolar–capillary membrane, is dependent on gravity, oxygen concentrations on the alveolar and capillary sides, and the availability of hemoglobin molecules for oxygen binding. Patients who are anemic will have fewer hemoglobin binding sites for oxygen. Also, if a patient's circulation is compromised by conditions such as shock or heart failure, the patient will not be able to exchange oxygen and carbon dioxide because blood flow is diverted from the alveoli and will not allow the exchange of gases to occur.

The nurse must be knowledgeable of the physiology of the pulmonary system and the physical integrity of the patient to be able to determine the ability of the patient to adequately exchange oxygen and carbon dioxide. Physical examination findings, diagnostic testing, and diagnostic criteria are described in this chapter for the nurse to assess the patient's current status and determine if current therapies are effective.

History

Components of the patient history include both objective and subjective data. Effective interviewing skills are necessary to elicit pertinent data regarding the symptoms and the effect the symptoms have on the patient's ability to carry out life functions. Biographic and demographic data assist the interviewer in determining if any cultural or educational factors figure importantly into the manner and style of the interview process.

The health history should begin with the complaint that caused the patient to seek care (the chief complaint), and what the patient thinks may have initiated the problem. The past medical history may provide clues as to the nature of the current problem. For example, a patient with a prior history of breast or testicular cancer may present with shortness of breath related to metastases from the primary site. The social history not only gives valuable clues regarding the availability of potential caregivers, but also may indicate potential occupational sources of the current patient problems.

One of the issues facing nurses caring for patients with respiratory disease is shortness of breath. Patients may not be able to verbally complete the health history due to **dyspnea**, the subjective feeling of shortness of breath or difficulty breathing. Therefore, it may be necessary for the nurse to obtain information from family members or the available medical record regarding the basic history, and limit the history obtained from the patient to focused responses and information not available from other sources. The nurse may need to focus on allowing the patient to rest and limit all forms of exertion during the history. Use of yes and no questions or allowing the patient to write or use a communication board may be useful. The nurse may need to provide supplemental oxygen for the patient to relieve distress and, in doing so, the nurse should follow established facility protocols. Patients with chronic respiratory diseases may respond adversely to increased oxygen levels, which can suppress their respiratory drive. Normally, hypoxia will cause an increase in respiratory drive. Patients with chronic hypoxia, such as that seen in chronic obstructive pulmonary disease (COPD), may no longer respond to hypoxia, and instead will respond to elevated carbon dioxide levels to stimulate breathing. Use of high-flow oxygen in this group may result in respiratory arrest.

Biographic and Demographic Data

Assessment of biographic and demographic data includes information regarding age, race, gender, and culture that can influence the patient's understanding, preconceptions, and susceptibility to some pulmonary disorders. In some instances, knowledge of the patient's place of birth or current address may give clues to the origin of the current complaints. For example, patients with a productive cough and night sweats who were born in or recently relocated from areas where tuberculosis (TB) is common should be isolated and appropriate precautions taken both during the interview and during discussions with the patient, family members, and continued care providers. If TB is suspected, testing measures such as sputum testing, chest x-ray, and/or intradermal tuberculin placement (PPD) testing must take place. Places of residence may also include areas with poor air quality or the presence of allergens and irritants that affect the respiratory system.

Gender no longer appears to be a factor in the development of pulmonary disease. Lung cancer, COPD, and emphysema occur only slightly more frequently in men than in women. Lymphangiomyomatosis is a disease affecting young women in their 20s and 30s that may have a genetic or hormonal component that causes changes in the smooth muscle tissue of the lung and cyst development. The symptoms and treatment of this disease are similar to those for emphysema. Normal aging may also play a part in activity-related shortness of breath. The nurse must utilize knowledge of age-related changes in the pulmonary vessels and tissue when performing a respiratory assessment.

Chief Complaint

The chief complaint is the patient's impression of what caused him to seek care. It should be recorded in the patient's own words. Often, by asking what exactly caused him to seek care, the patient will give information on both the symptoms and the impact the symptoms have had on his lifestyle and functional abilities. The chief complaint should direct a focused assessment of the patient's perception of the problem and the presenting symptoms.

Presenting Symptoms

A review of symptoms explores the patient's symptoms in a systematic fashion. The nurse may use any of a number of guidelines for this exploration. The PQRST (Dillon, 2003) or the COLDSA (Weber & Kelley, 2003) method may be helpful in performing a systematic analysis of symptoms. Each of these methods is used to describe a specific symptom in terms of location, onset, duration, quality, severity, aggravating and relieving factors, and related symptoms (Chart 33–1). The patient should be asked specifically when the symptoms began and how the symptoms progressed. Aggravating and relieving factors must be explored, as well as the timing at which the symptoms occur. For example, if shortness of breath occurs at night or with activity, the nurse must explore the possibility of a cardiovascular component to the presenting symptom.

Dyspnea, difficulty breathing, is a very common chief complaint for patients with respiratory illness. Because dyspnea is considered a subjective finding, current research is attempting to validate specific dyspnea scales so that they can be utilized in a manner similar to the analog and Wong-Baker pain scales. Orthopnea is shortness of breath that occurs in the supine position. Orthopnea may be related to gastrointestinal reflux, heart failure, or pulmonary disease. Exploration of symptoms with

---

CHART 33–1	**Symptom Assessment Mnemonics**

PQRST EVALUATION OF SYMPTOMS

P	**P**alliative and/or **P**rovocative
Q	**Q**uality and **Q**uantity
R	**R**adiation and location
S	**S**everity
T	**T**ime of day and duration

COLDSA EVALUATION OF SYMPTOMS

C	**C**haracter
O	**O**nset
L	**L**ocation
D	**D**uration
S	**S**everity
A	**A**ssociated factors

---

specific questions will aid the nurse in pinpointing the origin of the dysfunction. Presenting symptoms associated with pulmonary disease that should be explored with the patient include cough, sputum production, shortness of breath, chest, back or thoracic pain, activity intolerance, hemoptysis (bloody sputum), sleep disorders, and "noisy" respirations.

Past Medical History

The past medical history gives insight into the effect that prior illnesses and conditions may have on the current presenting symptom. For example, a prior history of prolonged intubation associated with cardiac surgery may indicate the risk of either cardiovascular system associated complications or preexisting pulmonary problems that can impact the patient's current condition. If the patient has received treatment for cardiac dysrhythmias, the nurse can explore the potential for medication-related pulmonary fibrosis such as occurs with the use of amiodarone. A history of thyroid disease may implicate myxedema or thyrotoxicosis as precipitating factors in the development of shortness of breath (see Chapter 52).

Childhood Diseases and Immunizations

Premature birth, childhood diseases, congenital pulmonary disease, and immunization (or lack thereof) are important to include in the history portion of the respiratory assessment. Current immunization status for influenza and pneumococcal pneumonia should also be assessed. Today, a number of adults present to health care systems with cystic fibrosis, often considered a childhood disease state. Asthma symptoms are frequently first seen during childhood. Cystic fibrosis and asthma are discussed in detail in Chapter 35 . Finally, the patient should be asked if she had frequent colds, episodes of wheezing, or shortness of breath during childhood.

Patients born prematurely who were mechanically ventilated for long periods in neonatal intensive care units (NICUs) may suffer from primary or secondary pulmonary disease. Pulmonary disease in this population may be related to lung injury such as barotrauma from ventilation pressures, to prolonged use of high oxygen levels, to primary pulmonary disease such as pulmonary atresia, to pulmonary hypertension, or to primary congenital heart disease or valvular dysfunction. Neonatal respiratory distress syndrome is caused by a lack of surfactant in the immature lungs of premature babies. Although synthetic exogenous surfactant is available today to treat this complication of preterm birth, adults currently presenting with pulmonary problems may not have had treatment with the medication and are at risk for long-term or chronic complications.

The nurse should also ask the patient if he suffered any childhood trauma. Swimming accidents during childhood could result in aspiration of water and resultant lung injury. Likewise, aspiration of foreign bodies in childhood may cause structural damage to airways.

Adults who work in areas where they will be exposed to flu, such as health care workers, the elderly, and patients with chronic conditions such as asthma and COPD, should receive yearly flu vaccination. The elderly and patients with chronic diseases should also receive pneumococcal vaccine to prevent pneumococcal pneumonia.

Previous Illnesses and Hospitalizations

The frequency of previous episodes of pneumonia, asthma exacerbations, and respiratory distress should be elicited from the patient as well as any hospitalizations associated with these conditions. This will give insight into the potential severity of the patient's condition or to the progression of the disease process. Treatment modalities, such as tracheostomy, chest tube insertion, intubation, and use of oxygen, should also be elicited. Information regarding hospitalizations and illnesses not necessarily related to the pulmonary system are also important. For example, a patient hospitalized with a bowel obstruction may have suffered aspiration related to reflux of gastric contents. Cardiac disease frequently has an adverse impact on the pulmonary system. Heart failure is a classic example of cardiac disease causing pulmonary symptoms and may result in residual pulmonary problems. Heart failure is discussed in detail in Chapter 42 👓. Mitral valve disease, or papillary muscle rupture associated with myocardial infarction may cause pulmonary congestion. Mitral valve abnormalities are discussed in Chapter 41 👓.

Treatment for thyroid disease may include local radiation therapy that could result in narrowing of the trachea due to goiter compression or tissue damage and edema from therapy. Patients who have been diagnosed with cancer may have metastases to the lung or a treatment that affects the pulmonary system. Thoracic trauma causing a rib fracture may impair the patient's ability to deep breathe and expectorate secretions. The patient with rib fractures is at risk for hypoventilation and pneumonia. Liver failure associated with alpha$_1$-antitrypsin (AAT) deficiency is also associated with the development of emphysema and pulmonary disease.

The patient's response to hospitalization and previous illness gives the nurse valuable information regarding prior experience with invasive and noninvasive testing and treatment. The analysis of previous illnesses and hospitalization also provides knowledge of comorbid conditions that may complicate diagnosis and care.

Diagnostic Procedures or Surgeries

The results of diagnostic procedures performed and the surgical history should be obtained by the nurse performing a respiratory assessment. Prior thoracic surgery, lung biopsy, or bronchoscopy indicates prior pulmonary dysfunction. Pulmonary function tests can give insight into the extent or nature of pulmonary disease. Chest x-rays give valuable information regarding the condition of pleural tissue, presence of rib fractures, pneumothorax, hemothorax, pulmonary edema, pneumonia, interstitial disease, and lung lesions. Electrocardiography (ECG) may indicate a cardiac component to the patient's condition or demonstrate changes related to pulmonary embolism. The ventilation and perfusion (V/Q) scan is the gold standard for diagnosis of pulmonary embolus determining lung perfusion status. Deep venous thrombosis (DVT), a precursor to pulmonary embolism, may be diagnosed from Doppler studies or suggested by a positive D-dimer blood test. Patient's who have had immobilizing illnesses and surgery of the abdomen or lower extremities are at risk for the development of DVT.

Arterial blood gas (ABG) analysis is utilized to determine oxygen and carbon dioxide levels and oxygen saturation. Laboratory tests such as the complete blood count (CBC) may give insight into an infectious process or anemia causing shortness of breath.

Carboxyhemoglobin levels should be obtained on patients exposed to smoke or fire, particularly if the exposure was in an enclosed space, or patients exposed to excessive automobile exhaust fumes. Sputum cultures are utilized to determine organisms causing pneumonia. In addition acid-fast bacilli testing of sputum cultures is utilized to determine if the patient has tuberculosis. Tuberculin skin testing is also used to determine exposure to tuberculosis. The AAT blood test is utilized to diagnose AAT deficiency, which is related to the development of pulmonary and liver disease in susceptible individuals. Allergy testing may be performed in patients exhibiting frequent occurrences of wheezing, pulmonary congestion, or chronic cough.

Medications

The patient should be encouraged to carry a list of all current medications. If possible, the medical record can also be explored for the use of medications prior to the present time. When discussing current medications with the patient, the nurse should inquire about dosage, frequency, and the last time the medication was taken. This is especially relevant if the patient is prescribed bronchodilators, anticholinergics, and steroids. Increased use of these medications may indicate that the patient's condition is worsening. Failure to take medications as directed may also increase pulmonary symptoms. The correct order in which to take inhaled medications is to take bronchodilators first to open the airways. Steroids should be taken after bronchodilators to improve absorption when the airways are dilated (open). Over-the-counter (OTC) medications such as cough suppressants, expectorants, antihistamines, or herbal supplements may be overlooked by patients in their report of medications taken. The nurse should specifically ask about OTC medication use.

If the patient is currently prescribed medications to treat tuberculosis, or antibiotics to treat pneumonia, the nurse should ensure that the patient is taking the medications as prescribed. Patients will frequently stop taking medications when they feel well. It should come as no surprise that symptoms return when patients fail to take medications as prescribed. When patients fail to complete a course of antibiotic therapy, the organism may develop a resistance and the antibiotic will no longer be effective in its treatment. Use of medications other than those prescribed for pulmonary disease may cause pulmonary symptoms. For example, angiotensin converting enzyme (ACE) inhibitors may cause cough, and amiodarone may cause pulmonary fibrosis. Respiratory medications are discussed in detail in Chapters 35 and 36 👓.

Patients who use inhalers should be requested to demonstrate their technique. If they are using metered-dose inhalers or spacers, the nurse should ensure that they are used correctly. Patients may assume that it is correct to use a spacer with all inhaled medications, when this is not true. For example, Advair, a combination inhaler, is not supposed to be taken with a spacer. Patients should be encouraged to bring all inhalers to their assessment. If patients bring inhalers that are no longer part of the prescribed regimen, they should be discarded to prevent the patient from potential overmedication with one of the inhaler components.

Allergies

Allergies frequently cause pulmonary symptoms ranging from simple congestion, coughing, and wheezing to anaphylactic reactions and airway obstruction. Patients should be instructed to report allergies to plant products, foods, medications, dusts, molds, and animal sources. Knowledge of *all* allergies is important to the nurse because patients frequently do not realize that the contents of some medications or OTC supplements may contain allergens to which they are susceptible. For example, Atrovent and Combivent (combination) inhalers should not be used in patients who are allergic to soy or nuts. Patients may recognize that they are allergic to certain plants or pollens, but not understand that most herbal supplements are made from plants and that they should carefully read the ingredients and understand the components of the supplement prior to taking them.

Use of Oxygen or Ventilatory Assist Devices

Outpatient oxygen therapy indicates that the patient has extensive or chronic pulmonary disease. Increased shortness of breath despite use of oxygen or ventilatory assistive devices should send up a red warning flag about the potential for imminent decompensation. The nurse should immediately assess the patient and determine if the health care provider needs to be notified or the patient requires immediate intervention such as airway suction. Prior need for oxygen therapy or assistive devices such as tracheostomy or mechanical ventilation may also indicate the existence of previous pulmonary problems.

Cough and Sputum Production

Coughing is a symptom associated with pulmonary congestion as well as reactive airway disease. It is a protective mechanism to rid the lungs of mucus in airways or to prevent inhalation of irritants. The nurse must evaluate the symptom of coughing in relation to its timing, frequency, duration, and the nature of sputum produced. Chronic cough is a classic warning sign of lung cancer. Patients who smoke may cough upon awakening. Cough at night may be related to heart failure, postnasal drip, or esophageal reflux, which occurs when supine. If decongestants and cough suppressants are utilized, the cough may have a specific pattern related to the timing of the dosage. Persistent or continuous coughing may be related to smoking, pneumonia, cancer, or chronic irritation.

The character and nature of sputum production gives valuable clues as to the potential cause of the cough. Hemoptysis may indicate a ruptured pulmonary blood vessel, pulmonary embolus, or cancer. Sputum that is thick is usually related to pneumonia. The color of the sputum also gives insight as to the cause or causative organism. Pink, frothy sputum is the hallmark of pulmonary edema. Bronchitis and pneumonia are associated with yellow, tan, green, or gray colored mucus. The color of the sputum does not indicate a particular organism nor should it influence the decision to obtain sputum cultures. Black or carbonaceous sputum may be related to burn trauma. A nonproductive cough may be related to ACE inhibitor use or irritation from dust or fumes. The amount of sputum production should be quantified as well.

Pain associated with cough may be related to musculoskeletal strain, pleurisy, or pneumothorax.

Family Health History

The family history gives information on potential genetic relationships associated with disease development as well as environmental and behavior-related risks for disease development. The family health history should include investigation of the presence of family members who smoke(d), and if any family members had pulmonary disease, lung cancer, or cardiovascular disease. Lung cancer and cardiovascular disease tend to run in families. The familial risk of lung cancer is likely related to the presence of cigarette smoke in the household. The occurrence of childhood asthma and preterm birth is greater in instances where the mother smoked. See Chapter 37 😊 for cardiovascular risk factors.

Risk Factors

Cigarette smoking, inactivity, cardiovascular disease, obesity, substance abuse, and trauma are some of the more common risk factors that contribute to the development of respiratory disorders. The *Healthy People 2010* initiative sites physical activity, obesity, tobacco use, and substance abuse as leading health indicators. The goal under respiratory diseases is to "Promote respiratory health through better prevention, detection, treatment, and education efforts" (U.S. Department of Health and Human Services, 2000).

Cigarette Smoking

The primary risk factor for the development of pulmonary disease is cigarette smoking. All patients should receive counseling on smoking cessation. The number of cigarettes smoked per day and the time in years a patient has smoked should be elicited from the patient (pack-years). Patients may be reluctant to accurately describe their smoking history to the nurse. After all, they know that it causes COPD, emphysema, and lung cancer. The risk for these three disorders increases with the number of cigarettes smoked and the length of time a patient has been a smoker. Patients ages 50 or older who have smoked a pack of cigarettes (20) per day are at highest risk of pulmonary complications (Dillon, 2003).

Inactivity

Patients who are physically inactive are at higher risk for DVT and pulmonary embolism. Immobility causes decreased venous return, venous stasis, and hypercoagulability. The longer the patient is inactive, the greater the risk for development of DVT. Patients with pulmonary disease may become short of breath with activity and become physically inactive to prevent development of shortness of breath. This starts a vicious cycle that further predisposes them to deconditioning, inactivity, and the potential for the development of thromboembolic disease. Recent weight loss unrelated to specific diet may indicate risk for tuberculosis or lung cancer.

Cardiovascular Disease

Patients with cardiovascular disease experience pulmonary complications related to the inability of the heart to effectively pump blood to the lungs due to pulmonary hypertension, or to the periphery due to hypertension, aortic disease, or diseases of the myocardium and valves. Frequently this results in a failure to adequately oxygenate or circulate oxygenated arterial blood to supply body tissues to meet metabolic demands. The result is activity intolerance, hypoxemia, and tachycardia, which further increase the myocardial oxygen demand and the potential for inadequate oxygen to supply these needs. A history of cardiovascular disease should alert the nurse to the potential for heart failure and pulmonary edema.

Obesity

Obesity is associated with a number of respiratory-related dysfunctions. There is hypoventilation related to restriction of thoracic expansion by excess adipose tissue. Upper airway changes related to fat deposits in the neck and poor muscle tone in the upper airway cause intermittent partial and complete airway obstruction (Jubber, 2004). In many obese patients, obstructive sleep apnea interrupts effective sleep patterns.

Patients with obstructive sleep apnea may wake up at night short of breath or may be unaware of breathing difficulties during sleep. A classic symptom is snoring, which is a form of partial airway obstruction (Merritt & Berger, 2004) Classically, the patient wakes up when the airway is completely obstructed, or when hypoxic or hypercapnic reflexes cause them to resume breathing. Obese patients with obstructive sleep apnea are also more prone to associated conditions such as diabetes, heart failure, dysrhythmias, hypercoagulability, coronary artery disease, and stroke (Shamsuzzaman, Gersh, & Somers, 2003).

Substance Abuse

Patients who abuse intravenous (IV) medications are at risk for a multitude of complications affecting almost every organ system. IV drug abusers are at high risk for pneumonia, pulmonary emboli, and pulmonary edema (Gotway et al., 2002). Inhaled drugs may cause pulmonary injury or pulmonary hemorrhage. CNS depression from alcohol or drugs can contribute to aspiration pneumonia, chemical pneumonitis, and respiratory arrest (Wilson & Saukkonen, 2004).

Trauma

Thoracic and abdominal traumatic injuries predispose patients to the development of pneumonias, hypoventilation, and atelectasis. Fractures of long bones are most closely associated with fat emboli, although they also can occur with other invasive fat-related procedures such as liposuction and lipid infusions. The clinical picture of the patient with fat emboli includes dyspnea, tachypnea, tachycardia, cyanosis, and petechiae (Harris, 2004). ABG analysis is very important in the patient with actual or potential fat emboli because the actual degree of hypoxemia may not be apparent until the patient decompensates (Peltier, 2004).

Both blunt and penetrating trauma may cause pneumothorax and/or hemothorax. Pneumothorax may be described as either open or closed. With an open pneumothorax, as a patient inhales, air enters the pleura, causing positive pressure and resultant lung collapse. In a closed pneumothorax, there is nowhere for the air to escape to, causing a rapid buildup of positive pressure and lung collapse, which can shift the trachea and mediastinal contents toward the uninjured lung side. This results in cardiovascular collapse if untreated. Treatment for pneumothorax may include high-flow oxygen if the pneumothorax is small or less than 10% of the lung. Large and symptomatic pneumothoraces are treated with needle thoracostomy, chest tube, or thoracic vent insertion. A hemothorax is treated with chest tube insertion.

Burn injury can occur in the pulmonary tree from inhalation of heated gases (see Chapter 68). The damaged lung tissue becomes edematous and the patient develops acute respiratory distress. Edema of the airways can cause upper airway obstruction. ABG studies are valuable in the early burn period because pulse oximetry values may be unreliable. The pulse oximeter is unable to recognize the difference between oxygenated hemoglobin and carboxyhemoglobin. The normal value for carboxyhemoglobin in a nonsmoking patient is <2.5%. A person who smokes may have a normal carboxyhemoglobin level of 4% to 5%; a heavy smoker 5% to 12% (Kee, 2005).

Trauma to the brain and spinal cord may also affect the respiratory system and assessment findings (see Chapters 29 and 32). The medulla and pons control respiratory rate and depth in response to changes in oxygen levels in the blood. Chemoreceptors relay information on blood pH to the cardiorespiratory centers in the brainstem. Spinal cord injuries above cervical level 3 will paralyze the muscles normally used in ventilation, including the diaphragm. Below cervical spine level 4, intercostal muscle paralysis may occur.

Social History

The social history includes information about patients' lifestyles and habits that may be relevant to their current state of health. For example, patients who smoke have increased risk for pulmonary disease, and patients who have allergies and engage in outdoor social activities such as golfing may have exacerbations of symptoms after participating in these activities. If patients frequent social events in which they are exposed to people with upper respiratory infections or poor hygienic conditions, they may be predisposed to the development of pulmonary infections.

Occupation

Many occupations are associated with exposure to airborne particles, vapors, and irritants. These occupational irritants can result in acute or chronic respiratory disease in susceptible individuals. The Occupational Safety and Health Administration (OSHA) sets and enforces standards in the work environment in the United States to ensure a safe work environment; however, it is impossible in many circumstances to prevent airborne or inhalation exposure, particularly in the out-of-doors. Farmers may be exposed to pesticides, and construction workers and masons may be exposed to cement dust. Even when personal protective equipment is available and recommended, it is each person's own decision to utilize precautions and the equipment.

Asbestos inhalation is associated with the development of pleurisy and pleural effusion up to 20 years after exposure. Mesothelioma is a rare form of asbestos-related malignancy in which symptoms may not appear for 40 years after exposure (Corbridge, Kamp, & Richlin, 2004). Patients at risk for asbestos-related pulmonary disease worked in naval shipyards, construction, and insulation prior to the 1970s. Today, firemen and demolition workers are at risk of asbestos-related pulmonary disease because older buildings still contain significant amounts of asbestos. Asbestos is also present in vehicle brake linings, placing auto mechanics at risk.

Occupational asthma may occur in many settings. Persons who work around animals are exposed to dander, hair, and allergens picked up from the environment. In the food industry, dust, proteins, and fumes may cause asthmatic reactions. Any occupation in which workers come into contact with fumes or vapors may provoke occupational asthma. This includes cleaning solvents that are utilized in work environments as well as the home. Symptoms associated with work-related asthma include wheezing, shortness of breath, and coughing when the worker is exposed to the allergen. The disease is progressive with each exposure. Initially the person may have symptoms only while at work, but as the airways become more reactive, symptoms occur in any setting.

Early recognition, diagnosis, and treatment of occupational asthma can prevent pulmonary complications.

Culture

Culture plays an important role in acceptance of diagnostic testing and treatment of respiratory symptoms (see the Cultural Considerations box). Cultural indoctrination may also influence the patient's responses to attempts to obtain the patient's history and to perform the physical examination. The nurse needs to have an understanding of cultural considerations specific to the patient's frame of reference. For example, East Indian patients may feel that eye contact is rude. The nurse must make allowances for this conception and not conclude that the lack of eye contact indicates deception or abuse.

Cultural practices such as the wearing of protective amulets may interfere with planned diagnostic testing. The nurse must respect the patient's belief and perhaps suggest an alternate placement of the amulet so that interference with diagnostic testing does not occur. For example, if an amulet is worn around the neck and would interfere with a chest x-ray, the nurse may suggest that the patient continue to wear the amulet but wrap it around the wrist during the diagnostic test. Refugees from countries that have been involved in civil conflict may have experienced traumatic injuries or toxic exposures.

Physical assessment of the patient may reveal cultural practices such as coining and cupping. Southeast Asian people may feel that respiratory illness is due to "wind illness" and traditionally treat the symptoms with "cupping." Cupping involves utilizing a cup applied to the skin to draw out the disease. This practice leaves circular marks on the skin. This traditional therapy is also practiced by people in Greece. "Coining" involves scraping the skin of the thorax with a coin or a spoon and is practiced in Southeast Asia, Italy, and Russia. Both coining and cupping may result in skin lesions or burns that may be mistaken as signs of abuse or cause complications that require medical treatment. Prior to coining or cupping, the skin may be treated with an herbal lotion or ointment (Kose, Karabagli, & Cetin, 2005; Snyder & Miska, 2003; Yoo & Tausk, 2004).

If the patient is experiencing respiratory symptoms, some cultures feel that the patient should avoid water or bathing because these may contribute to illness. Many cultures have herbal remedies for respiratory illness. A Native American herbal treatment for respiratory illness felt to boost the immune system is echinacea. Current research seems to vacillate regarding the effectiveness of this remedy. Among the Hmong (from Laos), opium is used as an analgesic. Smoking opium causes respiratory complications, and lung disease may be considered by the Hmong as an accepted part of life.

Environment

The nurse should explore the home and work environment for potential allergens or contributing factors for the development of pulmonary symptoms. If the environment contains allergens, they should be removed. Pets and mold allergens are easily removed. Patients with asthma should have allergy tests prior to suggestions that specific allergens and triggers be removed from the home environment. House dust mites are a common trigger for allergy and asthma symptoms. Weekly vacuuming and removal of stuffed products such as toys and pillows may help remove dust mites. Cockroach allergens may be removed with commercial cockroach insecticides as well as preventive measures such as disposing of trash daily to an area outside of the home. Although little can be done regarding workplace allergen containment, the workplace should be reviewed regarding patient triggers and accommodations made prior to specific activities such as painting, insecticide treatment, and use of specific cleansers. For persons with reactive airway disease who work outdoors, environmental agents such as cement dust and specific fumes that affect the patient may be avoided with appropriate communication.

Habits

Cigarette smoking is the most specific habit that should be avoided. Patients should be counseled regarding avoidance of situations in which cigarette smoking is present to prevent exposure to secondhand smoke. Personal hygiene habits should also be explored with the patient. Good oral hygiene can help prevent pulmonary disease. Oral infections can travel to the pulmonary tree to cause abscess formation or pneumonia. Hand hygiene is also important. Patients should be counseled to wash their hands frequently and always before eating and drinking. Proper clothing for the weather should be encouraged.

Exercise

Exercise tolerance is often decreased in patients with pulmonary disease. The nurse should obtain specific information regarding

---

CULTURAL CONSIDERATIONS Cultural Practices Related to Respiratory Disorders

Cultural Practice	Nursing Considerations
Use of amulets (many cultures)	May interfere with diagnostic testing such as x-rays, MRI, ultrasound. Suggest alternate placement of amulet for test duration or placement of amulet within eye contact but not in MRI.
Cupping (Southeast Asia, Greece)	May be mistaken for signs of abuse; may delay medical treatment. Burns or skin infections may occur and necessitate medical treatment.
Coining (Southeast Asia, Italy, and Russia)	May be mistaken for signs of abuse; may delay medical treatment. Burns or skin infections may occur and necessitate medical treatment.
Herbal remedies (used in many cultures)	Herbal remedies may be related to allergies because they are derived from plants that are associated with allergens. Herbal remedies may also interfere with the actions of medications and antibiotics or increase bleeding tendencies.

the distance that the patient can walk on a flat surface as well as specific activities that cause shortness of breath. Frequently, the distance a patient can ambulate independently will affect the level of care necessary for the patient on discharge from the hospital. For example, if the patient cannot ambulate 50 feet unassisted or without shortness of breath, she may need to be discharged to a skilled nursing facility. A specific plan for progressive exercise should be developed for the patient. Goals to be set for the patient on a daily basis require knowledge of the patient's baseline activity and exercise status.

Some forms of recreation and exercise predispose to pulmonary symptoms. Water sports such as wake boarding expose the rider to carbon monoxide fumes. Water sports that involve riding a ski or board in the exhaust path are the most frequent cause of carbon monoxide poisoning.

Nutrition

Frequently patients with shortness of breath have poor nutritional status. Obtaining, preparing, and consuming meals requires energy. Shortness of breath can interfere with the patient's abilities to shop for, prepare, and consume food. A typical body type is associated with pulmonary disease. The patient with chronic bronchitis or emphysema may be thin with muscle wasting. Inadequate nutrition places the patient at risk for infection. Nutrition is discussed in detail in Chapter 14 ☺.

Travel and Area of Residence

Area of recent travel may become an important aspect of the history in diagnosing potential respiratory problems. In 2003, a severe acute respiratory syndrome (SARS) outbreak demonstrated to the world that viral pulmonary disease could be traced to a specific location. Although there have been no subsequent episodes of SARS, recent travel and area of residence have been demonstrated to be an important factor in the history of respiratory symptoms and should be included in the interview process.

High-altitude pulmonary edema (HAPE) can occur in persons who are not acclimated and travel to altitudes greater than 5,000 feet. As altitude increases, atmospheric pressure decreases and the oxygen available in air also decreases. Persons with preexisting illness may develop rapid onset of hypoxemia related to the decreased oxygen levels. Compensatory increases in respiratory rate to compensate for the decreased available oxygen may contribute to fatigue and further respiratory insufficiency. Compensatory mechanisms cause initial pulmonary vascular vasoconstriction. Later, inflammatory mediators cause vasodilation. The alveolar–capillary membrane becomes more permeable in response to these mediators and engorges with fluid, causing pulmonary edema. HAPE is discussed in detail in Chapter 36 ☺.

■ Physical Examination

The physical examination of the patient begins with the first contact. All of the nurse's senses are utilized. Whether the patient is ambulating into a clinic or is a patient on a ventilator in the ICU, the nurse begins collecting data. The nurse may hear audible wheezes or stridor from a distance. When speaking with the patient, the nurse notes the amount of words in each sentence and if there is foul odor to the breath. Foul odor on the breath may be a sign of pulmonary infection or abscess. The

general appearance of the patient, the skin color, the presence of oxygen or assistive devices all provide data for the nurse in the assessment of the patient.

The assessment of any patient should be systematic and proceed from noninvasive data collection to invasive data collection. All available information should be elicited. If medical records are available, they should be obtained and included in data collection. Comparison of previous assessments should be applied to the patient's current physical status. If findings indicate new symptoms or an increase in symptoms of pathology, the nurse must document findings and take appropriate steps to ensure that the patient receives appropriate care. The nurse must pursue appropriate and complete evaluation of all physical findings and symptoms of respiratory dysfunction to assist in the determination of the cause and to prevent further compromise of the patient's ability to carry out activities essential to health and satisfaction with lifestyle.

Inspection

Inspection is the initial activity for any assessment of the patient. It involves observation of obvious physical characteristics that may indicate potential health problems or characteristics that indicate a need for more in-depth evaluation. Evaluation of the respiratory rate, pattern, and patient's ease of breathing should occur continually throughout the assessment of the patient.

General Appearance

The nurse should evaluate the patient's general appearance. Does the patient appear to have the physical capability to take care of himself? Does he appear comfortable or assume a tripod position to breathe easily? Is the patient in obvious distress?

The facial appearance may indicate that the patient is anxious, a symptom of hypoxia. Patients with COPD may exhibit facial flushing related to the effort of breathing. Pursed lip breathing during exhalation prolongs the expiratory phase of respiration. This maintains the smaller airways in an open position so that there is a longer period for exchange of oxygen and carbon dioxide and prevents collapse of the alveoli. Normal expiration time is twice the duration of inspiration. Nasal flaring may also be evident in the patient with pulmonary disease. Nasal flaring indicates that the patient is making a voluntary effort to inhale through the nostrils, which is a sign of increased work in breathing.

Patients may assume a posture that eases the work of breathing. The "tripod" position, in which the patient leans forward resting on both arms, allows expansion of the thorax and eases breathing. Sitting upright with the legs dependent may ease breathing in the patient with heart failure by decreasing venous return to the heart from the legs and allowing thoracic expansion.

Mentation

The brain relies on oxygen for function. Hypoxia causes changes in mental status including agitation, poor judgment, poor memory, and attention deficits. Symptoms of elevated carbon dioxide in the blood include lethargy, headache, and decreased level of consciousness. The nurse must assess the patient for orientation to person, place, and time as part of the assessment process.

 The nurse should first rule out hypoxia as the cause for changes in metal status in patients with changes in behavior or level of consciousness.

Rate, Depth, and Rhythm of Respirations

Respiratory rate should be counted for a full minute in patients with an irregular respiratory rhythm, and for 30 seconds in patients with a regular rhythm. The normal respiratory rate is 12 to 20 per minute. **Tachypnea** is considered to be a respiratory rate greater than 20 breaths per minute. A respiratory rate greater than 24 indicates respiratory distress. **Bradypnea** is considered to be a respiratory rate less than 12 breaths per minute. Bradypnea may be related to neurological disease or oversedation. Increased respiratory rate may be seen with fever, anxiety, and exercise. In general, for each increase in temperature of one degree, the heart rate will increase four beats per minute and the respiratory rate increase one breath per minute.

Hyperpnea refers to both increased rate and depth of respiration and is associated with metabolic acidosis. It is sometimes referred to as Kussmaul's breathing. Cheyne–Stokes breathing is a pattern of breathing in which the patient breathes rapidly then has a period of apnea. During deep inspiration, the lungs move downward to the 8th to 10th intercostal space anteriorly and the 10th to 12th space posteriorly. At the end of expiration, the lungs move upward to the 5th intercostal space anteriorly and the 9th to 10th intercostal space posteriorly. Shallow respirations may be seen with sedation, pneumonia, pain, or hypercalcemia. The respiratory pattern is normally rhythmic. Breathing patterns that are not rhythmic signal neurological dysfunction.

Thoracic Size and Shape

The thoracic size and shape provide important clues about risk for pulmonary disease. Structural abnormalities such as pectus excavatum (sternal depression) or pigeon chest (pectus carinatum), an outward bowing of the sternum, may indicate underlying structural abnormalities in the heart. Pectus excavatum may cause compression of the heart or great vessels. Barrel chest, an increased anterior-posterior diameter of the thorax, may indicate emphysema. Scoliosis and kyphoscoliosis (hunching and curvature of the spine) may prevent full expansion of the affected lung. These structural changes also prevent full lung expansion. Lung expansion is integral for oxygen and carbon dioxide exchange and for clearance of secretions. Cough may be ineffective to clear secretions in patients with structural deformities. This increases the risk of pneumonia.

Thoracic Expansion and Symmetry

During normal inspiration the diaphragm flattens and the lower rib cage expands. Although the lungs are paired, the right lung has three lobes and the left lung has two lobes. The liver causes the diaphragm on the right side to be higher than the left. In terms of overall expansion of the rib cage during inspiration, a 5 to 13 cm (2 to 5 in.) increase in diameter can be observed. In patients with COPD, the chest diameter during inspiration is decreased. Expansion is symmetrical, except when pneumothorax, structural abnormality, or pneumonia is present. Paradoxical movement may be present in flail chest. Flail chest occurs when two or more adjacent ribs are fractured in two or more places.

Use of Accessory Muscles

During normal inspiration the diaphragm and intercostal muscles contract, expanding the thorax and moving it upward. Patients with pulmonary disease may have difficulty with inspiration or expiration. **Accessory muscles** of inspiration include the trapezius, sternomastoid, and scalenus. During inspiration they may become pronounced in a patient with pulmonary dysfunction. Abdominal muscles may also be used in patients with pulmonary disease to force expiration.

Color and Appearance of Skin and Extremities

The color and appearance of the skin and extremities may give clues to the presence of hypoxia or anemia. Physical characteristics such as clubbing of the fingers may also indicate chronic hypoxia. Cardiovascular causes of pallor or skin changes must be explored as well. The nurse should corroborate findings of the physical examination with the patient to determine if they are familial characteristics or changes related to disease progression.

Pallor

Pallor can be related to vasoconstriction from cold ambient temperatures, melanin deficiencies, and heredity. It may also indicate that the patient is anemic. The nurse should check the mucous membranes and conjunctiva if pallor is suspected to be due to anemia. Ninety-eight percent of oxygen in the blood is bound to hemoglobin. In anemia there is a decrease in hemoglobin and a resultant decrease in the oxygen-carrying capacity. Patients with anemia tend to compensate for the decrease in oxygen-carrying capacity by increasing the heart rate. The hemoglobin moves through the vascular tree more rapidly, to the lungs to be oxygenated, to the body where it exchanges oxygen for carbon dioxide. Anemic patients are generally exercise intolerant because they cannot tolerate further increases in heart rate.

Cyanosis

Cyanosis is a very nonspecific and somewhat subjective sign. It is a bluish discoloration of the skin that occurs when oxygen levels are low in the presence of sufficient hemoglobin levels. It may also be seen in some patients with normal oxygen levels, polycythemia, and peripheral vascular disease. Ability to evaluate the presence of cyanosis also depends on available lighting and the eyesight and color discrimination of the person evaluating the patient's skin. Newborns may exhibit peripheral cyanosis when cold or agitated. Central cyanosis occurs when the mucous membranes, mouth, and lips are blue tinged. In the adult, central cyanosis indicates hypoxia.

The nail beds should be examined for the presence of cyanosis. Normally the nail beds are pink. Widening of the tips of the fingers and nail beds with loss of the normal angle, may indicate chronic hypoxia. This finding is known as clubbing.

Neck Inspection

The neck should be examined for tracheal deviation or the presence of goiter or lesions, which may cause upper airway obstruction and jugular venous distention. The trapezius, scalenus, and sternomastoid muscles may be enlarged in patients with COPD. **Tracheal deviation** occurs in pneumothorax and hemothorax. Deviation is usually away from the affected lung. Neck vein distention, or jugular venous distention, may be related to right heart failure. Right heart failure decreases flow of blood to the pulmonary tree for oxygenation. Jugular venous filling during expiration may be seen in COPD due to hyperinflation of the lungs.

Palpation of Skin and Extremities

Palpation of the thorax and dependent extremities helps determine if changes are due to cardiac, vascular, or pulmonary causes. Edema of the lower extremities points to heart failure as the cause for edema. Palpation of the thorax may uncover subcutaneous emphysema, step-off defects caused by rib fractures, and vibrations caused by respirations. Tactile **fremitus** is the palpation of vibrations in the thorax related to vocal speech. Capillary refill time can indicate a cardiovascular cause for dyspnea.

Edema

Edema of the lower extremities is generally related to right heart or heart failure. Right heart failure or combined left- and right-sided failure is common in patients with COPD. Right-sided failure is caused by pulmonary hypertension. Chronic distention of the lower airways makes forward blood flow more difficult. Over time, the right heart hypertrophies in an attempt to increase the force of blood through the pulmonary tree. Eventually the right heart fails, and fluid that cannot be accommodated is sequestered in dependent interstitial spaces (usually the lower extremities and coccyx) and causes edema. Edema is classified as pitting or nonpitting, and graded according to depth. Using one finger, the skin is depressed for 5 seconds and then released. If the nurse is able to depress the tissue up to 8 mm, the patient has 4+ edema; 6 mm, the patient has 3+ edema; 4 mm, 2+ edema; and 1+ edema measures 2 mm.

Skin Temperature and Moisture

The skin temperature and moisture status can give the nurse information on the patient's hydration, breathing effort, and temperature. Patients with COPD and asthma exacerbations may have very dry skin due to the loss of moisture through the respiratory tract. Shortness of breath with asthma and COPD exacerbations may prevent the patient from replacing fluids lost through rapid respiration, thus causing dehydration. Fever from pulmonary infections may increase skin temperature and moisture or cause cool, dry skin. Warm, moist skin may also be related to increased effort of breathing.

Clinical Reference Points

Although certain visible reference points, such as the trachea, nipple line, and sternum, are utilized in respiratory assessment, it is important to palpate and count ribs and interspaces for accuracy (Figure 33–1 ■). Landmarks utilized in the cardiorespiratory assessment include the anterior axillary line, the midaxillary line, and the midclavicular line. If a lesion is seen or adventitious breath sounds heard along one of these lines, it is then described further by its vertical location as delineated by the rib number or intercostal space.

Chest Excursion

Chest excursion is measured by placing the hands on the patient's back, equidistant from the spine or the center of the back, at the level of the 10th rib. When the patient takes a deep breath, the examiner's hands should move an equal distance laterally. This examination may also be performed on the anterior chest. The normal chest excursion (i.e., the distance between the thumbs with inspiration) should be 5 to 10 cm (2 to 4 in.). Elderly patients

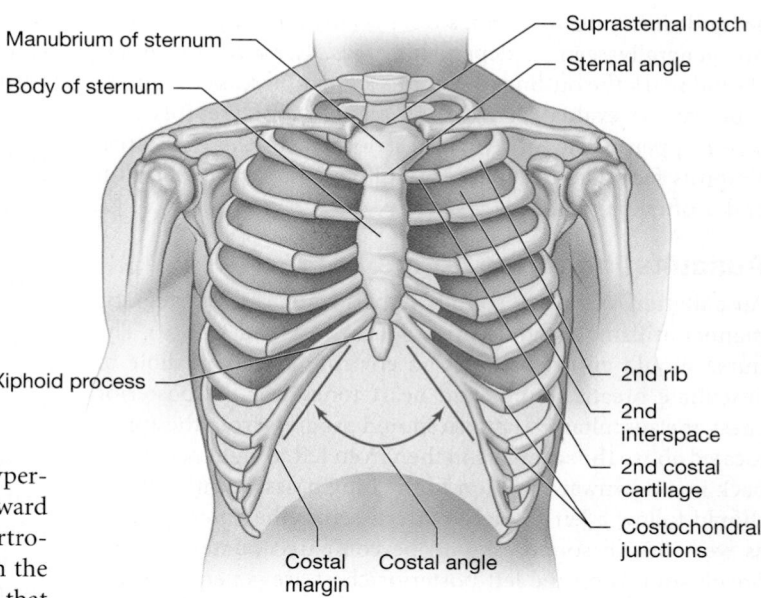

FIGURE 33–1 ■ In a respiratory assessment, it is important to palpate and count ribs and interspaces to accurately record the location of lesions or adventitious breath sounds.

may have decreased chest excursion as a normal finding. COPD patients may have decreased chest excursion due to anatomic flattening of the diaphragm from hyperinflation at the base of the lungs. Patients with rib fractures, pneumothorax, hemothorax, or pneumonia may also have decreased chest excursion.

Tactile Fremitus

Tactile fremitus is palpated over the thorax by having the patient vocalize the word "ninety-nine." Voice vibrations from the large airways are transmitted to the surface skin of the thorax. Start palpating with the ulnar side of the hand from the scapulae on the back and clavicles on the anterior chest, and move down bilaterally on each side of the thorax while the patient repeats "ninety-nine." The vibrations should be strongest over the large airways on the upper thorax and decrease in strength as you move down the thorax. Compare each side for symmetry. Unequal fremitus may be due to unilateral airway obstruction, pneumothorax, or pleural effusion causing a decrease in fremitus on the side with the defect. Increased fremitus is seen with consolidation or pneumonia and an increase in fremitus is felt over these areas.

Tenderness

Point tenderness may be seen in muscle strain or rib fracture. Excessive coughing may strain intercostals and thoracic muscles. Pneumonia and consolidation may also cause tenderness with deep inspiration. To avoid tenderness from any of these conditions, the patient may limit chest excursion and breathe shallowly. Shallow respirations promote atelectasis and may contribute to hypoxia.

Crepitus

Crepitus is also called **subcutaneous emphysema**. It is caused by air that escapes into the subcutaneous tissue. Crepitus may occur with rupture of pulmonary bullae, pneumothorax, or around chest tube insertion sites. Because air rises, crepitus is not generally seen in dependent areas. If noted, the nurse should mark the outline of crepitus so that increases in air escape can be evaluated. Excessive increases of crepitus may cause upper airway obstruction if located in the neck area. Crepitus feels like tiny packing bubble wrap under the skin and is often painless.

Auscultation of the Lungs

Auscultation of breath sounds is performed in a systematic manner utilizing a stethoscope (Figures 33–2 and 33–3 ■). The nurse should ensure as quiet an environment as possible to auscultate breath sounds and heart tones. On the posterior chest, the auscultatory pattern should progress from the apices located above the scapula and then from left to right across the back in a downward fashion to the lung bases. Breath sounds should follow a left-to-right pattern across the anterior chest as well. Breath sounds should be compared bilaterally. The breath sounds on the left posterior chest are generally heard about 2.5 cm (1 in.) lower than on the right side due to the location of the liver and increased height of the right diaphragm.

The diaphragm of the stethoscope is utilized to listen to breath sounds. Breath sounds are best auscultated with the pa-

Lobes of the lungs (anterior)

FIGURE 33–2 ■ Lobes of the lung—anterior.

Lobes of the lungs (posterior)

FIGURE 33–3 ■ Lobes of the lung—posterior.

tient in an upright position. Do not listen to breath sounds over clothing or hospital gowns. The movement of clothing causes rustling that will interfere with accurate auscultation of breath sounds.

Normal Breath Sounds

When listening for normal breath sounds, the patient should be upright so that the breath sounds can be auscultated bilaterally without interference and so that expansion is not restricted. Most texts advocate auscultating from the superior thorax at the level of C_7 posteriorly and anteriorly from above the clavicles. The diaphragm of the stethoscope should be used. The nurse should then move systematically from right to left and move steadily downward right to left toward the lung bases. Each site should be auscultated through both inspiration and expiration.

When the patient is obese, excess subcutaneous tissue may make it difficult to hear breath sounds because of the increased distance they must travel through the chest wall. Sometimes, having the patient stand so that gravity pulls subcutaneous tissue downward can aid in the auscultation of breath sounds in the obese person.

In the bedbound patient, the dependent areas are restricted from fully expanding by the pressure of the mattress. If the patient must remain supine, it is best to listen to the dependent areas before the superior areas because fluid and exudates will migrate to dependent areas with gravity. When the patient is turned so that these areas are no longer dependent, evidence of consolidation or fluid may disappear.

Tracheal Breath Sounds

Breath sounds auscultated over the trachea are called **tracheal breath sounds,** and they are loud and high pitched. The sounds heard in this location are caused by turbulent airflow through the tubular trachea. Because this is the largest airway, these sounds are also the loudest. As the airways become smaller, there is less turbulence and the sounds become softer and fainter. The duration of time that tracheal breath sounds are heard is equal during inspiration and expiration. They are best heard over the neck and trachea. Tracheal breath sounds should be auscultated if upper airway obstruction is suspected.

Bronchial Breath Sounds

Bronchial breath sounds are heard over the anterior chest on either side of the sternum, over the right and left main stem bronchus from the second to fourth intercostal spaces. On the back, they are best heard lateral to the spine between the third and sixth intercostal spaces. They are loud in pitch, harsh, less turbulent, and lower in frequency than tracheal breath sounds. A gap is heard between inspiration and expiration, and expiration is heard for a longer time than inspiration. The sounds over smaller airways are low pitched and softer.

Bronchovesicular Breath Sounds

Bronchovesicular breath sounds are heard during inspiration and expiration. They are midway in pitch and loudness between vesicular and bronchial breath sounds. They are best heard in the 1st and 2nd intercostal spaces of the anterior chest and between the scapulae of the posterior chest. Bronchovesicular breath sounds represent air movement in the moderate airways between the bronchi and the smaller airways.

Vesicular Breath Sounds

Vesicular breath sounds are heard over most of the thorax. The sounds are soft and low pitched, like a rustling, from air moving through small airways. Vesicular breath sounds are heard longer during expiration, because expiration generally lasts twice as long as inspiration.

Adventitious Breath Sounds

Abnormal breath sounds are decreased or absent sounds where normal breath sounds would normally occur. Diminished breath sounds indicate atelectasis, shallow respirations, pneumothorax, or decreased respiratory effort. These findings should be correlated with the patient's clinical condition and diagnoses. For example, a patient with myasthenia gravis who has diminished breath sounds should be assessed for respiratory muscle fatigue or paralysis. If the patient had a central venous line placed and develops diminished breath sounds, a pneumothorax should be suspected. Diminished breath sounds demonstrate decreased airflow and potentially decreased oxygen exchange. It is also abnormal for some breath sounds to occur where they should not be located. For example, bronchial breath sounds may be heard over consolidated areas or areas of pulmonary fibrosis because of increased tissue density.

Adventitious breath sounds are extra, abnormal sounds not normally heard during auscultation of breath sounds (Chart 33–2). They represent pathologic conditions of the heart or lungs, and indicate the presence of airway spasm, fluid, or secretions that disrupt airflow.

 Bronchial breath sounds over the large airways and diminished or absent breath sounds over smaller airways may indicate airway obstruction or pneumothorax.

Crackles

Crackles are sounds caused by fluid in the airways. They are described as intermittent or discontinuous, nonmusical, or popping sounds. They are caused by fluid, inflammation, infection, or secretions. (Note that the term *rales* is no longer used to describe fluid effects in the airways.) Crackles are described as either fine or coarse. Crackles occur when closed airways snap open during inspiration. Crackles may also be described as to timing, such as early inspiratory crackles or late inspiratory crackles. Sound is also produced when the airways close, but this sound is generally softer than heard on inspiration.

Wheezes

Wheezes are heard equally during inspiration and expiration. They are high-pitched musical sounds caused by air flowing across strands of mucus or swollen pulmonary tissue that narrows the airway or from bronchospasm. (Note that the term *rhonchi* is no longer used to describe harsh sounds caused by secretions in the airways.) Wheezes may be heard without a stethoscope. When auscultated, wheezes should be described as inspiratory or expiratory, continuous or discontinuous, and mild, moderate, or severe. Wheezing is typically heard in patients with asthma, allergic or reactive airway reactions, or after exercise. In patients who are experiencing acute asthma exacerbations, the absence of wheezing may indicate lack of airflow and is an ominous sign heralding respiratory arrest. Notify the health care provider or arrange for emergency care (911) immediately.

 *Absence of wheezing in a patient with asthma exacerbation indicates lack of airflow and impending respiratory arrest. Notify the health care provider immediately.*

Stridor

Stridor is heard only during inspiration, as air attempts to flow across an obstruction. Stridor may be heard without a stethoscope as a high-pitched, crowing sound. With a stethoscope it is heard best over the large airways, such as the trachea or bronchus. Stridor must be reported to the health care provider immediately and should alert the nurse to the presence of airway obstruction and the need for interventions to relieve the mechanical obstruction. Bronchoscopy may be necessary to remove the obstruction.

Pleural Friction Rub

Pleural friction rubs are low-pitched, creaking or squeaking sounds that occur when inflamed pleural surfaces rub together during respiration. They are most easily heard on inspiration. The pitch of the sound usually increases with chest expansion. To determine if the sound is due to pleural or pericardial friction, have the patient hold her breath. The pericardial friction rub will continue with each heartbeat, whereas the pleural friction rub will not occur when the patient is not actively breathing.

Percussion

Percussion is a skill rarely performed by nurses. Percussion is considered to be ultrasound without the technology, and helps

CHART 33–2	Adventitious Breath Sounds				
Breath Sound	**Inspiration**	**Expiration**	**Sound Description**	**Significance**	
Crackles	Louder	Softer	Discontinuous, nonmusical	Fluid in the pleural tissue, asthma, bronchitis, consolidation, pneumonia, congestive heart failure, pulmonary edema, fibrosis	
Wheeze	Yes	Yes	High-pitched, continuous musical sound	Bronchospasm, secretions, airway inflammation	
Stridor	Yes	No	High-pitched crowing	Airway obstruction	
Pleural friction rub	Yes	No	Rubbing or grating sound	Pleural inflammation	

assess whether the underlying tissues are air filled, fluid filled, or solid. Sounds produced by percussion are described as flat, dull, resonant, hyperresonant, or tympanic. The lungs are approximately 99% air filled; therefore, percussion over the lungs produces resonance. Decreased sounds indicate a lack of air.

Resonance should be heard throughout most lung fields during inspiration while they are air filled. **Resonance** is a low-pitched, clear sound that is heard over normal lung tissue.

Abnormal percussion sounds include hyperresonance and dullness. Tympany is not heard over lung tissue but may be heard over an air-filled cheek or abdomen. Hyperresonance is very loud, with a lower pitch and a longer sound than resonance and indicates hyperinflation of the airways, or an excess of air in the absence of lung tissue. Hyperinflation is seen and heard in emphysema. Pneumothorax causes the collapse of lung tissue and excess air in the pleural space.

Dullness is a percussive tone that is heard over solid tissue. Dullness occurs over the lungs when air is absent. This is heard over the lower thorax during expiration, when consolidation is present as in pneumonia, pleural effusion, hemothorax, or the presence of solid tumors. The sound elicited is a dull thumping sound without vibration.

Pain

Pain associated with breathing may be related to pulmonary embolism, pleural disease, pneumothorax, musculoskeletal injury, pericarditis, or pneumonia. Sudden onset of shortness of breath or pain may be related to pulmonary embolism or pneumothorax. Progressive development of pain may be related to heart failure, pneumonia, asthma, or conditions that cause coughing. Pain with respiration will decrease inspired tidal volumes and promote atelectasis. Pain medication should be provided to patients so that they can participate in pulmonary rehabilitation activities and breathe deeply to prevent pneumonia and atelectasis. Cough suppressants should be used with caution because the primary purpose of the cough is to remove secretions that block the airways.

Genetic Considerations

Cystic fibrosis is an autosomal recessive genetic disorder that produces multiple problems and pulmonary complications. Most patients with cystic fibrosis are diagnosed in childhood. Pulmonary complications are the primary cause of death in patients with cystic fibrosis. In the past, children with cystic fibrosis did not survive to adulthood. Today, approximately 60% of children with cystic fibrosis will reach adulthood (Crosier & Wise, 2001). They have ineffective airway clearance related to thick mucus. The thickness of the mucus is related to a defect in the cystic fibrosis transmembrane regulator (CFTR). CFTR affects the movement of sodium and water across epithelial tissues, producing thick mucus. Thick mucus is difficult to expectorate from the airways and promotes colonization of bacteria. The most common bacteria infection seen is *Pseudomonas aeruginosa.*

The patient with cystic fibrosis suffers from exacerbations of respiratory infection. Chest physical therapy and devices that support airway clearance may be used by both child and adult patients with cystic fibrosis. Rarely, cystic fibrosis has been diagnosed in adulthood. Children who survive to adulthood with cystic fibro-

sis may be unable to maintain employment and may have other physical and emotional challenges. Social isolation is not uncommon. In addition, as adult patients with cystic fibrosis leave their pediatricians and cystic fibrosis clinics, there are few adult health care providers who are as knowledgeable as the pediatricians about the problems associated with cystic fibrosis.

Gerontological Considerations

Respiratory function decreases with advancing age for a variety of reasons. Skeletal changes from osteoporosis may cause stooped posture and decreased rib expansion. The rib cage becomes more rigid and the anterior-posterior diameter increases. The alveolar surface area decreases with age. In addition, lung tissue becomes less elastic and reduced tidal volume and decreased exchange of oxygen and carbon dioxide result in lowered arterial oxygen values.

Geriatric patients are at higher risk for pneumonia because of ineffective coughing related to the aforementioned physiological changes and due to risk of disease states that increase risk for aspiration. Decreased subcutaneous fat may make the geriatric patient more susceptible to cool room temperatures during respiratory physical assessment, so care must be taken to provide heat or warmed blankets or sheets to promote comfort during the examination.

Health Promotion

Avoidance of cigarette smoking is a primary avenue to prevent the development of pulmonary disease. Adolescents and adults who do not smoke should not start and if they do smoke, should stop. Nurses in all realms of practice should offer smoking cessation information and support for patients to stop smoking.

Hand hygiene is recognized in health care settings as an important means to prevent the spread of infection. Frequent hand washing or the use of alcohol degermers in school settings and public places may prevent the spread of bacteria and decrease the spread of cold, flu, and pneumonia.

Flu vaccines and pneumococcal vaccines should be available to patients in high-risk populations. Frequently these frail patients are physically unable to go to local centers or wait in lines to obtain the vaccination. Insurance and health care providers should develop and execute plans to get the vaccines to the patients, instead of forcing these patients to "come to the vaccine."

Governmental agencies have been active in promoting healthy and safe workplaces. In occupations that commonly encounter environmental irritants and allergens, education in the use of personal protective equipment (PPE) should be provided in an ongoing basis. Although PPE may be uncomfortable at first, consistent insistence on its use should be provided. Construction workers have gotten used to hard hats; it is time for them to get used to respirator masks. Reduction of the effects of environmental allergens and irritants will prevent the development of chronic disease in this population.

Respiratory Monitoring

Whether the patient is on the medical–surgical ward, ICU, or postanesthesia recovery unit, respiratory monitoring includes observation, physical assessment, and the use of electronic monitoring devices. The nurse must be knowledgeable about the oxygen delivery method and the expected outcomes for the patient. If a patient is receiving supplemental oxygen, the nurse should expect that the patient will be able to maintain appropriate arterial oxygen levels. These are assessed using ABGs, physical assessment, and pulse oximetry. In a normal patient, with normal lungs, the nurse can expect that the FiO_2 delivered to the patient will increase the PaO_2 four times. That is why the PaO_2 in a normal patient inspiring room air that has an FiO_2 of approximately 24% is approximately 95%.

The standard of care for patients with cardiac and respiratory illness now includes continuous or intermittent observation of the patient's oxygen saturation and end-tidal carbon dioxide levels. The peak flow is utilized to trend treatment effectiveness in patients with asthma.

Pulse Oximetry

Pulse oximeters provide a digital readout of the percentage that the hemoglobin is saturated with oxygen (Figure 33–4 ■). Pulse oximeters use infrared light technology or reflectance photometry to reflect light off the hemoglobin molecules. The computer in the pulse oximeter then measures the absorption of light by hemoglobin during pulsatile arterial waves.

The oxygen saturation measured by infrared technology does not necessarily provide the same values obtained from the calculated oxygen saturation obtained from an ABG. Normal infrared oxygen saturation (SPO_2) and ABG saturations range from 95% to 100%. Nail polish color may interfere with the ability of the machine to read infrared pulsations. Pulse oximetry probes should not be placed on extremities with automated blood pressure cuffs, hemodialysis fistulas, or arterial lines, because these interfere with blood flow (Grap, 2002). Shock and hypovolemia also cause low-flow states that contribute to inaccurate pulse oximetry readings. Patient movement, ambient light, and venous pulsations may also cause inaccurate readings. The accuracy of the readout should be suspect if the waveform does not match the patient's pulse rate and amplitude. If ambient light is interfering with readings (producing results higher than suspected), cover the probe with a towel to see if the result is different.

Pulse oximetry does not distinguish methemoglobin or carboxyhemoglobin from oxygen-saturated hemoglobin. Fifty percent carboxyhemoglobin reads as 95% SpO_2 (Ford, 2002). Patients who have suspected thiocyanate toxicity or inhalation injury should have an ABG analysis to determine respiratory status and oxygen saturation.

Peak Flow

Peak flow meters are utilized to determine trends in a patient's condition or to evaluate air movement to determine severity of asthma exacerbation (Figure 33–5 ■). Many different types of meters and results graphs are available. Some peak flow meters are computerized so that the patient can provide a diary of results to the health care provider.

Peak flow meters measure the peak expiratory flow rate. Normal values for peak flow measurements are based on age and body size. Many peak flow meters utilize a red, yellow, and green zone to determine the severity of decrease in peak flow. Green is the "good zone," meaning that the patient meets at least 80% of normal. The yellow zone is a caution zone. Values in this area are below normal. The red zone means that the patient is in danger of respiratory complications and has a peak flow of less than 50% of the normal value. As a general rule, values of less than 400 L/min indicate poor airflow. The peak flow measures the peak expiratory flow rate, the amount of air the patient can exhale.

Arterial Blood Gas

ABG studies are utilized to provide information on arterial oxygen and carbon dioxide levels. The oxygen saturation, bicarbonate, and blood pH are also calculated. The carbon dioxide level is utilized as the major determinant for diagnosing respiratory alkalosis and respiratory acidosis. The bicarbonate level is the determinant of metabolic acidosis and alkalosis.

Low oxygen levels in the arterial blood may be due to a variety of pathologies. Oxygen travels in the arterial blood attached to hemoglobin. If the hemoglobin levels are decreased as in anemia, there are fewer sites to which oxygen can bind. Hemoglobin affinity for oxygen is affected by the blood pH. If the pH is elevated (alkalosis), less oxygen is delivered to tissues.

FIGURE 33–4 ■ Pulse oximetry monitor.
Source: Cheryl Wraa

FIGURE 33–5 ■ Peak flow meter.
Source: Courtesy of Monaghan Medical Corporation

		CHART 33–3 **Acute ABG Analysis**			
ABG	**Normal**	**Respiratory Acidosis**	**Respiratory Alkalosis**	**Metabolic Acidosis**	**Metabolic Alkalosis**
pH	7.35–7.45	<7.35	>7.45	<7.35	>7.45
PaO$_2$	80–100 mmHg	Normal or decreased	Normal	Normal	Normal
PaCO$_2$	35–45 mmHg	>45 mmHg	<35 mmHg	Normal	Normal
HCO$_3^-$	22–26 mEq/L	Decreased	Normal	Decreased	Increased

There is an increased affinity of hemoglobin for oxygen. In acidotic states, the affinity of hemoglobin for oxygen is decreased and it is readily released to tissues. Chart 33–3 outlines normal ABGs and the changes seen with acute respiratory and metabolic acidosis and alkalosis.

Capnography

Capnography is the measurement of exhaled carbon dioxide (Figure 33–6 ■). Small disposable capnographers are utilized to test endotracheal tube placement utilizing treated paper that changes color in the presence of an acid such as carbon dioxide. Some machines also measure amounts of carbon dioxide in exhaled breath through spectography. These analyzers also provide waveform readings corresponding to the patient's inspiratory and expiratory cycles. Capnography waveforms and CO$_2$ values are useful in determining the patient's ventilatory status and readiness for extubation or pulmonary vessel perfusion in patients with pulmonary embolus.

FIGURE 33–6 ■ End-tidal CO$_2$ monitoring.
Source: Cheryl Wraa

■ Summary

All nurses must be skilled in respiratory assessment because breathing is essential to life. The respiratory assessment must include pertinent data regarding the patient's history and current complaints. Acute changes in respiratory status must be acted on quickly to prevent patient compromise. Patients with chronic pulmonary disease will have abnormal physical findings, but the patients' usual and customary status must be ascertained by the nurse so that the progression of symptoms and the current status of the patient can be determined. This knowledge is also valuable in planning care for the patients. Data obtained from the respiratory assessment will determine if the current plan of care is adequate for a patient's needs. Is the patient getting better or worse? Utilizing the objective data from the respiratory assessment, the nurse can advocate for the patient with the health care provider to ensure an appropriate plan of care. Early recognition of symptoms by the nurse is important to provide education in risk reduction and to assist in determining possible environmental irritants and allergens that can then be eliminated and thus prevent chronic disease.

NCLEX® REVIEW

1. While auscultating a patient's lungs, the nurse hears intermittent popping sounds. The nurse would document this assessment finding as:
   1. Rales.
   2. Crackles.
   3. Wheezes.
   4. Rhonchi.

2. A patient tells the nurse that he just returned from visiting Asia and has had an upper respiratory infection for 2 weeks. Why is this information beneficial to aid in the care of this patient?
   1. It will help determine the patient's socioeconomic status.
   2. It will help determine the patient's occupation.
   3. It might help to know if there are any recent outbreaks of pulmonary disorders in the area of travel.
   4. It might help determine the patient's immunological status.

3. A patient, who is a nonsmoker, comes into the clinic with symptoms of a respiratory disorder. Which of the following should the nurse include regarding this patient's social history while conducting the assessment?

1. Do you have any heart problems?

2. Have you been to any activities or functions around other people with respiratory problems?

3. Do you have any family members with known respiratory problems?

4. Do you remember which immunizations you received as a child?

4. During the assessment of a patient with a respiratory disorder, the nurse observes lower extremity edema. This finding is important in respiratory disorders because:

1. It will indicate the patient's ability to ambulate.

2. Edema indicates the amount of fluid the patient can tolerate.

3. Edema indicates heart failure, a common finding in a patient with COPD.

4. It aids in determining if the patient will need assistance with activities of daily living.

5. A patient in the burn unit has a pulse oximetry reading of 98%. Which of the following should the nurse do about this reading?

1. Cover the probe to see if the reading is different.

2. Move the probe to another extremity.

3. Have an arterial blood gas analysis done to compare the readings.

4. Ask the patient to not move while doing another reading.

Answers for review questions appear in Appendix D

KEY TERMS

accessory muscles *p.872*
adventitious breath sounds *p.875*
bradypnea *p.872*
bronchial breath sounds *p.874*
bronchovesicular breath sounds *p.874*
capnography *p.878*
crackles *p.875*

crepitus *p.873*
dyspnea *p.865*
fremitus *p.873*
hypernea *p.872*
pleural friction rubs *p.875*
resonance *p.876*

subcutaneous emphysema *p.873*
tachypnea *p.872*
tracheal breath sounds *p.874*
tracheal deviation *p.872*
vesicular breath sounds *p.875*
wheezes *p.875*

PEARSON
EXPLORE **mynursingkit**™

MyNursingKit is your one stop for online chapter review materials and resources. Prepare for success with additional NCLEX®-style practice questions, interactive assignments and activities, web links, animations and videos, and more!

Register your access code from the front of your book at
www.mynursingkit.com

REFERENCES

Corbridge, S. J., Kamp, D. W., & Richlin, D. (2004). Asbestos related pulmonary diseases. *AAOHN Journal, 52,* 49–51.

Crosier, J., & Wise, L. C. (2001). Coming of age: Cystic fibrosis once a childhood disease makes its way to adulthood. *Nursing Management, 33*(11), 30–31.

Dillon, P. M. (2003). *Nursing health assessment: A critical thinking, case studies approach.* Philadelphia: F. A. Davis.

Ford, S. (2002). Common errors in clinical measurement. *Anesthesia and Intensive Care Medicine,* 3(12), 464–467.

Gotway, M. B., Marder, S. R., Hanks, D. K., Leung, J. W., Dawn, S. K., Gean, A. D., et al. (2002). Thoracic complications of illicit drug use: An organ system approach. *Radiographics, 22,* S119–S135.

Grap, M. (2002). Protocols for practice: Pulse oximetry. *Critical Care Nurse, 22*(3), 69–76.

Harris, H. (2004). Action stat fat embolism. *Nursing 2004, 34,* 96.

Jubber, A. S. (2004). Respiratory complications of obesity. *International Journal of Clinical Practice, 58,* 573–580.

Kee, J. L. (2005). *Handbook of laboratory & diagnostic tests* (5th ed.). Upper Saddle River, NJ: Pearson Prentice Hall.

Kose, A. A., Karabagli, Y., & Cetin, C. (2005). An unusual cause of burns due to cupping: Complications of a folk medicine remedy. *Burns, 33,* 126–127.

Merritt, S. L., & Berger, B. E. (2004). Obstructive sleep apnea-hypopnea syndrome. *AJN, 104,* 49–52.

Peltier, L. F. (2004). Fat embolism. *Clinical Orthopedics and Related Research, 422,* 148–153.

Shamsuzzaman, A. S., Gersh, B. J., & Somers, V. K. (2003). Obstructive sleep apnea implications for cardiac and vascular disease. *Journal of the American Medical Association, 290,* 1906–1914.

Snyder, M., & Miska, K. (2003). Cultural related complementary therapies: Their use in critical care units. *Critical Care Clinics of North America, 15,* 341–346.

U.S. Department of Health and Human Services. (2000). *Healthy people 2010: Understanding and improving health.* Washington, DC: Author.

Weber, J., & Kelley, J. (2003). *Health assessment in nursing* (2nd ed.). Philadelphia: Lippincott Williams & Wilkins.

Wilson, K. C., & Saukkonen, J. J. (2004). Acute respiratory failure from abused substances. *Journal of Intensive Care Medicine, 19,* 183–193.

Yoo, S. S., & Tausk, F. (2004). Cupping: East meets West. *International Journal of Dermatology, 43,* 664–665.

Caring for the Patient with Upper Airway Disorders

Ann Sievers

With contributions by:
Kathleen Osborn
Annita Watson

Outcome-Based Learning Objectives

After studying this chapter, the learner will be able to:

1. Compare and contrast nursing management of the most common facial fractures.
2. Explain nursing care for a patient with sinus disease.
3. Differentiate the essential components for developing a teaching plan for patients with infections of the upper airway.
4. Discuss the implications of the loss of the senses of smell, sight, and taste in patients with upper airway disorders and disfigurement.
5. Compare and contrast the nursing management of patients with partial versus total airway obstruction.
6. Identify the risk factors of head and neck cancer.
7. Explain the nursing management of a patient with head and neck cancer in the acute care setting related to airway, wounds, pain, and nutrition.

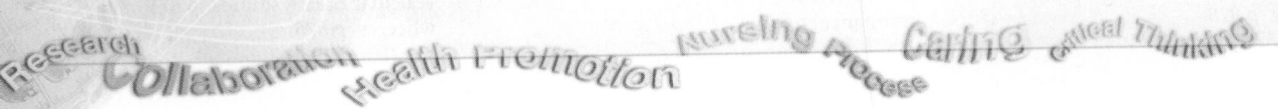

Otolaryngology, also called **otorhinolaryngology**, is the study of disorders of the head and neck, including the ears, nose, and throat. Disease and trauma that affect these structures impact a person's outlook on the world. They can change the way a person smells, tastes, breathes, sees, hears, and touches, and how a person is perceived by others.

Disorders of the head and neck area can not only be disfiguring, but also can involve vital tissues that function to meet the basic human needs of intake of air, fluids, and food. These tissues serve to assess the environment via the special senses of sight, hearing, taste, and smell. Speech also may be affected, as in the case of cancer and subsequent treatment. Any interference with facial appearance, basic human needs, or ability to communicate can be a devastating experience for the patient and family and is a meaningful component of caring for patients of this type. Nurses must be aware of the immense impact of otolaryngology disease and respond to their patients' needs accordingly. It is important for nurses to understand the physiological care needs of their patients and also to be sensitive to the impact on the patient's quality of life. Assisting and teaching patients how to cope with otolaryngologic illnesses and life changes is an essential part of the healing process.

This chapter focuses on disorders of the head and neck and is presented in discrete sections, each describing a specific type of disorder of the head and neck related to structure, function, and disease entities.

Structural, Traumatic, and Deformity Disorders of the Nose and Facial Structures

The facial skeleton serves to protect the brain, house and protect the sense organs of smell, sight, and taste, and provide a frame for the soft tissues of the face. It also helps to facilitate eating, facial expression, breathing, and speech. The primary bones of the face are the nasal bones, mandible, maxilla, zygoma, temporal bone, and frontal bone. Numerous types of deformities affect the facial structures of the head and neck, many of which deal with fractures. The head is the most frequently injured part of the body. Head injuries occur in approximately 75% of all motor vehicle crashes, with approximately 30% of head traumas resulting in skull fractures (Connell & Belafsky, 2005). The ear is the most frequently damaged sense organ.

Nasal Fractures

The skeletal structure of the nose is composed of paired nasal bones, the nasal process of the frontal bone and the maxilla, which form a framework to support the cartilaginous skeleton of the nose. The nasal bones rigidly support the upper portion of the nose between the eyes. The cartilages are flexible supports that maintain the shape of the rest of the nose. The septum divides the nostrils and is also made of both cartilage and bone. Figure 34–1 ■ shows the anatomical relationship between the nasal bones, cartilage, and septum. Underlying the framework of the nose are soft tissues, mucous glands, and nerves responsible for sensation and function of the nose. A "broken nose" may have injured bone, cartilage, nerves, skin, and/or mucosa (the nasal lining). Because the nose is the most prominent anterior feature of the face, nasal fractures account for approximately 40% of bone injuries (Bermant, 2007). According to Smith and Perez (2004), fracture of the nasal bones is the most common site-specific bone injury of the facial skeleton in the United States.

Epidemiology and Etiology

Nasal fractures typically are caused by a traumatic injury to the bone or cartilage of the nose. Although most of the nasal structure is made up of cartilage, the nasal bones usually are fractured in injury. Fights and sports injuries account for most nasal fractures in adults, followed by falls and vehicle crashes. Play and sports account foremost for nasal fractures in children. When nasal fractures are seen in children and women, physical abuse should be considered and appropriately ruled out (Smith & Perez, 2004). Nasal fractures occur more frequently in males than females (>2:1), with the incidence increasing in patients ages 15 to 30 years (Smith & Perez, 2004).

Laboratory and Diagnostic Procedures

Nasal fractures may be diagnosed by facial x-rays. If it is suspected that the ethmoid bone also is damaged due to its proximity to the nasal bones, neurological tests are indicated to assess cognition and response. The ethmoid bone lies posterior to the nasal bones and can be damaged from a direct trauma to the nose. A patient with this type of injury will have a profound headache and may have a cerebrospinal fluid (CSF) leak. Any clear fluid draining from the nose is highly suspect for CSF. Diagnosis is confirmed by allowing the fluid to drain on a clean white dressing. If a halo of red-tinged fluid is demonstrated (halo test), then a CSF leak is present.

Clinical Manifestations

Patients with a nasal fracture usually present with some combination of deformity, tenderness, hemorrhage, edema, ecchymoses,

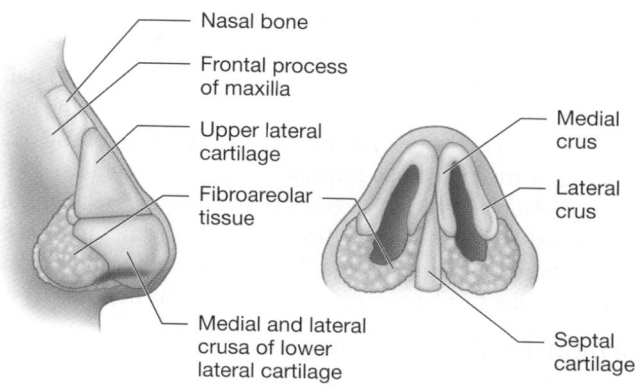

FIGURE 34–1 ■ Anatomical relationship between nasal bones, cartilage, and septum.

Labels: Nasal bone; Frontal process of maxilla; Upper lateral cartilage; Fibroareolar tissue; Medial and lateral crura of lower lateral cartilage; Medial crus; Lateral crus; Septal cartilage

instability, or crepitation. Nasal fractures can occur and not be displaced. In this case, no surgical treatment is indicated. Edema can mask underlying nasal bone displacement, which, if untreated, can result both in unfavorable appearance and function.

Air traveling through the nose normally is controlled by the position of the bones and cartilages and, if displaced, obstruction of the nose can occur. Mucosal swelling and clotted blood also will limit airflow. An injured nose can bleed from lacerations of the skin or from the mucosa inside the nose. These cuts may need to be evaluated and repaired. A septal hematoma can injure or thicken the septal structures, impairing airflow through the nose. Bruises often migrate around the eyes and eventually down the cheeks. Repositioning or moving fractured bones and cartilage typically results in additional swelling. The upper airway passages may be at risk for considerable edema and bruising.

Medical Management

With an uncomplicated (nondisplaced) acute nasal fracture, it is appropriate to prescribe pain medication and release the patient with instructions to rest, apply ice, and maintain head elevation. Follow-up evaluation and management can safely be scheduled after the swelling resolves, usually within 3 to 5 days. If there is displacement of the nasal bones, reduction should be accomplished between the 5th and 10th day after the injury, before the nasal bones start to fixate. Septal hematomas should be drained if possible to prevent nasal obstruction.

Most acute nasal fractures are able to be reduced in the primary care setting. However, for some fractures, open reduction in an operating room is necessary to obtain proper alignment of the nasal bones. Sometimes the aesthetic outcomes of closed-reduction techniques are less than optimal, and patients should be counseled that nasal reconstruction might eventually be necessary. A combination of medications inside the nose and injections around the nose lessens the discomfort of the reduction.

■ Nursing Management

Assessment is a key function of the nurse in caring for patients with a fractured nose. It is imperative that the nurse evaluate the patient for type and severity of injury, bleeding, swelling, patency of airway, skin discoloration, and pain. The immediate goals are to control bleeding, reduce swelling with application of ice, and provide pain control. The nurse will need to assess for further injury by testing the patient for facial numbness or tingling. The presence of tingling needs to be reported to the health care provider. An isolated nasal fracture does not require hospitalization.

Septal Deviation

The nasal septum is the wall dividing the nasal cavity into halves; it is composed of a central supporting skeleton covered on each side by mucous membrane. The front portion of this natural partition is a firm but bendable structure made mostly of cartilage and is covered by skin that has a substantial supply of blood vessels. The ideal nasal septum is exactly midline, separating the left and right sides of the nose into passageways of equal size. A septal deviation occurs when the septum is severely shifted away from the midline. Diagnosed septal deviations are a common occurrence in individuals, reportedly as high as 75%. Note, however, that the American Academy of Otolaryngology–Head and Neck Surgery (2007) has reported that 80% of all nasal septums are somewhat off-centered. The majority of diagnosed septal deviations that cause pathophysiological symptoms to patients are caused by trauma to the nose.

Epidemiology and Etiology

Deviations of the nasal septum may develop during growth or by trauma due to a fall, a blow to the nose, or surgery that further exaggerates the deviation. These deviations are common and, for the most part, cause no symptoms and require no treatment. However, the septal deviation may be severe enough to obstruct the passage of air through the nostrils. This obstruction predisposes the patient to sinusitis, infection, and epistaxis.

Pathophysiology and Clinical Manifestations

Although septal deviations usually present no problem for the individual, they may cause one or more of the following: blockage of one or both nostrils; nasal congestion, sometimes one sided; frequent nosebleeds; frequent sinus infections; at times, facial pain; headaches, postnasal drip; and noisy breathing during sleep, particularly in infants and young children.

In some cases, a person with a mildly deviated septum has symptoms only when an upper respiratory tract infection is also present. In these individuals, the respiratory infection triggers nasal inflammation that temporarily amplifies any mild airflow problems related to the deviated septum. Once the infection resolves, and the nasal inflammation subsides, symptoms of a deviated septum often also resolve.

Medical Management

It is easy to diagnose that a septum is deviated; it is more difficult to determine if that deviation needs correcting. A patient's complaint that she can breathe through only one nostril is the usual determinant of treatment. Decongestants, such as pseudoephedrine or phenylpropanolamine, will shrink the members and thereby enlarge the passages. Antihistamines, nasal cortisone spray, and other allergy treatments also may be temporarily beneficial. Normal saline drops and sprays are very helpful in loosening mucus in the obstructed side and preventing drying in the other side, where all of the air blows. These therapies are useful to take care of symptoms, but do not correct the problem.

If the patient complains of obstruction or has cosmetic complaints, a septoplasty, or surgical repositioning of the septum, may be performed. It is performed with a local anesthetic and conscious sedation. Some health care providers insert nasal splints and suture them into place as a temporary structural support. The splints are removed a few days after surgery. Surgical repair is curative and carries little risk. A nasospecific procedure in which a deflated balloon is inserted in the nostril and inflated to a large enough degree to adjust the septal deviation, can be an alternative to surgery. A practitioner trained in this nasospecific procedure is necessary.

◼ Nursing Management

Nursing management focuses on maintaining a clear air passage, detecting signs of infection, and maintaining patient comfort. The nurse is instrumental in teaching the patient how to instill nose drops and sprays and perform a saline lavage. In the event of a surgical repair, the nurse provides routine postoperative care and is alert for bleeding, swelling, and pain.

Epistaxis

Epistaxis is defined as any bleeding from the nostril, nasal cavity, or nasopharynx. Epistaxis is common due to the highly vascular linings of the nose. One of the primary causes of nosebleeds is traumatic nose injuries, although they may occur for other reasons. Air moving through the nose can dry and irritate the membranes lining the inside of the nose, forming crusts. These crusts bleed when irritated by rubbing, picking, or blowing the nose.

Epidemiology and Etiology

As noted, nosebleeds are very common. They tend to occur more frequently in the winter when viruses are common and heated indoor air dries out the nostrils. Common etiologies include injuries such as trauma; systemic problems, such as coagulation disorders or hypertension; environmental problems, such as dry air; irritation from nose picking; use of drugs and medications; or postoperatively with any nasal or sinus surgery. A foreign object in the nose or direct impact to the nose also can cause a nosebleed. A deviated septum also may make a person prone to nosebleeds.

The elderly are susceptible to nosebleeds for several reasons. As a person ages, the skin becomes more friable and retains less turgor. The same is true of the lining in the nose. Any mechanical irritation, such as nose picking or excessive rubbing, may cause a bleed. Individuals who use any type of inhaled drug also are at risk of damaging the nasal tissues and are highly prone to nosebleeds.

Pathophysiology

There are two areas within the nasal passage where a plexus of anastomotic vessels can be found. The anterior area is referred to as Kiesselbach's plexus (or Little's area), and the posterior area is known as Woodruff's plexus (Kucik, 2005). These areas often are implicated in nosebleeds. Anterior bleeds from Kiesselbach's plexus are the most common. They account for approximately 90% of nosebleeds. The bleeding erupts when the relatively thin nasal mucosa overlying a dilated septal vessel dries, scabs, and falls (or is picked) off. Posterior bleeds originating from Woodruff's plexus, which is located over the posterior middle turbinate, are less common. In these cases the site of bleeding is higher and deeper within the nose and the blood flows primarily down the back of the throat.

Only rarely is a nosebleed life threatening or actually fatal. In most cases of life-threatening nosebleeds, some underlying health problem, such as hypertension, a bleeding disorder, or use of anticoagulant medication, is impacting the patient's ability to clot (Pope & Hobbs, 2005). Hereditary hemorrhagic telangiectasia (also called HHT or Osler-Weber-Rendu syndrome) may be evidenced by nosebleeds. This is a disorder involving a blood vessel growth similar to a birthmark in the back of the nose.

Clinical Manifestations

The clinical manifestation of epistaxis consists of bleeding from the nose. There may be slight or profuse bleeding dependent on the cause of the nosebleed. If the bleeding does not stop after 20 minutes, it is imperative that the patient seek emergency care. If the nosebleed occurs after an injury to the head, this may indicate a skull fracture. It could also indicate a broken nose and x-rays should be taken no matter how trivial the blow seems to be at the time. Skull fractures are discussed in Chapter 29 &.

Laboratory and Diagnostic Procedures and Medical Management

Laboratory and diagnostic tests that may need to be performed include a complete blood count (CBC), partial thromboplastin time measurements, prothrombin (PT) measurements, and x-rays of the skull. Nasal endoscopy (examination of the nose using a camera) also may be called for.

Anterior bleeds generally resolve on their own by pinching the nares together and leaning forward for several minutes. The health care provider should apply cold packs to the face and have the patient lean forward or to the side to protect the airway and prevent swallowing of blood. This maneuver may prevent emesis. Electrocautery, chemical cautery, or anterior or posterior nasal packing may be used for any bleeding that does not quickly resolve (Figure 34–2 ■). Cryotherapy, laser therapy, embolization, or surgery may be used to ligate bleeding vessels (Pope & Hobbs, 2005).

Instruction for any patient recovering from a nosebleed should include refraining from picking or blowing of the nose, no heavy lifting, and no straining for 2 days to 2 weeks, as recommended by the health care provider. Stool softeners, pain medications, nasal emollients, or nasal saline spray may be prescribed.

■ Nursing Management

For patients with anterior epistaxis and anterior packing, a feeling of airway obstruction can arise. The nurse will need to take special note of the patient's concerns and provide reassurance as needed. The head of the bed should be elevated, and a face mask should be provided for humidity. In the event of surgery, routine postoperative care protocols should be followed. Pain medications should be provided as needed. The patient with posterior epistaxis, requiring posterior packing, should be observed in an intensive care unit (ICU). These patients are at risk

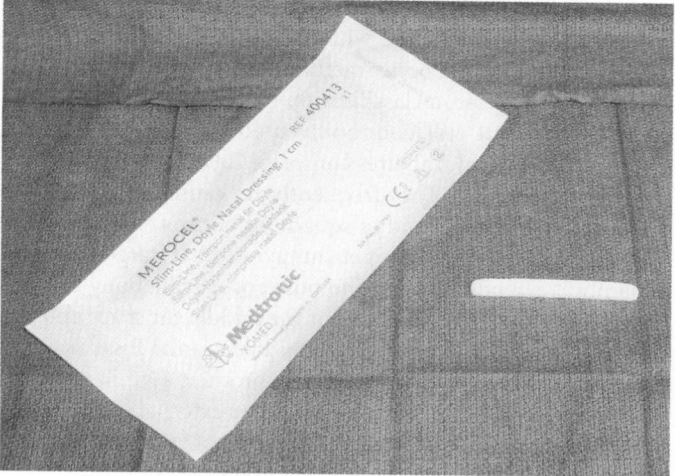

FIGURE 34–2 ■ Nasal tampon for the treatment of anterior epistaxis. This is placed in the anterior nasal cavity, impregnated with normal saline, and left in place for at least 5 days. Most nasal packing is bilateral to provide pressure support on either side of the nasal septum.
Source: University of California, Davis Medical Center

for airway obstruction if the packs slip. They also are at risk for developing bradycardia and hypercarbia due to the nasopulmonary reflex. Therefore, cardiac monitoring and pulse oximetry are mandatory.

The nurse also should advise patients of risk factors for nosebleeds, including a hot, dry climate, colds and allergies, a deviated septum, exposure to irritating chemicals, medical conditions, heavy alcohol use, and medications that interfere with blood clotting. Patient education should include advice on preventive measures that can be taken. These include not picking the nose, gently blowing the nose one nostril at a time, keeping mouth open when sneezing, not smoking, using a humidifier if indoor climate is dry, applying a dab of butter/petroleum jelly to the inside of the nostrils before bedtime, and avoiding aspirin and other medications that prolong the bleeding time.

Facial Fractures

Facial fractures refer to any injuries that result in a broken bone or bones of the face. Because nose fractures were discussed earlier, this discussion is restricted to the mandible, maxilla, zygoma, temporal bones, and the frontal bone. Multiple facial fractures may occur simultaneously, typically resulting from an injury to the face. Many situations can cause facial fractures. Motor vehicle crashes, sporting injuries, falls, and assault account for the majority, although injuries from gunshot wounds and stabbings occur as well. When dealing with facial fractures, the nurse should always be concerned that other injuries may exist. Other parts of the body may be injured, for example, if the patient has facial injuries caused by a motor vehicle crash.

Mandible Fractures

The mandible is a U-shaped bone; together with the maxilla, the mandible is the largest and strongest bone of the face. It forms the lower jaw and holds the lower teeth in place. The mandible consists of a curved, horizontal portion, referred to as the *body*; two perpendicular portions, the *rami*, which unite with the ends of the body nearly at right angles; the alveolar process; the tooth-bearing area of the mandible (upper part of the body of the mandible), the condyle; superior (upper) and posterior projection from the ramus, which makes the temporomandibular joint with the temporal bone; and the coronoid process, superior and anterior projection from the ramus, which provides attachment to the temporalis muscle.

The inferior alveolar nerve, a branch of the mandibular division of the trigeminal (V) nerve, enters the mandibular foramen and runs forward in the mandibular canal, supplying sensation to the teeth. At the mental foramen the nerve divides into two terminal branches: incisive and mental nerves. The incisive nerve runs forward in the mandible and supplies the anterior teeth. The mental nerve exits the mental foramen and supplies sensation to the lower lip (Babak & Blackwell, 2005). The mandible articulates with the two temporal bones at the temporomandibular joints. It is the only mobile bone of the facial skeleton, and since it houses the lower teeth, its motion is essential for mastication. Mandibular fractures often are accompanied by a "twin fracture" on the contralateral (opposite) side. The mandible may be dislocated anteriorly (to the front) and inferiorly (downward) but very rarely posteriorly (backward).

Maxilla Fractures

The maxilla forms the largest component of the middle third of the facial skeleton, and is a fusion of two bones along the palatal fissure that forms the upper jaw. This is similar to the mandible, which also is a fusion of two halves at the mental symphysis. The alveolar process of the maxilla holds the upper teeth and is referred to as the maxillary arch. The maxilla attaches laterally to the zygomatic bones (cheekbones) and assists in forming the boundaries of three cavities: the roof of the mouth, the floor and lateral side of the nasal antrum, and the floor of the orbit. The maxilla also enters into the formation of two fossae: the infratemporal and pterygopalatine, and two fissures, the inferior orbital and pterygomaxillary. The maxilla articulates with nine bones: two of the cranium (frontal and ethmoid) and seven of the face (nasal, zygomatic, lacrimal, inferior nasal, concha, palatine, vomer) and the adjacent fused maxillary bone. Sometimes it articulates with the orbital surface, and sometimes with the lateral pterygoid plate of the sphenoid. The maxilla is a key bone in the midface that is closely associated with adjacent bones providing structural support between the cranial base and the occlusal plane.

Fractures of the maxilla occur less frequently than those of the mandible or nose due to the strong structural support of this bone. The midface consists of alternating thick and thin sections of bone that are capable of resisting significant force. This structurally strong bone provides protection for the globes and brain, projection of the midface, and support for occlusion. Reestablishing the continuity of these buttresses is the foundation on which maxillary fracture treatment is based.

Le Fort Classification of Fractures

René Le Fort provided the earliest classification system of maxillary fractures in 1901. His model, which is still generally used, described "great lines of weakness in the face" using low-velocity impact forces directed against cadaver skulls. The categorization and assessment of Le Fort fractures are discussed next.

Le Fort I Fracture   Le Fort I fractures (horizontal) may result from a force of injury directed low on the maxillary alveolar rim in a downward direction. The Le Fort I fracture, or transverse fracture, extends through the base of the maxillary sinuses above the teeth, essentially separating the alveolar processes, palate, and pterygoid processes from the facial structures above. This transverse fracture across the entire lower maxilla separates the alveolus as a mobile unit from the rest of the midface. Fracture dislocations of segments of the alveolus may be associated with this fracture. With high-energy injuries, the palate may be split in the midline in addition to the Le Fort I fracture.

Le Forte II Fracture   Le Fort II fractures (pyramidal) may result from a blow to the lower or midmaxilla. A pyramidal fracture of the maxilla is synonymous with a Le Fort II fracture. This fracture pattern begins laterally, similar to a Le Fort I, but medially diverges in a superior direction to include part of the medial orbit as well as the nose. The fracture extending across the nose may be variable, involving only the nasal cartilage or being so extensive that the nasofrontal suture is separated. The fracture extends diagonally from the pterygoid plates through the maxilla to the inferior orbital rim and up the medial wall of the orbit to the nose. This separates the maxillary alveolus, the medial wall of the orbit and nose, as a separate piece.

Le Fort III Fracture   Le Fort III fractures (transverse) may result from impact to the nasal bridge or upper maxilla. A Le Fort III fracture, also referred to as a craniofacial disjunction, denotes a complete separation of the midface or facial bones from the cranium. This fracture transverses the zygomaticofrontal suture, continues through the floor of the orbit, and finally through the nasofrontal suture. The bones of the orbit are separated through the lateral wall, floor, and medial wall. It is unusual to have this fracture as a single segment of bone; more commonly, it comminutes with varying combinations of zygomatic, nasoethmoid, and orbital fractures. The fractures may not be symmetric on both sides and minimal mobility may be present.

Zygoma Fractures

The zygomatic bone (malar bone) is a paired bone of the human skull. It articulates with the maxilla, the temporal bone, the sphenoid bone, and the frontal bone. It forms part of the orbit, the lateral portion of the interior orbital rim, as well as the lateral rim and lateral wall of the orbit, and is commonly referred to as the cheekbone. It is situated at the upper and lateral part of the face, forming the prominence of the cheek, part of the lateral wall and floor of the orbit, and parts of the temporal and infratemporal fossae. This bone presents a malar and a temporal surface; four processes, the frontosphenoidal, orbital, maxillary, and temporal; and four borders.

Additionally, it forms the anterior zygomatic arch. The zygomatic arch is made up of three bone components: the zygomatic bone, coming off the zygomatic prominence of the maxilla, and the zygomatic process of the temporal bone. The masseter muscle also is suspended from the zygomatic arch. The masseter muscle acts to close the mandible for mastication and speech.

Temporal Bone Fractures

The temporal bones are situated at the sides and base of the skull. The temporal bone supports that part of the face known as the temple. It is considered by many to be the most complex bone in the human body (Connell & Belafsky, 2005). The temporal bone houses many vital structures, including the cochlear and vestibular end organs and the facial nerve, carotid artery, and jugular vein. It is possible that an involvement of all or some of the structures may occur with a temporal bone fracture.

Typically temporal bone fractures are classified into longitudinal and transverse, a classification originally set forth by Ullrich in 1926, but still commonly used (Connell & Belafsky, 2005). Longitudinal fractures comprise 70% to 90% of all temporal bone fractures. They frequently are caused by a blunt lateral force over the mastoid or squamous bone. The fracture line parallels the long axis of the petrous pyramid. It starts in the pars squamosa, extends through the posterosuperior bony external canal, continues across the roof of the middle ear space anterior to the labyrinth, and ends in the middle cranial fossa near the foramen spinosum. Oblique fractures produce a similar fracture line in the middle cranial fossa but differ externally. They cross the petrotympanic fissure, and longitudinal fractures are contained within it (Connell & Belafsky, 2005).

Frontal Bone Fractures

The frontal bone is the large bone that makes up the forehead and supplies the upper edge and roof of the orbit (eye socket). It resembles a cockle-shell in shape, and forms the anterior portion of the cranium. This bone consists of two portions: a vertical portion known as the squama frontalis, corresponding with the region of the forehead, and an orbital or horizontal portion, the pars orbitalis, which enters into the formation of the roofs of the orbital and nasal cavities (Babak & Blackwell, 2005). It articulates with a number of other bones including the parietal, nasal, ethmoid, maxillary, and zygomatic bones. The frontal sinus is a pyramid, air-filled cavity that lies between the lamina of the frontal bone. The anterior wall generally is considered the strongest of the tables. The posterior wall is much thinner and weaker, and separates the sinus from the dura of the frontal lobe of the anterior facial fossa. The eyebrows and the buttress of the supraorbital rim demarcate the lower anterior border of the frontal sinus. The sinus floor consists of membranous bone that is the thinnest of the sinus boundaries and the most vulnerable to injury. The floor also forms two-thirds of the medial orbital roof. The primary purpose of the frontal sinus is to serve as a mechanical barrier to protect the brain from trauma. The frontal sinuses are positioned more anteriorly than the other paranasal sinuses and are situated to absorb anterior cranial facial trauma.

Epidemiology and Etiology

All facial fractures usually occur as a result of an injury or trauma to the face. These injuries often are induced by motor vehicle crashes, motorcycle crashes, or from direct blows to the face.

A mandibular fracture generally is caused by trauma such as a direct blow or lateral blow to the face as a result of a motor vehicle crash, assault, fall, or contact sports. As with mandibular fractures, maxillary fractures also are often the result of motor vehicle crashes. The bones that make up the zygomatic arch frequently are fractured in collisions and as a result of blunt trauma. These high-velocity injuries many times produce fracture patterns not classified by the standard Le Fort system, but are described simply by the anatomic structure fractured and the degree of comminution present.

Temporal bone trauma usually is the sequelae of blunt head injury. Damage to the temporal bone typically requires the application of great force and may cause fracture, hemorrhage, nerve trauma, vascular damage, or disruption of the middle or inner ear structures. Associated intracranial injuries, such as extra-axial hemorrhage, shear (or diffuse axonal injury), and brain contusion, are common (Woodcock, 2007). Temporal bone injuries reportedly occur in 14% to 22% of all skull fractures, with motor vehicle crashes causing approximately 31% of temporal bone fractures (Connell & Belafsky, 2005).

Other causes, in descending order of frequency, are physical assaults, falls, motorcycle crashes, pedestrian injuries, bicycle crashes, and gunshot wounds. Males ages 21 to 40 years old comprise the most commonly involved group. Transverse temporal fractures are less common, comprising 10% to 30% of all temporal bone fractures. They usually are caused by a frontal or parietal blow, but may result from an occipital blow, producing a profound sensorineural hearing loss and severe ablative vertigo. Fractures may extend through the internal auditory canal and injure the nerves directly. Cochlear and vestibular structures usually are destroyed

Fractures involving the frontal region represent some of the least common injuries that affect the facial skeleton. The incidence is 5% to 15% of all facial fractures (Piccolino et al., 2007).

For purposes of initial evaluation, frontal sinus fractures should be regarded as head injuries. The majority of these patients are victims of automobile collisions with multiple injuries requiring a multiple-specialty team approach and complete evaluation. Skull fractures are discussed in detail in Chapter 29.

Laboratory and Diagnostic Procedures

The clinical exam, facial x-ray, or computed tomography (CT) scan is used to make the diagnosis of most facial fractures. The exact location and extent of injury for the majority of facial fractures determines the type of x-ray to be used. For example, the diagnosis of a mandibular fracture is by panorex, or CT scan, accompanied by presenting dental malocclusion, pain, and a history of trauma to the area.

As noted earlier, maxillary facial fractures are described by using the Le Fort categories. These fractures almost always require surgical repair and CT scans, and the more recent development of three-dimensional (3D) reconstructions has aided greatly in the diagnosis, classification, and preoperative planning of complex maxillary fractures.

A zygomatic fracture is diagnosed with a combination of a CT scan, a history of the trauma, and from the presenting signs and symptoms. In the case of temporal and frontal fractures high-resolution CT (HRCT) of the bones is useful in assessing injuries complicated by CSF leak or facial paralysis. If transient or persistent neurological deficits are present in a patient with basilar skull fracture, HRCT or temporal bone with CT angiography is indicated to evaluate for petrous carotid injury. With fractures of the temporal bones, it is necessary to test for hearing loss.

Clinical Manifestations

With most facial bone fractures there is some overt sign of the deformity, which may include bleeding, swelling, bruising, a change in the facial shape, and pain. With mandibular fractures, patients will have difficulty opening their mouths and chewing (masticating). A patient with a mandibular fracture will have pain and difficulty with talking and chewing. Paresthesia and numbness also may be present on the affected side due to swelling at the site of injury. With maxillary fractures, the face seems to be sunken in and, on palpation, irregularities and boney stepoffs, or misalignments, demonstrate free movement. Because of considerable and extensive facial edema, the nurse may not fully appreciate these assessments. Patients will have pain, difficulty on opening the mouth and chewing, and sometimes difficulty talking. They also may have paresthesia or numbness or a sensation of "pins and needles" on the affected side due to the proximity of the swelling to the trigeminal (CN V) and facial (CN VII) nerves. Of the three fracture types, the most extensive and life threatening is the Le Forte III. With this type of fracture, airway obstruction and severe bleeding are likely. The airway usually is supported with a temporary tracheotomy. A **tracheotomy** is a surgical airway. A **tracheostomy** is the opening created by the surgical procedure. In this chapter these terms are used interchangeably.

In zygomatic and orbital fractures, the orbital contents can become entrapped by bony fragments from the floor of the orbit. The patient will experience pain, diplopia, difficulty with eye movement, and sometimes blindness. Global entrapment must be surgically corrected very early on to prevent further visual damage. Swelling to the area may mask the fracture. Patients will have pain, difficulty on opening the mouth and chewing, and sometimes difficulty talking.

The two kinds of temporal bone fractures produce different findings. A longitudinal fracture runs vertically, usually causing injury to the tympanic membrane and ossicles. This produces conductive hearing loss (negative Rinne test, lateralization with Weber test), otorrhea of either blood or CSF, and, occasionally, facial nerve paralysis. Rinne and Weber tests evaluate hearing. The Rinne test distinguishes between conductive and sensorineural hearing loss and the Weber test evaluates bone conduction; both use a tuning fork. Other findings include headache, nystagmus, or vertigo. Some temporal bone fractures are difficult to see on x-ray. All clinical findings may not be present at the time of injury, but may develop later. Hearing impairment is discussed in detail in Chapter 70 ☺.

Medical Management

Medical management of all facial fractures includes airway support, pain control, and closed reduction or surgical repair depending on the type and severity of the fracture. The patient's airway should be assessed for patency because hemorrhage or edema can cause airway obstruction. Treatment generally consists of realigning the fractured pieces of bone with wires or repairing the break with metal plates and fine screws. If fragments of bone have pierced the skin or if teeth were lost or loosened, an antibiotic generally is ordered to reduce the risk of infection.

Maxillary fractures are treated by reduction and immobilization. Surgical repair of the fractures involves plating the bones together to stabilize the bony facial structure (Figure 34–3 ■). The maxilla and mandible also may be wired together for further stabilization. Establishment of preinjury occlusion and midface buttress alignment provides the foundation for this treatment.

The goals of treatment of Le Fort fractures are to reestablish preinjury occlusion with normal height and projection of the face. To accomplish this, the structural buttress of the maxilla must be aligned and stabilized to provide the necessary support and contour to the midface. The proper occlusal relationship between the dental arches is established with intermaxillary fixation (IMF), or more appropriately termed maxillomandibular fixation. Early placement of the patient in IMF can eliminate some of the secondary deformities caused by Le Fort fractures. IMF is established by securing arch bars to the upper and lower dental arches with individual wire ligatures around the teeth. The appropriate occlusion is then determined by wear facets, and the maxillary and mandibular arch bar are secured together. This is one of the simplest and most effective forms of treatment. However, IMF is more commonly used in conjunction with other immobilization and stabilization techniques.

Recent advances in the treatment of maxillary fractures include the use of extended open-reduction techniques with rigid plate and screw fixation of the facial buttresses. Bone grafts have been used to replace missing or comminuted bone with early treatment of these injuries. This more aggressive surgical approach has dramatically improved the aesthetic results now obtainable with fewer secondary deformities.

Zygomatic and mandibular fractures are usually treated surgically. Fractures are reduced by using screws, bars, wires, and plates. Following open-reduction internal fixation (ORIF) of the

FIGURE 34–3 ■ Plating facial fractures is the current method of internal fixation. Facial plates remain in place (or can be removed at a future surgery) for at least 6 to 8 weeks until the fractures heal. This plate demonstrates the fixation of an orbital rim fracture.
Source: University of California, Davis Medical Center

fractures, the jaws can be wired shut with or without plating of the fractures. Intermaxillary-mandibular fractures (IMMFs) are repaired with wires and bands, which are similar to braces, to maintain alignment during healing.

Management of temporal bone fractures generally is conservative. If the facial nerve (CN VII) is lacerated or impacted, the patient must undergo surgical facial nerve decompression. If a dural leak is suspected, systemic antibiotics are given to prevent meningitis. Transverse fractures across the middle ear produce pain, blood behind the eardrum (hemotympanum), and a sensorineural hearing loss resulting in a positive Rinne test, and showing lateralization in the Weber test due to vestibulocochlear (CN VIII) damage. Facial nerve (CN VII) injury or paralysis produces a facial droop, loss of a blink reflex, and paresthesia. The care of a patient with a temporal bone fracture and/or a temporal bone resection is similar; the focus is on care of the eye after facial nerve resection, cable grafting, or repair. Eye protection adding lubrication prevents corneal abrasions.

The long-range goals of treatment of frontal sinus fractures are cosmetic restoration and prevention of early and late complications including acute and chronic sinusitis, mucocele formation, brain abscess, and osteomyelitis. The first step, however, is to evaluate and manage more serious life-threatening injuries. Thus, in the case of frontal fractures, the standard trauma protocol must be followed with emphasis on ensuring an adequate airway, breathing, circulation, central nervous system (CNS) status, and C-spine. Frontal sinus fractures do not require immediate surgical attention unless they are associated with a neurosurgical or ophthalmologic emergency. The choice of treatment usually is dictated by the site and extent of the damage (Piccolino et al., 2007).

There are no uniform treatment guidelines for patients with fractures of the frontal sinus. Controversies exist regarding timing and indications for surgical intervention as well as the best types of surgical ablative materials to use. For anterior table fractures, displaced fractures require treatment to correct aesthetic deformity. With injury to the nasofrontal duct, an anterior table fracture is treated with duct occlusion and frontal sinus obliteration. Treatment of posterior table fractures is fraught with controversy. Some authors advocate sinus obliteration whenever there is a posterior table fracture in order to avoid complications with undetected nasofrontal duct injury or CSF leak. Other authors recommend treatment based on displacement, or the presence of CSF leak or nasofrontal duct injury. For nondisplaced fractures, surgical treatment is not required. For displaced fractures, sinus obliteration is only recommended if there is simultaneous injury to the nasofrontal duct and/or the presence of a CSF leak (Corey, 2006).

Nursing Management

With mandibular fractures, the patient's nutritional requirements and knowledge deficits should be determined regarding the planned procedure and self-care after discharge. Oral nutrition with a liquid diet high in protein and calories is essential. Weight loss should be avoided if possible to ensure nutritional adequacy for healing. A feeding nasogastric or oral gastric tube may be required for nutritional support for the patient with extensive facial swelling.

Assessment

For all patients with these types of fractures, it is critical for the nurse to observe for nausea and vomiting and to intervene to prevent aspiration when necessary.

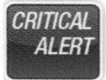 **CRITICAL ALERT** *Postoperatively give nausea medication to reduce the chances of vomiting. If, following surgery, the patient vomits and is unable to maintain his airway, the nurse, or family if at home, should cut the wires to open the mouth to protect the airway. The patient must then have the wires resecured to reestablish the fracture repair.*

Planning

Effective oral care is essential for healthy healing and prevention of dental complications. Patient education includes use of the water pick for mouth and teeth cleaning and dietary requirements. A nutritional consult can assess the patient's nutrition and home requirements for enteral feeding or an oral soft or liquid diet. Dental follow-up is important during and following the 6-week healing process. Chapter 14 🖉 includes a discussion of enteral feedings and their importance for maintaining nutritional balance.

Interventions and Rationales

Management of temporal bone fractures usually is conservative. The nurse must continually assess for nerve damage and hear-

ing loss. It is essential to test for any otorrhea (inflammation of the ear with purulent discharge), which may indicate a CSF leak. The nurse needs to institute CSF leak precautions which include the following:

- Keep the head of the patient's bed at 30 to 45 degrees at all times.
- Teach the patient not to bend over, strain, or lift heavy objects.
- Provide instruction about not straining during a bowel movement because this may prevent a CSF leak from healing or make it worse.

A lumbar drain is inserted to lessen the increased intracranial pressure at the site of injury and allow it to heal. If facial nerve injury is present, the nurse should provide eye care including artificial tears every 2 hours, ointment at night, and use of an eye shield to protect the eye from drying and corneal abrasion.

Patients who present with a frontal facial fracture have generally experienced other severe injuries as well. The nurse must be alert to patency of airway, bleeding, swelling, pain, and possible other injuries.

Inflammation, Infection, and Obstruction of the Nose and Paranasal Sinuses

Disorders affecting the nose and paranasal sinuses include inflammation, infection, and obstruction. The effect of these phenomena leads individuals to feel ill, tired, and irritable. Common disorders that fall within these categories are discussed following a review of the anatomy and physiology of the paranasal sinuses.

Anatomy and Physiology of the Paranasal Sinuses

The paranasal sinuses are the eight cavities in the skull that connect with the nasal cavity. They are arranged bilaterally in four pairs. The pairs are the maxillary sinuses in the maxillae, the frontal sinuses in the frontal bone, the sphenoid sinuses in the sphenoid bone behind the nasal cavity, and the ethmoid cells (sinuses) in the ethmoid bone behind and below the frontal sinuses. The exact function of the sinuses is not certain. They are believed to help the nose in circulating, warming, and moistening air as it is inhaled, thereby lessening the effect of cold, dry air to the lungs. They also are thought to have a role as resonating chambers for the voice (Miller-Keene & O'Toole, 2003). The anatomy of the sinuses varies tremendously from person to person. In some individuals, anatomical differences may affect breathing and block the normal nasal drainage.

The upper aerodigestive tract mucous membrane in the nose and sinuses acts to condition inhaled air. It warms, moisturizes, and filters the air. The mucous membrane creates clear, wet, slightly sticky mucus that gathers any dust, smoke, bacteria, or virus particles that may have been in the air. Tiny hairs along the membrane called cilia rotate to move the mucus along through the sinuses and out the nose. The mucous membrane also is one the body's frontline defense systems. It releases chemicals that help to destroy bacteria and viruses. If a virus, bacteria, allergen, or other irritant is strong enough to prevent the mucous membrane and cilia from functioning, an infectious obstruction can occur in any of the pairs of sinus.

Rhinitis

Rhinitis is an inflammation of the nasal mucous membrane and typically is classified as allergic or nonallergic (Quillen & Feller, 2006). Associated clinical symptoms of rhinitis include excessive mucous production, congestion, sneezing paroxysm, watery eyes, and nasal and ocular pruritus. Although the symptoms of both types of rhinitis may be similar, the etiology and treatment may vary, thus requiring a differential diagnosis.

Allergic rhinitis is considered a systemic illness and may be associated with generalized symptoms such as fatigue, malaise, and headache. It also may be a comorbidity in patients with asthma, eczema, or chronic sinusitis (Quillen & Feller, 2006). The three types of allergic rhinitis are (1) seasonal, which occurs particularly during pollen season, (2) perennial, which occurs throughout the year, and (3) occupational, which is triggered by exposure to irritants and allergens.

Nonallergic rhinitis usually is the result of a viral or bacterial infection. It resembles allergic rhinitis in symptoms and clinical manifestations, but not in etiology.

Epidemiology and Etiology

Rhinitis is common among individuals, affecting approximately 40 million people in the United States. Recent U.S. figures suggest a 20% cumulative prevalence rate (Sheikh, 2007). Allergic rhinitis occurs in persons of all races. A prevalence of allergic rhinitis seems to vary among different populations and cultures, which may be due to genetic differences, geographic factors, environmental differences, and/or other population-based factors. The prevalence of rhinitis is approximately equal between men and women in adulthood. The onset of rhinitis is common in childhood, adolescence, and early adulthood, with a mean age of onset of 8 to 11 years. However, allergic rhinitis may occur in persons of any age, with 80% of cases developing by age 20. In the geriatric population, rhinitis is less commonly allergic in nature (Sheikh, 2007).

Nonallergic rhinitis affects 5% to 10% of the population, and approximately half of these individuals seek treatment for relief of the symptoms (Ramakrishnan & Meyers, 2006). Nonallergic rhinitis has seven basic subclassifications: (1) infectious rhinitis, (2) vasomotor rhinitis, (3) occupational rhinitis, (4) hormonal rhinitis, (5) drug-induced rhinitis, (6) gustatory rhinitis, and (7) nonallergic rhinitis with eosinophilia syndrome (Ramakrishnan & Meyers, 2006).

- *Infectious rhinitis* is usually caused by an upper respiratory tract infection of viral origin. The most common causes are infections due to rhinovirus, coronavirus, adenovirus, parainfluenza virus, respiratory syncytial virus, or enterovirus. They are generally self-limiting, lasting between 7 and 10 days.
- *Vasomotor rhinitis* is believed to result from disturbed regulation of the parasympathetic and sympathetic systems in which the parasympathetic system dominates, resulting in

vasodilatation and edema of the nasal vasculature. Resulting symptoms of rhinorrhea are sneezing and congestion. Cold air, strong odors, stress, or inhaled irritants may exacerbate symptoms.

- *Occupational rhinitis* causes patients to have symptoms only in the workplace. These symptoms usually are due to an inhaled irritant, for example, metal salts, animal dander, latex, wood dusts, chemicals. Patients with occupational rhinitis frequently present with concurrent occupational asthma (Quillen & Feller, 2006).
- *Hormonal rhinitis* occurs during periods of hormonal imbalance. Estrogens are known to affect the autonomic nervous system by means of several mechanisms. Central parasympathetic activity, acetylcholine content, and activity of acetylcholine transferase are increased. The most common causes of hormonal rhinitis are pregnancy, menstruation, puberty, use of exogenous estrogen, and hypothyroidism.
- *Drug-induced rhinitis* is precipitated by several medications: angiotensin-converting enzyme inhibitors, reserpine, guanethidine, phentolamine, methyldopa, beta-blockers, chlorpromazine, gabapentin, penicillamine, aspirin, nonsteroidal anti-inflammatory drugs, inhaled cocaine, exogenous estrogens, and oral contraceptives. Rhinitis medicamentosa represents a different etiology. This is a drug-induced rhinitis resulting from prolonged use of nasal sympathomimetics.
- *Gustatory rhinitis* occurs after eating, particularly hot and spicy foods. The end results are profuse watery rhinorrhea secondary to nasal vasodilation that is vagally mediated and generally occurs within a few hours of oral ingestion. Symptoms of rhinitis rarely are secondary to ingestion of specific preservatives or dyes in food.
- *Nonallergic rhinitis with eosinophilia syndrome* (NARES) accounts for as many as 20% of the rhinitis diagnoses. Abnormal prostaglandin metabolism has been implicated as a cause of NARES. Eosinophil counts are elevated in approximately 20% of nasal smears in the general population; however, not everyone with eosinophilia has symptoms of rhinitis. A distinguishing feature of NARES is the presence of eosinophils, usually 10% to 20% on nasal smears. In general, patients with NARES present with nasal congestion, sneezing, rhinorrhea, nasal pruritus, and hyposmia.

Pathophysiology

An allergy is actually an inappropriate immune response to a substance in the environment that is normally harmless. When a person with allergies breathes in an allergen, histamine and other chemicals are released as part of the immune response, causing itching and swelling, mucous production, and in serious cases, hives and rashes, as well as other symptoms.

Allergic rhinitis involves inflammation of the mucous membranes of the nose, eyes, eustachian tubes, middle ear, sinuses, and pharynx. It is a reaction that occurs when airborne irritants (allergens) trigger the release of immune mediators. The mediators that are immediately released include histamine, tryptase, chymase, kinins, and heparin. These mediators act via various interactions and ultimately lead to the symptoms of rhinorrhea. Mucous glands are stimulated, leading to increased secretions.

Vascular permeability is increased, leading to plasma exudation. Vasodilation occurs, leading to congestion and pressure. Sensory nerves are stimulated, leading to sneezing and itching. Histamine causes inflammation and fluid production in the fragile linings of nasal passages, sinuses, and eyelids. All of these events can occur in minutes; hence, this reaction is called the early, or immediate, phase of the reaction.

Over 4 to 8 hours, these mediators, through a complex interplay of events, lead to the recruitment of other inflammatory cells to the mucosa, such as neutrophils, eosinophils, lymphocytes, and macrophages. This results in continued inflammation, termed the late-phase response. The symptoms of the late-phase response are similar to those of the early phase, but usually with less sneezing and itching, and more congestion and mucous production tend to occur. The late phase may persist for hours or days (Sheikh, 2007).

Nonallergic rhinitis follows the same path of symptom development as allergic rhinitis; however, autonomic stimuli have a greater effect on patients with nonallergic rhinitis than with those with allergic rhinitis. Autonomic imbalance favoring the parasympathetic system increases nasal blood flow, edema, and secretions, creating an overall presentation of rhinitis and nasal obstruction. Changes in body posture from erect to supine can increase nasal airway resistance. In the supine position pressure is lower in the right nostril than in the left nostril when the patient lies on the right side. Temperature also can affect nasal blood flow and compliance, both of which decrease in cold environments (Ramakrishnan & Meyers, 2006).

Clinical Manifestations

Patients with allergic rhinitis typically present with rhinorrhea, sneezing, pruritus, and conjunctivitis. Physical examination may demonstrate the "allergic shiner" (dark circles under the eyes that resemble bruises from a black eye) (Ramakrishnan & Meyers, 2006). Clinical manifestations of nonallergic rhinitis mimic those of allergic rhinitis (Chart 34–1). The usual symptoms of acute viral rhinitis include an initial profuse, clear, watery rhinorrhea (which often turns cloudy later in the course of the illness), nasal obstruction, postnasal discharge, and fever. Obstruction of the sinuses and/or eustachian tube causes referred facial pain or ear fullness. Many symptoms emanate from

the edema of the mucosal membranes. Rhinitis usually causes self-limiting, but annoying, symptoms that resolve in 7 to 10 days. The patient also may express feelings of fatigue, malaise, and headache (Quillen & Feller, 2006).

Laboratory and Diagnostic Procedures

The most common diagnostic tests for allergic rhinitis are the percutaneous skin test and the allergen-specific immunoglobulin E (IgE) antibody test. Less common diagnostic tools include nasal provocation testing, nasal cytology (e.g., blown secretions, scraping, lavage, and biopsy), nasolaryngoscopy, and intradermal skin testing. Skin testing involves introducing controlled amounts of allergen and control substances into the skin. Percutaneous testing is the most common type of skin testing and is preferred in primary care. It is conventional, safe, and widely accepted. Occasionally, intradermal testing is used because it is more sensitive, but less specific than percutaneous testing.

Allergic rhinitis can have an immediate or delayed response. Skin testing elicits both types of responses; however, the primary goal of skin testing is to detect the immediate allergic response caused by the release of mast cells or basophil IgE-specific mediators, which create the classic wheal and flare reaction after 15 minutes. The delayed response occurs 4 to 8 hours after exposure to the sensitizing allergen and is less useful in clinical diagnosis.

Other tests that may be used include, rhinoscopy, and imaging studies may include radiography, CT scanning, and magnetic resonance imaging (MRI). These latter studies are helpful in establishing possible structural abnormalities or for helping detect complications of comorbid conditions, such as sinusitis or adenoid hypertrophy. Imaging is particularly helpful in establishing obstruction of the ostiomeatal complex, and in delineating polyps, turbinate swelling, and septal and bony abnormalities, such as concha bullosa.

Medical Management

A wide variety of etiologies are involved in nonallergic rhinitis. Therefore, treatment options should not be implemented randomly. Instead, they should be aimed primarily at resolving the underlying causative physiology. The health care provider also must differentiate between acute and chronic rhinitis as well as allergic versus nonallergic rhinitis before a treatment method is chosen. Rhinitis is not a disease; it is simply a term used to describe the symptoms produced by nasal irritation or inflammation: a runny, itchy, or stuffy nose. If the rhinitis lasts less than 6 weeks, it is called acute rhinitis, which usually is caused by infections or chemical irritation and probably is classified as nonallergic rhinitis. If symptoms linger for longer than 6 weeks, the symptoms would be called chronic rhinitis. Chronic rhinitis may be caused by allergy or a variety of other factors.

It often is confusing to differentiate among the types of rhinitis, thus, a thorough and comprehensive history usually suggests the correct diagnosis. Health care providers should focus on symptoms (i.e., duration, exposures, magnitude of reaction, patterns, and chronicity) and triggers. The symptoms can be similar to allergic rhinitis, but with a less prominent nasal itch and conjunctiva irritation. Symptoms also tend to be consonant with seasonal variation, environmental influences, allergies, medical history (i.e., trauma, family and treatment histories) and current treatments. An acute onset of 1 week or less has a

| CHART 34–1 | Symptoms of Allergic Rhinitis |

Coughing

Headache

Itching (nose, mouth, eyes, palate, throat)

Runny nose

Impaired sense of smell

Sneezing

Stuffy nose (nasal congestion)

Sore throat

Tearing eyes

Wheezing

limited differential and usually suggests a viral etiology; an acute exacerbation of allergic rhinitis; or, less commonly, a foreign body, particularly when symptoms are unilateral with purulent discharge.

The goal of treatment is to reduce the allergy symptoms caused by the inflammation of affected tissues. The best "treatment" is to avoid what causes the allergic symptoms. It may be impossible to completely avoid all allergens that produce the sensitivity, but one can often take over-the-counter (nonprescription) medications, which relieve mild to moderate symptoms but tend to cause drowsiness. Longer acting antihistamines that require prescriptions and nasal corticosteroid sprays and decongestants are useful in relieving symptoms. Each individual must find the correct combination of medications to treat his specific symptoms. The use of antihistamines that have a rapid onset and a long duration of action with the least amount of side effects, especially drowsiness, is effective in maintaining a quality of life in people with seasonal allergic rhinitis (Hampel et al., 2003; Howarth, Stern, Roi, Reynolds, & Bousquet, 1999).

 CRITICAL ALERT *Sedating antihistamines may impair driving performance as seriously as alcohol. The first-generation antihistamine diphenhydramine may have an even greater impact than does alcohol on the complex task of operating an automobile (Weiler et al., 2000).*

In some cases people may outgrow an allergy as the immune system becomes less sensitive to the allergen. As a general rule, however, once a substance causes allergies for an individual, it can continue to affect the person over the long term. More severe cases of allergic rhinitis require immunotherapy (allergy shots) or removal of tissue in the nose (e.g., nasal polyps) or sinuses.

With allergy injections patients generally receive small amounts of diluted allergy products once or twice a week. Gradually the dose is increased to a maintenance concentration, which takes about 5 to 6 months. When at dose maintenance, the timing can be increased to every 2 weeks, then 3 weeks, and then to a maximum of 4 weeks. If an injection is missed, it may be repeated at the same dosage or the patient may need to back up a few doses. Most people notice improvement after they reach a maintenance dose. Patients may receive allergy injections for 3 to 5 years, predicated on symptoms.

To prevent complications, the health care provider should review a standard series of allergy questions with the patient prior to each injection. These questions include previous injection reactions, any new medications, any changes in health status, any increase in allergy/asthma (seasonal response), and determining if the patient has taken an antihistamine that day. Following the injection, the patient is monitored for reactions (Chart 34–2). After the injection is given, the patient is required to wait for 30 minutes. The risk for reaction is reduced by selecting low-risk patients and by educating patients about warning signs. Medical personnel are aware of symptoms and treatment and should educate patients about them (Hallet, 2006). Fatalities occur in less than 1 per million injections, but they do occur.

Treatment, dependent on etiology, generally consists of anticholinergics, nasal corticosteroids, antihistamines, sympathomimetics, capsaicin, and bacterially derived immunostimulants. Elderly patients typically are treated with antihistamines (e.g., fexofenadine, cetirizine, and loratadine) to avoid unwanted adverse effects such as loss of bladder control. One alternative therapy that may be helpful to patients with upper respiratory mucus and swelling is inhalation of peppermint oil, as discussed in the Complementary and Alternative Therapies box.

Patients also should be advised to take measures to stay away from any allergens that they know may trigger a reaction. These measures include:

- Reducing outdoor exposure during the season in which a particular type of pollen is present
- Limiting outdoor exposure by keeping the windows and doors of the house and car closed as much as possible during the pollen season

CHART 34–2 **Allergy Reactions and Treatments**

Reaction	Symptoms	Treatment	Medications
Local reaction	Erythema arm swelling of 2–3 cm, itchy eyes, slight body itching, transient local itching	Ice elevation. Observe closely until reaction resolves. Fill out anaphylaxis treatment record in patient chart.	Antihistamines, steroids Claritin, Zyrtec, Benadryl
Systemic reaction, anaphylaxis	Conjunctivitis, urticaria, chest tightness, problems breathing, syncope, wheezing, difficulty swallowing, shortness of breath, dyspneic hives, decrease in blood pressure	Maintain airway O₂ at 5 L/min. Place venous tourniquet above injection site. Check vital signs, peak flow, pulse ox every 5–10 min. Start two (14–16) IVs bolus 250–500 mL normal saline (NS). Repeat prn for BP stability. Continue to check vital signs every 5 min until reaction is resolved. Call 911 and transport to ED. Fill out anaphylaxis treatment record in patient chart.	1:1000 epinephrine up to 0.3–0.5 mL IM Chlorpheniramine 4 mg po or diphenhydramine 25–50 mg po or IM Albuterol 2.5 mg nebulizer or 8 puffs metered-dose inhaler if wheezing Prednisone 60 mg po or Solu-Medrol 125 mg IV Zantac 50 mg IV/Pepcid 20 mg IV Glucagon 1 mg (especially if on beta-blockers)

- Covering mattress and pillow with impermeable covers to reduce exposure to dust mites, washing linens every 2 weeks, and treating carpets and rugs as appropriate
- Reducing excessive humidity and removing standing water
- Practicing environmental controls for dust mites to help reduce mold spores
- Eliminating exposure to smoke, strong perfumes and scents, fumes, rapid changes in temperature, and outdoor pollution for patients with nonspecific triggers.

For animal allergies, complete avoidance is the best option. Confining the animal to a noncarpeted room and keeping it entirely out of the bedroom can be of some benefit. For occupational allergens, as with animal allergens, avoidance is the best measure. When this is not possible, using a mask or respirator might be helpful.

Patients with intermittent symptoms often are treated adequately with oral antihistamines, decongestants, or both as needed. Regular use of an intranasal steroid spray may be more appropriate for patients with chronic symptoms. Daily use of an antihistamine, decongestant, or both can be considered either instead of or in addition to nasal steroids. The newer second-generation (i.e., nonsedating) antihistamine drops usually are preferable to avoid sedation and other adverse effects as-

sociated with the older first-generation antihistamines. The second-generation oral antihistamines currently available in the United States are cetirizine, desloratadine, fexofenadine, and loratadine (Sheikh, 2007).

Nursing Management

Nursing management of patients with rhinitis is very similar to medical management. It is essential that during the assessment phase, the nurse secure a thorough history from the patient by asking questions such as these: What are the symptoms? When did they start? How long have they been occurring? Do you know what triggered the symptoms? Have they occurred before; if so, when and for how long? Is there a pattern that can be recognized?

If allergy medications are to be administered, this is typically the nurse's responsibility. The nurse should advise the patient of what the medication involves, and stay with the patient after the administration of the medication to determine any adverse effects.

Another major component of the nurse's role is education, helping the patient identify the known allergen and how to avoid subsequent allergic reactions. In many situations this is difficult because patients are being asked to change their lifestyles or elements within their life that are very important to them (e.g., pets). In these instances the nurse acts as a support

COMPLEMENTARY & ALTERNATIVE THERAPIES   **Peppermint Oil Inhalation**

Description:

The congestion caused by upper respiratory mucus and swelling is uncomfortable, and many seek relief from this discomfort. One CAM technique is the use of peppermint oil inhalation. This is an old Chinese healing technique in which a bowl is filled with steaming hot water. A few drops of peppermint oil are placed into the water. The patient immediately places a large towel over his or her head and leans over the vessel. The towel should cover both the head and the bowl, allowing the steam to rise directly into the nostrils. The patient then takes deep breaths through the nose, with the eyes and mouth closed. The menthol steam opens nasal passageways and loosens mucus. This is a safe technique, but the person should be careful to not make the water so hot that the steam burns. Although this technique is poorly documented in Western scientific literature, anecdotal evidence shows that it is an effective technique.

Research Support:

The peppermint (*Mentha piperita L.*) plant is one of the most widely used ingredients in herbal teas. Both peppermint tea, which is brewed from the plant leaves, and the essential oil of peppermint are used in traditional medicines. The acidic compounds (phenols) of the leaves include rosmarinic acid and several flavonoids, primarily eriocitrin, luteolin, and hesperidin. In the essential oil, the main volatile components are menthol and menthone. In vitro studies of peppermint show significant antimicrobial and antiviral properties, strong antioxidant and antitumor properties, and some antiallergenic properties. Animal model studies demonstrate that peppermint exerts a relaxation effect on gastrointestinal (GI) tissue, analgesic and anesthetic effects on the central and peripheral nervous system, immunomodulating properties, and chemopreventive properties. Human studies are limited; however, several clinical trials have been conducted that examine the effects of peppermint oil on irritable bowel syndrome (IBS) symptoms. No human studies have been conducted on peppermint tea. No

adverse reactions to peppermint tea have been reported. However, patients with GI reflux, hiatal hernia, or kidney stones should use peppermint oil with caution (McKay & Blumberg, 2006).

A literature review was performed to determine which herbs are most commonly used as CAM treatments for asthma, allergies, and immunologic conditions. Searches were conducted on the PubMed and OVID databases using the keywords that combined asthma, allergy, and CAM, plus the following herb names: echinacea (*Echinacea angustifolia, Echinacea pallida, and Echinacea purpurea*); garlic (*Allium*); angelica; chamomile; ephedra; gingko; grape seed extract; licorice root (*Glycyrrhiza*); St. John's wort (*Hypericum*); kava kava (*Piper*); peppermint oil and leaf (*Mentha*); stinging nettle (*Urtica*); and ginseng (*Panax*). The results showed that echinacea is one of the most common herbs used to treat symptoms of the "common cold" and upper respiratory tract allergies. Garlic is primarily used for cardiovascular health and relief of cough, colds, and rhinitis. Other herbs, including angelica, German chamomile flower, ephedra, gingko, grape seed extract, licorice root, St. John's wort, kava kava rhizome, peppermint, stinging nettle, and ginseng were also mentioned. The goal of this review was to alert practitioners of possible adverse effects, as the allergy and immunology fields have seen the second largest increase in CAM use (second only to practitioners who treat lower back pain). The most common adverse effect is in the form of a hypersensitivity reaction (Bielory, 2004).

References

Bielory, L. (2004). Complementary and alternative interventions in asthma, allergy, and immunology. *Annals of Allergy, Asthma, & Immunology, 93* (2 Suppl 1), S45–S54.

McKay, D. L., & Blumberg, J. B. (2006). A review of the bioactivity and potential health benefits of peppermint tea (Mentha piperita L.). *Phytotherapy Research, 20*(8), 619–633.

person to the patient. A person can prevent the symptoms of allergic rhinitis by avoiding known allergens. During the target season, people should remain indoors in an air-conditioned atmosphere whenever possible. It also is incumbent on the nurse to advise the patient of warning signs of an allergic reaction, and when and how to seek medical advice.

Sinusitis

Sinusitis is the inflammation of one or more of the paranasal and frontal sinuses, and occurs with obstruction of the normal drainage mechanism. It is traditionally subdivided into acute (symptoms lasting less than 3 weeks), subacute (symptoms lasting 3 weeks to 3 months), and chronic (symptoms lasting more than 3 months) (Kennedy, 2007).

Epidemiology and Etiology

More than 30 million patients in the United States are estimated to have sinus disease (Kennedy, 2007). A viral infection associated with the common cold is the most frequent etiology of acute sinusitis. Only a small percentage of viral sinusitis cases is complicated by bacterial sinusitis. The challenge is to differentiate a simple upper respiratory infection and allergic rhinitis from sinusitis.

Sinusitis can be caused by bacterial, viral, and fungal infections. Although the majority of community-acquired respiratory tract infections are viral in origin, bacteriologic causes are common (Chart 34–3). They include *Streptococcus pneumoniae, Haemophilus influenzae,* and *Moraxella catarrhalis* (File, 2005). Sinusitis may occur during an upper respiratory tract infection when infection in the nose spreads to the sinuses. It is sometimes encouraged by excessively strong blowing of the nose, thereby, disseminating bacteria. It also can occur as a complication of tooth infection, allergy, or certain infectious diseases such as pneumonia and measles. Basically, anything that causes swelling in the sinuses or keeps the cilia from moving mucus can cause sinusitis. Contributing factors, not causative, are air pollution, diving and underwater swimming, sudden extremes of temperature, and structural defects of the nose that interfere with normal breathing, such as a deviated septum (O'Toole, 2003).

Pathophysiology

The paranasal sinuses, a part of the upper respiratory tract, are in direct communication with the nasopharynx. Because of the proximity to nasopharyngeal flora, obstruction can cause bacterial infection. When sinusitis is caused by a bacterial or viral infection, a person develops a sinus infection.

CHART 34–3	**Common Causes of Sinus Disease**

Rhinoviruses

Influenza

Parainfluenza

Respiratory syncytial virus

Adenoviruses

Diseases that obstruct drainage can result in a reduced ability of the paranasal sinuses to function normally. For example, sinus and nasal tumors can block critical drainage pathways. When tumors, polyps, trauma, or benign growths occur near the sinus openings (ostia), the sinuses can become obstructed. When the ostia are obstructed, the normal flow of air into the sinuses and mucous drainage out of the sinuses is impeded. The mucociliary transport system becomes impaired, leading to more stagnation of secretion and epithelial damage, followed by decreased oxygen tension and subsequent bacterial growth. The reduced flow of air and mucus allows mucus to become stagnant, which, in turn, contributes to the growth of bacteria and infection. Once a bacterial infection is present, it causes inflammation and swelling, which leads to an increase in mucous production. The cycle continues and ultimately leads to sinusitis. Figure 34–4 ■ shows a picture of the sinuses that house sinusitis.

Clinical Manifestations

Symptoms of sinusitis can include fever, weakness, fatigue, cough, and congestion. Nasal congestion and discharge come first. The discharge typically is pus that is yellowish to yellow-green. There also may be mucous drainage in the back of the throat, called postnasal drip. A respiratory infection such as the common cold that starts to get better and then gets worse may be a sign of acute sinusitis. Pain or pressure in some areas of the face (forehead, cheeks, maxilla, or between the eyes) often is a sign of acute sinusitis. Pain in one's forehead that starts or becomes worse when the individual leans forward also can be a sign. Other symptoms may include a stuffy nose, fever, and an ache in the upper teeth, as well as increased fatigue.

Recurrent acute, chronic, and subacute sinusitis tend to take the following course. Symptoms are more vague and generalized than with acute sinusitis, and they last longer than 4 weeks. Subacute sinusitis lasts longer than 4 weeks but less than 8 weeks. Chronic sinusitis lasts 8 weeks or longer. Symptoms occur throughout the year, even during nonallergy seasons. Site-

Frontal sinus
Ethmoid sinus
Maxillary sinus
Sinusitis

FIGURE 34–4 ■ Sites of sinusitis.

specific symptoms also may occur depending on the location of the infection:

- Frontal sinusitis causes pain across the lower forehead.
- Pain from maxillary sinusitis occurs over the cheeks and may travel to the teeth, and the hard palate in the mouth sometimes becomes swollen.
- Ethmoid sinusitis causes pain behind the eyes and sometimes redness and tenderness in the area across the top of the nose.
- Sphenoid sinusitis rarely occurs by itself; when it does, the pain may be experienced behind the eyes, across the forehead, or in the face (University of Maryland Medical Center, 2006).

Laboratory and Diagnostic Procedures

Diagnosis of chronic sinusitis may be extremely difficult because patients commonly have vague symptoms. Unless sinusitis is suspected as a possible cause of symptoms, it may go undiagnosed. CT scans are commonly performed for the diagnosis of chronic sinusitis. In some cases, plain sinus films are adequate to make the diagnosis of acute sinusitis in the maxillary and sphenoid sinuses. A limited coronal CT scan allows visualization of all of the sinuses and potentially the ostiomeatal unit. It is also possible to visualize thickening of the lining of the sinuses, indicative of inflammation, on the CT scan (Kennedy, 2007).

Laboratory tests are sometimes useful. For example, a nasal smear may show polymorphonuclear leukocytes, which are suggestive of infection, versus eosinophils, which are suggestive of allergic rhinitis. Patients with chronic sinusitis that cannot be adequately controlled warrant immunologic testing for an immunodeficiency. Such testing should include immunoglobulin levels, IgG subtypes, antibody response to common bacterial antigens, and allergy testing by an allergist/immunologist.

Medical Management

Unlike a viral cold or an allergy, acute bacterial sinusitis requires antibiotic treatment to cure the infection. If sinus symptoms do not improve after 5 to 7 days, it becomes more likely that the infection is caused by bacteria and will respond to an antibiotic. The hallmark of any bacterial infection is fever and production of pus. However, about half of all bacterial sinus infections will resolve without antibiotics.

Chronic sinusitis symptoms can be difficult to treat, in part because treatment may require the coordinated efforts of several specialists to address all of the aspects of the disease. However, in general, treating chronic sinusitis is similar to treating acute sinusitis. If antibiotic treatment fails, allergy testing, desensitization, and or surgery may be recommended. Depending on the severity and duration of the sinusitis infection, there are five main treatments a health care provider may consider: oral antibiotics, nebulized antibiotics, topical rinses, intravenous antibiotics, and sinus surgery (Strong & Senders, 2003).

Functional Endoscopic Sinus Surgery

Currently, functional endoscopic sinus surgery (FESS) is the most common corrective surgery for chronic sinus inflammation (Strong, 2006). Performed under the magnification of a small telescopic endoscope, FESS is precise enough to remove diseased tissue and bone, open the sinuses, and help to restore the nose and sinus to health. FESS is much less invasive than older conventional surgical methods. The extent of sinus disease varies from person to person, and surgery may be a relatively minimal procedure or an extensive and prolonged operation. Endoscopic sinus surgery can correct chronic or severe blockages in one or more of the maxillary, ethmoid, frontal, or sphenoid sinuses.

With FESS the patient experiences very little postoperative discomfort and has an excellent chance of improvement in symptoms. Ongoing medical therapy controls the underlying causes of inflammation. After surgery severe chronic inflammation may take months or even years to disappear completely. Serious complications, such as blindness, are very rare, but because of the proximity of sinus structures to the eyes and the brain, risks are present. During the preoperative informed surgical consent meeting, the potential complication of blindness should be discussed.

Image-Guided Surgery

Image-guided surgery is surgery guided by CT registered guidance (Strong, 2006). Traditional sinus surgery is a complex procedure. The proximity of the sinuses to the brain, the eye, and major arteries can make the surgery risky. In addition the surgery can be disfiguring and painful because it involves making incisions in the mouth and face. Image-guided surgery, also known as stealth surgery, allows the surgeon to minimize the chances of sinus surgery complications, operate more thoroughly, and perform more difficult procedures.

A CT scan of the patient's head creates a "road map" of the patient's skull; the surgeon can then correlate the registered CT image with the position of the probe (Figure 34–5 ■). During the procedure, the surgeon places a handheld probe in the patient's nose while correlating the 3D position with the scan on a computer screen. This 3D image guidance system shows the location of the probe tip so the surgeon can safely navigate through trouble spots. Stealth technology is particularly useful if a patient's

FIGURE 34–5 ■ CT registered with probe for sinus surgery.

sinus anatomy is unusual, or for "revision" surgeries, when a patient has already had one or more sinus procedures.

Nursing Management

Nursing care of the patient relies heavily on assessment of signs and symptoms, which, in turn, is dependent on obtaining a thorough patient history. The history must include the onset and duration of the symptoms including site of pain or discomfort, redness of eyes, flushing of face across the nose, fever, weakness or fatigue, cough, congestion, sore throat, muscle ache, and sore teeth. It also is important to know if any particular event or incident triggered the patient's symptoms.

If the patient is experiencing acute sinusitis requiring surgical intervention, postoperative care becomes important. This care includes educating the patient about the signs and symptoms of potential complications contingent on the type of surgery that was performed. Patient education also includes information about the cause of the sinusitis and how to avoid the triggers: air pollution, diving, underwater swimming, and known allergens and irritants.

Nasal Obstruction

Nasal obstruction may be broadly described as any occurrence that blocks the flow of air in the nose. This feeling of blockage can result from many nasal disorders previously discussed in this chapter. These include those that cause a deformity of the cartilaginous or bony structures that make up the framework of the nose (e.g., fractures, a deviated nasal septum) and those that cause swelling and infections of the nasal lining and the turbinate bones (rhinitis and sinusitis). Two other common causes of nasal obstruction are nasal polyps and foreign bodies.

Nasal Polyps

Nasal polyps are small, saclike growths consisting of inflamed nasal mucosa and sinus linings. The nasal examination reveals a grayish, grapelike mass within the nasal cavity. Nasal polyps are smooth, pear-shaped growths of nasal mucosa that are gelatin-like, semitranslucent, and pale.

Epidemiology, Etiology, and Pathophysiology

Polyps are benign, can occur on one or both sides of the nose, and are more commonly seen in adults than in children. The polyps may originate near the ethmoid sinuses (located at the top of the nose) and grow into the sinus cavities. Large polyps can obstruct this part of the upper airway. The most common cause of polyps is allergy, followed by chronic sinus infection (Rosin, 1998). Aside from causing nasal blockage, polyps may plug up the normal sinus opening (ostia) and contribute to the development of sinus infection. Although nasal polyps in children are unusual, their occurrence before age 16 may indicate cystic fibrosis.

Nasal polyps are associated with a number of conditions, including asthma, hay fever, and sinus infections. In some patients, there is an association between asthma, nasal polyps, and aspirin intolerance known as Samter's triad (McClay, 2007; Rosin, 1998; Zitt, 2003). Almost one out of four patients with nasal polyps is intolerant to aspirin. In these individuals ingestion of aspirin is followed by wheezing, excessive watery nasal discharge, and swelling of the throat, which can be fatal if not treated immediately.

Medical Management

The initial treatment of polyps usually is medical. Polyps shrink after a course of cortisone (or other steroids). If there is significant shrinkage following cortisone, then an extended course of a cortisone-containing nasal spray may keep the nasal passages clear and prevent reformation of polyps. Cortisone-containing sprays have rare, minor side effects, so they can be used safely in most people for many months under a doctor's supervision. They do not cause rebound congestion as is seen with nonprescription decongestant sprays.

Despite appropriate medication, many polyp patients require surgery to remove polyps and open the nasal passages. Surgical polyp removal, or polypectomy, can be performed in an office or outpatient setting. Although, most polyps are not cancerous, once removed, they should be sent for pathologic examination to ensure that there is no malignancy present. Very infrequently these tissues may demonstrate abnormal growth patterns called inverting papillomas (adults) or juvenile angio neurofibromas (male teenagers) (Donald, Enepikedes, & Boggan, 2004).

Although most patients notice marked improvement in their breathing after removal of polyps, they should be aware that polyps often recur. If they start to grow back in a matter of months, then a more thorough search for the cause should be undertaken. This usually includes an allergy work-up and CT scan x-ray if they have not already been done. One way to prevent polyp regrowth after removal is to stay on topical steroid sprays for an extended period of time.

Nursing Management

Nurses assist in the examination of patients for polyps by assessing and documenting symptoms, including history, length of "stuffy nose" syndrome, and other related allergy symptoms. If surgical intervention is required, nurses are responsible for pre- and postoperative care of the patient. A major focus of nursing intervention and evaluation is education for the patient as to symptoms to look for, reasons to seek medical care, and relief of pain and difficulty breathing. It also is important to complete a health history to determine allergic patterns and any signs of genetic implications.

Foreign Bodies

The term *foreign bodies* refers to any foreign objects inserted into the nose. Common objects found in children include beads, buttons, crayons, small plastic toys, peanuts, raisins, popcorn, and pencil erasers. These objects, if allowed to remain in the nose, may lead to irritation, infection, and difficulty breathing. The symptoms are foul-smelling or bloody nasal discharge, difficulty breathing through the affected nostril, irritation, or a sensation of something in the nostril. It is important not to probe the nose with cotton swabs or other instruments. Doing so may push the object farther into the nose. The nurse should have the patient breathe through the mouth and avoid breathing in forcefully, which may force the object further inward.

Once it is determined which nostril is affected, the nurse should have the patient gently press the other nostril closed and have the patient gently blow through the affected nostril. Avoid blowing the nose too hard or repeatedly. Local or general anesthesia may be used for examination and object removal if conservative measures fail.

Anosmia

Anosmia is the loss or impairment of the sense of smell. To many people, the ability to sense thousands of different odors is a normal occurrence and something that may be taken for granted. However, to a minority, this natural skill is lost due to a disorder of the olfactory system. Odors bring both enhancement and improvement of life to an individual, whether it is the smell of food, fragrances, or a scent associated with a particular event or person. More than this, smell has other functions. Taste is to a great extent determined by smell, so a loss of smell often leads to a loss of taste.

Epidemiology, Etiology, and Pathophysiology

It has been estimated that 2 million Americans have smell and taste disorders and about 200,000 visit a doctor each year (Jafek, Murrow, & Linschoten, 2000). The loss of smell usually is the result of nasal congestion, a cold, or an obstruction, but sometimes it can indicate a neurological disorder. Loss of the sense of smell may be idiopathic (without any identifiable cause). Some diminution of smell occurs normally with aging, and in most cases, there are no obvious or immediate causes and there is no treatment (Medline Plus, 2006).

Temporary anosmia is common with colds and nasal allergies such as hay fever. It may occur following a viral illness. The sense of smell also is lost with disorders that prevent air from reaching the part of the nose where smell receptors are located (the cribriform plate located high in the nose). These disorders may include nasal polyps, nasal septal deformities, and nasal tumors. Other disorders that may cause anosmia include tumors of the head or brain, head trauma, endocrine and nutritional disorders, and neurological disorders.

Many medications may change or decrease the ability to detect odors. Most people who lose the sense of smell are unable to differentiate between salty, sweet, sour, and bitter tastes that are sensed on the ventral tongue. Individuals with such a disorder may not be able to distinguish other flavors. Some spices such as pepper may stimulate cranial nerves, but may be sensed rather than smelled. The olfactory nerve (CN I) is responsible for the sense of smell. This sensory organ is located in the roof of the nasal cavity.

Clinical Manifestations

There are many definitions of the various categories of smell dysfunction. The following definitions come from Seiden (1997):

- **Anosmia**—a complete loss of smell
- **Hyposmia**—a partial loss of smell
- **Hyperosmia**—enhanced smell sensitivity
- **Dysosmia**—distortion in odor perception (includes parosmia (distorted sense of smell) and phantosmia
- **Parosmia**—distortion of perception of external stimulus
- **Phantosmia**—smell perception with no external stimulus.

In all of the categories enumerated above, the patient experiences a change in the sense of smell. Changes in the sense of smell range from a lack of smell to smelling a perceived foul odor that no one else can smell; hence, the use of the word *phantom* as in *phantosmia*. It is necessary to determine, upon assessment, what the patient is experiencing.

Medical and Nursing Management

Several methods of diagnosis are used by primary care providers with respect to olfaction disorders. A thorough patient history and physical evaluation are essential for establishing the cause of the disorder (Jafek et al., 2000). In particular, when investigating the patient's history, identifying the time that the loss occurred and whether any other conditions may have contributed are fundamental for a diagnosis. It is important to distinguish between a smell-related disorder and a taste-related disorder because commonly they are misidentified or misunderstood.

It is important to identify events that occurred prior to the onset of the disorder. Some of the questions asked to do so are the length of time of olfactory loss and whether it is an intermittent or continuous olfactory loss. Fluctuation usually is a sign of conductive loss and hence may indicate a nasal or sinus disorder (Seiden, 1997).

A complete head and neck examination is essential to determine the cause of anosmia. The examination should focus on the nose to determine whether it is a conductive or sensorineural loss. An endoscope is used to provide reliable observations. Chemosensory testing and a neuroradiologic evaluation also are used to detect the type of dysfunction a patient is experiencing.

Treatment of underlying disorders may correct the loss of sense of smell. This includes antihistamines (if the condition is related to allergy), surgical correction of physical blockages, treatment of other disorders, and changes in medication. If loss of the sense of smell is permanent, dietary counseling may include use of highly seasoned foods and stimulation of taste sensations that remain. Caution should be taken to ensure safety around the home. Smoke detectors and electric appliances rather than gas appliances should be used as should technologies that detect the presence of gas fumes in the home. The health care provider is responsible for educating patients about these cautions.

Nurses are responsible for assessing the patent's symptoms, documenting and reporting them to the primary health care provider, and providing supportive care to the patient. Education as to the cause and alleviation of symptoms is primary for the nurse. The nurse also plays a key role in assessing and evaluating the patient's response to treatment and communicating this to the primary care provider.

Mucormycosis

Mucormycosis is a rare but often fatal disease caused by certain fungi. It is sometimes called zygomycosis or phycomycosis (Beers & Berkow, 2004). Mucormycosis is an opportunistic infection that typically develops in patients with weakened immune systems, diabetes, kidney failure, organ transplants, or chemotherapy for cancer. It also may develop in patients receiving an iron chelating drug called desferrioxamine (Desferal) as treatment for acute iron poisoning.

Epidemiology and Etiology

In the United States mucormycosis mostly occurs in patients who are immunocompromised, though cases in immunocompetent patients also are reported (Baugh & Earhart, 2006). It also is most likely that patients in the United States will develop mucormycosis in the nasal areas or in the lungs; however, it also may develop on the skin or in the digestive tract. Gastrointestinal disease usually develops only in severely malnourished patients. Cutaneous mucormycosis is most likely to develop under occlusive surgical dressings. Although occlusive dressings are intended to keep the air out of incisions and wounds, they also trap body heat and moisture.

Common fungi, frequently found in the soil among vegetation, cause mucormycosis. These fungi are prevalent in nature, but may be more prone to cause infection in moist, temperate climates (Baugh & Earhart, 2006). Most individuals are exposed to these fungi on a daily basis, but people with immune disorders or diabetes are at a higher risk for developing this rare infection. Aside from these, environmental spore exposure (from exposure to construction activities) also has led to clinical cases of mucormycosis. Other cases have been reported in patients with traumatic skin injury (as with the use of non-sterile adhesive tape or with the use of tongue depressors as splints in neonates). Exposure to voriconazole, which is not active against mucormycosis, is noted to be a risk factor in patients with cancer (Varman & Whaley, 2006). The incidence of the disease is difficult to evaluate because it is very rare; however, there is some indication that it is increasing (Beers & Berkow, 2004) (see the Risk Factors for Mucormycosis box).

Pathophysiology and Clinical Manifestations

Mucormycosis is caused by fungi of several different species, including *Mucor, Rhizopus, Absidia*, and *Rhizomucor*. The fungus gains entry into the body through the nasopharynx. It can be inhaled into the lungs, or it can extend to the sinuses, orbit, and brain, with mucormycosis development dependent on host immunity. Upon gaining access to the mucous membranes of the patient's nose or lungs, the organisms multiply rapidly and invade the nearby blood vessels. The fungi destroy soft tissue and bone, as well as the walls of blood vessels. Regardless of the anatomic site involved, characteristic histopathologic findings include angioinvasion with subsequent tissue infarction and necrosis leading to tissue destruction.

- With rhinocerebral mucormycosis, the fungus destroys the tissue of the nasal passages, sinuses, or hard palate, producing a black or pus-filled discharge and visible patches of dying tissue. The overt symptoms of rhinocerebral mucormycosis include acute sinusitis, fever, eye swelling and protrusion of the orbit (proptosis), dark nasal eschar (scabbing), and redness progressing to ecchymoses of the overlying skin. General symptoms also may include headache, nausea, and lethargy. Visual loss secondary to thrombosis of retinal artery or direct fungal invasion may occur. The fungus then invades the tissues around the socket and eventually the brain. At that point the patient may have convulsions or paralysis on one side of the body.

- Most patients with pulmonary mucormycosis are being treated for leukemia and are immunocompromised. The fungus enters the patient's lungs, where it eventually invades a major blood vessel, causing the patient to cough up blood or hemorrhage into the lungs. Early symptoms of pulmonary

RISK FACTORS for Mucormycosis

Diabetes mellitus	A risk factor particularly with poor glycemic control and acidosis as it relates to cellular immune dysfunction.
Iron overload	May be a risk factor as observed with hemochromatosis and deferoxamine treatment in patients receiving dialysis. Iron enhances fungal growth and leads to increased host susceptibility.
Burn patients	In burn patients, *Mucor* generally involves the skin and only rarely causes the rhinocerebral form.
Leukemia	Researchers estimate that the incidence in hematologic malignancy is approximately 1%.
Lymphoma	May result from immunosuppressions.
Transplantation	Infection may occur after solid organ (liver, kidney) and bone marrow transplants and in association with graft versus host disease (GvHD), severe neutropenia, or steroid therapy.
Immunosuppression	Those who are immunosuppressed are more susceptible to the fungal infection.
Prolonged neutropenia	The lowering of white blood cell count compromises immunity.
Chemotherapy	Neutropenia and immunosuppressions may result from administration of chemotherapeutic drugs.
High-dose steroids	Steroids affect metabolism and promote immunosuppressions thus facilitating the spread of mycormycosis.
Following donor leukocyte infusions	Infection may occur after donor infusions die to transfer of mucor fungi.
Acquired immunodeficiency syndrome (AIDS)	Immunosupression contributes to susceptibility of the fungal infection.
Intravenous drug use (embolic to brain)	Mucor hyphae, obtained from contaminated equipment, may invade the blood vessels and cause necrosis.

Source: Baugh, W. P., & Earhart, K. C. (2006). Rhinocerebral mucormycosis. *eMedicine.* Retrieved September 2, 2007, from the eMedicine website: http://www.emedicine.com/med/topic2026.htm.

mucormycosis include fever and difficulty breathing, with eventual bleeding from the lungs.

- The symptoms of gastrointestinal mucormycosis are not unique to the disease, which may complicate diagnosis. Patients typically complain of pressure or pain in the abdomen and nausea and vomiting.

Mucormycosis is a feared complication associated with diabetes. Diabetic ketoacidosis helps to potentiate the growth of mucormycosis. Patients with type II diabetes can present in ketoacidosis (Eledrisi, Alshanti, Shah, Brolosy, & Jaha, 2006; Linfoot & Bergstrom, 2005). The site of involvement is typically the nasopharyngeal region, but the infection can spread to involve soft tissues and bones of the face, orbit, skull, and brain. Rhinocerebral infection may start as a sinus infection and progress rapidly over hours to complete obtundation and coma. The disease may progress to involve inflammation of cranial nerves and blood vessels, causing blood clots that block blood supply to the surrounding tissue and brain (thrombosis). There is an increased incidence of cavernous sinus thrombosis and carotid involvement with rhinocerebral mucormycosis.

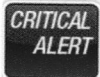 *Any patient who presents in diabetic ketoacidosis with findings of orbital cellulitis and vision changes must be evaluated immediately for mucormycosis. The progression of the disease occurs very quickly over a few hours. The time lapse between making an accurate diagnosis and instituting therapy is critical.*

Laboratory and Diagnostic Procedures

Diagnosis usually is based on a combination of the patient's medical history and a visual examination of the nose, throat, and eyes. Once mucormycosis is suspected, obtaining tissue for culture is vital. Specimens should be obtained from areas such as suggestive skin lesions, black eschars found in the nasopharynx, and nasal discharge that may appear like clotted blood. The tissue specimen reveals *Mucor* fungi and the species is oryzae. Serial CT scans and MRI scans are used to identify the extent of the disorder, the destruction of soft tissue of bone in patients with advanced disease. Chest x-rays sometimes reveal a cavity in the lung or an area filled with tissue fluid if the patient has pulmonary mucormycosis.

Medical Management

Treatment usually is begun without waiting for laboratory reports because of the rapid spread and high mortality rate of the disease (Beers & Berkow, 2004). The mainstay of treatment for mucormycosis is early aggressive surgical intervention to remove all dead and infected tissue along with intravenous and possibly intrathecal antifungal therapy of amphotericin and liposomal amphotericin. Surgery is disfiguring for rhinocerebral mucormycosis because it may involve the removal of the palate, nasal, and orbital structures. Reconstructive surgery is inevitable for those who have disfigurement due to severe rhinocerebral mucormycosis. Hyperbaric oxygenation (HBO) may be indicated and has proven to be very helpful in conjunction with long-term therapy with antifungal drugs. In addition, underlying comorbidities such as hyperglycemia, acidosis in diabetic patients, nutritional problems, neutropenia, lymphopenia, and immunosuppressions must be addressed.

■ Nursing Management

The nurse is responsible for assessing the patient for clinical manifestations of mucormycosis on the first interview with the patient. Obtaining an accurate and complete patient history is essential. Following diagnosis and treatment, the nurse assumes postoperative care of the patient. During this phase the nurse should be particularly sensitive to the fear and anxiety related to possible/potential disfigurement and high mortality rate of the disease. Follow-up care includes educating patients about the signs of recurrent mucormycosis, particularly facial swelling and a black discharge from the nose, and advising them to see a health care provider at once if they notice these symptoms.

Prevention also is critical to caring for patients with mucormycosis. It depends on protecting high-risk patients from contact with sugary foods, decaying plants, moldy bread, manure, and other breeding grounds for fungi. In addition, when caring for patients in the hospital, the nurse should be careful to change occlusive dressings frequently and check the underlying skin for any signs of possible fungal infection.

■ Disorders of the Pharynx and Oral Cavity

The oral cavity, tongue, and pharynx are the anatomic conduits to the esophagus and airway. The pharynx assists in speech and swallowing and begins the division of the airway from the esophagus. The oral cavity, which includes the tongue, is responsible for ingestion, taste, and other sensory responses to food, chewing, swallowing, speech, and respiration. The tongue is an articulator for speech, a propulsion device for swallowing, and a sensor for taste. These organs are susceptible to disease, which may affect an individual's ability to communicate and take in nutrition. Disorders specific to the pharynx and oral cavity are discussed in the following sections.

Sleep Apnea

Sleep apnea is a disorder in which a person stops breathing for more than 10 seconds, typically more than 20 to 30 times in an hour. The three main types of sleep apnea are central, obstructive, and a combination of central and obstructive.

Etiology, Epidemiology, Pathophysiology, and Clinical Manifestations

The cause of *central sleep apnea* is impairment in the respiratory center drive such that the brain fails to send the appropriate signal to the breathing muscles to initiate respirations. This is the less common form of sleep apnea. *Obstructive sleep apnea* (OSA) is caused by physical obstruction from tissues in the upper airway. Air cannot flow into or out of the person's mouth, despite continued efforts to breathe. Approximately 12 million Americans have obstructive sleep apnea. More than half the people who have sleep apnea are overweight or obese (National Heart, Lung, and Blood Institute [NHLBI], 2006). OSA is usually marked by recurrent sleep interruptions, loud snoring, choking and gasping spells on awakening, daytime drowsiness, loss of memory, and concentration caused by the lack of normal sleep. Alcohol consumption makes OSA worse. Patients usually wake up not feeling rested or refreshed. Individuals at risk for sleep apnea include those who:

- Are overweight.
- Have high blood pressure.
- Have a decreased airway size in the nose, throat, or mouth. This can be caused by the shape of these structures or by medical conditions causing congestion in these areas, such as hay fever or other allergies.
- Have a family history of sleep apnea (NHLBI, 2006).

Combination sleep apnea, also called *mixed*, starts as central sleep apnea, quickly followed by thoracoabdominal movements and upper airway obstruction. Mixed apnea occurs more often than central, but less often than OSA, and is treated the same way as OSA (Beers & Berkow, 2004).

Diagnostic Studies

For a formal diagnosis a patient should undergo a full ear, nose, and throat (ENT) examination and history, and a physical examination with fiber-optic endoscopy. An x-ray or CT scan of the head and neck is very helpful in identifying obstructive structures and checking the position of the tongue in relation to the jaw. The majority of patients with obstructive sleep apnea experience upper airway obstruction at the level of the soft palate (nasopharynx) or the level of the tongue and base of the tongue (oropharynx).

If a routine examination is inconclusive, the patient may require a formal sleep study or polysomnography. Although usually done in a controlled setting such as a sleep center, home sleep studies are being evaluated for their reliability. During a sleep study, several objective measurements are collected. These include oxygen saturation levels, electrocardiography (ECG) monitoring, air movement including chest wall and abdominal movements, electrical activity of the brain, eye movements, and airflow. These measures are evaluated for frequency of occurrence and physiological effect. These tests are used both to diagnose sleep apnea and to determine its severity.

Medical Management

Treatment for OSA varies depending on the degree of sleep apnea and the willingness and compliance of the patient. Behavioral changes such as weight loss are an important part of the treatment program. The individual should avoid the use of alcohol, tobacco, and sleeping pills. In some patients with mild sleep apnea, breathing pauses occur only when they sleep on their backs. In such cases, the use of pillows and other devices that help them sleep in a side-lying position is often helpful. In cases of mild sleep apnea, some patients may obtain relief from the use of a dental device that moves the tongue or mandible forward.

Severe symptoms of OSA need more aggressive treatment. **Continuous positive airway pressure (CPAP)** opens the airway and prevents airway collapse. It involves blowing air into the respiratory tract with just enough pressure to prevent the tissue collapse during sleep, reducing the number and severity of apneic episodes and significant oxygen desaturation. Although, CPAP is an effective treatment, many patients find it difficult to keep the device in place, especially if they are claustrophobic. The most common side effects of CPAP are dry mouth, rhinitis, and sinus congestion. Humidification and antihistamines effectively treat these side effects.

Patients also have several surgical options. Surgical intervention is available for those patients for whom CPAP has failed or those who are unable to comply with the rigors of home CPAP. An uvulovelopalatopharyngoplasty (UVPPP) is a surgical procedure in which a resection of the uvula and soft palate is done. This shortens and stiffens the palate. It is effective in about 40% of patients (Young et al., 2004). Another surgical approach involves the advancement of the tongue and maxillary/mandibular bone complex. This brings the pharynx forward and out of the airway path.

Tracheotomy

Tracheotomy, the surgical placement of an artificial airway, provides definitive correction because it bypasses the obstructive OSA. This still does not correct central apnea, but allows unrestricted airflow. All patients benefit from such a procedure, but it does cause significant changes in the lifestyle and quality of life of the OSA patient. Some patients require a tracheotomy to live, and extensive counseling is necessary before and after the procedure. A complete discussion of managing patients with a tracheostomy is provided later in the chapter.

■ Nursing Management

The nursing process guides the management of patients with sleep apnea. Nursing management of the patient with OSA after UVPPP focuses on airway patency. The outcome objective is to have normal airway function and relief of symptoms. Patients who undergo surgical intervention are placed on a pulse oximeter to monitor oxygen saturation level, and lung sounds are assessed for adventitious sounds. Patients who have had obstructive sleep apnea for an extended period of time develop higher pulmonary pressures due to the obstruction. Once the obstruction has been modified, the positive end-expiratory pulmonary (PEEP) pressures decrease. This can result in a condition called flash pulmonary edema, which is potentially life threatening. This change can happen very quickly; therefore, the patient is monitored closely for the first 24 hours after surgery. The integrity of the surgical site in the posterior pharynx and tonsillar pillars is monitored by direct observation with a tongue blade and flashlight. As with most oropharyngeal surgery, use of straws is prohibited so as not to disrupt clot formation with higher intraoral pressures.

Oral Cavity Disorders

Disorders of the oral cavity involve the teeth, tongue, and floor of the mouth, the maxilla, and tonsils. These affect chewing, taste, nutrition, and speech articulation. Nursing care should be directed toward maintaining the patient's oral health, nutrition, and control of pain.

Etiology and Clinical Manifestations of Hairy Tongue

Hairy tongue is a condition in which the tongue is covered with hairlike papilla due to the overgrowth of the fungus *Candida albicans* or *Aspergillus niger*. It usually is the result of antibiotic therapy that inhibits the growth of normal flora in the mouth. Antifungal agents, such as Diflucan, are used to treat the condition.

Etiology and Clinical Manifestations of Dental Caries

Dental caries are the result of the destruction of tooth enamel caused by dental plaque. Plaque, a substance formed by the interaction of saliva and food proteins, coats the teeth. Plaque breaks down tooth enamel. Deep crevasses in teeth, poor quality enamel, lack of fluoridated water, and poor dental hygiene also contribute to dental caries. Left untreated, dental caries can lead to a dental abscess and eventually loss of the affected tooth.

Etiology, Pathophysiology, Clinical Manifestations, and Medical Management of Ludwig's Angina

Ludwig's angina is a dental abscess that develops in the floor of the mouth. It is a deep neck infection involving the sublingual, submandibular, and submental spaces. Pus collects above the mylohyoid muscle in the sublingual space, pushing the tongue up and back. Posterior, superior displacement of the tongue results in obstruction of the oropharyngeal airway. This infection typically spreads rapidly through the anterior deep neck spaces. Immediate surgical intervention and tracheotomy often are necessary to maintain an airway. A neck incision is made, and surgical drains allow for external drainage of the abscess. Postoperatively, the wound is irrigated and packed with gauze to promote healing. Extraction of any abscessed teeth is important to control the infection.

Dental Abscess

A dental abscess (dentoalveolar abscess) is an acute lesion bacterial infection characterized by localization of pus in the structures that surround the teeth. Milder cases of a dental abscess result in painful swelling of the gums adjacent to the tooth in question. The tooth or, in some cases, multiple teeth have a large cavity or mandible fracture that infects the dental pulp (Schneider & Segal, 2006). Mandibular dental abscesses can progress to the floor of mouth, causing infection if not treated appropriately.

Pathophysiology

The term *dentoalveolar abscess* denotes three distinct processes as follows:

- A periapical abscess that originates in the dental pulp and usually is secondary to dental caries is the most common dental abscess in children. Dental caries erode the protective layers of the tooth (i.e., enamel, dentin) and allow bacteria to invade the pulp, producing a pulpitis. Pulpitis can progress to necrosis with bacterial invasion of the alveolar bone, causing an abscess.

- A periodontal abscess involves the supporting structures of the teeth (periodontal ligaments, alveolar bone). This is the most common dental abscess in adults but may occur in children with impaction of a foreign body in the gingiva.

- Pericoronitis describes the infection of the gum that overlies a partially erupted third molar.

Odontogenic infections are polymicrobial, with an average of four to six different causative bacteria. The dominant isolates are strictly anaerobic gram-negative rods and gram-positive cocci, in addition to facultative and microaerophilic streptococci. Anaerobic bacteria outnumber aerobes 2:1 to 3:1. In general, strictly anaerobic gram-negative rods are more pathogenic than facultative or strictly anaerobic gram-positive cocci (Schneider & Segal, 2006).

Epidemiology and Etiology

There are few epidemiological and etiological factors that are predictive of a dental abscess. No race predilection exists, nor is there a sex predilection. Dental abscesses are rare in infants because abscesses do not form until teeth erupt. In children, as noted, a periapical abscess is the most common type of dental abscess. This is because of the combination of poor hygiene, thinner enamel, and the primary dentition having a more abundant blood supply, which allows for an increased inflammatory response. In adults, periodontal abscess is more common than periapical abscess.

Laboratory and Diagnostic Procedures

An uncomplicated (i.e., simple) abscess does not require any laboratory or imaging studies, although x-rays may be taken. With a complicated abscess a CBC may reveal leukocytosis with neutrophil predominance. A blood culture may be taken to determine the bacteria before initiating parenteral antibiotics. A needle aspirate also may be done and is indicated for Gram stain and culture. There also are several levels of imaging, which may be completed for a complex abscess:

- Plain radiography represents the first level of investigation.

- Lateral and anterior-posterior neck views may be used to reveal a neck mass.

- A panoramic radiograph may be helpful to indicate whether bone or teeth are involved.

Clinical Manifestations

The main symptom of a tooth abscess is a severe, persistent, throbbing toothache. Initially, the tooth may be sensitive to heat and pressure with chewing or biting. Dependent on the age of the abscess, a patient also may have a fever, swelling in the face or cheek, and tender, swollen lymph nodes under the jaw or in the neck. If the abscess ruptures, the patient will experience a sudden rush of foul-smelling and foul-tasting fluid in the mouth.

Medical Management

A dental abscess is treated with antibiotics. If the abscess responds to treatment, no further intervention is needed. In larger abscesses surgical incision and drainage are done. General anesthesia may be necessary due to the size of the incision and the number of teeth involved or to be extracted. Intravenous (IV) antibiotic treatment continues postoperatively. Dental abscess infections have been known to spread upward to the face or distally into the neck and chest causing swelling, redness, drainage collection, and airway obstruction. These patients will require extensive surgery with wound debridement, a tracheotomy, aggressive frequent dressing changes, and antibiotic therapy. Management of an abscess also includes pain medicine to control the pain. Additional pain medication is given with antianxiety medicines during an incision and drainage of a larger abscess.

■ Nursing Management

Nursing assessment of the patient with a dental abscess is primarily focused on pain determination and observation of the wound, if present. Interventions include frequent oral dressing changes and oral packing after incision and drainage. The nurse must assess the patient for pain and administer medications as necessary or teach the patient when and how to take analgesics. Interventions include a strong educational component. It is necessary to teach the patient the importance of oral care especially after surgery. Prevention also is instrumental in patient education. The patient should be advised of how to recognize symptoms early and to seek treatment early before the abscess has a chance to become a major health problem.

Etiology, Pathophysiology, and Clinical Manifestations of Tonsillitis

The tonsils are masses of lymphoid tissue found in the root of the tongue (lingual tonsil), on both sides of the oropharynx (palatine tonsil, anterior and posterior), and on the superior wall of the nasopharynx (pharyngeal tonsil). **Tonsillitis** is an inflammation of the tonsils, most commonly caused by a virus, and occurs mainly in children. Symptoms are sore throat, red, swollen tonsils, dysphagia, odynophagia, fever, and enlarged, tender lymph nodes in the neck. Tonsillitis usually is self-limiting and treated symptomatically. However, if a throat culture reveals the cause as group A beta-hemolytic streptococci, then an antibiotic such as penicillin will be prescribed. Complications such as sinusitis, mastoiditis, rheumatic fever, or peritonsillar abscess may occur with tonsillitis. Surgery to remove the tonsils (tonsillectomy) may be necessary for individuals with repeated infections.

Etiology and Clinical Manifestations of Peritonsillar Abscess

Peritonsillar abscess, also known as Quinsy tonsillitis, is a rare complication of tonsillitis in which infection spreads to the tissue around the tonsillar capsule. Symptoms are severe throat pain, mouth breathing, drooling, and muffled voice. Physical examination reveals a large unilateral fullness of the affected tonsillar pillar and soft palate, and deviation of the uvula to the unaffected side. A peritonsillar abscess is treated with incision and drainage of the abscess and use of antibiotics. Four to 6 weeks after recovery a tonsillectomy may be necessary. This prevents recurrent infection and removes scar tissue from the tonsillar area. Nursing care should focus on antibiotic therapy, pain control, hydration, nutrition, and airway protection, during the acute episode.

Etiology of Pharyngitis

Pharyngitis is an inflammation of the pharynx, which results in a sore throat. Upper respiratory infections such as the common cold or flu may lead to pharyngitis. It occurs most frequently in the winter months and usually resolves on its own. For symptomatic comfort the patient should increase fluid intake, take analgesics, and gargle with warm saltwater. Pharyngitis from a *Streptococcus* infection requires antibiotics.

Etiology, Clinical Manifestations, and Medical Management of Epiglottitis

The epiglottis is a flap of tissue and cartilage that covers the opening of the trachea during swallowing. **Epiglottitis** is a life-threatening bacterial illness that may lead to airway obstruction. Epiglottitis is seen more frequently in children, but also occurs in adults. The cause of the infection usually is *Haemophilus influenzae* group B. The infection and inflammation affects the epiglottis and surrounding supraglottic structures. Symptoms are a cherry red epiglottis, drooling, inspiratory stridor, dyspnea, and high fever. **Stridor** is the raspy noise heard in the upper airway as the result of air attempting to move through a narrowed opening. Initial treatment focuses on maintaining a patent airway with conservative measures of oxygen, humidification, and inhaled respiratory therapy. Corticosteroids are given to reduce edema, antibiotics are prescribed to thwart the infection, and IV fluids are given for hydration. Only if the airway is in immediate jeopardy is a tracheotomy or endotracheal tube inserted. If a patient is suspected of having epiglottitis, avoid the use of a tongue blade or oral thermometer because either may cause further edema or laryngeal spasm and can obstruct the airway.

■ Disorders Related to the Larynx and Trachea

Caring for a patient with a disorder of breathing requires expert nursing care. Knowledge of airway anatomy and physiology is critical in the delivery of safe care. Nurses must advocate for these patients who often are unable to speak and breathe without assistance. Specific disorders related to the larynx and trachea are discussed below.

Anatomy and Physiology of the Larynx

The glottic structures include the larynx, epiglottis, the arytenoids, and the true and false vocal folds. The larynx and trachea are two major structures of the upper airway. The larynx is composed of four anatomic units: mucosa, skeleton, intrinsic muscles, and extrinsic muscles (Sataloff et al., 1998). The larynx, which connects the oropharynx to the trachea, is supported by firm cartilaginous structures that prevent collapse during inspiration. The larynx functions to protect the lungs from foreign substances and is needed for normal speech.

The epiglottis, which is located above the larynx, moves downward acting like a sphincter during swallowing to cover the larynx, thus, preventing food and fluid from entering the lungs. This same sphincter-type function is what allows for coughing, completion of a Valsalva maneuver, and vocalization. Closing of the glottis (vocal folds) creates a brief increase in intrathoracic pressure and intra-abdominal pressure. Rapid opening of the glottic opening allows quick upward movement of the air and produces a cough, or a bolus of air, that can be transformed into speech.

The cavity of the larynx is divided into two pairs of folds: upper vestibular folds and lower vocal folds. The vestibular folds function as protection, and the vocal folds vibrate to make vocal sounds (Porth, 2005). The vocal fold itself is composed of five layers: the epithelium, the superficial layer, the intermediate layer, the deep layers of the lamina propria, and the vocalis muscle (Figure 34–6 ■). The larynx, also referred to as the glottis, transmits air to and from the upper airway or the oropharynx

FIGURE 34–6 ■ Normal vocal cords in resting position.
Source: University of California, Davis Medical Center

and trachea and lungs. The vocal cords produce sound and the oral cavity, the palate, tongue, and lips function as articulators as the air passes through the oropharynx and mouth.

There are two synovial joints in the larynx that are of importance, the cricothyroid joint and the cricoarytenoid joint. The cricothyroid joint allows movement of the cords by changing the length of the vocal cords; thereby, controlling vocal pitch. The cricoarytenoid joint allows for the adduction (movement toward the midline) and abduction (movement away from the midline of the vocal cords during breathing, eating, and speaking. At the onset of inspiration, the recurrent laryngeal nerve is stimulated, which causes the vocal cords to abduct or open just before air is taken into the lungs.

These structures are vulnerable to trauma, disease, infection, inflammation, edema, and damage to the structures or to the nerves innervating these structures. This type of damage can result in respiratory, swallowing, and speaking disorders. The larynx is evaluated with fiber-optic laryngoscopy (Figure 34–7), stroboscopy, and voice evaluation (Leonard & Kendall, 2001).

The 10th cranial nerve (CN X), the vagus nerve, innervates the larynx. The superior laryngeal branch and the recurrent laryngeal branch are responsible for both motor and sensation to the larynx. The superior laryngeal nerve supplies sensation to the larynx above the vocal folds, and motor function to the cricothyroid muscle, which helps to control vocal pitch by lengthening the cords. The recurrent laryngeal nerve provides sensory innervation to the larynx below the vocal folds, and motor innervation to the posterior cricoarytenoid muscle,

which shortens and opens the vocal cords, the lateral cricoarytenoid muscle, which shortens and closes the vocal cords; and the thyroarytenoid muscle, which helps to create tension or resistance to airflow.

Damage to either one of these nerves can have a great impact on the quality of life for the patient. The location of these nerves makes them very vulnerable to damage by surgery or trauma to the neck and chest. Surgery of the larynx, thyroid, carotid, cardiac, or anterior cervical spine surgery and trauma to the chest or root of the neck may precipitate damage to these tissues. A patient with damage to the superior laryngeal nerve is at high risk for aspiration, because the loss of sensation above the vocal cords does not allow sensation of saliva, foods, or fluids as they are swallowed and drop into the airway. This is termed *silent aspiration* because patients may not be aware of aspirating until they develop pneumonia. Without the sensory innervation of the superior laryngeal nerve, the patient does not experience the typical reaction to aspiration, which is coughing while eating or drinking.

> **CRITICAL ALERT** *Any patient after laryngeal or thyroid surgery or anterior chest or neck trauma must be observed for airway and voice changes. The implication is a temporary or permanent injury to the larynx. These patients should also be observed eating and drinking and assessed for any difficulty with swallowing. This can include coughing, struggling while eating, or experiencing a foreign body sensation.*

Etiology, Epidemiology, Pathophysiology

Vocal cord paralysis is a disorder that occurs when one or both of the vocal cords (or vocal folds) do not open or close properly. This paralysis results in difficulty swallowing and coughing. Food or liquids slip into the trachea and lungs because the paralyzed cord or cords remain open, leaving the airway passage and the lungs unprotected.

Vocal Cord Paralysis

Vocal cord paralysis is a common disorder, and symptoms can range from mild to life threatening (National Institute on Deafness and other Communication Disorders, 2002).

Vocal cord/fold paralysis may occur at any age from birth to advanced age. It occurs equally in males and females from a variety of causes. It can be the result of an infectious process, trauma to the neck or chest area, neurological disorders, and cancer; however, transection of the recurrent laryngeal nerve during thyroidectomy remains a common cause (Bailey, Johnson, Newlands, Calhoun, & Deskin, 2006).

In total thyroidectomy surgery with dissection on both sides of the neck, there is a risk of damage to both recurrent laryngeal nerves, which could lead to bilateral vocal cord paralysis. Often the damage is apparent in the immediate postoperative period when the patient is extubated. The patient experiences respiratory difficulties and may require reintubation or a tracheostomy.

Due to the lengthy pathway of the vagus nerve to the recurrent laryngeal nerve, any surgery or injury involving the neck and chest area potentially can lead to vocal cord paralysis. The left recurrent laryngeal nerve is more susceptible to injury because of the course and location of the nerve through the chest. In addition to post-thyroid surgery, those patients having carotid endarterectomy, cervical spine surgery, surgery in the mediastinum, skull base surgery, or thoracic surgery are at high

FIGURE 34–7 ■ Fiber-optic scopes for upper airway endoscopy.
Source: University of California, Davis Medical Center

risk of vocal cord paralysis if the vagus or the recurrent laryngeal branch is damaged during the procedure. If the nerve is completely severed, there is little hope of regaining motion to the affected cord. However, if the nerve is stretched or bruised during the procedure, there may be slow return of vocal cord function over a period of up to 12 months. Airway obstruction usually is not a problem with unilateral vocal cord paresis, but voice changes and possible aspiration remain a concern.

Clinical Manifestations

The primary clinical manifestation of vocal cord paralysis is a change in the voice. It may become hoarse (croaky or rough); breathy, as though the individual is exhaling excessive air when speaking; and weakened. Other clinical manifestations include:

- Shortness of breath
- Noisy breathing
- Choking or coughing while swallowing food, drink, or saliva
- The need to take frequent breaths while speaking
- Inability to speak loudly
- Inability to "bear down" while lifting (Mayo Clinic, 2006).

If a patient indicates that she is breathing normally, but is unable to speak or is **aphonic** (without a voice), suspect bilateral vocal cord paralysis in the abducted (AB) or open position. Without cord closure, the patient will not be able to speak, produce an effective cough, or perform a Valsalva maneuver when lifting or straining for a bowel movement. If the patient has paralysis to only one of the vocal cords, the nurse can expect to hear a soft breathy or hoarse voice and minimal to no difficulty breathing. When the paralyzed cord is fixed in the lateral position, the mobile cord cannot meet with the other cord, and the air escaping through the cords when the patient talks creates the breathy sound. The severity of the patient's symptoms (breathy voice, ineffective cough, and dysphagia) is dependent on the position of the paralyzed cord, the degree of injury to the cord (paresis versus paralysis), and the ability of the opposite cord to compensate.

 CRITICAL ALERT *If the patient is able to speak and appears to be in respiratory distress, suspect vocal cord paralysis. With the cords closed together in the midline, it is difficult for the patient to move air in and out of the airway. These patients may require intubation or emergency tracheotomy to establish a safe airway. If the patient is able to breathe but not speak, suspect vocal cord paralysis. The airway is open for respiration, but the vocal cords are unable to move together to produce sound.*

Damage to the vagus nerve and its branches can have a significant impact on the patient's quality of life. Because the vocal cords have an integral role in the protection of the airway from aspiration, damage here can affect the patient's ability to eat and drink. This damage also may alter the sensation of the larynx, making the individual unable to sense the insults of aspiration. Persistent aspiration can be significant enough that the patient will not be able to eat orally. The larynx and the vocal cords must be able to close completely to prevent food and fluids from entering the airway and to allow the patient to build up sufficient intrathoracic and intra-abdominal resistance to be able to produce an effective cough. Additionally, the patient's ability to communicate is affected because this nerve is necessary to allow the open-

ing, closing, and vibration of the vocal cords as air moves up from the lungs. Without this ability the voice may be hoarse, weak, or nonexistent. Alteration in communication, method of eating, and body image are significant changes for any patient.

Laboratory and Diagnostic Procedures

Direct visualization of the vocal cord is done by endoscopy. The endoscope is a thin flexible tube with a light and camera that can be passed down the patient's throat for direct visualization of the cords to determine if one or both cords are affected. Additionally, laryngeal electromyography (LEMG) is a test that measures the electric currents in the cords. This will determine the degree of paralysis and what types of treatment may be most effective. During this test, the health care provider inserts small needles into the vocal cord muscles to measure the electric currents to the muscles.

Because other disorders can cause damage to the cords, additional tests may be needed to identify the cause of the paralysis. Tests may include blood work, x-rays, CT scans, or MRI of the head, neck, and chest. Referral to a neurologist may be necessary to rule out damage to nerves other than those of the vocal cords (Mayo Clinic, 2006).

Medical Management

Treatment alternatives to profound uncontrolled aspiration are a permanent enteral feeding option with placement of a gastrostomy tube and usually a tracheostomy. A gastrostomy or jejunostomy tube directs feeding through the anterior wall of the abdomen directly into the stomach or jejunum. Nutrition is taken as liquid supplements. However, if aspiration of oral secretions alone is causing recurrent pneumonias, this option is not realistic to prevent the problem as the insult to the larynx is not eliminated. Another alternative is to completely separate the larynx and the esophagus, similar to a total **laryngectomy**, the total removal of the larynx. This surgery provides the patient with the ability to eat without aspiration, but removes the ability to speak normally. Alternative speech is taught by speech pathologists trained in alaryngeal (without a larynx) speech.

In the patient with unilateral vocal cord paralysis with severe symptoms of aspiration and difficulty communicating, the surgeon may perform a procedure that medializes the paralyzed cord so that the two cords can meet in the midline to allow for vocalization and to prevent aspiration. The mobile cord still is able to move aside during breathing to allow adequate respiration. Different types of materials are used with this procedure to push the cord to the center. Silastic or fat from the patient's abdomen is used to plump up the vocal cord and bring it closer to midline. Patients with bilateral vocal cord paralysis may need a tracheostomy if the cords are adducted and a feeding tube if the cords are abducted, in the immediate period after injury, trauma, or surgery. Later in the healing process there may be surgeries that can be performed to open the space between the vocal cords (glottis) enough to allow air to pass through, so the patient will not require a tracheostomy, and without significantly affecting the voice quality. It is important for the patient to understand that the voice and airway will not return to normal with this procedure, but the goal is to communicate verbally and to breathe without a tracheostomy.

Nursing Management

The nursing process guides the management of patients with vocal cord paralysis.

Assessment

It is essential for the assessment to begin with identifying the patient's risk for aspiration.

Outcomes and Evaluation Parameters

The expected outcome is prevention of aspiration and the evaluation parameters include the following:

- Lungs are clear to auscultation.
- Oxygen saturation is greater than 95% or within normal range.
- There is no increase in respiration or work of breathing.
- The patient denies feeling short of breath.

These parameters need to be assessed regularly and after each oral intake.

Interventions and Rationales

Nursing interventions to prevent aspiration include having the patient sit upright in a chair to eat and staying with the patient to observe for coughing or frequent throat clearing after swallowing. If the patient appears to be having significant problems with fluids or foods, the tray should be taken away and the patient's response to eating should be reported to the health care provider and documented.

Evaluation

A formal evaluation by a health care provider and a trained speech pathologist should be done with fiber-optic laryngoscopy, and a dynamic swallow study should be completed to determine the safest and most appropriate diet for the patient. Liquid nutrition is discussed in detail in Chapter 14 . Patients with unilateral vocal cord paralysis are likely to have trouble with swallowing thin liquids safely. Solid foods, thickened fluids, or foods with a custard-like consistency seem to be less of a problem because the patient has more control of the food bolus, which stimulates sensation when swallowing thus decreasing the risk of aspiration.

For some patients their voice is their livelihood and damage to their vocal cords can create psychological as well as physical changes. Singers, teachers, preachers, and politicians who depend on their voices may be unable to return to their chosen profession.

The patient should be observed for signs and symptoms of depression and these should be discussed with the health care provider. Working with a speech therapist and learning how to maximize the remaining function of the vocal cords can help the patient physically by decreasing the risk of aspiration and mentally by increasing the patient's communication skills.

Etiology, Epidemiology, and Pathophysiology of Laryngeal Disorders

Hoarseness of the voice occurs because of the disruption of the normal vibration of the vocal cord. **Hoarseness** is defined as having difficulty producing sound when trying to speak. The voice may have a change in the pitch or quality and may sound weak, excessively breathy, scratchy, or husky (Medline Plus, 2005a). The causes are lesions on the vocal cords, lesions along the cranial nerves, vocal trauma, stiffness of the vocal cords, and a change in the mass of the cords due to swelling or growths or changes in the normal coordination of vocal cord movement.

A major cause of hoarseness is smoking and, hence, tobacco cessation is of the upmost priority (Rudy, 2006). Other common causes are acute and chronic laryngitis (Baitha, Raizada, Kennedy-Singh, Puttewar, & Chaturvedi, 2002). Any of these changes will affect the quality of the voice. Patients with hoarseness for more than 2 weeks should have a complete head and neck exam because this could be the presenting symptoms of vocal nodules or an early vocal cord cancer. Hoarseness in elderly patients is discussed in the Gerontological Considerations box.

Etiology, Pathophysiology, and Medical Management of Acute Laryngitis

Laryngitis is an inflammation of the larynx and vocal cords or just the larynx. The most common cause of acute laryngitis is a viral upper respiratory tract infection or acute vocal strain. When laryngitis occurs as part of an upper respiratory infection, the patient also may experience coughing, rhinorrhea, and a mild sore throat. The infection causes edema and inflammation of the vocal cords, which prevents them from vibrating properly.

The vocal cords may show submucosal hemorrhage and edema with any vocal strain such as after loud cheering for a sports team or trying to carry on a conversation over the dance music at a club. Any edema or changes to the surface of the vocal cords can disrupt the motion of the vocal cords and cause hoarseness.

Acute laryngitis secondary to a viral infection usually is self-limiting and does not require medical treatment. Antibiotics rarely are necessary unless there is evidence of a coexistent bacterial infection. Humidification, hydration, and voice rest usually are sufficient to allow the edema to resolve and the voice to return to normal. Symptomatic relief of sore throat, fever, and cough is appropriate.

Etiology, Pathophysiology, and Clinical Manifestations of Chronic Laryngitis

Chronic laryngitis is a result of long-standing inflammation to the larynx and vocal folds. Examination of the larynx usually

---

GERONTOLOGICAL CONSIDERATIONS for Hoarseness

In the elderly patient hoarseness can be a result of changes in the texture or shape of the vocal cords. It also can be the result of dehydration from poor nutritional intake and or medications. Bowing may occur which does not allow the cords to meet fully in the middle and stiffness decreases the normal vibratory action of the cords, resulting in a coarse and breathy voice. Arthritic changes in the cricoarytenoid joints can decrease the motion of the vocal cords. How the patient is affected by these changes depends on the severity of the decreased motion and how it manifests in the patient.

reveals redness of the true vocal cords and possibly edema. Causes include frequent inhalation of smoke, chemicals, and pollens, and exposure to gastric acids in patients with reflux disease, or mechanical irritation from frequent coughing or throat clearing, whether due to any of the just-mentioned exposures to irritants or simply as a bad habit.

Chronic irritation can lead to a chronic inflammatory state clinically presenting as a hoarse voice and a barking cough. Individuals who overuse and abuse their voices such as loud screaming sports fans or singers, teachers, preachers, and politicians who use their voice for long periods at a time day after day may develop forms of chronic irritation and inflammation to their vocal cords. Speech therapy is indicated for the person to learn to speak and project their voices in a nontraumatic method through education in the techniques of voice control.

Medical Management

The health care provider should obtain a thorough medical history from any patient presenting with a hoarse voice. This includes observing specific qualities of the voice such as coarse, raspy, breathy, or a quivering quality. Assessment of the patient's troublesome or stridorous breathing should be completed. It is essential to determine and report the use of any accessory muscles of respiration, because this indicates respiratory distress.

It is important to ask the patient how much difficulty he is having breathing and whether this has been a rapid or slow-onset change. The health care provider should attempt to elicit any potentially triggering events leading up to the change in voice. This is accomplished by inquiring if the patient has had a viral or bacterial illness or if this is a result of voice abuse or trauma. Assess smoking and secondhand smoke exposure and work history. Document the patient's environmental exposure to paint, chemicals, fertilizers, pets, or cleaning solutions. Answers to questions about these topics can assist in focusing in on the cause of hoarseness. Hoarseness is treated with voice rest, hydration, humidification, changes in voicing practices, or removal of the known inhaled irritant. Referral to a speech pathologist trained in voice is important.

Health Promotion

Instructions regarding voice rest must be reinforced for patients with laryngitis. Instruct the patients that if she must speak in an emergency to use a regular speaking voice and not whisper. Whispering is more strenuous on the vocal cords than speaking in a normal voice and, thus, can exacerbate the problem. The patient should be instructed to carry a notepad and pen or a hand-held communication device. If the patient is in the hospital for any condition that requires strict voice rest, a sign should be placed above the patient's bed indicating "Patient Is on Voice Rest." This alerts the staff and visitors entering the room that the patient is not to speak. If clerks at the nurses' station answering the call light understand that the patient is on voice rest, they can say "I know you cannot speak, therefore I am paging your nurse to come to your room now" to reassure patients that their call has been acknowledged.

Patients should be instructed to avoid inhaling irritants if this is the cause of the chronic inflammation. It also is important to stress the importance of smoking cessation (Rudy, 2006). Refer the patient to a smoking cessation program and instruct

to avoid exposure to secondhand smoke (Wynd, 2006). It may be necessary to wear a mask in the workplace if there are irritating substances in the environment. Encourage the patient to work with the occupational health nurse at the worksite and to find protective equipment to prevent further exposure to those substances.

Etiology and Clinical Manifestations of Edema of the Larynx

Laryngeal edema is defined as swelling in any region of the larynx. There are a variety of causes including allergic reactions, gastroesophageal reflux disease, laryngopharyngeal reflux disease, and endotracheal intubation. Allergic reaction is a common inflammatory response that potentially can lead rapidly to airway obstruction. Laryngeal edema usually is of sudden onset and results from exposure to a specific allergen. Common precipitators are bee stings, foods, or medicines. The edema may be mild at first, causing hoarseness and a scratchy sensation in the throat. Rapid progression to airway obstruction can develop if the patient is particularly sensitive to the allergen or has a significant exposure to a target food or medication. When airway obstruction occurs, it becomes a medical emergency.

Medical and Nursing Management

The priority for nursing management of edema to the larynx is to summon medical assistance and support the patient's airway until expert assistance arrives. The nurse should place a tracheostomy insertion tray at the bedside, elevate the head of the bed, monitor oxygen saturations, and provide supplemental oxygen. An IV line should be inserted to administer medications, which may include IV steroids and antihistamines. Epinephrine given subcutaneously or in aerosolized form via nebulizer treatments typically is effective. If the obstruction is severe and the patient does not respond rapidly enough to medications, a tracheotomy can establish an airway until the edema resolves.

Patients with allergies to medication should be given information on how to obtain a medic alert bracelet indicating the medication to which they are allergic. If they are taken ill and are unable to speak, the alert tag can speak for them. A patient with a bee sting allergy should, in addition to the medic alert information, be given an EpiPen auto-injector with instructions. An EpiPen is a dose of epinephrine that the patient or family injects into the subcutaneous tissue to help decrease the histamine release initiated by exposure to the allergen. The patient may feel better after the injection, but should still get medical help for follow-up treatment. EpiPen use is discussed in detail in Chapter 60 ☺.

Etiology, Pathophysiology, Clinical Manifestations, and Medical Management of Vocal Cord Pathology

Vocal cord nodules, also called "singer's" or "screamer's" nodes, are a result of chronic microtrauma from vocal strain, and generally can be thought of as scars or calluses on the vocal cords (Figure 34–8 ■). The nodules develop initially from submucosal hemorrhages resulting from an impact injury between the cords. The nodule may appear as a red edematous area on the cord, but

FIGURE 34–8 ■ Vocal cord nodules/vocal hemorrhage/abuse.
Source: University of California, Davis Medical Center

with continued trauma to the area, it becomes thick and fibrosed. Vocal cord nodules typically occur in individuals who abuse their voices such as cheerleaders, singers, teachers, bartenders, coaches, and politicians. These nodules, though painless, produce persistent hoarseness as they inhibit normal vibration and closure of the vocal cords. The patient will present with complaints of painless hoarseness, inability to sing in the higher ranges, inability to speak for a long period of time, or always have a breathy voice. Typically the nodules will resolve with humidification, hydration, voice rest, and treatment by a speech therapist to correct the underlying abuse issues. Some patients require surgical removal of the nodules.

Etiology, Pathophysiology, Clinical Manifestations, and Medical Management of Vocal Cord Polyps

A vocal cord polyp is a growth that typically occurs only on one side of the vocal cord, in a variety of shapes and sizes. Vocal cord polyps are a result of long-term vocal abuse or chronic irritation. The main causative factors include smoking, voice strain, and gastric reflux. What begins as microhemorrhages on the vocal folds turns into polyps, cystlike growths filled with a gelatinous material. Indirect laryngoscopy demonstrates significant vocal cord edema but no redness. Hoarseness occurs due to the disruption of the vibration of the cord, and breathiness develops due to incomplete closure of the cords due to the polyp. Treatment for polyps is voice therapy and often surgery with microlaryngoscopy to remove the polyp.

Because polyps may return after surgical removal if the same predisposing conditions exist, postoperative treatment must include treatment of the underlying etiologic factors to help prevent recurrence and speech therapy. Smoking cessation is encouraged; the patient must be offered information on programs and support groups at the health care facility or in the community.

Individuals who have polyps resulting from chronic vocal abuse should be instructed that humidification, hydration, and voice rest are necessary. These patients will benefit from an evaluation by a speech therapist, which serves to direct treatment at correcting the underlying causes for vocal strain. Patients who develop polyps as a result of laryngopharyngeal reflux, discussed later, require changes in diet and lifestyle, weight reduction, medical management, or surgical management.

Etiology, Epidemiology, Pathophysiology, and Medical Management of Laryngeal Papillomas

Laryngeal papillomas are benign laryngeal growths associated with the human papilloma virus. Although, laryngeal papillomas can affect any age group, it is children who seem to have the most aggressive form in terms of recurrence, spread, and requirements for frequent intervention. As the child approaches puberty, sometimes the severity and recurrences of the disease slow down.

The papillomas can be widespread, and patients present with hoarseness and, if severe, progressive respiratory distress. Treatment of this disorder involves carbon dioxide (CO_2) laser ablation of the papillomas during laryngoscopy. Despite frequent surgical interventions the papillomas may recur or spread. It is important to keep the papillomas from becoming large enough to cause airway obstruction. Placing a tracheostomy tube in a patient with laryngeal papillomas should be avoided to prevent spreading of the disease to the trachea. If the papillomas spread to the trachea, bronchial tree, and lungs, the disease usually is fatal.

Etiology, Pathophysiology, Clinical Manifestations, and Medical Management of Laryngeal Spasm

Laryngeal spasm is an abnormal reflexive response to a laryngeal insult. The laryngeal glottis reflexively closes with a swallow to protect the airway from aspiration of food or fluids. Laryngospasm is an abnormal response to this reflex. It may occur spontaneously or be triggered by certain foods, inhalants, or by reflux at night. After extubation of a laryngeal tube, patients also may experience laryngospasm. Although the episodes usually are transient (lasting several seconds to several minutes), this period of respiratory distress is quite disturbing to the patient. Although the patient may be stridorous and unable to speak (aphonic), these episodes usually are not associated with severe hypoxia or loss of consciousness.

Effective interventions include keeping the offending food or environmental stimulants (chemicals, cleaners, or perfumes) away from the patient in order to avoid triggering a spasm. If the laryngeal spasm occurs at night as a result of reflux, educate the patient regarding diet and lifestyle changes as discussed later in the section on laryngopharyngeal reflux disease.

Etiology and Clinical Manifestations of Laryngeal Injury

Laryngeal injury usually is the result of blunt trauma to the neck. Scenarios include a patient arriving in the emergency room after a motor vehicle crash, a child who has been thrown over and hits the handle bars of his bike, a softball player getting hit in the neck by a ball, a patient attempting suicide via hanging, or assault victims with strangulation injuries. The patient's symptoms and physical findings on examination may initially seem benign, and if the clinician is not aware of the potential complications of a direct blow to the larynx, a patient could conceivably be seen in the emergency department, discharged home, and then develop significant and life-threatening airway obstruction after discharge.

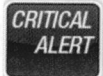 **CRITICAL ALERT** *Symptoms that have developed over a period of hours may progress to full obstruction very quickly.*

Initially patients presenting with no acute airway obstruction may develop obstruction hours later as the edema increases. In a stable patient with an adequate airway on admission, the initial evaluation includes a transnasal fiber-optic laryngoscopy to assess for fractures of the cartilage of the anterior neck and larynx, the functioning of the vocal cords, and any other internal damage from the trauma. Additional work-up may include a CT scan, a barium swallow, and an endoscopy.

If the blow is severe and the patient develops laryngeal edema rapidly, there may be a complaint of pain with swallowing, and a notable change in voice quality. The patient's breathing may be labored and sound stridorous, and the patient may complain of neck pain or coughing of blood (hemoptysis). On physical exam the thyroid cartilage notch or "Adam's apple" may not be visible and may be tender on palpation. Subcutaneous crepitus in the neck indicates leakage of air from the aerodigestive tract into the tissue of the neck, often due to a tear in the laryngeal mucosa. Hemoptysis is an ominous sign of mucosal tears and needs to be reported to the health care provider.

Swelling may come on slowly and progression to airway compromise or obstruction may be subtle. If a cartilage fracture of the larynx penetrates into or obstructs the airway or swelling occurs rapidly, the patient will immediately demonstrate signs of airway distress. Securing and maintaining an airway at this point is of utmost importance. When there is a strong suspicion of a fracture to the larynx, the nurse should prepare to assist with placement of a tracheostomy tube. Patients with suspected laryngeal injury should not be intubated because this may create further damage to the fragments of laryngeal cartilage or be difficult due to the vocal cord edema. It is critical to establish an effective airway first, then examine the larynx more thoroughly and stabilize the fracture for repair.

Laboratory and Diagnostic Procedures and Medical Management

Due to the vital structures and function in the anterior neck, any laryngeal injury must be fully investigated. The patient's ability to protect the airway must be determined as well as the ability to take in nutrition. The Diagnostic Tests for Laryngeal Injury and Disease box outlines the tests needed to determine injury and function.

A speech therapist trained in dysphagia can determine the type of diet, position for eating, and safety while eating. Examples of strategies include double swallowing, holding the breath while swallowing, coughing after each swallow, and positioning the head to the unaffected side to best protect the airway from aspiration. Sometimes just changing the thickness of the liquids the patient drinks can decrease the risk of aspiration. With thicker fluids, the patient has more control of the liquid as it is swallowed, thus helping to reduce the incidence of aspiration.

Although the majority of patients presenting to the emergency department (ED) with laryngeal trauma have experienced blunt trauma to the neck, patients may arrive in the ED with laryngeal injury secondary to intentional or accidental ingestion of caustic chemicals (lye, ammonia, bleach, Lysol), thermal burns from ingestion of hot food or liquids, or inhalation of hot air or gases. Patients should *not* be encouraged to vomit because aspiration of a caustic substance can lead to further damage to healthy airway tissues. Laryngeal injury after radiation treatment also can occur because radiation weakens the tissue and causes irritation; inflammation and stenosis also can occur as a result of the radiation therapy. Airway stabilization is the first priority in these patients because the most common

DIAGNOSTIC TESTS for Laryngeal Injury and Disease

Test	Expected Abnormality/Findings	Rationale for Abnormality
Flex scope	Revealed fixation of the left vocal cord in the open or abducted position. Decreased sensation throughout the left side of the larynx as evidenced by no response to touch with the scope.	Any injury to the anterior neck demands an inspection of the larynx.
Videostroboscopy	Decreased movement on the right side and no movement on the left side of the larynx. No mucosal wave.	Evaluate movement of the vocal folds. Test is done at postinjury day 14 to allow for swelling to dissipate and have a more accurate exam.
Dynamic swallow study	Timing delayed to 2.0 seconds (WNL 1.0 seconds). Oropharynx and oral cavity: normal transition of bolus to pharynx. Obvious pooling in the vallecula and pyriform sinus on the L side of the larynx and pharynx.	Objectively evaluate the patient's ability to protect her airway and ability to safely take oral nutrition. Establish safe methods of compensation and rehabilitation.
CT Scan	Injury to the structural support of the larynx, fracture of the thyroid cartilage. Significant soft tissue damage.	Evaluate the structure of the larynx used predominantly for soft tissue.
MRI scan	Injury to the structural support of the larynx. Fracture of the thyroid cartilage.	Evaluate the structure of the larynx used predominantly for bony structural and organ definition.

cause of severe respiratory distress in patients with caustic ingestion is supraglottic swelling (Calhoun, Eibling, & Wax, 2001). Endotracheal intubation with direct visualization by the oral route is preferred. The procedure of nasotracheal intubation is contraindicated because of the high risk of tracheal, pharyngeal, and esophageal perforation (Calhoun et al., 2001).

Endotracheal (ET) tube intubation may cause laryngeal trauma (Maktabi, Smith, & Todd, 2003). The placement of an ET tube may induce laryngeal swelling, which is a cause of upper airway obstruction after extubation (Tanaka, Isono, Ishikawa, Sato, & Nishino, 2003). Endotracheal intubation can result in laryngeal injury either at the time of insertion, or secondary to prolonged intubation or intubation with an inappropriately sized endotracheal tube. The acute complications include perforation or laceration of the trachea or esophagus, bleeding, and arytenoid dislocation. The arytenoid cartilages are attached to the upper edge of the cricoid cartilage and to the posterior cricoarytenoid muscles that are responsible for abducting, or opening, the vocal cords. Damage here can lead to speech and swallowing problems.

Routine tracheal intubation also produces mucosal changes in the airway (Tanaka et al., 2003). The long-term complications associated with endotracheal intubation include laryngeal, subglottic, and tracheal stenosis as well as vocal cord paralysis. Irritation and inflammation to the subglottic and upper tracheal mucosa most often are caused by the cuff on the ET tube. Before the advent of low-pressure endotracheal and tracheal cuffs, tracheal stenosis and tracheal esophageal fistulas were not uncommon in patients requiring long-term intubation. A **fistula** is a communication between two specific areas such as the oral cavity and the skin, or trachea and esophagus. Today, damage secondary to high cuff pressure is less of a problem than irritation and inflammation from the cuff on an improperly secured ET tube. This inflammation can cause subsequent scarring and subglottic stenosis.

To prevent any or all of the long-term complications of intubation, it is important that all health professionals who perform direct care of patients with ET tubes ensure the tube remains properly positioned and secured in place. Unnecessary movement of the tube can irritate and inflame the laryngeal tissue. Sedation of the patient may be necessary if the patient is restless due to withdrawal from alcohol or drugs or as a result of anxiety, pain, or head trauma. The risk of laryngeal or tracheal long-term complications can be reduced by changing the patient to a tracheostomy tube if intubation is anticipated to be necessary for longer than 7 to 14 days (Harris & Huntoon, 2007). Tracheostomy is an effective method of establishing an airway and has fewer complications than long-term endotracheal intubation.

Laryngopharyngeal Reflux Disease

Etiology, Pathophysiology, and Clinical Manifestations

The etiology of **laryngopharyngeal reflux disease (LPRD)** is reflux of gastric acid into the larynx. The reflux occurs when there is intermittent relaxation of the lower esophageal sphincter (LES). Patients with this problem most often seek medical care because of hoarseness and throat irritation rather than heartburn symptoms. Upon further questioning the patient may say,

"It feels like something is in my throat and I seem to be clearing my throat a lot." Typical clinical manifestations include:

- Hoarseness
- Chronic (ongoing) cough
- Frequent throat clearing
- Pain or sensation in throat
- Feeling of a lump in throat
- Problems while swallowing
- Bad/bitter taste in mouth (especially in morning)
- Asthma-like symptoms
- Referred ear pain
- Postnasal drip
- Difficulty with high notes when singing.

Laboratory and Diagnostic Procedures

Usually the diagnosis of LPRD is based on the patient's symptom history and examination of the larynx. Twenty-four-hour pharyngoesophageal pH monitoring is the gold standard for monitoring reflux events associated with LPRD (Belafsky, 2006). A tube with dual pH probes monitors the pH in the patient's esophagus. The pH monitor records values just below the upper esophageal sphincter and just above the LES. Patients are instructed to eat and drink normally and include foods that they know cause symptoms of indigestion. The patient wears the monitor for 24 hours and records any incidence of discomfort, throat irritation, or heartburn, and the time of occurrence. The recordings are reviewed to determine how many reflux episodes reached the upper pH monitor and how long and how acidic those exposures were.

If a patient complains of persistent hoarseness, a transnasal fiber-optic laryngoscopy or indirect laryngoscopy is used to assess the condition of the larynx. The vocal cords and arytenoids appear edematous and red on patients with this disease. During the fiber-optic exam, the health care provider or a specially trained speech pathologist can show the patient evidence of the irritation the gastric acid is having on her larynx. A videotape of the exam is an excellent teaching model.

Medical Management

The three major methods of treating LPRD are (1) behavioral and lifestyle changes, (2) medication, and (3) surgical intervention. It is necessary to teach the patient dietary and lifestyle changes that can decrease the incidence of laryngopharyngeal reflux. These include teaching the patient not to eat for 3 hours before bedtime and to avoid:

- Eating aggravating foods such as chocolate and peppermint (which are known to relax the LES)
- Fatty foods
- Substances that tend to increase the production of gastric acid such as caffeine, alcohol, milk, and nicotine
- Spicy, acidic, and tomato-based foods such as Mexican or Italian food
- Acidic fruit juices such as orange juice, grapefruit juice, or cranberry juice.

Elevating the head of the bed by 6 inches has been shown to decrease the incidence of reflux episodes and increase acid clearance (Belafsky, 2006). Using extra pillows to elevate the head actually may worsen the reflux by increasing intra-abdominal pressure. If the person is overweight, weight loss is imperative, and clothes that fit tightly around the waist should be avoided because this increases intra-abdominal pressure and, therefore, increases the incidence and severity of gastric acid reflux.

When diet and lifestyle changes are ineffective or when the edema and irritation are significant on physical exam, medications that neutralize the gastric acid, increase gastric emptying, or decrease the secretion of gastric acids help lessen the exposure of caustic acids to the sensitive tissues of the larynx. Medical management for LPRD is necessary for much longer than for gastroesophageal reflux disease because the tissues of the larynx are much more sensitive to the gastric acid and, therefore, take longer to respond to therapy and heal completely.

A surgical option is available for patients who fail dietary, lifestyle changes, and medical management, and who have a weak lower esophageal sphincter on esophageal manometry. Laparoscopic Nissen fundoplication tightens the LES, making it more difficult for the gastric acid to reflux into the esophagus and larynx. Combined medical and surgical treatment is curative for LPRD. The cessation of acid reflux into the larynx is the definitive goal of therapy.

■ Nursing Management

Nursing management of patients with laryngopharyngeal reflux disease depends on the severity of the disorder and the patient's general state of health. The nursing process guides the management of these patients.

Assessment

The nurse begins with an in-depth assessment of the patient with airway being the first priority. Any difficulty with breathing and gas exchange must be addressed immediately. Nursing assessment of the airway includes gathering both objective and subjective data. Objective data include lungs sounds, oxygen saturation levels, and respiratory rate and depth. Subjective data include a report of increasing difficulty breathing or shortness of breath.

Outcomes and Evaluation Parameters

Outcomes for these patients should be a treatment plan that allows for a resolution of the symptoms of laryngopharyngeal reflux disease. The patient should be experiencing clear lung sounds, respiratory rate and depth within normal limits, and O_2 sats within the normal range.

Evaluation

In the case of patients with intentional ingestion of caustic substances, it is imperative that plans for a psychiatric evaluation and follow-up be in place before patient discharge. It is essential for the patient to be allowed to communicate fears and concerns and for the nurse to provide comfort and reassurance as appropriate. Encourage patience when communication is difficult or not immediately understood, and share that this can be a frustrating experience for family and friends as well.

Nutritional evaluation by the dietician is important for the patient with LPRD. Patients with severe dysphagia or unhealed esophageal burns and erosions will need nutritional supplementation through a gastrostomy tube to allow the damaged tissue to heal and the patient to receive adequate nutrition to aid the healing process.

Health Promotion

Patients with LPRD have a difficult time understanding how they can have irritation in the throat without experiencing irritation in the esophagus. It needs to be explained that the tissue of the larynx is much more sensitive to the acids from the stomach than the esophagus; therefore, it does not take as much exposure to create irritation in the throat as it does in the esophagus. It is important for the patient to understand the correlation between reflux disease and hoarseness. If the patient does not understand this connection, there may be reluctance to initiate the medication and dietary and lifestyle modifications required to treat this disease.

Airway Obstruction

Airway obstruction is a potentially life-threatening event that requires immediate and skilled intervention. It is imperative to determine the cause of the obstruction in order to intervene and prevent a worsening of the obstruction. The obstruction could be caused by a variety of situations, such as a foreign object, allergy, lesions, stenosis, and swelling.

Etiology and Clinical Manifestations

Specific causes include viral and bacterial infections; fire or inhalation burns; allergic responses to foods, medications, or bee stings; and infections after dental extraction that have a large amount of swelling. Other causes include laryngeal trauma secondary to a motor vehicle crash, strangulation, nerve damage to the vocal cords during a surgical procedure or intubation, or a cancerous tumor large enough to press on the nerves or structures of the larynx or trachea or to physically narrow the airway opening. Aspiration of food material also is a cause of airway obstruction. Large boluses as well as small pieces of food, such as peanuts, can partially or totally obstruct the airway. In patients who have altered sensation or anatomy, talking while eating may cause aspiration. This can present acutely or as a chronic cough or infection.

The one clinical manifestation that is present in nearly all patients with partial airway obstruction is stridor. The patient's ability to speak must be determined. Ability to speak helps determine if the obstruction is partial or complete. With a complete obstruction, the patient is unable to speak. Labored respirations and use of accessory muscles is a common finding with airway obstruction. Mild obstruction may result in air hunger, whereas more severe obstruction can lead to cyanosis. Confusion and unconsciousness indicate a progression in the severity of the obstruction. If not treated a partial obstruction can lead to a complete obstruction, rapid suffocation, and death (Medline Plus, 2005b).

Diagnosis and Medical Management

If the patient is not in extreme distress as with a partial airway obstruction, obtain a medical and surgical history from the patient or the family regarding the onset and progression of the respiratory difficulty. Inquire about recent symptoms of an infection (sore throat, runny nose, fever, cough, dysphagia, or odynophagia), head and neck trauma, new medications, foreign body ingestion, or recent dental extractions. Ask the patient if he or she has recently been diagnosed and/or treated for a cancer of the head and neck, and determine whether the patient has had any prior experience with respiratory difficulty. Often patients presenting with partial obstruction secondary to a head or neck malignancy will relate recent weight loss, difficulty eating, coughing with meals, hoarseness, difficult or painful swallowing, or shortness of breath with minimal activity for a time before this more acute respiratory episode was significant enough for them to seek medical attention.

Surgical scars to the neck should be noted and the patient questioned about those past surgeries. It is necessary to determine if the patient had a thyroidectomy, carotid endarterectomy, goiter removal, tracheostomy, or cervical spine surgery with an anterior neck approach. This information can help the health care provider focus on possible causes of the airway distress.

It is imperative to keep the patient safe and provide oxygen. The patient should be placed in an upright position so as to straighten the airway and help alleviate the obstruction. Extending the patient's head and pulling the mandible forward to displace the tongue base away from the pharyngeal wall also may be helpful. This will straighten the airway and may improve air exchange until help arrives.

An IV line should be placed for medication and fluid administration, and oxygen and humidification are indicated. Administration of IV steroids to decrease swelling in the airway may be ordered by the health care provider. Even a small increase in the diameter of the airway can make a significant improvement in the patient's symptoms. Antibiotic therapy is indicated if the cause is a bacterial infection.

Patients with complete airway obstruction require immediate attention with endotracheal intubation, cricothyroidotomy, or tracheostomy to establish an airway. In the case of a full respiratory arrest secondary to airway obstruction, ventilating with a resuscitation bag will be futile. Therefore, it is critical to secure an emergency surgical airway.

Nursing Management of Airway Obstruction

The nursing process guides the management of patients with a partial or complete airway obstruction.

Assessment

The initial assessment of objective and subjective data includes:

- Presence of spontaneous breathing
- Rate, depth, and effort of respirations
- Presence of grunting or wheezing
- Use of accessory muscles of respiration
- Symmetry of chest expansion (determined through palpation) (Galler, Skinner, & Ng, 2005)
- Vital signs

- Oxygen saturation level
- Quality of the voice, such as hoarse, raspy, weak, muffled, normal, or nonexistent
- Stridor or any type of noisy breathing
- Patient complaint of "not getting enough air."

The patient's orientation, mentation, and general demeanor should be monitored on an ongoing basis. The patient may be cooperative and able to answer questions appropriately on arrival to the unit, but as the obstruction increases the patient may begin to appear anxious and agitated or confused. The patient who was cooperative initially may become disoriented and unable to follow directions. If the obstruction has been progressing gradually, the patient may not report as much discomfort breathing as his appearance belies.

Assessment also should include the patient's ability to handle oral secretions, and whether the patient is having pain with speaking or swallowing. Any frequent drooling or productive coughing to clear the airway should be noted. Drooling is an ominous sign that signifies an inability to swallow oral secretions, indicating near complete obstruction. It is essential to determine how long it has been since the patient has noticed voice or respiratory changes. Symptoms that have developed over a period of days may indicate a slower progressing airway problem.

 *Hoarseness and early respiratory distress are signs that must not be overlooked or discounted on initial exam. Patients with blunt neck trauma should be carefully assessed for hoarseness, respiratory distress, hemoptysis (bloody sputum), and dysphagia because these symptoms indicate airway injury and respiratory compromise.*

Planning

A patient with complete airway obstruction appears very anxious, agitated, and apprehensive, and progresses quickly to cyanosis and respiratory arrest. The chest wall may be moving in and out as the individual tries to breathe, but there will be no air exchange. As the patient becomes more hypoxic, agitation, combativeness, and loss of consciousness may ensue. There is no cough and the patient will be cyanotic and unable to speak. If the patient is unable to speak, a Heimlich maneuver should be performed in case the obstruction is from a foreign object or food or more information). Anticipation is the key to saving patients with a complete airway obstruction. Supplies should be kept at the bedside for creating an immediate artificial airway, such as tracheostomy insertion, cricothyroidotomy, or endotracheal intubation equipment. Resuscitation equipment should be brought to the bedside in case there is a subsequent cardiac arrest.

Outcomes and Evaluation Parameters

The outcome is relief of the obstruction and return of normal oxygenation. Evaluation parameters include an alert oriented patient who has normal oxygen saturation levels, respiratory rate and depth, and vital signs. It is necessary to continuously monitor vital signs and pulse oxygen saturations. It is the overall assessment of respiratory effort, stridor, body positioning, restlessness, agitation, cyanosis, and decreasing level of consciousness that will provide the true picture of how the patient is doing.

Tracheotomy

Patients with severe facial injuries, edema in the head and neck area, infection, surgery, large obstructive tumors, or neurological changes to the larynx may require an altered airway. A tracheotomy can be performed to provide an artificial airway.

Placement of a tracheostomy tube usually is temporary to support the patient through the initial period of obstructive swelling or to provide an airway in a patient with airway obstruction. Most health care providers recommend a tracheostomy for patients whom they expect to be intubated for longer than 7 to 10 days. This decreases the risk of permanent injury to the vocal cords or tissues in the larynx or upper airway. Patients with severe lung disease, as in chronic obstructive pulmonary disease (COPD), may have a tracheostomy to provide direct access to the lungs for vigorous pulmonary toilet. Another indication for tracheostomy is obstructive sleep apnea for those who have failed conservative therapy. Patients with short thick necks and large tonsils or a large amount of soft tissue in the posterior pharynx may have their airways obstructed as they relax to sleep. The tracheostomy allows the patient unobstructed breathing while sleeping.

The tracheostomy incision is below the prominent thyroid cartilage (Adam's apple) and below the cricoid cartilage, usually between the second and third, or third and fourth tracheal cartilages, and continues on through the anterior tracheal wall. The tracheostomy tube is placed into the tracheal stoma to keep the airway open. It is initially sutured into place to prevent inadvertent dislodgement. In addition, ties are placed through the faceplate of the tracheostomy tube and around the neck to further secure the tube. The tube remains sutured in place until the tract from the anterior neck into the trachea becomes well established. A post-tracheostomy tray is kept at the bedside or on the nursing unit; in it are instruments to help with reinsertion in the event of early accidental decannulation or early tube obstruction (Figure 34–9 ■). **Decannulation**, a term used to refer to the process of weaning toward the goal of removing the tracheostomy tube, is discussed later.

The tracheostomy tubes are usually made of silicone, plastic, stainless steel, or silver. The tube consists of an outer tube and a removable inner cannula. Remove the inner cannula for cleaning if it is a reusable one, or discard it if it is disposable. The inner cannula serves as a safety device. Remove the cannula if it becomes obstructed with crusts or thick secretions and the patient still has an adequate airway. The patient should always have an inner cannula in place except when cleaning it or when the tube is capped during weaning.

Tracheostomy tubes with a cuff are used for patients on mechanical ventilation to seal the airway around the tube (Figure 34–10 ■). The cuff is *not* intended to hold the tube in place. At best, it keeps the tube centered in the airway. Cuffed tubes may be used to minimize aspiration, although dependence on the cuff to prevent aspiration is not always successful (Tolentino-DelosReyes, Ruppert, & Shiao, 2007). The trachea expands during inhalation and often secretions can fall from around the cuff into the main stem bronchus. Sometimes special tubes must be used or customized to fit the patient appropriately. In patients with thick necks, the regular length tube

FIGURE 34–9 ■ Post-tracheotomy tray instruments are kept near the new tracheotomy patient for surgical access in the event of accidental decannulation.
Source: University of California, Davis Medical Center

may not be long enough to reach into the trachea, so a tube with a longer shaft must be used (Figure 34–11 ■).

■ Nursing Management of an Artificial Airway

The nursing process is used to guide the care of the patient with an artificial airway.

Assessment

Nursing assessment of the patient with a new tracheostomy includes auscultation of the lungs, monitoring of oxygen saturation, and assessment for any increase in amounts of blood in the sputum, subcutaneous emphysema in the neck, respiratory distress, and patency of the tracheostomy tube itself.

Most patients with a new tracheostomy will have some blood in their sputum and around the tracheostomy tube insertion site. If bleeding in and around the tracheotomy site is continuous and beyond mild oozing, the health care provider needs to be notified. The neck and thyroid area is rich with blood vessels, so trauma to this area during placement of the tracheotomy can lead to postoperative bleeding and may require some local cauterization or packing for control. Bleeding in the early postoperative period is usually from the thyroid vessels that are ligated during the proce-

FIGURE 34–10 ■ Shiley (A) cuffed and (B) uncuffed tracheotomy tube with disposable inner cannula.
Source: University of California, Davis Medical Center

FIGURE 34–11 ■ Shiley single-cannula tracheotomy tube used for patients who require an extra length to span the skin to trachea distance, or those who require a lower cuff placement. A single-cannula tube requires more aggressive nursing care to keep the single cannula free from lumen obstruction.
Source: University of California, Davis Medical Center

dure. Ligatures slip or the effect of local lidocaine and epinephrine is reversed. Hemorrhage seen very late in the postoperative period can be caused by erosion of the innominate artery by the tracheostomy tube through the anterior tracheal wall.

 CRITICAL ALERT *In all cases of bleeding, suction the tracheotomy tube to maintain patency of the patient's airway. Inflate the cuff if one is present. Request help to control a potentially very dangerous circumstance.*

If the patient has had a long-standing obstruction preoperatively, careful assessment of the lungs in the postoperative period is necessary. After placement of a tracheostomy, postobstructive pulmonary edema can occur in a patient with significant preoperative obstruction. Negative pressure is thought to be transmitted to the pulmonary interstitium, reducing the hydrostatic pressure around the pulmonary vessels and resulting in an increased hydrostatic pressure and interstitial water accumulation. This is referred to as postobstructive pulmonary edema (POPE) (Fidrose & Elamin, 2004). Signs and symptoms are frothy spu-

tum and moist rales on auscultation of the lungs. This condition is treated with a diuretic and ventilatory support if indicated by respiratory failure.

Interventions and Rationales

The patient should be encouraged to cough, deep breathe, and be suctioned as necessary. If the patient is able to take five to six deep breaths to maintain oxygenation, it is preferable to have the patient cough to clear secretions. The amount of tracheal suctioning should be limited, because excessive suctioning leads to irritation to the tracheal mucosa below the level of the tube. If necessary, give the patient supplemental oxygen and use a resuscitation bag prior to suctioning to prevent oxygen desaturation. The bagging should be timed to coincide with the patient's own inspiratory effort. The suction catheter should be inserted into the tube with the suction off and limited to 5 to 10 seconds, or as long as one can hold one's breath comfortably. Care should be exercised not to use suction greater than 100 mmHg pressure to prevent trauma to the tracheal mucosa. If the patient's oxygen saturation decreases after suctioning, the nurse can use the resuscitation bag with oxygen for a two- to six-breath interval to increase the patient's oxygen level, and further suctioning requires preoxygenation. If the patient is restless or agitated due to alcohol or drug withdrawal, upper extremity restraints may be necessary to keep the patient from removing the tube. When suctioning, the nurse must be careful not to injure the carina by inserting the suction catheter too far into the trachea. Suctioning a patient with a tracheostomy tube requires using only a small percentage of the suction catheter. The catheter may touch the delicate membrane of the carina and cause the patient to cough, but the catheter should not be inserted into the trachea and forcibly collide with the carina. Suctioning technique is discussed in detail in Chapter 36 .

Ensuring that the inner cannula is changed routinely to prevent occlusion is an important component of the nursing care. Depending on secretions the inner cannula can be changed every 8 to 12 hours or once a day. Care of the tracheostomy site itself involves cleaning around the tube with half-strength hydrogen peroxide on cotton swabs and rinsing with normal saline. Secretions under the tracheostomy plate can cause skin breakdown and can lead to infection if not cleaned regularly. Assess the area under the edges of the tracheostomy face plate for signs of skin breakdown. Keep the face plate flush with the skin of the neck.

Occasionally, due to the patient's anatomy, the lower edge of the plate puts pressure on the skin and can lead to skin breakdown if not assessed and protected. A split gauze dressing provides some padding, or some form of manufactured skin barrier such as DuoDerm or a stoma wafer can be used to protect the skin. The nurse needs to assess frequently for secretions undermining the barrier and change the barrier as necessary.

Outcomes and Evaluation Parameters

Outcomes for the patient with an artificial airway include lack of complications and normal oxygenation. Airway complication can occur from a variety of causes including bleeding, tube obstruction or dislodgement, and displacement into the subcutaneous tissue of the neck. Most complications of tracheotomies can be avoided by securing the tube well. Check the ties frequently and change them if they become wet or soiled. Cotton ties work well but do stretch as they become wet. The ties should be tied tightly enough so that only one finger can be placed between the skin and the ties.

The nurse should monitor the patient's oxygen and respiratory status and take note of changes in the patient's behavior. Increasing restlessness or agitation or changes in mentation (decreasing level of consciousness or increasing confusion) could indicate that the patient is not oxygenating well. If these symptoms occur remove the inner cannula and make sure the tracheostomy tube is clear; then suction the patient. If unable to pass a suction catheter down the tracheostomy tube, the tube may have become dislodged. If the tube becomes displaced or dislodged, the nursing priority is to stay with the patient and to position the patient with her head up and slightly extended. A health care provider who is able to reinsert the airway tube needs to be summoned, and the patient needs reassurance that help is on the way. If necessary the patient may need to be ventilated with a resuscitation bag until the airway is replaced. Acute respiratory distress is very frightening for the patient; therefore it is essential for the nurse to reassure the patient that everything is being done to rectify the situation. It is important to assemble the necessary equipment for reintubation or replacement of the tracheostomy tube. The obturator, which is used to guide the tracheostomy tube during insertion, should always be kept with the patient.

Decannulation

Decannulation, or removal of the tube, occurs with the resolution of the initial airway problem. This process typically begins by downsizing the size of the tracheostomy tube and/or capping the tracheostomy tube. A smaller tube allows enough air to pass around the tube and up into the natural larynx. This allows the patient to breathe in the normal physiological manner, taking in air through the nose and mouth and into the upper airway. Oxygen saturation is monitored continuously during and after this change. If the patient tolerates the downsizing, the tube is again downsized and a cap is placed over the end of the tracheostomy tube (Figure 34–12 ■).

> **CRITICAL ALERT** *If at any time the patient experiences respiratory distress during weaning, remove the cap and encourage the patient to cough. Suction if necessary, and recap the tube if the patient is able to tolerate.*

Teach the patient to occlude the end of the tracheostomy tube with a finger and to speak on exhalation. Instruct the patient to inhale through the tube, cover the tube, and exhale through the natural airway. Regaining communication can be very rewarding for the patient.

It also is critical to teach the patient how to uncap or remove the cap of the tube. This can help allay fears that may be associated with capping or the process of decannulation. Cap the patient's tube and monitor saturations for an extended period and while the patient is sleeping, before completely removing the tracheostomy. If the patient tolerates the capping throughout the night without episodes of oxygen desaturation, the health care provider removes the tracheostomy tube and places a dry sterile occlusive dressing over the site. Explain to the patient the importance of putting pressure on the site when coughing or talking to prevent air from passing through the stoma. The more consistent the patient is with this, the sooner the stomal incision will close. The incision is never closed with sutures. It is important for the wound to heal from the inside out. Closure of the skin edges before the tracheal incision itself closes can lead to subcutaneous emphysema in the neck. The dressing is changed as

FIGURE 34–12 ■ Shiley tracheotomy tube with red cap for weaning and eventual decannulation. If possible, the patient should be taught to uncap the tube if distress occurs. The nurse in the hospital must be vigilant for subtle and overt signs of distress during this process.
Source: University of California, Davis Medical Center

needed until there is no evidence of air passage through the incision and the skin edges are approximated. Wound care to the healing site is typically ordered twice a day and as needed, with half- or full-strength hydrogen peroxide and rinsing with normal saline before applying a dry dressing.

Oral communication is very important. If the patient cannot be decannulated for reasons such as vocal cord dysfunction, then the use of a speaking valve may help. These valves are one-way valves that allow the patient to breathe in through the valve; the valve then shuts and the patient then breathes out through his natural airway (Figure 34–13 ■). This flutter valve is very simple but very effective. Some types can be used inline and assist ventilator-dependent patients to speak.

Discharge Priorities for Patients with Tracheostomy

If a patient is to go home with a tracheostomy, the goal is for the patient to be safe at home, resume normal activities, and have an acceptable quality of life. Safety with an artificial airway is the priority for teaching. The patient and family must demonstrate safe care before discharge. This should include suctioning, saline instillation, wound care, inner cannula care, tracheostomy change, and emergency measures. Encourage the patient and family to participate in care early in the hospitalization to increase their confidence.

Total Laryngectomy Permanent Airway

Removal of the larynx or laryngectomy necessitates a permanent tracheal artificial airway. (Refer to the section on head and neck cancer for more information on causes for removal and management of patients who have had a laryngectomy.) A similar surgery called laryngotracheal separation is done for patients with severe aspiration resulting in repeated, frequent hospitalizations for aspiration pneumonia. In both surgeries the trachea is transected, and the distal portion of the trachea is brought to the skin surface in the anterior neck and sewn into

FIGURE 34–13 ■ The Shiley speaking valve with oxygen port is a one-way valve that allows airflow on exhalation upward into the larynx, thereby supporting speech. These valves are fragile and any secretions interfere with their operation.
Source: University of California, Davis Medical Center

place. This surgery completely separates the trachea from the esophagus and thus prevents problems with aspiration. However, because air no longer passes through the structures of the larynx, such as the vocal cords, the patient will not be able to speak in the normal way.

The loss of the ability to communicate verbally can be very frightening to the patient. Few things are as disabling as the impairment resulting from total loss of laryngeal speech. The impact of the total removal of the larynx is so dramatic that it may impact the patient's decision regarding treatment. Even though the total surgical removal of the larynx may provide the greatest chance of successfully controlling a malignancy, it is not unusual for a patient to knowingly compromise a chance for cure by choosing another form of treatment that would result in preservation of the larynx and the ability to speak (Bailey et al., 2006). Much time and care must be taken with these patients and their families during the diagnostic and preoperative phases. It is important for the health care provider to explain to the patient and family all of the risks and benefits of each form of treatment. It is equally important that the patient feel support in whatever decision is made—even though it might not seem the best choice for complete removal of the disease. Some patients opt for other treatments first, radiation or a combination of radiation and chemotherapy, or only a partial laryngectomy in order to preserve their voice. If cancer recurs or there is a significant problem with aspiration, then the patient may subsequently consent to a total laryngectomy.

■ Nursing Management

The nursing process guides the management of the postoperative laryngectomy patient. As always the airway is the first priority.

Interventions and Rationales

The laryngectomy stoma must be kept clean and free of crusts. It is a *life-threatening* situation if the laryngectomy stoma becomes obstructed with mucus or crusts. The outcomes for these patients are a patent airway and normal oxygenation as evidenced by normal oxygen saturation levels, lungs that are clear to auscultation, and unlabored respirations. Crusts of secretions and blood form when there is not enough humidity. The lungs are accustomed to heated, humidified, and filtered inspired air by the nose and upper airway. With the trachea positioned directly out to the neck now, this process is bypassed. It is important, therefore, to provide warm humidified mist to the patient's stoma to keep the airway moist. Occasionally the placement of a stoma button can keep the skin edges from contracting (Figure 34–14 ■, p. 914). Stoma buttons also can be used if a dressing around the stoma endangers the lumen of the airway.

Until the internal incision lines in the pharynx heal, the patient will not be able to eat orally. This typically takes 5 to 7 days postlaryngectomy. For this reason, a nasogastric feeding tube is placed intraoperatively. Before the patient resumes an oral diet, a barium swallow is completed to evaluate the internal suture lines of the pharynx, thereby ensuring that the suture lines are intact and there is no leak of barium through the incisions, referred to as internal dehiscence. Aspiration *cannot* be a problem for these patients because the esophagus and airway are

FIGURE 34–14 ■ Bivona stoma buttons for laryngectomy are placed into the laryngectomy stoma to prevent cicatricule (or circular) scarring and maintain the patient's only airway.
Source: University of California, Davis Medical Center

completely separated. There may be some swallowing issues initially as the patient learns to control food and fluids in the reconstructed esophagus.

Meticulous wound care includes cleaning incision lines with hydrogen peroxide and rinsing with normal saline to decrease infection and promote wound healing. Many times patients undergoing this surgery are poorly nourished. Difficulties eating and drinking due to tumor size and location lead to weight loss and malnourishment preoperatively. Patients with poor nutrition or patients with prior radiation to the area tend to take longer to heal and are at higher risk for complications, such as infection.

In the event an infection causing an abscess, called an oropharyngeal fistula, does develop, the health care provider may open the area widely to drain purulence, and begin wound packing with saline–soaked, wet-to-dry dressings. This allows the wound to heal from the inside outward to the skin.

CRITICAL ALERT *Notify the heath care provider if the temperature increases or there is swelling, pain, or redness at the suture line. Separation of the suture lines may be indicative of a wound infection or potential fistula formation.*

As with the patient with a tracheostomy or someone on voice rest, it is important to be patient with the new laryngectomy patient as he or she tries to communicate. This can be an extremely frustrating time for the patient and for the nurse if care is not taken to establish a workable form of communication. It is important to acknowledge the patient's frustration and to explain to her that writing and pantomiming, though tedious, are very effective communication tools. Some patients articulate well enough to read lips and use gestures so that writing may not be necessary all the time. For others, writing is the only way to communicate. Pen and paper or a dry erase board should be provided for this purpose.

Some individuals may not be able to write to communicate, which increases the frustration. Thus, the nurse should assess the patient's ability to read and write prior to surgery and establish a suitable form of communication. Remember that almost 50% of Americans are functionally illiterate, and it is difficult for low-literacy patients to read and understand such routine health information as dosage instructions on medication bottles, poi-

son warnings, appointment slips and consent forms, and written patient education information (Kutner, Greenberg, Jun, & Paulsen, 2006). Answering call lights promptly is extremely important for patients who cannot speak.

Health Promotion

Nursing assessment in the preoperative setting must include assessment of the patient's support systems. It is important to determine if the patient and spouse or other primary support person are able to read and write. Initially this will be the most used form of communication for the patient to express his needs and concerns. The Cultural Considerations box addresses the needs of patients who may not understand English.

It is important for the patient to understand that various options are available for vocal restoration procedures. Meeting with a speech therapist preoperatively and discussing these options may help the patient realize that having a total laryngectomy does not necessarily mean the end to communication with some form of speech. It may be helpful to have someone who has had the same procedure and has been trained to work with patients who have had laryngectomies visit with the patient to show him how to speak after surgery and how the voice sounds.

Tracheoesophageal puncture (TEP) is a procedure that can be done at the time of the original surgery or at a later date when healing is completed. This procedure provides voice restoration to patients who have had a total laryngectomy. A puncture is made through the posterior wall of the trachea into the anterior wall of the esophagus. A feeding tube is threaded through this puncture and used to help form a tract by acting as a stent. It also is used to feed the patient enterally while the surgical site heals. After the tract heals and matures, a one-way prosthetic valve is inserted into this tract for purposes of speech (Figure 34–15 ■). The purpose of the valve is to allow the patient to shunt air from the trachea into the esophagus, but not allow food and fluid from the esophagus to enter the trachea. The airflow through the one-way valve causes vibration in the upper esophagus when the stoma is occluded, and the mouth, tongue, and lips articulate the sound to produce speech.

Gerontological Considerations

One of the more common and difficult problems with the older patient is postoperative delirium. Family members become concerned when they see their loved ones picking and pulling at tubes, removing IV lines, attempting to get out of bed alone de-

CULTURAL CONSIDERATIONS for Patients with Total Laryngectomy

For patients with a total laryngectomy who speak a language other than English, communication can be even more difficult. It is helpful to have the family assist by making signs with words both in English and the patient's native language for things such as "pain," "bathroom," and "difficulty breathing." This allows the patient to just point to the appropriate sign. If no one in the family speaks English, use interpreting services. If a staff member speaks the patient's native language, assign her as one of the primary nurses. This can ease the patient's fears of not being understood.

FIGURE 34–15 ■ Bivona tracheoesophageal puncture speech prosthesis. This speech prosthesis is placed into the TEP to shunt air from the stoma (lungs) into the esophagus to produce speech after total laryngectomy.
Source: University of California, Davis Medical Center

spite frequent reminders to call for help, and generally behaving in an uncharacteristic manner (Jett, 2007). According to Kagan (personal communication, 2004), it is estimated that as many as 50% of hospitalized patients over the age of 65 experience some level of delirium during the course of their hospital stay.

Causes for the delirium include anesthesia, medications, stress, and/or an unfamiliar place with unfamiliar faces. It is important not to restrain the elderly physically or pharmacologically, unless absolutely necessary for safety. One-to-one supervision to prevent restraining the patient can help to decrease the length of the period of delirium. If possible, the number of new medications added to the patient's home regimen should be limited.

It is prudent to request a psychological evaluation to assess the patient and to perform the Mini-Mental State (State) Examination (MMSE) (Brannon, 2006). The MMSE is a nationally recognized tool that can be used to systematically and thoroughly assess mental status and separate patients with cognitive impairment from those without it. If used repeatedly the instrument is able to measure changes in cognitive status that may benefit from intervention. The MMSE is considered to be a standard diagnostic instrument by the American Psychiatric Association and, as such, is used in a variety of settings. Chart 34–4 (p. 916) provides more information about the MMSE. When used, the health care provider can assess orientation, memory attention, calculation, language, writing, and drawing. Preoperative cognitive function is an invaluable piece of information. If the delirium is not cleared by discharge, it is important to assess whether or not the family will be able to manage their loved one at home, or whether a temporary stay in a skilled nursing facility might be necessary until the patient clears mentally and can return safely to the home environment. Most likely if the patient is older, the spouse or primary caregiver also is elderly, so it is important to be realistic about how much he or she can do. Patient safety is the first priority.

Other issues with the older patient may be limited mobility, decreased manual dexterity, and decreased vision and hearing. Changing tracheostomy ties, managing tube feedings, and performing wound care can be difficult for someone with limited mobility and limited vision. Patients going home post-tracheostomy or with vocal cord paralysis may have decreased volume with their voice and if their spouse has impaired hearing, communication can be difficult.

Head and Neck Cancer

Head and neck cancer is one of the more uncommon cancers; however, the challenges the patient, family, and health care team face during diagnosis, treatment, and recovery are intense and persistent. Ablative surgery often is used to treat this type of cancer, leaving the patient with facial disfigurement and functional impairment. The use of an interdisciplinary team (early in diagnosis) will provide the patient with the clinical expertise that will optimize the patient's recovery potential and improve his quality of life.

If detected early head and neck cancer is treatable and curable. It is, however, an insidious disease and may not present itself until the patient has a large tumor burden. Discussions with family and significant others often help to explain the consequences of head and neck cancer and its treatment. Unfortunately, if not treated, this type of cancer is very disfiguring and alters the normal functions of breathing, eating, smelling, tasting, and facial attributes and expressions. Decisions regarding treatment must be informed decisions that include the outcome without treatment and the implications, risks, and benefits of surgery and radiation therapy.

Etiology

A variety of risk factors are associated with head and neck cancer, although some patients do not have any of the known risk factors, so it is not possible to know for sure how much they contributed to causing the cancer (American Cancer Society [ACS], 2006). The Risk Factors box (p. 917) lists the most common risk factors associated with head and neck cancer.

People of Asian heritage, predominantly first generation, can develop nasopharyngeal cancer from the Epstein–Barr virus. It seems that their culture-based risk factor for nasopharyngeal cancer from the consumption of salt-preserved fish decreases with each generation (Chang & Adami, 2006). The cessation of tobacco product (cigarettes, cigars, chewing tobacco, snuff) use and the limitation of alcohol in combination with tobacco is a goal for health promotion (Rudy, 2006).

Pathophysiology

The predominant cell type in head and neck cancer is squamous cell cancer. There are many other types, but in far less frequent occurrence. Squamous cells or epithelial cells line the aerodigestive tract and are irritated and altered by the environmental agents outlined earlier. Cells change from the normal fast growing and dividing cells into altered cells that grow along tissue planes and into adjacent structures. Chapter 64 ⊚ includes a complete discussion of the pathogenesis of cancer.

Laboratory and Diagnostic Procedures

Diagnosing head and neck cancer involves the accurate assessment of health history, physical condition, social factors, and presence of support systems. When a patient presents to an otolaryngologist, a thorough history is taken with emphasis on specific symptoms in the head and neck. Length of time each symptom has been present and sequence of symptom development also is documented. The 12 cranial nerves are evaluated carefully because they provide important clues to the invasion

CHART 34–4   The Mini-Mental State Examination

The MMSE is an 11-question measure that tests five areas of cognitive function: orientation, registration, retention and calculation, recall, and language. The maximum score is 30. A score of 23 or lower is indicative of cognitive impairment. The MMSE takes only 5 to 10 minutes to administer and is, therefore, practical to use repeatedly and routinely.

The MMSE is effective as a screening tool for cognitive impairment with older, community dwelling, hospitalized, or institutionalized adults. Assessment of an older adult's cognitive function is best achieved when it is done routinely, systematically, and thoroughly. Examples of questions included in the Mini-Mental State Examination are shown below.

MMSE Sample Items

Orientation to Time

"What is the date?"

Registration

"Listen carefully. I am going to say three words. You say them back after I stop.

Ready? Here they are…

APPLE (pause), PENNY (pause), TABLE (pause). Now repeat those words back to me."

[Repeat up to 5 times, but score only the first trial.]

Naming

"What is this?" [Point to a pencil or pen.]

Reading

"Please read this and do what it says." [Show examinee the words on the stimulus form.]

CLOSE YOUR EYES

Source: Reproduced by special permission of the Publisher, Psychological Assessment Resources, Inc., 16204 North Florida Avenue, Lutz, Florida 33549, from the Mini Mental State Examination, by Marshal Folstein and Susan Folstein, Copyright 1975, 1998, 2001 by Mini Mental LLC, Inc. Published 2001 by Psychological Assessment Resources, Inc. Further reproduction is prohibited without permission of PAR, Inc. The MMSE can be purchased from PAR, Inc. by calling (813) 968-3003

- *Tobacco Use*—Approximately 90% of people with oral cavity and oropharyngeal cancers use tobacco; risk is correlated with the length and amount smoked or chewed.
  - Tobacco smoke from cigarettes, cigars, or pipes can cause cancers anywhere in the mouth or throat, as well as causing cancers of the larynx (voice box).
  - Pipe smoking has a particularly significant risk for cancers in the area of the lips that touch the pipe stem.
  - Oral tobacco products (snuff or chewing tobacco) are associated with cancers of the cheek, gums, and inner surface of the lips. Long time snuff use poses an especially high risk.
- *Heavy Drinking*—Drinking alcohol strongly increases a smoker's risk of developing oral cavity and oropharyngeal cancers. Particularly heavy, non-smokers and alcohol drinkers also have a high risk of these cancers; however, the combination of drinking and smoking is the most dangerous.
- *Gender*—Oral and oropharyngeal cancers are about twice as common in men as in women, possibly due to the fact that men are more likely to use tobacco and alcohol, though this trend is changing.
- *Ultraviolet Light*—Cancers of the lip are more common in people who have prolonged exposure to sunlight.
- *Poor Nutrition*—A diet low in fruits and vegetables is linked with an increased risk of cancers of the oral cavity and oropharynx.
- *Human Papilloma Virus Infection*—HPV infection may contribute to oral and oropharyngeal cancers, 20–30% of such cancers.
- *Lichen Planus*—A severe case may slightly increase the risk of oral cancer in middle aged people.
- *Uncertain, Unproven or Controversial Risk Factors*
  - *Mouthwash*—Some studies have suggested that mouthwash with high alcohol content might be linked to a higher risk of oral and oropharyngeal cancers.
  - *Irritation From Dentures*—It has been suggested that long-term irritation of the lining of the mouth caused by poorly fitting dentures may be a risk factor for oral cancer.

Source: American Cancer Society. (2006). *Detailed guide: Oral cavity and oropharyngeal cancer. What are the risk factors for oral cavity and oropharyngeal cancer?* Retrieved August 23, 2007, from http://www.cancer.org/docroot/CRI/content/CRI_2_4_2X_What_are_the_risk_factors_for_oral_cavity_and_oropharyngeal_cancer_60.asp?rnav=cri

and location of the cancer. This information helps the health care provider better understand the patient's disease and recovery potential.

Integral to the complete evaluation of the patient and before a final decision for treatment is complete, the patient usually undergoes a panendoscopy. **Panendoscopy** includes tumor mapping and biopsy to confirm histologic diagnosis; it includes bronchoscope, esophagoscopy, nasal endoscopy, examination of the oral cavity, and anatomical mapping of the cancer. This tumor mapping directs the therapy that is recommended to the patient. From a surgical perspective this allows the surgeon to determine what must be removed and what can be saved during a surgical resection, and the method of reconstruction. The Diagnostic Tests box (p. 918) outlines specific tests for head and neck cancer.

Clinical Manifestations

Clinical manifestations of head and neck cancer include sore throat without fever, unilateral earache, change in voice or articulation, dental changes, and weight loss. Most symptoms are related directly to the location and invasion of the cancer, such as change in articulation with an oral tongue cancer, or hoarseness and dysphagia (difficulty swallowing) with a base of tongue or laryngeal cancer. Many people first recognize a mass in the neck, and may not even be aware of the site of the primary tumor. This neck mass represents nodal extent of the disease and the investigation must be done to locate the primary tumor.

Collaborative Management

A multidisciplinary team of experts including otolaryngologists, medical oncologists, radiation oncologists, social service providers, clinical nurse specialists, speech pathologists, nurses, and dentists or maxillofacial prosthodontists provides a collaborative approach to providing care for patients with head and neck cancer. This panel of experts reviews the patient's history, findings from the physical exam, and results of radiologic studies. This panel also examines the patient. The team develops a consensus opinion for the best chance for cure and develops a plan of therapy. Then, in a private session the plan is presented to patients so they can make their decisions. The nursing role is to participate as a team member, to act as an advocate for the patient, and to help interpret medical terms into lay terms for the patient and family.

The patient and family require assistance in understanding the choices and plan of care because many choices and decisions regarding treatment are available. Patients must understand that they may choose no treatment. Although unusual, some individuals elect no therapy as their option, with the ultimate outcome being death. When such a choice is made, it is important for the patient, family, friends, and significant others to understand that therapy is available for symptoms and palliative care (Meyers & Linder, 2003). Aggressive symptom control can be very powerful in life-threatening illnesses. Patients also must understand the process that lies ahead and the resources that are available to help. Aggressive palliative care and hospice can be an integral part of this process (Meyers, 1999).

Staging System

Head and neck cancer is defined by the organ or origins of the tumor, for example, the larynx, tongue, tonsil, and sinus, with subdefinitions within parts of that organ. Once a diagnosis is made, staging or evaluation is done to determine the size and extent of the solid tumor, using the American Joint Committee on Cancer guide (Greene et al., 2002). *Tumor staging* is an internationally recognized method of comparison of types, sizes, and locations of cancers (Greene et al., 2002). With this staging system, tumors are described by the acronym TNM. The *T* stands for tumor, which includes the size. The *N* represents the presence or absence of nodal extension, particularly into the cervical nodal system in the necks. The *M* represents metastatic disease to other organ systems, as described by clinical, laboratory, and radiographic investigations. Each section (TNM) has many subdivisions that further elucidate the extent of the tumor involvement. This staging system allows each health care practitioner to

DIAGNOSTIC TESTS for Head and Neck Cancer

Test	Expected Abnormality	Rationale for Abnormality
Fine-needle biopsy	Fine-needle aspirate of tumor or neck nodes. Taken with a very small needle, so as not to invade tissue planes.	To extract cells for microscopic evaluation, To determine cell type of tumors.
Fiber-optic laryngoscopy	Uses fiber-optic light bundle channel to transmit light. Local or no anesthesia required.	To look into the upper aerodigestive tract without using general anesthesia.
Panendoscopy	Includes laryngoscopy, nasopharyngoscopy, and esophagoscopy, examination of the oral cavity, tumor mapping, and biopsy. Conducted under general anesthesia.	To completely evaluate the upper aerodigestive tract with the patient asleep. Define the organ of origin. Map the extent or regions of the tumor and biopsy the tumor for pathologic conformation.
Blood tests	Chemistry 20. Complete blood count. Liver function tests.	To evaluate for alterations in liver function that may indicate metastatic disease and or liver failure.
CT head and neck	Computerized tomography.	To evaluate the extent of tumor involvement focusing on tissue.
CT chest	Computerized tomography.	To evaluate the lungs for metastatic disease or primary lung cancer.
MRI	Magnetic resonance imaging.	To evaluate the extent of tumor involvement and bony structures.
BTO	Balloon test occlusion.	To evaluate the carotid artery and assess the ability of the contralateral carotid artery to crossfill if the artery is resected.
SPECT scan	Single photon emission computerized tomography.	To evaluate brain activity before and after BTO. To assess for brain activity after carotid artery resection.
PET scan	Proton emission scan based on the uptake of glucose in tissues. Hypermetabolic tissues can be identified.	To measure the biological and metabolic changes associated with disease.
Doppler	This test uses Doppler technology to evaluate the blood flow in an artery or vein.	To assess the competency of an artery or vein for use in microvascular free flap reconstruction.

compare treatment results and survival with those of similar patients around the world. Chapter 64 includes a complete description of the TNM staging system.

Medical Management

Traditionally head and neck cancer has been treated with radiation alone, surgery alone, or the combination of surgery followed by radiation. Currently there also is the option of radiation with chemotherapy used to make the tumor more sensitive to the radiation therapy (Vokes & Stenson, 2003). The location and size of the tumor, patient choices, and the patient's general medical condition dictate most treatment recommendations (Forastiere et al., 2003). Ultimately, the choice is the patient's own. Chart 34–5 outlines the options for treatment of head and neck cancer.

Radiation is used not only as an attempt to cure, but also to save organ function and avoid debilitating surgery. Radiation has its own inherent side effects of permanent dry mouth, loss of taste or smell, and problems swallowing. Gene therapy is a very experimental, but promising, therapy and researchers hope it will be a viable frontline choice in the future (Merritt, Roth, & Logothetis, 2001; Nettelbeck & Curiel, 2003). Gene transfer is a new treatment modality that introduces new genes into a cancerous cell or the surrounding tissue to cause cell death or slow

CHART 34–5 **Treatment Options for Head and Neck Cancer**

Surgery, conventional or laser resection

Surgery and postoperative radiation therapy

Radiation therapy

Radiation and sensitizing chemotherapy

Radiation and conventional chemotherapy

Chemotherapy

Gene therapy

Combination of any of the above

Alternative therapies

No therapy; just palliative care and/or hospice

the growth of the cancer. This therapy technique is very flexible, and a wide range of genes and vectors are being evaluated in clinical trials (Cross & Burmester, 2006).

Early stage disease (stage I or II) typically is treated with either surgery or radiation therapy. In moderately advanced disease (stage III), those cases deemed resectable are treated with surgery plus postoperative radiation therapy; or radiation therapy with or without surgery, as feasible. Chemoradiation therapy is considered in select cases, based on the patient's choice and general medical condition. Advanced, unresectable disease is treated with chemoradiation therapy or definitive radiation therapy. The patient should be informed of all aspects of therapy including the pros and cons of each treatment. Chapter 64 ☺ includes a complete description of radiation and chemotherapy.

Surgical Resection

There are six general types of surgical resection: oral cavity resection, laryngectomy (partial or total), temporal bone resection, maxillary (with or without orbital exenteration) or bimaxillary resection, skull base resection, and the combination of each. Each surgery has its own subgroups based on the site of origin of the tumor. Each surgical resection presents with unique requirements because of the location of the tumor. Essentially all of the surgical approaches have similar needs in relation to airway, wound care, nutrition, self-image, self-care education, and recovery.

Neck dissection may accompany tumor resections. A neck dissection is necessary for metastatic disease in the lymph nodes of the neck or when there is a very high suspicion of tumor because of the behavior or tumor bulk at the primary site. A **neck dissection** includes lymph tissue, the jugular vein, the spinal accessory nerve, and the sternocleidomastoid muscle (SCM). Chart 34–6 outlines the various surgical approaches for head and neck cancer.

Reconstruction Flaps and Grafts

In otolaryngology cancer surgery, after the tumor is resected, the goal is to reconstruct the patient for optimum function and cosmetics. The surgical site can be primarily closed or left open to granulate by secondary intention. Frequently flaps and composite grafts of muscle, bone, and tissue are used for reconstruction. A **myocutaneous flap**, composed of muscle and skin, is used to reconstruct the defect caused by the tumor resection. A flap from the pectoralis major is commonly used for reconstruction. This rotation flap is supplied by its native blood supply, but rotated into the surgical defect. Free flaps that are harvested from a distant site also can be used for reconstruction. Common sites include the radial forearm, fibula, scapula, lateral arm, or lateral thigh. These flaps can include tissue, bone, and muscle as well as the artery and vein for the microvascular anastomosis (Figure 34–16 ■, p. 920).

A dermis graft may be harvested using the dermis layer of skin to cover the carotid artery or the bed of the resection. It acts as a watertight second layer seal. This allows the tissue to adhere and heal to the wound bed.

When assessing a reconstruction flap, myocutaneous or free, it should be pink and warm with brisk capillary refill (<2 seconds). A flap that is *blue* or cyanotic is a sign of venous congestion, *white* indicates no arterial supply, and *deep red* is a sign of partial venous congestion with a vigorous arterial supply. Tracheostomy and cupola ties should be positioned away from the graft to prevent pressure on the area, which may lead to impaired or decreased blood flow to the tissue and loss of the graft. The head position should be maintained straight or toward the operative side to prevent pressure or tension on the flap. The head of the bed is elevated to at least 30 degrees to facilitate drainage of fluid and to prevent edema of the head and neck area.

CHART 34–6	**Otolaryngology Surgical Resections for Head and Neck Cancer**	
Type of Surgery	**Major Areas Resected** *(Predicated on primary tumor location)*	**Major Implications**
Oral cavity resection	Tongue, buccal mucosa, mandible	Speech, articulation, chewing, swallowing, facial cosmesis
Oropharyngeal resections, bimaxillary resection	Tongue, base of tongue, tonsil, maxilla, mandible	Swallowing, speech, aspiration Facial cosmesis
Laryngectomy, partial (often called hemi or vertical hemi laryngectomy)	Larynx, partial	Speech, swallowing Aspiration (partial laryngectomy only) Cosmesis
Laryngectomy, total	Larynx, total	Speech, cosmesis *Complete* separation of airway and esophagus
Temporal bone resection	Temporal bone, parotid, maxilla, mandible	Hearing, balance Cosmesis Facial nerve impairment or paralysis Eye protection concerns
Maxillary, with or without orbital exenteration	Maxilla, orbit	Speech, swallowing, chewing, sight Cosmesis
Skull base resection (anterior, middle, posterior, or combination)	Skull base carotid artery	Cognition, speech, swallowing, balance Cosmesis
Neck dissection (radical, modified, *paired* with the above surgeries for lymph node involvement)	Lymph nodes, SCM, jugular vein, spinal accessory nerve CN XI	Impaired lymph drainage Trapezius muscle paralysis Facial edema (especially if bilateral neck dissections are performed at the same time) Cerebral edema with bilateral neck dissection
Combination of any of the above surgical resections	Any anatomical *combination* as required by tumor invasion for oncologic purposes	*All of the above* predicated on location of tumor and invasion

FIGURE 34–16 ■ Pectoralis major myocutaneous reconstruction flap.
Source: University of California, Davis Medical Center

The free flap is assessed for a pulse by Doppler per the surgeon's order, typically every 2 hours (Figure 34–17 ■). It also is important in the immediate postoperative period to maintain an adequate blood pressure with a mean arterial pressure (MAP) of at least 60 to ensure tissue perfusion to the graft.

■ Nursing Management

Nursing care management priorities for patients with head and neck cancer are airway maintenance, pain management, and nutrition. If surgery was done, these patients have special needs and consideration including wound management, drain assessment and care, oral care, wound complications, and carotid artery exposure assessment and management. There are also special nursing management priorities related to reconstruction flaps. The Nursing Process: Patient Care Plan outlines the care for a patient who has had an orbital exenteration and maxillectomy.

Airway Management

As always the patient's airway is the first priority. The outcome for these patients is to maintain a patent airway and normal gas

FIGURE 34–17 ■ Nursing care equipment for Doppler monitoring for arterial patency following microvascular free flap reconstruction.
Source: University of California, Davis Medical Center

exchange. Critical symptoms that need to be assessed on an ongoing basis are shortness of breath, stridor, blood-tinged sputum, and infection. Some blood may be present in the sputum, especially within the first 24 hours of having surgery and/or placement of a tracheostomy tube. Clinical manifestations of airway obstruction are increased work of breathing and increased use of accessory muscles, especially facial musculature that uses a higher amount of oxygen. There also may be an increased heart rate and decreased oxygen saturation levels. Nursing assessment of the airway needs to include the type of airway that is being used. There are many types and varieties of tracheotomy and endotracheal tubes. It is important for the nurse to become familiar with the different types and their uses. A complete discussion of airway assessment and management was presented earlier in this chapter.

Nursing interventions include securing the airway with the appropriate ties in order to prevent the possibility of the tube being dislodged or accidentally removed. The tracheostomy tube ties should be secured to the chest laterally with suspended ties. Circumferential ties can place pressure on the incision lines or reconstruction flaps or grafts. The ties should be changed every day or when soiled to decrease the possibility of infection. The tracheostomy site should be cleaned on a regular basis such as every 8 hours and more frequently as needed to remove crusts and secretions that could obstruct the airway. If the tracheostomy tube has an inner cannula, it should be changed if disposable or cleaned when every tie tracheostomy care is done. This will prevent the buildup of secretions in the tube and the possibility of airway obstruction. Frequent assessment is essential to patient safety when there are large amounts of secretions. (See earlier section for a complete description of the care of a patient with a tracheostomy tube.) If the patient is unable to clear the secretions from the airway independently, suctioning is indicated.

All patients who have an artificial airway require humidification to the airway because the normal upper airway passages that humidify sections are bypassed. This is done by tracheotomy cupola or collar. Many times in the early postoperative period, a patient is unable to clear her own secretions and may require bagging and deep suctioning. This procedure will mobilize mucous plugs, stimulate a cough, and clear the airway.

Patients who have had long surgical cases, large amounts of sedation, or have underlying lung conditions may require mechanical ventilation during the early postoperative period. Patients with head and neck cancer often have long histories of smoking with related chronic lung disease. Because their thorax or abdomen is not interrupted and their ventilation is not compromised, they usually wean early and easily from the ventilator. These patients need to be carefully but aggressively weaned as soon as they are awake and spontaneously breathing. Close monitoring is indicated including, pulse oximetry, arterial blood gases (ABGs), and respiratory rate and effort. The cuff of the tracheotomy tube should be deflated when the patient is off positive pressure ventilation. This will prevent serious complications that may include airway scarring and stenosis at the cuff site.

Other measures to improve airway and gas exchange include turning, coughing, and deep breathing, respiratory treatments with bronchodilators, and chest physiotherapy. Although very time consuming and labor intensive, early mobilization and

NURSING PROCESS: Patient Care Plan for Head and Neck Cancer

Assessment of Gas Exchange

Subjective Data:
Do you feel like you are getting enough air?
Are you short of breath?
Do you have any preexisting health problems such as heart, lung, or kidney disease?
Do you smoke? If so, for how long?

Objective Data:
Oxygen saturation
Work of breathing (e.g., gasping, increased rate, loudness)
Heart rate
Nail bed and skin color
Use of accessory respiratory muscles
Cough present, type of secretions
Level of consciousness and orientation
Lung sounds
Arterial blood gases

Nursing Assessment and Diagnoses	Outcomes and Evaluation Parameters	Planning and Interventions with *Rationales*
Nursing Diagnosis: *Risk for Impaired Gas Exchange* related to potential for airway obstruction due to cancer or surgery.	**Outcome:** Adequate gas exchange. *Evaluation Parameters:* Free of dyspnea: unlabored respirations < 24/min. Alert and oriented. Clear breath sounds. No restlessness, cyanosis, or fatigue. Oxygen saturation and ABGs are within normal limits.	**Interventions and *Rationales*:** Assess for adventitious or diminished breath sounds. *Indicates decreased gas exchange.* Note presence of cough and amount, color, and consistency of sputum *to assess for inhalation injury.* Monitor ABGs and oxygen saturation *to assess adequacy of gas exchange and level of shock state.* Monitor respiratory rate and depth *to assess for respiratory distress.* Monitor restlessness and confusion. *Indicators of inadequate gas exchange with resultant brain hypoxia.* Observe for cyanosis, especially in the mucous membranes. *Indicators of inadequate gas exchange with resultant tissue hypoxia.* Turn, cough, deep breathe, elevate head of bed, instruct on use of incentive spirometry. *Measures to promote gas exchange.* Administer humidified oxygen as prescribed *to loosen secretions and promote airway clearance.* Report respiratory distress to the health care provider. *Medical intervention may be indicated to prevent respiratory failure.* Assess need for suctioning and/or endotracheal intubation *to maintain adequate gas exchange.* **Tracheostomy:** • Cuff inflated while on ventilator • Always check cuff pressures • Cuff deflated at all other times • Position by securing from shoulders (not chest) Stomahesive and Elastoplast • Wound care • Remove crusts over suture lines • Spare tube at bedside (Bivona or similar stoma button if stoma contracts). *To maintain a patent airway.*

Assessment of Knowledge Regarding Diagnosis and Treatment

Subjective Data:
What do you understand about your diagnosis and treatment plan?
Do you have questions about the treatment program?
What would you like me to tell you about your diagnosis?

Objective Data:
Facial expressions
Verbalization of questions by patient and family

(continued)

Nursing Assessment and Diagnoses	Outcomes and Evaluation Parameters	Planning and Interventions with *Rationales*
Nursing Diagnosis: *Deficient Knowledge* related to diagnosis and treatment	**Outcome:** Adequate knowledge of treatment regimen. ***Evaluation Parameter:*** Patient and family will verbalize understanding of treatments and care.	**Interventions and *Rationales:*** Assess patient/family's readiness and ability to learn and individual learning needs. *The person must be psychologically ready to learn.* Determine level of existing knowledge. *Begin the teaching where existing knowledge ends.* Instruct patient and significant other about anatomic changes related to nasal and paranasal sinus surgery. *Preoperative education empowers the patient and decreases anxiety.* Provide factual information about diagnosis, treatments, and prognosis *to increase knowledge and understanding.* Explain all procedures in simple, concise language and allow for questions *to increase understanding.* Encourage questions. *Keeps open communication and augments understanding.* Provide ongoing education about treatment plan and rationale. *Ongoing education is necessary as situations and conditions change.* Document response to teaching *to assist health care team when implementing a teaching plan.*

Assessment of Cerebrospinal Fluid (CSF) Leak Related to Repair of Dural Defect

Subjective Data:
Do you have a headache or blurred vision?
Do you feel drowsy?

Objective Data:
Nasal drainage for presence of CSF

Nursing Assessment and Diagnoses	Outcomes and Evaluation Parameters	Planning and Interventions with *Rationales*
Nursing Diagnosis: *Risk for Injury* related to CSF leak	**Outcome:** Orbital graft site will heal without complications. ***Evaluation Parameter:*** No evidence of CSF leak.	**Interventions and *Rationales:*** Observe all nasal drainage for CSF leak with a halo test. CSF on a clean dressing demonstrates a halo of clear encircled with a red–tinged halo. Notify the surgeon when leak occurs. *This indicates an abnormal leak.* Instruct patient not to strain and to avoid excessive coughing *to minimize increased intracranial pressure.*

Assessment of Perioperative Anxiety Related to Diagnosis, Hospitalization, and Surgery

Subjective Data:
Tell me what you are feeling about your diagnosis and treatment plan?
Who are the people in your life that are your support system?
How have you handled fearful situations in the past?

Objective Data:
Facial expressions
Mood
Verbalization of fear regarding injury, impact on family, and future

Nursing Assessment and Diagnoses	Outcomes and Evaluation Parameters	Planning and Interventions with *Rationales*
Nursing Diagnosis: *Anxiety* related to changes in health status/role functioning; situational crisis	**Outcomes:** Patient will verbalize fears and concerns. Accurate preoperative teaching will help decrease patient's fear of the unknown. ***Evaluation Parameter:*** Patient states she is comfortable with care and interventions.	**Interventions and *Rationales:*** Assess and document level of anxiety *to track trends in anxiety levels.* Explore with the patient/family techniques to reduce anxiety. *This gives the patient a sense of control and opens communication about the subject.* Provide factual information concerning diagnosis, treatment, disfigurement, disabilities, and prognosis. *Truthful explanations increase trust and potentially decrease anxiety.* Explain all procedures and allow time for mental preparation. *This decreases fear and anxiety of the unknown.* Explore with patient effective ways to minimize anxiety. *This gives the patient a sense of control.* Instruct patient on use of relaxation techniques *to relieve anxiety.* Assess need for and administer antianxiety and pain medication. *If alternative measures are not effective, the patient may need antianxiety agents.* Assist patient/family in setting realistic goals for progress. *Indicates effectiveness of emotional adjustment.* Consider psychiatric counseling for patients/families who exhibit inability to accept situation. *Provide an ongoing plan and interventions to promote long-term relief of anxiety.*

NURSING PROCESS: Patient Care Plan for Head and Neck Cancer—*Continued*

Assessment of Impaired Skin Integrity Related to Surgery

Subjective Data:
Where are you hurting?

Objective Data:
Color, blanching, odor, bleeding from graft donor and surgical site
Size and depth of wound

Nursing Assessment and Diagnoses	Outcomes and Evaluation Parameters	Planning and Interventions with *Rationales*
Nursing Diagnosis: *Impaired Skin Integrity* related to surgery	**Outcome:** Suture lines will heal normally, without complications. **Evaluation Parameters:** On inspection of the graft, no areas of dehiscence are seen. Continuous airway maintenance. Gas exchange within normal limits.	**Interventions and *Rationales:*** Assess wound and incisions. Cleanse incisions and initiate oral care per surgeon's order. Assess nutritional intake. No tracheostomy ties over reconstruction flaps or grafts. *Preventing infection and promotion of wound healing.* Provide orocutaneous, pharyngocutaneous care: • Wet-to-dry dressing that is packed carefully into the wound per surgeon's order. Protect airway at all times *to prevent infection and maintain airway.* **Free Flap Care** • Do not change dressings. • Check neurovascular status. *Radial forearm free flap:* assess the fingers. *Fibular free flap:* assess the toes. *Assessment of blood supply distal to the flap site.* **Drain Care** Secure with Stomahesive and Elastoplast. • Strip to prevent clots. • Strict output recording. • Call surgeon if sudden increase or decrease in output or air leaks from the drains. Pressure dressing 24 hours after drain removal. **Internal Carotid Artery** Exposed external or intraoral: • Wet-to-wet dressing to keep carotid in a wet and clean environment. • Hespan at bedside. • Type and cross (or hold) two units of blood. • Two large–bore IV lines in place. • Alert operating room that the patient is on precautions. • If bleed occurs, apply DIRECT pressure do not remove. • Call surgeon and operating department emergently and prepare patient for transfer.

Assessment for Infection

Subjective Data:
Is your pain increasing in the surgical areas?
Do you feel weaker?

Objective Data:
Previously healed wounds are breaking down
Open wounds not healing
Partial thickness injuries/donor sites converting to full-thickness injuries
Increased odor and drainage from wound sites
Wound cultures positive for organisms
Fever
Increased WBC

(continued)

NURSING PROCESS:P atient Care Plan for Head and Neck Cancer—*Continued*

Nursing Assessment and Diagnoses	Outcomes and Evaluation Parameters	Planning and Interventions with *Rationales*
Nursing Diagnoses: *High Risk for Infection* related to loss of skin integrity and impaired healing	**Outcome:** Effective infection prevention. ***Evaluation Parameters:*** Surgical sites will not be colonized by organisms. Healing and reepithelialization will occur as noted by wound closure. Skin integrity will be restored.	**Interventions and *Rationales:*** Cleanse wounds per protocol *to prevent contamination.* Assess for infection and document with each dressing change *to prevent spread of infection.* Assess for drainage: exudate, color, odor, and amount. *These factors indicate infection.* Assess for undermining or sinus tract formation. *Indicates infection.* Use strict aseptic technique *to prevent infection.* Notify health care provider of presence of infection or wound enlargement *to facilitate medical intervention.* Monitor serum WBC daily. *Increased WBC indicates presence of infection.* Maintain nutritional therapies. *Malnutrition increases the risk of infection.* Monitor and record temperature. *Indicates infection.* Culture wounds and body secretions per protocol *to assess for infection.* Observe donor site for drainage, odor, and an increase in wound depth. Observe and document bolster orbital dressing for foul smell or purulence. *Indicates presence of infection.*

Assessment of Patient Safety

Subjective Data:
Do you feel safe when up walking?
How are you adapting to seeing out of only one eye?
What adjustments have been necessary?

Objective Data:
Is the patient able to navigate safely?
What assistive devices are necessary?

Nursing Assessment and Diagnoses	Outcomes and Evaluation Parameters	Planning and Interventions with *Rationales*
Nursing Diagnosis: *Risk for Falls* related to limited site and perception.	**Outcome:** Patient will adapt safely to monocular vision. ***Evaluation Parameter:*** Patient is able to navigate safely in hospital and home environment.	**Interventions and *Rationales:*** Explain anatomic changes and discuss implications for decreased vision. Discuss the implications of monocular vision and safety implications. *Patient has knowledge of limitations.* Encourage patient to wear glasses as soon as possible. *Helps improve vision.* Arrange for home evaluation to make needed adjustments to ensure fall prevention. *Improve the safety of the environment.*

Assessment of Psychological Adjustment to Facial Disfigurement

Subjective Data:
What impact does the change in your physical appearance have on your life?
How do you plan to cope with these changes?

Objective Data:
Does patient look at the changes in the mirror?
Does patient ask questions about the wounds?
Are the patient and family members willing to learn and participate in the required care after hospital discharge?
Is patient's perception realistic regarding body image changes?

NURSING PROCESS: Patient Care Plan for Head and Neck Cancer—*Continued*

Nursing Assessment and Diagnoses	Outcomes and Evaluation Parameters	Planning and Interventions with *Rationales*
Nursing Diagnoses: *Disturbed Body Image* related to facial disfigurement and formation and functional loss. *Anticipatory Grieving* related to body image change, risk of family role change, and possible occupational change	**Outcomes:** Acceptance of body image changes. Patient is safe and competent in wound care. Patient and family will cope with deficit. ***Evaluation Parameters:*** Patient will return to activities of daily living and social interactions. Patient verbalizes understanding of body changes.	**Interventions and *Rationales:*** Teaching will have begun preoperatively with patient education and informed consent. Teach patient and family about the anatomy, reconstruction, and prosthetic rehabilitation. Begin teaching wound care, orbital packing, and obturator care as soon as possible after packing removal. *To increase knowledge and potentially decrease anxiety of the unknown.* Have patient complete dressing with nurse's support, instruction, and understanding of the visual implications of self-image changes. *Begins the adjustment process and increases independence and autonomy.* Use eye patch (flesh tones) until orbital prosthesis is made. *More aesthetic and less visible.* Consider psychiatry or social service consults as needed. *May be necessary if patient is not adjusting to change in body image.* Arrange for home health nursing consult at discharge *to assist in the transition from hospital to home environment.* Assess patient's ability to participate in self-care of the orbital cavity. Assess need for psychiatric liaison support by consultation with social service, colleagues, and health care provider.

Assessment of Nutritional Intake

Subjective Data:

Does your stomach feel full?

Are you experiencing any nausea?

Objective Data:

Bowel sounds

Lung sounds

Residual volume

Nursing Assessment and Diagnoses	Outcomes and Evaluation Parameters	Planning and Interventions with *Rationales*
Nursing Diagnosis: *Risk for Imbalanced Nutrition; Less Than Body Requirements* related to surgery	**Outcomes:** Patient will have sufficient nutrition to heal. Home nutritional care plan is instituted as needed. ***Evaluation Parameters:*** No weight loss. Nutritional parameters at normal levels. Intake and output within normal limits. Prealbumin levels normal. No aspiration.	**Interventions and *Rationales:*** Observe ability to oral nourish self safely without aspiration. Arrange for nutrition consult for calorie and protein requirements and intake. Measure intake and output with calorie counts. *Nutrition is essential for wound healing.* Institute enteral nutrition by nasogastric (NG) or gastrostomy (GT) tube feeding as necessary. • If chyle leak, feed only no-fat formula (Vivonex TEN or similar). • Do not move NG tube. • Secure with Stomahesive and tape to nares. • Do not remove nasal stitch. • Do not attempt to replace NG without health care provider order. • Aspirate NG/GT tube at regular intervals to check residual volumes. Hold tube feeding if greater than amount specified by health care provider. *Safe administration of nasogastric feedings will prevent aspiration and not disturb suture lines.*

(continued)

NURSING PROCESS: Patient Care Plan for Head and Neck Cancer—*Continued*

Assessment of Pain

Subjective Data:
What is your pain level, using the 1 to 10 scale? (A 1 is very little pain; a 10 is the worst imaginable pain.)
What is your experience with pain?
Do you routinely take pain medications at home; if so, what for and what kind?
Are you allergic to any pain medication?
Do you have any cultural or religious beliefs that impact your pain control?

Objective Data:
Grimacing upon movement
Restlessness and irritability
Taut facial expression

Nursing Assessment and Diagnoses	Outcomes and Evaluation Parameters	Planning and Interventions with *Rationales*
Nursing Diagnosis: *Pain* related to surgery	**Outcome:** Comfort level maintained. ***Evaluation Parameters:*** Able to communicate pain level and therapies that help alleviate it. Pain reduced and/or absent as evidenced by patient report and no pain behaviors (i.e., no grimacing). Nonpharmacologic method of control is effective as evidenced by patient report and no pain behaviors. Reports satisfaction with pain management program.	**Interventions and *Rationales:*** Use pain scale (0–10) to quantify pain level. *Quantifying pain increases consistency.* Instruct patient to inform nurse if pain is not relieved. *Indicates need to change pain management plan.* Assess cultural and religious impact on patient's responses. *Different cultures and religions respond differently to pain.* Correct misconceptions about risk of addiction and overdose *to decrease anxiety related to medication addiction.* Explain, prepare, and medicate patient for painful procedures (dressing change) and anticipated discomforts *to control increased pain level related to procedure.* Provide a supportive environment where patient is able to express pain level. *Opens communication and facilitates pain management.* Use pain control measures before pain becomes severe. *This increases comfort and decreases need for medication.* Teach nonpharmacologic method of control (i.e., guided imagery, massage, breathing exercises). *These measures augment pain relief.* Cover wounds. *Covering areas where there is no skin decreases the pain.* Provide rest periods between procedures to assist with coping with ongoing pain. *Decreases the fatigue related to long-term pain.* Revise pain management plan as wounds heal and pain decreases *to prevent overmedication.* Plan diversional activities *to augment pain relief measures.*

Source: Adapted from Mulgrew and Dropkin, Memorial Sloan-Kettering Cancer Center. Mulgrew, B., & Dropkin, M. J. (1991). Coping with craniofacial resection: A case study. *ORL–Head and Neck Nursing, 9*(3), 8–18.

ambulation of the patient will greatly improve the respiratory status by stimulating coughing, encouraging greater lung expansion, recruiting lung fields, and mobilizing secretions. Early ambulation also benefits circulation and increasing muscle strength. The routine standards of turn, cough, and deep breathing are extremely important in this population.

Laryngectomy Stoma Care

Patients who have undergone surgery for cancer of the larynx and have had a total laryngectomy have a permanent change in their airway and their ability to speak naturally. These patients breathe *only* from their stoma because the aerodigestive tract has been separated and the trachea is sutured to the anterior neck. Care of the permanently reconstructed airway is similar to that of the patient with a temporary tracheostomy tube in place. Careful cleaning of the stoma should be done at least every 8

hours and as needed to prevent the buildup of secretions and debris around the suture line and to prevent scarring and narrowing of the airway. If edema causes narrowing of the airway, a stoma button can be inserted to open the airway and improve ease of breathing.

The patient's head should be positioned in a neutral position or slightly extended position so as not to occlude the airway and compromise breathing. Humidification must be provided and used after discharge from the hospital until the airway becomes used to unfiltered unwarmed air. Patients usually carry small spray bottles of normal saline to mist their stomas. A simple bedside humidification device is used at night.

Pain Management

One of the greatest fears for any patient undergoing cancer surgery is the fear of pain, and with patients with head and neck cancer their fear is augmented by their inability to communicate orally. Therefore, one of the highest nursing priorities and outcomes of care is to alleviate pain and anxiety related to pain. The pain of the cancer and the pain of the procedure must be defined and each treated together (Miaskowski, 2002). For many head and neck cancer patients, pain may have been the issue that brought them in to see the doctor in the first place. They may have been taking pain medications prior to the surgery. This is a key detail to ascertain, because normal pain relief measures may be ineffective for this type of patient.

It is important to do a very careful and exact assessment of the type and location of the pain. Have the patient set a goal pain level, using a pain rating scale, and use this scale to evaluate the effectiveness of the medication and intervention. This is a useful tool to use for a patient who is awake and alert and able to cooperate with the nurse. For patients who are uncooperative and unable to communicate, more subjective signs such as diaphoresis; restlessness; agitation; increased blood pressure, heart, and respiratory rates; facial grimacing; and lack of interaction may be clues to the need for pain medication. These signs also are useful for patients who are stoic and are not asking for pain medication.

The patient should be taught not to wait until the pain is unbearable to request pain medication because, once the pain sets in, it will take longer and require more medication to achieve relief. Nursing intervention for pain relief needs to occur early and frequently in the immediate postoperative period. The patient should receive small frequent doses of analgesia. Initially, the patient's pain is managed by morphine sulfate intravenously, the commonly preferred drug of choice. Increasing the dosage as the patient's respiratory status tolerates the higher doses may achieve the goal of pain relief. The use of patient-controlled analgesia (PCA) for alert cooperative patients can be considered. Transition to oral medications is predicated on the patient's ability to swallow safely and in sufficient quantity to sustain nutrition and medication. If a feeding tube is in place, as soon as tube feedings are tolerated the patient should start on acetaminophen with codeine or hydrocodone because the enteral route has a longer effect than the IV route.

Because head and neck oncology surgeries are very long, often exceeding 15 hours, many patients complain of joint pain. Particularly in the elderly, pain from immobility often is severe and not very responsive to opioids (White & Cohen, 2006). It is not appropriate to begin nonsteroidal medications in the early postoperative period because of the complication of bleeding. An excellent method of treating this pain is with mobility, frequent ambulation, or turning in bed, even as early as postoperative day 1.

Older adults may choose not to take pain medications, but instead opt for immobility as their treatment. They then have inadequate pain control and add the risk of immobility (Kemper, 2002). Patients should know that following surgical resection the cancer pain will be eliminated. The pain of surgical resection can be controlled by multiple methods. In-depth communication, ongoing evaluation, and documentation with the health care provider should be established (Miaskowski, 2001). Pain management is discussed in detail in Chapter 15 ⊙.

Nutrition Management

Many patients with head and neck cancer present with inadequate nutrition caused by the tumor burden, cancer cachexia, or the mechanical difficulty of eating because of tumor impingement into the aerodigestive tract. Early recognition of nutritional inadequacy and nutritional intervention is critical to ensure a positive nitrogen balance with enough calories and protein to heal following surgery and radiation therapy (van Bokhorst-de van der Schueren et al., 2000).

The preoperative evaluation will identify those patients who are at risk for malnutrition and outline interventions. Those at risk are patients presenting with significant weight loss (>10%) in the past few months and those presenting with low prealbumin levels. Body height and weight are included to calculate body mass index (BMI). BMI is a method of calculating a person's height-to-weight ratio (body mass index kg/m²). Rapid turnover proteins are the most practical window for viewing catabolic state and nitrogen loss despite the varying effects of kidney and liver failure and of steroids. The best test is serum prealbumin, transthyretin, or thyroxin-binding prealbumin (TBPA). Prealbumin is the laboratory measure of choice for assessing visceral protein status and should replace routine use of both albumin and transferrin for this purpose. Prealbumin is essential for monitoring nutrition status and nutritional therapy (Beck & Rosenthal, 2002; Bernstein et al., 1995).

The inclusion of a nutritionist in the multidisciplinary team is mandatory. Following cancer resection or during radiation therapy, nutrition consults are very helpful in targeting maintenance and replenishment goals. In the postoperative period a nutritional goal for caloric intake is estimated at 35 kcal/kg with specific attention to an increased need for hydration due to insensible water loss. Normal water loss per day is about 400 mL. In a patient with an artificial airway, water loss is about 500 to 600 mL insensible volume with an additional 600 to 700 mL per day with suctioning. Replacement requirements need to be carefully calculated in order to ensure proper hydration. The choice of feeding method, whether oral or enteral, is dependent on the patient's level of consciousness and ability to swallow. Feeding can proceed by an oral route, nasogastric route, gastrostomy, jejunostomy, or any combination thereof. Nutrition replacement must begin early and be continuous throughout the therapy for cancer. Most feeding can begin on postoperative day 1 and be advanced to goals as quickly as tolerated.

Dysphagia is a common issue that needs to be dealt with in patients with head and neck cancer. Swallowing is difficult because of tumor burden, invasion of the aerodigestive tract, and pain. Aspiration is a significant concern with patients who are unable to maintain their airway protection (Metheny, 2002; Metheny, Aud, & Wunderlich, 1999). See the Risk Factors for Aspiration box (p. 928).

Beginning as early as 1989, Logeman greatly advanced dysphagia research by directing the medical community to more accurately and objectively assess the amount, type, cause, and directed therapy for the treatment of swallowing problems and aspiration. Leonard and Kendall (1997) described an objective method of radiographic identification and quantification of aspiration. These more precise evaluations direct the process of intervention and swallow rehabilitation (Leonard & Kendall, 2007).

Enteral feeding routes are used because most patients with head and neck cancer have intact and functioning gastrointestinal systems. Once the patient is able to take oral food, the process needs to begin slowly with careful monitoring of tolerance and

RISK FACTORS for Aspiration

Documented previous episodes of aspiration

Decreased level of consciousness (sedation, increased intracranial pressure, coma)

Structural abnormalities of the aerodigestive tract (post head and neck cancer resection)

Neuromuscular disease

Endotracheal intubation

Vomiting

Persistently high gastric residual volumes

Need for prolonged supine position

Additional Factors

Presence of a nasoenteric tube

Noncontinuous or intermittent feeding

Abdominal/thoracic surgery or trauma

Delayed gastric emptying

Diabetes, hyperglycemia independent of diabetes, electrolyte abnormalities, drugs known to reduce gastroenteritis

Poor oral care

Age

Inadequate nursing staff

Large size or diameter of feeding tube

Malpositioned feeding tube

Transport

Source: McClave, S. A. et al. (2002). North American Summit of Aspiration in the Critically Ill Patient: Consensus statement. *Journal of Parenteral and Enteral Nutrition, 26* (6 Suppl.), S80–S85.

risk for aspiration. Sievers, Leonard, and McKenzie (1992) described a safe method for oral rehabilitation using an adaptive device (Figure 34–18 ■). All of these methods of nutritional support can and should be used to assist the patient with head and neck cancer to attain successful nutrition.

Wound Care

Gentle wound care is done with hydrogen peroxide to remove crusts, and normal saline is used to cleanse the skin wound and incisions. The surgeon dictates the frequency, but generally rou-

FIGURE 34–18 ■ Syringe with catheter for feeding placement for accurate placement of oral nutrition in the patient with oral tongue resections. Safe oral placement is critical to prevent aspiration.
Source: University of California, Davis Medical Center

tine care is considered to be every 4 hours and as needed (prn) to keep the wound clean and free from crusts. Depending on surgeon preference, the cleaning should be followed by the application of a thin layer of antibiotic ointment for the first 48 hours. This will help keep the incision clean and free from drainage and will aid in sealing the wound. Care of the suture lines also includes assessment for drainage, redness, odor, or other signs of infection. Any surgical incisions that are not well approximated or are draining pus, bile, saliva, or tube feedings must be reported to the health care provider at once because they indicate serious changes in the integrity of the surgical site. Oral care is included in wound care because many of the patients have intraoral incisions. The inside of the mouth should be very carefully cleaned on the side away from the internal suture lines using very soft toothbrushes and rinsing well.

The purpose of the placement of drains in the surgical site is to evaluate blood and other fluids from the surgical site. The assessment of the postoperative patient includes observing the drains for patency and the amount and type of drainage. Each drain is individually labeled and firmly secured, so the drain will not accidentally become dislodged or pulled out by the patient. Every drain is numbered, labeled, and documented precisely for position on the neck and chest. Document the color, type, and amount of output, and record each drain individually in the intake and output section of the nursing documentation record. The health care provider determines when the drain should be removed; typically this is done when there is less than 30 mL of drainage in a 24-hour period. A dressing is placed over the site for 24 hours following removal.

Wound Complications

A number of postoperative complications can occur in the patient with head and neck cancer. Patients who have a history of radiation therapy or have a poor nutritional status are at greater risk for alterations in wound healing and possible complications. Any type of excessive drainage may indicate a problem and, if caught early, treatment will mitigate complications. For example, a large amount of milky colored fluid (possibly up to 1 liter in 24 hours) is referred to as a chyle leak. A **chyle leak** is a disruption in the lymph system that causes lymphatic fluid to leak from the thoracic duct on the left side and the lymphatic duct on the right side. This condition should be reported to the health care provider immediately because it can result in serious fluid and electrolyte imbalances. Shifts in potassium, sodium, calcium, and magnesium can be life threatening with serious cardiac manifestations. The affected drain is placed to gravity drainage and a zero-fat diet is implemented. A decrease in fat in the diet will result in a decreased production of lymph. This is done with the hope that the leak will seal itself given the decrease in production of lymphatic fluid. The nurse must monitor fluid and electrolytes.

Bright red, excessive clots or large amounts of drainage indicate abnormal bleeding. Monitoring the patient's hematocrit (HCT) and hemoglobin (HBG) and carefully assessing vital signs are essential when bleeding occurs. A decrease in the HCT and HGB and/or an increase in the pulse rate and decrease in the blood pressure are reported to the surgeon. Each drain is milked or stripped according to the surgeon's orders to ensure patency. Stripping will remove excess fluid, drainage, and clots from the surgical area and tubing that may lead to problems of congestion, flap failure, and hematoma at the surgical site. The tube is stripped by first lubricating it with lotion or water-soluble jelly, then pinching the tube between two fingers and pulling down the length of the tubing, creating suction. Great care must be taken not to dislodge the tube from its position in the body. Any suspected problems with drain function should be reported to the surgeon for immediate intervention.

Other possible postoperative complications include the accumulation of fluid (seroma) or blood (hematoma) in the bed of the surgical wound, infection, fistulas, carotid artery exposure, and flap failure. As discussed earlier, fistulas are dehiscent wounds that traverse between two different tissue planes. In the head and neck, a fistula that occurs between the pharynx and the skin is termed a pharyngocutaneous fistula (Figure 34–19 ■).

A serious, potentially life-threatening complication is carotid artery exposure and potential rupture. This can occur in the patient who has problems with wound healing, fistula formation, poor nutrition, and/or a history of radiation therapy to the area. A tumor that has been removed close to the carotid artery leaves the artery in jeopardy of rupture, and if the tumor recurs or a fistula forms, the risk further increases. If the primary closure of the surgical incision fails and the artery is exposed to air, it can lead to drying and weakening of the arterial wall. If this occurs, place the patient on special alert for what is referred to as *carotid blowout* precautions. The patient should be in sight of a nurse at all times and specific supplies are placed in the patient's room that will be needed in the event of a rupture. A "herald" bleed (massive bleed), or prerupture sign, indicating an imminent bleed, can occur 24 to 48 hours prior to a major carotid bleed. If a rupture occurs, direct digital pressure should be placed on the vessel and the airway maintained with suctioning and positioning. The patient is transported to the operating room immediately to undergo carotid re-section. Never release direct pressure until surgical intervention has been secured. Chart 34–7 outlines typical health care provider orders for carotid artery precautions.

Physical Therapy

As the patient progresses through the hospital stay, it is important to include physical therapy in the plan of care. If the patient has had a neck dissection with the resection of CN XI, he will be unable to fully move the shoulder due to the enervation of the trapezius muscle. Physical therapy exercises help the patient to regain mobility, prevent a frozen shoulder, and improve general reconditioning. These exercises should be continued after hospital discharge either in the home or as an outpatient. Written instructions with pictures are very helpful for the patient and family to follow. This also gives the home health nurse and outpatient physical therapist goals for home therapy.

Discharge Priorities

Discharge priorities for patients with head and neck cancer are related to safety at home, airway maintenance, nutrition, wound care, follow-up therapy, compliance with the treatment regimen, and adaptation to illness (see Patient Teaching & Discharge Priorities box, p. 930). As these patients finish their hospital stay, it is the nurse's responsibility to become part of the team to help the patient transition from hospital to home. With the clinical nurse specialist, dietitian, speech therapist, discharge planner, physician, physical therapist, and social services providers, all efforts must be directed toward adaptation and safety. The most important part of the discharge process is to remember that discharge planning begins at the time of diagnosis.

FIGURE 34–19 ■ This post-laryngectomy patient developed a fistula on his left side just lateral to his laryngectomy stoma. Packing in place is changed four times a day to encourage healing and prevent saliva from entering his stoma.
Source: University of California, Davis Medical Center

CHART 34–7   Carotid Artery Precautions

1. Carotid tray at bedside
2. Four packages fluffs at bedside
3. Dual-suction machines with large oral suction at bedside
4. Portable suction on unit for transport
5. One-liter lactated Ringer's solution at bedside with connecting tubing
6. Two large-bore IVs at all times
7. Blood administration set at bedside
8. Type and antibody screen every 48 hours (1 adult clot tube) or per hospital protocol
9. Two units Hespan (or similar) at bedside
10. *Wound care:* saline-soaked dressings (Wet to wet every 2 hours. When stable and healing, advance to every 2 hours while awake and every 4 hours at night, with wetting of the dressing with normal saline every 2 hours.)
11. Frequent observation of patient for "herald" bleed (prerupture bleed), dry or dark area of artery or aneurysm formation
12. Call House Officer or Primary Care Provider immediately if any of the above occur.
13. Assess for higher level of care if other compounding problems are present.
14. Alert OR and blood bank that patient is on carotid precautions.

RESEARCH OPPORTUNITIES AND CLINICAL IMPACT RELATED TO UPPER AIRWAY DISORDERS

Research Area	Clinical Impact
What is the effect of anterior and posterior nasal packing on oxygenation and CO_2?	Currently patients who have anterior and/or posterior packing require cardiac monitoring and therefore advanced nursing care. What is the appropriate level of care required for these patients?
What is the effect of weight loss on the life of OSA patients?	Improved quality of life with OSA. Decreased hospitalizations and medical costs. Education of patients about the importance of weight control and OSA.
Insensible water loss with a tracheotomy.	Improved method of caring for patients with an artificial airway.
Use of normal saline in the ambulatory patient with an artificial airway.	Better hydration and fluid replacement techniques. Decreased frequency of dehydration.
Perceptions of patients with head and neck cancer.	Better adapted and better prepared patients.
Quality of life with patients and caregivers of those with head and neck cancer.	Improved quality of life.
What is safe staffing for an otolaryngology unit or clinic given the fragility of patients with artificial and at-risk airways?	Ability to define the appropriate staffing mix for an ENT nursing unit or clinic based on nursing decisions, patient education, and interventions.

PATIENT TEACHING & DISCHARGE PRIORITIES for Head and Neck Cancer Patients

Need	Teaching
Knowledge of home and self-care following surgery for head and neck cancer	Health care needs include verbal and written instructions for treatment plan and follow-up care. Assess patient and family understanding of disease process, surgical procedure performed, and health maintenance needs in the home setting.
Maintenance of airway	Patient and family or significant others are taught how to maintain an open airway by: • Providing verbal and written instructions on self-care needs, equipment usage, and indicators for emergency assistance. • Providing instructions on self-suctioning, wound care, change of tracheostomy tube, and safety precautions.
Nutrition	Patient and family are taught about nutritional needs by: • Instructing patient/family on nutritional needs, calories needed per day, and how to use enteral feedings. • Providing consultation from a dietitian as necessary.
Wound care	Ascertain patient/family's ability to care for the wound using aseptic technique: • Instruct patient/family on wound care and evaluate ability to complete by ensuring a return demonstration. • Providing all necessary supplies for wound care and ask patient/family to keep track of availability of necessary supplies.
Physical therapy	Assess patient's need for transportation to appointments. Determine patient's ability to perform exercises as directed by demonstrating exercises.
Speech therapy	Assess patient's need for transportation to appointments. Establish means of communication; practice speech. Instruct patient to keep track of therapy appointments and observe compliance to prescribed therapy.
Safety	Stress importance of safety precautions by: • Instructing to keep emergency numbers by phone. • Instructing to keep written instructions for self-care easily accessible. • Reinforcing instructions for airway maintenance. • Identifying ways to detect gas alerts if patient/family unable to smell.
Family/significant other support system	Assess availability, knowledge, and compliance with treatment regimen. Assess for need for professional home health needs. Establish a plan for caretaker rest and support. Establish a plan for assurance of meeting patient's rest needs. Discuss with patient and family independence goals and establish markers for advancement toward independence.
Follow-up therapy	Instruct patient on criticality of follow-up therapy. Assist patient in establishing a calendar of appointments with expected outcome that patient will keep appointments.
Compliance	Evaluate patient for knowledge of compliance needs in self-care with potential outcome of patient maintaining ongoing appointments as scheduled.
Adaptation to illness	Assess patient's coping needs and methods of coping. Encourage open discussion of feelings and concerns. Provide psychological counseling as needed.

Clinical Preparation

 Read

- History of Current Illness
- Past Medical History
- Physical Exam
- Admitting Medical Orders
- Laboratory Study Results

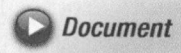 **Document**

- Summary of Hospitalization
- Pathophysiology Form
- Laboratory Values
- Laboratory Results Explanation

 Apply

- List of Potential Nursing Diagnoses
- Concept Map
- Critical Thinking Questions

Log on to MyNursingKit.com to download forms you will need and to complete further steps in the Clinical Preparation assignment.

HISTORY OF PRESENT ILLNESS

A 23-year-old female was brought in by ambulance to the emergency department (ED). She was transported because of an injury to her anterior neck after being hit by a softball during practice. The patient was responsive sitting in an upright forward position. She was initially evaluated by the ED physician. Otolaryngology was urgently consulted because the patient's airway distress was increasing as her neck swelling increased. There was too much swelling to safely view the vocal cords for intubation. With fluid resuscitation and stabilization, the patient was taken to the operating room where a tracheotomy was performed.

Following recovery from anesthesia, she was alert, cognitively intact, and could write to the staff. After 2 days in the ICU to rule out any other injuries such as closed head injury, the patient was stable and transferred to an acute care unit where you assumed care of her. The patient's tracheotomy was downsized from a cuffed #8 to an uncuffed #6 tracheotomy tube. The patient was taught to speak by covering the tube with finger occlusion. The patient's voice was very hoarse, and she coughed while drinking liquids. Aspiration precautions were initiated and otolaryngology speech therapy was called in to assess the patient's voice and swallowing. Otolaryngology continued to evaluate the patient's

hoarse, breathy voice and dysphagia. On fiber-optic examination it was apparent that she was not able to medialize her right vocal cord and her larynx was insensate, thus the hoarseness and inability to protect the airway during eating. The patient did not appear to be experiencing any further respiratory difficulties and her vital signs and oxygen (O_2) saturations were all within normal limits. She had a low-grade temperature (38°C), which was presumed to be a result of atelectasis from prolonged bed rest.

A dynamic swallow study was done in the speech lab to further assess the degree of difficulty the patient had protecting her airway while eating and to evaluate the patient's vocal cord status. The speech therapist worked with the patient with different types of food textures to determine which ones the patient could safely handle. It was determined that pureed food with thick liquids would be the safest diet for this patient.

Dietary was notified of the change in diet and a request was put in to have the diet tray left on the cart to be delivered to the patient by the nurse. That way, it was certain that the patient would be positioned properly in a chair or with the head of the bed at 90 degrees and that she would be observed for aspiration throughout the meal. Suction was available at the bedside for use as needed.

Medical–Surgical History

Appendectomy and tonsillectomy as a child

Social History

Married no children; attends graduate school
Travels frequently in the United States with her softball team

Physical Exam

Head: normocephalic, nontraumatic, no lacerations or bruising
Eyes: normal EOM bilaterally, PERL
Ears: WNL no hemotympanum or trauma
Nose: WNL

Mouth: WNL no evidences of trauma, tongue not swollen, occasional coughing of blood
Neck: Significant bruising was noted in the anterior of the neck; attributed to the direct injury of the softball
Cranial nerves: CN I not tested; CN X impairment on the L side; others WNL

Admitting Medical Orders

Otolaryngology Service
Admit to Medical–Surgical floor
Admitting diagnosis: 23-year-old woman admitted status postinjury to the neck by a softball; tracheotomy

Allergies: none known
Up ad lib with bathroom privileges
Head of bed at 90 degrees or up in chair for meals
Diet: pureed food with thick liquids
Vital signs and oxygen saturation q4h
Neuro assessment q4h
I&O
IV D51/2 NS at 75 mL/hr until tolerating fluids; then convert to
  saline lock: flush q8h with NS
Aspiration precautions
Routine tracheostomy care
Suction prn
O_2 per humidified trach collar to keep oxygen saturation > 92%
Call house officer: pulse < 60 and > 130/minute; BP < 90 and
  > 160 systolic; temperature > 38.5; urine output < 30 mL/hr
  for 2 hours; respiratory rate > 30/minute; oxygen saturation
  < 92%
Sequential compression devices (SCDs) to lower extremities while
  in bed

Scheduled Medications

Morphine sulfate PCA: 1 mg incremental dose q10min. If pain not
  well controlled, give morphine sulfate bolus 1–5 mg IV × 1

PRN Medications

Temazepam 15–30 mg po qhs prn insomnia
Droperidol 1.25–2.5 mg IV q6h prn nausea
Ativan 1 mg IV q6h prn anxiety
Milk of Magnesia 30 mL daily prn constipation
Tylenol 650 mg po/PR q4h prn for pain

Ordered Laboratory Studies

Chemistry 7 panel, CBC, ABGs, and magnesium daily
INR × 1

Ordered Diagnostic Studies

Flexible fiber-optic laryngoscopy
Videostroboscopy
Dynamic swallow study

LABORATORY STUDY RESULTS

Test	Day 1	Day 2	Day 3
Sodium	137 mEq/L	136 mEq/L	139 mEq/L
Potassium	3.8 mEq/L	3.8 mEq/L	3.7 mEq/L
Chloride	106 mEq/L	103 mEq/L	110 mEq/L
Blood urea nitrogen (BUN)	4 mg/dL	4 mg/dL	6 mg/dL
Creatinine	1.1 mg/dL	0.9 m/dL	0.7 m/dL
Blood glucose	143 mg/dL	120 m/dL	98 m/dL
Calcium	7.9 mEq/L	7.8 mEq/L	9.1 mEq/L
Total protein	6.3 g/dL	6.0 g/dL	5.8 mg/dL
Magnesium	2.1 mEq/L	1.9 mEq/L	2.4 mEq/L
White blood count	12,600 µL	19.1 µL	13.4 µL
Hemoglobin	9.8 g/dL	10.6 g/dL	12.5 g/dL
Hematocrit	28.1%	29.6%	31.5%
Red blood cells	3.35 million/ µL	3.26 million/µL	3.67 million/µL
Platelets	195,000 µL	189,000 µL	241,000 µL
INR	1.00 INR		
ABGs			
PaO_2	98 mmHg	112 mmHg	96 mmHg
O_2 sat	96	99	97
pH	7.44	7.46	7.56
$PaCO_2$	36 mmHg	35 mmHg	24 mmHg
HCO_3	25 mEq/L	25 mEq/L	20 mEq/L

CRITICAL THINKING QUESTIONS

1. Explain what the nurse's responsibility is to a patient who is unable to communicate by natural voice. What are the alternatives and what are the nurse's professional responsibilities?

2. Discuss the implications of nursing interventions used with a patient in airway obstruction following traumatic injury. How can the nurse help the patient adapt to a new airway?

3. Think of the quality-of-life implications for a 23-year-old athlete who has a tracheostomy and airway injury. Discuss the role of compassion and comportment in the nursing care of such a patient.

Answers to Critical Thinking Questions appear in Appendix D

NCLEX® REVIEW

1. The nurse is caring for a pediatric patient recovering from a fractured mandible. Which of the following should be included in this patient's plan of care?
   1. Provide system antibiotics to prevent meningitis.
   2. Once stable, instruct in the use of a water pik.
   3. Provide eye protection.
   4. Assess for facial droop every 2 hours.

2. Which of the following should the nurse include in a plan of care for a patient with acute sinusitis?
   1. Restrict fluids
   2. Administer antibiotics as prescribed
   3. Maintain on bedrest
   4. Dental consultation for gum and tooth pain

3. The nurse is planning instruction for a patient with seasonal allergic rhinitis. Which of the following should be included in this instruction?
   1. Expect to have allergy injections for 6 months.
   2. Spend time outdoors to increase immunity to the allergen.
   3. Boil a pan of water on the stove every day to increase environmental humidity.
   4. Avoid exposure to strong perfumes, smoke, and rapid changes in temperature.

4. During an assessment, an elderly patient tells the nurse that he "just doesn't smell things the way he used to." Which of the following should the nurse include in this patient's assessment?
   1. Presence of smoke detectors in the home and the type of cooking appliances used
   2. Mobility of head and neck
   3. Appetite
   4. Respiratory rate

5. A patient with obstructive sleep apnea is having difficulty using the CPAP device at home. Which of the following can the nurse instruct this patient?
   1. Only wear the device for a few hours every night.
   2. Assess the type of difficulty and provide recommendations accordingly.
   3. Sleep propped up with pillows instead of using the device.
   4. Use a dental device instead.

6. A patient diagnosed with neck cancer says he's never smoked and wants to know what caused the disease. Which of the following should the nurse respond to this patient?
   1. Most people deny a smoking history.
   2. Smoking is only one cause for the disease. Others include chronic mouth lesions and poor nutrition.
   3. You would be surprised to hear what can cause this type of cancer.
   4. It's because you drink alcohol.

7. The nurse is providing care to a patient with a tracheostomy because of neck cancer. Which of the following should be included in this patient's plan of care?
   1. Provide tracheostomy care every 24 hours.
   2. Change tracheostomy ties every 4 hours.
   3. Provide inner cannula care every day.
   4. Secure the tube ties laterally to the chest with suspended ties.

Answers for review questions appear in Appendix D

KEY TERMS

anosmia *p.895*
aphonic *p.902*
chyle leak *p.928*
continuous positive airway pressure (CPAP) *p.878*
decannulation *p.910*
epiglottitis *p.900*
epistaxis *p.882*
fistula *p.907*
hairy tongue *p.898*
hoarseness *p.903*

laryngeal spasm *p.905*
laryngectomy *p.902*
laryngitis *p.903*
laryngopharyngeal reflux disease (LPRD) *p.907*
Ludwig's angina *p.899*
mucormycosis *p.895*
myocutaneous flap *p.919*
nasal polyps *p.894*
neck dissection *p.919*
otolaryngology (otorhinolaryngology) *p.880*

panendoscopy *p.917*
peritonsillar abscess *p.900*
pharyngitis *p.900*
rhinitis *p.888*
sinusitis *p.892*
sleep apnea *p.897*
stridor *p.900*
tonsillitis *p.900*
tracheostomy *p.885*
tracheotomy *p.885*

REFERENCES

American Academy of Otolaryngology–Head and Neck Surgery. (2007). *Fact sheet: Deviated septum.* Retrieved May 19, 2008, from http://www.entnet.org/HealthInformation/deviatedSeptum.cfm

American Cancer Society. (2006). *Detailed guide: Oral cavity and oropharyngeal cancer. What are the risk factors for oral cavity and oropharyngeal cancer?* Retrieved August 23, 2007, from http://www.cancer.org/docroot/CRI/content/CRI_2_4_2X_What_are_the_risk_factors_for_oral_cavity_and_oropharyngeal_cancer_60.asp?rnav=cri

Babak, J., & Blackwell, K. (2005). *Facial bone anatomy.* Retrieved July 14, 2007, from http://www.emedicine.com/ent/topic9.htm

Bailey, B. J., Johnson, J. T., Newlands, S. D., Calhoun, K. H., & Deskin, R. W. (2006). *Head and neck surgery—otolaryngology.* Philadelphia: Lippincott Williams & Wilkins.

Baitha, S., Raizada, R. M., Kennedy-Singh, A. K., Puttewar, M. P., & Chaturvedi, V. N. (2002). Clinical profile of hoarseness of voice. *Indian Journal of Otolaryngology and Head and Neck Surgery, 54*(1), 554–558.

Baugh, W. P., & Earhart, K. C. (2006). *Rhinocerebral mucormycosis.* Retrieved September 2, 2007, from the eMedicine website: http://www.emedicine.com/med/topic2026.htm

Beck, F. K., & Rosenthal, T. C. (2002). Pre-albumin: A marker for nutritional evaluation. *American Family Physician, 65,* 1575–1578.

Beers, M. (Ed.). (2004). Neurological disorders. Section 14: Sleep disorders. In *The Merck manual of health and aging* (central ed.). West Point, PA: Merck Research Laboratories.

Beers, M. H. & Berkow, R. (2004). Mucormycosis. Section 13 Chapter 158. In *the merck manual of diagnoses and therapy.* Whitehouse Station, NJ: Merck Research Laboratories.

Belafsky, P. C. (2006). Empiric treatment with PPI's is not appropriate without testing. *American Journal of Gastroenterology, 101*(1), 6–8.

Bermant, M. (2007). *Nasal fractures.* Retrieved July 15, 2007, from http://www.plasticsurgery4u.com/procedure_folder/nasal_fx.html

Bernstein, L., et al. (1995). Measurement of visceral protein status in assessing protein and energy malnutrition: Standard of care prealbumin in nutritional care consensus group. *Nutrition, 11*(2), 169–171.

Brannon, G. E. (2006). *History and mental status examination.* Retrieved September 8, 2007, from http://www.emedicine.com/med/topic3358.htm

Calhoun, K., Eibling, D. E., & Wax, M. K. (Eds.). (2001). *Expert guide to otolaryngology.* Philadelphia: American College of Physicians and American Society of Internal Medicine.

Chang, E., & Adami, H. O. (2006). The enigmatic epidemiology of nasopharyngeal carcinoma. *Cancer Epidemiology, Biomarkers and Prevention, 15,* 1765–1777.

Connell, S., & Belafsky, P. C. (2005). *Temporal bone fractures.* Retrieved July 23, 2007, from http://www.emedicine.com/ent/topic477.htm

Corey, C. L. (2006). *Frontal sinus fractures.* Houston: Baylor College of Medicine, Bobby R. Alford Department of Otolaryngology–Head and Neck Surgery, Grand Round Archive.

Cross, D., & Burmester, J. (2006), Gene therapy for cancer treatment: Past, present and future. *Clinical Medicine & Research, 4*(3), 218–227.

Donald, P. J., Enepikedes, D., & Boggan, J. (2004). Giant juvenile nasopharyngeal angiofibroma: Management by skull-base surgery. *Archives of Otolaryngology—Head & Neck Surgery, 130,* 882–886.

Eledrisi, M. S., Alshanti, M. S., Shah, M. F., Brolosy, B., & Jaha, N. (2006). Overview of the diagnosis and management of diabetic ketoacidosis. *American Journal of the Medical Sciences, 331*(5), 243–251.

Fidrose, R., & Elamin, E. (2004). Pulmonary edema secondary to dynamic tracheal collapse. *Journal of Bronchology, 11*(2), 118–121.

File, T. M. (2005). Telithromycin new product overview. *Journal of Allergy and Clinical Immunology, 115*(2), S1–S13.

Forastiere, A. A., Goepfert, H., Maor, M., Pajak, T., Webers, R., Morrison, W., et al. (2003). Concurrent chemotherapy and radiotherapy for organ preservation in advanced laryngeal cancer. *New England Journal of Medicine, 349* (22), 2091–2098, and Correction, *350*(10),1049.

Galler, D., Skinner, A., & Ng, A. (2005). *Critical care considerations in trauma.* Retrieved January 25, 2006, from http://www.emedicine.com/med/topic3218.htm#section-neurotrauma

Greene, F. L., Page, D. L., Fleming, I. D., Fritz, A. G., Balch, C. M., Haller, D. G., et al. (Eds.). (2002). *AJCC cancer staging manual* (6th ed.). New York: Springer.

Hallet, R. (2006, October). *Allergy and immunology management.* Lecture given at the University of California Davis Medical Center.

Hampel, F., Ratner, P., Mansfield, L., Meeves, S., Liao, Y., & Georges, G. (2003, October). Fexofenadine hydrochloride exhibits equivalent efficacy to cetirizine with less drowsiness in patients with moderate-to-severe seasonal allergic rhinitis. *Annals of Allergy, Asthma and Immunology, 91*(4), 354–361.

Harris, L., & Huntoon, M. (Eds.). (2007). *Core curriculum for otorhinolaryngology head–neck nursing* (2nd ed.). New Smyrna Beach, FL: Society of Otorhinolaryngology and Head-Neck Nurses.

Howarth, P., Stern, M., Roi, L., Reynolds, R., & Bousquet, J. (1999). Double-blind, placebo-controlled study comparing the efficacy and safety of fexofenadine hydrochloride and cetirizine in seasonal allergic rhinitis. *Journal of Allergy and Clinical Immunology, 104*(5), 927–933.

Jafek, B. W., Murrow, B., & Linschoten, M. (2000). Evaluation and treatment of anosmia. *Current Opinion Otolaryngology & Head & Neck Surgery, 8,* 63–67.

Jett, K. F. (2007). Dementia, delirium and depression. *Advance for Nurses, 4*(6), 15–19.

Kemper, J. A. (2002). Pain management of older adults after discharge from outpatient surgery. *Pain Management Nursing, 3* (4), 141–153.

Kennedy, E. S. (2007). *Sinusitis.* Retrieved August 30, 2007, from http://www.emedicine.com/EMERG/topic536.htm

Kucik, C. J. (2005). Management of epistaxis. *American Family Physician, 71*(2), 305–311.

Kutner, M., Greenberg, E., Jun, Y., & Paulsen, C. (2006). *The health literacy of America's adults: Results from the 2003 National Assessment of Adult Literacy.* Washington, DC: National Center for Education Statistics, U.S. Department of Education.

Leonard, R., & Kendall, K. (Eds.). (1997). *Dysphagia assessment and treatment planning: A team approach.* San Diego: Singular Publishing.

Leonard, R., & Kendall, K. (2001). Phonoscopy: A valuable tool for otolaryngologists and speech language pathologists in the management of dysphonic patients. *Laryngoscope, 111*(10), 1760–1766.

Leonard, R., & Kendall, K. (Eds.). (2007). *Dysphagia assessment and treatment planning: A team approach.* San Diego: Singular Publishing.

Linfoot, P., & Bergstrom, C. (2005). Pathophysiology of ketoacidosis in Type 2 diabetes mellitus. *Diabetic Medicine, 22*(10), 1414–1419.

Maktabi, M., Smith, R., & Todd, M. (2003). Editorial views: Is routine endotracheal intubation as safe as we think or wish? *Anesthesiology, 99*(2), 247–248.

Mayo Clinic. (2006). *Nervous system: Vocal cord paralysis.* Retrieved August 28, 2007, from http://www.mayoclinic.com/health/vocal-cord-paralysis/DS00670/DSECTION=2

McClay, J. E. (2007). *Nasal polyps.* Retrieved May 29, 2008, from http://www.emedicine.com/PED/topic1550.htm

Medline Plus. (2005a). *Hoarseness or changing voice.* Retrieved August 28, 2007, from http://www.nlm.nih.gov/medlineplus/ency/article/003054.htm#Definition

Medline Plus. (2005b). *Upper airway obstruction.* Retrieved August 16, 2007, from http://www.nlm.nih.gov/medlineplus/ency/article/000067.htm

Medline Plus. (2006). *Smell—impaired.* Retrieved September 3, 2007, from http://www.nlm.nih.gov/medlineplus/ency/article/003053.htm

Merritt, J., Roth, J., & Logothetis, C. (2001). Clinical evaluation of adenoviral-mediated gene transfer: Review on INGN 201 studies. *Seminars in Oncology, 28* (5 Suppl. 16), 105–114.

Metheny, N. A. (2002). Risk factors for aspiration. *Journal of Parenteral and Enteral Nutrition,* S26–S31, and Discussion, S32–S3.

Metheny, N. A., Aud, M. A., & Wunderlich, R. J. (1999). A survey of bedside methods used to detect pulmonary aspiration of enteral formula in intubated tube-fed patients. *American Journal of Critical Care, 8,* 160–169.

Meyers, F. (1999). Perspectives on palliative care: A chair of medicine viewpoint. *Journal of Palliative Medicine, 2,* 371–375.

Meyers, F., & Linder, J. (2003). Simultaneous care: Disease treatment and palliative care. *Journal of Clinical Oncology, 21*(7), 1412–1415.

Miaskowski, C. (2001). Words with new meanings [Editorial]. *Pain Management Nursing, 2*(3), 73.

Miaskowski, C. (2002). The need to assess multiple symptoms [Editorial]. *Pain Management Nursing, 3*(4), 115.

National Heart, Lung, and Blood Institute. (2006). *Obstructive sleep apnea.* Retrieved August 16, 2007, from http://www.nhlbi.nih.gov/health/dci/Diseases/SleepApnea/SleepApnea_WhatIs.html

National Institute on Deafness and Other Communication Disorders. (2002). *Vocal cord paralysis.* Retrieved August 16, 2007, from http://www.nidcd.nih.gov/health/voice/vocalparal.htm

Nettelbeck, D., & Curiel, D. (2003, October). Tumor-busting viruses. *Scientific American,* 68–75.

O'Toole, M. T. (Ed.). (2003). *Miller-Keane encyclopedia and dictionary of medicine, nursing, and allied health* (7th ed.). Philadelphia: W. B. Saunders.

Piccolino, P., Vetrano, S., Mundula, P., Di Lella, G., Tedaldi, M., & Poladas, G. (2007). Frontal bone fractures: A new technique of closed reduction. Technical strategies. *Journal of Craniofacial Surgery, 18*(3), 695–698.

Pope, L. E. R., & Hobbs, C. G. L. (2005). Epistaxis: An update on current management. *Postgraduate Medical Journal, 81,* 309–314.

Porth, C. M. (2005) *Pathophysiology: Concepts of altered health status* (7th ed.). Philadelphia: Lippincott Williams & Wilkins.

Quillen, D. M., & Feller, D. B. (2006). Diagnosing rhinitis: Allergic vs. nonallergic. *American Family Physician, 73*(9), 1583–1590.

Ramakrishnan, V. R., & Meyers, A. D. (2006). *Nonallergic rhinitis.* Retrieved August 19, 2007, from http://www.emedicine.com/ent/topic402.htm

Rosin, D. (1998). Nasal obstruction. *The sinus source book.* Los Angeles: Lowell House.

Rudy, S. F. (2006). Staying motivated in providing tobacco cessation advice and counseling. *ORL—Head and Neck Nursing, 24*(4), 6–9.

Sataloff, R., et al. (1998). *Performing arts medicine.* San Diego: Singular Publishing.

Schneider, K., & Segal, G. (2006). *Dental abscess.* Retrieved July 29, 2007, from http://www.emedicine.com/ped/topic2675.htm

Seiden, A. M. (1997). *Taste and smell disorders.* New York: Thieme.

Sheikh, H. (2007). *Rhinitis, allergic.* Retrieved August 25, 2007, from http://emedicine.com/med/topic104.htm

Sievers, A., Leonard, R., & McKenzie, S. (1992). The safe use of an adaptative early feeding device for impaired patients. *ORL—Head and Neck Nursing, 10,* 17–19.

Smith, J. E., & Perez, C. L. (2004). *Nasal fractures.* Retrieved August 15, 2007, from http://www.emedicine.com/radio/topic468.htm

Strong, B. (2006). Image-guided functional endoscopic sinus surgery. *Current Opinion in Otolaryngology Head and Neck Surgery, 8*(1), 3–6.

Strong, E. B., & Senders, C. W. (2003). Surgery for severe rhinosinusitis. *Clinical Reviews in Allergy and Immunology, 2*(25),165–176.

Tanaka, A., Isono, S., Ishikawa, T., Sato, J., & Nishino, T. (2003). Laryngeal resistance before and after minor surgery. *Anesthesiology, 99*(2), 252–258.

Tolentino-DelosReyes, A. F., Ruppert, S. D., & Shiao, S.-Y. P. K. (2007). Evidence-based practice: Use of the ventilator bundle to prevent ventilator-associated pneumonia. *American Journal of Critical Care, 16*(1), 20–28.

University of Maryland Medical Center. (2006). *Sinusitis.* Retrieved August 30, 2007, from http://www.umm.edu/patiened/articles/what_symptoms_of_sinusitis_000062_4.htm

van Bokhorst-de van der Schueren M., et al. (2000).The impact of nutritional status on the prognoses of patients with advanced head and neck cancer. *Cancer, 86*(3), 519–527.

Varman, M., & Whaley, D. (2006). *Mucormycosis.* Retrieved September 2, 2007, from http://www.emedicine.com/ped/topic1488.htm

Vokes, E., & Stenson, K. (2003). Therapeutic options for laryngeal cancer. *New England Journal of Medicine, 349,* 2087–2089.

Weiler, J. M., Bloomfield, J. R., Woodworth, G. G., Grant, A. R., Layton, T. A., Brown, T. L., et al. (2000). Effects of fexofenadine, diphenhydramine, and alcohol on driving performance: A randomized, placebo controlled trial in the Iowa Driving Simulator. *Annals of Internal Medicine, 132* (5), 354–363.

White, H. K., & Cohen, H. J. (2006). The older cancer patient. *Medical Clinics of North America, 90*(5), 967–982.

Woodcock, R. (2007). *Temporal bone: Fractures.* Retrieved July 29, 2007, from http://www.emedicine.com/radio/topic678.htm

Wynd, C. A. (2006). Smoking patterns, beliefs, and the practice of healthy behaviors in abstinent, relapsed and recalcitrant smokers. *Applied Nursing Research, 19*(4), 197–203.

Young, T., Skatrud, J., & Peppard, P. E. (2004). Risk factors for obstructive sleep apnea in adults. *Journal of the American Medical Association, 291,* 2013–2016.

Zitt, M. J. (2003, November). *New developments in the medical management of rhinosinusitis. Current concepts in rhinosinusitis.* Program and abstracts of the American College of Allergy, Asthma & Immunology 2003 Annual Meeting, New Orleans, LA.

Caring for the Patient with Lower Airway Disorders

Ellen DeLuca
Kathleen Osborn

Annita Watson

Outcome-Based Learning Objectives

After studying this chapter, the learner will be able to:

1. Differentiate between restrictive and obstructive lung diseases.

2. Compare and contrast the etiology, pathophysiology, clinical manifestations, nursing management, and prevention of the various pulmonary infections and inflammatory disorders.

3. Explain the etiology, pathophysiology, and nursing management of COPD, chronic bronchitis, asthma, cystic fibrosis, pulmonary embolism, and cor pulmonale.

4. Compare and contrast the etiology and nursing management for patients with a variety of chest trauma and thoracic injuries.

5. Discuss the etiology, pathophysiology, and nursing management for patients with lung cancer and lung transplant.

6. Discuss the etiology, pathophysiology, and nursing management of occupational lung diseases.

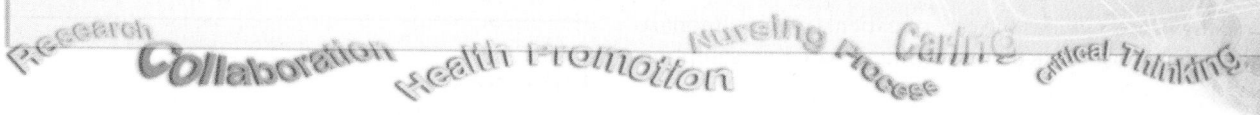

A VARIETY of pathologies can affect the respiratory system. These respiratory alterations include infections, obstructive diseases, occupational diseases, chest trauma, restrictive disorders, and pleural, vascular, and malignant disruptions. This chapter provides in-depth backgrounds for the common respiratory problems faced by individuals and families and also a thorough plan of care for nurses who are members of health teams that care for people with respiratory disorders.

Infections and Inflammatory Disorders

Respiratory infections are a common occurrence among Americans. For example, most individuals will experience symptoms of influenza during their lifetime. However, infections of the respiratory tract are potentially life threatening and a significant cause of morbidly and mortality (Esmond, 2000). The increasing number of resistant organisms enhances the complexity of treatments. The nurse's awareness of assessment, treatment, and prevention of respiratory infections is essential to nursing practice.

Acute Bronchitis

Acute bronchitis is defined as the sudden inflammation of the tracheobronchial tree, which comprises the trachea and the bronchi. Bronchitis can be acute or chronic (a discussion of chronic bronchitis occurs later in this chapter). Acute bronchitis is one of the most common conditions treated by primary care physicians.

Etiology and Epidemiology

Acute bronchitis is most prevalent in children and older adults, and its incidence is highest in the winter. Individuals who suffer from allergies, other respiratory illnesses such as chronic obstructive pulmonary disease (COPD), chronic sinusitis, chronic tonsillitis, or infected adenoids and smokers are at a higher risk (McCance & Huether, 2007; Pulmonology Channel, 2002). Chart 35–1 (p. 936) lists triggers of acute bronchitis.

Pathophysiology

When airways are assaulted by chemical agents or microorganisms, the result is an inflammation of the lower bronchial mucous membranes. Acute bronchitis commonly follows a respiratory viral illness and is usually self-limiting. Most often, its cause is viral; however, a wide variety of agents can produce acute bronchitis including viruses, bacteria, yeast, and fungi and noninfectious triggers (Knutson & Braun, 2002). In adult patients, the most common viral triggers include adenovirus, influenza virus, and respiratory syncytial virus (RSV). Parainfluenza virus, enterovirus, and rhinovirus infections most

MyNursingKit | Influenza

Triggers of Acute Bronchitis

- Viruses (e.g., adenovirus, rhinovirus, and influenza types A and B)
- Bacterias (e.g., *Streptococcus pneumoniae, Haemophilus influenzae*)
- Yeast and fungi (e.g., *Candida albicans*)
- Pollutants (e.g., asthma, air pollutants, ammonia, and tobacco)

commonly occur in the fall, whereas RSV and coronavirus occur in winter and spring. Other causes of acute bronchitis are pollutants, such as ammonia and tobacco. Common bacterial causes are *Streptococcus pneumoniae, Haemophilus influenzae*, and *Bordetella pertussis* (Knutson & Braun, 2002).

Clinical Manifestations

Many of the clinical manifestations (i.e., fever, cough, chills, and malaise) mimic pneumonia, but the physical exam and chest x-ray often are normal. Bacterial cultures are of limited use. The cough typically gets steadily worse for 10 to 12 days, is more profound at night, and becomes increasing loose over time. Most patients have a cough for less than 2 weeks; however, for some individuals, a cough may last for 6 to 8 weeks (Knutson & Braun, 2002). Shortness of breath and wheezing also are common manifestations.

 Nursing Management

The nursing process guides the care of patients with pulmonary infections. Diagnosis of acute bronchitis is based on symptom history.

Assessment

Assessment findings reveal a cough as the most commonly observed symptom in acute bronchitis. Individuals with viral bronchitis have a nonproductive cough. The cough often occurs in paroxysms and is aggravated by cold, dry, or dusty air (McCance & Huether, 2007). Patients with a bacterial bronchitis have a productive cough, and fever and pain behind the sternum that is aggravated by coughing.

Nursing Diagnoses

Priority nursing diagnoses for the patient with bacterial bronchitis include *Ineffective Airway Clearance, Impaired Gas Exchange*, and *Activity Intolerance*.

Outcomes

The outcomes of nursing management include relief of the clinical manifestations and a return to the previous level of functioning.

Interventions and Rationales

Nursing interventions focus on assisting patients with prescribed therapies. These include use of antitussives, analgesics, and bronchodilator medications; encouraging fluids; and teaching patients to cough effectively and avoid infections. Because viruses are the most common cause of acute bronchitis, treat-

ment in this case is focused on preventing the cough with antitussive therapy such as codeine or dextromethorphan or on making the cough more effective with protussive therapy. Terbutaline (Brethine), amiloride (Midamor), and hypertonic saline aerosols have been shown to be the most effective of these (Knutson & Braun, 2002).

In addition to administering these treatments, the nurse encourages an increase in fluid intake to 2 to 3 L/day for thinning secretions and offers mild analgesics such as aspirin or acetaminophen (Tylenol) for discomfort. Deep breathing exercises and use of an incentive spirometer help maintain oxygen and carbon dioxide exchange. For the patient who is wheezing or demonstrating asthmatic symptoms, bronchodilators such as albuterol are administered by the nurse. Antibiotics have not been shown to be effective with acute bronchitis except in patients with COPD (Hunter & King, 2001; Knutson & Braun, 2002). The American Thoracic Society (ATS) has recommended strategies for managing acute exacerbations of chronic bronchitis and emphysema (Voelkel & Tuder, 2000). These strategies include beta-2 agonists, the addition of anticholinergics, antibiotic therapy (when indicated), and the intravenous administration of corticosteroids or methylxanthines such as aminophylline.

Evaluation

Nursing evaluation of a patient with bronchitis includes relief of the respiratory symptoms, e.g., cough, wheezing, and shortness of breath. The patient needs teaching regarding prevention and avoidance of risk factors.

Influenza

Influenza, also known as the *flu,* is a contagious disease that is caused by the influenza virus. Most people recover from influenza in 2 weeks, but some develop life-threatening complications such as pneumonia. About 10% to 20% of people in the United States get influenza yearly. An average of 36,000 people per year die from influenza in the United States. People ages 65 years old and older and people of any age with chronic medical conditions are likely to have complications from the flu (Centers for Disease Control and Prevention [CDC], 2004b).

Epidemiology

Epidemics of influenza occur typically during winter months. Influenza A and B are the two types of influenza viruses that cause epidemic human disease. Influenza virus type C has not been classified and usually does not induce illness. Antigenic variations in influenza type A and B account for the yearly epidemics. These minor variations account for the yearly updating of vaccine strains to be employed (Fishman et al., 2002).

Yearly epidemics of influenza begin abruptly and last 5 to 6 weeks. Epidemics occur from December to April in the Northern Hemisphere. Immunocompromised individuals initially experience illness from influenza; this is the first indication of an impending epidemic followed by increasing numbers of febrile respiratory illnesses in children (Fishman et al., 2002). Worldwide pandemics occur when a new virus emerges for which there is no immunity. Three of the pandemics of the 20th century (1957, 1968, and 1977) began in China. One hypothesis for this geographic source is that influenza viruses can be isolated throughout the year in China and other parts of Asia where the proximity of birds, swine, and humans increases the opportunity for recombination of animal and human influenza viruses, leading to new antigenic shifts (Fishman et al., 2002).

Pathophysiology

Transmission of influenza occurs by small-particle aerosols. Viruses deposited in the lower respiratory tract attach to and infect epithelial cells (Fishman et al., 2002). This can happen when an infected person coughs or sneezes and droplets are propelled through the air and deposited on the mouth or nose of people nearby. Though a less frequent means of transmission, viruses also can be spread when a person touches respiratory droplets on another person or an object and then touches his own mouth or nose before washing his hands (CDC, 2006).

Clinical Manifestations

Typically, influenza has an abrupt onset and is characterized by fever, chills, headache, fatigue, dry, nonproductive cough, sore throat, nasal congestion, and myalgia. The cough may be associated with chest pain. Fever usually persists for 3 to 4 days and occasionally 1 week, at which point systemic symptoms abate. Lung sounds are usually normal, although the most common complication is pneumonia, which may be primary influenza pneumonia or a secondary bacterial pneumonia. The elderly and patients with COPD are at an increased risk for this complication (Fishman et al., 2002).

■ Nursing Management

The primary care goals are relief of symptoms and prevention of secondary infection. Patients are advised to rest, drink plenty of fluids, avoid using alcohol and tobacco, and take aspirin or acetaminophen (Tylenol) for symptom relief.

Medical Management and Health Promotion

The nurse works with the health care provider to ensure that medications are taken appropriately. Three antiviral drugs, amantadine, rimantadine, and oseltamivir, have been approved by the federal government and are commercially available for preventing flu. They are 70% to 90% effective for preventing illness in healthy adults (CDC, 2004b). Four antiviral drugs have been approved for treatment of the flu: amantadine, rimantadine, zanamivir, and oseltamivir. If taken within 2 days of getting sick, these drugs can reduce the symptoms of flu and shorten the time of illness by 1 or 2 days. Antiviral drugs most often are used to control flu outbreaks in institutions such as nursing homes or hospital wards where people are at high risk for complications (CDC, 2004b).

Pneumonia

Pneumonia is an inflammatory process that results in edema of the parenchymal lung tissue, such as alveoli and bronchioles. It also includes extravasation of fluid into the alveoli, thus causing hypoxemia. It is a condition that affects the terminal gas-exchanging portions of the lung primarily. Although at one time pneumonia was a major cause of death, antibiotics have reduced mortality significantly.

Epidemiology

Pneumonia is the sixth leading cause of death in the United States and the number one cause of death from an infectious disease (Niederman et al., 2001; Porth, 2007). The death rates from pneumonia and influenza increased by 59% in the 25-year period prior to 1994, perhaps reflecting an increased population of older Americans (Schultz, 2003). The incidence and mortality of pneumonia are highest in the elderly. Risk factors for pneumonia include advanced age, a compromised immune system, underlying lung disease, alcoholism, altered consciousness, smoking, endotracheal intubation, malnutrition, and immobilization (see the Risk Factors for Community-Acquired Pneumonia box). In general, nosocomial infections and those affecting immunocompromised individuals have a higher mortality rate than community-acquired pneumonias (McCance & Huether, 2007).

Pneumonia was a major cause of death in the 19th and early 20th centuries. The discovery of antibiotics has reduced mortality significantly. The most recent challenge in the treatment of pneumonia is the development of a variety of resistant strain organisms. This has occurred because of overuse and misuse of antibiotics, global transmission of resistant bacteria as a result of poverty and poor medical infection control practices in both developing countries and in the United States, increased world travel, and the increasing costs of developing new antibiotics (Wooten & Salkind, 2003).

Aspiration of oropharyngeal secretions is the most common route of lower respiratory infection. The nasopharynx and oropharynx constitute the first line of defense for most infectious agents. Another route of infection is through the inhalation of microorganisms that have been released into the air when an infected individual coughs, sneezes, or talks, or from aerosolized water, such as that from infected respiratory equipment. Pneumonia also can occur when bacteria are spread to the lungs in the blood from bacteremia, which can result from infection elsewhere in the body or from intravenous (IV) drug abuse (McCance & Huether, 2007).

Etiology

Pneumonia is an acute inflammation of lung tissue caused by inhalation of bacteria, viruses, fungi, protozoa, or parasites to the lung or transportation of these agents via the bloodstream. Other causes are radiation therapy; aspiration of water, food, fluid, and vomitus; and inhalation of toxic gases, chemicals, and smoke (McCance & Huether, 2007).

RISK FACTORS for Community-Acquired Pneumonia

- Advanced age
- Immunocompromised state
- Underlying lung disease
- Chronic disease
- Alcoholism
- Smoking
- Immobility
- Malnutrition
- Crowded living conditions
- Exposure to day care

Pneumonias are classified according to the type of agent causing the infection, the distribution of the infection (lobar or bronchopneumonia), and the setting (community or hospital). The causative microorganism influences the signs and symptoms with which the patient presents, the treatment methods to be used, and the prognosis. For example, bacterial pneumonia causes exudate to fill the alveoli, thereby interfering with oxygen and carbon dioxide exchange and resulting in more severe symptoms than viral and mycoplasmal infections, which involve the tissue surrounding the alveoli (Porth, 2007).

Acute bacterial pneumonias are further subdivided into their anatomic locations. Lobar pneumonia refers to consolidation of a part or all of a lung lobe, whereas bronchopneumonia indicates a patchy consolidation of more than one lobe. Pneumonias also are being classified according to the setting where they were acquired. Community-acquired pneumonia tends to be caused by different microorganisms than those infections acquired in the hospital (nosocomial) (McCance & Huether, 2007). Legionnaire's disease is a common community-acquired bronchopneumonia that is caused by a gram-negative rod, *Legionella pneumophila*. The organism is frequently found in warm standing water. Hospital-acquired pneumonia is defined as a lower respiratory infection that was not present or incubating on admission to the hospital (Porth, 2007).

Pathophysiology

In healthy individuals pathogens that reach the lungs are expelled. However, if a microorganism gets past the upper cough reflex and mucociliary clearance, the next line of defense is the alveolar macrophage. If the organism is virulent and overwhelms the macrophage, there is a full-scale activation of the body's defense mechanisms including the release of multiple inflammatory mediators, cellular infiltration, and immune activation. The end result is that bronchial mucous membranes become damaged, causing the acini and terminal bronchioles to fill with infectious debris and exudates. The accumulation of exudates leads to dyspnea, ventilation/perfusion mismatching, and hypoxemia (McCance & Huether, 2007).

Community-Acquired Pneumonia

Community-acquired pneumonia (CAP), which can be bacterial or viral, is defined as an infection that begins outside the hospital or is diagnosed within 48 hours after admission to a hospital in a person who has not resided in a long-term facility (Porth, 2007). The incidence of CAP is highest in winter months with smoking being an important risk factor (ATS, 2001).

In the outpatient setting, the mortality rate for pneumonia is low. Another feature associated with CAP is that drug resistance has been identified with increasing frequency among *Streptococcus pneumoniae, Haemophilus influenzae, Moraxella catarrhalis*, and a number of enteric gram-negative bacteria (Niederman et al., 2001). In general, CAP patients will be managed on an outpatient basis, but hospitalization may be necessary for persons who are acutely ill or for those at special risk for complications, such as the elderly (Schultz, 2003).

Types of Community-Acquired Pneumonias The most common community-acquired pneumonia is caused by *Streptococcus pneumoniae* (also known as pneumococcus), which has a low mortality rate, though higher in the elderly. *Mycoplasma pneu-*

moniae is a common cause of pneumonia in young people, especially those living in group dormitories or army barracks. Influenza is the most common viral CAP in adults.

Pseudomonas aeruginosa, other gram-negative organisms, and *Staphylococcus aureus* are the most common causes of nosocomial or hospital-acquired pneumonia. Immunocompromised individuals are especially susceptible to *Pneumocystis carinii*, mycobacterial infections, and fungal infections of the respiratory tract (Chart 35–2). In the compromised host, these infections can be difficult to treat and have a high mortality rate (McCance & Huether, 2007). Among patients with CAP who require hospitalization, the mortality rate averages 12% (Niederman et al., 2001). This is related to predisposing factors that include general debility, malnutrition, endotracheal intubation, and contaminated respiratory therapy equipment.

Hospital-Acquired Pneumonia

Pneumonia that occurs more than 48 hours after hospital admission is considered to be a hospital-acquired pneumonia (HAP) and has a mortality rate of 20% to 50% (Barnes, 2000). Ninety percent of the infections are bacterial, and individuals with compromised immune systems, chronic lung disease, and those requiring intubation and mechanical ventilation are at higher risk (Porth, 2007). See the Risk Factors for Hospital-Acquired Pneumonia box. Ventilator-associated pneumonia is discussed in detail in Chapter 36 ⊕. Some common microorganisms that cause HAP are *Pseudomonas aeruginosa, Staphylococcus aureus, Klebsiella pneumoniae*, and *Escherichia coli* (McCance & Huether, 2007).

Clinical Manifestations

Symptoms suggestive of pneumonia include fever, chills, increased respiratory rates, rusty, bloody sputum, crackles, and x-ray abnormalities. Patients who are immunocompromised,

---

CHART 35–2 **Microorganisms Associated with Pneumonia**

Community Acquired	Hospital Acquired
Streptococcus pneumoniae	*Pseudomonas aeruginosa*
Mycoplasma pneumoniae	Staphylococcal pneumonia
Haemophilus influenzae	*Klebsiella* pneumoniae
Oral anaerobic bacteria	
Influenza virus	
Legionella pneumophila	
Chlamydial pneumonia	

RISK FACTORS for Hospital-Acquired Pneumonia

- General debility and malnutrition
- Treatment in an ICU
- Depressed level of consciousness
- Endotracheal intubation
- Contaminated respiratory therapy equipment
- Mechanical ventilation
- Immunosuppressed state

hypothermic, or elderly may not have a fever, and in general 20% of all patients presenting with pneumonia are afebrile. Nonrespiratory symptoms include headache, abdominal pain, nausea and vomiting, diarrhea, and muscle aches. In general, elderly persons complain of fewer symptoms (Fishman et al., 2002). Chart 35–3 summarizes the clinical manifestations of pneumonia.

Laboratory and Diagnostic Procedures

Unfortunately, relatively few diagnostic tests can help the clinician clearly differentiate the pathogen specific to the diagnosis of pneumonia. See the Diagnostic Tests for Pneumonia box.

Medical Management

Antibiotics are the primary treatment for CAP. The fluoroquinolones have been very effective in the treatment of pneumonia. Currently available agents in addition to the quinolones ciprofloxacin and ofloxacin include levofloxacin, sparfloxacin, gatifloxacin, and moxifloxacin (Niederman et al., 2001). Use of the antipneumococcal fluoroquinolones is the recommended choice of treatment by the ATS (2001) for CAP because they are likely to be effective with both gram-negative and gram-positive pathogens. Resistance has been noted with both penicillin and ciprofloxacin (ATS, 2001). Other first-line antibiotics include doxycycline and the macrolides. Antibiotic therapy should be started while identifying the pathogen. When the causative organism is identified, drug therapy can be tailored to the specific pathogen (Schultz, 2003).

Therapy for HAP is empiric and uses combinations of broad-spectrum antibiotics. In some patients methicillin-resistant *Staphylococcus aureus* (MRSA) also is a consideration and vancomycin may be added to the combination antibiotic therapy (Fishman et al., 2002). Bronchodilators may be given via an aerosol route or with **metered-dose inhalers (MDIs)** when there is a significant degree of bronchospasm. A spacer is a device that may be added to the MDI to deliver medication more safely and efficiently. Figures 35–1 ■ and 35–2 ■ (p. 940) show various MDIs and how to use them.

The patient's oxygenation should be monitored so that the saturation is maintained at 93% unless otherwise specified by the health care provider. Pulse oximetry is the least invasive assessment tool, but arterial blood gas (ABG) studies should be done if the patient is suspected of being more severely hypoxemic. This may require that the patient be given supplemental oxygen via a nasal cannula or mask (Figure 35–3 ■, p. 940). In addition, the nurse monitors the patient for signs of hypoxemia.

CHART 35–3	Clinical Manifestations of Pneumonia

- Fever, chills, or hypothermia
- Respiratory rate greater than 20
- Heart rate greater than 100
- Crackles heard on auscultation
- Chest discomfort
- Dyspnea
- Rusty-colored sputum
- Cough
- Fatigue, muscle aches, headache, nausea

DIAGNOSTIC TESTS for Pneumonia

Test	Expected Abnormality	Rationale for Abnormality
Chest x-ray	Whiting out of areas of involvement.	Leukocytosis is present with a bacterial infection.
Sputum Gram stain and culture	Presence of pathogen.	Pathogens are present, and will be evident on the Gram stain.
Transtracheal aspiration	Presence of specific pathogen.	A single pathogen present on the Gram stain is indicative of pneumonia; mixed flora may indicate oral contamination of anaerobic infections.
Bronchoscopy with bronchoalveolar lavage	Presence of a specific pathogen or abnormalities of the trachea and bronchioles.	Bronchial washings specimens can be obtained. Protected brush and bronchoalveolar lavage can be performed for quantitative cultures.
CBC	Presence of leukocytosis.	Leukocytosis is present in pneumonia and infectious processes.
ABG study	Evidence of hypoxemia or hypercarbia, acid–base abnormalities.	Decreased oxygenation may be present if pneumonia is present.
Thoracentesis with pleural fluid sample	Presence of abnormal cells and bacteria.	Obtaining fluid from the pleural space for laboratory analysis allows for the differentiation between simple and complicated effusions. This is used to guide therapeutic intervention.
Urine sample	Hematuria, pyuria, or the presence of protein.	A urinary antigen test for pneumococcus is useful in determining the presence of Legionella serogroup 1.
Serum electrolytes, BUN, creatinine, liver function studies	Abnormal laboratory values in elderly individuals and in persons who are chronically ill for whom pneumonia is a secondary problem.	Serology is essential in the diagnosis of unusual causes of pneumonia such as Q fever and brucellosis.

MyNursingKit | Video: Respiratory: Asthma—Using Inhaler

FIGURE 35–1 ■ A variety of inhalers and their use.

Restlessness or increased pulse may be the first signs of hypoxia. Breathlessness and cyanosis are later signs.

Nursing Management

Priority nursing measures for the patient with pneumonia include airway maintenance oxygen saturation above 93% or the level specified by the health care provider. *Readiness for Enhanced Comfort* and *Readiness for Enhanced Nutrition* also are common nursing diagnoses. The nurse promotes nutrition and hydration as a component of care since patients may be anorexic because of the disease process. Small, frequent, high-carbohydrate and high-

FIGURE 35–2 ■ How to use a metered-dose inhaler.

(a) Simple face mask

(b) Plastic face mask with reservoir bag

Adjustable nose clip

Opening

Exhaled air

Venturi barrel

Room air

(c) Venturi mask

(d) Tracheostomy mask

(e) Face tent

(f) Standard nasal cannulas

FIGURE 35–3 ■ Use of an oxygen mask.

protein meals are provided and fluid intake is monitored closely. Oral hygiene is essential before and after meals. Promoting comfort also is a nursing role. The patient is monitored for chest pain and the character and location are noted. This may occur because of excessive coughing. Usually patients are most comfortable with the head of the bed elevated 45 to 90 degrees. Mild analgesics such as codeine, aspirin, and acetaminophen (Tylenol) are prescribed. Managing these patients is outlined in detail in the Nursing Process: Patient Care Plan for Pneumonia.

NURSING PROCESS: Patient Care Plan for Pneumonia

Assessment for Pneumonia

Subjective Data:
Do you have a cough, chills, or chest pain?
Describe the sputum you are coughing if any.
How are you treating the symptoms?
What seems to be most helpful?
Do you have any history of exposure to respiratory infections or pulmonary irritants?
Have you recently taken antibiotics?
Do you feel short of breath?
What triggers your discomfort?
Describe your sleeping pattern.

Objective Data:
Lung sounds
Vital signs
Sputum cultures
Chest x-ray
Spirometry
ABGs
Oxygen saturation

Nursing Assessment and Diagnoses	Outcomes and Evaluation Parameters	Planning and Interventions with *Rationales*
Nursing Diagnosis: *Ineffective Breathing Pattern* related to an infectious process in the lungs	**Outcomes:** The patient demonstrates effective coughing and breathing techniques. The patient drinks 3 liters of fluid per day. **Evaluation Parameters:** The patient's vital signs and temperature are within normal range. Upon auscultation, lung sounds in all fields are clear. The health care team, patient, and significant other(s) report that patient is drinking fluids as instructed. Sputum is easily expectorated and liquefied. Urine is clear light yellow.	**Interventions and *Rationales:*** Complete a physical assessment that includes vital signs, temperature, assessment of fever and or chills, tachycardia, and tachypnea *to detect early signs of infection and or exacerbation of infection.* Inspect for accessory muscle retraction, cyanosis, grunting on expiration, and restricted chest movement. In addition, auscultate for bronchial breath sounds, inspiratory crackles, increased vocal fremitus due to pleural effusion, unless the bronchus is completely plugged, which decreases vocal fremitus, and egophony due to consolidation. *These clinical signs are associated with hypoxemia, atelectasis, and pulmonary congestion. A baseline assessment is performed to ascertain the degree of pulmonary congestion and hypoxemia.* Assist the patient to perform controlled coughing and deep breathing, and place the patient in an upright position to do this. A small pillow used to splint the chest may facilitate coughing and increase comfort. When not sitting in a chair, the patient's position should be changed frequently. *This assists with mobilizing secretions.* Give mild analgesics for chest pain that the patient may experience *due to muscular fatigue as the result of frequent paroxysms of coughing. Coughing allows for expectoration of secretions and clearance of airways. A pillow supports the diaphragm and allows for deeper breaths.* Provide prescribed medications and teach the patient about the purpose of each. This may include the use of an MDI. Prior to discharge the patient should demonstrate accurate use of the MDI, inhalers, or other oxygen equipment, and state the purpose of each medication. In addition to bronchodilators the patient may be placed on antibiotic therapy. The nurse reviews the therapy regime with the patient and ascertains that he is able to take the medications correctly at home. *The patient is placed on bronchodilator medications as well as antibiotics to open airways and clear secretions. Providing teaching about medication and assessing the patient's ability ascertains that the patient will receive the prescribed dose at home.* Encourage fluids to 3 liters/day *to liquefy tenacious secretions and allow for easy expectoration.*

(continued)

NURSING PROCESS: Patient Care Plan for Pneumonia—*Continued*

Assessment of Oxygen Status

Subjective Data:
Do you have a cough, chills, or chest pain?
Describe the sputum you are coughing if any.
Do you have any history of exposure to respiratory infections or pulmonary irritants?
Have you recently taken antibiotics?
Do you feel short of breath?
Do you feel like you are getting enough air?
If not, what triggers your discomfort?

Objective Data:
Lung sounds
Vital signs
Sputum cultures
Chest x-ray
Spirometry
ABGs
Oxygen saturation

Nursing Assessment and Diagnoses	Outcomes and Evaluation Parameters	Planning and Interventions with *Rationales*
Nursing Diagnosis: *Impaired Gas Exchange* related to infectious process in the lungs	**Outcome:** The patient states she can breathe easily without distress. **Evaluation Parameter:** Pulse oximetry and or blood gas results are within normal range for the patient.	**Interventions and *Rationales:*** Assess the patient's dyspnea at rest, with exertion, and during sleep. Administer oxygen as ordered, usually via nasal cannula or mask, and position the patient in an upright position or with the head up at night. Explain the rationale for oxygen to patient and family members. *Perfusion abnormalities related to pulmonary congestion cause hypoxemia and dyspnea. Supplemental oxygen with a nasal cannula or a mask provides relief. Ventilation is improved in the upright position because it allows for maximal expansion of the lungs.*

Assessment of Ability to Perform ADLs

Subjective Data:
Can you perform the normal activities of daily living (ADL)?
What activities lead to fatigue?
How much activity can you do before needing to stop and rest? How is this different from your usual endurance?

Objective Data:
Exercise tolerance: How much activity can the patient tolerate before developing clinical manifestations?

Nursing Assessment and Diagnoses	Outcomes and Evaluation Parameters	Planning and Interventions with *Rationales*
Nursing Diagnosis: *Activity Intolerance* related to an infectious process in the lungs	**Outcome:** Patient is able to assist with ADLs and initiate short walks of one-quarter to one-half block without dyspnea. **Evaluation Parameter:** Patient's oxygen saturation remains normal during and after performance of ADLs and ambulation.	**Interventions and *Rationales:*** Assess the patient's ability to perform ADLs. Administering oxygen as necessary, encourage the patient to do partial completion of ADLs and assist to a chair position followed by ambulation at short distances until the goal is reached. *Dyspnea indicates increased work of breathing. In the hypoxemic patient, exercise should not be attempted without oxygen. Oxygen allows the patient to perform optimally by providing adequate oxygenation to the muscles and decreasing the work of breathing.*

Assessment of Patient/Family Knowledge

Subjective Data:
Tell me what you know about your health problems.
Do you have questions about your health care?

Objective Data:
Verbalizes education needs.
Identifies mode of receiving educational material.
Participates in education discussion.

Nursing Assessment and Diagnoses	Outcomes and Evaluation Parameters	Planning and Interventions with *Rationales*
Nursing Diagnosis: *Deficient Knowledge* related to disease process	**Outcomes:** Patient avoids risk factors related to pneumonia. Patient complies with follow-up care. **Evaluation Parameter:** Patient verbalizes understanding of health needs and importance of prevention.	**Interventions and *Rationales:*** Assess the patient's and family's learning needs, readiness to learn, and preferred method of education (verbal, written, audiovisual) to present information at a time and in a manner the patient and family can understand. The patient's understanding of the treatment measures decreases anxiety and promotes compliance. Instruct patient to seek immediate medical attention for return of clinical manifestations *to promote seeking early medical treatment of potential life-threatening illness.*

Discharge Priorities

Before discharging the patient recovering from pneumonia, the nurse emphasizes the importance of rest and a gradual increase in activity to avoid fatigue. Patients are instructed to maintain resistance to infection with proper nutrition and adequate fluid intake. They also are warned to avoid chilling and exposure to others with upper respiratory tract infections or viruses.

Health Promotion

The patient and family are made aware of the fact that one episode of pneumonia increases susceptibility to recurrent infections. The patient is taught about all medications that will be continued at home. The nurse provides written instructions as necessary. Patients should be reminded that they should continue deep breathing and coughing exercises 4 times a day for 6 to 8 weeks. They also are instructed to notify the health care provider if experiencing chills, fever, dyspnea, hemoptysis, increasing fatigue, or other respiratory complications.

Pulmonary Fungal Infections

The incidence of fungal infections of the lung has increased dramatically since the 1960s, particularly in immunocompromised patients (Haque, 1992; Mandanas, 2007). Fungal infections of the lung can be divided into those that occur in generally healthy individuals and those that occur in opportunistically immuno-suppressed patients (Chart 35–4). Both types are acquired by inhalation of contaminated soil resulting in pulmonary infections.

Etiology and Epidemiology

Fungal lung infections occur more frequently in areas where there are endemic fungi, which include the valleys of the Mississippi and Ohio rivers (histoplasmosis and blastomycosis), the southwestern United States, the San Joaquin valley in California, and northern Mexico (coccidioidomycosis), and Central and South America (paracoccidioidomycosis). The organisms grow in soil that has been enriched with bird excreta: old chicken coops, barns, pigeon nesting areas, and tress where birds roost (Porth, 2007). These infections affect men (75% to 95%) more often than women; estrogen-mediated inhibition of mycelium-to-yeast transformation may be responsible for the male predominance. Estrogen seems to have a protective effect against cryptococcal infection. Cryptococcosis has a male-to-female ratio of 2 to 3:1 (Mandanas, 2007). Known risk factors for the development of the fungal lung diseases include:

- Travel to an area where fungal pneumonia pathogens are endemic

- Regular exposure to bird, bat, or rodent droppings in endemic areas
- Immunocompromised patients who have an increased risk for opportunistic infections, such as cancer and human immunodeficiency virus (HIV)
- Males.

Endemic pneumonias are generally self-limiting in healthy patients. *Coccidioides immitis*, which causes coccidioidomycosis, is the most virulent, yet 90% of patients recover without treatment. However, in patients with acquired immunodeficiency syndrome (AIDS), the mortality rate is as high as 70%. Fungi that affect immunosuppressed individuals include *Aspergillus* and *Candida*, as well as *Cryptococcus neoformans* and fungi of the order *Mucorales* called mucormycosis. In patients with limited defense mechanisms these organisms can produce widespread systemic disease leading to death. A fungal etiology always should be considered in immunosuppressed patients with radiologic abnormalities (Amersham Health, 2004). Aspergillosis in patients who are neutropenic (from either leukemia chemotherapy or bone marrow transplantation) has a mortality rate of 50% to 85% (Mandanas, 2007).

Pathophysiology

Fungi can cause lung disease through direct infection of pulmonary tissue, through infection of pulmonary air spaces/lung cavities, or through their ability to trigger an immunologic reaction when fungal material is inhaled. Once in the lungs, the fungi elicit tissue responses ranging from acute exudative reactions to a prolonged chronic course, and disseminating to other organs and causing systemic infections. Additionally, individuals with fungal pneumonias may develop chronic pulmonary (e.g., cavitation, pleural effusions, bronchopleural fistulas) or extrapulmonary complications.

Clinical Manifestations

Clinical manifestations of fungal lung infections frequently resemble those of tuberculosis. The disease can take any of three forms depending on the host's resistance and immunocompetence:

- An acute primary disease
- A chronic (cavitary) pulmonary disease
- A disseminated infection.

The primary pulmonary lesions present with nodules containing macrophages that have engulfed microorganisms. These nodules may also be in the lymph nodes. Other clinical manifestations include a mild self-limiting flu-like syndrome (Porth, 2007).

When the individual is immunocompromised, chronic cavitary lesions develop, along with a productive cough, fever, night sweats, and weight loss. A disseminated fulminating infection most often occurs in the very young and very elderly who have compromised immune function. These patients present with a high fever, generalized lymph node enlargement, hepatosplenomegaly, muscle wasting, anemia, high white blood cell counts, and thrombocytopenia. Ulcerations of the tongue and mouth and voice hoarseness, nausea, vomiting, diarrhea, and abdominal pain may also occur. Frequently meningitis becomes the most pronounced manifestation (Porth, 2007).

CHART 35–4	**Fungal Infections of the Lung**

FUNGAL INFECTIONS OCCURRING IN IMMUNE COMPETENT INDIVIDUALS	FUNGAL INFECTIONS OCCURRING IN IMMUNE INCOMPETENT INDIVIDUALS
• Histoplasmosis	• Aspergillosis
• Coccidioidomycosis	• Candidiasis
• Blastomycosis	• Mucormycosis

Laboratory and Diagnostic Procedures

The diagnosis of a fungal infection depends on the demonstration of the organisms by culture or histology (Mandanas, 2007). The most characteristic chest x-ray presentation involves one or more nodular infiltrates that progress rapidly, cavitate, and cross lung fissures. Lung scans may demonstrate perfusion defects consistent with fungal disease. However, the patient may be symptomatic without radiologic findings. Skin tests similar to the tuberculin test are used to detect *Histoplasma* and *Coccidioides*.

Medical Management

Amphotericin B is the drug most commonly used in treating serious systemic fungal infections. It is given intravenously and considered a toxic drug with many possible side effects including fever, chills, malaise, nausea and vomiting, thrombophlebitis at the injection site, and renal dysfunction. Recent advances in amphotericin B include the development of lipid formulations, which demonstrate reduced nephrotoxicity when compared with the parent compound (American Lung Association, 2004; Crawford, 2004). Total treatment with the drug may last from 4 to 12 weeks. Many of the side effects can be avoided by premedication with hydrocortisone, an anti-inflammatory, or Benadryl. Renal function is monitored closely, and ensuring adequate hydration is essential. In addition to amphotericin, the oral agents currently available for treatment include the imidazoles, the triazoles, and the echocardins. More details on these agents are given in the Pharmacology Summary feature (p. 981).

◼ Nursing Management

Presenting symptoms are often dyspnea, nonproductive cough, and pleuritic chest pain. Fever and chills also may be present (Morrison & Lew, 2001).

Assessment

The nurse assesses the patient's breathing pattern, lung sounds, and presence of cough, sputum production, and pleuritic chest pain. Lung sounds can mimic those of bacterial pneumonia including signs of pulmonary consolidation, such as crackles, bronchial breath sounds, and increased fremitus. The nurse needs to monitor oxygen saturations and ABGs for evidence of respiratory failure. Fever and chills also may be present. Symptoms may range from mild to severe, including respiratory failure; therefore, the assessment must be done on an ongoing basis to monitor for trends in the clinical manifestations.

Outcomes and Evaluation Parameters

Outcomes and evaluation parameters for these patients include an absence of symptoms and an ability to perform activities of daily living (ADLs).

Interventions and Rationales

Nursing interventions depend on the clinical manifestations. The patient may just need to be encouraged and reminded to deep breathe and cough. Supplemental oxygen therapy and in some instances mechanical ventilation may be necessary. Administration of medications and patient education is a priority.

Pulmonary Tuberculosis

Pulmonary tuberculosis (TB) is a contagious bacterial infection caused by *Mycobacterium tuberculosis (M. tuberculosis)*. The lungs are primarily involved but the disease can spread to other organs. The disease can develop after inhaling droplets sprayed into the air from a cough or sneeze by someone infected with *M. tuberculosis*. The disease is characterized by the development of granulomas (granular tumors) in the infected tissues.

Epidemiology

In 1900, tuberculosis (TB) was the leading cause of death in the United States and Europe. In 2005, the total number of new cases of tuberculosis in the United States was 14,093. The annual decrease in tuberculosis cases has slowed from an average of 7.1% in the 1993–2000 period to the current average of 3.8% for the 2001–2005 period. In addition to those with active TB, an estimated 10 to 15 million people in the United States have latent tuberculosis. About 10% of these individuals will develop active TB at some time in their lives. Transmission of TB is rampant in crowded shelters and prisons where people weakened by poor nutrition, drug addiction, and alcoholism are exposed to *Mycobacterium tuberculosis* (Schoenstadt, 2006).

Noncompliance is a major cause of drug-resistant TB. Tuberculosis patients who do not complete drug treatment can stay infectious for longer periods of time and therefore can spread TB to more people. These treatment failures result in TB strains that are resistant to one or more of the standard medicines given to TB patients (Schoenstadt, 2006).

Many elderly people whose general health has declined develop active TB from TB infection that they had much earlier in life. Other elderly people, especially those with weak immune systems, become newly infected with *M. tuberculosis* and can develop active TB rapidly.

Cases of multidrug-resistant TB have declined sharply in the United States during the past decade. In 2003, the most recent year for which there is resistance rate reporting, 114 individuals were reported with multidrug-resistant TB—a 76.5% decline since 1993. Of these individuals, 28 were born in the United States, and 86 were born in other nations (Schoenstadt, 2006).

Etiology

The organism *Mycobacterium tuberculosis* is nonmotile, nonsporulating, and an acid-fast rod that secretes niacin. The tubercle bacillus is transmitted via aerosolization (i.e., an airborne route). Individuals who are most commonly infected are those having repeated close contact with an infected person who has not yet been diagnosed with TB.

TB also is one of the opportunistic infections common to persons with HIV/AIDS. According to the World Health Organization (WHO) (2003) the AIDS epidemic is considered a major factor in the increase of TB cases. The suppression of the immune system caused by HIV both opens the door to new active infection and permits activation of latent disease. One-third of the increase in global TB cases during the last five years can be attributed to HIV (WHO, 2003). Continuous assessment and intervention to prevent the spread of the disease must continue.

The newest form of TB is multidrug-resistant tuberculosis (MDR TB). It is resistant to two or more of the primary drugs (isoniazid and rifampin) used for the treatment of tuberculosis. Extensively drug-resistant TB (XDR TB) is TB resistant to isoniazid and rifampin among the first-line anti-TB drugs; and among the second-line drugs, it is resistant to any fluoroquinolone and at least one of three injectable drugs (Raviglione & Smith, 2007). Resistance occurs when bacteria develop the ability to withstand antibiotic attack and relay that ability to newly produced bacteria. Because that entire strain of bacteria inherits this capacity, resistance can spread from one person to another. Inadequate treatment of TB and/or improper use of antituberculosis medications is an important cause of drug-resistant tuberculosis. Drug-resistant TB is difficult and costly to treat and can be fatal (Raviglione & Smith, 2007).

Pathophysiology

TB is a highly communicable disease that is transmitted via aerosolization. When an infected person laughs, sneezes, or sings, droplet nuclei are produced and may be inhaled by others. When the tubercle reaches a suitable site (bronchi or alveoli), it multiplies freely. An exudative response occurs, causing a nonspecific pneumonitis. With the development of acquired immunity, further multiplication of bacilli is controlled in the majority of initial lesions. The lesions typically resolve and leave very little or no residual. A small percentage of those who are initially infected develop the disease (5% to 15%). Cell-mediated or type IV immunity develops 2 to 10 weeks after infection and is manifested by a significant reaction to a tuberculin test. A primary infection may be microscopic in size and may never appear on x-ray film.

The process of infection appears in the following way. The granulomatous inflammation created by the tubercle bacillus becomes surrounded by collagen, fibroblasts, and lymphocytes. In the center of the lesion (Ghon's tubercle), necrosis, which is called caseation necrosis, occurs. After this development, areas of caseation localize and undergo resorption, hyaline degeneration, and fibrosis. These necrotic areas may calcify (calcification) or liquefy (liquefaction). If the latter occurs, the liquid material then empties into a bronchus, and the evacuated area becomes a cavity (cavitation). Bacilli continue to proliferate in the necrotic cavity wall. The evacuated material leads to endobronchial spread of disease into new areas of the lung; this process can be a recurring one. A lesion also may progress by direct extension if bacilli multiply rapidly and there is marked exudative response. These lesions may extend into the pleura, which results in tuberculosis pleural effusion with a small number of organisms. Similarly, pericardial effusions may occur. Initial infection is seen more often in the middle or lower lobes of the lung. If a large number of organisms enter the bloodstream, disseminated disease, which is called miliary tuberculosis, occurs. Typically, many tiny discrete nodules scattered throughout the lung are visualized on x-ray film. If disseminated disease occurs through bloodborne foci, the brain, meninges, liver, kidney, and bone marrow are commonly involved.

Clinical Manifestations

The nurse inquires about presenting signs and symptoms such as dyspnea, weight loss, cough, sputum production, sleep disturbances, night sweats, and fatigue. The signs and symptoms of pulmonary TB are insidious and many patients do not become aware of symptoms until the disease is well advanced. Typically, the patient presents with lethargy, exhaustive fatigue, activity intolerance, nausea, irregular menses, and low-grade fever, which may have occurred for weeks or months. Fever also may be accompanied by night sweats. The patient finally notices a cough and the production of mucoid and mucopurulent sputum, which is occasionally streaked with blood. A dull aching chest pain may accompany the cough. The physical examination of the chest does not provide conclusive evidence of tuberculosis. The nurse may hear dullness with percussion over involved parenchymal areas, bronchial breath sounds, and increased transmission of spoken or whispered sounds. Wheezing related to obstruction may also be heard.

Laboratory and Diagnostic Procedures

The tuberculin skin test, chest x-ray, acid-fast bacillus smear, and sputum culture are used to diagnose TB. If the patient has had the bacille Calmette-Guérin (BCG) vaccine containing attenuated tubercle bacilli, which is used routinely in foreign countries to produce resistance to TB, she will have a positive skin test and should be evaluated via chest x-ray. See the Diagnostic Tests for Tuberculosis box (p. 946) for specific details.

Medical Management

Early detection of TB depends on subjective data rather than presentation of symptoms. Possible exposure and travel to foreign countries in which there is a high incidence of TB need to be determined. It is important to note whether the patient has had any prior tests for TB and what they were. There is a difference between being infected with TB and having TB disease. Someone who is infected with TB has the TB bacteria in his body and his body's defenses are protecting him from the bacteria and therefore the person is not sick. Someone with TB disease is sick and, if not properly treated, can spread the disease to other people. A person with symptoms of TB disease or evidence of infection needs to be seen by a health care provider.

Most patients are treated on an outpatient basis, and with effective drug therapy many individuals continue to work and lead normal lives. Medical management for TB centers on drug therapy (see the Pharmacology Summary, p. 981). Drug therapy is used for those who have clinical manifestations and for individuals who are infected. The patient receives instructions for the chemotherapy regime from the health care provider who follows up for at least a year during active treatment. The diagnosis also is reported to the local health department, which follows up on patient progress through treatment and provides resources.

The hospitalized patient with active TB or suspected active TB is placed in a negative pressure room with respiratory airborne isolation and use of standard precautions. Negative pressure is effective in moving airborne bacilli out into the atmosphere. The patient should remain in isolation until three consecutive sputum cultures have tested negative. Until the sputum cultures return negative, there is no certainty that an individual is not infectious.

Possible complications of TB include multidrug resistance, hemorrhage, and pleurisy; any of these complications may

DIAGNOSTIC TESTS for Tuberculosis

Test	Expected Results	Rationale
Mantoux test for TB (PPD)	A reaction at the injection site occurs 48–72 hours after injection of a small amount of intermediate strength purified protein derivative (PPD) given intradermally into the forearm. A reaction includes induration and erythema. The diameter of induration is measured at its widest part. An induration of 5 mm or greater may be significant for individuals at risk such as HIV patients. An induration of 10 mm or greater is significant in individuals with normal or mildly impaired immunity.	An individual with a positive PPD test has been exposed to TB and has developed antibodies. Also individuals who have received the BCG vaccine used routinely in Europe and South America to provide resistance to TB develop antibodies.
Chest x-ray	Visualizes tuberculosis lesions, cavities, and inflammation.	Visualizes the extent of lung involvement but does not confirm diagnosis. Used to assess patients with a positive PPD.
Sputum for acid–fast bacilli	Three sputum samples are positive on an acid-fast smear.	Confirms TB diagnosis.

indicate recurrence of tuberculosis activity, and the patient and family should be made aware of these complications.

■ Nursing Management

Nursing care for the TB patient focuses on preventing the spread of the infection, assisting the patient and family to manage the environment, and prescribed chemotherapy. The nurse addresses patient anxiety related to the disease and issues such as poor nutrition, pain, and fatigue (see Nursing Process: Patient Care Plan for Tuberculosis).

Health Promotion

The main focus of TB management is prevention of the spread of the infection. Most TB can be cured with drugs, but a patient must continually take the prescribed medication, usually for 9 months. Some patients require a year or more for successful treatment. If the drug is stopped before completion, the TB may come back more resilient than before. Surviving bacteria may become resistant to the drugs used to treat TB, causing MDR TB (ATS, CDC, and Infectious Disease Society of America, 2003). Finally, all persons who live with or have been in close contact with the infected individual must be tested and treated if necessary.

Atypical Mycobacterium

Atypical mycobacteria are a group of bacteria that are widely distributed in nature. They are found in water, soil, animals, and man, and usually do not produce disease. These are *Mycobacterium avium*, *M. intracellulare*, *M. kansasii*, *M. xenopi*, and *M. fortuitum*. Usually infections from these organisms are caused by exposure to infected water, soil, dust, or aerosols (Medical College of Wisconsin Healthlink, 2008).

Epidemiology and Etiology

The largest numbers of *M. avium* or mycobacterium avium complex (MAC) encounters have been among persons who were immunocompromised with HIV disease and other forms of immune compromise (Fishman et al., 2002). MAC disease is the second most commonly diagnosed opportunistic infection second to *Pneumocystis carinii*, commonly experienced by persons with HIV.

Clinical Manifestations

MAC and *Mycobacterium scrofulaceum* are associated with lymphadenitis in immunocompetent children. All nodes in the cervical chain can be affected, but the nodes of the submandibular region appear to be the most commonly involved. Disseminated infections are usually associated with HIV infection. Host immunity seems to play a major role because a low CD4+ lymphocyte count (fewer than 100 cells/μL for adults and age-appropriate decreases in children) is associated with an increased frequency of disseminated MAC disease (Dieudonne, 2008). Patients present with cough, increased sputum production, fever, weakness, and weight loss. A chest x-ray is likely to show abnormalities, and blood cultures or cultures of body fluids are likely to confirm the diagnosis.

Medical Management

Medical management involves administration of prescribed antibiotics and assessment of pulmonary status and oxygen saturation. Usually the patient is on two antibiotics. Common antibiotics include Zithromax, Biaxin, ciprofloxacin, and Mefoxin. Oxygen therapy is administered if the patient experiences dyspnea and low oxygen saturations. Family members and significant others are taught that there is no concern for person-to-person spread of these organisms so isolation is not necessary (Medical College of Wisconsin Healthlink, 2008). If the patient experiences weight loss or wasting syndrome, the nutritionist becomes very involved with meal planning. Patients may require follow-up with a home care nurse, respiratory therapist, and nutritionist upon discharge. Arrangements are also made for any respiratory therapy equipment or oxygen to be delivered and managed in the home setting.

Lung Abscess

A **lung abscess** is a localized area of lung destruction caused by liquefaction necrosis usually related to pyogenic bacteria.

Epidemiology and Etiology

The incidence of lung abscess is not well known due to it not occurring in isolation. It may be solitary or may occur in multiple discrete lesions. Most often such an abscess is secondary to anaerobic and aerobic organisms that colonize the upper respiratory tract and may be associated with periodontal disease (Fishman et al., 2002). Patients who present with this problem often have a history of pneumonia, possibly complicated by aspiration of oropharyngeal contents. Other causes of lung abscess include bacteremia seeding in the lungs, tricuspid endocarditis leading to septic pulmonary embolus, extension of hepatic abscess, associated with bronchial carcinoma, and bronchial obstruction (Patient UK, 2007). For example, an obstruction of a bronchus may cause a necrotizing process in the distal lung that eventually becomes an abscess. Formation of multiple abscesses and cavities occurs commonly in patients with TB or fungal infections of the lung.

Clinical Manifestations

Clinical manifestations are often insidious, although more acute if a lung abscess follows pneumonia. Typically the patient experiences spiking temperature with rigors and night sweats; a cough with sputum that is often foul tasting, foul smelling, and blood stained; pleuritic chest pain; tachycardia; and shortness of breath. Lung sounds are diminished and there is a dullness on percussion over the abscess. Depending on the size, oxygen saturation may be decreased.

Laboratory and Diagnostic Procedures

A CT scan is used if there is a question of cavitation not clearly seen. Pleural fluid and blood cultures may be obtained. Bronchoscopy may be used in the case of delayed drainage or suspected malignancy. If the health care provider is unable to obtain sputum, transtracheal aspiration via suction may be done to obtain a sample so that sputum can be cultured and appropriate organisms identified. The patient needs to be evaluated for signs of severe periodontal disease and infective endocarditis, as a possible cause of the lung abscess.

Medical Management

The type of organism isolated on sputum culture and the findings of the history, physical exam, and diagnostic work-up will determine the treatment required. Adequate drainage of the lung abscess can be achieved through postural drainage and chest physiotherapy. The patient should be assessed for adequate cough. Some patients may benefit from a percutaneous chest catheter placed for drainage of the abscess (Sharma, 2004). Intravenous antibiotic therapy with penicillin G or clindamycin is the pharmacologic therapy of choice followed by penicillin with metronidazole. The dose is continued until there is evidence of symptom improvement. Long-term therapy with oral antibiotics prevents relapse (Sharma, 2004). In addition, a diet high in protein is provided. Supportive care and emotional support for the long-term nature of this problem is necessary.

NURSING PROCESS: Patient Care Plan for Tuberculosis

Assessment of Airway and Gas Exchange

Subjective Data:

Have you been exposed to TB?

Have you had recent travel to foreign countries in which there is a high incidence of TB?

Have you had any prior tests for TB?

If so what were they?

Have you had the BCG vaccine?

Have you had dyspnea, weight loss, cough, sputum production, sleep disturbances, night sweats, or fatigue?

Objective Data:

Lung sounds

Vital signs

Sputum culture for acid-fast bacilli

Chest x-ray

Work of breathing

Oxygen saturation

Nursing Assessment and Diagnoses	Outcomes and Evaluation Parameters	Planning and Interventions with *Rationales*
Nursing Diagnosis: *Ineffective Airway Clearance* related to tracheobronchial secretions as evidenced by copious sputum production	**Outcome:** Upon auscultation of lung fields by the nurse, breath sounds are clear or with fewer adventitious sounds. *Evaluation Parameter:* Upon assessment by the nurse, vital signs are within normal range and the patient is afebrile.	**Interventions and *Rationales:*** Instruct the patient on methods to facilitate airway clearance. Teach proper coughing and deep breathing and postural drainage techniques. Encourage hydration with 2–3 liters of fluid daily. *Effective coughing and deep breathing techniques and good hydration promote liquefication of secretions and facilitate expectoration.* Assess respiratory status for changes, also observing for temperature spikes or recurrence of symptoms. The patient who is progressing well should show a remission of symptoms. *A temperature spike or changes in respiratory status may indicate a complication or drug resistance.*

(continued)

NURSING PROCESS: Patient Care Plan for Tuberculosis—*Continued*

Assessment of Patient/Family Knowledge of Disease

Subjective Data:
What is your understanding of TB?
Do you know who you got it from?
Do you know how it is spread?
Can you list your medications and how to take them and what precautions are necessary?
Do you understand the treatment of TB and how you can help clear your lungs?

Objective Data:
Can you give examples of when you would call your health care provider?
What are the best methods for preventing the spread of TB?

Nursing Assessment and Diagnoses	Outcomes and Evaluation Parameters	Planning and Interventions with *Rationales*
Nursing Diagnosis: *Deficient Knowledge about treatment regimen and preventive health measures* related to TB management as evidenced by inability to plan care without assistance	**Outcomes:** Patient demonstrates to the nurse accurate coughing and deep breathing techniques, positioning and postural drainage techniques, and proper use of humidification and hydration to facilitate airway clearance. **Evaluation Parameters:** Demonstrates an adequate level of knowledge with regard to the medication regime, side effects, and indications for contacting the health care provider. Describes methods for preventing the spread of TB. Describes methods for minimizing drug side effects such as regular checkups, laboratory evaluation, supplemental vitamins, and avoidance of alcohol and foods containing tyramine and histamine.	**Interventions and *Rationales:*** Review the necessary information regarding coughing and breathing techniques and drug therapy and provide written information and instructions. Information is repeated as needed, enlisting the support of family members. If the patient is not English speaking, an interpreter is sought as well as patient education materials in the appropriate language. The importance of scheduled laboratory evaluation of renal and liver function is stressed. Teach the patient that rifampin causes urine to become darker in color. In addition, rifampin can increase the metabolism of other medications, making them less effective. These include beta-blockers, oral anticoagulants, corticosteroids, digoxin, quinidine, oral hypoglycemic agents, oral contraceptives, theophylline, and verapamil. Patients taking isoniazid (also called isonicotinyl hydrazine or INH) are taught to avoid foods containing tyramine and histamine. These are tuna, aged cheese, red wine, soy sauce, and yeast extracts. Eating these foods while on INH causes headaches, flushing, hypotension, light-headedness, palpitations, and diaphoresis. Medications should be taken 1 hour before meals or on an empty stomach since food interferes with absorption. The patient is instructed to cover his or her mouth and nose when coughing and sneezing. The patient should alert the health care provider regarding any fever or recurrence of symptoms. He should avoid exposure to silicone or dust because these substances cause further lung damage. The patient also must understand that taking medications is the most effective method of preventing transmission. *The major reason treatment fails is that patients do not take medications regularly and for the prescribed duration. Adherence to the therapeutic regime is essential to recovery. Patients who are not compliant with medication regimes are likely to remain infectious, and also prone to developing resistant strains of TB that are much more difficult to treat.*

Assessment of Ability to Perform Activities of Daily Living (ADL)

Subjective Data:
What daily activities can you accomplish without assistance?
Describe your activity schedule.
Describe any physical symptoms you have while exercising or performing ADLs.

Objective Data:
Observation of physical status during exercise
Oxygen saturation pre- and postactivity
Lung sounds pre- and postactivity
Vital signs pre- and postactivity

Nursing Assessment and Diagnoses	Outcomes and Evaluation Parameters	Planning and Interventions with *Rationales*
Nursing Diagnosis: *Activity Intolerance* related to fatigue as evidenced by inability to engage in normal activities without dyspnea or fatigue	**Outcome:** Maintains an activity schedule without fatigue or dyspnea. **Evaluation Parameters:** Walks one-half block without experiencing dyspnea or fatigue. Completes ADLs independently and without dyspnea. Oxygen saturation is within normal range at rest and after completion of ADLs.	**Interventions and *Rationales:*** Plan a gradual progression of activity *to increase exercise tolerance and muscle strength.*

◼ Nursing Management

The nursing management of patients with lung abscess focuses on assessment, treatment, and evaluation. It is critical that the nurse assess the patient's recent past medical history, and plan interventions based on the patient's knowledge base and understanding. The nurse also must take into consideration the patient's support system and ability to care for self.

Assessment

It is important for the nurse to assess the patient's recent history of influenza, pneumonia, febrile illness cough, and sputum production. Physical assessment of the patient often reveals a febrile patient who appears pale and fatigued. The patient may complain of pleuritic chest pain, which is stabbing in nature when taking a deep breath. Auscultation of breath sounds may reveal decreased sounds in the involved area of the lung. Bronchial breath sounds and fine crackles are heard over the site of the lesion.

Nursing Diagnoses

Nursing diagnoses include *Impaired Gas Exchange* and *Ineffective Tissue Perfusion*, both of which are related to diminished gas exchange in the area of the abscess.

Outcomes

The nursing outcomes for the patient with a lung abscess include a relief of clinical manifestations and a return to the previous level of function.

Interventions and Rationales

Nursing interventions include management of the patient's clinical manifestations. Management of the oxygen status needs constant monitoring. The nurse assesses the oxygen saturation, the respiratory and heart rate, and the work of breathing. Nursing interventions also include administration of antipyretic, antibiotic, and pain medications, with a follow-up assessment of effectiveness. Physical care such as bathing needs to be spaced to allow for periods of rest between activities. If a catheter has been placed to drain the abscess, the amount and a description of the color, odor, and viscosity need to be assessed and documented.

Evaluation

Evaluation focuses on the ability or status of the patient in meeting the outcome parameters. If the desired outcomes are not met, an analysis of the reason why must be undertaken and different interventions must be considered.

Subdiaphragmatic Abscess

A subdiaphragmatic abscess is a collection of pus located in the left or right diaphragmatic space. The usual cause is infected fluid ascending from the pelvis. This movement is facilitated by the negative pressure caused by the movement of the right diaphragm.

Etiology, Clinical Manifestations, and Medical Management

A subdiaphragmatic abscess occurs more commonly on the right side where the right paracolic space provides an easy pathway for infected fluid. Changes in the level and configuration of the diaphragm and signs of pleural effusion or basal lung opacities on the side of the suspected abscesses are indirect signs observed on chest x-rays. Computed tomography (CT) scanning may be used to visualize the abscess. Drainage of the abscess may be accomplished percutaneously using an image-guided radiologic procedure. Nursing management is much the same as for a lung abscess.

◼ Collaborative Management for Pulmonary Infections

To optimize the patient care, the nurse collaborates with the health care provider for monitoring and adjusting medications, treatments, patient education, and the overall plan of care. The pharmacist is consulted regarding medication effectiveness and side effects, and the respiratory therapist assists with administration of the pulmonary toilet, including breathing and coughing techniques that allow for clearing pulmonary secretions.

The physical therapist may assist with ambulation and some physical rehabilitation if the patient is in a weakened state. The nurse provides adequate pain relief in advance of physical therapy. If anorexia is present, which is common with infections, especially with TB, the nutritionist plans for small frequent meals and nutritional supplements as needed. The treatment of anorexia is discussed in Chapter 14 🔗 . If monitoring is required after discharge, a social worker and home care nurse are enlisted. A community health nurse is likely to provide continuity of care.

Health Promotion for Pulmonary Infections

Patients should be taught principles of prevention. These include washing hands frequently, especially after using the bathroom, before meals, and after blowing the nose. Influenza vaccination is the primary method for preventing influenza and its severe complications. As indicated in a report from the Advisory Committee on Immunization Practices (ACIP) (MMWR, 2004 of the CDC), an annual influenza vaccination is now recommended for persons at high risk for influenza-related complications and severe disease, including children ages 6 to 59 months, pregnant women, persons 50 years or older, persons of any age with certain chronic medical conditions, and persons who live with or care for persons at high risk, including household contacts who have frequent contact with persons at high risk and who can transmit influenza to those persons at high risk, and health care workers who also have frequent contact with persons at high risk (CDC, 2006). A flu shot can be 70% to 90% effective in preventing the flu.

Elderly persons and those with chronic diseases such COPD and diabetes are at high risk for pneumonia and should avoid smoking (see the Gerontological Considerations box, p. 950). Exposure to environmental smoke, pollutants, and crowds also can be risk factors for these individuals. Those at risk should be inoculated with the influenza and pneumococcus vaccines. Individuals older than 65 years and younger patients who have chronic illnesses or are immunocompromised should also receive the pneumococcal vaccine, which is 60% effective in preventing bacterial pneumococcal infections in adults (Schultz, 2003). Gerontological considerations also are discussed at length in Chapter 10 🔗 .

GERONTOLOGICAL CONSIDERATIONS for Pulmonary Infections

Elderly patients are at high risk for acquiring pulmonary infections and pneumonia because they often experience risk factors such as immobility and chronic disease. They are more likely to be malnourished or immunosuppressed related to the aging process. In addition, the elderly experience a higher mortality rate from pneumonia. Research shows that pneumonia in the elderly can be the event that triggers a dangerous spiral of deterioration leading to death. Patients' families and health care providers need to be educated regarding these dangers (Kaplan et. al, 2003).

CRITICAL ALERT *Patients older than 50 years with a chronic disease, respiratory disease, or those who are immunocompromised should get a flu shot yearly and should be inoculated with the pneumococcal vaccine.*

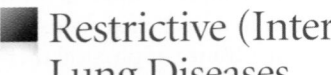

Restrictive (Interstitial) Lung Diseases

Restrictive lung diseases (also known as interstitial lung diseases) are those that result in reduced lung volumes, either because of an alteration in lung parenchyma or because of a disease of the pleura, chest wall, or neuromuscular apparatus. They are characterized by reduced total lung capacity, vital capacity, or resting lung volume. Accompanying characteristics are preserved airflow and normal airway resistance, which are measured as the functional residual capacity. If caused by parenchymal lung disease, restrictive lung disorders are accompanied by reduced gas transfer, which may be marked clinically by desaturation after exercise. The many disorders that cause reduction or restriction of lung volumes may be divided into two groups based on anatomic structures (Sharma, 2006b). These groups are classified as intrinsic lung diseases and extrinsic lung diseases.

Intrinsic lung diseases are diseases of the lung parenchyma. These diseases cause inflammation or scarring of the lung tissue (interstitial lung disease) or result in filling of the air spaces with exudate and debris (pneumonitis). These diseases can be characterized according to etiologic factors. They include idiopathic fibrotic diseases, connective tissue diseases, drug-induced lung disease, and primary diseases of the lungs (including sarcoidosis). Idiopathic pulmonary fibrosis and sarcoidosis are discussed independently in this chapter. Others are discussed throughout the text in Chapters 36 and 58 .

Extrinsic lung diseases are also called extraparenchymal diseases. Diseases of the chest wall, pleura, and respiratory muscles result in lung restriction, impaired ventilatory function, and respiratory failure (e.g., nonmuscular diseases of the chest wall and neuromuscular disorders).

Epidemiology and Etiology

For intrinsic lung diseases, studies cite an overall prevalence of 3 to 6 cases per 100,000 persons, with a prevalence of idiopathic pulmonary fibrosis (IPF) of 27 to 29 cases per 100,000 persons (Sharma, 2006b). The prevalence for adults ages 35 to 44 years is 2.7 cases per 100,000 persons. Prevalence exceeded 175 cases per 100,000 persons among patients older than 75 years. Exposure to dust, metals, or organic solvents and agricultural employment are associated with increased risk.

- In North America, the prevalence of sarcoidosis is 10 to 40 cases per 100,000 persons.
- The incidence of chronic interstitial lung diseases in persons with collagen vascular diseases is variable, but it is increasing for most diseases.
- Kyphoscoliosis is a common extrinsic disorder associated with an incidence of mild deformities amounting to 1 case per 1,000 persons, with severe deformity occurring in 1 case per 10,000 persons.
- Other nonmuscular and neuromuscular disorders are rare, and their incidence and prevalence are not well known.

The mortality and morbidity from various causes of restrictive lung disease are dependent on the underlying etiology of the disease process. For example, the median survival time for patients with IPF is less than 3 years. Factors that predict poor outcome include older age, male gender, severe dyspnea, history of cigarette smoking, severe loss of lung function, appearance and severity of fibrosis on radiologic studies, a lack of response to therapy, and prominent fibroblastic foci on histopathologic evaluation.

Although a familial variant of IPF exists, a genetic predisposition is not documented (Diaz & Quellette, 2008). U.S. prevalence of sarcoidosis is estimated to be 10 to 17 times higher among African Americans compared to Caucasian Americans (Diaz & Quellette, 2008). Lymphangioleiomyomatosis (LAM) and lung involvement in tuberous sclerosis occur exclusively in premenopausal women. Men are more likely to have pneumoconiosis because of occupational exposure, IPF, and collagen vascular diseases (e.g., rheumatoid lung). Worldwide, sarcoidosis is slightly more common in women (Sharma, 2006a).

Relative to age, IPF is rare in children. Some intrinsic lung diseases present in patients ages 20 to 40 years. These include sarcoidosis, collagen vascular–associated diseases, and histiocytosis X. Most patients with IPF are older than 50 years (Sharma, 2007).

Pathophysiology

Most restrictive (interstitial) lung diseases, regardless of the cause, have a common pathogenesis. It is thought that these disorders are initiated by some type of injury to the alveolar epithelium, followed by an inflammatory process that involves the alveoli and interstitium of the lung. As the inflammatory and immune cells accumulate, damage continues to develop and fibrous scar tissue replaces functioning lung tissue (Porth, 2007). Normally, air flows to and from the alveoli as lungs inflate and deflate during each respiratory cycle. Lung inflation is accomplished by a contraction of respiratory, diaphragmatic, and external intercostal muscles, whereas deflation is passive. Functional residual capacity (FRC) is the volume of air in the lungs when the respiratory muscles are fully relaxed and no airflow is present. The volume of FRC is determined by the balance of the inward elastic recoil of the lungs and the outward elastic recoil of the chest wall. Restrictive lung diseases are characterized by a reduction in FRC and other lung volumes because of pathology in lungs, pleura, or the structures of the thoracic cage.

The distensibility of the respiratory system is called compliance, the volume change produced by a change in the distending pressure. Lung compliance is independent of the thoracic cage, which is a semirigid container. The compliance of an intact respiratory system is an algebraic sum of the compliances of both of these structures; therefore, it is influenced by any disease of the lungs, pleura, or chest wall.

In cases of intrinsic lung disease, the physiological effects of diffuse parenchymal disorders reduce all lung volumes by the excessive elastic recoil of the lungs, in comparison to the outward recoil forces of the chest wall. Expiratory airflow is reduced in proportion to lung volume. Arterial hypoxemia in these disorders is primarily caused by ventilation/perfusion mismatching, with further contribution from an intrapulmonary shunt. The diffusion of oxygen is impaired, which contributes a little toward hypoxemia at rest, but is primarily the mechanism of exercise-induced desaturation. Hyperventilation at rest and exercise is caused by the reflexes arising from the lungs and the need to maintain minute ventilation by reducing tidal volume and increasing respiratory frequency.

In cases of extrinsic disorders of the pleura and thoracic cage, the total compliance by the respiratory system is reduced and, hence, lung volumes are reduced. As a result of atelectasis, gas distribution becomes nonuniform, resulting in ventilation/perfusion mismatch and hypoxemia. In kyphoscoliosis, lateral curvature, anteroposterior angulation, kyphosis, or several of these conditions are present. The Cobb angle, an angle formed by two limbs of a convex prime curvature of the spine, is an indication of the severity of disease. An angle greater than 100 degrees is usually associated with respiratory failure.

Neuromuscular disorders affect an integral part of the respiratory system, a vital pump. The respiratory pump can be impaired at the level of the central nervous system (CNS), spinal cord, peripheral nervous system, neuromuscular junction, or respiratory muscle. The pattern of ventilatory impairment is highly dependent on the specific neuromuscular disease.

Clinical Manifestations

Restrictive lung diseases may be acute or insidious in onset, depending on the causes. Symptoms of intrinsic diseases include progressive exertional dyspnea, which is the predominant symptom; a dry cough (a productive cough is an unusual sign in most patients); and hemoptysis or grossly bloody sputum, which occurs in patients with diffuse alveolar hemorrhage syndromes and vasculitis. Wheezing is an uncommon manifestation but can occur in patients with lymphangitic carcinomatosis, chronic eosinophilic pneumonia, and respiratory bronchiolitis. Chest pain also is uncommon, but pleuritic chest pain may occur in patients with rheumatoid arthritis, systemic lupus erythematosus, and some drug-induced disorders.

Symptoms of extrinsic disorders tend to occur in middle-aged patients who develop dyspnea, decreased exercise tolerance, and respiratory infections. The cause of respiratory failure is multifactorial and is secondary to spinal deformity, muscle weakness, disordered ventilatory control, sleep disordered breathing, and airway disease. As neuromuscular disorders occur and progress, the respiratory muscle weakness progresses. Patients develop dyspnea upon exertion, followed by dyspnea at rest, with their condition ultimately advancing to respiratory failure. Also, patients with neuromuscular diseases develop significant respiratory muscle weakness and may demonstrate fatigue, dyspnea, impaired control of secretions, and recurrent lower respiratory tract infections. Acute and chronic respiratory failure, pulmonary hypertension, and cor pulmonale eventually ensue (Sharma, 2006c).

From a physical examination perspective, patients with intrinsic lung disorders may exhibit distinguishing findings. Those with chest wall disorders:

- Show obvious massive obesity and an abnormal configuration of the thoracic cage.
- Have alveolar crackles.
- Have inspiratory squeaks or scattered, late, inspiratory high-pitched rhonchi.
- Demonstrate cyanosis at rest as a late manifestation of advanced disease.
- Have digital clubbing (in those with IPF) (Sharma, 2006a).

With extrinsic disorders, severe kyphoscoliosis and massive obesity easily are recognizable. The pleural disorders are associated with decreased tactile fremitus, dullness upon percussion, and decreased intensity of breath sounds. In cases of neuromuscular diseases, the physical examination findings may indicate accessory muscle usage, rapid shallow breathing, paradoxical breathing, and other features of systemic involvement (Sharma, 2006c).

Laboratory and Diagnostic Procedures

Routine laboratory evaluations are completed to reveal positive findings in intrinsic lung diseases. Though they often fail to reveal positive findings, anemia can indicate vasculitis, and polycythemia can indicate hypoxemia in advanced disease. Leukocytosis can suggest acute hypersensitivity pneumonitis. Additional tests should be directed by the findings of the clinical assessment. Extrinsic disorders rely on an elevated creatinine kinase level that may indicate myositis, which, in turn, may cause muscle weakness and restrictive lung disease.

Imaging studies consist of chest radiography and computed tomography of the chest to diagnose intrinsic disorders, whereas fluoroscopy often is used to diagnose extrinsic disorders. Other tests include pulmonary function testing and tests for extrinsic lung disorders, such as bronchoalveolar lavage, lung biopsy, and surgical lung biopsy.

Medical Management

Medical management depends on the specific diagnosis, which is based on findings from the clinical evaluation, imaging studies, and lung biopsy. Corticosteroids, immunosuppressive agents, and cytotoxic agents are the mainstay of therapy for many of the interstitial lung diseases. Ancillary therapies include supplemental oxygen therapy, which alleviates exercise-induced hypoxemia and improves performance. The treatment regime also may include antifibrotic therapies.

Relative to the treatment of extrinsic lung disorders, it is imperative that the cause of muscle weakness be identified. Preventive therapies are used to minimize the impact of impaired secretion clearance and the prevention and prompt treatment of respiratory infections. Patients who develop respiratory failure or have severe gas exchange abnormalities during sleep may be treated with non-invasive positive pressure ventilation via a nasal or oronasal mask. Patients in whom these devices fail may require a permanent tracheotomy and ventilator assistance with a portable ventilator.

Treatment for massive obesity consists of weight loss, which causes dramatic improvement in pulmonary function test findings but is harder to achieve. These patients require polysomnographic study because of the high incidence of nocturnal hypoventilation or upper airway obstructions. Either continuous positive airway pressure or noninvasive pressure ventilation helps correct hypoventilation and upper airway obstruction (Sharma, 2006c).

In advanced disease, when respiratory failure develops, patients are treated with mechanical ventilation. If they have copious secretions, cannot control their upper airway, or are not cooperative, invasive ventilation with a tracheotomy tube is indicated. If patients have good airway control and minimal secretions, noninvasive ventilation is used, initially nocturnally and then intermittently.

■ Nursing Management of Restrictive (Interstitial) Airway Diseases

Nursing management of patients with restrictive (interstitial) lung disease follows the protocols of patients with any type of lung disease. It is imperative that the nurse use the nursing process in determining what the patient's individual needs are and implement nursing interventions to ensure that the patient can meet individual health potential in carrying out normal daily activities without respiratory distress. Specific examples of nursing diagnoses, desired outcomes, and interventions are consistent with those for patients with obstructive pulmonary disease when airflow is lessened or restricted and are shown in the Nursing Process: Patient Care Plan for Chronic Obstructive Pulmonary Disease later in this chapter (p. 962).

■ Idiopathic Pulmonary Fibrosis

Idiopathic pulmonary fibrosis is a chronic, progressive, fibrosing interstitial lung disease of unknown etiology characterized by a poor prognosis and no proven effective treatment. Its pathogenesis remains unknown, but disordered fibroproliferation and alveolar epithelial cell function have been identified (Diaz & Quellette, 2008). The most common histologic pattern found in surgical lung biopsy specimens from patients with IPF is called usual interstitial pneumonia (UIP), making IPF and UIP interchangeable terms in most patients.

Epidemiology and Etiology

Idiopathic pulmonary fibrosis is a disease with unknown cause with a very severe prognosis. Typically, when detected, IPF is already in an advanced stage. Patients who have IPF cannot develop normally with pulmonary gas exchange and have a much reduced quality of life. Because of lack of an effective treatment, they rarely survive 5 years after being diagnosed. Idiopathic pulmonary fibrosis affects 13 out of 100,000 men and 7 out of 100,000 women,

normally over 40 years of age. Approximately 80,000 cases of IPF have been identified in the United States, with an estimated 30,000 new cases developing each year. England and Wales report a prevalence of 6 cases per 100,000 people.

The course of IPF is variable and unpredictable. Some patients exhibit a rapidly progressive fatal course over several months, whereas others demonstrate deterioration in lung function over a longer period. The median survival is 3 to 5 years from the onset of symptoms. IPF has no racial predilection (Patel, 2008).

More males than females have been reported to have IPF. Patients with IPF are often middle aged, usually between 40 and 70 years of age. Approximately two-thirds of patients with IPF are over the age of 60 years at the time of presentation, with a mean age at diagnosis of 66 years (Diaz & Quellette, 2008). The incidence of the disease increases with older age.

IPF has no distinct geographic distribution. It is reported worldwide in both rural and urban settings with no predilection by race or ethnicity. However, the age-adjusted mortality rates appear higher among Caucasians and lower among African Americans. The reason for this finding is unclear and likely relates to inadequate reporting rather than to differences in the disease course in Caucasians compared with African Americans (Diaz & Quellette, 2008). There is geographic variation in the age-adjusted mortality from pulmonary fibrosis. This variation may reflect differences in occupational or environmental exposures. In the United States, age-adjusted mortality rates due to pulmonary fibrosis are lowest in the Midwest and Northeast, and highest in the West and Southeast. In the United Kingdom, the highest rates of mortality secondary to IPF occur in the industrialized central areas of England and Wales (Antoniou et al., 2008).

It is documented that deaths from pulmonary fibrosis increase with increasing age (Verma & Slutsky, 2007). The mortality rate for IPF per 100,000 population is estimated to be 3.3 in men and 2.5 in women, with an overall rate of 3.0 in both sexes in Japan. A summary of various studies reports that the mean length of survival from the time of diagnosis of IPF varies between 3.2 and 5 years (Diaz & Quellette, 2008).

Potential risk factors for IPF include:

- Cigarette smoking
- Exposure to commonly prescribed drugs, such as antidepressants
- Chronic aspiration
- Environmental factors, such as metal dust and wood dust, solvents
- Infectious agents, such as Epstein–Barr virus, influenza, cytomegalovirus, hepatitis C, and HIV
- Genetic predisposition, based on familial cases of IPF, meaning at least two members of a primary biologic family (parent, child, sibling) (Dauber, 2006).

Pathophysiology

The pathogenesis of IPF remains unknown. It was once thought that intra-alveolar inflammation played a big role; however, anti-inflammatory agents and immune modulators have proved to be only minimally effective in the treatment of IPF. IPF is characterized by diffuse interstitial fibrosis with only mild inflammation, honeycomb cysts, and fibroblastic foci (areas of accumulation of fibroblasts and connective tissue). A disruption in the homeostasis of alveolar epithelial cells caused by unknown endogenous or environmental stimuli is thought to occur. This disruption in the homeostasis results in diffuse epithelial cell activation and aberrant epithelial repair, in which cytokines and dysfunctional apoptosis are involved (Verma & Slutsky, 2007).

Clinical Manifestations

Clinical manifestations of IPF consist of progressive dyspnea upon exertion, interstitial infiltrates on chest radiographs, and abnormal pulmonary function test results indicating restrictive disease (Patel, 2008). Symptoms depend on the extent of lung damage. Initially, patients present with shortness of breath on exertion, cough, and diminished stamina. Weight loss and fatigue are common. Complications include lung infections and cor pulmonale as the disease progresses (Merck, 2008). The definitive diagnosis should be made only after clinical, radiologic, and pathologic evaluations of the patient and only after excluding other causes of interstitial lung disease.

Laboratory and Diagnostic Procedures

Blood test results are not specific for IPF; however, some abnormal values can be related to the pathophysiology of IPF. For example, an elevated hemoglobin value may reflect chronic hypoxemia secondary to IPF. The erythrocyte sedimentation rate is elevated in 50% of patients. Serologic test results are nonspecific; however, high titers should raise the possibility of connective-tissue disorders.

Imaging studies may be used but are not specific to IPF. At the time of diagnosis of IPF, almost all patients have abnormal chest radiography findings of bilateral diffuse reticular or reticulonodular infiltrates at the periphery and the bases of the lungs.

Pulmonary function tests are conducted with a typical finding of a restrictive ventilatory defect. The most common abnormality found in patients with IPF is a decreased diffusing capacity. Bronchoalveolar lavage, echocardiography, and bronchoscopy also may be done to isolate or confirm diagnosis.

Lung biopsy of patients with IPF may be done. During the period of accelerated IPF, lung biopsy typically shows a combination of UIP with superimposed diffuse alveolar damage, characterized by fibroblast proliferation of the alveoli septa, hyperplasia of type 2 pneumocytes, and hyaline membrane remnants (Diaz & Quellette, 2008).

Medical Management

Medical management of IPF focuses on preserving as much lung function as possible, and enabling the patient to engage in normal activities as long as possible. In this regard, oxygen therapy should be prescribed for patients with documented hypoxemia; thereby, improving exercise tolerance. A pulmonary specialist generally is consulted to mange the patient with corticosteroids and cytotoxic or antifibrotic agents. Patients with acute respiratory failure may require mechanical ventilation, with consultation from a critical care specialist.

Maintaining adequate nutritional intake and immunizations is important for quality of life. Participation in a pulmonary rehabilitation should be encouraged in order to maintain functionality and address psychosocial aspects of this disease.

Patients with pneumothorax should be admitted to inpatient care as should patients with severe hypoxemia. Further outpatient care focuses on closely monitoring the patient for adverse drug effects and complications, maintaining functionality through pulmonary rehabilitation, encouraging smoking cessation, and recommending vaccines as appropriate.

Referral to a lung transplantation center should be instituted early in patients with histologic or radiographic evidence of UIP. Lung transplantation also should be considered, and a referral to an appropriate transplantation center may be appropriate. Referrals to a specialized center for any ongoing clinical trials for new treatments that may offer new hope for patients with IPF also should be considered.

■ Nursing Management

Nursing management of patients with IPF is based on the principles of caring for any patient with lung or respiratory disorders. The main focus is on assisting the patient to remain functional and to maintain as much self-care and life management as possible. The nurse works with the interdisciplinary health care team in carrying out treatment goals: identifying and removing the injurious agent, suppressing the inflammatory response, preventing progression of the disease, and providing supportive therapy for persons with advanced disease. The Nursing Process: Patient Care Plan for Chronic Obstructive Pulmonary Disease (p. 962) contains an approach to implementing the nursing process for IPF.

IPF does not have a positive prognosis, and the nurse must be aware of the psychosocial needs of the patient and family. These may become paramount in planning the care of the patient and in instituting discharge priorities. As noted under medical management, the nurse may assist the patient in referrals to transplant programs as well as pulmonary rehabilitation programs.

■ Sarcoidosis

Sarcoidosis is an inflammatory immune system disorder that affects multiple organ systems. It is characterized by noncaseating granulomas (small inflammatory nodules) that most often occur in the lungs or lymph nodes. They can clump together and form larger clumps that attack other organs including the skin, liver, eyes, spleen, bone marrow, kidneys, salivary glands, heart, endocrine system, and gastrointestinal system (Barreiro, DeMarco, Gemmel, & Schaub, 2005; Gould, 2006; Yakobi, 2007). Some people have signs and symptoms related to a specific organ, such as shortness of breath from lung problems, but others may have only a vague feeling of illness or no signs or symptoms at all.

Epidemiology, Etiology, and Pathophysiology

Although anyone can develop sarcoidosis, the disease mainly affects adults between the ages of 20 and 40. People of Scandinavian descent and African Americans are particularly at risk. African Americans also are more likely to have severe, chronic symptoms than are Caucasians. The annual incidence of sarcoidosis in the United States is approximately 10 cases in 100,000 among Caucasians, and 36 cases per 100,000 in the African American population. It is most commonly seen in the Mid-Atlantic States and in the South, rarely in the Southwest.

The disease does seem to run in families, particularly African Americans who present with a more aggressive course (Barreiro et. al., 2005).

Although the exact cause of sarcoidosis is unknown, it is believed to occur when a person's immune system overreacts to an unknown toxin, drug, or pathogen that enters the body through the airways (Mayo Clinic, 2008). Normally, a person's immune system helps protect the person's body from foreign substances and invading microorganisms, such as bacteria and viruses. But in sarcoidosis, T-helper lymphocytes—white blood cells that play a key role in the body's immune response—seem to respond too strongly to a perceived threat. This triggers small areas of inflammation called granulomas.

As the disease progresses, granulomas and scarring (fibrosis) may occur in the tissue between the air sacs, stiffening the lungs and reducing the amount of air the lungs can hold. Some experts speculate that the causative agent may be a nontuberculous mycobacterium, a noncontagious member of the family of bacteria that causes tuberculosis. In a small portion of people, sarcoidosis may have a genetic component. Studies are ongoing to investigate the genetic and environmental components of this disease (Gould, 2006).

Clinical Manifestations

Patients with symptoms of sarcoidosis most commonly present in winter and early spring, which suggests a possible environmental trigger. They may have no symptoms, having been diagnosed by chest x-ray, or they may have fever, night sweats, malaise, fatigue, weight loss, dry cough, wheezing, and dyspnea.

Sometimes sarcoidosis develops gradually and produces signs and symptoms that last for years. Or it may appear suddenly and then disappear just as quickly. In either case, signs and symptoms can vary, depending on which organs are affected and how long the individual has had the disease (American Lung Association, 2007). Ninety percent of patients present with pulmonary involvement, but if this is not the case they are likely to experience remission within 2 years or experience a milder disease presentation. Additional signs and symptoms of sarcoidosis that should be considered include small red bumps on the face, arms, or buttocks, a condition more common in African Americans than in Caucasians, and red, watery eyes. Arthritis in the ankles, elbows, wrists, and hands commonly is associated with bumps in the skin over a person's shins (erythema nodosum) (Gould, 2006; Yakobi, 2007).

Laboratory and Diagnostic Procedures

Chest x-rays are performed, but usually are nonspecific; CT scans and magnetic resonance imaging (MRI) are more helpful in confirming a diagnosis. Pulmonary function is assessed with pulmonary function studies, ABGs, and oxygen saturation. A fiber-optic bronchoscopy with transbronchial biopsies including culturing is helpful. A total chemistry and hematologic work-up is performed including liver function tests, and a TB skin test is administered to rule out TB (Barreiro et al., 2005).

Medical Management

Medical management of sarcoidosis is individualized, with the need for medical therapy varying based on the symptoms and organ systems involved in each patient. Many patients require no treatment; symptoms usually are not disabling and tend to disappear spontaneously. Because sarcoidosis can disappear even without therapy, health care providers may disagree on when to start treatment, what medication and dose to prescribe, and how long to continue the medicine. When therapy is recommended, the main goal is to keep the lungs and other affected body organs working and to relieve symptoms. The disease is considered inactive once the symptoms fade. The decision to initiate drug therapy depends on the organ system involved and how far the inflammation has progressed. If the disease appears to be severe, especially in the lungs, eyes, heart, nervous system, spleen, or kidneys, the doctor may prescribe medications.

Currently, corticosteroid drugs are the primary treatment for inflammation and granuloma formation. Prednisone probably is the corticosteroid most often prescribed today (Gould, 2006). Corticosteroid treatment usually results in improvement. However, symptoms often start up again when it is stopped. Treatment, therefore, may be necessary for several years. At present, there is no treatment to reverse the lung scarring (fibrosis) that might be present in advanced sarcoidosis.

Note also that more than one test is needed to diagnose sarcoidosis. Diagnostic tests also can determine if patients with sarcoidosis are getting better. Occasionally, a blood test will show a high blood level of calcium accompanying sarcoidosis. The reasons for this are not clear. When it does occur, the patient may be advised to avoid calcium-rich foods, vitamin D, or sunlight, or to take prednisone, as indicated earlier. Frequent checkups are important so that the health care provider can monitor the illness and, if necessary, adjust the treatment.

For example, corticosteroids can have side effects: mood swings, swelling, and weight gain because the treatment tends to make the body hold on to water; high blood pressure; high blood sugar; and a craving for food. Long-term use can affect the stomach, skin, and bones. This situation can bring on stomach pain, an ulcer, or acne or cause the loss of calcium from bones. However, if the corticosteroid is taken in carefully prescribed low doses, the benefits from the treatment usually are far greater than the problems.

■ Nursing Management

If the patient presents with pulmonary symptoms, the nurse monitors respiratory status frequently including oxygen saturation and lung sounds. Oxygen is administered if the patient is dyspneic or oxygen saturation falls below 90%. A total physical assessment is performed and may reveal abnormalities in vital signs, heart rhythm, skin, and eyes; cranial nerve damage may affect the gag reflex, causing swallowing difficulties, facial numbness, or unilateral drooping. If dyspnea is severe the patient may be started on prednisone 60 mg daily and gradually reduced to smaller doses of 10 to 30 mg as symptoms subside. The nurse educates the patient and family regarding administration of prednisone, the dangers associated with abrupt stoppage, and side effects such as weight gain, mood changes, hypokalemia, and muscle weakness.

Second-line drugs used include methotrexate and azathioprine (Imuran) for which patients are also educated. Persons with cardiac involvement may be on medications for dysrhythmias, hypertension, and congestive heart failure. Topical medications and eyedrops are administered for skin lesions or eye involvement. The nurse instructs the patient on all of these medications.

Discharge Priorities

Discharge priorities include patient education regarding medication, criteria for contacting the health care provider, and actions to be taken in an emergency. Referrals for home care and follow-up care are made if the patient and family require it.

Collaborative Management

The health care provider, nurse, respiratory therapist, physical therapist, and social worker are involved in the care of the patient. They discuss and implement the treatment plan. Frequently, patients with sarcoidosis, because of their younger age, are able to return home and manage care independently, but in the case of older patients and more extreme debilitation, referrals for physical therapy, respiratory therapy, and home care are required. If dyspnea is persistent, home oxygen may be prescribed and a referral is made to a home oxygen company.

Health Promotion

Because both prednisone and methotrexate decrease the immune response, the patient is counseled to avoid crowds and children or persons with colds or infectious illnesses and to receive the flu and pneumococcal vaccines. Symptoms of concern include increasing dyspnea, weight gain, more productive cough, and a change in the color of sputum from clear to yellowish brown.

Chronic Obstructive Pulmonary Diseases

Chronic obstructive pulmonary disease (COPD) refers to a group of respiratory disorders characterized by chronic and recurrent obstruction of airflow in the pulmonary airways (Porth, 2007). Two specific disorders, chronic bronchitis and emphysema, are encompassed in this definition, both of which are characterized by obstruction of airflow through the airways and out of the lungs. The obstruction generally is permanent and progressive over time (Sharma, 2006a). Chronic bronchitis is defined clinically as the presence of a chronic productive cough for 3 months during each of two consecutive years (other causes of cough being excluded). Emphysema is defined as an abnormal, permanent enlargement of the air spaces distal to the terminal bronchioles, accompanied by destruction of their walls and without obvious fibrosis. Chronic bronchitis is defined in clinical terms and emphysema in terms of anatomic pathology. Usually chronic bronchitis and emphysema are not seen as distinct clinical entities. Instead, they coexist in many patients, although one disease may be predominant. Unifying symptoms of these two entities are dyspnea, wheezing, and use of accessory muscles. These individuals have ventilation/perfusion mismatching and a decreased forced expiratory volume in 1 second (FEV_1) (McCance & Huether, 2007).

Chronic Bronchitis

Chronic bronchitis, as mentioned, is hypersecretion of mucus and chronic productive cough that continues at least 3 months of the year for at least two consecutive years. Symptoms are usually seen in the winter months (McCance & Huether, 2007). In chronic bronchitis infection, bronchial irritants contribute to increased secretions, edema, bronchospasm, and impaired mucociliary clearance. The mucous secretions are thicker and more tenacious than normal. Because of this, bacteria become embedded in the secretions where they reproduce rapidly.

Emphysema

Emphysema is identified by alteration of the lung architecture and destruction of alveolar walls. Lungs lose their elasticity and air spaces distal to the terminal bronchioles are abnormally enlarged or hyperinflated, causing limited airflow out of the lung.

Epidemiology and Etiology

Approximately 14.2 million people have COPD, with 12.5 million cases being from chronic bronchitis, and 1.7 million from emphysema. Prevalence in the United States is 8% to 17% for men and 10% to 19% for women, with a marked increase in women in the last decade (Sharma, 2007).

COPD is the fourth leading cause of death in America. The incidence of chronic bronchitis is increased 20-fold in smokers and even more so in workers exposed to air pollution. It is predominant in the elderly population (McCance & Huether, 2007). The primary cause of COPD is exposure to tobacco smoke. Clinically significant COPD develops in 15% of cigarette smokers. Age of initiation, total pack-years, and current smoking status predict COPD mortality. Smokers have a greater annual decline in FEV_1. Secondhand smoke or environmental tobacco smoke increases the risk of respiratory infections, augments asthma symptoms, and causes a measurable reduction in pulmonary function (Sharma, 2007). The rate of air pollution in the etiology of COPD is small when compared to cigarette smoking.

$Alpha_1$-antitrypsin (AAT) deficiency is the only known genetic risk factor for developing COPD, and it accounts for less than 1% of all cases in the United States (Sharma, 2007). Severe AAT deficiency leads to premature emphysema at the average age of 53 years for people who do not smoke and 40 years for people who do smoke. Usually primary emphysema is suspected in individuals who develop emphysema before age 40 and do not have a smoking history (McCance & Huether, 2007) as a result of insult to the lung from inhaled toxins such as cigarette smoke and air pollution.

In 2005 there were 4.1 million noninstitutionalized adults diagnosed with emphysema. The death rate from emphysema was 44.2 per 100,000 of the U.S. population or 130,933 (National Center for Health Statistics, 2006). Men have a higher mortality rate than do women (Sharma, 2007).

Pathophysiology

With chronic bronchitis, diffuse airway obstruction occurs because of inflammatory changes in the bronchial walls that cause them to thicken and impinge on the airway lumen (Figures 35–4 ■ and 35–5 ■, p. 956). Initially, chronic bronchitis affects

MyNursingKit | Video: Respiratory: Chronic Obstructive Pulmonary Disease—Etiology and Pathophysiology

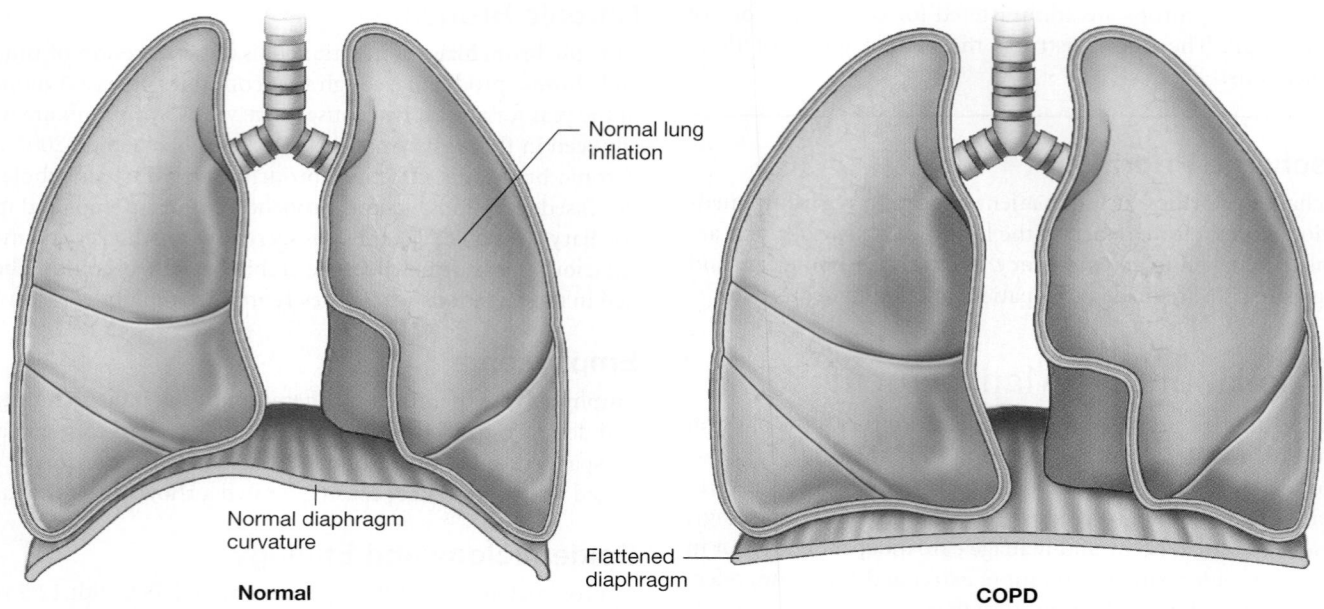

Normal lung inflation

Normal diaphragm curvature

Flattened diaphragm

Normal

COPD

FIGURE 35–4 ■ Flattened diaphragm in COPD.

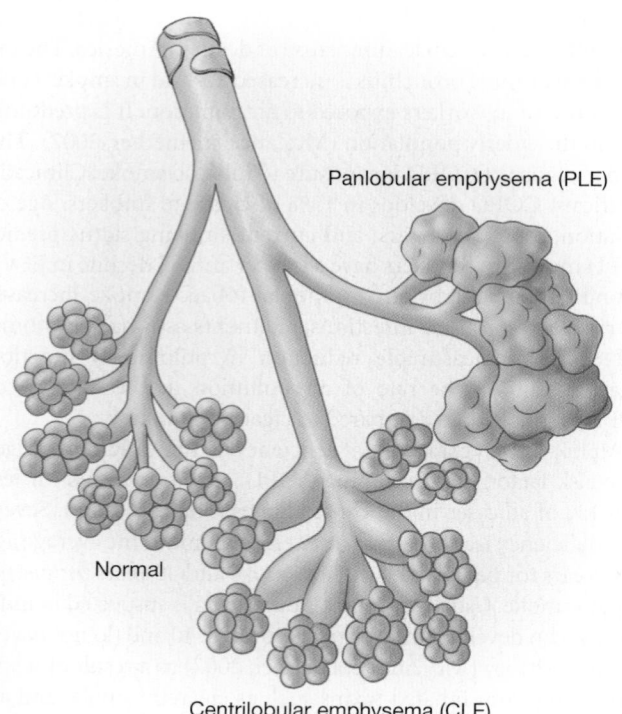

Panlobular emphysema (PLE)

Normal

Centrilobular emphysema (CLE)

FIGURE 35–5 ■ Changes in alveolar structure caused by various types of emphysema.

only the larger bronchi, but eventually all airways are involved. Obstructed airways are likely to close on expiration, causing air trapping in the distal portions of the lung. This leads to hypoventilation (increased $PaCO_2$), ventilation/perfusion mismatching, and hypoxemia (McCance & Huether, 2007).

Chronic bronchitis is characterized by an increase in mucous production with inspired irritants and by an increase in the size and number of mucous glands and goblet cells in the airway epithelium (Figure 35–6 ■). The mucous produced is thicker and more tenacious than normal. Because of this stickiness, bacteria become embedded in the airway secretions and reproduce there. Ciliary function is impaired, further reducing mucous clearance. The bronchial walls become inflamed and thickened from edema and the accumulation of inflammatory cells (McCance & Huether, 2007). Airway enlargement and loss of elastic recoil in the alveoli cause air trapping and limited airflow out of the lung.

In emphysema, the alveolar destruction is caused by abnormalities of lung enzymes, called proteases. These break down elastin. Researchers believe that inhaled oxidants such as cigarette smoke and air pollution tip the normal balance of elastases or lung enzymes. This is the same mechanism by which the AAT deficiency causes emphysema. The result is collapse or narrowing of the small airways including bronchioles and the walls of small alveoli. Portions of the pulmonary capillary bed necessary for gas exchange are eliminated. Airway enlargement and loss of elastic recoil and airway support structures combine to cause trapping of stagnant air. Airway resistance is increased because of compromised alveolar walls, or septa, especially during forced expiration. Hyperinflation of alveoli causes large air spaces (bullae) and air spaces adjacent to pleura (blebs) to develop. Additional airway narrowing can occur as a result of inflammatory hyperactivity of the bronchi with bronchoconstriction. This may be partially reversible with bronchodilators (McCance & Huether, 2007; Porth, 2007; Sharma, 2007).

Emphysema can be centriacinar (centrilobular) or panacinar (panlobular), depending on the site of involvement. In centriacinar emphysema, destruction of the alveolar walls occurs in the respiratory bronchioles and alveolar ducts in the upper lobes of the lung. The alveolar sac distal to the respiratory bronchiole remains intact. Panacinar emphysema involves the entire acinus with damage more randomly distributed and involving the lower lobes of the lung (McCance & Huether, 2007).

Normal bronchus

Smooth muscle

Open airway

Mucous gland

Chronic bronchitis

Inflammation

Excess mucus causing chronic cough

Increased number of mucous glands

FIGURE 35–6 ■ Bronchiolar changes as a result of chronic bronchitis.

Laboratory and Diagnostic Procedures

Laboratory assays are done initially to identify abnormalities of ventilation, oxygenation, and acid–base status. General laboratory tests are conducted to determine hematocrit levels as are tests to determine AAT levels in all patients younger than 40 years or in those with a family history of emphysema at an early age. Sputum is evaluated to determine organisms present. Imaging studies include chest radiograph and a CT scan. Pulmonary function tests also are completed. See the Diagnostic Tests for COPD box (p. 958).

Medical Management

The goal of medical management of COPD is to improve daily living and the quality of life by preventing symptoms and the recurrence of exacerbations by preserving optimal lung function (Sharma, 2007). Once the diagnosis has been established, patient education becomes of paramount importance, and the patient is encouraged to participate actively in therapy.

Smoking cessation is the most important therapeutic intervention. A smoking cessation plan is an essential part of a comprehensive management plan. This process typically involves multiple interventions.

The therapeutic regime for COPD includes medication, oxygen therapy, and physical therapy. Medications usually recommended for COPD include bronchodilators, theophylline, corticosteroids, and possibly magnesium (Kleinschmidt, 2004; Sharma, 2007). Antibiotics frequently become part of the regimen in patients who are colonized with *Haemophilus pneumoniae*, streptococcal pneumonia, and others. These aspects of the regime are discussed later.

Use of beta agonists and anticholinergic drugs are recommended, and research indicates that anticholinergic drugs have a particularly important role in acute exacerbations (Kleinschmidt, 2004). Commonly used beta agonists include terbutaline (Brethaire, Bricanyl) and albuterol (Proventil). Both are given as inhalers but terbutaline also may be given subcutaneously and is recommended in acute situations. Anticholiner-

gics include ipratropium bromide (Atrovent) and ipratropium and albuterol (Combivent), which combines ipratropium, a drug with antisecretory properties, with albuterol, a beta agonist.

Theophylline is a methylxanthine that increases respiratory muscle function. It is used cautiously because it precipitates arrhythmias. Its efficacy is controversial in the acute setting, but it should be continued in patients who are on it regularly. Aside from the mild bronchodilation it affords, it relieves diaphragmatic fatigue (Fishman et al., 2002). Tiotropium (Spiriva) is an ammonium compound that elicits anticholinergic effects leading to bronchodilation. It helps COPD patients by dilating narrowing airways and keeping them open for 24 hours. The most commonly used glucocorticoid is methylprednisolone (Solu-Medrol, Depo-Medrol) usually given intravenously to decrease the inflammatory response. Magnesium sulfate is thought to produce bronchodilation through counteraction of calcium-mediated smooth muscle constriction. This is given intravenously (Kleinschmidt, 2004). Because so many medications require inhalation with an MDI, patients are taught how to use an MDI before discharge to the home setting.

In an acute situation, adequate oxygen should be given to relieve hypoxia. The patient should be supplied with enough oxygen to maintain a near normal saturation of 90%. Kleinschmidt (2004) argues that there is a common belief that too much oxygen causes respiratory depression. This is not grounded in the research. With administration of oxygen, arterial oxygen (PO_2) and carbon dioxide (CO_2) rise but cause only minor changes in respiratory drive. If the patient becomes so sleepy that she is unable to hold a nebulizer in her hand, intubation is probably indicated (Kleinschmidt, 2004). Occasionally, large increases in CO_2 can lead to deterioration of mental status, causing stupor and obtundation. In such cases, decreasing oxygen delivery is the wrong action. The CO_2 narcosis inhibits respiratory drive to the point that decreasing oxygen delivery leads to worsening of hypoxia. The correct action is immediate intubation and oxygenation (Kleinschmidt, 2004).

DIAGNOSTIC TESTS for COPD

Test	Expected Abnormality	Rationale for Abnormality
Chest x-ray	Chest x-ray films usually show marked overinflation, a flattened diaphragm, and decreased lung markings. Other abnormalities include infiltrates and pneumothorax.	Overinflation results from air trapping, and a flattened diaphragm is a common clinical finding in chronic lung disease. Infiltrates are a common complication with infection and pneumonia.
Sputum Gram stain and culture	Identifies a specific pathogen.	Most often, an individual with COPD is admitted because of decompensation or exacerbation of the disease due to a respiratory tract infection. Colonization with *Haemophilus* pneumonia, streptococcal pneumonia, and others is common. Specific pathogens are treated with antibiotics according to guidelines.
Serum theophylline level	Elevated levels or subtherapeutic levels may occur (therapeutic range is 5–15 mg/L).	This is a weak bronchodilator with a narrow therapeutic window. It is used frequently in COPD patients for bronchodilation and to assist with increasing contractility of fatigued diaphragms. Because clearance may be affected by a variety of other medications, dosing regimens should be individualized and serum levels checked regularly (Fishman et al., 2002).
FEV_1 (volume of air that the patient can forcibly exhale in 1 second) to FVC (forced vital capacity)	Obstructive lung disease is defined as an FEV_1/FVC ratio of less than 70%.	COPD is classified from mild to severe and is diagnosed by pulmonary function tests or spirometry. This is used to evaluate airflow obstruction, which is determined by the FEV_1. With obstruction the patient has difficulty exhaling or cannot forcibly exhale from the lungs, reducing the FEV_1.
CBC	WBC count is likely to be elevated with infection.	Pulmonary infection commonly occurs related to copious mucous secretions and/or impaired airway clearance.
ABG study	Shows hypoxemia or hypercarbia, acid–base abnormalities.	Arterial oxygen of less than 60 mmHg or an oxygen saturation of less than 90% on room air indicates respiratory failure. An arterial oxygen of less than 50 mmHg, arterial carbon dioxide of greater than 70 mmHg, and a pH of 7.30 or less indicates life-threatening illness that needs intensive care management (Chojinowski, 2003).
Serum electrolytes, BUN, creatinine, liver function studies	Abnormalities occur in elderly individuals and in chronically ill persons for whom pneumonia is a secondary problem.	Abnormalities based on specific underlying causes.

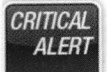 **CRITICAL ALERT** *Occasionally, large increases in carbon dioxide can lead to deterioration of mental status, causing stupor and obtundation. In such cases, decreasing oxygen delivery is the wrong action. The CO_2 narcosis inhibits respiratory drive to the point that decreasing oxygen delivery leads to worsening of hypoxia. The correct action is immediate intubation and oxygenation (Kleinschmidt, 2004).*

For the patient with COPD, oxygen therapy is long term and continuous. It relieves dyspnea, improves quality of life, and allows the patient to exercise without symptoms. (See Chart 35–5 for more on dyspnea.) Long-term continuous therapy means that the patient wears the supplemental oxygen at all times and sleeps with oxygen to maintain an oxygen saturation of 90% (National Institutes of Health [NIH], 2001). The nurse should instruct the patient regarding the benefits of this therapy, which include prevention of **polycythemia vera**, a condition that occurs when the hematocrit becomes elevated beyond the normal range as a compensatory mechanism of hypoxemia and the development of cor pulmonale, or an enlarged and weakened right

ventricle that causes right-sided heart failure known to increase mortality in COPD. These symptoms are also indicators for oxygen therapy. Prescriptions for oxygen therapy may include continuous therapy, therapy with exercise, or therapy at nighttime, depending on the severity of illness and factors affecting oxygen desaturation (NIH, 2001). The breathing pattern of most individuals with COPD is inadequate for maintaining proper ventilation. Patients are taught to use their diaphragm more effectively and to use a pursed-lip breathing technique to keep the airways open longer (Figure 35–7 ■).

An alternative treatment that can help patients clear mucus from their lungs is discussed in the Complementary and Alternative Therapies box.

■ Nursing Management

Nursing care goals involve assessment of the patient for dyspnea, muscle fatigue, increased work of breathing, and worsening

CHART 35–5 **Research on Assessment of Dyspnea**

Researchers Kendrick, Baxi, and Smith (2000, pp. 2–3) wished to answer the following questions: (1) Can patients with acute bronchospastic asthma or COPD adequately communicate their level of dyspnea using the modified Borg scale (MBS)? (2) Does subjective improvement in the patient's dyspnea using the MBS correlate with improvements in pulmonary functions as measured by the peak flow meter and cutaneous oxygen saturation (SaO$_2$)?

Four hundred male veterans ages 24 to 87 presented with a chief complaint of dyspnea. The assessing health care provider identified 102 of these patients as having acute bronchospasm, 42 were diagnosed with asthma, and 60 were diagnosed as COPD. All study patients were able to use the MBS to rate their perception of the severity of dyspnea. As the peak flow measurements increased, the MBS scores of difficulty breathing decreased. Researchers concluded that the MBS is a valid and reliable assessment tool for dyspnea. The emergency department triage and primary care nursing staff rated the MBS as highly satisfactory along with the patients. Respiratory assessment in the triage notes was streamlined to consistently include three measures: peak flow, MBS, and SaO$_2$. Long respiratory narratives were found to be unnecessary in many cases.

Source: This article was published in *Journal of Emergency Nursing 26*(3). Kendrick, K., Baxi, S., & Smith, R. Usefulness of the modified 0–10 Borg scale in assessing the degree of dyspnea in patients with COPD and asthma. pp. 216–222. Copyright Elsevier, 2000.

FIGURE 35–7 ■ Patient doing pursed lip breathing.

symptoms. The nurse monitors ABG results to determine the patient's status and make clinical decisions regarding treatment. The nurse assists the patient to manage the anxiety that often accompanies dyspnea related to asthmatic attacks or complications of chronic bronchitis and emphysema.

A major role of the nurse is patient and family education with the often complex therapies associated with chronic COPD. This may be in the form of a structured program or may incorporate

COMPLEMENTARY & ALTERNATIVE THERAPIES

Inhalation of Herbal Preparations

Description:
CAM use is increasingly popular for respiratory conditions, and is particularly well documented in German research. The aromatic components of herbal preparations are commonly used in a number of proprietary products to improve lung mucus clearance in patients with chronic airway obstruction.

Aromatics from nasturtium, horseradish root, ivy leaf, thyme, aniseed, and marshmallow and primrose root are used in many herbal products to improve mucus clearance.

Research Support:
A study conducted in the United Kingdom investigated the efficacy of inhaled aromatics on lung clearance. Twelve patients with chronic bronchitis were studied in a randomized, single-blind, placebo-controlled crossover trial. The mean age of the participants was 67. Relative to a baseline, airway mucus clearance observed during the first hour of testing was significantly correlated with the concentration level of aromatics (Hasani, Pavia, Toms, Dilworth, & Agnew, 2003).

A prospective cohort study was conducted in 251 German medical centers that involved 536 participants with acute sinusitis, bronchitis, or urinary tract infections (UTI) for 4 years or more. The participants were treated either with the herbal drug Angocin Anti-Infekt N (containing nasturtium and horseradish root) or with standard antibiotic therapy. The physician determined the treatment, dosage, and duration according to the patient's needs. Standard antibiotic therapy was found to be comparable to therapy with the herbal drug in treating acute sinusitis, acute bronchitis and acute urinary tract infection. In addition, the group treated with the herbal drug needed less supportive procedures and administration of concurrent medication, leading the investigators to conclude that there is a clear advantageous safety profile compared to the group treated with standard antibiotics (Goos, Albrecht, & Schneider, 2006).

A clinical trial involving 62 participants with common cold, bronchitis, or respiratory tract disease evaluated changes in the symptoms of cough

and tolerability after treatment with a combined herbal cough syrup preparation containing dry ivy leaf extract as the main active ingredient, decoctions of thyme and aniseed, and mucilage of marshmallow root (Weleda Hustenelixier, new formulation). At the end of the trial, there was an improvement in all symptom scores as compared to baseline, as well as good tolerability (Buechi, Vogelin, von Eiff, Ramos, & Melzer, 2005).

Another study of 150 outpatients with bronchitis evaluated the efficacy of a fixed combination of thyme fluid extract and primrose root tincture. The results showed a clinically relevant and more pronounced decrease of bronchitis symptoms (the primary outcome criterion) and a shortened duration of acute bronchitis (the secondary outcome criterion) when compared to placebo (Gruenwald, Graubaum, & Busch, 2005).

References
Buechi, S., Vogelin, R., von Eiff, M. M., Ramos, M., & Melzer, J. (2005). Open trial to assess aspects of safety and efficacy of a combined herbal cough syrup with ivy and thyme. *Forschende Komplementarmedizin und Klassiche Naturheilkunde, 12*(6), 328–332.

Goos, K. H., Albrecht, U., & Schneider, B. (2006). Efficacy and safety profile of a herbal drug containing nasturtium herb and horseradish root in acute sinusitis, acute bronchitis and acute urinary tract infection in comparison with other treatments in the daily practice/results of a prospective cohort study. *Arzneimittelforschung, 56*(3), 249–257.

Gruenwald, J., Graubaum, H. J., & Busch, R. (2005). Efficacy and tolerability of a fixed combination of thyme and primrose root in patients with acute bronchitis. A double-blind, randomized, placebo-controlled clinical trial. *Arzneimittelforschung, 55*(11), 669–676.

Hasani, A., Pavia, D., Toms, N., Dilworth, P., & Agnew, J. E. (2003). Effect of aromatics on lung mucociliary clearance in patients with chronic airways obstruction. *Journal of Alternative & Complementary Medicine, 9*(2), 243–249.

patient education and practice opportunities offered by the nurse, physical therapist, and respiratory therapist. Breathing retraining, use of postural drainage techniques, energy conservation, and physical reconditioning are the foci of education (Figures 35–8, 35–9, and 35–10 ■). The Nursing Process: Patient Care Plan for COPD (p. 962) depicts specific steps of the nursing process used in caring for the patient with COPD.

Health Promotion

Smoking cessation is the single most important factor in preventing COPD. The nurse refers the patient to a smoking cessation program or assists in a personal plan. Even for the patient who has COPD, quitting is likely to prevent future complications. The nurse educates the patient regarding the hazards of smoking and provides counseling opportunities as needed. In addition, it is important to teach the patient some of the subtle changes that may occur, such as fatigue, dyspnea, and change in sputum color, consistency, or amount, indicate a respiratory infection. To prevent infection, the nurse cautions patients to avoid extremes of temperature, exposure to crowds, poor air quality, or high pollen counts. These conditions may cause bronchospasm.

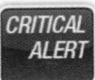 **CRITICAL ALERT** *Subtle changes indicating a respiratory infection are fatigue, dyspnea, and change in sputum color, consistency, or amount. To prevent infection, the nurse cautions patients to avoid extremes of temperature, exposure to crowds, poor air quality, or high pollen counts. These conditions may cause bronchospasm.*

■ Collaborative Management

Individuals with COPD will receive treatment from a team of professionals including nurses, respiratory therapists, physical therapists, social workers, pharmacists, and other health care

FIGURE 35–9 ■ Typical posture of patient with COPD.

providers. A social worker and or a psychologist also may assist with financial issues and vocational concerns.

It is likely that the COPD patient may require follow-up in a rehabilitation setting following discharge from an acute care setting. Follow-up with a home care nurse also is likely. Many patients and caregivers benefit from a formal or informal pulmonary rehabilitation program provided in the outpatient setting. Aside from assisting the patient with physical and respiratory rehabilitation and muscle strengthening, patients receive emotional support from staff and other participants. The Nursing Process: Patient Care Plan for COPD (p. 962) details nursing care priorities.

■ Asthma

Asthma is a chronic hyperreactive disorder of the airways (bronchioles) that is characterized by episodic reversible airflow obstruction and airway inflammation, persistent airway hyperreactivity, and airway remodeling (changes in wall structure) (Morris, 2007; Porth, 2007). The National Heart, Lung, and Blood Institute's (NHLBI's) Second Expert Panel on Management of Asthma defined bronchial asthma as "a chronic inflammatory disorder of the airways in which many cells and cellular elements play a role, in particular, mast cells, eosinophils, T lymphocytes, and epithelial cells" (NHLBI, 1997/2002). Morris (2007) notes that it is one of the most common chronic diseases worldwide and is the most common cause of hospitalization for children in the United States. This inflammatory process causes recurrent episodes of wheezing, breathlessness, chest tightness, and coughing, particularly at night or in the early morning, in

Normal adult

$$\frac{\text{A–P diameter}}{\text{Transverse diameter}} = \frac{1}{2}$$

(a)

Barrel chest

$$\frac{\text{A–P diameter}}{\text{Transverse diameter}} = \frac{2}{1}$$

(b)

FIGURE 35–8 ■ Barrel chest.

Right lung   Left lung

Lower lobes, anterior basal segment

Lower lobes, lateral basal segment

Lower lobes, superior segments

Upper lobes, anterior segment

Upper lobes, apical segment

Upper lobes, posterior segment

FIGURE 35–10 ■ Postural drainage positions.

susceptible individuals. These episodes are usually associated with widespread but variable airflow obstruction that is often reversible either spontaneously or with treatment. The inflammation also causes an associated increase in the existing bronchial responsiveness to a variety of stimuli.

Sometimes asthma is classified as intrinsic or extrinsic. Intrinsic asthma, also referred to as nonallergic asthma, is triggered by diverse nonimmune mechanisms, including respiratory tract infections, exercise, ingestion of aspirin, emotional upset, and exposure to bronchial irritants such as cigarette smoke, dust, chemicals, and fumes.

Extrinsic, or atopic, asthma is initiated by a type 1 hypersensitivity response to an extrinsic antigen, such as pollens and allergens. Although this distinction is considered helpful from a pathophysiological perspective, it is less helpful from a clinical

view because many people with asthma manifest overlapping characteristics of both extrinsic an intrinsic asthma (Porth, 2007). Note, however, that treatment of allergic asthma should include avoiding the primarily indoor and sometimes outdoor allergens to which the patient has become sensitized, and treatment of intrinsic asthma is aimed at avoiding respiratory infections (viral infections, colds, influenza, and all contact with smoke and fumes).

Epidemiology and Etiology

The prevalence of asthma appears to have increased continuously since the 1970s, and asthma now affects an estimated 4% to 7% of people worldwide (NHLBI, 2007). As the prevalence has increased, so has the mortality and morbidity. Although asthma occurs across races worldwide, in the United States,

NURSING PROCESS: Patient Care Plan for Chronic Obstructive Pulmonary Disease

Assessment of the COPD Patient

Subjective Data:

Do you experience cough, shortness of breath, or wheezing?

Describe the type of cough you experience. Is it dry hacking, productive, and/or triggered by smoking or other environmental, social, or emotional situations?

Is sputum clear or colored and how much would you say is expectorated per day?

Do you have any difficulty with sleeping and what position is most comfortable for you?

What is your current weight and eating habits? Has there been a change during the last month or year?

Do you or have you ever smoked any type of tobacco? If so, describe your smoking history.

Describe your medications and breathing treatments.

Do you use supplemental oxygen? If so, please describe.

Describe your activity tolerance. Has this changed during the last month or year?

If you experience wheezing or chest tightness, what situations seem to trigger this?

Objective Data:

Vital signs
Oxygen saturation with pulse oximetry
Spirometry results (FEV_1/FVC)
ABG results
Assessment of lung sounds and breathing pattern including use of accessory muscles
Presence or absence of clubbing
Presence or absence of barrel chest
Color of face, lips, and nail beds
Presence of cough
Color and amount of sputum production

Exercise tolerance
Oxygen requirements
Hemoglobin and hematocrit
Sputum culture and sensitivity results
Level of consciousness
Orientation
Note whether the patient responds with lucid answers and states them in compete sentences.
Breathlessness may be so severe that the patient can only respond with one- or two-word answers.

Nursing Assessment and Diagnoses	Outcomes and Evaluation Parameters	Planning and Interventions with *Rationales*
Nursing Diagnosis: *Ineffective Airway Clearance* related to inadequate cough and excessive mucous production	**Outcome:** Patient will demonstrate controlled cough and postural drainage. ***Evaluation Parameters:*** After completion of pulmonary toilet, lung sounds are clear or significantly improved upon auscultation. Oxygen saturation after pulmonary toilet is within normal range. Patient expectorates secretions effectively upon assessment by the nurse.	**Interventions and *Rationales:*** Assess the patient's ability to mobilize secretions. If unable to do so, suction as necessary to remove secretions *to clear the airway.* Teach use of postural drainage and chest physiotherapy or refer to respiratory therapist. Note characteristics of sputum. *Secretions can obstruct airways and cause respiratory complications.* Assess for presence of adventitious lung sounds every 4–8 hours. *Auscultation of lung sounds provides information on respiratory status.* Administer expectorants as ordered. Observe the patient for drug effectiveness. *Airway dilation is the result of medications.* Provide hydration of at least 2 L/day if not medically contraindicated. Administer vaporization therapy and perform physical therapy and postural drainage as ordered at least 1 hour before meals. *Hydration and vaporization help to liquefy secretions.*

Assessment of Anxiety and Coping with Disease

Subjective Data:

How do you think you are coping with episodes of dyspnea or chest tightness?
What are triggers for increasing anxiety?

Objective Data:

Facial expressions
Mood
Verbalization of fear regarding illness and its impact on family and the future

Nursing Assessment and Diagnoses	Outcomes and Evaluation Parameters	Planning and Interventions with *Rationales*
Nursing Diagnosis: *Anxiety* related to dyspneic episodes or asthmatic attacks	**Outcome:** Patient is able to identify activities that tend to decrease anxious behaviors. ***Evaluation Parameters:*** Demonstrates the ability to initiate purse-lipped breathing at the onset of dyspnea related to anxiety. Verbalizes anxious feelings and thoughts. Anxiety is relieved by consistently demonstrating aggression and anxiety control, coping, impulse control, self-mutilation restraint, and substantially effective social interaction skills. Verbalizes absence of sensory perceptual disorders. Verbalizes absence of physical manifestations of anxiety. Behavioral manifestations of anxiety absent.	**Interventions and *Rationales:*** Ask the patient to identify in writing various factors that elicit an anxious response. *Clarifying thoughts gives the patient control and may decrease anxiety.* Help the patient formulate a plan for coping with dyspneic and or wheezing episodes. *A plan allows the patient to prepare.* Encourage verbalization of feelings *to decrease anxiety.* Teach patient interventions for coping such as relaxation techniques and biofeedback. *These types of interventions decrease stress and anxiety.*

NURSING PROCESS: Patient Care Plan for Chronic Obstructive Pulmonary Disease—*Continued*

Assessment of Patient/Family Knowledge

Subjective Data:
Describe your disease history and the progression of symptoms. For example, has the shortness of breath worsened over time?

Objective Data:
Able to verbalize prevention techniques

Nursing Assessment and Diagnoses	Outcomes and Evaluation Parameters	Planning and Interventions with *Rationales*
Nursing Diagnosis: *Deficient Knowledge* related to COPD	**Outcome:** Patient and significant others describe breathing exercises and energy conservation techniques prior to discharge. ***Evaluation Parameters:*** Patient demonstrates breathing exercises and energy conservation techniques prior to discharge. Patient and family members describe the treatment regime with rationale prior to discharge. Patient discuses emotional reactions to lifestyle changes prior to discharge. Prior to discharge, the patient and caregiver verbalize issues that constitute an emergency and what actions they should take. Patient and caregiver describe the appropriate contacts to make in the case of an emergency.	**Interventions and *Rationales:*** Instruct the patient on prevention of infection. Discuss stress with the patient: avoidance of crowded rooms or contact with known cases of colds or flu, avoidance of irritants such as tobacco smoke, importance of receiving pneumococcal and influenza vaccines, importance of recognizing changes in sputum color and density. *These measures prevent complications of COPD.* The nurse, along with the respiratory therapist, physical therapist, and occupational therapist, teaches breathing techniques including breathing exercises and energy conservation strategies. Treadmills, weights, and bicycles may be used to improve muscle strength and endurance. Patients can incorporate use of portable oxygen systems into this exercise routine as needed. Inspiratory muscle training may be prescribed to strengthen muscles used in breathing. This requires that the patient breathe against resistance for 10–15 minutes a day, *thus conditioning muscles and increasing activity tolerance and ventilatory competence. Breathing exercises and physical reconditioning decrease the work of breathing and improve physical stamina.* Review the patient's treatment regime including medications, oxygen, breathing exercises, postural drainage, physical conditioning, and nutritional support. Attention to psychosocial issues is very important *since the patient with end-stage COPD is often discouraged because of immobility, and can easily become angry, depressed, and demanding. Making the necessary lifestyle changes requires that patients talk about the emotions associated with these changes.* Enlist family support and at the same time support caregivers who face these difficult issues daily. Attain resources for patient education from the American Lung Association, the American Association of Cardiovascular and Pulmonary Rehabilitation, the American Thoracic Society, and the American Association for Respiratory Therapy. The nurse plays a major role in educating the patient regarding the disease process and the medical regimen. *Enhancing the knowledge base of the patient and family is likely to facilitate health maintenance and prevention of complications.* Review what issues constitute an emergency and describes what action patients should take in a simulated situation offered by the nurse. The health care team arranges for oxygen, if ordered, to be available in the home setting. Plans for transfer to home should be made in consideration of oxygen needs. Instructions should be given in writing. Arrangements are made with the home oxygen distributor to provide specific education regarding home oxygen and respiratory equipment. *Discharge is a time of transition and anxiety. Repetition of information and visual cues such as written information reinforces what has been taught.* Give contact numbers for nursing and other care providers to the patient and caregiver. The patient and caregiver are instructed to place these near the phone for easy access in case of an emergency.

asthma prevalence, especially morbidity and mortality, is higher in African Americans than in Caucasians. Although genetic factors are of major importance in determining a predisposition to the development of asthma, environmental factors play a greater role than racial factors in the onset of the disease (Morris, 2007). Asthma occurs at all ages, but half of the cases occur during childhood and another third before age 40 (NHLBI, 2006).

During childhood, asthma predominantly occurs in boys with a male-to-female ratio of 2:1 until puberty, when the male-to-female ratio becomes 1:1. After puberty, the prevalence in females is greater, and the majority of adult-onset cases diagnosed in persons older than 40 years occurs in females. Boys are more likely than girls to experience a decrease in symptoms by late adolescence (Morris, 2007). Five percent of adults and 7% to 10% of children in the United States have asthma. It ranks among the most common chronic conditions in the United States, affecting an estimated 14.9 million persons in 1995 and causing 1.5 million emergency department visits (NHLBI, 2006).

The hygiene hypothesis also should be considered when discussing the increase in asthma diagnoses. This is a theory about the cause of asthma and other allergic disease that is supported by epidemiologic data for asthma. For example, asthma prevalence has been increasing in developed countries along with increased use of antibiotics, cesarean sections, and cleaning products (Martinez, 2007). All of these things may negatively affect exposure to beneficial bacteria and other immune system modulators that are important during development and, thus, may cause increased risk for asthma and allergy.

Asthma is caused by a complex interaction of genetic and environmental factors that is not yet fully understood (Martinez, 2007). These factors also can influence how severe a person's asthma is and how well one responds to medication (Choudhry et al., 2007). As with other complex diseases, many genetic and environmental factors have been suggested as causes of asthma, but not all of them have been replicated. In addition, as researchers detangle the complex causes of asthma, it is becoming more evident that certain environmental and genetic factors may only affect asthma when combined. It is likely that genes are inherited for increased interleukin-4 (IL-4) and immunoglobulin E (IgE). These cause responses to allergens and bronchial hyperresponsiveness. Environmental factors also increase the risk of asthma. In many individuals the symptoms of asthma are reversible, but fibrosis of the lung may occur in some patients with asthma and these changes cause abnormalities of lung function. This decreases lung compliance and initiates a restrictive component to the lung disease (McCance & Huether, 2007). See Risk Factors and Precipitating Factors for Asthma.

Pathophysiology

The pathophysiology of asthma involves the following components: (1) airway inflammation, (2) intermittent airflow obstruction, and (3) bronchial hyperresponsiveness (Figure 35–11 ■). The mechanism of inflammation in asthma may be acute, subacute, or chronic, and the presence of airway edema and mucous secretion also contributes to airflow obstruction and bronchial reactivity. Varying degrees of mononuclear cell and eosinophil infiltration, mucous hypersecretion, desquamation of the epithelium, smooth muscle hyperplasia, and airway remodeling are present (Morris, 2007; Porth, 2007).

Some of the principal cells identified in airway inflammation include mast cells, eosinophils, epithelial cells, macrophages, and activated T lymphocytes. T lymphocytes play an important role in the regulation of airway inflammation through the release of numerous cytokines. Other constituent airway cells, such as fibroblasts, endothelial cells, and epithelial cells, contribute to the chronicity of the disease. Factors such as adhesion molecules (e.g., selectins, integrins) are critical in directing the inflammatory changes in the airway. Finally, cell-derived mediators influence smooth muscle tone and produce structural changes and remodeling of the airway.

The presence of airway hyperresponsiveness or bronchial hyperreactivity in asthma is an exaggerated response to numerous exogenous and endogenous stimuli. The mechanisms involved include direct stimulation of airway smooth muscle and indirect stimulation by pharmacologically active substances from mediator-secreting cells such as mast cells or nonmyelinated sensory neurons. The degree of airway hyperresponsiveness generally correlates with the clinical severity of asthma.

Airflow obstruction can be caused by a variety of changes, including acute bronchoconstriction, airway edema, chronic mucous plug formation, and airway remodeling. Acute bronchoconstriction is the consequence of IgE-dependent mediator release upon exposure to aeroallergens and is the primary component of the early asthmatic response. Airway edema occurs 6 to 24

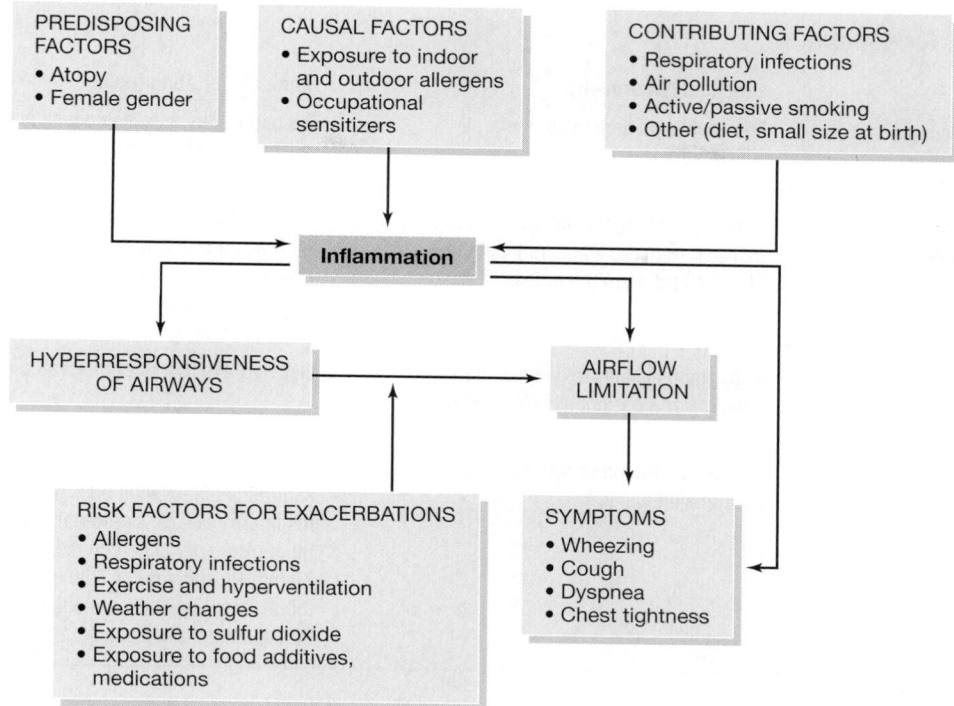

PREDISPOSING FACTORS
- Atopy
- Female gender

CAUSAL FACTORS
- Exposure to indoor and outdoor allergens
- Occupational sensitizers

CONTRIBUTING FACTORS
- Respiratory infections
- Air pollution
- Active/passive smoking
- Other (diet, small size at birth)

Inflammation

HYPERRESPONSIVENESS OF AIRWAYS

AIRFLOW LIMITATION

RISK FACTORS FOR EXACERBATIONS
- Allergens
- Respiratory infections
- Exercise and hyperventilation
- Weather changes
- Exposure to sulfur dioxide
- Exposure to food additives, medications

SYMPTOMS
- Wheezing
- Cough
- Dyspnea
- Chest tightness

FIGURE 35–11 ■ Pathophysiology of asthma.

hours following an allergen challenge and is referred to as the late asthmatic response. Chronic mucous plug formation consists of an exudate of serum proteins and cell debris that may take weeks to resolve. Airway remodeling is associated with structural changes due to long-standing inflammation and may profoundly affect the extent of reversibility of airway obstruction.

The pathogenesis of exercise-induced asthma (EIA) is controversial. The disease may be mediated by water loss from the airway, heat loss from the airway, or a combination of both. The upper airway is designed to keep inspired air at 100% humidity and body temperature at 37°C (98.6°F). The nose is unable to condition the increased amount of air required for exercise, particularly in athletes who breathe through their mouths. The abnormal heat and water fluxes in the bronchial tree result in bronchoconstriction, occurring within minutes of completing exercise. Results from bronchoalveolar lavage studies have not demonstrated an increase in inflammatory mediators. These patients generally develop a refractory period, during which a second exercise challenge does not cause a significant degree of bronchoconstriction (Morris, 2007; Porth, 2007).

Clinical Manifestations

Persons with asthma exhibit a wide range of signs and symptoms, from episodic wheezing and feelings of chest tightness to acute immobilizing attacks. Attacks vary from person to person, with many people being symptom free between attacks. The physical signs of bronchial asthma vary with the severity of the attacks. A mild attack may produce a felling of chest tightness, a slight increase in respiratory rate with prolonged expiration, and mild wheezing. A cough also may be present.

As attacks become more severe, the individual may exhibit signs of using accessory muscles for breathing, distant breath sounds caused by air trapping, and loud wheezing. Fatigue develops as the attack progresses, with the skin becoming moist and anxiety and apprehension becoming obvious. Dyspnea may be severe, and often the person is able to speak only one or two words at a time before taking a breath. At the point at which airflow is markedly decreased, breath sounds become inaudible with diminished wheezing, and the cough becomes ineffective despite being repetitive and hacking (NHLBI, 1997/2002; Porth 2007). Symptom patterns may vary according to:

- Perennial versus seasonal
- Continual versus episodic
- Duration, severity, and frequency
- Diurnal variations, for example, nocturnal and early-morning awakenings (Morris, 2007).

Despite variations in symptom patterns, clinical manifestations typically include cough, wheezing, shortness of breath, chest tightness, sputum production, and decreased exercise tolerance.

Laboratory and Diagnostic Procedures

The patient undergoes a detailed history to determine causes of airflow limitation in the environment as well as foods and stressful conditions. See Diagnostic Tests for Asthma (p. 966).

Medical Management

The goals for successful management of asthma as outlined in the NHLBI's 2007 Second Expert Panel report (NHLBI, 1997/2007) include the following:

- Achieve and maintain control of symptoms.
- Prevent asthma exacerbations.

DIAGNOSTIC TESTS for Asthma

Test	Expected Abnormality	Rationale for Abnormality
Sputum Gram stain and culture	Eosinophils present in sputum.	Eosinophils are associated with antigen–antibody reactions that occur commonly in allergic reactions and asthma.
FEV_1 (volume of air that the patient can forcibly exhale in 1 second) to FVC (forced vital capacity)	With obstruction, the patient has difficulty exhaling from the lungs, reducing the FEV_1/FVC ratio to 70% or less.	The FEV_1/FVC ratio is usually markedly decreased during an attack and improves with bronchodilator therapy. These spirometric results are expressed as an absolute volume and percent based on normal values for age, height, and weight.
CBC	WBC count is likely to be elevated with infection and eosinophils elevated with allergic response.	Elevated WBC count and elevated eosinophils.
ABG study	Shows hypoxemia or hypercarbia, acid–base abnormalities.	Arterial oxygen of less than 60 mmHg or an oxygen saturation of less than 90% on room air indicates respiratory failure. An arterial oxygen of less than 50 mmHg, arterial carbon dioxide of greater than 70 mmHg, and a pH of 7.30 or less indicates life-threatening illness that needs intensive care management (Chojinowski, 2003).

- Maintain pulmonary function as close to normal levels as possible.
- Maintain normal activity levels, including exercise.
- Avoid adverse effects from asthma medications.
- Prevent the development of irreversible airflow limitations.
- Prevent asthma mortality.

The long-term outpatient management of asthma is based on the Global Initiative for Asthma guidelines (2007). According to these guidelines, medical management should incorporate four treatment components: (1) objective measures of lung function, (2) environmental control measures and avoidance of risk factors, (3) compressive pharmacologic therapy, and (4) patient education. Two additional strategies include management of exacerbations and regular follow-up care (Morris, 2007). The severity of asthma should be classified based on symptom prevalence and measurement of lung function before therapy is initiated. Classification of severity and treatment options are listed here:

Step 1. Intermittent
- Intermittent symptoms occurring less than once a week
- Brief exacerbations
- Nocturnal symptoms occurring less than twice a month
- Asymptomatic with normal lung function between exacerbations
- No daily medication needed
- FEV_1 or Peak Expiratory Flow (PEF rate of greater than 80%, with less than 20% variability).

Step 2. Mild Persistent
- Symptoms occurring more than once a week, but less than once a day
- Exacerbations affect activity and sleep
- Nocturnal symptoms occurring more than twice a month

- Inhaled steroid (low dose), cromolyn (adult: 2 to 4 puffs tid/qid; child: 1 to 2 puffs tid/qid), or nedocromil (adult: 2 to 4 puffs bid/qid; child: 1 to 2 puffs bid/qid) (Children usually begin with a trial of cromolyn or nedocromil.)
- FEV_1 or PEF rate of greater than 80% predicted, with variability of 20% to 30%.

Step 3. Moderate Persistent
- Daily symptoms
- Exacerbations affect activity and sleep
- Nocturnal symptoms occurring more than once a week
- Anti-inflammatory, inhaled steroid (medium dose), or inhaled steroid (low-to-medium dose) and long-acting bronchodilator, especially for nighttime symptoms (either long-acting inhaled beta-2 agonist [adult: 2 puffs q12h, child: 1 to 2 puffs q12h], sustained-release theophylline, or long-acting beta-2 agonist tablets; if needed, give inhaled steroids in a medium-to-high dose)
- FEV_1 or PEF rate of 60% to 80% of predicted, with variability greater than 30%.

Step 4. Severe Persistent
- Continuous symptoms
- Frequent exacerbations
- Frequent nocturnal asthma symptoms
- Physical activities limited by asthma symptoms
- Anti-inflammatory or inhaled steroid (high dose) and long-acting bronchodilator (either long-acting inhaled beta-2 agonist [adult: 2 puffs q12h, child: 1 to 2 puffs q12h] and sustained-release theophylline or long-acting beta-2 agonist tablets and steroid tablets or syrup long term; make repeated attempts to reduce systemic steroid and maintain control with high-dose inhaled steroid)
- FEV_1 or PEF rate of less than 60%, with variability greater than 30% (Morris, 2007).

Medications usually are divided into two categories, quick relief and long-term control. Quick relief medications are used to relieve acute asthma exacerbations and to prevent EIA symptoms. These medications include short-acting beta agonists, anticholinergics (used for severe exacerbations), and systemic corticosteroids, which speed recovery from acute exacerbations. Long-term control inhaled medications include inhaled corticosteroids, cromolyn sodium, nedocromil, long-acting beta agonists, methylxanthines, and leukotriene antagonists. Use of these medications by the stepwise approach is outlined above in the four steps. Also, drug categories used in the treatment of asthma are described in the Pharmacology Summary table (p. 981).

Medical management also includes consultations, diet control, and activity control. It frequently is necessary to consult with a pulmonologist or allergist to ensure proper stepwise management of asthma, or referral for further evaluation to help rule out other diagnoses. Patients also may be referred to an otolaryngologist for treatment of nasal obstruction from polyps, sinusitis, or allergic rhinitis, or for the diagnosis of upper airway disorders.

The patient's diet also must be considered, because recent studies have suggested that there is an association between asthma and obesity. Patients with an elevated body mass index (BMI) have an increased risk for developing asthma (Morris, 2007). Activity generally is limited by patients' ability to exercise and their response to medications. No specific limitations are recommended for patients with asthma; however, they should avoid exposure to agents that may exacerbate their disease. A significant number of patients with asthma also have EIA, and baseline control of their disease should be adequate to prevent exertional symptoms. The ability of patients with EIA to exercise is based on their level of exertion, degree of fitness, and environment in which they exercise. Many patients have fewer problems when exercising indoors or in a warm, humid environment compared with outdoors or in a cold, dry environment (Morris, 2007).

Nursing Management

Nursing management of patients with asthma relies on a holistic approach to care through the nursing process. Immediate nursing care of patients with asthma depends on the severity of the symptoms and whether they are being treated as outpatients or inpatients. A major emphasis of all nursing care is patient and family education about the prevention of asthma attacks. Throughout the course of the illness, nurses also provide emotional support to the patient and family, who may be frightened and anxious because of the patient's dyspnea.

Assessment

Nursing responsibilities include a thorough assessment of symptoms and history of attacks, coordinating the plan of care as set forth by the health care provider. The nurse assesses the patient's respiratory status by monitoring the severity of symptoms, breath sounds, peak flow, pulse oximetry, and vital signs.

Interventions and Rationales

Administration of medications as ordered is inherent in the nursing role, having first obtained a history of any allergic responses to medications. Patient education is paramount in assisting the patient with taking medications. For example, regular use of anti-inflammatory medications via an MDI controls the symptoms of asthma (see Figures 35–1 and 35–2 ■, p. 940).

Corticosteroids are effective in improving symptoms and normalizing the FEV_1. The patient should use a spacer with this medication and rinse the mouth afterwards to prevent thrush. A spacer is a device that is attached to the inhaler, allowing medication to accumulate as the patient inhales and preventing medication from escaping outside of the patient's mouth. These are particularly helpful for elderly patients or patients with poor dexterity.

Other specific nursing responsibilities include fluid administration if the patient is dehydrated and performance of critical care procedures, such as assisting with intubation, if the patient is hospitalized.

As part of the educational approach to care, the patient should be encouraged to keep a diary regarding responses to triggers, in order to avoid known triggers as much as possible. The nurse teaches the patient to monitor peak flow measurements with a diary (Plaut, 2001).

See the Nursing Process: Patient Care Plan for Asthma feature (p. 968) for details on the nursing process for caring for asthma patients. The importance of patient education cannot be overemphasized. Patients do better the more they know about asthma—what triggers an attack, what drug to use when, proper inhaler technique, how to use a spacer with an MDI, and the importance of early use of corticosteroids in exacerbations. Every patient should have a written action plan for day-to-day management, especially for management of acute attacks that is based on the patient's best personal peak flow rather than on predicted normal value. Such a plan leads to much better asthma control, largely attributable to improved adherence to therapies.

Discharge Priorities

The nurse ensures that the patient is comfortable with the plan of care and is able to follow written instructions for medications and follow-up visits. When possible, the patients are taught to do their own peak flow measurements and can discuss plans for possible emergencies at home or work.

Health Promotion

Educating the public regarding the symptoms and dangers of asthma contributes to community well-being. This includes the role of environmental pollutants, smoking, allergens, chemicals, and inhalants. When the patient is diagnosed the nurse assists in preventing exacerbations by helping the patient and family to develop a health maintenance routine that includes regular checkups, regular assessment of peak flow rates and use of a peak flow meter (Figure 35–12 ■, p. 969), and awareness of individual triggers that cause bronchospasm or exacerbations.

Collaborative Management

In the care of the asthmatic patient, the nurse collaborates with the health care provider and the respiratory therapist, and patient and family education is essential. If there are financial issues related to maintenance care and equipment, the social worker becomes involved. Referral to the home care nurse is instituted if the patient is not able to manage outpatient clinic or office visits.

NURSING PROCESS: Patient Care Plan for Asthma

Assessment for Asthma

Subjective Data:

Do you have shortness of breath?
Do you have chest tightness?
Are you able to speak without effort?
Do you have a cough?
Do you produce sputum?
Could you describe the sputum?
At what times of day are your symptoms most evident?
Are there particular exposures that start the symptoms such as smoke, dust, or pollen?
Are there particular times of the year when you have symptoms?
Do any particular activities make you ill?
How long is it between attacks or is it continuous?
Do any family members have asthma?

Objective Data:

Lung sounds
ABGs
FVC and FEV_1
PERF
Vital signs
Chest x-ray
Work of breathing
Oxygen saturation
Observation of physical status during exercise
Oxygen saturation pre- and postactivity
Lung sounds pre- and postactivity
Vital signs pre- and postactivity

Nursing Assessment and Diagnoses	Outcomes and Evaluation Parameters	Planning and Interventions with *Rationales*
Nursing Diagnosis: *Impaired Gas Exchange* related to bronchoconstriction	**Outcome:** Patient will experience relief of chest tightness and dyspnea and will be able to exercise preventive strategies that alleviate frequency of symptoms. ***Evaluation Parameters:*** Patient will describe breathing as comfortable. Lung sounds will be clear upon auscultation. Pulse oximetry readings will show normal oxygen saturation. Patient or family member will describe the use of the PERF meter at home. Patient or family member will describe the purpose and administration of bronchodilators and anti-inflammatory drugs. Patient or family member will describe environmental or situational triggers she needs to avoid. Patient or family member will describe activities that will decrease stress, anxiety, and onset of symptoms. Patient or family member will describe symptoms that require immediate emergency care.	**Interventions and *Rationales:*** In the acute phase, monitor vital signs, lung sounds, oxygen saturation, and blood gases, noting improvement in air exchange. Later, the nurse plays a major role in prevention by doing patient and family education. After testing to determine triggers, encourage the patient to keep a diary regarding responses to triggers. *He should avoid known triggers as much as possible to prevent episodes of bronchospasm.* If symptoms persist for more than 2 days per week, revise the treatment plan. Teach the patient to monitor peak flow measurements with a diary PERF (Plaut, 2001). *Analysis of peak flow allows for evaluation of bronchoconstriction; a lowered peak flow indicates bronchoconstriction.* Regular use of anti-inflammatory medications via an MDI controls the symptoms of asthma. *Corticosteroids are effective in improving symptoms and normalizing the FEV_1.* The patient should use a spacer with this medication and rinse the mouth afterwards to prevent thrush. *A spacer is a device that is attached to the inhaler, allowing medication to accumulate as the patient inhales and preventing medication from escaping outside of the patient's mouth. These are particularly helpful for elderly patients or patients with poor dexterity. Corticosteroids can also be given orally to treat exacerbations. Cromolyn sodium is an anti-inflammatory agent used commonly in children but may be prescribed for adults. Long-acting beta-adrenergic agonists are used with anti-inflammatory agents to control symptoms* (Fishman et al., 2002; Wilson, Shannon, & Stang, 2006).

Cystic Fibrosis

Cystic fibrosis (CF) is the most common fatal recessive genetic disease among Caucasians (Sharma, 2006b). It affects mainly the exocrine (mucous) glands of the lungs, liver, pancreas, and intestines, causing progressive disability due to multiple-system failure. It is the most common fatal recessive genetic disease among Caucasians (Rowe, Miller, & Sorscher, 2005).

Epidemiology and Etiology

A person is born with CF, and it affects boys more than girls. It affects Caucasians five times more often than it does African Amer-

icans, and it is rare in Asian American children. Predictably, this disease affects 1 in 3,300 live births among Caucasians in the United States. In African Americans it affects 1 in 15,300. The frequency of unaffected carriers of Northern European ancestry is 1 in 25 (Fishman et al., 2002; Murray & Brown, 2007).

CF is caused by a mutation in a single gene, the cystic fibrosis transmembrane conductive regulator (CFTR). This gene controls the production of a protein that regulates how salt is carried across the membranes that separate cells. The gene disturbance leads to production of unusually thick mucus that blocks bodily passages, particularly in the digestive and respiratory systems. The disorder affects all exocrine glands. The pancreatic channel

FIGURE 35–12 ■ Use of a peak flow meter.
Source: © Dorling Kindersley

will be affected by sticky fluid, which may result in fibrosis and destruction of the gland. Pancreatic insufficiency may lead to malabsorption and diabetes. People with one copy of the defective gene carry it, but have no symptoms, which is the case for more than 10 million Americans. However, those who receive a copy of the defective gene from both parents will develop cystic fibrosis. The Risk Factors for Cystic Fibrosis box lists common risk factors.

Pathophysiology

The typical features of CF lung disease are mucous plugging, chronic inflammation, and infection. These lead to microabscess formation, bronchiectasis, patchy consolidation and pneumonia, peribronchial fibrosis, and cyst formation. These progressive changes cause gradual destruction of functional lung tissue. Peripheral bullae or blebs may develop because of obstruction and airway wall weakening. This occurs more frequently in older patients and often leads to the occurrence of

---

RISK FACTORS for Cystic Fibrosis

- About 30,000 people in the United States have cystic fibrosis (CF).
- About 1 in every 3,000 babies born in the United States has CF.
- It affects both males and females.
- It affects people from all racial and ethnic groups but is most common among Caucasians whose ancestors came from northern Europe. CF is one of the most common inherited diseases among Caucasians.
- CF also is common in Latinos and Native Americans, especially the Pueblo and Zuni.
- CF is much less common among African Americans and Asian Americans.
- About 12 million Americans are carriers of an abnormal CF gene. Many of them do not know that they are CF carriers.

---

pneumothorax. **Hemoptysis** (bloody sputum) may occur because of enlarged bronchial arteries that develop in response to the inflammation associated with bronchiectasis. Over a long period of time, localized hypoxia and arteriolar vasoconstriction cause pulmonary hypertension. This often leads to the development of cor pulmonale (McCance & Huether, 2007). Local factors in the CF airway environment favor bacterial colonization. *Staphylococcus aureus* is common and *Pseudomonas aeruginosa* ultimately colonizes in 75% of persons with CF. *Pseudomonas* acquisition has been linked with more rapid decline (McCance & Huether, 2007).

Clinical Manifestations

The most common symptoms are respiratory and gastrointestinal. Respiratory symptoms include persistent cough or wheeze and recurrent and severe pneumonia (McCance & Huether, 2007). In CF patients *S. aureus* and *P. aeruginosa* are rarely eradicated even with prolonged use of antibiotics. They often occur together in sputum samples (Fishman et al., 2002). An acute exacerbation is characterized by increasing breathlessness; change in sputum volume, color, and viscosity; tiredness; loss of appetite; and weight loss (Esmond, 2000). Physical signs developing over time include barrel chest (see Figure 35–8 ■, p. 960) and digital clubbing (McCance & Huether, 2007). Gastrointestinal manifestations in young adults include malabsorptive symptoms such as frequent loose and oily stools and abdominal cramping. About 10% of CF patients have no gastrointestinal symptoms or pancreatic abnormalities.

Endocrine function of the pancreas is usually preserved in children, but approximately 50% of adults are overtly diabetic by the age of 30. They experience signs and symptoms of diabetes including abnormal glucose tolerance, polydipsia, polyuria, and polyphagia (Fishman et al., 2002; Porth, 2007). Subtle manifestations of CF include chronic sinusitis, nasal polyps, and rectal prolapse (McCance & Huether, 2007). Infertility is common in males due to maldevelopment of the vas deferens. Women are fertile but frequently face a higher risk of complications with pregnancy. The trajectory of the disease varies among individuals, but death is usually caused by respiratory failure secondary to progressive lung involvement (Sharma, 2006b). Chart 35–6 (p. 971) lists additional clinical manifestations of CF.

Laboratory and Diagnostic Procedures

The standard method of diagnosis for CF is the sweat test, which will reveal a sodium chloride concentration in excess of 60 mEq/L. Other diagnostic studies include chest x-ray, pulmonary function studies, fecal analysis of fat, pancreatic enzyme studies, liver function studies, and semen analysis to determine infertility in males (see Diagnostic Tests for Cystic Fibrosis, p. 971). Genetic analysis can be used to confirm the diagnosis of CF (Fishman et al., 2002).

Medical Management

Early diagnosis and treatment are important in delaying the onset and severity of chronic illness in children with CF. CF has a remarkably variable clinical course, depending on the severity of the genetic mutation, the types of infections acquired, and the organs other than the lung that are affected. For all patients with CF, the median survival has risen steadily during the past four decades and is now approaching the age of 35.1 (Porth, 2007).

Environmental Causes of Asthma

Clinical Problem

It is known that people spend 90% of their time indoors in an increasingly technological environment. There has also been a major increase in respiratory illness in the past 40 years. The indoor environment, particularly the home, has been recognized as a major source of exposure to allergens and toxic chemicals that are associated with the development and exacerbation of asthma and other respiratory diseases (Richardson, Eick, & Jones, 2005). Therefore, Richardson and colleagues (2005) reviewed the literature to identify the factors in the environment that have an evidenced-based link to the development or exacerbation of asthma and to outline measures that health care professionals can use to reduce exposure to risk factors in the home.

Research Findings

The researchers concluded their meta-analysis by stating that there is currently evidence of a link between a small number of indoor environmental factors and the development and or exacerbation of asthma. They also concluded that there are measures to alleviate asthma that could be promoted by health care professionals, but the clinical evidence of symptom alleviation, with the exception of measures to isolate dust mites for atopic asthma in children, does not exist.

Variables associated with strong evidence for a causal relationship with exacerbation and development of asthma included house dust mites and environmental tobacco smoke. Cat allergen and cockroach antigen were associated with strong evidence of a causal relationship with exacerbation only and there is limited evidence regarding an association with exacerbation related to dog allergen. Regarding molds, there is sufficient evidence of an association with exacerbation but more data are needed in this area. Regarding nitrogen dioxide, carbon monoxide, general allergens, and formaldehyde, there is strong evidence of an association and strong evidence of low risk. Regarding pesticides, polycyclic aromatic hydrocarbons, endotoxins, and volatile organic compounds, there is insufficient evidence of an association.

Researchers found that most of the environmental controls that have been recommended lack clinical evidence of success via reduced risk of sensitization. The one exception is the use of mattress encasements with impermeable material such as polyurethane. This was shown to be effective with children, but ineffective with adults.

Other environmental controls include elimination of tobacco smoke, elimination of pets, particularly cats, use of feather-filled versus foam pillows, washing bedding regularly in hot water greater

EVIDENCE-BASED PRACTICE

than 55°C, use of a filtered ventilation system to reduce mold spores, use of a dehumidifier to reduce dampness and humidity, reduction of carpeted spaces, and restructuring of homes to eliminate leaks, dampness, and cold.

Implications for Nursing Practice

The results of this study indicate that there are a number of environmental controls individuals with asthma might initiate in their homes. Health professionals might review the evidence presented in this study as the basis for recommendations to clients. Consistent teaching standards can be developed for persons with asthma. More clinical trials need to be initiated with regard to the effect of molds, pesticides, and toxic chemicals as well as environmental controls that mitigate the effects of allergens and environmental pollutants in the development and exacerbation of asthma and other respiratory diseases.

Critical Thinking Questions

1. A good-quality indoor environment is important because
   a. most people spend 90% of time indoors.
   b. most people spend 50% of time indoors.
   c. molds are positively associated with asthma development.
   d. pesticides are positively associated with asthma exacerbations.

2. An implication of this study related to the development of asthma is
   a. tobacco smoke must be eliminated from the indoor environment.
   b. most houses need a total rehabilitation in order to be safe for persons with asthma.
   c. all rugs should be removed in order to prevent dust mites.
   d. pesticide use should be avoided.

3. There is currently not enough evidence to prove that
   a. reducing the exposure to indoor allergens and pollutants will reduce exacerbation of respiratory illness.
   b. reducing exposure to dust mites in children reduces symptoms.
   c. certain allergens are triggers for asthma and respiratory illness.
   d. molds are associated with dampness and humidity.

Answers to Critical Thinking Questions appear in Appendix D.

Source: From "How Is the Indoor Environment Related to Asthma?: Literature Review" by G. Richardson, S. Eick, and R. Jones, 2005, *Journal of Advanced Nursing, 52*(3), 328–339.

Diagnosis typically is based on the presence of respiratory and gastrointestinal manifestations typical of CF, a history of CF in a sibling, or a positive newborn screening test. Confirming laboratory tests are performed, the most common being the sweat test, as mentioned earlier (Murray & Brown, 2007).

At present, there are no approved treatments for correcting the genetic defects in CF or reversing the ion transport abnormalities associated with the dysfunctional CFTR. Thus, treatment measures are directed toward slowing the progression of secondary organ dysfunction and sequelae such as chronic lung infection and pancreatic insufficiency. Aggressive medical treatment is initiated prior to consideration of surgical interventions.

Medical treatments include the use of antibiotics to prevent and manage infections, the use of chest physical therapy (chest percussion and postural drainage) and mucolytic agents to prevent airway obstruction; and pancreatic enzyme replacement and nutritional therapy (Murray & Brown, 2007; Porth, 2007).

It is vital for patients to employ strategies to clear pulmonary secretions to prevent complications arising from airway plugging by viscous secretions. Chest physical therapy includes percussion and postural drainage performed regularly. Patients with CF should maintain a twice-daily routine of chest physical therapy. During periods of exacerbation, the regimen should be performed more frequently.

Clinical Manifestations of Cystic Fibrosis

CHART 35–6

PULMONARY SIGNS AND SYMPTOMS IN YOUNG ADULTS
- Persistent cough or wheeze
- *Pseudomonas aeruginosa* and/or *Staphylococcus aureus* in the sputum
- Hyperinflated lungs on chest x-ray
- Barrel chest and digital clubbing
- Chronic sinusitis
- Nasal polyps
- Recurrent episodes of pneumonia
- Chronic bronchitis

GASTROINTESTINAL MANIFESTATIONS
- Frequent loose and oily stools
- Pancreatic abnormalities
- Cramps and abdominal pain
- Rectal prolapse
- Malnutrition and weight loss

ENDOCRINE MANIFESTATIONS
- Glucose intolerance
- Polydipsia, polyuria, polyphasia

REPRODUCTIVE
- Infertility in males
- High risk of complications with pregnancy
- Delayed sexual development

Medical treatments are started whenever patients experience a subjective increase in nasal obstruction, cough, or drainage (Murray & Brown, 2007):

- **Antibiotic choices**—The bacteriology of sinonasal disease in patients with CF differs from that in patients without CF. This difference affects antibiotic choices. The most notable difference is the nearly consistent presence of *Pseudomonas* species in patients with CF.
- **Nasal toilet**—Because mucociliary clearance is chronically impaired, irrigations are critical and should be a daily routine as patients begin to develop condensed symptoms. Nasal saline irrigations serve to decrease bacterial colonization, wash away condensed secretions that lead to obstruction, and temporarily aid in ameliorating vasoconstriction. Irrigation is also required after any surgical intervention because surgery enlarges sinus ostia but does not address underlying defects in mucociliary clearance.
- **Irrigations**—Irrigations with antipseudomonal antibiotics such as tobramycin may be recommended.

The medication regime is a mainstay of treatment. Antibiotics can be used both prophylactically and for treatment of acute exacerbations. Other medications include bronchodilators and pancreatic enzymes. A detailed list can be found in the Pharmacology Summary (p. 981). Pancreatic enzymes are prescribed for patients with pancreatic insufficiency. These must be taken prior to meals and snacks. Fat-soluble vitamins (A, D, E, and K) must be supplemented. The Pharmacology Summary (p. 981) includes all the medications for CF.

Surgical care may be initiated if medical therapy is ineffective. However, surgical interventions for patients with CF must be carefully considered, because CF patients often are at risk for developing severe mucous plugging during general anesthesia,

DIAGNOSTIC TESTS for Cystic Fibrosis

Test	Expected Abnormality	Rationale for Abnormality
Sweat test	Sodium chloride concentration in excess of 60 mEq/L.	Mucous plugging of the sweat duct causes malabsorption of sodium chloride. This is a diagnostic indicator of CF.
Chest x-ray	Shows densities or whiteout in areas of consolidation.	This is a diagnostic indicator of CF.
Fecal fat	Fecal fat concentration is elevated.	Pancreatic enzymes such as amylase, lipase, and trypsinogen do not reach the intestine to digest ingested nutrients. There is malabsorption of fat, protein, and fat-soluble vitamins. This results in steatorrhea (fatty stool).
Pancreatic enzymes	Decreased.	Mucous plugging of the pancreatic duct results in fibrosis of the acinar glands of the pancreas. The exocrine function of the pancreas is altered and may be lost completely.
Pulmonary function studies	Show abnormal findings.	Tidal volume, vital capacity, and other functions are below normal related to the disease process.
Serum glucose	Elevated.	Diabetes mellitus may occur because the islets of Langerhans become fibrotic. CF-related diabetes affects 15% of patients with CF.
Semen analysis	Sperm count abnormally low.	Confirms infertility in males. CF causes maldevelopment of the vas deferens.
Genetic analysis	Positive for CF.	Confirms diagnosis.
Liver enzymes	Elevated.	Mucous plugging causes biliary cirrhosis late in the disease.

and this risk increases with duration of intubation. Indications for surgical intervention include the following:

- Persistent nasal obstruction associated with nasal polyposis and/or medial bowing of the lateral nasal wall following intensive medical management
- Medialization of the lateral nasal wall, as demonstrated by endoscopy or CT scanning
- Pulmonary exacerbations that appear to correlate with sinonasal disease exacerbations, worsening of pulmonary status, or diminished activity level, despite appropriate medical management
- Facial pain or headaches that have no other apparent cause and that adversely affect quality of life
- Desire for improvement in symptom profile beyond what medical management has achieved in a patient with significant nasal cavity and paranasal sinus symptoms (Murray & Brown, 2007).

According to Porth (2007), "up to 90% of patients with CF have complete loss of exocrine pancreas function and inadequate digestion of fats and proteins. They require diet adjustment, pancreatic enzyme replacement, and supplemental vitamins and minerals. Pancreatic enzyme dosage and product are individualized for each patient" (p. 508).

Nursing Management

Nursing management for the CF patient focuses on assisting the patient to maintain adequate airway clearance, reduce risk factors associated with infections, perform ADLs, prevent complications, and involve the patient and family in planning and implementing the therapeutic regimen.

Assessment

Objective and subjective data should be obtained from the patient and family. Subjective data includes obtaining a past health history of recurrent respiratory and sinus infection and persistent cough with excessive sputum production; use of and compliance with corticosteroids, bronchodilators, and antibiotics; functional health patterns, such as family history, diagnosis of cystic fibrosis in childhood; nutritional and metabolic needs and symptoms; elimination; activity patterns; cognitive perceptions of pain; and reproductive symptoms, such as menstrual irregularities.

Objective data includes assessment of general impression, such as mood, anxiety, depression, restlessness, failure to thrive; cyanosis of skin and nail beds; persistent runny nose, diminished breath sounds, sputum characteristics; tachycardia; protuberant abdomen, abdominal distention, foul and fatty stools; the possibility of abnormal ABGs and pulmonary function tests; and an abnormal sweat chloride test, chest x-ray, and fecal fat analysis. Determination of medications being used also is part of the assessment process.

Nursing Diagnoses

Nursing diagnoses may include:

- *Ineffective Airway Clearance* related to thick and abundant mucus, weakness, and fatigue

- *Ineffective Breathing Pattern* related to bronchoconstriction, anxiety, and airway obstruction
- *Impaired Gas Exchange* related to lung infections
- *Imbalanced Nutrition* related to dietary intolerances, intestinal gas, and altered pancreatic enzyme production.

Planning

Planning goals are focused on the patient having adequate airway clearance, reduced risk factors associated with respiratory infections and the ability to perform ADLs, freedom from complications from CF, and active participation in planning and implementing a restorative regime.

Outcomes and Evaluation Parameters

Outcomes and evaluation parameters include the following:

- The patient and family will show evidence of understanding the disease process, methods of maintaining a clear airway, and the ADL performance regime.
- The patient and family will demonstrate an understanding of a nutritional plan and a plan of continuous evaluation of the condition.

Interventions and Rationales

The goal of nursing implementations is to assist patients in gaining and maintaining independence by assuming responsibility for their own care. Active interventions include relief of bronchoconstriction, airway obstruction, and airflow limitation. The nurse is responsible for administering medications as ordered by the health care provider providing oxygen therapy, and instructing the patient and family on nutrition and exercise. Home care instruction consists of postural drainage techniques, aerosol-nebulation therapy, and breathing retraining. The patient also should be taught controlled coughing techniques, deep breathing exercises, and progressive exercise conditioning.

Psychosocial support regarding the financial and emotional burden of the disease should be provided to the patient and family.

Discharge Priorities

Fatigue and weakness related to an exacerbation of cystic fibrosis may render a young adult who was formerly an active and independent participant in care incapable of performing the treatment regime independently. Upon discharge he may need assistance with the treatment regime. Therefore, the family should be included in all patient education and discharge planning. This includes instruction regarding the chest physical therapy regime, oral or IV medications, and aerosols and breathing treatments.

Health Promotion

Because the adult with CF is extremely vulnerable to infection, the nurse should emphasize to the patient and family that the environment be kept as free from infection as possible. The patient is encouraged to wash her hands frequently, especially after coughing. Frequent mouth care is encouraged, especially after the chest physical therapy regime. Patients should avoid exposure to persons who are ill especially with upper respiratory infections. Patients with CF should be screened for

Mycobacterium tuberculosis infection with yearly PPD skin tests and treated prophylactically with the same regimen used for non-CF patients (Fishman et al., 2002).

Collaborative Management

Comprehensive multidisciplinary CF treatment programs have led to a dramatic increase in the median age of survival for those affected patients (Fishman et al., 2002). Care is managed by a multidisciplinary team including the health care provider, nurse, respiratory therapist, physical therapist, and nutritionist. The patient and family members work closely with the team to develop a regimen that is successful. Involvement of the patient is critical. Treatment depends on the severity of both the exacerbation and the underlying lung disease. The aim of treatment is to maintain lung function, which can be achieved by a regular regimen of chest physical therapy, early and effective antibiotic treatment of acute exacerbations, optimal bronchodilation, and attention to optimal nutrition (Esmond, 2000).

The dietitian can manage the caloric needs, which are high especially with advancing disease. High-calorie feedings or even gastrostomy feedings may be required (McCance & Huether, 2007). See Chapter 14 for details on nutritional management.

Lung transplant has emerged as an option for patients with end-stage CF. The outcome for those with CF who undergo lung transplantation is among the best reported with an average survival rate of 4 years in 50% of cases. Nutritional issues complicate post-transplantation management because 50% of those over age 30 are overtly diabetic, and the treatment with corticosteroids induces diabetes in another 10%. Patients are not considered for transplant unless their weight is greater than 75% of ideal (Fishman et al., 2002). Lung transplant is discussed later in the chapter.

Psychosocial Support

Careful attention should be paid to the social, emotional, and financial needs of the patient with CF and his or her family. Education regarding management of the disease should be ongoing and counseling resources should be available to the patient and family. Active participation in the therapeutic regimen is essential for the well-being of persons with CF. Other issues for young adults include building self-esteem, self-confidence, and meaningful friendships and relationships. The decision to have children should be considered carefully. The nurse might suggest genetic counseling because many men with CF are sterile and women may have difficulty with pregnancy (WHO, 1996). Any children produced will be carriers or have the disease. Britto et al. (2004) found in a study of adolescents with CF that the interpersonal aspects of nursing care were rated as very important and highly valued.

Pulmonary Embolism

Pulmonary embolism (PE) results when a thrombus breaks loose from an attachment and blocks a branch of the pulmonary artery. This produces widespread pulmonary vasoconstriction, which impairs ventilation and perfusion and, thus, produces life-threatening hypoxemia and the potential for ischemia and pulmonary infarction.

Epidemiology

In the United States, there are approximately 650,000 cases annually of PE, and as many as 50,000 patients die each year as a result of PE (Kavita, 2005; Wrong Diagnosis, 2008). PE is predominantly a disease of older individuals, and the highest incidence of recognized PE occurs in hospitalized patients. The incidence of venous thromboembolic events in the elderly is more common among men than women. In patients younger than 55 years, the incidence of PE is higher in females. Patients who survive an acute PE are at high risk for recurrent PE and the development of pulmonary hypertension or chronic cor pulmonale. Subtle population differences may exist in the incidence of deep venous thrombosis (DVT) and PE but the incidence is high in all racial groups. Although, the frequency of PE increases with age, age is not an independent risk factor (Feied & Handler, 2002).

Etiology

Pulmonary embolism is a complication of a DVT, which is a common occurrence after surgery or trauma, childbirth, stroke, heart failure, myocardial infarction, atrial fibrillation, cancer, and prolonged immobilization. Most emboli arise from thrombi in proximal deep veins. They also can originate from the pelvis, particularly with pregnant women and with pelvic fractures. Symptomatic pulmonary embolism occurs in 30% of cases of untreated DVT (McCance & Huether, 2007).

The most common risk factors for PE are a prior history of DVT or PE, recent surgery or pregnancy, prolonged immobilization, or underlying malignancy. Risks for PE include situations in which there is venous stasis or in which there is increased hypercoagulability or a clotting tendency of the blood. Aside from prolonged bed rest, inactivity may include long trips in planes, cars, and trains. Other causes are oral contraceptive use, surgery especially involving the pelvic area, massive trauma, burns, cancer, stroke, myocardial infarction, and fractures of the hips or femur (Fishman et al., 2002). Having an indwelling central venous catheter also increases risk (Morris, Morrison, & Yetsko, 2002). Genetic risk factors include mutations in Factor V, antithrombin III deficiency, protein C or protein S deficiency, and fibrinolysis defects (Kavita, 2005).

Pathophysiology

A pulmonary occlusion occurs when a bloodborne substance occludes a branch of the pulmonary artery and obstructs blood flow to the area that the artery feeds. The embolism can be a thrombus, air accidentally injected through an IV catheter, fat from bone marrow after a fracture, or amniotic fluid that has entered the mother's bloodstream after rupture of the membranes at birth (Porth, 2007). Pulmonary emboli can occur in a variety of ways: (1) a massive occlusion of the pulmonary circulation, (2) an embolus that is large enough to cause infarction of a portion of lung tissue, (3) an embolus without infarction, and (4) multiple pulmonary emboli that may be chronic or recurrent.

Depending on the pattern of occurrence and severity, the pulmonary embolism causes varying degrees of bronchoconstriction in the affected area of the lung, resulting in impaired gas exchange and loss of alveolar surfactant. Pulmonary edema and right heart failure may develop with massive vasoconstriction. **Atelectasis** (collapse of lung) and release of neurohumoral substances such as histamine, serotonin, and thromboxane also may occur. The embolus also may cause systemic hypotension, decreased cardiac output, and pulmonary hypertension, which when severe, results in acute right ventricular failure and death. If the clot does not cause infarction, it is dissolved by the fibrinolytic system (McCance & Huether, 2007).

Clinical Manifestations

The clinical manifestations of PE depend on its size, location, and the amount of obstruction. The classic triad of symptoms of PE is hemoptysis, dyspnea, and chest pain but they occur in fewer than 20% of patients. Many patients with PE are completely asymptomatic, and most of those who do have symptoms have an atypical presentation. Patients may present with pleuritic chest pain, chest wall tenderness, a pulmonary friction rub, or hypotension related to acute cor pulmonale, or they may have a completely normal physical exam. After 24 hours, loss of pulmonary surfactant causes atelectasis and alve-olar infiltrates that are indistinguishable from pneumonia on x-ray. In addition, patients with massive PE may have tachypnea, crackles, an accentuated second heart sound, tachycardia, fever, diaphoresis, S_3 or S_4 gallop, thrombophlebitis, lower extremity edema, cardiac murmur, and cyanosis (Feied & Handler, 2002).

Small emboli may be asymptomatic initially; however, repeated small emboli result in a gradual reduction in the pulmonary bed, ultimately resulting in pulmonary hypertension. Massive PEs typically present with sudden crushing substernal chest pain, shock, and loss of consciousness, and they are usually fatal (Porth, 2007).

Diagnostic Studies

Diagnosis of PE is particularly difficult because many of the diagnostic studies used to evaluate lung function may be normal in the patient with PE. See the Diagnostic Tests for Pulmonary Embolism box for details.

DIAGNOSTIC TESTS for Pulmonary Embolism

Test	Expected Abnormality	Rationale for Abnormality
ABGs	Abnormal in some cases.	Altered gas exchange secondary to PE.
Pulse oximetry	Abnormal in some cases, normal in most cases.	Altered oxygen saturation secondary to PE.
CBC	White blood cell count may be normal or elevated.	Atelectasis and infiltrates occur, causing elevated white count.
ECG	Specific abnormalities with PE are tachycardia, tall, peaked P waves in lead 2, right axis deviation, and right bundle branch block. Most significant finding is tachycardia.	Hypoxemia secondary to PE causes cardiac abnormalities.
Chest x-rays	Usually normal initially. Within 24–72 hours atelectasis or infiltrates may be apparent as well as a small pleural effusion.	Altered perfusion pattern not visible via chest x-ray. In massive embolus dilation of the pulmonary vasculature near the embolus may be seen. Infiltrates and pleural effusions are visible later.
D-Dimer test	Positive.	The D-dimer test is a degradation product of cross-linked fibrin generated by plasmin cleavage. When levels are above 500 mg/L, the test is positive. This indicates activation of the fibrolytic pathway, meaning the body is trying to break down clots. Therefore the D-dimer test will be elevated in any condition such as disseminated intravascular coagulation (DIC), PE, DVT, and myocardial infarction where clots are formed. If the D-dimer is positive and the patient also has tachycardia, crackles, dyspnea, pleuritic chest pain, and cough, a PE diagnosis can be confirmed (Woodruff, 1999).
V/Q scan	Diagnostic of abnormal perfusion pattern, or may be normal.	Perfusion pattern is altered by PE, but even if positive, this is not an acceptable end point in the diagnostic process.
Pulmonary angiogram	Positive.	Provides 100% certainty that an obstruction to pulmonary arterial blood flow does exist. A negative angiogram provides greater than 90% certainty in the exclusion of PE. This is still the most reliable diagnostic test for PE.
Ultrasonography and plethysmography	May detect presence of lower extremity DVT. Echocardiography reflects findings of right-sided heart failure.	Detection of lower extremity DVT helps confirm diagnosis of PE, but often cannot be visualized. Findings of right-sided heart failure consistent with PE (Porth, 2007).
Spiral CT scan	Positive.	This is a relatively new noninvasive diagnostic test that provides additional slices of the area visualized. In many patients a spiral or helical CT with intravenous contrast can visualize pulmonary vessels so well that an angiogram is not necessary.

Medical Management

Oxygen should be administered to any patient who is suspected of having a PE even if the arterial PO_2 is normal. Increased alveolar oxygen may help to promote pulmonary vascular dilation. Insertion of a pulmonary artery catheter is helpful to determine the condition of the heart and its ability to manage the circulating fluid volume. This catheter is inserted by a health care provider through the subclavian vein into the chambers of the heart and into the pulmonary artery. Readings are obtained regarding the patient's cardiac output and pressures within the right and left ventricles and within the pulmonary artery. Some pulmonary catheters can be manipulated to obtain sophisticated determinations such as the right ventricular ejection fraction and continuous cardiac output monitoring (Morton, Fontaine, Hudak, & Gallo, 2005). Pulmonary artery catheters are discussed in detail in Chapter 24 ☺. In the case of a cardiac arrest, CPR is not helpful since obstruction of the pulmonary circuit prevents oxygenated blood from reaching the peripheral and cerebral circulation. The only management approaches that are useful in these situations are an emergency cardiopulmonary bypass or emergency thoracotomy. If cardiopulmonary bypass with extracorporeal oxygenation is available, it may be lifesaving for patients with massive PE in whom cardiac arrest has occurred or appears imminent (Feied & Handler, 2002).

Compression stockings that provide a 30 to 40 mmHg compression gradient should be used, because they are a safe and effective adjunctive treatment that can limit or prevent extension of thrombus. Antiembolic or "Ted hose" produce a maximum compression of 18 mmHg, and because of this they have no value in the treatment of DVT or PE (Feied & Handler, 2002).

Fibrinolytic therapy has been the standard of care for patients with massive or unstable PE since the 1970s. Unless overwhelming contradictions are evident, a rapidly acting fibrinolytic agent should be administered immediately to any patient who has suffered any degree of hypotension or is significantly hypoxemic from PE (Feied & Handler, 2002). Fibrinolysis also should be considered in patients with PE who have any evidence of right heart strain and in all patients without contraindications to therapy because research studies have demonstrated that mortality rate, morbidity, and recurrence are reduced with its use (Feied & Handler, 2002). This should be followed immediately by treatment with heparin. Fibrinolytic medications are discussed in the Pharmacology Summary table in Chapter 40 (p. 1191) ☺.

Heparin is still the most effective treatment for PE because it slows or prevents clot progression and reduces the risk of further embolism. Early heparin anticoagulation should be started as soon as the diagnosis of pulmonary thromboembolism is considered seriously. Long-term anticoagulation is essential for patients who survive an initial DVT or PE. At least 6 months of anticoagulation is associated with significant reduction in recurrences and a net positive benefit (Feied & Handler, 2002). See the Pharmacology Summary table in Chapter 43 (p. 1349) ☺ for a complete description of heparin.

Surgical Therapy

Pulmonary embolectomy was the first definitive therapy for PE. This consists of an emergency thoracotomy; then while occluding the pulmonary artery and aorta, the emboli are removed through an incision into the pulmonary artery. When first discovered in 1908 it was considered an extreme therapy with very little hope of success. Two technical advances in the 1960s, cardiopulmonary bypass and pulmonary angiography, made pulmonary embolectomy a more feasible procedure. In spite of this it is only considered in patients with massive PE complicated by shock (Dalen, 2002).

Inferior vena cava (IVC) filters commonly are used in patients with venous thromboembolism who are concomitantly unable to tolerate anticoagulants. They also are indicated for patients who have recurrent PE in spite of anticoagulation. They may be used as an adjunctive therapy in patients undergoing embolectomy or with massive PE. Anticoagulant medications used for PE are outlined in the Pharmacology Summary table in Chapter 43 (p. 1349) ☺.

■ Nursing Management

The nursing process guides the nursing care for patients with a PE.

Assessment

Nursing assessment must include an evaluation of risk factors on admission and throughout the patient's hospital stay. The assessment includes: (1) an evalution of sudden onset chest pain that is usually described as sharp, (2) a cough that may produce blood, (3) anxiety, and (4) diminished breath sounds over the area of the clot.

Nursing Diagnoses

Nursing diagnoses related to PE include *Ineffective Tissue Perfusion* and *Impaired Gas Exchange*. Other nursing diagnoses are directly related to the specific clinical manifestations described earlier.

Outcomes and Evaluation Parameters

Nursing outcomes include supporting the patient through the acute period and resolution of the clinical manifestations. Evaluation parameters include normal vital signs, therapeutic blood levels for anticoagulation, and the absence of clinical manifestations.

Interventions and Rationales

Nursing interventions are aimed at assisting the patient to maintain the therapeutic regime during the acute period. Anticoagulant medication should be given at the same time each day. The nurse monitors hemoglobin, hematocrit, platelet, and the international normalized ratio (INR) levels, and other clotting studies as needed to assess the effectiveness of anticoagulants.

 CRITICAL ALERT *Anticoagulant medication should be given on time and at the same time each day. The nurse monitors hemoglobin, hematocrit, platelet, INR levels, and other clotting studies as needed to assess the effectiveness of anticoagulants.*

The nurse assesses for symptoms of bleeding and heparin-induced thrombocytopenia and teaches patients to do the same. Monitoring liver function is particularly important in elderly and critically ill patients receiving anticoagulants. The nurse has a major role in the prevention of DVT and PE. This is discussed further in the Health Promotion section below.

Discharge Priorities

Discharge priorities include educating the patient and family about risk factors and treatment regimes. The medication regimen is reviewed carefully with attention to the side effects of anticoagulation such as bleeding. Outpatient appointments for laboratory tests such as INR, clotting studies, and liver function studies should be stressed.

Health Promotion

Nurses should assess patients on admission for risks of PE and DVT. These can occur in young people as well as middle-aged people and the elderly. This assessment continues throughout the hospital stay. Orders for DVT prophylaxis should be obtained in patients with risk factors such as recent surgery, orthopedic surgery, injury, childbirth, stroke, cancer, heart failure and prolonged immobilization, indwelling central venous catheters, and older age. Patients who have had spinal cord injuries and spinal fractures are at increased risk often related to their postinjury status and immobilization (Kennedy, Zolot, & Sofer, 2001; Morris et al., 2002).

A number of deaths from pulmonary embolism caused by DVT have been attributed to long-distance airplane travel. Preventive strategies the nurse can stress for inpatients and outpatients include avoiding alcohol and caffeine before and during the flight, avoiding constrictive clothing, avoiding leg crossing, changing positions frequently while seated, not ingesting sleeping pills, not smoking, requesting bulkhead seating so as to stretch legs, staying well hydrated with water, noncaffeinated drinks, soft drinks, or juices, taking only short naps unless a normal sleeping position can be attained, and wearing compression stockings (Ball, 2003).

■ Pulmonary Hypertension

Pulmonary artery hypertension (PH) is a progressive disorder characterized by abnormally high blood pressure (hypertension) in the pulmonary artery. Hypertension develops when most of the very small arteries throughout the lungs narrow in diameter, thereby increasing the resistance to blood flow through the lungs. The increased pressure causes abnormally high and sustainable blood pressure elevations in the pulmonary arteries.

There are two types of PH: primary, also referred to as idiopathic, and secondary, that is, secondary to some other cause. Primary pulmonary artery hypertension (PPH) may be inherited (familial) or may occur for no known reason (idiopathic). Secondary pulmonary hypertension (SPH) is caused by or occurs either because of another condition, including chronic heart or lung disease or blood clots in the lungs, or a disease such as scleroderma (Porth, 2007).

Pulmonary artery hypertension is not curable, but it is treatable. Prognosis is compromised if the cause of SPH is not found and treated. Currently, many new treatments are being investigated that may help improve the quality of life for those patients experiencing PH (NHLBI, 2006).

Epidemiology and Etiology

Normal pulmonary circulation is a high-flow, low-resistance circuit capable of accommodating the entire right ventricular output at one-fifth the pressure of the systemic circulation level. The thin-walled right ventricle functions primarily as a flow-generator pump, and it is particularly sensitive to increases in its afterload. Increased pulmonary artery pressure and pulmonary vascular resistance characterize pulmonary hypertension. Pulmonary arterial hypertension is a mean pulmonary arterial pressure of greater than 25 mmHg at rest or greater than 35 mmHg during exercise (Merck, 2005b; Morton et al., 2005; Porth, 2007).

In accordance with the distinction between primary and secondary pulmonary arterial hypertension, the epidemiology and etiology of each is different. Idiopathic or primary pulmonary hypertension is the rarer of the two types, with an incidence of about 2 to 3 per million per year and a prevalence of about 15 per million (CDC, 2006). About 300 new cases of PPH are diagnosed in the United States each year, with a mean age of 35 to 37, but it can occur as late as age 60. SPH is much more common (NHLBI, 2006). Women are almost three times as likely to present with PPH as men (Sharma, 2006c). Although anyone can develop either type of pulmonary hypertension, older adults are more likely to have secondary pulmonary hypertension and young people are more likely to have idiopathic (primary) pulmonary hypertension.

PPH can be familial, meaning inherited or clustered, or sporadic. Most cases are sporadic, with approximately 10% being familial (Jassal & Sharma, 2004). In PPH, the precise etiology is unknown. However, presumed mechanisms include the following:

- **Endothelial dysfunction**—With impaired production of both prostacyclin and nitrous oxide, endothelium is overproduced. This overproduction results in vasoconstriction and remodeling of the pulmonary vasculature.
- **Voltage-gated K channel**—A defect in this ion channel changes the resting membrane potential, increasing intracellular calcium and leading to pulmonary vasoconstriction.
- **Thrombosis in situ**—Injury to the endothelial lining of the vessel wall, abnormal fibrinolysis, and platelet abnormalities may all contribute to thrombus formation (Sharma, 2006c, p. 1)

The etiologies and risk factors of PPH include the following:

- Use of appetite suppressants such as fenfluramine and dexfenfluramine; Fen-Phen produced an annual incidence of 25 to 50 per million per year.
- Genetic factors, for example, inheritance as an autosomal dominant trait, could play a role.
- Cocaine or amphetamine ingestion may be a contributing factor.

The specific genetic factors related to primary pulmonary hypertension are listed in the Genetic Considerations box.

Secondary pulmonary hypertension often is caused by several interactive disease processes. These causes may be categorized as pulmonary venous hypertension, chronic hypoxia

GENETIC CONSIDERATIONS Related to Primary Pulmonary Hypertension

Genetic factors, such as defects within the bone morphogenetic protein receptor type II gene, coding for a receptor member of the transforming growth factor-beta family, underlie familial primary pulmonary hypertension (Humbert & Trembath, 2002). About 20% of sporadic cases also have *BMPR2* mutations. Many people with PPH have increased levels of angiopoietin-1, which appears to downregulate *BMPR1A*, a sister receptor to *BMPR2*, and may stimulate serotonin production and endothelial smooth muscle proliferation.

Other possible contributing factors include abnormalities in serotonin transport and previous infection with human herpesvirus 8 (Humbert & Trembath; 2002; Merck, 2005b). Although achievements in determining the impact of genomic approaches on pulmonary hypertension have been made, additional research is indicated to identify specific molecular determinants for this disorder.

with secondary vasoconstriction of the pulmonary vasculature, pulmonary artery obstruction, and left-to-right shunts. Pulmonary venous hypertension is the most common form of pulmonary hypertension and usually due to left-sided heart disease. Pulmonary hypertension develops as a result of the obstruction of blood flow downstream from the pulmonary vein. Causes of pulmonary venous hypertension from distal to proximal of the pulmonary vasculature include coarctation of the aorta, aortic stenosis, aortic regurgitation, hypertrophic cardiomyopathy, constrictive pericarditis, restrictive cardiomyopathy, dilated cardiomyopathy, mitral stenosis, mitral regurgitation, and left atrial myxoma (Jassal & Sharma, 2004; Porth, 2007).

Chronic hypoxia with secondary vasoconstriction of the pulmonary vasculature induces vasoconstriction of the pulmonary vascular bed, causing high pulmonary resistance and hypertension with right ventricular failure. Causes include restrictive lung disease (obesity, pneumoconiosis, neuromuscular disorders) and obstructive lung diseases (asthma, COPD, bronchiectasis).

Concerning pulmonary artery obstruction, chronic major thromboembolic vessel disease is a treatable cause of pulmonary hypertension that results in anatomic obstruction of the arteries. Thrombotic disorders include sickle cell disease and other coagulation disorders. Embolic disease includes chronic thromboemboli, connective tissue disease, lupus, and schistosomiasis.

Individuals with pulmonary hypertension due to left-to-right shunts have high blood flow to the pulmonary vessels, which leads to increased pulmonary vascular resistance over time with reversal of the shunt (Eisenmenger complex). Extracardiac shunts include patent ductus arteriosus, and intracardiac shunts include ventricular and atrial septal defects.

Pathophysiology

Three predominant pathophysiological mechanisms may be involved in the development of SPH: (1) hypoxic vasoconstriction, (2) decreased area of the pulmonary vascular bed, and (3) volume/pressure overload (Sharma, 2006c). Chronic hypoxemia causes pulmonary vasoconstriction by a variety of actions

on pulmonary artery endothelium and smooth muscle cells, including downregulation of endothelial nitric oxide synthetase and reduced production of the voltage-gated potassium channel alpha subunit. Chronic hypoxemia leading to pulmonary hypertension can occur in patients with COPD, high-altitude disorders, and hypoventilation disorders (e.g., obstructive sleep apnea). COPD is the most common cause of SPH. These patients have worse than 5-year survival rates, more severe ventilation/perfusion mismatch than other diseases causing SPH, and nocturnal or exercise-induced hypoxemia. Other disorders, such as obstructive sleep apnea, neuromuscular disorders, and disorders of the chest wall, may lead to hypoxic pulmonary vasoconstriction and eventually SPH.

A variety of causes may decrease the cross-sectional area of the pulmonary vascular bed, primarily due to disease of the lung parenchyma. The pulmonary arterial pressure rises only when the loss of the pulmonary vessels exceeds 60% of the total pulmonary vasculature. Patients with collagen vascular diseases have a high incidence of SPH, particularly patients with systemic scleroderma or CREST (calcinosis cutis, Raynaud phenomenon, esophageal motility disorder, sclerodactyly, and telangiectasia) syndrome. A mild-to-moderate elevation in mean pulmonary artery pressure occurs secondary to acute pulmonary embolism. The peak systolic pressures usually do not rise above 50 mmHg, and they generally normalize following appropriate therapy. Chronic pulmonary emboli can result in progressive PH. HIV infection and several drugs and toxins are also known to cause PH.

Disorders of the left heart may cause SPH, resulting from volume and pressure overload. Pulmonary blood volume overload is caused by left-to-right intracardiac shunts, such as in patients with atrial or ventricular septal defects. Left atrial hypertension causes a passive rise in pulmonary arterial systolic pressure in order to maintain a driving force across the vasculature. Over time, persistent pulmonary hypertension accompanied by vasculopathy occurs. This may occur secondary to left ventricular dysfunction, mitral valvular disease, constrictive pericarditis, aortic stenosis, and cardiomyopathy.

Pulmonary venous obstruction is a rare cause of pulmonary hypertension. This may develop secondary to mediastinal fibrosis, anomalous pulmonary venous drainage, or pulmonary veno-occlusive disease.

Clinical Manifestations

Symptoms of pulmonary hypertension may develop very gradually and often are nonspecific. Thus, patients may delay seeing a health care provider for years, and when seen their disorder may be misdiagnosed and treated for more common conditions (Hegewald, Markewitz, & Elliott, 2007). Also, the clinical manifestations of SPH frequently are masked by the underlying etiology. Typically, the interval between the onset of symptoms of PH to diagnosis is about 2 years. The most common presenting symptoms are:

- Exertional dyspnea
- Fatigue and lethargy
- Angina
- Syncope
- Raynaud's disease
- Edema (Jassal & Sharma, 2004).

Less common symptoms include cough, hemoptysis, and hoarseness (due to compression of the recurrent laryngeal nerve by the distended pulmonary artery, i.e., Ortner's syndrome). In advanced disease, signs may include right ventricular heave; widely split second heart sound (S_2); accentuated, pulmonic component of S_2(P_2); pulmonary ejection click; right ventricular third heart sound (S_3); and jugular venous distention. Liver congestion and peripheral edema are common late manifestations (Sharma, 2006c).

Laboratory and Diagnostic Procedures

The diagnosis of PPH is suspected in patients with significant exertional dyspnea who are otherwise relatively healthy and have no signs of other diseases known to cause pulmonary hypertension. Patients usually undergo chest x-ray, spirometry, and electrocardiography (ECG) to identify more common causes of dyspnea, followed by Doppler ECG to assess right ventricular and pulmonary artery pressures as well as to detect structural heart disease causing secondary pulmonary hypertension.

The most common x-ray result in PPH is enlarged hilar vessels that rapidly prune into the periphery. Spirometry and lung volumes may be normal or show mild restriction, but diffusing capacity for carbon monoxide (DLCO) is usually reduced. Common ECG findings include right axis deviation, $R > S$ in V_1, $S_1Q_3T_3$, and peaked P waves.

Additional tests are obtained as indicated to diagnose secondary causes not apparent clinically. These include ventilation/perfusion scanning to detect thromboembolic disease, pulmonary function tests to identify obstructive or restrictive lung disease, and serum serologic tests to gather evidence for or against rheumatologic disease. Chronic thromboembolic pulmonary hypertension is suggested by CT or lung scan and is diagnosed by arteriography. Other tests, such as HIV testing, liver function tests, and polysomnography, are performed in the appropriate clinical context.

When initial evaluation reveals no conditions associated with secondary pulmonary hypertension, pulmonary artery catheterization is necessary to measure right atrial and ventricular, pulmonary artery, and pulmonary capillary wedge pressures and cardiac output. Right-sided O_2 saturation should be measured to exclude atrial septal defect. A mean pulmonary arterial pressure greater than 25 mmHg in the absence of an underlying cause defines PPH. However, most patients with PPH present with significantly higher pressure (e.g., 60 mmHg). Vasodilating drugs (e.g., inhaled nitric oxide, IV epoprostenol) often are administered during the procedure; a decrease in right-sided pressures in response to these drugs helps in the selection of drugs for treatment. Biopsy, once widely performed, is neither needed nor recommended because of high morbidity and mortality (Hegewald et al., 2007; Merck, 2005b; Sharma, 2006c).

Once PPH is diagnosed, the patient's family history is reviewed to detect possible genetic transmission, which is suggested by premature deaths in otherwise healthy members of the extended family. In familial PPH, genetic counseling is needed to advise family members of the risk of disease (about 20%) and to advocate serial screening with echocardiograms. Testing for mutations in the *BMPR2* gene in familial PPH may play a future role.

Medical Management

The treatment of SPH is primarily directed at treatment of the underlying disease. Effective therapy should be instituted in the early stages, before irreversible changes in pulmonary vasculature occur. Once the cause of SPH has been established, the management consists of specific interventional therapy, specific medical therapy, or general supportive therapy. Specific interventional and medical therapies are instituted for conditions such as atrial septal defects, mitral stenosis, sleep apnea, and chronic pulmonary thromboembolic disease. General supportive therapy is provided to patients who have right ventricular failure or to those patients in whom the cause cannot be addressed directly. General oxygen has a proven benefit in reducing patient mortality in selected patients with PH. Long-term oxygen is prescribed for those patients who have PaO_2 of less than 55 mmHg at rest from any cause and those who have decreased oxygen saturation during exercise.

Treatment of PPH is rapidly evolving. Oral calcium (Ca) channel blockers sustain reductions in pulmonary artery pressure or pulmonary vascular resistance in about 10% to 15% of patients and are the first drugs used. No differences in efficacy exist by Ca channel blocker type, although most specialists avoid verapamil because of its negative inotropic effects. Response to Ca channel blockers is a favorable prognostic sign, and patients who respond should continue this treatment. Those who do not respond are given other drugs. IV epoprostenol, a prostacyclin analog, improves function and lengthens survival even in patients who are unresponsive to a vasodilator during catheterization. Disadvantages are the need for continuous central catheter infusion and significant adverse effects, including flushing, diarrhea, and bacteremia due to the indwelling central catheter. Inhaled iloprost, oral beraprost, and subcutaneous prostacyclin analogs are under study as alternatives.

Other pharmacologic therapies for treating both primary and secondary pulmonary hypertension include anticoagulants, antidiuretics, anticoagulants, and digoxin. Anticoagulants are used regularly in patients with PPH because they help reduce symptoms and may provide a survival benefit. The role of anticoagulation has not been established in patients with SPH. Nonetheless, anticoagulation with warfarin is indicated in patients with chronic pulmonary emboli, pulmonary venoocclusive disease, and atrial fibrillation induced by left or right heart failure. Furthermore, long-term anticoagulation therapy should be considered in patients who are at high risk for developing venous thromboembolism (e.g., those with cor pulmonale and patients with immobility secondary to severe dyspnea).

Fluid removal with diuretics reduces hepatic congestion and pulmonary edema. It should, however, be instituted with caution to avoid hypokalemia, metabolic alkalosis, and a decrease in cardiac output. Phlebotomy should be considered if the patient's hematocrit value is greater than 60%. Digoxin has been shown to be beneficial for patients with supraventricular tachycardia or associated left ventricular dysfunction multifocal atrial tachycardia, but verapamil has been proven to be better than digoxin for controlling the heart rate.

Surgical Management

Lung transplantation offers the only hope of cure for PPH (Merck, 2005b). It is reserved for patients with New York Heart Association Class IV disease (defined as dyspnea associated with minimal activity, leading to bed to chair limitations) who have not been helped by prostacyclin analogs. Transplant surgery has a high morbidity due to the problems of rejection and infection and a 60% 5-year survival rate related to bronchiolitis obliterans (Sharma, 2006c).

Patients with an atrial septal defect, mitral stenosis, or chronic pulmonary thromboembolic disease should be considered for surgical management. PH resolves following successful surgical procedures, unless it is too far advanced. Although lung transplantation is reserved for patients with severe PPH, a subset of patients with SPH has undergone successful transplantation at several centers. These patients had SPH due to collagen vascular disease, drug-induced PAH, or pulmonary venous obstruction. Stability of the underlying causative disorder and the patient's ability to tolerate an extensive surgical procedure are prerequisites. Heart-lung transplantation has been performed in patients with SPH due to congenital cardiac disease or severe left ventricular dysfunction (Sharma, 2006c).

Nursing Management

The primary goal of nursing management is to identify those patients subject to or at high risk for pulmonary hypertension. There are numerous conditions, but primary diseases include cystic fibrosis, COPD, hypoventilation syndromes, pulmonary fibrosis, congenital heart disease, pulmonary emboli, mitral valve disease, and connective tissue diseases. See the Risk Factors for Secondary Pulmonary Hypertension for more details.

The nurse also must be alert to the foremost signs and symptoms of pulmonary hypertension: exertional dyspnea, fatigue and lethargy, angina, syncope, Raynaud's disease, and edema of ankles and legs. Nurses also are responsible for oxygen administration and medication administration as ordered. Patient education as to risk factors, activity tolerance, the use of oxygen, and discharge priorities is critical to the care of the patient. The remainder of the nursing management for pulmonary hypertension is covered under nursing management of restrictive pulmonary diseases.

RISK FACTORS for Secondary Pulmonary Hypertension

- Chronic high-altitude exposure
- Obstructive sleep apnea
- Vasculitis
- Infectious diseases
- HIV
- Drugs and toxins
- Amphetamines
- Anorexigens
- Cocaine
- Toxic rapeseed oil ingestion

Discharge Priorities

Discharge priorities are multifaceted and focus on self-care, education regarding medications and home equipment, and emergency needs. Fatigue and weakness related to the disease itself may render the patient dependent on others for self-care. Patients and families need to be advised about an activity regimen that the patient can safely assume. The physical environment also should be configured in order to provide easy and safe navigation, ambulatory or via a wheelchair. Precise instructions as to how and when to take medications should be given to the patient and family, and the patient should be instructed to keep the list in an easily accessible location along with emergency phone numbers to use if needed. Family members also should know the placement of these documents. Return medical appointments should be given to the patient, and the patient should indicate where these are recorded. If the patient is going to be on oxygen therapy at home, instruction should be provided as to how to use the equipment and how to secure replacement as necessary.

Psychological adjustment to the patient's illness also must be considered. The diagnosis carries with it an uncertain and historically very bleak prognosis. Although new oral and chronic parenteral (IV and subcutaneous) treatments have had a significant positive medical impact on the physical functioning of individuals with PAH, patients often struggle with new short- and long-term psychosocial challenges (Wryobeck, Lippo, McLaughlin, Riba, & Rubenfire, 2007).

Health Promotion

With regard to health promotion, patients with pulmonary hypertension should be made aware of risk factors that may exacerbate their disease, and cautioned to avoid them. Patients also may be on a variety of medications, including anticoagulants. They should be advised to avoid situations that would put them at risk for experiencing side effects of the medications. Counseling also is advised to help people cope with the serious and potentially life-threatening outcomes of their disease. Referral to a support group, locally or online, also may assist the patient in the coping process.

Collaborative Management

The health care provider, nurse, and social worker are involved in the care of the patient. They initiate the plan of care and assume responsibility for continuity. Various diagnostic tests, as previously described, are performed. These are essential to determine the cause of secondary hypertension. They also are essential to interrupting the self-perpetuation cycle responsible for the progress of this disease. Although there is no cure for PPH, treatment as prescribed by the health care provider can relieve symptoms, increase quality of life, and prolong life. The nurse is responsible for implementing and evaluating the plan of care. The social worker, occupational therapist, and dietitian may be called on to assist the patient in making appropriate plans for discharge, physical set-up of house that deters overexertion, self-care help, and dietary plans that reduce physiological stress.

Cor Pulmonale: Etiology, Epidemiology, and Pathophysiology

Cor pulmonale is defined as an alteration in the structure and function of the right ventricle caused by a primary disorder of the respiratory system. Pulmonary hypertension is the common link between lung dysfunction and the heart in cor pulmonale. Right ventricular disease caused by a primary abnormality of the left side of the heart or congenital heart disease is not considered cor pulmonale, but it can develop secondary to many cardiopulmonary diseases (Yunis & Crausman, 2006).

Cor pulmonale develops as a result of lung disorders such as chronic lung disease, pulmonary embolism, interstitial lung disease, idiopathic primary pulmonary hypertension, and blood disorders such as polycythemia vera, sickle cell disease, and macrohemoglobinemia (Yunis & Crausman, 2006). Blood disorders are discussed in detail in Chapter 63 . Cor pulmonale is estimated to account for 6% to 7% of all types of adult heart disease in the United States with COPD the causative factor in more than 50% of cases (Yunis & Crausman, 2006).

A variety of pathophysiological mechanisms lead to pulmonary hypertension and consequently, cor pulmonale. These include (1) pulmonary vasoconstriction due to alveolar hypoxia, (2) anatomic compromise of the pulmonary vascular bed, (3) increased blood viscosity secondary to blood disorders such as polycythemia vera and sickle cell disease, and (4) idiopathic primary pulmonary hypertension (Yunis & Crausman, 2006).

There are two forms of cor pulmonale, acute and chronic. Acute cor pulmonale usually results from a massive pulmonary embolus or from injury due to mechanical ventilation for acute respiratory distress syndrome. Chronic cor pulmonale is usually caused by COPD (chronic bronchitis, emphysema) and less often by extensive loss of lung tissue due to surgery or trauma, chronic unresolved pulmonary emboli, pulmonary veno-occlusive disease, scleroderma, pulmonary interstitial fibrosis, kyphoscoliosis, obesity with alveolar hypoventilation, neuromuscular disorders involving respiratory muscles, or idiopathic alveolar hypoventilation. In patients with COPD, an acute exacerbation or pulmonary infection may trigger right ventricular overload (Merck, 2005a).

Laboratory and Diagnostic Procedures

Diagnosis is based on the clinical manifestations and diagnostic tests such as echocardiography, which will give information about the size of the heart. Chest x-rays and computed axial tomography CAT scan of the chest are also used for this reason. Pulmonary function tests that evaluate ventilation/perfusion mismatch (Chapters 33 and 36) provide information about problems with gas exchange. ABG tests also help identify gas exchange and the presence of acidosis and alkalosis.

Clinical Manifestations

Cor pulmonale is asymptomatic initially, although patients usually have significant clinical manifestations related to underlying lung disorder (e.g., dyspnea, exertional fatigue). Later, as right ventricular (RV) pressures increase, physical signs commonly include a left parasternal systolic lift, a loud pulmonic component of the second heart sound (S_2), and murmurs of functional tricuspid and pulmonic insufficiency. Later, an RV gallop rhythm (third [S_3] and fourth [S_4] heart sounds) augmented during inspiration, distended jugular veins, hepatomegaly, and lower extremity edema may occur. The patient also may complain of fatigue, dyspnea or chest pain on exertion, and cough. In advanced stages hepatic congestion leads to anorexia, right upper quadrant abdominal discomfort, and jaundice (Yunis & Crausman, 2006).

Medical Management

Treatment is directed at the underlying illness. Oxygen therapy is a mainstay for patients with cor pulmonale because it relieves hypoxemic pulmonary vasoconstriction. Because the partial pressure of oxygen or PO_2 is likely to fall with exercise and sleep, oxygen is recommended during these times or continuously (Yunis & Crausman, 2006). Diuretics are used, particularly when the right ventricular filling volume is markedly elevated; however, they are used cautiously to prevent hypokalemia, metabolic acidosis, and a decline in cardiac output.

In addition to diuretics, vasodilator drugs including calcium channel blockers such as oral sustained-release nifedipine and diltiazem are effective. Theophylline has a weak inotropic effect and may improve right ventricular ejection as well as decrease pulmonary vascular resistance. Finally, anticoagulation with warfarin is recommended in patients who are high risk for thromboembolism (Yunis & Crausman, 2006). Phlebotomy is recommended for patients with severe polycythemia, which is defined as a hematocrit of over 65 (Yunis & Crausman, 2006). Cardiac medications are discussed in Chapter 40 and anticoagulants in Chapter 43 .

Nursing Management

Physical assessment findings include an increased chest diameter, labored respirations with retractions of the chest wall and use of accessory muscles, hyperresonance to percussion, diminished breath sounds, wheezing, and, rarely, cyanosis (Yunis & Crausman, 2006). Auscultation of the heart may reveal a split second heart sound, a systolic ejection murmur with a sharp ejection click over the pulmonary artery, along with a diastolic regurgitation murmur (Yunis & Crausman, 2006). There may be a third ventricular heart sound secondary to systemic venous congestion. This also may be reflected by distended neck veins (Yunis & Crausman, 2006). See the Diagnostic Tests for Cor Pulmonale box (p. 985) for relevant diagnostic studies.

The primary role of the nurse is managing dyspnea by administration of oxygen and medications to treat right ventricular hypertrophy and pulmonary hypertension. This includes medications that treat the underlying disease.

Patient education is another major role of the nurse. The nurse teaches the patient and caregiver to be comfortable managing oxygen equipment and medications. Referrals to home health and pulmonary rehabilitation are usually needed to ensure safe care in the home setting. A plan for regular assessment of oxygen needs and medications should be in place before discharge. The single most preventive measure is to encourage individuals to stop smoking and to avoid exposure to secondhand smoke and respiratory pollutants.

PHARMACOLOGY Summary of Medications to Treat Lower Airway Disorders

Medication Category	Action	Application/Indication	Nursing Responsibility
Mucolytics • Dornase alpha (Pulmozyme) • Acetylcysteine* (Mucomyst) • Amiloride**	Liquefies bronchial secretions by altering the structure of mucous molecule.	Cystic fibrosis, acute and chronic bronchitis, pneumonia, TB.	Monitor for adverse effects: nausea, vomiting. Observe for possible bronchospasm. Establish a routine for elimination of secretions post-treatment. Use with caution in patients with compromised ability to cough.
Decongestants • Sympathomimetics • Ephedrine (Efedron) • Oxymetazoline (Afrin 12 hour, Neo-Synephrine 12 hour) • Phenylephrine (Afrin 4–6 hour, Neo-Synephrine 4–6 hour) • Pseudoephedrine (Chlor-Trimeton, Drixoral, Sudafed) **Anticholinergic** • Intranasal ipratropium (Atrovent, Combivent)	Decreases nasal membrane edema by constricting nasal arterioles. Decreases rhinorrhea by blocking muscarinic receptors in nasal passages.	Common cold, sinusitis, allergic rhinitis, nasal congestion.	Monitor for adverse effects: insomnia, tremors, weakness, anxiety, hypertension, tachycardia, palpitations, arrhythmias. Observe for rebound nasal congestion with intranasal administration, CNS stimulation with oral administration. Monitor for severe reactions: hallucinations, convulsions. Be aware of drug interactions (MAOIs, methyldopa, tricyclic antidepressants and others).
Antitussives • Nonopioid dextromethorphan* (Benylin, Robitussin, Delsym) **Opioid** • Codeine** • Hydrocodone bitartrate (Hycodan, Mycodone)	Suppresses cough by direct action on the cough center in the medulla.	Nonproductive or hyperactive cough.	Monitor for adverse effects: drowsiness, sedation (especially patients on CNS depressants), nausea, vomiting, constipation, dizziness, **pruritus. *Be aware of drug interaction with MAOIs. Monitor for CNS stimulation, hypotension, hyperpyrexia.
Anti-infectives • Fluoroquinolones/quinolones • Ciprofloxacin (Cipro) • Ofloxacin (Floxin) • Levofloxacin (Levaquin) • Moxifloxacin (Avelox)	Exerts bactericidal effect by disrupting synthesis of gram-negative and gram-positive bacterial DNA.	Acute exacerbation of chronic bronchitis, community-acquired pneumonia, sinusitis.	Monitor for adverse effects: nausea, headache, diarrhea, some may cause dysrhythmias or liver failure. Monitor WBC count, liver and renal function. Monitor for signs of CNS toxicity especially if given in presence of epilepsy, cerebral artery disease, alcoholism. Be aware of drug interactions (warfarin, NSAIDs, theophylline, antacids, caffeine). Monitor for altered efficacy or toxicity. Do not give with antacids or vitamins containing calcium, magnesium, iron, or zinc.
Tetracyclines • Doxycycline (Vibramycin) • Tetracycline (Sumycin)	Exerts bacteriostatic effect by inhibiting bacterial protein synthesis in gram-positive and gram-negative bacteria. May be bactericidal at higher doses.	Respiratory tract infections, *Chlamydia*, gonorrhea, tetanus, *Helicobacter pylori*, Lyme disease.	Monitor for adverse effects: nausea, vomiting, diarrhea, signs of superinfection. Be aware of drug interactions (iron, calcium, magnesium, antacids, lipid lowering drugs, oral anticoagulants, oral contraceptives). Observe for decreased drug efficacy or toxicity. Do not give with milk products, iron, magnesium laxatives, or antacids. Warn patient of photosensitivity and need for sun block.

(continued)

PHARMACOLOGY Summary of Medications to Treat Lower Airway Disorders—*Continued*

Medication Category	Action	Application/Indication	Nursing Responsibility
Macrolides • Clarithromycin* (Biaxin) • Erythromycin (Erythrocin) • Azithromycin (Zithromax)	Exerts bacteriostatic effect by inhibiting bacterial protein synthesis in gram-positive and gram-negative organisms. May be bactericidal at higher doses.	Legionnaire disease, *Mycoplasma pneumoniae* pneumonia, diphtheria, chlamydial infections.	Monitor for adverse effects: urticaria, nausea, vomiting, diarrhea, abdominal cramping, *Clostridium* overgrowth. Observe for exacerbation of existing heart disease or, if given IV, torsades de pointes. Monitor hepatic function. Be aware of multiple drug interactions (warfarin, anticonvulsants, theophylline, and others). Monitor for toxicity or altered drug efficacy. Warn patient not to take OTC drugs without contacting physician. Do not give with fruit juice.
Aminoglycosides • Tobramycin (Nebcin) • Amikacin (Amikin) • Gentamicin (Garamycin)	Exerts bacteriocidal effect on gram-negative organisms and staphylococcus by altering bacterial protein synthesis.	TB, serious respiratory infections, sepsis, meningitis, osteomyelitis.	Monitor for adverse effects: signs of ototoxicity (dizziness, loss of balance, tinnitus, headache), superinfection. *Note:* Hearing loss is usually irreversible. Be aware of increased risk of nephrotoxicity and/or ototoxicity if given concurrently with amphotericin B, furosemide, acetylsalicylic, and others. Monitor renal function for signs of nephrotoxicity.
Sulfonamides • Trimethoprim-sulfamethoxazole (SMZ-TMP) (Bactrim, Septra)	Exerts bacteriostatic activity by inhibiting bacterial folic acid synthesis needed for cell growth.	Exacerbation of chronic bronchitis, pneumonia, traveler's diarrhea, urinary tract infections, otitis media.	Monitor for adverse effects: nausea, vomiting, urticaria. Be aware of drug interactions (warfarin, digoxin, phenytoin, and others). Observe for drug toxicity. Monitor CBC, renal function, urinalysis (crystalluria can occur). Increase fluid intake unless contraindicated.
Miscellaneous Antibiotics • Chloramphenicol (Chloromycetin)	Exerts broad-spectrum bacteriostatic activity by interfering with bacterial protein synthesis. May be bacteriocidal in some organisms.	Serious infections, cystic fibrosis regimes, bacteremia, meningitis, typhoid fever.	Monitor for adverse effects: nausea, vomiting, headache, fungal overgrowth. Monitor blood studies regularly. May cause blood dyscrasias and irreversible bone marrow depression. Increase monitoring of blood glucose in patients on oral antidiabetic agents. Monitor serum drug levels, especially in the presence of renal or hepatic impairment.

PHARMACOLOGY Summary of Medications to Treat Lower Airway Disorders—*Continued*

Medication Category	Action	Application/Indication	Nursing Responsibility
Antifungals • Polyene • Amphotericin B (Fungizone)	Causes fungal cell death by altering fungal cell membrane.	Progressive or potentially fatal systemic fungal or protozoal infections.	Monitor for anorexia, nausea, vomiting. May require premedication with antiemetic. During IV infusion, monitor vital signs, observe for infusion reaction: headache, fever, chills, nausea, vomiting, hypotension, bronchospasm (premedication with diphenhydramine and acetaminophen may reduce infusion reactions). Monitor input and output (I&O), renal function, appearance of urine, CBC, electrolytes, hepatic function. Monitor IV site for extravasation, thrombophlebitis. Be aware of multiple drug incompatibilities when given IV.
Azoles • Fluconazole (Diflucan) • Itraconazole (Sporanox)	Exerts fungistatic effect by interrupting fungal cell membrane function. May be fungicidal at higher concentrations.	Systemic candidiasis, pneumonia, esophageal candidiasis.	Monitor for adverse effects: headache, nausea, abdominal pain, diarrhea. Monitor liver function. Be aware of multiple drug interactions (oral hypoglycemics, Coumadin, phenytoin, theophylline, and others). Monitor for decreased drug efficacy or toxicity. Monitor for hypoglycemia in diabetic patients. Be aware of multiple drug incompatibilities when given IV.
Echocardins • Anidulafungin (Eraxis)	Exerts antifungal effect by inhibiting synthesis of major component of fungal cell wall.	Esophageal candidiasis, candidemia.	Monitor for adverse effects: nausea, vomiting, diarrhea, hypokalemia, rash. Monitor liver function.
Antiviral • Amantadine (Symmetrel) Rimantadine (Flumadine) • Oseltamivir* (Tamiflu) • Zanamivir* (Relenza)	Thought to exert antiviral effect by inhibiting early viral replication.	Prevention and treatment of influenza A. *Treatment of influenza A and B.	Monitor for adverse effects: dizziness, light-headedness, insomnia, nausea. Observe for increased seizure activity in presence of seizure disorder.
Carbapenem • Imipenem/Cilaseatin • Meropenem	Exerts antibacterial action against gram negative and positive and anaerobic pathogens. Inhibits cell wall synthesis by binding the penicillin binding proteins.	Treatments of lower resp track infections that are common with cystic fibrosis infections.	Observe for increased seizure activity in presence for seizure disorder and compromised renal function. Monitor for hypo tension, bradycardia, pruritus, elevated BUN and creatiniene, and liver enzymes.

(continued)

PHARMACOLOGY Summary of Medications to Treat Lower Airway Disorders—*Continued*

Medication Category	Action	Application/Indication	Nursing Responsibility
Anti–TB • Isoniazid* (INH, Nydrazid, Laniazid) • Rifapentine** (Priftin) • Pyrazinamide) • Ephambutol	Exerts bacteriostatic or bacteriocidal effects by disrupting synthesis of bacterial cell wall or impairing cell metabolism.	Prevention and treatment of pulmonary TB. Adjunct treatment when primary and secondary anti-TB drugs cannot be used or have failed.	Monitor for adverse effects: visual disturbances, orthostatic hypotension*, signs of hepatotoxicity (anorexia, fatigue, nausea, malaise), signs of peripheral neuropathy (burning, tingling, pain, numbness). Monitor hepatic function, CBC. Monitor for hyperglycemia in presence of diabetes. **Be aware of multiple drug interactions (phenytoin, warfarin, diazepam, theophylline and others). Monitor for altered drug efficacy. **Warn patient on oral contraceptives to use alternate birth control method. *Instruct patient to restrict alcohol and intake of foods rich in tyramine (dairy, beef, chicken, bananas, caffeine, and others) and histamine (tuna, yeast extract, brine).
Digestive Enzyme • Pancrelipase (Viokase)	Breaks down fats, proteins, and starches in the final stage of digestion for easier absorption.	Steatorrhea from malabsorption syndrome in cystic fibrosis.	Monitor for adverse effects: nausea, abdominal cramps, diarrhea. Assess for improved nutritional status and decreased steatorrhea. Be aware of religious considerations; drug is pork based.
Bronchodilators • Corticosteroids (see the Pharmacolgy Summary in Chapter 36 🔗)			

◼ Pleural Effusion

A **pleural effusion**, which affects 1.3 million people annually in the United States, is defined as the presence of fluid in the pleural space (Figure 35–13 ◼) (Abrahamian, 2008). This usually occurs secondary to other diseases. The source of the fluid usually is blood vessels or lymphatic vessels lying beneath either pleura. Occasionally, the source is an abscess or other lesion that drains into the pleural space.

Epidemiology and Etiology

Other common causes of pleural effusion include heart failure, TB, pneumonia, pulmonary infections, nephrotic syndrome, connective tissue disease, pulmonary embolism, fungal lung infections, and neoplastic tumors.

Pathophysiology

The pleura is a thin, transparent, serous permeable membrane that lines the thoracic cavity and encases the lungs. There are two layers: The parietal pleura lies adjacent to the chest wall, and the visceral pleura adheres to the outer surfaces of the lung. The small amount of serous fluid normally present between these two surfaces acts as a lubricant, thereby allowing the chest wall and lung to glide during inspiration and expiration. Fluids that accumulate in the lung can cross into the pleural space, causing a plural effusion (McCance & Huether, 2007). A pleural effusion can cause compression atelectasis and displacement of mediastinal contents. Because there is no communication between the pleural space and environmental air, pressure in the pleural space remains negative, and atelectasis is caused solely by pressure exerted by the effusion.

The effusion can be composed of a relatively clear fluid or it can be bloody or purulent. An effusion may be a transudate or an exudate. Transudates are clear in color, have a low protein content, and are secondary to underlying diseases. Some of these are caused by heart failure, cirrhosis, nephrotic syndrome, and/or medical disorders leading to hypoalbuminemia. Exudates have higher protein content and usually are caused by infection. Typ-

DIAGNOSTIC TESTS for Cor Pulmonale

Test	Expected Abnormality	Rationale
Chest x-ray	Enlargement of central pulmonary arteries; increased transverse diameter of the heart.	Changes in heart and pulmonary vessels are caused by pulmonary hypertension secondary to hypoxemia.
Echocardiography	Shows signs of chronic right ventricular pressure overload.	The right ventricle is strained by pulmonary hypertension.
ECG	Incomplete right bundle branch block, low-voltage QRS, signs of right ventricular hypertrophy, and atrial and junctional dysrhythmias.	ECG changes are secondary to right atrial enlargement and hypoxemia.
Cardiac catheterization	Assesses degree of pulmonary hypertension and differentiates cor pulmonale from occult left ventricular dysfunction.	Chronic hypoxemia causes pulmonary hypertension.
Hematocrit	Abnormally elevated.	Polycythemia developed secondary to hypoxemia.
Serum Alpha 1-antitrypsin	Decreased.	Deficiency of AAT causes COPD symptomatology and leads to cor pulmonale.

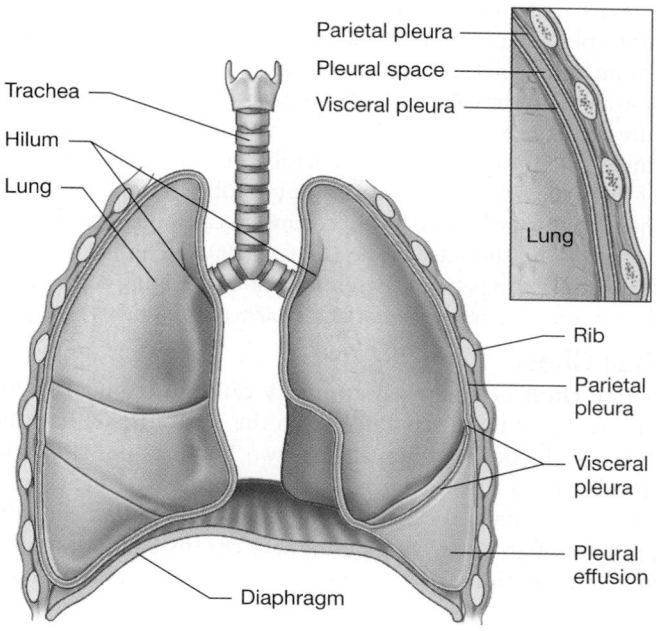

FIGURE 35–13 ■ Pleural effusion.

ically, they are deeper in color with a turbid appearance (Fishman et al., 2002). Causes are malignancy, collagen vascular disease, pneumonia, pancreatitis, or pulmonary embolism (Porth, 2007).

Clinical Manifestations

The symptoms of pleural effusion depend largely on the underlying disease and the size of the effusion. The patient may be asymptomatic if the effusion is small. However, if the effusion is large, clinical manifestations include severe breathlessness, pain, or both. Breath sounds are reduced on the affected side and the percussion note is dull. A pleural friction rub, which is described as a rubbing, grating, harsh, dry, and scratchy sound, may be present and best heard over the area of pleural inflammation. It will disappear with breath holding. There will be asymmetric ex-

pansion of the thoracic cage, with lagging expansion on the affected side. Mediastinal shift is seen only with massive effusions (usually >1,000 mL) and is noted on x-ray as displacement of the trachea and mediastinum to the contralateral side of the pleural effusion. Other important findings that provide clues to the cause of the pleural effusion are anasarca, distended neck veins, S_3 gallop rhythm, clubbing of the fingers, and breast nodule or intra-abdominal mass (Abrahamian, 2008).

Laboratory and Diagnostic Procedures

If more than 200 to 500 mL of fluid is present in the pleural space, the chest x-ray may show blunting of the costophrenic angle. As the volume of fluid increases, the hemidiaphragm becomes obscured as well. A lateral decubitus film may be helpful for showing fluid shifts. A CT scan, ultrasound, or thoracentesis also may be employed to make the final diagnosis. A sample of pleural fluid is obtained for biochemical, microbiologic, and cytologic analysis. Analysis of pleural fluid includes protein and glucose concentration, pH, and bacteria, including acid-fast bacilli and cell content. Cytologic testing reveals a malignant effusion about 80% of the time. Closed-needle biopsy is performed to identify tuberculosis and malignancies (Peek et al., 2000).

Medical Management

As with any other life-threatening condition, airway stabilization with adequate oxygenation and ventilation is the first priority. Administer supplemental oxygen to all unstable patients. Generally, any patient who requires thoracentesis is admitted to the hospital. A thoracentesis is a procedure to remove fluid from the space between the lungs and the chest wall called the pleural space. It is done with a needle (and sometimes a plastic catheter) inserted through the chest wall. This pleural fluid may be sent to a lab to determine what may be causing the fluid to accumulate in the pleural space.

Treatment of transudative effusions most commonly caused by heart failure differs from treatment of exudative effusions caused by infection and malignancy. In the case of a patient presenting with pleural effusion associated with congestive heart failure (CHF), the treatment involves controlling the patient's heart failure before considering thoracentesis (Coding Edge Archives, 2000).

Other treatment options include chemotherapy, radiation, intrapleural instillation of sclerosing agents, indwelling pleural catheters with intermittent drainage, chest tube drainage using the water seal system, pleuroperitoneal shunts, and pleurectomy. If thoracentesis provides relief, intermittent thoracenteses can be scheduled or a chest tube can be inserted to completely evacuate the pleural space. This is usually followed by pleurodesis or instillation of a sclerosing agent into the pleural cavity via the chest tube (Kvale, Simoff, & Prakash, 2003; Taubert, 2001).

When pleural effusion is related to a malignant cause, it may reaccumulate rapidly. Therefore, thoracentesis is done at frequent intervals to provide comfort and relieve dyspnea. The fluid is protein rich and hypoalbuminemia may result. Use of oral diuretics such as spironolactone has been suggested (Nevidjion & Sowers, 2000).

Nursing Management

Nursing assessment includes regular evaluation of the lung sounds. Pulse oximetry is used to assess oxygen saturation. The nurse provides symptomatic relief of dyspnea and pain. If a chest tube is placed, the nurse positions the patient and offers support during the thoracentesis procedure. Pain management is a priority, and the nurse assists the patient to assume positions of comfort and offers analgesics as needed. The nurse continues to assess levels of dyspnea and provides supplemental oxygen, bronchodilators, and opioid analgesics such as morphine for relief of dyspnea (Kvale et al., 2003). This procedure prevents reaccumulation of pleural fluid in the pleural space (Taubert, 2001).

If a chest tube and water seal system are used, the nurse monitors the system function and records the amount of drainage at frequent intervals. The patient is encouraged to turn frequently and ambulate to facilitate chest drainage. Care of the patient with a chest tube is discussed later in this chapter. The nurse also monitors electrolytes for imbalances and intake and output as indicated (see Chapter 18 ⊘).

Discharge Priorities

Patients may be discharged with a pleural catheter for drainage. The nurse is responsible for educating the patient and family regarding management and care of the catheter and drainage system. Another important issue for patient education is pain management. The patient and family should be given concrete instructions on medications to be taken for pain and what to do for breakthrough pain. Patients and families should be instructed to call the health care provider or health care team if dyspnea and discomfort are not relieved by the regimen suggested for discharge.

Chest Trauma and Thoracic Injuries

Chest trauma is the cause of nearly 16,000 deaths in the United States each year and the cause of death in 25% of all trauma patients. Chapter 73 ⊘ discusses chest trauma. Increased hand gun use has contributed to the rise in the number of penetrating injuries (Reeder & Danis, 2001). These injuries impair airway patency, breathing, and circulation so the role of the nurse in maintaining an excellent standard of care in these situations is paramount.

Rib and Sternal Fractures

Rib fractures are the most common blunt thoracic injury in adults. These are frequently associated with other injuries such as flail chest, pulmonary contusion, and pneumothorax.

Epidemiology and Etiology

Rib fractures usually are caused by a direct blow to the ribs. Another mechanism of injury may be due to a forceful compression of the rib cage, as can happen in a "pileup" during a football game (Cerro Coso Coyote Athletics [CCCA], 2004). The most important cause of significant blunt chest trauma is motor vehicle crashes (MVCs). MVCs account for 70% to 80% of such injuries (Sawyer, 2006).

Sternal fractures are most common in MVCs that result in a direct blow to the sternum via the steering wheel, and are most common in female patients over age 50 and those using shoulder restraints (Owens, Chaudry, Eggerstedt, & Smith, 2000). A fracture occurs because the pressure of an injury interrupts the bony integrity of the rib or the sternum. Ribs tend to break just in front of the angle, which is its weakest point. Ribs 4 through 9 are the most likely to be injured by direct blows because they are not protected by the shoulder girdle (CCCA, 2004). The incidence of fractured ribs in patients presenting to the operating department for emergency surgery is more than 60% (CCCA, 2004).

Flail Chest

A **flail chest** occurs when an injury causes a segment of the thoracic cage to be separated from the rest of the chest wall. This usually occurs when at least two fractures per rib occur (producing a free segment), in at least two ribs (Figure 35–14 ■). The significance of a flail chest is that it indicates the presence of an underlying pulmonary contusion, as described in a later section. The separated segment is unable to con-

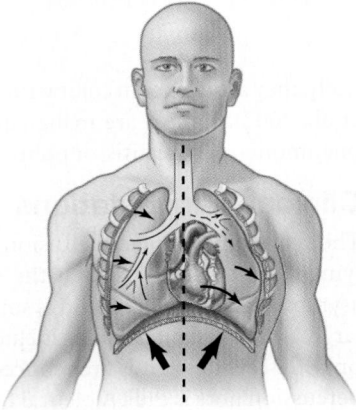

(a) Inspiration   (b) Expiration

FIGURE 35–14 ■ Flail chest.

tribute to lung expansion; in fact, during spontaneous ventilation the floating segment moves in the opposite direction or paradoxically to the chest wall. Large flail segments will involve a much greater proportion of the chest wall and may extend bilaterally or involve the sternum. In most cases, the severity and extent of the lung injury determine the clinical course and requirement for mechanical ventilation. Thus, the management of flail chest consists of standard management of the rib fractures and of the pulmonary contusions underneath (Trauma.org, 2004).

Laboratory and Diagnostic Procedures

Chest radiography should be obtained to detect rib fractures, but also to look for associated injuries such as pneumothorax, hemothorax, or pulmonary contusion (Devitt, 1995). The patient with a sternal fracture is evaluated closely for underlying cardiac injuries. An ECG should be done and the oxygenation should be monitored with pulse oximetry and ABGs.

No single condition confirms the diagnosis of flail chest. Chest x-ray and ABG measurements along with the patient's description of the pain along the ribs contributes to the diagnostic information. A CT scan also may be useful (Bjerke, 2002).

Clinical Manifestations

The clinical manifestations associated with rib fractures include severe localized pain, which is usually increased on movement of the ribs, deep breathing, coughing, or sneezing. An individual with a rib fracture usually will refrain from breathing deeply by taking shallow breaths, and may also hold the injured side in an attempt to restrict painful movement of the chest. Palpation of the ribs with gentle compression will indicate pain at the fracture site. If the fracture is displaced, there may be a palpable defect and crepitation on movement or coughing. Complications of a rib fracture also can occur with a puncture of the thoracic or visceral structures (Sawyer, 2006; Shahani, 2006). The signs and symptoms of a sternal fracture are similar to a rib fracture except that tenderness exists along the sternum (CCCA, 2004). There also may be anterior chest pain, tenderness, ecchymosis, swelling, and the potential for a chest wall deformity. If there are cardiac complications, crepitus may be detected upon auscultation and subcutaneous emphysema may be palpated.

The patient with flail chest engages in splinting with each breath because of pain, and intrusion of the flail segment on the contusion leads to increased work of breathing and pulmonary shunting with hypoxia (Devitt, 1995). As a result, the patient experiences severe respiratory distress.

Medical Management

The aim of medical management with a chest wall injury is directed toward protecting the underlying lung and allowing adequate oxygenation, ventilation, and pulmonary toilet. This approach will help prevent the most common complication, pneumonia. This is a particular concern in the elderly patient who is at a higher risk for the development of pneumonia and respiratory failure if not appropriately managed. Most commonly patients initially are placed on 100% oxygen via a nonrebreather face mask (Trauma.org, 2004). Oxygen saturation and ABGs are monitored regularly and when changes occur.

Analgesia is a crucial component in the management of rib fractures. Although strapping the chest to splint rib fractures may help with pain, the strapping impedes chest wall movement and prevents adequate inspiration and clearance of secretions. Sedation and pain management allow the patient to begin deep breathing and coughing in order to prevent the development of atelectasis, pneumonitis, and hypoxemia. Opioid analgesics are useful, but must be monitored carefully for respiratory depression, especially in the elderly. Patient-controlled administration of an opioid infusion is an effective method for cooperative patients. Chapter 15 ⊙ includes a complete discussion of patient-controlled analgesia (PCA) for pain management.

The addition of a nonsteroidal anti-inflammatory drug (NSAID) may provide adequate relief, but these should be withheld until other injuries have been excluded (e.g., traumatic brain injury) and used with caution in the elderly. Epidural analgesia for a severe chest wall injury is effective because it provides complete analgesia, allowing normal inspiration and coughing without the risks of respiratory depression. Alternative pain management strategies include intercostal nerve block, ice over the site, epidural analgesia, PCA, and nonopioid analgesia. The pain usually diminishes by the fifth to the seventh day, and healing occurs in 3 to 6 weeks.

Intubation and mechanical ventilation are rarely indicated for chest wall injury alone. Where ventilation is necessary, it is usually for hypoxia due to flail chest and underlying pulmonary contusions. Ventilation is usually necessary only until the resolution of the pulmonary contusion. Positive pressure ventilation may be required for severe chest wall instability that results in inadequate spontaneous ventilation. The patient also is evaluated for any injuries that are associated with the rib fractures. Surgical fixation usually is not necessary unless fragments pose a potential for further injury.

■ Nursing Management

Nursing management in the emergency setting for patients with rib fractures involves astute assessment for respiratory complications and diligent patient monitoring for dyspnea, hypoxemia, and pain. The nurse emphasizes pain management and gives specific instructions regarding medications for pain until the pain diminishes. The nurse administers pain medication and assesses for pain relief. The nurse assists the patient with coughing and deep breathing techniques, monitors patient response, and auscultates lung fields regularly for adventitious sounds. If the patient is receiving a narcotic and is using PCA, the nurse assesses the rate of breathing, level of alertness, and the presence of hypoxemia hourly. Research shows that patients with flail chest often continue to experience chronic pain, dyspnea, and disability for 6 months.

Discharge Priorities

The patient should be given written instructions regarding the plan of care. Patients and caregivers should be encouraged to call members of the health team for persistent problems such as pain or dyspnea. Patients may be reluctant to ask for more pain medication when it is needed, so the nurse stresses that healing will not occur unless the patient feels comfortable breathing and coughing. The patient should be well versed in situations that would constitute an emergency visit to the hospital and be given resources for handling problem situations. Patients should be aware of emergency contacts in case of increasing dyspnea and pain.

Pulmonary Contusion

A **pulmonary contusion** is an injury to the lung parenchyma, leading to edema and blood collecting in alveolar spaces and loss of normal lung structure and function.

This blunt injury develops over 24 hours, leading to poor gas exchange, increased pulmonary vascular resistance, and decreased lung compliance. There also is a significant inflammatory reaction to blood components in the lung, and 50% to 60% of patients with significant contusions develop bilateral acute respiratory distress syndrome (ARDS) (Wanek & Mayberry, 2004).

Epidemiology and Etiology

The most common cause of pulmonary contusion is trauma. It occurs in 20% of blunt trauma patients with significant injuries. The mortality ranges from 10% to 25%, and 40% to 60% for patients who require mechanical ventilation.

Clinical Manifestations

There are few clinical signs of contusion. Crackles may be heard on auscultation but are rarely heard in the emergency setting on admission. Rib fractures, flail chest, or bruising on the chest indicates the possibility of contusion. Frequently, if the patient has significant chest wall injury, pain will affect the ability to ventilate and clear secretions.

Laboratory and Diagnostic Procedures

Pulmonary contusions are rarely diagnosed on physical examination. Most significant contusions are diagnosed by chest x-ray; however, an x-ray will often underestimate the size of the contusion and lags behind the clinical picture. The true extent of injury may not be present on chest x-ray for 24 to 48 hours (Wanek & Mayberry, 2004). CT scan is very sensitive for identification of pulmonary contusion and may allow for differentiation from areas of atelectasis and or aspiration (2004). ABGs and/or pulse oximetry may be used to assess for hypoxemia and gas exchange.

Medical Management

The patient is monitored closely for hypoxemia. Supplemental oxygen is delivered as needed. If the patient has extreme difficulty with ventilation and clearing of secretions because of pain, intubation and mechanical ventilation are necessary. Patient management involves fluid restriction in order to prevent pulmonary edema and increasing respiratory insufficiency. Usually pulmonary contusions resolve in 3 to 5 days. The main complications are ARDS and pneumonia (Wanek & Mayberry 2004). (ARDS is discussed in Chapter 36 .) Careful discharge planning should allow for maximal supervision in the first few weeks after discharge. To accomplish patient care goals, the nurse collaborates with the health care provider and respiratory therapist. A referral to a home health nurse may be necessary if the patient is alone or without a supportive environment.

■ Nursing Management

The nurse focuses on assessment for hypoxemia and worsening pain or atelectasis. Management of pain is essential for pulmonary toilet. If fluid restrictions are in place, the nurse monitors fluids closely and frequently assesses the patient's respiratory status.

Pneumothorax

Under normal circumstances the pleural cavity is free of air. When air or gas enters the pleural space, it is referred to as a **pneumothorax**, which results in a partial or complete collapse of the lung on the affected side. It is caused by a rupture in the visceral pleura or the parietal pleura and chest wall. As air separates the pleura, it destroys the negative pressure of the pleural space, disrupting the normal state of equilibrium. Because it is no longer held in check by the recoil forces of the chest wall, the lung recoils and collapses toward the hilus (McCance & Huether, 2007). This may occur spontaneously or without obvious cause or as a result of trauma. Figure 35–15 ■ shows a tension pneumothorax.

Spontaneous Pneumothorax: Epidemiology, Etiology, and Pathophysiology

This anomaly occurs unexpectedly in healthy individuals between the ages of 20 and 40; therefore, it is referred to as spontaneous pneumothorax. It occurs more commonly in men who tend to be taller and thinner than most individuals (Fishman et al., 2002). Smoking also is a risk factor, due to disease it causes in the small airways. The cause of the pneumothorax is a ruptured, air-filled bleb or blister on the lung surface. Bleb rupture allows

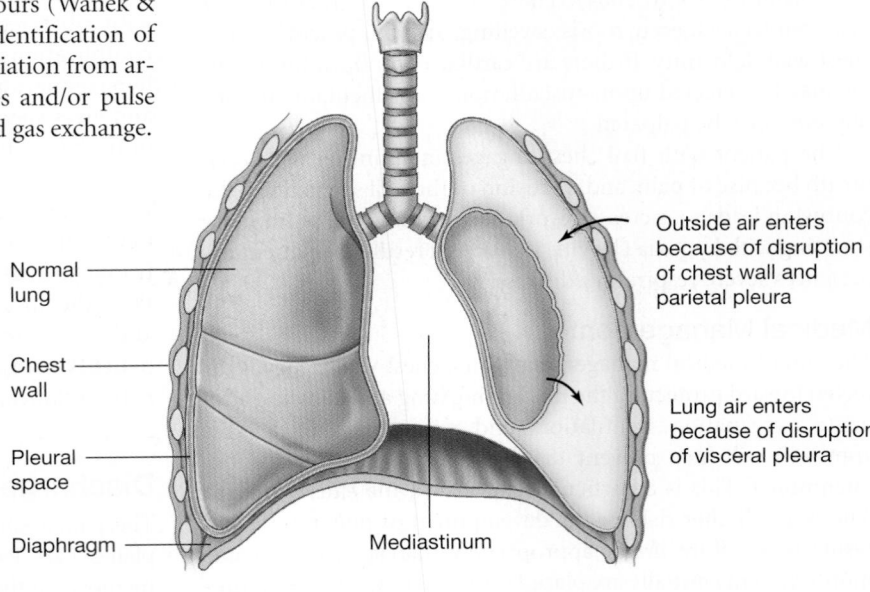

Normal lung

Chest wall

Pleural space

Diaphragm

Mediastinum

Outside air enters because of disruption of chest wall and parietal pleura

Lung air enters because of disruption of visceral pleura

FIGURE 35–15 ■ Tension pneumothorax.

atmospheric air to enter the pleural cavity, resulting in a loss of negative pressure and collapse of the lung (Porth, 2007). How the bleb ruptures is not fully understood but 80% of patients have emphysema-like changes in the lung whether they smoke or do not have blebs (McCance & Huether, 2007). Blebs on the visceral pleura rupture during sleep, rest, or exercise. These blebs usually are located on the apexes of the lung. Tension pneumothorax can develop with this rupture (McCance & Huether, 2007).

Traumatic Pneumothorax: Etiology

The most common causes of traumatic pneumothoraxes are penetrating chest injures such as bullets or stab wounds, and fractured ribs that penetrate the pleura. Hemothorax is frequently associated with these injuries. A traumatic pneumothorax may also occur with fracture of the trachea, bronchus, or esophagus (Porth, 2007).

Aside from trauma, tension pneumothorax can be caused by central venous catheterization and mechanical ventilation in which peak inspiratory pressure rises when the patient fights the ventilator. This more commonly occurs in patients with COPD receiving positive end-expiratory pressure (PEEP) during mechanical ventilation (Fishman et al., 2002).

Tension Pneumothorax: Epidemiology, Etiology, and Pathophysiology

A tension pneumothorax is one of the rapidly developing complications of blunt chest trauma and occurs as a result of an air leak in the lung or chest wall. It often is caused by blunt chest trauma in which the parenchymal injury has failed to seal and causes complete collapse of the lung. The air that enters the pleural space during expiration does not exit during inspiration due to the damaged tissue acting as a one-way valve. In addition to this mechanism, the positive pressure used with mechanical ventilation therapy can cause air trapping and increased intrapleural pressure. This increased pressure pushes the heart and mediastinal structures to the contralateral side. The mediastinum impinges on and compresses the contralateral lung. Hypoxia results as the collapsed lung on the affected side and the compressed lung on the contralateral side are compromised resulting in a diminished ability to effectively exchange gas. This hypoxia and decreased venous return caused by compression of the relatively thin walls of the atria impair cardiac function, thereby decreasing cardiac output and resulting in hypotension and, ultimately, hemodynamic collapse and death if untreated (Bowman, 2006).

Hemothorax: Epidemiology, Etiology, and Pathophysiology

Hemothorax is one of the most common problems encountered following blunt chest trauma. A simple hemothorax is defined as blood loss of less than 2,000 mL into the thoracic cavity. The absence of breath sounds over the lung and dullness to percussion are characteristic signs of a hemothorax (Fishman et al., 2002). Bleeding is caused by injuries to the lung parenchyma, such as pulmonary contusions and lacerations, which often are associated with rib and sternal fractures. Massive intrathoracic bleeding in blunt chest trauma usually stems from the heart, great vessels, or major systemic arteries. Chest surgery may cause what is classified as a traumatic pneumothorax as a result of air and fluid seeping into the pleural space. It also may emerge as a result of a malignancy that damages blood vessels. As air and blood separate the pleurae, it destroys the negative pressure of the pleural space disrupting the normal state of equilibrium. The lung recoils and collapses toward the hilus (McCance & Huether, 2007).

Pneumothorax and Hemothorax: Clinical Manifestations

Patients with pneumothorax or hemothorax present with pleuritic pain or breathlessness, or both, which can be life threatening. Respiratory distress, which can lead to respiratory arrest if untreated, is also present. The specific manifestations depend on the size of the pneumothorax. Patients may experience increasing levels of agitation especially if this is a sudden event. If cardiac output is affected blood pressure will drop and the patient will be tachycardic (Woodruff, 1999). Upon auscultation, breath sounds are unilaterally decreased or absent and the percussion note is hyperresonant or very loud. Hyperresonance and tracheal deviation are late findings (Woodruff, 1999). Hypotension is typically considered a key sign of a tension pneumothorax and typically occurs immediately before cardiovascular collapse (Bowman, 2006).

Laboratory and Diagnostic Procedures

Plain chest radiography is done and shows lung collapse and air in the pleural space (Ross, 2003). With hemothorax, chest radiography shows fluid accumulation in the pleural space or may show haziness if the quantity of blood in the chest is small. CT scanning is used after the individual is stabilized to determine the risk of recurrence. A CT scan is more sensitive than a chest radiograph in the evaluation of small pneumothoraxes. ABG analysis may be useful in evaluating for hypoxia, hypercarbia, and respiratory acidosis (Bowman, 2006).

Medical Management

The patient with a pneumothorax is experiencing dyspnea and anxiety. Pulse oximetry is used to document oxygen saturation. Based on this and the degree of dyspnea experienced by the patient, supplemental oxygen is given to treat hypoxemia. If a tension pneumothorax is present, the patient may experience severe air hunger and may require higher concentrations of supplemental oxygen. Lung reexpansion is accomplished by inserting a chest tube or chest drainage device. The patient may require mechanical ventilation.

Needle aspiration is a less invasive way of treating pneumothorax. A needle is inserted into the pleural space and air is withdrawn. This approach is not as successful as a chest tube, but it is less painful (Woodruff, 1999). Another approach to correcting a pneumothorax is to use a Heimlich valve, which is typically used as a stopgap measure until a tube can be placed. The valve attaches to a chest tube and is inserted into the chest. As the patient exhales, air and fluid drain through the valve into a plastic bag. When the patient inhales, the flexible tubing in the valve collapses, preventing secretions and air from reentering the pleura (Woodruff, 1999).

Nursing Management

The nurse must act promptly to assess pulmonary status quickly and to mobilize the health team to provide reexpansion of the lung via a chest tube. The nurse focuses on relieving dyspnea and supporting oxygenation. The patient may need supplemental oxygen and possibly mechanical ventilation.

Assessment, Interventions, and Rationales

Oxygen saturation and ABGs are monitored to assess the oxygen status. Equipment is prepared for insertion of a chest tube. The nurse explains the rationale for all treatments in advance and often assists with its preparation. Insertion of a chest tube is painful for the patient, so the nurse assists in providing a local anesthetic, IV pain medication, and a sedative (Woodruff, 1999).

The chest tube is attached to a water-controlled device, and usually suction is applied to 20 mmHg pressure. There should be gentle bubbling in the suction control chamber, the water column in the water seal should rise and fall unless air is escaping from the chest cavity, and there should be no kinks or dependent loops in the tubing (see Chapter 36). Bubbling in the water seal should occur during the initial reexpansion of the lung, but should then subside. In the case of a hemothorax, the nurse assesses vital signs regularly in order to establish blood loss and replenish blood and fluids. The nurse assesses for an excessive amount of bloody drainage in a short period and a repeat chest x-ray should be done in a few hours (Fishman et al., 2002).

Discharge Priorities

The patient should be given written instructions regarding the plan of care. Patients and caregivers should be encouraged to call members of the health team for persistent problems such as pain, dyspnea, congestion, or increasing sputum production. Patients may be reluctant to ask for more pain medication when it is needed, so the nurse needs to stress that healing will not occur unless the patient feels comfortable breathing and coughing. The patient should be made aware of symptoms that are emergency situations and receive resources for handling them.

Health Promotion

Once a patient has experienced a pneumothorax, he needs to understand that it could occur again. The nurse must stress that if the clinical manifestations reappear the patient must seek immediate medical help. The nurse reviews signs and symptoms of breathlessness and anxiety for which the patient and caregiver should seek emergency treatment. When a patient is admitted with a spontaneous pneumothorax, the individual should receive guidance from a pulmonary specialist regarding follow-up treatment and risk factors. The patient should be given information regarding the cause of the pneumothorax. If the health care provider believes pulmonary changes are related to genetic causes, the individual should be counseled regarding follow-up genetic testing and necessary lifestyle changes. The patient who smokes should be guided to quit smoking.

Nursing Management of a Patient with a Chest Tube

Many patients who are mechanically ventilated have chest tubes, and part of the nursing management is ensuring that the chest drainage system is intact and functioning properly. There are two types of chest tubes: pleural tubes and mediastinal tubes. A pleural tube is inserted in the pleural space in order to evacuate the air or blood and allow the lung to reexpand. The pleural tube re-creates the normal negative pressure in the chest that has been violated by trauma or surgery. Indications for insertion of a pleural tube include all the conditions listed in Chart 35–7.

A mediastinal tube is placed in the mediastinum after this area has been opened during cardiac or thoracic surgery. Mediastinal tubes prevent fluid and blood from collecting in the mediastinum and exerting pressure on the heart. These tubes do not look any different from pleural tubes. Usually they are inserted in the subxiphoid area, but only the surgeon or the operative report can alert the nurse to the difference in the two types of chest tubes.

Assessment

Pleural tubes are connected to underwater seal drainage or connected to a one-way valve. These devices, either the underwater seal or one-way valve, allow air to exit the chest but prevent air from entering the chest. Pleural tubes exhibit a characteristic called tidaling. With inspiration, the fluid in the tube can be seen moving with respiration. If there is no fluid in the tube, many chest drainage systems have a fluid diagnostic chamber. In this chamber the tidaling can be seen. It is important to assess this fluid movement either in the tube or in the diagnostic fluid chamber to ensure that the chest tube is in the thoracic cavity and there is no blockage.

Mediastinal tubes exhibit no tidaling because they are located in the mediastinal space and not the pleural space. Mediastinal tubes usually drain blood or other fluid. An important intervention with these tubes is to ensure that they are patent and draining freely. Most chest tube systems have available an autotransfusion unit attachment so that blood can be reinfused.

CHART 35–7 **Indications for Insertion of a Chest Tube**

INDICATIONS FOR A PLEURAL TUBE
- Hemothorax
- Pneumothorax
- Hemopneumothorax
- Pleural effusion
- Drainage of pus (empyema), bile (cholothorax), or chyle (chylothorax) from the pleural cavity
- Postoperative thoracostomy

INDICATIONS FOR A MEDIASTINAL TUBE
- Drainage of the mediastinal space after surgical procedure
- Cardiac surgery
- Pericardial window

Initially chest tubes are connected to suction to increase the drainage and to assist the lungs in reexpansion. The suction is most commonly set at 20 cm of water pressure. Though not recommended, disconnecting the chest tube from suction does not allow air to enter the chest but only stops the suction. As the drainage diminishes and the lung reexpands frequently, the heath care provider will discontinue the suction for a few hours prior to removal.

No chest tube should ever be clamped except under direct observation prior to removal. Clamping a chest tube can allow a tension pneumothorax to develop. The risk of a tension pneumothorax is increased when a patient is receiving positive pressure ventilation.

 Never clamp a chest tube except under direct observation prior to removing the tube.

Insertion of a Chest Tube

The equipment needed for insertion of a chest tube is listed in Chart 35–8. Pleural tubes commonly are inserted at the bedside, whereas mediastinal tubes are inserted in the operating room during surgery. The location on the chest of the tube is related to the reason for the chest tube insertion. If a chest tube is inserted to decompress a pneumothorax, it usually is inserted anteriorly, whereas a chest tube that is inserted to drain fluid or blood from the chest is inserted in a more posterior location on the chest wall. Air rises to the anterior surface of the chest when a patient is supine; therefore, placement of a chest tube is anterior if insertion is required because of a pneumothorax. However, if there is blood in the pleural space, a chest tube will be placed posteriorly because the blood will settle in the posterior of the chest cavity. Many different types of chest tube drainage systems are commercially available. Figure 35–16 ■ (p. 992) shows an example of one of those devices.

CHART 35–8	**Necessary Equipment for Insertion of a Chest Tube**

Chest tube insertion tray

Tube (size specified by health care provider)

Scalpel with size 11 blade

Several dissecting, such as curved Kelly clamps or artery forceps

A 10-mL syringe and a 20-ml syringe

One small-gauge needle (size 25)

A needle driver

Local anesthetic (Xylocaine)

Betadine (or other antiseptic)

Scissors

One packet of strong, non-absorbable, curved sutures of size 1.0 or larger, made from silk or nylon

Sterile gloves

4 × 4's

Suction setup

Suction tubing

Chest tube collection system

Vaseline gauze

Silk tape

Source: This article was published in *The AACN Procedure Manual,* 4th ed., p. 110, Lynn-McHale, D. & Carlson, K. Copyright W. B. Sanders, Philadelphia, 2001.

Near Drowning

Near drowning connotes an immersion episode of sufficient severity that it could lead to morbidity and death and, hence, warrants medical attention (Shepherd, 2003). To be categorized as a near drowning the patient must survive for at least 24 hours after submersion. Immersion in water causes laryngospasm and pulmonary injury resulting in hypoxemia and its effects on the brain and other organs.

Epidemiology and Etiology

Young adults typically drown in lakes, ponds, rivers, and oceans. Diving accidents are a common cause, and alcohol and recreational drugs have been implicated in many cases. Research shows that 30% to 50% of older adolescents and adults who drowned in boating accidents were inebriated (Shepherd, 2003). In the United States drowning deaths number more than 6,500 per year. The highest numbers are in toddlers and adolescent males. Drowning is second only to motor vehicle crashes as the most common cause of injury in children ages 1 month to 14 years. The true incidence of near drowning has yet to be reported, but it is estimated in the range of 20 to 500 times the rate of drowning (Shepherd, 2003).

Pathophysiology

After initial gasping, and possible aspiration, immersion stimulates hyperventilation, followed by involuntary apnea and laryngospasm leading to hypoxemia. The patient is likely to develop cardiac arrest and CNS ischemia. Asphyxia leads to relaxation of the airway, which permits the lungs to fill with water in many individuals (wet drowning). Approximately 10% to 20% of individuals maintain tight laryngospasm until cardiac arrest occurs. Inhalation of water causes pulmonary vasoconstriction, hypertension, destruction of surfactant, alveolar instability, and atelectasis (Shepherd, 2003).

Laboratory and Diagnostic Procedures

ABG analysis is the most reliable clinical parameter to assess level of hypoxia. In addition a complete blood count (CBC), electrolytes, and a coagulation profile are done. Lymphocytosis is commonly seen as well as elevated serum creatinine due to acute renal failure. A chest x-ray is done to determine evidence of aspiration, pulmonary edema, or atelectasis (Shepherd, 2003).

Medical and Nursing Management

Victims of submersion are classified into one of four groups:

1. Asymptomatic
2. Symptomatic
3. Cardiopulmonary arrest
4. Obviously dead.

Symptoms associated with near drowning are hypothermia, tachycardia, bradycardia, anxious appearance, tachypnea, dyspnea or hypoxia, metabolic acidosis, and altered level of consciousness.

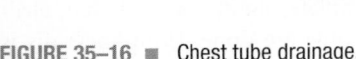

FIGURE 35–16 ■ Chest tube drainage.

In the emergency department phase of treatment, the patient in respiratory failure is intubated, mechanically ventilated, and rewarmed to 30°C (86°F). A nasogastric tube is inserted to decompress the stomach and prevent aspiration. The patient is treated for electrolyte imbalances, seizures, bronchospasm, atelectasis, dysrhythmias, and hypotension as necessary. Resuscitation efforts are not abandoned until the patient is rewarmed. Patients who are alert and oriented are observed in the emergency department until the ABGs become normal and there is an absence of dysrhythmias. If hypoxemia or other complications do not resolve, patients are admitted for observation and treatment (Shepherd, 2003). Possible complications are acute renal failure, ischemic cerebral injury, ARDS, pulmonary damage secondary to the drowning episode, and cardiac arrest.

Key health team members that the nurse collaborates with are the health care provider and respiratory therapist. If a social worker or liaison person is available to keep family members abreast of the patient situation, this is very helpful. The nurse obtains a history from the patient and family members to determine the cause of drowning and the type of water. The nurse assists the emergency department team in stabilizing the patient and communicates the patient status to family members. The major focus of nursing care is assessment and treatment of hypoxemia.

Carbon Monoxide Poisoning

Carbon monoxide poisoning occurs when an individual breathes carbon monoxide fumes that have built up in an enclosed space (CDC, 2004a). Carbon monoxide or CO is an odorless, colorless gas that can cause sudden illness or death. It is found in combustion fumes such as those produced by cars and trucks, small gasoline engines, stoves, lanterns, burning charcoal and wood, and gas ranges and heating systems. Persons who attempt suicide or are victims of smoke inhalation are poisoned with carbon monoxide (Fishman et al., 2002).

Epidemiology, Etiology, and Pathophysiology

Each year more than 500 Americans die from unintentional carbon monoxide poisoning and 2,000 commit suicide by intentionally poisoning themselves (CDC, 2004a). The ultimate injury that carbon monoxide produces is caused by hypoxia. Normally oxygen is carried to the tissues via the hemoglobin in red blood cells. Because carbon monoxide's affinity for hemoglobin is 300 times greater than that of oxygen, it quickly binds with hemoglobin, preventing oxygen molecules from doing so (McCance & Huether, 2007).

Laboratory and Diagnostic Procedures, Clinical Manifestations, and Medical and Nursing Management

Diagnostic tests are not as reliable as clinical assessment in the case of CO poisoning. Pulse oximetry is not valid because the hemoglobin is well saturated. ABG studies often are done to assess oxygen content as well as a chest x-ray to visualize the lung fields. Carboxyhemoglobin blood levels provide guidelines for treatment. Levels of greater than 40% are considered severe (Fishman et al., 2002). Symptoms related to CO poisoning include headache, giddiness, tinnitus, nausea, weakness, and vomiting. Persons at risk are smokers, coal miners, firefighters, unborn babies, and persons with chronic heart disease.

The nursing role is to participate with the emergency department team in stabilizing the patient and to communicate the patient status to family members. The major focus of nursing care is assessment and treatment of hypoxemia and management of mental status changes. The prognosis in carbon monoxide poisoning depends on the level of carbon monoxide inhaled. All persons who are victims of significant smoke inhalation should be resuscitated and transported on 100% oxygen. Hyperbaric oxygen therapy is the treatment of choice; this hastens clearance of carbon monoxide and decreases neurotoxicities, which include hallucinations, ataxia, visual disturbances, headaches, and psychoses (Fishman et al., 2002). The alternative treatment is treatment with 100% oxygen. This usually requires intubation and mechanical ventilation. Oxygen should be administered until the carbon monoxide level is less than 5%. In spite of this, mental status changes may persist and may be a sign of permanent brain damage.

Health Promotion

Educating the public regarding the dangers of smoking and the dangers of allowing exhaust fumes to be present in small enclosed places are preventive activities that increase awareness of the dangers of carbon monoxide. Advocating for the presence of smoke alarms and maintenance of fire safety regulations in all public and private buildings is another preventive strategy to promote community awareness of the problem. Nurses in home care and public health should make fire safety and the possibility of carbon monoxide escape a topic for environmental assessments. When unintentional carbon monoxide poisoning occurs, the health department should be contacted. Upon discharge, patients and families should be instructed to seek assistance if they experience dyspnea, confusion, altered levels of consciousness, hallucinations, weakness, or nausea.

■ Lung Cancer

Globally, lung cancer is the most common form of cancer; however, in the United States it is the second most common occurring malignancy (Parkin, Bray, & Ferlay, 2005). This disease accounts for the majority of cancer deaths among men since the 1950s and women since 1987 (ACS, 2006). In recent years the seriousness of lung cancer gained the public's attention as many Americans mourned the deaths of news anchorman Peter Jennings and Dana Reeve, wife of *Superman* star Christopher Reeve.

Epidemiology and Etiology

Efforts to combat the prevalence of lung cancer have been targeted at preventing exposure to known risk factors. Cellular genetic destruction results from repeated exposure to carcinogens such as tobacco smoke, radon, and asbestos. Smoking accounts for 87% of all lung cancer deaths (ACS, 2006); approximately 3,000 of these cases are due to environmental tobacco smoke (ETS) commonly referred to as "secondhand smoke." Exposure to radon, a colorless, odorless, radioactive gas, occurs in places where there is reduced air turnover and ventilation, as in underground mines.

Asbestos can still be found in products such as gaskets and roofing and friction items. Exposure occurs not only during the mining and manufacturing of these products but when we are at home, at the office, and in school (National Cancer Institute [NCI], 2005a). Other risk factors such as occupational hazards, air pollution, genetics, dietary factors, advancing age, and race are continuously being studied in an effort to determine more effective strategies to reduce mortality due to exposure. Chapter 64 ⊙ presents detailed information regarding cancer risk factors and recommended prevention programs.

Prevention of lung cancer has been primarily aimed at reducing the incidence of smoking. Persons who quit smoking reduce the risk of developing lung cancer over time. Those who refrain from smoking for approximately 10 years will reduce their risk of dying from this disease by 30% to 50% (NCI, 2005b). Multiple resources are now available for nurses and other clinicians as they develop programs designed to help patients and their families understand the importance of smoking cessation.

Pathophysiology

The World Health Organization has identified four major histologic types of lung cancer. These include small cell carcinoma, squamous cell carcinoma, adenocarcinoma, and large cell carcinoma. In the United States 85% of all lung cancers are non–small cell lung cancer (NSCLC) and 15% account for small cell lung cancer (SCLC) (National Comprehensive Cancer Network [NCCN], 2007). SCLC behaves differently from other cell types. Its unique ability to spread and be widely disseminated by the time of diagnosis leads to a poor prognosis, often survival ranging from only 2 to 4 months.

NSCLCs, including squamous cell carcinoma, adenocarcinoma, and large cell carcinoma, all have unique patterns of growth and clinical appearance. Squamous cell tumors typically originate in the proximal bronchi and account for 30% of all lung cancers (Hoffman & Gift, 2007). These malignancies have a tendency to be slow growing, such that a visible mass may not be detected for 3 to 4 years.

Adenocarcinoma is the most common form of lung cancer and the most common cell type in nonsmokers. Cancer cells can be found in the periphery of the lung and are known to present with fewer pulmonary symptoms than those that originate in the central portion of the lung parenchyma. Progression is slow; however, adenocarcinoma invades the lymphatic and blood vessels early in the disease, resulting in a worse prognosis compared to that for SCLCs. Large cell lung cancer commonly is located in the periphery of the lung, often times spreading to the subsegmental bronchi or larger airways. Because this cell type is poorly differentiated and possesses neuroendocrine features, the prognosis is often times very poor. Common metastatic sites for all types of lung cancer include liver, bone, adrenal glands, and the brain. For a more detailed discussion of the pathophysiology of cancer, refer to Chapter 64 .

Clinical Manifestations

Persons with lung cancer access the health care system when they have begun to experience multiple serious symptoms. This makes it very difficult for the patient to function physically, psychologically, and socially. A comprehensive history and physical includes obtaining an accurate history of risk factors. This information combined with the physical symptoms paints a more complete picture indicative of lung cancer. Respiratory symptoms include cough, dyspnea, sputum production, wheezing, hemoptysis, and chest pain. These symptoms need to be explored further so their origin can be identified. Additional manifestations include dysphagia, hoarseness, pain, fatigue, weakness, nausea, disturbed sleep, memory impairments, anorexia, and night sweats.

Lung cancers can produce complications that require the nurse to use sharp assessment skills and to have the ability to recognize manifestations that need immediate interventions. Examples of these complications include superior vena cava syndrome and paraneoplastic syndromes. Superior vena cava syndrome is an oncologic emergency that occurs when a tumor obstructs the superior vena cava, resulting in facial swelling, hands, arm, and neck swelling, distended neck veins, cyanosis of the upper torso, and dyspnea (Aurora, Milite, & Vander Els, 2000). Paraneoplastic syndromes (Cushing's syndrome, syndrome of inappropriate antidiuretic hormone [SIADH], and hypercalcemia) are considered metabolic emergencies that disrupt the homeostasis of vital body functions.

Laboratory and Diagnostic Procedures

Early diagnosis of lung cancer is difficult because most patients do not experience symptoms until the disease has begun metastasize. For those patients who have a localized malignancy without metastasis the likelihood of a 5-year survival rate is 50% (ACS, 2006). Initially, noninvasive tests are done to confirm the type of tumor, clinical stage, and additional information related to any preexisting conditions that may impact the recommended treatment plan (NCCN, 2007). Blood sampling for CBC, liver enzymes, and chemistries provides the clinician with information related to existing comorbidities, possible metasta-

tic disease, and complications commonly found with lung cancer (e.g., paraneoplastic syndromes).

An ECG and pulmonary function tests may be ordered to determine baseline pulmonary and cardiac function, especially if radiation therapy will be part of the treatment plan. Chest x-rays and chest CT scans are commonly used to assess the primary tumor, lymph node involvement, and the possible spread to other organs. Although MRI is infrequently done, it is helpful if there is suspected involvement of the CNS or spinal cord.

Invasive diagnostic tests are done to obtain tissue samples, which are used to diagnose the presence of lung cancer, determine the presence of cancer spread, and confirm whether lymph nodes are malignant or benign (Hoffman & Gift, 2007). Sputum cytology is useful to identify cancerous cells in those patients who experience hemoptysis. Direct tissue sampling is done via bronchoscopy. This test provides the clinician with information related to cell type and ultimately formalizing the diagnosis of lung cancer. Occasionally, transthoracic needle aspiration (TTNA) is necessary to confirm a diagnosis in those patients with peripheral lung masses that are not easily reached by the bronchoscope (Rivera, Detterbeck, & Mehta, 2003).

Medical Management

The medical management of lung cancer differs based on the cell type. Those patients with SCLC will likely receive chemotherapy, radiation therapy, or a combination of the two. Surgical intervention is saved for patients with a rare subset of SCLCs. Patients with NSCLC may receive surgery, chemotherapy, or radiation therapy. Depending on the staging of the disease, treatment options may be prescribed singly or in combination (Hoffman & Gift, 2007). For a better understanding of these three treatment options and the associated nursing responsibilities, refer to Chapter 64 .

▌ Nursing Management

Nursing management of patients with lung cancer is challenging and complex. The nurse must possess an appreciation of the care required for patients who have undergone surgical resection, those who receive chemotherapeutic agents, and those who receive radiation therapy.

Assessment

The surgical patient will need close postoperative observation for cardiac and pulmonary complications such as dyspnea, atelectasis, and atrial dysrhythmias due to surgical irritation of the vagus nerve (Quinn, 2003). Dyspnea is the most common postoperative symptom and can be attributed to decreased lung capacity and a thoracotomy incision. Effective pain management is crucial so the patient will be able to participate in progressive mobilization that, over time, will lead to decreased dyspnea.

Interventions and Rationales

Nurses who care for patients receiving chemotherapy and radiation therapy receive additional specialized training and certification. Regardless of the type of therapy prescribed, the patient may experience some common side effects (e.g., fatigue, nausea and vomiting, compromised immune function, pain, skin breakdown) that can severely impact their quality of life. Refer to Chapter 64 for a detailed discussion of the nursing care of the cancer patient.

Caring for patients with lung cancer often means caring for the older adult. Since the incidence of developing lung cancer increases with age, in the future, nursing will be faced with caring for more patients diagnosed with lung cancers. It is important for nurses to understand the effects of aging related to treatments and offer education and advocacy to patients and their families.

Lung Transplant

Lung transplantation has evolved as a viable alternative for patients with advanced pulmonary disease. Indications include AAT deficiency, bronchiectasis, cystic fibrosis, emphysema, idiopathic pulmonary fibrosis, interstitial lung disease, and pulmonary hypertension. The selection of patients is central to the success of the transplant and postoperative management. Persons more than 65 years of age are not recommended for a single lung transplant, and for bilateral lung transplants 60 is the recommended age based on international guidelines. These guidelines are more relaxed with pulmonary fibrosis because there is no pharmacologic treatment. The general guidelines for candidate selection for lung transplantation are shown in the International Guidelines box.

For patients with this terminal diagnosis, single lung transplants may be available to those over 65 years of age and double lung transplants for those over 60 years of age (Egan, 2004). Other circumstances that could jeopardize selection for this option are (1) colonization with antibiotic-resistant organisms, (2) noncompliance with medical regime, (3) inability to walk 600 feet (Egan, 2004), (4) diagnosis of a malignancy within 2 years, (5) renal or liver insufficiency, and (6) positive for HIV. Patients undergo an extensive evaluation for lung transplant and wait an average of 1 year for this procedure. The patient and family undergo psychological treatment to ensure that they can cope with a postoperative regimen that requires strict adherence to immunosuppressive therapy and continuous monitoring.

Infection postoperatively is the leading cause of morbidity and mortality. Viral infection with cytomegalovirus (CMV) and herpes simplex occurs frequently. The use of bronchodilator drugs and respiratory therapies to provide clearance of secretions is continued as a component of the patient routine. Acute rejection may occur as soon as 5 to 7 days after the transplant in spite of the patient's faithfulness to the regime. Symptoms of rejection include fever, chills, flu-like aches, shortness of breath, decreased urine output, and pain over the transplanted lung (ChestNet, 2004). Accurate diagnosis is by transtracheal biopsy and treatment is with corticosteroids. The body's response to organ transplant is discussed in detail in Chapter 60 and cardiac transplantation is discussed in Chapter 42.

Occupational Lung Disorders: Pneumoconiosis

Exposure to toxic dust and particulate matter may cause a variety of respiratory disorders. Depending on the degree of intensity of exposure, smoking history, and underlying pulmonary disease, individuals may experience irreversible effects of chronic pulmonary disease after long-term exposures. The dusts of silica, asbestos, and coal are the most common causes of pneumoconiosis. Others include talc, fiberglass, clays, mica, cement, cadmium, beryllium tungsten, cobalt, aluminum, and iron. The dust deposits are permanent. Treatment is palliative and focuses on preventing further exposure and improving workplace safety (McCance & Huether, 2007).

GUIDELINES for the Selection of Lung Transplant Candidates

Evaluation of patients for lung transplantation should include ensuring that patients have, or are receiving, optimal medical therapy for their disease, but are experiencing a decline in function. Candidates generally should have chronic disease for which no further medical or surgical therapy is available and survival is limited, or end-stage lung disease. Those who are acutely critically ill are seldom candidates for lung transplantation. Routine preventive medicinal measures, including mammograms, Pap smears, and colon cancer screening, should be completed where appropriate, and co-morbid medical conditions should be optimally treated as appropriate.

Older patients tend to have a significantly worse survival rate than younger patients.

There is no firm age restriction; people from birth to beyond 60 years have benefited from lung transplantation. The general age consideration is 70 years or younger. The International Guidelines for the selection of lung transplantation candidates suggest the following:

Age Limits
- Heart-lung transplants: ~55 years
- Single lung transplants: ~65 years
- Bilateral lung transplants: ~60 years.

Other general medical conditions may affect eligibility for lung transplantation. These include chronic ventricular dependence, current use of corticosteroids, significant chest wall deformity, cardiovascular abnormalities such as irreversible right ventricular dysfunctions, viral diseases, cancer, systemic hypertension, connective tissue disease, nutritional issues, substance abuse, psychological problems, and requirement for invasive ventilation.

Current contraindications for transplantation include the following:
- Dysfunction of major organs other than the lung
- Infection with HIV
- Hepatitis B antigen positivity
- Hepatitis C with biopsy-proven histologic evidence of liver disease.

Lung transplant is not contraindicated per se in patients with systemic disease (e.g., collagen vascular processes, diabetes mellitus). Each potential candidate is considered on an individual basis, with particular attention paid to the presence of any target organ damage outside the lung that might affect long-term outcome. This would constitute a relative or absolute contraindication.

Sources: American Thoracic Society. (1998). *International guidelines for the selection of lung transplant candidates.* Retrieved March 18, 2007, from http://patuents.uptodate.com/print.asp?print=&file=ats_guid/18053; Cedars-Sinai. (2000–2008). *Relative and absolute contraindications for lung transplantation.* Retrieved February 10, 2009, from http://www.csmc.edu/1247.html; Fallon Community Health Plan. (2003). *Lung transplant.* Retrieved February 10, 2009, from lungtransplant update.doc; Mayo Clinic. (2001–2009). *Lung transplant: criteria for lung transplant at Mayo Clinic.* Retrieved February 10, 2009, from http://www.mayoclinic.org/lung-transplant-criteria.html; Meyers, B.G., & Patterson, G.A. (1999). Lung transplantation-current issues and evolving concepts. *Seminar in Respiratory Critical Care Medicine.* 20(5), 429–436; Saint Barnabas Health Care System. (2009). Criteria for lung transplant. Retrieved February 10, 2009, from http://www.saintbarnabas.com/services/lungtransplant/criteria/index.html.

Occupational asthma can result from exposure to particulate matter in the workplace. Occupational asthma affects about 15% of the cases of adult asthma (American Lung Association [ALA], 2004). It is difficult to recognize because the patient continues to experience symptoms when away from the source of exposure. Symptoms experienced by the patient are dyspnea, wheezing, and chest tightness, which can occur within 12 hours of exposure or continue when the patient exercises, has a respiratory infection, and/or is undergoing emotional stress. Chemical irritants used in industry enzymes in food processing, detergents, pharmaceutical agents, and textile fibers may cause these symptoms. Exposure to workplace chemicals, gases, cereal grains, or irritants causes inflammation and edema of any portion of the respiratory tract, resulting in bronchospasm, hypersecretion of mucus from the bronchial mucosa, dyspnea, and wheezing. Nursing and medical management of occupational asthma is discussed under asthma.

Silicosis is a type of pneumoconiosis resulting from the inhalation of free silica and silica-containing compounds. It causes acute fibrosis of the lung tissue as well as fibrous nodules within the lung. Individuals are frequently asymptomatic. Between 1979 and 1995, 2,594 deaths were attributed to silicosis (McCance & Huether, 2007). Each year 200 people die of silicosis, a rate that has been stable since the 1990s. About 1.6 million workers are believed to have been exposed to silica dust and almost 60,000 are expected to suffer from some degree of silicosis. This occurs in coal mining and other industries involved in the extraction and processing of ore, preparation and use of sand, and manufacture of pipe building and roofing materials (McCance & Huether, 2007). Nursing management of silicosis is discussed under pulmonary fibrosis.

Coal miner pneumoconiosis (also called black lung or coal miner's lung) is caused by coal dust deposits in the lung. Its mild form is without symptoms except for chronic bronchitis. The disease affects about 4.5% of coal miners; about 2% have lung scarring causing restrictive disease. Between 1990 and 1999 there were more than 10,000 deaths and annual death counts increase by one-third. Its severe form consists of pulmonary fibrosis with dyspnea and wheezing often occurring. There is no specific treatment for the disease, and in complex cases patients may develop nodular lesions throughout the lungs. These enlarge and coalesce. Dense masses form in the upper portions of the lung, resulting in the loss of pulmonary volume. Patients experience a restrictive disease in which they cannot fully expand their lungs as well as an obstructive disease from secondary emphysema. Nursing management of restrictive lung disease is discussed in above sections of this chapter.

Asbestosis is a progressive lung disease caused by exposure to microscopic fibers of asbestos and resulting in a diffuse interstitial fibrosis with diaphragmatic calcification. Fibrous tissue eventually obliterates the alveoli. Between 1980 and 2002, 6,343 deaths were due to asbestosis (ALA, 2004). There is a considerable latency period between exposure and the development of symptomatology from about 10 to 20 years. Those at high risk for this disease are asbestos miners, millers, and those employed in building trades and shipyards, such as loggers, insulation workers, pipe fitters and steamfitters, sheet metal workers, and welders. Pulmonary function studies usually reveal a restrictive ventilatory defect and restricted lung volume as with silicosis. The patient experiences dyspnea and hypoxemia. The chances of arresting the disease are best in its early stages. Removal of the individual from the asbestos exposure is essential (Fishman et al., 2002).

Clinical Manifestations

Crackles of a dry quality can be auscultated in 70% to 90% of patients with diffuse interstitial fibrosis. Clubbing also is present frequently. Chronic cough and sputum production, similar to acute bronchitis, are often presenting signs. Shrinkage of the lung, which occurs with fibrotic changes, can cause a reduced vital capacity (Ross, 2003). Sputum is expectorated in large amounts and often contains varying amounts of black fluid, particularly with smokers. Eventually, respiratory failure and cor pulmonale result. There is no medical treatment for occupational lung diseases.

■ Nursing Management

The nurse provides supportive care and education to assist the patient and caregiver. Issues to be addressed are dyspnea, fatigue, and activity tolerance. Physical conditioning and breathing exercises are helpful. The oxygen prescription provides relief from dyspnea. Medications, including bronchodilators, glucocorticoids, and antibiotics, may be prescribed for the relief of bronchospasm and treatment of exacerbations. Fluids should be taken liberally to allow for liquefaction of sputum. The nurse addresses emotional issues such as depression, anxiety, and anger as the patient deteriorates in the end stage.

Discharge Priorities

Before the patient is discharged after an acute episode, she should have received education about all aspects of the treatment regime. Contact numbers for nursing and other care providers should be given to the patient and caregiver. The patient and caregiver should be able to verbalize issues that constitute an emergency. Oxygen, if ordered, should be available in the home setting. Plans for transfer to home should be made in consideration of oxygen needs and instructions should be given in writing.

Health Promotion

Workers who are exposed to these toxic agents must be fitted with appropriate safety equipment. In the industrial setting, the occupational health nurse advocates for the use of safety measures and reduced exposure to dust. The Occupational Safety and Health Administration (OSHA) issues regulations regarding dust control and ventilation that must be followed in the workplace. The nurse must be apprised of these regulations to advocate for workers. Environmental checks must be initiated as required by OSHA. Ongoing educational programs should be provided for workers so that they can be accountable for their own health. Refraining from smoking and receiving a yearly influenza vaccination contribute to pulmonary health.

Collaborative Management

Because there is no definitive treatment for the pulmonary fibrotic changes caused by occupational lung diseases, the health care team's focus is on the provision of supportive care and relief of dyspnea. The social worker often collaborates with the team to provide satisfactory care at home or in the community. Depending on the severity of disease, the patient may be discharged to a pulmonary rehabilitation program, home care, or hospice in the end stages of the disease. The health care provider collaborates with the nurse, physical therapist, and respiratory therapist on the plan of care after discharge. The physical therapist and a home care nurse may see the patient on an outpatient basis. Oxygen equipment along with patient and family education is provided by the medical equipment company.

Gerontological Considerations with Pulmonary Diseases

In the acute care setting, the nurse recognizes that elderly individuals may demonstrate confusion as well as agitation and breathlessness in the face of hypoxemia. This confusion is more likely to occur at night when the environment seems more unfamiliar. Elders also are at a higher risk for PE related to tendencies toward immobilization. They may be less tolerant of anticoagulants. Assessment for bleeding tendencies should be stressed and discharge planning should emphasize patient safety in this regard. Caution should be taken with positioning elders because of the possibility of osteoporosis and arthritis. Attention should be paid to alleviating pain during painful procedures such as the insertion of a chest tube. Attention also should be given to drug interactions and other systemic problems when pain medication is given to maintain the patient's comfort. Elderly individuals may require a lower dosage of medication. Upon ambulation with chest tubes or other equipment, an elderly person should be monitored closely because age and poor mobility constitute a risk for falls.

On discharge from the acute setting, elders benefit from an environmental assessment by a nurse. Hazards that could potentiate symptoms are wood-burning stoves, dust, or the presence of smoking or chemical fumes in the immediate environment. The nurse enlists the assistance of family or significant others to promote safety. Air conditioning in the summer and efficient heating in the winter will facilitate easy breathing for elders. Elderly patients with COPD and asthma should receive the influenza vaccine and the pneumococcal vaccine yearly. Refraining from smoking and staying indoors during extremes of temperatures is important. Written instructions are helpful for the elder person being discharged as is follow-up by a home health nurse to assist with the development of an individualized care plan and an emergency protocol.

Research

The treatment of lower airway disorders is aided by ongoing research on the topic, as outlined in the Research Opportunities and Clinical Impact box (p. 998). The research opportunities enumerated tend to focus on the use of complimentary and alternative medicine, stimulation of positive health behaviors in older adults, enhancement of nursing knowledge, and student nursing learning gaps in caring for asthmatic patients.

RESEARCH OPPORTUNITIES AND CLINICAL IMPACT RELATED TO LOWER AIRWAY DISORDERS

Research Area	Clinical Impact
What complementary therapies are used by asthma sufferers, and are they effective?	A study by Ernst (1999) referenced by Guthrie and Tingen (2002) stated that 60% of asthma sufferers use complementary therapies. Specific data on complementary therapies would add to the knowledge base about asthma treatment and could provide useful information for patient education. For example, "Which complementary modalities such as homeopathy, herbal remedies, and acupuncture, as examples, have been most useful?" Other research questions are: • Do persons who use complementary therapies have fewer exacerbations? • Is there a relationship between anxiety and use of complementary therapies?
Are students in university settings receiving adequate asthma care? (Knowledge base about asthma among college students and interventions for college students with asthma by the student health center)	McClennon, Holcroft, Faul, and Nicolosi (2002) stated that there is a research gap related to health behavior of college students with asthma and there is a need for better ways for a college health center to provide interventions and education for students. Questions that could be studied further are: • How do students' treatment regimes relate to the current asthma guidelines? • What is the relationship of stress and anxiety in the college environment to students' asthma exacerbations? • What is the relationship between the student with asthma and the college health center? Data obtained regarding these topics would add to the clinical nursing research on asthma in young adults and provide useful strategies for asthma management in college and university health centers.
Assessment of dyspnea (Dyspnea scales are currently being developed and tested.)	Kendrick and colleagues (2000) proposed use of a tool to measure dyspnea in patients by use of the Borg scale. Questions that could be studied further include: • How do nurses measure dyspnea in clinical settings? • What objective and subjective data are used by nurses to assess and evaluate severity of dyspnea? • How is the patient involved in assessing his own level of dyspnea? Obtaining survey and interview data regarding general nursing knowledge could be instrumental in framing clinical nursing education curricula and continuing education programs regarding standards of care for patients experiencing dyspnea. It could also provide guidelines for the formulation of dyspnea assessment tools that are practical for the clinical setting. Care algorithms may be developed based on dyspnea scores.
The effect of cues to promote positive health behaviors in older adults regarding obtaining flu shots.	McCall, Johnson, and Rothman (2002) tested the effectiveness of a variety of "cues to actions" or messages for elders regarding importance and availability of flu shots in North Dakota counties. This is an area for future research. Knowledge about effective cues that promote positive health behaviors among elders provides useful information for community health centers. Replication of the McCall et al. (2002) study would be useful since elders in rural settings such as North Dakota might respond to different "cues to action" than elders in other localities. Research regarding "cues to action" that are effective for diverse and poverty-laden populations of risk would be extremely useful as well. Aside from obtaining flu shots, "cues to action" for other positive health behaviors could also be established such as safe sex, weight loss, exercise, and quitting smoking.
Nursing knowledge base about chest drains.	According to Carroll (2000) chest drainage options are expanding and nurses need to know what is out there and when to use each type. Data could be collected regarding nursing knowledge about chest drains among cardiovascular nurses or emergency department nurses. These data could then be used as a basis for continuing education programs and training materials for nurses.
What is the effectiveness of various methods of smoking cessation?	Promotion of the most effective means of smoking cessation should aid patients in successful smoking cessation.
What is the effect of education on smoke avoidance in grade school on the rate of smoking in adolescence?	Early avoidance of primary and secondhand smoke should decrease the development of emphysema and COPD.

Clinical Preparation

 Read

- History of Current Illness
- Past Medical History
- Physical Exam
- Admitting Medical Orders
- Laboratory Study Results

 Document

- Summary of Hospitalization
- Pathophysiology Form
- Laboratory Values
- Laboratory Results Explanation

 Apply

- List of Potential Nursing Diagnoses
- Concept Map
- Critical Thinking Questions

*Log on to MyNursingKit.com to download forms you will need and to complete further steps in the Clinical Preparation assignment.

HISTORY OF PRESENT ILLNESS

Mr. H is a 70-year-old man admitted to the emergency department with complaints of intermittent chest tightness and dyspnea, which he states have gotten progressively worse in the past week. He states he is coughing up large amounts of thick, yellowish sputum and experiences muscle fatigue and dyspnea after bouts of coughing. Mr. H also indicates that he feels winded after a short walk to the bathroom of his apartment.

The patient is started on intravenous (IV) fluids equaling 3 liters per day. He is started on IV Solu-Medrol 200 mg every 6 hours, and he is continued on his captopril orally. The nurse maintains a record of intake and output. A respiratory physical therapist assists him with postural drainage and breathing and coughing exercises. He is maintained on 2 liters of nasal oxygen. He is also started on albuterol nebulization treatments four times a day. The physical therapist and nursing staff ambulate him in the hallway four times a day with oxygen. Because his glucose is controlled, his glipizide is discontinued and he is placed on glucometer checks four times a day. He is placed on an 1,800-calorie diabetic diet, which he tolerates well.

Medical–Surgical History

Mr. H has a history of chronic bronchitis, hypertension, and colon cancer. He has had two to three hospital admissions per year for exacerbations of chronic bronchitis. Past surgical procedures include a hernia repair at age 50 and a colon resection for colon cancer at age 65. He underwent chemotherapy at that time and is currently in remission. He sees an oncologist every 6 months for follow-up. He is also a non–insulin-dependent diabetic. Current medications include glipizide, captopril, and Atrovent three times a day.

Social History

Mr. H is married and lives with his wife. They have two children who live nearby in the same community. He has a history of smoking, but has quit within the last 5 years.

Physical Examination

Auscultation of lung sounds reveals crackles and a few expiratory wheezes throughout all lung fields. His breath sounds are decreased in the bases. He uses his accessory sternocleidomastoid muscles for breathing. While at rest, his respiratory rate is 30. His vital signs are as follows: blood pressure 160/100, pulse 100 beats per minute, and temp 100.6°F orally. Auscultation of the heart reveals he is tachycardic with an S_3. He seems most comfortable sitting forward in a chair and appears to have a barrel chest.

Admitting Medical Orders

Service: Medical floor
Diagnosis: dyspnea and shortness of breath
Allergies: none noted
Vital signs and O_2 sats q2h
Ambulate in hall with assistance and with oxygen four times daily
Diet: 1,800-calorie diabetic diet
Call house officer: HR < 60 or > 120, systolic blood pressure <100 or > 140, RR < 12 or > 30, temperature > 38°C, O_2 saturation < 92%, glucose < 70 or > 150 mg/dL
IV fluids: 0.45 normal saline at 125 mL/hr
I&O q shift
Respiratory care: maintain on 2 liters of nasal oxygen; postural drainage and breathing and coughing exercises by physical therapist q4h

Scheduled Medications

Albuterol nebulization treatments four times a day
IV Solu-Medrol 200 mg q6h
Captopril 50 mg PO twice daily, 1 hour before meals

PRN Medications

None noted

Ordered Laboratory Studies

Sputum culture × 1
ABGs, CBC, and Chem 7 panel daily
Accu-Chek q ac and hs

Ordered Diagnostic Studies

Anterior/posterior and lateral chest x-ray

Nursing Care Day 2

On day 2 Mr. H is started on a broad-spectrum antibiotic given intravenously in addition to the other therapies. His sliding scale insulin is discontinued and he is placed on oral glipizide. His dyspnea has eased and he is expectorating sputum more easily. Mr. H is tolerating ambulation and an increase in activity. His IV is changed to a saline lock through which he receives his antibiotic. His wife visits at his bedside regularly and is encouraged to assist with coughing and deep breathing exercises as well as a fluid intake of 8 glasses of water per day. Mr. H's vital signs are as follows: BP 130/70, HR 92, respiratory rate 24, and temperature 99.5°F.

LABORATORY STUDY RESULTS

Test	Day 1	Day 2	Day 3
O_2 saturation on room air	88%		
O_2 saturation on 2 L nasal O_2	92%	94%	94%
ABGs			
pH	7.40	7.40	7.40
PO_2	85 mmHg	90 mmHg	92 mmHg
PCO_2	50 mmHg	49 mmHg	49 mmHg
HCO_3	36 mEq/L	35 mEq/L	35 mEq/L
Hct	54%	50%	49%
Hgb	17 g/100 mL	16 g/100 mL	15 g/100 mL
Platelets	200,000 μL	210,000 μL	225,000 μL
RBCs	$4.6 \times 10^6/\mu L$	$5.0 \times 10^6/\mu L$	$5.2 \times 10^6/\mu L$
Sodium	148 mEq/L	128 mEq/L	139 mEq/L
Potassium	4.0 mEq/L	4.2 mEq/L	4.5 mEq/L
Chloride	105 mEq/L	100 mEq/L	100 mEq/L
HCO_3^-	35 mEq/L	35 mEq/L	32 mEq/L
Glucose	150 mg/dL	145 mg/dL	148 mg/dL
Sputum culture		*Staphylococcus aureus*	

CRITICAL THINKING QUESTIONS

1. As the nurse on the unit where Mr. H is admitted, what further assessment data do you plan to collect?

2. Your initial impression is that Mr. H has a barrel chest. How do you verify this with objective data? What is the etiology of a barrel chest in the patient with COPD?

3. Mr. H is placed on IV Solu-Medrol 200 mg every 6 hours. How will this drug alleviate Mr. H's symptoms? What are some potential side effects?

4. After 3 days Mr. H is to be discharged on 2 L nasal oxygen, which is to be administered continuously. His medications include glipizide, captopril, oral prednisone, an oral antibiotic to be taken for 3 more days, albuterol, and steroid inhalers to be taken three times a day. What patient education do you provide and what assessment do you want to make prior to discharge? Describe patient education strategies and use of visual aids.

5. What are some nutritional considerations for Mr. H?

6. What benefits will continuous oxygen therapy afford Mr. H in terms of quality of life?

Answers to Critical Thinking Questions appear in Appendix D.

NCLEX® REVIEW

1. A patient is seen in the emergency department with acute shortness of breath and chest tightness which started after exposure to a carpet cleaning agent in her home. The nurse realizes this patient is most likely experiencing:
   1. The flu.
   2. An acute asthma attack.
   3. COPD.
   4. Cystic fibrosis.

2. A patient with community acquired pneumonia is being discharged. Which of the following should the nurse include in this patient's discharge plan of care?
   1. Take the prescribed antibiotics until the coughing stops.
   2. Limit fluid intake to reduce secretions.
   3. Avoid smoking or environments with smoke.
   4. Resume normal activity level.

3. The nurse is providing care to a patient with chronic obstructive pulmonary disease. Which of the following should the nurse be prepared to administer to the patient?

   1. Pancreatic enzymes

   2. Ibuprofen

   3. Magnesium sulfate

   4. Pulmozyme

4. A patient is admitted with rib fractures after falling from a ladder while on the job. Which of the following is a priority for the care of this patient?

   1. Pain management

   2. Safety precautions

   3. Employment counseling

   4. Rehabilitation therapy

5. A patient with lung cancer is complaining of increasing arm pain. The nurse realizes the patient could be experiencing:

   1. Superior vena cava syndrome.

   2. Hypoxia.

   3. Hypercalcemia.

   4. Pain associated with the primary diagnosis.

6. A patient is admitted with asbestosis. Which of the following should be included in the assessment of this patient?

   1. Location of home and surrounding industrial community

   2. Current place of employment

   3. Place of employment 10 to 20 years prior to current admission

   4. Employment with roofing materials

Answers for review questions appear in Appendix D

KEY TERMS

acute bronchitis *p.935*
asbestosis *p.996*
asthma *p.960*
atelectasis *p.973*
carbon monoxide poisoning *p.992*
chronic bronchitis *p.955*
chronic obstructive pulmonary disease (COPD) *p.955*
coal miner pneumoconiosis *p.996*

cor pulmonale *p.980*
cystic fibrosis (CF) *p.968*
emphysema *p.955*
flail chest *p.986*
hemoptysis *p.969*
hemothorax *p.989*
influenza *p.936*
lung abscess *p.947*
metered-dose inhaler (MDI) *p.939*

near drowning *p.991*
occupational asthma *p.996*
pleural effusion *p.984*
pneumonia *p.937*
pneumothorax *p.988*
polycythemia vera *p.958*
pulmonary contusion *p.988*
pulmonary embolism (PE) *p.973*
silicosis *p.996*

EXPLORE mynursingkit

PEARSON

MyNursingKit is your one stop for online chapter review materials and resources. Prepare for success with additional NCLEX®-style practice questions, interactive assignments and activities, web links, animations and videos, and more!

Register your access code from the front of your book at
www.mynursingkit.com

REFERENCES

Abrahamian, F. M. (2008). *Pleural effusion.* Retrieved April 22, 2008, from http://www.emedicine.com/emerg/topic462.htm

American Cancer Society. (2006). *Cigarette smoking.* Retrieved from http://www.cancer.org

American Lung Association. (2004). *Fact sheet: Occupational lung disease.* Retrieved February 9, 2008, from http://www.lungusa.org/diseases/occupational_factsheet.html

American Lung Association. (2007). *Sarcoidosis.* Retrieved May 10, 2008, from http://www.lungusa.org/site/c.dvLUK9OOE/b.4061173/apps/s/content.asp?ct=5176723

American Thoracic Society. (2001). *Guidelines for the management of adults with community-acquired pneumonia.* Retrieved February 24, 2007, from http://ajrccm.atsjournals.org/cgi/content/full/163/7/1730

American Thoracic Society, Centers for Disease Control, and Infectious Diseases Society of America. (2003). Treatment of tuberculosis. *Morbidity and Mortality Weekly Report, 52*(RR-11), 1–77.

Amersham Health. (2004). *Pulmonary fungal infection.* Retrieved February 9, 2008, from http://www.amershamhealth.com/medcyclopeaedia/.../FUNGAL%20INFECTION%20PULMONARY.as

Antoniou, K. M., Hansell, D. M., Rubens, M. G., Marten, K., Desal, S. R., Siafakas, N. M., et al. (2008). Idiopathic pulmonary fibrosis:

Outcome in relation to smoking status. *American Journal of Respiratory Critical Care Medicine, 177*(2), 190–194.

Aurora, R., Milite, F., & Vender Els, N. J. (2000). Respiratory emergencies. Seminars in Oncology, 27(3).

Ball, K. (2003). Deep vein thrombosis and airline travel: The deadly duo. *AORN Journal, 77*(2), 346, 348–349, 351–352, 354, 357–358.

Barnes, P. J. (2000). Chronic obstructive pulmonary disease. *New England Journal of Medicine, 343,* 269–280.

Barreiro, T. J., DeMarco, R., Gemmel, D. J., & Schaub, C. R. (2005, October). Sarcoidosis: An enigmatic disease calls for a measured workup. *Patient Care for the Nurse Practitioner,* pp. 1–10.

Bjerke, S. (2002). *Flail chest.* Retrieved August 22, 2004, from http://www.emedicine.com/emerg/topic2813.htm

Bowman, J. G. (2006). *Pneumothorax, tension and traumatic.* Retrieved April 23, 2008, from http://www.emedicine.com/emerg/TOPIC470.HTM

Britto, M. T., DeVellis, R. F., Hornung, R. W., DeFriese, G. H., Atherton, H. D., & Slap, G. B. (2004). Health care preferences and priorities of adolescents with chronic illnesses. *Pediatrics, 114*(5), 1272–1280.

Carroll, P. (2000). Exploring chest drain options. *RN 63*(10), 50–54, 56.

Centers for Disease Control and Prevention. (2004a). *Carbon monoxide poisoning fact sheet.* Retrieved August 22, 2004, from http://www.cdc.gov/nceh/airpollution/carbonmonoxide/cofaq.htm

Centers for Disease Control and Prevention. (2004b). *Influenza: The disease.* Retrieved from http://www.cdc.gov/flu/about/disease.htm

Centers for Disease Control. (2006). Trends in tuberculosis—United States, 2005. *Morbidly and Mortality Weekly Report, 55*(11), 305.

Cerro Coso Coyote Athletics. (2004). *Chest injuries.* Retrieved May 12, 2008, from http://athletics.cerrocoso.edu/sportsmedicine/chest_injuries.htm

ChestNet. (2004). *A guide to lung transplantation.* Retrieved August 22, 2004, from http://www.chestnet.org/education/patient/guides/transplantation/p6.php

Chojinowski, D. (2003). "Gold" standards for acute exacerbation in COPD. *Nurse Practitioner, 28*(5), 26–39.

Choudhry, S., Seibold, M. A., Borrell, L. N., et al. (2007). Dissecting complex diseases in complex populations: Asthma in Latino Americans. *Proceedings of the American Thoracic Society, 4*(3), 326–333.

Coding Edge Archives. (2000). *Congestive heart failure and related cardiopulmonary conditions.* Retrieved June 5, 2005, from http://www.lagunamedsys.com/EdgeArchive/feature121500.htm

Crawford, S. (2004). *Current anti-fungal treatment in the ICU*. Retrieved February 9, 2008, from http://www.hospital_consult_pda.com?PDAcca44.htm

Dalen, J. (2002). Pulmonary embolism: What have we learned since Virchow? Treatment and prevention. *Chest, 122*(5), 1801–1818.

Dauber, J. H. (2006). *Risk factors for idiopathic pulmonary fibrosis.* Retrieved May 17, 2008, from University of Pittsburgh website: http://www.simmonsfund.pitt.edu/rishfactors.html

Devitt, H. (1995). *Blunt thoracic trauma: Assessment, management and anesthesia*. Retrieved August 22, 2004, from http://www.anesthesia.org/winterlude/w195_4.html

Diaz, J. I., & Quellette, R. R. (2008). *Pulmonary fibrosis, idiopathic*. Retrieved April 20, 2008, from http://www.emedicine.com/med/TOPOC1960.HTM

Dieudonne, A. (2008). *Atypical mycobacterial infection*. Retrieved February 12, 2008, from http://www.medicine.com/ped/TOPIC3034.HTM

Egan, J. (2004). The clinical practice of lung transplantation in America. *Chest, 125*(4), 1183–1184.

Ernst, E. (1999). Complementary/alternative medicine for asthma: We do not know what we need to. *Chest (American College of Chest Physicians), 115*, 1–3.

Esmond, G. (2000). *Respiratory nursing*. London: Harcourt Health.

Feied, C., & Handler, J. (2002). Pulmonary embolism. Retrieved February 28, 2008, from http://www.emedicine.com/EMERG/topic490.htm

Fishman, A. P., Elias, J. A., Fishman, J. A., Grippi, M. A., Kaiser, L. R., & Senior, R. M. (2002). *Fishman's manual of pulmonary diseases and disorders*. New York: McGraw-Hill.

Global Initiative for Asthma. (2007). *Global strategy for asthma management and prevention*. Retrieved July 29, 2008, from http://www.ginasthma.org

Gould, K. P. (2006). Sarcoidosis. *eMedicine*. Retrieved May 20, 2008, from http://www.emedicine.com/DERM/topic281.htm

Guthrie, C., & Tingen, M. S. (2002). Asthma: A case study. Review of pathophysiology and management strategies. *Journal of the American Academy of Nurse Practitioners, 14*(10), 457–462.

Haque, A. K. (1992). Pathology of common pulmonary fungal infections. *Journal of Thoracic Imaging, 4*, 1–11.

Hegewald, M. J., Markewitz, B., & Elliott, C. G. (2007). Pulmonary hypertension: Clinical manifestations, classification and diagnosis. *International Journal of Clinical Practice, 61*(Suppl. 156), 5–14.

Hoffman, A., & Gift, A. (2007). Lung cancer. In M. Langerhorne, J. Fulton, & S. Otto (Eds.), *Oncology nursing* (5th ed.). St. Louis: Mosby.

Humbert, M. and Trembath, R. C. (2002). Genetics of pulmonary hypertension: from bench to bedside. *European Respiratory Journal, 20*, 741–749.

Hunter, M., & King, D. (2001). COPD: Management of acute exacerbations and chronic stable disease. *American Family Physician, 64*, 603–612, 621–622. Retrieved February 24, 2007, from http://www.aafp.org/afp/20010815/603.html

Jassal, D., & Sharma, S. (2004). *Pulmonary hypertension*. Retrieved May 31, 2008, from http://www.emedicine.com/Radio/topic583.htm

Kaplan, V., Clermont, G., Griffin, M. F., Kasal, J., et al. (2003). Pneumonia: Still the old man's friend? *Archives of Internal Medicine, 163*(3), 317–324.

Kavita, G. (2005). Acute pulmonary embolism (helical CT). Retrieved April 21, 2008, from http://www.emedicine.com/RADIO/topic582.htm

Kendrick, K., Baxi, S., & Smith, R. (2000). Usefulness of the Borg scale in assessing the degree of dyspnea in patients with COPD and asthma. *Journal of Emergency Nursing, 26*(3), 216–222.

Kennedy, M., Zolot, J., & Sofer, D. (2001). Preventing thromboembolism after injury. *AJN, 101*(2), 18–19.

Kleinschmidt, P. (2004, June). *Chronic obstructive pulmonary disease and emphysema*. Retrieved August 1, 2004, from http://www.emedicine.com/emerg/topic99.htm

Knutson, D., & Braun, C. (2002). Diagnosis and management of acute bronchitis. *American Family Physician, 65*(10), 2039–2045.

Kvale, P. A., Simoff, M., & Prakash, U. B. (2003). Palliative care. *Chest, 123*(1), 284S–311S.

Mandanas, R. A. (2007). *Pneumonia, fungal*. Retrieved April 17, 2008, from http://www.emedicine.com/med/topic1853.htm

Martinez, F. D. (2007). Genes, environments, development and asthma: A reappraisal. *European Respiratory Journal, 29*(1), 179–184.

Mayo Clinic. (2008). *Sarcoidosis*. Retrieved May 10, 2008, from http://www.mayoclinic.com/health/sarcoidosis/DS00251

McCall, K., Johnson, R., & Rothman, A. (2002). The effects of framing and action instructions on whether older adults obtain flu shots. *Health Psychology, 21*(6), 624–628.

McCance, K., & Heuther, S. (2007). *Pathophysiology: The biological basis for disease in adults and children* (5th ed.). St. Louis: Mosby.

McClennon, S. R., Holcroft, C., Faul, N. Q., & Nicolosi, R. (2002). A look at asthma care in a university setting. *Nurse Practitioner, 27*(12), 35–42.

Medical College of Wisconsin Healthlink. (2008). *Atypical mycobacteria*. Retrieved February 12, 2008, from http://healthlink.mcw.edu/article/954973743

Merck. (2005a). *Cor pulmonale*. Retrieved April 24, 2008, from http://www.merck.com/mmpe/sec07/ch074/ch074c.html

Merck. (2005b). *Pulmonary hypertension*. Retrieved April 24, 2008, from http://www.merck.com/mmpe/sec05/ch058/ch058a.html

Merck. (2008). *Idiopathic pulmonary fibrosis*. Retrieved February 9, 2008, from http://www.merck.com/mmhe/sec04/ch050b.html

Morbidity and Mortality Weekly Report (MMWR): Recommendations and Reports, CDC. (2004). Prevention and control of influenza: recommendations of the advisory committee on immunization priorities (ACIP). Retrieved August 3, 2008 from http://www.cdc.gov/mmwr/preview/mmwrhtml/rr5306al.htm

Morris, B., Morrison, R. B., & Yetsko, C. (2002). Venous thromboembolism. *RN Magazine, 65*(10), 1–8.

Morris, M. J. (2007). Asthma. *eMedicine*. Retrieved July 29, 2008, from http://www.emedicine.com/med/topic177.htm

Morrison, C., & Lew, E. (2001). Aspergillosis. *AJN, 101*(8), 40–48.

Morton, P. G., Fontaine, D. K., Hudak, C. M., & Gallo, B. M. (2005). *Critical care nursing*. Philadelphia: Lippincott William & Wilkins.

Murray, L. N., & Brown, K. R. (2007). *Cystic fibrosis*. Retrieved May 6, 2008, from http://www.emedicine.com/ent/topic515.htm

National Cancer Institute. (2005a). *Asbestos exposure: Questions and answers*. Retrieved from http://cis.nci.nih.gov

National Cancer Institute. (2005b). *Small cell lung cancer*. Retrieved from http://cis.nci.nih.gov

National Center for Health Statistics. (2006). *Summary health statistics for U.S. adults: National health interview survey, 2006, Tables 3 and 4*. Retrieved May 16, 2008 from http://www.cdc.gov/nchs/fastats/copd.htm

National Comprehensive Cancer Network. (2007). *National comprehensive cancer network practice guidelines: Small cell lung cancer*. http://www.nccn.org

National Heart, Lung, and Blood Institute. (1997/2002). *Expert panel report 2: Guidelines for the diagnosis and management of asthma and Update on selected topics 2002*. Bethesda, MD: Author. Retrieved July 29, 2008, from http://www.nhlbi.nih.gov/guidelines/archives/epr-2/index.htm

National Heart Lung and Blood Institute (NHLBI). (2006). *What is pulmonary arterial hypertension?* Retrieved April 24, 2008, from http://www.nhlbi.nih.gov/health/dci/Diseases/pah/pah_what.html

National Heart Lung and Blood Institute. (2007). *Expert panel report 3: Guidelines for the diagnosis and management of asthma* (NIH Publication No. 09-5846). Retrieved from http://www.nhlbi.nih.gov/guidelines/asthma

National Institutes of Health. (2001). *Global initiative for chronic obstructive lung disease: Global strategy for the diagnosis, management and prevention of chronic obstructive lung disease* (NIH Publication No. 2701B). Bethesda, MD: Author.

Nevidjion, B., & Sowers, K. (2000). *A nurse's guide to cancer care*. Philadelphia: Lippincott Williams & Wilkins.

Niederman, M. S., Mandell, L. A., Anzueto, A., Bass, J. B., Broughton, W. A., Campbell, G. D., et al. (2001). Guidelines for management of adults with community-acquired pneumonia: Diagnosis, assessment of severity, antimicrobial therapy and prevention. *American Journal of Respiratory Critical Care Medicine, 163*(7), 1730–1754.

Owens, M., Chaudry, M. S., Eggerstedt, J. M., & Smith, L. M. (2000). In R. George, M. Light, M. Mathay, & R. Mathay (Eds.), *Chest medicine: Essentials of pulmonary and critical care medicine*. Philadelphia: Lippincott Williams & Wilkins.

Parkin, D., Bray, F., & Ferlay, J. (2005). Global cancer statistics 2002. *CA: A Cancer Journal for Physicians, 55*.

Patel, R. J. (2008). *Idiopathic pulmonary fibrosis*. Retrieved from http://www.emedicine.com/med/topic1960.html

Patient UK. (2007). *Lung abscess*. Retrieved April 21, 2008 from http://www.patient.co.uk/showdoc/40000608/

Peek, G., Morocos, G., & Cooper, T. (2000). The pleural cavity. *British Medical Journal, 320*, 1318–1330.

Porth, C. M. (2007). *Essentials of concepts of altered health states* (2nd ed.). Philadelphia: Lippincott Williams & Wilkins.

Pulmonology Channel. (2002). *Bronchitis: Overview, causes and risk factors*. Retrieved April 19, 2008, from http://www.pulmonologychannel.com/bronchitis/index.shtml

Quinn, K. (2003). Managing patients through thoracic surgery. In M. Hass (Ed.), *Contemporary issues in lung cancer: A nursing perspective* (1st ed.). Boston: Jones & Bartlett.

Raviglione, M., & Smith, I. (2007). XDR tuberculosis—Implications for global public health. *New England Journal of Medicine, 356*(7), 24–36.

Reeder, J., & Danis, D. (2001). Penetrating chest trauma: With careful assessment, rapid diagnosis, and relatively simple interventions, most patients with penetrating chest trauma will recover. *AJN, 101*(Suppl.), 15–18.

Rivera, M., Detterbeck, F., & Mehta, A. (2003). Diagnosis of lung cancer: The guidelines. *Chest, 123*(1 Suppl.).

Ross, R. (2003). The clinical diagnosis of asbestosis in this century requires more than a chest radiograph. *Chest, 124*(3), 1120–1129.

Rowe, S. M., Miller, S., & Sorscher, E. J. (2005). Cystic fibrosis. *New England Journal of Medicine, 352*, 1992–2001.

Sawyer, M. (2006). *Blunt chest trauma*. Retrieved May 12, 2008, from http://www.emedicine.com/med/TOPICS3658.HTM

Schoenstadt, A. (2006). *Tuberculosis statistics in the United States*. Retrieved May 13, 2008, from http://tuberculosis.emedtv.com/tuberculoosis-statistics-in-the-united-states.html

Schultz, P. (2003, September–October). Community-acquired pneumonia: Hunting the elusive respiratory infection. *Nursing 2003*, pp. 29–34.

Shahani, R. (2006). *Penetrating chest trauma*. Retrieved May 12, 2008, from http://www.emedicine.com/MED/topic2916.htm

Sharma, S. (2004). *Lung abscess*. Retrieved October 28, 2004, from http://www.emedicine.com/med/topic1332htm

Sharma, S. (2006a). Chronic obstructive pulmonary disease. *eMedicine*. Retrieved May 21, 2008, from http://www.emedicine.com/med/TOPIC373.HTM

Sharma, S. (2006b). Cystic fibrosis. *eMedicine*. Retrieved May 12, 2008, from http://www.emedicine.com/ped/topics535.htm

Sharma, S. (2006c). Pulmonary hypertension secondary. *eMedicine*. Retrieved April 26, 2008, from http://www.emedicine.com/MEd/topic2946.htm

Sharma, S. (2007). Chronic bronchitis. *eMedicine*. Retrieved May 16, 2008, from http://www.emedicine.com/med/TOPIC367.HTM

Shepherd, S. (2003). *Submersion injury: Near drowning*. Retrieved August 28, 2004, from http://www.emedicine.com/EMERG/topic744.htm

Taubert, K. (2001). Management of malignant pleural effusion. *Nursing Clinics of North America, 36*(4), 665–683.

Trauma.org. (2004). *Chest trauma rib fractures and flail chest*. Retrieved from http://www.trauma.org/archive/thoracic/CHESTflail.html

Verma, S., & Slutsky, A. S. (2007). Idiopathic pulmonary fibrosis—New insights. *New England Journal of Medicine, 356*(13), 1370–1372.

Voelkel, N. F., & Tuder, R. (2000). COPD: Exacerbation. *Chest, 117*, S376–S379.

Wanek, S. & Mayberry, J. C. (2004). Blunt thoracic trauma: flail chest, pulmonary contusion, and blast injury. *Critical Care Clinic, 20*(1), 71–81.

Wilson, B. A., Shannon, M., & Stang, C. L. (2006). *Nurse's drug guide*. Philadelphia: Pearson Prentice Hall.

World Health Organization. (1996). *Guidelines for the diagnosis and management of cystic fibrosis*. Retrieved February 24, 2007, from http://www.cf.org/WHO/guidelines

World Health Organization. (2003). *Global TB control report*. Retrieved from http://www.cf.org/WHO

Woodruff, D. (1999). Pneumothorax. *RN, 62*(9), 62–66.

Wooten, J., & Salkind, A. (2003). Superbugs: Unmasking the threat. *RN Magazine, 66*(3), 37–44.

Wrong Diagnosis. (2008). *Prevalence and incidence of pulmonary embolism*. Retrieved April 21, 2008, from http://www.wrongdiagnosis.com/p/pulmonary_embolism/prevalence.htm

Wryobeck, J. M., Lippo, G., McLaughlin, V., Riba, M., & Rubenfire, M. (2007). Psychosocial aspects of pulmonary hypertension: A review. *Psychosomatics, 28*, 457–475.

Yakobi, R. (2007). *Sarcoidosis*. Retrieved from http://www.emedicine.com/emerg/TOPIC516.HTM

Yunis, N. A., & Crausman, R. S. (2006). Cor pulmonale. *eMedicine*. Retrieved May 20, 2008 from http://www.emedicine.com/med/topic449.htm

Caring for the Patient with Complex Respiratory Disorders

Nancy Ames

With contributions by:
Kathleen Osborn

Outcome-Based Learning Objectives

After studying this chapter, the learner will be able to:

1. Describe the etiology, incidence, and types of acute respiratory failure as seen by nurses in acute care settings.
2. Define pulmonary edema and state three of the common etiologies of pulmonary edema that are seen in practice.
3. Differentiate between non-cardiogenic pulmonary edema and cardiogenic pulmonary edema, as it relates to patient symptomology.
4. Distinguish between acute respiratory distress syndrome (ARDS) and acute lung injury (ALI) in patients presenting in an acute care setting.
5. Identify the common ventilator modes and important nursing implications for each mode.
6. Define PEEP and state two complications of this therapy.
7. List the equipment needed for intubation, and explain how the equipment is used with a patient.
8. Review the procedure for suctioning and state two important nursing implications related to conducting this procedure.
9. State two indications for insertion of a chest tube in a patient in an acute care setting.

ONE OF THE most challenging groups of patients that nurses will likely care for are those patients who cannot breathe. These patients can be agitated and confused or unconscious and apneic. They might require emergency arterial blood gases (ABGs) or an immediate lifesaving intervention, such as intubation. Patients may need ventilator support and require immediate suctioning for a mucous plug or develop a tension pneumothorax that necessitates emergent placement of a chest tube.

This chapter addresses the different types of complex respiratory disorders that result in an alteration in oxygen perfusion to the tissues. Basic pulmonary physiology is important to understand in order to care for patients with these complex respiratory disorders. The relationship between oxygen and hemoglobin, ventilation/perfusion mismatching producing hypoxemia, and the role of the alveolar-capillary membrane in respiratory failure are reviewed. The reader is referred to other chapters to review such topics as ABG interpretation and other pertinent pulmonary physiology.

Before reviewing the pathophysiology of complex respiratory disorders, the reader is encouraged to review the chapter on acute coronary syndromes and other cardiac pathologies (Chapter 40 ☻). It is important to understand that the heart and lungs are inextricably linked and what affects one system eventually affects the other. An appreciation of this association

between the heart and the lungs will aid in understanding complex disorders of the respiratory system. Respiratory complications are frequently a result of a primary disorder somewhere else in the body. Therefore, determining the primary organ system failure and focusing on the treatment of this pathology are the goals for many of the complex respiratory disorders. The nursing management of patients with complex respiratory disorders focuses on airway management and maintaining oxygen for tissue perfusion. A description of the complex respiratory disorders follows. The nursing management for these disorders is similar; therefore, a discussion of nursing management is presented after the description of the disorders.

■ Respiratory Physiology

The *alveolar-capillary (A-C) membrane* is the central component of gas exchange in the lungs. The A-C membrane consists of many tissue layers through which gas diffuses. West (1998) describes the lungs as "a collection of 300 million bubbles, each 0.3 mm in diameter." (*Note:* One millimeter is equal to approximately 0.04 inch and 0.3 mm equals 0.0118 inch.) Figure 36–1 ■ (p. 1004) presents a section of the lung showing many alveoli. Visualize many of these clusters of alveoli arranged as groups around the terminal bronchioles in the lungs. These groups or

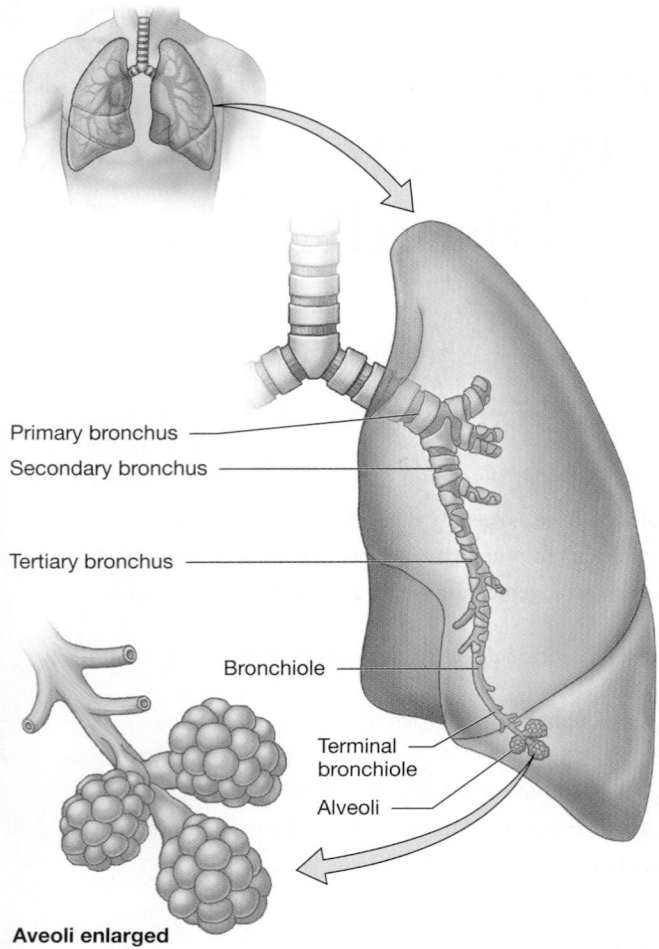

Aveoli enlarged

FIGURE 36–1 ■ Alveoli with bronchioles.

Primary bronchus
Secondary bronchus
Tertiary bronchus
Bronchiole
Terminal bronchiole
Alveoli

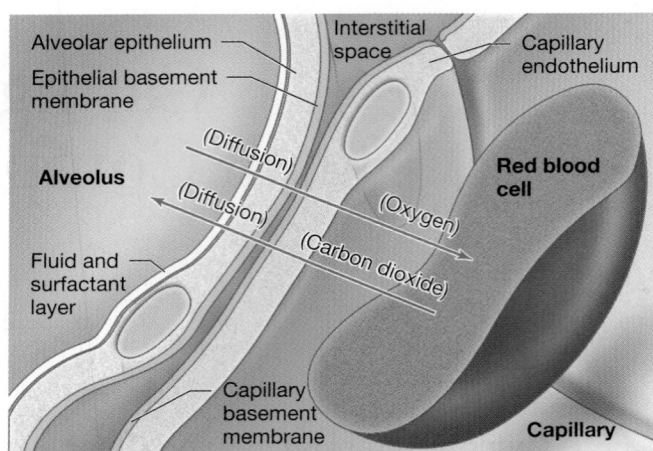

Alveolar epithelium
Epithelial basement membrane
Interstitial space
Capillary endothelium
Alveolus
(Diffusion)
(Diffusion)
(Oxygen)
(Carbon dioxide)
Red blood cell
Fluid and surfactant layer
Capillary basement membrane
Capillary

FIGURE 36–2 ■ Alveolar-capillary membrane.

acini permit 300 million alveoli to fit into the human thorax. The *acinus* is the functional unit of gas exchange and is the terminal respiratory unit of the lung. It is composed of all structures from the respiratory bronchiole to the alveolus, including alveolar ducts, alveolar sacs, and alveoli. This type of formation of the alveoli increases the surface area available for gas exchange in the lungs and makes the pulmonary organ system very efficient.

The 300 million "bubbles" or alveoli are uniquely structured to prevent fluid from filling their air-filled spaces. The distance between the alveolus and the capillary is less than 0.3 micron (a micron is one millionth of a meter). Oxygen diffuses from the alveolus into the pulmonary capillary, and carbon dioxide travels in the opposite direction because the partial pressure of CO_2 is higher in the pulmonary capillaries than it is in the alveoli. This multilayer lamination of tissues begins with the alveolar epithelium that lines the alveoli.

The alveolar epithelium is coated with a thin fluid layer. An important component of this fluid layer is surfactant. **Surfactant** is a surface-active agent that promotes alveolar stability and reduces the likelihood of alveolar collapse. Type II alveolar cells that line the alveoli and the small bronchioles produce surfactant. The alveolus basement membrane provides structure for the alveolus. The next structure, in the middle of the membranes that separate the alveoli from the pulmonary capillary, is a poten-

tial space, called the interstitial space (Figure 36–2 ■). In the normal A-C membrane, the interstitial space contains little or no fluid. In addition to the interstitial space, the pulmonary capillary is composed of a basement membrane and a capillary endothelium through which the gases diffuse. The oxygen diffuses into the red blood cells and attaches to hemoglobin. What is not shown in Figure 36–2 ■ is the lymphatic system in the lungs, which allows transudated fluid to drain from the lungs into the lymph system. Normal flow of this fluid in the lungs is approximately 20 mL/hr at rest (West, 1998). Normally, pressures exerted by water (hydrostatic) and proteins (oncotic) prevent fluid in the pulmonary capillaries and the lymphatics from entering the alveoli. Chart 36–1 describes the normal pressures present in the pulmonary capillaries that cause a net outward movement of a small amount of fluid from the pulmonary capillaries into the interstitial space where it is cleared by the lymphatics.

Oxyhemoglobin Dissociation Curve

The oxyhemoglobin dissociation curve is a commonly used tool for understanding how blood carries and releases oxygen

CHART 36–1	**Mechanisms of Pulmonary Edema**

Forces causing movement of fluid OUT of pulmonary capillaries into pulmonary interstitial space:

Pulmonary capillary hydrostatic pressure	7
Pulmonary interstitial colloid osmotic pressure (oncotic)	14
Negative pulmonary interstitial hydrostatic pressure	8
Total outward force	29

Forces causing adsorption of fluids INTO the pulmonary capillaries:

Pulmonary capillary colloid osmotic pressure	−28
Net outward flow	+ 1

As a result, flow is outward from the pulmonary capillaries into the interstitial space and is pumped away by the lymphatics.

Note: All pressures are in mmHg.

Source: This article was published in *Human Physiology and Mechanism of Disease.* Guyton, A. C., & Hall, J. E. (5 ed., p. 292). Copyright Elsevier 1992.

(Figure 36–3 ■). Specifically, the oxyhemoglobin dissociation curve shows the percentage of oxygen saturation (SO_2) at different oxygen pressures (PaO_2). This is determined by what is called "hemoglobin's affinity for oxygen," that is, how readily hemoglobin acquires and releases oxygen molecules from its surrounding tissue. Oxygen saturation does not change significantly with the higher PaO_2 (flat portion of the curve), but once 60 mmHg is reached, then, very little change in PaO_2 causes a rapid decline in oxygen saturation (steep portion of the curve). The curve can move to either the right or the left. When the curve shifts to the right, the hemoglobin has less affinity for oxygen and O_2 is released easily to the cells. Increased carbon dioxide, decreased pH, and hyperthermia are three conditions that cause a shift to the right. A shift to the left means that it is more difficult for hemoglobin to release oxygen to the tissues. Such a shift is caused by an increased pH, decreased carbon dioxide, and hypothermia (Kaplow & Hardin, 2007). A clear understanding of the association between oxygen and hemoglobin is important to understand the respiratory system pathophysiology. This curve will be referred to throughout this chapter.

Shunts and the Oxyhemoglobin Dissociation Curve

A **shunt** is a passage through which blood may pass or a connection between two locations. In pulmonary physiology, a shunt is present when deoxygenated blood passes through the pulmonary capillary without exchanging oxygen (Guyton & Hall, 2005). There are two types of shunts, physiological shunts and pathologic shunts. A physiological shunt occurs when a portion of the cardiac output goes through the regular pulmonary vasculature without becoming oxygenated in the alveolar sac. There is no abnormal connection between the blood vessels; rather, there is a severe redistribution of pulmonary blood flow due to some pathology. Physiological shunting is often seen in conditions such as pulmonary edema, pneumonia, and lobar atelectasis.

This physiological shunt prevents the SaO_2 (arterial saturation of oxygen) from ever reaching 100% and, for the same reason, prevents the upper arterial plateau of the oxyhemoglobin dissociation curve from reaching 100% saturation (see Figure 36–3).

The other type of shunt is a pathologic shunt. An example of this type of shunt could be a right-to-left septal defect, where deoxygenated blood passes from the right ventricle and flows directly into the left ventricle in a patient with this type of structural cardiac defect. Venous blood from the right heart mixes with oxygenated blood from the left. Breathing 100% oxygen cannot correct a shunt. This is an important diagnostic clue that assists the health care professional in determining the cause of the hypoxemia. Most patients with shunts do not have increased CO_2 levels in the blood because their respiratory center is responding to the hypoxemia by increasing the respiratory rate, therefore maintaining a near normal or low level of CO_2.

Ventilation/Perfusion Mismatching

Ventilation is the movement of air between the atmosphere and the alveoli that is accomplished by respirations, whereas **perfusion** is the movement of blood carrying oxygen and assisting in removing carbon dioxide. Usually there is a near equal relationship of ventilation (V) to perfusion in the lungs. The formula V/Q where ventilation is 4 L/min and perfusion is 5 L/min, explains this relationship. Normal ventilation to perfusion equals 4/5 or 0.8 (Porth, 2007; Shapiro, Peruzzi, & Templin, 1994). Figure 36–4A ■ shows an example of a unit where the perfusion is normal and the ventilation is also normal; that is, V/Q is equal to 0.8. Shapiro's classical example of ventilation and perfusion mismatching explains this principle. There exists a mismatch of ventilation and perfusion when this formula is not equal to 0.8. In Figure 36–4B ■ there is ventilation but no perfusion; note the air sac or alveoli without blood flow, hence no perfusion. This phenomenon is referred to as a dead space unit because there is ventilation and little if

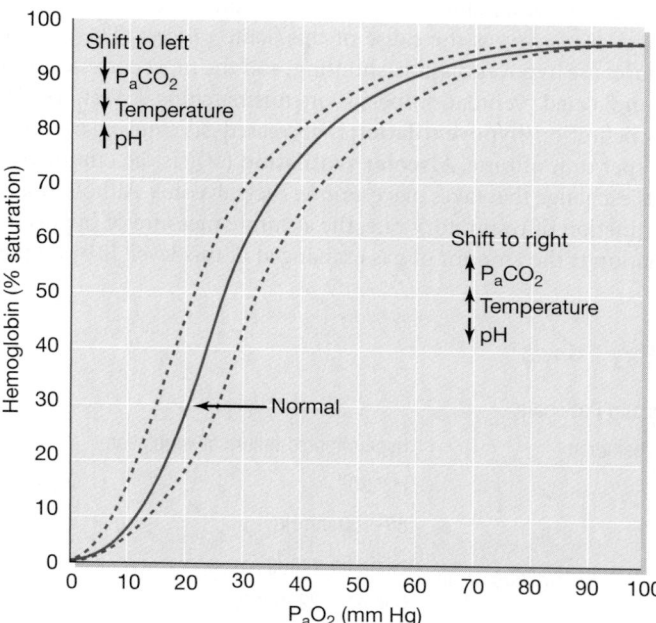

FIGURE 36–3 ■ Oxyhemoglobin dissociation curve.

(a) Normal unit

(b) Dead space unit

(c) Shunt unit

(d) Silent unit

FIGURE 36–4 ■ Ventilation/perfusion relationships: (A) normal unit; (B) dead space unit; (C) shunt unit; (D) silent unit.

any perfusion: V/Q > 0.8. Examples of diseases that are related to an increase in the ventilation-to-perfusion ratio are pulmonary emboli and cardiogenic shock. There is no abnormality in ventilation and the lungs may be normal, but tissues would become hypoxic because of lack of perfusion.

Figure 36–4C ■ (p. 1005) shows a shunt unit where V/Q < 0.8. There is perfusion but little or no ventilation—note that the air sac is collapsed. This occurs in pulmonary edema, pneumonia, and many other causes of respiratory failure. Figure 36–4D ■ (p. 1005) demonstrates both abnormalities producing neither ventilation nor perfusion. Increasing the oxygen concentration can correct some types of V/Q mismatch especially when V/Q < 0.8, but it will not correct other abnormalities caused by shunts. Shunting of blood across collapsed alveoli can cause a type of ventilation/perfusion mismatching that may produce hypoxemia. This "shunt effect" is a type of **ventilation/perfusion mismatch**. It should not be confused with the other main cause of hypoxemia, which was explained previously, even though the same term shunt is used to explain both conditions. Ventilation/perfusion mismatching is a common cause of acute respiratory failure.

■ Acute Respiratory Failure

Acute respiratory failure (ARF) is a condition defined as a failure of gas exchange (Hemmila & Napolitano, 2006). The lungs no longer meet the physiological needs of the body due to a failure of the heart, lungs, or both. The hallmark of ARF is respiratory difficulty with abnormal ABGs.

Epidemiology and Etiology

The purpose of the pulmonary system is to provide oxygen to the cells of the body and remove carbon dioxide and other waste products of metabolism. The inability of the respiratory system to accomplish this function is termed respiratory failure. The epidemiology of acute respiratory failure has recently been reported in four different European countries: Germany, Sweden, Iceland, and Norway (Lewandowski, 2003). The researchers found very similar incidences of ARF among the four countries, namely, a range of 77.6 to 88.6 and 77.6 cases per 100,000 population per year.

ARF results in a failure of oxygenation or ventilation or both (Fink, Abraham, Vincent, & Kochanek, 2005). Respiratory failure can be divided into three main categories, based on etiology: hypoxemic respiratory failure, hypercapneic respiratory failure, and failure of the respiratory centers in the central nervous system. The Diagnostic Tests box lists the normal values for ABGs and compares these normal values to ABGs representative of hypoxemic and hypercapneic respiratory failure.

A failure of oxygenation produces **hypoxemia**, which is defined as an arterial oxygen tension or pressure (PaO_2) that is below normal range. The normal range of PaO_2 is between 80 and 100 mmHg. Therefore, a PaO_2 of less than 60 mmHg and an arterial saturation of oxygen (SaO_2) of less than 90% while breathing room air is representative of hypoxemic respiratory failure. This value of 60 mmHg is located on the steep part of the oxyhemoglobin dissociation curve (see Figure 36–3 ■, p. 1005).

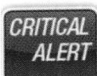 *The nurse should assess the patient carefully when:*
$PaO_2 < 60$ mmHg from ABGs
$SpO_2 < 90\%$.

Notify health care provider and increase oxygen delivery.

A failure of the respiratory system to ventilate produces the clinical sign of hypercapnia. Hypercapnia is an abnormal concentration of carbon dioxide ($PaCO_2$) in the blood above normal range. The normal range of $PaCO_2$ is between 35 and 45 mmHg. A $PaCO_2$ of greater than 50 mmHg represents hypercapneic respiratory failure with a pH of less than 7.3. Acute respiratory failure happens quickly, over hours to days, and is not characterized by a gradual worsening of symptoms that would portray chronic respiratory failure. Acute respiratory failure presents with no time for compensation by the renal system. The central and peripheral nervous systems are involved in the control and regulation of respiration. If these systems fail respiratory failure occurs. Chart 36–2 lists the major etiologies causing respiratory failure. This chart is divided into hypoxemic respiratory failure, hypercapneic respiratory failure, and a failure of the respiratory centers in the central nervous system (CNS). These three categories represent the three principal causes of acute respiratory failure.

Pathophysiology

Acute respiratory failure can be traced to three main pathophysiological reasons as the cause of this acute process. These three causes are hypoventilation, shunting, and the most common and complicated, ventilation/perfusion mismatching (West, 1998). By definition, **hypoventilation** is decreased gas entering the alveoli per unit of time. **Alveolar ventilation** (V_A) is the cumulative gas exchange that takes place among each alveolus. Although it is a function of respiratory rate, the accurate measure of hypoventilation is the amount of gas exchanged at this level. It is *not* the

DIAGNOSTIC TESTS for Hypoxemia and Hypercapneic Respiratory Failure

Test		Expected Abnormalities and Rationale	
ABGs	Normal	Hypoxemic-failure of oxygenation	Hypercapneic-failure of ventilation
pH	7.35–7.45	7.35–7.45	< 7.30
PaO_2	80–100 mmHg	< 60 mmHg	80–100 mmHg
$PaCO_2$	35–45 mmHg	35–45 mmHg	> 50–55 mmHg
HCO_3	22–27 mmHg	22–27 mmHg	Can be < 22 mmHg
SaO_2	95–99	< 90 %	> 90 %

CHART 36–2   Etiology of Acute Respiratory Failure

Type of Respiratory Failure	Diagnosis/Disease
Hypoxemic respiratory failure	Acute lung injury Acute respiratory distress syndrome Pneumothorax
Hypercapneic respiratory failure	Oversedation Obesity Diaphragmatic fatigue
Nervous system causes of respiratory failure	Cervical spinal cord injury Guillain-Barré syndrome Myasthenia gravis

CHART 36–3   Clinical Manifestations of Acute Respiratory Failure

System	Signs/Symptoms
Respiratory	Dyspnea Tachypnea Shortness of breath (SOB) Use of accessory muscles for breathing Adventitious lung sounds (crackles, rhonchi, wheezes) Decreased breath sounds Inspiratory/expiratory stridor Cough Increased secretions Orthopnea
Neurological	Agitation Confusion Disorientation Difficult to arouse, sleepiness (hypercarbic respiratory failure) Muscle twitching
Cardiac	Tachycardia Dysrhythmias (ventricular ectopy) Diaphoresis Hypertension or hypotension
Radiologic	Pulmonary infiltrates Atelectasis Pneumothorax Normal

quantity of gas that enters the large airways because the large airways, the trachea, and the bronchi down to the terminal bronchioles have no role in gas exchange. Their role is to transport ambient air beyond the terminal bronchioles where oxygen first meets the alveoli. These transporting airways compose the **anatomic dead space** because no gas exchange occurs. Ventilation of this anatomic region is defined as **dead space ventilation (V_D)**.

With hypoventilation, the level of CO_2 in the blood must rise because CO_2 is not exhaled adequately. Some common causes of hypoventilation are drugs that depress the respiratory center, such as morphine and barbiturates. Guillain-Barré syndrome, an immune-mediated disease that affects the peripheral nervous system and eventually causes respiratory depression and failure, respiratory paralysis from a spinal cord injury, and myasthenia gravis that affects the neuromuscular junction are all examples of diseases for which hypoventilation can be the major cause of respiratory failure (Hughes & Cornblath, 2005). Trauma with flail chest or multiple rib fractures, central and obstructive sleep apnea, and morbid obesity also can cause hypoventilation with increased CO_2 retention. Chapter 35 ☞ discusses flail chest, Chapter 34 ☞ discusses obstructive sleep apnea, and Chapter 19 ☞ discusses acid–base disturbances.

Hypoxemia is not a problem with pure hypoventilation and can be easily corrected by increasing the **fraction of inspired oxygen (FiO_2)** concentration. Oxygenation is defined as adding oxygen to any system. In the human body, hemoglobin increases the efficiency of this addition by associating with oxygen at the arterial level and releasing oxygen at the tissue level.

Clinical Manifestations

The presenting symptom in acute respiratory failure is shortness of breath, dyspnea, and increased work of breathing (WOB) with hypoxemia. Dyspnea is difficulty breathing and a subjective symptom (Wang, FitzGerald, Schulzer, Mak, & Ayas, 2005). In addition, the patient may be tachypneic, tachycardic, agitated, confused, and disoriented. There may be increased secretions with a productive cough. Chart 36–3 compares hypoxemic respiratory failure with hypercapneic respiratory failure. Many of the signs and symptoms are shared by both disorders. The central cyanosis of hypoxemic respiratory failure and the muscle twitching caused by the acidosis in hypercapneic respiratory failure are unique for each condition and provide some useful

clues for the nurse. The patient with hypoxemic respiratory failure will rarely become sleepy and usually will not have difficulty being aroused, but the patient who has high CO_2 levels commonly presents with somnolence and a decreased level of consciousness. This is an important diagnostic finding.

Laboratory and Diagnostic Procedures and Monitoring

A chest x-ray assists in determining the primary disorder that is contributing to the respiratory failure, but ABG levels are the most common test for assessing respiratory failure and are useful in predicting the type of respiratory failure the patient may be experiencing (see the Diagnostic Tests box earlier in the chapter for normal ABG values). In acute respiratory failure, no compensation in pH is seen because it takes the kidneys hours to days to compensate for altered pH. See Chapter 19 ☞ for a discussion of acid–base imbalance.

Medical Management

Correcting and treating the hypoxemia is the primary goal of treatment of acute respiratory failure. The secondary goal is to discover the cause. Supplemental oxygen devices should be used until treatment can reverse the hypoxemia. Chart 36–4 (p. 1008) outlines the common oxygen delivery devices and percentage of oxygen that they deliver.

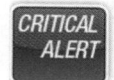 **CRITICAL ALERT** *To treat life-threatening hypoxemia that does not respond to supplemental oxygen, endotracheal intubation is necessary. The nurse must be able to assist with this procedure.*

CHART 36–4 Common Oxygen Delivery Devices, FiO₂, and Flow Rates

Device	FiO$_2$ (%)	Flow Rate (L/min)
Nasal cannula	24	1
	28	2
	32	3
	36	4
	40	5
	44	6
Simple face mask	35–55	5–10
Venturi mask	24	3
	26	3
	28	6
	31	6
	35	9
	40	12
	50	15
Nonrebreather mask	60–80	10–15

Note: FiO$_2$ = fraction of inspired oxygen. These are only approximations, not absolute FiO$_2$ values, because the delivery is via a mask or cannula.

If these devices fail to correct the hypoxemia, intubation and institution of mechanical ventilation are considered. Besides intubation, another intervention that is being used for more causes of acute respiratory failure is **noninvasive positive pressure ventilation (NPPV)**. This intervention uses a ventilator and mask attachment, either a nasal or full-face mask, to deliver the oxygen without requiring the use of an endotracheal tube and intubation. This intervention is discussed in more detail later in the chapter.

Gerontological Considerations

As the population of elderly patients increases, the potential exists for an increase in the incidence of acute respiratory failure. Nurses who care for the elderly must be aware of the important differences between the elderly patient with respiratory failure and those who are younger. There are some significant differences in the elderly person's respiratory system that predispose the elderly to developing respiratory failure. These differences have to do with the physiological effects of aging. Chart 36–5 outlines the physiological effects of aging on the pulmonary system.

A decrease in the forced expiratory volume in one second (FEV$_1$) begins after age 30 and is further pronounced if the patient smokes. The other criteria listed in Chart 36–5 include many important physiological parameters that are accentuated as the person ages and the muscles become deconditioned. Once the elderly patient has respiratory failure and is intubated and placed on mechanical ventilation, her outcome is not that different than that from of her younger counterparts. A recent study determined that the highest risks of death among patients who were 70 years or older were not related to age but to coexistent acute renal failure, shock, and limited functional status (Estebam et al., 2004). These predictors of death were more important than age. Age alone should not be a criterion for anticipating the success or failure of mechanical ventilation. However, age has a complex relationship with the most severe type of respiratory failure: acute respiratory distress disorder (ARDS). In a study of ARDS in trauma patients, patients 60 to 69 years of age showed increasingly higher risks for

CHART 36–5 Physiological Effects of Aging on the Pulmonary System

Widened alveolar arterial gradient

Reduced responsiveness to hypoxemia and hypercarbia

Decreased FEV$_1$

Decreased chest wall compliance

Decreased effectiveness of cough

Compromised mucociliary clearance

ARDS development (Johnston, Rubenfeld, & Hudson, 2003). Patients who were older had a decreased risk of ARDS. Although these results may be confusing, this study further emphasizes the importance of not predicting outcome by using age alone.

Acute Pulmonary Edema

Acute pulmonary edema is an abnormal accumulation of fluid in the lungs. This fluid accumulates because of a dysfunction with the lungs and/or the heart. Acute pulmonary edema may be attributed to many different etiologies and types of pulmonary edema, which are discussed below. These etiologies have different names but all can be traced back to a failure of the heart, lungs, or both. Heart failure is discussed in detail in Chapter 42 .

Epidemiology

Acute pulmonary edema is a common medical problem. Epidemiologic data on heart failure, which is the primary cause of cardiogenic acute pulmonary edema, demonstrates an incidence of 10 per 1,000 in persons more than 65 years old in the United States (Jessup & Brozena, 2003). Most patients with heart failure are admitted to the emergency department for life-saving treatment (Collins, Lindsell, Storrow, & Abraham, 2006). However, there is evidence that the number of patients who present with heart failure is declining because of improved hospital management (Fox et al., 2007). Heart failure, a chronic disease, affects about 5 million people in the United States with an incidence of 550,000 cases annually (Onwuanyi & Taylor, 2007). See Chapter 42 for a complete discussion of heart failure.

Etiologies

Acute pulmonary edema refers to the time frame during which the fluid accumulation develops. In acute pulmonary edema, this occurs quickly over minutes to hours. Some clinicians use the term *flash pulmonary edema* to define pulmonary edema that occurs within minutes of a precipitating event. Reported causes of flash pulmonary edema include the classic cardiac pathologies of left ventricular dysfunction as a result of a massive myocardial infarction or valve dysfunction with or without papillary muscle rupture. When the pulmonary capillary pressure rises quickly and reaches two to three times the normal pressures in the pulmonary arteries, edema fluid floods the interstitial space and the alveoli. The pulmonary lymphatic system and other vessels have no time to compensate, unlike in chronic pulmonary edema in which the pressure in the pulmonary arteries can be higher but the lungs have time to compensate. The etiology of pulmonary edema is divided into cardiogenic and noncardiogenic categories.

Cardiogenic pulmonary edema (CPE) is pulmonary edema that results from increased hydrostatic pressures in the pulmonary capillary bed secondary to increased pulmonary venous pressure due to heart failure (Jessup & Brozena, 2003). This pulmonary hypertension is related to many factors, the most common of which is cardiac dysfunction. But fluid overload and chronic hypoxemia also can contribute to this type of pulmonary edema. Pulmonary hypertension is a compensatory mechanism that develops as a result of hypoxemia and can lead to remodeling of the pulmonary vasculature. Pulmonary hypertension is discussed in detail in Chapter 35 ⊙.

Heart failure can be from cardiac muscle dysfunction or valvular problems. Dysrhythmias, especially tachydysrhythmias, such as supraventricular and ventricular tachycardias, can precipitate pulmonary edema (see Chapter 38 ⊙). Constrictive pericarditis is present when a thickened, fibrotic, and adherent pericardium restricts diastolic filling of the heart. It usually begins with an initial episode of acute pericarditis. Dressler's syndrome is a common type of pericarditis that occurs after an acute myocardial infarction. A large majority of cases of constrictive pericarditis are idiopathic or without a known cause (Talreja et al., 2003).

Noncardiogenic pulmonary edema (NCPE) is related to injury of the A-C membrane from numerous causes. Among the most important causes are sepsis, inflammation, inhaled toxins, and drugs. In NCPE usually there is no primary cardiac dysfunction. Chart 36–6 lists typical etiologies of pulmonary edema comparing the cardiac and noncardiac causes. Both types of pulmonary edema, cardiogenic and noncardiogenic, produce, as an end result, excess fluid in the lungs. This excess fluid in the alveoli decreases the number of alveoli available for gas exchange; however, the mechanism is very different. The initial insult in noncardiogenic pulmonary edema is caused by a change in the permeability of the A-C membrane caused by direct injury or as result of inflammation, whereas the initial insult in cardiogenic pulmonary edema is caused by heart failure.

One of the syndromes that is listed as a cause of NCPE is ARDS. Because of its prevalence and high mortality, this disease is discussed in more detail later in this chapter. Cardiogenic pulmonary edema, caused by an increased pressure in the pulmonary capillaries due to heart failure, is the major focus of this section. The next section discusses some common causes of noncardiogenic pulmonary edema other than ARDS.

Neurogenic Pulmonary Edema

Neurogenic pulmonary edema (NPE) is associated with direct insult to the CNS. Seizures, cerebral hemorrhage, and head injury are common precipitating factors to the development of pulmonary edema. The pathophysiology of the edema formation is not clear, but it might be related to disruption in sympathetic tone related to increased venous pressure and hypertension. The presenting symptom for these patients is dyspnea, but the other signs and symptoms of pulmonary edema—crackles, shortness of breath, and pink frothy sputum—also can be seen. Treatment includes treating the underlying events as well as supportive care (Fontes et al., 2003).

Negative Pressure Pulmonary Edema

Negative pressure pulmonary edema (NPPE) is caused by attempting to ventilate with an apparent airway obstruction. *Postobstruction pulmonary edema* and *airway obstruction pul-*

CHART 36–6 Common Causes of Acute Pulmonary Edema

Type of Acute Pulmonary Edema	Disease/Condition
Cardiogenic	Myocardial infarction
	Myocardial ischemia
	Hypertension
	Cardiomyopathies
	Viral myocarditis
	Acute dysrhythmias
	Valvular dysfunction
	Atrial myxomas
	Papillary muscle rupture
	Pericarditis
	Cardiac tamponade
Noncardiogenic	Acute lung injury (ALI)
	Acute respiratory distress syndrome (ARDS)
	Neurogenic pulmonary edema
	Excessive intravenous fluid administration
	Postoperative pulmonary edema
	Acute renal failure
	Pneumonia
	Drowning
Population or disease specific	High-altitude pulmonary edema
	Heroin-related pulmonary edema
	Transfusion-related acute lung injury
	Hyperbaric oxygen therapy
	Postanesthesia
	Postcardiopulmonary bypass
	Diving-related pulmonary edema
	Malaria
	Eclampsia
	Negative pressure pulmonary edema
Medication or chemical inhalant related	Certain chemotherapeutic agents
	Smoke and burn injuries
	Biowarfare agents (e.g., anthrax)
	Allergic reaction to IV contrast

monary edema are other names for the same disorder. This type of pulmonary edema develops because of the extreme pressures that are used to attempt to ventilate during the obstruction. These high pressures are transmitted to the pulmonary system, increasing transpulmonary pressures as well as pleural pressures. Once the airway obstruction is relieved, hydrostatic pressure forces fluid into the alveoli and pulmonary edema develops.

The most common cause of NPPE is laryngospasm during intubation or after extubation (Fremont, Kallet, Matthay, & Ware, 2007). NPPE has also been associated with oropharyngeal surgery and patients who have had head and neck surgeries. Symptoms of this type of pulmonary edema mimic other types of pulmonary edema with production of pink frothy sputum, difficulty breathing, tachypnea, and tachycardia. Treatment consists of positive pressure ventilation with positive end-expiratory pressure (PEEP). In some circumstances diuretics can be used. Hemodynamic monitoring will assist the health care provider in differentiating this type of noncardiogenic pulmonary edema from cardiogenic pulmonary edema (Tarrac, 2003).

High-Altitude Pulmonary Edema

High-altitude pulmonary edema (HAPE) is listed as a cause of pulmonary edema in a specific population: skiers and climbers. This type of pulmonary edema develops in persons who rapidly ascend to heights greater than 2,500 to 3,000 meters (8,202 to 9,842 feet). The pathogenesis of the formation of pulmonary edema is debated. The hypothesis is that a pulmonary vasoconstriction causes a relative hypoxemia. This increases the pressure in the pulmonary capillaries, thus forcing fluid into the interstitial space and the alveoli. A direct injury pattern from inflammatory mediators and oxygen free radicals also are believed to be responsible for some of the pulmonary capillary direct injury. Oxygen free radicals are components of oxygen that have an unpaired electron on an oxygen atom. These free radicals are believed to cause tissue injury at the cellular level. An example of an oxygen free radical is the one-electron reduction of O_2, which produces the superoxide radical, O_2. The most important treatment is removal from high altitudes. If this is done, the pulmonary edema should resolve. Other treatment measures include steroids and oxygen therapy (Gabry, Ledoux, Mozziconacci, & Martin, 2003).

Heroin-Related Pulmonary Edema

Another example of population-specific pulmonary edema is *heroin-related pulmonary edema* (HRPE). Heroin is one of the most commonly abused narcotics in the United States (Habal, 2006). This type of edema develops within 24 hours of the administration of heroin and has been reported in users of cocaine and methadone. One review reported that clinical symptoms appear immediately or within 4 hours of the administered dose of heroin and that 39% of patients who develop this type of pulmonary edema require mechanical ventilation (Frishman, Del Vecchio, Sanal, & Ismail, 2003).

Excessive Intravenous Fluid Administration

Any patient who has a continuous intravenous infusion and receives a large amount of fluid over a short period of time can develop pulmonary edema. If the patient has any comorbidities such as cardiac, pulmonary, or renal disease the risk of developing pulmonary edema increases. The pathophysiology of this type of pulmonary edema is very clear. Increased venous return of the excessive fluid contributes to increased pulmonary pressures that cause fluid to leak into interstitial spaces and then into the alveoli. A patient population that is at increased risk for this type of pulmonary edema is the dialysis-dependent patient. Fluid management for the patient who is in renal failure presents a challenge because underresuscitation of hypotension can be as harmful as overresuscitation. Failure of the dialysis-dependent patient to follow dietary restrictions (e.g., salt intake) predisposes this patient population to pulmonary edema.

The patient who is dialysis dependent is at risk for the development of pulmonary edema after excessive fluid administrative (Arieff, 1999; Fleischmann, Goldman, Young, & Lee, 2003). In Arieff's study 13 patients who died of postoperative pulmonary edema were analyzed for predictive factors. In the 13 patients each had retained greater than 67 mL · kg^{-1} · day^{-1} and there was no presenting sign. However, cardiorespiratory arrest was the most frequent clinical presentation.

Transfusion-Related Lung Injury

Patients who receive any type of transfusion are at risk for *transfusion-related acute lung injury* (TRALI), which can cause noncardiogenic pulmonary edema. Transfusions that can cause this syndrome include packed red blood cells, platelets, granulocytes, and fresh frozen plasma (Looney, Gropper, & Matthay, 2004). This syndrome has also been reported following allogeneic stem cell transplantation. The classic symptoms of dyspnea, hypoxemia, and bilateral pulmonary edema occur within 4 to 6 hours of administration of blood products. A large percentage of the patients require support with either intubation or noninvasive ventilation. An impressive feature of this type of NCPE is the speed of development and onset of pulmonary edema. The patient who has no respiratory problem receives a transfusion and within 4 to 6 hours requires maximal ventilation support in order to ventilate and oxygenate. TRALI is discussed in detail in Chapter 23 ⊕.

Hyperbaric Oxygen Therapy and Diving-Related Pulmonary Edema

Hyperbaric oxygen therapy and SCUBA (self-contained underwater breathing apparatus) diving can predispose this special population to pulmonary edema related to the increased pressure of oxygen used in both hyperbaric treatment and recreationally for SCUBA diving. Removal from the increased pressure resolves symptoms (Halpern, Gefen, Sorkine, & Elad, 2003).

Inhalation of Toxic Substances Related to Bioterrorism or Accidental Exposure

No discussion of the etiologies of noncardiogenic pulmonary edema would be complete without discussing the causes of NCPE related to inhalation of a toxic chemical or a bioterrorism agent. These agents can be bacteria, viruses, or biotoxins that are naturally occurring compounds, such as ricin, that are released for the purpose of inflicting harm or inciting terror. Many of the agents that are listed by the Centers for Disease Control and Prevention (CDC) as Category A agents cause death by attacking the lung parenchyma either directly or as a result of an inflammatory process. The CDC categorizes agents as A, B, and C based on their ability to inflict harm (CDC, 2007). Category A agents are those that can inflict the greatest harm and pose the greatest threat to the public. The Category A bioterrorism agents are listed in Chart 36–7. Anthrax and plague are discussed next because of their presenting symptoms and as examples of Category A agents. More information on these types of agents is given in Chapter 72 ⊕.

Bacillus anthracis is a gram-positive bacillus that is present in nature. Humans contract anthrax when they come in contact with animals or animal products. Three different sources of anthrax infections are known: gastrointestinal, cutaneous, and inhalation. Cutaneous anthrax is the most common type. Lesions on the skin develop a black eschar. With appropriate treatment deaths from cutaneous anthrax are rare (Inglesby et al., 2002). Gastrointestinal anthrax is uncommon. However, inhalation of the bacillus anthrax spores is the most deadly source of the types of anthrax. The various defense mechanisms of the respiratory system assist in activating the anthrax spores. As the spores are inhaled, the natural defense mechanism of the alveoli breaks down the spores. The alveolar macrophages destroy some of the inhaled spores, but others are transported in the lymph system to the mediastinal lymph nodes where they germinate. What causes this germination is not fully understood and the time range for activation of the spores can range in time from 2 to 43 days (Inglesby et al., 2002). Once the spores have germinated, clinical

CHART 36–7 Category A Bioterrorism Agents

Agent	Brief Description
Anthrax	Caused by *Bacillus anthracis*. Most severe form is inhalational anthrax, which produces fever, chills, malaise, widened mediastinum, pulmonary infiltrates, pleural effusion, and pulmonary edema (Ingelsby et al., 2002).
Plague	Caused by *Yersinia pestis*. Three types of plague: bubonic, septicemic, and pneumonic. Pneumonic plague is characterized by sudden-onset cough, fever, and chest pain (Cobbs & Chansolme, 2004).
Smallpox	Caused by *Variola* virus and is highly infectious. Produces a rash, fever, and chills. Contagious and because of vaccine has been eradicated as a natural occurring disease (Lupatkin, Lupatkin, & Rosenberg, 2004).
Botulism	Caused by *Clostridium botulinum*. Present in contaminated foods, but botulinum toxin can be used as an aerosolized agent in a bioterrorism attack. Bacillus produces neurotoxins that cause paralysis (Karwa et al., 2005).
Viral hemorrhagic fever	Caused by a diverse group of RNA viruses. Produces complex clinical syndrome of fever, chills, disturbances in regional circulation, and bleeding. Marburg and Ebola viruses are in this category (Karwa et al., 2005).
Tularemia	Caused by *Francisella tularensis*, a gram-negative bacterium. Patients present with fever, chills, and generalized weakness. Predisposes patients to pneumonia and ARDS (Karwa et al., 2005).

symptoms appear. Theses symptoms include fever, chills, and sweating with a nonproductive or minimally productive cough. Dyspnea and tachycardia are two other presenting symptoms.

At the presenting stage of the disease, the clinical symptoms for a case of acute febrile respiratory infection and inhalational anthrax are very similar. But as the disease progresses, pleural effusion, a widened mediastinum, and the presence of the bacillus in blood and other fluid cultures help the clinician differentiate the symptoms. The patient's clinical course deteriorates quickly with development of severe hypoxemia, ARDS, and shock. If recognized and treated early with antibiotics, mortality can be as low as 45% (Karwa, Currie, & Kvetan, 2005). Inhalational anthrax is not contagious. Normal universal precautions are all that is required for protection. A vaccine (Biothrax) is available but recommendations for its use are for the military and laboratory workers who are engaged in studying the bacillus (Karwa et al., 2005).

The "Black Death" or plague is really three diseases or clinical entities, namely, bubonic plague, septicemic plague, and pneumonic plague. All three diseases are caused by the bacterial pathogen *Yersinia pestis*. The disease is spread from the bite of a flea or direct contact with an animal that is infected. Two to 8 days after the contact, the person develops symptoms. The symptoms include fever, chills, and weakness. The other classic findings of bubonic plague are swollen and painful lymph glands. These are called buboes and are usually located in the

lymph node closest to where the contact occurred. These buboes appear as nonmovable masses. With antibiotic treatment the mortality is approximately 50% (Cobbs & Chansolme, 2004). Pneumonic plague is spread from infected droplets coughed by patients who are already infected. In this disease the microorganisms develop in the lung and spread systemically. Symptoms include cough, fever, chills, and chest pain. Pneumonia and lung consolidation occur rapidly. Without treatment with appropriate antibiotics, mortality is 100%. This type of plague is highly contagious and is spread from person-to-person contact through the aerosolized droplet. Because of the contagious properties and the mortality rate, pneumonic plague makes an excellent choice as an agent for bioterrorism.

Besides the viruses and bacteria that have been discussed, other agents such as chemicals can cause severe swelling of the respiratory tract, upper airways, and lungs. The subsequent pulmonary edema that develops from the injury caused by these agents produces dyspnea, shortness of breath, and death if the inhalation is severe. Chemical agents include ammonia, bromine, chlorine, hydrogen chlorine, phosgene, phosphine, and phosphorus. They can be inhaled as a result of an accidental exposure or because of bioterrorism. All of these agents produce an injury to the lung tissue and, if severe enough, death. Together these agents are termed pulmonary edemagens (Baker, 2005).

Two chemical agents, chlorine and phosgene, have similar injury patterns. Chlorine is one of the most common chemicals produced by man. It has many uses in bleaching and cleaning. If inhaled, chlorine gas is corrosive to the throat, lungs, eyes, and skin. When chlorine gas comes in contact with water, it forms hypochlorous acid and hydrochloric acid. These acids can cause damage to skin, eyes, and lung tissue. Therefore, water substantially enhances chlorine's oxidizing and corrosive effects. If exposed, washing and flushing of exposed mucous membranes is recommended. The symptoms depend on the amount of gas inhaled. Treatment is supportive.

Phosgene is a liquid and a vapor that is formed by the natural decomposition of chlorinated hydrocarbons. During World War I both sides used phosgene gas as a military weapon. Exposure to this gas causes pulmonary edema. The gas attacks the alveoli and the type I and II pneumocytes. Phosgene gas destroys the alveolar macrophages. The parenchymal lung injury produces platelet aggregation and vasoconstriction with increased capillary permeability. Treatment of phosgene gas inhalation includes supportive care and mechanical ventilation if the injury is severe. There is some information that supports steroid use in toxic gas inhalation (Baker, 2005).

The final category of substances that can be harmful if ingested or inhaled are those listed by the CDC as biotoxins. These naturally occurring proteins include ricin. Ricin is a glucoprotein that is extracted from the castor bean (*Ricinus communis*). Castor beans have been used for centuries all over the world for the oil that is used as a laxative and for lubricating. Ricin is produced from the mash of the castor bean after the oil is extracted. Ricin can be easily manufactured from a substance that is readily available, which makes it an excellent agent for bioterrorism. Ricin works by inhibiting protein synthesis in all cells with which it comes in contact. The toxin binds to the cell membrane and then is incorporated into the cell by a process termed receptor-mediated endocytosis (Doan, 2004). This process eventually destroys the cell. The liver and spleen are susceptible. There is a significant lag time between exposure and symptoms because of this process. Inhalation of ricin is rare but pulmonary symptoms would include increased permeability, pulmonary edema, shock, and death within 35 to 72 hours (Marks, 2004). Usually ingestion of the beans or parenteral injection of ricin is the method of contact. Symptoms include nausea, vomiting, diarrhea, and abdominal cramps with subsequent dehydration. Fever can be present. Treatment is supportive and a vaccine is under development (Doan, 2004).

Pathophysiology

The pathophysiology of acute pulmonary edema and the signs and symptoms of this dysfunction are related to the accumulation of fluid preventing adequate gas exchange across the alveolar-capillary membrane. This fluid accumulates in the interstitial space and floods the alveoli, thereby interfering with gas exchange. The three causes include (1) too much fluid being delivered to the delicate pulmonary capillaries; (2) increased pressure in the capillaries due to constriction, to such an extent that fluid is forced across the capillary into the alveolus; and (3) capillary injury, which causes a leaking of fluid, even if it is a normal amount.

Pathophysiology of Cardiogenic Pulmonary Edema

In cardiogenic pulmonary edema fluid enters the alveoli and prevents the diffusion of oxygen and carbon dioxide across the A-C membrane into the pulmonary capillaries. In CPE, this space is one of the first to fill with transudated fluid that is "pushed out" of the pulmonary capillaries. Transudated fluid is fluid that has decreased protein and cellular elements as compared to normal serum. This fluid shift occurs due to changes in the dynamics of the A-C membrane that are caused by increased pulmonary capillary pressure.

The fluid accumulates because of a primary cardiac etiology that causes the increased pulmonary capillary pressure. The interstitial edema occurs before the alveolar edema. Acute pulmonary edema develops when the pulmonary capillary pressure exceeds the pulmonary oncotic pressure. The increased pressure in the pulmonary capillary forces fluid into the interstitial space and the alveoli. The fluid that enters the interstitial space decreases the interstitial oncotic pressure. Increased fluid overwhelms the lymphatic drainage. Normally the pulmonary capillary oncotic pressure prevents fluid from flowing out of the pulmonary vessels, but this oncotic pressure is now lower than the pulmonary capillary pressure and fluid is forced to exit the pulmonary capillaries. The only place that this fluid can flow is into the interstitial space and then into the alveoli, producing pulmonary edema. Increased pulmonary capillary pressure, above the plasma oncotic pressure, is the central physiological event that causes fluid to follow this pathologic route. This interstitial edema is the first sign of pulmonary edema. As the fluid accumulates, it leaks into the spaces around the bronchi (peribronchial) and, finally, into the alveolus, preventing gas exchange. Eventually, if treatment is not instituted, more alveoli become flooded with fluid and collapse. Surfactant is washed out and deactivated. Lung compliance falls and the work of breathing increases as more and more of the lung becomes un-

available for gas exchange. Chart 36–8 lists the stages of cardiogenic pulmonary edema.

Systolic Dysfunction

Failure of the left ventricle to effectively propel blood into the aorta during systole is one the most common causes of pulmonary edema (Sanderson & Fraser, 2006). There are numerous causes of left ventricular dysfunction including acute myocardial infarction, valvular dysfunction, and viral cardiomyopathies. Chapter 42 🔗 reviews the pathophysiology of heart failure. Severe heart failure always produces pulmonary edema related to increased pressures in the pulmonary circuit. To compensate for decreased cardiac contractility and decreased ejection fraction, the left ventricle dilates and the pressures in the left ventricle at end diastole increase. This produces increased pressure in the left atrium and in the pulmonary circulation. This pressure is higher than the pulmonary oncotic pressure. The end result is that fluid develops in the interstitial space and then flows into the alveoli.

Diastolic Dysfunction

Another cause of heart failure is diastolic dysfunction (Brutsaert & De Keulenaer, 2006). Diastolic dysfunction produces slowed or decreased ventricular relaxation. This can be initiated by decreased venous return or preload and/or decreased compliance of the ventricle. The result of diastolic dysfunction is an increase in the pulmonary pressure and development of pulmonary edema (Andrew, 2003). Patients who develop acute hypertensive crisis

CHART 36–8	Stages of Cardiogenic Pulmonary Edema
Stages of Pulmonary Edema	**Physiological Abnormality**
Stage I	Fluid and colloids move into the lungs' interstitial space from the pulmonary capillaries. The lymphatics are able to increase flow and remove the fluid. Blood gas exchange does not deteriorate, or it may even be slightly improved.
Stage II	The lymphatics become overwhelmed with fluid and the efficient pump fails. The lung interstitial space becomes flooded. The interstitial space in the lungs is located around the bronchioles, arterioles, and venules in the dependent regions. The accumulation of liquid in the interstitium may compromise the small airways, leading to mild hypoxemia.
Stage III	Fluid continues to flow into the interstitial space. A large amount of fluid can be sequestered in this space in the lungs. With increasing fluid comes increasing pressure and fluid flows across the alveolar epithelium into the alveoli preventing gas exchange. The interstitial space can contain up to 500 mL of fluid. With further accumulations, the fluid crosses the alveolar epithelium into the alveoli, leading to alveolar flooding. This results in abnormalities in gas exchange and vital capacity, respiratory volumes are substantially reduced, and hypoxemia becomes more severe.

Source: Adapted from Sovari, A. A. (2008). Pulmonary edema: Cardiogenic. *eMedicine.* Retrieved June 4, 2008, from http://www.emedicine.com/med/topic1955.htm#.

can have diastolic dysfunction. Increased heart rate is the most common cause of decreased cardiac filling time. In the borderline cardiac patient, increasing the heart rate from 60 to 120 beats/min decreases diastolic filling time by approximately one-half the time the heart has to fill, resulting in cardiac diastolic dysfunction.

Other Cardiac Pathophysiological Causes

Pericardial tamponade from trauma or neoplasms produces increased fluid in the pericardium (Sagrista-Sauleda et al., 2006). This increased pressure around the heart prevents the heart from filling and contracting appropriately and can result in pulmonary edema. The force of the fluid in the pericardium produces increased pressures in the most distensible chambers of the heart, the atria. Again, this increased pressure results in pulmonary artery hypertension and, if not treated, pulmonary edema. This mechanical obstruction to the contraction of the heart usually is easily treated by removal of the fluid.

Valvular dysfunction, whether in a mitral or aortic valve, can cause pulmonary edema. See Chapter 41 for a discussion of the pathophysiology of valve dysfunction.

Another cause of pulmonary edema is atrial myxomas. Atrial myxoma usually is a benign primary tumor of the heart that develops either in the right or left atria. Seventy-five to 80% develop in the left atrium (Percell, Henning, & Siddique Patel, 2003). The myxoma is attached to the atrial wall by a stemlike structure. Myxomas can interfere with atrial function and produce pulmonary edema. If the myxoma becomes detached from the wall and occludes the atria, sudden death occurs. Treatment involves cardiac surgery for removal of the tumor.

Pathophysiology of Noncardiogenic Pulmonary Edema

In noncardiogenic pulmonary edema the fluid fills the alveoli because of direct injury to the membrane itself, not because of increased hydrostatic pressure as a primary event. When excess fluid collects in the interstitial space, special receptors are stimulated to help with clearing this fluid. These juxtacapillary receptors, or J receptors, increase respiratory rate and assist in increasing lymphatic drainage from the lungs.

Clinical Manifestations

The primary presenting clinical signs and symptoms of pulmonary edema are those of respiratory distress progressing to respiratory failure. The clinical manifestations include rapidly worsening dyspnea, shortness of breath, tachypnea, agitation, and adventitious lung sounds (Ware & Matthay, 2005). The other clinical signs are hypertension, tachycardia, and possibly S_3 or S_4 heart sounds. The chest x-ray demonstrates increased pulmonary infiltrates. ABGs are significant for hypoxemia and hypercarbia with a respiratory acidosis. Auscultation of the lungs provides the key assessment clue to the diagnosis of pulmonary edema. Crackles in the bases of the lungs bilaterally usually are an early sign of pulmonary edema. The crackles could advance to fill the entire lung field. Other adventitious lung sounds, such as wheezes and rhonchi, heard over the large airways also could be present. Cough and production of pink frothy sputum are the classic presenting signs of pulmonary edema. Central cyanosis and circumoral pallor, that is, a bluish tinge to the lips and mucous membranes, re-

flects worsening hypoxemia. Pulse oximetry (SpO_2) or the percent of saturation of oxygen demonstrates the hypoxemia with readings in the high 80s to low 90s, and ABGs could reflect a respiratory acidosis with increased carbon dioxide levels.

Chart 36–9 contrasts the assessment of cardiogenic pulmonary edema to noncardiogenic pulmonary edema. Notice that the respiratory assessment clues are identical for both types of pulmonary edema. In the cardiac assessment, some very subtle changes might assist the nurse in differentiating the two types of pulmonary edema. Tachycardia with hypotension and cool diaphoretic skin would be prognostic of a cardiogenic pathology, whereas tachycardia with hypertension bounding pulses and dry skin would be more predictive of a noncardiogenic cause. Jugular venous distention (JVD) occurs if there is right heart failure with a present hepatojugular reflex. JVD is a much more common finding in cardiogenic pulmonary edema than noncardiogenic. If a pulmonary artery catheter were placed, a pulmonary artery catheter wedge pressure (PCWP), or pulmonary artery occlusion pressure (PAOP) of greater than 18 mmHg would confirm a cardiogenic cause of the pulmonary edema. See Chapter 24 for a complete discussion of pulmonary artery catheters. Agitation and confusion are common symptoms of hypoxemia and sometimes are the first symptoms. The nurse should be alert to not discounting these important symptoms when assessing a patient with any type of respiratory distress.

Laboratory and Diagnostic Procedures

Increased interstitial markings on a chest x-ray can be a diagnostic finding of pulmonary edema. The chest x-ray also may reveal

CHART 36–9	Comparison of Cardiogenic Pulmonary Edema and Noncardiogenic Pulmonary Edema	
Assessment Parameters	**CPE**	**NCPE**
Cardiovascular	Tachycardia Hypotension (LV failure) Murmurs (valve dysfunction) Extra heart sounds present (S_3, S_4) PCWP > 18 mmHg Jugular venous distention	Tachycardia Hypertension Bounding pulses PCWP < 18 mmHg
Pulmonary	Dyspnea, orthopnea, shortness of breath Crackles bilaterally Wheezes and rhonchi SpO_2 and ABGs = hypoxemia and hypercapnia Central cyanosis Cough Pink frothy sputum	
Neurological	Agitation Confusion and disorientation If CO_2 high, difficult to arouse	
Skin	Cool and diaphoretic Pallor or mottling	Warm and dry
Chest x-ray	Diffuse bilateral or alveolar infiltrates	

Note: PCWP = pulmonary capillary wedge pressure; SpO_2 = saturation of oxygen obtained from plethysmograph signal amplitudes.

an enlarged heart. ABGs should be monitored at regular intervals for respiratory acidosis with increased carbon dioxide levels. An echocardiogram is indicated to detect a weak heart muscle, leaky or narrow heart valves, or fluid surrounding the heart. Serum testing for B-type natriuretic peptide has improved diagnostic accuracy (Mattu, Martinez, & Kelly, 2005).

Medical Management of Acute Pulmonary Edema

The most important treatment of pulmonary edema is to provide supplemental oxygen and, if necessary, intubation with mechanical ventilation to relieve the symptoms of hypoxemia. Recently, noninvasive positive pressure ventilation (NPPV) using full or partial masks has been used to treat acute pulmonary edema (Liesching, Kwok, & Hill, 2003). This mode of treatment removes the risks of intubation. Supplemental oxygen should be titrated to increase the SpO_2 and relieve air hunger. This treatment is the first line until the cause of the pulmonary edema is determined. Treatment also includes a short-acting diuretic such as furosemide. Medications to strengthen the heart muscle or to relieve the pressure on the heart may also be given. Specific medications are discussed next.

Medical Management of Cardiogenic Pulmonary Edema

After airway management, diuretics and vasodilators are the mainstay for treatment of cardiogenic pulmonary edema. Treatment should focus on aggressive preload and afterload reduction, not just diuretics. Intravenous (IV) furosemide is the diuretic of choice. Furosemide decreases venous return, reduces blood pressure, and decreases afterload. Diuresis should occur within 30 minutes of an intravenous dose. Morphine sulfate titrated to blood pressure relieves anxiety and decreases venous return, although, in higher doses, it can cause respiratory depression. Administering small doses of morphine sulfate, 2 to 4 mg IV, and titrating to blood pressure can prevent this side effect (Brunton, Lazo, & Parker, 2005). Continuous IV vasodilators, such as nitroglycerin, are useful in decreasing preload. In acute pulmonary edema, the IV route is preferred because of rapid onset of action and ability to relieve symptoms. The intravenous infusion can be discontinued and the effects of the drug are quickly reversed.

The safety and efficacy of the angiotensin-converting enzyme inhibitor (ACEI) enalapril were established in a randomized clinical trial to treat pulmonary edema (Annane et al., 1996). In this landmark study, 20 patients received either enalapril or placebo. Enalapril decreased PCWP, systemic blood pressure, and pulmonary shunt in these patients. Chapter 42 includes a summary of the medications used for the treatment of pulmonary edema.

Medical Management of Noncardiogenic Pulmonary Edema

Noncardiogenic pulmonary edema is a wide spectrum of diseases that is caused by either direct or indirect injury of the pulmonary capillary membrane that allows fluids to leak into the interstitial space and then into the alveoli. Another name for NCPE is nonhydrostatic pulmonary edema. This term emphasizes the etiology of this type of acute pulmonary edema, which results from permeability changes in the pulmonary capillaries, not increased hydrostatic pressure in the pulmonary capillaries.

Chart 36–6 (p. 1009) lists some common disease syndromes that are associated with noncardiogenic pulmonary edema (Martin et al., 2005). The first two causes, ALI and ARDS, are covered in the next section. However, some of the other diseases listed in Chart 36–6 (p. 1009) deserve a few words of explanation now. The medical management of these types of NCPE is mentioned if it relates to the etiology and is unique to that type of NCPE.

Acute Respiratory Distress Syndrome and Acute Lung Injury

Acute respiratory distress syndrome (ARDS) is a progressive form of respiratory failure that leads to alveolar capillary inflammation and damage. The term acute lung injury (ALI) is sometimes used when referring to ARDS, but ALI is less severe (Kaplow & Hardin, 2007). In 1994, the North American-European Consensus Conference outlined criteria for ALI and ARDS (Bernard et al., 1994). Chart 36–10 lists the criteria for both diseases. Both are reflections of the same mechanisms of lung injury, inflammation and pulmonary edema that results in hypoxemia (Wheeler & Bernard, 2007).

Epidemiology

The incidence of ARDS is difficult to predict because of the lack of a definitive diagnosis of the disease in most cases. Since 1994 when the definition for ARDS began to be used, most experts believe that ARDS is a major health problem (Ware, 2005). A large study group examining the disease noted its incidence as 64 per 100,000 population or approximately 150,000 cases per year (Goss, Brower, Hudson, & Rubenfeld, 2003). ARDS has a mortality rate of 40%, which is significantly decreased from previous years (Howard, Courtney-Shapiro, Kelso, Goltz, & Morris, 2004). Patients usually die from multiple-organ failure complications rather than from the respiratory failure. The lower mortality usually is seen in centers that are accustomed to treating patients with ARDS where the multidisciplinary team has a clear understanding of the goals of treatment and predicted outcomes. Some diseases and conditions increase the mortality of patients who acquire ARDS, as outlined in the Risk Factors box.

CHART 36–10 Criteria That Define Acute Lung Injury and Acute Respiratory Distress Syndrome

Type of Acute Lung Injury	Criteria
Acute lung injury	$PaO_2/FiO_2 < 300$ mmHg (regardless of PEEP level) Bilateral patchy infiltrates on chest x-ray PCWP < 18 mmHg or no evidence of left atrial hypertension
Acute respiratory distress syndrome	$PaO_2/FiO_2 < 200$ mmHg (regardless of PEEP level) Bilateral patchy infiltrates on chest x-ray PCWP < 18 mmHg or no evidence of left atrial hypertension

Source: Bernard, G. R., Artigas, A., Brigham, K. L., Carlet, J., Falke, K., Hudson, L., et al. (1994). The American-European Consensus Conference on ARDS. Definitions, mechanisms, relevant outcomes, and clinical trial coordination. *American Journal of Respiratory and Critical Care Medicine, 149* (3 Part 1), 818–824.

RISK FACTORS Predictive of Increased Mortality in Patients with ALI/ARDS

- Liver dysfunction
- Sepsis
- Nonpulmonary organ dysfunction
- Age
- Organ transplantation
- HIV infection
- Active malignancy
- Length of mechanical ventilation prior to ARDS
- Oxygenation index
- Mechanism of lung injury
- Right ventricular dysfunction
- PaO_2/FiO_2 ratio < 100
- Chronic alcoholism

Source: Adapted from TenHoor, T., Mannino, D.M., & Moss, M. (2001). Risk factors for ARDS in the United States: Analysis of the 1993 national mortality followback study. *Chest, 119,* 1179–1184.

Etiology

Acute injury to the lungs can be caused by many factors. Usually, these factors are divided into direct and indirect injury to the lungs. Chest trauma with lung contusions, aspiration, and infectious causes, such as pneumonia, are in the direct injury category. In fact, aspiration of gastric secretions is one of the most common causes of ALI (Murray & Nadel, 2005). These entities can cause direct injury to the airways and parenchyma of the lung. In the indirect category are many nonpulmonary etiologies that result in acute respiratory failure. These indirect causes of ALI require the action of intermediary substances that cause the lung injury. These intermediary substances are host defenses that are released when tissue is injured and when inflammation occurs. They include some of the substances listed in Chart 36–11. Their role is to protect the body from infection and disease, but in the case of ALI and ARDS these substances become "overactivated" and become part of the problem instead of the solution.

Systemic inflammatory response syndrome (SIRS) describes the syndrome when these substances of inflammation are activated. When SIRS is caused by infection, it is called sepsis, and with significant hypotension, septic shock as discussed in Chapter 61 ⊕. If other organ systems are involved such as the renal or cardiovascular system, then multiple-organ dysfunction syndrome (MODS) might develop. Severe sepsis with septic shock, acute pancreatitis, and even cardiopulmonary bypass can result in ALI, and if the injury is severe enough ARDS can develop. Acute lung injury associated with pancreatitis is referred to as *pancreatitis-associated acute lung injury* (Pastor, Matthay, & Frossard, 2003). There is a proposed link between sepsis and lung injury. ALI develops in 10% to 45% of patients who develop severe sepsis syndrome (Murray & Nadel, 2005). Chart 36–12 (p. 1016) lists some causes of ALI. This list is not all inclusive and, although it is varied and involves many different disease entities, it is important to realize that almost any disease process that generates a large-scale inflammation and injury pattern in the human body can cause ALI and ARDS. Apprecia-

CHART 36–11   Immune Cells and Cytokines Associated with ALI and ARDS

Type	Definition
Neutrophils or PMNs	White blood cells (WBCs) are part of the nonspecific rapid response to infection or inflammation.
Activated nuclear factor-kappa B in alveolar macrophages	Nuclear factor-kappa B/Rel transcription factors play an important role in the regulation of a variety of genes involved in the inflammatory responses of cells. Alveolar macrophages are monocytes that are located in the alveoli. These cells help the lungs fight infections.
Interleukins (ILs)	Cytokines or cell messengers; inter = between; leukins = white cells.
IL-1-beta	IL-1-beta, also known as lymphocyte activating factor (LAF), activates T-cell lymphocytes, which secrete IL-2, released primarily from macrophages, monocytes, and other cells.
IL-6	A protein that is directly involved in the responses that occur after infection and injury and is called the acute phase response. IL-6 is produced by fibroblasts, activated T cells, activated monocytes or macrophages, and endothelial cells.
IL-8	IL-8, formerly called monocyte-derived neutrophil chemotactic factor. Attracts WBCs.
Tumor necrosis factor-alpha	Tumor necrosis factor-alpha is a serum glycoprotein produced by activated macrophages and monocytes. It has the ability to destroy tumor cell lines and increases the ability to reject tumor transplants. Released early in sepsis, trauma, and other diseases.

Sources: Didier, D., Jean-Damien, R., & Georges, S. (2003). On the physiological and clinical relevance of lung-borne cytokines during ventilator-induced lung injury. *American Journal of Respiratory and Critical Care Medicine, 167,* 1467–1471; Roitt, I., & Delves, P. (2001). *Roitt's essential immunology* (10th ed.). London: Blackwell Scientific.

tion of this concept allows the nurse to recognize a worsening respiratory condition with a potential development of ALI and initiate treatment quickly to prevent further hypoxemia.

There is no cure for ALI/ARDS or treatment that prevents the patient from developing this disease (Vincent, Sakr, & Ranieri, 2003; Ware & Matthay, 2005).

Pathophysiology

ARDS is caused by injury to the alveolar-capillary membrane that allows fluids, proteins, and cell products to flow into the alveoli. Inflammation in the lungs adds to the damage. As alveoli collapse, the lungs become heavy and stiff and difficult to ventilate. Hypoxemia, low lung compliance, and increased **minute ventilation** (V_E) (volume of gas ventilated in 1 minute) are the classic features of respiratory failure caused by ARDS. ARDS is similar to the pathophysiology of pulmonary edema with injury to the A-C membrane. The injury to the A-C

Causes of Acute Lung Injury

Types of Disorders	Diagnoses/Clinical Causes
Infectious causes	Gram-negative sepsis or gram-positive sepsis: Bacterial pneumonia Viral pneumonia Mycoplasmal pneumonia Fungal pneumonia Parasitic infections Mycobacterial disease
Aspiration	Gastric acid: Food and other particulate matter Fresh or sea water (near drowning) Hydrocarbon fluids
Trauma	Lung contusion: Fat emboli Nonthoracic trauma Overdistention (mechanical ventilation) Blast injury (explosion, lightning) Thermal injury (burns) Inhaled gases (phosgene, ammonia)
Hemodynamic disturbances	Shock of any etiology: Anaphylaxis High-altitude pulmonary edema Reperfusion Air embolism Amniotic fluid embolism
Drugs	Suicide gesture (aspiration): Heroin Methadone Propoxyphene Naloxone Cocaine Barbiturates Colchicine Salicylates Ethchlorvynol Interleukin-2 Protamine Hydrochlorothiazide
Disseminated intravascular coagulation:	Incompatible blood transfusion Rh incompatibility Antileukocyte antibodies Leukoagglutinin reactions Postcardiopulmonary bypass pump oxygenator
Metabolic disorders	Pancreatitis Uremia Diabetic ketoacidosis
Neurological disorders	Head trauma Grand mal seizures Increased intracranial pressure (any cause) Subarachnoid or intracerebral hemorrhage
Miscellaneous disorders	Lung reexpansion Upper airway obstruction

membrane occurs when pro-inflammatory mediators, oxygen free radicals, and other cytokines are activated in response to injury. The injury is multifactorial and can be related to other diseases or can be related to increased pressures or volumes caused by mechanical ventilation. Injury from the ventilator is termed *ventilator-associated lung injury* or *ventilator-induced lung injury* (MacIntyre, 2005). The complexity, interrelatedness, and mechanism of action of these host defense mediators are reasons why no cure for ARDS has been found since the disease was first recognized as a syndrome.

Three phases have been identified in ARDS: the acute exudative phase, the proliferative phase, and a final fibrotic stage (Castro, 2006). Although theses phases may assist in categorizing and explaining the complex pattern of pathophysiological changes seen in ARDS, many researchers do not use them to explain the characteristics of this disease (Matthay et al., 2003).

Acute Exudative Phase

The acute exudative phase occurs within the first 7 to 10 days after injury. During this phase, extensive edema is produced in response to the lung injury. This edema fluid is high in protein content and floods the interstitial space, collapses alveoli, and causes hemorrhage. Further damage is done to alveolar ducts and other supporting structures of the alveoli. This diffuse alveolar damage is indicative of the early phase of ARDS.

The functional residual capacity (FRC) is the amount of gas in the lungs after a normal expiration. The FRC of the lungs decreases because the alveoli are no longer filled with air, but are filled with fluid instead. FRC is an important lung volume that can be measured as part of a pulmonary function test (PFT). It also can be measured in some diseases such as ARDS. It is a higher value in men than women (West, 1998).

In ARDS, because the lung is stiff and not as compliant and because alveoli have collapsed or are flooded with fluid, on expiration, the lung recoils to a smaller volume. More fluid and less air in the lungs decreases the ability of the lungs to exchange oxygen and carbon dioxide. One goal in the treatment of ARDS is to increase FRC. Because the lung is now filled with water, there is less room for air. Not every alveolus is collapsed or injured in this phase of ARDS, giving the disease one of its defining characteristics, heterogeneity (Marini & Gattinoni, 2004). That is, some alveoli remain normal in function and structure. If high pressures are used in an attempt to ventilate the patient, these pressures are transmitted to the "normal" alveoli injuring them.

Increased numbers of polymorphonuclear neutrophils (PMNs) also are found in the capillaries, in the interstitial spaces and in the alveoli, adding to the disruption of gas exchange at the A-C membrane (see Chart 36–11, p. 1015). Neutrophils are the body's nonspecific first responders to infection, injury, or inflammation. Once activated by lung injury, neutrophils produce pro-inflammatory cytokines such as interleukin-1-beta and tumor necrosis factor-alpha. PMNs also attract macrophages by producing specific chemical agents or chemokines that signal macrophages. The neutrophils cause damage by blocking the air spaces, and in their mission to destroy bacteria and limit inflammation, they destroy alveolar endothelial cells in the process (Abraham, 2003).

Neutrophils are not the only initiator of ARDS because this syndrome can occur without neutrophils. Patients who are neutropenic can still develop ARDS (Ognibene et al., 1986). As the disease progresses, the alveolar epithelium is swollen and lifted off the basement membrane. A hyaline membrane that is composed of plasma proteins, fibrin, and other cellular debris coats this basement membrane. This hyaline membrane is another mechanism that prevents normal gas exchange. The hyaline membrane is a collection of cells, proteinaceous materials, and necrotic epithelium that line the respiratory bronchioles, alveolar ducts, and unopened alveoli. In Chart 36–13 alveolar ducts (AD) are lined with hyaline membrane (HM). This hyaline membrane occurs because of decreased surfactant and increased lung injury, further compromising gas exchange at the alveolar-capillary membrane. The dense tissue surrounding this alveolar duct is collapsed alveoli.

Pulmonary hypertension can be another symptom that is seen in this phase caused by refractory hypoxemia and excretion of endothelin-1, a powerful vasoconstrictor (Moloney & Evans, 2003). Surfactant production by type II alveolar cells also is affected. Increased lung edema dilutes the surfactant in the alveoli, and the inflammation and damage to the type II cells produces a decrease in the amount of surfactant that is synthesized and recirculated. There also is some evidence that surfactant composition in patients with ARDS is structurally and chemically altered, preventing normal functioning of this essential ingredient of lung physiology.

Proliferative Phase

The next phase of ARDS begins approximately 7 to 10 days postinjury. It is difficult to distinguish between disease progression and pathophysiological abnormalities that occur because of the high ventilator pressures and oxygen toxicity that must be used at times to treat ARDS at this stage of the disease. The air spaces that have been filled with fluid are now narrowed and filled with fibroblasts, specialized cells that attempt to restructure the alveoli. Type I alveolar cells have been replaced by type II cells in the alveolar epithelium. The A-C membrane is thick and not efficient in gas exchange. This phase is marked by proliferation of these fibroblasts. Fibroblasts now are present in the interstitial spaces and even in the air spaces that continue to collapse at an alarming rate. The compliance of the lung is decreased now, and high pressures are needed to ventilate through narrowed air spaces and collapsed alveoli.

Fibrotic Phase

The final phase of ARDS is marked by fibrotic changes of the alveolar ducts, alveoli, and interstitial space (Hudson & Hough, 2006). This phase can begin as early as 10 days after initial insult. These stiff fibrotic structures can be seen on chest x-ray and their "honeycombed" appearance is a classic finding. This structure is a result of the body's attempt at repair. These pathologic changes still can be reversed if the patient's condition improves and the initial insult has been treated. Frequently, patients in this phase require long-term ventilator support until the lung damaged is repaired. Because of these fibrotic changes in the lungs, increased CO_2 retention can be seen at this phase of the disease. CO_2 retention usually is not present until this final stage of the disease.

Clinical Manifestations

The patient presents with all the symptoms of respiratory failure usually after a precipitating event. An early sign of respiratory failure is hyperventilation with a corresponding respiratory alkalosis. At this stage of ARDS, the chest x-ray may appear normal and this rapid respiratory rate is the only clinical sign that is present. As the hypoxemia increases, dyspnea, shortness of breath, and tachypnea with use of accessory muscles is a frequent finding. The skin may appear cyanotic or mottled, which does not improve with oxygen administration. Respirations are rapid, shallow, with intercostal and suprasternal retractions on inspiration only (Kaplow & Hardin, 2007).

In auscultating the lung fields, the nurse may hear bilateral crackles. These are heard in the bases or throughout the lung fields. Coarse rhonchi and wheezes, depending on the severity of the fluid that is flowing into the alveoli, also are heard. In some cases, the pink frothy sputum of classic pulmonary edema is seen. The hypoxemia quickly becomes refractory to standard oxygen therapies, and the patient requires intubation and mechanical ventilation to maintain oxygenation and ventilation. The ABGs frequently demonstrate a respiratory alkalosis in the early stage and respiratory acidosis in the advanced stage. The chest x-ray exhibits the bilateral patchy infiltrates that are characteristic of the disease. This "whiteout" can cover the entire lung field as the disease progresses. Finally, late findings include hypotension and decreased cardiac output.

Laboratory and Diagnostic Procedures

Once a patient is suspected of having ARDS, ABG values are used to detect and document hypoxemia and pH imbalances.

CHART 36–13	Hyaline Membrane Disease of the Newborn

Hyaline membrane disease of the newborn was the name given to the acute respiratory failure of infants who now are classified as having ARDS. The *A* in ARDS had previously been defined as *adult* but was recently changed to stand for *acute*.

The hyaline membrane is a collection of cells, proteinaceous materials, and necrotic epithelium that can line the respiratory bronchioles, alveolar ducts, and unopened alveoli. In the depiction here, the alveolus is lined with this hyaline membrane (arrow pointing to hyaline membrane). This hyaline membrane occurs because of decreased surfactant and increased lung injury. The hyaline membrane further compromises gas exchange at the alveolar-capillary membrane.

Source: Ware, L. B., & Matthay, M. A. (2005). Clinical practice: Acute pulmonary edema. *New England Journal of Medicine, 353*(26), 2788–2796. Photo © OJ Staats. MD/ Custom Medical Stock Photo.

three lumens of this "jet tube" are necessary in order to provide the jet ventilation, monitor airway pressures, and provide a connection for a conventional ventilator. As with HFOV, rates with jet ventilation are extremely rapid: from 240 to 660 breaths/min. HFJV is used in neonates and during surgical procedures that require immobilization of the chest (MacIntyre, 2005).

Experimental Medical Therapies

Many new and potential exciting therapies are being studied to determine if they are efficacious for treating patients with ARDS. Genetic susceptibility to ARDS is being studied by a group of researchers who have discovered a difference in the surfactant protein gene (Gong et al., 2004). Administration of surfactant to patients with ARDS has been attempted in the past with inconsistent results. Timing of the administration of surfactant is one facet of this therapy that is critical for success (Lewis & Brackenbury, 2003).

Extracorporeal gas exchange, either with total support, which is called *extracorporeal membrane oxygenation* (ECMO), or limited support, with just removal of CO_2, which is called *extracorporeal carbon dioxide removal* ($EC_{CO2}R$), remains a very invasive, expensive therapy that has a high mortality, but is used in some cases of ARDS. It is capable of supporting the patients until their lungs heal. Data from the ECMO Registry of the Extracorporeal Life Support Organization (ELSO) reported for the 1980–1995 period a total of 197 adult patients with a 41% survival rate. The neonatal cases number more than 10,000. Failure to respond to maximal ventilatory management was the most common indication for adult ECMO (ELSO Registry Information, 2008).

Fluorocarbon liquid–assisted gas exchange has been studied for many years. Fluorocarbon liquid–assisted gas exchange involves breathing an organic fluorocarbon liquid, which can dissolve 17 times more oxygen than water. This therapy potentially represents a way to oxygenate the lungs of a patient with ARDS without causing further damage to alveoli (Kaisers, Kelly, & Busch, 2003).

Research continues with medical therapies that are attempting to limit the inflammation and the activation of neutrophils and monocytes in ARDS. Exogenous surfactant, corticosteroids, and phosphodiesterase are examples of new medical therapies that could be administered to patients with ARDS to stop this cycle of inflammation (Calfee & Matthay, 2007).

◾ Nursing Management of Acute Respiratory Failure and ARDS

The nursing process guides the care of patients who are experiencing acute respiratory failure. It is imperative that the nurse be knowledgeable about the pathophysiology of the disease that caused the acute respiratory failure. The nurse also must recognize that the treatment for acute respiratory failure is based on supporting the patient until the underlying disease can be resolved. Prevention of the complications of hypoxemia is a primary goal.

Assessment

The nursing assessment begins with airway and oxygenation status. This includes both subjective and objective findings. The pa-

tient must be questioned about whether he is feeling short of breath. For example, ask the patient if he feels he is getting enough air. Objective assessment includes the respiratory rate, the work of breathing, oxygen saturation, and vital signs. Anxiety is frequently present with respiratory distress and must be evaluated in conjunction with the rest of the clinical manifestations. The skin and nail beds need to be assessed for cyanosis and pallor. Lung assessment is critical when evaluating for respiratory failure. Because respiratory status changes rapidly, it is imperative for the nurse to perform frequent and ongoing assessments. Specific clinical manifestations were discussed earlier in the chapter.

Nursing Diagnoses

Nursing diagnoses that apply to patients with respiratory compromise include:

- *Impaired Gas Exchange*
- *Ineffective Tissue Perfusion: Cardiopulmonary* and *Peripheral*
- *Deficient Knowledge* related to the disease process
- *Self-Care Deficit*
- *Ineffective Airway Clearance*
- *Ineffective Breathing Pattern.*

Outcomes and Evaluation Parameters

Outcomes include stable oxygen status and prevention of or resolution of respiratory failure. Evaluation parameters include vital signs and oxygen saturation within normal limits on room air. Lung sounds are clear and the patient denies shortness of breath or air hunger.

Interventions and Rationales

Nursing interventions include deep breathing and coughing, use of an incentive spirometer if ordered, and reporting to the health care provider when changes occur that may indicate a need for oxygen therapy and/or mechanical ventilation. Frequent turning and repositioning of patients has always been a standard component of the nursing care of the patient who is immobilized. In the patient with ARDS, turning is an important part of their care. The nurse should note if oxygen desaturation is correlated with turning from one side to the other or if desaturation is sustained if the patient is placed on a certain side. Patients with ARDS frequently have little respiratory reserve and develop hypoxemia when turned, suctioned, or bathed. Sometimes this desaturation is related to turning on a certain side or after an activity. The nurse can mitigate this hypoxemia by documenting this effect of the activity, so it is not repeated. Paying careful attention to preoxygenation prior to suctioning or to the grouping of nursing activities can prevent decreased SpO_2 and allow turning and other care activities.

Intubation and mechanical ventilation are two major interventions. Successful intubation is an important procedure that demands that the nurse know how to assist the health care provider, administer medications, demonstrate skill with suctioning and use of the **air-mask-bag unit (AMBU)** (a device used to deliver oxygen via a mask when a patient is not adequately ventilating or oxygenating), and document the event in the record.

The nursing care of the ventilated patient involves not only understanding the purpose of mechanical ventilation, its basic operation and common modes, but also the complications of mechanical ventilation. NPPV is being used to treat acute respiratory failure, especially with patients who have chronic obstructive pulmonary diseases and emphysema. Many of the complications of having an endotracheal tube in the airway are avoided with this type of ventilation. This type of mechanical ventilation support is becoming more available to patients who previously were intubated because of technological advances in ventilator design as well as the positive results of controlled studies.

Nursing Priorities During Endotracheal Intubation

The indications for intubation include inability of the respiratory system to maintain oxygenation and/or ventilation. Other indications for intubation include airway protection and elective surgery. Assisting with intubation requires that the nurse know what equipment is necessary and the proper operation of that equipment. It also requires that the nurse anticipate the needs of the health care professional who is performing the procedure. Prior to the procedure, the nurse should explain the procedure to the patient and the family. The patient is positioned on his or her back with a small blanket under the shoulder blades to hyperextend the neck and open the airway. The nurse also confirms that the equipment is working properly. Using an MRB and mask, the nurse preoxygenates the patient. During the procedure, the nurse provides suction as necessary and monitors the patient's SaO_2 by pulse oximetry, as well as the patient's heart rate and blood pressure. Orienting the patient to the need for the endotracheal tube and providing reassurance to the patient are primary nursing interventions.

Documentation of the intubation should include the size of the **endotracheal tube** (a tube used to deliver oxygen that is placed in the trachea) and where the tube is located in the airway. This is determined by the number of centimeters on the tube that is located at the teeth or gum line. The nurse should also document medication administered and how the patient tolerated the procedure. Chart 36–14 includes a list of equipment necessary for intubation.

Oral Endotracheal Intubation

An endotracheal tube located in the mouth produces many of the complications of patients with respiratory failure who require intubation. These complications can be reviewed by referring to Figure 36–6 ■ (Lanken, 2006). If the patient is not properly sedated, the patient can occlude the tube with teeth or gums (1 on the diagram) or remove the tube with her tongue (2). The tongue is a powerful muscle and it is not uncommon for a patient to "tongue-out" the endotracheal tube. The tube can cause pressure ulcers and erode the lips. The endotracheal tube can become kinked in the back of the throat (3).

The cuff of the endotracheal tube is important because it prevents most secretions from being aspirated into the lungs and prevents air from the ventilator from escaping from around the endotracheal tube into the upper airways instead of ventilating the lungs (4). The tube also can be too high in the trachea, which places the cuff in the vocal cords. This apparent herniation of the cuff can prevent the patient from being venti-

---

Equipment for Endotracheal Intubation

Personal protective equipment

Endotracheal tubes with intact cuff and 15-mm connectors
    Adult female: 7.5- to 8.0-mm tube
    Adult male: 8.0- to 9.0-mm tube

Laryngoscope handle with fresh batteries

Laryngoscope blades (straight or curved)

Spare bulbs for laryngoscope blades

Flexible stylet

Self-inflating resuscitation bag with mask connected to 100% oxygen

Oxygen source and connecting tubes

Swivel adapter

Nonsterile gloves

Luer-Lok 10-mL syringe for cuff inflation

Water-soluble lubricant

Rigid pharyngeal suction tip catheter (Yankauer)

Suction apparatus (wall or portable)

Suction catheters

Bite block or oropharyngeal airways

Endotracheal tube securing apparatus or tape

Stethoscope

Anesthetic spray or jelly (for nasal approach)

Sedating or paralyzing medication

Magill forceps

Ventilator

Source: This article was published in *The AACN procedure manual.* Lynn-McHale, D., & Carlson, K. (Eds.). (4th ed., p. 11). Copyright Elsevier 2001.

FIGURE 36–6 ■ Endotracheal tube.

lated properly. The pilot balloon (5) can leak and cause insufficient volumes to be delivered to the patient. Finally, the tip of the tube (6) itself can be blocked with secretions, bacteria, or blood that prevent delivery of adequate tidal volumes (Lanken, 2006).

There is increasing evidence that a biofilm develops on endotracheal tubes that are in place for any length of time. This biofilm is a complex matrix of bacteria that has been associated with ventilator-associated pneumonia (Rello et al., 2006).

Mechanical Ventilation

Indications for providing mechanical ventilation to the patient with acute respiratory failure include treating hypoxemia, hypercarbia, or both. Modern ventilators are termed positive pressure ventilators because they provide an increased pressure on inspiration to the lungs. This is the most common type of ventilator used in the acute care setting. There are devices, such as the chest cuirass and iron lung, that create a negative pressure around the chest and assist with exhalation. These devices are sometimes used in the home. Finally, a combined type of ventilator using negative and positive pressure to deliver the gas is used in some situations. The high-frequency oscillator used in pediatric and adult patients with decreased lung compliance produces an oscillating wave of pressures to deliver the gas. This type of ventilator was discussed earlier in the ARDS treatment section.

Figure 36–7 ■ displays the common components of a typical ventilator, and Chart 36–15 outlines common terms associated with ventilators. The ventilator circuit is connected to the patient and consists of a single plastic tube that fits directly onto the endotracheal tube or tracheostomy. The circuit divides at the wye into an inspiratory and expiratory circuit that connects directly to the ventilator. An important component of this system is humidification. Oxygen delivered without humidification can cause drying of the airways and solidification of secretions. Numerous types of humidification are available commercially.

The ventilator monitors rates, pressures, and volumes, and delivers the set volumes or pressures or a combination of the two to the patient during the inspiratory cycle. The ventilator accomplishes this monitoring and delivery of gas by using microprocessors to synchronize and detect when the patient inspires and expires and to time the delivery of machine support. Another necessary component of the ventilator is the compressor. In hospitals without compressed gas that is available piped in from the wall, a compressor is attached to the ventilator. The compressor provides the compressed air that is mixed with the percent of oxygen to deliver the ordered FiO_2. Some ventilators are equipped with the ability to monitor respiratory waveforms. These waveforms allow the health care team to assess the lung mechanics and

better adjust the ventilator to the patient's needs. The respiratory waveforms are monitored on a screen above the ventilator.

Providing nursing care to the patient on a ventilator has become increasingly complicated for two reasons. First, the complexities of ventilators in use today have increased dramatically with more and more of the functions becoming automatic within user-defined limits. Second, the variety and type of ventilators that are available have increased. The nurse who works on a pulmonary unit might have to learn the unique features of five to six different ventilators. Each ventilator manufacturer also uses many different terms to describe modes and ventilator operations.

In the next section, the most common ventilators and the modes they deliver as well as the implications for nursing care are reviewed. A discussion of specific ventilators and their modes is beyond the scope of this chapter. Many fine references and Internet resources are available that describe particular ventilators (Cairo & Pilbeam, 2004). The major resource for the nurse is the respiratory therapist who is responsible for the ventilator and for ensuring that the ventilator is meeting the respiratory needs of the patient. The nurse is responsible for knowing how the ventilator functions and the meaning of different modes to ensure that the patient receives an integrative approach and the best possible outcome. To ensure optimum care of a patient on a ventilator, the entire health care team must share a common goal, that is, to liberate the patient from the ventilator. But the respiratory therapist and the nurse have an added responsibility to work together in the care of the ventilated patient. The nurse and the therapist must ensure that they are communicating with each other with regard to changes in modes, sedation levels, and daily plans for weaning.

The ventilator decreases the work of breathing (WOB) for the patient. If the ventilator does all the work of breathing, that breath is called a mandatory breath. The ventilator starts the breath, controls inspiratory gas delivery, and determines the end of inspiration. Assisted breaths are those breaths that the patient initiates, but the ventilator controls the inspiratory gas delivery and time. If the ventilator provides any type of support during inspiration or expiration, that breath is defined as an assisted breath.

CHART 36–15	Common Respiratory Terms
Term	**Definition**
Fraction of inspired oxygen (FiO_2)	Amount of oxygen in the delivered gas; expressed as a percent or decimal
Minute ventilation (V_E)	Total ventilation per minute: Respiratory rate $\times V_T = V_E$
Tidal volume (V_T)	Amount of gas inspired with each breath
Functional Residual Capacity (FRC)	Total amount of gas left in the lungs after a normal expiration
Residual volume (RV)	Amount of gas remaining in the lungs after a maximal expiration
Rapid shallow breathing index (RSBI)	Parameter used for determining weaning success: Respiratory rate/spontaneous tidal volume

MyNursingKit | General Information on Ventilators

FIGURE 36–7 ■ Model of volume-cycled ventilator.

If the patient initiates the breath, the trigger or event that begins inspiration is termed patient triggered. If the trigger is not patient triggered, it is usually time triggered. For a respiratory rate of 12 times a minute, the ventilator triggers a breath every 6 seconds. This time-triggered breath also is called control ventilation because the breath is mandatory and the machine is controlling the rate and volume or pressure. Spontaneous breaths are those breaths for which the patient controls the change from inspiration to expiration. Another aspect of this breath delivery is related to the clinician controlling the volume delivered. This is called volume-targeted or volume ventilation. If the clinician wants to limit the pressure, it is called pressure-targeted or pressure ventilation. A debate about which mode is better or more comfortable for the patient began when the ventilator manufactures first gave the clinician a choice between volume ventilation and pressure ventilation. This debate continues today. The nurse should understand the difference between a volume and pressure mode. In volume ventilation, the clinician sets the volume and the pressure varies within certain parameters. In pressure ventilation, the pressure is set and the volume varies. The flow, or the way that the gas is delivered, is different between these two modes.

Nursing Management of the Ventilated Patient and Basic Modes of Ventilation

A mode describes the pattern of the breath delivery (Cairo & Pilbeam, 2004). The health care provider orders the mode that best meets the patient's needs. The mode is selected on the ventilator control panel. Figure 36–8 ■ shows a common ventilator used in critical care units and an enlarged drawing of the control panel, demonstrating the complexity of today's ventilators.

There is no common terminology used in naming the different modes. Different ventilator manufacturers use different names for the modes. Chart 36–16 (p. 1024) compares the modes, key features, and important nursing implications that are reviewed in this chapter.

Assist Control Mode and Nursing Implications

The definition of an assist control mode is one in which the patient can trigger a breath or the breath can be time triggered. Regardless of how the breath is initiated, the preset volume or preset pressure is delivered to the patient each time a breath is initiated. Each breath is a mandatory breath. Some ventilator manufacturers use the term CMV or controlled mandatory ventilation to define this mode. This is a common mode used in caring for the patient who requires ventilatory management. It typically is used with a preset volume instead of a set pressure. It is used in the postoperative patient who is recovering from anesthesia and is still heavily sedated.

Assist control mode allows the ventilator to deliver a set tidal volume for each breath. As the patient awakes and the level of sedation and analgesia decrease, the patient begins initiating breaths. The ventilator attempts to deliver the set tidal volume at a faster rate. Eventually as the rate increases, the ventilator can-

not deliver the set tidal volume and a high-pressure alarm occurs. The patient continues to attempt to initiate a breath because the patient is becoming hypoxemic and anxious because the ventilator continues to alarm without delivering the set tidal volume. There is no time for the full volume to be delivered. This phenomenon is called "stacking" and the high pressures that result from this can cause ventilated-associated lung injury. A simple solution to stacking is to change to a mode that allows the patient to breathe at a comfortable rate and set his own tidal volume. Synchronized mandatory ventilation mode, discussed next, would be one solution. The other option is to increase the level of sedation or analgesia that the patient is receiving.

The nurse who is caring for this patient should be able to assess the situation and intervene to ensure that the patient and the ventilator are working together to prevent patient–ventilator dyssynchrony. Respiratory alkalosis is not uncommon with assist control ventilation because of the patient's ability to increase his minute ventilation (V_E).

Synchronized Intermittent Mandatory Ventilation and Nursing Implications

The definition of synchronized intermittent mandatory ventilation (SIMV) is a mode of ventilation with a set rate during which the ventilator will deliver a set volume or pressure. This is the mandatory rate. Otherwise, patients can breathe between the set rates and receive whatever volume is determined by their effort. These spontaneous breaths also can be pressure supported. The synchronization means that the ventilator will wait for the patient to initiate a breath and then deliver the set mandatory breath in concert with the patient. If the patient does not inspire, the ventilator will initiate the breath.

SIMV is one of the most common modes used in the United States for patients on ventilators. Respiratory alkalosis is not much of a problem unless the set rate is too high. The nurse should record the set rate as well as the patient's rate to determine if the patient is breathing over the ventilator. Most health care providers want the patient to breathe over the set rate in order to use their respiratory muscles. If the patient does not breathe over the set SIMV rate, the team should evaluate the level of sedation and analgesia and consider decreasing it. Also, the set SIMV rate may be set too high. Decreasing the set rate will allow more opportunity for the patient to initiate a breath.

Pressure Support Ventilation and Nursing Implications

Pressure support ventilation (PSV) is an assisted form of ventilation. The patient must have a reliable respiratory effort because there is no set rate nor set tidal volume delivered by the ventilator. If the ventilator senses a negative pressure when the patient inspires, it delivers a set pressure, usually 5 to 10 cm of H_2O to assist with inspiration. Pressure support overcomes some of the resistance of the artificial airways, that is, an endotracheal tube or tracheostomy. It commonly is used in combination with SIMV but can be used as a stand-alone mode in stable ventilator patients who are weaning and have stable respiratory rates. In this situation, the pressure support decreases the work of breathing or at higher levels of pressure support (10 to 20 cm H_2O), the ventilator can assume much of the WOB.

VENTILATOR SETTINGS

| AREA PARAMETERS | AUTO PEEP | PRESSURE SUPPORT | DCI 2.0 | RESPIRATORY MECHANICS | FLOW BY 2:0 | GRAPHICS 2.0 | PRESSURE CONTROL | | | |

PATIENT DATA

AIRWAY PRESSURE cmH$_2$O

—60
—110
—50
—90
—40
—70
—30
—50
—20
—30
—10
—10
—0
—-10
—-10

PRESSURE SCALE HIGH/LOW

- ASSIST
- SPONTANEOUS
- SIGH
- PLATEAU

cmH$_2$O

24

MEAN AIRWAY PRESSURE   PEAK AIRWAY PRESSURE

PLATEAU PRESSURE

RATE I:E

1:2

RATE BPM   I:E RATE

LITERS

5.5

MINUTE VOLUME   SPONT MINUTE VOLUME

TIDAL VOLUME

TIDAL VOL liters

.450

PEEP/CPAP cm HO$_2$

5

SET RATE bpm

12.02%

PEAK FLOW lpm

1001 pm

O$_2$%

40

MESSAGE DISPLAY WINDOW

TIDAL VOLUME	RESPIRATORY RATE	PEAK RESPIRATORY FLOW
SENSITIVITY	O$_2$%	PLATEAU
HIGH PRESSURE LIMIT	LOW INSPIRATION PRESSURE	LOW PEEP/CPAP PRESSURE
LOW EXHALED TIDAL VOL	LOW EXHALED MINUTE VOL	HIGH RESPIRATORY RATE

7 8 9
4 5 6
1 2 3
0 . *
ENTER   CLEAR

CMV   SIMV   CPAP   + +

MANUAL INSPIRATION   MANUAL SIGH   AUTOMATIC SIGH   100% O$_2$ SUCTION   NEBULIZER

VENTILATOR STATUS

- HIGH PRESSURE LIMIT
- LOW INSPIRATORY PRESSURE
- LOW PEEP/CPAP PRESSURE
- LOW EXHALED TIDAL VOLUME
- LOW EXHALED MINUTE VOLUME
- HIGH RESPIRATORY RATE
- I:E
- APNEA
- LOW PRESSURE O$_2$ INLET
- LOW PRESSURE AIR INLET
- EXHALATION VALVE LEAK
- LOW BATTERY

VENT NOP
VENTILATOR ALARM
CAUTION
BACK UP VENTILATOR
SAFETY VALVE OPEN
NORMAL

LAMP TEST
ALARM SILENCE
ALARM RESET

Third-generation control panel for the 7200 ventilator displays potential patient settings. If the mean airway pressure button is selected, the cmH$_2$O could be 24. In the next section the inspiratory to expiratory ratio is 1:2. If the rate in breaths/minute is selected that will be displayed in this window. The center panel illustrates 5 ventilator settings. In the example the PEEP is 5 cm H$_2$O, the tidal volumne is .450 liters, and the rate is 12 with a peak flow of 100 liters and an oxygen concentration of 40%.

FIGURE 36–8 ■ Puritan-Bennett 7200 ventilator and control panel.

Source: Photo reprinted by permission from Nellcor Puritan Bennett LLC, Boulder Colorado, part of Corider. Photo Christelle Montichard.

PSV is commonly used in combination with SIMV. If the patient does not breathe over the set rate in the SIMV mode and has a set pressure support of 5 cm of H$_2$O, the patient does not receive any benefit from the pressure support (PS). Only when the patient initiates a breath does the PS, in this case 5 cm of H$_2$O, assist the patient in inspiration. The nurse should assess the patient and talk to the team regarding the fact that the patient is not breathing over the set rate and determine a course of action.

Another important factor with PS is assessing how much ventilator support the patient is requiring. Because PSV, when

CHART 36–16	Common Ventilator Modes	
Ventilator Mode	**Key Features**	**Nursing Implications**
Assist control (AC)	Each breath, whether patient or machine triggered, is a full pressure or volume breath.	You get "what you set." Patients can become tachypneic and the ventilator has no time to deliver a full breath. "Stacking breaths" can be a complication of this mode.
Synchronized mandatory ventilation (SIMV)	Machine (preset rate) breaths are interspersed with patient-initiated breaths. Patients set their own tidal volume when initiating breaths.	Standard mode used in most critical care units. Used in combination with PS.
Pressure support (PS)	Used in combination with SIMV on patient-initiated breaths. PS overcomes the resistance of the ETT and the ventilator tubing. Provides increased pressure on inspiration.	Only active when patient initiates a breath. If patient is too sedated and does not attempt to overbreathe the set rate, no PS is active. Can also be used in a stand-alone mode called PSV. Patient must have a reliable respiratory rate. The machine does not provide a rate.
Pressure control	A pressure-limited breath is delivered at a certain rate. This is a full control mode.	Usually used for patients who have restrictive disease and worsening lung function. This mode does not guarantee a set V_E (minute ventilation). This must be monitored.
Mandatory minute ventilation (MMV)	A pressure or volume breath that provides a minimum ventilation if the patient's spontaneous breaths do not achieve the set V_E.	Difficult to assess the amount of support the patient is receiving from the ventilator and how much effort is their own. Becomes problematic when attempting to liberate the patient from the ventilator.
Positive end-expiratory pressure (PEEP)	A pressure (usually 5 cm H_2O) that prevents the alveoli from returning to 0 pressure at the end of exhalation.	Increasing levels of PEEP can cause hypotension. All patients need some physiological PEEP.
Continuous positive airway pressure (CPAP)	The same as PEEP except that there is no rate set on the ventilator—the patient is spontaneously breathing.	Can be used with noninvasive ventilation as well as with an intubated patient.
Noninvasive positive pressure ventilation (NPPV)	Ventilation is provided without the benefit of an endotracheal tube.	Patient must be able to cooperate; must be alert and oriented and able to clear secretions.

used as a stand-alone mode, does not have a set rate nor volume delivery, the nurse might assume that the patient can be liberated from the ventilator when in fact, at the upper limits of pressure support, e.g., 20 cm, the ventilator is decreasing significantly the work of breathing. If the PS were removed, the patient would not be able to assume this WOB and would fail weaning. At this point in the patient's respiratory failure, assistance by the ventilator is still required.

Pressure-Controlled Ventilation and Nursing Implications

Pressure control (PC) or pressure-controlled ventilation (PCV) is a full control mode with a set rate and pressure. Sensitivity also is set that allows the patient to trigger a breath. Inspiratory time or the time the patient spends in inspiration is set. The tidal volume (V_T) varies from breath to breath. When the breath is triggered, a rapid flow of gas is delivered to reach the set pressure and then the flow is decelerated. This pattern of flow delivery is an important distinction between PCV and volume ventilation.

In most settings, the PCV is reserved for patients with noncompliant lungs whom it is difficult to ventilate and oxygenate. A patient in acute respiratory failure with ARDS is the perfect example. The nurse should trend the V_E and the expiratory volume over time. If the volume is decreasing, the lungs could be less compliant and the pressure would have to be changed to achieve the same volume.

Positive End-Expiratory Pressure and Continuous Positive Airway Pressure and Nursing Implications

Positive end-expiratory pressure and continuous positive airway pressure (CPAP) are not modes but a ventilator setting that prevents the pressure in the circuit from returning to zero pressure at the end of expiration. CPAP is PEEP when there is no set rate and the patient is breathing spontaneously. The ventilator accomplishes this task by applying resistance at the end of exhalation. There are three types of PEEP: physiological PEEP, which is 5 cm of H_2O; treatment PEEP, which is greater than 5 cm of H_2O; and auto-PEEP, which will be discussed further in the next section.

Most ventilated patients should have PEEP of at least 5 cm of H_2O to prevent the pressure in the alveoli from dropping to zero at the end of expiration. Without physiological PEEP there is a greater chance of alveoli collapsing and not opening again on the next tidal breath. To understand PEEP, it helps to think of pursed-lip breathing. When most people are short of breath, a compensatory mechanism is to breathe through pursed lips. Athletes do this forcibly and older adults use this technique to increase oxygenation after exertion. Obviously, when a patient is intubated the ability to purse-lip breathe is removed. PEEP is a method of allowing the ventilated patient to increase oxygenation. The use of PEEP and increasing the FiO_2 are two methods of increasing oxygenation. The complications of PEEP, that is, PEEP greater than 5 cm of H_2O, are decreased cardiac output, and at higher levels of PEEP, pneumothorax. These complications usually are not seen at PEEP set at 5 cm of H_2O. The nurse should be aware of the level of PEEP.

Prior to extubation, a common practice is to place the patient in CPAP alone on the ventilator. This means that the patient is not receiving any support from the ventilator except at the end of exhalation when the ventilator prevents the pressure from returning to zero.

Auto-PEEP, residual PEEP, or intrinsic PEEP is PEEP that is present in the ventilatory system at the end of expiration. This increased pressure is over and above the set PEEP that is ordered for the patient.

Auto-PEEP can be caused by increased respiratory rate where the patient has no time to expire before the next breath is delivered. This is common in patients with asthma who because of their increased airway resistance require long expiration times. With an increased respiratory rate, the ventilator is attempting to deliver a higher volume than is possible in a shortened respiratory cycle. Other pulmonary pathologies such as ARDS can cause the presence of auto-PEEP because of noncompliant lungs and gas trapping. The higher the set rate on the ventilator, the greater the potential for the development of auto-PEEP. The respiratory therapist can assess the level of auto-PEEP by a maneuver called an expiratory hold.

Finally, the clinician can cause auto-PEEP through the over-aggressive use of an AMBU. The patient is removed from the ventilator for transport or for suctioning. Rapid AMBU rates are used to bag the patient instead of the rate that was set on the ventilator. Treatment would involve disconnecting the patient from the AMBU or ventilator for a few seconds; this would allow the excess pressure to dissipate.

The modes that have been discussed can be seen on the ventilator panel in Figure 36–8 ■ (p. 1023). Note that the CMV mode on this particular ventilator is really Assist/Control as explained. This manufacture elected to call it CMV instead of A/C. There is no standard classification of terms used by manufacturers of ventilators when describing modes. This may create confusion and is especially difficult when the novice is attempting to understand the different modes and their implications for patient care.

Complications of Mechanical Ventilation and Nursing Implication

As soon as a patient is intubated and mechanical ventilation is initiated, the next moment is when the nurse should be activating a plan to liberate the patient from the ventilator. An endotracheal tube and positive pressure ventilation expose the patient to an increased risk of morbidity and mortality. The ventilator and endotracheal tube are necessary interventions to treat acute respiratory failure and other diseases where the patient's own pulmonary or cardiovascular system cannot support exchange of oxygen and removal of carbon dioxide. The ventilator provides this support but not without some risk. One way in which the nurse can prevent the occurrence of this increased risk is to coordinate the care of the patient who is ventilated to ensure timely extubation. Another way that the nurse can impact the care of the patient who is mechanically ventilated is to prevent the complications that can occur. The nurse caring for a patient on a ventilator must recognize the possible complications and work diligently to prevent them if at all possible. The important complications of mechanical ventilation are presented next and are organized by organ systems. This

is not an exhaustive list nor does it deal with some of the complications of long-term mechanical ventilation. Chatila and Criner (2002) present an excellent review of these complications. Nursing implications and prevention strategies also are discussed.

Cardiovascular Complications

Cardiovascular complications of mechanical ventilation are variable and depend on the amount of pressure used to ventilate the lungs, the amount of PEEP, and the underlying heart and lung dynamics. The heart and lungs are a system and what affects one component of that system will usually affect the other. In the setting of cardiac failure, mechanical ventilation can unload some of the stress exerted on the heart by decreasing preload and afterload. This assistance by the ventilator remains invisible until the patient is weaned, and then chest pain and other symptoms of heart failure may develop.

One of the most common complications of mechanical ventilation is hypotension. This can occur immediately after intubation and initiation of positive pressure ventilation or anytime during the course of treatment. This hypotension is related to decreased cardiac output, hypovolemia, and positive pressure delivered by the ventilator. This positive pressure changes the pressure in the thorax. Positive pressure ventilation can reduce ventricular filling by decreasing the amount of blood that flows into the atria (preload) and, therefore, decreasing filling during ventricular diastole. This decreased preload produces the hypotension. Compression of the pulmonary vessels can reduce blood flow into the left atrium or impede the ejection of blood from the right heart. The increased pressure in the chest produced by mechanical ventilation also can affect the dispensability of the chambers of the heart especially during diastole. The increased pleural pressure from the chest can be transmitted to the heart and prevent filling.

Assessment of heart failure and intervening with appropriate treatment in the patient on the ventilator is the primary role of the nurse in preventing cardiovascular complications. If hypotension is the presenting symptom without other indications of cardiac failure, fluid boluses can be ordered that usually correct hypovolemia and reverse the hypotension. The nurse should be prepared to intervene, report to the health care provider, and institute treatment for this common complication. The importance of recognizing the hypotension as potentially being related to the mechanical ventilation is important. The premedications used prior to intubation also can cause hypotension, but will respond to increasing intravascular volume. In some situations vasoactive medications, such as dopamine, might be required to support the blood pressure. Increased levels of PEEP, whether it is set PEEP or auto-PEEP, also can cause hypotension. Decreasing set PEEP levels if hypotension is a direct result of increased PEEP is an important intervention. Preventing auto-PEEP, by allowing time for the patient to exhale or preventing stacking of breaths by adequately sedating the patient or selecting the correct mode, also can prevent hypotension. In some patients, decreased cardiac output and decreased pH can predispose the patient to cardiac dysrhythmias. Careful attention to fluid and electrolyte replacement can help prevent this complication from occurring. Chapter 38 ☺ includes a complete description of cardiac dysrhythmias.

Gastrointestinal Complications

Abdominal distention is a common complication of mechanical ventilation. Gastric distention as a result of swallowed air from pressure ventilation necessitates the routine use of a nasal or oral gastric tube to decompress the stomach. Stress ulcer prevention is another important intervention to prevent gastrointestinal bleeding. Gastric ulcer formation is discussed in Chapter 45 .

Psychological Complications

Agitation, anxiety, and confusion are all complications of mechanical ventilation. It is very uncomfortable for a patient to be attached to a machine to breathe and unable to communicate simple wishes. In addition, lack of adequate sleep and use of analgesics and sedatives also may contribute to this state.

Providing periods of uninterrupted sleep is important in preventing agitation in the patient on a ventilator. Use of a speaking board, lip reading, or a special endotracheal tube that forces air through the vocal cords are all means that can assist the patient in communicating. Sedating appropriately using a sedation scale and individualizing sedation for each patient is key to providing good nursing care.

Pulmonary Complications

Barotrauma is defined as alveoli damage caused by increased pressure resulting from the ventilator. These high pressures are necessary in order to oxygenate the relatively noncompliant lungs of patients who are receiving mechanical ventilation. **Volutrauma** is similar but the lung damage is caused by increased volume that causes overdistention of alveoli. Generally, this lung injury is termed ventilator-induced lung injury (VILI) or ventilated-associated lung injury (VALI) (Suter, 2006). Alveolar damage and capillary leak can occur in the lungs from positive pressure ventilation and are recognized complications of using high pressures to ventilate. Besides the damage that these high pressures inflict on the alveoli, increased pressure can lead to pneumothorax, pneumomediastinum, or subcutaneous emphysema. Atelectasis or collapse of a segment of the lung can occur because of a mucous plug that obstructs the airway. It also can be the result of tidal volumes that are too low to ventilate the entire lung.

Severe airway injury can occur with high pressures, long-term ventilation, or with a predisposing abnormality. The endotracheal tube, the tape, or other devices used to secure the tube can cause nasopharyngeal injury. Ulcerations of the lips, nose, and mouth are too common in patients who have endotracheal tubes and can be prevented in most instances. Sinusitis is a common infection produced by the increase in secretions and the inability of drainage because of the location of the tube in the upper airway. Tracheal damage and tracheoesophageal fistulas have become less common with the universal use of low-pressure, high-volume cuffed endotracheal tubes. Trachea-innominate artery rupture, although almost always fatal, is a unique and rare complication of tracheostomies (Sue & Susanto, 2003).

Oxygen toxicity is another complication of mechanical ventilation that can occur with FiO_2 levels greater than 50% for long periods of time. Most health care providers who are managing patients on ventilators will attempt to reduce the FiO_2 to below 50% initially before decreasing other parameters (Pilbeam & Cairo, 2006).

In patients with severe ARDS, ventilating with high pressures is necessary to prevent hypoxemia. Plateau pressures should be less than 35 cm H_2O (Acute Respiratory Distress Syndrome Network, 2000). Plateau pressure is the true pressure that is transmitted to the alveoli that can cause lung damage. Plateau pressures are obtained by a maneuver that is performed by a respiratory thera-

pist called an inspiratory hold. Monitoring plateau pressures can alert the team to the increased risk of barotraumas. Keeping the plateau pressure to less than 35 cm H_2O can prevent barotrauma (Acute Respiratory Distress Syndrome Network, 2000). The ARDS Network, as previously described, correlated low tidal volumes (6 mL/kg) with improved outcomes versus higher tidal volumes in patients with ARDS. Note, however, that ventilating all patients with this low tidal volume is not adequate to prevent atelectasis. Adequate tidal volumes are necessary to ensure that the entire lung receives enough volume to prevent collapse.

Prevention of soft tissue injury of the lips, nares, and oral mucosal from the endotracheal tube and its attachment can be accomplished by paying careful attention to how the tube is secured. Many different types of tube holders are available besides the standard cloth tape used to secure the tube. Frequent changes of the device and assessment of underlying soft tissue is important. The nurse and the respiratory therapist working together can prevent the patient from acquiring an injury that is preventable.

Humidification of the entire ventilator circuit prevents excessive mucous plugging. There are many methods of humidification, such as heat and moisture exchanger (HME) and heater-humidifiers. Providing humidification is an important intervention when using any type of artificial airway that bypasses the natural humidification provided by the nose and upper airway. If this is not done, mucous plugging can be a common complication of mechanical ventilation.

Finally, prevention of oxygen toxicity can be accomplished by careful monitoring of ABGs and keeping the PaO_2 to less than 50 mmHg whenever possible.

Ventilated-Associated Pneumonia

Ventilated-associated pneumonia (VAP) has been the second most common hospital-associated infection after that of the urinary tract (CDC, 2005). The primary risk factor for the development of hospital-associated bacterial pneumonia is mechanical ventilation (with its requisite endotracheal intubation). Morbidity and mortality increase when an endotracheal tube is placed in a patient's airway. This is one of the most serious consequences of initiation of mechanical ventilation. This mortality ranges from 24% to 50% and, in the case of some high-risk pathogens, the mortality for VAP can be as high as 76% (Klompas, 2007). The rate of pneumonia for intubated patients is 3- to 10-fold that of patients who are not intubated. Along with the increased rates of pneumonia in intubated patients, the cost per admission is greater in patients who are intubated and the length of stay of these patients is significantly increased (Shorr & Kollef, 2005). The CDC (2003a) has published guidelines that are targeted toward medical and nursing staff for preventing VAP, as listed in the National Guidelines feature.

The most common etiology for a VAP is aspiration of contaminated oropharyngeal secretions. Microaspiration occurs commonly in everyone. A small amount of saliva is aspirated into the lungs but this saliva is not contaminated with the amount of bacteria that is common in the saliva of patients who are critically ill. In patients who require intubation, the saliva is commonly contaminated with pathogens that are not normally present in the mouth. The reason that the saliva is contaminated is multifactorial. Lack of appropriate mouth care, the immunecompromised state that accompanies critical illness, and relative xerostomia (dry mouth) are some of the important factors that

NATIONAL GUIDELINES for the Prevention of Health Care–Associated Bacterial Pneumonia

I. Staff Education and Involvement in Infection Prevention

Educate health care workers about the epidemiology of, and infection control procedures for, preventing health care–associated bacterial pneumonia.

II. **Infection and Microbiologic Surveillance**

A. Conduct surveillance for bacterial pneumonia in intensive care unit (ICU) patients who are at high risk for health-care–related bacterial pneumonia (e.g., patients with mechanically assisted ventilation or selected postoperative patients) to determine trends and help identify outbreaks and other potential infection-control problems. The use of the new National Nosocomial Infection Surveillance (NNIS) system's surveillance definition of pneumonia is recommended. Include data on the causative microorganisms and their antimicrobial susceptibility patterns. Express data as rates (e.g., number of infected patients or infections per 100 ICU days or per 1,000 ventilator days) to facilitate intrahospital comparisons and trend determination. Link monitored rates and prevention efforts and return data to appropriate health-care personnel.

B. In the absence of specific clinical, epidemiologic, or infection-control objectives, do not routinely perform surveillance cultures of patients or of equipment or devices used for respiratory therapy, pulmonary-function testing, or delivery of inhalation anesthesia.

III. Prevention of Transmission of Microorganisms

A. Sterilization or Disinfection and Maintenance of Equipment and Devices
1. Thoroughly clean all equipment and devices to be sterilized or disinfected.
2. Mechanical ventilators:
   - Do not routinely sterilize or disinfect the internal machinery of mechanical ventilators.
3. Breathing circuits, humidifiers, and heat-and-moisture exchangers (HMEs):
   - Do not change routinely, on the basis of duration of use, the breathing circuit (i.e., ventilator tubing and exhalation valve and the attached humidifier) that is in use on an individual patient. Change the circuit when it is visibly soiled or mechanically malfunctioning.
   - Periodically drain and discard any condensate that collects in the tubing of a mechanical ventilator, taking precautions not to allow condensate to drain toward the patient.
   - Wear gloves to perform the previous procedure and/or when handling the fluid. Decontaminate hands with soap and water (if hands are visibly soiled) or with an alcohol-based hand rub after performing the procedure or handling the fluid.
4. Humidifier fluids:
   - Use sterile (not distilled, nonsterile) water to fill bubbling humidifiers.
   - Ventilator breathing circuits with HMEs.
5. Changing an HME:
   - Change an HME that is in use on a patient when it malfunctions mechanically or becomes visibly soiled.
   - Do not routinely change more frequently than every 48 hours an HME that is in use on a patient.
   - Do not change routinely (in the absence of gross contamination or malfunction) the breathing circuit attached to an HME while it is in use on a patient.
6. Oxygen humidifiers:
   - Follow manufacturers' instructions for use of oxygen humidifiers.
   - Change the humidifier-tubing (including any nasal prongs or mask) that is in use when it malfunctions or becomes visibly contaminated.
7. Small-volume medication nebulizers: in-line and handheld nebulizers:
   - Between treatments on the same patient, clean, disinfect, and rinse with sterile water.
   - Use only sterile fluid for nebulization, and dispense the fluid into the nebulizer aseptically.
   - Whenever possible, use aerosolized medications in single-dose vials. If multidose medication vials are used, follow manufacturers' instructions for handling, storing, and dispensing the medications.
8. Other devices used in association with respiratory therapy:
   - *Respirometer and ventilator thermometer:* Between their uses on different patients, sterilize or subject to high-level disinfection portable respirometers and ventilator thermometers.
   - *Resuscitation bags:* Between their uses on different patients, sterilize or subject to high-level disinfection reusable hand-powered resuscitation bags.

B. Prevention of Person-to-Person Transmission of Bacteria
1. Standard Precautions
   - *Hand hygiene:* Decontaminate hands by washing them with either antimicrobial soap and water or with nonantimicrobial soap and water (if hands are visibly dirty or contaminated with proteinaceous material or are soiled with blood or body fluids) or by using an alcohol-based waterless antiseptic agent (e.g., hand rub) if hands are not visibly soiled after contact with mucous membranes, respiratory secretions, or objects contaminated with respiratory secretions, whether or not gloves are worn. Decontaminate hands as described previously before and after contact with a patient who has an endotracheal or tracheostomy tube in place, and before and after contact with any respiratory device that is used on the patient, whether or not gloves are worn.
   - *Gloving:* Wear gloves for handling respiratory secretions or objects contaminated with respiratory secretions of any patient.
   - Change gloves and decontaminate hands between contacts with different patients; after handling respiratory secretions or objects contaminated with secretions from one patient and before contact with another patient, object, or environmental surface; and between contacts with a contaminated body site and the respiratory tract of, or respiratory device on, the same patient.
   - When soiling with respiratory secretions from a patient is anticipated, wear a gown and change it after soiling occurs and before providing care to another patient.

(continued)

NATIONAL GUIDELINES for the Prevention of Health Care–Associated Bacterial Pneumonia—*Continued*

2. Care of patients with tracheostomy:
   - Perform tracheostomy under aseptic conditions.
   - When changing a tracheostomy tube, wear a gown, use aseptic technique, and replace the tube with one that has undergone sterilization or high-level disinfection.
3. Suctioning of respiratory tract secretions:
   - If the open-system suction is employed, use a sterile, single-use catheter.
   - Use only sterile fluid to remove secretions from the suction catheter if the catheter is to be used for reentry into the patient's lower respiratory tract.

IV. Modifying Host Risk for Infection
   A. Increasing Host Defense Against Infection: Administration of Immune Modulators
      1. *Pneumococcal vaccination:* Vaccinate patients at high risk for severe pneumococcal infections.
   B. Precautions for Prevention of Aspiration
      1. As soon as the clinical indications for their use are resolved, remove devices such as endotracheal, tracheostomy, and/or enteral tubes.
      2. Prevention of aspiration associated with endotracheal intubation:
         - Use noninvasive ventilation (NIV) to reduce the need for and duration of endotracheal intubation.
         - When feasible and not medically contraindicated, use noninvasive positive pressure ventilation delivered continuously by face or nose mask, instead of performing endotracheal intubation in patients who are in respiratory failure yet do not need immediate intubation (e.g., those who are in hypercapneic respiratory failure secondary to acute exacerbation of COPD or cardiogenic pulmonary edema).
         - When feasible and not medically contraindicated, use NIV as part of the weaning process (from mechanically assisted ventilation) to shorten the period of endotracheal intubation.
         - As much as possible, avoid repeat endotracheal intubation in patients who have received mechanically assisted ventilation.
         - Unless contraindicated by the patient's condition, perform orotracheal rather than nasotracheal intubation on patients.
         - If feasible, use an endotracheal tube with a dorsal lumen above the endotracheal cuff to allow drainage (by continuous or frequent intermittent suctioning) of tracheal secretions that accumulate in the patient's subglottic area.
         - Before deflating the cuff of an endotracheal tube in preparation for tube removal, or before moving the tube, ensure that secretions are cleared from above the tube cuff.
      3. Prevention of aspiration associated with enteral feeding:
         - In the absence of medical contraindication(s), elevate at an angle of 30 to 45 degrees the head of the bed of a patient at high risk for aspiration (e.g., a person receiving mechanically assisted ventilation and/or who has an enteral tube in place).
         - Routinely verify appropriate placement of the feeding tube.
      4. Prevention or modulation of oropharyngeal colonization:
         - *Oropharyngeal cleaning and decontamination with an antiseptic agent:* Develop and implement a comprehensive oral hygiene program (which might include the use of an antiseptic agent) for patients in acute care settings or residents in long-term care facilities who are at high risk for health care–associated pneumonia.
         - *Chlorhexidine oral rinse:* Use an oral chlorhexidine gluconate (0.12%) rinse during the perioperative period on adult patients who undergo cardiac surgery.
         - Oral decontamination with topical antimicrobial agents.
   C. Prevention of Postoperative Pneumonia
      1. Instruct preoperative patients, especially those at high risk for contracting pneumonia, about taking deep breaths and ambulating as soon as medically indicated in the postoperative period.
      2. Encourage all postoperative patients to take deep breaths, move about the bed, and ambulate unless medically contraindicated.
      3. Use incentive spirometry on postoperative patients at high risk for pneumonia.

Source: Centers for Disease Control and Prevention. (2003). *Prevention of health care–associated bacterial pneumonia.* Retrieved May 9, 2008, from http://www.cdc.gov/mmwr/preview/mmwrhtml/rr5303a1.htm.

predispose these patients to developing contaminated saliva that eventually is responsible for VAP (Safdar, Crnich, & Maki, 2005).

Prevention of Ventilated-Associated Pneumonia

What can a nurse do to prevent VAP? A device that has been shown to decrease the risk of VAP is a type of endotracheal tube that has an extra port that allows continuous suctioning of secretions from above the cuff. Secretions collect here and, because of a lack of complete seal between the endotracheal tube cuff and the trachea, drain into the lungs. This aspiration of subglottic secretions prevents the sputum from entering the lungs (O'Neal, Munro, Grap, & Rausch, 2007). The newest endotracheal tube is a silver-coated endotracheal tube that has been scientifically proven as a VAP-preventive device for patients at risk of intubation for 24 hours or longer that minimizes user dependence. In a multicenter clinical trial comparing the silver-coated device to an uncoated tube, the percentage of patients who developed microbiologically confirmed VAP was reduced by 36% for those who received the silver-coated endotracheal tube (Bard, 2008).

Some recommendations by the CDC (2003a) include:

- Hand hygiene using an alcohol-based antiseptic decreased the incidence of hand-transmitted infections.
- Gloving helps prevent cross-contamination. Personnel should use gloves properly and decontaminate their hands after gloves are removed.

- Proper cleaning and sterilization or disinfection of reusable devices used for respiratory therapy, pulmonary diagnostic tests, or delivery of anesthesia helps prevent infection transmission.

The other important intervention is providing oral care to patients who cannot perform their own oral care. Decontamination of the oral cavity either with toothbrushing or use of other interventions has shown a decrease in the rate of VAP in two recent studies (Koeman et al., 2006; Mori et al., 2006). The American Association of Critical Care Nurses (2006) recommends developing and implementing a comprehensive oral hygiene program for patients in critical care and acute care settings who are at high risk for health care–associated pneumonia. Interventions include:

- Brush teeth, gums, and tongue at least twice a day using a soft pediatric or adult toothbrush.
- Provide oral moisturizing to oral mucosa and lips every 2 to 4 hours.
- Use an oral chlorhexidine gluconate (0.12%) rinse twice a day during the perioperative period for adult patients who undergo cardiac surgery. Routine use in other populations is not recommended at this time.

The Complementary and Alternative Therapies box discusses some supportive measures, including the use of vitamin C, that patients can use at home when their pneumonia is not severe enough to warrant hospitalization.

COMPLEMENTARY & ALTERNATIVE THERAPIES

Supportive Measures Plus Vitamin C and Zinc for Pneumonia

Description:

PNEUMONIA is a significant problem in the elderly population. However, it is a condition that is particularly responsive to supportive care. If the patient's condition does not require hospitalization, there are a number of things the patient can do to improve symptoms. Heat is one method of supportive care. When applied in the form of a wrapped hot water bottle to the chest, it can loosen phlegm. Inhaling vapors is another method that can be beneficial in all respiratory conditions, both upper and lower. In addition, postural drainage moves phlegm from within the pulmonary lobes. The older method of postural drainage, cupping, involves a caregiver using a cupped hand patted on the patient's chest also works well. The caregiver should never perform postural drainage soon after the patient has eaten or if the patient has nausea or vomiting.

Vitamin C and zinc are also popular pneumonia treatment and prevention measures. Vitamin C is an antioxidant that protects cells against reactive oxygen species generated during the respiratory burst and in the inflammatory response. Likewise, zinc supports cellular mediators of immunity such as phagocytosis, natural killer cell activity, and the generation of oxidative burst. Both nutrients play important roles in immune function and resistance to infectious agents.

Research Support:

The prophylactic and therapeutic effects of vitamin C on pneumonia was assessed through a Cochrane database search. Researchers identified three prophylactic trials that recorded 37 cases of pneumonia in 2,335 people. In each of these trials, the participants who took vitamin C showed a statistically significant (80% or greater) reduction in pneumonia incidence. Based on these findings, investigators concluded that the prophylactic use of vitamin C to prevent pneumonia should be further studied in populations who have high incidence of pneumonia. This is particularly true for patients whose dietary vitamin C intake is low and who have low plasma vitamin C levels. In the general population, the current evidence is too weak to advocate widespread prophylactic use of vitamin C to prevent pneumonia. However, vitamin C is a low-cost and low-risk supplement, so therapeutic vitamin C supplementation may be reasonable for pneumonia patients who have low vitamin C plasma levels (Hemila & Louhiala, 2007).

A case study in the Netherlands described a 43-year-old male patient with acute sinistral pleuropneumonia and a pronounced thoracic pain syndrome. The patient refused antibiotic treatment, despite his painful ailments. The patient was treated with a complementary therapy comprised of physiotherapy, hydrotherapy, herbal therapy, vitamin C, cupping, and qi gong. A cantharidin blister was applied topically to the left thorax treat the pain syndrome. This combination of CAM treatments resulted in a rapid clinical and x-ray resolution of pneumonia. The cantharidin treatment effectively relieved pain (Rampp & Michalsen, 2006).

A Swiss study evaluated the effect of supplementation with vitamin C and zinc on human immune system function. The study found that vitamin C supplementation improved antimicrobial and natural killer cell activities, lymphocyte proliferation, chemotaxis, and delayed-type hypersensitivity. A large number of randomized controlled trials used intakes of up to 1 g of vitamin C and up to 30 mg of zinc. These trials show that adequate intakes of vitamin C and zinc ameliorate symptoms and shorten the duration of respiratory tract infections including the common cold. They also show that vitamin C and zinc reduce the incidence and improve the outcome of pneumonia (Wintergerst, Maggini, & Hornig, 2006).

A Finnish review evaluated the effect of vitamin C supplementation on respiratory infections in military personnel and other subjects living under conditions comparable to those of military recruits. Seven of the trials involved military personnel, three trials involved students in crowded lodgings, and two trials involved marathon runners. Eight of these trials were double blind and placebo controlled and seven were randomized. In five short, small trials with participants who were under heavy exertion, there was a statistically significant 45% to 91% reduction in common cold incidence. Three other trials found a statistically significant 80% to 100% reduction in the incidence of pneumonia in the vitamin C group (Hemila, 2004).

References

Hemila, H. (2004). Vitamin C supplementation and respiratory infections: A systematic review. *Military Medicine, 169*(11), 920–925.

Hemila, H., & Louhiala, P. (2007). Vitamin C for preventing and treating pneumonia. *Cochrane Database of Systematic Reviews, 24*(1), CD005532.

Rampp, T., & Michalsen, A. (2006). Complementary treatment of pneumonia with pleural effusion. *Forschende Komplementarmedizin und Klassiche Naturheilkunde, 13*(2), 116–118.

Wintergerst, E. S., Maggini, S., & Hornig, D. H. (2006). Immune-enhancing role of vitamin C and zinc and effect on clinical conditions. *Annals of Nutrition and Metabolism, 50*(2), 85–94.

Assessment and Care of the Ventilated Patient

Many of the interventions that are provided by nurses in caring for a patient on a ventilator determine the success of weaning and the prevention of complications. The attention to details and basic nursing care in this population affect the outcome of patients who require ventilators. Among the most important of these interventions is an accurate and detailed assessment. This section reviews the priorities of assessment and care of the patient on ventilation and will include a discussion of suctioning and weaning.

Inspection

Observing the patient and the patient–ventilator interactions is a highly underrated task. To observe the patient on a ventilator, the nurse stands at the foot of the bed and observes how the patient is breathing. The nurse should use a standardized method of observation. A head-to-toe method is one option. The nurse starts at the head of the patient and observes important structures in an organized manner. The endotracheal tube is checked for size and depth of insertion. The method of securing the tube is assessed. A tube that is loose can cause pressure ulcers or, worse, accidental extubation. Presence of an oral airway is noted. Oral airways usually are placed to prevent the patient from biting the tube, but an oral airway can cause significant oral trauma and prevent mouth care. The ventilator circuit is inspected to ensure that it is not pulling on the endotracheal tube or creating tension on the tube. The ventilator circuit should be free of fluid. If fluid is in the tubing, this fluid can lavage the trachea.

The amount and color of secretions in the endotracheal tube and the mouth and nose are noted. Position of the head is assessed. Some patients develop torsion of the neck muscles because they always keep their heads turned toward the side of the bed where the ventilator is situated. Agitation is assessed. Hypoxemia should be ruled out as a cause of agitation and restlessness, especially before administering medication for sedation and analgesia. Cyanosis present around the mouth and mucous membranes suggests central cyanosis and hypoxemia.

Observation of the chest wall for an adequate and symmetrical breathing pattern is crucial in assessing the patient on a ventilator. Assess for asymmetry between the right and left side of the chest. Observe for unusual movements. A tension pneumothorax or pleural effusion can change the size of the affected lung making it appear larger, or the side where an atelectatic segment is located can appear smaller. Both right and left sides of the chest should be symmetrical and rise equally with inspiration and fall with expiration. Paradoxical breathing can occur with trauma to the chest but also with muscle fatigue of the diaphragm. On inspiration the chest rises and the abdomen is drawn in because the fatigued diaphragm cannot descend on inspiration, as it should.

Look for use of accessory muscles of ventilation. Is the patient's WOB increased because of the ventilator mode or size of the endotracheal tube? Phrenic nerve injury or paralysis can affect the diaphragm and can be present on only one side of the chest, producing asymmetry in inspiration or paradoxical movement of the diaphragm, which is another etiology of paradoxical breathing that is described. Is the abdomen distended and protruding into the chest, preventing adequate ventilation? Are the upper extremities more swollen than the feet? Often, patients who have been on a ventilator for a significant period accumulate peripheral edema more in the upper extremities than in the feet. Is mottling present in the extremities? Is the patient shivering? Finally, is there any noise of escaping air heard on expiration that could be caused by too low a volume in the endotracheal tube cuff?

Palpation

Deviation of the trachea is seen in many defects such as tension pneumothorax, flail chest, and in patients who have had pneumonectomies. The nurse begins by palpating the trachea, checking for position as well as mobility. The chest wall is next, feeling for any abnormalities, bulging, or depressions. The point of maximal impulse (PMI) is palpated. Palpating for fremitus is another important component of the assessment. Pleural friction fremitus is a palpable vibration produced when the swollen, inflamed pleural surfaces come in contact with each other. Pleural friction fremitus can be felt during expiration and inspiration but sometimes is felt only during inspiration. Rhonchial fremitus is vibration produced when air is forced through thick secretions.

The chest wall and extremities also are checked for subcutaneous emphysema that is produced by air being forced into the tissue from a pneumothorax or other communication with the airway. Subcutaneous emphysema prompts the team to check for this apparent pathology but usually resolves without treatment. Subcutaneous emphysema is produced when small pockets of air are trapped under the skin.

Auscultation

Auscultation is the most significant component of the assessment in the patient who is ventilated. The frequency of assessment is patient specific and based on other assessment parameters. For example, if the pulse oximetry reading falls to 88% from 99%, after ensuring that the patient is receiving oxygen and ventilation from the ventilator, the nurse should immediately assess lung sounds. For example, absent lung sounds on the left could signal a pneumothorax. The endotracheal tube being advanced down the right main stem bronchus preventing air from entering the left lung also could cause the absence of lung sounds on the left.

The nurse should listen posteriorly as well as anteriorly, starting at the top of the thorax and moving down. It is important for the nurse to listen posteriorly. The importance of this exam cannot be overemphasized. When listening, the nurse should compare right against left lung and never listen through clothing or other material. The clinician should listen laterally in order to appreciate certain lung segments that can be heard in this position. For example, on the right side by listening laterally the nurse can auscultate the anterior basal segment of the right lower lobe. Assessing lung sounds in a ventilated patient can be assisted by performing manual breaths with the ventilator or removing the patient from the ventilator and having someone bag the patient while the other practitioner listens. Normal lung sounds heard in abnormal locations can alert the nurse to certain abnormalities. Bronchial or bronchovesicular sounds heard over the periphery can be indicative of consolidation caused by pneumonia. This sound can also be a result of atelectasis.

Adventitious or abnormal sounds are assessed to ascertain the apparent cause of the abnormality. Crackles occur first in the bases and without the posterior exam the majority of the lung fields cannot be assessed. Inspiratory or expiratory wheezes could be the result of a constriction of the bronchi. Initiation of a bronchodilatory treatment administered as a nebulization through the ventilator circuit might be indicated. Gurgles or rhonchi are low-pitched continuous sounds that are heard over the large airways and sometimes are so loud that the sound is transmitted throughout the lung field. This sound should prompt the nurse to assess the need for suctioning the endotracheal tube. Almost certainly there are secretions that need to be removed. Diminished lung sounds in the ventilated patient can be indicative of pleural fluid accumulation, pneumothorax, or obesity.

Usually, in the ventilated patient, when abnormal or absent sounds are observed, a portable chest x-ray is ordered. The reliance on the chest x-ray should not preclude an excellent clinical exam and an important component of this exam is auscultation of the lungs. Depending on the facility, portable chest x-rays can take minutes to take and even longer to produce the film. Some disorders such as tension pneumothorax can produce a fatal outcome in a few minutes. The nurse at the bedside must be able to quickly assess the change in the lung exam and alert the health care provider.

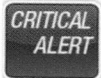 *Tension pneumothorax is more common in patients who are receiving positive pressure ventilation. Air enters the pleural space through a defect in the lung parenchyma and is trapped in the pleural space. As the pressure in the pleural space increases from the trapped air, the lung collapses and the pressure displaces the trachea and great vessels to the opposite side. If not relieved, the remaining lung collapses. This can occur very rapidly. Successful treatment is a needle thoracostomy and placement of a chest tube.*

Nutrition

Preventing malnutrition but at the same time not overfeeding and producing excess CO_2 in the patient who is mechanically ventilated is another important concern for care. Enteral feeding via a nasogastric or oral gastric feeding tube is the preferred method. Small lumen feeding tubes are being used more often than larger bore feeding tubes because of increased patient comfort. Aspiration and other complications including malposition can be prevented by instituting standard protocols and by monitoring problems associated with these tubes at the unit level (Metheny, Meert, & Clouse, 2007). Careful assessment of abdominal distention and bowel frequency can decrease the risk of aspiration. Most patients who are enterally fed in critical care units do not meet their nutritional needs for multiple reasons such as excessive residuals, stopping feeding because of procedures, and loss of access. Interventions to prevent aspiration include keeping the head of the bed elevated and administering medications to assist with gastric motility. Instillation of blue food coloring in the enteral feeding is not recommended because of possible contamination of the tube feeding. A complete description of enteral feedings is presented in Chapter 14 ⊙.

Communication and Sleep

One of the important needs of all patients is to be able to communicate their needs to the people who are caring for them. Inability to communicate because of mechanical ventilation is a concern for the patient and should be recognized by the nurse. Many devices are now available to assist with allowing the patient to communicate. Some are sophisticated such as a speak-

ing tracheostomy tube that allows a patient on a ventilator to communicate. This special tracheostomy tube has a port that can be connected directly to another oxygen source. The port exits near the vocal cords and with some training, the patient can learn to speak. Simple devices that allow patients to communicate include a message board with an alphabet or symbols that they can point to if they are unable to write. The concept is to provide some method for communication.

Lack of sleep is another concern for the patients who are receiving mechanical ventilation. Periods of rest and interrupted sleep should be addressed in the plan of care for the patient. Hospitalized patients typically receive very little uninterrupted sleep and patients who are in critical care units or in other specialty units receiving mechanical ventilation are more likely to be suffering from lack of sleep. Noise level also is a concern (Freedman, Gazendam, Levan, Pack, & Schwab, 2001). One unique intervention for dealing with this issue was a "quiet time" introduced by nurses in a neurocritical care unit. This quiet time was instituted to ensure that patients had some time during the 24-hour period during which the noise level was at a minimum and patients were allowed to rest (Reishtein, 2005).

Weaning from Mechanical Ventilation

Difficulty in discontinuation of mechanical ventilation is associated with critical illness, long-term mechanical ventilation, and lung disease. Patients who have been critically ill or "chronically critically ill" and required prolonged mechanical ventilation have difficulty being liberated from the ventilator (Ely et al., 2001). *Weaning* is the process of discontinuation of a patient from the ventilator. The best process of weaning patients from the ventilator is not known. Some researchers believe that weaning is a process that is provided by a multidisciplinary team of health care providers, nurses, respiratory therapists, dieticians, physical therapists, and others who coordinate the process based on a detailed care pathway in order to be successful (Burns et al., 2003). Other researchers and clinicians believe that health care provider directed–weaning with structured rounds and high availability of health care providers is what is needed (Krishnan, Moore, Robeson, Rand, & Fessler, 2004).

How does the nurse know that a patient is ready to be discontinued from the ventilator? There are two tests that have some ability to predict weaning and extubation success. They are the rapid shallow breathing index (RSBI) and the CROP index (Agency for Healthcare Research and Quality [AHRQ], 2000). The CROP index is an integrated scale that includes a thoracic **C**ompliance **R**espiratory rate, **O**xygenation, and maximal inspiratory **P**ressure. This scale is much more involved and difficult to obtain than the RSBI. Chart 36–17 (p. 1032) illustrates the RSBI scale and gives a clinical example.

Other more multidisciplinary screens such as the Burns' Weaning Assessment Tool (Figure 36–9 ■, p. 1032) have been developed that include other patient characteristics such as fever, strength, endurance, and other nonpulmonary system criteria.

Once the decision to wean the patient has been made, there are many different ways to attempt to wean. The use of pressure support with CPAP on the ventilator is one method. If the endotracheal tube is large enough (i.e., if it has a greater than 7-mm internal diameter), another method is to place the patient on a

CHART 36–17 **Rapid Shallow Breathing Index**

Definition	Clinical Example
Ratio of respiratory frequency f (breaths/minute) to V_T (liters). If $f/V_T < 105$, successful weaning is likely.	Calculate the RSBI for a patient whose respiratory rate is 28 breaths per minute and V_T is 250 mL or 0.25 liters: $28/0.25 = 112$ This patient is probably not ready to wean.

Source: Yang, K., & Tobin, M. (1991). A prospective study of indexes predicting the outcome of trials of weaning from mechanical ventilation. *New England Journal of Medicine*, 324(21),1445–1450.

T-piece with oxygen for 1 hour and then extubate if the patient tolerates the procedure (Krishnan et al., 2004). In a classic study by Esteban and colleagues (1995), four different methods of weaning were compared. A once-daily trial of spontaneous breathing accomplished weaning faster than the other three methods. In fact, this method of weaning is supported as a best practice that is recommended by the Agency for Healthcare Research and Quality (AHRQ, 2000). Use of NPPV in some patients with COPD to facilitate weaning was reviewed in five studies. The results were that NPPV might be associated with some clinical benefit (Burns et al., 2003).

When actively weaning the patient, the nurse should monitor SpO_2, respiratory rate, heart rate, and blood pressure closely and be able to return the patient to the ventilator if the patient is in acute distress.

BURNS' WEAN ASSESSMENT PROGRAM (BWAP)
Copyright Burns 1990

Patient Name _____   Patient History
                                        Number _____

    Patient Weight _____ kg

I. GENERAL ASSESSMENT

YES   NO   NOT ASSESSED

___   ___   1. Hemodynamically stable? (Pulse rate, cardiac output)

___   ___   2. Free from factors that increase or decrease metabolic rate (seizures, temperature, sepsis, bacteremia, hypo/hyperthyroid)?

___   ___   3. Hematocrit > 25% (or baseline)?

___   ___   4. Systematically hydrated? (weight at or near baseline, balanced intake and output)?

___   ___   5. Nourished? (albumin > 2.5, parenteral/enteral feedings maximized) If albumin is low and anasarca or third spacing is present, score for hydration should be "no."

___   ___   6. Electrolytes within normal limits? (including Ca++, Mg+, PO_4). Correct Ca++ for albumin level.

___   ___   7. Pain controlled? (subjective determination)

___   ___   8. Adequate sleep/rest? (subjective determination)

___   ___   9. Appropriate level of anxiety and nervousness? (subjective determination)

___   ___   10. Absence of bowel problems (diarrhea, constipation, ileus)?

___   ___   11. Improved general body strength/endurance? (i.e., out of bed in chair, progressive activity program)?

___   ___   12. Chest x-ray improving or returned to baseline?

Figure 2. Burns Wean Assessment Program (BWAP), RR respiratory rate; ETT, endotracheal tube; ID, inner diameter; NIP, negative inspiratory pressure; PEP, positive expiratory pressure; STV, spontaneous tidal volume; VC, vital capacity: MV, mechanical ventilation.

FIGURE 36–9 ■ Burns' Weaning Assessment Tool.

II. RESPIRATORY ASSESSMENT

Gas Flow and Work of Breathing

		NOT	
YES	NO	ASSESSED	

YES	NO	NOT ASSESSED	
___	___	13.	Eupnic respiratory rate and pattern (spontaneous RR <25, without dyspnea, absence of accessory muscle use). *This is assessed off the ventilator while measuring #20–23. RR = ___
___	___	14.	Absence of adventitious breath sounds? (rhonchi, rales, wheezing)
___	___	15.	Secretions thin and minimal?
___	___	16.	Absence of neuromuscular disease/deformity?
___	___	17.	Absence of abdominal distention/obesity/ascites?
___	___	18.	Oral ETT > #7.5 or trach > #6.0 (I.D.)

Airway Clearance

___	___	19.	Cough and swallow reflexes adequate?

Strength

___	___	20.	NIP <−20 (negative inspiratory pressure) NIP = ___
___	___	21.	PEP >+30 (positive expiratory pressure) PEP = ___

Endurance

___	___	22.	STV . 5 ml/kg (spontaneous tidal volume)? Spont VNT = ___ STV/BW in kg =
___	___	23.	VC > 10–15 ml/kg (vital capacity)? VC =

ABCs

___	___	24.	pH 7.30–7.45
___	___	25.	PaCO$_2$ - 40 mmHg (or baseline) with M.V. <10 L/min * This is evaluated while on ventilator. PaCO$_2$ - ___ MV =
___	___	26.	PaO$_2$ >60 on FiO$_2$ <40%

Figure 2. Continued.

FIGURE 36–9 ■ Burns' Weaning Assessment Tool—*Continued.*

Source: From Burns, S., Earven, S., Fisher, C., Lewis, R., Merrell, P., Schubart, J., Trawit, J., Bleck, T., University of Virginia Long Term Mechanical Ventillation Team. (2003). Implementation of an institutional program to improve clinical and financial outcomes of mechanically ventilated patients: One-year outcomes and lessons learned. *Critical Care Medicine, 31*(12): 2752–2763.

 CRITICAL ALERT *During weaning, if the patient exhibits any adverse symptoms, the nurse should request that the patient be returned to the ventilator and to the settings that the patient had been on before weaning. Symptoms that might prompt the nurse to terminate weaning include:*

Increase in respiratory rate and complaints of dyspnea

Increase in blood pressure

Increase in heart rate

Decrease in SpO$_2$.

Other symptoms might include diaphoresis, nausea, and increased anxiety.

Chart 36–18 (p. 1034) is an example of a weaning plan from a recent study that lists criteria for terminating weaning (Krishnan et al., 2004).

Successful weaning is important to patients in order to ensure continued recovery from their respiratory failure whatever the etiology. The nurse can assist with this process by being knowledgeable regarding the factors that are involved in weaning even though the "best practice" regarding weaning has not been fully clarified. As always, the most important nursing action is assessment of the patient's tolerance to ventilator changes and ultimately being off mechanical ventilation. Vital signs,

CHART 36–18	**Example of Weaning Plan**

RAPID SHALLOW BREATHING TEST (RSBT) SCREENING

f/V_T where f = frequency and V_T = tidal volume.

Patient is not advanced to f/V_T measurement if any of the following are present:

- Known or suspected increased intracranial pressure
- Unstable coronary artery disease
- Heart rate > 140
- Wean screen prohibited by health care provider
- SpO_2 < 92%
- PEEP > 5 cm H_2O
- FiO_2 > 0.5
- Receiving paralytics
- Absent cough and gag reflex
- Unresponsive to noxious stimuli

RSBT PERFORMED AND F/V_T <105

Patient is returned to ventilator if, within 1 hour of initiating spontaneous breathing trial (SBT), any of the following occurs:

- Heart rate > 20 beats per minute above rate before initiating SBT, persisting > 5 minutes.
- Systolic blood pressure < 90 torr (12 kPa) or > 30 torr (4 kPa) change after initiating SBT, persisting > 5 minutes.
- Chest pain or ECG changes (ischemia or new arrhythmia).
- SpO_2 < 88% or PaO_2 < 60 torr (8 kPa), persisting > 5 minutes.
- Marked distress or agitation.

Source: From Krishnan, J. A., Moore, D., Robeson, C., Rand, C. S., & Fessler, H. (2004). A prospective, controlled trial of a protocol-based strategy to discontinue mechanical ventilation. *American Journal of Respiratory and Critical Care Medicine, 169,* 673–678.

FIGURE 36–10 ■ Example of NPPV: BiPAP.
Source: Image courtesy of Respironics, Inc., Murrysville, PA

ABGs, and oxygen saturation levels are measured continuously. The patient may tire after being off the ventilator for an extended period of time and therefore need to be placed back on it to rest. Typically when the patient tires while on the ventilator, the heart and respiratory rate increase, while the blood pressure and oxygen saturation decrease. It is essential for the nurse to intervene when changes occur in order to prevent complications such as a myocardial infarction due to the physiological stress of trying to maintain oxygenation.

■ Noninvasive Positive Pressure Ventilation

Noninvasive positive pressure ventilation is the administration of pressure support and PEEP delivered via a face mask or nasal mask (Liesching et al., 2003). Ventilators designed to deliver NPPV can perform many options. Figure 36–10 ■ shows an example of a ventilator used for NPPV. The patient can have just CPAP without any set respiratory rate or the patient can have a combination of pressure support and CPAP. In patients without a stable respiratory drive or who require more support to maintain oxygenation and ventilation, it is possible to set a rate and two levels of CPAP. This mode of ventilation is referred to as **BiPAP**, an inspiratory level, which is called IPAP or inspiratory positive airway pressure and EPAP or expiratory airway pressure, is set.

The potential benefits of NPPV are that many of the complications of mechanical ventilation with placement of an endotracheal tube are avoided. Among these complications are infections, upper airway trauma, sinusitis, and increased ventilator days related to weaning. It is important to remember that the longer the patient is intubated, the greater the chance of complications related to the endotracheal tube. Psychosocial issues that are avoided by administering NPPV instead of administering ventilator support with an endotracheal tube are another important aspect of this therapy. Patients who are on NPPV can communicate, eat, and require very little, if any, sedation. Figure 36–11 ■ illustrates one type of interface, an oronasal mask that is used to initiate NPPV.

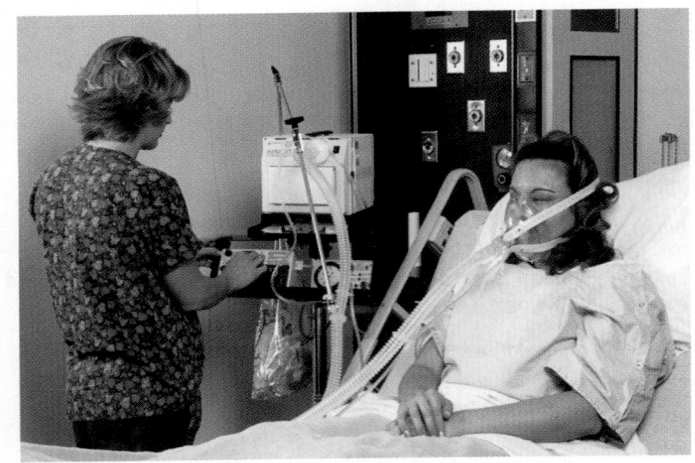

FIGURE 36–11 ■ Oronasal mask.

Nursing Management of the Patient with NPPV

Noninvasive positive pressure ventilation is a mode of supporting the patient with acute respiratory failure by using a mask and ventilator instead of an endotracheal tube. NPPV is an intervention that can be successful in preventing intubation but only when a comprehensive approach to the patient is followed. Patients receiving NPPV require many of the continuous monitoring devices that patients who are intubated require. The nurse should be aware that the most serious potentially fatal complication of NPPV is aspiration. Because the airway is not protected as in the patient who is intubated, patients receiving NPPV typically require more frequent assessments. Continuous heart rate, pulse oximetry (SpO_2), and especially trained nurses and respiratory therapists who are experienced with NPPV are essential for these patients. Two other common complications of NPPV include facial trauma related to the tight-fitting mask and abdominal distention. Chart 36–19 outlines the contraindications for NPPV.

A comprehensive approach to the patient who is a candidate for NPPV is outlined in the Nursing Process: Patient Care Plan for the Patient Receiving Noninvasive Positive Pressure Ventilation (p. 1037). This care plan applies the nursing process beginning with a diagnosis of altered respiratory status. Key interventions with rationales are listed for selection, initiation, and assessment of the patient on NPPV.

Discharge Priorities for Patients with Respiratory Failure/ARDS

Quality-of-life research has helped to focus the discharge priorities for patients with ARDS and respiratory failure who spend weeks to months in hospitals receiving mechanical ventilation. Quality of life is an important but elusive outcome measure in many diseases especially after critical illness. It is elusive because it is difficult to define and measure. Quality of life means many different things to patients. Quality of life has important implications for the nurses who care for patients as they recover from

ARDS. It is important for the nurse who discharges these patients home or to a rehabilitation facility to understand how this quality-of-life issue affects this group of patients.

What is life like for the patient after surviving ARDS? Studies have suggested that quality of life after ARDS is reduced. Some researchers (Orme et al., 2003) believe that patients' decreased quality of life is related to physical functioning caused by the chronic lung injury after recovering from the acute disease. Others believe that the emotional component, depression or a syndrome not unlike post-traumatic stress, decreases the quality of life. One study has followed these patients for 2 years following ARDS and found significant neurocognitive and emotional impairment besides decreased quality of life (Hopkins et al., 2005).

The nurse should be aware of the following implications for rehabilitation in patients recovering from respiratory failure:

- Recognize that depression, anxiety, and post-traumatic stress syndrome may occur after ARDS and obtain treatment and follow-up with appropriate resources, such as psychiatric consults.
- Inform the patient that crying and depression after recovering from ARDS are common reactions.
- Provide pulmonary rehabilitation for the patients after ARDS with a goal of improving lung function.
- Ensure adequate follow-up of patients with their family health care providers or pulmonologists after discharge from the hospital.

The Discharge Priorities chart summarizes the discharge needs of patients who have had ARDS and respiratory failure.

Health Promotion

Teaching the patient how to remove the ventilator mask and what the different alarms on the ventilator mean helps decrease patient anxiety. The nurse and therapist work closely together to accomplish this patient teaching. It is important to determine if the patient and spouse or primary support person are knowledgeable about the reason for the mask and the limitations the patient will experience while wearing it.

After removal of the mask, the patient is reminded that she should continue deep breathing and coughing exercises at least every 2 hours. Before discharging the patient, the nurse emphasizes the importance of rest and a gradual increase in activity to avoid fatigue. Patients are instructed to maintain resistance to infection with proper nutrition and adequate fluid intake. They also are warned to avoid exposure to others with upper respiratory tract infections or viruses. The patient is taught about all medications that will be continued at home. The nurse provides written instructions as necessary.

Collaborative Care

One of the primary examples of collaborative care is the multidisciplinary team of health care providers, nurses, and respiratory therapists who work together to successfully initiate NPPV for a patient.

The health care provider's role is to assess the patient and make the decision that NPPV is an option for the patient. There are many contraindications for NPPV. Timing in initiation of NPPV is crucial. This therapy must be started before the patient

---

CHART 36–19 **Contraindications to Noninvasive Positive Pressure Ventilation**

- Cardiac or respiratory arrest
- Nonrespiratory organ failure
- Severe encephalopathy (e.g., GCS < 10)
- Severe upper gastrointestinal bleeding
- Hemodynamic instability or unstable cardiac arrhythmia
- Facial surgery, trauma, or deformity
- Upper airway obstruction
- Inability to cooperate/protect the airway
- Inability to clear respiratory secretions
- High risk for aspiration

Source: International Consensus Conferences in Intensive Care Medicine: Noninvasive Positive Pressure Ventilation in Acute Respiratory Failure. Organized jointly by the American Thoracic Society, the European Respiratory Society, the European Society of Intensive Care Medicine, and the Societé de Reanimation de Langue Française, and approved by ATS Board of Directors, December 2000. *American Journal of Respiratory and Critical Care Medicine, 163*(1), 288.

Noninvasive Positive Pressure Ventilation

Clinical Problem

Who should receive noninvasive positive pressure ventilation? There are some patient characteristics and some absolutes with regards to patient selection. These absolute contraindications to NPPV are listed in Chart 36–19 (p. 1035). They were established by an international consensus conference on NPPV (Evans, 2001).

But how does the health care provider, nurse, or respiratory therapist decide who would be a good candidate for NPPV? It is difficult to predict which patient will tolerate NPPV. Some patients who are agitated and anxious when placed on NPPV become calm and relaxed. These patients relax because the cause of the agitation was hypoxemia that was resolved by application of the NPPV. If the patient does have any potential contraindications to NPPV, attempting a trial of this therapy is probably the best course for deciding if the patient will tolerate NPPV. However, there is some research that could assist the team in this regard.

Research Findings

Increased use of NPPV in the past 10 years has positively affected the outcome for many patients who present with acute respiratory failure (Hess & Fessler, 2007). Two surveys conducted in this country and in Canada reported that the most common reason for utilizing NPPV is for patients with COPD and congestive heart failure (Burns et al., 2005; Carlucci, Richard, Wysocki, Lepage, & Brochard, 2001). In fact, two meta-analyses demonstrated a survival benefit in patients who were place on NPPV with COPD (Keenan, Sinuff, Cook, & Hill, 2003; Lightowler, Wedzicha, Elliott, & Ram, 2003). Another meta-analysis of 15 trials compared NPPV or CPAP to conventional oxygen therapy in patients with acute cardiogenic pulmonary edema (Masip et al., 2005). This meta-analysis demonstrated a reduced mortality rate of close to 45% for those who received NPPV support. Another population that has benefited from NPPV are patients who present with acute hypoxemic respiratory failure and are immunocompromised (Antonelli et al., 2000; Hilbert et al., 2001). This therapy provides a bridge to prevent intubation in this high–risk, infection-prone population. Two studies have shown a positive benefit and decreased mortality in the NPPV group.

Some evidence supports NPPV as a tool to wean patients early from invasive ventilation. In other words, patients are extubated to NPPV before being transitioned to standard oxygen therapy. Five studies supported using NPPV to promote early weaning from invasive ventilation (Ferrer et al., 2003, 2006; Girault et al., 1999; Nava et al., 1998, 2005). Finally, in patients who have do-not-intubate orders, this method of ventilator support does not violate the patients' wishes, however, this approach is controversial (Curtis et al., 2007). In one study by Levy and others, they evaluated the outcome of 114 patients who had do-not-intubate orders. Forty-nine of these patients, or 43%, survived to hospital discharge (Levy et al., 2004).

Where is the best place to manage a patient on NPPV? Some experts have questioned the use of NPPV in the intensive care unit only (Kacmarek, 2006). One study demonstrated safe care of this patient population on a medical–surgical unit (Farha, Ghamra, Hoisington, Butler, & Stoller, 2006).

Implications for Nursing Practice

In the final analysis, if the patient does not meet any of the absolute contraindications and is cooperative, a trial of NPPV might be warranted if the clinical team feels that the patient might benefit from this therapy. The clinical judgment of health care providers, nurses,

and respiratory therapists is a key step toward ensuring a successful intervention. The research has provided evidence that patients with COPD, those with cardiogenic pulmonary edema failure, and immunocompromised patients might benefit from this therapy.

Critical Thinking Questions

1. An absolute contraindication to initiating NPPV is
   a. do-not-intubate orders.
   b. age greater than 75 years old.
   c. confused and not able to cooperate.
   d. There are no absolute contraindication to NPPV.

2. A common patient population that research has shown benefits from NPPV and that according to utilization surveys NPPV is used in most frequently is
   a. patients with acute asthma.
   b. patients with COPD.
   c. immunocompromised patients.
   d. None of the above.

Answers to Critical Thinking Questions appear in Appendix D.

References

Antonelli, M., Conti, G., Bufi, M., Costa, M. G., Lappa, A., Rocco, M., et al. (2000). Noninvasive ventilation for treatment of acute respiratory failure in patients undergoing solid organ transplantation: A random-ized trial. *Journal of the American Medical Association, 283*(2), 235–241.

Burns, K. E., Sinuff, T., Adhikari, N. K., Meade, M. O., Heels-Ansdell, D., Martin, C. M., et al. (2005). Bilevel noninvasive positive pressure ven-tilation for acute respiratory failure: Survey of Ontario practice. *Critical Care Medicine, 33*(7), 1477–1483.

Carlucci, A., Richard, J. C., Wysocki, M., Lepage, E., & Brochard, L. (2001). Noninvasive versus conventional mechanical ventilation. An epidemiologic survey. *American Journal of Respiratory and Critical Care Medicine, 163*(4), 874–880.

Curtis, J. R., Cook, D. J., Sinuff, T., White, D. B., Hill, N., Keenan, S. P., et al. (2007). Noninvasive positive pressure ventilation in critical and palliative care settings: Understanding the goals of therapy. *Critical Care Medicine, 35*(3), 932–939.

Evans, T. W. (2001). International Consensus Conferences in Intensive Care Medicine: Non-invasive positive pressure ventilation in acute respiratory failure. *Intensive Care Medicine, 27*(1), 166–178.

Farha, S., Ghamra, Z. W., Hoisington, E. R., Butler, R. S., & Stoller, J. K. (2006). Use of noninvasive positive-pressure ventilation on the reg-ular hospital ward: Experience and correlates of success. *Respiratory Care, 51*(11), 1237–1243.

Ferrer, M., Esquinas, A., Arancibia, F., Bauer, T. T., Gonzalez, G., Carrillo, A., et al. (2003). Noninvasive ventilation during persistent weaning failure: A randomized controlled trial. *American Journal of Respira-tory and Critical Care Medicine, 168*(1), 70–76.

Ferrer, M., Valencia, M., Nicolas, J. M., Bernadich, O., Badia, J. R., & Tor-res, A. (2006). Early noninvasive ventilation averts extubation failure in patients at risk: A randomized trial. *American Journal of Respira-tory and Critical Care Medicine, 173*(2), 164–170.

Girault, C., Daudenthun, I., Chevron, V., Tamion, F., Leroy, J., & Bonmarc-hand, G. (1999). Noninvasive ventilation as a systematic extubation and weaning technique in acute-on-chronic respiratory failure: A prospective, randomized controlled study. *American Journal of Res-piratory and Critical Care Medicine, 160*(1), 86–92.

EVIDENCE-BASED PRACTICE

Hess, D. R., & Fessler, H. E. (2007). Should noninvasive positive-pressure ventilation be used in all forms of acute respiratory failure? *Respiratory Care, 52*(5), 568–581.

Hilbert, G., Gruson, D., Vargas, F., Valentino, R., Gbikpi-Benissan, G., Dupon, M., et al. (2001). Noninvasive ventilation in immunosuppressed patients with pulmonary infiltrates, fever, and acute respiratory failure. *New England Journal of Medicine, 344*(7), 481–487.

Kacmarek, R. M. (2006). NPPV in acute respiratory failure: Is it time to reconsider where it may be applied? *Respiratory Care, 51*(11), 1226–1227.

Keenan, S. P., Sinuff, T., Cook, D. J., & Hill, N. S. (2003). Which patients with acute exacerbation of chronic obstructive pulmonary disease benefit from noninvasive positive-pressure ventilation? A systematic review of the literature. *Annals of Internal Medicine, 138*(11), 861–870.

Levy, M., Tanios, M. A., Nelson, D., Short, K., Senechia, A., Vespia, J., et al. (2004). Outcomes of patients with do-not-intubate orders treated with noninvasive ventilation. *Critical Care Medicine, 32*(10), 2002–2007.

Lightowler, J. V., Wedzicha, J. A., Elliott, M. W., & Ram, F. S. (2003). Noninvasive positive pressure ventilation to treat respiratory failure resulting from exacerbations of chronic obstructive pulmonary disease: Cochrane systematic review and meta-analysis. *BMJ, 326*(7382), 185.

Masip, J., Roque, M., Sanchez, B., Fernandez, R., Subirana, M., & Exposito, J. A. (2005). Noninvasive ventilation in acute cardiogenic pulmonary edema: Systematic review and meta-analysis. *Journal of the American Medical Association, 294*(24), 3124–3130.

Nava, S., Ambrosino, N., Clini, E., Prato, M., Orlando, G., Vitacca, M., et al. (1998). Noninvasive mechanical ventilation in the weaning of patients with respiratory failure due to chronic obstructive pulmonary disease. A randomized, controlled trial. *Annals of Internal Medicine, 128*(9), 721–728.

Nava, S., Gregoretti, C., Fanfulla, F., Squadrone, E., Grassi, M., Carlucci, A., et al. (2005). Noninvasive ventilation to prevent respiratory failure after extubation in high-risk patients. *Critical Care Medicine, 33*(11), 2465–2470.

 NURSING PROCESS: Patient Care Plan for Patient Receiving Noninvasive Positive Pressure Ventilation

Assessment for Selection, Initiation, and Assessment of Patient on NPPV

Subjective Data:
Do you think you could attempt a trial of NPPV?
Which interface would you prefer?
Are you experiencing any episodes of nausea or vomiting?
Have you ever had problems with claustrophobia?

Objective Data:
Level of consciousness
Hemodynamic stability
Ventilation
Work of breathing
Oxygen saturation
Abdominal and genitourinary assessment
Vital signs
ABGs

Nursing Assessment and Diagnoses	Outcomes and Evaluation Parameters	Planning and Interventions with *Rationales*
Nursing Diagnosis: *Ineffective Breathing Pattern* that can be treated with noninvasive pulmonary pressure ventilation (NPPV) related to *Impaired Gas Exchange, Ineffective Airway Clearance,* and *Ineffective Breathing Pattern*	**Outcomes:** Patient is candidate for NPPV. Improved gas exchange on NPPV. ***Evaluation Parameters:*** Arterial blood gases improved within 3 hours of NPPV. Decreased work of breathing as exhibited by the patient. Alert and oriented.	**Interventions and *Rationales:*** Assess level of consciousness and ability to follow commands and cooperate *to determine the presence of cerebral hypoxia.* Assess compliance with keeping the mask in place *to determine if the treatment is being tolerated.* Assess level of sedation *to determine if more or less is needed to keep the patient comfortable.*

Assessment for Level of Consciousness and Patient's Ability to Communicate and Procedural Tolerance

Subjective Data:
What is your name, where are you, what is the date, and why are you here?

Objective Data:
Glasgow Coma Scale
Follows commands

Nursing Assessment and Diagnoses	Outcomes and Evaluation Parameters	Planning and Interventions with *Rationales*
Nursing Diagnosis: *Tissue Perfusion Ineffective: Cerebral* related to decreased oxygenation and increased CO_2 levels	**Outcome:** Tolerance of NPPV until it is not needed. ***Evaluation Parameters:*** Able to follow commands. Responds correctly to questions of time and place. *Glasgow Coma Scale (GCS) < 10 and/or inability to follow commands would disqualify patient from receiving NPPV.*	**Interventions and *Rationales:*** Assess neurological status frequently after initiating NPPV. Increasing confusion related to increased CO_2 levels would signify failure of NPPV.

(continued)

NURSING PROCESS: Patient Care Plan for Patient Receiving Noninvasive Positive Pressure Ventilation—*Continued*

Assessment of Level of Comfort

Subjective Data:

What is your pain level at, using the 1–10 scale? A 1 is very little pain and a 10 is the worst imaginable pain.

What is your experience with pain?

Do you routinely take pain medications at home; if so, what for and what kind?

Are you allergic to any pain medication?

Do you have any cultural or religious beliefs that impact your pain control?

Does the pain get worse with deep inspiration?

Describe the pain: burning, sharp, aching, or any other term that is descriptive of it.

Objective Data:

Grimacing on movement

Restlessness and irritability

Taut facial expression

Nursing Assessment and Diagnoses	Outcomes and Evaluation Parameters	Planning and Interventions with *Rationales*
Nursing Diagnosis: *Pain* related to ventilation or other preexisting conditions	**Outcomes:** Pain controlled with analgesia. Level of sedation is adequate. **Evaluation Parameters:** Appears relaxed. Expresses relief of pain.	**Interventions and *Rationales*:** Assess pain and sedation level. *Increasing levels of pain would require increased analgesics that might decrease respiratory drive.* Provide adequate sedation. *Increasing anxiety would prevent patient from tolerating NPPV. Too much sedation could decrease respiratory rate and prevent ability to cooperate.*

Assessment of Hemodynamic Stability

Subjective Data:

Do you become light-headed or pass out?

Do palpitations or light-headedness occur at the same time?

Do your feet swell and, if so, under what circumstances.

Objective Data:

Vital signs: BP and HR

Oxygen saturation

Level of consciousness

ECG

Lab values: electrolytes and measures of acidosis

Cardiac output

Lung/cardiac

Urine output

Nursing Assessment and Diagnoses	Outcomes and Evaluation Parameters	Planning and Interventions with *Rationales*
Nursing Diagnosis: *Decreased Cardiac Output* related to heart failure and hypotension	**Outcome:** Hemodynamically stable. **Evaluation Parameters:** Adequate blood pressure. Heart rate less than 100 beats per minute. Respiratory rate less than 18 breaths per minute while resting. Urine output minimum of 30 mL/hr. Lungs clear to auscultation. Intake and output within normal limits.	**Interventions and *Rationales*:** Monitor blood pressure and heart rate. *Hemodynamic instability, severe tachycardia, and/or hypotension (shock) would exclude patient. Uncontrolled ischemia or arrhythmias would also disqualify patient.* Auscultate heart sounds. Palpate pulses. Assess cardiac rhythm if patient is on monitor. Obtain 12-lead ECG to *further evaluate rhythm.* Administer antiarrhythmic and or beta-blockers as prescribed. Assess extremities for edema. Assess fluid status and JVD. Weigh patient. Administer diuretics. Monitor intake and output. *Fluid overload can prevent adequate gas exchange.*

Assessment of Respiratory Effort

Subjective Data:

Do you feel short of breath?

Is it becoming worse or better?

How long have you been experiencing shortness of breath?

Do you have it at rest or just with activities?

Objective Data:

Oxygen saturation

ABGs

Skin color and temperature

Respiratory rate

Lung sounds

NURSING PROCESS: Patient Care Plan for Patient Receiving Noninvasive Positive Pressure Ventilation—*Continued*

Nursing Assessment and Diagnoses	Outcomes and Evaluation Parameters	Planning and Interventions with *Rationales*
Nursing Diagnoses: *Ineffective Breathing Pattern,* related to lung constriction, lung collapse, low tidal volumes	**Outcome:** Improved ventilation after application of NPPV. ***Evaluation Parameters:*** Decrease in respiratory rate, decreased use of accessory muscles, and decreased dyspnea. Oxygen saturation and ABGs within normal limits. Patient denies increased work of breathing.	**Interventions and *Rationales:*** Assess respiratory status for appropriateness of application of NPPV. *The following respiratory parameters would prompt the provider to **not** attempt NPPV:* *Inability to clear secretion* *Excessive secretions* *No cough or gag* *Impaired swallowing* *Respiratory arrest or unreliable respiratory drive.* Assess facial trauma or anatomic abnormalities that would prevent adequate mask fit. Assess breathing pattern, rate, and depth. Monitor respiratory rate and quality *to assess improvement in ventilation with NPPV.* Assess chest expansion. Note paradoxical respirations. Assess cough and ability to clear secretions. Assess use of accessory muscles during inspiration or prolonged expiratory phase. Assess nasal flaring or pursed-lip breathing.

Assessment for Sufficient Oxygen Saturation Related to Altered Blood Gas

Subjective Data:
Do you have any preexisting health problems such as heart or lung disease?

Objective Data:
Lung sounds
Oxygen saturation
Work of breathing, e.g., gasping, increased rate, loudness
Vital signs
Skin and nail bed color
ABGs
Oxygen saturation

Nursing Assessment and Diagnoses	Outcomes and Evaluation Parameters	Planning and Interventions with *Rationales*
Nursing Diagnosis: *Impaired Gas Exchange* related to pulmonary disease/infection	**Outcome:** Improved oxygen saturation after application of NPPV. ***Evaluation Parameters:*** $SpO_2 > 92\%$ on room air. No increased work of breathing. Lungs sounds clear.	**Interventions and *Rationales:*** Review ABGs and monitor SpO_2. *Ensure that initial ABG/SpO_2 value does not require immediate intervention such as endotracheal intubation.* Severe acidosis ($pH < 7.2$) and hypoxemia ($PaO_2 < 60$) would require invasive intubation. Auscultate breath sounds. Note any adventitious sounds such as wheezes or crackles in the bases. Assess pulse oximetry for absolute value as well as adequacy of waveform. *Waveform should always be monitored with SpO_2 to ensure that SpO_2 is accurate. Dampened waveform can reflect probe displacement.* Maintain $SpO_2 > 92\%$ *to provide appropriate level of oxygen therapy via mask.* Obtain chest x-ray as ordered. Compare film to previous studies *to assess lungs.* Administer bronchodilators if appropriate to increase ventilation.

Assessment of Patient's Coping Abilities

Subjective Data:
How are you feeling about your health and illness?
Tell me what you are feeling about your illness and being on NPPV.
Who are the people in your life that are your support system?
How have you handled fearful situations in the past?

Objective Data:
Facial expressions
Mood
Verbalization of fear regarding injury, impact on family, and future

(continued)

NURSING PROCESS: Patient Care Plan for Patient Receiving Noninvasive Positive Pressure Ventilation—*Continued*

Nursing Diagnosis: *Anxiety* related to discomfort, inability to communicate, lack of adequate sleep, and use of analgesics and sedatives	**Outcome:** Reduced anxiety and confusion. *Evaluation Parameters:* Calm demeanor; acceptance of therapy. Patient can communicate and eat. Mask fits appropriately.	**Interventions and *Rationales:*** Provide constant observation and coaching of patient once NPPV therapy is instituted. *Explaining procedure to patient and coaching will decrease anxiety and promote acceptance of therapy.* Select appropriate mask for patient. Examine patient and note face size. Discuss interfaces and plan for initiation with patient and team (health care provider, respiratory therapist, and patient). *Use of an oronasal or full-face mask with gel mask improves compliance and is more efficient for gas exchange and allows mouth breathing.* Transition to nasal mask if appropriate as patient improves.

Assessment of Soft Tissue Injury of Skin, Nose, Mouth, and Nasopharynx

Subjective Data:
Are you experiencing any pain around, under, or near the mask?

Objective Data:
Skin breakdown near and under mask

Nursing Assessment and Diagnoses	**Outcomes and Evaluation Parameters**	**Planning and Interventions with *Rationales***
Nursing Diagnosis: Risk for impaired skin integrity of face and nose related to poor fitting mask	**Outcome:** Absence of soft tissue injury. *Evaluation Parameters:* No tissue breakdown noted. Skin and soft tissue clear and intact.	**Interventions and *Rationales:*** Apply protective device on bridge of nose *to prevent skin breakdown.* Provide frequent oral care *to prevent mouth dryness and to prevent increase in plaque.* Keep dentures in place *to assist with mask fit.*

Assessment for Abdominal Pain

Subjective Data:
Are you having any abdominal pain?
Do you feel like you are swallowing air?
Are you nauseated?

Objective Data:
Abdominal girth   Vomiting
Oxygen saturation   Bowel sounds

Nursing Assessment and Diagnoses	**Outcomes and Evaluation Parameters**	**Planning and Interventions with *Rationales***
Nursing Diagnosis: *Risk for Injury and Abdominal Distention* related to high pressures, long-term ventilation, and predisposing abnormality	**Outcome:** No abnormal abdominal distention noted. *Evaluation Parameters:* Abdomen soft and nontender. Bowel sounds present. Patient free of nausea and vomiting.	**Interventions and *Rationales:*** Assess abdomen for distention, pain, or tenderness. Assess presence of bowel sounds in all four quadrants. *Persistent nausea and vomiting would be a contraindication to NPPV. Lack of bowel sounds and/or a distended abdomen might increase risk of aspiration with NPPV* If abdomen is distended, consider obtaining order for placement of nasogastric tube *to decompress stomach.* Stop all feeding and oral intake until patient is stable on NPPV. Position patient with head of bed > 30 degrees.

Assessment for Aspiration Related to Insecure Airway

Subjective Data:
Are you feeling like you are getting enough air?
Do you feel more short of breath?

Objective Data:
Lung sounds   Increased work of breathing
Oxygen saturation   Bowel sounds
Vital signs   Abdominal distention

Nursing Assessment and Diagnoses	**Outcomes and Evaluation Parameters**	**Planning and Interventions with *Rationales***
Nursing Diagnosis: *Risk for Aspiration*	**Outcome:** Free of aspiration. *Evaluation Parameters:* Clear lungs. Oxygen saturation within normal limits.	**Interventions and *Rationales:*** Instruct patient how to remove mask if vomiting occurs. *Aspiration is a significant risk for patients with NPPV.*

NURSING PROCESS: Patient Care Plan for Patient Receiving Noninvasive Positive Pressure Ventilation—*Continued*

Assessment of Knowledge Deficit

Subjective Data:

What are your concerns about the diagnosis of respiratory disease in terms of prognosis, changes in lifestyle, and progression of disease?
Do you understand how to take medications and their potential side effects?
Do you understand what symptoms you might have and how to monitor them at home and when to contact the health care provider?

Objective Data:

Patients may be anxious, confused, and need repeated information.

Nursing Assessment and Diagnoses	Outcomes and Evaluation Parameters	Planning and Interventions with *Rationales*
Nursing Diagnosis: *Deficient Knowledge* related to the diagnosis, treatments, and long-term management	**Outcomes:** Patient/family understand: The diagnosis of respiratory disease. Their prognosis and treatments. Lifestyle changes. Symptoms to monitor. *Evaluation Parameters:* Patient/family will: Ask appropriate questions. Follow appropriate medication regimen. Call when their symptoms worsen for urgent evaluation when needed.	**Interventions and *Rationales:*** Discuss with patient/family the cause and prevention of respiratory disease. *This will enhance their understanding of risk factors and prevention.* Discuss how the NPPV works and how to prevent complications. *This will provide the fundamental treatment strategies and should increase compliance.* Discuss the common symptoms of respiratory disease with the patient and family, describing shortness of breath, cough, fatigue, activity intolerance, weight gain/edema, palpitations, chest tightness, and poor concentration. *This will enable patients to recognize their symptoms and reinforce calling early when their symptoms worsen, so they can be seen and have adjustments made in their medications, preempting an urgent hospitalization.*

PATIENT TEACHING & DISCHARGE PRIORITIES for a Patient with ARDS

Need	Teaching
Respiratory care: Patient/family Family support/system Setting	Provide supplemental oxygen if appropriate.
	Instruct use of oxygen therapy and safety measures when using oxygen tanks.
	Provide pulse oximetry in order to assess oxygenation.
	Use values for SpO_2 that are individualized for patient. Document these parameters.
	Provide incentive spirometer if appropriate. Document frequency per day.
	Respiratory medication administration: • Have patient/family demonstrate use of inhalers. • Document frequency for administration of meds.
	Ensure that when to notify health care provider is clear.
	Schedule appointment with pulmonologist and other health care providers.
	Assess availability and knowledge with treatment regime.
	Assess respite needs.
	Assess discharge placement needs: home, rehabilitation, or extended facility.
Emotional and psychological needs, quality of life: Patient/family Setting	Encourage verbalization of frustration with inability to increase activity because of decreased lung function.
	Encourage increase in independent activity as appropriate.
	Stress that depression is common after a serious illness.
	Assess need for psychological counseling.
	Encourage participation in support groups.
Nutritional: Patient/family	Maintain a diet that is balanced.
	Continue vitamins or supplements as appropriate.
	Observe for weight loss and/or loss of appetite.
	Prevent weight gain.
	Institute an exercise program with professional consultation.
Pain management: Patient/family Setting	Assess pain level and report any increase in pain.
	Instruct about the timing and frequency of analgesia medications.
	Assess environment for safety.

Source: Reprinted from *Clinics in Geriatric Medicine, 19*(1), Sevransky, J. E. & Haponik, D. F., Respiratory failure in elderly patients, 205–294. Copyright 2003, with permission from Elsevier.

is exhausted and unable to sustain a reliable respiratory effort. The respiratory therapist and nurse work hand in hand to select the appropriate interface or mask that will fit the patient and prevent large air leaks. The mask needs to be comfortable but tight enough to allow a flow of air to the patient. Coaching the patient and explaining the goal of NPPV is another important role of the nurse and therapist. Nutrition is an important aspect of care and can be maintained with the help of a registered dietitian.

■ Nursing Management of the Patient with a Tracheostomy

Nursing care of patients with acute respiratory failure involves not only care of the ventilated patient but also care of patients with a tracheostomy. Suctioning is a major intervention that is necessary to perform appropriately to prevent airway injury and cause minimal discomfort. Insertion of chest tubes and assessment of the patient with a chest tube is another skill the nurse must master to care for patients with respiratory compromise. Finally, certain medications that affect the pulmonary system and delivery of these medications are another facet of the care of patients with acute respiratory failure.

Interventions and Rationales
Tracheostomy Tube
There is very little information of when is the optimum time for performing a tracheostomy on a patient who is mechanically ventilated. A tracheostomy is an elective surgical procedure. The surgeon creates a small incision in the skin and opens the lower

trachea in order to place a small tube, called a tracheostomy tube. This tube is more stable and secure and has less dead space than an endotracheal tube. Some experts suggest 2 weeks on mechanical ventilation as the optimum time before this surgical procedure is performed (Engoren, Arslanian-Engoren, & Fenn-Buderer, 2004). The benefits to the patient include patient comfort, a secure airway, effective airway suctioning, decreased airway resistance and dead space, better patient mobility, increased opportunities for communication, and the ability to eat.

On the other side, the patient faces some risks with this procedure. The major risks of tracheostomy include bleeding, inappropriate incision location, thyroid injury, pneumothorax, tracheoesophageal fistula, hypoxemia, and infection (Sue & Susanto, 2003). The ability to insert a tracheostomy tube at the bedside percutaneously also has increased the potential frequency of tracheostomies (Polderman et al., 2003).

As the patient improves and is liberated from the ventilator, the tracheostomy tube may be changed and decreased in size until the patient can be decannulated. The first tracheostomy tube change should not be performed until 7 to 10 days after the procedure in order to allow the stoma and tracheostomy tract to mature. In some clinical situations, a fenestrated tracheostomy tube is used (see Figure 36–12 ■). This allows the patient to breathe around

FIGURE 36–12 ■ Tracheostomy tube with inner cannula and fenestrated outer cannula.

FIGURE 36–13 ■ Passey Muir valve used on end of tracheostomy tube.
Source: Courtesy of Passy-Muir, Inc.

the tube more easily when the cuff is deflated. With the addition of a one-way valve on the end of the tracheostomy tube, the patient can inspire from the tracheostomy tube and expire, forcing air into the larynx around the vocal cord to produce audible sounds. Two devices that are available are the Passey-Muir valve (Figure 36–13 ■) or Olympic Trach-Talk one-way valve. This is a great advantage for the patient who feels elated that he can now communicate directly with the staff. Nursing management of the tracheostomy tube is discussed in detail in Chapter 34 ☞.

Suctioning

Another important component of the care of the patient who is ventilated is assessing the need for suctioning and performing this procedure appropriately. Chart 36–20 (p. 1044) reviews the suctioning procedure. Some key points of this procedure need to be emphasized:

- Suctioning is only performed based on clinical assessment; it is never ordered routinely.

- Complications of suctioning include hypoxemia, bronchospasms, cardiac arrhythmias, tissue injury, and increased risk of infection.

- Hyperoxygenation prior to and after suctioning is essential to limit hypoxemia.

- Normal saline should *not* be instilled routinely into the airway prior to suctioning.

- Closed suctioning systems (Figure 36–14 ■) should be used in patients with high PEEP and/or FiO_2 and patients who cannot tolerate suctioning with an open system or have an infectious disease that could be spread by aerosolization of secretions.

■ Administration of Common Respiratory Medications

A variety of respiratory medications are delivered through the aerosolized route using many different types of devices. Two of the most common devices are metered-dose inhalers (MDIs) with and without spacers and small-volume nebulizers (SVN).

FIGURE 36–14 ■ Ballard catheter.
Source: © 2007 Kimberly-Clark Worldwide Inc. Used with permission.

The nurse should be knowledgeable about the medication that is being administered and the important side effects. The nurse should understand how to administer an MDI and how to teach patients to administer their medication appropriately.

Medication is administered via the aerosolized route for many reasons. Because the medication is not given systemically, the ratio of dose to effect is high. Medication given via this route can be dosed at a lower level because the medication is delivered directly to the lungs. Because of the lower dose, fewer side effects will occur. Delivering medication directly to the lungs also is convenient and less expensive than other routes (Karwa et al., 2005).

Health Promotion

Teaching patients about the proper use and side effects of medication is a basic nursing function. The importance of this teaching is emphasized in teaching patients about respiratory medications. Improper timing and overuse of respiratory medications can prevent the medications from working properly and in a worst case scenario cause increasing symptoms and respiratory failure. For example, one of the most common devices that is used to deliver bronchodilators is the MDI. However, this device must be used correctly and patients must be taught how to use it.

One of the most effective methods of teaching patients about MDIs is for a member of the health care team to demonstrate use of the device and then to ask the patient to perform a return demonstration. This teaching can be accomplished in an acute care setting and usually takes less than 10 minutes. A recent study examined teaching time in an emergency setting and found that the mean teaching time was 6.5 minutes (Numata, Bourbeau, Ernst, Duquette, & Schwartzman, 2002). The majority of the patients in this study reported satisfaction with the teaching and treatment. To teach the patient correctly, the nurse must follow the steps described in Chart 36–21 (p. 1045).

CHART 36–20   Suctioning Procedure

EQUIPMENT

Sterile suction catheter

Sterile gloves

Sterile normal saline for irrigation, when indicated

Sterile disposable container

TECHNIQUE

1. Perform routine procedures before suction. Administer medication, assemble equipment, explain the procedure to the patient, adjust bed to comfortable working position, prepare suction pressure, wash hands, and don gloves.

2. Hyperoxygenate the patient with 100% oxygen, using a manual resuscitation bag (MRB) or the ventilator. If the ventilator method is used, preoxygenation must last at least 3 minutes. Return to the previous oxygen setting after suctioning is completed. (Clinical research shows that the use of the patient's ventilator for preoxygenation delivers higher oxygen concentrations and lower peak pressures than those generated with an MRB (Doering, 1993). In patients who do not tolerate suction with hyperoxygenation, a positive end-expiratory pressure (PEEP) attachment should be on the MRB at the appropriate setting, or in-line suctioning should be used to avoid loss of PEEP and desaturation.

3. Quickly, but gently, insert the catheter as far as possible into the artificial airway without application of suction.

4. Withdraw the catheter 1–2 cm, and apply intermittent suction while rotating and removing the catheter. Limit suction pressure to −80 to −120 mm Hg. Aspiration should not exceed 10 to 15 seconds. (Prolonged aspiration can lead to severe hypoxia, hemodynamic instability, and ultimately, cardiac arrest.

5. Hyperoxygenate the patient before and after each subsequent pass of the catheter for at least 30 seconds, and before reconnection to the ventilator.

6. Monitor heart rate and rhythm and pulse oximetry during and after suctioning.
   Discontinue the procedure if the patient does not tolerate it as evidenced by dysrhythmias, bradycardia, or a drop in SaO_2.

7. Remove equipment.

8. Perform oral hygiene.

9. Clean suction tubing.

10. Wash your hands.

11. Document procedure.

Source: Doering, L. V. (1993). The effect of positioning on hemodynamics and gas exchange in the critically ill: a review. *American Journal of Critical Care, 2,* 208–216. Used with permission; Morton, P. G., Fontaine, D. K., Hudak, C. M., & Gallo, B. M. 8th ed. *Critical care nursing. A holistic approach.* (2005) Philadelphia, Lippincott, Williams & Wilkins.

RESEARCH OPPORTUNITIES AND CLINICAL IMPACT RELATED TO COMPLEX RESPIRATORY DISORDERS

Research Area	Clinical Impact
ARDS and proning in adults	Improving oxygenation and preventing further lung injury
Ventilator management for the treatment of ARDS: 　Ventilator settings 　Mode selection 　Pressure versus volume 　Noninvasive ventilation in the treatment of ARDS 　HFOV	
Liquid ventilation	
ECMO for the treatment of ARDS	
Fluid management in ARDS	
Use of hemodynamic monitoring in the patient with ARDS	
Ventilated-associated pneumonia	Preventing VAP
Role of mouth care in decreasing pathogenic organisms in the oral plaque biofilm	
Other methods of preventing VAP: 　Patient positioning 　Use of subglottic endotracheal tube 　Antibiotic-coated endotracheal tube	
Quality of life in patients with lung disease	Improving quality of life after discharge Appropriate discharge criteria
Use of NPPV and weaning	Improving weaning
Incorporate this mode of weaning into weaning strategies	
NPPV and indications for instituting this mode of ventilation in cardiac failure and respiratory failure	Wider use of NPPV for many types of cardiac and respiratory failure
NPPV interfaces: 　Improved masks 　Improved ventilators that compensate for leaks	Improved interfaces that will improve patient compliance

CHART 36–21 Steps for Teaching a Patient How to Use a Metered-Dose Inhaler

The nurse should demonstrate this technique and then evaluate the patient's technique using the following checklist:

1. Removes cap from the MDI device.
2. Shakes the MDI.
3. Correctly inserts the MDI into the chamber.
4. Exhales prior to actuation.
5. Places chamber into mouth and closes lips around chamber.
6. Properly times actuation by beginning actuation and inhaling dose.
7. Holds breath for more than 5–10 seconds after dose.
8. Waits at least 30 seconds before administering next dose.

Sources: Numata, Y., Bourbeau, J., Ernst, P., Duquette, G., & Schwartzman, K. (2002). Teaching time for metered-dose inhalers in the emergency setting. *Chest, 122*(2), 498–504; Resnick, D. J., Gold, R. L., Lee-Wong, M., Feldman, B. R., Ramakrishnan, R., & Davis, W. J. (1996). Physicians' metered dose inhaler technique after a single teaching session. *Annals of Allergy and Asthma Immunology, 76*(2), 145–148.

■ Research

Research on complex respiratory disorders has led to tremendous advances in diagnosis and treatment, ultimately saving lives and improving the quality of life. The treatments outlined earlier in the chapter represent evidenced-based practice that resulted from ongoing research. There continue to be unanswered questions related to all aspects of complex respiratory disease. Therefore, research continues to strive to answer these questions in order to decrease the morbidity and mortality associated with these life-threatening disorders. The Research Opportunities feature outlines future directions in research studies related to complex respiratory diseases.

Clinical Preparation

 Read

- History of Current Illness
- Past Medical History
- Physical Exam
- Admitting Medical Orders
- Laboratory Study Results

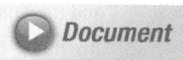 **Document**

- Summary of Hospitalization
- Pathophysiology Form
- Laboratory Values
- Laboratory Results Explanation

 Apply

- List of Potential Nursing Diagnoses
- Concept Map
- Critical Thinking Questions

Log on to MyNursingKit.com to download forms you will need and to complete further steps in the Clinical Preparation assignment.

HISTORY OF PRESENT ILLNESS

Mr. A is a 52-year-old man admitted to your unit with a diagnosis of pneumonia with increasing shortness of breath during the past several days. He is admitted from the emergency department receiving oxygen via nasal cannula at 6 L/min. Three days ago Mr. A stated that he "didn't feel right" and stayed home from work. He thought he had a cold and was congested and sneezing. He reported not being able to sleep lying flat. Last night he was awakened by an episode of severe shortness of breath. He called 911 and was transported to the hospital. On admission to the emergency department he was febrile at 39.4°C (102.9°F) with a pulse oximeter of 88% on room air. Oxygen via nasal cannula was instituted, which increased the pulse oximetry reading to 92%. A portable chest x-ray demonstrated consolidation of the right middle and lower lobe. Blood, sputum, and urine cultures were obtained and antibiotics were initiated. The patient was admitted to the special respiratory unit for further treatment. Continuous pulse oximetry, coughing and deep breathing encouragement, and Tylenol for fever are the nursing priorities for Mr. A on admission. Careful attention to the timing of his antibiotic doses also is a priority.

Medical–Surgical History

He has never been hospitalized before, but has a history of hypertension that is being treated with the angiotensin-converting enzyme inhibitor irbesartan (Avapro), 150 mg, and hydrochlorothiazide, 12.5 mg, each once a day.

Social History

Mr. A is a sedentary business executive who is 76 inches tall and weighs 250 pounds. He lives by himself, and has no close relatives locally.

Physical Examination

On physical exam, Mr. A is alert and oriented but anxious. His cardiac exam reveals bounding pulses with normal heart sounds and no jugular venous distention. He denies any chest pain or any type of pain except discomfort related to breathing and shortness of breath. His respiratory rate is rapid but his chest excursion is equal bilaterally. He is using accessory muscles for respiration and is sitting straight up in bed. On auscultation, he has decreased breath sounds on the right side with wet crackles heard posteriorly over the entire right lung field. His cough is productive for sputum that is thick, yellow, and tenacious. His blood pressure is 150/90; heart rate is 100 beats per minute with a respiratory rate of 34 to 36 per minute, and pulse oximetry fluctuating between 90% and 92% on 6 liters nasal cannula. His temperature is running 38° to 40°C (100.4° to 104°F). Abdomen is large but soft and nontender. He denies any problems with urination or defecation. His last bowel movement was yesterday. Skin is warm and dry with no areas of breakdown noted. An intravenous infusion is present in his left forearm with antibiotics infusing.

Admitting Medical Orders

Admit to MIC
Service: MICU
Condition: guarded
Admitting diagnosis: pneumonia
Allergies: no known drug allergies
Vital signs and O_2 sats q1h
Activity: bed rest
Diet: regular
Daily weight
Continuous cardiac monitor
Continuous pulse oximetry
Call house officer: HR < 60 or >120, systolic blood pressure < 90 or > 160, RR < 12 or > 30, temperature > 38.5°C, urinary output less than 30 mL/hr × 2, O_2 sat < 92%
IV: D5½ NS @ 50 mL/hr
Strict I/O q1h
Oxygen: via 6 liters nasal cannula; maintain oxygen saturation > 92%
Respiratory Care: Incentive Spirometer q1 hours when awake
Sequential compression stockings to lower extremities while in bed

Scheduled Medications

Irbesartan (Avapro) 150 mg PO once a day
Hydrochlorothiazide 12.5 mg PO once a day
Ceftazidime 2 grams every 8 hours IV

PRN Medications

Tylenol 650 mg po q4h for fever
Morphine 0.3–5 mg IV q4h prn pain
Temazepam 15–30 mg po at bedtime prn insomnia
Droperidol 1.25–2.5 mg IV q4–6h prn nausea

Ordered Laboratory Studies

CPK-MB q8h × 3
Chemistry panel, CBC, and magnesium daily
ABGs daily and prn for respiratory distress

Ordered Diagnostic Studies

Chest x-ray q a.m.

Nursing Priorities

Six hours later, the nurse is called to Mr. A's room. His dinner tray is on his bedside stand. He is cyanotic with pulse oximetry reading in the 70s. He is coughing sporadically with a respiratory rate in the high 40s. Lung sounds are decreased but bronchial sounds are heard throughout the lung fields except for the right side, which is very decreased. The health care provider is called and an emergency chest x-ray is ordered. Oxygen is changed to a face mask, 100% nonrebreather. His pulse oximetry increases to 85%. ABGs are obtained. (The ABGs are listed below with the laboratory results.)

The chest x-ray reveals a new infiltrate in the posterior segment of the left upper lobe and an increasing pattern of consolidation in the right lung. A presumptive diagnosis of worsening pneumonia with possible aspiration pneumonia is considered. On questioning, Mr. A. states that he had difficulty swallowing his dinner and after drinking some of the milk remembers that his coughing increased and he vomited. Presently he can barely talk because he is so short of breath and is increasingly anxious with nasal flaring. Respiratory rate has increased to 45 breaths/min, heart rate has increased to the 120s, and the blood pressure is 150/100. Other laboratory tests are ordered with electrolytes and troponin to rule out any cardiac involvement.

Mr. A's status is deteriorating. His respiratory rate is increasing and he is complaining of becoming tired. A repeat ABG is drawn (see below) and shows increasing hypoxemia. The health care provider recommends a trial of noninvasive positive pressure ventilation (NPPV). Mr. A is placed on an NPO regimen and fitted for a mask. A noninvasive ventilator is brought into the room. The mode selected was BiPAP (two levels of CPAP) with an inspiratory pressure or IPAP of 15 cm of H_2O and an expiratory pressure or EPAP of 5 cm of H_2O.

An hour after being placed on the NPPV, Mr. A is less anxious. His respiratory rate is 24 to 26. An ABG examination demonstrates improvement in his hypoxemia. The nurse continues to monitor his progress.

LABORATORY FINDINGS

Test	Day 1	Day 2	Day 3
Sodium	135 mEq/L	136 mEq/L	135 mEq/L
Potassium	4.1 mEq/L	4.0 mEq/L	4.0 mEq/L
Chloride	103 mEq/L	104 mEq/L	95 mEq/L
Carbon dioxide	26 mEq/L	25 mEq/L	25 mEq/L
Blood urea nitrogen (BUN)	16 mg/dL	15 mg/dL	14 mg/dL
Creatinine	1.2 mg/dL	1.3 mg/dL	1.2 mg/dL
Glucose	134 mg/dL	123 mg/dL	120 mg/dL
Phosphorus	2.2 mg/dL	3.4 mg/dL	3.8 mg/dL
Calcium	9.1 mg/dL	8.7 mg/dL	9.1 mg/dL
Albumin	3.7 g/dL	3.7 g/dL	3.5 g/dL
Alkaline phosphatase (ALP)	70 units/L	76 units/L	77 units/L
Bilirubin	0.8 mg/dL	1.0 mg/dL	1.0 mg/dL
Alanine transaminase (ALT)	15 units/L	20 units/L	30 units/L
Magnesium	2.0 mg/dL	1.9 mg/dL	1.9 mg/dL
Creatine kinase	64 units/L	67 units/L	62 units/L

Test	Day 1	Day 2	Day 3
CK-MB	0 ng/mL by immunoassay	0 ng/mL by immunoassay	0 ng/mL by immunoassay
Troponin I	0 mcg/mL	0.2 mcg/mL	0.1 mcg/mL
Troponin T	0 mcg/mL	0.1 mcg/mL	0.1 mcg/mL
WBC	4500/µL	5000/µL	8000/µL
RBC	4.89×10^6/µL	5.09×10^6/µL	4.92×10^6/µL
Hemoglobin	15.9 g/dL	16.5 g/dL	15.9 g/dL
Hematocrit	45.5%	47.8%	45.6%
Platelets	295,000/µL	256,000/µL	300,000/µL
ABGs	Admission	After Aspiration	After NPPV
pH	7.35	7.30	7.35
PaO_2	70 mmHg	53 mmHg	76 mmHg
$PaCO_2$	47 mmHg	50 mmHg	39 mmHg
HCO_3	26 mmHg	25 mmHg	24 mmHg
SpO_2	93%	86%	92%
Oxygen delivery	6 liters nasal cannula	100% FiO_2 via nonrebreather mask	NPPV with BIPAP; IPAP of 15 and EPAP of 5

CRITICAL THINKING QUESTIONS

1. What are the risks of placing Mr. A on NPPV versus intubating him and placing him on conventional ventilation?

2. What types of devices are available for administering NPPV and what are the benefits of each?

3. What are the nursing priorities involved with monitoring Mr. A?

Answers to Critical Thinking Questions appear in Appendix D.

NCLEX® REVIEW

1. A patient with acute respiratory failure is complaining of shortness of breath. Which of the following would be most effective to help this patient?
   1. Administer oxygen 2 liters nasal cannula.
   2. Maintain oxygen saturation above 85%.
   3. Administer a cholinergic medication.
   4. Educate to avoid crowds and poor air quality.

2. A patient comes into the emergency department with new onset of dyspnea, SOB, tachypnea, and increased anxiety. The nurse notes increased crackles, coarse rhonchi and pink frothy sputum. Which of the following should the nurse suspect this patient is experiencing?
   1. Heroin–related pulmonary edema (HRPE)
   2. Neurogenic pulmonary edema
   3. Pulmonary edema
   4. High altitude pulmonary edema (HAPE)

3. The nurse is caring for a patient with non-cardiogenic pulmonary edema. The nurse should notify the physician if the patient develops which of the following?
   1. Heart rate 124 bpm
   2. 3+ pulses in the lower extremities
   3. B/P 152/88
   4. PCWP > 30 mmHg

4. A patient, admitted with respiratory failure, develops ARDS and requires intubation. Which of the following clinical manifestations are usually consistent with this stage of ARDS?
   1. Chest x-ray showing absence of infiltrates
   2. Temperature of 99°F
   3. Arterial blood gases showing respiratory acidosis
   4. B/P 124/76 Pulse 86 Respiratory rate 18

5. While caring for a patient on a ventilator, the nurse notes that the patient is experiencing acute distress with a decrease in oxygen saturation to 82%. The nurse's initial intervention would be to:
   1. Call the respiratory therapist stat to assess the problem.
   2. Remove the patient from the ventilator and use the AMBU bag with 100% oxygen.
   3. Call the physician stat regarding the patient's drop in oxygen saturation.
   4. Administer a sedative per physician's orders to reduce the patient's anxiety.

6. A patient on a ventilator with 5 cm of H_2O PEEP develops severe hypotension when disconnected from the ventilator. The nurse realizes that:
   1. The patient cannot be removed from the ventilator when PEEP is used.
   2. The patient is hypovolemic as a result of the PEEP setting.
   3. The patient is anxious about being removed from the ventilator.
   4. When the patient is removed from the ventilator and the AMBU is used it causes over inflation from the AMBU aggressive rates.

7. A patient with severe respiratory failure has just been intubated. Which of the following should the nurse do first after the intubation?

  1. Auscultate lungs for bilateral breath sounds.

  2. Obtain a pulse oximeter reading to assess oxygenation.

  3. Call for a portable chest x-ray to verify placement.

  4. Secure the ET tube to maintain the patency of the ET tube.

8. The nurse has instructed a family on how to perform tracheostomy suctioning. Which of the following would indicate that the family needs more instruction on the procedure?

  1. Donning sterile gloves in preparation for suctioning

  2. Hyperoxygenating the patient with 100% oxygen prior to suctioning

  3. Placing the head of the bed in a semi-Fowlers position prior to suctioning

  4. Applying suction when passing the catheter into the patient's tracheostomy

9. The nurse has received a change of shift report. Which of the following patients would be of the highest priority for the nurse to assess first?

  1. A patient with oxygen at 2 liters N/C with an oxygen saturation of 96%

  2. A patient with a chest tube on the right side with bubbling in the water seal chamber

  3. A patient who is to receive postural drainage every four hours

  4. A patient being discharged and needs education on how to use a metered-dose inhaler

Answers for review questions appear in Appendix D

KEY TERMS

acute lung injury (ALI) *p.1014*
acute pulmonary edema *p.1008*
acute respiratory distress syndrome (ARDS) *p.1014*
acute respiratory failure (ARF) *p.1006*
air-mask-bag unit (AMBU) *p.1019*
alveolar ventilation (V_A) *p.1006*
anatomic dead space *p.1006*
barotrauma *p.1026*
BiPAP *p.1034*
cardiogenic pulmonary edema (CPE) *p.1009*
dead space ventilation (V_D) *p.1006*

endotracheal tube *p.1020*
fraction of inspired oxygen (FiO_2) *p.1007*
high-altitude pulmonary edema (HAPE) *p.1010*
hypoventilation *p.1006*
hypoxemia *p.1006*
minute ventilation (V_E) *p.1015*
negative pressure pulmonary edema (NPPE) *p.1009*
neurogenic pulmonary edema (NPE) *p.1009*
noncardiogenic pulmonary edema (NCPE) *p.1009*

noninvasive positive pressure ventilation (NPPV) *p.1008*
perfusion *p.1005*
shunt *p.1005*
surfactant *p.1004*
ventilated-associated pneumonia (VAP) *p.1026*
ventilation *p.1005*
ventilation/perfusion mismatching (V/Q) *p.1006*
volutrauma *p.1026*

REFERENCES

Abraham, E. (2003). Neutrophils and acute lung injury. *Critical Care Medicine, 31*(4 Suppl.), S195–S199.

Acute Respiratory Distress Syndrome Network. (2000). Ventilation with lower tidal volumes as compared with traditional tidal volumes for acute lung injury and the acute respiratory distress syndrome. *New England Journal of Medicine, 342,* 1301–1308.

Agency for Healthcare Research and Quality. (2000, June). *Criteria for weaning from mechanical ventilation. Summary, evidence report/technology assessment: Number 23* (AHRQ Publication No. 00-E028). Retrieved January 10, 2004, from http://www.ahrq.gov/clinic/epcsums/mechsumm.htm

American Association of Critical Care Nurses. (2006). *Practice alert: Oral care in the critically ill.* Retrieved May 6, 2008, from http://www.aacn.org/AACN/practiceAlert.nsf/Files/ORAL%20CARE/$file/Oral%20Care%20in%20the%20Critically%20Ill%208-2006.pdf

Andrew, P. (2003). Diastolic heart failure demystified. *Chest, 124*(2), 744–753.

Annane, D., Bellissant, E., Pussard, E., Asmar, R., Lacombe, F., Lanata, E., et al. (1996). Placebo-controlled, randomized, double-blind study of intravenous enalaprilat efficacy and safety in acute cardiogenic pulmonary edema. *Circulation, 94*(6), 1316–1324.

Antonelli, M., Conti, G., Esquinas, A., Montini, L., Maggiore, S. M., Bello, G., et al. (2007). A multiple-center survey on the use in clinical practice of noninvasive ventilation as a first-line intervention for acute respiratory distress syndrome. *Critical Care Medicine, 35*(1), 18–25.

Arieff, A. I. (1999). Fatal postoperative pulmonary edema: Pathogenesis and literature review. *Chest, 115*(5), 1371–1377.

Baker, D. J. (2005). Critical care requirements after mass toxic agent release. *Critical Care Medicine, 33*(1 Suppl.), S66–S74.

Bard, (2008). Agento I.C. endotracheal tube. Retrieved May 6, 2008, from http://www.bardmedical.com/products/loadProduct.aspx? prodID=391

Bernard, G. R., Artigas, A., Brigham, K. L., Carlet, J., Falke, K., Hudson, L., et al. (1994). The American-European Consensus Conference on ARDS. Definitions, mechanisms, relevant outcomes, and clinical

trial coordination. *American Journal of Respiratory and Critical Care Medicine, 149*(3 Part 1), 818–824.

Brower, R. G., Ware, L. B., Berthiaume, Y., & Matthay, M. A. (2001). Treatment of ARDS. *Chest, 120*(4), 1347–1367.

Brunton, L. B., Lazo, J. S., & Parker, K. L. (Eds.). (2005). *Goodman Gilman's pharmacological basis of therapeutics* (11th ed.). New York: McGraw-Hill.

Brutsaert, D. L., & De Keulenaer, G. W. (2006). Diastolic heart failure: A myth. *Current Opinions in Cardiology, 21*(3), 240–248.

Burns, S. M., Earven, S., Fisher, C., Lewis, R., Merrell, P., Schubart, J. R., et al. (2003). Implementation of an institutional program to improve clinical and financial outcomes of mechanically ventilated patients: One-year outcomes and lessons learned. *Critical Care Medicine, 31*(12), 2752–2763.

Cairo, J. M., & Pilbeam, S. P., I. (2004). *Mosby's respiratory care equipment.* St. Louis: Mosby.

Calfee, C. S., & Matthay, M. A. (2007). Nonventilatory treatments for acute lung injury and ARDS. *Chest, 131*(3), 913–920.

Castro, C. Y. (2006). ARDS and diffuse alveolar damage: A pathologist's perspective. *Seminars in Thoracic and Cardiovascular Surgery, 18*(1), 13–19.

Centers for Disease Control and Prevention. (2003a). *Prevention and control of ventilator-associated pneumonia guidelines.* Retrieved May 6, 2008, from http://www.cdc.gov/ncidod/dhqp/dpac_ventilate_pc.html

Centers for Disease Control and Prevention. (2005). *An overview of ventilator-associated pneumonia.* Retrieved June 4, 2008, from http://www.cdc.gov/ncidod/dhqp/dpac_ventilate.html

Centers for Disease Control and Prevention. (2007). *Bioterrorism overview.* Retrieved June 4, 2008, from http://emergency.cdc.gov/bioterrorism/overview.asp

Chan, K. P., & Stewart, T. E. (2005). Clinical use of high-frequency oscillatory ventilation in adult patients with acute respiratory distress syndrome. *Critical Care Medicine, 33*(3 Suppl.), S170–S174.

Chatila, W. M., & Criner, G. J. (2002). Complications of long-term mechanical ventilation. *Respiratory Care Clinics of North America, 8*(4), 631–647.

Cobbs, C. G., & Chansolme, D. H. (2004). Plague. *Dermatologic Clinics, 22*(3), 303–312, vi.

Collins, S. P., Lindsell, C. J., Storrow, A. B., & Abraham, W. T. (2006). Prevalence of negative chest radiography results in the emergency department patient with decompensated heart failure. *Annals of Emergency Medicine, 47*(1), 13–18.

Doan, L. G. (2004). Ricin: mechanism of toxicity, clinical manifestations, and vaccine development. A review. *Journal of Toxicology–Clinical Toxicology, 42*(2), 201–208.

ELSO Registry Information. (2008). Retrieved August 9, 2008 from http://www.elso.med.umich.edu/Registry.htm

Ely, E. W., Meade, M. O., Haponik, E. F., Kollef, M. H., Cook, D. J., Guyatt, G. H., et al. (2001). Mechanical ventilator weaning protocols driven by nonphysician health-care professionals: Evidence-based clinical practice guidelines. *Chest, 120*(6 Suppl.), 454S–463S.

Engoren, M., Arslanian-Engoren, C., & Fenn-Buderer, N. (2004). Hospital and long-term outcome after tracheostomy for respiratory failure. *Chest, 125*(1), 220–227.

Esteban, A., Alia, I., Gordo, F., de Pablo, R., Suarez, J., Gonzalez, G., et al. (2000). Prospective randomized trial comparing pressure-controlled ventilation and volume-controlled ventilation in ARDS. *Chest, 117*(6), 1690–1696.

Estebam, A., Anzueto, A., Frutos-Vivar, F., Alia, I., Ely, E. W., Brochard, L., et al. (2004). Outcome of older patients receiving mechanical ventilation. *Intensive Care Medicine, 30* (4), 639–646.

Esteban, A., Frutos, F., Tobin, M. J., Alia, I., Solsona, J. F., Valverdu, I., et al. (1995). A comparison of four methods of weaning patients from mechanical ventilation. *New England Journal of Medicine, 332*(6), 345–350.

Fink, M. P., Abraham, E., Vincent, J., & Kochanek, P. (2005). Acute respiratory failure. In *Textbook of critical care* (Chap. 9). Philadelphia: W. B. Saunders.

Fleischmann, K. E., Goldman, L., Young, B., & Lee, T. H. (2003). Association between cardiac and noncardiac complications in patients undergoing noncardiac surgery: Outcomes and effects on length of stay. *American Journal of Medicine, 115*(7), 515–520.

Fontes, R. B., Aguiar, P. H., Zanetti, M. V., Andrade, F., Mandel, M., & Teixeira, M. J. (2003). Acute neurogenic pulmonary edema: Case reports and literature review. *Journal of Neurosurgical Anesthesiology, 15*(2), 144–150.

Fox, K. A., Steg, P. G., Eagle, K. A., Goodman, S. G., Anderson, F. A., Jr., Granger, C. B., et al. (2007). Decline in rates of death and heart failure in acute coronary syndromes, 1999–2006. *Journal of the American Medical Association, 297*(17), 1892–1900.

Freedman, N. S., Gazendam, J., Levan, L., Pack, A. I., & Schwab, R. J. (2001). Abnormal sleep/wake cycles and the effect of environmental noise on sleep disruption in the intensive care unit. *American Journal of Respiratory and Critical Care Medicine, 163*(2), 451–457.

Fremont, R. D., Kallet, R. H., Matthay, M. A., & Ware, L. B. (2007). Post-obstructive pulmonary edema: A case for hydrostatic mechanisms. *Chest, 131*, 1742–1746.

Frishman, W. H., Del Vecchio, A., Sanal, S., & Ismail, A. (2003). Cardiovascular manifestations of substance abuse. Part 2: Alcohol, amphetamines, heroin, cannabis, and caffeine. *Heart Disease, 5*(4), 253–271.

Gabry, A. L., Ledoux, X., Mozziconacci, M., & Martin, C. (2003). High-altitude pulmonary edema at moderate altitude (< 2,400 m; 7,870 feet): A series of 52 patients. *Chest, 123*(1), 49–53.

Gong, M. N., Wei, Z., Xu, L. L., Miller, D. P., Thompson, B. T., & Christiani, D. C. (2004). Polymorphism in the surfactant protein-B gene, gender, and the risk of direct pulmonary injury and ARDS. *Chest, 125*(1), 203–211.

Goss, C. H., Brower, R. G., Hudson, L. D., & Rubenfeld, G. D. (2003). Incidence of acute lung injury in the United States. *Critical Care Medicine, 31*(6), 1607–1611.

Guyton, A., & Hall, J. (2005). *Textbook of Medical Physiology* (11th ed.). Philadelphia: W. B. Saunders.

Habal, R. (2006). *Toxicity, heroin.* EMedicine. Retrieved August 13, 2008 from http://www.emedicine.com/med/TOPIC1003.HTM

Halpern, P., Gefen, A., Sorkine, P., & Elad, D. (2003). Pulmonary oedema in SCUBA divers: Pathophysiology and computed risk analysis. *European Journal of Emergency Medicine, 10*(1), 35–41.

Hemmila, M. R., & Napolitano, L. M. (2006). Severe respiratory failure: Advanced treatment options. *Critical Care Medicine, 34*(9 Suppl.), S278–S290.

Hopkins, R. O., Weaver, L. K., Collingridge, D., Parkinson, R. B., Chan, K. J., & Orme, J. F., Jr. (2005). Two-year cognitive, emotional, and quality-of-life outcomes in acute respiratory distress syndrome. *American Journal of Respiratory and Critical Care Medicine, 171*(4), 340–347.

Howard, A., Courtney-Shapiro, C., Kelso, L., Goltz, M., & Morris, P. (2004). Comparison of three methods of detecting acute respiratory distress syndrome: Clinical screening, chart review and diagnosis coding. *American Journal of Nursing, 13*, 59–64.

Hudson, L. D., & Hough, C. L. (2006). Therapy for late-phase acute respiratory distress syndrome. *Clinics in Chest Medicine, 27*(4), 671–677; abstract, ix–x.

Hughes, R. A., & Cornblath, D. R. (2005). Guillain-Barre syndrome. *Lancet, 366*(9497), 1653–1666.

Inglesby, T. V., O'Toole, T., Henderson, D. A., Bartlett, J. G., Ascher, M. S., Eitzen, E., et al. (2002). Anthrax as a biological weapon, 2002: Updated recommendations for management. *Journal of the American Medical Association, 287*(17), 2236–2252.

Jessup, M., & Brozena, S. (2003). Heart failure. *New England Journal of Medicine, 348*(20), 2007–2018.

Johnston, C. J., Rubenfeld, G. D., & Hudson, L. D. (2003). Effect of age on the development of ARDS in trauma patients. *Chest, 124*(2), 653–659.

Kaisers, U., Kelly, K. P., & Busch, T. (2003). Liquid ventilation. *British Journal of Anaesthesia, 91*(1), 143–151.

Kaplow, R., & Hardin, S. R. (2007). *Critical care nursing: Synergy and optimal outcomes.* Boston: Jones & Bartlett.

Karwa, M., Currie, B., & Kvetan, V. (2005). Bioterrorism: Preparing for the impossible or the improbable. *Critical Care Medicine, 33*(1 Suppl.), S75–S95.

Klompas, M. (2007). Does this patient have ventilator-associated pneumonia? *Journal of the American Medical Association, 297*(14), 1583–1593.

Koeman, M., van der Ven, A. J., Hak, E., Joore, H. C., Kaasjager, K., de Smet, A. G., et al. (2006). Oral decontamination with chlorhexidine reduces the incidence of ventilator-associated pneumonia. *American Journal of Respiratory and Critical Care Medicine, 173*(12), 1348–1355.

Krishnan, J. A., Moore, D., Robeson, C., Rand, C. S., & Fessler, H. E. (2004). A prospective, controlled trial of a protocol-based strategy to discontinue mechanical ventilation. *American Journal of Respiratory and Critical Care Medicine, 169*(6), 673–678.

Lanken, P. N., Ed. (2006). *The intensive care unit manual* (3rd ed.). Philadelphia: W. B. Saunders.

Lewandowski, K. (2003). Contributions to the epidemiology of acute respiratory failure. *Critical Care, 7*(4), 288–290.

Lewis, J. F., & Brackenbury, A. (2003). Role of exogenous surfactant in acute lung injury. *Critical Care Medicine, 31*(4 Suppl.), S324–S328.

Liesching, T., Kwok, H., & Hill, N. S. (2003). Acute applications of noninvasive positive pressure ventilation. *Chest, 124*(2), 699–713.

Looney, M. R., Gropper, M. A., & Matthay, M. A. (2004). Transfusion-related acute lung injury: A review. *Chest, 126*(1), 249–258.

Lupatkin, H., Lupatkin, J., & Rosenberg, A. (2004). Smallpox in the 21st century. *Anesthesiology Clinics of North America, 22*(3), 541–561.

MacIntyre, N. R. (2005). Current issues in mechanical ventilation for respiratory failure. *Chest, 128*(5 Suppl. 2), 561S–567S.

Marini, J. J., & Gattinoni, L. (2004). Ventilatory management of acute respiratory distress syndrome: A consensus of two. *Critical Care Medicine, 32*(1), 250–255.

Marks, J. D. (2004). Medical aspects of biologic toxins. *Anesthesiology Clinics of North America, 22*(3), 509–532, vii.

Martin, C. M., Doig, G. S., Heyland, D. K., Morrison, T., & Sibbald, W. J. (2004). Multicentre, cluster-randomized clinical trial of algorithms for critical-care enteral and parenteral therapy (ACCEPT). *CMAJ, 170*(2), 197–204.

Martin, M., Salim, A., Murray, J., Demetriades, D., Belzberg, H., & Rhee, P. (2005). The decreasing incidence and mortality of acute respiratory distress syndrome after injury: A 5-year observational study. *Journal of Trauma, 59*(5), 1107–1113.

Matthay, M. A., Zimmerman, G. A., Esmon, C., Bhattacharya, J., Coller, B., Doerschuk, C. M., et al. (2003). Future research directions in acute lung injury: Summary of a National Heart, Lung, and Blood Institute working group. *American Journal of Respiratory and Critical Care Medicine, 167*(7), 1027–1035.

Mattu, A., Martinez, J. P., & Kelly, B. S. (2005). Modern management of cardiogenic pulmonary edema. *Emergency Medical Clinics of North America, 23*(4), 1105–1125.

Metheny, N. A., Meert, K. L., & Clouse, R. E. (2007). Complications related to feeding tube placement. *Current Opinions in Gastroenterology, 23*(2), 178–182.

Moloney, E. D., & Evans, T. W. (2003). Pathophysiology and pharmacological treatment of pulmonary hypertension in acute

respiratory distress syndrome. *European Respiratory Journal, 21*(4), 720–727.

Mori, H., Hirasawa, H., Oda, S., Shiga, H., Matsuda, K., & Nakamura, M. (2006). Oral care reduces incidence of ventilator-associated pneumonia in ICU populations. *Intensive Care Medicine, 32*(2), 230–236.

Murray, J., & Nadel, J. (Eds.). (2005). *Textbook of respiratory medicine* (4th ed.). Philadelphia: W. B. Saunders.

Numata, Y., Bourbeau, J., Ernst, P., Duquette, G., & Schwartzman, K. (2002). Teaching time for metered-dose inhalers in the emergency setting. *Chest, 122*(2), 498–504.

O'Neal, P. V., Munro, C. L., Grap, M. J., & Rausch, S. M. (2007). Subglottic secretion viscosity and evacuation efficiency. *Biological Research for Nursing, 8*(3), 202–209.

Ognibene, F. P., Martin, S. E., Parker, M. M., Schlesinger, T., Roach, P., Burch, C., et al. (1986). Adult respiratory distress syndrome in patients with severe neutropenia. *New England Journal of Medicine, 315*(9), 547–551.

Onwuanyi, A., & Taylor, M. (2007). Acute decompensated heart failure: Pathophysiology and treatment. *American Journal of Cardiology, 99*(6B), 25D–30D.

Orme, J., Jr., Romney, J. S., Hopkins, R. O., Pope, D., Chan, K. J., Thomsen, G., et al. (2003). Pulmonary function and health-related quality of life in survivors of acute respiratory distress syndrome. *American Journal of Respiratory and Critical Care Medicine, 167*(5), 690–694.

Pastor, C. M., Matthay, M. A., & Frossard, J. L. (2003). Pancreatitis-associated acute lung injury: New insights. *Chest, 124*(6), 2341–2351.

Percell, R. L., Jr., Henning, R. J., & Siddique Patel, M. (2003). Atrial myxoma: Case report and a review of the literature. *Heart Disease, 5*(3), 224–230.

Pilbeam, S. P. & Cairo, J. M. (2006). *Mechanical ventilation: Physiological and clinical applications* (4th ed.). Philadelphia: Mosby.

Polderman, K. H., Spijkstra, J. J., de Bree, R., Christiaans, H. M., Gelissen, H. P., Wester, J. P., et al. (2003). Percutaneous dilatational tracheostomy in the ICU: Optimal organization, low complication rates, and description of a new complication. *Chest, 123*(5), 1595–1602.

Porth, C. (2007). *Essential of Pathophysiology* (2nd ed.). St. Louis: Lippincott Williams & Wilkins.

Reishtein, J. L. (2005). Sleep in mechanically ventilated patients. *Critical Care Nursing Clinics of North America, 17*(3), 251–255.

Rello, J., Kollef, M., Diaz, E., Sandiumenge, A., del Castillo, Y., Corbella, X., et al. (2006). Reduced burden of bacterial airway colonization with a novel silver-coated endotracheal tube in a randomized multiple-center feasibility study. *Critical Care Medicine, 34*(11), 2766–2772.

Safdar, N., Crnich, C. J., & Maki, D. G. (2005). The pathogenesis of ventilator-associated pneumonia: Its relevance to developing effective strategies for prevention. *Respiratory Care, 50*(6), 725–739; discussion, 739–741.

Sagrista-Sauleda, J., Angel, J., Sambola, A., Alguersuari, J., Permanyer-Miralda, G., & Soler-Soler, J. (2006). Low-pressure cardiac tamponade: Clinical and hemodynamic profile. *Circulation, 114*(9), 945–952.

Sanderson, J. E., & Fraser, A. G. (2006). Systolic dysfunction in heart failure with a normal ejection fraction: Echo-Doppler measurements. *Progress in Cardiovascular Disease, 49*(3), 196–206.

Shapiro, B., Peruzzi, W., & Templin, R. (Eds.). (1994). *Clinical applications of blood gases.* St. Louis: Mosby.

Shorr, A. F., & Kollef, M. H. (2005). Ventilator-associated pneumonia: Insights from recent clinical trials. *Chest, 128*(5 Suppl. 2), 583S–591S.

Sue, R. D., & Susanto, I. (2003). Long-term complications of artificial airways. *Clinics in Chest Medicine, 24*(3), 457–471.

Suter, P. M. (2006). Reducing ventilator-induced lung injury and other organ injury by the prone position. *Critical Care, 10*(2), 139.

Talreja, D. R., Edwards, W. D., Danielson, G. K., Schaff, H. V., Tajik, A. J., Tazelaar, H. D., et al. (2003). Constrictive pericarditis in 26 patients with histologically normal pericardial thickness. *Circulation, 108*(15), 1852–1857.

Tarrac, S. E. (2003). Negative pressure pulmonary edema—a postanesthesia emergency. *Journal of Perianesthesia Nursing, 18*(5), 317–323.

Vincent, J. L., Sakr, Y., & Ranieri, V. M. (2003). Epidemiology and outcome of acute respiratory failure in intensive care unit patients. *Critical Care Medicine, 31*(4 Suppl.), S296–S299.

Wang, C. S., FitzGerald, J. M., Schulzer, M., Mak, E., & Ayas, N. T. (2005). Does this dyspneic patient in the emergency department have congestive heart failure? *Journal of the American Medical Association, 294*(15), 1944–1956.

Ware, L. B. (2005). Prognostic determinants of acute respiratory distress syndrome in adults: Impact on clinical trial design. *Critical Care Medicine, 33*(3 Suppl.), S217–S222.

Ware, L. B., & Matthay, M. A. (2005). Clinical practice: Acute pulmonary edema. *New England Journal of Medicine, 353*(26), 2788–2796.

West, J. B. (1998). *Pulmonary pathophysiology: The essentials* (5th ed.). Baltimore: Williams & Wilkins.

Wheeler, A. P., & Bernard, G. R. (2007). Acute lung injury and the acute respiratory distress syndrome: A clinical review. *Lancet, 369*(9572), 1553–1564.

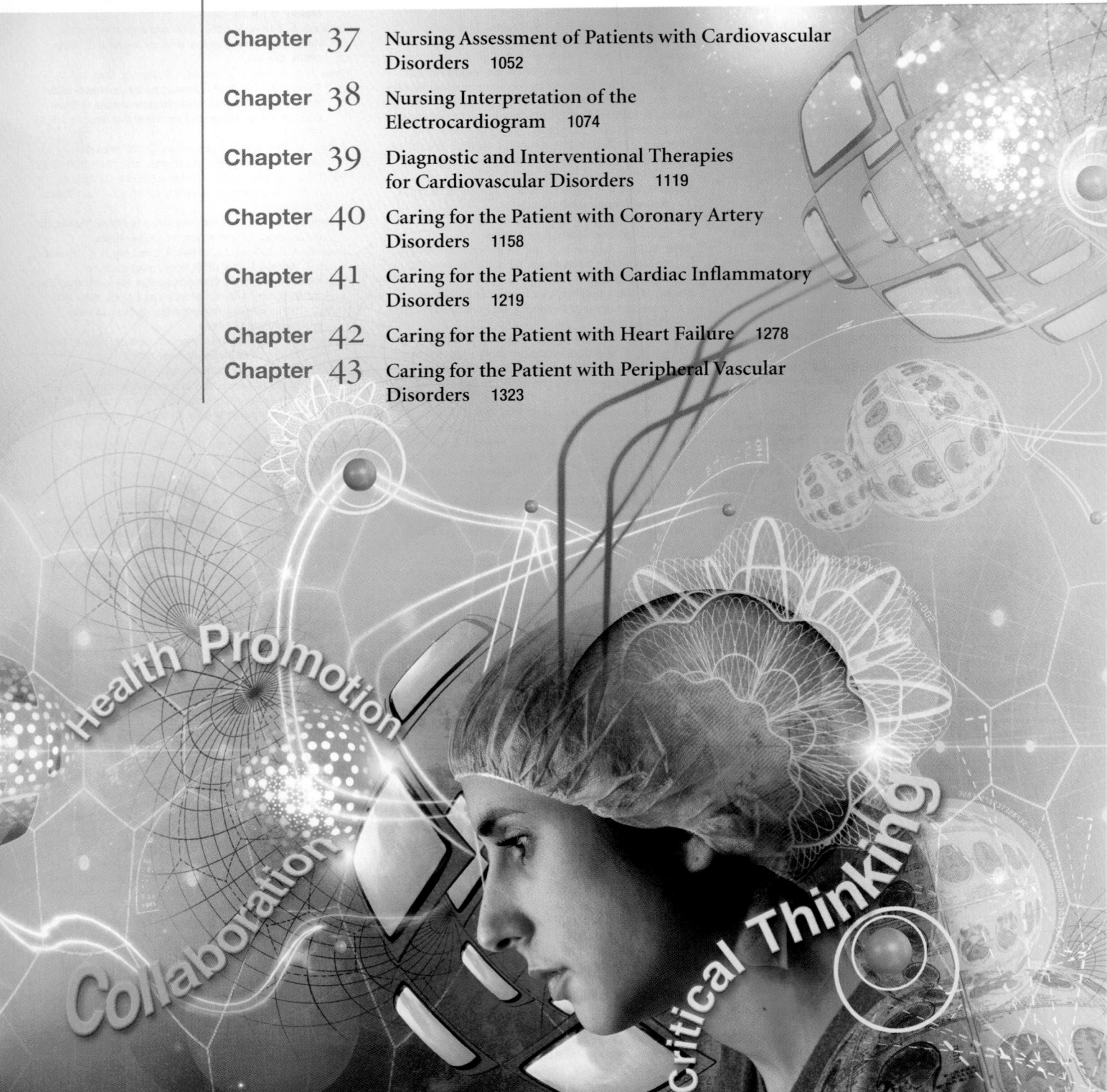

UNIT

8 Nursing Management of Patients with Cardiovascular Disorders

Health Promotion

Collaboration

Critical Thinking

JACKIE My name is Jackie and I am a registered nurse on the Cardiothoracic Progressive Care Unit at UC Davis Medical Center. Our typical patients are postoperative and have had coronary artery bypass graft surgery (CABG), valve replacements, and thoracotomies. We also have a wide variety of patients who are experiencing respiratory failure, alcohol withdrawal, and multiple system failures—all of which require telemetry monitoring. To be competent, all nurses on the unit are required to complete Advanced Cardiac Life Support (ACLS) certification and ECG monitor training.

On a typical day I have three patients. I will obtain report, research each patient's laboratory results, and check their telemetry, making sure that each patient is hemodynamically stable. I will then introduce myself to my patients, assess them and, with confidence, report anything pertinent to the health care team. I listen with compassion to any needs or concerns the patient and family may have. Postoperative patients can have many concerns and questions regarding their future health status. I answer their questions and let them know that I will help them in any way that I am able. As the day progresses, I will educate my patients about their disease process, wound care management, and any discharge needs. It is particularly important to have cardiac patients understand the disease process. The surgery may have reestablished blood flow to the heart muscle, but unless the patient makes lifestyle changes such as a healthy diet and exercise, the arteries can occlude again. It is important to have patients and their family participate in their care early to allay any fears they may have about being able to care for themselves after discharge from the hospital. I also watch for any changes in my patients and their telemetry monitoring. Are they having increased ectopy? Are their electrolytes within normal limits? Is the patient having an increase in pain or chest tube output? These are just a few things that I continually monitor. As the primary nurse I spend the most time with the patient and may be the first to observe subtle changes in their condition. Early recognition of complications can keep them from becoming severe.

Nursing is a rewarding career. Remember to be happy and keep humor in your daily routine—patients like a happy nurse who comports herself well. Always be kind, caring, and compassionate, and treat patients the way you would want your loved ones to be treated.

"It is important to have patients and their family participate in their care early to allay any fears they may have about being able to care for themselves after discharge from the hospital."

Nursing Assessment of Patients with Cardiovascular Disorders

Kristine L'Ecuyer
With contributions by:
Kathleen Osborn

Outcome-Based Learning Objectives

After studying this chapter, the learner will be able to:

1. Compare and contrast the significance of cardiovascular assessment findings.
2. Evaluate the relationship of current health status and the presence of cardiac risk factors.
3. Describe the relationship of clinical manifestations to data obtained from the review of a patient's social history.
4. Describe the essential components of a cardiovascular physical assessment.

Research   Collaboration   Health Promotion   Nursing Process   Caring   Critical Thinking

NURSES NEED in-depth knowledge and skills in order to assess the cardiovascular status of their patients rapidly. Although the cardiovascular system is complex, its purpose is simple: to deliver oxygen and nutrients to the tissues and cells of the body. An understanding of cardiovascular anatomy and physiology is essential for cardiovascular assessment. Additionally, it is important to gather data about the patient's medical history as well as the presenting symptoms, because they can provide clues to cardiac status. The relationship between the existence of risk factors and the patient's susceptibility for disease is an important concept this chapter presents.

A thorough physical examination, including inspection, palpation, and ausculation, helps to define an individual's ability to carry out the physiological function of the cardiovascular system. Nurses should be able to recognize normal assessment findings and, more importantly, to identify subtle abnormalities or deviations from normal that might indicate worsening of the patient's condition. Accuracy in monitoring and reporting of data is essential, and nurses have access to a wide variety of noninvasive and invasive technological devices that assist in cardiovascular monitoring and assessment.

Anatomy and Physiology of the Cardiovascular System

An in-depth cardiovascular assessment requires knowledge of cardiovascular anatomy and physiology, and an ability to integrate that knowledge into the current condition of each patient. As seen in Figure 37–1 ■, the heart is housed directly behind the central section of the thorax referred to as the mediastinum. Two-thirds of the heart lies to the left of the midline. The apex lies just above the diaphragm and the base of the heart lies approximately at the level of the third rib. The exact size of the heart varies among individuals, but on the average it is approximately 5 inches long and about 3 inches wide, resembling the size of a closed fist.

The heart is a four-chambered muscular organ composed of two separate pumps, each having one atrium and one ventricle. The upper chambers (atria) of the heart are separated by the interatrial septum, and the ventricles are separated by the interventricular septum. The two atria are located at the base or top of the heart, and the lower chambers are located at the bottom or apex of the heart. The upper chambers are thin walled and re-

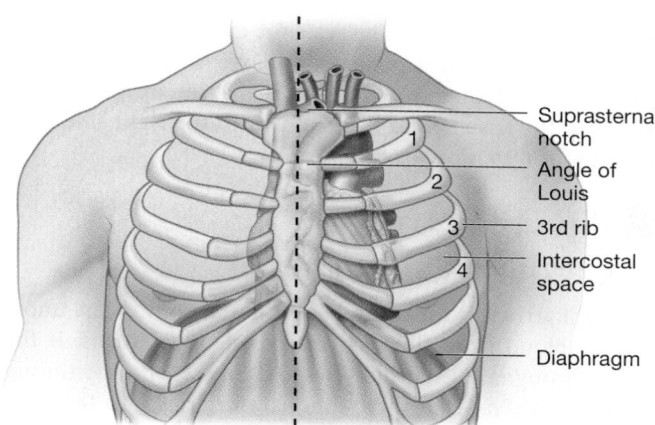

FIGURE 37–1 ■ Diagram of heart in chest.

FIGURE 37–2 ■ Cross section of heart.

ceive blood as it returns to the heart. The right atrium receives blood from the systemic venous circulation, while the left atrium receives blood from the pulmonary circulation. The lower chambers have thicker walls and pump blood out of the heart. The right ventricle pumps blood into the pulmonary circulation, while the left ventricle pumps blood into the systemic circulation. Although each ventricle pumps the same volume of blood, the left ventricle has a larger, stronger muscle. This increased strength is needed because the left ventricle has to pump blood into the systemic circulation, which has five times greater pressure than the pulmonic circulation. The heart wall is composed of the three layers:

1. The epicardium: the smooth outer serous layer.
2. The myocardium: the middle muscular layer, which is the thickest of the three layers and is responsible for the heart's ability to contract.
3. The endocardium: the inner lining of the heart, which is composed of thin connective tissue. This smooth inner surface and the valves allow blood to flow more easily throughout the heart.

Cardiac Valves

There are four valves in the heart (Figure 37–2 ■). The purpose of the valves is to ensure that blood travels in only one direction as it passes through the heart. The valve opens to fill a chamber and then closes when the pressure in the chamber builds, thereby allowing blood to continue to flow in one direction. The atrioventricular (AV) valves are located between the atria and the ventricles (see Figure 37–2 ■). These valves are referred to as the tricuspid valve and the bicuspid or mitral valve. The tricuspid valve lies between the right atrium and the right ventricle and is so named because it has three cusps. The mitral or bicuspid valve has only two cusps and is located between the left atrium and the left ventricle. The cusps of both the mitral and the tricuspid extend into the ventricles where they attach to the chordae tendineae. Chordae tendineae are cords of dense connective tissue that attach to the papillary muscles (see Figure 37–2 ■). The chordae tendineae and the papillary muscle work

together to prevent the valve cusps from fluttering back into the atrium and thereby interrupting forward blood flow. The semilunar valves are the pulmonic and the aortic valves. Each semilunar valve contains moon-shaped cusps (semilunar). The pulmonic valve is located between the right ventricle and the pulmonary artery. The aortic valve is located between the left ventricle and the trunk of the aorta.

As blood is filling the ventricular chamber, pressure is rising. The ventricular muscle fibers respond to an increase in blood volume by stretching to allow more fluid into the chamber (Starling law). As pressure in the ventricles increases, the ventricular muscles stretch. When the pressure in the right ventricle is greater than the pressure in the pulmonary system, and likewise, when the pressure in the left ventricle is greater than the pressure in the aorta, the AV valves (tricuspid and mitral) snap together to close as the semilunar valves (pulmonic and aortic) open. The ventricular muscles contract, and blood is ejected through the open pulmonic valve to the pulmonary artery and the pulmonary circuit, and through the open aortic valve to the aorta and the systemic circulation.

Surrounding the heart is a two-layered sac referred to as the pericardial sac (Figure 37–3 ■, p. 1054). The outer layer, called the parietal pericardium, is in direct contact with the pleura (lung). This layer consists of a tough, nonelastic, fibrous connective tissue and serves to prevent overdistention of the heart. The thin, serous inner layer of the pericardium, called the visceral pericardium, lays directly on the epicardium or outer layer of the heart. There is a small amount of fluid between the heart wall and the pericardial sac (approximately 10 mL). This fluid acts as a lubricant to prevent friction during contractions.

Cardiac Circulatory System

The heart has its own circulatory system allowing for constant nourishment of blood to the cardiac muscle. The heart's circulatory system consists of coronary arteries and veins

Transverse section of the heart

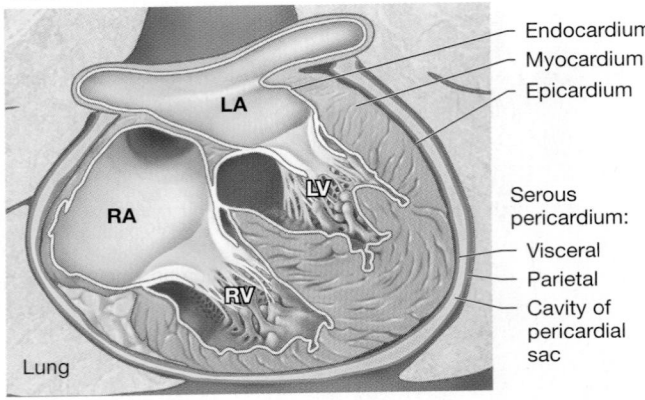

FIGURE 37–3 ■ Layers of heart.

(Figure 37–4 ■). The sinuses or openings into the coronary arteries lie at the base of the aorta, just above the aortic valve. As blood leaves the heart with each beat, it travels through the coronary sinus to supply the cardiac muscle. The two main arteries are the right and left coronary arteries. The right coronary artery and its branches normally supply the right atrium and ventricle and a portion of the posterior wall of the left ventricle. The left coronary artery branches into the left anterior descending and the circumflex arteries, both of which feed the left atrium and the massive walls of the left ventricle. The left coronary artery carries 85% of the blood flow to the myocardium. The left anterior descending (LAD) artery feeds the anterior wall of the left ventricle and the interventricular septum. The circumflex artery feeds the lateral and posterior portions of the left ventricle.

The pulmonary circulation consists of blood flow between the heart and lungs. Blood leaves the right ventricle, enters the

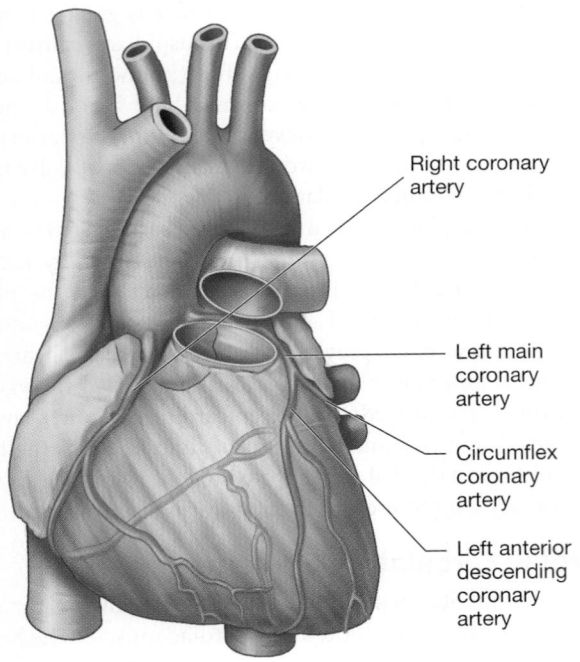

FIGURE 37–4 ■ Coronary arteries.

pulmonary artery and lungs, picks up oxygen, and travels to the left side of the heart. The systemic circulation consists of a network of arteries, capillaries, and veins. Blood leaves the heart, travels through these vessels delivering oxygen and nutrients to the tissues, and then returns to the right side of the heart to pick up more oxygen.

Physiology of the Cardiovascular System

The right atrium is the central point in the body where unoxygenated blood from the systemic circulation returns. It then travels through the tricuspid valve to the right ventricle, through the pulmonic valve to the pulmonary arteries into the lungs, through the pulmonary alveolar-capillary network into the pulmonary veins, into the left atrium, through the mitral valve into the left ventricle, and finally out the aortic valve to the systemic circulation.

Freshly oxygenated blood, traveling through the aortic valve, also enters into the coronary arteries to supply the myocardium with oxygen. Normally the myocardium extracts 75% of the available oxygen from the coronary arteries. This is more than is extracted from any other tissue in the body; the rest of the body extracts about 40%. If oxygen needs are not met from this near maximal extraction, then blood flow must be increased. With a healthy heart, blood flow is increased in two ways. First, the arteries are able to dilate, thereby increasing their capacity, and second, the myocardial muscle increases the force of the contraction, pumping more blood into the arteries. These two mechanisms result in an increase in the cardiac output and blood flow to the myocardium.

Cardiac Cycle

The pumping action of the heart consists of contraction and relaxation of the myocardial layer of the heart wall. Each contraction and relaxation is one cardiac cycle. During relaxation or diastole blood flows into the ventricles and the contraction that follows, termed systole, propels blood out of the heart. The heart functions as a unit because both atria contract simultaneously, and then both ventricles contract. When both atria contract the ventricles are filled to capacity, and then the ventricles contract and blood is ejected into both the pulmonary and the systemic circulation. At the time of ventricular contraction, the mitral and tricuspid valves are closed by the pressure from the contraction while the pulmonic and aortic valves are opened. The cardiac cycle represents the actual time sequence between ventricular contraction and ventricular relaxation.

Autonomic Nervous System

The autonomic nervous system is a built-in control center for the body. Its purpose is to regulate functions of the body that are not under conscious control. There are two major divisions: the sympathetic and the parasympathetic nervous systems. Most of the organs of the body are innervated with both systems, although the blood vessels are innervated with only the sympathetic nervous system. The sympathetic nervous system (SNS) prepares the body for activity (flight or fight), whereas the parasympathetic nervous system (PSNS) regulates the calmer (rest and digest) functions. Because the sympathetic nervous system (SNS) and the parasympathetic nervous system (PSNS) innervate the heart, neural impulses are not needed to maintain the cardiac cycle. In other words, the heart will beat in the absence of any nervous system connection. The SNS and the PSNS affect only the speed of the cardiac cycles and the diameter of the coronary arteries. It is said that these nervous systems only "fine-tune" the cardiac cycle.

Receptors and Neurotransmitters

The nerve endings of both the SNS and the PSNS secrete neurotransmitters. The SNS has two types of receptors at the nerve endings, the alpha- and the beta-receptors. These nerve endings are called adrenergic. The neurotransmitter for the SNS is norepinephrine, which causes an increase in heart rate and contractile force of the cardiac fibers. The PSNS nerve endings are known as cholinergic, and the neurotransmitter is acetylcholine, which causes the heart rate and blood pressure to go down.

History

A thorough history will help the nurse identify cardiovascular symptoms as well as current or potential problems that may affect cardiovascular function. Information learned from a thorough history and physical exam could help prevent undesirable responses to current therapies and treatment plans. The essential assessment data included in the cardiovascular history are outlined in this section.

Biographic and Demographic Data

Assessment of biographic and demographic data includes information regarding age, race, gender, and ethnicity, which can impact the susceptibility to some cardiovascular disorders. For example, African Americans have a higher incidence of hypertension than Caucasians (American Heart Association, 2006), and premenopausal women have a lower incidence of atherosclerotic coronary artery disease than men (American Heart Association, 2008b). Additionally, the presenting symptoms of cardiovascular diseases in women are often atypical, which may either delay diagnosis or make diagnosis more difficult. For example, women more frequently present with shortness of breath.

Chief Complaint

During the assessment process the nurse obtains a complete description of the present illness, paying particular attention to the chief complaint, or the reason the patient is seeking health care. The chief complaint focuses the history-taking process and prioritizes treatment regimens. For example, if the patient is complaining of chest pain, then the history should include information regarding the nature of the pain, associated symptoms, exacerbating and alleviating factors, as well as radiation of the pain and intensity of the pain. It also is important to determine what brings the pain and what relieves it.

Presenting Symptoms

Symptomatology is the review of symptoms the patient is experiencing. A review of symptoms helps define the current functional status of the patient. The nurse needs to ask questions about the date and mode of onset of the symptoms to find out when and how the symptoms first began. For example, has the shortness of breath been a problem for many weeks, or is it a new occurrence? Have the symptoms changed in intensity or duration? Additionally, questions about the exacerbations, or what causes the symptoms to worsen, and alleviating factors are important.

Specific Cardiovascular Clinical Manifestations

Patients with cardiovascular disease often present to the health care professional with typical or common cardiovascular symptoms. Knowledge of these common symptoms, their usual presentation, and their etiology can help focus and guide the exam process.

1. *Nurses should be particularly aware of the following common cardiovascular symptoms: chest pain, palpitations, dyspnea, orthopnea, cough, and nocturia.*
2. *The most severe symptoms should be assessed in greater depth and reported to the health care provider, if indicated.*

The most life-threatening symptoms should be addressed first. If the patient is complaining of shortness of breath, it needs to be assessed immediately. Airway management and oxygen status must be stabilized before the remainder of the assessment is completed. The management of airway is discussed in Chapters 34, 35, and 36 . Next, the patient is asked about the presence, site, and intensity of pain. The primary cardiovascular concern is pain associated with cardiac muscle ischemia, referred to as angina pectoris. The clinical manifestations of angina vary among patients; therefore, specific questions must be asked during the assessment in order to ascertain the cause of the pain. Pain may be described as indigestion, burning, numbness, tightness, or pressure in the midchest, or as epigastric or substernal pain, which can radiate to the shoulder, neck, arms, jaw, or back. It is essential that the nurse inquires about what brings the "pain on" and what makes it go away. An in-depth discussion of angina-type chest pain, the assessment data, and treatment is included in Chapter 40 . Patients might deny the presence of chest pain but admit to sensations of chest discomfort; therefore, it is important to allow patients to present their symptoms in their own words prior to analyzing their symptoms.

Palpitations are typically described by the patient as sensations of a racing heartbeat, irregular beats, or skipped beats. These sensations may be normal, or they may signify cardiac rhythm disturbances. The presence of **dyspnea**, or shortness of breath, may indicate an imbalance of arterial oxygen supply and demand. **Orthopnea**, the presence of dyspnea when the patient lies flat, is frequently a manifestation of cardiac disease. Often the degree of orthopnea is measured by the number of pillows (for example, 2- to 3-pillow orthopnea) necessary for the patient to use to breathe comfortably while sleeping. A cough may suggest pulmonary congestion resulting from fluid accumulation in the lungs due to either cardiac pump failure or fluid overload. If the patient has **nocturia,** the need to urinate often at night, it may indicate heart failure, although there are other disorders that cause frequent urination, such as an enlarged prostate. During the day as a patient is up and moving, fluid shifts to extremities and extravascular spaces, which serves to decrease fluid workload on a decompensated heart. At night, however, when the patient lies flat, fluid is returned to the central intravascular column, thereby increasing the amount of fluid to the kidneys. Patients with heart failure may report paroxysmal nocturnal dyspnea, which is acute dyspnea caused by lung congestion and edema that occurs suddenly at night, usually an hour or two after falling asleep.

Edema, or fluid accumulation in the extravascular spaces of the body, may be due to decreases in venous return. Fluid retention is manifested by weight gain, a feeling of being bloated, or clothes or shoes that no longer fit comfortably. Changes in weight should be specifically addressed. Large, sudden weight gains correlate with volume overload. Dizziness, **syncope** (fainting), or light-headedness may be experienced with sudden changes of position, and all are related to decreased cardiac output, which decreases blood to the brain.

Fatigue is a common complaint with cardiovascular patients. Fatigue is due to a decreased supply of oxygen to the tissues. Metabolic demands are higher in chronic cardiovascular conditions; however, due to a lowered cardiac output, demands are not met and the result is fatigue. The fatigue is usually progressive over time, and the patient may report decreased ability to complete usual activities of daily living. Additionally, patients may report a lack of energy or the need for more rest than usual. Medications such as diuretics, beta-adrenergic blockers, calcium channel blockers, digoxin, and antihypertensives have long been thought to contribute to fatigue. For example, beta-adrenergic blockers block the response from the beta nerve receptors, which serves to slow down the heart rate and lower the blood pressure. This desired physiological change, which decreases the myocardial oxygen demand, also may cause an undesired side effect of fatigue. Interestingly, clinical trials have not supported the notion that beta-adrenergic blocker therapy is associated with substantial risks of side effects. In a quantitative review of randomized trials that tested beta-adrenergic blockers in myocardial infarction, heart failure, and hypertension, the authors found no significant increased risk of depressive symptoms and only small increased risks of fatigue and sexual dysfunction (Ko et al., 2002). Therefore, the risks of adverse effects (fatigue) should be considered in context with the well-documented benefits of medications such as beta-adrenergic blockers.

Problems with the peripheral vascular system are frequently manifested with intermittent claudication. The patient reports pain in the muscles of the lower extremities associated with activity, which may be due to arterial insufficiency. Chapter 43 ⊙ includes a complete discussion of both venous and arterial peripheral vascular disorders.

Past Medical History

Past medical history should be reviewed because many past illnesses or disorders of other systems of the body can affect the cardiovascular system directly or indirectly. Additionally, the clinical manifestations of other diseases may mistakenly be attributed to cardiovascular disorders. For example, it is important to determine the presence of respiratory disorders to assess a patient's complaint of dyspnea properly, or a history of rheumatic heart disease may have damaged the heart valves. Unit 7 ⊙ discusses respiratory management, and Chapter 41 ⊙ discusses rheumatic fever and valve disorders.

Childhood Illnesses and Immunizations

Childhood illnesses, congenital heart diseases, history of murmurs, cyanosis, streptococcal infections, anemia, and rheumatic fever should all be assessed. They can either exacerbate current cardiovascular conditions or contribute to the development of additional cardiovascular problems and disease states. Nurses should question the status of immunizations and make sure they are up-to-date.

Previous Illnesses and Hospitalizations

Heart failure, coronary artery disease (CAD), stroke, heart valve disease, mitral valve prolapse, previous myocardial infarction (MI), peripheral vascular disease (PVD), diabetes mellitus (DM), hypertension (HTN), hyperlipidemia, dysrhythmias, murmurs, endocarditis, psychiatric illnesses, thrombophlebitis, deep vein thrombosis (DVT), and systemic or pulmonary emboli are all important components of or contributors to cardiovascular disease. Their presence, or a history of their presence, and the potential impact on the present health state must be assessed.

Diagnostic/Interventional Cardiac Procedures or Surgeries

Data from previous diagnostic tests, particularly for cardiovascular symptoms, should be obtained. The patient should be asked whether he had any cardiac studies or interventions in the past such as cardiac catheterizations, cardiac ultrasounds, electrocardiograms (ECGs), exercise tolerance tests (stress tests), or myocardial imaging. Previous chest x-rays or ECGs may be helpful to view for baseline data.

Past surgeries, treatments, or hospital admissions should be explored. Assess for a history of previous percutaneous transluminal coronary angioplasty (PTCA), atherectomy stent placement, or valvuloplasty. See Chapter 39 ⊙ for more information on diagnostic and interventional therapies for heart disease.

Medications

The patient's current and past medications should be reviewed. This includes over-the-counter (OTC) and any prescription medications. A medication list with the name and dose of each medication and the patient's understanding of its purpose is helpful. The consumption of herbal remedies or dietary supplements should be specifically assessed because some cardiovascular complications have been linked to these substances. Consideration is made of other common medications and their potential side effects on cardiovascular status. Chart 37–1 outlines common medications and their side effects that affect the cardiovascular system.

Cultural Considerations

Health and well-being of a culturally diverse population can be promoted by incorporating the therapies that patients have traditionally used. The basis for many complementary therapies is to promote harmony, promote health, reduce anxiety, and increase comfort (Snyder & Miska, 2003). During the assessment phase, nurses must be able to gather information on the use of all therapies being used by a patient, including complementary and nontraditional therapies, as discussed in the Complementary and Alternative Therapies box, in order to plan care that is safe and comfortable.

CHART 37–1	Common Medications and Side Effects That Affect Cardiovascular Status

Medication	Side Effect
Anabolic steroids	Increased total cholesterol, decreased HDL, hypertrophy
Antihistamines	Dysrhythmias, syncope
Aspirin	Prolonged blood clotting time
Corticosteroids	Sodium and fluid retention
Decongestants	Hypertension and arrhythmias
Doxorubicin (Adriamycin)	Cardiomyopathy
Lithium	Dysrhythmias
Oral contraceptives	Thrombophlebitis
Phenothiazines	Dysrhythmias, hypotension
Recreational or abused drugs	Tachycardia, dysrhythmias
Theophylline preparations	Tachycardia, arrhythmias
Tricyclic antidepressants	Dysrhythmias

Allergies

Certain diagnostic tests to evaluate heart disease use contrast media and medications, so the presence of any allergies, especially to radiographic contrast agents or iodine, should be assessed. Drug interactions or intolerance should also be noted. Information as to the nature of allergic reactions, such as rash, anaphylaxis, or dyspnea, is essential.

Family History

The link between familial history of cardiovascular disease and the risk for similar events is well established (Williams et al., 2001). Specifically, the patient should be asked whether blood relatives have suffered from any of the following: coronary artery disease (CAD) at or under age 55, myocardial infarction, hypertension, stroke, diabetes mellitus, and/or lipid disorders. Collagen vascular diseases such as lupus or scleroderma may be important, because they are linked to the development of cardiac disease or pericarditis. Additionally, a family health history of noncardiac conditions such as asthma, renal disease, and obesity should be noted due to their impact on cardiovascular function.

Risk Factors

It is necessary to assess for the presence of risk factors to anticipate the likelihood of the development of cardiovascular disorders. Risk factors can be classified as either nonmodifiable or modifiable. Nonmodifiable risk factors are not subject to interventions to decrease their significance yet play an important role in the development of cardiovascular diseases. Nonmodifiable risk factors include such things as age, gender, family history, and race. Modifiable risk factors are those that can be treated with interventions to decrease their impact on the development of the disorder. Modifiable risk factors include cigarette smoking, hypertension (HTN), hypercholesterolemia, physical inactivity, diabetes, stress, and obesity. Chapter 40 📀 includes a complete description of cardiac risk factors. Additionally, recent dental work or infection may put the patient at risk for development of cardiac complications such as endocarditis. Another risk factor associated with cardiovascular disorders is metabolic syndrome, as discussed in the Risk Factors box (p. 1058).

Social History

An assessment of social history is important because of the relationship between social history and the development of, acceleration of, and response to cardiovascular diseases. Risk factor assessment and history taking are done simultaneously. While taking a social history, nurses can gain valuable information from the patient about the presence of risk factors. Nurses then

MyNursingKit | Center for Disease Control

COMPLEMENTARY & ALTERNATIVE THERAPIES   **Herbal Products**

ONE OF THE MOST important complementary therapies that should be addressed during assessment is the use of herbal products. There is a known risk of interaction between herbal products and conventional medications.

Research Support:
A study by Yoon and Claydell (2001) explored the use of herbal products for medicinal purposes and compared differences in demographic characteristics and health status of herbal product users and nonusers among community-dwelling older women. In 1998, a random sample of 86 women aged 65 years and older who lived independently in a north central Florida county was selected. Questionnaires were completed for the 86 subjects. Findings indicated that herbal products had been used by 45% of the sample in the previous 12 months. The average number of herbal products used by the 45% was 2.5. Herbal products were used to prevent health problems (41%), to treat illness (23%), and for both prevention and treatment (36%). The three most commonly used herbal products were ginkgo biloba or ginkgo biloba with other combinations, garlic tablets and cloves, and glu-

cosamine with chondroitin. The women reported using an average of 3.2 prescribed medicines and 3.8 nonprescribed medicines. The most frequently used nonprescribed medicines taken regularly were multivitamins, calcium, vitamin E, vitamin C, and aspirin. Interestingly, there were no differences in demographic characteristics and health status for users and nonusers of herbal products except that herbal product users were more concerned with memory problems than were nonusers (Yoon & Claydell, 2001). The implications for nurses are that it is important for health care providers to be knowledgeable about the use of herbal products to provide comprehensive health care. In order to make these needed adaptations of care, nurses must be knowledgeable and committed to provide culturally competent care.

References
Yoon, S., & Claydell, H. (2001). Herbal products and conventional medicines used by community-residing older women. *Journal of Advanced Nursing, 33*(1), 51–59.

RISK FACTORS Related to Metabolic Syndrome

The metabolic syndrome describes a cluster of risk factors that significantly increases the incidence of an acute cardiac event and other diseases related to plaque buildup in artery walls (e.g., stroke and peripheral vascular disease) and type II diabetes. The metabolic syndrome has become increasingly common in the United States. It is estimated that over 50 million Americans have it (American Heart Association [AHA], 2008a). The *Third Report of the National Cholesterol Education Program Expert Panel on Detection, Evaluation, and Treatment of High Blood Cholesterol in Adults (Adult Treatment Panel III)* (ATP III) defines and describes the importance of metabolic syndrome. Individuals having three or more of the following criteria are defined as having the metabolic syndrome (National Institutes of Health, 2001; AHA, 2006):

- Abdominal obesity: waist circumference > 102 cm in men and > 88 cm in women
- Hypertriglyceridemia: > 150 mg/dL (1.69 mmol/L)
- Low high-density lipoprotein (HDL) cholesterol: < 40 mg/dL (1.04 mmol/L) in men and < 50 mg/dL (1.29 mmol/L) in women
- High blood pressure: > 130/85 mmHg
- High fasting glucose: > 110 mg/dL (>6.1 mmol/L)
- Prothrombotic state (e.g., high fibrinogen or plasminogen activator inhibitor–1 in the blood)
- Proinflammatory state (e.g., elevated C-reactive protein in the blood).

Abdominal obesity, elevated triglycerides, and insulin resistance (a metabolic disorder in which the body is unable to use insulin efficiently) are major features in metabolic syndrome and have a complex relationship. Fat accumulation in the lower body (pear-shaped) is subcutaneous, whereas fat accumulation in the abdominal area (apple-shaped) is largely visceral fat. Excess abdominal fat disrupts the normal balance and functioning of several hormones, including lipids and insulin. Abdominal fat and circulating triglycerides both increase with age, and recent studies have confirmed their relationship as major metabolic risk factors (Kahn & Valdez, 2003). Therefore, waist circumference measurement, as a measure of abdominal fat, is a useful tool in physical assessment and is a reliable, inexpensive indicator that helps identify those at risk for lipid accumulation. While assessing risk factors, nurses should be aware that individuals with metabolic syndrome are at a greater risk for developing cardiovascular disease than are individuals without metabolic syndrome (Kahn, Buse, Ferrannini, & Stern, 2005). Other conditions commonly associated with metabolic syndrome include physical inactivity, aging, hormonal imbalance, and genetic predisposition. Metabolic syndrome is discussed in depth in Chapter 40 🔗.

have an important role in assisting patients to recognize unhealthy habits that require education in order to modify or change to prevent the progression and complications associated with the development of cardiovascular disorders. As nurses develop relationships with patients, they are in a unique position to offer assistance in risk factor analysis and lifestyle modification. The identification of the presence of modifiable risk factors, as well as the patient's ability and interest in adopting lifestyle changes, forms a framework for the nursing discharge teaching plan discussed in the subsequent cardiac disorder chapters.

Occupation

Job stress is a common condition that promotes the occurrence of cardiovascular events. Previous and recent job-related stres-

sors should be explored. Stress and tension regardless of their etiology cause vasoconstriction, which increases afterload, oxygen consumption, and release of catecholamines, which in turn can contribute to the development of cardiac symptoms. Another occupational hazard that should be considered is exposure to noxious or harmful substances, and the potential effect of them on the cardiovascular system.

Culture

Nurses should be prepared to care for a diverse group of people, because the numbers of patients from other cultures in the health care system have increased. There is a great deal of variation in cultural consistency of different demographic areas. Beliefs and values related to health, illness, and death, as well as daily habits, nutritional preferences, and health practices, may exist that are culturally important to the patient, but conflict with the health care environment or even the function of the cardiovascular status. Nurses may need to ask questions about upcoming religious celebrations or rituals that might affect dietary patterns or preferences (Smith-Stoner, 2006). For example, the patient should be asked about the salt content in the food, because an increased amount may precipitate an episode of heart failure and/or high blood pressure. As nurses are caring for more diverse populations, they need to be knowledgeable about the health practices of other cultures and religions.

Environment

Environment and lifestyle issues are also strongly correlated with the risk for cardiovascular disease. Environmental conditions such as living conditions and the presence of any cardiovascular toxins may need to be addressed. It is understood that heart disease develops as a result of complex interactions between genes and the environment in which we live (Bhatnagar, 2006). Environmental risk factors are not limited to the better known risk factors of smoking, poor diet, and lack of exercise, but also include exposure to pollutants and chemicals. Similarly to the response to secondhand smoke, cardiovascular tissues are extremely sensitive to environmental chemicals and pollutants; therefore, environmental exposures should be routinely considered during cardiovascular assessment. Specifically, nurses should assess for exposure to particulate matter, arsenic, or metals. Further research is needed to determine the relationship of environmental chemicals and cardiovascular toxicity (Bhatnagar, 2006).

Habits

Lifestyle habits and dietary habits such as the use of tea, coffee, alcohol, recreational drugs, over-the-counter drugs, and smoking should be discussed and documented. If the patient smokes, the number of pack years of smoking (packs smoked per day multiplied by the years smoked) should be calculated. The patient's attitude about smoking and any attempts to stop smoking should be documented. The presence of secondhand smoke also must be assessed. Alcohol use, including type of beverages, amount, frequency, and any change in the reaction to it should be assessed. The use of habit-forming drugs and recreational drugs should be noted.

Exercise

The practice of engaging in physical activity has long been known to reduce the risk of cardiovascular events. Low levels of physical activity as well as consumption of excess calories, combined with inherited genes, cause obesity. Obesity, especially abdominal obesity, is a predisposing factor for the development of cardiovascular disease as well as hypertension and type II diabetes mellitus. The physical activity patterns of a patient, including the type of exercise, the duration and frequency of the exercise, and the presence of any cardiovascular symptoms, should be documented. Any decrease in previous abilities or changes in the response to physical activity should be noted, because they may be indications of the advent or progression of heart disease.

In 1996 with revisions in 1999, the Surgeon General of the United States Public Health Service published a report on physical activity and health. This report contains a comprehensive review of scientific evidence about the relationship between physical activity and health status in an attempt to heighten America's awareness of this important public health issue. The report makes it clear that current levels of physical activity among Americans remain low; however, the emphasis is that people can benefit from even moderate levels of physical activity, and that even greater health benefits can be achieved by increasing the amount (duration, frequency, or intensity) of physical activity (Centers for Disease Control and Prevention [CDC], 2008). The report suggests that adults should strive to meet either of the following physical activity recommendations.

- Adults should engage in moderate-intensity physical activities for at least 30 minutes on 5 or more days of the week (Centers for Disease Control and Prevention, 2008).

OR

- Adults should engage in vigorous-intensity physical activity 3 or more days per week for 20 or more minutes per occasion (U.S. Department of Health and Human Services [DHHS], 2004).

Nutrition

It is important to assess the patient's weight and diet history. An assessment of weight in comparison to height and build must be completed. Being overweight or underweight either may be related to certain cardiovascular disorders or may put the patient at risk for developing certain cardiac problems. Usual dietary intake including amounts of salt, saturated fats, triglycerides, and fluids should be determined. It may be important to identify which dietary habits are related to cultural preferences and which habits are the results of the environment or social situations. For example, an executive may consume many meals at restaurants while out with clients, and a construction worker might eat many meals at fast-food restaurants. In addition, the patient's attitudes and plans in relation to diet should be discussed. Food intake patterns should be accountable to exercise patterns and should be complementary.

The National Guidelines box outlines the dietary guidelines for Americans released by the American Heart Association in 2000. Choosing healthy foods can help to prevent the three major risk factors for heart attack—high blood cholesterol, high blood pressure, and excess body weight. Because heart disease and high blood pressure are major risk factors for stroke, these dietary guidelines also help prevent stroke (American Heart Association, 2006).

Personal Factors

Baseline cognitive functioning, recent life changes especially within the last 12 months, sleep-rest patterns, and relationship

---

NATIONAL GUIDELINES for Diet

American Heart Association 2006 Diet and Lifestyle Recommendations

Achieve an Overall Healthy Eating Pattern

- Choose an overall balanced diet with foods from all major food groups, emphasizing fruits, vegetables, and grains.
- Consume a variety of fruits, vegetables, and grain products.
- Eat at least 5 daily servings of fruits and vegetables.
- Eat at least 6 daily servings of grain products, including whole grains.
- Include fat-free and low-fat dairy products, fish, legumes, poultry, and lean meats.
- Eat at least 2 servings of fish per week.

Achieve a Healthy Body Weight

- Maintain a level of physical activity that achieves fitness and balances energy expenditure with caloric intake; for weight reduction, expenditure should exceed intake.
- Limit foods that are high in calories and/or low in nutritional quality, including those with a high amount of added sugar.

Achieve a Desirable Cholesterol Level

- Limit foods with a high content of saturated fat and cholesterol. Substitute with grains and unsaturated fat from vegetables, fish, legumes, and nuts.
- Limit cholesterol to 300 milligrams (mg) a day for the general population and 200 milligrams a day for those with heart disease or its risk factors.
- Limit *trans* fatty acids. Trans fatty acids are found in foods containing partially hydrogenated vegetable oils such as packaged cookies, crackers, and other baked goods; commercially prepared fried foods; and some margarines.

Achieve a Desirable Blood Pressure Level

- Limit salt intake to less than 6 grams (2,400 milligrams sodium) per day, slightly more than 1 teaspoon a day.
- If you drink, limit alcohol consumption to no more than one drink per day for women and two drinks per day for men.

Source: American Heart Association. (2006). *Dietary guidelines: At-a-glance.* Retrieved January 21, 2008, from http://www.americanheart.org/presenter.jhtml?identifier=851.

---

issues should all be considered. Emotional state, such as the evidence of psychological stress, anger, anxiety, or depression, causes the release of catecholamines, which results in vasoconstriction, thereby increasing cardiac workload and potentially resulting in a decreased cardiac output. Perception of illness and its meaning for the future should also be noted.

Personality type may also be a consideration for cardiovascular assessment. Type A personality behavior has been associated with increased incidence of cardiovascular disease. Researchers have found conflicting evidence to support or refute this notion. Gallacher, Sweetman, Yarnell, Elwood, and Stansfeld (2003) suggest that increased exposure to circumstances that induce extreme cardiovascular activity, as seen in type A personality behavior, may be a "trigger" that precipitates coronary events rather than affecting the process of atherosclerosis. The role of stress and the manner in which an individual deals with life stressors may also have an important role. Individuals with type

A personality may respond to stress with hostility or aggression, which may exaggerate sympathetic and hemodynamic responses leading to greater cardiovascular reactivity (Schroeder et al., 2000).

Physical Examination

A thorough physical examination is the foundation for accurate assessment of the cardiovascular system and encompasses skills of inspection, palpation, and ausculation. Percussion is not utilized for assessment of the cardiovascular system.

Inspection of Skin and Extremities

A great deal of information can be obtained about the status of the cardiovascular system by simply observing and touching the patient. An experienced nurse is able to assess general appearance quickly, including facial expressions, body posture and mentation, as well as color and temperature, and clubbing of the nail beds. Then it is necessary to relate the findings to the patient's current cardiovascular status.

General Appearance

General appearance includes a brief visual inspection of a patient's physical appearance. Observations of a patient who looks unwell, lethargic, exhausted, or breathless are important findings and may indicate reduced cardiac output or heart failure. An obese person who has fat evenly distributed over the body is vulnerable for serious cardiovascular health consequences. Additionally, an accumulation of abdominal (visceral) fat, measured by waist circumference, is a known risk factor for cardiovascular and other diseases.

Interestingly, recent studies suggest that variances in fat distributions (abdominal vs. peripheral) may exhibit different influences on lipid metabolism. Laszlo et al. (2004) studied 1,356 women aged 60 to 85 years and found that abdominal fat mass promoted atherogenesis, whereas peripheral fat deposits actually counteracted atherogenesis. The women with peripheral fat deposits rather than central fat deposits showed a negative correlation with glucose and lipid metabolites. The authors concluded that the localization or distribution of the fat mass is an important consideration in obese patients and should be considered during any risk appraisal.

Observation of facial expression may indicate important findings, such as the assessment of apprehension, pain, or fear. Body posture may indicate the amount of effort it takes to breathe. For example, a patient in acute heart failure may need to sit upright, whereas a patient with pericarditis may lean forward in order to breathe comfortably (Urden, Lough, & Stacy, 2006).

Mentation

Adequate functioning of all subsystems of the body indicates the individual organ is receiving adequate cardiac output. For example, normal neurological function indicates adequate cerebral perfusion. A quick and easy method to estimate baseline cognitive function is to assess the patient's orientation to person, place and time, and situation. Confusion could indicate hypotension or low cardiac output.

Color and Appearance of Skin and Extremities

The skin and mucous membranes are inspected for color and temperature. Extremities should be assessed bilaterally for equal temperature and appearance. The extremities are inspected for signs of peripheral arterial or venous vascular disorders. Arterial vascular disease is suspected when the skin is pale, shiny, with sparse hair growth. Venous vascular diseases cause an edematous limb with deep red rubor, brown discoloration, and leg ulcerations (Urden, Lough, & Stacy, 2006). Chapter 43 includes an in-depth description of peripheral vascular disease.

Cyanosis

Cyanosis is a bluish tinge to the skin due to deoxygenated hemoglobin in the blood vessels close to the skin surface; it can be either central or peripheral. Central cyanosis, which is noted on the lips or tongue, is often characteristic of impaired gas exchange. Central cyanosis may result from a cardiac right-to-left shunt due to septal defects, in which deoxygenated venous blood mixes with blood from the left heart and is ejected into the systemic circulation. In heart failure with significant pulmonary congestion, oxygenation of blood in the pulmonary vascular bed can be impaired, which leads to deoxygenated blood returning to the left heart and being pumped out into the systemic circulation. Peripheral cyanosis, which occurs in the extremities or under the nail beds, may indicate poor circulation. The room where the examination is taking place must have a comfortable temperature because nail beds can become cyanotic with cold temperatures.

Pallor

Pallor suggests poor perfusion, which may be related to peripheral vascular disease (a narrowing in the blood vessels outside the heart); a release of catecholamines and subsequent vasoconstriction; or a low hemoglobin and hematocrit. All of these conditions should be thoroughly assessed. Additionally, temperature changes such as generalized warmth or coolness may indicate altered peripheral perfusion.

Nail Beds

Clubbing of nail beds is easily assessed and appears as swelling of the subcutaneous tissue over the base of the nail and absence of the normal angle between the nail and the nail base. The presence of clubbing indicates long-term oxygen deficiencies such as congenital heart defects or pulmonary diseases with hypoxemia.

Neck Veins

The right external and internal jugular veins (Figure 37–5 ■) are used to assess for jugular venous distention (JVD) and **jugular venous pressure (JVP)** or pulse. Although these terms are often used interchangeably, there is a physiological significance in distinguishing between JVD and JVP. Anatomically, the right jugular veins drain blood from the head into the right atrium of the heart. Both veins reflect activity on the right side of the heart. The internal jugular vein lies in a straight path to the right atrium, but because it is buried beneath the sternomastoid muscle, it is difficult to visualize. The external jugular vein curves a few times before entering the right atrium, and because it is located closer to the skin it is easier to visualize. Findings from neck vein assessment are helpful in confirming suspicions of heart failure; however, the information must be put in context of the presenting symptoms and current health status. The importance of volume status and cardiovascular function is an important hemodynamic concept. Chapter 42 includes an in-depth discussion of the significance of distended neck veins with heart failure.

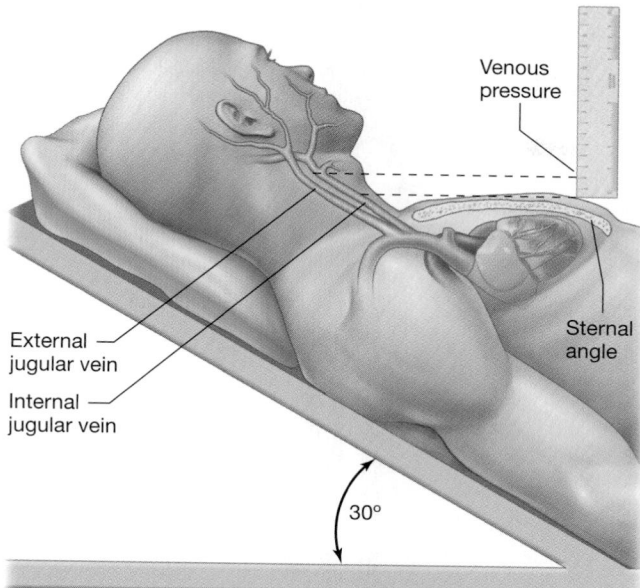

External jugular vein

Internal jugular vein

Venous pressure

Sternal angle

30°

FIGURE 37–5 ■ Jugular veins.

Jugular Venous Distention

Jugular venous distention (JVD) is assessed by visually observing the right external jugular (REJ) vein. Generally noting that this vein is full or overdistended is sufficient for the nursing assessment and provides useful information pertaining to hemodynamic volume status of the cardiovascular system. The REJ vein is always distended when the patient is lying flat and is eliminated as the patient becomes more upright. From a flat position, slowly elevate the head of the bed and observe the right external jugular vein, noting the degree of elevation at which the distention is eliminated (30, 45, 60, or 90 degrees). The finding is reported by noting the highest height of the head of the bed (HOB) when JVD was appreciated; for example, "presence of JVD was noted with HOB elevated to 45 degrees" (Urden et al., 2006).

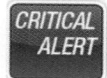 **CRITICAL ALERT** *The finding of JVD during inspection of the neck veins can contribute to diagnosis of right heart failure. Treatment to reduce volume, such as diuretics or vasodilators, may be needed. The finding of JVD may also help to explain other findings noted during the exam, such as shortness of breath (SOB), diaphoresis, or confusion.*

Jugular Venous Pressure

The right internal jugular (RIJ) vein is used to assess jugular venous pulses and jugular venous pressure. The RIJ lies deep in skin and soft tissues, and its pulsations are transmitted to the overlying tissues. These pulsations are produced by the right atrial and right ventricular activity (Garg & Garg, 2000). Changes in pulsations can be a diagnostic tool for the skilled practitioner. Assessment of RIJ for jugular venous pressure (JVP) provides valuable information as well; and it is a more reliable indicator of central venous pressure (CVP), or the pressure that exists in the central venous system, than is the right external vein assessment. To examine the JVP, stand on the patient's right side, and turn the patient's head slightly to the left. The neck muscles should be relaxed. The head of the bed should be elevated high enough to visualize the top of the

column of blood in the internal jugular vein. Observe the highest point of pulsation during exhalation. The vertical difference between this location and the sternal angle (see Figure 37–5 ■) is measured in centimeters. The normal measurement should be 4 centimeters or less. A measurement of more than 4 centimeters suggests increased JVP, an increase in pressure in the right heart, and therefore an increased CVP. Because the distance between the sternal angle and the mid-right atrium is approximately 5 centimeters, to measure CVP, 5 centimeters is added to the measurement of JVP. The upper limit of normal is a CVP measurement of 9 centimeters (JVP of 4 plus 5 centimeters) (Garg & Garg, 2000). An example of how this finding is reported is "JVP estimated at 9 centimeters with the head of the bed elevated to 45 degrees."

Abdominojugular Reflux

The assessment of the abdominojugular reflux (sometimes called hepatojugular reflux) can also be used as a noninvasive technique to assess cardiovascular volume status. In heart failure, or volume overload, blood volume that normally is pumped proficiently by the heart begins to be displaced throughout the body as a mechanism to minimize cardiac workload. Volume may be displaced in the abdomen, particularly the hepatic system, which has a large capacity to hold fluid. The technique to observe **abdominojugular reflux** is done by compressing the right upper abdomen for 15 to 30 seconds. Observe for JVD before, during, and after abdominal compression. This pressure causes volume in the abdomen to be pushed back to the right atrium. The failing heart will not be able to accommodate this increase in volume, and the pressure will be reflected in the jugular veins. Sustained JVD (longer than 10 seconds) with abdominal compression is another indicator that aids the diagnosis of cardiac failure (Urden et al., 2006).

Palpation of Skin and Extremities

Palpation of the skin and extremities during a cardiovascular assessment includes an assessment of edema, skin turgor, capillary refill, and the arterial pulses for abnormalities associated with cardiovascular disorders.

Edema

Edema is defined as an increase in interstitial fluid that is clinically evident. Although there are many types of edema, cardiovascular patients typically experience edema associated with the accumulation of fluid in the extracellular spaces, particularly the skin of the extremities, as seen earlier. Edema of the skin can be painful, and it interferes with normal blood circulation. Edema is an important assessment finding because it is indicative of an underlying disease process and requires treatment.

Normally two-thirds of the body's water is in the cells (intracellular), while one-third is outside the cells (extracellular). Extracellular fluid consists of water in the plasma and in the tissues (interstitial). Fluid exchange between these compartments is governed by a balance of hydraulic and oncotic pressures as well as the permeability of the capillary wall that separates them. When any of the factors are altered, excess fluid may be moved into the plasma and interstitial spaces. Changes in capillary hydraulic pressure can occur with heart failure. Capillary permeability can be increased as a consequence of the inflammatory process, which can be initiated as a response to numerous events including exposure to allergens. The kidneys play an important role in body fluid distribution as the kidneys respond to changes in blood pressure and volume by adjusting retention of sodium. Therefore, sodium balance is of utmost importance in cardiovascular disease processes involving the development or potential development of edema.

The skin can feel puffy and tight. Edema can be localized in one area of the body or can be generalized throughout. Dependent edema occurs when there is an increase in extracellular fluid volume in a dependent limb or area. Edema is assessed by firmly placing a thumb against a dependent area of the body (arms, hands, legs, feet, ankles). When the pressure is released, an indentation on the skin may be observed. When the indentation remains on the skin after releasing pressure, it is referred to as pitting edema. The degree of pitting edema can be rated on a 4-point scale (Chart 37–2).

Skin Turgor

Palpation of the skin **turgor**, or elasticity, reflects the skin's state of hydration. A small section of the patient's skin (anterior chest, under clavicle, or abdomen) is pinched between the examiner's thumb and forefinger. As the skin is slowly released, the speed at which the skin returns to its original contour is observed. It should return to normal rapidly. If there is poor skin turgor, the skin returns to its original contour very slowly. Dehydration, scleroderma, or aging can decrease skin turgor.

Capillary Refill

Capillary refill, the rate at which blood refills empty capillaries, is a quick method of assessing blood flow to the peripheral microcirculation. The tip of the finger is compressed until blanching of the nail bed is noted. When pressure is released, a return of color should be noted within 2 to 3 seconds. A delayed return of color is a sign of vasoconstriction or poor peripheral perfusion. A delayed capillary refill may be observed in heart failure, peripheral vascular disease (PVD), or shock.

Arterial Pulses

Palpation of the pulses in the neck and extremities provides information about arterial blood flow, particularly volume and pressure within the vessels. Arterial pulses are palpated bilaterally to compare characteristics of the arteries on the right and left sides of the body (Figure 37–6 ■). The volume of the pulsations is judged and recorded as normal, bounding, thready, or absent. Additionally, a common scale can be used for documentation of pulses. A score of 0 indicates an absent pulse. A score of 1+ indicates a pulse is present, but it is weak and thready. A score of 2+ indicates a pulse is present and normal in amplitude. A score of 3+ indicates a full and bounding pulsation. A normal

Systemic Circulation

FIGURE 37–6 ■ Arterial pulses.

pulse feels like a tap, whereas a vessel that is narrowed or bulging will vibrate. The rate and rhythm of arterial pulses are palpated. The examiner counts the number of pulsations in a minute to determine the heart rate. At the same time, a judgment is made as to the regularity of the pattern of pulses and the intervals between pulses. Pulses can be normal or abnormal. Abnormalities in rate and rhythm of arterial pulses may indicate inadequate cardiac output or cardiac dysrhythmias.

Inspection and Palpation of the Precordium

Inspection and palpation of the bony structures of the thorax, including the sternoclavicular joints, the manubrium, and the upper part of the sternum, are performed using clinical reference points. The precordium is assessed for pulsations, heaves, and thrills described on page 1063, which may indicate vessel abnormalities.

Clinical Reference Points

The normal clinical reference points or landmarks of the chest wall, as well as specific auscultatory areas, should be noted on every patient during cardiovascular assessment in a consistent manner. Experience enhances the ability to identify abnormalities and their significance to cardiovascular disorders (Figures 37–7 ■ and 37–8 ■).

Point of Maximal Impulse (PMI)

The mitral valve area of the thorax is palpated for the point of maximal impulse (PMI). This pulsation is normally located at the left fifth intercostal space (ICS) at the midclavicular line (MCL) (see Figure 37–7 ■). With the patient in a sitting position, the nurse uses fingertips to identify the PMI. Sometimes having the patient lean slightly forward enhances the PMI. The

CHART 37–2	**Scale for Rating Edema**
+0″	No pitting
+1	0″ – ¼″ pitting (mild)
+2	¼″ – ½″ pitting (moderate)
+3	½″ – 1″ pitting (severe)
+4	Greater than 1″ pitting (severe)

FIGURE 37–7 ■ Clinical reference points for palpation.

Right sternal border (RSB), 2nd intercostal space (ICS)

Left sternal border (LSB), 2nd ICS

LSB, 3rd ICS

LSB, 4th ICS

Midclavicular line (MCL), 5th ICS

Point of maximal impulse

PMI is normally felt as a single pulsation or light tap, and is 1 to 2 centimeters in diameter. The position and the diameter of the PMI should be recorded in relation to the MCL and ICSs. If the patient has an enlarged heart (cardiomegaly) due to heart failure, ventricular hypertrophy, or pregnancy, the PMI may be enlarged or displaced laterally and downward. The PMI may also be visualized as a pulsation on the chest in a patient with cardiovascular disease.

Heaves and Thrills

The precordium is inspected for pulsations, heaves, and thrills. Although rare, pulsations may be visualized on the chest wall, particularly in thin patients, and may be caused by pulmonary hypertension or a significant aneurysm. **Heaves** or lifts, which are normally not seen or felt over the precordium, are sustained lifts of the chest wall in the precordial area due to forceful cardiac contractions that cause a slight to vigorous movement of the sternum and ribs. Heaves may be caused by ventricular enlargement or hypertrophy. A **thrill** describes a palpable vibra-

tory sensation from turbulent blood flow across cardiac valves. Thrills are typically described as the throat of a purring cat.

Findings in various clinical reference points may indicate specific cardiac disorders. The respiratory system is observed simultaneously, because the purpose of the cardiovascular system is to deliver oxygen to the tissues that was received from the respiratory system. Alterations in rate and depth of respirations may indicate cardiovascular, respiratory, or neurological disorders.

Ausculation of the Precordium

Ausculation involves listening to the sounds produced by different body areas. Cardiac auscultation is an efficient, noninvasive manner to assess both normal and abnormal heart sounds. Although the technique is simply performed with only a stethoscope, a great deal of practice and expertise is required to appreciate and differentiate cardiac abnormalities associated with valvular alterations. The art of auscultation includes the ability to discriminate subtle differences in intensity, pitch, location, radiation, duration, timing, and intervals of heart sounds (O'Connor, 1998). Generally, nurses should be able to perform the technique proficiently, be able to recognize normal ausculatory sounds, and most importantly be alert to variations from normal that can provide valuable clinical clues and may indicate a change or deterioration in cardiac status.

The skill of auscultation begins with good technique and a quiet environment. The stethoscope should be of good quality with a bell, a diaphragm, and comfortable earpieces. The stethoscope must be applied directly to the skin; listening over clothing will obscure the sound. The patient should be in a comfortable position and asked to lie still and not talk. Imagine the position of the heart and the cardiac valves under the chest wall (see Figure 37–8 ■). Find the angle of Louis, felt as a ridge just below the suprasternal notch (see Figure 37–1 ■, p. 1053). Feel the ribs on each side of this angle and the intercostal space below each rib. Using the bell and the diaphragm of the stethoscope, listen to heart sounds at each ausculatory area (see Figure 37–8 ■), first with the diaphragm for high-pitched sounds and then with the bell with very light pressure for low-pitched sounds at each ausculatory

FIGURE 37–8 ■ Ausculatory areas.

site. Listen for the normal S_1 and S_2 heart sounds at each site, and note the intensity, the presence of split sounds, and the effect of the respiratory cycle on the regularity of the sounds. Also note the time between the S_1 and S_2 for regularity. Listen for extra heart sounds and abnormal heart sounds at each site. If abnormal sounds are heard, note the timing, pitch, loudness, duration, and location on the chest wall. If a murmur is heard, note where it can be heard best and whether it is a low-, medium-, or high-pitched sound. The presence of any pericardial friction rubs should also be noted.

Requirements for Ausculation

In order to understand cardiac ausculation, nurses need to have knowledge of the physiology of the cardiac cycle, the normal landmarks of the chest (see Figure 37–7 ■, p. 1063), and the ausculatory sites on the chest wall that correspond to specific valve sounds (see Figure 37–8 ■, p. 1063). When listening to dynamic blood flow across cardiac valves, the sounds associated with the closure of the valves are not heard directly over that valve area, but rather in the direction of the flow of blood. It is helpful to imagine the physical position of the heart under the chest wall, as well as the path or direction of blood flow (Figure 37–9 ■). Because sound is not transmitted through bone, the best ausculatory area of a particular valve would be the nearest tissue area in line with the path of blood flow. The key to a good ausculatory exam is to listen to one sound at a time in each ausculatory area. The nurse should be in the habit of listening to all the ausculatory areas with the diaphragm and then again with the bell.

Normal Heart Sounds: S_1 and S_2

Normal heart sounds are created by the turbulence of blood flow as the cardiac valves open and close during the cardiac cycle. As the valves move, some turbulence in blood flow is created. (See the Cardiac Valves section at the beginning of the chapter.) Two heart sounds can be heard with each cardiac cycle. The first heart sound is referred to as S_1 and the second heart sound, S_2. S_1 is a called a systolic sound because it signals the beginning of systole. When the pressures in the pulmonary artery and the right ventricle begin to equalize, and the pressures in the aorta and the left ventricle begin to equalize, systolic ejection tapers off and the semilunar valves snap shut. This signals the beginning of diastole, which allows the AV valves to open and diastolic ventricular filling to begin. The closing of the AV valves is heard as the S_2, or second heart sound (Chart 37–3). The S_1 and the S_2 are both high-pitched sounds heard best with the diaphragm. The S_1 is normally loudest over the apex or mitral area, while the S_2 is best heard over the base of the heart, or the aortic area.

Distinguishing S_1 from S_2

It is helpful during ausculation to differentiate the S_1 from the S_2. When there is an abnormality, it must be described as a sys-

Cardiac blood flow paths

Systemic venous circulation

Pulmonary circulation

Pulmonary circulation

Right atrium

Left atrium

Right ventricle

Left ventricle

Interventricular septum

Systemic venous circulation

Systemic atrial circulation

FIGURE 37–9 ■ Cardiac blood flow path.

CHART37–3 Summary of Heart Sounds

Heart Sounds	Cardiac Cycle Timing	Ausculation Site	Position	Pitch
S₁ (LUB — dub)	Start of systole	Best at apex with diaphragm	Position does not affect the sound	High
S₂ (lub — DUB)	End of systole	Both at 2nd intercostal space (ICS); pulmonary component best at left sternal border (LSB); aortic component best at RBS with diaphragm	Sitting or supine	High
Split S₁	Beginning of systole	If normal, at 2nd ICS, LSB abnormal if heard at apex	Better heard in the supine position	High
Fixed Split S₂	End of systole	Both at 2nd ICS: pulmonary component best at LSB; aortic component best at right sternal border (RSB) with diaphragm	Better heard in the supine position	High
Paradoxial Split S₂	End of systole	Both at 2nd ICS; pulmonary component best at LSB; aortic component best at RSB with diaphragm	Better heard in the supine position	High
Wide Split S₂ (Expiration / Inspiration)	End of systole	Both at 2nd ICS; pulmonary component best at LSB; aortic component best at RSB with diaphragm	Better heard in the supine position	High
S₃	Early diastole right after S₂	Apex with the bell	Ausculated better in left lateral position or supine	Low
S₄	Late diastole right before S₁	Apex with the bell	Ausculated better in left lateral position or supine	Low

tolic sound (occurring with or after the S₁) or a diastolic sound (occurring with or after the S₂). By determining where in the cardiac cycle the abnormality occurs, the listener can better estimate which cardiac valve is affected. For example, if the nurse hears an abnormality of the S₁ sound, she would know there is an alteration in either the mitral or the tricuspid valve. The S₁ and the S₂ sounds can be differentiated by three methods. The first is timing. During the cardiac cycle, the amount of time spent in diastole is longer than the amount of time spent in systole. Therefore, there should be a pause between the S_2 and the next S_1 (Chart 37–3, p. 1065). Of course this method is accurate only when the heart rate is slow enough to appreciate the diastolic pause. If, however, the heart rate is accelerated, the S_1 can be identified by palpating either the PMI (point of maximal impulse) or the carotid arterial pulsation. As the practitioner is listening with the stethoscope on the chest wall to the heart sound, she should be palpating these pulsation points. When the pulsation is felt, the S_1 is heard. Pulse points, further downstream, such as the radial artery should not be used to establish correlation, because they are too far away from the heart and are not likely to correspond with the S_1.

Split Heart Sounds: Split S_1 and Split S_2

Because the right and left heart are two separate pumps that function simultaneously, it is normal to hear the closure of two valves, the right and left AV valves, and the right and left semilunar valves, as one sound. Many conditions can alter the timing of the cardiac cycle on the right or left side of the heart causing one valve to close slightly later than normal. When this happens, the sounds of S_1 (closure of the tricuspid and mitral valves) or the sounds of S_2 (closure of the pulmonic and aortic valves) are heard separately, referred to as a split heart sound.

The S_1 is normally heard as a single sound, although there might be a slight split between the mitral component (M_1) and the tricuspid component (T_1) of the S_1. The S_2 exhibits a normal split on inspiration. This is called a *physiological split*, because it is associated with a normal physiological pattern. This physiological split S_2, heard best over the pulmonic area, is a result of asymmetry with the closure of the aortic (A_2) and pulmonic (P_2) valve sounds that make up the S_2 (A_2P_2). On inspiration, there is an increase in intrathoracic pressure that causes an increase in venous return to the right heart. The increased volume causes a delay in ventricular emptying, and thus the pulmonic valve closure (P_2) is slightly delayed. This effect is removed, however, during expiration; the A_2 and P_2 should be closer in synchrony, and the two components of the second heart sound are heard as one. Numerous other conditions, such as ventricular septal defects (VSDs), bundle branch blocks, and ventricular failure, can cause abnormal splitting of the S_2.

Extra Heart Sounds

Extra heart sounds are classified in relation to their timing in the cardiac cycle. Although the presence of an S_3 or S_4 can be normal, these extra heart sounds often signify cardiac disorders. Therefore, nurses should be knowledgeable about these sounds, as well as their significance in relation to heart disease, in order to detect and report their presence. Third and fourth heart sounds, if present, are both heard during diastole. S_3 and S_4 are low-frequency soft sounds, which are best heard by applying the stethoscope softly on the skin or just firmly enough to create a skin seal. It is easier to detect the S_3 or the S_4 by positioning the patient in the left lateral position, which brings the heart closer to the heart wall. S_3s and S_4s are not affected by respirations and are heard as single sounds.

S_3

S_3 is heard early in diastole just after the S_2 and is heard best in the apex (see Chart 37–3, p. 1065). One cardiac cycle (S_1, S_2, S_3,

sounds like lub-dub-dee or "Ken-tuc'-ky." S_3s are heard early in diastole because they are associated with abnormalities of ventricular filling, and they are sometimes called ventricular gallops. S_3s are markers of systolic dysfunction. When there is ventricular systolic dysfunction, the ventricle is not able to empty sufficiently with each systolic contraction. During each consecutive diastolic filling period, turbulence occurs as the "new" load of blood attempts to enter when the previous load of blood has not completely left the ventricle.

An S_3 heard over the left ventricle in children and young adults is normal, although after ages 35 to 40, the presence of a third heart sound is usually abnormal and may indicate systolic dysfunction. An S_3 and the presence of increased JVD are regarded as specific signs of heart failure. The presence of an S_3 in an older person may be the only clue to abnormal left ventricular function (O'Connor, 1998).

S_4

S_4 occurs late in diastole just before the S_1 and is heard best in the apex (Chart 37–3, p. 1065). One cardiac cycle (S_4, S_1, S_2) sounds like dee-lub-dub or "Ten-nes-see." S_4s are heard late in diastole because they are associated with the atrial kick component of diastole, and they are sometimes called atrial gallops. S_4s are markers of diastolic dysfunction. An S_4 occurs when the atria attempt to pump blood into a stiff, noncompliant ventricle that is resistant to further volume expansion.

Diastolic dysfunction may occur with ventricular hypertrophy associated with hypertension, with aortic stenosis, or with altered ventricular compliance associated with ischemia. Normal fourth heart sounds are common in older adults and are associated with an age-related decrease in left ventricular compliance (O'Connor, 1998). A fourth heart sound is almost always abnormal in children and may contribute to a decrease in ventricular compliance. An S_4 cannot be heard during atrial fibrillation, because S_4s are associated with atrial contraction against a noncompliant ventricle.

Summation Gallop

Summation gallops occur when both an S_3 and an S_4 are heard (S_4, S_1, S_2, S_3) (Chart 37–3, p. 1065); in other words, there is a combined ventricular and atrial gallop. A summation gallop is associated with advanced heart failure. The S_3 and S_4 may be heard as two distinct sounds in diastole or, in the case of tachycardia, as a single mid-diastolic sound. Summation gallops are sometimes described as galloping hooves.

Pericardial Friction Rubs

Pericardial friction rubs are due to inflammation of the pericardial sac surrounding the heart in conditions such as pericarditis. Pericarditis is described in detail in Chapter 41 ☞. Pericardial friction rubs are a transient high-pitched sound heard best at the left sternal border. The sound that is produced is a squeaky, rubbing, muffled sound. Pericardial friction rubs are heard best with the patient leaning forward or lying on the left side. Pericardial friction rubs may be a transient assessment finding.

Abnormal Heart Sounds: Murmurs

Murmurs are audible vibrations heard over the heart and great vessels. Murmurs are caused by turbulent blood flow across a diseased valve (stenosis or regurgitation), turbulence caused by increased blood flow through normal structures, or blood flow into a dilated chamber (Chart 37–4). Whereas murmurs are aus-

CHART37-4 Classification of Murmurs

TIMING
- Timing within the cardiac cycle.
- Systolic or diastolic (early, mid, late, continuous).
- Systolic murmurs are often benign.
- Diastolic murmurs are never benign.

LOCATION Auscultatory area the murmur is best heard.
- Aortic, pulmonic, mitral, tricuspid.
- Presence of murmurs at specific valve sites leads to the identification of the affected valve.

FREQUENCY
- High-pitched or low-pitched sound.
- Low-pitched murmurs are caused by a low velocity of blood flow.
- High-pitched murmurs are caused by a rapid velocity of blood flow.

QUALITY
- Descriptive quality of the sound.
- Harsh, rumbling, musical, soft, blowing, gurgling.
- Quality may indicate regurgitation or stenosis.

PATTERN
- Configuration of sound if one were to draw it.
- Crescendo, decrescendo, diamond shaped.

RADIATION
- Sounds may be radiated to the neck, back, shoulders, sternal border, jaw, arm, or left axilla.
- Some murmurs radiate in the direction of the bloodstream, by which they are produced.

INTENSITY Grading scale of loudness
- I/VI Very soft, barely audible.
- II/VI Soft, but loud enough to be appreciated.
- III/VI Loud, easily heard, no thrills or vibrations.
- IV/VI Loud, soft palpable thrill.
- V/VI Loud, heard with stethoscope barely touching chest wall; palpable thrill.
- VI/VI Very loud, can be heard with stethoscope fully off chest wall, pronounced palpable thrill.

culatory sounds caused by vibrations or turbulence in the heart and great vessels, **bruits** are auscultatory sounds associated with vibrations or turbulence in a blood vessel outside the heart.

Murmur Etiology

Murmurs are due to valve abnormalities of stenosis or regurgitation. Many different physiological conditions can lead to these alterations. A stenotic valve is one whose valve leaflets are hardened, calcified, or narrowed. Blood flow is obstructed as it is forced through a narrowed, stenotic valve orifice. Valve regurgitation occurs when the valve leaflets fail to close completely. This causes valve insufficiency, and a portion of the systolic blood volume is allowed to flow backward. Causes of abnormal valves are discussed in Chapter 41 ⊙. As blood flows through these two different types of valve alterations, the sounds generated are very distinct. For example, blood flowing through a stenotic valve would sound very harsh because blood is being forced through a narrow opening, whereas blood flowing through a regurgitant valve would sound softer and have more of a gurgling quality. The sounds associated with particular valve disorders

would be best heard at the corresponding valve's auscultatory site (Chart 37–5). When a murmur is auscultated, the etiology can be suggested by understanding the physiology of the cardiac cycle and heart sounds. For example, during systole the aortic valve is open, allowing blood to flow from the left ventricle through the aortic valve to the aorta, and the mitral valve is closed, preventing blood from flowing back into the left atrium. If the aortic valve were stenotic, the sound would be a harsh murmur during systole over the aortic valve area. Likewise, if the mitral valve were regurgitant, one would typically hear a gurgling sound over the mitral valve area. During the assessment the nurse should evaluate for head bobbing up and down in synchrony with the heartbeat, because this is characteristic of severe aortic regurgitation (D'Amico & Barbarito, 2007).

Systolic murmurs, heard during systole, include mitral regurgitation, tricuspid regurgitation, aortic stenosis, and pulmonic stenosis. Diastolic murmurs, heard during diastole, include mitral stenosis, tricuspid stenosis, aortic regurgitation, and pulmonic regurgitation.

Innocent Murmurs

Some murmurs may be classified as innocent or functional murmurs. An innocent murmur is a sound made by the blood circulating in the heart chambers or valves, or through the blood vessels near the heart. Innocent murmurs are often soft and may vary or disappear with position changes, whereas pathologic murmurs are generally louder and seldom disappear with position changes. Innocent murmurs are harmless, asymptomatic, and are commonly heard in children. Further diagnostic tests may be performed to rule out other conditions.

When a murmur is heard, it is important to describe the sound properly. Murmurs should be described in terms of their timing in the cardiac cycle, the auscultatory location they are heard best, frequency, intensity, radiation, and quality. A summary of murmurs associated with valve disorders is presented in Chart 37–6 (p. 1068).

Gender Implications/Gender Differences

Before the 1980s, it was believed that cardiovascular disease (CVD) affected primarily men. This was due in large part to the fact that most research studies involved men. It is now well known that women respond uniquely to CVD as well as to other diseases. Women experience the signs and symptoms associated with CVD differently than men. More women have asymptomatic and undiagnosed CVD. It is difficult to apply preventive cardiovascular care to women who have not been identified as having CVD. Mortality

CHART37-5 Valve Opening and Closing with Cardiac Cycle

	Open	Closed	Abnormality
SYSTOLE	Pulmonic Aortic (stenosis)	Tricuspid Mitral (regurgitation)	Regurgitation is unable to completely close
DIASTOLE	Tricuspid Mitral (stenosis)	Pulmonic Aortic (regurgitation)	Stenosis is unable to completely open

CHART 37–6 Summary of Murmurs Associated with Valve Disorders

AORTIC STENOSIS

1. Midsystolic, crescendo-decrescendo
2. Harsh
3. Usually heard best in the aortic area
4. Often heard widely over the chest
5. Often radiates to the carotid arteries
6. Loudness unrelated to severity

AORTIC REGURGITATION

1. Present in early diastole
2. Decrescendo configuration
3. High-pitched blowing
4. Heard best with the patient leaning forward; often faint
5. Loudness along Left Lower Sternal Border (LLSB)

MITRAL STENOSIS

1. Long, rumbling diastolic murmur
2. Low pitched
3. Heard best with bell
4. Localized to mitral area (apex)
5. Often accompanied by a diastolic thrill in the area
6. Crescendo occurs in late diastole

MITRAL REGURGITATION

1. Pansystolic
2. Loudest in mitral area (apex)
3. Radiates to left axilla
4. Usually blowing in quality
5. Systolic thrill usually present in mitral area

INNOCENT MURMUR

1. Short, soft, systolic
2. Normal S_1 and S_2
3. Normal ECG and chest x-ray
4. Crescendo-decrescendo
5. Heard in primary aortic area

rates of CVD, particularly from sudden death, are currently higher in women than in men (D'Amore and Mora, 2006). D'Amore and Mora (2006) suggest that women previously deemed at intermediate risk for the development of CVD from standard available guidelines, but who have concerning features in their medical history such as a strong family history, may benefit from stress testing, which may provide further gender-specific prognostic information. Further studies are needed to identify gender-specific predictors of cardiac disease, and more comprehensive approaches to CVD prevention and treatment are needed for women. Although, many of the gender-specific differences in CVD are not well explained, it is well understood that postmenopausal women are at greater risk of developing CVD than are premenopausal women.

This is due to the cardioprotective effect of estrogen in premenopausal women. (Genetic predispositions to cardiovascular disease are discussed in the Genetic Considerations box.)

Gerontological Considerations

The number of elderly people over age 65 in the population of the United States has been steadily increasing. Therefore, it stands to reason that the number of elderly patients cared for in health care settings will also increase. The gerontological population has unique considerations, which are important in cardiovascular assessment. Physiological changes associated with aging include myocardial hypertrophy; an increase in collagen and scarring; a decrease in elasticity; fibrotic and sclerotic changes of the atria and ventricles; calcification, sclerosis, or fibrosis of the cardiac valves; and rigidity and fibrosis of the vessels of the arterial system. These changes can lead to a drop in cardiac output, systolic or diastolic murmurs, increased frequency of dysrhythmias, and altered blood flow dynamics, all of which affect tissue perfusion. For example, elderly persons may have elevations in systolic or diastolic blood pressures. Additionally, in the response to injury or shock, the heart becomes less able to respond or initiate the stimulation of catecholamines needed to increase heart rate and contractility (Whetstone & Boswell, 2002). It is not uncommon to hear an S_4 in an elderly person due to decreased compliance of the left ventricle or a systolic murmur due to aortic or mitral valve abnormalities. Thickened myocardial fibers can also affect the conduction system of the heart and cause cardiac irritability and dysrhythmias. Diseases affecting other body systems can

GENETIC CONSIDERATIONS for Cardiovascular Disease

A great deal is known about the independent risk factors for the development of cardiovascular disease. Advances made in the area of genetics since the Human Genome Project in 1988 have helped scientists understand the genetic causes of cardiovascular disease. It has become clear that most cardiovascular diseases result from various genetic causes (Allen, 2000). Gene mutations and the interaction of genes and the environment are currently being examined. For example, polygenic disorders, such as hypertension, are caused by the combined effect of more than one mutated gene. Interestingly, the nature and severity of polygenic disorders vary significantly and are unpredictable in nature (Allen, 2000).

Coronary artery disease is an example of a multifactorial disorder. Multifactorial disorders may have a genetic component, but the presentation is largely affected by environmental factors. For example, multifactorial disorders may include an interaction of genetic factors (genetic abnormalities that result in lipid disorders, hypertension, and obesity) with nongenetic factors such as smoking, increasing age, and physical activity.

Through a thorough cardiovascular assessment, and potentially future genetic testing, inherited cardiovascular diseases or the susceptibility to diseases can be identified. The hope is that early detection and diagnosis will identify individuals at risk. Then prevention or modulation of the effects can be undertaken by the implementation of a treatment plan, education, and counseling. The goal of genetic testing would be to save lives through preventive treatment and therapeutic interventions. Nurses can complete family history assessments and initiate appropriate referrals for genetic counseling.

affect the heart and blood vessels. Diabetes mellitus is one example of a disease that can have damaging effects on the peripheral vasculature, and another is chronic obstructive lung disease, which contributes to right-sided heart failure.

Normal physiological changes in the elderly can contribute to the significance of cardiovascular signs and symptoms. For example, loss of muscle mass is a normal physiological change but can contribute to symptoms of weakness of fatigue. It is essential to encourage a healthy diet and regular exercise program. The gerontological population is more susceptible to cognitive impairments that make them more vulnerable to the effects of cardiac diseases and their treatments (Garrett, 1997). Dementia and delerium are common cognitive impairments found in the geriatric population. Cognitive losses of dementia affect the overall ability of an individual to interact successfully with the environment. The way the individual responds to stimuli from touch or stimuli from the environment may vary among individuals and should be considered prior to the exam (Garrett, 1997). The nurse needs to understand that there may be limitations in the patient's abilities to learn and apply new knowledge. It will be much more difficult for the individual who is cognitively impaired to manage the complexities of his cardiovascular disease and its treatment. Changes in cerebral perfusion due to atherosclerosis may also be present. When cognitive impairments such as dementia or delerium are suspected, the ability to provide accurate information for the health history will be altered (Garrett, 1997).

Critical Thinking Related to Cardiovascular Assessment

Critical thinking is essential in order to prioritize the most significant clinical manifestations that need further investigation. Cardiovascular clinical manifestations can range from conditions as benign as an innocent murmur to life-threatening disorders such as heart failure. It is imperative that the nurse be able to distinguish normal from abnormal, benign from serious. The nurse must rely on critical thinking skills in interpreting the patient's symptoms and assessment findings to determine possible and potential patient diagnoses and to consider the appropriate actions to take. Analysis of these data allows the nurse to make a diagnosis and then follow up with an intervention. It is imperative that the nurse communicate and collaborate with other members of the health care team in developing and implementing a plan of care.

Because cardiac disease manifestations can mimic other abnormalities such as pulmonary disease, the nurse must question each symptom and then compare and contrast symptoms. For example, when the patient reports a sudden onset of chest pain, the nurse must possess knowledge of the difference in manifestations between the causes of cardiac versus pulmonary chest pain and assess the patient for each of them. Making an assumption that the pain is cardiac in nature would be inappropriate and shortsighted. Effective critical thinking skills include being curious and not making any assumptions. Regardless of the health problem, each symptom identified should be thoroughly described in order for the nurse to gain a full understanding. The nurse can say to the patient, "Tell me more about the problem," or "How did it start?" The patient usually proceeds with a discourse about the symptoms. The nurse uses skillful interview techniques to explore and investigate each symptom further. Any symptom analysis would be incomplete without a thorough description of its characteristics.

Implications for Health Promotion

A good time to discuss the concept of health promotion with a patient is during a cardiovascular exam. Assessment can be a time to review current health status, examine problem areas, identify risk factors that need to be modified, identify possible health goals, discuss options, and potentially develop a plan of care. During a health assessment nurses need to provide health education and supply the patient with educational materials. Nurses are in a unique position to help patients recognize health problems or potential health problems. When abnormalities or positive findings are discovered during the health history process, an opportunity exists to discuss the issue in greater detail. Nurses should also recognize their role in promoting healthy lifestyles and their abilities to empower a patient and her family to make needed changes in their lives. Be aware that certain health topics are very personal, and some nurses have difficulty discussing these sensitive issues with patients.

As the populations that are served in health care settings continue to change and nurses are caring for more diverse populations, they need to be knowledgeable about the health practices of other cultures. Integrating culturally competent care includes incorporation of complementary therapies into the plan of care that will ultimately help nurses accomplish the goal of health promotion for all patients.

Cardiovascular Monitoring

Cardiovascular monitoring is an integral part of nursing management and includes many technologies used to augment the physical exam. Monitoring devices range from simple noninvasive monitoring, including assessment of heart rate, blood pressure, and pulse oximetry, to more invasive monitoring, such as hemodynamic monitoring using indwelling pulmonary artery catheters and arterial catheters. Chapter 24 ∞ includes a complete discussion of invasive hemodynamic monitoring. The goal of cardiovascular monitoring is to obtain the data needed to complete the cardiovascular assessment in a timely fashion, in the safest, most cost-efficient manner.

Assessment of Heart Rate

Counting the number of pulsations of the heart per minute determines heart rate. Assessment of heart rate should be performed when the patient is at rest in a calm environment. Many factors can alter the heart rate. For example, exercise, pain, and anxiety can cause an increase in circulating catecholamines, which may elevate heart rate and blood pressure. Endocrine and metabolic conditions can also affect the heart rate. The heart normally beats 60 to 100 times per minute. Heart rates less than 60 beats per minute (bradycardia) may be caused by hypoxia, parasympathetic stimulation, or beta-adrenergic blocker medication (Docherty, 2002a), although many well-conditioned athletes have resting heart rates well below 60 beats per minute. Bradycardia may not be clinically significant, unless accompanied by systolic blood pressure of less than 90 mmHg, which would indicate that the slow rate is compromising cardiovascular function (Docherty, 2002b).

Heart rates over 100 beats per minute are termed *tachycardia*, and some causes are exercise, pyrexia, hypovolemia, anxiety, and pain. Other clinical conditions that increase oxygen demand, such as myocardial ischemia or respiratory distress, may also cause tachycardia (Docherty, 2002a). Tachycardia can compromise cardiovascular status by decreasing diastolic filling time and increasing oxygen consumption, which may cause a reduction in stroke volume and eventually a drop in cardiac output. The regularity of the pulse should also be assessed. Irregularities suggest an alteration in cardiac conduction and should be further evaluated. Electrocardiogram (ECG) monitoring is a noninvasive method used to assess the heart rate and rhythm, and is commonly utilized in acute care settings. Interpretation and analysis of the ECG is discussed in Chapter 38 .

Assessment of Blood Pressure

Arterial blood pressure (BP) is a measure of the pressure exerted by blood against the walls of the arterial system as it is ejected from the left ventricle. Blood pressure is a dynamic, multidimensional indicator of a person's cardiovascular state (Thomas, Liehr, DeKeyser, Frazier, & Friedmann, 2002). Assessment of blood pressure reflects the events of the pulsatile cardiac cycle and is expressed as systolic/diastolic. The systolic blood pressure (SBP) is the peak pressure exerted against the arteries when the heart ventricles contract during systole. The diastolic blood pressure (DBP) is the residual pressure existing in the arterial system at the end of diastole when the ventricles are relaxed and are filling with blood from the atria.

The recording of blood pressure can provide important information about blood volume, cardiac output, and peripheral resistance. It is a critical component of vital signs and therefore is a basic parameter for nurses' physical assessments (Thomas et al., 2002). When the systolic and diastolic blood pressures are elevated, so is the risk of developing cardiovascular disorders. High blood pressure causes the heart to work harder and directly damages the smooth muscle that lines the cardiovascular system (see Chapter 21 and Chapter 40). Hypertension must be treated promptly to prevent complications such as the development of atherosclerotic cardiovascular disease, myocardial infarction, and stroke.

Blood pressure can be measured in several ways: either indirectly by use of ausculatory methods such as mercury column or aneroid (clock-face) sphygmomanometers or by use of oscillatory methods such as the electronic automatic blood pressure cuffs that produce a digital readout, or directly by use of invasive monitoring devices.

In many clinic and hospital settings the most common way to obtain blood pressure recordings is by ausculation with the use of an indirect sphygmomanometer. Pressure is exerted on the main artery of the arm by the inflated blood pressure cuff. The stethoscope is used to listen for Korotkoff's sounds, which change in tone and volume as the cuff is deflated and blood flow is gradually restarted. The first sound heard is the systolic blood pressure, which represents the highest blood pressure that occurs each time the heart beats. The second recording is the diastolic blood pressure, which represents the lowest blood pressure that occurs when the heart relaxes between beats.

Accuracy in the measurement of BP is imperative because these data often guide medical and nursing practice. Many ther-

apeutic decisions are made based on BP recordings. Although the skill of measuring blood pressure appears simple, there are many possible causes of errors and inaccuracies (Chart 37–7). Inaccuracies in BP assessment can lead to underestimation or overestimation of blood pressure, causing errors in the diagnosis and treatment of cardiovascular conditions. The American Heart Association has published standard recommendations and a step-by-step protocol for the indirect measurement of blood pressure (Chart 37–8). Guidelines provide a consistent, uniform technique for measuring blood pressure. However, nurses should be periodically retrained in determination of blood pressure. Retraining of blood pressure observers has been shown to reduce variability of blood pressure due to human error (Jones, Apperl, Sheps, Roccella, & Lenfant, 2003).

It is important for nurses to understand that the BP in an artery is a dynamic number and changes throughout the day. It is the lowest during sleep. It rises on waking and can rise with excitation, nervousness, or activity. Therefore, a single reading of high blood pressure is not used to make a diagnosis of hypertension. Treatment of hypertension includes lifestyle management including dietary changes and exercise as well as a variety of medications (angiotensin converting enzyme inhibitors, angiotensin receptor blockers, beta-blockers, calcium channel blockers). Chapter 21 contains an in-depth discussion of hypertension guidelines and treatment.

Classification of Blood Pressure

The National Heart, Lung, and Blood Institute (NHLBI) has classified two levels of high blood pressure. A blood pressure reading below 120/80 mmHg is considered normal. Blood pressures under 140/90 mmHg are classified as either normal or prehypertension. Prehypertension is systolic blood pressures between 120 and 137, or diastolic readings between 80 and 89. Hypertension is considered when the blood pressure reading is 140/90 mmHg. These clas-

---

CHART 37–7	**Inaccuracies in Measurement of Blood Pressure**

Inaccuracies in measurement of blood pressure are common clinical problems and can occur due to human error or device error for numerous reasons:

Inappropriately sized cuffs (too wide or too narrow)

Incorrect cuff positioning

Incorrect cuff wrapping (too loose or uneven)

Failure to allow a rest period before measurement

Deflating the cuff too quickly or too slowly

Inaccurate inflation level

Not measuring in both arms

Failure to palpate maximal systolic pressure before ausculation

Improper position of the arm (above or below heart level)

Poor observer concentration

Lack of repeated measurements

Poorly fitting stethoscope.

Sources: Jones, D. W., Apperl, L. J., Sheps, S. G., Roccella, E. J., & Lenfant, C. (2003). Measuring blood pressure accurately: New and persistent challenges. *JAMA, 289*(8), 1027–1030; McAlister, F. A., & Straus, S. E. (2001). Measurement of blood pressure: An evidenced based review. *British Medical Journal, 322*(7291), 908–911.

> ### CHART 37–8 Technique for Measurement of Blood Pressure
>
> The intent and purpose of the measurement should be explained to the subject in a reassuring manner, and every effort should be made to put the subject at ease.
>
> The sequential steps for measuring the blood pressure in the upper extremity, as for routine screening and monitoring purposes, should include the following:
>
> 1. Have paper and pen at hand for immediate recording of the pressure.
>
> 2. Seat the subject in a quiet, calm environment with her bared arm resting on a standard table or other support so the midpoint of the upper arm is at the level of the heart.
>
> 3. Estimate by inspection or measure with a tape the circumference of the bare upper arm at the midpoint between the acromion and olecranon process (between the shoulder and elbow), and select an appropriately sized cuff. The bladder inside the cuff should encircle 80% of the arm in adults and 100% of the arm in children under 13 years old. If in doubt, use a larger cuff. If the available cuff is too small, this should be noted.
>
> 4. Palpate the brachial artery and place the cuff so that the midline of the bladder is over the arterial pulsation; then wrap and secure the cuff snugly around the subject's bare upper arm. Avoid rolling up the sleeve in such a manner that it forms a tight tourniquet around the upper arm. Loose application of the cuff results in overestimation of the pressure. The lower edge of the cuff should be 1 inch (2 centimeters) above the antecubital fossa (bend of the elbow), where the head of the stethoscope is to be placed.
>
> 5. Place the manometer so that the center of the mercury column or aneroid dial is at eye level and easily visible to the observer, and the tubing from the cuff is unobstructed.
>
> 6. Inflate the cuff rapidly to 70 mmHg, and increase by 10 mmHg increments while palpating the radial pulse. Note the level of pressure at which the pulse disappears and subsequently reappears during deflation. This procedure, the *palpatory method*, provides a necessary preliminary approximation of the systolic blood pressure to ensure an adequate level of inflation when the actual, auscultatory measurement is made. The palpatory method is particularly useful to avoid underinflation of the cuff in patients with an auscultatory gap and overinflation in those with very low blood pressure.
>
> 7. Place the earpieces of the stethoscope into the ear canals, angled forward to fit snugly. Switch the stethoscope head to the low-frequency position (bell). The setting can be confirmed by listening as the stethoscope head is tapped gently.
>
> 8. Place the head of the stethoscope over the brachial artery pulsation, just above and medial to the antecubital fossa but below the lower edge of the cuff, and hold it firmly in place, making sure that the head makes contact with the skin around its entire circumference. Wedging the head of the stethoscope under the edge of the cuff may free up one hand but results in considerable extraneous noise.
>
> 9. Inflate the bladder rapidly and steadily to a pressure 20 to 30 mmHg above the level previously determined by palpation, and then partially unscrew (open) the valve and deflate the bladder at 2 mm/s while listening for the appearance of the Korotkoff's sounds.
>
> 10. As the pressure in the bladder falls, note the level of the pressure on the manometer at the first appearance of repetitive sounds (Phase I), at the muffling of these sounds (Phase IV), and when they disappear (Phase V). During the period the Korotkoff's sounds are audible, the rate of deflation should be no more than 2 millimeters per pulse beat, thereby compensating for both rapid and slow heart rates.
>
> 11. After the last Korotkoff's sound is heard, the cuff should be deflated slowly for at least another 10 mmHg, to ensure that no further sounds are audible, and then rapidly and completely deflated. The subject should be allowed to rest for at least 30 seconds.
>
> 12. The systolic (Phase I) and diastolic (Phase V) pressures should be immediately recorded, rounded off (upward) to the nearest 2 mmHg. In children, and when sounds are heard nearly to a level of 0 mmHg, the Phase IV pressure should also be recorded. All values should be recorded together with the name of the subject, the date and time of the measurement, the arm on which the measurement was made, the subject's position, and the cuff size (when a nonstandard size is used).
>
> 13. The measurement should be repeated after at least 30 seconds, and the two readings averaged. In clinical situations additional measurements can be made in the same or opposite arm, and in the same or an alternative position.
>
> *Source:* Perloff, D., Grim, C., Flack, J., Frohlich, E., Hill, M., McDonald, M., et al. (Writing Group). (1993). *Human blood pressure determination by sphygmomanometry* (American Heart Association, Product Code: 2460-2467). Dallas, TX: American Heart Association.

sifications are for adults over age 18 who are not on medicine for high blood pressure, are not having a short-term serious illness, and do not have other conditions such as diabetes or kidney disease. An exception to this classification is that a blood pressure of 130/80 mmHg or higher is considered high blood pressure in persons with diabetes and chronic kidney disease (NHLBI, 2008). Classifications, prevention, and management of hypertension are discussed in detail in Chapter 21 ☺.

Health Promotion: Preventing Hypertension

The National High Blood Pressure Education Program (NHBPEP), established in 1972, is a cooperative effort among professional and voluntary health agencies, state health departments, and many community groups. The NHBPEP is administered and coordinated by the National Heart, Lung, and Blood Institute (NHLBI). The goal of the NHBPEP is to reduce death and disability related to high blood pressure through programs of professional, patient, and public education. Another goal of the NHBPEP is to achieve the *Healthy People 2010* heart disease and stroke objectives for the nation (DHHS, 2004). Strategies to meet the program's goal include developing and disseminating science-based educational materials and developing partnerships among the program participants.

Assessment of Oxygen Delivery

Pulse oximetry allows noninvasive estimation of hemoglobin oxygen saturation, or SpO_2, which is the amount of hemoglobin saturated with oxygen (Figure 37–10 ■). These devices work by using a light sensor containing two sources of light (red and infrared) that are absorbed by hemoglobin and then transmitted through the tissue to a photodetector. The amount of light transmitted through the tissue is converted to a digital value, which represents the percentage of hemoglobin saturated with oxygen (Lynn-McHale & Carlson, 2005).

Normal oxygen saturation values are 97% to 99% in a healthy individual, but a value of 95% is clinically acceptable in a patient with a normal hemoglobin level (Lynn-McHale & Carlson, 2005). It should be reinforced that tissue oxygenation is not reflected by oxygen saturation because the affinity of hemoglobin to oxygen may actually either impair or enhance the way oxygen is released at the tissue level. Additionally, oxygen saturation does not reflect a patient's ability to ventilate, and thus its clinical use is limited in patients with obstructive pulmonary disease (Lynn-McHale & Carlson, 2005). SpO_2 values, however, are often monitored to allow for observations of trends and changes over time. For example, in a patient with emphysema, an SpO_2 of 93% might be considered a normal baseline. If however, he had an exacerbation of symptoms and his SpO_2 dropped to 90% or lower, the finding would be significant and reportable.

Oxygen saturation can be measured from several sites, including fingers, toes, and earlobes. It is important to remember that some situations—such as low perfusion, low temperature, anemia, discoloration of the nail bed, and even carbon monoxide poisoning,—will affect the ability of the sensor to estimate venous oxygen saturation accurately. The device should not be used on the same extremity as a blood pressure cuff, which may interrupt blood supply (Docherty, 2002b). The accuracy of the measurement is dependent on peripheral circulation, which may be compromised in a critically ill adult. Pulse oximetry, as a simple, noninvasive monitoring device, can be used continuously to assess adequacy of oxygen delivery. It may also be employed as a substitute for frequent arterial blood gas analysis, which involves needlesticks to obtain arterial blood (Docherty, 2002b). Therefore, pulse oximetry is efficient in that it can save nursing time, cost, and patient discomfort.

FIGURE 37–10 ■ Pulse oximeter.

can lead to early identification of potentially life-threatening conditions and provide an opportunity for timely application of preventative measures and treatment modalities. Cardiovascular assessment skills are mandatory in acute care as well as in many other nursing settings. Experience with cardiovascular assessment allows a nurse to validate and interpret findings in order to implement appropriate therapeutic interventions. Nurses may implement preventative strategies, initiate treatment plans, or provide education or counseling.

■ Summary

A thorough and accurate cardiovascular assessment is an important nursing tool. Findings from cardiovascular assessments

NCLEX® REVIEW

1. The nurse determines a male patient with hypertension and hypertriglyceridemia meets the criteria for metabolic syndrome when the cardiovascular assessment demonstrates which finding?

   1. Random blood sugar is 150 mg/dL.
   2. Waist circumference is 110 cm.
   3. High density lipids, HDLs, are 52 mg/dL.
   4. Fasting blood sugar is 100 mg/dL.

2. When assessing the medication history of a patient with heart disease the nurse would be most concerned when the patient reports frequent use of which medication?

   1. Proton pump inhibitor
   2. Antacids
   3. Bulk forming laxatives
   4. Decongestants

3. A patient reports having difficulty sleeping at night secondary to becoming short of breath when lying down. In order to further assess the degree of orthopnea, the nurse should ask which question.

1. "How often do you wake up at night?"
2. "How many pillows do you sleep on?"
3. "Do you experience palpitations that awaken you?"
4. "How often do you get up to urinate during the night?"

4. When ausculating heart sounds the nurse hears a third heart sound and recognizes the patient has which condition?

1. Diastolic dysfunction
2. Systolic dysfunction
3. Conduction defect of the SA node
4. Dysfunctional mitral valve

Answers for review questions appear in Appendix D

KEY TERMS

abdominojugular reflux *p.1061*
auscultation *p.1063*
bruits *p.1067*
cyanosis *p.1060*
dyspnea *p.1055*

edema *p.1056*
heaves *p.1063*
jugular venous pressure (JVP) *p.1060*
murmurs *p.1066*
nocturia *p.1055*

orthopnea *p.1055*
palpitations *p.1055*
syncope *p.1056*
thrills *p.1063*
turgor *p.1062*

EXPLORE mynursingkit™

MyNursingKit is your one stop for online chapter review materials and resources. Prepare for success with additional NCLEX®-style practice questions, interactive assignments and activities, web links, animations and videos, and more!

Register your access code from the front of your book at
www.mynursingkit.com

REFERENCES

Allen, J. K. (2000). Genetics and cardiovascular disease. *Nursing Clinics of North America, 35*(3), 653–661.

American Heart Association. (2006). *Our 2006 Diet and Lifestyle Recommendations.* Retrieved July 2, 2008, from http://www.americanheart.org/presenter.jhtml?identifier=851

American Heart Association. (2008a). *Metabolic syndrome.* Retrieved January 22, 2008, from http://www.americanheart.org/presenter.jhtml?identifier=4756

American Heart Association. (2008b). *Women and coronary artery disease.* Retrieved February 22, 2008, from http://www.americanheart.org/presenter.jhtml?identifier=2859

Bhatnagar, A. (2006). Environmental cardiology: Studying mechanistic links between pollution and heart disease. *Circulation Research, 99*, 692–705.

Centers for Disease Control and Prevention. (2008). *Physical activity for everyone.* Retrieved July 2, 2008 from http://www.cdc.gov/nccdphp/dnpa/physical/everyone/index.htm

D'Amico, D., & Barbarito C. (2007). *Health and physical assessment in nursing.* Upper Saddle River, NJ: Pearson Prentice Hall.

D'Amore, S., & Mora, S. (2006). Gender-specific prediction of cardiac disease: Importance of risk factors and exercise variables. *Cardiology in Review, 14*(6), 281–285.

Docherty, B. (2002a). Cardiorespiratory physical assessment for the acutely ill: 1. *British Journal of Nursing, 11*(11), 750–758.

Docherty, B. (2002b). Cardiorespiratory physical assessment for the acutely ill: 2. *British Journal of Nursing, 11*(12), 800–807.

Gallacher, J. E., Sweetman, P. M., Yarnell, J. W., Elwood, P. C., & Stansfeld, S. A. (2003). Is type A behavior really a trigger for coronary heart disease events? *Psychosomatic Medicine, 65*, 339–346.

Garg, N., & Garg, N. (2000). Jugular venous pulse: An appraisal. *Journal of Indian Academy of Clinical Medicine, 1*(3), 260–269.

Garrett, A. P. (1997). Assessing cardiovascular status in the older adult with cognitive impairments. *Journal of Cardiovascular Nursing, 11*(4), 1–11.

Jones, D. W., Apperi, L. J., Sheps, S. G., Roccella, E. J., & Lenfant, C. (2003). Measuring blood pressure accurately: New and persistent challenges. *JAMA, 289*(8):1027–1030.

Kahn, H. S., & Valdez, R. (2003). Metabolic risks identified by the combination of enlarged waist and elevated triacylglycerol concentration. *American Journal of Clinical Nutrition, 78*(5), 928–934.

Kahn, R., Buse, J., Ferrannini, E., & Stern, M. (2005). The metabolic syndrome: Time for a critical appraisal. *Diabetes Care, 28*(9), 2289–2304.

Ko, D. T., Hebert, P. R., Coffey, C. S., Sedrakyan, A., Curtis, J. P., & Krumholz, H. M. (2002). B-Blocker therapy and symptoms of depression, fatigue, and sexual dysfunction. *JAMA, 288*(3), 351–357.

Laszlo, B. et al. (2004). Novel Associations Between Bioavailable Estradiol and Adipokines in Elderly Women with Different Phenotypes of Obesity: Implications for Atherogenesis. *Circulation. 110:*2246–2252.

Lynn-McHale, D. J., & Carlson, K. K. (2005). *AACN procedure manual for critical care* (5th ed.). Philadelphia: W. B. Saunders.

National Heart, Lung, and Blood Institute. (2008). What Is High Blood Pressure? Retrieved January 25, 2008, from http://www.nhlbi.nih.gov

National Institutes of Health. (2001). *Third Report of the National Cholesterol Education Program Expert Panel on Detection, Evaluation, and Treatment of High Blood Cholesterol in Adults (Adult Treatment Panel III)* (NIH Publication 01-3670). Bethesda, MD: Author.

O'Connor, D. L. (1998). The art of auscultation. *Patient Care, 32*(20), 35–36, 38, 41–2.

Schroeder, K. E., Narkiewicz, K., Kato, M., Pesek, C., Phillips, B., Davison, D., et al. (2000). Personality type and neural circulatory control. *Hypertension, 36*, 830–833.

Smith-Stoner, M. (2006). Caring for patients of diverse religious traditions; Considerations for Buddhist clients in home care. *Home Healthcare Nurse, 24*(7), 459–466.

Snyder, M., & Miska, K. (2003). Cultural related complementary therapies: Their use in critical care units. *Critical Care Clinics of North America, 15*, 341–346.

Thomas, S. A., Liehr, P., DeKeyser, F., Frazier, L., & Friedmann, E. (2002). A review of nursing research on blood pressure. *Journal of Nursing Scholarship, 34*(4), 313–321.

Urden, L. D., Lough, M. E., & Stacy, K. M. (2006). *Thelan's critical care nursing: Diagnosis and management* (4th ed.). St. Louis: Mosby.

U.S. Department of Health and Human Services. (2004). *Healthy People 2010.* Retrieved on July 10, 2006, from http://www.health.gov/healthypeople/document/

Whetstone, G., & Boswell, S. (2002). The geriatric heart: Nurses need to be aware of how aging and disease affect the myocardium. *American Journal of Nursing, 102*(Suppl.), 22–24.

Williams, R. R., Hunt, S. C., Heiss, G., Province, M. A., Bensen, J. T., Higgins, M., et al. (2001). Usefulness of cardiovascular family history data for population-based preventive medicine and medical research. (The Health Family Tree Study and the NHLBI Family Heart Study). *American Journal of Cardiology, 87*(2), 129–135.

38

Nursing Interpretation of the Electrocardiogram

Kathleen Osborn
Annita Watson

Outcome-Based Learning Objectives

After studying this chapter, the learner will be able to:

1. Describe the configuration of the normal electrocardiogram (ECG).
2. Identify and calculate heart rate, rhythm, PR interval, QRS complex, and QT interval for normal and abnormal cardiac rhythms.
3. Discuss the etiology and significant ECG features of the following dysrhythmia classifications: sinus, atrial, junctional, block, ventricular, and asystole.
4. Interpret the significance of each of the dysrhythmias and formulate nursing responsibilities for each dysrhythmia.

Research Collaboration Health Promotion Nursing Process Caring Critical Thinking

THE ELECTROCARDIOGRAM (ECG) is the most important and definitive noninvasive diagnostic procedure that shows a graphic depiction of the electrical activity of the heart. It is used to assist the health care team in diagnosing and monitoring cardiac electrical system function. The ECG was first used less than a century ago, in the early 1900s. Initially the equipment was large and cumbersome and had limited use. As equipment improved, ECG bedside monitoring became possible in the 1960s. Today, due to increased patient acuity levels, the use of ECGs has become widespread, moving outside the traditional critical and emergent care settings. Thus, so has the expectation for nurses to have the knowledge and understanding of ECG interpretation. Nurses are expected to read and interpret ECGs when planning, providing, and evaluating patient care (Holtschneider, McBroom, & Patterson, 2006). In order to orient the learner to the cardiac conduction system, this chapter provides a brief overview of the anatomy and electrophysiology of the heart. This review is followed by information on how to obtain the graphic representation of the electrical activity of the heart, the ECG (also referred to as EKG). The equipment and skills needed to obtain an ECG are described. The learner is guided in the necessary steps for interpretation of both normal and abnormal cardiac rhythms. This is followed by a description of the appropriate nursing interventions and evaluation criteria.

■ Anatomy of the Heart

Recognition of common cardiac rhythms measured by an electrocardiogram requires a basic understanding of cardiac anatomy and physiology. A complete description of the cardiac anatomy is outlined in Chapter 37 ⊙ . Knowledge of the cardiac conduction system needed for ECG interpretation is presented here.

Cardiac Conduction System

The heart contains its own **cardiac conduction system** composed of specialized cell fibers called either **nodes** or **bundles.** These fibers enable the heart to generate and transmit action potentials without stimulation from the body's nervous systems. The heart's conduction system is responsible for the electrical activity that controls each normal heartbeat. The special cells and fibers called nodes or bundles are located beneath the endocardium, or inner lining of the heart, in the cardiac conduction system. These are referred to as the sinoatrial (SA) node, the atrioventricular (AV) node, and the Purkinje network (Figure 38–1 ■). Although the sympathetic nervous system (SNS) and the parasympathetic nervous system (PSNS) innervate the heart, these external neural impulses are not needed to maintain the cardiac cycle. The pacemaker cells are capable of initiating electrical activity automatically and act as a pacemaker; there-

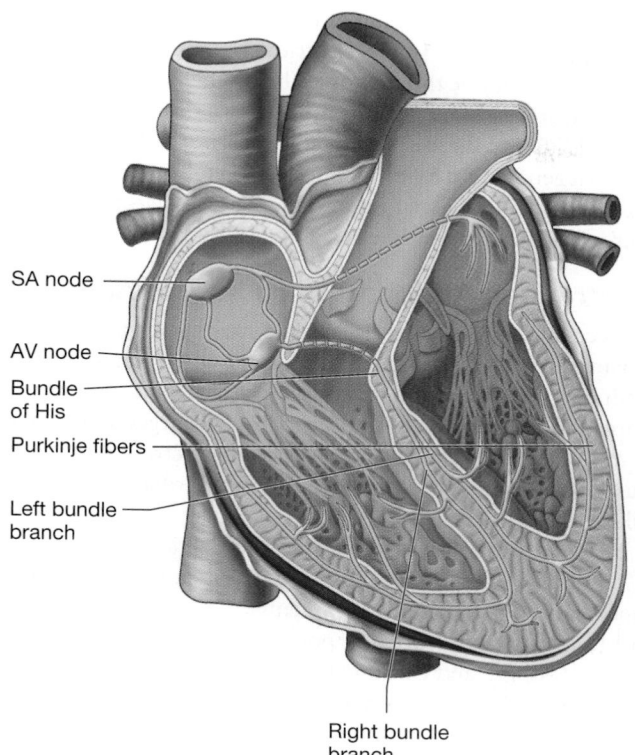

SA node

AV node

Bundle
of His

Purkinje fibers

Left bundle
branch

Right bundle
branch

FIGURE 38–1 ■ Electrical conduction system of the heart.

fore, the heart will beat in the absence of any nervous system connection. The SNS and the PSNS affect only the speed of the cardiac cycles and the diameter of the coronary arteries. It is essential to understand the heart's electrical conduction system in order to be able to understand an ECG strip interpretation. Each component of the system follows.

Sinoatrial (SA) Node

The **sinoatrial (SA) node** is located in the upper posterior portion of the right atrial wall, near the opening of the superior vena cava. The node is made up of hundreds of cells that compose a knot of modified heart muscle. The SA node is capable of generating impulses that travel throughout the muscle fibers of both atria, resulting in atrial depolarization. The SA node is commonly called the primary pacemaker of the heart because under normal conditions it depolarizes more consistently, frequently, and reliably than other normal pacemaker cells. The normal firing rate of the SA node is 60 to 100 beats per minute. Depolarization of the atria occurs as the impulse leaves the SA node and travels in a downward or waterfall fashion through the conduction pathways. If the SA node (pacemaker) fails to fire due to some abnormality, other pacemaker cells are able to take over, that is, the AV node or the Purkinje network. The emergence of a pacemaker that is lower in the heart, which sustains a heart rate when the SA node fails, is referred to as an **escape** mechanism or rhythm. During an escape rhythm, the heart rate is slower than the dominant pacemaker. If the rhythm originates in the junctional tissue, it is referred to as a junctional escape rhythm. If the rhythm originates in the ventricle, it is referred to as a ventricular escape rhythm.

Intra-Atrial Pathways

The **intra-atrial pathways,** located in the atria, transport impulses from the SA node to the AV node. There are three pathways: the anterior, middle, and posterior intranodal or intra-atrial pathways, and Bachmann bundle. **Bachmann bundle,** which is a part of the anterior pathway, is a group of fibers contained in the left atrium. All of the intranodal pathways and Bachmann bundle receive electrical impulses as they exit the SA node, distribute these impulses throughout the atria, and transmit them to the AV node (Beasley, 2003).

Atrioventricular (AV) Node and AV Junction

The **atrioventricular (AV) node** is located on the floor of the right atrium just above the tricuspid valve. Electrical activity at the AV node is delayed approximately 0.05 second to allow for atrial contraction, which increases the amount of blood reaching the ventricles. Atrial contraction, commonly referred to as **atrial kick,** augments the blood supply going to the ventricles and ultimately cardiac output. This delay also serves to stop the transmission for a very rapid succession of impulses that can occur under abnormal conditions. These abnormalities, called atrial flutter/fibrillation, are discussed later in the chapter.

The AV junction contains fibers that can polarize spontaneously, forming an impulse that can spread through the heart chambers. This means that if the SA node fails or falls below its normal range, the AV node can take over, thus assuming the role of a secondary pacemaker. Under normal conditions the AV junction is the only pathway for the conduction of atrial impulses to the ventricles.

Bundle of His and Bundle Branches

The **bundle of His** is approximately 15 millimeters long and lies on top of the interventricular septum, between the right and left ventricles. This area, also referred to as the common bundle, contains pacemaker cells that have the ability to self-initiate electrical activity at a rate of 38 to 60 beats per minute. At the top of the interventricular septum, the bundle of His divides into two bundle branches, the right and left bundles. The right bundle, a long, thin structure that lies beneath the endocardium, runs down the right side of the interventricular septum and terminates at the papillary muscles in the right atrium. The left bundle is shorter than the right bundle and divides into pathways that spread from the left side of the interventricular septum throughout the left ventricle. The two pathways of the left bundle branch are called **fascicles,** one being anterior and the other posterior. The anterior fascicle carries electrical impulses to the anterior wall of the left ventricle. The posterior fascicle spreads electrical impulses to the posterior ventricular wall. The bundle branches continue to divide until they finally terminate in the Purkinje network fibers.

Purkinje Network Fibers

Purkinje network fibers consist of a network of fibers that carry impulses directly to the ventricles. The rapid spread of the electrical impulse through the left and right bundle branches, the Purkinje network fibers, and the ventricular muscle initiates ventricular contraction. Purkinje fibers also may be pacemaker cells; they fire at an intrinsic rate of 20 to 40 beats per minute.

Cardiac Cells

There are two basic cardiac cell groups: the myocardial working cells and the specialized pacemaker cells of the electrical conduction system. The atria and the ventricles are constructed of myocardial working cells, which have an abundance of contractile filaments needed to generate cardiac muscle contraction. The cardiac muscle contraction is what actually pumps the blood through and out of the heart into the pulmonic and the systemic circulation. The myocardial working cells have the ability to contract in response to chemical, electrical, or mechanical stimuli.

The second type of cardiac cell is the specialized **pacemaker cell** whose primary function is to generate and conduct electrical impulses (stimuli). These cells found in the heart wall and septum (membrane dividing the right and left sides of the heart) control the heart rate and rhythm by coordinating regular cardiac muscle depolarization (contraction) (see Figure 38–1 ■, p. 1075). The myocardial contractions pump the blood through and out of the heart.

The term **threshold** refers to the point at which an electrical stimulus produces a cell response. When a stimulus is strong enough for cardiac cells to reach this threshold, all of the cells will respond to the stimulus and cause a muscle contraction. This is called the "all-or-none phenomenon"; in other words, either all the cells respond, or none of the cells respond. This principle allows for a coordinated muscle contraction and greater efficiency in pumping blood. Cardiac cells possess four primary characteristics: automaticity, excitability, conductivity, and contractility. These characteristics are described next.

Automaticity

Automaticity is the ability of the pacemaker cells to generate their own electrical impulses without depending on nervous system stimulation external to the heart. This spontaneous activity is what produces regular depolarization of the cardiac muscle. This characteristic is specific to only certain pacemaker cell sites within the conduction system. These cell sites are the sinoatrial (SA) node, the atrioventricular (AV) node, and the Purkinje network fibers.

Excitability

Excitability is the ability of the electrical cell to respond to a stimulus. This ability also is referred to as irritability, and all electrical cardiac cells possess this property. When cardiac cells are highly irritable, a cell other than the normal pacemaker may cause a contraction. Cell irritability can be caused by a number of problems, including cardiac muscle ischemia due to hypoxia, or a lack of oxygen. This is the most common cause of cardiac dysrhythmias, the abnormal rhythms of the heart.

Conductivity

Conductivity is the ability of the cardiac cell to accept and then transmit a stimulus to other cardiac cells. All cardiac cells share this characteristic, thereby portraying the all-or-none property of the heart muscle; the cardiac cells function as a unit.

Contractility

Contractility is the ability of the cardiac cells to shorten and cause the muscle to contract in response to an electrical stimulus. This ability also is referred to as rhythmicity. Contractility is the only mechanical function of the heart. Excitability, conductivity, and automaticity are electrical functions of the heart. Contractility may be thought of as the mechanical coordination of cardiac muscle contractions producing a heartbeat.

In addition to these cell characteristics, normal cardiac function is dependent on maintaining electrolyte concentrations inside and outside the cell membrane. Specific electrolytes and their relationship to cardiac function are described next.

Electrolytes Affecting Cardiac Function

An electrolyte is a substance or compound whose molecules dissociate into charged components, or **ions,** when placed in water, producing positively and negatively charged ions. A positively charged ion is called a **cation.** A negatively charged ion is called an **anion.** Myocardial cells are bathed in electrolyte solutions; thus, both the mechanical and the electrical cardiac functions are influenced by electrolytes.

The major cations that affect cardiac function are potassium (K), sodium (Na), and calcium (Ca). Magnesium (Mg) also is an important cation, but is not as influential as K, Na, and Ca with regard to stimulating the action potential discussed here. Magnesium, potassium, and calcium are intracellular cations, meaning they reside within the cell; whereas Na is an extracellular cation, residing outside the cell. Chloride (Cl) is a major anion in electrocardiac function. Chloride provides electroneutrality in relation to Na. Transport of chloride is passive and follows the active transport of sodium (Na).

Abnormally high or low levels of electrolytes, especially K, can potentiate very serious, life-threatening ventricular dysrhythmias. Therefore, monitoring and maintaining normal electrolyte values is essential. Nurses have a responsibility to report immediately any significant abnormal values to the health care provider.

 Assessing laboratory values is an essential nursing responsibility. Each time laboratory results are completed on a patient the nurse needs to compare the new results with reference normal values and previous findings, if applicable, and report significant changes and/or trends.

Cardiac Depolarization and Repolarization

When impulses travel through the myocardial muscle, they cause changes in the muscle fibers referred to as depolarization and repolarization. **Cardiac depolarization** refers to cardiac muscle contraction resulting from an electrolyte exchange in the cardiac cells, which then changes the electrical charge. As with all cells of the body, cardiac cells are electrically charged, with the inside of the cell more negative than the outside. To move Na and K across the cell membrane requires active transport by a mechanism referred to as the sodium-potassium adenosine triphosphatase (ATP) pump (Na-K pump). The Na-K pump is an energy-driven mechanism by which 3 Na ions are pumped out for every 2 K ions. Two enzymes, adenosine triphosphate (ATP) and adenosine triphosphatase (ATPase), are involved in the energy production for the pump (Porth, 2004).

Prior to depolarization the cells must be in a resting state, referred to as the **resting membrane potential.** In this state the myocardial cell is negatively charged to −90 millivolts (mV). This negative state is maintained until depolarization occurs.

When a muscle cell receives a stimulus due to the Na-K pump exchange, a rapid change occurs in the resting membrane potential, known as the **action potential,** which is measured in **millivolts** (a unit of electrical voltage or potential difference equal to one-thousandth of a volt). Once the action potential occurs, the cell moves toward a positive charge. The four phases (0–4) of the action potential are shown in Figure 38–2 ■. Phase 0 is rapid depolarization, phase 1 is rapid repolarization, phase 2 is the plateau, phase 3 is final repolarization, and phase 4 is the resting state. To generate this action potential and the resulting muscle depolarization, the threshold potential must be reached, which is phase 0. To initiate phase 0, Na enters the cell causing a sharp positively charged rise of the intracellular ions. The cell moves from -90 millivolts (mV) in its resting state to a positive 15 to 30 millivolts, causing myocardial depolarization to occur. When the threshold is reached, the cell will continue to depolarize with no further stimulation; this phenomenon is referred to as automaticity. During phase 1, the depolarized stage, the interior of the cell has a net positive charge. In this effort to continue to make the inside of the cell more positive, Ca enters; this is phase 2, the plateau phase. During phase 3 the calcium channels close, and Na is pulled from the cell by the Na-K pump; thus the cell is returning to its polarized negative resting membrane potential state (phase 4) (Figure 38–3 ■). The first area of the cardiac muscle to be depolarized is the first area that is repolarized. For example, after the atria depolarize they repolarize while the ventricles are depolarizing. Thus, when the SA node fires again, the muscle will be ready to respond with a new action potential.

Cardiac repolarization is the process whereby the depolarized cell is polarized, causing a return to the resting membrane potential (see Figure 38–2 ■). Repolarization also is referred to as the recovery phase that every cardiac cell must go through in order to be ready to accept another stimulus. It is a slower process than that of depolarization. During repolarization the

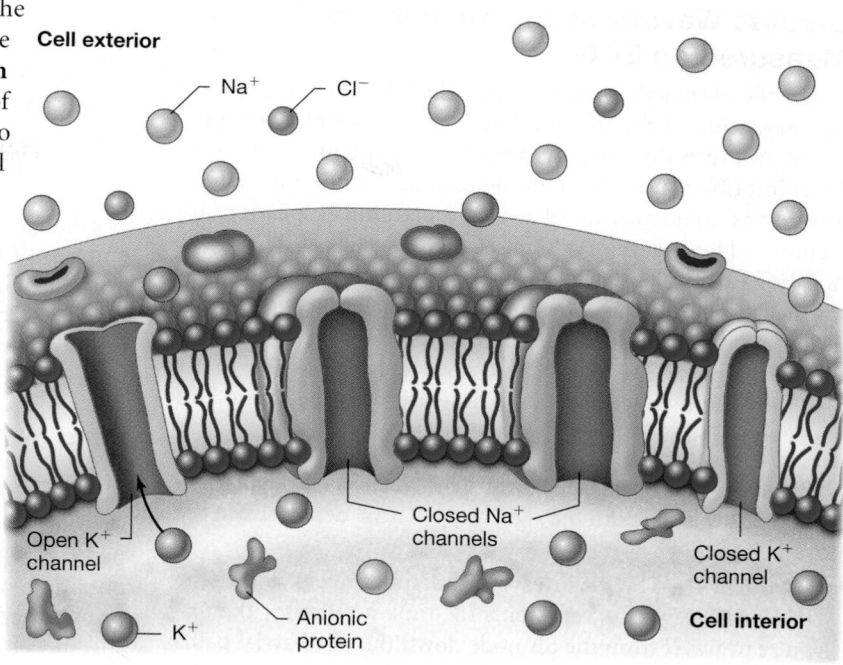

FIGURE 38–3 ■ Electrolyte movement during an action potential.

muscle is *refractory* (resistant) to stimulation. This **refractory period** consists of two stages; the absolute and the relative refractory periods. During the **absolute refractory period,** which is the majority of time for repolarization, the cardiac cell is unable to respond to any stimulus and thus cannot spontaneously depolarize (see Figure 38–2 ■).

The **relative refractory period** is a period when repolarization is almost complete (see Figure 38–2 ■). This period is known as the vulnerable period of cardiac cell repolarization. If a stimulus is strong enough, it can cause depolarization that can be life threatening. These situations are discussed later in this chapter. The refractory periods play a major role in either causing or preventing cardiac dysrhythmias. Further discussion of their role is explained regarding the various dysrhythmias and throughout the chapter.

Summary of the Cardiac Conduction System

The electrical impulse begins in the SA node located in the upper right atrium, causing atrial contraction. The impulse then travels through the atria along intra-atrial pathways to the AV node located near the center of the heart. After leaving the AV node the impulse moves down into the bundle of His, through the right and left bundle branches, and into the Purkinje network fibers, causing ventricular contraction followed by repolarization (see Figure 38–1 ■, p. 1075). Then the cycle begins again.

When caring for patients with actual or potential cardiac conduction abnormalities, it is essential that the nurse understand how the cardiac conduction system described here is graphically depicted on an electrocardiogram. Recognizing and interpreting these electrical impulses and their relationship to heart disease is an essential nursing responsibility. A discussion of how the electrical conduction system is depicted in an ECG follows.

FIGURE 38–2 ■ Action potential.

Cardiac Waveform and Time Intervals Measured on ECG

When the electrical impulse leaves the SA node, a graphical representation of the signal referred to as a waveform is produced and recorded with monitoring equipment. As the electrical impulse travels through the cardiac conduction system, waveforms characteristic of a given anatomical location are recorded. These waveforms are referred to as P, Q, R, S, and T. Additionally, time intervals, which represent the time it takes for the impulse to travel from one anatomical location in the heart to another, are recorded. These time intervals are called PR, QRS, and QT. One complete cardiac cycle has five to six waveforms and time intervals. These are described here and depicted in Figure 38–4 ■.

- **P wave**—The **P wave** represents contraction or depolarization of the atria. Both the right and left atria depolarize at the same time.
- **PR interval**—The **PR interval,** sometimes referred to as the PRI or PR segment, represents the time it takes for the impulse to travel from the SA node down the intra-atrial pathways to the ventricles. In other words, it represents the beginning of the atrial contraction to the beginning of the ventricular contraction.
- **QRS complex**—The **QRS complex** consists of the Q, R, and S waves, and represents the conduction of electrical impulses from the bundle of His near the AV junction to the Purkinje network fibers located in the ventricles, causing them to depolarize.
- **J point**—The point at which the QRS meets the ST segment is called the J point.
- **ST segment**—The **ST segment** is a line extending from the S wave that gradually curves upward to the T wave, represented on the ECG as an almost isoelectric line. The ST segment signifies ventricular repolarization.
- **T wave**—The **T wave** is ventricular recovery or repolarization. This is often referred to as the resting phase of the car-

diac cycle. Both the absolute and the relative refractory periods are in place during the T wave.
- **U wave**—The **U wave** is present only on some people's ECG. It follows the T wave. Its etiology is unknown, but it is frequently seen in exercise, in drug toxicity, and most frequently with low potassium levels.

Changes in the configuration of the waveforms or lengthening and/or shortening of time intervals may indicate an abnormality in the heart. These abnormalities are discussed in detail in Chapters 40, 41, 42, and 43 ☺. The following sections discuss the method used to evaluate waveforms and time intervals.

■ ECG Monitoring Equipment

Electrocardiography detects cardiac electrical impulses at various points on the surface of the body. The graphical depiction of these impulses, waveforms, and time intervals is obtained either with an electrocardiograph (ECG machine) or on a bedside cardiac monitor. To obtain an ECG tracing, specific equipment is needed including an electrode, lead wire, and monitor or oscilloscope. An **electrode** is most commonly a round adhesive pad that is impregnated with conducting gel in the center and is attached to a lead wire. Electrodes are sensing devices that detect the electrical activity of the heart and conduct the electrical impulses from the skin surface back to the ECG machine, where they are converted into waveforms. An electrode is much like a camera in that it takes pictures of the electrical activity in the heart. The electrodes are connected to a cardiac monitor by lead wires. Typically, these wires are color coded according to machine manufacturer, and these colors assist the provider in attaching the lead wires to the appropriate electrode. The cardiac monitor records the electrical impulses and provides a real-time visual tracing of the waveforms on the screen and/or a printed version on specialized ECG graph paper, described next. The printed version is called a rhythm strip or ECG strip. The rhythm strip gives the health care provider information about where the pathological processes are occurring in the heart. Figure 38–5 ■ shows the electrodes, lead wire, and cardiac monitor.

The term *lead* is used in different contexts when discussing ECGs. In addition to using the term as just described, as a connector from the electrode to the cardiac monitor, the term also is used when discussing a view or picture of the heart from a particular angle or vantage point. In this respect one can think of the lead as the "eye of the camera."

Lead Placement

Body tissues and fluids surround the heart; therefore, the electrical action potentials produced in the heart are widely conducted throughout the body via these tissues and fluids. The impulses or action potentials can be detected from any point in the body. Electrodes must be placed in certain positions on the body in order to obtain a clear picture of the electrical impulses in the heart, and there must always be a positive, a negative, and a ground electrode/lead. The ground lead minimizes outside

FIGURE 38–4 ■ Waveform relationship to cardiac conduction system.

FIGURE 38–5 ■ Electrodes, lead wire, and cardiac monitor.

electrical interference. Each electrode senses the flow of current in the heart in relation to the lead axis. The **lead axis** refers to the imaginary line drawn between the positive and negative electrodes. If the axis is directed toward the positive lead, there is an upward or **positive deflection** on the ECG tracing (above the isoelectric line). If the axis is directed toward the negative lead, there is a **negative deflection** on the ECG tracing (below the isoelectric line) Figure 38–6 ■. Multiple leads, as seen with a **12-lead ECG,** view cardiac electrical conduction from different perspectives. Think of the heart on a pedestal that one is able to move around while a camera takes pictures from various angles. This gives the provider 12 different views of the cardiac electrical activity.

For bedside monitoring it is not practical or necessary to have a 12-lead ECG or 12 continuous views of the heart. Therefore, 1 or 2 of the 12 possible leads from the entire 12-lead ECG are chosen for constant bedside monitoring because they give a clear view of cardiac activity and abnormalities. To obtain a single bedside ECG rhythm strip, a minimum of three electrodes is required: one positive, one negative, and one ground. Either lead II or modified chest lead$_1$ (MCL$_1$) is commonly used for three-

electrode bedside monitoring. The MCL$_1$ is one of the V leads from the 12-lead ECG that is modified for bedside monitoring. The lead chosen is dependent on the unit policy and nurse and/or health care provider preference. The specific dysrhythmia being monitored or anticipated may dictate the type of lead chosen.

No single monitoring lead is ideal for every patient. Therefore, if more than one lead or picture of the heart is required, five electrodes are placed to increase the monitor's capability beyond the three-electrode monitoring system. The five-electrode monitoring system has an exploring chest electrode that allows one to obtain the same 12 views as a 12-lead ECG when needed. However, at the bedside typically only two simultaneous leads are used to view the heart with the five-electrode system. Commonly the two leads that are run simultaneously are lead II and MCL$_1$. However, the lead or leads chosen depend on the desired view of the heart. Figure 38–6 ■ shows a cardiac rhythm strip that has simultaneous lead II and MCL$_1$ ECG views.

These two leads provide different perspectives of the various normal and abnormal ECG configurations. For example, lead II produces easily identifiable upright P waves and clear QRS

FIGURE 38–6 ■ Lead II and MCL$_1$ ECG configurations.

complexes. An MCL$_1$ lead is useful for evaluating abnormalities in the ventricles.

Placement of the electrodes depends on the lead being monitored and whether a three- or five-lead system is being used. Figure 38–7 ■ shows the position of the electrodes for both lead II and MCL$_1$.

The color coding on the lead wire gives the nurse information about whether the lead is positive or negative. Typically the color black is negative, white is positive, and green is ground. In the five-lead system red and brown colors also are used and their polarity changes depending on the lead being monitored (Morton, Fontaine, Hudak, & Gallo, 2005).

12-Lead Electrocardiogram (ECG)

The rhythm strips that have been used to demonstrate dysrhythmias throughout this chapter have all been from a single lead. A single-lead ECG rhythm strip gives one view of the electrical activity of the heart, whereas a 12-lead ECG provides 12 individual views or "snapshots" of the heart's electrical patterns. These added views provide a complete picture of the cardiac electrical system, both top to bottom and front to back. A 12-lead ECG is useful in evaluating not only the presence of damage but also the location in the heart where that damage occurred. Frequently, to assess damage accurately requires viewing the area with more than one lead. Chart 38–1 provides the indications for a 12-lead ECG.

There are 3 bipolar and 9 unipolar leads in a 12-lead ECG. A **bipolar lead** has electrodes with opposite polarity, one positive and one negative. A **unipolar lead** has only a positive polarity (Walraven, 2006). Both bipolar and unipolar leads provide information in one direction only—between two points. The two

---

CHART 38–1 **Indications for a 12-Lead ECG**

Evaluation of:

- Axis deviation
- Cardiac valve disease
- Chamber dilation or hypertrophy
- Chest pain/angina
- Dysrhythmias
- Effect of cardiac drugs
- Electrolyte imbalance
- Hypothermia
- Myocardial ischemia
- Myocardial patterns of ischemia, necrosis, and infarction
- New versus old myocardial infarction
- Pericarditis
- Pulmonary embolism
- Bundle branch block

---

dimensions on the chest in which leads can be placed are the frontal plane (up and down) and the horizontal plane (around the chest). Figure 38–8 ■ shows the horizontal plane and the frontal plane views.

The axis of a lead is the imaginary line drawn between the positive and the negative electrode in a bipolar lead and between the positive electrode and the zero reference point in a unipolar lead. Thus, depending on where a given lead is placed, it provides

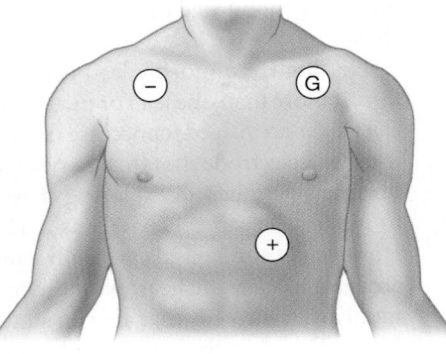

Lead II: Positive electrode left abdomen
        Negative electrode right shoulder
        Ground electrode left shoulder

MCL$_1$: Positive electrode 4th ICS RSB
       Negative electrode left shoulder
       Ground electrode right shoulder

MCL$_1$ is modified chest lead 1. It's like V$_1$.

FIGURE 38–7 ■ Electrode placement for bedside cardiac monitoring.

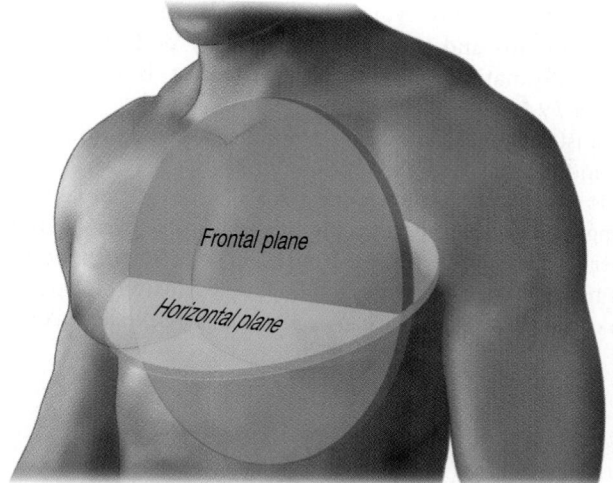

FIGURE 38–8 ■ Horizontal and frontal planes.

a picture of the electrical activity from that vantage point within the heart. Electrical current flowing toward a positive electrode creates a positive deflection on the ECG paper, whereas electrical current flowing toward a negative electrode creates a negative deflection on the ECG paper (Walraven, 2006).

The standard bipolar limb leads—I, II, III—are applied to the right arm (RA), left arm (LA), and left leg (LL). Each lead records the following electrical conduction pattern:

• Lead I records conduction from RA to LA.
• Lead II records conduction from RA to LL.
• Lead III records conduction from LA to LL.

The right leg electrode acts as a grounding electrode.

Three more frontal plane, unipolar augmented limb leads can be created by using a central terminal. Augmented leads are

so named because they generate such small waveforms that the ECG machine must augment, or increase, their size so they will show up on the ECG paper (Ellis, 2002a). These leads are aVR, aVL, and aVF. Each lead records the following electrical conduction pattern:

• aVR: central terminal to right arm
• aVL: central terminal to left arm
• aVF: central terminal to left leg.

The standard bipolar leads and the augmented limb leads provide the 6 frontal plane leads of the 12-lead ECG, whereas the 6 chest (precordial) unipolar leads, V1—V6, evaluate the horizontal plane of the heart. The positive electrode is placed on 6 different sites across the chest as shown in the diagram in Figure 39–1 ■ (p. 1121). These chest leads provide the 6 horizontal leads of the 12-lead ECG. Chart 38–2 describes the procedure for obtaining a 12-lead ECG.

For example, lead V1 evaluates the right ventricle; leads V2 and V3 span the interventricular septum; lead V4 is over the cardiac apex; and leads V5 and V6 evaluate the lateral wall. The Q wave, T wave, and ST segment are used to evaluate the presence of damage, and the lead placement is used to identify the area of damage. Chapter 40 ☞ discusses the myocardial damage associated with changes in the Q wave, T wave, and ST segment.

When performing an ECG, the nurse must have knowledge of the lead placement for each of the 12 leads. Improper placement may result in inaccurate information and treatment. The electrodes must have firm, unbroken contact with the skin. The limb leads are placed on the flat surfaces just above the wrists and ankles. If there is an amputation, the lead is placed on the remaining stump. Chest hair may interfere with skin contact and, if so, should be shaved. The type and sophistication of ECG machines varies; some can record only one lead at a time, whereas others can record 3, 6, or all 12 leads simultaneously.

CHART 38–2	**12-Lead ECG Procedure**
Electrode Placement	• Bring the portable ECG machine to the patient's bedside in any type of patient care setting. • Use 10 electrodes for the standard 12-lead ECG: 6 on the chest and 4 on the limbs. Figure 39–1 ■ (p. 1121) shows the correct placement of the electrodes. • Place limb electrodes away from bony prominences and areas of significant muscle movement to prevent interference of other muscle activity. • Palpate the intercostal spaces along the sternal border, until the fourth one is reached, for placement of the first chest electrode.
Cable Connection and Machine Operation	• Connect the cable that is attached to each of the electrodes to the ECG machine. • Adjust the ECG machine to obtain a clear picture of the cardiac electrical activity. • After completing the ECG, remove electrodes and clean the skin as necessary. • Leave the electrodes in place if the patient is going to have serial ECGs to ensure consistency of multiple readings.
Patient Instructions	• Explain the procedure and the rationale for the test prior to performing an ECG. • Advise the patient to lie still, breathe normally, and refrain from speaking while obtaining the ECG.
Documentation	• Document patient's height, weight, and use of cardiac medications. • Document current clinical manifestations if present and chief complaint. • Document reason for the ECG. • Record patient's response to procedure, if any.

Each ECG machine has its own method of identifying specific lead names (V1, V2, etc.) and a diagram of where to place them. The nurse must be cognizant when obtaining an ECG about which rhythms require immediate notification of the health care provider for emergent treatment. The significance and severity of the individual rhythms are presented under each rhythm discussed throughout the chapter.

Signal Averaged Electrocardiogram

Certain abnormal impulses are conducted during diastole, or when the heart is filling with blood, which is late into the QRS complex and ST segment. These impulses may be present in a patient who has survived an acute myocardial infarction and, if present, can result in ventricular tachycardia and sudden cardiac death. These signals, referred to as late potentials, are low-amplitude, high-frequency spikes that occur at the end of the QRS complex and extend into the ST segment. With the assistance of a computer, a signal averaged ECG is able to distinguish low-level signals not detected by the traditional ECG. Therefore, the risk for lethal dysrhythmias can be assessed. A signal averaged ECG also is used to evaluate His bundle activity, presence of a left ventricular mass, effects of thrombolysis, and surgical repair of congenital heart disease.

Cardiac Monitoring Systems

The purpose of continuous ECG monitoring is to detect new and changing abnormal heart rhythms and to trend data relatively to frequency and duration of dysrhythmias. When continuous ECG monitoring is necessary, it can be accomplished by two methods. First, the patient can be hardwired to a monitor whereby the leads are connected directly from the bedside monitor to the patient. The hardwired system has an oscilloscope at the bedside and in a central location such as the nurses' station. This system typically is able to monitor more than one lead simultaneously, and depending on the lead used the system also is able to visualize ST segment depression and elevation. Hardwired systems have the capability to print a rhythm strip and provide visual and audible alarms when abnormalities in the heart rhythm occur. These systems are computerized and therefore are able to interpret and store dysrhythmias in a memory bank. Hardwired monitoring is done in critical care areas.

The second method for continuously monitoring patients is with radio waves from a battery-operated transmitter. The transmitter, worn by the patient, transmits the rhythms to a central bank of monitors, which is typically at the nurses' station. This system allows the patient to ambulate about the unit while still being monitored.

Whichever system is being used, the patient must be informed of its purpose and any necessary precautions. Because it may be stressful and frightening for a patient to have his heart be continuously monitored, patient education is essential. The patient needs to understand that this system does not report clinical manifestations such as angina, dyspnea, or weakness. It is necessary, therefore, that the patient report these conditions as they occur.

Another form of continuous ECG monitoring is typically done in the outpatient setting. This system, referred to as a Holter monitor, records the heart electrical activity on a magnetic tape for 24 to 48 hours while the patient goes about normal activities of daily living. The patient keeps a diary of signs and symptoms and the associated activity performed. Additional information on the Holter monitor is discussed in Chapter 39 🔗.

Transtelephonic monitoring is another method of outpatient ECG monitoring. With this type of monitoring, a specific lead system is used for transmitting the signals and is accomplished by having the patient place a telephone mouthpiece over the transmitter box. The ECG is recorded and evaluated at another location. This method often is used as a follow-up evaluation for patients with cardiac pacemakers. Chapter 39 🔗 discusses pacemakers.

■ Nursing Management of the Monitored Patient

Prior to placing the patient on ECG monitoring, the nurse needs to explain the procedure and why it is necessary. It is essential that the patient understand that the heart is *just* being monitored, not controlled, by the equipment. Describe the electrodes, where they are placed, and how they are connected to the monitor. Skin preparation, electrode placement, and monitor connection are described in Chart 38–3.

The nurse needs to be knowledgeable about electrode placement for the lead that has been designated for monitoring the patient. Some manufactures have the electrode and the lead wire attached, whereas others produce them separately. The electrode placement should be as comfortable as possible for the patient. Documentation of the lead used needs to be included in the patient's record.

 Precise lead placement is critical to accurate continuous cardiac monitoring. The nurse must verify lead placement at the beginning of each shift. Once a transient cardiac problem has occurred it is too late to change lead placement so that an accurate analysis can be performed.

All cardiac monitors have alarm systems built into them to alert the nurse when abnormalities occur. Alarm systems have both a high and a low setting so that the nurse is alerted when the heart rate goes above or below the set parameters. The nurse must ensure at the beginning of the shift that the monitor alarms are on and set with the appropriate parameters established for the patient (see Chart 38–3). The nurse needs to explain to the patient that these alarms may also go off with excessive movement or if the lead wire falls off. The patient needs to be told the nurse will respond to the alarm each time it goes off and must be reassured that it does not necessarily mean there is a problem with her heart. The nurse must stress that excessive movement will cause the alarm to sound frequently.

 *When the monitor alarms it is essential that the nurse evaluates the clinical status of the patient prior to any other activities in order to assess for the presence of cardiac abnormalities and the patient's clinical response to the abnormalities.*

Nursing responsibility for monitored patients includes knowledge of the patient's specific rhythm in order to assess for changes. The more familiar the nurse is with the patient and the monitoring system, the quicker problems can be diagnosed

CHART 38–3 Procedure for Continuous ECG Monitoring

Electrode Attachment

- Choose an area to place the electrodes where there are no bony prominences, thick muscles, or skin folds, because these areas are prone to produce noncardiac waveforms and interference.
- Prepare the skin for electrode placement by making sure that it is clean, dry, and free of hair. It may be necessary to shave the chest area of male patients.
- Remove dead skin cells to improve electrical conductivity by rubbing the skin with the rough patch on the back of the electrode, a dry washcloth, or a gauze pad. The skin will become reddened with the rubbing; be careful not to cause skin breakdown.
- Wipe the skin with an alcohol sponge if skin is oily or a moist wipe; allow it to air dry.
- Make sure that the electrode pads are moistened with conducting gel prior to placing them on the chest to increase electrical conductivity. A dry electrode is not effective for conducting the electrical activity. When the electrode becomes dry or loose, it needs to be replaced. If the skin around the electrode becomes irritated the electrode must be removed and relocated.
- Position electrodes on the chest wall at prescribed locations depending on the lead or leads being monitored.
- Change electrodes when wet, poor contact, unclear tracing, and/or every 48 hours to avoid skin irritation.

Lead Wire and Cable Connection

- Connect the electrode to the lead wire, which is approximately 16 inches long. Typically a snap attaches the lead wire to the electrode.
- The lead wires are color coded to represent positive, negative, and ground leads.
- Attach the opposite end of the lead wire to the cable. The cable has individual color-coded receptacles or holes for each lead wire.

Monitor Connection and Adjustment

- Attach the cable to the monitor.
- Adjust the monitor to increase the size of the PQRST complex for more accurate interpretation.
- Read the operating instructions for the specific brand of monitor prior to use.

Alarm Setting

- Always leave the alarm on.
- Recognize that the alarms have upper and lower heart rate limits.
- Set the alarm approximately 20 beats above and below the patient's resting intrinsic heart rate.
- Follow institutional policy, if present, to determine different alarm limits.
- Be aware that when the alarm sounds, the first nursing responsibility is to check the patient.
- Recognize that movement by the patient may cause the alarm to sound falsely.

Documentation

- Document lead used.
- Document PR interval, QRS width, QT interval, ectopic beats, and type of rhythm/dysrhythmia.
- Record ECG changes and patient's response to changes.

---

and appropriate action taken. Assessment of patient tolerance of rhythm changes is the first nursing action, prior to assessing for problems with the equipment.

 When abnormalities appear on a cardiac rhythm strip it is an essential nursing responsibility to assess the patient's tolerance of the rhythm, especially if it is a new abnormality. The nurse needs to be knowledgeable about what changes need to be reported to the health care provider. The rhythm needs to be documented on the patient's record.

Tolerance to the rhythm is assessed by obtaining and evaluating vital signs, neurological status, and the presence of signs and symptoms of decreased cardiac output, for example, angina. After determining patient status and stability, the nurse then troubleshoots the equipment for problems such as a dry electrode or a disconnected wire. The problem could be as simple as the patient's tapping the electrode, and no action would be necessary. It also is essential that the nurse is knowledgeable of which cardiac disturbances are reportable and/or life threatening.

Communication with all personnel caring for the patient and observing the monitor is critical. They must be kept informed of when the patient needs to be off the monitor or of physical activities, such as bathing, occurring that may sound the alarms. For example, if there is a monitor technician, that person must be informed of the patient's leaving the floor and increased physical activities.

ECG Graph Paper

ECG **graph paper** is specialized paper on which the ECG pattern is recorded. The paper is designed to allow the measurement of various calculations related to the electrical activity of the heart. It is standard nursing protocol to measure these calculations when a patient is on a cardiac monitor. These measurements help determine whether the rhythm falls within the time limits of normal cardiac activity. Abnormal measurements may indicate a malfunction of the cardiac conduction system and will be discussed later in conjunction with the various dysrhythmias.

The ECG graph paper is arranged as a series of horizontal and vertical lines. This paper is standardized to allow for consistency in ECG measurement and strip analysis. Both the amplitude and the voltage may be measured on the paper. The vertical axis measures the amplitude and is stated in millivolts (mV). Two large squares on this axis equal 1 millivolt. This measurement is rarely used because the size of the picture or millivolts can be adjusted at the monitoring station, thereby reducing the consistency of this measurement.

The horizontal axis is divided into small squares. The squares on the ECG paper are used to measure the length of time required for the electrical impulse to traverse a specific part of the heart. Figure 38–9 ■ shows an example of ECG graph paper.

These squares are used to measure time intervals as follows:

- The smallest square is 1 millimeter (mm) in length and represents 0.04 second in time.
- The large square is 5 mm in length and represents 0.20 second in time.
- The large square equals 5 small squares.
- Five large squares represent 1 second.

ECG Measurements

When assessing either a rhythm strip or a 12-lead ECG, both the individual PQRST complexes need to be evaluated as well as the relationship of each individual complex to the overall rhythm. The assessment of an ECG configuration includes the following:

- **P wave**—There should be one P wave for every QRS complex.
- **PR interval**—This is measured from the beginning of the P wave to the beginning of the QRS complex. The normal PR interval is from 0.12 to 0.20 second or 3 small boxes to 1 large box.
- **QRS complex**—The QRS complex is measured from the beginning of the Q wave to the end of the S wave. The normal range is from 0.06 to 0.12 second or 1.5 boxes to 3 boxes. The shape of the QRS complex varies from individual to in-

dividual and also depends on the ECG lead being used. For example, QRS complexes are mostly positive in the lead II and mostly negative in the MCL₁ lead (see Figure 38–6 ■, p. 1079). Not everyone has a discernable Q wave.

- **QT interval**—This is measured from the Q wave to the end of the T wave. The normal QT interval is 0.34 to 0.43 second or 8.5 to 11 boxes.
- **Heart rate**—This is measured by using the very top of the ECG paper, which is marked off in 3-second intervals with tick marks. The tick mark is a small straight line or hash mark above the tracing. Count up the number of PQRST complexes that occur in 6 seconds and multiply that number by 10. This method provides a general estimate of the heart rate. A more accurate method for measuring heart rate is to count the number of small squares between two R waves and divide the total into 1,500. The normal HR is 60 to 100 beats per minute.
- **Heart rhythm**—This is determined by measuring the distance between P waves for atrial rate and two R waves for ventricular rate and then measuring each subsequent R wave to ensure it is the same distance apart as the previous ones. With a regular rhythm, the distance between R waves is equal.

Calipers (Figure 38–10 ■) are the instrument used to take all these measurements. Figure 38–11 ■ demonstrates where each measurement begins and ends.

FIGURE 38–10 ■ Calipers.

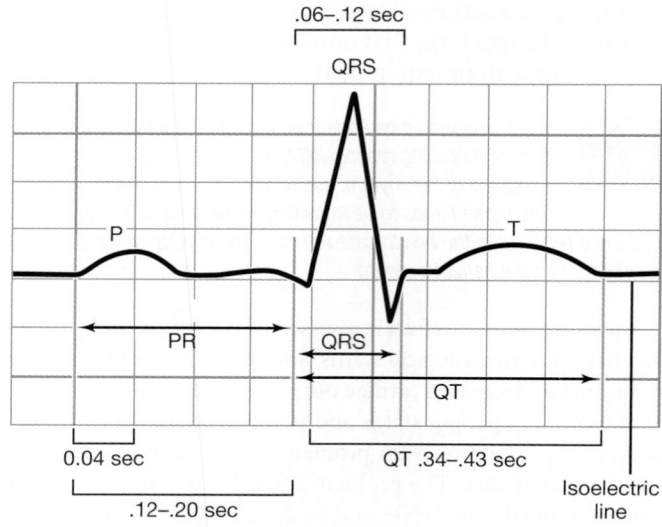

FIGURE 38–11 ■ ECG measurement.

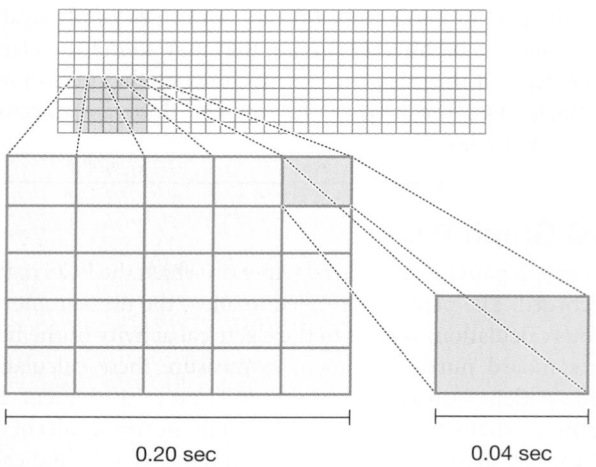

FIGURE 38–9 ■ ECG graph paper.

0.20 sec   0.04 sec

FIGURE 38–12 ■ Artifact.

Isoelectric Line

The **isoelectric line** marks the beginning and ending point of all waves. When the SA node fires, the **ECG waveform** (the actual tracing on the graph paper) begins and moves away from the isoelectric line (see Figure 38–12 ■). Any wave that has an upward deflection, which is above the isoelectric line, is referred to as a positive deflection, and any waveform that goes below the line is referred to as a negative deflection. Depending on the lead, certain waves normally are positive and certain ones are negative. In a lead II the normal P wave has a positive deflection, the PR interval is isoelectric, the Q wave is the first negative deflection, the R wave is positive, the S wave is negative, the ST segment is isoelectric, and the T wave is positive.

Artifact

Artifact is defined as an ECG pattern caused by sources outside the heart creating a false and abnormal pattern on the ECG graph paper. This interference is due to several causes:

- Malfunction of electrodes possibly due to dry conductive gel, clammy skin, or dense chest hair
- Patient movement, which precipitates a fluctuating isoelectric line that corrects itself when the patient lies still
- Improper grounding, which occurs when a patient is in contact with an outside source of electricity, such as poorly grounded beds and/or IV infusion pumps
- Equipment failures, such as broken wires or cables on the ECG equipment, which need to be exchanged for new equipment.

Because of this interference or artifact, the baseline or isoelectric line becomes fuzzy. When artifact is present, it is difficult to diagnose cardiac abnormalities, making it is necessary to correct the cause of the artifact. Figure 38–12 ■ depicts artifact.

Ectopic Focus

Ectopic focus is a heartbeat originating from a site other than the primary cardiac pacemaker tissue. Ectopic foci may affect cardiac output and must be assessed and documented carefully for their impact on the hemodynamic stability of the patient. The terms *dysrhythmia, arrhythmia,* and *ectopic focus* all mean the same thing and are used interchangeably.

ECG Rhythm Strip Evaluation and Documentation

When evaluating an ECG rhythm strip, using a simple stepwise process provides a consistent method for rhythm strip evaluation. This is shown in Chart 38–4. If the rhythm strip falls out of the normal parameters, then there is a high probability of an ab-

CHART 38–4	**Stepwise Process for ECG Strip Evaluation**
P Waves	Are the P waves regular? Is there one P wave for every QRS and one QRS for every P wave? Is the P wave in front of the QRS or behind it? Is the P wave normal and upright in lead II? Do all the P waves look alike? Are the abnormal P waves associated with ectopic beats?
PR Interval	Are all the PR intervals constant? Is the PR interval measurement within normal range (0.12 to 0.20 second)? If the PR interval varies, is there a pattern to the changing measurements?
QRS Complex	Are all the QRS complexes of equal duration? What is the measurement of the QRS complex size? Is the QRS complex measurement within normal limits (0.06 to 0.12 second)? Do all the QRS complexes look alike? Are the unusual QRS complexes associated with ectopic beats?
QT Interval	What is the length of the QT interval? Is it normal or prolonged? Is the patient on a treatment that prolongs the interval?
Rate	Atrial: how many P waves in 6 seconds times 10. Ventricular: how many R waves in 6 seconds times 10. A second method is to count the number of large boxes between two R waves and divide by 300. Both methods work best when the rhythm is normal. What is the heart rate?
Regularity (also called rhythm)	Is it regular? Is it irregular? Are there any patterns to the irregularity? Are there any ectopic beats; if so, are they early or late?
Ectopic Beats	Are they present? What are they? How is the patient tolerating them? Do they require treatment?

normality occurring in the conduction system. These abnormalities are discussed at length throughout the remainder of the chapter.

Normal Sinus Rhythm

Normal sinus rhythm (NSR) is a cardiac rhythm initiated from the SA or sinus node that has all the normal waveforms (PQRST) and normal time intervals (PR, QRS, QT) (Figure 38–13 ■).

The following criteria must be present to be NSR:

- P wave has a normal and consistent shape and appears before every QRS complex.
- There is a 1:1 ratio of P wave to QRS complex.
- PR interval is between 0.12 and 0.20 second.
- QRS complex is between 0.06 and 0.12 second.
- QT interval is between 0.34 and 0.43 second.
- Atrial and ventricular rate is between 60 and 100 beats per minute (beats/minute).
- Atrial and ventricular rhythm is regular.

Nursing Management

When the patient is on a cardiac monitor, it is the nurse's responsibility to measure, assess, and document the patient's rhythm strip at least every shift and more frequently depending on the patient's condition and agency protocol. Whenever changes occur in the heart rhythm, the nurse must begin the same process again: measure, assess, and document the rhythm strip. The nurse needs to understand when it is appropriate to report a change in the ECG to the health care provider.

Nursing Documentation

When documenting the heart rhythm in the patient's record, most institutions require that a rhythm strip is attached to the patient's chart once every shift and/or when a change in the rhythm occurs. The patient's name, the date and time of rhythm strip collection, and the ECG lead used for the rhythm strip should be documented. Additionally, the electrical features of the rhythm should be documented including the presence of a P wave, the PR interval, the width of the QRS complex, the QT interval, the heart rate, and rhythm (regular verses irregular), and the presence of ectopy (ectopic focus). Corresponding clinical manifestations associated with a given rhythm also need to be documented in the record. For exam-

ple, change in blood pressure, pulse, level of consciousness, and urine output.

Dysrhythmias

When the cardiac muscle does not receive enough blood, it becomes ischemic and irritable, causing cardiac dysrhythmias to occur. A **dysrhythmia** is an abnormal disturbance of the electrical conduction system of the heart. There are a number of dysrhythmias, which originate in different parts of the heart. This chapter addresses dysrhythmias according to location in the heart, beginning at the top with the atrial dysrhythmias. As the dysrhythmias occur anatomically lower in the heart, the severity is greater due to their impact on cardiac output. The cardiac output decreases as the severity of the dysrhythmia increases.

Heart rhythms are categorized according to the cardiac structure in which they begin, or their site of origin. The most common dysrhythmias begin at the top of the heart with the SA node. These types of dysrhythmias are called sinus dysrhythmias due to their origin in the SA, or sinus, node. The next area in the heart where dysrhythmias may occur is in the intra-atrial pathways, referred to as atrial dysrhythmias. Moving anatomically down to the next area of the conduction system, the AV node or junction is where junctional dysrhythmias occur. The final area of the heart where dysrhythmias may occur is in the ventricles. These ventricular dysrhythmias are considered to be the most dangerous because they precipitate the most profound decrease in the cardiac output.

When observing, assessing, and treating dysrhythmias, it is critical for the nurse to remember that it is the patient being treated, not the dysrhythmia. Treatment is always based on the hemodynamic impact of the dysrhythmia.

Sinus Dysrhythmias

The four common dysrhythmias associated with the sinus area of the heart are sinus bradycardia, sinus tachycardia, sinus arrhythmia/dysrhythmia, and sinus arrest.

Sinus Bradycardia

Sinus bradycardia, often called "sinus brady," occurs when the SA node is firing at a rate of less than 60 beats per minute. Sinus means the rhythm originated in the SA node; therefore, P waves are present. The only difference between sinus bradycardia and normal sinus rhythm (NSR) is the heart rate, but because of this variable, sinus bradycardia is not normal. Sinus bradycardia may result in decreased cardiac output, because while there is adequate time for the heart to fill up with blood, there are not enough contractions per minute to pump the amount of blood needed for normal cardiac output. Significant slowing of the heart rate predisposes the patient to an ectopic focus assuming the role of pacemaker in order to generate sufficient cardiac output. This condition may lead to serious dysrhythmias and warrants careful monitoring. An ECG strip showing sinus bradycardia is in Figure 38–14 ■.

P Wave: Present 1 P wave/QRS complex; PR Interval: 0.18 second; QRS Complex: 0.06 second; QT Interval 0.36 second; Heart Rate: Atrial: 90 beats per minute (bpm); Ventricular: 90 bpm; Rhythm: Regular, Ectopic Beats: None

FIGURE 38–13 ■ Normal sinus rhythm.

6 seconds

P Wave: Present, 1 P wave/QRS Complex; PR Interval: .16 second;
QRS Complex: 0.08 second; QT Interval: 0.32 second; Heart Rate: Atrial:
40 bpm; Ventricular: 40 bpm; Rhythm: Regular; Ectopic Beats: None

FIGURE 38–14 ■ Sinus bradycardia.

Significant ECG features of sinus bradycardia include:

- Both atrial and ventricular rates are less than 60 beats per minute.
- The QT interval tends to lengthen.

The etiology, physical assessment findings, and treatment for sinus bradycardia are outlined in Chart 38–5.

Sinus Tachycardia

Sinus tachycardia is defined as a firing of the (SA) node at a rate greater than 100 beats per minute. It is called *sinus* tachycardia because there is a P wave present, although it may be related to an abnormality of the SA node itself. For example, an acute myocardial infarction (AMI) may cause a decrease in the blood supply to the SA node, resulting in an abnormal response such as tachycardia.

Sinus tachycardia results in increased oxygen consumption, increased workload of the heart, and decreased cardiac output. Whenever the heart rate increases, more oxygen is required to nourish the muscle, resulting in increased work of the heart and increased oxygen consumption. Decreased cardiac output occurs when the heart rate is fast enough to lose the period of time needed for blood to enter the heart, referred to as **fill time.** An ECG strip showing sinus tachycardia is in Figure 38–15 ■ (p. 1089). Significant ECG features of sinus tachycardia include:

- Atrial and ventricular heart rates are over 100 beats per minute.
- As the sinus rate accelerates, both the PR interval and the QT interval tend to shorten slightly.
- The rhythm may be slightly irregular as the rate begins to accelerate, but then becomes a rapid regular rhythm.

The etiology, physical assessment findings, and treatment for sinus tachycardia are outlined in Chart 38–5.

Sinus Arrhythmia/Dysrhythmia

Sinus arrhythmia/dysrhythmia resembles normal sinus rhythm, except for the slight irregularity in the heart rhythm. The rate of impulse formation and conduction varies with the respiratory cycle; thus, the P to P and R to R intervals change with respiration. The heart rate increases during inspiration and decreases with expiration. This dysrhythmia is common in young children and tends to disappear as they grow older (Garcia & Miller, 2004). Additionally, it tends to disappear when the heart increases, for example, with exercise. Typically there is no clinical significance with this dysrhythmia; it is considered a variant of normal. However, the cyclic decreased heart rate may make the heart muscle

CHART 38–5   **Sinus Dysrhythmias: Etiology, Physical Assessment, and Treatment**

Dysrhythmia	Etiology	Physical Assessment	Treatment
Sinus bradycardia	Decreased sympathetic tone, or anatomic changes Hypothermia Drugs, such as morphine, digoxin, verapamil, and some sedatives Toxins Vagal stimulation, as with vomiting or Valsalva maneuver Hypothyroidism Infectious diseases Acidosis Hypovolemia Hypo/hyperkalemia Hypoglycemia Cardiac tamponade Tension pneumothorax Thrombosis: coronary and/or pulmonary Trauma Increased intracranial pressure Normal conditions: sleeping and a well-conditioned athlete's heart	Pulse: Less than 60 beats per minute and typically regular. Blood pressure (BP): Lower than usual if for pathological conditions. If cardiac output is decreased, the following clinical manifestations may occur: • Angina • Syncope • Generalized weakness • Dizziness • Shortness of breath. Altered mental state may be present, although rare.	Treat *only* if symptomatic. Treatment is typically instituted when syncope and/or alteration in consciousness occurs. If symptomatic, it means there is a significant drop in cardiac output. Attempt to identify and treat the cause. Assess for changes in vital signs. Observe for other dysrhythmias. With poor perfusion, typical treatment includes: • Oxygen • IV access • Drug therapy (atropine) • Epinephrine or dopamine • Pacemaker evaluation.

(continued)

CHART 38–5	Sinus Dysrhythmias: Etiology, Physical Assessment, and Treatment—*Continued*		
Dysrhythmia	**Etiology**	**Physical Assessment**	**Treatment**
Sinus tachycardia	Exercise Smoking Alcohol Caffeine Cocaine Fever Blood loss/anemia Hypovolemia Early sepsis Hypermetabolic state, e.g., burn injury Heart failure Allergic reactions Emotions Anxiety Pain Decreased PSNS Increased SNS stimulation Drug side effect of many over-the-counter cold drugs and drugs used to treat asthma and sinus conditions Compensatory response to a decreased cardiac output	Pulse: Greater than 100 beats per minute. BP: Lower than normal. If cardiac output is decreased, the following clinical manifestations may occur: • Angina • Syncope • Generalized weakness • Dizziness • Shortness of breath. Altered mental state may be present, although rare.	Treat *only* if symptomatic. Attempt to identify and treat the cause. Treatment may include: • Drug therapy, such as beta-adrenergic blockers, adenosine, diltiazem, and digoxin • Carotid massage/vagal maneuvers • Cardioversion • Anxiety medications • Fluid replacement. If causes are identified and managed, generally the rhythm converts back to NSR.
Sinus arrhythmia/ dysrhythmia	Common and normal finding, especially in children and young adults Pathological causes include underlying cardiac disease, such as sick sinus syndrome and myocardial infarction Digoxin Factors that cause heart rate variability including exercise, mental stress, and circadian rhythms	Pulse: irregular.	Not treated unless the bradycardic phase causes clinical manifestations described under bradycardia. Atropine for bradycardia. Provide reassurance that this rhythm is not dangerous, but it needs to be evaluated to rule out more serious dysrhythmias.
Sinus arrest	Hypoxemia Cardiac muscle ischemia Damage to the SA node Digoxin Aspirin Abnormal potassium levels Myocardial infarction Vagal dominance Hypersensitive carotid sinus reflex, e.g., tight shirt collar	Pulse: irregular. BP: Lower than normal depending on number of pauses per minute. If cardiac output is decreased, the following clinical manifestations may occur: • Angina • Syncope • Generalized weakness • Dizziness • Shortness of breath. Altered mental state may be present, although rare.	Treat *only* if patient is symptomatic and/or condition is complicated by other dysrhythmias. Ascertain and treat cause, if possible. Typical treatment may include permanent or temporary artificial pacemaker for repeated episodes, depending on the prognosis, age, and presence of clinical manifestations.

Source: Adapted from American Heart Association. (2006). *Handbook of emergency cardiovascular care for healthcare providers.* Dallas, TX: Author.

more susceptible to other dysrhythmias. Figure 38–16 ■ shows an ECG strip of sinus arrhythmia/dysrhythmia. Significant ECG features of sinus arrhythmia/dysrhythmia include:

• PR interval may change slightly as the heart rate changes.
• QT interval changes with the heart rate, becoming longer during the slow phase of the rhythm.
• Heart rate is 60 to 100 beats per minute; however, the slow phase may drop below 60 beats per minute.

• Heart rhythm is regularly irregular, with a variance of more than 0.08 second in the acceleration and deceleration phases.
• Ectopic beats may occur during the slow phase of the rhythm.

The etiology, physical assessment findings, and treatment for sinus arrhythmia/dysrhythmia are outlined in Chart 38–5.

Sinus Arrest

Sinus arrest is a momentary cessation of sinus impulse formation (SA node failure), causing a pause in the cardiac rhythm

6 seconds

P Wave: Present, 1/QRS Complex; PR Interval: 0.14 second; QRS Complex: 0.08 second; QT Interval: 0.36 second; Heart Rate: Atrial: 140 bpm, Ventricular: 140 bpm; Rhythm: Regular; Ectopic Beats None

FIGURE 38–15 ■ Sinus tachycardia.

6 seconds

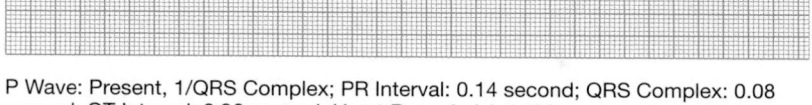

P Wave: Present 1/QRS Complex; PR Interval: 0.18 second; QRS Complex: 0.08 second; QT Interval: 0.40 second; Heart Rate: Atrial: 80 bpm, Ventricular: 80 bpm; Rhythm: Irregular; Ectopic Beats: None

FIGURE 38–16 ■ Sinus arrhythmia/dysrhythmia.

followed by spontaneous resumption of electrical activity. Sinus arrest also is called sinus pause. With a sinus pause there will be an absence of the PQRST complex on the ECG strip and a loss of cardiac output. Figure 38–17 ■ shows an ECG strip of sinus arrest (pause). Significant ECG features of sinus arrest include:

- There is an absence of one entire PQRST complex.
- QT interval changes with the heart rate, becoming longer during the slow phase of the rhythm.
- There may be marked bradycardia due to long sinus pauses.
- Underlying heart rhythm is regular except when the pauses occur.

The etiology, physical assessment findings, and treatment for sinus arrest are outlined in Chart 38–5.

■ Nursing Management for Sinus Dysrhythmias

The nurse should first evaluate the patient's response to and tolerance of any dysrhythmia. Depending on the type of dysrhythmia, the patient may or may not be symptomatic. However, if the abnormal rhythm results in a decreased cardiac output, it is important to assess for the changes outlined on Chart 38–6 (p. 1090).

The psychological impact of having a dysrhythmia also must be addressed. It is frightening to most patients when they experience the clinical manifestations of cardiac dysrhythmias, such as angina, dizziness, syncope, diaphoresis, and disorientation. The nurse should reassure the patient that all appropriate treatment is being provided and offer comfort

Pause

6 seconds

P Wave: Present 1/QRS Complex; PR Interval: 0.20 second; QRS Complex: 0.10 second; QT Interval: 0.40 second; Heart Rate: Atrial: 90 bpm, Ventricular: 90 bpm; Rhythm: Regular except for the pause; Ectopic Beats: None
Conclusion: Sinus arrest (pause)

FIGURE 38–17 ■ Sinus arrest (pause).

CHART 38–6	Clinical Manifestations of Decreased Cardiac Output
Lower than usual blood pressure	Exercise intolerance
Decreased or increased heart rate	Dizziness
Syncope	Alteration in consciousness
Generalized weakness	Angina

Note: Clinical manifestations depend on the degree of decreased cardiac output.

measures. Supply the patient with a quiet environment and treatments to alleviate clinical manifestations. Also provide support by actively listening to the patient's concerns and including family in the plan of care.

The cause of the dysrhythmia, as outlined in Chart 38–5 (p. 1087), must be evaluated and corrected, if possible. Typically the patient is treated only if he becomes symptomatic and/or the condition is complicated by other more serious dysrhythmias. When a dysrhythmia occurs, the nurse needs to do an in-depth assessment of the patient to determine the clinical manifestations. A dysrhythmia may not always occur due to an abnormality in the heart, but may be due to a variety of reasons not associated with a cardiac abnormality. For example, pain and anxiety are two noncardiac causes of tachycardia. Therefore, treatment may consist of pain medications or, if the patient is anxious, providing support, such as talking with the patient. If the patient is hemodynamically unstable, the health care provider should be notified. Chart 38–5 (p. 1087) outlines the standard treatments for each of the sinus dysrhythmias.

Atrial Dysrhythmias

Atrial dysrhythmias usually result from an irritable focus in the atria that initiates an electrical impulse before the SA node has fired in a normal fashion. Because the electrical impulse does not come from the SA node, the P wave configuration of the ECG is different. However, the QRS complex is normal because the electrical impulse travels down the normal pathway from the AV node through the ventricle. Seven different atrial dysrhythmias are discussed next: premature atrial contraction, atrial flutter, atrial fibrillation, supraventricular tachycardia, Wolff-Parkinson-White syndrome, wandering atrial pacemaker, and sick sinus syndrome.

Premature Atrial Contraction

Premature atrial contraction (PAC) is an ectopic focus in the atria that occurs early, before the next expected SA node impulse, causing depolarization and contraction of the cardiac muscle. This electrical impulse originates outside the SA node. It frequently occurs when the underlying rhythm is normal sinus rhythm (NSR), and the only abnormality is the PAC. When there are more than 5 to 6 PACs per minute, they are termed frequent and have more clinical significance. Whenever beats are premature, there is a loss of the time needed for blood to flow into the heart (fill time), which decreases the amount of blood pumped out of the heart, the cardiac output. Thus, if the beats occur frequently cardiac output is decreased. An increase in the frequency of the dysrhythmia also indicates irritability of the atrial muscle and becomes a cause for concern as it tends to increase the risk for other dysrhythmias occurring. Figure 38–18 ■ is a rhythm strip showing premature atrial contractions. Significant ECG features of PACs include:

- P wave is present and is premature.
- P wave configuration (shape) may look different because electrical impulses do not come from the SA node.
- PR interval may be shorter or longer than regular beats.
- PACs are premature, making the rhythm irregular.
- P wave after the PAC falls earlier than expected because of the early electrical discharge, which then resets the SA node rhythm, referred to as a noncompensatory pause.
- Heart rate and rhythm are typically within normal limits, except when the PAC occurs.

The etiology, physical assessment findings, and treatment of PACs are outlined in Chart 38–7.

Atrial Flutter

Atrial flutter is a rapid, regular, atrial rhythm with an *atrial* rate of 200 to 400 beats per minute (Garcia & Miller, 2004). There is loss of SA node dominance, which is the preferential pacemaker. Only a fraction of the atrial impulses are conducted through the AV node to the ventricle. Most of the atrial beats fall during the AV node refractory period when the cardiac cell is unable to respond to any stimulus, thus preventing conduction of the impulse. This makes the AV node the "gatekeeper" for the ventricles by prohibiting all of the atrial impulses from reaching the ventricles, thereby limiting ventricular rate. Atrial flutter also causes a decreased cardiac output due to the loss of the atrial kick or

Noncompensatory pause

P Wave: Premature; PR Interval: 0.16 second; QRS Complex: 0.10 second; QT interval: 0.40 second; Heart Rate: Atrial: 70 bpm; Ventricular: 70 bpm; Rhythm: Regular except for premature beats. Ectopic Beat PAC. Conclusion: One premature atrial contraction.

FIGURE 38–18 ■ Premature atrial contraction.

CHART 38–7	Atrial Dysrhythmias: Etiology, Physical Assessment, and Treatment		
Dysrhythmia	**Etiology**	**Physical Assessment**	**Treatment**
Premature atrial contraction	Mitral stenosis Mitral valve prolapse Cor pulmonale Underlying cardiovascular disease including ischemia and myocardial infarction Hypoxia Infectious diseases Electrolyte imbalance Increased sympathetic tone Stimulants Drug toxicity, e.g., digoxin Stress Anxiety	Pulse: Irregular BP: If frequent PACs, may be decreased. If cardiac output is decreased the following clinical manifestations may occur: Angina Syncope Generalized weakness Dizziness Shortness of breath Altered mental state may be present, although rare.	Observe the frequency of the PACs, and observe for decreased cardiac output (Chart 38–6). Treat the underlying cause, e.g., stress, anxiety, electrolyte imbalance. Frequent PAC's or those that cause sustained tachycardia may require treatment with drugs that prolong atrial refractoriness, such as digoxin, verapamil, or propranolol.
Atrial flutter	Coronary atherosclerosis Valvular disease; Cor pulmonale Pulmonary edema Myocardial infarction SA node disease Pulmonary embolism Digitalis toxicity ETOH abuse Postsurgical complication: one of the common dysrhythmias following open heart surgery. On rare occasions it may occur with normal healthy hearts.	Pulse: May be regular or irregular BP: Lower than normal if cardiac output is decreased. If cardiac output is decreased the following clinical manifestations may occur: Angina Syncope Generalized weakness Dizziness Shortness of breath Altered mental state may be present, although rare.	Cardioversion is a common intervention. Drug therapy is used to reduce AV conduction: digitalis, propranolol, diltiazem. If a chronic situation the patient may be placed on anticoagulants like warfarin.
Atrial fibrillation	Acute myocardial infarction Left atrial stretch due to mitral stenosis and mitral regurgitation May be a chronic rhythm associated with heart failure Transient after open-heart surgery Long-standing hypertension Digoxin toxicity Alcohol intake, chronic or acute, moderate to heavy Idiopathic	Pulse: Irregular (hallmark feature) BP: Lower than normal If cardiac output is decreased the following clinical manifestations may occur: Angina Syncope Generalized weakness Dizziness Shortness of breath Altered mental state may be present, depending on the ventricular rate.	Control the ventricular response, i.e., heart rate. If a rapid ventricular response control with drugs: digoxin is still the drug of choice; beta-blockers (propranolol) and calcium channel blockers (verapamil, diltiazem). Calcium channel blockers work the fastest, and are the drug of choice when medically unstable. Prevent thromboembolic events with anticoagulant therapy, e.g., warfarin, Cardioversion: Is used if new onset, especially when hemodynamic instability is present. If successful, digoxin is used to prevent reoccurrence.
Supraventricular tachycardia includes paroxysmal Atrioventricular node reentry tachycardia AVNRT Atrial tachycardia	Heart disease Rheumatic heart disease Coronary artery disease (CAD) Hypoxia May be precipitated by a premature atrial contraction (PAC) May occur in healthy adults from a variety of causes: Overexertion Stress Excessive use of stimulants Smoking Hypokalemia	Pulse: Very fast. BP: Decreased if drop in cardiac output. If cardiac output is decreased the following clinical manifestations may occur: Angina Syncope Generalized weakness Dizziness Shortness of breath Altered mental state may be present, although rare.	It is necessary to find and treat the cause, e.g., stress, hypokalemia. Vagal maneuvers, i.e., bearing down, coughing, and carotid artery massage. Specific treatment may include: oxygen therapy and cardioversion. Drug therapy: adenosine is used to briefly terminate the rhythm for differential diagnosis. Verapamil is a calcium channel blocker; decreases heart rate. Cardioversion is performed if drug therapy and vagal maneuvers are unsuccessful.

(continued)

CHART 38–7	Atrial Dysrhythmias: Etiology, Physical Assessment, and Treatment—*Continued*		
Dysrhythmia	**Etiology**	**Physical Assessment**	**Treatment**
Wolff-Parkinson-White (WPW) syndrome	Congenital in origin: twice as common in males, and occurs in 0.1 to 0.3% of the general population.	Pulse: Rapid. Frequent episodes of palpitations. BP: May be decreased due to fast heart rate. If cardiac output is decreased the following clinical manifestations may occur: Angina Syncope Generalized weakness Dizziness Shortness of breath Altered mental state may be present, although rare.	Same as that for supraventricular tachycardia. Radiofrequency ablation to terminate the accessory pathway.
Wandering atrial pacemaker	Frequently seen in normal individuals and is of no consequence. Digoxin toxicity	Pulse: 40–60 bpm BP: Lower than normal If cardiac output is decreased the following clinical manifestations may occur: Angina Syncope Generalized weakness Dizziness Shortness of breath Altered mental state may be present, although rare.	Treat only if symptomatic. Treatment typically is instituted when syncope and/or alteration in consciousness occurs. Attempt to identify and treat the cause. Administer oxygen. Establish IV access Drug therapy: Atropine Evaluate for transcutaneous or permanent pacemaker depending on impact on cardiac output
Sick sinus syndrome	Coronary artery disease Drugs: Cardiac glycoside, Antihypertensive agents, Calcium channel blockers Frequently, intermittent and unpredictable, may occur in the absence of heart disease Myocardial infarction Inflammatory or degenerative processes	Pulse: Bradycardia that alternates with tachycardia, referred to as brady-tachy syndrome. BP: May decrease due to decreased cardiac output. If cardiac output is decreased the following clinical manifestations may occur: Angina Syncope Generalized weakness Dizziness Shortness of breath Altered mental state may be present, although rare.	Clinical manifestations and ECG findings determine treatment. Anticoagulants are used because of blood stasis if atrial flutter/fibrillation is present. The only definitive treatment is a permanent pacemaker to replace the SA node.

normal atrial contraction. Atrial kick forces more blood into the ventricle, which augments cardiac output. With atrial flutter the atria are just fluttering instead of contracting, resulting in a decreased cardiac output by as much as 30% (Shade & Wesley, 2007). Additionally, with the loss of the atrial contraction, blood stasis and pooling occur, leading to an increased incidence of clot formation. Finally, due to the rapid atrial rate myocardial oxygen consumption increases, which eventually leads to the development of hypoxia of the myocardial muscle and predisposes the left ventricular to fail. Figure 38–19 ■ is a rhythm strip showing atrial flutter. Significant ECG features of atrial flutter include:

- P waves are not identifiable; instead there are flutter waves (F waves), creating a "sawtooth" baseline on the ECG strip.

- PR intervals are not measurable.
- QT interval is not measurable because the T waves are buried in the F waves.
- Atrial and ventricular rhythms typically are regular, but they may be irregular depending on how often the AV node allows impulses to travel to the ventricle.

The etiology, physical assessment findings, and treatment of atrial flutter are outlined in Chart 38–7.

Atrial Fibrillation

Atrial fibrillation, also referred to as "atrial fib" or "a-fib," is a common dysrhythmia. The Evidence-Based Practice box outlines the genetic considerations of atrial fibrillation.

P Wave: None, flutter waves; PR interval: None; QRS Complex: 0.08 second; QT Interval: unable to obtain; Heart Rate: Atrial: about 300 bpm, Ventricular: 90 bpm; Rhythm: Regular; Ectopic Beats: Flutter waves.

FIGURE 38–19 ■ Atrial flutter.

It is characterized by a disorganized, very rapid, and irregular atrial rhythm resulting in an irregular ventricular rhythm, the hallmark feature. Rapid or slow ventricular heart rate, referred to as the ventricular response, depends on the rate that the AV node allows impulses to be conducted to the ventricles. The cells in the atria have an increased irritability typically due to cardiac muscle hypoxia, which causes many sites in the atria to become pacemakers and initiate electrical impulses. The firing of these multiple sites causes the atria simply to quiver instead of contracting effectively. Atrial fibrillation causes three significant clinical manifestations: (1) loss of SA node pacemaker dominance, which is the most reliable pacemaker; (2) decreased cardiac output due to loss

of atrial kick; and (3) increased myocardial oxygen consumption. The immediate concern for atrial fibrillation is the ventricular response because it determines cardiac output. A heart rate that is too slow or too fast impacts cardiac output.

With the loss of the atrial kick, blood stasis and pooling occur, leading to an increased incidence of clot formation. Therefore, those individuals with atrial fibrillation are at high risk for a cardiovascular accident (CVA) and/or pulmonary emboli. The rapid atrial firing also increases the workload on the heart, eventually causing hypoxia of the myocardial muscle. Long-term hypoxia predisposes to left ventricular failure. Figure 38–20 ■ (p. 1096) is a rhythm strip showing atrial fibrillation.

Genetic Considerations

Clinical Problem

A conservative estimate of the number of people who are affected by atrial fibrillation (AF) is approximately 2 million. It is the most common dysrhythmia that causes an irregular heart rate, palpitations, unexplained rapid heart rate, and a sensation of "missed" beats. The incidence of AF increases with age, with less than 1% of the population experiencing it before age 60 years, while it is present in 1 in 10 individuals at age 80 years and over. Elderly white men compose the largest group that is affected by AF.

Research Findings

A new study conducted by the National Heart, Lung, and Blood Institute (2004) assessed the prevalence of AF in individuals who had it in their family history. The study evaluated 2,243 individuals whose parents were in the original Framingham Heart Study. The participants were at least 30 years of age and had no history of AF. Seventy of the subjects developed AF within four years. If individual participants had a history of one parent with AF they were twice as likely to develop the dysrhythmia as subjects who had no family history of AF. If both parents had AF before 75 years of age, the risk tripled. Further research continues to determine which genes are involved and what steps are necessary to enhance early diagnosis and treatment.

Implications for Nursing Practice

Implications for nursing practice begin with the nursing assessment. It is important to specifically question the family history for the presence of AF. This is especially essential if the patient has clinical manifestations and new onset irregular pulse. It needs to be documented in the patient's record that there is a family history of the disease. The nurse also must assess the presence of other risk factors for the development of AF including:

Cardiomyopathy

Hypertension

Heart failure

Excessive alcohol consumption

Previous myocardial infarction

Diabetes

Rheumatic heart disease

Mitral valve disorders such as prolapse, regurgitation, and annular calcification

Smoking

Caffeine

The need for patient/family counseling about the increased risk for the development of AF is necessary along with instructions about the need for medical attention if clinical manifestations described above occur. A major emphasis needs to be placed on increasing public awareness of AF and its many causative factors. Patients with a family history require more frequent and diligent testing. Treatment for AF is outlined on Chart 38–7 (p. 1091).

Critical Thinking Questions

1. When assessing a patient with new onset atrial fibrillation, what types of questions would assist the nurse to determine if there is a risk for a genetic predisposition?

2. When teaching a newly diagnosed patient how to live with AF, in order of priority what must be included in the teaching plan?

Answers to Critical Thinking Questions appear in Appendix D.

Sources: Fox, C. S., Parise, H., D'Agostino, R.B., et al. (2004). Parental atrial fibrillation as a risk factor for atrial fibrillation in offspring. *JAMA: 291*(23): 2852-2856; Pavlovich-Dannis, S.J. (2005). Mom's eyes and dad's atrial fibrillation. *Nurse Week:* 23–24. National Heart, Lung, and Blood Institute (NHLBI), National Institutes of Health. (2004). Parental atrial fibrillation increases risk in offspring, finds NHLBI's Framingham Heart Study. NIH News. Retrieved August 8, 2008 from http://www.nhlbi.nih.gov/new/press04-06-15.htm

EVIDENCE-BASED PRACTICE

P Wave: None; PR Interval: None; QRS Complex: 0.10 second; QT Interval: unable to obtain; Heart Rate: Ventricular: 80 bpm; Rhythm: Irregular; Ectopic Beats: f waves.

FIGURE 38–20 ■ Atrial fibrillation.

Significant ECG features of atrial fibrillation include:

- P waves are not identifiable due to the atrial quivering, referred to as "f" waves, occurring at 350 to 750 beats per minute.
- PR intervals are not measurable.
- QT interval is not obtainable because the T waves are buried in the f waves.
- Irregularly irregular rhythm occurs, meaning that there is no pattern to the irregularity.
- f waves are ectopic beats.

The etiology, physical assessment findings, and treatment of atrial fibrillation are outlined in Chart 38–7 (p. 1091).

Supraventricular Tachycardia

Supraventricular tachycardia (SVT) is a tachycardia that is generated somewhere above the ventricles. This general term encompasses all fast (tachy) rhythms with normal QRS complexes and heart rates greater than 100 beats per minute. Rhythms included under the SVT umbrella include sinus tachycardia, paroxysmal atrial tachycardia (PAT), and paroxysmal junctional tachycardia (PJT). Clinicians use the term *supraventricular tachycardia* when it is impossible to identify the source of the tachycardia.

Usually this rhythm is benign and is self-limiting when the cause is removed. If sustained, loss of blood *fill time* (diastole) causes a drop in cardiac output. Prolonged episodes of supraventricular tachycardia increase myocardial oxygen demand and also

may result in a conversion to atrial flutter or fibrillation. Eventually, signs and symptoms of congestive heart failure will be present. Figure 38–21 ■ is a rhythm strip showing supraventricular tachycardia (SVT).

Significant ECG features of supraventricular tachycardia include:

- Heart rate is 100 to 250 beats per minute.
- P wave is not seen; it is buried in the QRS complex.
- PR interval is not discernable.
- QRS complex is within normal limits unless distorted by the buried P waves.
- QT interval is not obtainable because the T waves are buried.
- Heart rhythm may be regular or irregular due to varying conduction rates through the AV node.
- Ectopic beats may or may not be present, depending on the pacemaker site.

The etiology, physical assessment findings, and treatment of supraventricular tachycardia are outlined in Chart 38–7 (p. 1091).

Atrioventricular Nodal Reentry Tachycardia

One phenomenon that can cause supraventricular tachycardia is atrioventricular nodal reentry tachycardia (AVNRT). Normally people are born with only a single electrical pathway at the base of the right atrium where impulses travel to the AV node. However, some individuals are born with two separate electrical pathways leading to the AV node, each with its own respective

P Wave: None; PR Interval: None; QRS Complex: 0.10 second; QT Interval: unable to obtain; Heart Rate: ⟶ Atrial rate rapid, Ventricular: 200 bpm; Rhythm: Regular; Ectopic Beats: Depends on pacemaker site.

FIGURE 38–21 ■ Supraventricular tachycardia (SVT).

properties. Each pathway has its own refractory period, one fast (beta) and one slow (alpha). The fast track has a long refractory period, and the slow track has a fast refractory period. Impulses travel the two separate pathways simultaneously. When the impulse begins down these two pathways, because of its speed, the one in the fast track stimulates the AV node and bundle of His, causing ventricular depolarization and a normal-width QRS complex. The fast track impulse also travels retrograde (backward transmission) back through the slow track, meeting the impulse coming down the slow track. When the two impulses meet, 99.9% of the time, they cancel each other out and the rhythm is normal. If for any reason, such as the presence of a refractory period in the fast track, the fast track will be unable to transmit the impulse, then the slow track transmits the impulse, causing depolarization of the ventricles. The QRS complex would still be within normal limits, but the PR interval would be longer than the ones coming from the fast track. This creates rhythm strips

that have identical QRS complexes but two different PR interval lengths. These beats still are considered to be sinus complexes, as opposed to coming from another atrial ectopic focus. The PR interval length differences are a result of the conduction alternating intermittently between the two functioning tracks.

The AVNRT phenomenon occurs when a reentrant circuit or loop is created along the two pathways and the AV node (Figure 38–22 ■). An early impulse such as a PAC hits the two pathways; the fast track is in refractory and therefore cannot accept the impulse, but the slow track can. The impulse travels from the slow track, to the AV node, and then retrograde up the fast track because this track has recovered, is no longer in a refractory state, and can accept the impulse. The impulses are now able to continue to cycle the circuit or loop and initiate ventricular depolarization at a fast rate; this is referred to as AVNRT (Garcia & Miller, 2004).

It is estimated that AVNRT occurs in 60% of patients presenting with paroxysmal (sudden onset) SVT and occurs in

(a) **Macro re-entry circut: antegrade through AV node and retrograde across an assessory pathway.**

(b) **Micro re-entry at the cellular level in the AV node and Purkinje fibers.**

FIGURE 38–22 ■   Reentrant circuit.

approximately several cases per thousand persons worldwide. It is more predominant in women, may occur with individuals of any age, and is common in young adults. AVNRT is usually well tolerated; it often occurs in patients with no structural heart disease. Clinical manifestations are the same as with any tachy dysrhythmia, although AVNRT may cause angina or myocardial infarction in patients with coronary artery disease. Prognosis for patients without heart disease is usually good (Olshansky et al., 2006). Treatment is aimed at breaking the reentrant cycle with the use of vagal maneuvers such as breath holding, stimulating gag reflex, and carotid sinus massage.

Wolff-Parkinson-White Syndrome

Wolff-Parkinson-White syndrome (WPW) is a genetic AV conduction disorder characterized by the presence of two AV conduction pathways, one normal and one abnormal. An impulse leaving the atrium may travel down one or the other pathway without any specific pattern. The abnormal pathway, called the Kent bundle, is composed of an extra muscle bundle made up of working myocardial tissue. This extra muscle bundle forms a connection between the atria and the ventricles outside the normal conduction system, referred to as an accessory pathway. This allows impulses coming from the atrium to bypass the normal AV connection. The hallmark feature on the ECG strip for the abnormal pathway is the presence of a delta wave, a slurred upstroke at the beginning of the QRS complex (Figure 38–23 ■). The delta wave occurs when the impulse travels via the accessory pathway to the ventricles. Because the conduction is outside the normal conduction system, it takes longer for the impulse to travel through the ventricles, thus creating an abnormally wide, bizarre QRS complex (Garcia & Miller, 2004).

Atrial flutter, atrial fibrillation, and supraventricular tachycardia that results in heart rates of greater than 250 beats per minute, are common dysrhythmias in patients with WPW. The increased heart rate increases the workload and oxygen consumption of the heart, predisposing to heart failure, and therefore could cause sudden cardiac death. When the patient does not exhibit any dysrhythmias, but has the delta wave, this is called WPW pattern. When the patient becomes symptomatic or develops dysrhythmias, then the correct terminology is WPW syndrome. Figure 38–23 ■ is a rhythm strip showing Wolff-Parkinson-White dysrhythmia. Significant ECG features of Wolff-Parkinson-White syndrome include:

- PR interval shortens to less than 0.12 second because the AV node is bypassed and delta waves appear just prior to the beginning of the R wave.

P Wave: Present and irregular; PR Interval: 0.12 second; QRS Complex: 0.16 second. QT Interval 0.52 second, 40-50 bpm, Ventricular: 40-50 bpm; Rhythm: Regular Ectopic Beats: None.

FIGURE 38–23 ■ Wolff-Parkinson-White syndrome.

- QRS complex is greater than 0.12 second due to the delta waves.
- QT interval shortens if tachycardia occurs and lengthens with bradycardia.
- Heart rate frequently tachycardic.
- Heart rhythm is regular, except during heart rate changes.

The etiology, physical assessment findings, and treatment of WPW syndrome are outlined in Chart 38–7 (p. 1091).

Wandering Atrial Pacemaker

Wandering atrial pacemaker is a pacemaker from at least three different sites above the bundle of His acting as the heart's pacemaker. These pacemaker sites may include the SA node, the AV junction, an atrial ectopic site, and/or any combination of these areas. This abnormality occurs because of SA node slowing, which permits an atrial ectopic focus and junctional escape rhythms to "jump in" as atrial pacemakers. Figure 38–24 ■ is a rhythm strip showing wandering atrial pacemaker. Significant ECG features of wandering atrial pacemaker include:

- P waves have multiple shapes, due to multiple atrial sites initiating the conduction.
- QT interval usually is normal, but may be prolonged due to a slow heart rate.
- Heart rhythm is irregular due to changing pacemakers.
- Atrial rate and ventricular heart rate typically are slow.
- Ectopic beats may be present due to the slow rhythm.

The etiology, physical assessment findings, and treatment of wandering atrial pacemaker are outlined in Chart 38–7 (p. 1091).

Sick Sinus Syndrome

Sick sinus syndrome (SSS) encompasses a broad range of abnormalities, including disorders of impulse generation and conduction, failure of pacemakers, and a susceptibility to paroxysmal or

P Wave: Multifocal; PR Interval: 0.16 second; QRS Complex: 0.06 second; QT Interval: 0.04 second; Heart Rate: Atrial: Approximately 60 bpm; Ventricular: 50 bpm; Rhythm: Irregular; Ectopic Beats; Multifocal P waves.

FIGURE 38–24 ■ Wandering atrial pacemaker.

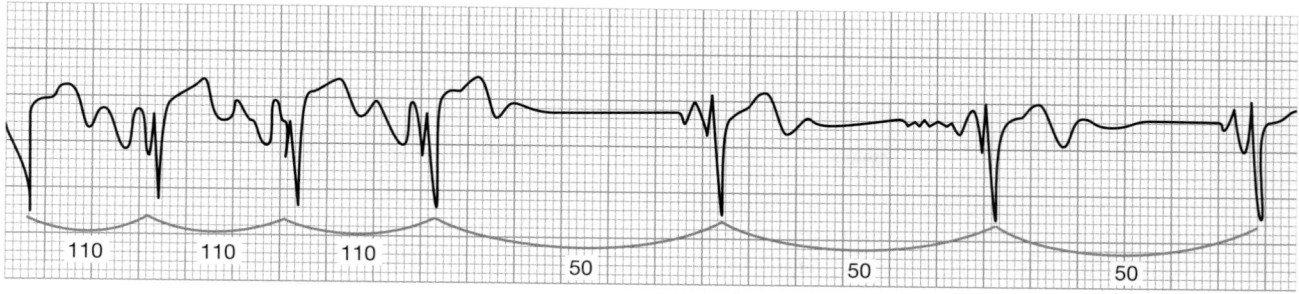

P Wave: Present, but variable configuration; PR Interval: 0.14 second; QRS Complex: 0.08 second; QT Interval: 0.40 second;
Heart Rate: Atrial: 60 bpm, Ventricular: 60 bpm; Rhythm: Irregular; Ectopic Beats: May occur with slow rate.

FIGURE 38–25 ■ Sick sinus syndrome.

chronic atrial tachycardia. This disorder also is referred to as sinoatrial disease and sinoatrial dysfunction. The cause is a severely depressed nonreliable SA node due to heart disease or the side effect of certain cardiac drugs, such as cardiac glycosides, sympatholytic antihypertensive agents, beta-adrenergic blockers, calcium channel blockers, and membrane active antiarrhythmic agents. When the tachycardia occurs with SSS there is increased oxygen consumption and workload for the myocardium. Profound sinus bradycardia with SSS may progress to sinus pauses or arrest, thereby decreasing cardiac output. Figure 38–25 ■ is a rhythm strip showing sick sinus syndrome. Significant ECG features of sick sinus syndrome include:

- P waves may be present or absent depending on which dysrhythmia is occurring.
- PR interval varies due to changing P wave sites.
- QT interval varies due to rate changes.
- Heart rate may be rapid or slow, or a combination of both.
- Heart rhythm is irregular and highly variable.
- Ectopic beats may be present when a slow rate occurs.

The etiology, physical assessment findings, and treatment of sick sinus syndrome are outlined in Chart 38–7 (p. 1091).

■ Nursing Management for Responsibilities for Atrial Dysrhythmias

Nursing responsibility when any dysrhythmia occurs is to assess the patient's response to the rhythm. This is especially true if it is a new onset dysrhythmia and/or if the dysrhythmia causes a drop in the cardiac output. The atrial dysrhythmias do not have the impact on cardiac output that the more serious ventricular dysrhythmias do, but any change in cardiac output may cause clinical manifestations, and therefore, requires an in-depth assessment. The patient is evaluated for the clinical manifestations of reduced cardiac output as outlined in Chart 38–6 (p. 1090). Vital signs and clinical manifestations must be monitored frequently to assess tolerance of the rhythm, especially if it is sustained. The health care provider needs to be notified, especially if this is a new rhythm, because medical intervention must be initiated to convert the rhythm back to normal sinus rhythm.

Atrial flutter and fibrillation may occur as a transient dysrhythmia in healthy young individuals. If these conditions are chronic they are typically associated with heart disease including atrial muscle disease or atrial distention with disease of the sinus node. Atrial fibrillation also is seen in congenital heart disease. If the atrial flutter and/or atrial fibrillation are chronic conditions, and normal sinus rhythm cannot be reestablished, the patient often is placed on an anticoagulant, such as warfarin. This treatment is indicated because a fluttering/fibrillating atrium creates blood stasis, which increases the risk of clot formation. If these clots travel out of the atrium they tend to lodge in the brain, and, on rare occasions in the lung, causing an alteration in normal function in these areas.

Treatment of atrial fibrillation/flutter may include cardioversion, which is the delivery of electrical voltage in order to stop unwanted electrical activity and allow the SA node to resume the heart's pacemaker. Cardioversion is discussed in detail in Chapter 39 ⊙ . This treatment increases risk for myocardial infarction, cerebral vascular accident (CVA), and pulmonary embolus. The nurse needs to assess the patient post-cardioversion for clinical manifestations of these disorders. Myocardial infarction is discussed in detail in Chapter 40 ⊙ . Cardiovascular accident (CVA) is discussed in Chapter 30 ⊙ , and pulmonary embolus is discussed in Chapters 35 and 36 ⊙ .

Besides heart disease frequently there are other causes for atrial cardiac dysrhythmias that must be evaluated and treated, e.g., stress, pain, and anxiety. The treatment may be narcotics for pain relief or an antianxiety medication for stress and increased anxiety. The nurse may need only to sit and listen to the patient and provide emotional support.

Junctional Dysrhythmias

Junctional dysrhythmias also referred to as nodal rhythms result from either an irritable focus in the junctional tissue that discharges before the SA node has had a chance to or because the SA node has failed to fire and the junctional node becomes the secondary pacemaker. AV junctional dysrhythmias may occur if the impulse from the SA node is blocked as it exits the SA node or if it is not conducted through the atria. AV junctional dysrhythmias have a distinctive pattern on ECG tracings because the impulse is not initiated in the SA node. The impulse is initiated in the AV junctional tissue and must travel in a backward (retrograde) direction to activate the atria. Therefore, the P wave is inverted or negatively deflected, due to this retrograde conduction, and may occur before, after, or buried in, the QRS complex. Retrograde conduction means that the impulse originates in the AV junction so it stimulates the atria from the bottom up instead of the top down. The impulse simultaneously initiates both atrial and ventricular contractions. The location of the P wave is, therefore, dependent on the speed with which the impulses travel in both chambers. The QRS complex configuration is normal in appearance because the impulse travels the normal pathway from the AV junctional node through the ventricles. AV junctional dysrhythmias are not considered lethal or life threatening, but as always, the most important indicator of the clinical significance of any dysrhythmia is the patient's response to or tolerance of the rhythm. The three AV junctional dysrhythmias discussed in this chapter are: junctional escape rhythm, premature junctional contractions, and paroxysmal junctional tachycardia.

Junctional Escape Rhythm

Junctional escape rhythm occurs when there is a problem with normal SA node function, either fails to produce an impulse, or when the SA node's rate of firing falls below the intrinsic rate of the AV node. At this time the AV node will assume the role of the pacemaker. The ability of the AV node to assume this role is a safety measure in that it becomes the pacemaker for the heart when the SA node fails to do so. When an isolated beat from the AV junction occurs it is called a junctional escape beat or complex, as compared to a series of beats that then is called a junctional rhythm. When a rhythm is generated from the junction, the rate is between 40 and 60 beats per minute. If the rate is greater than 60 but less than 100 it is referred to as an accelerated junctional rhythm. If the rate is greater than 100 typically it is called junctional tachycardia.

Figures 38–26 ■ and 38–27 ■ are ECG rhythm strips that show junctional escape rhythm and accelerated junctional rhythm, respectively. Significant ECG features of junctional escape rhythms include:

- P wave is inverted, negatively deflected, due to retrograde conduction, and either occurs before, after, or buried in the QRS complex.
- PR interval is dependent on the location of P wave; thus, the PR interval may or may not be present or normal.
- QRS complex is normal in duration and shape, unless distorted by a buried P wave.
- QT interval is within normal range, unless impacted by the heart rate. It is prolonged with slow heart rate or shortened with increased heart rate.
- Heart rate is usually within normal range for a rhythm generated from the AV junction and is 40 to 60 beats per minute. For an accelerated junctional rhythm the rate is 60 to 100 beats per minute and for junctional tachycardia the heart rate is greater than 100 bpm.
- Heart rhythm is typically regular.
- Entire rhythm is composed of ectopic beats because they all come from the AV junction instead of the SA node. Other ectopic beats may occur with slow heart rate.

The etiology, physical assessment findings, and treatment of junctional escape rhythms are outlined in Chart 38–8.

Premature Junctional Contraction

A **premature junctional contraction (PJC)** originates as an ectopic beat that is initiated in the atrioventricular (AV) junction. It discharges before the next expected SA node impulse causing simultaneous atrial and ventricular contraction to occur. This is not a dangerous dysrhythmia, although it does indicate that some degree of cardiac ischemia is occurring. Figure 38–28 ■ (p. 1100) is

P Wave: None, or buried in QRS Complex; PR Interval: Not measurable; QRS Complex: 0.10 second; QT Interval: 0.40 second; Heart Rate: Atrial: Not measurable, Ventricular: 40 bpm; Rhythm: Regular; Ectopic Beats: None.

FIGURE 38–26 ■ Junctional escape rhythm.

P Wave: Inverted and regular; PR Interval: 0.14–0.16 second; QRS Complex: 0.08 second: QT Interval: 0.44 second; Heart Rate: Atrial: 80 bpm, Ventricular: 80 bpm; Rhythm: Regular: Ectopic Beats: none.

FIGURE 38–27 ■ Accelerated junctional rhythm.

CHART 38–8	Junctional Dysrhythmias: Etiology, Physical Assessment, and Treatment		
Dysrhythmia	**Etiology**	**Physical Assessment**	**Treatment**
Junctional escape rhythm	SA node disease Myocardial infarction Hypoxia and ischemia Heart failure Increased vagal tone Certain cardiac drugs: such as digoxin, beta adrenergic blockers, and calcium channel blockers Sinus bradycardia Digoxin toxicity Hyperkalemia Valve disease	Pulse: rhythm is regular with a usual rate of 40 – 60 bpm unless it is an accelerated rhythm of > 100 bpm If cardiac output is decreased the following clinical manifestations may occur: Angina Syncope Generalized weakness Dizziness Shortness of breath Altered mental state may be present, although rare.	Observe for other dysrhythmias if a slow rate is present. Generally this condition is asymptomatic; however, if symptomatic, typical treatment includes: Oxygen Drug therapy: (atropine, dopamine) Pacemaker Cardioversion
Premature junctional contraction (PJC)	Irritability of the AV junctional tissue caused by: SA node disease Myocardial infarction Sinus bradycardia Mitral stenosis Mitral valve prolapse Cor pulmonale Hypoxia Ischemia Infectious diseases Increased vagal tone Increased sympathetic tone Electrolyte imbalances Digoxin Stimulants Stress Anxiety May precede AV block	Pulse: Irregular BP: Normal unless PJCs occur frequently enough to decrease cardiac output.	Rarely causes symptoms, thus typically not treated. Find and treat the underlying cause, if possible. If it initiates a more serious dysrhythmia, such as tachycardia, therapy becomes more aggressive, contingent on the type of dysrhythmia. If occurring frequently, more than 5 times per minute, they can drop cardiac output, and predispose the patient to other dysrhythmias. Oxygen Drugs such as stimulants, sympathomimetics, and digitalis may be discontinued.
Paroxysmal junctional tachycardia (PJT)	May occur at any age with no prior history of underlying heart disease. Digoxin toxicity (most common cause) Inferior wall myocardial infarction Myocarditis Ischemia Untoward response to open heart surgery Frequent ingestion of stimulants Anxiety Increased catecholamine secretion	Pulse: Rapid, with patient experiencing a fluttering sensation. BP: Lower than usual due to decreased cardiac output. If cardiac output is decreased the following clinical manifestations may occur: Angina Syncope Generalized weakness Dizziness Shortness of breath Altered mental state may be present, although rare.	Find and treat the cause as PJTs may be a predisposition to lethal dysrhythmias, heart failure, and shock. Vagal maneuvers may be applied. Oxygen Drug therapy initiated: includes: amiodarone or beta-adrenergic blockers. Cardioversion may be initiated if necessary.

a rhythm strip showing premature junctional contraction. Significant ECG features of premature junction contractions include:

- P wave is inverted and occurs before, after, or buried in the QRS complex.
- PR interval is dependent on the location of P wave; thus, the PR interval may or may not be present or normal.
- QRS complex is normal in duration and shape, unless distorted by a buried P wave.

- QT interval also is normal unless impacted by the heart rate.
- Heart rate is that of the underlying rhythm.
- Heart rhythm is irregular when PJCs are present; or it may be described as regular with premature beats.
- Ectopic beat is the PJC.

The etiology, physical assessment findings, and treatment of PJCs are outlined in Chart 38–8.

P Wave: Present and regular except for premature beat; PR Interval: 0.16 second; QRS Complex: 0.08 second; second; Heart Rate: Atrial: 110 bpm, Ventricular: 110 bpm; Rhythm: Regular except for premature beats: Ectopic Beats: none

FIGURE 38–28 ■ Premature junctional contraction (PJC).

Paroxysmal Junctional Tachycardia

The **paroxysmal junctional tachycardia (PJT)** rhythm is defined as an irritable focus in the AV junction that assumes the pacemaker role by discharging impulses more rapidly than the SA node. It begins and ends abruptly, which is why it is called paroxysmal. If it is a sustained rhythm, and greater than 60 beats per minute, it may be referred to as junctional tachycardia. The term *junctional tachycardia* sometimes is used interchangeably with the term accelerated junctional rhythm, which was discussed previously. This rhythm produces a junctional rate of over 60 beats per minute. Figure 38–29 ■ is a rhythm strip showing paroxysmal junctional tachycardia. Significant ECG features of paroxysmal junctional tachycardia include:

- Heart rate usually is 160 to 240 beats per minute and constant. It may, however, be as low as 110 beats per minute or exceed 240 beats per minute.
- P wave is inverted and occurs before, after, or buried in the QRS complex.
- PR interval is dependent on the location of P wave; thus, the PR interval may or may not be present or normal.
- QRS complex is normal in duration and shape, unless distorted by a buried P wave.
- QT interval shortens due to increased heart rate.
- Heart rhythm is essentially regular. It may become irregular as the rate increases.
- Entire rhythm is composed of ectopic beats because they all come from the AV junction instead of the SA node.

The etiology, physical assessment findings, and treatment of PJTs are outlined in Chart 38–8 (p. 1099).

■ Nursing Management for Junctional Dysrhythmias

Like atrial dysrhythmias, junctional dysrhythmias generally are not life threatening. However, the decreased and/or increased heart rate does have an impact on cardiac output. This is especially true in the presence of heart disease when the heart is unable to significantly increase the force of the muscle contraction to compensate for the rate changes. Therefore, the nurse must evaluate the patient for clinical manifestations of decreased cardiac output (Chart 38–6, p. 1090). When rhythm is slow other ectopic foci may attempt to become the heart's pacemaker, therefore, the nurse must assess the rhythm for other aberrancies. The health care provider needs to be notified, especially if it is a new onset dysrhythmia in order to determine cause and treatment. It is essential that the nurse assist the health care provider in determining the cause and treatment of dysrhythmias. Since some prescribed medications, e.g., digoxin, cause significant dysrhythmias, the patient's medical history should be reviewed to determine if the dysrhythmia is medication related. Serum drug levels should be ordered as indicated. For symptomatic junctional tachycardia, treatment also may include applying vagal maneuvers, initiating drug therapy, and completing cardioversion if necessary. As always any significant rhythm change or the appearance of new onset dysrhythmias needs to be reported to the health care provider.

P Wave: Inverted and regular; PR Interval: 0.08 second; QRS Complex: 0.06 second; QT Interval: 0.32 second; Heart Rate: Atrial: 130 bpm, Ventricular: 130 bpm. Rhythm: Regular; Ectopic Beats: None.

FIGURE 38–29 ■ Paroxysmal junctional tachycardia.

Due to the clinical manifestations of these dysrhythmias, the patient and family may experience anxiety. Thus, the nurse also must assess and treat the anxiety by use of supportive measures, such as listening to the patient's concerns, offering reassurance, providing a calm environment, and medicating for anxiety and pain relief as appropriate.

Conduction Block Dysrhythmias

Cardiac conduction block dysrhythmias occur due to an interruption in the continuity of the cardiac electrical conduction system. This discontinuity is caused by a loss of blood supply to the conduction system as a result of ischemic heart disease or coronary artery disease. Heart blocks are classified according to the degree of the block, either partial or complete obstruction of the electrical conduction pathway. These disorders may be either permanent or transient, and minor or significant. The clinical significance of an AV block depends on the degree (severity) of the block, the rate of the escape pacemaker (junctional vs. ventricular), and the patient's response to that ventricular rate. There are four types of heart block dysrhythmias discussed next: first-degree AV block; Mobitz I/Wenckebach/ Type I second-degree heart block; Mobitz II second-degree block; and third-degree AV block (complete).

First-Degree AV Block

First-degree AV block represents a conduction disturbance in which electrical impulses flow normally from the SA node through the atria, but are delayed at the AV node. There is a prolongation or slowing of conduction rather than an actual block. Because of this consistent delay the PR interval is greater than 0.20 second, making it abnormal. First-degree AV block is not actually a dysrhythmia. Its presence only indicates a delay at the AV node, rather than a definite block. Figure 38–30 ■ is a rhythm strip showing first-degree AV block. Significant ECG features of first-degree AV block include:

- P waves are present and normal in size and shape.
- PR interval is prolonged, greater than 0.20 second, but constant.
- QRS duration usually is normal.
- QT interval is normal unless there is an abnormal rate.
- Heart rate is usually within normal range.
- Heart rhythm is regular.

The etiology, physical assessment findings, and treatment of first-degree AV blocks are outlined in Chart 38–9 (p. 1102).

Mobitz I/Wenckebach/Type I Second-Degree Heart Block

The terms Mobitz I/Wenckebach/Type 1 second-degree heart block, are used interchangeably to refer to the same abnormality. This abnormality is depicted as a progressive prolongation of the electrical impulse delay in the AV node until there is a complete loss of the QRS complex, and thus, no ventricular contraction. This dysrhythmia is characterized by progressive lengthening of the PR interval until a QRS complex fails to appear after a P wave (Beasley, 2003). **Mobitz I/Wenckebach** is one of the two types of second-degree block that occurs in the AV node. Figure 38–31 ■ (p. 1104) is a rhythm strip showing Mobitz I/Wenckebach dysrhythmia. Significant ECG features of Mobitz I/Wenckebach dysrhythmia include:

- P waves are present, and they precede the QRS complexes.
- PR interval progressively prolongs until there is a dropped QRS complex and then the progressive prolongation begins again.
- QRS complexes are normal in shape and duration.
- QT interval is within normal limits, unless no QRS complex occurs.
- Atrial heart rate is normal and regular; ventricular heart rate is less than that of the atrial rate.
- Atrial rhythm is regular; the ventricular rhythm is irregular.

The etiology, physical assessment findings, and treatment of Mobitz I/Wenckebach/Type I second-degree heart block are outlined in Chart 38–9 (p. 1102).

Mobitz II Second-Degree Block

Mobitz II second-degree block results from an intermittent block of the AV node, the bundle of His, or bundle branches. This dysrhythmia occurs when this block causes an intermittent interruption in the electrical conduction system near or below the AV node, which prevents the sinus or atrial impulses from getting to the ventricles. On the ECG strip the P wave (atrial contraction) is present at regular intervals because the SA node is generating impulses in a normal manner; however when the block occurs, the P wave is not followed by a QRS complex. An AV conduction ratio of 2 Ps for every 1 QRS; 3Ps for every 1 QRS, or greater is common, with or without a bundle branch block

P Wave: Present and regular; PR Interval: 0.24 second; QRS Complex: 0.06 second; QT Interval: 0.40 second; Heart Rate: Atrial: 60 bpm, Ventricular: 60 bpm; Rhythm: Regular; Ectopic Beats: None.

FIGURE 38–30 ■ First-degree AV block.

CHART 38–9 AV Block Dysrhythmias: Etiology, Physical Assessment, and Treatment

Dysrhythmia	Etiology	Physical Assessment	Treatment
First-degree AV block	May occur without any underlying heart disease May occur in athletes Occurs in about 13% of the population Drug reactions to digoxin, beta-blockers, and CA channel blockers Cardiac related causes include: Ischemia Myocardial infarction Rheumatic heart disease Coronary artery disease	Pulse: Within normal limits BP: Within normal limits	This is not a dangerous rhythm in itself and usually is asymptomatic. May progress to a more advanced heart block, especially in the presence of a myocardial infarction. Observe closely and place on an ECG monitor to detect additional signs and symptoms.
Mobitz I / Wenckebach/ Type I second-degree heart block	Conduction delay within the AV node Most commonly associated with AV nodal ischemia secondary to occlusion of the right coronary artery Other causes may be: Myocardial infarction Inferior/right ventricular structural heart disease or an anatomical abnormality Myocarditis Transient side effect of open heart surgery Increased vagal activity Drug toxicity, e.g., digoxin	Pulse: Irregular BP: May be decreased with frequently dropped beats due to decreased cardiac output. If cardiac output is decreased the following clinical manifestations may occur: Angina Syncope Generalized weakness Dizziness Shortness of breath Altered mental state may be present, although rare.	This is often a transient rhythm and will revert to normal rhythm without treatment. Usually asymptomatic because the ventricular rate often remains nearly normal and cardiac output is not significantly affected. If symptomatic, and is a result of medications, they should be withheld. If the heart rate is slow and serious clinical manifestations such as low BP, angina, shortness of breath, occur, atropine or temporary pacing is considered. When occurs in conjunction with acute myocardial infarction, observe for increasing AV block.
Mobitz II second-degree AV block	Septal wall necrosis Acute inferior or right ventricular MI Myocarditis Advanced coronary artery disease (general ischemia) Electrolyte imbalance Digitalis toxicity Reaction to amiodarone, beta-blockers, or calcium channel blockers	Pulse: slow and typically irregular, depending on ventricular response BP: Decreased due to low cardiac output If cardiac output is decreased the following clinical manifestations may occur: Angina Syncope Generalized weakness Dizziness Shortness of breath Altered mental state may be present.	Often considered an emergent situation. The health care provider should be notified at once. May progress to a third-degree AV block and ventricular asystole, thus, a standby cardiac pacemaker is indicated for asymptomatic patients, and temporary cardiac pacing is required for symptomatic patients. For sustained permanent block, a permanent pacemaker is inserted.
Third-degree AV block (complete)	Ischemic damage Septal wall necrosis Acute inferior or right ventricular MI due to the effect of vagal tone and ischemia on the AV node Acute anterior MI Myocarditis Coronary artery disease Cardiomyopathies Cardiac muscle diseases Rheumatic heart disease Drug toxicity, reaction to amiodarone, beta-blockers, or calcium channel blockers Electrolyte imbalance Rheumatic heart disease Congenital condition usually located at the level of the AV junction	Pulse: Slow and usually irregular BP: Lower than usual If cardiac output is decreased the following clinical manifestations may occur: Angina Syncope Generalized weakness Dizziness Shortness of breath Altered mental state may be present.	Treatment is essential as third-degree block is potentially lethal. If an AV junctional or ventricular escape pacemaker does not take over following a sudden onset of third-degree AV block, asystole will occur. Clinical manifestations depend on the ventricular heart rate, especially for slow rates. If the QRS is narrow and the patient is symptomatic, initial management is atropine and/or transcutaneous pacing. If the QRS is wide and the patient is symptomatic, transcutaneous pacing is started. A temporary pacemaker is inserted, and may be followed by a permanent pacemaker.

CHART 38–9	AV Block Dysrhythmias: Etiology, Physical Assessment, and Treatment—*Continued*		
Dysrhythmia	**Etiology**	**Physical Assessment**	**Treatment**
Bundle branch block (BBB)	Causes vary depending on whether it is the right or left BBB Right BBB may be present in healthy individuals with apparently normal hearts without any apparent underlying cause Common pathological causes include: Coronary artery disease Cardiac tumors Cardiomyopathy Myocarditis Atrial septal defect Cardiac surgery Congenital RBBB Acute anterioseptal MI Acute pulmonary embolism or infarction Acute heart failure Unlike RBBB, LBBB always indicates a diseased heart and generally is more common in individuals with diseased hearts Common causes include: Hypertensive heart disease Cardiomyopathy Myocarditis Syphilitic, rheumatic, and congenital heart disease Cardiac tumors Idiopathic degenerative disease of the electrical conduction system Aberrant ventricular conduction associated with supraventricular premature contractions and tachycardia	Pulse: Within normal limits BP: Within normal limits	Specific treatment usually is not indicated if it is present alone and is not the result of an acute MI. Temporary cardiac pacing is indicated for the treatment of a right or left bundle branch block under the following conditions: results from an acute MI is complicated by a first- or second-degree AV block, or both, especially in the setting of an acute MI if the block progresses to a complete AV block.

(Beasley, 2003). In other words there are 2, 3, or 4 P waves for every QRS complex. Thus, with this dysrhythmia there may be enough dropped QRSs to significantly impact cardiac output. Therefore, Mobitz II is a more serious dysrhythmia than either first-degree AV block or Mobitz I (Wenckebach/ Type I second-degree heart block) because of the impact on the cardiac output and an increased risk of progression to third-degree block or complete heart block. Figure 38–32 ■ (p. 1104) is a rhythm strip showing Mobitz II/second-degree block. Significant ECG features of Mobitz II/second-degree block include:

- QRS complexes are intermittently absent; they may be normal to prolonged when present; and they are usually prolonged due to bundle branch block.
- P waves are present and regular.
- PR intervals are constant with conducted beats.
- QT intervals are within normal limits.
- Atrial heart rate is usually normal; ventricular heart rate is less than the atrial rate.

- Atrial rhythm is regular; ventricular rhythm may be regular or irregular. The ventricular rhythm is irregular when the AV block is intermittent; thereby, causing a varying AV conduction ratio.
- Ectopic beats may be present due to the slow heart rate.

The etiology, physical assessment findings, and treatment of Mobitz II heart block are outlined in Chart 38–9.

Third-Degree AV Block (Complete)

Third-degree AV block, or **complete block,** is the independent excitation and contraction of the atria and ventricles due to the inability of any atrial impulses to reach the ventricles. In other words, the top and bottom of the heart are not communicating; they are beating independently. This dysrhythmia also is referred to as **AV dissociation** because of the independent function of the atria and the ventricles. The SA node fires at regular intervals, producing P waves at a normal rate of 60 to 100 beats per minute; whereas, the ventricles are paced by either a pacemaker site in the ventricles themselves or in the junctional

P Waves: Present and regular; PR Interval: Progressively prolonged until one P wave is not conducted and the sequence begins again; QRS Complex: 0.10 second; QT Interval: 0.42–0.60 second; Heart Rate: Atrial: 70 bpm, Ventricular 50 bpm; Rhythm: Atrial: Regular, Ventricular: Irregular due to dropped beat; Ectopic Beats: None. Conclusion: Mobitz I/Wenckeback Second-Degree Heart Block.

FIGURE 38–31 ■ Mobitz I/Wenckebach/second-degree heart block.

P Waves: Present and regular; PR Interval: 0.24 second; QRS Complex: 0.06 second; QT Interval: 0.48 second; Heart Rate: Atrial: 100 bpm, Ventricular 50 bpm; Rhythm: Atrial: Regular, Ventricular: Irregular due to dropped beat; Ectopic Beats: None.

FIGURE 38–32 ■ Mobitz II/second-degree heart block.

tissue. If the QRS complex is narrow the pacemaker is in the junctional tissue with a rate of 40 to 60 beats per minute. However, if the QRS complex is wide the pacemaker is in the Purkinje network and the heart rate ranges from 20 to 40 beats per minute; this is referred to as an idioventricular rhythm. Complete AV block associated with an inferior myocardial infarction is thought to be a block in the bundle of His, and often occurs after progression from first-degree AV block or second-degree AV

block, type I. Third-degree heart block is the most serious type of heart block because it may progress to asystole (a complete cessation of electrical activity), and the slow ventricular heart rate results in decreased cardiac output. Since the ventricular rhythm may not be able to sustain adequate cardiac output, third-degree heart block is referred to as a lethal dysrhythmia. Figure 38–33 ■ is a rhythm strip showing third-degree or complete heart block. Significant ECG features of third-degree heart block include:

P Waves: Present and regular; PR Interval: None; QRS Complex: 0.12 second; QT Interval: 0.38 second; Heart Rate: Atrial: 90 bpm, Ventricular: 40–50 bpm; Rhythm: Regular; Ectopic Beats: None.

FIGURE 38–33 ■ Third-degree (complete) heart block.

- Atrial and ventricular rhythms are independent of one another (dissociated). Atrial rhythm usually is regular, depending on underlying sinus, atrial, or junctional rhythm. Ventricular rhythm may be regular or irregular.
- P waves are present and regular; however there is no relationship to QRS complexes.
- PR interval is absent.
- QRS complex may be narrow with a junctional rhythm, or wide with an idioventricular rhythm.
- QT interval may change with the rate change, but is not directly affected.
- Atrial heart rate is regular, 60 to 100 beats per minute; nodal rate is 40 to 60 beats per minute; and ventricular rate is 20 to 40 beats per minute.
- Atrial and ventricular rhythms are independent of one another (dissociated). Atrial rhythm usually is regular, depending on underlying sinus, atrial, or junctional rhythm. Ventricular rhythm may be regular or irregular.
- Ectopic beats usually are present due to slow rate.

The etiology, physical assessment findings, and treatment of Mobitz II heart block are outlined in Chart 38–9 (p. 1102).

Bundle Branch Block

Bundle branch block, also referred to as intraventricular conduction defect, is a discontinuity of conduction, complete or incomplete, in one branch of the bundle of His, which affects normal transmission of the impulse through the ventricles. When one bundle is blocked, the ventricles depolarize asynchronously. Bundle branch block is characterized by a delay of exci-

tation to one ventricle; therefore, an abnormal spread of electrical activity through the ventricles occurs. This delayed conduction causes a widening of the QRS complex to more than 0.12 second. When measuring the QRS complex, it is necessary to observe the axis of the complex to determine whether it is right or left bundle branch block. Figure 38–34 ■ is a rhythm strip showing a bundle branch block. Significant ECG features of bundle branch block include:

- QRS complex is more than 0.12 second if a complete bundle branch block is present. P waves are present and regular.
- PR interval is 0.12 to 0.20 second.
- QRS measuring 0.10 to 0.12 second is called an incomplete right or left bundle branch block.
- QT interval is within normal limits.
- Heart rate is 60 to 100 beats per minute.
- Heart rhythm is regular.

The etiology, physical assessment findings, and treatment of bundle branch block are outlined in Chart 38–9 (p. 1102).

■ Nursing Management for Conduction Block Dysrhythmias

The type of heart block determines the severity of the dysrhythmia, and therefore, nursing responsibilities. As with any dysrhythmia the patient's tolerance to the rhythm must be evaluated when heart block develops. First-degree heart block and bundle branch block in isolation, do not impact cardiac output, therefore, patients are not symptomatic. With first-degree heart block, the nurse must observe the cardiac monitor for any changes in the rhythm indicating a progression to a more severe type of heart block.

Mobitz I/Wenckebach often does not require treatment, however, the ECG monitoring and patient assessment are necessary because this type of block may lead to a more serious Mobitz II or complete heart block. It is necessary, therefore, that the nurse frequently checks the monitor to identify potential changes. As with any new dysrhythmia, Mobitz I/Wenckebach needs to be reported to the health care provider.

P Wave: Normal sinus rhythm; PR Interval: 0.16 second; QRS Complex: 0.20 second; QT Interval: 0.40 second. Heart Rate: Atrial: 90 bpm, Ventricular: 90 bpm; Rhythm: Atrial: Regular, Ventricular: Regular; Ectopic Beats: None.

FIGURE 38–34 ■ Bundle branch block.

The onset of Mobitz II and complete heart block are emergent situations that require immediate intervention. Mobitz II is described as a "treacherous and unpredictable" rhythm that can deteriorate to become a complete heart block. If untreated, these rhythms may progress to cardiac asystole and sudden death. At any indication of rhythm changes indicative of Mobitz II or complete heart block, the health care provider should be notified at once. The nurse should prepare for a temporary pacemaker insertion (Chapter 39 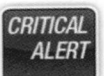), which generally is indicated for these types of dysrhythmias. A permanent pacemaker may be necessary if the block persists. It is the nurse's responsibility when working with monitored patients to be familiar with equipment location and operation.

CRITICAL ALERT *Signs and symptoms of third-degree AV block are the same as those in symptomatic sinus bradycardia. AV block can be more ominous, especially when associated with wide and bizarre QRS complexes. If an AV junctional or ventricular escape pacemaker does not take over the pacing of the heart following a sudden onset of third-degree AV block or ventricular asystole will occur. Temporary cardiac pacemaker is required immediately for treatment of symptomatic third-degree block with wide QRS complexes. The nurse must report this rhythm immediately to the health care provider in order to initiate treatment before a significant drop in cardiac output occurs.*

Ventricular Dysrhythmias

Ventricular dysrhythmias are caused by ectopic or irritable foci in the walls of the ventricles. The pacemaker cells in the ventricles may, in certain circumstances, serve as the heart's pacemaker. When the SA node fails or the impulse does not get through the AV node, the ventricles take over the pacing role. In this situation, an electrical impulse may be instigated from both the bundle of His and the Purkinje network. The intrinsic ventricular rate is only 20 to 40 beats per minute; therefore, cardiac output is severely compromised. Also, if the atrium is not contracting there is no atrial kick, causing further decrease in cardiac output. Because the rhythm originates in the ventricle there is no P wave, and because it is an abnormal conduction pathway the QRS is wide and distorted. Ventricular dysrhythmias are considered to be very serious dysrhythmias mainly due to their im-

pact on cardiac output. The various types of ventricular dysrhythmias are discussed next: premature ventricular contraction, ventricular tachycardia, torsade de pointes, ventricular fibrillation, pulseless electrical activity, and asystole.

Premature Ventricular Contraction

A **premature ventricular contraction (PVC)** is caused by an irritable focus within the ventricle that discharges before the next sinus impulse, stimulating the ventricle directly, and causing a contraction. PVCs are more likely to occur during bradycardia when there is more time for them to emerge. Premature ventricular contractions (PVCs) are individual beats, one ectopic beat, not a rhythm. PVCs have a wide and bizarre QRS complex that is more than 0.12 second in length. Because the activation begins outside the normal conduction system, it takes longer to travel the ventricular conduction pathways, thereby prolonging the QRS length. PVCs are followed by a full compensatory pause, meaning the SA node rate and rhythm are unaffected by the PVC. In other words, the rate prior to the PVC resumes, following the PVC. A compensatory pause is measured by:

- Measuring the two beats preceding the PVC
- Moving the calipers along, and marking where the next beat should have fallen
- Then placing the calipers on the spot where the beat should have occurred, measure the distance to the next beat, there should not be a change in the cadence of the rhythm.

The full compensatory pause is one of the factors used when evaluating and diagnosing PVCs. To distinguish PVCs from atrial and junctional ectopic beats, the full compensatory pause is present. Typically, atrial and junctional ectopic beats do not have a full compensatory pause, they are said to be non-compensatory or partially compensatory, meaning that there is a rhythm change following these dysrhythmias. Figure 38–35 ■ is a rhythm strip showing premature ventricular contractions (PVCs) with a full compensatory pause.

Unifocal and Multifocal PVCs

Premature ventricular contractions (PVCs) occur in various patterns. Each pattern differs in its severity and prognosis. First, if the PVC configuration (size and shape) remains the same

P Wave: Present and regular, except where absent (PVC); PR Interval: 0.20 second; QRS Complex: 0.08 second; QT Interval: 0.42 second; Heart Rate: Atrial: 70 bpm, Ventricular: 80 bpm; Rhythm: Atrial: Regular, Ventricular: Regular except for premature beat; Ectopic Beats: One PVC.

FIGURE 38–35 ■ Premature ventricular contractions (PVCs).

consistently, the dysrhythmia is coming from one irritable focus in the ventricle. These are referred to as unifocal PVCs. If PVCs occur with every other beat the rhythm is referred to as **bigeminy.** If PVCs occur every third beat, the rhythm is called **trigeminy,** and occurrence every fourth beat is **quadrigeminy.** The more often the PVC occurs, the greater the drop in cardiac output, and therefore, the more serious the dysrhythmia. The drop in cardiac output is due to the premature occurrence of the rhythm which does not allow for sufficient diastole or ventricle filling time. As cardiac muscle ischemia increases the muscle becomes more irritable, causing PVCs to be initiated in more than one place in the ventricle. This is referred to as multifocal PVCs. When multifocal, the morphology (shape) of the QRSs varies. Multifocal PVCs are more serious than unifocal PVCs because they indicate that there is more ischemia occurring in the myocardium.

PVC Patterns

When PVCs occur for two or more consecutive beats this is referred to as paired salvos. When there are three or more consecutive PVCs salvos, it is defined as ventricular tachycardia. Ventricular tachycardia may be life threatening due to the severe drop in cardiac output.

The most serious or dangerous time for a PVC to occur is during the relative refractory period, which is the top of the T wave on the ECG. This is referred to as an R on T phenomenon, and this occurrence may precipitate a run of ventricular tachycardia. Significant ECG features with PVCs include:

- QRS complex is premature, 0.12 second or greater in width, complexes are larger than the normal beats, with the T wave always occurring on the opposite side of the isoelectric line from the R wave.
- P waves are not present or are buried in the PVCs.
- PR interval-none.
- QT interval is prolonged for the ectopic beat only.
- PVC occurs prematurely.
- Heart rate usually is within normal range, but depends on underlying rhythm.
- Heart rhythm is irregular because the PVCs are premature.
- Ectopic beats are the PVCs.

The etiology, physical assessment findings, and treatment of premature ventricular contractions are outlined in Chart 38–10 (p. 1108).

Ventricular Tachycardia

Ventricular tachycardia (VT), often referred to as v-tach is a life threatening ventricular rhythm arising from an excitable ventricular focus in the tissue distal to the bifurcation of the bundle of His. In general, ventricular tachycardia affects the diseased heart, although it has been described in patients with apparently normal hearts. It is a rhythm that discharges repetitively, acting as the dominant pacemaker. It is present when three or more PVCs occur in a row at a rate of greater than 100 beats per minute (American Heart Association, 2006a). This dysrhythmia frequently begins rapidly, and is initiated by a PVC which then becomes the heart's pacemaker. A sustained ventricular tachycardia is a rhythm that lasts longer than 30 seconds and usually requires ter-

mination by antiarrhythmic drugs, antitachycardia pacing techniques, or electrical cardioversion. If the rhythm lasts less than 30 seconds it is a non-sustained rhythm or simply a run of ventricular tachycardia (three beats or longer) that terminates spontaneously. Ventricular tachycardia is an emergent situation, requiring urgent evaluation to assess cardiac output and the presence or absence of the pulse. Treatment is guided by published advanced cardiac support (ACLS) guidelines and varies based on the presence of a pulse. Ventricular tachycardia when sustained but hemodynamically stable (with pulse) is treated with pharmacologic agents such as lidocaine, procainamide or amiodarone (AHA, 2006a). Ventricular tachycardia that is hemodynamically unstable and pulseless is treated using the ACLS guidelines for pulseless cardiac arrest (AHA, 2006b). These guidelines dictate that the nurse assess the patient for a pulse, if none is present, cardiopulmonary resuscitation (CPR) is initiated and help is requested. Oxygen is administered and the patient is placed on a monitor/defibrillator when available. The nurse must be prepared to shock the patient per AHA guideline joules, CPR is resumed for 5 cycles, and then rhythm is checked. The patient is re-shocked if VT persists. Vasopressors are administered when intravenous access has been established. CPR and defibrillation cycles are repeated per ACLS guidelines until a viable rhythm is established or death occurs. Figure 38–36 ■ (p. 1110). Significant ECG features of ventricular tachycardia and ventricular fibrillation include:

- QRS complexes are uniform in appearance, usually wide and bizarre, measuring 0.12 second or greater, with the T wave occurring on the opposite side of the isoelectric line from the R wave.
- P waves in rapid VT are usually not recognizable. At slower ventricular rates, P waves may be recognized and may represent normal sinus node depolarization at a rate slower than VT, but the electrical activities do not affect one another.
- PR interval is not discernable.
- QT interval is not measurable.
- Heart rate is greater than 100 beats per minute and usually not faster than 200 beats per minute.
- Heart rhythm is essentially regular but may be irregular.
- Entire rhythm is ectopic beats.

The etiology, physical assessment findings, and treatment of ventricular tachycardia are outlined in Chart 38–10 (p. 1108).

Torsade de Pointes

Torsade de pointes, frequently referred to as "torsades," is a form of ventricular tachycardia that is usually accompanied by prolongation of the QT interval. The QT interval usually is more than 0.50 second in the beats preceding the onset of the rhythm. Once the rhythm has occurred the QRS complexes have varying morphology or shape and width that usually begin after a pause in the rhythm or bradycardia. The name, torsade de pointes, is derived from the French term that signifies the "twisting of the points." The name characterizes the rhythm in that it resembles a turning about or twisting motion along the baseline or isoelectric line. This form of VT, which is rare, is due to age, gender, drug toxicity, or an idiosyncratic reaction to certain cardiac drugs such as

CHART 38–10	Ventricular Dysrhythmias: Etiology, Physical Assessment, and Treatment		
Dysrhythmia	**Etiology**	**Physical Assessment**	**Treatment**
Premature ventricular contraction (PVC)	Organic heart disease Coronary artery disease Myocardial ischemia/irritability and infarction Cardiac valve disease Mitral valve prolapse Heart failure Primary electrical instability Fever Fluid volume deficit Electrolyte imbalance, e.g., hypokalemia, hypercalcemia, hypomagnesemia Acid/base imbalance Drug excess: e.g. Tricyclic antidepressants; digitalis, sympathomimetic amines, and antiarrhythmic agents Moderate to excessive alcohol intake Increase in catecholamine release and sympathetic tone as in emotional stress Sarcoidosis Change in posture Exercise Emotional excitement Vagal stimulation Normal variation that increases with age	Pulse: May be irregular due to asynchronous firing of the ventricles. The corresponding QRS complex may be detected on the monitor while contractions are felt as a peripheral pulse. BP: Normal or lower than usual due to decreased cardiac output leading to decreased perfusion. Thumping sensation in chest/throat Palpitations If cardiac output is decreased the following clinical manifestations may occur: Angina Syncope Generalized weakness Dizziness Shortness of breath Altered mental state may be present.	PVCs may be isolated when there is no underlying heart condition. Usually, then, they have no significance and require no treatment. Treatment depends on the cause and clinical manifestations. It is essential to identify and treat the underlying cause. When provoked by fast or slow heart rate, correcting the rate can abolish PVCs. Treatment usually is not required. Treatment is directed at uncovering the etiology and providing adequate oxygenation, pain relief, and rapid identification of causes. Antidysrhythmic drugs such as amiodarone and lidocaine should be administered as ordered per frequency of occurrence.
Ventricular tachycardia (VT)	Precipitated by the same conditions as premature ventricular contractions (see above)	Pulse: Rapid and weak BP: Hypotensive Cardiac output is decreased therefore the following clinical manifestations occur: Angina Syncope Generalized weakness Dizziness Shortness of breath Changes in mental status, starting with confusion and restlessness, leading to unconsciousness. Conscious sensation of ineffective cardiac activity often accompanied by anxiety. Presence and severity of the signs and symptoms depends on rhythm duration.	Initial treatment is based on the presence or absence of a palpable pulse. If hemodynamically stable, with a pulse, drug intervention is appropriate e.g., procainamide, amiodarone, lidocaine. If hemodynamically unstable (pulseless) defibrillation and cardiopulmonary resuscitation (CPR) is indicated. After initial stabilization other treatments which may be considered include: Implantable cardioverter defibrillator Electrophysiology Studies (EPS): ventricles are stimulated to produce VT: then antiarrhythmic drugs are administered, followed by a second attempt to produce the VT. If unable to reproduce the dysrhythmia, the drug is considered effective and continuous therapy is instituted. Drugs used include: procainamide, amiodarone, and lidocaiane. Radio-frequency ablation, burning the area or focus in the ventricle where the VT is coming from may also be considered. Chapter 39 ⊖ has a complete description of EPS and ablation.

CHART 38–10 **Ventricular Dysrhythmias: Etiology, Physical Assessment, and Treatment—*Continued***

Dysrhythmia	Etiology	Physical Assessment	Treatment
Torsade de pointes (TdP)	Prolonged QT interval, which may be congenital or acquired Severe bradycardia Electrolyte imbalance, e.g., hypokalemia, hypomagnesemia Central nervous system lesions Tricyclic antidepressants Antidysrhythmic drugs, e.g., quinidine, procainamide, amiodarone Antihistamines, e.g., seldane Antibiotics, e.g., erythromycin Diuretics Liquid protein diets Starvation Or any combination of the above	Pulse: Rapid, palpitations felt, often the first symptom BP: Low due to decreased cardiac output If cardiac output is decreased the following clinical manifestations may occur: Angina Syncope Generalized weakness Dizziness Shortness of breath Changes in mental status, starting with confusion and restlessness, leading to unconsciousness. Seizures may be present with a prolonged rhythm. Clinical manifestations are related to the decreased cardiac output caused by the dysrhythmia.	Assessment of QT interval for prolongation. Magnesium is the treatment of choice to shorten the QT interval. If unsuccessful, overdrive ventricular pacing to keep the heart rate up and the QT interval within normal limits. Stress testing and Valsalva will prolong QT interval and can be used to diagnose congenital prolonged QT interval. All agents that cause torsade de pointe are immediately discontinued. Administer potassium intravenously if QT interval is abnormal. Cardioversion and overdrive pacing are used to terminate torsades, but only may be temporary. Drugs are modified or discontinued if QT interval is prolonged.
Ventricular fibrillation (VF)	Severe myocardial ischemia Coronary heart disease Myocardial infarction Advanced heart block Abnormal repolarization Vagal stimulation Drug toxicity, e.g., psychotropics, digoxin Metabolic abnormalities, e.g., hypokalemia, hypomagnesemia Hypoxia Trauma Terminal event in many disease states Electrical shock	Pulse: None palpable and heart sounds usually absent BP: None Unconscious Seizures Apnea Death, if untreated	Initiate CPR and defibrillation per ACLS guidelines.
Pulseless electrical activity	Profound hypovolemia Massive myocardial damage Excessive vagal tone due to loss of sympathetic tone Obstruction of blood flow to or from the heart, e.g., severe pulmonary embolism Pericardial tamponade Myocardial rupture Massive cardiac trauma resulting in cardiac tamponade and/or tension pneumothorax Severe acidosis Hyperkalemia Hypothermia Drug overdose, e.g., tricyclics, beta-blockers, calcium channel blockers, digoxin	Pulse: None palpable BP: None Unconscious Seizures may occur Death, if untreated	Assess for pulse and blood pressure; initiate CPR protocol per ACLS guidelines. Find cause and treat.
Asystole	Cardiac standstill from massive cardiac muscle damage	Pulse: None palpable BP: None Unconscious Death, if untreated	Check the rhythm in two leads in order to rule out the possibility of fine ventricular fibrillation. Also, check the lead placement to make sure it has not fallen off. Initiate CPR and ACLS protocols. Administer drugs per ACLS guidelines, agency protocol or health care provider's orders.

P Wave: Two normal P waves present; PR Interval: Not discernable during dysrhythmia; QRS Complex: Wide and distorted during dysrhythmia; QT Interval: Not discernable during dysrhythmia; Heart Rate: Atrial: Not discernable, Ventricular: Rapid; Rhythm: Both regular and irregular; Ectopic Beats: PVCs, ventricular tachycardia/fibrillation.

FIGURE 38–36 ■ Ventricular tachycardia.

quinidine, procainamide, disopyramide, or other agents that prolong the QT interval. Electrolyte imbalance such as hypokalemia and hypomagnesemia also can initiate torsade de pointes (Garcia & Miller, 2004).

In addition to being a life-threatening dysrhythmia, torsade de pointes tends to recur repeatedly. It is, therefore, essential to find and treat the underlying cause. Figure 38–37 ■ is a rhythm strip showing torsade de pointes. Significant ECG features of torsade de pointes include:

- QRS complex height varies and undulates.
- P waves are not discernable.
- PR interval is not measurable.
- QT is not measurable.
- Heart rate varies; approximately 200 to 250 beats per minute.
- Heart rhythm may be regular or irregular.
- Entire rhythm is ectopy.

The etiology, physical assessment findings, and treatment of torsade de pointes are outlined in Chart 38–10 (p. 1108).

Ventricular Fibrillation

Ventricular fibrillation (VF), often referred to as v-fib, is a dysrhythmia marked by rapid, disorganized depolarization of the ventricles. There are no organized electrical impulses, and therefore, no coordinated atrial or ventricular contraction or palpable pulse. The myocardial cells appear to quiver rather than depolarize normally. With this dysrhythmia multiple ventricular sites initiate electrical impulses that are not transmit-

ted through the normal conduction pathway. There are no waveforms apparent on the ECG strip. The rhythm appears disorganized, rapid, and irregular with waves whose morphology varies greatly. Ventricular fibrillation may be classified further as coarse and fine, just like atrial fibrillation. Coarse waveforms are more easily visible and are greater than 3 mm; those that are less than 3 mm frequently are referred to as fine VF. Coarse VF responds better to treatment than does fine VF. Also, coarse VF typically progresses to fine VF unless treatment is initiated in a timely manner. Fine VF indicates that the rhythm has been present for an extended period of time. Figure 38–38 ■ is a rhythm strip showing ventricular fibrillation.

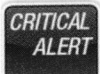 *Ventricular fibrillation (VF) is an ineffective quivering of the heart muscle that results in no blood delivery to tissues, thus, VF must be treated immediately. Detection of VF on a monitor requires immediate patient evaluation by the nurse to begin prompt treatment and to rule out equipment malfunctions that mimic VF such as ECG artifacts produced by loose or dry electrodes, broken ECG leads, or patient movements or muscle tremors.*

Significant ECG features of ventricular fibrillation include:

- P waves, PR intervals, QRS complexes, and QT intervals are all absent.
- Heart rate is not discernable because there are no waves or complexes to measure.
- Heart rhythm is irregular.
- Entire rhythm is ectopy.

P Waves: Not discernable; PR Interval: Not discernable; QRS Complex: Wide, distorted, and varying heights; QT Interval: not discernable; Rate: Rapid; Rhythm: Both regular and irregular; Ectopic Beats: All.

FIGURE 38–37 ■ Torsade de pointes.

P Waves: Not discernable; PR Interval: Not discernable; QRS Complex: Wide, distorted, and varying heights; QT Interval not discernable; Heart Rate: Not discernable; Ectopic Beats: All.

FIGURE 38–38 ■ Ventricular fibrillation.

The etiology, physical assessment findings, and treatment of ventricular fibrillation are outlined in Chart 38–10 (p. 1108).

Pulseless Electrical Activity

Pulseless electrical activity (PEA) is a clinical phenomenon that occurs when the heart muscle loses its ability to contract even though cardiac electrical activity is present. Cardiac electrical activity is seen on the monitor, but the patient has no detectable pulse or blood pressure. Though the electrical activity is represented as an organized rhythm (other than VT or VF) on the cardiac monitor, (e.g., bradycardia, heart block), the heart muscle is unable to respond to the electrical stimuli. Due to a variety of cardiac and noncardiac disorders such as acidosis, electrolyte imbalance, trauma, and cardiac rupture, the muscle is unable to respond to the stimuli, causing cardiac output and tissue perfusion to cease, and clinical death to occur. When PEA occurs biological death follows within minutes unless the cause is identified and treated (Beasley, 2003). Formerly, pulseless electrical activity was called electromechanical dissociation (EMD). The clinical outcome usually is poor despite aggressive life support measures. Significant ECG features of pulseless electrical activity include:

- P waves may or may not be present dependent on rhythm.
- PR intervals may or may not have a relationship to QRS complexes.
- QRS complex may be narrow or wide.
- QT interval is variable.
- Heart rate and rhythm are variable, usually bradycardia.
- Ectopic beats may be present.

The etiology, physical assessment findings, and treatment of pulseless electrical activity are outlined in Chart 38–10 (p. 1108).

Asystole

Asystole is a complete termination of all cardiac electrical activity. Without an electrical impulse, the atria and ventricles do not contract causing immediate loss of oxygen supply to the brain and tissues. In hospital settings efforts are usually made to reestablish cardiac activity but, often are futile. Figure 38–39 ■ is a rhythm strip showing asystole. In asystole, no measurable electrical activity exists and the rhythm strip appears as a straight line on the ECG monitor. The etiology, physical assessment findings, and treatment of asystole are outlined in Chart 38–10 (p. 1108).

■ Nursing Management for Ventricular Dysrhythmias

As with any dysrhythmia, the first nursing responsibility for ventricular dysrhythmias is to assess the patient's response to

No measurable electrical activity

FIGURE 38–39 ■ Asystole.

the specific abnormality. Nurses need to complete a health history to assess the risk factors related to the occurrence of ventricular dysrhythmias that are outlined in Chart 38–10 (p. 1108). Cultural awareness of populations that are at increased risk for ventricular dysrhythmias is discussed in the Cultural Considerations box.

Ventricular dysrhythmias have the greatest impact on cardiac output and are, therefore, the most serious. Depending on the variation in configuration and the frequency of occurrence, ventricular dysrhythmias require a variety of interventions from simple observation, to drug intervention, to advanced life support treatments. Generally, in monitoring units the health care providers provide protocols or "standing orders" for treating each type of ventricular dysrhythmia. The nurse must be knowledgeable of the treatment regimens required for each of the ventricular dysrhythmias based on the standing orders, basic cardiac life support (BCLS), advanced cardiac life support (ACLS), and agency specific protocols. When reporting ventricular dysrhythmias, the nurse needs to give a detailed description of the dysrhythmia pattern and the patient's clinical response to the health care provider, so treatment is tailored to the specific dysrhythmia. The seriousness and treatment of ventricular dysrhythmias depend on the duration and the impact on hemodynamic stability (blood pressure and cardiac output).

If the resuscitation efforts are initiated it is imperative that family and significant others be kept informed and be allowed to participate in the decision-making process. Research in the United States and the United Kingdom revealed that most family members wished to be present during the attempted resuscitation of a loved one (Boyd, 2000). The research concluded that even family members with no medical background found it comforting to be with their loved one during the final moments of life. It is imperative that the health care team offer this opportunity and be sensitive to the family during this crisis period. If possible, it is optimal to have a health care team member be assigned to the family to answer questions, clarify information, and provide comfort (AHA 2005a). Since the nurse is at the bedside it typically becomes a nursing responsibility to keep the family informed, act as a liaison, and advocate for the patient. Chapter 17 ⊙ includes a complete description of end of life issues.

National Guidelines for Cardiopulmonary Resuscitation and Emergency Cardiovascular Care

Since 1974 the American Heart Association has been publishing guidelines for cardiopulmonary resuscitation and emergency cardiovascular care. The guidelines were most recently updated in 2005 and are based on evidenced evaluation from the 2005 International Consensus Conference on Cardiopulmonary Resuscitation and Emergency Cardiovascular Care with Treatment Recommendations (International Liaison Committee on Resuscitation, 2005). These 2005 guidelines supersede the published 2000 guidelines for cardiovascular resuscitation and emergency cardiovascular care. The current guidelines contain recommendations designed to improve survival from sudden cardiac arrest and acute life-threatening cardiopulmonary disorders. These guidelines are based on the most extensive evidence review of CPR yet published. They confirm the safety and effectiveness of many treatments and recommend new treatments that have undergone evidence evaluation. Given that the guidelines do not apply to all situations, the leader of the resuscitation attempt may need to adapt application of the guidelines to unique circumstances. Finally, the guidelines also have streamlined the amount of information that rescuers need to learn and remember, and have clarified the most important skills that rescuers need to perform (American Heart Association, 2006b). Future goals of the AHA are to continue to improve the guidelines based on new and evolving research and practice evidence. Foci will be placed on CPR education, and improving the effectiveness and efficiency of instruction, skill retention, and a reduction in barriers to action for basic and advanced life support providers (Chamberlain & Hazinski, 2003). Continuous quality improvement issues focus on reducing time to CPR and shock delivery and improving the quality of CPR provided (Jacobs et al, 2004; Peberdy et al, 2003). The National Guidelines box outlines the 2005 AHA national guidelines for selected CPR and emergency cardiovascular care.

Nursing Management of Patients with Dysrhythmias

Nursing responsibilities when caring for patients experiencing cardiac dysrhythmias have been discussed throughout this chapter. To assist the learner, the patient care plan outlines a systematic approach to assessing and providing nursing care for

---

CULTURAL CONSIDERATIONS Brugada Syndrome

The term *Brugada sign* is an abnormal finding on an electrocardiogram (ECG) that refers to distance of at least 0.10 second from the onset of the QRS complex or the bottom of the S wave. Its presence may indicate Brugada syndrome which is an abnormality in the heart's electrical system that causes life-threatening heart rhythm disturbances such as ventricular fibrillation. It occurs in patients with a structurally normal heart, and few or no coronary artery disease risk factors, and a family history of sudden cardiac death. It's possible to have a Brugada sign without having Brugada syndrome. This syndrome occurs most often in young adults. It also occurs with increased frequency in Asians. The cause isn't clear, but it appears to be inherited in some cases.

Nursing implications are to assess young patients and patients of Asian decent who are having ventricular dysrhythmias with little to no risk of heart disease, for a family history of sudden cardiac death. Those considered at risk have:

- A family history of sudden cardiac death in young relatives
- A personal history of serious heart rhythm problems
- A personal history of severe fainting spells

Immediate treatment for ventricular fibrillation is outlined in the American Heart Association ACLS guidelines for 2005. Long-term treatment includes antidysrhythmic medication therapy and an implantable defibrillator.

Source: Adapted from: *Brugada Syndrome* (2005). MayoClinic.com. http://www.mayoclinic.com/health/brugada-syndrome/AN00551. Retrieved July 13, 2006.

NATIONAL GUIDELINES for Cardiopulmonary Resuscitation and Emergency Cardiovascular Care

Adult basic life support

Advanced cardiac life support

Electrical therapies

CPR techniques and devices

Adjuncts for airway control and ventilation

Management of cardiac arrest

Management of symptomatic bradycardia and tachycardia

Monitoring and medications

Post-resuscitation support

Stabilizing of the patient with acute coronary syndromes

Source: Adapted from American Heart Association. (2006). *2005 international consensus on CPR and ECC science with treatment recommendations.* Retrieved June 30, 2006, from http://www.americanheart.org/presenter.jhtml?identifier=3022512.

these patients. Beginning with the assessment the nurse needs to identify what type of information is necessary to help find the risk factors and causes that precipitate the occurrence or progression of cardiac dysrhythmias. The nursing diagnosis is generated from the assessment data and guides the nurse toward desired patient outcomes and an intervention plan (see Nursing Process: Patient Care Plan for Dysrhythmias).

To assist the nurse in the comprehensive assessment and interpretation of cardiac dysrhythmias, Chart 38–11 (p. 1114) summarizes the characteristics of each type of dysrhythmia.

Health Promotion

As with any disorder the primary focus is on prevention of the onset and progression of the disease. Health teaching about risk factors and life style habits that cause the disorders that underlie the occurrence of cardiac dysrhythmias is essential for prevention. Once an individual has been diagnosed with heart disease the best way to prevent dysrhythmias is to have the patient closely follow a treatment plan and make the necessary life style habit changes. Life style habits most closely associated with heart disease and the occurrence of dysrhythmias include:

- Smoking
- Alcohol use
- Caffeine intake
- Sedentary life style
- Stress
- Overweight/obesity
- Diet.

The nurse needs to develop a teaching plan that will effectively assist the patient in reducing or eliminating these risk factors. Additionally, the patient needs to be told to note if there is a pattern as to when the dysrhythmias occur, what brings them on and what makes them go away. For example, does it take a long time for the heart rate to return to normal after exercise or exertion? Instruct the patient to identify high-stress situations that bring on the dysrhythmias and examine with the patient how to diminish or avoid them as much as possible. All aspects of life including professional as well as personal relationships need to be examined.

Since the Human Genome Project ongoing research has focused on gaining a better understanding of how genetic disorders can predispose to dysrhythmias. For example, a mutation of gene ankyrin-B is now known to cause cardiac arrhythmia syndrome (Hamby, Mittal, & Stein, 2006). The goal is to use gene-based therapies in the future to better treat dysrhythmias as well as identifying those individuals who are susceptible to dysrhythmias. Nurses will assist in identifying whether or not the patient has a family history of dysrhythmias. This in turn will aid in the early diagnosis, treatment, or prevention of the occurrence of life-threatening dysrhythmias.

NURSING PROCESS: Patient Care Plan for Dysrhythmias

Assessment	Nursing Diagnosis	Expected Outcomes/Evaluation	Interventions
Health history	*Alteration in Tissue Perfusion*	Maintain adequate cardiac output	Monitoring and managing the dysrhythmia
Social Habits	*Altered Cardiac Output*	Free of clinical manifestations	Finding the cause
Psychosocial assessment	*Anxiety* related to fear of the unknown	Reduced anxiety	Reducing risk factors through patient teaching
Physical assessment	*Knowledge Deficit* related to dysrhythmias and their treatment	Verbalizes understanding of disorder and treatments	Controlling incidence
Coexisting conditions:			Minimizing anxiety
Heart disease			Promoting home and community-based care
Chronic obstructive pulmonary disease			
Prescription and over-the-counter medications			
Clinical manifestations:			
Syncope			
Dizziness			
Fatigue			
Chest discomfort			

| CHART 38–11 | **ECG Measurements for Cardiac Rhythms** | | | | | | |

ECG Rhythm	P Wave	PR Interval	QRS	QT Interval	Rate	Rhythm	Ectopic Beats
Normal Sinus Rhythm	Present and Regular	0.12–0.21	0.06–0.12	0.34–0.43	60–100 bpm	Regular	None
Sinus Bradycardia	Present and Regular	Normal limits	Normal	Lengthens to greater than normal	40–60 bpm	Regular	None
Sinus Tachycardia	Present and Regular	As the sinus rate accelerates, the PR interval tends to shorten slightly.	Normal	Usually shortens	100–180 bpm	May be slightly irregular as rate accelerates; then becomes a rapid regular rate.	None
Sinus Arrhythmia	Present and Irregular	Normal limits	Normal limits	Changes with the heart rate, becoming longer during the slow phase of the rhythm	60–100 bpm	Regularly irregular, with a variance of more than 0.08 seconds in the acceleration and deceleration phases.	May occur during the slow phase of the rhythm
Sinus Arrest (Pause)	Present and Irregular	May be the same before and after sinus pauses.	Normal limits	Changes with the heart rate, becoming longer during the slow phase of the rhythm.	There may be marked bradycardia due to long sinus pauses.	Underlying regular rhythm except where the sinus pauses occur.	Possible during sinus pauses
Premature Atrial Contraction (PAC)	Present and Irregular when PAC occurs.	Normal limits. May change with PAC only.	Normal limits	Normal if rate is normal.	60–100 bpm	Regular except for premature PAC which may reset rhythm.	PAC
Atrial Flutter	No P wave f waves	None	Normal limits	Unable to obtain as T waves are buried in F waves	Depends on the AV conduction ratio. There may be a slow ventricular response, or there may be a fast ventricular response.	Atrial rate regular. Ventricular rate may be regular or irregular.	Flutter waves
Atrial Fibrillation	No P wave f waves	None	Normal limits	Unable to obtain because the T waves are buried in the f waves.	T waves are buried in the f waves.	Irregular	Fibrillation waves
Supraventricular Tachycardia (SVT)	Not seen –buried in QRS complex	Not discernable	Within normal limits, unless distorted by buried P waves.	Unable to obtain as T waves are buried.	100–250 bpm	Regular or irregular due to varying conduction through the AV node.	Rapid ectopic focus takes over rhythm
Paroxysmal Atrial Tachycardia (PAT)	At onset of rhythm, shape of P waves different from sinus P waves.	Varies with rhythm change	Within normal limits, unless distorted by buried P waves.	T waves buried, so unable to obtain with fast rhythm.	100–250 beats/minute dependent on reference source.	Irregular due to varying heart rates.	Ectopic focus at onset of rapid rhythm

CHART 38–11   **ECG Measurements for Cardiac Rhythms—*Continued***

ECG Rhythm	P Wave	PR Interval	QRS	QT Interval	Rate	Rhythm	Ectopic Beats
Wolff-Parkinson White Syndrome	Present and Regular	Less than 0.12 second because the AV node is bypassed and contains presence of delta wave	Greater than 0.10 seconds due to delta waves created by the abnormal conduction pathway	Shortens with tachycardia and lengthens with bradycardia	High incidence of tachy-dysrthrymias	Regular, except during heart rate changes	Delta waves: Occur just prior to R wave
Wandering Atrial Pacemaker	Present and Irregular Multiform	Usually normal	Normal limits	Normal. May be prolonged due to slow heart rate	Atrial: Slow, bradycardic Ventricular: Slow, bradycardic	Irregular due to changing pacemakers	May be present due to the slow rhythm
Sick Sinus Syndrome	Present or absent depending on which dysrhythmia is occurring	Variable depending on the rhythm	Normal limits	Variable due to rate change	Bradycardia to tachycardia	Atrial: Irregular Ventricular: Irregular	May be present with slow rate
Junctional Escape Rhythm	May occur before, after, or buried in, the QRS complex	Less than 0.12 second if the P wave occurs before the QRS complex	Normal unless distorted by P wave	Normal unless impacted by rate	Usually 40–60 (normal intrinsic rate for junctional tissue)	Regular	May occur with slow rates
Premature Junctional Contraction (PJC)	May occur before, after, or buried in, the QRS complex	Less than 0.12 second if P wave occurs before QRS complex for the ectopic beat All others normal	Normal unless distorted by P wave for the ectopic beat All others normal	Normal	That of underlying rhythm	Regular except for the premature beat	PJC
Junctional Tachycardia	May occur before, after, or buried in, the QRS complex	Less than 0.12 second if P wave occurs before QRS complex for the ectopic beat	Normal unless distorted by P wave for the ectopic beat	No specific change unless it is heart rate related	Greater than 100 beats per minute	Appears regular, but may increase its rate	May occur due to muscle irritability
First Degree AV Block	Present and Regular	Greater than 0.20 second	Normal	Normal	Variable	Regular	None
Mobitz I/Wenckeback	Sinus P waves	Progressively prolonged until one P wave is not conducted and the sequence begins	Within normal limits	Within normal limits	Atrial rate within normal limits; ventricular rate slower than atrial	Atrial rhythm is regular; ventricular rhythm is irregular	Usually none unless they occur during period when no QRS has occurred and there is a long pause
Mobitz II/Second-Degree Block	Present Not always followed by QRS	Constant with conducted beats	Intermittently absent; may be normal (AV node) or prolonged when present	Within normal limits	Atrial rate is regular; ventricular rate irregular and bradycardic	Atrial is regular; ventricular is irregular	May occur due to slow rate

(continued)

CHART 38–11 **ECG Measurements for Cardiac Rhythms—*Continued***

ECG Rhythm	P Wave	PR Interval	QRS	QT Interval	Rate	Rhythm	Ectopic Beats
Third-Degree (Complete) Heart Block	Present and Regular	P wave has no relationship to QRS complexes; therefore no PR interval is present.	May be narrow (junctional rhythm), or wide (idioventricular rhythm)	May be rate related, but not directly affected.	Atrial rate is regular, 60–100 bpm; nodal rate is 40–60 bpm; ventricular rate is 20–40 bpm.	Atrial is regular; ventricular may be regular or irregular.	May occur due to slow rate.
Bundle Branch Block	Present and Regular sinus P waves	0.12–0.20 second.	Greater than 0.12 second. If notch higher on right, indicates right bundle branch block; if notch higher on left, indicates left bundle branch block.	Within normal limits.	60–100 beats/minute.	Regular	None
Premature Ventricular Contraction (PVC)	None with PVC.	None with PVC.	Broad and premature and has increased amplitude. R and T waves opposite sides of isoelectric line.	Prolonged with PVC.	Underlying rate may be normal or abnormal.	Irregular because PVCs are premature.	PVC more likely to occur during bradycardia when there is more time to emerge.
Ventricular Tachycardia	None visible	Not discernible	Wide and bizarre, measuring > 0.12 seconds. R and T waves opposite sides of isoelectric line	Not discernible.	100–250 beats/minute.	Essentially regular.	All waves are ectopy
Torsade de Pointes	Not discernible	Not discernible	Height undulates	Usually > 0.50 seconds in the beats preceding the onset of the rhythm	Rates vary 200–250 beats/minute.	Typically regular.	All waves are ectopy
Ventricular Fibrillation	None	None	None	None	Atrial: Absent Ventricular: Absent	Irregular	All waves are ectopy
Pulseless Electrical Activity	May or may not be present.	May or may not have a relationship to QRS complexes	May be narrow or wide complex.	Variable.	Variable, depends on rhythm; usually bradycardic.	Variable depends on rate.	May be present but none of the beats perfuse
Asystole	None	None	None	None	None	None	None

Source: Megan Redeen, (2007). California State University, Sacramento.

NCLEX® REVIEW

1. After reviewing the electrocardiogram of a patient, the nurse believes the tracing is normal. Which of the following did the nurse assess on this patient's ECG?

   1. PR interval less than 0.8 second
   2. QRS complex 0.10 second
   3. Absent PR interval
   4. QT interval greater than 0.50 seconds

2. The nurse is assessing the QRS complexes on a patient's electrocardiogram. The complex spans 3 small boxes on the ECG paper. The nurse would identify this patient's QRS complex to be:

   1. 0.03 second
   2. 0.06 second
   3. 0.12 second
   4. 0.15 second

3. A patient comes into the emergency department to be seen for chest pain that started after learning that his brother was killed in an accident. The electrocardiogram shows a normal heart rate with shorter PR intervals. Which of the following should be included in this patient's plan of care?

   1. Plan for cardioversion.
   2. Observe and treat the patient for anxiety.
   3. Medicate with calcium channel blockers.
   4. Provide carotid artery massage.

4. A patient is diagnosed with a junctional dysrhythmia. Which of the following should be included in this patient's plan of care?

   1. Have a serum digoxin level drawn.
   2. Implement ACLS protocols.
   3. Prepare to administer magnesium.
   4. Prepare to administer lidocaine.

Answers for review questions appear in Appendix D

KEY TERMS

absolute refractory period *p.1077*
action potential *p.1077*
anion *p.1076*
artifact *p.1085*
asystole *p.1111*
atrial dysrhythmia *p.1090*
atrial fibrillation *p.1092*
atrial flutter *p.1096*
atrial kick *p.1075*
atrioventricular (AV) node *p.1075*
automaticity *p.1076*
AV dissociation *p.1103*
Bachmann bundle *p.1075*
bigeminy *p.1107*
bipolar lead *p.1080*
bundle branch block *p.1105*
bundle of His *p.1075*
bundles *p.1074*
cardiac conduction system *p.1073*
cardiac depolarization *p.1076*
cardiac repolarization *p.1077*
cation *p.1076*
conductivity *p.1076*
contractility *p.1076*
dysrhythmia *p.1086*
ECG waveform *p.1085*
ectopic focus *p.1085*
electrode *p.1078*
escape *p.1075*
excitability *p.1076*

fascicles *p.1075*
fill time *p.1087*
first-degree AV block *p.1101*
graph paper *p.1083*
intra-atrial pathways *p.1075*
ion *p.1076*
isoelectric line *p.1085*
J point *p.1078*
junctional dysrhythmia *p.1097*
junctional escape rhythm *p.1098*
lead axis *p.1079*
millivolts *p.1077*
Mobitz I/Wenckebach *p.1101*
Mobitz II/second-degree block *p.1101*
negative deflection *p.1079*
nodes (bundles) *p.1074*
normal sinus rhythm (NSR) *p.1086*
P wave *p.1078*
pacemaker cell *p.1076*
paroxysmal junctional tachycardia
    (PJT) *p.1100*
positive deflection *p.1079*
PR interval *p.1078*
premature atrial contraction (PAC) *p.1090*
premature junctional contraction
    (PJC) *p.1098*
premature ventricular contraction
    (PVC) *p.1106*
pulseless electrical activity (PEA) *p.1111*
Purkinje network fibers *p.1075*

QRS complex *p.1078*
QT interval *p.1084*
quadrigeminy *p.1107*
refractory period *p.1077*
relative refractory period *p.1077*
resting membrane potential *p.1076*
sick sinus syndrome (SSS) *p.1096*
sinoatrial (SA) node *p.1075*
sinus arrest *p.1088*
sinus arrhythmia/dysrhythmia *p.1087*
sinus bradycardia *p.1086*
sinus tachycardia *p.1087*
ST segment *p.1078*
supraventricular tachycardia (SVT) *p.1094*
T wave *p.1078*
third-degree AV block (complete
    block) *p.1103*
threshold *p.1071*
torsade de pointes *p.1107*
trigeminy *p.1107*
12-lead ECG *p.1079*
U wave *p.1078*
unipolar lead *p.1080*
ventricular dysrhythmia *p.1106*
ventricular fibrillation (VF) *p.1110*
ventricular tachycardia (VT) *p.1107*
wandering atrial pacemaker *p.1096*
Wolff-Parkinson-White syndrome
    (WPW) *p.1096*

EXPLORE PEARSON **mynursingkit**™

MyNursingKit is your one stop for online chapter review materials and resources. Prepare for success with additional NCLEX®-style practice questions, interactive assignments and activities, web links, animations and videos, and more!

Register your access code from the front of your book at
www.mynursingkit.com

REFERENCES

American Heart Association. (2005a). *Handbook of emergency cardiovascular care for healthcare providers.* Dallas, TX: Author.

American Heart Association. (2005b). Part 5: Electrical therapies: Automated external defibrillators, defibrillation, cardioversion, and pacing. *Supplement to Circulation: Journal of the American Heart Association, 112*(24), IV-35–IV-46.

American Heart Association. (2005c). 2005 American Heart Association guidelines for cardiopulmonary resuscitation and emergency cardiovascular care: Part 2. Ethical issues. *Circulation, 112,* IV-6–IV-11.

American Heart Association. (2006a). *BLS guidelines for healthcare providers.* Dallas, TX: Author.

American Heart Association. (2006b). *2005 International Consensus on CPR and ECC Science with Treatment Recommendations.* Retrieved June 30, 2006, from http://www.americanheart.org/presenter .jhtml?identifier=3022512

Beasley, B. M. (2003). *Understanding EKGs: A practical approach* (2nd ed.). Upper Saddle River, NJ: Prentice Hall.

Boyd, R. (2000). Witnessed resuscitation by relatives. *Resuscitation, 43,* 171–176.

Chamberlain, D. A., & Hazinski, M. F. (2003). Education in resuscitation: An ILCOR symposium: Utstein Abbey: Stavanger, Norway: June 22–24, 2001. *Circulation, 108,* 2575–2594.

Ellis, K. M. (2002a). *EKG plain and simple: From rhythm strips to 12-leads.* Upper Saddle River, NJ: Prentice Hall Health.

Ellis, K. M. (2002b). *Q & A review of EKG.* Upper Saddle River, NJ: Prentice Hall Health.

Garcia, T. B., & Miller G. T. (2004). *Arrhythmia recognition: The art of interruption.* Sudbury, MA: Jones and Bartlett.

Hamby, R. L., Mittal, S., & Stein, K. M. (2006). *Arrhythmia.* Retrieved July 17, 2006, from http:// heart.healthcentersonline.com/ arrhythmia/arrhythmia8.cfm

Holtschneider, M. E., McBroom, K. G., & Patterson, A. (2006). ECG everywhere. *Advance for Nurses, 3*(13), 20.

International Liaison Committee on Resuscitation. (2005). International consensus on cardiopulmonary resuscitation and emergency cardiovascular care with treatment recommendations. *Circulation,* 2005, 112: III-I-III-136.

Jacobs, I., et al. (2004). Cardiac arrest and cardiopulmonary resuscitation outcome reports: Update and simplification of the Utstein templates resuscitation registries. A statement for health care professionals from a task force of the international liaison committee on resuscitation (AHA, European Resuscitation Council, Australian Resuscitation Council, New Zealand Resuscitation Council, Heart and Stroke Foundation of Canada, interAmerican Heart Foundation, Resuscitation Council of Southern Africa). *Resuscitation, 63,* 233–249.

Morton, P. G., Fontaine, D. K., Hudak, C.M. & Gallo, B. M. (2005). *Critical care nursing: A holistic approach* (8th ed.). Philadelphia: Lippincott Williams & Wilkins.

Olshansky, B. et al. (2006). Atrioventricular nodal reentry tachycardia (AVNRT). *eMedicine from WebMD.* Retrieved July 13, 2006, from http://www.emedicine.com/med/topic2955.htm

Peberdy, M. A. et al. (2003). Cardiopulmonary resuscitation of adult in the hospital: A report of 14720 cardiac arrests from the National Registry of Cardiopulmonary Resuscitation. *Resuscitation, 58,* 297–308.

Porth, C. M. (2004). *Essentials of pathophysiology: Concepts of altered health states.* Philadelphia: Lippincott Williams & Wilkins.

Shade, B., & Wesley, K. (2007). *Fast and easy ECGs: A self-paced learning program.* Boston: McGraw-Hill.

Walraven, G. (2006). *Basic arrhythmias* (6th ed.). Upper Saddle River, NJ: Prentice Hall Health.

Diagnostic and Interventional Therapies for Cardiovascular Disorders

Sue Apple
Joseph Lindsay, Jr.

Outcome-Based Learning Objectives

After studying this chapter, the learner will be able to:

1. Define sensitivity and specificity as they relate to diagnostic testing.
2. Describe the major noninvasive and invasive diagnostic tests to detect coronary disease.
3. Identify the appropriate screening test and associated nursing management for a given patient population.
4. Compare and contrast major advantages and limitations for each test.
5. Prioritize the nursing management for patients receiving percutaneous coronary interventional procedures.

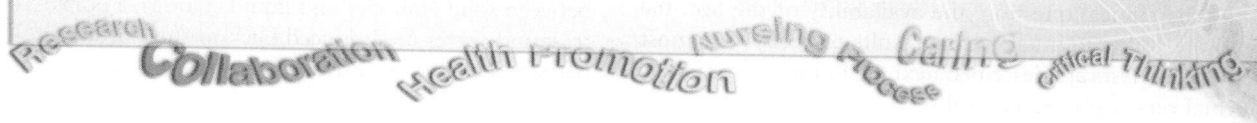

ALTHOUGH MUCH information is gained at the bedside by a detailed history and physical examination, health care providers also need results from both noninvasive and invasive diagnostic tests to determine the presence or absence of heart disease in their patients. For persons with known disease, such as the patient who has had a myocardial infarction, these tests provide the basis for determining functional status, treatment, and long-term prognosis.

The heart can be evaluated using x-rays (radiography, angiography, computed tomography [CT]), gamma rays (radionuclide imaging), sound waves (echocardiography), and magnetic properties of the body (magnetic resonance imaging [MRI]) (Thomas, 2002). Given the ever-widening array of tests, choosing the most appropriate test for an individual can be challenging. To be most beneficial, it is important to consider the cost, safety, accuracy, and availability of the particular test.

Certain basic concepts apply to nearly all cardiovascular testing. Each test may be assessed for its *sensitivity* against a known standard. In the case of coronary heart disease the "gold standard" is usually the detection of atherosclerotic plaque by coronary angiography (Baim & Grossman, 2000b). For practical purposes, if the standard is a valid one (and not "fool's gold") and as long as the criteria for discriminating a positive from a negative test remain constant, sensitivity will be constant. It may

be defined by means of population testing. **Sensitivity** describes the ability of a test to identify patients with disease (Greenland & Gaziano, 2003). It may be calculated by dividing the number of true positive tests by the sum of true positives plus false negatives. For example, positive tests in subjects with coronary disease are "true positives" whereas negative tests in subjects with disease are "false negatives." Similarly, negative tests in patients who are free of disease are "true negatives" and positive tests in patients without disease are "false positives." **Specificity** is calculated by dividing the number of true negatives in the population by the sum of true negatives plus false positives. Thus, specificity describes the frequency with which the test is normal in subjects who are free of disease (Kadish et al., 2001).

An understanding of test characteristics is only part of the information necessary for the clinician who will apply the test result in an individual subject. The clinician needs to know how often the *single* result reflects accurately the presence or absence of disease. For this interpretation he must understand an additional concept, **predictive accuracy** of a positive and of a negative test; that is, how well the results of the test predict the presence or absence of disease.

The sensitivity and specificity of most diagnostic tests are known for a given disease in a specific population. What is not always known is the **pretest probability,** which is the likelihood that disease is present in the patient before testing. Therefore, choosing the appropriate test requires knowledge of the test, including indications, advantages, and disadvantages, combined with clinical knowledge of the disease and the individual patient (Chart 39–1).

To be useful a positive test should substantially increase the **post-test probability** (likelihood that disease is present), and a negative test should lower the post-test probability.

This chapter will provide an overview of current diagnostic tests used to screen patients for the presence of heart disease as well as determine functional status, treatment outcomes, and long-term prognosis. A brief overview of cardiac pacemakers and percutaneous coronary interventions also will be provided.

Diagnostic Procedures

The choice of diagnostic procedure depends on several factors, including the clinical question, the availability of the test, the cost, and the ability to interpret the results correctly. The most frequently used tests are described next, including the rationale and normal versus abnormal results.

Electrocardiogram

The **electrocardiogram** (ECG) is a body surface recording of the electrical activity of the heart. Introduced in 1902 by Willem Einthoven, the ECG not only is the oldest but also remains the most frequently performed cardiac diagnostic test (Kadish et al., 2001; Rosen, 2002). The standard 12-lead ECG derives its name from the 12 leads that provide 12 different "views" of the electrical activity as it traverses the myocardium. These views are derived from the four limb and six precordial (chest) electrodes attached to the patient (Figure 39–1 ■).

Examining the electrical signals from the heart in different leads provides the clinician with accurate information about a variety of cardiac conditions (Chart 39–2, p. 1122). An in-depth discussion of electrocardiography is covered in Chapter 38 .

Drew (2002) noted that the ECG continues to be the gold standard for the detection and evaluation of cardiac dysrhythmias and ischemia. Because it is useful in many clinical situations and relatively easy to perform, the nurse at the bedside is frequently expected to obtain the 12-lead ECG. To improve the accuracy of the test, care must be taken to ensure correct positioning of the leads and firm contact with the skin (Drew & Ide, 1999; Kadish et al., 2001). Patient factors that can negatively influence the quality of the tracing include motion artifact, morbid obesity, and chronic obstructive pulmonary disease. Motion artifact distorts the baseline, introducing error into the interpretation. Morbid obesity and obstructive lung disease interfere with transmission of the electrical activity of the heart.

Although the ECG alone gives the clinician much valuable information, the tracing must always be interpreted at the bedside. That is, the ECG should be interpreted in the context of the patient's symptoms, laboratory values, and likely diagnosis.

Echocardiography

If the ECG is the most frequently performed diagnostic test, the echocardiogram (echo) is a close second (Smith & Thomas, 2002). This is not surprising because the echo exam provides a rapid, safe, and relatively inexpensive detailed examination of the heart. **Echocardiography** refers to the noninvasive assessment of the structures and function of the heart and great vessels utilizing high-frequency (ultrasound) sound waves. The first application of ultrasound, or sonar technology, to the clinical arena occurred almost 100 years ago in Sweden, where Edler and Hertz published their work on the utility of ultrasound to record the movements of the heart (Weyman, 2004). Since that time the definition of echocardiography has broadened to include not only traditional M-mode echocardiography but also two-dimensional transthoracic echocardiography, Doppler analysis and transesophageal echocardiography are explained later (Cheitlin et al., 2003).

Echocardiographic imaging relies on the generation of ultrasound waves (Armstrong & Feigenbaum, 2001; Hall, 2005). These waves are emitted from a transducer placed in standard positions on the chest wall. As the waves encounter an interface between solid (muscle) and liquid (blood), a portion of the ultrasound waves are bounced back to the transducer. Interfaces perpendicular to the ultrasound beam reflect echoes much more effectively than those that are not perpendicular. Because the speed of sound traveling in the body is known, the time it takes for the echo to return to the transducer allows determination of the depth of the structure. The fast rate of travel of the ultrasound waves allows for almost instantaneous or real-time recording of the cardiac structures in motion. The three noninvasive types of echocardiography are M-mode, two-dimensional, and Doppler ultrasound.

M-mode (motion) echocardiography was the earliest form of clinical ultrasound. Images are transmitted from a single narrow line of ultrasound and recorded as moving lines that do not resemble cardiac structures, and therefore can be difficult to interpret. M-mode provides information about the distance of each object (valve leaflet, pericardium, etc.) from the transducer and can be used to assess valvular motion and chamber wall thickness and motion.

Two-dimensional (2D) echocardiography came into use in the 1970s. 2D echo provides an anatomically recognizable image of the heart by sending out pulsed ultrasound waves in a fan or arc-shaped configuration, and today the transthoracic 2D echo is considered the mainstay of the echo evaluation (Armstrong & Feigenbaum, 2001).

Doppler ultrasound relies on analysis of frequency shifts as the beam encounters moving targets. In the heart, sound waves are reflected off moving red blood cells. The Doppler effect shifts the sound frequency as the cells move toward or away from the transducer; these shifts are viewed as color changes.

Midclavicular line
Anterior axillary line
Midaxillary line
Horizontal plane of $V_4 - V_6$

$V_1 V_2 V_3$ V_4 V_5 V_6

RA
LA

RL
LL

V_{6R} V_{5R} V_{4R} V_{3R} V_{2R} V_{1R}
Supplemental right precordial leads

ECG strip
ECG machine

Right and left arm leads should be placed outwardly on the shoulders (preferentially over bone rather than muscle)

V_1 and V_2 are positioned in the fourth intercostal space

V_4 should be placed in the fifth intercostal space on the midclavicular line

RA
LA

Anterior axillary line
Midaxillary line
Directly between leads V_2 and V_4

V_1 V_2 V_3
V_4 V_5 V_6

V_4, V_5, and V_6 should be placed on a horizontal line—this line does not necessarily follow the intercostal space

The right leg lead (ground lead) should be placed below the umbilicus

RL
LL

The left leg lead should be placed just below the umbilicus

FIGURE 39–1 ■ Position of the electrodes in the 12-lead electrocardiogram.

This ability to measure blood flow through the heart and great vessels provides hemodynamic data to supplement the anatomic information obtained from M-mode and 2D echo. Hemodynamic data include the amount and speed of blood flow through the valves, enabling the noninvasive detection and follow-up of stenotic or regurgitant heart valves, and measure-ment of intracardiac pressures, which can be used to detect ab-normal flow states such as shunts across the atrial or ventricu-lar septum.

The echocardiogram can also assess the pumping action of the cardiac muscle. This measure is known as an ejection frac-tion, or EF. A normal EF is around 55% to 65%. Numbers below

Clinical Conditions Detectable from the 12-Lead Electrocardiogram

1. Myocardial ischemia, injury, and infarction
2. Cardiac dysrhythmias
3. Electrical conduction abnormalities
4. Cardiac hypertrophy
5. Medication effects (i.e., digitalis toxicity)
6. Electrolyte abnormalities

45% usually represent some decrease in the pumping strength of the heart, whereas numbers below 30% to 35% are representative of an important decrease.

Currently a complete echocardiography exam incorporates all three modalities: M-mode, 2D, and Doppler (Cheitlin et al., 2003). Together they provide the clinician with detailed information about the structure and function of the heart and great vessels (Chart 39–3).

In certain populations the standard transthoracic examination (TTE) has limitations that require the use of further tests to establish the diagnosis or determine the therapeutic course of action. Because ultrasound waves cannot travel through air, echocardiography performed on patients who have chronic obstructive lung disease or who are on mechanical ventilators may

Indications for Echocardiography

ASSESSMENT OF THE HEART AND GREAT VESSELS
1. Size of the cardiac chambers
2. Size of the cardiac walls
3. Structure and function of the valves
4. Location and quantification of cardiac shunts (i.e., patent foramen ovale or a ventricular septal defect)
5. Cardiac tumors
6. Estimates of left ventricular functioning

ESTABLISHMENT OF CLINICAL DIAGNOSES
1. Aortic dissection
2. Location and quantification of pericardial effusions
3. Cardiac tamponade
4. Endocarditis
5. Murmurs
6. Stroke: identification of intracardiac sources of embolization

TIMING OF THERAPEUTIC INTERVENTIONS
1. When to repair/replace defective cardiac valves
2. Rule out intra-atrial thrombus before cardioversion for atrial fibrillation
3. Intraoperative TEE guidance
4. Ischemic heart disease

result in suboptimal or even inadequate images. Likewise, ultrasound cannot image through bone or heavily calcified structures. In the adult this limits the transducer placement to the intercostal and subxiphoid positions. Finally, excess adipose tissue can make visualization of the borders of the heart difficult.

Transesophageal Echocardiography

Transesophageal echocardiography (TEE) can overcome some of the limitations of TTE (Armstrong & Feigenbaum, 2001; Milani, Lavie, Gilliland, Cassidy, & Bernal, 2003; Peterson, Brickner, & Reimold, 2003). During TEE, the miniaturized transducer is advanced down the esophagus. Because the esophagus passes directly behind the posterior surface of the heart, it affords excellent views of the posterior structures of the heart and great vessels. Because TEE is minimally invasive and usually performed using conscious sedation, it is associated with a slight risk (<0.02%) of complications such as trauma to the structures of the mouth or throat or adverse reactions to the conscious sedation (Milani et al., 2003). Current guidelines recommend using TEE only when the information cannot be obtained from a standard TTE (Quiñones et al., 2003). TEE is frequently used to detect and assess endocarditis, aortic dissection, intracardiac masses such as thrombi or tumors, valvular pathology, and congenital disorders in both children and adults (Quiñones et al., 2003). TEE also is helpful in critically ill patients requiring ventilator support because the posterior images are not distorted by the constant motion of the lungs as the ventilator cycles. Finally, the role of TEE intraoperatively is expanding as evidence mounts that TEE guidance during procedures such as valvular repair improves clinical outcomes (improved valve function after surgery, less need for valve replacement or reoperation) (Cheitlin et al., 2003).

Stress Echocardiography

Stress echocardiography refers to the use of echocardiography to detect coronary artery disease (Marwick, 2002). Although exercise electrocardiography is the standard noninvasive method of detecting CAD, in some settings this test is of limited value because of incomplete data or difficulty in interpreting the test results. These instances include patients who have baseline ECG abnormalities or who are unable or unwilling to exercise to their peak heart rate. The standard treadmill test may also be more difficult to interpret in women and patients with left ventricular hypertrophy (ECG is least reliable in these populations) (Marwick, 2003). In these instances stress echocardiography can be used to make the diagnosis because the test results are based on echo images and not on ECG changes. Stress echocardiography is also used to evaluate patients with known coronary or valvular heart disease, populations who often cannot exercise to their peak heart rate and/or have baseline ECG abnormalities (Quiñones et al., 2003).

Stress echocardiography can be performed using standard forms of exercise (treadmill or bicycle) or a pharmacologic agent such as dobutamine, to increase the heart rate (Quiñones et al., 2003). The normal response to exercise is an increase in heart rate and contractility. The development of a new myocardial wall motion abnormality (failure to contract normally in one or more segments of the heart) or failure of the heart to increase strength of contraction during the test is a positive indication of reversible ischemia.

Contrast agents have been explored as a method of improving visualization of the left ventricle during echocardiography (Mulvagh et al., 2000; Smith & Thomas, 2002; Stewart, 2003). Agitated saline, created by forcefully mixing normal saline with air, is the simplest contrast agent and still the standard by which to detect intracardiac shunts (Armstrong & Feigenbaum, 2001). Because agitated saline results in microbubbles too large to pass through the pulmonary circulation, the visualization of bubbles in the left side of the heart after intravenous injection is considered positive proof of a cardiac shunt (abnormal opening in the atrial or ventricular septum).

Newer contrast agents that possess smaller, more stable bubbles are under investigation (Mulvagh et al., 2000). These agents improve endocardial border detection and thus improve the ability of echocardiography to detect ischemic disease and possibly evaluate **myocardial perfusion** (blood flow to the heart muscle) (Mulvagh et al., 2000; Quiñones et al., 2003; Stewart, 2003).

Finally, the development of three-dimensional echocardiography (3D) allows the clinician to view the structures and valves of the heart in a three-dimensional view noninvasively. This technology, combined with other advances in echocardiography, is bringing diagnostic cardiology closer to having an all-inclusive noninvasive assessment of the anatomy and physiology of the heart.

The advantages of echocardiography—the amount of information obtained with a noninvasive test, its portability and safety, and its relative low cost—can also lead to overuse of this technology. Clinical guidelines for the use of echocardiography are published and should be used to identify appropriate indications for testing (Cheitlin et al., 2003). Another well-known limitation of echocardiography is operator variability in performing and interpreting the results (Armstrong & Feigenbaum, 2001; Smith & Thomas, 2002). Again, standards are published for the performance and interpretation of echocardiography (Quiñones et al., 2003). Adherence to these standards improves the reliability and validity of the test results.

Exercise Testing

Exercise testing is a "cardiovascular stress test that uses treadmill or bicycle exercise and electrocardiographic and blood pressure monitoring" (Gibbons et al., 2002, p. 2). It is the most common noninvasive test used to evaluate patients with suspected ischemic heart disease (Gibbons et al., 2002; Grech, 2003).

Indications

Exercise testing is useful in many situations and populations (Chart 39–4). It is a relatively inexpensive test that can be safely performed in the hospital or in an outpatient setting. As with other diagnostic tests, the value of the information obtained from the test is directly related to the expertise and experience of all the staff performing and interpreting the results. Standards have been established for the performance and interpretation of exercise tests (Fletcher et al., 2001; Gibbons et al., 2002).

In persons with normal cardiac function, upright exercise such as walking on a treadmill results in an increased heart rate that is largely responsible for the increased cardiac output. Sys-

CHART 39–4 Indications and Contraindications for Exercise Testing

INDICATIONS

1. Evaluation of chest pain
2. Evaluation of severity of myocardial disease
3. Risk stratification, especially after a myocardial infarction
4. Prognosis in patients with known or suspected heart disease
5. Detection of exercise-related symptoms, such as syncope due to dysrhythmias
6. Evaluation after revascularization procedures, such as percutaneous coronary interventions or coronary artery bypass surgeries
7. Evaluation for cardiac rehabilitation
8. Patient reassurance

CONTRAINDICATIONS

1. Myocardial infarction within 2 days
2. Unstable angina
3. Aortic stenosis
4. Uncontrolled dysrhythmias
5. Symptomatic heart failure
6. Active endocarditis
7. Uncontrolled hypertension
8. Any acute disorder that may affect exercise (infection, renal failure)
9. Inability to obtain informed consent

Sources: Adapted from Fletcher, G. F., Balady, G. J., Amsterdam, E. A., Chaitman, B., Eckel, R., Fleg, J., et al. (2001). Exercise standards for testing and training. *Circulation, 104,* 1694–1740; Grech, E. D. (2003). ABC of interventional cardiology: Pathophysiology and investigation of coronary artery disease. *British Medical Journal, 326,* 1027–1030; and Myers, J. (2005). Exercise testing. In S. L. Woods, E. S. S. Froelicher, S. A. Motzer, & E. J. Bridges (Eds.), *Cardiac nursing* (5th ed., pp. 439–458). Philadelphia: Lippincott Williams & Wilkins.

tolic blood pressure increases as work increases, but there is minimal or no change in diastolic blood pressure (Fletcher et al., 2001; Myers, 2005).

During exercise there is an increase in heart rate along with increased myocardial oxygen need and thereby a demand for increased coronary blood flow (Myers, 2005). The maximal heart rate that a person can attain at peak exercise declines with age and can be roughly calculated from this formula: 220 − age (years) (Chaitman, 2001). Oxygen uptake is usually expressed in **metabolic equivalents (MET),** whereby 1 MET is a unit of sitting/resting oxygen uptake ($\approx$ 3.5 milliliters of O_2 per kilogram of body weight per minute). Maximal oxygen consumption, the greatest amount of oxygen a person can take in while exercising at maximum capacity, is considered the best measure of a person's exercise capacity (Fletcher et al., 2001).

Factors that influence a person's ability to exercise include age, gender, physical conditioning, heredity, and cardiovascular status (Fletcher et al., 2001). Cardiovascular disease causes maximal heart rate and systolic blood pressure, as well as maximal exercise capacity, to be reduced.

Protocols and Patient Preparation

Exercise tests are conducted according to established protocols that usually include a warm-up phase, progressive exercise to a maximal heart rate or prespecified end points, and a recovery phase. Several different exercise protocols are available. Selection of protocol will depend on the purpose of the test, the physical condition of the patient, and of course the equipment and personnel available. The most suitable protocols for clinical testing last 6 to 12 minutes (Fletcher at al., 2001; Myers, 2005).

Patients are usually asked not to eat or smoke for 3 hours before the exam. They should also be instructed about their medications; most centers do not stop cardiac medications before the test. During the test, heart rate, blood pressure, electrocardiographic changes, exercise capacity, and patient symptoms are monitored. The electrocardiogram is the cornerstone of the exercise test; therefore, skin preparation and lead placement are extremely important in order to obtain high-quality results.

Interpretation

The test is usually continued until the patient achieves a maximal level of exertion or displays clinical indications for stopping (Chart 39–5).

The results of the exercise test include both objective and subjective data. Objective information includes blood pressure measurements, heart rate, and exercise capacity reported in METs, or exercise stage achieved, and ECG findings. Failure to achieve 85% of the predicted heart rate is associated with an increased risk of mortality in patients with previously diagnosed coronary artery disease (CAD) (Chaitman, 2001; Fletcher et al., 2001). Numerous ECG criteria are used to diagnose CAD. Patients with exercise- or dobutamine-induced myocardial ischemia often develop ST segment depression. In patients with a normal baseline ECG, the traditional criteria include the development of 1 millimeter or greater ST segment depression (horizontal or downsloping) occurring for at least 60 to 80 milliseconds after the J point—the point on the ECG where the QRS complex ends and the ST segment begins (Fletcher et al., 2001; Myers, 2005) (Figure 39–2 ■). ECG abnormalities at baseline make interpretation of the stress tracing difficult or impossible.

CHART 39–5	**Selected Indications for Stopping Exercise Testing**

1. Target heart rate achieved (>85% of maximum predicted heart rate)
2. ST segment elevation (>1.0 millimeter) in leads without Q waves (except leads V$_1$ and aVR)
3. Decrease in systolic blood pressure (>10 mmHg) accompanied by other evidence of ischemia
4. Moderate to severe angina
5. Dizziness or near syncope
6. Sustained ventricular tachycardia

Sources: Adapted from Fletcher, G. F., Balady, G. J., Amsterdam, E. A., Chaitman, B., Eckel, R., Fleg, J., et al. (2001). Exercise standards for testing and training. *Circulation, 104,* 1694–1740; Grech, E. D. (2003). ABC of interventional cardiology: Pathophysiology and investigation of coronary artery disease. *British Medical Journal, 326,* 1027–1030; and Myers, J. (2005). Exercise testing. In S. L. Woods, E. S. S. Froelicher, S. A. Motzer, & E. J. Bridges (Eds.), *Cardiac nursing* (5th ed., pp. 439–458). Philadelphia: Lippincott Williams & Wilkins.

Subjective measurements include the development of any chest pain, excessive fatigue, general appearance, and perceived exertion, that is, shortness of breath. Classic symptoms of angina as a result of the test are predictive of coronary artery disease, especially when associated with ST segment depression (Fletcher et al., 2001).

The probability that a patient with a positive exercise test actually has significant coronary artery disease depends in part on the sensitivity and specificity of the test. Sensitivity, or the ability of the test to detect patients with CAD, is relatively low, ranging from 50% to 75%. Specificity in patients who do not have CAD is much higher; that is, the test will be negative in 77% to 90% of cases. The relatively high specificity is the real value of the exercise test in diagnosing CAD (Gibbons et al., 2002; Grech, 2003; Myers, 2005). However, remember that the most important factor affecting the results is the estimation of pretest probability of the patient actually having CAD. Tables are available that estimate the likelihood of CAD based on gender, age, and symptoms (Gibbons et al., 2002); nonetheless, the history and physical examination, as well as the experience of the health care provider, are critically important in deciding who is an appropriate candidate for exercise testing.

Radionuclide Imaging

Nuclear clinical cardiology is a relatively recent field, beginning in the early 1970s with the introduction of the scintillation camera and radioactive potassium to image the heart and great vessels (Iskandrian & Verani, 2002). Today nuclear cardiology techniques are used to establish the diagnosis, assess the severity of disease, calculate risk assessment, and evaluate outcomes of therapy in patients with acute and chronic coronary syndromes and heart failure (Klocke et al., 2003).

Perfusion Imaging

Exercise **myocardial perfusion imaging** (**MPI**) is the most common application of nuclear imaging techniques. In patients who do not have a normal baseline ECG, or who for other reasons such as physical limitations are not suitable candidates for a standard exercise test, imaging techniques combined with a basic stress test improve the ability to detect significant CAD (Fletcher et al., 2001; Klocke et al., 2003; Wackers, Soufer, & Zaret, 2001). In addition, imaging provides information regarding the location of ischemic myocardium, as well as an estimation of the amount of myocardium at risk. MPI is most useful in patients who have an intermediate risk of CAD (Greenland & Gaziano, 2003; Klocke et al., 2003).

During MPI a radioactive tracer is administered intravenously and given time to circulate in the bloodstream. Areas of the myocardium with normal coronary blood flow (normal perfusion) will absorb relatively large amounts of the tracer, whereas areas with compromised blood flow will absorb less. A gamma camera is placed over the precordium to record the amount of radioactive tracer emissions. Because most significant coronary plaques are associated with normal blood flow at rest, it is necessary to image the heart during a period of maximal exercise. A perfusion defect imaged only during exercise, termed a reversible defect, denotes an area of viable (functioning) but ischemic myocardium. If a defect is present during both exercise and rest, it is termed a fixed defect and probably indicates

FIGURE 39–2 ■ Positive electrocardiographic ischemic response to exercise.

an area of infarction (defect is not reversible). If the patient is unable to exercise to maximum capacity, pharmacologic agents such as dipyridamole or adenosine can be used to invoke a physiological response in coronary blood flow similar to physical exercise. The results obtained with these methods appear to be as accurate as the results obtained with traditional stress tests (Klocke et al., 2003).

Three perfusion tracers are currently approved for routine clinical use: thallium 201 (t. 201), technetium (Tc) 99m sestamibi, and Tc 99m tetrofosmin (Chart 39–6).

Although t. 201 was the first commercially available tracer and has been the standard for diagnosing CAD, it does appear that any of the three tracers can be used to diagnose CAD accurately (Klocke et al., 2003).

ECG single photon emission computed tomography (SPECT), performed in 80% to 90% of perfusion imaging studies, is considered state of the art (Klocke et al., 2003; Wackers et al., 2001). **Tomography** is the display of images within a single plane (slice) of the heart. SPECT images are obtained with a rotating gamma camera that stops at preset angles to record images. The results are displayed as views of the heart on three different axes (Figure 39–3 ■). SPECT images offer better resolution and better separation of overlapping myocardial segments than do traditional planar images.

SPECT images are often obtained by a technique referred to as **gating,** in which image acquisition is timed to the ECG. The cardiac cycle is divided into segments that, when viewed in cine mode, allow the clinician to evaluate wall motion and systolic thickening in all areas of the left ventricle (Iskandrian & Verani, 2002). This technique allows for more accurate interpretation because the perfusion image can be correlated with the gated image of ventricular contraction.

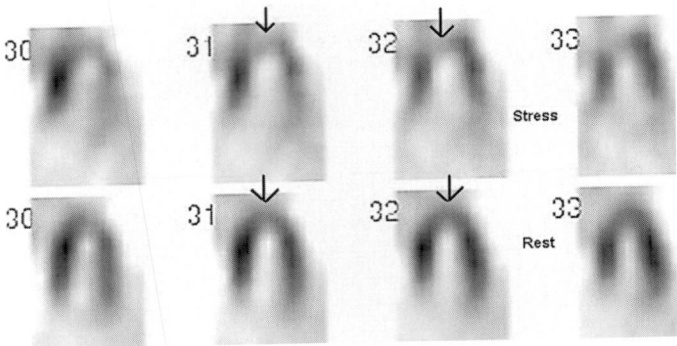

FIGURE 39–3 ■ Exercise–rest myocardial perfusion images.
Source: Courtesy of Dr. Guy Weingold, Director of Cardiac CT, Washington Hospital Center, Washington, DC

CHART 39–6 Radionuclide Tracers

THALLIUM 201 (t. 201)

- Uptake similar to potassium in living cells; after injection rapidly taken up by myocardial tissue in proportion to myocardial blood flow
- Half-life 74 hours; only small amounts can be administered
- Need for immediate imaging after injection because it redistributes in the myocardium over time (images obtained late do not reflect blood flow at time of injection)
- Not useful in evaluating chest pain in the emergency department
- Usual imaging protocol involves immediate imaging after injection during exercise; followed in 2 to 4 hours by imaging at rest to evaluate reversibility of any defects

TECHNETIUM 99m (Tc 99m) SESTAMIBI AND TETROFOSMIN

- Tracer trapped in myocardium and does not redistribute
- Less radiation exposure than thallium
- Sestamibi half-life 6 hours; larger doses can be administered
- Useful for imaging acute (emergency department) patients
- Useful for diagnosing coronary artery disease

Usual imaging protocol with sestamibi involves obtaining rest images first; after waiting 60 minutes after injection to allow for uptake and clearance from the liver, a second dose of sestamibi is administered during peak exercise.

Cardiac Magnetic Resonance Imaging

Magnetic resonance imaging (MRI) uses radiofrequency pulses from a large, powerful magnet to disrupt the normal spin of certain atoms within the body temporarily. When the pulses are stopped, the atoms emit small amounts of energy while returning to their original spin; this energy can be imaged and recorded as high-resolution images. These images allow detailed noninvasive assessment of both cardiac anatomy and physiology (Choudhury, Fuster, Badimon, Fisher, & Fayad, 2002; Schvartzman & White, 2002).

MRI can be used to evaluate patients with presumed congenital heart diseases, such as coarctation of the aorta or atrial septal defects (Pohost, Hung, & Doyle, 2003). It also is used to image structures of the heart such as the valves and the pericardium, and assessment of **myocardial viability.** This provides information about areas of the myocardium that appear to have normal functioning as well as areas that appear to be dysfunctional and may improve with revascularization.

Introduced in the late 1970s, the term *hibernating myocardium* defined areas of the heart that initially appeared dysfunctional but after restoration of blood flow (revascularization) were noted to have improved contractility (Wu & Lima, 2003). Similar improvements in function were noted in patients who had undergone successful thrombolytic therapy. Chapter 40 🔗 includes a complete discussion of thrombolytic therapy.

These areas were referred to as "stunned" myocardium by the sudden occlusion of the coronary artery during a myocardial infarction. An in-depth discussion of the pathophysiology of acute myocardial infarction is presented in Chapter 40 🔗.

Whether hibernating and stunned myocardium are different manifestations of the same process or distinct entities remains unknown (Kloner, Bolli, Marbán, Reinlib, & Braunwald, 1998).

However, the importance of identifying areas of the heart that could benefit from revascularization is self-evident.

MRI can identify viable myocardium through the use of low-dose dobutamine, with a sensitivity and specificity to identify functional recovery similar to echo (Wu & Lima, 2003). However, delayed hyperenhancement is rapidly challenging the conventional methods for assessing viability. Using gadolinium (Gd) based contrast agents increases the MRI signal of tissues, allowing characterization of specific areas of the myocardium. Gd is mainly an extracellular, interstitial agent. This property enables it to accumulate near acute infarcts where necrosis results in cell membrane rupture and interstitial edema. Gd also is increased in areas of chronic infarction. Compared to normal myocardium, areas of irreversibly damaged heart muscle appear hyperenhanced, allowing accurate quantification of the amount and location of nonviable myocardium (Higgins, 2002; Pohost et al., 2003; Wu & Lima, 2003).

The clinical uses of MRI are rapidly expanding. The application of this technology is limited by the size and expense of the magnet, the lack of dedicated cardiovascular MRI facilities, and the difficulty in imaging acutely ill patients (the nurse cannot remain with the patient during imaging). Additionally, patients with implanted metal devices such as pacemakers or defibrillators cannot be placed in the magnet (Chart 39–7) (Schvartzman & White, 2002).

Positron-Emission Tomography

Positron-emission tomography (PET) utilizes tracers that emit positrons (positively charged particles). When introduced into the body, these tracers travel only a short distance before interacting with electrons, which results in destruction of both particles and the release of a pair of high-energy photons. These photons travel in opposite directions, always 180 degrees apart. Two detectors positioned on opposite sides are programmed to recognize only simultaneous high-energy photons. Destruction of the tracer is assumed to have occurred somewhere along the straight line connecting the two detectors (Wackers et al., 2001).

The main advantage of PET scanning is the ability to label and image biologically active compounds such as glucose or drugs, which allows quantification of metabolic processes. PET scan is the current gold standard for assessment of myocardial viability. Cardiac metabolism is measured by uptake of tracers, which are analogues of glucose; viable heart muscle has normal or increased glucose uptake (Goldin, Ratib, & Aberle, 2000; Soine & Hanrahan, 2005; Wu & Lima, 2003). However, this technology has limited clinical availability because of the need for expensive equipment as well as the availability of other means of assessing viability.

Electron Beam Computed Tomography

Calcium deposits inside coronary arteries are part of the development of atherosclerosis; these deposits are not found in normal coronary arteries (O'Rourke et al., 2000). Thus the ability to quantify the amount of intracoronary artery calcium may identify asymptomatic individuals at risk for coronary events (Detrano & Carr, 2002; Fuseini, Goodwin, Ferris, & Mehta, 2003).

Computed tomography is very sensitive in detecting calcium, due to the increased absorption of x-rays by elements with high atomic numbers such as calcium. With the development of **electron beam computed tomography (EBCT),** which uses an electron gun and a stationary tungsten target to acquire rapidly ($\approx$ 90 seconds) multiple images of the heart during a single breath hold, detection and quantification of intracoronary calcium are now a clinical reality. Since the 1990s EBCT has become the accepted gold standard for assessing calcified plaques (Detrano & Carr, 2002; Fayad, Fuster, Nikolaou, & Becker, 2002; Greenland & Gaziano, 2003; O'Rourke et al., 2000).

The amount of calcium identified by EBCT is usually reported as a total calcium score (Agatson et al., 1990). A calcium score of zero is normal. There is no currently accepted standard for a high score, but values over 100 are usually considered to indicate high risk for the presence of CAD.

Many issues surround the measuring and reporting of calcium scores. First is the acknowledged low reproducibility rates; scores are influenced by the laboratory and the method of scoring (Detrano & Carr, 2002; Greenland & Gaziano, 2003; O'Rourke et al., 2000). Second, scores must be adjusted for age and gender (O'Rourke et al., 2000). Third, is the fact that a high calcium score is a sensitive but not specific marker for CAD. Sensitivity to detect CAD ranges from 80% to 90%, but specificity has been reported between 40% and 50% (Greenland & Gaziano, 2003; O'Rourke et al., 2000). Lack of data from controlled clinical trials makes it unclear at this time whether calcium scores have true incremental prognostic value.

In addition to lack of a standard reporting system for calcium scores, there is also uncertainty concerning the role of EBCT in detecting and evaluating CAD. Much of the controversy surrounding EBCT is attributable to the fact that, unlike most screening tests, EBCT is available to the public without a health care provider's order, and it has been aggressively marketed directly to consumers as a rapid, inexpensive screening tool to detect CAD (Lee & Brennan, 2002; O'Rourke et al., 2000). EBCT is a promising technology that needs clinical trials in order to assume its place as an important noninvasive, relatively inexpensive, rapid tool in the management of CAD.

Multislice Helical Computed Tomography

More recently, **multislice helical CT** has emerged as an exceptionally promising tool for visualization of general cardiac

---

CHART 39–7 **Advantages and Disadvantages of Cardiac Magnetic Resonance Imaging**

ADVANTAGES

- Noninvasive
- No exposure to radiation
- Can be repeated serially
- Provides high-resolution images of coronary artery vessel walls and lumen, allowing characterization of atherosclerotic plaque
- Allows noninvasive evaluation of acquired and congenital diseases affecting the heart, pericardium, and great arteries and veins of the thorax

DISADVANTAGES

- Relatively expensive
- Not portable
- Difficulty monitoring acutely ill patients during imaging
- Cannot be used for patients who have metal implants, such as pacemakers or implantable defibrillators

structures, the great vessels, and especially the coronary arteries (Figure 39–4 ■) (Detrano & Carr, 2002; Fayad et al., 2002; Nikolaou, Poon, Sirol, Becker, & Fayad, 2003; Schoepf, Becker, Hofmann, & Yucel, 2003).

Using 16-slice helical scanners, accompanied by ECG gating and the administration of 80 to 120 milliliters of iodinated contrast, it is possible to scan the entire volume of the heart, the proximal great vessels, and the coronary arteries with a single 25-second breath hold (Figure 39–5 ■). The spatial resolution of multislice helical CT is much higher than that of EBCT, allowing visualization of fine details of the coronary anatomy (Figure 39–6 ■), such as small side branches and atherosclerotic plaques, including "noncalcified" plaques. In addition, multislice helical CT can also detect coronary calcification using a noncontrast, low-radiation-dose scan.

The real advantage of multislice helical CT, however, is its ability to visualize the lumen of the coronary artery with high detail, allowing the interpreter to measure the degree of luminal stenosis, something that EBCT cannot do. In addition, some research suggests that identification of noncalcified plaque may be more significant as a marker of future coronary events, because calcified plaques may represent a more chronic and stable form of CAD (Choudhury et al., 2002).

Multiple-Gated Acquisition Scan (MUGA)

The MUGA scan is a useful noninvasive tool for assessing the function of the heart. The moving images of the beating heart that can be obtained provide important information about the motion of the ventricles. If muscle damage has occurred, as with a myocardial infarction, the MUGA scan can localize the portion of the heart muscle that has sustained damage and can assess the degree of damage. But more importantly, the MUGA scan is able to measure the ejection fraction of the cardiac ventricles. The left ventricular ejection fraction (LVEF), which is the proportion of blood

that is expelled from the ventricle with each heartbeat, is a commonly used measure of overall cardiac function (Fogorus, 2006).

A MUGA scan is performed by attaching a radioactive substance, technetium 99, to red blood cells and then injecting the red blood cells into the patient's bloodstream. The patient is

FIGURE 39–5 ■ Multislice helical computed tomography (CT) image of the heart.
Source: Courtesy of Dr. Guy Weingold, Director of Cardiac CT, Washington Hospital Center, Washington, DC

FIGURE 39–4 ■ Multislice helical computed tomography (CT) image of the heart.
Source: Courtesy of Dr. Guy Weingold, Director of Cardiac CT, Washington Hospital Center, Washington, DC

FIGURE 39–6 ■ Multislice helical computed tomography (CT) image of coronary arteries.
Source: Courtesy of Dr. Guy Weingold, Director of Cardiac CT, Washington Hospital Center, Washington, DC

then placed under a gamma camera, which is able to detect the technetium-labeled red cells. The image produced by the gamma camera is essentially an outline of those chambers, and after computer manipulation, the final product is a movie of the heart beating (Fogorus, 2006).

Nursing Management

Undergoing an evaluation for coronary artery disease, whether to detect new disease or to assess the progression or regression of a known clinical problem, can be stressful for the patient and her family. In order to provide optimum care during all phases of testing, the nurse must be knowledgeable about the particular test, including why it is ordered, what information is obtained, and how it is done. Explaining the procedure beforehand helps to calm the patient and may affect the results by improving patient compliance.

In many instances the nurse will actually perform the entire procedure, such as obtaining an ECG. In other situations the nurse may assist during portions of the test, such as monitoring the patient receiving conscious sedation during a TEE. Regardless, the nurse can play a critical role in ensuring a complete and accurate diagnostic exam.

Once the results are obtained, the nurse should be prepared to answer any further questions the patient or family may have regarding the outcome. This will be easier if the nurse if familiar with the standard report forms in her area of practice.

Many imaging techniques are currently available to health care professionals to identify and quantify CAD in their patients (Chart 39–8). There often is more than one appropriate test; factors such as the clinical assessment of the patient, the availability, the cost, and the experience of the professional with the current technology will all influence the choice of test.

Cardiac Catheterization

Cardiac catheterization is a procedure that is done in a special laboratory under sterile conditions. It consists of the insertion of a radiopaque catheter into the left or right side of the heart to provide anatomic and hemodynamic information about the heart and great vessels. This information is then utilized to assess the presence and severity of cardiac disease and assists to determine potential therapy and prognosis. Coronary angiography refers specifically to the use of radiopaque contrast media to image the coronary arteries. The first documented cardiac catheterization was done on a horse by Claude Bernard in 1844. The first human catheterization was performed by Werner Forssmann on himself in 1929. In 1959 Mason Sones accidentally cannulized the right coronary artery, thereby becoming the first person to perform coronary angiography on a human. In 2001 cardiac catheterizations were performed on over 1 million people, making it the second most frequent in-hospital procedure performed in the United States (American Heart Association, 2003; Deelstra & Jacobson, 2005; Grossman, 2000a; Scanlon et al., 1999).

Cardiac catheterization is indicated in a wide variety of clinical situations. Specifically it can provide information about:

- Hemodynamic pressures, which is used to evaluate cardiac and pulmonary function

---

CHART 39–8 | **Choosing the Appropriate Diagnostic Test**

Screening can be defined as the identification of previously unrecognized disease. How do you choose the most appropriate procedure?

1. Is the procedure rapid and accessible?
2. Can the results favorably alter the patient's quality or quantity of life?
3. Will the results of any intervention outweigh any potential adverse effects?
4. Does the disease have a clinically asymptomatic period during which the outcome of the disease can be altered?
5. Are acceptable treatments available?
6. Does the prevalence and seriousness of the disease justify the cost of the intervention?
7. Is the screening procedure relatively easy and inexpensive?
8. Are sufficient resources available?

- Heart chambers and the great vessels, which helps determine structural abnormalities
- Pressure gradients across valves to evaluate the extent of stenosis or regurgitation
- The patency of coronary arteries, which is used to evaluate the extent of coronary artery disease.

Chart 39–9 outlines the specific indications for cardiac catheterization.

Exact indications will vary depending on the aggressiveness of the institution in treating CAD (acute, chronic, or congenital). In addition, advances in other technologies such as cardiac MRI and multislice helical CT allow information previously available only by catheterization to be obtained in a noninvasive manner.

Right Heart Catheterization

Catheterization of the right atrium was first reported in the early 1940s. To access the right side of the heart, a catheter is advanced through a major vein into the right atrium (Figure 39–7a ■, p. 1130).

CHART 39–9 | **Indications for Cardiac Catheterization**

- Identify coronary artery disease and assess its extent and severity.
- Determine the treatment strategy in patients with acute coronary syndrome.
- Assess the consequences of coronary artery disease (CAD):
  - Ischemic mitral regurgitation
  - Left ventricular dysfunction
  - Ventricular aneurysm.
- In patients with known CAD:
  - Correlate symptoms with extent of CAD.
  - Evaluate response to acute pharmacologic intervention.
  - Assess left ventricular dysfunction in cardiomyopathy.
- Evaluate and determine the treatment strategy in patients with congenital heart disease.
- Obtain hemodynamic information such as shunt size or pulmonary vascular resistance.

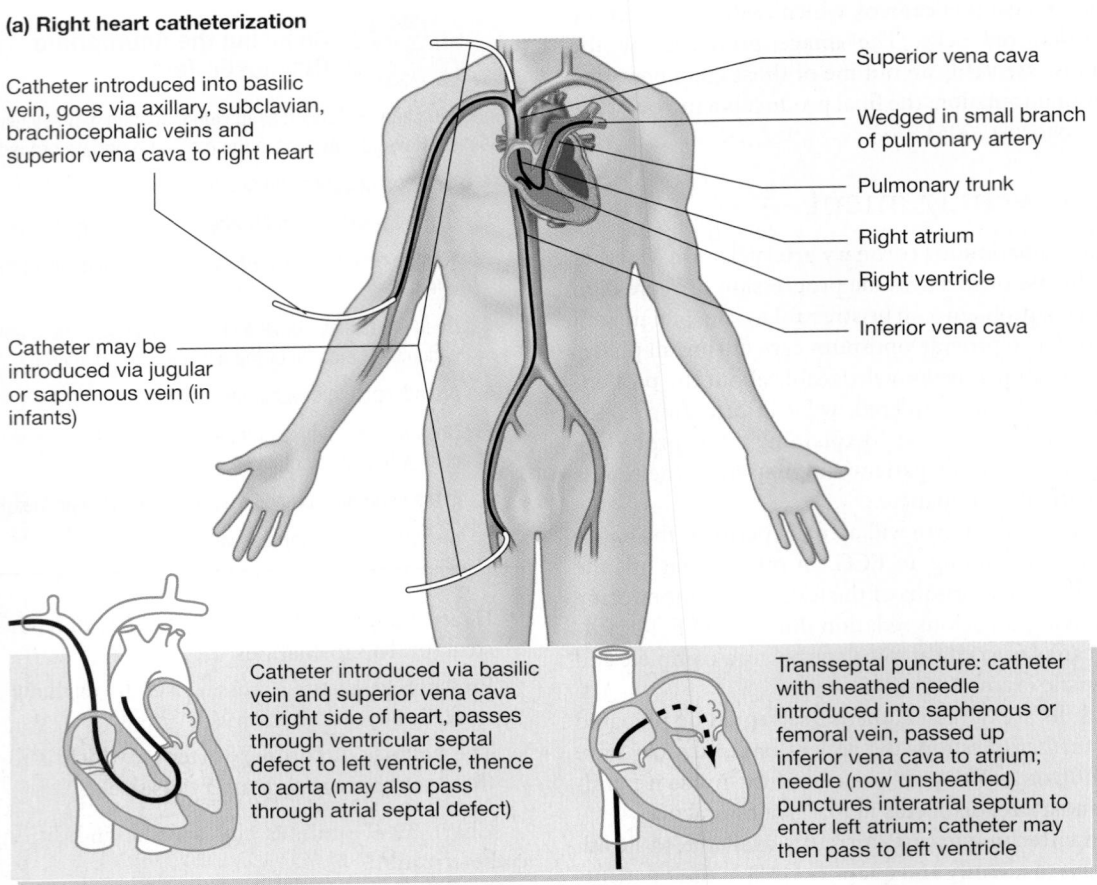

(a) **Right heart catheterization**

Catheter introduced into basilic vein, goes via axillary, subclavian, brachiocephalic veins and superior vena cava to right heart

Superior vena cava

Wedged in small branch of pulmonary artery

Pulmonary trunk

Right atrium

Right ventricle

Inferior vena cava

Catheter may be introduced via jugular or saphenous vein (in infants)

Catheter introduced via basilic vein and superior vena cava to right side of heart, passes through ventricular septal defect to left ventricle, thence to aorta (may also pass through atrial septal defect)

Transseptal puncture: catheter with sheathed needle introduced into saphenous or femoral vein, passed up inferior vena cava to atrium; needle (now unsheathed) punctures interatrial septum to enter left atrium; catheter may then pass to left ventricle

(b) **Left heart catheterization**

Catheter introduced into brachial, radial, or femoral artery and passed retrograde via aorta to left ventricle

FIGURE 39–7 ■ Heart catheterization.

Right heart catheterization allows for measurement and analysis of right heart pressures and oxygen saturations, pulmonary artery pressures including pulmonary capillary wedge pressures, screening for intracardiac shunts, and temporary ventricular pacing (Baim, 2000; Davidson & Bonow, 2001). Refer to

Chapter 24 ⚭ for more detail regarding hemodynamic measurements. Shunts, abnormal blood flow through an opening in the atrial or ventricular septum, can be detected by measuring oxygen saturation levels in the right heart. Clinically significant (needing closure) left-to-right shunts will be evident by a notable increase in the oxygen saturation levels in the right heart, as oxygenated blood from the left side of the heart crosses through the shunt and mixes with the desaturated blood in the right side (Grossman, 2000a).

Right heart catheterization is not a routine part of the evaluation of patients with CAD. In the 1990s several professional groups ruled that necessary information can be obtained with a left heart catheterization alone; since that time the number of right heart catheterizations has steadily declined (Baim, 2000).

Left Heart Catheterization

Left heart catheterization was first reported in the early 1950s. Today left heart catheterization is usually performed by accessing the femoral artery using the Judkins technique, named for Melvin Judkins, who perfected this percutaneous approach in the 1960s (Grossman, 2000). The catheter is inserted into a major artery, usually the femoral, and passed retrograde (opposite direction) to blood flow up the aorta to the openings of the coronary arteries at the base of the aorta, or it crosses the aortic valve to enter the left heart (see Figure 39–7b ■). Left heart catheterization allows for the direct measurement of left heart pressures and pressures on both sides of the aortic valve, ventriculography to measure cardiac output, and evaluation of both left ventricular function as well as the severity of any mitral or aortic valvular disease.

Coronary Angiography

Coronary cine-angiography remains the gold standard to detect significant coronary artery disease. Specialized catheters are inserted into the coronary arteries using the left heart catheterization just described. Then radiographic dye is injected into the arteries. The entire coronary vasculature (tree) is imaged, including any surgically placed saphenous vein or internal mammary artery grafts. Where plaque buildup has occurred, the lumen of the artery appears narrowed (Figure 39–8 ■) (Baim & Grossman, 2000a). See Chapter 40 🔗 for more information regarding coronary artery disease and coronary artery bypass surgery.

In addition to evaluating the extent of CAD, angiography also is used to define therapeutic options to treat CAD and to evaluate serial changes in the coronary lumen after revascularization or acute pharmacologic therapy (Baim & Grossman, 2000a; Deelstra & Jacobson, 2005; Popma & Bittl, 2001).

Percutaneous Coronary Interventions

Percutaneous transluminal coronary angioplasty (PTCA) refers to treatment of CAD using expandable balloons to crack (tear or rupture) atherosclerotic plaque, thereby enlarging the lumen of the coronary artery (Popma & Kuntz, 2001). The era of PTCA began with the first balloon angioplasty performed in a human by Andreas Grüntzig in 1977 (Grüntzig, 1978). During PTCA, a fluoroscopy-guided catheter with an expandable balloon mounted on the tip is passed into the coronary artery until it traverses the stenotic (narrowed by disease) area. The balloon is then inflated for several seconds, deflated, and then withdrawn. The procedure can be repeated until there is an increase in the diameter of the artery resulting in improved blood flow to the myocardium. Grüntzig's procedure marked the beginning of a period of rapid development in the percutaneous treatment of CAD, which continues even today (Kent, 2000;

(a)

(b)

FIGURE 39–8 ■ Coronary artery with contrast media: (A) before stent placement and (B) after stent placement.
Source: Dr. Walt Marquardt, Mercy Hospital

O'Neill & Dixon, 2004). Figure 39–9 ■ (p. 1132) shows a balloon-tipped catheter that is used to perform a PTCA.

Percutaneous coronary intervention (PCI) includes not only PTCA but also all other devices used either to remove plaque or to alter its morphology in the catheterization laboratory. Such devices include intracoronary lasers, which can be used to open totally occluded coronary arteries; intracoronary stents; and atherectomy devices, which shave the plaque and remove it. Coronary artery **stents,** first approved for elective angioplasty in 1993, are metallic mesh-like structures that are inserted permanently inside the coronary artery, compressing plaque and providing structural support of the vessel (Figure 39–10 ■, p. 1130).

Stents, either alone or in combination with PTCA, are the most frequently used device, with at least one coronary stent placed in over 70% of PCI procedures (Smith et al., 2001) (see Figure 39–8 ■). Currently over 500,000 PCIs are performed annually in the United States; worldwide the figure is estimated at over 1 million procedures (American Heart Association, 2003).

FIGURE 39–9 ■ Balloon-tipped catheter for PTCA.

FIGURE 39–10 ■ Intracoronary stent.

Indications for PCI are numerous and depend on the clinical history of the patient, the extent of coronary disease, the presence of any comorbidity, the left ventricular (LV) function, and the institution where the procedure is performed. Comorbidities such as diabetes, hyperlipidemia, renal failure, or hypertension are associated with higher morbidity and mortality rates during PCI. The same applies to patients with poor left ventricular (LV) function. See the National Guidelines for Class I Indications for Percutaneous Coronary Intervention (PCI) box.

Outcomes are measured in terms of success of the procedure and complications. A successful PCI procedure is usually defined as an angiographic success (minimal residual narrowing in the artery at the completion of the procedure) without any in-hospital major adverse cardiovascular event (MACE). A MACE is generally considered death, emergency bypass surgery, or myocardial infarction (MI), with MI defined as a significant elevation in cardiac enzymes even in the absence of new Q waves. Refer to Chapter 40 ⌘ for more information regarding MI. Clinical success includes angiographic and procedural success, as well as relief of any signs or symptoms of ischemia after the patient recovers from the procedure (short-term success) and ideally for more than 6 months after the procedure (long-term success) (Smith et al., 2001). Although outcomes are constantly changing in response to new technologies, improved operator skills, and changes in adjunct pharmacology, in general PCI angiographic success ranges from 96% to 99%, with MACE event rates from 0.2% to 3%, depending on the event measured. Long-term outcomes (5 to 10 years) are more difficult to measure, due to continuous changes in technology such as improved coronary stents, as well as clinical factors such as an increase in the number of elderly patients with poor left ventricular function undergoing PCI (Lindsay & Pinnow, 2000).

Restenosis, typically defined as a greater than 50% diameter stenosis at follow-up catheterization, has always been the Achilles' heel of PCI (Cannon, 2002; Smith et al., 2001; Waksman, 2000). Restenosis is an accumulation of smooth muscle cells at the site of the original procedure that occurs because of the artery's response to the injury from the PCI. Before the advent of stents, restenosis rates ranged from 30% to 50% within 6 to 12 months after the procedure.

Intracoronary stents marked a dramatic improvement in the incidence of restenosis, primarily by "tacking up" dissections and intimal tears as well as preventing the arterial recoil (tendency of the vessel wall to return to its original size weeks after the procedure) that commonly occurred with PCI. However, stents could not stop the smooth muscle cell proliferation that also occurred. Restenosis was occurring within the metal struts of the stent (in-stent restenosis) as well as near the ends of the device (Cannon, 2002; Carrozza & Baim, 2000; Waksman, 2000).

NATIONAL GUIDELINES for Class I Indications for Percutaneous Coronary Intervention (PCI)

1. Asymptomatic to mild angina
   a. Patients who do not have treated diabetes with one or more significant lesions in one or more coronary arteries and a high likelihood of successful PCI. The artery to be dilated must perfuse a large area of viable myocardium.

2. Moderate to severe symptoms, unstable angina, or non–ST segment elevation myocardial infarction
   a. Patients with one or more significant lesions in one or more coronary arteries suitable for PCI and a high likelihood of success. The artery to be dilated must perfuse a moderate or large area of viable myocardium.

3. Acute myocardial infarction (AMI)
   a. As an alternative to thrombolytic therapy in patients with ST segment elevation AMI or new left bundle branch block, if the

patient can undergo PCI ≤ 12 hours from the onset of ischemic symptoms or > 12 hours if symptoms persist and PCI can be performed quickly in a laboratory with experienced personnel and adequate equipment.
   b. In patients who are within 36 hours of an ST elevation AMI who develop cardiogenic shock, who are ≤ 75 years old, and revascularization can be completed within 18 hours of the onset of shock in a laboratory with experienced personnel and adequate equipment.

4. Prior coronary artery bypass surgery
   a. Patients with ischemia within 30 days of surgery

Note: Class I indications are "Conditions for which there is evidence and/or general agreement that the procedure or treatment is useful and effective."

Source: Adapted from ACC/AHA guidelines for percutaneous coronary intervention," by S. C. Smith, Jr., et al., 2001, *Journal of the American College of Cardiology, 39*, p. iii

Intracoronary **brachytherapy,** the use of localized radiation within the coronary artery, was the next development to treat in-stent restenosis (Teirstein & Kuntz, 2001; Weinberger, Lincoff, & Popma, 2002). The basis of this therapy is the assumption that restenosis is a benign process of smooth muscle cell prolifera-tion, and locally delivered radiation can halt or even prevent this process. Intracoronary brachytherapy has been approved in the United States for the treatment of in-stent restenosis, but its use in the future of PCI is questionable due to advances in coronary stents (Teirstein & Kuntz, 2001a).

Drug eluting stents (DESs) may have the potential to elimi-nate or at least dramatically reduce the problem of in-stent restenosis (O'Neill & Dixon, 2004; Sousa, Serruys, & Costa, 2003). DESs are bare metal stents coated with immunosuppres-sive agents such as sirolimus or paclitaxel that are eluted over a period of weeks to months to inhibit smooth muscle cell prolif-eration. Early clinical trials reported results that were almost too good: 0% restenosis. Although later trials in more complex pa-tients failed to duplicate the initial success, restenosis rates of less than 5% are common with the current DES. The result is that, despite the lack of long-term results, DES has captured the PCI market and become the standard of care worldwide (O'Neill & Dixon, 2004; Sousa et al., 2003; Squires, 2003).

Intravascular Ultrasound

Coronary angiography provides only a two-dimensional image of the coronary artery lumen (a "luminogram") and provides no information regarding the arterial wall. Intravascular ultra-sound (IVUS) fills that void. To obtain these images a small ul-trasound catheter is threaded into a coronary artery. From it ultrasound images that provide 360-degree cross-sectional im-ages of the artery can be obtained. Important information can be gathered regarding not only the coronary lumen but also the intima, media, and adventitia of the vessel wall. Peter Yock and colleagues recorded the first ultrasound images of human coro-nary arteries in 1988 (Chou, Fitzgerald, & Yock, 2000; Mintz & Walsh, 2000; Popma & Bittl, 2001).

IVUS can be used to detect vessel wall pathology, to help de-termine the choice of PCI, as well as to evaluate the results of the intervention, especially intracoronary stenting. IVUS is safe, rapid, and reproducible (results are consistent when performed by different clinicians). However, its use is not universal, owing to its steep "learning curve," additional cost of the equipment, and limited information linking IVUS to improved patient out-comes (Mintz & Walsh, 2000; Popma & Bittl, 2001). In addition, advances in technology such as multislice helical CT will allow similar information to be obtained noninvasively.

◼ Nursing Management

Patients undergoing PCI range from the stable person having an elective first procedure to the patient with an acute myocardial in-farction (AMI) who is hemodynamically unstable, requiring ven-tilatory and inotropic support during the procedure. The clinical status of the patient and the planned procedure will dictate the ex-act patient management.

Before the procedure the nurse should perform a complete assessment, with special attention to the cardiovascular and pe-ripheral vascular system. The patient and family should be ques-tioned about any medications taken today, including warfarin, metformin, diuretics, or insulin. Warfarin, an oral anticoagu-lant, could lead to increased bleeding during and after the pro-cedure. Metformin, a biguanide indicated in the treatment of non–insulin-dependent diabetes, has been associated with an increased risk of lactic acidosis after PCI. Diuretics in combina-tion with the patient's NPO status can lead to hypovolemia dur-ing or after the procedure. Baseline laboratory values include serum chemistries, coagulation factors, and a complete blood count. Finally, the nurse should review the patient and family's understanding of the planned procedure, including postproce-dure care. Explaining the purpose of the vascular access devices and monitoring equipment will help to decrease anxiety for everyone during the procedure.

Patients undergoing catheterization are told to have noth-ing to eat or drink for at least 6 hours before the test. There are a few contraindications to the procedure, which are outlined in Chart 39–10.

Patients with preexisting renal failure and a history of ana-phylactic reaction to contrast dye must be pretreated before the catheterization (Scanlon et al., 1999). Pretreatment for the pa-tient with a history of anaphylactic reaction to contrast dye in-cludes antihistamines and steroids. In the laboratory the patient will usually be given a mild sedative. Patients with renal failure (serum creatinine $\geq$ 1.5 mg/dL) should receive intravenous nor-mal saline for several hours before the procedure.

The length of the procedure will vary depending on the infor-mation needed; coronary angiography alone takes about 15 min-utes. The patient should be warned that during injection of any contrast medium he may feel hot and flushed; this will pass quickly. After the procedure the patient will have to remain on bed rest for a few hours unless a vascular closure device has been inserted.

Prior to the procedure the patient is given a mild sedative, but remains awake throughout the procedure. The nurse's role dur-ing PCI usually includes close monitoring of the patient to en-sure a safe environment for the procedure. The nurse must pay particular attention to the patient's airway and respiratory status during the administration of conscious sedation. Continuous assessment of the cardiovascular system, including vital signs and ECG, is also necessary to avoid complications. ECG changes such as ST segment elevation indicating myocardial injury may occur before the patient experiences chest pain. The nurse must always be alert for signs and symptoms of any allergic reaction, such as hypotension or difficulty breathing. Rapid identification of any potential problems is necessary to initiate treatment and to provide optimal care for the patient.

Adjunctive pharmacology is required for every patient un-dergoing PCI to maintain patency of the coronary artery. These

---

CHART 39–10 | **Relative Contraindications for Cardiac Catheterization**

- Severe congestive heart failure
- Severe electrolyte abnormalities
- Bleeding diathesis
- Serum creatinine $\geq$ 1.5 mg/dL
- Poor patient cooperation

drugs include antiplatelet agents, usually aspirin, and an adenosine diphosphate inhibitor (clopidogrel or ticlopidine). Intravenous antiplatelet drugs include the glycoprotein IIb/IIIa receptor inhibitors, abciximab, eptifibatide, or tirofiban. The dose and time of therapy will depend on the exact clinical status of the patient. Anticoagulants include either unfractionated heparin or low molecular weight heparin. Direct thrombin inhibitors such as bivalirudin or argatroban are increasingly used in place of heparins because of their more reliable anticoagulant effects, shorter half-lives, and lesser rates of complications (Smith et al., 2001). The drug, dose, and time of therapy will depend on the exact clinical status of the patient.

After the catheterization, patients are routinely observed in a holding area or observational unit for several hours, depending on the type of procedure, any anticoagulation administered, and the size of the sheath used for vascular access. The sheaths that are inserted to facilitate the passage of the catheters are usually removed immediately at the conclusion of the procedure. Hemostasis is obtained by manual compression; some institutions are utilizing compression or closure devices in an attempt to speed ambulation and decrease time to discharge (Koreny, Riedmuller, Nikfardjam, Siostrzonek, & Mullner, 2004). Regardless, all patients must have a complete nursing assessment, with special emphasis on the cardiovascular system including peripheral pulses and the vascular access site. This assessment, includes vital signs, ECG monitoring, and assessment of the vascular access site and pulses distal to the puncture site, should be done frequently until the patient is stable and ready for discharge. Evaluation of the access site includes inspection for any signs of bleeding or swelling and palpation for any tenderness. The arterial and venous sheaths (catheters through which the PCI devices are entered into the vascular system) may be removed in the catheterization laboratory or left in until the clotting times return to normal. Hemostasis at the access site can be achieved by manual compression or by a variety of external compression devices or patches. Patients are monitored for any complications such as hematoma, arteriovenous fistula, or retroperitoneal bleed (Apple, 2000).

Diagnosis of suspected arterial injuries is made through a careful physical assessment and confirmed through noninvasive vascular studies or arteriography. Physical examination of the femoral site is performed, assessing for the presence of localized tenderness, bruits, or a pulsatile mass. Hematomas are identified by swelling at the site of the arterial puncture. Large hematomas may need to be assessed by ultrasound to rule out the presence of pseudoaneurysms or arteriovenous fistulas.

A femoral pseudoaneurysm is an extravascular cavity communicating with the femoral artery by a channel or neck at the needle puncture site. Examination will reveal localized tenderness and a palpable, pulsatile mass, often associated with a bruit. Although rare, large pseudoaneurysms can compress the adjacent nerves causing significant discomfort for the patient. Diagnosis is confirmed through ultrasound with Doppler imaging that demonstrates a cavity communicating with the femoral artery as well as to-and-fro flow of blood through the neck. Treatment depends on the size of the pseudoaneurysm and the clinical assessment of the patient. Asymptomatic patients with a well-defined pseudoaneurysm (lumen < 2 centimeters in diameter) can initially be managed conservatively. External compression guided by ultrasound is the standard of treatment for

femoral artery pseudoaneurysms greater than 2 centimeters. Pseudoaneurysms associated with a rapidly expanding hematoma should be considered for urgent operative repair, because they can lead to rupture of the pseudoaneurysm or compression neuropathy.

An arteriovenous (AV) fistula is a direct communication between the artery and vein, resulting in a high-velocity jet from the artery into the vein. Fistulae are identified by the presence of a bruit over the access site. Diagnosis is confirmed by Doppler ultrasound. An AV fistula that is detected in clinically asymptomatic patients without evidence of expansion may be followed conservatively. If treatment is indicated, ultrasound-guided compression is usually attempted first. If this fails to close the fistulae, or there is evidence of clinical deterioration, the patient is referred for surgical repair.

Retroperitoneal hematomas are a rare but potentially fatal complication that accounts for significant morbidity, involving the need for blood transfusions and surgical repair. Bleeding into the retroperitoneal space can be difficult to detect until there has been significant blood loss. Early symptoms include flank or back pain, as well as nausea and vomiting, often associated with a vagal reaction (hypotension and bradycardia). Diagnosis is confirmed through abdominal CT scan. Small retroperitoneal hematomas in stable patients may be managed conservatively. However, surgical repair is indicated at the first sign of expansion of or deterioration in the patient's condition.

Infections at the access site are related to the length of sheath insertion, the need for repeat PCI, and the need for surgical repair. Organisms are typically gram-positive cocci, usually *Staphylococcus aureus*. Treatment may require several weeks of appropriate antibiotic therapy.

Contrast-induced nephropathy is a rare complication after PCI but remains the major cause of hospital-acquired renal failure (Apple, 2000; Smith et al., 2001). Patients with preexisting renal dysfunction and diabetes are at particular risk. Although the creatinine usually returns to baseline within a few days and hemodialysis is rarely required, nephropathy after PCI is a marker for the development of long-term adverse events (Lindsay et al., 2003). Complications from a catheterization are rare; the risk of major complications is less than 2% (Chart 39–11) (Baim & Grossman, 2000a; Scanlon et al., 1999).

Discharge criteria vary, but typically include stable vital signs, tolerating food and fluids, no evidence of complications at the access site, ability to ambulate without assistance, and void-

---

CHART 39–11 | **Potential Complications of Cardiac Catheterization**

- Death
- Myocardial infarction
- Neurological events
- Emergency surgery
- Cardiac perforation
- Dysrhythmias
- Vascular problems
- Vasovagal reactions
- Allergic reactions

ing without difficulty. Discharge instructions to patients and family members should include management of the access site; when to shower, drive, and return to work; and what to do if the patient develops chest pain.

In summary, the nursing management of patients with coronary artery disease who have undergone a PCI is challenging. The nurse must have an understanding of the procedure, including any complications that may arise and the typical medications that are crucial to optimum outcomes. Details of the nursing management of patients after PCI are given in the Nursing Process: Patient Care Plan After Percutaneous Coronary Intervention (p. 1136) feature. The following section will apply the nursing process to care of patients with coronary artery disease treated by PCI.

Collaborative Management

Care of patients with CAD undergoing urgent PCI requires a collaborative approach among all members of the health care team in different areas of the hospital, such as the emergency department, the cardiac critical care unit, the pharmacy, the catheterization laboratory, the cardiovascular operating room, and the step-down units. Staff in the emergency department must be aware of the need for urgent identification and treatment of any patient presenting with AMI. Medications including antiplatelet and antithrombotic agents need to be started as soon as the diagnosis is confirmed. The patient needs to be transported to the appropriate area for treatment (catheterization laboratory, operating room, or nursing unit) without delay. Catheterization laboratory personnel, including invasive cardiovascular professionals, health care providers, and nurses, must be prepared to treat AMI patients quickly, whether it is during the middle of a busy day or in the middle of the night. All health care team members must cooperate in order to meet the goal of restoring blood flow to the occluded artery as quickly as possible. Once the PCI is completed, the patient and family will require intensive education from the health care team regarding identification and management of all cardiac risk factors. For many patients, this procedure represents their first invasive cardiac procedure and usually requires significant changes in lifestyle. Because patients undergoing successful PCI may remain in the hospital for only a few days, this process should be started as soon as possible, because changes in lifestyle affect not only the patient but also the entire family.

Discharge Priorities

Patients are able to leave the hospital 24 to 36 hours after an uncomplicated PCI. Serum laboratory values are checked before discharge to verify that hemoglobin, hematocrit, and creatinine levels are within acceptable range and that there has been no abnormal elevation of cardiac enzymes. Physical examination includes a complete cardiovascular assessment, as well as auscultation and palpation of the vascular access site. If any tenderness, large hematoma, or bruit is noted, discharge must be postponed until the access site is stable.

Patients should be given written instructions regarding care of the access site, as well as what to do if they experience chest pain or other symptoms of CAD. All cardiac medications should be reviewed, with emphasis on the importance of not stopping any

medicine (especially antiplatelet and adenosine diphosphate inhibitor drugs) without first discussing this with the cardiologist. Finally, patients should be reminded of the need for careful follow-up with their health care provider. Comprehensive instructions are presented in the Patient Teaching & Discharge Priorities box (p. 1137).

Health Promotion

Patients should be discharged with instructions regarding risk factor modification and appropriate medical therapy. See Chapter 40 for a more detailed discussion of risk factors and medical therapy.

Depending on the patient's risk factors and clinical history, secondary prevention should include:

- Aspirin therapy
- Control of high blood pressure
- Control of diabetes
- Aggressive control of lipids
- Smoking cessation, if indicated
- Control of weight
- Physical exercise
- Angiotensin-converting enzyme (ACE) inhibitor therapy for patients with poor left ventricular function (ejection fraction < 40%).

The National Heart, Lung, and Blood Institute, the American Heart Association, the American College of Cardiology, and the National Cholesterol Education Program (NCEP) Expert Panel have jointly published national guidelines for the management of cardiovascular risk factors (Grundy et al., 2004). The importance of these guidelines is presented in the National Guidelines for the Management of Risk Factors for Cardiovascular Disease box (p. 1138).

Complementary and Alternative Therapies

Discharge teaching for patients with CAD is not complete without addressing complementary and alternative medicine (CAM). According the National Institutes of Health National Center for Complementary and Alternative Medicine, CAM is "a group of diverse medical and health care systems, practices, and products that are not presently considered to be part of conventional medicine" (National Institutes of Health, 2008). *Complementary* refers to therapies used together with conventional medicine; alternative therapies are used in place of conventional medicine. Estimates of the prevalence of CAM in patients with CAD range from 9% to over 60%; the wide variation is due in part to what exactly is considered CAM and the population surveyed (Bond & Heitkemper, 2005; Gold & Farnsworth, 2002).

Summary

Between 1987 and 2001 the number of PCI procedures in the United States increased by 266% (American Heart Association, 2003). Between the current epidemic of metabolic syndrome (type II diabetes mellitus, obesity, and hyperlipidemia), the aging of the population, and continued advances in technology, this

NURSING PROCESS: Patient Care Plan After Percutaneous Coronary Intervention

Assessment of Chest Pain

Subjective Data:
When did the pain start?
Is this pain like your typical angina?

Objective Data:
Vital signs including oxygen saturation.
12-lead electrocardiogram (ECG).
Heart and lung sounds.
Skin.
Peripheral pulses.

Nursing Assessment and Diagnoses	Outcomes and Evaluation Parameters	Planning and Interventions with *Rationales*
Nursing Diagnosis: *Acute Pain* related to transmission and perception of cutaneous, visceral, muscular, or ischemic impulses	**Outcome:** Management of chest pain and rapid initiation of appropriate treatment. *Evaluation Parameters:* 12-lead ECG—no change from previous ECG. Oxygen saturation within normal levels. Patient reports relief or lessening of chest pain. Laboratory values within normal levels. Patient/family are able to verbalize feelings.	**Interventions and *Rationales:*** Obtain 12-lead ECG. *To evaluate ischemic changes.* Administer oxygen as ordered; monitor oxygen saturation. *To assess adequacy of gas exchange.* Administer nitrates as ordered. Monitor vital signs and assess level of pain. *To assess relief of ischemia and prevent side effects, such as hypotension.* Administer analgesia as ordered. Monitor vital signs, and level of consciousness. *To assess relief of ischemia and prevent side effects such as respiratory depression.* Monitor laboratory values, especially cardiac enzymes and hematology. *Elevated cardiac enzymes after PCI may indicate reocclusion of the infarcted artery. A low hemoglobin/hematocrit may precipitate ischemic chest pain.* Assess level of anxiety of patient and family members. *Anxiety related to the procedure and diagnosis of AMI can precipitate nonischemic pain.*

Assessment of Cardiac Risk Factors

Subjective Data:
What are your risk factors for heart disease?
What medications are you taking?
Are you overweight?
How much physical exercise do you do in a typical week?
What type of food do you like to eat?

Objective Data:
Patient's body mass index (BMI) (weight/height^2, ideal < 25).
Blood pressure.
Lipid levels.
Smoking history.
Current medications.
Dietary habits.
Physical exercise.

Nursing Assessment and Diagnoses	Outcomes and Evaluation Parameters	Planning and Interventions with *Rationales*
Nursing Diagnosis: *Deficient Knowledge* related to current management of cardiac risk factors	**Outcome:** All appropriate cardiac risk factors are identified and patient/family verbalize understanding of discharge instructions. *Evaluation Parameters:* 1. Patient/family verbalize understanding of: Diet changes Regular exercise Weight control Medications	**Interventions and *Rationales:*** Measure patient's height and weight to calculate BMI. Evaluate results according to the American Heart Association guidelines. *People underestimate how much they weigh.* Evaluate multiple blood pressure readings after PCI. Evaluate results according to the American Heart Association guidelines. *Current guidelines indicate aggressive treatment of high blood pressure is necessary to decrease the risk of cardiac events. Family members may also need to be screened based upon the results.* Evaluate results of lipid profile with patient and family. *Treatment will depend on values and other risk factors. Family members may also need to be tested based on the results.* Assess patient's willingness to stop smoking, if this is indicated. *Goal for all people is no smoking. Include family members in this discussion in order to enhance compliance.* Assess current medications to ensure appropriate treatment of risk factors. *Patients often need written instructions at the appropriate reading level to enhance compliance.* Assess current dietary habits. Nutritional counseling may be indicated. *People frequently underestimate the amount of fat and calories consumed in an average meal.* Assess level of current physical exercise. *Before starting an exercise program, the patient will need to be cleared by her health care provider.*

PATIENT TEACHING & DISCHARGE PRIORITIES for Percutaneous Coronary Intervention and Heart Disease

Need	Teaching
Vascular Access Site Patient Family Setting	Assess the site daily. Some amount of bruising and firmness/tenderness at the site is normal. Patient should call her health care provider if the area of firmness gets bigger instead of smaller. The bruising should resolve by 4 to 6 weeks. • Shower or bathe as usual. • No special dressing is needed. • Take Tylenol for any discomfort at the site. If the access site was in groin, avoid bending over or straining for the first 48 hours. Avoid heavy lifting for the first week. • If patient experiences any of the following in her leg, toes, or foot, she should call her health care provider immediately: • Numbness • Tingling • Coolness. If patient experiences bright-red bleeding from the site, she should lie down and have someone apply firm pressure just above the site for 20 minutes and then gently release the pressure. If the bleeding cannot be controlled, call 911. If the access site was sealed using a special closure device, the patient will have received special instructions regarding the device. Usually no special care is required, but patient needs to keep these instructions containing the name of the device in case she or her health care provider has questions or concerns about the site. Assess availability, knowledge, and compliance with treatment regimen. Validate follow-up appointment with local health care provider. Assess availability of emergency health care.
Activity Patient	Patient should not resume or start an exercise program until he has been evaluated by his doctor. Regular exercise is a key component in maintaining a heart-healthy lifestyle. Patient must notify his health care provider immediately if he experiences any of the following during exercise: • Chest pain, especially pain similar to typical angina • Nausea, vomiting, or cool, clammy skin • Extreme or persistent fatigue not relieved by a short rest period • Shortness of breath, especially if it makes talking difficult • A change in heart rhythm. If patient has had a heart attack, he should be able to resume sexual relations in 4 weeks. Again, this should be discussed with his health care provider. Patient should notify his health care provider if he experiences any of the following: • Rapid heartbeat, palpitations, or shortness of breath persisting for 15 minutes after intercourse • Chest pain during or after intercourse • Extreme fatigue. Patient should be able to return to work very quickly. Discuss this with the health care provider.
Knowledge of Disease Process and Prognosis/Risk Factor Modification Patient Family Setting	It is critically important to obtain regular follow-up from one's health care provider. A heart-healthy lifestyle includes: • Weight control • Regular exercise • Smoking cessation • Diet high in fruits and vegetables and low in fat. Medications that may be prescribed include: • Aspirin therapy • Hypertensive control • Diabetes management • Lipid lowering agent. Other medications may be indicated, depending on the health of the patient's heart. Assess availability, knowledge, and compliance with treatment regimen. Assess need for lifestyle modification for all family members. Assess need for cardiac rehabilitation. Assess ability to obtain necessary medications after discharge.
Emotional Adjustment of Patient/Family Due to Chronic Nature of the Disease Patient Family Setting	Assess patient's understanding of need for lifelong medications and potential change in lifestyle. Assess family's ability to support necessary changes. Assess need for referrals to support therapeutic lifestyle changes.

number will certainly continue to increase. All members of the health care team will be challenged to keep up with the latest developments in order to continue to deliver the expert care required of all patients.

Evaluating and Treating Dysrhythmias

Cardiac dysrhythmias range from clinically insignificant (occasional premature atrial beats) to potentially lethal (ventricular fibrillation). An in-depth discussion of dysrhythmias is covered in Chapter 38. The significance of the dysrhythmia also depends on the clinical diagnosis; patients with severe coronary disease or valvular obstructions often cannot tolerate even minor dysrhythmias and require aggressive management. As always, the health care professional should begin with a careful history and physical examination before deciding which diagnostic test to utilize (Fenton, 2001; Miller & Zipes, 2001).

Ambulatory Electrocardiogram Monitoring

Ambulatory ECG monitoring, frequently called **Holter monitoring** after its inventor Norman Holter, was developed in the 1960s and first used clinically to detect ventricular dysrhythmias in patients recovering from acute myocardial infarction (Fenton, 2001; Holter, 1961). Today there are many indications for Holter monitoring, as it has become a valuable noninvasive tool with numerous clinical applications (Chart 39–12) (Crawford et al., 1999; Kadish et al., 2001).

CHART 39–12 Indications for Holter Monitoring

1. Assess symptoms that may be related to a dysrhythmia, such as syncope or palpitations.
2. Assess therapy response such as cardiac medications.
3. Monitor the rate of atrial fibrillation.
4. Analyze pacemakers or implantable cardioverter defibrillators.
5. Detect silent myocardial ischemia.
6. Assess heart rate variability.

Holter's original monitor was a 75-pound backpack that could record only a single ECG lead (Helena Cardiology Clinic, n.d.). Current Holter monitoring systems consist of leads placed on the chest that are connected to a small recording device, which can be worn around the waist or on a strap over the patient's shoulder. Typically two or three leads of ECG data are recorded, either continuously for 24 to 48 hours or when activated by the patient during periods of symptoms such as palpitations or dizziness. In general continuous recordings are indicated for assessment of frequent (at least once a day) symptoms that may be related to a dysrhythmia, syncope or near syncope, and unexplained palpitations (Kadish et al., 2001). If the symptoms occur very infrequently and other diagnostic tests have failed to provide a diagnosis, an implantable loop recorder can be utilized. Typically placed subcutaneously in the left subclavian or parasternal areas, these devices can be left in place for months or even years, increasing the probability of capturing the ECG during the time of the clinical event (Fenton, 2001; Futterman & Lemberg, 2002).

Holter monitoring is safe and relatively inexpensive. Because the electrodes must remain in place for 1 to 2 days, skin preparation is very important to ensure tracings free of artifact. Patients should be instructed not to pull at the electrodes, and to go about their normal daily activities. Frequently they are asked to keep a diary to record their activities and the occurrence of any symptoms during monitoring.

Electrophysiology Study

The **electrophysiology study (EPS)** is an invasive procedure that involves placing multiple multipolar catheter electrodes into the venous and sometimes the arterial side of the heart. These electrodes are positioned at various locations inside of the heart and they have two purposes: to record the electrical signal within the heart and to deliver an electrical stimulus at precisely timed intervals (programmed stimulation).

Developed in the 1960s, EPS originally recorded only intracardiac electrical activity during spontaneously occurring dysrhythmias in order to identify the location of the dysrhythmia, thereby determining treatment options. Currently EPS is the standard test for reproducing dysrhythmias in a controlled environment in order to diagnose and treat the disorder. EPS can include delivering programmed electrical stimulation in order to provoke dysrhythmias (a major indication for EPS), as well as pacing protocols to assess AV nodal function. During EPS catheters with several electrodes are advanced percutaneously and positioned within the heart; the exact location depends on the source of the dysrhythmia. Detailed recordings of the electrical activity of the heart are obtained, including interval measurements (time for the electrical activity to travel from one area of the conduction system to another) as well as the direction of conduction. Programmed electrical stimulation involves use of the catheters to deliver programmed stimulus in order to initiate the dysrhythmia. A series of impulses is delivered to the myocardium in an attempt to cause a tachyarrhythmia. If successful, the dysrhythmia is termed inducible. Treatment is instituted and the same procedure is repeated; if the tachy-arrhythmia cannot be induced, the treatment is successful. Medications to increase the heart rate such as epinephrine or isoproterenol also may be utilized to assess the conduction system (Blancher, 2005).

In addition, EPS can assess the function of SA and AV nodes and assess the effectiveness of specific antiarrhythmic medications. When assessing the cardiac conduction, the rate is turned up faster than the intrinsic rate, allowing the catheter to be the cardiac pacemaker. Then the stimulus is shut off and the time it takes for the SA node to take control is assessed. If the time is prolonged, the SA node is diseased.

During the 1980s EPS moved from strictly a diagnostic procedure to include multiple therapeutic and treatment regimens, such as radiofrequency catheter ablation, as permanent treatment for several dysrhythmias (Chart 39–13) (Blancher, 2005; Janosik, Quattromani, & Schiller, 2003; Miller & Zipes, 2001; Tracy, Akhtar, DiMarco, Packer, & Weitz, 2000). **Ablation** refers to destruction of an area of the myocardium through localized delivery of chemicals or electrical energy. Radiofrequency catheter ablation is one of the major advances in the treatment of supraventricular tachycardia (SVT). See Chapter 38 ⊘ for more detail about SVT. Prior to the development of radiofrequency catheter ablation, most patients required open-heart surgery to treat SVT. In the late 1980s catheters were developed that allowed the application of safe radiofrequency energy to heat the myocardium in very specific locations, thus destroying tissue responsible for dysrhythmia formation and propagation.

Patient preparation for EPS is similar to that for cardiac catheterization. The length of the procedure will vary greatly, depending on the indication for the test. The patient must be clear of severe infection before EPS and must be able to tolerate lying flat and relatively still for an extended period of time. Complications are very rare, but can include death (usually from intractable ventricular dysrhythmias), myocardial perforation (a risk any time catheters are introduced inside the heart), and thrombosis. The need for anticoagulation will depend on the length of the procedure and the position of the catheters. Conscious sedation may be required for long procedures.

Nursing management postprocedure includes a complete cardiovascular assessment, with special emphasis on the ECG as well as the access site. Specific parameters will depend on the type of procedure. Patients are usually discharged the same day after a diagnostic EPS. Discharge instructions include care of the access site, bathing, driving, and return to work. Specific instructions regarding the results of the EPS will depend on the indication for the test.

Electrical Treatment of Cardiac Dysrhythmias

Diagnosis and treatment of cardiac dysrhythmias are discussed in detail in Chapter 38 ⊘ . Cardioversion and defibrillation are common additional procedures used to treat cardiac dysrhythmias. Both of these procedures use a defibrillator that delivers a preset level of electrical voltage to the heart for the purpose of terminating an unwanted dysrhythmia. The electrical current depolarizes the myocardial cells, which is then followed by repolarization. During repolarization the sinus node usually is able to take over its role as the heart's natural pacemaker. Three major factors are assessed when deciding to do cardioversion versus defibrillation: timing of the delivery of the electrical current, rationale for use, and amount of voltage used. Cardioversion and defibrillation are discussed next. Chart 39–14 outlines safety rules when using a defibrillator.

Cardioversion

Cardioversion is defined as the delivery of electrical voltage in order to stop unwanted electrical activity and allow the SA node to

---

CHART 39–13 Selected Indications for Electrophysiology Studies

DIAGNOSTIC

Evaluate sinus and atrioventricular (AV) nodal function.

Confirm the mechanism of ventricular tachycardia.

Relate symptoms to potential dysrhythmias, such as bradycardia.

THERAPEUTIC

Evaluate and determine whether dysrhythmias are suitable for drug, device, or ablation therapy.

Assess effects of pharmacologic therapy.

INTERVENTIONAL

Ablation of AV node.

Ablation of atrial flutter or atrial tachycardias.

Ablation of accessory pathways such as found in Wolff-Parkinson-White.

Ablation of ventricular tachycardias.

PROGNOSTIC

Assess future risk of serious cardiac events.

Assess patient's predisposition to spontaneously occurring dysrhythmias.

Source: Adapted from O'Rourke, R. A., et al. (2000). American College of Cardiology/American Heart Association expert consensus document on electron-beam computed tomography for the diagnosis and prognosis of coronary artery disease. *Circulation, 102,* 126–140.

CHART 39–14 Safety Criteria When Using a Defibrillator

Use designated conductor pads or paddles.

Use designated conductor medium; gel, pastes, sheet.

Place pads or paddles so they are not in contact with the patient's clothes, bed linen, or near medication patches and monitor leads.

Do not place pads or paddles near a direct oxygen source to prevent a fire hazard.

For cardioversion, defibrillator must be set in a synchronous mode.

For defibrillation, defibrillator must be set in an asynchronous mode.

For cardioversion, make sure the monitor leads are attached to the patient.

Do not charge the defibrillator until ready to shock, and keep fingers off discharge buttons until ready to discharge voltage.

Exert enough pressure on the paddles to ensure adequate contact prior to discharging the voltage.

Call for everyone to clear the area prior to discharging the defibrillator.

Document entire procedure and effectiveness of the intervention.

Inspect skin for burns after the procedure, and report and treat per health care provider's orders.

resume as the heart's pacemaker. It is used for the treatment of tachyarrhythmias: atrial tachycardia, rapid atrial fibrillation, atrial flutter, and junctional tachycardia. The procedure typically is performed at the bedside in an area of the hospital where cardiac monitoring is available. The cardiac defibrillator is set on the synchronous mode, meaning it will discharge only on the down slope of the R wave or with the S wave of the QRS complex. Therefore, the electrical voltage will not discharge during the vulnerable period of ventricular repolarization (T wave), which could precipitate ventricular tachycardia and ventricular fibrillation; referred to as the R on T phenomenon. The patient is instructed not to eat or drink for at least 6 hours prior to the procedure, and digoxin is withheld for 48 hours prior to the procedure to ensure resumption of sinoatrial (SA) node activity and normal conduction to the atrioventricular (AV) node. The patient is sedated intravenously prior to the procedure and full resuscitation equipment is available, if necessary. The voltage on the defibrillator begins at 10 to 20 joules (J). If unsuccessful it is increased to 50 joules and increased at intervals to a maximum of 360 joules. The lower the joules, the less the chance of complications such as cardiac necrosis. Success is measured by conversion to normal sinus rhythm, with a normal heart rate and blood pressure. Nursing responsibilities include recording the postcardioversion rhythm, cardiac output, and vital signs for 2 to 3 hours after the procedure. Vital signs, level of consciousness, and oxygen saturation are measured until the patient recovers from the sedation. If the patient converts back to the unwanted rhythm, this must be reported to the health care provider immediately.

Defibrillation

Defibrillation is basically the same as cardioversion in that electrical voltage is delivered to the myocardium to terminate unwanted rhythms, except defibrillation is done in an emergency situation for life-threatening dysrhythmias. It is indicated for patients in ventricular tachycardia and ventricular fibrillation when they have lost consciousness and cardiopulmonary resuscitation is in progress. The defibrillator is usually set in an asynchronous mode unless there are discernable T waves. The voltage on the defibrillator is set at 360 joules. After each defibrillation, the rhythm is evaluated and voltage delivery is repeated as necessary until there is a viable rhythm or resuscitation is stopped. Between each defibrillation, cardiopulmonary resuscitation (CPR) is done to maintain oxygenation. Medications such as lidocaine, amiodarone, epinephrine, and vasopressin typically are administered during resuscitation to assist in conversion to normal sinus rhythm.

During both cardioversion and defibrillation, paddles or conductor pads are applied to the patient's chest and attached to the defibrillator. Figure 39–11 ■ demonstrates normal paddle placement using both the standard and anteroposterior placement.

Whichever type of pad is used, it must have a conducting medium to prevent burning the patient's skin.

Monophasic Versus Biphasic Defibrillation

Monophasic defibrillation is the traditional means by which electric voltage is delivered to patients in ventricular tachycardia

FIGURE 39–11 ■ Defibrillator paddle.

and fibrillation. These high-energy defibrillators deliver an electrical charge in one direction only. Side effects of monophasic defibrillation are the risks of burning the skin on the chest where the site of the voltage is delivered and postshock myocardial dysfunction manifested by prolonged ischemic ST segment changes. Having no other choice, clinicians historically believed that the benefits of monophasic defibrillation outweighed the side effects. In an attempt to reduce or eliminate side effects, researchers in the 1990s began evaluating low-energy biphasic defibrillation. **Biphasic defibrillation** delivers a charge in one direction for half of the shock and in the opposite direction for the second half. Biphasic shocks appear to achieve the same defibrillation success rates (most often defined as termination of ventricular fibrillation [VF] for at least 3 to 5 seconds) as monophasic waveforms, but with significantly lower energy levels (Amato-Vealey & Colonies, 2005). Therefore, fewer side effects such as burned skin and myocardial dysfunction have been noted.

Defibrillator manufacturers are able to achieve some technological advantages from these lower-energy devices in that they can be made smaller, lighter, less expensive, and less demanding of batteries, with fewer maintenance requirements.

Automated External Defibrillator

An **automated external defibrillator (AED)** is a small, lightweight device that can recognize and treat ventricular fibrillation (VF), also known as "sudden cardiac arrest" (SCA). The AED is designed for use by lay rescuers or "first responders" (Hallstrom, Ornato, Weisfeldt, Travers, 2004). If SCA is present, an AED will talk the responder through the very simple steps to defibrillate. These devices have been shown to decrease mortality when used in conjunction with cardiopulmonary resuscitation (CPR) (Federal Occupational Health, 2008). Once the domain of only highly trained emergency professionals, these technologically advanced defibrillators are now available on board airlines, on cruise ships, and in other public places. These defibrillators are appropriate for use with infants and children, as well as adults, as long as the appropriate pads are used. Typically, children over 55 pounds (25 kilograms) or 8 years of age are defibrillated as adults. Precautions when using AEDs include:

- Ensure pulseless criteria are met before AED is applied.
- Withhold unit analysis of the rhythm during cardiopulmonary resuscitation (CPR).

- Withhold unit analysis of the rhythm if the patient is seizing.
- Use caution with rhythm analysis in a moving vehicle.
- Stop frequently for rhythm analysis during transport.
- Place electrodes without shaving chest; not required for effective placement.
- Ensure skin is dry and free of nicks and cuts for effective electrode placement.
- Perform regular maintenance and battery placement according to manufacturer's recommendations.

Implantable Cardioverter Defibrillator

An **implantable cardioverter defibrillator (ICD)** is a device that can automatically terminate potentially lethal dysrhythmias of ventricular tachycardia and ventricular fibrillation. Developed by Dr. Michael Mirowski, the first ICD implanted in humans in 1980 was nonprogrammable and capable of defibrillating only the heart (Mirowski, 1985). Since that time ICDs, like all pacemakers, have become smaller, are programmable, and can combine a variety of therapies in one device, including:

- Tiered electrical therapy—the ability to deliver low-voltage cardioversion or high-voltage defibrillation
- Antitachycardia pacing—the ability to pace the heart at a faster rate than a tachycardia (supraventricular or ventricular), enabling the device to capture (control) the intrinsic heart rate and gradually slow it down to a normal heart rate
- Programmable ventricular or atrial pacing.

Current ICDs have been referred to as "an electrophysiology study (EPS) in a can" for their ability to analyze the ECG and deliver appropriate therapy, and then store this extensive information for later retrieval. Thus far these devices have effectively proven their lifesaving value, resulting in expanded indications for their use (Chart 39–15).

ICD System

The ICD system is similar to traditional pacemakers in that it consists of a pulse generator and defibrillation leads for both dysrhythmia detection and delivery of therapy (Jacobson & Gerity, 2005). Unlike early devices that required open thoracotomy, current ICDs are usually implanted transvenously with generator placement under the chest wall. Depending on the programmed functions of the ICD, the patient may have one, two, or three leads. A single-chamber ICD requires only one lead in the right ventricle. Combining ICD with biventricular pacing requires leads in the right atrium, in the right ventricle, and behind the left ventricle in a coronary vein. The ventricular leads are similar to pacemaker leads in their ability to sense and pace the heart; the difference is the large electrical surface area needed to deliver the shock.

Complications

Potential complications of ICD include those related to traditional pacemaker therapy, such as lead dislodgment or fracture and infection. Long-term potential complications unique to ICD include electromagnetic interference (electrocautery during surgery, radiofrequency transmitters, high-powered electromagnetic fields, etc.) that can result in inappropriate shocks or inhibition of the device (Jacobson & Gerity, 2005; Stone & McPherson, 2004).

CHART 39–15 **Selected Indications for Implantable Cardioverter Defibrillators**

CLASS I

1. Cardiac arrest due to ventricular tachycardia or ventricular fibrillation not due to a transient or reversible cause
2. Spontaneous sustained ventricular tachycardia associated with structural heart disease
3. Syncope of undetermined etiology associated with clinically significant ventricular tachycardia or ventricular fibrillation, and pharmacologic therapy is ineffective, not tolerated, or not preferred
4. Nonsustained ventricular tachycardia in patients with coronary artery disease, prior myocardial infarction, left ventricular dysfunction, and inducible ventricular fibrillation or sustained ventricular tachycardia during an electrophysiology study that is not suppressed by an appropriate antiarrhythmic medication
5. Spontaneous sustained ventricular tachycardia in patients without structural heart disease not amenable to other therapies

CLASS IIA

1. Patients with a left ventricular ejection fraction ≤ 30% at least 1 month after a myocardial infarction or 3 months after coronary artery bypass surgery

Note: According to the American Heart Association/American College of Cardiology, Class I indications are conditions for which there is evidence and/or general agreement that a given procedure or treatment is beneficial, useful, and effective. Class IIa indications are conditions for which conflicting evidence or a divergence of opinion exists, but the weight of the evidence/opinion favors its usefulness/efficacy.

Source: G. Gregoratos et al. (2002). ACC/AHA/NASPE 2002 guideline update for implantation of cardiac pacemakers and antiarrhythmia devices. Circulation, 106, 2145–2161+

If the patient requires external defibrillation, care must be taken not to position the paddles on or near the generator. In any event, the ICD must be thoroughly evaluated after any episode of external defibrillation.

■ Nursing Management

Nursing management of the patient immediately after ICD implantation is similar to care of the patient with a permanent pacemaker. However, most patients and their families need additional support in dealing with the emotional response to ICD implantation (White, 2002). The shock delivered by the ICD is lifesaving, but at the same time it is unpredictable and painful. Patients typically equate a shock to being kicked in the chest or being slammed to the ground. If the shock is delivered when the patient is at work or out in public, she may report feeling embarrassed at her reaction to the shock as well as her loss of control during the episode. Some patients report "phantom shocks," or reporting that a shock has been delivered when in fact the ICD has no record of delivering a shock. In addition, anyone touching the patient during an ICD firing will also feel the shock. The result is not fatal but can be painful. Continued emotional support for the ICD patient and her family before the device is implanted and during follow-up can promote acceptance of the technology and lead to improvement in quality of life.

Cardiac Pacemakers

Although the use of electricity to treat cardiac dysrhythmias dates back to the 16th century, it was not until the 1950s that electricity was successfully applied to clinical practice (Lüderitz, 1995). Following seminal publications by Zoll and others, Zoll successfully resuscitated a patient in full cardiac arrest using electrodes placed on the patient's chest to pace the heart (Zoll, 1952). By 1958 the first implantable cardiac pacemaker was placed by Elmquist and Senning. In 1960 the first battery-powered pacemaker with a myocardial lead was safely implanted by Chardack, and the modern era of cardiac pacemakers had begun. This section will review the basic principles of temporary and permanent artificial cardiac pacemakers.

A **cardiac pacemaker** is an electronic device that is capable of delivering an electrical stimulus to the heart. These devices are used to augment or replace the natural cardiac pacemaker when there is either a congenital abnormality or a disease of the cardiac conduction system. The earliest pacemakers stimulated one ventricle and were used to treat symptomatic bradycardia (heart rate of less than 60 beats per minute). Today pacemakers are capable of delivering impulses to multiple chambers of the heart in order to treat not only bradycardias but also tachydysrhythmias (greater than 100 beats per minute) originating from either the atria or the ventricles (Gregoratos et al., 2002; Obias-Manno, 2001). Current pacemakers also are able to vary the heart rate in accordance with a change in the patient's metabolic demand or activity level.

Pacemaker Components

A pacing system is composed of a generator and lead(s). The type of generator and type and number of leads will depend on the reason for implementing pacemaker therapy. There are basically two types of pacemakers, temporary and permanent, both of which are discussed below. Single-chambered devices pace a single chamber of the heart, such as the right ventricle. Dual-chambered pacemakers pace at least two chambers of the heart, such as the right atrium and the right ventricle, or both ventricles. A single-chambered right ventricular and a dual-chambered right atrium and right ventricular are shown in Figure 39–12 ■.

Generator

The generator contains the electronic circuitry and the power source, and is synonymous with the term *pacemaker* (Figure 39–13 ■).

Permanent pacemakers are small and usually implanted in the pectoral area. The generators of permanent pacemakers are typically composed of titanium and are hermetically (airtight) sealed to prevent erosion from contact with bodily fluids. Lithium-iodine batteries are contained within the generator, as well as the microprocessors that control the various functions of the pacemaker. Implanted generators last between 7 and 10 years, depending on multiple factors such as the amount of time the heart is actually paced (Jacobson & Gerity, 2005; Reynolds & Apple, 2001).

Generators of temporary pacing systems are connected to the pacemaker lead(s) but remain outside the body. They are powered by ordinary batteries and are manually programmed as needed (Figure 39–17 ■, p. 1146).

(a)

(b)

FIGURE 39–12 ■ (A) Single- and (B) dual-chambered pacemakers.

Leads

The pacemaker lead is the connection between the generator and the myocardium (Figure 39–13 ■). Permanent pacemaker leads may be placed inside the cardiac chambers (most common) or on the surface of the heart (epicardial leads). Leads contain tip electrodes, conductor, and insulation (Figure 39–14 ■).

Pacemaker lead

Implantable
generator

Left atrium

Right atrium

Right ventricle

Left ventricle

Anode

Cathode

FIGURE 39–13 ■ Pacemaker components.

Conductor

Tip
electrode

Insulation

Connector pin

FIGURE 39–14 ■ Pacemaker lead components.

The tip electrode is embedded directly into the cardiac tissue. The lead conducts the electrical stimulus between the negative and positive electrodes (poles). Electrical current flows between two metal poles. In a unipolar system, the tip of the electrode contains only the negative (cathode) electrode; the positive (anode) electrode is located in the generator. Most lead systems today are bipolar, meaning the distal tip of the electrode contains the negative pole; the positive pole is an exposed metal ring located a few

millimeters from the tip (see Figure 39–13 ■). The advantage of a bipolar system is that both electrodes are contained within the heart, making it less susceptible to sensing extraneous electrical activity. In addition, less battery power is needed with the bipolar system, thereby increasing the battery life.

Electrical impulses are carried from the generator to the tip electrode (Figure 39–14 ■) across a very thin wire conductor. The conductor also returns sensed intracardiac intrinsic electrical activity

Atrial Artifact

Ventricular Artifact

DDD (Dual: Paces both atria and ventricle, Dual: Senses both atria and ventricle: Dual: Can be programmed to be inhibited or triggered in response to intrinsic activity) pacemaker with evidence of 1:1 atrial and ventricular capture. Every pacing artifact is followed by depolarization. Note that pacemaker sensing can not be evaluated from this ECG because there is no intrinsic rhythm.

(a)

The first three beats exhibit 1:1 capture. After the 4th pacer artifact (arrow), there is no corresponding paced beat. The last QRS complex is an escape beat representing intrinsic ventricular activity.

(b)

FIGURE 39–15 ■ Pacemaker capture: (A) and (B) loss of ventricular capture.

to the generator. This conductor is covered with insulation, silicone or polyurethane, to prevent corrosion of the lead and to prevent current leaking into surrounding body tissues.

Assessment of Pacemaker Function

Information obtained from the ECG must be combined with knowledge of the specific type of pacemaker as well as a complete assessment of the patient in order to evaluate the pacemaker completely. The nurse should review the reason for the pacemaker, the date of insertion, the program settings, and the patient's intrinsic rate, if present.

The ECG should be examined in a systematic fashion regardless of the type of pacemaker (Chart 39–16).

CHART 39–16 ECG Assessment of the Patient with a Pacemaker

1. Assess for any intrinsic electrical activity (the patient's own rhythm). Look for intrinsic P waves or QRS complexes.

2. Assess for pacing spikes (pacer artifact). Pacemakers with bipolar pacing leads (most common) have smaller pacing artifacts than those with unipolar leads. Examine the ECG in more than one lead for evidence of pacing activity.

3. Determine the relationship between the P wave and the QRS complex, if any.

4. Look for capture beats (paced beats) with each pacemaker artifact (1:1 capture).

5. Calculate the heart rate. What is the pacemaker's programmed rate?

Pacemaker Capture

Capture is the depolarization of cardiac muscle after a paced electrical stimulus that results in myocardial contraction (Figure 39–15 ■). Loss of capture is noted when pacing artifact is present without depolarization, and is seen on the ECG as pacing artifact with no paced beat (see Figure 39–15 ■). Loss of capture can be continuous or intermittent.

Once loss of capture is identified, it is important to assess the patient because loss of capture can result in profound bradycardia and hypotension (Reynolds & Apple, 2001). Etiology for loss of capture in a temporary pacemaker includes lead dislodgment (most common), lead fracture, battery failure, altered pacemaker thresholds, perforation of the myocardium by the lead wire, and generator failure. Altered thresholds are the result of local inflammation at the site of the pacemaker wire, which interrupts the transmission of pacemaker signals. Typically, threshold levels will increase over several days after pacemaker insertion, sometimes increasing as much as three times the original level. The use of pacemaker wires containing small amounts of steroids that elute over a period of time, thereby suppressing inflammation, has greatly reduced this potential problem.

Pacemaker Sensitivity

Pacemaker sensitivity is the ability of the pacemaker to detect or "hear" intrinsic electrical activity and respond appropriately. Electrical activity also is generated by normal skeletal muscle activity. In order for the pacemaker to function properly, it must be programmed to detect only normal *cardiac* electrical activity. The sensitivity is usually set at two to three times higher than the threshold level (Chart 39–17).

Threshold levels increase during the first few days after implantation due to inflammation at the tip site. Threshold levels

CHART 39–17 Programming Temporary Pacemaker's Sensing

1. Set pacemaker programmed rate at least 10 beats per minute (beats/min) above the patient's intrinsic heart rate. Check that there is 1:1 capture; that is, every pacemaker spike is followed by a QRS complex and results in a palpable pulse.

2. Slowly decrease the programmed output (energy in milliamperes) until there is loss of capture.

3. Slowly increase the programmed output until there is 1:1 capture. This is the threshold value.

4. Set the programmed output to two to three times higher than the threshold value.

5. Slowly return pacemaker rate to original programmed value.

are usually checked daily while the temporary pacemaker remains in place (Jacobson & Gerity, 2005; Reynolds & Apple, 2001).

In order to evaluate sensing, there must be intrinsic beats on the ECG and the nurse must know the current pacemaker program. *Undersensing* occurs when the pacemaker fails to detect ("hear") intrinsic electrical cardiac activity and delivers inappropriate pacing artifacts (Figure 39–16A ■). Possible causes of undersensing include lead displacement or fracture, loose connections, or generator failure.

Oversensing (Figure 39–16B ■) occurs when the pacemaker is inhibited by inappropriate electrical artifact, such as extraneous muscle activity, or by the T wave on the ECG. A common cause of oversensing is airport security systems. The patient must be instructed not to go through airport security because the pacemaker will interpret the "electrical noise" as cardiac activity and inhibit itself. Depending on the length of exposure, the patient could experience a drop in cardiac output.

Temporary Pacemakers

Temporary pacing can be performed using transvenous, epicardial, or transcutaneous methods. The system used will depend on factors such as the clinical diagnosis and stability of the patient (elective or emergency situation). Temporary pacing is indicated in a variety of conditions (Chart 39–18).

Temporary Transvenous Pacing

Temporary transvenous pacing involves insertion of the lead through a major vein, such as the internal jugular, subclavian, or femoral. The pacing lead is threaded into the right side of the heart; the proximal end is sutured outside the body and connected to an external generator. If an epicardial lead is used, the lead is attached to the outside of the heart (typically during cardiac surgery) and is introduced through the chest wall. Temporary pacemakers can be either single chambered (lead in the ventricle only) or dual chambered (leads in both the atrium and the ventricle). Dual-chambered temporary pacemakers are not widely used at this time.

CHART 39–18 Indications for Temporary Pacemakers

Symptomatic sick sinus syndrome

Symptomatic second- or third-degree heart block

Drug refractory dysrhythmias

Prophylactic after cardiovascular surgery

Prior to insertion of a permanent cardiac pacemaker

Development of significant conduction disturbances after acute myocardial infarction

Overdrive tachydysrhythmias

During cardiac resuscitation

Undersensing. VVI pacemaker programmed at a rate of 60. Pacemaker fails to sense (hear) the intrinsic beat and delivers a pacing artifact into the ST segment of the intrinsic beat (arrow). Pacemaker artifact in this location has been noted to initiate a run of ventricular fibrillation (R on T phenomenon).

(a)

Oversensing. VVI pacemaker programmed at a rate of 60. Pacemaker is inhibited by extraneous electrical activity (arrows). When the pacemaker does fire, there is 1:1 capture.

Note: ECGs from Medtronics, Inc.

(b)

FIGURE 39–16 ■ Pacemaker sensing: (A) undersensing and (B) oversensing.

Programming the External Generator

Once the leads are connected to the generator, the system must be programmed. At a minimum this consists of setting the rate at which the pacemaker will fire, the amount of energy delivered with each paced beat (output), and the sensitivity (Figure 39–17 ■).

The programmed rate determines the patient's minimum heart rate. For example, a single-chamber temporary transvenous pacemaker (VVI) set at 60 beats per minute (beats/min) will deliver an electrical stimulus to the ventricle only when the patient's rate drops below 60. If the patient generates his own heartbeat faster than 60 beats per minute, the pacemaker will be inhibited (Figure 39–18 ■). This is referred to as a demand pacemaker.

The programmed output, the amount of energy delivered by the generator with each paced beat, is measured in milliamperes (ma). The amount of energy must be sufficient to cause capture, which means that a myocardial contraction has occurred.

Pacemaker sensitivity, the amount of electrical activity the pacemaker will sense or "hear," is measured in millivolts (mV).

A sensitivity of 2 millivolts is more sensitive than that of 5 millivolts, because the pacemaker will be able to hear smaller amounts of electrical activity. If the sensitivity is increased to the maximum, the pacemaker becomes asynchronous; that is, the pacemaker cannot sense any intrinsic electrical activity and will pace continuously at its programmed rate. A single-chamber ventricular pacemaker set to asynchronous would be designated VOO (paces the right ventricle, no chamber sensed, and no response to intrinsic beats). The sensitivity is usually set at two to three times higher than *threshold,* which is the minimum amount of current necessary for electrical capture and myocardial contraction (see Chart 39–17, p. 1145).

■ Nursing Management

Care of the patient with an external transvenous pacemaker includes a complete cardiovascular assessment, with special attention to the heart rate. The nurse needs to evaluate the

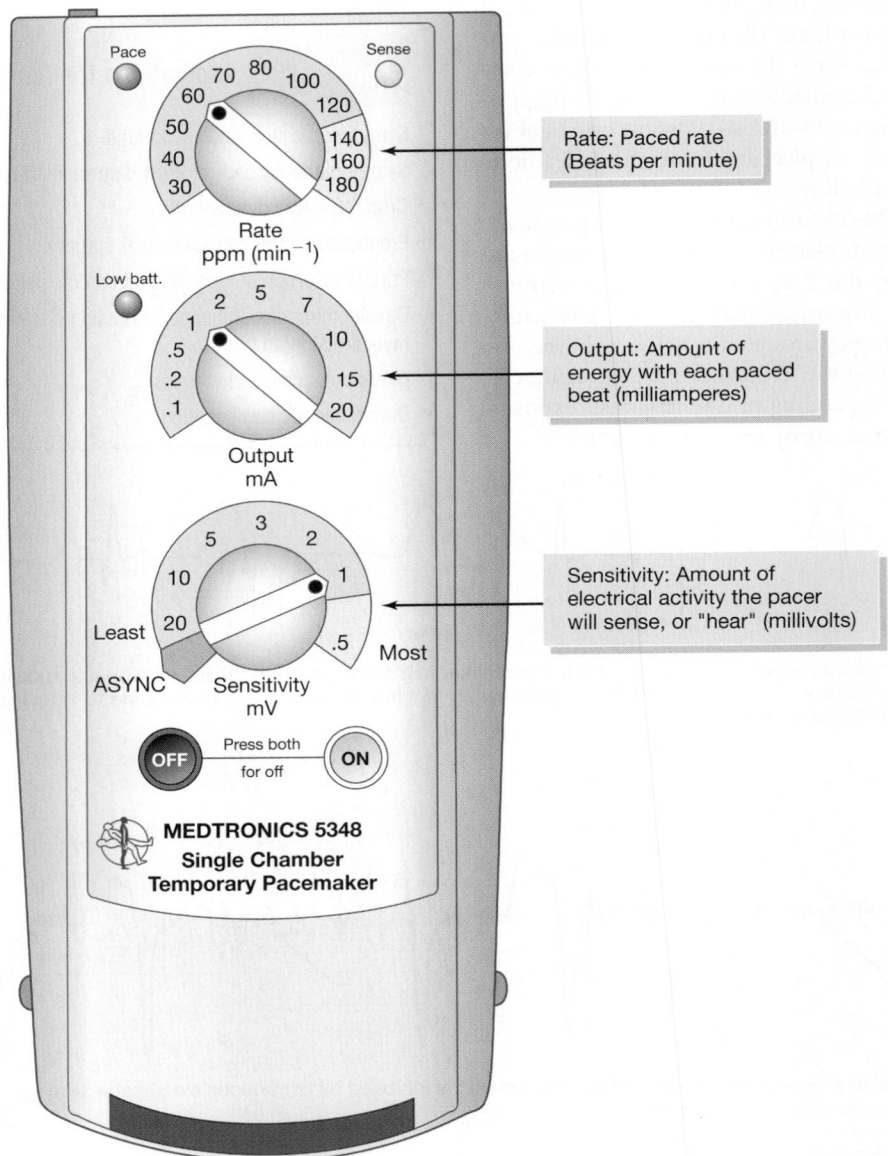

FIGURE 39–17 ■ Temporary pacemaker generator.

Paced ventricular beat. Similar in appearance to a PVC (premature ventricular beat) because like a PVC it also originates in the ventricle.

Pacemaker is "listening" for another intrinsic beat. The pacemaker will wait until the heart rate reaches 60; if there is no intrinsic beat (as in this ECG), it will deliver another paced beat.

Pacemaker artifact: The pacemaker has delivered an electrical current (fired) to the ventricle resulting in capture (paced beat).

Intrinsic (patient's own heart beat) beat: The VVI pacemaker appropriately senses ("hears") this beat and is inhibited (no pacemaker artifact present).

VVI Pacemaker: (Paces the ventricle; Senses the ventricle; Inhibited when it senses intrinsic electrical activity. This VVI pacemaker is set at a rate of 60.

FIGURE 39–18 ■ VVI pacemaker.

rhythm strip to determine whether capture is occurring appropriately. Thus, the nurse questions: If it is a single-chambered pacemaker, is there a QRS after each pacemaker spike, and if it is dual-chambered pacemaker, is there a P wave after the atrial spike and a QRS after the ventricular spike? Additionally, the nurse needs to assess for normal sensing. For example, does the pacemaker inhibit itself when there is intrinsic cardiac activity? Does the patient's heart rate and blood pressure indicate that the pacemaker rate is appropriate? Another important assessment is how often the pacemaker is pacing the heart. It typically is expressed in percentages and usually is a close approximation; for example, the patient is being paced 50% of the time. With a temporary pacemaker this will assist in determining the need for a permanent pacemaker.

In addition, electrical safety practices are critically important, because the leads are capable of carrying electrical current directly into the heart (Jacobson & Gerity, 2005; Overbay & Criddle, 2004).

1. *Always wear gloves when handling the pacemaker leads or connecting cables.*
2. *Verify that all connections are securely fastened.*
3. *Verify that all equipment in the room is electrically grounded.*
4. *If they are not connected to an external generator, keep epicardial leads covered in a disposable glove or a small tube.*
5. *Do not touch any of the pacemaker components on first entering the patient's room to avoid static electricity.*

Nurses should always wear gloves when handling any component of the pacemaker to avoid microshocks. The generator should be securely attached in order to avoid accidental dislodgment of the leads. Care of the access site should incorporate standards of care for any vascular access site.

Temporary Transcutaneous Pacing

Transcutaneous pacing (TCP) is accomplished by delivering the electrical stimulus directly through the chest wall. A variety

of devices is currently available; most portable defibrillators are now equipped with optional external pacing capabilities (Figure 39–19 ■).

Technological advances have resulted in TCP systems that are more reliable and safer to use, resulting in expanded indications for TCP (Chart 39–19, p. 1148).

Large-surface adhesive electrodes, similar to defibrillation electrodes, are placed on the anterior and posterior chest wall over the heart (Figure 39–20 ■, p. 1148).

If this is not feasible, the pads may be placed on the anterior chest wall on the right shoulder and over the left apex. Skin preparation is critical to optimize capture. If there is time the

FIGURE 39–19 ■ Temporary transcutaneous pacemaker.
Source: Courtesy of ZOLL Medical Corporation

FIGURE 39–21 ■ Permanent pacemakers.
Source: Reproduced with permission of Medtronic, Inc.

nurse should wash the skin with soap and water and thoroughly dry the chest, and avoid alcohol or benzoin. If there is significant body hair it may be trimmed carefully; shaving is avoided because this can leave small cuts, making TCP painful. The electrodes are placed firmly on the chest, avoiding the diaphragm and any metal on the patient, including permanent pacemakers. After the electrodes are applied, the programmed rate is set and the output increased until there is capture. Because TCP results in skeletal muscle movement, it is important to verify capture through palpation of a major vessel, preferably the femoral artery. Problems encountered with TCP include failure to capture, failure to sense, and painful stimulation of the chest wall. Newer systems have overcome many of these limitations.

Permanent Cardiac Pacemakers

The earliest pacemakers were implanted to treat symptomatic bradycardia; that is, "a documented bradydysrhythmia that is directly responsible for the development of the clinical manifestations of frank syncope or near syncope, transient dizziness or lightheadedness, and confusional states resulting from cerebral hypoperfusion attributable to slow heart rate" (Gregoratos et al., 2002, p. 4). Figure 39–21 ■ shows various pacemakers from the very first larger units to the current small, compact unit.

Although correcting symptomatic bradycardia remains the cornerstone of permanent pacemaker therapy, indications for implantation have greatly expanded. Technological advances have expanded the ability of pacemakers to detect and treat a variety of dysrhythmias as well as structural abnormalities such as cardiomyopathy (Gregoratos et al., 2002; Obias-Manno, 2001) (Chart 39–20).

Device Selection

Once the decision has been made to implant a permanent pacemaker, the clinician and patient are faced with a wide variety of choices (Chart 39–21).

Published guidelines exist to aid in the choice of the most appropriate therapy (Gregoratos et al., 2002). The nurse must be aware that there is frequently more than one treatment option. The choice of pacemaker will depend on the indication(s) for pacing, health care provider and patient preference, and availability and cost of the device.

Permanent Pacemaker Vocabulary

In order to understand pacemakers, the nurse must be familiar with basic pacemaker terminology and functions, which are outlined in Charts 39–22 and 39–23 (p. 1150).

In addition, a standard pacemaker code was originally developed in 1974 by the Inter-Society Commission for Heart Disease (ICHD) to describe the properties of any pacemaker. The original code contained three letters; however, with the advent of the more complex dual-chambered pacemakers, the code was expanded to five letters in 1987 (Chart 39–24, p. 1150).

It is not always necessary to use all five categories to identify clinically significant information. Two of the most commonly used pacing modes include VVI and DDD. The VVI pacemaker has the ability to pace the right ventricle (V), sense the intrinsic electrical activity in the right ventricle (V), and inhibit itself (does not deliver an electrical stimulus) when sensing intrinsic activity (I). The DDD pacemaker (also referred to as a dual-chambered or physiological pacemaker) has leads in both the right atrium and the right ventricle. The first D (dual) in the code indicates that these pacemakers can deliver atrial or ventricular paced beats, or both, depending on the settings. The second D indicates the ability to sense intrinsic electrical activity in both the right atrium and right ventricle. The third D indicates the ability of the

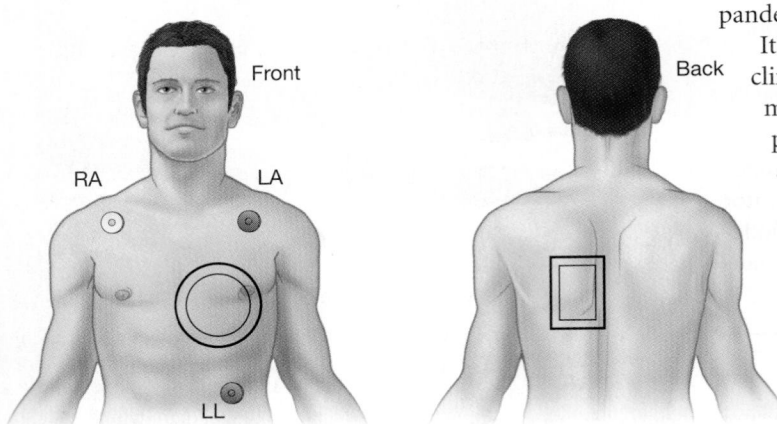

FIGURE 39–20 ■ Transcutaneous conductor pad placement.

Indications for Permanent Cardiac Pacemaker

1. Acquired atrioventricular block in adults
2. Chronic bifascicular and trifascicular block
3. Atrioventricular block associated with acute myocardial infarction
4. Sinus node dysfunction
5. Prevention and termination of tachydysrhythmias
6. Hypersensitive carotid sinus and neurocardiogenic syncope
7. Patients with congenital heart disease
8. In certain conditions:
   a. Hypertrophic obstructive cardiomyopathy
   b. Idiopathic dilated cardiomyopathy
   c. Cardiac transplantation.

Treatment of the preceding indications does not always require pacemaker implantation, and in many instances acceptable alternative therapies are available.

Source: "ACC/AHA/NASPE 2002 guideline update for implantation of cardiac pacemakers and antidysrhythmia devices." G. Gregortos et al., 2002, *Circulation,* 106: 2145–2161.

Selection of Pacemaker Device

GENERATOR

1. Single chamber versus dual chamber (Pace the atria, or ventricle, or both?)
2. Unipolar versus bipolar
3. Rate response; type of sensor for rate response (Pacer will have the ability to adapt to changing physiological needs, such as sleep or exercise.)
4. Advanced features
5. Battery capacity
6. Size of the generator
7. Cost

LEAD

1. Single or dual lead(s)
2. Polarity (bipolar or unipolar)
3. Type of insulation (silicone rubber or polyurethane)
4. Active or passive fixation (active fixation leads are permanently attached, usually by means of a small screw at the tip)
5. Steroid eluting tip (can result in lower thresholds for pacing and thus prolong battery life)

OTHER

1. Programming capabilities
2. Availability of technical support
3. Frequency and type of clinical follow-up required (clinic visits or transtelephonic monitoring)

Basic Pacemaker Vocabulary

Term	Definition
Anode	Positive electrode
Cathode	Negative electrode
Current	Volume of flow of the energy, measured in milliamperes (ma)
Voltage	Force of electrical energy from the generator through the lead to the electrode tip
Resistance	Function of lead integrity at the electrode and myocardial interface; opposes the flow of current; measured in ohms
Programmer	External device used to communicate with pacemaker for information stored in the pacer memory; enables the clinician to check settings and make changes
Rate modulation	Ability of pacemaker to vary its pacing rate automatically to adapt to physiological needs, such as exercise or sleep (also known as rate response)
Crosstalk	Inappropriate sensing of one lead or chamber activity by another
Tracking	Ventricular pacing in a 1:1 response to sensed atrial activity; that is, the ventricular rate will match the atrial rate

pacemaker to be either inhibited or triggered in response to a sensed activity. DDD pacemakers are commonly referred to as physiological pacemakers because of their ability to maintain atrial contraction followed by ventricular contraction, which most closely mimics normal intrinsic cardiac activity. The fourth letter of the code indicates programmability and rate modulation. In the United States, the overwhelming majority of modern permanent pacemakers have rate modulation, the ability to adjust the pacing rate automatically, as a programmable feature (Lamas, Ellenbogen, Hennekens, & Montanez, 2004).

Cardiac Resynchronization Therapy

Cardiac resynchronization therapy (CRT) refers to atrial-synchronized biventricular pacemakers (Abraham & Hayes, 2003; Auricchio & Abraham, 2004; Jacobson & Gerity, 2005; Leclercq & Hare, 2004; Legge & Leeper, 2002). The three leads necessary for this system are a right atrial lead, a right ventricular lead, and a left ventricular lead. The right leads are positioned inside the cardiac chambers; the left ventricular lead is usually placed in a left lateral vein via the coronary sinus.

Normally the right and left ventricles are activated almost simultaneously, resulting in synchronous systole and diastole. In patients with systolic heart failure, approximately 30% have a prolonged QRS complex (>120 milliseconds). A prolonged QRS results in a significant delay in the electrical activation of the left ventricle, resulting in ventricular dyssynchrony (left ventricular systole occurs after right ventricular systole). This dyssynchrony between the right and left ventricles results in a paradoxical motion of the interventricular septum; that is, instead of contracting with the left ventricle, the septal wall moves toward the right ventricle. Ventricular dyssynchrony forces a mechanical disadvantage

CHART 39–23 Basic Pacemaker Functions

Function	Definition
AV interval	The pacemaker's PR interval; the interval between the programmed or sensed P wave and the programmed or sensed QRS.
Capture	Myocardial contraction in response to the pacemaker firing; a palpable pulse is felt with every paced beat.
Hysteresis	The ability of a pacemaker to wait until a lower heart rate than the pacing rate before initiating pacing. For example, the pacemaker may be programmed to pace at a rate of 80, but the pacemaker will not start pacing until the patient's heart rate has dropped to 65.
Magnet rate	Rate of a pacer that is produced when a magnet is applied to the generator. The ability of the pacemaker to generate a magnet rate is a function of the battery and is useful in determining time to generator replacement.
Program	The parameters of the pacemaker; also refers to the ability to change or set the pacemaker's parameters noninvasively.
Pulse amplitude	Output voltage needed to stimulate the heart, measured in volts (V); how much current is needed to have capture.
Pulse width	The duration of the output, measured in milliseconds (ms); how long the electrical current is delivered to the heart.
Sensitivity	Pacemaker's ability to sense intrinsic cardiac activity (the patient's own heartbeat), measured in millivolts (mV).
Stimulation threshold	Minimum amount of energy required to capture the heartbeat consistently.

on an already failing heart (Jacobson & Gerity, 2005; Leclercq & Hare, 2004). This mechanical disadvantage results in a further drop in cardiac output and heart failure.

Biventricular pacemakers were first implanted in the early 1990s. However, the early systems required open-heart surgery and were plagued with high failure rates. Since that time technological advances have resulted in CRT systems that can be inserted percutaneously with a high rate of success. These devices are used for patients with severe systolic heart failure who have a prolonged QRS and remain symptomatic despite optimal medical management; these patients experience improved cardiac function with CRT. This therapy increases cardiac output and decreases ventricular filling pressures. In addition, CRT results in a decrease in heart failure symptoms and improved quality of life. In 2001 CRT was approved by the U.S. Food and Drug Administration (FDA) for use in this population (Abraham & Hayes, 2003; Leclercq & Hare, 2004). The latest advances in CRT devices include combining cardioverter/defibrillation capabilities with biventricular pacing, eliminating the need for a separate ICD in certain patients. In the fall of 2004, these combination devices were approved by the FDA for placement in patients who meet the criteria for CRT, regardless of whether they currently require an ICD. CRT is discussed in Chapter 42 as it relates to heart failure.

Nursing Management

Care of the patient with a new permanent pacemaker is similar to care of a patient with a temporary pacemaker. The nurse should be familiar with the type of pacemaker and current program settings. The patient should be assessed frequently for signs and symptoms of inadequate cardiac output that could be related to the pacemaker, such as hypotension, dizziness, or sudden syncope.

Discharge Teaching

Discharge instructions include care of the access site as well as providing the patient with the pacemaker information card provided by all pacemaker manufacturers. The patient should carry this information with her at all times. In addition, a letter from her health care provider and a medic alert bracelet will aid travel through systems such as airports that require screening by metal detectors. Finally, even though current technology has rendered pacemakers relatively easy to implant and maintenance free, careful long-term follow-up is necessary to avoid potential problems. The complexity of modern pacemakers makes it difficult to evaluate pacemaker function fully with only the ECG. Pacemaker device questioning by a trained professional is necessary to evaluate pacemaker function and settings completely (Jacobson & Gerity, 2005). This may occur in the office or by telephone.

CHART 39–24 Pacemaker Code

Chamber Paced	Chamber Sensed	Response of Sensing	Programmability	Antitachycardia Pacing Functions
0 = None	0 = None	0 = None	0 = None	0 = None
A = Atrium	A = Atrium	T = Triggered	P = Simple programmable	P = Antitachycardia pacing
V = Ventricle	V = Ventricle	I = Inhibited	M = Multiprogrammable	S = Shock
D = Dual (A and V)	D = A and V	D = Trigger and inhibited	C = Communicating	D = P and S
			R = Rate Modulation	

Sources: Code adapted from Parsonnet, V., Furman, S., & Smyth, N. P. D. (1974). Implantable cardiac pacemakers: Status report and resource guideline. *Circulation, 50,* 21A–35A; and Berstein, A. D., Camm, A. J., Fletcher, R. D., Gold, R. D., Rickards, A. F., Smyth, N. P., et al. (1987). The NASPE/BPEG generic pacemaker code for antibradycardia and adaptive-rate pacing and antitachyarrhythmia devices. *Pacing and Clinical Electrophysiology, 10,* 794–799.

Gerontological Considerations

Over 80% of pacemakers are implanted in patients over the age of 64 (Gregoratos et al., 2002). Because elderly patients already are at increased risk for falls due to a variety of natural physiological changes, health care professionals must be aggressive in providing careful pacemaker follow-up in order to prevent potential complications in this vulnerable population. The timing of follow-up evaluation depends on several factors, including clinical status of the patient, age of the pacemaker, and geographic location of the patient to a health care facility. Family members may need to be enlisted to ensure that patients adhere to their appointments. Telephone follow-up may be an option if patients have difficulty traveling.

Summary

Advances in pacemaker technologies have led to more complicated but reliable devices that have moved well beyond the ability of the first pacemakers to pace only the right ventricle at a fixed predetermined rate. Modern pacemakers are programmable, have the ability to modulate their rate in response to a variety of triggers, and are indicated not only for the treatment of dysrhythmias but also for clinical conditions such as heart failure. However, the decision to implant a pacemaker does not mean that the patient will not require long-term follow-up or be freed from medications. The pacemaker is just one component, albeit an important one, of comprehensive care for the cardiac patient and his family.

■ Research Opportunities Related to PCI

As with much of medicine and nursing, there is still a great deal to be learned in order to improve patient care and the quality of life for cardiac patients. Cardiac care is an ever-evolving science that requires continued research. The Research Opportunities and Clinical Impact box outlines areas of research that are still under investigation or need future trials.

RESEARCH OPPORTUNITIES AND CLINICAL IMPACT RELATED TO PERCUTANEOUS CORONARY INTERVENTION

Research Area	Clinical Impact
Physiological Research	
Long-term impact of drug eluting stents on restenosis.	Restenosis is the major cause of repeat revascularization procedures.
Vascular management techniques.	Potential to reduce length of stay and improve patient comfort and safety after PCI.
Length of time to continue antiplatelet agents after PCI.	Reduce complications associated with these medications.
Emotional and Psychological Research	
Denial of signs and symptoms of acute myocardial infarction.	Delaying treatment results in increased morbidity and mortality.
Risk factor modification.	Reduce incidence of CAD, as well as improve outcomes after PCI.
Use of alternative therapies such as guided imagery to reduce anxiety during PCI.	Lower stress during PCI while reducing need for sedatives/analgesics.
Effective teaching methods for discharge instructions.	Knowledge alone does not improve patient/family compliance.

Clinical Preparation

CRITICAL THINKING

 Read

- History of Current Illness
- Past Medical History
- Physical Exam
- Admitting Medical Orders
- Laboratory Study Results

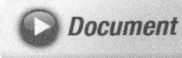 **Document**

- Summary of Hospitalization
- Pathophysiology Form
- Laboratory Values
- Laboratory Results Explanation

 Apply

- List of Potential Nursing Diagnoses
- Concept Map
- Critical Thinking Questions

Log on to MyNursingKit.com to download forms you will need and to complete further steps in the Clinical Preparation assignment.

HISTORY OF PRESENT ILLNESS

You are a nurse in a large hospital that is the referral center for cardiac patients needing urgent percutaneous coronary interventional (PCI) procedures or coronary artery bypass surgery. You have just received a report about Mr. W, a 52-year-old engineer who is having an acute myocardial infarction and is being transported to your hospital for urgent PCI. Mr. W went to work this morning despite not feeling well. After several episodes of nausea and chest pain, Mr. W's coworkers called 911. His wife and three children also were so notified and are on their way to your hospital.

Medical–Surgical History

Mr. W has a past medical history of hypertension, non–insulin-dependent diabetes, and hyperlipidemia. He states he is not currently under a doctor's care and is taking no medicines. He has had no prior surgeries. No known allergies.

Social History

Mr. W. lives with his wife and three young children. He works about 60 to 70 hours per week. He coaches his son's baseball team in the evening and weekends. He smokes 1 to 2 packs per day and drinks two to three beers every evening.

Physical Exam

When Mr. W arrives at the hospital, he is restless but able to answer questions appropriately, very anxious, and complaining of chest pain radiating down his left arm. He is diaphoretic and appears short of breath. Vital signs are temperature, 99.6°F; pulse, 118 beats per minute and regular; respiratory rate, 28 per minute; blood pressure, 90/50 mmHg; and his oxygen saturation is 92% on room air. He is 5'9" and weighs 220 pounds.

A 55-year-old man with 4 hours of "crushing" chest pain

FIGURE V–1 ■ Admission 12-lead ECG. ST segment elevation is present in leads II, III, and aVF, indicating acute inferior myocardial infarction. Note the ST segment depression in the posterior lead V₂, indicating possible posterior involvement. There is also ST segment depression in the lateral (I, and avL) leads. These are probably secondary changes related to the size of the infarct.

Mr. W has bilateral rales in both lung bases. He has a loud third heart sound, but no murmurs or rubs. Extremities are cool; all pulses are present and normal. His abdomen is soft and nontender with active bowel sounds. A Foley catheter has been placed; there is 90 milliliters of clear yellow urine in the bag. Mr. W has one peripheral line in his right arm; normal saline is infusing at 100 mL/hr. He has been given one adult aspirin and one dose of low-molecular-weight heparin. You accompany Mr. W as he is urgently transferred to the catheterization laboratory. Mr. W's admitting ECG indicates that he is experiencing an acute inferior/posterior myocardial infarction (Figure V–1 ■). This is usually related to a significant occlusion in the right coronary artery (RCA).

Mr. W's initial cardiac angiography revealed a total occlusion of the proximal RCA (Figure V–2 ■). After balloon angioplasty there was no blood flow to the artery, and significant thrombus (clot) had now formed in the distal portions of the artery (Figures V–3 ■ and V–4 ■). Despite the placement of multiple coronary stents, the artery remained blocked with thrombus. Eventually the decision was made to remove the thrombus directly with a mechanical thrombectomy device, in this case the AngioJet. This device creates suction at its tip that aspirates and then breaks up a clot, allowing it to be removed with almost no damage to the wall of the coronary artery. The final result was a patent RCA (Figure V–5 ■).

FIGURE V–4 ■ Angiogram after attempted balloon angioplasty. There is no blood flow and significant thrombus (clot) in the distal portions of the artery (arrows).

FIGURE V–2 ■ Cardiac angiography indicating a total occlusion in the midportion of the right coronary artery (arrow).

FIGURE V–3 ■ Balloon angioplasty of the occlusion in the RCA.

FIGURE V–5 ■ The patient eventually required the placement of multiple coronary stents, as well as direct removal of the clot by a mechanical thrombectomy device. The AngioJet catheter creates a vacuum at its tip that aspirates and removes thrombus and other material from within the artery. The final result is a widely patent RCA with excellent blood flow throughout.
Source: All catheterization images courtesy of Boston Scientific

Medications Before PCI

Aspirin 325 mg po daily (first dose at least 2 hours before the procedure)

Clopidogrel 300 mg po as a one-time loading dose, then 75 mg daily

Unfractionated heparin 70 international units/kg bolus IV, then 17 international units/kg per hour titrated to clotting time

Nitroglycerin, IV, titrated to maintain systolic blood pressure > 90 mmHg

Morphine, 3–5 mg IV q1h prn pain

Admitting Medical Orders

Admit to cardiology service, coronary care unit

Condition guarded

No known allergies

Diagnosis: acute inferior/posterior myocardial infarction; status postangioplasty, stent placement and thrombectomy

Vital signs and oxygen saturation q1h

Bed rest

Call house officer: pulse < 60 and > 110/minute; BP < 90 and > 160 systolic; temperature > 38.5; urine output < 30 mL/hr for 2 hours; respiratory rate > 30/minute; oxygen saturation < 92%

Diet: cardiac

Daily weight

Continuous cardiac monitor

Sequential compression devices (SCDs) to lower extremities

Strict in/out

Oxygen to 2 liters nasal cannula, maintain oxygen sat > 92%

IV: D51/2 NS @ 75 mL/hr

Scheduled Medications

Aspirin 81 mg po daily

Clopidogrel 75 mg po daily

Lipitor 10 mg po daily

ReoPro gtt @ 0.125 mcg/kg/minute for 12 hours

Lisinopril 10 mg po daily

Rosiglitazone 4 mg po daily

Metoprolol 25 mg po bid

PRN Medications

Nitroglycerin, IV, titrated to maintain systolic blood pressure > 90 mmHg

Morphine, 3–5 mg IV q1h prn pain

Temazepam 15–30 mg po qhs prn insomnia

Droperidol 1.25–2.5 mg IV q6h prn nausea

Ordered Laboratory Studies

Troponin I q8h × 3

CPK–MB q8h × 3

Chemistry panel 7 q a.m.

CBC q a.m.

Magnesium q a.m.

Lipid panel in a.m.

Ordered Diagnostic Studies

ECG q a.m.

Echocardiogram in a.m.

LABORATORY STUDY RESULTS

Test	Before PCI	Day 1 After PCI	Day 2 After PCI
WBC	5,000/mm³	8,000/mm³	5,000/mm³
RBC	4.89/mm³	4.69/mm³	4.38/mm³
Hemoglobin	13 g/dL	11 g/dL	11 g/dL
Hematocrit	35%	30%	29%
Platelets	120,000/mm³	100,000/mm³	130,000/mm³
Prothrombin time	10 seconds	10 seconds	10 seconds
Activated partial thromboplastin time	25 seconds	65 seconds (on heparin)	100 seconds (on heparin)
Glucose	156 mg/dL	130 mg/dL	130 mg/dL
BUN	10 mg/dL	15 mg/dL	10 mg/dL
Creatinine	0.5 mg/dL	0.9 mg/dL	0.7 mg/dL
Sodium	139 mEq/L	137 mEq/L	140 mEq/L
Potassium	3.8 mEq/L	4.9 mEq/L	4.9 mEq/L
Chloride	100 mEq/L	100 mEq/L	100 mEq/L
CO_2	25 mEq/L	25 mEq/L	25 mEq/L
Calcium	9.5 mg/dL	9.5 mg/dL	9 mg/dL
Magnesium	2.2mEq/L	2.0 mEq/L	2.0 mEq/L
Troponin I	0.8 ng/mL	30 ng/mL	25 ng/mL
CPK-MB	>250.00%	>300.00%	259.7%
Cholesterol	260 mg/dL		
High-density lipoproteins (HDL)	34 mg/dL		
Low-density lipoproteins (LDL)	190 mg/dL		
Very low-density lipoproteins (VLDL)	62%		
Apolipoproteins	161 mg/dL		
Triglycerides	200 mg/dL		

CRITICAL THINKING QUESTIONS

1. What factors in Mr. W's past medical history place him at high risk for complications from the planned PCI?

2. What is the rationale for taking Mr. W directly to the catheterization laboratory?

3. Why was Mr. W given an aspirin?

4. Mr. W is restless, tachycardic, with low blood pressure and urine output. What is the most likely cause of these findings?

Answers to Critical Thinking Questions appear in Appendix D

NCLEX® REVIEW

1. A patient with asthma is being treated with a glucocorticoid and has been told that his blood glucose level could increase, creating the picture that he has diabetes. The nurse has instructed the patient on which of the following types of sensitivity to tests?

1. True positive
2. False negative
3. True negative
4. False positive

2. A patient is demonstrating signs of cardiac valve stenosis. The nurse should be prepared to discuss which of the following diagnostic tests with this patient?

1. PET scan
2. MRI
3. TEE
4. Echocardiogram

3. A patient with a serum creatinine level of 2.8 mg/dL is scheduled for a cardiac catheterization. Which of the following should be done to assist this patient?

1. Provide an antihistamine prior to the procedure.
2. Provide intravenous normal saline prior to the procedure.
3. Provide an injection of steroids prior to the procedure.
4. Provide intravenous dextrose prior to the procedure.

4. A patient experienced an acute myocardial infarction the previous day. Of the following diagnostic tests planned for this patient, which of the following would be contraindicated at this time?

1. ECG
2. Echocardiogram
3. PCI
4. Stress test

5. While assessing a patient recovering from a cardiac catheterization, the nurse is unable to assess the pedal pulse on the limb used for the procedure. Which of the following should the nurse do?

1. Readjust the patient's foot.
2. Apply warm blankets to the patient's feet.
3. Assess the femoral site.
4. Ask the patient to move the foot.

Answers for review questions appear in Appendix D

KEY TERMS

ablation *p.1139*
automated external defibrillator (AED) *p.1140*
biphasic defibrillation *p.1140*
brachytherapy *p.1133*
capture *p.1144*
cardiac catheterization *p.1129*
cardiac pacemaker *p.1142*
cardiac resynchronization therapy (CRT) *p.1149*
cardioversion *p.1139*
defibrillation *p.1140*
ECG single photon emission computed tomography (SPECT) *p.1126*
echocardiography *p.1120*
electrocardiogram *p.1120*

electron beam computed tomography (EBCT) *p.1127*
electrophysiology study (EPS) *p.1138*
exercise testing *p.1123*
gating *p.1126*
Holter monitoring *p.1138*
implantable cardioverter defibrillator (ICD) *p.1141*
magnetic resonance imaging (MRI) *p.1126*
metabolic equivalent (MET) *p.1123*
monophasic defibrillation *p.1140*
multislice helical CT *p.1127*
myocardial perfusion *p.1123*
myocardial perfusion imaging (MPI) *p.1124*
myocardial viability *p.1126*
pacemaker sensitivity *p.1146*

percutaneous coronary intervention (PCI) *p.1131*
percutaneous transluminal coronary angioplasty (PTCA) *p.1131*
post-test probability *p.1120*
predictive accuracy *p.1119*
pretest probability *p.1119*
restenosis *p.1132*
sensitivity *p.1119*
specificity *p.1119*
stent *p.1131*
temporary transvenous pacing *p.1145*
tomography *p.1126*
transcutaneous pacing (TCP) *p.1147*
transesophageal echocardiography (TEE) *p.1122*

REFERENCES

Abraham, W. T., & Hayes, D. L. (2003). Cardiac resynchronization therapy for heart failure. *Circulation,108*, 2596–2603.

Agatston, A. S., Janowitz, W. R., Hildner, F. J., Zusmer, N. R., Viamonte, M., Jr., & Detrano, R. (1990). Quantification of coronary artery calcium using ultrafast computed tomography. *Journal of the American College of Cardiology, 15*, 827–832.

Amato-Vealey, E., & Colonies, P. A. (2005). Demystifying biphasic defibrillation. *Nursing2005, 35*(8, Suppl.), ED Insider, 6–11.

American Heart Association. (2003). *Heart disease and stroke statistics—2004 update.* Dallas, TX: Author.

Apple, S. (2000). Interdisciplinary management of the interventional patient. In S. Apple & J. Lindsay, Jr. (Eds.), *Principles and practice of interventional cardiology* (pp. 229–263). Philadelphia: Lippincott Williams & Wilkins.

Armstrong, W. F., & Feigenbaum, H. (2001). Echocardiography. In E. Braunwald, D. P. Zipes, & P. Libby (Eds.), *Heart disease* (6th ed., pp. 160–236). Philadelphia: W. B. Saunders.

Auricchio, A., & Abraham, W. T. (2004). Cardiac resynchronization therapy: Current state of the art cost versus benefit. *Circulation, 109*, 300–307.

Baim, D. S. (2000). Percutaneous approach, including transseptal and apical puncture. In D. S. Baim & W. Grossman (Eds.), *Grossman's cardiac catheterization, angiography, and intervention* (6th ed., pp. 69–100). Philadelphia: Lippincott Williams & Wilkins.

Baim, D. S., & Grossman, W. (2000a). Complications of cardiac catheterization. In D. S. Baim & W. Grossman (Eds.), *Grossman's cardiac catheterization, angiography, and intervention* (6th ed., pp. 35–65). Philadelphia: Lippincott Williams & Wilkins.

Baim, D. S., & Grossman, W. (2000b). Coronary angiography. In D. S. Baim & W. Grossman (Eds.), *Grossman's cardiac catheterization, angiography, and intervention* (6th ed., pp. 211–256). Philadelphia: Lippincott Williams & Wilkins.

Blancher, S. (2005). Cardiac electrophysiology procedures. In S. L. Woods, E. S. S. Froelicher, S. A. Motzer, & E. J. Bridges (Eds.), *Cardiac nursing* (5th ed., pp. 425–438). Philadelphia: Lippincott Williams & Wilkins.

Bond, E. F., & Heitkemper, M. M. (2005). Complementary and alternative medicine in cardiac and vascular disease. In S. L. Woods, E. S. S. Froelicher, S. A. Motzer, & E. J. Bridges (Eds.), *Cardiac nursing* (5th ed., pp. 974–985). Philadelphia: Lippincott Williams & Wilkins.

Cannon, R. O. (2002). Restenosis after angioplasty. *New England Journal of Medicine, 346*, 1182–1183.

Carrozza, J. P., Jr., & Baim, D. S. (2000). Coronary stenting. In D. S. Baim & W. Grossman (Eds.), *Grossman's cardiac catheterization, angiography, and intervention* (6th ed., pp. 639–666). Philadelphia: Lippincott Williams & Wilkins.

Chaitman, B. R. (2001). Exercise testing. In E. Braunwald, D. P. Zipes, & P. Libby (Eds.), *Heart disease* (6th ed., pp. 129–159). Philadelphia: W. B. Saunders.

Cheitlin, M. D., Armstrong, W. F., Aurigemma, G. P., Beller, G. A., Bierman, F. Z., Davis, J. L., et al. (2003). ACC/AHA/ASE 2003 guideline update for the clinical application of echocardiography—Summary article: A report of the American College of Cardiology/American Heart Association Task Force on Practice Guidelines. *Circulation, 108*, 1146–1162.

Chou, T. M., Fitzgerald, P. J., & Yock, P. G. (2000). Intravascular ultrasound. In D. S. Baim & W. Grossman (Eds.), *Grossman's cardiac catheterization, angiography, and intervention* (6th ed., pp. 423–444). Philadelphia: Lippincott Williams & Wilkins.

Choudhury, R. P., Fuster, V., Badimon, J. J., Fisher, E. A., & Fayad, Z. A. (2002). MRI and characterization of atherosclerotic plaque: Emerging application and molecular imaging. *Arteriosclerosis, Thrombosis, and Vascular Biology, 22*, 1065–1074.

Crawford, M. H., Berstein, S. J., Deedwania, P. C., DiMarco, J. P., Ferrick, K. J., Garson, A., Jr., et al. (1999). ACC/AHA guidelines for ambulatory electrocardiography—Executive summary and recommendations: A report of the American College of

Cardiology/American Heart Association Task Force on Practice Guidelines. *Circulation, 100*, 886–893.

Davidson, C. J., & Bonow, R. O. (2001). Cardiac catheterization. In E. Braunwald, D. P. Zipes, & P. Libby (Eds.), *Heart disease* (6th ed., pp. 359–386). Philadelphia: W. B. Saunders.

Deelstra, M. S., & Jacobson, C. (2005). Cardiac catheterization. In S. L. Woods, E. S. S. Froelicher, S. A. Motzer, & E. J. Bridges (Eds.), *Cardiac nursing* (5th ed., pp. 459–477). Philadelphia: Lippincott Williams & Wilkins.

Detrano, R., & Carr, J. J. (2002). Computed tomography of the heart. In E. J. Topol (Ed.), *Textbook of cardiovascular medicine* (2nd ed., pp. 1281–1296). Philadelphia: Lippincott Williams & Wilkins.

Drew, B. J. (2002). Celebrating the 100th birthday of the electrocardiogram: Lessons learned from research in cardiac monitoring. *American Journal of Critical Care, 11*, 387–389.

Drew, B. J., & Ide, B. (1999). Could inaccurate lead placement cause misdiagnosis of the culprit artery in patients with acute myocardial infarction? *Progress in Cardiovascular Nursing, 14*, 33–34.

Fayad, Z. A., Fuster, V., Nikolaou, K., & Becker, C. (2002). Computed tomography and magnetic resonance imaging for noninvasive coronary angiography and plaque imaging: Current and potential future concepts. *Circulation, 106*, 2026–2034.

Federal Occupational Health. (2008). *Automated external defibrillator program.* Retrieved February 24, 2008, from http://www.foh.dhhs.gov/Public/ProductFocus/Apr2006/AED.asp

Fenton, J. M. (2001). The clinician's approach to evaluating patients with dysrhythmias. *AACN Clinical Issues, 12*, 72–86.

Fletcher, G. F., Balady, G. J., Amsterdam, E. A., Chaitman, B., Eckel, R., Fleg, J., et al. (2001). Exercise standards for testing and training. *Circulation, 104*, 1694–1740.

Forgoros, R. N. (2006). *The MUGA scan. About heart disease.* Retrieved May 20, 2007, from http://heartdisease.about.com/cs/cardiactests/a/muga.htm

Fuseini, M., Goodwin, W. J., Ferris, E. J., & Mehta, J. L. (2003). Does electron beam computer tomography provide added value in the diagnosis of coronary artery disease? *Current Opinion in Cardiology, 18*, 385–393.

Futterman, L. G., & Lemberg, L. (2002). Ambulatory electrocardiographic monitoring: Use of the implantable loop recorder in the evaluation of syncope. *Journal of Cardiovascular Nursing, 16*, 24–33.

Gibbons, R. J., Balady, G. J., Bricker, J. T., Chaitman, B. R., Fletcher, G. F., Froelicher, V. F., et al. (2002). ACC/AHA 2002 guideline update for exercise testing: A report of the American College of Cardiology/American Heart Association Task Force on Practice Guidelines (Committee on Exercise Testing). Retrieved, May 10, 2008 from http://linkinghub.elsevier.com/retrieve/pii/S0735109702021642

Gold, M. E., & Farnsworth, N. (2002). Alternative medicines for cardiovascular diseases. *Journal of Cardiovascular Nursing, 16*, v–viii.

Goldin, J. G., Ratib, O., & Aberle, D. R. (2000). Contemporary cardiac imaging. *Journal of Thoracic Imaging, 15*, 218–229.

Grech, E. D. (2003). ABC of interventional cardiology: Pathophysiology and investigation of coronary artery disease. *British Medical Journal, 326*, 1027–1030.

Greenland, P., & Gaziano, J. M. (2003). Selecting asymptomatic patients for coronary computed tomography or electrocardiographic exercise testing. *New England Journal of Medicine, 349*, 465–473.

Gregoratos, G., Abrams, J., Epstein, A. E., Freedman, R. A., Hayes, D. L., Hlatky, M. A., et al. (2002). ACC/AHA/NASPE 2002 guideline update for implantation of cardiac pacemakers and antiarrhythmia devices—Summary article: A report of the American College of Cardiology/American Heart Association Task Force on Practice Guidelines (ACC/AHA/NASPE Committee to Update the 1998 Pacemaker Guidelines). *Circulation, 106*, 2145–2161.

Grossman, W. (2000a). Historical perspective and present practice of cardiac catheterization. In D. S. Baim & W. Grossman (Eds.), *Grossman's cardiac catheterization, angiography, and intervention* (6th ed., pp. 3–14). Philadelphia: Lippincott Williams & Wilkins.

Grossman, W. (2000b). Shunt detection and quantification. In D. S. Baim & W. Grossman (Eds.), *Grossman's cardiac catheterization, angiography, and intervention* (6th ed., pp. 179–191). Philadelphia: Lippincott Williams & Wilkins.

Grundy, S. M., Cleeman, J. I., Merz, C. N. B., Brewer, H. B., Jr., Clark, L. T., Hunninghake, D. B., et al. (2004). Implications of recent clinical trials for the National Cholesterol Education program Adult Treatment Panel III guidelines. *Circulation, 110*, 227–239.

Grüntzig, A. (1978). Transluminal dilation of coronary-artery stenosis. *Lancet, 1*, 263.

Hall, M. L. (2005). Echocardiography. In S. L. Woods, E. S. S. Froelicher, S. A. Motzer, & E. J. Bridges (Eds.), *Cardiac nursing* (5th ed., pp. 307–318). Philadelphia: Lippincott Williams & Wilkins.

Hallstrom, A. P., Ornato, J. P., Weisfeldt, M., & Travers, J. (2004). Public-access defibrillation and survival after out-of-hospital cardiac arrest: The public access defibrillation trial investigators. *New England Journal of Medicine, 351*(7), 637–646.

Helena Cardiology Clinic. (n.d.). *Holter monitoring.* Retrieved March 26, 2004, from http://www.helenacardiology.com/holtermonitor.htm

Higgins, C. B. (2002). Newer cardiac imaging modalities: Magnetic resonance imaging and computed tomography. In E. Braunwald, D. P. Zipes, & P. Libby (Eds.), *Heart disease* (6th ed., pp. 324–358). Philadelphia: W. B. Saunders.

Holter, N. J. (1961). New method for heart studies: Continuous electrocardiography of active subjects is now practical. *Science, 34*, 1214–1219.

Iskandrian, A. E., & Verani, M. S. (2002). Nuclear imaging techniques. In E. J. Topol (Ed.), *Textbook of cardiovascular medicine* (2nd ed., pp. 1192–1211). Philadelphia: Lippincott Williams & Wilkins.

Jacobson, C., & Gerity, D. (2005). Pacemakers and implantable defibrillators. In S. L. Woods, E. S. S. Froelicher, S. A. Motzer, & E. J. Bridges (Eds.), *Cardiac nursing* (5th ed., pp. 709–755). Philadelphia: Lippincott Williams & Wilkins.

Janosik, D. L., Quattromani, A., & Schiller, L. (2003). Electrophysiologic studies and ablation techniques. In M. J. Kern (Ed.), *The cardiac catheterization handbook* (4th ed., pp. 326–398). Philadelphia: Mosby.

Kadish, A. H., Buxton, A. E., Kennedy, H. L., Knight, B. P., Mason, J. W., Schuger, C. D., et al. (2001). ACC/AHA clinical competence statement on electrocardiography and ambulatory electrocardiography: A report of the American College of Cardiology/American Heart Association/American College of Physicians/American Society of Internal Medicine Task Force on Clinical Competence (ACC/AHA Committee to Develop a Clinical Competence Statement on Electrocardiography and Ambulatory Electrocardiography). *Circulation, 104*, 3169–3178.

Kent, K. M. (2000). Development of interventional cardiology. In S. Apple & J. Lindsay, Jr. (Eds.), *Principles and practice of interventional cardiology* (pp. 1–12). Philadelphia: Lippincott Williams & Wilkins.

Klocke, F. J., Baird, M. G., Bateman, T. M., Berman, D. S., Carabello, B. A., Cerqueria, M. D., et al. (2003). ACC/AHA/ASNC guidelines for the clinical use of cardiac radionuclide imaging: A report of the American College of Cardiology/American Heart Association Task Force on Practice Guidelines (ACC/AHA/ASNC Committee to Revise the 1995 Guidelines for the Clinical Use of Radionuclide Imaging). Retrieved March 4, 2004, from http://www.ncbi.nlm.nih.gov/pubmed/12975245

Kloner, R. A., Bolli, R., Marbán, E., Reinlib, L., & Braunwald, E. (1998). Medical and cellular implications of stunning, hibernation, and preconditioning: An NHLBI workshop. *Circulation, 97*, 1848–1867.

Koreny, M., Riedmuller, E., Nikfardjam, M., Siostrzonek, P., & Mullner, M. (2004). Arterial puncture closing devices compared with standard manual compression after cardiac catheterization: Systematic review and meta-analysis. *Journal of the American Medical Association, 291*, 350–357.

Lamas, G. A., Ellenbogen, K. A., with the assistance of Hennekens, C. H., & Montanez, A. (2004). Evidence base for pacemaker mode selection: From physiology to randomized trials. *Circulation, 109,* 443–451.

Leclercq, C., & Hare, J. M. (2004). Ventricular resynchronization: Current state of the art. *Circulation, 109,* 296–299.

Lee, T. H., & Brennan, T. A. (2002). Direct-to-consumer marketing of high-technology screening tests. *New England Journal of Medicine, 346,* 529–531.

Legge, D., & Leeper, B. (2002). Resynchronization therapy for the management of heart failure. *Critical Care Nursing Clinics of North America, 15*(4), 467–475.

Lindsay, J., Jr., Apple, S., Pinnow, E. E., Gevorkian, N., Gruberg, L., Satler, L. F., et al. (2003). Percutaneous coronary intervention–associated nephropathy foreshadows increased risk of late adverse events in patients with normal baseline serum creatinine. *Catheterization and Cardiovascular Interventions, 59,* 338–343.

Lindsay, J., Jr., & Pinnow, E. E. (2000). Outcomes of percutaneous transluminal coronary revascularization. In S. Apple & J. Lindsay, Jr. (Eds.), *Principles and practice of interventional cardiology* (pp. 277–286). Philadelphia: Lippincott Williams & Wilkins.

Lüderitz, B. (1995). *History of the disorders of cardiac rhythm* (2nd ed.). Armonk, NY: Futura.

Marwick, T. H. (2002). Stress echocardiography. In E. J. Topol (Ed.), *Textbook of cardiovascular medicine* (2nd ed., pp. 1115–1142). Philadelphia: Lippincott Williams & Wilkins.

Marwick, T. H. (2003). Stress echocardiography. *Heart, 89,* 113–118.

Milani, R. V., Lavie, C. J., Gilliland, Y. E., Cassidy, M. M., & Bernal, J. A. (2003). Overview of transesophageal echocardiography for the chest physician. *Chest, 124,* 1081–1089.

Miller, J. M., & Zipes, D. P. (2001). Management of the patient with cardiac dysrhythmias. In E. Braunwald, D. P. Zipes, & P. Libby (Eds.), *Heart disease* (6th ed., pp. 700–774). Philadelphia: W. B. Saunders.

Mintz, G. S., & Walsh, C. (2000). Intravascular ultrasound imaging. In S. Apple & J. Lindsay, Jr. (Eds.), *Principles and practice of interventional cardiology* (pp. 161–183). Philadelphia: Lippincott Williams & Wilkins.

Mirowski, M. (1985). The automatic implantable cardioverter-defibrillator. *American Journal of Cardiology, 6,* 461–466.

Mulvagh, S. L., DeMaria, A. N., Feinstein, S. B., Burns, P. N., Kaul, S., Miller, J. G., et al. (2000). Contrast echocardiography: Current and future applications. *Journal of the American Society of Echocardiography, 13,* 331–342.

Myers, J. (2005). Exercise testing. In S. L. Woods, E. S. S. Froelicher, S. A. Motzer, & E. J. Bridges (Eds.), *Cardiac nursing* (5th ed., pp. 439–458). Philadelphia: Lippincott Williams & Wilkins.

National Institutes of Health National Center for Complementary and Alternative Medicine. (2008). The use of complementary and alternative medicine in the United States. Retrieved August 20, 2008, from http://nccam.nih.gov

Nikolaou, K., Poon, M., Sirol, M., Becker, C. R., & Fayad, Z. A. (2003). Complementary results of computed tomography and magnetic resonance imaging of the heart and coronary arteries: A review and future outlook. *Cardiology Clinics, 21,* 639–655.

Obias-Manno, D. (2001). Unconventional applications in pacemaker therapy. *AACN Clinical Issues, 12,* 127–139.

O'Neill, W. W., & Dixon, S. R. (2004). The year in interventional cardiology. *Journal of the American College of Cardiology, 43,* 875–890.

O'Rourke, R. A., Brundage, B. H., Froelicher, V. F., Greenland, P., Grundy, S. M., Hachamovitch, R., et al. (2000). American College of Cardiology/American Heart Association expert consensus document on electron-beam computed tomography for the diagnosis and prognosis of coronary artery disease. *Circulation, 102,* 126–140.

Overbay, D., & Criddle, L. (2004). Mastering temporary invasive cardiac pacing. *Critical Care Nurse, 24,* 25–32.

Peterson, G. E., Brickner, E., & Reimold, S. C. (2003). Transesophageal echocardiography: Clinical indications and applications. *Circulation, 107,* 2398–2402.

Pohost, G. M., Hung, L., & Doyle, M. (2003). Clinical use of cardiovascular magnetic resonance. *Circulation, 108,* 647–653.

Popma, J. J., & Bittl, J. (2001). Coronary angiography and intravascular ultrasonography. In E. Braunwald, D. P. Zipes, & P. Libby (Eds.), *Heart disease* (6th ed., pp. 387–421). Philadelphia: W. B. Saunders.

Popma, J. J., & Kuntz, R. E. (2001). Percutaneous coronary and valvular intervention. In E. Braunwald, D. P. Zipes, & P. Libby (Eds.), *Heart disease* (6th ed., pp. 1364–1405). Philadelphia: W. B. Saunders.

Quiñones, M. A., Douglas, P. S., Foster, E., Gorcsan, J., III, Lewis, J. F., Pearlman, A. S., et al. (2003). American College of Cardiology/American Heart Association clinical competence statement of echocardiography: A report of the American College of Cardiology/American Heart Association/American College of Physicians/American Society of Internal Medicine Task Force on Clinical Competence. *Circulation, 107,* 1068–1089.

Reynolds, J., & Apple, S. (2001). A systematic approach to pacemaker assessment. *AACN Clinical Issues, 12,* 114–126.

Rosen, M. R. (2002). The electrocardiogram 100 years later: Electrical insights into molecular messages. *Circulation, 106,* 2173–2179.

Scanlon, P. J., Faxon, D. P., Audet, A., Carabello, B., Dehmer, G. J., Eagle, K. A., et al. (1999). ACC/AHA guidelines for coronary angiography: Executive summary and recommendations. *Circulation, 99,* 2345–2357.

Schoepf, U. J., Becker, C. R., Hofmann, L. K., & Yucel, E. K. (2003). Multidetector-row CT of the heart. *Radiologic Clinics of North America, 41,* 491–505.

Schvartzman, P. R., & White, R. D. (2002). Magnetic resonance imaging. In E. J. Topol (Ed.), *Textbook of cardiovascular medicine* (2nd ed., pp. 1213–1256). Philadelphia: Lippincott Williams & Wilkins.

Smith, R. L., & Thomas, J. D. (2002). Transthoracic echocardiography. In E. J. Topol (Ed.), *Textbook of cardiovascular medicine* (2nd ed., pp. 1091–1113). Philadelphia: Lippincott Williams & Wilkins.

Smith, S. C., Jr., Dove, J. T., Jacobs, A. K., Kennedy, J. W., Kereiakes, D., Kern, M. J., et al. (2001). ACC/AHA guidelines for percutaneous coronary intervention. *Circulation.* 2001;103:3019.

Soine, L., & Hanrahan, M. (2005). Nuclear and other imaging studies. In S. L. Woods, E. S. S. Froelicher, S. A. Motzer, & E. J. Bridges (Eds.), *Cardiac nursing* (5th ed., pp. 319–325). Philadelphia: Lippincott Williams & Wilkins.

Sousa, J. E., Serruys, P. W., & Costa, M. A. (2003). New frontiers in cardiology: Drug eluting stents. *Circulation, 107,* Part I, pp. 2274–2279, Part II, pp. 2383–2389.

Squires, S. (2003, September 16). The selling of the stent. *The Washington Post,* pp. F1, F5.

Stewart, M. J. (2003). Contrast echocardiography. *Heart, 89,* 342–348.

Stone, K. R., & McPherson, C. A. (2004). Assessment and management of patients with pacemakers and implantable cardioverter defibrillators. *Critical Care Medicine, 32,* S155–S165.

Teirstein, P. S., & Kuntz, R. E. (2001). New frontiers in interventional cardiology: Intravascular radiation to prevent restenosis. *Circulation, 104,* 2620–2626.

Thomas, J. D. (2002). Principles of imaging. In E. J. Topol (Ed.), *Textbook of cardiovascular medicine* (2nd ed., pp. 1031–1045). Philadelphia: Lippincott Williams & Wilkins.

Tracy, C. M., Akhtar, M., DiMarco, J. P., Packer, D. L., & Weitz, H. H. (2000). American College of Cardiology/American Heart Association clinical competence statement on invasive electrophysiology studies, catheter ablation, and cardioversion. *Circulation, 102,* 2309–2320.

Wackers, F. J. T., Soufer, R., & Zaret, B. L. (2001). Nuclear cardiology. In E. Braunwald, D. P. Zipes, & P. Libby (Eds.), *Heart disease* (6th ed., pp. 273–323). Philadelphia: W. B. Saunders.

Waksman, R. (2000). Restenosis. In S. Apple & J. Lindsay, Jr. (Eds.), *Principles and practice of interventional cardiology* (pp. 213–228). Philadelphia: Lippincott Williams & Wilkins.

Weinberger, J., Lincoff, A. M., & Popma, J. J. (2002). New techniques in interventional cardiology: Radiation, emboli protection, and therapeutic angiogenesis. In E. J. Topol (Ed.), *Textbook of cardiovascular medicine* (2nd ed., pp. 1677–1714). Philadelphia: Lippincott Williams & Wilkins.

Weyman, A. E. (2004). The year in echocardiography. *Journal of the American College of Cardiology, 43,* 140–148.

White, M. M. (2002). Psychosocial impact of the implantable cardioverter defibrillator: Nursing implications. *Journal of Cardiovascular Nursing, 16,* 53–61.

Wu, K. C., & Lima, J. A. C. (2003). Noninvasive imaging of myocardial viability: Current techniques and future developments. *Circulation Research, 93,* 1146–1158.

Zoll, P. M. (1952). Resuscitation of the heart in ventricular standstill by external electrical stimulation. *New England Journal of Medicine, 247,* 768–771.

Caring for the Patient with Coronary Artery Disease

Kori Harder
Kathleen Osborn
James Stotts

With Contribution By:
Gina Flaharty, Coronary Artery Bypass Graft
Surgery Section

Outcome-Based Learning Objectives

After studying this chapter, the learner will be able to:

1. Discuss the epidemiological factors of coronary artery disease (CAD) and define the risk factors.

2. Define and identify the etiology and pathophysiology of CAD/ischemic heart disease and explain the nursing assessment data and interventions used when evaluating a patient with angina pectoris.

3. Differentiate the three criteria used to evaluate ischemic heart disease and identify the pathologic significance of each criterion.

4. Compare and contrast the pathogenesis of unstable angina, a non Q wave, subendocardial, non–ST segment elevation myocardial infarction (MI), and a Q wave, transmural, ST segment elevation (MI).

5. Identify the complications of an MI and discuss the variables that affect the prognosis of the patient with an MI.

6. Identify which clinical manifestations and diagnostic finding are an indication for coronary artery bypass graft surgery (CABG).

7. Identify three possible complications of CABG and discuss nursing interventions that potentially reduce the incidence of these complications.

Research   Collaboration   Health Promotion   Nursing Process   Caring   Critical Thinking

A NEIGHBOR comes frantically knocking on the door saying that her husband is having chest pain and has just passed out. She is asking for help. A postoperative orthopedic patient is complaining of chest pressure. She has a history of myocardial infarction (MI), commonly referred to as a heart attack. A postoperative cholecystectomy patient shows dramatic ST segment elevation on the cardiac monitor. A 33-year-old with peripartum myocarditis complains of shortness of breath and palpitations. Each of these scenarios represents manifestations of coronary artery disease (CAD). The differences in settings highlight the fact that CAD is not gender, age, or specialty specific. Despite where one works the chances of caring for a patient, neighbor, or family member with CAD are high. This chapter discusses the clinical relevance to the prevalence, presentation, diagnostic work-up, and care guidelines for patients with manifestations of CAD.

Coronary Artery Anatomy

Coronary arteries are comprised of three concentric layers of differentiated cells separated by elastic membranes (Figure 40–1 ■). The **tunica intima** consists of endothelial cells, connective tissue, and smooth muscle cells. Once considered simply as a diffusing

FIGURE 40–1 ■ Normal artery layers.

barrier between blood and the subintimal, it is now recognized that the endothelium regulates vasomotor tone, pro- and anticoagulant stimulation, mediation of inflammatory and growth factors, and the adhesion and entry of inflammatory cells and lipids into the vessel wall. Adjacent to the intima is the internal elastic membrane (internal elastic lumina), a fenestrated sheet of elastic tissue that separates the intima from the medial layer.

The **tunica media**, the middle layer of the artery, consists of multiple layers of smooth muscle cells and connective tissue made up of elastic fibers, collagen, and proteoglycans (Figure 40–1 ■). The external elastic membrane (external elastic lumina) separates the medial layer from the adventitia. The external elastic membrane, comprised of interrupted layers of elastin, is thinner than the internal elastic membrane.

The **tunica adventitia**, the outer layer of the artery, is a flexible stratum consisting of fibrous tissue made of collagen and elastic fibers surrounded by collagen bundles (Figure 40–1 ■). The loose structure of the adventitia and the adjoining collagen bundles facilitates coronary vessel diameter changes during vasodilation and constriction. The adventitia also contains nerve fibers and, in larger vessels, the vasa vasorum, which is a network of arteries and veins that provide blood supply to the vessel wall.

Epidemiology of Coronary Artery Disease

Coronary artery disease (CAD) is defined as a progressive atherosclerotic disorder of the coronary arteries that results in narrowing or complete occlusion of the vessel lumen. This disease claims more lives each year in the United States than the next five leading causes of death combined (American Heart Association [AHA], 2006d). Coronary artery disease is responsible for approximately 50% of cardiovascular events in both men and women under the age of 75 (AHA, 2006d). CAD causes one-fifth of all deaths in the United States, making it the single largest killer of the American population. It is the leading cause of death in both males and females of white, African American, Hispanic, American Indian, and Asian Pacific Island ethnicities (AHA, 2006d). The overall risk of CAD is greater in men than in women, until menopause when it becomes more equal (AHA, 2006d).

The economic impact of CAD is significant. It is the leading cause of early, permanent disability in the U.S. labor force, with 22% of those over age 65 unable to return to work following a myocardial infarction (MI) (AHA, 2006d). Medical costs are significant with diagnostic testing of nearly 6 million patient visits to the emergency department annually for symptoms suspected of CAD and 2 million hospital discharges at an annual cost of $133 billion (AHA, 2006d). CAD is the leading cause of death, afflicts all ethnic groups and ages, and consumes the greatest portion of our national health dollars. The magnitude and pervasiveness of CAD provide sound rationale for advocating a greater allocation of research funds toward the prevention and treatment of CAD. Care providers, regardless of health care setting, are very likely to find that they are responsible for managing the care of a patient with CAD.

Etiology of Coronary Artery Disease

Coronary artery disease (CAD) is not an acute process but one that progresses over time and can begin as early in life as infancy. The rate of progression is related to risk factors such as genetic predisposition, gender, diet, sedentary lifestyle, and smoking.

Atherosclerosis affects the medium-size arteries perfusing the heart, brain, and kidneys and the large arteries branching off the aorta. Men predate women by about 10 years for CAD and 20 years for serious cardiac events such as an acute MI or sudden cardiac death. Because women present with CAD at an older age, they have a greater risk of overall mortality and developing serious complications that will be discussed throughout the chapter. Cardiovascular disease is the number-one killer of women over 40 years of age. According to the American Heart Association (AHA, 2008c), about 500,000 women die each year from heart disease. Recent national guidelines (AHA, 2006a) specifically target treating heart disease in women. The National Guidelines for Treating Women with Heart Disease box outlines these treatments.

Pathophysiology of Coronary Artery Disease

Coronary artery disease includes abnormal conditions such as arteriosclerosis, atherosclerosis, and arteritis of the coronary arteries, all of which result in reduced flow of oxygen and nutrients to the myocardium. **Arteriosclerosis** is characterized by thickening, reduced elasticity, and calcification of the arterial wall. **Atherosclerosis**, a type of arteriosclerosis, is the most common etiologic process that causes reduced myocardial blood flow. Atherosclerosis is coronary artery luminal obstruction caused by plaque buildup of cholesterol, lipids, and cellular debris infiltrating the intimal lining of the arterial wall, causing a reduced blood flow to the myocardium. Reductions in myocardial blood supply, especially in times of increased demand, are the cause of coronary syndromes,

---

NATIONAL GUIDELINES for Treating Women with Heart Disease

- Prevention should be tailored to a woman's level of risk.
- Quitting smoking, regular exercise, diet, and weight maintenance are strong priorities for all women.
- Aspirin is recommended as a preventive measure for all high-risk women; aspirin is not recommended for low-risk women. For intermediate-risk women, aspirin can be considered as long as blood pressure is controlled and the benefits outweigh the risk of side effects.
- Blood pressure–lowering drugs are recommended when blood pressure is greater than or equal to 140/90 mmHg. Blood pressure should be maintained at less than 130/80 mmHg for women with diabetes or with damage to target end organs related to blood pressure.
- Hormone therapy and antioxidant vitamin supplements are not recommended for heart disease prevention for women at any level of risk.
- Women with heart disease should be evaluated for depression and treated or referred for treatment when indicated.
- In addition to a heart-healthy diet, supplementation with omega-3 fatty acids and folic acid may be considered in some high-risk women.
- ACE inhibitors and beta-blockers are recommended for all high-risk women.

Source: American Heart Association. (2008c). Women and Coronary Heart Disease. Retrieved on July 18, 2008 from http://www.americanheart.org/presenter.jhtml?identifier=2859.

which include stable angina, unstable angina (UA), myocardial infarction (MI), and sudden cardiac death (SCD). These conditions depict a continuum of progressively worsening imbalances between the amount of oxygenated blood delivered and that which is required by myocardial tissues.

Normally the myocardium extracts 75% of the available oxygen from the coronary arteries, which is more than is extracted from any other tissue in the body (the rest of body extracts about 40% of available oxygen). If the oxygen needs are not met from this near maximal extraction, then myocardial blood flow must be increased. Normal coronary arteries are able to dilate, and normal hearts are able to increase the force of contraction, resulting in increased blood being delivered to the cardiac muscle and cardiac output. With CAD the arteries are unable to dilate because of the plaque buildup and subsequent calcification. In addition, because of the decrease in blood supply, the heart muscle has significant difficulty increasing the force of the contraction in order to increase the cardiac output. The result of all of the unmet oxygen needs is the shift to anaerobic metabolism and myocardial tissue hypoxia, which results in angina. The term myocardial **ischemia** or tissue hypoxia is a result of this oxygen imbalance. Ischemic heart disease, which is considered reversible, is insidious with prodromal anginal or chest pain symptoms present in only 20% of patients with MI and less than 50% of patients who suffer sudden cardiac death (SCD).

Certain factors, whether experienced internally or environmentally, such as stress or physical activity cause the heart to work harder and therefore increase oxygen demand. Whereas CAD decreases the blood supply to the myocardium, both abnormal demand and supply issues can cause angina to occur. Chart 40–1 outlines the most common factors that impact supply and demand.

The pathophysiology of plaque generation, development, composition, and injury provides the basis on which medical therapies for prevention of coronary artery disease and management of its sequelae have developed. The process of atherosclerotic development is described next.

Atherogenesis

An **atheroma** is an accumulation of plaque in the inner lining of an artery made up of cholesterol and other constituents. The cause of plaque generation is still unclear to researchers. One theory proposes that plaque pathogenesis is a response to injury to the vessel wall. Potential causes of injury include mechanical, chemical, immunologic, viral, bacterial, and subendothelial stressors. Some of these stressors as well as additional stressors are included in Chart 40–2. Once the endothelial lining has been injured, it undergoes a number of structural and functional changes. There is a disruption in cell-to-cell contact or cell to underlying connective tissue contact such that the once relatively impermeable endothelial monolayer can no longer protect or regulate the exposure of subendothelial constituents from elements in the circulating bloodstream. One effect of subendothelial cells coming in contact with blood is that there is a loss of endothelial vasodilatory control, as demonstrated by a decrease in focal endothelial-derived relaxing factor (EDRF) or nitric oxide (NO) synthesis and release, and increased sensitivity to catecholamines. Thus, rather than stimulating compensatory vasodilation, ischemia causes vasoconstriction in areas of vessel disruption. Endothelial injury also causes

CHART 40–1	Common Factors That Increase Oxygen Demand and Decrease Oxygen Supply
Increased Oxygen Demand	**Rationale**
Exercise	Increases the heart rate, which increases the workload of the heart, and diseased coronary arteries are unable to deliver an increased amount of oxygen to the heart muscle.
Eating	During digestion after a heavy meal, the blood is diverted to the gastrointestinal system, causing low blood flow to the coronary arteries.
Emotions	Stimulate the sympathetic nervous system and increase the workload of the heart by increasing heart rate and blood pressure.
Exposure to cold	Constricts blood vessels and increases metabolism, both of which put an extra workload on the heart.
Hypertension	Because the heart has to pump against greater pressure (afterload), it increases the workload and oxygen demands.
Sexual activity	Increases sympathetic nervous system stimulation, which increases the workload on the heart.
Decreased Oxygen Supply	**Rationale**
Coronary artery spasm	Causes a decrease in the size of the lumen of the artery, which decreases blood flow to the tissues. When combined with CAD, it markedly decreases blood flow to the tissues.
Coronary artery disease	Decreases vessel lumen, which decreases blood supply to the myocardium.
Hypotension	Decreases cardiac output.
Dysrhythmias	Decreases cardiac output if occurring in significant numbers and areas of the myocardium (ventricle).
Anemia	Decreases the oxygen-carrying capacity of the blood, which decreases oxygen to the myocardium.
Smoking	Causes vasoconstriction, which increases afterload and the workload of the heart.

stimulation of internal mechanisms that result in the smooth muscle extending into the inner layer of the vessel, thereby decreasing in the lumen of the artery and a loss of elasticity. Additionally, this process causes external recruitment of inflammatory and procoagulant cells (platelets, and coagulation factors), causing them to aggregate and further decrease the size of the lumen.

Stage I Lesion

Lesions in the coronary arteries develop in stages. In early atherosclerosis, stage I lesion has grossly visible yellow lesions, known as fatty streaks, in the intimal layer. This earliest form of plaque has been found in the aortas of newborns as well as in both the young and old. These streaks cause little or no obstruction to coronary blood flow; thus, the individuals are not symptomatic. Early fatty streaks consist primarily of macrophages, foam cells, and T lymphocytes, suggesting that plaque genesis may be a response to inflammation. The lesion develops with the migration of smooth muscle cells and the accumulation of macrophages, T lymphocytes, lipids, and foam cells. In response to injury, circulating monocytes

CHART 40–2   Causes of Intimal Vessel Wall Injury

Stressor	Source and Effect
Mechanical	Sheer stress from blood flow at vessel branches/bifurcation due to HTN; injury secondary to PCI procedures
Chemical	Hypercholesterolemia; homocystinemia; hydrocarbons, nicotine, and carbon monoxide from cigarettes; free fatty acids, oxygen radicals, angiotensin, hormones; oxidized lipids; oxidant stress caused by cigarette smoking, hypertension, and advanced glycation end products in diabetes mellitus; estrogen deficiency; vasoactive amines
Immunologic	Exposure to antigen–antibody complexes; virally induced injuries; exposure to bacteria; activated macrophages; infectious microorganisms such as herpesviruses, *Chlamydia pneumoniae*
Genetic	Alterations
Biologic	Advancing age

and platelets adhere to the damaged segment of endothelium. Activated platelets release their contents, and this release recruits and promotes adhesion of other platelets to the endothelium. This process then causes the release of growth factors, which inhibits cell proliferation and stimulates connective tissue formation, all of which cause a decrease in lumen size. Activated macrophages bind with lipoproteins to form foam cells. Macrophages and foam cells produce cytokines, growth factors, and other chemicals that induce and regulate the accumulation of lipids; the proliferation and migration of monocytes, T lymphocytes, possibly mast cells into the arterial wall, and smooth muscle cells from the media into the intima; and the synthesis of matrix components (Figure 40–2 ■).

Stage II Lesion

Over time, perhaps as a result of repeated injury, plaque lesions may mature with the organization of a lipid core and the formation of a fibrous cap (Figure 40–3 ■, p. 1162). This progression of the disease is referred to as a stage II lesion. During this stage the medial smooth muscle cells invade the intimal lesion, leading to a further buildup of plaque that obstructs luminal blood flow. These lesions contain an accumulation of smooth muscle cells, macrophages, T lymphocytes, intra- and extracellular lipids, foam cells, cellular debris from focal necrosis and foam cell apoptosis, and other blood components such as fibrin, fibrinogen, albumin, and white cells. The smooth muscle cells secrete collagen, elastin, and glycosaminoglycans that form a dense connective tissue matrix called the **fibrous cap**. Stage II lesions are grossly white in appearance and most frequently develop where arteries bifurcate. Figure 40–3 ■ (p. 1162) shows the fibrous cap. If the atheroma grows to occlude 40% to 45% of the vessel lumen, arterial remodeling occurs to maintain luminal diameter (Burke et al., 2002). *Remodeling* is a term used to describe how cells, tissue,

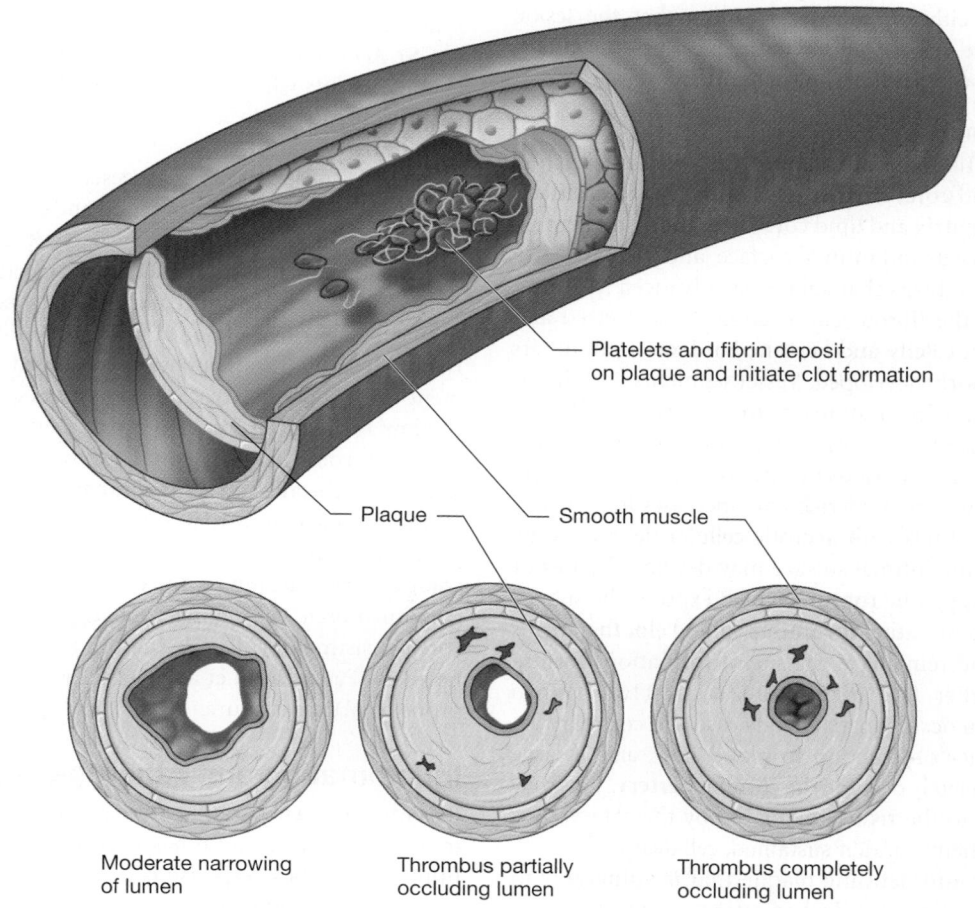

Platelets and fibrin deposit on plaque and initiate clot formation

Plaque — Smooth muscle

Moderate narrowing of lumen

Thrombus partially occluding lumen

Thrombus completely occluding lumen

FIGURE 40–2 ■ Stage of atheroma development in a coronary artery.

Lipid core

Thick fibrous cap

FIGURE 40–3 ■ Fibrous cap.

or organs react or change in response to injury that either serves to maintain function or structure (positive remodeling) or results in further disruption of normal processes (negative remodeling). With positive remodeling, despite increasing atheroma size within the intima, the vessel accommodates through expansion or stretching of the external elastic lumina. Over time, with continued plaque growth, negative remodeling occurs, which refers to shrinking or constriction of the external elastic lumina, resulting in increasing stenosis of the vessel lumen (Schoenhagen et al., 2002) (see Figure 40–3 ■). Once arterial diameter is reduced by 70%, whether due to plaque size or thrombosis, the patient develops symptoms of CAD such as angina. Coronary artery stenosis is described as either **eccentric,** meaning that the lesion occupies part of the vessel wall circumference, or **concentric,** whereby the lesion occupies the whole circumference.

Stage III Lesion

Advanced or stage III lesions are plaque with a well-established fibrous cap and lipid core. Further development and calcification of the fibrous matrix and lipid core, ulceration and hemorrhage of the fibrous cap and intimal surface, and increased risk of transluminal thrombosis characterize an advanced lesion.

In some lesions the fibrous cap becomes vascularized and grows in size; others calcify and become hardened; still others may be thin and poorly developed. Vessel segments with hardened fibrous caps are less responsive to ischemia-related vasodilatory compensatory mechanisms, which results in the vessel not dilating during periods of increased need for oxygen. In complicated lesions the lipid-rich core increases in size, may become calcified, and fills with necrotic cellular debris. As the atheroma enlarges, the intimal surface may develop fissures or cracks, referred to as plaque rupture, which exposes the subendothelial matrix and initiating **thrombus** (blood clot that forms in a blood vessel and remains at the site of formation) formation, described earlier (see Figure 40–2 ■, p. 1161). When thrombus formation occurs in an already diseased coronary artery, it causes further obstruction to blood flow, and if large enough it may completely occlude the coronary artery. This may stop all blood flow to the tissues being fed by the artery, thus leading to tissue ischemia and, if sustained, cell death.

Plaque anatomy and defining plaque that is vulnerable to rupture have received a great deal of attention. Studies have identified certain characteristics that suggest plaque instabil-

ity, which increases the risk for rupture (Pasterkamp, Fitzgerald, & de Kleijn, 2002). Plaque "prone to rupture" is associated with the following factors:

- Positive remodeling
- A thin fibrous cap
- A core rich in lipids, calcium deposits, macrophages, T lymphocytes, and mast cells
- A paucity of collagen and smooth muscle cells
- Of a size large enough to cause mild to moderate luminal obstruction (Pasterkamp et al., 2002).

Plaque injury occurs in lesions that are predominantly yellow in color with ragged edges. Unstable lesions are associated with areas of plaque hemorrhage and neovascularization (blood supply) within the fibrous cap. They are also associated with points of endothelial disruption or ulceration overlying the fibrous cap; sites where the fibrous cap is thinnest, typically at the shoulder where it attaches to the vessel; and sites where there is a dense concentration of matrix metalloproteinases (MMPs). Matrix metalloproteinases are proinflammatory substances that contribute to the breakdown of the fibrous cap. It is thought that MMPs play a role in plaque vulnerability. These lesions may be difficult to identify. Often there is not a flow-limiting stenosis and the patient is asymptomatic. Normal detection with conventional methods such as stress testing and angiography may be inconclusive.

Unstable angina (UA), non–ST segment elevation MI (NSTEMI), and ST segment elevation MI (STEMI) are the three syndromes that collectively describe **acute coronary syndrome (ACS).** Acute coronary syndrome, which is discussed later in the chapter, results when the plaque buildup in the artery becomes significant enough to cause ischemia that result in clinical manifestations.

A recent consensus paper suggests that when unstable plaque is conjoined with conditions of blood and myocardial maladies, the risk for ACS increases (Naghavi et al., 2003b). Blood abnormalities include abnormal platelet function or structure, hypercoagulable states, and/or reduced anticoagulation factors. Blood that is prone to coagulate because of one of these blood disorders increases the risk of thrombus formation when combined with plaque development or disruption. Myocardial maladies can be caused by dysrhythmias, reduced or abnormal ventricular function, and reduced myocardial perfusion. These patients are at higher risk of death from chronic and acute coronary artery occlusion.

In contrast, plaque that is more stable is associated with negative remodeling, a smooth surface with a predominant white color and no thrombi, a thick calcified fibrous cap with little smooth muscle cell or macrophage content, a smaller plaque core consisting of collagen, smooth muscle cells, and apoptotic necrosis (Pasterkamp et al., 2002). Lesions of this type are less prone to plaque rupture.

Inflammation and Atherogenesis

Recently the association between atherogenesis and the immune complex response has been described in the literature. Immune complex response is described in Chapter 60 ⬡. At every stage of plaque development, leukocytes act as instigators and regulators of many processes that are associated with plaque development, such as endothelial dysfunction, procoagulant activity, subendothelial macrophage and smooth muscle cell activity, fibrous cap matrix formation and degradation, and enhanced lipoprotein transfer in the vessel wall. Research studies have suggested that certain infectious organisms may stimulate an immune response that results in plaque disruption, plaque growth, or thrombosis in areas of existing atheroma (Higuchi et al., 2003; Pieniazek et al., 2001). Increased titers of antibodies to certain organisms such as cytomegalovirus, herpesvirus, *Chlamydia pneumoniae,* and *Helicobacter pylori* have been identified as possible predictors of elevated risk for coronary artery occlusions (Higuchi et al., 2003; Pieniazek et al., 2001). It is unclear what effect these organisms have on the cells of the vessel lining; however, these organisms have been found in atheromatous lesions and organs either at autopsy or from atheroma samples. In addition, patients with ACS demonstrate elevated levels of serum markers of inflammation, activated leukocytosis, and their by-products of cytokine, growth factor, and smooth muscle cell activation, which indicate a heightened inflammatory response (Aggarwal et al., 2004; Nomoto et al., 2003). These findings strongly suggest a role of inflammation in either propagating or promoting atherogenesis, or that inflammatory markers are signs that plaque disruption is ongoing and thus are considered markers of increased risk for future sentinel cardiac events (Porth, 2005; Rosenson & Koenig, 2003). Several serum markers of inflammation have been identified, including C-reactive protein (CRP).

Pathophysiology of Myocardial Injury and Death

Myocardial injury from ischemia begins in the subendocardium and progresses to the epicardium (Figure 40–4 ■). If blood flow is not restored within 20 minutes, cell death ensues, autodigestion of cells begins, and the inflammatory response is initiated. Rupture of the intracellular lysosomes is the final event signaling irreversible cell injury, cell death, and loss of muscle function. At this point the intracellular enzymes are released into the bloodstream. The dead nonfunctional tissue is referred to as the area of infarction, which has a central core comprised of nonfunctional cells with disorganized structures, which are surrounded by peripheral cells with varying amounts of disruption (Figure 40–5 ■, p. 1164). Within hours neutrophils infiltrate infarcted tissue, causing further endothelial damage, contraction of smooth muscles, and an increase in vascular permeability. Enzymes released by macrophages may lead to breakdown of connective tissue and cardiac muscle aneurysm formation or rupture, leaking of fluid into the pericardial space, and/or pericardial inflammation. Necrotic tissue is replaced by granulation tissue in 2 to 3 weeks, which can induce myocardial wall thinning and dilation. Fibroblasts eventually appear and synthesize a collagen matrix that provides the substrate for fibrous tissue and the formation of a mature scar in 2 to 3 months. Scarred or fibrotic myocardium becomes stiff and loses its ability to contract and relax, in other words, to function normally. Over time the myocardium may thin. Muscle cells around scarred tissue enlarge or hypertrophy. Myocardial stiffening, thinning, and hypertrophy also can cause contraction abnormalities. In addition myocardial scarring can cause abnormal conduction of cardiac impulses

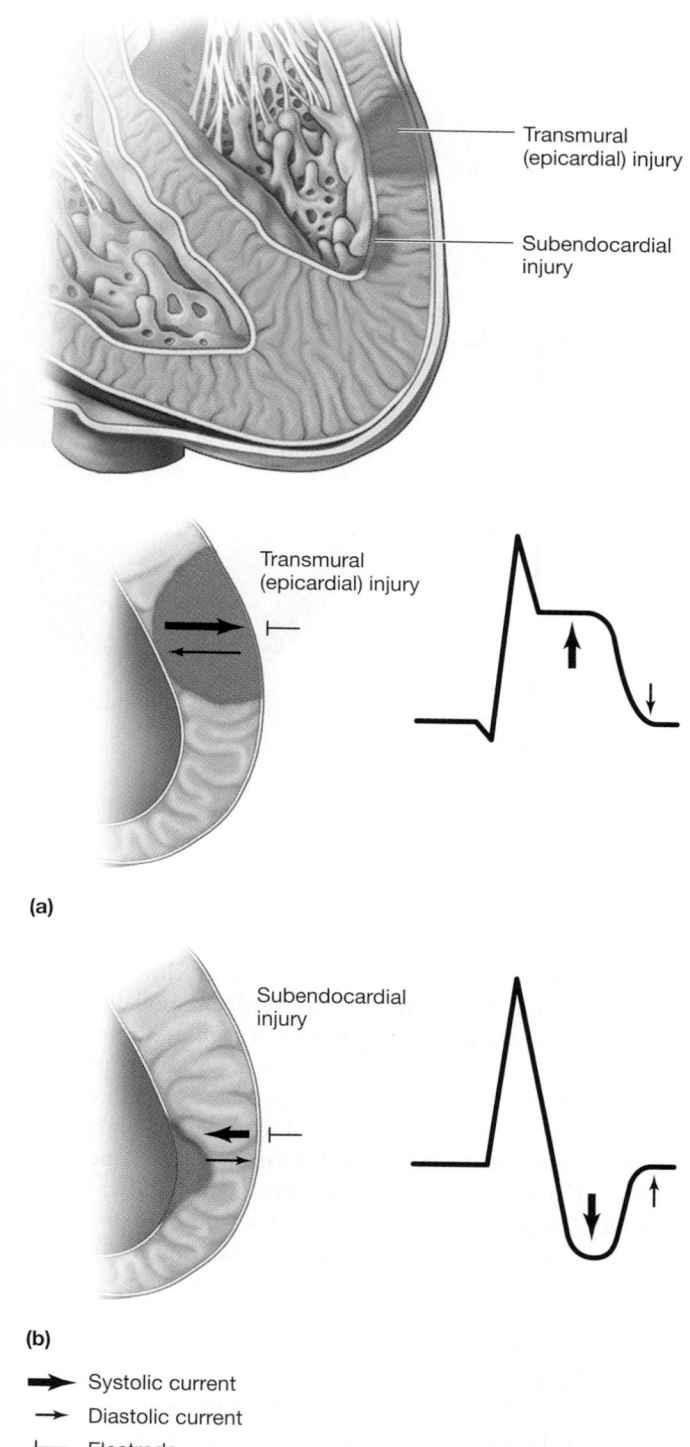

(a)

(b)

➡ Systolic current
→ Diastolic current
⊢ Electrode

FIGURE 40–4 ■ Subendocardial versus transmural damage.

from the sinoatrial (SA) node to the ventricles (Porth, 2005). The cardiac conduction system is discussed in Chapter 38 ☺.

Surrounding the area of infarction is the zone of injury and the zone of ischemia (see Figure 40–5 ■, p. 1164). These zones are made of potentially viable tissues. They can become necrotic and die, or be reperfused and remain functional. The goal of treatment for an AMI is to establish reperfusion as early as possible to prevent necrosis and salvage the myocardium.

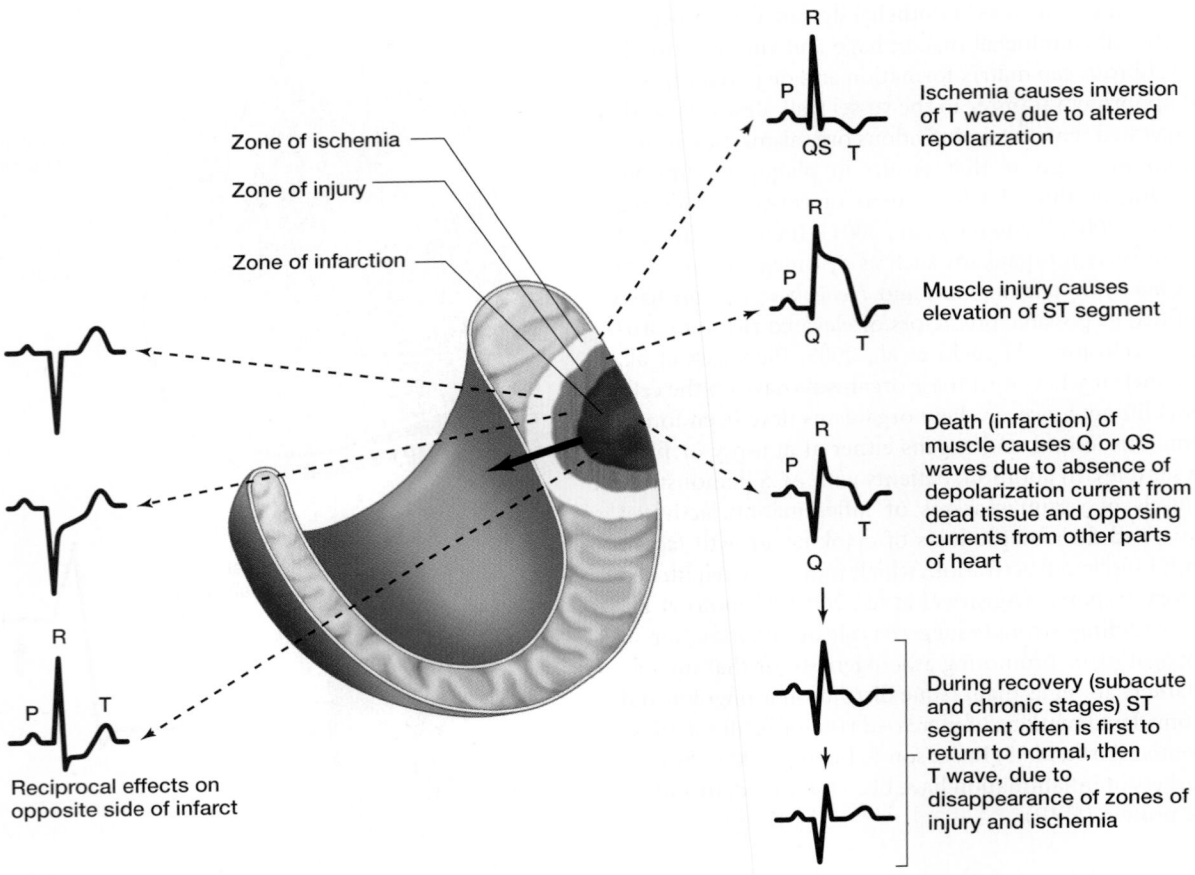

Ischemia causes inversion of T wave due to altered repolarization

Muscle injury causes elevation of ST segment

Death (infarction) of muscle causes Q or QS waves due to absence of depolarization current from dead tissue and opposing currents from other parts of heart

During recovery (subacute and chronic stages) ST segment often is first to return to normal, then T wave, due to disappearance of zones of injury and ischemia

Zone of ischemia
Zone of injury
Zone of infarction

Reciprocal effects on opposite side of infarct

FIGURE 40–5 ■ Zones of infarction and reciprocal ECG changes.

Prevention of cell death, reversing cell injury, limiting infarct size or extension, and preventing myocardial remodeling are all dependent on a number of adaptive responses to acute and chronic ischemia. These include the timing of reperfusion, the presence of ischemic preconditioning, the extent of collateral circulation, myocardial stunning and hibernation, and cellular apoptosis and oncosis (Henning & Olsson, 2001). Reperfusion within 20 minutes will abort cell death. Fibrinolytic, or clot-dissolving, agents (see the Pharmacology Summary of Medications to Treat Coronary Artery Disease box, p. 1199) have a window of less than 12 hours from symptom onset to achieve myocardial salvage. Vessels with chronic subacute thrombosis lasting a few minutes, precondition the tissue for periods of longer ischemia, protecting it from infarction. Chronic, progressive coronary obstruction also stimulates the development of coronary collateral vessels. It is unclear whether these vessels are indigenous and simply recruited in times of coronary insufficiency, or if collaterals represent neovascular development. Neovascular development can occur by angiogenesis, which is the growth of new microvessels budding from arteries in areas of healing infarcted tissue. Myocardial tissue stunning and hibernation are conditions of reversible muscle contractile dysfunction thought to be adaptive responses to chronic coronary occlusion. **Myocardial stunning** is a temporary dysfunction that occurs in response to artery occlusion of short duration or transient global hypoperfusion during a limited low flow state such as shock. The end result is that the myocardial muscle tem-

porarily has a limited ability to contract, whereas with **myocardial hibernation** the tissue actually undergoes cellular structural changes and progressive apoptosis (cell death) in response to prolonged ischemia (Henning & Olsson, 2001). Hibernating tissue is thought to recover contractile function fully once perfusion is reestablished (Brown, 2001).

Oncosis and apoptosis are two processes of cell death. **Oncosis** is cell swelling as a result of changes in membrane permeability. Apoptosis is a genetically derived and substrate controlled process of programmed cell death. Oncosis and apoptosis may contribute to the overall magnitude of ischemic necrosis and myocardial remodeling. Recent studies have identified apoptotic cells and myocyte proliferation in areas around the site of infarction (Barandon et al., 2004). Various hypotheses are the subject of ongoing research as to whether cells can be reprogrammed to limit apoptosis and/or enhance angiogenesis and myocyte regeneration as a means of altering the process of myocardial remodeling.

Cardiac Risk Factors

Cardiac risk factors are habits, lifestyles, and/or genetic factors that predispose an individual to the development of coronary artery disease. Risk factors have various categories, which are typically referred to as modifiable versus nonmodifiable, and contributing factors. The risk factors for coronary artery disease are outlined in the Risk Factors box. Modifiable risk factors are ones that an individual has some control over, such as physical

RISK FACTORS for Coronary Artery Disease

Modifiable Factors	Nonmodifiable Factors	Contributing Factors
Elevated low density lipoprotein cholesterol (LDL-C)	Increasing age	High-fat diet
Low high density lipoprotein cholesterol (HDL-C)	Heredity	Alcohol consumption
Triglycerides	Male gender	Increased stress
Elevated total cholesterol		Increased homocysteine level
Hypertension		Increased C-reactive protein
Tobacco smoke		Hormone replacement therapy
Diabetes		
Physical inactivity		
Overweight and obesity*		

*Normal weight = 18.5–24.9 kg/m²; overweight = 25–29 kg/m²; obesity = > 30.0 kg/m²; abdominal obesity is defined as waist circumference (men) > 102 centimeters (40 inches); (women) > 88 centimeters (35 inches)

activity, stress, and cigarette smoking, whereas nonmodifiable risk factors are not controllable. Nonmodifiable risk factors include advancing age, male sex, and heredity. The American Heart Association (2006c) recommends that all adults with or without established CAD be assessed for risk beginning at the age of 20. A review of lifestyle and predisposing factors at every annual physical evaluation or at least every 2 years should occur (AHA 2006c).

Since 1948 a longitudinal study has been conducted in Framingham, Massachusetts (Futterman & Lemberg, 2000). This study has been evaluating lifestyles and habits of the city's inhabitants. The results of this study have allowed researchers to identify factors that increase a person's risk for the development of CAD. The study is still going on and it is now evaluating the third and fourth generation of subjects. It continues to provide important information about the development of heart disease. Additionally, an abundance of other research continues to refine and add to the body of knowledge about the development of CAD. The modifiable risk factors include elevated serum total cholesterol, increased low density lipoprotein cholesterol (LDL-C), low levels of high density lipoprotein cholesterol (HDL-C), elevated blood pressure, tobacco smoke, physical inactivity, diabetes mellitus, and obesity/overweight (AHA, 2006c). Of these factors, high cholesterol, high LDL-C, high blood pressure, and smoking are most closely linked to development of atherosclerosis. Each of these factors is an independent predictor of CAD.

Research data from the last few decades have shown conclusively that it is possible to alter the natural history of atherosclerosis by either regression or stabilization of plaque with aggressive risk factor reduction (Naghavi et al., 2003a, 2003b). Risk factor reduction efforts focus on factors that are modifiable, specifically lifestyle changes aimed at promoting smoking cessation, blood pressure control, exercise, weight reduction, low-fat diets, and pharmacologic therapies that control dyslipidemia.

Modifiable Risk Factors

Modifiable risk factor identification is important for both assessment of risk and targets for intervention. The modifiable risk factors include hyperlipidemia, hypertension, tobacco smoke, diabetes, physical inactivity, and obesity/overweight.

 When educating patients about CAD, the nurse must stress that if the patient has nonmodifiable risk factors, it is essential to control the modifiable factors in order to prevent or slow the progression of CAD.

Hyperlipidemia

Hyperlipidemia, is defined as elevated cholesterol and/or triglyceride levels. These are lipids that permeate the arterial wall causing a narrowed lumen that ultimately decreases blood flow to the cardiac muscle. **Hypercholesterolemia** is defined as increased cholesterol level in the blood. **Cholesterol** is a steroid molecule produced primarily by the liver that is essential for the formation and maintenance of cell membranes. Cholesterol also is a building block for sex hormones; it aids in the production of digestive bile salts and enables the conversion of vitamin D in the skin. The serum cholesterol level is a potent indicator of risk for CAD. Approximately 85% of cholesterol in the blood is produced by the body. The other 15% is consumed through the diet. For a person with no cardiac history or risk factors, a total cholesterol level less than 200 mg/dL is considered low risk for the development of CAD. A total cholesterol level of 200 to 250 mg/dL is moderate risk, and levels greater than 250 mg/dL are considered high risk. For patients with known CAD or risk factors, the desired serum levels are lower (Chart 40–3).

 ### Laboratory Test Parameters That Prevent CAD

Patient teaching needs to stress that the following blood levels are the goal for prevention of CAD:

Total cholesterol/HDL-C ratio < 4

Total cholesterol < 200 mg/dL

LDL-C < 100 mg/dL

HDL-C > 40 mg/dL

Triglycerides < 150 mg/dL

Hs-C-reactive protein < 0.7 mg/dL = low risk

Homocysteine 4 to 14.

Source: Corbett, J. V. (2004). *Laboratory and diagnostic procedures with nursing diagnoses.* Upper Saddle River, NJ: Prentice Hall Health. Electronically reproduced by permission of Pearson Education, Inc., Upper Saddle River, New Jersey.

Hypercholesterolemia may be inherited as a genetic defect that leads to excessive production of low density lipoproteins or a decreased capacity for their removal. It also can be acquired through diet and lifestyle. Familial hypercholesterolemia is discussed in the Genetic Considerations box. Cultural variations on cholesterol levels have been noted as well. The Cultural Considerations box discusses cultural groups that have a lower rate of CAD. Cholesterol levels tend to increase with age. One correlation is resoundingly clear: The higher the elevated level of cholesterol, the greater the risk of future and acute cardiovascular adverse events. A 1% decrease in cholesterol results in a 2% to 3% decrease in the risk of MI (Castelli, 2001).

Cholesterol is carried in the blood via small proteins. When these carrier proteins join with cholesterol, they are called lipoproteins. The weight or density of lipoproteins depends on the amount of protein in the molecule. Total serum cholesterol is a composite value comprised of all the types of cholesterol carrying lipoproteins. The lipoproteins that alter one's risk for CAD are the low density lipoproteins, the high density lipoproteins, and possibly lipoprotein A. The American Heart Association (AHA) recommends that total cholesterol levels be drawn every 5 years. For men over 45 years, women over 55 years, and patients with elevated cholesterol, or low high density lipoprotein cholesterol (HDL-C), cholesterol levels should be drawn more often.

 **CRITICAL ALERT** *Patients need to be instructed that cholesterol and lipid panels should be drawn after a person has fasted overnight, including no alcohol.*

Low density lipoprotein cholesterol (LDL-C), the so-called "bad cholesterol," is the major cholesterol carrier in the blood. When circulating LDL-C becomes oxidized, it is modified such that it attaches to and migrates through the cell membrane into the intimal lining of the vessel. Once inside the cell membrane, LDL-C attracts immune complexes from the blood into the intimae. Smooth muscle cells from the medial layer of the vessel wall migrate into the intima, thus creating the substrate for plaque development. Oxidized LDL-C also causes endothelial dysfunction by inhibiting the release of endothelial nitric oxide, a compound that not only prevents LDL-C oxidation but also is necessary for vasodilation. Thus, vessel segments damaged by plaque do not vasodilate in response to local hypoxia caused from vessel occlusion the way undamaged vessel segments do. The optimal target goal for LDL-C is less than 100 mg/dL. Target ranges vary depending on the presence of CAD and the risk factor profile outlined in Chart 40–4.

GENETIC CONSIDERATIONS
for Hypercholesterolemia

Familial hypercholesterolemia (FH) is a dominantly inherited genetic disease that results in markedly elevated low density lipoproteins (LDL), the bad cholesterol, beginning at birth. This leads to premature coronary atherosclerosis, which increases the risk of suffering an acute myocardial infarction (AMI) or stroke at an early age. Men are more commonly affected, having their first AMI in their 40s to 50s, with 85% of them having an AMI by age 60. Women have an increased incidence of AMI, but it is delayed by 10 years.

Hypercholesterolemia has several alternative names including type II hyperlipoproteinemia, hypercholesterolemic xanthomatosis, and low density lipoprotein receptor mutation.

An individual can inherit two genes for this disorder, which magnifies the severity of the condition. The cholesterol level may exceed 600 mg/dL; and waxy plaques (xanthomas) of cholesterol develop beneath the skin over elbows, knees, and buttocks; in tendons; and around the cornea of the eye. Atherosclerosis begins before puberty, and AMI and death may occur before age 30.

Patient teaching for individuals with a strong family history includes stressing the risk of early AMI, and these patients should be evaluated with a lipid screen regularly. Proper diet, exercise, and the use of lipid lowering drugs to bring the cholesterol down to safer levels are also recommended.

Source: Leren, T. P. (2004). Cascade genetic screening for familial hypercholesterolemia. *Clinical Genetics: An International Journal of Genetics and Molecular Medicine. 66* (6). 483–487. Reproduced with permission of Blackwell Publishing Ltd.

CULTURAL CONSIDERATIONS for CAD
Development

Cultures vary in their tendency for high cholesterol levels and the development of CAD. This is dramatized by the fact that rural residents in the developing nations of Asia, Africa, and Latin America typically have low total cholesterol levels, in the range of 125 to 140 mg/dL, and they do not develop CAD (Castelli, 2001).

CHART 40–4	Factors That Affect the Lipid Profile	
HDL-C	Factors that ↑ HDL-C	Smoking cessation by 10% Exercise Weight reduction
	Factors that ↓ HDL-C	Smoking Trans fatty acids Sedentary Obesity Low-fat/high carbohydrate diet
LDL-C	Factors that ↑ LDL-C	Trans fatty acids Saturated fats Cholesterol
	Factors that ↓ LDL-C	Polyunsaturated fatty acids Monounsaturated fatty acids Soluble fiber Soy protein Weight reduction
Triglycerides	Factors that ↑ triglycerides	Excess body weight Reduced physical activity Increased intake of sugar and refined carbohydrates, particularly in the setting of insulin resistance and glucose intolerance Increased alcohol intake
	Factors that ↓ triglycerides	Exercise Weight reduction Reduced carbohydrate consumption

High density lipoprotein cholesterol (HDL-C) is heavier lipoproteins that bind to cholesterol, transporting it back to the liver, and may actually remove excess cholesterol from plaque in the arteries. High levels of HDL-C are thought to be cardioprotective. Levels greater than 40 mg/dL in men and greater than 50 mg/dL in women with no CAD and no risk factors are desirable. Even if one's HDL-C level is elevated above the target level, this does not negate the need to lower one's LDL-C level to target levels. The cardioprotection from HDL-C does not insulate one from the atherogenic effects of LDL-C. When determining one's risk of CAD, clinicians also use a comparison between the total cholesterol level and the HDL-C level. A total cholesterol/HDL-C ratio of 3.5:1 or less is optimal (AHA, 2006c). Methods used to alter lipid levels include dietary and lifestyle modifications, and/or pharmacologic intervention (Chart 40–5).

 CRITICAL ALERT *When teaching patients about dietary control of cholesterol and lipids, it is important for the nurse to inquire about food preferences and cultural factors. The teaching needs to be tailored to include these preferences and cultural considerations in order to increase compliance with the restrictions.*

Triglycerides are a form of fat derived from fats in food and produced by the body from other sources such as carbohydrates. Triglycerides are used as a partial building block for plasma lipids found in cell membranes. Elevated triglyceride levels are associated with high total cholesterol, high LDL-C, low HDL-C, heart disease, obesity, and diabetes (AHA, 2006e). Lowering levels to less than 150 mg/dL has become a part of risk prevention. Levels of 150 to 199 mg/dL are considered borderline high, levels of 200 to 499 mg/dL borderline high to high, and levels greater than 500 mg/dL very high (AHA, 2006e).

CHART 40–5	**Therapeutic Lifestyle Dietary Changes**
Nutrient	**Recommended Intake**
Saturated fat	Less than 7% of total calories
Polyunsaturated fat	Up to 10% of total calories
Monounsaturated fat—oils from olives, avocados, nuts	Up to 20% total calories
Total fat	25–35% of total calories
Carbohydrate—predominantly derived from foods rich in complex carbohydrates including grains, whole grains, fruits, and vegetables	50–60% of total calories, if > 60% of diet can cause reduced high density lipoproteins (HDL) and increased triglycerides
Fiber	20–30 grams/day
Protein	Approximately 15% of total calories
Cholesterol	Less than 200 milligrams/day
Total calories (energy)	Balance energy intake and expenditure to maintain desirable body weight/prevent weight gain

Source: Berra, K., & Klieman, L. (2003). National cholesterol education program. Adult treatment panel III—New recommendations for lifestyle and medical management of dyslipidemia. *Journal of Cardiovascular Nursing, 18*(2), 85–92.

Triglycerides are carried to tissues by many types of proteins such as very low density lipoprotein cholesterol (VLDL-C) and chylomicra. VLDL is converted to LDL-C after delivering triglycerides to the muscles and adipose or fat tissue. Chylomicra have the heaviest mass and richest triglyceride content of any lipid-containing particle. Chylomicra are metabolized or broken down into partial fragments or remnants by enzymes called apoproteins, such as lipoprotein A and apoprotein E. Elevated levels of VLDL, chylomicra and cylomicron remnants, and apoproteins have each been suggested as having an associated risk of atherogenesis (Nash, 2004).

Lipid Lowering Therapy

Lipid lowering drugs include hepatic hydroxymethyl glutaryl coenzyme A reductase inhibitors (HMG-CoA reductase inhibitors), also referred to as statins, and the newest generation, which are a combination of these drugs. The Pharmacology Summary (p. 1199) outlines the lipid lowering medications. Lipid lowering agents are considered in patients with CAD and fewer than two risk factors if their LDL-C is ≥ 190 mg/dL, in patients without CAD with two or more risk factors with an LDL-C ≥ 160 mg/dL, or in patients with known CAD with an LDL-C ≥ 130 mg/dL. Drug therapy is delayed in men under age 35 and premenopausal women with LDL-C of 190 to 219 mg/dL, except in high-risk patient groups such as patients with diabetes or patients who are obese or with hypertension. Patients with CAD and LDL-C between 100 and 129 mg/dL may still benefit from lipid lowering therapy. Additionally, lipid lowering therapy is indicated for familial dyslipidemia.

Hypertension

Maintaining a blood pressure within the recommended normal range reduces the mortality from CAD. Every 1 mmHg decrease in diastolic blood pressure results in a 2% to 3% decrease in the incidence of an MI (Diop & Aghababian, 2001). Research has demonstrated that with each age category well into the 80s there was significant reduction in risk of death from CAD or stroke with blood pressure lowering by 20 mmHg, even down to pressures as low as 115/75 mmHg (Lewington et al., 2002). African Americans have the highest overall mortality rate from CAD of all ethnic groups in the United States, which is attributed to the higher prevalence of certain coronary risk factors, among them hypertension and type II diabetes (Clark et al., 2001). A complete description of the cause, incidence, and treatment of high blood pressure is included in Chapter 21 .

Nonpharmacologic interventions aimed at lowering blood pressure focus on exercise, weight control, reduced salt intake, limited alcohol consumption, and a diet that emphasizes fruits, vegetables, and low-fat dairy products. Reducing sodium intake by 1.8 grams a day is associated with a 4 mmHg drop in systolic and a 2 mmHg drop in diastolic pressure in hypertensive patients. Salt intake should be limited to 2,400 milligrams a day, which is equivalent to a diet that includes no added salt and watching added salts in prepared foods. A weight reduction of 1.6 kilograms has shown to drop pressure by 1.1 mmHg averaged for both systolic and diastolic pressures. The American Heart Association advocates the use of antihypertensive medications if the following blood pressure targets cannot be reached after a 6- to 12-month trial of non-pharmacologic measures: blood pressure < 140/90 mmHg;

< 130/85 mmHg if the patient has heart failure or renal insufficiency; or < 130/80 mmHg if the patient has diabetes (Pearson et al., 2002). Age differences are an important consideration in the treatment of hypertension. According to new research published in the *Journal of the American Medical Association*, people age 60 and older should seek treatment when their systolic blood pressure rises above 160, even if the diastolic reading is less than 90. The researchers found "strong evidence" that treating systolic high blood pressure can decrease the likelihood of developing heart disease or having a stroke. High systolic blood pressure in people age 60 and over is a much more important heart disease risk factor than is high diastolic blood pressure (Sarwat, Krumholz, & Foody, 2004).

Tobacco Smoke

Tobacco smokers have a 50% greater chance of developing CAD with a 70% greater mortality than nonsmokers (Diop & Aghababian, 2001). Women who use oral contraceptives and smoke are at a greater risk of heart disease and stroke than are nonsmoking women who use oral contraceptives (Diop & Aghababian, 2001). Cardiovascular adverse effects are attributed to carbon monoxide and nicotine. Carbon monoxide displaces oxygen on the hemoglobin molecule, thus, reducing the blood's oxygen-carrying capacity. Carbon monoxide also may promote atherogenesis by causing endothelial damage. Nicotine increases myocardial oxygen demand by increasing blood pressure and heart rate, and is thought to promote thrombogenesis through platelet aggregation. Nicotine also causes vasospasm and endothelial dysfunction. The risk of cardiovascular adverse events in male and female smokers who successfully quit dramatically decreases. In fact their risk level approaches that of nonsmokers within 2 to 3 years of smoking cessation. HDL-C levels increase by 10% soon after smoking cessation.

Hospitalization presents a unique opportunity of social support for patients who want to stop smoking. A plan for assisting patients in smoking cessation should include the following: (1) Know that repeated attempts at cessation are often necessary; (2) encouragement by all of the patient's health care providers enhances success; (3) the greater the intensity of tobacco-dependence counseling, the higher the quit rate; (4) participation in a smoking cessation program encourages patients to be conscious of triggers for smoking, to develop diversional activities for cravings and rewards for successes, and to establish person–person contact via individual, group, or telephone support; and (5) pharmacotherapies including nicotine replacement with nicotine gum, patch, inhaler, and nasal spray as well as bupropion SR, clonidine, or nortriptyline may be necessary (Haskell, 2003). Useful contacts for more information on smoking cessation include the Agency for Healthcare Research and Quality and the American Lung Association.

Secondhand smoke, often also referred to as environmental tobacco smoke, is a mixture of the smoke given off by the burning end of a cigarette, pipe, or cigar and the smoke exhaled from the lungs of smokers (American Lung Association, 2006a). The residual smoke lingers in the air for hours, even after the tobacco has been extinguished and is involuntarily inhaled by nonsmokers, causing a wide range of adverse health effects, including cancer, respiratory infections, and asthma. Nonsmokers exposed to environmental smoke were 25% more likely to have coronary heart diseases as compared to nonsmokers not exposed to smoke (American Lung Association, 2006a). In 2005, 9 smoke-free states prohibited smoking in almost all workplaces, restaurants, and bars (American Lung Association, 2006a). Additionally, in 2006, 20 years after the first U.S. Surgeon General's report on the dangers of secondhand smoke, the Surgeon General reported that there is no safe level of exposure to secondhand smoke (American Lung Association, 2006b; United States Department of Health and Human Services, 2006a). The new report confirms that secondhand smoke is a cause of lung cancer and heart disease and has immediate adverse effects on the cardiovascular system. The report recommends eliminating smoking in all indoor spaces.

Diabetes

Various micro- and macrovascular changes are thought to be responsible for an overall higher rate of cardiovascular morbidity and mortality found in patients with diabetes. Women have twice the risk of men of developing cardiovascular events associated with diabetes (AHA, 2008b &c). These vascular changes are thought to be mediated through intimal proliferation and other pathologies of endothelial function. As a consequence, those with diabetes are at risk for developing the following conditions related to coronary artery disease:

- Cardiac autonomic neuropathy, resulting in a decreased perception of ischemic pain
- Arterial occlusion in the heart and peripheral vascular circulation
- Dyslipidemias
- Hypertension
- Increased platelet aggregation
- Elevated coagulation factors.

Heart failure because of myocyte hypertrophy, interstitial fibrosis, cardiomyopathy (Chapter 42 ⊚), and disease of the microcirculation called microangiopathy are other consequences of diabetes.

Reducing risk of CAD for patients with diabetes goes beyond controlling known cardiac risk factors. Even without additional risk factors those with diabetes are at greater risk for CAD (AHA, 2006c). Risk factor reduction focuses on aggressive treatment for diabetes including glycemic control (blood sugar) and lifestyle changes. Moderate changes in diet, exercise, and weight reduction can decrease the development of diabetes (National Guidelines and Tools for Cardiovascular Risk Reduction, 2006). Glycemic control has been shown to have an impact on decreasing overall CAD morbidity and mortality and reduces long-term mortality following an acute MI.

Physical Inactivity

Obesity, sedentary lifestyle, and lack of physical activity are mutually supporting cardiac risk factors that are the by-product of Western industrialized societies. Modern society is increasingly dependent on laborsaving technologies that once provided physical exercise or activity for the average person. These include transportation, work, computer- and video-based recreational outlets, and food products of supersized portions with flavor enhanced through fats, sugar, and salt.

Regular exercise ($\geq$ 5 times/week lasting $\geq$ 30 minutes) of moderate intensity (brisk walking) decreases heart attack risk by 10% to 50% in both men and women. Cardioprotection from exercise is attributed to improved functional work capacity, decreased heart rate, decreased platelet adhesiveness, enhanced fibrinolysis, attenuation of the sympathetic stress response, weight loss, lowered triglyceride levels, and increased HDL-C levels. The AHA recommends an exercise routine that totals 2.5 hours a week of any combination of days and hours per day. The recommended routine also includes resistance training of 8 to 10 different exercises, 1 to 2 sets per exercise, 10 to 15 repetitions per set, flexibility training, and habits that increase daily activity (AHA, 2006g). Exercise also may prevent obesity and insulin resistance.

Obesity and Overweight

Obesity has become a social stigma associated with Western civilizations and is destined to cause as much disease and preventable deaths as cigarette smoking. In fact obesity is second only to smoking in modifiable risk factors for all causes of death in the United States (National Guidelines for Treatment and Prevention of Obesity, p. 1170). Chronic obesity increases the risk of CAD in men and women and is antithetical to risk reduction in other areas. Obesity is attributed to increases in blood pressure, abnormal lipoprotein levels, insulin resistance, and platelet aggregation. The two units of measure associated with cardiovascular risk are body mass index (BMI) and abdominal circumference. BMI is a person's weight in kilograms divided by the square of one's height in meters, giving a measure of kg/m^2. Obesity is defined as a body mass index (BMI) > 30, whereas 25.0 to 29.9 is overweight, and 18.5 to 24.9 is normal weight. Abdominal obesity is defined as a waist circumference of > 40 inches (102 centimeters) in men and > 35 inches (88 centimeters) in women. Fat accumulation in the upper body, giving the body an appearance of an "apple," has been linked to a greater risk of CAD as opposed to a "pear" shape with body fat accumulation in the gluteofemoral region. Abdominal obesity is associated with elevated levels of cholesterol and greater risk for CAD.

Obesity is a product of overeating in relation to energy expenditure. General guidelines recommend that total energy intake match overall energy needs, and that activity level matches or exceeds energy intake. The Surgeon General has developed an action plan with specific activities as national priorities for immediate action for individuals, families, communities, schools, work sites, health care, media, industry, organizations, and government to take action to prevent and decrease overweight and obesity. These activities are presented in the National Guidelines for Treatment and Prevention of Obesity box (p. 1170).

 When counseling a patient in weight reduction, a multidisciplinary approach is typically most effective. In order to achieve lifetime changes in eating habits and adherence to an exercise program, the patient needs counseling from nutritionists, health care providers, nurses, physical therapists, and psychological counselors. Many cities have obesity clinics that provide these services.

Nonmodifiable Risk Factors

Nonmodifiable risk factors are those present that cannot be modified through lifestyle and habit changes. Meticulous attention in controlling the modifiable risk factors is recommended to mitigate the effects of the nonmodifiable risk factors. The nonmodifiable risk factors of increasing age, heredity, and male gender are discussed next.

Increasing Age

Cardiac aging results in stiffening of myofibrils, which cause a reduced ability of the muscle to relax, stretch, and contract. The number of myocytes decreases with age, cells enlarge or hypertrophy, they become less responsive to stimulation, and the rate of cellular apoptosis or death increases. As mentioned earlier, with advanced age cholesterol and triglyceride levels increase. Aging causes large arterial vessel walls to dilate and thicken, smooth muscle tone to increase, and increased vessel stiffness as elastic and collagen are replaced with fibrotic tissue. The consequences of these changes are an elevated systolic blood pressure, arteriosclerosis, atherosclerosis, and a decrease in cardiac performance. Age is an independent risk factor for CAD and should be a part of every risk assessment.

Heredity

A familial history of CAD dramatically increases the risk that aggregate family members will have cardiac disease as well. Adult offspring of parents with a CAD history also are more likely to have multiple risk factors for CAD and have greater likelihood of an acute cardiac event, even after correcting for other disease risk factors. First-degree relatives (children, parents, and siblings), families with greater prevalence meaning more than one person in the family have CAD, and families with early onset CAD are at greater risk. Reasons for this familial connection are not known. Possible mediators may be environmental or social factors, or genetic predisposition. Research in the area of genetic mapping is beginning to uncover links between the presence of specific genes or genetic mutations and CAD. For example, a gene called ABCC6 plays a role in keeping elastic fibers healthy. A mutation in this gene has been found to be associated with an increased risk of early CAD (Gene Analysis Service, 2005). Also, inherited variations in gene pairing of a gene that controls how beta-2 (β_2) adrenergic receptors influence blood flow may lower the risk of having a heart attack and dying from heart disease.

Health care personnel need to be mindful of the fact that family members are not always aware that others in their family have or are predisposed to heart disease, especially with regard to less obvious risk factors such as hypertension and hyperlipidemia. The good news is that family members predisposed to CAD who modify their risk in other ways, such as getting regular physical activity at a moderate level, have lower odds of developing CAD than those family members who do not modify their risk factors.

Race is also included under the category of heredity. African Americans have a higher overall CAD prevalence and mortality rate than do Caucasians in the United States (AHA, 2006c). Additionally, they also present with a disproportionate number of CAD risk factors such as hypertension, type II diabetes, metabolic syndrome, abdominal obesity, stress, and inactivity. Reasons for these disparities are unclear; however, ethnic, cultural, and physiological differences exist. Studies have highlighted that African Americans (1) perceive cardiac pain differently and often ascribe symptoms to other noncardiac causes; (2) less often seek, ask for, receive, and respond differently to appropriate preventive, diagnostic, and

NATIONAL GUIDELINES for Treatment and Prevention of Obesity

Overweight and Obesity: A Vision of the Future

The Surgeon General identifies specific activities as national priorities for immediate action. Individuals, families, communities, schools, work sites, health care, media, industry, organizations, and government must determine their role and take action to prevent and decrease overweight and obesity.

Communication

The Nation must take an informed, sensitive approach to communicate with and educate the American people about health issues related to overweight and obesity. Everyone must work together to:

Change the perception of overweight and obesity at all ages. The primary concern should be one of health and not appearance.

Educate all expectant parents about the many benefits of breastfeeding.

Breastfed infants may be less likely to become overweight as they grow older.

Mothers who breastfeed may return to prepregnancy weight more quickly.

Educate health care providers and health profession students in the prevention and treatment of overweight and obesity across the life span.

Provide culturally appropriate education in schools and communities about healthy eating habits and regular physical activity, based on the Dietary Guidelines for Americans, for people of all ages. Emphasize the consumer's role in making wise food and physical activity choices.

Action

The Nation must take action to assist Americans in balancing healthful eating with regular physical activity. Individuals and groups across all settings must work in concert to:

Ensure daily, quality physical education in all school grades. Such education can develop the knowledge, attitudes, skills, behaviors, and confidence needed to be physically active for life.

Reduce time spent watching television and in other similar sedentary behaviors.

Build physical activity into regular routines and playtime for children and their families. Ensure that adults get at least 30 minutes of moderate physical activity on most days of the week. Children should aim for at least 60 minutes.

Create more opportunities for physical activity at work sites. Encourage all employers to make facilities and opportunities available for physical activity for all employees.

Make community facilities available and accessible for physical activity for all people, including the elderly.

Promote healthier food choices, including at least 5 servings of fruits and vegetables each day, and reasonable portion sizes at home, in schools, at work sites, and in communities.

Ensure that schools provide healthful foods and beverages on school campuses and at school events by:

Enforcing existing U.S. Department of Agriculture regulations that prohibit serving foods of minimal nutritional value during mealtimes in school food service areas, including in vending machines.

Adopting policies specifying that all foods and beverages available at school contribute toward eating patterns that are consistent with the Dietary Guidelines for Americans.

Providing more food options that are low in fat, calories, and added sugars such as fruits, vegetables, whole grains, and low-fat or nonfat dairy foods.

Reducing access to foods high in fat, calories, and added sugars and to excessive portion sizes.

Create mechanisms for appropriate reimbursement for the prevention and treatment of overweight and obesity.

Research and Evaluation

The Nation must invest in research that improves our understanding of the causes, prevention, and treatment of overweight and obesity. A concerted effort should be made to:

Increase research on behavioral and environmental causes of overweight and obesity.

Increase research and evaluation on prevention and treatment interventions for overweight and obesity and develop and disseminate best practice guidelines.

Increase research on disparities in the prevalence of overweight and obesity among racial and ethnic, gender, socioeconomic, and age groups and use this research to identify effective and culturally appropriate interventions.

Source: United States Department of Health and Human Services. (2006). *Overweight and obesity: A vision for the future.* Retrieved September 17, 2006, from http://www.surgeongeneral.gov/topics/obesity/calltoaction/fact_vision.htm.

---

interventional therapy for CAD; (3) may be financially disenfranchised, which limits access to health care; (4) may experience psychosocial stress, racism, and frustration leading to suboptimal interactions with the health care system; and (5) may have genetic predisposition to vascular disease and atherosclerosis (Venkat, Hekstra, & Lindsell, 2003).

According to the AHA (2006c), CAD is also higher in Mexican Americans, American Indians, native Hawaiians, and some Asian Americans. This is thought to be due in part to higher rates of obesity and diabetes in these populations.

Male Gender

The literature is replete with references to how gender affects cardiovascular health and disease. Prevalence and mortality rates are higher in men than in women, especially men 45 to 70 years of age, surpassed by women only in older age (AHA,

2006c). Even when women's death rate from heart disease increases after menopause, it is not as great as that of men. Men are more likely to seek and receive diagnostic and therapeutic intervention related to differences in pain perception, treatment bias, and social roles. Men also respond differently to therapy with often separate prescription and guideline recommendations. As women achieve advanced financial and social status, there may be a change in CAD disease prevalence and mortality demographics.

 **CRITICAL ALERT**   *The American Heart Association has created a free online toolkit designed to educate women about cardiovascular disease. It was developed as part of the association's Go Red For Women campaign, which calls attention to the devastating effects of heart disease in women. Access this and other campaign resources through the American Heart Association's website.*

Contributing Risk Factors

Contributing risk factors include those factors that one may have a tendency or likelihood to have because of genetics, gender, habits, or other related causes. They are preventable risk factors that usually require self-discipline and motivation in order to avert. Contributing risk factors include high-fat diet, alcohol consumption, stress, homocysteine level, C-reactive protein, and hormone replacement therapy, all of which are discussed next.

High-Fat Diet

The term *heart-healthy diet* has undergone a metamorphosis over the years with on and off restrictive or liberal carbohydrate, protein, or fat portions. The cornerstone of cardiac nutrition stresses a diet low in calories; low in total fat (saturated fats, trans fatty acids, and cholesterol); moderate in protein; and high in fruits, vegetables, and other complex carbohydrates (see Chart 40–5, p. 1167). Limiting caloric intake aids in weight reduction and improves insulin resistance. Diets high in total fats are associated with excess body weight and elevated levels of circulating cholesterol and lipoproteins that are known to be atherogenic. Chapter 14 provides a complete description of heart-healthy diets.

Alcohol Consumption

In observational studies, alcohol consumption of 3 or more alcoholic drinks a day has been associated with elevated blood pressure, heart failure, and stroke (AHA, 2006c). Heavy use of alcohol also has been linked to CAD and related risk factors such as obesity, limited physical activity, diabetes, and malnutrition. Guidelines recommend limiting alcohol intake to no more than 2 drinks a day for men and 1 drink a day for women (AHA, 2006c). Within these limitations, reductions of 20% to 60% in risk have been observed (Diop & Aghababian, 2001). Alcohol in the form of red wine and dark beer may actually protect the heart in ways that have been recently discovered. Flavonals in red wine and dark beer, which are not as plentiful in other forms of alcohol or white wine, are thought to increase HDL-C, improve endothelial function, and reduce platelet aggregation (Goldfinger, 2003). However, drinking in excess of 1 glass of alcohol per day for women and 2 glasses for men, even red wine, is discouraged.

Stress

A number of psychosocial stressors appear to increase one's risk for CAD and morbidity and mortality following an acute MI. Anger, hostility, cynicism, anxiety, depression, lack of social support, type A personality, lack of spiritual support, and lack of financial resources have all been associated with increased risk of and morbidity and mortality from cardiovascular disease. Stress in general enhances autonomic stimulation. Sympathetic stimulation increases myocardial work, blood pressure, heart rate, dysrhythmia generation, and enhances platelet aggregation. Parasympathetic stimulation also predisposes one to dysrhythmias. Depression and lack of social support may affect autonomic impulses and may result in poor adherence to risk modification therapy. Spirituality includes a system of beliefs an individual has about the world and herself. People with greater spiritual awareness appear to display less distress, anxiety, and depression during times of personal turmoil, which may have a direct and indirect effect on CVD risk. The association between psychosocial stressors and CAD is based only on epidemiologic studies thus far. There is a complete discussion of the impact of stress on maladaptive or disease processes in Chapter 12.

Homocysteine Level

Homocysteine is an amino acid that is a by-product of the enzyme reactions from meat, dairy products, vitamin, and mineral metabolism (Coffey, Crowder, & Cheek, 2003). Homocysteine causes endothelial ulceration and scarring, and increases procoagulant properties of blood, all leading to an increase in the risk of thrombus formation. Elevated levels of homocysteine (Hyc > 15 µmol/L) are associated with an increased risk of CAD, as well as peripheral vascular disease, stroke, and venous thrombosis. A normal homocysteine level is 4 to 14 µmol/L. Vitamins B_6, B_{12}, and folic acid decrease the levels of homocysteine, which can be supplemented by either vitamins or foods such as fruits, vegetables, cereals, and legumes (Coffey, Crowder, & Cheek, 2003). Vitamin therapy including dosing is included in Chapter 14.

C-Reactive Protein

Inflammation as described earlier is thought to contribute to ACS, whether as a precursor to acute events because of plaque rupture, or as representative of ongoing endothelial and cell membrane damage. A serum marker of inflammation is C-reactive protein (CRP). C-reactive protein is produced and released by liver cells stimulated by activated macrophages. It is called an "acute phase" protein, meaning that within 24 to 48 hours after an inflammatory stimulus, as may occur during an acute coronary event, protein levels increase a thousandfold. CRP is a predictor of increased risk for heart attacks, strokes, and peripheral vascular disease, and is being used as a screening test for atherosclerosis for middle-aged and older people (AHA, 2006d). Elevated levels are present in patients with unstable angina and acute myocardial infarction (AMI) and appear to be predictive of higher risk for short- and long-term cardiovascular morbidity and mortality. A normal CRP value is < 0.9 mg/dL with levels > 1.6 mg/dL denoting risk and possibly a need for medical intervention such as coronary revascularization.

The standard CRP is not sensitive enough to detect small changes in the level of inflammation that occur in the cardiovascular system of individuals who appear free of CAD. A high-sensitivity CRP (hs-CRP) has been developed that can detect low-grade inflammatory activity within the cardiovascular system. An hs-CRP of < 0.7 mg/dL denotes low risk, 0.7 to 1.1 mg/dL mild risk, 1.2 to 1.9 mg/dL moderate risk, 2.0 to 3.8 mg/dL high risk, and 3.9 to 15 mg/dL very high risk. Aspirin, some forms of vitamin E, statin therapy, and weight loss have been shown to reduce CRP levels (AHA, 2006d).

Hormone Replacement Therapy

Recent studies have changed the thinking related to the benefits and risks of hormone replacement therapy (HRT) in women (AHA, 2006d). Menopause is associated with significant elevations in serum dyslipidemias and a threefold increase in risk of CAD. This is thought to be related to a decrease in the level of estrogen. However, studies have been inconclusive with regard to HRT conferring cardiac protection, and in fact it may increase the risk of CAD. Current recommendations dissuade the use of HRT as a CAD risk reduction strategy and suggest that women contact their health care provider to decide whether the therapeutic benefits of HRT outweigh the risks (AHA, 2006d). However, further research is needed to confirm or deny the more recent findings.

Metabolic Syndrome

Recently a cluster of cardiovascular risk factors, referred to as **metabolic syndrome**, has been defined as having three out of the five following conditions: (1) abdominal obesity, (2) high triglycerides, (3) low HDL-C, (4) high blood pressure, and (5) fasting glucose ($\geq$ 100 mg/dL). This cluster of conditions correlates with a higher risk for CAD and type 2 diabetes onset (Nash, 2004). Management of metabolic syndrome consists of targeting each abnormality with modification of corresponding risk factors, especially weight reduction and increased physical activity, and use of direct therapeutic interventions to lower blood pressure, serum glucose, and serum lipids. The American Heart Association recommends that adults over age 40 or those with two or more risk factors have a multirisk assessment score completed every 10 years.

Clinical Manifestations of Coronary Artery Disease

Coronary artery disease presents as clinical conditions of angina pectoris, unstable angina pectoris, myocardial infarction, and sudden cardiac death. These conditions depict a continuum of progressively worsening imbalances between the amount of oxygen delivered to and required by myocardial tissues. The underlying pathophysiology of each disorder is the same, atherosclerosis, as described earlier. However, as vessel stenosis intensifies, distinctions in the manifestations of signs and symptoms occur that are important for appropriate disease management. The clinical manifestations of ischemia are described next.

Electrocardiogram (ECG) Changes

When the heart muscle becomes ischemic, injured, or infarcted, depolarization and repolarization of cardiac cells are altered, causing changes in the ECG tracing. Figure 40–6 ■ depicts a normal ECG tracing. The ECG changes are manifested in three specific ways: ST segment elevation or depression, T wave extenuation or inversion, and QRS changes as in the development of pathologic Q waves (Figures 40–7 ■, 40–8 ■, 40–9 ■, p. 1174, 40–10 ■, p. 1175). A bundle branch block and cardiac dysrhythmias may also occur. The ECG is useful in identifying areas of injury or infarction, the infarct-related artery, in determining reperfusion following intervention, and in monitoring for cardiac dysrhythmias associated with myocardial damage. The ECG should be completed within the first 10 minutes of admission to the emergency department per national guidelines of the American College of Cardiology/American Heart Association (ACC/AHA) (Antman, Anbe, Armstrong, Bates, Green, Hand, et al. 2004).

ST Segment Changes

The ST segment begins at the end of the QRS complex and ends at the beginning of the T wave (see Figure 40–6 ■). The point marking the end of the QRS complex is referred to as the *J point* (see Figure 40–7 ■). Normally isoelectric, the ST segment represents the time during which the ventricles have been completely depolarized and are beginning to repolarize. When cardiac tissue

FIGURE 40–6 ■ Normal ECG waveforms.

becomes ischemic, the ST segment becomes abnormal and indicates a total reduction in localized blood flow. When the muscle ischemia involves only a portion of the heart wall, it is referred to as subendocardial injury, and ST segment depression occurs (see Figure 40–8 ■). When the ischemia traverses the entire width of the cardiac muscle, referred to as transmural ischemia, the ST segment becomes elevated (see Figure 40–7 ■). Prolonged, persistent ST segment elevation indicates acute ischemia and injury/infarction, and is associated with elevated cardiac blood markers. The greater the displacement of the ST segment and the more leads involved on the 12-lead ECG, the greater the amount of tissue damage (Morton, Fontaine, Hudak, & Gallo, 2005). The morphology (shape) of ST segment elevation is dependent on the lead. Figure 40–7 ■ depicts the various morphologies of ST segment elevation.

With transmural injury, the ST segment begins to rise almost immediately and can remain elevated for several hours to several days, as long as the ischemia continues. As the ischemia/injury subsides, the ST segment returns to the baseline. Once the ST segment has returned to the baseline, one of the main indicators of the acute MI is lost. Thus, obtaining a 12-lead ECG while the abnormality is present or the patient is having chest pain, is essential prior to treatment so that a diagnosis of a cardiac event can be made.

ST segment elevation greater than 1 millimeter or 1 small box on the ECG graph paper, or ST segment depression greater than 0.5 millimeter or one-half a small box, as determined on a 12-lead ECG, is considered a significant change. ST segment changes seen on continuous cardiac monitoring should be verified by obtaining a 12-lead ECG. The waveforms of continuous monitors are not calibrated and may be artificially enhanced by changes in the signal gain. Patients also may have a slight ST depression or elevation as a result of chronic cardiac disease, which can mimic an acute ECG change.

Coved (convex up)
ST segment elevation

Concave up
ST segment elevation

Junction (J point)
ST segment elevation

FIGURE 40–7 ■ ST segment elevation morphology differences.

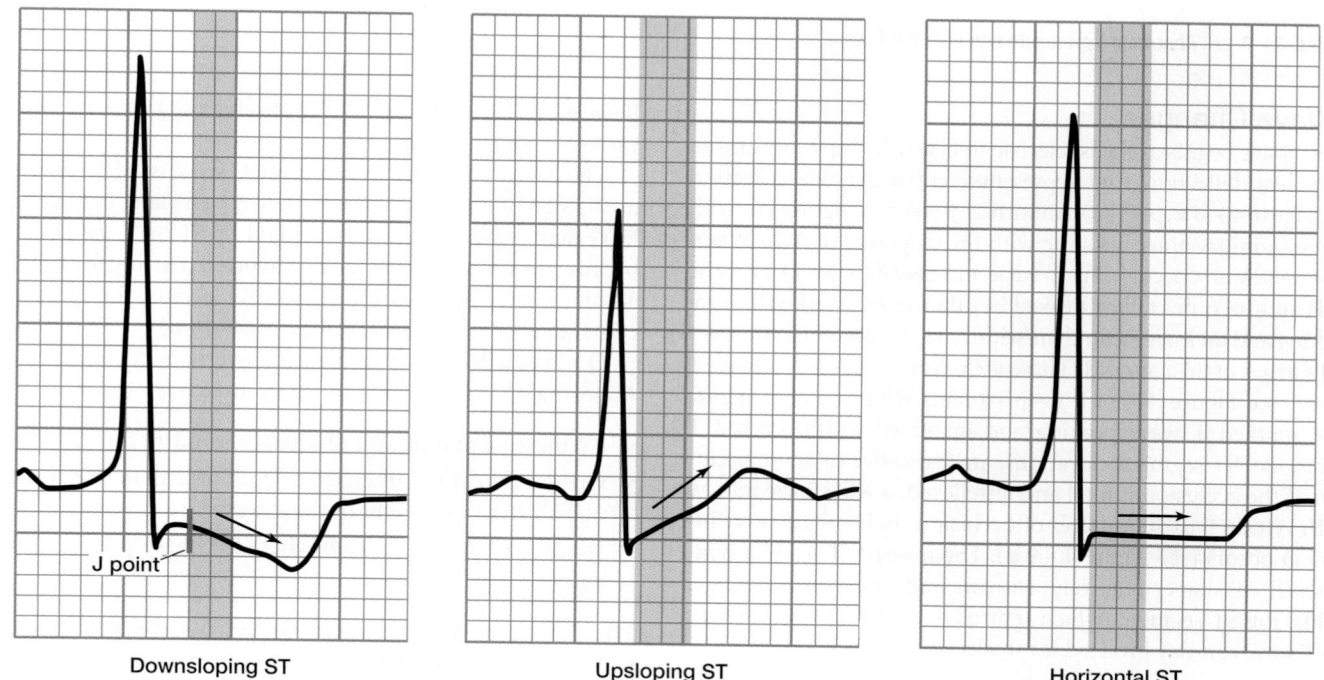

Downsloping ST

Upsloping ST

Horizontal ST

ST Segment Depression

The J point occurs at the end of the QRS complexes.
The ST segment begins at the J point and extends to a user defined interval.

FIGURE 40–8 ■ ST segment depression.

FIGURE 40–9 ■ Abnormal hyperacute and inverted T wave.

T Wave Changes

The T wave begins at the isoelectric line, gently slopes upward in a positive deflection, and represents ventricular repolarization (see Figure 40–6 ■, p. 1172). Abnormal T wave changes occur with ischemia/injury, thus, assisting with the diagnosis of ACS. When ischemia/injury occurs, the T wave inverts (flips over) in some leads and becomes tall or peaked in other leads. Marked T wave peaking and an increase in their width may be present in the very early stages of an acute MI. These are referred to as hyperacute T waves (see Figure 40–9 ■). Even patients with unstable angina have marked T wave peaking and increased width. Peaked T waves, like ST segment elevations, are indicative of acute occlusion. If the occlusion is total and unrelieved, it will evolve into an AMI. Within 5 to 30 minutes of occlusion/ ischemia, T wave inversion occurs (see Figure 40–9 ■). The inverted T wave is symmetrical in shape, relatively narrow, and somewhat pointed. Unlike the ST segment, which returns to normal rather quickly, the T wave can stay inverted for weeks after the ischemic event.

Q Wave Changes

The Q wave is the first component of the ventricular complex, and under normal conditions it is a negatively deflected wave (below the isoelectric line). It is small in size, is less than 0.04 second in duration, and is less than 25% of the amplitude of the R wave (see Figure 40–10 ■). The absence of Q waves is a normal variant of some people's ECG.

The development of an abnormal Q wave is a definitive diagnostic sign of myocardial necrosis. It appears later in time on the ECG than ischemia or injury evident by ST or T wave changes, because necrosis takes the longest to occur. During the first 24 to 48 hours after the AMI as the necrosis occurs, the Q wave becomes deeper and wider (see Figure 40–10 ■).

Q waves will develop in the leads overlying the affected area. Abnormal Q waves are identified in three ways:

- An increase in duration of > 0.04 second
- Greater than 4 millimeters in depth or > than one-fourth to one-third of the height of the R wave
- When they appear in leads where they have previously been absent.

The deep Q wave change seen on the ECG is due to necrosis, which is not reversible; therefore, Q wave changes on the ECGs are permanent, making previous MIs identifiable. The diagnosis of an "old" MI is made when there is a Q wave present in the absence of any ST segment elevation, patient symptoms, and positive blood markers. The ECG cannot determine how long ago the MI occurred; it could have been 2 weeks or 20 years.

Normal

Abnormal Q wave

FIGURE 40–10 ■ Normal and abnormal Q wave.

Angina Pectoris

Angina pectoris is defined as transient chest pain due to myocardial ischemia, caused by an inadequate supply of oxygen and nutrients for the myocardium. CAD is the most common cause of a decreased blood supply to the myocardium. In the United States approximately 6,400,000 people suffer from angina. The estimated age-adjusted prevalences of angina in women age 20 and older were 3.5 percent for non-Hispanic white women, 4.7 percent for non-Hispanic black women, and 2.2 percent for Mexican American women. Rates for men in these three groups were 4.5, 3.1, and 2.4 percent, respectively (AHA, 2006b). Angina accounts for 29% of all medical emergency department admissions, at the cost of billions of health care dollars, and has the highest risk for adverse events and death (Libby, Bonow, Zipes, & Mann, 2008). Angina typically appears in middle age, whereas the average age for first heart attacks is 65 years in men and 70 in women. Though considered mostly a white man's disease, incidence rates of angina have increased in Mexican American men and women, and African American women most significantly (AHA, 2006f).

Angina also can occur in people with normal coronary arteries without obstruction, as a result of vasospasm, endothelial dysfunction, valvular heart disease, hypertrophic cardiomyopathy, uncontrolled hypertension, exacerbations of heart failure, and noncardiac conditions of the esophagus, chest wall, or lungs. Angina in the presence of heart disease is a *warning sign* and needs to be treated emergently in an attempt to prevent an acute cardiac event, such as a myocardial infarction.

Clinical Manifestations of Angina

The clinical manifestations of angina pectoris include a sudden onset of discomfort in the chest, jaw, shoulder, back, or arm, aggravated by exertion or emotional stress, and relieved with rest or nitroglycerin (Figure 40–11 ■, p. 1176). Terms such as *burning, crushing, suffocating,* and *pressure* are typical descriptors of chest pain from myocardial ischemia, often with pain radiating to other areas of the upper torso. Cardiac chest pain usually is neither described as sharp nor localized to a defined spot.

Symptoms of chest pain alone are poor predictors of the presence of CAD and the severity of myocardial damage. In nearly one-third to one-half of individuals with myocardial ischemia, symptoms are not present at all. The clinician is faced with comparing data abstracted from the patient to a set of characteristics associated with diseases that have common presenting signs and symptoms. Charts 40–6 (p. 1177) and 40–7 (p. 1178) outline the presentation of patients with diseases that mimic chest pain associated with CAD.

Women, patients with diabetes, and elderly patients may not experience pain with myocardial ischemia. In addition, the characterization of pain by women may be different from that of men, with women expressing pain in less severe terms, if at all, and often ascribing the pain to causes other than cardiac issues.

Types of Angina Pectoris

There are several accepted classifications for angina pectoris that are based on what triggers the occurrence, how long it lasts, when it occurs, what makes it go away, and its seriousness. Angina is classified as either typical or atypical, depending on signs and symptoms and/or by its severity using the Canadian Cardiovascular Society's angina classification scale. It also is assigned various terms that describe its timing, location, and position. Chart 40–8 (p. 1180) outlines the classifications and descriptors of angina.

Two general categories or classifications include stable and unstable angina. Stable angina, the less serious type, is triggered by a predictable degree of exertion or emotions, and there is a pattern in relation to what brings it on, its duration, its intensity of symptoms, and how to relieve it. Stable angina subsides by taking away the precipitating factors and using sublingual nitroglycerin. Stable angina is differentiated from unstable angina pathologically by the absence of plaque disruption and thrombus formation in the lumen of the artery. Unstable angina is discussed in the next section under acute coronary syndrome.

Variant, Prinzmetal, or Vasospastic Angina   is the most serious type of angina. It occurs when single or multiple sites in major coronary arteries and their large branches have vasospasm. Most often the right coronary artery is involved. Sites of vasospasm generally occur over eccentric lesions. Causes of vasospasm are unknown but may be related to an imbalance of vasoactive agents derived from damaged coronary endothelial tissue, vessel segment hypersensitivity to sympathetic stimulation, allergy, or hypomagnesemia. Symptoms are usually episodic, may last several minutes, are often associated with exercise, and can occur frequently at night.

Medical Management of Angina Pectoris

The majority of patients with stable angina achieve symptom control by medical management alone. When patients with symptoms of angina present to a clinician's office or an emergency

(a) Upper chest

(b) Substernal radiating to neck and jaw

(c) Substernal radiating down left arm

(d) Epigastric

(e) Epigastric radiating to neck, jaw, and arms

(f) Neck and jaw

(g) Left shoulder and down both arms

(h) Intrascapular

FIGURE 40–11 ■ Location of anginal pain.

department, they must be taken seriously and evaluated thoroughly by the health care team. Routine evaluations of patients who complain of chest pain include a review of their symptoms, their medical/social history for associated diseases and risk factors, an assessment for physical signs, and diagnostic tests. Emergency department (ED) personnel use guidelines set forth by the American College of Cardiology and the American Heart Association (Antman et al., 2004) that dictate the patients' treatment. (See the Medical Management of Complications of Acute Myocardial Infarction section, p. 1198.)

Predictors of higher risk for complications generally include angina that has increased in duration, frequency, or at rest; associated ST segment or T wave changes on the ECG; and accompanying signs of heart failure such as the following: new or worsening mitral regurgitation murmur; skin changes such as cool, pale, or clammy; pulmonary edema or presence of an S_3 or S_4 heart sound; tachycardia; and hypotension. Patients classified at lower risk are generally treated on an outpatient basis. Goals for outpatient management include treating conditions that exacerbate angina such as anemia, thyrotoxicosis, dysrhythmias, and eliminating or suppressing symptoms through behavioral changes and prescribing antianginal agents.

Pharmacologic management for angina rests primarily on three classes of drugs: calcium channel blockers, nitrates, and beta-adrenergic blocking agents. Symptom characteristics, exer-

cise tolerance, and comorbid conditions dictate which antianginal agent to use. To date no one drug category has proven more effective at improving prognosis for patients treated for angina pectoris. Antianginal medications are outlined in the Pharmacology Summary (p. 1199). In addition to antianginal agents, management of angina includes ASA in daily doses of 81 to 325 milligrams.

Activity restriction and removing the precipitating factors also will help relieve angina due to decreasing the oxygen demand on the heart. Supplemental oxygen is frequently ordered during periods of pain.

■ Nursing Management

Nursing management of a patient who is experiencing angina requires critical thinking and decision-making skills. Angina pectoris is a warning that the myocardium is not getting enough oxygen, and increased perfusion of oxygen and nutrients is needed to prevent permanent myocardial muscle damage. The nursing process serves as the platform to manage the patients experiencing angina pectoris.

Assessment

The patient needs an in-depth nursing assessment of the pain, including the type of sensation, the location and transmission,

Differential Diagnosis of Chest Pain: Common Etiologies

Pain Description	Associated Findings	History
Angina/Myocardial Infarction		

• Usually retrosternal
• Can originate or radiate at the back, anterior chest, epigastric area, jaw, shoulder, elbow, forearm, wrist
• May be relieved with rest, lasts < 30 minutes
	• Tachycardia
	• Tachypnea, dyspnea
	• Weak heart sounds
	• Rhonchi
	• Diaphoresis
	• Abnormal precordial impulses
	• Evidence of dysrhythmias
		• Cardiac risk factors
		  • Smoking
		  • Male gender
		  • African American
		  • Sedentary lifestyle
		  • Social stressors
		  • High-fat diet.

• Heaviness, burning, tight pressure, aching, indigestion
• Is not relieved with position change
• May increase while supine
• Is not aggravated by deep breathing
	• Fever, elevated white blood count (WBC) count, elevated sedimentation rate
	• Anxiety, sense of impending doom
	• Nausea/vomiting
		• Cardiovascular disease
		  • Heart failure
		  • Dysrhythmias
		  • PVD
		  • Heart valve disease
		  • Angina, unstable angina, myocardial infarction (MI) cardiac interventions
		  • Cardiac surgery
		  • Catheter-based interventions.

Pulmonary Embolism		
• Sudden onset • Sharp • Pleuritic • Lateral chest • Increases on deep inspiration	• Shock • Syncope • Dyspnea, shortness of breath (SOB), cyanosis • Tachycardia • Hemoptysis • Pleural friction rub • Expiratory wheeze • Fever	• Hypercoaguable state • Immobility • Surgery • Trauma • DVT
Gastrointestinal Disorders		
• Burning, squeezing, gripping • Retrosternal without radiation • Lasts many hours or days, constant in nature • Precipitated by bending over, drinking very hot/cold liquids, meals • Relieved with food or beverage	• Reflux • Dysphagia • Dyspepsia	• GERD • Esophageal motility disorders • Esophageal malignancy
Costochondritis		
• Usually superficial and localized • Described as tender, ache, sharp • Can be in any location • Duration variable • Aggravated/provoked by movement or touch	• Sudden movement • Tachypnea, shallow breathing • Tachycardia • Elevated blood pressure	• Falls or trauma • Immobility • Chest tubes newly removed
Acute Anxiety		
• Dull, stabbing	• Breathlessness, hyperventilation	• Acute stress, phobia • Inability to cope

< = less than; PVD = peripheral vascular disease; DVT = deep vein thrombosis; GERD = gastroesophageal reflux disease; w/ = with; w/o = without; SOB = shortness of breath; MI = myocardial infarction; WBC = white blood count

Sources: Williams, J. L. (2003). Gastroesophageal reflux disease: Clinical manifestations. *Gastroenterology Nursing, 26*(5), 195–200; Zoorob, R. J., & Campbell, J. S. (2003). Acute dyspnea in the office. *American Family Physician, 68,* 1803–1810; Lissin, L. W., & Vagelos, R. (2002). Acute aortic syndrome: A case presentation and review of the literature. *Vascular Medicine, 7*(4), 281–287; Pope, J. H., & Selker, H. P. (2002). Diagnosis of acute cardiac ischemia. *Emergency Medical Clinics of North America, 21*(1), 27–59; and Kontos, M. C. (2001). Evaluation of the emergency department chest pain patient. *Cardiology Review, 9*(5), 266–275.

CHART 40-7 Differential Diagnosis of Chest Pain: Less Common Etiologies

Pain Description	Associated Findings	History
Pericarditis		
• Sudden, sharp	• Pulsus paradoxsus	• AMI
• Dull, aching	• Dyspnea	• Dressler's syndrome
• Stabbing, knife-like	• Low-grade erratic fever	• Tamponade
• Retrosternum or precordial	• Pericardial friction rub	• Pericardial effusion
• Can radiate to neck, left shoulder and arm, back, epigastrium	• Elevated neck veins	• Constrictive pericarditis
	• Tachycardia	• Myocardial/pericardial injury
	• Hiccups	• Connective tissue disease
• Aggravated by deep inspiration, cough, rotation of the chest	• Nausea/vomiting	• Infection
	• Dizziness	• Radiation therapy
	• Generalized malaise	• Neoplasm
• Alleviated by sitting up and forward	• Hoarseness	
	• Abdominal pain	
Dissecting Aortic Aneurysm		
• Acute sharp onset w/o warning	• Syncope	• Hypertension
	• Diaphoresis	• Congenital heart defects
• Tearing, ripping	• Tachycardia	• Syphilitic aortitis
• In synch w/heartbeat	• Hyper/hypotension	• Blunt trauma
• Lasts for hours or days	• Confusion	• Males > 50–70 years
• Upper back, anterior chest, epigastric, shoulders, retrosternal	• Fever	• Third trimester of pregnancy
	• Blood pressure different in each arm	
• Radiates to hips, groin, lower extremity, neck, shoulders, costovertebral area, epigastric area, jaw	• Absent or diminished pulses uni/bilateral	
	• Decreased level of consciousness	
• Settles in lower back	• Melena, hematemesis, nausea, vomiting	
Spontaneous Pneumothorax		
• Sudden	• Dyspnea	• Severe underlying lung disease
• Severe	• Tachycardia	• Necrotizing pneumonia
• Over lateral thorax	• Blood pressure difference in each arm	• ARDS
	• Hyperresonance and decreased breath sounds	• High airway pressures while on mechanical ventilation
		• Common ages 16–25 years
	• Tracheal deviation toward affected side	• COPD
		• Cystic fibrosis
	• Decreased respiratory excursion	• Blebs
	• Bulging intercostal muscles	
Cholecystitis		
• Severe abdominal pain	• Nausea/vomiting	
• Epigastric area	• Fever	
• Tenderness in abdomen, right upper quadrant	• Jaundice	
	• Changes in bowel habit	
• May radiate to back and scapula	• Intolerance to fatty foods	
Pancreatitis		
• Extreme epigastric pain, alternating with dull aching sensation	• Hypotension	
	• Fever	
	• Change in bowel habit	
• Radiates to back, flank	• Weight loss, malnutrition	

AMI = acute myocardial infarction; w/o = without; w/ = with; ARDS = acute respiratory distress syndrome; COPD = chronic obstructive pulmonary disease

Sources: Williams, J. L. (2003). Gastroesophageal reflux disease: Clinical manifestations. *Gastroenterology Nursing, 26*(5), 195–200. Zoorob, R. J., & Campbell, J. S. (2003). Acute dyspnea in the office. *American Family Physician, 68*, 1803–1810; Lissin, L. W., & Vagelos, R. (2002). Acute aortic syndrome: A case presentation and review of the literature. *Vascular Medicine, 7*(4), 281–287; Pope, J. H., & Selker, H. P. (2002). Diagnosis of acute cardiac ischemia. *Emergency Medical Clinics of North America, 21*(1), 27–59; and Kontos, M. C. (2001). Evaluation of the emergency department chest pain patient. *Cardiology Review, 9*(5), 266–275.

Coronary Heart Disease in Women

Clinical Problem

Coronary heart disease (CHD), resulting in an acute myocardial infarction, is the leading cause of death for American women. Many women believe that cancer is more of a threat, but nearly twice as many women in the United States die of heart disease and stroke as from all forms of cancer, including breast cancer. Heart disease and stroke claim more female lives than the next five causes of death combined (AHA, 2006a). Additionally, women have an overall poorer prognosis once they have had an acute myocardial infarction (AMI). According to the American Heart Association (2006a), 38% of women, as compared with 25% of men, will die within 1 year after a heart attack.

Diagnosing CHD in women is challenging, and yet few studies have focused on the scope of women's prodromal and acute CHD symptoms. For example, chest pain, a hallmark symptom of ischemia in men, is often not of significant prognostic value in women. No clear picture has emerged on women's typical prodromal symptoms and how they relate to the onset of an AMI. Currently, the description of typical cardiac symptoms is based primarily on what occurs in white, middle-class men. For nurses to improve patient teaching about prevention and occurrence of an AMI in women, it is imperative to identify prodromal and acute symptoms.

Research Findings

McSweeney et al. (2003) studied 515 women who were diagnosed with an AMI. These women were surveyed 4 to 6 months after hospital discharge. The research questionnaire targeted symptoms, comorbidities, and demographic characteristics. The results indicated that 95% of the women knew their symptoms were new or different a month or more before their AMI. The most common symptoms prior to the AMI were:

- Unusual fatigue (70%)
- Sleep disturbance (48%)
- Shortness of breath (42%)
- Indigestion (39%)
- Anxiety (35%).

Major symptoms during the AMI include:

- Unusual fatigue (43%)
- Weakness (55%)
- Shortness of breath (58%)
- Cold sweat (39%)
- Dizziness (39%).

Approximately 78% of women reported experiencing at least one prodromal symptom for more than 1 month either daily or several times a week before their AMI. Only 29.7% reported chest discomfort, which they described as aching (33%), tightness (33%), pressure (32%), sharpness (23%), burning (21%), fullness (18%), and tingling (18%) (McSweeney et al., 2003, p. 2).

Implications for Nursing Practice

This study indicates that there is still much to learn about women versus men experiencing AMIs. Education about heart disease in women began in 1997. To extend the effort that began in 1997, in 2004 the American Heart Association and other organizations began a series of national awareness campaigns to educate women about heart disease. At this time the American Heart Association launched its *Go Red For Women* movement to raise women's awareness of their risk for heart disease and to help them take action to reduce their risk. Today the association continues to play a leading role in educating women by providing them with heart-healthy tools through Go Red For Women (AHA, 2008b & c).

It is imperative that nurses educate women about the symptoms of heart disease at every opportunity. A study by Mosca et al. (2006) indicated that women's awareness of the risk of heart disease as the leading killer has risen from 30% in 1997 to 55% in 2006. The study also concluded that due to this awareness women are taking action to improve their own and their family's heart health. These changes in awareness and lifestyles can come about only through education. Nurses play a "key" role in this education process due to their close proximity to patients.

The downside of the study's results (Mosca et al., 2006) is that while 62% of white women surveyed were aware that heart disease was the leading cause of death, only 38% of African Americans and 34% of Hispanics had the same level of awareness. Given these statistics, efforts need to focus on educating the culturally diverse populations.

Teaching needs to include the risk for heart disease and well as the prodromal symptoms. Increasing awareness will ensure that women know whether they have healthy levels of risk factors and what their personal risk is. Mosca's study indicated that women's awareness of heart disease can positively influence their family. Therefore educational efforts for women can have a far-reaching impact.

Critical Thinking Questions

1. How can nurses adapt teaching materials and techniques for patients with limited or no English language skills?

2. When assessing a female patient suspected of having CHD, what types of questions would the nurse ask to help determine the presence of fatigue?

3. What facts would a nurse include in an education program to help increase the awareness of heart disease in women?

Answers to Critical Thinking Questions appear in Appendix D.

References

American Heart Association (2006a). *Facts about women and cardiovascular diseases.* Retrieved August 7, 2006, from http://www.americanheart.org/presenter.jhtml?identifier=2876.

American Heart Association. (2008). *Women and Coronary Heart Disease.* Retrieved July 18, 2008, from http://www.americanheart.org/presenter.jhtml?identifier=2859.

McSweeney, J., Cody, M., O'Sullivan, P., Elberson, K., Moser, D., & Garvin, B. (2003). Women's early warning symptoms of acute myocardial infarction. *Circulation, 108*(21), 2619–2623.

Mosca, L., Mochari, H., Christian, A., Berra, K., Taubert, K., Mills, T., et al. (2006). National study of women's awareness, preventive action, and barriers to cardiovascular health. *Circulation, 113,* 525–534.

EVIDENCE-BASED PRACTICE

CHART 40–8	**Angina Classifications and Descriptors**

Term	**Descriptor(s)/Definitions**
Typical angina, three key characteristics	1. Central/substernal chest or left arm pain, discomfort, pressure, tightness, heaviness 2. Provoked by exertion or emotional stress 3. Relieved by nitroglycerin
Atypical angina or ischemic equivalents, any two of the characteristics for typical angina	1. Jaw, neck, ear, arm, back 2. Weakness, dizziness, light-headedness, loss of consciousness, unexplained fatigue, diaphoresis 3. New or worsening dyspnea on exertion 4. Nausea/vomiting unexplained indigestion, belching, epigastric pain or discomfort 5. Burning, aching, cramping
Nocturnal angina	Occurs at night usually during sleep. May be relieved by sitting upright. Commonly associated with left venticular dysfunction.
Decubitus angina	Angina while lying down.
Preinfarction, postinfarction angina	Prior to or after infarction. Preinfarction angina may precondition the heart for episodes of subsequent infarction, resulting in a reduction in infarct size. Postinfarction angina denotes increased risk for death or recurrent myocardial infarction (MI).
Recurring/stuttering angina	Angina that comes and goes. Denotes instability, thrombus formation, and dissolution.
Canadian Cardiovascular Society Classification for Angina Pectoris	
Class I angina	Angina produced only with strenuous, rapid, or prolonged exertion. Patient is able to engage in ordinary physical activity such as walking and climbing stairs.
Class II angina	Angina that occurs with mild exertion such as climbing stairs rapidly; walking uphill, in the cold, against the wind; walking or stair-climbing after a meal. Angina that occurs under emotional stress or in the first few hours after awakening. Results in slight limitation of ordinary activity.
Class III angina	Angina that occurs during ordinary physical activities such as walking at a normal pace 1–2 blocks on level ground or climbing a flight of stairs under normal conditions. Results in marked limitation of ordinary physical activity.
Class IV angina	Angina at rest. Results in inability to carry on any physical activity without discomfort.

Source: Braunwald, E., Antman, E. M., Beasley, J. W., et al. (2002). ACC/AHA 2002 guideline update for the management of patients with unstable angina and non-ST-segment elevation myocardial infarction: A report of the American College of Cardiology/American Heart Association Task Force on Practice Guidelines (Committee on the Management of Patient with Unstable Angina). *Journal of the American College of Cardiology, 40*, 1366–1370. Retrieved July 15, 2008, from http://www.acc.org/clinical/guidelines/unstable/unstable.pdf. Retrieved July 15, 2008, from http://www.acc.org/qualityandscience/clinical/guidelines/unstable/appendix2.htm.

the duration, what brings it on, and what makes it go away. The nurse must inquire whether this is new onset pain or whether there is a history of anginal chest pain. If this pain has occurred before, is there a change in the pattern or intensity? For example, stable angina is predictable in what causes it, makes it go away, and its intensity, whereas unstable angina is more intense and less predictable in its pattern. The subjective and objective findings during an anginal attack may include tachycardia, increased or decreased blood pressure (BP), cardiac dysrhythmias, apprehension/anxiety, diaphoresis, and pallor. The nurse must assess vital signs, the ECG monitor, and the associated clinical manifestations. Typically the ECG is obtained during pain because the ischemic changes will resolve with treatment. It is also common to have cardiac dysrhythmias occur during angina, due to muscle irritability from the ischemia. Assessment for heart failure also is essential. Lung sounds, peripheral edema, increasing shortness of breath, and respiratory rate must be evaluated. Physical findings between periods of angina are usually normal and therefore not diagnostic.

Outcomes and Evaluation Parameters

The desired nursing outcome is to prevent the progression of ischemia to the myocardium, which would result in permanent cardiac muscle damage and worsening symptoms. The primary evaluation parameter is complete relief of the anginal pain, because this indicates that there is adequate blood supply to the myocardium. Associated outcome parameters include vital signs, cardiac output, activity tolerance, lungs, and mental orientation. The nurse must monitor the patient's vital signs both as the pain is beginning to subside and when it is totally relieved. The goal is for the heart rate and blood pressure to return to the patient's baseline. Normal ECG, absent or decreased dysrhythmias, and normal mentation also are outcomes that indicate an adequate blood supply to the myocardium. Absence of heart failure is an essential outcome because it is a serious long-term complication. Finally, once the pain is relieved, the patient will verbalize less fear and anxiety.

Planning and Interventions with Rationales

Nursing interventions must be instituted including prescribed antianginal medications, described under medical management, that dilate the coronary arteries, thereby increasing blood flow to the ischemic myocardium. Whatever activity was occurring that precipitated the pain must be stopped. The heart is unable to meet the oxygen needs, and stopping activity will decrease the need.

Supplemental oxygen is applied per health care provider orders, and vital signs and oxygen saturation levels are observed. The effectiveness of these interventions is assessed continuously until the patient is pain free and the heart rate and blood pressure are within normal range. If this is not achieved, it may indicate that there is a more serious problem, and the health care provider must be notified to order further interventions and testing.

 The nurse must stay with the patient who is experiencing angina and continue an ongoing assessment until the pain is gone or it is determined that the interventions are not effective and the health care provider needs to be notified.

Health Promotion

Because angina pectoris is an indicator of decreased cardiac reserve, it is imperative that a comprehensive education program be initiated on onset of the symptoms. The best prevention program would be instituted before the clinical manifestations, but often the patient is not seen prior to admittance to an emergency department (ED). The nurse is in an ideal position to begin education about lifestyle changes that will reduce or prevent a progression of the disease. The education needs to include risk factor management (see Charts 40–4, p. 1166 and 40–5, p. 1167), medication instructions, and avoidance of precipitating factors. The nurse must assess the patient/family's ability to understand and be receptive to education. There may be language or cultural barriers, and/or the anxiety level may interfere with the patient/family's ability to absorb the information. It is imperative that the teaching plan includes a review of medication regimens, side effects, symptoms of ischemia, and teaching about self-treatment and handling potentially emergent situations. The patients receiving beta-adrenergic blocking agents and calcium channel blockers need to be taught how to count their pulse and what rate must be reported to the health care provider. If taking nitrates, patients should be taught about safe storage, handling, and side effects of different nitrate preparations as well as how to take sublingual nitrates (see the Pharmacology Summary, p. 1199). Patients should also receive coaching on adaptation to and compliance with risk factor modification activities and be encouraged to seek assistance if therapy becomes a financial burden or creates conflicts within their support group. Families or significant others may need teaching about how to cope or help the patient deal with lifestyle and behavioral change, or referral to community services to learn bystander cardiopulmonary resuscitation.

◼ Acute Coronary Syndrome

Patients who present to the health care provider's office or the ED with a change in their previous pattern of angina or new onset angina, are evaluated for the likelihood that their symptoms represent an ACS secondary to CAD. They are evaluated for the presence of myocardial infarction, myocardial ischemia, and infarction-related complications, as well as a general state of hemodynamic stability. Disposition of patients to either outpatient management or admission to an inpatient unit, selection of therapy, and decisions about revascularization are based on these assessment data.

Categories of Acute Coronary Syndrome

Included under the umbrella of acute coronary syndrome (ACS) are the diagnoses of unstable angina (UA), non–ST segment elevation myocardial infarction (MI) (NSTEMI), and ST segment elevation MI (STEMI). *ACS* is a recent term that has emerged as research into the pathophysiology and optimal management of ischemic heart disease has progressed. Being admitted with a diagnosis of ACS just means there is a cardiac event going on, and after admission and further testing, a more definitive diagnosis is made. Pathogenesis of ACS involves fibrous plaque disruption and thrombosis formation, and can result in either a partial or a total occlusion of the lumen of the coronary artery. This process will either markedly decrease or completely cut off blood flow to the myocardium.

Unstable Angina Pectoris

Anginal symptoms controlled by rest or medical management are considered stable, as described earlier. **Unstable angina** depicts a transitory syndrome falling between stable angina and acute myocardial infarction (AMI) wherein thrombus forms in an area of arterial stenosis but is subsequently fully or partially lysed by endogenous antithrombotic mechanisms. Symptoms worsen such that the patient presents with the development of new onset exertion angina, angina present at rest for longer than 20 minutes, or symptoms that have accelerated in frequency, duration, or intensity (Diop & Aghababian, 2001). When the vessels are assessed with cardiac angiography (Chapter 39 ⊙), these patients most often show the presence of stenotic eccentric lesions, collateral circulation, and the absence of a totally occluded coronary artery. Blood markers indicating myocardial damage are normal, and ECG changes, if present, are transitory and will return to normal. Based on the assessment and physical findings, patients are categorized as low, intermediate, or high risk and triaged appropriately (Chart 40–9, p. 1182).

Non–ST Segment Myocardial Infarction

The term **myocardial infarction** (MI) denotes a loss of myocytes or myocardial cell death as a result of prolonged muscle ischemia. Cell death results in a permanent loss of myocardial muscle function. **NSTEMI** is a correlate syndrome to UA with a common pathogenesis and clinical presentation. Both usually occur as a result of transient subtotal occlusion of a coronary artery with reduced coronary blood flow resulting from plaque disruption and ensuing pathophysiological processes. The presence of serum blood markers and persistent ECG changes distinguishes a more severe myocardial injury associated with NSTEMI and thus a higher risk of death and MI, versus no blood marker release and transitory or no ECG changes seen with UA. See Figure 40–6 ◼ (p. 1172), which shows normal ECG waveforms, and compare it to Figure 40–8 ◼ (p. 1173) and to Figure 40–12 ◼ (p. 1183); the middle figure shows ECG changes associated with the partial obstruction seen with NSTEMI.

ST Segment Elevation Myocardial Infarction

ST segment elevation myocardial infarction (**STEMI**) refers to myocardial injury associated with ST segment elevation on the ECG (see Figure 40–7 ◼, p. 1173 & 40–12 ◼, p. 1183). Besides the ST segment, STEMI compares differently to NSTEMI in a number of ways. The presence of ST segment elevation means that myocardial tissue is undergoing severe anoxia and cellular damage. In

CHART 40–9   Short-Term Risk of Death or Nonfatal MI in Patients With UA/NSTEMI*£

Feature	Low Risk (No High or Intermediate risk features but may have any of the following)	Intermediate Risk (No High risk features, must have 1 of the following)	High Risk (At least 1 of the following features must be present)
History		Prior diagnosis of arterio-occlusive disease such as MI, PVD, CVD, or CABG; prior aspirin use	Accelerating tempo (increased frequency, severity, or duration) of ischemic symptoms over last 48 hours
Pain Characteristics	Increased frequency, severity, or duration of angina Angina provoked at a lower threshold New onset angina with onset 2 weeks to 2 months prior to presentation	Prolonged (> 20 minutes) rest angina, resolved at presentation, with likelihood of CAD Prolonged (> 20 minutes) angina relieved with rest or sublingual NTG Nocturnal angina New onset or progressive limitation of activity (walking 1–2 blocks, climbing 1–2 flights of stairs, pain with any physical exertion, angina at rest) in past 2 weeks without prolonged (> 20 minutes) rest pain but with likelihood of CAD.	Prolonged (> 20 minutes) ongoing at rest
Clinical Findings		Age > 70 years	Presence of any one of the following: pulmonary edema likely due to ischemia; new or worsening mitral regurgitation; S_3 or new/worsening rales; hypotension, bradycardia, tachycardia Age > 75 years
ECG	Normal or unchanged ECG	T wave changes Pathologic Qs or resting ST-segment depression > 1 mm in multiple lead groups (anterior, inferior, lateral)	Angina at rest with transient ST-segment changes > 0.5 mm BBB new or presumed new Sustained VT
Cardiac Markers	Normal	Slightly elevated TnT, TnI, or CK-MB	Elevated cardiac TnT, TnI, or CK-MB

Note: BBB-bundle branch block; CABG-coronary artery bypass graft surgery; CAD-coronary artery disease; CK-MB-creatine kinase, MB fraction; CVD-cerebral vascular disease; ECG-electrocardiogram; MI-myocardial infarction; NTG- nitroglycerin; PVD-peripheral vascular disease; TnI-troponin I; TnT- troponin T; UA/NSTEMI-unstable angina/non–ST-elevation myocardial infarction; VT-ventricular tachycardia.

*Estimation of risk for adverse events should be done with patients who present with a history and/or signs and symptoms of cardiac ischemia and considered in patient treatment.

£Adapted from Table 7 page e17 of Anderson et. al, ACC/AHA 2007 Guidelines for the Management of Patients With Unstable Angina/Non-ST-Elevation Myocardial Infarction: A Report of the American College of Cardiology/American Heart Association Task Force on Practice Guidelines. Content is meant to illustrate general guidelines and should not be used as practice algorithms.

most cases this is a result of complete coronary artery blockage from thrombotic occlusion over an underlying plaque lesion (Libby, Bonow, Zipes, & Mann, 2008). Unlike NSTEMI, the blockage is sustained. If blood flow is not reestablished in 20 minutes, cell death occurs. Ischemic damage traverses the myocardium vertically outward, starting with the subendocardial layer through to the epicardium (see Figure 40–4 ■, p. 1163). Prior to the current age of rapid revascularization therapies, ST segment elevation was usually associated with transmural myocardial infarction and the appearance of Q waves on the ECG days later. The Q wave changes indicate cell death and permanent loss of muscle function in the affected area. If the occlusion is treated early, a patient presenting with STEMI may suffer only subendocardial cell damage without subsequent Q waves.

Classifications of Myocardial Infarction

Both STEMI and NSTEMI are classified according to the coronary artery involved. Occlusion of the left anterior descending (LAD) artery is referred to as an anterior wall infarct. The LAD feeds the anterior left ventricle, anterior septum, papillary muscle, apex, bundle of His, and bundle branches. All or some of the function of these tissues is lost with an infarct to the LAD. Most infarcts affect the left ventricle.

Occlusion of the right coronary artery (RCA) results in an inferior wall MI. The RCA supplies the inferior left ventricle, inferior septum, papillary muscle, and right ventricle (the SA node in 60% of the population and the AV node in 90%). Occlusion of the circumflex artery results in a lateral wall infarct because it supplies the lateral wall of the left ventricle (the SA node in 40% of the population and the AV node in 10%).

Occlusion of the left main coronary (LMC) artery results in what is referred to as a massive MI because LMC supplies blood to over 70% of the left ventricle. Myocardial infarctions involving the LMC, often referred to as "widow makers," typically are associated with complications such as heart failure. Figure 40–13 ■ shows a thrombosis in the coronary arteries.

Stable angina or asymptomatic

Unstable angina or non ST segment elevation myocardial infarction (UA or NSTE-MI)

ST segment elevation myocardial infarction (STE-MI)

Lumen

Lipid core

Fibrous cap

Nonocclusive thrombus

Residual lumen

Occlusive thrombus

FIGURE 40–12 ■ Clot formation and ST segment ECG changes associated with ACS.

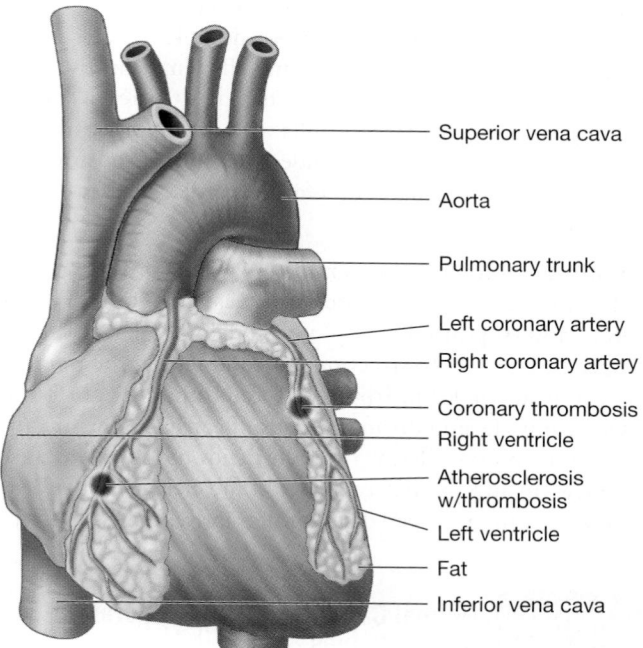

Superior vena cava

Aorta

Pulmonary trunk

Left coronary artery

Right coronary artery

Coronary thrombosis

Right ventricle

Atherosclerosis w/thrombosis

Left ventricle

Fat

Inferior vena cava

FIGURE 40–13 ■ Thrombosis in a coronary artery.

Silent Ischemia

Nearly 70% to 90% of daily life ischemic episodes are asymptomatic, and 25% of patients who experience an AMI have either no or atypical symptoms (Cohn, Fox, & Daly, 2003). The presence of silent ischemia predicts greater risk of adverse outcomes in patients with stable and unstable angina, and in patients follow-ing an AMI or revascularization therapies. Silent ischemia is more prevalent in the elderly, women, patients with diabetes, and patients with three-vessel disease. The lack of symptoms has been attributed to altered pain regulation or perception, higher pain tolerance, higher levels of circulating endorphins, or altered sensory secondary to pain pathway impairment (Cohn et al., 2003).

Sudden Cardiac Death

Sudden cardiac death (SCD) is cardiac arrest most often associated with abrupt coronary artery occlusion from plaque disruption over severely stenotic lesions in the setting of poorly developed collateral circulation. The abrupt occlusion triggers pulseless ventricular tachycardia, ventricular fibrillation, or asystole, which if not treated immediately is almost always fatal. Chapter 38 ⊙ includes an in-depth discussion of these dysrhythmias.

Clinical Manifestations of Acute Coronary Syndrome

Presenting signs and symptoms vary greatly from person to person experiencing acute coronary syndrome (ACS). Typical symptoms include chest pain, diaphoresis, shortness of breath, and generalized weakness. Patients describe the pain from an acute myocardial infarction (AMI) in the same terms as the pain from angina pectoris only usually more intense and longer in duration. If the chest pain lasts longer than 20 minutes, there is a concern that cardiac damage is occurring. The pain from an AMI is not relieved by rest and requires treatment with medications or interventions to open the occluded coronary artery.

Most frequently patients report that the anginal pain occurs in the mid to lower sternal areas of the chest. It also may radiate to the left arm, right arm, neck, jaw, and back areas. Atypical angina occurs in the stomach and back. Due to the close proximity to the epigastric region, many people mistake it for indigestion. Men having an AMI report the mid to lower sternal chest pain more often than women. Women who are having an AMI more typically report shortness of breath (57.9%), weakness (54.8%), and fatigue (40.9%); prodromal symptoms experienced 1 month prior to AMI include unusual fatigue (70.7%), sleep disturbance (47.8%), and shortness of breath (40.1%) (AHA, 2008c McSweeney et al., 2003). Figure 40–11 ■ (p. 1176) outlines the locations where angina occurs.

Other frequent signs and symptoms associated with AMI include nausea, vomiting, dyspnea, syncope, anxiety, and a feeling of impending doom. Approximately one-third of patients experiencing an AMI do not experience chest pain and initially exhibit other symptoms of decreased cardiac output such as shortness of breath and changes in sensorium, or syncope.

CRITICAL ALERT *Some patients are able to sense when a major cardiac event is occurring; and therefore, it is essential that the nurse pay close attention to patients who report impending doom.*

The physical assessment findings of a patient experiencing acute coronary syndrome are also variable. The blood pressure may be low due to a decreased cardiac output, or it may be elevated due to catecholamine release, fear, and anxiety. The heart rate may be bradycardic or tachycardic, depending on where in the heart the damage is occurring and the patient's anxiety level. There may be an S_3 or S_4 present and new systolic murmurs. Chapter 37 🔗 includes a description of S_3 and S_4. The lung sounds may be clear unless there is associated heart failure, in which case rales or crackles, and/or wheezes may be heard with an associated decrease in arterial oxygen saturation. Heart failure is described in Chapter 42 🔗.

■ Laboratory and Diagnostic Procedures to Diagnose Acute Coronary Syndrome

The clinical manifestations of CAD typically bring the patient to the ED or health care provider's office. The second indicators of acute coronary insufficiency are the laboratory tests and ECG changes that indicate the presence and extent of myocardial damage. As soon as the patient is admitted to the ED, laboratory tests are done to assist in determining the diagnosis. Many of the laboratory values are "time" sensitive, so it is essential that the blood is drawn immediately after admission. The initial laboratory and diagnostic workup includes blood serum markers and a 12-lead ECG. Chart 40–10 outlines normal laboratory values.

Blood (Serum) Markers of Myocardial Ischemia

Laboratory tests include myoglobin, cardiac enzymes (CK total, CK-MB), troponin (T or I), and possibly a C-reactive protein level. A rise in cardiac blood markers occurs when the myocardial cells become damaged from a lack of blood supply that occurs with myocardial injury and death. The cell membrane loses its integrity and intracellular enzymes are released. The extent of en-

zyme release is relative to the amount of tissue damage and, thus, the size of the infarct. Therefore, blood marker levels are useful to help confirm the diagnosis and the extent of tissue injury.

Myoglobin

Myoglobin is a heme-containing, oxygen-binding protein that is exclusive to striated and nonstriated muscle. Because of its very small molecular weight, it is released into the interstitial fluid as early as 2 hours following damage to muscle tissue. Unlike CK-MB, the presence of an elevated myoglobin level is not a specific indicator of just heart damage. Rather it is a sensitive indicator that muscle damage has occurred. For example, if a patient falls or has any type of muscle injury, the myoglobin will rise. In other words, if a patient has had an acute cardiac event, he will have an elevated myoglobin; however, the diagnosis cannot be made on myoglobin alone because of its lack of specificity.

Creatine Kinase

Creatine kinase (CK) is an enzyme found in high concentrations in the heart and skeletal muscle and in smaller concentrations in the brain. Laboratory studies are able to subdivide and analyze the total CK level into its three isoforms: CK-MM coming from damaged skeletal muscle, CK-BB from damaged brain tissue, and CK-MB from damaged cardiac tissue. Of the isoforms, only CK-MB, along with CK total and percentage of CK-MB of CK total, is relevant for determining cardiac ischemia and infarction. Other enzymes have been used in the past such as serum glutamic-oxaloacetic transaminase (SGOT), aspartate transaminase (AST), and lactic dehydrogenase (LDH) along with CK's isoforms. In the last 2 to 3 decades, CK and specifically CK-MB have proven to be more time-efficient, sensitive, and specific indicators of cardiac muscle damage. Currently, newer tests are providing even faster results with the same accuracy as the cardiac enzymes, which include troponin T and I. Chart 40–10 outlines the normal values for the cardiac markers.

Troponin

Troponin is a protein complex that is found in cardiac and skeletal muscle. There are three isotypes—**troponin T**, troponin C, and **troponin I**—all of which help regulate the force and speed of muscle contractions by modulating the interaction of actin and myosin. Troponin T and troponin I are found in cardiac muscle, and during periods of cardiac ischemia, intracellular troponin will leak from the inside of the cell because of changes in myocardial cell membrane permeability. Troponin levels can be detected soon after an ischemic event be-

CHART 40–10	Normal Cardiac Markers' Laboratory Normal Values	
Laboratory Test	**Normal Range**	
Creatine kinase (CPK)	0–250 U/L	
CPK-MB	<8.0 mcg/mL	
CPK-MB relative index	<3.2%	
Troponin I (cTnI)	0–.06 ng/mL	
Troponin T (cTnT)	0–.05 ng/mL	
Myoglobin	17–106 ng/mL	

CHART 40–11	**Cardiac Laboratory Markers' Pattern Consistent with Acute Myocardial Infarction**			
Laboratory Test	**Time to Elevation**	**Mean Time to Peak Elevation**	**Time to Return to Normal**	
Myoglobin	1–3 hours	6–7 hours	24 hours	
Troponin I	3–12 hours	24 hours	5–10 days	
Troponin T	3–12 hours	12 hours–2 days	5–14 days	
CK-MB	3–12 hours	24 hours	48–72 hours	
C-reactive protein	24 hours	2–3 days	2 weeks	

Source: This article was published in *Heart Disease: A textbook in Cardiovascular Medicine*, 5th ed., Antman E. M., Braunwald E. In: Braunwald E., ed., p. 1202. Copyright 1997, Philadelphia, PA: WB Saunders.

cause these proteins are very small and therefore leak out quickly. Normal and abnormal troponin T and troponin I laboratory markers are outlined in Chart 40–11.

ECG Changes
12-Lead ECG Changes with Acute Myocardial Infarction

The 12-lead ECG provides 12 different views of the electrical activity in the heart. When evaluating a 12-lead ECG, the Q wave, T wave, and ST segment are used to determine the presence of damage. Changes in specific leads reflect the specific location in the heart where the damage has occurred and which vessel(s) contain the culprit lesions. As the ischemia and injury evolve, so

do the ECG changes. Figure 40–12 ■ (p. 1183) demonstrates the ECG changes that occur with a transmural AMI.

The ST segment is the major focus when evaluating ischemic injury to the myocardium. As discussed earlier, the location of the AMI is identified by the involved coronary artery. Abnormal changes on the ECG correlate with the area in the myocardium where damage has occurred and, thus, identify the artery involved. Chart 40–12 outlines the artery, the associated 12-lead ECG changes, and complications.

For ST segment and T wave changes to be considered diagnostic, they must appear in two or more contiguous leads. This means that changes must be present in two or more leads that correspond to a given area of myocardium damage. For example,

CHART 40–12	**ECG Changes During an MI, Correlated with Coronary Anatomy**		
	Areas and Structures Supplied	**Type of MI and Leads Involved**	**Associated Symptoms and Complications**
Right Coronary Artery (RCA)	SA node (55%), AV node (90%) Bundle of His Right atrium and ventricle Inferior surface of left ventricle Posterior 1/3 of septum Left bundle branch Posterior/inferior division of right bundle branch	**INFERIOR MI (RCA)** II, III, aVF Reciprocal changes in I, aVL	Vagal symptoms: nausea and bradycardia AV blocks: most common = 1st degree and 2nd degree type I (Wenckebach); 3rd degree possible Usually transient; treat only if symptomatic
Left Anterior Descending (LAD)	Anterior wall of left ventricle Anterior 2/3 of septum Right bundle branch Anterior/superior division of left bundle branch	**ANTERIOR MI (LAD)** $V_1 - V_4$ Reciprocal changes in II, III, aVF **ANTEROLATERAL (LAD/CIRC)** $V_1 - V_4$ I, aVL, V_5, V_6 Reciprocal changes in II, III, aVF	Often associated with loss of large muscle mass If large myocardial infarction (MI), prone to develop diminished left ventricular branch function, signs and symptoms of heart failure (HF), cardiogenic shock Rhythm disturbances: atrial and ventricular dysrhythmias, bundle branch blocks, AV blocks with 2nd degree type II most common; may progress to 3rd-degree block (complete heart block)
Left Circumflex Artery (CIRC, CX)	SA node (45%), AV node (10%) Inferior surface of left ventricle Lateral wall of left ventricle Left atrium Posterior/inferior division of left bundle branch	**LATERAL MI (CIRC/LAD)** I, aVL, V_5, V_6 Reciprocal changes in V_1, V_3 **ANTEROLATERAL MI (LAD/CX)** I, aVL, V_5, V_6 $V_1 - V_4$ Reciprocal changes in II, III, aVF **POSTERIOR MI (RCA, CIRC)** Reciprocal changes only in V_1, V_2 unless 18-lead EKG is done	Frequently seen with large anterior MIs Occasionally seen with inferior MIs Least likely to alter hemodynamics or cause dysrhythmias Uncommon; involves both right coronary artery (RCA) and circumflex (CIRC) Hard to diagnose on traditional 12-lead; researchers developing 18-lead EKG Bradycardia with possible AV block; usually transient

in order for the ECG criteria to be met for an inferior wall MI, a patient would have to have ST segment elevation of 1 millimeter or greater in two of these three leads: II, III, and aVF.

Reciprocal ST Segment Abnormalities

When ST segment changes occur during an AMI, they are present in the leads on the 12-lead ECG that face the damaged myocardium and/or infarction, and are referred to as the indicative leads. Reciprocal (electrically opposite) leads are distant from the injury and reflect in an upside-down, mirror image of the changes or damage seen in the indicative leads. Reciprocal ST segment changes present as horizontal or downsloping of the ST segment. Other reciprocal changes include the absence of a Q wave, an increased height of the R wave in the QRS complex, and a tall, upright T wave. It is generally thought that the presence of reciprocal changes indicates more extensive damage and a worse prognosis. When looking at a 12-lead ECG for indicative and reciprocal changes, one has to keep in mind that ST segment depression interpreted as reciprocal changes may in fact reflect injury rising from a culprit lesion in another vessel (Morton et al., 2005).

Bundle branch block (BBB) is defined as a discontinuity of conduction (complete or incomplete) in one branch of the His bundle, which affects normal transmission of the impulse through the ventricles. The QRS is wider than the normal 0.12 second with BBB. When one bundle is blocked the ventricles depolarize asynchronously, which is characterized by a delay of excitation to one ventricle; therefore, an abnormal spread of electrical activity through the ventricles occurs. Spontaneous left bundle branch block or right ventricular pacing–induced left bundle branch pattern obscures the electrocardiographic diagnosis of an AMI.

ECG Signs of Reperfusion

The goal for the management of AMI is rapid restoration of blood flow to the infarct-related artery (IRA). The lack of reperfusion is an important predictor of cardiac morbidity and mortality following AMI. The amount of time to restoration of blood flow directly correlates to the morbidity and mortality associated with AMI. The resolution of ST segment deviation should occur within 90 minutes following revascularization for the therapy to be considered successful. "Time is muscle"; thus, immediate reperfusion must occur in order to salvage myocardium. Other markers of reperfusion include newly acquired T wave inversion within 4 hours after AMI, accelerated idioventricular rhythms of rates between 60 and 120 beats per minute, isolated premature ventricular contractions, and nonsustained asymptomatic runs of ventricular tachycardia. The emergence of polymorphic ventricular tachycardia and ventricular fibrillation is rare and more often represents reocclusion of the IRA. Chapter 38 has a complete description of ventricular tachycardia and ventricular fibrillation.

Cardiac Dysrhythmias Associated with Acute Myocardial Infarction

Premature atrial and ventricular contractions, conduction abnormalities, tachycardia, and bradycardia can all be seen with myocardial ischemia and infarction. Premature beats and tachycardias occur because of acute tissue hypoxemia and irritability, and derangement of electrical membrane potentials. Tachycar-

dia also is a by-product of elevated levels of circulating catecholamines due to the stress response. Atrial fibrillation may result from myocardial infarction because of enhanced vagal tone, increased atrial pressure, atrial infarction, or pericarditis. Conduction delays and bradycardia relate to the location of the infarct and the mass of involved myocardium.

In summary, although a significant number of patients do not have ECG changes indicative of AMI on admission, they are still considered an important diagnostic indicator when used in conjunction with the patient's history, presenting signs and symptoms, and blood markers indicative of cardiac ischemia.

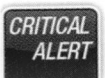 **CRITICAL ALERT** *Because the dysrhythmias that accompany an MI are common and varied, it is essential that the nurse understand the impact of each type on the cardiac output and the necessary interventions to terminate the abnormal rhythm.*

Medical Management of Coronary Artery Disease

The following case example represents the difficulty in evaluating the cause of a patient's complaint of chest pain:

A 42-year-old white female with no history of cardiac disease presents to the emergency department (ED) with substernal chest pain she has had for 10 hours. She describes her pain as feeling "like a weight" with nausea, dizziness, left arm numbness, and accompanied by dyspnea. Her medical history is positive for 10 pack/years of smoking, epigastric pain, gastric reflux disease, and black tarry stool. She has a negative family history for heart disease and no history of hypertension, diabetes, or hyperlipidemia. The patient is convinced her pain is epigastric, as she has had this same sensation before. She is given a GI cocktail consisting of Donnatal, viscous Lidocaine, and Maalox, which relieves her symptoms. Her initial set of cardiac markers were negative; her ECG showed ST depression of < 1 millimeter in leads II, III, and aVF.

Routine evaluation of patients who present with symptoms that may represent exacerbations of CAD includes a review of their symptoms, their medical/social history for associated diseases and risk factors, an assessment for physical signs, and diagnostic tests. In this case, the patient's description, history, physical signs, and initial diagnostic workup of her suspected anginal symptoms are compounded with those that are classic for gastric ulcer disease. Subsequent testing demonstrated that she was indeed having an AMI, but she could have easily been treated with antacids and sent home joining the cohort patients admitted to the emergency department with a nondiagnostic workup for CAD, discharged only to return later with ACS.

Tools used to determine the extent of myocardial perfusion depend on six indexes: the presence of physical signs and symptoms representative of tissue hypoxemia or heart failure, abnormal levels of blood serum markers indicating myocardial cell membrane damage, ECG changes consistent with myocardial injury and muscle death, the lack of uptake of substances by cardiac tissue, vessel patency as seen with angiography, and assessments of global intracardiac structure and function (Chapter 38). Signs and symptoms, blood markers, and ECG changes are completed expeditiously when a patient is admitted for suspected acute coronary ischemia. ECG testing is done either at rest during an acute event such as the presence of angina, or during exercise to determine the extent of stress on the heart during work. Angiography is used to confirm or define areas of critical stenosis or obstruction, referred to as culprit lesions, as well as for hemodynamic measurements. Viability studies employ the infusion of a radioactive indicator, typically technetium, that is taken up by tissue with good perfusion and is later "washed out" as perfusing blood dilutes the concentration of the isotope over time. Ventricular radiography done during coronary angiography identifies areas of abnormal heart contractility such as **dyskinesia** (impaired muscle movement), **akinesia** (severe loss or no muscle movement), and **hypokinesia** (hypoactive muscle movement) that can result from poor coronary perfusion. Echocardiography uses sonography to assess any damage to valve structure or chamber contractility at rest or during exercise that may result from chronic or acute myocardial ischemia. The studies discussed earlier are described in detail in Chapter 38 ☺. The Diagnostic Tests box (p. 1188) summarizes the laboratory studies that are used to diagnose the presence and extent of CAD.

Physical findings associated with CAD are not specific to just coronary artery disease but also may be associated with other diseases such as systemic arterial hypertension, hyperlipidemia, valvular heart disease, heart failure, diabetes, or peripheral atherosclerosis. Thus, findings such as the following are not diagnostic for CAD specifically: elevated blood pressure; presence of an S_3, S_4, or paradoxically split S_2; diminished peripheral pulses; murmurs of aortic stenosis or mitral insufficiency; enlarged cardiac silhouette; changes in pulse cadence and rate because of ventricular or atrial ectopic beats; and presence of crackles. However, they may represent exacerbations of associated diseases that result in coronary insufficiency or vice versa. The absence or presence of these findings also provides a baseline in the advent of complications, assists in excluding other conditions, and assists in stratifying risk for appropriate triage of patients who present with the clinical manifestations of CAD.

Pain is most effectively assessed using a systematic approach to help ensure that all aspects are assessed such as the following: aggravating and alleviating factors; timing related to frequency, duration, time of day, and relation to activity or rest; qualitative characteristics such as description, location, intensity, and radiation; and any other associated symptoms.

Medical Management of Acute Coronary Syndrome

Patients with unstable symptoms are at a greater risk and therefore warrant hospital admission for diagnostic workup and treatment. An estimated 5 million or more adults present each year to emergency departments with a primary complaint of chest pain (Libby, Bonow, Zipes, & Mann, 2008). More than 1.4 million Americans patients are subsequently hospitalized, of which one-third are found to have symptoms of cardiac disease (AHA, 2006f).

Patients with suspected cardiac ischemia but with nondefinitive results from the cardiac workup may be triaged to a cardiac observation unit located as part of an emergency department or inpatient unit. Observation units, also referred to as chest pain units, provide space for patients to be "ruled out" for ischemia

using specific protocols. These protocols involve serial ECGs, cardiac blood marker determinations, and possibly stress testing, echocardiography, or perfusion tests. These patients are not admitted to the hospital unless ischemia is "ruled in" or still suspected after 24 hours.

Patients with acute coronary syndrome should be evaluated in an environment where aggressive therapy can be initiated quickly, such as a hospital emergency department, which has advanced life support backup and personnel to provide continuous monitoring. On admission to the emergency department or critical care unit, patients are made NPO, put on bed rest, given supplemental oxygen, and undergo continuous cardiac and oxygen saturation monitoring. Blood chemistries including cardiac markers are drawn, a 12-lead ECG is obtained, and the patient is placed on a cardiac monitor.

The mnemonic **MONA**, cited in the Advanced Cardiac Life Support (ACLS) guidelines, describes a protocol for treatment of patients with suspected myocardial infarction. The mnemonic stands for morphine, oxygen, nitroglycerin, and aspirin. MONA does not, however, imply a correct sequencing of treatment. The platelet-inhibiting action of chewable aspirin in doses of 81 to 325 milligrams decreases platelet aggregation, and supplemental oxygen treatments are intended to increase oxygen supply to ischemic tissue. Nitroglycerin (NTG) dilates the large coronary arteries, thus increasing the blood supply to ischemic tissue. Initially NTG is administered sublingually, as spray, and with persistent symptoms it may be given intravenously. Intravenous morphine sulfate, a potent analgesic, is used to relieve angina, although it is also effective in reducing anxiety. Morphine along with nitroglycerin can cause the veins to dilate, resulting in a decrease in the amount of blood returning to the heart (preload). This reduced preload helps to decrease myocardial oxygen demand. Short-acting nitroglycerin and morphine can precipitate hypotension, especially in patients with a right ventricular infarction. Therefore, both drugs must be titrated cautiously to relieve pain without causing hypotension. For persistent symptoms of ischemia, IV or oral beta-blockers and heparin will be administered. Glycoprotein (GP) IIb/IIIa inhibitors may be added for unrelenting symptoms. A thrombolytic agent (see Pharmacology Summary, p. 1199) may be administered, or the patient is prepared for emergent percutaneous coronary intervention (PCI) (Chapter 39 ☺), as soon as the ECG and/or cardiac markers indicate the presence of STEMI. Thrombolytic medications are contraindicated in patients with unstable angina (UA) and non–ST segment elevation myocardial infarction (NSTEMI), because studies demonstrate a higher risk of bleeding and lower beneficial results compared to patients with MI (Libby, Bonow, Zipes, & Mann, 2008). Figure 40–14 ■ (p. 1189) is an algorithm for emergent management for patients with acute coronary syndromes.

Once medically stable (without recurrent ischemia, electrical instability [ECG], signs of heart failure, or other serious complications), patients with UA can be transferred to a non–critical care environment where oral nitrates, β-adrenergic blocker, or calcium channel blocker, and possibly low molecular weight heparin (LMWH) (i.e., Lovenox), therapy will be initiated or adjusted to maintain symptom control and hemodynamic stability. If minimal or no episodes of angina occur while the patient is transitioned off oxygen and to a normal activity level, discharge

DIAGNOSTIC TESTS for Coronary Artery Disease

Diagnostic Test and Normal Values	Expected Abnormality	Rationale for Abnormality
ECG: No ST segment elevation or depression. No T wave inversion. No Q waves.	ST segment elevation. ST segment depression. Q waves.	Identify ST segment or T wave abnormalities; and the presence of pathologic Q waves indicates myocardial ischemia, injury, and necrosis, which assists in the diagnosis of an AMI.
Stress test (exercise treadmill or bicycle): Induces abnormal ECG changes, which occur when myocardial oxygen demand increases due to exercise.	ST segment or T wave changes during stress.	Certain changes occur only when the heart is stressed due to the heart's inability to increase cardiac output during periods of high demand.
Nuclear myocardial perfusion imaging: Pharmacologic agent used to induce stress for those patients who cannot exercise.	ST segment or T wave changes during stress.	Identify both functional and nonfunctional myocardium when oxygen demand is increased.
Dobutamine stress echocardiography: Pharmacologic agent used to induce stress for those patients who cannot exercise.	ST segment or T wave changes during stress. Changes in ejection fraction.	Identify both functional and nonfunctional myocardium when oxygen demand is increased.
Electron beam computed tomography (EBCT)/multislice CT: Detect and quantify coronary artery calcification.	Calcium score is age dependent.	Coronary calcium is part of the development of atherosclerosis. It occurs exclusively in atherosclerotic arteries and is absent in the normal vessel wall. The presence of calcification in the coronary arteries indicates the presence of coronary atherosclerosis.
MRI: Identifies plaque size and composition.	Coronary artery stenosis.	Identifies area of plaque buildup from the presence and progression of coronary artery disease (CAD).
Cardiac catheterization: Confirms patency of coronary arteries, determines blood flow in chambers and great vessels, evaluates pressures across valves.	Coronary artery stenosis, valve damage, decreased ventricular function.	Identifies area of plaque buildup from the presence and progression of CAD.
Intravascular ultrasound:	Coronary artery stenosis	Quantify plaque burden and composition from the presence and progression of coronary artery disease.
Chest x-ray (CXR): Evaluate heart size. Identify congestion or effusions. Identify tumors or masses.	Enlarged heart and lung congestion. Pulmonary edema, congestive heart failure. Presence of lung tumor or mass.	Heart failure, cardiomyopathy, and coronary artery disease.
Echocardiogram, transthoracic or transesophageal.	Valvular damage; insufficiency, regurgitation, stenosis, or vegetation. Enlarged chamber size such as ventricular hypertrophy. Abnormal pressure gradients. Decreased ventricular function.	Measures diameters of the cardiac chambers, evaluates structural abnormalities, and identifies valvular vegetation and pressure gradients.
Hs-C-reactive protein: < 10 mg/L	>10 mg/L	Acute phase reactant protein used to indicate an inflammatory process.
Cardiac enzymes:	See Chart 40–10 (p. 1184)	See Chart 40–10 (p. 1184)
Magnesium: 1.3–2.1 mg/dL	<1.5 mg/dL >2.1 mg/dL	Electrolyte balance; decreases ventricular irritability.
Potassium: 3.5–5.0 mEq/L	<3.5 mEq/L >5.0 mEq/L	Electrolyte balance; decreases ventricular irritability.

can be expected in 1 to 3 days. For recurrent chest pain the patient should receive an immediate (stat) 12-lead ECG to document ischemia during pain, followed by sublingual NTG and IV NTG if pain persists. Noninvasive stress testing, perfusion scans, and/or cardiac catheterization may be scheduled to occur while in the hospital or as a follow-up procedure postdischarge. Discharge preparation includes teaching about cardiac risk factors, signs and symptoms of myocardial ischemia, how and when to access emergency medical services, and medication regimes. Patients diagnosed as having an AMI will receive either thrombolytic

CLINICAL PATHWAYS FOR EMERGENCY MANAGEMENT OF URGENT CHEST PAIN

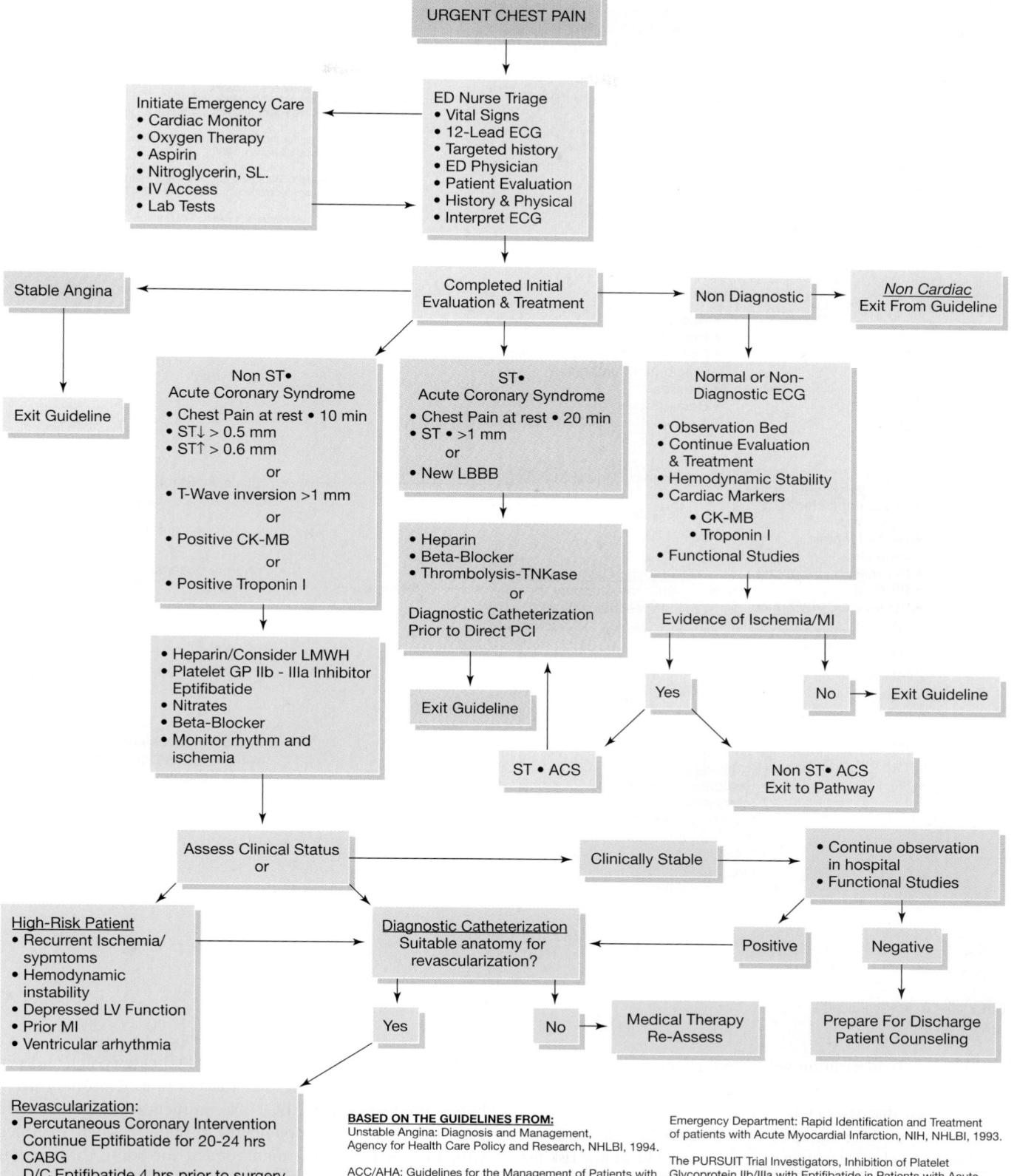

FIGURE 40–14 ■ Algorithm for emergent management of patients with acute coronary syndrome.

CLINICAL PATHWAYS FOR MANAGEMENT OF ACUTE CORONARY SYNDROMES

FIGURE 40–14 ■ Continued

therapy or revascularization with percutaneous coronary intervention (PCI) or coronary artery bypass graft (CABG) surgery. Chapter 39 😊 discusses PCI.

Thrombolytic drug therapy is recommended for patients suspected of AMI who are younger than 75 years old, at low risk for bleeding, with symptoms lasting less than 12 hours. PCI is indicated when thrombolytic therapy is contraindicated or in patients with cardiogenic shock. PCI is recommended as an alternative first-choice therapy only if intervention can be performed within 60 to 90 minutes, by skilled clinicians (performed 75 procedures/

year), in high-volume centers (>200 PCI cases/year), and with demonstrated acceptable PCI success rates. Coronary artery bypass graft surgery (CABG) is recommended for patients with persistent pain or hemodynamic instability when treatment with PCI or if medical management including thrombolytic therapy fails (Antman et al., 2004).

Patients with unrelieved chest pain and ECG changes, pulmonary edema, hypotension, or new mitral regurgitation indicate a need for intensive care unit monitoring. However, patients without these features may be admitted to a noncritical care en-

CLINICAL PATHWAYS FOR MANAGEMENT
OF ACUTE MYOCARDIAL INFARCTION

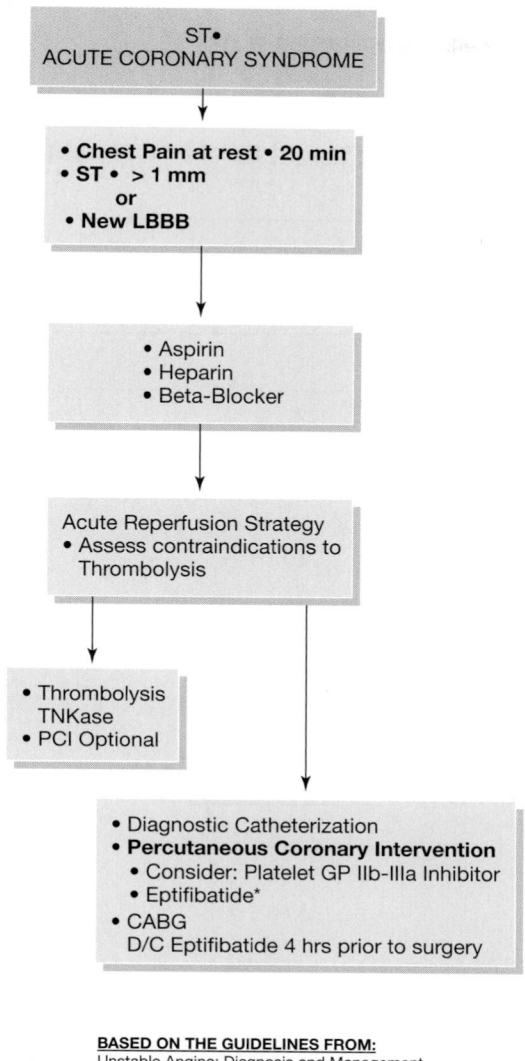

CLINICAL PATHWAYS FOR MANAGEMENT
OF ACUTE CORONARY SYNDROMES

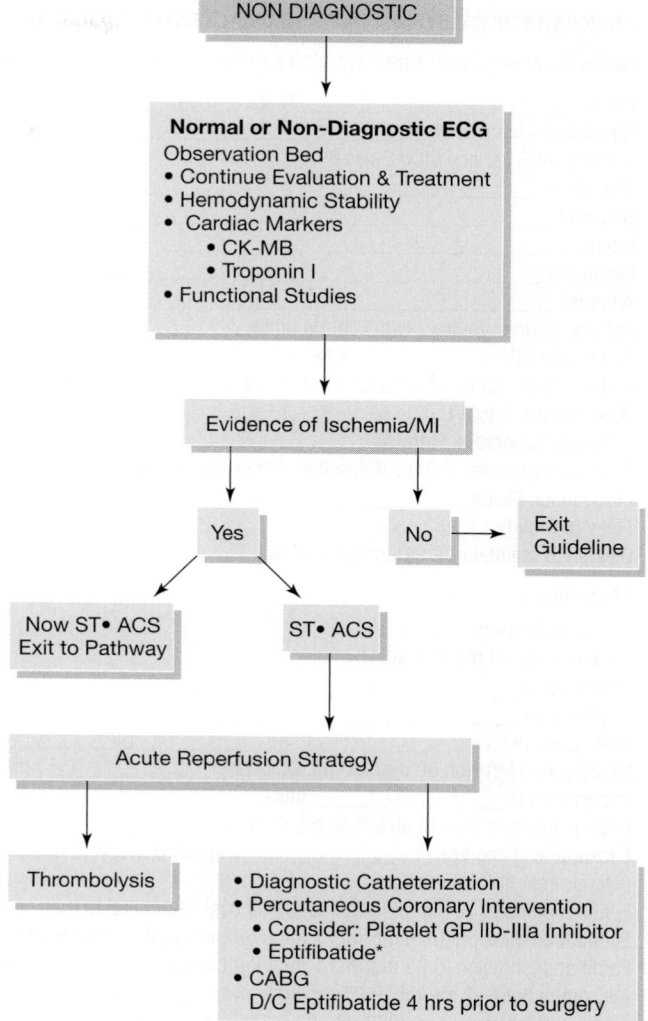

FIGURE 40–14 ■ Continued

vironment, depending on the health care provider's preference and hospital availability. Chart 40–13 (p. 1192) gives an example of a health care provider's orders used to treat ACS.

As part of the commitment to improving AMI outcomes, a number of studies have been conducted that bring teams of health care professionals together at the hospital and health system levels to evaluate treatment procedures, monitor resource utilization, identify patient-selection issues, and monitor outcomes. An example of this research is the National Registry of Myocardial Infarction (NRMI), sponsored by Genentech, Inc., which is one of the largest observational studies of acute myocardial infarction (AMI). As it is well known, AMI treatment

and intervention time is directly related to mortality. The faster the infarct-related artery is intervened on, the more myocardium is salvaged, thus, decreasing mortality. To track this, NRMI collects data on the four Ds: door, data, decision, and drug or dilation. From the time a patient presents to the emergency department door to the time the reperfusion drug is given should be 30 minutes or less, and the time from patient presentation to balloon dilation for reperfusion therapy should be 90 minutes or less. Since 1990, this study has collected data on more than 2.3 million AMI patients, helped more than 1,600 participating hospitals assess their approach to AMI treatment, and identified trends in patient outcome. Because of its size and

CHART 40–13   **Health Care Provider's Orders for Acute Coronary Syndrome**

UNIVERSITY OF CALIFORNIA DAVIS MEDICAL CENTER, SACRAMENTO, CALIFORNIA PHYSICIAN'S ORDERS USE PATIENT PLATE

Acute Coronary Syndrome Physician's Orders AM2036 (4/04) MR#03/04896

DATE: _____ TIME: _____

Directions: Check or fill in _____ for orders to be completed.

Admit to HRT Service CICU Davis 6

Attending _____   Fellow _____

Resident _____   Pgr PI# _____

Intern _____   Pgr PI# _____

Diagnosis _____   Condition _____

Allergies _____   Diet: NPO _____

Activity: Bedrest Bedrest with BRP Up ad lib

Call HO for SBP > _____ ; DBP > _____ < _____ ; HR > _____ < _____ ; Temp > _____ ; 02 Sat < _____

Call For Old Records Continuous Cardiac Monitor

Daily Weight Strict I/O

Initiate Collaborative Pathway

Establish IV Access, 2 Sites if Possible, Prefer 18 g–20 g

Intravenous Fluids _____ at _____ mL/hr

Foley to Gravity

Oxygen to Maintain 02 Saturation > 92%

Medications

ASA 325 PO daily

Pantoprazole 40 mg PO daily

Beta Blocker _____

Ace Inhibitor _____

HMG-CoA Inhibitor _____

Nitroglycerin Infusion 50 mg/250 mL D5W @ _____ mcg/min, titrate for chest pain, keep SBP > _____

Heparin bolus _____ units

Heparin Infusion 25,000 units/250 mL D5W drip @ _____ units/hour

Enoxaparin (1 mg/kg) _____ mg sub Q every 12 hours

Glycoprotein IIb/IIIa Inhibitor:

Eptifibatide bolus (2 mg/mL) 180 mcg/kg IV over 1–2 minutes then start drip

Eptifibatide infusion (0.75 mg/mL) 2 mcg/kg/min (creat. < 2.0 mg/dL) @ _____ mL/hr X _____ hrs

Eptifibatide infusion (0.75 mg/mL) 1 mcg/kg/min (creat. > 2.0 mg/dL, CRCL < 50 ml/min) _____ mL/hr X _____ hrs

Abciximab bolus (2 mg/mL) 0.25 mg/kg IV over 1–2 minutes

Abciximab Infusion (9 mg/250 mL NS) 0.125 mcg/kg/min @ mL/hr x 12 hrs

Additional Medications:

_____

_____

_____

_____

PRN Medications

Morphine 0.3–5 mg IV Q 3–5 min max 15 mg Q 3 hr PRN chest pain

Meperidine 5–20 mg IV Q 3–5 min max 125 mg Q 3 hr PRN pain

Temazepam 15–30 mg PO H at bedtime prn insomnia

Droperidol 1.25–2.5 mg IV q 4 hrs PRN nausea

Alprazolam 0.25 mg PO q 8 hrs PRN anxiety

Atropine 0.5–1.0 mg IV for HR < 40 if SBP < 90

NTG 0.4 mg SL PRN chest pain X 3 **(Do not use nitrates within 24 hours of Viagra, Levitra, and Cilias use)**

Tests/Procedures CPK-MB q _____ hrs or until peak

Basic Chemistry Panel qam Troponin q _____ hrs or until peak

CBC qam APTT qam

CBC w/auto diff Comprehensive Chemistry Panel

Magnesium qam CXR PA & Lateral

Lipid Panel ECG qam and prn chest pain, arrhythmias, or ST changes

Ordering Physician Signature _____ PI# _____ Pgr _____

Acute Coronary Syndrome

scope, NRMI has had a profound impact on AMI treatment practices. Although this is not a controlled, randomized clinical trial, it does not test the effectiveness between therapeutic interventions, and so comparisons of outcomes across treatment groups must be interpreted with caution.

Pharmacologic and Nonpharmacologic Treatment of Acute Coronary Syndrome

Oxygen fuels the metabolic processes that support myocyte contractility and heart pumping. Adequate oxygen supply to working cells is threatened during reductions in coronary blood flow. Because ACS causes a reduction in blood flow to the myocardium, the goal for the treatment of ACS is focused on reducing the myocardial oxygen demand or increasing the supply of oxygenated blood delivered to the injured cardiac tissue. Specific medical and nursing interventions will decrease the heart's need for oxygen, whereas others will increase the supply of oxygen to the cardiac muscle. Myocardial oxygen demand or myocardial consumption is affected most by increases in heart rate, contractility, and heart wall tension. Myocardial demand is decreased by modifying activity level; ameliorating the effects of the autonomic stress response; promoting rest; and reducing heart rate, contractility, and vascular resistance through drug and interventional therapies.

Efforts aimed at increasing oxygen supply to ischemic myocardium revolve around five strategies: (1) Raise the amount of oxygenated blood delivered to the tissues with supplemental oxygen and blood transfusions; (2) relieve coronary smooth muscle vasoconstriction or spasm with vasodilators; (3) reperfuse ischemic tissue by dissolving thrombus with thrombolytic agents; (4) prevent thrombus formation with anticoagulant therapy; and (5) reestablish blood flow through invasive revascularization procedures such as coronary artery bypass graft surgery (CABG) and percutaneous coronary intervention (PCI). An in-depth discussion of PCI is found in Chapter 39 .

Activity Progression

Activity for patients with ACS is dictated by the emergence of anginal symptoms. Patients are advised to avoid certain activities, to refrain from sudden exertion, and to stop what they are doing if symptoms occur. Activity prescriptions, based on ischemic thresholds determined during exercise testing, are recommended to maintain or enhance exercise tolerance, strengthen ventricular wall motion, or reduce ischemic episodes.

Activity guidelines for patients following acute ischemic events have changed dramatically over the past 20 years. Historically patients were kept on bed rest for up to 8 weeks to allow for myocardial healing and reduce complications. Today AMI patients, without clinical signs of ischemia or depressed ventricular function, get out of bed after a 24-hour pain-free period. Certain self-care activities are allowed, such as toileting, feeding, bathing, weighing, transferring, and positioning, which require minimal energy expenditure and do not cause undue strain on the recovering heart. For elimination needs, during the first 24 hours, patients may use either a bedpan or a bedside commode, as both are equivalent in energy expenditure. Barring other limitations patients admitted with UA can advance their activity after symptoms are controlled and hemodynamic stability is achieved for 8 hours. After 24 hours AMI patients should be up in a chair, during which time an assessment for orthostatic changes should be done. A drop in systolic pressure of 20 mmHg or more, or a heart

rate increase of 20 beats per minute or more represents a positive orthostatic change indicating that the patient is deconditioned. Muscle deconditioning, as it relates to cardiac function, refers to the delayed or inadequate response of the leg muscles to contract reflexively to increase return of peripheral blood volume as the patient progresses from a lying to standing position. When a patient is deconditioned, blood pools in the legs, dropping systemic blood pressure and causing syncope or dizziness, risk of falls, and possible recurrence of ischemia. Orthostatic BP and heart rate changes can be ameliorated by timing activity apart from administration times of vasodilating and diuretic medications, and having the patient warm up with in-bed isotonic exercises, such as extending and flexing the feet, prior to rising. The National Guidelines for Cardiac Rehabilitation box (p. 1194) outlines activity guidelines from the American Association of Cardiopulmonary Rehabilitation.

Reducing Autonomic Stress Responses

Norepinephrine and epinephrine levels are elevated during the first few hours after an AMI. These catecholamines increase heart rate and systemic vascular resistance (SVR), both resulting in increases in myocardial oxygen demand. To lessen the cardiovascular impact of autonomic system overstimulation, interventions for patients with angina and myocardial infarction are aimed at identifying and eliminating triggers of autonomic nervous system stimulation. Following an acute event, patients are monitored for signs of excessive sympathetic nervous stimulation such as dysrhythmias, diaphoresis, cool/clammy skin, and elevations in hemodynamic parameters such as pulmonary artery wedge pressure (PAWP), afterload, heart rate, and BP. Conditions that may cause or potentiate excessive catecholamine release such as abnormal electrolyte levels, hypoxemia, acidosis, hyper/hypotension, tachy/bradycardia, fever, anemia, volume depletion, immobility, discomfort, pain, or psychoemotional stress are avoided or treated quickly. Pain is treated with intravenous (IV) morphine sulfate. Morphine sulfate has the added benefit of being a vasodilator, thereby reducing both preload and afterload. Anxiety is treated with oral or IV benzodiazepine such as lorazepam (Ativan) or midazolam (Versed), although morphine sulfate also will help decrease anxiety. Family interaction is either liberal or restricted depending on patient preference; tolerance, defined in terms of cardiac signs and symptoms, is scheduled around adequate rest periods for the patient. Sleep is promoted by maintaining a quiet environment, keeping the lights off or low during the night, minimizing interactions with the patient during sleep periods, and pharmacologic sleeping aids. Dietary modifications that reduce sympathetic stimulation include avoidance of caffeinated beverages and beverages of extreme hot or cold temperature.

Overstimulation of the parasympathetic nervous system can be equally deleterious to recovering an ischemic heart. Valsalva maneuvers such as bearing down, pain, or heightened emotional responses may stimulate the vagus nerve, causing a decrease in heart rate and electrical conduction through the heart. As opposed to healthy hearts, myocardium scarred from ischemia with a concomitant reduced blood supply cannot compensate for a drop in heart rate and cardiac output. Pain from procedures such as chest tube insertion or sheath pulling from angiography can cause local excitation of the vagus nerve, resulting in bradycardia

NATIONAL GUIDELINES for Cardiac Rehabilitation from the American Association of Cardiopulmonary Rehabilitation

Cardiac rehabilitation is a combination of exercise training, lifestyle modification, and nutrition. Each patient's training program is individualized based on her own physical abilities.

Beginning Level, Weeks 1–4

Aerobic Training

Activities

Walking, cycling, etc.

Intensity

60–70% maximum capacity

Duration

5–10 minutes initially, adding 1–2 minutes per session as tolerated by patient

Frequency

3–5 times per week

Strength Training

Activities

Dumbbell exercise, water therapy

Intensity

1 set, 8–10 repetitions

Duration

5–10 minutes

Frequency

4 times per week

Flexibility Training

Stretching should be done before each workout period

Improvement Level, Months 1–5

Aerobic Training

Activities

Walking, cycling, jogging, etc.

Intensity

60–70% maximum capacity up to 85%

Duration

20–45 minutes, adding 1–2 minutes per session as tolerated by patient

Frequency

5 times per week

Strength Training

Activities

Dumbbell exercise, water therapy, exercise bands

Intensity

1 set, 12–20 repetitions

Duration

10–15 minutes

Frequency

4 times per week

Flexibilty Training

Stretching should be done before each workout period

Maintenance Level, 6 Months and Beyond

Aerobic Training

Activities

Walking, cycling, jogging, etc.

Intensity

60–85% maximum capacity

Duration

20–60 minutes

Frequency

3 times per week to maintain fitness, although 5 times per week is encouraged

Strength Training

Activities

Dumbbell exercise, water therapy, exercise bands

Intensity

1 set, 8 repetitions

Duration

5–10 minutes

Frequency

3 times per week

Flexibilty Training

Stretching should be done before each workout period

Source: University of California, Davis Medical Center, Sacramento, California (2005).

and hypotension called a vasovagal reaction. Precautionary treatments to avoid overstimulation of the parasympathetic nervous system include small frequent feedings, stool softeners and laxatives, analgesics prior to painful procedures, and avoiding Valsalva maneuvers. The avoidance of taking rectal temperatures in patients following an AMI is based on the misconception that the rectal mucosa has vagal innervation, and that stimulation will result in hemodynamic or electrophysiological instability. No study has demonstrated clinically significant cardiovascular changes resulting from rectal temperature taking. Chapter 24 ☞ describes all of the hemodynamic monitoring of cardiac patients.

Intra-Aortic Balloon Pump

Intra-aortic balloon pump (IABP) is used as an adjunct treatment for patients with ongoing ischemia, for those with complications related to AMI, and in high-risk patients who require prophylactic protection against ischemia prior to or during diagnostic, interventional, or surgical procedures. IABP employs a large catheter with a balloon, which is situated in the aorta between the left subclavian artery and the renal arteries takeoff branches. The balloon is inflated during the diastolic phase of the cardiac cycle and deflated right before systolic ejection. Inflating the balloon during diastole creates an elevated perfusion pressure back to the coronary artery located off the aortic route. This elevated perfusion pressure increases coronary blood flow, thereby enhancing oxygen delivery. The balloon is deflated during the contraction phase of the cardiac cycle so that ventricular pressure opens the aortic valve and blood is ejected out into the aorta. The deflation of the balloon just prior to systole creates a suction effect within the vessel that helps pull more blood from the left ventricle and decreases the resistance the blood encounters when leaving the heart (afterload). A lowered afterload resistance decreases workload on the heart and enhances forward ejection of blood. The goal when using an intra-aortic balloon pump is to increase the supply of oxygen to the myocardium and decrease the demand (Figure 40–15 ■).

Beta- (ß-) Adrenergic Blocking (ß-blockers) Agents

Inhibiting adrenergic stimulation by competitive binding sympathetic receptors with β-blocking agents has been shown to reduce myocardial ventilation oxygen consumption (MVO_2). β-blockers reduce heart rate at rest, attenuate heart rate with exercise, decrease myocardial fiber stretch and contractility, oppose platelet aggregation, and stabilize myocardial cellular membranes, thus,

reducing dysrhythmia occurrence. These actions slow the heart rate and decrease the oxygen demand. Patients with chronic stable angina, treated with β-blocker therapy, demonstrate reduced number, severity, and duration of ischemic episodes and increased exercise capacity (Adams, Josephsen, & Holland, 2005; Opie & Poole-Wilson, 2005). β-blockers are used to treat silent ischemia, angina associated with altered vasomotor tone, UA, and AMI. Whether administered IV or orally, early β-blocker therapy in the setting of AMI reduces infarct size, malignant ventricular dysrhythmia occurrence, chest pain, risk of cardiac arrest, and mortality without a greater incidence of heart failure or heart block. Because the risk of mortality is highest during the first year, therapy should begin soon after the first IV dose and continue for at least a year. When discontinuing β-blocker therapy, the drug should be weaned down with decreasing doses.

Therapeutic goals include reduction in frequency or suppression of anginal attacks, resting heart rate of 50 to 60 beats per minute, attenuated heart rate and BP response during exercise, and no adverse reactions. Contraindications and reasons for discontinuing therapy include hypotension, sinus bradycardia, bronchial asthma, AV nodal dysfunction, claudication or pain in legs from peripheral vascular disease, and hyperglycemia from diabetes. Patients should be advised against abruptly discontinuing β-blocking agents. Long-term therapy results in an increase in the number, affinity, and sensitivity of β-receptors. When no longer blocked, unopposed sympathetic stimulation is heightened, producing rebound tachycardia, hypertension, exacerbation of angina, ventricular ectopy, and greater risk of MI.

FIGURE 40–15 ■ Intra-aortic balloon pump catheter.

Angiotensin-Converting Enzyme Inhibitors

Low-dose angiotensin-converting enzyme inhibitors (ACEIs) started within 24 hours and continued indefinitely are part of the recommended therapy for patients suffering from an AMI because they reduce mortality and the incidence of left ventricular dysfunction and reinfarction (Antman et al., 2004). ACEIs are thought to be beneficial through a number of mechanisms: (1) increased production of superoxides by decreasing angiotensin II; (2) increasing endogenous nitric oxide, which increases vasodilation through ACEI inhibition of bradykinin degradation; and (3) positive influence on hemodynamic load, vascular function, myocardial remodeling, and neurohumoral regulation (Dendorfer, Dominiak, & Shunkert, 2005; Latini et al., 2003). Myocardial remodeling describes the process of replacing nonviable heart muscle tissue with nonelastic fibrinous collagen, which causes cardiac wall thinning, dilation, and subsequently an impaired ability for the ventricles to function normally. Side effects include hypotension, angioedema, persistent cough, and reduced creatinine clearance.

Angiotensin II Receptor Blockers in Myocardial Infarction

Angiotensin II receptor blockers (ARBs) have not been shown to be superior to ACEI alone, nor synergistic when added to ACEI, but are recommended for patients intolerant of ACEI therapy. The use of ACEI or ARBs is not advocated for patients with NSTEMI unless accompanied by persistent hypertension despite beta-blocker and nitrate therapy in patients with left ventricular dysfunction and in patients with diabetes (Libby, Bonow, Zipes, & Mann, 2008).

Nitrate Therapy

Once considered contraindicated in the setting of AMI, today nitrate therapy is a staple in drug management of occlusive coronary syndromes, regardless of the underlying mechanism triggering ischemia. Administration of nitrates causes the vascular smooth muscles to relax, resulting in dilation of venous, coronary, and, to a lesser degree, peripheral arterial vessels. Nitroglycerin dilates areas of arterial stenosis, especially in eccentric lesions, and can relieve spontaneous coronary vasospasm directly or possibly through the release of prostacyclin, another potent vasodilator, which improves collateral flow to ischemic areas. Nitroglycerin also has been shown to inhibit platelet aggregation, inhibit platelet adhesion, and cause disbursement of formed platelet clumps (Opie & White, 2005).

Nitrates are used alone or in combination with beta-blockers or calcium channel blockers to reduce the frequency and duration of angina symptoms, incidence of silent ischemia, and to improve exercise tolerance (Opie & White, 2005). Long-term benefits of nitrate therapy on mortality and incidence of AMI in patients with symptomatic and asymptomatic ischemia have not been determined. Short-term benefits of IV nitroglycerin with unstable angina and AMI are improved hemodynamics, decreased frequency and duration of symptoms, reduced infarct size, better patency rates following reperfusion therapy, greater residual left ventricular function, and decreased mortality. Long-acting nitrates such as oral, ointment, or patch preparations are used to treat patients with symptomatic CAD prophylactically. Faster acting nitrates such as sublingual tablets or spray-on nitroglycerin are used as needed to alleviate breakthrough angina. Patient are instructed to take up to 3 sublingual tablets or sprays spaced 5 minutes apart to relieve anginal attacks, which can be repeated in 30 minutes if symptoms return. If symptoms do not abate, or return despite rest and/or treatment, patients are instructed to activate the emergency medical system (EMS). Nitrates cannot be used within 24 hours after ingesting sildenafil citrate (Viagra) or like products because of the risk of severe vasodilation and death.

Other potential side effects of nitrate administration include reflex tachycardia, hypotension, headache, facial flushing, syncope, and cerebral ischemia. Over-the-counter analgesics usually relieve nitroglycerin-induced headaches. Patients should be cautioned about the potential for hypotension and reflex tachycardia when changing position from lying to standing. These same effects can be seem during IV nitroglycerin initiation and up-titration, especially in patients who present with hypovolemia, inferior wall MI, right ventricular infarction, or advanced age.

Vasodilator Therapy to Relieve Vasoconstriction or Vasospasm

Nitroglycerin is the drug of choice for relief of coronary vasoconstriction during chronic and acute myocardial ischemic syndromes. Sodium nitroprusside also produces coronary artery vasodilation. Unlike nitroglycerin, which is selective for venous and larger arterial beds, sodium nitroprusside affects only arterial vessels. Sodium nitroprusside is recommended as a second-line vasodilator if satisfactory blood pressure control is not obtained with nitroglycerin, and as the first-line therapy in the setting of AMI complicated with hypertension or acute heart failure.

Calcium channel blockers, such as diltiazem hydrochloride (Cardizem), are used in combination with nitrates in patients with Prinzmetal, or variant, angina to produce smooth muscle relaxation.

Thrombolytic Agents

Thrombus formation is an integral piece in the pathogenesis of myocardial ischemic syndromes. This has shifted treatment paradigms from simply supportive care and monitoring to rapid ischemia recognition, clot dissolution, and reperfusion of hypoxic tissue. Fibrinolytic therapy (treatment with thrombolytics) has been shown to establish reperfusion to the infarct-related artery successfully in a timely fashion. This has allowed myocardial muscle salvage, which has decreased the overall mortality rate for patients with a myocardial infarction.

Important general principles that guide the administration of thrombolytics are (1) contraindications, (2) timing of medication to time of event, and (3) monitoring for adverse reactions. Certain patient characteristics must be considered before administering thrombolytics. Essentially, patients who are at risk for bleeding because of a previous recent surgery, trauma, or history of recent bleeding complication, or who are hemodynamically unstable may be considered ineligible for thrombolytic therapy. An important aspect of administration is the delay from symptom onset to treatment. Every hour past symptom onset decreases the survival benefit of thrombolytic therapy. Past 12 hours, thrombolytic administration is associated with greater risk of complications (Antman et al., 2004).

Adverse reactions primarily focus on assessment of the patient for anaphylactic reactions, bleeding, and hemodynamic instability. Nurses need to watch for signs and symptoms of an allergic reaction, which include rash, wheezing, shortness of breath, flushing, and hypotension. Patients should be monitored for signs of bleeding from not only obvious sites such as IV catheter sites but also the mucous membranes of the oral pharynx, gums, nose, lungs, and rectum. Unnecessary catheter insertions and hypertensive states should be avoided. Neuro and vital sign checks should be performed according to institution protocol, monitoring for signs of intracranial hemorrhage and hemodynamic instability.

Anticoagulation Therapy

Procoagulant cells of the blood do not normally interact with the intact vascular endothelium. If vessel endothelium is injured or removed, blood contact with the elements of the subendothelial layer heralds the recruitment and activation of platelets and catalyzes the coagulation cascade. Anticoagulation therapies counteract thrombus formation in one or more of the following ways: deactivation of platelets, blocking of protein expression necessary for activation of the clotting cascade, and neutralization of thrombin generation or activity.

Plaque rupture causes the platelet surface glycoprotein (GP) Ib to adhere to subendothelial glycoproteins to form a monolayer of platelets over the plaque lesion. Additionally, activated platelets promote further platelet recruitment, aggregation, and activation by releasing stimulants from their granules and undergoing a change in shape, which allows expression of a binding protein. Activated platelets unleash other substances such as fibrinogen, thromboxane A_2, serotonin, and adenosine diphosphate (ADP) from granule stores, which in return attract and activate more platelets (Figure 40–16 ■). When a platelet is stimulated, it changes from a spherical contour to irregular shapes that result in the exposure of glycoprotein (GP) IIb/IIIa receptors and reactive phospholipids. The glycoprotein receptor sites bind with circulation fibrinogen to create a bridge between platelets, which then bind together to form a clot. Platelet surface phospholipids interact with plasma proteins of the clotting cascade, which also contributes to clot formation.

Antiplatelet agents deactivate platelets by either interfering with the production, release, or function of platelet-derived

stimulants or the binding of GP IIb/IIIa receptors. Acetylsalicylic acid (ASA), clopidrogrel bisulfate (Plavix), and GP IIb/IIIa inhibitors form the constellation of antiplatelet agents currently used to treat ACS. Aspirin (ASA) has proven to be the most cost effective and least adverse antiplatelet agent used to date. ASA inactivates cyclo-oxygenase, an enzyme responsible for arachidonic acid oxidation into thromboxane A_2 and prostaglandins. ASA therapy has been effective in risk reduction with MIs and sudden death in patients with angina; reduced recurrence of ischemic symptoms in patients with UA; and reduced infarct size, rates of reinfarction, and mortality in patients with MI (Antman et al., 2004). Optimal dosing of ASA has not been determined. Following an initial dose of at least 160 milligrams, all patients with CAD should begin daily doses of 81 to 325 milligrams indefinitely, unless contraindications exist. Absorption is better with the chewable form of ASA, especially in patients who have received opiates. ASA suppositories can be safely used if nausea, vomiting, or known upper-gastrointestinal disorders are present. Patients with hypersensitivity to ASA can be started on Plavix as a substitute. Although commonly used alone as prophylaxis against thrombus formation in patients with stable CAD, in circumstances where plaque rupture is a definite risk, ASA is frequently used in combination with other antiplatelet agents.

Clopidrogrel bisulfate (Plavix), a thienopyridine, inhibits the platelet-stimulating effects of ADP. Plavix may be more effective than ASA in preventing thrombus formation following endothelial injury in that it inhibits both platelet adhesion and intimal proliferation, although Plavix has few side effects. It is given as a daily dose of 75 milligrams and is currently recommended as a first-line drug in addition to or in place of ASA for patients who present with NSTEMI.

Platelet adhesion to one another is dependent on fibrinogen contact with GP IIb/IIIa. Three GP IIb/IIIa antagonists are used in clinical practice: abciximab (ReoPro), eptifibatide (Integrelin), and tirofiban hydrochloride (Aggrastat). Abciximab is different from the others in that it is a monoclonal antibody that binds irreversibly to the GP IIb/IIIa receptor. Because it is an antigenic protein, there is a slight risk of anaphylaxis following administration. Once given, the antiplatelet effects of abciximab cannot be reversed despite administration of new platelets. Abciximab not only lasts the 10-day life cycle of the platelet but also affects newly formed platelets; eptifibatide and tirofiban are synthetic nonpeptide antagonists that compete with fibrinogen to bind with GP IIb/IIIa receptors. Unlike abciximab, the antiplatelet effects of eptifibatide and tirofiban can be reversed by withholding administration for 2 to 4 hours. All three GP IIb/IIIa inhibitors are administered intravenously by an initial bolus dose followed by a continuous infusion. Bleeding is the major complication and requires close monitoring and patient education for prevention. One major disadvantage of the GP IIb/IIIa blocking agents is that there is currently no simple, inexpensive method to monitor the extent of receptor blockade, which would allow dose titration and possibly reduce side effects. The lack of an oral preparation also limits the use of these agents to acute thrombotic events only.

Coagulation via the intrinsic and extrinsic clotting pathways is a dynamic process of a series of linked and interdependent reactions wherein one protein converts and activates another along a defined cascade of reactions that ultimately leads to thrombin generation. Activated thrombin detaches from the

Platelet Aggregation

FIGURE 40–16 ■ Platelet aggregation.

phospholipids on the platelet surface and converts plasma fibrinogen to fibrin. Fibrin strands form a mesh that traps circulating blood elements to cause a clot. Inactivation of thrombin is achieved through the administration of (1) warfarin, which antagonizes the action of vitamin K–dependent clotting factors of the intrinsic clotting cascade; (2) unfractionated heparin, which when combined with the protein antithrombin III (AT III) adheres to and inactivates thrombin; (3) low molecular weight heparin (LMWH), which binds with factor X, effectively stopping the creation of thrombin through the clotting cascade; and (4) direct thrombin inhibitors such as hirudin, which bind directly to and inhibit thrombin activity.

Sodium warfarin (Coumadin) blocks an enzyme called vitamin K epoxide reductase necessary for the conversion of factors VII, IX, X, and II, and the proteins C and S into their activated forms. Wafarin's clinical use in the treatment of coronary syndromes is controversial and if used is limited to secondary prevention of thromboembolic complications following acute ischemic attacks and only in patients at low risk for serious bleeding complications. Because of this risk, warfarin therapy is not recommended in recent treatment guidelines for unstable angina or MI.

Intravenous heparin is an unfractionated combination of heparins with various densities and weights. The ability of heparin to bind with thrombin via the AT III protein depends on (1) the admixture of heparin molecules in the dose (high vs. low molecular weight), (2) circulating levels of AT III, (3) the presence of plasma proteins that inactivate heparin, and (4) the inability of heparin to reach thrombin sequestered within a fibrin clot. Plasma protein binding of unfractionated heparin contributes to a nonlinear, unpredictable, patient-specific anticoagulant response and heparin resistance. Using heparin doses adjusted according to patient weight and level of anticoagulation as measured by activated clotting time (ACT) or activated partial thromboplastin time (aPTT) produces better results with less bleeding complications. Most sources suggest a therapeutic aPTT range of 50 to 75 or 60 to 80 seconds with aPTT assessments drawn every 4 to 6 hours until a therapeutic range is achieved. Standardized nomograms, which prescribe how and when to adjust heparin dosage based on aPTT values, are extremely beneficial to nurses responsible for heparin titration (Figure 40–17 ■).

In summary, pharmacologic and nonpharmacologic measures to decrease oxygen demand and increase supply form the mainstay of initial management guidelines for patients with presenting signs of CAD, with resulting clinical manifestations of angina and ACS. Symptoms no longer controlled with pharmacologic agents are a clear indication of the need for more invasive procedures to revascularize the coronary arteries. These include either coronary artery angioplasty and/or surgical coronary revascularization. Decisions as to which treatment course is best, primarily depend on the severity of CAD and comorbid diseases, and their impact on the patient's lifestyle and risk for MI or death. Perhaps as important are patient preference and health care provider opinion in choosing treatment options. For emergent conditions, management may depend on the availability of cardiac catheterization and surgical services. See the Pharmacology Summary of Medications to Treat Coronary Disease box.

Medical Management of Complications of Acute Myocardial Infarction

Myocardial blood flow cut off for longer than 20 to 40 minutes initiates a dynamic process of cellular death, which extends over a period of several hours. Cell necrosis produces a loss of cell membrane integrity and degradation of connection tissue, which in turn causes cell swelling, protein leakage, and changes in cellular structure and function. In response, systemic catecholamine stimulation raises MVO_2 and taxes nonischemic tissue. With reestablishment of flow, initially cell necrosis continues and cell disruption and death ensue. Subsequent to cell death myocardial tissue undergoes remodeling characterized by the deposition of collagen in place of normal myocytes, muscle thinning, and dilation. These pathologic changes result in a myriad of complications that include recurrent angina, ventricular failure, dysrhythmias, and mechanical defects. Predictors of late major complications include the presence of early sustained ventricular tachycardia or fibrillation, presence of early sustained hypotension or cardiogenic shock, multivessel disease, and left ventricular dysfunction (Antman et al., 2004).

Recurrent Chest Pain from Ischemia

Chest pain that reemerges 12 hours to 6 days after an AMI, waxes and wanes, and is sometimes called stuttering or recurrent chest pain, may represent infarct extension. Recurrence of angina during recovery from AMI may depict coronary flow instability within the infarct-related artery. Pain, the most sensitive indicator

ACC/AHA Nomogram for Heparin Dosing

aPTT (s)	Bolus dose (u)	Stop infusion (min)	Rate change (mL/h)	Rate change (u/hr)	Repeat aPTT
<40	3,000	0	+1	100	6h
40–49	0	0	+0.5	50	6h
50–70	0	0	0	0	Next am
71–85	0	0	−0.5	50	Next am
86–100	0	30	−1	100	6h
101–150	0	60	−1.5	150	6h
>150	0	60	−3	300	6h

FIGURE 40–17 ■ Standardized nomograms for heparin dosage based on aPTT values.

PHARMACOLOGY Summary of Medications to Treat Coronary Artery Disease

Medication Category	Action	Application/Indication	Nursing Responsibility
Medical Management of Acute Coronary Syndrome (ACS)			

Calcium channel blockers:
  Diltiazem (Cardizem)
  Amlodipine (Norvasc)
	Inhibits calcium ion movement across the cell membrane in cardiac and vascular muscle, thereby relaxing the smooth muscle and dilating coronary and peripheral arteries.	Chronic stable angina.
		Vasospastic angina.
		Unstable angina.
		Hypertension.
		Postcoronary intervention.
		Dysrhythmias.
			Monitor blood pressure, heart rate, and rhythm. Monitor electrocardiogram (EKG) intervals. Monitor for response; i.e., decrease in angina, blood pressure, and dysrhythmias. Assess for increase in heart failure (HF), as edema may increase.

Nitrates:
  Nitroglycerin (NTG)
  Nitro-Bid
  Nitro-Dur
  Tridil
	Dilates coronary and systemic arteries, thereby decreasing preload and afterload.	Angina: chronic, unstable, or vasospastic.	Monitor blood pressure.
			Monitor for response; i.e., decrease in anginal pain, decrease in blood pressure. Assess patient for headache (known to cause headaches in some patients). Store drug in dark container, as it is sensitive to light. Do not administer within 24 hours of Viagra, Cialis, or Levitra.

Beta-adrenegic blockers:
  Metoprolol (Lopressor)
  Atenolol
	Selective: completely blocks beta-1 receptor stimulation in cardiac smooth muscle.
	Nonselective: causes a decrease in blood pressure through a mixture of beta-blocking effects but does not cause reflex tachycardia or decreased heart rate.
		Hypertension. Ventricular dysrhythmias.	Closely monitor blood pressure and heart rate. Monitor for response; i.e., decreased blood pressure, heart rate decreased, ventricular dysrhythmias. Monitor blood chemistries, especially those related to renal function. Use with caution in patients with chronic obstructive pulmonary disease (COPD), asthma, renal disease, or diabetes mellitus.

Angiotensin-converting enzyme inhibitors (ACE inhibitors):
  Benazepril (Lotensin)
  Captopril (Capoten)
  Enalapril (Vasotec)
	Inhibits the conversion of angiotensin I to angiotensin II; suppresses renin-angiotensin-aldosterone system.	Hypertension.
		Congestive heart failure.
			Monitor blood chemistries, specifically renal function and electrolytes. Monitor lower extremity edema. Monitor signs and symptoms of heart failure. Monitor response; i.e., decreased blood pressure, decreased shortness of breath (SOB), decreased rhonchi. Weigh patient every day.

Angiotensin II receptor blockers (ARBs):
  Candesartan (Atacand)
  Eprosartan (Teveten)
  Irbesartan (Avapro)
	Blocks the vasoconstrictor and aldosterone-secreting effects of angiotensin.	Hypertension.	Monitor for response; i.e., decrease in blood pressure (BP). Monitor blood chemistries.

Lipid Lowering Therapy			

HMG-CoA reductase inhibitors (statins):
  Atorvastin (Lipitor)
  Lovastatin (Mevacor)
  Simvastatin (Zocor)
  Pravastatin (Pravachol)
  Fluvastatin (Lescol)
  Rosuvastatin (Crestor)
	Inhibits HMG-CoA reductase enzyme, thereby preventing the formation of cholesterol in the liver. Statins lower total cholesterol, low density lipoproteins-cholesterol (LDL-C), and triglycerides while increasing high density lipoprotein-cholesterol (HDL-C). Statins have also been connected with stabilizing *rupture-prone* atherosclerotic plaque, improving vasomotor tone, decreasing levels of proinflammatory proteins, decreasing factors that contribute to thrombosis, and improving myocardial perfusion.	Hypercholesterolemia.	Monitor liver function studies. Monitor lipid panel. Monitor patient for myalgias. Administer medication in the evening to take advantage of the fact that the liver produces more cholesterol at nighttime than during the day. Patients may experience abdominal discomfort from gas or constipation, which usually subsides with continued therapy. Rarely causes elevated liver enzymes and muscle soreness, pain, and weakness, which may require changes in dose or discontinuance of statin therapy. Monitor liver function tests (LFT).

(continued)

PHARMACOLOGY Summary of Medications to Treat Coronary Artery Disease—*Continued*

Medication Category	Action	Application/Indication	Nursing Responsibility
Resins, or bile acid sequestrants: Cholestyramine (Questran) Colestipol (Colestid) Colesevelam (WelChol)	Binds with cholesterol-containing bile acids in the intestines and are then eliminated via stool.	Hypercholesterolemia.	Monitor lipid panel. Administered orally as powders or tablets and taken with water or fruit juice once, twice, or three times a day. May interfere with the absorption of other medications and, like statins, can cause constipation, bloating, nausea, and gas.
Fibrates: Gemfibrozil (Lopid) Fenofibrate (Tricor)	Fibrates lower triglycerides and can increase HDL-C levels.	Hypercholesterolemia.	Monitor serum LDL, very low density lipoprotein (VLDL), total cholesterol, and triglycerides. Monitor for gastrointestinal upset and bleeding. Assess for bloody stools, nosebleeds, cloudy or bloody urine, bleeding gums, and ecchyomoses.
Antihyperlipidemics: Ezetimibe (Zetia) Ezetimibe/Simvastatin (Zetia and Zocor) Combination drugs: Ezetimibe and Simvastatin (Vytorin) Work best when given with statin.	Ezetimibe: reduces blood cholesterol by inhibiting the absorption of cholesterol at the small intestine. This will decrease the level of cholesterol delivered to the liver. Simvastatin: inhibits HMG-CoA reductase enzyme, thereby decreasing cholesterol production; increases HDL-C and decreases VLDL and triglycerides.	Hypercholesterolemia.	Monitor liver function studies. Monitor lipid panel. Monitor patient for myalgias and headaches. Administer medication in the evening.
Niacin B vitamin	In high doses lowers triglycerides and LDL-C levels, and increases HDL-C.	Hypercholesterolemia. Increased triglycerides.	Patients should be advised not to start taking megadoses without being under the care of a clinician. Dose levels need to be gradually increased over time. Flushing or hot flashes (due to vasodilation) may occur, often requiring changes in antihypertensive medication dosage. Gastrointestinal symptoms of nausea, indigestion, gas, vomiting, diarrhea, and aggravation of peptic ulcers, liver problems, gout, and elevated blood sugar. Aspirin can be prescribed 30 minutes prior to the dose to decrease flushing.
Fibrinolytic (thrombolytic therapy) TNK	Modified human tissue plasminogen activator that binds to fibrin and converts plasminogen to plasmin. It is fibrin specific, thus decreasing the systemic activation of plasminogen.	Acute myocardial infarction.	Do not administer if the patient has active internal bleeding; history of cerebrovascular accident; intracranial or intraspinal surgery or trauma within 2 months; intracranial neoplasm, arteriovenous malformation, or aneurysm; known bleeding diathesis; or severe uncontrolled hypertension. Monitor for bleeding postdrug infusion. Administered as single bolus.
RPA	Nonglycoslated deletion mutein of tissue plasminogen activator, made by recombinant DNA technology.	Same as above.	Same as above. Administered as double bolus.

PHARMACOLOGY Summary of Medications to Treat Coronary Artery Disease—*Continued*

Medication Category	Action	Application/Indication	Nursing Responsibility
Antiplatelet Agents			
Acetylsalicylic acid aspirin (ASA)	Powerfully inhibits platelet aggregation by impairing hepatic synthesis of blood coagulation factors VII, IX, and X and possible inhibiting action of vitamin K.	Acute myocardial infarction and prevention of recurrence.	Monitor for gastrointestinal upset and bleeding. Assess for bloody stools, nosebleeds, cloudy or bloody urine, bleeding gums, and ecchyomoses. Administer with food. Do not administer if the patient has active internal bleeding. Discontinued use if ringing in ears. Maintain adequate fluid intake. Avoid medications with aspirin in them.
ADP receptor blockers: Clopidrogrel (Plavix) Ticlopidine (Ticlid)	Inhibits platelet aggregation by selectively preventing the binding of adenosine diphosphate to its platelet receptor.	Secondary prevention of myocardial infarction. Reduction in restenosis after stent placement.	Monitor for gastrointestinal upset and bleeding. Assess for bloody stools, nosebleeds, cloudy or bloody urine, bleeding gums, and ecchyomoses. Do not take other drugs that inhibit platelet aggregation.
Glycoprotein IIb/IIIa blockers: Eptifibatide (Integrilin) Abciximab (ReoPro) Tirofiban (Aggrastat)	Binds the IIb/IIIa receptor sites on platelets, preventing fibrinogen and von Willebrand factor from adhering to the platelet.	Treatment of acute coronary syndrome.	Monitor for bleeding. Stop infusion if bleeding occurs. Avoid invasive procedures including needle sticks.

Sources: Adams, M. P., Josephen, D. L., & Holland, L. N. (Eds.). (2005). *Pharmacology for nurses: A pathophysiologic approach.* Upper Saddle River, NJ: Prentice Hall Health; and Wilson, B. A., Shannon, M. T., & Stang, C. L. (2005). *Nurse's drug guide.* Upper Saddle River, NJ: Prentice Hall Health.

of infarct extension, may be accompanied by ECG changes, myocardial serum marker elevation (CK-MB, troponin I, and troponin T), hemodynamic instability, dysrhythmias, or worsening heart failure. Medical management for recurrent ischemic pain includes IV nitroglycerin (NTG), beta-adrenergic blockers, and calcium blockers. Refractory ischemic symptoms necessitate angiography to discern whether coronary occlusion is the cause and determine the appropriateness of repeat reperfusion therapy. Angiography is discussed in Chapter 39 .

Pericarditis

Extension of myocardial wall necrosis through to the epicardium causes pericardial inflammation in some post-MI patients. Early or acute pericarditis occurs 48 to 72 hours after an AMI and is associated with larger infarcts and lower ejection fractions. Pericarditis often presents with pain accompanied by the following: pericardial friction rub, pericardial effusion, dyspnea, fever, elevated erythrocyte sedimentation rate (ESR), leukocytosis, and ECG changes of J point elevation with concave upward ST segment elevation in all leads except aVR and V_1, PR depression, persistently elevated T waves, or inverted T wave reversal. Absence of elevated CK-MB levels, symptom qualities, and ECG characteristics help differentiate pericarditis from ischemic pain. Pericarditis is discussed in detail in Chapter 41 . The treatment of choice is the use of nonsteroidal anti-inflammatory drugs (NSAIDS) such as ibuprofen (Zipes et al., 2005). The use of indomethacin is discouraged because it can reduce coronary flow.

Dressler's syndrome (post-MI syndrome) connotes pericarditis that occurs 2 to 12 weeks after MI; it is thought to be an autoimmune or immunologic response to antimyocardial antibodies produced by myocardial necrosis (Zipes et al., 2005). Symptomology, diagnosis, and treatment are the same for early and late pericarditis except that symptoms developing later may reappear several times before resolving. The incidence of Dressler's syndrome has decreased with the era of thrombolytic therapy. Dressler's syndrome is discussed in detail in Chapter 41 .

Heart Failure

Ischemia to myocardial tissue may cause transient or prolonged ventricular dysfunction requiring inotropic and vasodilation therapy to reduce myocardial oxygen demand and augment forward flow of blood. Reductions in blood flow to the myocardium trigger compensatory mechanisms whereby an ischemic muscle's ability to contract is lessened or down-regulated. Brief ischemic episodes, lasting less than 15 minutes, followed by reperfusion may not result in cellular necrosis but can produce a reversible transient depression of ventricular contraction that persists for hours or days called myocardial stunning (Zipes et al., 2005). Prolonged ischemia can produce compensatory down-regulation of contractile tissue, called myocardial hibernation, wherein oxygen debt requirements are matched to reduced oxygen supply (Zipes et al., 2005). (See the Pathophysiology of Myocardial Injury and Death section earlier in this chapter.) Partial or complete function is restored once reperfusion improves blood supply or therapy reduces myocardial oxygen demand. On cardiac imaging stunned and hibernating myocardium are reflected as areas of hypokinetic, akinetic or dyskinetic ventricular wall movement resulting in heart failure. This results in a temporary ventricular dysfunction without permanent myocyte damage, which may or may not present clinically as symptoms of ventricular failure. Prolonged ischemia without down-regulation of contractile ventricular function and reperfusion of ischemic tissue may cause cell membrane destruction, impaired cellular function and integrity, and eventually tissue necrosis. Heart failure is discussed in detail in Chapter 42 ☺.

Cardiogenic Shock

The incidence of cardiogenic shock in the setting of AMI is 7% and occurs when more than 40% of the left ventricle is infarcted, usually with severe three-vessel disease (Hochman et al., 2006). In patients presenting with AMI complicated by cardiogenic shock, survival has been reported between 20% and 50% when treated with thrombolytic agents, 40% and 70% with PCI, and 58% and 91% with emergency bypass surgery (Hochman et al., 2006). Emergency CABG is recommended for AMI patients with multivessel disease or cardiogenic shock who are not candidates for or have not undergone unsuccessful thrombolytic therapy and/or PCI, and who are within 4 to 6 hours from onset of AMI (Antman et al., 2004). Cardiogenic shock is discussed in Chapter 63 ☺.

Dysrhythmias

It is not uncommon for most patients with myocardial ischemia to experience some type of dysrhythmia. Dysrhythmia type depends on the location of arterial occlusion and the underlying electrical conduction tissue, which becomes ischemic. These dysrhythmias may be related to increased catecholamine activity, drug therapies, altered electrophysiological properties from hypokalemia, hypomagnesemia, intracellular hypercalcemia, and acidosis (Antman et al., 2004). Relative importance of each factor is unknown as is the efficacy of prophylactic treatments. Chapter 38 ☺ describes the cause and treatment of each of the dysrhythmias discussed next.

Supraventricular Tachycardia

The most common type of supraventricular tachycardia (SVT) that affects patients who have experienced an AMI is atrial fibrillation (AF); sinus tachycardia, premature atrial contractions, atrial flutter, atrial tachycardia, and accelerated junctional rhythms also occur. SVTs are managed by treating the underlying cause first. Additional treatments that may be necessary are synchronized cardioversion if the patient is severely compromised, slowing the rate with overdrive pacing or pharmacotherapy using primarily amiodarone, β-adrenergic blockers, calcium blockers, digoxin, or other antiarrhythmics.

Bradycardia

Bradycardia occurring from either an underperfused inferior wall myocardium or a heart block is treated using atropine, or cardiac pacing and withholding drugs that decrease the heart rate. Atropine is the drug of choice for treatment of symptomatic sinus bradycardia, ventricular asystole, and symptomatic heart block (Antman et al., 2004). Though cardiac pacing has not been shown to reduce mortality specifically, its use is recommended for patients with symptomatic bradycardia unresponsive to drug therapy (Antman et al., 2004).

Ventricular Dysrhythmias

Ventricular dysrhythmias, including premature ventricular contractions (PVCs), idioventricular and accelerated idioventricular rhythms, and nonsustained ventricular tachycardia (VT), can be expected in most patients early and within 48 hours during the course of recovery from AMI. Emergence of these dysrhythmias has not been shown to increase mortality nor warn of impending ventricular fibrillation (VF), unless the patient that is symptomatic is not treated.

Infarct Expansion, Ventricular Remodeling

Infarct expansion is the process of ventricular wall thinning and elongation of the infarct zone, which produces ventricular dyskinesia. Ischemia causes cellular inflammation, edema, and side-to-side cell slippage resulting in myocardial fibril changes. Ischemia causes myocardial cell fibers to become soft, distensible, and to rearrange in a wavy pattern, which results in a paradoxical fiber lengthening and wall bulging during systole and shortening during diastole. Eventually fibroblast proliferation causes collagen deposition and scar formation. Myofibrils are stretched and elongated and new fibrils are added, resulting in ventricular hypertrophy. The two processes of infarct expansion and ventricular hypertrophy cause ventricular remodeling, which can lead to development of heart failure and/or left ventricular rupture (Takemura & Fuiwara, 2004). Myocardial remodeling begins in the early stages of infarction and can continue for months and years. It is a predictor of increased mortality. Topographic changes from remodeling are identified using echocardiography and magnetic resonance imaging, described in Chapter 39 ☺. Limiting infarct size and maintaining patency of the infarct-related artery with reperfusion therapies are two primary strategies for preventing ventricular remodeling. Clinicians should avoid the administration of drugs that inhibit healing and scar formation, such as steroids, indomethacin, and ibuprofen. Reducing ventricular wall stress by decreasing preload with NTG and afterload with IABP and ACE inhibition is another means of limiting the extent of ventricular remodeling. Reduction in afterload and preload limits myocardial wall stress and subsequently infarct expansion and ventricular hypertrophy.

Left Ventricular Aneurysm and Thrombus Formation

Left ventricular aneurysm is a potential consequence of infarct expansion and remodeling. Aneurysm formation is associated with a greater risk of death, heart failure, angina, ventricular dysrhythmias, and embolization. Symptomatic patients may require temporary medical measures such as inotropic and afterload reducing agents, followed by surgical resection and/or endoventricular patching of the aneurysm, provided their remaining myocardial function is normal.

Mitral Valve Disruption

Papillary muscle ischemia can cause valve leaflet regurgitation or complete rupture, which accounts for 5% of deaths from MI (Massad & Geha, 2004). The posterior medial papillary muscle is affected more frequently because it receives blood supply only from the posterior descending artery (Figure 40–18 ■). Rupture can be complete, in which case rapid hemodynamic collapse ensues, or partial, with variable hemodynamic effects. Diagnosis of mitral valve disruption is made by two-dimensional echocardio-

FIGURE 40–18 ■ Structures supporting the valves.

Av

S

P

B
(M)

T

A

Atrioventricular valves:
Tricuspid
Bicuspid (Mitral)

Semilunar valves:
Pulmonic
Aortic

Chordae tendineae

Papillary muscle

graphy, cardiac catheterization, and ventriculography (Chapter 39 ☜). Afterload reduction with vasodilation therapy and IABP, preload reduction using nitrates and diuretics, and inotropic support may be necessary to stabilize the patient medically. Intermittent ischemic episodes may be treated with coronary artery bypass graft (CABG) surgery. Severe mitral valve disruption is treated with mitral valve repair or complete valve replacement. The diagnosis and treatment of valve disease is discussed in Chapter 41 ☜ .

Ventricular Free Wall Rupture

Often fatal, rupture of the myocardial wall can be a result of an acute tear or a slow, incomplete rupture. It occurs in 1% to 3% of AMI patients and accounts for 10% of deaths from MI (Massad & Geha, 2004). Administration of thrombolytic therapy and intravenous β-adrenergic blockers has been linked to a decreased incidence of myocardial rupture following MI. Surgical repair is the only definitive treatment.

Ventricular Septal Defect (VSD)

Rupture of the ventricular septum results in a left-to-right shunting of the blood with symptoms of chest pain, syncope, and hypotension. Medical treatment includes the use of diuretics, vasodilators, inotropic agents, and IABP aimed at decreasing the amount of blood shunted from left to right and increasing forward flow. Emergency surgical repair involves debridement of infarcted tissue and suture of a septal patch to healthy septal tissue. This is indicated in the presence of pulmonary edema and cardiogenic shock.

■ Nursing Management

Nurses caring for AMI patients need to understand when and how to intervene to decrease the workload of the heart by increasing oxygen supply and decreasing oxygen demand. Nursing management of patients admitted to an intensive care unit depends on

which method was used to reestablish coronary blood flow. Care of the patient following PCI is reviewed in Chapter 39 ☜ . For patients treated medically, care is aimed at reducing myocardial oxygen demand, monitoring for signs indicative of adequate myocardial oxygen supply, administering and titrating medications to balance demand and supply, monitoring for and managing complications, and patient teaching. Hemodynamic monitoring with a balloon-tipped pulmonary artery (PA) catheter and intra-arterial pressure line is warranted for patients presenting with severe or progressive heart failure or pulmonary edema, cardiogenic shock or progressive hypotension, suspected mechanical/structural complications, or who are treated with vasoactive agents that affect blood pressure and therefore require titration. Pulmonary artery catheters and arterial lines are discussed in Chapter 24 ☜ . Continuous cardiac monitoring in leads that will show ischemia or dysrhythmias is required. IABP therapy may be needed to reduce myocardial oxygen demand in the presence of heart failure, cardiogenic shock, or complications following an AMI. Serum tests such as complete blood count, chemistry panels, and coagulation profiles will be ordered to prevent complications and monitor response to treatments. Serial ECGs and serum cardiac markers are done to confirm the diagnosis of AMI and to determine the extent of infarction. Patients who have received thrombolytic therapy should be monitored for clinical signs of reperfusion including chest pain and ST segment elevation. Patients should be encouraged to inform the nurses of any new onset of chest pain or symptoms that were the same that occurred with the AMI. Anginal-type pain such as burning and pressure must be communicated between care providers. Commonly health care providers provide the nursing staff with "standing orders," which include contingency orders should certain complications such as a change in blood pressure or cardiac dysrhythmias occur. It is the nurse's responsibility to understand when to use these orders and how to assess the patient for effectiveness of the treatment.

 It is not uncommon with cardiac patients for the health care provider to give a series of contingency orders that are implemented for a given clinical manifestation. An example is nitroglycerin (NTG) and 12-lead ECG orders for the occurrence of chest pain. It is important that the nurse obtain the ECG prior to administering the NTG because the medication will cause the ST segment to return to normal, thus, losing important diagnostic information.

Patients are categorized as either high or low potential for complications, as well as either actual presence or absence of adverse sequelae. These categories determine the degree and duration of care and aggressiveness of the required treatment. For example, patients with no complications are low risk and can be fast-tracked within 24 to 48 hours to a lower level of care and discharged early. Patients with secondary complications and active comorbid diseases are at higher risk and will require longer hospital stays in areas with cardiac and hemodynamic monitoring capabilities.

No empiric data define the level of care the patient should receive once discharged from an area of intensive monitoring. Given that risk of sudden death is highest during the first 48 hours post-AMI and that intrahospital transfers can precipitate dysrhythmias, continuous cardiac monitoring for the first 48 hours of hospital stay and/or first 24 hours post–intensive care unit discharge is warranted. Other care needs required during convalescence on a step-down, telemetry, or intermediate unit for the AMI patient are the same as outlined for patients with unstable angina, with the exception of added attention to monitoring patient response to progressive activity.

The assessment data, which include sample questions specific to ACS, are found in the Nursing Process: Patient Care Plan for Acute Coronary Syndrome feature. Nursing diagnoses are developed from the assessment data and follow the assessment in the first column of the Nursing Process/Nursing Care Plan feature. This care plan applies the nursing process to the relevant nursing diagnoses and provides a comprehensive care plan for a patient with ACS in the acute period.

NURSING PROCESS: Patient Care Plan for Acute Coronary Syndrome

Assessment of Activity Tolerance

Subjective Data:
Are you able to complete your activities of daily living without fatigue?
Are you able to walk up a flight of stairs without getting short of breath?
Do you exercise on a regular basis?

Objective Data:
Monitor vital signs before and after walking in hall.
Assess heart sounds.
Monitor vital signs after completion of activities of daily living (ADLs).

Nursing Assessment and Diagnoses	Outcome and Evaluation Parameters	Planning and Interventions with *Rationales*
Nursing Diagnosis: *Activity Intolerance* related to insufficient oxygenation secondary to decreased cardiac output	**Outcomes:** Patient enrolls in cardiac rehabilitation program and attends post-MI lectures. *Evaluation Parameters:* Patient uses exercise log to record distances walked and symptoms experienced. Patient is able to monitor vital signs and adjust activity accordingly.	**Interventions and *Rationale:*** Encourage participation in cardiac rehabilitation program. Teach patient to use exercise log to monitor distances walked and symptoms. Teach patient how to monitor heart rate, blood pressure, and respirations as response to activity. *To increase endurance and strength and prevent weight gain.*

Assessment of Cardiac Output

Subjective Data:
Do you ever feel your heart beat fast, beat irregularly, or skip beats?
Do you ever feel light-headed?
Do you get short of breath when you walk distances?

Objective Data:
Assess heart rate and rhythm for abnormalities.
Monitor medications given and evaluate their response, especially those given for tachy/bradydysrhythmias.
Monitor blood pressure and respirations.

Nursing Assessment and Diagnoses	Outcome and Evaluation Parameters	Planning and Interventions with *Rationales*
Nursing Diagnosis: *Decreased Cardiac Output* related to dysrhythmias secondary to acute myocardial ischemia and infarction	**Outcomes:** Patient maintains normal and regular heart rate and rhythm. Patient verbalizes less fear and anxiety. *Evaluation Parameters:* Vital signs within normal limits. Exercise endurance increases. No anginal-type chest pain. Cardiac output within normal limits. No clinical manifestations of heart failure. Alert and oriented. Lungs clear.	**Interventions and *Rationales:*** Administer and teach antiarrhythmic medications, as ordered by health care provider *to ensure proper dosages and time intervals.* Provide comfort measures to patient and assurance *to decrease fear and anxiety.*

Assessment of Patient Ability to Cope

Subjective Data:
How are you feeling about your heart attack?
What are your thoughts about your future health?

Objective Data:
Evaluate patient response to written and verbal teaching materials about the patient's heart attack.
Evaluate patient response to discussion about current and future health concerns.

Nursing Assessment and Diagnoses	Outcome and Evaluation Parameters	Planning and Interventions with *Rationales*
Nursing Diagnosis: *Ineffective Coping* secondary to denial related to decreased physical status after myocardial infarction	**Outcome:** Patient verbalizes a decrease in problems and concerns. *Evaluation Parameters:* Vital signs within normal limits. Denies apprehension. Able to state an understanding of disease process.	**Interventions and *Rationale:*** Determine degree of denial; do not directly confront patient's denial; support patient's behavior. Provide active listening *to ensure patient you are working with her, not against her.*

NURSING PROCESS: Patient Care Plan for Acute Coronary Syndrome—*Continued*

Assessment of Pain
Subjective Data:

Do you have chest pain?

Does your jaw hurt or throat hurt?

Does it radiate anywhere on your body?

Does it go away with a deep breath?

What makes the pain better or worse?

Objective Data:

Use pain scale (0–10) to quantify pain level.

Assess cultural or religious impact on the patient's response.

Assess location, duration, and onset of pain.

Nursing Assessment and Diagnoses	Outcome and Evaluation Parameters	Planning and Interventions with *Rationales*
Nursing Diagnosis: *Acute Pain* related to cardiac ischemia	**Outcome:** Pain free or controlled with medication. ***Evaluation Parameters:*** Patient notifies nurse immediately on experiencing pain. Patient's ECG is normal and pain is relieved with sublingual NTG. Patient is able to verbalize how to take sublingual NTG and its side effects.	**Interventions and *Rationale:*** Instruct patient to notify nurse immediately of chest pain. Implement health care provider's orders; i.e., ECG, sublingual NTG, morphine, oxygen. Teach patient about how to take sublingual nitroglycerin and its side effects. *This encourages the patient to participate in his own care and teaches one of the most important interventions for patients with CAD.*

Assessment of Fluid Status
Subjective Data:

Are you short of breath?

Do you monitor your weight?

Do you eat a lot of salt?

Objective Data:

Assess lung sounds for rales or crackles.

Monitor blood pressure, jugular venous distension (JVD), vital signs, urine output, daily weight, and peripheral edema.

Nursing Assessment and Diagnoses	Outcome and Evaluation Parameters	Planning and Interventions with *Rationales*
Nursing Diagnosis: *Excess Fluid Volume* related to fluid retention secondary to impaired myocardial contractility	**Outcomes:** Patient's body weight is within normal range; electrolytes will be maintained in normal range. ***Evaluation Parameters:*** Weight. Electrolyte values daily until stable. Lungs clear. No peripheral edema. Neck vein distention not present. Cardiac index and ejection fraction with normal limits.	**Interventions and *Rationales:*** Administer diuretics as ordered and teach patient rationale and side effects of medication. Weigh patient daily and stress to patient the importance of daily weights. Instruct patient to notify health care provider with greater than 2–3 pound gain. *This will allow the patient to identify weight gain from fluid.* Fluid restriction and low-sodium diet as ordered in order *to decrease excess fluid accumulation.*

Assess Patient/Family Knowledge of Disease and Treatment
Subjective Data:

Tell me what you know about your problems with your heart.

Tell me what you are doing about your risk factors.

Tell me about your dietary intake and your exercise program.

When do you develop chest pain and what makes it go away?

What medications are you on, when are you supposed to take them, and what are the side effects you should watch for?

When are you supposed to see your doctor?

Are you participating in a cardiac rehabilitation program?

Objective Data:

Patient/family may be anxious, confused, and need repeated information.

Mistakes being made with treatment plan.

Self-care deficit.

Nursing Assessment and Diagnoses	Outcome and Evaluation Parameters	Planning and Interventions with *Rationales*
Nursing Diagnosis: *Deficient Knowledge* related to disease and treatment plan	**Outcome:** Patient/family have an understanding of and comply with treatment plan. ***Evaluation Parameters:*** Patient and family understand treatment plan and safely become compliant. Patient and family understand the importance of risk factor control in preventing a progression of the disease. Patient and family participate in a cardiac rehabilitation program.	**Interventions and *Rationales:*** Describe the required diet, medications, activity, and limitations *to increase knowledge of disease and treatment.* Describe what clinical manifestations need to be reported to the health care provider and when to access the emergency medical system *to ensure immediate care when necessary.* Have patient/family repeat instructions *to assess understanding.* Provide information about the type, setting, and cost of a cardiac rehabilitation program, and assist with contacting the program *to decrease anxiety about the process.*

Sources: Wilkinson, J. M., & Ahearn, N. R. (2009). *Prentice Hall Nursing Diagnosis Handbook,* 9/E. Upper Saddle River, NJ: Prentice Hall.

Documentation of patient conditions is essential in order to assess normal progress following an AMI. Many institutions have developed a collaborative pathway as a mechanism for assessing this progress. The National Guidelines for an ACS Collaborative Pathway box includes an example of this pathway.

▪ Collaborative Management

Patients who have experienced an acute myocardial infarction often recover best when a multidisciplinary approach is put into place. These patients benefit from several subspecialties such as physical therapy, respiratory therapy, dieticians, social workers, and of course the cardiologist and nurse. If a patient has suffered a large myocardial infarction he can spend several days to a few weeks in the hospital. When this happens the patient becomes weak from being in bed for such a long period of time as well as because his heart is not able to function at its previous level. Physical therapists can help bridge this gap and get the patient ambulating and performing activities of daily living before discharge so

that he may function at home. Furthermore, they can help transition the patient into a cardiac rehabilitation program. Associated with prolonged bed rest comes the high risk of developing a respiratory infection. The respiratory therapist plays a key role in daily pulmonary toileting to prevent any nosocomial respiratory infections in these patients. The dietician focuses on proper in-hospital nutritional support as well as preparing the patient for dietary changes at home. The dietician emphasizes the need for a cardiac diet that is low in fat, cholesterol, and sodium intake. The social worker and discharge planner cannot go unnoticed in this collaborative approach. Oftentimes the myocardial infarction patient has a type A behavior pattern, is in denial, and is suffering from depression. Although the cardiologist can order some pharmacologic intervention, it is the social worker who can work best with these patients to help them understand their situation and learn effective coping mechanisms. They can assist these patients with behavior modification. The constant and consistent care provided by the nurse is the main link to these other disciplines. Only the nurse can provide an ongoing assessment of the patient

---

NATIONAL GUIDELINES for a portion of an ACS Collaborative Pathway

Acute Coronary Syndrome Collaborative Pathway

Collaborative Care Path Guidelines

Acute Coronary Syndrome
The **Collaborative Pathway** is part of the patient's medical record. For this reason, the physician, Registered Nurse, and other health-care professionals must collaborate together to insure that this Pathway is appropriately implemented. Utilizing the collaborative pathway supports the multi-disciplinary approach to patient care.

Upon admission, the RN will assess if the patient meets the criteria to be placed on this Pathway:

In general, any patient admitted with chest pain of unknown origin should be placed on the pathway.

Eligible Patients: *Chest pain of suspected cardiac origin, Angina Pectoris, Prinzmetal Angina, Unstable Angina/Rule-Out MI, MI.*

1. The RN is responsible to initiate the pathway and notify appropriate team members who will be involved in implementing patient care

2. The RN should collaborate with the admitting physician(s) regarding the patient's plan of care. This should be based on the pathway's standard of care while taking into consideration individualized patient care

3. It is the responsibility of the RN caring for the patient on each shift to:
   a. Review and document the progress of nursing and medical care as it occurs
   b. Review the pathway and evaluate whether the patient has met the expected outcomes
   c. Check off completion of care at the end of each day on the collaborative pathway
   d. Complete the "educational assessment" and "educational record" sections of the pathway
   e. Sign and date each page of the pathway
   f. Report to the upcoming shift the progress of the patient on the pathway, identify areas of concern, and outcomes that have not been met

4. It is the responsibility of the RN caring for the patient to document a Nursing Note on the Patient's progress on the pathway. A focus note is required if any pathway activity/outcomes are not met for any given day of the pathway.

Educational Record
Method of Teaching (MOT) Response (R)

AV – Audio-Visual V – Verbal 1 – Verbalizes/Indicates Understanding
2 – Further Instructions Needed

W – Written I – Interpreter 3 – Demonstrates Task 4 – Unable to Comprehend

D – Demonstration 5 – Refuses any information on Topic 6 – Other (see focus note for comments)

Teaching Topic Date Initials MOT Response Date Initials MOT Response

Explain Rationale For Admit to Hospital

Explain Reason for Tests and Procedures

Explain Chest Pain Scale of 1–10

Discuss Symptoms of Ischemia to Report to Nurse

Explain Collaborative Pathway

Provide Applicable Education Packet (Angina or MI)

Define ACS and Explain Causes
View AHA educational videos for condition
Discuss risk factors for CAD
Discuss feelings pt./significant other experiencing
Provide applicable printed information on discharge medications
Review DC instructions: Activity level, clinic appt., prescriptions and symptoms to report
Initials Signature Print Name Initials Signature Print Name
Patient Addressograph

Source: University of California, Davis Medical Center.

COMPLEMENTARY & ALTERNATIVE THERAPIES   Music Therapy

Description:

The prevention and psychosocial influences of cardiovascular diseases have been a focus for many in behavioral medicine, psychology, and nursing for the past 30 years. Music therapy is one method that provides a viable collaborative and complementary method to reduce risks for, and motivate rehabilitation from, cardiac events. During music therapy, the patient listens to music using headphones during hospitalization. Cardiac units should stock headphones, CD or other types of players, and a wide selection of musical CDs to fit patient preference, such as country-western, rock and roll, and classical. Prior to discharge, patients can be encouraged to continue listening to their music of choice at home during the recovery period.

Research Support:

Studies have shown that music modulates heart health measurements such as heart rate and blood pressure, enhances exercise programs, and relieves stress symptoms. In one study, a music therapy survey was administered to determine patients' current use and preference for music. The patients, who were in a cardiac rehabilitation program in a large city hospital, completed a survey on which they rated their level of use of music for exercise, relaxation, and enjoyment. The survey also gathered information on patients' musical preferences, musical experiences, and pertinent demographics. The patients, who were mostly white males over the age of 60, had positive, pleasurable responses to the aesthetic aspects of music. The researchers concluded that the use of music therapy in a cardiac rehabilitation program is warranted (Metzger, 2004).

A German study involved 15 patients in a coronary sport unit who listened to relaxation music while performing exercises adapted to their heart frequency. The patients' blood pressures were measured and their beta-endorphin blood levels were determined before the exercises and after listening to music. At the same time as having their blood samples collected, the participants had to perform two psychometric tests: Levenstein's perceived stress experience questionnaire (PSQ) to measure the graduation of subjective perceived stress and Spielberger's state-anxiety inquiry (STAI) as an indicator of coping. This protocol was performed 1 week prior to the mean trial, but the patients did not listen to music and had no blood collections or blood pressure measurements. There were no significant changes in PSQ-data in the test trial without music. However, in the mean trial (in which the participants listened to music), values in the section "worries" decreased. In addition, the STAI values were significantly lower, which indicates reduced anxiety after listening to music. Other results showed that beta-endorphin concentration and systolic blood pressure decreased significantly after participants listened to music. Researchers concluded that patients benefit from lower levels of worry and anxiety after music therapy (Vollert, Stork, Rose, & Mockel, 2003).

In patients having surgical procedures, music therapy has also been shown to reduce pain, anxiety, and physiological parameters. One study compared the effects of music therapy versus a quiet, uninterrupted rest period on pain intensity, anxiety, physiological parameters, and opioid consumption after cardiac surgery. Two randomized groups in a sample of 86 patients received either 20 minutes of music (intervention), or 20 minutes of rest in bed (control). The group that received music experienced a significant reduction in anxiety and pain as compared to the control group. However, there was no difference in systolic blood pressure, diastolic blood pressure, heart rate, nor a reduction in opioid usage in the two groups. (Sendelbach, Halm, Doran, Miller, & Gaillard, 2006).

References

Metzger, L. K. (2004). Assessment of use of music by patients participating in cardiac rehabilitation. *Journal of Music Therapy, 41*(1), 55–69.

Sendelbach, S. E., Halm, M. A., Doran, K. A., Miller, E. H., & Gaillard, P. (2006). Effects of music therapy on physiological and psychological outcomes for patients undergoing cardiac surgery. *Journal of Cardiovascular Nursing, 21*(3), 194–200.

Vollert, J. O., Stork, T., Rose, M., & Mockel, M. (2003). Music as adjuvant therapy for coronary heart disease. Therapeutic music lowers anxiety, stress and beta-endorphin concentrations in patients from a coronary sport group. *Deutsche Medizinische Wochenschrift, 128*(51–52), 2712–2716.

---

and the patient's response to these interventions. It is important that the nurses recognize they are the link and help collaborate all of these services, which will provide excellent patient care.

Health Promotion and Discharge Planning

The term *time is muscle* cannot be stressed enough in the care of the myocardial infarction patient. It is well known that the faster the infarct-related artery is opened, the more myocardium is salvaged. One reason early reperfusion is not established is because patients do not come into the hospital fast enough. The nurse is in a unique position to help with early treatment in a number of ways. First, nurses can collaborate with the community and establish educational programs that bring community awareness around the subject of timely treatment. Included in this is early recognition of symptoms and prompt initiation of emergency medical services. Nurses also can participate by teaching cardiopulmonary resuscitation so that, when an individual is suffering a heart attack, measures are being taken to ensure survival. A perfect place to offer these educational programs is in retirement communities because advanced age alone is a risk factor.

Once the patient enters the hospital system, the nurse again plays a key role in ensuring timely treatment. She can advocate on behalf of her patient to the health care provider. The nurse's physical assessment, as well as her interpretation of the ECG and laboratory tests, is vital in deciding the appropriate reperfusion strategy for these patients. Once the patient is discharged, again it is the nurse who plays a vital role in educating the patient and family in their recovery process. It is often the cardiac rehabilitation nurse who walks patients through lifestyle changes, behavior modification, and an exercise program to promote a full recovery. The nurse in this role teaches classes to small groups to educate them on topics such as nutrition, exercise, stress reduction, and even some new alternative therapies such as yoga, herbal medicines, and even acupuncture. It is important to include the family or another support system the patient has in this process so that others also can support optimal recovery. The Patient Teaching & Discharge Priorities box (p. 1208) presents the discharge needs for patients who have experienced a cardiac event.

■ Gerontological Considerations

The elderly population makes up the fastest growing portion of the American population. By the time a person reaches age 65, his heart has accomplished an amazing amount of work. To be specific the "adult heart beats more than 100,000 times a day,

PATIENT TEACHING & DISCHARGE PRIORITIES for Coronary Artery Disease/Acute Coronary Syndrome

Need	Teaching
Knowledge of disease process and prognosis	Written and verbal instructions for: • Specific diagnosis/treatment; i.e., angioplasty, stent, heart attack, congestive heart failure, CAD • Follow-up labs, test, health care provider appointment • Medications • Diet • Activity. These instructions will reinforce the need to comply with therapy.
Understanding of medications	The patient and family are taught what the purposes of the medications are, their side effects, and their timing. These instructions will reinforce medication compliance and prevent over- or underdosing.
Safety	Stress the importance of wearing an identification bracelet to identify a heart problem to health care workers. Carry stent identification card in wallet to identify implant information to health care workers.
Disease prevention	Teach about dietary consumption. Stress the importance of a low-fat, low-cholesterol, low-salt diet. Teach about an exercise program. Stress the importance of exercise to prevent further CAD and keep current CAD from progressing. Offer cardiac rehabilitation program resources. Teach about behavior modification; decrease stress environment. Stress importance of smoking cessation and offer resources for community programs.
Reportable clinical manifestations	Teach to report chest pain or anginal equivalent. Stress how to take sublingual nitroglycerin should patient experience angina. Stress importance of using 911 emergency response system instead of driving self to emergency department (ED). Teach about fatigue and shortness of breath, as they too may be indicators of an unstable plaque or valve problem exacerbating. Teach about dental prophylaxis if patient was diagnosed with valve problem or had invasive coronary procedure.
Family/support system	Assess availability, knowledge, and compliance with treatment regimen. Assess discharge needs; i.e., home placement, medications, driving. Involve discharge planning if specific needs are not met to offer community resources.
Emotional adjustment of patient/family	Answer questions honestly. Encourage verbalization of frustrations and anger. Encourage positive reinforcement from the family. Provide active listening. Provide additional hospital and community resources, as necessary.

pumping roughly 2,000 gallons of blood through 60,000 miles of blood vessels every 24 hours" (Young, 1992). As one ages, one's heart undergoes physiological changes. These changes include stiffer ventricles due to the lack of the ability for the muscle to relax completely, decreased pumping function, decreased response to adrenaline, and decreased elasticity of the arteries. These changes can occur even in the absence of CAD but can be magnified in the presence of CAD.

CAD is the leading cause of death in the elderly. In fact, over half the people who suffer a heart attack are over age 65 (Young, 1992). Although men usually have a higher rate of CAD as compared to women during most of their lifetime, women have an equal, if not higher, rate after menopause. This may be due to the decrease in estrogen production. When one experiences a heart attack as an older individual, it may result in more complications and a longer hospital stay. Recovery is slower and presents many challenges. It may involve multiple systems in the body beyond just the cardiovascular system. This is often seen in patients with diabetes. The elderly also have a higher incidence of heart failure

and rhythm disturbances as a result of CAD alone or in conjunction with an AMI. For this reason it is imperative that the patient is monitored via a cardiac monitor and nursing management is directed appropriately to these changes.

Silent heart attacks are not uncommon in the elderly. This is attributed to the decreased sensation of pain. This is especially true again in the diabetic population, where it can occur at any age but increases in the elderly population. Instead of the typical "I feel like an elephant is sitting on my chest" symptoms, these patients may experience atypical symptoms such as heartburn or gastrointestinal discomfort and shortness of breath. Older individuals grow accustomed to illness and discomfort and thus frequently will overlook these otherwise overt symptoms. It is especially important to educate not only the elderly about these symptoms but also those who help with their daily care. Simple knowledge of this may prevent untoward outcomes among the elderly population.

Treatment options for the elderly often present challenges. Different considerations are given to the elderly when deciding on treatment options. For example, a patient who presents with a myocardial infarction who might otherwise meet the criteria for thrombolytics may in fact not meet the criteria simply based on age. For example, a patient who is 75 years or older is at a higher risk for an intracranial hemorrhage than is a 50-year-old patient. The health care provider critically assesses the risk benefit ratio in this instance, and the patient may or may not receive fibrinolytic therapy. The 50-year-old patient usually would receive fibrinolytic therapy because this is not as great a concern among the nonelderly population. Another example that demonstrates the differences in treating the elderly is a patient who presents with a ventricular dysrhythmia that might be treated with prophylactic lidocaine. Lidocaine can cause confusion and other side effects in elderly patients, thus negating its use in this patient population.

The management of these patients may also be different because they may be willing to accept a decrease in their quality of life. They may choose to refuse further invasive testing such as coronary angiography or bypass surgery. Instead they may accept some degree of limitation and just be managed through medications.

Should patients choose a more invasive treatment strategy, they must be willing to accept longer hospitalizations and complicated recovery patterns. Elderly patients often have other medical problems besides CAD disease. They may have multiple cardiac problems as well that include hypertension, atherosclerosis, calcified valves, and rhythm disturbances. These patients may have a more complicated recovery from procedures or surgery due to renal impairment, mobility limitations, mental status changes, and poor nutrition. All of this must be considered when deciding the pathway of care for these patients.

Lifestyle changes must not go unrecognized in the elderly. Risk factor modification such as smoking cessation, weight reduction, and proper diet may have a dramatic impact on their quality of life. Age-appropriate measures to help promote a healthy lifestyle have been suggested by the American Heart Association (AHA, 2008a). Physical inactivity is a modifiable risk factor for developing coronary artery disease. Lack of exercise also contributes to obesity, high blood pressure, a low level of HDL ("good") cholesterol, and diabetes. Even modest levels of physical activity are beneficial. The AHA states that a moderate amount of physical activity, preferably daily, is recommended for older adults. Healthy moderate activity for older persons includes:

- Longer sessions of moderately intense activities such as walking or swimming
- Shorter sessions of more vigorous activities such as fast walking or stair-climbing.

■ Coronary Artery Bypass Graft Surgery

For more than three decades, coronary artery bypass grafting (CABG) has been a mainstay for the treatment of coronary artery disease. During this time period, great advancements have occurred in both technique and technology. However, the basic concept of providing the heart with alternative methods of circulation has remained the same.

Prior to the advent of percutaneous coronary intervention (PCI), CABG was the only method of revascularization that

showed success in alleviating symptoms, improving lifestyle, and improving mortality in select patient populations. PCI is discussed in detail in Chapter 39 ⊚ . Now that PCI is a widely accepted alternative, several research studies comparing the outcomes of CABG and PCI have helped develop an outline of which procedure is the most appropriate for different types of patients (Bypass Angioplasty Revascularization Investigation [BARI] 1996; Serruys et al., 2001). In short, the advantage of CABG is that it can provide more complete revascularization and show better long-term relief of symptoms. Less than 10% of patients who undergo CABG will need subsequent revascularization within 5 to 7 years (BARI, 1996). However, CABG patients also have more procedural-related pain, longer hospital stays, and more periprocedural myocardial infarctions (BARI, 1996). The final decision of CABG versus PCI is dependent on a number of factors and is important to review.

Indications

Patients who present with only mild symptoms of angina or who are even asymptomatic may benefit from CABG. However, there must be substantial evidence that CABG will prolong survival. In this scenario, a noninvasive test will show a very large area of myocardial ischemia. Despite the patient's being relatively asymptomatic, the test would suggest that the patient's anatomy is placing her at high risk. According to the American College of Cardiology (ACC) and the American Heart Association (AHA) guidelines for coronary artery bypass surgery, the following patients with mild or no symptoms are appropriate for CABG and are considered class 1 recommendations (Eagle et al., 2004):

- Significant left main coronary artery stenosis
- Left main equivalent: significant (greater than or equal to 70%) stenosis of the proximal left anterior descending artery (LAD) and proximal left circumflex artery
- Three-vessel disease. Survival benefit greater in patients with abnormal left ventricular function (less than 50%) or large areas of demonstrable myocardial ischemia.

Class 1 conditions are those for which there is evidence and/or general agreement that a given procedure or treatment is useful and effective. Patients with stable angina require a careful decision-making process as well. It is important that maximal medical therapy has been instituted and that risk factors have been addressed. The decision to proceed with surgery is driven by the likelihood that survival will be prolonged and symptoms will be relieved. It also is important to examine comorbidities. If a patient has diabetes or a reduced ejection fraction, a greater case can be made to proceed with surgery. According to the ACC/AHA guidelines, the following patients with stable angina are appropriate for CABG and are considered class 1 recommendations (Gibbons et al., 2002):

- Significant left main coronary artery stenosis
- Left main equivalent: significant (greater than or equal to 70%) stenosis of the proximal left anterior descending artery (LAD) and proximal left circumflex artery
- Three-vessel disease. Survival benefit greater in patients with abnormal left ventricular function (less than 50%)
- Two-vessel disease with significant proximal LAD stenosis and either left ventricular ejection fraction of less than 50% or demonstrable ischemia on noninvasive testing

- One- or two-vessel disease without significant proximal LAD stenosis but with a large area of viable myocardium and high-risk criteria on noninvasive testing
- Disabling angina despite maximal noninvasive therapy when surgery can be performed with acceptable risk.

The indications for CABG in a patient with unstable angina or non–ST segment elevation MI are similar to those in patients with stable angina. The critical factor that has to be considered with an unstable patient is the timing of the surgery. If a patient's symptoms are refractory and they are hemodynamically unstable, then revascularization should occur immediately. However, if a patient can be stabilized, there is some evidence that suggests a waiting period before performing surgery may improve outcomes. The following are class 1 recommendations for CABG by the ACC/AHA for unstable angina or non–ST segment elevation MI:

- Significant left main coronary artery stenosis
- Left main equivalent: significant (greater than or equal to 70%) stenosis of the proximal left anterior descending artery (LAD) and proximal left circumflex artery
- When percutaneous revascularization is not optimal or possible
- When ongoing ischemia not responsive to maximal nonsurgical therapy (Libby, Bonow, Zipes, & Mann, 2008).

The last group of patients would be those who are necessitating urgent intervention. Patients with ST elevation MI require immediate revascularization. These patients typically receive thrombolytics or undergo urgent PCI. In some cases PCI may fail or complications may occur. Performing surgery amid an acute MI greatly increases the risks of perioperative complications. Before the decision to undergo CABG is made, other acute therapies must be exhausted. The ACC considers the following to be class 1 recommendations for a patient with ST segment elevation MI to receive an urgent CABG:

- Failed angioplasty with persistent pain or hemodynamic instability in patients with coronary anatomy suitable for surgery
- Persistent or recurrent ischemia refractory to medical therapy in patients who have coronary anatomy suitable for surgery, who have a significant area of myocardium at risk, and who are not candidates for PCI
- If undertaking surgical repair of postinfarction ventricular septal rupture or mitral insufficiency
- Cardiogenic shock in patients less than 75 years old with ST segment elevation or left bundle branch block who develop shock within 36 hours of MI and are suitable for revascularization that can be performed within 18 hours of shock
- Life-threatening ventricular dysrhythmias in the presence of greater than or equal to 50% left main stenosis and/or triple vessel disease.

Standard Operative Techniques

Standard coronary artery bypass surgery is done via a median sternotomy using cardiopulmonary bypass (CPB), cold cardioplegia, and systemic hypothermia (28° to 32°C). CPB is a means to divert blood away from the heart and return it to the arterial system. The CPB machine temporarily performs the functions of the heart (circulation of blood) and lungs (gas exchange). This is accomplished by drainage of systemic venous blood directly to the CPB machine, usually via cannulation of the right atrium. The venous blood is then processed by the CPB machine. This entails a heat exchanger, which regulates the temperature of the blood; a filter, which does not permit air or atheroembolization to pass; and finally an oxygenator. Once the blood is oxygenated, it is then returned to the body via the arterial cannula, which usually is placed in the aorta. Further protection of the heart is achieved by cooling the heart with a cardioplegic solution. Infusions of cardioplegia allow surgeons to interrupt coronary flow safely for up to 20 minutes.

Once on CPB, anastomosis of the conduits will ensue (Figure 40–19 ■). The number of grafts usually varies from two to six. With the heart stopped, the surgeon can identify the obstructed artery and perform an arteriotomy to an area beyond the obstruction. An end-to-side anastomosis is then carried out with the chosen conduit. The proximal end of the graft is then anastomosed to the aorta using a similar technique.

Some surgeons perform coronary artery bypass without using CPB. This is generally referred to as beating heart bypass. Because CPB is not utilized, the heart remains beating. Mechanical stabilizers are placed on the area of the heart being bypassed to reduce motion. The advantage of this technique is the reduction of complications that can occur from CPB. The disadvantage is that the bypasses are more difficult to place accurately on a moving heart, which may lower the graft patency rate.

The left internal thoracic artery (ITA) is the preferred conduit as a graft to the LAD. The ITA (also commonly referred to as the IMA, or internal mammary artery) is the graft of choice due to its resistance to atherosclerosis and the ability to graft it as an *in situ* pedicle graft. This means that the artery remains connected proximally to the native subclavian artery. The 10-year patency rate for the ITA has been cited as 85% to 95% (Fitzgibbon et al., 1996; Goldman et al., 2004; Loop et al., 1986; Lytle et al., 1985). Because of the success of the ITA graft and its superiority over vein grafts, some surgeons are now performing bilaterally ITA grafting in nondiabetic patients. It is still too early to tell whether this will become common practice.

Vein grafts are typically the conduits used for the remaining bypasses. In most cases the greater saphenous vein is harvested from the leg. If the greater saphenous vein is not of good quality, the lesser saphenous vein and cephalic vein can be used. Up until just recently, a patient who required multiple bypasses would require an incision that extended over the entire length of the leg. A new technique wherein the vein is retrieved using an endoscope with one to three incisions is now being used in most large medical centers. The use of this technique has great advantages, including a decrease in incidence of leg wound infections and less pain.

Due to the success of ITA grafts, surgeons are exploring the use of other arteries as conduits. The most common arterial conduit other than the ITA is the radial artery. Before using the radial artery, Doppler studies must be done to assure adequate flow to the hand will resume with the radial artery gone. Unlike the ITA, the radial artery is used as a free graft. There is a greater incidence of spasm in radial artery grafts. The use of radial arteries has not replaced the use of vein grafts because most surgeons are waiting for more long-term data. Other arterial conduits that are being experimented with are the right gastroepiploic artery and the inferior epigastric artery. Use of these

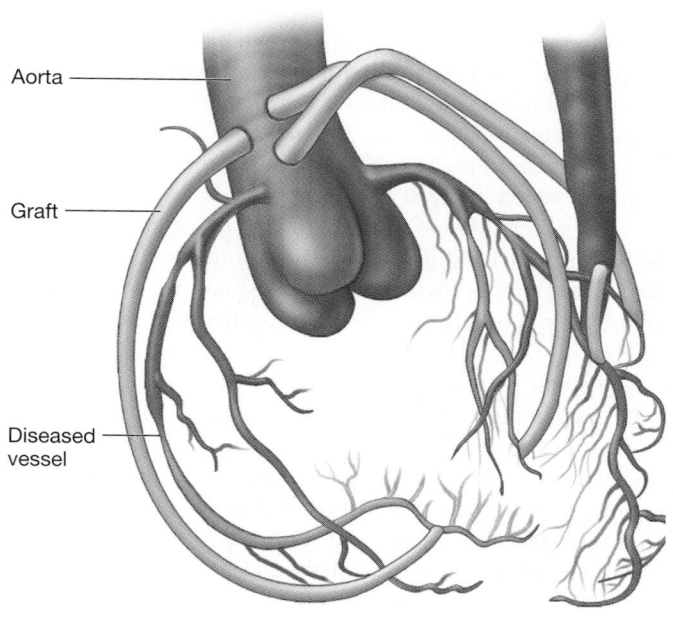

Arterial graft

Venous graft

Aorta

Graft

Diseased vessel

FIGURE 40–19 ■ Heart surgery grafts.

will require more research before determining whether they can be used as alternatives to vein grafts.

New Surgical Techniques

Advances in cardiac surgery have introduced new techniques. Although the use of these new techniques is not widespread, initial

results seem to be encouraging. Minimally invasive direct coronary artery bypass surgery (MIDCAB) was first done in Europe but quickly spread to the United States. MIDCAB is done via only a small left anterior thoracotomy incision. Using a thoracoscope and mechanical stabilizers, the left internal thoracic artery can be directly harvested and anastomosed. Similar to beating heart bypass, this procedure is done off CPB so the heart remains beating. Medications are used to the slow the heart and the stabilizers to reduce motion. The advantage of this approach may be that it will reduce recovery time and potential postoperative complications such as CPB-related complications and wound infections. As with beating heart bypass, the disadvantage is that the bypasses are more difficult to place accurately on a moving heart, which may lower the graft patency rate. This technique is also usually limited to only one or two types of bypasses.

The latest development in cardiac surgery is called port-access technique. This procedure combines a minimally invasive approach with an endovascular cardiopulmonary bypass–cardioplegic arrest system. This technique uses peripheral CPB via femoral vessels with an endaortic occlusion device. The heart can then be bypassed and stopped without opening the chest. This allows for more accurate anastomosis as well as use of multiple grafts. This technique has also been used on patients with mitral valve disease for valve repair or replacement.

Postoperative Considerations

The overall rate of mortality for CABG is between 1% and 3%, with the risk increasing according to the number of risk factors a patient may have (Society of Thoracic Surgeons, 2006). As with any surgical procedure, complications can occur. Chapter 27 ☞ includes an in-depth discussion of common postoperative complications. Serious complications include stroke, myocardial infarction, and bleeding. Stroke can be a devastating complication that greatly affects recovery. Stroke is usually caused by an embolus from the ascending aorta or aortic arch. Surgeons are now employing the use of intraoperative echo to help detect irregularities within the aorta and avoid them while cannulating or clamping the aorta. Other postoperative complications to consider after CABG include tamponade, renal failure, respiratory failure, dysrhythmias, wound infection, and both pericardial and pleural effusions.

A patient with a completely uncomplicated postoperative period can be discharged as soon as 4 days. Most patients, however, will leave the hospital within 5 to 7 days. Once home, patients will gradually increase their activity levels and should be able to resume regular activity after 6 to 12 weeks. The amount of time is individualized and is dependent on a patient's age and other health problems. Risk factor modification is imperative, and all patients should be counseled on diet, exercise, weight control, and smoking cessation. Patients with hypertension, diabetes, and hyperlipidemia need aggressive management of these conditions.

■ Nursing Management

Skilled postoperative nursing management for the CABG patient is crucial for a successful recovery and prevention of complications. In the immediate postoperative period, patients are typically taken directly from the operating room to a specialized intensive care unit (ICU) with nurses who are trained in postcardiac surgery care. Depending on the institution and the patient's condition, some patients are extubated (removal of endotracheal tube) prior to leaving the operating room (OR). On arrival to the ICU, it is imperative for the nurse to receive a report from the OR on the patient, which should include the following: a summary of the surgery performed, amount of time the patient was "on pump," any intravenous drips that are running, recent laboratory values including arterial blood gases (ABG), any problems that occurred in surgery, and any coexisting illnesses that are pertinent. Knowing the type of surgery performed and the amount of time a patient was on cardiopulmonary bypass (CPB) are crucial to a patient's care. Prolonged bypass induces cytokine activation and an inflammatory response that results in red cell damage and hemoglobinuria, thrombocytopenia, clotting abnormalities, reduced pulmonary gas exchange, and cerebrovascular accidents.

Nursing Diagnoses

1. Pain related to surgery
2. Deficient knowledge related to disease and surgery
3. Potential for ineffective tissue perfusion related to fluid balance
4. Infection potential related to altered skin integrity

Assessment

Nursing assessment includes close monitoring of the patient's hemodynamic status. Continuous monitoring of cardiac output, cardiac index, pulmonary artery pressure, central venous pressure, and arterial pressure are assessed at regular intervals. Chapter 24 ⊘ includes an in-depth discussion of these parameters. Close observation of the patient's heart rhythm, blood pressure, and oxygen saturation can detect new imbalances or hypoxia. Serum electrolytes and complete blood counts are assessed at regular intervals in order to intervene before complications occur. For example, an abnormal potassium or magnesium level can precipitate life-threatening cardiac dysrhythmias, and a low hemoglobin and hematocrit can decrease the oxygen-carrying capacity of the blood. Additionally, ventilator settings, chest tube drainage, and urine output are all assessed regularly.

Outcomes and Evaluation Parameters

Removal of the endotracheal tube (extubation) is an early outcome, and most hospitals will have protocols to wean the patient from ventilation as soon as possible. As a patient begins to wake up, it is important to prevent self-extubation and soft wrist restraints are usually required. Once a patient is extubated and hemodynamic parameters have remained stable, the next outcome is to get the patient weaned off all intravenous drips as tolerated and converted to oral medications. The patient's Swan-Ganz catheter is typically removed on postoperative day 1 if the patient is stable.

Neurological status is an essential evaluation parameter to establish, and once a patient begins to wake it is necessary to ask him to move each extremity and respond to simple questions. Early mobilization is important to reduce postoperative complications. It is standard for a patient to be out of bed and to a chair on post operative day 1 and transferred out of ICU if he is stable.

Planning and Interventions with Rationales

When the patient arrives to the ICU, laboratory work including chemistries, a complete blood count (CBC), arterial blood gases (ABGs), a chest x-ray, and an ECG should be done as soon as possible so a baseline can be established. Titration of intravenous drips will be employed to maintain adequate hemodynamic status such as cardiac output and blood pressure. Any abnormal change in a patient's status should be reported immediately to the surgeon. Depending on the institution and surgeon, a patient will have between 2 and 4 chest tubes. The chest tube output should be documented hourly. Any increase in output of greater than 100 milliliters per hour should be reported and serial CBCs should be done because postoperative bleeding most commonly occurs in the early postoperative period. Some patients will have temporary pacemaker wires placed, and a temporary pacemaker should be connected and tested to assure proper function (Chapter 36 ⊘). These will be removed later when it is established that the patient will not need them. It is common for patients to develop dysrhythmias such as atrial fibrillation on postoperative days 2 through 5. Should a patient develop a dysrhythmia, an ECG should be done and the surgeon is notified.

Once a patient is out of ICU, he should remain on a telemetry floor to continue monitoring of his heart rhythm. While on telemetry, aggressive mobilization and physical therapy must be a focus. Adequate pain control management is important to encourage ambulation as well as deep breathing and coughing. Common postoperative complications include pneumonia, deep vein thrombosis, and pulmonary embolism. Each of these complications can be minimized or prevented by ambulation and deep breathing exercises. As a patient's chest tube output begins to decrease, the chest tubes will be removed and the amount of pain a patient has will also decrease.

Close observation of wounds for any sign of infection should be performed each shift. Changes in wounds should be reported to the health care provider. Poor glucose control will greatly increase the risk of infection, so it is important to monitor glucose levels.

A patient with an uncomplicated postoperative course will usually go home on postoperative day 4 or 5. Discharge medications most always include aspirin, beta-adrenergic blockers, cholesterol-lowering medications, and ACE inhibitors, described earlier. Detailed discharge instructions include medication management, signs and symptoms of infection and bleeding, risk factor management, and progression of activity levels. These instructions can be the deciding factor of whether a patient will succeed as an outpatient and should be reviewed thoroughly with the patient and his family.

Health Promotion

Discussing risk factors and employing secondary prevention measures will reduce the number of patients who have recurrent events after CABG. Patients will usually take medications such as cholesterol drugs, aspirin, beta-blockers, and ACE inhibitors long term. Daily exercise and adequate weight control will help reduce the risk of further coronary disease. If a patient smokes, it is imperative to use every measure possible to encourage cessation. Patients with diabetes are at a higher risk for recurrent cardiac events and should be monitored for this closely. A patient should be instructed on the signs and symptoms of angina and advised to report changes promptly.

Most patients will require repetitive counseling to change risk factors that have taken a lifetime to develop. Therefore, frequent follow-up with their primary health care provider and cardiologist is important to review risk factors and to monitor blood pressure, blood sugar, and cholesterol levels.

■ Research

Research is essential to improve the care, quality of life, and survival of patients with coronary artery disease. The goal of research is to identify areas where practice could improve and evaluate and test methods for these improvements. The research topics related to CAD are included in the Research Opportunities and Clinical Impact box. The list provides both medical and nursing research topics still under investigation. Electronic databases are a source for finding specific studies related to these topics.

RESEARCH OPPORTUNITIES AND CLINICAL IMPACT RELATED TO CORONARY ARTERY DISEASE

Research Area	Clinical Impact
Stem cell injection after acute myocardial infarction.	Stimulate new growth of myocardial cells and increase myocardial viability.
Gene therapy for chronic CAD patients who have no other alternatives.	Stimulate angiogenesis, thereby decreasing symptoms and increasing quality of life.
Facilitated percutaneous intervention for acute myocardial infarction.	Conjoined mechanical and pharmacologic interventions for AMI will decrease mortality and increase myocardial salvage.
Establish heart-healthy food supplements.	Decrease hyperlipidemia, thereby providing risk factor modification for some predisposed risk factors.
Identify predictors of vulnerable plaque and their impact.	Provide ability to manage plaque and prevent plaque rupture, thus future coronary events.
Establish standard of providing fibrinolytic therapy in the field.	Increase survival for acute myocardial infarction patient.
Effect of community awareness programs on patients with ACS emphasizing early symptom recognition and treatment.	Decrease adverse cardiovascular events and increase survival from out-of-hospital events.
Effect of immediately triaging women with ACS-like symptoms to chest pain unit.	Increase survival in the female population and bring awareness because their symptoms are often missed.
Behavior modification techniques and their effect on CAD and its events.	Lower all modifiable risk factors, thereby decreasing cardiovascular events in a high-risk population.
Effect on established grammar and high school education program teaching about CAD; i.e., signs and symptoms, treatments, outcomes.	Establish an aware and healthier population early on, thereby decreasing total cardiovascular events.

Clinical Preparation

CRITICAL THINKING

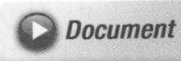 Read

- History of Current Illness
- Past Medical History
- Physical Exam
- Admitting Medical Orders
- Laboratory Study Results

 Document

- Summary of Hospitalization
- Pathophysiology Form
- Laboratory Values
- Laboratory Results Explanation

▶ Apply

- List of Potential Nursing Diagnoses
- Concept Map
- Critical Thinking Questions

Log on to MyNursingKit.com to download forms you will need and to complete further steps in the Clinical Preparation assignment.

HISTORY OF PRESENT ILLNESS

You are a nurse in the coronary care unit (CCU) and have been notified that you will be receiving a patient from the cardiac catheterization lab with the diagnosis of ST segment elevation myocardial infarction (STEMI). You receive the following report from the nurse in the catheterization lab: Mr. Ray is a 43-year-old male with a history of hypertension, hypercholesterolemia, gastroesophageal reflux disease (GERD), and hepatitis C. He developed substernal chest pain while doing some yard work at approximately 1 p.m. today. His pain radiated to his left arm and was accompanied by shortness of breath, nausea, and vomiting. He rated his pain as a 10/10 in severity. He presented to the emergency department, and his first electrocardiogram

(ECG) showed ST elevation in the anterolateral leads. He was initially treated with aspirin, nitro paste, morphine, and intravenous heparin. He was then emergently taken to the cardiac catheterization lab.

His cardiac catheterization showed a 100% thrombotic occlusion of his proximal left anterior descending artery. A drug eluting stent was placed, and the patient was placed on a ReoPro infusion.

On arrival to the CCU, the patient is awake and alert and denies any chest pain or shortness of breath. The patient denies any previous cardiac history. He is a pleasant man who appears in no acute distress.

Medical/Surgical History
No known allergies
Medications: none
Hypertension
GERD
Hepatitis C
Surgeries: knee and hip had "pins" placed

Social History
Family history: no premature heart disease; parents both alive and in good health
Last used tobacco 20 years ago and denies any ethanol use. He did use intravenous drugs approximately 15 years ago. He is employed as a landscaper.

Physical Exam
Temp: 97.6 BP 120/83 HR 80 RR: 14
Young Caucasian man with multiple tattoos, in no apparent distress
HEENT: scleras anicteric, oropharynx clear
Neck: supple, no lymphadenopathy
Lungs: clear to auscultation bilaterally
Cardiovascular: JVP not elevated; normal S_1 and S_2; regular rate and rhythm, no significant murmur, rub, or gallop; carotids 2+ without bruits
Abdomen: soft, nontender, nondistended, normoactive bowel sounds

Extremities: no edema
Neurological: normal, alert, and oriented × 3
CXR: normal
ECG: see history of present illness

Admitting Medical Orders
Admit to cardiology, coronary care unit
Condition guarded
Admitting diagnosis: acute coronary syndrome
Diagnosis: acute anterolateral STEMI
Vital signs and oxygen saturation q1h
Bed rest
Call house officer: pulse < 60 and > 100/minute; BP < 90 and > 160 systolic; temperature > 38.5; urine output < 30 mL/hr for 2 hours; respiratory rate > 30/minute; oxygen saturation < 92%
Sequential compression devices (SCD) to lower extremities
Diet: cardiac
Daily weight
Continuous cardiac monitor
Strict in/out
Foley to gravity
Oxygen per nasal cannula to maintain oxygen sat > 92%
IV: D5½NS @ 50 mL/hr

Scheduled Medications

ASA 325 mg po daily
Pantoprazole 40 mg po daily
Metoprolol 25 mg po bid
Lisinopril 20 mg po daily
Plavix 75 mg po daily
ReoPro gtt @ 0.125 mcg/kg/min for 12 hours
Lipitor 20 mg po daily

PRN Medications

Morphine 3–5 mg IV q3–5min, max 15 mg q3h prn pain
Temazepam 15–30 mg po qhs prn insomnia
Droperidol 1.25–2.5mg IV q6h prn nausea

Ordered Laboratory Studies

Troponin I q8h × 3
CPK–MB q8h × 3
Basic chemistry panel q a.m.
CBC q a.m.
Magnesium q a.m.
Lipid panel in a.m.

Ordered Diagnostic Studies

ECG q a.m.
Echocardiogram in a.m.

LABORATORY STUDY RESULTS

Test	Day 1	Day 2	Day 3
Sodium	135 mEq/L	136 mEq/L	137 mEq/L
Potassium	4.1 mEq/L	4.0 mEq/L	4.0 mEq/L
Chloride	103 mEq/L	104 mEq/L	103 mEq/L
Carbon dioxide (CO_2)	26 mEq/L	25 mEq/L	25 mEq/L
Blood urea nitrogen (BUN)	16 mg/dL	15 mg/dL	14 mg/dL
Creatinine	1.2 mg/dL	1.3 mg/dL	1.2 mg/dL
Glucose	85 mg/dL	96 mg/dL	89 mg/dL
Phosphorus	2.2 mg/dL	3.4 mg/dL	3.8 mg/dL
Calcium	9.1 mg/dL	8.7 mg/dL	9.1 mg/dL
Albumin	3.7 g/dL	3.7 g/dL	3.5 g/dL
Alkaline phosphorus	70 units/L	76 units/L	77 units/L
Aspartate aminotransferase	70 units/L	76 units/L	77 units/L
Bilirubin	1.8 mg/dL	1.4 mg/dL	1.2 mg/dL
Alanine phosphatase (ALT)	87 units/L	67 units/L	54 units/L
Magnesium	2.0 mEq/L	1.9 mEq/L	1.9 mEq/L
Creatine kinase	4368 units/L	2812 units/L	2000 units/L
Relative index	>6.9%	>10.7%	>9.4%
CK-MB	>300.00%	>300.00%	259.7%
Troponin I	>100 ng/mL	82.86 ng/mL	52.00 ng/mL
WBC	11.5/mm³	10.9/mm³	9.3/mm³
RBC	4.89/mm³	5.09/mm³	4.92/mm³
Hemoglobin	15.9 g/dL	16.5 g/dL	15.9 g/dL
Hematocrit	45.5%	47.8%	45.6%
Platelets	295/mm³	256/mm³	300/mm³
Cholesterol	280 mg/dL		
High-density lipoproteins (HDL)	22 mg/dL		
Low-density lipoproteins (LDL)	198 mg/dL		
Very low-density lipoproteins (VLDL)	68%		
Apolipoproteins	162 mg/dL		
Triglycerides	210 mg/dL		

CRITICAL THINKING QUESTIONS

1. What is the purpose of Plavix for this patient?

2. Why were cardiac markers ordered?

3. What is the purpose of ReoPro in this patient?

4. When reviewing the ECG, what leads can you expect to be elevated with an acute anterolateral MI?

5. If the patient complains of chest pain that mimics the pain that he had before during the next couple of days, what steps would you take and anticipate?

Answers to Critical Thinking Questions appear in Appendix D.

NCLEX® REVIEW

1. Which of the following information reported by a patient indicates a non-modifiable risk to develop coronary heart disease?
   1. "I am trying to quit smoking, but it is difficult."
   2. "My blood sugars sometimes run a little high."
   3. "I walk at least one mile every day."
   4. "My father died of a heart attack at age 70."

2. A patient reports a history of having substernal chest pain. To help establish a diagnosis of stable angina, the nurse should ask which question.
   1. "Does your pain last for at least 15 minutes?"
   2. "Did your pain occur at rest?"
   3. "Was your pain precipitated by activity?"
   4. "Does your pain always radiate to the jaw?"

3. A patient seen in the clinic reports having episodes of left arm pain and chest tightness that started after having an argument. The nurse concludes the pain was most likely typical angina pain when the client also reports:
   1. The pain was relieved by taking nitroglycerin.
   2. Having just eaten a large meal prior to having the pain.
   3. Feeling very anxious when having the pain.
   4. Experiencing weakness and dizziness.

4. Because the electrocardiogram, ECG, of a patient admitted with acute coronary syndrome shows ST segment elevations, the nurse recognizes the patient has experienced:
   1. Mild cardiac ischemia.
   2. A myocardial infarction in the past.
   3. Subendocardial injury.
   4. Transmural ischemia.

5. A patient admitted with complaints of epigastric pain is evaluated for a myocardial infarction. Blood markers are negative but the electrocardiogram, ECG, shows deep Q wave changes without ST segment elevation. The nurse recognizes these changes indicate:
   1. Occurrence of an old myocardial infarction.
   2. Very recent myocardial ischemia.
   3. Pacemaker dysfunction.
   4. Ventricular hypertrophy.

6. The nurse concludes a patient has most likely experienced a myocardial infarction, MI, when blood work drawn four days following an episode of substernal pain with shortness of breath shows elevation of:
   1. Troponin I levels.
   2. Myoglobin levels.
   3. C-reactive protein.
   4. CK-MB.

7. A patient with severe three vessel disease experiences myocardial infarction, MI, causing occlusion to the left ventricle. The nurse places high priority on monitoring for sign of:
   1. Pericarditis.
   2. Cardiogenic shock.
   3. Dressler's Syndrome.
   4. Premature ventricular contractions.

8. The nurse recognizes a patient who is currently asymptomatic for cardiac ischemia may benefit from having coronary artery bypass graft, CABG, surgery since the patient has:
   1. A 50% occlusion of the circumflex artery.
   2. Been hospitalized with angina three times in the past year.
   3. Significant stenosis of the left anterior descending, LAD, and circumflex artery.
   4. A history of heart failure following a myocardial infarction a year ago.

9. Chest tube drainage output measures 200 mL in one hour in a patient recovering from a CABG. Which action should be taken by the nurse initially?
   1. Continue to monitor hourly outputs.
   2. Have the patient do cough and deep breathing exercises.
   3. Check the chest tube dressing for drainage.
   4. Report the findings to the primary care provider.

Answers for review questions appear in Appendix D

KEY TERMS

acute coronary syndrome (ACS) *p.1162*
akinesia *p.1187*
angina pectoris *p.1175*
arteriosclerosis *p.1159*
atherosclerosis *p.1159*
atheroma *p.1160*
cardiac risk factors *p.1164*
cholesterol *p.1165*
concentric *p.1162*
coronary artery disease (CAD) *p.1159*
creatine kinase (CK) *p.1184*
dyskinesia *p.1187*
eccentric *p.1162*
fibrous cap *p.1161*

high density lipoprotein *p.1167*
hypercholesterolemia *p.1165*
hyperlipidemia *p.1165*
hypokinesia *p.1187*
ischemia *p.1160*
low density lipoproteins *p.1166*
metabolic syndrome *p.1172*
MONA *p.1187*
myocardial hibernation *p.1164*
myocardial infarction (MI) *p.1181*
myocardial stunning *p.1164*
myoglobin *p.1184*
NSTEMI *p.1181*
oncosis *p.1164*

STEMI *p.1181*
sudden cardiac death (SCD) *p.1183*
thrombus *p.1162*
triglycerides *p.1167*
troponin *p.1184*
troponin I *p.1184*
troponin T *p.1184*
tunica adventitia *p.1159*
tunica intima *p.1158*
tunica media *p.1159*
unstable angina *p.1181*
variant, Prinzmetal, or vasospastic
   angina *p.1175*

REFERENCES

Adams, M. P., Josephen, D. L., & Holland, L. N. (Eds.). (2005). *Pharmacology for nurses: A pathophysiologic approach*. Upper Saddle River, NJ: Prentice Hall Health.

Aggarwal, A., Schneider, D. J., Terrien, E. E., et al. (2004). Increased coronary arterial release of Interleukin-1 receptor antagonist and CD40 ligand indicative of inflammation associated with culprit coronary plaques. *American Journal of Cardiology, 93*(1), 6–9.

American Heart Association. (2008). *Inflammation markers signal rapidly advancing coronary disease*. Retrieved July 18, 2008, from http://www.americanheart.org/presenter.jhtml?identifier=3008009

American Heart Association. (2005a). Second International Conference on Women, Heart Disease, and Stroke. Orlando, FL, February 16–19.

American Heart Association. (2006a). *Facts about women and cardiovascular diseases*. Retrieved August 7, 2006, from http://www.americanheart. org/presenter.jhtml?identifier=2876

American Heart Association. (2006b). JAMA study: Incidence and prognostic implications of stable angina pectoris among women and men: American Heart Association Media Advisory. Retrieved July 18, 2008 from http://www. americanheart.org/presenter. jhtml?identifier=3038582

American Heart Association. (2006c). *Risk factors and coronary heart disease*. Retrieved August 16, 2006, from http://www. americanheart.org/presenter.jhtml?identifier=500

American Heart Association. (2006d). *Inflammation, heart disease and stroke: The role of C-reactive protein*. Retrieved August 16, 2006, from http://www.americanheart.org/presenter.jhtml?identifier=4648

American Heart Association. (2006e). *Triglycerides*. Retrieved August 16, 2006, from http://www. americanheart.org/presenter .jhtml?identifier=4778

American Heart Association. (2006f). *Heart disease and stroke statistics—2006 update*. Dallas, TX: Author. Retrieved August 8, 2006, from http://www.americanheart.org/presenter.jhtml? identifier=1928

American Heart Association. (2006g). *Physical activity and a healthy heart*. Retrieved September 17, 2006, from http://www.americanheart.org/ presenter.jhtml?identifier=1518

American Heart Association. (2008a). *Exercise (physical activity) for older people and those with disabilities*. Retrieved August 10, 2006, from http://www.americanheart.org/presenter.jhtml?identifier=4557

American Heart Association. (2008b). *Women, heart disease, and stroke*. Retrieved on July 18, 2008 from http://www.americanheart.org/ presenter.jhtml?identifier=4786

American Heart Association. (2008c). *Women and Coronary Heart Disease*. Retrieved on July 18, 2008 from http://www.americanheart.org/ presenter.jhtml?identifier=2859

American Lung Association. (2006a). *Secondhand smoke fact sheet*. Retrieved August 16, 2006 from http://www.lungusa.org/ site/pp.asp?c= dvLUK900E&b=35422

American Lung Association. (2006b). *Statement on release of U.S. Surgeon General report on health consequences of secondhand smoke*. Retrieved August 16, 2006, from http://www.lungusa.org/ site/apps/nl/content3.asp?c=dvLUK900E&b=40407&ct=2689673

Antman, E. M., Anbe, D. T., Armstrong, P. W., Bates, E. R., Green, L. A., Hand, M., et al. (2004). ACC/AHA guidelines for the management of patients with ST-elevation myocardial infarction – Executive summary: A report of the American College of Cardiology/American Heart Association Task Force on Practice Guidelines (Committee to Revise the 1999 Guidelines for the Management of Patients with Acute Myocardial Infarction). *Circulation, 110*, 588.

Barandon, I., Couffinhal, I. T., Dufourcq, P., et al. (2004). Frizzled A, a novel angiogenic factor: Promises for cardiac repair. *European Journal of Cardiothoracic Surgery, 25*(1), 76–83.

Brown, T. A. (2001). Hibernating myocardium. *American Journal of Critical Care, 10*(2), 84–92.

Burke, A. P., Kolodgie, F. D., Farber, A., et al. (2002). Morphologic predictors of arterial remodeling in coronary atherosclerosis. *Circulation, 105*, 297.

Bypass Angioplasty Revascularization Investigation (BARI). (1996). Comparison of coronary bypass surgery with angioplasty in patients with multivessel disease. *New England Journal of Medicine, 335*, 217–225.

Castelli, W. P. (2001). Making practical sense of clinical trial data in decreasing cardiovascular risk. *American Journal of Cardiology, 88*(4), 16–20.

Clark, L.T., Ferdinand, K. C., Flack, J. M., et al. (2001). Coronary heart disease in African Americans. *Heart Disease, 3*, 97–108.

Coffey, M., Crowder, G. K., & Cheek, D. J. (2003). Reducing coronary artery disease by decreasing homocysteine levels. *Critical Care Nurse, 23*(1), 25–30.

Cohn, P. F., Fox, K. M., & Daly, C. (2003). Silent myocardial ischemia. *Circulation, 108*,1263–1277.

Dendorfer, A., Dominiak, P., & Schunkert, H. (2005). ACE inhibitors and angiotensin II receptor antagonists. *Handbook of Experimental Pharmacology, 170*, 407–442.

Diop, D., & Aghababian, R. V. (2001). Definition, classification, and pathophysiology of acute coronary ischemic syndromes. *Emergency Medicine Clinics of North America, 19*, 259–267.

Eagle, K. A., Guyton, R. A., et al. (2004). ACC/AHA guideline update for coronary artery bypass surgery. Retrieved July 15, 2008 from http://www.acc.org/qualityandscience/clinical/guidelines/news/bypass.htm

Fitzgibbon, G. M., Kafka, H. P., Leach, A. J., et al. (1996). Coronary bypass graft fate and patient outcome: Angiographic follow-up of 5,065 grafts related to survival and reoperation in 1,388 patients during 25 years. *Journal of the American College of Cardiology, 28*(3), 616–626.

Futterman, L. G., & Lemberg, L. (2000). The Framingham heart study: A pivotal legacy of the last millennium. *American Journal of Critical Care, 9*(2), 147–152.

Gene Analysis Service. (2005). Retrieved July 15, 2008 from http://www.gene-analysis-service.de/abcc6.htm

Gibbons, R., et al. (2002). *ACC/AHA guideline update for the management of patients with chronic stable angina*. Retrieved July 15, 2008 from http://www.acc.org/qualityandscience/clinical/guidelines/stable/update%5Findex.htm

Goldfinger, T. M. (2003). Beyond the French paradox: The impact of moderate beverage alcohol and wine consumption in the prevention of cardiovascular disease. *Cardiology Clinics, 21*(3), 449–457.

Goldman, S., Zadina, K., Moritz, T., et al. (2004). Long-term patency of saphenous vein and left internal mammary artery grafts after coronary artery bypass surgery: Results from a Department of Veterans Affairs Cooperative Study. *Journal of the American College of Cardiology, 44*(11), 2149–2156.

Haskell, W. L. (2003). Cardiovascular disease prevention and lifestyle interventions: Effectiveness and efficacy. *Journal of Cardiovascular Nursing, 18*(4), 245–255.

Henning, R. J., & Olsson, R. A. (2001). Coronary blood flow and myocardial ischemia. In C. Rosendorff (Ed.), *Essential cardiology. Principles and practice*. Philadelphia: W. B. Saunders.

Higuchi, M. L., Reis, M. M., Sambiase, N. V., et al. (2003). Co-infection with *Mycoplasma pneumoniae* and *Chlamydia pneumoniae* in ruptured plaque with acute myocardial infarction. *Arquivos Brasileiros de Cardiologia, 81*(1), 12–22.

Hochman, J. S., Sleeper, L. A., Webb, J. G., et al. (2006). Early revascularization and long-term survival in cardiogenic shock complicating acute myocardial infarction. *Journal of the American Medical Association, 295*(21), 2511–2515.

Latini, R., Staszewsky, L., Maggioni, A., et al. (2003). Beneficial effects of angiotensin-converting enzyme inhibitor and nitrate association on

left ventricular remodeling in patients with large acute myocardial infarction: The delapril remodeling after acute myocardial infarction (DRAMI) trial. *American Heart Journal, 146*(1), 133–140.

Lewington, R., Clarke, N., Qizilbash, R., et al. (2002). Age-specific relevance of usual blood pressure to vascular mortality: A meta-analysis of individual data for one million adults in 61 prospective studies. *Lancet, 360*, 1903–1913.

Libby, Bonow, Zipes, & Mann. (2008). Braunwald's Heart Disease, 8th Edition—*A Textbook of Cardiovascular Medicine*. W. B. Saunders. Philadelphia.

Loop, F. D., Lytle, B. W., Cosgrove, D. M., et al. (1986). Free (aorta-coronary) internal mammary artery graft. Late results. *Journal of Thoracic and Cardiovascular Surgery, 92*(5), 827–831.

Lytle, B. W., Loop, F. D., Cosgrove, D. M., et al. (1985). Long-term (5 to 12 years) serial studies of internal mammary artery and saphenous vein coronary bypass grafts. *Journal of Thoracic and Cardiovascular Surgery, 89*(2), 248–258.

Massad, M. G., & Geha, A. S. (2004). Surgical repair of mechanical complications of myocardial infarction. *World Journal of Surgery, 28*(9), 847–856.

McSweeney, J., Cody, M., O'Sullivan, P., Elberson, K., Moser, D., & Garvin, B. (2003). Women's early warning symptoms of acute myocardial infarction. *Circulation, 108*(21), 2619–2623.

Morton, P. G., Fontaine, D. K., Hudak, C. M., & Gallo, B. M. (2005). *Critical care nursing: A holistic approach* (8th ed.). Philadelphia: Lippincott Williams & Wilkins.

Naghavi, M., Libby, P., Falk, E., et al. (2003a). From vulnerable plaque to vulnerable patient. A call for new definitions and risk assessment strategies: Part I. *Circulation, 108*, 1664–1672.

Naghavi, M., Libby, P., Falk, E., et al. (2003b). From vulnerable plaque to vulnerable patient. A call for new definitions and risk assessment strategies: Part II. *Circulation, 108*, 1772–1778.

Nash, D. (2004). Cardiovascular risk beyond LDL-C levels: Other lipids are performers in cholesterol story. *Post Graduate Medicine: online, 116*(3). Retrieved July 15, 2008 from http://www.postgradmed.com/issues/2004/09_04/nash.shtml

National Guidelines and Tools for Cardiovascular Risk Reduction. (2006). *Preventive cardiovascular nurses associations*. Philips Healthcare Communications.

Nomoto, K., Oguchi, S., Watanabe I., et al. (2003). Involvement of inflammation in acute coronary syndromes assessed by levels of high sensitivity C-reactive protein, matrix metalloproteinase-9 and soluble vascular-cell adhesion molecule-9. *Journal of Cardiology, 42*(5), 201–206.

Opie, L. H., & Poole-Wilson, P. A. (2005). β-Blockers. In L. H. Opie & B. J. Gersh (Eds.), *Drugs for the heart* (6th ed.). Philadelphia: W. B. Saunders.

Opie, L. H., & White, H. D. (2005). *Nitrates*. In L. H. Opie & B. J. Gersh, B. J. (Eds.), *Drugs for the heart* (6th ed.). Philadelphia: W. B. Saunders.

Pasterkamp, G., Fitzgerald, P. F., & de Kleijn, D. P. (2002). Atherosclerotic expansive remodeled plaques: A wolf in sheep's clothing. *Journal of Vascular Research, 39*, 514.

Pearson, T. A., Blair, S. N., Daniels, S. R., et al. (2002). *American Heart Association guidelines for primary prevention of cardiovascular disease and stroke: 2002 update*. Retrieved July 18, 2008 from http://circ.ahajournals.org/cgi/content/full/106/3/388

Pieniazek, P., Karczewska, E., Stepien, E., et al. (2001). Incidence of Chlamydia pneumoniae infection in patients with coronary artery disease subjected to angioplasty or bypass surgery. *Medicine Science Monitor, 7*(5), 995–1001.

Porth, C. M. (2005). *Pathophysiology: Concepts of altered health status* (7th ed.). Philadelphia: Lippincott Williams & Wilkins.

Rosenson, R. S., & Koenig, W. (2003). Utility of inflammatory markers in the management of coronary artery disease. *American Journal of Cardiology, 92*(1A), 10i–18i.

Sarwat, I., Krumholz, H., & Foody, J. A. (2004). Systolic hypertension in older persons. *Journal of the American Medical Association, 292,* 1074–1080.

Schoenhagen, P., Vince, D. G., Ziada, K. M., et al. (2002). Relation of matrix metalloproteinase 3 found in coronary lesion samples retrieved by directional coronary atherectomy to intravascular ultrasound observations on coronary remodeling. *American Journal of Cardiology, 89,* 1354–1359.

Serruys, P. W., Unger, F., Sousa, J. E., et al. (2001). Comparison of coronary-artery bypass surgery and stenting for the treatment of multivessel disease. *New England Journal of Medicine, 344*(15), 1117–1124.

Society of Thoracic Surgeons. (2006, Spring). *Adult cardiac database executive summary.* Retrieved July 15, 2008 from http://www.sts.org/documents/pdf/STS-ExecutiveSummarySpring2006.pdf

Takemura, G., & Fuiwara, H. (2004). Role of apoptosis in remodeling after myocardial infarction. *Pharmacology and Therapeutics, 104*(1), 1–16.

United States Department of Health and Human Services. (2006). *New Surgeon General's report focuses on the effects of secondhand smoke.* Retrieved August 16, 2006, from http://www.hhs.gov/news/press/2006pres/20060627.html

Venkat, A., Hekstra, J., & Lindsell, C. (2003). The impact of race on the acute management of chest pain. *Academic Emergency Medicine, 10*(11), 1199–1208.

Young, L. H. (1992). Yale University School of Medicine heart book. *Yale University School of Medicine, 21,* 263–271.

Zipes, D. P., Libby, P., Bonow, R. O., et al. (2005). *Heart disease: A textbook of cardiovascular medicine* (7th ed.). Philadelphia: W. B. Saunders.

Caring for the Patient with Cardiac Inflammatory Disorders

Kathleen Osborn

Outcome-Based Learning Objectives

After studying this chapter, the learner will be able to:

1. Compare and contrast the etiology, pathophysiology, clinical manifestations, and medical and nursing management for the four inflammatory/infectious disorders.

2. Integrate the etiology, pathophysiology, clinical manifestations, and treatment for valve stenosis, regurgitation, and mitral valve prolapse.

3. Explain the rationale and type of preventive therapy necessary for patients with valve disease.

4. Differentiate valve repair and replacement procedures in terms of patient care and education needs.

5. Compare and contrast the four types of cardiomyopathy in terms of etiology, pathophysiology, clinical manifestations, and medical and nursing management.

6. Apply nursing diagnoses and the nursing process to the care of the patient with inflammatory and structural heart disease.

Research   Collaboration   Health Promotion   Nursing Process   Caring   Critical Thinking

CARDIAC DISORDERS caused by inflammation or structural changes and abnormalities impact tissue perfusion due to altered myocardial pumping ability or abnormal blood flow through the heart. All three layers of the heart, the pericardium, myocardium, and endocardium, can be subject to inflammation and structural abnormalities. The manifestations differ depending on which layer is involved in the pathologic process. In recent years the incidence of cardiac structural disorders has increased due in part to advancements in the prevention and treatment of coronary artery disease. People are living long enough to develop the structural changes often associated with advanced age. An in-depth discussion of disorders affecting each layer of the heart is presented in this chapter.

INFLAMMATORY DISORDERS

The heart is susceptible to bacteria and microbes that may be infecting other organs of the body. The infection causes an inflammatory response that impacts the heart's ability to maintain a normal cardiac output. In the acute stages these infections are serious and potentially lethal. Additionally, damage to the heart during the infectious process can be long term and disabling. The inflammatory conditions affecting the heart—rheumatic heart disease, pericarditis, myocarditis, and endocarditis—are discussed next.

Rheumatic Heart Disease

Rheumatic heart disease is a complication of rheumatic fever. The pathologic process of **rheumatic fever** begins with a pharyngeal infection caused by Lancefield group A beta-hemolytic streptococcus (strep). If left untreated, approximately 3% of these pharyngeal infections result in rheumatic fever. The resulting rheumatic heart disease is thought to be caused by an abnormal autoimmune response to the original infection, but the exact pathogenesis remains unclear (Chin, 2006). The primary long-term damage is scarring and malfunction of the heart valves.

Epidemiology and Etiology

Until recently rheumatic fever was thought to be nearly eradicated from developed countries, although it continues to be a challenge because of its high prevalence in the developing world. It was the leading cause of death 100 years ago in the United States in people 5 to 20 years of age. Antibiotics and early treatment have made rheumatic fever rare in developed countries, although in recent years it has made a comeback in poor inner-city neighborhoods. Rheumatic fever occurs most frequently in children from 5 to 15 years of age and tends to affect connective tissues, especially those of the heart, brain, skin, and joints. The risk factors associated with the development and spread of streptococcal infections are outlined in the Risk Factors box. Rheumatic fever occurs equally among men and women, but the prognosis is worse for females because they are more likely to develop other conditions such as mitral valve prolapse (Chin, 2006).

Worldwide, chronic rheumatic heart disease is estimated to exist in 5 to 30 million children and young adults. Approximately 90,000 people die from this disease each year and the mortality rate remains 1% to 10% (Chin, 2006). Once rheumatic fever has occurred, a person is more susceptible to recurrent infections. With each infection more damage to the heart valve occurs.

Pathophysiology

As mentioned, rheumatic fever develops following pharyngitis from Lancefield group A beta-hemolytic streptococcus. The infecting organisms attach to the epithelial cells in the upper respiratory tract and produce enzymes that damage and invade other tissues of the body. These organisms elicit an acute inflammatory response after an incubation period of 2 to 4 days. Several weeks after the initial infection resolves, rheumatic fever results. Only infections of the pharynx initiate and reactivate rheumatic fever. Patients remain infected for weeks after the resolution of symptoms and may serve as a reservoir for infecting others.

In greater than half of the cases of rheumatic fever, an abnormal autoimmune response is thought to occur. It is theorized that the invading organism produces toxins that precipitate an antigen–antibody response. The antibodies appear to cross-react with connective tissues and bind to receptor sites on the heart, joints, skin, brain, and subcutaneous tissue, causing an acute inflammatory response. In the heart, all three layers, the endocardium, myocardium, and pericardium, become inflamed, giving rise to the term **pancarditis**. Microscopic lesions, referred to as Aschoff nodules are composed of a collection of lymphocytes and histocytes, are found in the fibrinous interstitial septa of the myocardium. Additionally, wartlike raised fibrinous lesions develop on the closure lines of the valve cusps. As Aschoff nodules age, they become more fibrinous scar tissue, contributing to the transient heart failure associated with rheumatic fever. As the inflammation subsides there is typically no long-term damage to the myocardium and pericardium. The long-term sequela of the inflammation is to the heart valves.

The inflammatory process causes swelling of the valves, and small bacterial vegetations form on the valve surface (Figure 41–1 ▪), which leads to fibrous thickening and fusion of the valve leaflets, causing valve dysfunction. Damaged valves either do not completely open (stenosis) or close (regurgitation). The severity of the symptoms is dependent on the valve involved and the degree of dysfunction. Valve stenosis and regurgitation, described later in this chapter, cause an increase in the workload of the heart. The symptoms typically become worse over time with the most advanced condition leading to heart failure.

Clinical Manifestations

Clinical manifestations of rheumatic fever typically begin about 1 to 6 weeks after a bout of strep throat (pharyngitis), although in some cases the infection may have been too mild to be recognized. The diagnosis of rheumatic fever and rheumatic heart disease is based on a cluster of clinical manifestations and laboratory findings. Clinical manifestations of acute rheumatic fever and rheumatic heart disease are outlined in Chart 41–1.

The diagnosis of rheumatic fever and rheumatic heart disease is made by clustering signs and symptoms and analysis of laboratory and diagnostic tests. Carditis is the most significant manifestation of rheumatic fever. New or changing murmurs are one of the major signs of cardiac involvement. The murmur is caused by valve insufficiency or regurgitation. Murmurs typically found with acute rheumatic fever are (1) the apical pansystolic, high-pitched murmur, which has a blowing quality that radiates to the left axilla, indicating mitral regurgitation; (2) the apical diastolic murmur, which is low pitched and rumbling and is present with active carditis and accompanies severe mitral in-

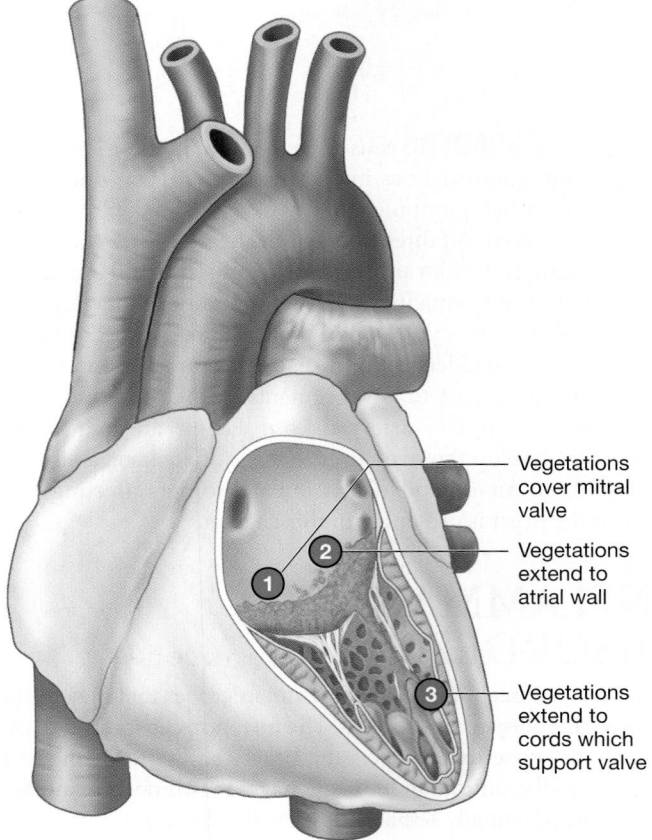

FIGURE 41–1 ▪ Vegetative growth on a heart valve.

RISK FACTORS for Rheumatic Fever

Poor inner-city neighborhoods
Damp weather
Crowded living conditions
Malnutrition
Immunocompromised state
Poor access to health care

CHART 41–1	Clinical Manifestations of Acute Rheumatic Fever and Rheumatic Heart Disease
Clinical Manifestations of Acute Rheumatic Fever	**Clinical Manifestations of Rheumatic Heart Disease**
Fever	Chest pain
Malaise	Development of a new murmur or change in an existing murmur
Headache	Tachycardia and cardiac dysrhythmias
Erythema marginatum: red, raised, lattice-like rash, usually on the chest, back, and abdomen	Electrocardiogram (ECG) changes: prolonged PR interval
Swollen tender joints with small bony protuberances with or without the presence of subcutaneous nodules	Pericardial friction rub
May have weakness and shortness of breath	Symptoms of heart failure
Sydenham chorea: sudden, irregular, aimless involuntary movements that are self-limiting with no permanent damage	Cardiomegaly
Elevated white blood count (WBC)	Mitral and aortic stenosis

sufficiency; and (3) the basal diastolic murmur, a high-pitched, blowing, decrescendo murmur associated with aortic regurgitation (Chin, 2006). A complete description of murmurs is outlined in Chapter 37 .

 CRITICAL ALERT *If a new murmur is noted during the assessment of a patient with rheumatic fever, the nurse needs to report this to the health care provider. It may indicate the onset of rheumatic heart disease and requires further diagnostic testing. Where the murmur is heard depends on the valve that is involved.*

Heart failure may develop secondary to myocarditis or valve insufficiency. Another manifestation of cardiac involvement during rheumatic heart fever is pericarditis. A pericardial friction rub, distant muffled heart sounds, chest pain, and evidence of pericardial effusion are all consistent clinical manifestations of pericarditis.

Polyarthritis is the most common symptom and in 70% to 75% of the cases is the earliest manifestation of acute rheumatic fever (Chin, 2006). The arthritis typically begins in large joints of the lower extremities, such as the knees and ankles, and then migrates to other large joints of the lower and upper extremities. The affected joints are painful, swollen, erythematous, and have decreased range of motion. The arthritis reaches its most intense severity 12 to 24 hours after onset and persists for 2 to 6 days. Polyarthritis is not associated with any permanent disability.

Sydenham chorea is the major central nervous system (CNS) manifestation and may occur in patients with rheumatic fever (Chin, 2006). It is characterized by difficulty writing, involuntary grimacing, purposeless movements of the arms and legs (choreiform), speech impairment, generalized weakness, and emotional lability. Sydenham chorea is slightly more common in females under age 18 than males.

Laboratory and Diagnostic Procedures

When evaluating the patient with suspected rheumatic heart disease, a complete history and physical is necessary in order to evaluate the risk factors and the extent of the disease process. In addition to the clinical findings, a number of laboratory tests are useful when making the diagnosis. The Diagnostic Tests box (p. 1222) describes the laboratory and diagnostic tests and abnormalities associated with rheumatic fever and rheumatic heart disease.

Medical Management

Prevention is the primary goal in the management of rheumatic heart disease. Early treatment of the streptococcal infection with antibiotics will usually prevent the development of rheumatic fever. People with previous attacks are more susceptible to future episodes and each attack increases the amount of heart damage. Therefore, aggressive early treatment is essential in this population.

An antibiotic, typically penicillin, is used in the treatment of rheumatic fever. Oral penicillin V is the drug of choice, although erythromycin may be used when there is a penicillin allergy. Following the acute stage, prophylactic antibiotics are indicated to prevent further damage to the valves. The recommendation in the United States is that after the initial course of antibiotics, an intramuscular injection of penicillin G be given every 4 weeks. Although controversial, this schedule is continued indefinitely for high-risk patients or recurrent infections. Additional prophylactic antibiotics are indicated before and after any dental work or any surgical procedure.

Aspirin and nonsteroidal anti-inflammatory drugs (NSAIDs) are used to treat joint pain and fever. If symptoms of moderate to severe carditis are present as evidenced by cardiomegaly and heart failure, steroid administration is typically added to the therapy and continued for 2 to 4 weeks (Chin, 2006).

If heart failure with left ventricular dysfunction (ejection fraction less than 40%) occurs as a consequence of rheumatic fever, cardiac medications, such as angiotensin converting enzyme (ACE) inhibitors (or angiotensin receptor blockers), beta-adrengeric blockers, digoxin, or diuretics for congestion are indicated. See Chapter 42 for pharmacologic management of heart failure. See the Pharmacology Summary (p. 1236) for medications to treat inflammatory heart disease.

Bed rest is prescribed to reduce cardiac workload, especially during the acute phase. Once the carditis subsides the patient may begin a gradual schedule of increasing activity. Activity levels are dictated by the presence or absence of symptoms.

Nursing Management

Nursing management of the patient with rheumatic heart disease begins with an in-depth assessment of the clinical

DIAGNOSTIC TESTS for Cardiac Inflammatory Disorders

Test and *Normal Values*	Expected Abnormality	Rationale for Abnormality
White blood cells (WBC): *5000–10,000/mm³*	Elevated with rheumatic fever, pericarditis, and myocarditis. Mild elevation with infective endocarditis (IE).	Elevated levels are associated with inflammation and infection.
Red blood cells (RBC): *Male: 4.7–6.1 mm³* *Female: 4.2–5.4 mm³*	Mild to moderate decrease with rheumatic fever.	Occurs due to the inflammatory inhibition of erythropoiesis.
Erythrocyte sedimentation rate: *Male: up to 15 mm/hour* *Female: up to 20 mm/hour*	Elevated rheumatic fever, pericarditis, IE, and myocarditis.	The test measures inflammation. Chronic inflammation and infection cause an elevation.
C-reactive protein: *<10 mg/L*	Elevated rheumatic fever, pericarditis, IE, and myocarditis.	Acute-phase reactant protein used to indicate an inflammatory illness.
Antistreptolysin O titer (ASO): *<160 units/mL*	>250 unit/mL with rheumatic fever.	Streptococcal antibody test used to determine whether a previous streptococcal infection has caused a poststreptococcal infection such as rheumatic fever.
Cardiac marker: creatinine kinase MB (CK–MB), troponin T, and troponin I *CPK–MB: <3% or 0–7.5 ng/mL* *Troponin T: <0.2 ng/mL* *Troponin I: <0.35 ng/mL*	Elevated if carditis is present with all of the inflammatory disorders.	May be transiently elevated during the acute stages of myocardial cell damage.
BNP: *<100 pg/mL or <100 ng/L*	Elevated with ventricular hypertrophy, severe hypertension, and heart failure.	Marker of ventricular systolic and diastolic dysfunction. Useful to determine presence of heart failure.
Throat culture: *Negative or normal flora*	Positive for A beta-hemolytic streptococci with rheumatic fever.	Quantifies and differentiates bacterial from viral throat infections.
ECG: *Normal conduction time intervals* (see Chapter 38)	Prolonged PR interval with rheumatic fever. Diffuse ST segment abnormalities, T wave changes, dysrhythmias and heart block with myocarditis. ST segment changes associated with myocardial ischemia and the conduction delays typical of IE.	Conduction delays may be present with inflammation. ST segment changes may be present when myocardial ischemia is occurring.
Chest x-ray: *Clear lungs and normal heart size*	Enlarged heart and lung congestion with pancarditis and heart failure. May show cardiac enlargement if a pericardial effusion is present. Diagnoses of heart failure and in right-sided IE may show evidence of septic pulmonary emboli.	Cardiac enlargement occurs with inflammation, heart failure, and pericardial effusion. Congestion occurs with heart failure.
Echocardiogram (ultrasound): *Normal chamber size and normal cardiac structures*	Valve damage and dilated chamber size, abnormal pressure gradients, decreased ventricular function, and/or pericardial effusion with structurally abnormal valves. Depressed systolic function, dilated chambers, and mild to no pericardial effusion may occur with myocarditis. Determines the presence of pericardial fluid, motion of the heart walls, and the presence of restriction with pericarditis. Presence of thickening and calcification of the pericardium for IE.	The inflammation causes structural changes in cardiac chambers and function.
Cardiac catheterization: *Normal coronary arteries, chambers, and valve pressures*	Valve damage, enlarged chamber size, decreased ventricular and/or function with rheumatic fever. Valvular and ventricular function abnormalities, and assists in evaluating need for valve replacement surgery.	Inflammation causes changes in chamber size and valve function. Valve stenosis disrupts blood flow causing enlarged chamber size. Valve regurgitation causes a backflow of blood into the previous chamber.

DIAGNOSTIC TESTS for Cardiac Inflammatory Disorders—*Continued*

Test and *Normal Values*	Expected Abnormality	Rationale for Abnormality
Blood cultures: *Negative for organisms*	Positive and organism specific in 90–95% of cases with IE and therefore guide antibiotic therapy.	Organisms enter the bloodstream, adhere to the valve surface, and multiply.
Viral titers: *Negative*	Elevated.	Viral titers are present for 8 to 10 days after onset of illness.
Endomyocardial biopsy: *Normal tissue*	Presence of patchy cell necrosis and inflammatory changes confirm the diagnosis.	Often done within 6 weeks of acute illness while lymphocytic infiltration and myocyte damage is present.
Autoimmune serum markers: *Negative*	Presence of intracellular adhesion molecules on cardiac myocytes.	Intracellular adhesion molecules on cardiac myocytes is specific to autoimmune myocarditis.

Source: From *Laboratory Tests and Diagnostic Procedures with Nursing Diagnosis,* 6th edition, by J. V. Corbett, 2004, Upper Saddle River, NJ: Pearson Prentice Hall.

manifestations outlined in Chart 41–1, p. 1221. Further subjective and objective data related to clinical manifestations are outlined in the Nursing Process: Patient Care Plan for Inflammatory Heart Disease feature (p. 1224). The nurse must specifically note and report to the health care provider any progression of the clinical manifestations related to heart failure. In addition, any change in the loudness of the murmur must be documented and reported because this may indicate a progression of cardiac valve disorders.

The outcome for the patient with rheumatic fever is to make a full recovery with no residual cardiac pathology. As outlined in the nursing process patient care plan, nursing management focuses on resting the heart, pain relief, eradication of the infecting organism, and emotional support. Nursing interventions require critical thinking and sound clinical judgment because not all patients present with the same manifestations. It is essential to stress the importance of decreasing myocardial oxygen demand and cardiac workload. Strict bed rest is typically ordered, especially in the acute stages of these illnesses. The nurse must explain the importance of bed rest and activity restriction to the patient and family. Spacing care and activities to allow for periods of rest will decrease oxygen demand and, thus, cardiac workload.

Health Promotion

Prevention of a recurrence of the disease requires patient/family education about the need for prophylactic antibiotics, vigilant hygiene, good nutrition, and rest. The patient needs to be instructed to avoid individuals with upper respiratory infections to minimize exposure. The nurse should stress the risk for recurrence if a streptococcal infection occurs. A list of clinical manifestations that would indicate a need to seek medical help must be provided. It should be stressed that cardiac valve disease could develop and will require medical intervention. The Patient Teaching & Discharge Priorities box (p. 1227) outlines specific discharge priorities.

■ Pericarditis

Pericarditis, an inflammation of the pericardial sac, is the most common pathologic process affecting the pericardium. The pericardium or pericardial sac is a double-walled mem-

branous sac that encloses the heart and the roots of the great vessels. The purpose of the pericardial sac is to prevent excessive dilation during diastole, to act as a barrier from infections in adjacent tissues, and to prevent displacement of the myocardium and great vessels. The inner serous layer of the pericardium is the visceral pericardium or epicardium and the outer layer is the parietal pericardium (Figure 41–2 ■, p. 1228). The space between these two layers is referred to as the pericardial space and normally it contains approximately 50 mL of fluid. The fluid serves to lubricate and decrease friction while the heart is moving during systole and diastole. Due to the inflammatory process, the two layers of the pericardium become inflamed and roughened, and the amount of fluid in the pericardial sac increases. Pericarditis can be acute and/or chronic constrictive (recurrent) and has several causes.

Epidemiology and Etiology

There are three general causes of pericarditis: infectious, noninfectious, and hypersensitive or autoimmune. These causes are listed in the Risk Factors box (p. 1228). If infectious, often the infection starts in some other organ in the body, usually the lungs and upper respiratory tract. The most common cause of pericarditis is caused by the coxsackie virus B and is referred to as Bornholm disease. People in their 20s and 30s who have had a recent upper respiratory infection and men ages 20 to 50 years are most likely to be affected. Frequently the cause of pericarditis is idiopathic. Noninfectious causes include uremia, which affects 6% to 10% of patients with advanced renal failure before initiation of dialysis. When patients with large effusions are studied, uremia may account for up to 20% of cases in some series. The widespread availability of dialysis has reduced the incidence of uremic pericarditis (Gowda, 2008). Noninfectious pericarditis also occurs after acute myocardial infarction (AMI) and following open heart surgery (postcardiotomy).

Hypersensitive or autoimmune responses are the third category of causes of pericarditis. This category includes connective tissue disorders, drug reactions, and rheumatoid diseases that affect the heart (Chart 41–5, p. 1250). **Dressler's syndrome**, also referred to as late pericarditis, occurs in 5% to 15% of the patients typically 1 to 4 weeks after an AMI. It is characterized by fever, pericarditis, chest pain, and pericardial friction rub and pleural

NURSING PROCESS: Patient Care Plan for Inflammatory Heart Disease

Assessment of Respiratory Status

Subjective Data:
Do you feel short of breath?
When does it occur?
How far can you walk before you have to rest due to shortness of breath?
Do you have a cough and, if so, do you cough anything up?
Do you become more short of breath when lying down?

Objective Data:
Acid–base balance.
Lung sounds.
Respiratory rate.
Assess for adventitious or diminished breath sounds.
Note presence of cough, and amount and color of sputum.
Monitor ABGs and oxygen saturation.
Monitor respiratory rate and depth.
Monitor restlessness and confusion.
Observe for cyanosis, especially in the mucous membranes.

Nursing Assessment and Diagnoses	Outcomes and Evaluation Parameters	Planning and Interventions with *Rationales*
Nursing Diagnosis: *Impaired Gas Exchange* related to heart failure	**Outcome:** Adequate gas exchange achieved. **Evaluation Parameters:** Normal arterial blood gases. No dyspnea: unlabored respirations < 24/minute. No ischemic ECG changes such as ST segment changes and dysrhythmias. Alert and oriented. Clear breath sounds. No restlessness, cyanosis, or fatigue. Oxygen saturation is within normal limits.	**Interventions and *Rationales*:** Monitor: ABG's, oxygen saturation, respiratory rate, lung sounds, and ECG Turn, cough, deep breathe, elevate head of bed. instruct on use of incentive spirometry. *Measures to promote gas exchange.* Administer humidified oxygen as prescribed *to increase oxygen levels.* Report respiratory distress to the health care provider. *Medical intervention may be indicated to prevent respiratory failure.* Assess need for suctioning and/or endotracheal intubation *to maintain adequate gas exchange.* Monitor fluid status *to assess heart failure.*

Assessment of Pain

Subjective Data:
Do you have problems with pain?
Where is the pain (joints, chest)?
What brings the pain on; what makes it go away?
What do you use to relieve it and is it effective?
Is the pain getting worse?

Objective Data:
Use pain scale (0–10) to quantify pain level.
Assess cultural and religious impact on patient's responses.
Assess the onset of increased pain to evaluate the presence of disease progression and/or an embolic event.

Nursing Assessment and Diagnoses	Outcomes and Evaluation Parameters	Planning and Interventions with *Rationales*
Nursing Diagnosis: *Pain, acute* related to fluid build up and inflammatory response	**Outcome:** Comfort level maintained. **Evaluation Parameters:** Patient able to communicate pain level and therapies that help alleviate it. Pain reduced and/or absent as evidenced by patient report and no pain behaviors: grimacing. Nonpharmacologic method of control is effective as evidenced by patient report and no pain behaviors. Patient reports satisfaction with pain management program. Patient is compliant with both antibiotics and pain medication schedule. Reports understanding of need to report a change in pain level to health care provider.	**Interventions and *Rationales*:** Instruct patient to inform nurse if pain is not relieved. *Indicates need to change pain management plan.* Obtain a clear description of source of discomfort. *This will assist in developing a pain management plan.* Correct misconceptions about risk of addiction and overdose *to decrease anxiety related to medication addiction.* Provide a supportive environment where patient is able to express pain level. *Opens communication and facilitates pain management.* Use pain control measures before pain becomes severe. *This increases comfort and decreases need for medication.* Teach nonpharmacologic method of control, i.e., guided imagery and massage, and breathing exercises. *These measures augment pain relief.* Teach the patient/family the correct dosage and time intervals for medication administration *to increase compliance and prevent complications.*

NURSING PROCESS: Patient Care Plan for Inflammatory Heart Disease—*Continued*

Assessment of Anxiety Related to Inflammatory Heart Disease

Subjective Data:
Has anyone explained your health problems to you?
Would you tell me what you know about your disease?
How does this disease affect your daily life?
Do you feel anxious about your health problems?
Do you have family members or close friends who provide emotional support?

Objective Data:
Observe for manifestations of anxiety: restlessness, apprehension, withdrawal.

Nursing Assessment and Diagnoses	Outcomes and Evaluation Parameters	Planning and Interventions with *Rationales*
Nursing Diagnosis: *Fear* and *Anxiety* related to inflammatory heart disease	**Outcomes:** Anxiety level minimized and manageable. **Evaluation Parameters:** Verbalizes anxious feelings. Verbalizes what relieves anxiety. Verbalizes absence of sensory perceptual disorders. Verbalizes absence of physical manifestations of anxiety. Behavioral manifestations of anxiety absent.	**Interventions and *Rationales*:** Provide factual information concerning diagnosis, treatment, disfigurement, disabilities, and prognosis. *Truthful explanations increase trust and potentially decrease anxiety.* Explain all procedures and allow time for mental preparation. *This decreases fear and anxiety of the unknown.* Allow time and encourage verbalization of fears related to illness *to assist in relieving anxiety.* Explore with the patient/family techniques to reduce anxiety. *This gives the patient a sense of control and opens communication about the subject.* Explore with patient effective ways to minimize anxiety. *This gives the patient a sense of control.* Instruct patient on use of relaxation techniques *to relieve anxiety.* Assess need for and administer antianxiety and pain medication. *If alternative measures are not effective, may need antianxiety agents.*

Assessment of Cardiac Output

Subjective Data:
Do you become short of breath at rest or with activity?
Has your shortness of breath become worse?
Do your legs become swollen at any time during the day?
Have you noticed a blue tinge in your nail beds?

Objective Data:
Determine heart rate and rhythm.
Assess:
Blood pressure
Lung sounds
Urine output

Capillary refill
Right-sided heart failure (JVD, hepatomegaly, peripheral edema).

Nursing Assessment and Diagnoses	Outcomes and Evaluation Parameters	Planning and Interventions with *Rationales*
Nursing Diagnoses: *Decreased Cardiac Output* and *Ineffective Tissue Perfusion* related to infection, incompetent valves, and heart failure	**Outcome:** Sufficient cardiac output to perfuse organs. **Evaluation Parameter:** Minimal valve damage that decreases cardiac output.	**Interventions and *Rationales*:** Auscultate heart sounds for murmur and S_3, S_4 *to evaluate valve function and onset of heart failure.* Provide oxygen per order *to increase oxygen to the heart and peripheral tissues.* Administer diuretics, inotropics, and a low sodium diet *to treat heart failure.* Plan rest period *to reduce cardiac workload.*

Assessment of Tissue Perfusion

Subjective Data:
Do you have any pain in either leg?
Have you noticed any swelling or hard reddened areas?
Have you had any sudden chest pain that becomes worse when you take a deep breath?
Have you had any headaches, loss of consciousness, or dizzy spells?

Objective Data:
Assess:
Lung congestion
Urine output and color
Abdominal pain
Neurological function

Skin and eyes
Nail beds
Calf Deep Vein Thrombosis (DVT)
Glasgow Coma Scale.

(continued)

NURSING PROCESS: Patient Care Plan for Inflammatory Heart Disease—*Continued*

Nursing Assessment and Diagnoses	Outcomes and Evaluation Parameters	Planning and Interventions with *Rationales*
Nursing Diagnosis: *Ineffective Tissue Perfusion* related to dislodging of vegetative growths and immobility-related thrombophlebitis	**Outcome:** Occurrence of emboli diagnosed early and treatment instituted. ***Evaluation Parameter:*** Effective prevention of DVT.	**Interventions and *Rationales:*** Apply elastic compression stocking *to provide venous support.* Teach leg exercises *to promote venous return and decrease risk of DVT.* Report any new abnormal clinical manifestations to the health care provider. Monitor for therapeutic levels of anticoagulant therapy. Monitor for bleeding.

Assessment of Knowledge of Health Problems

Subjective Data:
What have you been told about your health problems?
Tell me what you know about your health problems.
What do you do when symptoms occur?
Do you see your health care provider on a regular basis?
Do you know what symptoms are important to report to your health care provider immediately?

Objective Data:
Assess knowledge of need to rest the heart and decrease the oxygen needs.
Explore patient's understanding of purpose of preventive antibiotic therapy.

Nursing Assessment and Diagnoses	Outcomes and Evaluation Parameters	Planning and Interventions with *Rationales*
Nursing Diagnosis: *Deficient Knowledge* related to disease process and prognosis	**Outcome:** Verbalizes understanding of prevention. ***Evaluation Parameter:*** Reports regular dental appointments and follow-up visits. Verbalizes adherence and compliance to therapy.	**Interventions and *Rationales:*** See Patient Teaching & Discharge Priorities feature for home care and remainder of teaching needs.

Assessment of Activity Tolerance

Subjective Data:
What type of activity fatigues you?
Has it been getting progressively worse?
Does activity increase joint tenderness and swelling?
Are you able to complete your ADLs without fatigue or shortness of breath?

Objective Data:
Assess for joint tenderness, swelling, and decreased range of motion.
Monitor vital signs during activity.

Nursing Assessment and Diagnoses	Outcomes and Evaluation Parameters	Planning and Interventions with *Rationales*
Nursing Diagnosis: *Activity Intolerance* related to decreased cardiac output, fatigue, and inflammation	**Outcome:** Able to complete ADLs without fatigue. ***Evaluation Parameter:*** Able to increase activity level with resolution of clinical manifestations.	**Interventions and *Rationales:*** Take 30- to 60-minute rest periods between all activities *to decrease cardiac workload.* Perform only essential activities until endurance improves *to decrease cardiac workload during the healing process.*

Assessment of Fever

Subjective Data:
Do you feel hotter than normal?
If so, how long have you been feeling that way?
Have you had the chills?

Objective Data:
Monitor temperature and WBC count.

Nursing Assessment and Diagnoses	Outcomes and Evaluation Parameters	Planning and Interventions with *Rationales*
Nursing Diagnosis: *Hyperthermia* related to the infection	**Outcomes:** Normal temperature. Absence of chills. ***Evaluation Parameters:*** Effective antibiotic treatment. Resolution of infection.	**Interventions and *Rationales:*** Administer antipyretics *to decrease temperature.* Administer antibiotics *to treat causative organism.* Cover patient *to prevent shivering and subsequent temperature elevation.*

PATIENT TEACHING & DISCHARGE PRIORITIES for Inflammatory Heart Disease

Need	Teaching
Knowledge of disease process and prognosis	Home care needs include verbal and written instructions for: • Treatment plan • Follow-up care • Activity restriction
	These instructions will reinforce need to comply with therapy.
Understanding of medications	The patient/family are taught to administer the antibiotics and to care for the infusion site using aseptic technique.
	Teach the purpose, dose, and possible side effects of all medications to increase compliance and prevent over/underdosing.
Oral hygiene	Emphasize the importance of good dental hygiene and regular checkups to decrease the risk of pathogen entry via the mouth.
Disease prevention	Explain the need for antibiotic prophylaxis before invasive procedures to prevent reoccurrence.
	Encourage avoidance of people with upper respiratory infections to prevent an increased risk of infection.
	Avoid IV drug use.
Safety	Stress the importance of a medic alert bracelet to identify a heart problem to health care workers.
Reportable clinical manifestations	Instruct patient/family to report: • Change of exercise tolerance • New onset chest pain and fever • Clinical manifestations of heart failure
Family/Support system	Assess availability, knowledge, and compliance with treatment regimen.
	Assess respite needs and resources.
	Assess discharge placement needs: • Home • Rehabilitation facility • Extended care facility
	Assess home environment for need for assistive devices.
	Assess for need for professional home health needs.
	Assess need for follow-up appointments.
Emotional adjustment of patient/family due to the chronic nature of the disease.	Answer questions honestly.
	Encourage verbalization of frustrations and anger.
	Encourage positive reinforcement from the family.
	Stress that it is not uncommon to feel let down or depressed after discharge.

effusions. Dressler's syndrome may persist for weeks or even months after an AMI (Mayo Clinic, 2005a). Because it is thought to be an inflammatory process, treatment focuses on decreasing inflammation and treating the pain. NSAIDs such as aspirin treat the inflammation, and opioids are used to treat the pain.

Pathophysiology

With the infectious form of pericarditis, microbes causing the infection form an exudate of fibrin, white blood cells (WBCs), and endothelial cells. This exudate covers the pericardium, causing further inflammation of the surrounding tissues. Acute pericarditis can be either dry or exudative. If exudative, the pericardial sac fills with the serofibrinous exudate. Anywhere from 100 to 3,000 mL of fluid or exudate has been known to accumulate in the pericardial sac. This excess fluid accumulation restricts cardiac filling and emptying, therefore decreasing cardiac output and tissue perfusion. Without prompt treatment, shock and death will occur.

A number of causes of noninfectious pericarditis are listed in the accompanying Risk Factors box (p. 1228). Blunt trauma to the chest and heart surgery cause inflammation of the cardiac tissues. Small blood vessels may leak due to trauma, and the inflammation caused by tissue injury causes fluid to accumulate in the pericardial sac.

Chronic **constrictive pericarditis** occurs when the pericardial layers adhere to each other as a result of fibrosis of the pericardial sac. This usually occurs as a result of tuberculosis, typically found in the immigrant and prison populations, and people with acquired immunodeficiency syndrome (AIDS). Constrictive pericarditis also may develop secondary to surgery, uremia, or radiation. The fibrosis causes scarring and thickening of the pericardium, which decreases cardiac filling and contracting, leading to decreased cardiac output and heart failure.

Clinical Manifestations

Pain from pericarditis varies among patients with symptoms, ranging from mild to severe. The pain usually comes on suddenly,

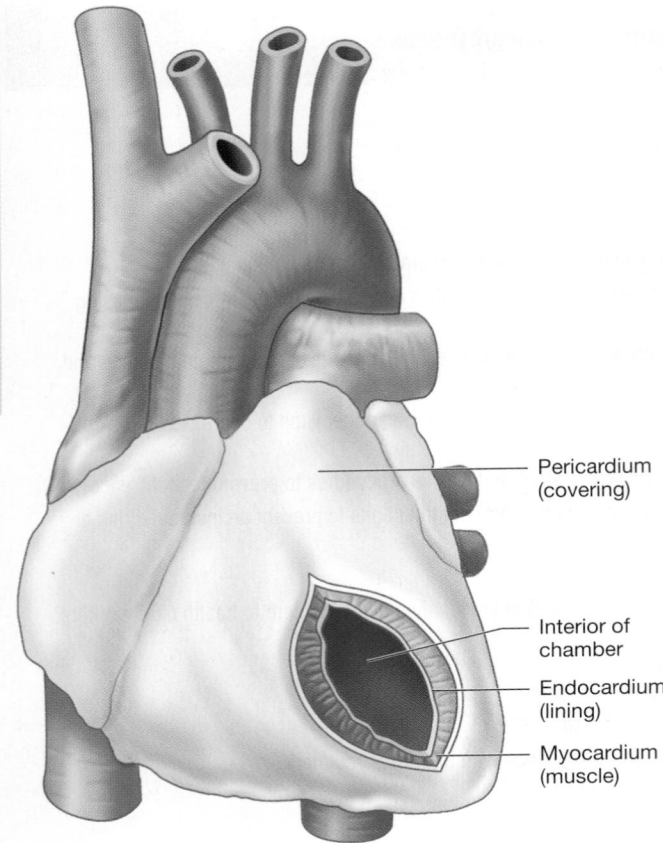

- Pericardium (covering)
- Interior of chamber
- Endocardium (lining)
- Myocardium (muscle)

FIGURE 41–2 ■ Layers of the heart wall.

often on the left side of the chest and radiates to the left shoulder, neck, and back. Some patients describe the pain in the same terms as anginal-type chest pain, while others describe it as a sharp pleuritic type pain. One way to differentiate the pain of pericarditis from angina is that it becomes worse with inspiration, coughing, movement of the trunk, and deep breathing. It also typically is worse when the patient is lying flat and tends to decrease when sitting up and leaning forward, when the heart is moved away from the diaphragmatic side of the lung pleura. This is often the key to the diagnosis. The chest pain often causes the patient to have dyspnea. Other causes of dyspnea also include compression of the bronchioles from the inflamed heart and fever.

The onset of bacterial pericarditis is associated with high fever (39.4°C [103°F]), chills, leukocytosis, malaise, joint pain, and a rise in the erythrocyte sedimentation rate (ESR). Anorexia, weight loss, and nausea also accompany the acute stages of the disease.

Electrocardiogram (ECG) changes also occur with pericarditis. ECG changes may include transient PR interval depression, tachycardia, bradycardia, and atrial fibrillation. Concurrent with the onset of chest pain, ST segment elevation in leads I, II, aVF, V_4, and V_6 occurs, followed by T wave inversion without Q wave changes. The T wave remains inverted for weeks to months later. ECG changes evolve over a period of weeks to months and are thought to be caused by superficial myocardial inflammation or epicardial injury. See Chapter 38 🔗 for a complete description of these ECG changes. Finally, the overall amplitude of the QRS complexes is typically decreased.

RISK FACTORS for Pericarditis

Infectious	Bacterial: tuberculosis, streptococcus, staphylococcus, meningococcus, syphilis, pneumococcus, Lyme disease Viral: coxsackie virus B, echoviruses, endoviruses, adenoviruses, HIV, hepatitis Fungal Parasitic
Noninfectious	Chest trauma or injury Cardiac surgery Uremia Radiation therapy Cancer that has metastasized to the pericardium Acute myocardial infarction (AMI) (48–72 hr) Dissecting aortic aneurysm
Hypersensitive or autoimmune	Systemic lupus erythematosus Rheumatoid arthritis Scleroderma Polyarteritis nodosa Ankylosing spondylitis Myxedema MI (1–4 weeks, Dressler's syndrome) Drug reactions: procainamide, hydralazine, minoxidil

Source: American Heart Association. (2006c). *Sudden cardiac death.* Retrieved June 14, 2006, from http://www.americanheart.org/presenter.jhtml?identifier=4741.

A **pericardial friction rub** is a key factor in the diagnostic assessment of a patient being evaluated for pericarditis. Friction rubs are described as a grating, scraping, squeaking, or crunching sound that is the result of friction between the roughened, inflamed layers of the pericardium. These sounds are best heard over the left sternal border in the 2nd, 3rd, or 4th intercostal space with the diaphragm of the stethoscope. The sounds become louder when the patient is sitting up and leaning forward. One way to distinguish it from a pleural friction rub is to ask the patient to momentarily hold her breath; if the rub persists, it is cardiac in nature. Pericardial friction rubs are often transient and may vary in intensity from hour to hour (Desai, 2002).

Pericardial effusion, an excess of pericardial fluid, is a threat to normal cardiac function. The fluid buildup in the pericardial sac is a result of an accumulation of infectious exudates or toxins, and/or blood. The clinical manifestations depend on the rate and amount of fluid collecting in the area. If the buildup is gradual, the pericardial sac will stretch and accommodate 1 to 2 liters without causing cardiac compression. Conversely, a rapid buildup of fluid does not allow the pericardial sac to stretch and, therefore, cardiac compression will occur with only 80 to 200 mL of fluid. If a pleural effusion is present, heart sounds are typically muffled and may be difficult to auscultate. Large effusions compress adjoining structures in the pleural cavity (e.g., pulmonary compression causes coughing, dyspnea, and tachypnea). Compression of the laryngeal nerve causes hoarseness, and compression of the phrenic nerve may induce hiccups (Desai, 2002).

Cardiac tamponade occurs when there is a rapid and large accumulation of fluid in the pericardial space. This is a medical emergency that is caused most frequently by bleeding, either from postoperative complications (thoracic surgery) or trauma. It also can be from an accumulation of pus or air and may be present with any type of pericarditis. This large collection of fluid raises the pressure in the pericardial sac, compressing the cardiac chambers, and prevents blood from entering the heart. Blood backs up into the venous system, raising venous pressure, while cardiac output and blood pressure fall because of a lack of blood filling the heart (decreased preload). See Chapter 24 for a complete explanation of preload. The drop in cardiac output and subsequent loss of tissue perfusion make this a life-threatening situation. The nurse must have knowledge of the clinical manifestations of cardiac tamponade and know how to intervene to prevent shock and death.

Clinical manifestations associated with tamponade are related to the decreased cardiac output and increased systemic venous congestion. A narrowing of the pulse pressure (systolic minus diastolic blood pressure to less than 30 mmHg) and tachycardia are hallmark signs of cardiac tamponade. The heart is attempting to compensate for the drop in cardiac output by increasing the rate. Without adequate preload, the increased rate cannot maintain a normal cardiac output, and the increased cardiac workload will lead to failure. Classic assessment findings for the patient with cardiac tamponade are referred to as **Beck's triad**, consisting of decreased blood pressure (BP), muffled heart sounds, and jugular venous distention. Additionally, weak peripheral pulses, and pulsus paradoxus are also present. A **pulsus paradoxus** is a greater than 10 mmHg drop in systolic BP during inspiration. The BP normally decreases during inspiration but does so by less than 10 mmHg. A paradox of greater than 10 mmHg is present when there is increased thoracic pressure as a result of pericardial swelling. This is an important diagnostic clue most frequently picked up by the nurse. The patient typically becomes restless and may have a decreased level of consciousness as the fluid accumulates and the cardiac output drops. Finally, the amplitude of the QRS complex of the ECG is low.

 CRITICAL ALERT *The sudden onset of pulsus paradoxus is an indication that cardiac tamponade is occurring. The patient needs to be assessed for other signs of tamponade: tachycardia, diminished heart sounds, narrowed pulse pressure, and distended neck veins. The health care provider needs immediate notification to institute diagnosis and treatment. Cardiac tamponade is a life-threatening complication of pericardial effusion.*

Laboratory and Diagnostic Procedures

The patient's clinical manifestations and diagnostic and laboratory tests are used to confirm the diagnosis of pericarditis. There are no specific laboratory tests to diagnose pericarditis, but tests are performed to rule out other possible causes of the symptoms. The earlier box titled Diagnostic Tests for Cardiac Inflammatory Disorders (p. 1223) outlines the typical tests that are done to assist in confirming the diagnosis. In addition to the tests outlined in that box, antibody titers, blood urea nitrogen (BUN), and TB testing also are used to help determine the cause. An ECG and serial troponin and cardiac isoenzymes are done to rule out a myocardial infarction (Chapter 40). Computed tomography (CT) scans and

magnetic resonance imaging (MRI) also are used to identify pericardial effusions and/or the pericardial thickening characteristics of constrictive pericarditis (Chapter 39).

Hemodynamic monitoring is used with acute pericarditis to assess pulmonary artery pressures and cardiac output. Elevated central venous pressures and pulmonary artery pressures are seen due to inflammation. Cardiac output is decreased especially in the presence of cardiac tamponade.

A pericardiocentesis, the removal of fluid from the pericardial sac, is both diagnostic and therapeutic when effusion is present. The procedure is performed under sterile conditions with ECG, and hemodynamic monitoring capabilities. A health care provider inserts an 8-inch, 16- to 18-gauge needle into the pericardial sac and the fluid is aspirated (Figure 41–3). The needle is attached to an ECG monitor to guide the depth of needle insertion. Once the needle touches the epicardial surface, ECG changes occur. The health care provider and the nurse observe the ECG monitor for ST segment and T wave changes that indicate the epicardial surface has been reached, and the needle is withdrawn slightly. When the needle is in the proper position, a catheter is placed, and the pericardial fluid is withdrawn. As the fluid drains, the pressures decrease and the clinical manifestations of tamponade begin to resolve. To assist in determining the cause of the pericardial effusion, the pericardial fluid is sent to the laboratory for culture and sensitivity analysis and cytology. If fluid buildup persists, the health care provider may choose to leave a catheter in the pericardium attached to a bag to allow for continuous draining of the fluid.

Medical Management

Medical management is directed toward finding the cause and instituting treatment to prevent complications. Because treatment is specific to the cause, it is essential that the cause of the pericarditis be determined. The diagnostic studies and clinical manifestations outlined above assist with determining the cause.

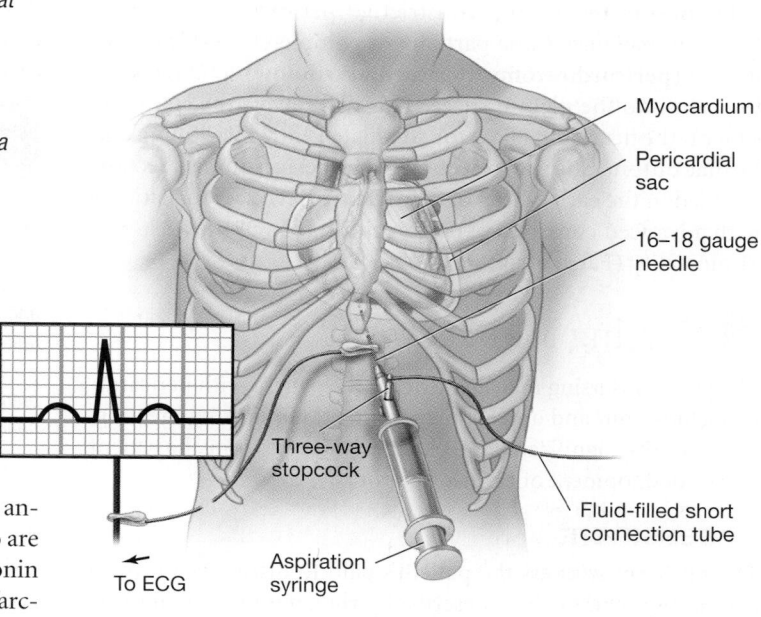

FIGURE 41–3 ■ Pericardiocentesis.

Myocardium
Pericardial sac
16–18 gauge needle
Three-way stopcock
Fluid-filled short connection tube
Aspiration syringe
To ECG

Antibiotic treatment is indicated if it is a bacterial infection and steroids are used when the pericarditis is secondary to systemic lupus erythematosus (SLE), a myocardial infarction (MI), or other immune system conditions. There is no specific curative treatment for viral pericarditis. It typically clears in 2 weeks to 3 months and symptom control treatments are indicated. Drugs known to treat tuberculosis are indicated if that is the cause of the pericarditis. If renal failure is the cause, more frequent and intense dialysis treatments are needed.

Pain must be assessed in order to differentiate pericarditis from a myocardial infarction, because treatment for myocardial infarction is time sensitive and would be contraindicated with pericarditis (Chapter 40 ☺). Pain control is managed with NSAIDs such as indomethacin (Indocin), ibuprofen, and aspirin in large doses. In addition to their analgesic properties, these medications reduce swelling. See the Pharmacology Summary (p. 1236) on medications to treat inflammatory heart disease.

Activity restriction is necessary until the swelling begins to subside and the pain is effectively managed. Bed rest is indicated with the head of the bed elevated to reduce cardiac workload. Symptoms and activity tolerance will dictate when increased activity is appropriate. Oxygen may be needed in the acute stages or in the presence of pericardial effusion. ECG monitoring is necessary to monitor for cardiac dysrhythmias and myocardial injury.

Because cardiac tamponade is a life-threatening complication of pericarditis, assessing for it is critical to patient survival. A pericardiocentesis is done to relieve the constricting effects of cardiac tamponade, and is indicated when the patient's blood pressure has decreased by 30 mmHg. Hemodynamic and ECG monitoring are necessary during and after the procedure to assess the patient's hemodynamic status. The amount of fluid removed is recorded on the output record in the patient's chart. Fluid replacement after pericardiocentesis is needed to increase cardiac output and tissue perfusion. Complications from a pericardiocentesis include dysrhythmias, pneumothorax, myocardial laceration, cardiac tamponade, and gastric fistula.

If recurrent effusions and tamponade occur or if there are adhesions from chronic constrictive pericarditis, the pericardium may have to be partially or completely surgically removed (**pericardiectomy**, **pericardial window**) to allow fluid to drain into the pleural space. This will relieve the compression on the heart and allow for adequate ventricular filling and cardiac output. Surgical resection of the pericardium is recommended in the early stages of constrictive pericarditis. Patients with advanced constrictive pericarditis have a 5% to 15% risk of mortality (Fauci et al., 1998).

◼ Nursing Management

The goals of nursing management for the patient with pericarditis include pain and anxiety management; monitoring, treating, and reporting significant ECG changes; and evaluating the patient for the development of cardiac tamponade.

Assessment

The nurse must assess the patient's pain to distinguish it from angina-type chest pain as described earlier. It is important to assess the pain for the amount, quality, and location, to differenti-

ate it from the pain of an acute myocardial infarction. The ECG is monitored during pain because ST segment changes seen with an AMI are only seen in certain leads depending on the location of the infarction, whereas ST segment changes seen with pericarditis are present in all leads except aVR and V_1. Additionally, the patient is assessed for the clinical manifestations of cardiac tamponade including a decreased BP, muffled heart sounds, jugular venous distention, weak peripheral pulses, and pulsus paradoxus.

Nursing Diagnosis

Actual and potential nursing diagnoses related to pericarditis include:

- *Cardiac Output, Decreased*
- *Tissue Perfusion, Ineffective*
- *Anxiety*
- *Activity Intolerance*
- *Pain, Acute*

Outcomes and Evaluation Parameters

The desired outcomes for the patient with pericarditis include absence of pain and normal cardiac output. Finding and treating the cause will result in a relief of symptoms. Medical intervention with a pericardiocentesis, as described earlier, may be a lifesaving measure. Evaluation parameters include normal heart rate and blood pressure as well as a balanced intake and urine output. There should be an absence of any unusual fatigue and shortness of breath.

Planning, Interventions, and Rationales

Administration of the anti-inflammatory analgesics is essential, and helping the patient find a position of comfort also helps relieve the pain. Sitting up and leaning forward on a table in order to give the heart more room in the pleural cavity is typically the most comfortable position. A warm heating pad or hot water bottle also may help relieve the pain. Pain relief measures include elevating the head of the bed and administering anti-inflammatory agents as ordered.

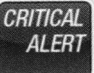 **CRITICAL ALERT** *When a patient complains of chest pain, it is essential that an assessment be done to determine if the pain is anginal-type pain associated with myocardial ischemia or if the pain is due to pericarditis. Anginal pain is typically described as a burning, pressure-type pain that is not associated with position change or deep breathing. It is relieved by nitroglycerin and rest.*

The chest pain associated with pericarditis is often described as sharp and gets worse with deep breathing. It is relieved by sitting up and taking anti-inflammatory drugs.

The ECG needs to be assessed for ST segment changes associated with both types of pain. If the pain is unrelieved, the nurse needs to notify the health care provider for further orders.

Nursing management of the patient during and following a pericardiocentesis includes monitoring the patient's response to the procedure. The nurse monitors the pulmonary artery, right atrial central venous pressure (CVP), pulmonary wedge pressures (Chapter 24 ☺), and the ECG during and after the procedure. As the effusion is relieved, the CVP and pulmonary artery wedge pressure will decrease and the blood pressure will increase. The amplitude of the QRS complex also increases as the pressure is relieved. Vital signs and urine output provide information about cardiac output and typically are monitored every 15 to 30 minutes for the first hour, then every 30 minutes for 1 hour, and then every hour for the first 24 hours. The amount of fluid removed is recorded on the output record and, if ordered, a specimen is sent to the laboratory for analysis. It is essential that the patient be monitored closely for a recurrence of tamponade. If the clinical manifestations prior to the pericardiocentesis return, a recurrence is suspected and the health care provider is immediately notified. The patient's anxiety is typically reduced when they are informed of what to expect in terms of clinical manifestations and treatment. The patient may require an antianxiety agent.

The remainder of the care is outlined in the Nursing Process: Patient Care Plan for Inflammatory Heart Disease feature (p. 1224).

Health Promotion

Health teaching for patients with pericarditis focuses on prevention. Teaching about the return clinical manifestations and when to seek medical help is essential. Identifying risk factors specifically related to the cause and outlining how to mitigate them will also help with disease prevention. The Patient Teaching & Discharge Priorities for Inflammatory Heart Disease box outlines specific patient teaching and discharge priorities (p. 1227).

◼ Myocarditis

Myocarditis, a focal or diffuse inflammation of the myocardium or heart muscle, is an uncommon disorder that is frequently associated with pericarditis. The myocardium is the middle muscular layer of the heart. Its function is to provide the pumping action that propels the blood through the heart and into the peripheral circulation. Cardiac muscle contraction, referred to as systole, is when the blood is pumped out of the heart. Systole is followed by muscle relaxation or diastole, when blood flows into the cardiac chambers. Myocardial dysfunction can be systolic, diastolic, or both. Myocarditis affects the heart's ability to pump blood normally, thereby affecting cardiac output. Most cases of myocarditis originate from a viral infection, and often remain undiagnosed, due to the general lack of initial symptoms. In some cases the disease presents as an acute catastrophic illness requiring immediate attention. Myocarditis may be mistaken for ischemic, valvular, or hypertensive heart disease and can be both acute and chronic.

Epidemiology and Etiology

The incidence of myocarditis in the United States is estimated to be 1 to 10 per 100,000 people. It can occur at any age and is more common in men. Viral infections are the most common cause of myocarditis, followed by bacterial and fungal infections. Approximately 1% to 5% of patients with acute viral infections have myocardial involvement (Howes, 2008). A genetic predisposition for myocarditis is under investigation. Immunosuppressed patients are at a higher risk. Approximately 10% of patients with HIV develop myocarditis because the virus infiltrates the myocardium. The Risk Factors box outlines the infectious and noninfectious risk factors and causes of myocarditis. The occurrence of myopericarditis following a smallpox vaccination was investigated

RISK FACTORS and Causes of Myocarditis

Risk Factors	Autoimmune and connective tissue diseases
	Drug hypersensitivity or toxicity
	Sarcoidosis
	Hypersensitive immune reactions such as rheumatic fever
	Postcardiotomy syndrome
	Toxins
	Chemicals
	Alcohol use
	Nosocomial infections
	Large doses of radiation to the chest for treatment of malignancy
Causes	
Viral Infection	Coxsackie B virus accounts for 50% of the cases
	Coxsackie A virus
	Adenovirus
	Echovirus
	Mumps
	Rubella
	Influenza A and B
	Epstein-Barr
	Hepatitis
	HIV
	Hepatitis C
	Poliovirus
Bacterial infection	Diphtheria
	Typhoid fever
	Staphylococcus
	Pneumococcus
	Tuberculosis
	Tetanus
Fungal infection	Chagas' disease (South and Central America)
	Toxoplasmosis

using a sample of 230,734 first-time vaccinees. The results indicated that there were 18 cases of confirmed myopericarditis after a smallpox vaccination, an incidence of 7.8 cases per 100,000 per 30 days. No cases of myocarditis occurred in the group of 95,662 vaccinees who had previously been vaccinated. All cases were white males, ages 21 to 33 years, who presented with acute myocarditis 14 to 21 days after the vaccination (Halsell et al., 2003).

Pathophysiology

Myocarditis is an inflammatory disorder resulting from the causes outlined in the Risk Factors and Causes of Myocarditis box that typically occurs several weeks after the initial infection. The inflammatory process causes an infiltrate to build up in the cardiac myocytes, resulting in injury to the myocardial cells. Infectious agents infiltrate myocardial tissues, forming abscesses, and an autoimmune injury may occur when the immune system destroys both the invading organism and myocardial cells. The extent of damage determines the long-term effect on heart function. The majority of infections are self-limiting, and often subclinical, although severe or repeated infections may cause progressive deterioration in cardiac function. The most severe cases develop into cardiomyopathy, described later in this chapter.

Clinical Manifestations

The clinical manifestations of myocarditis vary, ranging from no overt clinical symptoms to severe heart involvement. Mild signs and symptoms include fatigue, malaise, shortness of breath, fever, gastrointestinal upset, and aching joints—very similar to flu symptoms. In contrast, myocarditis may appear suddenly with manifestations of heart failure or sudden cardiac death without prior symptoms. Symptoms of heart failure are discussed more thoroughly in Chapter 42 ⬛. When myocarditis and pericarditis occur simultaneously, manifestations may include a pericardial friction rub, chest pain, and a pericardial effusion. Blood clots on the heart wall (mural thrombi) may develop if blood stasis is present. Early cardiac symptoms typically appear 7 to 10 days after the initial infection.

Laboratory and Diagnostic Procedures

Several laboratory tests are done to diagnose both the cause and extent of the disease process with myocarditis. An evaluation of presenting symptoms followed by a thorough history and physical will determine the need for diagnostic and laboratory studies. The tests that assist in determining a definitive diagnosis are discussed in the Diagnostic Tests for Cardiac Inflammatory Disorders box (p. 1223). The WBCs must be monitored for elevations when diagnosing the disorder as well as periodically if symptoms reappear or worsen. Mild to moderate leukocytosis with atypical lymphocytes is common.

Medical Management

The primary aim of medical management for myocarditis is early diagnosis and treatment to mitigate the damage to the myocardial cells. Finding the cause and instituting timely and appropriate treatment is the cornerstone of the medical management for the patient with myocarditis. A complete history and physical including an assessment of the risk factors is indicated along with the diagnostic studies described above. Bed rest, a quiet environment, and a semi-Fowler's position are measures that decrease metabolic demand and reduce myocardial workload. Activity restrictions of varying levels depending on clinical manifestations may continue for up to 6 months. Oxygen may be needed when heart failure symptoms are present in the setting of hypoxemia. Medications for treating myocarditis include the following:

- Immunosuppressive therapy includes the use of steroids to prevent cardiac damage when the cause is autoimmune myocarditis.
- Antimicrobial medications are used when the myocarditis is caused by a bacterial infection.
- ACE inhibitors (or angiotensin receptor blockers), beta-adrenergic-blockers, digoxin, and diuretics are used if heart failure with left ventricular dysfunction occurs. See the Critical Alert regarding the use of digoxin with myocarditis.
- Antidysrhythmic medications are indicated to treat the dysrhythmias.
- Anticoagulants are used to prevent thromboembolism from mural wall blood clots.
- Antianxiety agents may be necessary for patients who are anxious due to the sudden onset heart disease and its impact on the quality of their life.

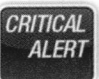 **CRITICAL ALERT**
- Digoxin: *Patients with myocarditis are sensitive to the effects of digoxin. Digoxin increases the force of cardiac contractions, thus, increasing the workload and oxygen demand of the heart muscle. These patients must be monitored closely for heart failure. Vital signs, lungs sounds, increasing shortness of breath, and peripheral edema need to be monitored on a frequent and ongoing basis.*
- NSAIDs: *The use of NSAIDs with myocarditis is contraindicated because they appear to increase cardiac damage.*

See the Pharmacology Summary of medications to treat inflammatory heart disease (p. 1236).

The prognosis for myocarditis caused by viral infections is excellent. Scarring and permanent myocardial damage from myocarditis vary from none to severe heart failure leading to death or requiring a heart transplant.

⬛ Nursing Management

The aim of nursing management is to rest the heart as much as possible. These patients are placed on strict bed rest and allowed minimal activities until the cause has been identified and treatment instituted. Increasing the level of activity can only progress when the symptoms subside with successful treatment.

Assessment and Nursing Diagnosis

Nursing assessment focuses on the clinical manifestations of heart failure. Alteration in cardiac output and altered tissue perfusion are the two sentinel nursing diagnoses for these patients.

The majority of patients experiencing myocarditis make a complete recovery without residual complications. Note, however, that cardiomyopathy can be a long-term complication of myocarditis. Nursing management and patient education are pivotal in preventing complications.

Outcomes and Evaluation Parameters

The desired outcomes for the patient with myocarditis include absence of pain and normal cardiac output. Finding and treating the cause will result in a relief of symptoms. Evaluation parameters include normal heart rate and blood pressure as well as a balanced intake and urine output. There should be an absence of any unusual fatigue and shortness of breath.

Planning, Interventions, and Rationales

As with other cardiac inflammatory diseases, resting the heart by spacing activities and by providing pain relief, emotional support, and a quiet environment will promote healing and assist in preventing compactions. As the patient's condition allows, active and passive range-of-motion exercises will help the patient regain strength and joint motion and should be performed regularly until activity levels increase. The nurse must teach the patient to avoid excessive fatigue and stop all activities immediately when light-headedness, dyspnea, or faintness occurs. Changes in activity restrictions are based on the patient's tolerance and the occurrence of clinical manifestations.

The remainder of the nursing management is outlined in the Nursing Process: Patient Care Plan for Inflammatory Heart Disease feature (p. 1224).

Health Promotion

Patient teaching goals focus on having the patient make a full recovery and preventing long-term complications. Gradually increasing activity levels promotes muscle tone and strength. The patient must be taught to stop activity and revise the plan if clinical manifestations recur. Additionally, it is essential for the nurse to outline the specific manifestations of heart failure and reinforce that the patient must seek medical care when they occur. Discharge medications need to be discussed and the nurse must assess the patient's understanding of the regimen. Specific discharge planning is outlined in the Patient Teaching & Discharge Priorities for Inflammatory Heart Disease box (p. 1227).

■ Endocarditis

Infective endocarditis (IE), previously known as bacterial endocarditis, is an infection of the cardiac endocardial layer of the heart, which may include one or more heart valves, the mural endocardium, and/or a septal defect. The endocardium is the inner lining of the heart and it is contiguous with the heart valves. Thus, an infection or inflammation of the endocardium affects the heart valve function. Figure 41–2 ■ (p. 1228) identifies the endocardium. IE is a life-threatening disease that occurs most often in persons with structural abnormalities of the heart or great vessels, but it also can occur with normal hearts.

There are two types of IE, acute and subacute. With acute IE the onset of symptoms is rapid, often in individuals with normal heart valves, and if untreated can lead to death within days to weeks. Acute IE is usually caused by a virulent organism and is more likely to follow infections of the respiratory, gastrointestinal, and genitourinary tracts, and following open heart surgery.

Subacute IE is the more common form and is usually caused by organisms of low virulence that have a limited ability to infect other organs. It is present in an inactive state for long periods of time in people with preexisting valve disease. It often becomes symptomatic after dental work or with an invasive procedure, but usually responds well to treatment.

Infective endocarditis is classified according to the causative organism, with hemolytic streptococci being the most common. Other causes and predisposing factors are outlined later in the Risk Factors box (p. 1234). The increasing use of contaminated needles by individuals using illegal intravenous (IV) drugs has increased the number of cases of IE in recent years. There is a high risk of bacteremia for these individuals due to the insertion of a contaminated needle into the venous blood. The tricuspid valve is the most frequently affected valve with IV drug use, especially cocaine use.

Epidemiology and Etiology

The incidence of IE continues to rise, with 15,000 to 20,000 new cases reported annually. Thus, IE is now the fourth leading cause of life-threatening infectious disease syndromes (after urosepsis, pneumonia, and intra-abdominal sepsis) (American Heart Association [AHA], 2006a). Internationally, the incidence of the disease is similar throughout developed countries. The greatest risk factor for the development of IE is preexisting heart damage. Infective endocarditis affects males twice as often as females and is distributed throughout all age groups. The mean age of patients has gradually risen during the last 50 years and cur-

rently more than 50% of the patients are greater than 50 years of age (Brusch, 2005). Infective endocarditis can develop in anyone and the most frequent bacteria are usually found in the mouth, intestinal tract, or urinary system. Nosocomial infections occur most often in patients who are debilitated and have long-term urinary and IV catheters. Patients who are immunosuppressed or who are receiving immunosuppressive therapy are at a higher risk for developing yeast or fungal IE. This population would include both cancer patients, people with human immunodeficiency virus, and IV drug users.

 CRITICAL ALERT Healthy People 2010 *(DHHS, 2004) established an important goal related to U.S. policy for the prevention of substance abuse among youth. The goal is to increase the percentage of young persons who reach adulthood without using tobacco, illicit drugs, or alcohol. Their focus is to strengthen the ability of children and teenagers to reject all such substances. To achieve overall prevention goals,* Healthy People 2010 *supports comprehensive community-based programs that include interventions that influence individual behavior and attitudes through education, and interventions that change environments through controls on the availability of substances. They recommend comprehensive programs that must be applied universally to the general population and in a more intensive fashion to selected and indicated groups and persons known to be at high risk for serious drug problems or to targeted groups of persons already exhibiting early signs of drug use. The prevention programs require coordination among schools, state and local governments, businesses, the faith community, civic groups, and other elements of the community.*

Prosthetic heart valve IE, which may develop in the early postoperative period (60 days or less) or later on (greater than 60 days), accounts for 10% to 20% of the cases. Common infecting organisms for early IE development are staphylococcus, gram-negative bacilli, and *Candida albicans*. *Staphylococcus epidermidis*, streptococci, and enterococci cause the later infections (Marill, 2006). Infective endocarditis affects males over 60 years old most frequently, and occurs most often with mitral valve replacements. Early prosthetic valve IE, usually due to a contaminated valve or preexisting bacteremia, has a rapid onset and high mortality. Late prosthetic valve IE follows the course of subacute IE. The Risk Factors box (p. 1234) outlines the risk factors and Chart 41–2 lists the organisms that cause IE.

Increased mortality is associated with increased age, infection of the aortic valve, development of heart failure, CNS

CHART 41–2	**Etiologic Organisms that Cause Infective Endocarditis**

Staphylococci (*Staphylococcus aureus, S. epidermidis*)

Streptococci (hemolytic streptococci, enterococci, *Streptococcus bovis, S. pneumoniae*)

Gram-negative bacteria (*Escherichia coli, Klebsiella*, pseudomonas)

Haemophilus

Actinobacillus

Cardiobacterium

Eikenella

Kingella

Aspergillus fumigatus

Candida albicans

complications, and other underlying diseases. Mortality rates also vary with infecting organism.

Pathophysiology

Several mechanisms are thought to contribute to the development of endocarditis. First a bacteremia (infection in the blood) occurs usually as a complication of an infection originating somewhere in the body (e.g., urinary tract infection, pneumonia, and cellulitis). Surgical procedures, dental work, and invasive diagnostics such as a colonoscopy also may allow bacteria to enter the bloodstream. Secondly, the narrowed orifice of a damaged valve reduces the movement of blood from the atria to the ventricle, allowing time for bacteria to grow and multiply. This increases the risk of bloodborne bacteria lodging on the endocardial valve surface, forming vegetative growths that adhere to the valve surface. These vegetative growths consist of fibrin, leukocytes, platelets, and the infecting microbe.

The infection spreads and becomes imbedded in the valve matrix, producing thinning and destruction of the valve and its supporting structures and ultimately causing valve dysfunction. Mechanical complications may occur, including rupture of chordae tendineae (Figure 41–4 ■; also see Figure 41–1 ■ (p. 1220) for vegetative growths on a valve surface), development of valve stenosis due to overgrowth of large vegetations, and perforation of a valve leaflet. The organisms then spread from the valve to the myocardium, culminating in myocardial dysfunction and heart failure.

The infection can be on either the right side or the left side of the heart or, in severe cases, both sides. Left-sided IE, which af-

FIGURE 41–4 ■ Cardiac valves, chordae tendineae, and papillary muscle.

fects the mitral valve most often, is more common with bacterial infections and patients with underlying heart disease. Right-sided IE, which affects the tricuspid valve, is primarily a result of IV drug use, and most often is caused by *Staphylococcus aureus*.

The friable vegetative growths on the valves may break off into the circulation causing embolization. Left-sided emboli travel to the systemic circulation affecting the brain, kidneys, spleen, and causing limb infarction. Right-sided emboli travel to the lungs causing pulmonary complications. When the emboli become trapped in the organ, abscesses may form, further spreading the infection and impacting organ function.

Clinical Manifestations

Endocarditis may mimic almost any systemic disease depending on the infecting organism and the associated complications. The signs and symptoms of IE can be nonspecific but may involve many organs, often making it difficult to differentially diagnose. Fever occurs in about 90% of the patients and is typically accompanied by tachycardia, fatigue, malaise, anorexia, weight loss, headache, and chills (Candela, 2002). Bacterial IE is associated with high fevers, shaking chills, and night sweats. Arthralgias, myalgias, back pain, abdominal discomfort, headache, clubbing of fingers, anorexia and weight loss, and a low-grade fever often accompany subacute IE.

The cardiac assessment reveals a heart murmur, usually on the aortic or mitral valves. The mitral murmur is typically a midsystolic regurgitant type, whereas the aortic murmur may be early diastolic. Murmurs are uncommon with right-sided IE, because the pressures on the right side are too low to transmit the sound. (See Chapter 37 ☜ for a complete description of murmurs.) Dyspnea, cough, and chest pain are common complaints, especially if heart failure and decreased cardiac output have occurred. The accumulation of serous, purulent, and/or

RISK FACTORS for Infective Endocarditis

Recent dental surgery

Bleeding gums

Invasive procedures: oral surgery, gynecologic procedures, implantation of a cardioverter-defibrillator, hemodynamic catheters, insertion of an indwelling urinary catheter, or renal shunts

Illegal intravenous drug use

Long-term central line placement

Weakened cardiac valves

Prosthetic heart valve

Previous history of endocarditis

Complex cyanotic congenital heart disease

Urinary tract infection

Pneumonia

Cellulitis

Narrowed valve orifice

Rheumatic fever

Mitral valve prolapse with murmur

Marfan's syndrome

Degenerative valvular lesions

Aortic valve leaflet abnormalities

Asymmetric septal hypertrophy (hypertrophic cardiomyopathy)

Nosocomial infections

HIV

Chest trauma

hemorrhagic fluid in the pericardial sac causes a pericardial effusion and possibly tamponade. Tamponade causes a decrease in cardiac output, leading to shock, heart failure, and death. Heart failure occurs in approximately 50% of the patients with IE. ECG changes may include conduction delays (first-, second-, and third-degree heart blocks), diffuse ST segment changes, and PR interval depression. (Chapter 38 ⊙ describes these and other ECG abnormalities.)

Vascular changes also may occur with IE including these:

- Splinter hemorrhages are black longitudinal streaks on the nail beds.
- Petechiae on the lips, buccal mucosa, palate, ankles, feet, antecubital space, and popliteal areas occur as a result of microembolization of vegetative lesions in these areas.
- Painful, red or purple, pea-size lesions, referred to as Osler's nodes, may be present on the fingertips or toes.
- Janeway's lesions, flat, painless, small, red spots, are found on the palms of the hand and soles of the feet.
- Roth's spots, round white spots surrounded by hemorrhage, may appear on the retina.

Finally, tiny emboli often break off of the heart valve and travel to distant organs, causing clinical manifestations associated with the specific organ: brain, heart, lungs, kidney, and/or spleen. Emboli also may travel to the limbs, interrupting peripheral perfusion. As many as 20% of the cases of IE have focal neurological complaints and stroke syndromes (Marill, 2006).

Laboratory and Diagnostic Procedures

The diagnosis of IE is typically based on a constellation of clinical findings. The history of clinical manifestations is variable, often with vague symptoms, making it difficult to diagnose. The Diagnostic Tests for Cardiac Inflammatory Disorders box (p. 1223) includes the tests used to diagnose IE. In addition to the standard tests described in that box, a positive rheumatoid factor and proteinuria are evaluated because they are present in some cases of IE. The echocardiogram evaluates the presence of thickening and calcification of the pericardium occurring most commonly with bacterial and fungal IE. Transesophageal echocardiography (TEE) is more sensitive than the traditional transthoracic echocardiogram particularly for detecting small vegetative growths and extension of the infection into the myocardial tissue and for assessing prosthetic valve function (Marill, 2006). A description of the TEE procedure and patient preparation is included in Chapter 39 ⊙ . If right-sided IE is suspected, a ventilation/perfusion (V/Q) scan may be useful to evaluate pulmonary function. A CT scan also is useful for localizing the area of the abscess.

Medical Management

Due to the complex nature of IE and its ability to mimic other diseases, diagnosing it is often difficult. Underdiagnosis can lead to clinical catastrophe and death, while overdiagnosis may result in weeks of unnecessary antimicrobial therapy with excessive costs and potentially avoidable drug-related side effects. It is imperative to make a definitive diagnosis and begin a treatment plan in a timely manner. Clinical management is both curative and supportive in nature. The priorities for management of IE are finding the cause and starting treatment to eradicate the infecting organism, minimize valve damage, and prevent heart failure. A thorough health history is required to evaluate risk factors including recent high-risk procedures (see earlier Risk Factors box) that may have precipitated an episode of IE. Most clinicians agree that patients who present with symptoms compatible with IE should be evaluated using the following criteria:

- When symptoms appear, blood cultures are obtained from separate sites that are repeated two to three times over a 24-hour period, and may be kept for up to 3 weeks to determine if the causative organism is slow growing. The cultures may be negative if the patient is currently on antibiotic therapy.
- TEE confirms a mass, abscess, or prosthetic valve damage.
- Clinical manifestations as outlined above include evidence of endocardial involvement.

Hospitalization is usually required for intravenous antibiotics and to administer supportive treatments for the clinical manifestations. Following the blood cultures, antibiotic therapy is initiated with drugs known to be specific to the organisms based on the laboratory sensitivity reports. Various classifications of antibiotics are used, including the penicillins, the cephalosporins, the aminoglycosides, and the antitubercular medications. If the cause is fungal, antifungal agents are used. Often a combination of these drugs is necessary to completely eradicate the organism.

Intravenous antibiotics are continued for 2 to 8 weeks depending on the organism, the blood culture, and the resolution of symptoms. The fibrin covering the vegetative growths protects the colonies from antibiotic therapy; therefore, an extended course of multiple antibiotics is typically required. Prosthetic heart valve IE usually requires combination antibiotic treatment for 6 to 8 weeks. Changes in antibiotic therapy may be necessary if allergic drug-related reactions occur and/or resistance to the medication develops. Resistance is measured by a repeated blood culture and sensitivity. The sensitivity portion of the test provides information about the medications' ability to kill the organism. Peak and trough drug levels also are measured to ensure that therapeutic levels of the drug are being given. Periodic blood cultures are done throughout the course of the illness. If the cultures remain positive, this indicates inappropriate therapy. Medications used to treat inflammatory heart disease are outlined in the Pharmacology Summary feature (p. 1236).

Surgical intervention is required for the following reasons: (1) to repair valvular regurgitation, which causes heart failure and is the most common reason for surgery; (2) to remove large vegetative growths that are at risk for embolization; (3) to treat fungal infections; (4) to replace a severely damaged valve; and (5) to remove a valve (native or prosthetic) that is a continuing source of infection and does not respond to antibiotic treatment. No response after 7 to 10 days of antibiotics is an indication that valve replacement is necessary.

Home care is appropriate once the symptoms are under control and the patient has adequate support systems at home. Intravenous antibiotic therapy can be continued at home once the patient/family has been taught the skills. Outpatient management is not advised for IV drug users due to issues with noncompliance. Patients with prosthetic valves typically stay in the hospital until the infection has resolved.

PHARMACOLOGY Summary of Medications to Treat Inflammatory Heart Disease

Medication Category	Action	Application/Indication	Nursing Responsibility
Inflammatory Heart Disease **Antibiotics** Erythromycin Penicillin Specific type depends on the organism	Inhibits protein synthesis of microorganisms by binding reversibly to a ribosome, thus interfering with transmission of genetic information.	*Rheumatic fever:* treats Lancefield group A beta-hemolytic streptococcus. *Pericarditis and myocarditis:* indicated if it is a bacterial infection. *Endocarditis:* indicated if infecting organism is bacterial and prophylactic for invasive procedures and dental work.	Assessment of history of drug allergies prior to administration. Assessment of clinical manifestations of allergic reaction. Assessment of relief of clinical manifestations to determine drug effectiveness. Patient education regarding need to complete the entire regimen and report any clinical manifestations of drug allergy.
Nonsteroidal Anti-Inflammatory Agents (NSAIDs) Indomethacin (Indocin) Ibuprofen Aspirin	Inhibits cyclooxygenase, an enzyme responsible for the formation of prostaglandins. When cyclooxygenase is inhibited, inflammation and pain are reduced.	*Rheumatic fever:* joint pain and fever. *Pericarditis:* chest pain and swelling. *Myocarditis:* pain. *Endocarditis:* fever.	Assess pain before and after administration to determine effectiveness. Medications should not be taken on an empty stomach. Monitor renal and liver function tests for abnormalities related to drug side effects. Assessment of bleeding and gastric ulcer development.
Steroids Solu-Cortef Cortisone Solu-Medrol	Stabilizes leukocyte lysosomal membrane; inhibits phagocytosis and release of allergic substances; reduces capillary dilation and permeability. Modifies immune response to various stimuli.	*Myocarditis:* to prevent cardiac damage when the cause is autoimmune.	Careful assessment of relief of clinical manifestations. Assessment of side effects: Infection due to depressed immune response. Blood glucose monitoring. Gastric bleeding. Emotional lability. Lack of wound healing. Patient education regarding need to eventually reduce dosage.
Cardiac Medications ACE inhibitors: Lisinopril Enalapril Ramipril Captopril	ACE inhibitor: Lowers peripheral resistance and reduces blood volume by enhancing the excretion of sodium by inhibition of angiotensin-converting enzyme.	*Myocarditis:* heart failure. *Rheumatic fever, pericarditis, and myocarditis:* to control atrial and ventricular dysrhythmias caused by inflammation and stretching of myocardium.	Monitor blood pressure carefully after first dose for hypotension. Educate patient that it takes 2 weeks for therapeutic effect. May experience dizziness.
Antiarrhythmic Agents Adenosine Amiodarone Atropine sulfate Sotalol	Alters the electrophysiological properties of the heart by either blocking flow through the channels or altering autonomic activity.	To control dysrhythmias.	There is a narrow margin between therapeutic effect and toxicity; therefore, careful and ongoing cardiac monitoring is essential. Patient teaching includes avoiding the use of alcohol, drugs, and tobacco.
Diuretics Furosemide Torsemide	Blocks reabsorption of sodium and chloride in the loop of Henle. Reduces edema associated with heart failure.	*Myocarditis:* heart failure.	Potassium levels also need monitoring because low levels are a side effect of certain diuretics, especially furosemide. May need potassium replacement. Measure urine output prior to administration to gauge the response to the medication.

PHARMACOLOGY Summary of Medications to Treat Inflammatory Heart Disease—*Continued*

Medication Category	Action	Application/Indication	Nursing Responsibility
Anticoagulant Therapy Coumadin Heparin Aspirin	Can either inhibit specific clotting factors in coagulation cascade or diminish the clotting action of platelets.	*Myocarditis:* to prevent thromboembolism from mural wall blood clots.	Ongoing assessment of therapeutic blood level per health care provider orders. Assess for bleeding including nosebleeds, bruising, "coffee-grounds" emesis, tarry stools, fatigue, and pale skin. Assess for decreases in hemoglobin, hematocrit, RBCs, and platelets.
Antianxiety Agents Valium Versed Xanax	Acts by binding with the gamma-aminobutyric acid (GABA) receptor-chloride channel molecule. This intensifies the effect of GABA, which is a natural inhibitory neurotransmitter.	*Rheumatic fever, pericarditis, myocarditis, and endocarditis:* may be necessary for anxiety-onset heart disease and its impact on the quality of life.	Assess patient's anxiety levels and ability to sleep. Assess for excessive sleepiness and respiratory depression as side effects.

Sources: Adams, M. P., Josephen, D. L., & Holland, L. N. (Eds.). (2005). *Pharmacology for nurses: A pathophysiologic approach.* Upper Saddle River, NJ: Pearson Prentice Hall; American Heart Association. (2005). *Handbook of emergency cardiovascular care for health providers.* Dallas, TX: Author; Wilson, B., Shannon, M., & Stang, C. (Eds.). (2005). *Nurses drug guide.* Upper Saddle River, NJ: Pearson Prentice Hall.

Prophylactic treatment for all persons who have the medical indications outlined on Chart 41–3 is critical to preventing an episode of IE. Moreover, other behaviors such as IV drug use need to be discussed with a patient who is at high risk for the development of IE. The use of an identification band would be helpful if an emergency situation occurred in which the patient was unable to speak for himself.

CRITICAL ALERT *Education of patients and families needs to stress the importance of informing health care providers of a valve disorder, history of infective endocarditis, or a prosthetic valve each time dental or invasive diagnostic procedures are performed. A medic alert bracelet would be useful.*

The emotional cost to the family and patient also cannot be overemphasized. This is a life-threatening illness, with the potential for permanent cardiac damage that has a significant impact on the quality of life.

Nursing Management

The goals of nursing management for a patient with IE include rest, pain management, and instituting the pharmacologic treatment and measures needed to reduce fever and other associated symptoms such as tachycardia, fatigue, malaise, anorexia, weight loss, headache, and chills. Patients with IE require a comprehensive plan of care. The nursing process serves as a template to develop the plan.

Assessment

Nursing care required for the patients with infective endocarditis includes an ongoing, in-depth physical assessment focusing on the patient's hemodynamic status, level of comfort, coping ability, and support from family or significant others. Nursing assessment is essential in order to prevent life-threatening complications. Frequent monitoring and assessment of trend changes in the vital signs and clinical manifestations will provide the most reliable information about the progress of these diseases. Careful monitoring of cardiac output and oxygenation also is necessary.

Nursing assessments specific to IE include murmurs, embolic events, and skin manifestations. Assessment for new and changing murmurs is essential because such changes indicate valve malfunction and are reportable to the health care provider. Heart sounds are assessed every 8 hours or more frequently if ordered by the health care provider. Assessing for embolic events also is

---

CHART 41–3 **Indications for Prophylactic Antibiotic Therapy with Infective Endocarditis**

Medical Indications	Procedural Indications
Prosthetic heart valve	A dental procedure in which bleeding is likely, including cleaning and extractions
Previous episodes of IE	Periodontal procedures/dental implants
Rheumatic heart disease	Bronchoscopy and/or pulmonary biopsy
Hypertrophic cardiomyopathy	Cystoscopy/colonoscopy
Mitral valve prolapse with regurgitation and murmur	Urinary catheterization when infection is present
Sclerotic aortic valve	Incision and drainage of infective tissue, especially soft tissue
Most congenital heart malformations	Vaginal delivery if infection is present
Surgically constructed systemic-pulmonary shunts or conduits	Most surgeries

Source: Eble, B. E., Reyeds, G., and Wiewall-Winkellmann, J. eMedicine—Endocarditis, Bacterial. http://intranet.santa.lt/thesaurus/REZIDENTUI/Valvular/endocarditis%20bacterial%20child.htm.

essential in that they may be life/organ threatening. Embolization of the spleen is manifested in localized abdominal tenderness and rigidity, sharp upper left quadrant pain, and splenomegaly. Emboli to the kidneys often cause flank pain, hematuria, and azotemia. Small peripheral blood vessels also may be affected by emboli, causing gangrene. Neurological deficits occur when emboli lodge in the brain, and finally, pulmonary emboli are common with right-sided IE. Skin assessment includes evaluating for splinter hemorrhages on the nail beds; petechiae on the lips, buccal mucosa, palate, ankles, feet, antecubital space, and popliteal areas; Osler's nodes, and Janeway's lesions (late finding).

Nursing Diagnosis

Nursing diagnoses that apply to patients with IE include:

1. Pain, acute
2. Fatigue
3. Altered cardiac output
4. Hyperthermia
5. Infection
6. Tissue perfusion ineffective

Outcomes and Evaluation Parameters

The desired outcomes for the patient with IE include absence of pain and normal cardiac output. Finding and treating the cause will result in relief of symptoms. Evaluation parameters include normal heart rate and blood pressure as well as a balanced fluid intake and urine output. There should be an absence of any unusual fatigue and fever. Education about prevention of a reoccurrence is critical. The patient/family needs to understand the importance of the preventive measures discussed next.

Planning, Interventions, and Rationales

The focus of nursing management is to provide an environment that supports decreasing myocardial oxygen demand and cardiac workload. The patient is encouraged to eat nutritious meals, drink lots of fluid, and rest both mentally and physically. Strict bed rest is only indicated with heart failure but restricted activity is necessary to decrease cardiac workload especially if there is valve incompetence. The nurse must explain the importance of bed rest and activity restriction to the patient and family. The nurse teaches the patient to avoid excessive fatigue and stop all activities immediately when chest pain, light-headedness, dyspnea, or faintness occurs. Changes in activity restrictions are based on the patient's tolerance and the occurrence of clinical manifestations. Fever, which typically persists for several days, is treated with antipyretics, forced fluids, cooling measures, and rest. Intravenous antibiotics and fluids are administered and as the antibiotics treat the infection, the discomfort level will decease.

Emotional support is essential for patients with IE. The patient needs to be given an opportunity to verbalize fears and concerns about a potentially life-threatening cardiac disorder that may cause permanent damage to the heart. Education about the clinical manifestations of heart failure and when it is necessary to seek medical attention also is essential. The Nursing Process: Patient Care Plan for Inflammatory Heart Disease feature (p. 1224) includes an in-depth care plan for patients with IE.

Health Promotion

Patient education includes information on how to avoid infection and making sure the patient knows that health care providers need to be informed that prophylactic antibiotics are necessary prior to the procedures outlined in Chart 41–3 (p. 1237). Patients are taught to use a soft toothbrush and to floss their teeth regularly to protect the gums from bleeding. Overall good hygiene will help prevent the reoccurrence of IE in high-risk patients. The patient must be taught the importance of seeking medical help if there is a return of clinical manifestations. In addition, it is important to stress seeking medical assistance if neurological or pulmonary symptoms occur, because these may indicate a serious complication. The specific education needed for management of the patient at home is outlined in the Patient Teaching & Discharge Priorities for Inflammatory Heart Disease box (p. 1227).

■ Collaborative Management

A collaborative care approach is optimal for management of patients with inflammatory heart disease. These conditions tend to be chronic with recurring remissions and exacerbations, thereby requiring lifelong management. Utilizing a multidisciplinary team approach, including health care providers, nurses, physical and occupational therapists, psychologists/psychiatrists, and pharmacists, will facilitate the best possible quality of life for the patient and the family.

In terms of medical care, in addition to the role of the cardiologist and surgeon, the patient may need psychiatric counseling to assist in lifestyle adjustments necessitated by a chronic disease process. The occupational therapist helps facilitate realistic occupational goals, while the physical therapist assists in the maintenance of optimum conditioning given the activity restrictions. Because much of the treatment for inflammatory cardiac disorders centers on medication, the role of the pharmacist is essential in educating the patient about how to manage the medications and their side effects. In addition to the nursing care described above, the nurse plays a pivotal role in coordinating the efforts of the health care team. In the inpatient setting the nurse facilitates communication between the members of the team and the patient/family. The nurse may also want to explore alternative therapies with the patient, such as music therapy, as discussed in the Complementary and Alternative Therapies box.

STRUCTURAL HEART DISEASE

Abnormalities in the physical structure of the heart impair blood flow and cardiac pumping ability. Therefore, these abnormalities result in decreased cardiac output and tissue perfusion. Structural abnormalities that affect the cardiac valves and heart muscle itself are discussed next.

CARDIAC VALVULAR DISORDERS

There are four valves in the heart: two semilunar valves, the aortic and the pulmonic; and two atrioventricular valves, the tricuspid and the mitral (Figure 41–5 ■). Each valve is located in a strategic position to provide unidirectional blood flow through

COMPLEMENTARY & ALTERNATIVE THERAPIES Music Therapy

Description:

MUSIC THERAPY is a technique that involves multiple senses, including the hands, voice, emotions, mind, and spirit. There are two branches of music therapy: active and passive. An example of active music therapy is a patient with an inflammatory cardiac disorder who plays a musical instrument, or sings alone or with a choir. Active musical expression utilizes both motor and emotional responses. An example of passive music therapy is listening to specific music and/or sounds in order to relax, stimulate, motivate, or soothe the body and mind. Music therapy provides a simple, safe, and effective way to reduce potentially harmful physiological and psychological responses that arise from pain, fear, and anxiety.

Music therapy has been used successfully to decrease patient anxiety and provide better patient outcomes prior to diagnostic cardiac catheterization. Patient anxiety may have various causes, including feeling a lack of caring for them as individuals, excessive wait time before the procedure, and physical discomfort (McCaffrey & Taylor, 2005).

Research Support:

A Chinese study investigated the effect of music on the level of pain in patients undergoing C-clamp application after percutaneous coronary interventions. Surgical pain may create stress that affects physical and mental health. This randomized controlled study was conducted on 43 patients in the intensive care units of two acute care hospitals. Researchers collected both physiological and psychological variables at baseline and at 15, 30, and 45 minutes. At 45 minutes, the music group showed statistically significant reductions in heart rate, respiratory rate, and oxygen saturation than the control participants. The control group did not show these effects. The baseline comparison of the two groups showed no statistically significant differences; however, statistically significant differences in pain scores were found at 45 minutes for participants in the music group compared with the control group. The control group showed statistically significant increases in pain at 45 minutes compared with baseline (Chan et al., 2006).

Recovery time is prolonged due to the effects of anxiety experienced before, during, and after surgery, as this anxiety increases cardiovascular workload. Studies of music therapy as a nursing intervention have shown its ability to reduce anxiety. One randomized control trial evaluated the effect of music therapy on 60 postoperative adults older than 65 years of age. The experimental group listened to music during and after surgery, while the control group received standard postoperative care. Researchers administered the Spielberger State Trait Anxiety Inventory to both groups before surgery and 3 days postoperatively. In addition, mean intubation time was measured in both groups. The group that listened to music had lower anxiety scores and significantly fewer minutes of postoperative intubation after cardiovascular surgery. Researchers concluded that older adults undergoing cardiovascular surgery who listen to music have less anxiety and reduced intubation time than those who do not (Twiss, Seaver, & McCaffrey, 2006).

Children with cardiac disease can also benefit from music therapy. A Brazilian randomized clinical trial with placebo assessed 84 children during the first 24 hours of their postoperative period. The children's ages ranged from 1 day to 16 years. Each child received a 30-minute music therapy session with classical music. The child was then observed at the start and end of the session, and researchers recorded the child's heart rate, blood pressure, mean blood pressure, respiratory rate, temperature and oxygen saturation, plus a facial pain score. The two groups showed statistically significant differences in subjective facial pain scale and the objectives parameters of heart and respiratory rate after the intervention (Hatem, Lira, & Mattos, 2006).

References

Chan, M. F., Wong, O. C., Chan, H. L., Fong, M. C., Lai, S. Y., Lo, C. W., et al (2006). Effects of music on patients undergoing a C-clamp procedure after percutaneous coronary interventions. *Journal of Advanced Nursing, 53*(6), 669–679.

Hatem, T. P., Lira, P. I., & Mattos, S. S. (2006). The therapeutic effects of music in children following cardiac surgery. *Jornal de Pediatria, 82*(3), 186–192.

McCaffrey, R., & Taylor, N. (2005). Effective anxiety treatment prior to diagnostic cardiac catheterization. *Holistic Nurse Practitioner, 19*(2), 70–73.

Twiss, E., Seaver, J., & McCaffrey, R. (2006). The effect of music listening on older adults undergoing cardiovascular surgery. *Nursing in Critical Care, 11*(5), 224–231.

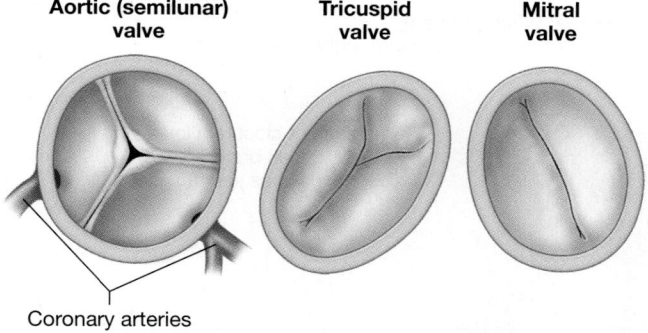

Aortic (semilunar) valve   **Tricuspid valve**   **Mitral valve**

Coronary arteries

FIGURE 41–5 ■ Normal cardiac valve shapes.

the heart (Figure 41–4, p. 1234). According to the AHA (2004), cardiac valve disease is the fifth most common cardiovascular disorder; the first four are coronary artery disease, heart failure, stroke, and hypertension. Although the incidence of rheumatic heart disease, a common causative factor in valve disease, has declined, no significant changes in the prevalence of valve disease have occurred (AHA, 2004). Three factors influence this lack of change:

(1) improvement in the assessment of valvular disorders, (2) an increased number of elderly, and (3) a greater number of recognized cases due to improvement in diagnostic testing technology.

Valvular heart disease is classified according to the valve involved and the functional alterations, which include stenosis and regurgitation. A regurgitant valve is one that is unable to close normally, causing a backward flow of blood, while a stenotic valve is unable to open normally, causing an impedance of blood flow. Valve regurgitation also is referred to as insufficiency or incompetence. When the valve is only mildly regurgitant or stenotic, the heart is initially able to adapt and maintain, but in time, chamber dilation and myocardial muscle hypertrophy occur, causing decreased contractility, reduced cardiac output, and finally heart failure. Valvular heart disease can be congenital or acquired, and it affects people of all ages (Wiegand, 2003). Most congenital valve repairs are performed immediately after birth or during early childhood. Significant advances have been made in the assessment and treatment of both congenital and acquired valve disease in the last several decades. Innovative diagnostic tools, pharmacologic developments, and improved invasive and surgical procedures have enhanced the quality of life for patients with valvular heart disease (Wiegand, 2003). The focus of medical and surgical intervention is to prevent heart failure and serious cardiac muscle damage.

Valvular Stenosis

Valvular stenosis is defined as a fibrotic thickening of the heart valve that causes fusion and calcification of the valve leaflet, resulting in a decrease in the size of the valve orifice (Figure 41–6 ■). The thickened leaflets interfere with the valve's ability to completely open, thus obstructing blood flow through the valve orifice and decreasing cardiac output. Valvular stenosis can occur in the mitral, aortic, and tricuspid valves. The degree of stenosis will determine the reduction in cardiac output and the presence and severity of clinical manifestations. Patients with mild to moderate stenosis are able to maintain cardiac output at rest but become symptomatic with exercise because the heart is unable to respond to the increased need for oxygen.

Valvular Regurgitation

Valvular regurgitation is defined as the inability of a valve to completely close during systole, resulting in a back flow of blood through the incompetent valve orifice into the previous chamber. In response to this, both of the chambers dilate and hypertrophy due to extra workload and the hypoxemia. This leads to progressive chamber failure and a decreased cardiac output. The development of failure is slow but it is the eventual outcome. Valve competence depends on normal leaflets, chordae tendineae, papillary muscles, and the valve annulus. A malfunction in any one of these structures will cause valvular regurgitation. Valvular regurgitation primarily affects the aortic, mitral, and on rare occasions the tricuspid valve and pulmonic valve.

MITRAL VALVE DISEASE

The mitral valve lies between the left atrium and the left ventricle, and controls blood flow between these two structures. Three diseases affect the mitral valve: stenosis, regurgitation, and prolapse. Each of these disorders is discussed next.

Mitral Valve Stenosis

Mitral valve stenosis (MVS), a common disorder of the mitral valve, is a progressive and chronic disease. The mitral valve assumes an abnormal funnel shape due to thickening and shortening of the valve structures as a result of calcification.

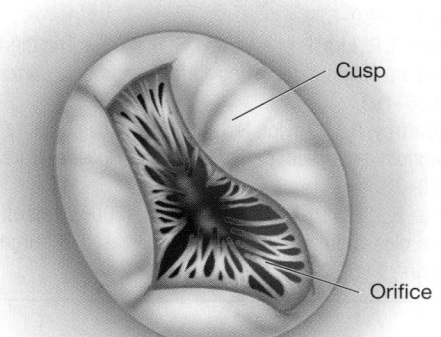

Normal Valve (open)
Normal valve opens widely and blood moves through freely.

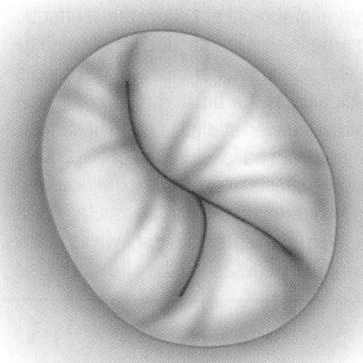

Normal Valve (closed)
Normal valve closes "water tight."

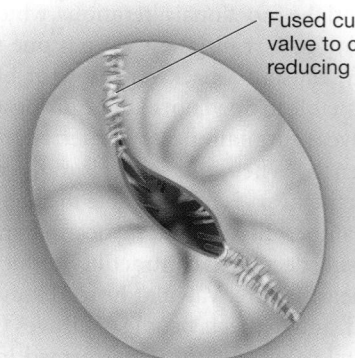

Fused cusps allow the valve to open only partly, reducing blood flow.

Stenosis (open valve)
Stenotic valve is thickened and bound down by scar tissue.

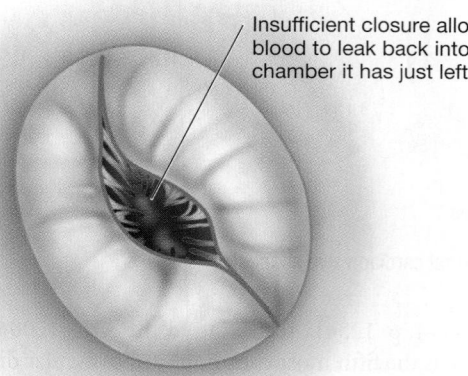

Insufficient closure allows blood to leak back into chamber it has just left.

Regurgitation (closed valve)
Valve leaflets are puckered and pulled apart by scar tissue—valve cannot close.

FIGURE 41–6 ■ Normal versus abnormal stenosed valve.

Contractures develop between the junctions or commissures (leaflets) of the valve (see Figure 41–6 ■). The stenosis narrows the opening of the valve, which obstructs blood flow from the left atrium to the left ventricle. The obstruction may be mild or severe. The normal orifice of a mitral valve is 4 to 6 cm and with stenosis it can become less than 1 cm.

Epidemiology/Etiology/Pathophysiology

Forty percent of persons with rheumatic heart disease develop mitral stenosis, making it the most common cause of this disease. Less common causes include infectious endocarditis, congenital mitral stenosis, rheumatoid arthritis, thrombus formation, calcification of the annulus, atrial myxoma (tumor), and SLE. Mitral stenosis is more common in women (66%) than men (Braunwald et al., 2005).

The inflammatory process caused by the infection results in fibrinous changes in the valve leaflet and chordae tendineae. The chordae tendineae shorten, causing narrowing of the outflow tract. The valve leaflets become fused, immobile, and are unable to completely open. The narrowed opening causes an obstruction to blood flow from the left atrium to the left ventricle during diastole, creating a pressure gradient. The obstruction causes the volume of blood and therefore the pressure to build up in the atrium, eventually backing up into the pulmonary system and causing increased pressure in the pulmonary vasculature. Consequently, it takes more pressure to pump blood and, thus, increases the workload of the heart. Eventually the prolonged rise in pressure and increased cardiac workload causes dilation and hypertrophy of the left atrium. Initially the heart is able to compensate, but eventually pulmonary capillary congestion occurs, causing pulmonary hypertension and subsequent backup into the right side of the heart. The increased pressure in the pulmonary vasculature causes fluid leakage across the alveolar membrane, leading to pulmonary edema. Finally, the increased pressure causes dilation and hypertrophy of the right ventricle and, if untreated, will lead to heart failure.

Clinical Manifestations

The size of the opening of the valve orifice determines the acuity of symptoms, and clinical manifestations depend on cardiac output and pulmonary vascular pressures. The most frequent complaint with mitral stenosis is dyspnea, which results from the pulmonary involvement.

Symptoms typically appear gradually over the course of a 20- to 30-year period and typically begin late in the fifth decade of life. In some cases, if rapid progression occurs, it usually takes 2 to 5 years for symptoms to appear. The early symptoms appear with exercise and in the later stages with rest. Specific clinical manifestations of mitral stenosis are outlined on Chart 41–4 (p. 1242).

■ Mitral Valve Regurgitation

Mitral valve regurgitation (MVR) or mitral insufficiency is defined as an inability of the mitral valve to close due to an abnormality in the structure and function of the valve. Fibrotic changes and calcification of the valve result in an inability to close completely during systole (see Figure 41–6 ■). There are two types of MVR, chronic and acute. In chronic MVR, the left atrium, left ventricle, and pulmonary vasculature dilate to accommodate the chronic volume overload. With acute MVR

there is no chamber or vessel dilation so pressures rise in both the left atrium and ventricle, ultimately backing up into the pulmonary system, causing pulmonary edema.

Epidemiology/Etiology/Pathophysiology

Rheumatic heart disease is the primary cause of MVR and since it is on the decline with early and effective antibiotic treatment, the incidence of MVR also is declining. Mitral valve regurgitation from rheumatic heart disease is more common in women, although MVR from nonrheumatic causes is more common in men. Mitral valve regurgitation often is present with mitral valve stenosis. Other causes of MVR include connective tissue disorders (Marfan's syndrome), congenital valve malformation, coronary artery disease, endocarditis, dilated cardiomyopathy, mitral valve prolapse, amyloidosis, ankylosing spondylitis, and myocardial infarction.

With MVR there is an abnormality of one or more of the valve structures: leaflets, annulus (the valve ring that attaches to the leaflets), chordae tendineae, or papillary muscle. Valve leaflets and the chordae tendineae may shorten or tear, and the annulus may be stretched by heart enlargement to dilation and hypertrophy. Ventricular dilation and scarring from a myocardial infarction cause the papillary muscle to rupture, stretch, or be pulled out of position.

Due to the inability of the mitral valve to close, there is a backward flow of blood into the left atrium during systole. During diastole both the regurgitant blood and the normal blood flow into the ventricle, causing the left ventricle to be overfilled and dilated. This backward movement also increases the pressure in the left atrium and the pulmonary vasculature, resulting in varying degrees of chamber and vessel dilation and hypertrophy. The degree of involvement of these structures is determined by the etiology, severity, and duration of the MVR. For example, the acute MVR that occurs with myocardial infarction causes rupture of the papillary muscle and a sudden increase in left atrial distention and pressure. This increased pressure is transmitted to the pulmonary vasculature, resulting in rapid pulmonary edema and shock. In addition, cardiac output drops, thereby affecting organ and peripheral tissue perfusion. Conversely, in chronic MVR the volume overload on the left ventricle, left atrium, and the pulmonary vasculature allows for dilation and hypertrophy of these structures. Patients typically remain symptom free for several years until the development of left ventricular failure.

Clinical Manifestations

The clinical manifestations of mitral regurgitation depend on the cause and the degree of incompetence. In acute regurgitation, the left atrium has not had time to dilate and therefore the symptoms of pulmonary edema and shock appear quickly. The clinical manifestations of chronic MVR often take years to appear. Atrial fibrillation is a common and potentially deadly dysrhythmia associated with MVR (AHA, 2004). The remainder of the clinical manifestations for both acute and chronic MVR are outlined on Chart 41–4 (p. 1242).

■ Mitral Valve Prolapse

Mitral valve prolapse (MVP) is the most common form of heart valve disease in the United States (also referred to as Barlow's syndrome and floppy valve syndrome). Mitral valve prolapse occurs

CHART 41–4	**Clinical Manifestations of Cardiac Valve Disorders**
Valve/Disorder	**Clinical Manifestation**
Mitral valve stenosis	Atrial fibrillation (occurs 50% of the time), when present, causes an irregular, often weak pulse and a drop in cardiac output and blood pressure.
	Dyspnea, dyspnea on exertion, orthopnea, all due to pulmonary hypertension.
	Low-pitched rumbling crescendo–decrescendo diastolic murmur heard best with the bell of the stethoscope.
	Mural thrombi and stagnate blood found with atrial fibrillation causing embolization.
	Loud first heart sound heard (S_1). An opening snap reflecting high atrial pressures. Sound is best heard with the diaphragm of the stethoscope at the apex of the heart.
	Dry cough, dysphasia, and bronchitis occur due to bronchial irritation from the left atrial enlargement.
	Fatigue and weakness due to decreased cardiac output.
	Clinical manifestations of right-sided heart failure (Chapter 42 ☺).
	Palpitations and angina.
	Crackles in the lung bases.
	Hemoptysis.
Mitral valve regurgitation, acute	Sudden onset of dyspnea, thready peripheral pulses, and cool clammy skin.
	Pulmonary crackles.
	Decreased cardiac output.
	Atrial fibrillation with thrombus formation (occurs 75% of the time).
	Blowing high-pitched, systolic murmur.
	Left- and right-sided heart failure (Chapter 42 ☺).
Mitral valve regurgitation, chronic	Gradual onset of dyspnea, weakness, and fatigue gradually progressing to orthopnea, paroxysmal nocturnal dyspnea, and peripheral edema.
	S_3 and pansystolic (both systole and diastole) murmur at the apex radiating to the left axilla.
	Cough, pulmonary crackles.
	Atrial fibrillation with thrombus formation (occurs 75% of the time).
Mitral valve prolapse	Palpitations and irregular heartbeat.
	Sharp stabbing chest pain, especially during periods of stress.
	Paroxysmal atrial tachycardia, premature ventricular contractions, and ventricular tachycardia, precipitated by stress, caffeine, alcohol, and over-the-counter stimulants.
	Sharp stabbing chest pain usually occurs at rest but may occur with exercise.
	Panic attacks, anxiety, and impending doom.
	Fatigue, weakness, dyspnea.
	Chronically cold hands and feet and paresthesia (numbness and tingling) of arms and legs.
	Pansystolic murmur.
	Midsystolic to late-systolic click heard between S_1 and S_2.
	Light-headedness, dizziness, especially with position change; low blood pressure.
Aortic valve stenosis	Dyspnea, angina, fatigue, and syncope, which increase with exertion and are due to the fixed cardiac output.
	Harsh crescendo–decrescendo systolic murmur heard best in the second intercostal space on the right sternal border and the sound radiates to the carotid arteries. Palpable thrill is present.
	Increased pulmonary artery pressure and decreased cardiac output.
	Prominent S_4.
	Lung congestion.
	Left- and right-sided heart failure (Chapter 42 ☺).
	Palpitations.
Aortic valve regurgitation	High-pitched blowing, crescendo–decrescendo diastolic murmur.
	Decreased diastolic pressure and a widening of the pulse pressure.
	Pistol-shot pulse auscultated over the femoral arteries.
	Some patients have head bobbing with each heartbeat (Musset's sign).
	Palpitations and exaggerated carotid artery pulsations.
	Sudden sharp pulse, followed by a swift collapse of the diastolic pulse (waterhammer pulse).
	Exertional dyspnea, orthopnea, and paroxysmal nocturnal dyspnea.
	Nocturnal angina with diaphoresis.
	Bounding atrial pulse. Apical pulse is displaced to the left.
	Widened pulse pressure with an increased systolic pressure and a decreased diastolic pressure.
	Dizziness and exercise intolerance.
	Angina that occurs mostly at night and may not respond to conventional therapy.
	Left- and right-sided heart failure (Chapter 42 ☺).

CHART 41–4	Clinical Manifestations of Cardiac Valve Disorders—*Continued*
Valve/Disorder	**Clinical Manifestation**
Tricuspid valve stenosis (TVS) and regurgitation (TVR)	TVR: high-pitched blowing systolic murmur heard over the xiphoid area. TVS: low-pitched rumbling diastolic murmur heard best in the fourth intercostal space of the left sternal border. Right-sided heart failure (Chapter 42 🔵). Low cardiac output. Fatigue and weakness. Atrial fibrillation. Prominent waves in the neck veins due to vigorous atrial contraction. If in normal sinus rhythm, there are tall P waves.
Pulmonic valve stenosis (PVS) and pulmonic valve regurgitation (PVR)	Dyspnea and fatigue. PVR: high-pitched diastolic blowing murmur along the left sternal border. PVS: systolic crescendo–decrescendo murmur heard in the second left intercostal space (pulmonic area). Right-sided heart failure (Chapter 42 🔵). PVS: ECG has tall peaked T waves from atrial hypertrophy. Atrial fibrillation is common.

when one or more of the valve leaflets bulge or prolapse into the left atrium during systole (Figure 41–7 ■). This prolapse of the valve essentially results in valvular regurgitation. Varying degrees of valvular incompetence occur depending on the extent of the disorder. In many patients the disease is benign and they remain asymptomatic and undiagnosed; in others, serious complications result.

Epidemiology/Etiology/Pathophysiology

Mitral valve prolapse affects approximately 2% to 6% of the population, is eight times more common in women than men, and may be genetically inherited as a dominant gene (Grau, Pirelli, Yu, Galloway, & Ostrer, 2007). (Genetic predispositions to MVP are discussed in the Genetic Considerations box.) Other causes of MVP include endocarditis, coronary artery disease, myocarditis, connective tissue disorders, cardiomyopathy, hyperthyroidism, and cardiac trauma. The cause can also be idiopathic.

GENETIC CONSIDERATIONS for Mitral Valve Prolapse

There is a genetic predisposition with some forms of mitral valve prolapse. It is associated with Marfan's syndrome, a disorder present from birth, Graves' disease, and connective tissue disorders (University of Maryland, 2005).

MVP can result from abnormalities of the valve leaflets, chordae tendineae, papillary muscles, and left ventricular dysfunction. With MVP the leaflets of the valve are displaced upward into the left atrium during systole when the valve needs to be sealed shut to prevent a back flow of blood (see Figure 41–9 ■, p. 1248). The blood then regurgitates into the left atrium, as seen with mitral regurgitation. Severe mitral regurgitation is a complication of MVP. If progressive worsening of the regurgitation occurs, it can lead to heart failure.

Clinical Manifestations

Sixty percent of patients with MVP never have symptoms, 25% have mild clinical manifestations, 14% have moderate symptoms, and only 1% demonstrates severe symptoms (Orhon-Jech, 1999). Often the onset of symptoms is due to a major physiological stressor such as childbirth, or emotional situations such as divorce or death of a family member. The chest pain that accompanies MVP, which is described as sharp, is not due to inadequate blood flow to the heart muscle, but instead may be due to a stretching of the chordae tendineae and papillary muscle during prolapse. The chest pain may last for hours or days and is not brought on by exertion. Many patients experience panic attacks and a feeling of intense anxiety, and some feel an overwhelming sense of impending doom. The cause of these symptoms is unknown, but some clinicians believe that the anxiety felt during palpitations makes the body more sensitive to the stress hormones, which in turn increase palpitations and release of more stress hormone (Fung, 1999; Woods, Froelicher, & Motzer, 2000). These symptoms can last from a few seconds to a few minutes.

A: Normal

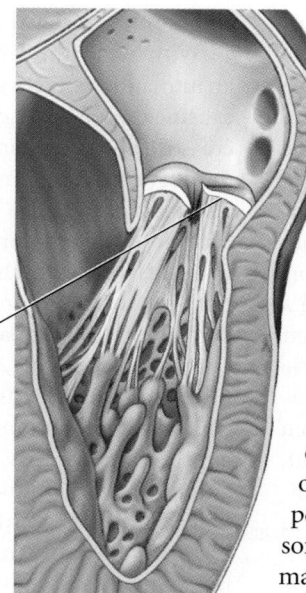
B: Valve prolapse

FIGURE 41–7 ■ Mitral valve prolapse.

If mitral regurgitation is present the patient will present with the associated symptoms. Patients with MVP have no activity restrictions except those mandated by the clinical manifestations. Patient teaching needs to include antibiotic prophylaxis for dental procedures and invasive testing (see Chart 41–3, p. 1237).

AORTIC VALVE DISEASE

The aortic valve lies at the root of the aorta in the left ventricle. It controls blood flow from the left ventricle through the aortic outflow tract into the systemic circulation. Diseases of the aortic valve include stenosis and regurgitation, both of which are discussed next.

◼ Aortic Valve Stenosis

Aortic valve stenosis (AVS) is similar to mitral stenosis in that there is a narrowing of the aortic valve orifice (see Figure 41–6 ◼, p. 1240). This stenosis results in an obstruction to blood flow from the left ventricle to the aorta during systole. AVS is a progressive, chronic disease, and if left untreated has a poor prognosis. Death is caused by sudden cardiac death (10% to 20% of cases) (Braunwald et al., 2005).

Epidemiology/Etiology/Pathophysiology

Causes of aortic stenosis include congenital leaflet malformation, rheumatic endocarditis, and degenerative changes associated with the aging process. It may also be idiopathic. Idiopathic aortic stenosis is typically mild and does not decrease cardiac output. Aortic stenosis is more common in males (80%) than females (Braunwald et al., 2005). In patients less than 30 years old, aortic stenosis is typically caused by a congenital malformation. When aortic stenosis is caused by rheumatic heart disease, typically the mitral valve also is involved and it occurs in persons between the ages of 30 and 70 years. Rheumatic heart disease destroys both valve leaflets with calcification and fibrosis, causing them to become scarred and rigid. In people older than 70 years of age, in the absence of rheumatic heart disease, atherosclerosis and degenerative calcification are the primary causes of aortic stenosis.

With aortic stenosis there is progressive narrowing of the valve orifice, typically over a period of several years or even decades (see Figure 41–6 ◼, p. 1240). The narrowed orifice makes it more difficult for the left ventricle to eject its load of blood. As the valve stenosis progresses, the left ventricle contracts more slowly and less forcibly in an attempt to maintain normal cardiac output. Even though the left ventricle attempts to increase blood flow, the stenotic valve blocks it, producing a fixed cardiac output. Prolonged increased pressure in the left ventricle causes hypertrophy, which is another cardiac muscle compensatory mechanism to maintain cardiac output. The increased cardiac workload results in increased cardiac oxygen consumption. Additionally, due to the decreased cardiac output, coronary artery blood flow is decreased. Thus, both the increased oxygen need and the decreased cardiac output result in myocardial ischemia. As ventricular end-diastolic pressure rises, the left atrial pressure increases and, over time, backs up into the pulmonary vasculature. Pulmonary vascular congestion and pulmonary edema eventually occur. If untreated, eventually pulmonary hypertension and right ventricular failure develop. With fixed cardiac output, the heart is unable to meet the oxygen demands during periods of increased activity and clinical manifestations begin to appear.

Clinical Manifestations

As aortic stenosis progresses, usually over several years, compensation fails, and symptoms begin to appear. Typically, the clinical manifestations begin to appear between the ages of 50 and 70 years and are a result of increased narrowing of the valve orifice and the onset of left ventricular failure. Symptoms generally develop when the valve orifice becomes one-third its normal size. Like mitral stenosis, dyspnea is the most frequent complaint and is usually accompanied by angina and exertional syncope. The clinical manifestations of aortic stenosis are outlined in Chart 41–4 (p. 1242).

◼ Aortic Valve Regurgitation

Aortic valve regurgitation (AVR) is similar to mitral valve regurgitation in that the blood regurgitates back into the left ventricle through a valve that is unable to completely close. This valve incompetence may be due to abnormal valve cusps or aortic root. The increased blood in the left ventricle causes dilation, hypertrophy, and eventually left ventricular dysfunction. Aortic valve regurgitation can be either chronic or acute.

Epidemiology/Etiology/Pathophysiology

The common causes of chronic AVR are rheumatic heart disease (67%), congenital valve malformation, and cardiomyopathy (Braunwald et al., 2005). Less common causes of chronic AVR include connective tissue disorders (Marfan's syndrome), rheumatoid arthritis, ankylosing spondylitis, chronic hypertension, and syphilitic aortitis. Abrupt dilation of the aortic root most commonly caused by a descending dissecting aortic aneurysm causes acute AVR. Other causes of acute AVR are blunt chest trauma and endocarditis. Except in cases caused by rheumatic heart disease, AVR is more common in men (75%) than women. In females it is commonly associated with coexisting mitral valve disease.

With AVR, the left ventricle receives blood from the left atrium and the regurgitant blood coming back from the aorta, causing the left ventricular end-diastolic volume to gradually increase. The regurgitant blood flow is caused by an inability of the aortic valve to close due to inflammation, scarring, and calcification of the valve leaflets from the causes listed earlier. With chronic AVR, as a compensatory mechanism, the left ventricle increases stroke volume in an attempt to increase cardiac output. The increased pressure causes ventricular dilation and hypertrophy (to increase muscle strength). As the condition progresses over time, the left ventricle loses its ability to compensate for the increased workload and cardiac output falls. The clinical manifestations of left ventricular heart failure begin to appear. Untreated, AVR will lead to increased left atrial pressures and dilation, pulmonary hypertension and congestion, and finally right-sided heart failure.

Much like acute mitral valve regurgitation, in acute AVR the left ventricle has not had time to develop the compensatory mechanisms. Therefore, with the extra blood volume the dramatic increase in cardiac workload results in a rapid decline in hemodynamic status, and patients develop fulminant pulmonary edema. If heart failure occurs rapidly, these patients often require emergent lifesaving measures.

Clinical Manifestations

Patients with chronic AVR may remain asymptomatic for as long as 20 years. The first complaints are typically an uncomfortable awareness of a heartbeat or palpitation. This bounding heartbeat is due to the large ventricular stroke volume and rapid diastolic runoff. The hallmark clinical manifestation of AVR is a diastolic murmur heard best at the second right intercostal space (aortic area) and radiating to the left sternal border. The remainder of the clinical manifestations for AVR are listed in Chart 41–4 (p. 1242).

▣ Tricuspid Valve Disease

Tricuspid valve stenosis, which obstructs blood flow between the right atrium and the right ventricle, is an extremely rare and uncommon disorder (see Figure 41–6 ▪, p. 1240). **Tricuspid valve regurgitation** is usually the result of pulmonary hypertension that increases right ventricular volume causing the ventricle to dilate and stretch. This stretching distorts the leaflets, chordae tendineae, and papillary muscle, preventing complete closure of the valve. The low pressure on the right side of the heart decreases the risk of inflammatory changes and calcification associated with high-pressure areas of the heart (left side).

Etiology/Epidemiology/Pathophysiology

Tricuspid stenosis occurs with rheumatic heart disease, IV drug use, and concurrently with mitral stenosis. Like aortic and mitral stenosis, the scarred and fibrosed valve leaflets are unable to completely open, creating the obstruction to blood flow. Right ventricular filling is decreased and right atrial pressure is increased due to the obstruction to blood flow. The right atrium enlarges and increased right atrial pressure is reflected backward into the systemic circulation causing congestion and clinical manifestations of right-sided heart failure. The decreased volume in the right ventricle reduces the blood flow to the lungs and left heart, resulting in a decreased cardiac output and tissue perfusion.

Like aortic and mitral regurgitation, with tricuspid regurgitation there is an inability of the valve to completely close during systole. The valve and its supporting structures become damaged by rheumatic heart disease, inferior myocardial infarction, blunt chest trauma, and infective endocarditis. Volume overload occurs in both the right atrium and right ventricle, causing a decreased cardiac output and right-sided heart failure.

Clinical Manifestations

Tricuspid stenosis increases the pressure in the right atrium, backing blood up into the venous circulation and resulting in right-sided heart failure. Atrial fibrillation is common due to the stretching of the atrium. If present, the patient is at a high risk for thrombus formation. The murmurs heard with both stenosis and regurgitation become more intense with inspiration.

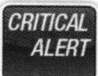
Atrial fibrillation decreases cardiac output by 20% to 25%. If new-onset atrial fibrillation occurs, the nurse needs to assess tissue perfusion in the presence of a decreased cardiac output. Blood pressure, heart rate, respiratory rate, and presence of cyanosis need to be monitored frequently. Notification of the health care provider is necessary so measures can be instituted to terminate the abnormal rhythm (Josephson & McMullen, 2003).

▣ Pulmonic Valve Disease

Like aortic and mitral stenosis, **pulmonic valve stenosis** (PVS) restricts blood flow due to an inability of the valve to completely open (see Figure 41–6 ▪, p. 1240). The blood from the right ventricle is obstructed from flowing into the pulmonary vasculature during systole. With **pulmonic valve regurgitation** (PVR) the valve is unable to completely close, causing blood to regurgitate back into the right ventricle (see Figure 41–6 ▪, p. 1240). Like tricuspid disorders, the pulmonic valve is on the low-pressure right side of the heart; therefore, it is at a lower risk for developing the inflammatory changes and calcification associated with the high-pressure areas of the left side of the heart.

Epidemiology/Etiology/Pathophysiology

Disorders of the pulmonic valve are rare, and are usually caused by a congenital valvular malformation, although endocarditis, tumors, and rheumatic heart disease also have been implicated as causes. Pulmonic regurgitation is slightly more common than pulmonic stenosis and is typically caused by infective endocarditis, pulmonary artery aneurysm, syphilis, and pulmonary hypertension. The pulmonary hypertension dilates the pulmonary orifice, preventing complete valve closure.

With PVS the blood backs up into the right ventricle because of obstruction to blood flow through the narrowed valve orifice. Pulmonic valve regurgitation allows the blood in the pulmonary artery to regurgitate back into the right ventricle due to an inability to completely close. Therefore, both PVS and PVR prevent the blood from reaching the left side of the heart, thereby decreasing cardiac output. The increased blood volume in the right ventricle caused by both disorders increases ventricular volume and pressure, causing dilation and eventually hypertrophy. The final consequence of both disorders is right-sided heart failure (see Chapter 42 ☜).

Clinical Manifestations

Pulmonic valve disease is frequently associated with diseases of other valves. Therefore, the clinical manifestations may be complicated by multiple valve involvement. The clinical manifestations specifically associated with pulmonic valve disease are listed in Chart 41–4 (p. 1242).

CLINICAL MANAGEMENT FOR VALVE DISORDERS

Despite differences in pathophysiology the clinical management of patients with valve disease is similar. As always, the first priority is to find and treat the cause of the disorder and prevent complications and ultimately death. Treatment is based on the involved valve and the severity of the clinical manifestations and disease. Specifically, treatment focuses on preventing recurrent infective endocarditis, heart failure, and thromboembolism. Initially the patient is treated medically, but as the clinical manifestations become more disabling, surgical intervention is considered. Outlined next are the diagnostic studies and medical and surgical interventions for the treatment of valve disease.

Laboratory and Diagnostic Procedures for Cardiac Valve Disease

A heart murmur is usually the first indication of valve disease and once it has been identified by auscultation, diagnostic studies are done to determine the specific valve or valves involved and to confirm the progression of the disease. The most sensitive diagnostic test for valve disease is the echocardiogram because it provides information about the structure and function of the heart valves and enlargement of the chambers that is often a result of malfunctioning valves. It is able to identify thickened valve leaflets, vegetative growths, thrombus, myocardial function, and chamber size. In addition, the echocardiogram is able to measure pressure gradients across valves and pulmonary artery pressures can be estimated. Transesophageal echocardiography (Chapter 39 ✐) is particularly useful not only for diagnosing but also for tracking the progression of the disease (AHA, 2004). A discussion of additional diagnostic tests for cardiac valve disease is included in the Diagnostic Tests box.

Medical Management

Medical management begins with an in-depth history and physical. It is important to remember that a patient with valve disease may suddenly become ill or may slowly develop the symptoms over several years. The history needs to include information about the patient's health history, genetic factors, and social habits, such as IV drug use, that would increase the risk for developing valve disease. Specific questions need to be asked about a history of rheumatic fever and infective endocarditis. Each episode of these infections further increases valve dysfunction. The patient's fatigue level and ability to perform activities of daily living (ADLs), as well as the other clinical manifestations of valve disease need assessment during the physical exam.

After the cause has been identified and treatment begun, the medical management focuses on maintaining cardiac output, activity tolerance, and preventing complications. The treatment plan includes rest and medication. Pharmacologic management depends on the clinical manifestations and the progression of the disease. If heart failure is present with left ventricular dysfunction, ACE inhibitors (or angiotensin receptor blockers), digoxin, diuretics, and fluid and sodium restrictions are typically prescribed. See Chapter 42 ✐ for a complete description of the management of heart failure. For the remainder of the patient's life antibiotics are used prophylactically for dental work and invasive diagnostic studies as well as for the treatment of endocarditis. See the Pharmacology Summary of medications to treat cardiac valve disease (p. 1254).

Antidysrhythmic medications are used to manage the dysrhythmias that are common with valve disease. If atrial fibrillation occurs, every effort is made to terminate the dysrhythmia because it decreases cardiac output by as much as 25% in patients who may already have a compromised cardiac output due to their valve disease. Conversion to normal sinus rhythm is done with either drug

DIAGNOSTIC TESTS for Cardiac Valve Disease

Test and *Normal Values*	Expected Abnormality	Rationale for Abnormality
Echocardiogram and transesophageal echocardiography (TEE) Echocardiogram (ultrasound): *Normal chamber size and normal cardiac structures*	Abnormal structure and function of heart valves, able to identify thickened valve leaflets, vegetative growths, myocardial function, and chamber size. TEE is particularly useful not only for diagnosing but also for tracking the progression of the disease.	Vegetative growths and infection cause a thinning of valve leaflets leading to abnormal function.
Chest x-ray: *Clear lungs and normal heart size*	Pulmonary congestion, cardiac hypertrophy, chamber and great vessel enlargement, and calcification of the valves.	Abnormal valve function causes a change in blood flow leading to changes in chamber size and valve structure.
Cardiac catheterization: *Normal coronary artery blood flow, chamber size, and valve function*	The size of the valve opening and pressure gradients across valve surfaces is abnormal. Pressure in the heart chambers and pulmonary system is increased. Cardiac output typically is decreased.	Abnormal valve structure causes changes in openings leading to increased pressures in the cardiac chambers and decreased cardiac output.
Electrocardiogram (ECG): *Normal conduction time intervals*	Conduction delays, atrial and ventricular dysrhythmias, and the presence of cardiac ischemia. Is useful in detecting increased ischemia and the presence of life-threatening dysrhythmias.	Changes occur due to diminished blood flow to the myocardium due to decreased cardiac output caused by abnormal valvular function.
Cardiac MRI (CMR): *Normal heart valve function*	Valve size and competence.	Abnormal valve structure causes changes in openings, leading to increased pressures in the cardiac chambers and decreased cardiac output.

therapy (calcium channel blockers) or, if unsuccessful, synchronized cardioversion. After conversion, digoxin is typically prescribed to prevent further episodes of atrial fibrillation and control the heart rate. Chapter 38 describes atrial fibrillation. If atrial fibrillation persists, the blood stagnates in the quivering atrium and the patient is at a high risk for thrombus formation. Anticoagulant therapy is necessary to prevent strokes, pulmonary emboli, and deep venous thrombosis. Oral nitrates are prescribed for patients with aortic valve disease to increase peripheral dilation and decrease preload. This will decrease the pressure gradient in the left ventricle, thereby allowing it to pump more effectively and decreasing myocardial oxygen demand. Additionally, nitrates dilate the coronary arteries to increase perfusion to the myocardium.

The fixed and/or decreased cardiac output associated with valve disease limits physical activity. As the disease progresses the need for surgical intervention is in part determined by the patient's ability to perform the ADLs. Patients with asymptomatic aortic stenosis are placed on prophylactic antibiotics and instructed to get an echocardiogram every 6 months (Clarkston & Waldman, 2001). The echocardiogram serves as a guide for appropriate surgical intervention. Medical management of patients with aortic regurgitation includes prophylactic antibiotics, vasodilators to decrease ventricular afterload, and an echocardiogram every 6 months (Clarkston & Waldman, 2001).

In 1997, an association between diet medications (fenfluramine and phentermine) and valve regurgitation was identified in both left- and right-sided heart valves. The development of a new murmur in patients with no previous heart disease was noted, along with other symptoms of valve regurgitation. Based on these findings the federal Food and Drug Administration withdrew the drugs from the market.

Invasive Management of Valve Disease

When medical management is no longer effective and the hemodynamic status becomes unstable, invasive intervention is necessary to cure the problem or at least relieve symptoms. The need for intervention is determined in part by the impact of the clinical manifestations on the quality of life, the type and severity of valvular damage, and the patient's ability to tolerate the procedure. Options include either valve repair (annuloplasty, valvulo-

plasty, or commissurotomy) or valve replacement with a prosthesis. The reparative procedures do not result in a normal valve leaflet, but are associated with fewer side effects than valve replacement. The repaired valve functions more normally and cardiac output is improved, in essence buying the patient more time.

> **CRITICAL ALERT** *The patient is instructed to report to the health care provider when it is becoming too difficult to perform ADLs. This is one important indicator of the need for valve repair or replacement surgery.*

Annuloplasty

An **annuloplasty** corrects valve regurgitation by repairing the enlarged **annulus**, which is the fibrous ring at the junction of the valve leaflets and the muscular wall. This procedure is done when the valve leaflets are normal, but the valve fails to close due to this enlargement. The surgical procedure involves tightening the annulus with a prosthetic ring sutured in place, which reduces the size of the annulus (Figure 41–8 ■). Open heart surgery and cardiopulmonary bypass are required for an annuloplasty.

Valvuloplasty

The repair of the valve leaflet rather than replacement is referred to as a **valvuloplasty**. The torn or damaged leaflet, chordae tendineae, or papillary muscle is surgically repaired under general anesthesia and cardiopulmonary bypass. This procedure is primarily performed to treat mitral and aortic stenosis, although it has been used to treat tricuspid and pulmonic stenosis.

The most common valvuloplasty is a **commissurotomy**. The objective of this procedure is to separate fused valve leaflets. The site where leaflets meet each other is referred to as a **commissure**. With stenosis these commissures are abnormally fused either congenitally or due to calcification and scarring from inflammatory heart diseases. A closed commissurotomy requires general anesthesia but not cardiopulmonary bypass. After a midsternal incision is made a small hole is cut into the heart and the surgeon's finger or a dilator is used to break open the commissure. This procedure is useful for mitral, aortic, tricuspid, and pulmonic valve stenosis.

An open commissurotomy is performed with general anesthesia and cardiopulmonary bypass. This gives the surgeon direct

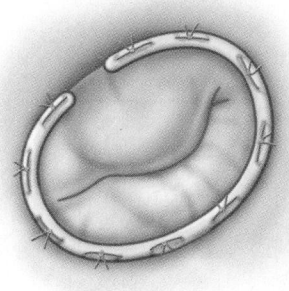

FIGURE 41–8 ■ Annuloplasty.

visualization of the valve and has the added advantages of allowing any thrombi to be removed and the degree of valve calcification to be identified. Additionally, if necessary, the chordae tendineae and papillary muscle can be repaired. The goals of this procedure are to improve leaflet mobility and to increase the size of the valve orifice. The procedure is most effective when the valve leaflets are thin and pliable (Wiegand, 2003).

Percutaneous Transluminal Balloon Valvuloplasty

Percutaneous transluminal balloon valvuloplasty (PTBV) is an invasive, nonsurgical commissurotomy used to dilate stenosed mitral and aortic valves (Figure 41–9 ■). In the heart catheterization

(a)

(b)

(c)

FIGURE 41–9 ■ Valvuloplasty.

laboratory with the patient under local anesthesia, a balloon-dilating catheter is inserted and positioned across the valve. To reach the mitral valve, the catheter is advanced through the femoral vein into the right atrium through the atrial septum and into the left atrium and across the mitral valve. The balloon is repeatedly inflated and deflated with dilute angiographic solution in order to dilate the stenosis. The valve is not completely occluded during inflation, thereby allowing some blood to flow to the left ventricle. The most common approach to treating aortic stenosis is to feed the catheter retrograde to blood flow in the femoral artery into the aorta until the valve is reached. To reach the tricuspid and pulmonic valves, a right-sided venous approach is used.

A balloon valvuloplasty will open the stenosis by 1 or 2 cm and reduce the pressure gradient across the valve. The aortic valve procedure is not as successful as that of the mitral valve. The rate of restenosis is approximately 50% in the first 12 to 15 months after the procedure (Braunwald et al., 2005). Some centers are reporting valve patency after 1 year and 60% to 70% required no intervention after 5 years. This procedure is useful to relieve symptoms in patients who are too high a surgical risk (Wiegand, 2003). Some degree of mitral regurgitation is present after the procedure. Other complications include emboli and rarely a left to right arterial shunt through the opening created by the catheter.

Prosthetic Heart Valves

Patients with cardiac valve disease must be monitored regularly by a cardiologist to determine the best time for valve replacement surgery. The general clinical state of the patient is usually appraised using the New York Heart Association classification system for functional disability (see Chapter 42 ☺). The goal is to replace the valve before permanent left ventricular damage occurs. Valve replacement is indicated when leaflets are calcified and immobile and when the clinical manifestations impact the patient's ability to perform ADLs.

Newer valves and improved surgical techniques have made valve replacement surgery safer. The goal for a valve is to be non-thrombogenic, durable, and create the least amount of stenosis. The type of valve used for a given patient is determined by the anatomic suitability, ease of insertion, the patient's age, contraindications to anticoagulant therapy (pregnancy), and patient preference. Valve replacement surgery is done under general anesthesia using cardiopulmonary bypass. After removal of the diseased valve, the new valve is sutured into the site of the native valve (Figure 41–10 ■). There are basically two different types of valves: mechanical and biological (Figure 41–11 ■).

Mechanical Valves **Mechanical valves** are commercially made valves. With the caged-ball valve, the ball floats up and occludes the valve opening when the pressure from the blood rises (Figure 41–11A ■). The tilting disk valve operates on the same principle except the disk closes when the pressure from the blood rises (see Figure 41–11B & D ■). There are two types of disk valves: single disk and double disk. The valve must have good hemodynamic design with the least amount of blood turbulence possible. The most frequently cited complications of mechanical valves are thromboembolism and anticoagulation-related problems (Aurigemma & Gaasch, 2002). Conversely, structural failure is relatively rare with mechanical valves as compared to

Sutures ready to be placed through valve's ring

Sutures already placed through valve's ring

Valve orifice

Prosthetic tissue valve

(a)

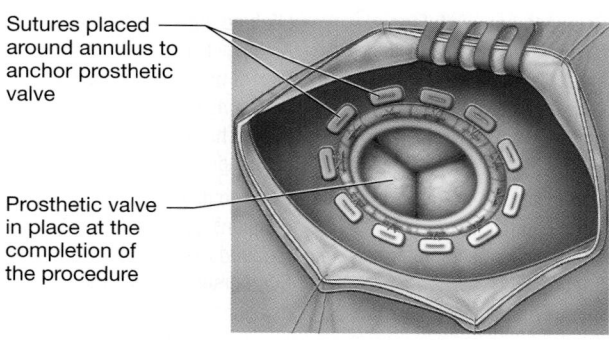

Sutures placed around annulus to anchor prosthetic valve

Prosthetic valve in place at the completion of the procedure

(b)

FIGURE 41–10 ■ Valve replacement surgery.

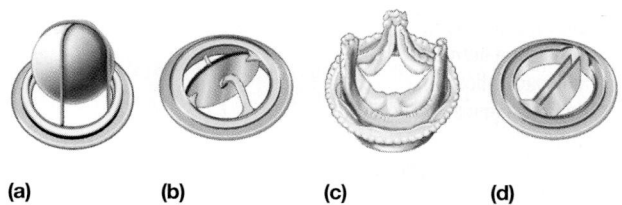

(a)   **(b)**   **(c)**   **(d)**

FIGURE 41–11 ■ Valve types: (A) caged-ball valve, (B) & (D) tilting-disc valve, and (C) porcine heterograph valve.

biological valves. Most mechanical valves are expected to last 20 to 30 years (Aurigemma & Gaasch, 2002). The specific valve description, advantages, and disadvantages are listed on Chart 41–5 (p. 1250).

Biological Valves   **Biological valves**, most commonly come from pigs (porcine valves; see Figure 41–11C ■), although cow valves (bovine), and human valves also are used. Biological valves have a decreased incidence of clot formation compared to mechanical valves; therefore, long-term anticoagulation is not necessary. Biological valves do tend to wear out faster (7 to 10 years), especially in the younger populations who have increased amounts of calcium in the blood that break down the valve.

Note, however, that biological valves are useful for women of childbearing age because long-term anticoagulation is not feasible, preventing bleeding complications associated with menses, pregnancy, and childbirth. Biological valves also are used for the elderly population (greater than 70 years of age) and for patients with a history of peptic ulcer disease when anticoagulants are contraindicated.

There are two major types of biological valves: homograft valves and autograft valves. **Homograft** or **allograft valves** come from human cadaver donations and are used primarily to replace the aortic and pulmonic valves. The valves are harvested from a cadaver and stored cryogenically, although they are not readily available and are very expensive.

Autograft valves or autologous valves are obtained from the patient's own pulmonic valve and pulmonary artery. The pulmonic valve replaces the diseased aortic valve, and then the pulmonic valve is either replaced with a homograft or left without a valve. If the pulmonary pressures are normal, the surgeon may elect not to replace the valve.

■ Nursing Management

Nursing care of the patient with valve disease is aimed at assessing the clinical manifestations and progression of the disease, and conserving energy. The physical assessment begins with an in-depth history and an assessment of risk factors. Any episodes of rheumatic fever, endocarditis, or habits that increase the risk of valve disease are evaluated. The physical assessment includes vital signs, dysrhythmias, fluid status, anxiety, lung sounds, and the clinical manifestations of right- and left-sided heart failure, as described in Chapter 42 ∞.

Nursing care focuses on conserving energy in order to maintain normal cardiac output and prevent the manifestations of heart failure and pulmonary congestion. Activity intolerance is a significant factor; therefore, the nurse spaces activities and visitors to allow for periods of rest. Because valve disease is a chronic debilitating disorder, it is important for the nurse to assess the patient's support systems. The Nursing Process: Patient Care Plan for Valve Disease (p. 1251) provides a comprehensive plan of care for a patient with valve disease. The Patient Teaching & Discharge box (p. 1253) outlines the patient teaching and discharge needs for a patient with valve disease.

The chronicity of valve disease and its atmosphere of uncertainty may produce anxiety, fear, and depression for the patient and family/significant others. A nursing assessment of the patient's ability to handle the situation and its impact on the quality of life is essential. The assessment findings are necessary in order to develop a comprehensive plan and help with the adjustment to the disease. The patient needs to be given an opportunity to express concerns and fears in a nonthreatening environment. Explanation of the medical regimen with rationales often decreases fear and frustration in patients.

The postoperative nursing care of the valve surgery patient includes monitoring for the usual complications such as hemorrhage, wound infection, and pulmonary complications. Additionally, the hemodynamic status and cardiac output must be closely monitored. For the first 24 to 48 hours after surgery, the patient is admitted to the critical care area where the ECG, cardiac

CHART 41–5	**Types of Prosthetic Heart Valves**			
Valve Type	**Types**	**Description**	**Advantage**	**Disadvantage**
Mechanical valve	Caged-ball: Starr-Edwards Smeloff-Cutter MaGovern-Cromie	Metal cage with struts mounted on ring, ball on inside of cage (Figure 41–11A ■, p. 1249).	Occupies less space in the ventricle. Requires less force to move the ball. Long-term durability up to 20 years. Hemodynamically efficient.	Lifetime anticoagulation. Audible click. Risk of thromboembolism. Infections harder to treat. Risk of hemorrhage from anticoagulants. Very large size.
	Tilting disc: Bjork-Shiley Lilehei-Kaster Medtronic Hall	Mobile disk attached to a circular ring by two struts (Figure 41–11B, D ■, p. 1249).	Produces central blood flow through orifice, like native valves. Long-term durability. Hemodynamically efficient.	Lifetime anticoagulation. Audible click. Risk of thromboembolism under pivoting points as a result of blood stasis. Infections harder to treat. Risk of hemorrhage from anticoagulants.
	Bileaflet valve: St. Jude Medical Duromedics	Two pivoting disks that open centrally attached to a ring.	Compact size, useful for children and patients with small aortic roots. Long-term durability. Hemodynamically efficient.	Lifetime anticoagulation. Audible click. Risk of thromboembolism. Infections harder to treat. Risk of hemorrhage from anticoagulants.
Biological tissue valve	Xenograft, porcine (pig): Hancock Carpenter-Edwards Medtronic	Harvested aortic valve from pig that is mounted on a sewing ring (Figure 41–11C ■, p. 1249).	Low incidence of thromboembolism. Need anticoagulation for only 3 months. Hemodynamically efficient. Quiet. Easier to treat infections.	Prone to deterioration. Frequent replacement required (5–7 years). Cumbersome structural design.
	Xenograft, bovine (cow): Ionescu-Shiley Carpenter-Edwards	Three leaflets composed of the pericardium of a 16- to 18-month-old calf that is mounted on a Dacron-covered frame.	Less resistant to blood flow. Useful for patients with small aortic roots. Low incidence of thromboembolism. Need short-term anticoagulation. Hemodynamically efficient. Quiet. Easier to treat infections.	Limited durability.
	Homograft/allograft: Cadaver	Harvested aortic valve from human cadaver that is sewn in place with special mounting material.	Low incidence of thromboembolism. Only rare need for anticoagulation. Excellent hemodynamics.	Limited durability. Not useful for mitral or tricuspid valve replacement. Not readily available. Very expensive.
Autograft valve	Autologous	Excised pulmonic valve and portion of pulmonary artery from patient.	Lasts 20 years. Nonthrombogenic, anticoagulation is unnecessary. Will grow with child. Useful for women in childbearing years, young adults, and for those who cannot tolerate anticoagulation.	Only possible if the aortic valve is normal. May require double valve replacement.

NURSING PROCESS: Patient Care Plan for Valve Disease

Assessment of Anxiety and Fear Related to Cardiac Valve Disease

Subjective Data:
What do you know about your disease process?
How do your health-related issues impact your daily life?
Do you feel anxious about your health?
Do you have family members or close friends who provide emotional support?

Objective Data:
Observe for manifestations of anxiety: restlessness, apprehension, withdrawal.

Nursing Assessment and Diagnoses	Outcomes and Evaluation Parameters	Planning and Interventions with *Rationales*
Nursing Diagnosis: *Anxiety* and *Fear* related to chronic disease process	**Outcome:** Anxiety level minimized and manageable. *Evaluation Parameters:* Verbalizes anxious feelings. Verbalizes what relieves anxiety. Demonstrates relief from anxiety by consistently controlling aggression, impulsiveness control, and self-mutilation restraint; and by improving coping and social interaction skills. Verbalizes absence of sensory perceptual disorders. Verbalizes absence of physical manifestations of anxiety. Behavioral manifestations of anxiety absent.	**Interventions and *Rationales:*** Provide factual information concerning diagnosis, treatment, disfigurement, disabilities, and prognosis. *Truthful explanations increase trust and potentially decrease anxiety.* Explain all procedures and allow time for mental preparation. *This decreases fear and anxiety of the unknown.* Allow time and encourage verbalization of fears related to illness *to assist in relieving anxiety.* Explore with the patient/family techniques to reduce anxiety. *This gives the patient a sense of control and opens communication about the subject.* Explore effective ways to minimize anxiety. *This gives the patient a sense of control.* Instruct the patient in the use of relaxation techniques *to relieve anxiety.* Assess need for and administer antianxiety and pain medication. *If alternative measures are not effective, may need antianxiety agents.*

Assessment of Activity Tolerance

Subjective Data:
What level of activity fatigues you?
Have you been becoming more fatigued with less activity recently?
Are you able to complete your ADLs without fatigue?

Objective Data:
Monitor tolerance to activities while on bed rest in order to obtain a baseline to plan activities.
Monitor for changes in symptoms and vital signs (VS) during activity.
Determine if pulse, respirations, and blood pressure (BP) return to normal within 3 minutes after stopping activity.

Nursing Assessment and Diagnoses	Outcomes and Evaluation Parameters	Planning and Interventions with *Rationales*
Nursing Diagnosis: *Fatigue* and *Activity Intolerance* related to decreased or fixed cardiac output	**Outcome:** Energy conservation. *Evaluation Parameters:* Endurance maintained. Balanced diet. Reports increased energy levels. Absence of clinical manifestations at rest.	**Interventions and *Rationales:*** Identify activities that increase fatigue *to avoid increasing cardiac workload.* Discontinue activity if chest pain, dyspnea, cyanosis, dizziness, hypotension, sustained tachycardia, or dysrhythmias develop *to aid in evaluating tolerance to activities.* Explore sedentary activities that the patient may enjoy *to provide a diversion that does not place a demand on the heart.* Maintain balanced nutrition to ensure adequate calories *to increase energy.*

(continued)

NURSING PROCESS: Patient Care Plan for Valve Disease—Continued

Assessment of Tissue Perfusion

Subjective Data:
Do you become short of breath? What causes it to occur?
How far can you walk before becoming short of breath?
Do you experience leg pain? If so, what brings it on and is it getting worse?
Do your hands and feet feel cold on a warm day?

Objective Data:
Assess:
Acid–base balance.
The presence of and/or change in a murmur.
Lung sounds.
Respiratory rate.
ECG.
Peripheral pulses.
Capillary refill.

Nursing Assessment and Diagnoses	Outcomes and Evaluation Parameters	Planning and Interventions with *Rationales*
Nursing Diagnosis: *Ineffective Tissue Perfusion* related to decreased cardiac output as a result of valve disease.	**Outcomes:** Maintenance of cardiac output. Adequate tissue perfusion. ***Evaluation Parameters:*** Absence of heart failure. Absence of atrial fibrillation and/or successful conversion to normal sinus rhythm.	**Interventions and *Rationales:*** Assess for adventitious or diminished breath sounds. *Indicates decreased gas exchange and heart failure.* Note presence of cough and amount and color of sputum. *Assessing for heart failure.* Monitor ABGs and oxygen saturation *to assess adequacy of gas exchange.* Monitor respiratory rate and depth *to assess for respiratory distress.* Monitor fluid status *to assess heart failure.* Monitor ECG for dysrhythmias, especially atrial fibrillation *to determine impact on cardiac output and risk for sudden death.* Monitor restlessness and confusion. *Indicators of inadequate gas exchange with resultant brain hypoxia.* Assess need for suctioning and/or endotracheal intubation. Suction when necessary *to maintain adequate gas exchange.* Observe for cyanosis, especially in the mucous membranes. *Indicators of inadequate gas exchange with resultant tissue hypoxia.* Turn, cough, deep breathe, elevate head of bed, instruct on use of incentive spirometry. *Measures to promote gas exchange.* Administer humidified oxygen as prescribed *to increase oxygen levels.* Report respiratory distress to the health care provider. *Medical intervention may be indicated to prevent respiratory failure.* Encourage low-sodium diet *to reduce fluid retention and heart failure.*

output, and pulmonary artery pressures can be monitored and ventilatory support can be provided if necessary.

Following repair or replacement of the valve, the heart requires time to adjust to the improved hemodynamic function. Vasoactive agents may be necessary in the immediate postoperative period to optimize cardiac output. Inotropic agents may be necessary to improve cardiac contractility, and vasodilators may be needed to decrease afterload (Wiegand, 2003). Continuous monitoring for cardiac dysrhythmias is essential because the mitral and aortic valves lie close to the conduction pathway. Transient or permanent heart blocks may occur due to edema, ischemia, or damage to the conduction pathway. A temporary or permanent pacemaker may be required. Additionally, atrial dysrhythmias are a common complication of cardiac surgery and are even more common after valve surgery (Wiegand, 2003). If indicated based on valve type, anticoagulant therapy is started within 48 hours of valve surgery.

 **CRITICAL ALERT** *Report to the health care provider an INR and/or PT that is either too low or too high. If the values are too low, there is increased risk of clot formation. If the values are too high there is an increased risk of excessive bleeding.*
Monitor and report decreases in hemoglobin and hematocrit, which may indicate bleeding. If the platelet count is less than 50,000/mm³, there also is an increased risk of bleeding.

PATIENT TEACHING & DISCHARGE PRIORITIES for Cardiac Valve Disease

Need	Teaching
Knowledge of disease and progression of clinical manifestations	Detailed teaching materials about the disease process, medical regimen, and possible complications to increase knowledge and compliance.
Prevention	Antibiotics for dental work to prevent valve infection and repeated endocarditis.
Assess need for valve surgery	Seek medical help when unable to perform ADLs.
Safety	Medication dosages, frequency, side effects, and special considerations need to be explained to both the family and patient.
Postoperative learning needs to prevent complications	Anticoagulant therapy teaching needs to include: • Drug and dosage • Monthly International Normalized Ratio (INR) to determine correct dosage (ratio typically 2.0 to 3.0 depending on the diagnosis and health care provider preference). Prothrombin time (PT) also may be used to monitor anticoagulants (1.2 to 2 times greater than normal). Report bruising, bleeding, epistaxis, and hemoptysis. Avoid large amounts of yellow and dark green vegetables and fatty foods, which increase the absorption of vitamin K (clots blood). Avoid alcohol, aspirin, and anti-inflammatory drugs (NSAIDs). Inform health care providers of anticoagulant therapy. Test stools and vomitus for blood. Use soft-bristled toothbrush and an electric razor. To maintain an adequate level of anticoagulation without side effects.
Follow-up care	Medical follow-up continues for about a year to assess for complications, valve function, and compliance to therapy.

Source: From *Laboratory Tests and Diagnostic Procedures with Nursing Diagnosis,* 6th edition, by J. V. Corbett, 2004, Upper Saddle River, NJ: Prentice Hall.

A clinical pathway (Chapter 6) is frequently used during the early postoperative period as a guideline to achieve established outcomes within a prescribed length of stay for patients who are recovering from valve surgery. The protocols and guidelines outlined on the pathway provide useful tools for facilitating the coordination of care (Zevola, Raffa, & Brown, 2002).

Health Promotion

Due to the progressive nature of the disease, health promotion begins as soon as the patient is diagnosed with a valve abnormality. Patient/family education focuses on controlling the clinical manifestations, reducing physical activity, and preventing reoccurrences of an infection in the valve. Education includes information on medications, lifestyle choices, and preventive care. The patient needs to be given specific instructions about when to seek medical advice for surgical intervention. When the patient is no longer able to perform the ADLs, generally surgical intervention is discussed.

Once surgical intervention has occurred, formulating a teaching plan for the postoperative valve surgery also is an essential nursing function. The plan needs to include information about medications, activity, and the signs and symptoms that need to be reported to the health care provider.

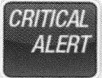 *Following valve replacement surgery the patient is taught that if fever, increased heart rate, fatigue, malaise, anorexia, weight loss, headache, and chills, or night sweats occur, the patient needs to notify the health care provider. The clinical manifestations are a sign of postoperative infective endocarditis, which needs immediate medical attention.*

Collaborative Management

Due to the chronic and progressive nature of cardiac valve disease, a collaborative care approach is optimal for management. Utilizing a multidisciplinary team approach, including health care providers, nurses, physical and occupational therapists, psychologists/psychiatrists, dieticians, and pharmacists, will facilitate the best possible quality of life for the patient and family. It is essential that the health care provider monitor the progress of the valve disease and determine when surgical intervention is necessary. Psychiatric counseling may be necessary to assist in lifestyle adjustments necessitated by a chronic disease process. The occupational therapist helps facilitate realistic occupational goals, while the physical therapist assists in the maintenance of optimum conditioning given the activity restrictions.

Because medication is an essential part of the management of valve disorders, the role of the pharmacist is crucial in educating the patient about how to manage the medications and their side effects. When cardiac valve disease is complicated by the presence of heart failure symptoms of congestion, diet and fluid restriction counseling are necessary. The dietitian can educate the patient/family about salt restrictions and help them learn about satisfying meals that do not increase the risk of fluid retention. In addition to the nursing care described earlier, the nurse plays a pivotal role in coordinating the efforts of the health care team. In the inpatient setting the nurse facilitates communication between the members of the team and the patient/family. The nurse also must include in the patient teaching the coordination of care after discharge (see Patient Teaching & Discharge Priorities box).

PHARMACOLOGY Summary of Medications to Treat Cardiac Valve Disease

Medication Category	Action	Application/Indication	Nursing Responsibility
Cardiac Medications Digoxin Calcium channel blockers: Diltiazem (Cardizem) Verapamil (Calan) ACE inhibitors Antiarrhythmic agents	Increases force and velocity of myocardial systolic contraction. Decreases conduction through AV node. Reduces automaticity in the SA node and slows impulse conduction through the AV node. Used for supraventricular dysrhythmias. ACE inhibitor: Lowers peripheral resistance and reduces blood volume by enhancing the excretion of sodium by inhibition of angiotensin-converting enzyme. Alters the electrophysiological properties of the heart by either blocking flow through the channels or altering autonomic activity.	Convert and then control atrial fibrillation. Control atrial fibrillation. Manage heart failure if present. To manage the dysrhythmias that are common with valve disease.	Digoxin requires periodic laboratory testing to ensure therapeutic drug level. Assess pulse prior to administration of digoxin. The pulse rate needs to be >60 beats/min. Never given if heart block, sick sinus syndrome, severe hypotension, and shock are present. Assess heart rate, blood pressure, lung sounds, and ECG monitor regularly. Monitor for hypotension especially when being given intravenously. Monitor blood pressure carefully after first dose for hypotension. Educate patient that it takes 2 weeks for therapeutic effect. May experience dizziness. There is a narrow margin between therapeutic effect and toxicity; therefore, careful and ongoing cardiac monitoring is essential. Patient teaching includes avoiding the use of alcohol, drugs, and tobacco.
Diuretics	Blocks reabsorption of sodium and chloride in the loop of Henle. Reduces edema associated with heart failure.	To manage heart failure if present.	Potassium levels also need monitoring because low levels are a side effect of certain diuretics, especially furosemide. May need potassium replacement. Measure urine output prior to administration to gauge the response to the medication.
Antibiotics	Inhibits protein synthesis of microorganisms by binding reversibly to a ribosome, thus interfering with transmission of genetic information.	Prophylactically for dental work and invasive diagnostic studies as well as for the treatment of acute endocarditis episodes.	Assessment of history of drug allergies prior to administration. Assessment of clinical manifestations of allergic reaction. Assessment of relief of clinical manifestations to determine drug effectiveness. Patient education regarding need to complete the entire regimen and report any clinical manifestations of drug allergy.
Anticoagulant Therapy Warfarin (Coumadin) Heparin	Can either inhibit specific clotting factors in coagulation cascade or diminish the clotting action of platelets.	Prevent strokes, pulmonary emboli, and deep venous thrombosis, especially if atrial fibrillation is occurring.	Ongoing assessment of therapeutic blood level per health care provider orders. Assess for bleeding including nosebleeds, bruising, "coffee-grounds" emesis, tarry stools, fatigue, and pale skin. Assess for decreases in hemoglobin, hematocrit, RBCs, and platelets.
Nitrates (nitroglycerin)	Relaxes both atrial and venous smooth muscle, causing decreased preload and afterload.	Used with aortic valve disease to increase peripheral dilation and decrease preload, thereby allowing the heart to pump more effectively, hence decreasing myocardial oxygen demand. Dilate the coronary arteries to increase perfusion to the myocardium.	Assess blood pressure before and during therapy. Hypotension could result. Should be given with other vasodilators. Patient education includes: No alcohol use. Rotate patches. Keep medication with you at all times and away from excessive heat and light. Report blurred vision, dry mouth, and severe headache.

Sources: Adams, M. P., Josephen, D. L., & Holland, L. N. (Eds.). (2005). *Pharmacology for nurses: A pathophysiologic approach.* Upper Saddle River, NJ: Pearson Prentice Hall; American Heart Association. (2005). *Handbook of emergency cardiovascular care for health providers.* Dallas, TX: Author; Wilson, B., Shannon, M., & Stang, C. (Eds.). (2005). *Nurses drug guide.* Upper Saddle River, NJ: Pearson Prentice Hall.

Cardiomyopathy

Cardiomyopathies (CMPs) are defined as diseases of the myocardial muscle fibers. The diseases result in progressive structural and functional abnormalities of the myocardium. The term *cardiomyopathy* was first introduced in 1957 and was defined simply as noncoronary artery heart disease of unknown etiology (Brigden, 1957). Currently, the World Health Organization defines cardiomyopathies as "diseases of the myocardium associated with cardiac dysfunction" (Richardson, 1996).

Cardiomyopathies are classified as primary and secondary. With primary CMPs, the etiology of the disease is unknown and the only abnormality is in the heart muscle itself. Secondary CMPs are caused by other disease processes such as ischemia, viral infections, alcohol intake and drug abuse, inherited disorders, and pregnancy. There are four types of CMPs: dilated, hypertrophic, restrictive, and arrhythmogenic. Each type is identified by differences in pathology, clinical manifestations, and treatment. All types of cardiomyopathy can lead to cardiomegaly and heart failure.

Dilated Cardiomyopathy

Dilated cardiomyopathy (DCM), the most common form of cardiomyopathy, is a disorder of the myocardium characterized by dilation and impaired contraction of one or more ventricles. When dilation becomes severe it may be accompanied by heart wall hypertrophy, which is an increase in myocardial wall thickness. Figure 41–12 ■ compares the ventricle size for each type of cardiomyopathy.

Epidemiology and Etiology

Dilated or congestive cardiomyopathy accounts for approximately 87% of all cardiomyopathies and is distributed throughout all age groups with the majority in the elderly population (Porth, 2005). The risk factors for the development of DCM are outlined in the Risk Factors box (p. 1256), although for 50% of cases no cause can be identified. Coronary artery disease is the most common cause of DCM in the United States, comprising 50% to 75% of patients with heart failure (Felker, Thompson, & Hare, 2000). This type of cardiomyopathy most frequently develops following a myocardial infarction and ventricular tissue remodeling. Prolonged ischemia causes a loss of myocytes that are replaced by noncontractile scar tissue, thereby leading to heart failure. These changes lead to irreversible myocardial dysfunction.

After initial diagnosis and onset of clinical manifestations, 50% of patients with DCM are alive in 5 years, and 25% are alive in 10 years. Mortality rates from DCM are highest in older persons, males, and the black race (Porth, 2004).

Pathophysiology

Some forms of DCM are idiopathic, but a genetic cause is present in as many as 30% of these patients (Hunt et al., 2005). Known risk factors for the development of DCM are outlined in the Risk Factors box (p. 1256). These factors cause the myocardial fibers to degenerate, become necrotic, and eventually be replaced by fibrotic tissue, referred to as tissue remodeling. Dilation of the cardiac chambers occurs due to the constant stress from overfilling. The stretching of the myocardial fibers increases the compliance of the ventricles but results in hypocontractility, reduced stroke volume, ejection fraction, and ultimately decreased cardiac output. Blood flows more slowly through the enlarged heart, causing mural thrombi (blood clots on the heart wall) to form, increasing the risk of atrial and ventricular emboli formation. Additionally, the extra blood that stays in the chambers after each contraction eventually backs up into the pulmonary system, causing heart failure symptoms and ultimately reducing blood flow to the tissues.

Cardiomyopathy during pregnancy or after pregnancy, referred to as peripartum cardiomyopathy (PPCM), is thought to be caused by an interaction of pericardium physiology with either infectious agents leading to myocarditis or by inflammatory, genetic, hormonal, or metabolic factors, and accounts for

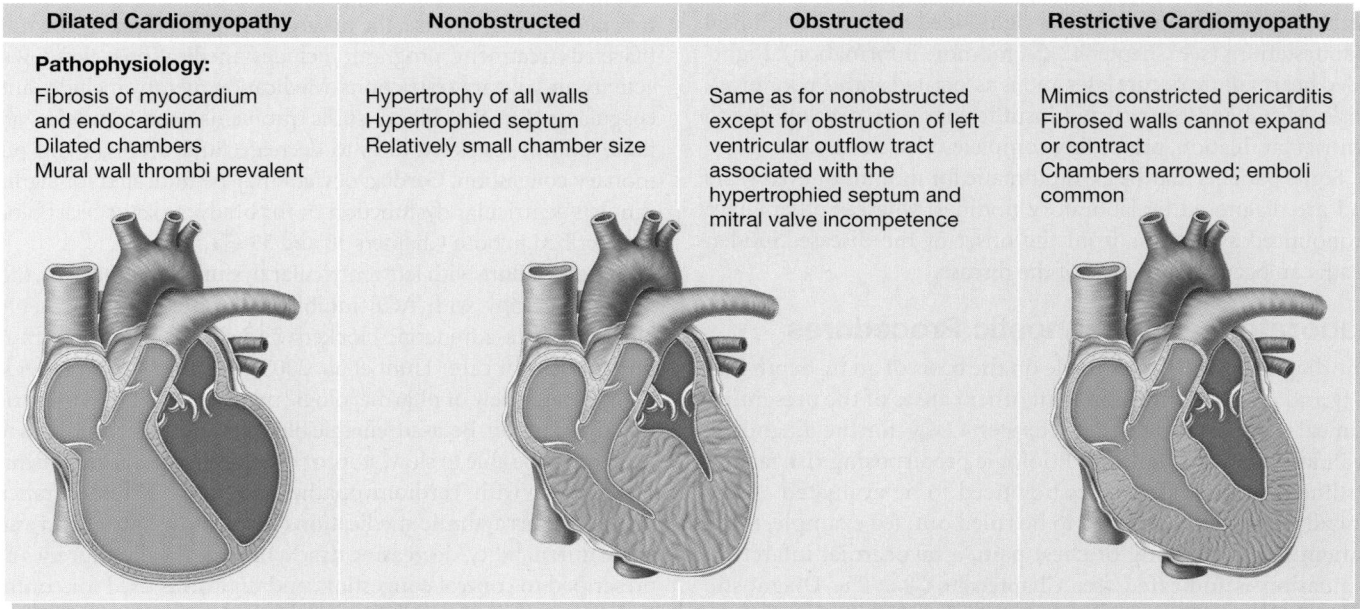

Dilated Cardiomyopathy	Nonobstructed	Obstructed	Restrictive Cardiomyopathy
Pathophysiology: Fibrosis of myocardium and endocardium Dilated chambers Mural wall thrombi prevalent	Hypertrophy of all walls Hypertrophied septum Relatively small chamber size	Same as for nonobstructed except for obstruction of left ventricular outflow tract associated with the hypertrophied septum and mitral valve incompetence	Mimics constricted pericarditis Fibrosed walls cannot expand or contract Chambers narrowed; emboli common

FIGURE 41–12 ■ Types of cardiomyopathy.

RISK FACTORS for Cardiomyopathy

Long-term uncontrolled hypertension	Neuromuscular disorders (Duchenne's muscular dystrophy)
Cardiac valve disease	Endocrine disorders (diabetes, Cushing's disease)
Coronary artery disease	Electrolyte abnormalities (hypocalcemia, hypophosphatemia, uremia)
Congenital heart disease	Antiviral medications (zidovudine, didanosine)
Viral myocarditis	Radiation therapy
Toxins (lead, mercury, carbon monoxide, arsenic)	Calcium overload
Pregnancy and postpartum period	Amyloidosis and sarcoidosis
Connective tissue disorders (SLE, scleroderma, giant cell arthritis)	Hyperlipidemia
Alcohol abuse	Sedentary lifestyle
Stress and sedentary lifestyle	Obesity
Genetic predisposition	Smoking
Nutritional deficiency (decreased thiamine, selenium, carnitine)	Diabetes mellitus
Sleep apnea	Familial cardiomyopathies
Cocaine	Idiopathic
Chemotherapeutic agents	Cardiac surgery
Bacterial/parasitic infections	

Source: Afridi, H. R., & Hartnell, G. G. (2002). *Cardiomyopathy, dilated.* Retrieved August 3, 2006, from http://www.emedicine.com/radio/topic128.htm.

approximately 4% of the cases (Flutterman & Lemberg, 2000). The diagnosis of PPCM is based on (1) no other identifiable causes of heart failure, (2) heart failure within 5 months of delivery, (3) absence of heart disease prior to the last month of pregnancy, and (4) ECG revealing abnormal left ventricular systolic function. The majority of the cases of PPCM occur in the postpartum period, with up to 50% of the related deaths occurring within 3 months after delivery (Flutterman & Lemberg, 2000).

Clinical Manifestations

The clinical manifestations of DCM have an insidious onset. Findings depend on the area and the degree of structural dysfunction. Initial complaints typically include a complaint of increasing fatigue, dyspnea, and activity intolerance, classic symptoms of heart failure. The failing heart may include one or both sides of the heart, manifesting both left- and right-sided heart failure clinical manifestations (see Chapter 42 ☺ for more information). Right-sided heart failure occurs later and is associated with a poor prognosis. Mitral and/or tricuspid insufficiency may develop due to ventricular dilation, preventing complete valve closure.

Some patients may be asymptomatic for months or even years and are diagnosed by laboratory findings, whereas others have pronounced symptoms from the onset of the disease. Sudden death can occur at any stage of the disease.

Laboratory and Diagnostic Procedures

The diagnosis of DCM is made on the basis of an in-depth history and physical and ruling out other causes of the presenting clinical manifestations. (See Chapter 42 ☺ for the diagnostic evaluation of heart failure.) Etiologic predisposing risk factors outlined in the Risk Factors box need to be evaluated. Additionally other diseases need to be ruled out; for example, if the patient is complaining of chest pain, a myocardial infarction evaluation is indicated (see Chapter 40 ☺). The Diagnostic Tests box outlines the tests that are usually done to evaluate

DCM. Because DCM is a progressive disease, frequent and ongoing monitoring is necessary. Clinical manifestations typically dictate the need for further testing and evaluation.

Medical Management

Because DCM is a chronic noncurable disease, management focuses on control of the disease, identifying precipitating factors, and control of clinical manifestations. Interventions are aimed at controlling progression of structural dysfunction that leads to heart failure, when possible. Treatment aims are more palliative than curative, and focus on decreasing cardiac workload.

The overall goals of medical management are to find the cause, improve contractile efficiency, and manage the symptoms and complications. If the cause can be identified and terminated, such as illicit drugs or alcohol, stopping these substances will help control, and possibly reverse, the progression of the disease. The multifaceted treatment program includes medications along with activity and dietary restrictions. Medication therapy includes anticoagulants for the blood stasis problems, and diuretics and fluid/sodium-restricted diets to decrease fluid overload and pulmonary congestion. Cardiac devices may be indicated for significant left ventricular dysfunction or for bradycardia or heart block as described in both Chapters 38 and 39 ☺ .

If heart failure with left ventricular dysfunction is present, then medical therapy with ACE inhibitors (or angiotensin receptor blockers), beta-adrenergic blockers, and aldosterone blockers are the standard of care (Hunt et al., 2005). Chapter 42 ☺ provides a complete review of pharmacologic management for left ventricular dysfunction. Beta-adrenergic blockers and ACE inhibitors together may be able to slow, stop, or even reverse tissue remodeling that occurs with cardiomyopathy and heart failure (Francis, 2004). Antiarrhythmic medications help control atrial and ventricular irritability, decreasing dysrhythmias. Finally, diuretics are prescribed to control congestion, and digoxin is used for continued symptoms of heart failure.

DIAGNOSTIC TESTS for Dilated Cardiomyopathy

Test with *Normal Values*	Expected Abnormality	Rationale for Abnormality
Chest x-ray: *Clear lungs and normal heart size*	DCM: Cardiomegaly and enlargement of the heart. Lung fields have pulmonary congestion and edema.	Cardiomyopathy causes an increase in heart size and predisposes heart failure.
Electrocardiogram (ECG): *Normal conduction time intervals* (see Chapter 38 🔗)	Dysrhythmias. Axis deviation. Left bundle branch block. ST segment changes. Sinus tachycardia.	Stretching of the myocardium may also cause conduction disturbances. Heart failure causes abnormal axis deviation. Ischemia associated with heart failure causes the dysrhythmias and ST segment changes.
Echocardiogram (ultrasound): *Normal chamber size and normal cardiac structures*	Enlarged chamber size, ventricular wall, and septum thickness. Sluggish wall motion. Decreased systolic and diastolic function.	The disease causes enlargement of the chamber, which results in sluggish wall motion and decreased systolic and diastolic function.
Cardiac catheterization to rule out coronary artery disease, assess hemodynamic status, and chamber size and function: *Normal coronary arteries, chambers, and valve pressures*	Enlarged chambers and decreased cardiac output.	The disease causes enlargement of the chamber, which results in a decreased force of muscle contraction leading to decreased cardiac output.
Endomyocardial biopsy occasionally done to rule out other causes of the clinical manifestations: *Normal myocardial tissue*	Myocardial cells positive for pathologic evidence of infiltration, fibrosis, or inflammation.	Changes due to disease process.
Radionuclide study: *Normal chamber volumes and blood perfusion to cardiac muscle*	Abnormally increased ventricular volume and deficits in myocardial muscle perfusion.	The disease causes enlargement of the chamber, which results in a decreased force of muscle contractions leading to an increase in blood being left in the chambers and thereby decreasing myocardial perfusion.

If left ventricular dysfunction is present with an ejection fraction of less than 35%, despite optimizing medications, an implantable cardioverter defibrillator (ICD) may be implanted (Chapter 39 🔗). A pacemaker with a lead in both ventricles, referred to as a biventricular pacemaker (or cardiac resynchronization therapy), is being used to treat heart failure when the ejection fraction is less than 35%, the QRS duration is greater than 120 milliseconds, and patients remain symptomatic despite optimal heart failure medicines. There are three leads, one in the right atrium and two in the ventricles. The pacemaker is able to synchronize cardiac contraction, beginning with atrial depolarization and ending with left ventricular depolarization. This produces significantly improved left ventricular performance, which results in an improved ejection fraction and cardiac output. Early studies have shown that because of improved blood flow and better emptying of the ventricles, the remodeling of tissue is reversing itself. The end result is an improved heart failure status. See Chapter 39 🔗 for complete descriptions of biventricular pacemakers. See the Pharmacology Summary of medications to treat cardiac valve diseases (p. 1254).

Activity restriction is essential during the acute illness, but over time, resuming activities that increase strength and endurance should be promoted. Early in the disease process patients may find the activity restrictions difficult to accept. Thus, patient/family education needs to stress that physical and emotional stress exacerbate the disease. As the disease progresses, most patients experience severe clinical manifestations that limit activity. Alcohol is discouraged for patients with DCM because it depresses myocardial contractility and further decreases cardiac output. End-stage therapies for patients who have progressive and refractory disease include heart transplantation or permanent mechanical assist devices. These therapies are fully described in Chapter 42 🔗.

In 2003 the Centers for Disease Control and Prevention reported that two patients contracted dilated cardiomyopathy 3 months after receiving the smallpox vaccine. Smallpox vaccinations have not been previously associated with DCM. The AHA (2004) advises that these two adverse events should raise awareness that an inflammatory reaction from the vaccine could be a potential mediating factor in cardiomyopathy. Myocarditis, which involves an inflammatory reaction, has been seen in increased numbers in patients receiving smallpox vaccination.

■ Nursing Management

Nursing management begins with a detailed history and in-depth physical assessment. The nurse must inquire about possible risk factors and other diseases that may mimic DCM. Continuous monitoring of assessment parameters of the patient for changes in systemic perfusion include mental status, heart rate and rhythm, peripheral perfusion, oxygenation, fluid status, and vital signs. Since this is a progressive disease, an ongoing assessment is necessary to note significant trends.

The Impact of Repeated Episodes of Recurrent Tachycardia in Patients with Tachycardia-Induced Cardiomyopathy

Clinical Problem

Sudden death from cardiac arrest is a major health problem worldwide. Sudden cardiac death (also called sudden arrest) is death resulting from an abrupt loss of heart function (cardiac arrest). It occurs unexpectedly in individuals who may or may not have diagnosed heart disease. It occurs within minutes after symptoms appear. The most common underlying reason for patients to die suddenly from cardiac arrest is coronary heart disease although there is a significant incidence in both hypertrophic (HCM) and arrhythmogenic right ventricular cardiomyopathy (ARVC) (American Heart Association, 2006). For these patients, early detection, treatment, and prevention of sudden death are the focus of both patient and family education. Nurses must understand how to apply evidence-based findings when caring for patients with all types of cardiomyopathy, especially the younger population with HCM and ARVC because of the increased risk of sudden cardiac death.

Research Findings

Nerheim, Birger-Botkin, Piracha, and Olshansky (2004) conducted a study to assess the impact of repeated episodes of recurrent tachycardia in patients with tachycardia-induced cardiomyopathy. These authors hypothesized that although left ventricular ejection fraction measurements normalize after heart rate or rhythm control in patients with tachycardia-induced cardiomyopathy, recurrent tachycardia may have abrupt and deleterious consequences. The sample consisted of patients with tachycardia-induced cardiomyopathy that developed over years. Tachycardia episodes and outcomes were assessed. Twenty-four patients were identified, of which one-third were heart transplant candidates.

Within 6 months of rate control or correction of the rhythm, left ventricular ejection fraction improved or normalized and symptoms abated in all of the subjects. In the five patients who had tachycardia recur, the left ventricular ejection fraction dropped precipitously and heart failure ensued within 6 months, even though the initial impairment took years. Rate control eliminated heart failure and improved or normalized ejection fraction in 6 months. Three of 24 patients died suddenly and unexpectedly. The authors concluded that tachycardia-induced cardiomyopathy develops slowly and appears reversible by left ventricular ejection fraction improvement, but recurrent tachycardia

causes rapid decline in left ventricular function and development of heart failure and the risk of sudden death increases.

Implications for Nursing Practice

This study clearly indicates a need for nurses to educate cardiomyopathy patients about the importance of maintaining a normal heart rate and rhythm. It appears from the study that controlling the heart rate and rhythm will slow the progression of the disease and reduce the risk for sudden cardiac death. Because both HCM and ARVC tend to occur in the younger population, which is more physically active, it is imperative that the importance of activity restriction be emphasized and reinforced. The family and significant others need to be included in the education process. Additionally, nurses need to understand that, when caring for this patient population, spacing of activities, allowing for rest periods, and careful monitoring of cardiac rhythms are essential. Ongoing nursing assessment of the heart rate and rhythm with activity will assist the patient and family in establishing parameters for a safe level of activity. The nurse needs to understand the importance of reporting the first signs of tachycardia so that treatment can be instituted.

Critical Thinking Questions

1. In order of priority, what are the most important points that would be included in an education plan for patients with cardiomyopathy and their families?

2. What method(s) would be effective in increasing compliance with activity limitations of young people with HCM and ARVC?

3. Identify nursing measures that would decrease the risk of tachycardia occurring.

Answers to Critical Thinking Questions appear in Appendix D.

References

American Heart Association. (2006e). *Sudden cardiac death.* Retrieved June 14, 2006, from http://www.americanheart.org/presenter.jhtml?identifier=4741.

Nerheim, P., Birger-Botkin, S., Piracha, L., & Olshansky, B. (2004). Heart failure and sudden death in patients with tachycardia-induced cardiomyopathy and recurrent tachycardia. *Circulation, 110* (3), 247–252.

The physical assessment focuses on an evaluation of the clinical manifestations and their impact on the patient's ability to perform ADLs. The basic assessment includes vital signs, fluid status, auscultation of a S_3, S_4, a murmur, pulmonary congestion, and an evaluation of peripheral perfusion. Typically the patient is on a cardiac monitor to detect dysrhythmias, conduction delays, and ST segment changes. The progressive nature of the disease requires that the patient have frequent ongoing nursing assessment in order to pick up ominous changes and worsening signs of heart failure.

Nursing care focuses on decreasing the workload of the heart. Pacing activities, restricting activity, positioning, and oxygen therapy will help conserve energy and diminish cardiac workload. Details of the nursing care for patients with cardiomyopathy are given in the Nursing Process: Patient Care Plan for Cardiomyopathy feature. The impact of repeated episodes of recurrent tachycardia in patients with tachycardia-induced cardiomyopathy is outlined in the Evidence-Based Practice feature.

Hypertrophic Obstructive Cardiomyopathy

Hypertrophic cardiomyopathy (HCM) is a disorder of the sarcomere, the contractile element of the cardiac muscle that is characterized by left ventricular and occasionally right ventricular hypertrophy, with greater hypertrophy occurring in the septum. This disorder is also referred to as idiopathic hypertrophic subaortic stenosis (IHSS) and hypertrophic obstructive cardiomyopathy (HOCM). The rationale for the variation in names is described below. Figure 41–13 ■ (p. 1262) demonstrates the difference between a normal ventricular wall and a hypertrophied wall.

Epidemiology and Etiology

Hypertrophic cardiomyopathy occurs in about 1 in 500 people in the general population, and it is the most common cause of sudden death in young people. In more than 50% of the cases, HCM is a genetic disorder, manifested by a defect in cardiac muscle development.

NURSING PROCESS: Patient Care Plan for Cardiomyopathy

Assessment of Knowledge of Disease

Subjective Data:

What have you been told about your health?

What is your understanding of the treatments you are on?

Do you drink alcohol or use any recreational drugs?

Do you take rest periods during the day?

What is your level of activity?

Do you feel any change in your ability to perform your activities of daily living (ADLs)?

How much activity can you do before you become short of breath?

What symptoms need to be reported to your health care provider?

Objective Data:

Assess:

Level of understanding of disease and treatment.

Compliance with therapy.

High-risk behaviors.

Lung sounds.

Vital signs.

Peripheral edema.

Shortness of breath.

Cough—type of sputum.

Nursing Assessment and Diagnoses	Outcomes and Evaluation Parameters	Planning and Interventions with *Rationales*
Nursing Diagnosis: *Deficient Knowledge* related to disease process, care needs, and complications	**Outcomes:** Understanding of disease process, care needs, and importance of compliance with treatment. **Evaluation Parameters:** Compliance with treatment plan. Activity level appropriate for cardiac workload.	**Interventions and *Rationales:*** Avoid high-risk behaviors (alcohol, cocaine). Report any increases in clinical manifestations to your health care provider. *To retard the progression of the disease.* Comply with therapy *to prevent progression of the disease.* Activity restriction *to decrease cardiac workload.*

Assessment of Heart Failure

Subjective Data:

How much activity are you able to do before becoming short of breath?

Do you have a cough? If so, is it productive?

Do your feet swell?

Objective Data:

Assess:

Vital signs.

Lung sounds.

Jugular venous distention.

Dyspnea.

Confusion.

Decreased urine output.

Orthopnea.

Pink frothy sputum.

Skin temperature.

Peripheral edema.

Nursing Assessment and Diagnoses	Outcomes and Evaluation Parameters	Planning and Interventions with *Rationales*
Nursing Diagnosis: *Tissue perfusion ineffective* related to hypercontractility and aortic outflow obstruction	**Outcome:** Prevention of heart failure. **Evaluation Parameters:** Lungs clear. Patient denies shortness of breath. Patient verbalizes understanding and willingness of treatment plan.	**Interventions and *Rationales:*** Monitor BUN, creatinine, liver enzymes, bilirubin *to assess blood supply to liver and kidneys.* Monitor fluid balance and record as prescribed *to assess fluid retention that would exacerbate the symptoms of heart failure.* Report significant imbalances to the health care provider *to obtain the necessary intervention(s) to correct the imbalance.*

Assessment of Anxiety

Subjective Data:

What do you know about your disease process?

How do your health-related issues impact your daily life?

Do you feel anxious about your health?

Do you have family members or close friends who provide emotional support?

Objective Data:

Observe for manifestations of anxiety: restlessness, apprehension, withdrawal.

(continued)

NURSING PROCESS: Patient Care Plan for Cardiomyopathy—*Continued*

Nursing Assessment and Diagnoses	Outcomes and Evaluation Parameters	Planning and Interventions with *Rationales*
Nursing Diagnosis: *Fear* and *Anxiety* related to disease process and sudden cardiac death	**Outcome:** Anxiety level minimized and manageable. ***Evaluation Parameters:*** Verbalizes anxious feelings. Verbalizes what relieves anxiety. Demonstrates anxiety-relief by consistently controlling aggression, impulsiveness, and self-mutilation, and by improving coping and social interaction skills. Verbalizes absence of sensory perceptual disorders. Verbalizes absence of physical manifestations of anxiety. Behavioral manifestations of anxiety absent.	**Interventions and *Rationales:*** Allow time and encourage verbalization of fears related to illness *to assist in relieving anxiety.* Explore with the patient/family techniques to reduce anxiety. *This gives the patient a sense of control and opens communication about the subject.* Provide factual information concerning diagnosis, treatment, disfigurement, disabilities, and prognosis. *Truthful explanations increase trust and potentially decrease anxiety.* Explain all procedures and allow time for mental preparation. *This decreases fear and anxiety of the unknown.* Explore effective ways to minimize anxiety. *This gives the patient a sense of control.* Instruct patient on use of relaxation techniques *to relieve anxiety.* Assess need for and administer antianxiety and pain medication. *If alternative measures are not effective, may need antianxiety agents.*

Assessment of Ability to Function in Usual Role

Subjective Data:
What is your role in your family?
Are you able to perform that role?
Who takes over your role function when you are not able to?
How do you feel about your inability to function in your role?

Objective Data:
Determine knowledge of health status (see *Deficient Knowledge* nursing diagnosis).
Assess level of functioning.
Assess alternatives or alterations in role function.

Nursing Assessment and Diagnoses	Outcomes and Evaluation Parameters	Planning and Interventions with *Rationales*
Nursing Diagnosis: *Powerlessness* over altered role function due to chronic progressive illness	**Outcomes:** Verbalizes a realistic perception of control. Verbalizes realistic perception of abilities to perform. ***Evaluation Parameters:*** Identifies health outcome priorities. Verbalizes powerlessness. Identifies actions that are within his/her control and demonstrates ability to perform those actions. Reports adequate support from staff and family.	**Interventions and *Rationales:*** Discuss realistic options for self-care. *Gives patient hope and realistic view of limitations.* Reinforce personal strengths. *Decreases sense of powerlessness.* Encourage verbalization of feeling of powerlessness. *Opens communication.* Assist patient to increase independence when realistic. *Decreases powerlessness.* Allow control over surroundings and schedule when possible. *Decreases powerlessness.* Keep items within reach. *Decreases powerlessness.* Set short-term realistic goals. *Decreases powerlessness.* Explore patient's support mechanisms: family, church, and friends. *Needed as a source of support.*

Assessment of Compliance with Treatment Regimen

Subjective Data:
What do you understand about your treatment plan?
Are you able to comply with the restrictions necessary to prevent further progression of your disease?
What can the health care team do to help you with treatment compliance?

Objective Data:
Assess motivation and willingness to comply with therapy.
Assess where health care team can assist with barriers to compliance.

NURSING PROCESS: Patient Care Plan for Cardiomyopathy—*Continued*

Nursing Assessment and Diagnoses	Outcomes and Evaluation Parameters	Planning and Interventions with *Rationales*
Nursing Diagnosis: *Noncompliance* with medication and activity restrictions	**Outcomes:** Shows willingness to comply with therapy. **Evaluation Parameters:** Accepts imposed restrictions and complies with treatment plan.	**Interventions and *Rationales:*** Suggest alternative solutions to barriers *to determine interventions that will increase compliance.* Monitor and evaluate compliance with therapy *to determine patient's ability to sustain treatment.*

Assessment of Fatigue

Subjective Data:

What level of activity fatigues you?
Have you been becoming more fatigued with less activity recently?
Are you able to complete your ADLs without fatigue?

Objective Data:

Monitor tolerance to activities while on bed rest in order to obtain a baseline to plan activities. Monitor for changes in symptoms and vital signs (VS) during activity.

Determine if pulse, respirations, and BP return to normal within 3 minutes after stopping activity.

Nursing Assessment and Diagnoses	Outcomes and Evaluation Parameters	Planning and Interventions with *Rationales*
Nursing Diagnosis: *Fatigue* and *Activity Intolerance* related to decreased cardiac output	**Outcomes:** No increase in fatigue or decrease in activity levels. **Evaluation Parameters:** Absence of or no progression of peripheral edema, congested lungs, decreased CO, dyspnea, pink frothy sputum, diaphoresis, and decreased renal and liver perfusion.	**Interventions and *Rationales:*** Identify activities that increase fatigue *to avoid increasing cardiac workload.* Discontinue activity if chest pain, dyspnea, cyanosis, dizziness, hypotension, sustained tachycardia, or dysrhythmias develop *to aid in evaluating tolerance of activities.* Explore sedentary activities the patient may enjoy *to provide diversion that does not place a demand on the heart.*

Assessment of Tissue Perfusion

Subjective Data:

Do you become short of breath? If so, what causes it to occur?
How far can you walk before becoming short of breath?
Do you experience leg pain? If so, what brings it on and is it getting worse?
Do your hands and feet feel cold on a warm day?

Objective Data:

Assess:
Acid–base balance.
Lung sounds.
Respiratory rate.

Nursing Assessment and Diagnoses	Outcomes and Evaluation Parameters	Planning and Interventions with *Rationales*
Nursing Diagnosis: *Ineffective Tissue Perfusion* related to decreased cardiac output	**Outcome:** Adequate gas exchange. **Evaluation Parameters:** Normal ABGs. No dyspnea: unlabored respirations < 24/minute. Alert and oriented. Clear breath sounds. No restlessness, cyanosis, or fatigue. Oxygen saturation is within normal limits.	**Interventions and *Rationales:*** Assess for adventitious or diminished breath sounds. *Indicates decreased gas exchange and heart failure.* Note presence of cough, and amount and color of sputum. *Assessing for heart failure.* Monitor ABGs and oxygen saturation *to assess adequacy of gas exchange.* Monitor respiratory rate and depth *to assess for respiratory distress.* Monitor fluid status *to assess heart failure.* Monitor restlessness and confusion. *Indicators of inadequate gas exchange with resultant brain hypoxia.* Assess need for suctioning and/or endotracheal intubation *to maintain adequate gas exchange.* Observe for cyanosis, especially in the mucous membranes. *Indicators of inadequate gas exchange with resultant tissue hypoxia.* Turn, cough, deep breathe, elevate head of bed, instruct on use of incentive spirometry. *Measures to promote gas exchange.* Administer humidified oxygen as prescribed *to increase oxygen levels.* Report respiratory distress to the health care provider. *Medical intervention may be indicated to prevent respiratory failure.*

(continued)

NURSING PROCESS: Patient Care Plan for Cardiomyopathy—*Continued*

Assessment of Cardiac Output

Subjective Data:

Do you feel weak or light-headed with activity?

Do you become short of breath? If so, what causes it to occur?

Is the shortness of breath getting worse?

Objective Data:

Assess:

Vital signs.

Lung sounds.

Weight.

Cardiac output.

Fluid intake and output.

Nursing Assessment and Diagnoses	Outcomes and Evaluation Parameters	Planning and Interventions with *Rationales*
Nursing Diagnosis: *Decreased Cardiac Output* related to hypercontractility and obstruction to outflow	**Outcomes:** Patient able to tolerate decreased cardiac output. Stabilization of cardiac output. **Evaluation Parameters:** Clear lung sounds. No dyspnea. Normal vital signs. Skin warm and dry. Normal heart rate and rhythm. No abnormal heart sounds (S_3 and S_4). No jugular venous distention, peripheral edema, and ascites. Normal urine output.	**Interventions and *Rationales*:** Monitor vital signs, lung sounds, skin, heart rate and rhythm, edema, JVD, and ascites *in order to monitor response and tolerance of altered cardiac output (CO).* Administer negative inotropic medications as ordered *to decrease the hypercontractility.* Avoid a Valsalva maneuver *because it impedes venous return (preload).*

(a) Normal septum

(b) Hypertrophied septum

FIGURE 41–13 ■ (a) Normal heart wall and (b) hypertrophied heart wall.

Close blood relatives (parents, children, or siblings) of someone with HCM often also have enlarged ventricular septums. In the majority of patients, hypertrophic cardiomyopathy is transmitted as an autosomal dominant trait.

Hypertrophic cardiomyopathy also can be caused by hypertension or hypoparathyroidism, and it frequently is idiopathic.

This condition is most commonly found in young adults, but it can also occur in the very young and in the aged population. Men and the black population are affected more by HCM. It is usually diagnosed in young adulthood in more active athletic individuals.

Hypertrophic obstructive cardiomyopathy has the same etiology as HCM, although these patients have the additional problem of having the left ventricular aortic outflow tract obstructed. This form of cardiomyopathy occurs in 1 in 500 persons with HCM in the United States (Lakkis, Nagueh, & Klieman, 1998). The pathophysiology of this type of cardiomyopathy is described next.

Pathophysiology

With HCM the walls of the ventricle hypertrophy or remodel, without an increase in the chamber size. Fibrotic infiltrates in the myocardium produce left ventricular stiffness and add to the hypertrophy of the wall and septum. One unique feature of HCM is that the cardiac muscle may not hypertrophy "equally." The interventricular septum, especially the upper portion, tends to have a greater increase in size than the free wall of the left ventricle. These changes result in a decreased ventricular chamber size and cause the ventricles to take a longer period of time to relax. The end result is diastolic dysfunction because the loss of ventricular compliance decreases the amount of blood that will flow into the ventricle during diastole. This has a direct negative effect on cardiac output and, thus, tissue perfusion. Another characteristic of HCM is hypercontractility of the muscle, rather than hypocontractility as seen in dilated cardiomyopathy. The hypercontractility occurs particularly in the intraventricular system.

A third characteristic of HCM is obstruction to the outflow tract of the left ventricle (LV) leading into the aorta. The site and extent of hypertrophy dictates the degree of obstruction. The hypertrophy distorts the septum, and in some patients, the anterior leaflet of the mitral valve is distorted, causing it to meet the septum, thus narrowing the left ventricular outflow tract during systole (Barkman & McCay, 2002). This occurs because of the inward movement of the septum during systole, which narrows the LV outflow and increases blood velocity. This increased velocity then pulls the mitral leaflet toward the septum (the venturi effect). Figure 41–14 ■ demonstrates how the septum and the anterior leaflet narrow the left ventricular outflow tract into the aorta.

Significant LV outflow obstruction is present in some patients at rest, while in others it is only evident during increased activity such as exercise. Reduced preload decreases chamber size and increased heart rate will increase LV outflow obstruction. Dehydration and suddenly sitting upright (orthostatic hypotension) are two examples of factors that will decrease preload, and fever and exercise are two factors that increase heart rate. The end result is a reduction in cardiac output that may range from minimal to severe and may lead to syncope, serious cardiac arrhythmias (ventricular tachycardia), and sudden death. Heart failure is the eventual outcome as the disease progresses. Not all individuals with HCM have obstruction to outflow, but if present, HCM is further classified as hypertrophic obstructive cardiomyopathy. If the obstructive process is present, the disorder is also referred to as idiopathic hypertrophic subaortic stenosis (see Figure 41–14 ■).

Clinical Manifestations

Clinical manifestations most commonly begin in late adolescence or early adulthood, but may appear at any age. Many of the clinical manifestations of HCM are similar to dilated cardiomyopathy. The most frequently reported manifestation is

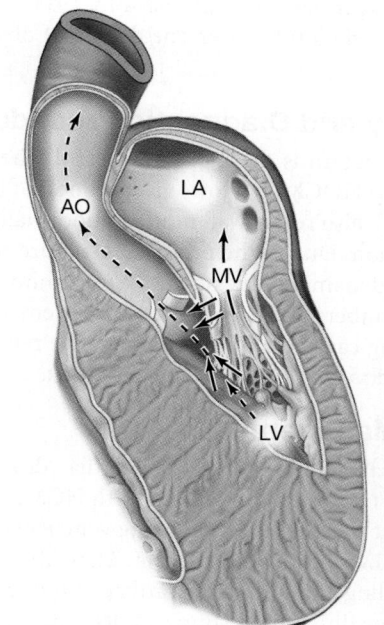

FIGURE 41–14 ■ Hypertrophic obstructive cardiomyopathy.

dyspnea, which is due to high pulmonary pressures created by the backup of blood from the restricted left ventricle. This type of cardiomyopathy also may occur without symptoms, although other frequently reported symptoms include chest pain, dizziness, presyncope or syncope, fatigue, orthopnea and paroxysmal nocturnal dyspnea, and palpitations. The symptoms appear gradually, will progress over time, and are associated with deterioration of LV function. Exercise tends to precipitate the symptoms and increases the risk of sudden death. But in some individual's sudden death or severe heart failure are the first clinical manifestations of the disease. Right- and left-sided heart failure may be present. The risk of sudden death, which appears most often in young adults, can be decreased by avoiding strenuous exercise. Sudden death is the most common cause of death for individuals with HCM.

Both supraventricular (primarily atrial fibrillation) and ventricular (tachycardia and fibrillation) dysrhythmias occur with HCM, along with sudden death. Additionally, it is common to have an abnormally forceful LV apical pulse, S_4, and a harsh crescendo–decrescendo systolic murmur of varying intensity that is heard best at the left lower sternal border and the apex. A systolic thrill may be palpated at the apex or lower left sternal border.

In severe cases of HOCM, pulmonary artery pressures are elevated because of increased backward pressure due to an inability of the left ventricle to empty. This eventually increases right ventricular pressure, causing the interventricular septum to shift to the left. The leftward shift causes further obstruction to the ventricular outflow tract (Barkman & McCay, 2002).

Adults with HCM were followed for 9 to 11 years by a group of researchers. The researchers found that patients who were asymptomatic had a lower cardiac mortality rate and a lower incidence of sudden cardiac death than those individuals with symptoms (Takagi, Yamakado, & Nakano, 1999). There is not a predictable correlation between the degree of obstruction and symptoms.

Laboratory and Diagnostic Procedures

The echocardiogram is the most useful tool when diagnosing both HCM and HOCM. It allows visualization of the LV hypertrophy and will also reveal wall motion abnormalities and diastolic dysfunction. Due to the progressive nature of the disease, bedside hemodynamic studies are done to monitor the pressures in cardiac chambers and the pulmonary system as well as providing ongoing cardiac output readings. The remainder of the tests are described in the Diagnostic Tests box.

Medical Management

Preventing heart failure and sudden cardiac death are the primary goals of treatment for patients with HCM. Improving the cardiac output is achieved by reducing ventricular contractility and relieving LV outflow obstruction. These measures improve ventricular filling and ultimately cardiac output and the quality of life. It is often difficult for young adults to adhere to a regimen of decreased activity. Emotional support and education are essential by both the nurses and the health care providers to help the individual understand and comply with the reduced activity levels.

If possible, finding and treating the underlying cause is the first priority of medical management. The remainder of medical care is directed toward controlling clinical manifestations, preventing progression of the disease, and improving the quality of life for the individual. The treatment plan, described below, consists of medications, activity restriction, fluid stabilization, surgical interventions, and possibly implanting electronic devices. Genetic testing for HCM is discussed in the Genetic Considerations box.

Negative inotropic medications, such as beta-adrenergic blocking agents and calcium antagonists, provide the mainstay of medical therapy and are used to decrease the hypercontractility and outflow obstruction. These medications also decrease the heart rate, which decreases cardiac workload and oxygen consumption. If the patient is in atrial fibrillation, anticoagulant medications are prescribed to assist in the prevention of clot formation. Antiarrhythmic medications are used to prevent life-threatening dysrhythmias and improve cardiac output and ICDs are used to prevent sudden cardiac death. Finally, HCM predisposes patients to endocarditis. Therefore, the health care

GENETIC CONSIDERATIONS for Hypertrophic Cardiomyopathy

Due to the genetic link of hypertrophic cardiomyopathy, the health care provider needs to test close family members for the disease. Family teaching needs to include CPR classes (National Institute on Alcohol Abuse and Alcoholism, 2002).

DIAGNOSTIC TESTS for Hypertrophic and Hypertrophic Obstructive Cardiomyopathy

Test with *Normal Values*	Expected Abnormality	Rationale for Abnormality
Chest x-ray: *Clear lungs and normal heart size*	Cardiac enlargement (cardiomegaly) specifically left atrial enlargement. If heart failure is present, pulmonary congestion and edema.	Due to progression of the disease process.
Resting and ambulatory ECG: *Normal conduction time intervals* (see Chapter 38)	*Resting:* Increased voltage and duration of the QRS complex. Both atrial and ventricular dysrhythmias. *Ambulatory:* ST segment changes that occur with increased activity. Increased hypercontractility that increases with activity.	Due to the ventricular hypertrophy and myocardial ischemia.
Echocardiogram (ultrasound): *Normal chamber size and normal cardiac structures*	Left ventricular hypertrophy. Hypercontractility. Asymmetrical wall size. Diastolic dysfunction.	The disease causes enlargement of the chamber and septum and hypercontractility, which results in abnormal valve function and cardiac output.
Cardiac catheterization to rule out coronary artery disease, assess hemodynamic status, and chamber size and function: *Normal coronary arteries, chambers, and valve pressures*	Increased chamber size and may see changes in valve function and cardiac output.	Tissue hypertrophy and hypercontractility cause abnormal valve motion, resulting in obstruction of the aortic outflow tract.
Radionuclide study: *Normal chamber volumes and blood perfusion to cardiac muscle*	Increased left ventricular and septal wall size. Asymmetrical hypertrophy. Hypercontractility.	Tissue hypertrophy and hypercontractility related to disease process.
Cardiac biopsy may be performed in order to analyze myocardial tissue: *Normal cellular size and function*	Tissue positive for infiltrations and fibrosis.	Changes due to disease process.

provider typically orders prophylactic antibiotics before dental work or invasive procedures (AHA, 2004).

Dehydration needs to be avoided because it will decrease preload and cardiac output. Patient and family education needs to stress the importance of consistent normal hydration. Activities, foods, and drinks (alcohol) that cause dehydration must be avoided. Surgical management is indicated for HCM if the patient has not responded positively to medical therapy and if marked obstruction to the aortic outflow tract is present due to the mitral valve meeting the enlarged septum. The surgical procedure is termed a ventriculomyotomy and involves excising some of the hypertrophied septal muscle. This widens the LV outflow tract, improves cardiac output, and relieves symptoms. Clinical manifestations and exercise tolerance are improved after this surgery in about 75% of cases (Braunwald, et al., 2005). A second surgical procedure sometimes used to decrease obstruction is the removal of the mitral valve, chordae tendineae, and the papillary muscle (see Figure 41–4 ■, p. 1234). The mitral valve is then replaced by an artificial valve. This procedure substantially reduces the space taken up by the mitral valve and supporting structures, allowing blood to move more easily around the enlarged septum. In addition to surgical complications, the primary problem of both of these procedures is dysrhythmias.

A nonsurgical treatment for HCM is alcohol ablation involving injection of alcohol down a small branch of the coronary artery feeding the area of muscle hypertrophy (septum). The alcohol destroys the extra cardiac muscle without having to surgically remove it, in effect causing an intentional myocardial infarction (Lewis, Boyd, Hubert, & Steele, 2001; Steinbis, 2003).

An implantable cardioverter defibrillator is useful for patients with HCM to treat ventricular tachycardia, ventricular fibrillation, and sudden death (American College of Cardiology [ACC], 2006; Saxton, Kumar, & DeMarco, 2006). If left ventricular dysfunction and ejection fraction less than 35% are present, a cardiac resynchronization therapy (CRT) (biventricular pacemaker) may help increase cardiac output (ACC, 2006; Saxton et al., 2006). Some experts believe with advanced heart failure a combination of an ICD and CRT is indicated (Saxton et al., 2006). Chapter 39 🔗 provides complete descriptions of both the ICD and the pacemaker. Heart transplantation is the only long-term cure for the disease. Heart transplantation is described in Chapter 42 🔗.

■ Nursing Management

The primary goals of nursing care are to assess and monitor progress of the disease and to provide patient education and emotional support for individuals with this chronic progressive disease. The nursing process provides a framework for the care of these patients. A complete plan of care for HCM is outlined in this chapter in the Nursing Process: Patient Care Plan for Cardiomyopathy (p. 1259).

Assessment

Nurses must monitor and report changes in the assessment that indicate complications and progression of the disease. Specific nursing assessment data, interventions, rationales, and outcomes are outlined in the Nursing Process: Patient Care Plan for Cardiomyopathy (p. 1259) and are also reviewed in Chapter 42 🔗.

Monitoring the patient's hemodynamic status is essential as the disease progresses. Pulmonary artery pressure increases indicate the onset of heart failure, which increases the risk of further ventricular outflow obstruction. Moreover, the cardiac output needs ongoing monitoring to evaluate oxygenation and adequate tissue perfusion. The nurse needs to space activities for the hospitalized patient in order to allow for periods of rest.

The nursing diagnoses that apply to HCM include:

1. *Activity Intolerance, Risk for*
2. *Tissue Perfusion Ineffective, Cardiac and Peripheral*
3. *Coping*
4. *Fatigue*

Outcomes and Evaluation Parameters

Due to the risk of cardiac sudden death, both HCM and HOCM have a grave prognosis. End-stage therapies such as cardiac transplantation may be a viable option. The patient and family need to be given all options and the nurse must assess their understanding of the situation. Evaluation parameters would include a verbalization of the options including the lifestyle changes that would be necessary with organ transplantation.

Planning, Interventions, and Rationales

Providing emotional support for the patient with HCM is essential when planning the management of these patients, since this is a progressive chronic disease that could cause sudden death at anytime. Identifying perceived stressors for both the family and patient and assisting them in alleviating them will decrease the emotional stress. The patient and family need to feel free to verbalize fears and concerns and be reassured that these concerns are legitimate and that there are resources available to provide assistance. Providing realistic hope helps reduce anxiety and increase self-esteem; the patient needs to be encouraged to accomplish a goal no matter how small. If the patient is facing imminent death or waiting for a donor heart, an environment must be created in which the patient and family can openly express concerns and acknowledge fears. Encouragement, a caring touch, and a listening ear will improve the quality of life for patients and families dealing with HCM. See the Nursing Process: Patient Care Plan for Cardiomyopathy (p. 1259) for a complete nursing care plan to guide the care of patients with HCM and HOCM.

CRITICAL ALERT *Families of patients with HCM and HOCM should be encouraged to learn CPR and how to access emergency care near their home.*

■ Restrictive Cardiomyopathy

Restrictive cardiomyopathy (RCM) is the least common type found in the United States. This disorder is characterized by endocardial scarring that usually affects one or both ventricles and restricts filling of blood, resulting in systolic dysfunction. The ventricle has normal wall thickness, but the walls are rigid, producing elevated filling pressures and dilated atria. Involvement of the valve is common, but the outflow tract is spared (see Figure 41–12 ■, p. 1255).

Epidemiology and Etiology

The cause of restrictive cardiomyopathy is divided into two classifications, primary and secondary. The cause of primary restrictive cardiomyopathy is idiopathic, whereas secondary cardiomyopathy is thought to be caused by a number of pathologic processes outlined below. Idiopathic restrictive cardiomyopathy can present at any age, but its incidence is increased in the elderly and is more common in women (Ammash, Seward, & Bailey, 2000).

The incidence of cocaine-related restrictive cardiomyopathy is on the rise. Cocaine causes both coronary artery and peripheral vasoconstriction and high levels of circulating catecholamines. The combined effect causes an increased workload for the myocardium and a decreased supply of oxygen, leading to myocardial ischemia and infarction. The cells of the myocardium become damaged, producing cardiomyopathy. These patients typically have a poor prognosis.

Pathophysiology

The development and progress of secondary RCM may be caused by amyloidosis, endomyocardial fibrosis, disorders in glycogen storage, hemochromatosis, and sarcoidosis or it may be idiopathic. With amyloidosis, a deposition of eosinophilic fibrinous protein buildup occurs in the heart, causing loss of an ability to stretch. Idiopathic restrictive cardiomyopathy is a poorly recognized entity of unknown cause characterized by nondilated, nonhypertrophied ventricles with diastolic dysfunction, resulting in dilated atria, with or without systolic dysfunction (Ammash et al., 2000). Contractility is unaffected by restrictive cardiomyopathy.

Microscopically, the endometrial changes that occur with restrictive cardiomyopathy include nonspecific patchy endocardial and interstitial fibrosis with increased collagen deposition and molecular hypertrophy. These changes result in the ventricle losing its ability to stretch, thereby decreasing compliance and an ability to fill, and causing a drop in cardiac output. As intraventricular pressures increase and cardiac output decreases,

manifestations of heart failure begin to appear. These manifestations typically progress rapidly, resulting in high mortality.

Clinical Manifestations

Patients with RCM have signs of pulmonary and systemic congestion. The most common symptom is dyspnea. In addition, patients complain of palpitations, fatigue, syncope, angina, generalized weakness, and exercise intolerance. In the advanced stages, clinical manifestations of either or both right- or left-sided heart failure are present. An S_3 is frequently present, and a systolic murmur from mitral and tricuspid regurgitation is common.

Laboratory and Diagnostic Procedures

As with all of the cardiomyopathies, the echocardiogram is the most useful diagnostic test for the diagnosis of restrictive cardiomyopathy. It reveals a thickened cardiac wall, a small ventricular chamber size, and dilated atria. This test also is able to evaluate diastolic filling changes as the disease progresses. The echocardiogram is also useful in distinguishing restrictive cardiomyopathy from constrictive pericarditis, the major disorder that mimics restrictive cardiomyopathy. Hemodynamic studies identify elevated left atrial and left ventricular pressures. The Diagnostic Tests box describes the remainder of the diagnostic tests for restrictive cardiomyopathy.

Medical Management

Currently there is no specific treatment or cure for RCM. Therefore, therapy is aimed at controlling symptoms to improve the quality of life. Like hypertrophic cardiomyopathy, restrictive cardiomyopathy patients are taught to avoid situations that impair venous filling, causing a further drop in cardiac output. The patient and family need to have a clear understanding that activity such as strenuous exercise, as well as any situation that causes dehydration, needs to be avoided.

Medical management is aimed at reducing pulmonary and systemic congestion and reducing the workload of the heart to di-

---

DIAGNOSTIC TESTS for Restrictive Cardiomyopathy

Test with *Normal Values*	Expected Abnormality	Rationale for Abnormality
Chest x-ray: *Clear lungs and normal heart size*	Cardiomegaly, specifically atrial enlargement. Pulmonary venous congestion. Pleural effusions may be present with heart failure.	Restriction of blood flow leading to pulmonary venous backup of blood and resulting in cardiac enlargement heart failure.
Electrocardiogram (ECG): *Normal conduction time intervals* (see Chapter 38)	Atrial fibrillation. Complex serious ventricular dysrhythmias. Tachycardia.	Distortion of the cardiac conduction system due to cardiomegaly. Cardiac ischemia causing dysrhythmias.
Echocardiogram: *Normal chamber size and normal cardiac structures*	Thickened cardiac wall. Small ventricular chamber size. Dilated atria. Decreased diastolic filling as disease progresses.	Restrictive nature of disease increases wall thickness and prevents myocardial fiber stretch to accommodate blood volumes. Blood backs up in atria causing it to dilate.
Radionuclide study: *Normal chamber volumes and blood perfusion to cardiac muscle*	Increased ventricular volume mass, decreasing chamber size. Areas of decreased perfusion.	Restrictive nature of disease prevents myocardial fiber stretch to accommodate blood volumes, causing decreased cardiac output and tissue perfusion.
Endomyocardial biopsy: *Normal myocardial tissue*	Presence of amyloidosis and/or sarcoidosis.	Causative agents for disease.

minish heart failure. There is not a medical cure for this disease, although treatment of the underlying cause of secondary restrictive cardiomyopathy may be beneficial.

The cornerstone of the medical treatment for RCM is drug therapy. Antiarrhythmic medications are prescribed, depending on the specific dysrhythmia. Diuretics are used to decrease pulmonary congestion, although the patient has to be monitored closely to prevent dehydration. Calcium channel blockers and beta-adrenergic blockers will decrease the heart rate, which then increases ventricular filling time. Anticoagulants are indicated for patients in atrial fibrillation to prevent thromboembolism (p. 1270). A low-sodium diet will decrease fluid retention and pulmonary congestion.

As with dilated cardiomyopathy, the heart failure from restrictive cardiomyopathy may be treated with a biventricular pacemaker. An implantable cardioverter defibrillator may be indicated to prevent sudden cardiac death (Chapter 39).

Both primary and secondary restrictive cardiomyopathies have a poor prognosis. Death is most frequently due to heart failure, sudden death, dysrhythmias, or stroke. End-stage heart failure strategies are more fully discussed in Chapter 42 .

PHARMACOLOGY Summary of Medications to Treat Cardiomyopathy

Medication Category	Action	Application/Indication	Nursing Responsibility
Cardiomyopathy			

Cardiac Medications
ACE inhibitors, angiotensin receptor blockers:
  Losartan
  Candesartan
  Irbesartan
  Valsartan
  Beta-adrenergic blockers
  Metoprolol tartrate (Carvedilol)
  Calcium channel blockers
  Antiarrhythmic agents
  Amiodarone
  Dofetilide
	ACE inhibitor: Lowers peripheral resistance and reduces blood volume by enhancing the excretion of sodium by inhibition of angiotensin-converting enzyme.
	Slows the heart rate. Decreases conduction through AV node.
	Increases force and velocity of myocardial systolic contraction. Reduces automaticity in the SA node and slows impulse conduction through the AV node. Used for supraventricular dysrhythmias.
		Dilated cardiomyopathy (DCM): slows or stops tissue remodeling and heart failure.
		Decreases preload and afterload.
		Arrhythmogenic right ventricular cardiomyopathy (ARVC): heart failure.
		DCM: reduces heart failure symptoms; lower risk of mortality, sudden death; and delays need for transplant. Slow or stop tissue remodeling.
		Hypertrophic cardiomyopathy/ hypertrophic obstructive cardiomyopathy (HCM/HOCM): decreases hypercontractility and outflow obstruction.
		Also decreases the heart rate, which decreases cardiac workload and oxygen consumption.
		Restrictive cardiomyopathy (RCM): decreases heart rate, which then increases ventricular filling time.
		ARVC: tachyarrhythmias.
		HCM/HOCM: decreases the hypercontractility and outflow obstruction.
		Also decreases the heart rate, which decreases cardiac workload and oxygen consumption.
		RCM: decreases heart rate, which then increases ventricular filling time.
		DCM: helps control atrial and ventricular irritability, decreasing dysrhythmias.
		HCM/HOCM/RCM: to prevent life-threatening dysrhythmias and improve cardiac output.
		ARVC: tachyarrhythmias.
			Monitor blood pressure carefully after first dose for hypotension.
			Educate patient that it takes 2 weeks for therapeutic effect.
			May experience dizziness.
			Monitor vital signs; observe for bradycardia, heart failure, or pulmonary edema.
			Monitor orthostatic hypotension.
			Assess fatigue and weakness.
			Monitor intake and output.
			Assess heart rate, blood pressure, lung sounds, and ECG monitor regularly.
			Monitor for hypotension especially when being given intravenously.

Diuretics	Blocks reabsorption of sodium and chloride in the loop of Henle. Reduces edema associated with heart failure.	*DCM /HCM/HOCM/RCM:* to decrease pulmonary congestion. *ARVC:* right heart failure.	Potassium levels also need monitoring because low levels are a side effect of certain diuretics, especially furosemide. May need potassium replacement. Measure urine output prior to administration to gauge the response to the medication.

(continued)

PHARMACOLOGY Summary of Medications to Treat Cardiomyopathy—*Continued*

Anticoagulant Therapy Coumadin Heparin	Can either inhibit specific clotting factors in coagulation cascade or diminish the clotting action of platelets.	*HCM/HOCM/RCM:* if atrial fibrillation present, used to decrease clot formation.	Ongoing assessment of therapeutic blood level per health care provider orders. Assess for bleeding including nosebleeds, bruising, "coffee-grounds" emesis, tarry stools, fatigue, and pale skin. Assess for decreases in hemoglobin, hematocrit, RBCs, and platelets.
Nitrates (nitroglycerin)	Relaxes both atrial and venous smooth muscle, causing decreased preload and afterload.	*DCM:* decreases preload and afterload.	Assess blood pressure before and during therapy. Hypotension could result. Should be given with other vasodilators. Patient education includes: No alcohol use. Rotate patches. Keep medication with you at all times and away from excessive heat and light. Report blurred vision, dry mouth, and severe headache.
Antibiotics	Inhibits protein synthesis of microorganisms by binding reversibly to a ribosome, thus interfering with transmission of genetic information.	*HCM/HOCM:* predisposed to endocarditis so prophylactic antibiotics before dental work or invasive procedures are prescribed.	Assessment of history of drug allergies prior to administration. Assessment of clinical manifestations of allergic reaction. Assessment of relief of clinical manifestations to determine drug effectiveness. Patient education regarding need to complete the entire regimen and report any clinical manifestations of drug allergy.

Sources: Adams, M. P., Josephen, D. L., & Holland, L. N. (Eds.). (2005). *Pharmacology for nurses: A pathophysiologic approach.* Upper Saddle River, NJ: Pearson Prentice Hall; American Heart Association. (2005). *Handbook of emergency cardiovascular care for health providers.* Dallas, TX: Author; Wilson, B., Shannon, M., & Stang, C. (Eds.). (2005). *Nurses drug guide.* Upper Saddle River, NJ: Pearson Prentice Hall.

■ Nursing Management

Nursing management focuses on decreasing the workload of the heart and conserving energy. Nursing care is similar to the care of the patient with the other types of cardiomyopathy. The Nursing Process: Patient Care Plan for Cardiomyopathy (p. 1259) outlines the care for all types of cardiomyopathy and the discharge priorities are presented in the Patient Teaching & Discharge Priorities box.

■ Arrhythmogenic Right Ventricular Cardiomyopathy

Arrhythmogenic right ventricular cardiomyopathy (ARVC) is a newly recognized heart disease. It is defined as an electrical disturbance that develops when the muscle tissue in the right ventricle is replaced with fibrous scar and fatty tissues. In approximately 30% of patients, the left ventricle also is involved (Bruce, 2006).

ARVC has several different names, all of which refer to the same condition. These names include arrhythmogenic right ventricular dysplasia/cardiomyopathy (ARVD/C) and arrhythmogenic right ventricular dysplasia (ARVD). It is becoming usual practice for the disease to be known as ARVC (Cardiomyopathy Association, 2006).

Epidemiology and Etiology

The precise cause of ARVC is unknown, although it has a possible familial link in some patients. The onset of the disease typically is between the late teens to early 20s. It is rare for it to develop in early childhood or after age 40. It appears that men and women of any ethnic origin can be affected. When more than one member of the family is affected, the mode of inheritance appears to be an autosomal dominant gene (Bruce, 2006; Cardiomyopathy Association, 2006).

Because little is known about the disease, it is difficult to estimate how many people are affected. It is reasonable to estimate in the light of current knowledge that approximately 1 in 3,000 to 1 in 10,000 people are affected (Cardiomyopathy Association, 2006). Certain areas of the world have a higher incidence of the disease; these include Venice, Italy, and parts of Greece.

Pathophysiology

Patchy areas of fat develop primarily on the right ventricle, replacing functional cardiac muscle. The specific reason for this occurrence is under investigation. One theory suggests that an abnormal gene or genes leads to heart muscle cell damage and loss. The fibrous and fatty tissues are thought to replace these heart muscle cells as an attempt by the body to repair the dam-

PATIENT TEACHING & DISCHARGE PRIORITIES for Cardiomyopathy

Need	Teaching
Prevention of disease progression	Teach the importance of following a treatment plan that includes medications (that slow disease progression) and lifestyle changes. Teaching includes: • Timed rest periods between activities. • Space activities to prevent dyspnea. • Avoid alcohol and drug use (cocaine). • Restrict sodium and fluid intake to prevent fluid overload.
Compliance with therapy	Teach the importance of complying with the treatment plan in order to slow the progress of the disease and prevent sudden death. Determine motivation factors for individual patients and create a plan that utilizes these factors. Comply with follow-up health care provider visits.
Prevent exacerbation of heart failure	Explain to patient/family what clinical manifestations to monitor and report to the health care worker: • Sudden increase in weight in a short period of time; i.e., greater than 2–3 lb in a few days • Shortness of breath at rest, possibly with chest pressure • Increased shortness of breath with activities • Persistent productive cough • Swelling ankles, feet, or abdomen • Waking breathless at night. Diet therapy: limit sodium to 2–3 g and 2 liters of fluid daily. Eat small, frequent meals. Plan rest periods between activities.
Reportable clinical manifestations	Clinical manifestations of heart failure (Chapter 42 ⊘). Clinical manifestations of infective endocarditis. New onset chest pain.

age. Once the muscle has been replaced, the areas become hypokinetic. Given the patchy nature of ARVC, abnormal areas may be surrounded by normal ones. Right ventricular thickening occurs early in the disease, and as the disease progresses it may involve the left ventricle. The patchy disorganized structure of the myocardium areas of the right ventricle may lead to one or more sites of abnormal electrical activity, accounting for abnormal ECG rhythm disturbances and abnormal contractile ability.

Clinical Manifestations

The degree and type of clinical manifestations and the risk of complications vary greatly among individuals with ARVC. Many patients report little to no difficulties or manifestations, whereas others have life-threatening problems. Typically, patients seek help for palpitations, light-headedness, and fatigue. More serious symptoms include syncope and symptoms of heart failure. The ECG exhibits complete or incomplete right bundle branch block. A signal-averaged ECG is abnormal. Patients may present with ventricular tachycardia that generally has a left bundle branch block contour, with T waves inverted over the right precordial leads. The ventricular tachycardia may be due to reentry. Supraventricular arrhythmias also can occur, and exercise can induce the ventricular tachycardia in some patients. Chapter 38 ⊘ provides an in-depth description of these dysrhythmias. Sudden cardiac death is the most serious complication of ARVC and at times the very first sign of the disease. It is generally believed that sporting activities do not cause ARVC, although the condition is reported more frequently among athletes compared to other groups of people (Cardiomyopathy Association, 2006).

Heart failure is a less common complication of ARVC and appears to occur later in the disease. Typically, right heart failure first is more common than left heart failure and is manifested by prominent visible veins in the neck; distention of the liver, which may lead to a sensation of fullness or discomfort in the upper abdomen; and swollen legs or ankles. Left heart failure occurs late when the disease is in the advanced stages and is manifested by fatigue and shortness of breath (see Chapter 42 ⊘).

Laboratory and Diagnostic Procedures

Research is showing that an MRI is a useful noninvasive test for diagnosis detection of right ventricular myocardial fibro-fatty changes in ARVD/C (Cardiomyopathy Association, 2006). The MRI has a strong correlation with histopathology and predicted inducible ventricular tachycardia (VT) on programmed electrical stimulation (Tandri et al., 2005). It has the unique ability to characterize tissue, specifically by differentiating fat from muscle. The echocardiogram also is a useful tool to assist in the diagnosis because it allows for visualization of the right ventricle and assessment of wall motion abnormalities. Due to the cardiac conduction changes that are associated with ARVC, serial ECGs are indicated to detect rhythm changes and serious life-threatening dysrhythmias. The remainder of the tests are described in the Diagnostic Tests box (p. 1270).

Medical Management

Other than heart transplant, there is no cure for ARVC, so medical management is aimed at controlling clinical manifestations and progression of the disease. Due to the familial nature of

DIAGNOSTIC TESTS for Arrhythmogenic Right Ventricular Cardiomyopathy

Test with *Normal Values*	Expected Abnormality	Rationale for Abnormality
Electrocardiogram (ECG): *Holter monitor:* ambulatory recording of the ECG over 24 to 48 hours. Exercise ECG: *Normal conduction time intervals* (see Chapter 38 💿)	Repolarization and depolarization abnormalities. Intraventricular conduction delay. Complete or incomplete right bundle branch block. Lethal ventricular dysrhythmias.	Dysrhythmias occur due to changes in the structure of the myocardial tissue causing abnormal conduction patterns. To detect exercise-induced ventricular dysrhythmias and assess functional capacity.
Cardiac catheterization and electrophysiological study (EPS)	Able to rule out coronary artery disease. Right ventricular dilation and dysfunction. *EPS:* able to induce the dysrhythmias. (Chapter 39 💿 discusses these tests.)	Determines the presence of other causes for the clinical manifestations. Fatty infiltration changes to myocardium cause ventricular dilation. Determines which drug will control the dysrhythmias.
Endomyocardial biopsy: *Normal cardiac tissue*	Fibrous scars and fatty infiltration changes to right ventricular myocardium.	Due to disease process.
Echocardiogram: *Normal chamber size and normal cardiac structures*	Dilated right and left ventricles with diminished contractility.	Due to fibrous scarring and fatty infiltrations to the myocardium.
Magnetic resonance imaging (MRI): *Normal cardiac tissue and chamber size*	Right ventricular myocardial fibro-fatty change.	Due to fibrous scarring and fatty infiltrations to the myocardium.
Exercise radionuclide study: *Normal chamber volumes and blood perfusion to cardiac muscle*	To detect exercise-induced ventricular dysrhythmias and assess functional capacity.	Detects changes that occur only with exercise.
Chest x-ray: *Clear lungs and normal heart size*	Cardiomegaly.	Due to fibrous scarring and fatty infiltrations to the myocardium.

Sources: Bruce, J. (2006). Getting to the heart of cardiomyopathy: Find out about the four types of cardiomyopathies. *Cardiac Insider*, pp. 16–20; Tandri, H., Saranathan, M., Rodriguez, E. R., Martinez, C., Bomma, C., Nasir, K., et al. (2005, January 4). Noninvasive detection of myocardial fibrosis in arrhythmogenic right ventricular cardiomyopathy using delayed-enhancement magnetic resonance imaging. *Journal of the America College of Cardiology, 45*(1), 98–103.

ARVC, medical management begins with an in-depth medical and family history. The heath care provider needs to assess any personal or family history of palpitations, light-headed sensation, or collapse.

Because the clinical manifestations and risk of sudden cardiac death vary with ARVC, there are no precise guidelines to determine which patients need to be treated and which is the best management approach. Established therapeutic options include beta-adrenergic blockers, antiarrhythmic drugs, catheter ablation, and an ICD. Pharmacologic therapy is the first choice of treatment for patients with well-tolerated and non–life-threatening ventricular arrhythmias. Treatment includes beta-adrenergic blockers and class I and III antiarrhythmic drugs (sotalol or amiodarone) alone or in combination with beta-adrenergic blockers. If heart failure is present, the patient is treated with diuretics and vasodilators. Typically, medication efficacy is based on symptom improvement, although a more reliable approach is the use of 24-hour Holter monitoring or stress testing to determine the effect of life activities and stress on arrhythmic events. Chapter 38 💿 discusses Holter monitoring.

Due to the risk for sudden cardiac death, in patients with sustained ventricular tachycardia (VT) and/or ventricular fibrillation (VF), antiarrhythmic drug treatment is indicated. Additionally, the need for electrophysiology (EPS) guided drug testing must be evaluated. The EPS is an invasive procedure that is done in the cardiac catheterization laboratory. It involves placing multiple multipolar catheter electrodes into the venous and sometimes the arterial side of the heart. These electrodes are positioned at various locations inside of the heart and they have two purposes: to record the electrical signal within the heart and to deliver an electrical stimulus at precisely timed intervals (programmed stimulation), which may or may not result in the initiation of VT/VF. This procedure identifies the location of the dysrhythmia. Antiarrhythmic drugs are administered followed by a second attempt to induce the dysrhythmia. If the dysrhythmia is not inducible, the drug is considered effective. Currently EPS is the standard test for reproducing dysrhythmias in a controlled environment in order to diagnose and treat the dysrhythmias.

Nonpharmacologic treatment is reserved for those patients with life-threatening ventricular dysrhythmias in whom drug treatment is either ineffective, is not applicable because of the inability to induce the clinical ventricular arrhythmias during EPS, or is associated with serious side effects. If the dysrhythmia remains inducible in patients with sustained VT and/or VF during EPS, other options are available. Pace mapping directed radio-frequency catheter ablation and ICD are the current options. Radio-frequency catheter ablation is a procedure done in the cardiac catheterization laboratory in which areas in the myocardium that initiate dysrhythmias are identified and destroyed with chemicals or electrical energy. The goal is to eliminate sites in the myocardium that initiate the dysrhythmia, thereby eliminating the dysrhythmia (AHA, 2006b). The implantable cardioverter defibrillator Radio-frequency ablation is a device that can automatically terminate potentially lethal dysrhythmias of VT and VF. It is considered safe and improves the long-term prognosis of ARVC patients at high risk of sudden death (Wichter et al., 2004). A complete description of ICDs is given in Chapter 39 . When all medical options have been exhausted, ARVC patients may be candidates for heart transplantation (Bruce, 2006).

Nursing Management

As with all types of cardiomyopathy, nursing management focuses on decreasing the workload of the heart and conserving energy. Additionally, these patients need to be monitored carefully for cardiac dysrhythmias. Nursing care is similar to the care of the patient with the other types of cardiomyopathy. The Nursing Process: Patient Care Plan for Cardiomyopathy feature (p. 1259) outlines the care of all four types of cardiomyopathy, and the discharge priorities are presented in the earlier Patient Teaching & Discharge Priorities box (p. 1269).

Health Promotion for the Cardiomyopathies

The chronicity of a cardiomyopathy has an impact on the quality of life for both the patient and the family/significant others. The nurse needs to evaluate the impact of the disease on the patient's role within the family and community. Additionally, the nurse needs to involve the family in the treatment plan and educational program. It is essential to identify stressors and attempt to work with the patient and family to relieve them.

Providing appropriate explanations of all treatments and interventions will increase compliance by both the patient and family. Home health nurses can provide the patient and family with an ongoing assessment of the effectiveness of the treatment plan and facilitate changes when necessary. The goal of therapy is to keep the patient functional and out of the hospital, and home health nurses are essential in the accomplishment of that goal.

When educating patients nurses must be knowledgeable about cultural factors that impact the development of cardiomyopathy. The dietary customs and social habits of certain cultures increase the risk for the development and progression of the disease. For example, excessive alcohol intake is a risk factor for the development and progression of dilated cardiomyopathy. Excessive alcohol intake is common in certain cultures. When developing a teaching plan, the nurse needs to evaluate the need for education related to alcohol intake and its impact on DCM. The Cultural Considerations box discusses cultural groups that have a higher rate of alcoholism.

For HCM and ARVC, patient education includes information on the importance of avoiding strenuous exercise in preventing symptoms, dehydration, and possibly lethal complications. Compliance with activity restriction is often difficult for the young adult with these disorders. Education also is necessary for increasing compliance with the medication regimen and dietary sodium restrictions. Patient compliance will help prevent the progression of the disease process and potentially improve the quality of life for the chronic disease. The Pa-

---

CULTURAL CONSIDERATIONS Alcoholism

Cultural Groups with the highest level of alcohol intake include:

American Indians

Alaska Natives

Native Hawaiians

Asian Americans

Note also that:

Alcohol use is increasing significantly among Hispanic adolescents.

Among all age and ethnic groups, men are more likely to drink than are women, and to consume large quantities in a single sitting.

---

tient Teaching & Discharge Priorities box (p. 1269) discussed the discharge priorities and learning needs for patients with cardiomyopathy. Due to the genetic predisposition of HCM and ARVC, family members need to be educated about being tested for the disease.

Collaborative Management

Due to the chronic and progressive nature of cardiomyopathy, a collaborative care approach is optimal for management. Utilizing a multidisciplinary team approach, including health care providers, nurses, physical and occupational therapists, psychologists/psychiatrists, dieticians, and pharmacists, will facilitate the best possible quality of life for the patient and the family. It is essential that the health care provider monitor the progression of the cardiomyopathy to determine the treatment plan. Psychiatric counseling may be necessary to assist in lifestyle adjustments necessitated by a chronic disease process. The occupational therapist helps facilitate realistic occupational goals, while the physical therapist assists in the maintenance of optimum conditioning given the activity restrictions.

Because medication is an essential part of the management of cardiomyopathy, the role of the pharmacist is crucial in educating the patient about how to manage the medications and their side effects. Given that heart failure is a common result of cardiomyopathy, the patient/family needs to consult with the dietician about dietary changes needed to control congestion that is exacerbated by excess salt and fluid intake. In addition to the nursing care described above and in the Patient Teaching & Discharge Priorities box (p. 1269) that discusses cardiomyopathy, the nurse plays a pivotal role in coordinating the efforts of the health care team. In the inpatient setting the nurse facilitates communication between the members of the team and the patient/family.

End-of-Life Issues with Cardiomyopathy

Due to the severity and progressive nature of the disease, the risk of sudden cardiac death increases as the disease progresses. Families and significant others need to be encouraged to learn cardiopulmonary resuscitation (CPR) and how to access emergency care near their home. When patients become end stage and are refractory to available therapies, they should be considered for advanced therapies such as cardiac transplantation or permanent mechanical assist devices or for palliative care and hospice. These options are discussed in Chapter 42 🔗 . Finally, the patient needs to be asked about end-of-life wishes and an advance directive should be signed in advance of a sentinel life-threatening event.

National Guidelines for Cardiomyopathy

Controlling risk factors, healthy habits, and medication and device therapy will assist in the slowing and perhaps preventing the progress of all four types of cardiomyopathy. *Healthy People 2010* (U.S. Department of Health and Human Services [DHHS], 2004) serves as a prevention agenda for the nation with published guidelines for educating this patient population about risk factors such as substance abuse, blood pressure control, diet, and activity restrictions. Nurses need to be knowledgeable about these guidelines and use them for educating patients and families with cardiomyopathy. The National Guidelines box outlines the *Healthy People 2010* guidelines for two controllable causes of DCM.

■ Gerontological Considerations

The effects of rheumatic fever and episodes of infective endocarditis are often not manifested until later in life. If valve stenosis or regurgitation occurs as a result of these infective processes, symptoms typically follow a slow stable course. In developed countries there is a latent period of 20 to 40 years from the occurrence of rheumatic fever to the onset of symptoms (AHA, 2006a,b). Then it is usually another decade before symptoms become disabling. Once significant limiting symptoms appear, however, survival rates drop to less than 3 years. This progression of the disease places the manifestations and need for treatment in the final decades of life. A decreased immune response and the existence of other debilitating diseases increase the risk for both medical and surgical complications in the elderly population. The stress of the illness and the normal physiological changes of aging put this group at risk for functional decline during hospitalization. Changes in cardiovascular, respiratory, and renal systems and the prevalence of comorbidities have been cited as possible causes (Cope & Hawley, 2001; Roche, Kramer, Hester, & Welsh, 1999).

Dilated cardiomyopathy is also a disease of the elderly. With the increasing geriatric population, more attention is being given to understanding diastolic failure induced by uncontrolled hypertension and cardiomyopathies. Researchers have demonstrated that the compensatory mechanisms associated with left ventricular diastolic dysfunction lead to elevated right heart pressures and eventually to right heart failure. When heart failure is present, the patient needs to be evaluated to differenti-

---

NATIONAL GUIDELINES for Two Controllable Causes of Dilated Cardiomyopathy

Risk Factor	Guideline
Alcohol intake	Moderate alcohol intake is defined as no more than 1 drink per day for women and no more than 2 drinks per day for men. However, some people should not drink any alcohol, including those who are: • Pregnant or trying to become pregnant • Taking prescription or over-the-counter medications that may cause harmful reactions when mixed with alcohol • Under the age of 21 • Recovering from alcoholism or are unable to control the amount they drink • Suffering from a medical condition that may be worsened by alcohol • Driving, planning to drive, or participating in other activities requiring skill, coordination, and alertness. Over time, excessive alcohol use can lead to the development of chronic diseases, neurological impairments, and social problems. These include cardiomyopathy.
Substance abuse	Expand research to identify and locate any genetic components that would predispose individuals to the risk of alcoholism and drug addiction. Encourage middle/junior high and senior high schools to use science classes to instruct students about the deleterious effects of alcohol and drug abuse on the body. Adopt strategies to counter and prevent substance abuse in young people that recognize various risky behaviors on their part as making up a complex whole, to which integrated and congruent approaches are required. Ensure that parents are integrated into national strategies against substance abuse by young people as partners on an equal footing with schools, communities, and other concerned elements of society. Support studies to determine the long-term biologic consequences for children who are born to mothers addicted to drugs or alcohol. Urge all agencies and individuals involved in acting to control substance abuse to begin interventions as soon as possible after the first offense, when success in preventing recurrence is more likely. Direct studies toward establishing whether youth exposure to advertisements for alcoholic beverages is altering attitudes about underage drinking and whether this in turn increases underage alcohol use. Increase research to explicate the nature and persistence of biologic and electrophysiologic changes in the brains of adolescent and adult abusers of alcohol and drugs.

Source: U.S. Department of Health and Human Services. (2004). *Healthy People 2010 progress report: Substance abuse.* Retrieved June 3, 2006, from http://www.healthypeople.gov/data/2010prog/focus26/holisticonline.com/remedies/Heart/cm causes-of-cardiomyopathy.

ate between ventricular systolic and ventricular diastolic origins of the disease process. This is done to both understand the origins of the heart failure and to guide clinical management. Treatment goals must be directed toward controlling both systolic and diastolic pressures in order to achieve optimum outcomes (Bollinger & Sadar, 2003; Hunt et al., 2005). End-stage cardiomyopathy patients benefit from hospice support (see Chapter 42 ⊙). Chapter 17 ⊙ includes a complete description of services provided by hospice.

■ Research

Research is essential to improve the care, quality of life, and the survival of patients with both inflammatory and structural heart diseases. The goal of research is to identify areas where practice could improve and evaluate and test methods in these areas. The research topics related to inflammatory and the structural heart diseases are listed in the Research Opportunities and Clinical Impact box. The list includes both medical and nursing research topics under investigation. Electronic databases are a source for finding specific studies related to these topics.

RESEARCH OPPORTUNITIES AND CLINICAL IMPACT RELATED TO INFLAMMATORY AND STRUCTURAL HEART DISEASE

Research Area	Clinical Impact
Effect of immunosuppressive treatment on myocarditis.	Improvement in left ventricular ejection fraction and evidence of healed myocarditis.
Identify predictors of embolic risk among the clinical and laboratory data obtained on hospital admission in patients diagnosed as having definite infective endocarditis (IE).	To identify high-risk individuals for embolic events associated with IE.
Lyme carditis and the incidence of myocarditis and/or pericarditis.	Diagnostic and complication guidelines.
Identify link between teeth brushing and infective endocarditis.	Identification of safer methods of teeth cleaning for patients with IE.
Herbal and complementary medicine to treat heart disease.	Lowers cholesterol, saturated fats, low-density lipoproteins, triglycerides, and blood pressure.
Heart valves that are durable, nonthrombogenic, with a low incidence of endocarditis.	Decreases need for multiple valve replacement and decreases complications of valve replacement surgery.
Septal ablation for hypertrophic obstructive cardiomyopathy.	Decreases obstruction of blood flow from the left ventricle to the aorta.
Prevention of sudden cardiac death with hypertrophic cardiomyopathy.	Increases survival of patients with HCM.
Stem cell homing and tissue regeneration in ischemic cardiomyopathy.	Repair of damaged tissue from ischemia.
Alcohol consumption's impact on heart failure.	Determine amount that is cardioprotective.
Use of beta-blockers in the treatment of heart failure.	Slow the progression of heart failure and reduce mortality, including sudden cardiac death.
Thiamin status, diuretic medications, and the management of heart failure.	
Relationship of heart failure severity, left ventricular loading conditions, and repolarization length in advanced heart failure secondary to ischemic or idiopathic dilated cardiomyopathy.	
Nonsustained ventricular tachycardia in hypertrophic cardiomyopathy: an independent marker of sudden death risk in young patients.	Determine predictors of sudden death risk to institute preventive therapy, such as implantation of an ICD.
Improvement in hypertrophic cardiomyopathy after significant weight loss.	Associated with striking improvement in cardiac functional indices, which could have profound implications for long-term cardiovascular risk.

Clinical Preparation

CRITICAL THINKING

▶ Read
- History of Current Illness
- Past Medical History
- Physical Exam
- Admitting Medical Orders
- Laboratory Study Results

▶ Document
- Summary of Hospitalization
- Pathophysiology Form
- Laboratory Values
- Laboratory Results Explanation

▶ Apply
- List of Potential Nursing Diagnoses
- Concept Map
- Critical Thinking Questions

Log on to MyNursingKit.com to download forms you will need and to complete further steps in the Clinical Preparation assignment.

HISTORY OF PRESENT ILLNESS

You are the nurse on the telemetry floor and you have been notified that you will be receiving a new patient from the emergency department (ED). The ED nurse calls the following report. Mr. H is a 26-year-old male brought in by ambulance, unconscious in the driveway of his home. He is initially seen by ED health care providers and the trauma team. Initial work-up included normal CT head, chest x-ray showing no pneumothorax, C-spine x-ray with no fractures, complete blood count (CBC), chemistry 7 panel, INR, UA; all were normal. ECG showed sinus tachycardia, low voltage, and nonspecific ST wave changes. Drug toxicology is still pending. A medicine consult was requested by the trauma service, for persistent shortness of breath (SOB) and an abnormal ECG.

At present, the patient is awake and alert. He feels weak and is short of breath. He denies assault. He denies a history of syncope and chest pain. He denies abdominal pain but has mild nausea. He denies fever, chills, and night sweats. He states he has a poor appetite but thinks he has gained weight due to swelling in his legs. He denies smoking cigarettes and denies crack/cocaine use. He states he drinks socially.

Of note, upon interviewing family, his mother states he is in good health and lives a very clean life. He is single, unemployed, and lives above her garage. She states he has no chronic health problems, but was told in his youth that he had a heart murmur. To her knowledge, the patient does not use any illegal drugs but does drink occasional alcohol. The patient's sister reports a very different story; she states the patient drinks at least six beers per day and frequently uses cocaine.

Medical–Surgical History
No known allergies
Medications: none
Illness: "heart murmur," no clinical problems
Surgeries: none

Social History
Family history: mom and dad healthy. The mother states that the patient does not use any illegal drugs but does drink occasional alcohol. The patient's sister reports a very different story; she states the patient drinks at least six beers per day and frequently uses cocaine.

Physical Exam
Young male overweight, mild discomfort due to SOB
Oxygen sat 90% on RA
BP 160/90 HR 115 RR 26
HEENT: normal but poor dentition
Neck: +JVD, no bruits
Heart: NL S_1, S_2, soft systolic murmur heard at PMI, S_3 present
Lungs: mild bibasilar rales
Abdomen: obese, soft, nontender
1+ lower extremity edema
Strong pulses throughout. Good cap refill
Normal neuro exam
No rash

Chest x-ray: cardiomegaly, mild interstitial edema
ECG: in history of present illness

Admitting Medical Orders
Admit to Cardiology–Telemetry Floor
Condition guarded
No known allergies
Admitting diagnosis: syncope unknown etiology: R/O dysrhythmia, ischemia, valvular disease; CHF probably due to cardiomyopathy via cocaine + alcohol abuse
Final diagnosis: cardiomyopathy and heart failure due to cocaine and alcohol abuse
Oxygen at 2–3 liters nasal cannula, keep oxygen saturation > 92%
Bed rest with bathroom privileges
Vital signs q2h with continuous ECG monitoring
Sequential compression device (SCD) to lower extremities
Incentive spirometry q hour while awake
Daily weight
Strict in/out
IV: saline lock; flush with NS q8h
Fluid restrict 1500 mL/day
Low Na diet
Call house officer: Pulse < 60 & > 110/minute; BP < 90 & > 160 systolic; temperature > 38.5; urine output < 30 mL/hr for 2 hours; respiratory rate > 30/minute; chest pain

Scheduled Medications

Lasix 40 mg IV every 12 hours for 2 days, then once a day
Nitropaste 1 inch q6h to chest wall topically
KCl 20 mEq po now and 20 mEq in 3 hours
Lisinopril 12.5 mg po daily
Lovenox 30 mg SQ bid
Magnesium sulfate 3 g IV dilute in 100 mL and give over 1 hour
    for a Mg level of less than 1.5 mEq/L × 1 now

PRN Medications

Phenergan 25 mg IV q6h prn nausea
Mylanta 30 mL q4–6h po prn dyspepsia
Triazolam 0.125–0.25 mg po q noc, prn sleep
Ativan 0.5–2 mg IV q6–8h prn anxiety (not to exceed
    10 mg /24 hours)
Milk of Magnesia 30 mL daily, po prn constipation
Tylenol 650 mg po/pr q4h prn for pain

Ordered Laboratory Studies

Troponin I q3h × 3 days
Myoglobin q3h × 3 days
CPK–MB q8h × 3 days
Chemistry 20 and PO_4 on admission and Chemistry 7 q12h for first
    2 days then daily
CBC q a.m.
Mg^{2+} q a.m.

Ordered Diagnostic Studies

Chest x-ray on admission and with adverse changes in O_2
    saturation, increased shortness or breath, and/or increasing
    rales
Echocardiogram
Cardiac catheterization
12-lead ECG daily

LABORATORY STUDY RESULTS

Test	Day 1	Day 2	Day 3
Sodium	132 mEq/L	137 mEq/L	140 mEq/L
Potassium	3.0 mEq/L	4.0 mEq/L	3.8 mEq/L
Chloride	90 mEq/L	92 mEq/L	95 mEq/L
Calcium	8.6 mg/dL		
Venous carbon dioxide	25 mEq/L	24 mEq/L	26 mEq/L
Blood urea nitrogen (BUN)	28 mg/dL	25 mg/dL	22 mg/dL
Creatinine	2.0 mg/dL	1.7 mg/dL	1.2 mg/dL
Blood glucose	150 mg/dL	138 mg/dL	112 mg/dL
Total proteins	5.2		
Magnesium	1.0 mEq/L	2.0 mEq/L	2.0 mEq/L
Phosphorus	3.2 mg/dL		
Troponin I	0.26/0.23/0.28 ng/mL		
Myoglobin	110 µg/L		
Albumin	3.5 g/dL		
GGT	48 units/L		
T. Bilirubin	1.1 mg/dL		
CPK total	212 units/L		
CPK MB	1.8%		
LDH	166 units/L		
AST	38 units/L		
ALT	28 units/L		
WBC	14,000/mm³	12,000/mm³	11,000/mm³
Hemoglobin	10.2 g/dL	12.2 g/dL	13.8 g/dL
Hematocrit	32%	37%	40%
RBC	5/mm3		
Platelets	395/mm³	325/mm³	250/mm³
ABGs			
PO2	70 mmHg	78 mmHg	80 mmHg
O_2 saturation	90%	91%	93%
pH	7.30	7.34	7.38
PCO_2	50 mmHg	48 mmHg	43 mmHg
HCO_3	24 mEq/L	26 mEq/L	24 mEq/L

CRITICAL THINKING QUESTIONS

1. What is the purpose of the echocardiography for this patient?

2. Why did the doctor order cardiac marker laboratory tests?

3. Why was a cardiac catheterization done?

4. What is the importance of assessing the potassium level frequently?

5. The teaching plan for this patient needs to include specific information about lifestyle changes that will not cause a worsening of the heart disease. What information does this patient need to know and what referrals would be appropriate?

6. What is the goal of medical therapy for this patient? This answer drives much of the patient teaching and helps the nurse anticipate complications and potential problems with the patient as well as additional orders.

Answers to Critical Thinking Questions appear in Appendix D.

NCLEX® REVIEW

1. A patient's history indicates a past history of rheumatic fever. The nurse plans to assess the client for signs of:
1. Pericarditis.
2. Endocarditis.
3. Mitral stenosis.
4. Pulmonary fibrosis.

2. A patient presents to the emergency department with complaints of increasing dyspnea and chest pain. The nurse suspects the symptoms reflect aortic stenosis when the patient states:
1. "I had a coronary artery bypass graft done five years ago."
2. "I had rheumatic heart disease when I was a child."
3. "I take a calcium channel blocker to treat an irregular heart rate."
4. "I frequently experience palpitations."

3. The nurse should include the following teaching for a patient diagnosed with mitral valve prolapse.
1. Avoid having any dental work until the valve is replaced.
2. Plan for rest periods throughout the day.
3. Take your oral temperature every morning.
4. Keep a diary of all the high fat foods you eat.

4. A patient is scheduled for open surgical valvuloplasty of the mitral valve. When preparing the patient for surgery the nurse includes the following information.
1. Cardiopulmonary bypass will not be required for this procedure.
2. Anticoagulation therapy will not be necessary in the postoperative period.
3. The valve will be repaired, but not replaced.
4. This procedure will prevent the need for future valve surgeries.

5. A patient is diagnosed with restrictive cardiomyopathy secondary to cocaine abuse. The nurse plans nursing care recognizing treatment for this type of cardiomyopathy usually involves:
1. Alcohol ablation.
2. Insertion of an implantable automatic defibrillator, ICD.
3. Aortic valve repair.
4. Supportive therapy with medications.

6. The nurse suspects a patient having frequent episodes of chest pain has pericarditis. To help confirm the suspicion the nurse should ask which question.
1. "Is the pain relieved by lying flat?"
2. "Do you only experience the pain during the night?"
3. "Does the pain become worse if you take a deep breath?"
4. "Is the pain preceded by an episode of heart palpitations?"

Answers for review questions appear in Appendix D

KEY TERMS

EXPLORE PEARSON **mynursingkit**™

MyNursingKit is your one stop for online chapter review materials and resources. Prepare for success with additional NCLEX®-style practice questions, interactive assignments and activities, web links, animations and videos, and more!

Register your access code from the front of your book at
www.mynursingkit.com

REFERENCES

American College of Cardiology. (2006). *American College of Cardiology/European Society of Cardiology Clinical Expert consensus document on hypertrophic cardiomyopathy. A report of the American College of Cardiology Foundation Task Force on Clinical Expert Consensus Documents and the European Society of Cardiology Committee for Practice Guidelines.* Retrieved June 15, 2006, from http://www.acc.org/media/releases/highlights/2003/aug03/hcm.htm

American Heart Association. (2004). *2002 Heart disease and stroke statistics update.* Dallas TX: Author. Retrieved October 12, 2004, from http://www.americanheart.org/presenter.jhtml?identifier=4468

American Heart Association. (2006a). *Diagnosis and management of infective endocarditis and its complications—conclusions.* Retrieved June 15, 2006, from http://www.americanheart.org/presenter.jhtml?identifier=9350

American Heart Association. (2006b). *Endocarditis guidelines.* Retrieved August 7, 2006, from http://www.americanheart.org/presenter.jhtml?identifier=11078

American Heart Association. (2006c). *Pericardium and paricarditis.* Retrieved August 7, 2006, from http://www.americanheart.org/presenter.jhtml?identifier=4683

Ammash, N., Seward, J., & Bailey, K. (2000). Clinical profile and outcome of idiopathic restrictive cardiomyopathy. *Circulation, 101,* 2490–2494.

Aurigemma, G. P., & Gaasch, W. H. (2002). *Management of patients with prosthetic heart valves.* Retrieved June 6, 2006, from http://store.utdol.com/app/index.asp

Barkman, A., & McCay, J. (2002). Cardiogenic shock in a patient with hypertrophic obstructive cardiomyopathy after insertion of a pacemaker. *American Journal of Critical Care,* 11(6).

Bollinger, K., & Sadar, A. M. (2003). Care and management of the patient with right heart failure secondary to diastolic dysfunction: An advanced practice perspective and case review. *Critical Care Nursing Quarterly, 26*(1), 22–27.

Braunwald, E., Fauci, A. S., Kasper, D. L., Hause, S. L., Longo, D. L., & Jamison, J. L. (2005). *Harrison's principles of internal medicine* (16th ed.). New York: McGraw-Hill.

Brigden, W. (1957). Uncommon myocardial diseases. *Lancet, 2,* 1179.

Bruce, J. (2006). Getting to the heart of cardiomyopathy: Find out about the four types of cardiomyopathies. *Cardiac Insider,* pp. 16–20.

Brusch, J. L. (2005). *Infective endocarditis.* Retrieved August 2, 2006, from http://www.emedicine.com/med/topic671.htm

Candela, L. (2002). Caring for a patient with listeria endocarditis: Use of antibiotics desensitization. *Critical Care Nurse, 22*(5), 38–48.

Cardiomyopathy Association. (2006). *Arrhythmogenic right ventricular cardiomyopathy (ARVC).* Retrieved June 8, 2006, from http://www.cardiomyopathy.org/html/which_card_arvc_text.htm

Chin, T. K. (2006). Rheumatic heart disease, eMedicine. Retrieved on May 29, 2008 from http://www.emedicine.com/ped/topic2007.htm

Clarkston, N., & Waldman, A. R. (2001). Aortic valve replacement. *RN,* 64(1), 58–63.

Cope, S., & Hawley, R. (2001). Needs of the older patient in the intensive care unit following heart surgery. *Progressive Cardiovascular Nursing,* 16(2), 44–48.

Desai, K. (2002). Pericardiocentesis. Retrieved June 10, 2003, from http://www.emedicine.com/topic3560.htm

Fauci, A. S., Braunwald, E., Isselbacher, K. J., Wilson, J. D., Martin, J. B., Kasper, D. L., et al. (1998). *Harrison's principles of internal medicine* (14th ed.). New York: McGraw-Hill.

Felker, C. M., Thompson, R. E., & Hare, J. M. (2000). Underlying causes and long-term survival in patients with unexplained cardiomyopathy. *New England Journal of Medicine, 342,* 1077.

Flutterman, L. G., & Lemberg, L. (2000). Peripartum cardiomyopathy: An ominous complication of pregnancy. *American Journal of Critical Care,* 9(5).

Francis, G. (2004). *Halting remodeling in congestive heart failure.* The Cleveland Clinic Foundation, American College of Cardiology. Retrieved October 14, 2004, from http://www.chfpatients.com/heartbytes.htm#remodel

Fung, G. L., associate clinical professor of cardiology, University of California at San Francisco Medical School. (1999, June 7). Interview by Arlene Orhon-Jech.

Gowda, A. (2008). Pericarditis, uremic. *eMedicine Web MD.* Retrieved February 23, 2008, from http://www.emedicine.com/med/byname/pericarditis-uremic.htm

Grau, J.B., Pirelli, L., Yu, J.P., Galloway, A.C., & Ostrer, H. (2007). The genetics of mitral valve prolapse. *PubMed.* Retrieved on May 29, 2008 from http://www.ncbi.nlm.nih.gov/pubmed/17850623?ordinalpos=3&itool=EntrezSystem2.PEntrez.Pubmed.Pubmed_ResultsPanel.Pubmed_RVDocSum

Halsell, J. S., Riddle, J. R., Atwood, J. E. et al. (2003). Myopericarditis Following Smallpox Vaccination Among Vaccinia-Naive US Military Personnel. *JAMA: 289*(24):3283-3289.

Howes, D. S. (2008). Myocarditis. *eMedicine.* Retrieved on May 28, 2008 from http://www.emedicine.com/emerg/TOPIC326.HTM

Hunt, S. A., et al. (2005). ACC/AHA 2005 guideline update for the diagnosis and management of chronic heart failure in the adult: Summary article: A report of the American College of Cardiology/American Heart Association Task Force on Practice Guidelines (Writing Committee to Update the 2001 Guidelines for the Evaluation and Management of Heart Failure). *Journal of the American College of Cardiology, 46,* 1116–1143.

Jospehson, L., & McMullen, P. (2003). Atrial fibrillation: Beyond irregularly irregular. *Critical Care Choices: A Supplement to Nursing 2003 and Nursing Management,* pp. 6–10.

Lakkis, N. M., Nagueh, S. F., & Klieman, N. S. (1998). Echocardiography-guided ethanol septal reduction for hypertrophic obstructive cardiomyopathy. *Circulation,* 98, 1750–1755.

Lewis, P. S., Boyd, C. M., Hubert, N. E., & Steele, M. C. (2001). Ethanol-induced therapeutic myocardial infarction to treat hypertrophic obstructive cardiomyopathy. *Critical Care Nurse,* 21(2), 20–34.

Marill, K. (2006). *Endocarditis.* Retrieved August 3, 2006, from http://www.emedicine.com/emerg/topic164.htm

Mayo Clinic. (2005a). *Dressler's syndrome.* Retrieved August 2, 2006, from http://www.mayoclinic.com/health/dresslers-syndrome/DS00666

National Institute on Alcohol Abuse and Alcoholism. (2002, January). *Alcohol Alert,* No. 55. Retrieved August 3, 2006, from http://pubs.miaaa.nih.gov/publications/aa55.htm

Orhon-Jech, A. (1999). Mitral valve prolapse: What you need to know. *Nurse Week,* 16–17.

Porth, C. M. (2004). *Essential in pathophysiology: Concepts of altered health states.* Philadelphia: Lippincott Williams & Wilkins.

Porth, C. M. (2005). Pathophysiology: *Concepts of altered health states.* (7th ed.). Philadelphia: Lippincott Williams & Wilkins.

Richardson, P. (1996). Report of the World Health Organization/International Society and Federation of Cardiology Task Force on the Definition and Classification of the Cardiomyopathies. *Circulation,* 93, 841.

Roche, V. M. L., Kramer, A., Hester, E., & Welsh, C. H. (1999). Long-term functional outcome after intensive care. *Journal of the American Geriatrics Society,* 47(1), 18–24.

Saxton, L. D., Kumar, U. N., & DeMarco, T. (2006). *Cardiac resynchronization therapy (biventricular pacing) in heart failure.* Retrieved June 3, 2006, from Up to Date website: http://www.utdol.com/utd/store/index.do

Steinbis, S. (2003). Hypertrophic obstructive cardiomyopathy and septal ablation. *Critical Care Nurse, 23*(3), 47–58.

Takagi, E., Yamakado, T., & Nakano, T. (1999). Prognosis of completely asymptomatic adult patients with hypertrophic cardiomyopathy. *Journal of American College of Cardiology, 33,* 296.

Tandri, H., Saranathan, M., Rodriguez, E. R., Martinez, C., Bomma, C., Nasir, K., et al. (2005, January 4). Noninvasive detection of myocardial fibrosis in arrhythmogenic right ventricular cardiomyopathy using delayed-enhancement magnetic resonance imaging. *Journal of the America College of Cardiology, 45*(1), 98–103.

University of Maryland Medical Center (2005). *Mitral valve prolapse.* Retrieved May 28, 2006, from http://www.umm.edu/ency/article/000180.htm

U.S. Department of Health and Human Services. (2004). *Healthy People 2010 progress report: Substance abuse.* Retrieved June 3, 2006, from http://www.healthypeople.gov/data/2010prog/focus26/holisticonline.com/remedies/Heart/cm causes-of-cardiomyopathy

Wichter, T., Paul, M., Wollmann, C., Acil, T., Gerdes, P., Ashraf, O., et al. (2004). Implantable cardioverter/defibrillator therapy in arrhythmogenic right ventricular cardiomyopathy: Single-center experience of long-term follow-up and complications in 60 patients. *Circulation, 109*(12), 1445–1447.

Wiegand, D. L. (2003). Advance in cardiac surgery: Valve repair. *Critical Care Nurse, 23*(2): 72–91.

Woods, S. L., Froelicher, E. S. S., & Motzer, S. U. (2000). *Cardiac nursing.* (4th ed.). Philadelphia: Lippincott Williams & Wilkins.

Zevola, D. R., Raffa, M., & Brown, K. (2002). Using clinical pathways in patients undergoing cardiac valve surgery. *Critical Care Nurse, 22*(1), 31–50.

42

Caring for the Patient with Heart Failure

Kismet Rasmusson
Jill Hall

Outcome-Based Learning Objectives

After studying this chapter, the learner will be able to:

1. Evaluate the etiology, incidence, and prevalence of heart failure.
2. Distinguish between systolic and diastolic dysfunction.
3. Describe the pathophysiology of heart failure and the compensatory neurohormonal responses that occur.
4. Compare and contrast right-sided versus left-sided symptoms of heart failure.
5. Evaluate the diagnostic workup used to determine the presence of heart failure.
6. Describe a comprehensive treatment plan including the medical, device, and surgical components to treatment, using the multidisciplinary team approach.
7. Describe the self-management concepts necessary for patients with heart failure.
8. Compare and contrast potential comorbidities associated with heart failure.
9. Describe components of end-of-life care for end-stage heart failure.

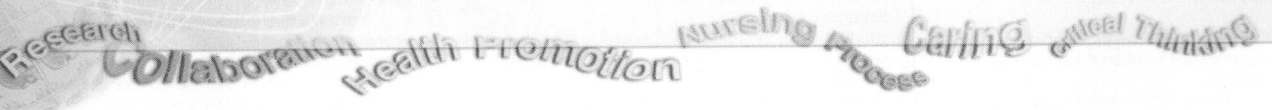

HEART FAILURE is a common, chronic condition that has a significant impact, not only on patients living with the disease but also on care delivery systems. Current understanding of heart failure has matured from what was once thought to be a hemodynamic condition, to an understanding of complex neurohormonal changes resulting in an impairment of cardiac filling and/or ejection of blood. If left untreated, the disease will progress resulting in increased symptoms, hospitalizations, and possibly death. Leaders in heart failure care, such as the Heart Failure Society of America and the American Heart Association with the American College of Cardiology, have updated guidelines to help providers with delivering appropriate, evidence-based care.

Heart failure treatments have expanded significantly over the last 20 years and have been able to improve symptoms and reduce morbidity, mortality, and hospitalizations. Today, heart failure is treated with therapies of growing complexity: medications, cardiac devices, and surgical/interventional approaches. Special attention to controlling comorbid conditions and volume status is paramount. Medical therapy is aimed to reduce the detrimental neurohormonal cascade. Cardiac devices have an expanding role to prevent sudden cardiac death, to resynchronize dyssynchronous ventricles, and even to aid in the assessment of fluid status. End-stage therapies may offer the promise of extended life with modalities such as cardiac transplantation or mechanical assist devices for select patients. Palliative care and hospice will be essential for patients whose prognosis is poor.

Multidisciplinary teams providing care by using established disease management strategies improve outcomes. Nurses have been pivotal in patient care in providing self-management instruction, telephone management, and more (Rasmusson et al., 2006). The future of heart failure will come with understanding genetic implications and integrating clinical research into practice. Genetic implications are discussed in the Genetic Consderations box.

Epidemiology

Heart failure is a major public health problem affecting 5 million Americans (American Heart Association [AHA], 2006b). With over 550,000 new cases diagnosed each year in the United States, heart failure is reaching epidemic proportions. Contributing to the rising prevalence of heart failure are the aging U.S. population and increased survival rates among patients with hypertension and coronary artery disease (AHA, 2006b; Baker, 2002). Individuals who would have succumbed to an acute cardiac event in the past are now more likely to survive,

GENETIC CONSIDERATIONS for Heart Failure

Risk factors	Family history of early coronary artery disease (CAD), idiopathic or hypertrophic cardiomyopathy, sudden cardiac death. Virus exposure. African American race. Potential for thromboembolic events: atrial fibrillation, pulmonary embolism, intra-cardiac thrombi, or deep vein thrombosis.
Research	Familial Dilated Cardiomyopathy Research Project.[a] Viral genome; studying parvovirus B19. A-HeFT: African-American Heart Failure Trial: showed increased response to hydralazine and nitrates in addition to standard heart failure therapy. Genetic testing to assess warfarin dosing.
Counseling/screening	Counsel patients that their condition might pose a risk to their first-degree relatives. Appropriate screening would be recommended, then starting treatment if left ventricular dysfunction is found. To screen those with risk factors or a family history suggests simple screening of first-degree family members with a limited history, physical examination, 12-lead ECG, and echocardiogram. Genetic screening by blood testing is not yet well understood but may guide future treatment.

[a] Website: http://www.fdc.to.

Sources: Burkett, E. L., & Hershberger, R. E. (2005). State of the art: Clinical and genetic issues in familial dilated cardiomyopathy. *Journal of the American College of Cardiology, 45,* 969–981; Taylor, A. L., Ziesche, S., Yancy, C., et al. (2004). For the African-American heart failure trial investigators. Combination of isosorbide dinitrate and hydralazine in blacks with heart failure. *The New England Journal of Medicine, 351,* 2049–2057; and Wilson-Tang, W. H., & Francis, G. S. (2005). The year in heart failure. *Journal of the American College of Cardiology, 46,* 2125–2133.

albeit with impaired cardiac function (AHA, 2006b; Baker, 2002). With the rise of conditions such as diabetes, obesity, and the metabolic syndrome, increases in the risk of developing heart failure are significant (Hunt et al., 2005).

Mortality

Despite advances in heart failure treatments, mortality rates increased by 20.5% from 1993 to 2003. Nearly 290,000 people die annually of heart failure in the United States (AHA, 2006b). More than 75% of patients diagnosed with heart failure die within 8 years. Those with heart failure are six to nine times more likely than the general population to suffer from sudden death (AHA, 2006b).

Medical Impact

Heart failure is the most common diagnostic-related group (DRG) used for hospital admissions in the United States among the Medicare population (Hunt et al., 2005). Since 1979, the rate

of hospital discharges for patients with heart failure has increased by 174%, totaling more than 1 million annually (AHA, 2006b). Recurrences or exacerbations of symptoms are likely, particularly as the disease advances. An exacerbation often results in an acute crisis, leading to either emergency department visits or hospitalizations. Between 30% and 50% of patients discharged with acute heart failure are readmitted with an exacerbation to the hospital within 6 months. Although hospital readmissions may be preventable, such prevention is often accomplished at the expense of increasing resources, such as office visits and home monitoring by experienced nurses. Health delivery systems across the continuum of care are challenged to provide appropriate care to all patients, while limiting resource utilization. See the National Guidelines box (p. 1280) for the diagnosis and management of heart failure.

Economic Impact

Heart failure also is the most costly DRG in the United States with more dollars spent on it than on any other condition for the Medicare population (Hunt et al., 2005). Direct and indirect costs associated with heart failure amount to nearly $30 billion in the U.S. (AHA, 2007). Therapeutic pharmacologic advances in the treatment of heart failure, such as angiotensin-converting enzyme (ACE) inhibitors and beta-adrenergic blockers, have been shown to be cost-effective therapies. However, more complex and costly cardiac devices are adding to the expense of overall management. End-stage therapies, such as mechanical circulatory support and cardiac transplantation, in reality represent failures of early prevention and treatment, yet are used in selected, but few, patients. If the current trajectory of rising costs continues, heart failure expenditures could financially drain current health care resources.

Pathophysiology

Heart failure is best defined as a complex and debilitating clinical syndrome whereby there is "loss or dysfunction of the cardiac muscle" (Adams et al., 2006) or an "inability of the ventricle to fill or eject blood" (Hunt et al., 2005). The heart muscle is simply unable to pump adequately to supply enough blood to meet the body's metabolic needs, leading to significant impairment and often disability (Hunt et al., 2005). The syndrome of heart failure ultimately leads to common symptoms of poor activity tolerance, fluid retention, and fatigue, that limit quality of life.

Heart failure, the syndrome, should be distinguished from structural or functional causes, such as cardiomyopathy (any disease that affects the structure and function of the heart). The diagnosis, cause, and treatment of all cardiomyopathies are discussed in Chapter 41.

Etiology

The leading etiologies of heart failure include hypertension, coronary artery disease, and dilated cardiomyopathies. Other factors that contribute to developing heart failure include well-established risk factors for cardiovascular disease or exposure to substances that are toxic to the cardiac muscle. Risk factors that may lead to heart failure are summarized in the Risk Factors box (p. 1280).

NATIONAL GUIDELINES for Heart Failure

Name of Guideline	Guideline Objectives
2005 American College of Cardiology and American Heart Association (ACC/AHA) Chronic Heart Failure Guidelines[a]	Characterizing the syndrome of heart failure. Initial and ongoing assessment. Therapies; stage based. Treating special populations. Treating concomitant disorders. End-of-life considerations. Implementation of practice guidelines.
Heart Failure Society of American (HFSA) 2006 Comprehensive Heart Failure Practice Guideline	Define heart failure. Discuss prevention strategies. Evaluating patients for heart failure. Managing asymptomatic patients. Nonpharmacologic treatments. Managing symptomatic patients. Disease management. Device therapies. Surgical therapies. Managing patients with preserved ventricular function. Managing acute decompensated heart failure. Managing patients with ischemic disease. Managing patients with hypertension. Managing special populations. Managing myocarditis.

[a] Website:http://www.hfsa.org/hf_guidelines.asp.

Sources: Adams, K. F., Lindenfeld, J., Arnold, J. M., et al. (2006). Executive summary: HFSA 2006 comprehensive heart failure practice guideline. *Journal of Cardiac Failure, 12*(1), 10–38; Hunt, S. A., Abraham, W. T., Chin, M. H., Feldman, A. M., Francis, G. S., Ganiats, T. G., et al. (2005). ACC/AHA 2005 guideline update for the diagnosis and management of chronic heart failure in the adult: Summary article: A report of the American College of Cardiology/American Heart Association Task Force on Practice Guidelines (Writing Committee to Update the 2001 Guidelines for the Evaluation and Management of Heart Failure). *Journal of the American College of Cardiology, 46,* 1116–1143.

RISK FACTORS for Heart Failure

Modifiable Risk Factors	Nonmodifiable Risk Factors
Atherosclerosis	Age
Cardiotoxic drug use (alcohol, illicit drugs, anthracyclines)	Positive family history of CAD
	Gender
Diabetes	Genetics
Hyperlipidemia	
Hypertension	
Metabolic syndrome	
Obesity	
Sedentary lifestyle	
Smoker	
Valvular abnormalities	

Sources: Adams, K. F., Lindenfeld, J., Arnold, J. M., et al. (2006). Executive summary: HFSA 2006 comprehensive heart failure practice guideline. *Journal of Cardiac Failure, 12*(1), 10–38; Hunt, S. A., Abraham, W. T., Chin, M. H., Feldman, A. M., Francis, G. S., Ganiats, T. G., et al. (2005). ACC/AHA 2005 guideline update for the diagnosis and management of chronic heart failure in the adult: Summary article: A report of the American College of Cardiology/American Heart Association Task Force on Practice Guidelines (Writing Committee to Update the 2001 Guidelines for the Evaluation and Management of Heart Failure). *Journal of the American College of Cardiology, 46,* 1116–1143.

Two very different pathologic processes may lead to heart failure as a result of a wide range of left ventricular functional abnormalities commonly referred to as systolic and diastolic dysfunction, discussed next. Both systolic and diastolic dysfunction may occur simultaneously and usually result in the same set of symptoms.

Systolic Dysfunction

Systolic dysfunction, also referred to as left ventricular systolic dysfunction (LVSD), is characterized by impaired ventricular function, which results in volume overload and decreased contractility. In the U.S., the most common cause of LVSD is coronary artery disease (CAD), followed by hypertension (Nohria, Lewis, & Stevenson, 2002). In an era of improved therapies to treat coronary artery disease and acute myocardial infarction, people now survive such events, but many remain with a dysfunctional ventricle. This may lead to the syndrome of heart failure. Other causes of systolic dysfunction include idiopathic, valvular, hypertrophic, and cardiotoxic substance use. LVSD is diagnosed when the **left ventricular ejection fraction (LVEF)** (the proportion of blood ejected during each ventricular contraction compared with the total ventricular filling volume) is below 40% to 45% (Cohn, 2000). A normal LVEF ranges from

55% to 70%. Chart 42–1 outlines the etiologies of heart failure. Once LVSD occurs, progressive adverse structural and neurohormonal changes occur within the heart, leading to deteriorating cardiac function and symptoms of low cardiac output and congestion (Jessup & Brozena, 2003). Neurohormones such as norepinephrine, endothelin, and cytokines are released, leading to an adverse condition called cardiac remodeling. This detrimental effect on the myocardium results from volume overload or cardiac injury and causes myocytes to revert to a fetal-type expression, ultimately changing the geometry from elliptical to spherical. These changes result in molecular, cellular, and interstitial changes of the cardiac muscle and are manifested clinically as changes in size, shape, and function of the heart, which leads to a reduction in ventricular function. Regardless of the etiology, once systolic dysfunction occurs, the heart is unable to pump enough blood to sustain the metabolic demands of the body. Right, left, and/or biventricular heart failure can occur, depending on the extent and anatomy of the damage (Figure 42–1 ■, p. 1282). Tissue remodeling is described in detail in Chapter 40 ☙.

Left-sided heart failure, as the name suggests, is an abnormal cardiac condition characterized by the impaired pumping ability of the left side of the heart, which eventually backs the blood up into the pulmonary circulation. Elevated pressure and congestion in the pulmonary veins and capillaries result as the disease progresses. Symptoms that eventually follow impaired left ventricular function include fatigue, activity intolerance, shortness of breath, and cough. Often, orthopnea (an abnormal condition in which a person must sit or stand to breathe deeply or comfortably) and paroxysmal nocturnal dyspnea (a disorder characterized by sudden attacks of respiratory distress that awakens the person usually after several hours of sleep in a reclining position) will occur (Greenberg & Hermann, 2002; Nohria et al., 2002).

Right-sided heart failure is an abnormal cardiac condition characterized by the impairment of the pumping ability on the right side of the heart, leading to a backup of blood, followed by congestion and elevated pressure in the systemic veins and capillaries. The most common cause of right-sided dysfunction is left-sided dysfunction (Nohria et al., 2002). Other causes include a pathologic process in the lungs whereby blood cannot flow into the pulmonary vasculature, or result from an isolated right ventricular myocardial infarction. Symptoms of right heart failure result from volume overload leading to ascites and edema. Patients may complain of abdominal bloating and discomfort, often with a poor appetite and sometimes nausea and vomiting. Lower extremity edema occurs in many, but the absence of edema does not exclude volume overload in patients with heart failure.

Biventricular heart failure refers to a global inability of both ventricles of the heart to pump blood effectively. Forward blood flow is compromised, leading to right and left heart failure symptoms (Greenberg & Hermann, 2002). Symptoms are typically a combination of those from both right and left heart failure. Generalized malaise, activity intolerance, and even poor concentration are common as the disease progresses.

Diastolic Dysfunction

Diastolic dysfunction, also known as heart failure with preserved left ventricular ejection fraction (LVEF), is diagnosed when ventricular relaxation is slowed, with elevated filling pressures in the setting of normal ventricular volume and contraction (Hunt et al., 2005). Diastolic dysfunction is usually diagnosed when the clinical symptoms of heart failure are present with a normal LVEF (Jessup & Brozena, 2003). Diastolic dysfunction may account for 40% to 70% of all heart failure diagnosis (Jessup & Brozena, 2003). Patients with diastolic dysfunction are primarily elderly women, frequently with hypertension, diabetes, obesity, and atrial fibrillation (Adams at al., 2006). Although current understanding of diastolic dysfunction is limited due to a small body of research, it appears to have a burden similar to systolic dysfunction on health care resources

---

CHART 42–1 Etiologies of Heart Failure

Heart failure is a syndrome of symptoms that occurs from two pathologic processes: systolic dysfunction (when the heart is unable to contract normally) and diastolic dysfunction (when the heart is unable to relax normally). The etiologies leading to either process are noted here.

Systolic Dysfunction	Diastolic Dysfunction
Hypertension	Hypertrophic cardiomyopathy
Coronary artery disease (CAD)	Acute coronary insufficiency
Myocardial infarction	Systemic hypertension with hypertrophy
Ischemia (hibernating myocardium, stunned myocardium)	Acute and chronic CAD
Diabetes	Infiltrative cardiomyopathy
Alcoholic cardiomyopathy	Obstructive or nonobstructive disease
Peripartum cardiomyopathy	
Valvular cardiomyopathy	
Drug-induced cardiomyopathy	
Idiopathic cardiomyopathy	

Sources: Adams, K. F., Baughman, K. L., Dec, W. G., Elkayam, U., Forker, A. D., Gheorghiade, M., et al. (1999). Heart Failure Society of America (HFSA) practice guidelines. *Journal of Cardiac Failure, 5*(4), 357–382; Braunwald, E., Zipes, D. P., & Libby, P. (2001). *Heart disease: A textbook of cardiovascular medicine* (6th ed.). Philadelphia: W. B. Saunders; Greenberg, B. H., & Hermann, D. D. (2002). *Contemporary diagnosis and management of heart failure.* Newtown, PA: Handbooks in Health Care: Hunt, S. A., Abraham, W. T., Chin, M. H., Feldman, A. M., Francis, G. S., Ganiats, T. G., et al. (2005). ACC/AHA 2005 guideline update for the diagnosis and management of chronic heart failure in the adult: Summary article: A report of the American College of Cardiology/American Heart Association Task Force on Practice Guidelines (Writing Committee to Update the 2001 Guidelines for the Evaluation and Management of Heart Failure). *Journal of the American College of Cardiology, 46,* 1116–1143.

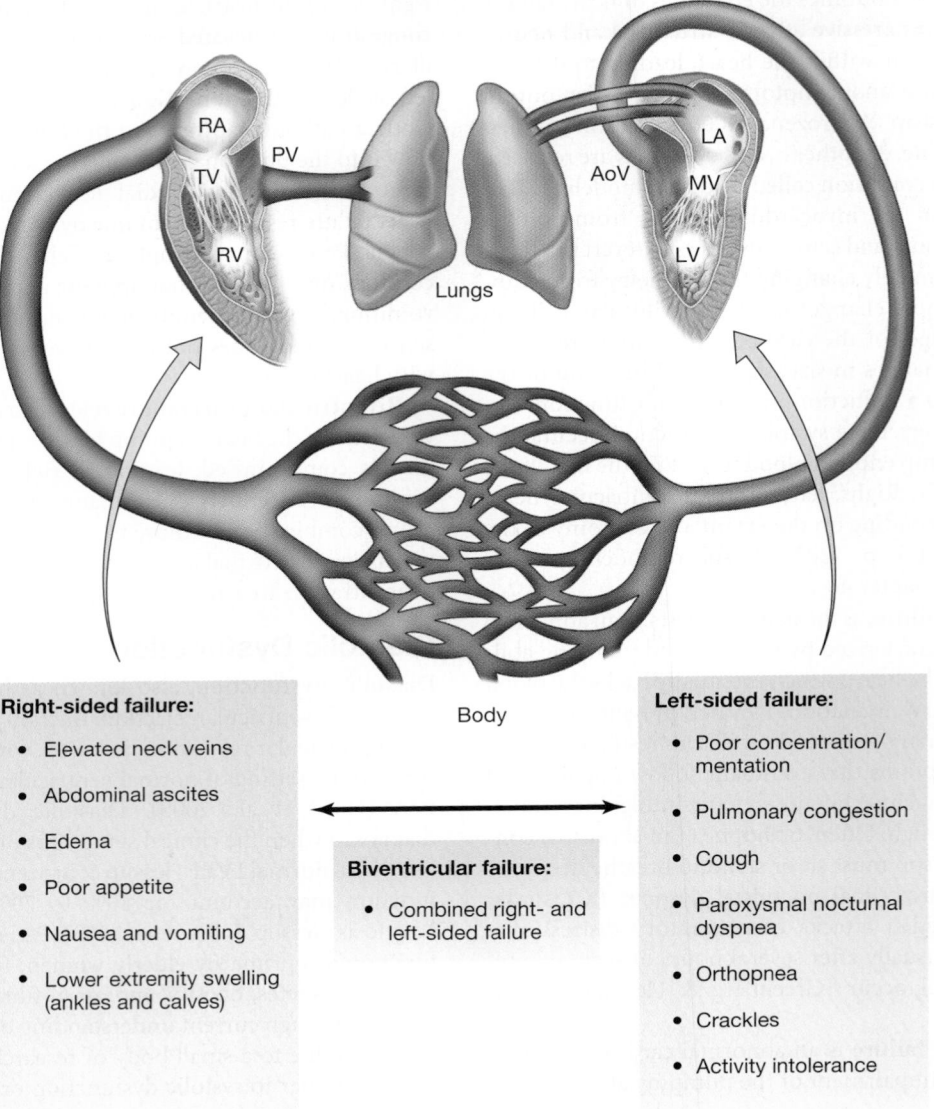

Right-sided failure:

- Elevated neck veins
- Abdominal ascites
- Edema
- Poor appetite
- Nausea and vomiting
- Lower extremity swelling (ankles and calves)

Body

Biventricular failure:

- Combined right- and left-sided failure

Left-sided failure:

- Poor concentration/mentation
- Pulmonary congestion
- Cough
- Paroxysmal nocturnal dyspnea
- Orthopnea
- Crackles
- Activity intolerance

FIGURE 42–1 ■ Right, left, and biventricular failure.

in terms of risk of admission, disability, and symptoms after hospitalization (Smith, Masoudi, Vaccarino, Radford, & Krumholz, 2003). Diastolic dysfunction seems to be related to a stiff, noncompliant heart with prolonged relaxation. The result is decreased filling, increased left ventricular end diastolic pressure, and reduced stroke volume at rest or during exercise (McKelvie, 2001). The increased susceptibility to changes in volume results in symptoms of "congestive" heart failure (Jessup & Brozena, 2003). Some causes of diastolic dysfunction include restrictive, obstructive, nonobstructive, hypertrophic, and infiltrative cardiomyopathies (see Chart 42–1, p. 1281). Principles of treatment focus on controlling hypertension, ischemia, and the ventricular rate when atrial fibrillation is present and on minimizing congestion (Adams et al., 2006). Given the robust data on systolic dysfunction and the lack of a standardized approach to treating diastolic dysfunction, this chapter focuses primarily on systolic dysfunction.

Neurohormonal Response

A series of compensatory mechanisms are triggered when the heart's pumping action is compromised. Regardless of the etiology of LVSD, the initial response to decreased cardiac output (the volume of blood expelled by the ventricles of the heart equal to the amount of blood ejected at each beat multiplied by the heart rate per minute) is the activation of the sympathetic nervous system (SNS) and the renin-angiotensin-aldosterone system (RAAS). Substances released with eventual detrimental cardiac effects include norepinephrine, angiotensin II, aldosterone, endothelin, vasopressin, and cytokines. Circulating levels play an important role in vasoconstriction, sodium retention, and toxic effects on the architecture of the heart described earlier (Hunt et al., 2005). In the early stages of heart failure, SNS and RAAS activation augments preload (the volume of blood being returned to the heart causing the stretch of myocardial fibers at end diastole), ventricular contractility, and heart rate, thereby maintaining cardiac output especially during exercise. But as cardiac function progressively worsens, these compensatory mechanisms are no longer able to maintain cardiac output and further compromise ventricular function (Greenberg & Hermann, 2002). Ventricular remodeling will result unless halted, which is a process by which detrimental effects are noted on the cardiac myocyte level.

Sympathetic Nervous System Activation

Increased SNS activity leads to elevated levels of norepinephrine. Norepinephrine causes vasoconstriction in the pulmonary and systemic vasculature and enhances venous tone, causing vasoconstriction. This initially maintains blood pressure and increases ventricular preload. Norepinephrine also causes renal vasoconstriction that allows for the glomerular filtration rate to remain stable despite decreased perfusion of renal blood flow. Circulating norepinephrine also increases sodium absorption leading to fluid retention that initially increases intravascular volume with subsequent temporary improvements in cardiac output and blood pressure. In addition, myocardial contractility and heart rate also are stimulated and therefore increase cardiac output. These neurohormonal effects provide short-term, necessary support to maintain cardiac output. In the long term, these deleterious effects cause increased cardiac wall stress, **hypertrophy** (an increase in the size of an organ caused by an increase in the size of the cells rather than in the number of cells), chamber dilation, increased myocardial oxygen consumption, worsening myocardial ischemia (a decreased supply of oxygenated blood to a body organ or part), and pulmonary and systemic congestion (Greenberg & Hermann, 2002).

Renin-Angiotensin-Aldosterone System Activation

Decreased renal perfusion triggers activation of the renin-angiotensin-aldosterone system (RAAS). Renin is released from the kidneys, causing a conversion of inactive angiotensin I into active angiotensin II. Angiotensin II is a potent vasoconstrictor that enhances venous tone and increases afterload (the load or resistance against which the left ventricle must eject its volume of blood during contraction). Angiotensin II also stimulates the secretion of aldosterone, causing sodium and fluid retention. In the short term, preload, cardiac output, and blood pressure are increased. However, long-term effects include increased cardiac workload, pulmonary and systemic congestion, and chamber dilation. Abnormal cell growth manifested by myocardial hypertrophy and adverse remodeling is also triggered by angiotensin II (Greenberg & Hermann, 2002).

Other Hormone Activation and Cytokine Release

Additional hormones that appear to be activated include the following: arginine vasopressin (from the pituitary hormone, which regulates free water clearance), endothelin (which is a potent vasoconstrictor released from endothelin cells), natriuretic peptides (released from cardiac tissue and vasculature, which cause vasodilation and natriuresis, which is the excretion of sodium), and cytokines, which have deleterious effects on cardiac remodeling (Greenberg & Hermann, 2002; Sha, Ali, Lamba, & Abraham, 2001).

Course of Heart Failure

Once diagnosed, heart failure disease progression follows a predictable course (Figure 42–2 ■). Formal diagnosis usually occurs when symptoms develop and functional status is compromised. Treatment of patients with heart failure, regardless of their course, involves providing supportive care for presenting symptoms and addressing needs for patients with chronic disease. Once standard heart failure therapies including medications and/or devices are initiated, functional status is usually improved for a period of time. As the disease progresses, after a period of stability of unknown duration, many patients experience episodes of exacerbations followed by some periods of stabilization. Often, they are unable to regain their prior level of functional ability. Exacerbations become increasingly more frequent and stabilization more difficult, eventually leading to death unless the patient is a candidate for end-stage therapies.

Understanding the course of heart failure can help guide not only therapeutic decisions, but also discussions with patients and families for a comprehensive approach to care. Even those who respond to medical or device therapies with improvement of cardiac function may eventually decompensate, with a select few eligible for advanced therapies such as cardiac transplantation or mechanical circulatory support. End-of-life care is essential for those with a poor prognosis, who are otherwise not candidates for advanced therapies. Therefore, both patients and health care providers may better anticipate treatment options and the trajectory of the disease when they understand the course of heart failure.

Chronic Heart Failure

The onset of heart failure can either be insidious or acute. Clinical challenges relate to diagnosing and treating heart failure along the continuum from inpatient to outpatient settings. Chronic heart failure is recognized by patients as having a mixture of good and bad days, with ongoing dyspnea, fatigue, and activity intolerance. Patients typically complain of weight gain (despite a decreased appetite), nausea, vomiting, and slow changes in their ability to perform activities of daily living (ADLs). Patients may also complain of irritability, restlessness,

········ Sudden death event

- - - - Transplant or ventricular assist device

—·—·— Non responders to medical management

FIGURE 42–2 ■ Course of heart failure.

or profound fatigue causing them to have poor energy. Increased urinary frequency and nighttime urination also are common (Greenberg & Hermann, 2002; Nohria et al., 2002). Symptoms will wax and wane in the majority of patients (Nohria et al., 2002). Heart failure is a chronic condition and, with suboptimal or lack of treatment, will lead to progressive cardiac dysfunction, progressive symptoms, and eventually death (Chart 42–2).

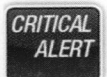

Subtle symptoms of heart failure include the following:

1. *Crackles are absent in over 80% of those with elevated filling pressures.*
2. *Edema in the elderly is often unrelated to filling pressures.*
3. *The easiest vital sign used to assess perfusion is blood pressure.*
4. *Patients who fall asleep while interviewed may have poor perfusion.*
5. *Cool forearms and legs may be more specific of low cardiac output than are cold hands and feet.*

Stages of Heart Failure

The stages of heart failure, as defined and created by the American College of Cardiology (ACC) and the AHA (Figure 42–3 ■) (Hunt et al., 2005), have better defined the evolution and progression of heart failure, which in turn helps direct treatment strategies to assist in halting disease progression. Criteria were set forth for Stages A through D to (1) identify risk factors for developing heart failure, (2) detect the presence or absence of

---

CHART 42–2	Heart Failure Symptoms
Dyspnea	Abdominal distention
Exertional dyspnea	Right upper quadrant pain
Orthopnea	Swelling
Paroxysmal nocturnal dyspnea	Nocturia
Dyspnea at rest	Fatigue
Cough	Restlessness
Hemoptysis	Agitation
Decreased urine output	Weight gain or loss
Nausea	Poor energy
Anorexia	Poor exercise tolerance
Bloating	

A thorough patient history includes asking directed questions that may glean important information about the type and extent of symptoms individuals have. These questions will help guide assessment of volume and perfusion status, so that treatment may be optimized.

Sources: Adams, K. F., Baughman, K. L., Dec, W. G., Elkayam, U., Forker, A. D., Gheorghiade, M., et al. (1999). Heart Failure Society of America (HFSA) practice guidelines. *Journal of Cardiac Failure, 5*(4), 357–382; Braunwald, E., Zipes, D. P., & Libby, P. (2001). *Heart disease: A textbook of cardiovascular medicine* (6th ed.). Philadelphia: W. B. Saunders; Greenberg, B. H., & Hermann, D. D. (2002). *Contemporary diagnosis and management of heart failure.* Newtown, PA: Handbooks in Health Care; Hunt, S. A., Abraham, W. T., Chin, M. H., Feldman, A. M., Francis, G. S., Ganiats, T. G., et al. (2005). ACC/AHA 2005 guideline update for the diagnosis and management of chronic heart failure in the adult: Summary article: A report of the American College of Cardiology/American Heart Association Task Force on Practice Guidelines (Writing Committee to Update the 2001 Guidelines for the Evaluation and Management of Heart Failure). *Journal of the American College of Cardiology, 46,* 1116–1143.

FIGURE 42–3 ■ The American College of Cardiology/American Heart Association (ACC/AHA) stages of heart failure vs. the New York Heart Association (NYHA) classes.

structural disease, and (3) treat based on well-proven strategies throughout the stages. The stages are described next.

Stage A

Stage A includes those at risk for developing the disease, but no structural abnormalities exist and no symptoms are present (Hunt et al., 2005). Risk factors for developing heart failure are similar to those for coronary artery disease: advancing age, diabetes, hypertension, hyperlipidemia, sedentary lifestyle, obesity, smoking, and excessive alcohol use (Greenberg & Hermann, 2002; Hunt et al., 2005). Risk factors for the development of coronary artery disease are described in detail in Chapter 40 ☞. Interventions for those in Stage A, aimed at reducing the risk of developing coronary artery disease, will likely prevent heart failure.

Stage B

Stage B includes asymptomatic patients who have structural heart disease. This is a difficult group to identify because symptoms are usually what will lead to the diagnosis of heart failure. Indiscriminately screening for heart failure is generally not recommended (Hunt et al., 2005) but could be selectively undertaken if risk factors were present. Persons with a prior myocardial infarction or significant coronary artery disease (CAD) or valvular disease are at particular risk in this stage. Evidence of structural disease can be detected on certain diagnostic tests including a 12-lead ECG (showing left ventricular hypertrophy); a chest x-ray showing **cardiomegaly** (enlargement of the heart); or an echocardiogram, chest CT, or MRI (showing ventricular hypertrophy or valvular dysfunction).

Evaluating a B-type natriuretic peptide (BNP) could be considered if there were clinical suspicions of heart failure, but an abnormally elevated value alone is not sufficient to diagnose heart failure. BNP is a 32-amino-acid polypeptide secreted by the ventricles of the heart in response to excessive stretching of myocytes in the ventricles. Levels of BNP are elevated in patients with left ventricular dysfunction, and levels correlate with both the severity of symptoms and the prognosis in congestive heart failure. BNP may also be elevated with acute myocardial infarction, acute pulmonary embolus, and renal failure; it also elevates some with age alone. The BNP is most useful in its ability to exclude heart failure as a diagnosis, if the value is normal. Elevations in BNP values have correlated with significant heart failure symptoms and increased risk of mortality. Reducing BNP has been shown to improve clinical status, yet the role of serial BNP measurements to guide therapy remains unclear (Hunt et al., 2005). Treatments for Stage B patients include ACE inhibitors, angiotensin receptor blockers, and beta-blockers (and aspirin and a statin if CAD is present). Such treatments prevent further damage of the myocardium and delay progression to symptomatic disease. Treatments from Stage B should be coupled with the recommended preventive measures of Stage A (Hunt et al., 2005; Jessup & Brozena, 2003).

Stage C

Stage C refers to patients with symptomatic, structural heart disease. Recommended therapies include ACE inhibitors, angiotensin receptor blockers, beta-blockers, and digoxin. (See the Pharmacologic Management section (p. 1294) for more detail.) Diuretics are used to relieve congestive symptoms, and aldosterone blockade is added for persistent symptoms. Cardiac devices, such as internal cardioverter defibrillators and biventricular pacemakers, are used in appropriate candidates either to reduce the incidence of sudden cardiac death or to improve the synchronous contraction in the ventricles, or both. Chapter 39 ⊚ discusses the pacemakers used for patients with heart failure.

Stage D

Stage D refers to patients with end-stage heart failure. When little hope of recovery exists, advanced interventions including heart transplantation, implantation of mechanical circulatory devices, enrollment in heart failure research studies, or hospice may be warranted (Hunt et al., 2005).

New York Heart Association Classification System

One measure used to quantify the degree of limitation and clinical symptoms of heart failure that are present in patients is the **New York Heart Association (NYHA) classification system**, a functional classification system that categorizes a patient's subjective degree of symptoms into NYHA classes I through IV (Cohn, 2000). It places patients in one of four classes dependent largely on the degree of dyspnea present when activities are performed (Hunt et al., 2005).

Class I: Patient has no symptoms.

Class II: Patient has symptoms with ordinary exertion.

Class III: Patient has symptoms with less than ordinary exertion.

Class IV: Patient has symptoms at rest.

Diagnosing Heart Failure

Heart failure is a complex clinical syndrome for which no standalone test has been able to establish the diagnosis (Adams et al., 2006; Hunt et al., 2005). Obtaining a full history, physical examination, and laboratory and diagnostic testing will help to understand the etiology, to assess the severity of symptoms, and to project the patient's prognosis.

History

A careful history of the onset, severity, and nature of symptoms will be critical in the initial evaluation when heart failure is suspected. Determine the patient's baseline ability to complete ADLs and his NYHA class. A patient with heart failure tends to present with symptoms of volume overload and low cardiac output (Chart 42–3, p. 1286).

Dyspnea continues to remain the most common presenting symptom, which patients largely identify as the key factor limiting their ADLs (Adams et al., 2006; Greenberg & Hermann, 2002; Hunt et al., 2005). Past medical history should include inquiring about potential comorbid conditions, such as coronary artery disease and the use of cardiotoxic substances. A thorough family history should also be reviewed to identify possible familial tendencies. Patients diagnosed with familial dilated cardiomyopathy may have up to a 30% chance of the same process in a first-degree relative (Burkett & Hershberger, 2005) (Charts 42–4 and 42–5, p. 1286).

◼ Clinical Manifestations

The physical examination focuses largely on identifying signs of volume overload and decreased peripheral perfusion. As cardiac output deteriorates, specific physical manifestations become evident (Nohria et al., 2002) (Chart 42–6, p. 1287). General assessment may reveal a confused or disoriented patient due to low cardiac output and poor oxygen perfusion to the brain, but more commonly, patients complain of forgetfulness and loss of concentration. Patients with chronic heart failure may appear to have cardiac cachexia (general ill health and malnutrition marked by weakness and emaciation usually associated with severe disease). Evaluation of the neck may reveal **jugular venous distention** (blood pressure in the jugular vein, which reflects the volume and pressure of venous blood) if volume overload is present. Upon auscultation of the lungs, **crackles** (a common abnormal sound heard on auscultation of the lungs from the movement of fluid or exudate) may or may not be present for those in chronic heart failure. A cough may be present due to an elevation in pulmonary venous pressure. A cough may or may not be productive, but if pink frothy sputum is present, one should suspect pulmonary edema as a potential cause. Dull breath sounds may be heard in the presence of a pleural effusion.

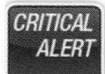 **CRITICAL ALERT**   *Signs of abrupt decline in cardiac output include:*

1. *Narrow pulse pressure*
2. *Cool extremities*
3. *Altered mentation*
4. *Hypotension*
5. *Cheyne–Stokes respiration*
6. *Resting tachycardia*
7. *Rise in BUN/creatinine*
8. *Oliguria.*

Patients may also have **tachypnea** (an abnormally rapid rate of breathing, more than 20 breaths per minute) while being examined. Palpation of the chest may reveal that the apical pulse is

CHART 42–3 Symptoms of Congestion Versus Symptoms of Low Cardiac Output

Heart failure symptoms typically are manifested in two categories: those of congestion, or excess fluid retention, and those of poor perfusion, resulting from diminished cardiac output. These symptoms can be categorized by body system or function, as noted here.

Organ System of Symptoms	Symptoms of Congestion	Symptoms of Low Cardiac Output
Pulmonary	Dyspnea, rest or exertional Paroxysmal nocturnal dyspnea Orthopnea Cough	
Cardiac	Chest pain/tightness/discomfort	Chest pain/tightness/discomfort Decreased urination
Abdominal	Epigastric distention General discomfort Discomfort with bending Abdominal distention Nausea or anorexia Early satiety	Nausea or anorexia
Extremities	Swelling; pedal, leg, sacral, scrotal/vulvar	Weakness, instability with ambulation
Cognitive	Fatigue	Impaired memory or concentration Confusion
Sleep	Sleep disturbance; air hunger, anxiety during sleep, need to sleep with head of bed elevated or in upright position	Sleep disturbance Daytime sleepiness
General	Fatigue Lack of energy Malaise	Lack of energy Easy fatigability Weight loss Malaise Decreased exercise tolerance Decreased urination

Sources: Braunwald, E., Zipes, D. P., & Libby, P. (2001). *Heart disease: A textbook of cardiovascular medicine* (6th ed.). Philadelphia: W. B. Saunders; Greenberg, B. H., & Hermann, D. D. (2002). *Contemporary diagnosis and management of heart failure.* Newtown, PA: Handbooks in Health Care; and Nohria, A., Lewis, E., & Stevenson, L. W. (2002). Medical management of advanced heart failure. *Journal of the American Medical Association, 287* (5), 628–640.

CHART 42–4 Past Medical History

Coronary artery disease

Prior myocardial infarctions

Hypertension

Diabetes

Hyperlipidemia

Valvular disease

Peripheral vascular disease

Rheumatic fever

Chest irradiation

Cardiotoxic agents

Alcohol consumption

Tobacco use

Obesity

Diabetes mellitus

Illicit drug use

Collagen vascular disease

Bacterial or parasitic infection

Thyroid disease

Pheochromocytoma

Interviewing patients for a thorough past medical history will help the nurse understand what may be the leading etiology of heart failure. Once the etiology is known, treatment is based on treating or alleviating pre-cipitating causes, instituting standard heart failure medications, and teaching self-management strategies.

Sources: Hunt, S. A., Abraham, W. T., Chin, M. H., Feldman, A. M., Francis, G. S., Ganiats, T. G., et al. (2005). ACC/AHA 2005 guideline update for the diagnosis and management of chronic heart failure in the adult: Summary article: A report of the American College of Cardiology/American Heart Association Task Force on Practice Guidelines (Writing Committee to Update the 2001 Guidelines for the Evaluation and Management of Heart Failure). *Journal of the American College of Cardiology, 46,* 1116–1143; Greenberg, B. H., & Hermann, D. D. (2002). *Contemporary diagnosis and management of heart failure.* Newtown, PA: Handbooks in Health Care.

CHART 42–5 Family History

Coronary artery disease

Hypertension

Diabetes

Hypercholesterolemia

Sudden cardiac death

Cardiomyopathies

Valvular disease

Peripheral vascular disease

Conduction system disease

Skeletal myopathies

Collagen vascular disease

A thorough interview of a patient's history includes the medical history of the patient's family. This information will be important so the nurse can understand the risk factors posed to patients who may have a genetic or familial tendency for developing disease.

Sources: Adams, K. F., Baughman, K. L., Dec, W. G., Elkayam, U., Forker, A. D., Gheorghiade, M., et al. (1999). Heart Failure Society of America (HFSA) practice guidelines. *Journal of Cardiac Failure, 5* (4), 357–382; Greenberg, B. H., & Hermann, D. D. (2002). *Contemporary diagnosis and management of heart failure.* Newtown, PA: Handbooks in Health Care; and Hunt, S. A., Abraham, W. T., Chin, M. H., Feldman, A. M., Francis, G. S., Ganiats, T. G., et al. (2005). ACC/AHA 2005 guideline update for the diagnosis and management of chronic heart failure in the adult: Summary article: A report of the American College of Cardiology/American Heart Association Task Force on Practice Guidelines (Writing Committee to Update the 2001 Guidelines for the Evaluation and Management of Heart Failure). *Journal of the American College of Cardiology, 46,* 1116–1143.

CHART 42–6	**Clinical Manifestations**
Hypotension	Engorged liver
Jugular venous distention	Positive hepatojugular reflux
Rales	Splenomegaly
Pleural effusion	Cyanosis
Wheezing	Cool extremities
Tachypnea	Cachexia
Tachycardia	Confusion
Third heart sound	Disorientation
Ascites	

The physical examination of patients with heart failure should be focused on a thorough assessment of the entire body. Assessment of vital signs, lungs, heart, abdomen, extremities, and mental status will often provide physical evidence of the abnormalities noted here, although their absence does not mean heart failure is not present.

Sources: Braunwald, E., Zipes, D. P., & Libby, P. (2001). *Heart disease: A textbook of cardiovascular medicine* (6th ed.). Philadelphia: W. B. Saunders; Greenberg, B. H., & Hermann, D. D. (2002). *Contemporary diagnosis and management of heart failure.* Newtown, PA: Handbooks in Health Care; Hunt, S. A., Abraham, W. T., Chin, M. H., Feldman, A. M., Francis, G. S., Ganiats, T. G., et al. (2005). ACC/AHA 2005 guideline update for the diagnosis and management of chronic heart failure in the adult: Summary article: A report of the American College of Cardiology/American Heart Association Task Force on Practice Guidelines (Writing Committee to Update the 2001 Guidelines for the Evaluation and Management of Heart Failure). *Journal of the American College of Cardiology, 46,* 1116–1143.

displaced laterally due to left ventricular hypertrophy. On auscultation an S_3 (abnormal third heart sound in the cardiac cycle) may be present with volume overload. An S_4 (abnormal fourth heart sound in the cardiac cycle) may be heard when patients have significant hypertension. With increasing sympathetic stimulation, tachycardia (a condition in which the myocardium contracts at a rate greater than 100 beats per minute) may be present. Abdominal examination may reveal **ascites** (an abnormal intraperitoneal accumulation of fluid containing large amounts of protein and electrolytes) and also an engorged liver and spleen. A positive **hepatojugular reflux** (an increase in jugular venous pressure when pressure is applied over the abdomen suggestive of right-sided heart failure) may also be present if volume overload is found in the periphery. The extremities may exhibit edema measured by the degree of **pitting** (an indention that remains for a short time after pressing edematous skin with the finger). Cyanosis (bluish discoloration of the skin and mucous membranes caused by an excess of deoxygenated hemoglobin in the blood) and cooling of the extremities with a poor capillary refill can occur with shunting of blood to vital organs (Braunwald, Zipes, & Libby, 2001). Chapter 37 discusses cardiac assessment.

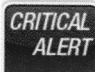 Assessment of tachypneic patients includes the following:

1. *Obtain oxygen saturation.*
2. *Assess extremities for temperature and appearance of cyanosis.*
3. *Assess neurological status.*
4. *Place oxygen and notify provider.*
5. *If patient is currently on oxygen, assess connections, and, if correct, increase oxygen level and notify provider.*

Assessment of cyanotic patients includes the following:

1. *Obtain oxygen saturation.*
2. *Assess extremities for temperature and appearance of cyanosis.*
3. *Assess neurological status.*
4. *Place oxygen and notify provider.*
5. *If patient is currently on oxygen, assess connections, and, if correct, increase oxygen level and notify provider.*

Laboratory and Diagnostic Procedures

Laboratory tests are obtained to evaluate for underlying disease or conditions that can cause or exacerbate heart failure. Other specific laboratory tests should be done to help the health care provider understand the etiology of heart failure, precipitating factors, and/or the degree of organ compromise when heart failure is present. Applicable tests are shown in the Diagnostic Tests box (p. 1288). Recommended blood work may give clues about the etiology and/or comorbidities of heart failure using a complete blood count, ferritin, troponin, lipid panel, and thyroid function tests. Other laboratory values may give an indication of the severity of the disease by assessing liver function tests, BNP, and renal function (Adams et al., 2006; Hunt et al., 2005).

Various cardiac imaging techniques are employed to identify structural abnormalities of the heart (see the Diagnostic Tests box, p. 1288). An echocardiogram, 12-lead electrocardiogram, and chest x-ray are indicated for all patients undergoing an evaluation for heart failure (Hunt et al., 2005). These are the least expensive and most accessible tests in many institutions. Further cardiac testing will provide information on the etiology of heart failure, extent of disease, measure of cardiac function, ejection fraction (EF), cardiac anatomy, and hemodynamics. Other means to assess ventricular function may be used, such as cardiac magnetic imaging (CMR). Both types of methods also examine cardiac wall motion, wall thickness, hypertrophy or enlargement of the ventricles, and valvular dysfunction, and may determine presence of infiltrative disease and estimate pulmonary pressures. Patients with angina should have an angiogram, but noninvasive imaging to detect myocardial ischemia may be used in patients for whom the diagnosis is less clear. An endomyocardial biopsy may be helpful in heart failure caused by infiltrative disease, collagen vascular disease, toxin exposure, or myocarditis, in which the diagnosis will guide specific treatment (Hunt et al., 2005). Other testing such as maximal oxygen consumption may be done to determine whether the symptoms are pulmonary in origin, as opposed to a cardiac etiology, or when assessing prognosis. Sleep disordered breathing should also be screened for, because this has increasingly become recognized as a common contributing factor of heart failure (Adams et al., 2006; Hunt et al., 2005).

Hemodynamic Monitoring

Hemodynamic monitoring has played an important role in assessing and guiding therapy in patients with acutely decompensated heart failure (Greenberg & Hermann, 2002). The ACC has recommended guidelines for the proper use of monitoring in the acute setting (Greenberg & Hermann, 2002). Hemodynamic monitoring has been found to be an adjunct to astute clinical assessment for the use of objective measures of cardiac

DIAGNOSTIC TESTS for Heart Failure

Test	Expected Abnormality	Rationale for Abnormality
LABORATORY TEST Complete blood count	Anemia Infection	Can determine whether anemia or infection is present, which can exacerbate heart failure symptoms. Anemia affects the oxygen carrying capacity, which could result in tissue hypoxia.
Serum electrolytes and creatinine	Renal insufficiency Electrolyte deficiencies	Can determine whether underlying renal disease or electrolyte deficiencies are present and also can obtain baseline measurements prior to the initiation of diuretic therapy.
Liver function tests	Hepatic congestion	Can determine the presence of hepatic congestion.
Urinalysis	Renal dysfunction Infection Diabetes	Can determine whether underlying renal disease, infection, or diabetes is present.
Thyroid function tests	Hypo-/hyperthyroidism	Can determine whether the etiology or the exacerbation of heart failure is related to hypo- or hyperthyroidism.
Serum ferritin	Hemochromatosis	Can determine whether the etiology of heart failure is related to iron overload.
B-type natriuretic peptide	Fluid volume overload	May be useful when the diagnosis is uncertain or to assess prognosis.
Lipid panel	Hypercholesterolemia Hyperlipidemia	May indicate the presence of coronary artery disease.
BNP	Elevated with left ventricular dysfunction	Levels correlate with both the severity of symptoms and the prognosis in congestive heart failure.
DIAGNOSTIC TEST Chest x-ray	Cardiomegaly Pleural effusion	Can determine presence of cardiac or great vessel enlargement, abnormal thoracic calcification, and pulmonary congestion.
Electrocardiogram	Left ventricular hypertrophy Left bundle branch block Pathologic Q waves	Can determine presence of dysrhythmias, left ventricular hypertrophy, and myocardial ischemia or insult.
Echocardiogram	Left ventricular dysfunction Myocardial infarction Diastolic dysfunction	Can determine size and function of atria and ventricles, segmental wall motion abnormalities, wall thickness, valvular structure and function.
Viability study	Coronary disease	Can determine extent of myocardial ischemia and viability.
Cardiac catheterization: right heart catheterization	Increased filling pressures, pulmonary artery pressures, cardiac output, and mixed venous blood gas	Can determine presence of volume overload or pulmonary hypertension.
Cardiac catheterization; left heart catheterization and selective coronary angiography	Evaluation of coronary arteries and assessment of ventricular function	Can determine whether coronary artery disease is present and whether intervention is possible.

Sources: Adams, K. F., Lindenfeld, J., Arnold, J. M., et al. (2006). Executive summary: HFSA 2006 comprehensive heart failure practice guideline. Journal of Cardiac Failure, 12(1), 10–38; Greenberg, B. H., & Hermann, D. D. (2002). Contemporary diagnosis and management of heart failure. Newtown, PA: Handbooks in Health Care; and Hunt, S. A., Abraham, W. T., Chin, M. H., Feldman, A. M., Francis, G. S., Ganiats, T. G., et al. (2005). ACC/AHA 2005 guideline update for the diagnosis and management of chronic heart failure in the adult: Summary article: A report of the American College of Cardiology/American Heart Association Task Force on Practice Guidelines (Writing Committee to Update the 2001 Guidelines for the Evaluation and Management of Heart Failure). Journal of the American College of Cardiology, 46, 1116–1143.

output, filling pressures, and systemic vascular resistance (Nohria et al., 2002).

Pulmonary artery occlusion pressure and cardiac output are both obtained with a pulmonary artery (Swan-Ganz) catheter. These readings give the heath care team information about the fluid volume and the patient's response to therapy such as diuretics. Specific values are discussed in the Nursing Process: Patient Care Plan for Heart Failure feature (p. 1302). Hemodynamic monitoring is discussed in detail in Chapter 24 .

Medical Management

Heart failure treatment options have evolved tremendously over time. Treating "dropsy," as it was referred to in the 1600s, with early forms of digitalis from the foxglove plant to advanced medications and device therapy to aid the failing heart (Figure 42–4 ■). The rapid growth of heart failure treatment in the 21st century includes a combination of pharmacologic measures, cardiac devices, and surgical approaches. The most significant advances in heart failure management have occurred since 1985,

Evolution of Heart Failure Therapies

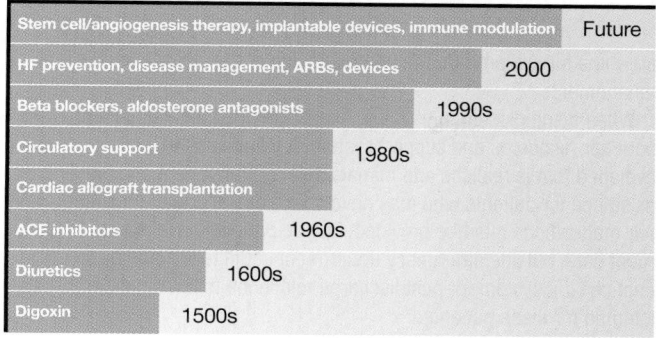

FIGURE 42–4 ■ Evolution of heart failure therapies.

taking the role of medications as palliation for heart failure symptoms to those that improve that natural history of the disease (Konstam, 2004). Medications, such as ACE inhibitors and beta-adrenergic blockers, have become the current standard of care for their role in not only decreasing morbidity and mortality but also decreasing heart failure hospitalizations. Additionally, heart failure device therapies such as the biventricular pacemakers have a significant role, because they address the impact of sudden cardiac death and cardiac dyssynchrony. Chapter 39 ⊛ discusses biventricular pacemakers in detail. Self-management and health promotion strategies will complete the heart failure treatment plan. Although a number of treatments have been shown to improve outcomes in patients with heart failure, the prognosis of these patients remains poor (Stewart, MacIntyre, Capewell, McMurray (2003), resulting in frequent readmission to the hospital. Research is currently looking at the efficacy of using multidisciplinary strategies to improve outcomes for HF patients. This research is discssed in the Evidence-Based Practice Box (p. 1290).

Pharmacologic Management

Heart failure has no cure, but effective pharmacologic treatments have shown clear benefits of patient quality and length of life in both acute and chronic heart failure. Optimal pharmacologic management for patients with LVSD includes a combination of ACE inhibitors or angiotensin receptor blockers, beta-adrenergic blockers, diuretics, digoxin, and aldosterone antagonists. Despite advances in heart failure management, utilization of these proven therapies remains poor (Stafford & Radley, 2003). Strategies to keep patients on lifesaving medications are paramount, such as providing medication assistance programs to those in need, educating patients about the role of medical therapy, and addressing side effects that may limit quality of life.

The primary targets of pharmacologic therapies in chronic heart failure focus largely on inhibiting the neurohormonal response invoked by left ventricular dysfunction in addition to relieving the symptoms of congestion. Treatment goals for chronic heart failure include:

- Alleviate symptoms of congestion.
- Improve perfusion.
- Increase activity tolerance.
- Improve quality of life.

- Decrease hospitalizations.
- Reduce readmissions.
- Slow or reverse progression of cardiac dysfunction.
- Improve survival.
- Minimize risk factors.
- Provide palliative care.
- Decrease heart failure–related costs.
- Track outcomes (Greenberg & Hermann, 2002; Jessup & Brozena, 2003; McKelvie, 2001).

In acute heart failure, primary pharmacologic therapy is based on a rapid and thorough assessment of volume status, the extent of peripheral and organ perfusion, and the presence of precipitating and life-threatening conditions (Fonarow, 2001). Treatment goals are usually aggressive for acute heart failure and are aimed at:

- Relieving symptoms
- Stabilizing hemodynamic parameters
- Improving organ function
- Eliminating precipitating or exacerbating causes (Fonarow, 2001; Greenberg & Hermann, 2002; Nohria et al., 2002).

Angiotensin-Converting Enzyme (ACE) Inhibitors

All patients with left ventricular dysfunction, with evidence of an ejection fraction less than 40%, should be placed on an ACE inhibitor unless they have a known contraindication (Adams et al., 2006). This class of medication has shown improved survival, delayed progression of heart failure, and improved exercise tolerance (Hunt et al., 2005). ACE inhibitors work within the renin-angiotensin-aldosterone system (RAAS) to prevent the conversion of inactive angiotensin I into active angiotensin II, thus inhibiting the vasoconstricting action of angiotensin II and the angiotensin-mediated secretion of aldosterone (Teerlink & Massie, 2003). In preventing the vasoconstrictive properties of angiotensin II from occurring, blood vessels dilate and systemic vascular resistance is decreased. A decrease in systemic vascular resistance is generally referred to as *afterload reduction* (Teerlink & Massie, 2003). By blocking the effects of angiotensin II, ventricular hypertrophy and remodeling are inhibited and cardiac output is moderately improved (Teerlink & Massie, 2003). By lowering levels of aldosterone, which is responsible for sodium retention, intravascular volume is decreased, leading to a decreased preload.

Adverse effects from ACE inhibitors include cough, angioedema, renal insufficiency, and hyperkalemia. Hypotension may occur, and should be monitored for, as doses are increased. An ACE inhibitor–induced cough, due in large part to ACE inhibitor interference with the breakdown of bradykinin, is the most common cause for withdrawal. However, this occurs in only 5% to 10% of the population (Hardman & Limbird, 2001; Hunt et al., 2005). Switching from an ACE inhibitor to an angiotensin receptor blocker (ARB) is reasonable when a cough is thought to be related to the ACE inhibitor. Angioedema, a rare, potentially life-threatening condition, in which excessive mucous membrane edema occurs, will require withdrawal from the ACE inhibitor. Renal function and serum electrolytes must be

EVIDENCE-BASED PRACTICE

Heart Failure

Clinical Problem

Heart failure (HF) remains the most common discharge diagnosis in elderly patients, accounting for almost a quarter of all cardiovascular hospitalizations (Stewart et al., 2002). Heart failure patients commonly experience readmissions due to noncompliance, lack of understanding of self-management principles, inadequate treatment, and/or progressive disease. Although a number of pharmacologic treatments have been shown to improve outcomes in patients with HF (Jessup & Brozena, 2003), the prognosis of these patients remains poor (MacIntyre et al., 2000), resulting in frequent readmission to the hospital. Thus, there is a need for other approaches to management.

Research Findings

McAlister, Stewart, Ferrua, & McMurray (2004) conducted a study to determine whether multidisciplinary strategies improve outcomes for HF patients. The researchers searched electronic databases, bibliographies, and contacted experts to find multidisciplinary management programs in HF. Twenty-nine trials (5,039 patients) were identified. The researchers independently reviewed the results of the search strategy and selected all studies reporting the impact of outpatient-based multidisciplinary management strategies on mortality or hospitalization rates in patients with HF. Each type of intervention was then independently assigned to one of four groups: (1) multidisciplinary HF clinic; (2) multidisciplinary team providing specialized follow-up but not in a hospital or practice-based clinic; (3) telephone follow-up or telemonitoring and enhanced communication with primary health care provider (including advice to deteriorating patients to see their regular health care provider); or (4) educational programs designed to enhance patient self-care activities.

The study results reveal that these programs are associated with a 27% reduction in HF hospitalization rates and a 43% reduction in total number of HF hospitalizations. Those strategies that incorporate specialized follow-up by a multidisciplinary team or in a multidisciplinary HF clinic also reduce all-cause mortality by approximately one-quarter and all-cause hospitalizations by one-fifth.

Implications for Nursing Practice

In order to assist the patient in getting ready for discharge from the hospital, it is essential that the nurse have an understanding of the symptoms, diagnosis, and management (medical, device, and self-management). The nurse must stress the importance of compliance with every aspect of care. If the patient has been cared for using a multidisciplinary approach, the nurse typically coordinates each member of the team. The nurse must reinforce teaching and determine the patient/family's understanding of the disease and its management.

When doing discharge planning, the nurse must ask the patient about her resources and support system. A plan needs to be developed that is realistic and manageable for the patient and family. Assistance for patients who may have difficulties taking or obtaining their medications must be provided. Ensure patients have access to urgent care, outside emergency department settings. It could be beneficial if a system for postdischarge telephone follow-up were instituted for these patients.

Critical Thinking Questions

1. Your patient was discharged from the hospital 3 days ago after a heart failure hospitalization. You are the nurse calling him to see how he is feeling since discharge. He states that his daughter was supposed to pick up his medications, but had a family emergency and forgot. He still does not have his medications, and he was discharged 5 days ago. What do you do?

2. You are the nurse in a clinic, and a patient with heart failure says she is taking her medications appropriately and following a low-salt, fluid-restricted diet. Your patient's weight continues to rise, and symptoms are worsening. What do you do to help this patient?

3. Your patient is readmitted for heart failure 2 weeks after his last heart failure hospitalization. What can you do to understand what went wrong at home, and how you can prevent a third admission?

Answers to Critical Thinking Questions appear in Appendix D.

References

Jessup, M., & Brozena, S. (2003). Medical progress heart failure. *The New England Journal of Medicine, 348,* 2007–2018.

MacIntyre, K., Capewell, S., Stewart, S., et al. (2000). Evidence of improving prognosis in heart failure trends in case fatality in 66,547 patients hospitalized between 1986 and 1995. *Circulation, 102,* 1126–1131.

McAlister, F. A., Stewart, S., Ferrua, S., & McMurray, J. J. (2004). Multidisciplinary strategies for the management of heart failure patients at high risk for admission: A systematic review of randomized trials. *Journal of the American College of Cardiology, 44*(4), 810–819.

Stewart, S., Jenkins, A., Buchan, S., McGuire, A., Capewell, S., & McMurray, J. J. V. (2002). The current cost of heart failure to the National Health Service in the UK. *European Journal of Heart Failure, 4,* 361–371.

monitored within a week of initiating an ACE inhibitor and periodically thereafter, because hyperkalemia (serum levels greater than 5) and worsening renal insufficiency may occur (Hardman & Limbird, 2001; Hunt et al., 2005).

Blood pressure should be monitored frequently in patients started on ACE inhibitors. If a systolic blood pressure is found to be consistently less than 90 mmHg or if the patient complains of light-headedness, it generally warrants either a reduction in dose or stopping it completely. These symptoms may occur, especially in the setting of concomitant diuretic therapy. Initiation of ACE inhibitors is usually with short-acting agents, at low dose, with slow up-titration (Adams et al., 2006; Greenberg & Hermann, 2002).

Angiotensin II Receptor Blockers (ARB)

The RAAS system is only partially suppressed by the use of ACE inhibitors because angiotensin II is also produced by other pathways. ARBs cause inhibition by blocking RAAS activation at the angiotensin II receptor site. Angiotensin receptor blockers have been found to have clinical effects similar to those of ACE inhibitors with regard to the interference with the RAAS, yet they have not demonstrated superior results to ACE inhibitors in clinical trials. ARBs remain second-line therapy and may be considered when patients exhibit an ACE inhibitor–induced cough or angioedema (Hunt et al., 2005).

Beta-Adrenergic Blockers

Beta-adrenergic blockers, commonly referred to as beta-blockers, act primarily by blocking the sympathetic nervous system (SNS) in patients with heart failure and have been a major advance in heart failure treatment (Hunt et al., 2005). Patients placed on beta-adrenergic blockers who have had a myocardial infarction and/or left ventricular ejection fraction (LVEF) < 40% in addition to standard therapy of an ACE inhibitor, digitalis, and a diuretic, have been found to have an improved survival and reduced symptoms (Adams et al., 2006; Hunt et al., 2005). Other benefits include improved clinical status, decreased risk of sudden death, and improved overall exercise tolerance. Beta-adrenergic blockers have been found to be effective in all classes of heart failure, including patients with severe, but stable heart failure (Hunt et al., 2005).

Initially, sympathetic nervous system (SNS) activation assists the heart in maintaining a stable cardiac output. But eventually, these effects can cause increased vasoconstriction, decreased exercise capacity, decreased left ventricular efficiency, myocardial ischemia, increased potential for dysrhythmias, and worsening cardiac dysfunction. By blocking these effects, there is an improvement in coronary blood flow and less ischemia. There also is a decreased workload on the heart and less myocyte hypertrophy. Adverse cardiac remodeling is inhibited and the risk of sudden death by dysrhythmia is lessened (Sackner-Bernstein & Mancini, 1995).

Patients must be clinically stable prior to the initiation of a beta-adrenergic blocker because fluid retention may be precipitated (Hunt et al., 2005). Adjustments of diuretic management may be necessary if signs and symptoms of increasing congestion are noted. Beta-adrenergic blockers are generally initiated at low doses and increased slowly over time until target doses are achieved (Adams et al., 2006; Hunt et al., 2005). Beta-adrenergic blockers can also cause fatigue that may resolve spontaneously or be persistent enough to require the discontinuance or reduction of the medication (Hunt et al., 2005).

Nursing assessment includes observing for signs of hypotension, bradycardia, or congestion, because these conditions may require adjustment to the beta-adrenergic blocker dose or other background medications. Diabetic patients with recurrent hypoglycemia or those with resting leg ischemia should be educated to monitor for any increase of related symptoms. It is also imperative that nurses instruct patients on how to monitor their pulse, blood pressure, and symptoms of congestion, including helping them recognize when they should notify their health care provider for worrisome symptoms (Hardman & Limbird, 2001). Beta-adrenergic blockers can worsen bronchospasm in patients with reactive airway disease. If on nursing assessment wheezing is present, this may prompt the health care provider to discontinue beta-blocker therapy or then change to a beta-1 selective agent (type of beta-adrenergic blocker with less bronchospastic characteristics) at a low dose (Hardman & Limbird, 2001; Hunt et al., 2005). If patients experience hypotension while on both ACE inhibitors and beta-blockers, they might try

splitting the doses, or alternating the time of day one is taken in relation to the other. Smaller doses of the combination of ACE inhibitors and beta-blockers are preferred to higher doses of either medication alone.

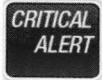 *Symptoms requiring adjustment of background medications or beta-blocker dose include:*

1. *Worsening shortness of breath*
2. *Weight gain*
3. *Fatigue*
4. *Hypotension*
5. *Light-headedness or syncope.*

Diuretics

The most effective method to relieve heart failure symptoms is to remove excess fluid with loop diuretics (Adams et al., 2006; Hunt et al., 2005). Patients with advanced heart failure needing enhanced diuresis may require the addition of chlorothiazides, such as metolazone, to loop diuretics. Hospitalized patients or those refractory to oral diuretics may require intravenous diuretics for rapid relief of congestive symptoms. The majority of diuretic agents work within the renal tubules to prevent sodium reabsorption and thereby cause natriuresis. Patients are started on a low diuretic dose, titrating subsequent doses to achieve the desired weight loss and symptom improvement. Primary management when using a diuretic will require the nurse to obtain laboratory work for close monitoring of serum electrolytes (because hypokalemia is common), to assess volume status (by evaluating symptomatology), to observe for excessive volume depletion (to ensure hypovolemia is prevented), and to monitor the response to diuretics (urine output and weight loss). Excessive volume depletion can also activate the RAAS system, negating the effect of the ACE inhibitor and ARB.

Patients placed on a diuretic will need nursing education regarding the mechanism of diuretic function and the importance of maintaining a euvolemic or "dry" weight (Greenberg & Hermann, 2002). If patient compliance with sodium and fluid restriction is poor, escalating diuretic doses may be needed to maintain **euvolemia** (when the body is in a state of equal fluid balance, without fluid retention). Often, by teaching patients the principles of diuretic self-adjustments, they are able to adjust their own dose, based on daily weights and symptoms, thus reducing the chance of volume overload. Patients who self-adjust diuretics must clearly understand how, when, and if their corresponding potassium supplementation is also increased. Patients who are unable to follow medication instructions, who are noncompliant, or who are challenged with more complicated multidrug regimens may not be candidates for adjusting their own diuretic dose due to the risk of dehydration or hypokalemia/hyperkalemia. A crucial point of education for congested patients is to emphasize the importance of sodium and fluid restriction (Greenberg & Hermann, 2002). Generally, a low-sodium diet of less than 2 to 3 grams combined with ingesting less than 2 liters of fluid per day is recommended.

Digitalis

Digitalis is a weak, positive inotrope that increases the contractility of the weakened heart muscle, thus, improving the volume of cardiac output (Teerlink & Massie, 2003). It has also been found to act as an antagonist to SNS activation (Greenberg & Hermann, 2002). It has been well studied and found to improve symptoms and exercise tolerance in patients with heart failure (Packer et al., 1993). Although there has been no mortality benefit identified with this medication, there is a decrease in hospitalizations with the greatest benefit in patients with NYHA class III and IV symptoms (Digitalis Investigation Group, 1997). Adverse effects of digitalis use are largely related to toxic serum concentrations, and therefore, patients should be placed on a low dose and be monitored to maintain a target therapeutic level < 1.0 ng/mL (Adams et al., 2006). Nursing assessment for patients on digitalis include monitoring for toxic drug levels that can cause cardiac dysrhythmias and conduction disturbances, bradycardia, gastrointestinal symptoms, and neurological complaints (Hardman & Limbird, 2001; Hunt et al., 2005). Certain medications can increase digitalis levels (Chart 42–7), and therefore, more frequent monitoring of serum concentrations is important in this subset of patients (Hardman & Limbird, 2001; Hunt et al., 2005).

Aldosterone Antagonists

Aldosterone antagonists are recommended for patients with heart failure and/or postmyocardial infarction with continued NYHA class III or IV symptoms treated with standard therapy of ACE inhibitors, beta-blockers, and diuretics. When the RAAS is activated, aldosterone release occurs. Aldosterone is a potent hormone secreted by the adrenal glands that, when activated in heart failure, causes sodium and fluid retention (Weber, 1999). Aldosterone also has neurohormonal effects including SNS activation and cardiac remodeling. Aldosterone antagonists provide a more complete blockade of the RAAS and reduce aldosterone release, resulting in a mortality benefit and a reduction in hospitalizations (Adams et al., 2006). Cautious use, with low doses of aldosterone antagonists, is encouraged. Strict monitoring of serum potassium and renal function is essential. It will

be necessary to reduce or discontinue potassium supplementation to maintain serum potassium at less than 5 mEq/L, and it should be discontinued if the serum creatinine is greater than 2.5 mg/dL (Adams et al., 2006). Gynecomastia (breast tenderness) is a troublesome adverse effect with spironolactone that is reversible when the medication is discontinued (Hunt et al., 2005). Eplerenone may be used as an alternative, due to its lower risk of causing gynecomastia. Because of the risk of hyperkalemia, aldosterone antagonists are not recommended in patients who are also on ACE inhibitors and ARBs.

Antiarrhythmic/Dysrhythmic Agents

Antiarrhythmic or dysrhythmic agents should not be used routinely to treat heart failure, but may be used for recurrent atrial fibrillation or symptomatic ventricular dysrhythmias (Hunt et al., 2005). Amiodarone, while effective in treating dysrhythmias, is associated with significant side effects such as thyroid and liver abnormalities, skin and visual abnormalities, pulmonary fibrosis, and nausea and vomiting. Careful monitoring during the course of therapy must be documented. Patients should be educated about increasing shortness of breath, bluish hue to nose or face, or other new symptoms.

Anticoagulant and Antiplatelet Agents

In patients with severe left ventricular dysfunction and an ejection fraction ≤ 35%, there is a potential for stasis within the ventricular chamber that could lead to the development of thrombi. It may be reasonable to anticoagulate such patients with warfarin therapy in the absence of a contraindication (Hunt et al., 2005). Patients with atrial fibrillation, mechanical heart valves, some mechanical assist devices, pulmonary embolism, transient ischemic attacks or cerebral vascular accidents, or other deep venous thrombosis also are candidates for anticoagulation therapy. Patients who have had a large anterior wall myocardial infarction or ventricular thrombus will often require anticoagulation therapy for 3 months (Hunt et al., 2005). Anticoagulation with warfarin requires frequent monitoring of the prothrombin time to keep patients in a therapeutic range measured by the international normalization ratio (INR) (Hardman & Limbird, 2001).

Nurses must assess a patient's "fall risk" because of potential bleeding in those taking oral anticoagulants and be sure the patient understands she may have an increased risk of bleeding. Patients must also receive instruction that frequent laboratory testing is required to maintain the INR in the desired target range. They should be instructed to call their health care provider with any signs of bleeding or with changes in their current medications, thus prompting additional assessment of changes that may occur to the INR. Antiplatelet agents, such as aspirin and clopidogrel, are indicated for patients with coronary artery, cerebral vascular, and peripheral vascular disease. Because patients may develop stomach upset and have increased bleeding risk with these agents, they should be alerted to associated warning signs.

CHART 42–7	**Medications That Increase Serum Digitalis Levels**
Quinidine	Captopril
Verapamil	Diltiazem
Spironolactone	Nifedipine
Flecainide	Nitrendipine
Propafenone	Cyclosporine
Amiodarone	

Any medication may have the potential of having an effect with other medications, leading to increased serum levels of one or both drugs. Even toxicity may result. This list includes those medicines known to increase serum digitalis levels. When digitalis levels become > 1.2, there is an associated increased risk of mortality. Those with levels > 2 are at risk of symptoms of digitalis toxicity, including nausea, vomiting, visual disturbance, or neurological changes.

Sources: Braunwald, E., Zipes, D. P., & Libby, P. (2001). *Heart disease: A textbook of cardiovascular medicine* (6th ed.). Philadelphia: W. B. Saunders; Hardman, J. G., & Limbird, L. E. (Eds.). (2001). *Goodman and Gilmans's The Pharmacological basis of therapeutics* (10th ed.). New York: McGraw-Hill; Hunt, S. A., Abraham, W. T., Chin, M. H., Feldman, A. M., Francis, G. S., Ganiats, T. G., et al. (2005). ACC/AHA 2005 guideline update for the diagnosis and management of chronic heart failure in the adult: Summary article: A report of the American College of Cardiology/American Heart Association Task Force on Practice Guidelines (Writing Committee to Update the 2001 Guidelines for the Evaluation and Management of Heart Failure). *Journal of the American College of Cardiology, 46,* 1116–1143.

CRITICAL ALERT

1. *Elderly patients with heart failure frequently void at night and therefore are at risk for falling if they arise suddenly.*

2. *Consider discussion with the health care provider about the different modalities to eliminate fall risks, including the use of indwelling catheter, bedside commode, or call light for assistance (for patients in the hospital) and home health and home needs–assessment for those at home.*

Potential risks of anticoagulation therapy include the following:

1. *When international normalization ratio (INR) levels are supratherapeutic, bleeding may occur (hemoptysis, hematuria, bloody stool, epistaxis, or excessive bleeding from lacerations).*
2. *When INR levels are subtherapeutic, thrombi may form.*
3. *Discuss the risks and benefits of anticoagulant therapy, including what to watch for, dietary suggestions, and recommendations for monitoring.*
4. *Encourage compliance with medication dose changes and with the treatment plan.*
5. *Adverse effects may result if either of these is not followed closely.*

Inotropic, Vasopressor, and Vasodilator Therapeutic Agents

In patients with acute decompensated heart failure and critical hypoperfusion, intravenous diuretics, inotropes, vasopressor, or vasodilator agents have been found to be beneficial in improving hemodynamics, including stroke volume and cardiac output, and thereby improving blood pressure and perfusion to organs and tissues (Fonarow, 2001; Stevenson, 2003). When a patient presents with acute decompensated heart failure, the ideal drug would support blood pressure and improve cardiac hemodynamic pressures; that is, decrease pulmonary artery occlusion pressure and right atrial pressure, and increase cardiac output (Stevenson, 2003). Acute reduction in cardiac filling pressures is associated not only with symptomatic improvement but also with a reduction in mortality rates, whereas acute improvements in measured cardiac output or ejection fraction are not as closely associated with improved survival (Fonarow, 2001).

Intravenous inotropes, such as milrinone and dobutamine, have been found to improve hemodynamic pressures in the acute setting. However, when used chronically, they have been found to lead to increased mortality (Abraham et al., 2005). Inotropic agents may have use in a subset of patients with reduced blood pressure and severe symptoms with poor end-organ perfusion (Adams et al., 2006). Chronic inotropes may have a role in palliating symptoms for patients with end-stage disease, but are not recommended for intermittent use. Agents with vasodilating properties, such as intravenous nitroglycerine, sodium nitroprusside, and nesiritide, may be an alternative in select, diuretic-resistant patients to reduce ventricular filling pressures, decrease afterload, and improve symptoms of acute decompensation (Adams et al., 2006; Hunt et al., 2005).

Medications for Select Patients

Hydralazine/nitrates had been used in combination until ACE inhibitors showed superior results in patients with heart failure. Now, this combination is recognized as a reasonable alternative for patients who are unable to take an ACE inhibitor, ARBs, and/or beta-adrenergic blockers for whatever reason (Adams et al., 2006). African Americans patients with continued NYHA class III or IV symptoms, despite standard medical management with an ACE inhibitor or ARB and beta-adrenergic blockers, have improved outcomes with hydralazine/nitrates, which should be added if blood pressure allows. The Pharmacology Summary (p. 1294) reviews all of the medications used to treat heart failure.

Complementary and Alternative Therapies

Surveys have shown that at least 50% of patients with heart failure take some type of vitamins or herbal supplements to treat their disease or prevent other diseases (Greenberg & Hermann, 2002). The Complementary and Alternatives Therapies feature (p. 1296) presents a range of alternative therapies that are available. Although over 40 products are touted for cardiovascular benefits, little randomized-controlled clinical research supports claims, and safety and efficacy are not known. Despite the fact that supplemental therapies are widely used, there remains little understanding of how they interact with prescribed heart failure medications. Potentially harmful results may occur, especially in the elderly or those with impaired metabolism (Greenberg & Hermann, 2002). Chronically ill patients, especially those on diuretic therapy, should take a standard multivitamin daily (Hunt et al., 2005).

Patients may ask their health care providers questions such as the following about herbal medicine:

1. *Will this alternative or herbal therapy interfere with my heart failure medicines?*
2. *How much of this alternative or herbal therapy is safe for me to take?*
3. *Has this alternative or herbal therapy been tested for safety in people with heart failure?*
4. *Have research studies proven that this alternative or herbal therapy helps people with heart failure?*

A particularly dangerous supplement that patients with heart failure should avoid is *ma huang* (commonly known as ephedra), because it has been shown to be associated with deaths (Young, 2001). Garlic, ginseng, and *ginkgo biloba* may alter antiplatelet and anticoagulant effects, so those taking aspirin, other antiplatelet agents, or warfarin should be cautioned about bleeding (American Society of Consultant Pharmacists, 1999). Ongoing research is under way to learn whether hawthorn and coenzyme Q10 (CoQ10) have any role in heart failure, because they have been touted as effective treatments in improving symptoms. For a discussion of CoQ10 supplementation, see the Complementary and Alternative Therapies feature (p. 1296).

In summary, multiple medications are used in the management of heart failure with different indications, side effects, costs, and interaction profiles. The entire health care team must share the responsibility of emphasizing the importance of medical therapy to patients, their families, and their caregivers. The complexity of the heart failure medication regimen increases the risk of noncompliance and medication errors. Using creative methods to reinforce medication use with patients at every encounter, during the hospitalization, at discharge, and in outpatient venues will lead to the best possible outcomes.

Device Therapies for Heart Failure

Cardiac devices have a well-established role in the management of systolic dysfunction. These revolutionary devices have improved both length and quality of life when added to medical therapy for those with heart failure. Cardiac pacemakers and the expanded use of implantable cardioverter defibrillators (ICDs) have become the standard of care in select patients. Internal cardioverter defibrillators have shown superiority over medical

PHARMACOLOGY Summary of Medications to Treat Heart Failure

Medication Category	Action	Application/Indication	Nursing Responsibility
Angiotensin-converting enzyme (ACE) inhibitors: Benazepril Captopril Enalapril Lisinopril Quinapril Ramipril	Works within the renin-angiotensin-aldosterone system (RAAS) to inhibit the vasoconstricting action of angiotensin II and the angiotensin-mediated secretion of aldosterone, thus causing blood vessels to dilate, and systemic vascular resistance is decreased. Results in decreased afterload, decreased sodium resorption, and increased contractility.	Use in all patients with reduced ventricular function; left ventricular ejection fraction (LVEF) < 40%. HF patients on ACE inhibitors have improved survival and delayed progression of heart failure due to the favorable blockade of the RAAS.	Monitor for ACE inhibitor-induced cough, dizziness, hypotension, hyperkalemia, and worsening renal insufficiency. Angioedema may also occur in rare settings.
Angiotensin II receptor blockers (ARBs): Candesartan cilexetil Eprosartan mesylate Irbesartan Losartan potassium Telmisartan Valsartan	Causes inhibition by blocking RAAS activation at the angiotensin II receptor site. Angiotensin receptor blockers have been found to have similar clinical effects as ACE inhibitors with regard to the interference with the RAAS. They decrease afterload, decrease sodium resorption, and increase contractility.	Use in heart failure (HF) patients who are intolerant to ACE inhibitors with an LVEF < 40%. HF patients on ARBs have improved survival and delayed progression of heart failure due to the favorable blockade of the RAAS.	Monitor for dizziness, hypotension, hyperkalemia, and worsening renal insufficiency.
Beta-adrenergic blockers: Carvedilol Metoprolol succinate	Acts primarily by blocking the sympathetic nervous system (SNS) in patients with heart failure. By blocking these effects, there is an improvement in coronary blood flow and less ischemia. There also is a decreased workload on the heart and less myocyte hypertrophy resulting in decreased myocardial ischemia and hypertrophy.	Use in HF patients with LVEF < 40% or postmyocardial infarction. HF patients on beta-blockers have been found to have improved survival, improvement in symptoms, a decrease in the risk of sudden death, and improved overall exercise tolerance.	Observe for signs of hypotension or bradycardia, as either condition may require adjustment to the beta-adrenergic-blocker dose or other background medications. Patient education is imperative about the initial response or up-titration of this drug, which can cause fatigue, dizziness, fluid retention, and worsening heart failure. It is also imperative that nurses instruct patients on how to monitor their pulse and blood pressure and to help them recognize when they should notify their provider if these parameters become too low. Beta-adrenergic blockers can worsen bronchospasm in patients with reactive airway disease and therefore should be monitored.
Diuretics: Bumetanide Furosemide Metolazone Torsemide	Interferes with the sodium retention of HF by inhibiting the reabsorption of sodium or chloride at specific sites in the renal tubules.	Use in HF patients exhibiting signs and symptoms of fluid overload. Diuretic drugs increase urinary sodium excretion and decrease physical signs of fluid retention in patients with HF.	Nursing assessment for patients on diuretics includes monitoring for signs of hypokalemia, hypotension, and dehydration. It is also imperative that nurses provide patient self-management instruction, including daily weights, sodium and fluid restrictions, and instruction on when to notify their health care provider about worsening symptoms.

PHARMACOLOGY Summary of Medications to Treat Heart Failure—*Continued*

Medication Category	Action	Application/Indication	Nursing Responsibility
Digitalis Digoxin	A weak, positive inotrope that increases the contractility of the weakened heart muscle thus, improving the volume of cardiac output. It has also been found to have an impact on enzyme inhibition in noncardiac tissues, thus, eventually leading to a suppression of renin secretion from the RAAS.	Use in HF patients with New York Heart Association (NYHA) class III or IV symptoms. This medication has been found to decrease hospitalizations and to improve symptoms, quality of life, and exercise tolerance.	Nursing assessment for patients on digitalis includes monitoring for toxic drug levels that can cause cardiac dysrhythmias and conduction disturbances, gastrointestinal symptoms, and neurological complaints.
Aldosterone antagonists: Spironolactone	Blocks the release of aldosterone hormone secreted by the adrenal glands that, when activated in heart failure, causes sodium and fluid retention.	Use in HF patients with continued symptoms, despite therapies listed above. Found to have a favorable mortality benefit and has shown to decrease hospitalizations. These benefits are greatest in those patients with NYHA class IV symptoms.	Monitor for signs of hyperkalemia and renal dysfunction. Should not be used in combination with ACE inhibitors and ARBs. Side effect of some aldosterone antagonists is gynecomastia, which may require a change in antagonist used. Nursing instruction should include a discussion with the health care provider regarding the reduction or discontinuation of potassium supplements and also the avoidance of high-potassium-containing foods. Nonsteroidal anti-inflammatory drugs and cyclooxygenase-2 inhibitors should be avoided, which can worsen hyperkalemia and renal dysfunction.
Hydralazine and isosorbide dinitrate	This combination of vasodilators acts on both arteries and veins. Theoretically, it may act as an antioxidant on nitric oxide.	African American HF patients on standard therapy (i.e., ACE inhibitors or ARBs) and beta-blockers may benefit when this combination is added. Patients unable to tolerate ACE inhibitor or ARB therapy may consider this alternative combination. This combination has shown improved survival, reduced hospitalizations, and improved quality of life.	Monitor for headache, hypotension, and gastrointestinal complaints. Should not be used in patients that have not had a trial of ACE inhibitor or ARBs. Compliance must be reinforced due to the multidose schedule required.

Antiarrhythmics:
  Amiodarone
  Bretylium
  Dofetilide
  Ibutilide
  Sotalol
	This class III antiarrhythmic agent has sympatholytic (or antiadrenergic) effects on the heart and AV nodal blocking properties.	May be used for rate and rhythm control for patients in atrial fibrillation, and to suppress significant ventricular dysrhythmias, or may suppress implantable cardioverter defibrillator (ICD) shocks.	Possible side effects include pulmonary toxicities, skin discoloration, hepatic and/or thyroid derangements, corneal deposits, optic neuropathy, and interactions with warfarin and digoxin. May be proarrhythmic; monitor cardiac rhythm.

Sources: Adams, K. F., Lindenfeld, J., Arnold, J. M., et al. (2006). Executive summary: HFSA 2006 comprehensive heart failure practice guideline. *Journal of Cardiac Failure, 12*(1), 10–38; Crawford, P. A., & Lin, T. L. (2004). *The Washington manual cardiology subspecialty consult* (pp. 122–126). Philadelphia: Lippincott Williams & Wilkins; and Hunt, S. A., Abraham, W. T., Chin, M. H., Feldman, A. M., Francis, G. S., Ganiats, T. G., et al. (2005). ACC/AHA 2005 guideline update for the diagnosis and management of chronic heart failure in the adult: Summary article: A report of the American College of Cardiology/American Heart Association Task Force on Practice Guidelines (Writing Committee to Update the 2001 Guidelines for the Evaluation and Management of Heart Failure). *Journal of the American College of Cardiology, 46,* 1116–1143.

therapy alone in reducing sudden cardiac death. Cardiac pacemakers and ICDs are discussed in detail in Chapter 39 .

Cardiac Resynchronization Therapy

Cardiac resynchronization therapy (CRT), also known as biventricular pacing, is useful in the treatment of heart failure in selected patients. The CRT device paces both ventricles simultaneously, thereby helping to restore a synchronized contraction that had been lost with the emergence of conduction abnormalities and dyssynchrony, which is present in approximately 25% to 30% of patients with heart failure (Abraham, 2003). CRT is most effective in patients with moderate to severe symptoms, despite optimal heart failure medication, with a LVEF < 35% and QRS duration > 120 milliseconds (Hunt et al., 2005). In a healthy heart, electrical impulses are generated from the sinus node in the right atrium, travel through the atrioventricular (AV) node, and then almost simultaneously down each bundle branch to cause a coordinated contraction of the left ventricle and efficient movement of blood through the heart. Heart failure patients with myocardial damage often have conduction abnormalities such as a bundle branch block, in which there is a delay in the transmission of the electrical impulse down one or the other bundle branch, causing a wide QRS complex on the ECG. This intraventricular conduction delay results in dyssynchronous movements between the ventricles, abnormal septal wall motion, suboptimal filling during diastole, poorly coordinated ventricular contraction, decreased left ventricular ejection fraction, and even impaired mitral valve function (Bakker et al., 2000;

Kerwin et al., 2000). Clinically, patients with a bundle branch block experience limited exercise tolerance, impaired quality of life, and poor functional capacity.

For CRT implantation, a pacemaker box is inserted surgically under the skin, usually in the left upper chest wall, and pacemaker leads are placed directly in the right ventricle and through a lateral vein into the left ventricle. These leads are programmed to coordinate contraction times between the ventricular leads while optimizing AV delay. Patients with atrial fibrillation may undergo AV junction ablation (rendering cells nonfunctional) and receive simple biventricular pacing (Abraham, 2003; Linde et al., 2002). The mechanical improvements seen with this kind of pacing in-

COMPLEMENTARY & ALTERNATIVE THERAPIES

Types of Therapies

Type of Therapy	Proposed Clinical Use	Evidence
Meditation	Inhibits sympathetic activation Improves quality of life (QOL)	In 17 elderly patients treated medically for heart failure, meditation led to a reduction in norepinephrine levels and improved QOL compared to control.
Relaxation	Improves some aspects of QOL	95 patients with moderately severe heart failure were randomized to 15 weeks of relaxation response therapy, to 15 weeks of cardiac education, or to usual care. Aspects of QOL that improved related to peace–spiritual and emotional scores, but not physical for the intervention group.
Inspiratory muscle training	Improves inspiratory muscle use, functional capacity, ventilatory response to exercise, and QOL	32 patients with heart failure with inspiratory muscle weakness were randomly assigned to either 12 weeks of inspiratory training or placebo training. Intervention group had improved inspiratory muscle strength, functional capacity, response to exercise, and QOL.
T'ai chi	Improves QOL Improves 6-minute walk test	30 patients with heart failure on standard therapy were randomized to 12 weeks of either t'ai chi or usual care. The intervention group had enhanced QOL and functional capacity.
Acupuncture	Inhibits sympathetic activation	15 advanced patients with heart failure underwent mental stress testing before and after (1) real acupuncture, (2) nonpoint acupuncture, and (3) no-needle acupuncture control. Acupuncture was found to attenuate sympathoexcitation during mental stress.
Nutraceuticals	Proposed to reduce risk of heart disease through antioxidant action	American College of Cardiology/American Heart Association (ACC/AHA) Chronic Heart Failure Guidelines 2005 ✓ **Not recommended to prevent or treat heart failure**
Hawthorn	Improved heart failure symptoms	A meta-analysis including 13 trials using hawthorn extract vs. placebo in chronic patients with heart failure showed significantly improved symptoms of dyspnea and fatigue.
Chelation therapy	Proposed to treat coronary artery disease	American Heart Association [a] ✓ **Not recommended for treating coronary artery disease**

[a] As per http://www.americanheart.org/presenter.jhtml?identifier=4493

Sources: Chang, B. H., et al. (2005). A relaxation response randomized trial on patients with chronic heart failure. *Journal of Cardiopulmonary Rehabilitation, 25*(3), 149–157; Curiati, J. A., et al. (2005). Meditation reduces sympathetic activation and improves the quality of life in elderly patients with optimally treated heart disease. *Journal of Alternative and Complementary Medicine, 11*(3), 465–472; Dall'Ago, P., Chiappa, G. R., Guths, H., Stein, R., & Ribeiro, J. P. (2006). Inspiratory muscle training in patients with heart failure and inspiratory muscle weakness: A randomized trial. *Journal of the American College of Cardiology, 47*(4), 757–763; Hunt, S. A., Abraham, W. T., Chin, M. H., Feldman, A. M., Francis, G. S., Ganiats, T. G., et al. (2005). ACC/AHA 2005 guideline update for the diagnosis and management of chronic heart failure in the adult: Summary article: A report of the American College of Cardiology/American Heart Association Task Force on Practice Guidelines (Writing Committee to Update the 2001 Guidelines for the Evaluation and Management of Heart Failure). *Journal of the American College of Cardiology, 46*, 1116–1143; Jeffrey, S. (2002). No evidence of benefit from chelation therapy. *HeartWire News.* Retrieved October 9, 2006, from http://www.theheart.org/article/277715.do; Middlekauff, H. F., Hui, K., Yu, J. L., Hamilton, M. A., Fonarow, G. C., Moriguchi, J., et al. (2002). Acupuncture inhibits sympathetic activation during mental stress in advanced heart failure patients. *Journal of Cardiac Failure, 8*(6), 399–406; Pittler, M. H., Schmidt, K., & Ernst, E. (2003). Hawthorne extract for treating chronic heart failure: Meta-analysis of randomized trials. *American Journal of Medicine, 114*(8), 665–674; and Yeh, G. Y., Wood, M. J., Lorell, B. H., Stevenson, L. W., Eisenberg, D. M., Wayne, P. M., et al. (2004). Effects of tai chi mind–body movement therapy on functional status and exercise capacity in patients with chronic heart failure: A randomized controlled trial. *American Journal of Medicine, 117*(8), 541–548.

COMPLEMENTARY & ALTERNATIVE THERAPIES

Coenzyme Q10 (CoQ10) Supplementation

Description:

Coenzyme Q10 (CoQ10) is an enzyme produced by the body that is a co-factor in mitochondrial energy production (Sander, Coleman, Patel, Kluger, & White, 2006). It is a solid, waxlike substance that is abundant in healthy heart tissue. Deficiencies of CoQ10—from 50% to 75% of normal levels—have been found in heart tissue biopsies of people with various heart diseases. The body produces less CoQ10 as a person ages and some cholesterol-lowering drugs also reduce levels of this vital enzyme. Supplement doses of CoQ10 range from 30 to 200 mg per day.

Heart failure (HF) is a condition that is greatly impacted by CoQ10 levels. HF impairs the heart's ability to maintain normal cardiac output. Following an initial cardiac insult, remodeling ensues, which results in left ventricular dilation and hypertrophy. Oxidative stress also increases after a cardiac insult, while CoQ10 levels decrease. This and other data led researchers to the hypothesis that CoQ10 may decrease oxidative stress, impair remodeling, and improve cardiac function (Weant & Smith, 2005)

Research Support:

A meta-analysis of trials by one team of researchers evaluated the impact of CoQ10 therapy on ejection fraction and cardiac output. The team conducted a systematic literature search to identify randomized, controlled trials of CoQ10 in heart failure between 1966 and June 2005. Researchers conducted a subgroup analysis to assess clinical heterogeneity between trials. The team identified 12 trials in which 10 evaluated ejection fraction and 2 evaluated cardiac output. Doses ranged from 60 to 200 mg/day, and treatment periods ranged from 1 to 6 months. Overall, ejection fraction showed a 3.7% net improvement. In addition, cardiac output increased an average of 0.28 L/minute. The researchers concluded that CoQ10 enhances systolic function in chronic heart failure; however, they noted that its effectiveness may be reduced with concurrent use of current standard treatments (Sander et al., 2006).

An Italian team conducted a double-blind, placebo-controlled crossover study of 23 patients with stable CHF secondary to ischemic heart disease. Researchers assigned patients to the following treatments, each of which lasted 4 weeks: oral CoQ10 (100 mg tid), CoQ10 plus supervised exercise training (ET) (60% of peak VO$_2$, five times a week), placebo, and placebo plus ET. There was significant improvement in both peak VO$_2$ and endothelium-dependent dilation of the brachial artery (EDDBA) after CoQ10 and after ET as compared with placebo. The researchers concluded that oral CoQ10 improves functional capacity, endothelial function, and LV contractility in CHF with no side effects. In addition, patients showed higher plasma CoQ10 levels and more pronounced effects on all the abovementioned parameters with a combination of CoQ10 and ET (Belardinelli et al., 2006).

The same research team, in a related study, found that CoQ10 supplementation resulted in a threefold increase in plasma CoQ10 level. Systolic wall thickening score index (SWTI) and left ventricular ejection fraction improved both at rest and peak dobutamine stress echo after CoQ10 supplementation (Belardinelli et al., 2005).

A New Zealand study examined 24 patients with stable, symptomatic heart failure and a left ventricular ejection fraction less than 40%. Each patient was randomized to 40 mg atorvastatin or placebo for 6 weeks, then the patient was crossed over to the other treatment arm for a further 6 weeks. Coenzyme Q10 was shown to be the significant variable that predicted improvement in endothelial function after adjusting for LDL-cholesterol levels (Strey et al., 2005).

References

Belardinelli, R., Mucaj, A., Lacalaprice, F., Solenghi, M., Principi, F., Tiano, L., et al. (2005). Coenzyme Q10 improves contractility of dysfunctional myocardium in chronic heart failure. *BioFactors, 25*(1–4), 137–145.

Belardinelli, R., Mucaj, A., Lacalaprice, F., Solenghi, M., Seddaiu, G., Principi, F., et al (2006). Coenzyme Q10 and exercise training in chronic heart failure. *European Heart Journal, 27*(22), 2675–2681.

Sander, S., Coleman, C. I., Patel, A. A., Kluger, J., & White, C. M. (2006). The impact of coenzyme Q10 on systolic function in patients with chronic heart failure. *Journal of Cardiac Failure, 12*(6), 464–472.

Strey, C. H., Young, J. M., Molyneux, S. L., George, P. M., Florkowski, C. M., Scott, R. S., et al. (2005). Endothelium-ameliorating effects of statin therapy and coenzyme Q10 reductions in chronic heart failure. *Atherosclerosis, 179*(1), 201–206.

Weant, K. A., & Smith, K. M. (2005). The role of coenzyme Q10 in heart failure. *Annals of Pharmacotherapy, 39*(9), 1522–1526.

clude less restrictive ventricular filling patterns, decreased mitral valve regurgitation, improved cardiac muscle contractile synchrony, increased LVEF, and improved cardiac index (Molhoek et al., 2002). Clinical improvements include improved NYHA class, peak oxygen uptake, quality-of-life scores, and 6-minute walk test scores (Abraham, 2003). The algorithm in Figure 42–5 ■ (p. 1298) illustrates how patients may be selected for CRT/automatic implanted cardioverter defibrillator (AICD) therapy. Cardiac resynchronization therapy is discussed in detail in Chapter 39 .

Implantable Cardioverter Defibrillators

Implantable cardioverter defibrillators (ICDs) are indicated for patients with heart failure at risk for sudden cardiac death due to significant reductions in ventricular function (LVEF < 35%). ICD implantation consists of a small generator box inserted surgically under the skin with leads extending into the heart. These programmable devices detect lethal ventricular dysrhythmias and respond by administering either overdrive pacing or an electric shock directly to the heart for sustained dysrhythmias. Mortality rates with the use of an ICD have decreased, even in the absence of a history of lethal ventricular dysrhythmias (Moss et al., 2002; Teerlink & Massie, 2003). Patients determined to be at risk of sudden death

who also need a pacemaker can receive a combined pacemaker/ICD (Abraham, 2003; Bristow, Feldman, & Saxon, 2000; Teerlink & Massie, 2003). Selection criteria for identifying those appropriate for ICD implantation are summarized in Figure 42–5 ■ (p. 1298). Newer devices have advanced capabilities that couple diagnostic and treatment modes. Currently patients can be monitored from remote locations for their volume status, activity levels, and more. Chapter 39 discusses the indications for implantation of ICDs.

■ Nursing Management

Implantation of a pacemaker, ICD, or combined device is usually a less invasive procedure, requiring a simple incision to insert the control box and vascular insertion of the leads. Patients are usually admitted overnight for observation and then discharged after receiving a chest x-ray to ensure lead placement and to rule out a postprocedure pneumothorax. Recovery after placement of a pacemaker or ICD occurs over weeks, and patients should expect to experience some soreness of the chest wall and bruising. Appropriate pain management should be considered. Patients need instruction on wound care, to keep the site clean, and to

Notes:
** = Excluding risk of sudden cardiac death
# = ACE inhibitors or ARBs, beta blockers, diuretics, digoxin, spironolactone

FIGURE 42–5 ■ Algorithm for cardiac pacemaker and defibrillator.

monitor for signs and symptoms of infection or bleeding. An office visit to the health care provider to inspect the site usually occurs 1 week after implantation. To minimize the risk of dislodging the ventricular leads, patients are instructed not to raise the affected arm above the head and to avoid lifting of more than 10 to 15 pounds for approximately 3–4 weeks. Over time, they may resume usual activities.

Patients usually follow up with their electrocardiologist 1 month after their device implantation, and then every 6 to 12 months thereafter to ensure that the device is functioning properly and to have the battery life assessed. The device should be interrogated after any ICD discharges, to ensure that it is responding appropriately to a dysrhythmia, and then generally every 6 months. Patients are advised to carry their device identification card with them at all times and to avoid strong magnets, particularly those used in magnetic resonance imaging (MRI), and to alert airport security personnel. The Patient Teaching & Discharge Priorities box shows key points of the discharge plan after such procedures.

Percutaneous and Surgical Treatments for Coronary Artery Disease

Treating heart failure may include various catheter-based procedures. Procedures in the cardiac catheterization laboratory can provide diagnostic information (to assess the coronary tree, to assess for the presence of life-threatening dysrhythmias, and to assess hemodynamic measurements) and often provide opportunities

for treatment (revascularization for patients with coronary disease and treatments for dysrhythmia management). Balloon valvuloplasty (a percutaneous, catheter-based technique to relieve valvular stenosis) is sometimes considered for patients with a high mortality risk with surgical repair (Cohn, 2000; McKelvie, 2001). Balloon valvuloplasty is discussed in detail in Chapter 41 ☯.

One of the leading causes of left ventricular dysfunction resulting in heart failure is from significant coronary artery disease. Percutaneous and surgical treatments will be employed based on the nature of the coronary lesions, the likelihood of achieving revascularization, and the patient's risk profile.

Percutaneous Coronary Interventions

Spanning from 1987 to 2003, cardiac catheterizations increased 326%, with 664,000 procedures performed on 652,000 patients (AHA, 2006b). Men accounted for 65% of these procedures, and 52% of the patients were over the age of 65. Percutaneous coronary interventions (PCIs) have become a modality of revascularization that is less invasive than coronary artery bypass graft (CABG) surgery, are associated with shorter recovery time, and have shown outcomes comparable to CABG (McKelvie, 2001). The elderly patient and those with significant left ventricular dysfunction may be better candidates for PCI over bypass surgery due to faster recovery rates and subsequent lower mortality rates.

PCIs include percutaneous transluminal coronary angioplasty (PTCA), atherectomy, laser angioplasty, implantation of intracoronary stents, and other catheter devices for treating CAD (Feldman et al., 2006). Patients with multivessel coronary disease treated with PTCA have 5-year survival rates, similar to those who undergo CABG, although patients with diabetes have a better survival rate when treated with CABG (McKelvie, 2001).

Adjunctive thrombolytic therapies (e.g., abciximab, tirofiban, and eptifibatide) with PTCA (and intracoronary stenting) have led to lower restenosis rates, fewer complications, and improved mortality (McKelvie, 2001). New directions in PCI will focus on the strategies to improve safety, reduce restenosis rates, and broaden eligibility criteria for patients with subsets of CAD that are currently excluded. Chapter 39 ☯ discusses in detail PCI procedures.

Coronary Artery Bypass Graft Surgery

Coronary artery bypass graft surgery competes with PCI to revascularize patients with significant coronary artery lesions. CABG surgery has been effective in treating significant CAD that is not amenable to catheter-based techniques in 50% to 70% of patients with heart failure (Nohria et al., 2002) (Figure 42–6 ■). As of 2003, 467,000 procedures were completed on 268,000 patients in the United States (AHA, 2006b). CABG may be considered in those with compensated heart failure with an ejection fraction greater than 20%. This procedure should be considered when there is a high likelihood that revascularization will decrease the amount of ischemic myocardium by improving blood flow and thereby improving cardiac muscle function (Kouchoukos, Blackstone, Doty, Hanley, & Karp, 2003). A complete description of CABG surgery is included in Chapter 40 ☯.

Signs of stable heart failure include:
1. On stable medications requiring little change
2. Normal hemodynamic parameters
3. Without recent acute decompensation
4. Acceptable blood pressure.

PATIENT TEACHING & DISCHARGE PRIORITIES for Pacemaker/Implantable Cardioverter Defibrillator Devices

A nursing care plan made for patients after implantation of cardiac devices includes monitoring patients postimplantation, teaching patients about the device, postoperative care, monitoring for adverse complications, and appropriate follow-up.

Need	Teaching
Patient/family • Provide patient education related to device and need for scheduled follow-up.	• Heart failure medical therapy will augment device therapy and will continue indefinitely. • Limit arm movement to affected side for 1 to 2 weeks (use of sling as needed). • No lifting with affected side for 3 to 4 weeks. • Assess site for signs and symptoms of infection/drainage/bleeding. • Call for abnormal sensation of chest wall muscle movement (indication of dislodged lead or diaphragmatic/pectoral pacing). • Follow-up will be in 1 week to assess site, at 1 month, and then every 6 months and as needed for device interrogation and battery life assessment.
Family/support system • Patients with an automatic implanted cardioverter defibrillator (AICD) may be shocked by the device.	• Family/supports need to understand this is the intended purpose, and that the patient will need follow-up with his cardiologist to assess appropriateness of device. • Patients may need support for anxiety due to the potential or real shocks from an implantable cardioverter defibrillator (ICD).
Setting • In hospital and at home: assess postoperative pain. • In hospital and at home: assess incision site.	• Have patient rate pain. • Provide pain medicines as ordered. • Continue to assess level of responsiveness and relief of pain. • Call cardiologist for unrelieved or new pain. • Assess for bleeding, other drainage. • Hematoma. • Call cardiologist for changes.

Sources: Bakker, P. F., Meijburg, H. W., de Vries, J. W., Mower, M. M., Thomas, A. C., Hull, M. L., et al. (2000). Biventricular pacing in end-stage heart failure improves functional capacity and left ventricular function. *Journal of Interventional Cardiac Electrophysiology, 4*(2), 395–404; and Vesty, J., Rasmusson, K. D., Hall, J., Schmitz, S., & Brush, S. (2004). Cardiac resynchronization therapy and automatic implantable cardiac defibrillators in the treatment of heart failure: A review article. *Journal of the American Academy of Nurse Practitioners, 16*(10).

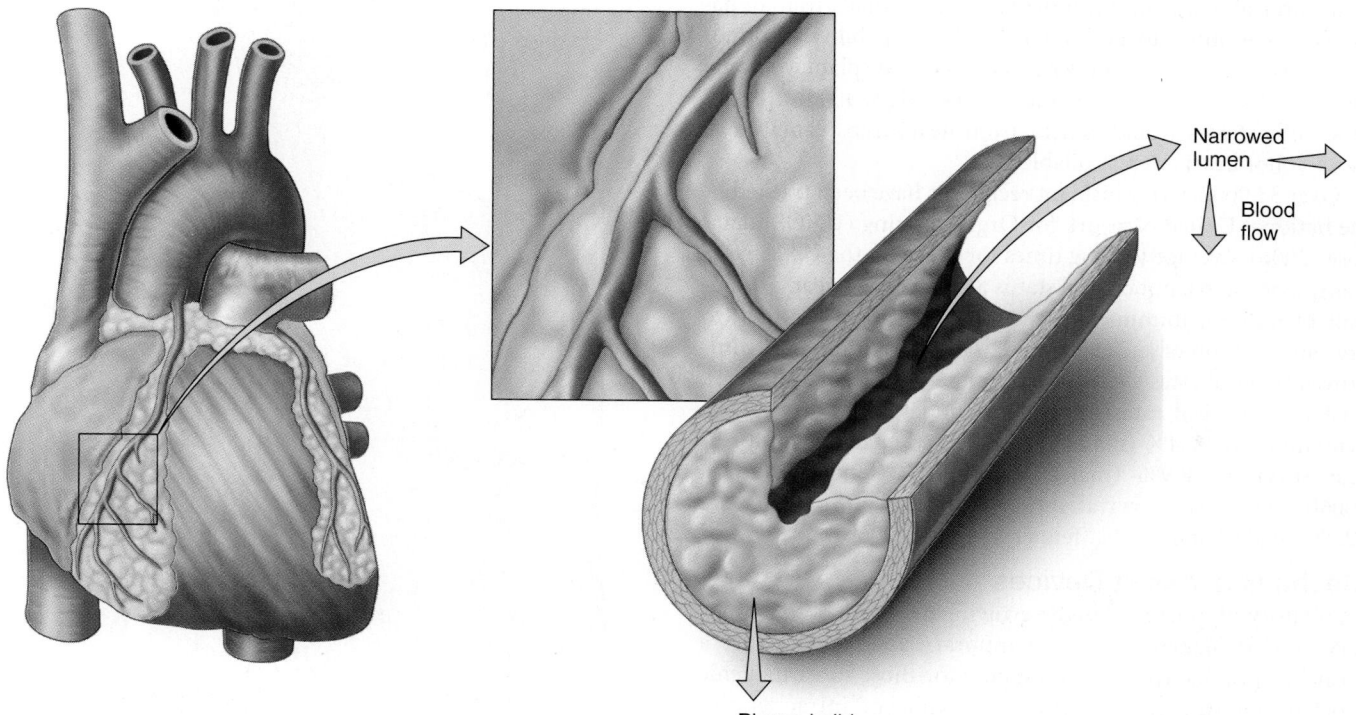

FIGURE 42–6 ■ Coronary artery disease.

Other Surgical Treatments for Systolic Heart Failure

Specific surgical procedures are utilized if they are likely to improve left ventricular function, clinical manifestations, and survival. The more chronically ill heart failure patient with significant comorbidities of renal, lung, and other vascular disease, however, will be placed at a higher surgical morbidity and mortality risk (Nohria et al., 2002). Surgical techniques to treat heart failure beyond CABG surgery include valve replacement or repair, cardiac transplantation, long-term mechanical assist devices, and investigational surgical therapies (Kouchoukos et al., 2003).

Valve Replacement or Repair

For those with significant cardiac valvular disorders, valve replacement or repair surgery may be performed to optimize hemodynamic parameters, limit symptoms, and improve survival (McKelvie, 2001). Timely consideration for valve replacement is the key to successful outcomes. When systolic dysfunction is severe, mitral regurgitant valve lesions are typically not replaced, because the advantage in this population has not been established (Nohria et al., 2002). Once the left ventricle becomes dilated with poor function, there is little hope for recovery by replacing the valve alone. Conversely, replacement or repair of stenotic valvular lesions is generally recommended. Chapter 41 🔗 discusses the surgical management of valvular disorders.

Cardiac Transplantation

Heart transplant surgery was pioneered in 1967, leading to its widespread use for the treatment of end-stage cardiomyopathy in the early 1980s. Heart transplantation is a highly successful treatment for a select patient population whose 1- to 2-year prognosis is estimated to be less than 50% (Renlund & Taylor, 2002). Although heart transplantation remains the best long-term surgical treatment for heart failure in a small group of patients, it continues to be limited by the availability of donor hearts. An average of just over 2,000 heart transplantations are performed annually in the United States (AHA, 2006b). Thousands of patients would benefit from heart transplantation if more donor hearts were available.

Over 33,000 heart transplant recipients have been tracked by the national United Network for Organ Sharing (UNOS) database (2006). Average waiting times for those on the U.S. UNOS transplant list in a noncritical status are just over 1 year. The advent of modern immunosuppression (drug therapies used to prevent rejection of a transplanted organ) has dramatically improved survival rates over time (Greenberg & Hermann, 2002). First-year survival rates for patients undergoing heart transplantation are 86.4% (males) and 84.6% (females); and for 3-year survival, 78.9% (males) and 76.1% (females) (AHA, 2006b). Five-year survival rates for transplant patients are 72.2% (males) and 68.5% (females) (AHA, 2006b).

Mechanical Assist Devices

Circulatory support remains an evolving field with both temporary and permanent devices. Temporary assist devices are a means to provide circulatory support for those in cardiogenic shock or when difficulties occur when coming off intraoperative cardiopulmonary support (Greenberg & Hermann, 2002). Such support includes intra-aortic balloon pumps, centrifugal right and left ventricular assist devices (VADs), and percutaneous ventricular assist devices (PVADs). Longer term devices used to "bridge" patients who are declining as they await cardiac transplantation, or those for long-term or permanent use, include left ventricular assist devices (LVADs), total artificial hearts (TAHs), and right ventricular assist devices (RVADs).

Implantation of permanent or "destination" VADs has emerged as a promising surgical treatment option for those with end-stage heart failure (Figure 42–7 ■). Patients with such devices are able to return to their home settings, living with a significant improvement in length and quality of life. Implantable LVADs have been used since the mid-1980s in transplant candidates who continue to deteriorate in the setting of long waits for suitable donor hearts (Nohria et al., 2002). The devices were designed for short-term use for those needing a bridge to heart transplantation or as a bridge to myocardial recovery (Greenberg & Hermann, 2002). In 2001, results were published of the Randomized Evaluation of Mechanical Assist Treatment for Congestive Heart failure (REMATCH) trial, a landmark trial showing mortality and quality-of-life benefits for patients implanted with an LVAD versus those in the medical management arm (Rose et al., 2001). LVADs, as destination therapy, have been approved by the Food and Drug Administration for treating patients with end-stage heart failure who are not transplant candidates (Blue Cross Blue Shield Association, 2002). The future and success of this technology will be based on appropriate patient selection, improved devices durability, and coordinated teams who are able to provide long-term management to this specific population.

Investigational Surgical Therapies

Surgical techniques that reconfigure the heart's muscular geometry have had mixed results. Batista and other colleagues have

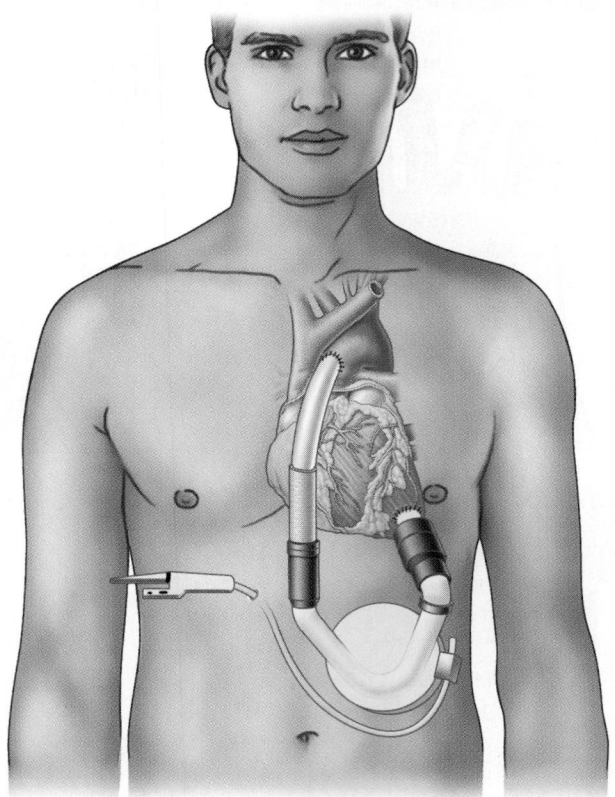

FIGURE 42–7 ■ Ventricular assist device.

performed a procedure of partial left ventriculectomy (Kouchoukos et al., 2003). This procedure involves resecting a segment of the left ventricle base on the premise that reduction in ventricular size will lead to improved function. Now known as the Batista procedure, it has grown out of favor as a treatment option for cardiomyopathy (Hunt et al., 2005; Nohria et al., 2002).

In contrast to the Batista procedure, in which weakened yet functional tissue is removed, ventricular aneurysm resection involves removal of nonfunctional myocardium (Kouchoukos et al., 2003). Ventricular restoration surgery is thought to reshape the misshapen geometry that occurs with systolic dysfunction. The future of this technique for patients with heart failure remains to be defined.

Research continues that examines the use of constraint devices that may change and support ventricular geometric configuration, thus leading to improved cardiac function. The Acorn cardiac support device is one such experimental device that is thought to cause improvements in function, symptoms, and degree of mitral valve regurgitation (Kouchoukos et al., 2003). Stem cell injection therapy during CABG is also under investigation.

Acute Decompensated Heart Failure

Acute heart failure contributes considerable expense to health care systems due to the need for frequent hospitalizations and has become a leading public health issue (Greenberg & Hermann, 2002; Jessup & Brozena, 2003; Nohria et al., 2002). Acute presentations of heart failure are manifestations of elevated ventricular filling pressures causing sudden congestion in the pulmonary vasculature and periphery, decreased cardiac output leading to poor perfusion of the periphery and kidneys, and increased systemic vascular resistance causing increased work for the heart (see Chart 42–1, p. 1281) (Adams et al., 2006; Fonarow, 2001; Greenberg & Hermann, 2002; Hunt et al., 2005; Nohria et al., 2002). Severe dyspnea (shortness of breath) is the leading symptom resulting in hospitalizations for heart failure, and its relief is usually a treatment priority (Greenberg & Hermann, 2002; Nohria et al., 2002). Paroxysmal nocturnal dyspnea, orthopnea, productive or nonproductive cough, bloating, right upper quadrant pain due to hepatic congestion, and palpitations due to excess volume in the atria may also present in the acute setting (Adams et al., 2006; Hunt et al., 2005; Nohria et al., 2002).

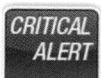
Nursing assessment of acute decompensated heart failure includes:

1. *Quick assessment of severity of symptoms*
2. *Vital signs*
3. *Hemodynamic status (peripheral pulses, temperature of skin, capillary refill time, and invasive hemodynamic parameters when available)*
4. *Oxygenation and work of breathing.*

Acute heart failure requiring intensive care monitoring:

1. *Evidence of myocardial infarction*
2. *Significant ventricular or supraventricular dysrhythmia*
3. *Compromised respiratory function*
4. *Evidence of low cardiac output*
5. *Anticipated need for hemodynamic monitoring*
6. *Severe comorbid disease.*

Acute decompensated heart failure can be precipitated by many conditions and situations (Chart 42–8). Cardiac decompensation generally may be attributed to issues with compliance, new or worsening comorbid conditions, and/or progressive disease (Greenberg & Hermann, 2002; McKelvie, 2001). Compliance issues that contribute to decompensated heart failure relate to failing to take medications at all or inappropriately, excess sodium and fluid intake, inadequate outpatient treatment, or inadequate follow-up, and they also may lead to acute decompensated symptoms (Greenberg & Hermann, 2002; Nohria et al., 2002). If acute decompensated heart failure is not treated, cardiogenic shock, multiorgan failure, and death may result. Patients with acute heart failure should be queried to understand better what circumstance(s) led to their decompensated state:

- Had they been self-monitoring at home?
- Did they know what actions to take if their clinical condition worsened?
- Did they have adequate access to outpatient care?
- Did they know who and when to call?
- Had they been taking medicines as prescribed?
- Did they understand how to follow a sodium and fluid restriction?
- Had they started any new medications recently?
- Had any other new medical problems been recently diagnosed?

Goals of acute decompensated heart failure include the following: to determine the reason for the decompensated state, relieve congestive symptoms, reverse hemodynamic compromise, treat dysrhythmias, assess for exacerbating comorbid conditions, use prognosis-altering medications, assess for their candidacy for cardiac devices or end-stage therapies, provide self-management education, and document that appropriate heart failure care was provided as mandated by regulatory entities. In preparing patients for life with heart failure outside the

CHART 42–8 | **Precipitating or Exacerbating Factors for Developing Acute Heart Failure**

Noncompliance	Renal or hepatic insufficiency
Silent or overt ischemia	Pulmonary embolism
Dietary indiscretion	Substance abuse
Fluid indiscretion	Worsening valvular or cardiac function
Untreated hypertension	
Acute or chronic infection	Over-the-counter supplementation
Uncontrolled hyperglycemia	
Thyroid dysfunction	Iatrogenic factors
Inadequate follow-up	Pregnancy
Atrial fibrillation, new or rapid	Anemia
Other dysrhythmias	

Factors that may precipitate or exacerbate heart failure are numerous and may be related to new or poorly controlled comorbid conditions, noncompliance, iatrogenic causes, or lack of adequate follow-up.

Sources: Braunwald, E., Zipes, D. P., & Libby, P. (2001). *Heart disease: A textbook of cardiovascular medicine* (6th ed.). Philadelphia: W. B. Saunders; Greenberg, B. H., & Hermann, D. D. (2002). *Contemporary diagnosis and management of heart failure.* Newtown, PA: Handbooks in Health Care; and Nohria, A., Lewis, E., & Stevenson, L. W. (2002). Medical management of advanced heart failure. *Journal of the American Medical Association, 287*(5), 628–640.

hospital, one should consider which patients might benefit from the organized structure of a heart failure disease management program. On presentation, the patient can be classified based on degree of perfusion and volume status: well perfused and either hyper- or hypovolemic, or poorly perfused and either hyper- or hypovolemic (Figure 42–8 ■) (Nohria et al., 2002).

Nursing Management

The nursing care needs of a patient admitted with heart failure are directed at treating congestion and monitoring the patient's response to therapy. Fluid retention is the primary reason most patients with heart failure are admitted or readmitted to the hospital. Goals of treatment for acute decompensated heart failure include assessing response to diuresis, monitoring intake/output and daily weights, assessment of cardiac output, monitoring for dysrhythmias, encouraging increased levels of activity, performing ADLs, and enhancing patient knowledge of the disease process. Application of the nursing process will facilitate a comprehensive ap-

Cold/Wet	**Warm/Wet**
Consider: Inotropes and/or diuretics	Consider: Diuretics
Cold/Dry	**Warm/Dry**
Consider: Volume and/or inotropes	Consider: volume

FIGURE 42–8 ■ Volume versus perfusion.

proach to patient assessment and care. The Nursing Process: Patient Care Plan feature applies the nursing process to the relevant nursing diagnosis of congestion and provides a comprehensive care plan for a patient with heart failure during hospitalization.

NURSING PROCESS: Patient Care Plan for Heart Failure

Assessment of Hypervolemia
Subjective Data:
Are you having difficulties breathing at rest or with activity?
How long have you had shortness of breath (SOB)?
Do you need to sleep with your head propped up, or do you awaken short of breath in the middle of the night?
Do you have a cough?
Do you have abdominal bloating or lower extremity swelling?
Have you had recent weight increase over a short period of time (2–3 days)?

Objective Data:
Vital signs: weight
blood pressure, heart rate (HR)
Oxygen saturation.
Dyspnea with exertion.
Lethargy.
Anxiety.
Lung sounds: crackles/wheezes.
Restlessness.
Elevated neck veins.
Ascites and/or lower extremity edema.
Daily weight.
Hemodynamic parameters:
1. Right atrial pressure (RAP) or central venous pressure (CVP)
2. Pulmonary artery pressure (PAP mean)
3. Pulmonary artery occlusion pressure (PAOP)
4. Cardiac output (CO) or cardiac index (CI).
Peripheral circulation:
1. Peripheral pulses
2. Presence of edema using the edema scale
3. Color and temperature
4. Capillary refill time.
Intake and output:
1. Assess volume of fluid intake by any route (e.g., oral, intravenous).
2. Assess volume of fluid expelled by any route (e.g., urinary, nasogastric (NG), drainage, blood).
Evaluate laboratory/diagnostic findings associated with hypervolemia:
1. Serum sodium (may be decreased, normal, or elevated based on cause of hypervolemia)
2. BUN (may be normal to decreased)
3. Urine specific gravity (may be decreased)
4. Hematocrit (may be decreased)
5. Chest x-ray (may show pulmonary congestion or cardiomegaly)
6. Right heart catheterization (may indicate elevated filling pressures).

NURSING PROCESS: Patient Care Plan for Heart Failure—*Continued*

Nursing Assessment and Diagnosis	Outcomes and Evaluation Parameters	Planning and Interventions with *Rationales*
Nursing Diagnosis: Fluid volume excess related to ventricular dysfunction and sodium/water retention	**Outcomes:** Diuresis: improved volume status (i.e., euvolemia) and improved symptoms. *Evaluation Parameters:* Blood pressure target: 120/80 mmHg. Heart rate target: 60–100 beats/min. Improved New York Heart Association (NYHA) class. No signs of pulmonary congestion: airway patent; respiratory rate < 20 breaths/min; pattern regular and unlabored; lungs clear to auscultation all lobes bilaterally. Oxygen saturation > 90% in patients breathing room air. Hemodynamic parameters (normals): 1. RAP 1–7 mmHg or CVP 2–8 cm H_2O 2. PAP 10–20 mmHg 3. PCWP 6–12 mmHg 4. CO 3.5–5.5 L/min or CI 2.0–3.2 L/min/m². Peripheral circulation: 1. Pulse 2–3+ on pulse grading scale 2. No edema 3. Skin warm, natural color 4. Capillary refill time less than 3 seconds. Intake and output: 1. Intake/output difference greater than 1,000 mL/24 hours or as defined for diuresis per provider 2. Urinary output average of greater than or equal to 30mL/hr. Daily morning weight less than the day prior. Abdomen soft, nondistended; no ascites. Laboratory/diagnostic workup indicates: 1. Serum sodium 135–140 mEq/L 2. Blood urea nitrogen (BUN) 10–20 mg/dL 3. Urine specific gravity 1.005–1.030 4. Hematocrit, male: 42–52%, female: 37–47%.	**Interventions and *Rationales:*** Insert intravenous catheter. *To facilitate intravenous medication administration.* Administer and titrate intravenous (IV) medications. *To facilitate diuresis.* Record amount of Intravenous (IV) fluid infused. *To monitor intake.* Assess vital signs and urine output regularly (every hour or less). *To assess adequacy of diuresis.* Monitor central venous pressure and pulmonary artery occlusion pressure (PAOP), if possible. *To assess response to diuresis.* Obtain and track daily morning weight. *To monitor adequacy of diuresis.* Monitor serum electrolytes, hematocrit, serum creatinine, and report critical abnormalities to the provider. *To monitor hematological changes associated with hypervolemia, possibly hypovolemia, electrolyte changes, and diuresis.* Instruct patient on fluid and sodium restrictions. *To prevent excess oral intake, which negates the effect of diuresis.*

Assessment of Cardiac Output

Subjective Data:

How is your energy level?
Are symptoms limiting your level of activity?
Are you light-headed?
Are you having memory problems or trouble concentrating?
Are you making the same amount of urine as usual?

Objective Data:

Cardiovascular system:
1. Heart rate
2. Heart rhythm
3. Blood pressure
4. Peripheral pulses
5. Presence of edema using the edema scale
6. Color and temperature
7. Capillary refill time.
Heart sounds: murmurs, clicks, rubs, splitting.
Pulmonary status.
Oxygen saturation.
Hemodynamic parameters (as applicable):
1. Right atrial pressure (RAP) or central venous pressure (CVP)
2. Pulmonary artery pressure (PAP mean)
3. Pulmonary artery occlusion pressure (PAOP)
4. Cardiac output (CO) or cardiac index (CI).
Intake and output:
1. Assess volume of fluid intake by any route (e.g., oral, intravenous).
2. Assess volume of fluid expelled by any route (e.g., urinary, NG, drainage, blood).
ECG waveform (rhythm and intervals) as ordered (including cardiac rhythm, PR interval, QRS interval, QT/QTc interval, dysrhythmias).
Obtain weight.

(continued)

NURSING PROCESS: Patient Care Plan for Heart Failure—*Continued*

Evaluate laboratory/diagnostic findings associated with decreased cardiac output:

1. Serum BUN and creatinine (may be elevated)
2. Serum hematocrit, hemoglobin (may be decreased)
3. Echocardiogram (may show depressed ventricular function, pericardial effusion)
4. 12-lead ECG (may show dysrhythmias, myocardial infarction, heart block, tachycrdia, or bradycardia)
5. Blood gases (may show acidosis, hypoxemia)
6. Arterial–mixed venous blood gases may show an increased SaO_2/SvO_2 ratio.

Nursing Assessment and Diagnosis	Outcomes and Evaluation Parameters	Planning and Interventions with *Rationales*
Nursing Diagnosis: *Decreased Cardiac Output* related to ventricular dysfunction	**Outcome:** Adequate cardiac output as seen by improved organ, tissue, and cerebral perfusion related to ***Evaluation Parameters:*** Cardiovascular system: 1. Heart rate: 60–100 beats/min 2. Regular rhythm or patient's normal asymptomatic rhythm 3. BP: 120/80 mmHg 4. Pulses 2–3+ on pulse grading scale 5. No edema 6. Skin warm and natural color 7. Capillary refill time less than or equal to 3 seconds. Heart sounds: normal S_1 and S_2. Airway patent; respiratory rate < 20 per minute, pattern regular and unlabored; lungs clear to auscultation all lobes bilaterally. Oxygen saturation > 90% in patients breathing room air. Hemodynamic parameters: 1. RAP 1–7 mmHg or CVP 2–8 cm H_2O 2. PAP 10–20 mmHg 3. PCWP 6–12 mmHg 4. CO 3.5–5.5 L/min or CI 2.0–3.2 L/min/m². Intake and output: 1. Intake/output difference greater than 1,000 mL/24 hours or as defined for diuresis per provider 2. Urinary output average of greater than or equal to 30 mL/hr. ECG is stable, with regular rhythm or patient's normal asymptomatic rhythm, without evidence of ischemia, myocardial infarction, tachycardia/bradycardia, or heart block. Cardiac intervals are within normal limits: • PR interval: 0.12–0.20 second • QRS interval: < .10 second • QTc interval: 0.37–.047 second. Daily morning weight less than the day prior. Laboratory/diagnostic findings: 1. BUN 10–20 mg/dL 2. Creatinine 0.8–1.3 mg/dL 3. Hematocrit, male: 42–52%, female 37–47%; hemoglobin, male: 14–18 g/dL, female 12–16 g/dL 4. May show depressed ventricular function 5. Sinus rhythm, sinus dysrhythmia, or patient's normal asymptomatic rhythm 6. pH 7.35–7.45, PCO_2 35–45 mmHg, HCO_3 21–28 mEq/L, PO_2 80–100 mmHg, O_2 saturation 95–100%. 7. Normal SaO_2/SvO_2 ratio.	**Interventions and *Rationales:*** Insert intravenous catheter. *To facilitate intravenous medication administration.* Administer and titrate IV medications. *To facilitate diuresis and inotropic support.* Record amount of IV fluid infused. *To monitor intake.* Assess vital signs and urine output regularly (every hour or less). *To assess adequacy of diuresis and inotropic support.* Monitor hourly urine output. *To assess adequacy of diuresis.* Monitor central venous pressure and pulmonary artery occlusion pressures (PAOP, CO/CI), if possible. *To assess adequacy of diuresis and inotropic support of cardiac output.* Monitor integument and neurological status. *To assess for adequacy of tissue and cerebral perfusion.* Administer oxygen. *To ensure proper oxygenation and tissue perfusion.* Administration of medications. *To improve cardiac output, tissue perfusion, and diuresis.*

NURSING PROCESS: Patient Care Plan for Heart Failure—*Continued*

Assessment of Activity Tolerance

Subjective Data:

How much activity are you able to do (i.e., walk for 5, 10, 30+ minutes, or not at all)?

Are you more or less active now than 1, 3, and 6 months ago?

Are you able to walk up 1 or 2 flights of stairs without stopping?

Do you have symptoms during exercise (chest pain, shortness of breath, palpitations, and light-headedness)?

Objective Data:

Vital signs: blood pressure (BP) and heart rate (HR).

Oxygen saturation.

NYHA classification for heart failure assessment.

Pain scale.

6-minute walk.

Nursing Assessment and Diagnosis	Outcomes and Evaluation Parameters	Planning and Interventions with *Rationales*
Nursing Diagnosis: *Risk for Activity Intolerance* related to impaired cardiac function secondary to chronic heart failure	**Outcomes:** Activity tolerance stabilizes or improves as seen by improved NYHA classification for heart failure, and decreased symptoms. ***Evaluation Parameters:*** Normal vital signs. Oxygen levels are within normal range: oxygen saturation >= 90%. Patients have clear plan for activity, with reasonable goals. Patients have access to activity. Patients understand what symptoms to monitor during activity: increased shortness of breath, chest pain, palpitations, light-headedness. Symptoms during activity are minimal. Patients have action plan for symptoms that occur. NYHA classification for heart failure has improved. Indexes of quality of life are improved. Pain scale improves. Strength and balance improve. Nutrition improves. Weight reduction occurs (if needed). Stress is reduced. Smoking cessation is successful.	**Interventions and *Rationales*:** Monitor vital signs at rest and with activity and 3 minutes after activity (heart rate, BP, respiratory rate). *To obtain a baseline for comparison.* Monitor oxygenation before, during, and after activity. *To obtain a baseline for comparison.* Assess baseline activity level (including strength and balance) and tolerance to activity. *To use as basis for individualized plan.* Assess symptoms at rest and with activity. *To use as a baseline for comparison.* Monitor level of pain. Assess degree of symptoms (NYHA class). *To use as a baseline for comparison.* Assess quality of life (QOL). *To use as a baseline for comparison.* Promote activity: Start with reasonable daily plan, increasing slowly, set reachable goal, plan around periods of rest, and reassure that small improvements will lead to physical, emotional, and psychosocial benefits. *An individualized plan of care will promote change.* Promote exercise prescription: type, activity, duration, intensity. Monitor level of strength. *To individualize each patient's plan.* Teach appropriate diet to accompany activity plan. Assess body mass index (BMI). Monitor current level of nutrition and calorie content. *To enhance balance nutrition and promote weight loss as needed.* Teach strengthening exercises. *To promote muscular strength to improve balance.* Discuss level of stress and anxiety. Teach stress reduction techniques. *To facilitate well-being and foster activity plan.* Stress smoking cessation. *Smoking decreases oxygenation to muscles during activity.* Teach heart failure symptoms to monitor: shortness of breath, chest pain, light-headedness, and passing out, palpitation. *To obtain a baseline for comparison.*

(continued)

NURSING PROCESS: Patient Care Plan for Heart Failure—*Continued*

Assessment of Dysrhythmias

Subjective Data:

Do you experience palpitations or feel that your heart races?
Do you become light-headed or pass out?
Do palpitations or light-headedness occur at the same time?

Objective Data:

Vital signs: BP and HR.
Oxygen saturation.
Level of consciousness.
ECG.
Lab values: electrolytes and
measures of acidosis.

Lung/cardiac.
Abdomen.
Integument.
Urine output.
Cardiac devices (if present).

Nursing Assessment and Diagnosis	Outcomes and Evaluation Parameters	Planning and Interventions with *Rationales*
Nursing Diagnosis: Cardiac output decreased due to dysrhythmias related to impaired cardiac function related to secondary to ischemia, acidosis, hypoxemia, electrolyte abnormalities, structural/conduction abnormalities, or device implantation.	**Outcome:** Absence of hemodynamically significant dysrhythmias. ***Evaluation Parameters:*** Heart rate is within normal range (60–80, or not > 100 beats per minute). Breath sounds are normal and clear, without respiratory distress. Oxygen levels are within normal range: Oxygen saturation >= 90%. Patient has no altered level of consciousness (LOC) or anxiety. ECG is stable, with regular rhythm or patient's normal asymptomatic rhythm, without evidence of ischemia, myocardial infarction, tachycardia/bradycardia, or heart block. Cardiac intervals are within normal limits: • PR interval: 0.12–0.20 second • QRS interval: < 0.10 second • QTc interval: 0.33–0.47 second. Lab values are within normal limits: 1. Potassium 3.5–5.1 mEq/L 2. Magnesium 1.3–2.1 mEq/L 3. Digoxin level, optimal = < 1.1 ng/mL, toxic: > 2.0 ng/mL 4. pH 7.35–7.45 5. $PaCO_2$ 35–45 mmHg 6. HCO_3 21–27 mEq/L 7. Base excess +/− 2 mEq/L Abdomen is soft, without pain, ascites, organomegaly. Urine output remains normal. Integument is dry, warm, well perfused. Cardiac device interrogation: shows properly functioning device with settings optimized and optimal battery life with leads intact.	**Interventions and *Rationales*:** Assess cardiovascular status: heart rate, regularity of rhythm (pattern), and blood pressure. *To assess baseline, monitor for changes and response to therapy.* Assess lung sounds. *To assess for presence of lung fluid from increased dysrhythmias.* Assess oxygenation saturation. *To monitor baseline, for changes with dysrhythmias and response to therapy.* Assess level of consciousness (LOC). *To assess for tissue perfusion.* Assess ECG and waveforms (rhythm, PR, QRS, and QTc intervals, dysrhythmias). *To establish a baseline, determine degree of abnormality and response to therapies.* Assess lab and blood gas values (potassium, magnesium, calcium, digoxin level, presence of acidosis). *To establish a baseline, determine degree of abnormality and response to therapies.* Assess abdomen. *To assess for ascites, abdominal pain, presence of bowel sounds, organomegaly.* Assess urine output. *To assess for decreases that may occur with dysrhythmias.* Assess integument. *To assess for cyanosis, pallor, or diaphoresis.* Assess cardiac device if present (i.e., pacemaker, cardiac defibrillator). *To assess proper position of leads and for appropriate device function.*

Assessment of Knowledge Deficit

Subjective Data:

Patient/family express concerns about the diagnosis of heart failure, in terms of prognosis, changes in lifestyle, and progression of disease.
Patient/family express lack of understanding of therapies to treat heart failure.
Patient/family express concerns about how to take medications and their potential side effects.
Patient/family express concerns what symptoms they might have and how to monitor them at home.
Patient/family express concerns about continuing a sexual relationship.
Patient/family express concerns about treatment options if medicines fail.
Patient/family express concerns about the mode of death.

Objective Data:

Patients may be anxious, confused, and may need repeated information.

NURSING PROCESS: Patient Care Plan for Heart Failure—*Continued*

Nursing Assessment and Diagnosis	Outcomes and Evaluation Parameters	Planning and Interventions with *Rationales*
Nursing Diagnosis: *Deficient Knowledge* related to the diagnosis of heart failure.	**Outcomes:** Patient/family understand: The diagnosis of heart failure. Their prognosis. Treatments for heart failure. Lifestyle changes. Progression of the disease. Symptoms to monitor. Sexuality. End-stage treatment options. Mode of death. ***Evaluation Parameters:*** Patient/family will: • Ask appropriate questions about the course of heart failure. • Follow appropriate medication adjustments, and consider recommendations for surgical procedures and devices. • Come in with a completed self-care diary, following instructions between visits. • Call when their symptoms worsen for urgent evaluation when needed. • Express attempts at maintaining a sexual relationship. • Understand which end-stage therapies are available and for which they qualify. • Understand the usual mode of death of heart failure and have made appropriate plans with their health care team and family regarding their wishes. Advanced directives and power of attorney will have been filled out.	**Interventions and *Rationales:*** Discuss with patient/family the course of heart failure, using the diagram. *This will enhance their understanding of the chronic and progressive nature of the disease, which usually presents with periods of exacerbation and stabilization.* Discuss how heart failure is treated with the patient and family. *This will provide the fundamental treatment strategies for heart failure including medications, surgical strategies, and devices.* Discuss with patients/family the MAWDS-based curriculum of self-management support (see Figure 42–9 ■, p. 1311). *This will teach the basic concepts that will help them to understand their medications, about activity, the importance of daily weights, their diet, and what to do when their symptoms worsen.* Discuss the common symptoms of heart failure with the patient and family, describing shortness of breath, cough, fatigue, activity intolerance, weight gain/edema, palpitations, chest tightness, and poor concentration. *This will enable the patient to recognize her symptoms and reinforce calling early when her symptoms worsen, so she can be seen and have adjustments made in her medications, preempting an urgent hospitalization.* Discuss ways for the patient and significant other to maintain a sexual relationship. *Patients will understand that having sexual intercourse is about the amount of effort in climbing 2 flights of stairs. If they are able to complete this activity without significant symptoms, then sexual intercourse will likely be safe. Patients will understand other means of sexual intimacy and will understand what to do if symptoms worsen during sexual activities.* Describe end-stage treatment options to the patient and family. Those who fail standard therapy might be considered for cardiac transplantation, mechanical assist devices, and heart failure research studies or for hospice care. *The patient and family will understand which of the preceding end-stage therapies they might be considered for and why they might not be a candidate for others.* Describe the mode of death for patients with heart failure. *Most patients with heart failure die either by a sudden dysrhythmia (caused by ventricular tachycardia or fibrillation) or by progressive deterioration of the cardiac muscle and its function. Dying suddenly will be a fast, typically painless, way to die. Dying of progressive disease is typically associated with more symptoms that will require an individualized plan for symptom relief by medicines such as narcotics, anxiolytics, nitrates, diuretics, and oxygen.*

PATIENT TEACHING & DISCHARGE PRIORITIES for Heart Failure

Patients discharged from the hospital have multiple needs. Teaching strategies should be based on these needs, with the goal to prevent readmissions, decrease disease progression, and improve quality of life.

Need	Teaching
Patient/family • Prevent recurrent symptoms of congestion.	MAWDS self-management instruction (medications, activity, weights, diet, symptoms).
• Optimize medical therapy for heart failure and comorbid conditions.	Provide list of current medications to patients with dose and schedule, with clear instructions on changes from prehospitalization. Instruct purpose of medications; refill prescriptions before running out; do not double up for missed doses; call with adverse effects.
• Increase activity tolerance.	Increase activity as tolerated, monitoring for symptoms; become active most days; call with new or worsened symptoms.
• Minimize risk factors.	Review health maintenance strategies: smoking cessation, limited ethyl alcohol (ETOH), regular exercise, stress reduction, eating balanced diet, and optimally treating comorbid conditions.
• Provide palliative care.	Discuss chronic nature of disease; encourage multidisciplinary team meeting regarding overall plans for care.
Family/support system • Assess resources to assist with chronic illness in the home setting.	Provide resources based on individual's needs: home health, hospice, family/friends/neighbors to help with home care, meals, transportation.
Setting • Assess home needs.	Assess safety from falls for those who are weak and at risk for falling; use occupational therapy to assess home safety and for home aids for debilitated patients.

Once the patient is ready for discharge, it is essential that a teaching plan be implemented that will help prevent a recurrence of the heart failure. A practical approach, tailored to individual patients, will be needed to help patients integrate self-management strategies at home. The Patient Teaching & Discharge Priorities box outlines discharge care for patients with heart failure. It is also essential that cultural considerations be addressed because they potentially impact the patient's ability to prevent progression of the disease. The Cultural Considerations box presents necessary considerations related to various cultures.

Collaborative Management

Patients with heart failure need a multidisciplinary team approach to achieve optimal recovery and return to society. Nurses at all levels collaborate with health care providers, health care provider assistants, dietitians, pharmacists, social workers, and cardiac rehabilitation specialists across various care settings. Close scrutiny is required by the team to provide optimal, evidence-based care. Nursing assessment of subjective and objective measures of adequate diuresis will allow for a prompt notification to the health care provider if adjustments to the medical plan are needed. Nursing staff also can focus on the essential aspects of patient self-management, including instruction on medications, activity, daily weights, dietary guidance, and symptom management. A comprehensive nutritional plan should include helping patients follow a restricted salt and liquid diet. Dietitians help patients and families with a greater understanding of appropriate food and fluid guidelines. When hypervolemia is present, patients generally have a decline in physical activity, with dyspnea being their primary source of limitation in activity. Cardiac rehabilitation specialists help mobilize pa-

tients with monitored physical activity during their hospitalization and may provide a plan to follow after discharge. Social workers can evaluate and instruct on the psychosocial aspects of this diagnosis and also address any financial concerns.

Hospital Clinical Pathway

A focused clinical pathway, individualized to each patient, should be initiated at the beginning of a heart failure admission, guiding inpatient care in preparation for postdischarge management (Chart 42–9, p. 1310) (Greenberg & Hermann, 2002).

 Clinical discharge criteria include:

1. *Achievement of euvolemia*
2. *Twenty-four-hour stability of fluid status, blood pressure, and renal function on oral medications*
3. *Walks without dyspnea*
4. *No complaints of light-headedness*
5. *Optimal blood pressure defined*
6. *Stable cardiac rhythm.*

Starting in 2002, the Joint Commission has mandated that patients admitted to the hospital with heart failure have documentation on their care related to the following: (1) a measure of ventricular function; (2) those with an LVEF less than 40% receive an ACE inhibitor (or ARB) unless contraindicated; (3) patients receive self-management instruction before discharge; and (4) smoking cessation counseling is provided to smokers. Adhering to these core measures has shown reductions in heart failure mortality (Kfoury, Hall, Rasmusson, Horne, & Renlund, 2006). Plans for optimal outpatient management should focus on ways to prevent readmissions for heart failure, to improve prognosis, to

CULTURAL CONSIDERATIONS for Risk Factors of Heart Failure

- At least 46% of African Americans and American Indians/Alaska Natives have at least two or more cardiovascular disease risk factors; and therefore, nursing care should include a thorough evaluation of their risk factors.

- The African-American Heart Failure Trial (A-HeFT) results suggest that African Americans have improved outcomes when isosorbide dinitrate and hydralazine are added to standard heart failure medications; and therefore, nursing care should entail a thorough review of their medications.

- Heart failure is more common in African Americans and appears to be of worse severity. The strongest risk factor for heart failure among African Americans is hypertension, which can also contribute to the pathology of their heart failure disease. African Americans experience a higher incidence of hospitalization. Nursing care for African American patients with heart failure may include hypertension education and also self-management strategies to prevent further rehospitalization.

- African Americans and Native Americans have higher incidences of renal disease than do Caucasians and Asians; and therefore, nursing care for these groups should include close monitoring of renal function because their heart failure management may need adjustment.

- Diabetes has been found to be the strongest risk factor for heart failure. The prevalence of diabetes in the American Indian or Alaska Native adult population was more than twice that of U.S. adults overall; and therefore, nursing care and management of patients with heart failure who are American Indians should entail an evaluation for diabetes.

- Cardiovascular disease is not a "man's" disease. It is the number-one killer of women and has killed more women than men, causing the death of over 500,000 women annually. Nursing care of both male and female patients should be consistent and thorough.

- Cardiovascular disease has been shown to cause an increased incidence of premature deaths greatest among American Indians or Alaska Natives (36%) and African Americans (31.5%), and the lowest among Caucasians (14.7%). Premature death was also higher among Hispanics (23.5%). Nursing care of these "at-risk" populations must be thorough, in particular with their discharge instructions, because cardiovascular mortality risk is greater among these populations.

Nursing care can be significantly enhanced when considering a patient's cultural background. This list describes pertinent cultural considerations that may need to be addressed.

Sources: American Heart Association. (2006a&b). *Heart and stroke statistics—2006 update.* Dallas, TX: Author; Smith, G. L., et al. (2005). Race and renal impairment in heart failure: Mortality in blacks versus whites. *Circulation, 111*(10), 1270–1277; Taylor, A. L. (2003). The African-American heart failure trial (A-HeFT): Rationale and methodology. *Journal of Cardiac Failure, 9,* S216–S219; Thomas, K. L., et al. (2005). Outcomes by race and etiology of patients with left ventricular systolic dysfunction. *American Journal of Cardiology, 96*(7), 1001–1013; Yancy, C. W. (2004). The prevention of heart failure in minority communities and discrepancies in health care delivery systems. *Medical Clinics of North America, 88*(5), 1347–1368; and Yancy, C. W., & Strong, M. (2004). The natural history, epidemiology, and prognosis of heart failure in African Americans. *Congestive Heart Failure, 10*(1), 15–18.

decrease mortality, to foster adherence, and to restore functional capacity (McKelvie, 2001). The power of educating patients with heart failure with standardized self-management techniques has led to reductions in mortality and should also be a focus prior to discharge (Hall et al., 2005).

Health Promotion

Heart failure management would be incomplete without the vital need for patients to receive self-management instruction and education from nurses and other members of the health care team. Research supports the importance self-management has on indexes such as quality-of-life, readmission rates, and functional status (Krumholz et al., 2002). Not only have heart failure medications altered patients' prognoses, but evidence exists showing the addition of self-management education can reduce mortality as well. Essential principles that focus on living with heart failure couple medications with nonpharmacologic therapies. Nonpharmacologic management strategies include appropriate diet and nutrition, health maintenance, and psychosocial/ lifestyle changes (Greenberg & Hermann, 2002).

The key concepts that patients must learn to incorporate into their daily lives can be summarized by an acronym called MAWDS: medications, activity, weights, diet, and symptoms, as depicted in Figure 42–9 ■ (p. 1311). If these concepts are followed, reductions in readmissions and costs associated with heart failure may occur (Krumholz et al., 2002). One community-based study has shown that patients who attended a MAWDS-based curriculum have improved knowledge of heart failure and an improved sense of quality of life (Rasmusson, Hall, Hofmann, Moore, & Renlund, 2002). This MAWDS-based self-management

education has even shown mortality benefits when documented during a heart failure admission (Hall et al., 2005).

Self-management plan includes:

1. *Patient and family education about MAWDS (medications, activity, daily weights, low-sodium diet, fluid restriction, and changes in symptoms)*

2. *Understands when to call provider with worsening symptoms*

3. *Follow-up appointment scheduled.*

Medications

Patients need instruction about their medications' action to improve symptoms, prevent hospitalizations, and prevent death. The typical patient with heart failure is on a complicated medical regimen for his heart condition along with therapy for his comorbid conditions. The more medications a person takes in a day, the more he is at risk for noncompliance or mistakes with his regimen. Patients need to understand the names of the medications, the time of the day they should be taken, their purpose, and what to do in case of missed doses and/or adverse reactions. Strategies aimed to increase long-term compliance and access to medications for those with limited resources must be planned.

Activity

Activity was long discouraged for those living with heart failure (Nohria et al., 2002). Exercise was thought to put an undue burden on the already weakened heart muscle. Now, it is increasingly evident that an optimal amount of activity can have significant benefits. Hemodynamic parameters, quality-of-life

CHART 42–9 **Heart Failure Clinical Pathway**

Once patients are hospitalized with heart failure, they need comprehensive care using a multidisciplinary approach such as the clinical pathway proposed here. Each day noted, progress should be made, looking forward to the anticipation of discharge. Planning should focus on medical and nursing therapies, education, physical therapy and dietary needs, consultations that may be needed, and discharge goals.

Aspect of Care	Day 1	Day 2	Day 3	Day 4
Inpatient Care	Admission weight vital signs (VS) q4h input and output (I & O) Physical assessment IV access Urinary catheterization optional Cardiac monitoring Oxygen Telemetry Begin admission medications to include IV diuretics Pain assessment	Daily weight by 0600 VS q4h I & O Physical assessment Continue meds: IV diuretics, change as indicated Increase ACEI if BP stable Adjust potassium supplementation Pain management	Daily weight by 0600 VS q4h I & O Physical assessment Continue meds/consider changing to oral diuretics if approaching euvolemia Increase ACEI, if tolerated Consider discharge urinary cath, cardiac monitor Pain management	VS q4h I & O Physical assessment Administer meds Increase ACEI Weigh on patient's home scale for discharge baseline Discharge IV access Pain management
Education	Self-management module I introduced Assess patients knowledge of heart failure (HF) (pre-test) Review: What is HF	Review HF pretest Teach self-management module I	Complete self-management module I Schedule patient/family conference	Post-test and review discharge instructions Smoking cessation
Nutrition/ Dietary	Notify dietary of: Na+ restriction Fluid restriction	Reinforce: Low Na+ foods Fluid restriction	Reinforce: Low Na+ foods Fluid restriction	Reinforce: Low Na+ foods Fluid restriction
Laboratory/ Diagnostics	Admit labs on admit orders Consider diagnostic tests: x-ray, ECG, MUGA, Echo, Pulse oximetry, etc.	Chem 7 PT/INR (if appropriate)	Chem 7 PT/INR	Chem 7 PT/INR
Activity	Bed rest/BP with assistance Initial Cardiac Rehab consult	OOB at least 30 minutes Cardiac Rehab	OOB for meals AMB qid Cardiac Rehab	OOB for meals AMB qid Cardiac Rehab

Consults	CONSULTS:
	  Pharmacist
	  Social Worker
	  Dietitian
	  Cardiac Rehab
	  Other
		CONSULT VISITS:
		  Pharmacist
		  Social Worker
		  Dietitian
		  Cardiac Rehab
			CONSULT VISITS:
			  Pharmacist
			  Social Worker
			  Dietitian
			  Cardiac Rehab
				F/U APPOINTMENTS WITH CONSULTS ARRANGED

Discharge Planning	Identify issues in the home setting	Assess self-care ability	Immunizations: pneumovax and influenza	Home scale Home health nursing Oxygen need Medications: ACEI, digoxin, spironolactone Follow up with CHF Clinic CHF support group referrals
Outcomes	Establish NYHA class Diagnostic evaluation of heart failure complete Estimate goal for baseline weight Establish extent of lung congestion Measurement of JVP HF pretest given Pain assessment complete	Improved NYHA class Relief of symptoms: improved breathing, lung sounds, decreased edema, weight Vital signs stable Improved JVP MAWDS understanding increased Pain management begun	Improved NYHA class Continued relief of symptoms Increase activity as tolerated Labs WNL for this patient Improved JVP MAWDS understanding increased Improved pain management	DISCHARGE CRITERIA: Symptoms improvement Without lung congestion Optimal JVP Decreased edema Decreased weight Stable labs Baseline weight achieved Cardiac rehab goal achieved Pain management has occurred Passed post-test Discharge instructions understood

FIGURE 42–9 ■ Heart failure self-care diary.

indexes, functional status, and depression scores are all improved as persons with heart failure exercise on a consistent basis (Adams et al., 2006). The reality of living with heart failure, however, is that the syndrome is fraught with a cycle of inactivity that leads to further deconditioning. The challenge is, therefore, to encourage a reasonable exercise program that will lead to clinical benefits. Cardiac rehabilitation may be started during a hospitalization in stable patients, but coverage by the Centers for Medicare & Medicaid Services (CMS) for outpatient cardiac rehab for heart failure remains limited. An exercise prescription given to patients must include the following components: type, frequency, duration, and intensity (Chart 42–10, p. 1312). Setting reasonable goals with patients is critical so that success with an exercise prescription may be achieved. Assessing behavioral and motivational issues is important for those patients who have struggled with maintaining an active lifestyle.

Weight

One of the most important aspects for patients to understand is to record their weight daily and know what to do when it deviates from a dry weight. The ultimate goal is to maintain a state of euvolemia, or when they are not retaining fluid, which means less congestion and fewer symptoms. As easy as this concept sounds, it is quite a challenge to health care providers to work out a plan with patients related to their weight. Some terms used to describe a "goal" weight when there is an absence of congestion are *optivolemic* and *euvolemic*. This weight needs to be determined in conjunction with the health care provider and may change over time with weight gain or loss from other causes than fluid. Patients not only feel better when they are not congested but also will likely stay out of the hospital (Greenberg & Hermann, 2002; Nohria et al., 2002).

Patients should be instructed to call their health care provider when their weight increases 2 or more pounds overnight, or more than 5 pounds from their "goal" weight.

Conversely, patients who lose too much weight are at risk of dehydration and possibly syncope. A 5-pound or greater drop below their goal weight should prompt a call to their health care team. Patients should have an individualized plan for self-adjusted diuretic dosing regimens to achieve relief of congestion and limit the chance of readmission.

Diet

Activation of the RAAS leads to sodium and water retention. Patients need instruction to help them understand that treating congestion with diuretics offers the best result when coupled with limiting dietary sodium (Greenberg & Hermann, 2002). Patients with heart failure with congestive symptoms should be counseled to ingest less than 2 grams of sodium daily (Silver, 1998). Those with persistent evidence of volume overload should also ingest less than 2 quarts (or liters) of all fluids per day (Silver, 1998). Following a low-sodium diet is challenging, because the American diet usually consists of 6 to 10 grams of sodium daily (Greenberg & Hermann, 2002). Most complain about food lacking in flavor when they change to the reduced sodium preparation, yet herbs and spices should be encouraged to add flavor to foods to enhance their flavor. See Chart 42–11 (p. 1312) for a list of foods that are commonly know to be high in sodium content with recommended alternatives. Patients often need help to understand how to read food labels, how to calculate their sodium intake, and how to make wise food selections when eating out. Meeting with a dietitian and others to share shopping and food preparation tips will likely heighten success and compliance. Chapter 14 🔗 includes a specific discussion of low-sodium diets.

Many patients with heart failure complain of "thirst." This mechanism is a neurohormonal response that tries to trick the body into seeking and retaining more fluids so that blood volume will increase, leading to increased flow to the renal system. Unfortunately, when heart failure is present, the heart is unable to keep

CHART 42–10 **Exercise Prescription**

Patients with heart failure usually fall into a cycle of inactivity, thus leading to further deconditioning. Exercise is usually limited by symptoms of congestion or poor perfusion. It is important to provide thorough instructions to patients on how to exercise safely as they live with heart failure.

Exercise Prescription	Recommendation to Patients	Caution to Patients
Type of exercise	Walk, run, bike, swim, hike. Factors such as personal preference, location, orthopedic challenges, and so on will help plan type. Choosing a type of exercise patient will enjoy should help her continue this activity over the long term.	Do not pursue an activity known to exacerbate certain conditions: e.g., walking downhill, which causes more knee pain.
Intensity of exercise	Discuss in terms of being able to maintain a conversation while exerting, yet having a high enough amount of energy expenditure.	Having significant symptoms of dyspnea, chest pain, or light-headedness means patient should back off or stop the activity.
Duration of exercise	Will depend on baseline level of fitness. Start slowly and increase the duration of their activity over time.	Reduce duration and intensity if the day following an activity, patient is too tired to perform activities of daily living (ADLs).
Frequency of exercise	Be active most days of the week.	Patient should not worry if he needs to skip a day occasionally. Just remember to try being active most days.

Sources: Adams, T. D., Fisher, A. G., Hansen, S. F., & Yanowitz, F. G. (2001). *Maintaining the miracle and owner's manual for the human body* (3rd ed.). Salt Lake City, UT: CAPP Publishing.

up with the body's demands and backward flow results in "volume-overloaded" patients and worsened symptoms. Low sodium intake, coupled with fluid restriction, will assist patients in maintaining their goal weight and may often lead to reductions in diuretic dosing (Greenberg & Hermann, 2002; Nohria et al., 2002).

Symptoms

Patients need to understand the typical symptoms of heart failure including exertional dyspnea, orthopnea, paroxysmal nocturnal dyspnea (PND), cough, edema, fatigue, and activity intolerance. Symptoms of heart failure lead to a poorer quality of life and re-

CHART 42–11 **Dietary Sodium Recommendations**

The sodium-restricted diet (2 g/day) is a well-known part of the heart failure patient's self-management, although the patient's ability to understand this diet and to comply with it remains a challenge in her care.

Food Group	High-Sodium Choice	Lower Sodium Alternative
Meats/fish/poultry	Cured meats (bacon, ham) Processed meats: jerky, salami, sausage Stews, casseroles, anchovies, pickled herring, King crab, canned meat/fish/poultry	Fresh lean meat seasoned with herbs/spices, roasted, baked, boiled, or poached
Fruits	Canned fruits, fresh fruit with salt added	Fresh fruit, no added salt, fruit juices
Vegetables	Canned soups or vegetables; canned vegetable juices; those in sauce or au gratin; canned beans: refried beans, pork and beans, kidney beans	Any vegetables; stewed, steamed, fresh, or boiled
Carbohydrates	Pretzels, potato chips, peanuts, popcorn, bagels, croissants, English muffins, oyster crackers, pita pockets, pancakes, stuffing, packaged puddings, pastries, cream pies, ice cream, creamed potatoes, noodles in cream sauce, fried rice	Fresh fruit, angel food cake, sherbert, frozen/nonfat yogurt, ice milk, gelatin, hard or soft rolls, plain bread or toast, unsalted crackers, breadsticks, mashed/baked/steamed/boiled potatoes, boiled or steamed rice, boiled noodles
Dairy/fats	Cottage cheese, Parmesan cheese, other hard and/or processed cheeses	Mozzarella
Condiments	Canned gravies, salad dressings, canned sauces, soy sauce, ketchup, mustard, olives, pickles, bouillon	Homemade gravy, other herbs/spices, oil and vinegar dressing, low-salt dressings
Fast foods	Hamburger, cheeseburger, fried chicken, pizza, onion rings, fish sandwich, burrito	Salad bars, baked potatoes, broiled chicken sandwich without sauce, fresh fruits/vegetables, sandwiches with low-salt meat and cheese options and limited spreads
Other	Frozen foods, milk shakes, chocolate or whole milk, cocoa, alcoholic drinks	Fruit juices, skim milk, soft drinks, tea, or coffee

Sources: Nephrogenic Diabetes Insipidus Foundation. (2006). *Low sodium diet basics.* Retrieved December 6, 2006, from http://www.ndif.org/pages/5-Low_Sodium_Diet_Basics; Silver, M. A. (1998). *Success with heart failure; Success and hope for those with congestive heart failure.* Reading, MA: Perseus Books.

sult in frequent hospitalizations (Nohria et al., 2002). Each patient should receive clear instruction on how to track her own symptoms and when to call if symptoms worsen. If a patient calls early enough, the issue may be managed on an outpatient basis, preventing an emergency room visit or hospitalization. Patients with heart failure need to understand that their symptoms will wax and wane, resulting in a combination of good and bad days. Listening to their bodies and keeping track of objective information (such as weight, blood pressure, and heart rate) that should be reported is critical. See Figure 42–9 ■ (p. 1311) for an example of a tool to help assist patients monitor and record weights, which may be used to communicate with their health care team about changes that occur outside predetermined parameters of weight and symptoms.

Family/Significant Other Support

Heart failure, like other chronic diseases, requires support from family, significant others, and also members of the community. Heart failure can pose both emotional and physical challenges to patients and those surrounding them. When patients are initially diagnosed, during times of exacerbations, and as they approach the end-of-life stage, patients with heart failure may need a significant amount of emotional and physical support. Patients and their loved ones need to understand the chronicity of the disease with which they live so they can make foreseeable adjustments to their daily activities to ensure an acceptable quality of life. This may include adjustments in all family-related activities such as family meal preparation and home maintenance. Meals should be planned that adhere to the sodium and fluid restrictions instructed for the patient. It also remains important for family members to encourage compliance with MAWDS recommendations (p. 1311). Available Internet resources, such as through the American Association of Heart Failure Nurses can help both patients and families better understand how to live with this common condition.

Lifestyles and Habits

Promoting healthy lifestyles is critical for all patients and is no different for patients with heart failure. General health promotion strategies that should be age and gender focused include:

- Smoking cessation
- Regular physical activity and weight control
- Limiting alcohol use and discouraging illicit drug use
- Stress management
- Dental care.

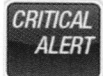 *Health maintenance recommendations include:*

1. *Vaccination for influenza and pneumonia*
2. *Regular exercise*
3. *Stress reduction techniques*
4. *Limitation of alcohol use*
5. *Discontinuance of nonsteroidal anti-inflammatory drugs (NSAIDs)*
6. *Regular health care follow-up.*

Patients with a chronic disease, such as heart failure, are recommended to follow additional disease prevention strategies for the following conditions: infection, CAD, hypertension, dia-

betes, hyperlipidemia, obesity, and malnutrition. Infection prevention includes recommendations for an annual influenza vaccination and a current pneumococcal vaccination. For those with valvular heart disease, endocarditis prophylaxis should be followed for dental and other invasive procedures. Primary prevention strategies for CAD include smoking cessation, regular exercise, and maintaining a healthy body weight. Additionally, CAD secondary prevention strategies focus on tight control of comorbid conditions that may influence the development or worsening of heart failure including diabetes, hypertension, hyperlipidemia, and obesity.

Hypertension and hyperlipidemia screening and treatment not only may prevent the development of CAD but also may prevent systolic dysfunction. Lifestyle changes including more exercise and better dietary choices will also help reduce hypertension and hyperlipidemia. Aggressively treating diabetes, targeting an optimal hemoglobin A_{1C} and prevention of target organ damage, will limit the risk of developing CAD and subsequent systolic dysfunction. Regular exercise and an improved diet will also prevent obesity and malnutrition.

Heart Failure Resources for Patients and Families

Many resources are available to help assist the nurse in educating the patient. It is also vital for nurses to instruct patients on how to access educational materials. In this multimedia era, patients with heart failure have numerous resource options available to them. The Internet alone has over 2 million sites to choose from on "congestive heart failure" for a search done through Google. Web-based sites for heart failure represent many different entities providing information: organizations specific to heart failure and cardiology, hospital systems providing heart failure care, governmental agencies with guidelines for treatment, drug and device companies with their product information and patient education, patients with their own websites, studies done on heart failure, and more. Help patients with tips about some of the more credible Internet sites, which are those ending in (dot) .edu, .gov, and .org. Well-established organizations providing valuable resources include the Heart Failure Society of America, the American Association of Heart Failure Nurses, and the American Heart Association.

Other resources on heart failure can be obtained through books from bookstores and hospital, university, or public libraries. Many companies have produced videos for patients to help them better understand heart failure. Drug and device companies and hospital systems often produce tools that focus on heart failure improvements. Community-based resources that are available include health care fairs, community lecture series, the local health department, the local chapter of the American Heart Association, and hospitals and care providers in the community. Patients with heart failure need resources sensitive to various cultures, in multiple languages, and at various levels of literacy.

Comorbidities of Heart Failure

Patients with heart failure commonly have comorbid conditions, requiring thoughtful and optimal treatment (Jessup & Brozena, 2003). The need for the evaluation of other comorbidities in the progression of heart failure has become increasingly more evident. Depression, anemia, renal insufficiency, diabetes, coronary artery disease, hypertension, and sleep apnea have all been found not only to worsen prognosis and increase morbidity and mortality rates, but also to confound heart failure treatment (Jessup & Brozena, 2003).

Depression

Depression is increasingly common among the elderly and especially in those with heart failure (Havranek, Ware, & Lowes, 1999). Patients with heart failure with untreated depression are at risk for increases in morbidity and mortality and also have reported poorer quality of life and functional capacity (Havranek et al., 1999; Nohria et al., 2002). A comprehensive treatment strategy, including counseling and the use of antidepressants, is important in managing patients with depression (Greenberg & Hermann, 2002). Counseling patients to enhance their understanding of the course of heart failure and helping the patient understand their treatment plan can significantly assist to decrease anxiety levels and to empower patients to be more proactive in their self-management. Drug therapy primarily involves antidepressants known as selective serotonin reuptake inhibitors (SSRIs) that are generally felt to be safe and therapeutic in patients with heart failure and do not alter hemodynamics (Greenberg & Hermann, 2002).

Anemia

Anemia is defined by the World Health Organization (WHO) as a hemoglobin of <12 g/dL in women or <13 g/dL in men (WHO, 1968). The prevalence of anemia is significant and increases with age, detected in up to 48% of the heart failure population (Kosiborod et al., 2003). Blood loss; iron, folate, or B_{12} deficiencies; infections; and medications have been common sources of anemia in patients with heart failure. Most commonly, chronic renal insufficiency leads to decreased erythropoietin production, resulting in anemia. The risk with anemia in patients with heart failure includes myocardial ischemia and increased need for higher cardiac output to maintain tissue metabolic oxygen requirements (which, in turn, can trigger the deleterious effects of the SNS system) (Greenberg & Hermann, 2002). Patients with heart failure and anemia have been found to have an increased risk of mortality (Horwich, 2002) and poorer prognosis (Dries, Exner, Domanski, Greenberg, & Stevenson, 2000). The treatment of choice is to correct the underlying disorder (Greenberg & Hermann, 2002). The use of blood transfusions or erythropoietin administration has not been supported in improving mortality but has been shown to improve clinical status (Greenberg & Hermann, 2002; Silverberg et al., 2001). Chapter 63 discusses anemia.

Renal Insufficiency

Renal insufficiency, as defined by a creatinine clearance of <60 mL/min, is prevalent in as many as 50% of patients with heart failure. It is present in at least 25% of patients hospitalized with heart failure (Krumholz et al., 2000). Poor renal perfusion, actual renal disease, or drug-induced disease have all been identified as sources of renal insufficiency in heart failure (Hunt et al., 2005). Renal insufficiency can cause increased activity by the RAAS system, triggering the vasoconstrictive properties of an-

giotensin II, causing blood vessels to constrict, and resulting in increased systemic vascular resistance and afterload (Braunwald et al., 2001). Renal insufficiency may prompt thoughtful reductions in heart failure medication therapies due to the greater risk of potential toxicities, such as with digitalis (Hunt et al., 2005). Worsening renal function can also be a prognostic indicator in heart failure and may require reductions in ACE inhibitors and beta-blocker therapies (Weinfeld, Chertow, & Stevenson, 1999). Treating renal insufficiency involves optimizing heart failure therapy (including ACE inhibitors, diuretics, and digitalis), optimizing renal hemodynamics, eliminating adverse medication use, and reversing identifiable causes if able (Braunwald et al., 2001). Chapter 47 discusses renal insufficiency.

Diabetes

There are 23.6 million children and adults in the United States, or 7.8% of the population, who have diabetes. While an estimated 17.9 million have been diagnosed with diabetes, unfortunately, 5.7 million people (or nearly one quarter) are unaware that they have the disease (American Diabetic Association, n.d.). Diabetes has a significant impact on cardiovascular function because of microvascular (endothelial proliferative changes of the arterioles) and macrovascular (atherosclerosis) changes in the vasculature promoted by the disease, leading to worsening ventricular dysfunction (Braunwald et al., 2001). Patients with diabetes are at greater risk of coronary artery disease, myocardial infarction, renal disease, hypertension, and heart failure (Braunwald et al., 2001). Patients who have strict glycemic control of their diabetes can significantly decrease their risk for coronary disease and subsequent risk of heart failure. Patients with diabetes and heart failure may halt the deleterious effects diabetes has on heart muscle function when optimal control is attained (Heart Outcomes Prevention Evaluation Study Investigators, 2000; Iribarren et al., 2001; Stratton et al., 2000). The cornerstone of diabetic therapy includes adjustments to diet and the use of insulin or oral hypoglycemic agents (Braunwald et al., 2001). Chapter 53 discusses diabetes.

Coronary Artery Disease

Coronary artery disease (CAD) is prevalent in over 13 million individuals in the United States (AHA, 2006b). It is the number-one killer of women and men alike. Coronary artery disease contributes to two-thirds of patients with heart failure (He et al., 2001). Approximately 22% of men and 46% of women will be disabled with heart failure postmyocardial infarction (AHA, 2006b). Coronary artery disease causes plaque buildup, which decreases perfusion to cardiac tissue (myocardial ischemia) and eventual inflammatory occlusion in the coronary arteries (myocardial infarction). Left ventricular pump function can be impaired, causing a depression in cardiac output and stroke volume that induces RAAS and SNS activation and their deleterious effects (Hunt et al., 2005). Therefore, primary prevention of coronary artery disease by preventing hypercholesterolemia becomes essential in preventing left ventricular dysfunction (Hunt et al., 2005). Secondary prevention of coronary disease with the use of hydroxy-methylglutaryl-coenzyme A (HMG-CoA, or "statins") medications and aspirin can significantly decrease the risk of heart failure by as much as

19% (Scandinavian Simvastatin Survival Study, 1994). Cardiovascular disease is not a "man's" disease. It is the number-one killer of women and has killed more women than men since 1984, causing the death of over 500,000 women annually (AHA, 2006a). While all cancers combined kill only 260,000 females annually, 40,000 of these deaths are attributed to breast cancer (AHA, 2006a). The fear of developing breast cancer has led to a successful awareness campaign that has yet to be matched by a campaign to alert women of their even higher risk for heart disease. Chapter 40 discusses CAD.

Hypertension

Hypertension is prevalent in over 50 million individuals in the United States (Chobanian et al., 2003). It is the primary diagnosis in 35 million office visits (Chobanian et al., 2003). It is a major risk factor for heart failure and is present in 10% of patients with diagnosed heart failure (Chobanian et al., 2003; He et al., 2001; Levy, Larson, Vasan, Kannel, & Ho, 1996). Hypertension causes increased workload on the heart due to increased systemic vascular resistance, leading to hypertrophy and dilation, and eventual worsening ventricular dysfunction (Braunwald et al., 2001). Patients who have their hypertension treated have demonstrated as high as a 51% risk reduction for developing heart failure (Dahlof et al., 1991; Kostis et al., 1997; Neal, MacMahon, & Chapman, 2000). Patients with hypertension are treated not only with pharmacologic agents but also with lifestyle modifications such as exercise, especially for weight reduction, a low-salt diet, and reducing alcohol consumption (Chobanian et al., 2003). Patients with heart failure along with persistent hypertension are placed on medications that not only control blood pressure but also treat heart failure (Adams et al., 2001; Baker, 2002). These medications include diuretics, ACE inhibitors, and also beta-adrenergic blockers (Baker, 2002). Chapter 21 discusses hypertension.

Sleep Apnea

Sleep disordered breathing, including central or obstructive sleep apnea, has prevalence rates estimated as high as 50% in patients with heart failure (Javaheri, 2000; Javaheri et al., 1998; Sin et al., 1999). Sleep apnea can subsequently increase mortality rates in patients with heart failure (Hanly & Zuberi-Khokhar, 1996; Naughton 2006). Episodes of **apnea** (cessation of airflow for more than 10 seconds) and **hypopnea** (a reduction but not complete cessation of airflow to less than 50% of normal) while sleeping may result in oxygen desaturation, which causes transient increases in SNS activation leading to vasoconstriction, elevation of systemic blood pressure, and increased heart rate, all leading to ventricular hypertrophy, systolic dysfunction, and interstitial pulmonary edema (Bradley & Floras, 2003a, 2003b; Leung & Bradley, 2001). Patients may complain of irritability, excessive daytime fatigue, poor concentration, light or disrupted sleep, persistent PND, and orthopnea even when euvolemic on physical exam (Bradley & Floras, 2000; Naughton, 2006). Patients who present with these complaints should be screened for sleep apnea that is performed by overnight **polysomnography** (multichannel electrophysiological recording used to detect disturbances of breathing during sleep), evaluating for at least 10 to 15 episodes of apnea and hypopnea per hour of sleep (Bradley & Floras, 2003a & b). Treatment includes a continuous positive airway pressure (CPAP) mask, which has been found to be beneficial in alleviating symptoms and improving abnormal respiratory patterns by reducing the degree of negative intrathoracic pressure required for respiration and decreasing left ventricular afterload, resulting in an improvement in left ventricular function (Kaneko et al., 2003; Naughton, 2006; Yan, Bradley, & Liu, 2001).

Gerontological Considerations

Heart failure is generally a condition of the elderly, with the aging baby boomers contributing to the rise in heart failure incidence. There is little guidance in the literature on heart failure in the elderly, yet as the baby boomers continue to age and improvements are made in the treatment of CAD, those over age 65, living with heart failure will continue to grow. Although heart failure is the number-one discharge diagnosis in the elderly (Ahmed, 2003; Nohria et al., 2002), persons over age 65 are underrepresented in heart failure clinical trials (Heiat, Gross, & Krumholz, 2002; Jessup & Brozena, 2003). Although one epidemiologic study showed the average age at the time of first diagnosis to be 75 years of age, a review of randomized, controlled heart failure trials showed that only 3 of 59 studies included individuals in this age group (Heiat, Gross, & Krumholz, 2002). Some studies went so far as to exclude those over age 65 in the trial. Few studies have been done specific to the needs of this patient population; thus, the treatment approach comes from studies done in younger age groups (Heiat, Gross, & Krumholz, 2002; Nohria et al., 2002).

Due to the incidence of CAD and hypertension in the elderly, they are more likely to have heart failure with preserved systolic function. Logically, it follows that they will have more comorbid conditions and are thus victim to "polypharmacy," more so than those in younger age groups (Heiat, Gross, & Krumholz, 2002; McKelvie, 2001). Diastolic dysfunction is particularly common in obese, elderly women (Greenberg & Hermann, 2002; Jessup & Brozena, 2003). Whether the cause of heart failure is systolic dysfunction or diastolic dysfunction, the prognosis is poor once hospitalized, although mortality trends for systolic dysfunction have been found to be double those for diastolic dysfunction (McKelvie, 2001). The Gerontological Considerations box (p. 1316) summarizes prognostic predictors of increased mortality for those elderly patients with systolic dysfunction.

The common symptoms of heart failure are similar to those of any age: dyspnea (especially with exertion), cough, orthopnea, and dependent edema. The elderly, however, may present with less common or overt symptoms, such as fatigue, poor concentration, disorientation, and failure to thrive (McKelvie, 2001). Often, their symptoms may be confused with other disease processes or other concomitant comorbidities such as CAD, infection, or depression. A normal part of age-related changes of cardiac function may include modest decreases in systolic function and decreases in cardiovascular response with increased work load. As a result, stressors in the elderly may precipitate heart failure symptoms that might not present themselves in the younger population. These stressors include infection, hypothyroidism, hyperthyroidism, anemia, cardiac ischemia, hypoxia, hypothermia, hyperthermia, renal failure, nonadherence to drug or diet regimens, and potentially the use of certain drugs (nonsteroidal anti-inflammatories, beta-blockers, and some calcium channel blockers) (McKelvie, 2001).

Given the limited available data in the literature related to treating diastolic dysfunction, most of the therapies should be aimed at treating CAD, hypertension, and volume overload (Ahmed, 2003; Jessup & Brozena, 2003). Therapeutic approaches for systolic dysfunction in the elderly should be based on general guidelines in the literature; start at low doses and titrate medications slowly to maximum tolerated doses (McKelvie, 2001). Because the elderly are at risk of hypotension in the setting of volume depletion, cautious use of antihypertensive agents that have vasodilatory properties is recommended in the setting of diuretic use (McKelvie, 2001) (see Chart 42–4, p. 1286). Toxicities to medications may occur in the elderly with renal insufficiency. Digoxin should be started at low doses (0.125 milligram daily) for those over the age of 70, monitoring levels because patients may be prone to toxicity because of reduced renal clearance (McKelvie, 2001; Nohria et al., 2002).

Coping with Heart Failure and End-of-Life Planning

Many challenges present themselves to those diagnosed with heart failure. There is the uncertainty related to prognosis, expectations related to response to medications, and possible loss of earning potential for those in the workforce. As with many chronic conditions, the impact of depression on heart failure is significant (Nohria et al., 2002). Persons diagnosed with heart failure need family or loved ones who participate actively in their life for the physical, psychological, and emotional support that is needed.

Despite medicine's best treatment options, those with heart failure will likely die from this disease process, as displayed in the course of heart failure (see Figure 42–2 ■, p. 1283). As usage

rates of medications that can alter the prognosis of heart failure improve, internal cardioverter defibrillators offer corresponding reductions in mortality. Using medications such as beta-adrenergic blockers can lead to a 5% to 15% increase in ejection fraction or even its normalization, which improves the patient's prognosis (Greenberg & Hermann, 2002). Many factors contribute to the unpredictability of a given patient's course, such as response to prognosis altering medications, compliance, and timing and level of care (Greenberg & Hermann, 2002).

When heart failure reaches a terminal stage and treatment options are limited, care should be geared toward comfort measures and reducing symptoms typically manifested as respiratory distress and pain (Albert, Davis, & Young, 2002). Palliative care is treatment done to reduce symptoms and suffering in end-of-life planning (Albert et al., 2002). Only recently has research focused on how best to treat patients in the final stages of heart failure (Albert et al., 2002; Brush, Zambroski, & Rasmusson, 2006). Optimally, palliative care should be included in the management of heart failure from the time of diagnosis, designed as part of comprehensive care across the continuum. Discussions about the level of care should be planned ahead of time, not during times of crisis. Advance directives, resuscitation wishes, living wills, formalizing estate planning, and discussing wishes with family and health care providers will lead to the best laid plans. Forward planning of this nature, however, is not often done.

Care providers have struggled with the ability to predict when death is near for patients with heart failure. It has become clear that patients with hypotension that require dose reductions of ACE inhibitors (or ARBs) and beta-adrenergic blockers, as well as increasing creatinine, and anemia, are all predictors of a poor prognosis. Albert and colleagues (2002) have proposed an algorithm with a scoring system based on identifiable criteria, as a means to assess readiness for palliative care. The criteria suggestive of a poor prognosis include NYHA class IV symptoms, tachycardia (heart rate > 100 beats per minute), serum sodium < 134 mmol/L, serum creatinine > 2.0 mg/dL, prior decompensation, use of inotropic infusion for hemodynamic stability, serious comorbid conditions, and dependence on others for assistance with ADLs. Others have used similar and additional prognostic indicators such as severe reductions in objective assessment of functional and exercise capacity. Those with 6-minute walk performance at 300 meters have higher mortality than those who can reach 450 meters (Greenberg & Hermann, 2002). Still, more evidence may be predictive of higher mortality (2 years; 60%) for those with left ventricular dimension > 85 millimeters (Nohria et al., 2002).

Patients and loved ones deserve an honest discussion related to caring for those who are near the end of life. Patients with heart failure will likely die of a sudden dysrhythmic event (if an ICD has not been implanted or has been deactivated) or the slower, progressive cardiac pump dysfunction (Nohria et al., 2002). Clear decisions should be made regarding symptom management (often done with narcotics, diuretics, nitrates, and anxiolytics) and can be planned ahead so medications are ready for use when needed (Albert et al., 2002; Nohria et al., 2002). Engaging home care, family and loved ones, community resources, and hospice can assist with facilitating the patient's individual preferences (Nohria et al., 2002). Discussing plans for turning off mechanical devices (pacemakers, defibrillators, ventricular assist devices) that may prolong life when little hope is present is often difficult, but will be necessary as their use becomes increasingly more common in treating heart failure (Albert et al., 2002). Planning for the end of life must account for the patient's spiritual, psychological, physical, social, and cultural needs. Ethical issues regarding heart failure care that must be considered thoughtfully are outlined in the Ethical Issues box.

Research

Cardiovascular research has led to tremendous advances in diagnosis and treatment. The Framingham Heart Study continues to be one of the research landmarks on which epidemiologic data on heart disease and treatment are based. In the past 30 years, studies that have been done on all the forms of heart failure treatment mentioned in this chapter have led to treatment guidelines for care. There has been an explosion of heart failure studies striving to find new treatments, hoping for methods to reduce mortality, to improve quality and length of life, and to reduce the cost. Understanding heart failure management will include a sensitivity and awareness of cultural aspects (see the Cultural Considerations box, p. 1309).

Comprehensive disease management strategies have been shown to improve outcomes associated with chronic heart failure. Such strategies include telephone follow-up with decision support software and protocol-driven pharmacologic management with close telephone nurse follow-up (Reigel et al., 2002; Whellen et al., 2001). Future directions for heart failure research studies can be found in the Research Opportunities and Clinical Impact feature (p. 1318).

ETHICAL ISSUES Related to Heart Failure

Specific ethical issues for heart failure (HF) patients and their families include:

- Quality of life after the initial onset of left ventricle (LV) dysfunction
- Employability after clinical stabilization
- When to withhold or withdraw care
- Dignified and comfortable death
- Psychological adjustment
- Considerations of futility
- Financial costs of end-stage therapies (i.e., transplant, mechanical circulatory support, intravenous medications)
- Turning off an implantable cardioverter defibrillator (ICD) device in chronic, severe, refractory HF patient
- Pregnancy in female HF patients
- Therapeutic potential of embryonic stem cells in HF
- Differences of care between male and female HF patients.

Sources: Adams, K. F., Lindenfeld, J., Arnold, J. M., et al. (2006). Executive summary: HFSA 2006 comprehensive heart failure practice guideline. *Journal of Cardiac Failure, 12*(1), 10–38; Kirkpatrick, J. N., & Kim, A. Y. (2006). Ethical issues in heart failure: Overview of an emerging need. *Perspectives in Biological Medicine, 49,* 1–9; and Lerou, P. H., & Daley, G. Q. (2005). Therapeutic potential of embryonic stem cells. *Blood Review, 19*(6), 321–331.

Genetic Considerations

Understanding genetic mechanisms of cardiomyopathy will broaden treatment approaches (Tang & Francis, 2005). Studies will evaluate genetic risk factors, therapies, legal implications, counseling, and screening issues. The Genetic Considerations box provides a more thorough review of genetic implications (p. 1279).

RESEARCH OPPORTUNITIES AND CLINICAL IMPACT RELATED TO HEART FAILURE CARE

Research Area	Clinical Impact
Depression and anxiety in patients with mechanical cardiac devices	Patients with heart failure are increasingly having cardiac devices implanted to prevent cardiac death or to improve contractility, or both. Understanding optimal treatment for anxiety or depression will be critical given the growing use of device therapy.
Caregiver support for end-stage heart failure	Heart failure is increasing in incidence and prevalence; thus, learning how to support the caregiver will be imperative.
Cost-effectiveness of heart failure therapies	Given the increasing evidence to support the use of cardiac devices, such as ICDs, pacemakers, and left ventricular assist device (LVADs), continual cost analysis of these therapies is essential.
Respiratory support for sleep disordered breathing	Patients with HF frequently experience abnormal respiratory patterns. Treatment or prevention of these abnormal respiratory patterns may lead to a reduction in the incidence of heart failure (HF).
External counterpulsation	This involves the use of a device that inflates and deflates around a patient's legs. This therapy has been shown to decrease the frequency of ischemic attacks in coronary artery disease (CAD) patients. Larger trials are underway to determine its routine use in HF care.
Implantable hemodynamic monitors	Implantable monitors are able to monitor ventricular filling pressures. This form of technology may be able to prevent HF exacerbations prior to their occurrence.
Cardiac support devices	Several surgical devices are currently in design stages to assist in the reduction of physical stresses on the left ventricle.
Myocardial regeneration by activation of stem cells	The possibility of reconstituting dead myocardium by activation of stem cells is a promising area of research.
Understanding the knowledge deficits of patients with heart failure	Patient understanding of his course of heart failure and self-management strategies is essential. Identifying the most significant barriers to patient understanding of his disease and self-management may likely improve outcomes.
Self-management strategies in heart failure	Identifying what improves patient compliance with self-management strategies may lead to improved outcomes.
The role of culture in patients with advanced heart failure	Identifying cultural barriers in providing patient care can help providers in formulating a comprehensive treatment plan.
Anthracycline-induced cardiomyopathy	Anthracyclines used to treat malignancies have been known to cause left ventricular dysfunction. More study is needed to learn how to prevent this, and to monitor and optimally treat this patient population.

Sources: Cohn, J. N., et al. (1997). Report of the National Heart, Lung, and Blood Institute special emphasis panel on heart failure research. *Circulation, 95,* 766–770; Garry, D. J., Masino, A. M., Naseem, R. H., & Martin, C. M. (2005). Ponce de Leon's fountain: Stem cells and the regenerating heart. *American Journal of Medical Science, 329*(4), 190–201; and Hunt, S. A., Abraham, W. T., Chin, M. H., Feldman, A. M., Francis, G. S., Ganiats, T. G., et al. (2005). ACC/AHA 2005 guideline update for the diagnosis and management of chronic heart failure in the adult: Summary article: A report of the American College of Cardiology/American Heart Association Task Force on Practice Guidelines (Writing Committee to Update the 2001 Guidelines for the Evaluation and Management of Heart Failure). *Journal of the American College of Cardiology, 46,* 1116–1143.

Clinical Preparation

 Read

- History of Current Illness
- Past Medical History
- Physical Exam
- Admitting Medical Orders
- Laboratory Study Results

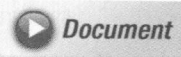 **Document**

- Summary of Hospitalization
- Pathophysiology Form
- Laboratory Values
- Laboratory Results Explanation

 Apply

- List of Potential Nursing Diagnoses
- Concept Map
- Critical Thinking Questions

Log on to MyNursingKit.com to download forms you will need and to complete further steps in the Clinical Preparation assignment.

HISTORY OF PRESENT ILLNESS

As the on-coming nurse on a telemetry cardiovascular care unit, you receive report about Mr. X, who was admitted with a diagnosis of heart failure 48 hours ago. He is a 56-year-old male who presented to his primary care provider with a 2-month history of worsening symptoms of dyspnea on exertion, a nonproductive cough, general fatigue, and decreased activity tolerance. Initially, the patient thought he had the flu, but when the symptoms persisted longer than expected, he sought medical attention. At the office Mr. X was found to have profound jugular venous distention, rhonchi in his lungs, and lower extremity swelling. After admission, he had an echocardiogram and a serum BNP that was 1,560 pg/mL. Coronary angiography was performed to provide a definitive diagnosis that revealed no evidence of coronary artery disease. Echocardiogram shows moderate concentric hypertrophy of the ventricles, moderate left ventricular dysfunction, ejection fraction 33%, mild to moderate mitral regurgitation. Angiogram: normal coronary arteries, ejection fraction 33%, confirmed reduction in ventricular function with a ventriculogram.

Medical Surgical History

Hyperlipidemia: diagnosed 3 years ago
Hypertension: diagnosed this past year
Type II diabetes: diagnosed this past year
Obesity: over 20 years
Hypothyroidism: diagnosed 12 years ago
Tonsillectomy: 40 years ago
Cholecystectomy: 4 years ago

Current Medications

Simvastatin 20 mg po qhs
Levothyroxine 0.125 mg po daily
Glipizide 500 mg po bid
Hydrochlorothiazide 25 mg po daily

Physical Exam

Vital signs: HR: 84 beats per minute; BP: 146/84 mmHg; temperature: 36.8°C; oxygen sat: 94% on 2 liters of oxygen.
He is a well-nourished male with appropriate affect and no apparent distress
All extremities have palpable pulses, are warm to touch, and have a capillary refill of less than 3 seconds.
3+ pitting edema is present in his lower ankles bilaterally, which extends to his midcalf; his lungs have bibasilar crackles without wheezing or retractions; he also has a nonproductive cough.
Normal S_1 and S_2 are present. S_3, and the point of maximal impulse is displaced laterally, into the anterior axillary line of his chest.
Positive hepatojugular reflux.
Bowel sounds present and palpation is nontender.

Admitting Medical Orders

Cardiology Service
Diagnosis: acute heart failure
Telemetry floor
Condition guarded
No known allergies
Full code
Bed rest with bathroom privileges
Call house officer: pulse < 60 and > 100/minute; BP < 90 and > 160 systolic; temperature > 38.5; urine output < 30 mL/hr for 2 hours; respiratory rate > 30/minute; oxygen saturation < 92%; Blood sugar < 60 or >120
Continuous cardiac monitor
Oxygen per nasal cannula to maintain oxygen sat > 92%
Vital signs and oxygen saturation q4hours
Daily a.m. weights
IV: saline lock-flush with NS q8h
Blood sugars ac and hs
Cardiac rehab evaluation and management
Low-sodium (< 2,000 mg/day), fluid-restricted (< 2 L/day) diet
Strict I&O
Sequential compression devices (SCD) to lower extremities when in bed
Incentive spirometry 2 hours while awake and q4 at night

Scheduled Medications

Simvastatin 20 mg PO qhs
Levothyroxine 0.125 mg PO daily
Glipizide 500 mg PO bid
Furosemide 80 mg PO bid
Potassium 40 mEq PO bid
Lisinopril 2.5 mg PO daily

PRN Medications

Morphine 3–5 mg IV q3–5min, max 15 mg q3h prn chest pain
Temazepam 15–30 mg PO qhs prn insomnia
Droperidol 1.25–2.5 mg IV q 6hours prn nausea

Ordered Laboratory Studies

Chemistry 7 panel daily
CBC now

BNP daily × 3
Lipid panel

Ordered Diagnostic Studies

Chest x-ray in a.m.
Echocardiogram
Angiogram

LABORATORY STUDY RESULTS

Test	Day 1 Admission	Day 1 Evening	Day 2 Morning
Potassium	4.8 mEq/L	3.5 mEq/L	3.8 mEq/L
Sodium	136 mEq/L	138 mEq/L	137 mEq/L
Chloride	103 mEq/L	104 mEq/L	103 mEq/L
Carbon dioxide (CO_2)	26 mEq/L	25 mEq/L	25 mEq/L
Calcium	8.8 mg/dL	8.7 mg/dL	9.1 mg/dL
Creatinine	1.8 mg/dL	1.4 mg/dL	1.2 mg/dL
(BUN)	30 mg/dL	24 mg/dL	18 mg/dL
Glucose	110 mg/dL	108 mg/dL	102 mg/dL
Hematocrit	40%	39%	44%
Hemoglobin	13.9 g/dL	13.5 g/dL	14.9 g/dL
Platelets	285/mm³	266/mm³	289/mm³
WBC	8.5/mm³	7.9/mm³	8.3/mm³
RBC	4.89/mm³	5.02/mm³	4.96/mm³
BNP	1,560 pg/mL	662 pg/mL	422 pg/mL
Cholesterol	260 mg/dL		
High-density lipoproteins (HDL)	36 mg/dL		
Low-density lipoproteins (LDL)	187 mg/dL		
Very-low-density lipoproteins (VLDL)	70%		
Apolipoproteins	160 mg/dL		
Triglycerides	196 mg/dL		

CRITICAL THINKING QUESTIONS

1. When reviewing Mr. X's orders when coming on shift, list them in order of priority.
2. Why would the patient receive daily a.m. weights?
3. Which laboratory values may require notification to the ordering provider?
4. What should you monitor for after giving lisinopril 2.5 mg PO daily?
5. Why is a beta-adrenergic blocker not listed on the ordered medications?

Answers to Critical Thinking Questions appear in Appendix D.

NCLEX® REVIEW

1. The nurse identifies the following risk factors in a patient admitted with symptoms of heart failure.
   1. A recent episode of acute pancreatitis
   2. Chronic fatigue syndrome
   3. Aortic stenosis
   4. Pleural effusion
2. When caring for a patient with systolic dysfunction the nurse anticipates the patient will exhibit symptoms related to which cardiac condition?
   1. Decreased cardiac output
   2. Aortic stenosis
   3. Mitral regurgitation
   4. Bradycardia
3. The nurse understands when a patient with heart failure experiences a decrease in cardiac output, the following neurohormonal responses will occur.
   1. Activation of the sympathetic nervous system, SNS
   2. Activation of the parasympathetic nervous system, PNS
   3. Inactivation of the renin angiotensin system, RAS
   4. Suppression of cytokine release
4. Which of the following symptoms should the nurse expect to see in a patient with left-sided heart failure?
   1. Weight gain
   2. Anorexia
   3. Dyspnea
   4. Peripheral edema

5. The nurse checks the brain naturietic peptide, (BNP) levels of a patient admitted with dyspnea and activity intolerance. Because the levels are normal, the nurse concludes:

   1. A diagnosis of heart failure can be excluded.

   2. The client has long standing heart failure.

   3. The client is most likely experiencing cardiac ischemia.

   4. The symptoms are related to pulmonary tissue damage.

6. The nurse should anticipate the treatment of a patient with stage B heart failure will include:

   1. ACE inhibitors and beta-blockers.

   2. Use of diuretics only.

   3. Insertion of an implantable cardiac defibrillator.

   4. Possible referral to hospice.

7. The nurse should incorporate the following key issues of a self-management program for a patient with heart failure:

   1. Medications, diet restrictions, weight reduction, and financial concerns.

   2. Medications, activity, weight, diet, and symptoms.

   3. Diet management, psychosocial concerns, and medications.

   4. Weight management, symptoms, social support, spirituality, and medications.

8. Because the following comorbidities can increase the mortality rate of patients with heart failure, the nurse assesses the patient for symptoms of:

   1. Diabetes and liver failure.

   2. Hypovolemic shock and anemia.

   3. Depression and anemia.

   4. Sleep apnea and deep vein thrombosis (DVT).

9. A patient is in end stage heart failure and the family asks what they should anticipate. The nurse recognizes the need to address the following:

   1. The lack of hearts available for heart transplants.

   2. Plans for treatment in the final stages of heart failure.

   3. Long-term home care management.

   4. Surgical interventions to correct structural abnormalities of the heart.

Answers for review questions appear in Appendix D

KEY TERMS

apnea *p.1315*
ascites *p.1287*
biventricular heart failure *p.1281*
cardiomegaly *p.1284*
crackles *p.1285*
diastolic dysfunction *p.1281*
euvolemia *p.1291*
heart failure *p.1279*

hepatojugular reflux *p.1287*
hypertrophy *p.1283*
hypopnea *p.1315*
jugular venous distention (JVD) *p.1285*
left-sided heart failure *p.1281*
left ventricular ejection fraction (LVEF) *p.1280*
New York Heart Association (NYHA) classification system *p.1285*

pitting *p.1287*
polysomnography *p.1315*
right-sided heart failure *p.1281*
S_3 (third heart sound) *p.1287*
S_4 (fourth heart sound) *p.1287*
systolic dysfunction *p.1280*
tachypnea *p.1285*

EXPLORE PEARSON **mynursingkit**™

MyNursingKit is your one stop for online chapter review materials and resources. Prepare for success with additional NCLEX®-style practice questions, interactive assignments and activities, web links, animations and videos, and more!

Register your access code from the front of your book at
www.mynursingkit.com

REFERENCES

Abraham, W. T. (2003). Electrophysiological aids in congestive heart failure: Supporting and synchronizing systole. *Medical Clinics of North America, 87*(2), 509–521.

Abraham, W. T., Adams, K. F., Constanzo, M. R., Berkowitz, R. L., Cheng M. L., Fonarow, G. C., et al. (2005). In-hospital mortality in patients with acute decompensated heart failure requiring intravenous vasoactive medications. *Journal of the American College of Cardiology, 46*, 57–64.

Adams, K. F., Lindenfeld, J., Arnold, J. M., et al. (2006). Executive summary: HFSA 2006 comprehensive heart failure practice guideline. *Journal of Cardiac Failure, 12*(1), 10–38.

Adams, T. D., Fisher, A. G., Hansen, S. F., & Yanowitz, F. G. (2001). *Maintaining the miracle and owner's manual for the human body* (3rd ed.). Salt Lake City, UT: CAPP Publishing.

Ahmed, A. (2003). American College of Cardiology/American Heart Association chronic heart failure evaluation and management

guidelines: Relevance to the geriatric practice. *Journal of American Geriatric Society, 51*(1), 123–126.

Albert, N. M., Davis, M., & Young, J. (2002). Improving the care of patients dying of heart failure. *Cleveland Clinic Journal of Medicine, 69*(4), 321–327.

American Association of Heart Failure Nurses. (2007). *Patients are the heart of what we do.* Retrieved January 22, 2008, from http://www.aahfn.org/

American Diabetic Association. (N/D). *All about diabetes.* Retrieved July 23, 2008 from http://www.diabetes.org/about-diabetes.jsp.

American Heart Association. (2006a). *Facts about women and cardiovascular diseases.* Retrieved August 7, 2006, from http://www.americanheart. org/presenter.jhtml?identifier=2876

American Heart Association. (2006b). *Heart and stroke statistics—2006 update.* Dallas, TX: Author.

American Society of Consultant Pharmacists. (1999). *Consultant pharmacist forum; Herbal products and drug interactions.* Retrieved November 10, 2006, from http://www.ascp.com/public/pubs/tcp/ 1999/aug/forum.shtml

Baker, D. (2002). Prevention of heart failure. *Journal of Cardiac Failure, 8*(5), 333–346.

Bakker, P. F., Meijburg, H. W., de Vries, J. W., Mower, M. M., Thomas, A. C., Hull, M. L., et al. (2000). Biventricular pacing in end-stage heart failure improves functional capacity and left ventricular function. *Journal of Interventional Cardiac Electrophysiology, 4*(2), 395–404.

Blue Cross Blue Shield Association. (2002). *Left-ventricular assist devices as destination therapy for end-stage heart failure.* Assessment Program, 17(19). Retrieved November 10, 2006, from http://www.bcbs.com/tec/vol17/17_19.html

Bradley, T. D., & Floras, J. S. (2003a). Sleep apnea and heart failure: Part I. Obstructive sleep apnea. *Circulation, 107*, 1671–1678.

Bradley, T. D., & Floras, J. S. (2003b). Sleep apnea and heart failure: Part II. Central sleep apnea. *Circulation, 107*, 1822–1826.

Bradley, T. D. & Floras, J. S. (2000). Pathophysiologic interactions between sleep apnea and congestive heart failure. In T. D. Bradley & J. S. Floras (Eds.), *Sleep apnea: Implications in cardiovascular and cerebrovascular disease. Lung biology in health and disease* (Vol. 146, pp. 385–414). New York: Marcel Dekker.

Braunwald, E., Zipes, D. P., & Libby, P. (2001). *Heart disease: A textbook of cardiovascular medicine* (6th ed.). Philadelphia: W. B. Saunders.

Bristow, M. R., Feldman, A. M., & Saxon, L. A. (2000). Heart failure management using implantable devices for ventricular resynchronization: Comparison of medical therapy, pacing, and defibrillation in chronic heart failure (COMPANION) trial. *Journal of Cardiac Failure, 6*(3), 276–285.

Brush, S., Zambroski, C. H., & Rasmusson, K. (2006, Summer). Palliative care for the patient with end-stage heart failure. *Progress in Cardiovascular Nursing*, 166–170.

Burkett, E. L., & Hershberger, R. E. (2005). State of the art: Clinical and genetic issues in familial dilated cardiomyopathy. *Journal of the American College of Cardiology, 45*, 969–981.

Chobanian, A. V., Bakris, G. L., Black, H. R., Cushman, W. C., Green, L. A., Izzo, J. L., Jr., et al. (2003). The seventh report of the Joint National Committee on Prevention, Detection, Evaluation, and Treatment of High Blood Pressure. *Hypertension, 42*(6), 1206–1252.

Cohn, J. N. (2000). Pathophysiology and clinical recognition of heart failure. In J. T. Willerson & J. N. Cohn (Eds.), *Cardiovascular medicine* (2nd ed.). Philadelphia: Churchill Livingstone.

Dahlof, B., Lindholm, L. H., Hansson, L., Schersten, B., Ekborm, T., & Wester, P. O. (1991). Morbidity and mortality in the Swedish Trial in Old Patients with Hypertension (STOP-Hypertension). *Lancet, 338*, 1281–1285.

Digitalis Investigation Group. (1997). The effect of digoxin on mortality and morbidity in patients with heart failure. *The New England Journal of Medicine, 336*, 525–533.

Dries, D. L., Exner, D. V., Domanski, M. J., Greenberg, B., & Stevenson, L. W. (2000). The prognostic implications of renal insufficiency in asymptomatic and symptomatic patients with left ventricular systolic dysfunction. *Journal of the American College of Cardiology, 35*, 681–689.

Feldman, T. E., Hirshfeld, J. W., Jacobs, A. K., Kern, M. J., King, S. B., Morrison, D. A., et al. (2006). ACC/AHA/SCAI 2005 guideline update for percutaneous coronary intervention. *Journal of the American College of Cardiology, 47*, 216–235.

Fonarow, G. C. (2001). The treatment targets in acute decompensated heart failure. *Reviews in Cardiovascular Medicine, 2*(2), S7–S12.

Greenberg, B. H., & Hermann, D. D. (2002). *Contemporary diagnosis and management of heart failure.* Newtown, PA: Handbooks in Health Care.

Hall, J. A., Rasmusson, K. D., Kfoury, A. G., French, T. K., Rimmasch, H. L., Hofmann, L. C., et al. (2005). Successful implementation of heart failure self-management improves survival. *Journal of Heart and Lung Transplantation, 24*(Suppl. 2S), S68–S79.

Hanly, P. J., & Zuberi-Khokhar, N. S. (1996). Increased mortality associated with Cheyne–Stokes respiration in patients with congestive heart failure. *American Journal of Respiratory Critical Care Medicine, 153*, 272–276.

Hardman, J. G., & Limbird, L. E. (Eds.). (2001). *Goodman and Gilman's The Pharmacological basis of therapeutics* (10th ed.). New York: McGraw-Hill.

Havranek, E. P., Ware, M. G., & Lowes, B. D. (1999). Prevalence of depression in congestive heart failure. *American Journal of Cardiology, 84*, 348–350.

He, J., Ogden, L. G., Bazzano, L. A., Vupputuri, S., Loria, C., & Whelton, P. K. (2001). Risk factors for congestive heart failure in US men and women: NHANES I epidemiologic follow-up study. *Archives of Internal Medicine, 161*, 996–1002.

Heart Outcomes Prevention Evaluation Study Investigators. (2000). Effects of ramipril on cardiovascular and microvascular outcomes in people with diabetes mellitus: Results of the HOPE study and MICRO-HOPE sub study. *Lancet, 355*, 253–259.

Heiat, A., Gross, C. P., & Krumholz, H. M. (2002). Representation of the elderly, women, and minorities in heart failure clinical trials. *Archives of Internal Medicine, 162*, 1682–1688.

Horwich, T. B. (2002). Anemia is associated with worse symptoms, greater impairment in functional capacity and a significant increase in mortality in patients with advanced heart failure. *Journal of the American College of Cardiology, 39*(11), 1780–1786.

Hunt, S. A., Abraham, W. T., Chin, M. H., Feldman, A. M., Francis, G. S., Ganiats, T. G., et al. (2005). ACC/AHA 2005 guideline update for the diagnosis and management of chronic heart failure in the adult: Summary article: A report of the American College of Cardiology/American Heart Association Task Force on Practice Guidelines (Writing Committee to Update the 2001 Guidelines for the Evaluation and Management of Heart Failure). *Journal of the American College of Cardiology, 46*, 1116–1143.

Iribarren, C., Karter, A. J., Go, A. S., Ferrara, A., Liu, J. Y., Sidney, S., et al. (2001). Glycemic control and heart failure among adult patients with diabetes. *Circulation, 103*, 2668–2673.

Javaheri, S. (2000). Effects of continuous positive airway pressure on sleep apnea and ventricular irritability in patients with heart failure. *Circulation, 101*, 392–397.

Javaheri, S., Parker, T. J., Liming, J. D., Corbett, W. S., Nishiyama, H., Wexler, L., et al. (1998). Sleep apnea in 81 ambulatory male patients with stable heart failure: Types and their prevalences, consequences, and presentations. *Circulation, 97*, 2154–2159.

Jessup, M., & Brozena, S. (2003). Heart failure. *The New England Journal of Medicine, 348*, 2007–2018.

Kaneko, Y., Floras, J. S., Phil, D., Usui, K., Plante, J., Tkacova, R., et al. (2003). Cardiovascular effects of continuous positive airway pressure in patients with heart failure and obstructive sleep apnea. *The New England Journal of Medicine, 348*, 1233–1241.

Kerwin, W. F., Botvinick, E. H., O'Connell, J. W., Merrick, S. H., DeMarco, T., Chatterjee, K., et al. (2000). Ventricular contraction abnormalities in dilated cardiomyopathy: Effect of biventricular pacing to correct interventricular dyssynchrony. *Journal of the American College of Cardiology, 35*(5), 1221–1227.

Kfoury, A. G., Hall, J. C., Rasmusson, K. D., Horne, B., & Renlund, D. G. (2006). Incremental survival benefit with adherence to JCAHO heart failure measures. *Supplement to the Journal of Heart and Lung Transplant.*

Konstam, M. A. (2004). Heart failure training: A call for an integrative, patient-focused approach to an emerging cardiology subspecialty. *Journal of Cardiac Failure, 10*(5), 366–367.

Kosiborod, M., et al. (2003). The prognostic importance of anemia in patients with heart failure. *American Journal of Medicine, 114*, 112–119.

Kostis, J. B., Davis, B. R., Cutler, J., Grimm, R. H., Jr., Berge, K. G., & Cohen, J. D. (1997). Prevention of heart failure by antihypertensive drug treatment in older persons with isolated systolic hypertension. SHEP Cooperative Research Group. *Journal of the American Medical Association, 278*, 212–216.

Kouchoukos, N. T., Blackstone, E. H., Doty, D. B., Hanley, F. L., & Karp, R. B. (2003). *Kirklin/Barratt-Boyes cardiac surgery* (3rd ed., Vol. 2). Philadelphia: Churchill Livingstone.

Krumholz, H. M., Amatruda, J., Smith, G. L., Mattera, J. A., Roumanis, S. A., Radford, M. J., et al. (2002). Randomized trial of an education and support intervention to prevent readmission of patients with heart failure. *Journal of the American College of Cardiology, 13*(1), 83–89.

Krumholz, H. M., Chen, Y. T., Vaccarino, V., et al (2000). Correlates and impact on outcomes of worsening renal function in patients > or = 65 years of age with heart failure. *American Journal of Cardiology, 85*, 1110–1113.

Leung, R. S. T., & Bradley, T. D. (2001). Sleep apnea and cardiovascular disease. *American Journal of Respiratory and Critical Care Medicine, 164*, 2147–2165.

Levy, D., Larson, M. G., Vasan, R. S., Kannel, W. B., & Ho, K. K. (1996). The progression from hypertension to congestive heart failure. *The Journal of the American Medical Association, 275*, 1557–1562.

Linde, C., Leclercq, C., Rex, S., Garrigue, S., Lavergne, T., Cazeau, S., et al. on behalf of the Multisite Stimulation in Cardiomyopathies study group (MUSTIC). (2002). Long-term benefits of biventricular pacing in congestive heart failure: Results from the Multisite Stimulation in Cardiomyopathy (MUSTIC) study. *Journal of the American College of Cardiology, 40*(1), 111–118.

McKelvie, R. (2001). *Clinical evidence concise.* Kingsport, TN: BMJ Publishing Group.

Molhoek, S. G., Bax, J. J., van Erven, L., Bootsma, M., Boersma, E., Steendijk, P., et al. (2002). Effectiveness of resynchronization therapy in patients with end-stage heart failure. *American Journal of Cardiology, 90*(4), 379–383.

Moss, A. J., Zareba, W., Hall, W. J., Klein, H., Wilber, D. J., Cannom, D. S., et al. for the Multicenter Automatic Defibrillator Implantation Trial II Investigators (MADIT-II). (2002). Prophylactic implantation of a defibrillator in patients with myocardial infarction and reduced ejection fraction. *The New England Journal of Medicine, 346*(12), 877–883.

Naughton, M. T. (2006). The link between obstructive sleep apnea and heart failure: Underappreciated opportunity for treatment. *Current Heart Failure Reports, 3*(4), 183–188.

Neal, B., MacMahon, S., & Chapman, N. (2000). Effects of ACE inhibitors, calcium antagonists, and other blood pressure-lowering drugs: Results of prospectively designed overviews of randomized trials. Blood Pressure Lowering Treatment Trialists' Collaboration. *Lancet, 356*, 1956–1964.

Nohria, A., Lewis, E., & Stevenson, L. W. (2002). Medical management of advanced heart failure. *Journal of the American Medical Association, 287*(5), 628–640.

Packer, M., Gheorghiade, M., & Young, J. B., et al., for the RADIANCE Study. (1993). Withdrawal of digoxin from patients with chronic heart failure treated with angiotensin-converting-enzyme inhibitors. *The New England Journal of Medicine, 397*, 1–7.

Rasmusson, K. D., Hall, J. A., Hofmann, L. C., Moore, S. V., & Renlund, D. G. (2002). Patient self-management knowledge and perceptions improve through community based heart failure teaching. *Journal of Cardiac Failure, 8*(4).

Rasmusson, K. D., Hall, J. A., & Renlund, D. G. (2006). Heart failure epidemic boiling to the surface. *Nurse Practitioner, 31*(11), 12–21.

Renlund, D. G., & Taylor, D. O. (2002). *Cardiac transplantation. Textbook of cardiovascular medicine* (2nd ed.). Philadelphia: Lippincott Williams & Wilkins.

Riegel, B., Carlson, B., Kopp, Z., LePetri, B., Glaser, D., & Unger, A. (2002). Effect of a standardized nurse case-management telephone intervention on resource use in patients with chronic heart failure. *Archives of Internal Medicine, 162*, 705–712.

Rose, E. A., Gelijns, A. C., Moskowitz, A. J., Heitjan, D. F., Stevenson, L. W., Dembitsky, W., et al. (2001). Long term use of a left ventricular assist device for end-stage heart failure. *The New England Journal of Medicine, 345*(20), 1435–1493.

Sackner-Bernstein, J. D., & Mancini, D. M. (1995). Rationale for treatment of patients with chronic heart failure with adrenergic blockage. *Journal of the American Medical Association, 274*, 1462–1467.

Scandinavian Simvastatin Survival Study. (1994). Randomised trial of cholesterol lowering in 4444 patients with coronary heart disease: The Scandinavian Simvastatin Survival Study (4S). *Lancet, 344*, 1383–1389.

Sha, M., Ali, V., Lamba, S., & Abraham, W. (2001). Pathophysiology and clinical spectrum of acute congestive heart failure. *Reviews in Cardiovascular Medicine, 2*(2), S2–S6.

Silver, M. A. (1998). *Success with heart failure; Success and hope for those with congestive heart failure.* Reading, MA: Perseus Books.

Silverberg, D. S., Wexler, D., Sheps, D., et al (2001). The effect of correction of mild anemia in severe, resistant congestive heart failure using subcutaneous erythropoietin and intravenous iron: A randomized controlled study. *Journal of the American College of Cardiology, 37*, 1775–1780.

Sin, D. D., Fitzgerald, F., Parker, J. D., Newton, G., Floras, J. S., & Bradley, T. D. (1999). Risk factors for central and obstructive sleep apnea in 450 men and women with congestive heart failure. *American Journal of Respiratory and Critical Care Medicine, 160*, 1101–1106.

Smith, G. L., Masoudi, F. A., Vaccarino, V., Radford, M. J., & Krumholz, H. M. (2003). Outcomes in heart failure patients with preserved ejection fraction. *Journal of the American College of Cardiology, 41*(9), 1510–1517.

Stafford, R. S., & Radley, D. C. (2003). The underutilization of cardiac medications of proven benefit, 1990–2002. *Journal of the American College of Cardiology, 41*(1), 56–61.

Stevenson, L. W. (2003). Clinical use of inotropic therapy for heart failure: Looking backward or forward. *Circulation, 108*, 367–372.

Stewart, S., MacIntyre, S., Capewell, S., McMurray, J. J. (2003). Heart failure and the aging population: An increasing burden in the 21st century? *Heart.* <javascript:AL_get (this,'jour', 'Heart.');>. 2003 Jan; 89 (1): 49–53. <http://www.ncbi.nlm.nih.gov/entrez/utils/fref. fcgi?rid=3051&itool=AbstractPlus-def&uid=12482791&db=pubmed&url=http://heart.bmj.com/cgi/pmidlookup?view-long&pmid=12482791> <http://www.ncbi.nlm.nih.gov/entrez/utils/fref.fcgi?rid=3494&itool=AbstractPlus-nondef&uid=12482791&db=pubjed&url=http://www.pubmedcentral.nih.gov/articlerender.fcgi?tool=pubmed&pubmedid=12482791> Retrieved November 3, 2008 from http://www.ncbi.nlm.nih.gov/pubmed/1248279

Stratton, I. M., Adler, A. I., Neil, H. A., Matthews, D. R., Manley, S. E., & Cull, C. A. (2000). Association of glycaemia with macrovascular and microvascular complication of type 2 diabetes (UKPDS 35): Prospective observational study. *British Medical Journal, 321*, 405–412.

Tang, W. H., & Francis, G. S. (2005). The year in heart failure. *Journal of the American College of Cardiology, 46*(11), 2125–2133.

Teerlink, J. R., & Massie, B. M. (2003). Late breaking heart failure trials from the 2003 ACC meeting: EPHESUS and COMPANION. *Journal of Cardiac Failure, 9*(3), S163–S163.

United Network for Organ Sharing. (2006). *It is all about life.* Retrieved December 1, 2006, from http://www.unos.org

Weber, K. T. (1999). Aldosterone and spironolactone in heart failure. *The New England Journal of Medicine, 341*, 753–755.

Weinfeld, M. S., Chertow, G. M., & Stevenson, L. W. (1999). Aggravated renal dysfunction during intensive therapy for advanced chronic heart failure. *American Heart Journal, 138*, 285–290.

Whellan, D. J., Gualden, L., Gattis, W. A., Granger, B., Russell, S. D., Blazing, M. A., et al. (2001). The benefit of implementing a heart failure disease management program. *Archives of Internal Medicine, 161*, 2223–2228.

World Health Organization. (1968). *Nutritional anaemias: Report of a WHO scientific group.* Geneva, Switzerland: Author.

Yan, A. T., Bradley, T. D., & Liu, P. P. (2001). The role of continuous positive pressure in the treatment of congestive heart failure. *Chest, 120*, 1675–1685.

Young, J. B. (2001). New therapeutic choices in the management of acute congestive heart failure. *Reviews in Cardiovascular Medicine, 2*(2), S19–S24.

Caring for the Patient with Peripheral Vascular Disorders

Brenda McCulloch

Outcome-Based Learning Objectives

After studying this chapter, the learner will be able to:

1. Describe the risk factors and clinical findings in peripheral arterial disease.
2. Develop a nursing care plan for the patient with peripheral arterial disease.
3. Compare and contrast the clinical findings and management of Raynaud's disease and Buerger's disease.
4. Discuss signs and symptoms of common potential complications of endovascular repair and surgery of the aorta, and appropriate nursing interventions for each.
5. Identify the risk factors, diagnosis, medical management, and nursing care for deep venous thrombosis.
6. Explain the actions of commonly used anticoagulants and antiplatelet agents used for patients with peripheral arterial disease and nursing management of the patient receiving them.
7. Identify the risk factors, diagnosis, medical management, and nursing care for varicose veins.
8. Identify the risk factors, diagnosis, medical management, and nursing care for aortic aneurysm and aortic dissection.

VASCULAR DISORDERS include disorders of the arterial, venous, and lymphatic systems of the body. Peripheral arterial disease includes occlusive, aneurysmal (dilated), and vasospastic disorders affecting the arterial system of the neck, abdomen, and extremities. Peripheral venous disease predominantly involves the legs and is usually due to thrombosis or insufficiency of the veins. Lymphatic disease leads to abnormal fluid collection, edema, and fibrosis. These peripheral vascular diseases may cause serious complications such as loss of limb or even loss of life.

Anatomy and Physiology Review

The peripheral vascular system is a network of branching blood vessels carrying oxygenated blood from the heart to the tissues of the body and returning deoxygenated blood to the lungs. The peripheral vascular system is made up of arteries, veins, and capillaries. The lymphatics, also considered part of the peripheral vascular system, help maintain adequate blood volume by returning tissue fluid to the bloodstream.

Arteries consist of three distinct layers: the tunica intima, the tunica media, and the tunica adventitia. The innermost lining of the tunica intima consists of the endothelium, which provides a smooth surface for flowing blood. The middle layer, or the tu-nica media, is made up of smooth muscle cells, collagen, and elastin, providing elasticity and strength to the vessel. The tunica adventitia, or the outermost layer of the artery, consists of connective tissue and anchors the vessel in the surrounding tissue.

The largest artery in the body is the aorta. It ascends from the aortic root of the heart, passes through the chest, and descends into the abdomen, where it bifurcates about the level of the umbilicus. It branches off to various vital organs along the way. The major arteries are shown in Figure 43–1 ■ (p. 1324). Arteries branch sequentially from large to medium to the smallest arteries called arterioles, eventually reaching the capillary bed.

Capillaries are thin-walled structures consisting of a single layer of endothelial cells. Capillaries help facilitate rapid nutrient and waste product transport and removal. Venules are formed when several capillaries join together. Small venules form progressively larger veins and return blood from the periphery to the right atrium. The major veins are shown in Figure 43–2 ■ (p. 1325). Veins are thin-walled structures in contrast to arteries, and the venous system is comparably low pressure.

The lymphatic system is a network of vessels that transports lymph—a clear fluid that comes from the blood and bathes the tissues. Lymph contains water, protein, minerals, and white blood cells. Functions of the lymphatic system include the absorption of excess fluid and its return to the bloodstream, the

External carotid artery
Internal carotid artery
Vertebral artery
Brachiocephalic artery
Axillary artery
Ascending aorta
Brachial artery
Abdominal aorta
Superior mesenteric artery
Gonadal artery
Inferior mesenteric artery
Common iliac artery
External iliac artery
Digital arteries
Femoral artery
Popliteal artery
Anterior tibial artery
Posterior tibial artery

Common carotid arteries
Subclavian artery
Aortic arch
Coronary artery
Thoracic aorta
Branches of celiac trunk:
• Left gastric artery
• Common hepatic artery
• Splenic artery
Renal artery
Radial artery
Ulnar artery
Internal iliac artery
Deep palmar arch
Superficial palmar arch

FIGURE 43–1 ■ Major arteries of the body.

Dural sinuses

External jugular vein
Vertebral vein
Internal jugular vein
Superior vena cava
Axillary vein

Great cardiac vein

Hepatic veins
Hepatic portal vein
Superior mesenteric vein
Inferior vena cava

Ulnar vein

Radial vein

Common iliac vein
External iliac vein
Internal iliac vein

Digital veins

Femoral vein

Great saphenous vein

Popliteal vein

Posterior tibial vein

Anterior tibial vein

Peroneal vein

Subclavian vein

Right and left
brachiocephalic veins

Cephilic vein

Brachial vein

Basilic vein

Renal vein

Median cubital vein

Splenic vein

Inferior mesenteric vein

FIGURE 43–2 ■ Major veins of the body.

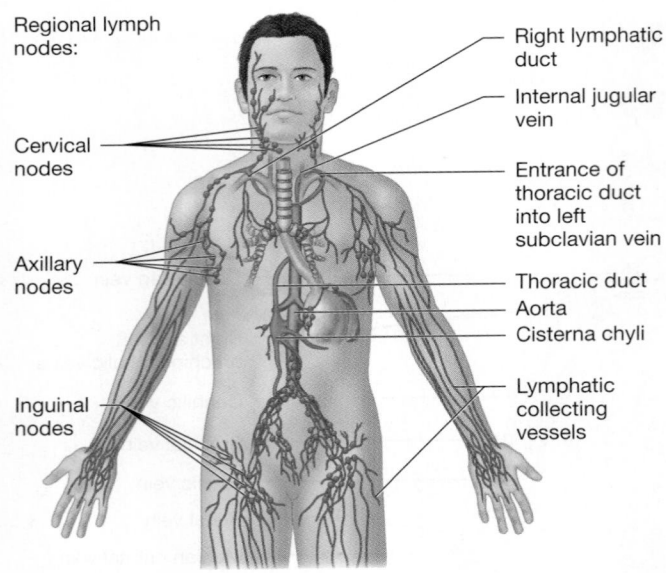

Regional lymph
nodes:

Cervical
nodes

Axillary
nodes

Inguinal
nodes

Right lymphatic
duct

Internal jugular
vein

Entrance of
thoracic duct
into left
subclavian vein

Thoracic duct

Aorta

Cisterna chyli

Lymphatic
collecting
vessels

FIGURE 43–3 ■ The lymphatic system.

absorption of fat, and an immune system function. The lymphatic system is shown in Figure 43–3 ■.

■ Peripheral Arterial Disease

The American College of Cardiology (ACC) and the American Heart Association (AHA) define **peripheral arterial disease (PAD)** as "vascular disease caused primarily by atherosclerosis and thromboembolic pathophysiological processes that alter the normal structure of the aorta, its visceral arterial branches, and the arteries of the lower extremities." This chronic and progressive disorder is a largely underrecognized and underdiagnosed disease affecting 12 million Americans (AHA, 2007). Atherosclerosis has been defined as the process of fatty substances, cholesterol, cellular waste products, calcium, and fibrin building up in the inner lining of an artery, resulting in plaque buildup and a narrowing of the lumen of the artery (AHA, 2008b). PAD is defined as the development of this atherosclerotic process at various levels in the aortic bifurcation and the iliac arteries and the lower extremities, including the femoral, popliteal, peroneal, and tibial arteries. Atherosclerosis is further discussed in Chapter 40 ⚭.

Etiology and Epidemiology

The incidence of PAD increases with age, and approximately 5% of people 55 and older and 20% of those 70 and older have signs and symptoms. The incidence in men is slightly higher than in women, and it is more common in the African American population (Criqui et al., 2005). The risk factors, similar to those of heart disease and stroke, include cigarette smoking, diabetes, hyperlipidemia, hypertension, elevated C-reactive protein, and hyperhomocysteinemia (Hirsch et al, 2006; Sontheimer, 2006). Screening for PAD is recommended for patients with exertional leg pain, patients over age 50 who have associated risk factors such as smoking and diabetes, patients who have had diabetes for more than 20 years, and all patients over the age of 70 (Oka, 2006).

Pathophysiology

Atherosclerosis is a disease process that occurs over many years, usually beginning in childhood. Lipids (fats) collect under the inner lining of damaged artery walls, eventually narrowing or blocking the artery and obstructing blood flow. Over time, this fatty tissue can erode the wall of the artery, diminish its elasticity, and interfere with blood flow. Plaque deposits also can rupture, causing debris to migrate downstream within an artery. Clots can also form around the plaque deposits, further interfering with blood flow and posing added danger if they break off.

Clinical Manifestations

Signs and symptoms of PAD may include intermittent claudication, muscle/limb weakness with use, absent or diminished pulses, poor hair growth, cool skin, resting limb pain, **paresthesia** (an abnormal physical sensation such as prickling, tingling, or numbness), and poor healing of sores or ulcers.

Intermittent claudication (IC), or exercise-induced leg pain, is the most common symptom of peripheral arterial disease (Oka, 2006). The word *claudication* is derived from the Latin word for limp, or *claudico*. Descriptors patients may use about their pain include aching, cramping, tiredness, and/or fatigue. This pain can occur in the buttocks, hip, thigh, or calf, depending on the portion of the arterial tree affected by atherosclerotic disease. The muscle group distal to a stenotic (narrowed) or occluded (completely blocked) artery is affected by the decreased circulation. For example, more proximal lesions, such as aortoiliac lesions, will produce the pain of intermittent claudication in the hip, buttocks, or thigh, whereas the pain from lesions lower in the femoral or popliteal arteries produces calf pain. When a muscle is at rest, the metabolic needs are minimal, and even diseased arteries can provide adequate blood supply to maintain perfusion. With exercise, such as walking, metabolic demands are increased, and the diseased arteries are unable to deliver the needed oxygen to the muscles or to dispose of the metabolic byproduct lactic acid. The buildup of lactic acid causes pain in the affected muscle group of the leg. When the walking ceases, or shortly afterward, the pain resolves and exercise may resume.

Reproducibility of the ischemic pain is a hallmark finding of intermittent claudication. The pain occurs consistently at the same distance, and after resting, the pain subsides and exercise may continue. Time and distance to claudication, for example, the number of blocks a patient can walk before the pain starts, is useful information to obtain during the nursing assessment and can be used as a subjective measure of improved function after intervention.

Intermittent claudication can remain stable for years, and walking can improve muscle endurance, especially if the patient stops smoking tobacco. The atherosclerotic process can, however, progress to a point at which the patient experiences pain in the foot at rest. Rest pain is a sign of severe ischemia or lack of sufficient oxygen supply to the tissues. It is characterized by pain in the forefoot and toes, usually worse at night when lying flat in bed, and can either awaken a person from sleep or prevent sleep altogether. Patients will usually be more comfortable with the leg in a dependent position, such as dangling over the edge of the bed or chair, because gravity can enhance arterial circulation. Narcotic pain medicines, such as opiates, are indicated but may not control the pain well due to the severe nature of the ischemic rest pain.

Ulceration (skin breakdown) can occur as a result of poor blood supply, pressure, or trauma to an ischemic limb. A non-healing area of tissue injury is prone to necrosis or gangrene and infection. Arterial ulceration accounts for about 20% of all leg ulcers and is most likely to occur at the distal-most point of arterial flow. The toes are a common site for arterial ulceration (Sieggreen & Kline, 2004a). In arterial ulcerations, the base is pale, gray, or yellowish in color with little drainage and regular borders. Wounds are described in detail in Chapter 67 🔗. The foot pulses are diminished or absent, and the skin is pale and cool to touch. The patient typically complains of a burning, throbbing pain, unless he has peripheral neuropathy, most commonly seen in long-standing diabetes. Pain management can be challenging, requiring narcotics for relief (Sieggreen, 2005a).

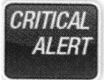 *Ongoing and regular nursing assessment of ulcerations and wounds in the patient with peripheral vascular disorders are essential, so that early signs and symptoms of infection can be detected and treated. Assessment finding in early localized infection can include low-grade temperature, warmth, tenderness, pain, edema, erythema, and new or increased drainage that may have a foul odor. If the patient develops mental status changes, hyperventilation, tachycardia, fever, chills, elevated white blood count, fatigue, or malaise, systemic infection (sepsis) may be occurring. These changes need to be reported to the health care practitioner.*

Laboratory and Diagnostic Procedures

The diagnosis of peripheral arterial disease is typically based on the patient's history; physical examination findings; and resting **ankle-brachial index (ABI)** results, which is a simple to perform, noninvasive test that detects peripheral arterial disease of the legs (Figure 43–4 ■). To determine the ABI, check the blood pressure of both arms with a Doppler and take the higher reading. Using a Doppler over the posterior tibial and dorsalis pedis pulses, determine the blood pressure in the foot, and take the higher of the two. It is the ratio of the highest ankle systolic pressure to the highest arm systolic pressure. An ABI ≥ 1.0 is considered normal, whereas a finding of ≤ 0.90 indicates peripheral arterial disease. A result less than 0.4 indicates severe arterial ischemia (Oka, 2006; Sieggreen, 2005a). The ABI may be falsely elevated in patients with diabetes (Olson & Treat-Jacobson, 2004). The Diagnostic Tests box (p. 1328) outlines the diagnostic tests performed for peripheral arterial disease.

Medical Management

According to the Seventh American College of Chest Physicians (ACCP) Conference on Antithrombotic and Thrombolytic Therapy (Hirsh, Guyatt, Alberts, & Schünemann, 2004), patients with PAD should receive lifelong antiplatelet therapy with aspirin. Aspirin has antithrombotic effects and inhibits platelet aggregation. Ticlopidine (Ticlid), clopidogrel (Plavix), and cilostazol (Pletal) or pentoxifylline (Trental) also may be indicated for some patients. Ticlopidine and clopidogrel are thienopyridine derivatives and inhibit adenosine diphosphate (ADP)-induced platelet aggregation. Cilostazol inhibits phosphodiesterase III, but its exact mechanism of action is not fully understood. It suppresses platelet aggregation and is a direct ar-

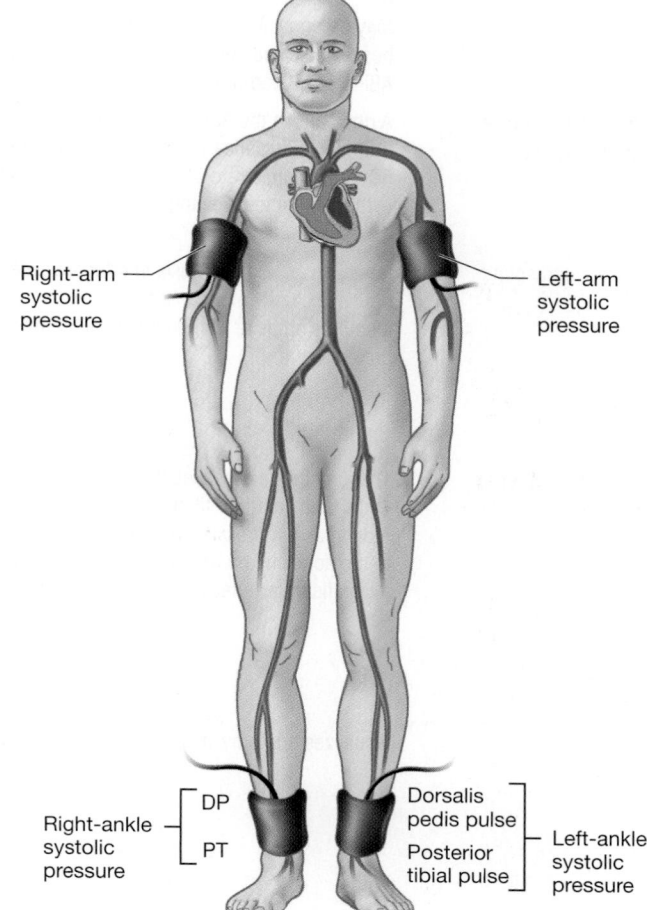

Right ABI	$\dfrac{\text{Average right ankle pressure}}{\text{Average brachial artery pressure}}$		Interpretation of ABI	
			>1.30	Noncompressible
			0.91–1.30	Normal
Left ABI	$\dfrac{\text{Average left ankle pressure}}{\text{Average brachial artery pressure}}$		0.41–0.90	Mild-to-moderate peripheral arterial disease
			0.00–0.40	Severe peripheral arterial disease

Right-arm systolic pressure

Left-arm systolic pressure

Right-ankle systolic pressure — DP / PT

Dorsalis pedis pulse / Posterior tibial pulse — Left-ankle systolic pressure

FIGURE 43–4 ■ Ankle-brachial index chart.

terial vasodilator. Pentoxifylline has weak antithrombotic effects and lowers blood viscosity (Lipsitz & Kim, 2005). Additionally, cardiovascular risk reduction strategies are important for the patient with PAD and include the use of beta-adrenergic blockers, angiotensin receptor blockers, and lipid lowering agents. The Pharmacology Summary feature (p. 1335) provides a detailed list of pharmacologic therapies used to treat PAD.

Endovascular repair is the treatment of vascular disease from inside the blood vessel (endoluminal). It started as percutaneous balloon angioplasty for peripheral arterial disease in the 1960s and was further refined for coronary artery intervention 10 years later. Today, various endovascular options are available including angioplasty, stenting, and radiation therapy. Percutaneous transluminal angioplasty (PTA) is indicated for those patients who are limited by their pain, and there is a reasonable likelihood of

DIAGNOSTIC TESTS for Peripheral Arterial Disease (PAD)

Test	Expected Abnormality	Rationale for Abnormality
Ankle-brachial index (ABI)	0.95–1.1 normal. ≤0.9 indicative of PAD. ≤0.4 advanced ischemic disease with impending loss of tissue. Segmental arterial pressures and ankle-brachial indexes (ABIs) can be falsely elevated if the patient has calcified, noncompressible arteries. May be unreliable in patients with diabetes or patients with heavily calcified vessels. Suspect calcified arteries if the ABI is > 1.3 and/or if the ankle pressure is > 300 mmHg.	Noninvasive. Simple to perform. Cost effective. ABI compares ankle pressure with arm pressure. ABI is obtained by dividing the ankle pressure by the highest brachial blood pressure. Can also be assessed before and after exercise testing to evaluate arterial insufficiency.
Treadmill exercise arterial studies	A decrease in the ABI following exercise indicates arterial insufficiency. Patients with intermittent claudication (IC) will demonstrate 20 mmHg or more decrease in ABI within 1 minute following exercise.	Measures the lower extremity circulation's response to exercise. May be used to index severity of disease and assess a patient's response to an intervention, as well as for follow-up.
Duplex ultrasound	Identifies areas of stenosis in arterial vessels and defines severity of stenoses. Identifies areas of turbulent flow and abnormal flow patterns.	Noninvasive. Widely available. Portable. Uses sound waves reflected off of moving red blood cells and other tissues to evaluate the flow of blood. The different vascular beds have unique waveforms and variations from normal indicate disease.
Segmental arterial pressures	This procedure assesses the femoral, popliteal, dorsalis pedis, and posterior tibial arteries. A decrease in pressure of 20–30 mmHg from one segment to the adjacent, more distal segment implies a significant arterial obstruction in the vessels between the cuffs.	Noninvasive. More time-consuming than ABI to perform. Provides information about the anatomic location of vascular disease. Uses a sphygmomanometer and a Doppler at several areas, or segments, of the lower extremity. Pressures are recorded at the thigh, below the knee, and at the ankle and are compared to the brachial blood pressure. The blood pressure in the leg should equal the blood pressure in the arm.
Angiography	Visualizes anatomy, areas of stenosis, and/or occlusion.	Definitive method for anatomic evaluation. Invasive. Requires vascular access. Requires iodine-based contrast administration. Requires x-ray exposure. Accurate diagnosis. Requires skilled interpretation.
Computed tomography (CT)	Visualizes anatomy, areas of stenosis, and/or occlusion.	Noninvasive. Requires iodine-based contrast administration. Requires x-ray exposure. Expensive. Requires skilled interpretation. Less readily available. Useful for patients who cannot undergo magnetic resonance testing (pacemakers, defibrillators).
Magnetic resonance imaging (MRI) and magnetic resonance angiography (MRA)	Visualizes anatomy, areas of stenosis, and/or occlusion. Provides excellent anatomic detail. May be inaccurate in arteries treated with metal stents.	Noninvasive. Does not require vascular access. Does not require iodine-based contrast administration. Expensive. Requires skilled interpretation. Not widely available. May be difficult for claustrophobic patients. Cannot be used for some patients (pacemakers, defibrillators).

improvement with intervention. PTA is an invasive percutaneous procedure that can be done using local anesthesia with sedation. It is performed in the interventional radiology suite or in the cardiac catheterization laboratory by vascular surgeons, interventional radiologists, and/or cardiologists. A balloon-tipped catheter is inserted into the arterial vasculature, usually the femoral artery, and positioned at the area of obstruction. The balloon is then inflated, disrupting the plaque and stretching the media of the artery, thereby enlarging the opening. Stents—tubular metal devices made of stainless steel, nitinol, or titanium—are inserted to act as a mechanical scaffolding to hold a vessel open in the diseased area. Stents and other interventional devices are further discussed in Chapter 39 ☺.

PTA is indicated for the treatment of arterial occlusive disease. It is most successful when performed for shorter lesions that are <5 cm (2 in.) in the iliac artery and <10 cm (4 in.) in the superficial femoral artery. PTA of lesions longer than these is more likely to restenose and also may be done in the smaller tibial vessels if the lesion is <2 cm (<1 in.)(Singh & Cousin, 2005). The long-term results of PTA for these lesions are less than optimal, but performing this procedure may allow enough improved blood flow to permit wound healing and/or limb salvage and to prevent or delay amputation.

Complications of percutaneous transluminal angioplasty are uncommon (2% to 5%) and include bleeding and hematoma at the access site, distal embolization, arterial dissection, or occlusion at the dilation site (Singh & Cousin, 2005). Other complications can include contrast allergy and contrast-induced renal failure. Following PTA, patients are discharged on aspirin and/or clopidogrel. Although the long-term results of this procedure are unknown at this time, PTA is rapidly becoming the initial intervention for revascularization of the lower extremities. The PTA technique is further discussed in Chapter 39 ☺. Other adjunctive interventional techniques such as lasers, cutting balloons, atherectomy devices, and thermal devices can be useful in the iliac, femoral, popliteal, and tibial arteries.

Gene therapy may emerge as a treatment for peripheral arterial disease. Gene therapy, or therapeutic angiogenesis, augments collateral artery development by stimulating capillary growth and enhancing blood flow. Three growth factors are being studied in clinical trials: acidic fibroblast growth factor (aFGF), basic fibroblast growth factor (bFGF), and vascular endothelial growth factor (VEGF). The agents are delivered via intravascular catheter or intramuscular injection. Additional study is needed to determine the most effective agent and dosing (Hirsch et al., 2006).

Surgical Management

Arterial bypass is the surgical revascularization procedure performed for debilitating peripheral arterial disease. Surgery is done when a patient has disabling claudication and/or limb-threatening ischemia due to blocked arteries in the lower extremities. These reconstructive procedures are performed by a vascular surgeon and involve bypassing areas of occlusion with the patient's own vein (autogenous) or a synthetic graft. Numerous types of surgical procedures are available for the treatment of peripheral arterial disease, depending on the level of the disease within the aorta and distal leg arteries, and include aortoil-

iac bypass; aortobifemoral bypass; iliac endarterectomy, or iliofemoral bypass; femorofemoral bypass; and femoropopliteal bypass, the most commonly performed arterial bypass (Figures 43–5 through 43–9 ■, pp. 1330–1331). Following arterial bypass surgeries, frequent and careful assessment of circulation to the leg and foot is essential. Pulselessness distal to the graft site indicates decreased or no blood flow.

Amputation may be indicated for uncontrolled infection, uncontrolled pain, extensive tissue loss, and in cases in which adequate revascularization cannot be accomplished (Sieggreen & Kline, 2004a). Chapter 57 ☺ discusses amputation.

■ Nursing Management

Peripheral arterial disease (PAD) is a systemic process, and the majority of patients with PAD also have coronary artery disease (Oka, 2006). When assessing patients for PAD, the nurse needs to obtain subjective information from the patient about the

FIGURE 43–5 ■ Aortoiliac bypass.

FIGURE 43–6 ■ Aortobifemoral bypass.

FIGURE 43–7 ■ Iliac endarterectomy.

Iliofemoral bypass graft

(a)

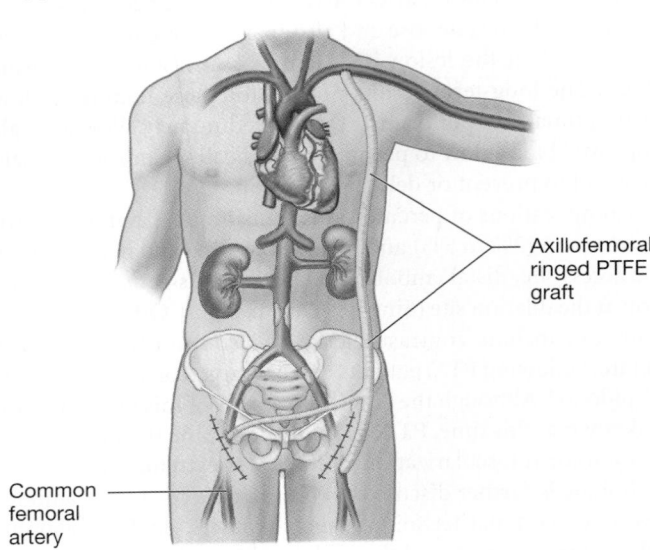

Axillofemoral bypass graft

(b)

FIGURE 43–8 ■ Femorofemoral bypass types: (A) iliofemoral bypass graft and (B) axillofemoral bypass graft.

present illness and symptoms, as well as the past medical history, especially previous cardiac diagnoses, such as myocardial infarction, hypertension, heart failure, and stroke. Obtaining information regarding the patient's history of smoking, hyperlipidemia, diabetes, family history, and activity level is important for planning necessary risk-reduction patient teaching.

Assessment

When assessing the patient for peripheral arterial disease, a thorough evaluation is essential. The measurement of bilateral blood pressure should be taken and documented. Differences between the right and left arms may indicate **aortic coarctation** (narrowing of the lumen of the aorta) or a lesion in a large vessel such as the subclavian artery. The carotid should be auscultated for vascular bruits, or abnormal sounds heard over areas of turbulent blood flow. The abdomen, flank area, and femoral arteries also should be auscultated for bruits. Additionally, the abdomen should be palpated to assess for signs of a pulsatile abdominal mass, indicating abdominal aortic aneurysm.

Assess fingers of each hand for capillary refill by depressing the nail until it blanches, then releasing it. The color should return to normal within 3 seconds (Sieggreen, 2005a). An Allen test (done to assess blood supply to the hand) should be performed to assess

for patency of the radial and ulnar arteries before the radial artery is cannulated for arterial blood gases or an arterial line insertion. To perform an Allen test, ask the patient to tightly clench her fist to produce blanching of the palm. While the fist is clenched, the nurse should occlude both the radial and the ulnar flow with his fingers or thumbs. While holding occlusive pressure, ask the patient to relax her fist and then release pressure over one of the arteries. Note the time it takes the palm to return to normal color. Repeat this while releasing pressure over the other artery. Failure of the color to return or a delay in return of color longer than 6 seconds is an abnormal finding that indicates narrowing or occlusion of the artery not being compressed. The Allen test also is discussed in Chapter 24 .

Peripheral pulses are assessed in a systemic manner. Pulses—including the brachial, radial, femoral, popliteal, dorsalis pedis, and posterior tibial—are assessed for presence, rate, equality, regularity, and strength and are assessed and recorded as absent,

FIGURE 43–9 ■ Femoropopliteal bypass.

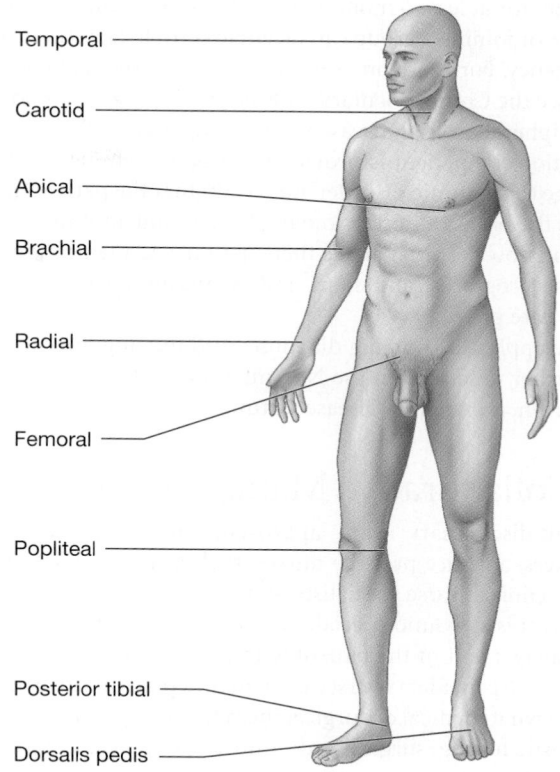

FIGURE 43–10 ■ Peripheral pulses.

diminished, normal, or bounding (Figure 43–10 ■). Occlusive arterial disease can impair blood flow and obliterate pulses in the affected extremity. Congenitally absent dorsalis pedis pulses occur in 10% of the population (Sieggreen, 2005a). Socks and shoes should be removed so that the feet can be inspected thoroughly. Note the color, temperature, and integrity of the skin, including any ulcerations. If ulcerations are present, ask the patient how long they have been there. Inspect the lower extremities for pallor, cyanosis, trophic changes—which include hair loss; thin, smooth, shiny skin; thick, brittle nails with or without fungal infection; tapering of toes or fingers—and any skin breakdown. Skin color should be examined carefully and with the patient in various positions. If arterial disease is present, pallor may be present when the legs are elevated. When patients hang their legs over the side of the exam table or bed, the legs become a deep red in color (dependent ruber) because blood is pooling in the arterioles. Hyperpigmentation of the skin is associated with venous, rather than arterial, disease. Additional physical findings may include decreased capillary refill, increased venous filling time, skin discoloration, decreased warmth, muscle or limb weakness with use, and poor healing. Pulse assessment is discussed in depth in Chapter 37 😔.

Nursing Diagnoses

Peripheral arterial disease results in decreased blood flow to the extremities causing tissue damage that can lead to ulceration, gan-

grene, infection, and amputation, causing disability and affecting quality of life. Many nursing diagnoses apply to these patients, including *Impaired Physical Mobility, Ineffective Tissue Perfusion, Impaired Skin Integrity, Readiness for Enhanced Comfort,* and *Deficient Knowledge.*

Interventions, Outcomes and Evaluation Parameters

Outcomes of nursing care of the patient with PAD include adequate vascular perfusion resulting in palpable pulses and warm extremities, sufficient tissue perfusion to promote healing of ulcers and reduce pain, and adequate knowledge of PAD so that the patient understands the disease process, how to manage her risk factors, and the current treatment plan.

It can be difficult to manage pain for some patients with PAD. The "six Ps" of arterial ischemia include the sudden onset of pain, pallor, pulselessness, poikilothermia (same as room temperature), paresthesia (sensation such as prickling, tingling, or numbness), and paralysis of the affected extremity. Patients with chronic pain may benefit from learning nonpharmacologic methods of pain control, such as intermittent rest periods while walking, guided imagery, and breathing exercises in addition to pharmacologic agents that may be prescribed.

Research has shown that regular structured exercise significantly improves the patient's functional capacity and is recommended as an initial treatment modality for patients with intermittent claudication. The most improvement was found when patients walked at least 30 minutes three times per week, walked until near maximal pain was reached, and continued this program for at least 6 months (Oka, 2006). Recruiting a walking partner or joining a group can facilitate compliance and increase consistency. For more on exercise as a way to help patients with PAD, see the Complementary and Alternative Therapies box.

Peripheral arterial disease is a lifelong disease. The more information the patient is provided, the better equipped he is to manage this chronic disorder. Be certain that the patient understands the basic pathophysiology of PAD, contributing risk factors and how best to manage them, prescribed medications and exercise programs, and signs and symptoms to report to his health care provider.

The applicable nursing diagnoses and nursing interventions are further described in the Nursing Process: Patient Care Plan for Peripheral Arterial Disease feature.

■ Collaborative Management

A multidisciplinary team approach, including health care providers, advance practice nurses, such as nurse practitioners and/or clinical nurse specialists, staff nurses, pharmacists, physical therapists, wound specialists, and dietitians, is important in the management of the patient with peripheral arterial disease. Health care providers oversee the patient's plan of care by determining what medical or surgical therapies are needed, including diagnostic testing, surgical procedures, and pharmacologic and nonpharmacologic interventions. Nurses implement the plan of care and are responsible for ongoing monitoring, assessment, and evaluation of interventions. Pharmacists oversee the patient's pharmacologic profile, assessing for appropriateness of dosing, drug-to-drug interactions, and potential adverse reactions of medications. Physical therapists are essential in assisting patients in gaining and maintaining strength and mobility, especially after surgical interventions.

Wound specialists are a helpful resource for those patients who have sustained injury or infection and have wounds on their extremities. The wound care specialist assists with specialized treatments and dressings that promote healing. Whenever a patient has skin breakdown or wounds, a nutritional assessment by a dietitian can provide helpful insight into the patient's nutrition and hydration status. The dietitian can offer recommendations for foods or supplements that may promote healing. Patients with advanced PAD, who are dealing with pain, altered mobility, and/or potential amputation, may also benefit from interactions with social workers and hospital chaplains.

Health Promotion

Patient and family education is important in managing the patient with PAD. Begin with educating the patient and family about pathophysiology, intermittent claudication, and the mechanism by which the pain sensation occurs with walking,

COMPLEMENTARY & ALTERNATIVE THERAPIES   Exercise

Description:
An active exercise program can improve symptoms in patients with early peripheral vascular disease. A variety of exercises can improve peripheral vascular circulation, such as the use of treadmills, elliptical machines, plus walking and organized exercise classes.

Research Support:
While exercise rehabilitation has been effective, it is an underused therapy. Currently, however, exercise rehabilitation is the subject of several large research projects. Such projects are investigating mechanisms by which exercise therapy could benefit people with claudication and are also directly comparing exercise with other therapies (Regensteiner & Stewart, 2006).

One nonrandomized controlled study assessed the clinical and cost effectiveness of a supervised exercise program (SEP) in two groups of patients with intermittent claudication (IC). Thirty-seven patients (median age 69) received conservative medical therapy (CMT). Thirty-three patients (median age 67) received CMT plus a 3-month program of graduated physical exercise for 60 minutes, three times each week. Both groups of patients were assessed prior to and at 6 months following treatment. Patients were assessed using the SF36 questionnaire, which included walking distances (PRWD), treadmill claudication and maximal distances (ICD and MWD), ankle brachial pressure indices (ABPI) pre- and postexercise, and quality of life (QoL). Prior to intervention, the two groups reports on these areas were very similar. Following treatment, CMT patients demonstrated no significant change in PRWD or ICD; however, they did record a small but significant improvement in MWD. The exercise program patients demonstrated significant improvement in PRWD, ICD, and MWD. The researchers concluded that, compared to the conservative medical treatment group, the exercise program group increased walking distances, improved QoL, and was a highly cost-effective treatment for IC (Lee, Mehta, Ray, Heng, McCollum, & Chetter, 2006).

An effective treatment to improve walking capacity for individuals with peripheral arterial disease (PAD) is supervised treadmill-walking training. Another study examined the effect of a supervised treadmill-walking program on calf-muscle strength and endurance in individuals with PAD over the course of two stages. The first stage, a 12-week period, was a nonexercise, within-subject control stage. The second stage, a 12-week period, was an exercise training stage. Twenty-two subjects trained in the laboratory, 3 sessions per week for 12 weeks. Researchers measured walking capacity, calf-muscle strength and endurance, and peak oxygen uptake at the baseline and the end of each stage. The supervised treadmill-walking program significantly increased calf-muscle strength and endurance. There were also significant improvements in walking capacity and peak oxygen uptake following the training program. The results showed a significant correlation between the improved calf-muscle endurance and walking capacity (Wang, Zhou, Bronks, Graham, & Myers, 2006).

References
Lee, H. L., Mehta, T., Ray, B., Heng, M. S., McCollum, P. T., & Chetter, I. C. (2006, December 1). A non-randomised controlled trial of the clinical and cost effectiveness of a supervised exercise programme for claudication. *European Journal of Vascular and Endovascular Surgery,* Epub ahead of print.

Regensteiner, J. G., & Stewart, K. J. (2006). Established and evolving medical therapies for claudication in patients with peripheral arterial disease. *Nature Clinical Practice. Cardiovascular Medicine, 3*(11), 604–10.

Wang, J., Zhou, S., Bronks, R., Graham, J., & Myers, S. (2006). Effects of supervised treadmill-walking training on strength and endurance of the calf muscles of individuals with peripheral arterial disease. *Clinical Journal of Sport Medicine, 16*(5), 397–400.

Assessment of Vascular Status

Subjective Data:

How far can you walk without stopping before you have pain?

Does leg discomfort or pain keep you from sleeping?

Does the pain wake you from your sleep?

Do you use an aid for walking such as a cane, walker, or wheelchair?

Do you need assistance to do your daily activities?

How many blocks (stairs) does it take to produce your pain?

Is the pain worse with elevation? Worse with cool temperatures?

Objective Data:

Peripheral pulses, temperature, and color of extremities.

Signs of ulceration, impaired healing, and trauma.

Walking distance.

Nursing Assessment and Diagnoses	Outcomes and Evaluation Parameters	Planning and Interventions with *Rationales*
Nursing Diagnosis: *Impaired Physical Mobility* related to disease and pain	**Outcome:** Adequate vascular perfusion. *Evaluation Parameters:* Palpable pulses. Warm extremities.	**Interventions and *Rationales:*** Teach patient importance of regular and structured ambulation *to enhance circulation and promote collateral development.* Teach patient importance of smoking cessation *to reduce the adverse vasospastic effects of nicotine.*

Assessment of Peripheral Vascular Perfusion and Skin Integrity

Subjective Data:

Do your extremities feel cold?

Do you have pain in your extremities?

Do you have any areas of sores or ulcerations?

Objective Data:

Assess extremities for perfusion: warmth, color, bilateral pulses, and edema.

Assess extent of wounds, if applicable.

Nursing Assessment and Diagnoses	Outcomes and Evaluation Parameters	Planning and Interventions with *Rationales*
Nursing Diagnoses: *Ineffective Peripheral Tissue Perfusion* and *Impaired Skin Integrity* related to diseased arteries	**Outcomes:** Sufficient tissue perfusion to perfuse extremities. Skin intact or ulcers healing. *Evaluation Parameters:* Warm extremities, palpable pulses, reduction in pain, and prevention of ulceration. No wounds or no signs of infection of the lower extremities. Demonstrates good foot care techniques. Eats well-balanced diet. Does not smoke or use smokeless tobacco.	**Interventions and *Rationales:*** Notify the heath care provider immediately if any of the six Ps of arterial ischemia occur abruptly: pain, pallor, pulselessness, poikilothermia (coldness), paresthesia, and paralysis of the affected extremity *to prevent tissue damage and loss.* Explain the importance of smoking cessation *to promote understanding and compliance.* Encourage patient to keep legs in dependent position *to enhance arterial perfusion.* Encourage patient to walk regularly and progressively *to promote conditioning and blood flow.* Teach patient risk factor modification *to prevent worsening of the atherosclerotic process.* Initiate wound care as directed *to promote healing and prevent infection and further tissue loss.* Teach patient to avoid trauma, heat, and sunburn to feet/legs *to prevent wounds and infection.* Teach patient about foot care: Keep feet and toes clean, mild soap only; dry well between toes; use lanolin emollient; inspect feet daily; clip toenails straight; wear proper fitting shoes; avoid walking barefoot. Avoid extremes in temperature to the extremities (hot baths, heating pads, cold water) *because sensation may be diminished.* Teach patient signs and symptoms of infection. Teach patient about good nutrition *to promote healing and prevent skin breakdown.* Smoking cessation counseling *to avoid detrimental effects of nicotine.*

Assessment of Discomfort

Subjective Data:

Do you have problems with pain when you are at rest?

Do you have problems with pain during activity, or when in a cold environment?

Where is the pain, what brings it on, and what makes it go away?

Is the pain getting worse?

Objective Data:

Use pain scale (0–10) to quantify pain.

Assess cultural and religious impact on patient's responses.

Assess the onset of increased pain to evaluate for disease progression or acute arterial obstruction.

(continued)

NURSING PROCESS: Patient Care Plan for Peripheral Arterial Disease—*Continued*

Nursing Assessment and Diagnoses	Outcomes and Evaluation Parameters	Planning and Interventions with *Rationales*
Nursing Diagnosis: *Readiness for Enhanced Comfort* related to tissue ischemia	**Outcome:** Comfort level maintained. **Evaluation Parameter:** Patient states adequate pain control has been obtained.	**Interventions and *Rationales*:** Assess pain so appropriate pain interventions can be initiated. Encourage periods of rest when walking *for pain relief*. Provide a supportive environment where patient is able to express pain level. Instruct patient to inform nurse if pain is not relieved. Use pain control measures before the pain becomes severe *to intervene early and with less medication*. Teach nonpharmacologic methods of pain control; that is, guided imagery and breathing exercises *to augment other treatments*.

Assessment of Knowledge of Self-Care Needs

Subjective Data:
How much do you smoke?
Are you willing to quit?
Has anyone explained your health problems to you?
How does this disease affect your daily life?
Are you able to care for yourself independently? If not, how much assistance do you need?

Objective Data:
Assess knowledge of disease process and progression, risk factors, and impact of smoking cessation.
Assess knowledge of patient's understanding of treatment plan, including medications and wound care, if indicated.
Assess needs for assistance.

Nursing Assessment and Diagnoses	Outcomes and Evaluation Parameters	Planning and Interventions with *Rationales*
Nursing Diagnosis: *Deficient Knowledge* of self-care needs and treatment plan related to tobacco use	**Outcome:** Adequate knowledge level. **Evaluation Parameters:** Patient/family are able to discuss disease process, risk factors, and current treatment plan. Verbalizes adherence to and compliance with treatment plan. Assistance is provided where deficiency exists. Patient/family verbalize understanding of disease, management, and prevention.	**Interventions and *Rationales*:** Provide factual information about diagnosis, treatment, risk factor modification, medications, and treatment plan *to ensure compliance*. Explain all procedures and allow patient to ask questions *to promote his understanding*. Provide information about care assistance *to ensure adequate help to provide a safe environment*.

and the important and ongoing need for risk factor modification. Compliance with the treatment plan is essential to help prevent the possible complications such as ulceration, gangrene, amputation, and myocardial infarction.

It is vital that the patient understand the risk factors that worsen PAD. Cigarette smoking is the single most important risk factor, and smoking cessation decreases the progression of PAD and improves the patient's functional status (Sieggreen, 2005a). Smoking cessation is fundamental because of the detrimental effects of tobacco on the arterial system. Endothelial function, lipoprotein metabolism, coagulation pathways, and platelet function are adversely affected by smoking tobacco. Smoking cessation decreases the risk of cardiovascular morbidity and mortality to levels that approach those who have never smoked. Abstinence from smoking as little as 8 weeks causes a gradual normalization of blood and plasma viscosity. Smoking cessation increases long-term survival in patients and decreases the amputation rate for patients with PAD (Cahall, 2004; Lu & Creager, 2004). The Agency for Healthcare Research and Quality (AHRQ, 2008) published "Treating Tobacco Use and Dependence," which is a set of evidence-based guidelines for treatment of nicotine dependence. The major steps of the AHCR guidelines to successful intervention are termed

the "five As": ask, advise, assess, assist, and arrange. Ask your patient if she smokes. If the patient is not a current smoker, ask about a past history of smoking or tobacco use. Advise her to quit in a clear, strong nonjudgmental manner. Assess her willingness to stop. Assist with counseling and pharmacotherapy. Arrange follow-up, preferably within the first week of quitting (Cahall, 2004).

Smokers trying to quit should receive pharmacotherapy and counseling. Approved medications for aiding smoking cessation include bupropion (Zyban), a nontricyclic antidepressant; nicotine replacement, available in gum, oral inhaler, nasal spray, and transdermal patch forms; and varenicline (Chantix), a drug that binds to nicotine receptors in the brain, blocking the full reinforcing effects of inhaled nicotine. Additionally, it slows the release of dopamine, which normally provides the feelings of pleasure from smoking. Nicotine replacement therapy is well tolerated and safe. The use of these agents doubles the rate of successful smoking cessation. Pharmacologic therapy alone is not enough; counseling also is needed. This can take the form of group meetings or individual behavioral therapy. Many hospitals and associations such as the American Lung Association and the American Heart Association offer ongoing group therapy for smoking cessation. For patients who are unwilling to quit, employ the five Rs: relevance of quitting, risks of smoking, rewards of quitting, roadblocks to quitting, and repetition. The Pharmacology Summary feature (p. 1337) outlines the pharmacologic agents that are used for smoking cessation.

For patients with diabetes, control of blood glucose is recommended. While there is no evidence that tight glycemic control (defined as a level of glycosylated hemoglobin < 7%) decreases intermittent claudication or critical limb ischemia, tight control of blood sugar levels has been demonstrated to decrease microvascular complications and the risk of myocardial infarction.

For PAD patients with hypertension, blood pressure control should be consistent with the evidence-based Seventh Report of the Joint National Committee on Prevention, Detection, Evaluation, and Treatment of High Blood Pressure (National Heart, Lung, and Blood Institute, 2004) recommendations of systolic blood pressure < 130 mmHg and diastolic blood pressure < 90 mmHg. Good blood pressure management has been found to decrease the risk of stroke, coronary artery disease, and mortality (Jacoby & Mohler, 2004). Chapter 21  discusses blood pressure guidelines and management.

Patients also need to be taught to avoid trauma, heat, and/or sunburn to their legs and feet to prevent the development of wounds and possible infection. Foot care information is essential for patients with PAD. The patient/caregivers need to be taught to keep feet and toes clean using mild soap. Thoroughly drying the feet and toes, and the use of a lanolin emollient regularly will help prevent skin breakdown. The feet need to be assessed daily for areas of potential pressure or breakdown. Toenails should be clipped straight across. Patients should not walk barefooted to avoid injury. Shoes should be properly fitted. Regular visits to a podiatrist may be beneficial for many patients with PAD.

Clinical trials have demonstrated the benefit of lipid lowering agents for patients who have PAD and coexisting cardiovascular and/or cerebrovascular disease (Gey, Lesho, & Manngold, 2004; Jacoby & Mohler, 2004; Rehring, Sandhoff, Stolepart, Merenich, & Whitton-Hollis, 2005). Normalizing lipid levels has been shown to reduce disease progression and the severity of intermittent claudication. According to the evidence-based National Cholesterol and Education Program III (2002 update), PAD patients should be managed the same as patients with coronary artery disease, whereby the primary goal is to lower the LDL-C levels to below 100 mg/dL. Coronary artery disease and dyslipidemia are discussed in Chapter 40.

Complications

Acute arterial ischemia occurs when trauma, thrombosis, or embolism abruptly stops or greatly diminishes arterial flow. The most common cause is thromboembolism from the atrial appendage that occurs in patients with chronic atrial fibrillation, or from the left ventricle in the patient following acute myocardial infarction or chronic heart failure due to clot formation from stagnant blood.

CRITICAL ALERT *Acute arterial ischemia is an emergency. Assessment findings in acute arterial ischemia include the "six Ps": pain, pallor, pulselessness, poikilothermia (coldness), paresthesia, and paralysis of the affected extremity.*

Immediate contrast angiography may be performed to determine the cause of the ischemia accurately. Management of the patient is dependent on the cause of the ischemia. If trauma, such as fractures or penetrating injuries, is the cause of the ischemia,

PHARMACOLOGY Summary of Medications to Treat Hypercholesterolemia

Medication Category	Action	Application/Indication	Nursing Responsibility
HMG-CoA reductase inhibitors (statins): Atorvastatin (Lipitor) Lovastatin (Mevacor) Simvastatin (Zocor) Pravastatin (Pravachol) Fluvastatin (Lescol) Rosuvastatin (Crestor)	Inhibits HMG-CoA reductase enzyme, thereby preventing the formation of cholesterol in the liver. Statins lower total cholesterol, LDL-C, and triglycerides while increasing HDL-C. Statins have also been connected with stabilizing *rupture-prone* atherosclerotic plaque (see the Etiology and Epidemiology of Carotid Artery Disease section later in this chapter), improving vasomotor tone, decreasing levels of proinflammatory proteins, decreasing factors that contribute to thrombosis, and improving myocardial perfusion.	Hypercholesterolemia.	Monitor liver function studies. Monitor lipid panel. Monitor patient for myalgias. Administer medication in the evening to take advantage of the fact that the liver produces more cholesterol at nighttime than during the day. Patients may experience abdominal discomfort from gas or constipation, which usually subsides with continued therapy. Rarely causes elevated liver enzymes and muscle soreness, pain, and weakness, which may require changes in dose or discontinuance of statin therapy. Monitor liver function tests (LFT).
Fibrates: Gemfibrozil (Lopid) Fenofibrate (TriCor)	Fibrates lower triglycerides and can increase HDL-C levels.	Hypercholesterolemia.	Monitor serum low density lipoprotein (LDL), very low density lipoprotein (VLDL), total cholesterol, and triglycerides. Monitor for gastrointestinal upset and bleeding. Assess for bloody stools, nosebleeds, cloudy or bloody urine, bleeding gums, and ecchymoses.

surgical repair is often required. Ischemia due to thrombosis or embolism is generally treated by immediate heparin therapy to stop the propagation of new clot and removal of the clot, either pharmacologically with catheter-based thrombolysis (streptokinase, urokinase, alteplase, reteplase) or mechanically with **embolectomy**, or mechanical removal of the clot.

Raynaud's Disease

Raynaud's disease (RD), first described in 1862, is an arterial vasospastic disorder caused by emotional distress or cold. The fingers and hands are most commonly affected, but the toes and feet also can be involved.

Etiology and Epidemiology

Individuals can have Raynaud's without any underlying disease associated with it, in which case it is called Raynaud's disease or primary Raynaud's. Or it can be part of another disease, in which case it may be referred to as Raynaud's phenomenon or secondary Raynaud's. Raynaud's disease is more prevalent in women and the typical onset is before age 30 (Mayo Clinic, 2006).

Pathophysiology

The precise pathophysiology of RD is unclear. It is caused by a transient spasm of the small cutaneous and subcutaneous arteries and arterioles, which results in a decreased blood flow to the affected extremity. Abnormalities of the endothelium may be responsible for initiating the vasospasm. RD is classified as primary or secondary. Primary or idiopathic RD has no known cause. Secondary RD is associated with many diseases, including connective tissue diseases, such as rheumatoid arthritis, scleroderma, and systemic lupus erythematosus (SLE), and myeloproliferative diseases, such as leukemia and polycythemia rubra vera. Occupational and environmental conditions are also associated with RD, particularly cold exposure, repetitive trauma, and vibration injury (chain saws, pneumatic drills).

Clinical Manifestations

The diagnosis of RD is made based on the patient's clinical manifestations. Usually during times of high stress/emotions or exposure to the cold, patients develop vasoconstriction of the arterial blood vessels causing cooling of the temperature of fingers, toes, and earlobes. As the temperature decreases, the skin color of the affected parts changes. There are three color changes that occur with RD (1) pallor (whiteness) in response to the vasospasms; (2) cyanosis (blue) due to the reduction of oxygenation of the blood; and (3) finally rubor (redness) when the vasospasms stop and the arterial blood returns (Reilly & Snyder, 2005). Other factors that may trigger ischemia include smoking, alcohol use, caffeine intake, cocaine, and amphetamines. The vascular changes also cause paresthesia to the affected parts. The episode ends when the arterial spasm relaxes and perfusion normalizes. Digits appear normal between attacks.

Diagnosis

A cold stimulation challenge may be administered to induce symptoms. The patient is exposed to cold temperatures by placing the hands in a basin of cold water. Patients with Raynaud's disease will quickly develop pallor and possibly cyanosis. When warmed, the patients experience redness and pain in their hands.

Nail-fold capillaroscopy can be performed to distinguish between primary and secondary Raynaud's disease (Reilly & Snyder, 2005). The nail bed is examined using a stereoscopic microscope or handheld ophthalmoscope to assess for the presence of enlarged, distorted, or deformed capillaries that may be associated with secondary RD.

Medical Management and Surgical Management

It is critical for the health care provider to obtain a complete history of the patient's past medical history to find out whether the patient has other connective tissue disorders, such as SLE and scleroderma. The signs and symptoms are vague: (1) malaise, (2) light sensitivity, (3) joint pain, and (4) skin lesions. Because the symptoms are vague, it is difficult to diagnosis. Treatment is based on signs and symptoms presented. Nonpharmacologic management of RD is directed toward avoiding known stressors (cold, emotional stress); controlling exposure to extremes in climate; dressing warmly in cold weather; and limiting tobacco, caffeine, and alcohol intake. Some patients may benefit from learning relaxation techniques. Regular physical exercise is important because it improves circulation and warms the body temperature. If pharmacologic treatment is needed to manage symptoms, the dihydropyridine calcium channel blocking agents, such as nifedipine, isradipine, amlodipine, and nicardipine, are used. Other agents that have been used to treat RD include prazosin (Minipress), fluoxetine, losartan, pentoxifylline, captopril, and topical nitroglycerin.

Surgical **sympathectomy**, removal of the sympathetic ganglia, has been performed for patients with severe symptoms of RD. It interrupts sympathetic nervous system stimulation to the affected vessels, decreasing vasoconstriction and spasm. Following this procedure, patients may experience relief of pain, decreased tissue loss, and improved wound healing. There is no cure for RD.

Complications

Complications of RD are not common. Digital ulcers may occur as a result of the disorder. Most digital ulcers will heal over several weeks to months with conservative therapy, provided the patient cares for his hands and/or feet carefully and seeks prompt treatment for signs and symptoms of infection. Surgery may be required when there is the threat of loss of a digit because of a nonhealing ulceration or gangrene.

Nursing Management

Careful history taking is important when assessing the patient with Raynaud's. Determine the patient's particular stressors and characteristics of attacks such as pain, numbness, color changes of the extremities, and frequency of attacks. The skin of the hands and toes should be assessed for the presence of ulcers and gangrene. Some medications, such as beta-adrenergic blockers, ergot alkaloids, and hormones, can precipitate episodes of vasospasm. It is important to obtain a detailed list of medications that the patient takes to assess for drug-induced vasospasm.

PHARMACOLOGY Summary of Medications for Smoking Cessation

Medication Category	Action	Application/Indication	Nursing Responsibility
Antidepressants Nontricyclic: Bupropion (Zyban, Wellbutrin)	Antidepressant neurochemical effect unknown.	Smoking cessation (off-label use for addiction to smokeless tobacco), depression.	Monitor for adverse effects: dry mouth, insomnia, sweating, blurred vision, weakness, vomiting, constipation, weight loss, or gain. Monitor for increased seizure potential if increasing dose, dose > 300 mg/day, or in presence of seizure disorder; head trauma history. Monitor for treatment-induced hypertension. Warn patient to avoid alcohol (increases seizure risk) and not to stop drug abruptly. Check hepatic and renal function for dose determination.
Tricyclic: Nortriptyline (Pamelor)	Antidepressant effect may be due to inhibition of norepinephrine reuptake.	Depression, smoking cessation (off-label use).	Monitor for adverse effects: orthostatic hypotension, urinary retention, constipation, confusion, or dry mouth. Monitor vital signs when initiating drug. Withhold and notify health care provider for systolic BP decrease is > 20mmHg or sudden increase in pulse. Be aware of drug interactions (alcohol, antihypertensives, hypnotics, and others). Monitor for adverse reactions. Contraindicated in patients during or within 14 days of treatment with monoamine oxidase inhibitor (MAOI).
Anxiolytic Alprazolam (Xanax)	Central nervous system (CNS) depressant effect may be due to limbic, thalamic, or hypothalamic action.	Anxiety disorders; short-term relief from anxiety symptoms.	Monitor for adverse effects: drowsiness, insomnia, and paradoxical excitement. Be aware of drug interactions (alcohol, CNS depressants, anticonvulsants, cimetidine, and others). Monitor for altered drug effect. Be aware drug should be reduced gradually when discontinued.
Smoking Deterrents Nicotine: Gum (Nicorette) Lozenge Transdermal patch (Habitrol, NicoDerm, Nicotrol) Nasal spray (Nicotrol NS) Vapor inhaler (Nicotrol inhaler)	Replaces nicotine.	Symptom reduction of nicotine-dependent smoker during cigarette withdrawal.	Monitor for adverse effects: headache, dizziness, and nausea. Monitor for route-specific adverse effects: gum: tongue, mouth, throat irritation; jaw pain; patch: skin irritation; nasal spray: nasal, throat irritation, or rhinorrhea. Be aware of drug interactions (theophylline, insulin, acetaminophen, and others). Monitor for decreased drug efficacy. Warn patient against smoking cigarettes or using smokeless tobacco while on replacement therapy.
Varenicline (Chantix)	Provides some nicotine effects through nicotine receptor agonist activity; blocks pleasurable effects of nicotine.	Nicotine withdrawal symptoms.	Monitor for adverse effects: nausea, diarrhea, anxiety, headache, sleep disturbance, arthralgia, and lethargy. Monitor for mood disturbances (depression, suicidal ideation).

Because the treatment of RD is supportive and there is no cure, patient and family teaching is very important to assist the patient in preventing and managing vasospastic episodes. It is important that patients clearly understand the disease process to avoid aggravating and alleviating events, such as cold environments and emotional stress. Smoking cessation counseling is essential. Patients may benefit from referrals for stress management class or relaxation techniques.

Health Promotion

Most patients have only mild to moderate symptoms and can manage sufficiently by avoiding exposure to cold and tobacco. Teach the patient to wear warm clothes and gloves, mittens, and/or hand warmers when required to be in cold environments. Exposure to cigarette smoke can cause symptoms. Patients with RD should avoid oral contraceptives, beta-adrenergic blockers, and ergot preparations because they have been known to exacerbate the symptoms of RD. Behavioral modification therapy may be helpful for some patients who have an emotional component to their RD.

◼ Buerger's Disease (Thromboangiitis Obliterans)

Buerger's disease, or **thromboangiitis obliterans (TAO)**, is a nonatherosclerotic inflammatory vascular disease first described in 1879. It causes thrombus formation and occlusion bilaterally of the small vessels of the feet and hands. It is most common in young men who are heavy cigarette smokers.

Etiology and Epidemiology

The incidence of TAO has decreased overall in the last 50 years, but the incidence is increasing in women, most likely because of increased cigarette smoking among women (Arkkila, 2006). Although the cause of TAO is unknown, it is clearly associated with tobacco exposure.

Pathophysiology

In TAO, recurring inflammation of intermediate and small arteries and veins occurs predominantly in the lower extremities. This results in thrombus formation leading to occlusion of the vessels. Buerger's disease is thought to be an autoimmune disease. Immune assessment is discussed in Chapter 59 ◎ and immune disorders are discussed in Chapter 60 ◎ .

Clinical Manifestations

Patients typically present with distal toe and/or finger ischemia and may have foot claudication. In advanced stages, ulcerations and gangrene of the fingers and toes may be present. Patients may also have superficial thrombophlebitis of the affected limb. Paresthesias of the feet and hands may also be present.

Diagnosis, Medical Management, and Surgical Management

There is no specific diagnostic testing for TAO, although an abnormal Allen test may be present. The diagnosis of TAO is based on clinical findings, and criteria for its diagnosis include smoking history, onset before age 50, ischemic ulcers, and pain. There is no cure for TAO. The primary treatment is directed toward smoking cessation and avoidance of secondhand smoke. Various medications are used, including steroids, antiplatelet agents, and anticoagulants, but there is no strong evidence of their effectiveness. Surgical revascularization is typically not feasible, although sympathectomy may be an option. Toe and finger ulceration, nonhealing wounds, and gangrene can occur, and amputation is required in up to 25% of patients (Arkkila, 2006). Chapter 67 ◎ discusses the incidence and care of ulcerations and non-healing wounds.

Complications

Complications of TAO include progressive ischemia and gangrene, leading to amputation. Infection of wounds can occur and patients can become septic. On rare occasion TAO also can affect other parts of the vasculature and cause occlusion of the cerebral, coronary, renal, splenic, or mesenteric arteries.

◼ Nursing Management

Supportive nursing care of the patient with TAO is indicated. Smoking cessation counseling is essential for these patients, because continued smoking will keep the disease process progressing. Patients who continue smoking will likely require amputation. Nursing assessment of the patient with TAO is similar to that of the patient with peripheral arterial disease. The extremities should be closely assessed for abnormal findings such as pale or cyanotic skin, diminished or absent pulses, or skin ulcerations. Outcomes of care are directed toward improving circulation to the affected areas and to teach the patient to protect the limbs from injury and infection. Pain management and wound management may be indicated for patients with advanced stages of the disease. Pain management is discussed in detail in Chapter 15 ◎ and wound management in Chapter 67 ◎ .

Health Promotion

Smoking cessation and the avoidance of all tobacco products, including chewing tobacco, are essential. Patient education is needed to teach the importance of avoiding injury to the feet and hands. Additionally, avoiding cold environments and medications that may cause vasoconstriction is required. If ulceration occurs, close monitoring for signs of infection is important to avoid subsequent gangrene and amputation. Skin assessment is discussed in Chapter 65 ◎ and wound management in Chapter 67 ◎ .

◼ Thoracic Outlet Syndrome

The thoracic outlet is a space between the thorax and the clavicle through which the main blood vessels and nerves pass from the neck and thorax into the arm. Thoracic outlet syndrome (TOS) is a rare disorder, more common in females, in which there is compression of the nerves and arteries of the arm in the thoracic outlet. It may be due to an extra first rib or an old fracture of the clavicle, which reduces the space of the outlet. Compression may occur with repetitive activities that require the arms to be held overhead.

Clinical manifestations include pain, paresthesias, muscular weakness and fatigue or swelling, and coldness in the arm and hand. The symptoms can be confused with those of other conditions, such as a herniated disk in the neck, carpal tunnel syndrome, and even bursitis of the shoulder.

The diagnosis of thoracic outlet syndrome is usually based on history and physical examination. Many patients will have history of an accident or trauma. To diagnose TOS, the elevated arm stress test (EAST) may be conducted. This is done by having the patient place both arms in 90 degrees of abduction and external rotation, then opening and closing her hands for 3 minutes. A positive EAST study is reproduction of symptoms (Chang, 2008). Other noninvasive testing that may be useful in diagnosing thoracic outlet syndrome includes cervical and chest x-ray to assess skeletal abnormality, color flow duplex scanning, MRI, and ulnar nerve conduction or electromyography. Invasive testing that may be performed includes an arteriogram and venography.

Treatment of TOS is initially directed toward nonsurgical interventions including physical therapy and pain management strategies. Physical therapy involves specific exercises aimed at strengthening the supporting muscles of the thoracic outlet structures. Muscle relaxants, nonsteroidal anti-inflammatory drugs such as aspirin or ibuprofen, moist heat, massage, analgesics, and short courses of steroids may be recommended. Surgical decompression of the thoracic outlet to remove the point of compression is indicated for patients with severe symptoms that limit their lifestyle.

Carotid Artery Disease

Stroke is a significant cause of death and disability in the United States and is the second leading cause of death worldwide. Stroke rates are higher for women and African Americans. Risk factors for stroke include hypertension, smoking, diabetes, atrial fibrillation, hyperlipidemia, physical inactivity, obesity, and illicit drugs, such as cocaine (American Stroke Association, 2006).

Etiology and Epidemiology

Stroke occurs when there is a sudden cessation of blood flow to an area of the brain resulting in cell death and loss of function to the involved area of the brain. The right and the left carotid and vertebral arteries supply blood to the brain.

Pathophysiology

The most common cause of stroke is atherosclerosis. The atherosclerotic process has previously been described in this chapter and in Chapter 40. The bifurcation of the carotid artery and its branches is a common site for vascular turbulence and atherosclerotic plaque buildup, causing an obstruction to blood flow. When these plaques rupture, thrombosis can occur, causing altered blood flow to the area. This process can cause small thrombic clots to form, embolize, and occlude the carotid artery or branches of the carotid artery causing stroke.

Clinical Manifestations

A stroke may be preceded by a **transient ischemic attack (TIA)**. A TIA is a "warning stroke" or "mini-stroke" that produces stroke-like symptoms but no lasting damage. It occurs when the blood supply to part of the brain is briefly interrupted. Symptoms include numbness or weakness in the face, arm, or leg, especially on one side of the body; confusion or difficulty in talking or understanding speech; trouble seeing in one or both eyes; and difficulty with walking, dizziness, or loss of balance and coordination, which usually disappear within 1 to 5 minutes (American Stroke Association, 2006).

Neurological deficits associated with a stroke are dependent on where the damage to the brain has occurred. The clinical manifestations may include the abrupt onset of severe headache, confusion, transient monocular blindness, blindness, changes in speech such as slurring of words, and mono- or hemiparesis. Chapter 30 provides a complete description of the pathophysiology, clinical manifestations, and treatment of stroke.

Diagnosis

Carotid artery disease may initially be found on physical exam when a bruit is auscultated over the artery. Patients who are experiencing clinical manifestations of carotid artery disease are typically referred for noninvasive testing with duplex ultrasound. Patients who are found on ultrasound to have significant lesions and are symptomatic may be further referred for invasive studies. Magnetic resonance imaging and/or computed tomography angiography (CTA) are replacing contrast angiography, once the gold standard for defining anatomy.

Medical Management

Medical therapy for patients with carotid disease includes antiplatelet therapy with aspirin. Endovascular therapy for carotid disease may be an option for patients who are not otherwise surgical candidates. It is a controversial procedure that requires skilled operators and careful patient selection. Carotid artery balloon angioplasty and stenting can be performed in the neurointerventional radiology laboratory or the cardiac catheterization laboratory. Using local anesthesia and minimal sedation, a balloon or stent is placed percutaneously across the lesion in the carotid artery to restore flow. Various cerebral protection devices have been developed and are being used to filter embolic particles that can break off during angioplasty or stent placement to decrease the risk of complications.

Surgical Management

Standard treatment for symptomatic carotid disease is **carotid endarterectomy (CEA)**, a surgical repair of carotid artery disease, which has been performed in this country since 1953. It is a commonly performed procedure done to prevent stroke in which atherosclerotic plaque and fatty deposits are removed from the carotid artery to restore blood flow to the brain. Operative stroke-death mortality has been reported to be 2.3% up to 7.4% for high-risk patients with severe coronary artery disease, chronic obstructive lung disease, and renal disease (Sullivan, 2005). Complications of CEA include perioperative stroke, blood pressure instability, cranial nerve injury, infection, restenosis, and death. Hyperperfusion syndrome, a rare complication of CEA, may occur in patients with bilateral carotid stenosis; it is the occurrence of ipsilateral temporal or frontal throbbing headache with or without nausea, vomiting, ipsilateral focal seizures, or focal neurological deficit without evidence of cerebral infarction (Abou-Chebl et al.,

2006). Contraindications to carotid endarterectomy surgery include acute hemorrhagic or major stroke, anatomy not accessible to the surgeon, and other technically challenging patients, such as those who have had prior radical neck dissection, radiation therapy, or severe cervical arthritis (LaMuraglia & Nigri, 2004).

Nursing Management

Following carotid endarterectomy, patients are monitored in various inpatient settings including neurological observation units, step-down units, or intensive care units.

Assessment

Beginning with assessment, the nursing process guides the care for the postoperative patient. In the immediate postoperative period, frequent cardiovascular and neurological assessments are done to monitor for complications such as carotid artery occlusion, cerebral embolization, or cranial nerve damage as well as incision site assessment and donor site assessment, if a venous graft was used. Frequent neurological assessment is aimed at assessing for cerebral ischemia, which may be evidenced by agitation, lethargy, visual disturbances, slurred speech, and paresthesias or paralysis. Nursing assessment includes facial symmetry, ability to swallow, tongue deviation, and shoulder strength to evaluate cranial nerve function.

Careful assessment of the patient's mental status, level of consciousness, pupillary responses, and motor/sensory function is needed to assess for perioperative stroke. In the event of stroke, motor and sensory changes would be noted on the contralateral side of the body. CEA may also interfere with cranial nerve function, which can be temporary or permanent. To assess for cranial nerve damage, observe for difficulty with speech, dysphagia, and upper airway obstruction, which may indicate hypoglossal nerve damage. Monitor facial muscles to assess the facial nerve. Ask the patient to shrug his shoulders and raise his arms to assess the accessory nerves. Loss of gag reflex and hoarseness may indicate damage to the vagus nerve or the recurrent laryngeal nerve. Nursing intervention includes notifying the health care provider promptly of changes in neurological status.

Nursing Diagnoses

The nursing diagnoses related to the postoperative carotid endarterectomy patient include:

- *Tissue Perfusion, Ineffective, Peripheral*
- *Risk for Infection*
- *Gas Exchange, Impaired.*

Interventions, Outcomes, and Evaluation Parameters

Careful monitoring for respiratory obstruction from edema or expanding hematoma at the surgical site is essential. If respiratory distress develops in the postoperative phase, nursing interventions include elevating the head of the bed, loosening the neck dressing if it appears to be constricting the neck, and administering oxygen as ordered. Stridor or deviation of the trachea from midline indicates an impending respiratory emergency and immediate intervention is required. Notification of the health care provider is done while suction supplies and equipment and a tracheostomy tray are being assembled. Outcomes of care include prevention of respiratory distress due to edema, and evaluation parameters include normal oxygen saturation levels, arterial blood gases, and no increased work of breathing.

Close monitoring of blood pressure is required in the early postoperative phase. Hypotension can occur because of stimulation of the carotid sinus during surgery. Hypertension can lead to bleeding or damage the arterial reconstruction.

Following CEA, patients are maintained on daily aspirin. The Patient Teaching & Discharge Priorities box provides discharge priorities for patients following carotid artery procedures. Nursing management of the stroke patient is discussed in detail in Chapter 30 .

PATIENT TEACHING & DISCHARGE PRIORITIES for Carotid Artery Procedures

Need	Teaching

Knowledge of disease process	Home care needs include verbal and written instructions for:
	    Treatment plan, including wound care
	    Continued risk factor modification
	    Follow-up care
	    Activity instruction.

Understanding of medications	Teach the purpose, dose, and possible adverse effects of all medications to increase compliance and prevent over/underdosing.

Reportable clinical manifestations	Instruct patient/family to report:
	    Signs and symptoms of stroke, including sudden onset severe headache, visual disturbances or visual loss, weakness or paralysis of arms and/or legs
	    New onset fever, signs of wound infection.

Family/support system	Assess availability of, knowledge of, and compliance with treatment plan. Assess respite needs and resources. Assess discharge placement needs: home, skilled nursing care, rehabilitation facility, extended care facility. Assess for need for professional home health needs. Assess need for follow-up appointments.

Health Promotion

Patient teaching includes the importance of continuing daily aspirin, adequate blood pressure control, and risk factor modification. Patients and their families need to be instructed about reportable signs and symptoms, which include unilateral headache, neurological deficits, and seizure activity.

Subclavian Steal Syndrome

Subclavian steal syndrome is a form of a transient ischemic attack (Chapter 30) that is caused by an obstruction of an extracranial artery that impairs blood flow to the vertebrobasilar arterial system. If the subclavian artery is occluded near its origin, the flow of blood in the vertebral artery is diverted or stolen from the basilar artery in the brain and shunted into the brachial circulation. Subclavian steal syndrome also can occur in the patient following coronary artery bypass grafting when a **stenosis**, or narrowing in the subclavian artery, is not corrected prior to use of the internal mammary artery as a bypass, causing the patient to have recurrent angina.

Clinical manifestations include complaints of dizziness, syncope, and vertigo due to the decreased circulation of the posterior cerebral circulation. Arm claudication also may occur. A difference in blood pressure between the right and left arm is found. It would be reduced on the same side as the subclavian stenosis. Blood pressure difference greater than 20 mmHg suggests subclavian stenosis. A carotid bruit may be audible as well.

Repair of the subclavian stenosis may be required for the symptomatic patient. Balloon angioplasty and stenting or carotid-subclavian bypass and axilloaxillary bypass may be done, depending on the patient's anatomy and surgical risk (Eisenhauer & Shaw, 2004).

Renovascular Disease

Renovascular diseases are disorders of the arteries of the kidneys, which result in systemic hypertension and kidney dysfunction.

Etiology and Epidemiology

Two disorders primarily affect the renal arteries: atherosclerotic renal artery stenosis (AS-RAS) and fibromuscular dysplasia (FMD). FMD is more common in girls and women between the ages of 15 and 50 and frequently involves the main renal artery and its branches (American Urological Association [AUA], 2002; Porth, 2007).

Atherosclerosis accounts for approximately 70% to 90% of renovascular disease (AUA, 2002). It is the cause of 1% to 2% of all cases of hypertension, making it the most common cause of secondary hypertension (Porth, 2007). The prevalence of AS-RAS increases with age, particularly in patients with diabetes, aortoiliac occlusive disease, coronary artery disease, or hypertension. However, many cases are never detected because hypertension or kidney failure does not develop (AUA, 2002). Hypertension is discussed in detail in Chapter 21 .

Pathophysiology

Patients with AS-RAS have progressive abnormal narrowing of the renal artery that occurs in 51% of the cases within 5 years after the initial diagnosis has been made. Anywhere from 3% to 16% of the arteries eventually become totally blocked, and shrinkage of the kidney occurs in approximately 20% of patients. The resulting hypertension is caused by reduced renal blood flow and activation of the renin-angiotensin-aldosterone mechanism. The diminished blood flow to the kidney causes a release of excessive amounts of renin, which increases the circulating levels of angiotensin II. Angiotensin II vasoconstricts the peripheral vessels and acts as a stimulus to increase aldosterone levels and sodium retention. The result of all of these changes is systemic hypertension. One or both kidneys may be affected (Porth, 2007). The renin-angiotensin-aldosterone system is discussed in detail in Chapter 21 .

Fibromuscular dysplasia is a noninflammatory, nonatherosclerotic disease that also can affect the renal arteries, which causes alterations in the intimal and/or medial layer leading to obstruction of blood flow and accounts for 10% to 25% of renovascular disease. This disorder is seen almost exclusively in women (Caulfield, Fernando, & Rosenfield, 2005; Porth, 2005). Unlike AS-RAS, FMD rarely leads to total renal artery blockage. The cause of FMD is unknown; a genetic predisposition, smoking, hormonal factors, and disorders of the blood supply to the renal artery itself are some of the causal theories associated with the disease.

Clinical Manifestations

Patients with renovascular disease present with significantly elevated blood pressure that is difficult to control, although it is not readily distinguishable from other forms of hypertension. Certain classic features such as lack of family history of hypertension, recent onset of hypertension, or onset of hypertension before age 50 are more suggestive of renovascular hypertension than of other forms of high blood pressure. It is frequently higher than 180/100 mmHg and may be resistant to two or more medications.

Diagnosis

The goal of diagnostic studies is to assess perfusion to the kidneys and the renin-angiotensin-aldosterone system. Duplex ultrasonography is recommended as the screening test to establish the presence of renal artery stenosis. CTA and magnetic resonance angiography (MRA) may also be used as screening tests. Contrast angiography may be performed to assess the renal-arterial vasculature. Angiographic findings of fibromuscular dysplasia demonstrate a very characteristic "string of beads" appearance in the lumen of the artery (Dickinson, Krishnan, Houlihan, & Walker, 2004).

Medical and Surgical Management

Medical therapy of atherosclerotic renal artery disease is directed toward careful blood pressure control, antiplatelet therapy, lipid management, smoking cessation, and weight reduction. Angiotensin-converting enzyme (ACE) inhibitors may be indicated in the presence of renal stenosis (Porth, 2007).

Endovascular therapy may be an option for select patients. Patients with fibromuscular dysplasia have good outcomes with renal angioplasty, obtaining improvements or cure in over 90% of patients. Percutaneous ballooning and stenting of renal artery atherosclerotic lesions have success rates of near 100% when performed by an experienced health care provider (Dickinson et al., 2004). Complications of renal artery angioplasty and stenting may include cholesterol embolization, vessel rupture, renal infarction, temporary deterioration in renal function, retroperitoneal hemorrhage, and access site vascular complications such as bleeding and hematoma (Dickinson et al., 2004).

Surgical management for renovascular disease is limited to those patients who present with severe hypertension in spite of maximal medical therapy and ischemic nephropathy. Procedures that may be performed include aortorenal bypass, the most common surgery performed for patients with renovascular disease, and renal artery thromboendarterectomy or renal artery reimplantation.

Health Promotion and Complications

Patients need to be instructed on the importance of regular and continuing medical follow-up. Close monitoring of blood pressure is required. Changes to the antihypertensive medication regime will likely be needed following stenting or surgical repair. Patients must be monitored for progression of renovascular disease and decline in renal function. Complications of untreated renovascular disease can include severely elevated blood pressure, stroke, renal insufficiency and failure, heart failure, retinopathy, and death.

■ Nursing Management

Caring for the patient who has undergone renal artery stenting is similar to the care of the patient who has undergone other types of peripheral angioplasty. Monitoring of blood pressure and urinary output is essential. Because renal stenting is performed by percutaneous arterial access, careful monitoring of the access site is needed, along with regular assessment of distal pulses. Follow-up laboratory testing of blood urea nitrogen (BUN) and creatinine levels is important to assess renal function.

Patients who have undergone surgical treatment of their renovascular disease, such as reconstruction of the renal arteries or aortorenal bypass, may require intensive care monitoring for several hours postoperatively. Postoperative monitoring includes frequent and ongoing assessment of the blood pressure. The remainder of postoperative nursing management is discussed in Chapter 27 ☞ .

■ Aortic Aneurysm

An **aneurysm** is a diseased segment of an artery that becomes thin and dilated because of degenerative changes in the tunica media layer.

Etiology and Epidemiology

Arterial aneurysms can occur throughout the body. Aortic aneurysms can be saccular (extending over only part of the vessel circumference), projecting from one side of the aorta only, or fusiform (involving the entire circumference), which is symmetrical involvement of the aorta. The prevalence of aortic aneurysm in the United States varies with advancing age, family history, male gender, and tobacco use. The condition is more common in men, especially between ages 50 and 70. The incidence increases with age and develops more frequently in smokers. Additionally,

aortic aneurysms tend to have familial tendencies. The most common causes of aortic aneurysms are atherosclerosis and degeneration of the vessel media (Porth, 2005).

Pathophysiology

Aortic aneurysms can occur anywhere in the aorta, although the majority of them occur below the level of the renal arteries (infrarenal). These are referred to as abdominal aortic aneurysms (AAA). Thoracic aneurysms account for only 10% of the occurrences. The pathogenesis of an aortic aneurysm is not well understood. It is a localized area of the aorta that is weakened because of decreased elastin in the medial layer, loss of medial smooth muscle cells with thinning of the vessel wall. Inflammatory changes may also play a part. Causes include congenital weakness, trauma, and disease. Once the aneurysm is initiated, it will grow larger as the tension on the vessel wall increases. The pressure may increase to the point that it is putting pressure on the adjacent organs and interrupting blood flow. If a growing aneurysm is left untreated, it may rupture due to the increased tension (Porth, 2007).

Clinical Manifestations

The clinical manifestations of an aortic aneurysm depend on its size and location. Aneurysms of the thoracic area present with substernal, back, and neck pain. These patients also may have dyspnea, stridor, and brassy cough due to pressure on the trachea. If the laryngeal nerve is compressed, hoarseness may occur (Porth, 2007). Abdominal aortic aneurysms are typically asymptomatic. Frequently, an unknown aortic aneurysm is discovered during abdominal imaging performed for some other reason or during routine physical exam. Visual inspection may reveal a pulsatile abdominal mass near the umbilicus in the lean patient. Auscultation of this mass reveals a bruit (Chapter 37 ☞), caused by the turbulent flow in the widened area of the aorta.

Diagnosis

Diagnostic testing performed for aortic aneurysms includes abdominal ultrasound, CT scan, abdominal angiography, and MR angiography. The aortic aneurysm is followed by serial diagnostic tests to evaluate growth and impedance of surrounding organs. To be considered an AAA, the size must exceed 3 centimeters in diameter.

Medical Management

Medical management of the stable AAA includes ongoing surveillance with abdominal ultrasound performed every 6 months to assess the amount of aneurysmal growth, as well as smoking cessation, optimal blood pressure control, monitoring, and controlling fasting lipid values and discontinuance of steroids, if possible.

Endovascular stent graft covered with a thin layer of Dacron may be an option for some patients with an AAA. In endovascular repair of an AAA, the graft is placed into the aorta via access from the femoral artery. This procedure is performed in the operating room or in the cardiac catheterization laboratory using general, regional, or local anesthesia with sedation. Several endovascular stent graft systems are currently available (Figure 43–11 ■). Advantages for the patient include no long abdominal incisions, faster recovery time, and shorter length of stay. This ap-

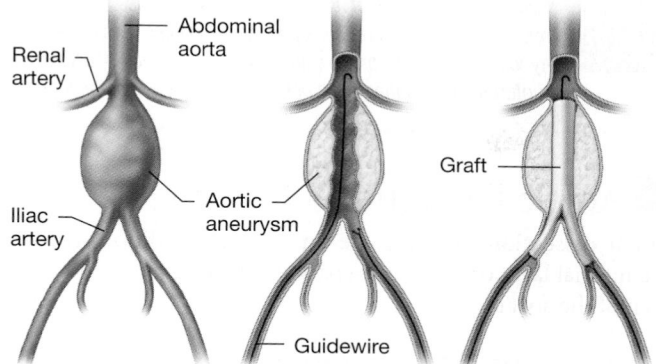

FIGURE 43–11 ■ Endovascular stent graft.

Abdominal aortic aneurysm surgical repair

FIGURE 43–12 ■ Repair of abdominal aneurysm.

proach may be an option for the patient at very high risk for open-heart surgery because of extensive comorbidities, such as cardiac and or pulmonary disease. Complications of endovascular stent graft repair of an AAA include **endoleaks** (continued leaking of blood into the aneurysmal sac), arterial trauma, occlusion of the renal or hypogastric arteries, renal impairment due to contrast administration, device migration, structural failure, and/or infection. The long-term durability of these stent grafts is not known; lifelong follow-up is needed for these patients. The early mortality rate for endograft repair generally has been less than 3% (Hirsch, Haskal, Hertzer, Bakal, Creager, Halperin, et. al., 2006).

Surgical Management

Options for treating AAA are open surgical repair and endovascular repair. Surgical intervention for AAA has been performed for over 50 years. Patients with infrarenal AAAs measuring 5.5 centimeters or larger should undergo repair to eliminate the risk of rupture (Hirsch, Haskal, Hertzer, Bakal, Creager, Halperin, et. al., 2006). Elective AAA repair is a major surgical procedure with mortality rates reported between 2% and 6% and postoperative complication rates up to 32.4%. Cardiac complications are most common (Fleming, Whitlock, Beil, & Lederle, 2005). The perioperative administration of beta-adrenergic blockers, if not contraindicated, reduces the risk of adverse cardiac events and mortality in patients with coronary artery disease undergoing repair of atherosclerotic aortic aneurysms (Hirsch, Haskal, Hertzer, Bakal, Creager, Halperin, et. al., 2006).

The surgical approach is dependent on the location of the aneurysm, but the traditional approach is a midline or transverse incision with retroperitoneal dissection of the aneurysm. The aneurysm is resected, or removed, and replaced with Dacron graft material. The aneurysm wall is usually left in place to cover the Dacron graft. Aneurysms that extend above the renal arteries and into the thoracic aorta are more difficult to repair. If the ascending aorta is involved, cardiopulmonary bypass is required. Chapter 40 discusses cardiopulmonary bypass surgery. Figure 43–12 ■ shows the repair approach for AAA.

Immediate surgical repair is indicated for the patient who presents with expanding aneurysm or rupture. The mortality rate for emergency surgery for ruptured AAA is as high as 40% (Upchurch & Schaub, 2006).

Complications that can occur following open AAA repair include hemodynamic instability due to postoperative bleeding, hypothermia, myocardial ischemia and/or infarction, hypoxia due

to atelectasis, fluid and electrolyte disturbances due to renal insufficiency, massive transfusions, inadequate hydration, ileus and abdominal distention due to ischemia or surgical manipulation of the bowel, and spinal cord ischemia due to interrupted blood flow during cross-clamping.

Complications

Complications that can occur from AAA include rupture, thrombosis, and embolization. The risk of rupture is related to the size of the aneurysm and is very high if the aneurysm is larger than 5.5 centimeters. Factors that can increase the risk of rupture include hypertension, smoking, and family history of ruptured AAAs. Embolization from the aneurysm can decrease perfusion to the lower extremities and is referred to as "blue toe syndrome." This syndrome, caused by emboli, is an indication for surgical repair of the AAA.

■ Nursing Management

Careful in-depth nursing assessment is essential for the patient undergoing surgical or endovascular repair of an abdominal aortic aneurysm. Prior to repair, the nurse needs to monitor the patient closely for signs and symptoms of impending rupture: restlessness, abdominal pain and tenderness, hypotension, and shock. Any of these symptoms should be reported immediately to the health care provider and the patient should be prepared for emergent surgery.

> **CRITICAL ALERT** *The unstable patient who has experienced rupture of an abdominal aortic aneurysm (AAA) requires immediate fluid and blood resuscitation, blood pressure control with propranolol (Inderal) or nitroprusside (Nipride), and pain management while being prepared for emergency surgery.*

The nursing process guides the postoperative care of the patient immediately following the open AAA surgery. Nursing diagnoses that pertain to these patients include *Tissue Perfusion, Ineffective* related to the surgical procedure; *Decreased Cardiac Output,* and *Risk for Deficient Volume; Gas Exchange, Ineffective* related to anesthesia, possible fluid overload, and blood transfusions; *Readiness for Enhanced Comfort* related to surgical pain, immobility, and fear and anxiety; *Risk for Infection* related to the surgery; and *Deficient Knowledge* of postoperative care and discharge needs.

The postoperative patient is typically monitored in the intensive care setting for 6 to 24 hours. Priority nursing interventions include blood pressure and hemodynamic support, aggressive pulmonary toilet, and prevention and early detection of surgical complications. Hemodynamic instability can occur in the immediate postoperative phase, and patients are generally monitored invasively using an arterial line and central venous catheter and/or pulmonary artery catheter. Frequent and careful assessment of pulses and neurological function in the lower extremities is essential because normal blood flow may have been interrupted during surgery. Urine output also must be monitored closely if the aneurysm occurred above the renal arteries.

Postoperative complications can be caused by bleeding, hypovolemia, and third spacing of fluid, myocardial ischemia/infarction, hypertension, and hypothermia. Vasoactive drugs may be required in the immediate postoperative phase to support and control the blood pressure and other hemodynamic parameters. Patients are placed on bedside ECG monitors to assess cardiac dysfunction and the presence of dysrhythmias. The nurse should compare the postoperative cardiac rhythm to the preoperative ECG to assess for new changes that may indicate myocardial ischemia or infarction, such as ST segment depression or elevation. Hypothermia causes an increase in the systemic vascular resistance. Patients should be rewarmed 1 degree per hour until the core body temperature exceeds 36°C. Rewarming can be accomplished by using forced warm air blankets, administering warmed IV fluids/blood, warming the inspired ventilator air, and covering the patient's head with warm blankets.

Patients who have undergone open AAA repair require frequent assessment of their pulmonary status, including signs of poor oxygenation and ventilation as evidenced by abnormal arterial blood gases, cyanosis, sluggish capillary refill, use of accessory muscles to breathe, nasal flaring, and decreased level of consciousness. Regular assessment of the patient's airway is essential. Adequate pain management, frequent repositioning, and the regular use of incentive spirometry are essential to promote oxygenation and ventilation and prevent atelectasis.

Impaired renal function can occur due to decreased blood flow to the kidneys during surgery and with episodes of hypotension and hypovolemia. Monitor the urine output, BUN, and serum creatinine closely. Gastrointestinal disturbances can occur postoperatively because of ischemia and/or manipulation of the bowel during surgery. Assess for nausea, vomiting, abdominal pain/tenderness, distention, presence/absence of bowel sounds, blood in stools, and diarrhea. Spinal cord ischemia can occur because of an interruption of blood supply during cross-clamping of the aorta and cause sensory and motor deficits.

Health Promotion

Prior to surgery, patients should be taught the importance of blood pressure control and compliance with their medication regime. Risk factor reduction is important. Patients should be counseled to stop smoking. Following surgery, risk factor modification teaching is reinforced. Additionally, patients are taught wound care, activity restrictions, medication regime, and reportable symptoms, such as changes in sensation to the legs, which may indicate thrombosis of the graft, or gastrointestinal bleeding, which may indicate erosion of the graft into the duodenum.

 *Spontaneous rupture of an aortic aneurysm causes sudden onset of abdominal and back pain accompanied by signs of hypotension, shock, and collapse. Once the aortic aneurysm ruptures, many patients die before arriving at a hospital for care.*

■ Aortic Dissection

Aortic dissection (AD) is a life-threatening condition whereby the intimal layer of the aorta separates, creating a tear in the lumen of the aorta.

Etiology and Epidemiology

Blood flows into this space, referred to as a "false lumen," and diminishes the blood supply distal to the area of dissection. A dissection can occur anywhere in the aorta, although two-thirds of the dissections occur in the ascending aorta (Porth, 2005). As the dissection increases in size, pressure is placed on the surrounding organs, which may impact organ function. Risks for the development of AD include hypertension, degeneration of the medial layer of the vessel wall, trauma, Marfan's syndrome, and iatrogenic (treatment-induced) dissection caused by catheter-based interventions and aortic clamping during surgery. It occurs most frequently in those ages 40 to 60 and is more prevalent in males (Porth, 2007).

Pathophysiology

The exact cause of AD is unknown. Chronic stress from hypertension may play a significant role in the deterioration of the aortic wall. An aortic dissection begins with a tear in the intima, which allows blood to enter the aortic wall, stripping the intima from the adventitia of the aorta. Aortic dissection is classified according to its location. Dissection that involves the ascending aorta, which is the most common, is classified as Stanford type A or DeBakey type I. This type requires immediate surgical repair. Dissections that involve only the descending aorta are classified as Stanford type B or DeBakey type III. They do not generally require immediate surgery and are stabilized medically.

Clinical Manifestations

Most patients with AD present with sudden, sharp, shifting chest or back pain that can mimic acute myocardial infarction, pulmonary embolus, or ruptured AAA. The patient may describe it as "ripping" or "tearing." The pain is not affected by position changes and it may wax and wane. These patients also may have syncope or altered level of consciousness. About 25% of patients with AD present with signs of ischemia from blood flow obliterated by the dissection, such as stroke, anuria, and mesenteric and/or extremity ischemia that occurs because of the altered blood flow to the brain, kidneys, gut, and legs.

 Rapid identification of aortic dissection is key in preventing death. Signs and symptoms of aortic dissection (AD) can mimic other disorders such as acute myocardial infarction and pulmonary embolus, making the diagnosis difficult. The most classic symptom of AD is the abrupt onset of severe, tearing chest pain that may radiate to the back. Patients may also present with sudden onset aortic insufficiency, neurological changes, and cardiac tamponade.

Diagnosis

The diagnosis of aortic dissection begins with taking the patient's history and doing a physical examination. An assessment of risk factors is essential. Because aortic dissection is a life-threatening situation, prompt and careful assessment of the clinical manifestations also is essential. Diagnostic tests that will assist with the diagnosis include aortic angiography, transesophageal echocardiography, CT scan, and MRI studies. The Diagnostic Tests box outlines the diagnostic tests used to evaluate AD.

Medical Management

Medical therapy is recommended for type B dissections or those that are in the descending aorta, although surgery may be required when there is poor blood pressure control, inadequate pain relief, and/or progression of the dissection. Control of hypertension is essential for the patient with AD. Aggressive control of blood pressure is managed using beta-adrenergic blockers such as esmolol (Brevibloc), labetalol (Normodyne, Trandate), propranolol (Inderal), metoprolol (Lopressor), and nitroglycerine or nitroprusside (Nipride).

Endovascular repair of AD may also be an option for select patients. Because these procedures are less invasive, the patients have a shorter recovery period and a shorter length of stay. Complications, such as endoleaks, are similar to those seen in endovascular repair of AAA. Endovascular procedures are typically done with local anesthesia and procedural sedation.

Surgical Management

Surgical intervention is indicated for type A dissections, which are those that involve the ascending aorta when the patient develops ischemic complications and/or when medical management fails. If the proximal aorta is involved, the aortic valve may need to be replaced and the coronary arteries may need to be reimplanted. Surgical complications may include myocardial ischemia or infarction, arrhythmias, pulmonary atelectasis, renal failure, ischemic bowel, prolonged ileus, and leg ischemia.

Complications

The disruption of the aorta can cause life-threatening complications or death if not rapidly recognized and treated. Abnormal blood flow into the false lumen of the aorta results in occlusion of the branches of the aorta. If the dissection occurs proximally in the aorta, there is risk of shearing of the aortic valve and the coronary arteries, causing serious complications including myocardial infarction, acute aortic insufficiency, and pericardial tamponade. If the dissection moves distally in the aorta, there is risk of damage to the arteries that supply the kidneys, spine, abdomen, and legs.

■ Nursing Management

The nursing management of the patient following open AD repair is complex and very similar to the nursing management of

DIAGNOSTIC TESTS for Aortic Dissection

Test	Expected Abnormality	Rationale for Abnormality
ECG	May have ST segment changes if coronary arteries are affected in ascending aortic dissection.	Easily performed. Provides rapid information about coronary ischemia.
Chest x-ray	Widened mediastinum may be seen.	Easily performed. Not diagnostic.
TEE	Detects cardiac tamponade, involvement of coronary arteries, and damage to aortic valve.	Relatively easy to perform. Requires sedation.
CT scan	Quickly confirms location and extent of dissection.	Noninvasive. Requires contrast administration. Requires x-ray exposure. Expensive. Requires skilled interpretation. Less readily available. Provides no information about aortic valve involvement.
Angiography	Visualization of true and false lumen possible. Identification of coronary artery anatomy.	Invasive. Requires vascular access. Requires contrast administration. Requires x-ray exposure. Accurate diagnosis. Requires skilled interpretation.
MRI/MRA	Shows intimal tear, type and extent of dissection, and involvement of aortic valve.	Noninvasive. Does not require vascular access. Does not require contrast administration. Expensive. Requires skilled interpretation. Not widely available. May be difficult for claustrophobic patients.

the patient who has had open AAA repair. Patients spend the first 1 to 2 days in the intensive care unit for careful monitoring. Goals of therapy are directed toward airway and blood pressure management, and pain control. Care of the postoperative patient is discussed in detail in Chapter 27 ☺ .

Health Promotion

Patients must be instructed to control their blood pressure carefully for the rest of their lives. Compliance with their medication regime is essential.

Venous Disorders

Venous disease is more likely to affect the lower extremities. The patient may experience intermittent swelling, tightness, and discomfort in one or both lower extremities due to a venous disorder. Unilateral extremity swelling may be associated with **deep venous thrombosis (DVT)**. Bilateral or diffuse edema may indicate that the patient has heart failure, valvular venous incompetence, or **lymphedema**, which is swelling due to obstruction of the lymphatic system.

The venous system of the lower extremities has two components: the superficial and the deep systems. Perforating of communicating veins transports blood from the skin and subcutaneous tissues from the superficial system to the deeper venous channels where it is then transported to the heart. The veins contain valves, which prevent retrograde flow, thereby maintaining normal flow of blood back to the heart. Muscle

function also assists in moving the blood back to the heart. There are more venous valves located in the lower legs than in the upper legs. Loss of valve function causes venous insufficiency, and venous hypertension can occur.

Varicose Veins

Varicose veins are dilated, tortuous veins that occur in the lower extremities as a result of the incompetence of valves of the deep and superficial venous system leading to valve reflux.

Etiology and Epidemiology

Risk factors for the development of varicose veins include older age, family history, female gender, occupations that requires standing, obesity, and history of phlebitis or clot. Other potential risk factors include constipation/low-fiber diet, smoking, hypertension, and injury. Pregnancy is likely a contributing factor for the increased incidence in females (Beebe-Dimmer, Pfeifer, Engle, & Schottenfeld, 2004). Varicose veins are subcutaneous veins that remain dilated when the patient is standing or sitting. Figure 43–13 ■ shows a normal venous structure and a varicose venous structure. In the general population, the incidence of varicose veins is between 5% and 30%, with a higher incidence in females (Eberhardt & Raffetto, 2005).

Clinical Manifestations

Some patients may have no symptoms whereas other patients experience sensations of heaviness, tiredness, itching, burning,

(a)

(b)

FIGURE 43–13 ■ (A) normal venous structure and (B) varicose veins.

or aching in their leg(s). Symptoms may intensify by the end of the day, especially after standing for long periods of time. Varicose veins may be prominent during pregnancy or menstruation.

Diagnosis, Medical Management, and Surgical Management

Diagnosis is made by physical examination and the patient's report of clinical manifestations. A frequent site of varicose veins is the greater saphenous vein. Doppler ultrasound may be used to assess blood flow in the large vessels, and angiography is used to assess valve function. Treatment may be required for patients with extensive varicose veins or those who are severely symptomatic. Interventional therapy, or nonsurgical alternatives to treatment for varicose veins, such as sclerotherapy, is performed less frequently because of the high incidence of reoccurrence. In sclerotherapy, generally reserved for small varicose veins and spider veins, the vein is injected with an irritating chemical, causing fibrosis and occluding the vessel lumen, which results in reduction of the varicose vein.

Surgical therapy for varicose veins may include ligation, stripping, laser therapy, or radiofrequency ablation of the vein, usually the saphenous vein (Teruya & Ballard, 2004). This is performed in the outpatient setting and the patient's recovery is generally a few days to 3 weeks at the most. Following venous sclerotherapy or surgery, patients must wear compression stockings to help prevent further varicosities. Complications of surgical repair of varicose veins may include hemorrhage, thrombophlebitis, edema, and infection.

Complications

Complications of untreated varicose veins can include increased risk of DVT and chronic venous insufficiency (CVI) leading to hyperpigmentation and ulceration of the feet and legs. This can increase the patient's susceptibility to injury and infection.

■ Nursing Management

Repair of varicose veins is generally scheduled as outpatient surgery, in either a hospital or a surgical clinic. Bed rest is suggested for the first 24 hours, with the foot of the bed elevated; then the patient is encouraged to walk short distances every 2 hours. Compression stockings are usually worn for several days following surgery. Surgical incisions should be inspected daily for signs of infection such as redness, tenderness, warmth, and drainage.

Patients should avoid showering or bathing the legs the first 24 hours and should avoid the use of lotions and creams on the legs until the incisions are fully healed.

Health Promotion

Prior to discharge, the patient should be taught to avoid activities that cause venous pooling, such as sitting for long periods of time and standing in one position for long periods of time. The nurse needs to explain the proper method for applying and wearing compression stockings. The patient should be encouraged to develop a walking program and to lose weight, if needed.

■ Venous Thromboembolism

Venous thromboembolism (VTE) consists of two conditions: deep venous thrombosis and pulmonary embolism (Tapson, 2005).

Etiology and Epidemiology

VTE is a common cardiovascular disorder affecting over 2 million in the United States each year, and an estimated 200,000 deaths in this country alone result from VTE (AHA, 2007). **Virchow's triad**—venous stasis, damage of the endothelium, and hypercoagulability—first described in 1846, remains the theory behind the thrombus formation of VTE. Multiple risk factors for the development of VTE are outlined in the Risk Factors box. **Pulmonary embolism (PE)** in this context is defined as the presence of a thrombus or blood clots in the pulmonary vessels, which obstructs blood flow and impedes gas exchange. The diagnosis and treatment of PE is discussed in detail in Chapter 36 ☺.

Deep Venous Thrombosis

A deep venous thrombosis is defined as a clot that forms in the deep veins, usually those of the lower extremities and pelvis, although these clots can also occur in the upper extremities. Factors that contribute to the development of DVT include venous stasis, hypercoagulability, immobility, and thrombus formations. Figure 43–14 ■ (p. 1348) shows common locations for DVT occurrence. Risk factors for DVT are outlined in the Risk Factors for Venous Thromboembolism box.

Most hospitalized patients are at risk of developing DVT due to immobility, making risk assessment and prophylaxis extremely important. Medical and general surgery patients have a 10% to 40% risk of developing DVT during hospitalization, whereas orthopedic surgery patient have a 40% to 60% risk

---

RISK FACTORS for Venous Thromboembolism (VTE)

- Major abdominal, thoracic, gynecologic, and/or urologic surgeries
- Major orthopedic surgeries such as total hip or total knee procedures
- Spinal cord injuries; paresis
- Fracture of the pelvis, hip, or long bones
- Multiple trauma; burns
- Malignancy
- Myocardial infarction, heart failure, respiratory failure, sepsis, ulcerative colitis
- Intensive care unit admission

- Previous DVT/ Pulmonary embolism (PE)
- Age > 40 years
- Obesity
- Prolonged immobility of 3 days or more
- Varicose veins
- Pregnancy/postpartum
- Oral contraceptive use
- Acquired and inherited disorders of coagulation
- Presence of central venous catheters

Sources: Geerts, W. H., Pineo, G. F., Heit, J. A., Bergqvist, D., Lassen, M. R., Colwell, C. W., et al. (2004). Prevention of venous thromboembolism: The seventh ACCP conference on antithrombotic and thrombolytic therapy. *Chest, 126,* 338S–400S.

Internal iliac
External iliac

Common femoral vein

Deep femoral vein

Femoral vein

Popliteal vein

Peroneal vein

Greater saphenous vein

Popliteal vein

Posterior tibial vein

Peroneal vein

(a)   (b)   (c)

FIGURE 43–14 ■ Common locations of venous thrombosis.

(Kehl-Pruett, 2006). In 2004, the American College of Chest Physicians published its Seventh ACCP Conference on Antithrombotic and Thrombolytic Therapy guidelines (Hirsh et al., 2004) providing recommendations for DVT prophylaxis and treatment in medical and surgical patients. Despite these detailed guidelines, many hospitalized patients are not receiving adequate treatment to prevent DVT (Kehl-Pruett, 2006).

Clinical Manifestations

Signs and symptoms of DVT are variable, and the presence of a DVT may not be known until the patient develops a PE. Most DVTs begin in the deep veins of the calf. Some patients have no discomfort, whereas others may complain of unilateral extremity discomfort and pain, edema, warmth, tenderness, and redness. A palpable vein cord may be present. Homans' sign, or pain in the calf when the foot is dorsiflexed, is not a reliable indicator of DVT (Walsh & Rice, 2004).

Diagnosis, Medical Management, and Surgical Management

A number of diagnostic tests assist in identifying the presence and location of DVT. These tests are outlined in the Diagnostic Tests for Deep Venous Thrombosis box (p. 1350).

Pharmacological agents that can be added to the DVT prophylaxis regime include anticoagulants, such as intravenous or subcutaneous unfractionated heparin, subcutaneous low molecular weight heparin, intravenous or subcutaneous direct thrombin inhibitors, and oral warfarin. Aspirin has not been demonstrated to be effective in preventing DVT and is not recommended (Geerts

et al., 2004). According to the Seventh ACCP Conference on Antithrombotic and Thrombolytic Therapy guidelines (Hirsh et al., 2004), strict bed rest for confirmed DVT is not needed and patients may ambulate as tolerated. Additional interventions for confirmed DVT include extremity elevation 10 to 20 degrees above the level of the heart, local application of moist heat, avoidance of massaging affected extremity to prevent clot from breaking loose, and compression stockings. Anticoagulation with short-term intravenous or subcutaneous unfractionated heparin or subcutaneous low molecular weight heparin followed by long-term warfarin therapy for 3 to 6 months is initiated. The goal for the international normalized ratio (INR) is 2 to 3 (Rectenwald & Wakefield, 2005). Treatment regimes for DVT can be done in the outpatient setting as well as for the hospitalized patient. The Pharmacology Summary box outlines the pharmacologic treatment of VTE/DVT. The Evidence-Based Practice feature (p. 1356) discusses medications that prevent DVTs.

Some patients may require surgical intervention to prevent PE from occurring. Procedures include venous thrombectomy and interruption of the vena cava. Thrombectomy is not commonly performed. Vena cava interruption is done percutaneously by placement of an inferior vena cava filter device that captures thrombi, yet allows blood to flow through it. (Figure 43–15 ■, p. 1351). This is indicated for patients who have a contraindication to anticoagulation for DVT prophylaxis and treatment, such as the trauma patient or patients who have failed therapy by developing a clot while on anticoagulation (Marr, 2006). Complications of filter placement are rare. Trapped clots can eventually lead to venous

PHARMACOLOGY Summary of Medications to Treat Peripheral Vascular Disease

Medication Category	Action	Application/Indication	Nursing Responsibility
Anticoagulants			
Unfractionated heparin	Prevents clot formation by inhibiting thrombin, preventing the conversion of fibrinogen to fibrin.	Prevention of clot formation and extension in venous thrombosis and pulmonary embolism; prevention of postoperative DVT; treatment of DIC; maintenance of venous access device patency.	Monitor for adverse effects: bleeding, thrombocytopenia. Monitor aPTT, blood count, platelet count. Assess for presence of beef or pork allergy, history of heparin-induced thrombocytopenia (HIT), or active bleeding (contraindicated in these patients). Be aware of drug interactions (cephalosporins, penicillins, nitroglycerin (NTG), salicylate). Monitor for increased risk of bleeding. Preferred over low molecular weight heparin (LMWH) in presence of renal failure.
Low molecular weight heparin (LMWH): Enoxaparin (Lovenox) Dalteparin (Fragmin) Tinzaparin (Innohep)		Treatment of pulmonary embolism, DVT; prevention of venous thromboembolism.	Monitor for adverse effects: bleeding. Monitor for increased risk of bleeding in presence of reduced creatinine clearance. Contraindicated in patients who have or will receive epidural or spinal anesthesia or puncture.
Warfarin (Coumadin)	Inhibits hepatic synthesis of the vitamin K–dependent coagulation factors II, VII, IX, and X.	Long-term prophylaxis for thrombus formation; e.g., mitral valve replacement, atrial fibrillation, hypercoagulability disorders.	Monitor for adverse effects: bleeding, nausea, vomiting, and diarrhea. Monitor international normalized ratio (INR) and/or prothrombin time (PT). Be aware of multiple drug and food interactions (green leafy vegetables, alcohol, NSAIDs, acetaminophen, phenytoin, barbiturates, and many others). Assess current drug regime prior to initiating warfarin.
Antiplatelet Drugs			
Aspirin (acetylsalicylic acid, ASA)	Inhibits platelet aggregation.	Prevention of recurrent thromboembolism in MI, stroke; reduces progressive arterial obstruction in peripheral arterial disease (PAD).	Monitor for adverse effects: dyspepsia, nausea, heartburn, abdominal pain, gastrointestinal bleeding. Monitor for signs of toxicity (tinnitus, altered hearing). Increase blood sugar monitoring in presence of diabetes. Give with food. Warn patient to avoid alcohol and other drugs containing salicylates.
Clopidogrel (Plavix) Ticlopidine[a] (Ticlid) Cilostazol[b] (Pletal)	Inhibits adenosine diphosphate (ADP)-induced platelet aggregation. Promotes vasodilation.	Prevention of atherosclerotic event (e.g., myocardial infarction (MI), stroke, vascular death); intermittent claudication; may improve arterial ulcer healing.	Monitor for adverse effects: bleeding, abdominal pain, diarrhea, nausea, and headache. Monitor blood count, bleeding time, platelet function. Check neutrophil count if infection develops. Be aware of drug interactions (NSAIDs, diltiazem, vitamin A, anticoagulants, and others). Monitor for altered drug efficacy. Give with food.
Hemorheologic Drugs			
Pentoxifylline (Trental)	Prevents thrombus formation by decreasing blood viscosity; improves microcirculation by decreasing platelet aggregation.	Intermittent claudication.	Monitor for adverse effects: dyspepsia, nausea, vomiting, tremors, dizziness, and headache. Monitor for toxicity in presence of impaired renal function. Be aware of drug interactions (cimetidine, insulin, and theophylline). Monitor for drug toxicity or reduced efficacy. Give with food.

[a]Monitor for hematologic adverse reactions: agranulocytosis, aplastic anemia, thrombotic thrombocytopenic purpura.

[b]Warn patient to avoid grapefruit and grapefruit juice.

DIAGNOSTIC TESTS for Deep Venous Thrombosis

Test	Expected Abnormality	Rationale for Abnormality
Duplex ultrasound	Location and extent of clot or noncompressibility of the vein. Can identify floating, or unstable clot. May be difficult to perform in obese patient.	Most common diagnostic testing for deep venous thrombosis (DVT). 90% sensitive in the setting of symptomatic DVT. Noninvasive. Readily available; portable. Operator dependent.
Venography (also called phlebography)	Defines location and extent of the clot, which is seen as a filling defect. Identifies collateral circulation, if present.	Provides most accurate diagnosis of presence, location, and extent of clot. Invasive. Requires contrast administration. Costly. Risk of procedure induced thrombophlebitis. Invasive. Requires vascular access. Requires contrast administration. Requires x-ray exposure. Accurate diagnosis. Requires skilled interpretation.
CT scan	Useful to evaluate possible pelvic or abdominal thrombus. Useful for obese patients.	Noninvasive. Requires contrast administration. Requires x-ray exposure. Expensive. Requires skilled interpretation. Less readily available. May equal ultrasound in accuracy.
MRI	Useful for suspected iliac vein or inferior vena caval thrombosis.	Noninvasive. Sensitive for both acute and chronic DVT. Does not require vascular access. Does not require contrast administration. Expensive. Requires skilled interpretation. Not widely available. May be difficult for claustrophobic patients.
D-dimer	Elevated in DVT/PE due to release of degradation products released into the circulation when fibrin undergoes fibrinolysis.	Used to rule out the disorder, not confirm. A positive D-dimer test indicates that a DVT or pulmonary embolism (PE) is possible. Not diagnostic for DVT/PE, because the D-dimer is also elevated with recent surgery, trauma, and inflammation or any condition where clots may form.
Venous duplex imaging	Provides anatomic extent of venous disease. Detects DVT or venous obstruction. Provides information about valve function.	Noninvasive. Widely available. Portable. Uses sound waves reflected off of moving red blood cells and other tissues to evaluate the flow of blood. The different vascular beds have unique waveforms, and variations from normal indicate disease.
Photoplethysmography	A venous refill time < 20 seconds is indicative of venous disease.	Noninvasive testing. Provides overall assessment of venous physiology.
Venography	Determines venous patency.	Invasive testing. Requires contrast administration. Largely replaced by duplex scanning.
Ambulatory venous pressure	Pedal vein pressure measured before and after exercise to assess severity of venous disease.	Invasive testing. Seldom used in clinical practice.

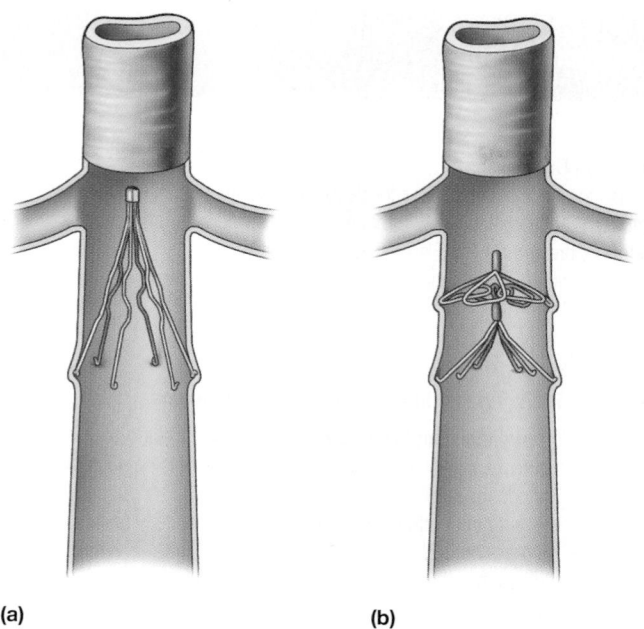

(a)   **(b)**

FIGURE 43–15 ■ Vena cava filters.

congestion and obstruction of the vena cava. Collateral vessels develop to maintain venous flow.

Nursing Management

Nurses play an active and important role in DVT prophylaxis and prevention. Nursing interventions include early ambulation whenever possible, active and passive range of motion exercises, extremity elevation, and mechanical methods of prophylaxis such as graduated compression stockings, intermittent pneumatic devices, and venous foot pumps. These mechanical devices increase venous outflow and/or reduce stasis in the leg veins (Geerts et al., 2004; Kehl-Pruett, 2006). Accurate leg length and calf circumference measurements are required to size graduated compression stockings correctly. Knee-high stockings are effective, less expensive, and easier to apply than are thigh-high stockings, which may enhance patient compliance with wearing stockings. Graduated compression stockings apply 18 mmHg at the ankle level and 8 mmHg at the thigh level. Intermittent and sequential compression devices decrease venous stasis and are often used in conjunction with graduated compression stockings (Figure 43–16 ■). Patients with underlying peripheral arterial disease should use compression stockings carefully. Complications of compression devices are rare and may include skin blisters. It is important that these devices are correctly sized and applied and that they are removed for only short periods of time.

The Nursing Process: Patient Care Plan (p. 1352) for Venous Thromboembolism feature outlines the nursing diagnoses and patient care needs that will provide a comprehensive plan of care for a patient experiencing a DVT.

Collaborative Management

A multidisciplinary team approach including health care providers, nurses, pharmacists, physical therapy, and dietitians is needed in providing care for the patient with VTE. Patients may benefit greatly from a nurse/pharmacist-directed antico-

FIGURE 43–16 ■ Intermittent and sequential compression devices.
Source: Cheryl Wraa

agulation program to assist them in taking and monitoring their warfarin, if prescribed. Home health visits may be necessary for the patient undergoing outpatient treatment of DVT.

Health Promotion

To prevent DVT, patients should be taught the importance of regular walking, foot and ankle exercises, and foot elevation when hospitalized and during their recovery from hospitalization. If patients are discharged home on a pharmacologic prophylaxis plan such as unfractionated heparin, warfarin or enoxaparin, or direct thrombin inhibitors, they need to be taught their medication regime, which may include learning how to do injections, follow-up monitoring, and reportable adverse effects. The Patient Teaching & Discharge Priorities for Use of Anticoagulant Medications box (p. 1354) presents suggestions for teaching the patient who is on anticoagulating medications. The most common complications of these medications include bleeding and heparin-induced thrombocytopenia. Compression stockings should be worn to prevent venous pooling. The nurse needs to stress to patients to avoid prolonged sitting, standing, and to avoid crossing their legs. The Patient Teaching & Discharge Priorities for Deep Venous Thrombosis (p. 1355) outlines the discharge priorities that the nurse needs to include in the discharge teaching plan.

NURSING PROCESS: Patient Care Plan for Venous Thromboembolism

Assessment of Peripheral Vascular Status

Subjective Data:
Do you have pain, tenderness, or swelling in your legs or arms?
When did this occur and how long have you had it?
What is your activity level?
Have you traveled long distances recently?
Are you feeling short of breath?
Do you have pain in your chest?

Objective Data:
Assess for contributing factors for deep vein thrombosis (DVT)/pulmonary embolism (PE) development: immobility, major surgery, trauma, paralysis, history of previous DVT/PE episodes, and so on.
Assess extremities for pain, tenderness, erythema, and swelling.

Nursing Assessment and Diagnoses	Outcomes and Evaluation Parameters	Planning and Interventions with *Rationales*
Nursing Diagnosis: *Impaired Tissue Perfusion* related to DVT	**Outcomes:** Patient has adequate blood flow to extremities. Patient does not develop pulmonary clinical manifestations. Patient/family verbalize understanding of disease, management, and prevention. **Evaluation Parameters:** Warm skin, absence of edema, and absence of pain. Normal respiratory patterns, normal heart rate, and absence of chest pain.	**Interventions and *Rationales:*** Apply properly fitting compression stockings *to promote venous return and decrease venous stasis.* For confirmed DVT: Measure circumference of affected extremity daily *to monitor progression and/or resolution of DVT.* Maintain activity per order with affected limb elevated 10–20 degrees above the level of the heart *to reduce venous pooling and edema.* Maintain hydration *to prevent increased blood viscosity.* Explain the risk factors of venous thromboembolism (VTE), and the need for bed rest, limb elevation, compression stockings, and sequential compression; avoid rubbing/massaging calf *to prevent reoccurrences.* Monitor results of lab testing and noninvasive studies *to assess treatment effectiveness.*

Assessment of Pain Related to Impaired Circulation

Subjective Data:
On a scale of 0–10, how would you rate your pain at this time?
Where is your pain?
What brings it on?
What makes it go away?
How long have you had it, and is it getting worse or better?

Objective Data:
Use pain scale (0–10) to quantify pain.
Assess cultural and religious impact on patient's responses.
Assess the onset of increased pain to evaluate for disease progression or acute arterial obstruction.

Nursing Assessment and Diagnoses	Outcomes and Evaluation Parameters	Planning and Interventions with *Rationales*
Nursing Diagnosis: *Readiness for Enhanced Comfort* related to impaired circulation	**Outcome:** Relief of pain. **Evaluation Parameters:** Patient states adequate relief of pain. Patient understands measures necessary to prevent pain.	**Interventions and *Rationales:*** Obtain a clear description of source of discomfort. Provide moist heat *to help relieve pain and inflammation.* Keep affected extremity elevated above the level of the heart *to promote venous return and decrease venous stasis.* Provide a supportive environment where patient is able to express pain level. Instruct patient to inform nurse if pain is not relieved *in order to revise the care plan.* Use pain control measures before the pain becomes severe *to enhance comfort.* Teach nonpharmacological methods of pain control; that is, guided imagery and breathing exercises *to assist in relaxation and pain control.* Pain relief *to promote comfort.*

Assessment of Bleeding Related to Anticoagulant Therapy

Subjective Data:
Do your gums bleed when you brush your teeth?
Do you notice any blood in your urine or stool?
Do you notice any increased or unusual bruising?

Objective Data:
Assess aPTT or INR, and report subtherapeutic values and over therapeutic range.
Stool guaiac negative.
Assess for bleeding in mouth, nose, and urine.

NURSING PROCESS: Patient Care Plan for Venous Thromboembolism—*Continued*

Nursing Assessment and Diagnoses	Outcomes and Evaluation Parameters	Planning and Interventions with *Rationales*
Nursing Diagnosis: *Fluid Volume Deficient, risk for*	**Outcomes:** Therapeutic aPTT or INR maintained in therapeutic range. No bleeding. **Evaluation Parameters:** No signs of bleeding in mouth, nose, urine, or stool.	**Interventions and *Rationales:*** Initiate and continue anticoagulant therapy *to prevent further clot development.* Monitor aPTT and/or INR prior to adjusting heparin or administering Coumadin *to optimize anticoagulation.* Assess for signs of bleeding *to ensure prompt identification and treatment.* Teach dietary restrictions of vitamin K *to avoid interactions with Coumadin.*

Assessment of Pulmonary Embolus Related to Embolization of Thrombus

Subjective Data:
Are you feeling short of breath?
Are you having chest pain? Are you coughing up blood-tinged sputum?
When did these symptoms begin?

Objective Data:
Rate, depth, and ease of respiration.
Assess lung sounds for adventitious or diminished sounds.
Assess sputum for blood.
Assess oxygen saturation levels.

Nursing Assessment and Diagnoses	Outcomes and Evaluation Parameters	Planning and Interventions with *Rationales*
Nursing Diagnosis: *Impaired Gas Exchange* related to VTE	**Outcomes:** No respiratory distress. Normal arterial blood gases. Normal oxygen saturation levels. **Evaluation Parameters:** No signs or symptoms of respiratory distress. No blood in sputum. No shortness of breath. No pain.	**Interventions and *Rationales:*** Instruct patient of reportable conditions: signs and symptoms of pulmonary embolus. Auscultate breath sounds for *assessment of crackles, rhonchi, or diminished sounds.* Provide oxygen per order *to increase oxygen to the heart, lungs, and periphery.* Administer anticoagulants or thrombolytic therapy *to treat VTE.*

Assessment of Self-Care Activities

Subjective Data:
Has anyone explained your health problems to you?
How does this disease affect your daily life?

Objective Data:
Assess knowledge of disease process and progression, risk factors, and need for compression stockings.
Assess knowledge of patient's understanding of treatment plan, including medications, if indicated.

Nursing Assessment and Diagnoses	Outcomes and Evaluation Parameters	Planning and Interventions with *Rationales*
Nursing Diagnosis: *Deficient Knowledge* of self-care needs related to disease	**Outcome:** Adequate knowledge level. **Evaluation Parameters:** Patient is able to discuss disease process, risk factors, and current treatment plan. Verbalizes adherence to and compliance with treatment plan.	**Interventions and *Rationales:*** Provide factual information about diagnosis, treatment, risk factor modification, medications, and treatment plan *to ensure compliance.* Explain all procedures and allow patient to ask questions *to promote his understanding.*

Complications

One of the complications of DVT is pulmonary embolism, which is described in Chapter 36 . Most thrombus come from the deep veins of the legs and can break loose spontaneously or be jarred loose by mechanical forces such as sudden standing and Valsalva. Pulmonary embolism may occur despite adequate anticoagulation. Clinical findings in PE may include dyspnea, tachypnea, pleuritic chest pain, cough, wheezing, syncope, hypotension, and cardiovascular collapse. The mortality associated with a large pulmonary embolism is 30% or more. A majority of patients with PE die within the first hour of symptom onset. Hypoxia occurs in these patients because of the imbalance or mismatch between blood flow and alveolar ventilation (Cardin & Marinelli, 2004).

> **CRITICAL ALERT**
>
> *Signs and symptoms of pulmonary embolism (PE) include dyspnea, tachypnea, anxiety, apprehension, tachycardia, chest pain, hemoptysis, hypoxia, collapse, shock, and cardiac arrest. Right ventricular failure is the cause of death in patients who die of PE.*

A second complication following acute DVT is postphlebitic syndrome, which is chronic venous insufficiency (CVI). As many as 50% of patients develop this disorder following a DVT (Fahey, 2004; Rectenwald & Wakefield, 2005). To prevent postphlebitic syndrome from occurring, the use of elastic compression stockings with a pressure of 30 to 40 mmHg at the ankle is recommended for at least 2 years following the acute DVT episode (Büller et al., 2004). Chronic venous insufficiency occurs from

PATIENT TEACHING & DISCHARGE PRIORITIES for Use of Anticoagulant Medications

Medication Need	Teaching
All anticoagulant/antiplatelet agents	Take as directed by the health care provider. Do not skip doses. Consider an alert bracelet/necklace. Avoid activities that can cause injury or falling. Early warning signs of bleeding include bruising, nosebleeds, or bleeding gums. Serious bleeding can occur and includes: • Pink or brown urine • Red or black stool • Spitting up or coughing up bloody secretions or secretions that look like coffee grounds • Severe headache • Dizziness, fatigue, or weakness. Report any excessive bruising or bleeding to the health care provider.
Heparin	Patients need to be taught subcutaneous injection techniques.
Low molecular weight heparin	Patients need to be taught subcutaneous injection techniques. Frequent monitoring of lab work is generally not required for patients on low molecular weight heparin.
Warfarin/Coumadin	Patients need to take the exact dose as prescribed by their health care provider or pharmacist. They may need to take different doses of warfarin/Coumadin on different days of the week. Many patients taking warfarin are monitored by an interdisciplinary anticoagulation clinic rather than their health care provider. Instruct patients to know who is monitoring their warfarin/Coumadin. If patients miss two or more doses in a row, they should call whoever is managing their medication for further instructions. Regular blood testing of the INR level is required. Instruct patients to know their optimal INR range. For many cardiovascular patients, it is between 2 and 3. Drug interactions can occur. Patients should use care when taking many over-the-counter drug preparations. The most likely drugs to affect the INR include aspirin, ibuprofen, cold remedies, antacids, and vitamin supplements. Herbal supplements can impact the INR, especially dan shen, garlic, *Ginkgo biloba,* ginseng, green tea, or kava. Food interactions can occur. Because the drug reduces the liver's ability to use vitamin K, any foods that change the amount of vitamin K in the body can affect the INR. These foods include brussels sprouts, kale, green tea, asparagus, avocado, broccoli, cabbage, cauliflower, collard greens, liver, soybean oil, soybeans, certain beans, mustard greens, peas (black-eyed peas, split peas, chick peas), turnip greens, parsley, green onions, spinach, and lettuce. Patients may be advised to limit their alcohol intake. Warfarin/Coumadin can cause birth defects; it should NOT be taken by patients planning to become pregnant.

vein pathology, such as venous valvular incompetence, causing venous stasis and increased venous pressure in the lower extremities. Symptoms of CVI include dependent swelling, pain, and skin changes. Typical findings include hyperpigmentation, or brownish discoloration of the skin, edema, dermatitis, ulcerations, or scarring from healed ulcerations (Figure 43–17 ■). Patients may complain of cramping, heaviness, or aching of their legs.

Venous ulcerations are typically located near the medial malleolus or the lateral malleolus of the ankle, but can occur anywhere below the knee, including the foot (Brem, Kirsner, & Falanga, 2004). They are shallow, irregularly shaped, exudative wounds that are typically difficult. Pain may be worse when the legs are in a dependent position. Walking or elevating the legs may improve the pain of venous ulcers. Venous ulcers, which often recur, impact the patient's quality of life by causing pain and discomfort, decreased mobility, increased visits to the health care provider, or

hospitalizations, as well as the negative impact of managing a chronic condition: anxiety, fear, and depression.

Prior to treating venous ulcers, concomitant peripheral arterial disease must be ruled out. Compression therapy is the primary therapy used to treat venous ulcers. It is contraindicated in peripheral arterial disease; therefore, an ankle-brachial index (ABI) should be performed prior to compression therapy. A finding of ≤0.9 indicates peripheral arterial disease.

Compression therapy is provided using elastic or nonelastic dressings or wraps. An elastic dressing stretches with changes in leg size but will continue to compress, whereas a nonelastic dressing resists stretching. A rigid bandage, such as the **Unna's boot,** commonly used to treat venous ulcers, prevents edema while promoting healing and is worn for several days at a time.

The Unna's boot is being replaced in clinical practice by multilayer wrap compression, which is available in high and low compression pressures. An example of a multilayer wrap that

PATIENT TEACHING & DISCHARGE PRIORITIES for Deep Venous Thrombosis

Need	Teaching
Knowledge of disease process	Home care needs include verbal and written instructions for: Treatment plan, including anticoagulation Follow-up care Activity restrictions, if any.
Understanding of medications	Teach the purpose, dose, and possible adverse effects of all medications to increase compliance and to prevent over/underdosing.
	Anticoagulant teaching: reason and importance, how to perform injections (if low molecular weight heparin prescribed), taking medications at the same time each day, not to skip a dose, frequent follow-up and lab testing, avoiding anything that might cause trauma/bleeding such as vigorous toothbrushing, contact sports.
Disease prevention	Explain the risk factors for DVT/PE development to prevent reoccurrences. The Risk Factors box (p. 1347) presents a detailed list of risk factors for venous thromboembolism.
	Avoid prolonged immobility, standing for long periods of time, car/airline flights > 6 hours; avoid constrictive clothing.
	Wear properly fitting and applied graduated compression stockings. If these stockings are recommended long term, teach patient to replace them every 3 months, because they lose their elasticity.
Reportable clinical manifestations	Instruct patient/family to report: Increase in pain, tenderness, swelling of affected extremity New onset pain, tenderness, swelling in another extremity New onset shortness of breath, chest pain, anxiety, restlessness New onset bleeding, headache, mental status changes.
Family/support system	Assess availability of, knowledge of, and compliance with treatment plan.
	Assess discharge placement needs.
	Assess for need for professional home health needs.
	Assess need for follow-up appointments.

FIGURE 43–17 ■ Chronic venous insufficiency.
Source: Ribotsky/Custom Medical Stock Photo, Inc.

provides graded compression is Profore (Hunter, Langemo, Hanson, Anderson, & Thompson, 2005; Sieggreen, 2005a).

Venous ulcers require treatment using absorbent compresses, compression dressings, topical steroids, topical zinc oxide, or a broad-spectrum antifungal cream (rarely). The wound should be cleansed at each dressing change. The patient should be instructed to avoid known skin irritants and allergens. The application of eutectic mixture of local anesthetics (EMLA) cream may produce pain relief for sharp debridement, if needed. Adhesive hydrocolloid dressings have been found to be effective in healing venous ulcers. Topical antibiotics are generally not effective; a short course with a topical antimicrobial such as silver sulfadiazine may be beneficial. If signs of infection occur such as pain, fever, and drainage from the ulcer, a culture should be obtained and the appropriate systemic antibiotic started. Infections most commonly include gram-positive organisms such as *Staphylococcus* and *Streptococcus,* and gram-negative organisms such as *Pseudomonas* (Brem et al., 2004; Davis & Gray, 2005; Wound, Ostomy, and Continence Nurses Society, 2005).

An important component of wound assessment is ongoing photography of the wound and measurement of the wound size. This can readily be achieved by using a digital camera and single-use rulers that are available from various manufacturers. Having this objective history of the wound appearance and size makes it easier to follow trends in therapy and healing (Brem et al., 2004). An in-depth discussion of wound healing is presented in Chapter 67 ⬤.

Patients with venous leg ulcers need to maintain adequate nutritional status to promote healing. A dietary consultation may be indicated. If indicated, the patient should be counseled about weight loss. Sufficient amounts of protein, vitamins A and C, and zinc are important. Decreased sodium intake is important to assist with managing edema. For patients with diabetes, tight

Medications for the Prevention of Deep Vein Thrombosis (DVT)

Clinical Problem

Homocysteine is a sulfur-containing amino acid found in the blood. Elevated levels of homocysteine have been linked to increased risk of premature coronary artery disease, stroke, and thromboembolism (venous blood clots), even among people who have normal cholesterol levels. Abnormal homocysteine levels appear to contribute to atherosclerosis in at least three ways: (1) direct toxic effect that damages the cells lining the inside of the arteries, (2) interference with clotting factors, and (3) oxidation of low density lipoproteins (LDL) (Barrett, 2003).

Elevated homocysteine levels also are associated with an increased risk of deep vein thrombosis and pulmonary embolism. According to den Heijer, Lewington, and Clarke (2005), up to now 24 case-control studies have been published with an overall relative risk for venous thrombosis of 1.60 (95% CI 1.10–2.34) for a 5 µmol/L higher homocysteine level. Moreover, three prospective studies showed an overall relative risk for venous thrombosis of 1.27 (95% CI 1.01–1.59), for a difference of 5 µmol/L. Recent meta-analyses on the effect of the MTHFR 677TT genotype on cardiovascular disease and venous thrombosis showed a modest increase in risk, supporting a hypothesis that homocysteine levels are causally related to thrombotic risk (den Heijer et al., 2005; Klerk et al., 2002; Wald, Law, & Morris, 2002).

Plasma homocysteine levels are strongly influenced by diet, as well as by genetic factors. The dietary components with the greatest effect in lowering the levels of homocysteine are folic acid and vitamins B_6 and B_{12}. Folic acid and other B vitamins help break down homocysteine in the body. Several studies have found that higher blood levels of B vitamins are related, at least partly, to lower concentrations of homocysteine (American Heart Association, 2008). Daily use of folic acid gives a 25% reduction in homocysteine levels, even at low doses of 0.5 milligram. The question is whether lowering of homocysteine by use of B vitamin supplementation also lowers the risk for venous thrombosis.

Research Findings

In 2006 den Heijer et al. (2007) conducted the VITRO (Vitamins and Thrombosis) study to investigate the effect of a combination preparation of 5 mg of folic acid, 50 mg of pyridoxine, and 0.4 mg of cyanocobalamin in the secondary prevention of deep venous thrombosis and pulmonary embolism in patients with a first event of venous thrombosis and hyperhomocysteinemia in a randomized, double-blind, and placebo-controlled setting. A secondary aim was to study the effect of vitamin supplementation in patients with a first event of venous thrombosis and a "normal" homocysteine concentration in an identical setting. The study concluded that B vitamin supplementation lowers homocysteine values, but it does not show a risk reduction in recurrent venous thrombosis. Elevated homocysteine blood levels remain a modest risk factor for recurrent thrombotic events.

Implications for Nursing Practice

The implication for nursing practice is that patients with elevated homocysteine levels are at a higher risk for DVT, a form of venous thromboembolism. Hospitalized patients are already at an increased risk of developing DVT due to immobility, advanced age, acute medical illness, and central venous catheters. Individuals who develop DVT are at further risk for serious complications such as pulmonary embolism and death. If a homocysteine level has been done, and the

nurse is aware that the level is evaluated, it is imperative to institute timely nursing measures.

Treatment options, including high-dose anticoagulants and thrombolytics, may be contraindicated in certain inpatient populations; therefore, other methods of preventing DVT are imperative. Foot and ankle exercises encourage plantar and dorsiflexion, a very basic, natural technique. For those patients who are unable to perform foot and ankle exercises, passive range of motion is an appropriate substitute to reduce venous pooling by passively exercising muscles. Other measures for DVT prevention include active range of motion, early ambulation, graduated stockings, and pneumatic compression devices. Each improves venous return and reduces venous stasis in the leg veins. These measures are simple to use and do not increase the risk of bleeding, making them ideal for most hospital patients.

Nurses play key role in the prevention of DVT and its complications. Nursing management includes assessing every patient for risk factors for the development of the DVT. Admission assessments are an opportune time to evaluate risk factors such as mobility, age, previous history of DVT, and medical conditions that increase the risk of developing DVT in hospital patients. Patient risk assessment should be ongoing throughout hospitalization but especially with condition changes. Nurses must advocate for timely prevention and treatment measures. Following the intuition of these measures, the nurse must then evaluate their effectiveness (Kehl-Pruett, 2006).

Critical Thinking Questions

1. When a patient is admitted with an elevated homocysteine level, in order of priority, what nursing measures are essential?

2. Identify measures that would decrease the risk for the development of DVT.

3. What is the primary reason for instituting measures that prevent the development of DVT?

Answers to Critical Thinking Questions appear in Appendix D.

References

American Heart Association. (2008). *What is homocysteine?* Retrieved March 11, 2008, from http://www.americanheart.org/presenter .jhtml?identifier=535.

Barrett, S. (2003). *Homocysteine: A cardiovascular risk factor worth considering.* Retrieved March 11, 2008, from http://www.quackwatch .com/03HealthPromotion/homocysteine.html.

den Heijer, M., Lewington, S., & Clarke, R. (2005). Homocysteine, MTHFR and risk of venous thrombosis: A meta-analysis of published epidemiological studies. *Journal of Thrombosis Haemostasis, 3,* 292–299.

den Heijer, M., Williams, H. P. J., Blom, H. J., Gerrits, W. B. J., Cattaneo, M., Eichinger, S., et al. (2007). Homocysteine lowering by B vitamins and the secondary prevention of deep-vein thrombosis and pulmonary embolism. A randomized, placebo-controlled, double blind trial. *Blood, 109*(1), 139–144.

Kehl-Pruett, W. (2006). Deep vein thrombosis in hospitalized patients: A review of evidence-based guidelines for prevention. *Dimensions of Critical Care Nursing, 25*(2), 53–59.

Klerk, M., Verhoef, P., Clarke, R., Blom, H. J., Kok, F. J., & Schouten, E. G. (2002). MTHFR 677C->T polymorphism and risk of coronary heart disease: a meta-analysis. *JAMA, 288,* 2023–2031.

Wald, D. S., Law, M., & Morris, J. K. (2002). Homocysteine and cardiovascular disease: Evidence on causality from a meta-analysis. *British Medical Journal, 325,* 1202–1208.

EVIDENCE-BASED PRACTICE

glycemic control is essential to reduce infection and promote healing. An in-depth discussion of the nutritional aspects of wound healing is presented in Chapter 14 ☞. Surgical intervention for venous ulcers is rarely required because no definitive procedure has been found for treatment.

Research into causes and treatment of DVT continues. See the Evidence-Based Practice box.

Lymphatic Disorders

The lymphatic system is composed of lymphatic vessels, lymph nodes, the spleen, and the thymus. This system filters bacteria and other particulate matter, thereby providing defense against disease. **Lymphangitis** is an acute inflammation of the lymphatic channels most commonly caused by an infection in one of the extremities. The associated lymph nodes become enlarged and tender. Recurrent episodes of lymphangitis can be associated with progressive lymphedema. The Diagnostic Tests box outlines the typical tests that are done to assist in confirming the diagnosis. Lymphedema can be primary or secondary. Primary lymphedema is inherited as an autosomal dominant trait. Secondary lymphedema occurs as a result of an acquired disorder, such as a malignancy, radiation, surgical removal of a component of the lymphatic system, trauma, or infection. Malignancy is the most common cause of secondary lymphedema in the United States (Sieggreen & Kline, 2004b). Figure 43–18 ■ shows lower extremity severe lymphedema.

Pathophysiology

Lymphedema occurs when there is an obstruction causing excess lymph buildup within the system, which ultimately overloads the transport capacity of the lymphatic system. This can progress to fibrosis and irreversible tissue damage. Lymphedema is classified into three stages. In Stage I, the edema is pitting and is reversible with elevation of the affected limb. In Stage II, fibrosis has occurred and the edema is nonpitting and nonreversible. In Stage III, the affected limb is greatly enlarged and the skin is thickened.

Clinical Manifestations

Lymphedema is the interstitial accumulation of lymph fluid that occurs when the lymphatic system is impaired. The affected

FIGURE 43–18 ■ Severe lymphedema.
Source: MSNB/Custom Medical Stock Photo, Inc.

limb(s) become edematous with thickened skin. Patients may complain of heaviness or fullness of the affected extremity.

Diagnosis and Medical Management

Diagnosis of lymphedema is based on the patient's history and clinical presentation. The patient should be asked about previous surgeries, radiation treatment, trauma, and infection. Medical therapy of lymphedema is directed toward controlling the fluid accumulation, maintaining skin integrity, and preventing infections. Bed rest, compression therapy, manual lymphatic drainage, short stretch compression wrapping, and limb elevation are the primary interventions for lymphedema.

Complications

Complications of lymphedema include recurrent cellulitis and/or lymphangitis, deep venous thrombosis, severe functional impairment, cosmetic embarrassment, and amputation (rare). Complications following surgery are common and include partial wound

DIAGNOSTIC TESTS for Lymphedema

Test	Expected Abnormality	Rationale for Abnormality
Lymphangiography	Obstructions in lymphatic communication visualized.	Requires contrast administration by injection into a small lymph channel in the dorsum of the foot. Complications of lymphangiography include acute lymphangitis. Rarely performed.
Lymphoscintigraphy	Obstructions in lymphatic communication visualized.	Most commonly performed diagnostic test for lymphedema. Requires injection of technetium 99m labeled colloid in the web spaces of the fingers or toes, and images are obtained at preset intervals. Complications are uncommon.

separation, seroma, hematoma, skin necrosis, and exacerbation of foot or hand edema. Patients with chronic lymphedema have a risk of developing lymphangiosarcoma. Although rare, this cancerous tumor is highly aggressive, requires radical amputation of the involved extremity, and has a very poor prognosis.

Nursing Management

Patients with lymphedema require limb elevation; compression garments (Figure 43–19 ■), which are custom fit garments that apply compression and prevent fluid from accumulating in the limb; and manual drainage, or the use of a lymph pump to reduce edema. The affected extremity is placed into the sleeve of the lymph pump, and it is then inflated to a preset pressure to help drain the extremity. The lymph pump may be used daily to reduce edema. Surgical options include resection of skin and subcutaneous tissue, skin grafting, drainage procedures, removal of tissue containing abnormal lymphatics, and less commonly, transplant of tissue from areas with normal lymphatic tissues to areas with abnormal lymphatic drainage. Rarely, bypass of abnormal lymphatic tissue is attempted, in some cases using vein grafts. Such procedures, which are frequently unsuccessful, are usually performed only under experimental protocols. Surgery has met with limited success and requires significant experience and technical expertise. Complications of surgery include poor healing, infection, prolonged hospitalization, poor cosmetic results, and failure to reduce the edema (Sieggreen & Kline, 2004b).

Health Promotion

Instruct patients on the importance of excellent skin hygiene and infection prevention. Good skin care with mild soaps and moisturizing creams is needed. Because patients with lymphedema are at risk of infection, particularly fungal infections, they need to be taught to inspect regularly for signs and symptoms of infection and to report them promptly.

FIGURE 43–19 ■ Compression garment for lymphedema.
Source: © Gottfried Medical, Inc., used with permission

Gerontological Considerations

The prevalence of peripheral arterial disease, abdominal aortic aneurysm, deep venous thrombosis, and chronic venous insufficiency increases with age. Peripheral arterial disease, stroke, and myocardial infarction are the principal causes of death and disability in patients over age 50. Elderly patients with peripheral arterial disorders are at higher risk of coronary and cerebrovascular events, such as myocardial infarction and stroke. Elderly patients with acute and chronic venous disease are at higher risk of pulmonary embolus and death (AHA, 2006; Oka, 2006).

Peripheral vascular disease can cause functional limitations in the elderly, greatly affecting their quality of life. Physical training, strength training, and exercise programs can improve functional status. Low-intensity exercise programs, such as walking, golf, and shuffleboard, can be of great benefit for the elderly. Patients should be encouraged to continue to modify their risk factors for peripheral vascular disease by smoking cessation and controlling their blood pressure and blood sugar levels.

Special nursing care considerations for the elderly include a careful assessment of the cardiovascular and cerebrovascular systems. Myocardial ischemia and infarction can occur, leading to decompensation of the cardiovascular system. Stroke is a leading cause of death and disability in the elderly. The risk of having a stroke more than doubles for each decade of life after age 55. Following stroke, 25% of the elderly die and 25% will not be able to care for themselves. Teaching the patient and family members the signs and symptoms of TIA/impending stroke is essential (Federman, Bravata, & Kirsner, 2004).

Recovery from major vascular surgical procedures, such as abdominal aortic aneurysm repair or femoropopliteal bypass, can be prolonged in the elderly. Wound healing may be delayed and the elderly may be more likely to develop surgical complications, such as atelectasis, pneumonia, and wound infection. Elderly patients are more likely to develop complications of immobility, so turning, repositioning, and ambulating the patient as early as possible to maintain pulmonary function and promote independence also are important aspects of care. Careful assessment of the patient's nutritional intake is essential, in that it impacts wound healing and survival. Strict asepsis is critical because of the diminished immune response and increased susceptibility to infection.

Research

Peripheral vascular disorders affect millions of Americans, and the effects of these diseases can be limiting and potentially devastating. Research that further explores and defines nursing interventions and therapies for patients with peripheral vascular disease is needed. Nursing research in the area of peripheral vascular disorders and the application of evidence-based practice is essential for the continued refinement of care for the patients with peripheral vascular disorders. The research topics related to peripheral vascular disorders are outlined in the Research Opportunities and Clinical Impact box.

RESEARCH OPPORTUNITIES AND CLINICAL IMPACT RELATED TO PERIPHERAL VASCULAR DISORDERS

Research	Clinical Impact
Effects of gene therapy on peripheral arterial disease	Decrease in tissue loss and enhanced healing
Herbal and complementary medicine to treat peripheral arterial disease	Lowers blood lipids and blood pressure
Wound care in arterial and venous ulcers	Rapid and enhanced healing
Pressure reduction surfaces and devices	Rapid and enhanced healing; prevention of skin breakdown in patients with peripheral arterial disease (PAD) and other high-risk patients

Clinical Preparation

CRITICAL THINKING

 Read

- History of Current Illness
- Past Medical History
- Physical Exam
- Admitting Medical Orders
- Laboratory Study Results

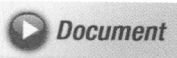 **Document**

- Summary of Hospitalization
- Pathophysiology Form
- Laboratory Values
- Laboratory Results Explanation

 Apply

- List of Potential Nursing Diagnoses
- Concept Map
- Critical Thinking Questions

Log on to MyNursingKit.com to download forms you will need and to complete further steps in the Clinical Preparation assignment.

HISTORY OF PRESENT ILLNESS

As the on-coming nurse on the medical–surgical unit, you receive a report on Mr. Davis, a 68-year-old retired school-teacher admitted 2 days ago with peripheral arterial disease, rest pain in the right forefoot, and a nonhealing ulcer on the distal aspect of the right great toe. He was admitted from the ED and gave a 2-week history of persistent and severe pain, which has kept him from sleeping at night. He also noted redness and drainage from what had previously been a stable callus over the distal great toe.

You are told by the night nurse that Mr. Davis was stable throughout the night, was able to sleep at short intervals, although his pain level never decreased below 5/10 despite use of a morphine sulfate patient-controlled analgesia (PCA) pump and bolus doses of 5 mg twice.

Medical/Surgical History

His past medical history includes intermittent claudication after walking two blocks, type II diabetes, hypertension, hypercholes-terolemia, and coronary artery disease. He is allergic to penicillin. Currently, he is a nonsmoker for 1 year after smoking 1 pack per day for 50 years. He has an alcohol intake of one glass of red wine with dinner. Past surgeries include three-vessel coronary artery bypass grafting 8 years prior and percutaneous transluminal angioplasty (PTA) and stenting of the right external iliac artery 1 year ago.

Social History

He is married with two grown children and a 2-year-old grand-daughter. He is active in his church group and plays golf three times per week, although he is unable to walk the course because of leg pain and now uses a cart.

Current Medications
Atorvastatin (Lipitor) 40 mg po daily
Cilostazol (Pletal) 100 mg po bid
Aspirin 325 mg enteric-coated po daily
Metformin (Glucophage) 500 mg po bid
Benazepril (Lotensin) 20 mg po daily
Nitroglycerine 0.4 mg sublingual prn

Physical Exam
Physical exam findings reveal that Mr. Davis is alert and cooperative and oriented × 3. He currently rates his pain as 5/10 in the right foot. Vital signs: Blood pressure is 150/90 in the left arm, 160/100 in the right arm; heart rate 72; respiratory rate 18; temperature 37.5°C. His weight is 200 pounds. His height is 5'10". He has a left carotid bruit. His neurological exam is normal. He has a well-healed midline sternal incision. Heart tones are regular with no murmur heard. Lungs are clear with diminished breath sounds at the bases bilaterally. His abdomen is soft, nontender with active bowel sounds. He has bilateral femoral bruits. His femoral pulses are faintly palpable bilaterally and his popliteal, dorsalis pedis, and posterior pulses are absent bilaterally.

Dependent rubor is noted in the right foot, which blanches with elevation. Skin of the feet is dry and intact, except for the right great toe ulcer, which measures 1 cm. Capillary refill of the other toes is sluggish. Slight erythema is noted on the surrounding skin, and there is a small amount of serous drainage on the dressing. His toenails are thickened. 12-lead ECG: sinus rhythm with nonspecific ST segment changes.

Admitting Medical Orders
Vascular service
Admit to telemetry with continuous cardiac monitoring
Diagnosis: Peripheral arterial disease with ulceration, right toe
Allergy: penicillin
Vital signs q4h
Bilateral lower extremity pulse checks q4h
Bed rest with bathroom privileges
1,800-calorie ADA diet
Accuchecks ac and hs
Call house officer: pulse < 60 and > 130/minute; BP < 90 and > 160 systolic; temperature > 38.5; urine output < 30 mL/hr for 2 hours; respiratory rate > 40/minute; glucose > 150
IV saline lock: flush with NS q8h
NS wet-to-dry dressing changes to right great toe q8h

Scheduled Medications
Atorvastatin (Lipitor) 40 mg po daily
Cilostazol (Pletal) 100 mg po bid
Aspirin 325 mg enteric-coated po daily
Metformin (Glucophage) 500 mg po bid
Benazepril (Lotensin) 20 mg po daily
Nitroglycerine 0.4 mg sublingual prn chest discomfort/angina
Mylanta 30 mL q4h prn dyspepsia
Zolpidem (Ambien) 5 mg po qhs prn for sleep
Ativan 1 mg IV q6h prn anxiety
Milk of Magnesia 30 mL daily prn constipation
Tylenol 650 mg po/pr q4h prn for pain
Morphine sulfate PCA: 1 mg incremental dose q10min; if pain not well controlled, give morphine sulfate bolus 1–5 mg IV × 1

Ordered Laboratory Studies
CBC, basic metabolic panel, daily
Culture drainage right toe

Ordered Diagnostic Studies
12-lead ECG
PA and lateral chest x-ray
Carotid duplex today; also have vascular lab perform bilateral ABI
NPO at midnight for aortic angiography with runoff

LABORATORY STUDY RESULTS

Test	Admit	Day 2	Day 3
WBC	13.4/mm³	14.0/mm³	17.1/mm³
RBC	3.66/mm³	3.93/mm³	3.67/mm³
Hemoglobin	11.4 g/dL	12.1 g/dL	11.6 g/dL
Hematocrit	33.6%	35.8%	33.3%
Platelet count	172/mm³	192/mm³	221/mm³
Sodium	137 mEq/L	134 mEq/L	135 mEq/L
Potassium	3.7 mEq/L	3.8 mEq/L	3.8 mEq/L
Chloride	101 mEq/L	96 mEq/L	97 mEq/L
Calcium	7.9 mg/dL	8.6 mg/dL	8.2 mg/dL
Blood sugar	306 mg/dL	255 mg/dL	203 mg/dL
BUN	34 mg/dL	36 mg/dL	34 mg/dL
Creatinine	1.7 mg/dL	1.8 mg/dL	1.7 mg/dL

CRITICAL THINKING QUESTIONS

1. What are the priorities of care for Mr. Davis?
2. What additional objective data would be helpful in assessing Mr. Davis?
3. What is the significance of the smoking history?
4. After morning rounds, Mr. Davis' health care provider orders an angiogram of the aorta and lower extremities. What is the rationale for these tests?
5. How will you prioritize Mr. Davis' nursing care following his angiogram?

Answers to Critical Thinking Questions appear in Appendix D.

NCLEX® REVIEW

1. A patient with a 30-year history of smoking tells the nurse that he can only walk a few blocks before the pain becomes severe in his lower legs. The nurse realizes this patient is describing:
   1. Intermittent claudication.
   2. Deep vein thrombosis.
   3. Peripheral neuropathy.
   4. Exercise intolerance.

2. A patient with peripheral arterial disease has intermittent claudication. Which of the following should the nurse include in this patient's plan of care?
   1. The use of moist heat.
   2. Keep legs elevated above the level of the heart.
   3. Teach importance of regular and structured ambulation.
   4. Remind that the legs will feel cool to the touch.

3. The nurse is instructing a patient with Raynaud's disease on self-management. Which of the following should be included in this instruction?
   1. Smoking cessation is the only treatment for this disease.
   2. Dress warmly in cold weather and limit alcohol intake.
   3. Avoid physical exercise.
   4. Prescribed medications have no effect on the disease.

4. A patient is having an endovascular stent graft to repair for an aortic abdominal aneurysm. Which of the following should the nurse include when assessing post-operative complications for this patient?
   1. Cerebrovascular embolus
   2. Abdominal surgical site infection
   3. Deep vein thrombosis associated with a longer hospital stay
   4. Renal impairment due to alterations in blood flow

5. A patient recovering from orthopedic surgery has developed a deep vein thrombosis in the left calf. Which of the following should the nurse include when instructing this patient?
   1. The need for early ambulation, use of compression stockings, and range of motion exercises.
   2. Avoid the use of compression stockings.
   3. Complete bed rest with the left leg elevated.
   4. Avoid unnecessary exercise.

6. A patient diagnosed with a deep vein thrombosis is started on low molecular weight heparin. Which of the following should the nurse instruct the patient about this medication?
   1. The need to avoid foods high in vitamin K
   2. The signs and symptoms of bleeding
   3. The need to have blood drawn to measure the INR
   4. Why this is the preferred medication for anyone with kidney failure

7. A patient with varicose veins is scheduled for radiofrequency ablation of the vein. Which of the following should the nurse include when providing pre-operative teaching to this patient?
   1. Complete bed rest will be required for 72 hours following this procedure to avoid stressing the suture line.
   2. Compression stockings will be worn to decrease venous stasis.
   3. Avoid showering until a week following the procedure to allow for maximum wound healing.
   4. Anticipate the use of anticoagulants to decrease the viscosity of the blood.

8. An elderly patient is assessed as having a pulsatile mass near the umbilicus. The nurse realizes that treatment will be according to which of the following?
   1. If an aortic aneurysm is diagnosed that is larger than 6 centimeters, surgery will be performed.
   2. If the abdominal ultrasound and CAT scan reveal a 4 centimeter abdominal aortic aneurysm, surgery will be performed.
   3. If diagnostic testing reveals the presence of an abdominal aortic aneurysm, steroids will be added to decrease the inflammatory response.
   4. If an abdominal aortic aneurysm is identified in the infrarenal area, the surgical approach is contraindicated.

Answers for review questions appear in Appendix D

KEY TERMS

aneurysm *p.1342*
ankle-brachial index (ABI) *p.1327*
aortic coarctation *p.1330*
aortic dissection (AD) *p.1344*
carotid endarterectomy (CEA) *p.1339*
deep venous thrombosis (DVT) *p.1346*
endoleaks *p.1343*

intermittent claudication (IC) *p.1326*
lymphangitis *p.1357*
lymphedema *p.1346*
paresthesia *p.1326*
peripheral arterial disease (PAD) *p.1326*
pulmonary embolism (PE) *p.1347*
stenosis *p.1341*

sympathectomy *p.1336*
thromboangiitis obliterans (TAO) *p.1338*
transient ischemic attack (TIA) *p.1339*
Unna's boot *p.1354*
varicose veins *p.1346*
venous thromboembolism (VTE) *p.1347*
Virchow's triad *p.1347*

PEARSON
EXPLORE **mynursingkit™**

MyNursingKit is your one stop for online chapter review materials and resources. Prepare for success with additional NCLEX®-style practice questions, interactive assignments and activities, web links, animations and videos, and more!

Register your access code from the front of your book at
www.mynursingkit.com

REFERENCES

Abou-Chebl, A., Yadiv, J. S., Reginelli, J. P., Bajzer, C., Bhatt, D., & Kreiger, D. W. (2006). Intracranial hemorrhage and hyperperfusion syndrome following carotid artery stenting. *Journal of the American College of Cardiology, 43,* 1596–1601.

Agency for Healthcare Research and Quality. (2008). *Treating tobacco use and dependence: 2008 update.* Rockville, MD: Author. Retrieved July 22, 2008, from http://www.ahrq.gov/path/tobacco.htm

American Heart Association. (2006). American Heart Association. Home Page Retrieved March, 28, 2006, from http://www.americanheart.org

American Heart Association. (2007). *Few Americans aware of dangerous peripheral arterial disease.* Retrieved on July 24, 2008 from http://www.americanheart.org/presenter.jhtml?identifier=3050383

American Heart Association. (2008b). *Atherosclerosis.* Retrieved July 24, 2008 from http://www.americanheart.org/presenter.jhtml?identifier=4440

American Stroke Association. (2006). *Learn to recognize a stroke.* Retrieved March 28, 2006, from http://www.strokeassociation.org/presenter.jhtml?identifier=1020

American Urological Association. (2002). *Renovascular disease.* Retrieved November 13, 2006, from http://www.urologyhealth.org/adult/index.cfm?cat=02&topic=126

Arkkila, P. E. (2006). Thromboangiitis obliterans (Buerger's disease). *Orphanet Journal of Rare Diseases, 1,* 14.

Beebe-Dimmer, J. L., Pfeifer, J. R., Engle, J. S., & Schottenfeld, D. (2004). The epidemiology of chronic venous insufficiency and varicose veins. *Annals of Epidemiology, 15,* 175–184.

Brem, H., Kirsner, R. S., & Falanga, V. (2004). Protocol for the successful treatment of venous ulcers. *The American Journal of Surgery, 188* (Suppl. 1A), 1S–8S.

Büller, H. R., Agnelli, G., Hull, R. D., Hyers, T. M., Prins, M. H. & Raskob, G. E. (2004). Antithrombotic therapy for venous thromboembolic disease: The seventh ACCP conference on antithrombotic and thrombolytic therapy. *Chest, 126*(3), 401S–428S.

Cahill, E. J. (2004). Assisting with tobacco cessation. *Journal of Vascular Nursing, 22,* 117–123.

Cardin, T., & Marinelli, A. (2004). Pulmonary embolism. *Critical Care Nursing Quarterly, 27*(4), 310–322.

Caulfield, M. T., Fernando, D., & Rosenfield, K. (2005). Renal and iliac intervention. In H. C. Herrmann (Ed.), *Interventional cardiology: Percutaneous noncoronary intervention* (pp. 295–320).Totowa, NJ: Humana Press.

Chang, A. K. (2008). *Thoracic outlet syndrome.* Retrieved July 25, 2008 from http://www.emedicine.com/emerg/TOPIC578.HTM

Criqui, M. H., Vargas, V., Depenberg, J., Ho, E., Allison, M., Langer, R. D., et al. (2005). Ethnicity and peripheral arterial disease: The San Diego population study. *Circulation, 112,* 2703–2707.

Davis, J., & Gray, M. (2005, May/June). Is the Unna's Boot bandage as effective as the four-layer wrap for managing venous leg ulcers? *Journal of Wound, Ostomy and Continence Nursing,* 152–156.

Dickinson, M. G., Krishnan, U., Houlihan, G., & Walker, C. M. (2004). Renal artery stenosis: Diagnosis and management. In G. S. Abela (Ed.), *Peripheral vascular disease: Basic diagnostic and therapeutic approaches* (pp. 270–282). Philadelphia: Lippincott Williams & Wilkins.

Eberhardt, R. T., & Raffetto, J. D. (2005). Chronic venous insufficiency. *Circulation, 111,* 2398–2409.

Eisenhauer, A. C., & Shaw, J. C. (2004). Atherosclerotic subclavian artery disease and revascularization. In G. S. Abela (Ed.), *Peripheral vascular disease: Basic diagnostic and therapeutic approaches* (pp. 283–294). Philadelphia: Lippincott Williams & Wilkins.

Fahey, V. A. (Ed.). (2004). *Vascular nursing* (4th ed.). Philadelphia: Elsevier.

Federman, D. G., Bravata, D. M., & Kirsner, R. S. (2004). Peripheral arterial disease: A systemic disease extending beyond the affected extremity. *Geriatrics 59*(4), 26–34.

Fleming, C., Whitlock, E. P., Beil, T. L., & Lederle, F. A. (2005). Screening for abdominal aortic aneurysm: A best-evidence systematic review for the U.S. Preventative Services Task Force. *Annals of Internal Medicine, 142*(3), 203–211.

Geerts, W. H., Pineo, G. F., Heit, J. A., Bergqvist, D., Lassen, M. R., Colwell, C. W., et al. (2004). Prevention of venous thromboembolism: The seventh ACCP conference on antithrombotic and thrombolytic therapy. *Chest, 126,* 338S–400S.

Gey, D. C., Lesho, E. P., & Manngold, J. (2004). Management of peripheral arterial disease. *American Family Physician, 69,* 525–533.

Hirsch, A. T., Haskal, Z. J., Hertzer, N. R., Bakal, C. W., Creager, M. A., Halperin, J, L., et al. (2006). ACC/AHA guidelines for the management of patients with peripheral arterial disease (lower extremity, renal, mesenteric, and abdominal aortic): A collaborative report from the American Association for Vascular Surgery/Society for Vascular Surgery, Society for Cardiovascular Angiography and Interventions, Society of Interventional Radiology, Society for Vascular Medicine and Biology, and the American College of Cardiology/American Heart Association Task Force on Practice Guidelines (Writing Committee to Develop Guidelines for the Management of Patients with Peripheral Arterial Disease). *Journal of the American College of Cardiology, 47,* 1–192.

Hirsh, J., Guyatt, G., Alberts, G. W., & Schünemann, H. J. (2004). The Seventh ACCP Conference on Antithrombotic and Thrombolytic Therapy: Evidence-based guidelines. *Chest, 126,* 172S–173S.

Hirsh, J., & Raschke, R. (2004). Heparin and low molecular weight heparin: The seventh ACCP conference on antithrombotic and thrombolytic therapy. *Chest, 126*(3), 188S–203S.

Hunter, S., Langemo, D., Hanson, D., Anderson, J., & Thompson, P. (2005). Compression therapy for venous ulcers. *Advances in Skin & Wound Care, 18*(8), 404–408.

Jacoby, D. S., & Mohler, E. R. (2004). Peripheral arterial disease: Risk factor identification and modification. In G. S. Abela (Ed.), *Peripheral vascular disease: Basic diagnostic and therapeutic approaches* (pp. 190–199). Philadelphia: Lippincott Williams & Wilkins.

Kehl-Pruett, W. (2006). Deep vein thrombosis in hospitalized patients: A review of evidence-based guidelines for prevention. *Dimensions of Critical Care Nursing, 25*(2), 53–59.

LaMuraglia, G. M., & Nigri, G. R. (2004). Surgery for peripheral vascular disease. In G. S. Abela (Ed.), *Peripheral vascular disease: Basic diagnostic and therapeutic approaches* (pp. 365–373). Philadelphia: Lippincott Williams & Wilkins.

Lipsitz, E. C., & Kim, S. (2005). Antithrombotic therapy in peripheral arterial disease. *Clinics in Geriatric Medicine, 22* 183–198.

Lu, J. T., & Creager, M. T. (2004). The relationship of cigarette smoking to peripheral arterial disease. *Reviews in Cardiovascular Medicine, 5*(4), 189–193.

Marr, W. L. (2006). Deep venous thrombosis recommendations. *Journal of Vascular Nursing, 24*(3), 91–93.

Mayo Clinic. (2006) *Raynaud's disease.* Retrieved October 15, 2007, from http://www.mayoclinic.com/health/raynauds-disease/DS00433

National Heart, Lung, and Blood Institute. (2004). *Seventh report of the Joint National Committee on Prevention, Detection, Evaluation, and Treatment of High Blood Pressure* (NIH Publication No. 04-5230, pp. 1–104). Bethesda, MD: Author.

Oka, R. K. (2006). Peripheral arterial disease in older adults: Management of cardiovascular risk factors. *Journal of Cardiovascular Nursing, 21*(55), S15–S20.

Olson, K. W., & Treat-Jacobson, D. (2004). Symptoms of peripheral arterial disease: A critical review. *Journal of Vascular Nursing, 22*(3), 72–77.

Porth, C. M. (2005). *Pathophysiology: Concepts of altered health status* (7th ed.). Philadelphia: Lippincott Williams & Wilkins.

Porth, C. (2007). *Essentials of pathophysiology* (2nd,ed.). St. Louis: Lippincott Williams & Wilkins.

Rectenwald, J. E., & Wakefield, T. W. (2005). The treatment of deep venous thrombosis, including the newer agents. *Disease of the Month, 51,* 104–111.

Rehring, T. F., Sandhoff, B. G., Stolepart, R. S., Merenich, J. A., & Whitton-Hollis, H. (2005). Atherosclerotic risk factor control in patients with peripheral arterial disease. *Journal of Vascular Surgery, 41*(5), 816–822.

Reilly, A., & Snyder, B. (2005). Raynaud's phenomenon. *American Journal of Nursing, 105*(8), 56–65.

Sieggreen, M. (2005a). Lower extremity arterial and venous ulcers. *Nursing Clinics of North America, 40,* 391–410.

Sieggreen, M. (2005b). Venous disorders: Overview of current practice. *Journal of Vascular Nursing, 23*(1), 33–35.

Sieggreen, M. Y., & Kline, R. A. (2004a). Arterial insufficiency and ulceration: Diagnosis and treatment options. *Nurse Practitioner, 29*(9), 46–52.

Sieggreen, M. Y., & Kline, R. A. (2004b). Current concepts in lymphedema management. *Advances in Skin & Wound Care, 17*(4), 174–180.

Singh, V. N., & Cousin, A. (2005). *Angioplasty, Peripheral.* eMedicince. Retrieved on July 24, 2008 from http://www.emedicine.com/radio/topic754.htm

Sontheimer, D. L. (2006). Peripheral vascular disease: Diagnosis and treatment. *American Family Physician, 73*(11), 1971–1976.

Sullivan, T. M. (2005). Surveillance and follow-up after carotid angioplasty and stenting. In M. A. Mansour & N. Labropoulos (Eds.), *Vascular diagnosis* (pp. 183–191). Philadelphia: Elsevier Saunders.

Tapson, V. F. (2005). The diagnosis of venous thromboembolism. *Disease of the Month, 51,* 86–93.

Teruya, T. H., & Ballard, J. L. (2004). New approaches for the treatment of varicose veins. *Surgical Clinics of North America, 84,* 1397–1417.

Upchurch, G. R., & Schaub, T. A. (2006). Abdominal aortic aneurysm. *American Family Physician, 73*(7), 1198–1204.

Walsh, M. E., & Rice, K. L. (2004). Venous thromboembolic disease. In V. A. Fahey (Ed.), *Vascular nursing* (4th ed.). Philadelphia: Elsevier.

Wound, Ostomy, and Continence Nurses Society. (2005). *Guideline for management of wounds in patients with lower-extremity venous disease.* Glenview, IL: Author.

APPENDIX A   2009–2011 NANDA-APPROVED NURSING DIAGNOSES

Activity Intolerance
Activity Intolerance, Risk for
Activity Planning, Ineffective
Airway Clearance, Ineffective
Anxiety
Anxiety, Death
Aspiration, Risk for
Attachment, Parent/Infant/Child, Risk for Impaired
Autonomic Dysreflexia
Autonomic Dysreflexia, Risk for
Bleeding, Risk for
Blood Glucose, Risk for Unstable
Body Image, Disturbed
Body Temperature: Imbalanced, Risk for
Bowel Incontinence
Breastfeeding, Effective
Breastfeeding, Ineffective
Breastfeeding, Interrupted
Breathing Pattern, Ineffective
Cardiac Output, Decreased
Caregiver Role Strain
Caregiver Role Strain, Risk for
Childbearing Process, Readiness for Enhanced
Comfort, Impaired
Comfort, Readiness for Enhanced
Communication: Impaired, Verbal
Communication, Readiness for Enhanced
Confusion, Acute
Confusion, Acute, Risk for
Confusion, Chronic
Constipation
Constipation, Perceived
Constipation, Risk for
Contamination
Contamination, Risk for
Coping: Community, Ineffective
Coping: Community, Readiness for Enhanced
Coping, Defensive
Coping: Family, Compromised
Coping: Family, Disabled
Coping: Family, Readiness for Enhanced
Coping (Individual), Readiness for Enhanced
Coping, Ineffective
Decisional Conflict
Decision Making, Readiness for Enhanced
Denial, Ineffective
Dentition, Impaired
Development: Delayed, Risk for
Diarrhea
Disuse Syndrome, Risk for
Diversional Activity, Deficient
Electrolyte Imbalance, Risk for
Energy Field, Disturbed
Environmental Interpretation Syndrome, Impaired
Failure to Thrive, Adult
Falls, Risk for

Family Processes, Dysfunctional: Alcoholism
Family Processes, Interrupted
Family Processes, Readiness for Enhanced
Fatigue
Fear
Fluid Balance, Readiness for Enhanced
Fluid Volume, Deficient
Fluid Volume, Deficient, Risk for
Fluid Volume, Excess
Fluid Volume, Imbalanced, Risk for
Gas Exchange, Impaired
Grieving
Grieving, Complicated
Grieving, Risk for Complicated
Growth, Disproportionate, Risk for
Growth and Development, Delayed
Health Behavior, Risk-Prone
Health Maintenance, Ineffective
Health Management, Ineffective Self
Health-Seeking Behaviors (Specify)
Home Maintenance, Impaired
Hope, Readiness for Enhanced
Hopelessness
Human Dignity, Risk for Compromised
Hyperthermia
Hypothermia
Identity, Disturbed Personal
Immunization Status, Readiness for Enhanced
Infant Behavior, Disorganized
Infant Behavior: Disorganized, Risk for
Infant Behavior: Organized, Readiness for Enhanced
Infant Feeding Pattern, Ineffective
Infection, Risk for
Injury, Risk for
Insomnia
Intracranial Adaptive Capacity, Decreased
Knowledge, Deficient (Specify)
Knowledge (Specify), Readiness for Enhanced
Latex Allergy Response
Latex Allergy Response, Risk for
Liver Function, Impaired, Risk for
Loneliness, Risk for
Maternal/Fetal Dyad, Risk for Disturbed
Memory, Impaired
Mobility: Bed, Impaired
Mobility: Physical, Impaired
Mobility: Wheelchair, Impaired
Moral Distress
Motility, Dysfunctional Gastrointestinal
Motility, Risk for Dysfunctional Gastrointestinal
Nausea
Neonatal Jaundice
Neurovascular Dysfunction: Peripheral, Risk for
Noncompliance (Specify)
Nutrition, Imbalanced: Less than Body Requirements
Nutrition, Imbalanced: More than Body Requirements

Nutrition, Imbalanced: More than Body Requirements, Risk for
Nutrition, Readiness for Enhanced
Oral Mucous Membrane, Impaired
Pain, Acute
Pain, Chronic
Parenting, Impaired
Parenting, Readiness for Enhanced
Parenting, Risk for Impaired
Perfusion, Ineffective Peripheral Tissue
Perfusion, Risk for Decreased Cardiac
Perfusion, Risk for Impaired Renal
Perfusion, Risk for Ineffective Cerebral Tissue
Perfusion, Risk for Ineffective Gastrointestinal Tissue
Perioperative Positioning Injury, Risk for
Personal Identity, Disturbed
Poisoning, Risk for
Post-Trauma Syndrome
Post-Trauma Syndrome, Risk for
Power, Readiness for Enhanced
Powerlessness
Powerlessness, Risk for
Protection, Ineffective
Rape-Trauma Syndrome
Relationship, Readiness for Enhanced
Religiosity, Impaired
Religiosity, Readiness for Enhanced
Religiosity, Risk for Impaired
Relocation Stress Syndrome
Relocation Stress Syndrome, Risk for
Resilience, Impaired Individual
Resilience, Readiness for Enhanced
Resilience, Risk for Compromised
Role Conflict, Parental
Role Performance, Ineffective
Sedentary Lifestyle
Self-Care, Readiness for Enhanced
Self-Care Deficit: Bathing/Hygiene
Self-Care Deficit: Dressing/Grooming
Self-Care Deficit: Feeding
Self-Care Deficit: Toileting
Self-Concept, Readiness for Enhanced
Self-Esteem, Chronic Low
Self-Esteem, Situational Low
Self-Esteem, Risk for Situational Low
Self-Mutilation
Self-Mutilation, Risk for
Self Neglect
Sensory Perception, Disturbed (Specify: Auditory, Gustatory, Kinesthetic, Olfactory, Tactile, Visual)
Sexual Dysfunction
Sexuality Pattern, Ineffective
Shock, Risk for
Skin Integrity, Impaired
Skin Integrity, Risk for Impaired
Sleep Deprivation

Sleep Pattern, Disturbed
Sleep, Readiness for Enhanced
Social Interaction, Impaired
Social Isolation
Sorrow, Chronic
Spiritual Distress
Spiritual Distress, Risk for
Spiritual Well-Being, Readiness for Enhanced
Spontaneous Ventilation, Impaired
Stress, Overload
Sudden Infant Death Syndrome, Risk for
Suffocation, Risk for
Suicide, Risk for
Surgical Recovery, Delayed
Swallowing, Impaired
Therapeutic Regimen Management: Family, Ineffective

Therapeutic Regimen Management, Ineffective
Therapeutic Regimen Management, Readiness for Enhanced
Thermoregulation, Ineffective
Tissue Integrity, Impaired
Tissue Perfusion, Ineffective (Specify: Cerebral, Cardiopulmonary, Gastrointestinal, Renal)
Tissue Perfusion, Ineffective, Peripheral
Transfer Ability, Impaired
Trauma, Risk for
Trauma, Risk for Vascular
Unilateral Neglect
Urinary Elimination, Impaired
Urinary Elimination, Readiness for Enhanced
Urinary Incontinence, Functional
Urinary Incontinence, Overflow

Urinary Incontinence, Reflex
Urinary Incontinence, Stress
Urinary Incontinence, Urge
Urinary Incontinence, Risk for Urge
Urinary Retention
Ventilatory Weaning Response, Dysfunctional
Violence: Other-Directed, Risk for
Violence: Self-Directed, Risk for
Walking, Impaired
Wandering

Source: NANDA Nursing Diagnoses: Definitions and Classification, 2007–2008. Philadelphia: North American Nursing Diagnosis Association. Used with permission.

Standard precautions are designed to reduce the risk of transmission of microorganisms from both recognized and unrecognized sources of infection. They are the primary strategies for preventing nosocomial infections within institutions, and are important to protect health care workers as well. Standard precautions apply to (1) blood; (2) all body fluids, secretions, and excretions except sweat, regardless of whether or not they contain visible blood; (3) nonintact skin; and (4) mucous membranes. Standard precautions are applied to all patients receiving care in hospitals, regardless of their diagnosis or presumed infection status. These precautions are specifically designed for hospitals; however, they also may be implemented in extended and long-term care facilities, and to a more limited extent in providing home care or in other community-based care settings.

Hand Washing

- Wash your hands (a) after touching blood, body fluids, secretions, excretions, and contaminated items, whether or not gloves are worn; (b) immediately after removing gloves, even if gloves appear to be intact; (c) between contacts with patients; and (d) when otherwise indicated to prevent transfer of organisms to other patients. You may need to wash your hands between tasks and procedures on the same patient to prevent cross-contaminating different body sites.
- Use soap and warm water for hand washing when hands are visibly dirty or contaminated with blood or other body fluids.
- If hands are not visibly soiled, use an alcohol-based hand rub for routinely decontaminating hands in all other situations.

Gloves

- Wear clean, nonsterile gloves when touching blood, body fluids, secretions, excretions, and contaminated items.
- Put on clean gloves just before touching mucous membranes and nonintact skin.
- Change your gloves between tasks and procedures on the same patient after contacting material that may contain a high concentration of microorganisms.
- Wear gloves for all invasive procedures such as performing venipuncture or other vascular or surgical procedures.
- Wear gloves if you have cuts, scratches, or other breaks in the skin.
- Remove gloves promptly after use, before touching noncontaminated items and surfaces, and before going to another patient; wash hands immediately after removing gloves.

Mask, Eye Protection, Face Shield

Wear a mask and eye protection or a face shield to protect mucous membranes of your eyes, nose, and mouth during procedures and patient care activities that are likely to generate splashes or sprays of blood, body fluids, secretions, or excretions.

Gown

Wear a gown (clean, disposable) to protect your skin and prevent soiling of clothing during procedures and patient care activities that are likely to generate splashes or sprays of blood, body fluids, secretions, or excretions. Remove soiled gowns promptly, washing your hands immediately after gown removal.

Equipment

Handle used patient care equipment that is soiled with blood, body fluids, secretions, and excretions in a way that prevents exposing your skin and mucous membranes, contaminating your clothing, and transferring microorganisms to other patients or environments. Ensure that reusable equipment is cleaned and appropriately reprocessed before using for the care of another patient.

Environmental Control

Follow hospital procedures for routine care, cleaning, and disinfecting environmental surfaces, beds, bed rails, bedside equipment, and other frequently touched surfaces.

Linen

Handle and transport linens soiled with blood, body fluids, secretions, and excretions in a manner that prevents exposing your skin and mucous membranes, contaminating your clothing, and transferring microorganisms to other patients and environments. Place soiled linen in leakage-resistant bags at the location where it is used.

Occupational Health and Bloodborne Pathogens

- Take care to prevent injuries when using needles, scalpels, and other sharps; when handling sharp instruments after procedures; when cleaning used instruments; and when disposing of used needles.
- Never recap used needles, manipulate them using both hands, or handle them in a manner that directs the point of a needle toward any part of your body. If it is necessary to protect the needle prior to disposal, use a one-handed "scoop" technique or mechanical device to hold the needle sheath.
- Do not remove used needles from disposable syringes by hand; do not bend, break, or otherwise manipulate used needles by hand.
- Place used disposable syringes and needles, scalpel blades, and other sharp items in appropriate puncture-resistant containers located as close as practical to the area in which the items were used.
- Place reusable syringes and needles in a puncture-resistant container for transport to the reprocessing area.

- Use mouthpieces, resuscitation bags, or other ventilation devices as an alternative to mouth-to-mouth resuscitation methods whenever possible.

Patient Placement

Place patients who contaminate the environment or who do not (or are not expected to) assist in maintaining appropriate hygiene or environmental control (e.g., an ambulatory, confused patient with fecal incontinence) in a private room.

Sources: Centers for Disease Control and Prevention. (2002). Guidelines for hand hygiene in health-care settings: Recommendations of the Healthcare Infection Control Practices Advisory Committee and the HICPAC/SHEA/APIC/IDSA Hand Hygiene Taskforce. *MMWR, 51*(RR-16), 1–56; Hospital Infection Control Practices Advisory Committee. (1997). Part II. Recommendations for isolation precautions in hospitals. Atlanta: Public Health Service, U.S. Department of Health and Human Services, Centers for Disease Control and Prevention.

APPENDIX C Units of Measurement in Metric and Household Systems

ABBREVIATIONS

Volume

Metric		Household	
milliliter	mL	microdrop	mcgtt
liter	L	drop	gtt
cubic centimeter	cc	teaspoon	t or tsp
		tablespoon	T or tbs
		fluid ounce	oz
		pint	pt
		quart	qt

Weight

Metric		Household	
microgram	mcg	ounce	oz
milligram	mg	pound	lb
gram	g		
kilogram	kg		

Length

Metric		Household	
centimeter	cm	inch	in
meter	m	foot	ft

Area

Metric	
square meter	m^2

Evidence-Based Practice Boxes

Chapter 10
Evidence-Based Practice #1 Answers
1. In this scenario, the nurse will need to perform a digital rectal exam to assess for hardened stool in the rectal vault. If the patient is uncooperative, a provider's order for any abdominal x-ray to assess for fecal impaction would be indicated.
2. Because narcotics can cause a slowing of the intestine, with constipation as a result, the nurse will need to consider adding a stool softener or laxative to the patient's medication regimen.
3. Yes, patients often have fecal impaction of stool in the rectum but have small amounts of liquid stool that are expelled around the impaction. The nurse will need to facilitate removal of the hardened stool through the use of either a suppository or an enema or via manual disimpaction, if needed.

Evidence-Based Practice #2 Answers
1. Ask the daughter why she feels her mother should have a mammogram now, when she has refused them in the past. This allows the daughter to verbalize her concerns about her mother, which may reflect the daughter's greater concerns as to her mother's overall medical condition.
2. If the daughter is the patient's appointed spokesperson, share with her your findings. She may already know about the mass and have decided to take no further action, or it may be new information to her. Either way, notify the patient's provider with your findings for further action, if indicated.
3. Call the breast imaging center in advance to determine whether it has the equipment available to accommodate this patient. If the patient is frail, the breast imaging center may want to schedule a longer appointment than usual to give the patient extra time to complete the mammogram.

Evidence-Based Practice #3 Answers
1. The nurse should diplomatically remind the health care provider that Darvocet (propoxyphene) can cause adverse central nervous system effects in the elderly, with little analgesic advantage over acetaminophen. The nurse can suggest a medication more appropriate in this population, such as acetaminophen with a short-acting opiate if necessary for pain control. It is also helpful to know what is available in your facility's emergency medication kit so that you will be able to give a medication without having to order it from the pharmacy and wait for delivery.
2. Diphenhydramine can cause urinary retention, especially in elderly males who may have a baseline prostate hypertrophy. Diphenhydramine should not be used as a sleeping agent; safer alternatives exist. The nurse should notify the health care provider of the patient's symptoms and then discuss a plan of treatment, including addressing the patient's urinary retention as well as insomnia.
3. Her health care provider needs to know about her diazepam use because this medication should be avoided in the elderly due to its extremely long half-life. The nurse needs to discuss with both the patient and the health care provider a plan of care to address the patient's "nerves." Obtaining medications from multiple providers is a dangerous practice, especially for the aging patient.

Chapter 12
1. The perception and chronicity of stress causes a cellular response and an increase in oxidative stress. The cellular response includes a reduction in the number of telomeres and telomerase, a decrease in the ability of the cells to divide, and a decrease in the DNA component, which precipitates genetic damage and eventually cell death. Over time, the tissues comprising the affected cells also die, producing the effects of aging: muscles weaken; skin wrinkles; hair grays; eyesight; hearing; and organs fail; and thinking abilities diminish.
2. Young adults have higher telomerase levels and a greater ability for the enzyme to repair the cell by regenerating telomeres. The telomerase levels decrease with normal aging. This process is accelerated with high levels of chronic psychological stress, thus precipitating premature aging. It is important to know this information to assist in the assessment process. Understanding the age differentiation helps the nurse to know which type of patient is the most vulnerable candidate for cellular response to chronic perceived stress.
3. a. Sleep.
   b. Social connections.
   c. Exercise.
   d. Quiet time alone.
   e. Rest and relaxation.
   f. Meditation/contemplation.
   g. Hobbies.
   h. Nutrition.
   i. Journaling.
   j. Yoga.

Chapter 14
1. Postpyloric placement of a feeding tube into the small bowel can be useful to minimize the risk of high gastric residuals. If it is not contraindicated, elevation of the head of the bed to a 45-degree angle may decrease risk of aspiration.
2. Feedings should not be held until there are two or more consecutive gastric residual volumes greater than 250 mL.

Chapter 15
1. Is this new onset pain?
   What is the patient's perception of discomfort?
   Has this type of pain occurred before?

What has been effective in the past for pain relief?
Drug allergies or unwanted side effects such and nausea and vomiting.
2. Facial grimacing.
Increased movement.
Increased heart rate and blood pressure.
Ask family members and caregivers what the usual response to pain is.

Chapter 17

1. Ask and identify open-ended questions to clarify how they are feeling.
2. Listen carefully to what they are saying. Let them know that you are available to answer questions. Advocate for the patient and family by contacting other members of the health care team as needed.

Chapter 20

1. a. Ensure an adequate diet with vitamins A and C, iron, and zinc.
   b. Avoid exposure to others with infection.
   c. Instruct the patient to wash hands after toileting and before eating.
   d. Report to the surgeon all medications taken.
2. a. Check color; redness may indicate infection.
   b. Check temperature; warmth may indicate infection.
   c. Check for swelling.
   d. Check for drainage from the wound. If present, check the color and amount of drainage.
3. a. Wash hands before and after touching the patient.
   b. Wear gloves when providing wound care.
   c. Keep the patient well hydrated and provide foods that are high in protein.
4. a. Instruct patients to take their prescriptions as directed, including the prescribed frequency and duration.
   b. Educate patients on when antibiotics are appropriate and not appropriate.

Chapter 21

1. Ask the patient an open-ended question to describe what insights have become apparent during the interview.
2. Listen carefully to the story of the patient. Use nonverbal cues to support the patient.

Chapter 23

1. f. b & c
2. a. Slow the transfusion.
   b. Take vital signs and oxygen saturation.
   c. Call the health care provider.

Chapter 25

1. These questions are designed to get one to think about issues that may influence the generalizability of research findings and the need to replicate research studies using subjects of both genders, varying ages, and multiple ethnicities and cultures. In thinking about this study, one might wonder how culture, specifically the Chinese culture, might influence things such as attitudes toward pain and pain expression as well as attitudes toward taking pain medication or using nonpharmacologic therapies for pain control. Culture may also play a role in how the subjects respond to being part of a research study. One needs to know more fully about Chinese culture to theorize about how these research results will generalize to a Western culture. Similarly, it is helpful to know about national health insurance in China. The economics of health care in a country influence aspects of care, such as what kind of preoperative teaching is available, what pain medications are used, how medications are administered, and what nonpharmacologic approaches are covered by the insurance. These may, in turn, influence attitudes.

2. Pain is a subjective experience, and the use of a visual analog scale is a valid and reliable measure of a person's pain experience. The researchers could include objective indices of pain or of physiological stress, with physiological stress serving as a marker for pain. Examples of objective measures might include blood pressure (elevation or changes correlating with pain ratings), heart rate (elevation or correlation with pain rating), respiratory rate (elevation), and plasma cortisol levels (elevation). Objective markers have limitations because they are nonspecific; nevertheless, they could contribute to the discussion of pain reduction. The authors could also use functional performance as indirect markers of pain reduction. Physical performances that often improve with pain relief include ability and distance of ambulation, amount of time spent out of bed, and ability and frequency of deep breathing or ability to perform coughing exercises.

Chapter 26

1. a. Communication with surgical team for timing of antibiotic administration and to maintain surgical asepsis guidelines.
   b. Institute measures to maintain normothermia throughout surgery and postanesthesia care unit.
   c. Develop policies that ensure that standards regarding warning procedures are used by all members of the surgical team.

Chapter 27

1. It is not known which aspects of the protocol accounted for the change in the patient outcomes. One could explain, using Maslow's hierarchy of needs, that the protocol was effective because it helped patients to meet basic needs of comfort: toileting, repositioning, and pain management. These needs were met on a regular basis without the patient having to ask. The protocol also increased patients' sense of personal control over their environment by ensuring that important objects were close by and by giving information about care schedules. Perhaps the consistency of the schedule met higher levels of human need by allowing patients to feel safe and cared for. Several nursing theories can be used to explain the outcomes of this study. Hildegard Peplau's interpersonal relationships theory that puts the nurse–patient relationship at the center of nursing practice or Jean Watson's theory of caring are both appropriate, as are many

nursing theories. Katherine Kolcaba's theory of comfort is particularly relevant to the protocol of nursing rounds. In her theory, enhanced comfort is an immediate and desirable outcome of nursing interventions.

2. It seems as if any number of patient outcomes might be influenced by a nursing round protocol (the protocol used in the study or one that is tailored for specific nursing units). Examples of specific patient outcomes include reduction in urinary or bowel incontinence, reduction in the incidence of decubiti, improved pain management, increased mobility, and increased oral fluid intake.

3. The study could be replicated using a larger number of nursing units and varied types of units (medical, cardiac, oncology, neurology, surgical specialties, etc.). The protocol could be lengthened from the 4 weeks that was used. The nursing rounds protocol could be adapted for specific patient populations (e.g., it could include a reminder to use the incentive spirometry on a surgical unit).

Chapter 29

1. a. Difficulty with concentration.
   b. Family observations of irritability.
   c. Memory impairment.
2. a. A recent motor vehicle accident, with or without loss of consciousness.
   b. Participation in sporting events.
   c. Difficulty in school or work environment.
3. a. Consults for therapies, such as speech and occupational therapies.
   b. Family teaching and support.

Chapter 30

1. The elderly, any patient with uncontrolled hypertension, any patient on Coumadin.
2. Severe headache, difficulty with speech, decreased motor function of either side of the body, sudden loss of consciousness.
3. Close control of blood glucose, careful monitoring of blood pressure, vigilant neurological assessment.

Chapter 31

1. a. Disease process.
   b. Disease and symptom management.
   c. Community resources for assistance at home.
2. a. Verbalize instructions back to the nurse.
   b. Demonstrate the skill back to the nurse.
3. a. Get regular medical checkups.
   b. Get regular physical activity, such as walking.
   c. Use stress management techniques such as pleasurable activities, praying, or meditating.

Chapter 32

1. a. Immobility due to paralysis and spinal precautions.
   b. Ineffective cough.
   c. Use of a cervical orthosis.
   d. Abnormalities in the mechanics of swallowing.
2. a. Frequent coughing with oral intake.
   b. Wet vocal quality.

c. Difficulty managing oral secretions.
3. a. Sitting patient in an upright position for meals once cleared for activity.
   b. Avoid talking while eating.
   c. Avoidance of large boluses of food at one time.
   d. Monitor patient to ensure that food is cleared from the oropharynx.

Chapter 35

1. a. Most people spend 90% of their time indoors.
2. a. Tobacco smoke must be eliminated from the indoor environment.
3. a. Reducing the exposure to indoor allergens and pollutants will reduce exacerbation of respiratory illness.

Chapter 36

1. c. Confused and not able to cooperate.
2. b. COPD.

Chapter 38

1. a. Has anyone in your family, including parents, grandparents, siblings, aunts, and uncles, ever been diagnosed with AF?
   b. Have you ever been diagnosed with any cardiac disorder, such as heart failure, valve disease, heart attack, or rheumatic fever?
   c. Do you smoke, drink caffeine, or drink alcohol, and if so, in what quantity?
   d. Are you diabetic?
2. a. Report light-headedness, dizziness, shortness of breath, or chest pain to your health care provider as soon as they occur.
   b. Stop smoking and drinking alcohol and caffeine.
   c. Consistently take prescribed medications.
   d. Have family members tested if the AF is genetically induced.

Chapter 40

1. a. Use of interpreters.
   b. Instructions written in native languages.
   c. Use of family or friends who can assist with interpretation.
2. a. Are you noticing any changes in your energy level when performing your daily activities?
   b. Is there a change in the number of hours of sleep needed to feel rested?
   c. Has the need to rest during the day increased recently?
3. a. Statistics about the prevalence of heart disease in women.
   b. The types of clinical symptoms that women experience compared to those experienced by men.
   c. Lifestyle changes that would prevent or slow the progress of heart disease.

Chapter 41

1. a. Understand when it is important to seek medical help for the tachycardia.
   b. How to avoid activities that bring on the tachycardia.

    c. How to slow the heart rate when tachycardia occurs.

    d. List of ideas and activities that would be safe.

2.   a. Education about the relationship between tachycardic episodes and the progression of the disease.

    b. Providing alternative activities that interest the young person to decrease the frustration associated with the limitations of the disease.

    c. Evaluate the presence of social support and educate these significant individuals about the need for activity restriction.

3.   a. Space activities to allow for periods of rest.

    b. Medicate with antianxiety per orders when necessary.

    c. Control the environment and visitors to diminish stress.

    d. Evaluate current measures and the need for further intervention when necessary.

Chapter 42

1.   a. Notify the patient's health care provider.

    b. Ask to talk to another member of the family to see if it is possible to get the patient his medications.

    c. Have the patient explore the possibility of having the medications delivered by the pharmacy.

    d. Ask the patient if he can afford to have a taxi deliver the medications.

2.   a. Ask the patient specific questions about her diet, in terms of food types and amounts.

    b. Ask the patient to keep track of the amount of fluids consumed each day.

    c. Discuss with the patient/family the implications associated with failure to comply with therapy.

    d. Ascertain the patient/family understanding of failure to comply with medical management.

    e. Report clinical manifestations to the health care provider.

3.   a. Ask the patient about diet, fluid intake, and compliance with medications.

    b. Ask the patient about support system and availability of help with cooking and procurement of medications.

    c. Assess patient motivation with compliance with treatment plan.

    d. Assess patient/family understanding of treatment needs and ability to comply.

Chapter 43

1. Assessment of other risk factors for the development of DVT. Reporting homocysteine and risk factors to the health care provider. Instating health care provider orders to prevent DVT. Assessment for the effectiveness of the interventions.

2. Active and passive range of motion. Foot and ankle exercises. Graduated stocking, pneumatic compression devices.

3. Prevent venous pooling of blood.

Chapter 45

1. A, C, E, F

2. Visual inspection of the oral mucosa.

3. When assessing the oral cavity, the nurse should note any subjective complaints, such as soreness or pain of the lips or gums, reports of increased salivation, toothache, or earache. The objective assessment findings of concern would include indurations or painless ulcer on the lips, ulcerations, areas of thickening, increased salivation, leukoplakia, erythroplakia, rough areas, slurred speech, dysphagia, or difficulty chewing or speaking.

Chapter 46

1. Most medications are metabolized by the liver. Decreased hepatic blood flow and shunting of blood slows the metabolism of medications and creates a higher bioavailability. Also, the shifts in body fluids that occur with decreased serum albumin will change the volume of distribution for the medications.

2. The nurse should check the medication information to see if the pharmacologic half-life is affected by liver failure. Because the metabolism of morphine is greatly affected, the nurse should review the dosage and frequency with the health care team to ensure the safety of the patient.

Chapter 47

1. Nonadherence with fluid restrictions may cause fluid overload with symptoms of shortness of breath, muscle cramping, dizziness, anxiety, panic, pulmonary edema, and hypertension. Nonadherence with dietary restrictions and medication regimens may result in chronically elevated serum levels of phosphate, which contribute to the development of coronary artery disease and the development of secondary hyperparathyroidism.

2. Implement adherence-enhancing interventions with the goal of improving the clinical outcome.

Chapter 49

1. c

2. a

3. a

Chapter 50

1. Meeting the needs of the spouse will improve the quality of life for both the patient and the spouse.

2. d. Involve spouses in medical decision making along with the patient.

Chapter 53

1. The best answer would be "b." This is an adolescent who is not focused so much on the future as on his current lifestyle. It is important to look at what is going on around him to try to find the reason why he is not checking his blood glucose. There may be a variety of reasons as to why he does not test his glucose, including feeling self-conscious about his diabetes. At this point, the nurse can help to explore practical ways to integrate glucose testing into his lifestyle, regardless of whether he really understands the long-term complications or not.

2. The best answer would be "a." The point that you want to emphasize is that regardless of the type of diabetes, the relationship between glucose control and the development of

complications is a primary mediator of complications (chronically elevated blood glucose levels are associated with the development of diabetes-related complications). The nurse may also want to explore whether there are financial or other concerns that are influencing one's ability to check blood glucose levels.

3. Of the two responses, the second is the best. This is because it involves a systematic approach to the problem while recognizing that if the patient and family decide to continue multiple daily injections, the plan will be in place to recognize and prevent hypoglycemia.

Chapter 55

1. Identifying high-risk individuals allows the health care team, patient, and family to develop a plan and implement preventive measures to decrease the chance of a fall and subsequent fracture.

2. Moderate exercise such as walking, swimming, or riding a stationary bike helps to strengthen muscles, slows the loss of calcium from the bone, and helps to maintain balance. Exercise such as yoga helps to strengthen core muscles, which helps with maintenance of balance and flexibility.

Chapter 56

1. The pin site will become infected. Skeletal traction pins are exposed to the environment where they protrude through the skin, and bacteria can travel down to the bone. Moisture creates an area for bacteria, always present at the pin–skin interface, to accumulate and grow.

2. Signs and symptoms of infection include pain, redness, edema, and drainage from the site.

Chapter 57

1. Early control of pain is more effective in controlling pain than is medication administered after pain becomes severe. With amputation, pain normally begins to diminish in intensity 3 or 4 days after surgery.

2. Phantom limb pain is the sensation of pain in the amputated body part. The cause of the phenomenon is unknown, but the perception of pain can interfere with the patient's rehabilitation.

Chapter 58
Critical Thinking Application #1 Answers
1. a. Have the patient take the medication with food.
   b. Encourage small frequent meals.
   c. Drink milk when taking medication.
2. a. Xanthine oxidase inhibitors.
   b. Nonsteroidal anti-inflammatory drugs.
   c. Steroids.
   d. Uricosuric agents.

Critical Thinking Application #2 Answers
1. a. Compliance with multiple treatments, such as medication and lifestyle changes.
   b. What impact can the nursing profession make on improving patient care with gout?

c. Providing an understanding of the risks and pathophysiology of the disease process.
   d. Teaching the patient ways to improve lifestyle choices and reduce gout attacks.
   e. Educating the patient on medication therapy.

Chapter 60
1. b. Ease of availability and financial resources.
2. a. Diminished or absent diarrhea.
   c. Absence of candidiasis.
   d. No painful swallowing.

Chapter 61
1. a. Hypotension after infusion of 2 liters of isotonic crystalloid infusion.
2. b. Infusing 7 liters of crystalloid solution through a central line.
3. 1. Suctioning blood from the patient's airway.
   2. Initiating a large-caliber IV for fluid resuscitation.
   3. Stabilizing the patient's pelvis with a sheet.
   4. Applying 100% oxygen by mask to the patient.

Chapter 63
Evidence-Based Practice #1 Answers
1. Pain, short duration of inspiration, and frustration.
2. a. Provide patient education regarding the relationship between lung inspiration, oxygenation, and pulmonary complications.
   b. Provide instruction on proper use of IS, including length of inspiration, volume goals, and frequency.
   c. Recruit family to encourage patient.
   d. Provide adequate pain management.
   e. Provide frequent encouragement and progress assessments/reports to patient.
3. a. Lung sounds.
   b. Chest expansion.
   c. Pain level with inspiration.
   d. Oxygenation status.
   e. Incentive spirometry volume and frequency of use.

Evidence-Based Practice #2 Answers
1. a. Assessment.
   b. Regular flushing.
   c. Solution based on clinical assessment.
2. Benefits include prevention of clot formation. However, risks are increased HIT.

Chapter 64
1. a. Understanding at what point during the course of treatment there is a potential to develop fatigue.
   b. Explanation of how the patient may feel as he or she becomes fatigued.
   c. A list of strategies to reduce energy consumption.
   d. Dietary suggestions to optimize nutrition during and after treatment.
2. a. Report presence of fatigue to health care team so that recommendations can be offered.

b. Encourage the patient and family to discuss the impact of fatigue on their daily lives.

c. Referral to social services or psychiatry as needed.

d. Acknowledge the potential for fatigue to alter sexuality.

3. a. Provide information about interventions available to treat fatigue.

b. Accurate assessment and prompt treatment for fatigue.

c. Encourage patients to maintain adequate activity to increase energy stores.

Chapter 67

1. e. All of the above.

2. a. It would combine to form the compound silver chloride and the silver would no longer be bioavailable to perform its function because ionic silver is the element that is effective against bacteria.

3. e. All of the above.

Chapter 68

1. a. Obtain immediate medical care when injuries occur.

b. Understand that there is an increased risk for complications and prolonged hospitalization.

c. Daily foot inspection for breakdown.

d. Avoidance of extreme temperatures when bathing.

e. No exposure to heaters to help keep feet warm.

2. a. Fireplaces.

b. Poorly controlled heaters.

c. Living alone.

d. Confusion and poor memory.

e. Little to no social support.

f. Inadequate nutrition.

g. Inadequate blood sugar control.

3. a. Blood sugar control.

b. Adequate nutritional support.

c. Strict aseptic technique for wound care.

d. Reporting of the first signs of infections.

Chapter 70
Evidence-Based Practice #1 Answers

1. Know which noises can cause damage (those above 85 decibels). Wear earplugs or other hearing protection devices when involved in a loud activity. Be alert to hazardous noise in the environment. Protect children who are too young to protect themselves. Make family, friends, and colleagues aware of the hazards of noise. Have a medical examination by an otolaryngologist, a physician who specializes in diseases of the ears, nose, throat, head, and neck, and a hearing test by an audiologist, a health professional trained to identify and measure hearing loss and to rehabilitate persons with hearing impairments.

2. Everyone is exposed to hazardous sound levels at one time or on a regular basis—individuals of all ages, including children, adolescents, young adults, and older people. Exposure occurs in the workplace, in recreational settings, and at home.

3. A variety of activities can predispose an individual to NIHL. It may occur from only a one-time exposure to loud sound as well as from repeated exposure to sounds at various loudness levels over an extended period of time. Examples of activities are listening to loud iPods, radios, or TV. Examples of workplace noises are jackhammers and explosive sounds. Participation in recreational activities, such as flying loud model airplanes, snowmobiling, go-carting, woodworking, target shooting, and hunting, may even be a factor.

Evidence-Based Practice #2 Answers

1. Culturally deaf adults are at risk for health-related behaviors that address nutrition, psychological well-being, stress management, physical activity and exercise, activities of daily living, and responsible health care practices.

2. Culturally deaf adults may use a variety of interventions to help them adjust to their environments. The following is just a small list of such activities: learning sign language; having communities provide street warning signs for adults with hearing impairments; using devices that help with communication, such as flashing lights for doorbells or visual readings for telephone communication; and participating in educational activities that will inform society of ways to prevent hazards that cause hearing impairment or hearing loss.

3. School nurses not only are helpful in identifying those adolescents with hearing problems through screening programs, but they may act as advocates for educational activities that inform adolescents of hazardous activities that may lead to NIHL.

Chapter 71

1. a. Inform the patient as to what AMD is and how it impacts the vision and general well-being of the patient, with a return demonstration of gained knowledge.

b. Advise patient about possible ways to decrease the advancement of AMD with prevention.

c. Teach the patient about when it is important to seek medical direction for vision changes from AMD, with a return demonstration of information gained.

d. List the problem stages of treatment or management of AMD.

2. a. Educating about the relationship of possible aging, genetics, ultraviolet light, air pollution, smoking, comorbidities, blood thinners, zinc, luteins, antioxidants, and VEGF toward the advancement of AMD.

b. Providing alternative activities that interest older adults to decrease the frustration associated with the limitations of vision with AMD and general well-being.

c. Incorporating a significant other in the relationship and care, depending on the degree of visual impairment, to prevent social isolation.

d. Providing possible activities that would be beneficial and safe in adding to the prevention or stabilization of visual impairment from AMD.

3. a. Educate on maintaining good general health and avoiding comorbidities that may affect or advance a decline in vision health.

b. Educate on self-vision testing, for example, Amsler grid, and coping with vision loss and maintaining quality of life.

c. Control the environment by adding more independence activities with visual impairment.

d. Evaluate current measures and the need for further intervention as needs present.

Chapter 73

1. b. A policy and procedure should be present to assist in the implementation of family presence. Staff members need education and support.
2. d. All of the above.

Chapter 74

1. f. All of the above.
2. b. It decreases the risk of coagulopathy.

Clinical Preparation Boxes

Chapter 14

1. a. Obesity (BMI 33).
   b. Obesity, family history, hypercholesterolemia, hypertension, hyperglycemia, decreased serum HDL cholesterol, sedentary activity level.
2. a. Assess readiness to lose body weight.
   b. Educate on health benefits of losing weight.
   c. Assist in development of short-term goals toward losing 1 to 2 pounds/week:
      - Increase physical activity. Begin with sitting for fewer hours in the day and gradually add activity.
      - Decrease intake by 500 to 100 kcal/day; assist patient with identifying ways to do this, such as decreased intake of alcohol and empty calories (e.g., change cream in coffee to fat-free half and half, snack on fruit instead of chips).
   d. Educate about the DASH diet for hypertension (reduced sodium, saturated fat, and cholesterol; moderate alcohol; adequate dairy; ample fruits, vegetables, and whole grains).
   e. Refer to registered dietitian.
3. a. Fat intake.
   b. Alcohol intake.
   c. Caffeine intake.
   d. Large meals.
   e. Eating large meals late in the evening, close to bedtime (lying flat with increased gastric pressure).
   f. Overweight/obese.
4. Reduced intake of fat, moderating alcohol intake, weight loss.

Chapter 15

1. Sensory, affective, cognitive, and behavioral.
2. Discuss concerns about pain management and discuss reasons for behavior when wife is present.
3. PCA demand doses attempted/given, medication side effects, renal function, patient's current and acceptable level of pain.

Chapter 19

1. This patient has a respiratory acidosis—the $PaCO_2$ is increased and the pH is acid. The HCO_3^- is higher than normal, with a base excess of $+5$.
2. Age, 50 pack/year smoking history, emphysema, history of coronary artery disease.
3. Emphysema and pneumonia.
4. Coughing and deep-breathing exercises. Up in chair and walking at regular intervals.

Chapter 20

1. Room 122—apparent best immune system.
2. Yes—open draining leg wound that is positive for *S. aureus*.
3. Diabetes, living in the woods, age, and smoking.
4. *Body Image, Disturbed.*
   Fatigue.
   Mobility: Physical, Impaired.
   Pain, Acute.
   High Risk for Self-Care Deficit: Toileting.
   Skin Integrity, Impaired.
   Tissue Perfusion, Ineffective, Risk for.

Chapter 21
Part 1

1. *Assessment:* The nurse's initial assessment of Ms. Bell began at the time of her first visit to the health care center. The nurse began to collect the database concerning the characteristics that Ms. Bell was demonstrating. The subjective database suggested depression and distortion of reality concerning her health and work problems. The objective database was anger, agitation, and intolerance for the environment and the reporting of psychosomatic symptoms.
   Related Factors: Ms. Bell has highly ambivalent feelings concerning her family and the loss of employment.
   Nursing Diagnosis: Coping: Family Disabled (Wilkinson, 2005, p. 117).
   Alternative Diagnosis: Management of Therapeutic Regimen: Families/Individual, Ineffective (Wilkinson, 2005, p. 118).
   NOC Outcomes (Wilkinson, 2005):
   - Aggression control.
   - Depression control.
   - Neglect recovery.
   Goals/Evaluation Criteria:
   - Ms. Bell will use *Disabled Family Coping* as demonstrated by satisfactory status in aggression control, depression control, and neglect of recovery.
   - *Family and Individual Coping* with:
     Demonstrates role flexibility.
     Manages problems.
     Receives care and cares for the needs of family members.
     Secures financial stability.
     Asks for assistance when appropriate (Wilkinson, 2005, p. 119).
   NIC Interventions:
   - Coping enhancement: Assist Ms. Bell to adapt to the real and perceived stress and changes that were interfering with her life goals.

- Normalization promotion: Assist Ms. Bell with adaptation to a chronic disease, diabetes mellitus. Encourage her to accept that her life experience is a reality (Wilkinson, 2005).

Nursing Activities:

- Obtain a history of the family's patterns of behavior and changes that have occurred.
- Assess the interaction between Ms. Bell and her family.
- Determine the physical, emotional, educational, and spiritual resources of Ms. Bell.
- Assess Ms. Bell's motivation for resolving the crisis.
- Discuss with Ms. Bell the most effective ways to assist her with becoming familiar with her multiple health needs. Ms. Bell needs referrals to other agencies such as social services, nutrition counseling, support groups, and the Council on Aging.

Part 2

The strategies essential to controlling Ms. Bell's hypertension were an adequate knowledge base of what the disease is, how it may be controlled, the use of lifestyle changes, and weight control. Ms. Bell was encouraged to participate in the plan of care, and her questions can be answered through the use of the office hotline.

Part 3

If Ms. Bell relapses into noncompliance, the nurse will assess the problems interfering with Ms. Bell's following through with her plan of care. With this information, the plan of care can be modified by removing the element that was keeping her from following through. At times, the patient may not understand how and why a particular segment of the plan was important to the management and control of the disease. The use of totally illustrated brochures and conferences within the location may assist in the understanding of hypertension. In addition, the teaching appointments can be recorded on audio tape for the patient's review at home.

2. • Acceptance of the diagnosis of high blood pressure.
   • Enabling Ms. Bell in seeking information about high blood pressure and how the diagnosis is made.
   • Partnership with the nurse as the treatment plan is established, maintained, and revised.
   • Use of the plan and the ability to negotiate changes in the treatment plan as the physiological situation need modification.
   • Understands the reason for keeping appointments with the health care provider. Ms. Bell will report self-screening results at each visit.
   • Ms. Bell monitors herself for the treatment response.
   • Ms. Bell performs self-screening tests such as blood pressure, weight, and glucose monitoring.
   • Ms. Bell seeks to reinforce her lifestyle changes.

3. When the nurse listens to Ms. Bell in a therapeutic manner, the nurse will engage in an assessment of the patterns of communication and as a self-interpreting person. This means listening to the individual for his or her interpretation and the embedded meaning of the situation. This activity, the process of active listening, is "attending to and

attaching significance to a patient's verbal and nonverbal messages" (Wilkinson, 2005, p. 82).

4.

Nursing Assessment of Loss

Nursing Assessment and Diagnoses	Outcomes and Evaluation Parameters	Planning and Interventions with Rationale
Subjective: "I'm standing under a very dark cloud." "How much more can or must I tolerate?"	**Outcome:** Practice effective coping strategies. **Evaluation Parameters:**	**Interventions and Rationales** Discusses importance of participating in the high blood pressure support group in the community.
Objective: Death of husband of 35 years Loss of employment due to downsizing Daughter lives 250 miles away	Documented improvements in self-reports. States reasons for changes in lifestyle and coping styles.	Discusses changing role in her home, community, and church. Reviews changes in lifestyle.
Nursing Diagnosis: Chronic Losses related to chronic illness and Ineffective Coping with lifestyle related to chronic illness		*Lifestyle changes and modification of role within family, community, and church have positive value in fostering effective coping strategies.*

Chapter 23

1. ASA and Celebrex.
2. Rehydration, undetected bleeding.
3. Transfusion reactions, lung sounds. Identification of patient, vital signs, and signs and symptoms of transfusion reactions.
4. Fluid overload due to his age and cardiac history.
5. History of taking Lopressor, a beta-blocker that decreases heart rate.
6. The Na and Cl levels are elevated (concentrated blood solutes). The BUN is elevated, but the creatinine is normal. Values return to normal after rehydration.
7. To rule out pancreatitis, which can cause GI bleed.
8. Vitamin K absorption by the intestine is decreased in GI bleed, and vitamin K is needed for clotting. Vitamin K affects the part of the clotting cascade that is measured by the PT and INR.

Chapter 27

1. *Pain:* Abdominal incisions are painful, and Mr. Landry's pain ratings show that he is not getting adequate pain relief. Pain is a likely factor in his reluctance to ambulate and to use the incentive spirometer.

   Impaired Gas Exchange: Mr. Landry is on 4 liters of oxygen but has only marginal oxygen saturation. He is not performing deep breathing or coughing as needed to open the airways and alveoli and to clear respiratory secretions.

Fluid Volume, Deficient: Mr. Landry is losing fluid through the NGT and because he has a fever. The low urine output, tachycardia, dry skin, thirst, and vertigo when standing suggest that he is dehydrated.

Anxiety: Mr. Landry demonstrates anxious behaviors and he reports feeling anxious. Anxiety is an uncomfortable state, and it can influence all aspects of his care and recovery.

Activity Intolerance: Mr. Landry has vertigo, tachycardia, and tachypnea with activity.

2. Pain: Evidenced by high pain ratings and reluctance to do IS, cough, and ambulate.

Atelectasis: Evidenced by fever, crackles, shallow breathing.

Dehydration: Evidenced by tachycardia, low urine output, warm skin, thirst.

Orthostatic hypotension: Likely, given his complaints of vertigo on standing.

Ileus: Evidenced by no passing of flatus (expected finding for the first several days postop following surgery on colon).

Nausea: Evidenced by complaints of nausea.

Anemia: Evidenced by a low hematocrit and hemoglobin.

Vital Signs: Part of routine nursing care. The data are used to monitor for a variety of postoperative complications, including fever, bleeding, dehydration, abnormal cardiac rhythm.

NPO: To prevent abdominal distention and nausea and vomiting.

NGT to low continuous suction: Used to decompress the stomach. Prevents abdominal distention until peristalsis returns to the bowel. Abdominal distention would place tension on the sutures.

IS: A mechanism used to encourage deep breathing. Deep breathing increases lung volumes and stimulates surfactant. This intervention is used to treat hypoxia and to prevent atelectasis and pneumonia.

Foley: Used to get an accurate, hourly measurement of urine output.

I&O: Used to estimate fluid balance. Many patients are slightly dehydrated at the end of surgery. In this case, Mr. Landry is continuing to lose fluid as a result of a fever and drainage from the NGT.

Pneumatic compression boots: Increase venous return from the legs, helping to prevent deep venous thrombus (DVT).

Ambulate: Ambulation is the single most important intervention to prevent postoperative complications. Ambulation increases respiratory rate, minute ventilation, tidal volume, and inspiratory flow rates, helping to prevent atelectasis and pneumonia. Ambulation increases blood flow to organs and tissues, helping with wound healing, restoring peristalsis, and preventing venous stasis and DVT.

Cardiac telemetry: Used to monitor for bradycardia and dysrhythmia because Mr. Landry is receiving Metoprolol intravenously.

Dextrose 5% and 0.45 sodium chloride with 20 mEq KCl: This is an isotonic solution used to replace routine fluid loss and to cover fluid loss through the NGT. Mr. Landry requires potassium replacement because he is NPO and unable to replace routine loss of potassium in the urine and additional potassium losses from gastric drainage.

3. The most pressing nursing activities are the treatment of Mr. Landry's pain and nausea. Until pain and nausea are controlled, Mr. Landry will be unable to concentrate on learning to use incentive spirometry or participate in morning care. The nurse should first change the syringe in the PCA pump (this activity is entirely within the nurse's control) to make sure that Mr. Landry has uninterrupted pain medication. Second, the nurse should empty and record urine output and then call the surgeon for the antiemetic. Calling for the antinausea medication is important, but Mr. Landry has been having a low urine output that, if it continues, will require intervention (calling the surgeon and administration of a fluid bolus), and measuring urine output will only take a minute. Third, the nurse calls the surgeon for an antiemetic order (and reports the urine output if low). Once Mr. Landry is comfortable, he should receive teaching on use of the incentive spirometry. A.M. care is important to helping patients feel better, but most patients will decline morning care if they are uncomfortable with either pain or nausea.

4. Treatment for cancer, including colon cancer, depends on the stage of the cancer. Although surgery is a treatment for colon cancer, it is also part of the staging process because the tissue and lymph nodes removed will be examined for evidence of cancer cells. Mr. Landry may need adjunctive treatment (chemotherapy or radiation) once the stage of the cancer is determined. The nurse's best response in this situation is to explore with Mr. Landry his understanding of his disease and the treatment plan. The nurse can help clarify information provided by the surgeon and encourage Mr. Landry to ask the surgeon about questions he has regarding further treatment. The nurse can also help clarify for Mr. Landry the roles of the various people who are or will be involved in his care (e.g., the surgeon, the oncologist, the primary health care provider). The nurse should encourage Mr. Landry to keep the appointment with the oncologist.

Chapter 29

1. An injury to the left temporal area may result in speech difficulties, motor and/or sensory deficits to the right side of the body, and/or confusion.

2. The first sign that Jose's neurological status had changed was when he became restless and agitated and tried to climb over the rails. Though a subtle sign, restlessness and/or agitation may be the first sign that the level of consciousness has deteriorated.

3. The significance of this subtle neurological change is the probability that the size of the subdural hematoma may

be expanding. Subdural hematomas are space-occupying lesions; therefore, an expanding lesion has the potential to increase ICP, with neurological deterioration to follow.

4. With a decrease in the patient's neurological assessment, the nurse might expect the size of the subdural hematoma to have increased, causing more mass effect and increasing ICP.

5. Although the change in the patient's level of consciousness is usually the first sign of neurological deterioration, Jose had other signs to support his decrease in status. His severe headache and projectile vomiting were signs of increasing ICP. He also was more confused than on prior examination. The nurse could expect to see further signs of deterioration if the hematoma is not evacuated. If the hematoma continues to increase in size, without treatment, further deterioration of this patient's neurological condition might occur. An increase in the size of the hematoma would result in increased mass effect and cerebral edema. Clinical manifestations of increasing ICP were discussed earlier in this chapter and include further depression of the level of consciousness, continuing through stupor, lethargy, coma, and possibly death from herniation.

Chapter 30

1. The rupture of an aneurysm with hemorrhage into the subarachnoid space produces severe pain. The complaint of "worst headache of my life" is a hallmark complaint of subarachnoid hemorrhage.

2. Motor and speech deficits in a right-handed person usually indicate a left side lesion; hemiparesis of both upper and lower extremities indicates that the middle cerebral artery probably is affected.

3. The patient showed several signs of decreased neurological function. She was agitated, indicating increased ICP. She also had a decrease in her speech function, indicating decreased blood flow to the left middle cerebral artery territory.

4. Resume triple H therapy: Increase IV fluids; raise blood pressure, including the use of vasopressors, if necessary, for the treatment of vasospasm. Hyponatremia is often seen in the presence of vasospasm and must be corrected. The addition of supplemental salt tablets and hypertonic saline should be administered judiciously to increase serum sodium to a normal level.

Chapter 31

1. Stroke, seizure, CSF leak, infection, and prevention of venous thrombotic events (rate is higher in cases >4 hours).

2. Motor status, for improvement of symptoms—tremor, rigidity, bradykinesia. Also complications from overstimulation of dopaminergic neurons: dyskinesia, dystonia, confusion, hallucination.

3. Depression, anxiety, body image.

4. Orthostatic blood pressures; history of nausea with administration; orders for antiemetic other than prochlorperazine; motor status and mental status.

Chapter 32

1. History of smoking, history of submersion, dyspnea, tachypnea, hypoxia on ABGs. Also, patient has a lower cervical spinal cord injury, which may affect the ability to use respiratory accessory muscles.

2. An order should be obtained for prophylactic anticoagulation therapy such as low-molecular-weight heparin. Antiembolic stockings and pneumatic compression devices should be worn by the patient. Mobilization of the patient should be instituted as soon as the patient is medically stable.

3. Ileus, stress ulcer, constipation, bowel incontinence.

4. Lack of social support, refusal to open eyes, poor interaction with staff, diagnosis of a complete cervical spinal cord injury.

5. Severe hypertension, bradycardia, patient complaint of pounding headache, blurred vision, skin flushing, piloerection, and nasal congestion. Sit the patient upright and place lower extremities in a dependent position. Find and eliminate the cause. Common causes include bladder distention, stool impaction, and pressure ulcer formation. If blood pressure remains elevated, an order for a quick-acting antihypertensive may be needed.

Chapter 34

1. The nurse is responsible for recognizing the frustration and concern that this may cause the patient. The nurse also is responsible for assisting the patient in finding ways to communicate. This may take several forms: having the patient use a chalk board to write on, pantomiming, using signs and symbols that the patient can point to, and assisting the patient in lip reading. If the tracheostomy still is in place, a speaking (flutter) valve may be used to assist the patient in speaking.

2. Maintaining an open airway is the first priority for the nurse and patient. The nurse should instruct the patient on keeping the airway open through suctioning and wound care. It is important to instruct the patient on how to keep the stoma clean and free of crusts. It also is important to reassure the patient that he or she can maintain an open airway and adequate oxygenation by following the instructions for keeping the stoma clean and free of crusts. Normal oxygenation is evidenced by normal oxygen saturation levels, lungs that are clear to auscultation, and unlabored breathing. The patient can be taught to assess these critical elements and take appropriate or emergency action if adequate oxygenation is not present.

   It is helpful to remember that the patient has made a difficult decision in opting to have the total larynx removed. The nurse's attitude and approach to helping the patient speak should be one of caring and compassion.

3. The patient is dealing with a major change in self-image and, in all probability, a major change in lifestyle, including recreational activities, at least for the present. The nurse, through his or her attitude and approach to the patient, or demeanor, should convey understanding of the

patient's situation and feelings. For example, if the patient reacts with anger or by withdrawing, the nurse should recognize these symptoms as ones of depression and adjustment to the changes the patient is experiencing; they are not directed at the nurse or other health care providers.

If the patient and/or family members can express their feelings, it is helpful for the nurse to listen, to not pass judgment, and to offer resources that may be available to help the patient adjust. Specifically, relative to comportment, the nurse should assume an interested, unhurried approach to patient care, with the nurse's posture and demeanor communicating interest and concern.

Chapter 35

1. The nurse evaluates the spirometry values when available as a measure of lung function and continues to evaluate all lab values daily. Physical assessments with a focus on respiratory status are done twice a shift. The nurse obtains information related to the home environment, such as the presence of stairs or safety hazards and dust or environmental pollutants, average daily exercise and activities of daily living, support systems, family or significant others, the patient's understanding of the disease and treatments, use of oxygen and use and cleaning of oxygen equipment at home, and financial status and insurance. This information will be needed to individualize the discharge plan and identify teaching needs.

2. A barrel chest is one in which the anterior-posterior (A-P) diameter is twice that of the transverse diameter. The normal chest has an A-P diameter of half of the transverse diameter. This manifestation is caused by inflation of alveoli due to emphysema.

3. Solu-Medrol alleviates symptoms of inflammation and may relieve wheezing and chest tightness. Because it is a glucocorticoid, it raises serum blood sugar. It may also cause retention of sodium, with a lowering of potassium. It causes gastric irritation, so it should be taken with an antacid or food. It also depresses the immune response, so the patient is more prone to infections. In some patients it may cause mood swings.

4. Mr. H and his wife should be given plenty of written material to reinforce teaching content. Blood sugars should be checked at least twice a day with a glucometer. The patient and/or spouse should demonstrate this to the nurse before discharge. Usually, if the glucose reading is consistently above 200 g/dL, the health care provider should be notified. Because prednisone depresses the immune system, the patient should avoid crowds and/or individuals with infections. He should be observed using an inhaler and taught to rinse his mouth after using each medication to prevent thrush. If he experiences side effects such as "feeling hyper," palpitations, or a fast heart rate after using Atovent, he should call his health care provider. He should be taught to take his blood pressure and should be given the acceptable range. This should be 100/70 to 140/80. If he experiences dizziness, weakness, or headache, he should call his provider. In addition, the patient should describe reasons for taking an antibiotic and possible side effects, such as gastrointestinal disorders. A representative from the oxygen company should meet Mr. H in the hospital if possible for an introductory information session on his oxygen prescription and needed equipment and follow-up on teaching at home after discharge.

5. Mr. H should receive a balanced diet and high-protein, high-potassium foods. If he is retaining sodium, this will be restricted in the diet to 1 to 4 grams daily. He must adhere to his diabetic meal plan as well. He should drink 8 to 10 glasses of water daily. Dairy products should be used in moderation because they may interfere with mobilization of secretions. He should use his supplemental oxygen during meals because eating requires energy, and this will support his additional oxygen needs at mealtime. While at home, he should continue this routine. Prednisone and any potential exacerbation of his condition are likely to raise his glucose level, so his general physical condition, diet, exercise, fluid intake, and glucose levels should be continually monitored.

6. Use of continuous therapy can prevent the development of cor pulmonale and pulmonary hypertension. This increases the survival rate and general quality of life because the patient is able to lead a more normal, active life without the onset of these cardiopulmonary complications of COPD.

Chapter 36

1. a. Inability to maintain adequate oxygen levels for normal tissue perfusion.
   b. Increased risk of aspiration.
   c. Two other common complications of NPPV include facial trauma related to the tight-fitting mask and abdominal distention. Chart 36-19 outlines the contraindications for NPPV.

2. a. CPAP mask: Holds airways open in order to increase resistance and increase oxygenation.
   b. BiPAP mask: Has IPAO for inspiratory positive airway pressure and EPAP or expiratory airway pressure. Numerous full masks and nasal masks.
   c. Patients who are on NPPV can communicate and eat and require very little, if any, sedation.
   d. The benefit of NPPV is that Mr. A does not have an endotracheal tube in his throat and the further mortality and morbidity associated with intubation and ventilator-associated pneumonia (VAP) are absent.
   e. Patient comfort and prevention of skin breakdown are the indications for selection.

3. a. The nurse should be aware that the most serious potentially fatal complication of NPPV is aspiration. Therefore, the airway must have frequent assessments.
   b. Continuous heart rate, pulse oximetry (SpO_2), and specially trained nurses and respiratory therapists who are experienced with NPPV are essential for these patients.
   c. An NG tube might be considered to empty his stomach and decrease the risk of gastric distention and aspiration of gastric contents.

Chapter 39

1. Hypertension, non–insulin-dependent diabetes, hyperlipidemia, current smoker.
2. Urgent PCI in the setting of AMI is the treatment of choice in eligible patients who can be transported to an appropriate hospital in a timely manner.
3. To inhibit platelet activation resulting from the AMI.
4. Impending cardiogenic shock from the AMI.

Chapter 40

1. Because this patient had a drug-eluting stent placed, it is imperative to have adequate antiplatelet therapy to prevent subacute stent thrombosis, which will then cause a subsequent heart attack, as well as to prevent restenosis.
2. This patient had a STEMI, so it is crucial to follow his cardiac enzymes to know the extent of damage as well as to measure against possible reinfarction.
3. ReoPro will provide maximal protection against platelet activation and aggregation to prevent additional thrombus burden after stent placement. This drug is in the classification of GPIIB/IIIA inhibitors and blocks the final common pathway of the clotting cascade.
4. V_1–V_4.
5. Do a 12-lead ECG, apply oxygen, give nitroglycerin sublingual, and call the doctor. Anticipate changes on the ECG that would be similar to his initial ECG and reflect changes in leads V_1–V_4 representing his left anterior descending artery.

Chapter 41

1. To diagnose problems with heart structure and function in the presence of cardiomegaly in a young person. He has a questionable history of a heart murmur, and he reportedly uses cocaine and drinks alcohol, both of which have an adverse effect on the cardiac structure and function. He will most likely have four-chamber dilation.
2. The patient is complaining of clinical manifestations similar to those of a myocardial infarction; therefore, the enzyme tests are done to rule out a myocardial infarction.
3. To rule out coronary artery disease and any other possible reason for cardiomyopathy.
4. Cardiac dysrhythmias are also frequently associated with cardiomyopathy. Lasix is potassium depleting, thus further increasing the risk of cardiac dysrhythmias.
5. Stop cocaine or alcohol intake due to the increased risk of myocardial ischemia caused by these two substances. Diet and fluid intake changes, medication schedule, and activity restriction. Referral to Alcoholics Anonymous and Narcotics Anonymous; this patient needs to understand that if lifestyle changes do not occur, life expectancy is about 5 years.
6. Forward blood flow and improved pump function as a result of the ACE inhibitors, nitropaste, and Lasix therapy. Decreased preload and afterload will result in decreased cardiac workload and decreased stretch on the myocardial fibers.

Chapter 42

1. • Vital signs every 4 hours, including blood pressure, heart rate, oxygenation saturation, temperature.
   • Medications: simvastatin 20 mg po qhs, levothyroxine 0.125 mg po daily, glipizide 500 mg po bid, furosemide 80 mg po bid, potassium 40 mEq po bid, lisinopril 2.5 mg po daily.
   • Low sodium (<2,000 mg/day), fluid-restricted (<2 liters/day) diet.
   • Intake and output tracking.
   • Blood sugars ac and at bed time.
   • Daily A.M. weights.
2. To assess for an objective measure of fluid volume loss with weight changes in response to diuretic therapy.
3. Day 2 serum potassium.
4. Hypotension, worsened renal function, hyperkalemia.
5. Because the patient is fluid volume overloaded and therefore at risk of further congestion if initiated.

Chapter 43

1. Improved pain management, improved sleep and rest patterns, maintaining skin integrity, preventing injury/infection, improving control of blood sugar, preventing complications of immobility, and emotional and spiritual support.
2. Additional information that would be helpful would include an ankle-brachial index measurement, arterial duplex ultrasonography, and aortic angiogram with run-off.
3. Cigarette smoking is a significant risk factor for developing PAD. Avoiding all nicotine products is essential for the patient with PAD to decrease the risk of complications of vasospasm and poor healing.
4. Angiography of the aorta and lower extremities is performed to visualize anatomy and locate areas of stenosis and/or occlusion. It is an invasive procedure, requiring arterial access and contrast administration.
5. Preventing bleeding from the access site, monitoring for complications, maintaining hydration, providing pain management, accessing neurovascular status of the affected extremity, vital signs, and keeping the affected extremity straight for 4–6 hours.

Chapter 45

1. Aspirin inhibits prostaglandin E_2, which is part of the mucosal barrier that protects the gastric mucosa from the digestive actions of the gastric secretion.
2. Proton pump inhibitors effectively inhibit acid secretion and promote healing of the gastric ulcer.
3. Acute hemorrhage will decrease the hemoglobin, hematocrit, and RBCs and will cause an increase in the release of immature RBCs, as indicated by the increase in the reticulocyte count.

Chapter 46

1. Confusion, irritability, asterixis, and hyperactive reflexes.
2. Continuous damage and regeneration of liver tissue leads to fibrosis and scarring, which can affect liver function and cause structural changes in the liver so that blood and bile

flow is impeded/obstructed, leading to esophageal varices (blood flow) and jaundice (bile). Because the liver function is impaired, the serum albumin may be decreased, contributing to the formation of ascites. The liver converts ammonia to urea and when this function is impaired, ammonia levels increase, leading to neurological symptoms such as irritability, confusion, and asterixis.

3. Ammonia is a by-product of protein metabolism and the liver is unable to convert ammonia to urea, so the diet should provide less protein so that there is less ammonia.

4. Lactulose changes the acidity of the stool, which converts ammonia to ammonium ion, which is not absorbable. It also decreases the number of ammonia-forming bacteria.

Chapter 47

1. The patient was underresuscitated, causing decreased fluid volume. This reduced the perfusion to the kidneys, causing ischemic injury to the tubular epithelium and preventing normal concentration of urine, filtration of waste products, and regulation of acid–base balance, electrolyte hemostasis, and fluid balance.

2. Due to the impaired filtration, the nurse would expect to see elevated serum creatinine, blood urea nitrogen (BUN), potassium, and phosphate.

Chapter 49

1. Donning gloves and assessing the site where the blood is coming from. Observe the site for the amount of drainage, the suture line, and any disrupted sutures or signs of dehiscence. Take a full set of vital signs, including oxygen saturation and temperature, and notify the health care provider if medical intervention is needed. Apply pressure to the oozing incision site with sterile gauze until the oozing has stopped, and then apply a reinforcing dressing to the incision. Maintain very close observation.

   If the nurse chooses to remove the abdominal dressing as top priority, that is an error: The occlusive dressing is adding pressure to the oozing incision and should remain in place.

   If the nurse chooses to leave the patient's bedside, that is an error: Leaving the patient's bedside when vital signs are bordering on shock and she appears very tired, with a bleeding incision, would not be advised.

2. Asking for the health care provider to be notified using the patient call light is a correct action.

   Continue holding pressure on the dressing site.

   Ask another nurse to monitor vital signs and oxygen saturation.

   Apply oxygen to the patient who is hypotensive, tachycardic, or tachypneic.

   Put the head of the bed flat.

   Stay with the patient until the health care provider arrives.

3. **Indicates priorities.

   The incision has just been assessed, so the nurse can wait 30 minutes for the next assessment.

   **The patient has lost a reasonable amount of blood and needs the increased fluids from the IV.

**Oxygen should be applied because the oxygen-carrying capacity has been decreased secondary to drop in hemoglobin and hematocrit.

**The patient is in pain, 7/10, and needs analgesics. The Unasyn will need to be prepared, so there is leeway before having to give it.

Vital signs are ordered every 4 hours and were done just prior to the retention sutures being inserted.

**CBC is essential due to blood loss.

Calling laboratory results to the health care provider will occur when results received.

**Educating the patient on safety is an important consideration to prevent injury.

**Changing the linens is important because the patient has blood on her sheets, which is unsightly, can increase emotional discomfort, and can cause skin breakdown from the wetness against the patient.

The increased IV rate will take care of fluids temporarily, and the diet change can be implemented at the next meal.

Chapter 50

1. Pain.

2. If the catheter is occluded in any way, the patient will experience increased pain.

3. There is no significance as to the drainage itself because urine often seeps around a suprapubic catheter. There is significance in respect to potential damage to skin tissues from a wet dressing.

4. Low hemoglobin provides decreased oxygen to the patient for healing and it decreases the patient's overall energy level, which can decrease the patient's desire to ambulate and to eat. Oxygen, nutrition, and ambulation contribute to the patient's healing and recovery. The diabetes can alter wound healing, and glucose levels should be kept in good control to increase the ability of the body to heal. Nurses should also track hemoglobin trends to detect internal bleeding. This hemoglobin level is trending downward, and the cause of it needs to be sought.

5. It is not unusual to see a low-grade fever within 24 hours of a significant surgical event. The fever is the body's response to trauma. If the temperature is above 100.4°F or is elevated after 24 hours, it is more indicative of an infection.

Chapter 52

1. Prevailing symptoms include weight gain, constant fatigue, cold intolerance, dry skin, thinning hair, and difficulty concentrating. The patient also expresses that she does not feel as alert as usual and is experiencing a decline in work performance and task completion. These symptoms are indicative of low thyroxine levels and circulating hormone levels and hypothyroidism.

2. A high level of TSH is caused by the pituitary responding to an underproduction of thyroid hormone that, in turn, results in lower thyroxine (T_4). Measurement of the T_4 serum level reflects the amount of unbound thyroxine in the blood and is considered the best clinical measure of thyroxine levels. Low levels of T_4 in the presence of high

levels of TSH indicate that the problem is due to disease of the thyroid gland.

3. The main focus of the plan of care should be symptom management. This includes the following key elements:
   - Instruction in hormone replacement therapy. It is important to understand the prescribed medication and to take it precisely according to directions in order to return the patient to a euthyroid or normal thyroid state.
   - Assessment of fatigue and activity tolerance to determine ability to provide self-care.
   - Assessment of skin, nails, and hair condition because patient is at risk for impaired skin integrity and alopecia.
   - Assessment of bowel function because patient is at risk for constipation and abdominal pain due to the reduced activity (lethargy) and hypometabolic state.
   - Assessment of body temperature and ability to tolerate ambient temperatures. Patient may be prone to hypothermia due to hypometabolic state.
   - Assessment of cognition and thought processes because patient may experience disturbed thought processes due to hypothyroidism. Is patient oriented to time, place, person, and circumstances?

Chapter 53

1. The major biochemical deficits include (1) hyperglycemia, (2) metabolic acidosis, and (3) fluid and (4) electrolyte imbalance.

2. Polyuria, polydipsia, weight loss, and fatigue primarily result from hyperglycemia. The poor skin turgor, dry mucous membranes, and sinus tachycardia primarily result from the fluid imbalance (dehydration). The increasing lethargy, facial flushing, deep rapid breathing, and fruity odor of breath result from the metabolic acidosis (ketosis). The nausea and vomiting are thought to result from the metabolic acidosis (ketosis). The patient's sodium is low and his potassium is high; however, he appears to have no symptoms related to hyponatremia or hyperkalemia.

3. The nursing interventions derived from these treatments include (1) general assessment of patient's response to therapy, (2) evaluation of the patient's response to insulin therapy (e.g., monitoring for changes in blood glucose level; monitoring for signs and symptoms of hypoglycemia; monitoring for correction of metabolic acidosis [ketosis]), (3) evaluating patient's response to fluid replacement, and (4) evaluating the patient's response to electrolyte replacement therapy.

4. Severe DKA is a medical emergency. In terms of clinical signs and symptoms, the most significant difference is that the patient with severe DKA is more likely to present in an obtunded or comatose state. In terms of laboratory values, the most significant differences in the laboratory values between mild and severe DKA are related to the degree of metabolic acidosis: arterial pH < 7.0; serum bicarbonate < 10; anion gap > 12. Although the basic fluid and electrolyte treatments would be the same, the patient may present with more pronounced fluid and electrolyte imbalances (e.g., hyperkalemia, hyperosmolality). The fluid and electrolyte imbalances may reflect renal insufficiency and/or renal failure. As such, the fluid and electrolyte treatment of severe DKA may become highly individualized.

5. The general discharge plan for this patient includes (1) general teaching about the pathophysiology of type 1 diabetes; (2) basic dietary instruction; (3) instruction on insulin injection techniques; (4) instruction on signs and symptoms of hypoglycemia; (5) instruction on blood glucose monitoring—patients should be provided with a meter or provisions should be made to purchase a blood glucose monitor at discharge; and (6) follow-up appointment with health care provider—patient should be given phone number of person to contact for questions prior to appointment.

Chapter 55

1. Other questions may include these: (1) Is there a history of past fractures? (2) How did her accident occur? (3) What type of activities does she participate in at home? (4) Has she had a bone density study? (5) Has she ever taken hormones?

2. This patient is an older adult, which would lead to suspicion of osteoporosis. This patient's risk factors include the following: (1) age, (2) postmenopausal, and (3) family history of fractures. These risk factors would warrant further investigation.

3. Alkaline phosphate is found in the bone, liver, vascular endothelium, lung, kidney, and intestinal mucosa. Increased levels may be a warning sign and indicate the need for further investigation. An elevated alkaline phosphate can be observed when the body attempts to form new bone (i.e., metastatic cancer) (Corbett, 2004).

4. Serum calcium and phosphate.

5. The goal is to restore function and independence. In the acute phase, the goal of medical management would be to align and stabilize the hip fracture. This is achieved through surgical intervention. Older patients are at a greater risk for postop complications (i.e., infection, pulmonary complications, and thrombophlebitis). Following surgery, medical management would direct treatment in the prevention of postop complications and restoring function.

6. Nursing diagnoses:
   a. *Pain* related to edema and inflammatory response.
   b. *Risk for Impaired Skin Integrity* related to immobility.
   c. *Risk for Infection* related to invasive procedure.
   d. *Deficient Knowledge* related to unfamiliarity with surgical procedure.

7. In the postoperative phase it will be important for the nurse to know the patient's past medical–surgical history. It will be important for the patient to understand that her past medical–surgical history may help the team anticipate and prevent problems. Postoperative teaching should focus on reviewing strategies for preventing postop complications. She should be instructed regarding pain medication and the importance of progressively increasing her activity. Physical therapy is critical to her recovery, so reviewing some of the expectations might be helpful. The patient will need to understand that the Foley catheter may remain in her bladder until she is able to ambulate to the bathroom.

Other topics might include the use of TED, sequential decompression devices, incentive spirometry, and an abduction pillow.

Chapter 56

1. Postoperative complications can include hypovolemic shock, compartment syndrome, and rhabdomyolysis. The nurse should complete a neurovascular exam of the injured extremity that consists of assessing the color, temperature, capillary refill, pulses, edema, sensory and motor function, and pain level.
2. The right leg should be elevated and supported in correct anatomic position.

Chapter 57

1. Compartment syndrome pain is not relieved by narcotic pain medication, and the affected part is swollen and tense. Normal postoperative incisional pain is located only in the surgical site and is relieved by administration of pain medication.
2. Immediately upon admission to the nursing unit, the nurse should assess the patient for airway patency, breathing effectiveness, and evidence of bleeding at the surgical site and perform a neurovascular assessment of structures distal to the surgical site.
3. The type of surgical approach impacts the type of precautions necessary after hip replacement surgery. In the posterior approach, body positions that cause backward action or actions that cause the hip joint to swivel inward will stress the prosthesis and increase the potential for dislocation. Posterior hip precautions include not bending forward greater than 90 degrees and not moving the operative leg across the body midline. Anterior hip precautions include not moving the hip backward and not turning the leg and foot outward.
4. Postoperative pulmonary complications are prevented by early ambulation and use of pulmonary exercises such as coughing and deep breathing and use of incentive spirometry every 2 hours while awake.
5. The nurse must determine whether the patient is exhibiting confusion related to hypoxia, pain, infection, or hypotension or as an adverse effect of medications. The nurse should assess the patient's respiratory status, vital signs, and oxygen saturation. If these are within normal parameters, the nurse should determine whether the patient is in pain and medicate the patient if indicated. Medications can contribute to delirium, and the nurse should assess the medications ordered for the postoperative elderly person for their potential to contribute to confusion.

Chapter 58

1. Weight and pain in the toe.
2. Food with increased purines. Foods that should be avoided are organ meats, meat extracts, anchovies, sardines, herring, mackerel, scallops, game meats, and gravy. Patients should consume a moderate amount of protein and limit meat, fish, and poultry to 4 to 6 ounces per day. Diet should include low-fat dairy products, tofu, and eggs. Alcohol consumption should be limited to one drink three times a week, although beer ingestion should be completely discontinued because it has a high purine count and increases gout risks regardless of amount.
3. Excruciating pain in his right great toe. Stress. Weight.
4. With gouty arthritis, there is an imbalance with purine metabolism. Instead of the uric acid crystals being excreted through the kidneys, they accumulate in the joints. These crystals are needle-like, causing excruciating pain, usually in the joints of the elbows, wrists, fingers, knees, ankles, and toes, with 75% of patients affected in the great toe.

Chapter 60

1. Mr. B is relatively young and has symptoms consistent with significant immune insufficiency evidenced by oral and esophageal candidiasis. Mr. B also has HIV risk factors: history of sexually transmitted infection, indicating unprotected sex, multiple partners, and IV drug use. He currently uses alcohol and tobacco, which are gateway drugs for other forms of illegal substance abuse.
2. HIV testing is often very frightening and overwhelming to a patient. Therapeutic communication includes expressing feelings of caring, empathy, and understanding that HIV testing is frightening because the potential diagnosis is very serious. This should be balanced with calm and direct provision of information on the process of testing. Testing information should include information on consent for testing, confidentiality of test results, process of drawing blood and confirming any positive test with a second blood test, importance of testing to enable diagnosis, and appropriate treatment and the availability of antiretroviral medications that can help control the progression of HIV if the test is positive.
3. The CD4 receptor is the small protein found on T-helper cells and other cells that allows the HIV virus into the cell. Because the receptor was first isolated on T-helper cells and is found there in abundance, T-helper cells are also called CD4. HIV infection results in a progressive decline in the number of CD4 T-helper cells. The role of these CD4 cells in the immune response is critical because they initiate and regulate the process of stimulating other cells to initiate the immune response and attack an invading antigen such as virus or bacteria. They also stimulate B cells to make antibodies. Additionally, T-helper 1 cells (CD4) are responsible for the initiation of a response to a tumor or mutant cells. Therefore, when CD4 cells decline with HIV infection, the patient is at great risk of developing opportunistic infections and some cancers, such as lymphoma.
4. Yes, a CD4 count < 200/mL is a category C3 AIDS defining CD4 count according to CDC Guidelines described in Chapter 59, Chart 59–10.
5. Triple antiretroviral therapy, possibly including zidovudine + lamivudine (Combivir) and indinavir (Crixivan). Triple therapy interferes with HIV replication at different points in the replication process, thus more effectively controlling HIV replication and decreasing viral load levels. Additionally, triple therapy has a lower incidence of viral resistance than monotherapy.

Chapter 61

1. David should be assessed for hyperthermia from infection, seizure activity that may result from meningeal irritation, hypotension and hypoxia, and the development of hypotension that will lead to an altered mental status because of altered circulation. This hypotension can result from the sepsis and the body's inflammatory response.
2. Meningitis can be transmitted from droplet contamination from respiratory exposure. Respiratory isolation should be instituted. The nurse and anyone who has contact with David should wash their hands before and after leaving his room. Chemoprophylaxis may be recommended for any close contacts that David may have had. The local health department and college campus should be notified about David's infection in order to ensure that appropriate precautions are taken to prevent further spread of the disease. Some health care providers recommend a prophylactic vaccination of all college students.
3. Toxins from the bacteria causing David's meningitis will cause vasodilation and hypotension. Levophed has been found to be very beneficial in the early management of sepsis to maintain an adequate blood pressure and end-organ perfusion.

Chapter 63

1. Anemia and thrombocytopenia.
2. The low level of reticulocytes shows that erythropoiesis has not accelerated.
3. Petechiae, conjunctival hemorrhage, GI bleeding, positive guaiac.
4. Shortness of breath, pallor, activity intolerance.
5. Bleeding precautions, ambulation with assistance, reinforcement of patient education to prevent additional injury and falls.

Chapter 64

1. Infection, nutritional status, pain, and coping.
2. Calculate the ANC: 1,050.
3. Perform hand hygiene, assess invasive devices for redness and drainage, assess urine for sign of infection, assess for worsening respiratory status, instruct visitors to avoid contact with patient if they are ill, provide private room.
4. Listen attentively, demonstrate compassion and caring, offer resources as needed, collaborate with health care provider to determine further medical interventions.

Chapter 66

1. Hypotension, decreased level of consciousness, increased wound size, fever, renal failure.
2. Spread through breaks in the skin and contaminated hands. Contact isolation, strict aseptic technique.
3. There will be some scarring, but the goal is to return the leg to normal function, and the extent of the injury is still being determined.

Chapter 68

1. Grief, circulation, gas exchange.
2. Increase circulation distal to the burn injury. Loss of circulation and possible loss of limb.

3. Delays wound healing.
4. Fluid resuscitation will decrease these values.

Chapter 70

1. The nurse can contact environmental services/housekeeping to obtain a device that can be attached to the patient's bed to control the volume on the television. The nurse can instruct Mrs. M to place this device close to her best hearing ear so as to hear the television and not disturb the roommate.
2. Mrs. M most likely is experiencing hearing loss from the ototoxic medication streptomycin, which she took in 1955 for tuberculosis treatment. In addition, she was given the diagnosis of presbycusis. The first course of treatment for her hearing disturbance would be a hearing aid.
3. A hearing aid would be the first step to correcting Mrs. M's hearing disturbance. Because she also has some degree of nerve damage, a cochlear implant might be suggested if the hearing aid proves to be nonbeneficial to restoring her hearing.
4. Four specific discharge instructions for the family with regard to Mrs. M's hearing disorder include:
   a. Face Mrs. M when speaking.
   b. Do not shout.
   c. Drop the pitch of the voice.
   d. Speak slowly and enunciate, avoid slurring, avoid speaking rapidly.

Chapter 71

1. Vitreous hemorrhage, proliferative diabetic retinopathy, diabetic retinopathy with macula edema, retinal detachment.
2. Cholesterol, BUN, perfusion time.
3. Blood sugar under control, blood pressure under control, laser photocoagulation, vitrectomy.
4. Insulin dependent, blood sugar control, weight control, blood pressure control, regular eye examination referrals, and regular exercise.
5. Regular dilated eye examinations once a year if there are no vision problems and more often if there are problems, blood sugar and blood pressure controls, diet, exercise, and staying healthy.

Chapter 74

1. To identify and intervene with life-threatening injuries.
2. Patterns of injury that are anticipated are as follows:
   - Cervical spine fracture
   - Traumatic brain injury
   - Anterior flail chest
   - Myocardial contusion
   - Pneumothorax
   - Traumatic aortic disruption
   - Fractured spleen or liver
   - Posterior fracture/dislocation of the hip, knee, and/or ankle.
3. No, the CT will reveal solid organ injury but may not identify bowel injury.
4. Decreased core temperature with an inflammatory response leads to increased coagulopathy.

End-of-Chapter NCLEX-Style Review Questions

Chapter 1

1. Answer: 1. Health promotion and maintenance
   Rationale: Health promotion and maintenance are emphasized in nursing education. Advocacy is a characteristic of the role in which the nurse acts on behalf of patients in order to protect their rights and assist in obtaining information and services. Complementary therapies are strategies used in conjunction with traditional treatment. Physiological adaptation is the management and provision of care to patients with acute, chronic, or life-threatening physical health conditions.
   Congnitive Level: Analysis
   Nursing process: Implementing
   Client needs: Health Promotion and Maintenance
2. Answer: 2. Psychological and spiritual
   Rationale: Adding the aspects of caring enables nursing to meet psychological and spiritual needs. Without caring, nursing is a scientific and technical profession. The physiological needs will be met without the aspects of caring through the utilization of the technical body of knowledge. Ethical and moral needs are personal values.
   Cognitive level: Application
   Nursing process: Assessment
   Client needs: Psychosocial Integrity
3. Answer: 4. Total patient care nursing
   Rationale: Total patient care refers to a delivery model in which the nurse assumes total responsibility for meeting the needs of assigned patients during their time on duty. Functional nursing is an adaptation of the industrial model and is work assignment based on functions and tasks to be completed within a specific time frame. Modular nursing is the utilization of mini teams who stay near the bedside; it involves assigning a wider range of responsibilities. Primary care nursing has a professional nurse assigned to plan and coordinate care from admission to discharge.
   Cognitive level: Application
   Nursing process: Implementation
   Client needs: Safe, Effective Care Environment
4. Answer: 3. Variety of patient diagnoses and complexities of patient care
   Rationale: A variety of patient diagnoses and complexities of patient care require that the staff nurse incorporate organization and coordination into the practice role. The need to support the achievement of practice standards is a nursing administration level responsibility. Patient advocacy would require coordination but not necessarily organization as an inherent role. The nurse manager has 24-hour accountability for the unit.
   Cognitive level: Application
   Nursing process: Implementation
   Client needs: Safe, Effective Care Environment
5. Answer: 1. Cultural encounters
   Rationale: Cultural encounters are the fourth component of Campinha-Bacote's model. Cultural study is a process that would increase cultural knowledge. Cultural diversity refers to the variations among groups of people with respect to habits, values, preferences, beliefs, taboos, behaviors, and social interaction. Culture refers to a complex of learned patterns of behavior, beliefs, and values that can be attributed to a particular group of people.
   Cognitive level: Application
   Nursing process: Evaluation
   Client needs: Psychosocial Integrity

Chapter 2

1. Answer: 2. Advanced beginner
   Rationale: The novice stage begins in the first year of education to become a nurse. The advanced beginner is a new graduate. There is a level of trust in the environment and legitimacy of coworkers' knowledge. There is freedom with learning, mainly because of no responsibility for situations with which they have no experience. Competency is evidenced by exhilaration with good personal performance as opposed to remorse when performance could have been more precise or effective. Proficiency is evidenced by a change in the perspective of a situation or being able to read and respond to a patient's needs. This nurse was functioning at the level of advanced beginner.
   Cognitive level: Analysis
   Nursing process: Evaluation
   Client needs: Physiological Integrity: Physiological Adaptation
2. Answer: 4. The patient's hemoglobin and hematocrit levels are low.
   Rationale: There is a difference between practical knowledge and theoretical knowledge. With practical knowledge, practice is shaped by one's knowledge of the discipline, the science and technology relevant to the situation at hand. Theoretical knowledge is scientific, formal knowledge that is needed prior to the development of practical knowledge. This patient's hemoglobin and hematocrit levels were low, which could mean bleeding. A reduction in hemoglobin means a lesser amount of oxygen will reach the body organs. This patient's condition is changing, even though the vital signs are not yet reflecting the change.
   Cognitive level: Analysis
   Nursing process: Implementation
   Client needs: Physiological Integrity: Physiological Adaptation
3. Answer: 2. Return the patient to the bed.
   Rationale: Clinical knowledge is knowledge necessary to perform proficiently in the clinical setting. Clinical judgment is clinical reasoning, across time, about a particular patient. Techne is something that can be standardized and replicated. Even though the care map states a day 2 total knee replacement patient should be transferred from the bed to a chair with minimal weight bearing, the sudden onset of bright red bleeding would indicate that this patient be immediately returned to

bed and be prepared for further intervention. The care map, or standardized care, should not be followed in the best interest of the patient.

Cognitive level: Application

Nursing process: Implementation

Client needs: Physiological Integrity: Physiological Adaptation

4. Answer: 2. Repeat the questions to evaluate the patient's hearing.

Rationale: Phronesis is a form of rationality and skill-based character. It is similar to clinical judgment, which is clinical reasoning across time about a patient. The nurse should determine if the patient understands the health-related questions before assuming the patient is in acute distress or has a worsening condition.

Cognitive level: Analysis

Nursing process: Implementation

Client needs: Physiological Integrity: Reduction of Risk Potential

5. Answer: 3. Further explore the patient's breathlessness.

Rationale: To make good clinical judgments, the nurse must be skillful in moral and clinical perception. Even though conceptual knowledge is needed, it is not sufficient to ensure the nurse will notice and correctly identify a change in a patient's condition even though the nurse may know conceptually what the formal characteristic of the patient condition is in principle. The most important thing for the nurse to do to help this patient is to further explore the patient's breathlessness. Culturing the leg wounds and elevating the legs could theoretically wait until a later time. The patient should not be ambulated to the bathroom but rather should be provided with a bedpan.

Cognitive level: Analysis

Nursing process: Evaluation

Client needs: Physiological Integrity: Physiological Adaptation

Chapter 3

1. Answer: 2. It is a proven process that produces consistent, high-quality results.

Rationale: Best practices are defined as proven processes that produce consistent, high-quality results. Evidence-based practice can be described as an approach that integrates current research evidence with clinical expertise and patient's needs. Benchmarking offers qualitative or quantitative measurement of specific data related to reported outcome information. The Leapfrog Group focuses on collecting data about medical errors and setting standards that will reduce errors.

Cognitive level: Analysis

Nursing process: Planning

Client needs: Safe, Effective Care Environment: Management of Care

2. Answer: 4. Volume

Rationale: Volume for hospitals overall is based on units of services. The overall hospital generally looks at patient days, and departments look at relative statistics for the

type of work they do. Volume is a component of the revenue category. Salaries/wages is a component of controllable operating expenses. Supplies is a component of operating expenses. Overhead is considered an operating expense.

Cognitive level: Application

Nursing process: Planning

Client needs: Safe, Effective Care Environment: Management of Care

3. Answer: 2. Select supplies that can be used over a period of time for less cost.

Rationale: It is important for nurses to take an active role in containing costs through judicial use of supplies. The nurse should select supplies that can be used over a period of time for less cost. Using supplies already charged to another patient is unethical and can lead to contamination issues. Selecting too many supplies or stocking supplies in a patient's room for future use is not a judicial use of supplies.

Cognitive level: Application

Nursing process: Planning

Client needs: Safe, Effective Care Environment: Management of Care

4. Answer: 2. The Joint Commission

Rationale: The Joint Commission conducts accreditation surveys every 3 years. Beginning in 2004 the "tracer" methodology process was implemented that monitors a specific patient through his or her hospitalization and evaluates policies along with the patient's interactions and experience with all services. Effective in 2005, the Commission started making unannounced survey visits. The Occupational Safety and Health Administration (OSHA) is an agency that oversees environmental safety and works through federal and state partnerships to inspect and enforce safety standards in the workplace. The Centers for Disease Control and Prevention (CDC) is an agency that focuses on protecting the health and safety of people within and outside of a health care environment by development and application of disease prevention and control, promotion of environmental health, and education. The state board of nursing is an agency that oversees the practice of professionally licensed care providers by setting specific requirements for initial licensure, ongoing or continuing education hours and courses, the scope of practice for the particular discipline, and the disciplinary action processes.

Cognitive level: Application

Nursing process: Evaluation

Client needs: Safe, Effective Care Environment: Safety and Infection Control

5. Answer: 3. Health care power of attorney

Rationale: A health care power of attorney is a legal document that establishes a surrogate decision maker to make medical treatment decisions for an individual should that individual become incapacitated. A living will is a formal written document that communicates the wishes of the individual about life-sustaining medical treatments should he become terminally ill. An advance directive is instructions about future health care if

the patient cannot speak for herself. An oral advance directive includes instructions given to a health care provider during the course of treatment, illness, or stay in the hospital. This directive is documented in the patient's medical record. A written advance directive is a witnessed document, which requires the individual's signature and those of the witnesses.
Cognitive level: Application
Nursing process: Evaluation
Client needs: Safe, Effective Care Environment: Management of Care

Chapter 4

1. Answer: 2. Principlism
   Rationale: Principlism is an emerging theory that incorporates existing ethical principles and attempts to resolve conflicts by applying one or more of the ethical principles. Four principles form the basis for decision making: respect for autonomy, nonmaleficence, beneficence, and justice. In deontology, a sense of duty consists of rational respect for the fulfilling of one's obligations to other human beings, rather than looking at the rewards of one's actions. Rule utilitarianism seeks the greatest happiness for all; it appeals to public agreement as a basis for objective judgment about the nature of happiness. Act utilitarianism tries to determine in a particular situation which course of action will bring about the greatest happiness, or the least harm and suffering, to a single person.
   Cognitive level: Analysis
   Nursing process: Evaluation
   Client needs: Safe, Effective Care Environment: Management of Care

2. Answer: 3. Options
   Rationale: The M stands for massage or identify the issues and all of the people involved. The O stands for examining options. The R stands for resolving the dilemma. The A stands for act by applying the chosen option. And the L stands for look back and evaluate the success of achieving desired outcomes.
   Cognitive level: Application
   Nursing process: Planning
   Client needs: Safe, Effective Care Environment: Management of Care

3. Answer: 2. Social justice model
   Rationale: The social justice model considers broad social issues that may arise within an institution and within this model; many ethics committees hold ethical grand rounds. The autonomy model facilitates decision making for the competent patient. The patient benefit model uses substituted judgment and facilitates decision making for the incompetent patient. Fidelity model does not exist.
   Cognitive level: Application
   Nursing process: Planning
   Client needs: Safe, Effective Care Environment: Management of Care

4. Answer: 1. Read the state nurse practice act.

Rationale: The state nurse practice act sets educational and examination requirements, provides for licensing by individuals who have met these requirements, defines the functions of each category of nurse, and may include a section on mandatory continuing education hours for renewal of licenses. Reading the organization's standards of patient care and contacting the school in which she earned her nursing education would not be appropriate for the nurse to do. Assuming she can provide all aspects of care is also something this nurse should not do.
Cognitive level: Analysis
Nursing process: Assessment
Client needs: Safe, Effective Care Environment: Management of Care

5. Answer: 4. Tort
   Rationale: Tort law is defined as a wrongful act committed against another person or the person's property. Common law is based on justice, reason, and common sense. It represents law made by judges through decisions in specific cases; these case-by-case decisions are used again and again in similar cases and, thereby, become customary or common to all people living under the authority of the court of law. Civil law starts with abstract rules, which judges must then apply to the various cases before them. Contracts are promises that the law will enforce. Contract law is that which governs the formation of these promises or agreements between two or more parties, in relation to a particular subject.
   Cognitive level: Application
   Nursing process: Planning
   Client needs: Safe, Effective Care Environment: Management of Care

Chapter 5

1. Answer: 1. Case method
   Rationale: The case method of nursing care is one in which the registered nurse is responsible for the patient and has total care responsibility for the patient during the shift worked. Functional nursing is task oriented and nurses perform assigned tasks but are not given a patient assignment. In team nursing, patients are assigned to a team that is led by a registered nurse. In primary nursing, each patient is assigned to a nurse who has 24-hour responsibility for the nursing care provided to a particular patient.
   Cognitive level: Analysis
   Nursing process: Assessment
   Client needs: Safe, Effective Care Environment: Management of Care

2. Answer: 4. Intentional fragmentation of care
   Rationale: The functional nursing model of care is an industrial efficiency model that intentionally fragments care because of the increased number of personnel performing specific tasks for individual patients. Holistic and comprehensive care are characteristics of the case method of care delivery. Maximum use of individual caregivers' strengths for a large number of patients is a characteristic

of the team nursing care delivery system. Better care outcomes and greater nurse satisfaction are characteristics of the primary nursing care delivery system.

Cognitive level: Analysis
Nursing process: Assessment
Client needs: Safe, Effective Care Environment: Management of Care

3. Answer: 2. Team
Rationale: Responsibility for the delegation of tasks within team nursing is the same as in the functional nursing care delivery system. In the case method care delivery system, the entire caregiving staff consists of registered nurses. Unlicensed assistive personnel are not used. Within primary nursing, other caregivers are considered associate caregivers and the primary nurse is responsible for delegating responsibilities to these caregivers. Primary care is relationship-based care and is a blend of primary nursing with a professional nursing practice environment.

Cognitive level: Application
Nursing process: Implementation
Client needs: Safe, Effective Care Environment: Management of Care

4. Answer: 1. Highest quality for lowest cost
Rationale: The cost-effective measurement of nursing care delivery systems is difficult to achieve. Identifying the best care for the lowest cost may be deemed a cost-effective choice. The characteristics of job autonomy and nurse accountability are measurements of nurse job satisfaction. Patient acuity is the measurement of patient severity of illness and the amount of nursing care required to care for the patient.

Cognitive level: Analysis
Nursing process: Evaluation
Client needs: Safe, Effective Care Environment: Management of Care

5. Answer: 2. Functional
Rationale: Organizations that follow a functional approach to patient care avoid high labor costs by using lower paid workers and will not change the system to improve coordination and increase costs by adding advanced practice nurses or case managers. In the case method of care delivery, advanced practice nurses and case managers aid in the coordination of care. Advanced practice nurses and case managers are used as consultants within the team nursing care delivery system. Advanced practice nurses are used in the primary nursing care delivery system to add clinical expertise and education; however, the use of case managers is redundant in this model of care delivery.

Cognitive level: Application
Nursing process: Planning
Client needs: Safe, Effective Care Environment: Management of Care

Chapter 6

1. Answer: 3. The Joint Commission
Rationale: Each year the Joint Commission publishes patient safety goals that need to be addressed by health care facilities to improve patient care. They are listed on the Joint Commission website for the current and subsequent years. Medicare and Medicaid do not publish annual patient safety goals but expect organizations to comply with the Joint Commission's goals and standards. State boards of nursing control the practice of nursing by development of state nursing practice acts that establish guidelines to ensure safe practice. The standards set by the practice acts are based on the nursing process, which is a systematic method of planning and providing care to the patient, and requires compliance as evidenced in documentation.

Cognitive level: Analysis
Nursing process: Planning
Client needs: Safe, Effective Care Environment: Management of Care

2. Answer: 2. Draw a single line through the entry, write the word *error,* date, time, and sign the entry.
Rationale: When a documentation error occurs, correct it immediately by drawing a single line through the entry, identify it as an error with the date and time, and sign it. Never try to obliterate the error with ink or correction fluid because this can appear as if the documenter is trying to hide something.

Cognitive level: Application
Nursing process: Implementation
Client needs: Safe, Effective Care Environment: Management of Care

3. Answer: 4. There is a tendency to document everything.
Rationale: A disadvantage to narrative documentation is the tendency to chart everything that happens. The disadvantage of the CBE system is the time it takes to develop the guidelines and standards of care. Listing problems in chronological order is a disadvantage to the problem-oriented system. Having to evaluate each problem once per shift is a disadvantage of the PIE system.

Cognitive level: Application
Nursing process: Implementation
Client needs: Safe, Effective Care Environment: Management of Care

4. Answer: 2. Concept Map
Rationale: The concept map assists the learner in the development of the nursing plan of care using the nursing process. The Kardex contains information regarding the patient's name, age, religion, medical diagnoses, past medical history, surgeries and major procedures since admission, current medications, treatments, diet, intravenous therapy, and diagnostic tests and procedures. The medication administration record includes the usual dose, route, frequency, class, and action of the drug, rationale for administration, side effects with nursing implications, and assessment data that indicate effectiveness. The past medical history is data found within the Kardex.

Cognitive level: Analysis
Nursing process: Planning
Client needs: Safe, Effective Care Environment: Management of Care

Chapter 7

1. Answer: 1. Assessing the wound

    Rationale: Independent activities are those that nurses perform, prescribe, and or delegate based on their education and skills. Examples are assessing, analyzing and diagnosing, planning, implementing, and evaluating. Interdependent activities are those activities that overlap with other health team members, physicians, social workers, pharmacist, nutritionist, and therapists (physical, speech, occupational) and require coordination and planning with these various health team members. Dependent activities are those that are prescribed by the physician and carried out by the nurse. They include implementing the physician's orders to administer medications or treatments.

    Cognitive level: Analysis

    Nursing process: Evaluation

    Client needs: Safe, Effective Care Environment: Management of Care

2. Answer: 1. Assessment

    Rationale: A definition of assessment as it relates to nursing is "the act of reviewing a situation for the purpose of diagnosing the patient's problems." Planning is done after the formulation of nursing diagnoses and is prioritized according to the patient's needs. Implementation is the "doing" or intervening phase of the nursing process. It involves organization and actual delivery of nursing care, which leads to achievement of stated goals and objectives. Evaluation focuses on the patient's behavioral changes and compares them with the criteria stated in the objectives. It consists of both the patient's status and the effectiveness of the nursing care.

    Cognitive level: Application

    Nursing process: Implementation

    Client needs: Health Promotion and Maintenance: Prevention/Early Detection of Health Problems

3. Answer: 3. Psychomotor

    Rationale: To conduct a comprehensive nursing assessment, the nurse must utilize cognitive, affective, and psychomotor skills. Conducting a fingerstick to assess a blood glucose level is utilizing the psychomotor skill. There is no psychosocial skill level utilized to conduct a comprehensive nursing assessment.

    Cognitive level: Analysis

    Nursing process: Implementation

    Client needs: Health Promotion and Maintenance: Prevention/Early Detection of Health Problems

4. Answer: 4. Determining a nursing diagnosis

    Rationale: Goal setting is done during the planning phase of the nursing process. Planning of interventions is done during the planning phase of the nursing process. Nursing diagnoses are clinical judgments about an individual, family, or community response to actual or potential health problems and life processes. Nursing diagnoses are different from collaborative problems such as medical diagnoses because nurses' accountability differs for nursing diagnoses and collaborative problems. Nurses ultimately are accountable for formulating nursing diagnoses and intervening appropriately.

    Cognitive level: Application

    Nursing process: Evaluation

    Client needs: Health Promotion and Maintenance: Prevention/Early Detection of Health Problems

5. Answer: 2. Planning

    Rationale: The use of critical thinking with the nursing process enhances the validity, reliability, and effectiveness of outcomes to patients. It is essential in nursing when the nurse is assessing, diagnosing, implementing, and evaluating the patient and developing the care plan. Getting a better understanding of something or someone else is part of the assessment phase of the nursing process. Reducing the risk of getting undesirable results is part of the implementation phase of the nursing process. Increasing the likelihood of achieving beneficial results is part of the evaluation phase of the nursing process. Making decisions about an action is part of the planning phase of the nursing process.

    Cognitive level: Analysis

    Nursing process: Evaluation

    Client needs: Health Promotion and Maintenance: Prevention/Early Detection of Health Problems

Chapter 8

1. Answer: 3. The effectiveness of a type of wound dressing

    Rationale: Basic research is done to extend the knowledge base in a discipline or to formulate or refine a theory. This would include studying how Orem's theory can be applied to the nursing process. Applied research focuses on finding solutions to existing problems such as wound dressings, side effects of medications, or outcomes of teaching.

    Cognitive level: Analysis

    Nursing process: Planning

    Client needs: Safe, Effective Care Environment: Management of Care

2. Answer: 3. Collect numerical values within a controlled situation.

    Rationale: Quantitative research is characterized by the collection of numerical values, under a controlled situation, that yield data, which can be generalized. Qualitative research describes events as they occur naturally. It is a systematic, subjective approach used to describe life experiences and give them meaning. This type of research uses methods that are more subjective, a smaller sample size, and fewer research controls. The design of the qualitative study tends to evolve over time during the study. Qualitative studies do not follow the same linear progression of quantitative studies; instead, the process tends to resemble a circle more than a line.

    Cognitive level: Analysis

    Nursing process: Implementation

    Client needs: Safe, Effective Care Environment: Management of Care

3. Answer: 4. In a laboratory

    Rationale: Quantitative designs typically are descriptive, correlational, quasi-experimental, and experimental. An experimental design is used to find the effects of an intervention, is highly controlled, and most often occurs in a laboratory setting.

Cognitive level: Application

Nursing process: Planning

Client needs: Safe, Effective Care Environment: Management of Care

4. Answer: 2. Identify the problem to be studied.

Rationale: The first step in any research process is to identify a researchable problem. A researchable problem is a situation in need of a solution, alteration, or improvement. It is an area of concern for a particular population that requires investigation and that is derived from a topical area. Determining the patients who will participate in the study, assigning data collection roles, and setting the time frame for the study are all steps involved in research but occur later in the process.

Cognitive level: Analysis

Nursing process: Planning

Client needs: Safe, Effective Care Environment: Management of Care

5. Answer: 4. Write out the research problem or question.

Rationale: The research design is the overall plan for the study and should be described in detail. The research design includes data collection methods and methods to analyze the data. It doesn't matter if the research is quantitative or qualitative. The research question or problem statement is the primary guide for the design of the study.

Cognitive level: Application

Nursing process: Planning

Client needs: Safe, Effective Care Environment: Management of Care

Chapter 9

1. Answer: 2. Data about the patient's physical, social, cultural, environmental, and emotional statuses

Rationale: Assessment, the first step of the nursing process, is when the nurse gathers initial data. It is a systematic process that assists the nurse in identifying current health status, actual and potential problems, and areas that need health promotion. It also provides a baseline on which future comparisons can be made. The assessment includes data about the physical, emotional, mental, spiritual, and cultural factors that impact health. It consists of both objective and subjective data.

Cognitive level: Application

Nursing process: Assessment

Client needs: Health Promotion and Maintenance: Prevention/Early Detection of Health Problems

2. Answer: 4. Address the patient including the surname.

Rationale: When beginning the interview, nurses should address patients using their surnames and then introduce themselves and their role in the agency. They should state if they are students. Finally, nurses should tell patients the purpose for the interview.

Cognitive level: Application

Nursing process: Planning

Client needs: Health Promotion and Maintenance: Prevention/Early Detection of Health Problems

3. Answer: 2. What makes you think that you have cancer?

Rationale: The nurse should ask more probing questions in efforts to have the patient explain his or her fears of cancer. Responses that are nonproductive and should be avoided by the nurse include providing false reassurance, using authoritarian language, giving unwanted advice and not allowing patients to make their own decisions, talking too much, using professional jargon that the patient will not understand, and using avoidance language or euphemisms to avoid reality.

Cognitive level: Application

Nursing process: Implementation

Client needs: Health Promotion and Maintenance: Prevention/Early Detection of Health Problems

4. Answer: 3. Inspection

Rationale: Inspection is the deliberate, systematic examination of the patient using both sight and smell. It begins with the first encounter and continues during the entire time the nurse is with the patient. The nurse observes gait, mannerisms, stature, and other physical attributes. The inspection begins by assessing the patient's appearance and comparing the right and left side of the body for symmetry. Palpation uses touch in order to collect data to determine specific characteristics of the body. Such characteristics as temperature, texture, moisture, tenderness, pain, vibrations, and edema are assessed using palpation. Percussion is the creation of sound vibrations by pushing, tapping, or using a device to generate a vibration. The vibrations produced will help in determining position of organ structures. Auscultation is the technique of listening to body sounds. The nurse must use both the unassisted sense of hearing and, where needed, a stethoscope.

Cognitive level: Analysis

Nursing process: Assessment

Client needs: Health Promotion and Maintenance: Prevention/Early Detection of Health Problems

5. Answer: 1. Analysis of the situation

Rationale: The five components of critical thinking related to health assessment include collection of information, analysis of the situation, generation of alternatives, selection of alternatives, and evaluation. Collection of information begins with the interview and continues throughout the entire health assessment. The second skill is analysis of the situation. During this phase the nurse must distinguish normal from abnormal. The patient's age, gender, genetic background, and culture affect the analysis. The nurse must utilize laboratory findings, diagnostic tests, charts, and measures related to development and aging. Generation of alternatives includes identifying options and establishing priorities. It begins with identification of options and then the nurse and patient work together to establish the priorities. The next step is the selection of alternatives. The critical thinking skills needed for this step are the ability to develop outcomes and plans. The outcome is the final result of what the patient will attain, and the plan is the activities that will lead to that outcome. The last step in critical thinking is evaluation. Evaluation requires the nurse to determine if the expected outcomes have been achieved.

Cognitive level: Analysis

Nursing process: Assessment

Client needs: Health Promotion and Maintenance: Prevention/Early Detection of Health Problems

Chapter 10

1. Answer: 3. Point of maximal impulse may be at the sixth left intercostal space, midclavicular line.

    Rationale: Inspiration tends to be shallower in the elderly patient, but accessory muscle use is often noted during expiration. Thus, vital capacity is decreased while residual capacity is increased. The taste sensation is decreased due to the atrophy of papillae on the outer edges of the tongue. Peristalsis decreases in the elderly client, and a decreased thirst sensation may lead to decreased fluid intake. Enlargement or decreased rigidity of the heart muscle may cause displacement of the point of maximal impulse at the fifth or sixth left intercostal space at the midclavicular line.

    Cognitive level: Analysis

    Nursing process: Assessment

    Client needs: Health Promotion and Maintenance; Physiological Integrity

2. Answer: 2. Elderly patients who are hospitalized may be immunized according to the recommendations, as this can decrease both pneumonia and its resultant death rates.

    Rationale: The United States Preventive Services Task Force guidelines do not address the specific needs for the frail patient, those with functional decline, or those with limited life expectancy. The pneumococcal and influenza vaccines may be given at the same time in separate arms because there is no decreased antibody response or increased reaction severity when given together. Doses of the varicella-zoster virus vaccine should be 14 times greater than the vaccine for the varicella virus in order to boost immunity against shingles and its sequelae, such as post-herpetic neuralgia. When elderly patients are already hospitalized, this may provide an opportunity to update them on their immunizations. Studies have shown that vaccinations for older adults are 50% to 60% effective in preventing hospitalizations from pneumonia and 80% effective in preventing death.

    Cognitive level: Analysis

    Nursing process: Assessment

    Client needs: Safe, Effective Care Environment; Health Promotion and Maintenance; Physiological Integrity

3. Answer: 4. As an adjunct for researchers to evaluate the quality of drug prescribing, utilization, and education in the nursing home

    Rationale: The Beers criteria were initially developed to aid researchers in evaluating the quality of prescribing, utilization, and education related to medications in the nursing home setting, but now it includes the identification of medications or medication classes that may be either ineffective or potentially harmful among elderly patients, even in home or community settings. Approximately 5% to 15% of hospital admissions among elderly patients may be linked to adverse drug reactions or toxic drug effects. Polypharmacy includes the administration of excessive amounts of medications or numbers of medications together. Polypharmacy is best prevented by a thorough assessment of medication history. The United States Preventive Services Task Force is a panel of independent preventive and primary care specialists whose purposes include making recommendations about preventive services to be included in routine primary care and documenting evidence for the effectiveness and outcomes of screening, counseling, and preventive medications.

    Cognitive level: Analysis

    Nursing process: Assessment

    Client needs: Safe, Effective Care Environment; Health Promotion and Maintenance; Physiological Integrity

4. Answer: 2. Ensure confidentiality and inquire directly about the contusion.

    Rationale: This scenario suggests possible elder abuse. With any abuse situation, the patient should be ensured confidentiality. It is possible that the incident requires reporting to law enforcement or some other appropriate agency, and nurses should be aware of laws regarding mandatory reporting. The patient is a victim and should not be blamed or accused of causing the event, and a questionable situation of abuse or neglect should never be ignored. It is not the nurse's job to contact the news media or make implications or allegations regarding abuse or neglect cases.

    Cognitive level: Application

    Nursing process: Implementation

    Client needs: Safe, Effective Care Environment; Health Promotion and Maintenance; Physiological Integrity

5. Answer: 3. Residential Care Facility.

    Rationale: Residential care facilities can be covered by some long-term care policies and offer assistance with ADLs and medications. These facilities are not usually medically focused. Skilled nursing care facilities provide long-term intermediate or skilled nursing care and are usually covered by insurance for short periods of time. The types of clients who require 24-hour-a-day supervision, special diets or moderate assistance with ADLs need this type of residence. Adult day care programs may not be covered by insurance and offer few to no health services. Senior supported housing is not covered by insurance and includes low-income housing for seniors that may also include social activities and help with meals and laundry. They offer no health services.

    Nursing process: Analysis

    Category of client need: Safe, effective care environment/ Health promotion and maintenance/Psychosocial integrity

Chapter 11

1. Answer: 4. Patients who know they are heterozygous for coronary artery disease can initiate medications and lifestyle changes to help lower cholesterol.

   Rationale: Although legislation to protect patients with genetic disorders is pending, sometimes insurance and employer discrimination exists. Sometimes patients are afraid that being diagnosed as having or carrying the trait for a disease or disorder will make it more difficult, not easier, to find health coverage or employment. The nurse should be able to counsel the parents who are carriers of phenylketonuria that the disease is autosomal recessive and, thus, the chance of having offspring with the disease is 25%, not 50%. Again, the nurse should be able to counsel the parents of a patient with Turner syndrome, but the nurse should inform them about the monosomy cause. Patients who are heterozygous for coronary artery disease can reduce cholesterol levels by means of appropriate medication and lifestyle regimens.

   Cognitive level: Analysis

   Nursing process: Assessment

   Client needs: Health Promotion and Maintenance; Psychosocial Integrity; Physiological Integrity

2. Answer: 2. "There is always either an abundance or deficiency of genes within the chromosome."

   Rationale: The nurse should always remain professional and never give a nonchalant answer to a patient. It is the nurse's responsibility to appropriately educate the patient. A variation in genes, in combination with environmental factors, causes complex disorders; and gene mutation results from a change in the DNA sequence of an individual gene. Chromosomal disorders are caused by an abundance or deficiency of genes in the chromosome, but there is no abnormality with an individual gene.

   Cognitive level: Analysis

   Nursing process: Implementation

   Client needs: Health Promotion and Maintenance

3. Answer: 1. "The primary function of introns is to code for proteins using transcription and translation."

   Rationale: The upregulation, or increased transcription, of mRNA causes a subsequent increase in activity and production of more proteins. A codon codes for a single amino acid. Through transcription and translation, the amino acid will form a protein. The double-helix shape of DNA is formed by the alignment of purines and pyrimidines that forms two polynucleotide chains. Introns are noncoding regions within the gene. The exons code for proteins using transcription and translation.

   Cognitive level: Analysis

   Nursing process: Implementation

   Client needs: Health Promotion and Maintenance

4. Answer: 2. Cystic fibrosis

   Rationale: A mutant gene located on an autosome instead of the X chromosome is an autosomal disorder. The fact that two copies of the mutation are required for expression instead of one makes the disorder recessive. Marfan syndrome is an autosomal dominant disorder where only one copy of the mutation is required for expression of the disorder or disease. Color blindness is not autosomal at all, but rather it is X-linked. However, the disorder is recessive. Leigh disease follows an atypical pattern of inheritance, in which a defect in mtDNA is inherited maternally. Cystic fibrosis is the only disorder included that is both autosomal and recessive.

   Cognitive level: Analysis

   Nursing process: Assessment

   Client needs: Health Promotion and Maintenance

5. Answer: 3. To assist in identifying disease risk and developing a customized prevention program for some conditions

   Rationale: Carrier genetic tests are done to determine if unaffected or healthy individuals are carriers of disease-causing genes that could be passed to offspring. Genotype is the genetic makeup of the individual and not visible by outward signs. Genomic imprinting is caused by a chromatin alteration that affects gene expression but not DNA sequence. Differences in gene expression between maternal and paternal alleles are often caused by genomic imprinting. Core genetic conditions are screened for in newborns, and prenatal genetic testing is often done when the child is at risk for a genetic disorder. Pedigrees are used by health care professionals such as nurses, physicians, and genetic counselors to help identify disease risk and develop a personalized prevention and treatment program for certain genetic conditions.

   Cognitive level: Application

   Nursing process: Planning

   Client needs: Safe, Effective Care Environment; Health Promotion and Maintenance; Physiological Integrity

Chapter 12

1. Answer: 3. Long commute to work each day

   Rationale: Stress may be caused by internal and external sources. Internal stressors originate within a person. They include lifestyle choices, such as the use of caffeine; an overloaded schedule; negative self-talk, such as self-criticism and overanalyzing; and stressful personality traits, such as being a perfectionist, workaholic, or pleaser. External stressors originate outside the body. They are precipitated by changes in the external environment. They may be triggered by the actual physical environment, the social environment, the organizational environment, major life events, or other catastrophic events such as hurricanes, floods, and fires. Daily hassles, such as commuting long distances, misplacing keys, and experiencing mechanical breakdowns, also act as external stressors.

   Cognitive level: Analysis

   Nursing process: Assessment

   Client needs: Psychosocial Integrity: Coping and Adaptation

2. Answer: 2. Attributed to hardiness

   Rationale: According to the stimulus-based theory of stress, stress is defined as a stimulus, a life event, or a set of circumstances that arouses physiological and/or psychological reactions that result in a disrupted response that may increase the individual's vulnerability to illness. The patient is not demonstrating this response to the stressors. Daily hassles are experiences and conditions of daily living that have been appraised as relevant and harmful or threatening to an individual's well-being. Uplifts, the counterpart to hassles, are defined as positive experiences that are likely to occur in everyday life. This patient is demonstrating hardiness. Some individuals who experience high scores in terms of life-event changes do not experience illness. The hardy person has a clear sense of personal values and goals, a strong tendency toward interaction with the environment, a sense of meaningfulness, and an internal rather than an external locus of control.

Cognitive level: Analysis

Nursing process: Assessment

Client needs: Psychosocial Integrity: Coping and Adaptation

3. Answer: 1. Elevated blood pressure

Rationale: The general adaptation syndrome has three phases: alarm, resistance, and exhaustion. Physical signs and symptoms of the alarm reaction generally are those of the sympathetic nervous system stimulation. They include increased blood pressure, increased heart and respiratory rate, decreased gastrointestinal motility, pupil dilation, and increased perspiration. The patient also may complain of such symptoms as increased anxiety, nausea, fatigue, anorexia, and weight loss. There are fewer signs and symptoms of the resistance stage. The bodily symptoms of the alarm reaction disappear, and resistance rises above normal. Instead of continuing to lose weight, such as occurred in the alarm phase, the person returns to a "normal" weight. In the exhaustion phase, physical symptoms of the alarm reaction may reappear briefly in a final attempt by the body to survive. This is exemplified by a terminally ill person whose vital signs become stronger just before death. The individual in the stage of exhaustion usually becomes ill and may die if assistance from outside sources is not available.

Cognitive level: Analysis

Nursing process: Assessment

Client needs: Psychosocial Integrity: Coping and Adaptation

4. Answer: 3. The additional stresses of daily life add more stress hormones to the body, which can lead to disease.

Rationale: In our modern society with stressful daily events, hassles, and relationships, stress does not always let up. The stress hormones continue to wash through the system at high levels, never leaving the blood and tissues. Long-term activation of the stress system can have hazardous effects on the body, increasing the risk of obesity, heart disease, depression, and a variety of other illnesses. Repressed stressful emotions can predispose to a variety of diseases, from rheumatoid arthritis to cancer.

Cognitive level: Analysis

Nursing process: Evaluation

Client needs: Physiological Integrity: Physiological Adaptation

5. Answer: 4. Improve nutritional intake including foods containing vitamin E

Rationale: Oxidative stress is a physiological response to both internal and external stressors. Although it is not a disease, it is a condition that can lead to or accelerate disease development. Oxidative stress occurs when the available supply of the body's antioxidants is insufficient to handle and neutralize free radicals of different types. Free radicals have useful functions in the body under controlled conditions and it is not wise to strive to remove all free radicals from the body. Water-based foods have not been linked to the formation of free radicals. Ingesting high doses of vitamin C has not proven to effect free-radical production. Oxygen free radicals are neutralized by antioxidants such as vitamin E. Poor nutrition contributes to oxidative stress.

Cognitive level: Application

Nursing process: Planning

Client needs: Physiological Integrity: Physiological Adaptation

6. Answer: 1. Increased heart rate and blood pressure

Rationale: The physiological effects of stressors include increased heart rate, increased blood pressure, loss of appetite, sweating, and dilated pupils. Additional signs are pale skin, increased rate and depth of respirations, decreased urine output, dry mouth, and decreased intestinal peristalsis.

Cognitive level: Analysis

Nursing process: Assessment

Client needs: Physiological Integrity: Physiological Adaptation

Chapter 13

1. Answer: 2. Freud

Rationale: This patient is demonstrating the concept of denial, which is considered an ego defense mechanism within Freud's psychoanalytical theory. Erikson's theory addresses how persons develop across the life span. Maslow's theory focuses on the hierarchy of human needs. Piaget's theory focuses on the cognitive development of children.

Cognitive level: Analysis

Nursing process: Assessment

Client needs: Psychosocial Integrity: Psychosocial Adaptation

2. Answer: 3. Asking the patient if more information is needed to help in the decision-making process

Rationale: Certain actions foster the nurse–patient relationship. Conveying respect for the person's uniqueness, being nonjudgmental, showing attentiveness, and being empathic all create the building blocks of a therapeutic nurse–patient relationship. Patients need to feel safe, secure, and understood. Also pivotal is that the nurse is perceived as knowledgeable, trustworthy, sensitive, and unambiguous. There is also an emphasis on problem solving and a mandatory duty to accountability, responsibility, and confidentiality. Integral to the nurse–patient relationship is the concept of empowerment. When we empower persons, we assist them in developing the resources they need in which to make informed decisions about their health care based on their own priorities. The nurse should ask the patient if more information is needed to help in the decision-making process.

Cognitive level: Analysis

Nursing process: Assessment

Client needs: Psychosocial Integrity: Coping and Adaptation

3. Answer: 2. Sit with the patient and encourage him to explain to the best of his ability.

Rationale: Cultural competence is defined as the nurse continually striving to provide culturally appropriate care to patients and families. Nurses must convey empathy, show respect, build trust, establish rapport, listen actively, provide appropriate feedback, and demonstrate genuine interest. Barriers to effective transcultural communication include nurses' lack of knowledge, bias, ethnocentrism, prejudice, and stereotyping. Language differences, differences in the understanding of terminology, and differences in perceptions and expectations also create barriers.

Cognitive level: Analysis

Nursing process: Implementation

Client needs: Psychosocial Integrity: Coping and Adaptation

4. Answer: 1. I will do my best to learn how to do this. I have to.

Rationale: The nurse must assess the emotional and experiential readiness of the patient or family to learn. The following factors are to be considered when assessing the readiness to learn: level of emotional health, motivation to learn, self-concept and body image, social and economic stability, past experiences with learning, and attitude toward learning. The response that best identifies this patient's readiness to learn is the one that positively shows the patient's willingness to learn the skill.

Cognitive level: Analysis

Nursing process: Assessment

Client needs: Safe, Effective Care Environment: Management of Care

5. Answer: 1. Sit with the patient and be prepared to answer any questions.

Rationale: Nurses are often in contact with individuals and families when they are vulnerable or in crisis and, therefore, nurses become a valuable resource. Early intervention is essential to reduce the effects of the crisis. Providing information and resources sometimes serves to prevent a full-blown crisis from occurring. Rapport needs to be established quickly. It is important to understand the meaning the event has for the patient and, further, to allow for free expression of feelings, which can be cathartic. Once these things are accomplished, the nurse can then help the patient clarify the events of the crisis.

Cognitive level: Application

Nursing process: Implementation

Client needs: Psychosocial Integrity: Coping and Adaptation

Chapter 14

1. Answer: 1. Body mass index (BMI), weight, and waist circumference

Rationale: Anthropometric measurements are physical measurements that include height, weight, BMI, waist circumference, body composition, and measurement of fat and muscle. Food diaries provide valuable information, but are not anthropometric measurements. Blood pressure and pulse are measures of cardiovascular status.

Cognitive level: Application

Nursing process: Implementation

Client needs: Health Promotion and Maintenance

2. Answer: 4. Explain importance of adhering to scheduled mealtimes.

Rationale: The nurse should focus on interventions that will help to interrupt the binge–purge cycle. Regular mealtimes help to establish a pattern and avoid hunger that is brought on by long periods without eating. Finger foods should be avoided because portion control is difficult. Avoiding hunger should be stressed since this can lead to overeating. Regular exercise is encouraged, but excessive exercise may prompt the bulimic patient to view the exercise as a compensation for binging.

Cognitive level: Application

Nursing process: Implementation

Client needs: Physiological Integrity: Reduction of Risk Potential

3. Answer: 3. Maintain your carbohydrate intake by eating noodles, toast, and sports drinks.

Rationale: During periods of illness the need for insulin continues, so the patient should try to maintain a carbohydrate intake of 150 to 200 g/day. Some suggested types of carbohydrates that are easy to digest include ginger ale, cranberry and apple juice, sports drinks, toast, noodles, chicken noodle soup, gelatin, and pudding. Carbohydrates should not be restricted or be sugar free. Insulin is still needed during illness; doses may be adjusted but not stopped.

Cognitive level: Application

Nursing process: Implementation

Client needs: Physiological Integrity: Reduction of Risk Potential

4. Answer: 2. The wound drains large amounts of exudates.

Rationale: A large wound draining large amounts of exudates, which are rich in protein, will contribute to further protein losses. Antibiotic therapy should contribute to protein losses. Dairy products are often high in protein and could help to restore protein levels. A need for surgical debridement indicates there is necrotic tissue in the wound.

Cognitive level: Analysis

Nursing process: Diagnosis

Client needs: Physiological Integrity: Physiological Adaptation

5. Answer: 1. Burn injuries
   Rationale: Patients recovering from burn injuries have a high caloric requirement that often necessitates intermittent enteral feedings, either in addition to oral feedings or as the sole source of nutrition. The other conditions should not require the need for enteral feedings.
   Cognitive level: Application
   Nursing process: Assessment
   Client needs: Physiological Integrity

Chapter 15

1. Answer: 1. Is a common symptom to most illnesses, disease processes, and traumatic injuries
   Rationale: Although pain is recognized by all cultures, the expression and response to that pain can vary greatly among different cultures. Today's health care system can be very unfriendly at times to patients experiencing pain. Many health care providers lack the knowledge to or are unwilling to treat pain. Also, because of the widespread and undertreated nature of pain today, many patients experience significant personal, social, or economic distress. Pain is, however, a common symptom to most illnesses, disease processes, and traumatic injuries.
   Cognitive level: Analysis
   Nursing process: Assessment
   Client needs: Safe, Effective Care Environment
2. Answer: 3. Recognize the fundamental responsibility of all nurses to help alleviate patient suffering and relieve pain.
   Rationale: Chronic nonmalignant pain is not usually proportional to objective disease severity. A ban on opiate use in chronic nonmalignant pain is not ethically acceptable, even when patients are being assessed and treated for concurrent psychiatric disorders. A psychiatric disorder does not mean that these patients are not entitled to pain relief. Patients, their families, and even health care providers may have concerns about dependence or addiction associated with chronic opiate use, and disciplinary actions do exist for some nurses who administer inappropriate amounts of pain-controlling medications. However, being prescribed and receiving opiates for pain control does not subject patients to potential legal sanctions. Nurses do have the legal and ethical responsibility to help alleviate patient pain and suffering.
   Cognitive level: Analysis
   Nursing process: Implementation
   Client needs: Safe, Effective Care Environment
3. Answer: 4. "My pain may last for months, years, or for my whole life."
   Rationale: Pain of short duration with complete resolution is known as transient pain, whereas pain associated with a recent event, such as surgery, illness, or trauma, is acute pain. Recurrent pain is short in duration but recurs after a pain-free period. Chronic pain usually lasts in excess of 3 to 6 months but may last for years or even a lifetime.
   Cognitive level: Analysis
   Nursing process: Evaluation
   Client needs: Health Promotion and Maintenance

4. Answer: 2. The McGill Pain Questionnaire and the patient interview.
   Rationale: The patient's self-report of pain intensity, behavioral assessment, numeric rating system, simple verbal descriptive scale, Critical-Care Pain Observation Tool, and visual analog scale are all examples of unidimensional pain assessment methods. Within the choices given, only the McGill Pain Questionnaire and patient interview are credited with assessing the multidimensional pain experience.
   Cognitive level: Application
   Nursing process: Assessment
   Client needs: Health Promotion and Maintenance

Chapter 16

1. Answer: 2. "There is a potential for the baby to have birth defects."
   Rationale: According to genetic theories, each partner contributes on the genetic level and drug use impacts the sperm and egg health. The husband's cocaine use may impact fetal development; birth defects are more commonly linked to paternal DNA damage than maternal DNA damage. Telling the mother the infant should be fine provides false reassurance. It will not help to use barrier contraception at this point because the fetus has already formed. Sociocultural and environmental factors do have an influence on substance abuse, but the biologic and genetic influence also play a large role and at this point in the pregnancy have the greatest influence.
   Cognitive level: Application
   Nursing process: Implementation
   Client needs: Physiological Integrity
2. Answer: 4. Impulsive and extroverted
   Rationale: A number of personality traits are associated with disruptive substance abuse, including extroversion, impulsivity, social conformism, anxiousness, tenseness, and being less satisfied with present life situation. Being gregarious, quiet, studious, independent, and loyal are not characteristics usually associated with substance abuse.
   Cognitive level: Application
   Nursing process: Assessment
   Client needs: Psychosocial Integrity
3. Answer: 3. Diaphoresis
   Rationale: Symptoms associated with alcohol withdrawal usually develop around 62 hours after the last drink and include elevated temperature, severe diaphoresis, hypertension, and tachycardia. Behavioral symptoms include confusion, agitation and tremors, and altered sensory perception.
   Cognitive level: Analysis
   Nursing process: Assessment
   Client needs: Physiological Integrity
4. Answer: 1. Cardiac arrhythmias
   Rationale: Inhalants and solvents can cause life-threatening arrhythmias, such as ventricular fibrillation. Withdrawal of some amphetamines may cause severe depression and

suicidal tendencies. Methamphetamine withdrawal may produce outbursts of rage. Hallucinations can occur with the use of hallucinogens and alcohol withdrawal.

Cognitive level: Application
Nursing process: Implementation
Client needs: Physiological Integrity

5. Answer: 3. Diazepam, Valium

Rationale: Treatment of PCP intoxication includes the use of diazepam to treat the seizures, muscle spasms, and agitation that occur. Naloxone is the antidote for opiate overdoses. Prochlorperazine is a phenothiazine and would be contraindicated because PCP is an anticholinergic. Amitriptyline, a tricyclic antidepressant, is often used to help a patient withdrawing from cocaine because such patients often experience depression.

Cognitive level: Application
Nursing process: Planning
Client needs: Physiological Integrity

Chapter 17

1. Answer: 1. Integrating the goals and expertise of many different disciplines encourages the development of the most comprehensive plan of care.

Rationale: Patients and their families may receive conflicting information with increasing numbers of medical teams. Advance directives may provide civil and criminal immunity for health care personnel meeting certain conditions, but solely being part of or using an interdisciplinary approach to palliative care does not. Also, the patient's goals of care should guide the utilization of technology in end-of-life care, not vice versa. An interdisciplinary approach does, however, offer the patient the most comprehensive plan of care because of the variety of experience and expertise it brings.

Cognitive level: Application
Nursing process: Implementation
Client needs: Safe, Effective Care Environment; Psychosocial Integrity

2. Answer: 4. "The family usually finds it easier to withdraw life-sustaining treatments than to withhold them."

Rationale: End-of-life, palliative care is always focused on symptomatology rather than cure. All patients have the rights of autonomy, privacy, and decision making regarding their own health care. However, it is often more emotionally difficult for a family to withdraw life-sustaining treatments once they have been initiated than to withhold them.

Cognitive level: Application
Nursing process: Evaluation
Client needs: Safe, Effective Care Environment; Psychosocial Integrity

3. Answer: 2. "By signing the advance directive my appointed family member will have the ability to make health care decisions for me if I become ill."

Rationale: An advance directive directs the health care team in the decision-making process for the incapacitated patient, and the patient's own wishes regarding treatment are followed. The living will, a type of advance

directive, also describes the patient's desires for any life-prolonging treatments. Signing the advance directive does not grant proxy for a friend or family member to make health care decisions. Only by signing a medical durable power of attorney may decision-making rights be granted to the person of the patient's choosing.

Cognitive level: Application
Nursing process: Evaluation
Client needs: Safe, Effective Care Environment

4. Answer: 1. "We will continue to increase the pain medication until the symptoms are relieved."

Rationale: Efforts to control pain in the hospice patient are of great importance. Nonpharmacologic methods such as providing room for the patient's family and reducing excess light and noise may help make the patient more comfortable, and concerns surrounding physical or psychological dependencies related to increased opiate or benzodiazepine use are inappropriate. Conversely, when being titrated for pain control in the hospice patient, opiates have no maximum dose. Dosages are continuously titrated to achieve symptom relief.

Cognitive level: Application
Nursing process: Implementation
Client needs: Physiological Integrity

5. Answer: 2. "Some Russians may make their elderly family members a DNR so they will die comfortably and without life-sustaining treatments."

Rationale: Followers of Judaism believe the dying person should not be left alone. Baha'i law forbids the body from being cremated, but in Buddhism organ donation is encouraged and cremation is common. People from South Asia tend to express grief openly, whereas American Indians grieve privately. Russians do tend to encourage DNR orders to promote a comfortable death and prevent artificial life support.

Cognitive level: Analysis
Nursing process: Evaluation
Client needs: Psychosocial Integrity

Chapter 18

1. Answer: 3. Extracellular fluid volume deficit

Rationale: The intracellular fluids (ICFs) are fluids that exist within the cell cytoplasm and nucleus. The extracellular fluids (ECFs) are fluids that exist outside the cell, such as interstitial fluid between cells, fluid in the bloodstream (serum), cerebrospinal fluid (CSF) in the central nervous system, gastrointestinal secretions, sweat, and urine. Two-thirds of the body's water is ICF and one-third is ECF.

Cognitive level: Analysis
Nursing process: Assessment
Client needs: Physiological Adaptation: Physiological Integrity

2. Answer: 2. Prepare to administer a hypotonic intravenous solution.

Rationale: This patient is dehydrated as evidenced by the elevated hemoglobin and serum sodium and potassium levels. A hypertonic solution would exacerbate the dehydration and would not be indicated. The nurse should prepare to administer a hypotonic solution, which has a lower osmolality to hydrate the patient. An isotonic intravenous solution has the osmolality of blood and would most likely not serve to rehydrate the patient very effectively. This patient is dehydrated and a sodium and fluid restriction would be detrimental to this patient's care.

Cognitive level: Analysis

Nursing process: Planning

Client needs: Physiological Integrity: Physiological Adaptation

3. Answer: 1. Na+: 115 mEq/L

Rationale: Of the four electrolytes presented, the Na+ of 115 is out of range because normal values for sodium are 135 to 145 milliequivalents/liter (mEq/L). Ninety-eight percent of potassium is found within cells. Small amounts are found in blood (3.5 to 5.0 millimoles/liter [mmol/L]) and bone. Ninety-eight percent of calcium in the body is found in the bones and teeth. Two percent is in the blood serum (8.5 to 10.5 mg/dL; 50% ionized and 45% bound to albumin). More than 50% of body magnesium is stored in muscle and bone, and only 1% is in the blood (1.4 to 2.1 mg/dL).

Cognitive level: Analysis

Nursing process: Assessment

Client needs: Physiological Adaptation: Reduction of Risk Potential

4. Answer: 1. Hypokalemia

Rationale: Diarrhea may increase excretion of potassium to 200 mEq/day. Vomiting and/or nasogastric suction can increase loss through GI fluids removed. Typical circumstances leading to hypocalcemia include primary hyperparathyroidism, bone malignancy, and drug toxicity. Hypermagnesemia is often associated with renal failure. Hypophosphatemia causes include vitamin D deficiency, bowel disorders that lead to malabsorption, excessive use of phosphate-binding antacids, alcoholism, or diabetic ketoacidosis.

Cognitive level: Analysis

Nursing process: Assessment

Client needs: Physiological Integrity: Physiological Adaptation

5. Answer: 1. Dependent edema

Rationale: With fluid volume excess, the patient would likely show dependent edema, increased blood pressure, decreased urine output, shortness of breath, and adventitious breath sounds. An example of this condition is a patient with congestive heart failure.

Cognitive level: Analysis

Nursing process: Assessment

Client needs: Physiological Integrity: Physiological Adaptation

6. Answer: 4. Obtain an electrocardiogram

Rationale: Obtaining an ECG is a priority because serum potassium levels greater than 6.0 mEq/L can be life threatening due to the decreased ability of the heart to repolarize as evidenced by the tented T wave, loss of the P wave, and a wide, bizarre QRS with a depressed ST segment. Evaluating the level of consciousness would be associated with hyponatremia; measuring urine output hourly would be fruitless for a patient with renal failure; and the ABGs, although likely abnormal, would not serve as a priority intervention.

Cognitive level: Analysis

Nursing process: Implementation

Client needs: Physiological Integrity: Physiological Adaptation

7. Answer: 3. Eat a balanced diet including tomato juice and potatoes.

Rationale: Discharge teaching of patient/family with regard to hypokalemia includes properly taking potassium supplements such as K-Dur. In addition, increasing potassium-rich foods in the diet and recognizing/reporting increased muscle weakness are critical teaching points. Kayexalate enemas are used for hyperkalemia and, therefore, would not be an appropriate measure.

Cognitive level: Application

Nursing process: Planning

Client needs: Physiological Integrity: Physiological Adaptation

Chapter 19

1. Answer: 1. Increasing

Rationale: Because it is a negative log, as the hydrogen ion concentration increases, the pH decreases. Conversely, as the hydrogen ion concentration goes down, pH goes up. The hydrogen ion is the smallest ionic particle and it is extremely reactive. The hydrogen ion combines with alkali/bases or other negatively charged ions at low concentrations.

Cognitive level: Analysis

Nursing process: Assessment

Client needs: Physiological Integrity: Physiological Adaptation

2. Answer: 3. Increase the secretion of hydrogen ions.

Rationale: The main metabolic acids are lactic acid, pyruvic acid, ketoacids seen in diabetic acidosis, acetoacetic acid, and beta-hydroxybutyric acid. These acids are eliminated by the kidneys or they are metabolized by the liver. The capacity for elimination of these metabolic acids is much less than that of the lungs. In respiratory acidosis and most cases of metabolic acidosis, the kidneys excrete hydrogen ion and conserve bicarbonate to correct the pH.

Cognitive level: Analysis

Nursing process: Assessment

Client needs: Physiological Integrity: Physiological Adaptation

3. Answer: 4. 10 L/min

Rationale: The amount of ventilation is generally quantified by how much air the lungs move in 1 minute, referred to as the minute ventilation. Minute ventilation is the product of respiratory rate and depth, referred to as the tidal volume. Normal resting respiratory rate is about 12 breaths per minute. Normal resting depth tidal volume is about 500 mL. This yields a normal minute ventilation of

6 L/min: 12 breaths/min × 500 mL = 6,000 mL or 6 L. This patient's respiratory rate is 20 breaths per minute. The minute ventilation would be 10 L/min.
Cognitive level: Application
Nursing process: Assessment
Client needs: Physiological Integrity: Physiological Adaptation

4. Answer: 2. Deep rapid respirations
Rationale: In a state of metabolic acidosis, such as that which exists during diabetic ketoacidosis, the medullary centers will stimulate the lungs to increase the minute ventilation to blow off CO_2, even if that level is normal. These rapid, deep respirations, referred to as Kussmaul's respirations, are an attempt to correct the arterial pH by decreasing respiratory acid. This process is referred to as compensation.
Cognitive level: Analysis
Nursing process: Assessment
Client needs: Physiological Integrity: Physiological Adaptation

5. Answer: 1. Ammonia
Rationale: In the face of a high load of metabolic acids, the kidneys also increase their production of the urinary buffer, ammonia. Under normal circumstances, ammonia excretion is about 30 mmol/day, or about 0.5 mmol/kg. This excretion can increase to about 280 mmol/day, but this response takes several days to be completed.
Cognitive level: Analysis
Nursing process: Assessment
Client needs: Physiological Integrity: Physiological Adaptation

6. Answer: 4. pH
Rationale: The steps to analyze an arterial blood gas results are as follows: Step 1: Assess the pH; Step 2: Assess the $PaCO_2$; Step 3: Assess the bicarbonate and the base excess; Step 4: Evaluate compensation.
Cognitive level: Application
Nursing process: Assessment
Client needs: Physiological Integrity: Physiological Adaptation

7. Answer: 3. Place the patient in high Fowler's position.
Rationale: The patient is in respiratory acidosis. The main treatment for respiratory acidosis is correction of the underlying disorder that led to its development. For a patient with pneumonia, this would include antibiotic therapy, improving oxygenation, and management of fever. Placing the patient in high Fowler's position will improve air flow. Breathing into a paper bag and/or giving a sedative are indications of respiratory alkalosis. Sodium bicarbonate administered intravenously is a controversial treatment for metabolic acidosis.
Cognitive level: Analysis
Nursing process: Implementation
Client needs: Physiological Integrity: Physiological Adaptation

8. Answer: 3. Slow, shallow respirations
Rationale: Whenever excretion of CO_2 via the lungs fails to keep up with the body's CO_2 production, respiratory acidosis will occur such as with a drug overdose. Kussmaul's respirations (rapid, deep breaths) occur with metabolic acidosis, seizures are associated with respiratory alkalosis, and hyperreflexia is a symptom of metabolic alkalosis.
Cognitive level: Analysis
Nursing process: Assessment
Client needs: Physiological Integrity: Physiological Adaptation

9. Answer: 3. "I will take a stress management class or seek counseling."
Rationale: Respiratory alkalosis is characterized by a lower than normal $PaCO_2$ accompanied by an elevated pH. Respiratory rate is a major determinant of the $PaCO_2$ level. Excessively fast or deep ventilation "blows off" the carbon dioxide, decreasing the level and increasing the pH, causing alkalosis. Psychological conditions such as anxiety and panic or severe pain can also cause overventilation. Patients with psychological hyperventilation syndromes should benefit from reassurance and methods to decrease stress.
Cognitive level: Application
Nursing process: Evaluation
Client needs: Physiological Adaptation: Reduction of Risk Potential

Chapter 20

1. Answer: 1. Response of white blood cells to the cellular injury
Rationale: The inflammatory process involves a vascular phase and a cellular phase. The cellular phase includes the responses and actions of the white blood cells. Neutrophils then die, releasing proteolytic enzymes that liquefy the dead cells and bacteria, resulting in the formation of pus. The vascular phase would include such responses as temporary vasoconstriction followed by vasodilation and leakage of fluid into the interstitial space.
Cognitive level: Analysis
Nursing process: Assessment
Client needs: Physiological Integrity: Physiological Adaptation

2. Answer: 1. Inadequate nutrition
Rationale: A balanced diet helps the body maintain an effective immune system by providing the nutrients needed for growth of new, healthy tissue. With age, the immune system weakens as a result of decreasing thymus gland function and some lymphocytes become less responsive in the elderly, while others function normally. A personality disorder or urban living would not necessarily increase risk for infection.
Cognitive level: Application
Nursing process: Assessment
Client needs: Health Promotion and Maintenance: Prevention/Early Detection of Health Problems

3. Answer: 2. Airborne
Rationale: Tuberculosis is spread by airborne transmission, which occurs when the organism is expelled from the

infected person and remains suspended in the air in tiny droplets no larger than 5 microns. Contact transmission can occur by direct contact or indirect contact, such as with sneezing or coughing. Vehicle transmission occurs when the organism's life is maintained on something outside the reservoir until it is passed to the susceptible host. Vector-borne transmission occurs when a disease-producing organism is carried by a living intermediate host that transfers the organism to a susceptible host.

Cognitive level: Analysis
Nursing process: Assessment
Client needs: Physiological Integrity: Physiological Adaptation

4. Answer: 4. Wash for at least 15 seconds covering all surfaces.

Rationale: Guidelines for hand washing include the following: Vigorously rub hands together for 15 seconds, generating friction on all surfaces including between the fingers and under fingernails. Wet hands under running water using tepid, not hot, water. Artificial nails are not to be worn due to high risk for microorganism growth. Avoid the use of petroleum-based moisturizers because they can lead to a deterioration of latex gloves.

Cognitive level: Application
Nursing process: Implementation
Client needs: Safe, Effective Care Environment: Safety and Infection Control

5. Answer: 4. *Staphylococcus epidermidis*

Rationale: *Staphylococcus epidermidis* is found commonly on the skin, nasopharynx, and lower GU tract. Infection occurs with indwelling devices that are inserted through the skin, such as catheters. Group A beta-hemolytic streptococci are found in the nose and throat, respiratory secretions, and the hands. This bacteria is the cause of acute pharyngitis, cutaneous impetigo, and systemic infection. *Staphylococcus aureus* is found in the nasopharynx, skin, and clothing. This bacteria can be found in subcutaneous and cutaneous abscesses, and foreign devices such as IVs. *Neisseria meningitidis* is found in the nasopharynx and transported through the respiratory tract; it causes meningitis.

Cognitive level: Analysis
Nursing process: Assessment
Client needs: Physiological Integrity: Physiological Adaptation

6. Answer: 3. Injecting already formed antibodies into the body

Rationale: Active immunization involves the introduction of live, killed, or attenuated toxin of a disease organism into the body. The immune system responds by producing antibodies. Active immunization provides long-term and possibly lifelong immunity. Some vaccines require boosters to maintain the immunity. Examples of active immunizations include measles, mumps, hepatitis B, and hepatitis A. Passive immunity provides immunity for a short period of time, usually around 6 to 12 weeks. This involves already formed antibodies injected into the body. The individual may still have the disease but it will be a less severe case. An example of this type of immunity is immunoglobulin injections given to people exposed to hepatitis A.

Cognitive level: Analysis
Nursing process: Assessment
Client needs: Health Promotion and Maintenance: Prevention/Early Detection of Health Problems

7. Answer: 2. Increase the proportion of all tuberculosis patients who complete curative therapy within 12 months.

Rationale: Increasing compliance with medication treatment for tuberculosis is an actual *Healthy People 2010* goal. Eradication of the disease is not realistic. No immunization for health care workers is currently available. The rural population is not targeted for focus with avoidance of tuberculosis spread; an overcrowded condition such as that found in urban living is a risk factor however.

Cognitive level: Analysis
Nursing process: Planning
Client needs: Health Promotion and Maintenance: Prevention/Early Detection of Health Problems

8. Answer: 3. Have you received chemotherapy for cancer, psoriasis, or rheumatoid arthritis?

Rationale: The patient should be asked about any preexisting conditions that might affect the immune system such as the use of steroids, chemotherapy, transplants, or other chronic illnesses. Employment history, recreational activities, and exercise routine would not generate information about infectious diseases.

Cognitive level: Analysis
Nursing process: Assessment
Client needs: Health Promotion and Maintenance: Prevention/Early Detection of Health Problems

Chapter 21

1. Answer: 2. Prehypertension

Rationale: The term *prehypertension* describes those individuals with a blood pressure finding on two or more office visits of 130–139/80–89 mmHg as being at twice the risk to develop hypertension as those with lower values. Hypertension stage I is a BP of 140–159 mmHg systolic or 90–99 mmHg diastolic, whereas stage II would be multiple measurements of a systolic pressure greater than 160 mmHg or a diastolic pressure exceeding 100 mmHg.

Cognitive level: Analysis
Nursing process: Diagnosis
Client needs: Physiological Integrity

2. Answers:
   1. Cardiac output
   2. Peripheral vascular resistance
   3. Baroreceptors
   4. Chemoreceptors
   5. Body fluid volume

Rationale: Cardiac output × peripheral vascular resistance equals blood pressure (CO × PVR = BP). Baroreceptors, located in carotid sinuses and the wall of the left ventricle, monitor arterial BP and counteract rising pressure by vasodilation through stimulation of the vagus nerve. Chemoreceptors regulate ventilation and communicate

with the brainstem and cardiovascular centers to cause widespread vasoconstriction. Fluid balance is essential to maintaining normal blood pressure. When hypovolemia and hypervolemia occur, it is reflected in the systemic blood pressure. Adrenocorticotropic hormone (ACTH) functions as an aid to growth and development, not affecting blood pressure.
Cognitive level: Analysis
Nursing process: Evaluation
Client needs: Physiological Integrity

3. Answer: 3. 56-year-old male, African American, insulin-dependent diabetic
Rationale: Age (older than 55 for men and 65 for women) is considered a risk factor for hypertension along with being of male gender. African American individuals have two times greater possibility of developing high blood pressure than Caucasian Americans. Environmental factors such as obesity, cigarette smoking, sedentary lifestyle, use of illegal drugs, and excessive alcohol consumption create risk. Stress such as job stresses, economic position, losses and/or gains of any kind, and many other issues of life are risk factors for hypertension.
Cognitive level: Analysis
Nursing process: Assessment
Client needs: Health Promotion and Maintenance

4. Answer: 3. Not crush, break in half, or chew the extended release form of the drug
Rationale: Instruct the patient taking a sustained-action capsule or tablet, such as nifedipine (Procardia XL), a calcium channel blocker, that it cannot be crushed, broken up, or chewed. Adding potassium would be necessary with a loop diuretic; dry cough is most associated with angiotensin-converting enzyme inhibitors. Beta-adrenergic blocking agents require teaching blood pressure and pulse taking prior to medication. If pulse is below 60, inform the health care provider prior to taking the medication.
Cognitive level: Application
Nursing process: Implementation
Client needs: Safe, Effective Care Environment

5. Answers:
1. Asian populations undergoing Westernization will have significant increases in high blood pressure.
2. Individuals living in the southeastern region of the United States have a higher percentage of high blood pressure.
Rationale: African Americans have a 3 to 4 times higher risk of angioedema and cough attributed to ACE inhibitors than Caucasians. American Indian and Asian populations undergoing Westernization will have significant increases in high blood pressure. Individuals living in the southeastern region (sometimes called the Salt Belt) of the United States have a higher percentage of high blood pressure. Compliance with the DASH diet and exercise to prevent/control hypertension is not culture dependent.
Cognitive level: Application
Nursing process: Evaluation
Client needs: Health Promotion and Maintenance

6. Answers:
1. Developing a diet plan that is low in saturated fats and sodium
2. Eliminating or reducing alcohol consumption to one ounce a day
Rationale: A diet rich in fruits, vegetables, and whole grains and low in sodium and saturated fats is recommended with all stages of hypertension. Alcohol consumption will elevate arterial blood pressure and adds "empty" calories to the patient's diet. A sedentary lifestyle is avoided; aerobic exercise 3 to 5 times per week reduces stress and blood pressure. Smoking cessation is encouraged, not reduction of nicotine. Coping with stress-producing situations is the goal, because total avoidance is not possible. A realistic weight loss goal is 1 to 2 pounds per week.
Cognitive level: Analysis
Nursing process: Planning
Client needs: Health Promotion and Maintenance

7. Answer: 2. Verbalizing the warning signs and symptoms of cerebral vascular accident
Rationale: High blood pressure, referred to as the "silent killer," often goes undetected until signs and symptoms of other organ involvement are present. High blood pressure is the leading contributing cause of cerebral vascular accident; therefore, knowing the warning signs is the priority outcome. Generic brands of antihypertensive drugs are acceptable and a cost-saving method for long-term use. Positive personal relationships help with stress reduction, but are not the priority. Stage II hypertension warrants monitoring of blood pressure more often than once a month.
Cognitive level: Application
Nursing process: Planning
Client needs: Health Promotion and Maintenance

Chapter 22

1. Answer: 3. A midline catheter
Rationale: A midline catheter is the best peripheral vascular access device for parenteral therapy up to 4 weeks. A peripheral short catheter is for infusions that last between 72 and 96 hours. A winged steel infusion set is for infusions of less than 4 hours in duration. A PICC line is a central venous access device and not a peripheral vascular access device.
Cognitive level: Application
Nursing process: Planning
Client needs: Physiological Integrity: Pharmacological and Parenteral Therapies

2. Answer: 4. Secondary administration set
Rationale: A stop cock and extension set are add-on devices that might not be necessary for the infusion of the medication. An elastomeric balloon is a one-time-use device seen most frequently in home care. The secondary administration set is the device used to administer an intravenous medication when the patient is already receiving parenteral therapy. This administration set is piggybacked into the main infusion line.

Cognitive level: Application
Nursing process: Implementation
Client needs: Physiological Integrity: Pharmacologic and Parenteral Therapies

3. Answer: 2. Preserve the patient's right to safe quality care and protect the nurse who administers infusion therapy.

Rationale: The primary goal of the Infusion Nursing Standards of Practice is to preserve the patient's right to safe quality care and protect the nurse who administers infusion therapy. Even though it is important for nurses to follow Standard Precautions, be in compliance with all regulatory agencies, and have adequate skill levels, these are not Standards of Practice of the Infusion Nursing organization.

Cognitive level: Application
Nursing process: Planning
Client needs: Physiological Integrity; Pharmacologic and Parenteral Therapies

4. Answer: 4. Review the procedure with the patient and obtain consent.

Rationale: The first thing the nurse should do is review the procedure with the patient or conduct education. Obtain the patient's consent to have the access device inserted. Once this has been done, the nurse can then gather equipment and prepare flushes all using standard precautions.

Cognitive level: Application
Nursing process: Planning
Client needs: Physiological Integrity: Pharmacologic and Parenteral Therapies

5. Answer: 2. Stop the infusion and remove the catheter.

Rationale: This patient is complaining of an infiltration of the parenteral fluids. The nurse should discontinue the infusion immediately and remove the catheter. The nurse should then elevate the affected extremity to relieve patient discomfort and assist in absorption of excess fluids and improving circulation. The nurse should not take the time to check for a blood return, reposition the catheter, or change the dressing and observe the site.

Cognitive level: Application
Nursing process: Evaluation
Client needs: Physiological Integrity: Pharmacologic and Parenteral Therapies

Chapter 23

1. Answer: 1. Increase plasma colloidal osmotic pressure and plasma volume.

Rationale: Albumin will increase colloidal osmotic pressure and plasma volume. Albumin does not impact platelets or coagulation and does not include red blood cells.

Cognitive level: Analysis
Nursing process: Planning
Client needs: Physiological Integrity: Pharmacologic and Parenteral Therapies

2. Answer: 2. The youngest age for a blood donor is 17.

Rationale: There are specific guidelines for being a blood donor. Vital signs need to be within normal limits. Blood pressure needs to be less than 180/100 mmHg.

Blood count or hemoglobin needs to be greater than 12.4 mg/dL for a female. A blood donor needs to be between the ages of 17 and 65. There are no guidelines or restrictions about family members donating to other family members.

Cognitive level: Application
Nursing process: Implementation
Client needs: Physiological Integrity: Pharmacologic and Parenteral Therapies

3. Answer: 4. Patient provides informed consent for the transfusion.

Rationale: A history of blood transfusion reactions and the patient's circulatory and respiratory status are included in the assessment phase of blood administration. Assembling appropriate equipment is part of the implementation phase of blood administration. The patient providing informed consent for the transfusion is part of the planning phase of blood administration.

Cognitive level: Application
Nursing process: Planning
Client needs: Physiological Integrity: Pharmacologic and Parenteral Therapies

4. Answer: 1. Stop the blood transfusion.

Rationale: Circulatory overload can occur with transfusions when the blood is infused too rapidly or in too large a quantity, causing hypervolemia. High-risk patients include the elderly and those individuals who already have increased circulatory volume or who have a history of heart failure. Clinical manifestations of circulatory overload include dyspnea, tachycardia, distended neck veins, crackles in the lungs, and a rise in blood pressure. If the transfusion is not slowed down or stopped, pulmonary edema will result. Administering an antipyretic or epinephrine and flushing the access device are inappropriate actions.

Cognitive level: Planning
Nursing process: Implementation
Client needs: Physiological Integrity: Pharmacologic and Parenteral Therapies

5. Answer: 2. Stop the transfusion, call for help, and begin life-supporting measures.

Rationale: The sudden onset of chest pain is seen in an acute hemolytic reaction. This is a life-threatening situation. Slowing the transfusion rate and administering epinephrine or antipyretics are not appropriate actions for this level of transfusion reaction.

Cognitive level: Application
Nursing process: Implementation
Client needs: Physiological Integrity: Pharmacologic and Parenteral Therapies

Chapter 24

1. Answer: 2. Help with diagnosis, treatment, and evaluation of care.

Rationale: The three purposes of hemodynamic monitoring are aiding in the diagnosis of various disorders, assisting in guiding therapies to minimize or correct dysfunction, and evaluating the patient's response to therapy. There are noninvasive ways to ensure a correct blood pressure reading. The use of hemodynamic monitoring does not reduce the amount of patient care required. Although hemodynamic monitoring will provide information about the patient's status, it is not used individually to determine if a patient is stable enough for transfer.

Cognitive level: Application

Nursing process: Planning

Client needs: Physiological Integrity: Physiological Adaptation

2. Answer: 3. Find out if the correct type of tubing was used.

Rationale: High-pressure tubing instead of flexible intravenous tubing is necessary to withstand the external pressure exerted by the sleeve and to decrease the distortion of the waveform. The nurse should find out which type of tubing was used.

Cognitive level: Analysis

Nursing process: Assessment

Client needs: Physiological Integrity: Physiological Adaptation

3. Answer: 4. Advance the catheter into the pulmonary artery.

Rationale: This patient is having a pulmonary artery catheter placed. As the pulmonary artery catheter passes through the right ventricle, the tip of the catheter can irritate the ventricle. Patients may exhibit premature ventricular contractions. This rhythm usually ceases when the catheter is advanced into the pulmonary artery or withdrawn from the right ventricle.

Cognitive level: Analysis

Nursing process: Implementation

Client needs: Physiological Integrity: Physiological Adaptation

4. Answer: 4. Compare the result with other measurements.

Rationale: A venous pressure of 2 to 6 mmHg is adequate; however, patients may be hemodynamically stable or unstable with lower or higher pressures. Monitoring the trend in pressure readings, either increasing or decreasing, is of more importance than one observed value. The findings should also be correlated with a patient assessment.

Cognitive level: Application

Nursing process: Assessment

Client needs: Physiological Integrity: Physiological Adaptation

5. Answer: 2. Eliminate any values that differ by 10%.

Rationale: When using the thermodilution method of obtaining a cardiac output, a specified amount of solution, typically 5 to 10 mL, is injected through the proximal injectate port of the PA catheter. This process is commonly referred to as "shooting" a cardiac output. The injectate should be at room temperature when it enters the right atrium and mixes with blood. The cardiac output computer calculates the time required for the solution of a different temperature to reach the thermistor, located at the end of the catheter in the pulmonary artery. The change of temperature occurs over time to produce a cardiac output curve. Hesitation or starting and stopping during a CO injection would yield an invalid curve. The injectate should be injected smoothly and in less than 4 seconds. Injecting less than or greater than the recommended amount of injectate invalidates the measurement. Any cardiac output value that is questionable based on the curve or two CO measurements that differ by 10% should be discarded.

Cognitive level: Analysis

Nursing process: Evaluation

Client needs: Physiological Integrity: Physiological Adaptation

6. Answer: 1. Fluid volume overload or ventricular failure

Rationale: Excess preload may indicate hypervolemia or ventricular failure. Excessive circulating volume strains the heart and compromises adequate tissue oxygenation. Excess preload increases the workload of the heart and increases myocardial oxygen demands. Diuretics and venodilators are ordered if the cause is hypervolemia. If patients do not respond to diuretic therapy or renal failure is diagnosed, then continuous renal replacement therapy utilizing ultrafiltration or dialysis may be considered. If ventricular failure is determined to be the cause, inotropic medications are prescribed.

Cognitive level: Analysis

Nursing process: Assessment

Client needs: Physiological Integrity: Physiological Adaptation

7. Answer: 4. Closure of the pulmonic valve

Rationale: As the pulmonary artery catheter enters the right atrium, the waveform appears similar to a central venous pressure waveform: the *a* wave correlates with the P wave or atrial contraction (systole); the *c* wave may not be visible on the tracing and reflects retrograde swelling of the tricuspid valve into the right atrium, which occurs during ventricular contraction; and the *v* wave represents atrial diastole and the increased pressure against the closed tricuspid valve in early diastole. As the catheter enters the pulmonary artery, the waveform resembles an arterial pressure waveform with not only systolic and diastolic pressures but also a dicrotic notch. The dicrotic notch represents closure of the pulmonic valve.

Cognitive level: Analysis

Nursing process: Assessment

Client needs: Physiological Integrity: Physiological Adaptation

Chapter 25

1. Answer: 1. Reduce allergic reactions to medications or to latex.

Rationale: Allergies and allergic reactions to medications, chemicals, and foods must always be identified and prominently displayed on the patient's wristband, in the chart, and in the medication record. Patients with histories of allergic reactions have a greater risk of hypersensitivity to anesthesia, so the type of allergic reaction is very important. They also are much more likely to develop latex allergies.

Cognitive level: Application
Nursing process: Planning
Client needs: Physiological Integrity: Reduction of Risk Potential

2. Answer: 3. Antibiotic prophylaxis
Rationale: Patients with valvular disorders may require antibiotic prophylaxis to reduce the risk of bacterial endocarditis. Monitoring fluid and electrolyte status and a BNP level would be indicated for a patient with heart failure.
Cognitive level: Application
Nursing process: Planning
Client needs: Physiological Integrity: Reduction of Risk Potential

3. Answer: 2. Stop all NSAIDs 2 weeks before the scheduled surgery.
Rationale: NSAIDs increase the risk of intraoperative and postoperative bleeding. Aspirin inhibits platelet aggregation and the effect lasts the duration of the thrombocyte life span, 7 to 10 days. Preoperative arterial blood gas and recent hemoglobin A1c level are not indicated for this patient. Routine preoperative electrocardiograms are needed for patients over the age of 55.
Cognitive level: Analysis
Nursing process: Planning
Client needs: Physiological Integrity: Reduction of Risk Potential

4. Answer: 1. Encourage deep breathing and coughing
Rationale: To reduce the risk of pulmonary complications, the patient should be instructed and encouraged to breathe deeply and to cough. Monitoring of oxygen saturation levels would be indicated for a cardiovascular complication. Monitoring intake and output would be indicated for cardiovascular and genitourinary complications. Aspiration precautions would be indicated for a gastrointestinal complication.
Cognitive level: Analysis
Nursing process: Planning
Client needs: Physiological Integrity: Reduction of Risk Potential

5. Answer: 2. Can you explain to me what you mean by cauterized?
Rationale: Preoperative teaching is best accomplished in a calm, quiet, and private environment that facilitates discussion and questions and reduces the patient's anxiety or embarrassment. The nurse needs to be sensitive to the patient's level of anxiety, the patient's ability to understand instructions and express himself, and to cultural issues. Written instructions are important for reinforcing teaching and serving as a reference. When written instructions are given to patients, they should avoid medical jargon, be written at a level that is easy to understand, and be available in various languages. The nurse assesses whether or not a patient is literate in English or in another language before giving written instructions.
Cognitive level: Application
Nursing process: Implementation

Client needs: Physiological Integrity: Basic Care and Comfort

6. Answer: 2. Assess the patient's understanding of the procedure to supplement any areas not reviewed through the Internet.
Rationale: The use of the Internet has altered the amount and focus of preoperative teaching. It may also affect the type and amount of information desired. The best approach for the nurse to take would be to assess the patient's understanding of the procedure and to supplement any areas not reviewed through the Internet. Documenting that the patient had preoperative teaching through the Internet might be appropriate, however the nurse should do more. The nurse should not end the preoperative teaching session or leave the patient with instructions to call the nurse in case of questions.
Cognitive level: Analysis
Nursing process: Implementation
Client needs: Physiological Integrity: Reduction of Risk Potential

Chapter 26

1. Answer: 3. Conduct an interview.
Rationale: Preoperative holding is a semirestricted area usually just inside of the surgical area. This area provides a quiet, calm transition area for the patient to wait immediately before surgery. It provides a shield from the sights and sounds of the busy surgical suite and allows personnel to interview the patient and verify the documentation. Inspecting and ensuring the correct operation of surgical instruments is done in the surgical suite. Inserting an indwelling urinary catheter would be done after anesthesia has been provided to the patient, within the surgical suite.
Cognitive level: Application
Nursing process: Implementation
Client needs: Physiological Integrity: Reduction of Risk Potential

2. Answer: 4. Collaborating with the surgeon and suturing the wound closed
Rationale: The RNFA collaborates with the surgeon and performs the role of first assistant during the operation. This role includes handling tissue, providing exposure, using instruments, suturing the wound closed, and providing hemostasis. The anesthesia care provider administers anesthetic agents. Serving as the patient advocate is the role of the circulating nurse. Providing the surgeon with instruments is a role of the scrub nurse.
Cognitive level: Analysis
Nursing process: Implementation
Client needs: Physiological Integrity: Physiological Adaptation

3. Answer: 2. Anesthesiologist
Rationale: The anesthesiologist is the health care provider who is responsible for maintaining the patient's airway; monitoring and ensuring gas exchanges, respiration, and circulation; estimating and replacing blood and

fluid losses; administering medications to maintain hemodynamic stability; managing care in the event of a physiological crisis; and constantly communicating with the surgical and nursing team.

Cognitive level: Application

Nursing process: Implementation

Client needs: Physiological Integrity: Physiological Adaptation

4. Answer: 4. Stop all preparations until it can be verified which knee is the site of surgery.

Rationale: According to the AORN and American College of Surgeons guidelines, if any verification process fails to identify the correct site, all activities should be halted until verification is accurate.

Cognitive level: Application

Nursing process: Planning

Client needs: Physiological Integrity: Reduction of Risk Potential

5. Answer: 2. Examine the leg for possible injury or extent of injury and document the event.

Rationale: The most important role of the perioperative nurse is that of patient advocate. Protecting patients from harm is the essence of the advocacy role of nurses, and it is a critical component for patients whose family members are not readily accessible and whose only possible advocate is the nurse. The essence of the advocacy in the perioperative role is defined as protection, giving a voice, providing comfort, and caring. The nurse should examine the leg for injury and document the event.

Cognitive level: Analysis

Nursing process: Implementation

Client needs: Physiological Integrity: Reduction of Risk Potential

6. Answer: 2. Stop the surgery or deepen the anesthesia.

Rationale: Malignant hyperthermia is an emergency. The surgery should be stopped or the anesthesia deepened. The agent responsible for the hyperthermia should be stopped. Once stabilized, the patient should be transferred to the ICU for postoperative care. Calcium channel blockers should not be administered. One hundred percent oxygen should be delivered to the patient.

Cognitive level: Analysis

Nursing process: Implementation

Client needs: Physiological Integrity: Physiological Adaptation

7. Answer: 4. Respiratory therapist

Rationale: The anesthesiologist heads the anesthesia team and might be assisted by a respiratory therapist, by an anesthesia resident or fellow in a university teaching hospital, or by a certified registered nurse anesthetist (CRNA). The CRNA is an advance practice nurse, educated with a master's degree from an accredited nurse anesthesia educational program. CRNAs administer anesthesia and anesthesia-related care and work under the supervision of the anesthesiologist. The scrub nurse would not be working with the patient's oxygen. The RN first assistant would be assisting the surgeon.

Cognitive level: Analysis

Nursing process: Implementation

Client needs: Physiological Integrity: Reduction of Risk Potential

Chapter 27

1. Answer: 1. Bleeding

Rationale: In the patient who is bleeding postoperatively, initially the heart rate increases in an attempt to maintain a normal cardiac output and blood pressure; thus, it is an early sign of bleeding.

Cognitive level: Analysis

Nursing process: Assessment

Client needs: Physiological Integrity: Physiological Adaptation

2. Answer: 2. Easily arousable and moving all four extremities

Rationale: These activities support the second phase of postanesthesia, which begins when the patient is more alert and functional. The use of an oral airway to maintain an airway would not indicate the patient is ready to be discharged to another inpatient care area. Reduced or lack of motor response of the lower extremities after spinal anesthesia would indicate that the patient has not yet recovered from the anesthesia and should not be transferred to another care area at this time. It would be best to help control the vomiting before transferring the patient to another care area.

Cognitive level: Analysis

Nursing process: Planning

Client needs: Physiological Integrity: Reduction of Risk Potential

3. Answer: 3. Ambulate three times a day.

Rationale: Abdominal distention or a postoperative ileus is common with bowel surgery, anesthesia, narcotics, and decreased mobility. The patient should be kept NPO until flatus returns. If vomiting, the patient should have a nasogastric tube placed and put to suction. The patient should also be ambulated three times a day. The patient should not be given a full diet, should not be placed on a fluid restriction, and should not receive an antiemetic.

Cognitive level: Application

Nursing process: Implementation

Client needs: Physiological Integrity: Physiological Adaptation

4. Answer: 2. Keep the wound open to air and permit the Steri-Strips to fall off on their own.

Rationale: It is theorized that postoperative recovery includes four dimensions: physiological recovery, marked by a return of bodily functions; psychological recovery, a return of well-being; social recovery, a return to social activities and independence; and habitual recovery, a point at which the person returns to a full range of normal activities. Patients need to know that recovery takes time. Staples and sutures are often removed 7 to 10 days after the surgery in a follow-up appointment with the nurse or health care provider. If Steri-Strips cover the wound, they are left in place until they fall off naturally.

Cognitive level: Application

Nursing process: Implementation
Client needs: Physiological Integrity: Reduction of Risk Potential

5. Answer: 3. Nurse's ability to manage postoperative pain
   Rationale: A study that looks at nurses' ability to manage postoperative pain would provide a basis for understanding how nurses develop clinical judgment. Factors that influence anxiety levels in the older surgical patient would be a topic of study about the psychological well-being of postoperative patients. Strategies to increase the patient's ability to manage symptoms at home and adjustment of discharge teaching to accommodate cultural differences are both topics of study about how to increase patients' competence in managing their own recovery.
   Cognitive level: Analysis
   Nursing process: Planning
   Client needs: Physiological Integrity: Reduction of Risk Potential

Chapter 28

1. Answer: 1. Central nervous system
   Rationale: Neuroglia comprise a major cellular component of the nervous system. Neuroglia do not directly transmit information. There are three main types of neuroglia: oligodendrocytes, astrocytes, and microglia. Oligodendrocytes form the myelin sheath covering many neuronal axons. Multiple sclerosis is a disorder that affects the myelin sheath.
   Cognitive level: Analysis
   Nursing process: Implementation
   Client needs: Physiological Adaptation: Reduction of Risk Potential

2. Answer: 3. Medication history
   Rationale: The presenting problem is the reason the individual is seeking care. The presenting problem is followed by the history of the present problem. The nurse should begin with the initial presentation of the symptom and proceed to the present. The medication history should include all medications the patient currently is taking or historically has taken. Herbal, over-the-counter, home remedies, and supplements need to be listed as well as prescribed medications. The past medical history includes major illnesses, including all hospitalizations, surgeries, ambulatory procedures, and both acute and chronic illnesses. In addition, childhood diseases, immunizations, medications, and allergies are explored.
   Cognitive level: Application
   Nursing process: Assessment
   Client needs: Physiological Adaptation: Reduction of Risk Potential

3. Answer: 3. Spinal accessory
   Rationale: The spinal accessory nerve has motor function only. This nerve innervates the sternocleidomastoid and trapezius muscles. Damage to this nerve can result in impaired strength in lifting the shoulders, or difficulty in turning the head to either side. The vagus nerve controls swallowing and speaking by innervating the larynx

and pharynx. The hypoglossal nerve innervates the tongue. The facial nerve has a sensory and motor function. The facial nerve innervates the sense of taste in the anterior two-thirds of the tongue and the motor functioning of the face.
   Cognitive level: Application
   Nursing process: Assessment
   Client needs: Physiological Adaptation: Reduction of Risk Potential

4. Answer: 1. Level of consciousness
   Rationale: The mental status examination assesses the higher cortical functions of thinking and reasoning as well as level of consciousness, orientation, speech and language, memory, attention, fund of knowledge, and abstraction. The Glasgow Coma Scale is the most widely recognized level of consciousness assessment tool and is commonly used in emergency departments, trauma units, and intensive care areas. This tool evaluates three areas: eye opening, verbal response, and best motor response.
   Cognitive level: Application
   Nursing process: Assessment
   Client needs: Physiological Adaptation: Reduction of Risk Potential

5. Answer: 3. Normal
   Rationale: Reflexes are graded from 0 to +4. A 0 means there is no muscle reflex response. A +1 indicates a diminished response. A +2 is indicative of a normal reflex response. A +3 is more brisk but can be normal for the patient. A +4 indicates hyperactivity and possibly the presence of disease.
   Cognitive level: Analysis
   Nursing process: Assessment
   Client needs: Physiological Adaptation: Reduction of Risk Potential

6. Answer: 2. Handle of the reflex hammer
   Rationale: The Babinski reflex is tested by using a moderately sharp object, such as the handle of a percussion hammer, and stroking the lateral aspect of the sole of the foot from the heel to the ball of the foot, curving medially across the ball. The rubber triangle end of the reflex hammer is used to assess the four major reflex areas. A safety pin is not used to assess reflexes. A cotton swab is used to assess a corneal reflex.
   Cognitive level: Application
   Nursing process: Planning
   Client needs: Physiological Adaptation: Reduction of Risk Potential

7. Answer: 4. Nothing; this can be a normal finding.
   Rationale: When assessing cranial nerves III, IV, and VI in an elderly patient, the pupils are generally smaller and reflexes to light and accommodation become slower. This is due to aging changes in the muscles of the pupil sphincter and lens, not neurological changes.
   Cognitive level: Analysis
   Nursing process: Assessment
   Client needs: Physiological Adaptation: Reduction of Risk Potential

Chapter 29

1. Answer: 4. Increasing absorption of CSF

   Rationale: Increased CSF absorption is one mechanism to maintain a constant relationship between the three brain components. Brain tissue does not expand; it is compressed. Autoregulation ensures that the brain receives required sufficient oxygen and glucose to meet metabolic needs; this may be inhibited, but it is not blocked as a normal compensatory mechanism.

   Cognitive level: Application

   Nursing process: Assessment

   Client needs: Physiological Integrity

2. Answer: 3. Complaints of a "different" headache and projectile vomiting

   Rationale: Complaints of a "different" headache and projectile vomiting may be an early indication of increasing ICP. Changes in cranial nerve III, the oculomotor nerve, result in changes in papillary response and are early signs of ICP. Decorticate movements are a late sign. Cushing's triad is a late sign of ICP.

   Cognitive level: Application

   Nursing process: Assessment

   Client needs: Physiological Integrity

3. Answers:

   1. Normocapnia levels (PaCO$_2$ levels of 35–40 mmHg)
   2. Euglycemic levels of 80–120 mg/dL
   3. Normothermia and interventions for body temperatures >99.5°F rectally

   Rationale: Normocapnia levels (PaCO$_2$ levels of 35–40 mmHg) are best for the brain; also good are euglycemic levels of 80–120 mg/dL, because the brain is adversely impacted by both hypoglycemia and hyperglycemia, and normothermia and interventions for body temperatures >99.5°F rectally. Pulse oximetry and supplemental oxygen should be used to maintain saturations of 95% or greater.

   Cognitive level: Analysis

   Nursing process: Assessment

   Client needs: Physiological Integrity

4. Answer: 2. A CAT scan of the head to rule out skull fracture

   Rationale: A CAT scan of the head to rule out skull fracture must be performed before wound closure is undertaken. A complete neurological assessment may indicate symptoms suggestive of a cerebral contusion, but a CAT scan is the diagnostic tool. A cerebral arteriogram is not appropriate in this case because the vessel is outside of the skull. A skull series is used to identify bone placement and continuity and, if a hematoma was suspected, a CAT scan would be the appropriate diagnostic test.

   Cognitive level: Application

   Nursing process: Assessment

   Client needs: Physiological Integrity

5. Answer: 1. In the spinal fluid, protein levels will be high and glucose levels will be low.

   Rationale: With bacterial meningitis, the spinal fluid protein levels will be high and glucose levels will be low. The spinal fluid will be clear in viral meningitis. Option 3 is false. The spinal fluid will be bloody if there has been a bleed within the cranium. If bleeding occurred as a result of the puncture, the fluid would clear.

   Cognitive level: Application

   Nursing process: Application

   Client needs: Physiological Integrity

6. Answer: 3. Benign tumors may be surgically difficult to remove and may compress vital structures.

   Rationale: If the tumor is deep within the brain structure, it may be extremely difficult or impossible to remove surgically. Tumors may not invade surrounding tissue, but their growth will compress them and may interfere with their function. Benign tumors can progress into malignant tumors.

   Cognitive level: Application

   Nursing process: Assessment

   Client needs: Physiological Integrity

7. Answer: 4. A flexible approach due to the changing resistance patterns to specific drugs

   Rationale: Brain tissue has no lymph drainage and this can interfer with clearing drugs and debris. Many chemotherapeutic agents cannot cross the blood–brain barrier. Malignant cells are heterogeneous and their sensitivity to the drugs is variable.

   Cognitive level: Application

   Nursing process: Implementation

   Client needs: Physiological Integrity

8. Answer: 3. Provide answers to questions honestly as they arise, educate them about the treatment plan, and involve them in discussions of the rehabilitation process.

   Rationale: Providing answers to questions honestly as they arise, educating patients and family about the treatment plan, and involving them in discussions of the rehabilitation process is important in keeping families informed and involved and provides as much control as possible and appropriate. The role of the nurse extends beyond teaching about the early detection of cognitive impairment because this would severely limit the family's knowledge and support. The early implementation of rehabilitative therapies does not alter the importance of family teaching. Family teaching should offer encouragement and realistic hope.

   Cognitive level: Application

   Nursing process: Implementation

   Client needs: Physiological Integrity

Chapter 30

1. Answer: 3. The strokes are commonly caused by atherosclerosis.

   Rationale: Eighty percent of all strokes are ischemic in nature and most are caused by atherosclerosis. Hemorrhagic strokes are commonly associated with hypertension. Patients experiencing ischemic strokes are generally older than those experiencing hemorrhagic strokes.

   Cognitive level: Analysis

   Nursing process: Assessment

   Client needs: Physiological Integrity

2. Answers:
   1. Plaque formation that alters the internal diameter of a cerebral artery
   2. Thrombus formation as a result of plaque formation.
   3. Lipohyalinosis, a vascular abnormality, caused by hypertension

   Rationale: Plaque formation that alters the internal diameter in a cerebral artery is a common cause of ischemic stroke. The fragmentation of a clot in the venous system of the leg cannot enter the arterial circulation of the brain unless there is a defect in the heart. The plaque disrupts the integrity of the arterial lining, causing blood to enter the clot and ultimately forming a thrombus. Lipohyalinosis is a process that results in a vascular abnormality in small vessels and is normally associated with hypertension.

   Cognitive level: Application
   Nursing process: Planning
   Client needs: Physiological Integrity

3. Answer: 2. Ischemic cascade further extends the area of infarction.

   Rationale: The ischemic cascade further propagates cerebral edema, cerebral ischemia, cerebral infarction, and cell death. Tissues surrounding the necrotic area have undergone tissue hypoxia and may be viable if perfusion is restored before anoxia occurs. The functional ability of the tissue has not been permanently impaired until cell death occurs. The penumbra is the area surrounding the necrotic core.

   Cognitive level: Application
   Nursing process: Planning
   Client needs: Physiological Integrity

4. Answer: 2. Assessing lung and heart sounds to detect fluid overload

   Rationale: With hypervolemic therapy, plasma expanders may cause pulmonary compromise or congestive heart failure. Cerebral salt wasting is a complication of subarachnoid hemorrhage not associated with vasospasm. The nidus is a concentration of abnormal vessels located at the center of an arteriovenous malformation. Seizures may be generalized or focal depending on the area of the brain involved.

   Cognitive level: Application
   Nursing process: Assessment
   Client needs: Physiological Integrity

5. Answer: 3. Endovascular coiling is associated with the patient being able to return to his activities of normal living and work earlier than patients who had undergone neurosurgical clipping.

   Rationale: Endovascular coiling is associated with a shorter, not longer length of hospital stay. Endovascular coiling, not neurosurgical clipping, is associated with a higher survival and lower morbidity rates 1 year after the procedure. Although the availability of an interventional neuroradiologist is important, if the patient is a candidate for endovascular coiling, this is the option of choice.

Cognitive level: Application
Nursing process: Implementation
Client needs: Physiological Integrity

Chapter 31

1. Answer: 2. Alzheimer's disease
   Rationale: A person with Alzheimer's disease will demonstrate multiple cognitive deficits, including aphasia, apraxia, agnosia, and disturbances with executing functioning. Specific cognitive deficits are not typically seen in multiple sclerosis, Parkinson's disease, or myasthenia gravis.
   Cognitive level: Analysis
   Nursing process: Assessment
   Client needs: Physiological Integrity: Reduction of Risk Potential

2. Answer: 2. Myasthenia gravis
   Rationale: Multiple sclerosis is a neuroimmunologic disease that affects myelin, the protective sheath surrounding nerve fibers. Demyelinating lesions or plaques form along nerve fibers in the brain and spinal cord, producing symptoms related to the location of damage. The brain of a patient with Alzheimer's disease shows a profusion of amyloid plaques and neurofibrillary tangles, which form in the hippocampus and other parts of the brain critical to memory. Myasthenia gravis is a disease of muscle weakness as the result of dysfunction at the neuromuscular junction where the transmission of nerve impulses is blocked. Parkinson's disease is a disease of poor dopamine production, which leads to difficulty with movement, tremor, rigidity, and difficulty maintaining posture.
   Cognitive level: Analysis
   Nursing process: Assessment
   Client needs: Physiological Integrity: Reduction of Risk Potential

3. Answer: 4. Instruct to avoid prolonged exposure to hot temperatures to include showers, baths, and environmental temperatures.
   Rationale: A patient with multiple sclerosis will have episodes of fatigue. Fatigue is exacerbated with exposure to hot temperatures, including showers, baths, and environmental temperatures. The use of assistive devices will decrease fatigue. Voiding patterns will not affect a patient's level of fatigue.
   Cognitive level: Application
   Nursing process: Planning
   Client needs: Physiological Integrity: Reduction of Risk Potential

4. Answer: 2. Increase dietary fiber
   Rationale: Interventions to assist a patient with Parkinson's disease who is experiencing constipation include increasing dietary fluid and fiber and avoiding the use of laxatives. Limiting protein is not recommended to help with constipation. Because protein can interfere with levodopa absorption in a small percentage of patients, patients might be instructed to take levodopa at least 30 minutes before eating or 1 hour after eating.

Cognitive level: Application

Nursing process: Planning

Client needs: Physiological Integrity: Reduction of Risk Potential

5. Answer: 2. Encourage talking about advance directives

Rationale: The physical and mental health of the primary family caregiver is critical to the care of the Alzheimer's patient. One health promotional activity that can optimize both patient and caregiver health is to encourage talking about advance directives for management of advanced stages of AD. Involvement in clinical research studies is often done by patients with Parkinson's disease as a way of advancing science while managing their condition with the latest, most promising treatments. Physical and emotional stress can exacerbate the symptoms of multiple sclerosis, so patients should be instructed to avoid extreme temperatures and exposure to infections. People with ALS do maintain careers and interests; however, referral for psychological and/or spiritual counseling may help the patient and family come to terms with the disease and its prognosis.

Cognitive level: Application

Nursing process: Planning

Client needs: Physiological Integrity: Reduction of Risk Potential

6. Answer: 3. Would you like to talk about things that can help you and your husband?

Rationale: People can live with Parkinson's disease for many years. The chronic and progressive nature of the disease can significantly impact older, spousal caregivers, who may not have the physical strength to handle the weight of a patient with limited mobility. Caregiver stress and burden have been shown to increase as the disease progresses. The nurse should encourage the patient to talk about things that can help both the patient and the husband. Minimizing the patient's concerns would not be an appropriate response. Suggesting the patient discuss the concern with her physician is also not an appropriate response.

Cognitive level: Application

Nursing process: Implementation

Client needs: Physiological Integrity: Reduction of Risk Potential

7. Answer: 4. Impact of meditation and prayer on disease management and experience

Rationale: The impact of meditation and prayer on disease management and experience is a topic that addresses complementary/alternative approaches to neurodegenerative disease processes. Interventions that improve the quality of life focus on quality of life research. Topics about literacy address patient/family education research. Anticipatory grief is a topic within emotional and psychological research.

Cognitive level: Analysis

Nursing process: Planning

Client needs: Physiological Integrity: Basic Care and Comfort

Chapter 32

1. Answer: 4. "A sudden deceleration injury, such as a head-on motor vehicle collision, is frequently the cause of hyperflexion injuries."

Rationale: Hyperextension injuries are caused by a sudden forceful extension of the head and neck, for instance, during a forward fall where the chin or forehead strikes the ground. These injuries can cause spinal ligaments to stretch, can compress the spinal cord, and can fracture the posterior spinous processes, but these injuries usually do not cause dislocations. Axial pressure loaded onto the spine may cause compression injuries, which include vertebral body fractures and spinal cord compression. Rotational injuries are associated with lateral flexion or rotation of the spine, causing posterior ligaments to rupture and facets to dislocate and fracture. Sudden deceleration injury, such as a head-on motor vehicle collision, is often the cause of hyperflexion injuries. These injuries can cause anterior vertebral body fractures and posterior spinal column facet fracture and dislocation.

Cognitive level: Application

Nursing process: Evaluation

Client needs: Safe, Effective Care Environment; Health Promotion and Maintenance; Physiological Integrity

2. Answer: 2. Central cord syndrome

Rationale: Central cord syndrome is often caused by hyperextension injuries, such as a rear-impact motor vehicle collision. This syndrome is caused by central spinal cord damage, which, in turn, causes damage to the more centrally located fibers leading to the upper extremities. The fibers leading to the lower extremities are more laterally located, producing less motor and sensory problems in the lower versus upper extremities. Anterior cord syndrome is caused by direct insult to the anterior portion of the spinal cord. Compression or hyperextension injury may produce this problem, but paralysis and loss of pain and temperature sensations are evident below the level of the injury. Also, light touch, vibration, and proprioception are preserved. Cauda equina syndrome is caused by compression of the lumbar nerve roots below the first lumbar vertebra. The associated signs and symptoms can vary based on the specific nerve root involved, but they often involve motor and sensory loss to the pelvic organs and lower extremities. Brown-Séquard syndrome is usually the result of penetrating trauma that causes hemisection of the spinal cord. The ipsilateral side experiences paralysis and proprioception loss, and the contralateral side experiences pain and temperature sensation loss.

Cognitive level: Analysis

Nursing process: Assessment

Client needs: Physiological Integrity

3. Answer: 3. Use of a reclining wheelchair to gradually progress the patient into an upright position so as not to cause orthostatic hypotension

Rationale: A reclining wheelchair or tilt table gradually places the patient into an upright position, decreasing the development of orthostatic hypotension. The use of an abdominal binder and compression stockings does decrease blood pooling in the peripheral veins, but these interventions are used to help improve venous return to the heart and to prevent orthostatic hypotension as well. A duplex Doppler ultrasound is a highly sensitive screening tool for detecting deep venous thrombosis. It does not dissolve clots. Good nutrition is important is aiding bowel evacuation, but increased caloric, protein, and micronutrient intake is used to aid in wound healing and the promotion of good skin integrity. Increased fiber and fluid intake would help prevent constipation.

Cognitive level: Analysis

Nursing process: Intervention

Client needs: Health Promotion and Maintenance; Physiological Integrity

4. Answer: 1. The patient's family will need ongoing education to help them deal with the stress of any role changes associated with the injury.

Rationale: Role changes within the family are a very real possibility following spinal cord injury, and the family will require ongoing support and education to help deal with this change. Elation and jubilation are not negative emotions; however, patients who experience spinal cord injury often do have negative feelings. They may exhibit denial, anger, grief, hopelessness, and depression. Patients should be encouraged to openly discuss their feelings, but they should also be allowed the opportunity to make their own health care decisions when possible. It is because of the physical challenges caused by the spinal cord injury that the patient usually faces significant psychosocial challenges as well.

Cognitive level: Analysis

Nursing process: Planning

Client needs: Psychosocial integrity

5. Answer: 1. Information regarding support systems that can help the patient and their family adjust to the changes in lifestyle and roles.

Rationale: It is important to put patients and their families in touch with support that can help them cope with the often difficult physical and psychological changes associated with spinal cord injury. Rehabilitative programs that maximize function following spinal cord injury should be multidisciplinary and comprehensive. Infrequent position changes predispose the patient to the development of pressure ulcers, but frequent position changes with good skin care regimens can help with pressure ulcer prevention. Suppository medications, digital bowel stimulation, and disimpaction of stool can aid in the prevention of hyperreflexia.

Cognitive level: Application

Nursing process: Planning

Client needs: Psychosocial Integrity

6. Answer: 4. Ineffective airway clearance related to the loss of spinal innervation of the respiratory and accessory muscles.

Rationale: Airway (with cervical spine immobilization in trauma situations) is always the first priority for any patient. When compared with the other nursing diagnoses listed for this patient, ineffective airway clearance would be the primary diagnosis. *Anxiety* is important and should be attended to, but airway issues should be dealt with first. *Risk for Imbalanced Nutrition* and *Risk for Ineffective Peripheral Tissue Perfusion* are potential problems, and actual problems, such as ineffective airway clearance, should be treated before these other diagnoses are addressed.

Cognitive level: Application

Nursing process: Planning

Client needs: Safe, Effective Care Environment

Chapter 33

1. Answer: 2. Crackles

Rationale: Crackles are sounds caused by fluid in the airways. They are described as intermittent or discontinuous, nonmusical, or popping sounds. They are caused by fluid, inflammation, infection, or secretions. The term *rales* is no longer used to describe fluid effects in the airways. Crackles occur when closed airways snap open during inspiration. Wheezes are high-pitched musical sounds caused by air flowing across strands of mucous, swollen pulmonary tissue that narrows the airway, or from bronchospasm. The term *rhonchi* is no longer used to describe harsh sounds caused by secretions in the airways.

Cognitive level: Application

Nursing process: Assessment

Client needs: Health Promotion and Maintenance: Prevention/Early Detection of Health Problems

2. Answer: 3. It might help to know if there are any recent outbreaks of pulmonary disorders in the area of travel.

Rationale: Area of recent travel may become an important aspect of the history in diagnosing potential respiratory problems. In previous years, the severe acute respiratory syndrome outbreak demonstrated to the world that viral pulmonary disease could be traced to a specific location. Recent travel and area of residence have been demonstrated to be an important factor in the history of respiratory symptoms and should be included in the interview process. The other options would not help in figuring out where the patient might have been exposed to an upper respiratory infection.

Cognitive level: Analysis

Nursing process: Assessment

Client needs: Health Promotion and Maintenance: Prevention/Early Detection of Health Problems

3. Answer: 2. Have you been to any activities or functions around other people with respiratory problems?

Rationale: The social history includes information about the patient's lifestyle and habits that may be relevant to his or her current state of health. Patients who smoke have increased risk for pulmonary disease and patients who have allergies and engage in social activities in the out-of-doors such as golfing may have exacerbations of symptoms after participating in these activities. Also, if patients frequent social events where they may be exposed to people with upper respiratory infections or poor hygienic conditions, they may be predisposed to the development of pulmonary infections. The other choices focus on either the patient's health history, family history, or history of immunizations.

Cognitive level: Application

Nursing process: Assessment

Client needs: Health Promotion and Maintenance: Prevention/Early Detection of Health Problems

4. Answer: 3. Edema indicates heart failure, a common finding in a patient with COPD.

Rationale: Edema of the lower extremities is generally related to right heart or congestive heart failure. Right heart failure and combined left- and right-sided failure are common in patients with COPD. Right-sided failure is caused by pulmonary hypertension. Chronic distention of the lower airways makes forward blood flow more difficult. The right heart hypertrophies in an attempt to increase force of blood through the pulmonary tree. The right heart fails and fluid unable to be accommodated is sequestered in dependent interstitial spaces and causes edema.

Cognitive level: Analysis

Nursing process: Assessment

Client needs: Health Promotion and Maintenance: Prevention/Early Detection of Health Problems

5. Answer: 3. Have an arterial blood gas analysis done to compare the readings.

Rationale: The oxygen saturation measured by infrared technology does not necessarily provide the same values obtained from the calculated oxygen saturation obtained from an ABG. Normal infrared oxygen saturation and ABG saturations range from 95% to 100%. Pulse oximetry probes should not be placed on extremities with automated blood pressure cuffs, hemodialysis fistulas, or arterial lines because these interfere with blood flow. Shock and hypovolemia also cause low-flow states that contribute to inaccurate pulse oximetry readings. Patient movement, ambient light, and venous pulsations may also cause inaccurate readings. If ambient light is interfering with readings (producing results higher than suspected), cover the probe with a towel to see if the result is different. Pulse oximetry does not distinguish methemoglobin or carboxyhemoglobin from oxygen-saturated hemoglobin. Fifty percent carboxyhemoglobin reads as 95%. Patients who have suspected thiocyanate toxicity or inhalation injury should have an ABG analysis to determine respiratory status and oxygen saturation.

Cognitive level: Analysis

Nursing process: Assessment

Client needs: Physiological Integrity: Physiological Adaptation

Chapter 34

1. Answer: 2. Once stable, instruct in the use of a water pik.

Rationale: With mandibular fractures, good oral care is essential for healthy healing and prevention of dental complications. Patient education should include use of the water pik and dietary requirements. The use of systemic antibiotics to prevent meningitis is indicated in the management of temporal bone fractures. The use of eye protection is indicated in the patient with a temporal bone fracture. Facial nerve injury is seen in temporal bone fractures.

Cognitive level: Application

Nursing process: Planning

Client needs: Physiological Integrity: Reduction of Risk Potential

2. Answer: 2. Administer antibiotics as prescribed.

Rationale: Nursing care of the patient relies heavily on assessment of signs and symptoms, which, in turn, is dependent on obtaining a thorough patient history. The history must include the onset and duration of the symptoms including site of pain or discomfort, redness of eyes, flushing of face across the nose, fever, weakness or fatigue, cough, congestion, sore throat, muscle ache, and sore teeth. It also is important to know if any particular event or incident triggered the patient's symptoms. There is no reason to restrict fluids, maintain on bed rest, or consult with a dentist.

Cognitive level: Application

Nursing process: Planning

Client needs: Physiological Integrity: Reduction of Risk Potential

3. Answer: 4. Avoid exposure to strong perfumes, smoke, and rapid changes in temperature.

Rationale: With allergy injections, the dose is gradually increased to a maintenance concentration, which takes about 5 to 6 months. Patients may receive allergy injections for 3 to 5 years, depending on symptoms. The patient should be instructed to stay away from allergens that create a reaction. This means limiting outdoor exposure. Excessive humidity should be reduced and standing water should be removed. The patient should be instructed to eliminate exposure to smoke, strong perfumes and scents, fumes, rapid changes in temperature, and outdoor pollution for patients with nonspecific triggers.

Cognitive level: Application

Nursing process: Planning

Client needs: Health Promotion and Maintenance: Prevention/Early Detection of Health Problems

4. Answer: 1. Presence of smoke detectors in the home and the type of cooking appliances used

Rationale: Caution should be taken to ensure safety around the home. Smoke detectors and electric appliances rather than gas appliances should be used as should technologies that detect the presence of gas fumes in the home.

Cognitive level: Analysis

Nursing process: Assessment

Client needs: Health Promotion and Maintenance: Prevention/Early Detection of Health Problems

5. Answer: 2. Assess the type of difficulty and provide recommendations accordingly.

Rationale: The nursing process guides the management of patients with sleep apnea. The nurse should first assess the patient's description of "difficulty" and then make suggestions accordingly. The nurse should not alter the patient's prescribed treatment without health care provider involvement and should not recommend changing the use of the CPAP machine or not using the device.

Cognitive level: Application

Nursing process: Implementation

Client needs: Health Promotion and Maintenance: Prevention/Early Detection of Health Problems

6. Answer: 2. Smoking is only one cause for the disease. Others include chronic mouth lesions and poor nutrition.

Rationale: A variety of risk factors are associated with head and neck cancer, although some patients do not have any known risk factors; therefore, it is not possible to know for sure how much they contributed to causing the cancer. Some risk factors include alcohol intake, ultraviolet light exposure, tobacco use, mouth irritation, poor nutrition, HPV infection, immune system suppression, male gender, and exposure to Epstein–Barr virus if a first-generation Asian.

Cognitive level: Application

Nursing process: Implementation

Client needs: Psychosocial Integrity: Coping and Adaptation

7. Answer: 4. Secure the tube ties laterally to the chest with suspended ties.

Rationale: Nursing interventions include securing the airway with the appropriate ties in order to prevent the possibility of the tube being dislodged or accidentally removed. The tracheostomy tube ties should be secured to the chest laterally with suspended ties. Circumferential ties can place pressure on the incision lines or reconstruction flaps or grafts. The ties should be changed every day or when soiled to decrease the possibility of infection. The tracheostomy site should be cleaned on a regular basis such as every 8 hours and more frequently as needed to remove crusts and secretions that could obstruct the airway. If the tracheostomy tube has an inner cannula, it should be changed if disposable or cleaned when every tie tracheostomy care procedure is done.

Cognitive level: Application

Nursing process: Implementation

Client needs: Physiological Integrity: Physiological Adaptation

Chapter 35

1. Answer: 2. An acute asthma attack

Rationale: Asthma is a chronic inflammatory disorder of the airways in which many cells and cellular elements play a role, in particular, mast cells, eosinophils, T lymphocytes, macrophages, neutrophils, and epithelial cells. In susceptible individuals, this inflammation causes recurrent episodes of wheezing, breathlessness, chest tightness, and coughing, particularly at night or in the early morning. These episodes usually are associated with widespread but variable airflow obstruction that is often reversible, either spontaneously or with treatment. The inflammation also causes airway hyperresponsiveness or bronchospasm related to a variety of stimuli.

Cognitive level: Analysis

Nursing process: Assessment

Client needs: Physiological Integrity: Physiological Adaptation

2. Answer: 3. Avoid smoking or environments with smoke.

Rationale: The incidence of community-acquired pneumonia is highest in winter months with smoking being an important risk factor. The nurse should emphasize the importance of rest and a gradual increase in activity to avoid fatigue. Instructions should include ways to maintain resistance to infection with proper nutrition and adequate fluid intake. The patient should also be taught about all medications that will be continued at home.

Cognitive level: Application

Nursing process: Planning

Client needs: Physiological Integrity: Physiological Adaptation

3. Answer: 3. Magnesium sulfate

Rationale: Magnesium sulfate is thought to produce bronchodilation through counteraction of calcium-mediated smooth muscle constriction in the patient with COPD. This is given intravenously. Pancreatic enzymes are provided to the patient with cystic fibrosis because of failure of the pancreas to produce these enzymes. Ibuprofen is often used to reduce inflammation in the patient with cystic fibrosis. Pulmozyme decreases sputum viscosity in cystic fibrosis. Its use also has been shown to improve FEV_1 and decrease incidence of exacerbations.

Cognitive level: Application

Nursing process: Planning

Client needs: Physiological Integrity: Physiological Adaptation

4. Answer: 1. Pain management

Rationale: Rib fractures are treated by controlling the patient's pain. Sedation and pain management allow the patient to begin deep breathing and coughing in order to prevent the development of atelectasis, pneumonitis, and hypoxemia. A chest binder may decrease pain on movement. Usually the pain diminishes by the fifth to the seventh day, and healing occurs in 3 to 6 weeks. The nurse emphasizes pain management and gives specific instructions regarding medications for pain until the pain diminishes.

Cognitive level: Analysis

Nursing process: Planning

Client needs: Physiological Integrity: Physiological Adaptation

5. Answer: 4. Pain associated with the primary diagnosis

Rationale: The patient with lung cancer may complain of hoarseness, dysphagia, or vague complaints that have persisted longer than normally expected. Chest pain, tightness, or an ill-defined sensation of fullness may be experienced. This may be accompanied by pleuritic pain on inspiration or a subscapular pain radiating to the arm.

Cognitive level: Analysis

Nursing process: Assessment

Client needs: Physiological Integrity: Physiological Adaptation

6. Answer: 3. Place of employment 10 to 20 years prior to current admission

   Rationale: There is a considerable latency period of about 10 to 20 years for asbestosis between exposure and the development of symptomatology. Those at high risk for this disease are asbestos miners, millers, and those employed in the building trade and shipyards, such as loggers, insulation workers, pipe fitters and steamfitters, sheet metal workers, and welders. Working within the roofing materials industry is linked to silicosis.

   Cognitive level: Application

   Nursing process: Assessment

   Client needs: Physiological Integrity: Reduction of Risk Potential

Chapter 36

1. Answer: 1. Oxygen 2 liters nasal cannula

   Rationale: Acute respiratory failure results in a failure of oxygenation or ventilation or both. A failure of oxygenation produces hypoxemia, which is defined as a decreased arterial oxygen tension or pressure in the blood below normal range. The administration of oxygen would be the most effective in treating this type of patient. The patient's arterial saturation of oxygen level of less than 90 while breathing room air is representative of hypoxemic respiratory failure. Correcting and treating hypoxia is always a primary goal. Presenting symptoms in acute respiratory failure are shortness of breath, dyspnea, and increased work of breathing with hypoxemia and should always be addressed initially. Educating the patient and family is always important, but addressing the airway is always a priority.

   Cognitive level: Application

   Nursing process: Implementation

   Client needs: Physiological Integrity: Physiological Adaptation

2. Answer: 3. Pulmonary edema

   Rationale: The classic clinical presentation of acute pulmonary edema includes rapidly worsening dyspnea, shortness of breath, tachypnea, agitation, increased crackles, and possibly coarse rhonchi in all lung fields. Pink, frothy sputum may also be present. The other clinical signs are hypertension, tachycardia, and possibly S_3 or S_4 heart sounds. The pathophysiology of acute pulmonary edema and the signs and symptoms of this dysfunction are related to the accumulation of fluid, which prevents adequate gas exchange across the alveolar-capillary membrane. Cardiogenic pulmonary edema is pulmonary edema that results from increased hydrostatic pressures in the pulmonary capillary bed secondary to increased pulmonary venous pressure. Noncardiogenic pulmonary edema is related to injury of the alveolar-capillary membrane from numerous causes. Among the most important causes are sepsis, inflammation, inhaled toxins, and drugs. Usually in noncardiogenic pulmonary edema there is no primary cardiac dysfunction.

   Cognitive level: Analysis

   Nursing process: Assessment

   Client needs: Physiological Integrity: Physiological Adaptation

3. Answer: 4. PCWP > 30 mmHg

   Rationale: The patient with noncardiogenic pulmonary edema will develop tachycardia, hypertension, bounding pulses, and a drop in PCWP. If the patient's PCWP increases, the health care provider should be notified because this could indicate the development of cardiogenic pulmonary edema where the PCPW > 18 mmHg.

   Cognitive level: Application

   Nursing process: Assessment

   Client needs: Physiological Integrity: Physiological Adaptation

4. Answer: 3. Arterial blood gases showing respiratory acidosis

   Rationale: The hypoxemia of a patient with ARDS quickly becomes refractory to standard oxygen therapies, and the patient will require intubation and mechanical ventilation to maintain oxygenation and ventilation. The arterial blood gases frequently demonstrate respiratory acidosis. The chest x-ray exhibits the bilateral patchy infiltrates that are characteristic of the disease instead of the absence of infiltrates. This "white-out" observed on the chest x-ray can cover the entire lung field as the disease progresses. The vital signs are within normal range and will not usually be noted with a patient who has ARDS.

   Cognitive level: Application

   Nursing process: Assessment

   Client needs: Physiological Integrity: Physiological Adaptation

5. Answer: 2. Remove the patient from the ventilator and use the Ambu bag with 100% oxygen.

   Rationale: When the patient is experiencing hypoxia, it is imperative that the nurse remove the patient from the mechanical ventilator and administer 100% oxygen until the problem can be detected. Once the oxygenation returns to an acceptable range, the nurse should continue the assessment process. It is also important for the nurse to listen anteriorly and posteriorly in all lung fields. The importance of this exam cannot be overemphasized. When listening, the nurse should compare the right against the left lung and never listen through clothing or other material. The clinician should listen laterally in order to appreciate certain lung segments that can be heard in this position.

   Cognitive level: Application

   Nursing process: Implementation

   Client needs: Physiological Integrity: Physiological Adaptation

6. Answer: 4. When the patient is removed from the ventilator and the Ambu is used it causes overinflation from the Ambu aggressive rates.

Rationale: Most ventilated patients should have PEEP of at least 5 cm of H_2O to prevent the pressure in the alveoli from dropping to zero at the end of expiration. The nurse can cause auto-PEEP with overaggressive rates with an air-mask-bag unit. The patient is removed from the ventilator for transport or for suctioning. Rapid rates are used to bag the patient instead of the rate that was set on the ventilator. The patient might become hypotensive. Treatment would involve disconnecting the patient from the Ambu or ventilator for a few seconds; this would allow the excess pressure to dissipate. PEEP does not have any correlation with hypovolemia.

Cognitive level: Implementation

Nursing process: Assessment

Client needs: Physiological Integrity: Physiological Adaptation

7. Answer: 1. Auscultate lungs for bilateral breath sounds.

Rationale: The nurse as well as other members of the health care team should verify proper placement of the ET tube. The importance of this exam cannot be overemphasized. When listening, the nurse should compare the right against the left lung and never listen through clothing or other material. The clinician should listen laterally in order to appreciate certain lung segments that can be heard in this position. The endotracheal tube being advanced down the right main stem bronchus preventing air form entering the left lung also could cause the absence of lung sounds on the left, so accurate assessment is very important. Securing the ET tube, assessing oxygen saturation, and obtaining a chest x-ray are all important steps that need to be performed after the initial auscultation of breath sounds.

Cognitive level: Application

Nursing process: Implementation

Client needs: Physiological Integrity: Physiological Adaptation

8. Answer: 4. Applying suction when passing the catheter into the patient's tracheostomy

Rationale: To perform tracheostomy suctioning, the nurse or caregiver should use sterile gloves in order to prevent nosocomial infections. The patient should be oxygenated prior to suctioning and the patient's head should be elevated. The patient should always be preoxygenated to prevent hypoxemia as well. The nurse/caregiver should never suction going into the tracheostomy, only when withdrawing the catheter.

Cognitive level: Application

Nursing process: Evaluation

Client needs: Physiological Integrity: Physiological Adaptation

9. Answer: 2. A patient with a chest tube on the right side with bubbling in the water seal chamber

Rationale: The nurse should initially see the patient with the chest tube. A pleural tube is inserted in the pleural space in order to evacuate the air or blood and allow the lung to reexpand. The pleural tube re-creates the negative pressure in the chest that has been violated by trauma or surgery. A pleural chest tube should not bubble in the water seal chamber.

Cognitive level: Application

Nursing process: Assessment

Client needs: Physiological Integrity

Chapter 37

1. Answer: 2. Waist circumference is 110 cm.

Rationale: The patient already has two of the criteria for the metabolic syndrome: hypertension and hypertriglyceridemia. The third factor is a waist circumference of greater than 102 cm in males and 88 cm in females. The fasting blood sugar would need to be greater than or equal to 110 mg/dL. The HDL would need to be less than 40 mg/dL in males. Random blood sugars are not part of the criteria for metabolic syndrome.

Cognitive level: Application

Nursing process: Assessment

Client needs: Physiological Integrity: Physiological Adaptation

2. Answer: 4. Decongestants

Rationale: Decongestants cause vasoconstriction and can contribute to hypertension and cardiac arrhythmias. The other medications would not present a cardiac risk.

Cognitive level: Application

Nursing process: Assessment

Client needs: Physiological Integrity: Physiological Adaptation

3. Answer: 2. "How many pillows do you sleep on?"

Rationale: The degree of orthopnea is best measured by the number of pillows that are needed to help the patient breathe comfortably. Frequency of waking up could be caused by many factors and is not specific to orthopnea. Palpitations can occur for many reasons or even be normal and do not correlate with orthopnea. Nocturia may indicate congestive heart failure, but does not correlate with a diagnosis of orthopnea.

Cognitive level: Application

Nursing process: Assessment

Client needs: Physiological Integrity: Physiological Adaptation

4. Answer: 2. Systolic dysfunction

Rationale: S_3 sounds are a marker of systolic dysfunction. They are heard early during diastole and are associated with ventricular dysfunction. S_4 sounds are indicative of diastolic dysfunction. Conduction defects are not heard as heart sounds. Alterations in the mitral valve are heard as abnormal S_1 sounds.

Cognitive level: Application

Nursing process: Assessment

Client needs: Physiological Integrity: Physiological Adaptation

Chapter 38

1. Answer: 2. QRS complex 0.10 second

Rationale: The following criteria must be present to be a normal electrocardiogram: P wave has a normal and consistent shape and appears before every QRS complex; there is a 1:1 ratio of P wave to QRS complex; PR interval is between 0.12 and 0.20 second; QRS complex is between 0.06 and 0.12 second; QT interval is between 0.34 and 0.43 second; atrial and ventricular rate is between 60 and 100 beats per minute; and atrial and ventricular rhythm is regular.

Cognitive level: Analysis

Nursing process: Assessment

Client needs: Physiological Integrity: Reduction of Risk Potential

2. Answer: 3. 0.12 second

Rationale: Each "small box" is 0.04 second. This patient's QRS complex should be documented as being 0.12 second.

Cognitive level: Application

Nursing process: Assessment

Client needs: Physiological Integrity: Reduction of Risk Potential

3. Answer: 2. Observe and treat the patient for anxiety.

Rationale: This patient is demonstrating premature atrial contractions (PACs) that started after learning of a stressful and/or anxiety-producing event. This patient should be observed for the frequency of the PACs and the anxiety should be treated. Cardioversion is a treatment for atrial flutter. Calcium channel blockers are used with atrial fibrillation. Carotid artery massage is a treatment used for supraventricular tachycardia.

Cognitive level: Analysis

Nursing process: Planning

Client needs: Physiological Integrity: Physiological Adaptation

4. Answer: 1. Have a serum digoxin level drawn.

Rationale: Because some prescribed medications, such as digoxin, cause significant dysrhythmias, the patient's medical history should be reviewed to determine if the dysrhythmia is medication related. Serum drug levels should be ordered as indicated. ACLS protocols would be indicated in some cases of ventricular dysrhythmias. Magnesium is the treatment of choice for torsade de pointes. Lidocaine is used in the treatment of premature ventricular contractions.

Cognitive level: Analysis

Nursing process: Planning

Client needs: Physiological Integrity: Physiological Adaptation

Chapter 39

1. Answer: 4. False positive

Rationale: Sensitivity describes the ability of a test to identify patients with disease. It may be calculated by dividing the number of true positive tests by the sum of true positives plus false negatives. For example, positive tests in subjects with coronary disease are "true positives," whereas negative tests are "false negatives." Similarly, negative tests in patients who are free of disease are "true negatives," and positive tests in patients without disease are "false positives."

Cognitive level: Application

Nursing process: Implementation

Client needs: Health Promotion and Maintenance: Prevention/Early Detection of Health Problems

2. Answer: 4. Echocardiogram

Rationale: With an echocardiogram, hemodynamic data include the amount and speed of blood flow through the valves, enabling the noninvasive detection and follow-up of stenotic or regurgitant heart valves. TEE is frequently used to detect and assess endocarditis, aortic dissection, intracardiac masses such as thrombi or tumors, valvular pathology, and congenital disorders in both children and adults. MRI can be used to evaluate patients with presumed congenital heart diseases, such as coarctation of the aorta or atrial septal defects. PET scan is the current "gold standard" for assessment of myocardial viability.

Cognitive level: Application

Nursing process: Planning

Client needs: Health Promotion and Maintenance: Prevention/Early Detection of Health Problems

3. Answer: 2. Provide intravenous normal saline prior to the procedure.

Rationale: Patients with preexisting renal failure and a history of anaphylactic reaction to contrast dye must be pretreated before the catheterization. Pretreatment for the patient with a history of anaphylactic reaction to contrast dye includes antihistamines and steroids. In the laboratory the patient will usually be given a mild sedative. Patients with renal failure (serum creatinine ≤1.5 mg/dL) should receive intravenous normal saline for several hours before the procedure.

Cognitive level: Application

Nursing process: Planning

Client needs: Physiological Integrity: Reduction of Risk Potential

4. Answer: 4. Stress test

Rationale: A stress test is contraindicated for myocardial infarction within 2 days, unstable angina, aortic stenosis, uncontrolled dysrhythmias, symptomatic heart failure, active endocarditis, uncontrolled hypertension, any acute disorder that may affect exercise, and the inability to obtain informed consent. The ECG is helpful in determining the overall electrical functioning of the patient's heart. The echocardiogram is useful to determining the patient's ejection fraction in addition to the functioning of other cardiac structures. The PCI can be done to prevent further myocardial damage.

Cognitive level: Analysis

Nursing process: Planning

Client needs: Physiological Integrity: Reduction of Risk Potential

5. Answer: 3. Assess the femoral site.

Rationale: All patients must have a complete nursing assessment, with special emphasis on the cardiovascular system including peripheral pulses and the vascular access site. This assessment includes vital signs, ECG monitoring, and assessment of the vascular access site and pulses distal to the puncture site. Evaluation of the access site includes inspection for any signs of bleeding or swelling and palpation for any tenderness. Diagnosis of suspected arterial injuries is made through a careful physical assessment, and confirmed through noninvasive vascular studies or arteriography. Physical examination of the femoral site is performed assessing for the presence of localized tenderness, bruits, or a pulsatile mass. Hematomas are identified by swelling at the site of the arterial puncture. Large hematomas may need to be assessed by ultrasound to rule out the presence of pseudoaneurysms or arteriovenous fistulas.

Cognitive level: Application

Nursing process: Assessment

Client needs: Physiological Integrity: Reduction of Risk Potential

Chapter 40

1. Answer: 4. "My father died of a heart attack at age 70."
   Rationale: Genetics, sex, and age are nonmodifiable risk factors, or those that cannot be changed. Smoking, hypertension, diabetes, obesity, and a sedentary lifestyle are modifiable risk factors. The patient's smoking and high blood sugars reflect modifiable risk factors. Walking provides exercise to modify the risk factor of a sedentary lifestyle.

   Cognitive level: Application

   Nursing process: Assessment

   Client needs: Physiological Integrity: Reduction of Risk Potential

2. Answer: 3. "Was your pain precipitated by activity?"
   Rationale: Stable angina is frequently precipitated by activity, emotional stress, cold weather, or large meals. Pain lasting 15 minutes would be indicative of a myocardial infarction; angina pain usually lasts 5 to 10 minutes. Anginal pain radiates to the jaw, but not always.

   Cognitive level: Application

   Nursing process: Implementation

   Client needs: Physiological Integrity: Physiological Adaptation

3. Answer: 1. The pain was relieved by taking nitroglycerin.
   Rationale: The three key characteristics of typical angina include pain, pressure, tightness, or heaviness that is substernal, central chest, or in the left arm that is provoked by exertion or emotional stress and that is relieved by nitroglycerin. Angina may be precipitated by eating a large meal, but relief with nitroglycerin provides stronger support for a diagnosis of typical angina. Angina may also cause anxiety and dizziness, but again, these do not provide the best support.

   Cognitive level: Application

   Nursing process: Assessment

   Client needs: Physiological Integrity: Physiological Adaptation

4. Answer: 4. Transmural ischemia
   Rationale: When ischemia traverses the entire width of cardiac muscle, it is called transmural and the ST segment

is elevated. The more leads in which the ST segment is elevated indicate greater damage. Mild ischemia of subendocardial injury would be reflected as ST segment depression. Past myocardial infarction damage is diagnosed by the presence of a Q wave.

Cognitive level: Analysis

Nursing process: Assessment

Client needs: Physiological Integrity: Physiological Adaptation

5. Answer: 1. Occurrence of an old myocardial infarction
   Rationale: An old MI is diagnosed when a Q wave is present in the absence of ST elevation, patient symptoms, and blood markers. The Q-wave changes are due to necrosis and are irreversible, so they allow for identification of MIs. They cannot determine how long ago the necrosis occurred, so it would not be safe to conclude the damage was recent. Q waves do not reflect pacemaker function or ventricular hypertrophy.

   Cognitive level: Analysis

   Nursing process: Assessment

   Client needs: Physiological Integrity: Physiological Adaptation

6. Answer: 1. Troponin 1 levels
   Rationale: Troponin 1 levels are specific to cardiac muscle and are released from the myocardial cell within 3 to 12 hours of cellular injury and may stay elevated for 5 to 14 days. Myoglobin levels are not a specific indicator of heart damage and only stay elevated for 24 hours. C-reactive protein is also not specific to cardiac muscle. CK-MB levels are specific to myocardial tissue, but return to normal within 72 hours.

   Cognitive level: Application

   Nursing process: Assessment

   Client needs: Physiological Integrity: Physiological Adaptation

7. Answer: 2. Cardiogenic shock
   Rationale: Cardiogenic shock is an acute condition that must be detected and treated immediately to improve survival. An infarction of greater than 40% of the left ventricle and three-vessel disease place the patient at greater risk to develop cardiogenic shock. Pericarditis is associated with large infarctions and low ejection fractions but is not the highest priority. Dressler's syndrome is indicative of pericarditis that occurs 2 to 12 weeks following an MI. PVCs can occur following any cardiac ischemic event, but are not the highest priority.

   Cognitive level: Analysis

   Nursing process: Planning

   Client needs: Physiological Integrity: Physiological Adaptation

8. Answer: 3. Significant stenosis of the left anterior descending, LAD, and circumflex artery
   Rationale: Class I recommendations indicate a CABG is indicated when the patient has significant stenosis of the proximal LAD and left circumflex artery even though the patient is asymptomatic. A 50% occlusion of the circumflex artery is not part of the criteria. Recent history of angina and heart failure are also not qualifying criteria.

Cognitive level: Application
Nursing process: Assessment
Client needs: Physiological Integrity: Physiological Adaptation

9. Answer: 4. Report the findings to the primary care provider.
Rationale: An output of greater than 100 mL/hr reflects postoperative bleeding and should be reported. Output should continued to be monitored but is not the first priority. Having the patient cough and deep breathe does not address the problem of bleeding. Although the chest tube dressing should be checked, the chest tube output reflects internal bleeding and must be reported immediately.
Cognitive level: Analysis
Nursing process: Implementation
Client needs: Physiological Integrity: Physiological Adaptation

Chapter 41

1. Answer: 3. Mitral stenosis
Rationale: Rheumatic fever produces an inflammatory process that often causes valvular heart damage, leading to stenosis of heart valves. Pericarditis and endocarditis may be experienced during the initial inflammatory process, but should not persist after treatment is done. Pulmonary fibrosis is not caused by rheumatic fever.
Cognitive level: Application
Nursing process: Planning
Client needs: Physiological Integrity: Physiological Adaptation

2. Answer: 2. "I had rheumatic heart disease when I was a child."
Rationale: Aortic stenosis is often caused by rheumatic heart disease, which destroys valve leaflets with calcification and fibrosis, which leads to the stenosis. As the narrowing of the valve increases, clinical manifestations are exhibited; dyspnea is the most frequent complaint and is often accompanied by angina and exertional syncope. Having had a CABG or having a dysrhythmia are not contributing factors for aortic stenosis. Palpitations are associated with mitral valve prolapse and stenosis or aortic regurgitation.
Cognitive level: Application
Nursing process: Assessment
Client needs: Physiological Integrity: Physiological Adaptation

3. Answer: 2. Plan for rest periods throughout the day.
Rationale: Excessive exercise and exertion place demands for increased circulation and oxygen to the heart. Allowing time for rest reduces the workload and therefore oxygen demands on the heart. The valve may not need to be replaced; the patient should be taught to take prophylactic antibiotics before dental work, but not to avoid dental work. An elevated temperature could be a sign of endocarditis, but it is not necessary to take the temperature daily. A diet high in fatty foods should be avoided, but it is not necessary to keep a food diet.
Cognitive level: Application

Nursing process: Implementation
Client needs: Physiological Integrity: Physiological Adaptation

4. Answer: 3. The valve will be repaired, but not replaced.
Rationale: An open procedure involves surgical repair under general anesthesia and cardiopulmonary bypass. Valvuloplasty involves repair of the torn or damaged leaflets, chordae tendineae, or papillary muscle, but the valve is not replaced. Anticoagulation therapy will be needed in the postoperative period to prevent thrombus formation at the surgical site. A valvuloplasty does not guarantee that future repairs or valve replacement will not be necessary.
Cognitive level: Application
Nursing process: Implementation
Client needs: Physiological Integrity: Physiological Adaptation

5. Answer: 4. Supportive therapy with medications
Rationale: Because the prognosis for this type of cardiomyopathy is poor, management is focused at reducing the workload of the heart and diminishing heart failure with use of diuretics, calcium channel blockers, beta-blockers, and antiarrhythmic medications. Alcohol ablation and ICDs are sometimes used in the treatment of hypertrophic cardiomyopathy. Aortic valve repair is not indicated for treatment.
Cognitive level: Application
Nursing process: Planning
Client needs: Physiological Integrity: Physiological Adaptation

6. Answer: 3. "Does the pain become worse if you take a deep breath?"
Rationale: Chest pain associated with pericarditis is often described as sharp and gets worse with deep breathing; it is relieved by sitting up. Anginal pain is not associated with position changes or deep breathing. It is relieved by sitting up, not lying flat. Pericarditis does not occur at any particular time of day and is not associated with palpitations.
Cognitive level: Application
Nursing process: Implementation
Client needs: Physiological Integrity: Physiological Adaptation

Chapter 42

1. Answer: 3. Aortic stenosis
Rationale: Risk factors for heart failure include a history of hypertension, coronary heart disease, obesity, diabetes, and structural and valvular disorders, such as aortic stenosis. Pancreatitis, chronic fatigue syndrome, and pleural effusions are not risk factors for heart failure.
Cognitive level: Application
Nursing process: Assessment
Client needs: Physiological Integrity: Physiological Adaptation

2. Answer: 1. Decreased cardiac output
Rationale: Systolic dysfunction occurs when the ventricle is unable to contract forcefully during systole and often

hypertrophies in an effort to compensate. As a result, the percentage of blood ejected from the heart is decreased. Aortic stenosis and mitral regurgitation may contribute to the development of heart failure and may be manifested by the presence of a murmur. Systolic dysfunction primarily affects cardiac output, not heart rate.
Cognitive level: Application
Nursing process: Assessment
Client needs: Physiological Integrity: Physiological Adaptation

3. Answer: 1. Activation of the sympathetic nervous system, SNS
Rationale: Activation of the SNS and RAS systems occurs when cardiac output falls, in an effort to increase blood volume and rate of heart contractility. The parasympathetic system is not activated because this would further decrease the heart rate. Cytokines are also released, not suppressed.
Cognitive level: Application
Nursing process: Assessment
Client needs: Physiological Integrity: Physiological Adaptation

4. Answer: 3. Dyspnea
Rationale: Dyspnea is seen secondary to pulmonary congestion, which occurs most with left-sided heart failure. Fluid accumulates in the pulmonary bed as it backs up from the left ventricle. Right-sided failure causes venous congestion with fluid accumulation in the interstitial spaces, manifested by weight gain, anorexia, nausea, and peripheral edema.
Cognitive level: Application
Nursing process: Assessment
Client needs: Physiological Integrity: Physiological Adaptation

5. Answer: 1. A diagnosis of heart failure can be excluded.
Rationale: The BNP is very useful in ruling out a diagnosis of heart failure if the level is normal. Elevated levels correlate with heart failure, increased risk of mortality, acute MI, PE, and renal failure. Because they are not elevated, the patient does not have long-standing heart failure, cardiac ischemia. Pulmonary tissue damage would not be diagnosed with BNP levels.
Cognitive level: Application
Nursing process: Evaluation
Client needs: Physiological Integrity: Physiological Adaptation

6. Answer: 1. ACE inhibitors and beta-blockers
Rationale: Treatment of stage B heart failure is aimed at reduction afterload with ACE inhibitors and reduction of workload on the heart with beta-blockers, as well as antihypertensives and diuretics. Insertion of a defibrillator may be done for stage C heart failure. A patient with stage D heart failure may need hospice referral.
Cognitive level: Analysis
Nursing process: Application
Client needs: Physiological Integrity: Physiological Adaptation

7. Answer: 2. Medications, activity, weight, diet, and symptoms

Rationale: The most important key concepts that patients with heart failure should learn to incorporate into their daily lives follow the acronym MAWDS: medication, activity, weight, diet, and symptoms. Although finances, psychosocial concerns, social support, and spirituality are also important, they are not the key issues.
Cognitive level: Application
Nursing process: Implementation
Client needs: Physiological Integrity: Physiological Adaptation

8. Answer: 3. Depression and anemia
Rationale: Depression, anemia, renal insufficiency, hypertension, coronary heart disease, and sleep apnea have all been shown to worsen the prognosis of patients with heart failure. Patients with heart failure usually experience hypertension, not hypovolemic shock. Liver failure and DVTs are not identified as factors that will increase mortality of heart failure.
Cognitive level: Application
Nursing process: Assessment
Client needs: Physiological Integrity: Physiological Adaptation

9. Answer: 2. Plans for treatment in the final stages of heart failure
Rationale: Discussion about the level of care should occur ahead of time, not at the time of crisis. The nurse needs to address issues of patient comfort and dignity during the terminal stage of heart failure. In end-stage disease, a heart transplant and surgical interventions are not options. Long-term home care management may not be an option for the family and patient.
Cognitive level: Application
Nursing process: Planning
Client needs: Physiological Integrity: Physiological Adaptation

Chapter 43

1. Answer: 1. Intermittent claudication
Rationale: The risk factors, similar to those of heart disease and stroke, include cigarette smoking, diabetes, hyperlipidemia, hypertension, elevated C-reactive protein, and hyperhomocysteinemia. Intermittent claudication, or exercise-induced leg pain, is the most common symptom of peripheral arterial disease. This pain can occur in the buttocks, hip, thigh, or calf, depending on the portion of the arterial tree affected by atherosclerotic disease. With exercise, such as walking, metabolic demands are increased, and the diseased arteries are unable to deliver the needed oxygen to the muscles or to dispose of the metabolic by-product lactic acid. The buildup of lactic acid causes pain in the affected muscle group of the leg. When the walking ceases, or shortly afterward, the pain resolves and exercise may resume.
Cognitive level: Application
Nursing process: Assessment
Client needs: Physiological Integrity: Physiological Adaptation

2. Answer: 3. Teach importance of regular and structured ambulation.

Rationale: The patient with impaired mobility would benefit from being taught the importance of regular and structured ambulation to enhance circulation and promote collateral development. The use of moist heat would aid in comfort for a venous occlusion. Legs should be kept in the dependent position to enhance arterial perfusion. Cool skin to the touch is one of the six Ps of arterial ischemia and should be reported to a health care professional immediately.

Cognitive level: Application

Nursing process: Planning

Client needs: Physiological Integrity: Physiological Adaptation

3. Answer: 2. Dress warmly in cold weather and limit alcohol intake.

Rationale: Nonpharmacologic management of Raynaud's disease is directed toward avoiding known stressors; controlling exposure to extremes in climate; dressing warmly in cold weather; and limiting tobacco, caffeine, and alcohol intake. Some patients may benefit from learning relaxation techniques. Regular physical exercise is important because it improves circulation and warms the body temperature. Some medications, such as beta-blockers, ergot alkaloids, and hormones, can precipitate episodes of vasospasm. There is no cure for Buerger's disease. The primary treatment is directed toward smoking cessation and avoidance of secondhand smoke.

Cognitive level: Application

Nursing process: Planning

Client needs: Physiological Integrity: Physiological Adaptation

4. Answer: 4. Renal impairment due to alterations in blood flow

Rationale: Interruption in blood flow may occur with the endovascular stent or the open approach and the nurse would monitor urine output and BUN and serum creatinine levels. If an embolus were to follow this procedure, the legs are the most common site for perfusion problems. The insertion site for the stent is through a femoral stick and not through an abdominal incision. The hospital stay for this procedure is shorter than for the traditional surgical approach.

Cognitive level: Application

Nursing process: Assessment

Client needs: Physiological Integrity: Physiological Adaptation

5. Answer: 1. The need for early ambulation, use of compression stockings, and range-of-motion exercises

Rationale: Early ambulation, use of compression stockings, and performance of range-of-motion exercises are important nursing processes for this patient. Patients with a deep venous thrombosis with arterial involvement may still use carefully applied compression stockings. Patients benefit from early ambulation.

Cognitive level: Application

Nursing process: Implementation

Client needs: Physiological Integrity: Physiological Adaptation

6. Answer: 2. The signs and symptoms of bleeding

Rationale: Avoiding foods high in vitamin K is indicated for warfarin sodium therapy. Having an INR drawn is indicated for warfarin sodium therapy. Unfractionated heparin is preferred for patients with kidney failure. When low molecular weight heparin is being administered, the patient should be instructed on signs and symptoms of bleeding.

Cognitive level: Application

Nursing process: Implementation

Client needs: Physiological Integrity: Pharmacologic and Parenteral Therapies

7. Answer: 2. Compression stockings will be worn to decrease venous stasis.

Rationale: Bed rest is recommended for the first 24 hours following surgery. The patient may shower the next day following the procedure. Anticoagulants are not a part of the treatment for varicose veins unless there is a condition that warrants these medications.

Cognitive level: Application

Nursing process: Planning

Client needs: Physiological Integrity; Physiological Adaptation

8. Answer: 1. If an aortic aneurysm is diagnosed that is larger than 6 centimeters, surgery will be performed.

Rationale: The physician will monitor the growth of an AAA and will surgically correct when it has reached 5.5 centimeters. If a patient is on steroids, they are discontinued if possible in the medical management of this patient. The infrarenal area is the most common site for the development of an AAA and is repaired with either the surgical or endovascular option.

Cognitive level: Analysis

Nursing process: Assessment

Client needs: Physiological Integrity: Physiological Adaptation

Chapter 44

1. Answer: 4. Diverticulitis

Rationale: This pain pattern in the adult is suggestive of diverticulitis. The pain of acute appendicitis is predominantly in the right lower quadrant. Intussusception and pyloric stenosis are not seen in the adult.

Cognitive level: Analysis

Nursing process: Assessment

Client needs: Physiological Integrity: Reduction of Risk Potential

2. Answer: 1. Inspection

Rationale: The correct order for examination is inspection, auscultation, percussion, and palpation. Bowel sounds should be auscultated prior to percussion to avoid changing the frequency or rate. Light palpation in all quadrants precedes deep palpation.

Cognitive level: Application

Nursing process: Assessment

Client needs: Health Promotion and Maintenance: Prevention/Early Detection of Health Problems

3. Answer: 4. A full bladder

Rationale: Percussing the abdomen will elicit different sounds. There should be a hollow sound, similar to that of tapping on a watermelon, over the epigastric area and sometimes over the bowels. If this hollow sound is throughout the entire abdomen, it is called tympany and is indicative of an obstruction or distention of the abdomen. This sound is produced by air in the intestine. The liver and a full bladder give off a dull sound, similar to that when percussing a piece of meat.

Cognitive level: Application

Nursing process: Assessment

Client needs: Health Promotion and Maintenance: Prevention/Early Detection of Health Problems

4. Answer: 3. Inflammatory process in the abdomen

Rationale: Rebound tenderness describes pain that is more prominent when pressure is released and is indicative of an inflammatory process in the abdomen. A negative obturator's sign is a normal finding and further testing may be warranted depending on the initial complaint. A positive Murphy's sign is seen in inflammation of the gallbladder.

Cognitive level: Application

Nursing process: Assessment

Client needs: Health Promotion and Maintenance: Prevention/Early Detection of Health Problems

5. Answer: 2. Ask the patient what caused the abdominal scar.

Rationale: When obtaining a medical history from patients with gastrointestinal symptoms, past surgeries play a major role. It is also important to correlate this information with the physical exam. At times, patients will forget a surgery, especially if it was many years ago. Therefore, correlating the history with the scars on the abdomen is a helpful tool. When doing the abdominal examination, confirm which operation relates to which scar. This can also trigger more information from the patient. Pay particular attention to the area around the umbilicus, because laparoscopic scars are small and can be very faint.

Cognitive level: Application

Nursing process: Assessment

Client needs: Physiological Integrity: Reduction of Risk Potential

Chapter 45

1. Answer: 1. Increased salivation and bad breath

Rationale: Vincent's stomatitis, also known as acute necrotizing stomatitis or trench mouth, is a bacterial infection characterized by erythematous ulceration and necrosis of the gingival margins, red gingival papilla, a purulent gray exudate, increased salivation, bad breath, bleeding gums, and pain. Painful red maculae with erythematous halos are seen in the early stage of contact stomatitis, and ulcers covered with a grayish membrane develop in the ulcerative phase of contact stomatitis. Curd-like patches on the tongue and cheek are characteristic of oral candidiasis.

Cognitive level: Application

Nursing process: Assessment

Client needs: Physiological Integrity: Physiological Adaptation

2. Answer: 1. Premalignant tissue in the esophagus

Rationale: With repeated exposure of erosive stomach contents, an inflammatory response is initiated. When the inflammation becomes chronic, normal squamous epithelial cells are replaced with columnar epithelium. This new epithelium is called Barrett's epithelium and is a premalignant tissue that increases the risk of esophageal cancer. Esophageal strictures and fine tears may occur with achalasia. Ulcers and inflamed tissue are associated with exacerbations of GERD.

Cognitive level: Application

Nursing process: Assessment

Client needs: Physiological Integrity: Physiological Adaptation

3. Answer: 4. Biopsy of the small intestine

Rationale: A biopsy of the small intestine is considered the gold standard and currently the most definitive test to diagnose celiac disease. Stools are not Gram stained. The antigliadin antibody is a new test being used, but still not the most definitive. Gastric pH analysis is done when diagnosing GERD.

Cognitive level: Analysis

Nursing process: Implementation

Client needs: Physiological Integrity: Physiological Adaptation

4. Answer: 3. Malabsorption of nutrients often occurs.

Rationale: Malabsorption of nutrients is more specific to Crohn's. The inflamed tissue occurs most frequently in the jejunum and ileum, which impairs absorption of nutrients. In ulcerative colitis the inflammation occurs in the rectum and sigmoid colon. The loss of exudates from ulcerated tissues in Crohn's further leads to protein losses. Loose watery stools can occur with both disorders. Abdominal pain is usually present in both conditions. Rectal urgency and incontinence can also occur with both conditions.

Cognitive level: Application

Nursing process: Planning

Client needs: Physiological Integrity: Physiological Adaptation

5. Answer: 3. Drinks citrus juice with meals

Rationale: Foods with a high acidic content or that are spicy will reduce the lower esophageal sphincter tone, causing reflux of acidic stomach contents into the esophagus. A BMI of 21 is normal; obesity can contribute to reflux. Patients who are lactose intolerant often experience abdominal cramping and bloating after eating, not heartburn. Eating high-fiber foods does not cause GERD.

Cognitive level: Application

Nursing process: Assessment

Client needs: Physiological Integrity: Physiological Adaptation

6. Answers:
   1. Daily alcohol intake
   2. A history of irritable bowel disease (IBD)

Rationale: Recent research indicates that daily alcohol consumption increases the risk for colon cancer. IBD causes a chronic inflammation of the bowel, leading to local tissue injury and cancer. A high-fat diet, not low-fat, causes increased deposition of fatty acids within cell membranes and increases intestinal prostaglandins, which stimulate cell proliferation, contributing to cancer. Intake of folic acid, selenium, vitamin D, and calcium reduce the risk for colon cancer. Daily use of NSAIDs helps to reduce inflammation, which in turn reduces cancer risk.

Cognitive level: Application
Nursing process: Planning
Client needs: Physiological Integrity: Reduction of Risk Potential

7. Answer: 4. Place the tube at the shoulder level of patient.

Rationale: Placing the tube at shoulder level reduces the pull of gravity and fluid into the port. The port should be open and patent to allow for air inflow. The port should never be irrigated or plugged. Placing the patient in a high Fowler's position will not correct the problem if the tube is also not positioned higher.

Cognitive level: Application
Nursing process: Implementation
Client needs: Physiological Integrity: Reduction of Risk Potential

8. Answer: 1. Check for signs of hypoglycemia 2 hours after a meal.

Rationale: When the hyperosmolar load of a meal is dumped into the jejunum, there is a rapid rise in blood sugar followed by a release of excessive amounts of insulin. The insulin then causes a secondary hypoglycemia about 2 to 3 hours after eating. Patients with dumping syndrome should rest or even lie down if tolerated for 30 minutes after a meal; ambulation would not be encouraged. Liquids should be taken between meals to reduce the load entering the jejunum. The diet should be low in simple carbohydrates; protein and fats will help to slow transit time and reduce symptoms.

Cognitive level: Analysis
Nursing process: Implementation
Client needs: Physiological Integrity: Physiological Adaptation

9. Answer: 1. Beefy red and moist

Rationale: A stoma should be pink or beefy red and moist without obvious cyanosis or bleeding. It should extend about 2 to 3 cm from the abdominal wall. A slightly purple or pale pink color could be indicative of impaired circulation to the stoma.

Cognitive level: Application
Nursing process: Planning
Client needs: Physiological Integrity: Physiological Adaptation

Chapter 46

1. Answer: 3. "Have you ever had a tattoo?"

Rationale: Hepatitis C is found predominantly in blood, blood products, and transplanted tissue and it has been transmitted by percutaneous exposures, such as tattooing, body piercing, barbering, and folk medicine practices. Traveling in areas where hepatitis A is endemic and eating uncooked shellfish are risks for exposure to hepatitis A. Sharing utensils with a person infected with hepatitis A put the person at risk for hepatitis A, not hepatitis C.

Cognitive level: Application
Nursing process: Implementation
Client needs: Physiological Integrity: Physiological Adaptation

2. Answer: 4. Constant epigastric pain

Rationale: The prodromal phase of hepatitis occurs between exposure to the virus and appearance of jaundice. Symptoms are often vague and include anorexia, nausea, vomiting, malaise, arthralgias, and mild, but constant abdominal, RUQ or epigastric pain. Hyperthermia, not hypothermia, would occur. Appetite is decreased, not increased. Dark-colored urine would be seen during the icteric phase, as serum bilirubin levels rise.

Cognitive level: Application
Nursing process: Assessment
Client needs: Physiological Integrity: Physiological Adaptation

3. Answer: 1. Peripheral edema

Rationale: An albumin level of 2.5 g/dL reflects hypoalbuminemia, which causes a decrease in colloidal osmotic pressure, leading to leakage of fluid into the tissues and is manifested as ascites or peripheral edema in cirrhosis. Lack of vitamin K and prothrombin production by the liver would cause prolonged blood coagulation. The liver's inability to conjugate bilirubin properly would lead to jaundice. Vitamin A may not be absorbed when bile is not produced or released into the duodenum, which may be seen with gallbladder disease or advanced cirrhosis.

Cognitive level: Application
Nursing process: Assessment
Client needs: Physiological Integrity: Physiological Adaptation

4. Answer: 2. Oxazepam, Serax

Rationale: Serax is a benzodiazepine that is not metabolized by the liver, but is still used cautiously to treat agitation. Lactulose is an osmotic laxative and is given to treat elevated ammonia levels and constipation. Protonix is a proton pump inhibitor given to reduce gastric acidity. Vitamin K is stored in the liver and is given to aid in blood clotting since it may be deficient in the patient with cirrhosis.

Cognitive level: Application
Nursing process: Implementation
Client needs: Physiological Integrity: Physiological Adaptation

5. Answer: 1. Provide supportive and comfort measures to the patient and family.

Rationale: An elevated AFP level is indicative of advanced hepatocellular carcinoma and rapid tumor growth.

Survival rates are short term and so quality of life should be provided with supportive and comfort measures. A TIPS is done to treat portal hypertension and ascites that has been refractory to treatment. Liver transplants are only indicated for small tumors without evidence of spread. Protein restriction is sometimes ordered to treat hepatic encephalopathy associated with cirrhosis, and salt restriction is indicated when ascites is present.
Cognitive level: Application
Nursing process: Implementation
Client needs: Physiological Integrity: Physiological Adaptation

6. Answer: 3. The patient has had rapid weight loss secondary to crash dieting.
Rationale: Risk factors for developing gallstones include obesity, high estrogen states, diabetes, hyperlipidemia, cirrhosis, Crohn's disease, rapid weight loss, and bariatric surgery. A high-fiber diet helps to utilize bile and cholesterol and would not predispose the patient to stones. Some drugs, such as oral contraceptives, clofibrate, and hormone replacement therapy can increase the risk of gallstones, but not aminoglycosides. Native American people have a higher risk; people of northern European descent are at greater risk for osteoporosis.
Cognitive level: Application
Nursing process: Assessment
Client needs: Physiological Integrity: Reduction of Risk Potential

7. Answer: 3. Examine abdomen for rigidity and tenderness.
Rationale: Increasing abdominal pain and tenderness may be a sign of intra-abdominal leak of bile or blood so the patient should first be assessed for abdominal tenderness and rigidity, since the opioid analgesia should have been effective in relieving postoperative pain. Administering a second dose of analgesia without first further assessing the pain could mask the cause of the pain. Ambulating the patient could be done after it has been determined the cause of pain is not peritonitis. A side-lying fetal position is helpful for patients with acute pancreatitis.
Cognitive level: Analysis
Nursing process: Implementation
Client needs: Physiological Integrity: Reduction of Risk Potential

8. Answer: 2. Amylase level is normal.
Rationale: In chronic pancreatitis, amylase levels are not always elevated, whereas amylase is usually always elevated with acute pancreatitis. Stools may be clay colored and the abdomen would be tender in both acute and chronic pancreatitis. The blood sugar would most likely be elevated in chronic pancreatitis due to loss of endocrine function with progressive destruction of the gland.
Cognitive level: Analysis
Nursing process: Assessment
Client needs: Physiological Integrity: Reduction of Risk Potential

9. Answer: 2. Clay-colored stools
Rationale: Jaundice occurs in patients with pancreatic cancer when the bile duct becomes blocked from the tumor.

The bilirubin pigment does not enter the duodenum to be changed and excreted in the stool and so the stools are clay colored. The urine becomes dark, not pale, from the pigment. Patients with pancreatic cancer usually lose, not gain, weight. Easy bruising is seen more with liver cirrhosis and cancer.
Cognitive level: Application
Nursing process: Assessment
Client needs: Physiological Integrity: Physiological Adaptation

10. Answer: 2. Eat a diet low in fat.
Rationale: A low-fat diet is indicated because the pancreas is unable to produce the pancreatic enzyme lipase, which is needed for the breakdown of fats. A replacement enzyme such as Viokase may be prescribed. It is not necessary to avoid all analgesics; acetaminophen may be used, but aspirin is usually contraindicated since it may produce gastric irritation. Abstinence from alcohol is mandatory to prevent future attacks of pancreatitis. Eating utensils can be shared.
Cognitive level: Application
Nursing process: Planning
Client needs: Physiological Integrity: Reduction of Risk Potential

Chapter 47

1. Answer: 3. Sodium level is 152 mg/dL.
Rationale: The elevated sodium level would best substantiate a diagnosis of acute renal failure. In acute renal failure the kidneys are unable to excrete electrolytes properly, resulting in the elevated sodium level. A BUN level of 16 is WNL. A calcium level of 8.7 mg/dL is slightly low. A potassium level of 4.8 is WNL and it would be expected to be elevated in ARF.
Cognitive level: Analysis
Nursing process: Assessment
Client needs: Physiological Integrity: Physiological Adaptation

2. Answer: 3. Casts in the urine
Rationale: Pyelonephritis is a sudden inflammation of the kidney and renal pelvis caused by bacteria. Expected abnormalities in the urine include a low specific gravity, high leukocyte count, and casts in the urine. Counts of 100,000 bacteria or greater are often found. A finding of protein in the urine is associated with hydronephritis and glomerulonephritis.
Cognitive level: Application
Nursing process: Assessment
Client needs: Physiological Integrity: Physiological Adaptation

3. Answer: 3. Congestive heart failure
Rationale: Congestive heart failure causes a decrease in cardiac output, which leads to poor renal perfusion, or blood flow coming into the kidney. Contrast dyes can cause acute tubular necrosis, an intrarenal or intrinsic cause of renal failure. Crushing injuries cause breakdown of muscle cells, which can also cause acute tubular necrosis within the kidney. Urinary calculi are a cause of postrenal failure.

Cognitive level: Application
Nursing process: Assessment
Client needs: Physiological Integrity: Physiological Adaptation

4. Answer: 4. Restrict fluid and salt intake.
   Rationale: In chronic renal failure (CRF) the kidneys are unable to excrete sodium and water, leading to fluid retention, which contributes to hypertension and increases the workload of the heart. Applying lotion will help to relieve the dry skin and pruritus associated with CRF, but is not specific to the cardiovascular system. A low-fat, low-sodium diet is indicated. Ankles should be evaluated for edema to identify if fluid is being retained, but this is not the best measure to prevent cardiovascular problems.
   Cognitive level: Application
   Nursing process: Implementation
   Client needs: Physiological Integrity: Physiological Adaptation

5. Answer: 3. Self-catheterization
   Rationale: A neobladder is formed by creating an internal urine collection reservoir formed from the small intestine and connected to the urethra. Because the neobladder does not empty fully, self-catheterization should be done twice daily. Kegel exercises are taught as part of bladder training to strengthen the muscles when incontinence is a problem. Crede's method is a done to aid in bladder evacuation by applying manual pressure over the lower abdomen. A stoma wafer change would be necessary if the patient had an ileoconduit done.
   Cognitive level: Application
   Nursing process: Planning
   Client needs: Physiological Integrity: Physiological Adaptation

6. Answer: 3. The leg cramps are because of the extra water and salt that is being removed.
   Rationale: One complication of hemodialysis is the onset of muscle cramps, which result from the rapid removal of water and sodium. The muscle cramps are not associated with blood transfusions, infections, or amount of protein ingested.
   Cognitive level: Analysis
   Nursing process: Implementation
   Client needs: Physiological Integrity: Physiological Adaptation

Chapter 48

1. Answer: 2. The uterine lining becomes thicker because of estrogen.
   Rationale: The menstrual cycle is a complex physiological process that involves the hypothalamus, pituitary gland, ovaries, and endometrium. The cycle begins with the first day of menses. Menses, or vaginal bleeding, occurs when the thickened endometrial lining that was constructed during the previous cycle is sloughed off or shed. As this occurs, the hypothalamus recognizes a need to secrete gonadotropin-releasing hormone. This hormone stimulates the anterior pituitary to release follicle-stimulating

hormone (FSH), which in turn stimulates a few of the follicles that exist on the ovary. From the follicles that first respond to the FSH, one becomes dominant. This growing follicle produces and secretes estrogen. When estrogen peaks, it signals the anterior pituitary to release luteinizing hormone. When LH peaks, ovulation occurs. The dominant follicle extrudes the ovum. The ovum travels to the fallopian tube and into the uterus. Under the influence of estrogen, the uterine lining has been thickening before ovulation. After ovulation, the lining begins to proliferate, that is, it gets thicker.
   Cognitive level: Application
   Nursing process: Implementation
   Client needs: Health Promotion and Maintenance: Growth and Development Through the Life Span

2. Answer: 1. Any other chronic illnesses such as diabetes
   Rationale: Medical comorbidities that may impact the reproductive system would include diabetes, hypertension, hepatitis, and HIV. The male with diabetes or hypertension treated with certain antihypertensive drugs may experience impotence. The childhood disease of concern for men is mumps. This viral illness has the potential to affect the testicles, causing sterility. Sexually transmitted infections do not typically cause impotence. The date of first sexual experience would not contribute to the assessment of the patient's current health concern.
   Cognitive level: Application
   Nursing process: Assessment
   Client needs: Health Promotion and Maintenance: Prevention/Early Detection of Health Problems

3. Answer: 2. Occupations and hobbies
   Rationale: There is evidence from cohort and case-control research that cigarette smoking and secondhand smoke increase the risks for cervical cancer. Occupations or hobbies where patients have been exposed to hazardous materials increase the risks of male and female infertility. Ask the patient if she has worked around hazardous materials such as excessive heat, radiation, heavy metals, or organic solvents and how she protects herself. There is no evidence to suggest that the amount of exercise or rest/sleep has an impact on fertility.
   Cognitive level: Application
   Nursing process: Assessment
   Client needs: Health Promotion and Maintenance: Growth and Development Through the Life Span

4. Answer: 1. Smegma, a normal finding
   Rationale: The examination of the male external genitalia is completed by inspection followed by palpation. If the male is not circumcised, ask the patient to retract the foreskin so that the glans can be inspected. Lesions that may be seen include chancres or ulcers of syphilis, abnormal contour of the scrotum, cancer, warts, herpetic vesicles, or infestation by lice or other insects in the pubic hair. Smegma or a white, cheesy material is a normal finding under the foreskin. Inflammation of the glans is called balanitis. If the patient has reported discharge, but it is not visible, he

should be asked to strip the penis to bring discharge to the meatus for culture.

Cognitive level: Analysis

Nursing process: Assessment

Client needs: Health Promotion and Maintenance: Prevention/Early Detection of Health Problems

5. Answer: 2. Hair loss over the mons and vulva is a normal part of the aging process.

Rationale: Over time, decreased estrogen levels in females will contribute to the loss of muscle mass and bone, and increased fat on the abdomen. The breasts will atrophy as the glandular tissue is replaced by fat. The vulva will lose fat and the mons and vulva will lose hair. There may also be graying of the pubic hair.

Cognitive level: Application

Nursing process: Assessment

Client needs: Health Promotion and Maintenance: Growth and Development Through the Life Span

6. Answer: 2. Routine screening for prostate cancer can lead to unnecessary anxiety.

Rationale: For older men, the United States Preventive Services Task Force has found that there is insufficient evidence to recommend for or against routine screening for prostate cancer with serum levels of prostate specific antigen and digital rectal examination of the prostate. Routine screening has been shown to cause unnecessary anxiety, biopsies, and treatments with severe side effects for a cancer that may never have affected the patient. In addition, there continue to be many false-positive PSAs.

Cognitive level: Analysis

Nursing process: Assessment

Client needs: Psychosocial Integrity; Coping and Adaptation

Chapter 49

1. Answer: 3. Doryx

Rationale: Penicillin G is used to treat syphilis. Flagyl is used to treat trichomoniasis. Cleocin is used to treat bacterial vaginosis. Doryx and Zithromax are both used to treat a chlamydia infection.

Cognitive level: Application

Nursing process: Planning

Client needs: Physiological Integrity: Pharmacologic and Parenteral Therapies

2. Answer: 4. Have children before the age of 30

Rationale: Modifiable risk factors for the development of breast cancer include having no children or having children after the age of 30, both of which will increase the risk. The use of underarm antiperspirants and dietary fat intake are considered uncertain, controversial, or unproven risk factors for the development of the disease.

Cognitive level: Application

Nursing process: Implementation

Client needs: Health Promotion and Maintenance: Prevention/Early Detection of Health Problems

3. Answer: 2. Use a mirror to examine the shape and size of each breast.

Rationale: The nurse should instruct the patient to establish a regular schedule of examining and not just at any time during the month. The patient should use a mirror to examine the shape and size of each breast. The breasts should be examined standing (in front of a mirror and in the shower) and lying down on a flat surface. The nurse should include that many lumps are benign and that early detection increases the survival rate.

Cognitive level: Application

Nursing process: Implementation

Client needs: Health Promotion and Maintenance: Prevention/Early Detection of Health Problems

4. Answer: 2. Decreased estrogen production

Rationale: Fibroid tumors of the uterus, also known as leiomyomas and myomas, occur in more than 30% of women 40 to 60 years of age but are almost always benign. The lesions are growths arising from the tissue of the uterine muscle for unknown reasons. They develop slowly in women ages 25 through 40, and tend to enlarge during pregnancy and after menopause; fibroids often decrease on their own, due to decreased estrogen production. Fibroids often cause no symptoms, so many are undiscovered unless the patient has dysfunctional uterine bleeding, pelvic pain, and infertility or pregnancy loss.

Cognitive level: Analysis

Nursing process: Assessment

Client needs: Physiological Integrity: Reduction of Risk Potential

5. Answer: 2. Methotrexate

Rationale: A pessary is a device that, when inserted into the vagina, will help support the vaginal walls, reducing the bulging into the vagina. It is used for management of pelvic support defects such as cystocele, rectocele, and uterine prolapse. Cystoceles and rectoceles are repaired using a procedure called a colporrhaphy. Medical treatment of ectopic pregnancy is preferred over surgical treatment. Methotrexate, a drug often used in cancer treatment, is the current drug of choice and will act on the ectopic cells as it does in cancer treatment: to destroy the cells. It is given if the ectopic pregnancy is unruptured and the patient is in stable condition. It is given intramuscularly and often as an outpatient procedure. Successful treatment may require more than one dose of methotrexate. If surgery is indicated with a ruptured ectopic pregnancy, it consists of repair of the tube if future pregnancies are desired. Removal of the tube may be necessary if repair is not possible or may be desired if future pregnancies are not planned.

Cognitive level: Analysis

Nursing process: Planning

Client needs: Physiological Integrity: Physiological Adaptation

6. Answer: 1. Type 1 diabetes mellitus

Rationale: Female-related causes of infertility are most commonly related to ovulatory dysfunction. Other

causes may include hormone imbalance, ovarian cysts, or pelvic infections. Age has also been associated with fertility difficulties. The woman reaches peak fertility in her early 20s, and the likelihood of conceiving after age 35 or 40 is less than 10% per month. In addition to age-related factors, couples at risk for infertility include those with multiple sexual partners, those with a sexually transmitted infection, endometriosis, men with a history of orchitis or a history of undescended testicles, a past history of diethylstilbestrol exposure for both men and women, and those with chronic diseases such as diabetes or thyroid disorders.
Cognitive level: Analysis
Nursing process: Assessment
Client needs: Health Promotion and Maintenance: Growth and Development Through the Life Span

7. Answer: 2. Ambulate
Rationale: An exploratory laparoscopy is a minimally invasive procedure that involves a small incision through which a laparoscope is inserted that allows visualization of the internal organs and structures to assess for disease processes. Carbon dioxide is instilled into the abdomen to elevate the abdominal wall and create a larger work area. After the procedure, the incision is sutured to secure the edges for healing. The patient may experience shoulder pain as the carbon dioxide dissipates from the abdomen. Instruct the patient to sit up and walk to promote gas diffusion and reduce pain.
Cognitive level: Application
Nursing process: Implementation
Client needs: Physiological Integrity: Physiological Adaptation

8. Answer: 4. Locate a SANE immediately.
Rationale: Readily available rape advocates, specially trained law enforcement personnel, and sexual assault nurse examiners (SANEs) should be involved with the patient from the very beginning of the patient's presentation. The importance of careful and meticulous evidence collection is the second priority after ensuring the patient's safety and treatment of injuries. The victim of a sexual assault must consent to the collection of evidence in total or in part. No unnecessary personnel should be involved in handling evidence.
Cognitive level: Application
Nursing process: Implementation
Client needs: Psychosocial Integrity; Psychosocial Adaptation

Chapter 50

1. Answer: 3. Sexually transmitted infections
Rationale: Infection of the epididymis in men younger than 35 years is more likely to be the result of gonococcal, chlamydial, or ureaplasma organisms. A sports injury does not contribute to this condition, mumps can lead to orchitis, and in older men, infection is more likely to be the result of prostatitis, instrumentation of the urinary system, or a structural lesion such as carcinoma of the testis.

Cognitive level: Application
Nursing process: Assessment
Client needs: Physiologic Integrity: Reduction of Risk Potential

2. Answer: 2. Testicular
Rationale: Cancer that forms in the tissue of the testis usually occurs in men between the ages of 20 and 39. It is the most common form of cancer in white men between the ages of 15 and 34.
Cognitive level: Analysis
Nursing process: Assessment
Client needs: Health Promotion and Maintenance: Prevention/Early Detection of Health Problems

3. Answer: 4. Quantifying the symptoms of benign prostatic hypertrophy
Rationale: The American Urological Association (AUA) has developed a symptom index tool that can be used to quantify the symptoms of benign prostatic hypertrophy (BPH) for each patient. The AUA Symptom Score is used both in diagnosing and monitoring therapeutic response. It is a seven-question exploration of symptoms that the patient can answer while waiting to be seen. The score allows the doctor to match treatment options with the severity of the symptoms for each patient. It would focus on sexual dysfunction, urinary tract malignancy, or incontinence.
Cognitive level: Application
Nursing process: Assessment
Client needs: Physiologic Integrity: Reduction of Risk Potential

4. Answer: 4. Checking the drainage tubing for kinks on a regular basis
Rationale: Postsurgical care following a TURP will include maintenance of continuous bladder irrigation to decrease clot formation and bleeding. A three-way catheter is placed after surgery and a steady flow of saline is used to flush the bladder; the amount is determined by the color of outflow and presence of clots. The nurse should be sure that the catheter is secured to the patient's thigh, rather than the bed rail, with a Velcro strap to prevent injury to the urethra and bladder neck. The irrigation and drainage tubing should be checked often for kinks that would block flow. Clot formation will cause obstruction and fluid retention. If a clot should occlude the catheter, the system can be opened and direct irrigation with saline can be done, but this should be a sterile procedure and avoided unless absolutely necessary.
Cognitive level: Application
Nursing process: Planning
Client needs: Physiological Integrity: Reduction of Risk Potential

5. Answer: 3. *Disturbed Body Image*
Rationale: With orchiectomy, the surgery is quick and recovery usually goes well. The loss of the testicles, however, may have a profound effect on the patient. The loss of masculinity can mean depression due to disturbed body image and function with an empty scrotal sac.

Therefore, risk for infection is minimal, mobility should not be affected, nor would impaired urinary elimination be expected.

Cognitive level: Analysis

Nursing process: Planning

Client needs: Psychosocial Integrity: Coping and Adaptation

6. Answer: 1. Encourage to receive a DRE and PSA test annually.

Rationale: It has been recommended that men older than age 50 receive DRE and PSA tests every year. Testicular self-exam should be primarily focused for males under the age of 40. A man's lifetime risk for prostate cancer is 1 in 6, making this disease the most common cancer in men in the United States and the second leading cause of death.

Cognitive level: Application

Nursing process: Implementation

Client needs: Health Promotion and Maintenance: Prevention/Early Detection of Health Problems

Chapter 51

1. Answer: 4. Insulin is a hormone and works through the bloodstream.

Rationale: Because glands are ductless, hormones are released directly into the circulation. The hormone then travels through the bloodstream where it will exert its action on target cells or receptors. A feedback system is a regulatory system that keeps certain activities of body function within a prescribed range to sustain homeostasis. Feedback systems can be positive or negative. In negative feedback, alterations in hormone levels stimulate a series of changes to return the level to normal.

Cognitive level: Application

Nursing process: Implementation

Client needs: Physiological Integrity: Pharmacologic and Parenteral Therapies

2. Answer: 3. Autocrine functioning

Rationale: The endocrine system's functioning is intimately connected to that of the nervous system. Together, they provide a mechanism for communication between cells and organs. This connection is referred to as neuroendocrine regulation. Hormones also function in other ways. If hormones affect cells within the vicinity of their release, it is known as paracrine functioning. Hormones are said to have autocrine functioning when the hormones produced act on the cells that created them. In basal hormone release, small amounts of hormones are released continuously.

Cognitive level: Application

Nursing process: Implementation

Client needs: Health Promotion and Maintenance: Growth and Development Through the Life Span

3. Answer: 3. Epinephrine

Rationale: The adrenal glands have two distinct layers with specialized functions. The outer layer is known as the adrenal medulla. The adrenal medulla produces the catecholamines epinephrine and norepinephrine, substances that play an important role in the body's physiological response to stress. The adrenal cortex secretes corticosteroids of which there are two types, mineralocorticoids and glucocorticoids.

Cognitive level: Analysis

Nursing process: Assessment

Client needs: Physiological Integrity: Physiological Adaptation

4. Answer: 4. Does anyone in your family have diabetes?

Rationale: Exploration of the patient's history is essential. Questioning should seek to assess the onset, characteristics, and severity of symptoms. Along with a review of the entire medical history, family, occupational, and social histories are evaluated. Disorders of the endocrine system tend to occur in a familial pattern. There is a high correlation of diabetes, thyroid disorders, and obesity among families. Knowing this information should assist the interviewer in targeting a more focused assessment. Dietary patterns and involuntary weight losses and gains should be explored. Exposure to chemicals, use of drugs and alcohol, smoking, coping with stress, and behavioral patterns are all areas to be explored.

Cognitive level: Application

Nursing process: Assessment

Client needs: Physiological Integrity: Physiological Adaptation

5. Answer: 3. It checks for ovarian function and might indicate if you are approaching menopause.

Rationale: FSH controls the growth and maturation of ovarian follicles in women and the production of sperm in men. An increased level is seen in ovarian failure of menopause. Blood tests used for adrenal functioning include ACTH stimulation, serum adrenocorticotropic hormone level, serum cortisol level, and urinary cortisol level. The hormones produced from the thyroid include thyroxine, triiodothyronine, and calcitonin. Growth hormone, from the anterior pituitary gland is responsible for the metabolism of carbohydrates, fats, and protein.

Cognitive level: Application

Nursing process: Implementation

Client needs: Physiological Integrity: Physiological Adaptation

Chapter 52

1. Answer: 2. Enterogastrone

Rationale: Enterogastrone is a hormone produced in the gastrointestinal tract. This hormone inhibits secretion and motility. Progesterone is a hormone produced by the placenta and is responsible for gestational support. Angiotensinogen is a hormone produced by the liver that supports the constriction of blood vessels and raises blood pressure. Calcitriol is a hormone produced by the kidney that stimulates calcium absorption from the gastrointestinal tract.

Cognitive level: Analysis

Nursing process: Assessment

Client needs: Physiological Integrity: Reduction of Risk Potential

2. Answer: 1. Giantism

Rationale: Growth hormone is produced by the anterior pituitary gland. An excessive amount of this hormone can lead to giantism in children and adolescents. Acromegaly is the outcome of an excessive amount of growth hormone in adults. Sheehan's syndrome and infertility are seen when there is an underproduction of growth hormone.

Cognitive level: Analysis

Nursing process: Assessment

Client needs: Physiological Integrity: Physiological Adaptation

3. Answer: 2. Take the medication first thing in the morning on an empty stomach.

Rationale: To ensure maximum absorption of the hormone, it is advised that levothyroxine be taken in the early morning on an empty stomach. Synthetic thyroid hormone can be taken safely concurrently with some medications, but patients taking medications such as anticoagulants, beta-blockers, cholesterol-lowering drugs, or seizure control drugs should check with the pharmacist for potential drug interactions. Although administration of levothyroxine will bring thyroid hormone levels within normal limits, it may suppress TSH, which increases the risk of osteoporosis, a side effect that can be avoided by the ingestion of calcium carbonate. However, if the two preparations are taken together, the calcium can interfere with absorption of thyroid hormone. Patients should be advised to take any over-the-counter vitamins, minerals, and antacids at least 4 hours earlier or later than thyroid hormone. Patients also need to be advised that they will be taking thyroid replacement hormone for life. Symptoms of hypothyroidism gradually fade over a period of 3 to 6 weeks as therapy is initiated.

Cognitive level: Application

Nursing process: Implementation

Client needs: Physiological Integrity: Pharmacologic and Parenteral Therapies

4. Answer: 2. Hyperthyroidism

Rationale: Neurological effects of hyperthyroidism include insomnia, jitteriness, shaking, nervousness, irritability, hand tremors, muscle weakness, myalgia, and muscle cramps. Neurological effects of hypothyroidism include drowsiness, fatigue, mental lethargy, forgetfulness, depression, muscular weakness, emotional lability, and paranoia. Patients with pheochromocytoma may experience hypertension, headache, tachycardia, and palpitations. Diabetes insipidus (DI) is characterized by polyuria and polydipsia. Patients with DI present with dry mucous membranes, poor skin turgor, and other signs of dehydration.

Cognitive level: Analysis

Nursing process: Assessment

Client needs: Physiological Integrity: Physiological Adaptation

5. Answer: 2. Strategies to have access to fluids at all times

Rationale: Discharge priorities focus on patient instruction regarding the nature of the disease and the importance of hydration and strategies to ensure the availability of fluid at all times. Medic alert jewelry and a medical identification card should always be carried by the patient so that the patient's condition is known and in emergency situations the treatment is efficient. Patients should be made aware of community resources, including organizations that promote education and research on diabetes insipidus.

Cognitive level: Application

Nursing process: Planning

Client needs: Physiological Integrity: Physiological Adaptation

6. Answer: 3. Consider the onset of myxedema coma and contact the physician.

Rationale: Hypothyroidism is seen clinically at an increasing rate in women over age 50. Clinical manifestations, unless severe, may be too subtle to easily recognize, thus making diagnosis and intervention more difficult. In rare cases, myxedema coma, a rare life-threatening complication in which there is overwhelming cardiopulmonary failure, may be seen in elderly patients, usually precipitated by some untoward event such as infection, trauma, surgery, or neurological disorder. Patients present with all the usual, but exacerbated and serious symptoms of hypothyroidism, and they typically have body temperatures below normal as well. Hypothermia, with body temperature lower than 35°C (95°F), is a key sign that myxedema coma may be impending.

Cognitive level: Analysis

Nursing process: Implementation

Client needs: Physiological Integrity: Physiological Adaptation

7. Answer: 1. What part of your life is terrible?

Rationale: Improvement in clinical management of endocrine diseases is another important frontier in research. Although medical and surgical interventions, as well as hormone replacement therapy, have reaped big rewards in patient management and outcomes, some patients report decreased quality of life despite treatment. This suggests that although hormone levels may appear to be normal after therapy is initiated in endocrine disease, other complex physiological and psychological factors are at play in restoring patients to optimal health. Nurses in ambulatory clinics could play a role in investigating quality of life issues for patients with endocrine disease.

Cognitive level: Application

Nursing process: Assessment

Client needs: Psychosocial Integrity; Coping and Adaptation

Chapter 53

1. Answer: 2. Approximately 20% of Americans over age 60 have diabetes.

Rationale: Approximately 20.9% of the U.S. population over the age of 60 has diabetes. Type 1 accounts for 5% to 10% of diabetes, with type 2 being the most common form. Native Americans, Mexican Americans, and Native Alaskans have a higher incidence of diabetes than

Caucasians, and the highest incidence worldwide occurs in India and China.

Cognitive level: Analysis

Nursing process: Assessment

Client needs: Health Promotion and Maintenance

2. Answer: 3. Fasting blood sugar (FBS) level is 130 mg/dL.

Rationale: Pre-diabetes is determined in two ways: an FBS above normal (80 to 110 mg/dL) or abnormal results of an oral glucose tolerance test. Diabetes is no longer classified by age or treatment regimens. A patient on an oral hypoglycemic agent is classified as having type 2 diabetes. Gestational diabetes does not ensure the patient has pre-diabetes, but it does place her at an increased risk to develop type 2 diabetes later in life.

Cognitive level: Analysis

Nursing process: Assessment

Client needs: Physiological Integrity: Physiological Adaptation

3. Answer: 3. A toddler with a monozygotic twin who has type 1 diabetes.

Rationale: Type 1 diabetes is frequently diagnosed before the age of 20 and it has many genetic, viral, and autoimmune risk factors. There is a 25% to 50% incidence of type 1 diabetes in monozygotic twins, but only a 6% incidence among dizygotic twins. There is an epidemiologic association between viral infections, such as mumps and rubella, and the development of type 1 diabetes, but not bacterial infections. The offspring of a mother with type 1 diabetes has a 3% risk of developing diabetes.

Cognitive level: Analysis

Nursing process: Assessment

Client needs: Physiological Integrity: Reduction of Risk Potential

4. Answer: 2. Abdominal obesity and decreased HDL level

Rationale: The primary abnormalities associated with metabolic syndrome include central or abdominal obesity, insulin resistance, glucose intolerance (which is often manifested as elevated blood sugar levels), increased triglycerides, decreased HDL cholesterol, and hypertension.

Cognitive level: Application

Nursing process: Evaluation

Client needs: Physiological Integrity: Physiological Adaptation

5. Answer: 2. "Avoid doing any isometric exercises."

Rationale: Isometric exercises can raise intraocular pressure and worsen the proliferative retinopathy, so they should be avoided. A dilated eye exam should be done yearly. Protein does not need to be restricted with retinopathy, but may be restricted if renal impairment is present. An ideal target for blood sugar is 80 to 110 mg/dL.

Cognitive level: Application

Nursing process: Implementation

Client needs: Physiological Integrity: Reduction of Risk Potential

6. Answer: 4. Instruct patient to eat within 20 minutes of taking the medication.

Rationale: Patients should eat within 20 minutes of taking a meglitinide to prevent hypoglycemia. They cause a rapid release of insulin, which can lead to hypoglycemia. They should be given before a meal. It is not necessary to check for sulfa allergies; patients taking sulfonylureas should be checked for sulfa allergies.

Cognitive level: Application

Nursing process: Implementation

Client needs: Physiological Integrity: Pharmacologic and Parenteral Therapies

7. Answer: 3. "Exercise may lower your blood sugar for several hours after completing the activity."

Rationale: During exercise, glucose is transported into the muscle for energy use. Patients taking oral hypoglycemic agents and insulin are at increased risk for hypoglycemia following exercise and this may last for several hours. If the blood sugar is 100 mg/dL or less before starting exercise, the patient should consume carbohydrates. If hypoglycemia occurs, the patient should eat complex carbohydrates that will provide a longer supply of energy.

Cognitive level: Application

Nursing process: Implementation

Client needs: Physiological Integrity: Reduction of Risk Potential

8. Answer: 1. Abdominal bloating and diarrhea

Rationale: Alpha glucosidase inhibitors delay the absorption of carbohydrates in the small intestine, which helps to prevent the normal sharp rise in postprandial blood sugar. They cause a number of gastrointestinal side effects, such as diarrhea, flatulence, bloating, and softer stools. They do not cause an elevated temperature. Tremors, palpitations, and fatigue are associated with hypoglycemia, which is seen more with sulfonylureas and meglitinides.

Cognitive level: Application

Nursing process: Evaluation

Client needs: Physiological Integrity: Pharmacologic and Parenteral Therapies

9. Answer: 1. Face is flushed and red.

Rationale: Patients experiencing DKA often have Kussmaul respirations to help correct the acidotic state; the increased levels of $PaCO_2$ have a vasodilating effect, which causes a red, flushed face. Inelastic skin turgor, lethargy, and hypotension can be seen with both DKA and HHS.

Cognitive level: Analysis

Nursing process: Assessment

Client needs: Physiological Integrity: Physiological Adaptation

10. Answer: 3. A male patient with chronic renal failure (CRF).

Rationale: Factors that have been associated with an increased risk for lower extremity ulcers and amputation include patients who have had diabetes for more than 10 years, male gender, poor glucose control, and the presence of cardiovascular, retinal, or renal complications. According to these risk factors, the male patient with CRF is more at risk than a female with cardiovascular disease. The elderly female has fairly

well controlled blood sugar and the patient just diagnosed 2 years ago does not meet these criteria.
Cognitive level: Application
Nursing process: Assessment
Client needs: Physiological Integrity: Reduction of Risk Potential

Chapter 54

1. Answer: 3. Flat
   Rationale: The long bones of the body include the femur, tibia, fibula, humerus, radius, ulna, clavicle, metacarpals, metatarsals, and phalanges. The short and irregular bones include those within the vertebral column and the carpal and tarsal bones. The flat bones include the ribs, scapula, sternum, and the ilium.
   Cognitive level: Analysis
   Nursing process: Assessment
   Client needs: Physiological Integrity: Reduction of Risk Potential

2. Answer: 2. Social
   Rationale: A social history provides additional information about the patient's lifestyle that may affect his or her potential disorder or complaint. The nurse should consider a variety of questions including "Do you use an assistive device such as a cane, walker, or brace?" Characteristics, lengths, exacerbation or diminishment of symptoms, and what is wrong or feared by the patient define the chief complaint. Demographic data may be helpful in determining causes of injury. Biographical data should include age, gender, culture, and educational background.
   Cognitive level: Application
   Nursing process: Assessment
   Client needs: Physiological Integrity: Reduction of Risk Potential

3. Answer: 3. Inspection
   Rationale: When inspecting compare corresponding paired joints for symmetry. The nurse should observe for skin color, scars, shape of the site, deformities, muscle atrophy, masses, or swelling. Palpation is used to determine skin temperature, the presence of any nodules, or muscle or joint tenderness and swelling. The assessment technique of percussion is not used for the musculoskeletal status. Range of motion is used to determine the functionality of joints.
   Cognitive level: Application
   Nursing process: Assessment
   Client needs: Health Promotion and Maintenance: Prevention/Early Detection of Health Problems

4. Answer: 2. Shoulder
   Rationale: The nurse should explain that testing the range of motion of the shoulders involves having the patient perform seven movements, one of which is testing for adduction by asking the patient to raise the arms above the head with the palms facing each other. The elbow is not assessed by having the patient raise the arms above the head. The wrist and hands are not assessed by ask-

ing the patient to raise the arms above the head with the palms facing each other.
   Cognitive level: Application
   Nursing process: Assessment
   Client needs: Health Promotion and Maintenance: Prevention/Early Detection of Health Problems

5. Answer: 4. Toes pointing inward
   Rationale: A normal finding when assessing the feet would be the toes pointing straight and in alignment with the feet, though some may point slightly inward or slightly outward. Abnormal findings include a great toe that is deviated medially and abducted to the first metatarsal with an inflamed bursa or bunion on the medial side or a hallux valgus; an abnormally high arch or a cavus foot; or a wart located over the thick skin of the sole of the foot or a verruca vulgaris.
   Cognitive level: Analysis
   Nursing process: Assessment
   Client needs: Health Promotion and Maintenance: Prevention/Early Detection of Health Problems

6. Answer: 3. External rotation 45 degrees
   Rationale: A normal finding is that the patient is able to externally rotate the hip to 45 degrees. Additional normal findings on assessment of the range of motion of the hip include ability to raise the legs to at least 90 degrees of flexion with the knee straight and 120 degrees of flexion with the knee flexed; adduct leg to 20 to 30 degrees and abduct 45 to 50 degrees; internally rotate to 40 degrees and externally rotate to 45 degrees; hyperextend the leg at least 15 degrees; move the extremities against resistance.
   Cognitive level: Analysis
   Nursing process: Assessment
   Client needs: Health Promotion and Maintenance: Prevention/Early Detection of Health Problems

Chapter 55

1. Answer: 3. Stress and strain
   Rationale: Two concepts are important to remember: stress and strain. First, stress results when mechanical force is applied to a stretched or compressed bone. Compressive stressors are those of the body weight pushing the bone down, and tensile stresses are from the muscles pulling the bones away from each other. Strain, the second concept, is expressed in length/original length and results as a force that is applied, causing an amount of deformation in the bone relative to its original length.
   Cognitive level: Analysis
   Nursing process: Assessment
   Client needs: Health Promotion and Maintenance

2. Answer: 2. Diet low in calcium and vitamin D
   Rationale: A diet low in calcium and vitamin D is a risk factor for both men and women. Low body weight and low body mass index, along with a history of maternal hip fracture, are risk factors affecting men. Anorexia applies to females only.
   Cognitive level: Application
   Nursing process: Assessment
   Client needs: Health Promotion and Maintenance

3. Answer: 1. "Living at my own home increases my chance of a fracture."

Rationale: In addition to gender (being a female), another factor that increases the risk of hip fracture is living in institutional care, rather than one's own home. Other factors include significant cognitive impairment, certain medications (e.g., anticonvulsants, corticosteroids), personal history and lifestyle factors, certain medical conditions (e.g., type 2 diabetes in women) and low bone mineral density.

Cognitive level: Application

Nursing process: Assessment

Client needs: Safe, Effective Care Environment

4. Answer: 3. Muscle membranes have a protein deficiency or absence of dystrophin.

Rationale: Muscular dystrophies are a group of genetic myopathies caused by a protein deficiency in muscle membranes. In other words, a person's DNA is not producing a particular protein named dystrophin that is required by muscles and muscle membranes to function properly. Cardiomyopathy leads to heart failure, which is a major cause of death in patients with muscular dystrophy or respiratory failure. The course of Duchenne muscular dystrophy is progressive and usually fatal in the teens or early 20s. The child/adolescent generally has a normal IQ for age with Becker's dystrophy.

Cognitive level: Analysis

Nursing process: Evaluation

Client needs: Health Promotion and Maintenance

5. Answer: 1. Hypokalemic

Rationale: Hypokalemic myopathy is common in the elderly and is due to a low serum potassium level caused by long-term diuretic use. Other causes of hypokalemic myopathy include potassium deficiency in the diet, excessive alcohol consumption, aldosteronism, intestinal wasting of potassium (malabsorption), and licorice intoxication.

Cognitive level: Analysis

Nursing process: Evaluation

Client needs: Health Promotion and Maintenance

6. Answer: 4. Subjective symptoms

Rationale: The diagnosis of fibromyalgia is based on the patient's subjective symptoms, as well as a medical and surgical history. Patients with fibromyalgia do not have any other associated musculoskeletal disorder; therefore, arthritis, inflammations, and bursitis should be ruled out. Depression is not uncommon. Family tendency is not used as a diagnostic tool.

Cognitive level: Application

Nursing process: Assessment

Client needs: Health Promotion and Maintenance

Chapter 56

1. Answer: 2. Prevention of injuries

Rationale: Prevention is the only method to decrease the effects of injuries to the muscles, tendons, ligaments, and bones. Half of all sports-related injuries are preventable. Education and awareness surrounding protective equipment, safer playing environments, and rules designed to prevent injury are important in reducing the frequency and severity of sports injuries. Stretching, warm-up exercises, and strengthening and balance training regimens are key in preventing sports injuries.

Cognitive level: Application

Nursing process: Planning

Client needs: Health Promotion and Maintenance: Prevention/Early Detection of Health Problems

2. Answer: 4. Ossification

Rationale: A fracture or break in the bone causes a healing cascade beginning with the blood that leaks out at the fracture site. This hematoma is rich in osteoblasts, which make bone. Clotting factors that remain due to the hematoma initiate the formation of a fibrin meshwork that serves as a framework for the fibroblasts and new capillary buds. During cellular proliferation and callus formation, the osteoblasts, or bone-forming cells, multiply and differentiate into the fibrocartilaginous callus. This process begins distal to the fracture where there is greater blood supply. Within a few days a cartilage "collar" is evident around the fracture site. Initially the callus is soft but within the third to fourth week of fracture healing, the bone calcifies as mineral salts are deposited. Ossification is the final lying down of bone after the fracture has been bridged and the fragments are united. Mature bone replaces the callus, and the fracture site feels firm and appears united on radiograph. It is at this point that a cast may be removed.

Cognitive level: Analysis

Nursing process: Assessment

Client needs: Physiological Integrity: Physiological Adaptation

3. Answer: 3. Decrease the potential for contamination.

Rationale: The important concept is that all open fractures have the potential to be contaminated and this increases the morbidity and mortality of the injury. The time frames vary by institution but many consider 6 to 8 hours to be the maximum time that a contaminated fracture can wait to be taken to the operating room and be "washed out," often referred to as an I&D (i.e., inspection and debridement). Pain relief, assessing, treating injury to surrounding tissue, and casting of the fracture would follow this goal.

Cognitive level: Analysis

Nursing process: Planning

Client needs: Physiological Integrity: Physiological Adaptation

4. Answer: 1. Monitoring hemodynamic status

Rationale: The nurse should monitor the patient for signs that would indicate the onset of hypovolemic shock and the need for resuscitative measures. An orthopedic trauma patient who has experienced fractures of the pelvis or long bones is at risk for significant bleeding. The nurse should monitor the patient's hemodynamic status including vital signs and laboratory values. A patient may lose as much as 20% of his or her blood volume before exhibiting signs and symptoms of shock. The nurse should monitor the vital signs for an increase in heart rate, decrease in blood pressure, increase in respiratory rate, and a decrease in urine output. Laboratory results will show a decrease in the hemoglobin and hematocrit. Arranging for traction can be delegated, and explaining care is important, however, this is a psychosocial need that should follow hemodynamic stability. Most patients will require intravenous narcotics, such as a patient-controlled analgesic pump.

Cognitive level: Application

Nursing process: Planning

Client needs: Physiological Integrity: Physiological Adaptation

5. Answer: 2. Dark-colored urine

Rationale: Complications associated with rhabdomyolysis include acute renal failure. This occurs due to renal tubular obstruction from the filtration of the released myoglobin. The patient may also exhibit respiratory distress due to muscle weakness and fluid and electrolyte imbalances. Signs and symptoms of rhabdomyolysis may include pain, tenderness, swelling, bruising, and weakness within the affected muscles. Upon assessment the muscles involved may feel soft and flabby. The patient's urine will also become dark in color, referred to as myoglobinuria, as the renal system attempts to filter the myoglobin. They may also develop systemic symptoms including general malaise, fever, nausea and vomiting, confusion, agitation, and anuria as the acute renal failure progresses.

Cognitive level: Analysis

Nursing process: Assessment

Client needs: Physiological Integrity: Physiological Adaptation

6. Answer: 2. You are experiencing something called phantom sensations.

Rationale: There are as many physical/mobility issues to deal with as there are emotional for the patient with an amputation. The patient may have trouble just looking at it, or may have bizarre sensations such as feeling that the foot is cold or itchy when it is not even there. These are called phantom limb sensations and are not caused by narcotic use. The other responses do not acknowledge the patient's concerns or provide a reason.

Cognitive level: Application

Nursing process: Implementation

Client needs: Psychosocial Integrity; Coping and Adaptation

Chapter 57

1. Answers:
   1. Pain level
   2. Pulse quality
   3. Sensation and movement
   4. Color of extremity
   5. Use of muscles

Rationale: The neurovascular assessment should be performed bilaterally so that the affected extremity can be compared to the unaffected extremity. The neurovascular assessment includes assessment of the five "Ps": pain, pulse, paresthesia, paralysis, and pallor. A complete assessment of circulation and motor and sensory function must be performed. Neurovascular compromise or deterioration should be reported to the surgeon immediately. The nurse should anticipate performing the neurovascular assessment in conjunction with vital signs. Level of consciousness is part of a neurological assessment.

Cognitive level: Application

Nursing process: Assessment

Client needs: Health Promotion and Maintenance

2. Answer: 4. Use an elevated toilet seat in the main bathroom at home.

Rationale: Discharge teaching should include precautions to avoid adduction, flexion, or any movement that may dislocate the hip prosthesis. Precautions include use of an elevated toilet seat, use of a hip abductor pillow while in bed, not bending the hip greater than 90 degrees, not sitting in low chairs, not twisting or turning the body toward the operative side, not turning the leg or foot inward, and keeping the operative leg straight when getting up using arms to push.

Cognitive level: Application

Nursing process: Planning

Client needs: Physiological Integrity: Reduction of Risk Potential

3. Answer: 1. Ace bandages to wrap around the bivalved cast

Rationale: Treatment of compartment syndrome requires release of the constriction to accommodate swelling. If a cast is causing the restriction, it should be bivalved (cut down both sides) with ace wraps or wide tape placed around it to hold it in place. If the constriction is at the fascia level, the patient will require surgery. If the nurse suspects compartment syndrome is present, the surgeon should be notified immediately to prevent permanent disability or loss of limb. If compartment syndrome in an extremity is suspected, the extremity should not be elevated, but should be maintained at the level of the heart to improve perfusion. As edema and engorgement increase, pain increases and is unrelieved by narcotic pain medication administration.

Cognitive level: Application

Nursing process: Implementation

Client needs: Physiological Integrity: Reduction of Risk Potential

4. Answer: 2. A "reacher" tool

Rationale: It is important for the patient not to bend over or flex the affected extremity. A "reacher" tool can be very helpful for picking up an item off the floor, or overhead to avoid standing on a step stool, which requires flexion. A heel lift boot is used to offset development of pressure ulcers for an immobilized patient and the CPM would be indicated following a total knee replacement. Generally, after hip replacement, the patient would use a walker or cane to assist ambulation and avoid flexion by prolonged sitting rather than a wheelchair.

Cognitive level: Application

Nursing process: Assessment

Client needs: Physiological Integrity: Reduction of Risk Potential

5. Answer: 2. "Every hour 2 mg of morphine is delivered continuously."

Rationale: Patient-controlled analgesia (PCA) or around-the-clock pain medication is often utilized in the early postoperative period. The PCA can be set to deliver a constant or basal rate; in addition, the patient is able to self-administer a preset dose at prescribed intervals to achieve pain control. In this scenario, the patient would receive 2 mg of morphine every hour regardless of intermittent use of the pump.

Cognitive level: Analysis

Nursing process: Evaluation

Client needs: Physiological Integrity: Basic Care and Comfort

Chapter 58

1. Answer: 3. It's a common connective tissue disorder.

Rationale: Common connective tissue disorders include lupus erythematosus, gout, and Lyme disease. A term used to describe rheumatic disease is arthritis. A chronic inflammatory process that affects joints is rheumatoid arthritis. An inflammation associated with psoriasis is psoriatic arthritis.

Cognitive level: Application

Nursing process: Implementation

Client needs: Physiological Integrity: Physiological Adaptation

2. Answer: 4. Prevent deformities

Rationale: During the planning stage, goals for a patient with rheumatoid arthritis include prevention of contractures and deformities and provision of health teaching.

Cognitive level: Application

Nursing process: Planning

Client needs: Physiological Integrity: Physiological Adaptation

3. Answer: 1. Reactive arthritis

Rationale: Reactive arthritis is caused by a reaction to an infection somewhere else in the body. Reactive arthritis most commonly causes secondary conditions such as arthritis, uveitis, and urethritis. Other symptoms that may occur are dactylitis, inflammation of the neck and low back, and painless skin lesions termed circinate balanitis.

Cognitive level: Analysis

Nursing process: Assessment

Client needs: Physiological Integrity: Physiological Adaptation

4. Answer: 3. *Imbalanced Nutrition: More than Body Requirements*

Rationale: For the patient with osteoarthritis, priority nursing diagnoses include *Chronic Pain, Impaired Physical Mobility, Risk for Falls, Disturbed Body Image, Readiness for Enhanced Self-Care, Imbalanced Nutrition: More than Body Requirements,* and *Powerlessness.*

Cognitive level: Application

Nursing process: Planning

Client needs: Physiological Integrity: Physiological Adaptation

5. Answer: 2. Gravies

Rationale: Because gouty arthritis is caused by indulging in foods high in purines, it can be controlled by eating a well-balanced, low-calorie, low-purine diet and by reducing alcohol consumption. Foods to be avoided are alcohol, organ meats, and rich foods such as gravies, dried legumes, and anchovies. These foods will increase uric acid in the blood and can lead to uric acid crystal buildup, most often resulting in uric acid crystals located in the joint of the great toe.

Cognitive level: Application

Nursing process: Implementation

Client needs: Physiological Integrity: Physiological Adaptation

6. Answer: 3. Dermatomyositis

Rationale: Myositis may be triggered by an injury, infection, or an autoimmune disease. Polymyositis consists of muscle weakness. Dermatomyositis has the same symptoms as polymyositis except for a distinctive rash over the face, shoulders, arms, and bony prominences. This purplish blue rash can also appear on the eyelids, bridge of the nose, neck, elbows, knees, knuckles, and upper chest.

Cognitive level: Analysis

Nursing process: Assessment

Client needs: Physiological Integrity: Physiological Adaptation

Chapter 59

1. Answer: 3. Bone marrow

Rationale: Deficiencies in functional bone marrow and stem cells can lead to immune deficiency disorders. Lymph nodes and lymph tissue filter debris from the breakdown of cells, bacteria, virus, and fungal antigens. Adenoids are consolidated lymph tissue located in the throat. They function to remove and filter debris, bacteria, and viruses from the upper airways and mouth. The spleen plays a significant role in immune function as part of the lymphatic system. It is comprised of white and red pulp and is involved in hematologic filtration, sequestering of red and white cells, and immune response.

Cognitive level: Analysis

Nursing process: Assessment

Client needs: Physiological Integrity: Physiological Adaptation

2. Answer: 1. The body reacting to self receptors as an antigen

Rationale: Immune tolerance is defined as the ability of the immune system to tolerate all self antigens while retaining the ability to mount an immune response to non-self antigens. Immune tolerance begins during embryonic development of the immune system. Lymphocytes that react with self antigens are selectively eliminated as the immune system develops. This leaves the newborn with B-cell and T-cell lines that do not attack self antigens. Self antigens include HLAs and MHC, as well as several other antigenic particles that are often cell receptors. When the body reacts to self receptors or other cell parts as an antigen, autoimmune disease may result.

Cognitive level: Analysis

Nursing process: Assessment

Client needs: Physiological Integrity: Physiological Adaptation

3. **Answer: 1. Produce antibodies in response to exposure to an antigen**

Rationale: Plasma cells are differentiated B cells that are found in the plasma and are responsible for production of specific antibodies. Plasma cells produce the antibodies in response to a primary or initial exposure to an antigen. The most common groups of antibodies, also known as immunoglobulins, include immunoglobulin G (IgG), immunoglobulin A (IgA), immunoglobulin M (IgM), immunoglobulin D (IgD), and immunoglobulin E (IgE). Suppressor T cells, also called CD8 cells, slow or stop the immune response. This downregulation is the primary role of suppressor T cells, and is an important part of regulation of the immune system because the ability to stop the production of antibodies and cell destruction is important once the threat of infection has been overcome. Natural killer cells, also referred to as "null cells," are types of T cells that lack CD4 or CD8 external receptors, but are able to directly kill cells or send cytokine messages to start the process of programmed cell death. T-helper 1 cells help regulate immune activity and produce chemicals called cytokines that stimulate cytotoxic cells to destroy mutant and cancer cells.

Cognitive level: Analysis

Nursing process: Assessment

Client needs: Physiological Integrity: Physiological Adaptation

4. **Answer: 3. Complement**

Rationale: Complement is a group of small proteins made in the liver and present in blood that can interact with cells and each other for a variety of functions. Complement proteins are important in the inflammatory and immune responses. Tumor necrosis factor is a small peptide that is produced by a variety of cells, including granulocytes and lymphocytes. Interferons are proteins made and released by T cells when the invading organism is a virus. Interleukins are lymphokines, chemical mediators released by lymphocytes, that enable the cells of the immune system to communicate and coordinate the immune response.

Cognitive level: Analysis

Nursing process: Assessment

Client needs: Physiological Integrity: Physiological Adaptation

5. **Answer: 2. The vaccine is made from killed flu organisms.**

Rationale: Acquired immunity involves lymphocyte cells and chemicals that can confer long-term permanent

protection against the disease for which the antibodies have been produced. Immunization is a term often used interchangeably with vaccination or inoculation and involves the process of stimulating the immune system to create active immunity for protection against a disease. A vaccine, a preparation that contains an infectious agent or its components, is administered to stimulate the production of antibodies that can prevent infection or create resistance to infection from that agent. Antigens used in vaccines to stimulate an immune response may be inactivated (whole-killed microorganisms or purified products derived from them), live-attenuated (live virus weakened through chemical or physical processes), or recombinant (artificially manufactured from segments of DNA from different sources). Vaccines against influenza, diphtheria, and tetanus use inactivated antigens. Attenuated vaccines include vaccines for measles, mumps, rubella, polio, yellow fever, and varicella. Vaccines are most commonly administered by needle injections, but also can be given by mouth and by aerosol.

Cognitive level: Application

Nursing process: Implementation

Client needs: Health Promotion and Maintenance: Prevention/Early Detection of Health Problems

6. **Answer: 2. Antigen presentation**

Rationale: B cells must be activated or told to make specific antibodies; this is accomplished through the mechanism of antigen presentation. When a foreign antigen enters a host, the macrophages found in tissue, or monocytes found in blood, ingest the bacterium or virus and then digest the antigen. The macrophage expresses a portion of the digested antigen on its cell surface in the form of a small protein receptor with a part of the bacterial wall attached. T cells are often found near macrophages and can chemically bind to the receptor and accept the antigen onto their surface. T cells then present the antigen to the B cells that have a receptor to match the shape of the antigen. Linking of the T cell and B cell at the site of the antigen activates the B cell to make the appropriately shaped antibody to attach to the antigens.

Cognitive level: Analysis

Nursing process: Assessment

Client needs: Physiological Integrity: Physiological Adaptation

7. **Answer: 2. Decreased primary and secondary production of antibodies**

Rationale: The effects of aging on the immune system include decreased percentage of suppressor T cells, which means the body cannot downregulate the immune system as quickly; decreased primary and secondary production of antibodies, which means the body has a reduced response to infectious organisms leading to more severe infection; increased auto-antibody production, which means the body shows evidence of more exacerbations of autoimmune disease; and a delayed hypersensitivity response, which means the body has a decreased allergic response.

Cognitive level: Application
Nursing process: Assessment
Client needs: Physiological Integrity: Physiological Adaptation

8. Answer: 4. The patient is at risk for malnutrition.

Rationale: Fatigue and weight loss may be associated with chronic disease processes. Inadequate nutrition affects the ability of the immune cells to function normally and causes immunosuppression. Rapid and significant weight loss that is unintentional is a serious concern because it is a symptom of malignancy. An unintentional weight loss of 10 pounds or more in a month is also an indicator of a need for a nutritional consult. Lymphedema, or nonpitting edema at the site of lymph nodes, indicates inadequate drainage from lymphatic vessels and excessive accumulation of fluid in the interstitial spaces around the lymph vessels. Percussion is helpful in determining if there is inappropriate fluid or a mass in an organ, indicating disease. Symptoms of infection include redness, inflammation, streaking lines, edema, or drainage. Signs of rash or petechiae indicate an allergic response or infection.

Cognitive level: Analysis
Nursing process: Assessment
Client needs: Physiological Integrity; Basic Care and Comfort

9. Answer: 1. Erythrocyte sedimentation rate

Rationale: The erythrocyte sedimentation rate is a serum test that is used to diagnose acute and chronic inflammation, as well as rheumatoid and autoimmune diseases. In the presence of inflammatory mediators, blood proteins are altered and red blood cells stick together and then fall out of solution when the blood sample is spun. This results in an elevated sedimentation rate. This test is ordered when an autoimmune disease is suspected such as rheumatoid arthritis. A protein called rheumatoid factor is often present in the serum of patient's with rheumatoid disease in greater quantities than individuals without autoimmune diseases. Antinuclear antibodies are immunoglobulins (IgG, IgM, IgA) that react with the nuclear portion of leukocytes, forming auto-antibodies against the host's DNA and ribonucleic acid. The presence of these antibodies is indicative of systemic lupus erythematosus. The enzyme-linked immunosorbent assay and the Western blot tests detect the presence of antibodies created in response to infection with the HIV antigen.

Cognitive level: Analysis
Nursing process: Assessment
Client needs: Physiological Integrity: Reduction of Risk Potential

Chapter 60

1. Answer: 2. Hypersensitive reactions are determined by the type of antigen, the time sequence of the reaction, and the immunological response.

Rationale: When the immune system loses self-tolerance, immune hypersensitivity reactions result. The primary mechanism of an immune deficiency is a genetic disorder that occurred during the embryonic development of the immune system. Immune deficiency is associated with opportunistic infections.

Cognitive level: Analysis
Nursing process: Assessment
Client needs: Physiological Integrity: Physiological Adaptation

2. Answer: 3. The trigger for an autoimmune response is a self-antigen.

Rationale: The primary trigger for a hypersensitive reaction is an environmental antigen. An alloimmune reaction is triggered by antigens from another individual. The symptoms of different categories of hypersensitive responses vary according to the origin of the antigen.

Cognitive level: Analysis
Nursing process: Assessment
Client needs: Physiological Integrity: Physiological Adaptation

3. Answers:
   1. AIDS is a syndrome of opportunistic infections that occurs as a final stage in patients infected with HIV.
   2. HIV transmission is limited to contact with infected body fluids that have lymphocytes that can harbor HIV.

Rationale: A syndrome of opportunistic infections, AIDS occurs as a final stage in patients infected with HIV. Transmission of HIV is limited to contact with infected body fluids that have lymphocytes that can harbor HIV. AIDS is the end disease manifestation of HIV. HIV precedes AIDS and is associated with the virus's entry into the host's lymphocytes.

Cognitive level: Analysis
Nursing process: Assessment
Client needs: Physiological Integrity, Physiological Adaptation

4. Answers:
   1. Subjective assessment to promote the early detection of infection from any body region.
   2. Health care providers and family members wash hands before and after patient contact to reduce the risk of opportunistic infection cross-contamination.
   3. Encourage hydration and maintenance of weight to support the immune system.

Rationale: Cultures should be obtained prior to starting antibiotics to ensure the appropriate therapy is initiated in a timely manner.

Cognitive level: Application
Nursing process: Assessment
Client needs: Physiological Integrity: Physiological Adaptation

Chapter 61

1. Answer: 2. Anaphylactic

Rationale: Anaphylactic shock is most likely caused by insect bites, medication allergies, food allergies, latex allergies, and idiopathic reactions. Cardiogenic shock is most often caused by myocardial infarction/contusion, ruptured ventricles or papillary muscles, and cardiomyopathy. Neurogenic shock is most often caused by spinal cord or medulla trauma, anesthetic agents, severe emotional stress, or severe pain. Septic shock is most often caused by bacterial or viral infections, immunosuppression, technological causes, or antibiotic misuse.

Cognitive level: Analysis
Nursing process: Assessment
Client needs: Physiological Integrity: Physiological Adaptation

2. Answer: 1. The stress response
   Rationale: Glucose metabolism is impaired in a manner similar to that of oxygen metabolism. The result of this impaired metabolism is insulin resistance. This phenomenon has been observed in patients with sepsis and those who are critically ill or injured. The stress response that is initiated by an illness or injury triggers gluconeogenesis to supply glucose energy to heal. The liver and kidneys produce more glucose in response to epinephrine, norepinephrine, glucagons, and cortisol, which are part of the body's stress response. Insulin resistance is unresponsiveness of anabolic processes to the normal effects of insulin and possibly tissue insensitivity to insulin.

Cognitive level: Analysis
Nursing process: Assessment
Client needs: Physiological Integrity: Physiological Adaptation

3. Answer: 2. Low circulating blood volume or hypoglycemia
   Rationale: The brain is dependent on both oxygen and glucose. When either of these is not sufficient, an alteration in cerebral perfusion occurs. The patient will suffer an altered mental status, which will eventually lead to coma and even death.

Cognitive level: Analysis
Nursing process: Assessment
Client needs: Physiological Integrity: Physiological Adaptation

4. Answer: 2. 86-year-old female with abdominal injuries
   Rationale: Patient risk factors such as significant injuries, catastrophic illness, age, and allergies must be quickly acknowledged. It is interesting that both the very young and aged share similar risk factors for developing shock including compromised immune systems due to age, fluid shifts, and an integumentary system that may not afford needed protection.

Cognitive level: Analysis
Nursing process: Assessment
Client needs: Physiological Integrity: Physiological Adaptation

5. Answer: 1. Normal saline
   Rationale: Fluids that are used for resuscitation include lactated Ringer's solution or normal saline. The type of fluid used will depend on the provider's preference, because at present the research has not clearly defined one more favorably over the other. The initial amount of fluid will range from 2 to 3 liters for an adult if the cause

of the shock is unknown. If the patient has sustained blood loss, then administration of blood and blood products will be needed; however, patients who have sustained blood loss greater than 2 liters should not receive excessive fluid resuscitation from either colloids or crystalloids until surgical management of bleeding has been initiated because it dilutes the existing volume and further diminishes oxygen-carrying capacity.

Cognitive level: Application
Nursing process: Implementation
Client needs: Physiological Integrity: Physiological Adaptation

6. Answer: 2. Nitroprusside sodium
   Rationale: Dopamine and dobutamine hydrochloride improve cardiac contractility. Nitroprusside sodium and nitrates decrease afterload. Epinephrine and norepinephrine bitartrate increase afterload.

Cognitive level: Application
Nursing process: Planning
Client needs: Physiological Integrity: Physiological Adaptation

7. Answer: 1. Systemic inflammatory response syndrome
   Rationale: Systemic inflammatory response syndrome (SIRS) is an organized immune response that can be triggered by infectious or noninfectious clinical insults including burns, pancreatitis, acute respiratory distress syndrome, surgery, and trauma. Sepsis is a clinical syndrome defined as the presence of SIRS associated with a confirmed infectious process. Septic shock is a state of acute circulatory failure characterized by persistent hypotension unexplained by other causes, for example, despite the fact that adequate fluids have been administered. Severe sepsis is defined as sepsis or the presence of a confirmed infection and a systemic inflammatory response, and single or multiple organ failure. The patient is hypotensive, which causes hypoperfusion abnormalities such as arterial hypoxemia, acute oliguria, and coagulation abnormalities.

Cognitive level: Analysis
Nursing process: Assessment
Client needs: Physiological Integrity: Physiological Adaptation

8. Answer: 4. Central venous pressure 10 mmHg
   Rationale: Fluid resuscitation should be directed to achieve a central venous pressure reading of 8 to 12 mmHg, a mean arterial pressure of greater than or equal to 65 mmHg, a urine output of greater than or equal to 0.5 mL/kg, and a central venous or mixed venous oxygen saturation of greater than or equal to 70%.

Cognitive level: Analysis
Nursing process: Evaluation
Client needs: Physiological Integrity: Physiological Adaptation

9. Answer: 1. MODS
   Rationale: Reperfusion injury, which results from the reestablishment of blood flow after ischemia, causes conversion of the enzyme xanthine dehydrogenase to xanthine oxidase to form oxygen free radicals with oxygen when hypoperfused tissues are reperfused. These

oxygen radicals attack already damaged tissues and can lead to MODS.

Cognitive level: Analysis

Nursing process: Assessment

Client needs: Physiological Integrity: Physiological Adaptation

10. Answer: 4. Frequent assessment of vital signs and clinical status

Rationale: Frequent monitoring and assessment to trend changes in vital signs and clinical manifestations will provide the most reliable information about early signs of MODS. Nursing care needs to be focused on decreasing oxygen demand, which includes pain and anxiety management as well as spacing activity to allow for long periods of rest. The nurse should assess for signs of pain and anxiety and medicate as needed. Tachycardia related to pain and anxiety increases oxygen consumption due to the stress imposed on the body by pain. Positioning of the patient is important to prevent the complications that occur with immobility such as skin breakdown, pulmonary congestion, and pooling of blood and secretions. Hypermetabolism causes loss of muscle, so it is important to prevent additional loss of movement. Patients should receive active and passive ROM exercises to retain strength and joint motion.

Cognitive level: Application

Nursing process: Planning

Client needs: Physiological Integrity: Physiological Adaptation

Chapter 62

1. Answer: 1. The stem cell is a primitive cell located in the bone marrow that is the precursor of red blood cells, white blood cells, and platelets.

Rationale: Stem cells are primitive cells located in the bone marrow that are the precursor to all blood lines. When stimulated these cells undergo a series of cell divisions and differentiations to become the appropriate respective cell in a process known as hematopoiesis. However, when the bone marrow has been destroyed, as with certain diseases or medications, the liver and spleen can produce blood cells in a process known as extramedullary hematopoiesis. Although the blood is considered to be a type of connective tissue, it has two important functions. The first is to transport oxygen, nutrition, secretory products, and waste products, but the second is to house and transport the immunologic products that are critical to the body's defense against infections. The proportion of red bone marrow diminishes and is replaced by yellow bone marrow as the patient ages. However, in the healthy individual the active red bone marrow can replace the fatty yellow bone marrow if an increase in blood cell production is required.

Cognitive level: Analysis

Nursing process: Assessment

Client needs: Health Promotion and Maintenance; Physiological Integrity

2. Answer: 3. "The cells of the reticuloendothelial system facilitate blood clotting and initiate the inflammatory and immune responses."

Rationale: White blood cells are only found in small amounts in the blood unless they are needed. Instead, they can be found in the bone marrow, lungs, liver, spleen, and lymph nodes as developing and mature cells. Reticulocytes are small, immature red blood cells that are released whenever there is an increased demand for red cells. The red blood cells, or erythrocytes, are responsible for transporting, maintaining the chemical integrity of, and distributing oxygen-carrying hemoglobin to the body's tissues. One function of the reticuloendothelial system is to provide phagocytic cells for the inflammatory and immune responses, but these cells do not facilitate blood clotting.

Cognitive level: Application

Nursing process: Evaluation

Client needs: Physiological Integrity; Physiological Adaptation

3. Answer: 4. MCH, MCV, MCHC

Rationale: The PT (prothrombin time) and aPTT (activated partial thromboplastin time) are useful coagulation studies, and the PLT determines the numbers of platelets. The HGB (hemoglobin) and HCT (hematocrit) can be reduced with anemia, but this does not help classify the type of anemia. The ANC (absolute neutrophil count) is helpful when measuring the proportion of white blood cells that are available for an initial immune response. Red blood cell (RBC) count alone is not a reliable indicator of RBC function or adequacy. The RDW (red blood cell distribution width) measures the consistency of RBC size, and the white blood cell (WBC) count determines the number of leukocytes. The MCH (mean corpuscular hemoglobin), MCV (mean corpuscular volume), and MCHC (mean corpuscular hemoglobin concentration) are used primarily for the classification of anemia and delineating the likely cause.

Cognitive level: Application

Nursing process: Planning

Client needs: Physiological Integrity

4. Answer: 1. HCT 28%

Rationale: A HCT level of 28% is dangerously low for any patient and should immediately be reported to the health care provider. The other values, PLT 400,000/μL, WBC 10,000/μL, and MCH 30 pg/dL, are all within normal limits for either a male or female patient.

Cognitive level: Application

Nursing process: Analysis

Client needs: Health Promotion and Maintenance; Physiological Integrity

5. Answer: 2. An increase in the total white blood cell count because of the proliferation of juvenile band and immature blast cells

Rationale: A shift to the left indicates that the total white blood cell count has increased because of the proliferation of juvenile band and immature blast cells. This phenomenon is the result of bone marrow stimulation to release large amounts of leukocytes, usually in response to severe infection. The absolute neutrophil count (ANC) measures the proportion of white blood cells that are available for use in a first response immune reaction. The mean corpuscular hemoglobin (MCH) and mean corpuscular hemoglobin concentration (MCHC) measure the hemoglobin proportion in an erythrocyte, indicating the efficacy of interaction between the hemoglobin molecule and the red cell. Numerous clotting studies are used to indicate problems within the clotting cascade, and these are not related to a shift to the left.

Cognitive level: Analysis
Nursing process: Assessment
Client needs: Physiological Integrity

6. Answer: 2. Vascular contraction, intrinsic adenosine diphosphate release, prothrombin conversion into thrombin, fibrinogen conversion into fibrin

Rationale: The first step in primary hemostasis is vascular contraction, followed by platelet adhesion and formation of a soft aggregate plug, respectively. The initial platelets that respond to the site of insult release intrinsic adenosine diphosphate, which causes more platelets to aggregate together. Once the short-lived primary hemostasis has occurred, secondary hemostasis begins through either the intrinsic or extrinsic pathway. During these mechanisms Factor XII activates Factor XI; active Factor VII and active Factor XI start a cascade of events that eventually activate Factor X; and active Factor X, along with Factor III, Factor V, Ca^{2+}, and platelet thromboplastic factor, activates prothrombin activator. Also, prothrombin activator converts prothrombin into thrombin, and thrombin converts fibrinogen into fibrin.

Cognitive level: Analysis
Nursing process: Assessment
Client needs: Physiological Integrity

7. Answer: 3. "What medications are you currently taking?"

Rationale: Medications that are myelosuppressive in nature or those that affect bleeding times, such as aspirin, can suppress or alter blood cell production or function, respectively. The patient's allergies to shellfish or IV contrast material are irrelevant to hematologic function. Cholecystectomy, assuming minimal blood loss or complications, is also unrelated to hematologic function. A widened pulse pressure or tachycardia may indicate compensatory mechanisms during states of hypoxia, such as with anemia, but heart disease is not known to cause or be caused by a primary hematologic issue.

Cognitive level: Application
Nursing process: Assessment
Client needs: Health Promotion and Maintenance

Chapter 63

1. Answer: 3. Reduction in hematopoietic stem cells
Rationale: Hematopoietic stem cells (HSCs) reside largely in the spongy bone marrow of the femurs, hips, ribs, sternum, and other long bones, while a small volume of HSCs circulates in the peripheral blood. HSCs may be thought of as the common ancestor cell of all of the blood cell lines. Although HSCs eventually give rise to mature red blood cells, platelets, and white cells, they themselves do not possess the full capabilities of oxygen transportation, clotting, or immune response associated with their more mature progeny, the erythrocytes, platelets, and leukocytes.

Cognitive level: Analysis
Nursing process: Assessment
Client needs: Physiological Integrity: Reduction of Risk Potential

2. Answer: 1. Reduced red blood cell production
Rationale: Dietary elements play a key role in red blood cell production. Deficiencies in any of these elements can negatively affect erythropoiesis. This blood cell development is highly dependent on sufficient quantities of metals such as iron, cobalt, and manganese, vitamins B_{12}, B_6, C, E, folate, riboflavin, pantothenic acid, and thiamin, amino acids, and carbohydrates. Although cellular growth requires all of these elements, vitamin B_{12}, folate, and iron play particularly pivotal roles in erythropoiesis. Folate and vitamin B_{12} are required for the extensive DNA synthesis that occurs with erythropoiesis. All proliferating cells require iron, but the iron requirements of erythroid cells in the late basophilic erythroblast through reticulocyte stages, when hemoglobin is synthesized and accumulates, are much greater than for all other cell types. Disease such as megaloblastic anemia and iron deficiency anemia result when sufficient supplies do not exist to support erythropoiesis.

Cognitive level: Analysis
Nursing process: Assessment
Client needs: Physiological Integrity: Reduction of Risk Potential

3. Answer: 4. Glossitis
Rationale: Because the highly efficient iron storage system provides a rich reservoir for active metabolic needs, early iron deficiency anemia often does not produce bothersome symptoms. As with all anemia, the severity of the symptoms correlates with the degree of hemoglobin deficiency, which in turn correlates with the volume of total iron body stores. As erythropoiesis becomes increasingly hampered, the patient may present with the general manifestations of anemia such as fatigue, pallor, shortness of breath, cold intolerance, headache, and activity intolerance. When iron stores fall critically low as to impact epithelial cell production, the patient may present with symptoms uniquely indicative of iron deficiency anemia including pica or clay eating, glossitis or tongue inflammation, gastric atrophy, stomatitis, ice eating or pagophagia, and leg cramping.

Cognitive level: Application
Nursing process: Assessment
Client needs: Physiological Integrity: Physiological Adaptation

4. Answer: 2. RBC mass being lost at the same rate as total blood volume

Rationale: For sudden blood loss, hematocrit values may not accurately indicate the severity of the problem because RBC mass is lost at the same rate as total blood volume, thus the percentage of RBCs in the blood is unaffected. After 2 to 3 days when then body is able to initiate the compensatory mechanism of increasing plasma volume, RBCs become diluted as reflected by decreasing erythrocyte, hemoglobin, and hematocrit values.

Cognitive level: Analysis

Nursing process: Assessment

Client needs: Physiological Integrity: Physiological Adaptation

5. Answer: 4. Frequent skin and oral mucosa assessment

Rationale: Nursing interventions for a patient with thrombocytopenia should focus on reducing the risk for bleeding. This would include assessing the color and presence of blood in the urine and stool. Additional interventions would include frequent vital signs, breath sounds, and abdominal and neurological assessments.

Cognitive level: Application

Nursing process: Planning

Client needs: Physiological Integrity: Physiological Adaptation

6. Answer: 3. Persistent and last for days or weeks

Rationale: The hallmark clinical presentation of hemophilia is prolonged bleeding and inability to form clots in response to injury, both of which can appear and persist for days to weeks. For patients with severe disease completely lacking any Factor VIII or Factor IX, such bleeding can have serious life-threatening consequences. Distinguished from the disease of primary hemostasis, which causes increased bruising and superficial hemorrhages in the integumentary, people with hemophilia typically suffer from bleeding deep in the tissues. Typically, bleeding sites include joints and organs. If left uncontrolled the internal bleeding can cause severe pressure on closed compartments. Serious consequences of internal bleeding into closed spaces include increased intracranial pressure, hemiarthrosis leading to compartment syndrome, and oropharyngeal bleeding. The eventual sequelae following each of these situations can cause lifetime disability. Increased intracranial pressure can cause ischemia and brain tissue damage. Bleeding into the joints predisposes the patient to arthritis, synovial tissue damage, and joint malformation. Oropharyngeal bleeding may occlude the airway so severely as to require intubation.

Cognitive level: Analysis

Nursing process: Planning

Client needs: Physiological Integrity: Physiological Adaptation

Chapter 64

1. Answer: 2. Instruct in the avoidance of tobacco, excessive alcohol, and a high-fat diet.

Rationale: The risk factors for the development of cancer can be divided into endogenous and exogenous causes. Endogenous causes include increasing incidence with age, an occasional genetic link, and the need for immunocompetence to identify antigens. Exogenous causes include exposure to drugs, chemicals, and tobacco smoke; a diet high in fat and low in fiber; multiple sex partners; large consumption of ethyl alcohol; exposure to ultraviolet and ionizing radiation; and exposure to viruses that have been linked to cancer. The effects of psychosocial stress have yet to be linked specifically to the development of cancer.

Cognitive level: Application

Nursing process: Implementation

Client needs: Health Promotion and Maintenance: Reduction of Risk Potential

2. Answer: 3. Angiogenesis

Rationale: Mechanisms of metastasis include angiogenesis, migration, cell attachment, cell invasion, and growth factors. Angiogenesis is the creation of new blood vessels due to migration and proliferation of endothelial cells from existing blood vessels. New blood vessels provide nutrients, protein growth factors, and oxygen to the tumor mass.

Cognitive level: Application

Nursing process: Implementation

Client needs: Physiological Integrity: Physiological Adaptation

3. Answer: 2. Prostate

Rationale: The treatment for prostate cancer includes surgery or a radical prostatectomy, radiotherapy to include external beam or brachytherapy, cryotherapy, chemotherapy, and expectant management or "watchful waiting."

Cognitive level: Analysis

Nursing process: Assessment

Client needs: Physiological Integrity: Physiological Adaptation

4. Answer: 3. Use strict aseptic technique when caring for venous access devices.

Rationale: The patient with cancer is at risk for the development of an infection. Care for this patient should include the avoidance of rectal procedures, including taking rectal temperatures. Foods that could harbor bacteria should be avoided such as raw meat and fresh fruits and vegetables. Intramuscular injections should be avoided. Strict aseptic technique should be used at all times when caring for venous access devices, urinary catheters, and other monitoring devices.

Cognitive level: Application

Nursing process: Planning

Client needs: Physiological Integrity: Reduction of Risk Potential

5. Answer: 1. Cluster care activities to increase rest periods.

Rationale: Many patients who receive radiotherapy experience fatigue. The exact causative mechanism is unknown, although it is thought to be due to the result of tumor breakdown, which releases by-products into the bloodstream. Another explanation for the development of fatigue is the increase in basal metabolic rate consuming the body's energy stores. Fatigue typically begins during the third or fourth week of treatment and will gradually wane once the treatment is over. The loss of energy and feeling of tiredness tend to be cumulative and have a significant impact on patients' quality of life. Patient education regarding the side effects of radiation begins before treatment and needs to continue once it is over. Teaching patients that side effects should be expected may decrease their fear that treatment is ineffective. Nursing care needs to be designed with energy conservation in mind. Clustering patient care activities together will allow for prolonged periods of rest for patients who are experiencing fatigue. Teaching patients and their caregivers these principles will assist the patient in coping with the tiredness experienced with fatigue while at home.

Cognitive level: Application

Nursing process: Implementation

Client needs: Physiological Integrity: Physiological Adaptation

6. Answer: 3. Alter the immunologic relationship between the tumor and the patient.

Rationale: Biotherapy is known as treatment with agents whose origin, mostly mammal, is from biologic sources and/or affecting biologic responses. Biotherapy has emerged since the 1980s as another treatment option for patients with cancer who are receiving high-dose chemotherapy and transplantation. Nurses caring for patients receiving biotherapy need to possess an understanding of the immune system before they can begin to comprehend the rationale behind this unique treatment modality and the primary agents currently used. Although the mechanism of action varies with each type of biologic response modifier, the goal is the same: to destroy or halt the malignant growth of a tumor. A therapeutic effect is accomplished by altering the immunologic relationship between the tumor and the patient.

Cognitive level: Analysis

Nursing process: Planning

Client needs: Physiological Integrity: Physiological Adaptation

Chapter 65

1. Answer: 4. Vitamin D deficiency

Rationale: Functions of the skin include retarding the loss of body heat and fluids, assisting in the control of body temperature, functioning as an excretory organ, and functioning as a synthesizer of vitamin D when sunlight reacts with cholesterol.

Cognitive level: Analysis

Nursing process: Assessment

Client needs: Health Promotion and Maintenance: Prevention/Early Detection of Health Problems

2. Answer: 3. Biographic and demographic data

Rationale: Biographic and demographic data include data such as the patient's name, address, telephone number, Social Security number, contact person, age, gender, race or ethnic origin, marital status, birthplace, occupation, level of education, and religious affiliation. Examples of biographic and demographic data that may be significant to assessment of the skin include travel to different environments such as when camping or travel to rural areas of the world. The patient's current issue or the reason for seeking health care is referred to as the chief complaint. The reason for obtaining information about the past medical history is to identify the patient's entire past relevant health problems. Past illnesses could possibly have some effect on the patient's current health. The nursing assessment includes questions about major illnesses such as diabetes, cardiovascular disease, and infectious diseases. Patients with diabetes are prone to skin breakdown and delayed wound healing. Patients with cardiovascular disease may have clubbed nail beds. Infectious diseases such as cellulitis have skin manifestations, which assist with the diagnosis.

Cognitive level: Application

Nursing process: Assessment

Client needs: Health Promotion and Maintenance: Prevention/Early Detection of Health Problems

3. Answer: 4. Social history

Rationale: Social history includes use of alcohol or street drugs that can have adverse effects on the condition of the patient's skin. The presence of certain cutaneous lesions in a patient should prompt an investigation into the patient's drinking and drug habits. If drug use is suspected due to the presence of a cutaneous lesion, the nurse needs to inquire about skin popping. Skin popping is a technique used by individuals to administer illicit drugs. Skin popping is a significant risk factor in skin and soft tissue infections, which are common among injection drug users.

Cognitive level: Application

Nursing process: Assessment

Client needs: Physiological Integrity: Physiological Adaptation

4. Answer: 3. Inspect and palpate the skin at the same time.

Rationale: The assessment should proceed in an orderly fashion, beginning with an examination of the most frequently exposed areas such as the face, hands, arms, legs, and feet. The nurse inspects the skin while the patient is in a sitting or lying position with all clothes removed except an examination or hospital gown. The nurse will inspect and palpate simultaneously.

Cognitive level: Application

Nursing process: Assessment

Client needs: Health Promotion and Maintenance: Prevention/Early Detection of Health Problems

5. Answer: 4. Normal findings

Rationale: The nail surface is normally slightly curved with the posterior and lateral folds smooth and rounded. The nail edges should be smooth, rounded, and clean. The normal nail bed angle is 160 degrees. The nail base is firm to palpation. A nail bed with greater than a 160-degree angle suggests a clubbed nail. Clubbing of nails indicates a state of chronic hypoxia and is often seen with congenital and adult heart disease and chronic obstructive pulmonary disease. The surface of the nail should be smooth and nonbrittle, with no splitting. Pits, transverse grooves, or lines may indicate a nutritional deficiency. Patients with arterial insufficiency may have thickened, ridged nails.

Cognitive level: Application

Nursing process: Assessment

Client needs: Health Promotion and Maintenance: Prevention/Early Detection of Health Problems

6. Answer: 3. Keloid

Rationale: A fissure is a linear crack or break from the epidermis to the dermis. A scale is an abundance of dry or oily keratinized cells. A keloid results from the overproduction of scar tissue that extends laterally beyond the initial wound; it is usually raised and smooth in appearance. A cherry angioma is a distinct benign vascular lesion.

Cognitive level: Analysis

Nursing process: Assessment

Client needs: Physiological Integrity: Reduction of Risk Potential

7. Answer: 4. Vitiligo

Rationale: Jaundice is a yellowish discoloration of the skin, sclera, and mucous membranes that is often associated with increased amounts of bilirubin in the blood. Pallor is paleness of the skin that occurs when the red-pink tones from the oxygenated hemoglobin in the blood are lost. Petechiae are pinpoint purpuric lesions of the skin. Vitiligo is the absence of pigmentation in a circumscribed area.

Cognitive level: Analysis

Nursing process: Assessment

Client needs: Physiological Integrity: Reduction of Risk Potential

Chapter 66

1. Answer: 1. Atopic dermatitis

Rationale: Atopic dermatitis is characterized by severe itching. Treatment involves controlling the aggravating factors and treating the rash. It is important to moisturize the skin to maintain the skin barrier. Bathing should be held to a minimum; however, when bathing, the patient should use tepid water and mild, unscented soap such as Cetaphil or Dove.

Cognitive level: Analysis

Nursing process: Implementation

Client needs: Physiological Integrity: Basic Care and Comfort

2. Answer: 2. Eat foods high in vitamin C, iron, and zinc.

Rationale: The nurse should instruct the patient to maintain a high-calorie, high-protein, well-balanced diet. Include vitamin C, iron, and zinc in the diet. Avoid foods that cause hypersensitivity reactions.

Cognitive level: Application

Nursing process: Implementation

Client needs: Physiological Integrity: Physiological Adaptation

3. Answer: 4. Instruct in the use of sunscreen.

Rationale: The sun, along with other pollutants in the air, can irritate and damage the skin, with most of the damage occurring before the age of 18. Nearly 80% of this damage can be prevented if sunscreen is applied properly in those first 18 years of life.

Cognitive level: Application

Nursing process: Implementation

Client needs: Health Promotion and Maintenance: Prevention/Early Detection of Health Problems

4. Answer: 1. Rub the medication into wet skin thoroughly.

Rationale: Topical corticosteroids should be applied in a thin layer and rubbed in thoroughly on wet skin. Retinoic acid can be irritating to the skin and produce phototoxicity. Systemic antihistamines can cause drowsiness.

Cognitive level: Application

Nursing process: Implementation

Client needs: Physiological Integrity: Pharmacologic and Parenteral Therapies

5. Answer: 1. Signs of infection

Rationale: The focus of nursing care is to prevent problems or recognize complications early so they can be successfully treated. The nurse must assess the patient frequently, noting changes in skin color, texture, wound size, drainage, and temperature. Analysis of the data collected during assessment will provide a basis for determining a treatment plan and assessing response to treatment. Patients with skin disorders may develop problems with hydration, fluid balance, or nutrition. Fluid loss through wounds leads to dehydration and electrolyte imbalances. The skin also provides protection against infection, so when its barrier is broken, infection becomes more likely. It is very important to assess for signs of infection both in the wound and systemically. Clinical manifestations of infection include fever, increased redness or drainage, increased pain, changes in odor or color of drainage, increased white blood cell count, and increased tissue erosion. If the infecting organism is contagious, such as occurs with staphylococcus, isolation procedures may be needed.

Cognitive level: Application

Nursing process: Assessment

Client needs: Physiological Integrity: Reduction of Risk Potential

6. Answer: 3. There are light materials that you could wear to protect your arms while still enjoying the summer activities.

Rationale: Psychological assessment needs to be uppermost in the mind of the nurse as care is given to patients with skin disorders. The appearance of the skin affects self-esteem and body image. Skin disorders can cause the patient to withdraw from social situations. Society can be unkind to people who have scars or rashes with an unpleasant appearance. Some individuals may withdraw from the patient, fearing the disorder is contagious. Patients should be provided with an open, supportive environment in which they are comfortable voicing their concerns.

Cognitive level: Application

Nursing process: Implementation

Client needs: Psychosocial Integrity: Coping and Adaptation

7. Answer: 2. This is a normal part of aging.

Rationale: Many anatomic changes occur during the aging process: Skin loses elasticity and water content; the texture and turgor of the skin change; the retaining ligaments of the soft tissue of the face weaken; the face loses volume as a result of decreased subcutaneous adipose stores and muscle mass; facial bones undergo resorption; the eye orbit changes shape, allowing for positional changes of the eye globe; the face becomes elongated and flattened; and smoking, genetics, and sun exposure contribute to the loss of skin elasticity and wrinkle formation.

Cognitive level: Application

Nursing process: Implementation

Client needs: Health Promotion and Maintenance: Growth and Development Through the Life Span

Chapter 67

1. Answer: 3. Proliferation

Rationale: Homeostasis is the tendency of the human body to maintain stability, and maintaining stability is the first reaction when a wound occurs. The inflammatory phase of wound healing begins at the time of the injury or surgery. The purpose of this critical phase is to prepare the site for growth of new tissue. The proliferative phase is the next phase in the healing process. Reconstruction occurs at this phase. It can last up to 3 weeks after the inflammatory phase in a normal, healthy person. Growth factors originating from injured vessels stimulate the formation of vascular buds and regrowth of vascular loops. Stimulated endothelial cells multiply and form tubular structures, differentiating into arterioles or venules, a process referred to as angiogenesis. These new blood vessels can begin to form in a wound within 3 days of injury, provided there is sufficient blood circulation to the wound bed. Remodeling, the third and final phase of wound healing, occurs after the wound is closed. It begins about 3 weeks after the injury and can still be in progress from 6 months to 2 years later.

Cognitive level: Analysis

Nursing process: Assessment

Client needs: Health Promotion and Maintenance: Prevention/Early Detection of Health Problems

2. Answer: 3. Using the clock face method

Rationale: A sinus tract is an area, sometimes referred to as a tunnel, where there is nonhealed detached tissue under intact skin. Sinus tracts are measured in centimeters. Referring to location, the area of tunneling is defined on a clock face with 12 o'clock being the head of the body. For example, if a wound located on the anterior aspect of the leg has tunneling on the medial side of the left leg, the measurement would be x amount of centimeters at the 9 o'clock position. There is also a measurement for undermining. Undermining is like a cliff without tissue below and more broad than a sinus tract. It is measured from each point or side using the clock face method. The surface area of the wound is the length multiplied by the width in centimeters squared (cm^2). The volume is the length multiplied by the width and the depth in centimeters cubed (cm^3).

Cognitive level: Application

Nursing process: Assessment

Client needs: Physiological Integrity: Physiological Adaptation

3. Answer: 2. Use the rule of 30 to reposition the patient every two hours.

Rationale: Positioning is important in the prevention of pressure ulcers. The goal is to get the patient mobile and active as soon as possible; however, when mobility is physically impossible, the patient's position should be changed a minimum of every 2 hours. A sufficient number of people should be available to move the patient so that shearing and friction during movement can be avoided. Assistive devices such as transfer boards or mechanical lifts may be helpful to minimize tissue injury during movement. The "rule of 30" is used for positioning. This rule states that the head of the bed should be elevated 30 degrees or less and the body placed in a 30-degree laterally inclined position when placed on either side. These positions avoid pressure directly over the trochanter and promote improved circulation to the skin over the sacrum and ischial tuberosities. Pillows or foam wedges may be used to keep the patient properly positioned. The prone position may also be used if the patient is able to tolerate it. Attention should be focused on maintaining proper alignment so that functional ability can be maintained.

Cognitive level: Application

Nursing process: Planning

Client needs: Physiological Integrity: Reduction of Risk Potential

4. Answer: 3. Apply a moisture barrier and secure with gauze.

Rationale: Compression is used for venous wounds. Surgery is indicated for arterial wounds. Debridement is appropriate for wounds with eschar. Appropriate care for a skin tear wound includes avoiding the use of adhesive dressings or tapes, applying a moisture barrier, wrapping a gauze bandage around the extremity, using hydrogel sheet dressings or foam, and/or using zinc-impregnated gauze and cotton.

Cognitive level: Application

Nursing process: Implementation

Client needs: Physiological Integrity: Physiological Adaptation

5. Answer: 1. Autolytic debridement

Rationale: Autolytic debridement allows the body to utilize its phagocytes to destroy the necrotic tissue. This is often a preferred method of debridement for those persons for whom daily or more frequent dressing changes would be a hardship; that is, patients who are critically ill and cannot be turned. Autolytic debridement is a slow and nonaggressive treatment. Sharp debridement is done with a scalpel, scissors, or nippers. Anesthetics or the operating room may be required depending on wound size and depth. Mechanical debridement is the

dislodging of necrotic tissue, which is accomplished by wet-to-dry dressings, the whirlpool, or pulse lavage. Enzymatic debridement is chemically induced by prescriptive ointments that contain papain-urea or collagenase, which penetrates the slough and eschar causing them to soften and "melt down." Once softened, the slough and eschar are mechanically debrided.
Cognitive level: Analysis
Nursing process: Planning
Client needs: Physiological Integrity: Physiological Adaptation

6. Answer: 2. Tell me why you think the wound is ugly.
Rationale: Depression can occur when a patient has a wound. It may affect the way she sees herself or the way she perceives that others see her, especially if the wound is easily visible. Not only does the patient have an emotional response to her wound, but almost everyone the patient encounters has an emotional response to her wound. Wounds are perceived as unpleasant, disgusting, scary, and a nuisance. Depression may affect the patient's ability to perform the daily activities she desires to do, and it may limit patient independence. It can be very costly for the treatments and medications. The patient may have to wear some special type of shoe or device that makes her self-conscious. The nurse needs to assess the patient for her feelings about her wound and associated treatment. Empathize with the patient, and try to devise a plan that is least intrusive and yet realistic.
Cognitive level: Application
Nursing process: Assessment
Client needs: Psychosocial Integrity: Coping and Adaptation

7. Answer: 2. Healing rate
Rationale: Poor nutrition will negatively impact the healing rate of a wound. Wound dressings impact the risk of infection. Mechanisms to preventing scar formation impact wound appearance. Appropriate pain management impacts the patient's comfort level.
Cognitive level: Analysis
Nursing process: Evaluation
Client needs: Physiological Integrity: Physiological Adaptation

Chapter 68

1. Answer: 3. Major burn injury
Rationale: This patient has experienced a major burn injury. The classifications are minor, moderate, and major, not medium. Electrical burns and burns involving the feet are always considered major injuries, even though the dermal injuries only appeared as 2% or less.
Cognitive level: Application
Nursing process: Assessment
Client needs: Physiological Integrity

2. Answer: 4. "Liquid at 140°F requires five minutes to cause a full-thickness burn."
Rationale: Liquids at 120°F require 5 minutes to cause a full-thickness burn. At 140°F liquids can cause a burn

injury in 5 seconds or less. Sunscreens help prevent radiation burns from the sun and help decrease the risk of skin cancers. Children's sleepwear should be made from fire retardant materials, and every home should have smoke alarms that are clean and in working order.
Cognitive level: Application
Nursing process: Evaluation
Client needs: Safe and Effective Care Environment

3. Answer: 1. "With bacterial translocation the gastrointestinal mucosal atrophy that occurs causes intraluminal bacteria to migrate to extraluminal sites."
Rationale: Paralytic ileus and gastrointestinal mucosal atrophy are not uncommon with severe burn injuries. This allows opportunity for the intraluminal bacteria to migrate to extraluminal sources in a process called bacterial translocation. Decreased cardiac output can occur early after a burn injury because of the vasoconstriction caused by the sympathetic nervous system. When damaged erythrocytes and muscle tissue cause the release of excess hemoglobin and myoglobin, respectively, the liver is unable to handle this increased load. Therefore, these substances must be excreted through the urine and can clog the renal tubules, causing renal failure. Leukocytes are not transfused, although their stores may be depleted within 48 hours following a burn. Decreased circulating iron causes a resultant low red blood cell count, and it is not uncommon to replace red blood cells or platelets in patients with major burns.
Cognitive level: Application
Nursing process: Assessment
Client needs: Physiological Integrity

4. Answer: 2. The acute care period
Rationale: The emergency and resuscitative periods are the same and include the initial treatment with airway and hemodynamic stabilization with fluid resuscitation. The rehabilitative period begins when the open burn wound size is less than 20% and the patient is at his or her highest level of functioning since admission. This phase focuses on physical and psychological restoration, including increased strength, function, flexibility, and cosmetic restoration. The acute care period begins once the patient is hemodynamically stable. The focus is on wound care, prevention of infection and other complications, and pain control.
Cognitive level: Analysis
Nursing process: Implementation
Client needs: Physiological Integrity

5. Answer: 1. A 35-year-old with a history of migraines and 40% TBSA full-thickness thermal burns to the neck, left upper extremity, and circumferentially around the chest. Vital signs are HR 116, BP 90/68, RR 26 and shallow, SpO$_2$ 90%.
Rationale: The 35-year-old patient has a major burn injury. The size and location of the burn, as well as the circumferential nature of the wound, have the potential to cause increased morbidity and mortality in this patient. The vital signs reflect possible cardiopulmonary

compromise. The 70-year-old patient is older and has a chronic medical condition, but partial-thickness wounds of less than 15% and full-thickness wounds of less than 1% are considered minor. Also, the burns do not involve the head, neck, chest, hands, feet, or perineum nor are the vital signs abnormal. The 12-year-old patient is younger, but not an infant or young child. A partial-thickness burn of 20% is moderate, and it is important to note that while the injury to the foot is significant, it is not full thickness nor would it take precedence over an injury that could compromise airway, breathing, or circulation. The history of astigmatism is unremarkable to the emergent burn treatment, and the vital signs are normal. The 44-year-old patient does have a significant chronic medical condition, as exemplified by the blood pressure reading. However, an 8% full-thickness injury and 15% partial-thickness injury are moderate injuries. It is also important to note that none of the burns are classified as circumferential.
Cognitive level: Analysis
Nursing process: Planning
Client needs: Physiological Integrity

6. Answer: 2. Fluid volume deficit related to increased capillary permeability
Rationale: After airway and breathing, the priority during emergency care is cardiovascular assessment with fluid resuscitation. Therefore, of the choices given, fluid volume deficit would be the priority nursing diagnosis during the emergency phase. Altered skin integrity is addressed during the emergency phase, but it is the basis for care during the acute care phase. Acute pain should certainly be addressed, but it will not take precedence over fluid volume deficit. A potential problem, such as high risk for infection, will also be attended to after actual problems.
Cognitive level: Application
Nursing process: Planning
Client needs: Physiological Integrity

7. Answer: 4. "My pressure garments should be removed one to four times a day to allow for adequate circulation."
Rationale: Exercise programs for burned patients should be progressive in nature so as to improve strength and endurance. These programs may also include stretching exercises to elongate shortened tissues. These exercises are providing adequate stretch when the burn scar blanches. Also beneficial to helping healed burn wounds is scar massage. The massage should be performed daily, from one to four times a day. The massage helps improve the cosmetic appearance and hypertrophy of the scar, as well as increase circulation and possibly range of motion. Pressure garments should be worn continuously for 23 hours a day, not removed several times to promote circulation.
Cognitive level: Analysis
Nursing process: Evaluation
Client needs: Physiological Integrity

8. Answer: 3. Heart rate 114
Rationale: The heart rate is tachycardic, indicating possible hypovolemia. The blood pressure appears normal, but this is a poor early indicator because the increased systemic vascular resistance that occurs causes the blood pressure to be maintained regardless of volume status. A central venous pressure of 6 indicates adequate fluid volume, as does a urine output of 30 mL/hr.
Cognitive level: Analysis
Nursing process: Assessment
Client needs: Physiological Integrity

Chapter 69

1. Answer: 2. Normal
Rationale: The inside of the ear is inspected with an otoscope. An otoscopic examination includes inspection of the auditory canal and tympanic membrane. Look for inflammation, exudates, lesions, and foreign bodies. Check for narrowing of the ear canal, nodules, redness, scales, edema, drainage, and foreign objects. Normally the eardrum is slightly conical, shiny, smooth, and pearl gray. Cerumen should be moist and may vary in color from brown to white, but hardened, dry, or foul-smelling cerumen may indicate infection. In a majority of Asians and Native Americans, cerumen is dry, white, and flaky. In African Americans and Caucasians, cerumen is brown, wet, and sticky.
Cognitive level: Analysis
Nursing process: Assessment
Client needs: Health Promotion and Maintenance: Prevention/Early Detection of Health Problems

2. Answer: 4. Do you think that there is something in the room causing you to sneeze?
Rationale: The nurse needs to inquire about a history of upper respiratory infection. Sneezing, particularly at specific times of the year or under specific environmental circumstances, should be investigated for the possibility of allergies or respiratory infection. Allergic rhinitis is an inflammation of the nasal mucosa caused by an allergic substance, for example, hay fever or pollen. The nurse needs to inquire if the allergies are related to a specific time of year. Does the patient regularly take medications for allergic rhinitis, sinus infections, stuffy nose, or frequent respiratory infections? Some nasal sprays and decongestants may cause rebound nasal swelling. Over-the-counter oral decongestants may have an adverse effect on patients with diabetes, hypertension, hyperthyroidism, and cardiac illnesses.
Cognitive level: Analysis
Nursing process: Assessment
Client needs: Health Promotion and Maintenance: Prevention/Early Detection of Health Problems

3. Answer: 2. Even though you have dentures, seeing a dentist regularly is necessary for good oral health.
Rationale: Poorly fitting dentures or orthotic appliances and inadequate dentition can cause difficulty chewing,

nutritional problems, and mouth sores. To maintain good oral health, the patient should see the dentist at regular intervals and use good oral hygiene measures.

Cognitive level: Analysis

Nursing process: Assessment

Client needs: Health Promotion and Maintenance: Prevention/Early Detection of Health Problems

4. Answer: 3. Social isolation because of hearing loss

Rationale: Age impacts hearing ability. For example, presbycusis, hearing loss in the high-frequency range, is the most common sensorineural hearing loss in older people. The patient experiencing the gradual hearing loss of aging may limit social interactions as it becomes so difficult to understand the spoken word. During the assessment the nurse should inquire about functional ability and social interactions. Loss of hearing also can be perceived as mental status changes. Nurses need to be more aware of the impact of hearing loss on the elderly.

Cognitive level: Analysis

Nursing process: Assessment

Client needs: Psychosocial Integrity: Coping and Adaptation

5. Answer: 1. Normal

Rationale: With the voice whisper test the examiner stands approximately 1 to 2 feet in back of the patient and whispers several words near each ear. The patient should be able to hear bilaterally and equally.

Cognitive level: Analysis

Nursing process: Assessment

Client needs: Health Promotion and Maintenance: Prevention/Early Detection of Health Problems

Chapter 70

1. Answer: 3. Sound transmission

Rationale: The tympanic membrane or eardrum, comprised of tissue that makes up the ear canal, is the final structure within this portion of the outer ear anatomy. It is this structure that transmits sounds from the outer to the middle ear. The cochlea is responsible for hearing, whereas the vestibular system is responsible for balance. Within the inner ear are found the semicircular canals, specifically the horizontal, anterior, and posterior canals, which help with balance and movement. The acoustic nerve consists of two separate parts, the vestibular and cochlear branches. This eighth cranial nerve controls hearing and equilibrium.

Cognitive level: Analysis

Nursing process: Assessment

Client needs: Health Promotion and Maintenance: Prevention/Early Detection of Health Problems

2. Answer: 2. Air conduction

Rationale: There are actually two mechanisms involved with hearing: bone conduction and air conduction. Bone conduction is the conduction of sound to the inner ear through the bones of the skull. Air conduction begins the process when noise enters the external ear and travels to the middle ear. Once inside the middle

ear, the sound is transmitted through the three auditory bones, the malleus, incus, and stapes. Once the sound or noise reaches the stapes, it is then transmitted to the inner ear where it reaches the acoustic nerve and is transmitted to the brain for interpretation. Hearing disorders can be caused by an alteration anywhere within the auditory structures.

Cognitive level: Analysis

Nursing process: Assessment

Client needs: Health Promotion and Maintenance: Prevention/Early Detection of Health Problems

3. Answer: 3. Conductive

Rationale: In conductive hearing loss, sound waves cannot reach the inner ear for processing and interpretation. With sensorineural hearing loss, the cause is damage to the auditory nerve or possibly damage to the small hair cells within the inner ear. Mixed hearing loss refers to both conductive and sensorineural hearing loss caused by a dysfunction of both air and bone conduction processes. Acoustic hearing loss would refer to a damaged acoustic nerve.

Cognitive level: Analysis

Nursing process: Assessment

Client needs: Health Promotion and Maintenance: Prevention/Early Detection of Health Problems

4. Answer: 3. The baby should be tested now.

Rationale: Within the *Healthy People 2010* "Objectives for Reducing Hearing Loss," it is recommended that newborns should have a first hearing examination by 1 month of age. Babies with a hearing loss should have additional testing by 3 months of age. And if hearing loss continues, the baby should be enrolled in a rehabilitative program by 6 months of age. Hearing loss in the newborn can be linked to birth trauma, toxicity, infection, fetal anoxia during delivery, premature or low birth weight, genetics, or an elevated serum bilirubin level. In addition, deafness upon birth has been seen in those women who have been exposed to highly communicable diseases such as rubella and syphilis or who have ingested known ototoxic medications while pregnant. The presence of hearing can be assessed as early as 2 to 3 days of life. Hearing loss is one of the most common developmental abnormalities present at birth. If left undiagnosed, it will impede speech, language, and cognitive developments. Individuals with hearing impairment at this early age will face a lifetime of challenges. Learning how to communicate with sign language and lip reading are just two ways to aid the person born without the sense of hearing.

Cognitive level: Analysis

Nursing process: Assessment

Client needs: Health Promotion and Maintenance: Prevention/Early Detection of Health Problems

5. Answer: 1. Mechanical

Rationale: The causes of hearing impairment or loss can be categorized as mechanical, inflammatory, or an obstructive disorder. One mechanical cause of hearing loss is due to otosclerosis or a primary bone dyscrasia that leads to conductive hearing loss. Otosclerosis is a condition in which the structures of the ear begin to harden. Seen as a common cause of conductive hearing loss, treatment options are limited to a stapedectomy.

Cognitive level: Analysis

Nursing process: Assessment

Client needs: Physiological Integrity: Physiological Adaptation

6. Answer: 3. Mechanism to ensure a visual alert in the event of a home fire

   Rationale: The home needs to have services or mechanisms that make the environment safer; for instance, visual fire safety provisions and access to alerting and telephone services, and TVs with teletext ability.

   Cognitive level: Application

   Nursing process: Planning

   Client needs: Health Promotion and Maintenance: Prevention/Early Detection of Health Problems

7. Answer: 2. Drop the tone of the voice when talking.

   Rationale: When providing care to an elderly patient with a hearing deficit or balance disorder, the nurse needs to include specific items in the assessment process. First the method of communication must be determined. A loud voice does not ensure successful hearing or comprehension. Depending on the cause and degree of hearing loss, the nurse might simply drop the tone of the voice to be successful with vocal communication with an elderly patient who has a hearing impairment because the loss of high-frequency sounds occurs first.

   Cognitive level: Application

   Nursing process: Implementation

   Client needs: Physiological Integrity: Reduction of Risk Potential

8. Answer: 1. Assure the patient that the call light will be answered as soon as possible.

   Rationale: The nurse should implement strategies to reduce the patient's anxiety such as responding to the call light as soon as possible, answering questions, teaching about medications/treatments, and providing emotional support to the patient having difficulty coping with the new sensory deficit.

   Cognitive level: Application

   Nursing process: Implementation

   Client needs: Psychosocial Integrity: Coping and Adaptation

Chapter 71

1. Answer: 3. Floaters

   Rationale: The vitreous body is the largest chamber of the eye that maintains the shape of the eyeball. The vitreous gel is made up mainly of water with a collagen framework, which includes collagen, hyaluronic acid, proteins, and solutes. Due to aging, the collagen network can be aggregated by vitreous collapse that forms vitreous opacities, which cast shadows on the retina. These shadows are referred to as floaters.

Cognitive level: Analysis

Nursing process: Assessment

Client needs: Health Promotion and Maintenance: Prevention/Early Detection of Health Problems

2. Answer: 2. The uncovered eye is fixated outward.

   Rationale: When conducting the cover–uncover test for tropia, the patient is to wear his own corrective lenses, if he has them. Have the patient fixate on a target about 20 feet away for far and 16 inches for near; it can be a visual acuity chart, picture chart, E chart, or toy. The tester is to sit in front of the patient, but does not block target view. Note the eye that is fixating cover that eye with an occluder, and note what the fellow eye does. If the uncovered eye moves to pick up fixation, note the direction it moves: If toward the nose, then it was fixated outward, so it is exo; if toward the ear, then it was fixated inward, so it is eso. If the uncovered eye does not move and has steady fixation, no strabismus exists. The eye would move up and down to indicate vertical tropia.

   Cognitive level: Analysis

   Nursing process: Assessment

   Client needs: Health Promotion and Maintenance: Prevention/Early Detection of Health Problems

3. Answer: 4. Eye muscle surgery

   Rationale: Adult strabismus may be treated with eye muscle exercises, eyeglasses containing prisms, botulinum toxin (Botox) injections, and eye surgery. Eye muscle exercise usually is used when treating a form of adult strabismus, called convergence insufficiency, in which eyes cannot align themselves for close work or reading. These exercises can retrain eyes to focus inward together. Prism eyeglasses can be used to correct the mild double vision associated with adult strabismus. Botox injections are an effective treatment when overactive eye muscles are causing strabismus. Eye muscle surgery is the most common treatment; it is used to loosen or tighten the muscles around the eye in order to correct the misalignment.

   Cognitive level: Analysis

   Nursing process: Planning

   Client needs: Psychosocial Integrity: Coping and Adaptation

4. Answer: 2. The correct use of eyedrops

   Rationale: Nursing assessment and education include patient compliance with regular use of eyedrops and follow-up, which is one of the main goals in treating glaucoma. The major reason for the cause of blindness from glaucoma, besides not knowing one has glaucoma, is noncompliance in using eyedrops and not considering glaucoma to be a serious disease. It is imperative that patients understand that the long-term goal of treatment is to lower intraocular pressure to prevent optic nerve damage, and only with continued use of drops can this goal be reached. Patient education includes information on risk factors for glaucoma such as family history, myopia, previous eye trauma, low blood pressure, African ancestry, diabetes, longtime exposure to steroids, and aging. The patient is taught how to instill eyedrops properly for the full benefit of treatment.

Cognitive level: Application

Nursing process: Planning

Client needs: Physiological Integrity: Physiological Adaptation

5. Answer: 2. Explain that whatever decision they make, they have freedom of choice.

Rationale: The decision to donate corneal tissue for transplantation can have ethical considerations. It is important for the family that is being asked to donate a cornea for the benefit of someone else's vision that the decision be a well-informed one, one that is freely chosen, and one that is compatible with the ethical beliefs of the individuals concerned. It is important for the family members to know that whatever decision they make, to donate or not to donate, they have freedom of choice. Under the circumstances of facing the loss of a loved one, any decision they make is the right decision for them. Usually the decision is one of three choices: Donate all organs, donate only the cornea, or do not donate at all. The two most common reasons not to donate are (1) the fear of something being done before the person is dead, and (2) the fear that the health care provider may hasten the death to benefit another. Thoughts that the family should consider include these: Donation is an ethical decision to benefit another person; with treatment of the body after death, respect is the greatest issue, especially for psychological, religious, spiritual, moral, and cultural reasons; donation is the last giving act the person donor does to reflect his life; and the family knows that the loved one still lives on in another person.

Cognitive level: Application

Nursing process: Implementation

Client needs: Psychosocial Integrity: Coping and Adaptation

Chapter 72

1. Answer: 3. "When the group responsible for committing the violence has connection to a foreign country like al Queda in the Middle East."

Rationale: Terrorist acts use force, destruction, and violence to coerce and intimidate and cause disruption, terror, and panic. When the group or individual is operating independently from within the United States or Puerto Rico with acts of terrorism that are directed at the U.S. government or its population, then it is said to be an act of "domestic" terrorism. Terrorist acts committed across international boundaries or by groups with foreign ties are said to be acts of "international" terrorism.

Cognitive level: Analysis

Nursing process: Assessment

Client needs: Safe and Effective Care Environment

2. Answer: 1. "The outbreak of an intentionally caused food-borne illness in Oregon during the early 1980s was attributed to *Shigella sonnei*."

Rationale: In 1979 the nuclear power plant at Three Mile Island in the United States did experience an accidental radiation leak. However, there were never any effects on physical health reported. In both 1994 and 1995, sarin gas was released into the Tokyo subway system by the Aum Shinrikyo cult, making the resultant disaster the largest peace-time event involving nerve gas. Rye ergot was used in the 6th century B.C. by the Assyrians who would use it to poison the water wells of their enemies. In 1984, in The Dalles, Oregon, a religious group known as the Rajneeshees intentionally contaminated a salad bar at a local restaurant with *Salmonella typhimurium*.

Cognitive level: Analysis

Nursing process: Evaluation

Client needs: Safe and Effective Care Environment

3. Answer: 4. Inhalation anthrax

Rationale: Although the patient clearly has an infectious process manifesting with signs of shock, tachypnea, dyspnea, and fever with chills, the complaint of chest pain with radiologic confirmation of a widened mediastinum several days following possible biologic agent exposure are classic for inhalation anthrax. Septicemic plague may also present with signs of sepsis or septic shock, but it also usually includes gastrointestinal symptoms such as vomiting and diarrhea. Also known as the "Black Death," septicemic plague causes purpuric lesions, distal gangrene, and disseminated intravascular coagulopathy. Undulant fever is also called brucellosis. It presents much like the flu, with generalized body aches, fever, headache, and malaise. Patients may also have gastrointestinal symptoms. The onset of typhoidal tularemia is abrupt and progressive. Patients may experience fever, chills, and chest pain, but they usually also have severe body aches, low back pain, sore throat, and pneumonia. They may also have nausea, vomiting, diarrhea, and weight loss.

Cognitive level: Analysis

Nursing process: Assessment

Client needs: Physiological Integrity

4. Answer: 1. Ineffective airway clearance related to copious secretions and ineffective cough

Rationale: Although all of the nursing diagnoses are appropriate for the patient with known nerve agent exposure, the priority for any patient is airway. Nursing diagnoses that relate to actual problems would always take precedence over potential problems, such as increased risk for altered cardiac output or for fluid and electrolyte imbalance. Also, physiological issues should be addressed prior to any psychosocial problems this patient may be experiencing.

Cognitive level: Application

Nursing process: Planning

Client needs: Physiological Integrity

5. Answer: 2. Prodromal phase

Rationale: The prodromal phase is the initial phase after exposure and has an onset of minutes to hours and lasts from hours to days. In this phase the onset of symptoms is rapid and may include nausea, vomiting, and fatigue. Fever, hypotension, and diarrhea may occur with high-level exposure. The rapid onset in this case, within half an hour, is bleak. The latent phase follows the prodromal phase, and during this time, the patient is relatively symptom free. Once the patient has recovered from an exposure, the acute symptoms should not occur. The illness phase is marked by overt illness. Signs and symptoms may be more systemic, involving the hematopoietic, gastrointestinal, central nervous, and dermatologic systems in any combination.

Cognitive level: Analysis

Nursing process: Assessment

Client needs: Safe, Effective Care Environment/Physiological Integrity

6. Answer: 3. This flexible plan allows for only necessary positions and functions to be activated on an as-needed basis during the incident.

Rationale: The Incident Commander is in charge of four areas: operations, planning, logistics, and finance. Although the HICS plan does outline a clear chain of command and responsibilities for each position involved, the positions do not have to have a sole commander nor must they remain independent of other positions. If needed, the positions may be combined under the leadership of one individual. Media use is very helpful if the HICS is activated. Its utilization can decrease mass hysteria by increasing public awareness of the situation. The plan is flexible, allowing for only necessary positions and functions to be activated on an as-needed basis during the incident.

Cognitive level: Analysis

Nursing process: Planning

Client needs: Safe and Effective Care Environment

7. Answer: 1. It helps augment the local and state resources so as to help decrease the morbidity and mortality in the civilian population following a large-scale disaster.

Rationale: The SNS maintains a national repository of pharmaceutical agents, vaccines, and medical supplies and equipment to be delivered to an area after a large-scale disaster. It helps augment the local and state resources so as to help decrease morbidity and mortality in the civilian population. This program is organized with a five-tiered approach that includes 12-hour Push Packs, vendor-managed inventory (VMI), storage of and rapid vaccine deployment, buying power with surge capacity, and technical assistance. The 12-hour Push Packs can be shipped within 12 hours of the decision to do so. They contain critical supplies and pharmaceuticals that might be needed in the event of a large-scale disaster. The VMI is designed to be used to provide pharmaceuticals and medical supplies for treatment of a known agent or for smaller scale events. The Technical Advisory Response Unit is a group of logistical, public health, communications, operations, and emergency preparedness experts who assist state and local authorities with supply receiving, distribution, dispensing, and replenishing.

Cognitive level: Analysis

Nursing process: Planning

Client needs: Physiological Integrity

8. Answer: 4. "Critical incident defusings are formal, confidential group sessions where the stressful event and its experiences and reactions are reviewed."

Rationale: Critical incident stress debriefings are formal sessions run by trained counselors that are held within 72 hours of a critical event. Group information briefings are also called demobilizations. This is a short informal meeting that helps with rumor control, possible reactions, and self-help guidelines. The fact phase of CISD allows for each participant to describe the stressful event from his or her own perspective on a cognitive level. Critical incident defusings give mutual reassurance and assess the need for more help. Critical incident defusings are formal, confidential group sessions where the event and its experiences and reactions are reviewed. Each session consists of six to eight people with similar job descriptions, and each session lasts 20 to 45 minutes.

Cognitive level: Analysis

Nursing process: Evaluation

Client needs: Safe and Effective Care Environment

Chapter 73

1. Answer: 2. It can describe patient care for perceived, actual, or undiagnosed health problems.

Rationale: Emergency nursing does involve episodic patient care, but the care is usually acute or critical in nature. Florence Nightingale has long been associated with the origins of emergency nursing because of her care of wounded soldiers out in the field. Judith Kelleher and Anita Dorr are credited with establishing the Emergency Department Nurses Association in 1970. The patients seeking emergency care are becoming increasingly diverse in culture and ethnicity. Thus, it is important for emergency nurses to also become more educated about, sensitive to, and competent in these diversities and how they affect patient care. Emergency nursing is patient care for perceived, actual, or undiagnosed physical and mental health conditions.

Cognitive level: Analysis

Nursing process: Assessment

Client needs: Safe and Effective Care Environment

2. Answer: 3. A patient having a possible allergic reaction with facial edema, drooling, stridor, and severe urticaria with pruritus

Rationale: Patients requiring immediate airway or cervical spine intervention are always identified and treated first in the emergency department. The patient having an allergic reaction is demonstrating signs of possible airway obstruction (i.e., facial edema, drooling, and stridor). This patient should be treated first among the other patients listed. The patient with chest pain and shortness of breath has signs of a possible cardiac or respiratory event that would require urgent intervention without delay in care, but issues pertaining to airway or cervical spine would be treated emergently. The patients with the urinary condition and the laceration also need intervention, but they are not experiencing life-threatening issues at this time and would be treated after the patients with the airway problem and the cardiopulmonary event, respectively.

Cognitive level: Application

Nursing process: Planning

Client needs: Physiological Integrity

3. Answer: 4. Level IV – Nonurgent

Rationale: The patient's complaint is nontraumatic and chronic, having been an issue for 4 months. Also, the patient has sought previous medical treatment from his or her primary care provider, who now refuses to give the patient access to more prescription analgesics, and the triage assessment is benign. Because the patient's condition does not require immediate resuscitative efforts nor is the patient unstable, categorizing him or her as a Level I or Level II, respectively, would be inappropriate. The Level III category would also be incorrect in this case, because the patient does not have an urgent problem that requires timely intervention. Level IV, nonurgent, is the best choice for this patient in the four-level triage system.

Cognitive level: Application

Nursing process: Evaluation

Client needs: Physiological Integrity

4. Answer: 1. General consent and informed consent.

Rationale: Both general and informed consents should be obtained prior to this patient's treatment. The general consent would be for any treatment, such as evaluation by the staff, and noninvasive procedures, such as radiographs. The informed consent would be for the procedures of conscious sedation and reduction of the dislocation. This consent states that the patient has been fully informed about these procedures and their risks. Implied consent is used only in emergency situations when it is presumed that the patient would give permission for treatment if she or he were able. Blood product consent would be used prior to administration of any blood or blood products.

Cognitive level: Application

Nursing process: Implementation

Client needs: Physiological Integrity

5. Answer: 2. "I am glad that emergency nurses do not have to deal with obstetrical issues because they can call the labor and delivery nurses."

Rationale: Emergency nurses must be prepared for all types of emergencies, including obstetrical issues. Additional preparation for new graduates or nurses who are new to the field of emergency nursing should include instruction in psychiatric emergencies and trauma assessment. The Trauma Nursing Core Course is just one course that is recommended for these nurses. Time management and the ability to care for multiple patients simultaneously are also learned skills that are imperative to emergency nursing.

Cognitive level: Analysis

Nursing process: Evaluation

Client needs: Safe and Effective Care Environment

Chapter 74

1. Answer: 4. Spinal

Rationale: Spinal cord injury is commonly noted in patients following rear-impact motor vehicle crashes.

Cognitive level: Analysis

Nursing process: Assessment

Client needs: Physiological Integrity: Physiological Adaptation

2. Answer: 3. Utilize a rigid cervical collar to stabilize the cervical spine.

Rationale: When assessing and treating patients with trauma, the priorities of the primary survey must be recognized. The first priority is airway with simultaneous cervical spine immobilization. A rigid cervical collar is one way to stabilize the cervical spine in an emergent situation. Controlling bleeding should be performed during the circulation portion of the primary survey. This falls after the priority of airway and cervical spine treatment. A neurological exam would come after dealing with airway, cervical spine, and circulation. Although the patient may need a CT scan to determine if there is a head injury, this is not a priority initially. This intervention would be a portion of the secondary survey that is performed after the primary survey is complete.

Cognitive level: Application

Nursing process: Assessment

Client needs: Health Promotion and Maintenance: Prevention/Early Detection of Health Problems

3. Answer: 1. It will include a comprehensive medical record review to help ensure all injuries and treatments for the patient with trauma have been properly addressed.

Rationale: The tertiary trauma survey includes a comprehensive medical record review, repetition of the primary and secondary surveys, and reviews of all lab and radiologic results to help ensure that all injuries and treatments for the patient with trauma have been properly addressed. It is done within 24 hours of admission and repeated once the patient is awake, responsive, and able to communicate and helps to make certain that all injuries have been properly identified, catalogued, and treated. The Eastern Association for the Surgery of Trauma formed a work group to develop evidence-based guidelines for practice regarding the best and most important nutritional recommendations for the patient with trauma. The primary and secondary surveys provide a systematic approach to initial trauma assessment, helping the health care team identify injuries, provide appropriate interventions, and prioritize patient care. Trauma rehabilitation is a multidisciplinary plan of care developed to help increase the patient's quality of life and maximize the impaired patient's function by minimizing any deficits.

Cognitive level: Analysis

Nursing process: Planning

Client needs: Health Promotion and Maintenance: Prevention/Early Detection of Health Problems

4. Answer: 3. Assess for bleeding into the chest, abdomen, pelvis, or around long bones.

Rationale: Hemorrhage is the predominant cause of preventable death in the injured patient. During the primary survey, hypotension should be considered hypovolemic in origin until proven otherwise. If external hemorrhage is identified, measures to control the bleeding should be taken immediately. The easiest way to do this is to apply direct manual pressure on the wound.

The major sources of occult blood loss are hemorrhage into the chest or abdominal cavities, into the soft tissue surrounding a major long bone fracture, or into the retroperitoneal space from a pelvic fracture. Control of bleeding may require immediate operative intervention.

Cognitive level: Application

Nursing process: Assessment

Client needs: Physiological Integrity: Physiological Adaptation

GLOSSARY

12-lead ECG Standard surface ECG with 12 leads, 3 bipolar and 9 unipolar.

2,3-diphosphoglycerate (2,3-DPG) Substance produced by red blood cells during hypoxic states that sustains the deoxyhemoglobin configuration.

abdominojugular reflux An indicator of jugular venous distention that becomes visible as a result of the displacement of excess blood volume when the upper abdominal region is compressed.

abduction Movement of a body part away from the midline (center) of the body.

aberration Deviation from the normal.

ablation Destruction of a specific area of the myocardium through localized delivery of chemicals or electrical energy.

abortion The ending of a pregnancy before the age of fetal viability.

absolute iron deficiency Physiological state indicating insufficient amounts of total body iron.

absolute neutrophil count (ANC) A useful measurement that reveals that proportion of the white blood cells that can be utilized in first-response immune interactions; the most accurate measurement of circulating neutrophils within white blood cells.

absolute refractory period Period of time during which a cardiac cell is unable to respond to any stimulus and cannot spontaneously depolarize. Corresponds with the beginning of the QRS complex and ends at the peak of the T wave on an ECG tracing.

absorption The process by which a medication leaves the site of administration to cross membranes as it journeys to the site of action.

academic nurse educator A nurse who is responsible for designing, implementing, evaluating, and revising academic and continuing education programs for nurses.

accessory muscles The sternocleidomastoid, scalene, and trapezius muscles, which are normally not necessary to respiration, but are utilized by patients who require extra effort to move air in and out of the lungs.

accommodation (1) Process a child goes through to modify existing schema because the incorporation of new knowledge does not fit into existing schema. (2) The ability of the lens to focus up-close or near; to focus a clear image on the retina.

accreditation Process of evaluating an organization against performance standards.

acculturative stress Job-related stress that is exacerbated by cultural differences such as diverse assumptions, values, and beliefs among the participants.

acetylcholine A neurotransmitter critical to the process of memory formation.

achalasia A motor disorder of the esophagus that is characterized by failure of the lower esophageal sphincter to relax properly and by impaired peristalsis.

achlorhydria Lack of hydrochloric acid in the stomach.

acids Compounds in solution that have a pH of less than 7.40. They form hydrogen ion in solution and are proton donors.

acne vulgaris A chronic skin disorder with an increased production of sebum from the sebaceous glands and the formation of comedones that plug the pores.

acoustic neuroma A benign tumor of the eighth cranial (acoustic) nerve.

acquired immunity Type of immunity that occurs after birth and includes antibodies, immune-competent T cells and B cells, and cytokines that act to remove antigens that are considered non-self.

acquired immunodeficiency syndrome (AIDS) The disease resulting from infection by the human immunodeficiency virus; manifested by loss of T cells and opportunistic infections.

acromegaly A hypermetabolic condition of the pituitary gland, characterized by enlargement of the extremities, particularly the hands, feet, and other body parts such as the face, in which excess pituitary hormones (somatotropin and growth hormone) are secreted.

actinic keratosis A skin disorder caused by the sun that leads to proliferation of abnormal, dystrophic cells.

action potential Response of the resting membrane potential to a stimulus that exceeds the membrane threshold value. Carries signals along the muscle cell and conveys information from one cell to another, resulting in cardiac muscle depolarization.

active acquired immunity Type of immunity that involves the production of antibodies by the immune system in response to specific foreign antigens, such as bacteria. This immunity is considered acquired because the body develops the ability to regulate the immune system and produce antibodies after birth and after exposure to antigens in the environment, such as bacteria or viruses.

active immunization Immunization that involves the introduction of a live, killed, or attenuated toxin of a disease organism into the body. The immune system responds by producing antibodies.

activity theory of aging Theory of aging based on the premise that decreased activity later in life leads to meaninglessness and life dissatisfaction, and maintaining activity tends to increase life satisfaction.

acuity The measurement of severity of illness in a patient and the amount of nursing care required to care for the patient.

acute angle-closure glaucoma (AACG) Disorder characterized by the angle in the anterior chamber closing suddenly as a result of iris blockage; prevents aqueous flow through the trabecular meshwork, causing the intraocular pressure to rise suddenly, usually to greater than 40 mmHg.

acute bronchitis Inflammation of the tracheobronchial tree, usually in association with a respiratory infection.

acute care nurse A nurse who works with patients experiencing sudden illness or trauma, usually in the prehospital, hospital, or emergency department.

acute coronary syndrome (ACS) Syndrome collectively described by unstable angina, non–ST segment elevation myocardial infarction (MI), and ST segment elevation MI.

acute graft rejection A type IV cell-mediated immune response that occurs between 2 weeks and 1 month after transplant. This occurs when a recipient's T cells are activated against unmatched HLA antigens in the transplanted tissue.

acute lung injury (ALI) Sometimes used when referring to acute respiratory distress syndrome, but is less severe.

acute pain Pain of relatively short duration that coincides with injury, surgery, or illness.

acute pulmonary edema An abnormal accumulation of fluid in the lungs.

acute radiation syndrome An acute illness caused by irradiation of the whole body. The phases of the illness are prodromal, latent, illness, and recovery or death.

acute respiratory distress syndrome (ARDS) A progressive form of respiratory failure that leads to alveolar capillary inflammation and damage.

acute respiratory failure (ARF) A condition defined as a failure of gas exchange.

acute retroviral syndrome A group of generalized symptoms seen in some individuals during the period of primary infection with the human immunodeficiency virus (1 to 3 months). Symptoms include fever, malaise, lymphadenopathy, and skin rash.

acute stress A reaction to an immediate threat; commonly triggers the fight-or-flight response.

acute stressor One that is brief and involves a tangible threat that is readily identified as a stress.

acute wounds Recent wounds that are either traumatic or iatrogenic in etiology that progress through the stages of wound healing normally.

adaptation A reaction to stress that signifies that the person is able to cope with the stressor or change.

adapter Portion of a catheter that is used to affix infusion equipment to a vascular access device. Also known as the *hub*.

Addisonian crisis (adrenal crisis) A rare, life-threatening disease in which a deficiency of adrenal hormones is exacerbated by stress or trauma.

Addison's disease A rare condition caused by severe or total deficiency of hormones produced by the adrenal cortex.

add-on devices Any extra equipment such as filters, stopcocks, extensions, connectors, and injection ports or caps added to the primary intervenous set.

adduction Movement of a body part toward the midline (center) of the body.

adenomatous polyps Polyps that result from a mutation on chromosome 5. They are long thin projections of tissue arising from the mucosal epithelium and are considered premalignant tissue. Most colorectal cancers develop from this type of polyp.

adjuvant medications Medications that are not primarily indicated for treatment of pain, but are used to augment pain relief medications.

administration set Infusion-specific tubing that delivers parenteral fluid via a sterile pathway from its container to the patient via a vascular access device.

adrenal insufficiency Condition in which the body fails to produce an adequate amount of adrenal hormones.

advanced practice nurse (APRN) A nurse who has been trained to practice beyond the scope defined for a registered nurse by the state nurse practice act. Advanced practice nurses are qualified through postgraduate education and practice through the use of standardized procedures or by indirect supervision of a physician.

advanced practice nursing Specialized type of nursing practice in which nurses diagnose and treat illnesses and provide health care. Most advanced practice nurses are also certified to prescribe medication.

adventitious breath sounds Abnormal lung sound indicating a pathologic process.

adverse drug event (ADE) Noxious and unintended patient event caused by a drug accompanied by various symptoms, signs, and laboratory abnormalities.

adverse drug reaction (ADR) *See* adverse drug event (ADE).

aerophagia The swallowing of air; may lead to intestinal bloating.

affective dimension of pain Describes the emotions patients assign to their pain.

affective learning Involves changes in attitudes, values, and feelings.

afferent Ability to transport toward a center; for example, a sensory nerve that carries impulses from the peripheral nervous system to the central nervous system.

afterload The amount of pressure or resistance the ventricles must overcome to eject blood during systole.

agglutination The surrounding and attaching of antibodies to an antigen, causing the antigens to clump together and stimulate the immune cells to locate the complex and consume it or destroy it.

aging The process of growing old and maturing.

agonist Opioid that is often referred to as morphine-like, or as a mu agonist, because it binds to the mu, kappa, and delta receptors of cells located in the central nervous system, peripheral nervous system, and the gastrointestinal tract.

agonist-antagonist Opioid that is a kappa- or mu-receptor partial agonist; generally considered to be less efficacious than a pure mu agonist.

AIDS indicator conditions Indicates an HIV-infected individual has been diagnosed with opportunistic infections such as *Pneumocystis carinii* pneumonia or AIDS-defining cancer, such as Kaposi's sarcoma, or that the individual's CD4 count has fallen below 200 mL/μL.

air conduction Process of sound waves reaching the inner ear for interpretation.

air embolism Obstruction of a blood vessel by an air bubble.

air-mask-bag unit (AMBU) A device used to deliver oxygen via a mask when a patient is not adequately ventilating or oxygenating.

airway obstruction Obstruction that occurs most often because medications used in anesthesia cause the muscles to relax.

akinesia Condition characterized by areas of abnormal heart contractility where there is loss of or no muscle movement.

alanine aminotransferase (ALT) An enzyme released from hepatocytes when liver injury occurs.

albumin A commercially prepared product that is derived from the plasma portion of blood.

aldosterone A hormone secreted by the adrenal cortex in response to the conversion of angiotensinogen to angiotensin II. Aldosterone causes sodium reabsorption from the renal tubules and thus causes the body to retain water.

alkaline phosphatase (ALP) An enzyme found mostly in the liver and bone. It is released when liver injury or inflammation occurs and when abnormal osteoblastic activity is present in the bone.

alkalis Compounds in solution that have a pH of greater than 7.40, which is caused by either an increase of base/alkali or a loss of acid. There is more base and less acid, thus raising the 20:1 ratio of bicarbonate to carbonic acid.

allele An alternate or variant form of a gene. On a gene pair, one allele is inherited from the father and the other allele from the mother. The maternal and paternal alleles may be identical or homozygous or they may be different forms of the same gene (heterozygous).

Allen's test Test performed prior to arterial line insertion to test the patency of the palmar arch.

allergen An antigen, or protein, from the external environment. Common allergens include dust, food, pollen, and pet dander.

allergic rhinitis Inflammation of the nasal mucosa caused by an allergic substance such as pollen.

allergy A form of type I hypersensitivity reaction that occurs when an external antigen, or allergen, attaches to IgE antibodies. IgE antibodies attach to mast cells and result in degranulation and release of histamine. Symptoms are the result of the activity of histamine.

allogeneic bone marrow Bone marrow from a histocompatible donor.

allograft Grafting of skin to a wound that was harvested from human cadavers.

allograft valve A valve obtained from human cadaver donations; used primarily to replace the aortic and pulmonic valves. Also called a *homograft valve*.

alloimmune response A hypersensitivity response of the immune system to antigens from another human; usually occurs when tissue is transplanted or grafted.

allopathic medicine Method of treating disease with remedies that produce effects different from those caused by the disease itself.

alopecia Loss of hair, which can be a result of familial patterns of baldness, disease, medications, or a pathologic condition.

alpha-amylase An enzyme mainly in the pancreas; aids in the digestion of carbohydrates.

alternative therapy A therapy used instead of conventional or mainstream therapy. Also called *unconventional therapy*.

alveolar ventilation (V_A) The cumulative gas exchange that takes place within each alveolus.

Alzheimer's disease (AD) A chronic, progressive, irreversible brain disorder found most frequently in adults age 65 and older.

amblyopia Disorder in which a person has an eye with decreased or impaired vision with no obvious anatomic explanation, usually from childhood. Also known by the lay term *lazy eye*.

ametropia A general term used to indicate a refractive error that can usually be corrected with glasses, contact lenses, or possibly refractive surgery.

amputation Surgical removal of an anatomic part.

amyotrophic lateral sclerosis (ALS) A rare, progressive neurological disease characterized by loss of motor neurons.

anal canal The last part of the large intestine situated between the rectum and the anus. It is about 2.5 to 4 cm long.

analog A compound that is structurally similar to another with some slight differences in composition.

analytical preciseness Measure of how findings emerge from the data, how the data collection process is made flexible, and how themes emerge from the data.

anaphylaxis A severe form of type I hypersensitivity response that is systemic. Symptoms can include hives, severe bronchoconstriction, and loss of airway.

anasarca Total body edema.

anatomic dead space Area in the transporting airways or upper airways and bronchi that results when no gas exchange occurs. The amount of the tidal volume taken in that remains in the trachea and bronchi. The amount of anatomic dead space can be estimated as 1 mL per pound of ideal body weight. A person with an ideal body weight of 150 pounds has an anatomic dead space of about 150 mL.

androgenetic alopecia Physiological baldness in which androgen levels are normal; however, there is a genetic predisposition to balding.

androgenic alopecia Loss of hair related to excessive androgen production that causes a decrease in size of the hair follicles, leading to hair loss in central and frontal areas.

andropause A decrease in testosterone associated with aging.

anemia Disorder that results when the total body red blood cell volume is decreased; usually measured by hemoglobin, hematocrit, and red blood cell count.

anemic hypoxia Physiological state of decreased oxygen availability due to decreased concentration of hemoglobin or red blood cells.

anergy Impaired or absent ability to react to common antigens.

aneuploidy Having too many or too few chromosomes in a cell or any number other than 46 chromosomes in somatic or body cells or other than 23 chromosomes in germ cells or the eggs and sperm.

aneurysm Localized diseased segment of an artery that becomes thin and dilated because of degenerative changes in the tunica media layer.

angina pectoris Transient chest pain due to myocardial ischemia.

angiogenesis Process in which stimulated endothelial cells multiply and form tubular structures differentiating into arterioles or venules.

anion A negatively charged ion.

anion gap Represents the concentration of all unmeasured anions in plasma. It is comprised of negatively charged proteins as well as the acid anions produced during metabolism such as lactate. It is calculated by subtracting the sum of the chloride and bicarbonate levels from the sodium level, and its reference range is 8 to 16 mEq.

anisocoria Inequality of the size of the pupils; may be congenital or associated with aneurysms, head trauma, diseases of the nervous system, brain lesion, paresis, or locomotor ataxia.

ankle-brachial index (ABI) Ratio of arterial pressure at the ankle to the pressure at the brachial artery; used to predict the severity of peripheral arterial disease that may be present. A decrease in the ABI result with exercise is a sensitive indicator that significant pulmonary arterial disease is probably present.

ankylosing spondylitis A type of arthritis that affects the spine and the sacroiliac joint.

annuloplasty A surgery done to correct valve regurgitation by repairing the enlarged annulus.

annulus The fibrous ring at the junction of the cardiac valve leaflets and the muscular wall.

anorexia Loss of appetite.

anorgasmia Difficulty reaching orgasm.

anosmia The loss or impairment of the sense of smell.

antagonist Substance that displaces and replaces an opioid at the receptor, reversing the opioid's pharmacologic effect and side effects such as respiratory depression.

anterior circulation Describes the areas of the brain supplied by the right and left carotid arteries and their branches, including circulation in the arteries in the anterior portion of the circle of Willis.

anteriorly Front plane of the body.

anthropometric measurements Any physical measurement of the body.

antibody Proteins made by B cells and found in the plasma that are capable of attaching to antigens and stimulating immune responses.

antidiuretic hormone (ADH) A small peptide molecule released by the pituitary gland at the base of the brain. It has an antidiuretic action that prevents the production of dilute urine.

antigen Any foreign substance (bacterium, virus, protein) that elicits an immune response.

antigen–antibody complex The attachment of the FAB portion of an antibody to an antigen, resulting in the stimulation of a strong immune response; each FAB portion of the antibody is specifically shaped for only one type of antigen. Attracts other phagocytic cells such as neutrophils and macrophages to help eliminate the antigen; stimulates creation of B memory cells for long-term protection.

antigenicity The ability of a pathogen to elicit an immune defense in its host. It affects the ability of the host to develop a long-term immunity.

anti-infectives Drugs that are used to treat infections and include antibiotics, antivirals, and antifungals.

antiplatelet therapy Therapy that inhibits platelet adhesion and aggregation.

antrum Any nearly closed cavity or chamber.

anuria Total loss of urine production.

aortic coarctation Narrowing of the lumen of the aorta.

aortic dissection (AD) Weakening of the layers inside the aorta, which can result in tears in the aortic wall and leakage of blood into the chest or abdomen.

aortic valve regurgitation Incomplete closure of the aortic valve, which causes blood to regurgitate back into the left ventricle through a valve; results from abnormal valve cusps or aortic root.

aortic valve stenosis A narrowing of the aortic valve orifice, which results in an obstruction to blood flow from the left ventricle to the aorta during systole.

apathetic Indifferent; showing a lack of emotion.

aphasia The disorder of speech and language due to cerebral dysfunction. The three primary aphasic deficits are in comprehension of spoken language, expressive language, and naming.

apheresis A technology in which the blood of a donor or patient is passed through a machine that separates out one specific particle and returns the remainder of the blood to circulation.

aphonic Without a voice.

aphthous stomatitis (contact stomatitis) A common ulcerative condition limited to the oral cavity. Also known as *canker sores*.

apnea Cessation of airflow for more than 10 seconds.

apoptosis Programmed cell death in a multicellular organism; process by which cells can self-destruct when infected or mutated.

applied research Research that focuses on finding solutions to existing problems.

apudomas A rare tumor of the islets of Langerhans in the pancreas.

areflexia Loss of reflexive activity.

arrhythmogenic right ventricular cardiomyopathy (ARVC) An electrical disturbance that develops when the muscle tissue in the right ventricle is replaced with fibrous scar and fatty tissues.

arterial line An indwelling catheter inserted into an artery in order to monitor blood pressure.

arterial-venous shunts Shunts placed using surgical anastomosis of venous and arterial structures to facilitate dialysis procedures.

arteriosclerosis Thickening, reduced elasticity, and calcification of arterial walls.

arteriovenous malformation (AVM) A mass of abnormal blood vessels in which arterial blood flows directly into the venous system.

arthrodesis Surgical fusion of bone.

arthroplasty Restoration of a joint either by total joint replacement surgery or by resurfacing bone and removing damaged bone and cartilage.

artifact An ECG pattern from sources outside the heart; creates an abnormal pattern on ECG graph paper. This interference causes the baseline or isoelectric line to become fuzzy; this fuzzy baseline is referred to as 60 cycle.

asbestosis Diffuse lung fibrosis caused by exposure to asbestos.

ascites An abnormal intraperitoneal accumulation of fluid containing large amounts of protein and electrolytes.

aspartate aminotransferase (AST) An enzyme found in the liver, heart, skeletal muscle, and kidneys that is released when cellular injury occurs.

asphyxiates Chemical agents that cause injury, illness, and death by damaging the lungs. Also called *choking agents*.

assault Any action that places another person in apprehension of being touched in a manner that is offensive, insulting, or physically injurious without consent or authority.

assessment The act of evaluating or appraising.

assignment The transfer of a task and the accountability for the outcome.

assimilation Incorporation of new concepts into existing schemas.

assisted living A residential setting in which patients are provided long-term assisted care.

assistive device Device required by a patient to assist with ambulation (e.g., cane, crutches, walker).

associate caregiver An LVN/LPN or unlicensed assistive personnel assigned to provide care to patients according to the plan established by the primary nurse.

associate nurse A registered nurse who assists the primary nurse during off-duty hours and provides care consistent with the plan developed by the primary nurse.

asterixis A flapping tremor of the hands when the arms are outstretched; believed to be caused by the accumulation of substances normally detoxified by the liver.

asthma A disease with multiple precipitating factors resulting in reversible airflow obstruction.

astigmatism An optical defect.

asymmetry Unequal.

asystole Complete termination of ventricular activity with no measurable cardiac electrical activity. Represents cardiac standstill from massive cardiac muscle damage.

ataxia A failure of muscle coordination, resulting in loss of balance and coordination, as well as speech difficulties including dysarthria or slurred and scanning speech.

atelectasis Collapse or airless condition of the alveoli caused by hypoventilation and obstruction of airways by secretions.

atherogenesis The development of atherosclerosis.

atheroma Condition characterized by an accumulation in the inner lining of an artery of a plaque of cholesterol and other constituents.

atherosclerosis A type of arteriosclerosis; the most common etiologic process that causes reduced myocardial blood flow.

atopic dermatitis A chronic inflammatory skin disorder characterized by dry skin related to water loss in the epidermis and decreased skin lipid levels.

atrial dysrhythmia Dysrhythmia that generally results from an irritable focus in the atria that fires off an electrical impulse before the SA node has had a chance to fire in a normal fashion. Results in a P-wave

configuration on the ECG that is different from that of a normal P wave; however, the QRS complex is normal.

atrial fibrillation A disorganized, very rapid, and irregular atrial rhythm resulting in an irregular ventricular rhythm. The rhythm is usually described as either course or fine fibrillation.

atrial flutter A rapid, regular atrial rhythm with a rate of about 300 beats per minute. Only a fraction of the impulses are transmitted through the AV node as a protective mechanism. Most of the atrial beats fall during the refractory period of the AV node so they are not conducted.

atrial kick Atrial contraction, which augments the blood supply going to the ventricles and ultimately cardiac output.

atrial natriuretic peptide (ANP) A hormone secreted by the right atrium in response to fluid overload that causes the excretion of sodium, which results in loss of the excess fluid; however, most regulation of excess volume is through decreased aldosterone secretion.

atrioventricular (AV) node Node located on the floor of the right atrium just above the tricuspid valve. The AV node has three regions: the AV junctional tissue between the atria and the node; the nodal area between the junctional tissue and the bundle of His; and the AV junction, the region where the AV node joins the bundle of His.

atrophy A reduction in the size of a cell and tissues or in muscle size.

auscultation Technique of listening to the sounds produced by different body areas.

autoantibodies An antibody produced in response to a self protein. Antinuclear antibodies, antibodies that bind to the nucleus of cells and result in cell destruction, are one example of autoantibodies.

autoantibody tests Tests that measure the amount or presence of antibodies to self proteins. Examples include the antinuclear antibody test and anti-IgG serum test.

autocrine functioning Secretion of cells that act to influence only their own growth.

autograft valve Valve obtained from the patient's own pulmonic valve and pulmonary artery. Also called *autologous valve*.

autografting Grafting of the patient's own skin to somewhere else on the patient's body.

autoimmune diseases Diseases that result from hypersensitivity responses and produce tissue damage and destruction. Examples include Goodpasture's syndrome and systemic lupus erythematosus; in both of these diseases, tissue is damaged by the production of antibodies to self-antigens.

autoimmune hemolytic anemia Red blood cell disorder characterized by destruction of cells by antibodies of the host.

autoimmune response Occurs when the body fails to recognize self cells or proteins and mounts an immune response against the self. Autoantibodies result in immune complexes that stimulate phagocytosis and destruction of cells and tissue.

autologous BMT Procedure in which bone marrow is collected from the patient and frozen. It is then reinfused into the patient following high-dose chemotherapy, with or without radiation.

autologous transfusion The process of collecting and reinfusing a patient's own blood.

automated external defibrillator (AED) A small, lightweight device that can recognize and treat ventricular fibrillation.

automaticity Ability of pacemaker cells to generate their own electrical impulses without depending on nervous system stimulation external to the heart.

autonomic hyperreflexia A syndrome characterized by severe hypertension, bradycardia, vasoconstriction below the level of injury, and vasodilation above the level of injury resulting from unchecked stimulation of the sympathetic nervous system triggered by a noxious stimulus.

autonomy Personal freedom to make choices or decisions.

autoregulation The ability of the brain to change its vessel size to accommodate changes in intracranial pressure.

autosomal dominant inheritance A Mendelian pattern of inheritance in which an affected individual has one copy of a mutant allele and one normal allele. Individuals who have autosomal dominant disorders have a 50–50 chance of passing the mutant allele and disorder to their children. This is in contrast to autosomal recessive disorders in which the individual must have two copies of the mutant allele.

autosomal recessive inheritance A Mendelian pattern of inheritance in which an affected individual receives two copies of a mutant allele, one from each parent, or the phenotype is expressed only when two copies of the mutant allele are present.

autosome A single chromosome from any 1 of 22 pairs of the chromosomes that is not a sex chromosome (XX or XY). Disorders caused by mutation in an autosomal gene or gene pair shows autosomal inheritance.

AV dissociation Independent function of the atria and the ventricles.

avascular necrosis (AVN) Condition in which bone tissue dies due to a temporary or permanent loss of blood supply to the bone.

avulsion fracture Fracture that occurs when a ligament is pulled away from its attachment point at the bone and takes a small piece of the bone with it.

azotemia An increase in blood urea nitrogen (BUN) caused when the kidneys are unable to excrete normally.

B cells White blood cells that are produced in the bone marrow and develop into plasma cells that are responsible for the creation and release of antibodies and development of long-term immune protection.

B lymphocytes Type of white blood cell that make antibodies against antigens, perform the role of antigen in presenting cells, and eventually develop into memory cells after activation by antigen interaction.

Bachmann bundle Part of the electrical conduction system of the heart composed of a group of interatrial fibers contained in the left atrium that conduct electrical impulses from the SA node to the left atrium.

bacterial meningitis Inflammation of the meninges caused by a bacterial pathogen.

bacterial phlebitis Inflammation of a vein associated with an infectious process.

bacterial vaginosis (BV) The most common bacterial infection in women of childbearing age. The cause is not clearly understood.

barium enema Type of enema used to obtain an x-ray of the large intestines. Radiographs are taken after the patient receives barium sulphate through an enema tube.

barotrauma Alveoli damage caused by the increased pressure resulting from use of a ventilator. Physical injury or rupture of tympanic membrane, resulting from changing air pressure.

Barrett's epithelium Columnar epithelial tissue that replaces the normal squamous epithelium in the esophagus after prolonged exposure to gastric juice. It is resistant to gastric acid, supports the healing of the esophagus, and is premalignant.

basal skull fracture A fracture of the skull that extends into the base of the skull.

base excess Part of the blood gas report, this is a calculated value that is based on the bicarbonate and carbon dioxide levels and the hematocrit. It expresses the number of milliequivalents of bicarbonate per liter of extracellular fluid that one has too much of (a base excess) or too little of (a base deficit). It is used as a guide by clinicians as they consider how much bicarbonate to administer to a patient with a severe metabolic acidosis.

basement membrane A thin, acellular layer between the dermis and epidermis that acts as scaffolding for the epidermis. Blood supply and nutrients reach the epidermis by passing through the basement membrane.

bases Compounds that combine with hydrogen ion in solution. A proton acceptor.

basic human needs As defined by Abraham Maslow, needs on the first four rungs of Maslow's hierarchy.

basic research Research undertaken to extend the knowledge base in a discipline or to formulate or refine a theory.

basophil A component of the white blood cell differential; actual function is not well known.

battery Contact with another or with another's immediate "personage" (clothes, car keys, cane, purse, etc.) without consent or authority; the touching of another without permission.

Battle's sign Bogginess of the temporal or postauricular region of the head, which indicates fracture of the basilar area of the skull.

Beck's triad Classic assessment findings for the patient with cardiac tamponade, consisting of decreased blood pressure, muffled heart sounds, and jugular venous distention.

behavioral dimension of pain Includes responses to pain that may be situational, developmental, or learned.

beneficence The ethical duty to do good.

benign Lacking malignant cells.

benign prostatic hyperplasia (BPH) Term applied to age-related benign enlargement of the prostate gland where there is no cancerous growth involved.

berry aneurysm Saccular-shaped aneurysm.

bevel The slanted or angled part of a needle or stylet.

Bier block Process in which an IV catheter is inserted in the extremity at the most distal site possible. A pneumatic tourniquet is applied proximal to the surgical site and inflated higher than the patient's systolic blood pressure. When a local anesthetic (lidocaine) is injected intravenously, the obstruction of blood by the tourniquet prevents it from leaving the surgical area.

bigeminy Premature ventricular contraction that occurs every other beat.

bile A substance produced in the liver containing bile salts, cholesterol, bilirubin, electrolytes, and water. It is concentrated and stored in the gallbladder, where it is released in response to a meal to aid in the emulsification and absorption of dietary fat.

bile canaliculi Small channels adjacent to the hepatocytes that move bile toward the common bile duct.

biliary dyskinesia Motility disorders of the gallbladder.

bilirubin A product in the breakdown of hemoglobin. It is conjugated by the hepatocytes and is excreted in bile.

binge-eating disorder (BED) Disorder characterized by the same type of binge eating as bulimia nervosa, but without the compensatory purging.

bioavailable Pertaining to a molecular form that can be readily used by the body.

bioavailable testosterone Free testosterone and testosterone that is loosely bound to albumin.

biologic agent Viruses, bacteria, and toxins that can be weaponized to cause disease, illness, and/or death.

biologic aging theory General theory of aging comprised of programmed theories and error theories. *See error theories of aging and programmed theory of aging.*

biologic dressing Heterografts such as pigskin or allografts obtained from living or deceased humans.

biologic valve Valve obtained from other species, most commonly from pigs (porcine valves), although cow valves (bovine) also are used. Also referred to as *xenografts*.

biopsy A portion of tissue examined for the presence of abnormal cells.

biosynthetic dressing A combination of biologic and synthetic materials that are effective as temporary covering for a variety of wounds.

biotherapy Treatment with agents whose origin, mostly mammal, is from biologic sources and/or affecting biologic responses.

biotransformation The process of changing a medication's structure in preparation for elimination. Metabolism occurs primarily in the liver, but also in the kidneys and, to a very small degree, other organ systems. Once a medication is metabolized, it is no longer the same and effectively discontinues its pharmacologic activity.

BiPAP Stands for *bi-level positive airway pressure*, which is a breathing apparatus that helps people get more air into their lungs. The air is delivered through a mask that can be set at two different pressures, one for inhaling (IPAP or inspiratory positive airway pressure) and another for exhaling (EPAP or expiratory airway pressure).

biphasic defibrillation Defibrillation procedure that delivers a charge in one direction for half of the shock and in the opposite direction for the second half.

bipolar lead ECG leads that have electrodes with opposite polarity, one positive and one negative.

biventricular heart failure A global inability of the heart muscle to pump blood effectively from both ventricles, compromising forward flow leading to right and left heart failure symptoms.

blackouts Amnesia for short-term events; can occur in patients with alcohol abuse problems.

bladder suspension A procedure designed to correct urinary incontinence. It is done to suspend the bladder and correct urinary incontinence that is often caused by weakened ligaments due to childbirth. Also called a *Burch procedure*.

blepharoplasty Surgical procedure to fix ptosis or drooping of the eyelid.

blister agent Chemical agent that can cause redness and irritation of the skin and blistering. Also called a *vesicant*.

blood pressure The pressure created by blood circulating through the arteries and veins and the chambers of the heart.

blood transfusion The process of infusing blood products in order to restore circulating volume and therefore increase oxygen carrying capacity.

blunt percussion Technique of placing the palm of the nondominant hand over a body area (such as the kidney) and striking the palm with the closed fist of the dominant hand.

bone conduction Process of sound vibrations reaching the inner ear for interpretation.

bone marrow transplantation Procedure in which hematopoietic cells from the bone marrow of one person are transferred into another person; used to treat a variety of diseases.

Botox Botulism toxin that has been purified and is injected into the lower esophageal sphincter to relax the muscle.

Bouchard's nodes Hard, painless nodules at the joints of the fingers; may indicate osteoarthritis (progressive loss of cartilage at a joint). Bouchard's nodes are found over the proximal interphalangeal joints.

boutonnière deformity Flexion of the proximal interphalangeal joint.

Bowman's capsule A thin, double-walled capsule encasing the glomerulus.

brachytherapy The use of localized radiation within the coronary artery to increase the size of the lumen of the artery.

bradykinesia Slowed movement; primary symptom of Parkinson's disease.

bradypnea A respiratory rate of less than 12 breaths per minute.

brain abscess A localized infection carried from other sites of the body and extending into the cerebral tissue.

breach of confidentiality Failure to prevent the disclosure of all or parts of a patient's medical record without the proper authority to do so.

breakthrough pain A transitory exacerbation of pain that occurs on a background of otherwise stable pain in a patient receiving chronic opioid therapy.

breast cancer The formation of a malignant glandular tumor, which over time destroys normal breast tissue and can spread to other parts of the body.

Brief Pain Inventory (BPI) Questionnaire that asks multiple questions regarding pain and its impact on patient function and addresses the multidimensionality of the pain experience.

bronchial breath sounds Breath sounds normally heard over the right or left bronchus of the lung.

bronchovesicular breath sounds Breath sounds normally heard between the bronchus and the smaller airways.

bruits The sound heard with a stethoscope of blood flowing through a narrowed blood vessel that is outside of the heart.

bubo Acutely swollen and usually painful lymph node seen in plague near the site of the flea bite.

Buck's boots traction A foam boot used for traction.

buffer A compound that minimizes the change in hydrogen ion concentration (and also the pH) when ions are added to or removed from solution. Think of a buffer as a sponge. When there is too much hydrogen ion, the sponge soaks up the extra. When the level of hydrogen ion is decreased, the sponge can be squeezed out to return hydrogen ions to the blood.

bundle branch block Discontinuity of conduction (complete or incomplete) in one branch of the bundle of His that affects normal transmission of the impulse through the ventricles. When one bundle is blocked, the ventricles depolarize asynchronously. Characterized by a delay of excitation to one ventricle; therefore, an abnormal spread of electrical activity through the ventricles occurs.

bundle of His Part of the conduction system that lies on top of the interventricular septum, between the right and left ventricles; it contains pacemaker cells. Also referred to as the *common bundle*.

bursae Sac containing synovial fluid that cushions joints during movement.

burst fracture Fracture that occurs when an axial load is placed on the spine and vertebrae.

cachexia Wasting of skeletal muscle and adipose.

café-au-lait spot Pigmented macules that are light brown in color.

calciphylaxis A condition during severe serum calcium excess, as in renal failure, in which calcium is deposited into the soft tissues of the body. This can be reflected in irregular purple lesions on the lower extremities that may lead to necrosis and gangrene.

calcium The most abundant cation in the body, primarily found in bones and teeth. Serum calcium plays a role in neuromuscular transmission (including cardiac) and cell membrane permeability. Normal serum levels are 8.5 to 10.5 mg/dL, 50% ionized and 40% bound to albumin.

caloric test Assesses abnormal nystagmus, tinnitus, or hearing loss as a result of vestibular dysfunction from eighth cranial nerve lesions by inserting water into the ear.

cancellous (trabecular) bone Bone with a hard outer casing and an interior that is porous, spongy, and meshwork-like in structure.

cancer Common term for all malignant neoplasms.

cancer pain Pain associated with malignancy; can be acute and chronic in nature.

candidiasis A common fungal infection caused by the *Candida* species of fungus; more commonly known as a yeast infection.

capnography Use of a device to measure exhaled or end-tidal carbon dioxide.

capture Term used to indicate that sufficient voltage has been put out by a pacemaker to make a myocardial contraction occur.

caput medusae A term used to describe the engorged, tortuous, and visible blood vessels radiating from the umbilicus in patients with severe liver disorders. In mythology, Medusa's hair was a tangle of snakes.

carbon dioxide An atmospheric gas composed of one carbon atom and two oxygen atoms. Produced as a by-product of metabolism, carbon dioxide can be thought of as a potential acid because, when it is dissolved in water, it forms carbonic acid.

carbon monoxide poisoning Occurs when an individual breathes carbon monoxide fumes that have built up in an enclosed space.

carbonic acid A weak acid formed by water reacting with carbon dioxide. If carbonic acid loses one proton, it becomes the bicarbonate ion.

carboxypeptidase An enzyme that breaks away the end amino acids on protein molecules.

carbuncle An infection of the skin composed of a cluster of boils caused by *Staphylococcus aureus*.

carcinoembryonic antigen (CEA) A glycoprotein found in embryonic gastrointestinal epithelium, but also found in tumors of the adult gastrointestinal tract. It is used to detect colon cancer, most specifically adenocarcinoma.

carcinogenesis Pertaining to the production of cancer.

carcinoma *in situ* Disorder in which neoplasms have not invaded the basement membrane of the epithelial site, thus the surrounding tissues are left untouched by malignant cells.

cardia The upper orifice of the stomach connecting with the esophagus.

cardiac catheterization A term used to describe a variety of invasive procedures used to identify atherosclerotic disease as well as provide anatomic and hemodynamic information about the heart and great vessels using radiopaque catheters.

cardiac conduction system Conduction system unique to the myocardium that is composed of specialized cells that enable it to generate and transmit action potentials without stimulation from the nervous system. The specialized cells are concentrated in the sinoatrial and atrioventricular nodes, and the Purkinje network.

cardiac depolarization Muscle contraction of the heart resulting from electrolyte exchange in the cardiac cells.

cardiac index (CI) Individualized measurement of cardiac output by taking into account the body surface area.

cardiac output (CO) The amount of blood leaving the left ventricle per minute.

cardiac pacemaker An electronic device that is capable of delivering an electrical stimulus to the heart.

cardiac repolarization Process whereby a depolarized cell is polarized, causing a return to the resting membrane potential. Also referred to as the recovery phase that every cardiac cell must go through in order to be ready to accept another stimulus.

cardiac resynchronization therapy (CRT) Therapy that uses atrial-synchronized biventricular pacemakers.

cardiac risk factors Habits, lifestyles, and/or genetic factors that predispose an individual to the development of coronary artery disease.

cardiac tamponade Bleeding into the pericardial sac. As the accumulation of blood increases, it compresses the atria and ventricles decreasing venous return and filling pressure, which leads to decreased cardiac output, myocardial hypoxia, and cardiac failure.

cardioesophageal Pertaining to the junction of the esophagus and the stomach.

cardiogenic embolism Blood clots from cardiac sources.

cardiogenic pulmonary edema (CPE) An abnormal accumulation of fluid in the lungs caused by cardiac failure; results from increased hydrostatic pressures in the pulmonary capillary bed secondary to increased pulmonary venous pressure.

cardiomegaly Enlargement of the heart.

cardiomyopathies (CMPs) Diseases of the myocardial muscle fibers that result in progressive structural and functional abnormalities of the myocardium.

cardioversion The timed delivery of an electrical current to depolarize cardiac muscle in order to terminate tachyarrhythmias, atrial tachycardia, rapid atrial fibrillation, atrial flutter, and junctional tachycardia.

caring The core of nursing; constitutes the essence of nursing regardless of the level at which nursing is practiced.

carotid endarterectomy (CEA) Surgical procedure to correct carotid stenosis by opening the carotid artery, removing plaque, and restoring blood flow in the lumen.

carpal tunnel syndrome Compression of the median nerve in the carpal tunnel, just below the palm dorsally.

carrier People or animals that do not have symptoms of infection but carry an active pathogenic microorganism.

case management An approach to coordinating care for patients in the hospital or in an outpatient setting.

case manager A person who collaboratively plans, coordinates, and evaluates services for cost effectiveness, but does not provide direct patient care.

case method A nursing care delivery system in which total patient care is delivered by a registered nurse who has shift responsibility for the patient.

cast A rigid circumferential encasement device made of plaster or fiberglass.

cataracts The opacity of the natural crystalline lens.

catheter A device that is introduced through the skin, into the vascular network, for the purpose of infusing parenteral solutions and medications.

catheter embolism Occurs when a piece of catheter is fractured and enters the circulatory system. The catheter may block a major vein, causing loss of circulation, or may travel to the heart, causing cardiac irritability and cardiac arrest.

cation A positively charged ion. Major cations affecting cardiac function are potassium (K), sodium (Na), and calcium (Ca).

cauda equina syndrome The bundle of nerve roots in the lower portion of the spinal canal, below the conus medullaris, which when compressed or inflamed causes symptoms of pain, altered reflexes, decreased strength, and decreased sensation. When extreme, can cause paralysis of the lower extremities, bowel and bladder dysfunction, and loss of the Achilles reflex; most commonly seen with large disk herniations at L_4/L_5, causing mass effect on the nerve roots as they descend through the spinal canal.

cavernous malformation Low-flow, cluster-type nodular lesion, not separated by brain tissue.

CBRNE Acronym suggested for common use by the Department of Justice to describe weapons of mass destruction. The acronym stands for chemical, biologic, radiologic, nuclear, and explosive devices.

CD4+ T cells T lymphocytes with cluster of differentiation 4 (CD4) receptors. The HIV particle can attach and enter T-helper (CD4) cells via the CD4 receptor.

celiac disease An autoimmune disorder involving a sensitivity to gluten, a protein found in wheat, that results in an immune-mediated response that causes a histologic change in the villi of the small intestine, resulting in malabsorption.

celiac sprue A lifelong condition affecting the small intestine in which the villi morphology is damaged because of the presence of gluten in the diet.

cell-mediated immune response Immune responses that are initiated through specific antigen recognition by the T cells; important in identifying and destroying cells that are already infected and providing protection against fungi, and has major involvement in rejection of transplant tissues, tumor immunity, and hypersensitivity reactions.

cellulitis A diffuse inflammatory process of the dermis and subcutaneous tissue layers characterized by erythema, edema, and pain; usually caused by staphylococcus or streptococcus infections.

Centers for Disease Control and Prevention (CDC) Agency under the U.S. Department of Health and Human Services whose function is to protect the health and safety of the public with regard to disease prevention and control.

central retinal artery occlusion (CRAO) Blockage of the central retinal artery, usually by an embolism. Its symptom is sudden, painless, unilateral blindness.

central vascular access device (CVAD) A vascular access device that is inserted into a centrally located vein with the tip residing in the vena cava.

central venous pressure (CVP) Measurement of venous return to the right atrium after insertion of a central venous catheter.

centromere The narrowed portion near the center of a human chromosome where the two sister chromatids or spindle traction fibers attach during mitosis or meiosis.

cerebral aneurysm A balloon-like outpouching, or widening, of an artery.

cerebral blood flow (CBF) The measurement of blood flow in the brain.

cerebral edema An increase in water content of the brain; swelling.

cerebral infarction A condition in which brain tissue dies due to lack of oxygen.

cerebral ischemia A condition in which brain tissue is oxygen deprived.

cerebral perfusion pressure (CPP) The pressure gradient that drives cerebral blood flow.

cerebral salt wasting Electrolyte abnormality characterized by loss of sodium and loss of extracellular fluid volume.

certified nurse midwife (CNM) An advanced practice nurse with postgraduate training and state certification to deliver healthy babies without direct supervision by a physician.

certified registered nurse anesthetist (CRNA) An advanced practice nurse with postgraduate training and state certification to administer anesthesia without direct supervision by a physician.

cerumen Earwax.

chain of infection Consists of a causative agent, reservoir, portal of exit, mode of transmission, portal of entry, and susceptible host.

Chance fracture A fracture through the body and posterior elements of the vertebrae of the spine; caused by forward flexion, causing a distraction injury.

chancres Ulcers of syphilis.

chancroid A bacterial, sexually transmitted infection that is rare outside of the tropics.

chemical agent Chemicals that can be used as weapons to cause injury, illness, and death. They are roughly divided by their mechanism of action into blood agents, blister agents, choking agents, irritants, and nerve agents.

chemical burns Burns that occur when the skin is in contact with caustic chemical compounds such as strong acids, alkalis, or organic compounds.

chemical phlebitis Inflammation of a vein associated with infusates of varying ranges of pH or osmolarities.

chemotaxis The movement of white blood cells to an area of inflammation or infection in response to the release of chemical mediators from neutrophils, macrophages, T cells, and injured tissue.

chief complaint Information about what brought the patient to the health care provider in the patient's own words.

chlamydia Most frequently reported sexually transmitted infection in the United States. It is caused by *Chlamydia trachomatis* and is treatable with antibiotics.

chloride A primary anion in extracellular fluid; its normal serum level is 95 to 108 mEq/L. Chloride is usually found in combination with sodium to create electrical neutrality in the body; it assists in the reabsorption of sodium in the kidneys and combines with hydrogen ion to form hydrochloric acid for digestion.

choking agent Chemicals that cause injury, illness, and death by damaging the lungs. Also called an *asphyxiate*.

cholangiocarcinoma Cancer of the gallbladder.

cholecystectomy Surgical removal of the gallbladder either through an open incision or with a laparoscope.

cholecystitis Inflammation of the gallbladder; most commonly caused by gallstones.

cholecystokinin A hormone secreted by the gastrointestinal mucosa that stimulates the gallbladder to eject bile and the pancreas to secrete alkaline fluid.

choledocholithiasis A gallstone in the common bile duct.

cholelithiasis Disorder in which stones form in the gallbladder that may be composed of cholesterol or calcium.

cholesterol A steroid molecule produced primarily by the liver that is essential for the formation and maintenance of cell membranes.

cholinergic crisis A life-threatening condition associated with myasthenia gravis; results from excess acetylcholine.

chromosomal disorder Condition caused by an abnormal chromosome makeup in which there is duplication, loss, or rearrangement of chromosomal material.

chromosome Threadlike structures in the nucleus of a cell that contain the genes. Chromosomes occur in pairs, with a typical human cell containing 46 chromosomes: 22 pairs of autosomes, and 2 sex chromosomes.

chronic bronchitis Hypersecretion of mucus and chronic productive cough that continues at least 3 months of the year for at least 2 consecutive years.

chronic graft rejection Occurs months to years after graft transplant and involves the slow, progressive failure of a transplanted organ.

chronic lymphocytic thyroiditis An autoimmune condition characterized by high titers of the circulating antibodies thyroid peroxidase and thyroglobulin that destroy thyroid cells and may lead to hypothyroidism. It is the most common thyroid disease in the United States. Also known as *Hashimoto's thyroiditis.*

chronic obstructive pulmonary disease (COPD) A disease state characterized by airflow limitation that is not fully reversible.

chronic pain Pain that does not resolve within the expected time frame, and is persistent beyond 3 to 6 months.

chronic stress Stress that occurs on a daily basis and is the result of an ongoing situation.

chronic wounds Wounds that do not follow the expected sequence of repair in a timely and uncomplicated manner.

Chvostek's sign Spasm of facial muscles; latent tetany, which can be demonstrated by tapping the inferior portion of the zygoma resulting in facial spasms.

chyle Lymphatic system drainage; a milky fluid comprised of serous fluid, white cells, and fatty acids, arising from the interstitial fluid of the gastrointestinal tract. It contains a high proportion of fat and proteins.

chyle leak A disruption in the lymph system into the tissues of the neck and chest.

chymotrypsin An enzyme that aids in the breakdown of large protein molecules by breaking the interior bonds of the amino acids.

circadian rhythm Pertinent to events that occur at approximately 24-hour intervals.

circinate balanitis Inflammation surrounding the circular muscle around the penis.

circulating nurse Nurse in the operating room whose duties are performed outside the sterile field. They encompass responsibilities of nursing care management within the operating room to create and maintain a safe, comfortable environment for surgery.

cirrhosis An inflammatory disease of the liver in which normal structure and function are disrupted.

civil law Rules and regulations that form the bases of legal actions; branch of law that pertains to contracts, torts, patents, and the like.

clinical judgment A complex skill involving several cognitive phases and integrative processes; clinical reasoning across time about a particular patient.

clinical knowledge Knowledge necessary to perform proficiently in the clinical setting, including recognizing signs and symptoms, applying skilled know-how in titrating an intravenous rate, recognizing signs of physiological distress and changes in patient's vital signs, and using clinical judgment.

clinical nurse leader (CNL) An advanced practice nurse with postgraduate training with the responsibility to integrate care among other disciplines and manage care at the bedside.

clinical nurse specialist (CNS) An advanced practice nurse with postgraduate training in a clinical disease specialty. The CNS may schedule clinic visits with patients, provide specialized inpatient or nurse education, or case manage a group of patients.

coal miner pneumoconiosis A chronic lung disease leading to pulmonary fibrosis. It is caused by inhalation of coal dust.

code of ethics A formal statement by a group that expresses the group's ideals, values, and ethical principles, which have been agreed on by the group's members to reflect their moral judgments and serve as a standard for their professional actions.

codon The sequence of three nucleotides in mRNA that specifies a single amino acid.

cognitive dimension of pain Includes the impact of personal beliefs, attitudes, and meanings attached to pain.

cognitive reappraisal The process of allowing for changes in the person's evaluation of an event or a relabeling of the cognitive appraisal.

coiling An endovascular procedure in which an aneurysm is filled with a soft coil. Also referred to as a *GDC (Guglielmi detachable coil)*.

collaborative problems Problems that are identified by other health care workers, such as physicians, in contrast to nursing problems, which are identified by nurses. The nurse is accountable for monitoring for changes in the status of the problem and initiating the appropriate interventions.

collagen synthesis Multistep process in which fibrin proteins form a matrix to support the newly forming tissue.

colon The large intestine from the end of the ileum to the anal canal that surrounds the anus.

colon cancer Disease in which malignant tissue arises from the cells in the colon; it is frequently associated with adenomatous polyps. When there is an allelic deletion on chromosomes 5, 17, or 18, the transformation from normal to malignant colon tissue is promoted.

colonoscopy Visualization of the lower gastrointestinal tract, usually through the insertion of an endoscope through the anus.

colposcopy A test in which the health care provider looks at the cells of the cervix through a special magnifying scope that is placed near the opening of the speculum that is inserted into the vagina.

comminuted skull fracture The fragmented interruption of the skull resulting from multiple linear fractures.

commissure The site where cardiac valve leaflets meet each other.

commissurotomy Surgical procedure used to separate fused heart valve leaflets.

common law System of law derived from principles rather than rules and regulations; consists of principles based on justice, reason, and common sense.

community-acquired infection An infection acquired outside a health care facility.

community-based care A setting for practice outside of acute care institutional walls. Care is directed toward individuals and families within any community setting and is designed to assist patients as they move among health care settings. Also describes a philosophy of care in settings that reflect *how* nursing care is provided, not *where*.

community health nursing Type of nursing practice for registered nurses who work in various health district programs. RNs provide follow-up care, immunizations, health education, and referrals of clients to appropriate agencies for assistance.

compact (cortical) bone Bone that is resistant to compression, is dense, and is laid down in concentric layers.

compartment syndrome An acute problem following injury or surgery caused when pressure within the muscles builds to dangerous levels. The resulting increased pressure within the fascial compartment impairs blood supply.

compensation Correction of the blood pH by the system that is *not* the cause of abnormal levels of carbon dioxide or bicarbonate. For example, when an excess of metabolic acid leads to metabolic acidosis, the lungs increase their ventilation to "blow off" carbon dioxide and reduce its level below normal, thus helping bring the pH back toward normal. Metabolic compensation for a respiratory problem is slower; it takes days to weeks to retain the bicarbonate.

complement A group of proteins in the blood that stimulates the inflammatory response and serves as a primary chemical mediator of the antigen–antibody reactions of the B-cell immune response.

complementary therapy A therapy used in addition to a conventional therapy.

complete spinal cord injury Permanent loss of all neurological function below the level of injury.

comprehensive exam A head-to-toe assessment usually performed on new patients who will be seen on a routine basis by various clinicians.

compression injuries Injuries that occur when pressure is applied to the spinal cord as a result of mass effect from bone fragments, disk herniation, tumor, abscess, or blood clot.

Compromised Family Coping Nursing diagnosis that refers to the inability of a family to function optimally.

concentric When referring to coronary artery stenosis, the term used to describe a lesion that occupies the whole circumference.

concussion A recognized collection of symptoms that result from a mild head injury.

conductive hearing loss Type of hearing loss in which sound waves cannot reach the inner ear for processing and interpretation; caused by diseases such as external ear infections.

conductivity Ability of the cardiac cell to accept and then transmit a stimulus to other cardiac cells.

configuration Refers to the pattern of arrangement or position of lesions.

congenital Present at birth or prenatally.

conjugate gaze Paired or joined eyes moving in tandem in the cardinal fields of gaze.

conscious A mental state that encompasses all things that are easily remembered.

conscious sedation A minimally depressed level of consciousness and satisfactory analgesia that allows the patient to retain the ability to maintain an airway independently and to respond to physical stimulation and verbal commands, obtained through the administration of a combination of pharmacologic agents.

constrictive pericarditis Occurs when the pericardial layers adhere to each other as a result of fibrosis of the pericardial sac.

contact dermatitis An inflammation of the skin related to exposure to an irritant or allergen in the environment.

continent ileostomy (Kock ileostomy or Kock pouch) During ileostomy surgery, the procedure in which the terminal ileum is folded back on itself and the inner wall removed, thereby forming a reservoir and a nipple valve that prevents leakage of fecal contents through the stoma.

continuity theory of aging Theory of aging based on the premise that successful aging is obtained by maintaining values, habits, and behaviors from adult life.

continuous passive motion device Machine into which an extremity is placed to perform continuous passive range of motion.

continuous positive airway pressure (CPAP) Procedure that delivers air into a patient's airway through a specially designed nasal mask or pillows.

continuous subcutaneous infusion (CSI) The uninterrupted infusion of small-volume parenteral medication via the subcutaneous route.

continuous subcutaneous insulin infusion (CSII) A method of exogenous insulin delivery that uses an external "insulin pump," which allows for programmed delivery of insulin into subcutaneous tissue.

contractility A mechanical function that enables the cardiac cells to shorten and cause the muscle to contract in response to an electrical stimulus. Also referred to as *rhythmicity*.

contrast sensitivity (CS) The function of being able to distinguish subtle gradations of grayish patterns between targets and background.

contusion An injury to soft tissue caused by trauma; a bruise.

convalescent phase In viral hepatitis, the phase that occurs approximately 6 to 8 weeks after exposure to the virus and lasts up to 10 weeks when liver function returns to normal. Also called the *recovery phase*.

convenience sampling Type of statistical sampling in which the most available persons or units are selected for inclusion in the study; the researcher has no control over the characteristics of the sample. Also referred to as *accidental sampling*.

coping A compensatory process with physiological and psychological components that allows the individual to adapt to a stressor.

cor pulmonale Enlargement of the right ventricle in response to pulmonary hypoxia; literally means "heart of the lungs."

coronary artery disease (CAD) A progressive atherosclerotic disorder of the coronary arteries that results in narrowing or complete occlusion of the vessel lumen.

correlational research design Research conducted to examine linear relationships between two or more variables.

corticosteroids A class of synthetic steroid hormones that decreases the inflammatory response and suppresses immune activity; used to prevent graft rejection. Examples include Solu-Medrol, Solu-Cortef, hydrocortisone, dexamethasone, and prednisone.

cosmetic surgery Surgery performed for the primary purpose of improving physical appearance.

cotton-wool spots (CWS) Soft exudates that appear as white cotton spots in the nerve fiber layer of the retina; caused by lack of blood supply to the tissue.

counterregulatory hormones Hormones that antagonize the actions of insulin. Examples include glucagon, cortisol, growth hormone, and catecholamines.

crackles When auscultating the lungs, common abnormal, short popping sounds heard on inspiration; caused by the movement of fluid or exudates.

C-reactive protein (CRP) A protein released from the liver in response to local inflammation or tissue injury; useful as a marker for inflammation and colon cancer.

creatinine kinase (CK) An enzyme found in high concentrations in the heart and skeletal muscle and in smaller concentrations in the brain.

cremasteric reflex Condition in which testicles rise in the scrotum to the abdominal cavity when the thigh is stroked or the room is cold.

crepitus Abnormal sounds (grating, snapping, crackling, rattling) emanating from a joint while in movement.

cretinism Condition caused by the congenital absence or atrophy of the thyroid gland, resulting in hypothyroidism and characterized by mental deficiency, large tongue, puffy facial features, and dwarfism.

criminal law Law pertaining to conduct that is offensive or contrary to the public good, such as murder, theft, and rape.

crisis The occurrence of an event or series of events that creates a situation that is perceived as threatening.

critical incident A stressful incident that is so markedly distressing and powerful as to overcome a person's normal feelings of control and coping.

critical incident stress debriefing (CISD) Formal event run by trained counselors to assist those involved in a critical incident to better cope with the incident.

critical incident stress management A comprehensive approach to the management of stress and critical incidents.

critical pathways Comprehensive plans of care for specific patient situations or disease processes. Critical pathways include nursing interventions, medical interventions, and expected timelines for patient outcomes.

critical thinking A purposeful, two-dimensional, goal-directed process that is context bound. Two dimensions are necessary for the development of critical thinking: the cognitive, which is reflective, reasoned thinking, and the affective, which is open-mindedness to divergent perspectives and an inquisitive spirit.

Crohn's disease An inflammatory bowel disease that involves all layers (transmural) of the intestinal wall and can occur anywhere from the mouth to the anus, but commonly affects the ileum.

cross-linking theory of aging Theory of aging based on the premise that the binding of glucose to protein causes various problems. Also referred to as the *glycosylation theory of aging*.

cryoprecipitates Clotting factors used to treat bleeding associated with hemophilia and disorders that cause a depletion of the clotting factors.

cryptorchidism Undescended testicle(s).

cultural competence The ongoing practice of knowing, respecting, and incorporating the values of others; being open to the cultural beliefs and behaviors of others.

cultural diversity Variety and differences in the customs and practices of defined social groups; refers to the variation among groups of people with respect to the habits, values, preferences, beliefs, taboos, and rules determined to be appropriative for individual and social interaction.

culture Learned patterns of behavior, beliefs, and values that can be attributed to a particular group of people.

curative procedures Surgeries performed for the primary purpose of curing a condition.

Cushing's syndrome A hypermetabolic state in which there is a chronic excess of corticosteroid hormones for a variety of reasons.

Cushing's triad Combination of widening pulse pressure, bradycardia, and irregular respiratory patterns; may indicate increasing intracranial pressure.

cyanosis Bluish-tinged skin or mucous membranes due to deoxygenated hemoglobin in blood vessels close to the skin.

cystic fibrosis (CF) A chronic disease in which the process of transportation of salt and water across cell membranes is disturbed, leading to production of unusually thick mucus that blocks bodily passages, particularly in the digestive and respiratory systems. This disorder affects all exocrine glands.

cystocele Occurs when the wall between the bladder and the anterior vagina weakens, often as a result of childbirth, and the bladder protrudes into the vaginal vault.

cytogenetics A specialization of genetics that involves the study of chromosomes.

cytokines Chemical signals released by white blood cells (predominately T cells) that act as messages between cells and instruct immune cells to proliferate, differentiate, or alter activities; more than 100 different cytokines have been identified.

cytotoxic edema The accumulation of intracellular water, causing brain swelling.

dactylitis A uniform swelling of the soft tissues between the metacarpophalangeal and interphalangeal joints.

DASH diet A diet low in saturated fat, cholesterol, and total fat. There are two versions of the DASH plan: Plan 1 limits the patient to 2,000 mg of sodium per day; plan 2 limits the patient to 1,500 mg of sodium per day.

data saturation Sampling to the point at which no new information is obtained and redundancy is achieved.

dawn phenomenon Situation in which a patient has fasting hyperglycemia that is not related to nocturnal hypoglycemia and rebound hyperglycemia.

dead space The portion of the tidal volume that does not reach the alveoli of the lungs or take part in the exchange of oxygen and carbon dioxide.

dead space ventilation (V_D) The portion of the tidal volume that is not participating in gas exchange.

decannulation Term used to refer to the process of weaning a patient toward the goal of removing a tracheotomy tube.

decerebrate posturing The characteristic posture of an individual with decerebrate rigidity. The extremities are stiff and extended, and the head is retracted.

decibel (dB) A measurement of sound. Sounds typically range from 0 to 140 dB or greater.

decontamination The reduction or removal of contaminating agents.

decorticate posturing The characteristic posture of a person with a lesion at or above the upper brainstem. The person is rigidly still with arms flexed, fists clenched, and legs extended.

deep venous thrombosis (DVT) The formation of a blood clot within a deep vein, commonly in the thigh or calf.

defamation of character Publication of anything that is injurious to the good name or reputation of another or that tends to bring another's reputation into question.

defibrillation Basically the same as cardioversion in that electrical voltage is delivered to cause depolarization of the myocardium to terminate unwanted rhythms, except it is done in an emergency situation when sudden cardiac arrest has occurred.

degenerative joint disease Progressive loss of cartilage at a joint.

delayed hypersensitivity reaction Occurs when the immune system responds to an antigen over several hours to days. An example is contact dermatitis.

delegation The assignment of work to others while maintaining accountability for the outcome of the work.

deletion The loss of a chromosome or DNA segment of any length.

delirium A disturbance in consciousness resulting in decreased attention and a change in cognition, or development of a perceptual disturbance that develops over a short period of time and tends to fluctuate throughout the day.

delirium tremens (DTs) Tremor and clouding of consciousness that can accompany physiological withdrawal from alcohol.

dementia A general term for brain dysfunction characterized by a decline in cognition and memory that causes loss of ability to carry out activities of daily living and communicate with others, ultimately resulting in death.

deontological theories In ethics, theories that derive norms and rules from the duties human beings owe one another by virtue of commitments that are made and roles that are assumed.

deoxyhemoglobin Configuration of hemoglobin stimulated by hypoxic states and characterized by rapid release of oxygen to peripheral tissues.

deoxyribonucleic acid (DNA) A complex protein present in the chromosomes of the nuclei of cells that is the basis of heredity and the carrier of genetic information for all organisms except RNA viruses.

dependent activities Activities prescribed by the physician and carried out by the nurse; includes implementing the physician's orders to administer medications or treatments.

depressed skull fracture Displacement of a comminuted skull fracture.

dermabrasion Process of removing the epidermis and upper dermis of the skin so that the skin can regenerate into a smooth surface.

dermatofibromas Common, fibrous, tumor-like nodules of the skin.

dermatomyositis Progressive inflammatory muscle condition that occurs with inflammatory skin changes.

dermatophyte A fungus parasite on the skin.

descriptive research design Type of research question, design, and data analysis that will be applied to a given topic.

descriptive vividness In qualitative research, the practice of describing the site, participants, experience of collecting data, and the thinking of the research so clearly that the reader has a sense of personally experiencing the event.

desensitization The process of introducing small amounts of a triggering allergen to an allergic individual in increasing amounts over time. The goal is to reduce the severity of the allergic response.

desquamation Shedding of the outer layer of epidermis (skin or mucosa).

developmental stressor Stressor that occurs during specific periods of the life span, for examples, as a child, adolescent, young adult, middle adult, or older adult.

Diabetes Control and Complications Trial (DCCT) A landmark research study in the United States and Canada which demonstrated that intensive management of type 1 diabetes (aimed at normal blood glucose levels) resulted in decreased occurrence and progression of development of microvascular complications (i.e., retinopathy, neuropathy, nephropathy).

diabetes insipidus (DI) A hypometabolic disorder of the adrenal gland in which there is excretion of a large volume of dilute urine due to deficiency of antidiuretic hormone (ADH) or an inability of the kidneys to respond to ADH.

Diabetes Prevention Program (DPP) A major clinical research trial of patients with pre-diabetes that clearly demonstrated that lifestyle modification was superior to pharmacologic therapy with metformin (an oral diabetes medication) in preventing diabetes.

diabetic ketoacidosis (DKA) An acute emergent complication of diabetes (usually type 1 diabetes) primarily characterized by hyperglycemia, dehydration, and metabolic acidosis.

diabetic peripheral neuropathy (DPN) A chronic complication of diabetes in which the nerves outside of the spinal cord are damaged. Diabetic peripheral neuropathy is associated with numbness, weakness, burning pain (which often worsens at night), and loss of reflexes in the extremities.

diabetic retinopathy (DR) Disorder characterized by weakened and damaged blood vessels (capillaries) that result in edema from leaking capillaries that hemorrhage.

diagnostic procedures Surgeries performed for the purpose of diagnosing a condition.

dialysis catheter A large-bore vascular access device used as a temporary means to facilitate dialysis procedures; its configuration is similar to that of a pheresis catheter.

diaphysis Shaft of a long bone, between both metaphysis.

diascopy Examination of superficial skin lesions with a diascope.

diastolic A blood pressure reading of the minimum pressure in the arteries, which occurs just prior to the next cycle of ventricular ejection of blood; reflects cardiac relaxation.

diastolic dysfunction Impaired relaxation, preventing the heart from filling appropriately at normal preload pressures.

differentiation Maturation process of blood cells during which cell generations gain increasing specialization; begins with the hematopoietic stem cell and goes to the fully mature peripheral cell.

diffuse axonal injury (DAI) A primary injury of diffuse white matter that results in tearing or shearing of axons and small blood vessels.

diffusion The movement of molecules from an area of high concentration to an area of low concentration in liquids, gases, and solids.

dilated cardiomyopathy A disorder of the myocardium characterized by dilation and impaired contraction of one or more ventricles; the most common form of cardiomyopathy.

diploid The number of chromosomes in most cells except the gametes. The diploid number in humans is 46.

diplopia Seeing double vision, when one object appears as two.

direct inguinal hernia Occurs when abdominal contents herniate through a weak point in the fascia of the abdominal wall and into the inguinal canal.

direct percussion Technique of using gentle tapping to illicit the presence or absence of fluid, which results in a dull sound; used to examine such areas as the sinuses.

direct question Question used to elicit specific information and to clarify specific details; for example, "Is the pain sharp or dull?"

discectomy Surgery to remove a diseased disk.

discrete lesion An individual or separate lesion.

disengagement theory of aging Theory of aging based on the premise that age-related changes bring about a mutual and reciprocal withdrawal of the individual from society.

dislocation Displacement of a bone from its normal position in a joint.

dissecting aortic aneurysm A localized dilation of the aorta that has a longitudinal dissection between the outer and middle layers of the vascular wall.

distribution (1) A description of the lesions on the skin according to location or body region affected. (2) The process of moving a medication into the bloodstream and the extracellular and intracellular compartments, as well as in the compartment that is the site of absorption.

diverticular disease Disease in which abnormal saclike outpouchings (diverticula) of the intestinal wall occur anywhere in the gastrointestinal tract except the rectum, but usually occurring in the distal large intestine.

diverticulitis Inflammation of a diverticulum.

diverticulosis The presence of one or more diverticula.

DMAT Acronym for disaster medical assistance team. A group of volunteer health care professionals and ancillary staff that can provide emergency medical services and relief in times of disaster.

DMORT Acronym for disaster mortuary operations response team. A team of volunteers that can assist with handling mass casualties in time of disaster.

doll's eye reflex *See* oculocephalic reflex.

donor site An area on the body where skin is surgically harvested to use for covering burn wounds.

dopamine A neurotransmitter necessary for ease of movement; loss of dopamine is a key factor in Parkinson's disease.

Dressler's syndrome Condition characterized by fever, pericarditis, chest pain, and pericardial and pleural effusions. Believed to be an autoimmune response, it occurs in 5% to 15% of patients 1 to 4 weeks after a myocardial infarction.

Dreyfus model of skill acquisition A learning model based on determining the level of practice evident in particular situations. It elucidates strengths as well as problems. In this model, situated practice capacities are described rather than traits or talents of the practitioners.

drip factor The number of drops equal to 1 mL of fluid.

drusen Yellowish, round, slightly elevated, different-sized subretinal pigment epithelial deposits in the macula.

dual-channel pump Pole-mounted electronic infusion devices that have multiple channels for infusion within a single device.

dullness A high-pitched tone of short duration that is soft in quality. It is heard over the large organs such as the liver and kidney.

duodenal ulcer An erosion of the duodenal lining resulting from *Helicobacter pylori* infection and hypersecretion of acid and pepsin.

Dupuytren's contracture Difficulty or an inability to extend the ring or fifth finger.

durable power of attorney for health care (DPAHC) A document that allows a patient to appoint a decision maker in the case of future incapacity. The DPAHC specifically states which powers the patient gives to the surrogate. The appointed person responsible for making medical decisions does not need consent from other family members or friends.

dwell The time period during which an infusion catheter remains in place.

dynamic response test A test to assess whether a transducer system is accurately transmitting pressures.

dysconjugate gaze Eyes moving separately from each other in the cardinal fields of gaze.

dyskinesia Involuntary, writhing movements that may involve limbs, trunk, face, and neck; results from overstimulation of dopamine receptors. Condition characterized by areas of abnormal heart contractility where muscle movement is impaired.

dysmenorrhea Painful menstruation.

dyspareunia Painful intercourse; can be a result of several factors such as endometriosis or menopause.

dysphagia Difficulty swallowing.

dysphoria An exaggerated feeling of depression and unrest without apparent cause; a mood of general dissatisfaction, restlessness, anxiety, discomfort, and unhappiness.

dysplasia Change in the appearance of cells after they have been subjected to chronic irritation.

dyspnea Subjective feeling of shortness of breath or difficulty breathing.

dysrhythmia A heartbeat originating from a site other than the primary cardiac pacemaker tissue. The terms *dysrhythmia*, *arrhythmia*, and *ectopic focus* all mean the same thing and are used interchangeably.

eccentric When discussing plaque buildup in a coronary artery, the term used to describe a lesion that occupies part of a vessel wall.

ecchymosis A lesion that is initially dark red or purple, but gradually fades to yellowish green before it disappears.

ECG single photon emission computed tomography (SPECT) A nuclear medicine technique that uses radiopharmaceuticals, a rotating camera, and a computer to produce images representing slices through the body in different planes.

ECG waveform Movement away from the baseline, or the isoelectric line, on an ECG tracing on graph paper.

echocardiography The noninvasive assessment of the structures and function of the heart and great vessels utilizing high-frequency (ultrasound) sound waves.

ectopic Implantation of the products of conception outside the uterine endometrium.

ectopic focus A heartbeat originating from a site other than the primary cardiac pacemaker tissue. Also called *dysrhythmia*.

edema Accumulation of fluid in the intercellular spaces that causes swelling of tissue.

efferent Ability to transport away from a central organ or section; conducts impulses from the brain or spinal cord to the periphery. In the nervous system, efferent nerves are known as motor or effector neurons that carry nerve impulses *away* from the central nervous system to effectors such as muscles or glands.

ego Mediates the drives of the id with a dose of reality.

ego defense mechanisms Utilized to alleviate anxiety by denying, distorting, and misinterpreting reality.

ejection fraction (EF) The amount of blood ejected from the left or right ventricle; calculated by comparing end-diastolic volume to stroke volume.

elastomeric balloon A portable, disposable mechanical infusion device that requires no power source to function.

elective procedures Procedure for which the timing is determined by the patient and the surgeon. A total knee replacement scheduled in advance is an example of an elective surgery.

electrocardiogram Surface recording of the electrical activity of the heart.

electrode An adhesive pad that contains conducting gel and is connected to a cardiac monitor by lead wires. Electrodes serve as sensing devices to detect changes in electrical activity of the heart. Electrodes must be placed in certain positions in order for the ECG machine to have a clear picture of the electrical impulse, and they must have a positive, a negative, and a ground lead.

electrolytes Ionized minerals (calcium, chloride, magnesium, phosphorus, potassium, and sodium) serving as energy transfer mechanisms in combinations of positive charges (cations) or negative charges (anions).

electromyelogram (EMG) A graphic recording that tests the contraction of muscles that have been electrically stimulated.

electron beam computed tomography (EBCT) Procedure that uses an electron gun and a stationary tungsten target to rapidly (about 90 seconds) acquire multiple images of the heart during a single breath hold.

electroneutrality The principle that asserts that the sum of all positive or cationic charges in plasma must equal the sum of all negative or anionic charges. The primary cations measured in venous plasma are sodium and potassium. The main anions are chloride and bicarbonate or serum carbon dioxide.

electronic infusion device (EID) An infusion device that can be portable, or pole mounted; requires a power supply (i.e., batteries or electric current) to function; used to control delivery of parenteral solutions or medications.

electrophysiology study (EPS) An invasive procedure that involves placing multiple multipolar catheter electrodes into the venous and sometimes the arterial side of the heart in order to evaluate the electrical activity of the heart and to identify areas of initiation and propagation of dysrhythmias.

elemental iron Amount of iron in a food substance that is available for absorption from the digestive tract.

elimination The process of excretion from the body that is generally accomplished in the renal system. Elimination can occur after medications are metabolized or medications may be eliminated in their primary form.

emancipated minors Persons under the legal age of adulthood who are no longer under the control and regulation of their parents and who may give valid consent for medical procedures.

embolectomy Mechanical removal of a clot in a blood vessel.

embolization Endovascular procedure in which an aneurysm is obliterated by filling it with a glue-type substance.

emergency doctrine Allows implied consent for treatment to exist in true emergency situations in which an individual is in danger of loss of life or limb.

Emergency Medical Treatment and Active Labor Act (EMTALA) A part of the 1986 COBRA laws and the 1990 OBRA amendment that defines the legal responsibilities of Medicare-participating hospitals in treating individuals who present with emergency medical conditions; ensures that patients have access to emergency services regardless of their ability to pay.

emergency nursing The care of individuals of all ages with perceived or actual physical or emotional alterations of health that are undiagnosed or require further interventions.

emergent (emergency) surgery Surgery that must be performed suddenly without advanced planning.

emmetropia The condition of the normal eye when parallel rays are focused exactly on the retina and vision is perfect. Normal refractive error or vision without any corrective optical devices.

emphysema A disease of the airways that involves destruction of the alveolar walls.

empiric therapy Therapy that is begun before culture results are available; physicians determine if empiric therapy is necessary based on the severity of the infection.

encephalitis Inflammation of brain tissue.

endocrine Glands that secrete directly into the bloodstream.

endoleaks Continued leakage of blood into the aneurysmal sac.

endometriosis Condition in which endometrial-like cells are found outside of the uterus. During the menstrual cycle, these cells respond to hormone production and may swell and bleed. In response, the body will surround these lesions with scar tissue, which can form adhesions on the area of attachment.

end-organ perfusion The blood perfusion of the end organs such as the integumentary system.

endorphins Endogenous, morphine-like substances that reduce or inhibit pain perception in the descending pathways.

endoscopic retrograde cholangiopancreatography (ERCP) Radiograph following injection of a radiopaque material into the papilla of Vater.

endoskeletal Pertaining to the cartilaginous and bony skeleton of the body.

endotoxins Produced by live bacteria and released when the bacteria are killed.

endotracheal tube Tube used to deliver oxygen that is placed in the trachea.

end-stage renal disease (ESRD) A patient is considered to have end-stage renal disease when the loss of filtration ability reaches approximately seven-eighths, at which point the survival of the patient depends on dialysis or, if an acceptable candidate, a kidney transplant.

engraftment Establishment of new bone marrow.

enkephalins Pentapeptides produced in the brain that act as an opiate.

enteral nutrition Use of the gastrointestinal tract for feeding.

enthesitis Upon palpitation, discomfort at the site of the attachment of bone to the tendon.

enzyme immunoassays (EIAs) Laboratory tests of blood to determine whether or not antibodies are present. A specific enzyme is used to link to antibodies, in this case, HIV antibodies. A positive test indicates antibodies are present.

eosinophil Acts as a phagocyte in inflammatory conditions, particularly allergic reactions.

ependymomas Tumors originating from the ependymal cells of the cerebral ventricles.

epididymitis Inflammation of the long, tubular structure that connects and carries sperm from the testicle to the vas deferens.

epidural anesthesia A type of regional anesthesia in which an anesthetic agent is injected in the epidural space.

epidural hematoma (EDH) Bleeding into the space between the skull and the dura.

epiglottitis Infection and inflammation of the epiglottis and surrounding supraglottic structures often resulting in airway obstruction. Usually caused by *Haemophilus influenzae* type B.

epiphysis The end of the bone beyond the physis.

epistaxis Bleeding from the nose.

epithelialization Process by which a wound closes from its margins, covering the defect with a layer of new skin.

erectile dysfunction (ED) The inability to achieve or maintain an erection sufficient to allow intercourse.

error theories of aging Theory of aging based on the premise that environmental factors negatively impact the human body, causing destruction and damage.

erysipelas A form of cellulitis characterized by inflammation and redness of the skin due to group A hemolytic streptococci.

erythrocyte Red blood cell.

erythropoiesis Process of red blood cell development.

erythropoietic stem cell (proerythroblast) The earliest of four stages in development of the normoblast. Ancestor cell giving rise to red blood cells.

erythropoietin Hormone that stimulates the production of red blood cells.

escape Term that applies to the emergence of a pacemaker that is lower in the heart and sustains a heart rate when the SA node fails.

eschar Nonviable burned tissue.

escharotomies Incisions made through burn tissue to relieve the constricting effects of the edema that accompanies circumferential injuries.

esophageal cancer Cancer that occurs anywhere in the esophagus, but more often occurs in the middle and distal portions; is usually squamous cell carcinoma.

esophageal varices Varicose veins in the distal esophagus that result most often from portal hypertension, a complication of cirrhosis of the liver.

esophagus The muscular tube that carries swallowed foods and liquids from the pharynx to the stomach.

esophoria Inward deviation of the eye.

ethical decision making Evaluating the principles and values of all persons involved in a decision before coming to a conclusion.

ethical dilemma A situation that involves two or more unfavorable alternatives to a given situation.

ethics Discipline relating to moral actions and moral values.

ethnography A form of research that focuses on the sociology of meaning through field observation and description of a sociocultural phenomenon.

ethos Notions of what counts as good nursing or good scientific practice.

euphoria An exaggerated feeling of well-being.

eustress Stress associated with positive events.

euthymia Normal, nondepressed, reasonably positive mood.

euthyroid Appearing to function as a normal thyroid gland.

euvolemia Term used when the body is in a state of equal fluid balance, without fluid retention.

evaluation Focuses on a patient's behavioral changes and compares them with criteria stated in predetermined patient outcomes. Evaluation is ongoing through all phases of the nursing process.

evidence-based practice (EBP) A problem-solving approach to clinical decision making that incorporates a search for the best and latest evidence, clinical expertise, and assessment, and a patient's preferences and values within a context of caring. This decision-making approach integrates clinical expertise with the best available evidence from systematic research in contrast to opinion-based health care decision making that is based primarily on values and resources.

excitability Ability of an electrical cell to respond to a stimulus. All cardiac cells possess this property. Also referred to as *irritability*.

exercise testing A cardiovascular stress test combining exercise (either physical or pharmacologic) and electrocardiographic and blood pressure monitoring, typically to evaluate patients with suspected coronary artery disease.

exocrine pancreas The portion of the pancreas that secretes enzymes for digestion into the duodenum.

exon The portion of a gene that contains the code for producing the gene's protein.

exophthalmos Abnormal protrusion of the eyeball; may be due to thyrotoxicosis, tumor of the orbit, orbital cellulitis, leukemia, or aneurysm.

exostosis A condition of the ear canal in which the bony lining under the skin develops a number of lumps that grow into the tube. Also called *surfer's ear*.

exotoxins Proteins released by bacterial cells during growth; they have very specific actions. Exotoxins modify cell enzymes and functions, leading to cell death or dysfunction. They are usually named for the site they affect.

experience An active process of gaining knowledge and skill, not just a passage of time.

experiential learning Requires a turning around of preconceptions, or an adding of nuances to one's understanding. Experiential learning requires openness and responsiveness by the learner to improve practice over time.

experimental research design Type of research in which the researcher attempts to maintain control over all factors that may affect the results of an experiment. In so doing, the researcher attempts to determine or predict what may occur when a hypothesis is tested and conclusions are drawn between independent and dependent variables.

exploratory surgery Surgery performed for the purpose of identifying abnormalities when the diagnosis of a condition is not established beforehand.

expressivity The degree or amount of symptomology to which an individual with a genotype is affected. For example, two individuals may have the same genotype, but one may have all of the symptoms of the disorder, while the second one has relatively few symptoms.

extension set Tubing that adds length and/or access ports to an administration set.

external fixation A treatment in which the bones or bone ends of a fracture are held in place by skeletal pins. The pins are screwed into the bone and attached to a frame worn on the outside of the body.

external locus of control An orientation in which a person believes that events in his or her life are controlled more by fate, luck, and external circumstances.

external stressor Stressor that originates outside the body.

extra-axial tumors Tumors originating from the supporting structures of the brain.

extracellular fluid (ECF) Fluid between the cells (interstitial fluids) and in plasma (serum).

extravasation Inadvertent administration of a vesicant solution or medication into surrounding tissues.

Factor VIII A clotting factor that may be administered intravenously for the treatment of hemophilia A.

false imprisonment The unjustified detention or confinement of a person without legal warrant.

familial intracranial aneurysms The presence of proven aneurysms in two or more family members among first- and second-degree relatives.

fascicles Anterior and posterior pathways that branch off the heart's left bundle branch. The anterior fascicle carries electrical impulses to the anterior wall of the left ventricle. The posterior fascicle spreads electrical impulses to the posterior ventricular wall.

fasciculation Involuntary contraction or twitching of a group of muscles or muscle fibers, visible under the skin.

fasciotomy Incisions made to release skin and muscle coverings.

FAST examination Focused assessment with sonography for trauma.

fast-tracking Term used to describe a situation in which a patient is transferred from the operating room to the postanesthesia care unit (PACU) phase II, bypassing PACU phase I. Fast-tracking is possible when surgical techniques are minimally invasive and anesthesia is of a short duration.

fat embolus Fat that enters the circulatory system after the fracture of a long bone.

ferritin A form of iron in the body acting as a supply reservoir.

fetal alcohol syndrome (FAS) Physical and mental defects found in babies of women who consumed alcohol during pregnancy.

fetid breath Halitosis or foul or putrid breath.

fever of unknown origin (FUO) A fever that lasts 2 weeks or more without identification of the cause.

fibroblasts Small cells that migrate along the fibrin network to produce the connective tissue and collagen fibers.

fibrocystic breast An increase in glandular and fibrous tissues in the breast; characterized by small, nodular cysts that are palpable in the breast.

fibroid tumor Growths arising from the tissue of the uterine muscle; they develop slowly in women ages 25 through 40 years of age.

fibrous cap A dense connective tissue matrix in the inner lining of an artery that is formed when smooth muscle cells secrete collagen, elastin, and glycosaminoglycans.

fidelity In ethics, keeping one's promises or commitments.

fill time Period of time needed for blood to enter the heart between contractions.

filter Add-on device used to screen particulate matter, bacteria, and toxins from the infusion system.

filtration The movement of molecules from an area of higher concentration through permeable membranes to an area of lower concentration as a result of hydrostatic pressure.

first-degree AV block Conduction disturbance in which electrical impulses flow normally from the SA node through the atria, but are delayed at the AV node. This results in a prolongation of conduction rather than an actual block. Due to this delay, the PR interval is greater than 0.20 second, making it abnormal.

Fisher grading scale Grading scale for subarachnoid hemorrhage referring to the amount of blood on a CT scan.

fissure Deep linear crack or furrow in the continuity of the epidermis.

fistula Dehiscent wound that traverses between two different tissue planes; a communication between two areas such as the oral cavity and the skin.

flail chest Occurs when a person sustains two or more rib fractures in two or more places such that the ribs are no longer attached to the thoracic cage, resulting in a free or floating segment of chest wall. As a result, during spontaneous ventilation the floating segment moves in the opposite direction or paradoxically to the chest wall. This condition is almost always associated with pulmonary contusion.

flame-shaped hemorrhages Retinal hemorrhages that occur in the nerve fiber layer.

flare A round area of redness surrounding the wheal of an allergic reaction on the skin.

flashback chamber Small space located after the hub of the catheter and attached to the stylet; used to collect blood.

flashes Sudden bright light noticed by a person; flashes appear as sparks or minuscule strands of light, almost like streaks of lightning across the sky that occur when the vitreous gel bumps, rubs, or tugs against the retina.

flatness A soft, high-pitched tone of short duration. It is heard over muscle and bone.

flexible sigmoidoscopy A sigmoidoscope that uses fiber optics to inspect the sigmoid colon.

floaters Deposits of various size, shape, consistency, refractive index, and motility within the eye's vitreous humor, which is normally transparent.

flow control device Device used to regulate fluid administration.

flushing Procedure performed to maintain device patency and prevent mixing of incompatible solutions or medications.

focused exam An exam performed in emergent or urgent situations that focuses on a specific problem.

folate Naturally occurring, water-soluble form of vitamin B critical for red blood cell formation.

folliculitis Inflammation of the hair follicles.

Folstein Mini-Mental State Exam A common screening tool used by clinicians to evaluate dementia.

foreign body sensation (FBS) A feeling in the eye of a "gritty" feeling, as if something is in the eye.

forensic evidence Something that is legally submitted to a court of law as a means of determining the truth related to an alleged crime.

foreseeability of harm Concept that certain actions are known to cause or create specific outcomes.

for-profit (proprietary) organization Organization that focuses on making a profit from operations and distributing those profits to the owners or investors in the organization.

fraction of inspired oxygen (FiO$_2$) The amount expressed as a number of oxygen in a gas mixture, 0 (0%) to 1 (100%). For example the FiO$_2$ of normal room air is 0.21 (21%).

fractures Discontinuities in bone that may be complete or incomplete.

fragment antigen binding (FAB) portion The section of an antibody that is capable of being shaped to receive a specific antigen. DNA within B cells is capable of creating many millions of combinations of FAB portions of antibodies to match an antigen and help protect the body against an invasion by pathogens.

fragment crystalline (FC) portion The section of an antibody that is capable of attaching to the cell membrane of infected or mutant cells or of foreign pathogens (bacteria, viruses) and assisting macrophages to eliminate them.

Frank-Starling law The ability of muscle fibers to stretch to accommodate filling during diastole.

free radical theory of aging Theory of aging that postulates that aging changes are caused by free radical reactions that cause cells and organs to lose function and reserve energy.

fremitus Tactile vibration felt over airways.

frequency The number of sound waves emanating per second; measured in hertz (Hz). Hearing frequencies from 500 to 2,000 Hz are needed to understand everyday speech.

fresh frozen plasma A process in which the plasma portion of blood is separated from the cells and frozen until needed. Units of fresh frozen plasma are used to increase the level of clotting factors in patients with demonstrated deficiency.

friable Easily damaged.

frozen RBCs Red blood cells coated in glycerol prior to freezing and then washed after thawing to remove the glycerol prior to administration. This is a method of storage.

full-thickness injury An injury that extends into the underlying structures and organs.

full-thickness skin graft Grafting of skin that is surgically removed by excising the entire thickness of the donor skin to the level of the subcutaneous tissue, typically 0.025 to 0.30 inch thick.

functional iron deficiency Physiological state characterized by failure to supply enough iron for erythropoiesis despite sufficient quantities.

functional nursing A task-oriented nursing care delivery system in which individual caregivers are not given patient assignments but are expected to perform specific assigned tasks within their capability for all patients in a given area.

furuncle A boil or a walled-off, deep, painful, firm inflammation of the skin that contains pus.

fusiform aneurysms Elliptically shaped aneurysm.

gait Walking.

galactogenesis Formation of breast milk from nutrients available from the bloodstream.

galactorrhea The spontaneous flow of milk in a breast unassociated with childbirth or nursing.

gamete Reproductive cell, ovum or sperm, with the haploid chromosome number.

gamma-glutamyltransferase (GGT) An enzyme found mostly in the liver that is released when cellular damage occurs.

gastric carcinoma Cancer in the stomach, most commonly in the antrum and distal portions; is usually an adenocarcinoma.

gastric outlet obstruction Results from edema, inflammation, or scarring and obstructs the flow of gastric contents from the stomach to the duodenum. Also called *pyloric obstruction*.

gastric ulcer An erosion of the stomach lining that develops most often in the antrum, which is adjacent to the body of the stomach. It is not associated with increased acid secretion, but rather, with a defect in the mucosal barrier to hydrogen ions, allowing the ions to permeate the mucosa.

gastroduodenostomy (Billroth I) A partial gastrectomy in which the lower portion of the stomach is removed and the remainder is anastomosed with the duodenum.

gastroesophageal reflux The backflow of gastric contents into the lower end of the esophagus.

gastroesophageal reflux disease (GERD) A common condition in which acid from the stomach flows back into the esophagus, causing discomfort and, in some cases, damage to the esophageal lining.

gastrojejunostomy (Billroth II) Procedure in which a larger distal portion of the stomach is removed than with the gastroduodenostomy (Billroth I) procedure, and the remainder is anastomosed to the jejunum.

gastroparesis Delayed emptying of food from the stomach into the small bowel.

gate control theory Proposes that the spinal cord has a gating mechanism that either permits or inhibits the transmission of pain information to the brain.

gating Dividing the cardiac cycle into segments so that images viewed in cine mode allow the clinician to evaluate wall motion and systolic thickening in all areas of the left ventricle.

gauge Needle or catheter size.

gene The functional unit of heredity that occupies a certain position on a chromosome and is passed from parent to offspring. Genes consist of DNA and most contain information for making a specific protein.

gene mutations Abnormal genes inherited from parents.

gene therapy Therapy that involves adding a functional gene or group of genes to a cell by gene insertion to correct a hereditary disorder.

general adaptation syndrome (GAS) Physical response to stress as defined by Selye. GAS is composed of three stages: alarm reaction, stage of resistance, and stage of exhaustion.

general anesthesia The production of complete unconsciousness, muscular relaxation, and absence of pain sensation.

genetic variance Variation in genotype that is associated with phenotype.

genital herpes An incurable condition caused primarily by the herpes simplex virus; it can be treated with antiviral drugs.

genital warts Sexually transmitted, cauliflower-like growths in the genital, anal, and vaginal areas. Also called *human papillomavirus*.

genome All of the DNA in an organism or cell to include the 44 autosomes, 2 sex chromosomes, and the mitochondrial DNA.

genomic imprinting Genetic inheritance process in which both maternal and paternal alleles are present, but one allele is expressed and the other remains silent.

genomics The field of genetics concerned with structural and functional studies of the genome.

genotype The genetic makeup of an individual that is not evident as outward or visible characteristics.

germ line cells The sex cell or gamete (egg or spermatozoan).

gerontological nurse practitioner (GNP) A registered nurse with a master's degree from a nurse practitioner program specializing in the care of older adults.

gestational diabetes mellitus (GDM) A specific type of diabetes that occurs during pregnancy in women who had no history of diabetes prior to the pregnancy.

gigantism Condition brought on by overproduction of pituitary growth hormone in youth before the long bones have closed. Characterized by abnormal height.

gingival hyperplasia Excessive proliferation of normal cells of the gingiva.

glaucoma A group of diseases of the optic nerve involving loss of retinal ganglion cells in a characteristic pattern of optic neuropathy. Raised intraocular pressure is a significant risk factor for developing glaucoma (above 22 mmHg).

glomerulus A compact tuft of capillaries in which blood is filtered.

glucagon A hormone produced by the alpha cells of the pancreas. Glucagon has several actions, the most important of which is (along with insulin) maintaining blood glucose levels within a normal range. In diabetes, elevated levels of glucagon contribute to hyperglycemia and ketosis.

gluconeogenesis The formation of glucose from noncarbohydrate organic molecules (i.e., lactate, glycerol, and amino acids); is a function of the liver.

glucose-6-phosphate dehydrogenase (G6PD) deficiency The most common enzyme deficiency contributing to hemolytic anemia. Enzymatic deficiencies in erythrocytes increase the red blood cell's sensitivity and susceptibility to oxidative stress. Deficiencies in the enzyme are genetically encoded and relatively common especially in persons of African American and Mediterranean descent.

glutamate An excitatory neurotransmitter implicated in cell death.

glycated serum proteins (GSPs) A test of short-term blood glucose control (14 to 20 days) obtained by measuring the glycosylation of total serum proteins or glycosylation of albumin. The most widely used method to measure GSPs is the hemoglobin A_{1c} (HbA_{1c}) test. A normal HbA_{1c} is less than 6%. This test is also known as glycated hemoglobin or glycosylated hemoglobin, and is frequently is referred to as "A1C."

glycogen A starch polysaccharide that is stored in the liver and muscles of humans and can be hydrolyzed to glucose.

glycogenolysis The conversion of glycogen to glucose.

glycolysis A biochemical pathway that results in the generation of high-energy compounds (e.g., ATP and NADH).

goal A broad statement of purpose that describes the aim of nursing care.

goiter Abnormal enlargement of the thyroid gland.

goitrogen A substance in a food or a drug that inhibits the production of thyroid hormone.

goniometer Used for measuring a patient's range of motion.

gonorrhea A sexually transmitted infection that is caused by the bacterium *Neisseria gonorrhoeae*, which infects the warm moist environment of the reproductive tract, along with any other mucous membranes in the body.

Gottron's sign Reddish raised rash or papules over the knuckles.

gouty arthritis Condition in which there is an imbalance in purine metabolism, which increases uric acid in the joints by the formation of uric acid crystals.

gouty joint Inflammation of the big toe, dorsum, ankles, heels, or elbows.

graduated compression stockings Elastic stockings that apply varying degrees of pressure on the lower leg with the greatest exertion of

pressure at the ankle and the lowest pressure at the thigh (or knee in shorter stockings).

graft versus host disease (GVHD) An alloimmune response in which the grafted tissue initiates an immune response against tissue of the host or recipient of the grafted tissue. An example of graft versus host disease is seen in transplanted bone marrow.

granulation tissue Tiny, round granule-like nodules that become beefy, red, and moist because of the dense revascularization process.

granulocyte White blood cell with numerous granules in the cytoplasm; granulocytes are divided into neutrophils, eosinophils, and basophils.

graph paper Paper specifically designed and used to measure various calculations related to the electrical activity of the heart; it is arranged as a series of horizontal and vertical lines and is standardized to allow for consistency in ECG tracing analysis.

Graves' disease A hypermetabolic condition caused by an autoimmune disease in which the thyroid gland produces too much thyroid hormone.

grounded theory The idea that conclusion of a qualitative study should be grounded in the data, that is, based on direct and careful observations of everyday life within the group.

growth factors A group of extracellular polypeptides (secreted by platelets and macrophages) that affect cell growth, reproduction, movement, or function.

growth needs The top levels of Maslow's hierarchy associated with psychological needs.

gynecomastia Male breast enlargement due to a hormonal imbalance.

hairy tongue A condition in which the tongue is covered with hairlike papilla due to the overgrowth of the fungus *Candida albicans* or *Aspergillus niger*.

haploid The number of chromosomes in an egg or sperm cell; it is half the diploid number.

hardiness Condition in which a person has a clear sense of personal values and goals, a strong tendency toward interaction with the environment, a sense of meaningfulness, and an internal rather than an external locus of control. It is a mediating factor in how people respond to stress.

Hashimoto's thyroiditis An autoimmune condition characterized by high titers of the circulating antibodies thyroid peroxidase and thyroglobulin that destroy thyroid cells and may lead to hypothyroidism. It is the most common thyroid disease in the United States. Also known as *chronic lymphocytic hypothyroidism*.

hassles Experiences and conditions of daily living that have been appraised as relevant and harmful or threatening to an individual's well-being.

Haversian canals Canals located in cortical bone; they contain one or two capillaries and nerve fibers that serve as the transport system for nutrients.

health care delivery system System that provides client-centered, comprehensive, interdisciplinary, integrated, and accessible health care that meets the needs of the clients.

Health Insurance Portability and Accountability Act (HIPAA) A federal law designed to improve the portability of health care coverage for people who lose or change employment, to simplify the administrative process through the use of electronic transactions, and to ensure the privacy of membership information.

health maintenance organization (HMO) Organization that provides coverage for medical care and controls costs through utilization review and management and by restricting access to a specific network of providers.

heart failure A complex and debilitating clinical syndrome in which there is loss or dysfunction of the cardiac muscle or an inability of the ventricle to fill or eject blood.

heaves Palpable sustained lifts of the chest wall due to forceful cardiac contractions.

Heberden's nodes Hard, painless nodules at the joints of the fingers; may indicate osteoarthritis. Heberden's nodes are found over the distal interphalangeal joints.

Helicobacter pylori (H. pylori) A bacterium that infects the stomach and duodenum and is associated with peptic ulcers.

hematocrit The ratio of the volume of erythrocytes (red blood cells) to that of the whole blood.

hematology The branch of biology (physiology), pathology, clinical laboratory, internal medicine, and pediatrics that is concerned with the study of blood, the blood-forming organs, and blood diseases.

hematoma An area of swelling or mass of blood confined to an organ, tissue, or space, due to a broken blood vessel.

hematopoiesis The formation and development of blood cells.

hematopoietic stem cell (HSC) Bone marrow cell that is the precursor to all hematologic cell types.

hematuria The presence of blood in the urine.

heme iron Form of dietary iron that is common in red meats and fish.

hemodynamic monitoring The monitoring of pressures and blood flow within the cardiovascular system.

hemoglobin The oxygen carrying pigment of the erythrocytes, formed by the developing erythrocyte in bone marrow.

hemoglobin A_{1c} (HbA_{1c}) test Refers to a series of stable minor hemoglobin components formed nonenzymatically from the glycosylation of the hemoglobin molecule. The amount of HbA_{1c} is directly proportional to the ambient glucose concentration, providing an estimation of blood glucose control during the previous 2 to 3 months. Sometimes also referred to as *glycohemoglobin*, *glycosylated hemoglobin*, or *A1C*.

hemoglobinopathies Red blood disorders characterized by abnormal hemoglobin.

hemolytic anemia Group of diseases characterized by increased red blood cell destruction.

hemophilia Genetic disorder resulting from mutated genes controlling Factors VIII or Factor IX; characterized by uncontrolled bleeding.

hemoptysis Coughing up of blood from the lower respiratory tract.

hemosiderin A form of iron in the body acting as a supply reservoir.

hemosiderin staining Occurs when the heme part of the red blood cell is deposited in the tissues as red blood cells get trapped and accumulate due to venous congestion. As the red blood cell dies, the heme is deposited and a brownish hue staining color results.

hemostasis Cessation of bleeding; a complex process that changes blood from a fluid to a solid state. Hemostasis occurs in two phases: primary and secondary. Primary hemostasis is characterized by vascular contraction, platelet adhesion, and formation of a soft aggregate plug. Secondary hemostasis is responsible for stabilizing the soft clot and maintaining vasoconstriction.

hemothorax Partial or complete collapse of the lung due to blood in the pleural space.

heparin-induced thrombocytopenia (HIT) Drug-induced, immune-mediated thrombocytopenia; caused by exposure to heparin therapy.

hepatic artery catheter A catheter inserted into the hepatic artery for targeted antineoplastic therapies.

hepatic encephalopathy A result of an increased level of circulating neurotoxins. The most abundant neurotoxin is ammonia and is the end product of protein digestion.

hepatic first pass Refers to the reduction of a medication's effect due to partial metabolism in the liver prior to distribution to the ultimate site of action.

hepatitis A virus (HAV) An RNA virus that causes hepatitis and is transmitted mainly through contaminated food and water.

hepatitis B virus (HBV) A DNA virus that causes hepatitis and is transmitted sexually and parenterally.

hepatitis C virus (HCV) An RNA virus that causes hepatitis and is transmitted mainly parenterally. The majority of the cases develop chronic hepatitis.

hepatitis D virus (HDV) An RNA virus that occurs only in the presence of HBV.

hepatitis E virus (HEV) An RNA virus that is transmitted mostly through the fecal–oral route and is endemic in Southeast Asia and parts of Africa.

hepatocellular Pertaining to the cells of the liver.

hepatojugular reflux An increase in jugular venous pressure when pressure is applied over the abdomen; is suggestive of right-sided heart failure.

hepatorenal syndrome Syndrome characterized by azotemia occurring in a patient with liver failure.

hepcidin Hormone produced in the liver that is responsible for iron supply regulation.

hereditary spherocytosis (HS) Hemolytic anemia disorder characterized by insufficient red blood cell membrane proteins.

hernia Protrusion of an anatomic structure through the wall that normally contains it.

herniation The displacement of brain structures under pressure, causing compression and damage of brain tissue.

herpetic stomatitis Inflammation of the oral cavity caused by the herpes simplex virus.

heterografts Biologic dressing made from animals such as pigs.

heterotropic ossification (OS) The development of bone tissue in areas where bone tissue is not normally present.

heterozygous Having two different alleles for a given gene, one inherited from each parent.

heuristic relevance Discovering or revealing a relationship that may lead to additional development along a particular line of research.

hiatal hernia Protrusion of the upper portion of the stomach into the thorax through the esophageal hiatus.

high-altitude pulmonary edema (HAPE) Type of pulmonary edema that develops in persons who rapidly ascend to heights greater than 2,500 to 3,000 meters (8,202 to 9,842 feet).

high density lipoprotein A type of lipoprotein that binds to cholesterol to transport it back to the liver; lipoproteins may actually remove excess cholesterol from plaque in the arteries.

highly active antiretroviral drug therapy (HAART) Combination therapy has the greatest effect in controlling HIV proliferation and minimizing the development of drug resistance. Antiretroviral drugs are grouped according to the mechanism of action against HIV.

hirsutism Abnormal growth of hair, especially in women.

histamine A protein produced by mast and other cells. Release of histamine results in vasodilation and bronchoconstriction. Symptoms associated with histamine release include shortness of breath, wheezing, itching, and hives.

histamine$_2$ (H$_2$)-receptor blockers Drugs that block the H$_2$-receptors located in the gastrointestinal tract and reduce acid secretion.

HIV antibody positive status An individual's status when enough HIV antibodies have been produced in response to infection by the HIV virus to be measured by antibody serology, usually after 3 weeks to 3 months. Symptoms may or may not be present.

hoarseness Condition that occurs when the normal vibration of the vocal cords is disrupted.

holding area A physical space located adjacent to the operating room where patients wait prior to an operation.

holism An idea based on the premise that the whole is more than the sum of its parts.

Holter monitoring Ambulatory electrocardiogram monitoring for an extended period of time.

homeostasis The tendency toward stability within an organism; it is the first reaction toward that stability when a wound occurs.

homograft valve *See* allograft valve.

homologous transfusion The process of collecting blood from a donor for transfusion into other individuals who are in need of blood.

homozygous Having identical alleles at a given location.

honeymoon period A transient period of time when newly diagnosed patients with type 1 diabetes have restoration of insulin production and thus a reduced requirement for exogenous insulin.

horizontal organization model Service structure of hospitals aligned to form a multihospital system; focuses on traditional acute care services.

hospice Palliative care and support services for patients with terminal illnesses and their families.

hospitalist Physician who concentrates her or his practice in the acute care environment.

host versus graft disease (HVGD) A type of alloimmune hypersensitivity response that involves transplanted organs or tissues; occurs when a recipient's immune system reacts against the foreign antigens on the cells of the graft.

human genome The complete DNA sequence that contains the entire genetic information for a human.

Human Genome Project (HGP) An international research project to map each human gene and completely sequence human DNA.

human immunodeficiency virus (HIV) The infective agent responsible for causing AIDS; HIV is a retrovirus that infects CD4 T cells and fatally impairs immune function. Two specific strains of HIV have been identified: HIV type 1 and HIV type 2.

human leukocyte antigens (HLAs) Genetic protein markers on the cell wall of white blood cells that alert the immune system to the appropriateness of a cell belonging to the system. HLAs can differentiate self from non-self. There are six different HLA markers: HLA-A, HLA-B, HLA-C, HLA-D, HLA-DR, and HLA-DQ. Each of these markers is capable of creating multiple different antigen subtype combinations. HLA matching between donor and recipient is key to preventing transplant graft rejection.

human papillomavirus (HPV) *See* genital warts.

humoral immune response Mechanism by which organisms gain immunity to previously encountered substances; involves B lymphocytes and antibody-mediated immunity. The term *humoral* comes from the Greek word "humor," which means body fluids; B cells are in the plasma.

Hunt-Hess classification Grading scale for subarachnoid hemorrhage.

hydrocele Swelling of the scrotum caused by fluid collection.

hydrogen ion A single, charged atomic proton that is not orbited by any electrons. It is the smallest ionic particle and is extremely reactive.

hydronephrosis Collection of urine in the pelvis of the kidney from obstructed outflow.

hydroxyapatite Inorganic hexagonal matrix of bone composed of calcium and phosphorus.

hyperacute rejection Occurs within the first hours after transplant when the recipient has a preexisting antibody to the antigen in the graft tissue. Blanching of the graft is one of the earliest signs of rejection.

hyperbaric oxygen therapy (HBOT) Refers to intermittent treatment of the entire body with 100% oxygen at greater than normal atmospheric pressures.

hypercarbic drive The stimulus for ventilation that occurs when elevated levels of carbon dioxide alter the pH of the blood and cerebrospinal fluid, making them more acid. Central chemoreceptors located in the brainstem react to this change in the pH and stimulate the body to breathe more deeply and more rapidly. It is the strongest stimulus of ventilation.

hypercatabolism Metabolic state in which degradation of protein stores is elevated.

hypercholesterolemia An increased cholesterol level in the blood.

hyperflexion injuries Increased flexion of a joint from trauma.

hyperglycemia Elevated blood glucose levels.

hypergranulation The formation of soft, pink fleshy projections as the body attempts to heal an enlarged wound track.

hyperkalemia An excess of potassium in the blood.

hyperlipidemia An elevated cholesterol and/or triglyceride level in the blood that is a modifiable risk factor for the development of coronary artery disease.

hypermetabolism Metabolic state in which resting energy expenditure is elevated.

hyperopia A defect in vision caused by an imperfection in the eye (often the eyeball is too short).

hyperosmolar hyperglycemic nonketotic syndrome (HHS) An emergent complication of diabetes characterized by serum hyperosmolarity, hyperglycemia, and dehydration.

hyperparathyroidism A hypermetabolic condition in which the parathyroid gland produces an excess of parathyroid hormone.

hyperplasia An increase in the number of new cells in an organ or tissue.

hyperpnea Refers to both the increased rate and depth of respiration associated with metabolic acidosis. It is sometimes referred to as *Kussmaul's breathing*.

hyperreflexia Exaggeration of the deep tendon reflexes.

hyperresonance A loud, low tone of longer duration than resonance. It is heard when air is trapped in a space such as the lungs.

hypertensive crisis A rare, sometimes fatal, occurrence that is characterized by the sudden onset of a diastolic blood pressure reading of 120 to 130; the clinical manifestation indicates target organ vascular damage and the presence of retinal exudates and hemorrhages.

hypertensive encephalopathy A very dangerous state of multifocal cerebral ischemia due to a severe acutely or subacutely elevated blood pressure.

hyperthyroidism A hypermetabolic condition in which the thyroid gland produces and the body responds to an excess production of thyroid hormones.

hypertonic Term used to identify a solution that contains a higher concentration of electrolytes than that found in body cells. If such a solution is allowed to enter the bloodstream, the osmotic pressure difference between the blood and the cells will cause water to flow out of the cells, which will then shrink.

hypertonic formula An enteral or parenteral nutrition formula with an osmolality, or concentration, that is greater than that of the body's plasma.

hypertrophic cardiomyopathy A disorder of the sarcomere, the contractile element of the cardiac muscle; characterized by left ventricular and occasionally right ventricular hypertrophy, with greater hypertrophy occurring in the septum. Also referred to as *idiopathic hypertrophic subaortic stenosis (IHSS)*.

hypertrophic scar Scar tissue that is an overgrowth of dermal tissue that remains within the boundaries of the wound.

hypertrophy An increase in the size of an organ caused by an increase in the size of the cells and tissues rather than the number of cells.

hyperventilation A state that exists when there is a lower than normal level of carbon dioxide in the blood. Also referred to as *hypocapnia*.

hyphema A collection of blood cells in the anterior chamber of the eye.

hypoalbuminemia Refers to low serum albumin, which most often results from liver damage.

hypochromic Term describing red blood cells that are paler in color than normal, suggesting iron deficiencies.

hypodermoclysis Continuous subcutaneous infusion of a large volume of isotonic parenteral fluids for purposes of rehydration.

hypoglycemia Decreased blood glucose levels.

hypoglycemic unawareness Condition that results from altered counterregulation, particularly deficient glucagon and epinephrine responses to hypoglycemia. This results in a loss of autonomic nervous system symptoms; for instance, tachycardia, palpitations, and tremors are absent. Patients are unaware that they are hypoglycemic and, without treatment, can progress rapidly into severe hypoglycemia.

hypokinesia Condition characterized by areas of abnormal heart contractility where muscle movement is hypoactive.

hypokinetic dysarthria Speech difficulty as a result of slowed, rigid muscles of tongue, mouth, and throat; associated with Parkinson's disease.

hypomimia Decreased facial expression due to rigid facial muscles.

hypoparathyroidism A hypometabolic condition in which the parathyroid gland fails to produce adequate parathyroid hormone.

hypophonia Soft, muffled voice.

hypopituitarism A hypometabolic condition in which the secretion of pituitary hormones is inadequate.

hypopnea A reduction but not complete cessation of airflow to less than 50% of normal.

hypopyon White layer of inflammatory cells in the anterior chamber.

hypospadias Opening of the urinary meatus on the ventral or bottom of the penis, between the penis and scrotum.

hypothalamic–pituitary–adrenal (HPA) axis A feedback loop by which signals from the brain trigger the release of hormones needed to respond to stress. Because of its function, the HPA axis also is referred to as the *stress circuit*.

hypothermia A core body temperature of less than 96.8°F (36°C) or a condition, regardless of body temperature, in which a person experiences shivering, peripheral vasoconstriction, piloerection, and feelings of cold.

hypothesis A statement that predicts a certain relationship between two or more variables.

hypothyroidism A metabolic condition in which the thyroid gland fails to produce adequate thyroid hormones.

hypotonia The absence of muscle tone, resulting in flaccidity of the muscles.

hypotonic Term used to identify a solution in which the concentration of electrolyte is below that found in body cells. In this situation osmotic pressure leads to the migration of water into the cells in an attempt to equalize the electrolyte concentration inside and outside the cell walls.

hypoventilation Decreased ventilation, which causes an increased $PaCO_2$; exists when there is a higher than normal level of carbon dioxide in the blood. Also referred to as *hypercapnia*.

hypoxemia Insufficient oxygen content in the blood.

hypoxia Physiological state of decreased blood oxygen levels.

hypoxic drive The stimulus to ventilation that occurs when peripheral chemoreceptors located in the carotid arteries and the aorta sense a decrease in the oxygen concentration in the blood.

hypoxic hypoxia Physiological state of decreased oxygen availability due to cardiac or pulmonary causes.

hysterectomy A surgical procedure to remove the uterus.

iatrogenic wounds Include intravenous puncture sites, incisions, radiation-induced skin damage, and grafts that occurred while a patient was in the hospital.

icteric phase The phase of acute hepatitis in which jaundice occurs, usually 1 to 2 weeks after the prodromal phase.

id Represents all of a person's biological and psychological drives.

IgE antibodies A class of antibodies produced by the B-lymphocyte plasma cells in response to exposure to a foreign antigen or allergen. They create an antibody–antigen complex that connects to receptors on mast cells and causes degranulation of mast cells and release of histamine; they are the major factor in type I hypersensitivity reactions.

ileal pouch anal anastomosis (IPAA) Procedure in which the entire colon, including the rectum, is removed and a pouch formed from the terminal ileum, which is then attached to the anus.

ileostomy Procedure in which a stoma is formed from the ileum. In a permanent ileostomy, the entire colon is removed and fecal material is collected in an external collection bag.

ileus A condition in which peristalsis does not return as expected postoperatively and the bowel remains hypoactive.

iliopsoas Refers to three muscles of the abdomen—psoas major, psoas minor, and iliacus—that pass from the abdomen through the pelvis and are partially responsible for hip flexion.

immediate hypersensitivity reaction An excessive response of the immune system that occurs in seconds to hours after exposure to an antigen. A systemic anaphylaxis is one example of an immediate hypersensitivity reaction response.

immune complex A substance formed when antibodies attach to antigens to destroy them.

immune deficiencies Deficiencies that occur when all or some part of the immune system fails to develop or is damaged through disease processes and, thus, cannot mount an appropriate immune response. There are two types, primary and secondary.

immune hypersensitivity response Occurs when the immune system overresponds to an antigen, either from the environment, from the individual himself, or from another individual. Disorders fall into three broad categories based on the type of triggering antigen, and include allergy, autoimmune, and alloimmune reactions.

immune tolerance The ability of the immune system to differentiate self from non-self and tolerate all self-antigens while retaining the ability to mount an immune response to non-self-antigens.

immunity The protective process of response to a foreign substance.

immunization The process of stimulating the immune system to create active immunity for protection against a disease by injection with a live or killed vaccine. Often used interchangeably with *vaccination* or *inoculation*.

immunoglobulin A diverse group of plasma proteins, made of polypeptide chains; one of the primary mechanisms for protection against diseases.

immunologic theory of aging Theory of aging based on the premise that the aging body is less able to distinguish its own cells from foreign cells.

impaired fasting glucose (IFG) A category of pre-diabetes in which the fasting glucose level is >100 mg/dL but <126 mg/dL.

impaired glucose tolerance (IGT) A category of pre-diabetes in which the blood glucose level following an oral glucose load of 75 grams is >140 mg/dL but <200 mg/dL.

impaired wound healing The disruption of the normal biochemical repair or regeneration process.

impetigo A common, contagious skin infection caused by *Staphylococcus aureus* and/or group A beta-hemolytic streptococcus that is characterized by vesicles that rupture and form yellow crusts.

implantable cardioverter defibrillator (ICD) Device that can automatically terminate the potentially lethal dysrhythmias of ventricular tachycardia and ventricular fibrillation. Currently these devices are incorporated into cardiac pacemakers.

implanted port A surgically placed central vascular access device; a chambered device comprised of a reservoir and an attached catheter; used for long-term or chronic infusion therapies.

implementation The "doing" or intervening phase of the nursing process.

implied consent Permission that is inferred by a person's conduct or by law.

impotence Refers to problems associated with ejaculation or orgasm, in addition to erectile dysfunction.

incapacitating agent Chemical agents that decrease acetylcholine at nerve synapses. They work in the opposite manner of nerve agents.

incidence The number of newly diagnosed cases of cancer in a specific time period in a defined population.

incident command system (ICS) A system of policies and procedures within a framework that allows for safe and effective management during a disaster.

INCMCE Acronym for International Nursing Coalition for Mass Casualty Education.

incomplete spinal cord injury Preservation of some degree of motor and/or sensory function below the level of a spinal injury.

incretin mimetics A class of medications that enhances glucose-dependent insulin secretion from the pancreatic β-cell resulting in a reduction in postprandial glucose levels. The incretins suppress elevated glucagon levels, promoting satiety, decreasing food intake, and slowing gastric emptying.

independent activities Activities that nurses perform, prescribe, and or delegate based on their education and skills. Assessing, analyzing, diagnosing, planning, implementing, and evaluating are independent activities.

independent practice association (IPA) Organization that contracts on the behalf of individuals or groups of physicians to provide health care to members of a health maintenance organization.

indirect calorimetry The measurement of energy expenditure by measuring oxygen intake and carbon dioxide output.

indirect inguinal hernia Occurs when abdominal contents protrude through the deep inguinal ring.

indirect percussion Technique that involves using the hyperextended middle finger of the nondominant hand (pleximeter) and then the finger tip of the middle finger of the dominant hand (plexor) to strike the pleximeter by using a wrist action that will elicit a sound.

Ineffective Coping Nursing diagnosis that refers to an inability to manage internal or environmental stressors appropriately as a result of inadequate physical, psychological, behavioral, or cognitive resources.

infarction An area of dead tissue.

infective endocarditis An infection of the cardiac endocardial layer of the heart, which may include one or more heart valves, the mural endocardium, and/or a septal defect; previously known as bacterial endocarditis.

infectivity The ability of a pathogen to enter a host and then live and grow within that host.

infiltration Inadvertent administration of a nonvesicant solution or medication into surrounding tissues.

inflammation A defensive mechanism of the body that is intended to neutralize, control, or eliminate an offending agent to prepare a site for repair. It is a nonspecific response that is meant to serve a protective function.

inflammatory bowel disease (IBD) An immunologic disease that results in idiopathic intestinal inflammation; includes Crohn's disease and ulcerative colitis.

inflammatory phase A phase of wound healing that begins at the time of the injury or surgery. The purpose of this phase is to prepare the site for growth of new tissue.

influenza A contagious disease that is caused by the influenza virus. Also known as the *flu*.

informatics The theory, science, and practice of the use of computer and informational technologies to store, retrieve, transmit, and manipulate data.

information technology Refers to those systems, including software programs and computer hardware, used to manage and process information.

informed consent Doctrine that mandates that individuals must be fully appraised of the nature, risks, benefits, alternative therapies, and potential consequences of procedures and therapies in health care settings.

infradian rhythm Rhythmic repetition of cycles lasting for more than a 24-hour period; an example is the female menstrual cycle.

infusate Parenteral fluid or medication.

inhalation injury Inhalation of smoke, causing injury to the lungs.

injection port or cap Device that allows entrance to a catheter's fluid pathway.

insensible fluid loss Water lost from the body carried as vapor in exhaled gases and evaporated from the body as sweat.

insomnia Difficulty falling or remaining asleep.

inspection The deliberate, systematic examination of a patient using both sight and smell.

Institute of Medicine (IOM) Organization that provides unbiased, evidence-based, authoritative information on medicine and health to policy makers, professionals, and the public at large in an effort to improve health.

insulin A hormone produced by the beta cells of the pancreas that has multiple effects. Insulin is necessary for glucose transport into insulin-sensitive tissues and storage of carbohydrates, fats, and proteins.

insulin resistance Unresponsiveness of anabolic processes to the normal effects of insulin and possibly tissue insensitivity to insulin.

intentional torts Wrongful conduct that is intentional in nature and designed to cause harm or damage to another.

interdependent activities Activities that overlap with other health care team members, physicians, social workers, pharmacists, nutritionists, and therapists, and require coordination and planning with those various team members.

interface pressure The pressure between a bony prominence and a surface such as a hospital bed or seating surface.

interferon (IFN) Protein made and released by T cells when the invading organism is a virus; functions to protect other cells from viral attack and stimulates the immune response; also inhibits the growth of certain tumor cells.

interleukin (IL) Chemical message produced by lymphocytes that enables the cells of the immune system to communicate and stimulate or slow an immune response. The various types of IL include IL-1 and IL-6, which are pro-inflammatory and stimulate B-cell production, whereas others, such as IL-12 and IL-13, help slow and inhibit the immune and inflammatory responses.

intermittent claudication (IC) Exercise-induced leg pain.

intermittent pneumatic compression devices Devices used to apply intermittent compression of the calf muscle, thereby increasing venous return.

internal locus of control An orientation in which a person believes that events in his or her life are controlled by his or her own actions and decisions.

internal stressor Stressor that originates within a person.

interphalangeal joint Joints between the fingers.

interstitial fluid Fluid between cells, but not in serum.

intervention An action designed to facilitate achievement of desired patient outcomes. It must be purposeful, must be supported by a rationale, and involve organization and actual delivery of nursing care, which ideally leads to achievement of stated patient goals and objectives.

intestinal obstruction The impairment of the forward movement of intestinal contents by mechanical causes (tumors), adhesions, or functional causes (surgery, anesthesia, medications); can occur anywhere from the pylorus to the rectum.

intra-atrial pathways Part of the electrical conduction system of the heart that consists of the internodal pathways and the Bachmann bundle.

intra-axial tumors Tumors originating from glial cells; found mostly in white matter.

intracellular fluid (ICF) Fluid contained within the cells.

intracranial pressure (ICP) The pressure exerted by cerebrospinal fluid within the ventricles.

intramedullary (I-M) rodding A method of fracture fixation that entails sliding a metal rod down the medullary canal of a long bone.

intraoperative During surgery.

intraosseous therapy Administration of parenteral fluids via the bone marrow; used in emergent situations when vascular access is not available.

intraspinal catheter A catheter used to access the intraspinal route.

intrathecal anesthesia A type of anesthesia in which a local anesthetic agent is inserted into the spinal fluid by penetrating the spinal dura.

intrathecal therapy Delivery of parenteral medications into the cerebrospinal fluid.

intrinsic factor (IF) Chemical secreted by the gastric mucosa required for vitamin B_{12} absorption.

intrinsic pathway Also known as the contact activation pathway, describes the clotting cascade branch initiated by the contact between circulating plasma proteins and the negatively charged surface of the injured subendothelial layer.

intron A noncoding segment of DNA that is transcribed into nuclear RNA, but removed in the subsequent processing into mRNA.

intussusception The slipping of one part of an intestine into another part just below it.

invasion of privacy Violation of the right to protection against unreasonable and unwarranted interference with one's solitude.

invasiveness Degree to which an organism can spread through the body.

ion Electrically charged components derived from the molecules of electrolytes. When placed in water the molecules dissociate into charged components or ions, producing positively and negatively charged ions.

iron deficiency anemia (IDA) Most common cause of anemia resulting from insufficient iron in the diet.

irregularly-irregular rhythm Heartbeats that occur when the R-to-R intervals exhibit no regularity in their distance from each other.

irritants Agents that generally cause pain, burning, lacrimation, or discomfort upon exposure to mucous membranes. Also called *riot control agents*.

ischemia Tissue hypoxia resulting from reduced blood flow to the tissues.

ischemia cascade A series of events that occurs as a compensatory mechanism in response to cerebral hypoxia. Also called *ischemic cascade*.

ischemia reperfusion injury A multifactorial process that occurs when anaerobic metabolism is initiated by hypoperfusion and hypoxia that leads to an oxygen deficit in endothelial, parenchymal, or immune competent cells.

ischemic cascade *See* ischemia cascade.

isoelectric line Straight line on the ECG graph paper that marks the beginning and ending point of all waves. Also referred to as the *baseline*.

isotonic Having the same osmolality as blood (275 to 295 mOsm/kg of body weight).

isotonic formula An enteral or parenteral nutrition formula with an osmolality, or concentration, that is approximately equal that of the body's plasma.

J point On an ECG tracing, the point at which the QRS meets the ST segment.

Joint Commission The accrediting body for hospitals and health care organizations; it is an independent, private, not-for-profit organization.

jugular venous distention (JVD) Increased blood pressure in the jugular vein that reflects the volume and pressure of venous blood, when volume overload is present.

jugular venous pressure (JVP) An indication of the hemodynamic events of the right atrium; derived from measurement of the pulsations of the right internal jugular vein.

junctional dysrhythmia Dysrhythmia resulting from an irritable focus in the junctional tissue that fires off before the SA node has had a chance to, or because the SA node has failed to fire. Three typical junctional dysrhythmias are junctional escape rhythm, premature junctional contraction, and junctional tachycardia.

junctional escape rhythm Dysrhythmia that occurs when the SA node fails to produce an impulse, or when the SA node's rate of firing falls below the intrinsic rate of the AV node. When this occurs, the AV node assumes the role of pacemaker.

justice In ethics, states that people should be treated fairly and equally.

Kaposi's sarcoma A malignancy involving the endothelial layer of blood and lymphatic vessels. Kaposi's is the most common cancer associated with AIDS.

karyotype A set of photographed, banded chromosomes of an individual, arranged from largest to smallest.

keloid scar Hypertrophic scar tissue that extends beyond the wound edges.

ketogenesis Condition in which an excessive amount of ketones are produced during diabetic ketoacidosis (DKA); is the cause of metabolic acidosis during DKA.

kinematics The predictive patterns of injuries.

KUB Abbreviation for kidney-ureter-bladder radiograph, and is also known as a "plain film of the abdomen." The radiograph helps to determine position, size, and structure of the kidneys and urinary tract. It is useful in evaluating for the presence of calculi and masses. This is also an excellent test for intestinal obstruction because it shows the air in the colon nicely.

Kupffer cells Cells that line the liver sinusoids and are phagocytic.

Kussmaul's respirations Deep, sighing respirations. Also called *hyperpnea*.

kyphosis Curvature of the spine that creates a stooped-over "humpback" appearance.

L'Hermite's sign Electric shock-like sensation throughout the body, elicited by flexing the neck.

labyrinthectomy Surgical procedure in which the labyrinth is excised to eradicate vertigo; results in complete hearing loss to the ear.

labyrinthitis Organ of balance within the middle ear.

lactase An enzyme that breaks down lactose, a sugar found in milk.

lactation Breast-feeding.

lactic dehydrogenase (LDH) An intracellular enzyme present in many cells, but high concentrations are found in the liver. The enzyme is released in response to liver injury.

lactose intolerance Results from a deficiency of lactase, the enzyme responsible for the breakdown of lactose, at the brush border of the small intestine, resulting in malabsorption.

lacunar stroke Thrombosis of a small penetrating artery, resulting in ischemia and infarction of deep white matter of the brain.

lamellar bone Mature bone.

laminectomy The removal of a vertebral posterior arch intended to remove a lesion or herniated disk.

laryngeal spasm An abnormal reflexive response to a laryngeal insult.

laryngectomy A permanent surgical airway with removal of the larynx, usually for cancer.

laryngitis Inflammation of the larynx and/or vocal cords.

laryngopharyngeal reflux disease (LPRD) Inflammation of the laryngopharynx as a result of gastric reflux into the pharynx and larynx.

laryngospasm Occurs when the muscles of the larynx contract forcefully, causing a closure or partial closure of the airway.

latent autoimmune diabetes in adults (LADA) An autoimmune form of diabetes that affects adults.

law Rules and regulation by which a society is governed.

lead axis Refers to the imaginary line drawn between the positive and negative electrodes.

leading health indicators Ten indicators from *Healthy People 2010* that reflect major public health concerns: (1) physical activity, (2) overweight and obesity, (3) tobacco use, (4) substance abuse, (5) responsible sexual behavior, (6) mental health, (7) injury and violence, (8) environmental quality, (9) immunization, and (10) access to health care.

Leapfrog Group A coalition of public and private organizations that provides health care benefits. The coalition provides public information on medical errors, health care standards, and health care provider quality performance measures.

left-sided heart failure An abnormal cardiac condition characterized by the impairment of the left side of the heart and elevated pressure and congestion in the pulmonary veins and capillaries.

left ventricular ejection fraction (LVEF) The proportion of blood ejected during each ventricular contraction compared with the total ventricular filling volume.

legal blindness The best-corrected visual acuity of 20/200 or a visual field of 20 degrees or less in both eyes.

leukemia Malignancy of the hematopoietic system.

leukocyte White blood cell.

leukocyte-poor RBCs A unit of packed red blood cells that had most of the white blood cells removed as soon as the blood was taken from the donor (i.e., prior to storage).

leveling Positioning of a transducer system in line with the chamber being monitored.

levodopa Precursor to dopamine; key drug used to treat Parkinson's disease.

licensed vocational/practical nurse (LVN/LPN) A nurse with 1 to 2 years of technical training to provide basic care.

licensure Process for approving a health care organization to provide medical care or services. Also refers to the certification process for professionals.

ligament A strong fibrous band of connective tissue.

limits of formalization In philosophy, the inability to make explicit or formal all elements of a social practice.

linear lesion Lesion that forms a line.

linear skull fracture A simple break in the continuity of the skull with no displacement of bone.

lipase An enzyme secreted by the pancreas that hydrolyzes triglycerides, cholesterol, and phospholipids.

lipodystrophy Abnormal deposition of adipose in the body.

lipohyalinosis Coating of the walls of small arteries with a lipid substance, causing narrowing of the arterial lumen.

lipolysis Breakdown of triglycerides to free fatty acids and glycerol.

lipoma Benign tumor consisting of fat cells.

liposuction Common type of cosmetic surgery, the purpose of which is to remove subcutaneous fat.

literature review A search of the latest research articles and scholarly studies.

lithotomy Position in which the patient lies on the back with the legs flexed at the hips and knees and the legs spread widely at the hip.

living wills A form of an advanced directive that describes a patient's preferences in case he or she becomes incapacitated. They usually describe what level of life-prolonging interventions the patient would or would not want and under what circumstances they should be completed, withheld, or withdrawn.

local adaptation syndrome (LAS) A local response to a stressor that proceeds through the same three stages as the general adaptation syndrome: alarm, resistance, and exhaustion.

locus of control The perception a person has about how much control he or she exerts over the events that happen in his or her life.

long-term care insurance Private insurance that covers the expenses of nursing care in a variety of settings, depending on the policy.

lordosis Excessive inward curvature of the spine.

low density lipoproteins A type of lipoprotein that transports cholesterol and triglycerides from the liver to peripheral tissues.

lower esophageal sphincter (LES) An area at the distal end of the esophagus that prevents the movement of gastric juice into the esophagus.

Ludwig's angina A deep neck infection involving the sublingual, submandibular, and submental spaces; usually the result of a dental abscess.

Luer-Lok™ Screw-type locking mechanism used to prevent accidental separation of infusion equipment.

lumen The bore or internal opening of a catheter.

lumpectomy Removal of a cancerous growth and a small amount of surrounding normal tissue.

Lund-Browder formula Formula for determining burn size that divides the body into percentage areas.

lung abscess An area of pulmonary infection with parenchymal necrosis.

Lyme disease A bacterial infection that affects the organs and joints; transmitted by black-legged ticks.

lymph nodes Lymph tissue that filters debris from the breakdown of cells, bacteria, viruses, and fungal antigens located throughout the body.

lymphangitis An acute inflammation of the lymphatic channels.

lymphatic system The circulatory system of the immune system that is comprised of the lymph vessels, lymph nodes, and lymph tissue and functions to drain lymph fluid (chyle) from throughout the body and return it to venous circulation in the chest.

lymphedema Edema due to the obstruction of the lymphatics.

lymphocyte Mature white cell; the two types of lymphocytes are T lymphocytes (T cells) and B lymphocytes (B cells).

lymphogranuloma venereum (LGV) A sexually transmitted infection caused by *Chlamydia trachomatis*. It is a rare condition, with only 200 cases reported each year.

lymphokines Cytokines that are made by lymphocytes; act as chemical messengers between cells and instruct immune cells to proliferate, differentiate, or alter activities. The major lymphokines are interleukins and interferons.

lymphoma Malignancy of the lymphatic system.

macrocephalic Abnormally large head size; found in acromegaly, hydrocephalus, rickets, osteitis deformans, leontiasis ossea, myxedema, leprosy, and pituitary disturbances.

macronutrients Nutritional components such as protein, carbohydrates, and fat that are needed in large quantities by living organisms.

macrovascular Pertaining to the large blood vessels of the arterial and venous system (e.g., coronary arteries).

macular degeneration (MD) The deterioration and mottling of the macula through the course of time.

magnesium An intracellular cation primarily in muscle and bone (only 1% is in the blood; 1.8 to 2.4 mg/dL).

magnet hospital A hospital designated by the American Nurses Credentialing Center as meeting the standards that result in excellence in delivery of nursing services and promoting a professional practice environment.

magnetic resonance cholangiopancreatography (MRCP) A noninvasive imaging test used to detect bile duct stones and pancreatic duct obstruction.

magnetic resonance imaging (MRI) Technique that uses radiofrequency pulses from a large, powerful magnet to temporarily disrupt the normal spin of certain atoms within the body. When the pulses are stopped, the atoms emit small amounts of energy while returning to their original spin; this energy can be imaged and recorded as high-resolution images that allow detailed noninvasive assessment of the both cardiac anatomy and physiology.

malabsorption The failure of the small intestine to absorb nutrients from digested food.

maladaptive coping mechanisms Those responses to stress that are not effective.

maldigestion The failure of chemical processes such as inadequate pancreatic enzymes or bile salts.

malignant Containing cancerous cells.

malignant hyperthermia (MH) A rare but life-threatening metabolic complication of anesthesia that usually occurs during the induction phase but could occur anytime during surgery. Certain people have a genetic predisposition to this illness. Immediate attention is vital to the recovery of the patient, and intensive care monitoring is mandatory following its occurrence.

malnutrition The physical consequences resulting from underconsumption of energy or nutrients compared to recommended amounts.

malpractice Professional misconduct; failure to meet the standards of care that a reasonably prudent member of the profession would employ.

mammography A low-dose x-ray procedure that allows visualization of the internal structure of the breast.

mandatory reporter A person required by law to report allegations and/or suspicions of abuse.

masked facies Immobile, expressionless facial appearance commonly seen in Parkinson's disease.

massive hemothorax An accumulation of 1,500 mL or more of blood in the thoracic cavity.

mastalgia Breast pain.

mastectomy Removal of the entire breast (total) or a modified radical mastectomy, which is removal of the entire breast along with the surrounding lymph nodes.

mastitis Inflammation of the breast tissue; occurs most frequently in breast-feeding women. Microorganisms invade the tissue through some portal of entry, such as a crack, fissure, or duct.

mastoidectomy Surgical procedure in which the mastoid process is excised in the event of infection.

mastoiditis Infection of the mastoid bone.

mature minors Persons under the legal age of adulthood who are legally able to give valid informed consent.

maturity onset diabetes of the young (MODY) Diabetes that has early onset (usually before the age of 25); it is inherited in an autosomal dominant manner and more closely resembles type 2 diabetes rather than type 1.

McGill Pain Questionnaire (MPQ) Assesses pain intensity, character, and location of pain using a body diagram, and also the duration of the pain experience.

mean arterial pressure (MAP) The average pressure in the arteries during one cardiac cycle.

mean corpuscular hemoglobin (MCH) Amount of hemoglobin per red blood cell.

mean corpuscular hemoglobin concentration (MCHC) Concentration of hemoglobin in each red blood cell.

mean corpuscular volume (MCV) Measure of the size of a red blood cell.

mechanical infusion device (MID) Infusion system that does not rely on an external power source.

mechanical phlebitis Inflammation of a vein associated with a catheter, its insertion, and the selected insertion site.

mechanical valves Commercially manufactured heart valves.

Medicaid Federally aided, but state-operated and -administered, program for providing medical care to qualifying low-income individuals.

medical durable power of attorney (MDPA) A document that sets out wishes for health care if an individual becomes too ill to make those decisions; a trusted person is designated to make health care decisions.

medical nutrition therapy (MNT) Meal planning approaches for patients with diabetes that combine clinical evidence, cultural, social, and ethnic approaches, and patient motivation.

medical record The legal document for all information regarding a patient's hospital course and evidence for the extent of care provided and the outcome of that care.

Medicare Federally sponsored health insurance program for people over age 65, some individuals with disabilities who are younger than age 65, and patients with end-stage renal disease. Medicare consists of Part A, hospital insurance, and Part B, general medical insurance and other options. Medicare also administers its own managed care plan.

medication nurse A registered nurse assigned the specific task of giving all patient medications under a functional nursing care delivery system.

medication reconciliation Process of identifying an accurate list of all medications the patient is taking, and using this list to provide correct medications for the patient anywhere in the health care system.

megakaryocytic stem cells Ancestor cells form giving rise to platelets.

megaloblast Large, immature red blood cells.

megaloblastic anemia Anemia resulting from impaired DNA synthesis of the red blood cells' ancestor cells.

melena Black or maroon, sticky, foul-smelling feces resulting from the digestion of blood.

menarche Beginning of menstruation or first menses.

Ménière's disease Inner ear disorder that affects hearing and balance.

meningiomas Tumors originating from the meninges.

meningismus Meningeal irritation.

menorrhagia Heavy bleeding during a menstrual period.

meshed skin graft Procedure of cutting holes in harvested skin, which allows it to be stretched over a greater surface area.

messenger ribonucleic acid (mRNA) RNA containing genetic information that is transcribed from DNA and translated to produce polypeptides.

metabolic equivalent (MET) A measure of oxygen consumption. One MET is the energy requirement for a person at rest while sitting: around 3.5 mL of oxygen per kilogram of body weight per minute.

metabolic syndrome The diagnosis given when a patient has a cluster of cardiac risk factors, including having three out of the five following conditions: abdominal obesity, high triglycerides, low HDL-C, high blood pressure, and high fasting glucose ($\geq$100 mg/dL).

metabolism All energy and material transformations that occur within a living cell.

metacarpophalangeal joints Joints at the knuckles.

metamorphopsia Condition characterized by vision distortion, that is, when straight lines, such as door frames or posts, look crooked or irregular.

metaphysis An area of widening between the diaphysis and physis.

metaplasia Cell transformation in which a highly specialized cell changes into a less specialized cell.

metastasis The spread of cancerous cells beyond the tumor to distant sites.

metastatic tumors Tumors that originate somewhere else in the body and migrate to another organ.

metered-dose inhaler (MDI) A device that helps deliver a specific amount of medication to the lungs, usually by supplying a short burst of aerosolized medicine that is inhaled by the patient. It is commonly used to treat asthma, chronic obstructive pulmonary disease, and other respiratory disorders.

metered-volume chamber set An administration set comprised of tubing, a semirigid metered chamber, and an access spike to be inserted in the fluid container.

methodological congruence Congruence among four dimensions of a research study: documentation rigor, procedural rigor, ethical rigor, and auditability.

metrorrhagia Bleeding between menstrual periods.

microalbuminuria Small amounts of protein (30 to 299 mg/24 hours) in the urine.

microcephalic Abnormal smallness of the head, often seen in mental retardation.

microcytic Term describing red blood cells that are smaller in size than normal.

micrographia Small, cramped handwriting.

micronutrients Nutritional components such as vitamins or minerals that are needed in small quantities by living organisms.

microvascular Pertaining to the small blood vessels of the arterial and venous system.

midline (ML) catheter A flexible catheter measuring not more than 8 inches with the distal tip dwelling in the basilica, cephalic, or brachial veins, level with the axilla and distal to the shoulder.

mild cognitive impairment (MCI) A term used to describe memory loss that appears greater than what is expected for a patient's age.

millivolts A unit of electrical voltage or potential difference equal to one-thousandth of a volt.

minute ventilation (V_E) A measurement of how much air the lungs move in 1 minute; it is equal to respiratory rate times tidal volume. A normal resting respiratory rate and a normal resting tidal volume of about 500 mL yield a normal minute ventilation of 6 L/min.

missense mutation A mutation that changes a codon specific for one amino acid to specify a different amino acid.

mitral valve prolapse Occurs when one or more of the valve leaflets bulge or prolapse into the left atrium during systole. This prolapse of the valve results in valve regurgitation.

mitral valve regurgitation An inability of the mitral valve to close due to an abnormality in the structure and function of the valve.

mitral valve stenosis Occurs when the mitral valve assumes an abnormal funnel shape due to thickening and shortening of the valve structures as a result of calcification. Contractures develop between the junctions or commissures (leaflets) of the valve. The stenosis narrows the opening of the valve, which obstructs blood flow from the left atrium to the left ventricle.

mixed hearing loss Type of hearing loss that is both conductive and sensorineural in cause.

mixed venous oxygen saturation Measurement of venous oxygen content in the pulmonary artery; used to assess oxygen consumption and metabolic needs of the tissues.

Mobitz I/Wenckebach One of the two types of second-degree block that occurs in the AV node, a progressive prolongation of the electrical impulse delay in the AV node until there is a complete loss of the QRS complex and, thus, no ventricular contraction. Depicted on an ECG tracing as a progressive lengthening of the PR interval until the P wave does not progress through the conduction system, resulting in a dropped QRS complex.

Mobitz II/second-degree block Periodic blocking of sinus impulses at the AV node, the bundle of His, or bundle branches. Occurs when there is an intermittent interruption in the electrical conduction system near or below the AV node and is a more serious dysrhythmia than either first-degree AV block or Mobitz I/ Wenckebach. This dysrhythmia indicates an increased risk of progression to third-degree, or complete, heart block.

mode of transmission Means by which an organism travels from a reservoir to a susceptible host.

modeling The process by which bone growth occurs and where there is a higher rate of bone formation relative to bone loss.

molecular mimicry A process in which peptides from proteins, such as viruses, become structurally similar to self-peptides and activate T-cell autoimmunity.

molimenal Symptoms of menstruation.

MONA A protocol for empirical treatment of patients with suspected myocardial infarction. Cited in the Advanced Cardiac Life Support guidelines, the mnemonic stands for *m*orphine, *o*xygen, *n*itroglycerin, and *a*spirin.

monocyte The largest of the white blood cells and makes up about 3% to 8% of the total leukocyte count. Monocytes are a part of the reticuloendothelial (or mononuclear phagocytic) system, whose function is to engulf and digest microbes and other foreign substances. Monocytes migrate from the blood to various tissues where they mature into macrophages, working to kill invading antigens.

monophasic defibrillation Traditional means by which electrical voltage is delivered to patients in ventricular tachycardia and fibrillation.

monosomy A chromosomal constitution in which one member of the chromosome pair is missing.

Monro-Kellie doctrine Doctrine that provides the foundation for understanding the implications of increased intracranial pressure. Incompressible structures within the cranial vault are in a state of volume equilibrium, such that any increase of the volumes of one component (i.e., blood, CSF, or brain tissue) must be compensated by a decrease in the volume of another. If this cannot be achieved then pressure will rise and once the expandable reserve of the intracranial space is exhausted then small changes in volume can lead to precipitous increases in pressure.

moral agency The ability to affect and influence situations.

MORAL model An ethical decision-making model based on a series of five steps that represent the acronym MORAL: *m*assage the dilemma; *o*utline the options; *r*esolve the dilemma; *a*ct by applying the chosen option; and *l*ook back and evaluate.

morality A code of conduct held to be authoritative in matters of right and wrong.

morphologic classification Classification of skin lesions in terms of type of lesion (primary, secondary, or vascular), size, shape or configuration, color, texture, elevation or depression, and pedunculation.

mortality The number of deaths from cancer in a specific period of time and within an identified population.

mosaicism Nondisjunction of a pair of chromosomes that occurs in a mitotic division after formation of the zygote, and leads to an individual with at least two cell lines differing in genotype or karyotype, derived from a single zygote.

mucormycosis A fungal infection often seen in the sinuses of patients with diabetes who do not have good glycemic control.

multichannel pump Electronic infusion device often used in critical care areas; used to administer multiple parenteral therapies simultaneously.

multiflow adapter Add-on device used to facilitate multiple administrations of fluids and medications via a single vascular access device.

multiple organ dysfunction syndrome (MODS) Diagnosed when two or more organ systems fail.

multiple sclerosis (MS) Disease in which the immune system attacks the nerve tissues in the central nervous system, causing damage to the neurons, which disrupts the body's ability to send signals and causes symptoms. Believed to be an autoimmune disease.

multislice helical CT Detailed, noninvasive imaging of the heart using 16-slice helical scanners, accompanied by ECG gating and iodinated contrast. This device can scan the entire volume of the heart, proximal great vessels, and the coronary arteries with a single 25-second breath hold.

murmurs Abnormal heart sounds produced by turbulent blood flow.

muscle atrophy Shortening of a muscle attached to a joint.

mutation A permanent structural change in DNA.

myasthenia gravis A chronic autoimmune neuromuscular disorder in which acetylcholine receptors at the neuromuscular junction are destroyed.

myasthenic crisis A life-threatening exacerbation of myasthenia gravis that requires mechanical ventilation.

myelin A soft, white coating that surrounds and protects nerve fibers. Myelin also helps nerve fibers conduct electrical impulses.

myeloid progenitor cell Ancestor cell that gives rise to granulocytes and monocytes.

myelopathy Motor, sensory, and reflex abnormalities due to an abnormality of the spinal cord.

myocardial hibernation Condition in which myocardial tissue undergoes cellular structural changes and progressive apoptosis (cell death) in response to prolonged cardiac ischemia.

myocardial infarction (MI) The loss of myocytes or myocardial cell death as a result of prolonged ischemia.

myocardial perfusion Blood flow to the heart muscle.

myocardial perfusion imaging (MPI) Use of a radioactive tracer and a gamma camera to detect blood flow to the myocardium.

myocardial stunning A temporary dysfunction that occurs in response to artery occlusion of short duration (artery spasm) or transient global hypoperfusion during a limited low-flow state such as shock.

myocardial viability Term applied to areas of the myocardium that appear to have normal functioning as well as areas that appear dysfunctional (hibernating or stunned) that might improve with revascularization.

myocarditis A focal or diffuse inflammation of the myocardium or heart muscle; an uncommon disorder that is frequently associated with pericarditis.

myocutaneous flap A piece of tissue, muscle or skin, used in reconstructive surgery; may be used for reconstructing breasts, large lateral temporal, scalp, or intraoral defects, and defects involving the trunk and chest wall.

myoglobin A heme-containing, oxygen-binding protein that is exclusive to striated and nonstriated muscle. Because of its very small molecular weight, it is released into interstitial fluid as early as 2 hours following damage to muscle tissue.

myopia Individuals see nearby objects clearly, but distant objects appear blurred.

myositis An uncommon disease in which the immune system inflames the body's own healthy muscle tissue.

myringotomy Surgical procedure in which tubes are placed in the ears to facilitate drainage and prevent the buildup of pressure within the inner ear and prevent ear infections.

myxedema A long-term consequence of hypothyroidism in which the facial features are coarsened and changed by puffiness, periorbital edema, and a mask-like appearance.

myxedema coma A rare, life-threatening complication of hypothyroidism.

nadir The point at which the lowest blood count is reached.

nasal polyps Small saclike growths inside the nasal cavity and sinuses.

national standards of care Statements of actions consistent with minimum safe professional conduct under specific medical conditions as determined by professional medical organizations.

natural immunity Type of immunity that is the responsibility of a group of body organs, cells, and chemicals that are present at birth or shortly after.

near drowning Condition that connotes survival for at least 24 hours after submersion.

neck dissection Surgical procedure to remove nodal disease in conjunction with the central part of the cancer surgery.

necrotizing fasciitis (NF) An infection of the superficial fascia or the connective tissue surrounding muscle and subcutaneous tissue leading to necrosis.

needleless system Components of infusion equipment that do not use needles.

negative deflection Any waveform that goes below the isoelectric line on ECG graph paper.

negative feedback A compensatory mechanism by which homeostasis is achieved in which the endocrine glands respond to a decrease in hormone levels, leading to gland stimulation and increased hormone production. When a normal level of hormone is reached, it feeds back to suppress the stimulating hormone and a normal state occurs.

negative pressure pulmonary edema (NPPE) A disorder caused by attempts to ventilate a person with an apparent airway obstruction. Also called *postobstruction pulmonary edema* and *airway obstruction pulmonary edema*.

negligence Failure to exercise the degree of care that a person of ordinary prudence would exercise under the same or similar conditions.

neoantigens Antigens created by the developing fetal immune system while it is in the process of eliminating autoreactive lymphocytes.

neoplasm New growth.

nephron The functional unit of the kidney.

nerve agents Chemicals that inactivate acetylcholinesterase at the receptor site. They cause symptoms of SLUDGE'M (*s*alivation, *l*acrimation, *u*rination, *d*efecation, *g*astric upset, *e*mesis, and *m*iosis).

network sampling Type of sampling in which participants refer other participants to the study. Also referred to as *snowball sampling*.

neurofibromatosis An autosomal dominant inherited disorder characterized by the formation of tumors of the peripheral nerves over the entire body.

neurogenic pulmonary edema (NPE) A rare type of pulmonary edema that develops after a neurological insult to the central nervous system.

neurogenic shock Occurs in spinal cord injuries above T_6 thoracic spine and results in interruption of the sympathetic change, causing bradycardia, hypotension, and vasodilation of the peripheral vascular system.

neuromatrix theory Addresses the brain's role in pain perception as well as other multiple determinants.

neuron A nerve cell; the structural and functional unit of the nervous system.

neuropathic pain Pain resulting from injury or dysfunction in one or more nerves.

neuroprotection Therapies used to arrest the sequence of events that occur during the ischemic cascade.

neutralization Action of antibodies that involves the process of changing the charge or shape of the antigen and blocking its ability to attach to another cell.

neutrophil Primary phagocytic defense; responds to bacteria, inflammation, injury, infection, and foreign objects.

nevi Well-circumscribed malformations of the skin. Also known as *moles*.

New York Heart Association (NYHA) classification system A functional classification system that categorizes cardiac patients' subjective degree of symptoms into NYHA classes I through IV.

nidus Refers to the focus of an arteriovenous malformation.

nits The eggs of a louse.

nociception The process by which tissue damage (noxious stimuli) activates sensory neurons to send a pain message to the central nervous system, resulting in a nociceptive pain response; literally means "pain sense."

nociceptive pain Pain resulting from the process of nociception.

nocturia The need to get up at night to urinate.

nodes (bundles) Special cells and fibers that make up the electrical conduction system of the heart.

nodules Small aggregation of cells formed in response to injury or inflammation.

noise-induced hearing loss (NIHL) Hearing loss caused by noises or sounds at a high decibel level for long periods of time.

noncardiogenic pulmonary edema (NCPE) An abnormal accumulation of fluid in the lungs caused by a noncardiac etiology.

noncoring needle Type of access needle required to access an implanted port or reservoir; used to prevent accidental coring of the port's septum.

nondisjunction The failure of two members of a chromosome pair to separate during meiosis or mitosis, resulting in daughter cells with either a missing or extra chromosome.

nonexperimental research design Research design in which the researcher collects data without introducing an intervention.

nongranulocyte White blood cell that is produced in the bone marrow and develops into a lymphocyte or monocyte; does not contain granules in its cytoplasm.

nonheme iron Form of dietary iron available in vegetables, cereals, and fortified food.

nonintentional torts Actions that result in harm to another, but intent is lacking; often synonymous with carelessness.

noninvasive positive pressure ventilation (NPPV) Procedure for delivering breaths to a patient without placement of an artificial airway, such as an endotracheal or tracheostomy tube.

nonmaleficence The duty to do no harm.

nonprobability sampling Type of sampling in which elements and participants are selected by nonrandom methods.

nonsense mutation A single base substitution in DNA that results in a chain-termination codon.

nontunneled and noncuffed device Type of central vascular access device; inserted by a puncture directly through the skin and to the intended location without passing through subcutaneous tissue.

normal sinus rhythm (NSR) A regular heart rate between 60 and 100 beats per minute that has all of the normal components of one cardiac cycle (PQRST) and normal time intervals between the waveforms.

normoglycemia Normal blood glucose levels.

normothermia A normal body temperature.

nosocomial infection An infection that occurs in a hospitalized patient.

not-for-profit organization Organization that reinvests profits from operations back into the organization.

notifiable disease Any of certain diseases or conditions that must be reported to local, county, or state public health departments.

noxious stimuli Tissue damage that activates sensory neurons to send a pain message to the central nervous system, resulting in a nociceptive pain response.

NSTEMI Non–ST segment elevation myocardial infarction is the result of transient subtotal occlusion of a coronary artery with reduced coronary blood flow resulting from plaque disruption and ensuing pathophysiological processes. Serum blood markers and persistent ECG changes are present with NSTEMI.

numeric rating scale (NRS) A horizontal line marked with the numbers 0 to 10 from left to right with three interval descriptors of pain located along the scale: "no pain," "moderate pain," and "worst pain."

nurse–patient relationship The means for applying the nursing process. It is the mechanism by which the nurse works with the patient.

nurse practice acts State guidelines that define the practice of nursing and give guidance in terms of scope of practice issues; they are designed to ensure safe practice.

nurse practitioner (NP) An advanced practice nurse with postgraduate training who is licensed by the state to provide basic medical care under standardized procedures.

nursing care delivery systems A set of concepts based on principles that involve clinical decision making, work allocation, communication, and management.

nursing diagnosis The end product of the nursing assessment. Describes an actual or potential health problem, based on gathered data, that a nurse can legally manage.

nursing process A thinking/doing approach to patient care that provides the nurse with a systematic means of identifying, preventing, and treating actual and potential health problems.

Nursing's Agenda for the Future The American Nurses Association statement outlining issues related to nursing practice. Issues include an expanded role for registered nurses and advanced practice nurses in the delivery of basic and primary health care, obtaining federal funding for nurse education and training, and helping to change and improve the health care workplace.

nutritional imbalance A deficiency or excess of one or more essential nutrients, resulting from inadequate nutrition or too much nutrition.

nystagmus A constant, involuntary tremor, oscillation, or jerky movement of the eyeball; the movement may be in any direction.

objective data Behaviors, activities, and events that can be observed or measured by another person using the senses of observation, palpation, auscultation, percussion, and smell. Objective data are factual: They can be seen, heard, touched, smelled, or tasted.

obstructive sleep apnea (OSA) Disorder of sleep with habitual snoring characterized by brief periods of breathing cessation or a marked reduction in tidal volume with a minimum of five episodes per hour during sleep with excessive daytime somnolence.

occupational asthma Occurs when a worker experiences asthmatic symptoms upon exposure to substances that trigger an asthma attack.

Occupational Safety and Health Administration (OSHA) Agency under the U.S. Department of Labor whose function is to inspect and enforce safety standards in the workplace.

oculocephalic reflex Reflex eye movement that stabilizes images on the retina during head movement by producing an eye movement in the direction opposite to the head movement that maintains the visual field or a more-or-less steady gaze. Also called *doll's eye reflex.*

oculovestibular reflex Reflex that stabilizes images on the retina during head movement by producing an eye movement in the direction opposite that of the head movement.

odontoid process The toothlike projection of C_2 (cervical spine), which sits behind the anterior portion of the ring of C_1.

oligoanalgesia Results when a patient complains of pain, but no interventions are provided for pain relief.

oliguria Decreased urine output of less than 400 mL in a 24-hour period.

Ommaya reservoir Nonvascular infusion device inserted with the catheter tip residing in the ventricles of the brain; used to deliver targeted therapies (i.e., pain and antineoplastic therapies) or to obtain cerebrospinal fluid.

oncosis Cell swelling as a result of changes in membrane permeability.

oncotic pressure In the circulatory system, the term refers to a form of osmotic pressure exerted by proteins in blood plasma that normally tends to pull water into the circulatory system. Also referred to as *colloid osmotic pressure.*

on–off phenomena Abrupt fluctuations in movement ability associated with Parkinson's disease.

open-ended questions Questions that ask for narrative information by stating a topic in general terms; for example, "What brought you to the hospital?"

open globe An open eyeball with a laceration, penetrating injury, or intraocular foreign body; usually results from blunt trauma or projectile injury.

open pneumothorax An open communication between the atmosphere and intrathoracic pressure; usually caused by penetrating trauma.

open reduction internal fixation (ORIF) A treatment in which a fracture is exposed by an incision in the skin directly over the fracture. Implants such as plates (strips of metal), screws, and wires are placed directly on or in the bone to anatomically stabilize a fracture.

opportunistic infections (OIs) Infections from microorganisms that are not usually considered pathogens, but cause disease if the immune system is impaired.

opsonization A chemical coating of an antigen by cytokines or antibodies that makes that cell more attractive to phagocytes.

oral cancer Cancer that arises from the flat cells that line the oral cavity and is slow growing; most often squamous cell carcinoma.

oral candidiasis An overgrowth of the yeast-like fungus *Candida albicans.*

oral glucose tolerance test (OGTT) A test in which the glycemic response to a prescribed dose of oral glucose is used to determine glucose tolerance status (i.e., normal glucose tolerance, impaired glucose tolerance, or diabetes).

orchiectomy Surgical removal of the testes.

orchiopexy Surgical fixation of a testis.

orchitis Inflammation of one or both testes.

orthopnea Shortness of breath relieved by sitting or standing erect.

osmolality Number of molecules of solute per kilogram of water.

osmosis The movement of water from one compartment of low solute concentration through a semipermeable membrane into a second compartment with high solute concentration.

osmotic diuresis Excessive urination caused by the presence of certain substances (such as glucose) in the renal tubules.

osteitis fibrosa cystica A complication of hypoparathyroidism in which the bone softens and becomes deformed or forms cysts.

osteoarthritis (OA) Chronic condition that accompanies aging, affecting the weight-bearing joints most commonly; is the most common form of arthritis.

osteoblasts Any cells that form bone within the body.

osteoclasts Large cells formed in bone marrow and originating from macrophage-like cells; designed to absorb and remove unwanted bone tissue, causing the bone to be "remodeled" or "destroyed."

osteocytes Mature osteoblasts that maintain the bony matrix and participate in the dynamic task of releasing calcium into the bloodstream.

osteoid Type I collagen and noncollagenous protein osteocalcin.

osteology The study of bones and the bone structure of the human body.

osteolysis Destruction of implanted synthetic or cement components of repaired bone segments.

osteonecrosis The death of bone tissue.

osteoporosis A skeletal disease that is characterized by low bone mass and deterioration of the bone tissue. This continued deterioration results in bone fragility and susceptibility to fractures.

otalgia Ear pain.

otitis externa Inflammation/infection of the external ear canal.

otitis media Inflammation/infection of the middle ear.

otolaryngology (otorhinolaryngology) The study of ear, nose, and throat disorders.

otosclerosis Abnormal bone growth within the middle ear that causes hearing loss.

ototoxic Something that, if ingested, causes damage to the auditory nerve, affecting hearing.

ototoxicity Harmful effect on the eighth cranial nerve or organs of hearing and balance.

outcome Individual, measurable patient objective; measurable criterion that indicates the patient's care objectives have been met; a change in patient behavior that results from nursing interventions.

outcome standards Quality standards that focus on whether the services provided by an organization make any difference to patients or to the health status of the patient population.

overnutrition The physical consequences resulting from overconsumption of energy or nutrients compared to recommended amounts.

over-the-needle peripheral-short catheter A catheter with a stylet needle housed in the catheter lumen.

oxidative stress Stress to the cells caused by a decrease in the removal of or an overproduction of oxygen free radicals, common in physiological disorders of the critically ill; the imbalance between reactive oxygen species and the body's defense system.

oxytocin Peptide hormone produced in the hypothalamus but secreted by the posterior pituitary gland. It causes uterine contraction and stimulates breast milk production.

P wave Part of the cardiac cycle; represents atrial contraction or depolarization on an ECG tracing.

pacemaker cell Cardiac cell found in the electrical conduction system, which lies in the heart wall and septum. It generates and conducts impulses.

pacemaker sensitivity Amount of electrical activity the pacemaker will sense or "hear"; measured in millivolts (mV).

packed RBCs Red blood cells that have had the plasma portion of the blood removed by a centrifuge process.

pain An unpleasant sensory and emotional experience associated with actual or potential tissue damage, or described in terms of such damage.

palliative The alleviation (not curative) of suffering from symptoms.

palliative care Comprehensive care focused on alleviating suffering and promoting the quality of remaining life of patients living with a chronic life-threatening or terminal illness; allows patients and families to guide treatment and set goals for care.

palliative procedures Surgeries performed for the primary purpose of alleviating symptoms rather than affecting a cure.

palpation Technique of using touch to collect data to determine specific characteristics of the body.

palpitations An awareness of the beating of the heart.

pancarditis Inflammation of all three layers of the heart: the endocardium, myocardium, and pericardium.

pancreatic beta cells Cells in the pancreatic islets of Langerhans that produce insulin.

pancreatic insufficiency A deficiency of pancreatic enzymes resulting in malabsorption of nutrients.

pancreatic polypeptide A complex peptide hormone secreted by the pancreatic islet cells whose role is not completely understood.

pancreaticoduodenal (Whipple) resection A radical surgical procedure to treat pancreatic cancer that involves removal of the head of the pancreas, the duodenum, the distal portion of the stomach, part of the jejunum, and the lower half of the common bile duct.

pancreatitis Inflammation of the pancreas.

panendoscopy Surgical procedure to evaluate the upper aerodigestive tract, locate the organ of origin, and obtain a cellular diagnosis.

panhypopituitarism Condition in which there is inadequate secretion of all of the hormones of the anterior pituitary.

paracentesis Removal of ascites fluid from the abdomen.

paracrine functioning Bioregulation of one cell type that influences the activity of an adjacent cell type by secreting chemicals that diffuse into the tissue and act specifically on cells in that area.

paraphimosis Condition in which the foreskin is retracted, but cannot be returned to its normal position covering the glans.

paraplegia Paralysis of the lower half of the body including both lower extremities and loss of bowel and bladder function.

parenteral Term used to describe fluids and medications that are administered via routes other than the alimentary canal.

parenteral nutrition Provision of nutrients and energy by means of intravenous access, without use of the gastrointestinal tract.

paresthesia An abnormal physical sensation such as prickling, tingling, or numbness.

Parkinson's disease (PD) A disease of the basal ganglia characterized by a slowing down in the innervation and executive of movement, increased muscle tone rigidity, tremors at rest, and impaired postural reflexes.

paronychia Inflammation of the folds of tissue surrounding the fingernail.

paroxysmal junctional tachycardia (PJT) An irritable focus in the AV junction that assumes the pacemaker role by discharging impulses more rapidly than the SA node. Begins and ends abruptly.

partial-thickness injury Injury in which the epidermis and part of the dermis are destroyed.

passive immunization Immunization that provides immunity for a short period of time, usually around 6 to 12 weeks; involves the injection of already formed antibodies into the body.

paternalism In ethics, policy that allows one to make decisions for another.

pathogenicity Disease-causing potential of a microorganism, the number of invading microorganisms, and the host defenses.

pathologic dead space A portion of the tidal volume that does reach the alveoli, but does not take place in gas exchange. Various lung pathologies and disease conditions can increase this dead space amount and affect the lungs' ability to oxygenate and ventilate.

pathologic fractures Fractures that occur without trauma due to bone thinning.

patient care plan A documented record of the nursing process, a plan designed to incorporate the patient's identified problems, outcomes, and actions to be implemented by the nurse.

patient-centered care An innovative approach to the planning, delivery, and evaluation of health care that is based on mutually beneficial partnerships among health care patients, families, and providers.

patient-controlled analgesia (PCA) pump A computerized machine that is attached to a patient's intravenous line and allows the patient to control the amount of medication that is administered based on his or her pain level.

pattern theory a group of theories that asserts that pain receptors share nerve pathways with other sensory pathways and that the intensity of the stimulus determines the frequency of firing of the receptor.

pediculosis Infestation with lice.

pedigree A diagram that shows the heredity of a particular trait or genetic disorder through many generations of a family.

pelvic inflammatory disease (PID) An infection of the internal reproductive organs, including the fallopian tubes. It is a very common and a very serious complication of many sexually transmitted infections.

The highest risk for the development of PID is seen in women of childbearing age who are sexually active.

penectomy Removal of part of or the entire penis.

penetrance The proportion of individuals with a genotype known to cause a genetic disorder who have signs and symptoms of the disorder.

peptic ulcer A generic term used for any ulceration in the digestive surfaces of the upper GI tract.

percussion Technique of either pushing, tapping, or using a device to generate a sound vibration. The vibrations produced will help in determining position of organ structures.

percutaneous angioplasty The use of mechanical widening when opening blood vessels other than coronary arteries.

percutaneous coronary intervention (PCI) The use of devices to either remove plaque or alter its morphology in the catheterization laboratory, including atherectomy devices, lasers, and intracoronary stents.

percutaneous transluminal coronary angioplasty (PTCA) Treatment of coronary artery disease (CAD) using expandable balloons to crack (tear or rupture) atherosclerotic plaque, thereby enlarging the lumen of the coronary artery.

percutaneously Passing through the skin.

perfusion The movement of blood carrying oxygen.

pericardial effusion An excess buildup of pericardial fluid that is a threat to normal cardiac function. The fluid buildup is the result of an accumulation of infectious exudates or toxins and/or blood.

pericardial friction rub A grating, scraping, squeaking, or a crunching sound that is the result of friction between the roughened, inflamed layers of the pericardium.

pericardial window An opening in the pericardial sac that allows fluid from effusion and tamponade to drain.

pericardiectomy Removal of the pericardial sac to allow fluid to drain from around the heart.

pericarditis Inflammation of the pericardial sac due to an inflammatory process in which the two layers of the pericardium become inflamed and roughened, causing fluid to build up.

perimenopause The time during which periods may increase, decrease, and become irregular as the function of the ovaries waxes and wanes.

perioperative A broad term that refers to the time period surrounding a surgical procedure. It includes the preoperative, intraoperative, and postoperative time periods.

perioperative blood salvage The process of collecting and reinfusing blood lost during both the intraoperative and early postoperative periods.

periosteum Fibrous membrane that covers bone.

peripheral arterial disease (PAD) Disease that affects the arteries of the extremities.

peripheral blood stem cell (PBSC) transplantation Transplantation of stem cells located in peripherally circulating blood.

peripheral nerve block An anesthesia technique in which a local anesthetic is injected into or around a nerve plexus to produce anesthesia of a selected area without inducing a systemic effect.

peripheral parenteral nutrition (PPN) Provision of nutrition intravenously through a peripheral vein.

peripheral-short catheter Type of vascular access device used for short-term infusion therapies.

peripheral vascular resistance The resistance in the pulmonary vasculature.

peripherally inserted central catheter (PICC) Central vascular access device that is inserted into an extremity, typically in the antecubital fossa, and advanced until the tip is positioned in the vena cava.

peristalsis A progressive wavelike movement that occurs involuntarily in hollow tubes of the body.

peritonsillar abscess A rare complication of tonsillitis in which the infection spreads to the tissue around the tonsillar capsule.

perivascular Situated around a blood vessel.

pernicious anemia Anemia caused by insufficiencies in intrinsic factor.

persistent The ability of a chemical agent to remain in an area. In general, the agent would have a low vapor pressure and a high vapor density.

pessary A device that, when inserted into the vagina, will help support the vaginal walls, reducing the bulging of those walls into the vagina.

Peyronie's disease Condition in which plaque forms on the erectile tissue of the penis, primarily in middle-aged or older men.

pH An indicator of hydrogen ion concentration; the negative logarithm of the hydrogen ion concentration expressed in nanomoles per liter. A normal pH of 7.4 is equivalent to 40 nmol/L of hydrogen ion (or 0.0004 mEq/L).

phagocytes Granulocytes, macrophages, and lymphocytes, which are attracted to an injured site by the complement factors and antigens.

phagocytosis The process by which phagocytes absorb and enzymatically degrade foreign matter and devitalized tissue.

phantom limb pain Pain appearing to come from an amputated limb.

pharmacogenetics Area of biochemical genetics concerned with drug responses and their genetically controlled variations.

pharmacogenomics The application of genomic information or methods to pharmacogenetics problems.

pharyngitis Inflammation of the pharynx caused by upper respiratory infection, which causes a sore throat.

pharyngoesophageal Pertaining to the pharynx and the esophagus.

phenomenology A qualitative research method that describes the meaning of a lived experience through the perspective of the participant.

phenotype Observable characteristics of an organism produced by the organism's genotype interacting with the environment.

pheochromocytoma A tumor (usually benign) that originates from the adrenal medulla.

pheresis catheter Central vascular access device used for plasma exchange therapies.

phimosis The inability to retract the foreskin over the penile glans.

phlebostatic axis Reference point used to level transducers.

phoria A tendency toward a functional deviation or defect that results from a break in visual fusion by covering an eye. Latent deviation meaning that the deviation is not apparent unless fusion of the eyes is broken.

phosphorus An abundant mineral used in all sources of energy (ATP, ADP, and AMP). Eighty percent is found bound to calcium in the bone as calcium phosphate. Normal serum levels are 2.5 to 4.5 mg/dL.

photodermatitis A common, inflammatory adverse reaction to sunlight in which the individual sunburns more easily than usual or develops papular or vesicular lesions with exposure to the sun.

phronesis A form of rationality and skill-based character that is similar to clinical judgment.

physes Growth plates.

physiological stress Metabolic conditions characterized by hypermetabolism and hypercatabolism.

pilosebaceous follicles A sebaceous cyst containing hair follicles.

pilot study A small preliminary study prior to conducting a larger study.

pitch Describes frequency; low pitch is 100 Hz and high pitch is 10,000 Hz.

pitting An indention that remains for a short time after pressing edematous skin with the finger.

planning Determining how expected patient outcomes can be achieved through nursing interventions by establishing priorities of care.

plasma The protein portion of blood that remains when cells have been removed.

plasma cells Differentiated B cells that are found in the plasma and are responsible for production of specific antibodies or immunoglobulins.

plasmapheresis A treatment used in some autoimmune diseases that involves removing blood from the body and filtering antibodies out of the plasma. The red blood cells and fluids are returned to the body. The removal of antibodies decreases immune stimulation and helps control clinical symptoms of some autoimmune diseases.

platelet Thrombocyte of blood that is small and colorless with no nucleus, which assists in blood clotting by adhering to other platelets and to damaged epethelium. Also called *blood platelet, thrombocyte.*

pleasure principle The principle of tension reduction.

pleural effusion Abnormal accumulation of fluid in the pleural space.

pleural friction rubs Harsh leathery sound created from inflamed pleural surfaces rubbing against each other.

pneumatoscope An otoscope with a bulb attachment that can be used to introduce air into the ear canal and middle ear to test for ruptured tympanic membrane.

Pneumocystis carinii **pneumonia (PCP)** An opportunistic fungal respiratory infection that can be seen in severely immune-compromised hosts.

pneumonia An inflammatory process that results in edema of interstitial lung tissue and extravasation of fluid into the alveoli, thus causing hypoxemia.

pneumothorax Partial or complete collapse of the lung.

point mutation A single nucleotide base-pair change in DNA.

polycythemia vera A hematocrit value that is elevated beyond normal values; frequent occurrence in chronic hypoxemia.

polymorphism A common variation in the sequence of DNA among individuals seen in more than 1% of the population.

polypharmacy The administration of many drugs together; also, the administration of excessive medications.

polysomnography Multichannel electrophysiological recording used to detect disturbances of breathing during sleep.

population Entire aggregation of cases in which a researcher is interested.

population-based care Care focused on aggregates and communities. A population is a collection of individuals who have in common one or more personal or environmental characteristics. As an aggregate, the members are defined in terms of geography, special interest, disease state, or other common characteristics.

portal hypertension Increased pressure in the hepatic circulation that is a complication of cirrhosis.

portal of entry The path by which an infective organism enters a susceptible host.

portal of exit Path in the chain of infection that allows a causative agent to escape from a reservoir.

positive deflection Any waveform that goes above the isoelectric line on ECG graph paper.

positive feedback Process by which a deviation from normal is reinforced or accelerated, producing an increased stimulus. For example, uterine contraction stimulates oxytocin secretion, which brings about increased contractions and increased oxytocin.

positive pressure infusion pump Electronic infusion device used to administer parenteral fluids and medications under preset pressures.

postacute withdrawal syndrome (PAWS) An enduring physical remnant of neurotransmitter production and/or receptor site damage. The mood is affected, as are interpersonal interactions and cognitive skills.

postanesthesia care unit (PACU) A physical space located adjacent to the operating room where patients are monitored closely as they recover from anesthesia.

postconcussion syndrome A condition that may follow mild head injury.

posterior circulation Refers to circulation in the arteries in the posterior portion of the circle of Willis.

posteriorly Back plane of the body.

postoperative blood salvage The process of salvaging blood in which blood is obtained from mediastinal and chest tubes, and then reinfused.

It is used following major surgeries, typically cardiovascular, thoracic, and some orthopedic procedures.

post-test probability The likelihood that a disease is actually present in a patient after testing (a positive test indicates disease).

postural instability Diminished postural reflexes, which contribute to difficulty maintaining balance.

potassium An intracellular cation with 98% found within cells. Small amounts are in blood (3.5 to 5.0 mEq/L) and bone. Its function is to maintain intracellular osmolality and participate in cellular depolarization and repolarization.

power analysis A research design's ability to detect relationships that exist among variables.

PPE Acronym for personal protective equipment, which is designed to protect the wearer from various hazards.

PR interval Part of the cardiac cycle; represents time from atrial depolarization to ventricular depolarization on an ECG tracing. Sometimes referred to as the *PRI* or *PR segment*.

practical knowledge Knowledge shaped by one's familiarity with the discipline and practice of the science and technology relevant to the situation at hand.

precipitation One of the actions of antibodies; occurs when an immune complex falls or precipitates out of circulation and is more easily located by neutrophils and monocytes for phagocytosis.

pre-diabetes A condition of glucose intolerance ranging between normal glucose tolerance and overt diabetes.

predictive accuracy Ability of a diagnostic test to predict the presence or absence of disease.

preferred provider organization (PPO) Organization that provides health care coverage through a coordinated plan for medical care that includes a network of contracted providers.

prehypertension A term used to describe those individuals who have a blood pressure finding on two or more office visits of 130 to 139/80 to 89 mmHg. These individuals are at twice the risk of developing hypertension as those with lower values.

preload The volume of blood in the ventricle at the end of diastole.

premature atrial contraction (PAC) An ectopic focus in the atria that occurs early, before the next expected SA impulse, causing depolarization and contraction of the atrial muscle.

premature junctional contraction (PJC) Dysrhythmia that originates in the AV junction. It discharges before the next expected sinus impulse and activates the ventricles in a normal manner. Due to retrograde conduction, the P wave is inverted and may appear before, buried, or after the QRS complex on an ECG tracing.

premature ventricular contraction (PVC) An irritable focus within the ventricle that discharges before the next sinus impulse; thereby, stimulating the ventricle directly and causing a contraction, which is followed by a full compensatory pause. Each contraction is an individual beat, not a rhythm.

premenstrual dysphoric disorder (PMDD) A severe form of premenstrual syndrome that includes five or more symptoms of depression for most of the time during the last week of the luteal phase and begins to remit within a few days after onset of the follicular phase of the menstrual cycle.

premenstrual syndrome (PMS) A complex, often misunderstood condition, involving physical, psychological, and behavioral symptoms associated with the menstrual cycle.

preoperative health evaluation An evaluation done within 30 days of a planned operation and must be documented in the patient's chart per the Joint Commission requirements.

presbycusis Hearing loss caused by changes in the middle and inner ear due to the aging process.

presbyopia Condition where the eye exhibits a progressively diminished ability to focus on near objects with age; also recognized as a symptom of aging.

pressure ulcer A localized injury to the skin and/or underlying tissue usually over a bony prominence, as a result of pressure or pressure in combination with shear and/or friction.

pretest probability The likelihood that a disease is actually present in a patient before testing.

prevalence The measurement of all cancer cases at a designated point in time.

priapism A persistent erection.

PRICE Acronym for *protection* (immobilize and prevent weight bearing), *rest, ice, compression,* and *elevation.*

primary adrenal insufficiency Condition in which 90% of the adrenal gland has been destroyed, resulting in an absence of adrenal hormones.

primary appraisal The process of evaluating the significance of a transaction as it relates to a person's well-being, based on Lazarus's theory of stress.

primary biliary cirrhosis An autoimmune disease in which there is inflammation and destruction of the intrahepatic biliary system, resulting in fibrosis.

primary immune deficiency Results from genetic abnormalities in immune system development and causes partial or total immune system dysfunction.

primary immune response The first exposure to a specific antigen; results in creation of B memory cells, which provide lifelong protection against the specific antigen.

primary injury Refers to mechanical injury to the brain.

primary intention A wound that is surgically closed or one with smooth, closely aligned margins.

primary lesion Lesion that results from the initial reaction to a pathologic condition.

primary nursing A primary nursing care delivery system is a system in which a registered nurse providing direct care to the patient has 24-hour responsibility for the planning, implementation, and outcomes of patient care.

primary set Infusion set with a single fluid pathway from the fluid container to a vascular access device.

primary tumors Tumors that are at the original site where it first arose. For example, a primary brain tumor is one that arose in the brain as opposed to one that arose elsewhere and metastasized to the brain.

principlism An emerging theory in ethics that incorporates the various ethical principles in attempting to resolve conflicts in clinical settings.

probability sampling Type of sampling that involves random selection when choosing the elements and participants.

process standards Quality standards that focus on whether the activities within an organization are being conducted appropriately.

prodromal phase The phase of acute hepatitis that occurs between exposure to the virus and the appearance of jaundice. It is characterized by fatigue, anorexia, malaise, nausea, vomiting, and a headache; often mistaken for the flu.

progenitor cells In development, a parent cell that gives rise to a distinct cell lineage by a series of cell divisions. Like stem cells, progenitor cells have a capacity to differentiate into a specific type of cell. In contrast to stem cells, however, they are already far more specific: They are pushed to differentiate into their "target" cell.

progesterone Steroid hormone produced by the ovaries and the placenta. It is responsible for uterine changes in the second half of the menstrual cycle.

programmed theory of aging Theory of aging based on the premise that aging follows a biological timetable.

prolactin Peptide hormone produced by the anterior pituitary gland. Stimulates breast development and breast milk during and after pregnancy.

prolapse Condition in which the uterus is unable to remain high in the vaginal canal and begins to protrude into the vagina; can occur if the structures supporting the uterus are weakened during childbirth.

proprioception The awareness of posture, movement, and changes in equilibrium and the knowledge of position, weight, and resistance of objects in relation to the body.

proptosis A downward displacement of the eyeball in exophthalmic goiter or in inflammatory conditions of the orbit.

prostaglandin A long-chain fatty acid that regulates platelet aggregation and controls inflammation.

prostatectomy Removal of the prostate and seminal vesicles.

prostatitis Inflammation of the prostate gland.

protein C A normal component of the coagulation system.

protein-calorie malnutrition Physical state resulting from the underconsumption of energy and protein specifically.

proteinuria The presence of protein in the urine.

proton pump inhibitor (PPI) Drug that blocks the proton pump in the stomach, thus reducing gastric acid secretion.

psoriasis A chronic, noncontagious inflammatory skin disorder; characterized by erythematous papules and plaques with silver-white scales that are sharply demarcated and the result of hyperproliferation of keratinocytes.

psoriatic arthritis An inflammatory process associated with psoriasis.

psychogenic polydipsia Condition in which excessive thirst occurs for psychogenic, rather than organic, reasons.

psychomotor learning Learning that occurs when a physical skill has been acquired.

psychosocial theories of aging Theories of aging that describe the changes that take place emotionally and socially as one enters the later years of life.

ptosis Drooping of the upper eyelid, generally due to paralysis.

pulmonary artery catheter (PAC) A flow-directed, balloon-tipped catheter used to measure intracardiac pressures.

pulmonary artery occlusion pressure (PAOP) Pressure obtained by inflating the balloon on a pulmonary artery catheter at the end of expiration to reflect left ventricular end-diastolic pressure.

pulmonary contusion Occurs when blunt thoracic trauma is applied through the chest wall to the parenchyma, causing disruption of alveolar capillary networks and usually resulting in hypoxemia; initially a hemorrhage into the lung tissue followed by alveolar and interstitial edema.

pulmonary embolism (PE) The presence of a thrombus or blood clot in the pulmonary vessels, which obstructs blood flow and impedes gas exchange.

pulmonic valve regurgitation The inability of the pulmonic valve to completely close, causing blood to regurgitate back into the right ventricle.

pulmonic valve stenosis A narrowing of the cardiac valve orifice that restricts blood flow due to an inability of the valve to completely open, thus, obstructing blood from the right ventricle from flowing into the pulmonary vasculature during systole.

pulse pressure The difference between the systolic and diastolic pressure, which is about 40 mmHg.

pulseless electrical activity (PEA) Absence of a detectable pulse and blood pressure in the presence of electrical activity in the heart as evidenced by some type of ECG rhythm other than ventricular fibrillation or ventricular tachycardia. It is not an actual rhythm, but represents a clinical condition wherein the patient is clinically dead, despite the fact that some type of organized rhythm appears on the ECG monitor.

pulsus paradoxus A greater than 10 mmHg drop in systolic blood pressure during inspiration.

Purkinje network fibers Part of the cardiac conduction system; a network of fibers that carries impulses directly to the ventricular muscle cells. Ventricular contraction is facilitated by the rapid spread of the electrical impulse through the left and right bundle branches, the Purkinje network fibers, and the ventricular muscle.

purposive sampling Type of sampling that implies that certain people or elements are deliberately selected for the study.

pyloric stenosis Narrowing of the pyloric orifice. In adults, frequently results from peptic ulcer disease, malignant compression of the gastric outlet, or pneumatosis intestinalis.

QRS complex Part of the cardiac cycle; represents ventricular contraction or depolarization on an ECG tracing.

QT interval Part of the cardiac cycle; is measured from the Q wave to the end of the T wave. The normal QT interval is 0.34 to 0.43 second.

quadrigeminy Premature ventricular contraction that occurs every fourth beat.

quadriplegia (*Latin*) Paralysis of all four extremities.

qualitative research A systematic, subjective approach used to describe life experiences and give them meaning.

quality Refers to characteristics of and the pursuit of excellence.

quality in fact Conforming to standards and meeting one's own expectations.

quality in perception Meeting the customer's expectations.

quality of care The degree to which health services for individuals and populations increase the likelihood of desired health outcomes and are consistent with current professional knowledge.

quantitative research Research characterized by the collection of numerical values, under a controlled situation, that yield data, which can be generalized.

quasi-experimental research design A study with an intervention, but one in which it is difficult to manipulate or control the setting, subjects, or variables, as is needed for a true experimental study.

quasi-intentional torts Volitional actions that result in harm to another, but intent is lacking.

quota sampling Type of sampling in which participants are selected by a researcher in a nonrandom manner using prespecified characteristics of the sample to increase their representation.

raccoon eyes Ecchymosis over the orbit of the eyes that is indicative of a basilar skull fracture. Also called *raccoon sign*.

radiation Waves and particles of energy. Radiation causes mutation of cells' DNA, which can weaken the cells' defense against a carcinogen or cause cell death.

radiation burns Burns that usually result from overexposure to the sun or are associated with radiation treatment for cancer.

radiologic agents Agents that are a source of alpha, beta, or gamma radiation that can be used as a weapon.

random assignment Subjects are randomly assigned to treatment versus control groups.

range of motion (ROM) Movement of a joint within its normal range.

rate of living theory of aging Considered one of the oldest theories on aging, it is based on the belief that individuals possess a finite amount of some "vital substance." When that substance is consumed, the individual dies.

rationality The ability to reason across time when changes in the patient's condition occurs. It includes noticing subtle changes, not limited to explicit vital signs and may not show up immediately in the vital sign trends.

RDD Acronym for radiation dispersal device, a device that can release radiation into the environment.

reactive arthritis A type of arthritis caused by a reaction to an infection somewhere else in the body. Also called *Reiter's syndrome* or *undifferentiated spondyloarthropathy*.

reactive oxygen species (ROS) Intermediary products, or species, that are produced in the metabolic production of energy; occur when oxygen is used to oxidize molecules and generate energy. A phenomenon that occurs during oxidative stress development and a major contributing factor in diseases in patients who are critically ill.

receptors Structure in a cell membrane or within a cell that combines with a hormone to alter an aspect of the functioning of the cell.

reconstructive surgery Surgery performed for the purpose of rebuilding tissues or body structures to achieve a more normal function and appearance.

rectocele Occurs when the posterior vaginal wall is weakened and the rectum bulges into the vagina.

rectum The lower part of the large intestine between the sigmoid colon and the anal canal.

recurrent pain Acute pain that completely resolves, leaving the patient free from pain for a period of time before the pain reoccurs.

red blood cell (RBC) A type of blood cell that transports oxygen and carbon dioxide. Also called an *erythrocyte*.

red blood cell distribution width (RDW) A direct measurement of the homogeneity (consistency) of red blood cell size.

refeeding syndrome Syndrome consisting of metabolic disturbances that arise from reinstitution of nutrition to patients who are severely malnourished.

refractory period Period of time that ensures the cardiac muscle is totally relaxed before another action potential or depolarization can be initiated.

regional anesthesia The production of insensibility of a part by interrupting the sensory nerve conductivity of any region of the body by local injection of a medication.

regional (locality) rule Existence of a prevailing community standard.

registered nurse (RN) An individual licensed by the state to practice nursing in accordance with the nurse practice act.

rehabilitation The multidisciplinary plan of care that maximizes an impaired individual's function by minimizing the deficits to achieve the highest quality of life possible.

relative refractory period Period when depolarization is almost complete, and corresponds with the top and the downslope of the T wave on an ECG tracing.

remodeling The fourth and final phase of wound healing that begins about 3 weeks after the injury and can still be in progress 6 months to 2 years later.

renal calculi Kidney stones.

renin An enzyme produced in the kidneys that converts angiotensinogen to angiotensin, which is an enzyme that helps elevate blood pressure.

repatriation Return of patients from one health care setting to another appropriate level of care or to a contracted institution.

reperfusion injury Injury to the cells after blood supply to an ischemic area is restored.

research A formal, systematic, and organized method of answering a question, solving a problem, validating and redefining existing knowledge, and developing new knowledge.

research critique A critical appraisal of a piece of completed research.

research design Overall plan or blueprint for a study; guides an investigator in planning and implementing a study.

research problem A situation or circumstance that requires a solution to be described, explained, or predicted.

research process Process of undertaking discrete steps to conduct a research study. Includes identifying a researchable problem, completing a literature review, creating the theoretical/conceptual framework, selecting an appropriate design, and collecting, analyzing, and distributing data/findings.

research purpose A concise, clear statement of the specific goal or aim of the study that is generated from the problem.

research question A research problem stated in an interrogative form.

research utilization (RU) The purposeful application of research findings to the clinical setting to improve patient care.

reservoir A place where an organism can survive and may or may not multiply.

resonance A low-pitched, clear, hollow tone of long duration. It is commonly heard over the lungs.

respect for others In ethics, the highest principle because it incorporates all other principles.

respiratory quotient (RQ) Ratio between carbon dioxide produced and oxygen consumed per molecule of fat, carbohydrate, and protein. Fat has an RQ of 0.7, protein 0.8, and carbohydrate 1.0.

restenosis Accumulation of smooth muscle cells at the site of the original percutaneous coronary intervention that occurs because of an artery's response to injury.

resting membrane potential The difference in electrical charge, or voltage, between the inside and outside of a cardiac cell.

restrictive cardiomyopathy A disorder characterized by endometrial scarring that usually affects one or both ventricles and restricts filling of blood, resulting in systolic dysfunction. The ventricle has normal wall thickness, but the walls are rigid, producing elevated filling pressures and dilated atria.

rete pegs Protrusions in the fifth layer of the epidermis that extend down into the dermis and help anchor the epidermis to the dermis. Also called *epidermal ridges*.

reticular activating system (RAS) Network of neurons that is involved with arousal and consciousness.

reticulocyte A biconcave, immature red blood cell disk without a nucleus.

reticuloendothelial system (RES) Part of the immune system; consists of the phagocytic cells located in reticular connective tissue, primarily monocytes and macrophages.

retinal detachment The separation of the sensory retinal layers from the retinal pigment epithelium, where subretinal fluid collects in the potential space.

retinopathy Degenerative changes in the retina.

retrograde ejaculation Backward ejaculation of semen into the bladder.

retroperitoneal space Area behind the peritoneum and outside the kidney.

reverse transcriptase An enzyme present is some classes of virus, including HIV, that is capable of replicating DNA from RNA, the reverse of normal replication of DNA.

Rh factor A protein substance made up of numerous complex antigens. When it is present on the surface of red blood cells, the person is Rh positive (Rh+); if not present, the person is Rh negative (Rh–). Also called *factor D*.

rheumatic fever A pharyngeal infection caused by Lancefield group A beta-hemolytic streptococci. In 3% of the cases it leads to rheumatic heart disease.

rheumatic heart disease An inflammatory disease of the heart that causes long-term damage, scarring, and malfunction of the heart valves.

rheumatoid arthritis (RA) Chronic inflammatory process that affects the peripheral joints and surrounding muscles, ligaments, tendons, and blood vessels.

rhinitis A collection of symptoms predominantly in the nose and eyes that occur after exposure to airborne particles of dust, dander, or the pollens of certain seasonal plants in people who are allergic to these substances.

rhinoplasty Plastic surgery of the nose.

rhytidectomy Surgical excision of skin to eliminate wrinkles of the face.

right-sided heart failure An abnormal cardiac condition characterized by impairment of the right side of the heart and congestion and elevated pressure in the systemic veins and capillaries.

rigidity Abnormal stiffness or inflexibility associated with Parkinson's disease.

Rinne test A hearing test that measures conduction of sound by bone when placing an activated tuning fork on the right and left mastoid sequentially.

riot control agent Agents that generally cause pain, burning, lacrimation, or discomfort upon exposure to mucous membranes. Also called an *irritant*.

risk management A comprehensive program for identifying and evaluating potential risks to the health care organization. Risks can be illness or injury related as well as financial.

robotics Electromechanical devices that are computer controlled and used to perform surgical tasks.

rolling (paraesophageal) hernia A protrusion of the greater curvature of the stomach through the esophageal hiatus.

Romberg test Assesses inner ear balance, proprioceptive ability, and visual and cerebellar system function by asking the patient to maintain an upright posture when arms are held out in front, with eyes open and eyes closed.

rotational injuries Injuries resulting from extreme lateral flexion or flexion-rotation of the spine, causing disruption of the posterior spinal ligaments and spinal instability.

rule of nines Divides the body into seven areas, which represent 9% or multiples of 9% of the body surface area; used to determine burn size.

S_3 (third heart sound) Abnormal third heart sound in the cardiac cycle; often heard when the ventricles are volume overloaded.

S_4 (fourth heart sound) Abnormal fourth heart sound heard in the cardiac cycle; often heard with heart failure and hypertension.

salience Having some things stand out as more or less important in a practical situation, it is a form of practical knowledge that is learned from many concrete clinical experiences in which a range of relevant clinical issues stand out as high priority.

same-day admission A hospital process in which the patient is not hospitalized prior to a surgical procedure but instead reports directly to the reception area of the operating room from home.

sample A portion selected from a population and interpreted to represent that population; a subset of the population.

sampling Process of selecting a portion of the population to represent the entire population.

scabies Contagious skin disease caused by a mite; commonly found in underdeveloped countries and places where there is overcrowding and poor hygiene.

scald burns Type of thermal injury that occurs from contact with hot foods or liquids, including steam.

schema Coordinated patterns of recurring actions that are created for the purpose of organizing and interpreting information.

Schilling test Procedure to identify anemia due to malabsorption.

Schwabach test Tests hearing for air and bone conduction by using an activated tuning fork on the mastoid process.

schwannomas Tumors of the Schwann cells (nerve sheath tumor).

sclerosing cholangitis An inflammatory disorder of the biliary tract that leads to fibrosis and strictures in the biliary system.

sclerotherapy A treatment for esophageal varices in which a bleeding vessel is sclerosed with a chemical agent.

scoliosis Lateral curvature of the spine.

scope of practice Refers to legally permissible boundaries of practice for a given health care profession.

scrub nurse Nurse in the operating room who works directly with the surgeon within the sterile field, passing instruments, sponges, and other items needed during the surgical procedure.

seborrheic keratosis A benign epidermal lesion seen predominantly in the middle-aged and elderly populations.

secondary adrenal insufficiency Condition in which the pituitary gland has insufficient secretion of ACTH, resulting in insufficient cortisol production by the adrenal glands.

secondary appraisal The process of evaluating the significance of a transaction between the person and his or her environment as it relates to available coping resources and options.

secondary immune deficiencies Impaired immune responses that result from a nongenetic cause such as aging, malnutrition, malignancies, immunosuppressive drug therapy, and infections such as the human immunodeficiency virus.

secondary immune response Second exposure to a specific antigen that triggers a stronger and quicker immune response than the first exposure, with production of greater amounts of antibodies due to the presence of memory B cells; results in a milder set of clinical symptoms or no observable response to the pathogen because the immune system quickly eliminates the pathogen.

secondary injury The body's response that can result from a primary injury.

secondary intention In the granulation process, healing that occurs when major tissue defects gradually close by epithelialization and contracture formation, and then form scar tissue.

secondary lesion Lesion that results from a change in the primary lesion or external trauma to the primary lesion.

secondary set Infusion set used to administer supplemental infusion therapies via the primary infusion system.

second-impact syndrome A condition characterized by a second concussion that occurs before the brain completely recovers from the first concussion.

secretion The active process of moving substances, such as H+ ion, from the blood into the tubular fluid against the concentration gradient.

self-antigen Receptors on cells that are recognized as unique to that individual.

self-sheathing Engineered safety mechanism in which a needle is encased in a protective chamber.

senile purpura A type of hemorrhaging under the skin that occurs most frequently in the elderly because their blood vessels are thinner and more fragile than those of younger people.

sense of coherence (SOC) Refers to how an individual sees the world and one's life in it.

sensitivity Describes the ability of a test to identify patients with disease; calculated by dividing the number of true positive tests by the sum of true positives plus false negatives.

sensitization The process of producing antibodies to an antigen present in the body.

sensorineural hearing loss Type of hearing loss attributed to damage to the eighth cranial nerve.

sensory dimension of pain Includes consideration of the location, intensity, quality, and temporal patterns of pain.

sentinel event Unexpected occurrence that has the potential to, or actually does, result in death or serious physical or psychological injury. Serious injury specifically includes loss of limb or function.

sepsis Clinical syndrome that is defined by the presence of infection and a systemic inflammatory response.

septic arthritis The most destructive form of acute arthritis; can result from trauma, direct inoculation of bacteria during joint surgery, spread of infection from another part of the body (hematogenous), or when an infection from an adjacent bone extends through the cortex into the joint space. Also called *nongonococcal bacterial arthritis*.

septic shock In adults, septic shock refers to a state of acute circulatory failure characterized by persistent hypotension unexplained by other causes. In pediatric patients, septic shock is defined as a tachycardia with signs of decreased perfusion. Hypotension is a late sign in children.

septum Material covering a portal; access point of an implanted port or reservoir, usually made of compressed silicon.

sequelae Residual problems that result from an illness.

seroma A mass caused by the accumulation of serum within a tissue or organ. It is similar to a hematoma except that instead of a collection of blood it is a collection of serous fluid.

serum immunoglobulin G (IgG) An antibody produced by the body that is an indicator of long-term immunity or resolving infection.

serum immunoglobulin M (IgM) An antibody produced by the body in response to an antigen; usually present during the acute phase of an infection.

setting The environment or place (locale) in which research is conducted; may be classified as natural, partially controlled, or highly controlled.

severe sepsis Sepsis with one or more organ system dysfunction.

sex chromosome One of the two chromosomes that determine an individual's genetic sex. The two kinds of sex chromosomes are X and Y. Normal females possess two X chromosomes and normal males one X and one Y.

sheet skin grafts Split-thickness grafts that have not been meshed.

shingles A viral infection that occurs because of the reactivation of latent varicella zoster virus or the virus that causes chickenpox. Also known as *herpes zoster*.

short bowel syndrome Syndrome in which the surface of the small intestine is reduced as a result of surgical resection of the small bowel, typically because of tumors, Crohn's disease, infarction, trauma, or radiation.

shunt A hole or passage that allows movement of fluid from one part of the body to another. Pulmonary shunts exist when there is normal perfusion to an alveolus, but ventilation fails to supply the perfused region.

sick role A set of expectations that people who are ill must meet and which society, including caregivers, expects of them.

sick sinus syndrome (SSS) Term that encompasses a broad range of abnormalities, including disorders of impulse generation and conduction, failure of pacemakers, and a susceptibility to paroxysmal or chronic atrial tachycardia. Also referred to as *sinoatrial disease* and *sinoatrial dysfunction*, a disorder in which the SA node is severely depressed due to heart disease or drugs.

sickle cell anemia Chronic erythrocyte disorder characterized by misshapen "sickle-shaped" red blood cells resulting from malfunctioning hemoglobin molecules.

silicosis Disease that results from exposure to free crystalline silica in mines, foundries, blasting operations, stone, clay, and glass manufacturing.

simple random sampling Type of sampling strategy in which each person in a population has an equal chance of being selected for a study.

simple verbal descriptive scale (SVDS) Scale that uses a horizontal line marked with the numbers 0 to 10 from left to right, but also includes interval descriptors of "no pain," "mild," "discomforting," "distressing," "horrible," or "excruciating pain."

single-gene disorder A disorder due to one or a pair of mutant alleles at a single locus.

sinoatrial (SA) node Part of the electrical conduction of the myocardium; located in the upper posterior portion of the right atrial wall near the opening of the vena cava. The SA node is commonly referred to as the primary pacemaker of the heart.

sinus arrest Momentary cessation of sinus impulse formation, causing a pause in the cardiac rhythm followed by spontaneous resumption of electrical activity. This dysrhythmia may be referred to as sinus pause, and is reflected as an absence of the PQRST complex on an ECG tracing and an absence of cardiac output.

sinus arrhythmia/dysrhythmia Dysrhythmia resembling normal sinus rhythm except for a slight irregularity in the heart rhythm.

sinus bradycardia Situation in which the SA node is firing at a heart rate of less that 60 beats per minute. Often called *sinus brady*.

sinus tachycardia Rapid firing of the sinus node at rates of more than100 beats per minute at rest. There may be a compensatory response to a decreased cardiac output state.

sinusitis Infection or inflammation of the sinuses.

situational stressor Stressor that is unpredictable and may occur at any time during life; such stressors can be positive or negative. The effect of the situational stressor may vary depending on the developmental stage of the individual experiencing the stress.

Sjögren's syndrome An autoimmune disease in which the immune system attacks and destroys the glands that produce tears and saliva.

skeletal traction Treatment that entails placement of a skeletal pin through the bone which is then attached to a weighted cord to maintain proper alignment of the fractured bone.

skills of involvement The skills of perceiving relevant changes or nuances in clinical situations; these skills are experientially learned and form part of a nurse's practical clinical knowledge.

skin testing Introduction of small amounts of various allergens into the skin of an allergic individual through either intradermal injection or a scratch or "prick test" technique to evaluate for a triggering allergen. Individuals sensitive or capable of producing immediate IgE response to allergens will show a wheal and flare when the allergen is introduced in a skin test.

skin traction Treatment that uses straps or foam boots secured to the lower extremity attached to a weighted cord that is pulling no more than 6 pounds to maintain proper alignment of the fractured bone.

sleep apnea A disorder in which a person stops breathing for more than 10 seconds, typically more than 20 to 30 times in an hour. The three main types of sleep apnea are central, obstructive, and a combination of central and obstructive.

sliding (direct) hiatal hernia Occurs when a portion of the fundus of the stomach moves upward through the esophageal hiatus into the thoracic cavity.

sodium Most numerous cation in extracellular fluid (ECF); maintains ECF volume through osmotic pressure, assists acid–base balance, and conducts nerve impulses via sodium channels. Normal blood values are 135 to 145 mEq/L.

sodium bicarbonate A base or alkali that removes hydrogen ion when added to the blood.

solar lentigo Lesions that develop due to a familial tendency and chronic sun exposure in Caucasians older than 60 years of age. They are macules that are darker and larger than freckles and do not fade during winter. Commonly referred to as *age spots* or *liver spots*.

Somogyi effect A response to the use of exogenous insulin, which results in nocturnal hypoglycemia. The hypoglycemia is accompanied by release of counterregulatory hormones; as a result patients awake in the morning with elevated blood glucose levels. This is often referred to as *rebound hyperglycemia*.

specific gravity (SG) An estimate of the solute concentration in a volume of liquid measured with a hydrometer which compares the liquid to an equal amount of distilled water. Normal urine values are 1.016 to 1.022.

specificity Describes the frequency with which a test is normal in subjects who are free of disease; calculated by dividing the number of true negatives in the population by the sum of true negatives plus false positives.

specificity theory Theory asserting that pain is directly related to the degree of injury. Once a noxious stimulus has occurred, the message is carried directly to the pain centers in the brain.

spermatocele Painless, sperm-containing cysts found on the testicle.

spermatogenesis Production of mature male germ cells.

Spetzler-Martin AVM grading scale A scale to grade arteriovenous malformations (AVMs) based on the degree of surgical difficulty in removing them.

spinal anesthesia An anesthesia technique in which a local anesthetic is injected into the subarachnoid space and directly into the cerebrospinal fluid. Also called *intrathecal anesthesia*.

spinal cord injury (SCI) Injury to the spinal cord that results in impairment or loss of motor, sensory, and autonomic functions.

spinal precautions Methods of immobilizing the spine and moving patients to prevent or avoid additional spinal injury. Spinal precautions are initiated at the trauma scene and maintained until spinal injury has been ruled out or appropriate treatment strategies have been implemented.

spinal shock A period of flaccid paralysis and absent reflexes lasting up to 6 weeks after spinal cord injury.

split-thickness skin graft Grafting of a partial layer of skin, including the epidermis and part of the dermis.

spondylitic disease A condition consisting of inflammation and degenerative changes of the spine including formation of osteophytes, calcification and hypertrophy of the ligaments, and degeneration of the intervertebral disks.

sprain An injury to a ligament.

spring-coil container Mechanical infusion device with a combination of a spring coil and collapsable disk; used to deliver small-volume parenteral solutions or medications.

spring-coil syringe Mechanical infusion device that uses a syringe to deliver parenteral solutions or medications.

ST segment Interval between the end of the QRS complex and the beginning of the T wave on an ECG tracing. Represents the time during which the ventricles have been completely depolarized and are beginning ventricular repolarization. Normally is isoelectric on ECG graph paper.

stage 1 hypertension A blood pressure of 140 to 159 mmHg systolic or 90 to 99 mmHg diastolic measured during multiple office visits following the guidelines for obtaining accurate blood pressure measurements.

stage 2 hypertension A blood pressure of greater than 160 mmHg systolic or greater than 100 mmHg diastolic measured during multiple office visits following the guidelines for obtaining accurate blood pressure measurements.

staghorn calculus A calculus or stone that remains in the renal pelvis and becomes so large that it fills the pelvis completely, blocking the flow of urine.

staging The portion of the tumor classification system that describes the extent of the tumor and evidence of metastasis throughout the body.

standards of care General standards of care and guidelines for nursing practice formulated in 1991 by the American Nurses Association.

standards of nursing practice Authoritative statements by which the nursing profession describes the common level of performance or care by which the quality of practice can be determined and responsibilities for which its practitioners are accountable.

standards of professional performance Standards that address the professional nursing role with regard to education, ethics, research, collegiality, and resource utilization.

stapedectomy Removal of the stapes bone and its replacement to restore hearing.

statistical significance A term indicating that the results from an analysis of sample data are unlikely to have been caused by chance, at some specified level of probability.

steady state Dynamic balance of the body's internal environment, even in the presence of change.

steatorrhea Feces that have a high fat content. The stool is typically foul-smelling, greasy, and floats.

stem cell Primitive cell in the bone marrow from which mature blood cells derive.

STEMI Acronym for ST segment elevation myocardial infarction; refers to myocardial injury associated with ST segment elevation on the ECG. ST segment elevation means that myocardial tissue is undergoing severe anoxia and cellular damage, in most cases resulting from complete coronary artery blockage from thrombotic occlusion over an underlying plaque lesion.

stenosis Narrowing of the lumen of a blood vessel.

stent A device used to secure a widened arterial lumen; it is inserted permanently inside the coronary artery, compressing plaque and providing structural support of the vessel. The two general type of stents are bare-metal stents, which do not have a coating, and drug-eluting stents, which are "coated" with medications, including heparin and various immunosuppressant agents, in such a manner that the medications diffuse (elute) into the vessel wall over a period of weeks to months.

Stevens-Johnson syndrome (SJS) A severe, acute, self-limiting skin reaction to infection or to certain medications; affects the epidermal layer of the skin and mucous membranes.

stomatitis Generalized inflammation of the oral mucosa; it is classified according to the etiology.

stopcock Manually operated add-on device used to direct the flow of an infusate.

strabismus A condition in which an individual's eyes do not look at the same object together. Also referred to as *cross-eyed*.

strain An injury to the muscle belly or its tendon attachment to bone.

strategic national stockpile (SNS) A national repository of pharmaceutical agents, vaccines, medical supplies, and equipment that can be delivered to the site of a large-scale disaster to augment local and state resources in order to reduce the morbidity and mortality in the civilian population.

stratified random sampling Type of sampling that gives individuals within designated categories an equal chance of selection. The population is first divided into two or more strata or subpopulations. The goal is to enhance representation.

stress An organism's response to stimulation or change; a state produced by a change in the environment that may be perceived as challenging, threatening, or damaging to the person's dynamic balance or equilibrium. These changes may be real or perceived, and they activate an organism's attempts to cope by means of neural and endocrine mechanisms.

stress perception Recognition of a stressor by the brain.

stress response Activation of physiological fight-or-flight-or-fright systems within the body.

stressor A stimulus that activates a stress response.

stridor A raspy noise heard in the upper airway as a result of air attempting to move through a narrowed opening.

stroke Syndrome characterized by a set of neurological deficits that fit a known vascular region.

stroke volume (SV) The amount of blood leaving a ventricle with each contraction.

structure standards Quality standards that focus on the internal characteristics of an organization and its personnel.

subarachnoid hemorrhage (SAH) A condition characterized by bleeding into the space below the arachnoid space.

subchondral bone The smooth tissue at the ends of bones that is covered with cartilage.

subconscious A mental state that encompasses things that have been forgotten but can easily be brought to consciousness.

subcutaneous emphysema Air that escapes into the subcutaneous tissue.

subcutaneous nodules Small, nontender swellings found over bony prominences on the hands and feet.

subdural hematoma (SDH) Bleeding between the dura and the arachnoid layers of the meninges.

subjective data Data that consists of information the patient or caretaker tells the nurse; information that can be perceived only by the patient and not by the observer.

substance abuse Repeated use of a substance despite significant and repeated negative substance-related consequences.

substance dependence A pattern of substance use that is continued despite significant consequences, usually with physiological tolerance effects and a withdrawal syndrome if the substance is withdrawn.

substance intoxication Reversible substance-specific changes in thinking, emotions, behavior, and/or physiological functions caused by recent substance ingestion.

substance withdrawal A substance-specific mental disorder that follows the cessation or reduced intake of a substance that has regularly been used to induce a state of intoxication.

substance withdrawal syndrome The symptoms that occur when drug use is reduced or discontinued.

substantia nigra Structure located in the midbrain beneath the basal ganglia.

substituted judgment A subjective determination of what a person would have chosen to do had that person been capable of making his or her opinion known.

sudden cardiac death (SCD) Type of cardiac arrest most often associated with abrupt coronary artery occlusion from plaque disruption over severely stenotic lesions in the setting of poorly developed collateral circulation.

superego An extension of the ego that represents an individual's early moral training and ideal values imparted by societal norms.

suppurative Pertaining to the formation of pus.

supraventricular tachycardia (SVT) Tachycardia that is generated somewhere above the ventricles. The term encompasses all fast rhythms with normal QRS complexes and heart rates greater than 100 beats per minute. Rhythms included in this category include sinus tachycardia, premature atrial tachycardia, and paroxysmal junctional tachycardia. This term may be used when it is impossible to identify the source of the tachycardia.

surfactant Surface-active agent that promotes alveolar stability.

surveillance The systematic and continuous assessment of patients for the recognition and management of potentially catastrophic events.

survival Observation of persons with cancer over time and the likelihood of their dying over several time periods; a link between incidence and mortality data.

Swan-Ganz catheter A pulmonary artery catheter that is inserted into the pulmonary artery via the right atrium and ventricle; used to measure cardiac output and pulmonary artery pressure and to infuse fluids.

sympathectomy Excision of a portion of the sympathetic division of the autonomic division of the autonomic nervous system.

synapse The space between the junction of two neurons in a neural pathway where the termination of the axon of one neuron comes into proximity with the cell body or dendrites of another.

syncope Temporary dizziness or loss of consciousness caused by low blood pressure and insufficient blood flow.

syndrome of inappropriate antidiuretic hormone (SIADH) A hypermetabolic state of the adrenal glands in which antidiuretic hormone is produced in excess, leading to the retention of fluid and hyponatremia.

syphilis A sexually transmitted infection (STI) that is caused by the *Treponema pallidum* bacterium; has been called the "great imitator" because its symptoms often mimic those of other STIs.

systemic inflammatory response (SIRS) A systemic response of the immune system that can be triggered by both infectious and noninfectious causes.

systemic lupus erythematosus (SLE) An example of a systemic type III hypersensitivity autoimmune disease characterized by damage to joints and soft organs as a result of the effects of autoantibodies and antibody–antigen activity (immune complex responses).

systemic vascular resistance The arterial systolic pressure; normal SVR is 900 to 1,400 · dyn s/cm^5.

systolic A blood pressure reading of the maximum pressure in the aorta and major arteries, which occurs when the left ventricle contracts and ejects blood onto the central vascular system.

systolic dysfunction Impaired ventricular function with volume overload and decreased contractility.

T cells White blood cells that are vital to initiating and regulating an immune response; produced in the bone marrow and mature and differentiate into various types of T cells in the thymus and other lymphatic tissue such as CD4 (cluster of differentiation, a type of receptor), CD8, T-memory, and T-suppressor cells. They are a crucial part of the immune response because they function as the regulatory cells of the immune system and are responsible for initiating and controlling immune processes such as phagocytosis, cytokine/lymphokine secretion, and activation of B cells.

T lymphocyte Lymphocytes that, when active, divide rapidly and secrete small proteins called cytokines that regulate or assist in the immune response.

T wave Represents ventricular recovery or repolarization in the cardiac cycle; often referred to as the resting phase of the cycle.

tachypnea Rapid respiratory rate.

tau A specialized protein that is a key component of the neurofibrillary tangles associated with Alzheimer's disease.

teaching Any deliberate act that involves the planning, implementation, and evaluation of instructional strategies that meet expected learner outcomes.

team nursing A nursing care delivery system in which a group of RNs, LVNs/LPNs, and unlicensed assistive personnel are assigned shift responsibility for a group of patients, with the RN assuming a leadership role in accordance with the nurse practice act.

techne Something that can be standardized and replicated.

telemedicine Systems or programs that use video or computer-based equipment to link providers or monitor patients electronically.

teleological theories Theories that derive norms or rules for conduct from the consequences of actions; looks merely at consequences to determine the rightness or wrongness of an action.

telomere The tip or end of each chromosome arm.

temporary transvenous pacing Procedure that involves insertion of a pacemaker wire through a major vein, such as the internal jugular, subclavian, or femoral. The pacemaker wire is then advanced into the heart for pacing.

tenosynovitis An infection of the flexor tendon sheaths.

tension pneumothorax Occurs when an injury perforates the chest or pleural space. During inspiration air enters the pleural space and becomes trapped. As more air is trapped, the pressure in the pleural space increases, collapsing the lung and causing the mediastinum to shift to the opposite side.

terrorism An act designed to disrupt daily life and cause terror and panic. The definition according to the FBI is "The unlawful use of force or violence against persons or property to intimidate or coerce a government, the civilian population, or any segment thereof, in furtherance of political or social objectives."

tertiary or third intention Healing that occurs in wounds that have not been sutured in a timely manner or have broken down and been sutured later.

testicular torsion Twisting of the spermatic cord.

tetraplegia (Greek) Paralysis of both upper and lower extremities.

thalassemia Class of hematologic disorders characterized by genetic inheritance of a mutated hemoglobin-coding gene; characterized by increased hemolysis.

T-helper cells A type of T cell that is identified and named by the kind of receptor that is on its surface, a CD4 receptor (cluster of differentiation receptor 4). T-helper cells regulate immune function by stimulating B lymphocytes to produce antibodies and chemically stimulate the cell-mediated response to viral and mutant cells.

theoretical connectedness Requires that the theoretical schema developed for the study be clearly expressed, logically consistent, reflective of the data, and compatible with the practice of nursing.

therapeutic alliance An alliance that involves the nurse and the patient consciously working together to reach mutually agreed-on goals.

therapeutic communication Purposeful communication that is designed to convey openness and caring.

therapeutic lifestyle changes (TLC) Dietary modifications recommended for treatment and prevention of disease.

thermal burns Injury from flames; the most common type of burn injury.

thermistor Thermometer imbedded in a pulmonary artery catheter that is used to detect core temperatures.

third-degree AV block (complete block) Independent excitation and contraction of the atria and ventricles due to the inability of any atrial impulses to reach the ventricles. The top and the bottom of the heart are not communicating; they are each beating independently. This dysrhythmia is referred to as AV dissociation because of the independent function of the atria and the ventricles.

threshold Point at which a stimulus will produce a cell response or depolarization.

thrills Palpable vibratory sensations from turbulent blood flow across cardiac valves due to cardiac murmurs.

thromboangiitis obliterans (TAO) A chronic inflammatory vascular occlusive disease most common in men who smoke. Also known as *Buerger's disease*.

thrombocyte Platelet.

thrombopoietin Hormone produced by the liver and kidneys; responsible for stimulating thrombopoiesis.

thrombus Blood clot that forms in a blood vessel and remains at the site of formation.

through-the-needle peripheral-short catheter Vascular access device in which the catheter is inserted into the vein by threading it through the lumen of an introducer.

thyroid storm A life-threatening, hypermetabolic condition in which excess production of thyroid hormones causes serious cardiac disorders.

thyroidectomy Full or partial surgical removal of the thyroid gland.

thyroiditis Inflammation of the thyroid gland.

thyromegaly Abnormal growth of thyroid tissue.

thyrotoxicosis A critical, hypermetabolic condition in which excess production of thyroid hormones threatens physiological stability and well-being.

tinnitus A buzzing, roaring, or ringing in the ears.

tissue factor (TF) Cytokine that is important in immune function and inflammation; released by a variety of injured tissue cells, macrophages, and platelets; stimulates platelets to stick together and form the beginning of a clot to stop bleeding when injury occurs.

tissue-specific antigens Proteins located in the cell membrane of some tissues such as blood, nerves, lungs, and kidneys that are involved in type II tissue-specific–mediated hypersensitivity reactions.

tolerance Physiological habituation to a substance, resulting in the need for progressively greater amounts to achieve intoxication and/or a diminished effect from continued use of the same amount of the substance.

toll receptors Part of the natural immune response; microcellular receptors on the surface of many types of immune and tissue cells that are able to initiate immune responses when pieces of bacterial cell walls attach to them. Functions include stimulation of a cell to release tumor necrosis factor or start the process of programmed cell death (apoptosis).

tomography Imaging technology that displays images of a single plane (slice) of the heart.

tonsillitis An acute or recurrent infection of the tonsils.

tophi Accumulation of uric acid crystals in the cartilage of the earlobe.

torsade de pointes Form of ventricular tachycardia in which the QRS complexes have varying morphology or shape and width. This dysrhythmia resembles a turning about or twisting motion along the baseline or isoelectric line and tends to recur repeatedly.

tort law A brand of civil law concerning legal wrongs committed by one person against another or against another's property.

total joint replacement A diseased or injured joint that is surgically removed, and replaced with an orthosis.

total parenteral nutrition (TPN) Provision of nutrition intravenously via a central vein.

total patient care Another name for the case method of nursing care delivery.

toxic epidermal necrolysis (TEN) Part of the same syndrome of diseases as Stevens-Johnson syndrome, but it is a more severe form of the disorder and is life threatening with more extensive skin detachment.

toxin Material produced by living organisms that has chemical properties that can cause injury, illness, and death.

tracheal breath sounds Breath sounds auscultated over the trachea; they are normally loud and high pitched.

tracheal deviation Shifting of the tracheal position to the right or left of midline due to the push or pull of thoracic structures.

tracheostomy Refers to the making of a semipermanent or permanent opening into the trachea, and to the opening itself.

tracheotomy A temporary surgical airway into the trachea.

transcription Formation of an RNA molecule on a DNA template in the cell nucleus.

transcutaneous electrical nerve stimulation (TENS) Low-voltage electrical stimulation through the skin; used to relieve pain.

transcutaneous pacing (TCP) Procedure that delivers an electrical stimulus directly through the chest wall.

transduction The transmission of pain from the periphery to the central nervous system.

transection Cutting across.

transesophageal echocardiography (TEE) Echocardiogram performed using a miniaturized transducer advanced down the esophagus. Because the esophagus passes directly behind the posterior surface of the heart, TEE affords excellent views of the posterior structures of the heart and great vessels.

transesophageal ultrasound A diagnostic test that uses an ultrasound device that is passed into the esophagus of a patient to create a clear image of the heart muscle and other parts of the heart.

transferrin Protein concentrated in the small intestine; responsible for transportation of iron from the gut to target cells.

transfusion-related acute lung injury (TRALI) A serious, life-threatening clinical syndrome that is a complication of blood transfusions. It is thought to be caused by the presence of granulocyte antibodies and biologically active lipids in the donor plasma to which the recipient reacts.

transient ischemia attack (TIA) An episode of neurological deficits resulting from temporary ischemia that produces strokelike symptoms but no lasting damage. It occurs when the blood supply to part of the brain is briefly interrupted. Also referred to as a *warning stroke* or *mini-stroke*.

transient pain Acute pain that is brief and then resolves completely such as is the case in a needlestick for phlebotomy or an intramuscular injection.

translation Formation of a polypeptide chain from its mRNA template.

translocation A chromosome aberration that results from a transfer of a segment of one chromosome to another chromosome.

traumatic brain injury (TBI) An acute brain disorder characterized by an injury to the brain secondary to trauma.

traumatic wounds Abrasions, blisters, cuts, bites, stab wounds, gunshot wounds, and first- and second-degree burns.

tremors Involuntary muscle movements of a body part or limb.

triage A process that is used to determine the severity of a patient's illness or injury.

trichomoniasis A sexually transmitted protozoan infection caused by *Trichomonas vaginalis*.

tricuspid valve regurgitation Inability of a heart valve to completely close, resulting in a backflow of blood from the right ventricle to the right atrium.

tricuspid valve stenosis Obstruction of blood flow between the right atrium and the right ventricle due to a narrowed valve orifice.

trigeminy Premature ventricular contraction that is evidenced every third beat.

triglycerides A form of fat derived from fats in food and produced by the body from other sources such as carbohydrates.

triple-H therapy A triad of medical treatments for vasospasm (hemodilution, hypervolemia, and hypertension).

trismus Restricted movement of the jaw.

trisomy The state of having three representatives of a given chromosome instead of the usual pair.

tropia Deviation of an eye from the normal position with respect to the line of vision when the eyes are open.

Trousseau's sign Contraction of the muscles when the nerves are mildly compressed; for example, inflating a blood pressure cuff and keeping it above systolic will induce carpal spasms.

trypsin A pancreatic enzyme that hydrolyzes the interior bonds of large protein molecules.

tumor necrosis factor (TNF) A small peptide produced by a variety of cells, including granulocytes and lymphocytes; critical in the stimulation of the initial inflammatory response, specifically the activity of macrophages and granulocytes; also stimulates cells to initiate programmed apoptosis when mutations occur, which is important in inhibiting tumor development and growth.

tunica adventitia The outer layer of an artery; flexible stratum that consists of fibrous tissue made of collagen and elastic fibers surrounded by collagen bundles.

tunica intima Layer of an artery that consists of a monolayer of connecting endothelial cells and a lamina of connective tissue and smooth muscle cells.

tunica media The middle layer of an artery that consists of multiple layers of smooth muscle cells and connective tissue made up of elastic fibers, collagen, and proteoglycans.

tunneled and cuffed device Long-term central vascular access device whose proximal end is tunneled subcutaneously from the insertion site and the remaining length is brought out through the skin at an exit site.

turgor The elasticity and mobility of the skin; reflects the skin's hydration status.

tympanic membrane Eardrum.

tympanoplasty Surgical repair of the eardrum or bones of the middle ear in an effort to restore hearing.

tympany (1) A high-pitched, drum-like tone of medium duration. It is commonly heard over the air-filled intestines. (2) Abdominal distention with gas.

type 1 diabetes mellitus Type of diabetes characterized by the destruction of pancreatic beta cells.

type 2 diabetes mellitus Type of diabetes characterized by insulin resistance and decreased insulin secretion.

type A blood Blood type for an individual with A antigen.

type AB blood Blood type for an individual with both A and B antigens.

type B blood Blood type for an individual with B antigen.

type I (IgE-mediated) allergic reactions Involve the production of antigen-specific IgE antibodies after exposure to a foreign antigen or allergen; most common of the immune hypersensitivity disorders.

type II (tissue-specific–mediated) hypersensitivity reactions Involve IgG and IgM antibody–antigen immune complexes; tissue-specific antigens on the surface of cells are not recognized as self by the immune system and are attacked and damaged or destroyed. Only tissues with the specific antigens are involved.

type III (immune complex–mediated) hypersensitivity reactions Involve IgG and IgM antibody–antigen immune complexes; differentiated from type II reactions in that such reactions are soluble in plasma and circulate in the blood and are not localized at a tissue-specific surface. The traveling antibody–antigen complexes can deposit in tissue or joints and precipitate phagocytosis and inflammation. Multiple body systems/locations can be involved and a variety of clinical symptoms may be observed.

type IV (cell-mediated) hypersensitivity reactions T-cell–mediated immune response, instead of an antibody response as is the case with type I, II, and III hypersensitivity reactions. Additionally, the response is delayed, with the onset of symptoms 24 to 48 hours after antigen exposure. One example of a type IV hypersensitivity response is poison ivy reaction.

type O blood Blood type for an individual with neither A or B antigens.

type-specific hypersensitivity reactions Four specific mechanisms of overreactive immunologic response (types I, II, III, and IV) to environmental allergens, self-antigens, or antigens from another human.

U wave Follows the T wave in the cardiac cycle and is present only in some people on an ECG tracing.

ulcerative colitis (UC) Disorder that involves chronic inflammation of the mucosal and submucosal layers of the colon and rectum.

unconscious A mental state that encompasses all of those things that cannot be remembered or brought to conscious thought.

undernutrition Synonym for *malnutrition*.

unipolar lead Lead with one positive electrode and one indifferent zero reference point; consists of standard leads and augmented limb leads. The leads provide the five frontal plane leads of a 12-lead ECG.

United Kingdom Prospective Diabetes Study (UKPDS) A large clinical research study in Great Britain of patients with type 2 diabetes which concluded that tight glucose control (i.e., maintaining blood glucose levels close to normal ranges) results in decreased microvascular complications.

unlicensed assistive personnel Health care personnel who are not licensed; they may be technicians or certified nurses' aides or nursing assistants.

Unna's boot A rigid bandage that prevents edema while promoting healing; it is worn for several days at a time. Commonly used to treat venous ulcers.

unstable angina A transitory syndrome falling between stable angina and myocardial infarction wherein thrombus forms in an area of arterial stenosis, but is subsequently fully or partially lysed by endogenous antithrombotic mechanisms.

uplifts Positive experiences that are likely to occur in everyday life.

urgent procedures Surgeries that must be performed sooner rather than later.

urticaria Raised, erythematous, intensely pruritic plaques or wheals that are surrounded by a white halo. Also known as *hives*.

U.S. Preventive Services Task Force (USPSTF) A group of health care experts that makes recommendations for appropriate preventive services and screening exams in adults ages 65 and over.

vaccine A preparation that contains an infectious agent (live or killed) or its components; administered to stimulate the production of antibodies that can prevent infection or create resistance to infection from that agent; a type of acquired artificial immunity.

vaginismus Condition in which the vaginal muscles at the introitus contract very tightly, making vaginal penetration painful.

values Freely chosen beliefs or attitudes about the worth of an individual or object.

valvular regurgitation Inability of a heart valve to completely close, resulting in a backflow of blood through the incompetent valve orifice into the previous chamber.

valvuloplasty A surgical procedure to repair torn or damaged leaflets, chordae tendineae, or papillary muscle.

variables Attributes of a person or object that vary, that is, take on different values. Examples include body temperature, age, and blood pressure.

variant, Prinzmetal, or vasospastic angina Condition characterized by a vasospasm occurring at a single or multiple sites in major coronary arteries and their large branches.

varicocele Varicosities of the veins of the scrotum.

varicose veins Dilated, tortuous, superficial veins most commonly seen in the lower extremities.

vascular access device (VAD) A catheter, tube, or device inserted into the vascular system.

vascular lesion Lesions that appear as red or purple pigmented.

vasectomy Male sterilization surgery.

vasodilator A substance that causes the dilation of blood vessels.

vasodilatory cascade A series of events triggered by hypoxia, resulting in increased intracranial pressure.

vasogenic edema A condition characterized by an alteration in vascular permeability with disruption of the blood–brain barrier.

vasospasm Refers to the transient narrowing of an artery, causing decreased blood flow.

venous thromboembolism (VTE) Includes the disorders of deep venous thrombosis and pulmonary embolism.

ventilated-associated pneumonia (VAP) Pneumonia that develops in mechanically ventilated patients after more than 48 hours of intubation, with no clinical evidence of pneumonia at the time of intubation.

ventilation The movement of air between the atmosphere and the alveoli accomplished by respirations or the ability of the lungs to remove carbon dioxide.

ventilation/perfusion mismatching (V/Q) Usually there is a near equal relationship of ventilation ($\dot{V}$) to perfusion ($\dot{Q}$) in the lungs. The formula $\dot{V}/\dot{Q}$, where ventilation is 4 L/min and perfusion is 5 L/min, explains this relationship. Normal ventilation to perfusion equals 4/5 or 0.8.

ventral hernia A hernia through the abdominal wall.

ventricular dysrhythmia Dysrhythmia that originates in the ventricle and is caused by ectopic or irritable foci in the wall of the ventricle. These are the most serious types of dysrhythmias.

ventricular fibrillation (VF) Dysrhythmia marked by rapid, disorganized depolarization of the ventricles. There are no organized electrical impulses or coordinated atrial or ventricular contractions or palpable pulse.

ventricular tachycardia (VT) Life-threatening excitable ventricular focus arising from the tissue distal to the bifurcation of the bundle of His. It discharges repetitively, acting as the dominant pacemaker. When present, three or more premature ventricular contractions occur in a row at a rate of 130 to 250 beats per minute.

veracity In ethics, truth-telling.

verrucae Viral epidermal eruptions caused by human papilloma virus. Also known as *warts*.

vertically integrated models Organizational service structure of hospitals and related health care services aligned along a continuum of care. This model includes the integration of physician, hospital, and ancillary services. Integrated systems can offer a broad range of services pre- and post-hospitalization from primary care to long-term care.

vertigo Subjective sensation of spinning; dizziness; the illusion of rotational movement, tilting, and swaying with feelings of imbalance during standing or walking; symptom of a balance disorder.

vesicant (1) Chemical agent that can cause redness and irritation of the skin and blistering. Also called a *blistering agent*. (2) Parenteral solution or medication known to cause tissue damage and possible necrosis if infiltrated.

vesicular breath sounds Breath sounds normally heard over most of the chest wall from the movement of air in small airways distal to the bronchioles.

vestibular nerve dissection Surgical procedure to cut the vestibular nerve in the event of constant vertigo or dizziness.

viability The ability of a pathogen to survive outside of its host.

Vincent's stomatitis An acute bacterial infection of the gingiva oral mucous membranes caused most often by the bacteria *Borrelia vincentii*. Also known as *acute necrotizing stomatitis* or *trench mouth*.

viral hepatitis Inflammation of the liver caused by several viruses: HAV, HBV, HCV, HDV, and HEV.

viral load The number of HIV viral particles in a sample of blood, expressed as *copies*. Used to monitor the virulence of HIV infection. Levels of >100,000 copies indicate increased risk of AIDS-related illness.

viral meningitis Inflammation of the meninges due to a viral pathogen.

Virchow's triad The three factors that contribute to thrombosis: damage to the venous wall, a change in flow, and blood hypercoagulability.

virulence Related to the severity of disease a pathogen is capable of causing; virulence can vary depending on the ability of the host to mount an immune response. It is expressed as the number of cases of infection that are serious or produce a disability in all those infected.

visual analog scale (VAS) Does not have numeric intervals; rather it uses "no pain" and "pain as bad as it can possibly be" as descriptors at either end of a horizontal line measuring 10 cm in length.

vital signs Temperature, pulse, respirations, blood pressure, and pain level. Used to monitor patients for infection and hemodynamic changes.

vitamin B$_{12}$ (cobalamin) Essential nutrient found in animal proteins; responsible for the activation of folate iron.

vitiligo Condition leading to a localized loss of melanocytes and, thus, patches of depigmentation.

voice whisper test A hearing test in which the examiner stands 1 to 2 feet in back of the patient and whispers.

volumetric pump Electronic infusion device that calculates the volume of solution delivered based on the amount displaced in the set's reservoir.

volutrauma Similar to barotrauma, but the lung damage is caused by increased volume that causes overdistention of alveoli.

vomiting agent Chemical agents that cause vomiting.

von Willebrand's disease Most common inherited bleeding disorder; characterized by deficiencies in von Willebrand factor.

wandering atrial pacemaker A pacemaker from at least three different sites above the bundle of His. Pacemaker sites may include the SA node, the AV junction, an atrial ectopic site, or any combination of these areas.

washed RBCs Red blood cells that have undergone a washing process that increases the removal of immunoglobulins and proteins that cause reactions. The use of washed RBCs is indicated when previous transfusion reactions have occurred.

wasting syndrome Involves the loss of lean tissue from increased protein metabolism, changes in metabolic rate, and anorexia and diarrhea. It is a hallmark of AIDS-related disease.

wear-and-tear theory of aging Theory of aging based on the premise that exposure to internal and external stressors results in the death of cells.

Weber test A hearing screening test that distinguishes whether hearing loss in an ear is conductive or sensorineural.

Western blot (WB) A specific and sensitive serum test that measures the presence of antibodies to HIV; generally done as a confirmation test when enzyme immunoassay tests for HIV are positive.

wheal A small, round, serous-filled raised blister on the skin that is the result of exposure to an allergen.

wheezes High-pitched musical sounds created by air moving over mucous strands.

white blood cell (WBC) A type of blood cell involved in protecting the body against foreign matter.

white coat phenomenon Phenomenon that occurs when a patient's blood pressure is susceptible to elevation as a result of apprehension and anxiety in a health care provider's office or during any other stressful situation.

whole blood Blood that is obtained from a donor, processed, and infused into a recipient.

wild type A normal allele of a gene or its normal phenotype.

window period The time between actual HIV infection and when HIV tests can detect the presence of the virus or antibodies to the virus in blood; usually 1 to 6 months.

winged steel infusion set A metal needle manufactured with flexible plastic attachments to facilitate insertion technique; used for phlebotomy procedures or for single-dose parenteral administrations and infusions of less than 4 hours duration.

withdrawal Uncomfortable and maladaptive physiological, cognitive, emotional, and behavioral changes associated with lowered blood or tissue concentrations of a substance after an individual has established some tolerance toward it, usually through heavy recent use.

WMD Acronym for weapons of mass destruction, which are agents that can cause massive damage and injury.

Wolff-Parkinson-White (WPW) syndrome AV conduction disorder characterized by two AV conduction pathways. This disorder generates an accessory conduction pathway.

wound dehiscence The separation of sutures or staples along the incision in a previously closed wound.

wound evisceration The protrusion of organs from a wound site.

xerosis A skin condition characterized by dry, pruritic, cracked, or fissured skin with scaling and flaking.

X-linked dominant Disorder in which a trait is dominant if it is phenotypically expressed in heterozygotes due to one or more genes located on the X chromosome.

X-linked recessive Disorder in which a trait is recessive if the trait is expressive only in homozygotes due to one or more genes located on the X chromosome.

Y set Devices used for administration of two or more infusates simultaneously. Access to the multiflow adapter is usually via a cap that maintains sterility of the fluid pathway.

zone of coagulation Area where the amount of injury to the tissue is the greatest.

zone of hyperthermia The outermost portion of an injured area where cell damage is minor.

zone of stasis Area surrounding the zone of coagulation that has potentially viable but injured cells.

zones; hot zone, warm zone, cold zone The hot zone, also called the exclusion or the red zone, is the area of highest contamination in a decontamination area. The warm zone, or yellow zone, is also called the contamination reduction corridor, and this is where actual decontamination takes place. The cold zone, or green zone, is also known as the support zone. No one is allowed in the cold zone without first being decontaminated. Those waiting to be decontaminated would be in the hot zone as well as the triage area.

zygote Fertilized egg.

INDEX

Page numbers followed by *f* indicate figures and those followed by *t* indicate tables, boxes, or special features. The titles of special features (e.g., Nursing Process: Patient Care Plans) are also capitalized. Trade names of drugs are capitalized and cross-referenced to their generic name.

A

for testicular cancer, 1570, 1585*t*
types, 2101*t*
Chenix. *See* chenodiol
chenodiol, 1449, 1457*t*
cherry angioma, 2144*t*
chest pain, differential diagnosis, 1177–78*t*
chest trauma, 986–87, 986*f*
chest tube:
drainage systems, 991*f*
equipment for, 991*t*
expected drainage, 680*t*
indications/purpose, 680*t*, 990, 990*t*
insertion, 991
nursing management, 990
assessment, 990–91
chest x-ray:
in aortic dissection, 1345*t*
in cardiac inflammatory disorders, 1222*t*
in cardiac valve disease, 1246*t*
in chronic obstructive pulmonary disease, 958*t*
in coronary artery disease, 1188*t*
in cor pulmonale, 985*t*
in cystic fibrosis, 971*t*
in heart failure, 1288*t*
in pneumonia, 939*t*
preoperative, 600*t*
in pulmonary embolism, 974*t*
in pulmonary hypertension, 978
in tuberculosis, 946*t*
chewing tobacco, 2072
chief complaint, 155
Chinese culture:
communication customs, 154*t*, 404*t*
death rituals, 404*t*
genetic testing and counseling, 207*t*
chiropractic, 26*t*, 1780*t*
chitosan, 285*t*
chlamydia infections, 1518–19, 1519*f*, 1551*t*, 1552*t*
Chlamydia trachomatis, 2355
chlorambucil, 2104*t*
chloramphenicol, 982*t*
chlordiazepoxide, 367*t*
chloride (Cl⁻), 432
functions, 432
imbalances. *See* hyperchloremia; hypochloremia
regulation, 432–33
serum levels
normal values, 420*t*
in overhydration/dehydration, 420*t*
chlorine gas, 1011, 2395–96
Chloromycetin. *See* chloramphenicol
chloroquine, 1840*t*, 1915*t*
chlorothiazide, 497*t*
chlorpheniramine, 183*t*, 890*t*
chlorpropamide, 1678*t*
Chlor-Trimeton. *See* pseudoephedrine
choking agents (asphyxiates), 2395
ammonia, 2395
chlorine, 2395–96
phosgene, 2396
cholangiocarcinoma, 1444. *See also* liver cancer
cholecystectomy, 1374*t*, 1449
laparoscopic, 623, 1449
Nursing Process: Patient Care Plan, 1451–52*t*
open, 604*t*
T-tube placement in, 1449, 1450*t*
cholecystitis, 1448
clinical manifestations, 1449
diagnostic procedures, 1449
differential diagnosis, 1178*t*

health promotion, 1450
medical management, 1449
complementary therapy, 1450
dietary and lifestyle management, 1449, 1449*t*
medications, 1449–50
surgery. *See* cholecystectomy
ultrasound therapy, 1450
nursing management
assessment, 1450
interventions, 1450
pathophysiology, 1448
cholecystokinin (CCK), 1427, 1616*t*
choledochojejunostomy, 1374*t*
choledocholithiasis, 1447
cholelithiasis. *See also* cholecystitis
clinical manifestations, 1448
ethnic/gender considerations, 1448*t*
etiology and epidemiology, 1447
pathophysiology, 1447–48
cholesterol, 1165, 1166. *See also* hyperlipidemia
serum levels
in cirrhosis, 1438*t*
in hypertension, 494*t*
normal values, 494*t*, 1165*t*
cholestyramine, 1200*t*, 1457*t*
cholinergic crisis, 820
cholinesterase inhibitors, 821, 822*t*
chondro–, 2066
chondrosarcoma, 1749, 1750
chordae tendineae, 1053, 1234*f*
Christianity, 402*t*
Christian Scientists, 543*t*
chromium, 285*t*
chromosomal disorders, 198–99
deletions, 199
nondisjunction, 199
translocations, 199
chromosomes, 193–94, 194*f*, 195*f*
chronic bronchitis, 955. *See also* chronic obstructive pulmonary disease
chronic glomerulonephritis, 1465
etiology, 1466
laboratory and diagnostic procedures, 1466, 1466*t*
medical management, 1466
nursing management
assessment, 1466
evaluation, 1467
interventions and rationales, 1467
nursing diagnoses, 1466
outcomes and evaluation parameters, 1466–67
planning, 1466
Patient Teaching & Discharge Priorities, 1468*t*
chronic graft rejection, 1913
chronic lymphocytic leukemia, 2080*t*
chronic lymphocytic thyroiditis, 1618. *See also* hypothyroidism
chronic myeloid leukemia, 2081*t*
chronic obstructive pulmonary disease (COPD), 955
chronic bronchitis, 955
collaborative management, 950
Complementary and Alternative Therapies, 959*t*
dyspnea assessment in, 959*t*
emphysema, 955
epidemiology and etiology, 955
health promotion, 950
laboratory and diagnostic procedures, 957, 958*t*
medical management, 957–58, 959*f*

medical nutrition therapy, 317–18, 318*t*
nursing management, 958–60, 960*f*, 961*f*
Nursing Process: Patient Care Plan, 962–63*t*
pathophysiology, 955–56, 956*f*, 957*f*
respiratory acidosis in, 443
chronic pain, 334, 342. *See also* pain assessment; pain management
chronic renal failure, 1480
clinical manifestations, 1481–82
collaborative management. *See* hemodialysis; peritoneal dialysis
laboratory and diagnostic procedures, 1481, 1482*t*
medical management
of complications, 1483–84
to slow disease progression, 1482–83
nursing management, 1484
Nursing Process: Patient Care Plan, 1485–86*t*
risk factors, 1480
stages, 1481
chronic stress, 225
chronic stressors, 215
chronic venous insufficiency, 1353–55, 1355*f*
chronic wounds, 2199
chronosystem, 254*t*
Chvostek's sign, 430, 1608, 1633
chyle, 1865, 1994
chyle leak, 928
chymotrypsin, 1427
CIAMPEDS mnemonic, for triage, 2418*t*
cigarettes. *See* smoking
cilostazol, 1327, 1349*t*
cimetidine, 1390*t*
cingulate herniation, 716
Cipro. *See* ciprofloxacin
ciprofloxacin:
for diverticulitis, 1409
for gastrointestinal disorders, 1384*t*
for infections, 478*t*
for lower airway disorders, 981*t*
for renal disorders, 1490*t*
for urinary tract infections, 1496*t*
circadian rhythms, 1597
circinate balanitis, 1847
circle of Willis, 764, 765*f*
circulating nurse, 620
circulatory overload, 550
circumduction, 1712*t*
cirrhosis, 1434
clinical manifestations, 1435–36, 1437*t*
Clinical Preparation, 1459–60*t*
complications
hepatic encephalopathy, 308–9, 309*t*, 1436
hepatorenal syndrome, 1436
portal hypertension, 1436
etiology, 1435*t*
health promotion, 1441
laboratory and diagnostic procedures, 1436, 1438*t*
medical management, 1436
ascites, 1439–40, 1440*t*
end-stage liver disease, 1441
esophageal varices, 1440–41
hepatic encephalopathy, 1440
medical nutrition therapy, 308
nursing management
assessment, 1441
interventions, 1441
Nursing Process: Patient Care Plan, 1442–43*t*
pathophysiology, 1434–35
Patient Teaching & Discharge Priorities, 1444*t*

head and neck:
  age-related disorders, 172
  assessment, 1719–20, 1999
head and neck cancer, 915
  clinical manifestations, 917
  collaborative management, 917
    medical management, 918–19, 918*t*
    reconstruction flaps and grafts, 919–20, 920*f*
    staging system, 917–18
    surgical resection, 919, 919*t*
  etiology, 915
  laboratory and diagnostic procedures, 915, 917, 918*t*
  nursing management, 920
    airway management, 920, 926
    aspiration risk factors, 928*t*
    carotid artery precautions, 929, 929*t*
    discharge priorities, 929, 930*t*
    laryngectomy stoma care, 926
    nutrition management, 927–28, 928*f*
    pain management, 926–27
    physical therapy, 929
    wound care, 928
    wound complications, 928–29, 929*f*
  Nursing Process: Patient Care Plan, 921–26*t*
    cerebrospinal fluid leak, 922*t*
    gas exchange, 921*t*
    infection, 923–24*t*
    knowledge regarding diagnosis and treatment, 921–22*t*
    nutritional intake, 925*t*
    pain, 926*t*
    patient safety, 924*t*
    perioperative anxiety, 922*t*
    psychological adjustment to facial disfigurement, 924–25*t*
    skin integrity, 923*t*
  pathophysiology, 915
  Patient Teaching & Discharge Priorities, 930*t*
  risk factors, 917*t*
healing, 499*t*
healing touch, 854*t*, 1819*t*
health and wellness promotion, 9–10, 209
health assessment:
  critical thinking in, 165–66
  health history, 110, 111*t*, 152. *See also* health history
  physical assessment
    behavior, 158
    functional assessment, 158
    height and weight, 158
    mental status, 158
    mobility, 158
    nutritional assessment, 158
    pain, 159–60
    physical appearance, 158
    physical assessment, 158
    vital signs, 159, 159*f*
  physical examination. *See* physical examination
health beliefs/practices, 155
health care:
  influences on
    advances in technology and genetics, 25–28
    aging population, 22–23
    changing disease patterns, 24–25
    complementary and alternative therapies. *See* complementary and alternative therapies
    cultural diversity, 23
    demand for quality care, 29
    economics, 28–29
    informed consumers, 23
    population demographics, 22

legal aspects
  advance directives. *See* advance directives
  case management, 62–63
  documentation. *See* documentation
  Health Insurance Portability and Accountability Act, 62
  nursing practice and, 59–60
health care–associated pneumonia, 938, 938*t*, 1027–28*t*
health care delivery system, 45. *See also* health care organizations
  future implications, 46
  hospital organizations, 46, 47*t*
  models, 45–46
health care durable power of attorney, 60*t. See also* advance directives
health care economics:
  future projections, 50–51
  historical development, 46–48
  insurance plan types, 48, 48*t*
  managed care and, 48. *See also* managed care
  reimbursement practices, 48
health care organizations:
  accreditation, 58–59
  budgeting process, 51–52, 52*t*
  financial structure, 51
  fire and life safety standards, 58
  infection and disease control, 58
  licensure, 57–58
  OSHA guidelines, 58
  professional practice oversight, 58
health care professionals:
  HIV exposure in, 1925–26
  substance abuse in, 380, 380*t*
health care trends:
  demand for quality care, 55–57
  emergency preparedness, 53–54
  evidence-based practice, 52
  gene therapy, 54–55
  hospitalist programs, 55
  hospital report cards, 53
  information technology, 55
  inpatient to outpatient shift, 55
  minimally invasive surgery, 54
  patient safety standards, 53
  robotics, 54
  telemedicine, 54
  worker shortages, 55
health history. *See also* specific body systems
  biographical data, 153–55
  conducting the interview, 152–53, 154*f*
  cultural beliefs and practices, 157
  Cultural Considerations, 154*f*, 698*t*
  documentation, 160, 161*f*
  family history, 156
  health beliefs and practices, 155
  health patterns, 155
  medications, 155–56
  past medical history, 155, 161*f*
  present health/illness, 155
  psychosocial history, 151*f*, 156–57
  sexual behavior, 150
  spiritual beliefs, 157
  stress and coping, 157
health insurance plans, 48, 48*t*
Health Insurance Portability and Accountability Act (HIPAA), 62
  documentation standards, 97
  nursing research and, 137, 137*t*
  overview, 76, 77*t*
health maintenance organization (HMO), 48*t*, 49–50, 86
health patterns, 155

Health Plan Employer Data and Information Set (HEDIS), 56
Healthy People 2010:
  cancer goals, 2069*t*
  focus areas, 10*t*, 149*t*
  goals, 148
  hypertension objectives, 489, 490*t*
  immunization and infectious disease guidelines, 469–70, 470*t*
  immunization guidelines for adults, 178*t*
  leading health indicators, 11*t*, 149
    access to health care, 152
    environmental quality, 152
    immunization, 152
    injury and violence, 152
    mental health, 150
    overweight and obesity, 150
    physical activity, 149–50
    responsible sexual behaviors, 150
    substance abuse, 150
    tobacco use, 150
  nutrition objectives, 279, 280*t*
  objectives for reducing hearing loss, 2318*t*
  objectives for reduction in injury, disability, and death due to unintentional injuries, 2426*t*
  tobacco use goals, 2073*t*
Healthy Vision 2010, 2327*t*
hearing:
  age-related changes, perioperative risk, and nursing implications, 601*t*
  assessment/screening
    in aging patient, 172, 179
    procedures, 2292–93, 2312*t*
  end-of-life issues, 2320–21
  mechanisms of, 2303
hearing aids, 2314–15, 2315*t*
hearing dogs, 2314
hearing loss/impairment:
  in adults, 2305
  assessment, 2291, 2319*t*
  in children, 2305
  Clinical Preparation, 2321–23*t*
  collaborative management, 2318
  conductive, 2287, 2303
  cultural considerations, 2319
  discharge priorities, 2317
  drug-related, 2290, 2292
  etiology and epidemiology, 2303–4, 2304*t*
  genetic implications, 2319, 2319*t*
  gerontological considerations, 2305, 2319–20
    assessment, 2320
    caregiver needs, 2320
    laboratory test alterations, 2320
    medications and compliance, 2320
    prognosis and complications, 2320
    psychosocial and economic needs, 2320
  health promotion, 2317
    adolescent, 2318
    adult, 2318
    neonate/baby/child, 2317–18
    patient, family, and community perspectives, 2318
  laboratory and diagnostic procedures, 2292–93
  mixed, 2303
  in newborn, 2305
  noise-induced, 2307
  nursing management, 2315–16
  Nursing Process: Patient Care Plan, 2316*t*
  pathophysiology and treatment, 2304–5
  Patient Teaching & Discharge Priorities, 2317*t*
  prevention, 2318–19, 2318*t*
  Research Opportunities and Clinical Impact, 2321*t*

pathophysiology, 1634
risk factors, 1634
hyperphosphatemia, 431
causes, 431
in chronic renal failure, 1483
complications, 431
nursing management
planning, interventions, and rationales, 432
hyperpigmentation, 2141t, 2158–59
hyperpituitarism:
clinical manifestations, 1639
Cultural Considerations, 1645t
discharge priorities, 1642
epidemiology and etiology, 1639
gerontological considerations, 1642
health promotion, 1642
laboratory and diagnostic procedures, 1639–40
medical management, 1640–41
nursing management, 1641
interventions and rationales, 1642
nursing diagnoses, 1641–42
pathophysiology, 1639
risk factors, 1639
hyperplasia, 227, 227t, 2063, 2063t
hyperpnea, 872
hyperpyrexia, 470
hyperreflexia, 837
hyperresonance, 162
hypersensitivity response:
allergic. See allergy(ies)
autoimmune. See autoimmune hypersensitivity
response
immune. See immune hypersensitivity response
hypertension:
assessment, 492. See also blood pressure,
assessment
in chronic renal failure, 1483
classification, 489–90, 490t
clinical awareness and monitoring, 487t
clinical manifestations, 492
Clinical Preparation, 507–8t
collaborative management, 499, 502–3
Complementary and Alternative Therapies,
495–96, 496t, 499t
complications
dissecting aortic aneurysm, 504
hypertensive crisis, 504
hypertensive encephalopathy, 504
target organ damage, 503–4, 503t
culture, environment, race, genetics, and history,
492, 492t, 499t
diagnostic tests, 493, 494t
epidemiology, 489
etiology, 492t
Evidence-Based Practice, 505t
Healthy People 2010 objectives, 489, 490t
heart failure and, 1315
increased intracranial pressure and, 749
induced, for cerebral vasospasm, 766
medical management, 493
nonpharmacologic therapy, 1167
alcohol consumption, 495
dietary modifications, 292–94, 293t,
294t, 493
exercise, 493
lifestyle modifications, 293, 293t, 493
stress reduction, 493, 495
weight control, 493
pharmacologic agents, 495, 497–98t
nursing management, 496
discharge priorities, 499
health promotion, 496

Nursing Process: Patient Care Plan, 500–501t
Patient Teaching & Discharge Priorities, 502t
postoperative, 659
psychosocial assessment, 492
research, 504–5
Research Opportunities and Clinical
Impact, 506t
risk factors, 490–92, 491t
hypertensive encephalopathy, 504
hyperthyroidism. See also Graves' disease
clinical manifestations, 1604, 1626
collaborative management, 1632
complementary and alternative therapies, 1632
complications, 1631t
Cultural Considerations, 1631t
discharge priorities, 1630–31
epidemiology and etiology, 1625–26
Genetic Considerations, 1625t, 1631t
Gerontological Considerations, 1631t
health promotion, 1631
laboratory and diagnostic procedures, 1620t,
1621–22t, 1626
medical management, 1618t, 1626–27, 1628t
nursing management, 1627–29, 1630
Nursing Process: Patient Care Plan, 1629–30t
pathophysiology, 1618t, 1626, 1907t
in pregnancy, 1626
risk factors, 1626t
hypertonic fluids, 419
hypertonic formula, enteral nutrition, 322
hypertrophic cardiomyopathy (HCM), 1258, 1262f.
See also cardiomyopathy(ies)
clinical manifestations, 1263–64
epidemiology and etiology, 1258, 1262–63
Genetic Considerations, 1264t
laboratory and diagnostic procedures,
1264, 1264t
medical management, 1264–65, 1267–68t
nursing management
assessment, 1265
outcomes and evaluation parameters, 1265
planning, interventions, and rationales, 1265
pathophysiology, 1263, 1263f
hypertrophic scar, 2157–58, 2157t, 2269, 2269f
hypertrophy, 226, 1283
cardiac, 1283
as growth pattern, 2063, 2063t
skin, 2144t
as stress response, 226, 227t
hyperventilation, 439
hyphema, 2353t, 2436
hypnosis, 499t
hypnotherapy, 1415t
hypoalbuminemia, 1436
hypocalcemia, 429
causes, 429–30
clinical manifestations, 1608
nursing management
planning, interventions, and rationales, 430
in parathyroid disorders, 1608
symptoms, 430
hypochloremia, 433
hypochromic, 2018
hypodermoclysis, 518, 519f
hypoglossal nerve (CN XII), 705, 711t
hypoglycemia:
clinical manifestations, 1691, 1692t
in diabetes mellitus, 300, 1663
etiology and precipitating factors, 1690t
laboratory and diagnostic procedures, 1691,
1692t, 1693
pathophysiology, 1691

hypoglycemia unawareness, 1690
hypokalemia, 427
causes, 427–28
metabolic alkalosis and, 448
nursing management
assessment, 428
evaluation, 428
planning, interventions, and rationales, 428
hypokalemic myopathy, 1759–60, 1759t. See also
myopathies
hypokinesia, 1187
hypokinetic dysarthria, 800
hypomagnesemia, 431
causes, 431
nursing management
planning, interventions, and rationales, 431
symptoms, 431
hypomimia, 800
hyponatremia, 424
causes, 424
acute brain disorders, 723t, 750
subarachnoid hemorrhage, 768
syndrome of inappropriate antidiuretic
hormone, 1644
nursing management, 424
Nursing Process: Patient Care Plan, 426t
symptoms, 424
hypoparathyroidism, 1617t, 1633
clinical manifestations, 1633–34
collaborative management, 1635
complementary and alternative therapies,
1635–36
discharge priorities, 1634
epidemiology and etiology, 1633
Genetic Considerations, 1633t
Gerontological Considerations, 1634t
health promotion, 1634
laboratory and diagnostic procedures,
1609t, 1634
medical management, 1634
nursing management, 1634
pathophysiology, 1633
risk factors, 1633t
hypophonia, 800
hypophosphatemia, 430
causes, 430
nursing management
assessment, 430
planning, interventions, and rationales, 430
symptoms, 430
hypopigmentation, 2159
hypopituitarism, 1637
clinical manifestations, 1638
Cultural Considerations, 1645t
discharge priorities, 1638
epidemiology and etiology, 1637
Gerontological Considerations, 1638t
health promotion, 1638
laboratory and diagnostic procedures, 1638
medical management, 1638
nursing management, 1638
pathophysiology, 1637–38
risk factors, 1637
hypopnea, 1315
hypopyon, 2355
hyposmia, 895
hypospadias, 1509, 1584
hypotension:
in mechanical ventilation, 1025
postoperative, 659
hypothalamic–pituitary–adrenal (HPA) axis, 231
responses to stress, 224–25, 231, 231f

priapism, 1587
PRICE acronym, sprains and strains, 1777
Priftin. *See* rifapentine
Prilosec. *See* omeprazole
primary adrenal insufficiency, 1648
primary appraisal, in transactional theory of stress, 220, 220*f*
primary biliary cirrhosis, 1441
primary chemotherapy, 2101*t*
primary immune deficiencies, 1890
primary immune response, 1874–75, 1877*f*
primary injury, 727
primary intention, 2212
primary lesion, skin, 2143, 2143*t*
primary nursing, 19–20, 91–93, 92*f*
primary set, 520
primary tumors, 735
principlism, 67
PR interval, 1078, 1084, 1084*f*, 1085*t*
Prinzmetal angina, 1175
PRIO staging system, sepsis, 1969*t*
Privacy Act of 1974, 135
privilege, 81
prn dosing, 350–51
probability sampling, 127
Pro-Banthine. *See* propantheline bromide
probenecid, 1844*t*
problem, intervention, evaluation (PIE) system, 101*t*, 102–3
problem-oriented medical record (POMR), 101–2, 101*t*, 102*t*
problem solving, versus nursing research, 122*t*, 123*t*
procainamide, 595*t*, 1761*t*
procarbazine, 733*t*
process standards, 57
prochlorperazine:
    in acute brain disorders, 733*t*
    in cerebral vascular disorders, 762*t*
    for postoperative nausea and vomiting, 661*t*
proctoscope, 2077*t*
prodromal phase, hepatitis, 1430
proerythroblasts, 2007
proficiency, 37*t*, 40–41
progenitor cells, 2007
progesterone, 1505
    for female reproductive system disorders, 1552*t*
    serum levels, 1551*t*
    targets and effects, 1616*t*
Prograf. *See* tacrolimus
programmed theory of aging, 168
Program of All-inclusive Care for the Elderly (PACE), 188–89
progression, 2063
projection, 252*t*
prolactin, 1505
    production, 1598*t*
    targets and effects, 1598*t*, 1615*t*, 1637*t*
prolactinoma, 1638–39
    clinical manifestations, 1639
    epidemiology and etiology, 1639
    laboratory and diagnostic procedures, 1639
prolapse, uterine, 1538–39
promethazine:
    in acute brain disorders, 733*t*
    in aging patient, 183*t*
    in cerebral vascular disorders, 762*t*
    in Ménière's disease, 2314*t*
    for postoperative nausea and vomiting, 661*t*
pronation, 1712*t*
Pronestyl. *See* procainamide
propantheline bromide, 1494

proparacaine, 2346*t*
Propionibacterium acnes, 2159
propofol, 625, 627*t*
    in acute brain disorders, 733*t*
    in increased intracranial pressure management, 719
propoxyphene, 183*t*, 359*t*
propranolol:
    for cocaine withdrawal, 375
    for hypertension, 497*t*
    preoperative use, 611*t*
    in thyroid disorders, 1628*t*
proprietary (for-profit) organization, 51
proprioception, 708
proptosis, 704
propylthiouracil, 1627, 1628*t*
pro re nata. *See* prn dosing
Proscar. *See* finasteride
prostate:
    disorders
        benign prostatic hyperplasia. *See* benign prostatic hyperplasia
        cancer. *See* prostate cancer
        prostatitis. *See* prostatitis
    physical examination
        in men age 65 and older, 179–80
        technique, 1514–15, 1515*f*
prostate cancer, 2078*t*
    clinical manifestations, 1577, 1578*t*, 2078*t*
    collaborative management, 1580
    diagnostic testing and staging, 1577–78, 1578*t*, 2078*t*
    epidemiology, 1576–77
    Evidence-Based Practice, 1573*t*
    medical management, 1578, 1580*t*, 1586*t*, 2078*t*
    nursing management, 1578–80
    Nursing Process: Patient Care Plan, 1581–83*t*
    pathophysiology, 1577
    Patient Teaching & Discharge Priorities, 1584*t*
    prognosis, 2078*t*
    risk factors, 1577*t*
    screening recommendations, 1515
prostatectomy, 1578
    Nursing Process: Patient Care Plan, 1581–83*t*
prostate-specific antigen (PSA), 2076*t*
prostatitis, 1572
    classification, 1572*t*
    clinical manifestations, 1572, 1572*t*
    etiology, 1572
    laboratory and diagnostic procedures, 1572–73
    medical management, 1573
    nursing management, 1573
    Patient Teaching & Discharge Priorities, 1574*t*
prosthetic heart valves, 1248, 1249*f*. *See also* cardiac valve disease
    autograft, 1250*t*
    biological, 1249, 1249*f*, 1250*t*
    mechanical, 1248–49, 1249*f*, 1250*t*
Prostigmin. *See* neostigmine
protanomaly, 2372*t*
protanopia, 2372*t*
protease inhibitors, 1937, 1938*f*, 1939*t*
protein buffers, 437–38
protein C, 1970
protein-calorie malnutrition, 277
proteinuria, 1464
proteolysis, 1662*t*
prothrombin time (PT):
    in liver disease, 1379*t*, 1438*t*
    normal values, 2002*t*, 2043*t*
    preoperative, 600*t*

in shock, 1962*t*
in SIRS/septic shock, 1971*t*
Protonix. *See* pantoprazole
proton pump inhibitors:
    applications/indications/actions
        gastroesophageal reflux disease, 1389, 1390*t*
        hiatal hernia, 1385
        spinal cord injury, 845*t*
    implications for surgery, 595*t*
    nursing responsibility
        in gastroesophageal reflux, 1390*t*
        in spinal cord injury, 845*t*
    preoperative use, 611*t*
proto-oncogene, 2074
Protopic. *See* tacrolimus
protozoa, 466
Prussian blue, 2402
pseudoaneurysm, femoral, 1134
pseudoephedrine, 1898*t*
pseudoephedrine disorders, 981*t*
Pseudomonas, 465*t*
Pseudomonas aeruginosa, 938, 2164
pseudophakic, 2352
psoriasis, 2160–61, 2160*f*, 2160*t*
psoriatic arthritis, 1842
    clinical manifestations, 1842
    epidemiology and etiology, 1842
    laboratory and diagnostic procedures, 1842–43
    medical management, 1843
    nursing management, 1843
    pathophysiology, 1842
PS (pressure support) ventilation, 1022–24, 1024*t*. *See also* mechanical ventilation
psychiatric hospital, 46, 47*t*
psychoanalytical theory, 251–52, 252*t*
psychomotor learning, 259, 262*t*
psychosocial history, 156–57
psychosocial issues:
    in illness and hospitalization
        anger, 268–70
        anxiety, 267–68
        crisis, 263
        depression, 265–67
        loss and grief, 264–65
        sick role behavior, 263–64
    preoperative assessment, 598
    Research Opportunities and Clinical Impact, 270*t*
    in teaching–learning process
        assessment of learning needs, 259
        developing a teaching plan, 262
        evaluating a teaching plan, 262
        implementing a teaching plan, 262, 262*t*
    theoretical foundations
        biopsychosocial model, 256
        cognitive development, 254, 255*t*
        cognitive theory, 254–55, 256*t*
        developmental, 252–53, 253*t*, 254*t*
        family systems, 255–56
        humanistic perspective, 254, 255*f*
        psychoanalytic perspective, 251–52, 252*t*
psychosocial theories of aging, 169–70
psyllium seed, 1410, 1410*t*, 1414*t*
PT. *See* prothrombin time
PTA (percutaneous transluminal angioplasty), 1327, 1329
PTCA (percutaneous transluminal coronary angioplasty), 1131, 1132*f*
pterygium, 2356*t*
ptosis, 704, 820
ptosis senilis, 2371*t*
PTT. *See* partial thromboplastin time

ultrasonography, *continued*
    in peripheral arterial disease, 1328*t*
    in pulmonary embolism, 974*t*
    in renal calculi, 1492*t*
    thyroid, 1622*t*
    transvaginal, 1551*t*
    urinary system, 1378
    in visual disorders, 2333*t*
ultraviolet radiation, 2074, 2138, 2152
umbilical cord blood, 2116
umbilicus, 1375
uncal herniation, 716–17
unconscious, 252
undernutrition, 272. *See also* eating disorders
undifferentiated spondylarthropathy. *See* reactive
        arthritis
undoing, 252*t*
unipolar lead, 1080
United Kingdom Prospective Diabetes Study
        (UKPDS), 1671
University of Texas Wound Classification
        System, 2200*t*
unlicensed assistive personnel (UAP), 89
    in functional nursing care delivery system, 89
    in primary nursing, 91
    in team nursing care delivery system, 90–91
Unna's boot, 1354
unstable angina, 1181. *See also* acute coronary
        syndrome
uplifts, 221
upper airway disorders:
    Clinical Preparation, 931–32*t*
    head and neck cancer. *See* head and neck cancer
    larynx. *See* larynx, disorders
    nose and facial structures
        anosmia, 895
        epistaxis, 882–83
        facial fractures. *See* facial fractures
        mucormycosis. *See* mucormycosis
        nasal fractures, 880–81
        nasal obstruction, 894–95
        septal deviation, 881–82
        sinusitis. *See* sinusitis
    pharynx and oral cavity
        dental abscess, 899
        dental caries, 898
        epiglottitis, 900
        hairy tongue, 898
        Ludwig's angina, 898, 899
        peritonsillar abscess, 900
        pharyngitis, 900
        sleep apnea. *See* sleep apnea
        tonsillitis, 900
    Research Opportunities and Clinical
        Impact, 930*t*
upper airway endoscopy, 901, 901*f*
uremic pericarditis, 1484
ureteral calculi. *See* renal calculi
urethral stricture, 1583–84
urethritis, 1493
urgent procedures, 587
uric acid, 1492*t*
urinalysis:
    in acute glomerulonephritis, 1465*t*
    in acute renal failure, 1477*t*
    in acute tubular necrosis, 1475*t*
    in bladder cancer, 1498*t*
    in chronic renal failure, 1482*t*
    in dehydration, 420*t*
    in heart failure, 1288*t*
    in hypertension, 494*t*
    normal values, 420*t*, 494*t*
    in overhydration, 420*t*

    in pneumonia, 939*t*
    preoperative, 600*t*
    in pyelonephritis, 1469*t*
    in reactive arthritis, 1848*t*
    in renal calculi, 1492*t*
    in renal infarction, 1472*t*
    in shock, 1962*t*
    in systemic lupus erythematosus, 1852*t*, 1910*t*
    in trauma, 2437*t*
urinary retention:
    in neurogenic bladder, 1494–95
    postoperative, 671*t*, 677
urinary system, 1370–71, 1371*f*. *See also* kidney
urinary tract disorders:
    assessment. *See* abdominal pain/complaints
    bladder cancer. *See* bladder cancer
    calculi. *See* renal calculi (stones)
    cystitis. *See* urinary tract infection
    medications affecting urination, 1575*t*
urinary tract infection (UTI):
    Complementary and Alternative
        Therapies, 1467*t*
    laboratory and diagnostic procedures, 1493
    nursing management, 1493
        interventions and rationales, 1493
    pathophysiology, 1493
urine:
    electrolyte levels
        normal values, 420*t*
        in overhydration/dehydration, 420*t*
    glucose testing, 1670
    ketone testing, 1670
    specific gravity
        in burn injuries, 2241*t*
        normal values, 420*t*
        in overhydration and dehydration, 419, 420*t*
urine amylase, 1379*t*
urine bilirubin, 1379*t*
urine creatinine clearance, 1465*t*
urine culture, 1469*t*
urine osmolality, 1379*t*
urine output, 658
urine urobilinogen, 1379*t*
urography:
    in bladder cancer, 1498*t*
    in renal calculi, 1492*t*
    in renal infarction, 1472*t*
Uroxatral. *See* alfuzosin
ursodiol, 1449, 1457*t*
urticaria, 2154, 2154*t*
U.S. Preventive Services Task Force (USPSTF), 175
Usher syndrome, 2319*t*, 2373*t*
uterine evacuation, 1553
uterine prolapse, 1538–39
uterus, fibroid tumors, 1535–36, 1536*f*
uveal tract, 2328
uveitis, 2353*t*, 2355, 2372*t*
U wave, 1078

V

vaccines, 1876. *See also* immunizations
    hepatitis, 1431
    herpes zoster, 178
    human papillomavirus, 1522
    influenza. *See* influenza vaccine
    pneumococcal, 178, 1878
    prostate cancer, 1578
vacuum aspiration, 1553
vacuum assisted closure (VAC), 2217, 2218*f*
VAD. *See* ventricular assist device
V agent (VX), 2391
vaginal cancer, 1540*t*

vaginismus, 1541
vaginitis:
    in bacterial vaginosis, 1523–24, 1551*t*, 1552*t*
    in candidiasis, 1524, 1551*t*
    health promotion, 1524
    in trichomoniasis, 1523, 1524*f*, 1551*t*, 1552*t*
vagotomy, 1374*t*
vagus nerve (CN X):
    in aging patient, 711*t*
    anatomy, 1367
    examination, 705
    injury, 901, 1367
valerian, 596*t*
Valium. *See* diazepam
Valsalva maneuver, 1495
valsartan:
    for cardiomyopathy, 1267*t*
    for heart failure, 1294*t*
    for hypertension, 498*t*
values, 12
valvular regurgitation, 1240, 1240*f*. *See also* cardiac
        valve disease
valvular stenosis, 1240, 1240*f*. *See also* cardiac valve
        disease
valvuloplasty, 1247
vanadium, 285*t*
vancomycin:
    for infectious disease, 477*t*
    preoperative use, 610
vanillylmandelic acid (VMA), 1610*t*
VAP. *See* ventilated-associated pneumonia
varenicline, 1334, 1337*t*
variables, 125
variant angina, 1175
variceal ligation, 1441
varicocele, 1514, 1599
varicose veins, 1346, 1346*f*
    clinical manifestations, 1346–47
    complications, 1347
    diagnosis, 1347
    etiology and epidemiology, 1346
    health promotion, 1347
    medical and surgical management, 1347
    nursing management, 1347
vascular access devices (VAD), 512. *See also*
        infusion therapy
    central
        implanted ports, 516–17, 516*f*, 517*f*
        nontunneled and noncuffed, 515–16,
            515*f*, 516*f*
        tunneled and cuffed, 516, 516*f*
    peripheral
        midline catheter, 514–15
        over-the-needle peripheral-shot catheters,
            514, 514*f*
        peripheral-short catheters, 513
        through-the-needle peripheral-short
            catheter, 514
        veins used for, 513*f*
        winged steel infusion set, 513–14, 514*f*
    specialized
        arterial-venous shunt, 518
        dialysis catheter, 518
        for hemodialysis, 1486–87, 1486*f*, 1487*t*
        hepatic artery catheter, 518
        intra-arterial. *See* intra-arterial catheters
        pheresis catheter, 518
        pulmonary artery. *See* pulmonary artery
            catheter
vascular circuit, 566*f*, 567
vascular (multiple-infarct) dementia, 176, 794*t*
vascular endothelial growth factor (VEGF), 2067
vascular lesions, 2143, 2144*t*

SPECIAL FEATURES